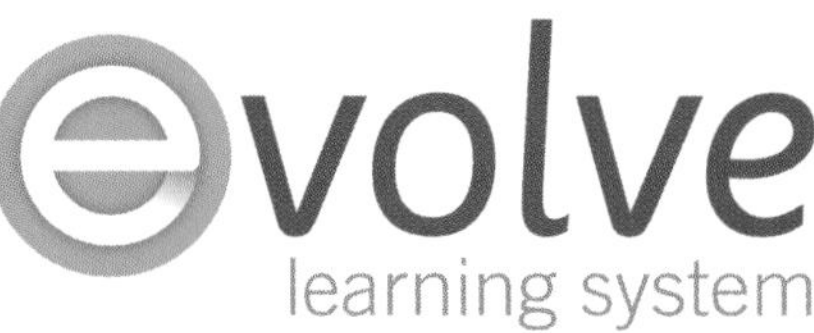

To access your Student Resources, visit:

http://evolve.elsevier.com/Perry/maternal/

Register today and gain access to:

- **Anatomy Reviews**
- **Animations**
- **Answers to Critical Thinking Exercises**
- **Assessment Videos**
- **Audio Glossary**
- **Audio Summaries**
- **Care Plan Constructor**
- **Case Studies**
- **Childbirth Videos**
- **Critical Thinking Exercises**
- **Developmental/Sensory Assessment**
- **Dietary Reference Intakes**
- **Growth Measurements**
- **Nursing Skills**
- **Patterns of Inheritance**
- **Resources**
- **Review Questions**
- **Spanish Guidelines**
- **Translation of FACES Pain Rating Scale**

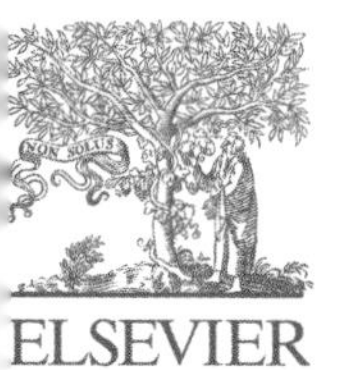

4th edition

Maternal Child Nursing Care

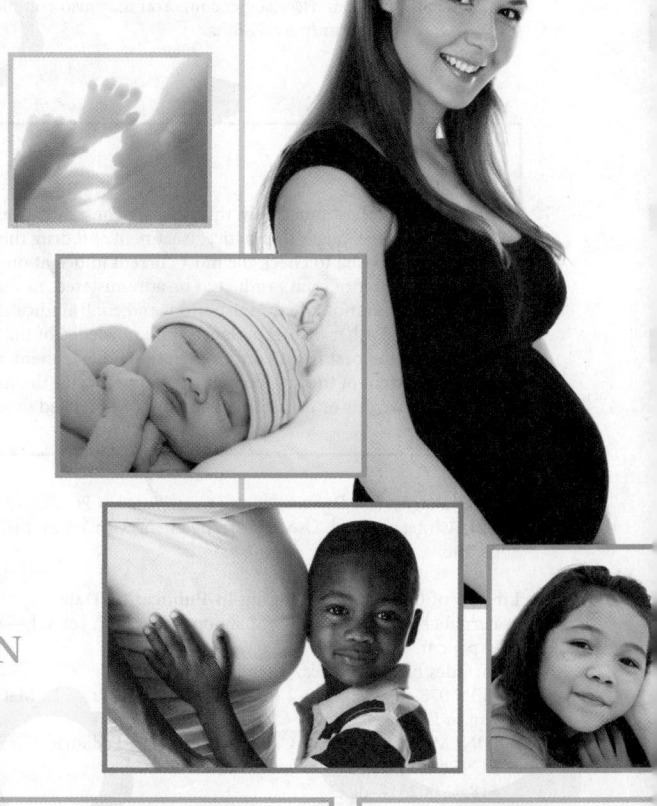

Shannon E. Perry, RN, CNS, PhD, FAAN
Professor Emerita, School of Nursing
San Francisco State University
San Francisco, California

Marilyn J. Hockenberry, PhD, RN-CS, PNP, FAAN
Director, Center for Research and Evidence-Based Practice
Nurse Scientist, Texas Children's Hospital;
Director of Nurse Practitioners
Texas Children's Cancer Center;
Professor, Department of Pediatrics
Baylor College of Medicine
Houston, Texas

Deitra Leonard Lowdermilk, RNC, PhD, FAAN
Clinical Professor Emerita, School of Nursing
University of North Carolina at Chapel Hill
Chapel Hill, North Carolina

David Wilson, MS, RNC
Faculty, School of Nursing
Langston University;
Staff, Pediatric Emergency Center
Saint Francis Hospital
Tulsa, Oklahoma

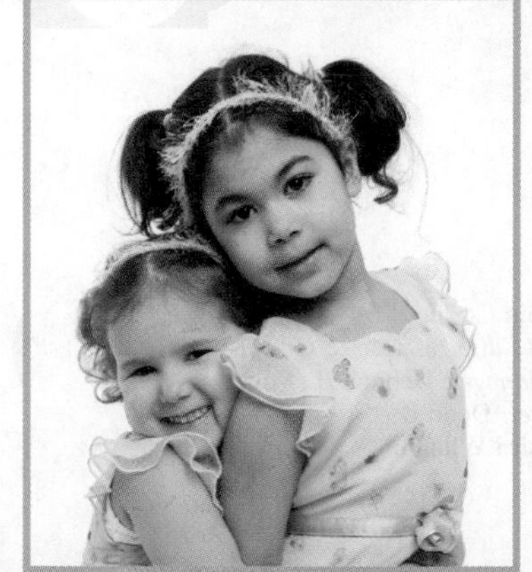

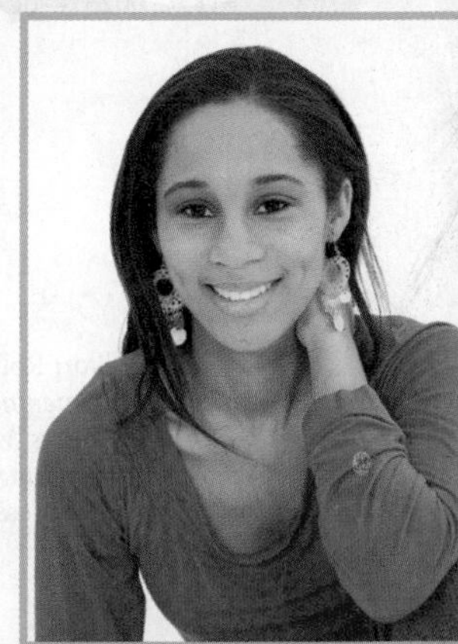

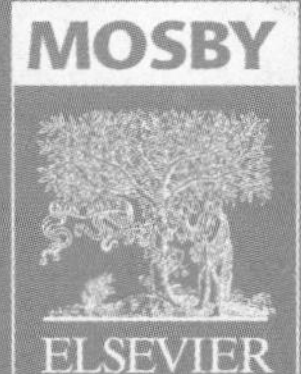

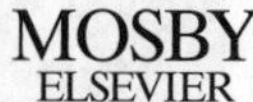

3251 Riverport Lane
Maryland Heights, Missouri 63043

MATERNAL CHILD NURSING CARE, FOURTH EDITION ISBN: 978-0-323-05720-2

Notice

Knowledge and best practice in this field are constantly changing. As new research and experience broaden our knowledge, changes in practice, treatment and drug therapy may become necessary or appropriate. Readers are advised to check the most current information provided (i) on procedures featured or (ii) by the manufacturer of each product to be administered, to verify the recommended dose or formula, the method and duration of administration, and contraindications. It is the responsibility of the practitioner, relying on his or her own experience and knowledge of the patient, to make diagnoses, to determine dosages and the best treatment for each individual patient, and to take all appropriate safety precautions. To the fullest extent of the law, neither the Publisher nor the Authors assume any liability for any injury and/or damage to persons or property arising out of or related to any use of the material contained in this book.

The Publisher

Library of Congress Cataloging-in-Publication Data
Maternal child nursing care / Shannon E. Perry ... [et al.].—4th ed.
p. ; cm.
Includes bibliographical references and index.
ISBN 978-0-323-05720-2 (hardcover : alk. paper) 1. Maternity nursing. 2. Pediatric nursing. I. Perry, Shannon E.
[DNLM: 1. Maternal-Child Nursing. 2. Pediatric Nursing. WY 157.3 M42543 2010]
RG951.W87 2010
618.92′00231—dc22

2009029198

Executive Editor: Robin Carter
Senior Developmental Editor: Laurie K. Gower
Publishing Services Manager: Deborah L. Vogel
Senior Project Manager: Deon Lee
Design Direction: Jessica Williams

Printed in Canada

Last digit is the print number: 9 8 7 6 5 4 3 2 1

Contributors

Contributing Editor

Patrick F. Barrera, BS
Assistant Director, Evidence-Based Clinical Decision Support
Center for Research and Evidence-Based Practice
Texas Children's Hospital
Houston, Texas

Contributors

Suzanne McMurtry Baird, MSN, RN
Assistant Professor, School of Nursing
Vanderbilt University
Nashville, Tennessee

Pat Mahaffee Gingrich, RN-C, MSN, WHNP
Clinical Assistant Professor, School of Nursing
University of North Carolina at Chapel Hill
Chapel Hill, North Carolina

Edward L. Lowdermilk, BS, RPh
Clinical Pharmacist
Piedmont Health Services
Siler City, North Carolina

INSTRUCTOR AND STUDENT ANCILLARIES

Test Bank, Audience Response Questions, Curriculum Guides, PowerPoint Slides
Barbara Pascoe, RN, BA, MA
Director, The Family Place
Concord Hospital
Concord, New Hampshire

Instructor's Manual, Study Guide
Karen A. Piotrowski, RNC, MSN
Associate Professor of Nursing
D'Youville College
Buffalo, New York

Study Guide, Review Questions
Julie White, RN, MSN
Clinical Instructor, Graduate Entry Program
College of Nursing, Maternal/Child Department
University of Illinois at Chicago
Chicago, Illinois

Reviewers

Martha Barry, RN, MS, CNM
Adjunct Clinical Instructor
University of Illinois at Chicago
Chicago, Illinois

Beverly Bowers, PhD, RN, CNS
Assistant Professor, College of Nursing
University of Oklahoma Health Sciences Center
Oklahoma City, Oklahoma

Diana C. Bridge, RN, BSN, MSN
Assistant Professor
Maranatha Baptist Bible College
Watertown, Wisconsin

Marsha Cannon, RN, BSN, MSN
Associate Professor, Department of Nursing
University of West Alabama
Livingston, Alabama

Kitty Cashion, RN, BC, MSN
Clinical Nurse Specialist
Department of Obstetrics and Gynecology
Division of Maternal-Fetal Medicine
University of Tennessee Health Science Center
Memphis, Tennessee

Denise Marshall, RN, MEd, EdD
Head, Department of Nursing
Wor-Wic Community College
Salisbury, Maryland

Jan Riordan, EdD, ARNP, IBCLC, FAAN
Professor of Nursing
Wichita State University
Wichita, Kansas

Johnett Benson Soros, MSN, RN, NP
Assistant Professor, College of Nursing
Kent State University
Ashtabula, Ohio

Charlotte Stephenson, RN, DSN, CLNC
Clinical Professor, College of Nursing
Texas Woman's University
Houston, Texas

Deborah A. Terrell, PhD, RN, CFNP
Associate Professor
Harry S Truman College
Chicago, Illinois

Kerstin I. West-Wilson, MS, RN, C, IBCLC
Eastern Oklahoma Perinatal Center
Saint Francis Children's Hospital
Tulsa, Oklahoma

About the Authors

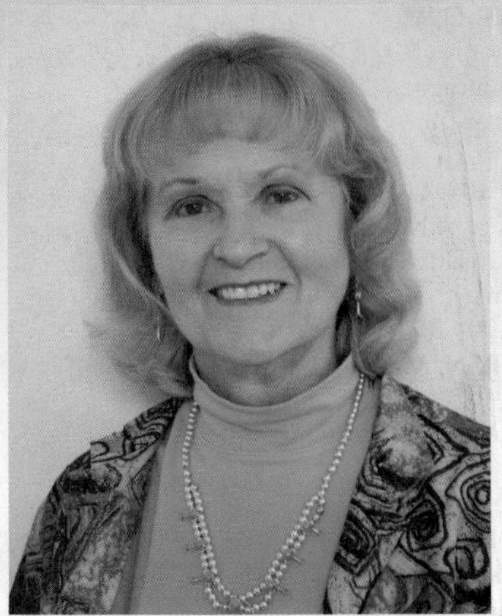

Shannon E. Perry is Professor Emerita, School of Nursing, San Francisco State University. She received her diploma in nursing from St. Joseph Hospital School of Nursing, Bloomington, Illinois; a Baccalaureate in Nursing from Marquette University; an MSN from the University of Colorado Medical Center; and a PhD in Educational Psychology from Arizona State University. She completed a 2-year postdoctoral fellowship in perinatal nursing at the University of California, San Francisco, as a Robert Wood Johnson Clinical Nurse Scholar.

Dr. Perry has had clinical experience as a staff nurse, head nurse, and supervisor in surgical nursing, obstetrics, pediatrics, gynecology, and neonatal nursing. She has served as expert witness and legal consultant. She has taught in schools of nursing in several states and was Interim Director and Director of the School of Nursing and Director of the Child and Adolescent Development Baccalaureate Program at SFSU. She was Marquette University College of Nursing Alumna of the Year in 1999 and the University of Colorado School of Nursing Distinguished Alumna of the Year in 2000, and she received the San Francisco State University Alumni Association Emeritus Faculty Award in 2005.

She is a Fellow in the American Academy of Nursing, a nursing consultant to the International Education Research Foundation, and co-chair of INESA, the International Nursing Education Services and Accreditation.

Dr. Perry's experience in international nursing includes teaching international nursing courses in the United Kingdom, Ireland, Italy, Thailand, Ghana, and China and participating in health missions in Ghana, Kenya, and Honduras. For her "exemplary contributions to nursing, public service, and selfless commitment and passion in shaping the future of international health," she received the President's Award from the Global Caring Nurses Foundation, Inc, in 2008.

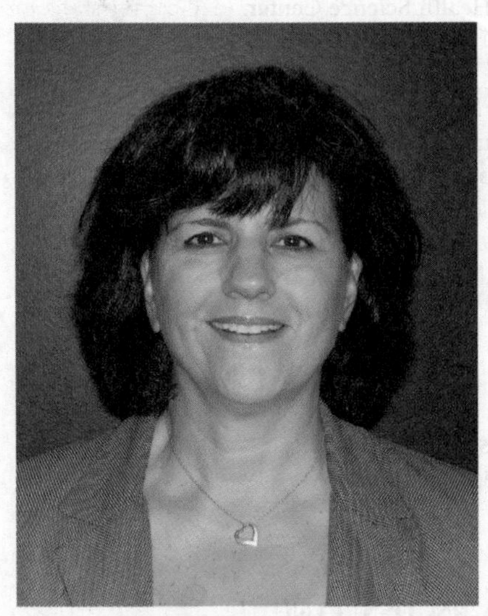

Marilyn J. Hockenberry is Professor of Pediatrics in the Hematology/Oncology Division at Baylor College of Medicine. She is the Director of the Center for Research and Evidence-Based Practice for Texas Children's Hospital in Houston, Texas, and the Director of the Pediatric Nurse Practitioner Program in the Texas Children's Cancer Center. Her research focuses on symptom management and treatment-related side effects experienced by children who have cancer. Dr. Hockenberry's current studies are evaluating treatment-related fatigue, sleep-related disturbances, and neurocognitive deficits of leukemia treatment. She has authored over 50 articles and has served as the senior editor on the Wong nursing textbooks for the past 10 years.

Dr. Hockenberry completed her prenursing education at Mt. Vernon Nazarene College and received her Bachelors of Science from Capital University. She received her Masters of Science from Texas Woman's University and her doctorate of philosophy with distinction from the Medical College of Georgia. She is a Fellow of the American Academy of Nursing.

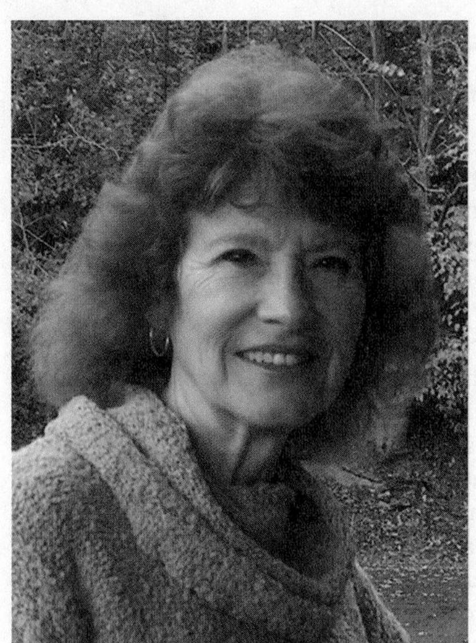

Deitra Leonard Lowdermilk is Clinical Professor Emerita, School of Nursing, University of North Carolina at Chapel Hill. She received her BSN from East Carolina University and her MEd and PhD in Education from UNC CH. She is certified in In-Patient Obstetrics by the National Certification Corporation. She is a Fellow in the American Academy of Nursing. In addition to being a nurse educator for over 34 years, Dr. Lowdermilk has clinical experience as a public health nurse and as a staff nurse in labor and delivery, postpartum, and newborn units, and she has worked in gynecologic surgery and cancer care units.

Dr. Lowdermilk has been recognized for her expertise in nursing education. She has repeatedly been selected as Classroom and Clinical Teacher of the Year by graduating seniors. She was a recipient of the Educator of the Year Award from both the District IV Association of Women's Health, Obstetric and Neonatal Nurses (AWHONN) and the North Carolina Nurses Association. She also received the 2005 AWHONN Excellence in Education Award.

She is active in AWHONN, having served as Chair of the North Carolina Section of AWHONN, and has served as chair and member of various committees in AWHONN at the national, district, state, and local levels. She has served as guest editor for the *Journal of Obstetric, Gynecologic, and Neonatal Nursing* and served on editorial boards for other publications.

Dr. Lowdermilk's most significant contribution to nursing has been to promote excellence in nursing practice and education in women's health through integration of knowledge into practice. In 2005 she received the first Distinguished Alumni Award from East Carolina University School of Nursing for her exemplary contributions to the nursing profession in the area of maternal-child care and the community.

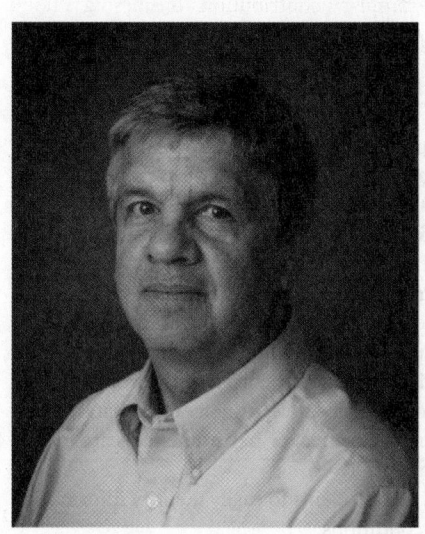

David Wilson is a graduate of Dallas Baptist College (now University) (BSN) and Texas Woman's University (MSN). He has more than 20 years of neonatal intensive care experience in Texas and Oklahoma. During his nursing career David has worked in a number of positions including staff nurse, neonatal educator, outreach educator, nutrition support coordinator, and BLS and Neonatal Resuscitation Program instructor. David was involved in medical missions in Costa Rica and Colombia for 2 years. David has also been nursing faculty at several universities, either on a full-time or adjunct basis for 15 years. Writing for nursing publications is an endeavor he has enjoyed for many years. He has authored several articles pertaining to neonatal and pediatric nursing, has served as a reviewer for two nursing journals, and has been an author and contributor with Mosby/Elsevier since 1993. David is currently a staff nurse in the Children's Hospital Pediatric Emergency Center at Saint Francis Hospital in Tulsa, Oklahoma, and serves as nursing faculty for Langston University, Tulsa, Oklahoma.

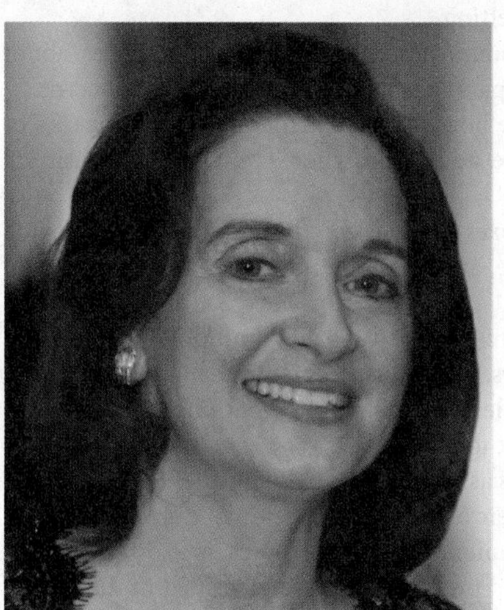

We remember **Donna Lee Wong**, PhD, RN, PNP, CPN, FAAN, who passed away on May 4, 2008, following complications of leukemia. Donna was the original co-author of this book. She co-developed the Wong-Baker FACES Pain Rating Scale, which is used worldwide to assess pain in children and adults and has been used in extensive research on pain.

For those of us who had the honor of knowing this remarkable individual, she is most remembered for her outstanding generosity and concern for others. Donna taught us that nursing is about providing the best care possible and that our patients will be the better for it. She led by example, always looking for ways to improve care for pediatric patients. Donna Wong was an example for all of us who strive for excellence in our nursing profession. We hold her dear to our hearts and will continue to work to carry on her outstanding legacy. She will never be forgotten.

Preface

This fourth edition of *Maternal Child Nursing Care* combines essential maternity and pediatric nursing information into one text. The text focuses on the care of women during their reproductive years and the care of children from birth through adolescence. Issues and concerns of childbearing women and the health care of children are the primary concentrations. The promotion of wellness and the management of common women's health problems and child development in the context of the family are also addressed. As we move further into the twenty-first century, this fourth edition of *Maternal Child Nursing Care* is designed to address the changing needs of women during their childbearing years and children during their developing years.

Maternal Child Nursing Care was developed to provide students with the knowledge and skills they need to become competent critical thinkers and to attain the sensitivity needed to become caring nurses. This fourth edition has been revised and refined in response to comments and suggestions from educators, clinicians, and students. It includes the most accurate, current, and clinically relevant information available.

Approach

Professional nursing practice continues to evolve and adapt to society's changing health priorities. The rapidly changing health care delivery system offers new opportunities for nurses to alter the practice of maternity and pediatric nursing and to improve the way care is given. Increasingly, nursing practice must be evidence based. It is incumbent on nurses to use the most up-to-date and scientifically supported information on which to base their care. To assist nurses in providing this type of care, **Evidence-Based Practice** boxes with implications for practice are included throughout the text.

Consumers of maternity and pediatric care vary in age, ethnicity, culture, language, social status, marital status, and sexual orientation. They seek care from a variety of health care providers in numerous health care settings, including the home. To meet the needs of these consumers, clinical education must offer students a variety of health care experiences in settings that include hospitals and birth centers, homes, clinics, private physicians' offices, shelters for the homeless or for women and children in need of protection, and other community-based settings.

Nursing Care Management has been used as an organizing framework for discussion in the nursing care chapters. This approach demonstrates how nursing must collaborate with other health care disciplines to provide the most comprehensive care possible to women and children. **Nursing Process** boxes include assessments, nursing diagnoses, expected outcomes, nursing care implementation, and evaluation of nursing care; these boxes are incorporated throughout the chapters. **Nursing Care Plans** reinforce the problem-solving approach to patient care. In chapters that focus on complications of childbearing, reproductive conditions, and childhood illnesses, medical interventions are presented first and are followed by nursing care management. Throughout the discussion of assessment and care, we alert the nurse to signs of potential problems and provide information boxes that highlight warning signs and emergency situations.

Patient education is an essential component of nursing care of women and children. The chapter on women's health promotion and screening emphasizes teaching for self-care to promote wellness and to encourage preventive care. The chapter on transition to parenthood focuses on teaching for new mothers and infants at home. Special boxes highlight community care throughout the text. **Family-Centered Care** boxes incorporate family considerations important to care of women and children. Issues concerning grandparents, siblings, and different family constellations are addressed. In the pediatric chapters, these boxes focus on the special learning needs of families caring for their child. **Legal Tips** are integrated throughout the maternity section to emphasize these issues as they relate to the care of women and infants.

This fourth edition features a contemporary design with logical, easy-to-follow headings and an attractive four-color design that highlights important content and increases visual appeal. Hundreds of color photographs and drawings throughout the text, many of them new, illustrate important concepts and techniques to further enhance comprehension. To help students learn essential information quickly and efficiently, we have included numerous features that prioritize, condense, simplify, and emphasize important aspects of nursing care. In addition, the text encourages students to think critically. The organizing framework, Nursing Care Management, is used consistently to discuss nursing care.

Special Features

- **Electronic Resources** providing additional information related to chapter content are placed at the beginning of each chapter and highlighted throughout the text.
- **Learning Objectives** focus students' attention on the important content to be mastered.
- **Critical Thinking Exercises** present students with real-life situations and encourage them to make appropriate clinical judgments. Answer guidelines are provided on the book's Evolve site.
- **Evidence-Based Practice** boxes are incorporated throughout the book. Findings that confirm effective practices or that identify practices with unknown, ineffective, or harmful effects are identified by an icon in the margin ( ).
- **Nursing Process** boxes help students to easily identify information on major diseases and conditions.
- **Home Care** boxes emphasize patient and family self-care and provide information to help students transfer learning from the hospital to the home setting.
- **Cultural Awareness** boxes describe beliefs and practices about pregnancy, childbirth, parenting, and women's health concerns.
- **Family-Centered Care** boxes highlight the needs or concerns of families that should be addressed when family-centered care is provided.
- **Community Focus** boxes emphasize community issues, provide resources and guidance, and illustrate nursing care in a variety of settings.
- **Nursing Care Plans** are provided for all commonly encountered situations and disorders. NANDA-accepted nursing diagnoses are included, as are rationales for nursing interventions that might not be immediately evident to students.
- **Patient Teaching** boxes assist students to help patients and families become involved in their own care with optimal outcomes.
- **Alternative and Complementary Therapies** are discussed for many pregnancy-related problems and are identified in the text by an icon in the margin ( ).

- **Atraumatic Care** boxes emphasize the importance of providing competent care while minimizing undue physical and psychologic distress for the child and family.
- **Emergency** boxes alert students to the signs and symptoms of various emergency situations and provide interventions for immediate implementation.
- **Nursing Alerts** call the reader's attention to critical information that could lead to deteriorating or emergency situations.
- During assessment, the nurse must be alert for **Signs of Potential Complications;** these are included in chapters that cover uncomplicated pregnancy and childbirth.
- **Guidelines** boxes provide students with examples of various approaches to implementing care.
- **Medication Guide** boxes include key information about medications used in maternity and newborn care, including their indications, adverse effects, and nursing considerations.
- **Legal Tips** are integrated throughout Part 1 to provide students with relevant information to deal with important legal areas in the context of maternity nursing.
- **Key Points,** located at the end of each chapter, help the reader summarize major points, make connections, and synthesize information. The Key Points are also available in a downloadable audio format and can be found on this book's Evolve site.
- **Resources,** including websites and contact information for organizations and educational resources available for the topics discussed, are listed throughout.
- A highly detailed, cross-referenced **index** allows readers to quickly access needed information.

Teaching and Learning Package

Several ancillaries to this text have been developed for instructors and students to use in classroom and clinical settings.

Evolve. Evolve is an innovative website that provides a wealth of content, resources, and state-of-the-art information on maternity and pediatric nursing. Evolve's wide array of information includes course resources for instructors (Instructor's Manual, Test Bank, Image Collection, PowerPoint slides, Audience Response Questions) and learning resources for students (Case Studies, NCLEX-style Review Questions, Nursing Skills, Assessment Videos, Animations, Nursing Care Plans, and more).

Instructor's Electronic Resource. The innovative electronic resources for the instructor (available online) contain the following components:

- *Instructor's Manual* contains learning objectives, chapter outlines and accompanying teaching strategies, learning activities, and curriculum guides for courses of varying lengths.
- *Electronic Test Bank* in ExamView format contains more than 1500 NCLEX-style test items, including new alternate-format questions. An answer key with page references to the text, rationales, and NCLEX-style coding is included.
- *Electronic Image Collection,* containing more than 500 full-color illustrations and photographs from the text, helps instructors develop presentations and explain key concepts. All images can be printed as acetates for overhead projection.
- *PowerPoint Slides,* with lecture outlines for each chapter of the text, assist in presenting materials in the classroom.
- Audience Response Questions for i-Clicker and other systems provide additional review of content in the classroom.

Study Guide. This comprehensive and challenging study aid presents a variety of questions to enhance learning of key concepts and content from the text. Multiple-choice and matching questions are included, as well as Critical Thinking Case Studies. Answers for all questions are included at the back of the study guide.

Virtual Clinical Excursions: CD and Workbook Companion. A CD-ROM and workbook have been developed as a virtual clinical experience to expand student opportunities for critical thinking. This package guides the student through a computer-generated virtual clinical environment and helps the user apply textbook content to virtual patients in that environment. Case studies are presented that allow students to use this textbook as a reference to assess, diagnose, plan, implement, and evaluate "real" patients using clinical scenarios. The state-of-the-art technologies reflected on this CD-ROM demonstrate cutting edge learning opportunities for students and facilitate knowledge retention of the information found in the textbook. The clinical simulations and workbook represent the next generation of research-based learning tools that promote critical thinking and meaningful learning.

Acknowledgments

Thanks to Pat Gingrich for preparing the Evidence-Based Practice boxes in Part 1; to Julie Perry Nelson, Loveland, CO, and Cheryl Briggs, RN, Annapolis, MD, for many new photographs; and to those parents who permitted us to use photos of their infants and families. Very special thanks to Laurie Gower and Robin Carter, whose support was crucial for the completion of this project, and to Deon Lee for her exceptional attention to detail.

Shannon E. Perry
Deitra Leonard Lowdermilk

Special thanks to Patrick Barrera for his continued support of the Wong legacy textbooks. We are so thankful for the supportive staff at Elsevier—Shelly Hayden, Heather Bays, Laurie Gower, and Deon Lee—for their continued devotion to excellence in pediatric nursing education.

Marilyn J. Hockenberry
David Wilson

The authors would like to acknowledge the following individuals for contributions to the eighth edition of *Wong's Essentials of Pediatric Nursing:* Debbie Fraser Askin, MN, RNC; Annette L. Baker, MSN, RN, PNP; Rose U. Baker, MSN, APRN, BC; Patrick Barrera, BS; Faye Blair, MSN, RN; Christine A. Brosnan, DrPH, RN; Terri L. Brown, MSN, RN, CPN; Rosalind Bryant, APRN, MN, BC, PNP; Lisa Creamer RN, BSN; Martha R. Curry, MS, RN, CPNP; Marsha L. Ellett, DNS, RN; Angela M. Ethier, DSN, RN, CNS, CPN, CT; Joy Hesselgrave, MSN, RN, CPON; Mary C. Hooke, PhD(C), APRN-BC, CPON; Eufemia Jacob, PhD, RN; Linda M. Kollar, MSN, RN; Shannon Stone McCord, MS, RN, CPNP, WOCN, CCRN; Mary A. Mondozzi, MSN, APRN, BC; Rebecca A. Monroe, MSN, RN, CPNP, CPON; Barbara A. Montagnino, MS, RN, CNS; Patricia O'Brien, MSN, RN, CPNP-AC; Patricia A. Ring, MS, RN, CPNP; Cheryl C. Rodgers, MSN, RN, CPNP, CPON; Jennifer Sanders, RN, BSN; Rebecca J. Schultz, MSN, RN, CPNP; Sandra L. Upchurch, PhD, RN; and Barbara J. Wheeler, MN, RN, IBCLC, RLC.

Contents

Part 1 Maternity Nursing

UNIT 1 INTRODUCTION TO MATERNITY NURSING, 3

Chapter 1 Contemporary Maternity Nursing, 3
Contemporary Issues and Trends, 5
Healthy People 2010 Goals, 5
Millennium Development Goals, 5
Integrative Health Care, 5
Problems with the U.S. Health Care System, 5
Trends in Fertility and Birthrate, 6
Low Birth Weight and Preterm Birth, 7
Infant Mortality in the United States, 7
International Trends in Infant Mortality, 7
Maternal Mortality Trends, 7
Increase in High Risk Pregnancies, 8
High Technology Care, 8
Care During Pregnancy and Childbirth, 8
View of Women, 8
Safe Motherhood, 9
Childbirth Practices, 9
Community-Based Care, 9
Involving Consumers and Promoting Self-Management, 10
Health Literacy, 10
Breastfeeding in the Workplace, 10
International Concerns, 10
Trends in Nursing Practice, 10
Evidence-Based Practice, 11
A Global Perspective, 12
Standards of Practice and Legal Issues in Delivery of Care, 12
Risk Management, 13
Sentinel Events, 13
Failure to Rescue, 14
Ethical Issues in Perinatal Nursing, 14
Research in Perinatal Nursing, 14
Ethical Guidelines for Nursing Research, 14

Chapter 2 The Family and Culture, 16
The Family in Cultural and Community Context, 16
The Family in Society, 16
Family Organization and Structure, 16
Family Dynamics, 17
Family Nursing, 17
Family Assessment, 18
Theoretic Approaches to Understanding Families, 18
Family Systems Theory, 18
The Calgary Family Assessment Model, 19
Using Theories to Guide Practice, 19
Cultural Factors Related to Family Health, 20
Cultural Context of the Family, 20
Childbearing Beliefs and Practices, 22
Developing Cultural Competence, 24
Integrating Cultural Competence with the Nursing Care Plan, 26
Nursing Care Management, 26

Chapter 3 Community and Home Care, 28
Community Health Promotion, 29
Levels of Preventive Care, 29
Assessing the Community, 29
Data Collection and Sources of Community Health Data, 30
Vulnerable Populations in the Community, 32
Women, 32
Individuals with Low Literacy, 34
Refugees and Immigrants, 34
Implications for Nursing, 34
Home Care in the Community, 34
Communication and Technology Applications, 35
Guidelines for Nursing Practice, 35
Perinatal Services, 36
Patient Selection and Referral, 37
Nursing Care Management, 37
Preparing for the Home Visit, 37
First Home Care Visit, 39
Nursing Considerations, 39
Safety Issues for the Home Care Nurse, 41
Personal Safety, 41
Patient's Home, 42
Infection Control, 42

UNIT 2 REPRODUCTIVE YEARS, 44

Chapter 4 Health Promotion and Illness Prevention, 44
Reasons for Entering the Health Care System, 44
Preconception Counseling and Care, 44
Pregnancy, 45
Well-Woman Care, 45
Fertility Control and Infertility, 46
Menstrual Problems, 46
Perimenopause, 46
Barriers to Receiving Health Care, 46
Financial Issues, 46
Cultural Issues, 47
Gender Issues, 47
Health Risks in the Childbearing Years, 47
Age, 47
Social and Cultural Factors, 49
Substance Use and Abuse, 49
Cigarette Smoking and Caffeine Consumption, 49
Alcohol Consumption, 50
Prescription Medication Use, 50
Illicit Drug Use, 50
Nutrition, 51
Physical Fitness and Exercise, 53
Stress, 54
Sexual Practices, 55
Medical Conditions, 56
Gynecologic Conditions, 56
Female Genital Mutilation, 56
Environmental and Workplace Hazards, 56

Anticipatory Guidance for Health Promotion and Illness Prevention, 57
Substance Use Cessation, 57
Health Screening Schedule, 58
Health Risk Prevention, 58
Health Protection, 58
Intimate Partner Violence, 60

Chapter 5 Health Assessment, 65
Female Reproductive System, 65
External Structures, 65
Internal Structures, 66
The Bony Pelvis, 68
Breasts, 68
Menstruation, 71
Menarche and Puberty, 71
Menstrual Cycle, 71
Prostaglandins, 73
Climacteric and Menopause, 74
Sexual Response, 74
Health Assessment, 75
Interview, 75
Women with Special Needs, 76
History, 78
Physical Examination, 79
Laboratory and Diagnostic Procedures, 85

Chapter 6 Common Health Problems, 86
Menstrual Disorders, 86
Amenorrhea, 86
Cyclic Perimenstrual Pain and Discomfort, 87
Alterations in Cyclic Bleeding, 93
Abnormal Uterine Bleeding, 95
Infections, 96
Sexually Transmitted Infections, 96
Sexually Transmitted Bacterial Infections, 99
Sexually Transmitted Viral Infections, 103
Vaginal Infections, 110
Infection Control, 113
Problems of the Breast, 113
Fibrocystic Changes, 115
Fibroadenomas, 115
Lipomas, 115
Nipple Discharge, 115
Mammary Duct Ectasia, 116
Intraductal Papilloma, 116
Malignant Conditions of the Breast, 117

Chapter 7 Infertility, Contraception, and Abortion, 129
Infertility, 129
Incidence, 129
Factors Associated with Infertility, 129
Nursing Care Management, 130
Contraception, 138
Nursing Care Management, 138
Methods of Contraception, 139
Abortion, 156
First-Trimester Abortion, 157
Second-Trimester Abortion, 158
Emotional Considerations, 158

UNIT 3 PREGNANCY, 160

Chapter 8 Genetics, Conception, and Fetal Development, 160
Genetics, 160
Relevance of Genetics to Nursing, 161
Genetic History Taking and Counseling Services, 162
The Human Genome Project, 163
Clinical Genetics, 165
Patterns of Genetic Transmission, 169
Nongenetic Factors Influencing Development, 170
Behavioral Genetics, 170
Conception, 172
Cell Division, 172
Gametogenesis, 172
Conception, 172
Fertilization, 173
Implantation, 174
The Embryo and Fetus, 174
Primary Germ Layers, 174
Development of the Embryo, 175
Membranes, 175
Amniotic Fluid, 175
Yolk Sac, 176
Umbilical Cord, 176
Placenta, 176
Fetal Maturation, 179
Multifetal Pregnancy, 183

Chapter 9 Assessment for Risk Factors, 189
Definition and Scope of the Problem, 189
Maternal Health Problems, 189
Fetal and Neonatal Health Problems, 190
Regionalization of Health Care Services, 190
Assessment for Risk Factors, 190
Antepartum Testing and Biophysical Assessment, 190
Daily Fetal Movement Count, 191
Ultrasonography, 192
Nursing Role, 199
Magnetic Resonance Imaging, 200
Biochemical Assessment, 200
Amniocentesis, 201
Indications for Use, 201
Percutaneous Umbilical Blood Sampling, 202
Chorionic Villus Sampling, 203
Maternal Assays, 203
Antepartal Assessment Using Electronic Fetal Monitoring, 204
Indications, 204
Fetal Responses to Hypoxia and Asphyxia, 204
Variability, 205
Nonstress Test, 205
Vibroacoustic Stimulation, 205
Contraction Stress Test, 206
Nursing Role in Antenatal Assessment for Risk, 207
Psychologic Considerations, 207

Chapter 10 Anatomy and Physiology of Pregnancy, 210
Gravidity and Parity, 210
Pregnancy Tests, 211
Adaptations to Pregnancy, 212
Signs of Pregnancy, 212
Reproductive System and Breasts, 212
General Body Systems, 218

Chapter 11 Nursing Care During Pregnancy, 229
Diagnosis of Pregnancy, 230
Signs and Symptoms, 230
Estimating Date of Birth, 230
Adaptation to Pregnancy, 230
Maternal Adaptation, 230
Paternal Adaptation, 233
Sibling Adaptation, 234
Grandparent Adaptation, 234
Nursing Care Management, 235
Reason for Seeking Care, 239
Current Pregnancy, 239
Obstetric and Gynecologic History, 239
Medical History, 239
Nutritional History, 239
History of Use of Drugs and Herbal Preparations, 239
Family History, 240
Social, Experiential, and Occupational History, 240
History of Physical Abuse, 240
Review of Systems, 240
Physical Examination, 240
Laboratory Tests, 241
Follow-Up Visits, 241
Nursing Care, 244
Variations in Prenatal Care, 259
Childbirth and Perinatal Education, 263
Perinatal Care Choices, 265
Childbirth Education, 265
Current Practices in Childbirth Education, 265
Strategies for Childbirth Education, 265
Options for Care Providers, 266
Birth Plans, 267
Birth Setting Choices, 268
Components of Perinatal Education Programs, 269
Preparation for Cesarean Birth, 270
Childbirth Education Outcomes, 271

Chapter 12 Maternal and Fetal Nutrition, 273
Nutrient Needs Before Conception, 273
Nutrient Needs During Pregnancy, 273
Energy Needs, 275
Protein, 279
Fluids, 279
Minerals, Vitamins, and Electrolytes, 280
Other Nutritional Issues During Pregnancy, 284
Nutrient Needs During Lactation, 285
Nursing Care Management, 286

Chapter 13 Pregnancy at Risk: Preexisting Conditions, 295
Metabolic Disorders, 295
Diabetes Mellitus, 295
Nursing Care Management, 299
Gestational Diabetes Mellitus, 306
Thyroid Disorders, 309
Maternal Phenylketonuria, 311
Cardiovascular Disorders, 311
Peripartum Cardiomyopathy, 312
Rheumatic Heart Disease, 312
Mitral and Aortic Valve Stenosis, 313
Mitral Valve Prolapse, 313
Eisenmenger's Syndrome, 313
Atrial and Ventricular Septal Defects, 313
Tetralogy of Fallot, 313
Marfan Syndrome, 313
Heart Transplantation, 314
Nursing Care Management, 314
Cardiopulmonary Resuscitation of the Pregnant Woman, 319
Anemia, 320
Iron Deficiency Anemia, 321
Folic Acid Deficiency Anemia, 322
Sickle Cell Hemoglobinopathy, 322
Thalassemia, 322
Pulmonary Disorders, 322
Asthma, 322
Cystic Fibrosis, 324
Gastrointestinal Disorders, 325
Cholelithiasis and Cholecystitis, 325
Inflammatory Bowel Disease, 325
Integumentary Disorders, 325
Neurologic Disorders, 326
Epilepsy, 326
Multiple Sclerosis, 326
Bell's Palsy, 327
Autoimmune Disorders, 327
Systemic Lupus Erythematosus, 327
Myasthenia Gravis, 327
Human Immunodeficiency Virus and Acquired Immunodeficiency Syndrome, 328
Preconception Counseling, 328
Pregnancy Risks, 328
Nursing Care Management, 329
Substance Abuse, 330
Barriers to Treatment, 330
Legal Considerations, 330
Nursing Care Management, 330

Chapter 14 Pregnancy at Risk: Gestational Conditions, 334
Hypertension in Pregnancy, 334
Significance and Incidence, 334
Morbidity and Mortality, 335
Classification, 335
Preeclampsia, 337
HELLP Syndrome, 338
Nursing Care Management, 338
Hyperemesis Gravidarum, 349
Etiology, 349
Clinical Manifestations, 349
Collaborative Care, 349

Hemorrhagic Disorders, 350
Early Pregnancy Bleeding, 350
Nursing Care Management, 353
Recurrent Premature Dilation of Cervix (Incompetent Cervix), 355
Ectopic Pregnancy, 356
Gestational Trophoblastic Disease, 358
Late Pregnancy Bleeding, 360
Nonobstetric Surgery During Pregnancy, 368
Appendicitis, 368
Intestinal Obstruction, 368
Gynecologic Problems, 369
Trauma During Pregnancy, 369
Significance, 369
Nursing Care Management, 372

UNIT 4 CHILDBIRTH, 376

Chapter 15 Labor and Birth Processes, 376
Factors Affecting Labor, 376
Passenger, 376
Passageway, 378
Powers, 384
Position of the Laboring Woman, 385
Process of Labor, 387
Signs Preceding Labor, 387
Onset of Labor, 387
Stages of Labor, 387
Mechanism of Labor, 388
Physiologic Adaptation to Labor, 390
Fetal Adaptation, 390
Maternal Adaptation, 390

Chapter 16 Management of Discomfort, 394
Discomfort During Labor and Birth, 394
Neurologic Origins, 394
Perception of Pain, 395
Expression of Pain, 395
Factors Influencing Pain Response, 395
Nonpharmacologic Management of Discomfort, 397
Childbirth Preparation Methods, 398
Childbirth Education Outcomes, 401
Relaxation and Breathing Techniques, 401
Pharmacologic Management of Discomfort, 406
Sedatives, 406
Analgesia and Anesthesia, 406
Nursing Care Management, 416

Chapter 17 Fetal Assessment During Labor, 422
Basis for Monitoring, 422
Fetal Response, 422
Uterine Activity, 423
Fetal Compromise, 423
Monitoring Techniques, 423
Intermittent Auscultation, 423
Electronic Fetal Monitoring, 424
Fetal Heart Rate Patterns, 427
Baseline Fetal Heart Rate, 427
Periodic and Episodic Changes in Fetal Heart Rate, 429
Nursing Care Management, 433
Electronic Fetal Monitoring Pattern Recognition, 433

Chapter 18 Nursing Care During Labor and Birth, 440
First Stage of Labor, 440
Nursing Care Management, 440
Second Stage of Labor, 466
Duration of Second Stage, 466
Nursing Care Management, 468
Maternal Position, 469
Birth in a Delivery Room or Birthing Room, 471
Birth in a Labor, Delivery, Recovery or Labor, Delivery, Recovery, Postpartum Room, 473
Water Birth, 473
Mechanism of Birth: Vertex Presentation, 473
Management of Infant Born in Meconium-Stained Fluid, 474
Use of Fundal Pressure, 475
Immediate Assessment and Care of the Newborn, 475
Perineal Trauma Related to Childbirth, 475
Emergency Childbirth, 477
Third Stage of Labor, 477
Maternal Physical Status, 479
Fourth Stage of Labor, 480
Postanesthesia Recovery, 480
Interactions with the Newborn, 483
Family-Newborn Relationships, 484

Chapter 19 Labor and Birth at Risk, 486
Preterm Labor and Birth, 486
Preterm Birth vs. Low Birth Weight, 486
Nursing Care Management, 488
Preterm Premature Rupture of Membranes, 496
Nursing Care Management: Home vs. Hospital, 497
Dystocia, 497
Nursing Care Management, 502
Postterm Pregnancy, Labor, and Birth, 518
Maternal and Fetal Risks, 518
Nursing Care Management, 518
Obstetric Emergencies, 519
Shoulder Dystocia, 519
Prolapsed Umbilical Cord, 520
Rupture of the Uterus, 522
Amniotic Fluid Embolism (Anaphylactoid Syndrome of Pregnancy), 522

UNIT 5 POSTPARTUM PERIOD, 525

Chapter 20 Maternal Physiologic Changes, 525
Reproductive System and Associated Structures, 525
Uterus, 525
Cervix, 527
Vagina and Perineum, 527
Abdomen, 527
Endocrine System, 528
Placental Hormones, 528
Pituitary Hormones and Ovarian Function, 528
Urinary System, 528
Urine Components, 528
Postpartal Diuresis, 528
Urethra and Bladder, 528
Gastrointestinal System, 529
Appetite, 529
Bowel Evacuation, 529

Breasts, 529
Breastfeeding Mothers, 529
Nonbreastfeeding Mothers, 529
Cardiovascular System, 529
Blood Volume, 529
Cardiac Output, 530
Varicosities, 531
Neurologic System, 531
Musculoskeletal System, 531
Integumentary System, 531
Immune System, 531

Chapter 21 Nursing Care During the Fourth Trimester, 533
Transfer from the Recovery Area, 533
Discharge—Before 24 Hours and After 24 Hours, 534
Laws Relating to Discharge, 534
Criteria for Discharge, 534
Nursing Care Management—Physical Needs, 535
Nursing Care Management—Psychosocial Needs, 547
Nursing Care Management, 549
Discharge Teaching, 550

Chapter 22 Transition to Parenthood, 554
Parental Attachment, Bonding, and Acquaintance, 554
Assessment of Attachment Behaviors, 556
Parent-Infant Contact, 557
Early Contact, 557
Skin-to-Skin Contact, 557
Extended Contact, 557
Communication Between Parent and Infant, 558
The Senses, 558
Entrainment, 559
Biorhythmicity, 559
Reciprocity and Synchrony, 559
Parental Role After Childbirth, 559
Transition to Parenthood, 560
Parental Tasks and Responsibilities, 560
Becoming a Mother, 561
Resuming Sexual Intimacy, 562
Postpartum Adjustment in the Lesbian Couple, 564
Becoming a Father, 564
Infant-Parent Adjustment, 565
Rhythm, 565
Behavioral Repertoires, 565
Responsivity, 566
Diversity in Transitions to Parenthood, 566
Age, 566
Social Support, 567
Culture, 568
Socioeconomic Conditions, 569
Personal Aspirations, 569
Parental Sensory Impairment, 569
Visually Impaired Parent, 570
Hearing-Impaired Parent, 570
Sibling Adaptation, 570
Grandparent Adaptation, 571
Nursing Care Management, 573
Recognizing Signs of Illness, 574

Chapter 23 Postpartum Complications, 576
Postpartum Hemorrhage, 576
Definition and Incidence, 576
Etiology and Risk Factors, 577
Nursing Care Management, 579
Hemorrhagic (Hypovolemic) Shock, 581
Coagulopathies, 583
Idiopathic Thrombocytopenic Purpura, 583
von Willebrand Disease, 583
Disseminated Intravascular Coagulation, 583
Thromboembolic Disease, 584
Incidence and Etiology, 584
Clinical Manifestations, 584
Medical Management, 584
Postpartum Infections, 585
Endometritis, 585
Wound Infections, 585
Urinary Tract Infections, 586
Mastitis, 586
Nursing Care Management, 586
Sequelae of Childbirth Trauma, 587
Uterine Displacement and Prolapse, 587
Cystocele and Rectocele, 588
Urinary Incontinence, 589
Genital Fistulas, 589
Postpartum Psychologic Complications, 592
Mood Disorders, 592
Loss and Grief, 598
Grief Responses, 598
Family Aspects of Grief, 600
Grandparents and Siblings, 600
Nursing Care Management, 601
Communicating and Caring Techniques, 601
Cultural and Spiritual Needs of Parents, 605
Maternal Death, 606

UNIT 6 NEWBORN, 609

Chapter 24 Physiologic Adaptations of the Newborn, 609
Transition to Extrauterine Life, 609
Physiologic Adjustments, 609
Physical Assessment, 625
General Appearance, 636
Vital Signs, 636
Baseline Measurements of Physical Growth, 637
Neurologic Assessment, 637
Behavioral Characteristics, 637
Sleep-Wake States, 637
Other Factors Influencing Behavior of Newborns, 639
Sensory Behaviors, 639
Response to Environmental Stimuli, 640

Chapter 25 Nursing Care of the Newborn, 643
Birth Through the First 2 Hours, 643
Nursing Care Management, 643
From 2 Hours After Birth Until Discharge, 649
Nursing Care Management, 649
Common Newborn Problems, 652
Physical Injuries, 652
Physiologic Problems, 653

Laboratory and Diagnostic Tests, 657
Collection of Specimens, 657
Supporting Parents in the Care of Their Infant, 662
Social Interactions, 662
Infant Feeding, 663
Therapeutic and Surgical Procedures, 663
Intramuscular Injection, 663
Therapy for Hyperbilirubinemia, 665
Circumcision, 667
Discharge Planning and Teaching, 669
Temperature, 671
Respirations, 671
Feeding Schedules, 671
Elimination, 671
Positioning and Holding, 671
Rashes, 672
Clothing, 673
Safety: Use of Car Seat, 673
Nonnutritive Sucking, 673
Bathing, Cord Care, and Skin Care, 674
Infant Follow-Up Care, 674
Immunizations, 674

Chapter 26 Newborn Nutrition and Feeding, 678
Recommended Infant Nutrition, 678
Benefits of Breastfeeding, 678
Contraindications to Breastfeeding, 679
Choosing an Infant Feeding Method, 679
Nutrient Needs, 680
Overview of Lactation, 682
Milk Production, 682
Unique Properties of Human Milk, 684
Nursing Care Management: The Breastfeeding Mother and Infant, 685
Role of the Nurse in Promoting Successful Lactation, 698
Formula Feeding, 700
Rationale for Formula Feeding, 700
Parent Education, 700

Chapter 27 Infants with Gestational Age–Related Problems, 706
The Preterm Infant, 706
Late Preterm Infant, 707
Nursing Care Management, 707
Parental Adaptation to Preterm Infant, 710
Growth and Development Potential, 726
Complications of Prematurity, 727
The Postterm Infant, 733
Meconium Aspiration Syndrome, 733
Persistent Pulmonary Hypertension of the Newborn, 733
Other Problems Related to Gestation, 734
Small-for-Gestational-Age Infants and Intrauterine Growth Restriction, 734
Large-for-Gestational-Age Infants, 735
Infants of Diabetic Mothers, 735
Discharge Planning, 737
Transport to a Regional Center, 738
Transport from a Regional Center, 739

Chapter 28 The Newborn at Risk: Acquired and Congenital Problems, 742
Birth Trauma, 742
Nursing Care Management, 743
Neonatal Infections, 745
Sepsis, 745
Nursing Care Management, 746
Perinatally Acquired Infections, 748
Substance Abuse, 755
Alcohol, 756
Tobacco, 758
Marijuana, 759
Cocaine, 759
Phencyclidine ("Angel Dust"), 760
Heroin, 760
Methadone, 760
Methamphetamine, 761
Phenobarbital, 761
Caffeine, 761
Nursing Care Management, 761
Hemolytic Disorders, 766
Hemolytic Disease of the Newborn, 766
Nursing Care Management, 767
Congenital Anomalies, 767
Central Nervous System Anomalies, 768
Cardiovascular System Anomalies, 769
Respiratory System Anomalies, 770
Gastrointestinal System Anomalies, 771
Musculoskeletal System Anomalies, 774
Genitourinary System Anomalies, 776
Nursing Care Management, 777

Part 2 **Pediatric Nursing**

UNIT 7 CHILDREN, THEIR FAMILIES, AND THE NURSE, 785

Chapter 29 Contemporary Pediatric Nursing, 785
Health Care for Children, 785
Health Promotion, 785
Nutrition, 786
Dental Care, 786
Immunizations, 786
Childhood Health Problems, 786
Obesity and Type 2 Diabetes, 786
Childhood Injuries, 787
Violence, 788
Substance Abuse, 789
Mental Health Problems, 789
Mortality, 790
Infant Mortality, 790
Childhood Mortality, 791
Morbidity, 791
Childhood Morbidity, 791
The Art of Pediatric Nursing, 791
Philosophy of Care, 791
Family-Centered Care, 792
Atraumatic Care, 792

Role of the Pediatric Nurse, 792
Therapeutic Relationship, 793
Family Advocacy and Caring, 793
Disease Prevention and Health Promotion, 793
Health Teaching, 793
Support and Counseling, 794
Coordination and Collaboration, 794
Ethical Decision Making, 794
Research, 794
Critical Thinking and the Process of Nursing Children and Families, 794
Critical Thinking, 794
Evidence-Based Practice, 795
Nursing Process, 795
Health Care Planning, 796
Future Trends, 797

Chapter 30 Community-Based Nursing Care of the Child and Family, 799
Nursing in the Community, 799
Community Concepts, 799
Community, 799
Demography, 800
Epidemiology, 800
Economics, 802
Community Nursing Process, 802
Community Needs Assessment and Diagnosis, 802
Community Planning, 803
Community Intervention, 804
Community Evaluation, 804

Chapter 31 Family Influences on Child Health Promotion, 806
General Concepts, 806
Definition of Family, 806
Family Nursing Interventions, 806
Family Roles, Relationships, and Strengths, 807
Parental Roles, 807
Role Learning, 807
Parenting, 810
Motivation for Parenthood, 810
Preparation for Parenthood, 811
Transition to Parenthood, 811
Parenting Behaviors, 812
Limit Setting and Discipline, 812
Special Parenting Situations, 814
Parenting the Adopted Child, 815
Parenting and Divorce, 816
Single Parenting, 818
Parenting in Reconstituted Families, 819
Parenting in Dual-Earner Families, 819
Foster Parenting, 819
Accommodating Contemporary Parenting Situations, 819

Chapter 32 Social, Cultural, and Religious Influences on Child Health Promotion, 822
Culture, 822
Social Roles, 823
Subcultural Influences, 824
The Child and Family in North America, 827
Cultural Shock and Cultural Competence, 828
Cultural and Religious Influences on Health Care, 829
Susceptibility to Health Problems, 829
Cultural Customs, 830
Health Beliefs and Practices, 833
Religious Beliefs, 835
Importance of Culture and Religion to Nurses, 837

Chapter 33 Developmental Influences on Child Health Promotion, 842
Growth and Development, 842
Foundations of Growth and Development, 842
Biologic Growth and Physical Development, 844
Physiologic Changes, 846
Temperament, 847
Development of Personality and Mental Function, 848
Theoretic Foundations of Personality Development, 848
Theoretic Foundations of Mental Development, 850
Development of Self-Concept, 852
Role of Play in Development, 853
Classification of Play, 853
Content of Play, 854
Social Character of Play, 855
Functions of Play, 856
Toys, 857
Selected Factors That Influence Development, 857
Heredity, 857
Neuroendocrine Factors, 857
Nutrition, 857
Interpersonal Relationships, 857
Socioeconomic Level, 859
Disease, 859
Environmental Hazards, 860
Stress in Childhood, 860
Influence of the Mass Media, 861

UNIT 8 ASSESSMENT OF THE CHILD AND FAMILY, 866

Chapter 34 Communication, History, Physical, and Developmental Assessment, 866
Guidelines for Communication and Interviewing, 866
Establishing a Setting for Communication, 866
Computer Privacy and Applications in Nursing, 867
Telephone Triage and Counseling, 867
Communicating with Families, 867
Communicating with Parents, 867
Communicating with Children, 870
Communication Techniques, 875
History Taking, 875
Performing a Health History, 875
Nutritional Assessment, 881
Dietary Intake, 881
Clinical Examination, 883
Evaluation of Nutritional Assessment, 886
General Approaches Toward Examining the Child, 886
Sequence of the Examination, 886
Preparation of the Child, 886

Physical Examination, 888
- Growth Measurements, 889
- Physiologic Measurements, 892
- General Appearance, 900
- Skin, 901
- Lymph Nodes, 902
- Head and Neck, 902
- Eyes, 903
- Ears, 907
- Nose, 910
- Mouth and Throat, 911
- Chest, 912
- Lungs, 914
- Heart, 915
- Abdomen, 917
- Genitalia, 919
- Anus, 921
- Back and Extremities, 921
- Neurologic Assessment, 922

Developmental Assessment, 923
- Denver II, 924
- Denver II Prescreening Developmental Questionnaire, 926

Chapter 35 Pain Assessment and Management, 929

Pain Assessment, 929
- Behavioral Measures, 929
- Physiologic Measures, 929
- Self-Report Measures, 930
- Multidimensional Measures, 931

Pain Assessment in Specific Populations, 933
- Pain in Neonates, 933
- Children with Communication and Cognitive Impairment, 934
- Cultural Issues in Pain Assessment, 934
- Children with Chronic Illness and Complex Pain, 935

Pain Management, 935
- Nonpharmacologic Management, 935
- Complementary Pain Medicine, 938
- Pharmacologic Management, 938

UNIT 9 HEALTH PROMOTION AND SPECIAL HEALTH PROBLEMS, 953

Chapter 36 The Infant and Family, 953

Promoting Optimum Growth and Development, 953
- Biologic Development, 953
- Psychosocial Development, 957
- Cognitive Development, 958
- Development of Body Image, 960
- Social Development, 961
- Temperament, 963
- Coping with Concerns Related to Normal Growth and Development, 965

Promoting Optimum Health During Infancy, 972
- Nutrition, 972
- Sleep and Activity, 976
- Dental Health, 978
- Immunizations, 978
- Injury Prevention, 991
- Anticipatory Guidance—Care of Families, 999

SPECIAL HEALTH PROBLEMS, 999

Feeding Difficulties, 999
- Regurgitation and "Spitting Up," 999
- Colic (Paroxysmal Abdominal Pain), 1001
- Growth Failure (Failure to Thrive), 1003

Disorders of Unknown Etiology, 1005
- Sudden Infant Death Syndrome, 1005
- Apnea and Apparent Life-Threatening Events, 1010

Chapter 37 The Toddler and Family, 1017

Promoting Optimum Growth and Development, 1017
- Biologic Development, 1017
- Psychosocial Development, 1019
- Cognitive Development, 1019
- Spiritual Development, 1021
- Development of Body Image, 1022
- Development of Gender Identity, 1022
- Social Development, 1022
- Coping with Concerns Related to Normal Growth and Development, 1024

Promoting Optimum Health During Toddlerhood, 1029
- Nutrition, 1029
- Sleep and Activity, 1031
- Dental Health, 1031
- Injury Prevention, 1033
- Anticipatory Guidance—Care of Families, 1040

Chapter 38 The Preschooler and Family, 1043

Promoting Optimal Growth and Development, 1043
- Biologic Development, 1043
- Psychosocial Development, 1044
- Cognitive Development, 1044
- Moral Development, 1045
- Spiritual Development, 1045
- Development of Body Image, 1045
- Development of Sexuality, 1045
- Social Development, 1046
- Coping with Concerns Related to Normal Growth and Development, 1048

Promoting Optimum Health During the Preschool Years, 1053
- Nutrition, 1053
- Sleep and Activity, 1054
- Dental Health, 1055
- Injury Prevention, 1055
- Anticipatory Guidance—Care of Families, 1055

Infectious Disorders, 1055
- Communicable Diseases, 1055

Child Maltreatment, 1066
- Child Neglect, 1066
- Physical Abuse, 1066
- Sexual Abuse, 1068
- Nursing Care of the Maltreated Child, 1069

Chapter 39 The School-Age Child and Family, 1077

Promoting Optimal Growth and Development, 1077
- Biologic Development, 1077
- Psychosocial Development, 1079
- Cognitive Development (Piaget), 1079
- Moral Development (Kohlberg), 1081
- Spiritual Development, 1081
- Social Development, 1081
- Developing a Self-Concept, 1084
- Coping with Concerns Related to Normal Growth and Development, 1085

Promoting Optimal Health During the School Years, 1089
Nutrition, 1089
Sleep and Rest, 1090
Exercise and Activity, 1090
Dental Health, 1091
Sex Education, 1092
School Health, 1093
Injury Prevention, 1093
SPECIAL HEALTH PROBLEMS, 1096
Health Problems Related to Sports Participation, 1096
Overuse Syndromes, 1096
Nurse's Role in Sports for Children and Adolescents, 1096
Altered Growth and Maturation, 1097
Tall or Short Stature, 1097
Sex Chromosome Abnormalities, 1098
Disorders with Behavioral Components, 1099
Attention-Deficit/Hyperactivity Disorder and Learning Disability, 1099
Enuresis, 1100
Encopresis, 1100
Posttraumatic Stress Disorder, 1101
School Phobia, 1101
Recurrent Abdominal Pain, 1101
Conversion Reaction, 1102
Childhood Depression, 1102
Childhood Schizophrenia, 1103

Chapter 40 The Adolescent and Family, 1105
Promoting Optimum Growth and Development, 1105
Biologic Development, 1105
Psychosocial Development, 1109
Cognitive Development (Piaget), 1110
Moral Development (Kohlberg), 1111
Spiritual Development, 1111
Social Development, 1111
Adolescent Sexuality, 1113
Development of Self-Concept and Body Image, 1115
Promoting Optimum Health During Adolescence, 1116
Immunizations, 1117
Nutrition, 1118
Sleep and Rest, 1119
Exercise and Activity, 1119
Dental Health, 1120
Personal Care, 1120
Stress Reduction, 1121
Sexuality Education and Guidance, 1122
Injury Prevention, 1122
Anticipatory Guidance—Care of Families, 1124
SPECIAL HEALTH PROBLEMS, 1125
Disorders Related to the Reproductive System, 1125
Amenorrhea, 1125
Dysmenorrhea, 1125
Vaginitis, 1126
Disorders of the Male Reproductive System, 1126
Gynecomastia, 1127
Eating Disorders, 1127
Obesity, 1127
Anorexia Nervosa and Bulimia Nervosa, 1132
Serious Health Problems with a Behavioral Component, 1136
Tobacco, 1136
Substance Abuse, 1137
Suicide, 1140

UNIT 10 SPECIAL NEEDS, ILLNESS, AND HOSPITALIZATION, 1146

Chapter 41 Chronic Illness, Disability, and End-of-Life Care, 1146
Perspectives on the Care of Children with Special Needs, 1146
Scope of the Problem, 1146
Trends in Care, 1147
The Family of the Child with Special Needs, 1149
Impact of the Child's Chronic Illness or Disability, 1149
Coping with Ongoing Stress and Periodic Crises, 1151
Assisting Family Members in Managing Their Feelings, 1152
Establishing a Support System, 1154
The Child with Special Needs, 1154
Developmental Aspects, 1154
Coping Mechanisms, 1154
Responses to Parental Behavior, 1155
Type of Illness or Disability, 1156
Nursing Care of the Family and Child with Special Needs, 1156
Assessment, 1156
Provide Support at the Time of Diagnosis, 1157
Support Family's Coping Methods, 1157
Educate About the Disorder and General Health Care, 1159
Promote Normal Development, 1160
Establish Realistic Future Goals, 1163
Perspectives on the Care of Children at the End of Life, 1164
Principles of Palliative Care, 1164
Decision Making at the End of Life, 1164
Nursing Care of the Child and Family at the End of Life, 1169
Fear of Pain and Suffering, 1169
Fear of Dying Alone or of Not Being Present When the Child Dies, 1170
Fear of Actual Death, 1170
Organ or Tissue Donation and Autopsy, 1172
Grief and Mourning, 1172
Nurses' Reactions to Caring for Dying Children, 1174

Chapter 42 Cognitive and Sensory Impairment, 1177
Cognitive Impairment, 1177
General Concepts, 1177
Nursing Care of Children with Impaired Cognitive Function, 1178
Down Syndrome, 1183
Fragile X Syndrome, 1185
Sensory Impairment, 1186
Hearing Impairment, 1186
Visual Impairment, 1191
Deaf-Blind Children, 1196
Retinoblastoma, 1197
Autism Spectrum Disorders, 1198

Chapter 43 Family-Centered Home Care, 1203
General Concepts of Home Care, 1203
Definition, 1203
Home Care Trends, 1203
Effective Home Care, 1205
Discharge Planning and Selection of a Home Care Agency, 1205
Care Coordination (Case Management), 1208
Role of the Nurse, Training, and Standards of Care, 1208

Family-Centered Home Care, 1209
- Respect for Diversity, 1210
- Parent-Professional Collaboration, 1211
- The Nursing Process, 1212
- Promotion of Optimal Development, Self-Care, and Education, 1214
- Safety Issues in the Home, 1215
- Family-to-Family Support, 1216

Chapter 44 Reaction to Illness and Hospitalization, 1219

Stressors of Hospitalization and Children's Reactions, 1219
- Separation Anxiety, 1219
- Loss of Control, 1221
- Effects of Hospitalization on the Child, 1223

Stressors and Reactions of the Family of the Hospitalized Child, 1224
- Parental Reactions, 1224
- Sibling Reactions, 1224
- Altered Family Roles, 1224

Nursing Care of the Hospitalized Child, 1225
- Preparation for Hospitalization, 1225
- Nursing Interventions, 1228

Nursing Care of the Family, 1236
- Supporting Family Members, 1236
- Providing Information, 1237
- Encouraging Parent Participation, 1237
- Preparing for Discharge and Home Care, 1238

Care of the Child and Family in Special Hospital Situations, 1239
- Ambulatory or Outpatient Setting, 1239
- Isolation, 1239
- Emergency Admission, 1239
- Intensive Care Unit, 1242

Chapter 45 Pediatric Variations of Nursing Interventions, 1245

General Concepts Related to Pediatric Procedures, 1245
- Informed Consent, 1245
- Preparation for Diagnostic and Therapeutic Procedures, 1247
- Surgical Procedures, 1251
- Compliance, 1253

General Hygiene and Care, 1256
- Maintaining Healthy Skin, 1256
- Bathing, 1257
- Oral Hygiene, 1258
- Hair Care, 1258
- Feeding the Sick Child, 1258
- Controlling Elevated Temperatures, 1259
- Family Teaching and Home Care, 1260

Safety, 1261
- Environmental Factors, 1261
- Infection Control, 1262
- Transporting Infants and Children, 1264
- Restraining Methods and Therapeutic Holding, 1265
- Positioning for Procedures, 1266

Collection of Specimens, 1267
- Urine Specimens, 1267
- Stool Specimens, 1270
- Blood Specimens, 1271
- Respiratory Secretion Specimens, 1272

Administration of Medication, 1273
- Determination of Drug Dosage, 1273
- Oral Administration, 1273
- Intramuscular Administration, 1275
- Subcutaneous and Intradermal Administration, 1278
- Intravenous Administration, 1279
- Nasogastric, Orogastric, or Gastrostomy Administration, 1282
- Rectal Administration, 1282
- Optic, Otic, and Nasal Administration, 1282
- Family Teaching and Home Care, 1284

Maintaining Fluid Balance, 1285
- Measurement of Intake and Output, 1285
- Parenteral Fluid Therapy, 1285

Procedures for Maintaining Respiratory Function, 1289
- Inhalation Therapy, 1289
- Bronchial (Postural) Drainage, 1291
- Artificial Ventilation, 1291

Procedures Related to Alternative Feeding Techniques, 1294
- Gavage Feeding, 1295
- Gastrostomy Feeding, 1296
- Nasoduodenal and Nasojejunal Tubes, 1298
- Total Parenteral Nutrition, 1298
- Family Teaching and Home Care, 1298

Procedures Related to Elimination, 1299
- Enema, 1299
- Ostomies, 1299
- Family Teaching and Home Care, 1300

UNIT 11 HEALTH PROBLEMS OF CHILDREN, 1303

Chapter 46 Respiratory Dysfunction, 1303

Respiratory Infection, 1303
- General Aspects of Respiratory Infections, 1303

Upper Respiratory Tract Infections, 1307
- Nasopharyngitis, 1307
- Pharyngitis, 1310
- Tonsillitis, 1311
- Influenza, 1313
- Otitis Media, 1314
- Infectious Mononucleosis, 1317

Croup Syndromes, 1318
- Acute Epiglottitis, 1318
- Acute Laryngitis, 1319
- Acute Laryngotracheobronchitis, 1320
- Acute Spasmodic Laryngitis, 1321
- Bacterial Tracheitis, 1321

Lower Respiratory Tract Infections, 1321
- Bronchitis, 1321
- Respiratory Syncytial Virus and Bronchiolitis, 1321
- Pneumonias, 1324

Other Respiratory Tract Infections, 1326
- Pertussis (Whooping Cough), 1326
- Tuberculosis, 1326
- Severe Acute Respiratory Syndrome, 1329

Pulmonary Dysfunction Caused by Noninfectious Irritants, 1330
- Foreign Body Aspiration, 1330
- Aspiration Pneumonia, 1330
- Acute Respiratory Distress Syndrome/Acute Lung Injury, 1331
- Smoke Inhalation Injury, 1332
- Environmental Tobacco Smoke Exposure, 1333

Long-Term Respiratory Dysfunction, 1334
Asthma, 1334
Cystic Fibrosis, 1346
Obstructive Sleep-Disordered Breathing, 1353
Respiratory Emergency, 1354
Respiratory Failure, 1354
Cardiopulmonary Resuscitation, 1355
Airway Obstruction, 1358

Chapter 47 Gastrointestinal Dysfunction, 1363
Nutritional Disturbances, 1363
Vitamin Imbalances, 1363
Complementary and Alternative Medicine, 1364
Mineral Imbalances, 1365
Vegetarian Diets, 1365
Nursing Care Management, 1366
The Dietary References Intakes (DRIs), 1366
Protein-Energy Malnutrition, 1368
Food Sensitivity, 1370
Gastrointestinal Dysfunction, 1380
Dehydration, 1380
Disorders of Motility, 1383
Diarrhea, 1383
Constipation, 1389
Hirschsprung Disease, 1391
Vomiting, 1393
Gastroesophageal Reflux, 1394
Intestinal Parasitic Diseases, 1395
General Nursing Care Management, 1395
Giardiasis, 1396
Enterobiasis (Pinworms), 1397
Inflammatory Disorders, 1398
Acute Appendicitis, 1398
Meckel's Diverticulum, 1400
Inflammatory Bowel Disease, 1401
Peptic Ulcer Disease, 1404
Hepatic Disorders, 1406
Acute Hepatitis, 1406
Cirrhosis, 1409
Biliary Atresia, 1410
Structural Defects, 1411
Cleft Lip or Cleft Palate, 1411
Esophageal Atresia with Tracheoesophageal Fistula, 1414
Hernias, 1417
Obstructive Disorders, 1417
Hypertrophic Pyloric Stenosis, 1417
Intussusception, 1420
Malrotation and Volvulus, 1422
Anorectal Malformations, 1422
Malabsorption Syndromes, 1423
Celiac Disease, 1423
Short-Bowel Syndrome, 1425
Ingestion of Injurious Agents, 1426
Principles of Emergency Treatment, 1426
Heavy Metal Poisoning, 1432
Lead Poisoning, 1432

Chapter 48 Cardiovascular Dysfunction, 1442
Cardiovascular Dysfunction, 1442
Congenital Heart Disease, 1445
Circulatory Changes at Birth, 1446
Altered Hemodynamics, 1446
Classification of Defects, 1447
Clinical Consequences of Congenital Heart Disease, 1453
Congestive Heart Failure, 1453
Hypoxemia, 1464
Nursing Care of the Family and Child with Congenital Heart Disease, 1467
Help Family Adjust to the Disorder, 1467
Educate Family About the Disorder, 1468
Help Family Manage the Illness at Home, 1468
Prepare Child and Family for Invasive Procedures, 1469
Provide Postoperative Care, 1469
Plan for Discharge and Home Care, 1471
Acquired Cardiovascular Disorders, 1472
Bacterial (Infective) Endocarditis, 1472
Rheumatic Fever, 1473
Hyperlipidemia (Hypercholesterolemia), 1474
Cardiac Dysrhythmias, 1476
Pulmonary Artery Hypertension, 1477
Cardiomyopathy, 1478
Heart Transplantation, 1478
Vascular Dysfunction, 1479
Systemic Hypertension, 1479
Kawasaki Disease (Mucocutaneous Lymph Node Syndrome), 1481
Shock, 1482
Anaphylaxis, 1485
Septic Shock, 1486

Chapter 49 Hematologic and Immunologic Dysfunction, 1490
Hematologic and Immunologic Dysfunction, 1490
Red Blood Cell Disorders, 1490
Anemia, 1490
Iron Deficiency Anemia, 1493
Sickle Cell Anemia, 1495
β-Thalassemia (Cooley Anemia), 1500
Aplastic Anemia, 1501
Defects in Hemostasis, 1502
Hemophilia, 1503
Idiopathic Thrombocytopenic Purpura, 1505
Disseminated Intravascular Coagulation, 1506
Epistaxis (Nosebleeding), 1507
Neoplastic Disorders, 1507
Leukemias, 1507
Lymphomas, 1514
Hodgkin's Disease, 1514
Non-Hodgkin's Lymphoma, 1516
Immunologic Deficiency Disorders, 1516
Human Immunodeficiency Virus Infection and Acquired Immunodeficiency Syndrome, 1516
Severe Combined Immunodeficiency Disease, 1519
Wiskott-Aldrich Syndrome, 1520
Technologic Management of Hematologic and Immunologic Disorders, 1520
Blood Transfusion Therapy, 1520
Hematopoietic Stem Cell Transplantation, 1522
Apheresis, 1523

Chapter 50 Genitourinary Dysfunction, 1526
Genitourinary Dysfunction, 1526
Genitourinary Tract Disorders and Defects, 1530
Urinary Tract Infection, 1530
Obstructive Uropathy, 1533
External Defects, 1534

Glomerular Disease, 1535
Nephrotic Syndrome, 1535
Acute Glomerulonephritis, 1538
Miscellaneous Renal Disorders, 1540
Hemolytic Uremic Syndrome, 1540
Wilms' Tumor, 1540
Renal Failure, 1542
Acute Renal Failure, 1542
Chronic Renal Failure, 1545
Technologic Management of Renal Failure, 1547
Dialysis, 1547
Transplantation, 1548

Chapter 51 Cerebral Dysfunction, 1551
Assessment of Cerebral Function, 1551
General Aspects, 1551
Increased Intracranial Pressure, 1552
Altered States of Consciousness, 1552
Neurologic Examination, 1553
Special Diagnostic Procedures, 1555
Nursing Care of the Unconscious Child, 1558
Respiratory Management, 1558
Intracranial Pressure Monitoring, 1559
Nutrition and Hydration, 1560
Medications, 1561
Thermoregulation, 1561
Elimination, 1561
Hygienic Care, 1561
Positioning and Exercise, 1561
Stimulation, 1561
Family Support, 1562
Cerebral Trauma, 1562
Head Injury, 1562
Near-Drowning, 1570
Nervous System Tumors, 1572
Brain Tumors, 1572
Neuroblastoma, 1574
Intracranial Infections, 1575
Bacterial Meningitis, 1575
Nonbacterial (Aseptic) Meningitis, 1578
Encephalitis, 1578
Rabies, 1579
Reye's Syndrome, 1580
Seizure Disorders, 1581
Epilepsy, 1581
Febrile Seizures, 1592
Cerebral Malformations, 1593
Cranial Deformities, 1593
Hydrocephalus, 1593

Chapter 52 Endocrine Dysfunction, 1600
Disorders of Pituitary Function, 1600
Hypopituitarism, 1600
Pituitary Hyperfunction, 1602
Precocious Puberty, 1603
Diabetes Insipidus, 1604
Syndrome of Inappropriate Antidiuretic Hormone, 1605
Disorders of Thyroid Function, 1605
Juvenile Hypothyroidism, 1605
Goiter, 1606
Lymphocytic Thyroiditis, 1606
Hyperthyroidism, 1607
Disorders of Parathyroid Function, 1609
Hypoparathyroidism, 1609
Hyperparathyroidism, 1610
Disorders of Adrenal Function, 1611
Acute Adrenocortical Insufficiency, 1611
Chronic Adrenocortical Insufficiency (Addison's Disease), 1612
Cushing's Syndrome, 1613
Congenital Adrenal Hyperplasia, 1614
Pheochromocytoma, 1615
Disorders of Pancreatic Hormone Secretion: Diabetes Mellitus, 1616

Chapter 53 Integumentary Dysfunction, 1632
Integumentary Dysfunction, 1632
Skin Lesions, 1632
Wounds, 1633
General Therapeutic Management, 1636
Nursing Care Management, 1639
Home Care and Family Support, 1641
Infections of the Skin, 1641
Bacterial Infections, 1641
Viral Infections, 1642
Dermatophytoses (Fungal Infections), 1643
Systemic Mycotic (Fungal) Infections, 1643
Skin Disorders Related to Chemical or Physical Contacts, 1646
Contact Dermatitis, 1646
Poison Ivy, Oak, and Sumac, 1647
Drug Reactions, 1648
Foreign Bodies, 1648
Skin Disorders Related to Animal Contacts, 1648
Arthropod Bites and Stings, 1648
Scabies, 1650
Pediculosis Capitis, 1651
Rickettsial Diseases, 1652
Lyme Disease, 1653
Mammal Bites and Scratches, 1654
Pet and Wild Animal Bites, 1654
Human Bites, 1654
Cat-Scratch Disease, 1654
Miscellaneous Skin Disorders, 1655
Skin Disorders Associated with Specific Age Groups, 1655
Diaper Dermatitis, 1655
Atopic Dermatitis (Eczema), 1656
Seborrheic Dermatitis, 1659
Acne, 1659
Thermal Injury, 1661
Burns, 1661
Sunburn, 1673
Cold Injury, 1674

Chapter 54 Musculoskeletal or Articular Dysfunction, 1676
The Immobilized Child, 1676
Physiologic Effects of Immobilization, 1676
Psychologic Effects of Immobilization, 1678
Effect on Families, 1678

Traumatic Injury, 1680
Soft-Tissue Injury, 1680
Fractures, 1681
The Child in a Cast, 1684
The Child in Traction, 1686
Distraction, 1690
Amputation, 1690
Congenital Defects, 1691
Developmental Dysplasia of the Hip, 1691
Congenital Clubfoot, 1693
Metatarsus Adductus (Varus), 1695
Skeletal Limb Deficiency, 1695
Osteogenesis Imperfecta, 1696
Acquired Defects, 1697
Legg-Calvé-Perthes Disease, 1697
Slipped Capital Femoral Epiphysis, 1698
Kyphosis and Lordosis, 1699
Idiopathic Scoliosis, 1700
Infections of Bones and Joints, 1703
Osteomyelitis, 1703
Septic Arthritis, 1704
Skeletal Tuberculosis, 1705
Bone and Soft-Tissue Tumors, 1705
General Concepts: Bone Tumors, 1705
Osteosarcoma, 1705
Ewing's Sarcoma (Primitive Neuroectodermal Tumor), 1707
Rhabdomyosarcoma, 1707
Disorders of Joints, 1708
Juvenile Idiopathic Arthritis (Juvenile Rheumatoid Arthritis), 1708
Systemic Lupus Erythematosus, 1711

Chapter 55 Neuromuscular or Muscular Dysfunction, 1716
Congenital Neuromuscular or Muscular Disorders, 1716
Cerebral Palsy, 1716
Spina Bifida (Myelomeningocele), 1724
Spinal Muscular Atrophy, 1731
Spinal Muscular Atrophy Type 1 (Werdnig-Hoffmann Disease), 1731
Spinal Muscular Atrophy Type 3 (Kugelberg-Welander Disease), 1732
Muscular Dystrophies, 1733
Duchenne (Pseudohypertrophic) Muscular Dystrophy, 1733
Acquired Neuromuscular Disorders, 1735
Guillain-Barré Syndrome (Infectious Polyneuritis), 1735
Tetanus, 1737
Botulism, 1739
Spinal Cord Injuries, 1740

APPENDIXES, 1745

A Relationship of Drugs to Breast Milk and Effect on Infant, 1745
B Developmental/Sensory Assessment, 1749
C Growth Measurements, 1751
D Common Laboratory Tests, 1753
E Pediatric Vital Signs and Parameters, 1762

Part 1

Maternity Nursing

Unit 1 Introduction to Maternity Nursing

Unit 2 Reproductive Years

Unit 3 Pregnancy

Unit 4 Childbirth

Unit 5 Postpartum Period

Unit 6 Newborn

Unit 1

1 Contemporary Maternity Nursing

Learning Objectives

On completion of this chapter the reader will be able to:

- Describe the scope of maternity nursing.
- Evaluate contemporary issues and trends in maternity nursing.
- Describe sociopolitical issues affecting the care of women and infants.
- Compare selected biostatistical data among races and countries.
- Examine social concerns in maternity nursing.
- Explain risk management and standards of practice in the delivery of nursing care.
- Debate ethical issues in perinatal nursing.
- Examine the *Healthy People 2010* goals related to maternal and infant care.

Electronic Resources

Additional information related to the content in Chapter 1 can be found on

Evolve the Companion Website at

http://evolve.elsevier.com/Perry/maternal/

- NCLEX Review Questions

Maternity nursing focuses on the care of childbearing women and their families through all stages of pregnancy and childbirth, as well as the first 4 weeks after birth. Throughout the prenatal period nurses, nurse practitioners, and nurse-midwives provide care for women in clinics and physicians' offices and teach classes to help families prepare for childbirth. Nurses care for childbearing families during labor and birth in hospitals, in birthing centers (e.g., *www.birthcenters.org*), and in the home. Nurses with special training may provide intensive care for high risk neonates in special care units and for high risk mothers in antepartum units, in critical care obstetric units, or in the home. Maternity nurses teach about pregnancy; the process of labor, birth, and recovery; and parenting skills. They provide continuity of care throughout the childbearing cycle. An excellent model for nurses who care for women and children is the International Confederation of Midwives' *(www.internationalmidwives.org)* Vision for Women and Their Health (Box 1-1).

Nurses caring for women have helped make the health care system more responsive to women's needs. Nurses have been critically important in developing strategies to improve the well-being of women and their infants and have led the efforts to implement clinical practice guidelines and to practice using an evidence-based approach. Through professional associations, nurses can have a voice in setting standards and influencing health policy by actively participating in the education of the public and of state and federal legislators (e.g., *www.nursingworld.org; www.can-nurses.ca; www.awhonn.org*). Some nurses hold elective office and influence policy directly.

Tremendous advances have taken place in the care of mothers and their infants during the past 150 years (Box 1-2).

BOX 1-1 The Vision for Women and Their Health

The International Confederation of Midwives envisions a world where:

- Women are respected and treated as persons in their own right in all societies.
- Women stand as equal partners with men in the world order.
- Women are recognized as crucial to the health of any nation.
- Women and their families are part of a health care system with high-quality care and easy access when needed.
- Women have the right to choose from among safe options for care throughout their lives, including high-quality, state-of-the-art care from competent providers who truly care about the woman and her health.
- Women are educated and empowered to delight in a strong sense of self, to trust their bodies, to plan their pregnancies, and to make wise choices in their health care.
- Women experience a reasonable standard of living, including a clean and safe environment, healthy food, and a reasonable place to live.
- No woman has to fear for her life or the life of her baby when she is pregnant.
- Women believe that birth is normal and prefer to avoid unnecessary intervention.

Source: The International Confederation of Midwives. Available at www.internationalmidwives.org/vision.htm (accessed April 11, 2008).

BOX 1-2 Historic Milestones in the Care of Mothers and Infants

1847—James Young Simpson in Edinburgh, Scotland, used ether for an internal podalic version and birth; first reported use of obstetric anesthesia
1861—Ignaz Semmelwies wrote *The Cause, Concept, and Prophylaxis of Childbed Fever*
1906—First program for prenatal nursing care established
1908—Childbirth classes started by the American Red Cross
1909—First White House Conference on Children convened
1911—First milk bank in the United States established in Boston
1912—U.S. Children's Bureau established
1915—Radical mastectomy determined to be effective treatment for breast cancer
1916—Margaret Sanger established first American birth control clinic in Brooklyn, NY
1918—Condoms became legal in the United States
1923—First U.S. hospital center for premature infant care established at Sarah Morris Hospital in Chicago
1929—The modern tampon (with an applicator) invented and patented
1933—Sodium pentothal used as anesthesia for childbirth; *Natural Childbirth* published by Grantly Dick-Read
1935—Sulfonamides introduced as cure for puerperal fever
1941—Penicillin used as treatment for infection
1941—Papanicolaou (Pap) tests introduced
1942—Premarin approved by the Food and Drug Administration (FDA) as treatment for menopausal symptoms
1953—Virginia Apgar, an anesthesiologist, published Apgar scoring system of neonatal assessment
1956—Oxygen determined to cause retrolental fibroplasia (now known as retinopathy of prematurity)
1958—Edward Hon reported on the recording of the fetal electrocardiogram from the maternal abdomen (first commercial electronic fetal monitor produced in late 1960s)
1958—Ian Donald, a Glasgow physician, was first to report clinical use of ultrasound to examine the fetus
1959—*Thank You, Dr. Lamaze* published by Marjorie Karmel
1959—Cytologic studies demonstrated that Down syndrome is associated with a particular form of nondisjunction now known as trisomy 21
1960—American Society for Psychoprophylaxis in Obstetrics (ASPO/Lamaze) formed
1960—International Childbirth Education Association formed
1960—Birth control pill introduced in the United States
1962—Thalidomide found to cause birth defects
1963—Title V of the Social Security Act amended to include comprehensive maternity and infant care for women who were low income and high risk
1965—Supreme Court ruled married people have the right to use birth control
1967—Rh_o(D) immune globulin produced
1967—Reva Rubin published article on Maternal Role Attainment
1968—Rubella vaccine available
1969—Nurses Association of the American College of Obstetricians and Gynecologists (NAACOG) founded; renamed Association of Women's Health, Obstetric and Neonatal Nurses (AWHONN) and incorporated as a 501(c)3 organization in 1993
1969—Mammogram became available
1972—Special Supplemental Food Program for Women, Infants, and Children (WIC) started
1973—Abortion legalized
1974—First standards for obstetric, gynecologic, and neonatal nursing published by NAACOG
1975—The Pregnant Patient's Bill of Rights published by the International Childbirth Education Association
1976—First home pregnancy kits approved by FDA
1978—Louise Brown, first test-tube baby, born
1987—Safe Motherhood Initiative launched by World Health Organization and other international agencies
1991—Society for Advancement of Women's Health Research founded
1992—Office of Research on Women's Health authorized by U.S. Congress
1993—Female condom approved by FDA
1993—Human embryos cloned at George Washington University
1993—Family and Medical Leave Act enacted
1994—DNA sequences of BRCA1 and BRCA2 identified
1994—Zidovudine guidelines published to reduce mother to fetus transmission of HIV
1996—FDA mandated folic acid fortification in all breads and grains sold in United States
1998—Newborns' and Mothers' Health Act put into effect
1998—First emergency contraception pill for pregnancy prevention in women who had unprotected sex approved by FDA
2000—Working draft of sequence and analysis of human genome completed
2006—HPV vaccine available

However, in the United States serious problems exist related to the health and health care of mothers and infants. Lack of access to prepregnancy and pregnancy-related care for all women and of reproductive health services for adolescents are major concerns. Sexually transmitted infections, including acquired immunodeficiency syndrome (AIDS), continue to affect reproduction adversely.

Racial and ethnic diversity is increasing within North America. It is estimated that by the year 2050 50% of the population will be European-American, 15% will be African-American, 24% will be Hispanic, and 8% will be Asian-American (U.S. Census Bureau, 2004). Significant disparity exists in health outcomes among people of various racial and ethnic groups despite the great strides in public health that the

United States has made. People may have lifestyles, health needs, and health care preferences related to their ethnic or cultural backgrounds. They may have dietary preferences and health practices that are not understood by caregivers. To meet the health care needs of a culturally diverse society, the nursing workforce must reflect the diversity of its patient population.

The focus of the first part of this book is maternity nursing. Chapter 1 presents a general overview of issues and trends related to the health and health care of women and infants during the maternity cycle. The second part, which begins with Chapter 29, addresses the issues and trends related to the health care of children.

Contemporary Issues and Trends

Healthy People 2010 Goals

Healthy People 2010 is the United States' agenda for improving health. It has two overarching goals: to increase the quality and years of healthy life and to eliminate health disparities. In *Healthy People 2010* the 467 objectives to improve health are organized into 28 specific focus areas, including one related to maternal, infant, and child health (Box 1-3). Current information about the goals of *Healthy People 2010* is available on the Internet *(www.health.gov/healthypeople)*.

Millennium Development Goals

The Millennium Development Goals (MDGs) are eight goals to be achieved by 2015 that respond to the world's main development challenges. The MDGs are drawn from the actions and targets contained in the Millennium Declaration that was adopted by 189 nations and signed by 147 heads of state and governments during the United Nations Millennium Summit in September 2000 *(www.un.org/millenniumgoals/goals.html)*. Goals 3 through 5 of the MDGs relate specifically to women and children (Box 1-4).

Integrative Health Care

Integrative health care encompasses complementary and alternative therapies in combination with conventional Western modalities of treatment. Many popular alternative healing modalities offer human-centered care based on philosophies that recognize the value of the patient's input and honor the individual's beliefs, values, and desires (Fig. 1-1). The focus of these modalities is on the whole person, not just on a disease complex. Patients often find that alternative modalities are more consistent with their own belief systems and allow for more patient autonomy in health care decisions. Complementary and alternative therapies are identified throughout the text with an icon. ( )

BOX 1-3 *Healthy People 2010*, Focus Area 16, Maternal, Infant, and Child Health

Goal: Improve the health and well-being of women, infants, children, and families

- Fetal, infant, and child deaths
- Maternal death and illness
- Prenatal care
- Obstetric care
- Risk factors
- Developmental disabilities and neural tube defects
- Prenatal substance exposure
- Breastfeeding, newborn screening, and service systems

From US Department of Health and Human Services: *Healthy People 2010* (conference edition, two volumes), Washington, DC, 2000, USDHHS.

Problems with the U.S. Health Care System

Structure of the Health Care Delivery System

The changing health care delivery system offers opportunities for nurses to alter nursing practice and improve the way care is delivered through managed care, integrated delivery systems, and redefined roles. There is increased consumer participation in health care decisions, information is available on the Internet, and care is provided in a technology-intensive environment (Tiedje, Price, & You, 2008).

The American Nurses Association (ANA) published *ANA's Health System Reform Agenda* (2008). ANA believes that the most critical elements of health care reform are access, quality, cost, and the workforce. Elements of access are affordability, availability, and acceptability. Care must be directed away from costly secondary and tertiary care and toward primary care.

BOX 1-4 The United Nations Millennium Development Goals

Goal 1—Eradicate extreme poverty and hunger
Goal 2—Achieve universal primary education
Goal 3—Promote gender equality and empower women
Goal 4—Reduce child mortality
Goal 5—Improve maternal health
Goal 6—Combat HIV/AIDS, malaria, and other diseases
Goal 7—Ensure environmental sustainability
Goal 8—Develop a global partnership for development

Source: UN Millennium Development Goals. Available at www.un.org/millenniumgoals/goals.html (accessed April 19, 2008).
AIDS, Acquired immunodeficiency syndrome; *HIV*, human immunodeficiency virus.

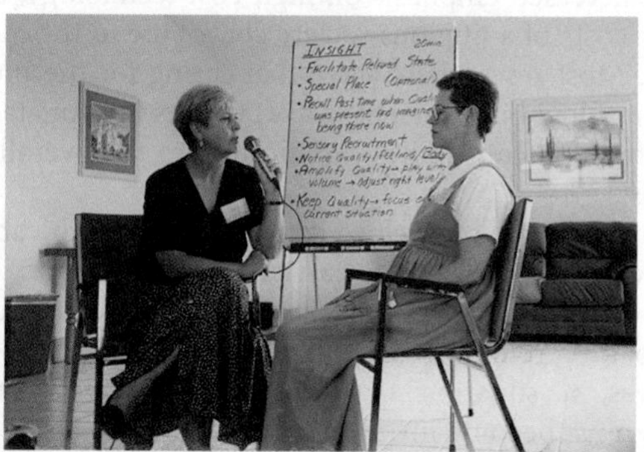

Fig. 1-1 Nurse and patient during guided imagery session. *(Courtesy Nurses Certificate Program in Interactive Imagery, Foster City, CA.)*

BOX 1-5 National Quality Forum "Never Events" Pertaining to Maternal and Child Health

- Infant discharged to the wrong person
- Maternal death or serious disability associated with labor or delivery in a low risk pregnancy while being cared for in a health care facility
- Death or serious disability (kernicterus) associated with failure to identify and treat hyperbilirubinemia in neonates
- Artificial insemination with the wrong donor sperm or donor egg

Source: The National Quality Forum: National Quality Forum Updates Endorsement of *Serious Reportable Events in Healthcare.* Available at www.qualityforum.org (accessed May 24, 2008).

Reducing Medical Errors

Medical errors are the leading cause of death in the United States and result in as many as 98,000 deaths per year (Gauthier & Serber, 2005). In Canada adverse events are implicated in up to 23,750 deaths per year (French, 2006). Since the Institute of Medicine released its 1999 report, *To Err Is Human: Building a Safer Health System*, there has been a concerted effort to analyze causes of errors and develop strategies to avoid them. In 2002 the National Quality Forum published a list of 27 events that should never occur in a health care facility (Shalo, 2007). The list was updated in 2006 with the addition of one event. Of these 28 events, four pertain to maternity and newborn care (Box 1-5).

Recognizing the multifaceted causes of medical errors, The Agency for Healthcare Research and Quality (20 Tips, 2000) prepared a *Patient Fact Sheet* with *20 Tips to Help Prevent Medical Errors* for patients and the public. Patients are encouraged to be knowledgeable consumers of health care and ask questions of providers, including physicians, midwives, nurses, and pharmacists.

High Cost of Health Care

Health care is one of the fastest-growing sectors of the U.S. economy. Currently 16% of the gross domestic product is spent on health care, with an expectation that the proportion will rise to 20% by 2016 (Roehr, 2008). A shift in demographics, an increased emphasis on high-cost technology, and the liability costs of a litigious society contribute to the high cost of care. Most researchers agree that caring for the increased number of low-birth-weight (LBW) infants in neonatal intensive care units contributes significantly to the overall health care costs.

Midwifery care has helped contain some health care costs. However, not all insurance carriers reimburse nurse practitioners and clinical nurse specialists as direct care providers. Nor do they reimburse for all services provided by nurse-midwives, a situation that continues to be a problem. Nurses must become involved in the politics of cost containment because they, as knowledgeable experts, can provide solutions to many health care problems at a relatively low cost.

Limited Access to Care

Barriers to access must be removed so pregnancy outcomes can be improved. The most significant barrier to access is the inability to pay. The number of uninsured people in the United States in 2006 was 47 million or 15.8% of the population (DeNavas-Walt, Proctor, & Smith, 2007). Lack of transportation and dependent child care are other barriers. In addition to a lack of insurance and high costs, a lack of providers for low-income women exists. Many physicians either refuse to take Medicaid patients or take only a few such patients. This presents a serious problem because a significant proportion of births are to mothers who receive Medicaid.

Efforts to Reduce Health Disparities

Significant disparities in morbidity and mortality rates are experienced by African-Americans, Native Americans, Hispanics, Alaska Natives, and Asians/Pacific Islanders. Shorter life expectancy, higher infant and maternal mortality rates, more birth defects, and more sexually transmitted infections are found among these groups. The disparities are thought to result from a complex interaction among biologic factors, environment, and health behaviors. Disparities in education and income are associated with differences in occurrence of morbidity and mortality. A broad public health perspective is needed to reduce these disparities (Satcher & Higginbotham, 2008).

The Health Resources and Services Administration (HRSA) Health Disparities Collaboratives is a national effort with the goal of eliminating disparities and improving delivery systems of health care for all people in the United States who are cared for in HRSA-supported health centers (Calvo, 2006). The National Institutes of Health has a commitment to improve the health of minorities and provides funding for research and training of minority researchers (*www.nih.gov*). The National Institute of Nursing Research (*www.ninr.nih.gov*) has included the goal of reducing disparities in its strategic plan and supports research for that purpose. The nation must make a concerted effort to eliminate health disparities.

Trends in Fertility and Birthrate

Fertility trends and birthrates reflect women's needs for health care. Box 1-6 defines biostatistical terminology useful in analyzing maternity health care. In 2006 the *fertility rate*, the number of births per 1000 women from 15 to 44 years of age, increased 3%, to 68.5 (Martin et al, 2008). The highest *birthrates* (number of births per 1000 women) were for women between ages 25 and 29 (116.8 per 1000), but the birthrate for women in their forties (9.4 per 1000) continues to increase (Martin et al, 2008). More than one third (38.5%) of all births in the United States in 2006 were to unmarried women, with much variation in proportion among racial groups (non-Hispanic Black 70.7%, Hispanic 49.9%, non-Hispanic white 26.6%) (Martin et al, 2008). Births to unmarried women are often related to less favorable outcomes such as LBW or preterm birth because there are typically a large number of teenagers in the unmarried group. In 2006 10.4% of all births were to women less than 20 years of age (Martin et al, 2008) (see Critical Thinking Exercise).

BOX 1-6 Maternal-Infant Biostatistical Terminology

Abortus—An embryo or fetus that is removed or expelled from the uterus at 20 weeks of gestation or less, weighs 500 g or less, or measures 25 cm or less

Birthrate—Number of live births in 1 year per 1000 population

Fertility rate—Number of births per 1000 women between the ages of 15 and 44 (inclusive), calculated on a yearly basis

Infant mortality rate—Number of deaths of infants under 1 year of age per 1000 live births

Maternal mortality rate—Number of maternal deaths from births and complications of pregnancy, childbirth, and puerperium (the first 42 days after termination of the pregnancy) per 100,000 live births

Neonatal mortality rate—Number of deaths of infants under 28 days of age per 1000 live births

Perinatal mortality rate—Number of stillbirths and number of neonatal deaths per 1000 live births

Stillbirth—An infant who at birth demonstrates no signs of life such as breathing, heartbeat, or voluntary muscle movements

CRITICAL THINKING EXERCISE

Prevention Programs for Teenage Pregnancy

The rate of teenage pregnancy in the United States is high. Many babies born to these young women are of low birth weight and/or are preterm. Many effective programs exist to provide education to decrease sexual activity among teens, the rate of sexually transmitted infections, and teen pregnancy (see Science and Success, Second Edition [available online at *www.advocatesforyouth.org*] or What Works 2008 [available on line at *www.thenationalcampaign.org/resources/pdf/pubs/What_Works.pdf*]). Access the website of the public health department in your community to determine the teen pregnancy rate in your community. Based on your knowledge of the community in which you reside, which one(s) of the programs described would likely be accepted? Consider the educational level, ethnicity, religious context, culture, and socioeconomic status of the people in the community.

1. Evidence—Is there sufficient evidence to determine the effectiveness of teenage pregnancy prevention programs?
2. List the assumptions that can be made about the acceptability of any of the programs in relation to:
   a. Age of the participants
   b. Cultural and ethnicity of the population in the community in which the program will occur
   c. Location of the programs
   d. Cultural and ethnicity of the presenter of the programs
3. What implications and priorities for nursing care can be drawn at this time?
4. Does the evidence objectively support your conclusion?
5. Are there alternative perspectives to your conclusion?

Low Birth Weight and Preterm Birth

The risks of morbidity and mortality increase for newborns weighing less than 2500 g (5 lb, 8 oz)—LBW infants. Multiple births contribute to the incidence of LBW. In 2006 the incidence of LBW was 8.3%, and the incidence of very low birth weight (VLBW; less than 1500 g) was 1.4% (Martin et al, 2008). There is racial disparity in the incidence of LBW. Non-Hispanic black babies are twice as likely as non-Hispanic white babies to be LBW and to die within the first year of life. By race the incidence of LBW for non-Hispanic black births was 14%; for non-Hispanic white births, 7.3%; and for Hispanic births, 6.9%. Cigarette smoking is associated with LBW, prematurity, and intrauterine growth restriction. In 2005 10.7% of pregnant women smoked, a proportion that declined slightly from 2004 (Martin et al, 2008).

The proportion of preterm infants (i.e., those born before 38 weeks of gestation) was 12.8% in 2006. There was racial variation in rates: 18.4% for non-Hispanic black births, 12.2% for Hispanic births, and 11.7% for non-Hispanic white births (Martin et al, 2008). Multiple births accounted for 3.4% of births in 2006, with most of the increase associated with increased use of fertility drugs and older age at childbearing (Martin et al, 2008).

Infant Mortality in the United States

A common indicator of the adequacy of prenatal care and the health of a nation as a whole is the *infant mortality rate*, the number of deaths of infants younger than 1 year of age per 1000 live births. The neonatal mortality rate is the number of deaths of infants younger than 28 days of age per 1000 live births. The perinatal mortality rate is the number of stillbirths plus the number of neonatal deaths per 1000 live births. The preliminary infant mortality rate for 2005 was 6.9 (Martin et al, 2008). The infant mortality rate continues to be higher for non-Hispanic black babies (13.60 per 1000) than for non-Hispanic white babies (5.66 per 1000) and Hispanic babies (5.55 per 1000) (Martin et al, 2008). Limited maternal education, young maternal age, unmarried status, poverty, and lack of prenatal care appear to be associated with higher infant mortality rates. Poor nutrition, smoking and alcohol use, and maternal conditions such as poor health or hypertension are also important contributors to infant mortality. To address the factors associated with infant mortality, there must be a shift from the current emphasis on high-technology medical interventions to a focus on improving access to preventive care for low-income families.

International Trends in Infant Mortality

The infant mortality rate of Canada (5.3 per 1000 in 2003 [data not available for 2004]) ranks twenty-fifth, and that of the United States ranks twenty-ninth (6.8 per 1000 in 2004) when compared with other industrialized nations (Martin et al, 2008). One reason for this is the high rate of LBW infants born in the United States compared with other countries.

Maternal Mortality Trends

The fifth Millennium Development Goal is to improve maternal health and reduce maternal mortality rate by 75% between

1990 and 2015. Worldwide approximately 1400 women die each day of problems related to pregnancy or childbirth, with hemorrhage being the leading cause of death. There are great disparities in maternal mortality rate between developing and developed countries. In the United States in 2004 the annual maternal mortality rate (number of maternal deaths per 100,000 live births) was 11.3 (National Center for Health Statistics, 2007), whereas the rate in Africa in 2005 was 820 (WHO, 2007).

In the United States there are significant racial differences in the rates: black or African-American women have a maternal mortality rate four times higher than that of non-Hispanic white women. The maternal mortality rate was 32.3 per 100,000 for black or African-American women, in contrast with 7.8 per 100,000 for non-Hispanic white women (National Center for Health Statistics, 2007). The *Healthy People 2010* goal of 3.3 maternal deaths per 100,000 poses a significant challenge. To achieve this goal, early diagnosis and appropriate intervention must occur. Worldwide strategies to reduce maternal mortality rates include improving access to skilled attendants at birth, providing postabortion care, improving family planning services, and providing adolescents with better reproductive health services.

Increase in High Risk Pregnancies

The number of high risk pregnancies has increased, which means that a greater number of women are at risk for poor pregnancy outcomes *(www.nlm.nih.gov/medlineplus/highriskpregnancy.html).* Escalating drug use (ranging from 11% to 27% of pregnant women, depending on geographic location) has contributed to higher incidences of prematurity, LBW, congenital defects, learning disabilities, and withdrawal symptoms in infants. Alcohol use in pregnancy has been associated with miscarriages, mental retardation, LBW, and fetal alcohol syndrome.

The twin birth rate was 32.2 per 1000 in 2005. The downward trend in the birthrate of higher-order multiples (triplet, quadruplet, and greater) continued in 2005 with a rate of 161.8 per 100,000 (Martin et al, 2008). The cesarean birthrate increased to 31.1% in 2006, with the primary cesarean rate rising and the number of vaginal births after cesarean dropping (Martin et al, 2008). This cesarean rate is significantly higher than the *Healthy People 2010* goal of 15%.

More than one third of women in the United States are obese (body mass index of 30 or greater), with adults ages 40 to 59 having the highest prevalence. There are significant racial disparities in obesity in women: 53% of non-Hispanic black women, 51% of Mexican-American women, and 39% of non-Hispanic white women ages 40 to 59 are obese *(www.cdc.gov/nchs/pressroon/07newsreleases/obesity.htm).* Almost 20% of women who give birth in the United States are obese. The two most frequently reported maternal medical risk factors are hypertension associated with pregnancy and diabetes, both of which are associated with obesity. Obesity in pregnancy is associated with use of more health care services and hospital stays that are longer (Chu et al, 2008).

Table 1-1 Percent of Women Receiving Six Obstetric Procedures

PROCEDURE	PERCENT
Induction of labor	22.3
Tocolysis	2.0
Cesarean birth	30.3
Forceps delivery	0.9
Vacuum extraction	3.9
Vaginal birth after cesarean	7.9

Data from Martin JA et al: Births: Final data for 2005, *Natl Health Stat Report* 56(6):1-104, 2007.

High-Technology Care

Advances in scientific knowledge and the large number of high risk pregnancies have contributed to a health care system that emphasizes high-technology care. Maternity care has extended to preconception counseling, more and better scientific techniques to monitor the mother and fetus, more definitive tests for hypoxia and acidosis, and neonatal intensive care units. Virtually all labors in hospital settings are monitored electronically; there are increasing numbers of assisted labors and births (Table 1-1). Internet-based information is available to the public that enhances interactions among health care providers, families, and community providers. Point-of-care testing is available. Personal data assistants are used to enhance comprehensive care; the medical record is increasingly in electronic form. Virtually all women are monitored electronically during labor despite the lack of evidence of the efficacy of such monitoring.

Telemedicine is an umbrella term for the use of communication technologies and electronic information to provide or support health care when the participants are separated by distance. Telemedicine permits specialists, including nurses, to provide health care and consultation when distance separates them from those needing care. This technology has the potential to save billions of dollars annually for health care, but these technologic advances have also contributed to higher health care costs. Nurses must use caution and prospective planning and assess the effect of the emerging technology.

Care During Pregnancy and Childbirth

View of Women

Women must be viewed holistically and in the context in which they live. Their physical, mental, and social factors must be considered because these interdependent components influence health and illness. Even the language health care professionals use to describe women and their problems needs to be examined. For example, practitioners describe women who have an "incompetent cervix," who "fail to progress," or who have an "arrest" of labor. They may describe a fetus as having intrauterine growth "retardation." They also "allow" women a "trial" of labor. The use of these phrases implies a failure or inadequacy of the woman. More positive language should be incorporated into the vocabulary.

Safe Motherhood

The Centers for Disease Control and Prevention (CDC) began working with national and international groups in 2001 to develop and implement programs to promote safe motherhood (Jones, 2008). Maternal mortality and morbidity is a measure of a nation's commitment to the status of women and their health. The leading causes of pregnancy-related deaths in the United States are hemorrhage, blood clots, hypertension, infection, stroke, amniotic fluid embolism, and heart muscle disease. It is estimated that over half of these deaths could be prevented with better access to care, better quality care, and positive changes in the health and lifestyle habits of women. The CDC continues to invest resources to improve positive outcomes and prevent negative outcomes of pregnancy (Jones, 2008).

Childbirth Practices

Prenatal care may promote better pregnancy outcomes by providing early risk assessment and promoting healthy behaviors such as improved nutrition and smoking cessation. In 2005 83.9% of all women received care in the first trimester. There is disparity in use of prenatal care by race and ethnicity; Native American, Hispanic, or non-Hispanic black women were more than twice as likely as non-Hispanic white women to receive late care (i.e., care beginning in the third trimester or no care at all) (Martin et al, 2008). In spite of this, there have been substantial gains in the use of prenatal care since the early 1990s; this is attributed to the expansion in the 1980s of Medicaid coverage for pregnant women.

Women can choose physicians or nurse-midwives as primary care providers. In 2005 physicians attended 92% and nurse-midwives attended approximately 8% of all births (Martin et al, 2008). Hospital births accounted for 99% of births. Of the out-of-hospital births, 67% were in the home, 27% in free-standing birth centers, 0.9% in clinics or doctor's offices, and 5% other or not specified (Martin et al, 2007).

Certified nurse-midwives are registered nurses with education in the two disciplines of nursing and midwifery. Certified midwives (direct-entry midwives) are educated only in the discipline of midwifery. In the United States certification of midwives is through the American College of Nurse-Midwives, the professional association for midwives in the United States. The Royal College of Midwives is the professional association for midwives in the United Kingdom. In Canada the Association of Ontario Midwives is the professional association, and the College of Midwives of Ontario is the regulatory body for midwives in Ontario; the other provinces of Canada have similar regulatory bodies. Many national associations belong to the International Confederation of Midwives, which comprises 83 member associations from 70 countries in the Americas and Europe, Africa, and the Asia-Pacific region.

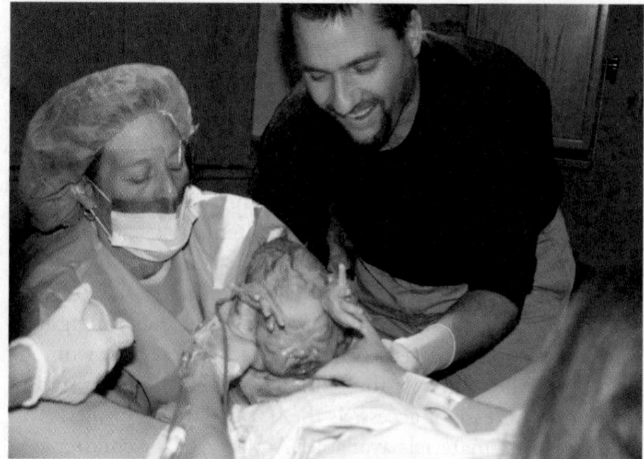

Fig. 1-2 Father "catching" newborn son. Mother is reaching down to help birth the baby. *(Courtesy Darren and Julie Nelson, Loveland, CO.)*

With family-centered care, fathers, partners, grandparents, siblings, and friends may be present for labor and birth. Fathers or partners may be present for cesarean births. Fathers may participate by "catching the baby" and/or cutting the umbilical cord (Fig. 1-2). Doulas—trained and experienced female labor attendants—provide a continuous, one-on-one caring presence throughout the labor and birth. Newborn infants remain with the mother and are encouraged to breastfeed immediately after birth. Parents participate in the care of their infants in nurseries and neonatal intensive care units.

Neonatal security in the hospital setting is of concern. A number of cases of "baby-napping" and of sending parents home with the wrong baby have been reported. Security systems are being placed in nurseries, and nurses are required to wear photo identification or some other security badge.

Discharge of a mother and baby within 24 hours of birth has created a growing need for follow-up or home care. Legislation has been enacted to ensure that mothers and babies are permitted to stay in the hospital at least 48 hours after vaginal birth and 96 hours after cesarean birth, although they may choose to leave earlier. Focused and efficient teaching is necessary to enable the parents and infant to make a safe transition from hospital to home.

Community-Based Care

A shift in settings from acute care institutions to the home has been occurring. Even childbearing women at high risk are cared for in the home. Technology previously available only in the hospital is now found in the home. This has affected the organizational structure of care, the skills required to provide such care, and the cost to consumers.

Home health care also has a community focus. Nurses are involved in caring for women and infants in homeless shelters; in caring for adolescents in school-based clinics; and in promoting health at community sites, churches, and shopping malls. Nursing education curricula are increasingly community based (see Community Focus box).

COMMUNITY FOCUS

Culturally Appropriate and Adequate Prenatal Care

Make an appointment with staff to visit a community health clinic that serves pregnant women. What are the qualifications of the staff (i.e., are there registered nurses, licensed practical/vocational nurses, nutritionists, social workers, childbirth educators, lactation consultants)? Is a laboratory available? What clientele does the clinic serve (i.e., what racial and/or ethnic groups are served)? Is the staff representative of those racial and/or ethnic groups? Is the staff bilingual? Are educational materials available in languages of the women served by the clinic? Is the clinic located near public transportation for ease of access? Is the setting "friendly" (i.e., Are there reading materials available? A play area for children? A restroom? A drinking fountain?) What could improve the setting? Would you be willing to seek care in that clinic?

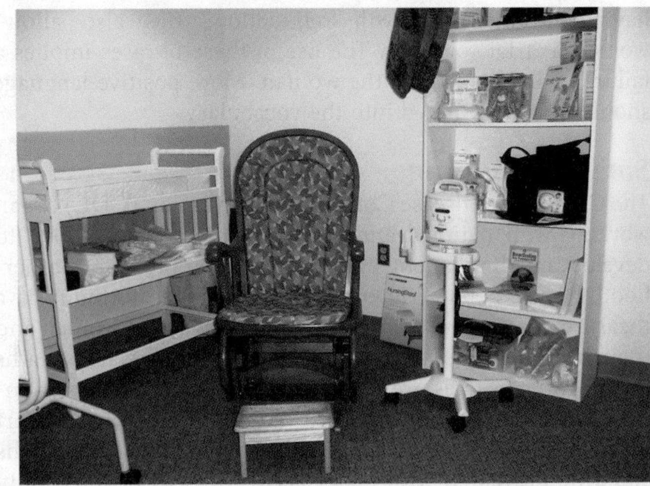

Fig. 1-3 Lactation room. Note the breast pump, rocking chair and nursing foot stool, changing table, books, and supplies. *(Courtesy Cheryl Briggs, RN, Annapolis, MD.)*

Involving Consumers and Promoting Self-Management

Self-management is appealing to both patients and the health care system because of its potential to reduce health care costs. Maternity care is especially suited to self-management because childbearing is essentially health focused, women are usually well when they enter the system, and visits to health care providers can present the opportunity for health and illness interventions. Measures to improve health and reduce risks associated with poor pregnancy outcomes and illness can be addressed. Topics such as nutrition education, stress management, smoking cessation, alcohol and drug treatment, prevention of violence, improvement of social supports, and parenting education are appropriate for such encounters.

Health Literacy

Health literacy involves a spectrum of abilities, ranging from reading an appointment slip to interpreting medication instructions. These skills must be assessed routinely to recognize a problem and accommodate patients with limited literacy skills. An excellent resource is *Teaching Patients with Low Literacy Skills,* second edition (Doak, Doak, & Root, 1996).

Individuals and groups for whom English is a second language often lack the skills necessary to seek medical care and function adequately in the health care setting. As a result of the increasingly multicultural U.S. population, there is an urgent need to address health literacy as a component of culturally and linguistically competent care. Health care providers can contribute to health literacy by speaking slowly and using simple, common words; avoiding jargon; and assessing whether the patient understands the discussion.

Breastfeeding in the Workplace

Women are a significant proportion of the workforce. Companies are recognizing that it is good business to retain good employees and are making provisions for women returning to work after childbirth. Lactation rooms that provide space and privacy for pumping are available at many work sites and on college campuses (Fig. 1-3). In some instances breastfeeding women bring their babies to work. Since 1999, by law women may breastfeed in federal buildings and on federal property. Some states have enacted legislation to ensure that mothers can breastfeed their babies in public places. These efforts may help mothers breastfeed longer and meet the recommendation of the American Academy of Pediatrics that breastfeeding continue for at least 1 year.

International Concerns

Female genital mutilation is the removal of part or all of the female external genitalia for cultural or nontherapeutic reasons (WHO Study Group, 2006). Worldwide, many women undergo such procedures. With the growing number of immigrants from Africa and other countries where female genital mutilation is practiced, nurses will increasingly encounter women who have undergone the procedure. Women who have undergone the procedure are significantly more likely to have adverse obstetric outcomes, resulting in one or two additional perinatal deaths per 100 births (WHO Study Group, 2006). The International Council of Nurses and other health professionals have spoken out against the procedures as harmful to women's health and a violation of human rights.

Trends in Nursing Practice

The increasing complexity of care for maternity and women's health patients has contributed to specialization of nurses working with these patients. This specialized knowledge is gained through experience, advanced degrees, and certification programs. Nurses in advanced practice (e.g., nurse practitioners and nurse-midwives) may provide primary care throughout a woman's life, including during the pregnancy cycle. In some settings the clinical nurse specialist and nurse practitioner roles are blended; and nurses deliver high-quality, comprehensive, and cost-effective care in a variety of settings. Lactation consultants provide services in the postpartum unit or on an outpatient basis, including home visits.

EVIDENCE-BASED PRACTICE Searching for and Evaluating the Evidence —*Pat Gingrich*

Throughout this text you will see Evidence-Based Practice boxes. These boxes provide examples of how a nurse might conduct an inquiry into an identified practice question. Curiosity and access to a virtual or real library are all the nurse needs to be confident that his or her practice has a sound foundation of evidence.

A literature search may reveal up to three levels of evidence. The first layer consists of primary studies. The strongest of these are randomized controlled trials. Well-designed studies, even small ones, each add another piece to the puzzle.

These primary studies may be combined into the second level of evidence. In systematic analyses such as those in the Cochrane Database, the researcher uses a methodology to identify all studies relevant to a particular question. If the data are similar enough, they can be pooled into a meta-analysis. If the evidence is strong, some analyses will form the basis for recommendations for practice and to guide further inquiry.

At the tertiary level professional organizations such as the Agency for Healthcare Research and Quality (AHRQ) *(www.ahrq.gov)* or the Academy of Breastfeeding Medicine (ABM) *(www.bfmed.org)* may decide to address a broad practice question by sorting through all the available primary and secondary evidence, plus consulting experienced clinicians. After thoughtful review the committee of experts in the organization then crafts its consensus statement. These recommendations for best practice stand on the shoulders of the systematic analysts, who stand on the many shoulders of the primary researchers.

Provided the professional organization is well respected and the process is rigorous, these guidelines in the consensus statement carry enormous authority. Individuals and institutions may choose to adopt these guidelines with confidence. An example of this is the Association of Women's Health, Obstetric and Neonatal Nurses (AWHONN) *(www.awhonn.org)* Late Preterm Infant Initiative. This initiative began in 2005 in response to the confusion that surrounded the care of infants who do not qualify for neonatal intensive care admission yet require extra vigilance. Nurseries can adapt these recommendations to their specific institutions, enabling nurses to become more effective at caring for the unique problems of this population of neonates. Like AWHONN, most professional organizations make their guidelines available free of charge on their websites.

Evidence-Based Practice

Evidence-based practice—providing care based on evidence gained through research and clinical trials—is increasingly emphasized. Although not all practice can be evidence based, practitioners must use the best available information on which to base their interventions. The Association of Women's Health, Obstetric and Neonatal Nurses (AWHONN) *(www.awhonn.org) Standards for Professional Nursing Practice in the Care of Women and Newborns* (2003) and the *Standards for Professional Perinatal Nursing Practice and Certification in Canada* (2002) include an evidence-based approach to practice. Discussion of nursing care and evidence-based nursing boxes throughout this text provide examples of evidence-based practice (see Evidence-Based Practice box).

AWHONN has conducted six research-based practice projects (Box 1-7). These projects were conducted in several states, and staff nurses were involved in their implementation and in data collection. The AWHONN practice guidelines incorporate evidence-based practices for second-stage labor management, continence for women, breastfeeding support, midlife well-being, perianesthesia care, neonatal skin care, and cardiac health. By using such guidelines and published reports, nurses can develop protocols and procedures based on published research and incorporate an evidence base into their own practice. AWHONN research priorities include the aforementioned topics, as well as family violence, fetal surveillance, genetics, infertility, and early parenting (Box 1-8).

BOX 1-7 Association of Women's Health, Obstetric and Neonatal Nurses Research-Based Practice Projects

- Transition of the Preterm Infant to an Open Crib
- Management of Women in the Second Stage of Labor
- Continence for Women
- Neonatal Skin Care
- Cyclic Pelvic Pain and Discomfort Management
- Late Preterm Infant Initiative

Source: Available at www.awhonn.org/awhonn/content.do?name=03_JournalsPubsResearch/3G_ResearchBasedPracticeProjects.htm (accessed May 25, 2008).

Cochrane Pregnancy and Childbirth Database

The Cochrane Pregnancy and Childbirth Database was first planned in 1976 with a small grant from the World Health Organization to Dr. Iain Chalmers and colleagues at Oxford. In 1993 the Cochrane Collaboration was formed, and the Oxford Database of Perinatal Trials became known as the Cochrane Pregnancy and Childbirth Database. The Cochrane Collaboration oversees up-to-date, systematic reviews of randomized controlled trials of health care and disseminates these reviews. The premise of the project is that these types of studies provide the most reliable evidence about the effects of care.

The evidence from these studies should encourage practitioners to implement useful measures and abandon those that are useless or harmful. Studies are ranked in six categories:

1. Beneficial forms of care
2. Forms of care that are likely to be beneficial
3. Forms of care with a trade-off between beneficial and adverse effects
4. Forms of care with unknown effectiveness
5. Forms of care that are unlikely to be beneficial
6. Forms of care that are likely to be ineffective or harmful

BOX 1-8 Association of Women's Health, Obstetric and Neonatal Nurses (AWHONN) Research Priorities for Women's and Neonatal Health

Research Priorities

The AWHONN theory-based women's and neonatal health research priorities focus on the development, dissemination, and utilization of knowledge to guide clinical nursing practice. They encompass nursing care of women across their lifespan, including childbearing and newborn care, as well as professional issues in nursing practice.

Clinical

Healthy lifestyles (obesity, nutrition, exercise, stress reductions, cancer screenings)
Preterm births
Access to care (barriers to care)
Mental health in women's health
Patient safety

Professional Practice

Community/environmental influence on women's health (violence)
Nursing sensitivity outcomes
Nursing leadership
Patient safety
Workplace environment (staffing, culture, etc.)
Models of care

Approved by AWHONN Board of Directors 2008.

Practices that have been reviewed by the Collaboration are identified with a symbol (❋) throughout this text.

Joanna Briggs Institute

Founded in 1995 as an initiative of the Royal Adelaide Hospital and the University of Adelaide in Australia, the Joanna Briggs Institute (JBI) uses a collaborative approach for evaluating evidence from a range of sources *(www.joannabriggs.edu.au)*. The JBI has formed collaborations with a variety of universities and hospitals around the world, including in the United States and Canada. It provides another source for perinatal nurses to access information to support evidence-based practice.

A Global Perspective

Advances in medicine and nursing have resulted in increased knowledge and understanding in the care of mothers and infants and reduced perinatal morbidity and mortality rates. However, these advances have affected industrialized nations predominantly. For example, most of the 3.2 million children living with human immunodeficiency virus (HIV) or acquired immunodeficiency syndrome acquired the infection through perinatal transmission and live in sub-Saharan Africa. This illustrates the inequities that exist between industrialized and resource-poor parts of the world. The World Health Organization and partners in nursing developed Strategic Directions for Nursing and Midwifery Services (Box 1-9).

BOX 1-9 Strategic Directions for Nursing and Midwifery Services

- Health and human resource planning
- Management of health personnel
- Evidence-based practice
- Education
- Stewardship and regulation

Source: Al-Gasseer N, Persaud V: Measuring progress in nursing and midwifery globally, *J Nurs Sch* 35(4):309-315, 2003.

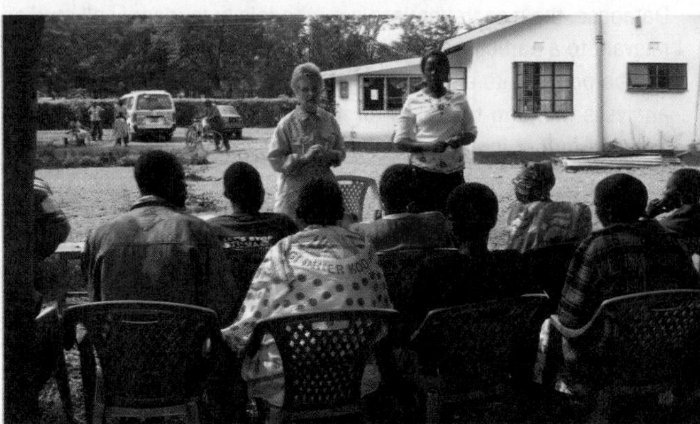

Fig. 1-4 Nurse teaching breast self-examination with the assistance of an interpreter to traditional birth attendants (TBAs) in a rural clinic in Kenya. (Both men and women serve as TBAs.) Women may detect lumps but usually don't seek care unless there is pain associated with the lump. *(Courtesy Shannon Perry, Phoenix, AZ.)*

As the world becomes smaller because of travel and communication technologies, nurses and other health care providers are gaining a global perspective and participating in activities to improve the health and health care of people worldwide (Perry & Mander, 2005). Nurses participate in medical outreach, providing obstetric, surgical, ophthalmologic, orthopedic, or other services; attend international meetings; conduct research; and provide international consultation (Fig. 1-4). International student and faculty exchanges occur. More articles about health and health care in various countries are appearing in nursing journals. Several schools of nursing in the United States are World Health Organization Collaborating Centers.

The Global Health eLearning Center *(www.globalhealthlearning.org)* of USAID currently has 22 free online courses that are useful for nurses and other health care providers who plan to work in developing countries. Of these 22 courses, 14 pertain to the health of women and infants (Box 1-10).

Standards of Practice and Legal Issues in Delivery of Care

Nursing standards of practice in perinatal nursing have been described by several organizations, including the ANA, which

BOX 1-10 Courses Related to Maternal and Infant Health Offered by the USAID Global Health eLearning Center

- Antenatal Care
- Emergency Obstetric and Newborn Care
- Essential Newborn Care
- Family Planning 101
- Family Planning Counseling
- Family Planning Legislative and Policy Requirements
- Immunization Essentials
- Intrauterine Device
- Maternal Survival—Programming Issues
- Mother-to-Child Transmission of Human Immunodeficiency Virus
- Postpartum Care
- Preventing Postpartum Hemorrhage
- Standard Days Method
- Youth Reproductive Health

Source: USAID Global Health eLearning Center. Available at www.globalhealthlearning.org/courses.cfm (accessed May 24, 2008).

publishes standards for maternal-child health nursing; AWHONN, which publishes standards of practice and education for perinatal nurses (Box 1-11); the American College of Nurse Midwives (ACNM), which publishes standards of practice for midwives; and the National Association of Neonatal Nurses (NANN), which publishes standards of practice for neonatal nurses. These standards reflect current knowledge, represent levels of practice agreed on by leaders in the specialty, and can be used for clinical benchmarking.

In addition to these more formalized standards, agencies have their own policy and procedure books that outline standards to be followed in that setting. In legal terms the standard of care is that level of practice that a reasonably prudent nurse would provide. In determining legal negligence, the care given is compared with the standard of care. If the standard was not met and harm resulted, negligence occurred. The number of legal suits in the perinatal area has typically been high. As a consequence, malpractice insurance costs are high for physicians, nurse-midwives, and nurses who work in labor and delivery.

LEGAL TIP Standard of Care When you are uncertain about how to perform a procedure, consult the agency procedure book and follow the guidelines printed therein. These guidelines are the standard of care for that agency.

Risk Management

Risk management is an evolving process that identifies risks, establishes preventive practices, develops reporting mechanisms, and delineates procedures for managing lawsuits. Nurses should be familiar with concepts of risk management and their implications for nursing practice. These concepts can be viewed as systems of checks and balances that ensure high-quality patient care from preconception until after birth. Effective risk management minimizes the risk of injury to patients and the number of lawsuits against nurses. Each facility or site develops site-specific risk management procedures based on accepted standards and guidelines. The procedures and guidelines must be reviewed periodically.

BOX 1-11 Standards of Care for Women and Newborns

Standards That Define the Nurse's Responsibility to the Patient

Assessment—Collection of health data of the woman or newborn
Diagnosis—Analysis of data to determine nursing diagnosis
Outcome Identification—Identification of expected outcomes that are individualized
Planning—Development of a plan of care
Implementation—Performance of interventions for the plan of care
Evaluation—Evaluation of the effectiveness of interventions in relation to expected outcomes

Standards of Professional Performance That Delineate Roles and Behaviors for Which the Professional Nurse Is Accountable

Quality of Care—Systemic evaluation of nursing practice
Performance Appraisal—Self-evaluation in relation to professional practice standards and other regulations
Education—Participation in ongoing educational activities to maintain knowledge for practice
Collegiality—Contribution to the development of peers, students, and others
Ethics—Use of Code for Nurses to guide practice
Collaboration—Involvement of patient, significant others, and other health care providers in the provision of patient care
Research—Use of research findings in practice
Resource Utilization—Consideration of factors related to safety, effectiveness, and costs in planning and delivering patient care
Practice Environment—Contribution to the environment of care delivery
Accountability—Legal and professional responsibility for practice

Source: Association of Women's Health, Obstetric and Neonatal Nurses (AWHONN): *Standards for professional nursing practice in the care of women and newborns,* ed 6, Washington, DC, 2003, AWHONN.

To decrease risk of errors in the administration of medications, The Joint Commission (formerly the Joint Commission on Accreditation of Healthcare Organizations) developed a list of abbreviations, acronyms, and symbols *not* to use (Table 1-2). In addition, each agency must develop its own list.

Sentinel Events

The Joint Commission describes a sentinel event as "an unexpected occurrence involving death or serious physical or psychologic injury, or the risk thereof. Serious injury specifically includes loss of limb or function." These events are called "sentinel" because they signal a need for an immediate inves-

Table 1-2 The Joint Commission "Do Not Use" List*

ABBREVIATION	POTENTIAL PROBLEM	PREFERRED TERM
U (for unit)	Mistaken as zero, four, or cc	Write "unit."
IU (for international unit)	Mistaken as IV (intravenous) or 10 (ten)	Write "international unit."
Q.D., QD, q.d., qd (daily)	Mistaken for each other; period after the Q mistaken for "I" and "O" mistaken for "I"	Write "daily."
Q.O.D., QOD, q.o.d., qod (every other day)		Write "every other day."
Trailing zero (X.0 mg)† Lack of leading zero (.X mg)	Decimal point is missed	Write X mg. Write 0.X mg.
MS	Can mean morphine sulfate or magnesium sulfate	Write "morphine sulfate."
MSO_4 and $MgSO_4$	Confused for one another	Write "magnesium sulfate."

*Applies to all orders and all medication-related documentation that is handwritten (including free-text computer entry) or on pre-printed forms.
†Exception: A "trailing zero" may be used only where required to demonstrate the level of precision of the value being reported, such as for laboratory results, imaging studies that report size of lesions, or catheter/tube sizes. It may not be used in medication orders or other medication-related documentation.
Source: The official "Do not use" list. Available at www.jointcommission.org/PatientSafey/DoNotUseList (accessed May 24, 2008).

tigation and response (Joint Commission, 2008a). Reportable sentinel events in perinatal nursing include any maternal death related to the process of birth, any perinatal death not related to a congenital condition in an infant with a birth weight greater than 2500 g, and infant discharge to the wrong family (Joint Commission, 2008b).

Failure to Rescue

Failure to rescue is used to "evaluate the quality and quantity of nursing care by comparing the number of surgical patients who develop common complications who survive versus those who do not" (Simpson, 2005). Because mothers and babies are generally healthy, complications leading to death in obstetrics are comparatively rare. Simpson (2005) proposes evaluating the perinatal team's ability to decrease risk of adverse outcomes by measuring processes involved in common complications and emergencies in obstetrics. Key components of failure to rescue are (1) careful surveillance and identification of complications, and (2) acting quickly to initiate appropriate interventions and activating a team response. For the perinatal nurse, this involves timely identification of complications, appropriate interventions, and efforts of the team to minimize client harm. Maternal complications that are appropriate for process measurement are placental abruption, postpartum hemorrhage, uterine rupture, eclampsia, and amniotic fluid embolism (Simpson, 2005). Fetal complications include nonreassuring fetal heart rate and pattern, prolapsed umbilical cord, shoulder dystocia, and uterine hyperstimulation (Simpson, 2005). Perinatal nurses can use these complications to develop a list of expectations for monitoring, timely identification, interventions, and roles of team members. The list can be used to evaluate the perinatal team's response.

Ethical Issues in Perinatal Nursing

Ethical concerns and debates have multiplied with the increased use of technology and with scientific advances. For example, with reproductive technology pregnancy is now possible in women who thought they would never bear children, including some who are menopausal or postmenopausal. Should scarce resources be devoted to achieving pregnancies in older women? Is giving birth to a child at an older age worth the risks involved? Should older parents be encouraged to conceive a baby when they may not live to see the child reach adulthood? Should a woman who is HIV-positive have access to assisted reproduction services? Should third-party payers assume the costs of reproductive technology such as the use of induced ovulation and in vitro fertilization? Questions about informed consent and allocation of resources must be addressed with innovations such as intrauterine fetal surgery, fetoscopy, therapeutic insemination, genetic engineering, stem cell research, surrogate childbearing, surgery for infertility, "test-tube" babies, fetal research, and treatment of VLBW babies. The introduction of long-acting contraceptives has created moral choices and policy dilemmas for health care providers and legislators (i.e., should some women [substance abusers, women with low incomes, or women who are HIV positive] be required to take the contraceptives?). With the potential for great good that can come from fetal tissue transplantation, what research is ethical? What are the rights of the embryo? Should cloning of humans be permitted? Discussion and debate about these issues will continue for many years. Nurses and patients, as well as scientists, physicians, attorneys, lawmakers, ethicists, and clergy, must be involved in the discussions.

Research in Perinatal Nursing

Research plays a vital role in the establishment of a maternity nursing science. Research can validate that nursing care makes a difference. For example, although prenatal care is clearly associated with healthier infants, no one knows exactly which nursing interventions produce this outcome. Many possible areas of research exist in maternity and women's health care. The clinician can identify problems in the health and health care of women and infants. Nurses should promote research funding and conduct research on maternity and women's health, especially concerning the effectiveness of nursing strategies for these patients.

Ethical Guidelines for Nursing Research

Research with perinatal patients may create ethical dilemmas for the nurse. For example, participating in research may cause additional stress to a woman concerned about outcomes of genetic testing or one who is waiting for an invasive procedure. Obtaining amniotic fluid samples or performing cordocentesis poses risks to the fetus. Nurses must protect the rights of human subjects (i.e., patients) in all of their research. For example, nurses may collect data on or care for patients who are participating in clinical trials. The nurse ensures that the participants are fully informed and aware of their rights as subjects. The nurse may be involved in determining whether the benefits of research outweigh the risks to the mother and the fetus. Following the ANA ethical guidelines in the conduct, dissemination, and implementation of nursing research helps nurses ensure that research is conducted ethically (Silva, 1995).

Key Points

- Maternity nursing focuses on women and their infants and families during the childbearing cycle.
- Nurses caring for women can play an active role in shaping health care systems to be responsive to the needs of contemporary women.
- Childbirth practices have changed to become more family focused and to allow alternatives in care.
- Canada ranks sixteenth and the United States ranks twenty-sixth among industrialized nations in infant mortality.
- Integrative medicine combines modern technology with ancient healing practices and encompasses the whole body, mind, and spirit.

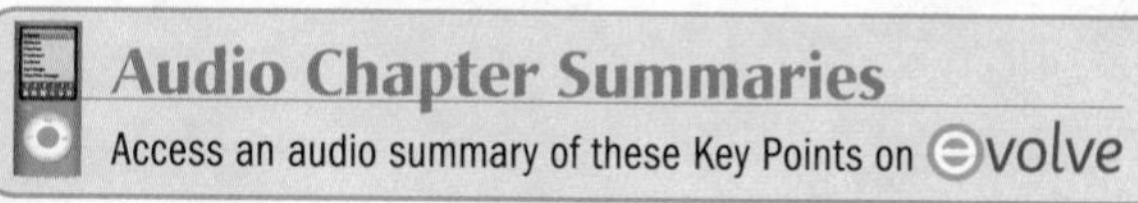
Audio Chapter Summaries
Access an audio summary of these Key Points on evolve

- Perinatal practice is increasingly evidence based.
- *Healthy People 2010* provides goals for maternal and infant health.
- Ethical concerns have multiplied with increasing use of technology and scientific advances.

References

ANA's Health System Reform Agenda, American Nurses Association, 2008, Silver Spring, Md. Available at www.nursingworld.org/MainMenuCategories/HealthcareandPolicyIssues/HSR/ANAsHealthSystemReformAgenda.aspx (accessed May 26, 2008).

Association of Women's Health, Obstetric and Neonatal Nurses (AWHONN): *Standards for professional nursing practice in the care of women and newborns*, ed 6, Washington, DC, 2003, AWHONN.

Association of Women's Health, Obstetric and Neonatal Nurses (AWHONN): *Standards for professional perinatal nursing practice and certification in Canada*, Washington, DC, 2002, AWHONN.

Calvo A: *HRSA Health disparities collaboratives: executive summary—September, 2006*. Available at www.healthdisparities.net/hdc/hdcsearch/isysquery/bea8637b-09f9-4d31-a92b-1ff4b0ecde8e/1/doc/ (accessed May 24, 2008).

Chu SY et al: Association between obesity during pregnancy and increased use of health care, *N Engl J Med* 358(14):1444-1453, 2008.

DeNavas-Walt C, Proctor BD, Smith J: *US Census Bureau, Current Population Reports, P60-233, Income poverty, and health insurance coverage in the United States: 2006*, Washington, DC, 2007, US Government Printing Office.

Doak CC, Doak LG, Root JH: *Teaching patients with low literacy skills*, ed 2, Philadelphia, 1996, Lippincott.

French J: Medical errors and patient safety in health care, *Can J Med Radiat Technol* 37(4):9-13, 2006.

Gauthier A, Serber M: A need to transform the US health care system: *Improving access, quality, and efficiency*, The Commonwealth Fund, October 3, 2005. Available at www.commonwealthfund.org/publications/publications_show.htm?doc_id=302833 (accessed May 25, 2008).

The Joint Commission (a): *Sentinel event*. Available at http://search.jointcommission.org/search?q=sentinel%20events&site=Entire-Site&client=jcaho_frontend&output=xml_no_dtd&proxystylesheet=jcaho_frontend (accessed May 24, 2008).

The Joint Commission (b): *Sentinel event statistics—March 31, 2008*. Available at www.jointcomission.org/SentinelEvents/Statistics/ (accessed May 24, 2008).

Jones WK: *Safe motherhood at a glance: promoting health for women before, during, and after pregnancy*, Atlanta, Ga, 2008, USDHHS, CDC. Available at www.cdc.gov/nccdphp/publications/aag/pdf/drh.pdf (accessed May 25, 2008).

Martin JA et al: Division of Vital Statistics: Births: Final data for 2005, *Natl Health Stat Report* 56(6):1-104, 2007.

Martin JA et al: Annual summary of vital statistics: 2006, *Pediatrics* 121(4):788-801, 2008.

National Center for Health Statistics: *Health, United States, 2007, with chart book on trends in the health of Americans*, Hyattsville, Md, 2007. Available at www.cdc.gov/nchs/data/hus/hus07.pdf (accessed April 18, 2008).

Perry SE, Mander R: A global frame of reference: learning from everyone, everywhere, *Nurs Educ Perspect* 26 (3):148-151, 2005.

Roehr B: Pressure mounts to cut US spending on health care, *BMJ* 336 (7638):236-237, 2008.

Satcher D, Higginbotham EJ: The public health approach to eliminating disparities in health, *Am J Public Health* 98(3):400-403, 2008.

Shalo S: In the news. The price of committing error, *Am J Nurs* 107(8):20, 2007.

Silva M: *Ethical guidelines in the conduct, dissemination, and implementation of nursing research*, Washington, DC, 1995, American Nurses Association.

Simpson K: Failure to rescue in obstetrics, *MCN Am J Matern Child Nurs* 30(1):76, 2005.

Tiedje LB, Price E, You M: Childbirth is changing. What now? *MCN Am J Matern Child Nurs* 33(3):144-150, 2008.

20 Tips to help prevent medical errors: patient fact sheet: AHRQ Publication No. 00-PO38, Rockville, Md, February 2000, Agency for Healthcare Research and Quality. Available at www.ahrq.gov/consumer/20tips.htm (accessed May 24, 2008).

US Census Bureau: *U.S. interim projections by age, sex, race, and Hispanic origin: 2000-2050*, 2004. Available at www.census.gov/population/www/projections/usinterimproj (accessed February 18, 2009).

WHO Study Group on Female Genital Mutilation and Obstetric Outcome; Banks E et al: Female genital mutilation and obstetric outcome: WHO collaborative prospective study in six African countries, *Lancet* 367(9525):1835-1841, 2006.

World Health Organization: *Maternal mortality in 2005: estimates developed by WHO, UNICEF, UNFPA, and the World Bank*, 2007. Available at www.unfpa.org/upload/lib_pub_file/717_filename_mm2005.pdf (accessed April 18, 2008).

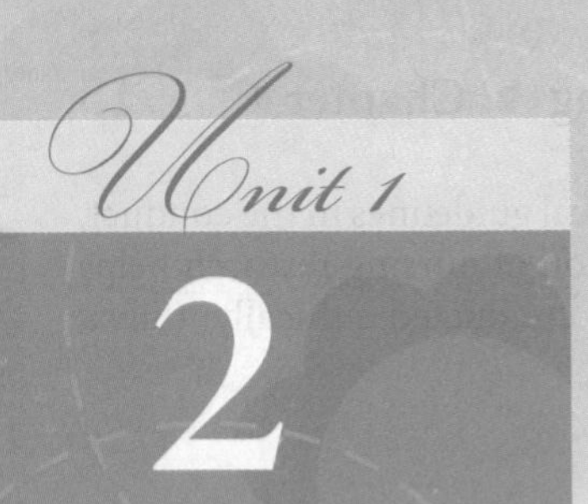

The Family and Culture

Learning Objectives

On completion of this chapter the reader will be able to:

- Describe the main characteristics of contemporary family forms.
- Identify key factors influencing family health.
- Explain family functions that contribute to the well-being of its members and society.
- Explain family dynamics and how family dynamics contribute to accomplishing family functions.
- Compare theoretic approaches for working with childbearing families.
- Relate the impact of culture on childbearing families.
- Discuss cultural competence in relation to one's own nursing practice.

Electronic Resources

Additional information related to the content in Chapter 2 can be found on

evolve the Companion Website at

http://evolve.elsevier.com/Perry/maternal/

- NCLEX Review Questions
- Critical Thinking Exercise—Cultural Health and the Family
- Nursing Care Plan—The Family Newly Immigrated from a Non–English-Speaking Country
- Nursing Care Plan—Incorporating the Infant into the Family

The Family in Cultural and Community Context

The family and its cultural context play an important role in defining the work of maternity nurses. Despite modern stresses and strains, the family forms a social network that acts as a potent support system for its members. Family care-seeking behavior and relationships with providers are all influenced by culturally related health beliefs and values. Ultimately all of these factors have the power to affect maternal and child health outcomes. Therefore it is important to recognize these influences, discuss current trends in families, and explore nursing implications. The current emphasis in working with families is on wellness and empowerment for families to achieve control over their lives.

The Family in Society

The social context for the family can be viewed in relation to social and demographic trends that define the population as a whole. Current U.S. census data indicate that the racial and ethnic diversity of the population has grown dramatically in the last three decades. This increased diversity—first manifested among children and soon to be evident in the older population—is projected to increase in the future.

Each family sets up boundaries between itself and society. People are conscious of the difference between "family members" and "outsiders," or people without kinship status. Some families isolate themselves from the outside community; others have a wide community network to whom they can turn for help in times of stress. Although boundaries exist for every family, family members set up channels through which they interact with society. These channels also ensure that the family receives its share of social resources.

Family Organization and Structure

The nuclear family has long represented the traditional American family in which male and female partners and their children live as an independent unit, sharing roles, responsibilities, and economic resources (Fig. 2-1). In contemporary society this idealized family structure actually represents only a relatively small number of families. The binuclear family is an alternate form of the traditional nuclear family arrangement that results from divorce. Children of remarried parents then become members of both the maternal and paternal nuclear households. In joint custody the court assigns divorcing parents equal rights to and responsibilities for the minor child or children.

Reconstituted or blended families (i.e., those formed as the result of divorce and remarriage) consist of unrelated family members (stepparents, stepchildren, and stepsiblings) who join together to create a new household. These family groups frequently involve a biologic or adoptive parent whose spouse has not adopted the child.

Many nuclear families have other relatives living in the same household. These extended family members may be

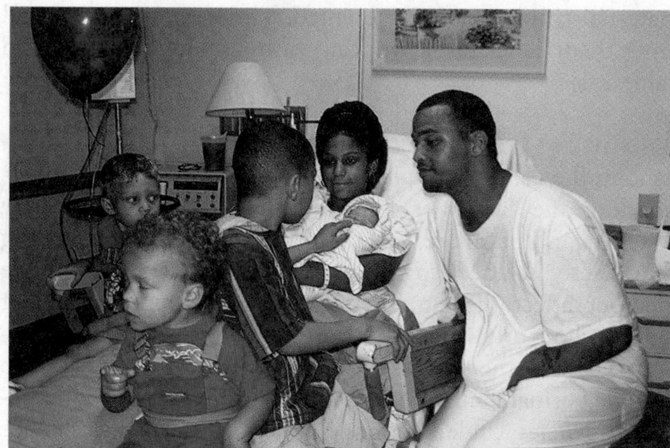

Fig. 2-1 Nuclear family. *(Marjorie Pyle, RNC, Lifecircle, Costa Mesa, CA.)*

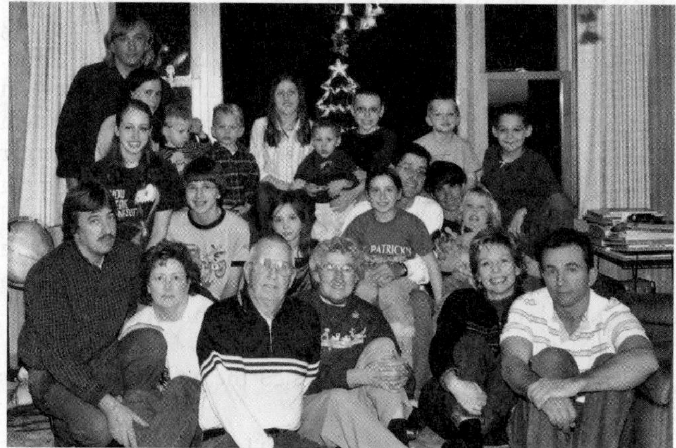

Fig. 2-2 Extended family. *(Rosemary Toohill, LeRoy, IL.)*

grandparents, aunts or uncles, or other people related by blood (Fig. 2-2). For some groups such as African-American and Latin-American women, the family network is an important resource in terms of preventive health behavior.

Single-parent families comprise an unmarried biologic or adoptive parent who may or may not be living with other adults. The single-parent family may result from the loss of spouse by death, divorce, separation, or desertion; from either an unplanned or a planned pregnancy; or from the adoption of a child by an unmarried woman or man. This family structure has become a common and acceptable choice in society, with current estimates at one fifth of Caucasian families, one third of Hispanic families, and more than half of African-American families in the United States. In many cases the single-parent family tends to be vulnerable economically and socially, creating an unstable and deprived environment for the growth potential of children. Single mothers are more likely to live in poverty and have poor perinatal outcomes.

Other family configurations, which are less well documented, include children in families whose parents are cohabiting and an increasing number of homosexual (lesbian and gay) families, who may live together with or without children. Children in homosexual families may be the offspring of previous heterosexual unions, conceived by one member of a lesbian couple through therapeutic insemination, or adopted.

Family Dynamics

Through family dynamics (interactions and communication), family members assume appropriate social roles. Social roles in the family are learned in pairs (e.g., mother-father, parent-child, and brother-sister). Role pairing enables social interactions to take place in an orderly, predictable manner; the roles are said to be complementary. Some families maintain a traditional pairing of roles, whereas other families change behavior patterns to suit a change in family lifestyle. Rather than mother-father, brother-sister, the roles may be mother-daughter, mother-son. Negotiation brings these pair roles into a new alignment. Negotiation is essential to maintain family equilibrium.

Ideally the family uses its resources to provide a safe, intimate environment for the biopsychosocial development of the family members. The family provides for the nurturing of the newborn and the gradual socialization of the growing child. Children form their earliest and closest relationships with their parents or parenting persons; these affiliations continue throughout a lifetime. For better or worse, parent-child relationships influence self-worth and the ability to form later relationships. The family also influences the child's perceptions of the outside world. The family provides the growing child with an identity that possesses both a past and a sense of the future. Cultural values and rituals are passed from one generation to the next through the family.

Over time the family develops protocols for problem solving, particularly regarding important decisions such as having a baby, buying a house, or sending children to college. The criteria used in making decisions are based on family values and attitudes about the appropriateness of the behavior and the moral, social, political, and economic events of society. The power to make critical decisions is given to a family member through tradition or negotiation. All families have strengths and potential for growth. It is important for the nurse to identify those strengths and potentials to facilitate the growth of the family (Black & Lobo, 2008).

Family Nursing

evolve Nursing Care Plan—Incorporating the Infant into the Family

Nurses are morally and ethically obligated to include families in health care. Their commitment to inclusion of the family influences the health and well-being of the family (Wright & Leahy, 2005). This necessitates that nurses must become competent in assessing and intervening with families through collaboration with the family. Family nursing must focus on relationships, not on individuals (Wright & Leahy, 2005). Family plays a pivotal role in health care, representing the primary target of health care delivery for maternal and newborn nurses. Most models of health behavior view family as a "system" within the larger social framework of a community. These understandings affect our approaches to health and health care of individuals within the family unit.

The core concepts of patient- and family-centered care are dignity and respect, information sharing, participation, and collaboration (Johnson et al, 2008). When treating the patient and family with respect and dignity, health care providers listen to and honor perspectives and choices of the patient and family. They share information with families in ways that are positive, useful, timely, complete, and accurate. The family is supported in participating in the care and decision making at the level of their choice. Collaboration in development, implementation, and evaluation of policy and programs, facility design, professional education, and delivery of care by all involved (i.e., patients and their families, health care providers, and hospital leaders) is essential for providing family-centered care (Johnson et al, 2008).

Family Assessment

When selecting a family assessment framework, an appropriate model for a perinatal nurse is one that is a health-promoting rather than illness-care model. The low risk family can be assisted in promoting a healthy pregnancy, childbirth, and integration of the newborn into the family. The high risk perinatal family has illness-care needs, and the nurse may be able to meet those needs while also promoting the health of the childbearing family.

Theoretic Approaches to Understanding Families

A family theory can be used to describe families and how the family unit responds to events both within and outside the family. Each family theory makes certain assumptions about the family and has inherent strengths and limitations. Most nurses use a combination of theories in their work with families. A brief discussion of a theory commonly used with families, systems theory, and the implications of this theory for maternal-child nursing is presented. A brief synopsis of several other theories useful in working with families is included in Table 2-1.

Family Systems Theory

Among the caring disciplines, a systems approach to understanding the family is almost universally applied. Many systems concepts are central to the delivery of holistic nursing care. These include recognition that changes occurring in one member affect the entire family and an appreciation that nurses who work with families also enter into a systemic relationship with them. This is especially true for nurses who provide perinatal nursing care through community- or home-based agencies. Understanding how family members influence and interact with one another can help the nurse develop empathy with and respect for different ways of functioning.

When applied to families, the systems theory allows nurses to "view the family as a unit and thus focus on observing the interaction among family members rather than studying family members individually" (Wright & Leahey, 2005). Within a systems framework the individual takes on several roles as a unique and important person in his or her own system and as part of one or more subsystems within the larger family. For example, an individual may belong to one of several subsystems such as a child subsystem or a parental subsystem. When considering more than one generation of a family, a married woman may belong to a parental subsystem in her own home and to a subsystem of children when considered in relationship to her own parents.

Wright and Leahy (2005) outlined the key characteristics of family systems theory:

- A family system is part of a larger suprasystem and is composed of many subsystems.

Table 2-1 Theories and Models Relevant to Family Nursing Practice

THEORY	SYNOPSIS OF THEORY
Family Life Cycle (Developmental) Theory (Carter & McGoldrick, 1999)	Families move through stages. The family life cycle is the context in which to examine the identity and development of the individual. Relationships among family members go through transitions. Although families have roles and functions, a family's main value is in relationships that are irreplaceable. The family involves different structures and cultures organized in various ways. Developmental stresses may disrupt the life cycle process.
Family Stress Theory (Boss, 2002)	This theory is concerned with ways families react to stressful events. Family stress can be studied within the internal and external contexts in which the family is living. The internal context involves elements that a family can change or control such as family structure, psychologic defenses, and philosophic values and beliefs. The external context consists of the time and place in which a particular family finds itself and over which the family has no control such as the culture of the larger society, the time in history, the economic state of society, the maturity of the individuals involved, the success of the family in coping with stressors, and genetic inheritance.
McGill Model of Nursing (Allen, 1997)	This model is a strength-based focus in clinical practice with families rather than a deficit approach. It identifies family strengths and resources, provides feedback about strengths, and assists the family to develop and elicit strengths and use resources.
Health Belief Model (Becker, 1974; Janz & Becker, 1984)	The goal of the model is to reduce cultural and environmental barriers that interfere with access to health care. Key elements of the Health Belief Model include the following: perceived susceptibility, perceived severity, perceived benefits, perceived barriers, cues to action, and confidence.
Human Developmental Ecology (Bronfenbrenner, 1979, 1989)	Behavior is a function of interaction of traits and abilities with the environment. Major concepts include ecosystem, niches (social roles), adaptive range, and ontogenetic development. Individuals are "embedded in a microsystem (role and relations), a mesosystem (interrelations between two or more settings), an exosystem (external settings that do not include the person), and a macrosystem (culture)" (Klein & White, 1996). Change over time is incorporated in the chronosystem.

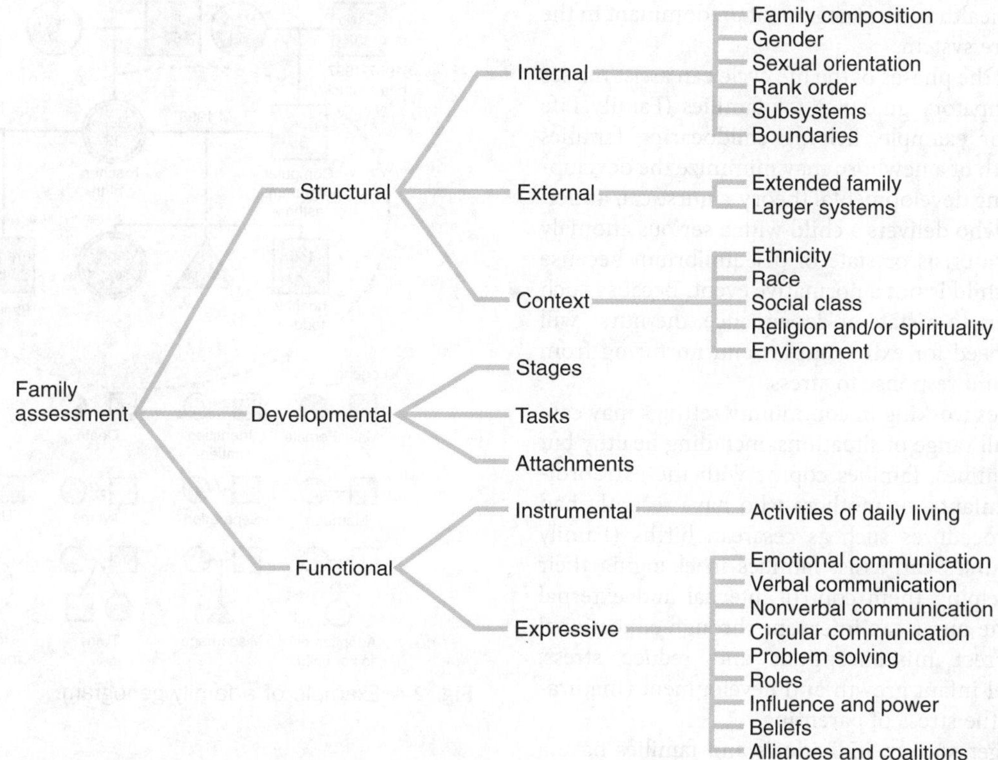

Fig. 2-3 Branching diagram of Calgary Family Assessment Model (CFAM). (From Wright LM, Leahy M: *Nurses and families: a guide to family assessment and intervention*, ed 4, Philadelphia, 2005, FA Davis.)

- The family as a whole is greater than the sum of its parts.
- A change in one family member affects all family members.
- The family is able to create a balance between change and stability.
- Family members' behaviors are best understood from a view of circular rather than linear causality.

The family systems theory encourages nurses to view individual family members as part of a larger family system influenced by and influencing others. Application of these concepts can guide assessment and interventions for the family. For example, the childbearing family interacts as a system with many elements in the environmental suprasystem, including the health care community. The extent to which this suprasystem influences the family in matters such as prenatal care, childbirth education, and infant care depends on the family's boundary permeability. A relatively closed family may want instructions only from others within the family, whereas a relatively open family may be more receptive to instructions from health care providers.

The Calgary Family Assessment Model

The Calgary Family Assessment Model (CFAM) is an example of a model that uses systems theory as well as other theories. Wright and Leahy (2005) described the CFAM as "an integrated, multidimensional framework based on the systems, cybernetics, communication, and change theoretical foundations and influenced by postmodernism and biology of cognition." CFAM is comprised of three major categories: structural, developmental, and functional. There are several subcategories within each category. The three assessment categories and the many subcategories can be conceptualized as a branching diagram (Fig. 2-3). These categories and subcategories can be used to guide the assessment that will provide data to help the nurse better understand the family and formulate a plan of care.

Using Theories to Guide Practice

To be effective in working with families, the nurse must possess a degree of personal openness and acceptance and be willing to work with families in a way that is respectful and adapts to their ways of learning and communicating. When interacting with family members, the nurse becomes part of a system with them (Family Systems Theory). The behaviors and interaction style of the nurse not only affect the individual who is identified as the "patient" but also contribute to family members' responses to each other. Finally, the quality of the nurse-family system strongly influences how the family will interact with the greater health care community in the future.

People interact effectively with each other in many ways. Countless factors influence ways in which family members relate among themselves and with the health care community. Some of these factors include the natural history of the family, culture, roles, values, beliefs, and traditional customs. Because so many variables affect ways of relating, the nurse must be aware that most family members will interact and communicate with each other in ways that are very different from those of the nurse's own family of origin. Most families will hold at least some beliefs about health that are very different from those of the nurse. In some instances their beliefs will conflict with principles of health care management predominant in the Western health care system.

Knowing about the phases of the life cycle can assist nurses in providing anticipatory guidance for families (Family Life Cycle Theory). For example, helping childbearing families prepare for the birth of a newborn may minimize the development of crises. Using developmental theory, a nurse can anticipate that a family who delivers a child with a serious anomaly might experience a crisis or state of disequilibrium because the birth of an ill child is not a normative event. Because such a family may revert to a state of dependence, the nurse will realize that their need for extra support and nurturing from the nurse is a natural response to stress.

Maternity nurses working in community settings may care for families in a full range of situations, including healthy but highly stressed families, families coping with the extraordinary stress of ill infants, or mothers who have recently had major surgical procedures such as cesarean births (Family Stress Theory). Nurses can assist families in changing their stress levels by helping them control internal and external context factors. The nurse can intervene through educational strategies to correct misconceptions and reduce stress. Explaining normal infant growth and development (maturation) may reduce the stress of parenting.

Within the larger society, individuals and families have a variety of stressors that affect their ability to function and to engage consistently in behaviors that promote health and wellness. These individuals and families fall into high risk or vulnerable populations. Their stresses relate to many aspects of life: ethnic and cultural minority status, immigration status, poverty, challenges with English language fluency and literacy, malnutrition, and limited access to housing. Some families have multiple stressors, placing them at especially high risk for poor health outcomes. Even those who are well educated and in a higher socioeconomic class can have life stressors that make them highly vulnerable to health problems. Nurses cannot make the assumption that a family is immune to vulnerability because its members live in an exclusive neighborhood, are well educated, and are fully employed. The concepts of high risk and vulnerability potentially apply to everyone.

By using the Health Belief Model as a guide to assessment, nurses can better address concerns specific to an individual from a cultural group different from that of the nurse and motivate the individual to take action on his or her own behalf. Understanding a woman's concerns from her own point of view can help the nurse provide interventions that will place women at ease in the health care setting. For example, the nurse can modify or adjust her care in assessing uterine involution as part of postpartum care for a woman who holds traditional Mexican beliefs and fears of having cold enter her uterus during a normal examination. The culturally competent nurse can close the door to the room, pull curtains to minimize air flow around the woman, position the woman so that the perineum is facing away from the door or air vents, and keep the perineum draped so that the examination takes place with a minimum of exposure.

A family genogram (family tree format depicting relationships of family members over at least three generations) (Fig. 2-4) provides valuable information about a family and can be placed in the nursing care plan for easy access by care providers. An ecomap, a graphic portrayal of social relationships of the patient and family, may also help the nurse understand the social environment of the family and identify support systems available to them (Fig. 2-5) (Rempel, Neufeld, & Kushner, 2007). Software is available to generate genograms and ecomaps (*www.interpersonaluniverse.net*).

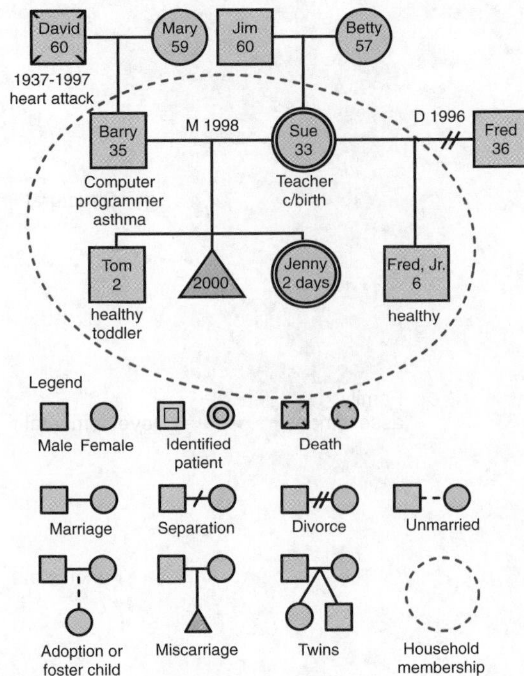

Fig. 2-4 Example of a family genogram.

Cultural Factors Related to Family Health

Cultural Context of the Family

Culture of an individual is influenced by religion, environment, and historic events and plays a powerful role in the individual's behavior and patterns of human interaction. Culture is not static; it is an ongoing process that influences people throughout their entire lives, from birth to death.

Cultural knowledge includes beliefs and values about each facet of life and is passed from one generation to the next. Cultural beliefs and traditions relate to food; language; religion; art; health and healing practices; kinship relationships; and all other aspects of community, family, and individual life. Culture also has been shown to have a direct effect on health behaviors. Values, attitudes, and beliefs that are culturally acquired may influence perceptions of illness, as well as health care–seeking behavior and response to treatment. The impact of these influences must be assessed by health professionals in providing health care and developing effective intervention strategies.

Many subcultures may be found within each culture. Subculture refers to a group existing within a larger cultural

evolve Critical Thinking Exercise–Cultural Health and the Family

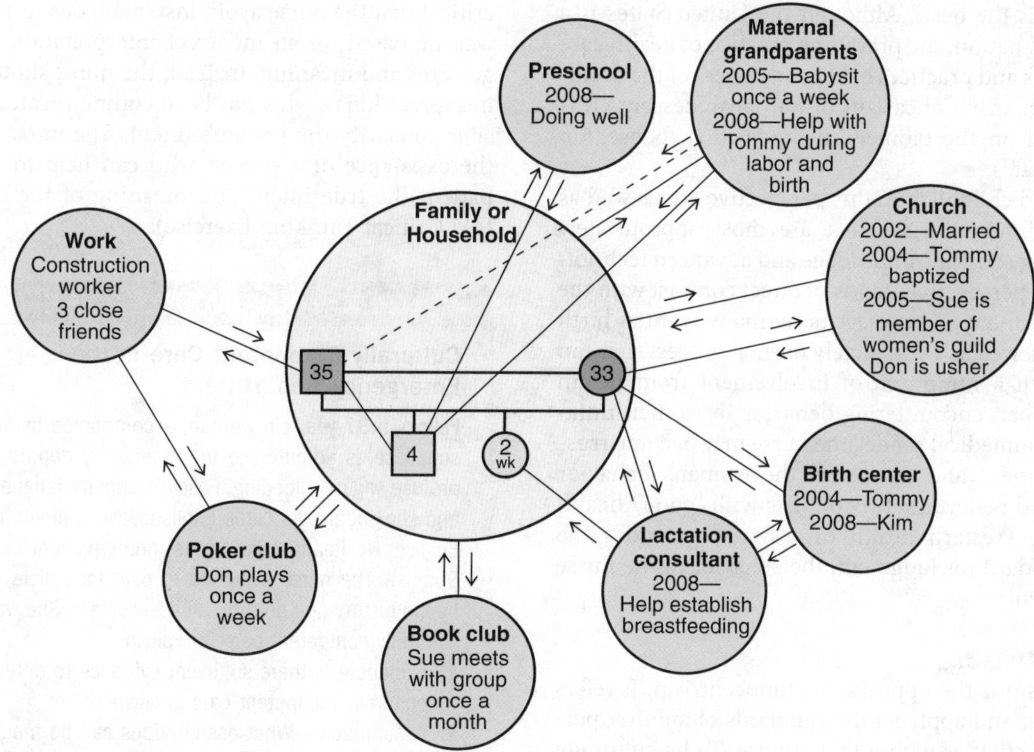

Fig. 2-5 Example of an ecomap. An ecomap describes social relationships and depicts available supports.

system that retains its own characteristics. A subculture may be an ethnic group or a group organized in other ways. Each subculture holds rich and complex traditions, including health practices that have proven effective over time. These traditions vary from group to group. In a multicultural society many groups can influence traditions and practices. As cultural groups come in contact with each other, acculturation and assimilation may occur.

Acculturation

Acculturation refers to changes that occur within one group or among several groups when people from different cultures come in contact with one another. People may retain some of their own culture while adopting some of the cultural practices of the dominant society. This familiarization among cultural groups results in some overt behavioral similarity, especially in mannerisms, styles, and practices. Dress, language patterns, food choices, and health practices especially show differences among cultural groups. In the United States acculturation generally is thought to take three generations. An adult grandchild of an immigrant is usually fully Americanized. An example of acculturation is the adoption of ethnic food practices in the United States.

During times of family transitions such as childbearing or during crisis or illness, a woman may rely on old cultural patterns even after she has become acculturated in many ways. This is consistent with family developmental theory that states that during times of stress people revert to practices and behaviors that are most comfortable and familiar.

Assimilation

Assimilation occurs when a cultural group loses its identity and becomes part of the dominant culture. Assimilation is the process by which groups "melt" into the mainstream, thus accounting for the notion of a "melting pot," a phenomenon that has been said to occur in the United States. This is illustrated by individuals who identify themselves as being of "Irish" or "German" descent, without having any remaining cultural practices or values linked specifically to that culture such as food preparation techniques, style of dress, or proficiency in the language associated with their reported cultural heritage. Spector (2009) asserts that in the United States, the melting pot, with its dream of a common culture, "has proved to be a myth and has faded; it is now time to identify the mosaic phenomenon and both accept and appreciate the differences among people."

The family process within its cultural context is a central concern in nursing, especially when the nurse is providing care to the childbearing family. A critical life experience such as childbearing is often bound by traditional beliefs and practices. Patients have the right to expect that their physiologic and psychologic health care needs will be met and that their cultural beliefs will be respected. Cultural sensitivity, compassion, and a critical awareness of family dynamics and social stressors that affect health-related decision making are critical components in developing an effective plan of care.

Ethnocentrism

Ethnocentrism is a belief in the rightness of one's culture's way of doing things. Essentially ethnocentrism supports the notion that "my group is the best." Although the United States is a culturally diverse nation, the prevailing practice of health care is based on beliefs and practices held by members of the dominant culture, primarily Caucasians of European descent. This practice is based on the biomedical model that focuses on curing disease states.

Pregnancy and childbirth in this perspective are viewed as processes with inherent risks that are most appropriately managed by using scientific knowledge and advanced technology. The medical perspective stands in direct contrast with the belief systems of many cultures. Among many women birth traditionally is viewed as a completely normal process that can be managed with a minimum of involvement from health practitioners. When encountering behavior in women unfamiliar with the biomedical model, the nurse may become frustrated and impatient and may label the woman's behavior inappropriate and believe that it conflicts with "good" health practices. If the Western health care system provides the nurse's only standard for judgment, the behavior of the nurse is called ethnocentric.

Cultural Relativism

Cultural relativism is the opposite of ethnocentrism. It refers to learning about and applying the standards of another person's culture to activities within that culture. To be culturally relativistic, the nurse recognizes that people from different cultural backgrounds comprehend the same objects and situations differently. In other words, culture determines a person's viewpoint.

Cultural relativism does not require nurses to accept the beliefs and values of another culture. Instead, nurses recognize that the behavior of others may be based on a system of logic different from their own. Cultural relativism affirms the uniqueness and value of every culture.

Childbearing Beliefs and Practices

Nurses working with childbearing families care for families from many different cultures and ethnic groups. To provide culturally competent care, the nurse must assess the beliefs and practices of patients. A nurse should consider all aspects of culture, including communication, space, time orientation, and family roles, when working with childbearing families.

Communication

Communication often creates the most challenging obstacle for nurses working with patients from diverse cultural groups. Communication is not merely the exchange of words. Instead it involves (1) understanding the individual's language, including subtle variations in meaning and distinctive dialects; (2) appreciation of individual differences in interpersonal style; and (3) accurate interpretation of the volume of speech, as well as the meanings of touch and gestures. For example, members of some cultural groups tend to speak more loudly, with great emotion, and with vigorous and animated gestures when they are excited; this is true whether their excitement is related to positive or negative events or emotions. Therefore it is important for the nurse to avoid rushing to judgment regarding a patient's intent when the patient is speaking, especially in a language not understood by the nurse. In these situations it is critical that the nurse avoid instantaneous responses that may well be based on an incorrect interpretation of the patient's gestures and meaning. Instead, the nurse should withhold an interpretation of what has been communicated until it is possible to clarify the patient's intent. The nurse needs to enlist the assistance of a person who can help to verify with the patient the true intent and meaning of the communication (see Critical Thinking Exercise).

CRITICAL THINKING EXERCISE

Culturally Competent Care in the Emergency Department

Felicia, a 37-year-old woman, accompanied by her 16-year-old son, Jose, is admitted to the emergency department (ED) with profuse vaginal bleeding. Felicia's primary language is Spanish, and she speaks very little English; Jose is fluent in Spanish and English. No health care professionals present in the ED speak Spanish. The nurse assigned to care for Felicia must obtain a health history and perform an assessment. She wants to provide culturally competent care for Felicia.

1. Evidence—Is there sufficient evidence to determine what culturally competent care consists of?
2. Assumptions—What assumptions can be made about culturally competent care and the role language plays in providing that care?
    a. How the nurse, who speaks no Spanish, might effectively communicate with Felicia
    b. How the nurse can obtain a health history with questions about vaginal bleeding, sexual activity, and pregnancy if Jose is the only person available who speaks Spanish
    c. How the nurse can provide culturally competent teaching
    d. Appropriate teaching materials and resources; appropriate questions to gain information about sexual activity and possibility of pregnancy
3. What implications and priorities for nursing care can be drawn at this time?
4. Does the evidence objectively support your conclusion?
5. Are there alternative perspectives to your conclusion?

Use of Interpreters

Inconsistencies between the language of patients and that of providers present a significant barrier to effective health care. Because of the diversity of cultures and languages within the United States and Canadian populations, health care agencies are increasingly seeking the services of interpreters (of oral communication from one language to another) or translators (of written words from one language to another) to bridge these gaps and fulfill their obligation for culturally and linguistically appropriate health care (Box 2-1). Finding the best possible interpreter in the circumstance also is critically important. A number of personal attributes and qualifications contribute to an interpreter's potential to be effective. Ideally interpreters should have the same native language and be of the same religion or have the same country of origin as the

BOX 2-1 Working with an Interpreter

Step 1: Before the Interview

A. Outline your statements and questions. List the key pieces of information you want/need to know.
B. Learn something about the culture so that you can converse informally with the interpreter.

Step 2: Meeting with the Interpreter

A. Introduce yourself to the interpreter and converse informally. This is the time to find out how well he or she speaks English. No matter how proficient or what age the interpreter is, be respectful. Some ways to show respect are to ask a cultural question to acknowledge that you can learn from the interpreter or learn one word or phrase from the interpreter.
B. Emphasize that you want the patient to ask questions because some cultures consider this inappropriate behavior.
C. Make sure that the interpreter is comfortable with the technical terms you need to use. If not, take some time to explain them.

Step 3: During the Interview

A. Ask your questions and explain your statements (see Step 1).
B. Make sure that the interpreter understands which parts of the interview are most important. You usually have limited time with the interpreter, and you want to have adequate time at the end for patient questions.
C. Try to get a "feel" for how much is "getting through." No matter what the language is, if in relating information to the patient the interpreter uses far fewer or far more words than you do, "something else" is going on.
D. Stop every now and then and ask the interpreter, "How is it going?" You may not get a totally accurate answer, but you will have emphasized to the interpreter your strong desire to focus on the task at hand. If there are language problems: (1) speak *slowly,* (2) use gestures (e.g., fingers to count or point to body parts), and (3) use pictures.
E. Ask the interpreter to elicit questions. This may be difficult, but it is worth the effort.
F. Identify cultural issues that may conflict with your requests or instructions.
G. Use the interpreter to help problem solve or at least give insight into possibilities for solutions.

Step 4: After the Interview

A. Speak to the interpreter and try to get an idea of what went well and what could be improved. This will help you to be more effective with this or another interpreter.
B. Make notes on what you learned for your future reference or to help a colleague.

Remember:

Your interview is a *collaboration* between you and the interpreter. *Listen* as well as speak.

Notes

1. The interpreter may be a child, grandchild, or sibling of the patient. Be sensitive to the fact that the child is playing an adult role.
2. Be sensitive to cultural and situational differences (e.g., an interview with someone from urban Germany will likely be different from an interview with someone from a transitional refugee camp).
3. Younger females telling older males what to do may be a problem for both a female nurse and a female interpreter. This is not the time to pioneer new gender relations. Be aware that in some cultures it is difficult for a woman to talk about some topics with a husband or a father present.

Courtesy Elizabeth Whalley, PhD, San Francisco State University.

evolve Nursing Care Plan—The Family Newly Immigrated from a Non-English-Speaking Country

patient. Interpreters should have specific health-related language skills and experience and help bridge the language and cultural barriers between the patient and the health care provider. The person interpreting also should be mature enough to be trusted with private information. However, because the nature of nursing care is not always predictable and because nursing care that is provided in a home or community setting does not always allow expert, experienced, or mature adult interpreters, ideal interpretive services sometimes are impossible to find when they are needed. In crisis or emergency situations or when family members are having extreme stress or emotional upset, it may be necessary to use relatives, neighbors, or children as interpreters. If this situation occurs, the nurse must ensure that the patient is in agreement and comfortable with using the available interpreter to assist.

When using an interpreter, the nurse respects the family by creating an atmosphere of respect and privacy. Questions should be addressed to the woman and not to the interpreter. Even though an interpreter will of necessity be exposed to sensitive and privileged information about the family, the nurse should take care to ensure that confidentiality is maintained. A quiet location free from interruptions is the ideal place for interpretive services to take place. In addition, culturally and linguistically appropriate educational materials that are easy to read, with appropriate text and graphics, should be available to assist the woman and her family in understanding health care information. When using interpretive services, the nurse demonstrates respect for the woman and helps her maintain a sense of dignity by taking care to do all of the following:

- Respect the woman's wishes
- Involve her in the decision about who will be the most appropriate person to interpret under the circumstances
- Provide as much privacy as possible
- Use culturally appropriate learning aids

Personal Space

Cultural traditions define the appropriate personal space for various social interactions. Although the need for personal space varies from person to person and with the situation, the actual physical dimensions of comfort zones differ from culture to culture. Actions such as touching, placing the woman in proximity to others, taking away personal possessions, and making decisions for the woman can decrease personal security and heighten anxiety. Conversely, respecting the need for distance allows the woman to maintain control over personal space and support personal autonomy, thereby increasing her sense of security. For example, many Asian groups have reserved attitudes about physical contact, and touching a woman may at times create anxiety when health care is delivered. Nurses must touch patients. However, they frequently do so without any awareness of the emotional distress they may be causing them.

Time Orientation

Time orientation is a fundamental way in which culture affects health behaviors. People in cultural groups may be relatively more oriented to past, present, or future. Those who focus on the past strive to maintain tradition or the status quo and have little motivation for formulating future goals. In contrast, individuals who focus primarily on the present neither plan for the future nor consider the experiences of the past. These individuals do not necessarily adhere to strict schedules and are often described as "living for the moment" or "marching to the beat of their own drummer." Individuals oriented to the future maintain a focus on achieving long-term goals.

The time orientation of the childbearing family may affect nursing care. For example, talking to a family about bringing the infant to the clinic for follow-up examinations (events in the future) may be difficult for the family that is focused on the present concerns of day-to-day survival. Because a family with a future-oriented sense of time plans far in advance and thinks about the long-term consequences of present actions, they may be more likely to return as scheduled for follow-up visits. Despite the differences in time orientation, each family may be equally concerned for the well-being of its newborn.

Family Roles

Family roles involve the expectations and behaviors associated with a member's position in the family (e.g., mother, father, grandparent). Social class and cultural norms also affect these roles, with distinct expectations for men and women clearly determined by social norms. For example, culture may influence whether a man actively participates in pregnancy and childbirth, yet maternity care practitioners working in the Western health care system expect fathers to be involved. This can create a significant conflict between the nurse and the role expectations of very traditional Mexican or Arab families, who usually view the birthing experience as a female affair. The way that health care practitioners manage such a family's care molds its experience and perception of the Western health care system.

In maternity nursing the nurse supports and nurtures the beliefs that promote physical or emotional adaptation to childbearing. However, if certain beliefs might be harmful, the nurse should carefully explore them with the woman and use them in the reeducation and modification process.

Table 2-2 provides examples of some cultural beliefs and practices surrounding childbearing. The cultural beliefs and customs in this table are categorized on the basis of distinct cultural traditions and are not practiced by all members of the cultural group in every part of the country. Women from these cultural and ethnic groups may adhere to some, all, or none of the practices listed.

In using Table 2-2 as a guide, the nurse should take care to avoid making stereotypic assumptions about any person based on sociocultural-spiritual affiliations. Nurses should exercise sensitivity in working with every family, being careful to assess the ways in which they apply their own mixture of cultural traditions.

Developing Cultural Competence

Cultural competence has many names and definitions, all of which have subtle shades of difference, but which are essentially the same: multiculturalism, cultural sensitivity, and intercultural effectiveness. Cultural competence involves acknowledging, respecting, and appreciating ethnic, cultural, and linguistic diversity. Culturally competent professionals act in ways that meet the needs of the patient and are respectful of ways and traditions that may be very different from their own. In today's society it is of critical importance that nurses develop more than technical skill. At every level of preparation and throughout their professional lives, nurses must engage in a continual process of developing and refining attitudes and behaviors that will promote culturally competent care.

CULTURAL AWARENESS

Questions to Ask to Obtain Cultural Expectations About Childbearing

1. What do you and your family believe you should do to remain healthy during pregnancy?
2. What are the things you can or cannot do to improve your health and the health of your baby?
3. Do you have any special dietary needs or foods that you cannot eat?
4. Do you or your family have concerns or fears about hospitalization for childbirth?
5. Whom do you want with you during your labor?
6. What actions are important for you and your family to take after the baby's birth?
7. What do you and your family expect from the nurse(s) caring for you?
8. How will family members participate in your pregnancy, childbirth, and parenting?

In addition to issues of preserving and promoting human dignity, the development of cultural competence is of equal importance in terms of health outcomes. Nurses who relate effectively with patients are able to motivate them in the direction of health-promoting behaviors. Rust and colleagues (2006) developed a CRASH Course in Cultural Competency for health care personnel. This course includes the essential components of culturally competent health care (Box 2-2).

Table 2-2 Traditional* Cultural Beliefs and Practices: Childbearing and Parenting

PREGNANCY	CHILDBIRTH	PARENTING
Hispanic (Based primarily on knowledge of Mexican-Americans; members of the Hispanic community have their origins in Spain, Cuba, Central and South America, Mexico, Puerto Rico, and other Spanish-speaking countries.)		
Pregnancy Pregnancy desired soon after marriage Late prenatal care Expectant mother influenced strongly by mother or mother-in-law Cool air in motion considered dangerous during pregnancy Unsatisfied food cravings thought to cause a birthmark Some pica observed in the eating of ashes or dirt (not common) Milk avoided because it causes large babies and difficult births Many predictions about sex of baby May be unacceptable and frightening to have pelvic examination by male health care provider Use of herbs to treat common complaints of pregnancy Drinking chamomile tea thought to ensure effective labor	*Labor* Use of "partera" or lay midwife preferred in some places; may prefer presence of mother rather than husband After birth of baby, mother's legs brought together to prevent air from entering uterus Loud behavior in labor *Postpartum* Diet may be restricted after birth; for first 2 days only boiled milk and toasted tortillas permitted (special foods to restore warmth to body) Bed rest for 3 days after birth Keep warm Delay bathing Mother's head and feet protected from cold air; bathing permitted after 14 days Mother often cared for by her own mother 40-day restriction on sexual intercourse	*Newborn* Breastfeeding begun after third day; colostrum may be considered "filthy" or "spoiled" Olive oil or castor oil given to stimulate passage of meconium Male infant not circumcised Female infant's ears pierced Belly band used to prevent umbilical hernia Religious medal worn by mother during pregnancy; placed around infant's neck Infant protected from "evil eye" Various remedies used to treat "mal ojo" (evil eye) and fallen fontanel (depressed fontanel)
African-American (Members of the African-American community, many of whom are descendants of slaves, have different origins. Today a number of black Americans have emigrated from Africa, the West Indian Islands, the Dominican Republic, Haiti, and Jamaica.)		
Pregnancy Acceptance of pregnancy depends on economic status Pregnancy thought to be state of "wellness," which is often the reason for delay in seeking prenatal care, especially by lower-income African-Americans "Old wives' tales" include beliefs that having a picture taken during pregnancy will cause stillbirth and reaching up will cause cord to strangle baby Craving for certain foods, including chicken, greens, clay, starch, and dirt Pregnancy may be viewed by African-American men as a sign of their virility Self-treatment for various discomforts of pregnancy, including constipation, nausea, vomiting, headache, and heartburn	*Labor* Use of "granny midwife" in certain parts of United States Varied emotional responses: some cry out, some display stoic behavior to avoid calling attention to selves Patient may arrive at hospital in far-advanced labor Emotional support often provided by other women, especially own mother *Postpartum* Vaginal bleeding seen as sign of sickness; tub baths and shampooing of hair prohibited Sassafras tea thought to have healing power Eating liver thought to cause heavier vaginal bleeding because of its high "blood" content	*Newborn* Feeding very important: "Good" baby thought to eat well Early introduction of solid foods May breastfeed or bottle-feed; breastfeeding may be considered embarrassing Parents fearful of spoiling baby Commonly call baby by nicknames May use excessive clothing to keep baby warm Belly band used to prevent umbilical hernia Abundant use of oil on baby's scalp and skin Strong feeling of family, community, and religion
Asian-American (Typically refers to groups from China, Korea, the Philippines, Japan, Southeast Asia [particularly Thailand], Indochina, and Vietnam.)		
Pregnancy Pregnancy considered time when mother "has happiness in her body" Pregnancy seen as natural process Strong preference for female health care provider Belief in theory of hot and cold May omit soy sauce in diet to prevent dark-skinned baby Prefer soup made with ginseng root as general strength tonic Milk usually excluded from diet because it causes stomach distress Inactivity or sleeping late may cause difficult delivery	*Labor* Mother admitted by other women, especially her own mother Father does not actively participate Labor in silence Cesarean birth not welcome *Postpartum* Must protect self from yin (cold forces) for 30 days Ambulation limited Shower and bathing prohibited Warm room Chinese mother avoids fruits and vegetables Diet: Warm fluids Some patients are vegetarians Korean mother served seaweed soup with rice Chinese diet high in hot foods	*Newborn* Concept of family is important and valued Father is head of household; wife plays a subordinate role Birth of boy is preferred May delay naming child Some groups (e.g., Vietnamese) believe colostrum is dirty; therefore they may delay breastfeeding until milk comes in

Continued

Table 2-2 Traditional* Cultural Beliefs and Practices: Childbearing and Parenting—cont'd

PREGNANCY	CHILDBIRTH	PARENTING
European-American		
(Members of the European-American [Caucasian] community have their origins in countries such as Ireland, Great Britain, Germany, Italy, and France.)		
Pregnancy Pregnancy viewed as a condition that requires medical attention to ensure health Emphasis on early prenatal care Variety of childbirth education programs available and participation encouraged Technology driven Emphasis on nutritional science Involvement of the father valued Written source of information valued	*Labor* Birth is a public concern Technology dominated Birthing process in institutional setting valued Involvement of father expected Physician seen as head of team *Postpartum* Emphasis or focus on early bonding Medical interventions for dealing with discomfort Early ambulation and activity emphasized Self-management valued	*Newborn* Increased popularity of breastfeeding Breastfeeding begins as soon as possible after childbirth *Parenting* Motherhood and transition to parenting seen as stressful time Nuclear family valued, although single parenting and other forms of parenting more acceptable than in the past Women often deal with multiple roles Early return to prenatal activities
Native American		
(Many different tribes exist within the Native American culture; viewpoints vary according to tribal customs and beliefs.)		
Pregnancy Pregnancy considered as a normal, natural process Late prenatal care Avoid heavy lifting Herb teas encouraged	*Labor* Prefers female attendant, although husband, mother, or father may assist with birth Birth may be attended by whole family Herbs may be used to promote uterine activity Birth may occur in squatting position *Postpartum* Herb teas to stop bleeding	*Newborn* Infant not fed colostrum Use of herbs to increase flow of milk Use of cradle boards for infant Babies not handled often

Data from Amaro H: Women in the Mexican-American community: religion, culture, and reproductive attitudes and experiences, *J Comp Psych* 16(1):6-19, 1994; Bar-yam NB: Learning about culture: a guide for birth practitioners, *Int J Childbirth Educ* 9(2):8-10, 1994; D'Avanzo CE: *Mosby's pocket guide to cultural health assessment*, ed 4, St Louis, 2008, Mosby; Galanti G: *Caring for patients from different cultures: case studies from American hospitals*, ed 2, Philadelphia, 1997, University of Pennsylvania Press; Mattson S: Culturally sensitive prenatal care for Southeastern Asians, *J Obstet Gynecol Neonatal Nurs* 24(4):335-341, 1995; Spector RE: *Cultural diversity in health and illness*, ed 7, Upper Saddle River, NJ, 2009, Prentice Hall Health; and Williams R: Issues in women's health care. In Johnson B (editor): *Psychiatric mental health nursing: adaptation and growth*, Philadelphia, 1989, Lippincott.

NOTE: Most of these cultural beliefs and customs reflect the traditional culture and are not universally practiced. These lists are not intended to stereotype patients but rather to serve as guidelines while discussing meaningful cultural beliefs with a patient and her family. Examples of other cultural beliefs and practices are found throughout this text.

*Variations in some beliefs and practices exist within subcultures of each group.

BOX 2-2 CRASH Course in Cultural Competency

- **C**ulture
- Show **R**espect
- **A**ssess/Affirm differences
- Show **S**ensitivity and Self-awareness
- Do it all with **H**umility

From Rust G et al: A CRASH-course in cultural competence, *Ethn Dis* 16(2 suppl 3):29-36, 2006.

One strategy to teach cultural competence in nursing education is to have international clinical placements or experiences (Perry & Mander, 2005; Sloand, Bower, & Groves, 2008). In such placements students may experience being in the minority, not knowing the language, eating unfamiliar foods, not having a ready source of safe drinking water, using primitive bathroom facilities, and having a shortage of equipment and supplies. Students come away with an appreciation for the problems of nonnative speakers having limited access to care and being dependent on health care workers who may not appreciate the stress and fears of being cared for in an unfamiliar environment.

Integrating Cultural Competence with the Nursing Care Plan

In many cultures family members make most of the decisions for the patient; therefore the central relationship between the nurse and patient is mediated directly by the family. The nurse must recognize the cultural importance of family in supporting the patient, guiding decision making, and preserving cultural integrity in the health care interaction.

Nursing care is delivered in multiple cultural contexts. These contexts include the cultures of the patient, the nurse, and the health care system, as well as the larger culture of the society in which health care is delivered. If any of these cultural groups is excluded from the nurse's assessment and consideration, nursing care may fail to achieve its goals and may be culturally insensitive.

Nursing Care Management

Effective communication is a critical element in the delivery of quality health care. Nurses must be aware of the attitudes, beliefs, biases, and behaviors of patients that may influence care (Markova & Broome, 2007).

Assessment

When nurses develop plans of care for patients who are culturally different from themselves or from the dominant culture of the community, they should be certain to include an assessment that addresses psychosocial issues related to that diversity. No nursing care plan is complete without attention to nursing diagnoses that address cultural diversity issues.

Nursing Diagnoses

- *Impaired verbal communication related to*
  — inability to speak or understand English
- *Coping, family, compromised related to*
  — inability to obtain culturally appropriate health care
- *Health-seeking behaviors related to*
  — keeping prenatal appointments
- *Powerlessness, risk for, related to*
  — lack of health insurance, limited access to care for family members

Expected Outcomes

Examples of expected outcomes for perinatal patients include that the woman/family will do the following:

- Verbalize (through an interpreter) understanding of treatments
- Use support systems to cope effectively with problems (e.g., pregnancy complications, newborn complications or treatments)
- Perform procedures accurately, as evidenced by return demonstration
- Access financial assistance for care

Plan of Care and Implementation

The nursing plan of care is developed in collaboration with the patient and family, based on their health care needs.

Evaluation

Evaluation is based on the expected outcomes of care. The plan is revised as necessary.

Key Points

- Contemporary American society recognizes and accepts a variety of family forms.
- The family is a social network that acts as an important support system for its members.
- Family theories provide nurses with useful guidelines for understanding family function.
- Family socioeconomics, response to stress, and culture are key factors influencing family health.
- The reproductive beliefs and practices of a culture are embedded in its economic, religious, kinship, and political structures.

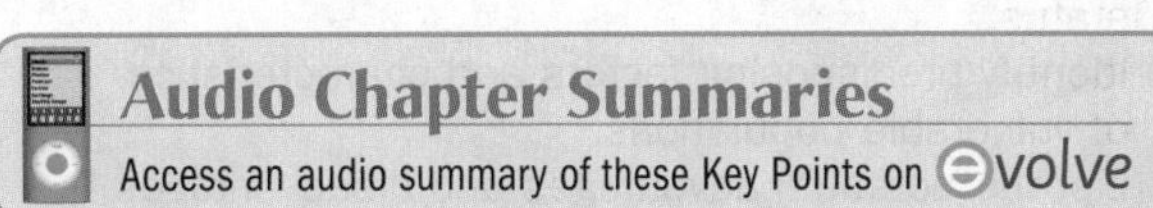
Audio Chapter Summaries
Access an audio summary of these Key Points on evolve

- To provide quality care to women in their childbearing years and beyond, nurses should be aware of the cultural beliefs and practices important to individual families.

References

Allen M: Comparative theories of the expanded role in nursing and implications for nursing practice: a working Paper, *Nurs Pap* 9(2):38-45, 1997.

Becker M: The Health Belief Model and sick role behavior, *Health Educ Monogr* 2:409-419, 1974.

Black K, Lobo M: A conceptual review of family resilience factors, *J Fam Nurs* 14(1):33-55, 2008.

Boss P: *Family stress management*, ed 2, Thousand Oaks, Calif, 2002, Sage.

Bronfenbrenner U: *The ecology of human development: experiments by nature and design*, Cambridge, Mass, 1979, Harvard University Press.

Bronfenbrenner U: Ecological systems theory. In Vasta R (editor): *Annals of child development*, vol 6, Greenwich, Conn, 1989, JAI, pp 187-249.

Carter B, McGoldrick M: The expanded family life cycle: individual, family, and social perspectives, ed 3, Boston, 1999, Allyn & Bacon.

Janz NK, Becker MH: The Health Belief Model: a decade later, *Health Educ Q* 11(1):1-47, 1984.

Johnson B et al: *Partnering with patients and families to design a patient- and family-centered health care system*, Bethesda Md, 2008, Institute for Family-Centered Care.

Klein D, White J: *Family theories: an introduction*, Newberry Park, Calif, 1996, Sage.

Markova T, Broome B: Effective communication and delivery of culturally competent health care, *Urol Nurs* 27(3):239-242, 2007.

Perry S, Mander R: A global frame of reference: learning from everyone, everywhere, *Nurs Ed Persp* 26(3):148-151, 2005.

Rempel G, Neufeld A, Kushner K: Interactive use of genograms and ecomaps in family caregiving research, *Fam Nurs* 13(4):403-419, 2007.

Rust G et al: A crash-course in cultural competence, *Ethn Dis* 16(2 suppl 3):29-36, 2006.

Sloand E, Bower K, Groves S: Challenges and benefits of international clinical placements in public health nursing, *Nurse Educ* 33(1):35-38, 2008.

Spector RE: *Cultural diversity in health and illness*, ed 7, Upper Saddle River, NJ, 2009, Prentice Hall Health.

Wright LM, Leahey M: *Nurses and families: a guide to family assessment and intervention*, ed 4, Philadelphia, 2005, FA Davis.

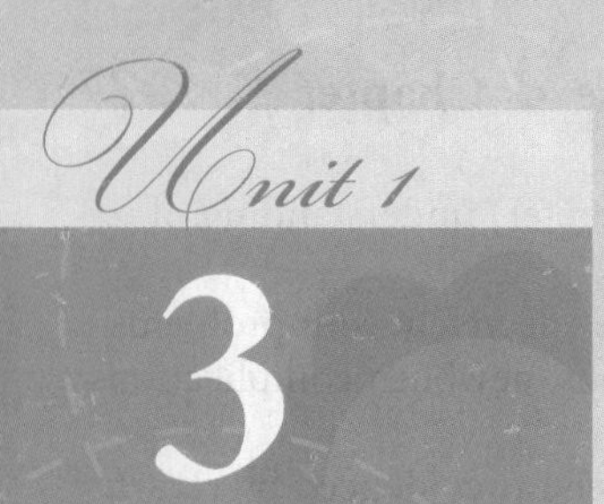

Unit 1 3 Community and Home Care

Learning Objectives

On completion of this chapter the reader will be able to:

- Compare community-based health care and community health (population- or aggregate-focused) care.
- Identify key components of the community assessment process.
- List indicators of community health status and their relevance to perinatal health.
- Describe data sources and methods for obtaining information about community health status.
- Identify predisposing factors and characteristics of vulnerable populations.
- List the potential advantages and disadvantages of home visits.
- Explore telephonic nursing care options in perinatal nursing.
- Describe how home care fits into the maternity continuum of care.
- Identify and define common perinatal conditions amenable to home care.
- Discuss safety and infection control principles as they apply to the care of patients in their homes.
- Describe the nurse's role in perinatal home care.

Electronic Resources

Additional information related to the content in Chapter 3 can be found on

evolve the Companion Website at
http://evolve.elsevier.com/Perry/maternal/

- NCLEX Review Questions
- Critical Thinking Exercise—Community Resources for Families
- Nursing Care Plan—Community and Home Care

Health care in the United States has evolved rapidly in recent years, with notable shifts in both the nature of health priorities and the ways that health care is delivered to populations, families, and individuals. Greater emphasis is placed on the prevention of disease and disability rather than the curative focus of past decades.

One major shift in health care delivery is an increased emphasis on brief hospital stays that serve to reduce the financial burden for individuals, agencies, and insurance carriers. Hospital stays after childbirth may be abbreviated. By minimizing inpatient length of stay, much of acute care nursing has been transferred to home-based nursing services in local communities.

Healthy People 2010 established national health priorities that focus on two major goals: (1) increased quality and years of healthy life, and (2) elimination of health disparities (U.S. Department of Health and Human Services [USDHHS], 2000) *(www.healthypeople.gov)*. National objectives for each maternal-child health indicator are used to track progress, highlight achievement, and identify areas for further action. Every 10 years the USDHHS examines insights and lessons learned from the previous 10 years and, with current data, includes assessments of major risks to health and wellness, the changes in public health priorities, and issues related to the nation's health preparedness and prevention. Objectives for the nation's health are developed based on these data. Reenvisioning the nation's goals is currently in process *(www.healthypeople.gov/hp2020)*.

Trends in maternal and infant health in the United States reveal that progress has been made in relation to reduced infant and fetal deaths and use of prenatal care (see Chapter 1), but notable gaps remain in many other target areas. Some critical measures such as the rates of low birth weight (LBW), very low birth weight, and preterm birth have increased. There are significant disparities in infant mortality rates that continue to fall short of *Healthy People 2010* target goals, with persistent disparities between non-Hispanic whites and other racial and ethnic groups in the United States. The cesarean birth rate is increasing. Despite favorable trends in early prenatal care, maternal mortality has not decreased significantly since 1982, with disproportionate rates among African-American and Hispanic women (Martin et al, 2008). That many of these outcomes are preventable through access to prenatal care and use of preventive health practices clearly demonstrates the need for comprehensive, community-based care that is culturally relevant for mothers, infants, and families. In the community, health care ranges from individual care to group and community services and from primary prevention to tertiary care experiences and home visiting. Depending on the needs of the individual family unit, independent self-management, ambulatory care, home care, low risk hospitalization, or specialized intensive care may be appropriate at different points along this continuum.

In community-based health care, both the aggregate (group of people who have shared characteristics) and the population become the focus of intervention. Health professionals are required not only to determine health priorities but also to develop successful plans of care to be delivered in the health clinic, the community health center, or the patient's home. This home- and community-based delivery system presents unique challenges for perinatal and maternity nurses.

Changing demands on the community-based nurse evolve out of these societal, economic, and health-related trends. Acuity of illness of home care patients may be far greater than in the past, requiring the community nurse to become more adept in maternal assessment, direct care, and teaching. Assessment of the neonate requires knowledge of parameters for measuring the health of a newborn within the first days of life. Skill in assisting with breastfeeding is essential. Knowledge of an ever-widening array of diverse family traditions, beliefs, and expectations related to childbearing becomes even more critical in order for the nurse to facilitate effectively the transition required when a family moves through the stages of incorporating a new family member.

Community and family cannot be considered separately. Furthermore, as population demographics change, nurses are assuming greater roles in assessing community health status and providing health promotion and disease prevention interventions across the perinatal health continuum. Chapter 2 contains an overview of family and cultural theory and assessment. In this chapter the integration of community and home care is discussed within the context of family-centered nursing in relation to *Healthy People 2010* and perinatal health outcomes. Methods of community assessment and the special perinatal health needs of vulnerable aggregates in the population are discussed.

Community Health Promotion

Best practices in community-based health initiatives involve both understanding of community relationships and resources and participation of community leaders. Empowerment of people, organizations, and communities working together is necessary for lasting change (Cottrell, Girvan, & McKenzie, 2006). A community-based framework helps to bring together multiple perspectives and diverse community resources to address a specific health priority.

The emphasis on community-based health promotion has grown in recent years, with recognition that many health issues require the collaborative efforts of a diverse community network to achieve public health goals (Cottrell et al, 2006). These efforts are particularly relevant in relation to maternal-newborn health, which is affected by multiple public health issues: lack of health insurance, teen pregnancy, substance abuse, and the consequences of inadequate prenatal care.

Levels of Preventive Care

Population-based care involves prevention activities focused on target needs identified in the community assessment process. These levels of prevention provide a framework for nursing interventions. *Primary prevention* involves health promotion and disease prevention activities to decrease the occurrence of illness and enhance general health and quality of life. Primary prevention precedes disease or dysfunction and encourages individuals to achieve the optimal level of health possible. Examples of primary prevention include health education and counseling about healthy lifestyle behaviors, including nutrition and exercise. Other examples are immunizations, injury prevention through the use of seat belts and safety helmets, and environmental modifications to improve air quality. Educational programs that teach sex practices that reduce risk or the dangers of smoking and drug use are also examples of primary prevention.

Secondary prevention is aimed at early detection of a disease and prompt treatment to either cure the disease or slow its progression and prevent subsequent disability (Maurer & Smith, 2005). Screening programs to detect disease while persons are asymptomatic are the most frequent forms of secondary prevention. Examples of this level of prevention are community blood pressure and cholesterol screenings that identify persons at high risk for heart attack and stroke and facilitate early treatment. The goal is to shorten disease duration and severity, thus enabling an individual to return to normal function as quickly as possible.

Tertiary prevention follows the occurrence of a defect or disability and is aimed at preventing disability through restoration of optimal functioning. Persons who have developed disease are provided with treatment and rehabilitation to prevent complications and further deterioration. Examples of tertiary prevention are early treatment and management of diabetes to reduce problems and rehabilitation of persons after a stroke.

Because most women are healthy during pregnancy, maternal-newborn nursing emphasizes primary and secondary prevention activities regardless of where care is provided. Tertiary prevention is frequently the focus for the ill pregnant patient at home or in the hospital.

Assessing the Community

Community assessment is a complex but well-defined process through which the unique characteristics of the populations and their special needs are identified to plan and evaluate health services for the community as a whole. The purpose of this process is to identify direct service and advocacy needs of the targeted aggregate or group and to improve health for the community.

In community health assessment, data are collected, analyzed, and used to educate and mobilize communities, develop priorities, garner resources, and plan actions to improve public health. Many models and frameworks of community assessment are available, but the actual process often depends on the extent and nature of the assessment to be performed, the time and resources available, and the way the information is to be used *(www.assessnow.info/resources/models-of-community-health-assessment).*

The community *asset mapping* approach provides an overview of community attributes and strengths that may facilitate long-term change and improved quality of life for community residents. Community *capacity* looks at a community's ability to address social and health problems or to develop knowledge, systems, and resources that contribute to a community health status. These approaches help to direct the health promotion process by identifying community priorities and areas of needed change.

Data Collection and Sources of Community Health Data

Data collection is often the most time-consuming phase of the community assessment process, but it provides an important definition and description of the community. Measures of community health include access to care, level of provider services available, and other social and economic factors. Consideration of individual, interpersonal, community, organizational, and policy-level data and the interaction of these factors are important in providing a comprehensive framework for community health promotion. A community assessment model (Fig. 3-1) is often used to provide a comprehensive guide to data collection.

The most critical community indicators of perinatal health relate to access to care; maternal mortality; infant mortality; LBW; first trimester prenatal care; and rates for mammography, Papanicolaou tests, and other similar screening tests (Agency for Healthcare Research and Quality [AHRQ], 2005; USDHHS, 2007). Nurses may use these indicators as a reflection of access, quality, and continuity of health care in a com-

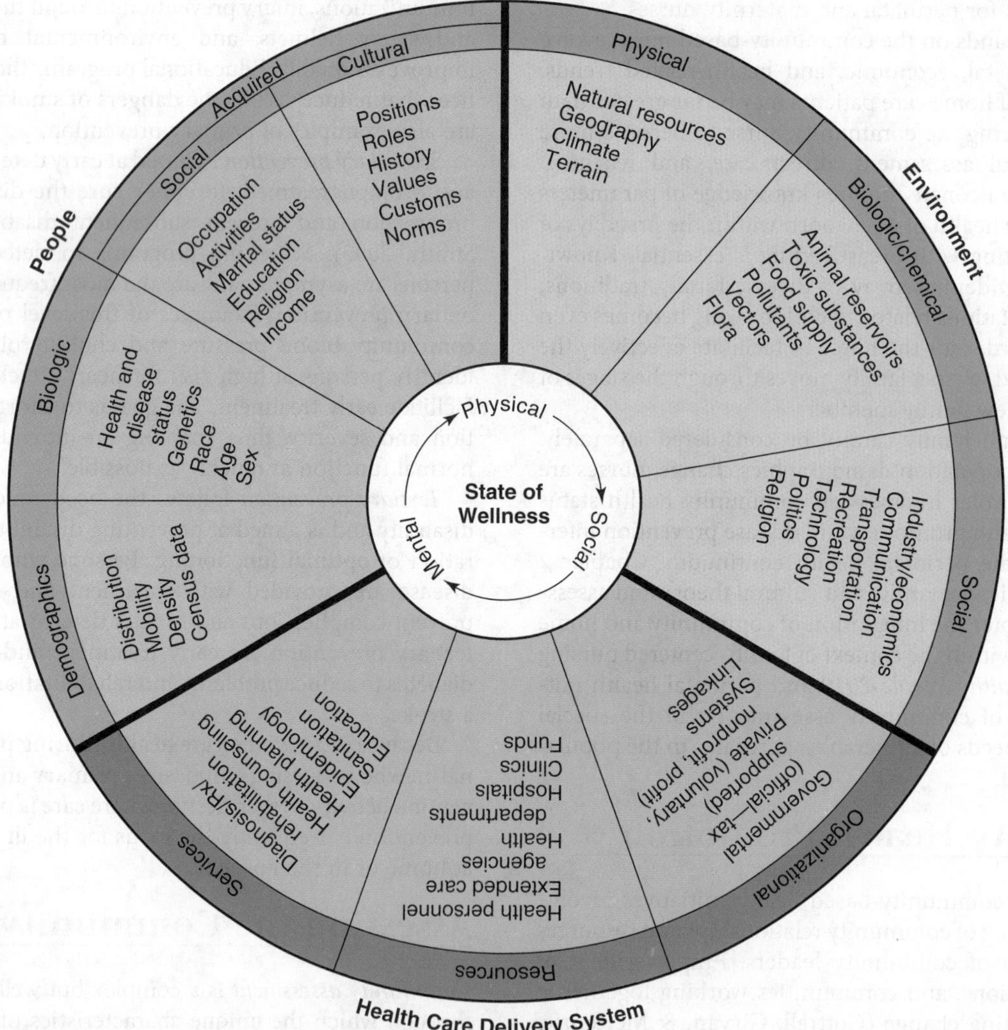

Fig. 3-1 Community health assessment wheel. (From Clemen-Stone S: Community assessment and diagnosis. In Clemen-Stone S, McGuire S, Eigsti D, editors: *Comprehensive community health nursing: family, aggregate, and community practice*, ed 6, St Louis, 2002, Mosby.)

munity. For women and infants, access to a consistent source of care is critical. Those with a regular source of care are more likely to use preventive services and receive timely treatment for illness and injury (USDHHS, 2007), but current statistics indicate that many women lack access to a usual source of care or rely primarily on emergency services.

Access to health care is also an important measure of community health. This indicator relates not only to the *availability* of health department services, hospitals, public clinics, or other sources of care, but also to *accessibility* of care. In many areas where facilities and providers are available, geographic and transportation barriers render the care inaccessible for certain populations. This is particularly true in rural areas or other remote locations. Other barriers to care should also be evaluated, including cultural and language barriers and lack of providers or specialty care. Local health departments provide varied levels and types of services, which may or may not meet the needs of the populations they serve. For example, primary care services are limited in many areas, although health education is offered by most health departments. There is a growing trend in the United States to have walk-in clinics in grocery and drug stores, which are easily accessible locations.

Health departments at the city, county, and state level are a valuable resource for annual reports of births and deaths. Maternal and infant death rates are particularly important since they reflect health outcomes that may be preventable. Local health departments also compile extensive statistics about the birth complications, causes of death, and leading causes of morbidity and mortality for each age group. Local and state health data are compiled and reported through the Centers for Disease Control and Prevention (CDC) (*www.cdc.gov*) to the National Center for Health Statistics (NCHS) (*www.cdc.gov/nchs*). The National Health Survey published annually from this source describes national health trends. However, national data are only as accurate and reliable as the local data on which they are based; thus caution is needed in interpreting the data and applying them to specific population groups.

The U.S. government census provides data on population size, age ranges, sex, racial and ethnic distribution, socioeconomic status, educational level, employment, and housing characteristics. Summary data are available for most large metropolitan areas, arranged by zip code and census tract, which usually correspond to a neighborhood comprising approximately 3000 to 6000 people. Looking at individual census tracts within a community helps to identify subpopulations or aggregates whose needs may differ from those of the larger community. For example, women at high risk for inadequate prenatal care according to age, race, and ethnic or cultural group may be readily identified; and outreach activities may be targeted appropriately.

Other sources of useful information are hospitals and voluntary health agencies. For example, the March of Dimes Birth Defects Foundation has supported perinatal needs assessments in many communities across the United States (*www.modimes.org*). Other community health resources include health care providers or administrators, government officials, religious leaders, and representatives of voluntary health agencies. Community or county health councils exist in many areas, with oversight of specific health initiatives or programs for that region. These key informants often provide a unique perspective that may not be accessible through other sources. Community gatekeepers who are at the forefront of addressing the social and health care needs of the population are also critical links to population-specific health information.

The perinatal health nurse also may explore existing community health program reports, records of preventive health screenings, and other informal data. Established programs often provide reliable indicators of the health promotion and disease prevention characteristics of the population.

Professional publications are a rich and readily accessible source of information for all nurses. In addition to nursing and public health journals, behavioral and social science literature offers diverse perspectives on community health status for specific populations and subgroups. The Internet has increased the availability and accessibility of national, state, and local health data as well. However, the use of Internet-based resources for health information requires some caution, since data reliability and validity are difficult to verify. (Some guidelines for evaluation of Internet health resources can be found at the Health on the Net website, *www.hon.org*.)

Data collection methods may be either qualitative or quantitative and may include visual surveys that can be completed by walking through a community, participant observation, interviews, focus groups, and analysis of existing data. Potential patients and health care consumers may be asked to participate in focus groups or community forums to present their views on needed community services and programs. Formal surveys conducted by mail, telephone, or face-to-face interviews can be a valuable source of information not available from national databases or other secondary sources. Several drawbacks exist with this method: surveys are generally expensive to develop and time-consuming to administer. In addition to the cost of such surveys, poor response rates often preclude a sufficiently representative response on which to base nursing interventions.

A walking survey is generally conducted by a walk-through observation of the community (Box 3-1), taking note of specific characteristics of the population, economic and social environment, transportation, health care services, and other resources. This method allows the nurse to collect subjective data and may facilitate other aspects of the assessment. Participant observation is another useful assessment method in which the nurse actively participates in the community to understand the community more fully and validate observations.

Finally, as part of the assessment process, nurses working in multiethnic and multicultural groups need an in-depth assessment of culturally based health behaviors.

Analysis and synthesis of data obtained during the assessment process help to generate a comprehensive picture of the community's health status, needs, and problem areas, as well as its strengths and resources for addressing these concerns. The goals of this process are to assign priorities to community health needs and to develop a plan of action for correcting them. A comparison of community health data with state and national statistics may be useful in identification of appropri-

BOX 3-1 Community Walk Through

As you observe the community, take note of the following:

Physical environment—Older neighborhood or newer subdivision? Sidewalks, streets, and buildings in good or poor repair? Billboards and signs? What are they advertising? Are lawns kept up? Is there trash in the streets? Parks or playgrounds? Parking lots? Empty lots? Industries?

People in the area—Old, young, homeless, children, predominant ethnicity, language? Is the population homogeneous? What signs do you see of different cultural groups?

Stores and services available—Restaurants: chain, local, ethnic? Grocery stores: neighborhood or chain? Department stores, gas stations, real estate or insurance offices, travel agencies, pawn shops, liquor stores, discount or thrift stores, newspaper stands?

Social—Clubs, bars, fraternal organizations (e.g., Elks, American Legion), museums?

Religious—Churches, synagogues, mosques? What denominations? Do you see evidence of their use other than on religious/holy days?

Health services—Drug stores, doctors' offices, clinics, dentists, mental health services, veterinarians, urgent care facilities, hospitals, shelters, nursing homes, home health agencies, public health services, traditional healers (e.g., herbalists, palmists)?

Transportation—Cars, bus, taxi, light rail, sidewalks, bicycle paths, access for disabled persons?

Education—Schools, before- and after-school programs, child care, libraries, bookstores? What is the reputation of the schools?

Government—What is the governance structure? Is there a mayor? City council? Are meetings open to the public? Are there signs of political activity (e.g., posters, campaign signs)?

Safety—How safe is the community? What is the crime rate? What types of crimes are committed? Are police visible? Is there a fire station?

Evaluation of the community based on your observations—What is your impression of the community? Is the environment pleasing? Are services and transportation adequate? How difficult is it for residents to obtain needed services (i.e., how far do they have to travel)? Would you want to live in this community? Why or why not?

ate target populations and interventions to improve health outcomes.

Vulnerable Populations in the Community

Assessment of population health includes indicators related to diverse groups and cultures, particularly disenfranchised or "vulnerable" community members *(www.crosshealth.com).* Vulnerability in terms of health status and health outcomes may take many forms, including sociocultural, economic, and environmental risk factors that contribute to disparities in health. Health disparities are conditions that disproportionately affect certain racial, ethnic, or other groups. African-Americans, Hispanics or Latinos, Native Americans, Pacific Islanders, and Asian-Americans are all considered vulnerable populations because they are more likely to have poor health and die prematurely.

Women

Women comprise 51% of the U.S. population, representing a very diverse and largely "at risk" group in relation to health (USDHHS, 2007). One of the primary factors compromising women's health is lack of access to acceptable-quality health care, which may take many forms: lack of health insurance, living in a medically underserved area, or an inability to obtain needed services, particularly basic services such as prenatal care. For example, some rural areas have few obstetricians, pediatricians, and nurse-midwives; women may have to travel hundreds of miles for this kind of care. Women often have lower incomes and less education and therefore are considered at high risk. Infant mortality is nearly two times higher for mothers without a high school education.

Within the larger group of vulnerable women, a number of subgroups present challenges to the community-based perinatal nurse.

Women in Racial and Ethnic Minorities

In addition to social, economic, and cultural barriers to optimal health, women who are in racial and ethnic minorities experience a disproportionate burden of disease, disability, and premature death. Whereas 63% of non-Hispanic white females reported that they are in excellent or good health, only 53% of Hispanic and 51% of non-Hispanic black women reported this level of health (USDHHS, 2007).

Significant health disparities continue to exist in terms of adult women's health and the health of their infants. There are persistent disparities within racial and ethnic groups in early prenatal care, infant mortality rates, LBW, preterm birth, and infant mortality. Infant mortality rates are highest among Native American, Alaska Native, and Puerto Rican women.

Minority women, many of whom live in poverty, also have higher rates of chronic disease, including heart disease, cancer, hepatitis, acquired immunodeficiency syndrome (AIDS), and mental health issues (USDHHS, 2007). Women with underlying health conditions are at especially high risk for poor obstetric outcomes for both themselves and their infants. They have high rates of preterm labor and gestational hypertension and often have intrauterine growth restriction, resulting in the birth of infants who are small for gestational age. These are the patients for whom the community-based perinatal nurse will be providing care, and their needs are complex, demanding high levels of expertise and skill.

Adolescent Girls

The adolescent population in the United States generally is considered healthy. Yet this group of women is often vulnerable because of high risk behaviors. Adolescent girls, especially those from minorities and low-income or disrupted families, are more likely to engage in early sexual activity and other high risk behaviors, with both immediate and long-term health consequences. Female adolescents in the United States also experience a high rate of teen pregnancy, with 4 out of 10 becoming pregnant before the age of 20 years. Sexually transmitted infection (STI) rates, primarily chlamydia and gonorrhea, are highest among adolescent and young adult females (USDHHS, 2007).

Adolescent health is another broad target area for community health promotion efforts, including both health education and policy initiatives. Because adolescents fail to perceive their own vulnerability, they need help navigating a complex environment and dealing with risk behaviors through preventive strategies that enhance decision making and increase protective factors.

Although adolescents are concerned about becoming pregnant, they still engage in unprotected sex. Adolescents also use a variety of sources for health information (i.e., the media, friends, and sex education); yet they are often misinformed, particularly about STIs and human immunodeficiency virus (HIV) transmission. These findings have significant implications for perinatal outcomes and emphasize the importance of aggressive prevention programs and community outreach related to sexuality, teen pregnancy, and substance abuse.

Older Women

In 2005 the U.S. population comprised 20.4 million women over the age of 65 years. This represents over 57% of the population ages 65 and older. Although women have a greater life expectancy than men, they are more likely to have chronic illnesses, less likely to use preventive services, and ultimately spend more on health care (USDHHS, 2007).

However, there is a great deal of emphasis on preventive interventions that are effective in delaying or controlling age-related changes. Improving self-management activities such as diet and exercise are important health-promotion elements for this population.

Incarcerated Women

The number of incarcerated women in the United States has continued to climb in recent years, increasing at a significantly greater rate than for men. In 2003 nearly 182,000 were in prison, with the highest number of these being black, non-Hispanic women (Harrison & Karlberg, 2004). Many of these women report a history of sexual and physical abuse.

Because their relationship histories are often unstable and because they often lack the support of family, incarcerated women or those with a history of repeated incarceration frequently have difficulty providing emotional stability, secure housing, and health promotion role modeling for their children.

The lifestyle choices of this group, including risky sexual relationships, illicit drug use, and smoking, place them at high risk for STIs, HIV, and AIDS; other chronic and communicable diseases; and complicated pregnancies (USDHHS, 2007).

Women and the Migrant Work Force

There are an estimated three million migrant and seasonal farm workers in the United States, 21% of whom are women. Diverse ethnic and cultural groups are represented among migrant workers; however, 75% of these workers were born in Mexico. The majority (81%) speak Spanish, their average age is 33, and seventh grade is the highest grade completed on average (U.S. Department of Labor National Agricultural Workers Survey, 2005).

Migrant workers in the United States are primarily in regions associated with agriculture, tobacco production, and fishing and mining industries. The three primary migrant streams are East Coast states, midwestern and western states, and West Coast states.

Migrant laborers and their families face many problems, including financial instability, child labor, poor housing, lack of education, language and cultural barriers, and limited access to health and social services. Poor dental health, diabetes, hypertension, malnutrition, tuberculosis, and parasitic infections are common health issues among migrant populations.

Numerous reproductive health issues exist for migrant women, including less consistent use of contraception and increased rates of STIs. Migrants are less likely to receive early prenatal care and have a greater incidence of inadequate weight gain during pregnancy than do other poor women.

Primary health care services are largely provided by a number of migrant health centers, of which there are over 400 throughout the United States. Routine prenatal care and screening and treatment for hypertension and diabetes are provided. Community health nurses frequently encounter the challenges of providing culturally and linguistically appropriate care while facing numerous health issues.

Homeless Women

Homelessness among women is an increasing social and health issue in the United States. Although exact numbers are unknown, it is estimated that women make up one third of America's two to three million homeless people. The Bureau of Primary Health Care (BPHC, 2006) identifies poverty, acute and chronic health problems, substance abuse, and domestic violence as major factors for homelessness. As women are increasingly affected by poverty, homelessness is becoming more prevalent for families and children, particularly among rural populations.

Health issues among the homeless are numerous and result primarily from a lack of preventive care and resources in general. Health problems, including chronic illness, asthma, circulatory problems, and diabetes are rampant. Homeless women face a number of health issues, related both to lifestyle factors and the vulnerability resulting from being homeless. In addition to extreme poverty, women are at increased risk for illness and injury; many have been victims of domestic abuse, assault, and rape.

In 2006 the Health Care for the Homeless Program, funded by the Health Resources and Services Administration (HRSA), a division of the USDHHS, served close to 829,000 persons, 42.6% of whom were women (Bureau of Primary Health Care, 2006). Although little is known about pregnancy in this population, about 20% of women do become pregnant while homeless. Conversely, pregnancy and recent birth are highly correlated with becoming homeless (American College of Obstetricians and Gynecologists [ACOG], 2005). In addition to risk factors related to inadequate nutrition, inadequate weight gain, anemia, bleeding problems, and preterm delivery, homeless women face multiple barriers to prenatal care: transportation, distance, and wait times. Most women also underuse available prenatal services. The unsafe environment and high risk lifestyles often result in adverse perinatal outcomes.

Individuals with Low Literacy

Individuals and groups for whom English is a second language often lack the skills necessary to seek medical care and function adequately in the health care setting. Communication barriers may affect access to care, particularly in such areas as making appointments, applying for services, and obtaining transportation.

Health literacy involves a spectrum of abilities, ranging from reading an appointment slip to interpreting medication instructions. There is growing evidence of the effects of low health literacy on adult health status *(www.hsph.harvard.edu/healthliteracy)*. Low health literacy may also be an independent contributor to a disproportionate disease burden among disadvantaged populations. Disparities in preventive care, early screening for cancer, and use of health care services, particularly among minority women, have also been linked to language barriers (Jacobs et al, 2005).

As the United States becomes increasingly multicultural, nurses will be required to interact with non–English-speaking groups or those with limited health literacy. Consequently, health literacy must be viewed as a component of culturally and linguistically competent care. These skills must be assessed routinely to recognize a problem and accommodate patients with limited literacy skills.

Refugees and Immigrants

Along with their profound resilience and determination, refugees and immigrants have brought rich diversity to the United States in several important dimensions, including cultural heritage and customs, economic productivity, and enhanced national vitality. At the same time, multiple challenges accompany the dramatic influx of individuals and families from other countries.

Immigrants differ from U.S.-born persons in demographics: overall they are younger, with lower incomes and educational attainments. Although 73% of immigrants are legal citizens, this population is disproportionately affected by health disparities related to cultural and language barriers, no usual source of care, and lack of insurance.

Women without U.S. citizenship are less likely to have a usual source of care (26.1%) and more likely to be without health insurance coverage (45.5%). Nearly 25% of these women have not seen a health care provider in the past year (USDHHS, 2007).

Refugee status imposes a particular type of vulnerability on affected individuals and groups. Of primary significance are the precipitating factors by which people are displaced suddenly or forced to leave their country of origin: persecution, civil unrest, or war. Families are forced from their own homes to seek residence and employment elsewhere. Often these groups are extremely impoverished and face extreme physical and emotional stress when they arrive in the United States.

In general, refugees are more likely to live in poverty than are immigrants. Over time, health disparities that adversely affect health and well-being actually decline for the immigrant population as they become part of American society. Many of the conditions or illnesses that both immigrants and refugees acquire contribute to the persistence of disparities in their maternal and neonatal health outcomes.

Implications for Nursing

Working in the community or in the home with the full spectrum of family organizational styles, vulnerable populations, and cultural groups presents challenges for the nurse. Whether it involves perinatal care focused on women and their newborns or women's health care directed toward treatment and prevention of other health conditions such as communicable diseases and STIs, nurses must exhibit a high degree of professionalism. Cultural sensitivity, compassion, and a critical awareness of family dynamics and social stressors that will affect health-related decision making are critical components in developing an effective plan of care.

Although the long-term consequences of contemporary immigration for American society are unclear, the successful incorporation of immigrant families depends on the resources, benefits, and policies that ensure their healthy development and successful social adjustment. Culturally competent health care and involvement of the immigrant community in health care programs are recommended strategies for improving the access to and effectiveness of health care for this population.

The use of camp volunteers has been effective in assisting families living in migrant worker camps to obtain prenatal, postpartum, and infant care. Working in partnership with health professionals such as nurses, lay camp aides have been used effectively for outreach and health education; however, more strategies are needed to link traditional practices with the formal health care system. Guidance and information about other health resources are available to health care providers through the National Migrant Resource Program and the Migrant Clinicians Network *(www.migrantclinician.org)*.

Nurses working with homeless women and families are challenged to treat them with dignity and respect to establish a therapeutic relationship. Case management is recommended to coordinate the services and disciplines that may be involved in meeting the complex needs of these families. Whenever possible, general screening and preventive services must be provided when the woman seeks treatment since this may be the only opportunity to provide health information and intervention. Building on existing coping strategies and strengths, the health care provider helps the woman and her family to reconnect with a social support system. Nurses also have an important role in advocating for funding to support homeless health services and to improve access to preventive care for all homeless populations.

Home Care in the Community

Modern home care nursing has its foundation in public health nursing, which provided comprehensive care to sick and well patients in their own homes. Specialized maternity home care nursing services began in the 1980s when public health maternity nursing services were limited and services had not kept pace with the changing practices of high risk obstetrics and emerging technology. Lengthy antepartal hospitalizations for such conditions as preterm labor and preeclampsia created nursing care challenges for staff members of inpatient units.

Many women expressed their concern for the negative effect of antepartal hospitalizations on the family. Although clinical indications showed that a new nursing care approach was needed, home health care did not become a viable alternative until third-party payers (i.e., public or private organizations or employer groups that pay for health care) pushed for cost containment in maternity services.

In the current health care system, home care is an important component of health care delivery along the perinatal continuum of care (Fig. 3-2 and Critical Thinking Exercise). The growing demand for home care is based on several factors:

- Interest in family birthing alternatives
- Shortened hospital stays
- New technologies that facilitate home-based assessments and treatments
- Reimbursement by third-party payers

CRITICAL THINKING EXERCISE

Home Care of a Woman in Preterm Labor

The home care agency receives a referral for a home visit to Mariana, a 30-year-old Hispanic woman. She is 26 weeks' pregnant with her third pregnancy and is experiencing preterm labor. Her physician has prescribed bed rest at home for her. She has 2½-year-old and 1-year-old children at home. Before visiting Mariana, the nurse establishes as priorities (1) to promote bed rest, (2) involve the father in child care, and (3) recommend activities to provide distraction during bed rest.

1. Evidence—Is there sufficient evidence to draw conclusions about the appropriateness of the nurse's plan of care?
2. Assumptions—What assumptions can be made about the needs of this family in regard to the following issues?
   a. The priorities for care
   b. Conditions for ensuring bed rest
   c. Feasibility of involving the father in child care
   d. Cultural relevancy of involving the father
3. What implications and priorities for nursing care can be drawn at this time?
4. Does the evidence objectively support your conclusion?
5. Are there alternative perspectives to your conclusion?

As health care costs continue to rise and because millions of American families lack health insurance, there is greater demand for innovative, cost-effective methods of health care delivery in the community. Large health care systems are developing clinically integrated health care delivery networks whose goals are (1) improved coordination of care and care outcomes; (2) better communication among health care providers; (3) increased patient, payer, and provider satisfaction; and (4) reduced cost. The integration of clinical services changes the focus of care to a continuum of services that are increasingly community based.

Communication and Technology Applications

As maternity care continues to consist of frequent and brief contacts with health care providers throughout the prenatal and postpartum periods, services that link maternity patients throughout the perinatal continuum of care have assumed increasing importance. These services include critical pathways, telephonic nursing assessments, discharge planning, specialized education programs, parent support groups, home visiting programs, nurse advice lines, and perinatal home care (Fig. 3-3). Some hospitals provide cross-training for hospital-based nurses to make postpartum home visits or to staff outpatient centers for postpartum follow-up.

Telephonic nursing care through services such as "warm lines," nurse advice lines, and telephonic nursing assessments is a valuable means of managing health care problems and bridging the gaps among acute, outpatient, and home care services. Some providers are using the Internet to communicate with patients who have an Internet service provider. Nursing care that occurs by telephone is interactive and responsive to immediate health care questions about particular health care needs. Warm lines are telephone lines that are offered as a community service to provide new parents with support, encouragement, and basic parenting education. Nurse advice lines, or toll-free nurse consultation services, often are supported by third-party payers or health maintenance organization/managed care organization nurse case managers and are designed to provide answers to medical questions. These nurses are prepared to guide callers through urgent health care situations, suggest treatment options, and provide health education. Telephonic nursing assessments, or nurse consultation, assessment, and health education that take place during a telephone conversation, can be added to the plan of care in conjunction with skilled nursing visits; or they may comprise a separate nursing contact for the woman. Telephonic nursing assessments are commonly used after a postpartum home care visit to reassess a woman's knowledge about the signs and symptoms of adequate hydration in breastfeeding or, after initiating home phototherapy, to assess the caregiver's knowledge regarding problems with equipment.

Guidelines for Nursing Practice

The Association of Women's Health, Obstetric and Neonatal Nurses (AWHONN, 2003) defined *home care* as the provision of technical, psychologic, and other therapeutic support in the patient's home rather than in an institution. The scope of nursing care delivered in the home is necessarily limited to practices deemed safe and appropriate to be carried out in an environment that is physically separated from a health care institution and its resources. Nursing practice at home is consistent with federal and state regulations that direct home care practice. The nurse demonstrates practice competence through formalized orientation and ongoing clinical education and performance evaluation in the respective home care agency. Standards for practice from key specialty organizations such as AWHONN *(www.awhonn.org)*, the National Association of Neonatal Nurses *(www.nann.org)*, ACOG *(www.acog.org)*, the American Academy of Pediatrics (AAP) *(www.aap.org)*, and the Intravenous Nurses Society (INS) *(www.ins1.org)* provide the basis for clinical protocols and pathways and organiza-

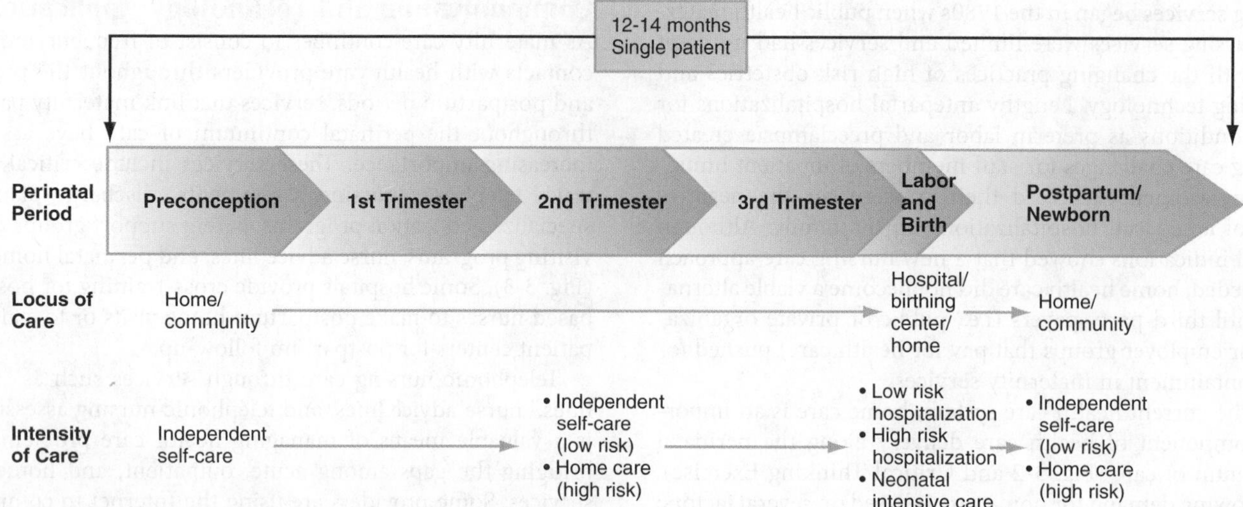

Fig. 3-2 Perinatal continuum of care.

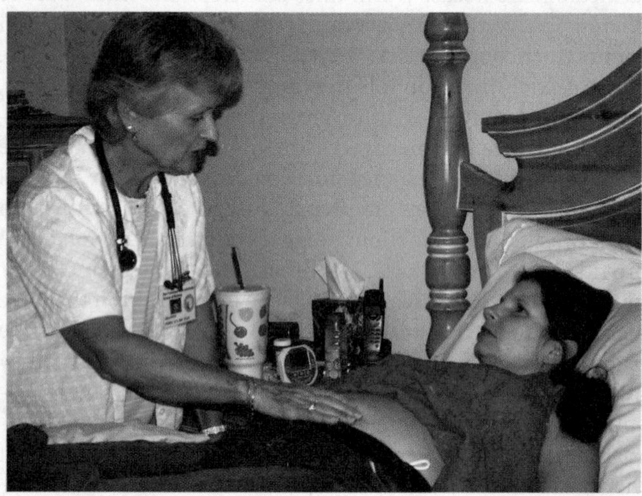

Fig. 3-3 Home care nurse visits with woman in preterm labor at home on bed rest. *(Courtesy Shannon Perry, Phoenix, AZ.)*

tional programs in home care practice. The Joint Commission *(www.jointcommission.org)* provides criteria for home care operations based on Centers for Medicare and Medicaid Services regulations.

A wide range of professional health care services and products can be delivered or used in the home by means of technology and telecommunication. For example, telehealth and telemedicine make it possible for patients in the home to be interviewed and assessed by a specialist located hundreds of miles away. Some view home health care as an extension of in-hospital care. Essentially the primary difference between health care in a hospital and home care is the absence of the continuous presence of professional health care providers in a patient's home. Generally, but not always, home health care entails intermittent care by a professional who visits the patient's home for a particular reason and/or provides care on site for fewer than 4 hours at a time. The home health care agency maintains on-call professional staff to assist home care patients who have questions about their care and for emergencies such as equipment failure.

Perinatal Services

Home care perinatal services may be provided by hospital-based programs, independent proprietary (for-profit) agencies or nonprofit home care agencies, and official or tax-supported agencies. Innovative programs may be supported by research grants for a period of years, but ultimately they must be sponsored by an agency with long-term funding.

Home visits have both advantages and disadvantages. The pregnant woman is able to maintain bed rest if indicated, and vulnerable neonates are not exposed to the weather or external sources of infection. The nurse can observe and interact with family members in their most natural and secure environment. Adequacy of resources and safety factors can be assessed. Teaching can be tailored to the actual home conditions, and other family members can be included.

A home visit is less expensive than a day's hospitalization, but a 60- to 90-minute visit requires 2.5 to 3 hours of nursing time, including travel and documentation. Travel time may be even greater when a patient resides in a rural area because of distance, travel, and weather-related factors. It is more cost-effective for the health care provider to see patients in an office, where professional time is not spent in travel. Availability of nurses with expertise in maternity care may be limited, and concerns about the nurse's physical safety in some communities may limit visits.

Visits for outreach and health promotion are an integral part of community (or public) health nursing. In countries with national health systems, a nurse or midwife may see all women during pregnancy and after birth. In the United States visits of this sort have been provided mainly to low-income families without health insurance and Medicaid recipients who use the clinics provided by local health departments. Until recently private insurers did not reimburse for health promotion visits. Managed care organizations now recognize that anticipatory guidance can be cost-effective, but for the most part home visitation programs still target specific high risk populations such as adolescents and women at risk for preterm labor.

Home care agencies are subject to regulation by governmental and professional organizations. They provide interdisciplinary services, including social work, nutrition, and occupational and physical therapy. Increasingly their case loads are made up of patients who require high-technology care such as infusions or home monitoring. Although the home health nurse develops the care plan, all care must be ordered by a physician. In addition, interventions must meet the insurer's criteria for reimbursement, and services are limited to registered patients. Preconception care and low risk antepartum care can usually be provided more efficiently in offices and are not currently reimbursable. High risk antepartum care can be provided by home care agencies. For example, women with hyperemesis gravidarum who require parenteral nutrition may be treated at home. Conditions requiring bed rest such as preterm labor and hypertension are other common indications for home care. Other conditions often managed with home care may include cardiac disease, substance abuse, and diabetes in pregnancy.

Some insurers reimburse for at least one postpartum visit to families after early discharge or in the presence of high risk factors. Home phototherapy is used for treatment of neonatal hyperbilirubinemia and to avoid separation of mother and infant. Many other neonates who require long-term high-technology care also are managed with home care.

Patient Selection and Referral

The office- or hospital-based nurse is often the key person in making effective referrals to home care. When considering a referral to home care, the following factors are evaluated:

- Health status of mother and fetus or infant: Is the condition serious enough to warrant home care? Is it stable enough for intermittent observation to be sufficient?
- Availability of professionals to provide the needed services within the patient's community
- Family resources, including psychosocial, social, and economic resources: Will the family be able to provide care between nursing visits? Are relationships supportive? Is third-party reimbursement available, or can it be negotiated with the insurer? Could a voluntary or tax-supported community agency provide needed care without payment?
- Cost-effectiveness: Is it more reasonable for the patient to receive these services at home or to go to a local outpatient facility to receive them?

Community referrals should not be limited to women with physiologic complications of pregnancy that require medical treatment. Patients at risk (e.g., young adolescents, families with a history of abuse, members of vulnerable population groups, developmentally disabled individuals) may need follow-up care at home. In consultation with the social worker, the hospital-based nurse should become familiar with agencies in the community that accept such referrals. When the patient lives in a rural area, hospital-based nurses should familiarize themselves with available formal and informal resources in that community since these may be different from those in a more populated setting (see Community Focus box).

COMMUNITY FOCUS

Availability of Home Care in Your Community

Consult the yellow pages of the telephone directory. How many home health agencies are in your area? Are any of these agencies located in the less affluent part(s) of your city? Call one of the agencies and ask the following questions: How many nurses are employed at the agency? How many of the nurses are bilingual? Does the agency accept patients on public assistance? Do they ever accept referrals for patients who cannot pay? What happens to patients who cannot pay? Based on the information you gathered, are there adequate and appropriate home care services in your area?

Standardized referral forms simplify the referral process and ensure that all needed information will be forwarded to the home health agency. The nursing assessment should include the woman's physical and psychologic status, her level of knowledge about self-management activities, her willingness to learn, the availability of caregivers and social support in the home, and her level of comfort with home care. If the referral is for a mother and infant home care visit, the nursing assessment should include newborn data.

High-technology home care requires that additional information be collected from the medical record and consultation with the referring physician and other members of the health care team before making a home care referral. These additional data include the medical diagnosis, medical prognosis, prescribed therapies, medication history, drug-dosing information, potential ancillary supplies, type of infusion access device, and the available systems of social support for the patient and family. The nursing assessment and therapies data provide baseline information for the home care nurse and other types of health care providers involved in the care plan.

Whenever a referral is called in to a home health care agency, a member of the nursing or admission staff determines the agency's ability to accept the patient for service. The use of telecommunication such as fax machines, cellular phones, and the Internet to transmit information has eliminated delays in initiating home care services, even in more remote rural areas.

Nursing Care Management

Preparing for the Home Visit

The home care nurse reviews the available clinical data, demographic information, and completed plan of care form and consults with the home care pharmacist or other health care team members who have previously contacted the woman to determine the goals of the visit. At this point, the nurse uses the medical diagnosis and the place on the perinatal continuum on which the case falls as a starting point to organize the woman's care. The nurse reviews agency policies and procedures, professional literature about diagnosis, and community resources as part of the previsit preparation work (Box 3-2).

Before going on a home visit, the nurse contacts the woman to make necessary arrangements and obtain detailed instructions on the location of the home. Contact by telephone has several goals in addition to establishing a convenient time to

BOX 3-2 Protocol for Perinatal Home Visits

Previsit Interventions

1. Contact family to arrange details for home visit.
   a. Identify self, credentials, and agency role.
   b. Review purpose of home visit follow-up.
   c. Schedule convenient time for visit.
   d. Confirm address and route to family home.
2. Review and clarify appropriate data.
   a. Review all available assessment data for mother and fetus or infant (i.e., referral forms, hospital discharge summaries, family-identified learning needs).
   b. Review records of any previous nursing contacts.
   c. Contact other professional caregivers as necessary to clarify data (i.e., obstetrician, nurse-midwife, pediatrician, referring nurse).
3. Identify community resources and teaching materials appropriate to meet needs already identified.
4. Plan the visit and prepare bag with equipment, supplies, and materials necessary for assessments of mother and fetus or infant, actual care anticipated, and teaching.

In-Home Interventions: Establishing a Relationship

1. Reintroduce self and establish purpose of visit for mother, infant, and family; offer family opportunity to clarify their expectations of contact.
2. Spend brief time socially interacting with family to become acquainted and establish trusting relationship.

In-Home Interventions: Working with Family

1. Conduct systematic assessment of mother and fetus or newborn to determine physiologic adjustment and any existing complications.
2. Throughout visit, collect data to assess the emotional adjustment of individual family members to pregnancy or birth and lifestyle changes. Note evidence of family-newborn bonding and sibling rivalry; note relationships among mother, father, children, and grandparents.
3. Determine adequacy of support system.
   a. To what extent does someone help with cooking, cleaning, and other home management tasks?
   b. To what extent is help being provided in caring for the newborn and any other children?
   c. Are support persons encouraging the new mother to care for herself and get adequate rest?
   d. Who is providing helpful information? Emotional support?
4. Throughout the visit, observe home environment for adequacy of resources:
   a. Space: privacy, safe play of children, sleeping
   b. Overall cleanliness and state of repair
   c. Number of steps pregnant woman/new mother must climb
   d. Adequacy of cooking arrangements
   e. Adequacy of refrigeration and other food storage areas
   f. Adequacy of bathing, toilet, and laundry facilities
   g. Arrangements in home for newborn: sleeping, bathing, formula preparation (if needed), layette items, and diapers
5. Throughout the visit, observe home environment for overall state of repair and existence of safety hazards:
   a. Storage of medications, household cleaners, and other substances hazardous to children
   b. Presence of peeling paint on furniture, walls, or pipes
   c. Factors that contribute to falls such as dim lighting, broken steps, scatter rugs
   d. Presence of vermin
   e. Use of crib or playpen that fails to meet safety guidelines
   f. Existence of emergency plan in case of fire; fire alarm or extinguisher
6. Provide care to mother, newborn, or both as prescribed by their respective primary care provider or in accord with agency protocol.
7. Provide teaching on basis of previously identified needs.
8. Refer family to appropriate community agencies or resources such as warm lines and support groups.
9. Ascertain that woman knows potential problems to watch for and whom to call if they occur.
10. Ensure that used disposable items have been handled appropriately and that reusable items are cleaned and repacked appropriately in the nurse's bag.

In-Home Interventions: Ending the Visit

1. Summarize the activities and main points of the visit.
2. Clarify future expectations, including schedule of next visit.
3. Review teaching plan and provide major points in writing.
4. Provide information about reaching the nurse or agency if needed before the next scheduled visit.

Postvisit Interventions

1. Document the visit thoroughly, using the necessary agency forms to serve as a legal record of the visit and allow third-party reimbursement, as possible.
2. Initiate the plan of care on which the next encounter with the woman/family will be based.
3. Communicate appropriately (by telephone, letter, progress notes, or referral form) with primary care provider, other health professionals, or referral agencies on behalf of woman/family.

visit and exact directions; it also sets the stage for the first home care visit.

The nurse identifies himself or herself by name, title, and agency. He or she then explains who referred the woman to the agency for home care and the purpose of the home care visits. The nurse briefly explains what will occur during the visit and approximately how long the visit will last. The woman should be asked to restrain any pets during the visit. Last, the nurse asks about health supplies that may be needed for the woman's care.

First Home Care Visit

Making the first home care visit can be stressful for the nurse and the woman. The home care nurse is faced with an unknown environment controlled by the woman and her family. The woman and her family also experience feelings about the unknown, such as anxiety about the way the nurse will treat them or what the nurse will do during the visit. The challenge for the home care nurse is to establish a nurse-patient relationship and provide the prescribed home care services within the time provided for the initial home visit. One of the most important roles of the home care nurse is modeling health-related behaviors for the patient and others who are in the home during the visit.

Introductions generally begin the visit; the nurse identifies himself or herself and the home care agency. The woman introduces herself and the other family members who are present. Sometimes the woman may feel uncertain of her role or be uncomfortable in taking the lead in introductions, so other people in the home may not be introduced to the nurse. In these situations the nurse can politely ask about other people in the home and their relationship to the woman.

In the first visit to the home, the home care nurse completes extensive documentation with the patient. Before performing any services, the nurse must obtain written agreement and consent for the home health care services. This consent-for-care serves two major purposes: agreement for care and authorization to release medical information. Many third-party payers require written documentation of the services provided; therefore the agency obtains authorization from the woman to give information to her physician and any individual or company involved in payment for the services. Agencies that bill third-party payers for the rendered services will include agreement language for assignment of benefits and financial remuneration. By agreeing to assign insurance benefits to the agency, the woman allows her insurance company to pay the home health care agency directly.

All patients have the right to participate actively in their plan of care. These patient rights and responsibilities should begin the discussion about the nurse and patient roles during this initial visit.

Assessment

The primary goals of the assessment phase are to develop a trusting relationship and collect data by various methods to obtain a comprehensive patient profile (see Nursing Process box). It may not be feasible or appropriate to collect in-depth information about all areas of assessment during the first visit. However, in many instances the nurse may be limited to one visit and must obtain information pertinent to the current situation in that hour.

Establishing a trusting relationship begins with the previsit telephone call. An interview style that reflects sensitivity; a nonjudgmental, accepting attitude; and respect for the woman's rights facilitates the development of that trusting relationship. A skillful interviewer avoids barriers to communication such as false reassurance, advice giving, excessive talking, and showing approval or disapproval. This nurse-patient relationship continues to develop over the course of home visits.

The nurse is a guest in the woman's home and should show respect for her and her belongings. Some adaptation of the home visit schedule may be made if numerous distractions interrupt a visit, such as caring for the needs of small children. The nurse may ask to have the volume of the television reduced or suggest moving to another room where it is more quiet and private.

Each plan of care has a different emphasis in the home environment. For example, women receiving infusion therapy for hyperemesis gravidarum need a safe place to store medications and infusion supplies that is out of reach of small children living in the home. The home care nurse should incorporate the agency's policies and procedures for the storage and handling of infusion supplies into her walk-through inspection. During the walk through the home care nurse looks at the potential storage areas that are dry and clean and where the temperature can be maintained. The home care nurse should include an inspection of work areas such as countertops, tabletops, sinks, and trash areas that the woman or caregiver may use for mixing medications, changing infusion tubing, handling supplies, or disposing of used equipment and supplies.

The homes of patients using electronic home health care equipment such as phototherapy equipment or infusion pumps require physical inspection of electrical outlets, electrical cords, and extension cords that will be used. Homes with faulty electrical wiring may place the patient at risk for being involved in an electrical fire. Faulty wiring may require inspection and repair by a professional electrician before electronic devices are used. Findings from the assessment are incorporated into the plan of care.

Plan of Care and Implementation

The nursing plan of care is developed in collaboration with the patient, based on the health care needs of the individual. Home care nurses working in home health care agencies regulated by the Centers for Medicare and Medicaid Services use a plan of care that includes patient demographics, the health care provider's orders, home care goals, and the patient's level of functioning. This document is initiated at the time of referral to the home care agency and must be updated every 60 days or as specified by state regulations.

The frequency of the skilled nursing visit may vary with the individual plan of care and reimbursement criteria established by the third-party payers.

Nursing Considerations

In home care the woman or family members are responsible for administration of medications in the absence of the nurse. A careful medication history should be obtained to see if the woman is taking her medications correctly and understands the desired action and potential side effects. Sometimes when orders are changed, women continue to take both the old and new prescriptions, which can lead to dangerous overdoses or medication interactions. The culturally competent nurse ensures that there is an adequate supply and a safe place for proper storage of medications to prevent deterioration or accidental ingestion by children or pets. The nurse inquires about any other medications that the woman might be taking con-

evolve Nursing Care Plan—Community and Home Care

NURSING PROCESS: HOME VISIT

Assessment

The major areas of the assessment are demographics, medical history, general health history, medication history, sociocultural assessment, home and community environment, and physical assessment. Some of this information can be obtained from patient records sent to the home care agency at the time of referral or from the previsit interview.

Social assessment includes information regarding the number in the family and the roles of each household member, which family members or individuals have taken on the roles of caregivers, and the woman's social support network (Box 3-3).

Nursing Diagnoses

Nursing diagnoses for perinatal home health care patients derived from data collected at the first home visit may include the following:

Deficient knowledge related to
- management of therapeutic regimen (e.g., nausea and vomiting, preterm labor, gestational diabetes)
- newborn care and feeding
- phototherapy

Compromised family coping related to
- lack of child care while mother is on bed rest
- care of newborn receiving oxygen therapy

Impaired parenting related to
- maternal immaturity and lack of family support

Deficient diversional activity related to
- prolonged bed rest

Planning

Examples of expected outcomes for perinatal patients include that the woman/family will do the following:

- Verbalize understanding of treatments
- Report decreased anxiety about performing procedures (e.g., blood glucose monitoring)
- Use support systems to cope effectively with problems (e.g., pregnancy complications, newborn complications or treatments)
- Perform procedures accurately, as evidenced by return demonstration
- Verbalize decreased role strain

Interventions

Interventions are described in the text on pp. 37-42.

Evaluation

Evaluation is a continuous process through which the nurse must reassess the women's and family's condition and any response to the interventions in relation to expected outcomes of care. The nurse, in collaboration with the woman and family, then revises the nursing diagnoses and plan of care as necessary to meet mutually determined goals.

BOX 3-3 Psychosocial Assessment

Language

Identify the primary language spoken in the home.
Assess whether there are any language barriers to receiving support.

Community Resources/Access to Care

Identify primary and secondary means of transportation.
Identify community agencies family currently uses for health care and support.
Assess cultural and psychosocial barriers to receiving care.

Social Support

Determine the people living with the pregnant woman.
Identify who assists with household chores.
Identify who assists with child care/parenting activities.
Identify who the pregnant woman turns to with problems or during a crisis.

Interpersonal Relationship

Identify the way decisions are made in the family.
Identify the family's perception of the need for home care.
Identify roles of adults in caring for family members.

Caregiver

Identify the primary caregiver for home care treatments.
Identify other caregivers and their roles.
Assess the caregiver's knowledge of treatments and care process.
Identify potential strain from the caregiver role.
Identify the level of satisfaction with the caregiver role.

Stress and Coping

Identify what the woman perceives as lifestyle changes and their impact on her and her family.
Identify the changes she and her family have made to adjust to her health condition and home health care treatments.

currently. Over-the-counter drugs or herbal supplements may not be considered medications by the women and not mentioned unless such information is specifically asked for. Even more important is ensuring that the patient and her caregivers fully understand the information that they are given by health care providers.

High-technology home care involves many diagnostic and therapeutic procedures. A focused physical assessment is always part of the visit. Nurses involved in perinatal home care must be skilled in prenatal, postpartal, and newborn assessment. Many women require additional diagnostic tests. The nurse may need to collect blood or other specimens. Portable fetal monitoring equipment or even ultrasound can be used in the home for fetal assessment. Home infusion for women with hyperemesis gravidarum often replaces hospitalization. Women with preterm labor may receive parenteral tocolytic therapy. Phototherapy or apnea monitors can be provided in the home for newborns. Family members may need to be taught to monitor equipment between nurse visits and to prevent accidental damage.

Medical emergencies may occur during or between the nurse's visits to the home. Prior planning and education can reduce the risk of problems. All parents of newborns should know infant cardiopulmonary resuscitation (CPR). There should be immediate telephone access to call for emergency medical assistance. Women and their families should be taught to recognize danger signs related to their condition. For example, women at risk for preterm labor should learn to palpate the uterus and recognize contractions in the absence of pain; women with diabetes must learn the signs of hypoglycemia and what to do if it occurs; women with preeclampsia must know the danger signs that indicate worsening of their condition and notify the health care provider immediately. In a more remote rural community that does not have an obstetrician in the region, the nurse may need to assist the patient's family to arrange for "boarding" somewhere that is closer to a medical specialist.

Patient and family education in home care includes information about the specific high risk condition(s) involved, implications for pregnancy outcome, and measures for self-monitoring. Verbal explanations should be supplemented with clearly written instructions. General information to promote well-being such as about nutrition and common discomforts of pregnancy also should be included. The need for preparation for childbirth can be addressed by using books or videos and supplemented by individual teaching at home. Coping with bed rest or other limitation of activity is a problem for many women with high risk pregnancies. The nurse may share strategies that others have used, help with time management, and provide information about support services. Teaching about infant care or the special needs of the preterm infant may be appropriate during the prenatal period.

Clear documentation of assessments, problems identified, treatments and interventions performed, and patient's responses is essential. Third-party payers base reimbursement on the nurse's written record of providing skilled nursing care and assessments that support the woman's continuing need for those services. The nurse must promptly inform the health care provider by telephone or facsimile of any significant changes. When new orders are transmitted by telephone, a written copy must be sent for the physician's signature.

Nursing documentation should reflect an objective description of the nursing assessment data collected at each visit. Statements such as "no change" or "same as last visit" do not accurately reflect the monitoring of the patient's condition that occurred during the skilled nursing visit. Once the home care outcomes are achieved and the patient is discharged from the home care agency, documentation should include information about the patient's status at the time of discharge, progress toward attaining health care goals, and plans for follow-up care.

The role of the clinical record in home care has been affected by social, economic, and legal health care changes. Appropriate care should be taken to complete the necessary home health care records accurately and in a timely manner. Documentation guidelines include writing or dictating notes or using a laptop computer at the patient's home or shortly after the visit.

Safety Issues for the Home Care Nurse

Nurse safety and infection control are two important aspects specific to home care. The nurse should be fully aware of the home environment and neighborhood in which the home care is being provided. Unlike hospitals, in which the environment is more predictable and controlled, the patient's neighborhood and home have the potential for uncertainty. Home care nurses should take necessary safety precautions and avoid dangerous areas.

Agencies that serve patients in high crime areas may conduct a violence potential assessment by telephone before the visit and enlist the patient's cooperation in minimizing risk. Others have hired full-time security personnel to accompany nurses on their visits. Personal strategies recommended for nurses visiting families with a history of violence or substance abuse include (1) self-awareness, (2) environmental assessment, (3) using listening and observation skills with patients to be aware of behavioral changes that indicate aggression or lack of impulse control, (4) planning for dealing with aggressive behavior (i.e., allowing personal space and taking a nonaggressive stance), (5) making visits in pairs, and (6) having access to a cellular phone at all times.

Personal Safety

The home care nurse must be aware of personal safety behaviors before going on a home visit. Dress should be casual but professional in appearance, with a name identification tag. Limited jewelry should be worn. Valuable personal items such as an expensive purse or coat should not be worn on a visit. Carrying an extra set of car keys in the nursing home care bag saves time and frustration if the nurse becomes locked out of the automobile. Automobile keys spread between the fingers with sharp ends outward can be used as a weapon if necessary. The same commonsense behaviors and precautions that guide a person's behavior when alone in any setting should be followed by home care nurses.

The agency should have a copy of the nurse's home care itinerary, including contact telephone numbers if a patient does not have a telephone and information on the nurse's car (make, model, color, and license plate number). Many home care nurses carry agency-provided pagers or cellular telephones that allow the agency to contact the nurse throughout the day to give information about patient updates, changes in orders or services, schedule changes, and new patients who require an initial visit. The telephone also is useful to notify patients when the nurse is delayed.

The automobile used for home care visits, whether a personal or an agency-owned vehicle, should have regular preventive maintenance checks, an adequate fuel level, and road safety items stored in the trunk. Items to carry in the vehicle include change for telephone calls and tolls, maps, emergency telephone numbers, a flashlight, a first-aid kit, flares, a blanket, and equipment for inclement weather conditions. When making a visit to a patient in a more remote rural setting, other travel considerations may be needed, including taking additional supplies or medication to the patient.

Home care nurses should park and lock their cars in a safe place that is visible from the street and the patient's home and away from hidden alleys. While driving to the patient's home, the nurse should assess the neighborhood for safety, especially if it is unfamiliar. All valuable items should be stored out of sight before leaving the office. While walking to the patient's home, nurses should not walk near groups of strangers hanging out in doorways or alleys, enter into vacant buildings, or enter a yard that has an unrestrained dog. The home or building should not be entered if the nurse has any safety concerns. All home care agencies should have policies to follow for such situations.

Patient's Home

Once inside the woman's home, the nurse may encounter unsafe situations such as the presence of weapons, abusive behavior, or health hazards. Each potentially hazardous situation must be dealt with according to agency policies and procedures. If abuse or neglect is reasonably suspected, the home care nurse should follow home care agency and state and federal regulations for reporting and documenting the situation. Nurses should maintain their own safety first and act accordingly throughout the visit.

Infection Control

The nurse carries the necessary supplies and equipment to provide nursing care to the woman. Home care bags should contain infection control supplies such as personal protection equipment; disposable nonsterile, sterile, and utility gloves; disinfectants; disposable CPR masks; gowns; shoe covers; caps; leak-proof and puncture-resistant specimen containers; sharps container; dry hand disinfectants; and leak-proof barriers. Proper infection control techniques should be used in stocking, storing, handling, and transporting this bag. When a procedure is to be performed, the nurse should set up a clean area for necessary supplies. A "dirty" area is designated with a trash bag for the collection of soiled equipment and supplies. Hands are washed before all supplies and equipment for the visit are removed from the bag and placed in a clean area.

The importance of infection control does not diminish because nursing care is provided in the patient's home rather than in a hospital. Patients are not likely to become infected because of their home environment, but the nurse may become exposed to an infectious disease.

Standard Precautions should be used whenever a treatment is performed because it is difficult to determine which patients have a communicable disease (see Box 6-7, p. 113).

Handwashing remains the single most important infection-control procedure, and the caregiver is in a position to educate about the importance of this practice in preventing disease. Hands should be washed before and after each patient contact. Wearing gloves does not eliminate the necessity for handwashing. If running water or clean facilities are unavailable, the hands can be cleaned with a self-drying antiseptic solution.

Using gloves reduces the incidence of exposure to bloodborne pathogens. Gloves should be selected according to the nursing activity to be performed. Nonsterile latex or vinyl gloves should be worn with each procedure that has the potential for contact with bodily substances (e.g., performing venipunctures, heel sticks on the newborn, perineal care). Sterile gloves should be worn with clinical procedures requiring sterile technique such as insertion of peripherally inserted central lines and certain dressing changes. General purpose utility gloves should be used for housekeeping activities such as cleaning equipment or spills. Nonsterile and sterile gloves should be discarded after each use in a leak-resistant waste receptacle. Utility gloves may be disinfected and reused.

Disposable personal protection equipment should be removed after each use and discarded in a plastic trash container. Safety glasses or goggles can be cleaned with soap and water after each use.

Whenever specimens are collected, Standard Precautions should be used. Any specimen of bodily fluids should be placed in a leak-proof bag and secured in a puncture-proof container. The outside of the container is washed, if it was soiled, before transporting it. Specimens should be labeled with the woman's or infant's name and additional identifying information according to the home health care agency or laboratory policies. If specimens are being transported, they should be placed in a container on a flat surface in the vehicle. An insulated container may be used to keep specimens cool in transit. The nurse should be aware of the time sensitivity for certain types of specimens and laboratory procedures.

Sharps containers are puncture-proof and leak-proof containers labeled with a biohazard sign on the outside and should be used to collect needles and sharp objects. Patients are instructed to fill containers between two-thirds and three-fourths full to prevent spillage of their contents. As part of the patient teaching process, information about storage and handling is covered by the home care nurse. When the container reaches its maximal capacity, it should be returned to the home health care agency and replaced. Medical waste such as urine and secretions can be discarded through the sewer or septic system.

Contaminated dressings and disposable supplies should be placed in a leak-proof plastic bag and securely fastened for disposal at the patient's home. The patient should be instructed regarding the proper disposal of medical waste in the home. Agency policies and procedures and local waste management ordinances should be consulted before the patient is instructed.

Key Points

- A community is defined as a locality-based entity composed of systems of societal institutions, informal groups, and aggregates that are interdependent and whose function is to meet a wide variety of collective needs.
- Of necessity, most changes aimed at improving community health involve partnerships among community residents and health workers.
- Methods of collecting data useful to the nurse working in the community include walking surveys, analysis of existing data, informant interviews, and participant observation.
- Vulnerable populations are groups who are at higher risk for developing physical, mental, or social health problems.
- Social and economic factors affect the scope of perinatal nursing practice.
- Perinatal home care is a unique nursing practice that incorporates knowledge from community health nursing, acute care nursing, family therapy, health promotion, and patient education.
- Perinatal home care can be provided for women and infants throughout the perinatal period, beginning before conception and ending in the postpartum period.
- Perinatal home care nurses should incorporate personal safety and infection control practices in the nursing plan of care.
- Telephonic nurse advice lines, telephonic nursing assessments, and warm lines are low-cost health care services that facilitate continuous patient education, support, and health care decision making, even though health care is delivered in multiple sites.

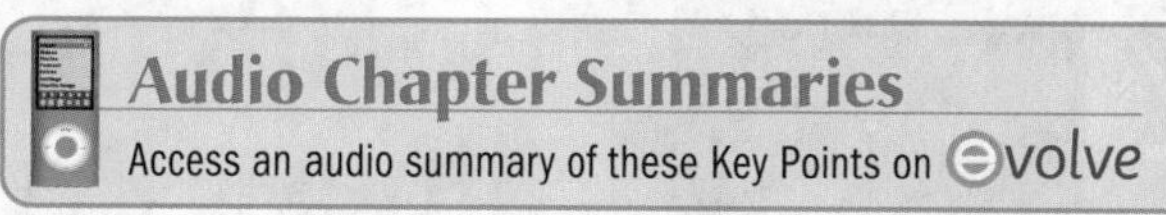
Audio Chapter Summaries
Access an audio summary of these Key Points on evolve

References

Agency for Health Care Research and Quality (AHRQ): *Women's health care in the United States: selected findings from the 2004 National Healthcare Quality and Disparities Report: Fact Sheet*, AHRQ Publication No. 05-P021, Rockville, Md, May 2005, AHRQ. Available at www.ahrq.gov/qual/nhqrwomen/nhqrwomen.htm (accessed June 11, 2008).

American College of Obstetricians and Gynecologists (ACOG): Health care for homeless women. ACOG Committee Opinion No. 312, *Obstet Gynecol* 106:429-434, 2005.

Association of Women's Health, Obstetric and Neonatal Nurses (AWHONN): *Standards and guidelines for professional nursing practice in the care of women and newborns*, ed 6, Washington, DC, 2003, AWHONN.

Bureau of Primary Health Care: *Homeless population statistics*, Washington, DC, 2006, Bureau of Primary Health Care. Available at www.bphc.hrsa.gov (accessed June 11, 2008).

Cottrell R, Girvan J, McKenzie J: *Health promotion and education*, ed 3, San Francisco, 2006, Pearson Benjamin Cummings.

Harrison P, Karlberg J: *Prison and jail inmates at midyear 2003*, Bureau of Justice Statistics Bulletin, Washington, DC, May 2004, US Department of Justice.

Jacobs E et al: Limited English proficiency and cervical cancer screening in a multiethnic population, *Am J Public Health* 95 (8):1410-1416, 2005.

Martin JA et al: Annual summary of vital statistics: 2006, *Pediatrics* 121(4):788-801, 2008.

Maurer F, Smith C: *Community public health nursing practice: health for families and populations*, ed 3, St Louis, 2005, Saunders.

US Department of Health and Human Services (USDHHS): *Healthy people 2010: understanding and improving health*, Washington, DC, 2000, US Department of Health and Human Services, US Government Printing Office.

US Department of Health and Human Services (USDHHS): Health Resources and Services Administration: *Women's health USA 2007*, 2007. Available at www.mchb.hrsa.gov/whusa_07/ (accessed June 10, 2008).

US Department of Labor: *National agricultural workers survey*, 2005. Available at www.doleta.gov/agworker/naws.cfm (accessed June 11, 2008).

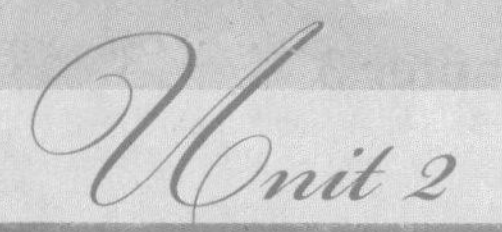

Unit 2

4 Health Promotion and Illness Prevention

Learning Objectives

On completion of this chapter the reader will be able to:

- Identify reasons women enter the health care delivery system.
- Analyze financial, cultural, and communication barriers that may affect a woman's decision to seek and follow through with health care.
- Analyze conditions and characteristics that increase health risks for women during their childbearing years.
- Evaluate programs of anticipatory guidance that promote health and prevention of disease.
- Suggest community resources to combat violence against women.
- Explain the cycle of violence and its use in assessment and intervention for battered women.
- Discuss the incidence of battering in pregnant women.
- Outline health-screening schedules for women in the childbearing years.

Electronic Resources

Additional information related to the content in Chapter 4 can be found on

evolve the Companion Website at

http://evolve.elsevier.com/Perry/maternal/

- NCLEX Review Questions
- Critical Thinking Exercise—Women's Health and Safety
- Nursing Care Plan—The Battered Woman
- Spanish Guidelines—Recognizing Violence in a Relationship

Reasons for Entering the Health Care System

Many women initially enter the health care system because of some reproductive system–related situation such as pregnancy, irregular menses, a desire for contraception, or an episodic illness such as a vaginal infection. Once the woman is in the system, it is important that health care providers recognize the importance of health promotion and preventive health maintenance and offer these services across the life span of women. This chapter addresses barriers to seeking health care and contains an overview of conditions and circumstances that increase health risks across the life span. Anticipatory guidance suggestions, including nutrition and stress management, are included. Intimate partner violence (IPV) and battering of women are discussed.

Preconception Counseling and Care

Preconception health promotion provides women and their partners with information that is needed to make decisions about their reproductive future. Preconception counseling and care guide couples on how to avoid unintended pregnancies, identify and manage risk factors in their lives and their environment, and identify healthy behaviors that promote the well-being of the woman and her potential fetus.

Activities that promote healthy mothers and babies must be initiated before the period of critical fetal organ development, which is between 17 and 56 days after fertilization. By the end of the eighth week after conception and certainly by the end of the first trimester, any major structural anomalies in the fetus are already present. Because many women do not realize that they are pregnant and do not seek prenatal care until well into the first trimester, the rapidly growing fetus may be exposed to many types of intrauterine environmental hazards during this most vulnerable developmental phase. Thus preconception health care should occur well in advance of an actual pregnancy.

Preconception care is important for women who have had a problem with a previous pregnancy (e.g., miscarriage or preterm birth). Although causes are not always identifiable, in many cases problems can be identified and treated and do not recur in subsequent pregnancies. Preconception care is also important to minimize fetal malformations. For example, the offspring of women who have type 1 diabetes mellitus have significantly more congenital anomalies than do children of

BOX 4-1 Components of Preconception Care

Health Promotion: General Teaching

Nutrition
- Healthy diet, including folic acid
- Optimum weight

Exercise and rest

Avoidance of substance abuse (tobacco, alcohol, "recreational" drugs)

Use of risk-reducing sex practices

Attending to family and social needs

Risk Factor Assessment

Medical history
- Immune status (e.g., rubella, hepatitis B)
- Family history (e.g., genetic disorders)
- Illnesses (e.g., infections)
- Current use of medications (prescription, nonprescription)

Reproductive history
- Contraceptive
- Obstetric

Psychosocial history
- Spouse/partner and family situation, including domestic violence
- Availability of family or other support systems
- Readiness for pregnancy (e.g., age, life goals, stress)

Financial resources

Environmental (home, workplace) conditions
- Safety hazards
- Toxic chemicals
- Radiation

Interventions

Anticipatory guidance/teaching

Treatment of medical conditions and results
- Medications
- Cessation/reduction in substance use/abuse
- Immunizations (e.g., rubella, tuberculosis, hepatitis)

Nutrition, diet, and weight management

Exercise

Referral for genetic counseling

Referral to and use of
- Family planning services
- Family and social needs management

mothers without diabetes. The rate of malformation is greatly reduced when the insulin-dependent woman with diabetes has excellent blood glucose control when she becomes pregnant and maintains euglycemia (normal blood sugar) throughout the period of organ development in the fetus. The incidence of neural tube defects such as spina bifida and anencephaly is decreased significantly with the intake of 400 mcg of supplemental folic acid.

Many examples illustrate effects of maternal age or illnesses; conditions that produce anomalies in the fetus (teratogenic agents) such as drugs, viruses, and chemicals; genetically inherited diseases; or other conditions that might be harmful to the woman should a pregnancy occur. In many instances counseling can allow for behavior modification before damage is done, or the woman can make an informed decision about her willingness to accept potential hazards. The components of preconception care such as health promotion, risk assessment, and interventions are outlined in Box 4-1.

Pregnancy

A woman's entry into health care is often associated with pregnancy, for either diagnosis or actual care. Early entry into prenatal care (i.e., within the first 12 weeks) allows for identification of the woman at risk for complications and initiation of measures to prevent problems or treat them if they arise. Major goals of prenatal care are listed in Box 4-2 and should be addressed in the first visit. Extensive discussion of pregnancy is found in Unit 3.

BOX 4-2 Major Goals of Prenatal Care

- Define health status of mother and fetus.
- Determine the gestational age of the fetus and monitor fetal development.
- Identify the woman at risk for complications and minimize the risk whenever possible.
- Provide appropriate education and counseling.

Well-Woman Care

Current trends in the health care of women have expanded beyond a reproductive focus. A holistic approach to women's health care goes beyond simple reproductive needs and includes a woman's health needs throughout her lifetime. This restructuring places women's health within the primary health care delivery system. Women's health assessment and screening focus on a multisystem evaluation emphasizing the maintenance and enhancement of wellness.

Many women first enter the health care delivery system for a Papanicolaou (Pap) test or for contraception. Visits to the nurse may be their only contact with the system unless they become ill. Some women postpone examination until a specific need arises such as pregnancy, infertility, pain, abnormal bleeding, or vaginal discharge.

Health care needs vary with culture, religion, age, and personal differences. The changing responsibilities and roles of women, their socioeconomic status, and their personal lifestyles also contribute to differences in the health and behavior of women. Employment outside of the home, physical disability, inadequate or no health insurance, divorce, single parenthood, and sexual orientation also can affect women's ability to seek and receive health care in clinical settings. As women age, many continue to address their primary health care needs within their established gynecologic care setting; therefore well-women's health care should include a complete history, physical examination, age-appropriate screening, and health promotion.

Fertility Control and Infertility

More than half of the pregnancies in the United States each year are unintended, and the majority of these occur in the 10% of women who do not use birth control (Trussel, 2007). Education is the key to encouraging women to make family planning choices based on preference and actual benefit-to-risk ratios. Providers can influence the user's motivation and ability to use the method correctly (see Chapter 7 for further discussion of contraception).

The concept of health promotion applies to contraception, as can be seen in Box 4-3. The nurse can provide information regarding the need for child spacing, methods of family planning that are consistent with religious and personal preferences, noncontraceptive benefits of certain methods, the appropriate use of methods selected, and the protection of future fertility when so desired.

Women also enter the health care system because of their desire to become pregnant. Approximately 15% of couples in the United States have some degree of infertility. Many couples have delayed starting their families until they are in their 30s or 40s, which allows more time to be exposed to situations that affect fertility negatively (including age-related infertility for the woman). In addition, sexually transmitted infections (STIs), which can predispose to decreased fertility, are becoming more common, and many women and men are in workplaces and home settings where they may be exposed to reproductive environmental hazards.

Infertility can cause emotional pain for many couples, and the inability to produce an offspring sometimes results in feelings of failure and places inordinate stress on the couple's relationship. Much time, money, and emotional investment can be used for testing and treatment in efforts to build a family.

BOX 4-3 Contraceptive Health Promotion

- Child spacing and quality maternity care improve perinatal outcomes and health in general of mother and children.
- Achieving desired family size enables a better sharing of all resources, with attendant increases in education, health care, and other positive societal parameters.
- Contraceptives themselves may positively affect future health. For example, use of condoms may prevent acquisition of human immunodeficiency virus infection; combined oral contraceptives may provide some protection against later development of cancer of ovary and endometrium; barrier methods decrease transmission of sexually transmitted infections, which can develop into pelvic inflammatory disease with resultant infertility or sterility and thus affect future childbearing capacity.

Steps toward prevention of infertility should be undertaken as part of ongoing routine health care, and such information is especially appropriate in preconception counseling. Primary care providers can undertake initial evaluation and counseling before couples are referred to specialists. For additional information about infertility, see Chapter 7.

Menstrual Problems

Irregularities or problems with the menstrual period are among the most common concerns of women and often cause them to seek help from the health care system. Common menstrual disorders include amenorrhea, dysmenorrhea, premenstrual syndrome, endometriosis, and menorrhagia or metrorrhagia. Simple explanation and counseling may handle the concern; however, history and examination must be completed, as well as laboratory or diagnostic tests, if indicated. Questions should never be considered inconsequential, and age-specific reading materials are recommended, especially for teenagers. See Chapter 6 for an in-depth discussion of menstrual problems.

Perimenopause

The body responds to this natural transition in a number of ways, most of which are caused by the decrease in estrogen. Most women seeking health care during the perimenopausal period do so because of irregular bleeding. Others are concerned about vasomotor symptoms (hot flashes and flushes). Although fertility is greatly reduced during this period, women are urged to maintain some method of birth control because pregnancies still can occur. All women need to have factual information, the dispelling of myths, a thorough examination, and periodic health screenings thereafter.

Barriers to Receiving Health Care

Financial Issues

Great variation in access to care occurs, depending on type and size of the system, source of payment for services, private versus public programs, availability of and accessibility to providers, individual preferences, and insurance coverage or ability to pay. The existing system continues to be oriented to treatment of acute or episodic conditions rather than the promotion of health and comprehensive care.

In the United States disparity among races and socioeconomic classes affects many facets of life, including health. With limited money and awareness, there is a lack of access to care, delay in seeking care, few prevention activities, and little accurate information about health and the health care system. Women use health services more often than men but are more likely than men to have difficulty in financing the services. They are twice as often underinsured (i.e., have limited coverage with high-cost co-payments or deductibles). Women make up the majority of Medicaid recipients; however, only 42% of poor women are eligible. Medicaid includes special benefits for pregnant women, but the benefits are limited to treatment of pregnancy-related conditions and terminate 60 days after birth. More and more states are requiring their Medicaid recipients to enroll in managed care programs; whether this improves access and outcomes is yet to be determined.

Insurance coverage varies significantly by age, marital status, race, and ethnicity. Caucasians of all ages are more likely than African-Americans and other racial or ethnic groups to have private insurance. Caucasians possess insurance 2.5 times more often than Hispanics and 1.8 times more often than African-Americans. Single, separated, or divorced individuals are less likely to have insurance. Often unmarried teenagers, who are usually covered by their parents' medical insurance, do not have maternity coverage because policies have exclusion statements and cover only the employee or spouse. Midwifery care has helped contain some health care costs, but reimbursement issues still exist in some areas. The existing health care system continues to be oriented to treatment of acute or episodic conditions rather than the promotion of health and comprehensive care.

Cultural Issues

As our nation becomes more racially, ethnically, and culturally diverse, the health of minority groups becomes a major issue. A variety of reasons are given to explain some of the differences in accessing care when financial barriers are adjusted. Some women experience racial discrimination or disrespectful, disillusioning, or discouraging encounters with community service providers such as social services and health care providers. A lack of cross-cultural communication also presents problems. Desired health outcomes are best achieved when the health care provider has knowledge of and understanding about the culture, language, values, priorities, and health beliefs of those in minority groups. Conversely, members of the group should understand the health goals to be achieved and the methods proposed to do so. Language differences can produce profound barriers between patients and providers. Even with an interpreter, misinformation can occur on both sides of the communication.

Providers must consider culturally based differences that could affect the treatment of diverse groups of women, and the women themselves must share practices and beliefs that could influence their management responses or willingness to comply. For example, women in some cultures value privacy to such an extent that they are reluctant to disrobe and as a result avoid physical examination unless absolutely necessary. Other women rely on their husbands to make major decisions, including those affecting the woman's health. Religious beliefs may dictate a plan of care, as with birth control measures or blood transfusions. Some cultural groups prefer folk medicine, homeopathy, or prayer to traditional Western medicine; and others attempt combinations of some or all practices. Although there is an increasing amount of health information on the Internet, information in languages other than English is limited.

Gender Issues

Gender influences provider-patient communication and may influence access to health care in general. The most obvious gender consideration is that between men and women. Researchers have reported significant male-female differences in receipt of major diagnostic and therapeutic interventions, especially with cardiac and kidney problems. Women tend to use primary care services more often than do men and, some believe, more effectively. The gender of the provider plays a role; studies have shown that female patients have Pap tests and mammograms more consistently if they are seen by female providers.

Sexual orientation may produce another barrier. Some lesbians may not disclose their sexual orientation to health care providers because they feel they may be at risk for hostility, inadequate health care, or breach of confidentiality. In many health care settings heterosexuality is assumed, and the setting may be one in which the woman does not feel welcome (magazines, brochures, and environment reflect heterosexual couples, or the health care provider shows discomfort interacting with the woman). Lesbians themselves may hold beliefs that are incorrect (e.g., that they have immunity to human immunodeficiency virus [HIV], STIs, and certain cancers [e.g., cervical]). The perceived lack of risk can result in lesbians avoiding medical care, as well as in health care providers giving incorrect advice or not providing appropriate cancer screening for these women. Not all gynecologic cancers are related to sexual activity; lesbians who have never had children may be more at risk for breast, ovarian, and endometrial cancer. Their risk for heart disease, cancer of the lung, and colon cancer is not different from that of the heterosexual woman. To offset stereotypes, it is necessary for providers to develop an approach that does not assume that all patients are heterosexual.

Health Risks in the Childbearing Years

Maintaining optimal health is a goal for all women. Essential components of health maintenance are the identification of unrecognized problems and potential risks and the education and health promotion needed to reduce them. This is especially important for women in their childbearing years because conditions that increase a woman's health risks not only are of concern for her well-being but also may be associated with negative outcomes for both mother and baby in the event of a pregnancy. Prenatal care is an example of prevention that is practiced after conception. However, prevention and health maintenance are needed before conception because many of the mother's risks can be identified and eliminated, or at least modified. An overview of conditions and circumstances that increase health risks in the childbearing years follows.

Age

Adolescents

As a female progresses through developmental ages and stages, she is faced with conditions that are age related. All teens undergo progressive development of sex characteristics. They experience the developmental tasks of adolescence such as establishing identity, developing sexual preference, emancipating from family, and establishing career goals. Some of these situations can produce great stress for the adolescent, and the health care provider should treat her very carefully. Female teenagers who enter the health care system usually do so for screening (Pap tests start at age 18 or when sexually active) or because of a problem such as episodic illness or accidents. Gynecologic problems are often associated with menses (either bleeding irregularities or dysmenorrhea), vaginitis or leukorrhea, STIs, contraception, or pregnancy. The adolescent is also at risk for use of street drugs, eating disorders, and depression.

Most young women begin having sex in the mid to late teens; for those who do not, the likelihood of having intercourse increases steadily with age. A sexually active teen who does not use contraception has a 90% chance of pregnancy within 1 year. Effective educational programs about sex and family life are imperative to control the rate of teen pregnancy and STIs (Box 4-4; see Community Focus box).

COMMUNITY FOCUS

Sex Education, Violence Prevention, Sexual Abuse, and Rape Awareness in the Schools

Contact the school nurse at a local high school. Find out what type of sex education, violence prevention, sexual abuse, and rape awareness is available at the school. Negotiate with the nurse to display a poster and pamphlets that provide accurate information about the extent of violence and what preventive measures the students might take. There may be a local violence against women coalition that can be consulted; alternatively you can use Internet resources to design your display.

BOX 4-4 Characteristics of Successful Sex and Family-Life Programs

- Focus clearly on reducing one or more sexual behaviors that lead to unintended pregnancy.
- Maintain age-appropriate and culturally relevant behavioral goals, teaching methods, and materials that coincide with the sexual experience level of the participants.
- Use theoretic approaches that have demonstrated effectiveness at reducing other health-related risky behaviors, such as social learning theory, social inoculation theory, and cognitive behavioral theory.
- Allow sufficient time for presentation of information and completion of activities.
- Involve the participants to personalize the information being presented.
- Provide basic and scientifically accurate information about the risks of engaging in sexual intercourse without protection and about ways to avoid participating in unprotected sexual intercourse.
- Address social pressures to engage in sexual activity.
- Model communication, negotiation, and refusal skills.
- Select teachers or peer leaders who are committed to the program and provide training to help them facilitate the program.
- Give and continually reinforce a clear message about abstaining from sexual activity and/or using birth control. (This appears to be one of the most important components of effective sexuality education programs.)

Source: The American College of Obstetricians and Gynecologists Committee on Adolescent Health Care: *Strategies for adolescent pregnancy prevention*, Washington, DC, 2007, Author.

Teenage Pregnancy

Pregnancy in the teenager who is 16 years of age or younger often introduces additional stress into an already stressful developmental period. The emotional level of such teens is commonly characterized by impulsiveness and self-centered behavior, and they often place primary importance on the beliefs and actions of their peers. In attempts to establish a personal and independent identity, many teens do not realize the consequences of their behavior; their thinking processes do not include planning for the future.

Teenagers usually lack the financial resources to support a pregnancy and may not have the maturity to avoid teratogens or have prenatal care and instruction or follow-up care. Children of teen mothers may be at risk for abuse or neglect because of the teen's inadequate knowledge of growth, development, and parenting. Implementation of specialized adolescent programs in schools, communities, and health care systems is demonstrating continued success in reducing the birth rate in teens.

Young and Middle Adulthood

Because women ages 20 to 40 have a need for contraception, pelvic and breast screening, and pregnancy care, they may prefer to use their gynecologic or obstetric provider as their primary care provider. During these years the woman may be "juggling" family, home, and career responsibilities, with resulting increases in stress-related conditions. Health maintenance includes not only pelvic and breast screening but also promotion of a healthy lifestyle (i.e., good nutrition, regular exercise, no smoking, moderate or no alcohol consumption, sufficient rest, stress reduction, and referral for medical conditions and other specific problems). Common conditions requiring well-woman care include vaginitis, urinary tract infections, menstrual variations, obesity, sexual and relationship issues, and pregnancy.

Parenthood After Age 35

The woman older than 35 years does not have a different physical response to a pregnancy per se, but rather has had health status changes as a result of time and the aging process. These changes may be responsible for age-related pregnancy conditions. For example, a woman with type 2 diabetes may not have had expression of her diabetes at age 22 years but may have full-blown disease when she is 38 years old. Other chronic or debilitating diseases or conditions increase in severity with time, and these in turn may predispose to increased risks during pregnancy. Of significance to women in this age group is the risk for certain genetic anomalies (e.g., Down syndrome). The opportunity for genetic counseling should be available to all (see Chapter 8).

Late Reproductive Age

Women of later reproductive age are often experiencing change and reordering personal priorities. In general, the goals of education, career, marriage, and family have been achieved; and now the woman has increased time and opportunity for new interests and activities. Divorce rates are high at this age, and children leaving home may produce an "empty nest syndrome," resulting in increased levels of depression. Chronic diseases also become more apparent. Most problems for the well woman are associated with perimenopause (e.g., bleeding irregularities and vasomotor symptoms). Health maintenance screening continues to be of importance because some conditions such as breast disease or ovarian cancer occur more often during this stage.

Social and Cultural Factors

Differences exist among people from different socioeconomic levels and ethnic groups with respect to risk for illness and distribution of disease and death. Some diseases are more common among people of selected ethnicity (e.g., sickle cell anemia in African-Americans, Tay-Sachs disease in Ashkenazi Jews, adult lactase deficiency in Chinese, β-thalassemia in Mediterranean peoples, and cystic fibrosis in northern Europeans). Cultural and religious influences also increase health risks because the woman and her family may have life and societal values and a view of health and illness that dictate practices different from those expected in the Judeo-Christian Western model. These may include food taboos or frequencies, methods of hygiene, effects of climate, care-seeking behaviors, willingness to undergo screening and diagnostic procedures, and value conflicts.

Socioeconomic status affects birth outcomes. The rates of perinatal and maternal deaths, preterm births, and low-birth-weight babies are considerably higher in disadvantaged populations (Martin et al, 2008). Social consequences for poor women as single parents are great because many mothers with few skills are caught in the bind of insufficient income to afford child care. These families generate fewer and fewer resources and increase their risks for health problems. Multiple roles for women in general produce overload, conflict, and stress, resulting in higher risks for psychologic illness.

Substance Use and Abuse

Use of illicit drugs and inappropriate use of prescription drugs continue to increase and are found in all ages, races, ethnic groups, and socioeconomic levels. Addiction to substances is seen as a biopsychosocial disease, with several factors leading to risk. These include biogenetic predisposition, lack of resilience to stressful life experiences, and poor social support. Women are less likely than men to abuse drugs, but the rate in women is increasing significantly. Substance-abusing pregnant women create severe problems for themselves and their offspring, including interference with optimal growth and development and addiction. In many instances the use of substances is identified through screening programs in prenatal clinics and obstetric units.

Legal Considerations

Because of the risks to the unborn children and financial concerns, pregnant women who abuse substances may now face criminal charges under expanded interpretations of child abuse and drug trafficking statutes (Lester, Andreozzi, & Appiah, 2004). At least 24 states have attempted to prosecute a pregnant woman on a variety of charges for suspected harm to the fetus. Some policymakers have proposed that pregnant women who abuse substances should be jailed, placed under house arrest, or committed to psychiatric hospitals for the remainder of their pregnancies (Stuart & Laraia, 2005). Nurses who screen for substance abuse in pregnancy and encourage prenatal care, counseling, and treatment will be of greater benefit to the mother and child than will prosecution.

LEGAL TIP **Drug Testing During Pregnancy** There is no requirement in the United States for a health care provider to test either the pregnant woman or the newborn for the presence of drugs. However, nurses need to know the practices of the states in which they are working. In some states a woman whose urine drug screen test is positive at the time of labor and birth must be referred to child protective services. If the mother is not in a drug treatment program or is judged unable to provide care, the infant may be placed in foster care. The U.S. Supreme Court has ruled that in all states it is unlawful to test for drug use without the pregnant woman's permission.

Cigarette Smoking and Caffeine Consumption

Tobacco use is the leading cause of preventable death and illness. Smoking is linked to cardiovascular heart disease, various types of cancers (especially lung and cervical), chronic lung disease, and negative pregnancy outcomes. Tobacco contains nicotine, which is an addictive substance that creates physical and psychologic dependence. About 24% of women ages 18 to 44 smoke (Centers for Disease Control and Prevention [CDC], 2007b). These are the major childbearing years with significant consequences for pregnancy and the fetus. Smoking in pregnancy is known to cause a decrease in placental perfusion and is one cause of low birth weight in infants (see Critical Thinking Exercise).

CRITICAL THINKING EXERCISE

Smoking Cessation During Pregnancy

Doreen is a 25-year-old who is 8 weeks pregnant. At her first prenatal visit a history is taken; she reports that she smokes about half a pack of cigarettes a day. She says she knows that she should probably try to cut down, but she has been smoking since she was 15. She has tried to quit smoking before and has not been successful. How would you respond to her statement?

1. Evidence—Is there sufficient evidence to draw conclusions about what the nurse should say?
2. Assumptions—What assumptions can be made about the following issues?
   a. Effects of smoking on pregnancy
   b. Cessation interventions for pregnant women
3. What implications and priorities for nursing care can be made at this time?
4. Does the evidence objectively support your conclusion?
5. Are there alternative perspectives to your conclusion?

Smoking rates vary among women in different U.S. ethnic groups. Of women smokers in the United States, Native American and Alaska Native women have the highest rates of all ethnic groups (29%), followed by Caucasian (20%) and African-American (19%). Hispanic (10%) and Asian (5%) have the lowest prevalence (CDC, 2007a).

Cigarette smoking impairs fertility in both women and men, may reduce the age for menopause, and increases the risk for osteoporosis after menopause. Passive, or secondhand, smoke (environmental tobacco smoke) contains similar hazards and presents additional problems for the smoker and harm for the nonsmoker.

Caffeine is found in society's most popular drinks: coffee, tea, and soft drinks. It is a stimulant that can affect mood and interrupt body functions by producing anxiety and sleep interruptions. Heart arrhythmias may be made worse by caffeine, and there can be interactions with certain medications such as lithium. Birth defects have not been related to caffeine consumption; however, high intake has been related to a slight decrease in birth weight and may also increase risk of miscarriage. The U.S. Food and Drug Administration recommends that pregnant women eliminate or limit their consumption of caffeine to less than 300 mg/day (three cups of coffee or cola).

Alcohol Consumption

Women ages 35 to 49 have the highest rates of chronic alcoholism, but women ages 21 to 34 have the highest rates of specific alcohol-related problems. About one third of alcoholics are women, and many relate the onset of their drinking problem to stressful events. Women who are problem drinkers are often depressed, have more motor vehicle injuries, and have a higher incidence of attempted suicide than do women in the general population. They are also at risk for alcohol-related liver damage. Early case finding and treatment are important in alcoholism for both the ill individual and family members.

Prenatal alcohol exposure is the single greatest preventable cause of mental retardation (Lester, Andreozzi, & Appiah, 2004). Alcohol use during pregnancy can cause high blood pressure, miscarriage, premature birth, stillbirth, and anemia (Lester, Andreozzi, & Appiah, 2004). In addition, women may experience nutritional deficiencies, pancreatitis, alcoholic hepatitis, deficient milk ejection (let-down), and cirrhosis (Cunningham et al, 2005). A 2010 national health objective is to have 94% of pregnant women abstain from alcohol use (U.S. Department of Health and Human Services [USDHHS], 2000).

Alcohol use during pregnancy can produce "fetal alcohol spectrum disorder" (FASD), which includes fetal alcohol syndrome (FAS), fetal alcohol effects, and alcohol-related neurologic developmental disabilities. Approximately 40,000 babies per year are born with FASD; however, recent research reveals that antioxidants may lessen the effects of prenatal alcohol exposure in the children of women who are unable or unwilling to curtail their alcohol abuse when pregnant (Lee et al, 2005). Low birth weight, mental retardation, behavioral problems, and learning and physical problems are some of the symptoms of FAS babies (see Chapter 28). Severe facial deformities of FAS occur at day 20 of conception when women may not even suspect that they are pregnant.

Prescription Medication Use

Psychotherapeutic medications such as stimulants, sleeping pills, tranquilizers, and pain relievers are used by an estimated 2% of American women. Such medications can bring relief from undesirable conditions such as insomnia, anxiety, and pain. Because the medications have mind-altering capacity, misuse can produce psychologic and physical dependency in the same manner as illicit drugs. Risk-to-benefit ratios should be considered when such medications are used for more than a very short period of time.

Depression is the most common mental health problem in women. Many kinds of medications are used to treat depression. All of these psychotherapeutic drugs can have some effect on the fetus and must be monitored very carefully.

Illicit Drug Use

Marijuana

Marijuana is a substance derived from the cannabis plant. It is usually rolled into a cigarette and smoked, but it also may be mixed into food and eaten. Marijuana produces an altered state of awareness, relaxation, mild euphoria, and reduced inhibition (Stuart & Laraia, 2005). Prolonged use may lead to apathy, lack of energy, loss of desire to work or be productive, diminished concentration, poor personal hygiene, and preoccupation with marijuana—the amotivational syndrome (Stuart & Laraia, 2005). Marijuana readily crosses the placenta and causes increased carbon monoxide levels in the mother's blood, which reduces the oxygen supply to the fetus. Research findings regarding the effects of marijuana on pregnancy are inconsistent; however, it may cause fetal abnormalities (Stuart & Laraia, 2005).

Cocaine

Cocaine is a powerful central nervous system stimulant that is addictive because of the tremendous sense of euphoria that it creates. It can be snorted, smoked, or injected. Crack or rock cocaine is a form of the drug that is exceedingly potent and even more highly addictive. (Some say that an individual is "hooked" after the first use or at least after two or three "hits.") After ingestion of cocaine, an intensely pleasurable high results that is followed by an uncomfortable low; this increases the urge to repeat the drug.

Predisposing factors and problems associated with cocaine use in pregnancy are polydrug use; poor nutrition; poverty; STIs; hepatitis B infection; dysfunctional family systems; employment difficulties; stress; anger; poor self-esteem; and previous or present physical, emotional, and sexual abuse. Cocaine use is especially concentrated among poor women of color. The clinical manifestations of cocaine use include tachycardia, pupillary dilation, and hypertension.

Cocaine affects all of the major body systems. Among other complications, it produces cardiovascular stress that can lead to heart attack or stroke, liver disease, central nervous system stimulation that can cause seizures, and even perforation of the nasal septum. Needle-borne diseases such as hepatitis B and acquired immunodeficiency syndrome (AIDS) are common among cocaine users. If the user is pregnant, there is an increased incidence of miscarriage, preterm labor, small-for-gestational-age babies, abruption of placenta, and stillbirth. Anomalies have been reported.

One of the promising treatments for cocaine abuse in pregnancy is acupuncture. A component of traditional Chinese medicine, acupuncture is used to redirect energy flow (chi) within the body, reduce cravings, and enhance well-being. The pace and location of the flow of chi can be influenced by the insertion of needles at certain points along the meridians to facilitate harmony (Otto, 2003). Evidence from controlled studies of the effectiveness of acupuncture alone or in combination with other therapies has been inconsistent (Vickers, Wilson, & Kleynen, 2002). Further investigation of this therapy is needed.

Opiates

The opiates include opium, heroin, meperidine, morphine, codeine, and methadone. Heroin is one of the most commonly abused drugs of this class. It is usually taken by intravenous injection but can be smoked or "snorted." The signs and symptoms of heroin use are euphoria, relaxation, relief from pain, "nodding out" (apathy, detachment from reality, impaired judgment, and drowsiness), constricted pupils, nausea, constipation, slurred speech, and respiratory depression.

The incidence of heroin use among pregnant women is unknown; however, women with a dependency on heroin may use multiple drugs. Possible effects on pregnancy include preeclampsia, intrauterine growth restriction, miscarriage, premature rupture of membranes, infections, breech presentation, and preterm labor. Possible effects on the mother include poor nourishment with subsequent vitamin, iron, and folic acid deficiencies; medical complications from frequent use of dirty needles; STIs; and hypertension (Stuart & Laraia, 2005).

The recommended treatment is methadone maintenance combined with psychotherapy. This well-documented approach improves outcomes for both the woman and her fetus (Stuart & Laraia, 2005). The other approach is slow medical withdrawal with methadone, but the safety of this second approach is questionable. In pregnancy methadone is metabolized more rapidly, leading to withdrawal symptoms in less than 24 hours in many women. Withdrawal symptoms can include fetal hyperactivity and, if severe, preterm labor or fetal death. Women may resort to heroin to alleviate the uncomfortable symptoms.

Methamphetamine

Described as the number one drug problem in America, "meth" has been tried by approximately 12 million Americans, and 1.5 million are regular users (Jefferson, 2005). Relatively cheap, this highly addictive stimulant is hooking more and more people across the socioeconomic spectrum. Methamphetamine makes many users feel hypersexual and uninhibited and thus leads to more sex and less protection from pregnancy. The use among fertile women is creating a new generation of "meth babies" (Jefferson, 2005).

The active metabolite of methamphetamine is amphetamine, a central nervous system stimulant known as both "speed" and meth. The crystalline form of methamphetamine is known as "ice." When smoked, it produces a potent, long-lasting high. Ice enables a person to go without rest or food for 24 hours, only to "crash" for the next 24 hours (Jefferson, 2005). The active ingredient is pseudoephedrine and is easily "cooked," using recipes readily available on the Internet (Jefferson, 2005).

Clinical manifestations of methamphetamine use are euphoria, abrupt awakening, increased energy, talkativeness, elation, agitation, hyperactivity, irritability, grandiosity, diaphoresis, weight loss, insomnia, hypertension, increased temperature, ectopic heartbeat, urinary retention, constipation, dry mouth, paranoid delusions, and violent behavior. Seizures, cardiac shock, and death may occur as a result of overdose (Stuart & Laraia, 2005). Most of the effects of amphetamines are similar to those of cocaine.

Although fewer maternal and neonatal complications have been attributed to this class of substances than to cocaine, the rates of preterm births and intrauterine growth restriction with smaller head circumference are higher in methamphetamine-exposed pregnant women than in pregnant women who abuse other substances.

Phencyclidine

Phencyclidine (PCP) is a synthetic drug known by various names ("peace pill," "elephant," "angel dust," "hog"). Its use is more prevalent among ethnic minorities and in people between the ages of 18 and 40. Its effects are unpredictable and include hostility, aggressiveness, and other bizarre behavior (Stuart & Laraia, 2005). Signs and symptoms of PCP use include confusion, disorientation, euphoria, hallucinations, paranoia, grandiosity, agitation, a tendency toward violence, and antisocial behavior; the severity of these symptoms depends on the dose. Clinical manifestations include red, dry skin; dilated pupils; nystagmus; ataxia; hypertension; rigidity; and seizures (Stuart & Laraia, 2005). Because some effects mimic the signs and symptoms of schizophrenia, a user may be admitted to a psychiatric unit.

The major concerns regarding PCP use in pregnant women are its association with polydrug abuse and the neurobehavioral effects on the neonate.

Other Illicit Drugs

A number of other street drugs pose risk to users. A few are derived from organic materials, but more and more are produced synthetically in laboratories. Sedatives such as "downers," "yellow jackets," or "red devils" are used to come off of "highs." Hallucinogens alter perception and body function. PCP ("angel dust") and LSD produce vivid changes in sensation, often with agitation, euphoria, paranoia, and a tendency toward antisocial behavior. Their use may lead to flashbacks, chronic psychosis, and violent behavior. Hallucinogens taken during pregnancy may have negative neurobehavioral effects on the newborn.

Nutrition

Good nutrition is essential for optimal health. A well-balanced diet helps prevent illness and also is used to treat certain health problems. Conversely, poor eating habits, eating disorders, and obesity are linked to disease and debility. *Dietary Guidelines for Americans 2005* provides evidence-based recommendations to promote health and reduce risks for chronic diseases through diet and physical activity. This guide contains resources for health professionals and consumers on dietary guidelines, the food guide pyramid *(www.MyPyramid.gov)*, food composition, dietary supplements, and resource lists *(www.nal.usda.gov/fnic/)*.

Nutritional Deficiencies

Overt disease caused by a lack of certain nutrients is rarely seen in the United States. However, insufficient amounts or imbalances of nutrients do pose problems for individuals and families. Overweight or underweight status, malabsorption, listlessness, fatigue, frequent colds and other minor infections, constipation, dull hair and nails, and dental caries are examples of problems that could be related to nutrition and indicate the need for further nutritional assessment. Poor nutrition, especially related to obesity and high fat and cholesterol intake, may lead to more serious conditions and contribute to 4 of the 10 leading causes of death in the United States: heart diseases, malignant neoplasms, cerebrovascular diseases, and diabetes.

Obesity

During the past 20 years there has been a dramatic increase in obesity in the United States. More than one third of women in the United States are obese (Body Mass Index [BMI] of 30 or greater), with adults ages 40 to 59 having the highest prevalence. The BMI is defined as a measure of an adult's weight in relation to his or her height, specifically the adult's weight in kilograms divided by the square of his or her height in meters (Box 4-5).

Overweight and obesity are known risk factors for premature death, diabetes, heart disease, stroke, hypertension, gallbladder disease, diverticular disease, some anemias, oral disease, constipation, osteoarthritis, gout, osteoporosis, respiratory dysfunction, sleep apnea, and some types of cancer (uterine, breast, colorectal, kidney, and gallbladder) (American Cancer Society, 2008). In addition, obesity is associated with high cholesterol, menstrual irregularities, hirsutism (excess body/facial hair), stress incontinence, depression, complications of pregnancy, increased surgical risk, and shortened life span. Pregnant women who are morbidly obese are at increased risk for hypertension, diabetes, gallbladder disease, postterm pregnancy, and musculoskeletal problems.

Other Considerations

Other dietary extremes also can produce risk. For example, insufficient amounts of calcium can lead to osteoporosis, too much sodium can aggravate hypertension, and megadoses of vitamins can cause adverse effects in several body systems. Fad weight-loss programs and yo-yo dieting (repeated weight gain and weight loss) result in nutritional imbalances and in some instances medical problems. Such diets and programs are not appropriate for weight maintenance. Adolescent pregnancy produces special nutritional requirements because the metabolic needs of pregnancy are superimposed on the teen's own needs for growth and maturation at a time when eating habits are less than ideal. Neural tube defects are more common in infants born of women with a diet poor in folate. In their childbearing years women should ingest at least 0.4 mg (400 mcg) of folic acid daily in addition to consuming a diet rich in folate-containing foods.

Anorexia Nervosa

Some women have a distorted view of their bodies and, no matter what their weight, perceive themselves to be much too heavy. As a result, they undertake strict and severe diets and rigorous extreme exercise. This chronic eating disorder is known as anorexia nervosa. Women can carry this condition to the point of starvation, with resulting endocrine and metabolic abnormalities. If not corrected, significant complications of arrhythmias, amenorrhea, cardiomyopathy, and congestive heart failure occur and in the extreme can lead to death. The condition commonly begins during adolescence in young women who have some degree of personality disorder. They gradually lose weight over several months, have amenorrhea, and are abnormally concerned with body image. A coexisting depression usually accompanies anorexia.

There are no specific tests to diagnose anorexia nervosa. A medical history, physical examination, and screening tests help identify women at risk for eating disorders. Several tools are available to use in primary care settings. The SCOFF questionnaire is easy to administer and can help the nurse decide whether an eating disorder is likely and if the woman needs further assessment and possibly psychiatric and medical intervention (Johnston et al, 2007; Parker, Lyons, & Bonner, 2005) (Box 4-6).

Bulimia Nervosa

Bulimia refers to secret, uncontrolled binge eating alternating with methods to prevent weight gain: self-induced vomiting, laxatives or diuretics, strict diets, fasting, and rigorous exercise. During a binge episode large numbers of calories are consumed, usually consisting of sweets and "junk foods." Binges occur at least twice per week. Bulimia usually begins

BOX 4-5 Ideal Body Weight with Body Mass Index

BMI 18.5 or less—Underweight
BMI 18.5 to 24.9—Normal weight
BMI 25.0 to 29.9—Overweight
BMI 30.0 to 34.5—Obese
BMI 35.0 to 40—Very obese

Source: Partnership for Healthy Weight Management: *Body Mass Index (BMI)*. Available at www.consumer.gov/weightloss/bmi.htm (accessed June 16, 2008).
BMI, Body mass index.

BOX 4-6 Screening for Eating Disorders: SCOFF Questions

Each question scores 1 point. A score of 2 or more indicates the person may have anorexia nervosa or bulimia.

1. Do you make yourself **S**ick (i.e., induce vomiting) because you feel too full?
2. Do you worry about loss of **C**ontrol over the amount you eat?
3. Have you recently lost more than **O**ne stone (6.4 kg [14 lbs]) in a 3-month period?
4. Do you think you are too **F**at even if others think you are too thin?
5. Does **F**ood dominate your life?

Source: Parker S, Lyons J, Bonner J: Eating disorders in graduate students: exploring the SCOFF questionnaire as a simple screening tool, *J Am College Health* 52(2):103-107, 2005.

in early adulthood (ages 18 to 25) and is found primarily in females. Complications can include dehydration and electrolyte imbalance, gastrointestinal abnormalities, and cardiac arrhythmias. Bulimia is somewhat similar to anorexia in that it is an eating disorder and usually involves some degree of depression. Unlike those with anorexia, individuals with bulimia may feel shame or disgust about their disorder and tend to seek help earlier. The SCOFF screening assessment also can be used (see Box 4-6).

Physical Fitness and Exercise

Exercise contributes to good health by lowering risks for a variety of conditions that are influenced by obesity and a sedentary lifestyle. It is effective in the prevention of cardiovascular disease and in the management of chronic conditions such as hypertension, arthritis, diabetes, respiratory disorders, and osteoporosis (Fig. 4-1). Exercise also contributes to stress reduction and weight maintenance. Women report that engaging in regular exercise improves their body image and self-esteem and acts as a mood enhancer. Aerobic exercise produces cardiovascular involvement because increasing amounts of oxygen are delivered to working muscles. Anaerobic exercise such as weight training improves individual muscle mass without stress on the cardiovascular system. Because women are concerned about both cardiovascular and bone health, weight-bearing aerobic exercises such as walking, running, racket sports, and dancing are preferred. However, excessive or strenuous exercise can lead to hormone imbalances, resulting in amenorrhea and its consequences. Physical injury is also a potential risk.

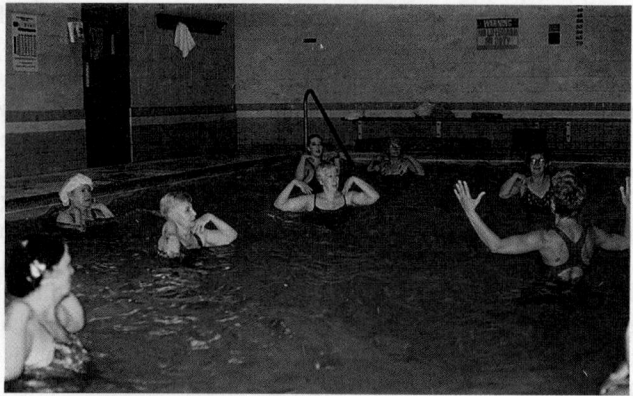

Fig. 4-1 Water aerobics improves cardiovascular function. *(Courtesy Jonas McCoy, Raleigh, NC.)*

Kegel exercise, or pelvic muscle exercise, is used to strengthen the muscles that support the pelvic floor and should be practiced regularly. Instructions for this exercise are in the Patient Teaching Box.

PATIENT TEACHING Kegel Exercises

Description and Rationale

Kegel exercise, or pelvic muscle exercise, is a technique used to strengthen the muscles that support the pelvic floor. This exercise involves regularly tightening (contracting) and relaxing the muscles that support the bladder and urethra. By strengthening these pelvic muscles, a woman can prevent or reduce accidental urine loss.

Technique

The woman needs to learn how to target the muscles for training and how to contract them correctly. One suggestion for teaching is to have the woman pretend she is trying to prevent the passage of intestinal gas. Have her use this tightening motion on the muscles around her vagina and the upper pelvis. She should feel these muscles drawing inward and upward. Other suggested techniques are to have the woman pretend she is trying to stop the flow of urine in midstream or to have her think about how her vagina is able to contract around and move up the length of the penis during intercourse.

The woman should avoid straining or bearing-down motions while performing the exercise. She should be taught how bearing down feels by having her take a breath, hold it, and push down with her abdominal muscles as though she were trying to have a bowel movement. Then the woman can be taught how to avoid straining down by exhaling gently and keeping her mouth open each time she contracts her pelvic muscles.

Specific Instructions

- Each contraction should be as intense as possible without contracting the abdomen, thighs, or buttocks.
- Contractions should be held for at least 10 seconds. The woman may have to start with as little as 2 seconds per contraction until her muscles get stronger.
- She should rest for 10 seconds or more between contractions so that the muscles have time to recover and each contraction can be as strong as she can make it.
- She should feel the pulling up and over the three muscle layers so that the contraction reaches the highest level of her pelvis.

Other Suggestions for Implementation

- At first the woman should set aside about 15 minutes a day to do the Kegel exercises.
- She may want to put up reminders such as notes on her bathroom mirror, her refrigerator, her TV, or a calendar to do the exercises.
- Guidelines for practicing Kegel exercises suggest performing between 30 and 80 contractions a day; however, positive results can be achieved with only 30 a day.
- The best position for learning how to do Kegel exercises is to lie supine with the knees bent. Another position to use is on the hands and knees. Once the woman learns the proper technique, she can perform the exercises in other positions such as standing or sitting.

Sources: Sampselle CM: Behavioral interventions for urinary incontinence in women: evidence for practice, *J Midwifery Womens Health* 45(2):94-103, 2000; Sampselle CM et al: Continence for women: evidence-based practice, *J Obstet Gynecol Neonatal Nurs* 26(4):375-385, 1997.

Physical activity and exercise counseling for persons of all ages should be undertaken at schools, work sites, and primary care settings. Specific recommendations include 20 to 30 minutes of moderate activity at least three times per week. Few Americans exercise this often, and physical inactivity increases with age, especially during adolescence and early adulthood. Even small increases in activity can be beneficial. During pregnancy an ongoing exercise regimen can be continued but should be decreased in intensity and duration (Fig. 4-2). Sedentary women should obtain medical clearance to initiate exercise during pregnancy and should begin with low-intensity and low-impact workouts (see Evidence-Based Practice box).

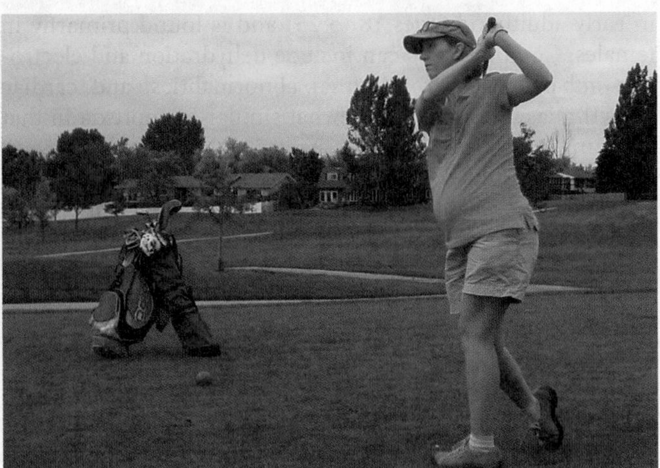

Fig. 4-2 Participation in physical activity is possible and important during pregnancy. A woman at 30 weeks of gestation enjoys a game of golf. *(Courtesy Julie Perry Nelson, Loveland, CO.)*

Stress

The modern woman faces increasing levels of stress and, as a result, is prone to a variety of stress-induced complaints and illnesses. Stress often occurs because of multiple roles in which coping with job and financial responsibilities conflicts with

EVIDENCE-BASED PRACTICE Exercise and Work in Pregnancy

—Pat Gingrich

Ask the Question

What sorts of work and leisure activities are safe for pregnant women?

Search for Evidence

Search Strategies

Professional organization guidelines, meta-analyses, systematic reviews, randomized controlled trials, nonrandomized prospective studies, and retrospective studies since 2006

Databases Searched

CINAHL, Cochrane, Medline, National Guideline Clearinghouse, TRIP Database Plus, and the websites for ACOG, AWHONN, and CDC

Critically Analyze the Evidence

Historically health care providers worried that exercise during pregnancy might lead to poor uteroplacental perfusion or increased inflammatory response, resulting in low birth weight, gestational hypertension, or prematurity. These concerns lead to restrictions on activity. However, exercise has been shown to have many physiologic and psychologic benefits. For example, in a randomized clinical trial of women with prior preeclampsia, walking and stretching promoted antioxidants and decreased recurrence of gestational hypertension (Yeo, 2008).

In a review of scientific literature on exercise in pregnancy, Gavard and Artal (2008) found that healthy women benefited from exercising, with no difference in birth weights or gestational age at birth when compared to sedentary women. Moderate leisure and work activity conferred a protective effect against preeclampsia and gestational diabetes, especially if the exercise predated the pregnancy. Even vigorous exercise such as running, bicycling, lap swimming, or racquetball did not make any difference in the outcomes of birth weight or gestational age. For a small group of very intense exercisers, birth weight decreased 200 to 400 g, which may reflect insufficient calories. Even previously sedentary women can initiate exercise during pregnancy, with no change in mean gestational age (Barakat, Stirling, & Lucia, 2008).

Occupational activities of prolonged hours, shift work, lifting, standing, and heavy physical work are not statistically associated with the outcomes of preterm delivery, low birth weight, or gestational hypertension according to a systematic review by Bonzini, Coggon, and Palmer (2007). However, the authors caution that these activities do not confer any protective benefits and recommend decreasing work hours, standing time, and physical labor in the third trimester.

Implications for Practice

The nurse can encourage healthy pregnant and nonpregnant patients to incorporate moderate exercise such as brisk walking for 30 minutes a day most days of the week. Benefits of regular exercise in pregnancy include weight control, psychologic well-being, and a protective effect against gestational hypertension and diabetes. The benefits are greater if the woman begins exercise before pregnancy, but even sedentary women can safely start to exercise during pregnancy. There is no evidence that moderate cardiovascular exercise leads to prematurity or low birth weight.

Strenuous exercisers or women whose jobs require heavy labor, prolonged hours, and shift work may need to consider modifying their activity in late pregnancy. This might be of particular interest to pregnant nurses, whose jobs can involve long hours and physical labor.

References

Barakat R, Stirling JR, Lucia A: Does exercise training during pregnancy affect gestational age? A randomised, controlled trial, *Br J Sports Med* 42(8):674-678, 2008.

Bonzini M, Coggon D, Palmer KT: Risk of prematurity, low birthweight, and pre-eclampsia in relation to working hours and physical activities: a systematic review, *Occup Environ Med* 67:228-243, 2007.

Gavard JA, Artal R: Effect of exercise on pregnancy outcome, *Clin Obstet Gynecol* 51(2):467-480, 2008.

Yeo S et al: A comparison of walking versus stretching exercises to reduce the incidence of preeclampsia: a randomized clinical trial, *Hypertens Pregnancy* 27(2):113-130, 2008.

parenting and duties at home. To add to this burden, women are socialized to be caretakers, which is emotionally draining in itself. They also may find themselves in positions of minimal power that do not allow them control over their everyday environments. Some stress is normal and contributes to positive outcomes. Many women thrive in busy surroundings. However, excessive or high levels of ongoing stress trigger physical reactions such as rapid heart rate, elevated blood pressure, slowed digestion, release of additional neurotransmitters and hormones, muscle tenseness, and a weakened immune system. Consequently, constant stress can contribute to clinical illnesses such as flare-ups of arthritis or asthma, frequent colds or infections, gastrointestinal upsets, cardiovascular problems, and infertility. Box 4-7 lists symptoms that may be related to chronic or extreme stress. Psychologic symptoms such as anxiety, irritability, eating disorders, depression, insomnia, and substance abuse have also been associated with stress.

BOX 4-7 Stress Symptoms

Physical

Perspiration/sweaty hands
Increased heart rate
Trembling
Nervous tics
Dryness of throat and mouth
Tiring easily
Urinating frequently
Sleeping problems
Diarrhea, indigestion, vomiting
Butterflies in stomach
Headaches
Premenstrual tension
Pain in neck and lower back
Loss of appetite or overeating
Susceptibility to illness
Behavior

- Stuttering and other speech difficulties
- Crying for no apparent reason
- Acting impulsively
- Startling easily
- Laughing in a high-pitched and nervous tone of voice
- Grinding teeth
- Increasing smoking
- Increasing use of drugs and alcohol
- Being accident prone

Psychologic

Feeling anxious
Feeling scared
Feeling irritable
Feeling moody
Having low self-esteem
Being afraid of failure
Being unable to concentrate
Embarrassing easily
Worrying about the future
Being preoccupied with thoughts or tasks
Forgetful

Modified from State University of New York Counseling Center: *Stress management*, Buffalo, NY, 2002, University of Buffalo, State University of New York.

Stress Management

Because it is neither possible nor desirable to avoid all stress, women must learn how to manage it. The nurse should assess each woman for signs of stress, using therapeutic communication skills to determine risk factors and the woman's ability to function.

Some women must be referred for counseling or other mental health therapy. Women are twice as likely as men to suffer from depression, anxiety, or panic attacks. Nurses must be alert to the symptoms of serious mental disorders such as depression and anxiety and make referrals to mental health practitioners when necessary. Women experiencing major life changes such as separation and divorce, bereavement, serious illness, and unemployment also need special attention.

Many centers offer support groups to help women prevent or manage stress. Social support and good coping skills can improve a woman's self-esteem and give her a sense of mastery. Anticipatory guidance for developmental or expected situational crises can help her plan strategies for dealing with potentially stressful events. Role-playing, relaxation techniques, biofeedback, meditation, desensitization, imagery, assertiveness training, yoga, diet, exercise, and weight control are all techniques nurses can include in their repertoire of helping skills.

Sexual Practices

Potential risks related to sexual activity include undesired pregnancy and STIs. The risks are particularly high for adolescents and young adults who engage in sexual intercourse at earlier and earlier ages. Adolescents report many reasons for wanting to be sexually active: peer pressure, desire to love and be loved, experimentation, to enhance self-esteem, and to have fun. However, many teens do not have the decision-making or values-clarification skills needed to take this important step. They may also lack knowledge about contraception and STIs. Many do not believe that becoming pregnant or getting an STI will happen to them.

Although some STIs can be cured with antibiotics, many cause significant problems. Possible sequelae include infertility, ectopic pregnancy, neonatal morbidity and mortality, genital cancers, AIDS, and even death. The incidence of STIs is increasing rapidly and reaching epidemic proportion. Choice of contraception has an impact on the risk of contracting an STI. No method of contraception offers complete protection. (See Chapter 6 for a discussion of STIs and Chapter 7 for a discussion of contraception.)

STI and HIV Prevention Counseling

Prevention of STIs is predicated on the reduction of high risk behaviors by educating toward a behavioral change. Behaviors of concern include multiple and casual sexual partners and unsafe sexual practices. Specific self-management measures to prevent STIs are listed in Box 4-8. The abuse of alcohol and drugs is a high risk behavior, resulting in impaired judgment and thoughtless acts. Behavioral changes must come from

BOX 4-8 STI and HIV Prevention

- Prevention of STIs and HIV is possible only if there is no oral, genital, or rectal exchange of body fluids or if a person is in a long-term, mutually monogamous relationship with an uninfected partner.
- Correct use of latex condoms, although greatly reducing risk, is not exclusively protective.
- Sexual partners should be selected with great care.
- Partners should be asked about history of STIs.
- Preexposure vaccination is one of the most effective methods for preventing transmission of some STIs (hepatitis A and B, human papilloma virus).
- A new condom should be used for each act of sexual intercourse.
- Abstinence from sexual intercourse is encouraged for persons who are being treated for an STI or whose partners are being treated.

Source: Adapted from Centers for Disease Control and Prevention: Sexually transmitted diseases treatment guidelines 2006, *MMWR* 55(RR-11):1-94, 2006.

STI, Sexually transmitted infection; *HIV*, human immunodeficiency virus.

within; therefore the nurse must provide sufficient information for the individual or group to "buy into" the need for change. Education is a powerful tool in health promotion and prevention of STIs and pregnancy. However, it works best when delivered in a way that takes into account the language, culture, and lifestyle of the intended listener.

Medical Conditions

Most women of reproductive age are relatively healthy. Heart disease; lung, breast, colon, and other nongynecologic cancers; chronic lung disease; and diabetes are all concerns for adult women because they are among the leading causes of death in women. Certain medical conditions present during pregnancy can have deleterious effects on both the woman and the fetus. Of particular concern are risks from all forms of diabetes, urinary tract disorders, thyroid disease, hypertensive disorders of pregnancy, cardiac disease, and seizure disorders. Effects on the fetus vary and include intrauterine growth restriction, macrosomia, anemia, prematurity, immaturity, and stillbirth. Effects on the woman also can be severe. These conditions are discussed in later chapters.

Gynecologic Conditions

Women are at risk throughout their reproductive years for pelvic inflammatory disease, endometriosis, STIs and other vaginal infections, uterine fibroids, uterine deformities such as bicornuate uterus, ovarian cysts, interstitial cystitis, and urinary incontinence related to pelvic relaxation. These gynecologic conditions may contribute negatively to pregnancy by causing infertility, miscarriage, preterm labor, and fetal and neonatal problems. Gynecologic cancers also affect women's health, although the risk for most cancers is low in pregnancy. Risk factors depend on the type of cancer. The impact of developing a gynecologic problem or cancer on women and their families is shaped by a number of factors, including the specific type of problem or cancer, the implications of the diagnosis for the woman and her family, and the timing of the occurrence in the woman's and the family's lives.

Female Genital Mutilation

Female genital mutilation is practiced in more than 45 countries, with the majority of these countries being in Africa. As emigrants from these countries arrive in North American, nurses in the United States and Canada will see patients who have had such procedures performed (see Cultural Awareness box).

CULTURAL AWARENESS

Female Genital Mutilation

It is estimated that 100 to 140 million girls and women have undergone female genital mutilation (FGM) (female circumcision, female genital cutting, "cutting"). FGM occurs in women of many different ethnic, cultural, and religious backgrounds. The procedure involves the removal of part or all of the female external genitalia. The procedure may involve removal of the entire clitoris and labia minora. In some instances the labia majora may be stitched together over the urethral and vaginal openings.

Although FGM is usually performed during childhood, some communities circumcise infants or older females. The practice is recognized internationally as a violation of human rights, and many countries have policies and legislation to ban it. The World Health Organization is working to eliminate FGM. Canada, the U.S. federal government, and 17 states have criminalized the practice.

The extent of the FGM site affects the seriousness of complications. Common complications include bleeding, pain, local scarring, keloid or cyst formation, and infection. Impaired drainage of urine and menstrual blood may lead to chronic pelvic infections, pelvic and back pain, and chronic urinary tract infections. On occasion the girl will die from complications. Some women may require surgery before vaginal examination, intercourse, or childbirth if the vaginal opening is obstructed. Cesarean birth may be necessary.

Nurses are providing care to a growing number of women who have emigrated from the Middle East, Asia, and Africa, where FGM is common. Nurses must be sensitive to the unique needs of these patients, especially if these women have concerns about maintaining or restoring the intactness of the FGM site after childbirth.

References: *Female genital mutilation (FGM). Legal prohibitions worldwide.* Available from www.reproductiverights.org/pdf/pub_fac_fgm_1.08.pdf (accessed June 12, 2008). World Health Organization: *Eliminating female genital mutilation: an interagency statement UNAIDS, UNDP, UNECA, UNESCO, UNFPA, UNHCHR, UNHCR, UNICEF, UNIFEM, WHO,* Geneva, 2008, World Health Organization.

Environmental and Workplace Hazards

Environmental hazards in the home, the workplace, and the community can contribute to poor health at all ages. Categories and examples of health-damaging hazards include the following: (1) pathogenic agents (viruses, bacteria, fungi, parasites); (2) natural and synthetic chemicals (natural toxins from animals, insects, and plants; consumer and industrial products such as pesticides and hydrocarbon gases; medical and diagnostic devices; tobacco; fuels; and drug and alcohol abuse); (3) radiation (radon, heat waves, sound waves); (4) food substances (added components that are not necessary for nutrition); and (5) physical objects (moving vehicles, machinery, weapons, water, and building materials).

Environmental hazards can affect fertility, fetal development, live birth, and the child's future mental and physical development. Children are at special risk for poisoning from lead found in paint and soil. Everyone is at risk from air pollutants such as tobacco smoke, carbon monoxide, smog, suspended particles (dust, ash, and asbestos), and cleaning solvents; noise pollution; pesticides; chemical additives; and poor preparation of food. Workers also face safety and health risks caused by ergonomically poor work stations and stress. It is important that risk assessments continue to be in effect to identify and understand environmental public health problems.

Anticipatory Guidance for Health Promotion and Illness Prevention

Over the last several decades women have made tremendous strides in education, careers, policy making, and overall participation in today's complex society. There have been costs for these advances; and, although women are living longer, they may not be living better. As a result, the health care system needs to pay greater attention to the health consequences for women. Women must be active participants in their own health promotion and illness prevention (see Community Focus box).

COMMUNITY FOCUS

Anticipatory Guidance for Health Promotion

Janie, a 30-year-old Navajo woman living on a reservation, comes to the clinic after attending a health fair in which she learned that her blood sugar is above normal, she is overweight, and her blood pressure is elevated. She informs the nurse that she doesn't want to end up like her grandmother who had to have her toes amputated as a result of diabetes. Prepare a plan that uses community resources to meet Janie's needs to reduce her blood sugar and blood pressure and lose weight.

- Ascertain her opinion regarding her health status.
- Identify need for counseling regarding nutrition, exercise, and stress management.
- Are physicians or nurse practitioners available on the reservation?
- What health education programs are available on the reservation?
- Working with Janie, develop an exercise program for her.
- What community resources are available to her?

Nurses have a major opportunity and responsibility to help women understand risk factors and motivate them to adopt healthy lifestyles that prevent disease. Lifestyle factors that affect health—and over which the woman has some control—include diet; tobacco, alcohol, and substance use; exercise; sunlight exposure; stress management; and sexual practices. Other influences such as genetic and environmental factors may be beyond the woman's control, although some opportunities for prevention exist (e.g., through environmental legislative activism or genetic counseling services).

Knowledge alone is not enough to bring about healthy behaviors. The woman must be convinced that she has some control over her life and that healthy life habits, including periodic health examinations, are a sound investment. She must believe in the efficacy of prevention, early detection, and therapy and in her ability to perform self-management practices such as breast self-examination. Many people believe that they have little control over their health, or they become so immobilized by fear and anxiety in the face of life-threatening illnesses such as cancer that they delay seeking treatment. The nurse must explore the reality of each woman's perceptions about health behaviors and individualize teaching if it is to be effective.

Substance Use Cessation

All women at all ages will receive substantial and immediate benefits from smoking cessation. However, this is not easy, and most people will attempt to stop several times before they accomplish their goal. Many are never able to do so.

New approaches are needed to increase cessation among smokers and discourage smoking among young women, especially in adolescence and during pregnancy. Health care providers can have an impact on smoking behavior and should attempt to motivate smokers to stop (Box 4-9). Raising questions about social consequences (e.g., stained teeth and foul-smelling breath and clothes) is sometimes effective with young people.

Those who wish to stop smoking can be referred to a smoking cessation program in which individualized methods can be implemented. At the very least, individuals should be guided to self-help materials available from the March of Dimes Birth Defects Foundation, the American Lung Association, and the American Cancer Society. During pregnancy women seem to be highly motivated to stop or at least to limit smoking to 10 or fewer cigarettes a day. Insult to the fetus can be reduced or even avoided if this is done by the end of the first trimester.

Alcohol and other drugs exact a staggering toll on society, not only in terms of personal health, but also in their association with poverty and homelessness, family disorganization, violence, crime, motor vehicle injuries, reduced productivity, and economic costs. The abuse of alcohol and other drugs increases the risk of victimization and date rape and of acquiring HIV through shared needles or sexual contact. Alcohol and drug use are the leading preventable causes of birth defects.

A national awareness of the seriousness of problems associated with substance abuse has led to raising the legal drinking age to 21 in all states and to tighter controls on advertising. Stronger regulation of advertising and tougher laws and law enforcement for alcohol- and drug-related offenses are being implemented. There is still much that must be done to increase the accessibility to care for low-income people, minorities, and

BOX 4-9 Interventions for Smoking Cessation: The Five A's

Ask

What was her age when she started smoking?

How many cigarettes does she smoke a day? When was her last cigarette?

Has she tried to quit?

Does she want to quit?

Assess

What are her reasons for not being able to quit before, or what made her start again?

Does she have anyone who can help her?

Does anyone else smoke at home?

Does she have friends or family who have quit successfully?

Advise

Give her information about the effects of smoking on pregnancy and her fetus, on her own future health, and on the members of her household.

Assist

Provide support; give self-help materials.

Encourage her to set a quit date.

Refer to a smoking cessation program or provide information about nicotine replacement products (not recommended during pregnancy) if she is interested.

Teach and encourage use of stress reduction activities.

Provide for follow-up with a phone call, letter, or clinic visit.

Arrange Follow-Up

Arrange to follow the woman to find out about smoking-cessation status.

Make a phone call around the time of her quit date. Assess her status at every prenatal visit.

Congratulate her on her success, or provide support for her if she relapses.

Referral to intensive treatment may be necessary.

Source: American College of Obstetricians and Gynecologists Committee on Health Care for Underserved Women; ACOG Committee on Obstetric Practice: ACOG Committee Opinion No. 316, October 2005, Smoking cessation during pregnancy, *Obstet Gynecol* 106(4):883-888, 2005.

BOX 4-10 Safety Guidelines to Reduce Risk

- Wear seat belts at all times in a moving vehicle.
- Wear safety helmets when riding a motorcycle or bicycle.
- Follow driving rules of the road.
- Have working smoke alarms in place throughout the home and workplace.
- Avoid secondhand smoke.
- Reduce noise pollution or safeguard against hearing loss.
- Protect skin from ultraviolet light via sunscreen and clothing.
- Handle and store firearms appropriately.
- Practice water safety.

young people. Women—especially pregnant women and the mothers of young children—have special needs that must be addressed.

All primary care providers should screen for alcohol and other drug use problems, with an understanding of the obvious problems in relying on self-reporting of these behaviors. The use of over-the-counter drugs by women should also be explored. Counseling women who appear to be drinking excessively or using drugs may include strategies to increase self-esteem and teaching new coping skills to resist and maintain resistance to alcohol abuse and drug use. Appropriate referrals should be made, with the health care provider arranging the contact and then following up to ensure that appointments are kept. General referral to sources of support should also be provided. National groups that provide information and support for those who are chemically dependent are listed in resources on the EVOLVE website for this text. Many of these organizations have local branches or contacts that are listed in the telephone book.

Anticipatory guidance includes teaching about the health and safety risks of alcohol and mind-altering substances and discouraging drug experimentation among preteen and high school students because the use of drugs at an early age tends to predict greater involvement later.

Health Screening Schedule

Periodic health screening includes history, physical examination, education, counseling, and selected diagnostic and laboratory tests. This regimen provides the basis for overall health promotion, prevention of illness, early diagnosis of problems, and referral for appropriate management. Such screening should be customized according to a woman's age and risk factors. In most instances it is completed in health care offices, clinics, or hospitals; however, portions of the screening are now being carried out at events such as community health fairs. An overview of health screening recommendations for women over 18 years of age is provided in Table 4-1. Consistent with information provided earlier in this chapter, it is important for the nurse to continually educate and counsel on diet, exercise, smoking cessation, alcohol moderation, help for drug abuse, and stress management.

Health Risk Prevention

Often simple safety factors are forgotten or perceived not to be important; yet injuries continue to have a major impact on the health status of all age groups. Awareness of hazards and implementation of safety guidelines will reduce risks. The nurse should regularly reinforce concepts that will protect the individual (Box 4-10). Taking necessary precautions and avoiding dangerous situations are imperative.

Health Protection

Nurses can make a difference in stopping violence against women and preventing further injury. Educating women that abuse is a violation of their rights and facilitating their access to protective and legal services constitute first steps. Encouraging health care institutions to implement appropriate

Table 4-1 Health Screening Recommendations for Women Age 18 Years and Older

INTERVENTION	RECOMMENDATION*
Physical Examination	
Blood pressure	Every visit, but at least every 2 years
Height and weight	Every visit, but at least every 2 years
Pelvic examination	Annually until age 70; recommended for any woman who has ever been sexually active
Breast examination	
Clinical examination†	Every 3 years for women in their 20s
High risk	Annually after age 18 with history of premenopausal breast cancer in first-degree relative
Skin examination	Family history of skin cancer or increased exposure to sunlight after age 40; every 3 years between ages 20 and 40; monthly self-examinations also recommended
Oral cavity examination	Mouth lesion or exposure to tobacco or excessive alcohol
Laboratory and Diagnostic Tests	
Blood cholesterol (fasting lipoprotein analysis)	Every 5 years
High risk	More often per clinical judgment with potential for cardiac or lipid abnormalities
Papanicolaou (Pap) test†	Initially 3 years after becoming sexually active but no later than age 21; annually with conventional Pap test or every 2 years with liquid-based Pap tests; after age 30 and after three normal test results in a row, every 2 to 3 years; after age 70 and no abnormal test results in 10 years, screening may be stopped
Mammography‡	Annually over age 50 Annually over age 40 Every 1 to 2 years between ages 40 and 49 and annually thereafter
Colon cancer screening	Fecal occult blood test annually and flexible sigmoidoscopy every 5 years after age 50; more often if family history of colon cancer or polyps
Risk Groups	
Fasting blood sugar	Annually with family history of diabetes, gestational diabetes, or significant obesity; every 3 to 5 years for all women older than 45 years of age
Hearing screen	Annually with exposure to excessive noise or when loss is suspected
Sexually transmitted infection screen	As needed with multiple sexual partners
Tuberculin skin test	Annually with exposure to persons with tuberculosis or in risk categories for close contact with the disease
Endometrial biopsy	At menopause for women at risk for endometrial cancer
Vision	Every 2 years between ages 40 and 64; annually after age 65
Bone mineral density testing	All women age 65 and older; younger women with risk for osteoporosis may need periodic screenings
Immunizations	
Tetanus-diphtheria	Booster is given every 10 years after primary series
Measles, mumps, rubella	Once if born after 1956 and no evidence of immunity
Hepatitis B	Primary series of three for all who are in risk categories
Influenza	Annually after age 65 or in risk categories such as chronic diseases, immunosuppression, renal dysfunction

*Unless otherwise noted, the recommended intervention should be performed routinely every 1 to 3 years.

†Sources: American Cancer Society: *Cancer facts and figures 2008,* New York, 2007, American Cancer Society; Centers for Disease Control and Prevention, Workowski KA, Berman SM: Sexually transmitted diseases treatment guidelines 2006, *MMWR* 55(RR-11):1-94, 2006; Howard F, Scott-Findlay S: Breast self-examination: when research contradicts accepted practice, *AWHONN Lifelines* 10(1):66-70, 2006; National Heart Lung and Blood Institute: *ATP III Update 2004: Implications of recent clinical trials for the ATP III guidelines.* Available at www.nhlbi.nih.gov/guidelines/cholesterol/atp3upd04.htm (accessed June 16, 2008); National Women's Health Report Online: *Preventive health screening for women,* National Women's Health Resource Center, 2007. Available at www.healthywomen.org/healthreport/december2007 (accessed June 16, 2008).

‡NOTE: There is no consensus regarding mammograms for women between 40 and 49 years of age; thus various recommendations are listed. Women are urged to discuss circumstances with their health care provider.

domestic violence screening programs is also of great value. Other measures that may help women avoid falling into abusive relationships are promoting assertiveness and self-defense courses; suggesting support and self-help groups that encourage positive self-regard, confidence, and empowerment; and recommending educational and skills-development classes that will enhance independence (or at least the ability to take care of oneself).

Many national and local organizations provide information and assistance for women in abusive situations. Nurses and victims may find these resources helpful (see Resources on the EVOLVE site). All nurses who work in women's health care should become familiar with local services and legal options.

Intimate Partner Violence

Intimate partner violence (IPV) is the most common form of violence experienced by women worldwide, with a reported incidence of one out of every six women having been a victim of domestic violence. In the United States IPV it is a significant social problem and a major health care problem that affects millions of women and men each year and costs millions of dollars in annual medical costs. It is estimated that 29% of all women and 22% of men will experience abuse—physical, sexual, threats, or emotional—in their lifetime. In 2004 there were 1544 deaths in the United States from IPV, 75% of which were of women (CDC, 2006). A *Healthy People 2010* objective is to decrease the rate of IPV to 4 per 1000 women older than 12 years (USDHHS, 2000).

Battered Women

Although IPV is the preferred term, *wife battering, spouse abuse,* and *domestic* or *family violence* are all terms that may be applied to a pattern of assaultive and coercive behaviors inflicted by a male partner in a marriage or other heterosexual, significant, intimate relationship. Relationship violence rarely consists of a single episode but is a pattern that may start with intimidation or threats (Fig. 4-3) and progress to more aggressive physical and sexual acts, resulting in injury to the woman. Common elements of IPV are physical abuse; psychologic or emotional abuse; sexual assault; isolation; and controlling all aspects of the victim's life, including money, shelter, time, and food (National Women's Health Information Center [NWHIC], 2007) (Box 4-11) (see Critical Thinking Exercise).

BOX 4-11 Signs of Intimate Partner Violence

- Overuse of health services
- Vague, nonspecific complaints
- Missed appointments
- Unexplainable injuries
- Untreated serious injuries
- Injuries not matching the description
- Intimate partner never leaving the patient's side
- Intimate partner insisting on telling the story of the injury

Source: Krieger CL: Intimate partner violence: a review for nurses, *Nurs Women's Health* 12(3):224-234, 2008.

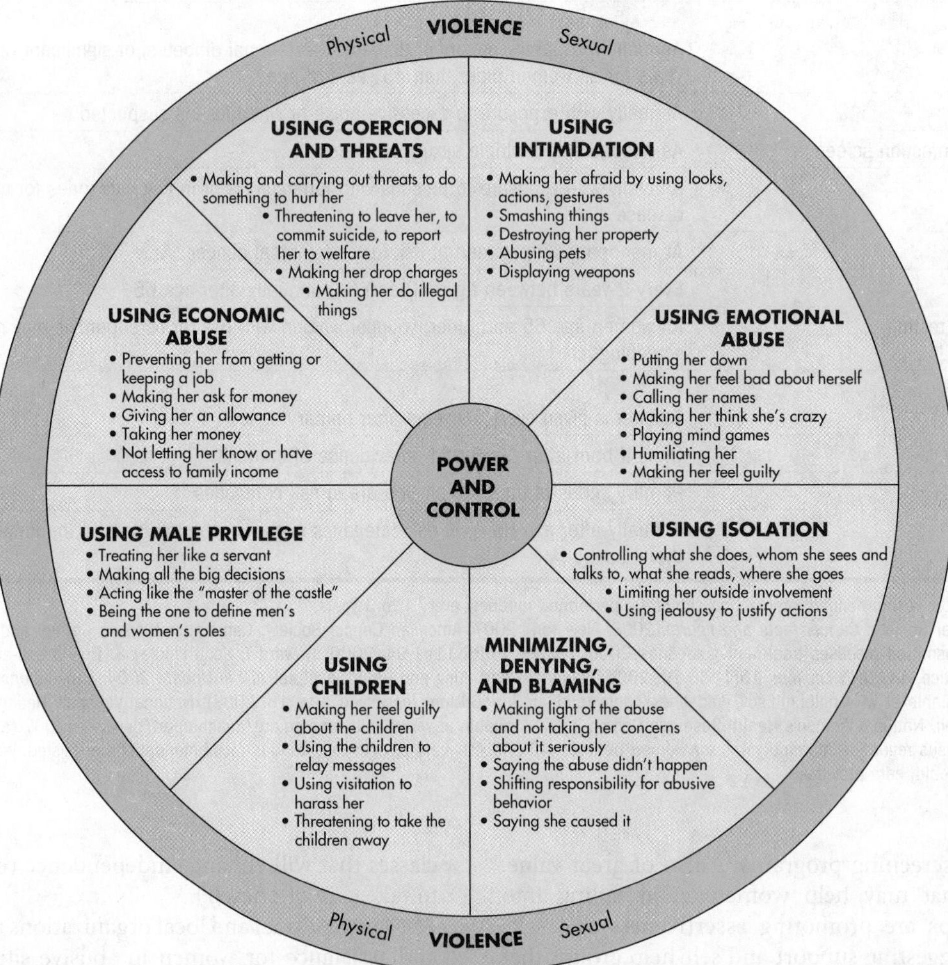

Fig. 4-3 Model of how power and control issues perpetuate battering. (From Duluth Domestic Abuse Intervention Project: *Power and control: tactics of men who batter*, Duluth, Minn, 1986, Author.)

CRITICAL THINKING EXERCISE

Intimate Partner Violence

Annette is a 35-year-old married woman who comes to the clinic for complaints of abdominal pain and headaches. The nurse notices that Annette has bruises on her left cheek, forearms, and upper back. When the nurse asks about the cause of the bruises, Annette says that "she ran into a door." It is obvious to the nurse that the injuries could not have been caused by running into a door. What is the nurse's responsibility in this instance regarding confidentiality, questioning Annette about domestic violence, risks to Annette of admitting she has been beaten by her husband, and reporting the incident to the police?

1. Evidence—Is there sufficient evidence to draw conclusions about the rights of Annette to privacy and the responsibility of the nurse to provide care for Annette and report the incident to the police?
2. Assumptions—What assumptions can be made about the following risks for Annette of disclosing the fact that her injuries were caused by her husband?
   a. Annette's right to privacy
   b. Safety for Annette if she discloses domestic violence
   c. Nurse's responsibility to discuss domestic violence and offer a safety plan
   d. Nurse's legal responsibility to report the incident to the police
3. What implications and priorities for nursing care can be drawn at this time?
4. Does the evidence objectively support your conclusion?
5. Are there alternative perspectives to your conclusion?

Cultural Considerations

Women of all races and all ethnic, educational, religious, and socioeconomic backgrounds are affected. In the United States Caucasian women report less IPV than do non-Caucasians. Native American/Alaskan Native women report significantly more instances of IPV than do women of any other racial background; Asian women report significantly less IPV than do other racial groups. Reporting rates may not reflect the magnitude of the problem since many women do not disclose violence because of fear, embarrassment, or not having been asked by those from whom they seek help. Poor and uneducated women tend to be disproportionately represented because they are seen in emergency departments (EDs), they are financially more dependent, they have fewer resources and support systems, and they may have fewer problem-solving skills.

Table 4-2 lists some myths and facts about abuse and battering.

Table 4-2 Myths and Facts About Intimate Partner Violence

MYTHS	FACTS
Battering occurs in a small percentage of the population.	One fourth of all women experience battering by an intimate partner.
Being pregnant protects the woman from battering.	From 4% to 8% of all women who are battered are battered during pregnancy. Battering frequently begins or escalates in frequency and intensity during pregnancy. Pregnancy may be the result of forced sex or of the man's control of contraception.
Battering occurs only in "problem" or lower-class families.	Intimate partner violence can occur in any family. Although lower-income families have a higher reported incidence of battering, it also occurs in middle- and upper-income families. Incidence is not accurately known because of the tendency of middle- and upper-income families to hide their battering.
Battered women like to be beaten and deliberately provoke the attack. They are masochistic.	Women are terrified of their assailants and go to great lengths to avoid a confrontation. In some cases, the woman may provoke her partner to release tension that, if left unchecked, might lead to a more severe beating and possible death.
Only men with psychologic problems abuse women.	Many batterers are successful professionals, including politicians, ministers, physicians, and lawyers. Research indicates that only a small number of abusers have psychologic problems.
Only people who come from abusive families end up in abusive relationships.	Most battered women report that their partners were the first person to beat them.
Alcohol and drug abuse cause battering.	Although alcohol may be involved in abusive incidents, it is not the cause. Many batterers use alcohol as an excuse to batter and shift the blame to the alcohol.
Women would leave the relationship if the abuse were really that bad.	Women who stay in the relationship do so out of fear and financial dependence. Shelters have long waiting lists.
Batterers and battered women cannot change.	Counseling may effectively help both batterers and battered women.

From Caetano R, Schafer J, Cunradi CB: Alcohol-related intimate partner violence among white, black, and Hispanic couples in the United States, *Alcohol and Violence* 25(1): 58-65, 2001; National Women's Health Information Center: *Violence against women,* 2007. Available at www.4woman.gov/violence/index.cfm (accessed June 16, 2008).

Cycle of Violence: The Dynamics of Battering

Battering is neither random nor constant; rather, it occurs in repeated cycles. A three-phase cyclic pattern to the battering behavior includes a period of increasing tension leading to the battery. The battery consists of slaps, punches to the face and head, kicking, stomping, punching, choking, pushing, breaking of bones, burns from irons, and mutilation from knives and guns. The honeymoon phase is characterized by a period of calm and remorse in which the male partner displays kind, loving behavior and pleas for forgiveness. This honeymoon phase lasts until stress or other factors cause conflict and tension to mount again toward another episode of battering. Over time the tension and battering phases last longer,

evolve Spanish Guidelines—Recognizing Violence in a Relationship and the calm phase becomes shorter until there is no honeymoon phase.

All women entering the health care system should be assessed for potential abuse. At least the following questions should be asked (American College of Obstetricians and Gynecologists [ACOG], 2009):

- Are you with a spouse or partner who threatens or physically hurts you?
- Within the past year or in this pregnancy has anyone hit, slapped, kicked, or otherwise hurt you?
- Has anyone forced you to have sexual activities that made you uncomfortable?

These questions give a woman permission to disclose sensitive information.

Battering During Pregnancy

Estimates of prevalence of battering in pregnancy vary, ranging from 4% to 8% to as many as 20%. Most women abused before pregnancy will be abused during the pregnancy, and the incidence may escalate. Abuse also may happen for the first time during pregnancy. Pregnant adolescents are abused at higher rates than are adult women; thus they should be considered at high risk. Battering during pregnancy in teenagers constitutes a particularly difficult situation. Adolescents may be more trapped in the abusive relationship than adult women because of their inexperience. They may ignore the violence because the jealous and controlling behavior is interpreted as love and devotion. Because pregnancy in young adolescent girls is frequently the result of sexual abuse, feelings about the pregnancy should be assessed.

During pregnancy the nurse should assess for abuse at each prenatal visit and on admission to labor. Battering episodes initiate or increase in pregnancy for a variety of reasons: (1) the biopsychosocial stresses of pregnancy may strain the relationship beyond the couple's ability to cope, and frustration is followed by violence; (2) the man may be jealous of the fetus, resenting the intrusion into the couple's relationship and the woman's displacement of attention; (3) the man may be angry at the unborn child or the woman; and (4) the beating may be the man's conscious or subconscious attempt to end the pregnancy. After birth the mother may be so physically and emotionally drained that she may have difficulty bonding with her infant. She may be at risk of becoming an abusive mother whether or not she remains in the abusive relationship.

In the United States a pregnant woman is often accompanied by her husband to the antepartum appointment if the woman does not speak English and the husband does. Unless an interpreter is available, it is difficult to interview the woman alone; in addition, asking questions about abuse through an interpreter is more difficult unless the interpreter is a woman and can communicate the nurse's sensitivity and concern accurately. See the Spanish Guidelines on the EVOLVE website for this text for descriptions of abusive relationships and how a woman can recognize whether she is in one.

A therapeutic relationship and skillful interviewing help women disclose and describe their abuse (Box 4-12). Language is important when talking with women. For example, using the term *victim* connotes powerlessness and hopelessness; a more empowering term is *survivor*. Women who have identified their abuse may appear passive, hostile, anxious, depressed, or hysterical because they may think they are at the mercy of the man's temper or that he is "out of control." In addition, they may be embarrassed, afraid, angry, sad, and shocked.

The most significant part of the intervention is to ensure that the woman has knowledge of the resources available to her and a plan of action should she stay with the battering partner. First, the nurse should provide services and telephone numbers of a hotline and the battered women's shelter or other safe haven. The woman can be offered a telephone to call the shelter if this is an option she chooses. If she chooses to go back to the abuser, a safety plan includes necessities for a quick escape: a bag packed with personal items for an overnight stay (can be hidden or left with a neighbor), money or a checkbook, an extra set of car keys, and any legal documents for identification. Legal options such as those for restraining orders or arrest of the perpetrator also are important aspects of the safety plan (Box 4-13). A restraining order can be obtained 24 hours a day from the county court or police department. Shelters also can be helpful with assistance in obtaining orders of protection. If the woman chooses not to act in the middle of a violent episode, she may use the hotline or shelter for some counseling when the threat of harm is no longer present.

BOX 4-12 What Not to Say to a Battered Woman and What You Can Say and Do

What *Not* to Say

1. Do not ask "why." This question "revictimizes" and blames the victim.
2. Do not talk negatively about the abuser to the victim. She may become defensive and stop talking.
3. Do not talk directly to the abuser about your suspicions of abuse. The abuser will assume the victim told you, and the victim risks retaliation.

What to Say

1. "I'm afraid for your safety (and the safety of your children)."
2. "I believe you."
3. "It is progressive and will only get worse."
4. "You deserve better than this. You deserve to be treated with respect."
5. "You are not alone."
6. "It is a crime."
7. "I'm here for you."

What to Do

1. Empower the victim.
2. Sit down with her.
3. Assure her of total privacy and confidentiality (but only if you can).
4. Use your best listening skills.
5. Call 911 and report any incident of imminent danger.
6. Give the woman the telephone number of the nearest battered women's shelter.

evolve Critical Thinking Exercise—Women's Health and Safety

BOX 4-13 Safety Strategies

Victims of intimate partner violence should try to maintain the following safety strategies:
- Always be aware of surroundings.
- Minimize time in kitchens, bathrooms, and closets when abuser is near.
- Shop and bank at different places.
- Drive to work multiple ways.
- Get a protection order.
- Never lunch alone.
- Cancel joint credit cards and old bank accounts with abuser.
- Provide a picture of abuser to security at workplace.
- Be escorted by workplace security to car or transportation.
- When in danger, go to a place of safety and call 911.
- Change locks on house if abuser has moved out.
- Get unlisted telephone number.
- Block caller ID.

Source: Krieger CL: Intimate partner violence: a review for nurses, *Nurs Women's Health* 12(3):224-234, 2008.

LEGAL TIP **Mandatory Reporting of Domestic Violence** Domestic violence is considered a crime in all states, but it varies between misdemeanor and felony offenses, the majority being misdemeanors. Forty states and the District of Columbia have laws that mandate reporting by health care providers in situations in which the woman has an injury that may be caused by a deadly weapon. Some states also require reports when there is a reason to believe that the woman's injury may have resulted from an illegal act or act of violence.

Because of the wide variation from state to state in mandatory reporting, nurses *must* be knowledgeable about the reporting requirements of the state in which they practice. Nurses can check the Family Violence Prevention Fund (2004) for a listing and evaluation of reporting laws, or they can call the local shelter for assistance.

Prevention

Nurses can make a difference in stopping the violence and preventing further injury. Educating women that abuse is a violation of their rights and facilitating their access to protective and legal services is a first step. Other helpful measures for women to discourage the risk of abusive relationships are promoting assertiveness and self-defense courses; suggesting support and self-help groups that encourage positive self-regard, confidence, and empowerment; and recommending educational and skills-development classes that will enhance independence or at least the ability to take care of oneself (Pennell & Francis, 2005). Classes for English language learners may be particularly helpful to immigrant women. Nurses can offer information on local classes.

Key Points

- Culture, religion, socioeconomic status, personal circumstances, the uniqueness of the individual, and the stage of development influence a person's recognition of need for care and the response to the health care system and therapy.
- Preconception counseling allows identification and possible remediation of potentially harmful personal and social conditions, medical and psychologic conditions, environmental conditions, and barriers to care before pregnancy occurs.
- Conditions that increase a woman's health risks also increase risks for her offspring.
- Periodic health screening provides the basis for overall health promotion, prevention of illness, early diagnosis of problems, and referral for management.

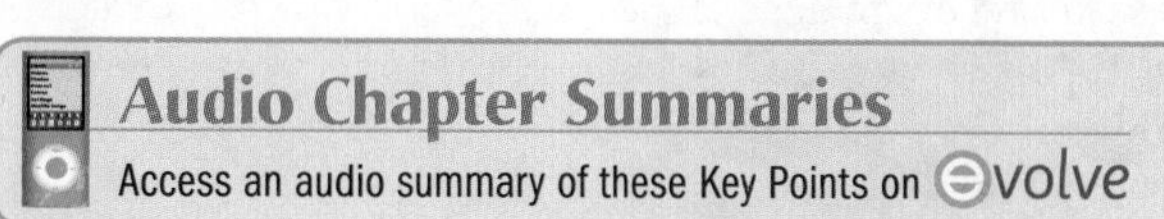
Audio Chapter Summaries
Access an audio summary of these Key Points on evolve

- Health promotion and prevention of illness assist women to actualize health potential by increasing motivation, providing information, and suggesting how to access specific resources.
- IPV against women is a major social and health care problem in the United States and includes physical, sexual, emotional, psychologic, and economic abuse.
- Battering affects all races; all socioeconomic, educational, and religious groups; and many pregnant women.

References

American Cancer Society (ACS): *Cancer facts and figures 2008*, New York, 2008, ACS.

American College of Obstetricians and Gynecologists (ACOG): *Screening tools for domestic violence*, ACOG violence against women home page, 2009. Available at www.acog.org (accessed February 17, 2009).

Centers for Disease Control and Prevention: *Understanding intimate partner violence: fact sheet*, 2006. Available at www.cdc.gov/ncipc/dvp/ipv_factsheet.pdf (accessed June 4, 2008).

Centers for Disease Control and Prevention: *Adult cigarette smoking in the United States: current estimates: fact sheet*, updated November 2007a. Available at www.cdc.gov/tobacco/data_statistics/Factsheets/adult_cig_smoking.htm (accessed June 13, 2008).

Centers for Disease Control and Prevention: Cigarette smoking among adults—United States, 2006, *MMWR* 56(44):1157-1161, 2007b.

Cunningham G et al: *Williams obstetrics*, ed 22, New York, 2005, McGraw-Hill.

Family Violence Prevention Fund (FVPF): *Mandatory reporting of domestic violence by health care providers*, San Francisco, 2004, FVPF. Available at www.endabuse.org/health/mandatoryreporting/tables1.pdf (accessed June 15, 2008).

Jefferson D: America's most dangerous drug, *Newsweek* pp 41-48, August 8, 2005.

Johnston O et al: Feasibility and acceptability of screening for eating disorders in primary care, *Fam Pract* 24(5):511-517, Epub Jun 24, 2007.

Lee R et al: Neurotoxic effects of alcohol and acetaldehyde during embryonic development, *J Toxicol Environ Health* (Part A) 68(23-24):2147-2162, 2005.

Lester B, Andreozzi L, Appiah L: Substance use during pregnancy: time for policy to catch up with research, *Harm Reduct J* 1(5):1-44, 2004.

Martin JA et al: Annual summary of vital statistics: 2006, *Pediatrics* 121(4):788-801, 2008.

National Women's Health Information Center: *Violence against women*, 2007. Available at www.4woman.gov/violence/types/domestic.cfm (accessed June 14, 2008).

Otto K: Acupuncture and substance abuse: a synopsis with indications for further research, *Am J Addict* 12(1): 43-51, 2003.

Parker S, Lyons J, Bonner J: Eating disorders in graduate students: exploring the SCOFF questionnaire as a simple screening tool, *J Am College Health* 52(2):103-107, 2005.

Pennell J, Francis S: Safety conferencing: toward a coordinated and inclusive response to safeguard women and children, *Violence Against Women* 11(5):666-692, 2005.

Stuart GW, Laraia MT: *Principles and practice of psychiatric nursing*, ed 8, St Louis, 2005, Mosby.

Trussel J: Choosing a contraceptive: efficacy, safety, and personal considerations. In Hatcher R et al, editors: *Contraceptive technology*, ed 19, New York, 2007, Ardent Media.

US Department of Health and Human Services: *Healthy people 2010: national health promotion and disease prevention objectives*, Washington, DC, 2000, US Department of Health and Human Services.

Vickers A, Wilson P, Kleynen J: Effectiveness Bulletin: acupuncture, *Qual Saf Health Care* 11(1):92-97, 2002.

Unit 2

5 Health Assessment

Learning Objectives

On completion of this chapter the reader will be able to:

- Identify the structures and functions of the female reproductive system.
- Differentiate the menstrual cycle in relation to hormonal, ovarian, and endometrial responses.
- Identify the four phases of the sexual response cycle.
- Investigate how the history and physical examination can be adapted for women with special needs.
- Identify indications of abuse, appropriate screening, and referral to community agencies.
- Describe components of taking a woman's history and performing a physical examination.
- Identify the correct procedure for assisting with and collecting Papanicolaou test specimens.
- Review patient teaching of breast self-examination.

Electronic Resources

Additional information related to the content in Chapter 5 can be found on

evolve the Companion Website at

http://evolve.elsevier.com/Perry/maternal/

- NCLEX Review Questions
- Anatomy Review—Adult Female Pelvis
- Anatomy Review—External Female Genitalia
- Anatomy Review—Female Breast
- Anatomy Review—Female Pelvic Organs
- Animation—Breasts
- Animation—External Female Genitalia
- Animation—Menstrual Cycle: Uterine
- Animation—Ovaries
- Animation—Ovulation
- Case Study—Health Assessment
- Skill—Breast Self-Examination
- Spanish Guidelines—Menstruation
- Spanish Guidelines—Physical Examination

The purpose of this chapter is to review female anatomy and physiology, the menstrual cycle, and gynecologic health assessment.

Female Reproductive System

The female reproductive system consists of external structures visible from the pubis to the perineum and internal structures located in the pelvic cavity. The external and internal female reproductive structures develop and mature in response to estrogen and progesterone. This process starts in fetal life and continues through puberty and the childbearing years. Reproductive structures atrophy with age or in response to a decrease in ovarian hormone production. A complex nerve and blood supply supports the functions of these structures. There is great variation among women in the appearance of the external genitalia. Heredity, age, race, and the number of children a woman has borne influence the size, shape, and color of her external organs.

External Structures

The external genital organs, or vulva, include all structures visible externally from the pubis to the perineum. These include the mons pubis, labia majora, labia minora, clitoris, vestibular glands, vaginal vestibule, vaginal orifice, and urethral opening. The external genital organs are illustrated in Fig. 5-1.

The mons pubis is a fatty pad that lies over the anterior surface of the symphysis pubis. In the postpubertal female the mons is covered with coarse, curly hair. The labia majora are two rounded folds of fatty tissue covered with skin that extend downward and backward from the mons pubis. The labia are highly vascular structures that develop hair on the outer surfaces after puberty. They protect the inner vulvar structures. The labia minora are two flat, reddish folds of tissue visible when the labia majora are separated. There are no hair follicles on the labia minora, but many sebaceous follicles and a few sweat glands are present. The interior of the labia minora is composed of connective tissue and smooth muscle and is supplied with extremely sensitive nerve endings. Anteriorly the labia minora fuse to form the prepuce (the hoodlike covering of the clitoris) and the frenulum (the fold of tissue under the clitoris). The labia minora join to form a thin, flat tissue called the *fourchette* underneath the vaginal opening at midline. The clitoris is located underneath the prepuce. It is a small structure composed of erectile tissue with numerous sensory nerve endings. During sexual arousal the clitoris increases in size.

The vaginal vestibule is an almond-shaped area enclosed by the labia minora that contains openings to the urethra, Skene glands, vagina, and Bartholin glands. The urethra is not a reproductive organ but is discussed here because of its location. It usually is found about 2.5 cm below the clitoris. Skene glands are located on each side of the urethra and produce

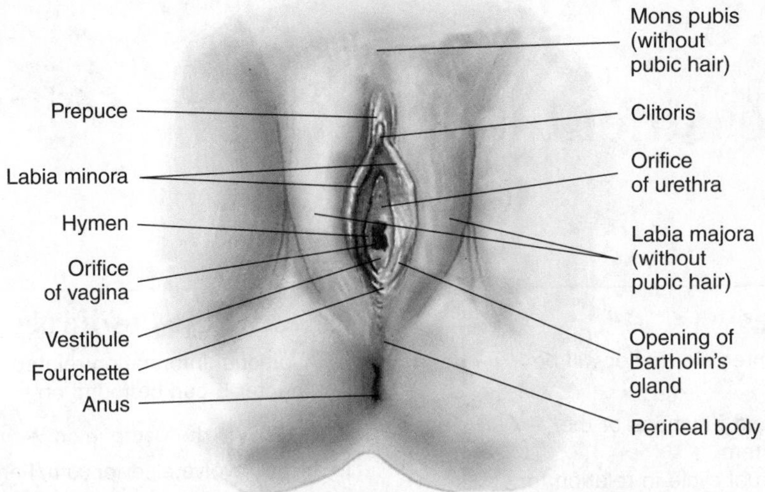

Fig. 5-1 External female genitalia.

mucus, which aids in lubrication of the vagina. The vaginal opening is in the lower portion of the vestibule and varies in shape and size. The hymen, a connective tissue membrane that surrounds the vaginal opening, can be perforated during strenuous exercise, insertion of tampons, masturbation, and vaginal intercourse. Bartholin glands lie under the constrictor muscles of the vagina and are located posteriorly on the sides of the vaginal opening, although the ductal openings usually are not visible. During sexual arousal the glands secrete clear mucus to lubricate the vaginal introitus.

The area between the fourchette and the anus is the perineum, a skin-covered muscular area that covers the pelvic structures. The perineum forms the base of the perineal body, a wedge-shaped mass that serves as an anchor for the muscles, fascia, and ligaments of the pelvis. The muscles and ligaments form a sling that supports the pelvic organs.

Internal Structures

The internal structures include the vagina, uterus, uterine tubes, and ovaries.

The vagina is a fibromuscular, collapsible, tubular structure that lies between the bladder and rectum and extends from the vulva to the uterus. During the reproductive years the mucosal lining is arranged in transverse folds called *rugae*. These rugae allow the vagina to expand during childbirth. Estrogen deprivation that occurs after childbirth, during lactation, and at menopause causes dryness and thinning of the vaginal walls and smoothing of the rugae. The vagina, particularly the lower segment, has few sensory nerve endings. Vaginal secretions are slightly acidic (pH 4 to 5) so that vaginal susceptibility to infections is limited. The vagina serves as a passageway for menstrual flow, as a female organ of copulation, and as a part of the birth canal for vaginal childbirth. The uterine cervix projects into a blind vault at the upper end of the vagina. There are anterior, posterior, and lateral pockets called fornices (singular: fornix) that surround the cervix. The internal pelvic organs can be palpated through the thin walls of these fornices.

The uterus is a muscular organ shaped like an upside-down pear that sits midline in the pelvic cavity between the bladder and rectum and above the vagina. Four pairs of ligaments support the uterus: cardinal, uterosacral, round, and broad. Single anterior and posterior ligaments also support the uterus. The cul-de-sac of Douglas is a deep pouch, or recess, posterior to the cervix formed by the posterior ligament.

The uterus is divided into two major parts, an upper triangular portion called the *corpus* and a lower cylindric portion called the *cervix* (Fig. 5-2). The fundus is the dome-shaped top of the uterus and is the site at which the uterine tubes enter the uterus. The isthmus, or lower uterine segment, is a short, constricted portion that separates the corpus from the cervix.

The uterus serves for reception, implantation, retention, and nutrition of the fertilized ovum and later of the fetus during pregnancy and for expulsion of the fetus during childbirth. It is also responsible for cyclic menstruation.

The uterine wall is made up of three layers: the endometrium, the myometrium, and part of the peritoneum. The endometrium is a highly vascular lining made up of three layers, the outer two of which are shed during menstruation. The myometrium is made up of layers of smooth muscles that extend in three different directions (longitudinal, transverse, and oblique) (Fig. 5-3). Longitudinal fibers of the outer myometrial layer are found mostly in the fundus, and this arrangement assists in expelling the fetus during the birth process. The middle layer contains fibers from all three directions, which form a figure-eight pattern encircling large blood vessels. These fibers assist in ligating blood vessels after childbirth and control blood loss. Most of the circular fibers of the inner myometrial layer are around the site where the uterine tubes enter the uterus and around the internal cervical os (opening). These fibers help keep the cervix closed during pregnancy and prevent menstrual blood from flowing back into the uterine tubes during menstruation.

The cervix is made up of mostly fibrous connective tissues and elastic tissue, making it possible for the cervix to stretch during vaginal childbirth. The opening between the uterine cavity and the canal that connects the uterine cavity to the vagina (endocervical canal) is the internal os. The narrowed opening between the endocervix and the vagina is the external

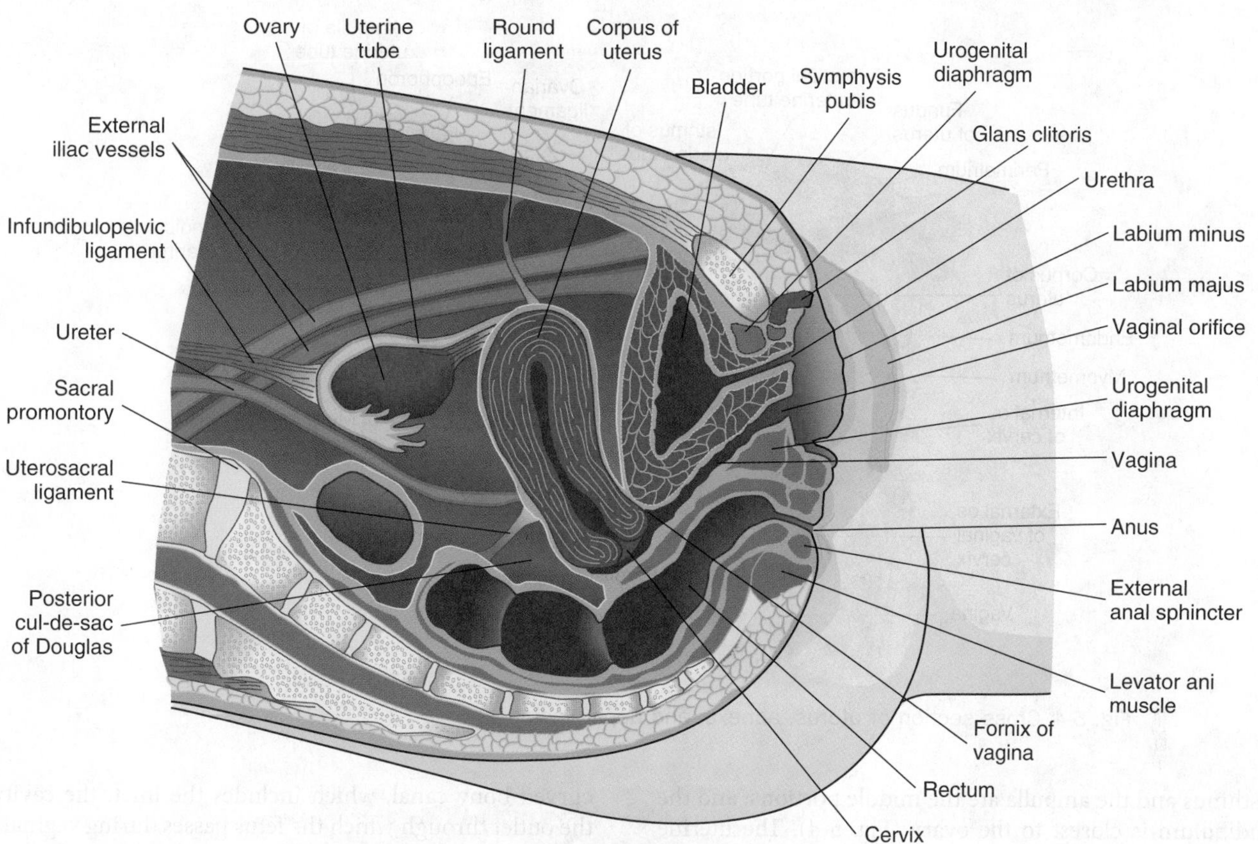

Fig. 5-2 Midsagittal view of female pelvic organs with woman lying supine.

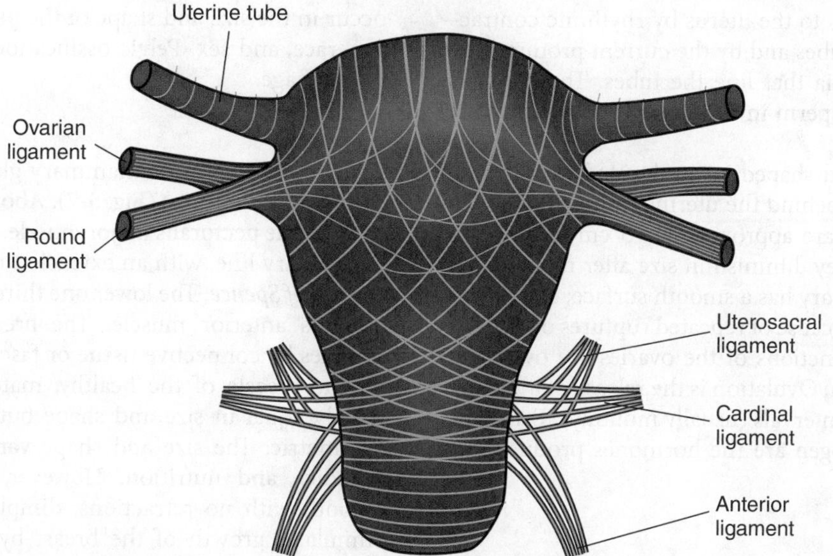

Fig. 5-3 Schematic arrangement of directions of muscle fibers. Note that uterine muscle fibers are continuous with supportive ligaments of uterus.

os, a small circular opening in women who have never been pregnant. The cervix feels firm (like the end of a nose) with a dimple in the center that marks the external os.

The outer cervix is covered with a layer of squamous epithelium. The mucosa of the cervical canal is covered with columnar epithelium and contains numerous glands that secrete mucus in response to ovarian hormones. The squamocolumnar junction, where the two types of cells meet, is usually located just inside the cervical os. This junction also is called the *transformation zone* and is the most common site for neoplastic changes. Cells from this site are scraped for the Papanicolaou (Pap) test (see later discussion).

The uterine tubes (fallopian tubes) attach to the uterine fundus. The tubes are supported by the broad ligaments and range from 8 to 14 cm in length. The tubes are divided into four sections: the interstitial portion is closest to the uterus;

evolve Anatomy Review—Female Pelvic Organs
evolve Animation—Ovaries

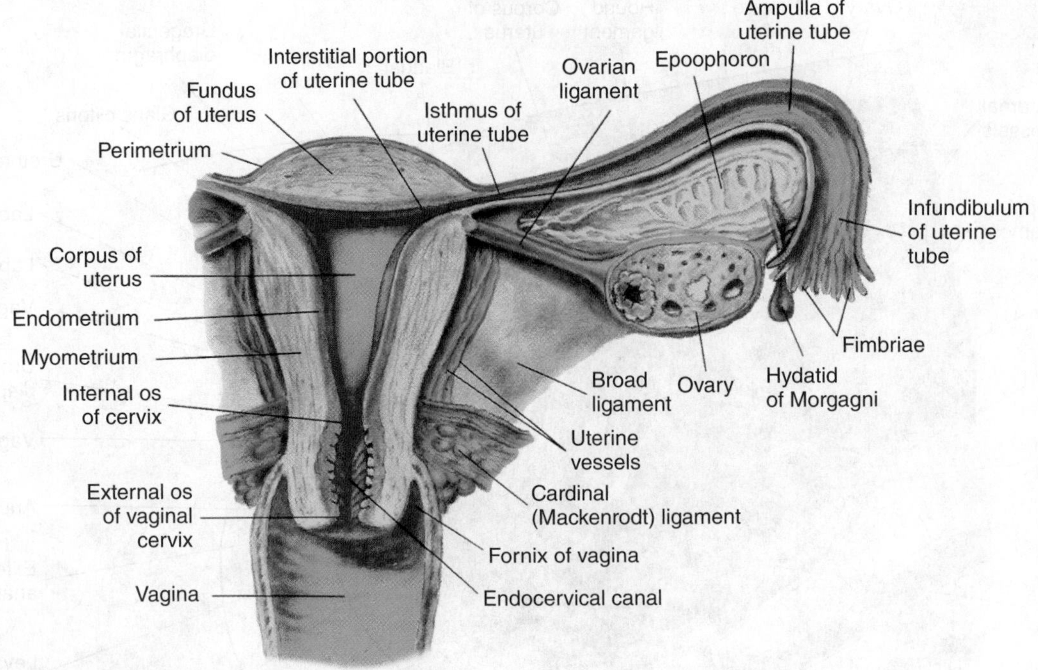

Fig. 5-4 Cross section of uterus, adnexa, and upper vagina.

the isthmus and the ampulla are the middle portions; and the infundibulum is closest to the ovary (Fig. 5-4). The uterine tubes provide a passage between the ovaries and the uterus for the movement of the ovum. The infundibulum has fimbriated (fringed) ends, which pull the ovum into the tube. The ovum is pushed along the tubes to the uterus by rhythmic contractions of muscles of the tubes and by the current produced by the movement of the cilia that line the tubes. The ovum is usually fertilized by the sperm in the ampulla portion of one of the tubes.

The ovaries are almond-shaped organs located on each side of the uterus below and behind the uterine tubes. During the reproductive years they are approximately 3 cm long, 2 cm wide, and 1 cm thick; they diminish in size after menopause. Before menarche each ovary has a smooth surface; after menarche they are nodular because of repeated ruptures of follicles at ovulation. The two functions of the ovaries are ovulation and hormone production. Ovulation is the release of a mature ovum from the ovary at intervals (usually monthly). Estrogen, progesterone, and androgen are the hormones produced by the ovaries.

The Bony Pelvis

The bony pelvis serves three primary purposes: protection of the pelvic structures, accommodation of the growing fetus during pregnancy, and anchorage of the pelvic support structures. The two innominate (hip) bones (consisting of ilium, ischium, and pubis), the sacrum; and the coccyx make up the four bones of the pelvis (Fig. 5-5). Cartilage and ligaments form the symphysis pubis, sacrococcygeal joint, and two sacroiliac joints that separate the pelvic bones.

The pelvis is divided into two parts: the false pelvis and the true pelvis (Fig. 5-6). The false pelvis is the upper portion above the pelvic brim or inlet. The true pelvis is the lower curved bony canal, which includes the inlet, the cavity, and the outlet through which the fetus passes during vaginal birth. The upper portion of the outlet is at the level of the ischial spines, and the lower portion is at the level of the ischial tuberosities and the pubic arch (see Fig. 5-5). Variations that occur in the size and shape of the pelvis are usually related to age, race, and sex. Pelvic ossification is complete at about 20 years of age.

Breasts

The breasts are paired mammary glands located between the second and sixth ribs (Fig. 5-7). About two thirds of the breast overlies the pectoralis major muscle, between the sternum and midaxillary line, with an extension to the axilla referred to as the *tail of Spence*. The lower one third of the breast overlies the serratus anterior muscle. The breasts are attached to the muscles by connective tissue or fascia.

The breasts of the healthy, mature woman are approximately equal in size and shape but often are not absolutely symmetric. The size and shape vary with the woman's age, heredity, and nutrition. However, the contour should be smooth with no retractions, dimpling, or masses. Estrogen stimulates growth of the breast by inducing fat deposition in the breasts, development of stromal tissue (i.e., increase in its amount and elasticity), and growth of the extensive ductile system. Estrogen also increases the vascularity of breast tissue.

Once ovulation begins in puberty, progesterone levels increase. The increase in progesterone causes maturation of mammary gland tissue, specifically the lobules and acinar structures. During adolescence fat deposition and growth of fibrous tissue contribute to the increase in the size of the glands. Full development of the breasts is not achieved until after the end of the first pregnancy or in the early period of lactation.

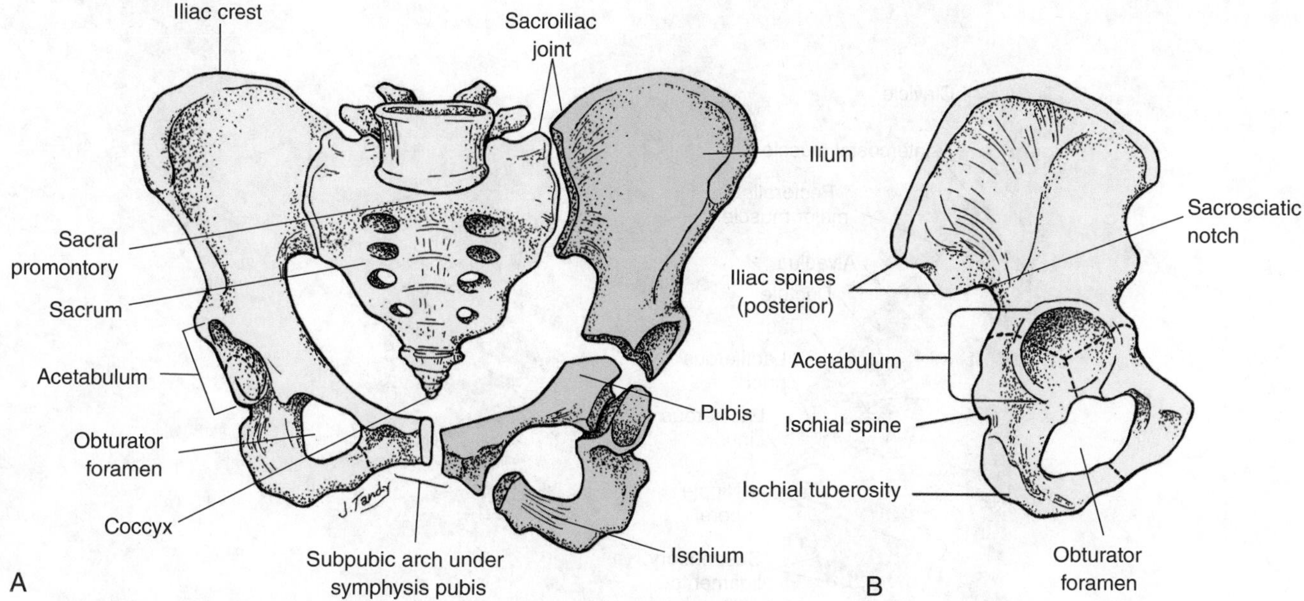

Fig. 5-5 Adult female pelvis. **A,** Anterior view. **B,** External view of innominate bone (fused).

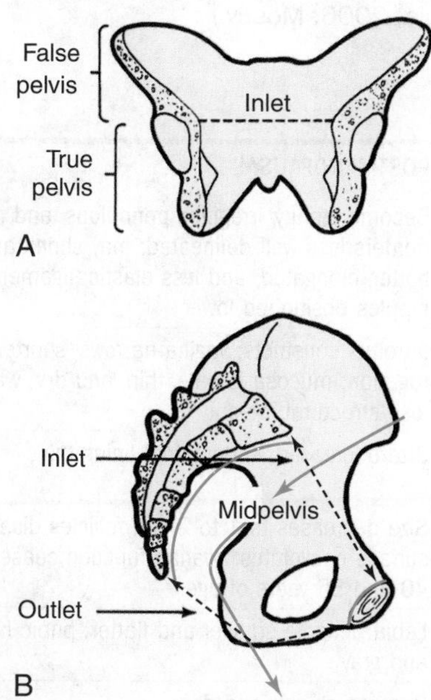

Fig. 5-6 Female pelvis. **A,** Cavity of false pelvis is shallow. **B,** Cavity of true pelvis is an irregularly curved canal *(arrows).*

Each mammary gland is made of 15 to 20 lobes, which are divided into lobules. Lobules are clusters of acini. An acinus is a saclike terminal part of a compound gland emptying through a narrow lumen or duct. In discussions of mammary glands, *acinus,* the correct anatomic term, is often used interchangeably with the term *alveolus.* The acini are lined with epithelial cells that secrete colostrum and milk. Just below the epithelium is the myoepithelium (*myo,* or muscle), which contracts to expel milk from the acini.

The ducts from the clusters of acini that form the lobules merge to form larger ducts draining the lobes. Ducts from the lobes converge in a single nipple (mammary papilla) surrounded by an areola. Just as the ducts converge, they dilate to form common lactiferous sinuses, which are also called *ampullae.* The lactiferous sinuses serve as milk reservoirs. Many tiny lactiferous ducts drain the ampullae and exit in the nipple.

The glandular structures and ducts are surrounded by protective fatty tissue and are separated and supported by fibrous suspensory Cooper's ligaments. Cooper's ligaments provide support to the mammary glands while permitting their mobility on the chest wall (see Fig. 5-7). The nipple is usually round, slightly elevated, and projects slightly upward and laterally. It contains 15 to 20 openings from lactiferous ducts. The nipple is surrounded by fibromuscular tissue and covered by wrinkled skin. Except during pregnancy and lactation, there is usually no discharge from the nipple.

The nipple and surrounding areola are usually more deeply pigmented than the skin of the breast. The rough appearance of the areola is caused by sebaceous glands, Montgomery tubercles, directly beneath the skin. These glands secrete a fatty substance thought to lubricate the nipple. Smooth muscle fibers in the areola contract to stiffen the nipple to make it easier for the breastfeeding infant to grasp.

The vascular supply to the mammary gland is abundant. In the nonpregnant state there is no obvious vascular pattern in the skin. The normal skin is smooth without tightness or shininess. The skin covering the breasts contains an extensive superficial lymphatic network that serves the entire chest wall and is continuous with the superficial lymphatics of the neck and abdomen. The lymphatics form a rich network in the deeper portions of the breasts. The primary deep lymphatic pathway drains laterally toward the axillae.

Besides their function of lactation, breasts function as organs for sexual arousal in the mature adult.

The breasts change in size and nodularity in response to cyclic ovarian changes throughout reproductive life. Increasing levels of both estrogen and progesterone in the 3 to 4 days

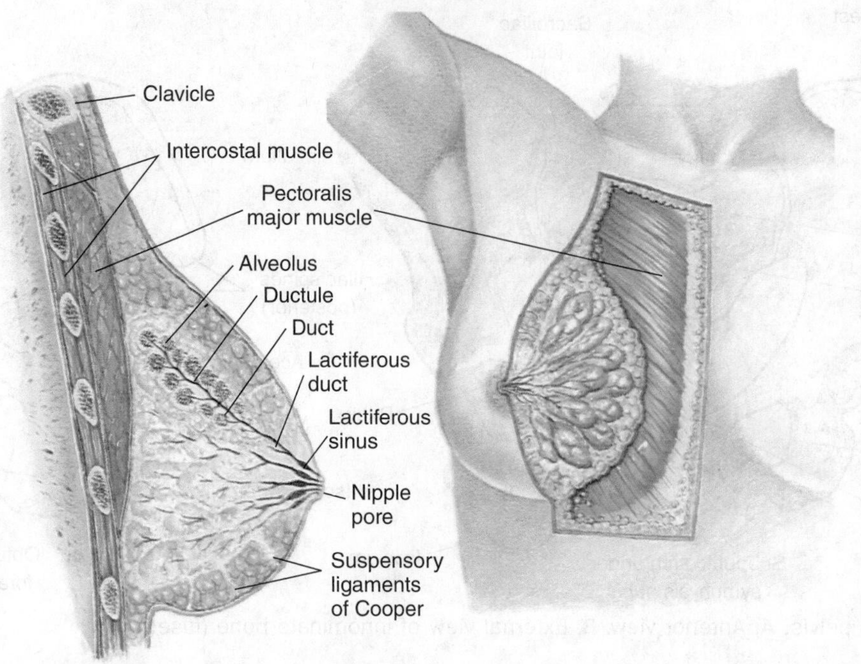

Fig. 5-7 Anatomy of the breast, showing position and major structures. (From Seidel HM et al: *Mosby's guide to physical examination*, ed 6, St Louis, 2006, Mosby.)

Table 5-1 Female Reproductive Physical Assessment Across the Life Cycle

	ADOLESCENT	ADULT	POSTMENOPAUSAL
Breasts	Tender when developing; buds appear; small, firm; one side may grow faster; areola diameter increases; nipples more erect	Grow to full shape in early adulthood; nipples and areola become pinker and darker	Become stringy, irregular, pendulous, and nodular; borders less well delineated; may shrink and become flatter, elongated, and less elastic; ligaments weaken; nipples positioned lower
Vagina	Vagina lengthens; epithelial layers thicken; secretions become acidic	Growth complete by age 20	Introitus constricts; vagina narrows, shortens, loses rugation; mucosa is pale, thin, and dry; walls may lose structural integrity
Uterus	Musculature and vasculature increase; lining thickens	Growth complete by age 20	Size decreases; endometrial lining thins
Ovaries	Increase in size and weight; menarche occurs between 8 and 16 years of age; ovulation occurs monthly	Growth complete by age 20	Size decreases to 1 to 2 cm; follicles disappear; surface convolutes; ovarian function ceases between 40 and 55 years of age
Labia majora	Become more prominent; hair develops	Growth complete by age 20	Labia become smaller and flatter; pubic hair sparse and gray
Labia minora	Become more vascular	Growth complete by age 20	Become shinier and drier
Uterine tubes	Increase in size	Growth complete by age 20	Decrease in size

before menstruation increase the vascularity of the breasts, induce growth of the ducts and acini, and promote water retention. The epithelial cells lining the ducts proliferate in number, the ducts dilate, and the lobules distend. The acini become enlarged and secretory, and lipid (fat) is deposited within their epithelial cell lining. As a result, breast swelling, tenderness, and discomfort are common symptoms just before the onset of menstruation. After menstruation cellular proliferation begins to regress, acini begin to decrease in size, and retained water is lost. After breasts have undergone changes numerous times in response to the ovarian cycle, the proliferation and involution (regression) are not uniform throughout the breast. In time, after repeated hormonal stimulation, small persistent areas of nodulations may develop. This normal physiologic change must be remembered when breast tissue is examined. Nodules may develop just before and during menstruation, when the breast is most active. The physiologic alterations in breast size and activity reach their minimum level about 5 to 7 days after menstruation stops. Therefore breast self-examination (systematic palpation of breasts to detect signs of breast cancer or other changes) is best carried out during this phase of the menstrual cycle (see Guidelines box). Table 5-1 compares the variations in physical assessment related to age difference in women.

GUIDELINES Breast Self-Examination

If you choose to do breast self-examination, the best time to examine your breasts is when breasts are not tender or swollen. Here's how to examine your breasts:

1. Lie down and put a pillow under your right shoulder. Place your right arm behind your head (Fig. 1).

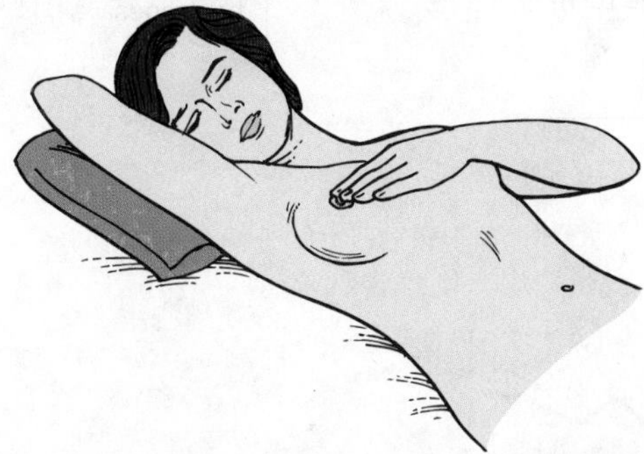

2. Use the finger pads of your three middle fingers on your left hand to feel for lumps or thickening. Your finger pads are the top third of each finger. Use circular motions of the finger pads to feel the breast tissue.
3. Press firmly enough to know how your breast feels. Use light pressure to feel the tissue just under the skin; medium pressure for a little deeper and firm pressure to feel the breast tissue close to the chest and ribs. A firm ridge in the lower curve of each breast is normal.
4. Move around the breast in an up and down pattern (Fig. 2). Go up to the collar bone and down to the ribs and from your underarm on the side to the middle of your chest. Do it the same way every time. It will help you to make sure that you've gone over the entire breast area and to remember how your breast feels.

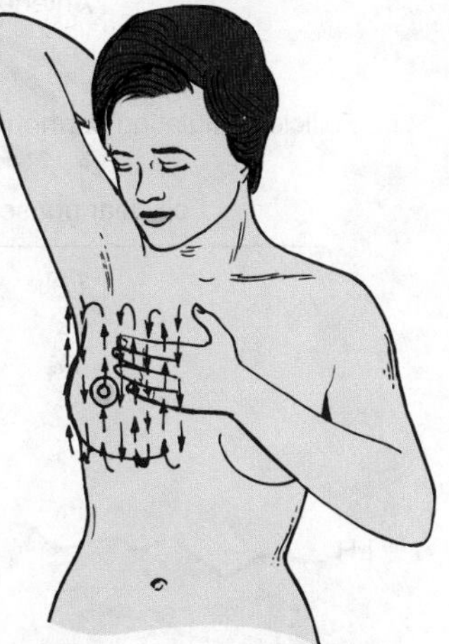

5. Now examine your left breast using the finger pads of your right hand.
6. Stand in front of a mirror and press down on your hips with your hands. See if there are any changes in the way your breasts look: dimpling of the skin, changes in the nipple, or redness or swelling.
7. Examine each underarm standing or sitting up with your arm lightly raised so that it is easy to feel in this area.
8. If you find any changes, see your health care provider right away.

Reference: American Cancer Society: *How to perform breast self-exam*, 2008. Available at www.cancer.org (accessed February 18, 2009).

evolve Skill—Breast Self-Examination

Menstruation

Menarche and Puberty

Although young girls secrete small, rather constant amounts of estrogen, a marked increase occurs between 8 and 11 years of age. The term *menarche* denotes first menstruation. *Puberty* is a broader term that denotes the entire transitional stage between childhood and sexual maturity. Increasing amounts and variations in gonadotropin and estrogen secretion develop into a cyclic pattern at least a year before menarche. In North America this occurs in most girls at about 13 years of age.

Initially menstrual periods are irregular, unpredictable, painless, and anovulatory (no ovum is released from the ovary). After 1 or more years a hypothalamic-pituitary rhythm develops, and the ovary produces adequate cyclic estrogen to make a mature ovum. Ovulatory (ovum released from the ovary) periods tend to be regular, monitored by progesterone.

Although pregnancy can occur in exceptional cases of true precocious puberty, most pregnancies in young girls occur after the normally timed menarche. All young adolescents of both sexes would benefit from knowing that pregnancy can occur at any time after the onset of menses.

Menstrual Cycle

Menstruation is the periodic uterine bleeding that begins approximately 14 days after ovulation. It is controlled by a feedback system of three cycles: endometrial, hypothalamic-pituitary, and ovarian. The average length of a menstrual cycle is 28 days, but variations are normal. The first day of bleeding is designated as day 1 of the menstrual cycle, or menses (Fig. 5-8). The average duration of menstrual flow is 5 days (with a range of 3 to 6 days), and the average blood loss is 50 ml (with a range of 20 to 80 ml), but these vary greatly.

For about 50% of women, menstrual blood does not appear to clot. The menstrual blood clots within the uterus, but the clot usually liquefies before being discharged from the uterus. Uterine discharge includes mucus and epithelial cells in addition to blood.

The menstrual cycle is a complex interplay of events that occur simultaneously in the endometrium, the hypothalamus, the pituitary glands, and the ovaries. The menstrual cycle prepares the uterus for pregnancy. When pregnancy does not occur, menstruation follows. A woman's age, physical and emotional status, and environment influence the regularity of her menstrual cycles.

evolve Spanish Guidelines—Menstruation

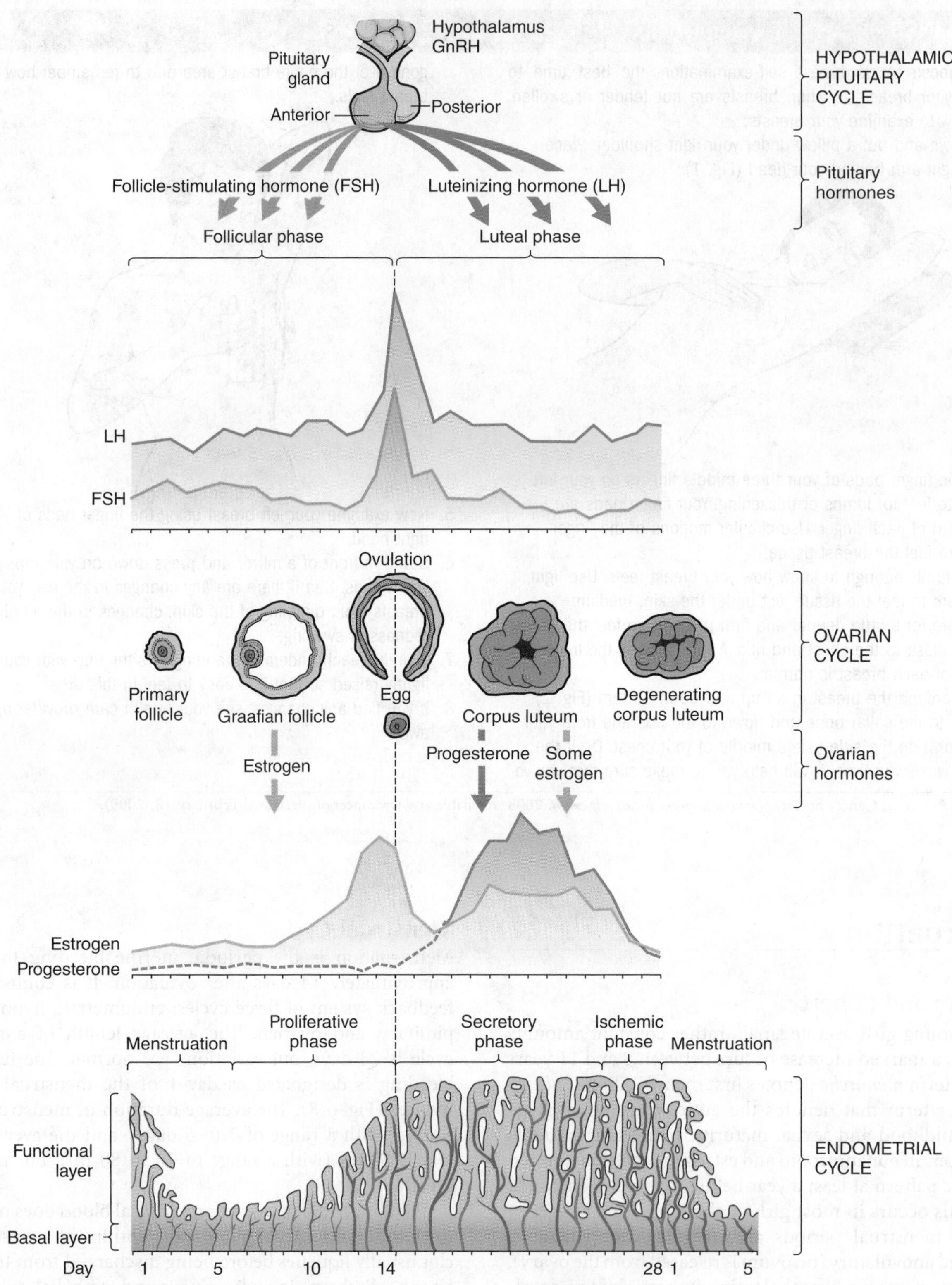

Fig. 5-8 Menstrual cycle: hypothalamic-pituitary, ovarian, and endometrial.

Endometrial Cycle

The four phases of the endometrial cycle are (1) the menstrual phase, (2) the proliferative phase, (3) the secretory phase, and (4) the ischemic phase (see Fig. 5-8). During the menstrual phase shedding of the functional two thirds of the endometrium (the compact and spongy layers) is initiated by periodic vasoconstriction in the upper layers of the endometrium. The basal layer is always retained, and regeneration begins near the end of the cycle from cells derived from the remaining glandular remnants or stromal cells in this layer.

The proliferative phase is a period of rapid growth lasting from about the fifth day to the time of ovulation. The endometrial surface is completely restored in approximately 4 days, or slightly before bleeding ceases. From this point on an eight-fold to tenfold thickening occurs, with a leveling off of growth at ovulation. The proliferative phase depends on estrogen stimulation derived from ovarian follicles.

The secretory phase extends from the day of ovulation to about 3 days before the next menstrual period. After ovulation larger amounts of progesterone are produced. An edematous, vascular, functional endometrium is now apparent. At the end of the secretory phase the fully matured secretory endometrium reaches the thickness of heavy, soft velvet. It becomes luxuriant with blood and glandular secretions, a suitable protective and nutritive bed for a fertilized ovum.

Implantation of the fertilized ovum generally occurs about 7 to 10 days after ovulation. If fertilization and implantation do not occur, the corpus luteum, which secretes estrogen and progesterone, regresses. With the rapid decrease in progesterone and estrogen levels, the spiral arteries go into spasm. During the ischemic phase the blood supply to the functional endometrium is blocked, and necrosis develops. The functional layer separates from the basal layer, and menstrual bleeding begins, marking day 1 of the next cycle (see Fig. 5-8).

Hypothalamic-Pituitary Cycle

Toward the end of the normal menstrual cycle, blood levels of estrogen and progesterone decrease. Low blood levels of these ovarian hormones stimulate the hypothalamus to secrete gonadotropin-releasing hormone (GnRH). In turn, GnRH stimulates anterior pituitary secretion of follicle-stimulating hormone (FSH). FSH stimulates development of ovarian graafian follicles and their production of estrogen. Estrogen levels begin to decrease, and hypothalamic GnRH triggers the anterior pituitary to release luteinizing hormone (LH). A marked surge of LH and a smaller peak of estrogen (day 12; see Fig. 5-8) precede the expulsion of the ovum from the graafian follicle by about 24 to 36 hours. LH peaks at about day 13 or 14 of a 28-day cycle. If fertilization and implantation of the ovum have not occurred by this time, regression of the corpus luteum follows. Levels of progesterone and estrogen decline, menstruation occurs, and the hypothalamus is once again stimulated to secrete GnRH. This process is called the hypothalamic-pituitary cycle.

Ovarian Cycle

The primitive graafian follicles contain immature oocytes (primordial ova). Before ovulation from 1 to 30 follicles begin to mature in each ovary under the influence of FSH and estrogen. The preovulatory surge of LH affects a selected follicle. The oocyte matures, ovulation occurs, and the empty follicle begins its transformation into the corpus luteum. This follicular phase (preovulatory phase) (see Fig. 5-8) of the ovarian cycle varies in length from woman to woman. Almost all variations in ovarian cycle length are the result of variations in the length of the follicular phase. On rare occasions (i.e., 1 in 100 menstrual cycles) more than one follicle is selected, and more than one oocyte matures and undergoes ovulation.

After ovulation, estrogen levels drop. For 90% of women only a small amount of withdrawal bleeding occurs, and it goes unnoticed. In 10% of women there is sufficient bleeding for it to be visible, resulting in what is termed *midcycle bleeding.*

The luteal phase begins immediately after ovulation and ends with the start of menstruation. This postovulatory phase of the ovarian cycle usually requires 14 days (range 13 to 15 days). The corpus luteum reaches its peak of functional activity 8 days after ovulation, secreting the steroids estrogen and progesterone. Coincident with this time of peak luteal functioning, the fertilized ovum is implanted in the endometrium. If no implantation occurs, the corpus luteum regresses, and steroid levels drop. Two weeks after ovulation, if fertilization and implantation do not occur, the functional layer of the uterine endometrium is shed through menstruation.

Other Cyclic Changes

When the hypothalamic-pituitary-ovarian axis functions properly, other tissues undergo predictable responses. Before ovulation the woman's basal body temperature is often less than 37° C; after ovulation, with increasing progesterone levels, her basal body temperature rises. Changes in the cervix and cervical mucus follow a generally predictable pattern. Preovulatory and postovulatory mucus is viscous (thick) so that sperm penetration is discouraged. At the time of ovulation cervical mucus is thin and clear. It looks, feels, and stretches like egg white. This stretchable quality is termed *spinnbarkeit.* Some women have localized lower abdominal pain called *mittelschmerz* that coincides with ovulation. Some spotting may occur.

Prostaglandins

Prostaglandins (PGs) are oxygenated fatty acids classified as hormones. The different kinds of PGs are distinguished by letters (PGE and PGF), numbers (PGE$_2$), and letters of the Greek alphabet (PGF$_{2\alpha}$).

PGs are produced in most organs of the body, including the uterus. Menstrual blood is a potent PG source. PGs are metabolized quickly by most tissues. They are biologically active in minute amounts in the cardiovascular, gastrointestinal, respiratory, urogenital, and nervous systems. They also exert a marked effect on metabolism, particularly on glycolysis. PGs play an important role in many physiologic, pathologic, and pharmacologic reactions. PGF$_{2\alpha}$, PGE$_4$, and PGE$_2$ are most commonly used in reproductive medicine.

PGs affect smooth muscle contractility and modulation of hormonal activity. Indirect evidence indicates that PGs have an effect on ovulation, fertility, changes in the cervix and cervical mucus that affect receptivity to sperm, tubal and uterine motility, sloughing of endometrium (menstruation), onset of miscarriage and induced abortion, and onset of labor (term and preterm).

After exerting their biologic actions, newly synthesized PGs are rapidly metabolized by tissues in such organs as the lungs, kidneys, and liver.

PGs may play a key role in ovulation. If PG levels do not rise along with the surge of LH, the ovum remains trapped within the graafian follicle. After ovulation PGs may influence production of estrogen and progesterone by the corpus luteum.

The introduction of PGs into the vagina or the uterine cavity (from ejaculated semen) increases the motility of uterine musculature, which may assist the transport of sperm through the uterus and into the oviduct.

PGs produced by the woman cause regression of the corpus luteum and regression and sloughing of the endometrium, resulting in menstruation. PGs increase myometrial response

evolve Animation—Ovarian Torsion

evolve Animation—Menstrual Cycle: Uterine

evolve Animation—Ovulation

to oxytocic stimulation, enhance uterine contractions, and cause cervical dilation. They may be a factor in the initiation of labor, the maintenance of labor, or both. They may also be involved in dysmenorrhea (see Chapter 6) and preeclampsia/eclampsia (see Chapter 14).

Climacteric and Menopause

The climacteric is a transitional phase during which ovarian function and hormone production decline. This phase spans the years from the onset of premenopausal ovarian decline to the postmenopausal time when symptoms stop. Menopause (from the Latin *mensis,* month, and Greek *pauses,* to cease) refers only to the last menstrual period. However, unlike menarche, menopause can be dated with certainty only 1 year after menstruation ceases. The average age at natural menopause is 51.4 years, with an age range of 35 to 60 years. Perimenopause is a period preceding menopause that lasts about 4 years. During this time ovarian function declines. Ova slowly diminish, and menstrual cycles may be anovulatory, resulting in irregular bleeding. The ovary stops producing estrogen, and eventually menses no longer occur.

Sexual Response

The hypothalamus and anterior pituitary glands in females regulate the production of FSH and LH. The target tissue for these hormones is the ovary, which produces ova and secretes estrogen and progesterone. A feedback mechanism between hormone secretion from the ovaries, the hypothalamus, and the anterior pituitary aids in the control of the production of sex cells and steroid sex hormone secretion.

Although the first outward appearance of maturing sexual development occurs at an earlier age in females, both females and males achieve physical maturity at approximately 17 years of age; however, individual development varies greatly. Anatomic and reproductive differences notwithstanding, women and men are more alike than different in their physiologic response to sexual excitement and orgasm. For example, the glans clitoris and the glans penis are embryonic homologues. Little difference exists between female and male sexual response; the physical response is essentially the same whether stimulated by coitus, fantasy, or masturbation. Physiologic sexual response can be analyzed in terms of two processes: vasocongestion and myotonia.

Sexual stimulation results in increase in circulation to circumvaginal blood vessels (lubrication in the female), causing engorgement and distention of the genitals. Venous congestion is localized primarily in the genitals, but it also occurs to a lesser degree in the breasts and other parts of the body. Arousal is characterized by myotonia (increased muscular tension), resulting in voluntary and involuntary rhythmic contractions. Examples of sexually stimulated myotonia are pelvic thrusting, facial grimacing, and spasms of the hands and feet (carpopedal spasms).

The sexual response cycle is divided into four phases: excitement, plateau, orgasmic, and resolution. The four phases occur progressively, with no sharp dividing line between any two phases. Specific body changes take place in sequence. The time, intensity, and duration for cyclic completion also vary for individuals and situations. Table 5-2 compares male and female body changes during each of the four phases of the sexual response cycle.

Table 5-2 Four Phases of Sexual Response

REACTIONS COMMON TO BOTH SEXES	FEMALE REACTIONS	MALE REACTIONS
Excitement Phase		
Heart rate and blood pressure increase. Nipples become erect. Myotonia begins.	Clitoris increases in diameter and swells. External genitals become congested and darken. Vaginal lubrication occurs; upper two thirds of vagina lengthen and extend. Cervix and uterus pull upward. Breast size increases.	Erection of the penis begins; penis increases in length and diameter. Scrotal skin becomes congested and thickens. Testes begin to increase in size and elevate toward the body.
Plateau Phase		
Heart rate and blood pressure continue to increase. Respirations increase. Myotonia becomes pronounced; grimacing occurs.	Clitoral head retracts under the clitoral hood. Lower one third of vagina becomes engorged. Skin color changes occur—red flush may be observed across breasts, abdomen, or other surfaces.	Head of penis may enlarge slightly. Scrotum continues to grow tense and thicken. Testes continue to elevate and enlarge. Preorgasmic emission of two or three drops of fluid appears on the head of the penis.
Orgasmic Phase		
Heart rate, blood pressure, and respirations increase to maximum levels. Involuntary muscle spasms occur. External rectal sphincter contracts.	Strong rhythmic contractions are felt in the clitoris, vagina, and uterus. Sensations of warmth spread through the pelvic area.	Testes elevate to maximum level. Point of "inevitability" occurs just before ejaculation and an awareness of fluid in the urethra. Rhythmic contractions occur in the penis. Ejaculation of semen occurs.
Resolution Phase		
Heart rate, blood pressure, and respirations return to normal. Nipple erection subsides. Myotonia subsides.	Engorgement in external genitalia and vagina resolves. Uterus descends to normal position. Cervix dips into seminal pool. Breast size decreases. Skin flush disappears.	Fifty percent of erection is lost immediately with ejaculation; penis gradually returns to normal size. Testes and scrotum return to normal size. Refractory period (time needed for erection to occur again) varies according to age and general physical condition.

Health Assessment

Trends in women's health have expanded beyond a reproductive focus to include a holistic approach to health care across the life span and place women's health within the scope of primary care. Women's health assessment and screening focus on a systems evaluation that begins with a careful history and physical examination. During assessment and evaluation the responsibility for self-management, health promotion, and enhancement of wellness is emphasized.

In a market-driven system such as managed care, specific guidelines may be provided for health screening by the insurer or the managed care organization. A nurse often takes the history, orders diagnostic tests, interprets test results, makes referrals, coordinates care, and directs attention to problems requiring medical intervention. Advanced practice nurses who have specialized in women's health such as nurse practitioners, clinical nurse specialists, and nurse-midwives perform complete physical examinations, including gynecologic examinations (see Community Focus box).

COMMUNITY FOCUS

Referral Resources

Identify resources in your community for referring the following women: a woman with severe physical disability without health insurance; a 72-year-old widow with diabetes who lives by herself; a 24-year-old with a body mass index greater than 30 desiring a fitness program. Evaluate the resources in terms of access, confidentiality, cost, and follow-up services. Develop a resource file for each.

Culturally competent nursing care should be delivered with an awareness of cultural diversity while respecting the unique qualities of each woman. Such care cannot be provided in the absence of self-awareness. Nurses must acknowledge their own values, beliefs, and communication styles to understand what they contribute to cross-cultural communication.

Interview

Contact with the woman usually begins with an interview. This interview should be conducted in a private, comfortable, and relaxed setting (Fig. 5-9). The nurse is seated and makes sure that the woman is comfortable. The woman is addressed by her title and name (e.g., Mrs. Martinez), and the nurse introduces herself or himself using name and title. It is important to phrase questions in a sensitive and nonjudgmental manner. Body language should match oral communication. The nurse is aware of a woman's vulnerability and assures her of strict confidentiality. For many women, fear, anxiety, and modesty make the examination a dreaded and stressful experience. Many women are uninformed, misguided by myths, or afraid they will appear ignorant by asking questions about sexual or reproductive functioning. The woman is assured that no question is irrelevant.

The history begins with an open-ended question such as, "What brings you into the office/clinic/hospital today?" and is furthered by other questions such as "Anything else?" and "Tell me about it." Additional ways to encourage women to share information include the following:

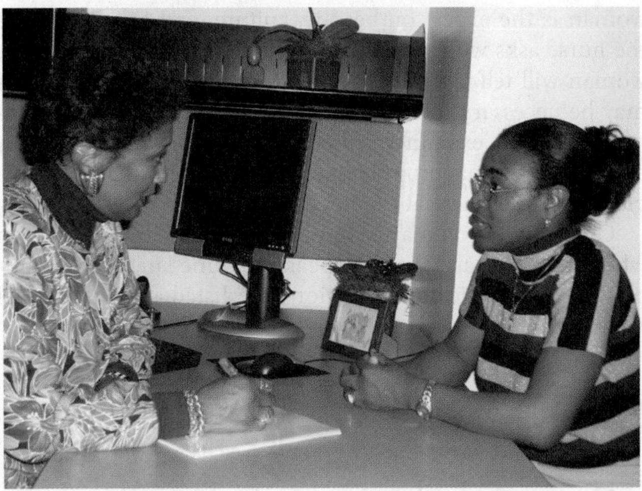

Fig. 5-9 Nurse interviews patient as part of annual physical examination. *(Courtesy Skip Davis, San Francisco, CA.)*

- **Facilitation**—Using a word or posture that communicates interest such as leaning forward, making eye contact, or saying "Mm-hmmm" or "Go on"
- **Reflection**—Repeating a word or phrase that a woman has used
- **Clarification**—Asking the woman what is meant by a stated word or phrase
- **Empathic responses**—Acknowledging the feelings of a woman by statements such as "That must have been frightening"
- **Confrontation**—Identifying something about the woman's behavior or feelings not expressed verbally or apparently inconsistent with her history
- **Interpretation**—Putting into words what you infer about the woman's feelings or about the meaning of her symptoms, events, or other matters

Direct questions may be necessary to elicit specific details. These should be worded in language that is understandable to the woman and expressed neutrally so that the woman will not be led into a specific response. The nurse asks about one item at a time and proceeds from the general to the specific (Seidel et al, 2006).

Cultural Considerations and Communication Variations

Recognizing signs and symptoms of disease and deciding to seek treatment are influenced by cultural perceptions. Culture evolves over time and is a system of symbols that are learned, shared, and passed on through generations of a social group. Cultural competence in nursing is a complex combination of knowledge, attitudes, and skills mixed with personal attributes of flexibility, empathy, and language facility. It is more than simply acquiring knowledge about another ethnic group. It is essential that a nurse have respect for the rich and unique qualities that cultural diversity brings to individuals. In recognizing the value of these differences, the nurse can modify the plan of care to meet the needs of each woman. Trust that the woman is the expert on her life, culture, and experiences. If the nurse asks with respect and a genuine desire to learn, the woman will tell the nurse how to care for her. Modifications may be necessary for the physical examination. In many cultures a woman examiner is preferred. In some cultures it may be considered inappropriate for the woman to disrobe completely for the physical examination.

Communication may be hindered by different beliefs, even when the nurse and woman speak the same language. Examples of communication variations are listed in the Cultural Awareness box.

CULTURAL AWARENESS

Communication Variations

Conversational style and pacing—Silence may show respect or acknowledgment that the listener has heard. In cultures in which a direct "no" is considered rude, silence may mean no. Repetition or loudness may mean emphasis or anger.

Personal space—Cultural conceptions of personal space differ. For example, based on one's culture, someone may be perceived as distant for backing off when approached or aggressive for standing too close.

Eye contact—Eye contact varies among cultures from intense to fleeting. Consistent with the effort to refrain from invading personal space, avoiding direct eye contact may be a sign of respect.

Touch—The norms about how people should touch each other vary among cultures. In some cultures physical contact with the same sex (embracing, walking hand in hand) is more appropriate than that with an unrelated person of the opposite sex.

Time orientation—In some cultures involvement with people is more valued than being "on time." In other cultures life is scheduled and paced according to clock time, which is valued over personal time.

Reference: Mattson S: Striving for cultural competence: providing care for the changing face of the U.S., *AWHONN Lifelines* 4(3):48-52, 2000.

Women with Special Needs

Women with Disabilities

Women with emotional or physical disorders have special needs. Women who have vision, hearing, emotional, or physical disabilities should be respected and involved in the assessment and physical examination to the full extent of their capabilities. The nurse should communicate openly, directly, and with sensitivity. It is often helpful to learn about the disability directly from the woman while maintaining eye contact. Family and significant others should be relied on only when absolutely necessary. The assessment and physical examination can be adapted to each woman's individual needs.

Communication with a woman who is hearing impaired can be accomplished without difficulty. Many of these women can read lips, write, or both. The interviewer who speaks and enunciates each word slowly and in full view may be easily understood. If a woman is not comfortable with lip reading, she may use an interpreter. In this case it is important to continue to address the woman directly, avoiding the temptation to speak directly with the interpreter.

The visually impaired woman needs to be oriented to the examination room and may have her guide dog with her. As with all patients, the visually impaired woman needs a full explanation of what the examination entails before proceeding. Before touching her, the nurse explains, "Now I am going to take your blood pressure. I am going to place the cuff on your right arm." The woman can be asked if she would like to touch each of the items that will be used in the examination to reduce her anxiety.

Many women with physical disabilities cannot comfortably lie in the lithotomy position for the pelvic examination. Several alternative positions may be used, including a lateral (side-lying) position, a V-shaped position, a diamond-shaped position, and an M-shaped position (Fig. 5-10). The woman can be asked what has worked best for her previously. If she has never had a pelvic examination or has never had a comfortable pelvic examination, the nurse proceeds slowly by showing her a picture of various positions and asking her which one she prefers. The nurse's support and reassurance can help the woman to relax, which will make the examination go more smoothly.

Abused Women

Nurses should screen all women entering the health care system for abuse. Abuse is a life-threatening public health problem that affects millions of women and their children. The risk for intimate partner violence increases during pregnancy and after separation or divorce. Help for the woman may depend on the sensitivity with which the nurse screens for abuse, the discovery of abuse, and subsequent intervention. The nurse must be familiar with the laws governing abuse in the state in which she or he practices.

Pocket cards listing emergency numbers (abuse counseling, legal protection, and emergency shelter) may be obtained from local police departments, women's shelters, or emergency departments. It is helpful to have these on hand in the setting where screening is done. An abuse assessment screen (Fig. 5-11) can be used as part of the interview or written history. If a male partner is present, he should be asked to leave the room because the woman may not disclose experiences of abuse in his presence, or he may try to answer questions for her to protect himself. The same procedure applies for partners of lesbians or the adult children of older women.

Fear, guilt, and embarrassment may keep many women from giving information about family violence. Clues in the history and evidence of injuries on physical examination should give a high index of suspicion. The areas most commonly injured in women are the head, neck, chest, abdomen, breasts, and upper extremities. Burns and bruises in patterns resembling hands, belts, cords, or other weapons may be seen, as well as multiple traumatic injuries. Attention should be given to women who repeatedly seek treatment for somatic complaints such as headaches; insomnia; choking sensations; hyperventilation; gastrointestinal symptoms; and pain in the chest, back, or pelvis. During pregnancy the nurse should assess for injuries to the breasts, abdomen, and genitalia. See Chapter 4 for further discussion of violence.

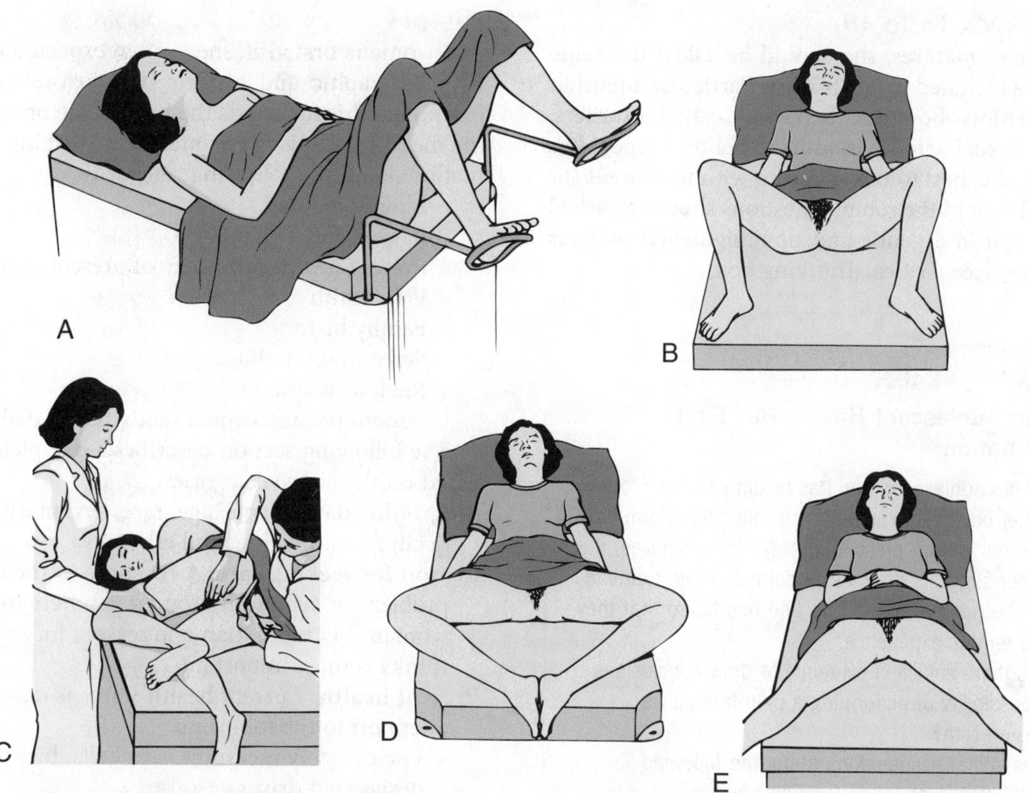

Fig. 5-10 Lithotomy and variable positions for women who have a disability. **A,** Lithotomy position. **B,** M-shaped position. **C,** Side-lying position. **D,** Diamond-shaped position. **E,** V-shaped position.

ABUSE ASSESSMENT SCREEN

1. Have you ever been emotionally or physically abused by your partner or someone important to you?

YES ☐ NO ☐

2. Within the last year, have you been hit, slapped, kicked, or otherwise physically hurt by someone?

YES ☐ NO ☐

If YES, by whom? ______________________

Number of times ______________________

Mark the area of injury on body map.

3. Within the last year, has anyone forced you to have sexual activities?

YES ☐ NO ☐

If YES, who? ______________________

Number of times ______________________

4. Are you afraid of your partner or anyone you listed above?

YES ☐ NO ☐

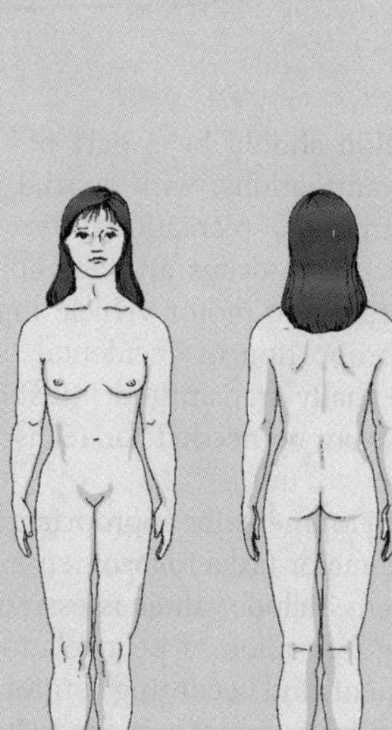

Fig. 5-11 Abuse assessment screen. *(Modified from the Nursing Research Consortium on Violence and Abuse, 1991.)*

Adolescents (Ages 13 to 19)

As a young woman matures, she should be asked the same questions that are included in any history. Particular attention should be paid to hints about risky behaviors, eating disorders, and depression. Sexual activity is addressed after rapport has been established. It is best to talk to a teen with the parent (or partner or friend) out of the room. Questions should be asked with sensitivity and in a gentle and nonjudgmental manner (Seidel et al, 2006) (see Critical Thinking box).

CRITICAL THINKING EXERCISE

Caring for an Adolescent Having Her First Pelvic Examination

Nita, a 16-year-old adolescent, who has recently had sex for the first time with her boyfriend, comes to the clinic for information about birth control. Before prescribing any contraceptives, the nurse practitioner suggests that she perform a pelvic examination. Nita said she has never had one and has heard that they hurt and are "a terrible experience."

1. Evidence—Is there sufficient evidence to draw conclusions about the possibility of performing a pain-free pelvic examination on Nita?
2. Assumptions—What assumptions about the following factors can be made about performing a pelvic examination on an adolescent?
   a. Need for confidentiality
   b. The nurse's usual assessment procedure
   c. Equipment needed for pelvic examination of a young girl or woman
   d. Necessary education about sexuality and prevention of sexually transmitted infections and pregnancy
3. What implications and priorities for nursing care can be drawn at this time?
4. Does the evidence objectively support your conclusion?
5. Are there alternative perspectives to your conclusion?

Injury prevention should be a part of the counseling at routine health examinations, with special attention to seat belts, helmets, firearms, recreational hazards, and sports involvement. The use of drugs and alcohol and the nonuse of seat belts contribute to motor vehicle injuries, accounting for the greatest proportion of accidental deaths in women. Contraceptives/sexually transmitted infection (STI) prevention information may be needed for teens who are sexually active.

To provide developmentally appropriate care, it is important to review the major tasks for women in this stage of life. Major tasks for teens include values assessment; education and work goal setting; formation of peer relationships that focus on love, commitment, and becoming comfortable with sexuality; and separation from parents. The teen is egocentric as she progresses rapidly through emotional and physical change. Her feelings of invulnerability may lead to misconceptions such as the belief that unprotected sexual intercourse will not lead to pregnancy.

History

At a woman's first visit, she is often expected to fill out a form with biographic and historic data before meeting with the examiner. This form aids the health care provider in completing the history during the interview. Most forms include information about the following categories:

- Biographic data
- Reason for seeking care
- Present health or history of present illness
- Past health
- Family history
- Screening for abuse
- Review of systems
- Functional assessment (activities of daily living)

The following section describes a complete health history based on the above categories.

Biographic data: Name, age, race, sex, marital status, occupation, religion, and ethnicity

Reason for seeking care: A response to the question, "What problem or symptom brought you here today?" If the woman lists more than one reason, focus on the one she thinks is most important.

Present health: Current health status is described with attention to the following:

- Use of safety measures: seat belts, bicycle helmets, designated driver
- Exercise and leisure activities: regularity
- Sleep patterns: length and quality
- Sexuality: Is she sexually active? With men, women, or both? STI/pregnancy prevention practices?
- Diet, including beverages: 24-hour dietary recall; caffeine: coffee, tea, cola, or chocolate intake
- Nicotine, alcohol, illicit or recreational drug use: type, amount, frequency, duration, and reactions
- Environmental and chemical hazards: home, school, work, and leisure setting; exposure to extreme heat or cold, noise, industrial toxins such as asbestos or lead, pesticides, diethylstilbestrol, radiation, cat feces, or cigarette smoke

History of present illness: A chronologic narrative that includes onset of the problem, the setting in which it developed, its manifestations, and any treatments received is recorded. The woman's state of health before the onset of the present problem is determined. If the problem is of long standing, the reason for seeking attention at this time is elicited. The principal symptoms should be described with respect to the following:

- Location
- Quality or character
- Quantity or severity
- Timing (onset, duration, frequency)
- Setting
- Factors that aggravate or relieve
- Associated factors
- Woman's perception of the meaning of the symptom

Past health:

- Infectious diseases: For example, measles, mumps, rubella, whooping cough, chickenpox, rheumatic fever, scarlet fever, diphtheria, polio, tuberculosis (TB), hepatitis

- Chronic disease and system disorders: arthritis, cancer, diabetes, heart, lung, kidney, seizures, thyroid, stroke, ulcers, sickle cell anemia
- Adult injuries, accidents
- Hospitalizations, operations, blood transfusions
- Obstetric history
- Allergies: medications, previous transfusion reactions, environmental allergies
- Immunizations: diphtheria; pertussis; tetanus; polio; measles, mumps, rubella; hepatitis B; varicella; influenza; pneumococcal vaccine; last TB skin test
- Last date of screening tests: Pap test, mammogram; stool for occult blood; sigmoidoscopy/colonoscopy; hematocrit; hemoglobin; rubella titer; urinalysis; cholesterol test; electrocardiogram; vision, dental, hearing examinations
- Current medications: name, dose, frequency, duration, reason for taking, and compliance with prescription medications; home remedies, over-the-counter drugs, vitamin and mineral or herbal supplements used over a 24-hour period

Family history: Information about age and health of family members may be presented in narrative form or as a family tree or genogram: age, health/death of parents, siblings, spouse, children. Check for history of diabetes; heart disease; hypertension; stroke; respiratory, renal, or thyroid problems; cancer; bleeding disorders; hepatitis; allergies; asthma; arthritis; TB; epilepsy; mental illness; human immunodeficiency virus (HIV); or other disorders.

Screen for abuse: Has she ever been hit, kicked, slapped, or forced to have sex against her wishes? Has she been verbally or emotionally abused? Does she have a history of childhood sexual abuse? If yes, has she received counseling or does she need referral?

Review of systems: It is probable that all questions in each system will not be included every time a history is taken. Some questions regarding each system should be included in every history. The essential areas to be explored are listed in the following head-to-toe sequence. If a woman gives a positive response to a question about an essential area, more detailed questions should be asked.

- General: weight change, fatigue, weakness, fever, chills, or night sweats
- Skin: skin, hair, and nail changes; itching, bruising, bleeding, rashes, sores, lumps, or moles
- Lymph nodes: enlargement, inflammation, pain, suppuration (pus), or drainage
- Head: trauma, vertigo (dizziness), convulsive disorder, syncope (fainting); headache: location, frequency, pain type, nausea/vomiting, or visual symptoms present
- Eyes: glasses, contact lenses, blurriness, tearing, itching, photophobia, diplopia, inflammation, trauma, cataracts, glaucoma, or acute visual loss
- Ears: hearing loss, tinnitus (ringing), vertigo, discharge, pain, fullness, recurrent infections, or mastoiditis
- Nose/sinuses: trauma, rhinitis, nasal discharge, epistaxis, obstruction, sneezing, itching, allergy, or smelling impairment
- Mouth/throat/neck: hoarseness, voice changes, soreness, ulcers, bleeding gums, goiter, swelling, or enlarged nodes
- Breasts: masses, pain, lumps, dimpling, nipple discharge, fibrocystic changes, or implants; breast self-examination practice
- Respiratory: shortness of breath, wheezing, cough, sputum, hemoptysis, pneumonia, pleurisy, asthma, bronchitis, emphysema, or TB; date of last chest x-ray
- Cardiovascular: hypertension, rheumatic fever, murmurs, angina, palpitations, dyspnea, tachycardia, orthopnea, edema, chest pain, cough, cyanosis, cold extremities, ascites, intermittent claudication (leg pain caused by poor circulation to the leg muscles), phlebitis, or skin-color changes
- Gastrointestinal: appetite, nausea, vomiting, indigestion, dysphagia, abdominal pain, ulcers, hematochezia (bleeding with stools), melena (black, tarry stools), bowel-habit changes, diarrhea, constipation, bowel-movement frequency, food intolerance, hemorrhoids, jaundice, or hepatitis; sigmoidoscopy, colonoscopy, barium enema, ultrasound
- Genitourinary: frequency, hesitancy, urgency, polyuria, dysuria, hematuria, nocturia, incontinence, stones, infection, or urethral discharge; menstrual history (e.g., age at menarche, length/flow of menses, last menstrual period, dysmenorrhea, intermenstrual bleeding, age at menopause or signs of menopause), dyspareunia, discharge, sores, itching
- Sexual health: sexual activity: with men, women, or both; contraceptive use; STIs
- Peripheral vascular: coldness, numbness and tingling, leg edema, claudication, varicose veins, thromboses, or emboli
- Endocrine: heat/cold intolerance, dry skin, excessive sweating, polyuria, polydipsia, polyphagia, thyroid problems, diabetes, or secondary sex characteristic changes
- Hematologic: anemia, easy bruising, bleeding, petechiae, purpura, or transfusions
- Musculoskeletal: muscle weakness, pain, joint stiffness, scoliosis, lordosis, kyphosis, range-of-motion instability, redness, swelling, arthritis, or gout
- Neurologic: loss of sensation, numbness, tingling, tremors, weakness, vertigo, paralysis, fainting, twitching, blackouts, seizures, convulsions, loss of consciousness or memory
- Mental status: moodiness, depression, anxiety, obsessions, delusions, illusions, or hallucinations

Functional assessment: Ability to care for self

Physical Examination

In preparation for the physical examination, the woman is instructed on undressing and given a gown to wear during the examination. She is usually given the opportunity to undress privately. Objective data are recorded by system or location. A general statement of overall health status is a good way to start. Findings are described in detail.

evolve Case Study—Health Assessment

- General appearance: age, race, sex, state of health, posture, height, weight, development, dress, hygiene, affect, alertness, orientation, cooperativeness, and communication skills
- Vital signs: temperature, pulse, respiration, blood pressure
- Skin: color; integrity; texture; hydration; temperature; edema; excessive perspiration; unusual odor; presence and description of lesions; hair texture and distribution; nail configuration, color, texture, and condition; presence of nail clubbing
- Head: size, shape, trauma, masses, scars, rashes, or scaling; facial symmetry; presence of edema or puffiness
- Eyes: pupil size, shape, reactivity, conjunctival injection, scleral icterus, fundal papilledema, hemorrhage, lids, extraocular movements, visual fields and acuity
- Ears: shape and symmetry, tenderness, discharge, external canal, and tympanic membranes; hearing—Weber should be midline (loudness of sound equal in both ears) and Rinne negative (no conductive or sensorineural hearing loss); should be able to hear whisper at 3 feet
- Nose: symmetry, tenderness, discharge, mucosa, turbinate inflammation, frontal or maxillary sinus tenderness; discrimination of odors
- Mouth and throat: hygiene; condition of teeth; dentures; appearance of lips, tongue, buccal and oral mucosa; erythema; edema; exudate; tonsillar enlargement; palate; uvula; gag reflex; ulcers
- Neck: mobility, masses, range of motion, trachea deviation, thyroid size, carotid bruits
- Lymphatic: cervical, intraclavicular, axillary, trochlear, or inguinal adenopathy; size, shape, tenderness, and consistency
- Breasts: skin changes, dimpling, symmetry, scars, tenderness, discharge, or masses; characteristics of nipples and areolae
- Heart: rate, rhythm, murmurs, rubs, gallops, clicks, heaves, or precordial movements
- Peripheral vascular: jugular vein distention, bruits, edema, swelling, vein distention, Homan sign, or tenderness of extremities
- Lungs: chest symmetry with respirations, wheezes, crackles, rhonchi, vocal fremitus, whispered pectoriloquy, percussion, and diaphragmatic excursion; breath sounds equal and clear bilaterally
- Abdomen: shape, scars, bowel sounds, consistency, tenderness, rebound, masses, guarding, organomegaly, liver span, percussion (tympany, shifting, dullness), or costovertebral angle tenderness
- Extremities: edema, ulceration, tenderness, varicosities, erythema, tremor, or deformity
- Genitourinary: external genitalia, perineum, vaginal mucosa, cervix; inflammation, tenderness, discharge, bleeding, ulcers, nodules, or masses; internal vaginal support, bimanual and rectovaginal palpation of cervix, uterus, and adnexa
- Rectal: sphincter tone, masses, hemorrhoids, rectal wall contour, tenderness, and stool for occult blood
- Musculoskeletal: posture, symmetry of muscle mass, muscle atrophy, weakness, appearance of joints, tenderness or crepitus, joint range of motion, instability, redness, swelling, or spine deviation
- Neurologic: mental status, orientation, memory, mood, speech clarity and comprehension, cranial nerves II to XII, sensation, strength, deep tendon and superficial reflexes, gait, balance, and coordination with rapid alternating motions

evolve Spanish Guidelines—Physical Examination

Pelvic Examination

Many women fear the gynecologic portion of the physical examination. The nurse can be instrumental in allaying these fears by providing information and assisting the woman to express her feelings to the examiner (Box 5-1).

The woman is assisted into the lithotomy position (see Fig. 5-10, *A*) for the pelvic examination. When she is in the lithotomy position, the woman's hips and knees are flexed, with buttocks at the edge of the table, and her feet are supported by heel or knee stirrups.

Some women prefer to keep their shoes or socks on, especially if the stirrups are not padded. Many women express feelings of vulnerability and strangeness when in the lithotomy position. During the procedure the nurse assists the woman with relaxation techniques.

BOX 5-1 Procedure: Assisting with Pelvic Examination (see Fig. 5-13)

1. Wash hands. Assemble equipment.
2. Ask woman to empty her bladder before the examination (obtain clean-catch urine specimen as needed).
3. Assist with relaxation techniques. Have the woman place her hands on her chest at about the level of the diaphragm, breathe deeply and slowly (in through her nose and out through her O-shaped mouth), concentrate on the rhythm of breathing, and relax all body muscles with each exhalation (Barkauskas, Baumann, & Darling-Fisher, 2002).
4. Encourage the woman to become involved with the examination if she shows interest. For example, a mirror can be placed so that she can see the area being examined.
5. Assess for and treat signs of problems such as supine hypotension.
6. Warm the speculum in warm water if a prewarmed one is not available.
7. Instruct the woman to bear down when the speculum is being inserted.
8. Apply gloves and assist the examiner with collection of specimens for cytologic examination such as a Pap test. After handling specimens, remove gloves and wash hands.
9. Lubricate the examiner's fingers with water or water-soluble lubricant before bimanual examination.
10. Assist the woman to a sitting position at completion of the examination.
11. Provide tissues to wipe lubricant from perineum.
12. Provide privacy for the woman while she is dressing.

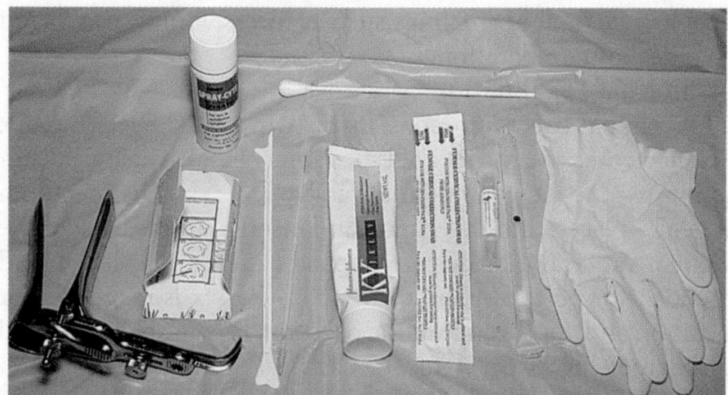

Fig. 5-12 Equipment used for pelvic examination. *(Courtesy Michael S. Clement, MD, Mesa, AZ.)*

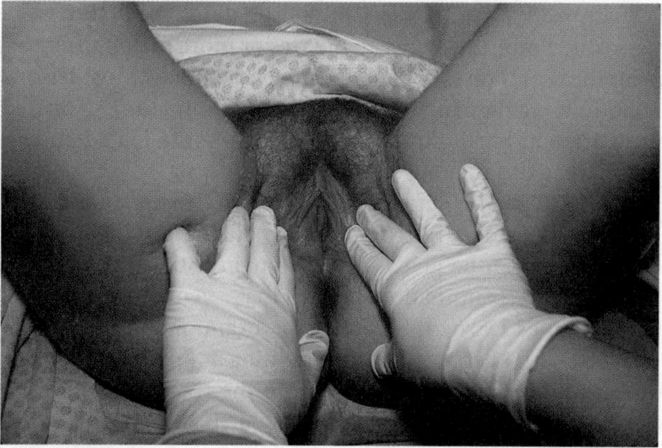

Fig. 5-13 External examination. Separation of the labia. (From Wilson SF, Giddens JF: *Health assessment for nursing practice*, ed 4, St Louis, 2009, Mosby.)

One method of helping the woman relax is to have her place her hands on her chest at about the level of the diaphragm, breathe deeply and slowly (in through her nose and out through her O-shaped mouth), concentrate on the rhythm of breathing, and relax all body muscles with each exhalation. This breathing technique is particularly helpful for the adolescent and for the woman whose introitus may be especially tight or for whom the experience is new or may provoke tension. Some women relax when they are encouraged to become involved with the examination with a mirror placed so that they can view the area being examined. This type of participation helps with health teaching as well. Distraction is another technique that can be used effectively (e.g., placing interesting pictures on the ceiling over the head of the table).

Many women find it distressing to attempt to converse in the lithotomy position. Most women appreciate an explanation of the procedure as it unfolds, as well as coaching for the type of sensations they may expect. Generally, however, women prefer not to have to respond to questions until they are again upright and at eye level with the examiner. Being asked questions during the procedure, especially if they cannot see their questioner's eyes, may make women tense.

A teen's first speculum examination is the most important because she will develop perceptions that will remain with her for future examinations. What the examination entails should be discussed with the teen while she is dressed. Models or illustrations can be used to show exactly what will happen. All of the necessary equipment should be assembled so there are no interruptions (Fig. 5-12). Pediatric specula that are 1 to 1.5 cm wide can be inserted with minimal discomfort. If the teen is sexually active, a small adult speculum may be used.

External Inspection

The examiner wears gloves and sits at the foot of the table for the inspection of the external genitals and the speculum examination. In good lighting external genitals are inspected for sexual maturity, clitoris, labia, perineum, and lesions indicative of STIs. After childbirth or other trauma there may be healed scars.

External Palpation

Before touching the woman, the examiner explains what is going to be done and what the woman should expect to feel (e.g., pressure). The examiner may touch the woman in a less sensitive area such as the inner thigh to alert her that the genital examination is beginning. This gesture may put the woman more at ease. The labia are spread apart to expose the structures in the vestibule: urinary meatus, Skene glands, vaginal orifice, and Bartholin glands (Fig. 5-13). To assess the Skene glands, the examiner inserts one finger into the vagina and "milks" the area of the urethra. Any exudate from the urethra or the Skene glands is cultured. Masses and erythema of either structure are assessed further. Ordinarily the openings to the Skene glands are not visible; prominent openings may be seen if the glands are infected (e.g., with gonorrhea). During the examination the examiner keeps in mind the data from the review of systems such as history of burning on urination.

The vaginal orifice is examined. Hymenal tags are normal findings. With one finger still in the vagina, the examiner repositions the index finger near the posterior part of the orifice. With the thumb outside the posterior part of the labia majora, the examiner compresses the area of Bartholin glands located at the 8 o'clock and 4 o'clock positions and looks for swelling, discharge, and pain.

The support of the anterior and posterior vaginal wall is assessed. The examiner spreads the labia with the index and middle finger and asks the woman to strain down. Any bulge from the anterior wall (urethrocele or cystocele) or posterior wall (rectocele) is noted and compared with the history, such as difficulty starting the stream of urine or constipation.

The perineum (area between the vagina and anus) is assessed for scars from old lacerations or episiotomies, thinning, fistulas, masses, lesions, and inflammation. The anus is assessed for hemorrhoids, hemorrhoidal tags, and integrity of the anal sphincter. The anal area is also assessed for lesions, masses, abscesses, and tumors. If there is a history of STI, the examiner may want to obtain a culture specimen from the anal canal at this time. Throughout the genital examination the examiner notes any odor, which may indicate infection or poor hygiene.

Vulvar Self-Examination

The pelvic examination provides a good opportunity for the practitioner to emphasize the need for regular vulvar self-examination (VSE) and to teach this procedure. Because there has been a dramatic increase in cancerous and precancerous conditions of the vulva in recent years, a VSE should be an integral part of preventive health care for all women who are sexually active or 18 years of age or older. VSE should be performed monthly between menses or more often if there are symptoms or a history of serious vulvar disease. Most lesions, including malignancy, condyloma acuminatum (wartlike growth), and Bartholin cysts, can be seen or palpated and are easily treated if diagnosed early.

The VSE can be performed by the practitioner and woman together by using a mirror. A simple diagram of the anatomy of the vulva can be given to the woman, with instructions to perform the examination herself that evening to reinforce what she has learned. She does the examination in a sitting position with adequate lighting, holding a mirror in one hand and using the other hand to expose the tissues surrounding the vaginal introitus. She then systematically examines the mons pubis, clitoris, urethra, labia majora, perineum, and perianal area and palpates the vulva, noting any changes in appearance or abnormalities such as ulcers, lumps, warts, and changes in pigmentation.

Internal Examination

A vaginal speculum consists of two blades and a handle. Specula come in a variety of types and styles. A vaginal speculum is used to view the vaginal vault and cervix. The speculum is gently placed into the vagina and inserted to the back of the vaginal vault. The blades are opened to reveal the cervix and are locked into the open position. The cervix is inspected for position and appearance of the os: color, lesions, bleeding, and discharge (Fig. 5-14, *A* to *D*). Cervical findings that are not within normal limits include ulcerations, masses, inflammation, and excessive protrusion into the vaginal vault. Anomalies such as a cockscomb (a protrusion over the cervix that looks like a rooster's comb), a hooded or collared cervix (seen in diethylstilbestrol daughters [Box 5-2]), or polyps are noted.

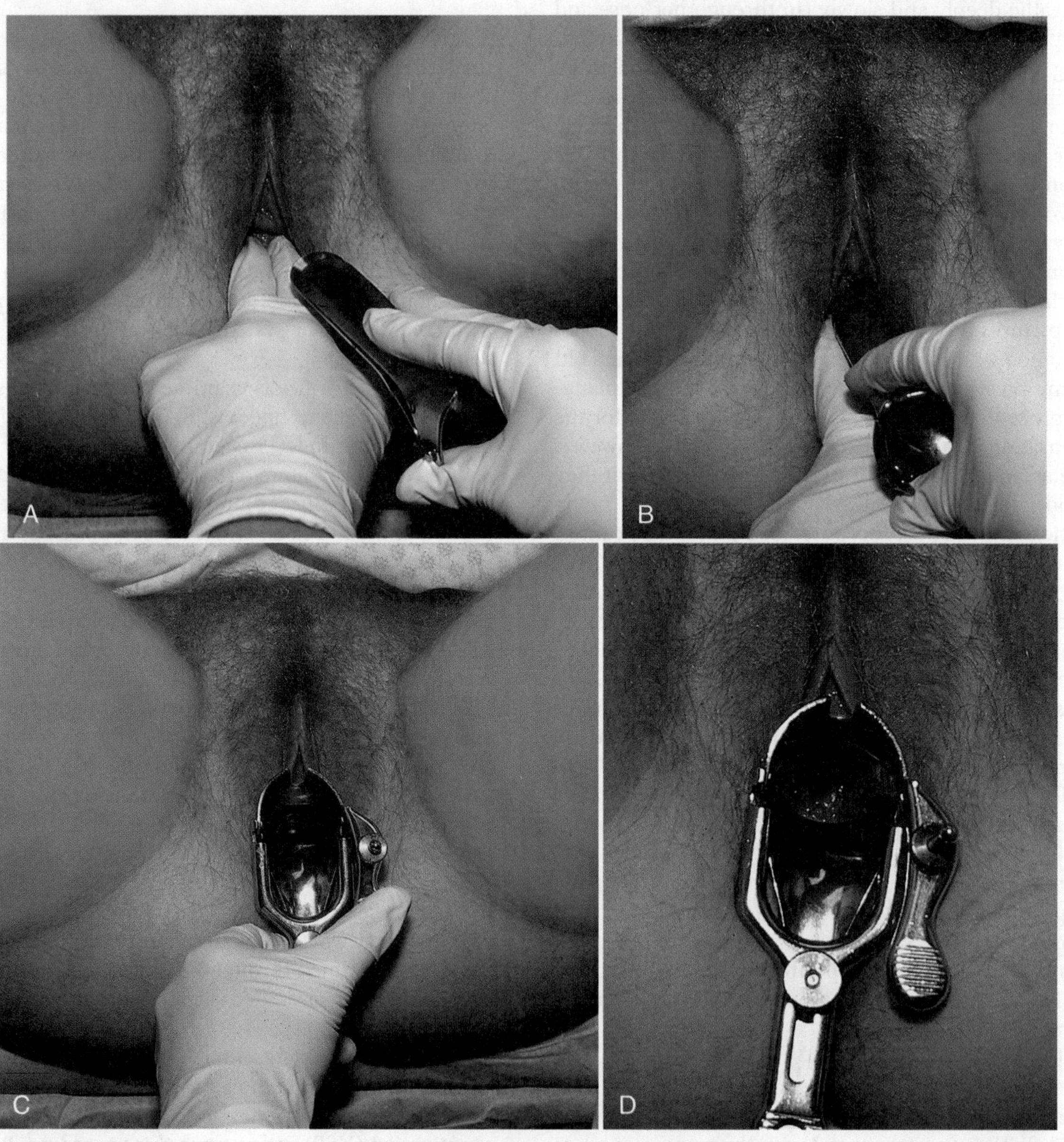

Fig. 5-14 Insertion of speculum for vaginal examination. **A,** Opening of the introitus. **B,** Oblique insertion of the speculum. **C,** Final insertion of the speculum. **D,** Opening of the speculum blades. (From Wilson SF, Giddens JF: *Health assessment for nursing practice*, ed 4, St Louis, 2009, Mosby.)

BOX 5-2 Diethylstilbestrol—Yesterday and Today

Between 1938 and 1971, 5 to 10 million pregnant women who had previously experienced a miscarriage or premature birth received diethylstilbestrol (DES) to improve their chances of having a successful pregnancy. In 1971 researchers discovered that prenatal exposure to DES increases the risk of clear cell adenocarcinoma of the cervix and vagina. At that time the Food and Drug Administration issued a warning and advised physicians to stop prescribing DES. Today researchers are discovering more adverse effects of exposure to DES. The women who received DES while pregnant have a moderate increase in the risk of breast cancer. DES daughters have an increased risk of pregnancy complications, infertility, and structural differences of the reproductive tract such as a T-shaped uterus. DES sons have an increased risk of noncancerous epididymal cysts. There are no known effects on granddaughters of women who received DES, but grandsons are 20 times more likely than those in the general population to have hypospadias.

Source: A drug of the past still haunts some, *Am J Nurs* 103(8):20, 2003.

Collection of Specimens

The collection of specimens for cytologic examination is an important part of the gynecologic examination. Infection can be diagnosed by examination of specimens collected during the pelvic examination. These infections include candidiasis, trichomoniasis, bacterial vaginosis, group B streptococcus, gonorrhea, chlamydia, and herpes simplex virus. Once the diagnoses have been made, treatment can be instituted.

Papanicolaou Test Carcinogenic conditions, whether potential or actual, can be determined by examination of cells from the cervix collected during the pelvic examination (i.e., a Pap test) (Box 5-3 and Fig. 5-15).

Vaginal Wall Examination

After the specimens are obtained, the vagina is viewed when the speculum is rotated. The speculum blades are unlocked and partially closed. As the speculum is withdrawn, it is rotated; the vaginal walls are inspected for color, lesions, rugae, fistulas, and bulging.

Bimanual Palpation The examiner stands for this part of the examination. A small amount of lubricant is placed on the first and second fingers of the gloved hand for the internal examination. To avoid tissue trauma and contamination, the

BOX 5-3 Procedure: Papanicolaou Test

1. In preparation make sure that the woman has not douched, used vaginal medications, or had sexual intercourse for at least 24 hours before the procedure. Reschedule the test if the woman is menstruating. Midcycle is the best time to test.
2. The woman is assisted into a lithotomy position. A speculum is inserted into the vagina.
3. Explain to the woman the purpose of the test and what sensations she will feel as the specimen is obtained (e.g., pressure but not pain).
4. The cytologic specimen is obtained before any digital examination of the vagina is made or endocervical bacteriologic specimens are taken with cotton swabbing of the cervix.
5. The Papanicolaou (Pap) test is done by using an endocervical sampling device (Cytobrush, Cervex-Brush, papette, or broom) (see Fig. 5-15). If the two-sample method of obtaining cells is used, the cytobrush is inserted into the canal and rotated 90 to 180 degrees, followed by a gentle smear of the entire transformation zone using a spatula. Broom devices are inserted and rotated 360 degrees five times. They obtain endocervical and ectocervical samples at the same time. If the patient has had a hysterectomy, the vaginal cuff is sampled. Areas that appear abnormal on visualization require colposcopy and biopsy. If using a one-slide technique, the spatula sample is smeared first. This is followed by applying the cytobrush sample (rolling the brush in the opposite direction from which it was obtained), which is less subject to drying artifact; the slide is then sprayed with preservative within 5 seconds.
6. The ThinPrep Pap Test is an improved method of preserving cells that reduces blood, mucus, and inflammation. The Pap specimen is obtained in the manner described previously, and the collection device (brush, spatula, or broom) is simply rinsed in a vial of preserving solution that is provided by the laboratory. The sealed vial with solution is sent off to the appropriate laboratory. A special processing device filters the contents, and a thin layer of cervical cells is deposited on a slide, which is then examined microscopically. Initial reports state that specimen adequacy is improved by 50% and detection of low-grade and more severe lesions is improved by 65%. The AutoPap and PapNet tests are similar to the ThinPrep test.
7. Label the slides with the woman's name and site. Include on the form to accompany the slides the woman's name, age, last menstrual period, parity, and chief complaint or reason for taking the cytologic specimens.
8. Send specimens to the pathology laboratory promptly for staining, evaluation, and a written report, with special reference to abnormal elements, including cancer cells.
9. Advise the woman that repeat tests may be necessary if the specimen is not adequate.
10. Instruct the woman concerning routine checkups for cervical and vaginal cancer. The American Cancer Society advises that women over 18 years of age and those under 18 who are sexually active have the test at least every 3 years, but only after they have had three negative Pap tests a year apart. A pelvic examination is recommended every 3 years from age 20 to 40 and every 1 to 3 years thereafter.
11. Record the examination date on the woman's record.

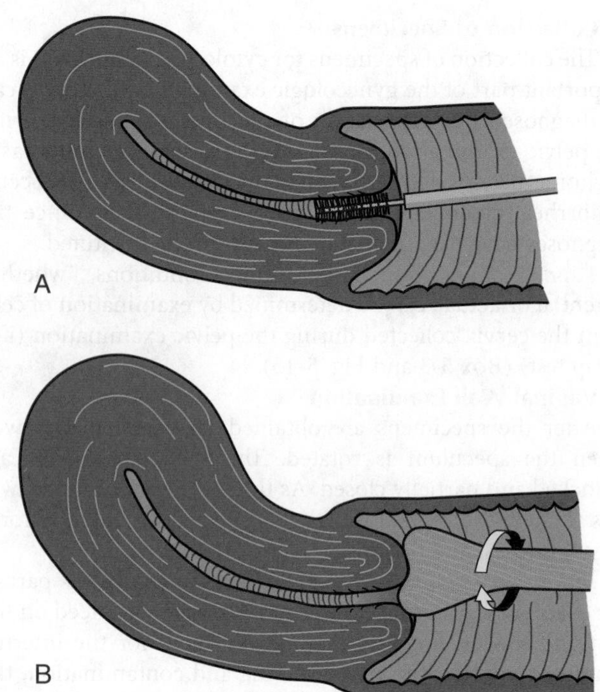

Fig. 5-15 Pap test. A, Collecting cells from the endocervix using a cytobrush. B, Obtaining cells from the transformation zone using a wooden spatula. (From Katz VL et al: *Comprehensive gynecology*, ed 5, Philadelphia, 2007, Mosby.)

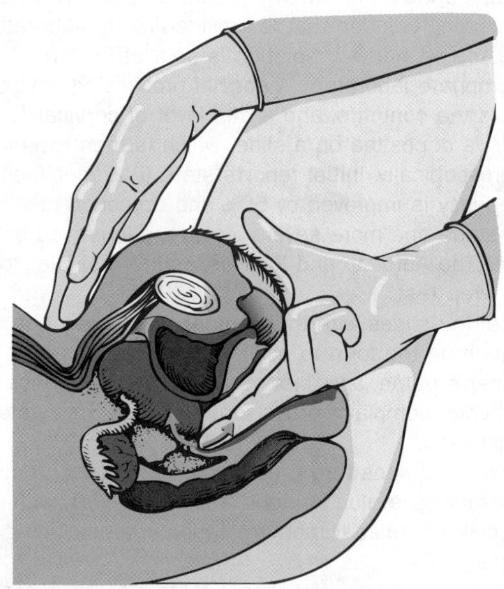

Fig. 5-16 Bimanual palpation of the uterus.

thumb is abducted, and the ring and little fingers are flexed into the palm (Fig. 5-16).

The vagina is palpated for distensibility, lesions, and tenderness. The cervix is examined for position, shape, consistency, motility, and lesions. The fornix around the cervix is palpated.

The other hand is placed on the abdomen halfway between the umbilicus and symphysis pubis and exerts pressure downward toward the pelvic hand. Upward pressure from the pelvic hand traps reproductive structures for assessment by palpation. The uterus is assessed for position, size, shape, consistency, regularity, motility, masses, and tenderness.

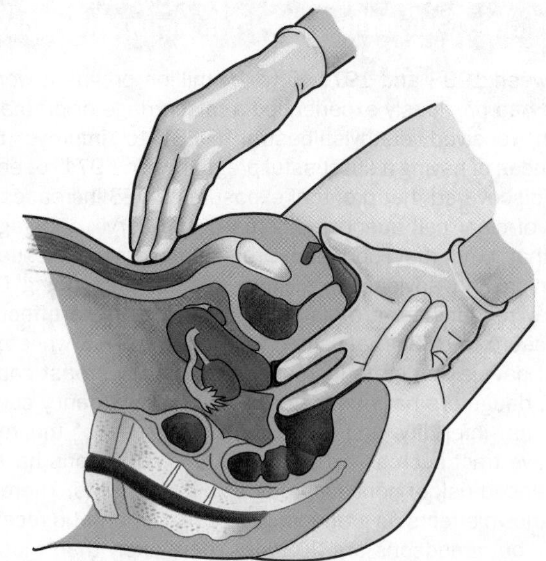

Fig. 5-17 Rectovaginal examination. (From Seidel HM et al: *Mosby's guide to physical examination*, ed 6, St Louis, 2006, Mosby.)

With the abdominal hand moving to the right lower quadrant and the fingers of the pelvic hand in the right lateral fornix, the adnexa is assessed for position, size, tenderness, and masses. The examination is repeated on the woman's left side.

Just before the intravaginal fingers are withdrawn, the woman is asked to tighten her vagina around the fingers as much as she can. If the muscle response is weak, the woman is assessed for her knowledge about Kegel exercises.

Rectovaginal Palpation To prevent contamination of the rectum from organisms in the vagina (such as *Neisseria gonorrhoeae*), it is necessary to change gloves, add fresh lubricant, and then reinsert the index finger into the vagina and the middle finger into the rectum (Fig. 5-17). Insertion is facilitated if the woman strains down. The maneuvers of the abdominovaginal examination are repeated. The rectovaginal examination permits assessment of the rectovaginal septum, the posterior surface of the uterus, and the region behind the cervix and the adnexa. The vaginal finger is removed and folded into the palm, leaving the middle finger free to rotate 360 degrees. The rectum is palpated for rectal tenderness and masses.

After the rectal examination the woman is assisted into a sitting position, given tissues or wipes to cleanse herself, and afforded privacy to dress. The examiner returns after the woman is dressed to discuss findings and the plan of care.

Pelvic Examination During Pregnancy The pelvic examination is done in the same way as it is during a routine examination on a nonpregnant woman. Pelvic measurements are completed, and uterine size is estimated. A Pap test may be done initially, and cytologic specimens collected to test for gonorrhea, chlamydia, human papillomavirus, herpes simplex virus, and group B streptococci. As the pregnancy progresses, the nurse inspects the woman's abdomen, palpates fetal size and position, auscultates fetal heart tones, and measures fundal height at each visit.

While the pregnant woman is in lithotomy position, the nurse must watch for supine hypotension (decrease in blood pressure) caused by the weight of the uterus pressing on the vena cava and aorta. Symptoms of supine hypotension include pallor, dizziness, faintness, breathlessness, tachycardia, nausea, clammy skin, and sweating. The woman should be positioned on her side until symptoms resolve and vital signs stabilize. The vaginal examination can be done with the woman in lateral position.

Pelvic Examination After Hysterectomy The pelvic examination is done much as it is done on a woman with a uterus. Vaginal screening using the Pap test is not recommended in women who have had a total hysterectomy with removal of the cervix for benign disease (American Cancer Society, 2008; National Comprehensive Cancer Network, 2008). Because of the epidemic of human papillomavirus, which causes vaginal intraepithelial neoplasia, sampling of the vaginal cuff and vaginal walls after hysterectomy may still be practiced, with schedules varying from every year to every 2 to 3 years.

Laboratory and Diagnostic Procedures

The following laboratory and diagnostic procedures are ordered at the discretion of the clinician, considering the patient and family history: hemoglobin, fasting blood glucose, total blood cholesterol, lipid profile, urinalysis, syphilis serology (Venereal Disease Research Laboratories [VDRL] or rapid plasma reagent [RPR]) and other screening tests for STIs, mammogram, tuberculosis skin testing, hearing, visual acuity, electrocardiogram, chest x-ray, pulmonary function, fecal occult blood, flexible sigmoidoscopy, and bone mineral density (dual energy x-ray absorptiometry [DEXA] scan). Results of these tests may be reported in person, by phone call, or by letter. Tests for HIV, hepatitis B, and drug screening may be offered with informed consent in high risk populations. These test results are usually reported in person.

Key Points

- Normal feedback regulation of the menstrual cycle depends on an intact hypothalamic-pituitary-gonadal mechanism.
- The female's reproductive tract structures and breasts respond predictably to changing levels of sex steroids across her life span.
- The myometrium of the uterus is uniquely designed to expel the fetus and promote hemostasis after birth.
- Health promotion and illness prevention assist women to actualize health potential by increasing motivation, providing information, and suggesting how to access specific resources.

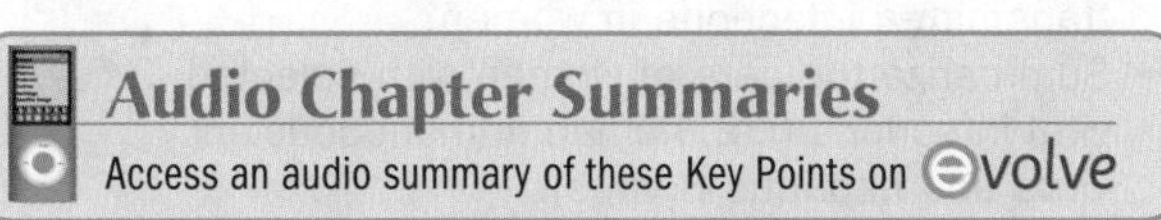
Audio Chapter Summaries
Access an audio summary of these Key Points on evolve

- Periodic health screening, including history, physical examination, and diagnostic and laboratory tests, provides the basis for overall health promotion, prevention of illness, early diagnosis of problems, and referral for management.
- Routine screening mammography and annual breast examinations by practitioners are recommended for early detection of breast cancer.

References

American Cancer Society (ACS): *Cancer facts and figures 2008*, New York, 2008, ACS.

Barkauskas VH, Baumann LC, Darling-Fisher CS: *Health and physical assessment*, ed 3, St Louis, 2002, Mosby.

National Comprehensive Cancer Network (NCCN): *NCCN practice guidelines in oncology: cervical cancer screening*, version 1.2009, 2008. Available at www.nccn.org/professionals/physician_gls/PDF/cervical_screening.pdf (accessed February 16, 2009).

Seidel HM et al: *Mosby's guide to physical examination*, ed 6, St Louis, 2006, Mosby.

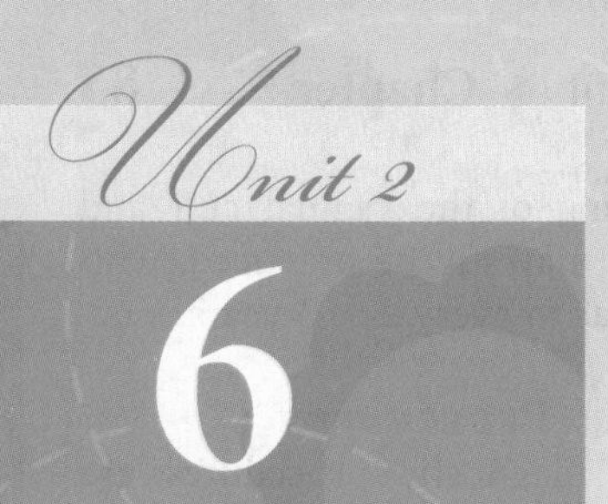

6 Common Health Problems

Learning Objectives

On completion of this chapter the reader will be able to:

- Develop a nursing care plan for the woman with primary dysmenorrhea.
- Outline patient teaching about premenstrual syndrome.
- Relate the pathophysiology of endometriosis to associated symptoms.
- Evaluate the use of alternative therapies for menstrual disorders.
- Describe prevention and treatment of sexually transmitted infections in women.
- Summarize the care of women with selected viral infections (i.e., human immunodeficiency virus and hepatitis B virus).
- Differentiate signs, symptoms, and management of selected vaginal infections.
- Review principles of infection control for human immunodeficiency virus and blood-borne pathogens.
- Discuss the pathophysiology and emotional effects of selected benign breast conditions and malignant neoplasms of the breasts found in women.

Electronic Resources

Additional information related to the content in Chapter 6 can be found on

evolve the Companion Website at
http://evolve.elsevier.com/Perry/maternal/

- NCLEX Review Questions
- Animation—Pelvic Inflammatory Disease
- Case Study—Breast Cancer
- Nursing Care Plan—Breast Cancer
- Nursing Care Plan—Endometriosis
- Nursing Care Plan—Premenstrual Syndrome
- Nursing Care Plan—Sexually Transmitted Infections

Problems may occur at any point in the menstrual cycle. Many factors, including anatomic abnormalities, physiologic imbalances, and lifestyle, can affect the menstrual cycle. The average woman is likely to have some concerns related to her menstrual and gynecologic health at some point in her life and will experience bleeding, pain, or discharge or infections associated with her reproductive organs or functions. This chapter provides information on common menstrual problems, sexually transmitted infections, and selected other infections that can affect reproductive functions. Benign breast conditions are also discussed. Breast cancer is included because it is the most common reproductive cancer occurring in women.

Menstrual Disorders

Normal menstrual patterns are averages based on observations and reports from large groups of healthy women. Generally a woman's menstrual frequency stabilizes at 28 days within 1 to 2 years after puberty with a range of 26 to 34 days. Although no woman's cycle is exactly the same length every month, the typical month-to-month variation in an individual's cycle is usually plus or minus 2 days. However, greater but still normal variations are commonly noted.

Women typically have menstrual cycles for about 40 years. Once a cyclic, predictable pattern of monthly bleeding is established, women may worry about any deviation from that pattern or from what they have been told is normal for all menstruating women. A woman may be concerned about her ability to conceive and bear children or believe that she is not really a woman without monthly evidence. A sign such as amenorrhea or excess menstrual bleeding can be a source of severe distress and concern for a woman.

Amenorrhea

Amenorrhea, the absence of menstrual flow, is a clinical sign of a variety of disorders. Generally the following circumstances should be evaluated: (1) the absence of both menarche and secondary sexual characteristics by age 14 years; (2) the absence of menses by age 16, regardless of normal growth and development (primary amenorrhea); or (3) a 3- to 6-month cessation of menses after a period of menstruation (secondary amenorrhea).

Amenorrhea is most commonly the result of pregnancy. Although amenorrhea is not a disease, it is often a sign of disease. It may occur from any defect or interruption in the hypothalamic-pituitary-ovarian-uterine axis. It may also result from anatomic abnormalities, other endocrine disorders such as hypothyroidism or hyperthyroidism, chronic diseases such as type 1 diabetes, medications such as phenytoin (Dilantin), illicit drug abuse (opiates, marijuana, cocaine), eating disorders, strenuous exercise, emotional stress, and oral contraceptive use.

Assessment of amenorrhea begins with a thorough history and physical examination. An important initial step is to be sure that the woman is not pregnant. Specific components of the assessment process depend on a patient's age—adolescent, young adult, or perimenopausal—and whether she has previously menstruated.

Hypogonadotropic Amenorrhea

Hypogonadotropic amenorrhea reflects a problem in the central hypothalamic-pituitary axis. In rare instances a pituitary lesion or genetic inability to produce follicle-stimulating hormone (FSH) and luteinizing hormone (LH) is at fault. Once pregnancy has been ruled out by a β-human chorionic gonadotropin (hCG) pregnancy test, diagnostic tests may include FSH level, thyroid-stimulating hormone (TSH) and prolactin levels, radiographic or computed tomography scan of the sella turcica, and a progestational challenge (Bielak & Harris, 2008).

Hypogonadotropic amenorrhea often results from hypothalamic suppression as a result of stress (in the home, school, or workplace) or a sudden and severe weight loss, eating disorders, strenuous exercise, or mental illness. Research on the interaction between nervous system or neurotransmitter functions and hormone regulation throughout the body has demonstrated a biologic basis for the relation of stress to physiologic processes. Women who are more than 20% underweight for height or who have had rapid weight loss may report amenorrhea, as may women with eating disorders such as anorexia nervosa. Amenorrhea is one of the classic signs of anorexia nervosa; and the interrelation of disordered eating, amenorrhea, and premature osteoporosis has been described as the female athlete triad (*www.femaleathletetriad.org*). A loss of calcium from the bone, comparable to that seen in postmenopausal women, may occur with this type of amenorrhea.

Exercise-associated amenorrhea can occur in women undergoing vigorous physical and athletic training and is thought to be associated with many factors, including body composition (height, weight, and percentage of body fat); type, intensity, and frequency of exercise; nutritional status; and presence of emotional or physical stressors. Women who participate in sports emphasizing low body weight are at greatest risk, including the following:

- Sports in which performance is subjectively scored (e.g., dance, gymnastics)
- Endurance sports favoring participants with low body weight (e.g., distance running, cycling)
- Sports in which body contour–revealing clothing is worn (e.g., swimming, diving, volleyball)
- Sports with weight categories for participation (e.g., rowing, martial arts)
- Sports in which prepubertal body shape favors success (e.g., gymnastics, figure skating)

Assessment of amenorrhea begins with a thorough history and physical examination. An important initial step, often overlooked, is to be sure that the woman is not pregnant. Specific components of the assessment process depend on a patient's age—adolescent, young adult, or perimenopausal—and whether she has previously menstruated.

Management

When amenorrhea is caused by hypothalamic disturbances, the nurse is an ideal health professional to assist women because many of the causes are potentially reversible (e.g., stress, weight loss for nonorganic reasons). Counseling and education are primary interventions and appropriate nursing roles. When a stressor known to predispose a woman to hypothalamic amenorrhea is identified, initial management involves addressing the stressor. Together the woman and nurse plan how the woman can decrease or discontinue medications known to affect menstruation, correct weight loss, deal more effectively with psychologic stress, address emotional distress, and alter exercise routine.

The nurse works with the woman to help her identify, cope with, and eliminate sources of stress in her life. Deep-breathing exercises and relaxation techniques are simple yet effective stress-reduction measures. Referral for biofeedback or massage therapy also may be useful. In some instances referrals for psychotherapy may be indicated.

If a woman's exercise program is thought to contribute to her amenorrhea, several options exist for management. She may decide to decrease the intensity or duration of her training or to gain 2% to 3% in body weight. Accepting this alternative may be difficult for one who is committed to a strenuous exercise regimen. The woman and nurse may have several sessions before the woman elects to try exercise reduction. Many young female athletes may not understand the consequences of low bone density or osteoporosis; nurses can point out the connection between low bone density and stress fractures. The nurse and woman should also investigate other factors that may be contributing to the amenorrhea and develop plans for altering lifestyle and decreasing stress.

A daily calcium intake of 1200 to 1500 mg, accomplished by drinking three glasses of skim milk or by taking a calcium supplement, is recommended for women experiencing amenorrhea associated with the female athlete triad. Some researchers have found that oral contraceptives have a positive effect on bone density in amenorrheic premenopausal women (Liu & Lebrun, 2006).

Cyclic Perimenstrual Pain and Discomfort

Cyclic perimenstrual pain and discomfort (CPPD) is a concept developed by a nurse science team for a research project for the Association of Women's Health, Obstetric and Neonatal Nurses (AWHONN, 2003; Collins Sharp et al, 2002). This concept includes dysmenorrhea, premenstrual syndrome (PMS), and premenstrual dysphoric disorder (PMDD), as well as symptom clusters that occur before and after the menstrual flow starts. CPPD is a health problem that can have a significant impact on the quality of life for a woman. The following discussion focuses on the three main conditions of CPPD.

Dysmenorrhea

Dysmenorrhea, pain during or shortly before menstruation, is one of the most common gynecologic problems in women of all ages. Most adolescents have dysmenorrhea in the first 3 years after menarche. Young adult women ages 17 to 24 are most likely to report painful menses. Dysmenorrhea improves in most women after a full-term pregnancy (Speroff & Fritz, 2005). Between 30% and 40% of women report some level of discomfort associated with menses, and 7% to 15% report severe dysmenorrhea. However, the amount of disruption caused in women's lives is difficult to determine. It has been estimated that up to 10% of women with dysmenorrhea have pain severe enough to interfere with their functioning for 1 to 3 days a month. Menstrual problems, including dysmenorrhea, are more common in women who smoke and who are obese. Traditionally dysmenorrhea is differentiated as primary or secondary. Symptoms usually begin with menstruation, although some women have discomfort several hours before onset of flow. The range and severity of symptoms differ from woman to woman and from cycle to cycle in the same woman. Symptoms of dysmenorrhea may last several hours or several days. Pain is usually located in the suprapubic area or lower abdomen. Women describe the pain as sharp, cramping, or gripping or as a steady dull ache; pain may radiate to the lower back or upper thighs.

Primary Dysmenorrhea

Primary dysmenorrhea, a condition associated with abnormally increased uterine activity, is caused by myometrium contractions induced by prostaglandins in the second half of the menstrual cycle. During the luteal phase and subsequent menstrual flow, prostaglandin $F_{2\alpha}$ ($PGF_{2\alpha}$) is secreted. The uterine muscle of both normal and dysmenorrheic women is sensitive to prostaglandins; however, the amount of prostaglandin produced is the major differentiating factor (Speroff & Fritz, 2005). Excessive release of $PGF_{2\alpha}$ increases the amplitude and frequency of uterine contractions and causes vasospasm of the uterine arterioles, resulting in ischemia and cyclic lower abdominal cramps. Systemic responses to $PGF_{2\alpha}$ include backache, weakness, sweating, gastrointestinal symptoms (anorexia, nausea, vomiting, and diarrhea), and central nervous system symptoms (dizziness, syncope, headache, and poor concentration). Pain begins at the onset of menstrual flow and lasts from 8 to 48 hours. The release of most prostaglandins during menstruation occurs in the first 48 hours, which coincides with the greatest intensity of symptoms.

Primary dysmenorrhea is not caused by underlying pathology. Rather it is the occurrence of a physiologic alteration in some women. Primary dysmenorrhea usually appears within 6 to 12 months after menarche when ovulation is established. Anovulatory bleeding, common in the first few months or years after menarche, is painless. Because both estrogen and progesterone are necessary for primary dysmenorrhea to occur, it is experienced only with ovulatory cycles. This problem is most common in women in their late teens and early twenties; the incidence declines with age.

Management Management of primary dysmenorrhea depends on the severity of the problem and an individual woman's response to various treatments. Education and support are important components of nursing care. Because menstruation is so closely linked to reproduction and sexuality, menstrual problems such as dysmenorrhea can have a negative influence on sexuality and self-worth. Nurses can correct myths and misinformation about menstruation and dysmenorrhea by providing facts about what is normal.

Often more than one alternative for alleviating menstrual discomfort and dysmenorrhea can be offered. Women can then try options and decide which ones work best for them. Heat (heating pad or hot bath) minimizes cramping by increasing vasodilation and muscle relaxation and minimizing uterine ischemia. Massaging the lower back can reduce pain by relaxing paravertebral muscles and increasing pelvic blood supply. Soft rhythmic rubbing of the abdomen (effleurage) may be useful because it provides distraction and an alternative focal point. Guided imagery, progressive relaxation, hatha yoga, and meditation also have been used successfully to decrease menstrual discomfort (Fig. 6-1).

Exercise helps relieve menstrual discomfort through increased vasodilation and subsequent decreased ischemia; release of endogenous opiates, specifically β-endorphins; suppression of prostaglandins; and shunting of blood flow away from the viscera, resulting in less pelvic congestion. A specific exercise that nurses can suggest to their patients is pelvic rocking.

In addition to maintaining good nutrition at all times, specific dietary changes may be helpful in decreasing some of the systemic symptoms associated with dysmenorrhea. Decreased salt and refined sugar intake in the 7 to 10 days before expected menses may reduce fluid retention. Increasing water intake may serve as a natural diuretic. Including natural diuretics such as asparagus, cranberry juice, peaches, parsley, and watermelon in the diet may help reduce edema and related discomforts. Decreasing red meat intake and switching to a low-fat diet may also help to minimize dysmenorrheal symptoms.

Medications used to treat primary dysmenorrhea in women not desiring contraception include prostaglandin synthesis

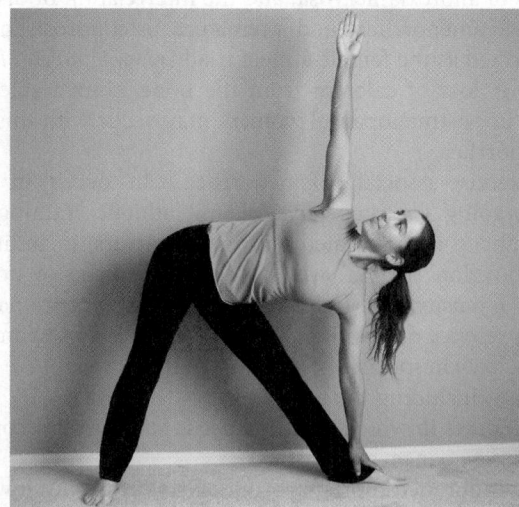

Fig. 6-1 Yoga asana: triangle pose. Helpful for assisting digestion and stretching and strengthening the spine; also used for dysmenorrheal and pelvic congestion. *(Courtesy Julie Perry Nelson, Loveland, CO.)*

Table 6-1 Medications Used to Treat Dysmenorrhea

DRUG	COMMON SIDE EFFECTS*	COMMENTS
Diclofenac (Cataflam Rx)	Nausea, diarrhea, constipation, abdominal distress, dyspepsia, flatulence	Enteric coated: immediate release
Fenoprofen† (Nalfon Rx)	Nausea, diarrhea, constipation, abdominal distress, dyspepsia, flatulence	Use for mild-to-moderate pain only if other NSAIDs are not effective; take with meals; avoid alcohol
Ibuprofen (Motrin Rx) (Advil OTC, Nuprin OTC, Motrin IB OTC)	Nausea, dyspepsia, rash, pruritus	If GI upset occurs, take with food, milk, or antacids; avoid alcoholic beverages; do not take with aspirin
Ketoprofen (Orudis Rx) (Orudis KT OTC) (Actron OTC)	Nausea, diarrhea, constipation, abdominal distress, dyspepsia, flatulence	See ibuprofen
Meclofenamate (Meclomen Rx)	Dizziness, headache, severe diarrhea, nausea, abnormal liver function tests	See ibuprofen
Mefenamic acid (Ponstel Rx)	Severe diarrhea, nausea, and vomiting	Very potent and effective prostaglandin-synthesis inhibitor Antagonizes already formed prostaglandins Increased incidence of adverse GI side effects
Naproxen (Naprosyn Rx)	See ibuprofen	See ibuprofen
Naproxen sodium (Anaprox Rx) (Aleve OTC)	See ibuprofen	See ibuprofen

Sources: Facts and Comparisons: *Loose-leaf drug information service,* St Louis, 2002, Facts and Comparisons; Parent-Stevens L, Burns E: Menstrual disorders. In Smith M, Shimp L (editors): *20 common problems in women's health care,* New York, 2000, McGraw-Hill.
NOTE: For all NSAIDs: Do not give if patient has hemophilia or bleeding ulcers; do not give if patient has had an allergic or anaphylactic reaction to aspirin or another NSAID; do not give if patient is taking anticoagulant medication.
GI, Gastrointestinal; *NSAID,* nonsteroidal antiinflammatory drug; *OTC,* over the counter; *Rx,* prescription.
*Risk with all NSAIDs is gastrointestinal ulceration, possible bleeding, and prolonged bleeding time. Incidence of side effects is dose related. Reported incidence, 3% to 9%.
†Unlabeled indications for use in treating dysmenorrhea.

inhibitors, primarily nonsteroidal antiinflammatory drugs (NSAIDs) (Table 6-1). NSAIDs are effective if begun 2 to 3 days before menses or with the first sign of bleeding. This regimen decreases the possibility of a woman taking these drugs early in pregnancy (Speroff & Fritz, 2005). Often if one NSAID is ineffective, a different one will be effective. All NSAIDs have potential gastrointestinal side effects, including nausea, vomiting, and indigestion. All women taking NSAIDs should be warned to report dark-colored stools, which may be an indication of gastrointestinal bleeding. Women with a history of aspirin sensitivity or allergy should avoid all NSAIDs. Approximately 80% of dysmenorrheic women obtain relief with prostaglandin inhibitors.

Oral contraceptive pills (OCPs) are a reasonable choice for women who want to use a contraceptive agent. The benefits of OCP use are attributed to decreased prostaglandin synthesis associated with an atrophic decidualized endometrium (Speroff & Fritz, 2005). No single OCP has been shown to be superior to another for the relief of primary dysmenorrhea. OCPs are a particularly good choice for therapy because they combine contraception with a positive effect on dysmenorrhea, menstrual flow, and menstrual irregularities. Since OCPs have side effects, women may not wish to use them for dysmenorrhea. OCPs may be contraindicated for some women. (See Chapter 7 for a complete discussion of OCPs.)

Over-the-counter (OTC) preparations that are indicated for primary dysmenorrhea contain the same active ingredients (e.g., ibuprofen or naproxen sodium) as prescription preparations. However, the labeled recommended dose may be subtherapeutic. Preparations containing acetaminophen are even less effective because acetaminophen does not have the antiprostaglandin properties of NSAIDs.

If dysmenorrhea is not relieved by one of the NSAIDs, further investigation into the cause of the symptoms is necessary. Conditions associated with dysmenorrhea include müllerian duct anomalies, endometriosis, and pelvic inflammatory disease (PID).

Alternative and complementary therapies are increasingly popular and used in developed countries. Therapies such as acupuncture, acupressure, biofeedback, desensitization, hypnosis, massage, reiki, relaxation exercises, and therapeutic touch have been used to treat pelvic pain (Dehlin & Schuiling, 2006; Proctor & Farquhar, 2004). Herbal preparations have long been used for management of menstrual problems, including dysmenorrhea (Table 6-2). Herbal medicines may be valuable in treating dysmenorrhea. However, it is essential that women understand that these therapies are not without potential toxicity and may cause drug interactions.

NURSING ALERT Nurses must routinely ask women about use of herbal and other alternative therapies and document their use.

Secondary Dysmenorrhea

Secondary dysmenorrhea is menstrual pain that develops later in life than primary dysmenorrhea, typically after age 25. It is associated with pelvic pathology such as adenomyosis, endometriosis, PID, endometrial polyps, or submucous or interstitial myomas (fibroids). Women with secondary dysmenorrhea often have other symptoms that may suggest the underlying cause. For example, heavy menstrual flow with dysmenorrhea suggests a diagnosis of leiomyomata, adenomyosis, or endometrial polyps. Pain associated with endometriosis often begins a few days before menses but can be present at ovulation and continue through the first days of menses or

Table 6-2 Herbal Medicinals Taken Orally for Menstrual Disorders

SYMPTOMS/INDICATIONS	HERBAL	ACTION	CONTRAINDICATIONS	ADVERSE REACTIONS	DRUG INTERACTIONS
Menstrual cramping	Black haw	Uterine anti-spasmodic; β_2-agonist activity	None known	None known	None known
	Ginger	Antiinflammatory			
Premenstrual discomfort (anxiety, tension, depression), dysmenorrhea	Black cohosh root	Estrogen-like LH suppressant, binds to estrogen receptors	Pregnancy	Gastric irritation, CNS side effects at high doses	None known
Tension, breast pain	Bugleweed	Antigonadotropic, antithyrotropic, decreased prolactin levels	Thyroid disease	Thyroid enlargement with prolonged high dose	Interferes with diagnostic radioactive isotopes
Mastodynia, premenstrual discomfort, menstrual cycle irregularities	Chaste tree fruit	Decreased prolactin levels	None known	Itching, urticaria	Possible antagonism of dopaminergic antagonists
Dysmenorrhea	Potentilla	Increased tonus and contraction frequency in uterus	Pregnancy and lactation	Gastric irritation	None known
	Dong quai	Stimulate/relax uterus; antiinflammatory; possibly analgesic activity	Phototoxicity Liver and renal damage in animal studies Abortifacient	Pregnancy	Coumarin components may increase risk of bleeding
Menorrhea and metrorrhagia	Shepard's purse	Increased uterine contractions	None known	None known	None known

Sources: Bascom A: *Incorporating herbal medicine into clinical practice,* Philadelphia, 2002, FA Davis; Fugh-Berman A, Awang D: Black cohosh, *Altern Ther Womens Health* 39(11):81-85, 2001; Dog L: *An integrative approach to dysmenorrhea,* Corrales, NM, 2000, Integrative Medicine Education Association; Dog L: *Endocrinology and women's issues*, Third Annual Conference on Clinical Relevance of Medicinal Herbs and Nutritional Supplements in the Management of Major Medical Problems, September 21-23, 2001; Schellenberg R: Treatment for the premenstrual syndrome with *Agnus castus* fruit extract: prospective, randomized, placebo controlled study, *BMJ* 322(7279):134-137, 2001; Stevinson C, Ernst E: Complementary/alternative therapies for premenstrual syndrome: a systemic review of random controlled trials, *Am J Obstet Gynecol* 185(1):227-235, 2001.

CNS, Central nervous system; *LH,* luteinizing hormone.

start after menstrual flow has begun. In contrast to primary dysmenorrhea, the pain of secondary dysmenorrhea is often characterized by dull, lower abdominal aching that radiates to the back or thighs. Often women experience feelings of bloating or pelvic fullness. In addition to a physical examination with a careful pelvic examination, diagnosis may be assisted by ultrasound examination, dilation and curettage (D&C), endometrial biopsy, or laparoscopy. Treatment is directed toward removal of the underlying pathology. Many of the measures described for pain relief of primary dysmenorrhea are also helpful for women with secondary dysmenorrhea.

Premenstrual Syndrome

PMS is a complex, poorly understood condition that includes a number of cyclic symptoms occurring in the luteal phase of the menstrual cycle. About 85% of women experience mood and/or somatic symptoms that coincide with their menstrual cycles. Between 5% and 14% of women report symptoms severe enough to be disabling. All age groups are affected, with women in their twenties and thirties most frequently reporting symptoms. Ovarian function is necessary for the condition to occur. PMS does not occur before puberty, after menopause, or during pregnancy (see Critical Thinking Exercise). The condition is not dependent on the presence of monthly menses;

evolve Nursing Care Plan—Premenstrual Syndrome

CRITICAL THINKING EXERCISE

Premenstrual Syndrome in Adolescents

Brandy, a 20-year-old college student, has been diagnosed with premenstrual syndrome (PMS). The week before her menses, she is irritable, cries easily, becomes angry over little things, has breast and abdominal discomfort, and in general, "feels terrible." She tells the nurse in the health center that her friends get mad at her when she just wants to be left alone and that she has trouble concentrating in class. She asks the nurse for ways to deal with her PMS. What advice can the nurse give Brandy?

1. Evidence—Is there an evidence base for practical suggestions for dealing with PMS?
2. Assumptions—What assumptions can be made about the following aspects of PMS?
   a. Physical symptoms
   b. Psychologic factors
   c. Behavioral changes
   d. Effective therapies
3. What implications and priorities for nursing care can be drawn at this time?
4. Does the evidence objectively support your conclusion?
5. Are there alternative perspectives to your conclusion?

women who have had a hysterectomy without bilateral salpingo-oophorectomy (BSO) still can have cyclic symptoms.

It is difficult to establish a universal definition of PMS because so many symptoms have been associated with the condition. However, Speroff and Fritz (2005) suggest that the simplest definition is a commonsense one: "The cyclic appearance of one or more of a large constellation of symptoms just prior to menses, occurring to such a degree that lifestyle or work is affected, followed by a period of time entirely free of symptoms." PMS symptoms include distressing physical, mood, and behavioral experiences.

Premenstrual Dysphoric Disorder

PMDD is a diagnostic term for a smaller percentage of women who suffer from severe PMS with an emphasis on mood symptoms (American Psychiatric Association [APA], 2000). Commonly symptoms occur in the final 7 to 10 days of the menstrual cycle. Symptoms commonly reported include abdominal bloating, anxiety, tension, breast tenderness, crying episodes, depression, fatigue and lack of energy, irritability, difficulty concentrating, appetite changes, thirst, and swelling of the extremities (Speroff & Fritz, 2005). The most common symptoms are those associated with mood disturbances.

A diagnosis of PMS is made only when the following criteria are met (AWHONN, 2003; Taylor, Schuiling, & Sharp, 2006):

- Symptoms occur in the luteal phase and resolve within a few days of onset of menses.
- A symptom-free period occurs in the follicular phase.
- Symptoms are recurrent.
- Symptoms have a negative impact on some aspect of a woman's life
- Other diagnoses that better explain the symptoms have been excluded.

For a diagnosis of PMDD, the following criteria must be met:

- Five or more affective and physical symptoms are present in the week before menses and absent in the follicular phase of the menstrual cycle.
- At least one of the symptoms is irritability, depressed mood, anxiety, or emotional lability.
- Symptoms interfere markedly with work or interpersonal relationships.
- Symptoms are not caused by an exacerbation of another condition or disorder.

These criteria must be confirmed by prospective daily ratings for at least two menstrual cycles (APA, 2000).

The etiology of PMS and PMDD is not clear, but there is general agreement that they are distinct psychiatric and medical syndromes rather than an exacerbation of an underlying psychiatric disorder. They do not occur if there is no ovarian function. A number of biologic and neuroendocrine etiologies have been suggested; however, none have been substantiated conclusively as the causative factor. It is likely that biologic, psychosocial, and sociocultural factors contribute to PMS and PMDD (Speroff & Fritz, 2005; Taylor, Schuiling, & Sharp, 2006).

Readers are encouraged to explore current feminist, medical, and social science literature for more information on PMS.

Management There is little agreement on management. A careful, detailed history and daily log of symptoms and mood fluctuations spanning several cycles may give direction to a plan of management. Any changes that assist a woman with PMS to exert control over her life have a positive impact.

Education is an important component of the management of PMS. Nurses can advise women that self-help modalities often result in significant symptom improvement. Women have found a number of complementary and alternative therapies to be useful in managing the symptoms of PMS. Diet and exercise changes are a useful way to begin and provide symptom relief for some women. Nurses can suggest that patients not smoke and limit their consumption of refined sugar (less than 5 tbsp/day), salt (less than 3 g/day), red meat (less than 3 oz/day), alcohol (less than 1 oz/day), and caffeinated beverages.

Women can be encouraged to include whole grains, legumes, seeds, nuts, vegetables, fruits, and vegetable oils in their diet. Use of natural diuretics (see the section on dysmenorrhea management earlier in this chapter) may help reduce fluid retention. Nutritional supplements may assist in symptom relief. Calcium (1200 mg/day), magnesium (300 to 400 mg/day), and vitamin E (100 to 150 mg/day) have been shown to be moderately effective in relieving symptoms, to have few side effects, and to be safe. For some women daily supplements of evening primrose oil decrease premenstrual mood symptoms, breast pain, and fluid retention. The safety of this herb is well established; however, approximately 2% of those taking evening primrose oil may have stomach distress, nausea, or headaches. Other herbal therapies have long been used to treat PMS; specific suggestions are found in Table 6-2.

Regular exercise (aerobic exercise three to four times a week), especially in the luteal phase, is widely recommended for relief of PMS symptoms. A monthly program that varies in intensity and type of exercise according to PMS symptoms is best. Women who exercise regularly seem to have less premenstrual anxiety than do nonathletic women. It is thought that aerobic exercise increases β-endorphin levels to offset symptoms of depression and elevate mood. Yoga, acupuncture, hypnosis, chiropractic therapy, and massage therapy have all been reported to have a beneficial effect on the woman with PMS.

Counseling in the form of support groups or individual or couple counseling may be helpful. Stress-reduction techniques may also assist with symptom management. If these strategies do not provide significant symptom relief in 1 to 2 months, medication is often begun. Many medications have been used in treatment of PMS, but no single medication alleviates all PMS symptoms.

Medications often used in the treatment of PMS include diuretics, prostaglandin inhibitors (NSAIDs), progesterone, and OCPs. Serotonergic-activating agents, including the selective serotonin reuptake inhibitors (SSRIs) fluoxetine (Prozac or Sarafem), sertraline (Zoloft), paroxetine (Paxil), and citalopram (Celexa), have been shown to decrease severe premenstrual symptoms, including depression (PMS Health Center, 2006). Common side effects are headaches, sleep disturbances, dizziness, weight gain, dry mouth, and decreased libido.

Endometriosis

Endometriosis is characterized by the presence and growth of endometrial tissue outside of the uterus. The tissue may be

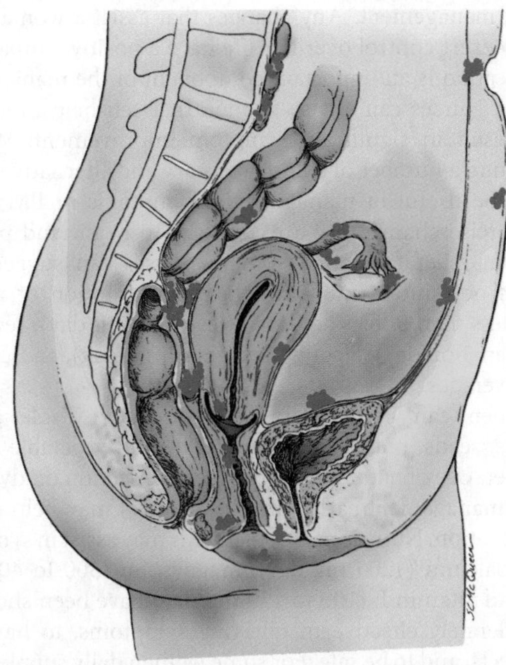

Fig. 6-2 Common sites of endometriosis. (From Katz VL et al: *Comprehensive gynecology*, ed 5, Philadelphia, 2007, Mosby.)

implanted on the ovaries; anterior and posterior cul-de-sac; broad, uterosacral, and round ligaments; rectovaginal septum; sigmoid colon; appendix; pelvic peritoneum; cervix; and inguinal area (Fig. 6-2). Endometrial lesions have been found in the vagina and surgical scars, as well as on the vulva, perineum, and bladder. Lesions have also been found on sites far from the pelvic area such as the thoracic cavity, gallbladder, and heart. A cystic lesion of endometriosis found in the ovary is sometimes described as a chocolate cyst because of the dark coloring of the contents of the cyst caused by the presence of old blood.

Endometrial tissue contains glands and stoma and responds to cyclic hormone stimulation in the same way that the uterine endometrium does but often out of phase with it. The endometrial tissue grows during the proliferative and secretory phases of the cycle. During or immediately after menstruation, the tissue bleeds, resulting in an inflammatory response with subsequent fibrosis and adhesions to adjacent organs.

The overall incidence of endometriosis is 3% to 10% in reproductive-age women, 20% to 40% in infertile women, and 5% to 20% in women with chronic pelvic pain (Speroff & Fritz, 2005). Although the condition usually develops in the third or fourth decade of life, endometriosis has been found in adolescents with disabling pelvic pain or abnormal vaginal bleeding. Endometriosis may worsen with repeated cycles, or it may remain asymptomatic and undiagnosed, eventually disappearing after menopause. However, endometriosis has been reported to occur in about 5% of postmenopausal women receiving menopausal hormone therapy. The condition appears equally in Caucasian, African-American, and Asian women. It occurs across all socioeconomic levels. There appears to be a familial tendency to develop endometriosis; the condition is six to seven times more prevalent in women who have a first-degree relative with endometriosis as compared to the general population (Speroff & Fritz, 2005).

evolve Nursing Care Plan—Endometriosis

Several theories concerning the cause of endometriosis have been suggested. However, the etiology and pathology of this condition continue to be poorly understood. One of the most widely accepted theories is transplantation or retrograde menstruation. According to this theory, endometrial tissue is refluxed through the uterine tubes during menstruation into the peritoneal cavity, where it implants on the ovaries and other organs. Retrograde menstruation has been documented in a number of surgical studies and is estimated to occur in 90% of menstruating women. For most women endometrial tissue outside the uterus is destroyed before it can implant or seed in the peritoneal cavity or elsewhere. Endometriosis may develop in only 10% to 15% of women because of differences in the functioning of an individual's immune system. It also may reflect differences in genetic makeup or environmental challenges (Speroff & Fritz, 2005).

Symptoms from nonexistent to incapacitating vary among women. Severity of symptoms can change over time and may not reflect the extent of the disease. The major symptoms of endometriosis are pelvic pain, dysmenorrhea, and dyspareunia (painful intercourse). Women may also have chronic noncyclic pelvic pain, pelvic heaviness, or pain radiating into the thighs. Many women report bowel symptoms such as diarrhea, pain with defecation, and constipation caused by avoiding defecation because of the pain. Less common symptoms include abnormal bleeding (hypermenorrhea, menorrhagia, or premenstrual staining) and pain during exercise as a result of adhesions. Women who have endometriosis may also have other conditions such as chronic fatigue syndrome, fibromyalgia, endocrine disorders, and autoimmune disorders (Conversations with Colleagues, 2002-2003).

Impaired fertility may result from adhesions around the uterus that pull the uterus into a fixed, retroverted position. Adhesions around the uterine tubes may block the fimbriated ends or prevent the spontaneous movement that carries the ovum to the uterus.

Management Treatment is based on the severity of symptoms and the goals of the woman or couple. Women without pain who do not want to become pregnant need no treatment. In women with mild pain who may desire a future pregnancy, treatment may be limited to use of NSAIDs during menstruation (see earlier discussion of these medications).

Suppression of endogenous estrogen production and subsequent endometrial lesion growth is the cornerstone of management of the disease. Two main classes of medications are used to suppress endogenous estrogen levels: gonadotropin-releasing hormone (GnRH) agonists and androgen derivatives. GnRH agonist therapy (leuprolide [Lupron] or nafarelin [Synarel]) acts by suppressing pituitary gonadotropin secretion. FSH and LH stimulation of the ovary declines markedly, and ovarian function decreases significantly. A medically induced menopause develops, resulting in anovulation and amenorrhea. Shrinkage of already established endometrial tissue, significant pain relief, and interruption in further lesion development follow. The hypoestrogenism results in hot flashes in almost all women. Trabecular bone loss is common, although most loss is reversible within 12 to 18 months after the medication is stopped.

Both leuprolide (3.75 mg intramuscular injection given once a month) and nafarelin (200 mg administered twice daily by nasal spray) are effective and well tolerated. Both medications reduce endometrial lesions and pelvic pain associated with endometriosis and have posttreatment pregnancy rates similar to that of danazol (Danocrine) therapy (Speroff & Fritz, 2005). Common side effects of these drugs are those of natural menopause—hot flashes and vaginal dryness. Occasionally women report headaches and muscle aches. Treatment is usually limited to 6 months to minimize bone loss. Although unlikely, it is possible for a woman to become pregnant while taking a GnRH agonist. Because the potential teratogenicity of this drug is unclear, women should use a barrier contraceptive during treatment.

Danazol, a mildly androgenic synthetic steroid, suppresses FSH and LH secretion, thus producing anovulation and hypogonadotropism. This results in decreased secretion of estrogen and progesterone and regression of endometrial tissue. Danazol can produce side effects severe enough to cause a woman to discontinue the drug. Side effects include masculinizing traits in the woman (weight gain, edema, decreased breast size, oily skin, hirsutism, and deepening of the voice), all of which often disappear when treatment is discontinued. Other side effects are amenorrhea, hot flashes, vaginal dryness, insomnia, and decreased libido. Migraine headaches, dizziness, fatigue, and depression are also reported. Danazol treatment has been reported to adversely affect lipids, with a decrease in high-density lipoprotein levels and an increase in low-density lipoprotein levels. Danazol should never be prescribed when pregnancy is suspected, and barrier contraception should be used with it because ovulation may not be suppressed. Danazol can produce pseudohermaphroditism in female fetuses. The medication is contraindicated in women with liver disease and should be used with caution in women with cardiac and renal disease.

Women who have early symptomatic disease and who can postpone pregnancy may be treated with continuous OCPs that have a low estrogen-to-progestin ratio to shrink endometrial tissue. Any low-dose OCPs can be used if taken for 15 weeks, followed by 1 week of withdrawal. This therapy is associated with minimal side effects and can be taken for extended periods.

Continuous combined hormone therapy (OCPs, estrogen/progestin patch, estrogen/progestin vaginal ring) for menstrual suppression and administration of NSAIDs are the usual treatment for adolescents under the age of 16 who have endometriosis. GnRH agonists are usually not used since the resultant hypoestrogenic state can affect bone mineralization (ACOG Committee on Adolescent Health Care, 2005).

Surgical intervention is often needed for severe, acute, or incapacitating symptoms. Decisions regarding the extent and type of surgery are influenced by a woman's age, desire for children, and location of the disease. For women who do not want to preserve their ability to have children, the only definite cure is total abdominal hysterectomy with BSO (TAH with BSO). In women who are in their childbearing years and who want children and in whom the disease does not prevent bearing children, reproductive capacity should be retained through careful removal by surgery or laser therapy of all endometrial tissue possible with retention of ovarian function.

Regardless of the type of treatment (short of TAH with BSO), endometriosis recurs in approximately 40% of women. Thus for many women endometriosis is a chronic disease with conditions such as chronic pain or infertility. Counseling and education are critical components of nursing care for women with endometriosis. Women need an honest discussion of treatment options, with potential risks and benefits of each option reviewed. Because pelvic pain is a subjective, personal experience that can be frightening, support is important. Sexual dysfunction resulting from dyspareunia is common and may necessitate referral for counseling. Support groups for women with endometriosis may be found in some locations. Resolve (*www.resolve.org*), an organization for infertile couples, or the Endometriosis Association (*www.ivf.com/endohtml.html*) may also be helpful. The nursing care discussed in the previous section on dysmenorrhea is appropriate for managing chronic pelvic pain and dysmenorrhea experienced by women with endometriosis.

Alterations in Cyclic Bleeding

Women often have changes in amount, duration, interval, or regularity of menstrual cycle bleeding. Often women worry about menstruation that is short, small in amount, or occurs too frequently.

Oligomenorrhea and Hypomenorrhea

The term *oligomenorrhea* often is used to describe decreased menstruation, in amount, time, or both. However, oligomenorrhea more correctly refers to infrequent menstrual periods characterized by intervals of 40 to 45 days or longer, and hypomenorrhea to scanty bleeding at normal intervals. The causes of oligomenorrhea are often abnormalities of hypothalamic, pituitary, or ovarian function. Oligomenorrhea also can be physiologic or part of a woman's normal pattern for the first few years after menarche or for several years before menopause.

Treatment is aimed at reversing the underlying cause, if possible. Hormone therapy using progestins, with or without estrogens, also may be used to prevent complications of unopposed estrogen production (endometrial hyperplasia or carcinoma) or of absent estrogen (vaginal dryness, hot flashes or flushes, osteoporosis).

Women with menstruation characterized by prolonged intervals between cycles need education and counseling. The cause of the condition and the rationale for a specific treatment should be discussed, as should advantages and disadvantages of hormone therapy. If a woman chooses medical intervention, she should be provided with written instructions, taught how to take the medications, and made aware of side effects of any medications. Teaching and counseling should emphasize the importance of the woman keeping careful records of her vaginal bleeding.

Metrorrhagia

Metrorrhagia, or intermenstrual bleeding, refers to any episode of bleeding, whether spotting, menses, or hemorrhage, that occurs at a time other than the normal menses. Mittlestaining, a small amount of bleeding or spotting that occurs at the time of ovulation (14 days before onset of the next menses), is considered normal.

Women taking OCPs may have midcycle bleeding or spotting. (See Chapter 7 for a discussion of the side effects of OCPs.) If the OCP does not sufficiently maintain a hypoplastic endometrium, the endometrium will begin to shed, usually in small amounts at a time, a process termed *breakthrough bleeding.* Breakthrough bleeding is most common in the first three cycles of OCPs. The reduced potency of OCPs (resulting in increased safety) has decreased the amount of available hormones, making it more important that blood levels be kept constant. Taking the pill at exactly the same time each day may alleviate the woman's problem. If the spotting continues, a different formulation that increases either the estrogen or progestin component of the pill can be tried.

Progestin-only contraceptive methods (oral and injectable) also may cause midcycle bleeding, especially in the first several cycles. Women should be advised of this and counseled to report continuation of breakthrough bleeding after the first three to six cycles to their health care provider.

Women with an intrauterine device (IUD) may have spotting between their periods and a heavier menstrual flow.

The causes of intermenstrual bleeding are varied (Box 6-1). It is important that the nurse always consider the possibility that any woman who has not undergone menopause and who seeks care for intermenstrual bleeding is or has recently been pregnant.

Treatment of intermenstrual bleeding depends on the cause and may include reassurance and education concerning mittlestaining, observation of three menstrual cycles for presumed functional ovarian cyst, adjustment of an OCP, removal of foreign bodies, and treatment for vaginal infections. More complex treatment may consist of removal of polyps; evaluation and treatment of an abnormal Papanicolaou (Pap) test, including colposcopy, biopsy, cautery, cryosurgery, or conization; and surgery, chemotherapy, or radiation treatment for malignancy. Important nursing roles include reassurance, counseling, education, and support.

BOX 6-1 Causes of Intermenstrual Bleeding

Reproductive Disorder
Functional ovarian cyst
Cervical erosion infection
Leiomyoma
Polyps, uterine or endocervix
Trauma
Foreign body
Malignancy of reproductive tract

Pregnancy Problems
Pregnancy: implantation
Miscarriage
Ectopic pregnancy
Molar pregnancy
Retained placenta: miscarriage or induced abortion
Retained placenta: birth

Infections
Endometritis
Sexually transmitted infections

Menorrhagia

Menorrhagia (hypermenorrhea) is defined as excessive menstrual bleeding in either duration or amount. A single episode of heavy bleeding may occur, or a woman may have regular flooding as a pattern in which she changes tampons or pads every few hours for several days. The causes of heavy menstrual bleeding are many, including hormonal disturbances, systemic disease, benign and malignant neoplasms, infection, and contraception (IUDs).

NURSING ALERT If the woman herself considers the amount or duration of bleeding to be excessive, the problem should be investigated.

Hemoglobin and hematocrit provide objective indicators to actual blood loss and should always be assessed.

A single episode of heavy bleeding may signal an early pregnancy loss. This type of bleeding is often thought to be a period that is heavier than usual, perhaps delayed, and is associated with abdominal pain or pelvic discomfort. When early pregnancy loss is suspected, a hematocrit and serum β-hCG pregnancy test should be done.

Uterine leiomyomas (fibroids or myomas) are a common cause of menorrhagia. Fibroids are benign tumors of the smooth muscle of the uterus, the etiology of which is unknown. They are estrogen sensitive and commonly develop during the reproductive years and shrink after menopause. Other uterine growths ranging from endometrial polyps to adenocarcinoma and endometrial cancer are other common causes of both heavy menstrual and intermenstrual bleeding.

Treatment for menorrhagia depends on the cause of the bleeding. Treatment options include medical and surgical management. Most fibroids can be monitored by frequent examinations to judge growth, if any, and correction of anemia, if present. Women with menorrhagia should be warned not to use aspirin because of its tendency to increase bleeding. Medical treatment is directed toward temporarily reducing symptoms, shrinking the myoma, and reducing its blood supply. This reduction is often accomplished with the use of a GnRH agonist.

If the woman wishes to retain childbearing potential, a myomectomy may be done. Myomectomy, or removal of the tumors only, is particularly difficult if multiple myomas must be removed. If the woman does not want to preserve her childbearing function or if she has severe symptoms (severe anemia, severe pain, considerable disruption of lifestyle), hysterectomy or endometrial ablation (laser surgery or electrocoagulation) may be done. Based on the assumption that control of arterial blood flow to the fibroid will control symptoms, uterine artery embolization has been reported to result in reduced menorrhagia, less dysmenorrhea, and reduced pelvic pressure and urinary symptoms. This method of treatment is used for women who have completed their childbearing since there is a risk for loss of fertility.

BOX 6-2 Possible Causes of Abnormal Uterine Bleeding

Pregnancy-Related Conditions
Threatened or spontaneous miscarriage
Retained products of conception after elective abortion
Ectopic pregnancy
Placenta previa/placenta abruptio
Trophoblastic disease

Lower Reproductive Tract Infections
Cervicitis
Endometritis
Myometritis
Salpingitis

Benign Anatomic Abnormalities
Adenomyosis
Leiomyomata
Polyps of the cervix or endometrium

Neoplasms
Endometrial hyperplasia
Cancer of cervix and endometrium
Hormonally active tumors (rare)
Vaginal tumors (rare)

Malignant Lesions
Cervical squamous cell carcinoma
Endometrial adenocarcinoma
Estrogen-producing ovarian tumors
Testosterone-producing ovarian tumors
Leiomyosarcoma

Trauma
Genital injury (accidental, coital trauma, sexual abuse)
Foreign body
Lacerations

Systemic Conditions
Adrenal hyperplasia and Cushing's disease
Blood dyscrasias
Coagulopathies
Hypothalamic suppression (from stress, weight loss, excessive exercise)
Polycystic ovary disease
Thyroid disease
Pituitary adenoma or hyperprolactinemia
Severe organ disease (renal or liver failure)

Iatrogenic Causes
Medications with estrogenic activity
Anticoagulants
Exogenous hormone use (oral contraceptives, menopausal hormone therapy)
Selective serotonin reuptake inhibitors
Tamoxifen
Intrauterine devices
Herbal preparation (ginseng)

Source: Albers JR, Hull SK, Wesley RM: Abnormal uterine bleeding, *Am Fam Physician* 69:1915-1926;1931-1932, 2004.

Abnormal Uterine Bleeding

Abnormal uterine bleeding (AUB) is any form of uterine bleeding that is irregular in amount, duration, or timing and not related to regular menstrual bleeding. Box 6-2 lists possible causes of AUB. Although often used interchangeably, the terms *AUB* and *dysfunctional uterine bleeding (DUB)* are not synonymous. DUB is a subset of AUB and is diagnosed by ruling out pregnancy, systemic conditions, genital tract pathology, and iatrogenic causes (Albers, Hull, & Wesley, 2004). DUB is most frequently caused by anovulation. When there is no LH surge or if the corpus luteum does not produce sufficient progesterone to support the endometrium, it will begin to involute and shed. This most often occurs at the extremes of a woman's reproductive years—when the menstrual cycle is just becoming established at menarche or when it draws to a close at menopause. DUB also can be found with any condition that gives rise to chronic anovulation associated with continuous estrogen production. Such conditions include obesity, hyperthyroidism and hypothyroidism, polycystic ovarian syndrome, and any of the endocrine conditions discussed in the sections on amenorrhea and oligomenorrhea.

Women also may unknowingly use medications with an impact on the endometrium (e.g., ginseng, an herbal root, has been associated with estrogen activity and abnormal bleeding). A diagnosis of DUB is made only after all other causes of abnormal menstrual bleeding have been ruled out (Albers, Hull, & Wesley, 2004).

Management

When uterine bleeding is severe and a woman's hemoglobin level is less than 8 g/100 ml (hematocrit of 23% or 24%), the woman may be hospitalized and given conjugated estrogens (Premarin), 25 mg, intravenously. The dose may be repeated until bleeding stops or slows significantly (usually within 1 to 5 hours (Dodd & Sinert, 2007). If bleeding continues after instituting intravenous estrogen, it can be tamponaded by inserting a pediatric Foley catheter into the cervical os and inflating it. The balloon is filled with saline until the bleeding stops. If blood exits through the catheter, the catheter should be clamped. The balloon may be left in place for 12 to 24 hours (Dodd & Sinert, 2007).

If the bleeding has not stopped in 12 to 24 hours, D&C may be done to control severe bleeding and hemorrhage. An endometrial biopsy may be done at the same time to evaluate endometrial tissue or to rule out endometrial cancer. After this treatment, oral conjugated estrogen is given for 21 days. During the last 7 to 10 days of this estrogen regimen, progesterone (e.g., medroxyprogesterone [Provera]) is added. Alternatively a combined OCP is given for 21 days after intravenous therapy.

Once the acute phase has passed, the woman is maintained on cyclic, low-dose OCPs for 3 to 6 months. Such long-term treatment will help prevent recurrence of the pattern of DUB and hemorrhage. If the woman wants contraception, she should continue to take OCPs. If the woman has no need for contraception, the treatment may be stopped to assess her bleeding pattern. If her menses does not resume, a progestin regimen may be prescribed after ruling out pregnancy. This is done to prevent persistent anovulation with chronic unopposed endogenous estrogen hyperstimulation of the endometrium, which can result in eventual atypical tissue changes.

If the recurrent, heavy bleeding is not controlled by hormone therapy or D&C, ablation of the endometrium through laser treatment may be performed. Nursing roles include informing patients of their options, counseling and education as indicated, and referring to the appropriate specialists and health care services (see Nursing Process box).

Infections

Sexually Transmitted Infections

evolve Nursing Care Plan—Sexually Transmitted Infections

Sexually transmitted infections (STIs), or sexually transmitted diseases, include more than 25 infectious organisms that cause infections or infectious disease syndromes primarily transmitted by close, intimate contact (Box 6-3). The terms STIs and sexually transmitted diseases have replaced the older designation, venereal disease, which primarily described gonorrhea and syphilis; we use only STIs in this text. Caused by a wide spectrum of bacteria, viruses, protozoa, and ectoparasites (organisms that live on the outside of the body such as a louse), STIs are a direct cause of tremendous human suffering, place heavy demands on health care services, and cost an estimated $14.7 billion annually to treat. The U.S. Surgeon General has targeted STIs as a priority for prevention and control efforts. Still, STIs are among the most common health problems in the United States. The Centers for Disease Control and Prevention (CDC) estimates that more than 19 million

BOX 6-3 Sexually Transmitted Infections

Bacteria
Chlamydia
Gonorrhea
Syphilis
Chancroid
Lymphogranuloma venereum
Genital mycoplasmas
Group B streptococci

Viruses
Human immunodeficiency virus
Herpes simplex virus, types 1 and 2
Cytomegalovirus
Viral hepatitis A and B
Human papillomavirus

Protozoa
Trichomoniasis

Parasites
Pediculosis (may or may not be sexually transmitted)
Scabies (may or may not be sexually transmitted)

NURSING PROCESS: THE WOMAN WITH A MENSTRUAL DISORDER

Assessment

Take a careful menstrual, obstetric, sexual, and contraceptive history.
Explore the woman's perceptions of her condition, cultural or ethnic influences, experiences with other caregivers, lifestyle, and patterns of coping.
Evaluate the amount of pain or bleeding experienced and its effect on daily activities.
Note home remedies and prescriptions to relieve discomfort.
A symptom diary, in which the woman records emotions, behaviors, physical symptoms, diet, and exercise and rest patterns, is a useful diagnostic tool.

Nursing Diagnoses

Ineffective individual or family coping related to
- insufficient knowledge of the cause of the disorder
- emotional and physiologic effects of the disorder

Deficient knowledge related to
- self-management
- available therapy for the disorder

Risk for disturbed body image related to
- menstrual disorder
- sexual dysfunction

Acute pain related to
- menstrual disorder

Planning

Expected outcomes are that the woman will do the following:
- Verbalize understanding of reproductive anatomy, etiology of her disorder, medication regimen, and diary use
- Develop personal goals that benefit her emotionally and physically
- Choose appropriate therapeutic measures for her menstrual problems
- Adapt successfully to the condition if cure is not possible

Interventions

Medical interventions are discussed on pp. 87-96.
- Express concern for and acceptance of the woman's symptoms as valid.
- Correlate data from the daily diary about emotional status, subjective feelings, and physical state with physiologic changes.
- The clinician facilitates insights and suggests therapeutic options. The woman (or couple) makes choices considered best for her (or them).
- Support groups are an important resource.

Evaluation

The nurse can be assured that care has been effective when the woman reports improvement in the quality of her life, skill in self-management, and a positive self-concept and body image.

Americans are infected with STIs every year, almost half of these are young people ages 15 to 24 (CDC, 2006b) (see Community Focus box). The most common STIs in women are chlamydia, human papillomavirus (HPV), gonorrhea, herpes simplex virus (HSV) type 2, syphilis, and human immunodeficiency virus (HIV) infection. These are discussed in this chapter. Neonatal effects of STIs are discussed in Chapter 28.

COMMUNITY FOCUS

Sexually Transmitted Infections

While in the clinic, interview a nurse about sexually transmitted infections commonly seen in the clinic.

- What are the most common infections seen in the clinic?
- Has the incidence of infections changed over the last 5 years? Which infections have increased and which have decreased in incidence during that time?
- Are adolescents seen in the clinic? Is there a special clinic for adolescents?
- How much independence does the nurse have in diagnosing and treating the sexually transmitted infections?
- What patient teaching guidelines are available in the clinic? Are the guidelines available in languages other than English?

Prevention

Preventing infection (primary prevention) is the most effective way of reducing the adverse consequences of STIs for women and for society. With the advent of serious and potentially lethal STIs that are either not readily cured or incurable, primary prevention becomes critical. Prompt diagnosis and treatment of current infections (secondary prevention) can prevent personal complications and transmission to others.

Preventing the spread of STIs requires that women at risk for transmitting or acquiring infections change their behavior. A critical first step is for the nurse to include questions about a woman's sexual history, sexual risk behaviors, and drug-related risky behaviors as a part of her assessment (Box 6-4). Effective techniques in providing prevention counseling include using open-ended questions, using understandable language, and reassuring the woman that treatment will be provided regardless of consideration such as ability to pay, language spoken, or lifestyle (CDC, Workowski, & Berman, 2006). Prevention messages should include descriptions of specific actions to be taken to avoid acquiring or transmitting STIs (e.g., refrain from sexual activity if STI-related symptoms are present) and should be tailored to the individual woman, with attention given to her specific risk factors (see Patient Teaching box).

To be motivated to take preventive actions, a woman must believe that acquiring a disease will be serious for her and that she is at risk for infection. Most individuals tend to underestimate their personal risk of infection in a given situation. Thus many women may not perceive themselves as being at risk for contracting an STI, and telling them that they should carry condoms may not be well received. Although levels of awareness of STIs are generally high, widespread misconceptions or specific gaps in knowledge also exist. Therefore nurses have a responsibility to ensure that their patients have accurate, complete knowledge about transmission and symptoms

BOX 6-4 Assessing Risk Behaviors for Human Immunodeficiency Virus and Other Sexually Transmitted Infections

Answer these questions for all the times in your life from 1977* to the present.

Sexual Risk

Are you sexually active now?
If no, have you had sex in the past?
Ever had an oral, vaginal, or anal sexual experience with another person?
With how many different people? One? Two or 3? Four to 10? More than 10?
Have your partners been men, women, both?
Ever thought that a sex partner put you at risk for AIDS/STI (intravenous drug user, bisexual)?
Ever had an STI (herpes, gonorrhea, genital warts, chlamydia)?
Ever had sex against your will?
What do you do to protect yourself from AIDS/STIs?
Do you use male condoms? Female condoms? Other barriers?

Drug Use–Related Risk

Ever injected drugs using shared equipment, including street drugs, steroids?
Ever had sex with a person who uses and shares?
Ever had sex while stoned, high, or too drunk to remember the details?
Ever exchanged sex for drugs, money, shelter?

Blood-Related Risks

Ever had a blood transfusion?
Ever had sex with a person who had a blood transfusion?
Ever had sex with a person with hemophilia?
Ever received donor semen, egg, transplanted organ or tissue?
Ever shared equipment for tattoo, body piercing?

Other

Ever had a test for HIV?
Ever worried about AIDS and would like to talk with someone about it?

Adapted from Marrazzo JM, Guest F, Cates W: Reproductive tract infections, including HIV and other sexually transmitted infections. In R Hatcher et al: *Contraceptive technology*, ed 19, New York, 2007, Ardent Media.
*Relates to risk of HIV—infection not known to exist in humans until this time.
AIDS, Acquired immunodeficiency syndrome; *HIV*, human immunodeficiency virus; *STI*, sexually transmitted infection.

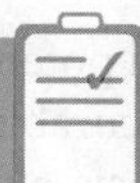

PATIENT TEACHING Prevention of Genital Tract Infections in Women

- Practice genital hygiene.
- Choose underwear or hosiery with a cotton crotch.
- Avoid tight-fitting clothing (especially tight jeans).
- Select cloth car seat covers instead of vinyl.
- Limit the time spent in damp exercise clothes (especially swimsuits, leotards, and tights).
- Limit exposure to bath salts or bubble bath.
- Avoid colored or scented toilet tissue.
- If sensitive, discontinue use of feminine hygiene deodorant sprays.
- Use condoms.
- Void before and after intercourse.
- Decrease dietary sugar.
- Drink yeast-active milk and eat yogurt (with lactobacilli).
- Do not douche.

of STIs and the behaviors that place them at risk for contracting an infection.

Primary preventive measures are individual activities aimed at avoiding infection. Risk-free options include complete abstinence from sexual activities that transmit semen, blood, or other body fluids or that allow for skin-to-skin contact (CDC, Workowski, & Berman, 2006). Involvement in a mutually monogamous relationship with an uninfected partner also eliminates risk of contracting STIs. When neither of these options is realistic for a woman, the nurse must focus on other, more feasible measures.

STI/HIV Prevention Strategies

An essential component of primary prevention is counseling the woman regarding sexual practices so that she can avoid acquiring or transmitting STIs, including attaining knowledge of her partner, reducing her number of partners, practicing low risk sex, and avoiding the exchange of body fluids.

Reducing the number of partners and avoiding partners who have had many previous sexual partners decreases a woman's chances of contracting an STI. Discussing each new partner's previous sexual history and exposure to STIs will augment other efforts to reduce risk; however, sexual partners are not always truthful about their sexual history. Women must be cautioned that measures to avoid transmission of infections are always advisable, even when partners insist otherwise. Critically important is whether male partners will accept wearing condoms. Women should be cautioned against making decisions about a partner's sexual and other behaviors based on appearances and unfounded assumptions such as the following (Marrazzo, Guest, & Cates, 2007):

- Single people have many partners and risky practices.
- Older people have few partners and infrequent sexual encounters.
- Sexually experienced people know how to avoid transmitting infections.
- Married people are heterosexual, low risk, and monogamous.
- People who look healthy are healthy.
- People with good jobs do not use drugs.

Sexually active persons also may benefit from carefully examining a partner for lesions, sores, ulcerations, rashes, redness, discharge, swelling, and odor before initiating sexual activity.

Women should be taught low risk sexual practices, as well as which sexual practices to avoid (see Box 4-8). Sexual fantasizing is safe, as are caressing, hugging, body rubbing, and massage. Mutual masturbation is low risk as long as there is no contact with a partner's semen or vaginal secretions. All sexual activities are safe when both partners are monogamous, trustworthy, and known (by testing) to be free of disease.

The physical barrier promoted for the prevention of sexual transmission of HIV and other STIs is the condom (male and female). The nurse should remind women to use a condom with every sexual encounter; to use latex or plastic male condoms rather than natural skin condoms for STI protection; to use a condom with a current expiration date; to use each one only once; and to handle it carefully to avoid damaging it with fingernails, teeth, or other sharp objects. Condoms should be stored away from high heat. Although it is not ideal, women may choose to safely carry condoms in wallets, shoes, or inside a bra. Women can be taught the differences among condoms: price ranges, sizes, and where they can be purchased. Explicit instructions for how to apply a male condom are included in Box 7-9.

The female condom—a lubricated polyurethane sheath with a ring on each end that is inserted into the vagina—has been shown in laboratory studies to be an effective mechanical barrier to viruses, including HIV. Studies suggest that the female condom is at least as effective as male condoms in preventing transmission of STIs (Hoffman et al, 2004). What is important and should be stressed by nurses is the consistent use of condoms for every act of sexual intimacy when there is the possibility of transmission of disease (Box 6-5).

There is concern about the potential for cervicovaginal epithelial disruption with nonoxynol-9 (N-9)–based spermicides (Wilkinson et al, 2002). Frequent use of spermicides containing N-9 has been associated with genital lesions and may increase HIV transmission; thus condoms lubricated with N-9 are not recommended (CDC, Workowski, & Berman, 2006).

Certain sexual practices should be avoided to reduce one's risk of infection. Abstinence from any sexual activities that could result in exchange of infective body fluids helps decrease risk. Anal-genital intercourse, anal-oral contact, and anal-digital activity are high risk sexual behaviors and should be avoided. Because enteric infections are transmitted by oral-fecal contact, avoiding oral-anal activities, "rimming" (licking the anal area), and digital-anal activities should reduce the likelihood of infection. Vaginal intercourse should never follow anal contact unless a condom has been used and then removed and replaced with a new condom.

Sexual transmission occurs through direct skin or mucous membrane contact with infectious lesions or body fluids. Because mucosal linings are delicate and subject to considerable mechanical trauma during intercourse, small abrasions often may occur, facilitating entry of infectious agents into the bloodstream. The rectal epithelium is especially easy to trau-

BOX 6-5 Strategies to Enhance a Woman's Negotiation and Communication Skills Regarding Condom Use

- Suggest that the woman talk with her partner about condom use at a time removed from sexual activity.
- Role play possible partner reactions with a woman and her alternative responses.
- Ask a woman who appears particularly uncomfortable to rehearse how she might approach the topic of condom use.
- Women may feel more comfortable and in control of the situation if they sort out their feelings and fears before talking with their partners. Women can be reassured that it is natural to be uncomfortable and that the hardest part is getting started.
- Clarify for herself what she will and will not do sexually.
- Suggest that the woman begin by saying, "I need to talk with you about something that is important to both of us. It's hard for me, and I feel embarrassed, but I think we need to talk about ways to reduce risk when we have sex."
- The partner may need time to think about what he has heard.
- If the partner resists risk-reducing sexual behaviors, the woman may wish to reconsider the relationship.

matize with penetration. Sexual practices that increase the likelihood of tissue damage or bleeding such as fisting (inserting a fist into the rectum) should be avoided. Deep kissing when lips, gums, or other tissues are raw or broken also should be avoided.

Sexually Transmitted Bacterial Infections

Chlamydia

Chlamydia trachomatis is the most common and fastest-spreading STI in American women, with an estimated 3 million new cases each year (CDC, 2006b). These infections are often silent and highly destructive. Their sequelae and complications can be very serious. In women chlamydial infections are difficult to diagnose; the symptoms, if present, are nonspecific, and culturing the organism is expensive.

Early identification of *C. trachomatis* is important because untreated infection often leads to acute salpingitis or PID. PID is the most serious complication of chlamydial infections, and past chlamydial infections are associated with an increased risk of ectopic pregnancy and tubal factor infertility. Chlamydial infection of the cervix causes inflammation that results in microscopic cervical ulcerations. These ulcerations may increase the risk of acquiring HIV infection.

Sexually active women younger than age 20 are two to three times as likely to become infected with chlamydia as women between ages 20 and 29. Women over age 30 have the lowest rate of infection. Risky behaviors, including multiple partners and failure to use barrier methods of birth control, increase a woman's risk of chlamydial infection. Lower socioeconomic status may be a risk factor, especially with respect to treatment-seeking behaviors.

Screening and Diagnosis

In addition to obtaining information about the presence of risk factors, the nurse should inquire about the presence of any symptoms. The CDC, Workowski, & Berman (2006) and the U.S. Preventive Services Task Force (USPSTF, 2001a) strongly urge screening of asymptomatic, high risk women in whom infection would otherwise go undetected. CDC guidelines recommend screening of all sexually active adolescents, women between ages 20 and 25, and women older than 25 who are at high risk (e.g., those with new or multiple partners). Whenever possible, all women with two or more risk factors for chlamydia should be cultured.

All pregnant women should have cervical cultures for chlamydia at the first prenatal visit. Culturing should be repeated late in the third trimester (36 weeks) if the woman was previously positive or if she is younger than age 25, has a new sex partner, or has multiple sex partners.

Although chlamydia infections are usually asymptomatic, some women may experience spotting or postcoital bleeding, mucoid or purulent cervical discharge, or dysuria. Bleeding results from inflammation and erosion of the cervical columnar epithelium. Women taking OCPs may have breakthrough bleeding.

Diagnosis of chlamydia is by culture (expensive and labor intensive), deoxyribonucleic acid (DNA) probe (less expensive but less sensitivity), enzyme immunoassay (less expensive but less sensitivity), and nucleic acid amplification (expensive but about 90% sensitivity). Special culture media and proper handling of specimens are important; thus the nurse should always know what is required in the individual practice site. Chlamydial culture testing is not always available, primarily because of expense.

Management

CDC recommendations for the treatment of urethral, cervical, and rectal chlamydial infections are doxycycline (100 mg orally twice a day for 7 days) or azithromycin (1 g orally in a single dose) (CDC, Workowski, & Berman, 2006). Azithromycin is often prescribed when compliance may be a problem because only one dose is needed; however, expense is a concern with this medication. If the woman is pregnant, erythromycin (500 mg orally four times a day for 7 days) or amoxicillin (500 mg orally three times a day for 7 days) is used. Women who have a chlamydial infection and are also infected with HIV should be treated with the same regimen as those who are not infected with HIV.

Because chlamydia is often asymptomatic, the woman should be cautioned to take all medication prescribed. All exposed sexual partners should be treated. Women treated with recommended or alternative regimens do not need to be retested unless symptoms continue. It is recommended that pregnant women be retested 3 weeks after completing the medication, although the validity of this practice has not been established (CDC, Workowski, & Berman, 2006).

Gonorrhea

Gonorrhea is probably the oldest communicable disease in the United States. An estimated 600,000 American men and women contract gonorrhea each year (CDC, Workowski, & Berman, 2006). The incidence of drug-resistant cases of gonorrhea, in particular penicillinase-producing *Neisseria gonorrhoeae*, is increasing dramatically in the United States.

Gonorrhea is caused by the aerobic, gram-negative diplococci *N. gonorrhoeae.* It is almost exclusively transmitted by sexual contact. The principal means of transmission is genital-to-genital contact during sexual activity; however, it is also spread by oral-genital and anal-genital contact. There is also evidence that infection may spread in females from vagina to rectum. Although the organism has been recovered from inanimate objects artificially inoculated with the bacteria, there is no evidence that natural transmission occurs this way.

Age is probably the most important risk factor associated with gonorrhea. In the United States the highest reported rates of infection are among sexually active teenagers, young adults, and African-Americans. The majority of those contracting gonorrhea are younger than 20 years of age and engage in sexual activities with multiple partners (CDC, 2005).

Women are often asymptomatic, with one third of infections in adolescent women going unnoticed. When symptoms are present, they are often less specific than the symptoms in men. Women may have a purulent endocervical discharge, but discharge is usually minimal or absent. Menstrual irregularities may be the initial symptom, or women may complain of pain: chronic or acute severe pelvic or lower abdominal pain or longer, more painful menses. Infrequently dysuria, vague abdominal pain, or low backache prompts a woman to seek care. Gonococcal rectal infection may occur in women after anal intercourse, with 10% to 30% of urogenital infections accompanied by rectal infection. Individuals with rectal gonorrhea may be completely asymptomatic or, conversely, have severe symptoms with profuse purulent anal discharge, rectal pain, and blood in the stool. Rectal itching, fullness, pressure, and pain are also common symptoms, as is diarrhea. A diffuse vaginitis with vulvitis is the most common form of gonococcal infection in prepubertal girls. There may be few signs of infection; or vaginal discharge, dysuria, and swollen, reddened labia may be present.

Gonococcal infections in pregnancy potentially affect both mother and infant. Women with cervical gonorrhea may develop salpingitis in the first trimester. Perinatal complications of gonococcal infection include premature rupture of membranes, preterm birth, chorioamnionitis, neonatal sepsis, intrauterine growth restriction, and maternal postpartum sepsis. Amniotic infection syndrome—manifested by placental, fetal, and umbilical cord inflammation following premature rupture of the membranes—may result from gonorrheal infection during pregnancy.

Screening and Diagnosis

Because gonococcal infections in women are often asymptomatic, the CDC recommends screening all women at risk for gonorrhea (CDC, Workowski, & Berman, 2006). All pregnant women should be screened at the first prenatal visit, and infected women and those identified with risky behaviors rescreened at 36 weeks of gestation. Gonococcal infection cannot be diagnosed reliably by clinical signs and symptoms alone. Individuals may have "classic" symptoms, vague symptoms that may be attributed to a number of conditions, or no symptoms at all. Cultures should be obtained from the endocervix, the rectum, and, when indicated, the pharynx. Thayer-Martin cultures are recommended to diagnose gonorrhea in women. Because coinfection is common, any woman suspected of having gonorrhea should have a chlamydial culture and serologic test for syphilis unless one has been done within the past 2 months.

Management

Management of gonorrhea is straightforward, and with appropriate antibiotic therapy the cure is usually rapid. Single-dose efficacy is a major consideration in selecting an antibiotic regimen for women with gonorrhea. Another important consideration is the high proportion (45%) of women with coexisting chlamydial infections. The treatment of choice for uncomplicated urethral, endocervical, and rectal infections in pregnant and nonpregnant women is cefixime (400 mg orally once) or ceftriaxone (125 mg intramuscularly once). The CDC recommends concomitant treatment for chlamydia because coinfection is common (CDC, Workowski, & Berman, 2006). All women with both gonorrhea and syphilis should also be treated for syphilis according to CDC guidelines (see discussion of syphilis later in this chapter).

Gonorrhea is highly communicable. Recent (past 30 days) sexual partners should be examined, cultured, and treated with appropriate regimens. Most treatment failures result from reinfection. The woman needs to be informed of this, as well as of the consequences of reinfection in terms of chronicity, complications, and potential infertility. Women are counseled to use condoms. All women with gonorrhea should be offered confidential counseling and testing for HIV infection.

LEGAL TIP Gonorrhea Gonorrhea is a reportable communicable disease. Health care providers are legally responsible for reporting all cases of gonorrhea to health authorities, usually the local health department in the patient's county of residence. Women should be informed that the case will be reported, told why, and informed of the possibility of being contacted by a health department epidemiologist.

Syphilis

Syphilis, one of the earliest described STIs, is caused by *Treponema pallidum,* a motile spirochete. Transmission is thought to be by entry through microscopic abrasions in the subcutaneous tissue, which can occur during sexual intercourse. The disease can also be transmitted through kissing, biting, or oral-genital sex. Transplacental transmission may occur at any time during pregnancy; the degree of risk is related to the quantity of spirochetes in the maternal bloodstream.

The rate of primary and secondary syphilis in the United States in 2006 was 3.3 per 100,000, an increase of 11% since 2005 (CDC, 2007). Among women rates were highest in the 20- to 24-year-old age group. Much of the increase in cases was observed in men having sex with men.

Syphilis is a complex disease that can lead to serious systemic disease and even death when untreated. Infection manifests itself in distinct stages with different symptoms and clinical manifestations. Primary syphilis is characterized by a primary lesion, the chancre, which appears 5 to 90 days after infection. This lesion often begins as a painless papule at the site of inoculation and then erodes to form a nontender,

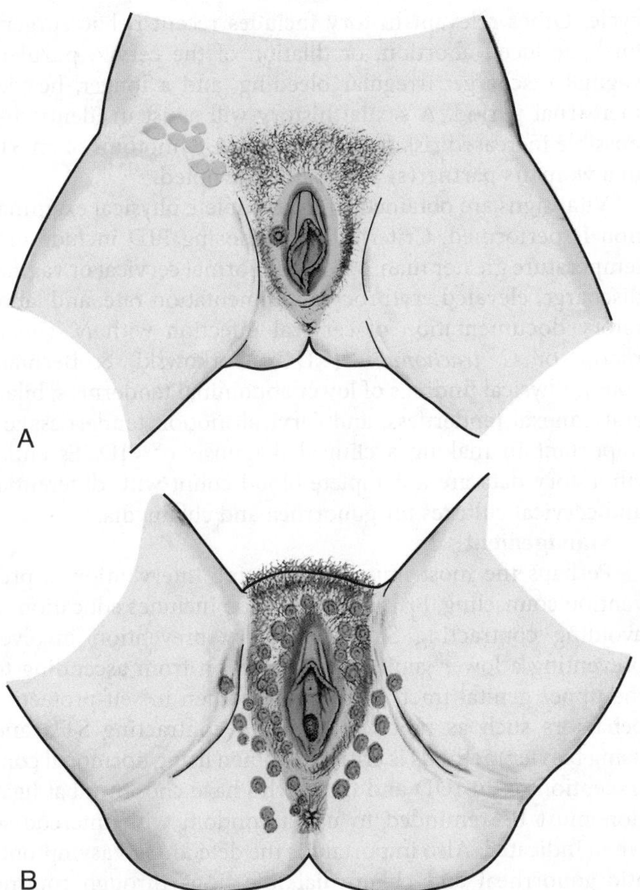

Fig. 6-3 Syphilis. **A**, Primary stage: chancre with inguinal adenopathy. **B**, Secondary stage: condylomata lata.

shallow, indurated, clean ulcer several millimeters to centimeters in size (Fig. 6-3). Secondary syphilis occurs 6 weeks to 6 months after the appearance of the chancre. It is characterized by a widespread, symmetric, maculopapular rash on the palms and soles and generalized lymphadenopathy. The infected individual also may experience fever, headache, and malaise.

Condylomata lata (broad, painless, pink-gray, wartlike infectious lesions) may develop on the vulva, perineum, or anus. If the woman is untreated, she enters a latent phase that is asymptomatic for the majority of individuals. Left untreated, about one third of these women will develop tertiary syphilis. Neurologic, cardiovascular, musculoskeletal, or multiorgan system complications can develop in the third stage.

Screening and Diagnosis

All women who are diagnosed with another STI or with HIV should be screened for syphilis. All pregnant women should be screened for syphilis at the first prenatal visit, again in the late third trimester, and at the time of giving birth if high risk (CDC, Workowski, & Berman, 2006). Diagnosis depends on microscopic examination of primary and secondary lesion tissue and serology during latency and late infection. A test for antibodies may not be reactive in the presence of active infection because it takes time for the body's immune system to develop antibodies to any antigens. Up to one third of people in early primary syphilis may have nonreactive serologic tests. Two types of serologic tests are used: nontreponemal and treponemal. Nontreponemal antibody tests such as VDRL (Venereal Disease Research Laboratories) and RPR (rapid plasma reagin) are used as screening tests. False-positive results are not unusual, particularly when conditions such as acute infection, autoimmune disorders, malignancy, pregnancy, and drug addiction exist, and after immunization or vaccination. The treponemal tests, fluorescent treponemal antibody absorbed and microhemagglutination assays for antibody to *T. pallidum,* are used to confirm positive results. Test results in patients with early primary or incubating syphilis may be negative. Seroconversion usually takes place 6 to 8 weeks after exposure; thus testing should be repeated in 1 to 2 months when a suggestive genital lesion exists.

Tests (e.g., wet preps and cultures) for concomitant STIs (e.g., chlamydia and gonorrhea) should be done, and HIV testing offered if indicated.

Management

Penicillin is the preferred drug for treating patients with syphilis. It is the only proven therapy that has been widely used for patients with neurosyphilis, congenital syphilis, or syphilis during pregnancy. Intramuscular penicillin G benzathine (2.4 million units intramuscularly once) is used to treat primary, secondary, and early latent syphilis. Women with syphilis of longer than 1 year's duration (late latent or tertiary stages) require weekly treatment of 2.4 million units of penicillin G benzathine for 3 weeks. Although doxycycline, tetracycline, and erythromycin are alternative treatments for penicillin-allergic patients, both tetracycline and doxycycline are contraindicated in pregnancy, and erythromycin is unlikely to cure a fetal infection. Therefore, if necessary, pregnant women should receive skin testing and be treated with penicillin or be desensitized (CDC, Workowski, & Berman, 2006). Specific protocols are recommended by the CDC.

NURSING ALERT Patients treated for syphilis may experience a Jarisch-Herxheimer reaction. This is an acute febrile reaction often accompanied by headache, myalgias, and arthralgias that develop within the first 24 hours of treatment. The reaction may be treated symptomatically with analgesics and antipyretics. If treatment precipitates this reaction in the second half of pregnancy, women are at risk for preterm labor and birth. They should be advised to contact their health care provider if they notice any change in fetal movement or have any contractions.

Monthly follow-up is mandatory so that repeated treatment may be given if needed. The nurse should emphasize the necessity of long-term serologic testing even in the absence of symptoms. The woman should be advised to practice sexual abstinence until treatment is completed, all evidence of primary and secondary syphilis is gone, and serologic evidence of a cure is demonstrated. Women should be told to notify all partners who may have been exposed. They should be informed that the disease is reportable. Preventive measures should be discussed.

Pelvic Inflammatory Disease

Pelvic inflammatory disease (PID) is an infectious process that most commonly involves the uterine tubes, causing salpingitis;

the uterus, causing endometritis; and, more rarely, the ovaries and peritoneal surfaces. Multiple organisms have been found to cause PID; most cases are associated with more than one organism. In the past the most common causative agent was thought to be *N. gonorrhoeae;* however, *C. trachomatis* is now estimated to cause one half of all cases of PID. In addition to gonorrhea and chlamydia, a wide variety of anaerobic and aerobic bacteria cause PID. It encompasses a wide variety of pathologic processes; the infection can be acute, subacute, or chronic and can have a wide range of symptoms.

evolve Animation—Pelvic Inflammatory Disease

Most PID results from the ascending spread of microorganisms from the vagina and endocervix to the upper genital tract. This spread most commonly happens at the end of or just after menses following reception of an infectious agent. During the menstrual period several factors facilitate the development of an infection: the cervical os is slightly open, the cervical mucus barrier is absent, and menstrual blood is an excellent medium for growth. PID also may develop after a miscarriage or an induced abortion, pelvic surgery, or childbirth.

Risk factors for acquiring PID are those associated with the risk of contracting an STI, including young age, multiple partners, high rate of new partners, and a history of STIs. Women who use IUDs may be at increased risk for PID if they have more than one sexual partner or if the partner has other sexual partners because they are at higher risk for acquiring an STI. Most of this risk occurs in the first months after IUD insertion. PID tends to recur.

Women who have had PID are at increased risk for ectopic pregnancy, infertility, and chronic pelvic pain. After a single episode of PID, a woman's risk for ectopic pregnancy increases sevenfold compared with the risk for women who have never had PID. Other problems associated with PID include dyspareunia, pyosalpinx (pus in the uterine tubes), tuboovarian abscess, and pelvic adhesions.

The symptoms of PID vary, depending on whether the infection is acute, subacute, or chronic. However, pain is common to all clinical presentations. It may be dull, cramping, and intermittent (subacute) or severe, persistent, and incapacitating (acute). The woman with acute PID also may complain of intermenstrual bleeding. Physical examination reveals adnexal tenderness, with or without rebound, and exquisite tenderness with cervical movement (Chandelier sign). Pelvic tenderness is usually bilateral. There may or may not be a palpable adnexal swelling or thickening. A urethral or cervical discharge, often purulent in nature, may be present. A fever of 39° C or above is characteristic. Significant laboratory data include an elevated white blood cell count and a markedly elevated erythrocyte sedimentation rate. Fever and peritonitis are more characteristic of gonococcal PID; PID caused by other organisms is more likely to be "silent." Because PID caused by chlamydia is more commonly asymptomatic, it more often results in tubal obstruction from delayed diagnosis or inadequate treatment.

Screening and Diagnosis

A careful history is necessary to distinguish between PID and other conditions that cause abdominal pain such as an ectopic pregnancy or appendicitis. A menstrual history is useful in establishing the relationship of onset of pain to menses and in identifying any variations from normal in the cycle. Other relevant history includes recent pelvic surgery, birth, induced abortion, or dilation of the cervix; purulent vaginal discharge; irregular bleeding; and a longer, heavier menstrual period. A sexual history will assist in identifying possible increased risk for STI exposure. Symptoms of an STI in a woman's partner(s) also should be noted.

Vital signs are obtained, and a complete physical examination is performed. Criteria for diagnosing PID include oral temperature greater than 38.3° C, abnormal cervical or vaginal discharge, elevated erythrocyte sedimentation rate, and laboratory documentation of cervical infection with *N. gonorrhoeae* or *C. trachomatis* (CDC, Workowski, & Berman, 2006). Physical findings of lower abdominal tenderness, bilateral adnexal tenderness, and cervical motion tenderness are important in making a clinical diagnosis of PID. Essential laboratory data are a complete blood count with differential and cervical cultures for gonorrhea and chlamydia.

Management

Perhaps the most important nursing intervention is prevention counseling. Primary prevention includes education in avoiding contracting STIs; secondary prevention involves preventing a lower genital tract infection from ascending to the upper genital tract. Instructing women in self-protective behaviors such as practices to avoid contracting STIs and using barrier methods is critical. Women using hormonal contraception or an IUD and those who have chosen tubal ligation must be reminded to use a condom with intercourse when indicated. Also important is the detection of asymptomatic gonorrheal and chlamydial infections through routine screening of women who practice risky behaviors or have specific risk factors such as age. Partner notification when an STI is diagnosed is essential to prevent reinfection.

When and if women with PID are hospitalized varies. Although many experts recommend that all women with PID be hospitalized so parenteral antibiotic treatment can be done, the CDC does not. The CDC recommends hospitalization in the following situations (CDC, Workowski, & Berman, 2006):

- Surgical emergencies such as appendicitis cannot be excluded.
- The woman has a tuboovarian abscess.
- The woman is pregnant.
- Severe illness precludes outpatient management.
- The woman is unable to tolerate or follow an outpatient oral regimen.
- The woman has failed to respond to oral outpatient therapy.

Although treatment regimens vary with the infecting organism, generally a broad-spectrum antibiotic is used. Several antimicrobial regimens have proved to be effective, and no single therapeutic regimen of choice exists. The woman with acute PID should be on bed rest in a semi-Fowler's position. Comfort measures include analgesics for pain and all other nursing measures applicable to a patient confined to bed. Few pelvic examinations should be done during the acute phase of the disease. During the recovery phase the woman should restrict her activity and make every effort to get adequate rest and a nutritionally sound diet. Follow-up laboratory work after treatment should include endocervical cultures for a test of cure.

Health education is central to effective management of PID. Nurses should explain the nature of the disease to women and encourage them to comply with all therapy and prevention recommendations, emphasizing the need to take all medication, even if symptoms disappear. Any potential problems (such as a lack of money for prescriptions or a lack of transportation to return for follow-up appointments) that would prevent a woman from completing a course of treatment should be identified, referrals made for assistance as needed, and the importance of follow-up visits stressed. Women should be counseled to refrain from sexual intercourse until their treatment is completed. Contraceptive counseling, including information on barrier methods such as condoms, the contraceptive sponge, and the diaphragm, should be provided. A woman with a history of PID should not use an IUD as her contraceptive method.

The woman with PID may be acutely ill or have long-term discomfort. Either or both take an emotional toll. Pain in itself is debilitating and is compounded by the infectious process. The potential or actual loss of reproductive capabilities can be devastating and can adversely affect the woman's self-concept. Part of the nurse's role is to help the woman adjust her self-concept to fit reality and to accept alterations in a way that promotes health. Because PID is so closely tied to sexuality, body image, and self-concept, the woman diagnosed with it will need supportive care. Her feelings should be discussed, and her partner(s) included when appropriate.

Sexually Transmitted Viral Infections

Human Papillomavirus

Human papillomavirus (HPV) infection, previously named genital or venereal warts, is an STI that was first described in 25 AD and is now the most common viral STI seen in ambulatory health care settings. HPV, a double-stranded DNA virus, has more than 30 serotypes that can be transmitted sexually: five of which are known to cause genital wart formation, and eight of which are currently thought to have oncogenic (tumor-causing) potential (CDC, Workowski, & Berman, 2006). HPV is the primary cause of cervical neoplasia (American Cancer Society [ACS], 2008a)

In women HPV lesions (also called *condylomata acuminata*) are most commonly seen in the posterior part of the introitus. Lesions also are found on the buttocks, vulva, vagina, anus, and cervix (Fig. 6-4). Typically the lesions are small (2 to 3 mm in diameter and 10 to 15 mm in height), soft, papillary swellings occurring singly or in clusters on the genital and anal-rectal region. Infections of long duration may appear as a cauliflower-like mass. In moist areas such as the vaginal introitus, the lesions may appear to have multiple fine, finger-like projections. Vaginal lesions are often multiple. Flat-topped papules, 1 to 4 mm in diameter, are seen most often on the cervix. Often these lesions are visualized only under magnification. Warts are usually flesh colored or slightly darker on Caucasian women, black on African-American women, and brownish on Asian women. The lesions are usually painless; but they may be uncomfortable, particularly when very large, inflamed, or ulcerated. Chronic vaginal discharge, pruritus, or dyspareunia can occur.

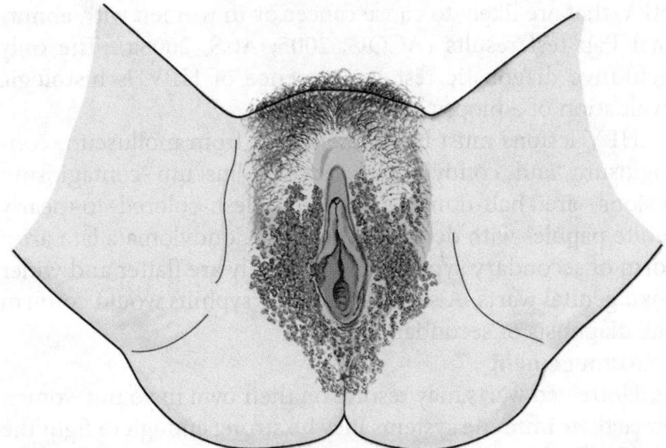

Fig. 6-4 HPV infection. Genital warts or condylomata acuminata.

HPV infections are thought to be more common in pregnant than in nonpregnant women, with an increase in incidence from the first trimester to the third. Furthermore, a significant proportion of preexisting HPV lesions enlarge greatly during pregnancy, a proliferation presumably resulting from the relative state of immunosuppression present during this period. Lesions may become so large during pregnancy that they affect urination, defecation, mobility, and fetal descent, although birth by cesarean is rarely necessary. Cesarean birth may be performed when extensive growths are present. Initial observation of large growths can be misleading, suggesting that the entire vagina is involved. However, all of the growth may derive from one stalk, and in such cases it may be possible to push the large mass to the side, allowing the baby to pass through.

Screening and Diagnosis

A woman with HPV lesions may complain of symptoms such as a profuse, irritating vaginal discharge, itching, dyspareunia, or postcoital bleeding. She also may report "bumps" on her vulva or labia. History of a known exposure is important; however, because of the potentially long latency period and the possibility of subclinical infections in men, the lack of a history of known exposure cannot be used to exclude a diagnosis of HPV infection.

Physical inspection of the vulva, perineum, anus, vagina, and cervix is essential whenever HPV lesions are suspected or seen in one area. Because speculum examination of the vagina may block some lesions, it is important to rotate the speculum blades until all areas are visualized. When lesions are visible, the characteristic appearance previously described is considered diagnostic. However, in many instances cervical lesions are not visible, and some vaginal or vulvar lesions also may be unobservable to the naked eye. Because of the potential spread of vulvar or vaginal lesions to the anus, gloves should be changed between vaginal and rectal examinations.

Viral screening and typing for HPV is available but not standard practice. History, evaluation of signs and symptoms, Pap test, and physical examination are used in making a diagnosis. The HPV-DNA test can be used in women over the age of 30 in combination with the Pap test to screen for types of

HPV that are likely to cause cancer or in women with abnormal Pap test results (ACOG, 2005; ACS, 2008a). The only definitive diagnostic test for presence of HPV is histologic evaluation of a biopsy specimen.

HPV lesions must be differentiated from molluscum contagiosum and condylomata lata. Molluscum contagiosum lesions are half-domed, smooth, flesh-colored–to–pearly white papules with depressed centers. Condylomata lata are a form of secondary syphilis and generally are flatter and wider than genital warts. A serologic test for syphilis would confirm the diagnosis of secondary syphilis.

Management

Untreated warts may resolve on their own in young women since their immune systems may be strong enough to fight the HPV infection. Treatment of genital warts, if needed, is often difficult. No therapy has been shown to eradicate HPV. Therefore the goal of treatment is removal of warts and relief of signs and symptoms, not the eradication of HPV (CDC, Workowski, & Berman, 2006). The patient often must make multiple office visits; frequently many different treatment modalities will be used. Eradication of the virus is not considered conclusive even after there is no visible evidence of wart tissue because of the high incidence of recurrence.

Treatment of genital warts should be guided by preference of the woman, available resources, and experience of the health care provider. No one of the treatments is superior to all other treatments, and no one treatment is ideal for all warts (CDC, Workowski, & Berman, 2006). Imiquimod, podophyllin, and podofilox are common treatments but should not be used during pregnancy. Because the lesions can proliferate and become friable during pregnancy, many experts recommend their removal using cryotherapy or various surgical techniques (CDC, Workowski, & Berman, 2006).

Women who have discomfort associated with genital warts may find that bathing with an oatmeal solution and drying the area with cool air from a hair dryer provides some relief. Keeping the area clean and dry also decreases the growth of the warts. Cotton underwear and loose-fitting clothes that decrease friction and irritation may lessen discomfort. Women should be advised to maintain a healthy lifestyle to aid the immune system and be counseled regarding diet, rest, stress reduction, and exercise.

Patient counseling should address how the virus is transmitted and stress that no immunity is conferred with infection and that reacquisition of the infection is likely with repeated contact. Women need to know that partners should be checked even if they are asymptomatic. Because HPV is highly contagious, the majority of women's partners will be infected and should be treated. All sexually active women with multiple partners or a history of HPV should be encouraged to use latex condoms and a vaginal spermicide for intercourse to decrease acquisition or transmission of condylomata.

Instructions for all medications and treatments must be detailed. Women should be informed before treatment of the possibility of posttreatment pain associated with specific therapies. The importance of thorough treatment of concurrent vaginitis or STI should be emphasized. The link between cervical cancer and HPV infections and the need for close follow-up should be discussed. Annual health examinations are recommended to assess disease recurrence and screening for cervical cancer.

Women should be counseled to have regular Pap screening as recommended for women without genital warts. The presence of genital warts is not an indication for a change in Pap test frequency or for cervical colposcopy (CDC, Workowski, & Berman, 2006).

Women with HPV infection may radically alter their sexual practices both from fear of transmission to and from a partner and from genital discomfort associated with treatment, which may have a negative impact on their sexual relationships. Unless the partner accepts and understands the necessary precautions, it may be difficult for the woman to follow the treatment regimen. The nurse can offer to discuss feelings that the woman may have. When indicated, joint counseling can be suggested.

Prevention

Preventive strategies that have been suggested include abstinence from all sexual activity, staying in a long-term monogamous relationship, and prophylactic vaccination (ACOG, 2005). A vaccine against HPV (types 6, 11, 16, 18) became available in 2006 and is recommended for females ages 9 to 26. Vaccines for other HPV types continue to be investigated (CDC, Workowski, & Berman, 2006). Practitioners should stay current with results of these clinical trials and make recommendations about vaccination based on the outcomes of the research.

Herpes Simplex Virus

Unknown until the middle of the twentieth century, herpes simplex virus (HSV) infection is now widespread in the United States, especially in women. HSV infection results in painful, recurrent ulcers. It is caused by two different antigen subtypes of HSV: HSV type 1 (HSV-1) and HSV type 2 (HSV-2). HSV-2 is usually transmitted sexually, and HSV-1 nonsexually. Although HSV-1 is more commonly associated with gingivostomatitis and oral labial ulcers (fever blisters) and HSV-2 with genital lesions, neither type is exclusively associated with the respective sites.

Although HSV infection is not a reportable disease, it is estimated that about 50 million people in the United States are infected with genital herpes and that up to one million new infections occur each year (CDC, Workowski, & Berman, 2006). Recurrent HSV infections are much more common. Most persons infected with HSV-2 have not been diagnosed, and most infections are transmitted by persons unaware that they are infected.

An initial HSV genital infection is characterized by multiple painful lesions, fever, chills, malaise, and severe dysuria and may last 2 to 3 weeks. Women generally have a more severe clinical course than do men. Women with primary genital herpes have many lesions that progress from macules to papules; they then progress to form vesicles, pustules, and ulcers that crust and heal without scarring (Fig. 6-5). These ulcers are extremely tender, and primary infections may be bilateral. Women also may have itching, inguinal tenderness, and lymphadenopathy. Severe vulvar edema may develop, and women may have difficulty sitting. HSV cervicitis is common with initial HSV-2 infections. The cervix may appear normal

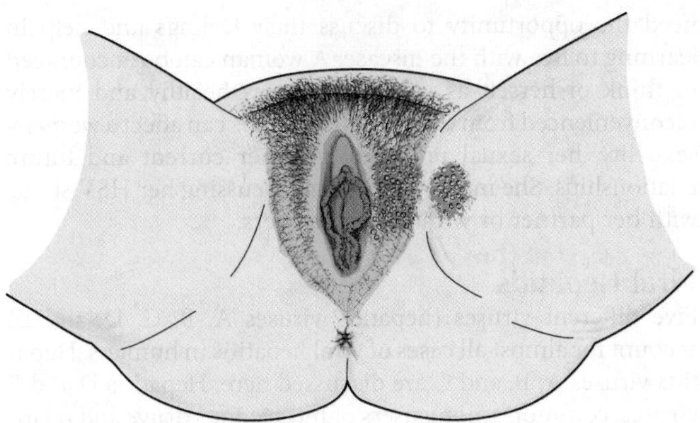

Fig. 6-5 Herpes genitalis.

or be friable, reddened, ulcerated, or necrotic. A heavy, watery-to-purulent vaginal discharge is common. Extragenital lesions may be present because of autoinoculation. Urinary retention and dysuria may occur secondary to autonomic involvement of the sacral nerve root.

Women with recurrent episodes of HSV infections commonly have only local symptoms that are usually less severe than those associated with the initial infection. Systemic symptoms are usually absent, although the characteristic prodromal genital tingling is common. Recurrent lesions are unilateral, are less severe, and usually last 5 to 7 days. Lesions begin as vesicles and progress rapidly to ulcers. Few women with recurrent disease have cervicitis.

During pregnancy maternal infection with HSV-2 can have adverse effects on both the mother and fetus. Viremia occurs during the primary infection, and congenital infection is possible although rare. Primary infections during the first trimester have been associated with increased miscarriage rates.

An association between cervical cancer and HSV-2 has been observed. It is theorized that genital herpes is a marker for high risk sexual behaviors that could transmit other STIs, including HPV.

Screening and Diagnosis

A diagnosis of herpes is facilitated by a careful history. A history of exposure to an infected person is important, although infection from an asymptomatic individual is possible. A history of having viral symptoms such as malaise, headache, fever, or myalgia is suggestive. Local symptoms such as vulvar pain, dysuria, itching, or burning at the site of infection and painful genital lesions that heal spontaneously are also highly suggestive of HSV infections. The nurse should ask about history of a primary infection, prodromal symptoms, vaginal discharge, and dyspareunia. Pregnant women should be asked whether they or their partner(s) have had genital lesions.

During the physical examination the nurse should assess for inguinal and generalized lymphadenopathy and elevated temperature. The entire vulvar, perineal, vaginal, and cervical areas should be carefully inspected for vesicles or ulcerated or crusted areas. A speculum examination may be very difficult for the woman because of the extreme tenderness often associated with herpes infections. Any suspicious or recurrent lesions found during pregnancy should be cultured to document HSV. Although a diagnosis of herpes infection may be suspected from the history and physical examination, it is confirmed by laboratory studies. A viral culture is obtained by swabbing exudate during the vesicular stage of the disease. In primary HSV infection viral shedding is prolonged, and HSV is more easily isolated.

Management

Genital herpes is a chronic and recurring disease for which there is no known cure. Management is directed toward specific treatment during primary and recurrent infections, prevention, self-help measures, and psychologic support.

Systemic antiviral medications partially control the symptoms and signs of HSV infections when used for the primary or recurrent episodes or when used as daily suppressive therapy. However, these medications do not eradicate the infection; nor do they alter subsequent risk, frequency, or recurrences after the medication is stopped. Three antiviral medications provide clinical benefit: acyclovir, valacyclovir, and famciclovir. Safety and efficacy have been clearly shown in persons taking acyclovir daily for up to 3 years. The safety of acyclovir, valacyclovir, and famciclovir therapy during pregnancy has not been established; however, acyclovir may be used to reduce the symptoms of HSV if the benefits to the woman outweigh the potential harm to the fetus (CDC, Workowski, & Berman, 2006). Continued investigation of HSV therapy with these medications during pregnancy is needed.

Cleaning lesions twice a day with saline helps prevent secondary infection. Bacterial infection must be treated with appropriate antibiotics. Measures that may increase comfort for women when lesions are active include warm sitz baths with baking soda; keeping lesions dry by using cool air from a hair dryer or by patting dry with a soft towel; wearing cotton underwear and loose clothing; using drying aids such as hydrogen peroxide, Burow's solution, or oatmeal baths; applying cool, wet, black tea bags to lesions; and applying compresses with an infusion of cloves or peppermint oil and clove oil to lesions.

Oral analgesics such as aspirin or ibuprofen may be used to relieve pain and systemic symptoms associated with initial infections. Because the mucous membranes affected by herpes are extremely sensitive, any topical agents should be used with caution. Nonantiviral ointments, especially those containing cortisone, should be avoided. A thin layer of lidocaine ointment or an antiseptic spray may be applied to decrease discomfort, especially if walking is difficult.

A diet rich in vitamin C, B-complex vitamins, zinc, and calcium is thought to help prevent recurrences. The amino acid L-lysine has been used in doses of 750 to 1000 mg daily while lesions are active and 500 mg during asymptomatic periods. It is thought that L-lysine has an inhibitory effect on the multiplication of the HSV.

Counseling and education are critical components of the nursing care of women with herpes infections. Information regarding the etiology, signs and symptoms, transmission, and treatment should be provided. The nurse should explain that each woman is unique in her response to herpes and emphasize the variability of symptoms. Women should be helped to understand when viral shedding and thus transmission to a partner are most likely. They should be counseled to refrain from sexual contact from the onset of prodrome until complete healing of lesions.

Some authorities recommend consistent use of condoms for all persons with genital herpes. Condoms may not prevent transmission, particularly male-to-female transmission; however, this does not mean that the partners should avoid all intimacy. Women can be encouraged to maintain close contact with their partners while avoiding contact with lesions. Women should be taught how to look for herpetic lesions using a mirror and good light source and a wet cloth or finger covered with a finger cot to rub lightly over the labia. The nurse should ensure that women understand that, when lesions are active, sharing intimate articles (e.g., washcloths or wet towels) that come into contact with the lesions should be avoided. Only plain soap and water are needed to clean hands that have come in contact with herpetic lesions; isolation is neither necessary nor appropriate.

The nurse should explain the role of precipitating factors in the reactivation of the latent virus and recurrent episodes. Stress, menstruation, trauma, febrile illnesses, chronic illness, and ultraviolet light have all been found to trigger genital herpes. Women may wish to keep a diary to identify stressors that seem to be associated with recurrent herpes attacks so that they can then avoid these stressors when possible. The role of exercise in reducing stress can be discussed. Referral for stress-reduction therapy, yoga, or meditation classes may be indicated. Avoiding excessive heat, sun, and hot baths and using a lubricant during sexual intercourse to reduce friction may also be helpful. Women in their childbearing years should be counseled regarding the risk of herpes infection during pregnancy. They should be instructed to use condoms if there is any risk of contracting an STI from a sexual partner. If they become pregnant while taking acyclovir, the risk of birth defects does not appear to be higher than for the general population; however, continued use should be based on whether the benefits for the woman outweigh the possible risks to the fetus. Acyclovir does enter breast milk, but the amount of medication ingested during breastfeeding is very low and is usually not a health concern (Organization of Teratology Information Services, 2003).

Because neonatal HSV infection is such a devastating disease, prevention is critical. Current recommendations include carefully examining and questioning all women about symptoms at onset of labor (CDC, Workowski, & Berman, 2006). If visible lesions are not present at onset of labor, vaginal birth is acceptable. Cesarean birth within 4 hours after labor begins or membranes rupture is recommended if visible lesions are present. Infants who are born through an infected vagina should be carefully observed and cultured. Some experts recommend presumptive treatment of infants who were exposed to HSV during birth. Because HSV infection may be associated with cervical dysplasia, women must be encouraged to have annual Pap tests and gynecologic examinations.

The emotional impact of contracting herpes is considerable. No cure is available, and most women experience recurrences. At diagnosis many emotions may surface—helplessness, anger, denial, guilt, anxiety, shame, or inadequacy. Women need the opportunity to discuss their feelings and help in learning to live with the disease. A woman can be encouraged to think of herself as someone who is healthy and merely inconvenienced from time to time. Herpes can affect a woman's sexuality, her sexual practices, and her current and future relationships. She may need help in discussing her HSV status with her partner or with future partners.

Viral Hepatitis

Five different viruses (hepatitis viruses A, B, C, D, and E) account for almost all cases of viral hepatitis in humans. Hepatitis viruses A, B, and C are discussed here. Hepatitis D and E viruses, common among users of intravenous drugs and recipients of multiple blood transfusions, are not included in this discussion.

Hepatitis A

Hepatitis A virus (HAV) infection is acquired primarily through a fecal-oral route by ingestion of contaminated food, particularly milk, shellfish, or polluted water, or person-to-person contact. Hepatitis A, like other enteric infections, can be transmitted during sexual activity. Women living in the western United States, Native Americans, Alaskan Natives, and children and employees in day care centers are at high risk.

HAV infection is characterized by flu-like symptoms with malaise, fatigue, anorexia, nausea, pruritus, fever, and upper right quadrant pain. Serologic testing to detect the immunoglobulin M (IgM) antibody is done to confirm acute infections. The IgM antibody is detectable 5 to 10 days after exposure and can remain positive for up to 6 months. Because HAV infection is self-limited and does not result in chronic infection or chronic liver disease, treatment is usually supportive. Women who become dehydrated from nausea and vomiting or who have fulminating hepatitis A may need to be hospitalized. Medications that might cause liver damage or that are metabolized in the liver (e.g., acetaminophen, ethyl alcohol) should be avoided. A well-balanced diet is recommended. Hepatitis A vaccine is recommended for women at high risk for being exposed to HAV infection. The safety of the vaccine has not been established in pregnancy; therefore immunoglobulin (γ-globulin) or immune-specific globulin is indicated for a pregnant woman exposed to HAV. All household contacts of the woman also should receive γ-globulin (CDC, Workowski, & Berman, 2006).

Hepatitis B

Hepatitis B virus (HBV) infection is an STI and is the virus most threatening to the fetus and neonate. It is caused by a large DNA virus and is associated with three antigens and their antibodies: hepatitis B surface antigen (HBsAg), HBV antigen (HBeAg), HBV core antigen (HBcAg), antibody to HBsAg (anti-HBs), antibody to HBeAg (anti-HBe), and antibody to HBcAg (anti-HBc). Screening for active or chronic disease or disease immunity is based on testing for these antigens and their antibodies.

Populations at risk include women of Asian, Pacific Island (Polynesian, Micronesian, Melanesian), or Alaskan-Eskimo descent and women born in Haiti or sub-Saharan Africa. Women who have a history of acute or chronic liver disease, who work or receive treatment in a dialysis unit, or who have household or sexual contact with a hemodialysis patient are at greater risk. Women who work or live in institutions for the mentally handicapped are considered to be at risk, as are women with a history of multiple blood transfusions. Health care workers and public safety workers exposed to blood in the workplace are at risk. Behaviors such as multiple sexual partners and a history of intravenous drug use increase the risk of contracting HBV infections.

HBsAg has been found in blood, saliva, sweat, tears, vaginal secretions, and semen. Drug abusers who share needles are at risk, as are health care workers who are exposed to blood and needle sticks. Perinatal transmission most often occurs in infants of mothers who have acute hepatitis infection late in the third trimester or during the intrapartum or postpartum periods from exposure to HBsAg-positive vaginal secretions, blood, amniotic fluid, saliva, and breast milk. HBV has also been transmitted by artificial insemination. Although HBV can be transmitted by blood transfusion, the incidence of such infections has decreased significantly since testing of blood for HBsAg became routine.

HBV infection is a disease of the liver and is often a silent infection. In the adult the course of the infection can be fulminating, and the outcome fatal. Symptoms of HBV infection are similar to those of hepatitis A: arthralgias, arthritis, lassitude, anorexia, nausea, vomiting, headache, fever, and mild abdominal pain. Later the woman may have clay-colored stools, dark urine, increased abdominal pain, and jaundice. Between 5% and 10% of individuals with HBV have persistent HBsAg and become chronic hepatitis B carriers.

Screening and Diagnosis All women at high risk for contracting HBV should be screened on a regular basis. Since screening only individuals at high risk may not identify up to 50% of HBsAg-positive women, screening for the presence of HBsAg is recommended on all women at the first prenatal visit, regardless of whether they have been tested previously. Testing should be repeated later in pregnancy or on admission for labor and birth for women with high risk behaviors (USPSTF, 2001a).

Testing for HBV is complex. Patients with acute hepatitis B generally have detectable serum HBsAg levels in the late incubation phase of the disease, 2 to 5 weeks before symptoms appear. Anti-HBs with a negative HBsAg test signals immunity. Anti-HBs with a positive antigen denotes a chronic carrier state. During this time the disease can be transmitted. During the recovery phase the patient may continue to be infectious, even though HBsAg cannot be detected. This is called the "window phase" and is identified by anti-HBc in the absence of anti-HBs. Women should be prepared for repeated testing because HBV screening tests may also be used to monitor the progression of the disease.

Components of the history to be obtained when hepatitis B is suspected include inquiry about the symptoms of the disease and risk factors outlined earlier. Physical examination includes inspection of the skin for rashes, inspection of the skin and conjunctiva for jaundice, and palpation of the liver for enlargement and tenderness. Weight loss, fever, and general debilitation should be noted. If the HBsAg is positive, further laboratory studies may be ordered (anti-HBe, anti-HBc, serum glutamic-oxaloacetic transaminase, alkaline phosphatase, and liver panel). If the HBsAg is negative in early pregnancy and the woman could be in the window phase or if high risk behaviors continue during pregnancy, a repeat HBsAg should be ordered in the third trimester.

Management There is no specific treatment for hepatitis B. Recovery is usually spontaneous in 3 to 16 weeks. Pregnancies complicated by acute viral hepatitis are managed on an outpatient basis. Women should be advised to increase bed rest; eat a high-protein, low-fat diet; and increase their fluid intake. They should avoid medications metabolized in the liver and alcohol. Pregnant women with a definite exposure to HBV should be given hepatitis B immunoglobulin and should begin the hepatitis B vaccine series within 14 days of the most recent contact to prevent infection (CDC, Workowski, & Berman, 2006). Vaccination during pregnancy is not thought to pose risks to the fetus.

All nonimmune women at high or moderate risk of hepatitis should be informed of the availability of hepatitis B vaccine. Vaccination is recommended for all individuals who have had multiple sex partners within the past 6 months (CDC, Workowski, & Berman, 2006). In addition, intravenous drug users, residents of correctional or long-term care facilities, persons seeking care for an STI, prostitutes, women whose partners are intravenous drug users or bisexual, and women whose occupation exposes them to high risk should be vaccinated. The vaccine is given in a series of three (four if rapid protection is needed) doses over a 6-month period, with the first two doses given at least 1 month apart. The vaccine is given in the deltoid muscle.

Patient education includes explaining the meaning of hepatitis B infection, including transmission, state of infectivity, and sequelae. The nurse should also explain the need for immunoprophylaxis for household members and sexual contacts. To decrease transmission of the virus, women with hepatitis B or who test positive for HBV should be advised to maintain a high level of personal hygiene (e.g., wash hands after using the toilet; carefully dispose of tampons, pads, and bandages in plastic bags; do not share razor blades, toothbrushes, needles, or manicure implements; have male partner use a condom if unvaccinated and without hepatitis; avoid sharing saliva through kissing or through sharing of silverware or dishes; and wipe up blood spills immediately with soap and water). They should inform all health care providers of their carrier state. Postpartum women should be reassured that breastfeeding is not contraindicated if the infant receives prophylaxis at birth and is currently on the immunization schedule.

Hepatitis C

"Hepatitis C virus (HCV) infection is the most common chronic blood-borne infection in the United States; approximately 2.7 million persons are chronically infected" (CDC, Workowski, & Berman, 2006). The most common risk factor for pregnant women is a history of intravenous drug use. Other risk factors include STIs such as hepatitis B and HIV, multiple sexual partners, and a history of blood transfusions. Hepatitis C is readily transmitted through exposure to blood.

Most patients with hepatitis C are asymptomatic or have general flu-like symptoms similar to those of hepatitis A. HCV infection is confirmed by the presence of anti-C antibody during laboratory testing. Routine HCV testing is recommended for women who have ever injected drugs; women who received a blood transfusion before July 1992; children of HCV-positive women; health care, emergency, medical, and public safety workers; and women with chronic liver disease (CDC, Workowski, & Berman, 2006). Counseling and testing should be offered to pregnant women with known risk factors.

Interferon alfa-2b and ribavirin for 6 to 12 months are the main treatment for HCV infection, although effectiveness of this treatment varies. Drug abuse treatment is an important adjunct for many persons with HCV (CDC, Workowski, & Berman, 2006).

Currently there is no vaccine to prevent hepatitis C. Transmission of HCV through breastfeeding has not been reported.

Human Immunodeficiency Virus

Although HIV has traditionally been thought to be a homosexual or gay disease, heterosexual transmission is now the most common means of transmission in women. An estimated 26% of new infections occur in women. Among women diagnosed with HIV/AIDS in 2007, 66% were African-American, 18% were Caucasian, 14% were Hispanic, less than 1% were Asian, less than 1% were Native Hawaiian/Other Pacific Islander, and less than 1% were American Indian/Alaska Native (CDC, 2009).

Transmission of HIV, a retrovirus, occurs primarily through exchange of body fluids (semen, blood, or vaginal secretions). Severe depression of the cellular immune system associated with HIV infection characterizes acquired immunodeficiency syndrome (AIDS). For both men and women the most commonly reported opportunistic diseases are *Pneumocystis carinii* pneumonia, candida esophagitis, and wasting syndrome. Other viral infections such as HSV and cytomegalovirus infections seem to be more prevalent in women than men. PID may be more severe in HIV-infected women, and rates of HPV and cervical dysplasia may be higher. The clinical course of HPV infection in women with HIV infection is accelerated, and recurrence is more frequent.

Once HIV enters the body, seroconversion to HIV positivity usually occurs within 6 to 12 weeks. Although HIV seroconversion may be totally asymptomatic, it usually is accompanied by a viremic, influenza-like response. Symptoms include fever, headache, night sweats, malaise, generalized lymphadenopathy, myalgias, nausea, diarrhea, weight loss, sore throat, and rash.

Laboratory studies may reveal leukopenia, thrombocytopenia, anemia, and an elevated erythrocyte sedimentation rate. HIV has a strong affinity for surface-marker proteins on T lymphocytes. This affinity leads to significant T-cell destruction. Both clinical and epidemiologic studies have shown that declining CD4 levels are strongly associated with increased incidence of AIDS-related diseases and death in many different groups of HIV-infected persons.

Transmission of the virus from mother to infant can occur throughout the perinatal period. Exposure may occur to the fetus through the maternal circulation as early as the first trimester of pregnancy, to the infant during labor and birth by inoculation or ingestion of maternal blood and other infected fluids, or to the infant through breast milk (Lawrence & Lawrence, 2005; Riordan, 2005).

Screening and Diagnosis

Screening, teaching, and counseling regarding HIV risk factors, indications for being tested, and testing are major roles for nurses caring for women today. A number of behaviors place women at risk for HIV infection. These include intravenous drug use, high risk sex partners, multiple sex partners, and a previous history of multiple STIs. HIV infection is usually diagnosed by using HIV-1 and HIV-2 antibody tests. Antibody testing is done first with a sensitive screening test such as the enzyme immunoassay. Reactive screening tests must be confirmed by an additional test such as the Western blot or an immunofluorescence assay. If a positive antibody test is confirmed by a supplemental test, it means that a woman is infected with HIV and is capable of infecting others. HIV antibodies are detectable in at least 95% of patients within 3 months after infection. Although a negative antibody test usually indicates that a person is not infected, antibody tests cannot exclude recent infection. Because HIV antibody crosses the placenta, definite diagnosis of HIV in children younger than 18 months is based on laboratory evidence of HIV in blood or tissues by culture, nucleic acid, or antigen detection (CDC, Workowski, & Berman, 2006).

CDC guidelines "advocate routine voluntary HIV testing as normal part of medical practice, similar to screening for other treatable conditions" (Branson et al, 2006). Recommendations for testing pregnant women and newborns are in Box 6-6.

The U.S. Food and Drug Administration (FDA) has approved six methods of rapid testing for HIV: variously using a blood sample obtained by finger stick or venipuncture, serum or plasma, or an oral fluid sample. The tests have accuracy rates of 98% to 99%. If the results are reactive, further testing is done (CDC, 2008; FDA, 2006). Quick results mean that patients don't have to make extra visits for follow-up standard tests, and the oral test provides an option for patients who do not want to have a blood test.

Counseling for HIV Testing

Counseling before and after HIV testing is standard nursing practice. It is a nursing responsibility to assess a woman's understanding of the information such a test would provide and ensure that the patient thoroughly understands the emotional, legal, and medical implications of a positive or negative test before she is ready to take an HIV test. One's life is profoundly altered by knowledge of HIV seropositivity. A unique stigma associated with HIV infection can have a profound impact on the quality of life of those infected. This stigma extends to those who are asymptomatic but seropositive.

Barriers to routine prenatal testing may be the requirement for lengthy HIV prevention counseling and documentation of informed consent for HIV testing. Testing rates are higher when opt-out testing is used with pregnant women rather then opt-in strategies with requirements for written documentation of informed consent for HIV testing (Branson et al, 2006).

Unless rapid testing is done, there is generally a 1- to 3-week waiting period after testing for HIV; this can be a very anxious time for the woman. It is helpful if the nurse informs her that this time period between blood drawing and test results is routine. Test results must always be communicated in person, and women should be informed in advance that

BOX 6-6 Human Immunodeficiency Virus Screening for Pregnant Women and Their Infants

Universal Opt-Out Screening

All pregnant women in the United States should be screened for human immunodeficiency virus (HIV) infection.

Screening should occur after a woman is notified that HIV screening is recommended for all pregnant patients and that she will receive an HIV test as part of the routine panel of prenatal tests unless she declines (opt-out screening).

HIV testing must be voluntary and free from coercion. No woman should be tested without her knowledge.

Pregnant women should receive oral or written information that includes an explanation of HIV infection, a description of interventions that can reduce HIV transmission from mother to infant, and the meaning of positive and negative test results. They should be offered an opportunity to ask questions and to decline testing.

No additional process or written documentation of informed consent beyond that required for other routine prenatal tests should be required for HIV testing.

If a patient declines an HIV test, this decision should be documented in the medical record.

Timing of HIV Testing

Women should be tested as early as possible in pregnancy.

A second HIV test during the third trimester, preferably before 36 weeks of gestation is cost effective.

Rapid Testing During Labor

Any woman with undocumented HIV status at the time of labor should be screened with a rapid HIV test unless she declines (opt-out screening).

Reasons for declining a rapid test should be explored.

Immediate initiation of appropriate antiretroviral prophylaxis should be recommended to women on the basis of a reactive rapid test result without waiting for the result of a confirmatory test.

Postpartum/Newborn Testing

When a woman's HIV status is still unknown at the time of birth, she should be screened with a rapid HIV test immediately after giving birth unless she declines (opt-out screening).

When the mother's HIV status is unknown, rapid testing of the newborn as soon as possible after birth is recommended so antiretroviral prophylaxis can be offered to HIV-exposed infants. Women should be informed that identifying HIV antibodies in the newborn indicates that the mother is infected.

The benefits of neonatal antiretroviral prophylaxis are best realized when it is initiated within 12 hours after birth.

Source: Branson BM et al: Revised recommendations for HIV testing of adults, adolescents, and pregnant women in health-care settings, *MMWR* 55(RR-14):1-17, 2006.

this is the procedure. Whenever possible, the person who provided the pretest counseling should also tell the woman her test results. The nurse should make sure that the woman understands what a positive test result means and review the reliability of the test results.

When some women are informed of negative results, they may escalate risk behaviors because they equate negativity with immunity. Others may believe that negative means "bad" and positive means "good." The woman's reaction to a negative test should be explored by asking, "How do you feel?" Counseling sessions for women with an HIV-negative result are another opportunity to provide education. Emphasis can be placed on ways in which a woman can remain HIV free. She should be reminded that, if she has been exposed to HIV in the past 6 months, she should be retested, and that she should have ongoing testing if she continues high risk behaviors.

Pregnancy and HIV

Pregnancy is not encouraged for women who are HIV positive. Preconception counseling is recommended; contraceptive counseling should be offered to HIV-positive women who do not desire pregnancy. HIV-infected women should be informed specifically about the risks for perinatal infection. Current evidence indicates that 25% to 30% of infants born to untreated HIV-infected women are infected with HIV, whereas the transmission rate in treated women is less than 2%.

Perinatal transmission of HIV has decreased by 67% since 1994 because of a three-part regimen consisting of (1) the administration of antiretroviral prophylaxis (zidovudine [ZDV]) to women during pregnancy, (2) intravenous ZDV during labor, and (3) ZDV to the newborn infant for 6 weeks. Subsequent studies using highly active antiretroviral therapy (HAART) demonstrated a reduction of perinatal transmission to less than 2% of births in women with HIV. The major side effect of ZDV is bone marrow suppression; periodic hematocrit, white blood cell count, and platelet count assessments should be performed.

Women who are HIV positive should also be vaccinated against hepatitis B, pneumococcal infection, *Haemophilus influenzae* type B, and viral influenza. To support any pregnant woman's immune system, appropriate counseling is provided about optimal nutrition, sleep, rest, exercise, and stress reduction. Use of condoms is encouraged to minimize further exposure to HIV if her partner is the source.

It is estimated that one third to one half of perinatal transmission occurs during breastfeeding. Thus in the United States, where safe and affordable substitutes are available, HIV-infected women should not breastfeed (CDC, 2006a). Giving nevirapine once daily to breastfeeding infants from days 8 to 42 of life helps the infants remain HIV negative. It is used more in developing countries where safe water and affordable substitutes are not available (National Institute of Child Health and Human Development, 2008). There is risk of liver toxicity in women with CD4 counts greater than 250 cells/mm^3 and thus nevirapine should be used with caution.

Cesarean birth performed before rupture of membranes and onset of labor has been shown to be of benefit for preventing vertical transmission of HIV in women who did not have antiretroviral therapy or had only ZDV in pregnancy. The benefits of cesarean birth for women who received combination therapy are less clear (CDC, 2006a). Complications after cesarean birth are more common in HIV-positive women than in uninfected women.

Management

During the initial contact with an HIV-infected woman, the nurse should establish what the woman knows about HIV infection and that she is being cared for by a medical practitioner or a facility with expertise in caring for persons with HIV infections, including AIDS. Psychologic referral also may be indicated. Resources such as counseling for financial assistance, suicide prevention, death and dying, and legal advocacy may be appropriate. All women who are drug users should be referred to a substance abuse program. A major focus of counseling is prevention of transmission of HIV to partners.

Nurses counseling seropositive women who wish to receive contraceptive information may recommend (1) oral contraceptives and latex condoms, or (2) tubal sterilization or vasectomy and latex condoms. The IUD is not appropriate for the HIV-infected woman because of increased risk of infection. Female condoms or abstinence can be offered to women whose partners refuse to use condoms.

Routine gynecologic care for HIV-positive women should include a pelvic examination every 6 months. Careful Pap screening is essential because of the greatly increased incidence of abnormal findings. In addition, HIV-positive women should be screened for syphilis, gonorrhea, chlamydia, and other vaginal infections.

No cure is available for HIV infection. Rare and unusual diseases are characteristic of HIV infection. Opportunistic infections and concurrent diseases should be managed vigorously with treatment specific to the infection or disease.

Discussion of the medical care of HIV-positive women and women with AIDS is beyond the scope of this chapter. The reader is referred to the Centers for Disease Control and Prevention (*www.cdc.gov*) and Internet websites such as HIV/AIDS Treatment Information Service (*www.hivatis.org*) for current information and recommendations.

Vaginal Infections

Vaginal discharge and itching of the vulva and vagina are among the most common reasons a woman seeks help from a health care provider. More women complain of vaginal discharge than of any other gynecologic symptom. Women who have adequate endogenous or exogenous estrogen will have vaginal secretions. Vaginal discharge resulting from infection must be distinguished from normal secretions. Normal vaginal secretions (or leukorrhea) are clear to cloudy in appearance. The discharge may turn yellow after drying; is slightly slimy; is nonirritating; and has a mild, inoffensive odor. Normal vaginal secretions are acidic, with a pH range of 4 to 5. The amount of leukorrhea differs with phases of the menstrual cycle, with greater amounts occurring at ovulation and just before menses. Leukorrhea is also increased during pregnancy. Normal vaginal secretions contain lactobacilli and epithelial cells.

Vaginitis, or abnormal vaginal discharge, is an infection caused by a microorganism. The most common vaginal infections are bacterial vaginosis (BV), candidiasis, and trichomoniasis. Although streptococcus B is considered normal vaginal flora, it may also cause infection. Vulvovaginitis, inflammation of the vulva and vagina, may be caused by vaginal infection; copious leukorrhea, which can cause maceration of tissues; and chemical irritants, allergens, and foreign bodies, which may produce inflammatory reactions.

Bacterial Vaginosis

BV, formerly called nonspecific vaginitis, *Haemophilus* vaginitis, or *Gardnerella,* is the most common type of vaginitis. BV is associated with preterm labor and birth. The exact etiology of BV is unknown. It is a syndrome in which normal H_2O_2–producing lactobacilli are replaced with high concentrations of anaerobic bacteria *(Gardnerella* and *Mobiluncus).* With the proliferation of anaerobes, the level of vaginal amines is raised, and the normal acidic pH of the vagina is altered. Epithelial cells slough, and numerous bacteria attach to their surfaces (clue cells). When the amines are volatilized, the characteristic odor of BV occurs.

Screening and Diagnosis

A careful history may help distinguish BV from other vaginal infections if the woman is symptomatic. Women with previous occurrence of similar symptoms, diagnosis, and treatment should be queried because women with BV often have been treated incorrectly because of misdiagnosis.

Most women with BV complain of a characteristic "fishy odor" in the vaginal area, although not all note it. The odor may be noticed by the woman or her partner after heterosexual intercourse because semen releases the vaginal amines. When present, the BV discharge is usually profuse; thin; and white, gray, or milky in appearance. Some women also may experience mild irritation or pruritus.

Microscopic examination of vaginal secretions is always done (Table 6-3). Both normal saline and 10% potassium

Table 6-3 Wet Smear Tests for Vaginal Infections

INFECTION	TEST	POSITIVE FINDINGS
Trichomoniasis	Saline wet smear (vaginal secretions mixed with normal saline on a glass slide)	Presence of many white blood cell protozoa
Candidiasis	Potassium hydroxide (KOH) prep (vaginal secretions mixed with KOH on a glass slide)	Presence of hyphae and pseudohyphae (buds and branches of yeast cells)
Bacterial vaginosis	Normal saline smear	Presence of clue cells (vaginal epithelial cells coated with bacteria)
	Whiff test (vaginal secretions mixed with KOH)	Release of fishy odor

hydroxide (KOH) smears should be made. The presence of clue cells confirmed by wet smear is highly diagnostic because the phenomenon is specific to BV (USPSTF, 2001b). Vaginal secretions should be tested for pH and amine odor. Nitrazine paper is sensitive enough to detect a pH of 4.5 or greater. The fishy odor of BV will be released when KOH is added to vaginal secretions on the lip of the withdrawn speculum.

Management

Treatment of BV with oral metronidazole (Flagyl) is most effective (CDC, Workowski, & Berman, 2006). Metronidazole is an antiprotozoal and antibacterial agent. Side effects of metronidazole are numerous and include a sharp, unpleasant metallic taste in the mouth; furry tongue; central nervous system reactions; and urinary tract disturbances. When oral metronidazole is taken, the patient is advised not to drink alcoholic beverages or she will experience severe side effects of abdominal distress, nausea, vomiting, and headache. Gastrointestinal symptoms are common whether alcohol is consumed or not. Treatment of sexual partners is not recommended because sexual transmission of BV has not been proven.

Several adverse outcomes are associated with BV during pregnancy: preterm labor and birth, premature rupture of the membranes, intraamniotic infection, and postpartum endometritis. Therefore pregnant women should be treated to relieve vaginal symptoms and the signs of infection. Consideration should also be given to evaluation and treatment of asymptomatic women at high risk for preterm birth (CDC, Workowski, & Berman, 2006).

Metronidazole is contraindicated if the woman is breastfeeding because high concentrations have been found in infants. If it is necessary to prescribe metronidazole for the lactating woman, she can suspend breastfeeding temporarily (pump and discard milk to maintain supply) and resume it 48 to 72 hours after taking the last dose.

Candidiasis

Vulvovaginal candidiasis, or yeast infection, is the second most common type of vaginal infection in the United States. Although vaginal candidiasis infections are common in healthy women, those seen in women with HIV infection are often more severe and persistent. Genital candidiasis lesions may be painful, and coalescing ulcerations necessitate continuous, prophylactic therapy.

The most common organism is *Candida albicans.* It is estimated that 80% to 95% of yeast infections in women are caused by this organism. However, in the past 10 years the incidence of non–*C. albicans* infections has increased steadily. Women with chronic or recurrent infections often are infected with a higher percentage of non–*C. albicans* species than are women with their first infection or who have few recurrences.

Numerous factors have been identified as predisposing a woman to yeast infections. These include antibiotic therapy, particularly broad-spectrum antibiotics such as ampicillin, tetracycline, cephalosporins, and metronidazole; diabetes, especially when uncontrolled; pregnancy; obesity; diets high in refined sugars or artificial sweeteners; use of corticosteroids and exogenous hormones; and immunosuppressed states. Clinical observations and research have suggested that tight-fitting clothing and underwear or pantyhose made of nonabsorbent materials create an environment in which a vaginal fungus can grow (see Patient Teaching box).

PATIENT TEACHING Yeast Infection—Inadequate Patient Education

Marcella, an 82-year-old widow, had a precancerous lesion excised from her forehead and was placed on a broad-spectrum antibiotic for 1 week. She later presented to the clinic with profuse, white vaginal discharge; severe itching; and excoriation on her labia, in her groin, and extending onto her buttocks and lower abdomen. When she expressed hesitance in talking to the physician, the nurse assured her that she would be with her during the examination. Marcella said that wasn't the problem. When the nurse examined Marcella, she said that her problem looked like a yeast infection and asked Marcella if she had been taking antibiotics. The nurse explained that yeast infections are common when taking antibiotics. The physician verified the diagnosis and prescribed Monistat. On further discussion the nurse determined that Marcella had thought that she picked up a sexually transmitted infection (STI) when she used a public restroom and was ashamed and embarrassed to discuss her problem, so had not told anyone or sought treatment earlier. When Marcella returned home and told her daughter that she had seen a physician, her daughter stated, "You have a yeast infection." When Marcella asked how she knew that, the daughter said that her friend and her daughter both had yeast infections when on antibiotics.

This situation could have been avoided if the physician who prescribed the antibiotic or the nurse had told Marcella that yeast infections are common when antibiotics are taken or if Marcella had discussed the condition with her daughter. Marcella can be counseled to discuss problems and seek care in the early stages of a problem, even when discussing the condition may be embarrassing. Had she discussed this with her daughter, treatment could have been started much sooner, and Marcella would have avoided the distress she experienced. Marcella also needs some teaching about the transmission of STIs.

The most common symptom of yeast infection is vulvar and possibly vaginal pruritus. The itching may be mild or intense, may interfere with rest and activities, and may occur during or after intercourse. Some women report a feeling of dryness. Others may have painful urination as the urine flows over the vulva. The latter usually occurs in women who have excoriations resulting from scratching. Most often the discharge is thick, white, lumpy, and cottage cheese like. The discharge may be found in patches on the vaginal walls, cervix, and labia. Commonly the vulva is red and swollen, as are the labial folds, vagina, and cervix. Although there is no odor characteristic of yeast infections, sometimes a yeasty or musty smell is noted.

Screening and Diagnosis

In addition to noting the woman's symptoms, their onset, and their course, the history is a valuable screening tool for identifying predisposing risk factors. Physical examination should include a thorough inspection of the vulva and vagina.

A speculum examination is always done. Commonly saline and KOH wet smear and vaginal pH are obtained. Vaginal pH is normal with a yeast infection; if the pH is greater than 4.5, trichomoniasis or BV should be suspected. The characteristic pseudohypha (bud or branching of a fungus) may be seen on a wet smear done with normal saline; however, they may be confused with other cells and artifacts.

Management

A number of antifungal preparations are available for the treatment of *C. albicans.* Many of these medications (e.g., miconazole [Monistat] and clotrimazole [Gyne-Lotrimin]) are available as OTC agents. The first time a woman suspects that she may have a yeast infection, she should see a health care provider for confirmation of the diagnosis and treatment recommendation. If she has another infection, she may wish to purchase an OTC preparation and self-treat. If she elects to do this, she should always be counseled to seek care for numerous recurrent or chronic yeast infections. If vaginal discharge is extremely thick and copious, vaginal debridement with a cotton swab followed by application of vaginal medication may be effective.

Women who have extensive irritation, swelling, and discomfort of the labia and vulva may find sitz baths helpful in decreasing inflammation and increasing comfort. Adding Aveeno powder to the bath may also increase the woman's comfort. Not wearing underpants to bed may help decrease symptoms and prevent recurrences. Completing the full course of treatment prescribed is essential to removing the pathogen. Medication should be continued even during menstruation. Women should be counseled not to use tampons during menses because the medication will be absorbed by the tampon. If possible, intercourse is avoided during treatment; if this is not feasible, the woman's partner should use a condom to prevent introduction of more organisms. Suggested measures to prevent genital tract infections are in the Patient Teaching box on p. 98.

Trichomoniasis

Trichomoniasis is a cause of up to 25% of all vaginal infections and is almost always a sexually transmitted infection. Trichomoniasis is caused by *Trichomonas vaginalis,* an anaerobic, one-celled protozoan with characteristic flagella. Although trichomoniasis may be asymptomatic, commonly women have yellowish-to-greenish, frothy, mucopurulent, copious, and malodorous discharge. Inflammation of the vulva, vagina, or both may be present; and the woman may complain of irritation and pruritus. Dysuria and dyspareunia are often present. Typically the discharge worsens during and after menstruation. Often the cervix and vaginal walls demonstrate the characteristic "strawberry spots" or tiny petechiae, and the cervix may bleed on contact. In severe infections the vaginal walls, cervix, and occasionally the vulva may be acutely inflamed.

Screening and Diagnosis

In addition to obtaining a history of current symptoms, a careful sexual history should be obtained. Any history of similar symptoms in the past and treatments used should be noted. The nurse should determine whether the patient's partner(s) were treated and if she has had subsequent sexual relations with new partners.

A speculum examination is always done, even though it may be very uncomfortable for the woman; relaxation techniques and breathing exercises may help the woman with the procedure. Any of the classic signs may or may not be present on physical examination. The typical one-celled flagellate trichomonads are easily distinguished on a normal saline wet prep. Trichomoniasis also may be identified on Pap tests. Because trichomoniasis is an STI, once diagnosis is confirmed, appropriate laboratory studies for other STIs should be carried out.

Management

The recommended treatment is metronidazole, 2 g orally in a single dose (CDC, Workowski, & Berman, 2006). Although the male partner is usually asymptomatic, it is recommended that he receive treatment also because he often harbors the trichomonads in the urethra or prostate. It is important that nurses discuss the importance of partner treatment with patients because it is likely that the infection will recur if partners are not treated.

Women with trichomoniasis need to understand the sexual transmission of this disease. The patient must know that the organism may be present without observable symptoms, perhaps for several months, and that it is not possible to determine when she became infected. Women should be informed of the necessity for treating all sexual partners and given suggestions about how to raise the issue with their partner(s).

Group B Streptococcus

Group B streptococcus (GBS) may be considered a normal vaginal flora in a woman who is not pregnant. It is present in 9% to 23% of healthy pregnant women. However, GBS infection is associated with poor pregnancy outcomes. GBS infections are an important factor in perinatal and neonatal morbidity and mortality, usually resulting from vertical transmission from the birth canal of the infected mother to the infant during birth.

Risk factors for neonatal GBS infection include positive prenatal culture for GBS in the current pregnancy; preterm birth of less than 37 weeks of gestation; premature rupture of membranes for longer than 18 hours; intrapartum maternal fever higher than 38° C; and a positive history for early-onset neonatal GBS.

To decrease the risk of neonatal GBS infection, it is recommended that all women be screened at 36 to 37 weeks of gestation for GBS using a rectovaginal culture and that intravenous antibiotic prophylaxis (IAP) be offered to all who test positive. If a culture is not available at onset of labor or if risk factors are present, IAP is also offered. IAP is not recommended before a cesarean birth if labor or rupture of membranes has not occurred. The recommended treatment is penicillin G, 5 million units in an intravenous loading dose, and then 2.5 million units intravenously every 4 hours during labor. Ampicillin, 2 g intravenous loading dose, followed by 1 g intravenously every 4 hours, is an alternative therapy (see Home Care box).

HOME CARE

Sexually Transmitted Infections

- Take your medication as directed.
- Use comfort measures for symptom relief as suggested by your health care provider.
- Keep your appointment for repeat cultures or checkups after your treatment to make sure that your infection is cured.
- Advise your sexual partner(s) to be tested and treated if necessary.
- Abstain from sexual intercourse until your treatment is completed or for as long as you are advised by your health care provider.
- Use practices to prevent infection when sexual intercourse is resumed.
- Call your health care provider immediately if you notice bumps, sores, rashes, or discharges.
- Keep all future appointments with your health care provider, even if things appear normal.

Infection Control

Infection control measures are essential to protect care providers and prevent nosocomial infection of patients, regardless of the infectious agent. The risk for occupational transmission varies with the disease. Even when the risk is low, as with HIV, the existence of any risk warrants reasonable precautions. Precautions against airborne disease transmission are available in all health care agencies. Standard Precautions (precautions to use in care of all persons for infection control) are listed in Box 6-7.

Problems of the Breast

Approximately 50% of women have a breast problem at some point in their adult lives. The most common sign of a breast problem is a palpable mass. Most of these lumps are benign, although finding them may produce anxiety for the woman, who may fear she has cancer. With the exception of skin

BOX 6-7 Standard Precautions

Assume that every person is potentially infected or colonized with an organism that could be transmitted in the health care setting and apply the following infection control practices during the delivery of health care.

Hand Hygiene

During the delivery of health care, avoid unnecessary touching of surfaces in close proximity to the patient to prevent both contamination of clean hands from environmental surfaces and transmission of pathogens from contaminated hands to surfaces. When hands are visibly dirty, contaminated with proteinaceous material, or visibly soiled with blood or body fluids, wash them with either a nonantimicrobial soap and water or an antimicrobial soap and water. If hands are not visibly soiled or after removing visible material with nonantimicrobial soap and water, decontaminate them. The preferred method of hand decontamination is with an alcohol-based hand rub. Alternatively hands may be washed with an antimicrobial soap and water. Frequent use of an alcohol-based hand rub immediately following handwashing with nonantimicrobial soap may increase the frequency of dermatitis. Perform hand hygiene: (a) Before having direct contact with patients; (b) after contact with blood, body fluids or excretions, mucous membranes, nonintact skin, or wound dressings; (c) after contact with a patient's intact skin (e.g., when taking a pulse or blood pressure or lifting a patient); (d) if hands will be moving from a contaminated body site to a clean body site during patient care; (e) after contact with inanimate objects (including medical equipment) in the immediate vicinity of the patient; and (f) after removing gloves. Wash hands with nonantimicrobial soap and water or with antimicrobial soap and water if contact with spores (e.g., *Clostridium difficile or Bacillus anthracis*) is likely to have occurred. The physical action of washing and rinsing hands under such circumstances is recommended because alcohols, chlorhexidine, iodophors, and other antiseptic agents have poor activity against spores. Do not wear artificial fingernails or extenders if duties include direct contact with patients at high risk for infection and associated adverse outcomes (e.g., ICUs) or operating rooms. Develop an organizational policy for the wearing of nonnatural nails by health care personnel who have direct contact with patients outside of the groups previously specified.

Personal Protective Equipment

Observe the following principles of use:

- Wear personal protective equipment (PPE) when the nature of the anticipated patient interaction indicates that contact with blood or body fluids may occur. Prevent contamination of clothing and skin during the process of removing PPE. Before leaving the patient's room or cubicle, remove and discard PPE.
- **Gloves**—Wear gloves when it can be reasonably anticipated that contact with blood or other potentially infectious materials, mucous membranes, nonintact skin, or potentially contaminated intact skin (e.g., of a patient incontinent of stool or urine) could occur. Wear gloves with fit and durability appropriate to the task. Wear disposable medical examination gloves for providing direct patient care. Wear disposable medical examination gloves or reusable utility gloves for cleaning the environment or medical equipment. Remove gloves after contact with a patient and/or the surrounding environment (including medical equipment), using proper

Continued

BOX 6-7 Standard Precautions—cont'd

Personal Protective Equipment—cont'd

technique to prevent hand contamination. Do not wear the same pair of gloves for the care of more than one patient. Do not wash gloves for the purpose of reuse since this practice has been associated with transmission of pathogens. Change gloves during patient care if the hands will move from a contaminated body site (e.g., perineal area) to a clean body site (e.g., face).

- **Gowns**—Wear a gown that is appropriate to the task to protect skin and prevent soiling or contamination of clothing during procedures and patient care activities when contact with blood, body fluids, secretions, or excretions is anticipated. Wear a gown for direct patient contact if the patient has uncontained secretions or excretions. Remove gown and perform hand hygiene before leaving the patient's environment. Do not reuse gowns, even for repeated contacts with the same patient. Routine donning of gowns on entrance into a high risk unit (e.g., ICU, NICU, HSCT unit) is not indicated.
- **Mouth, nose, eye protection**—Use PPE to protect the mucous membranes of the eyes, nose, and mouth during procedures and patient care activities that are likely to generate splashes or sprays of blood, body fluids, secretions, and excretions. Select masks, goggles, face shields, and combinations of each according to the need anticipated by the task performed. During aerosol-generating procedures (e.g., bronchoscopy, suctioning of the respiratory tract [if not using in-line suction catheters], endotracheal intubation) in patients who are not suspected of being infected with an agent for which respiratory protection is otherwise recommended (e.g., *Mycobacterium tuberculosis,* SARS, or hemorrhagic fever viruses), wear one of the following: a face shield that fully covers the front and sides of the face, a mask with attached shield, or a mask and goggles (in addition to gloves and gown).

Respiratory Hygiene/Cough Etiquette

Educate health care personnel on the importance of source control measures to contain respiratory secretions to prevent droplet and fomite transmission of respiratory pathogens, especially during seasonal outbreaks of viral respiratory tract infections (e.g., influenza, RSV, adenovirus, parainfluenza virus) in communities.

Implement the following measures to contain respiratory secretions in patients and accompanying individuals who have signs and symptoms of a respiratory infection, beginning at the point of initial encounter in a health care setting (e.g., triage, reception and waiting areas in emergency departments, outpatient clinics and physician offices). Post signs at entrances and in strategic places (e.g., elevators, cafeterias) within ambulatory and inpatient settings with instructions to patients and other persons with symptoms of a respiratory infection to cover their mouths/noses when coughing or sneezing, use and dispose of tissues, and perform hand hygiene after hands have been in contact with respiratory secretions. Provide tissues and no-touch receptacles (e.g., foot-pedal operated lid or open, plastic-lined wastebasket) for disposal of tissues. Provide resources and instructions for performing hand hygiene in or near waiting areas in ambulatory and inpatient settings; provide conveniently located dispensers of alcohol-based hand rubs and, where sinks are available, supplies for handwashing. During periods of increased prevalence of respiratory infections in the community (e.g., as indicated by increased school absenteeism, increased number of patients seeking care for a respiratory infection), offer masks to coughing patients and other symptomatic persons (e.g., persons who accompany ill patients) on entry into the facility or medical office and encourage them to maintain special separation, ideally a distance of at least 3 feet, from others in common waiting areas. Some facilities may find it logistically easier to institute this recommendation year-round as a standard of practice.

Safe Injection Practices

The following recommendations apply to the use of needles, the use of cannulas that replace needles, and, where applicable, intravenous delivery systems. Use aseptic technique to avoid contamination of sterile injection equipment. Do not administer medications from a syringe to multiple patients, even if the needle or cannula on the syringe is changed. Needles, cannulas, and syringes are sterile, single-use items; they should not be reused for another patient or to access a medication or solution that might be used for a subsequent patient. Use fluid infusion and administration sets (i.e., intravenous bags, tubing, and connectors) for one patient only and dispose appropriately after use. Consider a syringe or needle/cannula contaminated once it has been used to enter or connect to a patient's intravenous infusion bag or administration set. Use single-dose vials for parenteral medications whenever possible. Do not administer medications from single-dose vials or ampules to multiple patients or combine leftover contents for later use. If multidose vials must be used, both the needle or cannula and syringe used to access the multidose vial must be sterile. Do not keep multidose vials in the immediate patient treatment area and store in accordance with the manufacturer's recommendations; discard if sterility is compromised or questionable. Do not use bags or bottles of intravenous solution as a common source of supply for multiple patients.

Infection Control Practices for Special Lumbar Puncture Procedures

Wear a surgical mask when placing a catheter or injecting material into the spinal canal or subdural space (i.e., during myelograms, lumbar puncture, and spinal or epidural anesthesia).

Centers for Disease Control and Prevention: Standard Precautions: excerpted from Guideline for isolation precautions: preventing transmission of infectious agents in healthcare settings 2007, January 1996, updated October 12, 2007. Available from www.cdc.gov/ncidod/dhqp/gl_isolation_standard.html (accessed June 24, 2008).

HSCT, Hematopoietic stem cell transplant; *ICU,* intensive care unit; *NICU,* neonatal intensive care unit; *RSV,* respiratory syncytial virus; *SARS,* severe acute respiratory syndrome.

cancer, cancer of the breast is the most frequently diagnosed cancer in women in the United States (ACS, 2008b). The development of breast cancer can have a far-reaching impact on the woman and her family. Beyond the obvious physiologic alterations, the woman also may experience threats to her self-concept and her ability to cope. The condition and its treatments can affect a woman's concept of herself as a sexual being. A woman's family is also challenged in the way it responds to her diagnosis. When breast cancer occurs during or after pregnancy, it adds to the complexity of both physical and emotional responses to childbearing.

Fibrocystic Changes

The most common benign breast problem is fibrocystic change. Fibrocystic change is not a disease but a condition found in varying degrees in healthy women's breasts. Fibrocystic changes are palpable thickenings in the breast usually associated with pain and tenderness. The pain and tenderness fluctuate with the menstrual cycle and can become progressively worse until menopause. The histologic findings associated with fibrocystic changes are considered part of the spectrum of normal involutional patterns of the breast; thus the changes are not a disease.

Etiology

Fibrocystic changes tend to appear most commonly in women in their second and third decades of life. No known etiologic agent is responsible for benign breast disease, although an imbalance of estrogen and progesterone may be responsible. One theory is that estrogen excess and progesterone deficiency in the luteal phase of the menstrual cycle may cause changes in breast tissue. Risk factors associated with benign breast disease include nulliparity, low parity, late menopause, and estrogen therapy.

Clinical Manifestations and Diagnosis

The usual clinical presentation of fibrocystic change is lumpiness in both breasts; single simple cysts may also occur. Symptoms usually develop about a week before menstruation begins and subside about a week after menstruation ends. They include dull, heavy pain and a sense of fullness and tenderness that increases premenstrually. The woman with fibrocystic change may form cysts that manifest as painful enlarging lumps in her breasts. Cysts are common in premenopausal women who are not receiving estrogen therapy. The cysts are soft on palpation, well differentiated, and movable. Deeper cysts, especially aggregations of cysts, are indistinguishable by palpation from carcinomas, which are malignant growths that infiltrate surrounding tissue.

A first step in the workup of a breast lump is ultrasonography to determine if it is fluid filled or solid. Fluid-filled cysts are aspirated, and the woman is monitored on a routine basis for development of other cysts. If the lump is solid, mammography is obtained if the woman is older than 35 years. Fine-needle aspiration (FNA) is then performed, regardless of the woman's age, to determine the nature of the lump. In some cases a core biopsy may be needed after FNA to harvest adequate amounts of tissue for pathologic examination.

Management

Treatment for fibrocystic change is usually conservative, with diuretics and restriction of salt and fluid. Vitamin E supplements also have been recommended, although megadose therapy should be avoided. Even though no research support has been found, some advocate eliminating dimethylxanthines such as caffeine. Some women report relief of symptoms by avoiding smoking and consuming alcohol. Recommended pain relief measures include taking analgesics or NSAIDs such as ibuprofen, wearing a supportive bra, and applying heat to the breasts. Some women report relief while taking oral contraceptives, but others report worsening of symptoms. Women may need to try several approaches for a number of months before improvement is noted. Surgical removal of nodules is attempted only in select cases. In the presence of multiple nodules the surgical approach involves multiple incisions and tissue manipulation and may not prevent the development of more nodules.

Fibroadenomas

The next most common benign condition of the breast is fibroadenoma. Fibroadenomas occur in women from puberty through menopause. Masses are solid, encapsulated, nontender and are most often found in the upper outer quadrant of the breast.

The cause of fibroadenomas is unknown. Fibroadenomas are characterized by discrete, usually solitary lumps less than 3 cm in diameter. Occasionally the woman with a fibroadenoma experiences tenderness in the tumor during the menstrual cycle. Fibroadenomas increase in size during pregnancy and shrink as the woman ages. Fibroadenomas do not increase in size in response to the menstrual cycle (in contrast to fibrocystic cysts). The mass tends to remain the same size or increase in size slowly over time.

Diagnosis is made by a review of the history and physical examination. Mammography, ultrasonography, or magnetic resonance imaging may be used to determine the type of lesion. FNA may be used to determine the underlying disorder. Surgical excision may be necessary if the lump is suspicious or if the symptoms are severe. Fibroadenomas do not respond to either dietary changes or hormone therapy. Periodic observation of masses by professional physical examination or mammography may be all that is necessary for masses not needing surgical intervention.

Lipomas

A lipoma is a tumor composed of fat that is soft and has discrete borders. The cause of lipoma is unknown. Lipomas are often found in women over 45 years of age, usually on the chest wall and breast. They are characterized as palpable soft masses that are mobile and nontender. Mammography can be used to make a diagnosis; biopsy usually is not needed. Lipomas can be surgically excised if removal is desired.

Nipple Discharge

Nipple discharge is a common occurrence that concerns many women. Although most nipple discharge is physiologic, each woman who has this problem must be evaluated carefully. A small percentage of women are found to have a serious endocrine disorder or malignancy. Bilateral serous discharge expressed during nipple stimulation can be considered a normal finding. Patient education and reassurance are indicated.

Galactorrhea is another form of breast discharge not related to malignancy. Galactorrhea manifests as a bilaterally spontaneous, milky, sticky discharge. It is a normal finding in pregnancy. It can also occur as the result of elevated prolactin levels, which in turn may occur as a result of a thyroid disorder, pituitary tumor, or chest wall surgery or trauma. A complete medication history is essential because certain medications can precipitate galactorrhea (e.g., OCPs and neuroleptic drugs).

The optimal time to draw blood to determine a prolactin level is between 8 and 10 AM. Ideally prolactin levels should not be determined directly after a breast examination, sexual activity, or exercise session. Diagnostic tests that may be indicated include prolactin levels, microscopic analysis of the discharge, a thyroid profile, a pregnancy test, and a mammogram.

Mammary Duct Ectasia

Mammary duct ectasia is an inflammation of the ducts behind the nipple. The cause of mammary duct ectasia is unknown, although chronic inflammation and dilation of the lactiferous ducts has been suggested. It occurs most often in perimenopausal women and is characterized by a nipple discharge that is thick; sticky; and white, brown, green, or purple. Often the woman will experience a burning pain, itching, or a palpable mass behind the nipple.

The diagnostic workup includes a mammogram and aspiration and culture of fluid. Duct ectasia is usually self-limiting, requiring only reassurance of the woman. An infection in the inflamed area can occur and requires antibiotic therapy. Incision and drainage is necessary if an abscess develops. Treatment also may include a local excision of the affected duct(s) if the woman has no future plans to breastfeed.

Intraductal Papilloma

Intraductal papilloma is a rare benign condition that develops in the terminal nipple ducts. The cause is unknown. It usually occurs in women between ages 30 and 50. Usually too small to be palpated (less than 0.5 cm), this papilloma causes serous, serosanguineous, or bloody nipple discharge. The discharge is unilateral and spontaneous. After the possibility of malignancy is eliminated, the affected segments of the ducts and breasts are surgically excised.

Table 6-4 compares common manifestations of benign breast masses.

Care Management

Assessment should include a careful history and physical examination. The history should focus on risk factors for breast diseases, events related to the breast mass, and health maintenance practices. Risk factors for breast cancer are discussed later in this chapter. Information related to the breast mass should include how, when, and by whom the mass was discovered. The interval between discovery and seeking care is crucial. The answers to these questions can give clues about breast self-examination (BSE) practice and access to care. The nurse should document the following patient information: pain, whether symptoms increase with menses, dietary habits, smoking habits, use of oral contraceptives, regular BSE, and the examination technique used. The woman's emotional status, including her stress level, fears, and concerns, and her ability to cope should also be assessed.

Physical examination may include assessment of the breasts for symmetry, masses (size, number, consistency, and mobility), and nipple discharge.

Nursing actions might include the following:

- Demonstrate correct BSE technique.
- Discuss the intervals for and facets of breast screening, including professional examination and mammography. Women with breast implants may need special views of the breast and precautions taken to avoid rupture of the implant during mammography.
- Provide written educational materials in the woman's primary language.
- Encourage the verbalization of fears and concerns about treatment and prognosis.
- Provide specific information regarding the woman's condition and treatment, including dietary changes, drug therapy, comfort measures, stress management, and surgery.

Table 6-4 Comparison of Common Manifestations of Benign Breast Masses

FIBROCYSTIC CHANGES	FIBROADENOMA	LIPOMA	INTRADUCTAL PAPILLOMA	MAMMARY DUCT ECTASIA
Multiple lumps	Single lump	Single lump	Single or multiple	Mass behind nipple
Nodular	Well delineated	Well delineated	Not well delineated	Not well delineated
Palpable	Palpable	Palpable	Nonpalpable	Palpable
Movable	Movable	Movable	Nonmobile	Nonmobile
Round, smooth	Round, lobular	Round, lobular	Small, ball-like	Irregular
Firm or soft	Firm	Soft	Firm or soft	Firm
Tenderness influenced by menstrual cycle	Usually asymptomatic	Nontender	Usually nontender	Painful, burning, itching
Bilateral	Unilateral	Unilateral	Unilateral	Unilateral
May or may not have nipple discharge	No nipple discharge	No nipple discharge	Serous or bloody nipple discharge	Thick, sticky nipple discharge

- Describe pain-relieving strategies in detail and collaborate with the primary health care provider to ensure effective pain control.
- Encourage discussion of feelings about body image.
- Refer to a support group or stress management resource if needed to cope with long-term consequences of benign breast conditions.

Malignant Conditions of the Breast

The United States has one of the highest rates of breast carcinoma in the world. One in eight American women will develop breast cancer in her lifetime. The incidence of breast cancer is higher in Caucasian women than in African-American women, but the mortality rate for African-American women with breast cancer is higher (Fig. 6-6). Even though African-American women practice BSE and obtain clinical breast examinations and mammograms by a professional with a frequency the same as or greater than that of Caucasian women, more African-American women are initially diagnosed with a later stage of breast cancer.

Mortality rates from breast cancer have declined since 1990. The death rate increased by 0.4% annually between 1975 and 1990 but decreased by 2.2% between 1990 and 2004 (ACS, 2008b).

Etiology

Although the exact cause of breast cancer continues to elude investigators, certain factors that increase a women's risk for

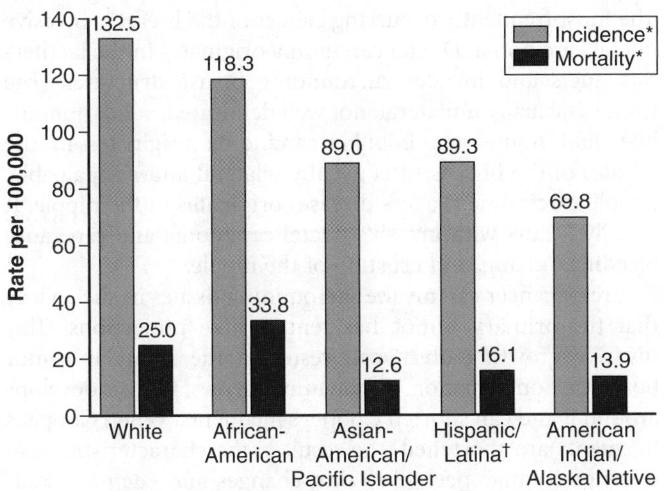
Incidence*
Mortality*
Rate per 100,000
140
120
100
80
60
40
20
0
132.5
25.0
118.3
33.8
89.0
12.6
89.3
16.1
69.8
13.9
White
African-American
Asian-American/Pacific Islander
Hispanic/Latina†
American Indian/Alaska Native
*Rates are age-adjusted to the 2000 U.S. standard population.
†Persons of Hispanic origin may be any race.
Data sources: Incidence – Surveillance, Epidemiology, and End Results (SEER) Program, SEER 17 Registries, 2000-2004, Division of Cancer Control and Population Science, National Cancer Institute, 2007. Incidence data for Hispanics exclude cases from the Alaska Native Registry and Kentucky. Mortality – National Center for Health Statistics, Centers for Disease Control and Prevention, 2007. For Hispanics, information is included for all states except Minnesota, New Hampshire, and North Dakota.
American Cancer Society, Surveillance Research, 2007

Fig. 6-6 Female breast cancer incidence and mortality rates by race and ethnicity, United States, 2000-2004. *(Courtesy American Cancer Society, Surveillance Research, 2007.)*

developing a malignancy have been identified. The factors are listed in Box 6-8.

The most important predictor of risk for breast cancer is age. A woman's risk of breast cancer increases as her age increases. Most of the other risk factors involve the effects of the menstrual-reproductive cycle (probably the effect of estrogen or progesterone) on the development of breast cancer. Fewer menstrual cycles and early childbearing appear to have a protective effect.

Although most breast cancers are not related to genetic factors, the identification of the BRCA1 and BRCA2 genes demonstrated the role of heredity and genetic mutations in this disease. Only about 5% to 10% of breast cancers are caused by a specific inherited mutation that confers a high risk of developing breast cancer. The American Society of Clinical Oncology identified the following as factors that place a woman at high risk for genetically transmitted breast cancer: a family with more than two breast cancer cases and one or more ovarian cancer cases diagnosed at any age; a family with more than three breast cancer cases diagnosed before 50 years of age; and sister pairs that have been diagnosed before age 50 with two breast cancers, two ovarian cancers, or a breast and ovarian cancer (Sakorafas, 2003).

Ethical Considerations of Genetic Testing

Although knowing whether one is hereditarily predisposed to breast cancer may have benefits, the extent to which an individual can benefit remains unclear. Confirming one's mutation status may provide a sense of control in life plans or it may create high levels of anxiety and distress. Genetic testing can alter decisions regarding family and intimate relationships, childbearing, body image, and quality of life. Regardless of whether results are positive or negative for BRCA1 and BRCA2 mutations, the results can have a highly negative impact on women's lives. Women at increased risk for breast cancer need comprehensive information about the benefits and limitations

BOX 6-8 Risk Factors for Breast Cancer*

- Age
- Previous history of breast cancer
- Family history of breast cancer, especially a mother or sister (particularly significant if before menopause)
- Previous history of ovarian, endometrial, colon, or thyroid cancer
- Early menarche (before age 12 years)
- Late menopause (after age 55 years)
- Nulliparity or first pregnancy after age 30 years
- Use of estrogen replacement therapy
- Daily alcohol use
- Obesity after menopause
- Previous history of benign breast disease with epithelial hyperplasia
- Race (Caucasian women have highest incidence)
- High socioeconomic status
- Sedentary lifestyle

*Risk factors are cumulative (i.e., the more risk factors present, the greater the likelihood of breast cancer occurring).

evolve Nursing Care Plan–Breast Cancer

of genetic testing to ensure that informed decisions about genetic testing can be made. Because decisions regarding genetic testing, genetic counseling, and breast cancer risk assessment are highly individualized, health care professionals should be careful regarding any generalizations about women at risk for breast cancer.

Some known and suspected environmental risk factors include exposure to organochlorine pesticides and other synthetic chemicals, hormonal factors (both exogenous and endogenous), diet, tobacco and alcohol use, radiation, and magnetic fields. However, definitive links between these factors and breast cancer have not been established.

Clinical outcomes of the Women's Health Initiative randomized controlled trial to assess the risks and benefits of estrogen and progestin in healthy postmenopausal women were released in May 2002. The safety monitoring board recommended that the trial be stopped because the overall health risks exceeded the benefits. These risks included 290 cases of breast cancer in the study group of about 8500 women (Writing Group for the Women's Health Initiative Investigators, 2002). Further evidence supports that combined estrogen and progestin increased the risk of breast cancer as well as the risk of heart disease, stroke, blood clots, and urinary incontinence more than estrogen alone among healthy users (National Cancer Institute [NCI], 2007).

In a study to determine whether HRT is safe for women with previous breast cancer, an unacceptably high number of women receiving HRT had a new breast cancer event, and the study was stopped. The researchers concluded that their findings indicated an unacceptable risk for these women (Holmberg, Anderson, HABITS steering and data monitoring committees, 2004).

Women considering HRT should be cautious and consult with their health care providers to determine their suitability for it. Maintaining normal weight, eating a diet rich in fruits and vegetables and low in fat, limiting intake of alcohol, not smoking, and regular exercise seem to exert a protective effect against the development of breast cancer (NCI, 2007).

Information about breast cancer risks can be confusing, and women can overestimate or underestimate their risks. The Breast Cancer Risk Assessment Tool can be used by women and health professionals to calculate risk. This tool was developed and verified by the NCI to predict the risk of breast cancer in 5 years and over the lifetime (to age 90 years) of a woman. The tool is available on the Internet at the NCI website (*www.nci.nih.gov*).

An accurate estimation of risk for breast cancer is needed so that women may be given rational management recommendations. During breast cancer risk counseling, facts should be presented to women by their physicians in a supportive, nondirective way, without personal opinions or preferences. Discussion should also include treatment options and prognosis of breast cancer, as well as risks and benefits of alternative methods of prevention and early diagnosis. A woman's recognition of having increased breast cancer risk can carry psychologic consequences such as anxiety, guilt, depression, and reduced self-esteem. Enormous guilt may be experienced by high risk women who pass specific genetic mutations on to their children. Psychologic intervention should be considered to assist individuals in coping with these significant adverse sequelae (Sakorafas, 2003).

Chemoprevention

Researchers from the NCI and other groups are investigating the role of tamoxifen and raloxifene, both of which protect bone health, in the prevention of breast cancer (NCI, 2006). Both tamoxifen and raloxifene reduce by 50% the risk of invasive breast cancer in postmenopausal women who are at risk for the disease. Raloxifene may be an ideal choice for the woman at high risk for both osteoporosis and breast cancer. Tamoxifen also reduces the recurrence of breast cancer in women with prior breast malignancies. Patients should be made aware of the risk of occasional serious side effects before taking tamoxifen (NCI, 2006) (see later discussion).

Pathophysiology

Breast cancer occurs when there are genetic alterations in the DNA of breast epithelial cells. Many types of breast cancer exist. Genetic alterations, either inherited or spontaneous, are found in the epithelial cells, compromising ductal or lobular tissue. Researchers are investigating which oncogenes (potentially cancer-inducing genes) may cause breast cancer or change its growth pattern and how the process can be stopped.

Breast cancer begins in the epithelial cells lining the mammary ducts of the breast. The rate of breast cancer growth depends on the effect of estrogen and progesterone. These cancers can be either invasive (infiltrating) or noninvasive (in situ). Invasive or infiltrating breast cancers can grow into the wall of the mammary duct and into the surrounding tissues. The most frequently occurring cancer of the breast is invasive ductal carcinoma. Ductal carcinoma originates in the lactiferous ducts and invades surrounding breast structures. The tumor is usually unilateral, not well delineated, solid, nonmobile, and nontender. Lobular carcinoma originates in the lobules of the breasts. It is usually bilateral and nonpalpable. Nipple carcinoma (Paget's disease) originates in the nipple. It usually occurs with invasive ductal carcinoma and can cause bleeding, oozing, and crusting of the nipple.

Breast cancer can invade surrounding tissues in such a way that the primary tumor has tentacle-like projections. This invasive growth pattern can result in the irregular tumor border felt on palpation. As the tumor grows, fibrosis develops around it and can shorten Cooper's ligaments. When Cooper's ligaments are shortened, the result is the characteristic peau d'orange (orange peel–like) skin changes and edema associated with some breast cancers. If the breast cancer invades the lymphatic channels, tumors can develop in the regional lymph nodes, often occupying the axillary lymph nodes. The tumor may invade the outer layers of skin, creating ulcerations.

Metastasis results from seeding of the breast cancer cells into the blood and lymph systems, leading to tumor development in the bones, lungs, brain, and liver.

Clinical Manifestations and Diagnosis

Breast cancer in its earliest form can be detected on a mammogram before it can be felt by the woman or her health care provider. However, approximately 90% of all breast lumps are detected by the woman. Of these, only 20% to 25% are malig-

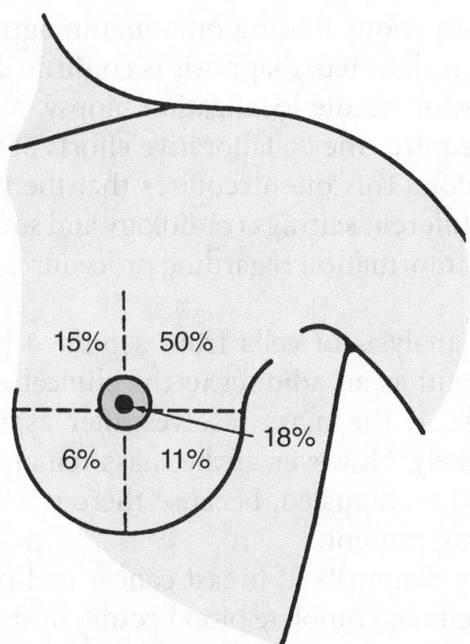

Fig. 6-7 Relative location of malignant lesions of the breast.

nant. More than half of all lumps are discovered in the upper outer quadrant of the breast (Fig. 6-7). The most common initial sign is a lump or thickening of the breast. The lump may feel hard and fixed or soft and spongy. It may have well-defined or irregular borders. It may be fixed to the skin, thereby causing dimpling to occur. A bloody or clear unilateral nipple discharge may be present.

Unilateral and spontaneous discharge (without nipple manipulation) is associated with mastitis, intraductal papilloma, and cancer. The discharge is usually intermittent and persistent and may be clear, serous, green-gray, purulent, serosanguineous, or sanguineous. Women with these findings need a complete diagnostic workup to determine the actual cause of their signs.

As a general principle, any unilateral breast sign or symptom (i.e., mass, discharge, pain, or itching) is a more ominous finding than a bilateral sign or symptom. However, all findings are carefully followed up to avoid missing a serious diagnosis such as cancer. Any delay in treatment can adversely affect the woman's subsequent prognosis and treatment options.

Early detection and diagnosis reduce the mortality rate because the cancer is found when it is smaller, lesions are more localized, and there tends to be a lower percentage of positive nodes. Therefore it is imperative that protocols for assessment and diagnosis be established. Regular clinical examination by a qualified health care provider and screening mammography (x-ray filming of the breast) (Fig. 6-8) can aid in the early detection of breast cancers. Table 6-5 lists the current recommendations of the ACS for breast cancer screening.

Major obstacles to breast cancer screening include older age; fiscal barriers (e.g., expense, lack of health insurance); knowledge, attitudinal, and behavioral barriers (e.g., fear, ignorance, lack of motivation); and organizational barriers (e.g., scheduling problems, lack of availability of mammography services, lack of physician referral). Strategies that may be helpful to health care providers in improving screening for breast cancer include education and encouragement of older women; continuing education of providers; provision of information about new, affordable screening options; use of reminder systems in office practice; use of patient-directed

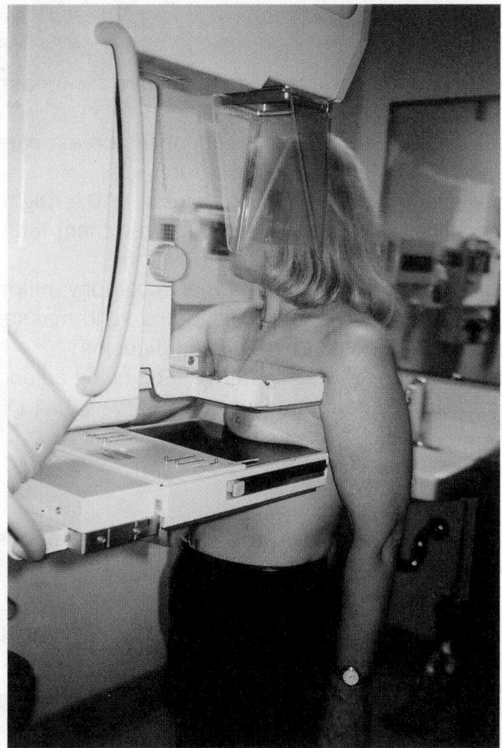
Fig. 6-8 Mammography. *(Courtesy Shannon Perry, Phoenix, AZ.)*

Table 6-5 Screening Guidelines for Breast Cancer: Detection in Asymptomatic Women Recommended by the American Cancer Society

AGE (yr)	EXAMINATION	FREQUENCY
20-39	Clinical breast examination	Every 3 yr
40 and older	BSE	Monthly
	Clinical breast examination	Annually
	Mammography	Annually
Women at increased risk	Talk with doctor about starting mammography screening earlier and having additional tests such as breast ultrasound and magnetic resonance imaging	More frequently as recommended by doctor

Source: American Cancer Society: *Cancer facts and figures, 2008,* Atlanta, 2008, American Cancer Society.

literature; and interventions that reward, support, and prompt desired screening behaviors. In addition, it is important for a practitioner to assess a woman's BSE technique and frequency at the annual visit.

Cultural factors may influence a woman's decision to participate in breast cancer screening. Knowledge of these factors and use of culturally sensitive tailored messages and materials that appeal to the unique concerns, beliefs, and reading abilities of identified groups of women who don't participate in breast screening may assist the nurse in helping women overcome barriers to seeking care (see Cultural Awareness box).

evolve Case Study–Breast Cancer

BOX 6-9 Technologies for Breast Cancer Screening

Screen-film mammography—Gold standard for breast cancer screening
Full-field digital mammography—Identifies breast cancers missed by screen-film mammography
Computer-aided detection and diagnosis (CAD)—Digitizes screen-film mammograms and analyzes them for abnormalities
Ultrasound—Valuable adjunct to mammography; helpful in distinguishing between fluid-filled and solid masses; useful in performing image-guided biopsies
Magnetic resonance imaging (MRI)—Screening adjunct to mammography and ultrasound.

A variety of technologies are used in breast cancer screening (Box 6-9).

CULTURAL AWARENESS

Breast Screening Practices

Certain minority women tend to have low compliance rates in the use of early screening methods for breast cancer. Many factors play a role in influencing the screening practices of these women. African-American women reported not participating in early breast cancer screening because of discomfort with impersonal care from providers; lack of health care insurance; lack of funds to pay for mammograms; lack of awareness of community assistance within the health care system; lack of access to transportation; and feelings of fatalism, fear, helplessness, and powerlessness. Hispanic women cited lack of a regular physician, lack of health insurance coverage, inaccessibility of screening facilities, lack of access to transportation, and being unable to obtain time off from work. Asian women cited unawareness of mammography tests, gender and modesty concerns unique to their cultural beliefs, and fear resulting from a sense of vulnerability to breast cancer.

Interventions that will encourage minority women to participate in early breast cancer screening practices begin with the development of culturally sensitive community education programs designed to help women overcome barriers to reaching optimal levels of health. Programs should be designed to educate small groups of woman about risk factors of breast cancer, prevention strategies, and early detection methods. Recruitment of women may be communicated through fliers in neighborhoods, women's groups, churches, clubs, and organizations. Use of incentives to reward participation may be helpful. Nurses and guest speakers of similar ethnicity as the attending group who are breast cancer survivors would be valuable in providing meaningful information and support and past, present, and future perspective to the educational content.

Source: Office of Minority Health, USDHHS, Office of Public Health and Science: *Breast cancer. A resource guide for minority women, 2005*. Available at www.4woman.gov/minority/africanamerican/bc.cfm (accessed February 19, 2009).

When a suspicious finding on a mammogram is noted or when a lump is detected, diagnosis is confirmed by FNA, core needle biopsy, or needle localization biopsy. Needle localization biopsy requires the collaborative efforts of the radiologist and the surgeon. This often requires that the procedure take place in two different settings (radiology and surgery). Patients need specific information regarding procedures, duration, and outcomes.

Cytologic analysis of cells from aspirated breast tissue is extremely useful as an adjunct to the clinical evaluation of a palpable mass. If the mass resolves after aspiration, malignancy is unlikely. However, if the mass remains after aspiration, it should be biopsied, because there is a greater chance of cancer being present.

Laboratory diagnosis of breast cancer and possible cancer metastasis includes complete blood count, liver enzyme levels, serum calcium level, and alkaline phosphatase level. Elevated liver enzyme levels indicate possible liver metastasis, and increased serum calcium and alkaline phosphatase levels may indicate bone metastasis.

Prognosis

Major advances in understanding the biology of cancer have occurred in the past 10 years. Many studies support the theory that breast cancer is a systemic disease; micrometastasis could be present at the initial presentation with or without nodal involvement. The area in which affected lymph nodes are located is also prognostic. The involvement of axillary lymph nodes worsens the prognosis of breast cancer. However, nodal involvement and tumor size remain the most significant prognostic criteria for long-term survival (Fig. 6-9).

Other biologic factors are helpful in predicting response to therapy or survival. These biologic factors include estrogen receptor assay, progesterone receptor assay, tumor ploidy (the amount of DNA in a tumor cell compared with that in a normal cell), S-phase index or growth rate (the percentage of cells in the S phase of cellular division done by flow cytometric determinations of the S-phase fraction), and histologic or nuclear grade. Estrogen and progesterone receptors are pro-

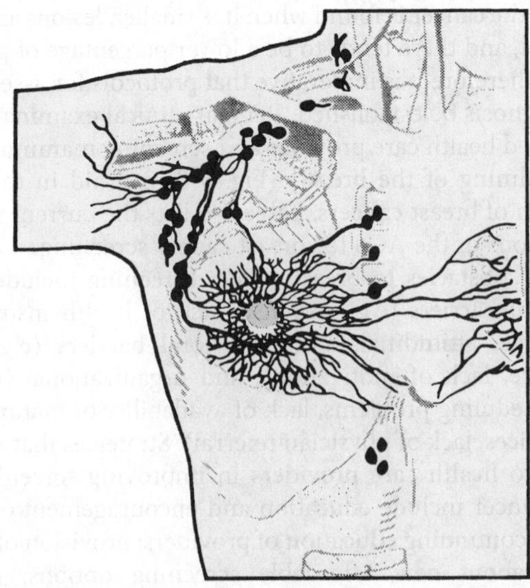

Fig. 6-9 Lymphatic spread of breast cancer.

teins in the cell cytoplasm and surface of some breast cancer cells. When these receptors are present, they bind to estrogen or progesterone, and binding promotes growth of the cancer cell. A breast cancer can have estrogen (ERs), or progesterone receptors (PRs) or both types. Knowledge of the ER status of the cancer is valuable in predicting which patients will respond to HRT.

Human epidermal growth factor receptor 2 (HER2), which is associated with cell growth, is overexpressed in 30% of all breast cancers and is associated with loss of cell regulation and uncontrolled cell proliferation. Thus a positive HER2 status is associated with aggressive tumors, poor prognosis, and resistance to some chemotherapeutic drugs.

Medical Management

Medical management of breast cancer includes surgery, breast reconstruction, radiation therapy, adjuvant hormone therapy, and chemotherapy.

Surgery

The most frequently recommended surgical approaches are lumpectomy and modified radical mastectomy (Fig. 6-10). Lumpectomy involves the removal of the breast tumor, a small amount of surrounding tissue, and a sampling of axillary lymph nodes, leaving the pectoralis major muscle intact. Partial mastectomy (see Fig. 6-10, *B*) includes tylectomy, wide excision, and quadrantectomy or segmental mastectomy and involves removal of differing amounts of tissue along with the tumor. Axillary lymph nodes are usually sampled through a separate incision at the time of these procedures, and surgery is usually followed by radiation therapy to the remaining breast tissue. Lumpectomy offers survival equivalent to that with modified radical mastectomy.

Axillary dissection is performed as a standard part of breast cancer treatment to obtain prognostic information and maintain local control in the axilla, and it is helpful in determining the need for adjunctive systemic treatment by indicating whether nodes are positive for metastatic cells. Lymphatic mapping and sentinel node biopsy is a minimally invasive technique that identifies women with axillary node involvement. The sentinel node is the first node that receives lymphatic drainage from the tumor and is identified by injecting vital blue dye or radioactive dye in the area surrounding the tumor. A small incision in the axilla allows for identification of the blue-stained lymphatic channel leading to the blue sentinel node, either visually or by gamma probe. This node then can be removed and examined for the presence of tumor cells, as opposed to an entire axillary dissection. Clinical trials have reported identification of the sentinel node in more than 95% of cases, with false-negative rates for predicting axillary nodal metastases of less than 5%.

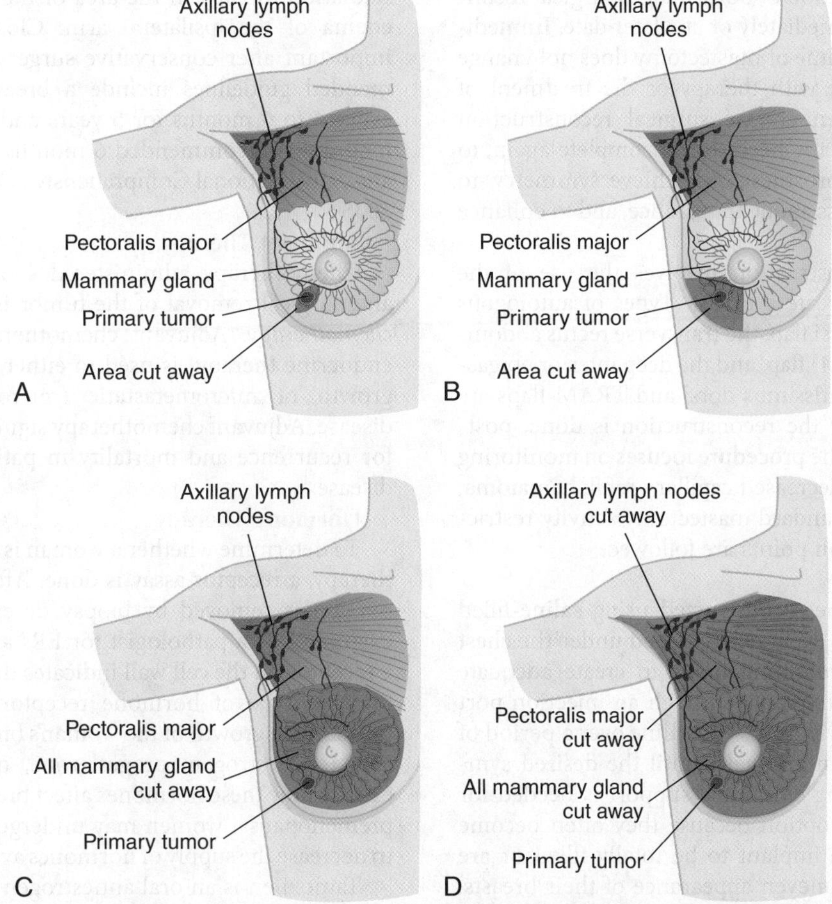

Fig. 6-10 Surgical alternatives for breast cancer. **A,** Lumpectomy (tylectomy). **B,** Quadrantectomy (segmental resection). **C,** Total (simple) mastectomy. **D,** Radical mastectomy.

Total mastectomy (see Fig. 6-10, *C*) (also called simple mastectomy) is the removal of all breast tissue, nipple, and areola; the axillary nodes and pectoral muscles are not removed. Modified radical mastectomy is the removal of the entire breast and a sample of axillary lymph nodes, sparing the pectoral muscles. A radical mastectomy (see Fig. 6-10, *D*), although rarely performed, removes the entire breast, axillary nodes, and the pectoral muscles.

Mastectomy is used for the treatment of early-stage breast cancer when (1) there are multiple tumors in different parts of the breast, (2) tumor removal alone would produce a cosmetically unacceptable result, (3) the breast had been radiated previously, (4) the woman is in the first or second trimester of pregnancy, (5) there are persistent positive margins after reasonable surgery, and (6) there is a possible history of collagen-vascular disease. Women who are found to have metastatic breast cancer at the time of diagnosis usually do not have a mastectomy because it does not offer increased chances of survival.

Women who have these surgeries experience cosmetic changes. Change in shape (because of lumpectomy) or loss of a breast results in a change in body image, which can cause significant alterations in perceptions of femininity and sexual image and interest.

Breast Reconstruction

The goals of surgical breast reconstruction are achievement of symmetry and preservation of body image. Surgical reconstruction can be done immediately or at a later date. Immediate reconstruction at the time of mastectomy does not change survival rates or interfere with therapy or the treatment of recurrent disease. Women choose surgical reconstruction for the following reasons: the need to feel complete again, to avoid using an external prosthesis, to achieve symmetry, to decrease self-consciousness about appearance, and to enhance femininity.

Autologous flap reconstruction involves the use of the woman's own tissue to create a breast. Types of autologous flaps are the latissimus dorsi flap, the transverse rectus abdominis myocutaneous (TRAM) flap, and the deep interior epigastric perforator flap. The latissimus dorsi and TRAM flaps are the most common. After the reconstruction is done, postoperative care specific to the procedure focuses on monitoring the skin flap for signs of decreased capillary refill, hematoma, infection, and necrosis. Standard mastectomy activity restrictions and patient education points are followed.

Breast Implants

The breast may also be reconstructed using saline-filled tissue expanders. A tissue expander is placed under the chest tissue to stretch the surrounding tissue to create adequate space for the permanent implant. Through an injection port the tissue expander is slowly filled with saline over a period of months to stretch the skin gradually until the desired symmetry is attained. Ongoing emotional support is needed for women who choose this option because they often become impatient waiting for the implant to be totally filled or are self-conscious about the uneven appearance of their breasts. Use of cotton padding to equalize the appearance of the breasts may be helpful during this time. After each saline injection the woman has mild discomfort, which is easily relieved with ibuprofen or naproxen. As with all implantation procedures, risks of surgical complications such as hematoma, infection, and delayed wound healing are possible, as well as capsular contractions from, or leakage of, the implant.

In 2006 the FDA approved use of silicone gels for implants (FDA, 2006). Women interested in these implants should be informed of all the risks before making a decision to have one.

After the woman has recovered from initial reconstructive surgery, she may choose to have nipple and areolar reconstruction. Nipple reconstruction is achieved by using an autologous skin graft to construct a nipple, either from tissue from the remaining nipple or from a donor site. Tiny flaps from the new breast itself also may be used. This outpatient procedure requires local anesthesia, intravenous sedation, or a combination of both, depending on how much sensation has returned to the breast. The procedure lasts about an hour, and 4 weeks later tattooing may be used to create an areola and match the color of the natural nipple.

Radiation

The standard therapy for early-stage breast cancer is lumpectomy followed by radiation therapy. Radiation to the breast destroys tumor cells remaining after manipulation and handling of the tumor during surgery. Side effects of radiation therapy include swelling and heaviness in the breast, sunburn-like skin changes in the treated area, and fatigue. Changes to the breast tissue and skin usually resolve in 6 to 12 months. Radiation therapy in the area of the axilla can cause lymphedema of the ipsilateral arm. Close medical follow-up is important after conservative surgery and radiation. Recommended guidelines include a breast physical examination every 4 to 6 months for 5 years and then annually. A mammogram is recommended 6 months after radiation and then annually (National Comprehensive Cancer Network [NCCN], 2005).

Adjuvant Therapy

Chemotherapy administered soon after initial diagnosis and surgical removal of the tumor is referred to as *adjuvant chemotherapy*. Adjuvant chemotherapy (chemotherapy and endocrine therapy) is used to either eradicate or impede the growth of micrometastatic (microscopic cell metastasis) disease. Adjuvant chemotherapy significantly reduces the risks for recurrence and mortality in patients with node-positive disease.

Hormone Therapy

To determine whether a woman is a candidate for hormone therapy, a receptor assay is done. After the entire tumor or a portion is removed by biopsy or excision, cancer cells are examined by a pathologist for ERs and PRs. The presence of a receptor on the cell wall indicates that the woman is positive for that type of hormone receptor. If these receptors are present, the growth of the woman's breast cancer may be influenced by estrogen, progesterone, or both. It is unknown exactly how these hormones affect breast cancer growth. Some premenopausal women may undergo bilateral oophorectomy to decrease the supply of hormones available for tumor growth.

Tamoxifen is an oral antiestrogen medication that mimics progesterone and estrogen. It attaches to the hormone receptors on cancer cells and prevents natural hormones from attaching to the receptors. When tamoxifen fits into the receptors, the cell is unable to grow. Adjuvant hormone therapy using tamoxifen is recommended for all postmenopausal women with breast cancer. In this group of women adjuvant tamoxifen therapy improves disease-free survival and in some cases length of survival. Women treated with hormone therapy should receive therapy for at least 5 years (NCCN, 2005). The side effects of hormone therapy include hot flashes, nausea, vomiting, fluid retention, weight gain, and thrombocytopenia. Tamoxifen therapy also increases the risk of endometrial cancer and deep vein thrombosis (see Medication Guide).

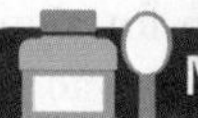

MEDICATION GUIDE

Tamoxifen (Nolvadex)

Action

Antiestrogenic effects; attaches to hormone receptors on cancer cells and prevents natural hormones from attaching to the receptors

Indication

For treatment of metastatic breast cancer, treatment of breast cancer in postmenopausal women after breast cancer surgery and radiation therapy, to reduce the incidence of breast cancer in women at high risk

Dosage

20 to 40 mg orally daily. Dosages greater than 20 mg should be given in divided doses (am and pm).

Adverse Reactions

Common side effects include hot flashes, nausea, vomiting, vaginal bleeding or discharge, menstrual irregularities, and rash. Hair loss is an uncommon effect. Serious side effects include deep vein thrombosis, increased risk of endometrial cancer, and stroke.

Nursing Considerations

The medication may be taken on an empty stomach or with food. Missed doses should be taken as soon as possible, but taking two doses at once is not recommended. A barrier or nonhormonal form of contraception is recommended in premenopausal women because tamoxifen may be harmful to the fetus.

Raloxifene is an oral selective ER modulator. It is used to prevent osteoporosis in postmenopausal women. Raloxifene works as well as tamoxifen in reducing breast cancer risk in women with a high risk for breast cancer. There is less risk of thromboembolic events, uterine cancer, and cataracts in women who take raloxifene than in those who take tamoxifen (see Medication Guide).

Aromatase inhibitors markedly suppress plasma estrogen levels in postmenopausal women by inhibiting or inactivating aromatase, the enzyme responsible for synthesizing estrogens from androgenic substrates. Aromatase inhibitors such as anastrozole, letrozole, and exemestane have shown to be effective agents in hormone therapy for breast cancer. Clinical trials indicate that letrozole is better than tamoxifen in treating advanced disease in postmenopausal women and anastrozole is at least as good. In early-stage breast cancer adjuvant therapy with anastrozole appears to be superior to adjuvant therapy with tamoxifen in reducing recurrence in postmenopausal women. The aromatase inhibitors appear to be well tolerated, with a lower incidence of adverse effects compared to tamoxifen. The adverse effects of aromatase inhibitors include hot flashes, vaginal dryness, musculoskeletal pain, and headache

MEDICATION GUIDE

Raloxifene hydrochloride (Evista)

Action

A selective estrogen receptor modulator, serving as an agonist and antagonist to estrogen receptor sites

Indications

Treatment and prevention of osteoporosis, reduction in the risk of invasive breast cancer in postmenopausal women with osteoporosis, reduction of risk of invasive breast cancer in postmenopausal women at high risk of invasive breast cancer

Dosage

60 mg orally daily

Adverse Reactions

Common side effects include hot flashes, nausea, vomiting, peripheral edema arthralgia, sweating. Serious and life-threatening side effects can occur from existing condition. Raloxifene is contraindicated in women with an active or past history of venous thromboembolism.

Nursing Considerations

The medication may be taken on an empty stomach or with food. Missed doses should be taken as soon as possible, but taking two doses at once is not recommended. Counsel woman to contact primary health care provider if leg pain or feeling of warmth in lower legs, swelling of hands and feet, sudden chest pain or shortness of breath, or sudden changes in vision occur. Calcium, 1500 mg plus vitamin D 400 to 800 units daily, is recommended.

Chemotherapy

Chemotherapy with multiple drug combinations is used in the treatment of recurrent and advanced breast cancer with positive results. Combination regimens and sequential single agents may be used (NCCN, 2005). Some chemotherapeutic agents provide additional treatment options for women with metastatic breast cancer.

Because chemotherapy drugs are designed to kill rapidly reproducing cells, normal body cells that rapidly reproduce (red and white blood cells, gastric mucosa, and hair) also can be affected during treatment. Thus chemotherapy can cause leukopenia, neutropenia, thrombocytopenia, anemia, gastrointestinal side effects (nausea, vomiting, anorexia, mucositis), and partial or full hair loss.

Chemotherapy treatments are usually given in ambulatory care settings once or twice per month. During the informed consent process, before the treatment is selected, the woman and her family members should be educated about the names of the medications, routes of administration, treatment schedule, timing and ordering of medications, length of time of administration, reimbursed and unreimbursed costs of therapy, potential side effects, management of side effects, possible changes in body image (e.g., full or partial hair loss), recovery time after treatment (necessitating lost work time), and need for a caregiver to transport the woman to treatment and care for her afterward.

Depending on the medications used, the treatments may include intravenous, subcutaneous, and oral medications. Often a long-term central venous catheter is inserted when the women will be receiving chemotherapy for an extended period or when she will receive medications that may damage the vein. Presence of a central venous catheter, hair loss, loss of part or all of her breast, menopause, and possible infertility all have the potential to cause a change in body image and increase emotional distress for the woman with breast cancer.

Breast cancer treatment often causes changes in reproductive function. The postmenopausal woman may have to cope with hair loss and other unpleasant side effects from chemotherapy and loss of part or all of her breast. The premenopausal woman may experience these changes along with symptoms of menopause and possible infertility. The young woman with breast cancer may become devastated by an early and abrupt menopause and the possibility of jeopardized reproductive function. These factors can seriously affect the quality of life of the young woman.

Chemotherapy agents are mutagenic and teratogenic. Any woman who is of childbearing age and receiving chemotherapy, even though no longer menstruating, must use a contraceptive. Birth control pills are not recommended because they contain hormones that may assist in the growth of cancer. A contraceptive method is chosen with the assistance of the gynecologist and the medical oncologist, and it must be used before chemotherapy begins and continue to be used until the medical oncologist and gynecologist believe it is safe to discontinue.

With the advance in monoclonal antibody technology, it is now possible to test for residual disease with a serum tumor marker, CA 15-3, if it is secreted by the patient's tumor. From 75% to 80% of women with breast cancer secrete this tumor marker. If the level of CA 15-3 is elevated at the time of diagnosis, circulating levels of CA 15-3 can be checked periodically through the treatment course to measure response. This technology is used to determine effectiveness of therapy for cancer without the need for second-look diagnostic surgery.

Care Management

Before surgery women need to be assessed for psychologic preparation and specific teaching needs. General preoperative teaching and care are given, including expectations regarding physical appearance, pain management, equipment to be used (e.g., intravenous therapy, drains), and emotional support. The emotional reaction to the diagnosis of cancer is always intense, and the many disruptions caused by the disease challenge the woman's and family's ability to cope. A visit from a woman who has had a similar experience may be beneficial both before and after surgery. The woman is reminded that, when she awakens after surgery, her arm on the affected side will feel tight.

Postoperative nursing care focuses on recovery. After recovery from anesthesia, the woman is returned to her room. Special precautions must be observed to prevent or to minimize lymphedema of the affected arm.

NURSING ALERT When vital signs are taken, never apply the blood pressure cuff on the affected arm.

The affected arm is elevated with pillows above the level of the right atrium. Blood is not drawn from this arm, and it is not used for intravenous therapy. Early arm movement is encouraged. Any increase in the circumference of that arm is reported immediately.

Nursing care of the wound involves observation for signs of hemorrhage (dressing, drainage tubes, and Hemovac or Jackson-Pratt drainage reservoirs are emptied at least every 8 hours and more frequently as needed), shock, and infection. Dressings are reinforced as necessary. The woman is asked to turn (alternating between unaffected side and back), cough (while the nurse or the woman applies support to the chest), and deep breathe every 2 hours. Breath sounds are auscultated every 4 hours. Active range-of-motion exercise of legs is encouraged. Parenteral fluids are given until adequate oral intake is possible. Emotional support is continued.

The woman is given self-management instructions and usually discharged to home after 24 hours or more, depending on the type of procedure done (see Home Care box). Lumpectomy is an outpatient procedure, and the patient returns home a few hours after surgery. A woman is discharged 24 to 48 hours after modified radical mastectomy. A referral for home nursing care can be made if the woman needs assistance caring for her incision. Through a referral to the ACS's Reach to Recovery program, a breast cancer survivor who has been trained in how to offer information will visit (see Community Focus box). The resources offered may include such things as a list of sources for prostheses and lingerie. Arm exercises are encouraged at least twice a day (see Patient Teaching box).

Exercise is increased as tolerated and stopped at the point of pain. Initially the woman alternately clenches and extends her fingers and then progresses to wrist and elbow exercises, gradually abducting her arm and raising it to and over her head. She is encouraged to exercise by assisting with her care—washing her face, brushing her teeth, and eating with

COMMUNITY FOCUS

Reach to Recovery

Check the Internet for the American Cancer Society's (*www.cancer.org*) Reach to Recovery program. Identify the services provided by the program and the requirements to become a volunteer. Visit the women's clinic in a local community health agency. Are materials about the Reach to Recovery program visible in the waiting areas? Talk to one of the nurses who work in the clinic (make an appointment for this conversation). What does she know about Reach to Recovery? Does she refer her patients to this program? What is her evaluation of the program? Has she met any of the volunteers? Do her patients have positive things to say about the program?

HOME CARE

After a Mastectomy

- Wash hands well before and after touching incision area or drains.
- Empty surgical drains twice a day and as needed, recording the date, time, drain site (if more than one drain is present), and amount of drainage in milliliters in a diary you will take to each surgical checkup until your drains are removed. (Before discharge you may receive a graduated container for emptying drains and measuring drainage.)
- Avoid driving, lifting more than 10 lb, or reaching above your head until given permission by surgeon.
- Take medications for pain as soon as pain begins.
- Perform arm exercises as directed.
- Call physician if inflammation of the incision or swelling of the incision or the arm occurs.
- Avoid tight clothing, tight jewelry, and other causes of decreased circulation in the affected arm.
- Until drains are removed, wear loose-fitting underwear (camisole or half-slip) and clothes, pinning surgical drains inside of clothing. (You will be taught how to do this safely.)
- After drains are removed and surgical sites are healing and still tender, wear a mastectomy bra or camisole with a cotton-filled, muslin temporary prosthesis. Temporary prostheses of this type are often available from Reach to Recovery.
- Avoid depilatory creams; strong deodorants; and shaving of affected chest area, axilla, and arm.
- Sponge bathe until drains are removed.
- Return to the surgeon's office for incision check, drain inspection, and possible drain removal as directed.
- Contact Reach to Recovery for assistance obtaining external prosthesis and lingerie when dressings, drains, and staples are removed and wound is healing and nontender.
- Contact insurance company for information about coverage of prosthesis and wig if needed. Obtain prescriptions for prosthesis and wig to submit with receipts of purchase for these items to the insurance company. If insurance does not pay for these items, contact hospital or agency social worker or local American Cancer Society for assistance.
- Continue with BSE of unaffected side and affected surgical site and axilla.
- Encourage mother, sisters, and daughters (if applicable) to learn and practice BSE and to have annual professional breast examinations and mammography (if appropriate).
- Keep follow-up visits for professional examination, mammography, and testing to detect recurrent breast cancer.
- Expect decreased sensation and tingling at incision sites and in the affected arm for weeks to months after surgery.
- Resume sexual activities as desired.

PATIENT TEACHING Exercises After Breast Surgery

It is important to talk to your doctor before starting any exercises. A physical or occupational therapist can help design an exercise program for you.

Exercises in Lying Position

These exercises should be performed on a bed or the floor while lying on your back with your knees and hips bent, feet flat.

Wand Exercise

This exercise helps increase the forward motion of the shoulders. You will need a broom handle, yardstick, or other similar object to perform this exercise.

- Hold the wand in both hands with palms facing up.
- Lift the wand up over your head (as far as you can), using your unaffected arm to help lift the wand, until you feel a stretch in your affected arm.
- Hold for 5 seconds.
- Lower arms and repeat five to seven times.

Elbow Winging

This exercise helps increase the mobility of the front of your chest and shoulder. It may take several weeks of regular exercise before your elbows will get close to the bed (or floor).

- Clasp your hands behind your neck with your elbows pointing toward the ceiling.
- Move your elbows apart and down toward the bed (or floor).
- Repeat five to seven times.

Exercises in Sitting Position

Shoulder Blade Stretch

This exercise helps increase the mobility of the shoulder blades.

- Sit in a chair very close to a table with your back against the chair back.
- Place the unaffected arm on the table with your elbow bent and palm down. Do not move this arm during the exercise.
- Place the affected arm on the table, palm down with your elbow straight.
- Without moving your trunk, slide the affected arm toward the opposite side of the table. You should feel your shoulder blade move as you do this.
- Relax your arm and repeat five to seven times.

Shoulder Blade Squeeze

This exercise also helps increase the mobility of the shoulder blade.

- Facing straight ahead, sit in a chair in front of a mirror without resting on the back of the chair.
- Arms should be at your sides with elbows bent.
- Squeeze shoulder blades together, bringing your elbows behind you. Keep your shoulders level as you do this exercise. Do not lift your shoulders up toward your ears.
- Return to the starting position and repeat five to seven times.

Continued

PATIENT TEACHING Exercises After Breast Surgery—cont'd

Exercises in Sitting Position—cont'd

Side Bending

This exercise helps increase the mobility of the trunk/body.

- Clasp your hands together in front of you and lift your arms slowly over your head, straightening your arms.
- When your arms are over your head, bend your trunk to the right while bending at the waist and keeping your arms overhead.
- Return to the starting position and bend to the left.
- Repeat five to seven times.

Exercises in Standing Position

Chest Wall Stretch

This exercise helps stretch the chest wall.

- Stand facing a corner with toes approximately 20.3 to 25.4 cm (8 to 10 inches) from the corner.
- Bend your elbows and place forearms on the wall, one on each side of the corner. Your elbows should be as close to shoulder height as possible.
- Keep your arms and feet in position and move your chest toward the corner. You will feel a stretch across your chest and shoulders.
- Return to starting position and repeat five to seven times.

Shoulder Stretch

This exercise helps increase the mobility in the shoulder.

- Stand facing the wall with your toes approximately 20.3 to 25.4 cm (8 to 10 inches) from the wall.
- Place your hands on the wall. Use your fingers to "climb the wall," reaching as high as you can until you feel a stretch.
- Return to starting position and repeat five to seven times.

Source: American Cancer Society: *Exercises after breast surgery*. Available at www.cancer.org/docroot/CRI/content/CRI_2_6x_Exercises_After_Breast_Surgery.asp?sitearea=CRI&viewmode=print& (accessed June 24, 2008).

NURSING CARE PLAN The Woman with Breast Cancer

Nursing Diagnosis: Pain related to surgical incision and surgical drains as evidenced by patient verbalizations

Expected Outcome

Patient will report minimal intensity and decreased number of painful episodes.

Nursing Interventions/*Rationales*

Use pain scale to assess for type and intensity of pain *to provide accurate database.*

Administer analgesics as ordered *to decrease perception of pain.*

Reposition patient with affected arm elevated *to promote comfort and lymphatic channel return.*

Nursing Diagnosis: Risk for infection related to disruption of skin integrity and removal of lymph nodes

Expected Outcome

Patient will experience no clinical manifestations of infection.

Nursing Interventions/*Rationales*

Assess for clinical manifestations of infection at the incision and drain sites that may include redness, swelling, localized heat, fever, increasing pain, and foul-smelling drainage *to facilitate prompt treatment.*

Demonstrate the procedure for emptying and recording the amount of drainage from the Jackson-Pratt drain(s) *to provide information to the surgeon as to the appropriate removal time of drains.* Drains are usually removed when 24 hours of drainage does not exceed 30 ml of fluid.

Explain the need to avoid trauma or irritation to the affected arm *to reinforce to the patient that alterations in sensation and removal of some lymph nodes may affect ability to sense irritation and prevent infection.*

Reinforce to patient the need to protect the arm from injury and to avoid venipunctures or blood pressures to be taken on the affected arm *to avoid trauma and infection since decreased sensation may be present as well as decreased lymphatic return.*

Explain the importance of reporting any clinical manifestations of infection to the caregiver as soon as possible *to provide identification and treatment of problem.*

Nursing Diagnosis: Disturbed body image related to loss of all or part of a breast as evidenced by patient statements

Expected Outcome

Patient will maintain a positive body image.

Nursing Interventions/*Rationales*

Provide opportunity through therapeutic communication to express feelings about body image changes *to clarify and validate feelings.*

Provide information about breast prostheses and other cosmetic devices *to assist in maintaining an intact body image.*

Encourage woman to speak to physician about the possibility of breast reconstructive surgery *to provide additional resources for body image enhancement.*

Refer to support groups *to facilitate verbalization of feelings with women who have similar concerns.*

her hand and arm on the affected side. Physical therapy may be prescribed to improve strength and mobility of the affected arm.

Concerns about appearance after breast surgery may affect the woman's self-concept. Before surgery the woman and her partner need information about what the woman's postoperative appearance will be like. Some women may not want to view their surgical site, but it is important to give them the opportunity to do so and to provide emotional support at that time. Both the woman and her partner need to be able to discuss feelings and concerns about accepting the changes. Information about community resources and support groups such as Reach to Recovery may be beneficial. Invaluable resources are the NCCN and the ACS, which provide specific, up-to-date recommendations on breast cancer treatments on the Internet.

Before discharge considerable time should be spent counseling the woman and her family about the aspects of self-management. Printed instructions should be given to the woman and her family (see Nursing Care Plan).

Key Points

- Menstrual disorders diminish the quality of life for affected women and their families.
- PMS is a disorder that begins in the luteal phase of the menstrual cycle and ends with the onset of menses.
- Endometriosis is characterized by secondary amenorrhea, dyspareunia, abnormal uterine bleeding, and infertility.
- Alternative therapies are beneficial in relieving some discomforts associated with menstrual disorders.
- Sex practices to prevent STIs are key strategies.
- STIs are responsible for substantial mortality and morbidity, great personal suffering, and heavy economic burden in the United States.
- Pregnancy confers no immunity against infection; both mother and fetus must be considered when a pregnant woman contracts an infection.

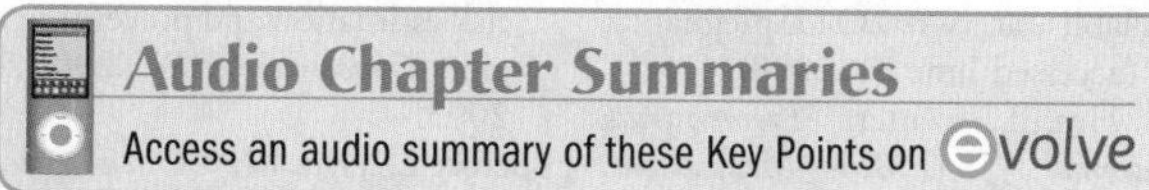
Audio Chapter Summaries
Access an audio summary of these Key Points on evolve

- Approximately 50% of women experience a breast problem at some point in their adult lives; the risk of an American woman developing breast cancer is one in eight.
- Annual clinical breast examinations by a health care provider and routine screening mammograms are recommended for early detection of breast cancer.
- Treatment for breast cancer includes surgery, radiation, and chemotherapy.

References

Albers JR, Hull SK, Wesley RM: Abnormal uterine bleeding, *Am Fam Physician* 69:1915-1926, 1931-1932, 2004.

American Cancer Society: *Cancer facts and figures 2008*, Atlanta, 2008a, American Cancer Society.

American Cancer Society: *Breast cancer facts & figures 2007-2008*, Atlanta, 2008b, American Cancer Society.

American College of Obstetricians and Gynecologists Committee on Adolescent Health Care: Endometriosis in adolescents, ACOG Committee Opinion No. 310, *Obstet Gynecol* 105(4):921-927, 2005.

American Psychiatric Association: *Diagnostic and statistical manual of mental disorders*, ed 4, text revision, Washington, DC, 2000, American Psychiatric Association Press.

Association of Women's Health, Obstetric and Neonatal Nurses (AWHONN): *Evidence-based clinical practice guideline: nursing management for cyclic perimenstrual pain and discomfort*, Washington, DC, 2003, AWHONN.

Bielak KM, Harris GS: *Amenorrhea*, updated March 12, 2008. Available at www.emedicine.com/ped/topic2779.htm (accessed June 24, 2008).

Branson BM et al: Revised recommendations for HIV testing of adults, adolescents, and pregnant women in health-care settings, *MMWR Morb Mortal Wkly Rep* 55(RR14): 1-17, 2006.

Centers for Disease Control and Prevention: *Sexually transmitted disease surveillance report 2004*, Atlanta, GA, 2005, U.S. Department of Health and Human Services.

Centers for Disease Control and Prevention: Achievements in public health: reduction in perinatal transmission of HIV infection—United States, 1985-2005, *MMWR Morb Mortal Wkly Rep* 55(21):592-597, 2006a.

Centers for Disease Control and Prevention: *Trends in reportable sexually transmitted diseases in the United States*, 2006b. Available at www.cdc.gov/std/stats/trends2006.htm (accessed June 19, 2008).

Centers for Disease Control and Prevention: *Standard precautions: excerpted from Guideline for Isolation Precautions: preventing transmission of infectious agents in healthcare settings 2007*, updated October 12, 2007. Available from www.cdc.gov/ncidod/dhqp/gl_isolation_standard.htm (accessed June 24, 2008).

Centers for Disease Control and Prevention: *FDA-approved rapid HIV antibody screening tests*, 2008. Available at www.cdc.gov/hiv/topics/testing (accessed February 19, 2009).

Centers for Disease Control and Prevention: *HIV/AIDS surveillance report, Vol 19*, 2009. Available from www.cdc.gov/hiv/topics/surveillance/resources/resports/2007report/table6a/htm (accessed February 18, 2009).

Centers for Disease Control and Prevention, Workowski KA, Berman SM: *Sexually transmitted diseases treatment guidelines 2006*, 2006. Available at www.cdc.gov/std/treatment/2006/hepatitis-c.htm (accessed June 21, 2008).

Collins Sharp B et al: Cyclic perimenstrual pain and discomfort: the scientific basis for practice, *J Obstet Gynecol Neonatal Nurs* 31(6):637-649, 2002.

Conversations with Colleagues: Endometriosis sufferers risk other diseases, *AWHONN Lifelines* 6(6):502-504, 2002-2003.

Dehlin L, Schuiling K: Chronic pelvic pain. In Schuiling K, Lokis F (editors): *Women's gynecologic health*, Boston, 2006, Jones & Bartlett.

Dodd N, Sinert R: *Dysfunctional uterine bleeding*, updated November 12, 2007. Available at www.emedicine.com (accessed June 18, 2008).

Food and Drug Administration: *FDA news. FDA approves silicone gel-filled breast implants after in-depth evaluation*, November 17, 2006. Available at www.fda.gov/bbs/topics/NEWS/2006/NEW01512.html (accessed February 19, 2009).

Hoffman S et al: The future of the female condom, *Perspect Sex Reprod Health* 36(3):120-126, 2004.

Holmberg L, Anderson H, HABITS steering and data monitoring committees: HABITS (hormonal replacement therapy after breast cancer—is it safe?) a randomized comparison: trial stopped, *Lancet* 363(9407):453-455, 2004.

Lawrence R, Lawrence R: *Breastfeeding: a guide for the medical profession*, ed 6, Philadelphia, 2005, Mosby.

Liu S, Lebrun C: Effect of oral contraceptives and hormone replacement therapy on bone mineral density in premenopausal and perimenopausal women: a systematic review, *Br J Sports Med* 40(1):11-24, 2006.

Marrazzo JM, Guest F, Cates W: Reproductive tract infections, including HIV and other sexually transmitted infections. In Hatcher R et al: *Contraceptive technology*, ed 19, New York, 2007, Ardent Media.

National Cancer Institute: *Menopausal hormone replacement therapy use and cancer: questions and answers: fact sheet*, 2007. Available at www.cancer.gov/cancertopics/factsheet/Risk/menopausal-hormones (accessed June 23, 2008).

National Cancer Institute: *Results of the study of tamoxifen and raloxifene (STAR) released: osteoporosis drug raloxifene shown to be as effective a tamoxifen in preventing invasive breast cancer*, National Cancer Institute News, April 17, 2006. Available at www.cancer.gov/newscenter (accessed June 23, 2008).

National Comprehensive Cancer Network: *Breast cancer treatment guidelines for patients*, 2005. Available at www.nccn.org (accessed June 24, 2008).

National Institute of Child Health and Human Development: *Extended nevirapine regimens reduce HIV transmission and death in breastfed infants of HIV-infected mothers,* February 6, 2008. Available at www.nichd.nih.gov/news/realeases/swennnn_pepi_020608.cfm?renderforprint=2 (accessed June 22, 2008).

Organization of Teratology Information Services: *Acyclovir (Zovirax)/valacyclovir (Valtrex) in pregnancy,* 2003. Available at www.OTISpregnancy.org (accessed June 21, 2008).

PMS Health Center: *Premenstrual syndrome (PMS)—Medications,* last updated July 7, 2006. Available at http://women.webmd.com/pms/premenstrual-syndrome-pms-medications (accessed June 24, 2008).

Proctor M, Farquhar C: Dysmenorrhoea, *Clin Evid* Dec(12):2524-2547, 2004.

Riordan J: *Breastfeeding and human lactation,* ed 3, Boston, 2005, Jones & Bartlett.

Sakorafas G: The management of women at high risk for breast cancer: risk estimation and prevention strategies, *Cancer Treat Rev* 29(2):79-89, 2003.

Speroff L, Fritz M: *Clinical gynecologic endocrinology and infertility,* ed 7, Philadelphia, 2005, Lippincott Williams & Wilkins.

Taylor D, Schuiling K, Sharp B: Menstrual pain and discomforts. In Schuiling K, Liskis F (editors): *Women's gynecologic health,* Sudbury, Mass, 2006, Jones & Bartlett.

US Preventive Services Task Force: Screening for chlamydial infection: recommendations and rationale, *Am J Prev Med* 20(3 Suppl):90-94, 2001a.

US Preventive Services Task Force: Screening for bacterial vaginosis in pregnancy: recommendations and rationale, *Am J Prev Med* 20(3 Suppl):59-61, 2001b.

Wilkinson D et al: Nonoxynol-9 spermicide for prevention of vaginally acquisition of HIV infection by women from men. In the *Cochrane Database of Systematic Reviews,* 2002, Issue 4, Art. No. CD003936. DOI: 10.1002/14651858.CD003936.

Writing Group for the Women's Health Initiative Investigators: Risks and benefits of estrogen plus progestin in healthy postmenopausal women: principal results from the Women's Health Initiative randomized controlled trial, *JAMA* 288(3):366-368, 2002.

Unit 2

7

Infertility, Contraception, and Abortion

Learning Objectives

On completion of this chapter the reader will be able to:

- List common causes of infertility.
- Discuss the psychologic impact of infertility.
- Describe common diagnoses and treatments for infertility.
- Compare reproductive alternatives for couples experiencing infertility.
- State the advantages and disadvantages of methods of contraception.
- Explain common nursing interventions that facilitate contraceptive use.
- Describe the techniques used for medical and surgical interruption of pregnancy.
- Recognize ethical, legal, cultural, and religious considerations of infertility, contraception, and elective abortion.

Electronic Resources

Additional information related to the content in Chapter 7 can be found on

evolve the Companion Website at http://evolve.elsevier.com/Perry/maternal/

- NCLEX Review Questions
- Critical Thinking Exercise—Patient Teaching: Contraception
- Nursing Care Plan—Infertility
- Nursing Care Plan—Sexual Activity/Contraception
- Spanish Guidelines—Contraception

This chapter addresses infertility, associated tests, and common therapies; contraception; and abortion. Available alternatives and psychosocial implications are discussed.

Infertility

Incidence

Infertility is a serious medical concern that affects quality of life and is a problem for 10% to 15% of reproductive-age couples (American Society for Reproductive Medicine [ASRM], 2008). Infertility implies subfertility, a prolonged time to conceive, as opposed to sterility, or the inability to conceive. Normally a fertile couple has approximately a 20% chance of conception in each ovulatory cycle. Primary infertility applies to a woman who has never been pregnant. Secondary infertility applies to a woman who has been pregnant in the past.

The prevalence of infertility is relatively stable among the overall population. It increases with the age of the woman, particularly in those older than 40 years of age. Probable causes of infertility include the trend toward delaying pregnancy until later in life, when fertility decreases naturally and the prevalence of diseases such as endometriosis and ovulatory dysfunction increases. There are questions regarding whether there has been an increase in male infertility or whether it is more readily identified because of improvements in diagnosis.

Diagnosis and treatment of infertility require considerable physical, emotional, psychologic, and financial investment over an extended period. Men and women often perceive infertility differently. Women have more stress from tests and treatments, place greater importance on having children, are more accepting of indicated treatments, and want children more than men (Sherrod, 2004).

In the United States feelings connected with infertility are many and complex. The origins of some of these feelings are myths, superstitions, misinformation, or magical thinking about the causes of infertility. Other feelings arise from the need to undergo many tests and examinations and from a perception of being "different" from others (RESOLVE, 2008). The attitude, sensitivity, and caring nature of those who are involved in the assessment and treatment of infertility lay the foundation for the couples' ability to cope with the many tests and treatments they must undergo. Team members must respect individuals' and couples' desires in choosing to stop treatment and to select other alternatives such as remaining childless or adoption. RESOLVE (*www.resolve.org*) is an organization that provides support, advocacy, and education about infertility for the infertility community as well as health care providers.

Factors Associated with Infertility

Many factors, both male and female, contribute to normal fertility. A normally developed reproductive tract in both the male and female partners is essential. Normal functioning of an intact hypothalamic-pituitary-gonadal axis supports gametogenesis (the formation of sperm and ova). The life spans of the sperm and the ovum are short. Although sperm remain viable in the female's reproductive tract for 48 hours or more, probably only a few retain fertilization potential for more than 24 hours. Ova remain viable for about 24 hours, but the optimal time for fertilization may be no more than 1 to 2 hours (Cunningham et al, 2005); thus timing of intercourse becomes critical. The couple should be taught about the menstrual cycle and the way to detect ovulation (see Chapter 6).

An alteration in one or more of these structures, functions, or processes results in some degree of impaired fertility. Causes of impaired fertility can lie with either the male or female. In general, about 20% of couples will have unexplained or idiopathic causes of infertility. Among the 80% of couples who have an identifiable cause of infertility, about 40% are related to factors in the female partner, 40% are related to factors in the male partner, and 20% are related to factors in both partners (Nelson & Marshall, 2007; Lobo, 2007). Boxes 7-1 and 7-2 list factors affecting female and male infertility.

Nursing Care Management

The nurse assists in the assessment (see Nursing Process Box). Some of the data needed to investigate impaired fertility are of a sensitive, personal nature. Obtaining these data may be viewed as an invasion of privacy. The tests and examinations are occasionally painful and intrusive and can take the romance out of lovemaking. A high level of motivation is needed to endure the investigation.

Because multiple factors involving both partners are common, the investigation of impaired fertility is conducted systematically and simultaneously for both male and female partners. Both partners must be interested in the solution to the problem. The medical investigation requires time (3 to 4 months) and considerable financial expense (Box 7-4). It causes emotional distress and strain on the couple's interpersonal relationship.

Assessment of Female Infertility

Investigation of impaired fertility begins for the woman with a complete history and physical examination. A complete general physical examination is followed by a specific assessment of the reproductive tract. Laboratory data, including routine urine and blood tests, are collected.

A woman may have an abnormal uterus and tubes (Fig. 7-1) as a result of in utero exposure to diethylstilbestrol (see Box 5-2). A history of infection of the genitourinary system is noted. Bimanual examination of internal organs may reveal lack of mobility of the uterus or abnormal contours of the uterus and adnexa.

Diagnostic Testing

The basic infertility survey of the female involves evaluation of the cervix, uterus, tubes, and peritoneum; detection

BOX 7-1 Factors Affecting Female Fertility

Ovarian Factors

Developmental anomalies

Anovulation—primary
- Pituitary or hypothalamic hormone disorder
- Adrenal gland disorder
- Congenital adrenal hyperplasia

Anovulation—secondary
- Disruption of hypothalamic-pituitary-ovarian axis
- Amenorrhea after discontinuing oral contraceptive pills
- Premature ovarian failure

Increased prolactin levels

Tubal/Peritoneal Factors

Developmental anomalies
Reduced tubal motility
Inflammation within the tube
Tubal adhesions
Endometriosis

Uterine Factors

Developmental anomalies
Endometrial and myometrial tumors
Asherman syndrome (uterine adhesions or scar tissue)

Vaginal-Cervical Factors

Vaginal-cervical infections
Cervical mucus inadequate
Isoimmunization (development of sperm antibodies)

Other Factors

Nutritional deficiencies (i.e., anemia)
Thyroid dysfunction
Idiopathic condition

BOX 7-2 Factors Affecting Male Fertility

Structural or Hormonal Disorders

Undescended testes
Hypospadias
Varicocele
Obstructive lesions of the epididymis and vas deferens
Low testosterone levels
Hypopituitarism
Endocrine disorders
Testicular damage caused by mumps
Retrograde ejaculation

Substance Abuse

Changes in sperm from cigarette smoking or use of heroin, marijuana, amyl nitrate, butyl nitrate, ethyl chloride, or methaqualone
Decrease in libido from use of heroin, methadone, selective serotonin reuptake inhibitors, or barbiturates
Impotence from use of alcohol or antihypertensive medications

Other Factors

Sexually transmitted infections
Exposure to workplace hazards such as radiation or toxic substances
Exposure of scrotum to high temperatures
Nutritional deficiencies
Antisperm antibodies
Idiopathic conditions

NURSING PROCESS: IMPAIRED FERTILITY

Assessment

Obtain data relevant to fertility through interview and physical examination.

Identify whether infertility is primary or secondary.

Note religious, cultural, and ethnic data because these may place restrictions on tests and treatments.

Obtain results from diagnostic tests (Box 7-3; see Cultural Awareness box).

Nursing Diagnoses

Disturbed body image or risk for situational low self-esteem related to

– impaired fertility

Decisional conflict related to

– therapies for impaired fertility
– alternatives to therapy (e.g., childfree living or adoption)

Sexual dysfunction related to

– loss of libido secondary to medically imposed restrictions

Social isolation related to

– impaired fertility, its investigation, and its management

Planning

Expected outcomes include that the woman/family will do the following:

- Verbalize understanding of the anatomy and physiology of the reproductive system
- Verbalize understanding of treatment for any abnormalities identified through various tests and examinations and be able to make an informed decision about treatment
- Resolve guilt feelings and not need to focus blame
- Conceive or, failing to conceive, decide on an alternative acceptable to both of them (childfree living or adoption)

Interventions

Teach, counsel, and reinforce information about tests and test results

Assist the couple to

- Express and discuss feelings.
- Separate concepts of success and failure of treatment for infertility from personal success and failure.
- Recognize infertility as a loss and resolve these feelings even if treatment is successful.

Explore support systems of the couple.

- Persons available to assist
- Relationship to couple
- Ages, availability
- Available cultural or religious support

Refer for mental health counseling as necessary.

Evaluation

Evaluation of the effectiveness of care of the couple experiencing impaired fertility is based on the previously stated outcomes.

CULTURAL AWARENESS

Fertility and Infertility

Worldwide cultures continue to use symbols and rites that celebrate fertility. One fertility rite that persists today is the custom of throwing rice at the bride and groom. Other fertility symbols and rites include passing out congratulatory cigars, candy, or pencils by a new father and baby showers held in anticipation of a child's birth.

In many cultures the responsibility for infertility is usually attributed to the woman. A woman's inability to conceive may be caused by her sins, evil spirits, or the fact that she is an inadequate person. The virility of a man in some cultures remains in question until he demonstrates his ability to reproduce by having at least one child (D'Avanzo, 2008).

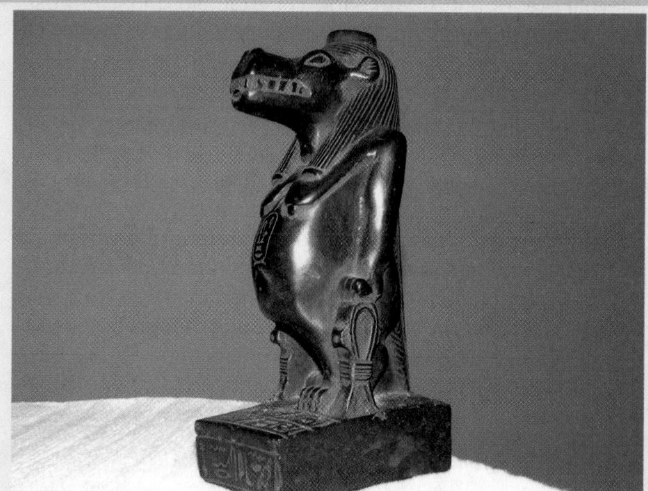

Taweret, goddess of fertility, Egypt. *(Courtesy Julie Perry Nelson, Phoenix, AZ.)*

of ovulation; hormone analysis; assessment of immunologic compatibility; and evaluation of psychogenic factors (Table 7-1). Ultrasonography (timed—during the luteal phase), endometrial biopsy, hysterosalpingography (x-ray examination of the uterine cavity and tubes after instillation of radiopaque contrast material through the cervix), and laparoscopy (to detect and possibly treat problems such as endometriosis or adhesions in the peritoneal cavity) may be performed. The nurse can alleviate some of the anxiety associated with testing by explaining the timing and rationale for each test. Test findings favorable to fertility are summarized in Box 7-5.

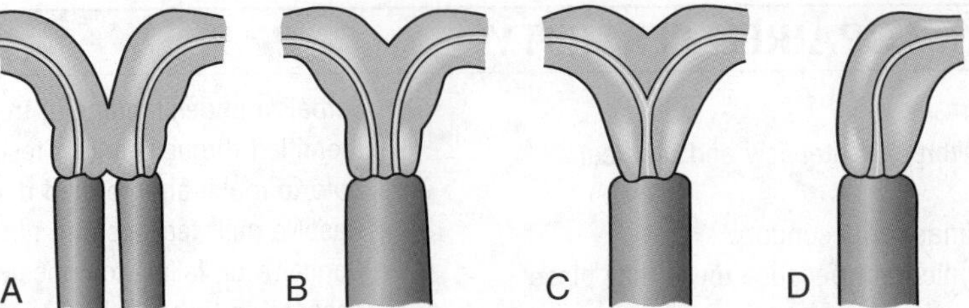

Fig. 7-1 Abnormal uterus. **A**, Complete bicornuate uterus with vagina divided by a septum. **B**, Complete bicornuate uterus with normal vagina. **C**, Partial bicornuate uterus with normal vagina. **D**, Unicornuate uterus.

BOX 7-3 Religious Considerations of Infertility

Civil laws and religious proscriptions about sex must always be kept in mind by the health care provider.

Conservative and reform Jewish couples are accepting of most infertility treatment; however, the Orthodox Jewish husband and wife may face problems in infertility investigation and management because of religious laws that govern marital relations. For example, according to Jewish law the Orthodox couple may not engage in marital relations during menstruation and through the following 7 "preparatory days." The wife then is immersed in a ritual bath *(Mikvah)* before relations can resume. Fertility problems can arise when the woman has a short cycle (i.e., a cycle of 24 days or fewer, when ovulation would occur on day 10 or earlier).

The Roman Catholic Church regards the embryo as a human being from the first moment of existence and regards as unacceptable technical procedures such as in vitro fertilization (IVF), therapeutic donor insemination, and freezing embryos.

Other religious groups may have ethical concerns about infertility tests and treatments. For example, most Protestant denominations and Muslims usually support infertility management as long as IVF is done with the husband's sperm, there is no reduction of fetuses, and insemination is done with the husband's sperm. These groups are less supportive of surrogacy and use of donor sperm and eggs. Christian Scientists do not permit surgical procedures or IVF but do permit insemination with husband and donor sperm.

Care providers should seek to understand the woman's spirituality and how it affects her perception of health care, especially in relation to infertility. Women may wish to seek infertility treatment but have questions about proposed diagnostic and therapeutic procedures because of religious proscriptions. These women are encouraged to consult their minister, rabbi, priest, or other spiritual leader for advice.

BOX 7-4 Insurance Coverage for Infertility

As of October 2005, only 14 states had mandated some form of insurance coverage for infertility. These mandates included in vitro fertilization in some states, whereas others only covered some diagnostic tests. Some states require health maintenance organizations (HMOs) to cover some costs, whereas in others HMOs are exempt. Patients need information about what they can expect from their insurers. For questions about an individual state, call the state's Insurance Commissioner's office. The website for the American Society for Reproductive Medicine *(www.asrm.org)* has more complete information.

Couples should be cautioned that everything can be normal and conception still may not occur. Unexplained infertility accounts for 20% of cases (ASRM, 2008). Conversely, even poor test results do not mean that pregnancy will not occur.

Assessment of Male Infertility

The systematic investigation of infertility in the male patient begins with a thorough history and physical examination. Assessment of the male patient proceeds in a manner similar to that of the female patient, starting with noninvasive tests.

Semen Analysis

The basic test for male infertility is semen analysis. A complete semen analysis, study of the effects of cervical mucus on sperm forward motility and survival, and evaluation of the sperm's ability to penetrate an ovum provide basic information. Sperm counts vary from day to day and depend on emotional and physical status and sexual activity. Therefore a single analysis may be inconclusive. A minimum of two analyses must be performed several weeks apart to assess male fertility.

Semen is collected by ejaculation into a clean container or a plastic sheath that does not contain a spermicidal agent. The specimen is usually collected by masturbation following 2 to 5 days of abstinence from ejaculation. The semen is examined at the collection site or taken to the laboratory in a sealed container within 2 hours of ejaculation. Exposure to excessive heat or cold is avoided. Commonly accepted values for semen characteristics are given in Box 7-6. If results are in the fertile range, no further sperm evaluation is necessary. If results are not within this range, the test is repeated. If subsequent results are still in the subfertile range, further evaluation is needed to identify the problem.

Hormone analyses are done for testosterone, gonadotropin, follicle-stimulating hormone (FSH), and luteinizing hormone (LH). The sperm penetration assay and other alternative tests can be used to evaluate the ability of sperm to penetrate an egg. Testicular biopsy may be warranted.

Table 7-1 Tests for Impaired Fertility

TEST OR EXAMINATION	TIMING (MENSTRUAL CYCLE DAYS)	RATIONALE
Hysterosalpingogram	7-10	Late follicular, early proliferative phase; will not disrupt a fertilized ovum; may open uterine tubes before time of ovulation
Postcoital test	1-2 days before ovulation	Ovulatory late proliferative phase; look for normal motile sperm in cervical mucus
Sperm immobilization antigen-antibody reaction	Variable, ovulation	Immunologic test to determine sperm and cervical mucus interaction
Assessment of cervical mucus	Variable, ovulation	Cervical mucus should have low viscosity, high spinnbarkeit
Ultrasound diagnosis of follicular collapse	Ovulation	Collapsed follicle is seen after ovulation
Serum assay of plasma progesterone	20-25	Midluteal midsecretory phase; check adequacy of corpus luteal production of progesterone
Basal body temperature	Chart entire cycle	Elevation occurs in response to progesterone, documents ovulation
Endometrial biopsy	21-27	Late luteal, late secretory phase; check endometrial response to progesterone and adequacy of luteal phase
Sperm penetration assay	After 2 days but ≤1 wk of abstinence	Evaluation of ability of sperm to penetrate an egg

BOX 7-5 Summary of Findings Favorable to Fertility

1. Follicular development, ovulation, and luteal development are supportive of pregnancy:
   a. Basal body temperature (presumptive evidence of ovulatory cycles) is biphasic, with temperature elevation that persists for 12 to 14 days before menstruation.
   b. Cervical mucus characteristics change appropriately during phases of the menstrual cycle.
   c. Laparoscopic visualization of pelvic organs verifies follicular and luteal development.
2. The luteal phase is supportive of pregnancy:
   a. Levels of plasma progesterone are adequate.
   b. Findings from endometrial biopsy samples are consistent with day of cycle.
3. Cervical factors are receptive to sperm during expected time of ovulation:
   a. Cervical os is open.
   b. Cervical mucus is clear, watery, abundant, and slippery and demonstrates good spinnbarkeit and arborization (fern pattern).
   c. Cervical examination does not reveal lesions or infections.
   d. Postcoital test findings are satisfactory (adequate number of live, motile, normal sperm present in cervical mucus).
   e. No immunity to sperm is demonstrated.
4. The uterus and uterine tubes are supportive of pregnancy:
   a. Uterine and tubal patency are documented by (1) spillage of dye into the peritoneal cavity; and (2) outlines of uterine and tubal cavities of adequate size and shape, with no abnormalities.
   b. Laparoscopic examination verifies normal development of internal genitals and absence of adhesions, infections, endometriosis, and other lesions.
5. The male partner's reproductive structures are normal:
   a. There is no evidence of developmental anomalies of penis, testicular atrophy, or varicocele (varicose veins on the spermatic vein in the groin).
   b. There is no evidence of infection in prostate, seminal vesicles, and urethra.
   c. Testes are more than 4 cm in largest diameter.
6. Semen is supportive of pregnancy:
   a. Sperm (number per milliliter) are adequate in ejaculate.
   b. Most sperm show normal morphology.
   c. Most sperm are motile, forward moving.
   d. No autoimmunity exists.
   e. Seminal fluid is normal.

Scrotal ultrasound is used to examine the testes for presence of varicoceles and to identify abnormalities in the scrotum and spermatic cord. Transrectal ultrasound is used to evaluate the ejaculatory ducts, seminal vesicles, and vas deferens.

Assessment of the Couple

Postcoital Test

The postcoital test (PCT) is one method used to test for adequacy of coital technique, cervical mucus, sperm, and degree of sperm penetration through cervical mucus. The test

BOX 7-6 Semen Analysis

Semen volume 2.5 ml
Sperm concentration/density ≥20 million/ml
Normal morphology ≥30%; normal shaped heads >14%
Motility
- Number of active cells as percentage of total number of cells ≥50%
- Quality of movement of sperm (rated 0-4) ≥2

Liquefaction <20 minutes

Source: RESOLVE: *The semen analysis*, 2008. Available at www.resolve.org/site/PageServer?pagename+lrn_wdigfh_tmwu_sa (accessed February 21, 2009).

is performed within several hours after ejaculation of semen into the vagina. A specimen of cervical mucus is obtained from the cervical os and examined under a microscope. The quality of mucus and the number of forward-moving sperm are noted. A PCT with good mucus and motile sperm is associated with fertility.

Intercourse is synchronized with the expected time of ovulation (as determined from evaluation of basal body temperature [BBT], cervical mucus changes, and usual length of menstrual cycle or use of LH detection kit to determine LH surge). Intercourse should occur only in the absence of vaginal infection. Couples may experience some difficulty abstaining from intercourse for 2 to 4 days before expected ovulation and then having intercourse with ejaculation on schedule. Sex on demand may strain the couple's interpersonal relationship. A problem may arise if the expected day of ovulation occurs when facilities or the physician is unavailable (such as over a weekend or holiday).

Plan of Care and Implementation

Psychosocial

Infertility is recognized as a major life stressor that can affect self-esteem; relations with the spouse, family, and friends; and careers. Psychologic responses to the diagnosis of infertility may tax a couple's capacity for giving and receiving physical and sexual closeness. The prescriptions and proscriptions for achieving conception may add tension to a couple's sexual functioning. Couples may report decreased desire for intercourse, orgasmic dysfunction, or midcycle erectile disorders.

To be able to deal comfortably with a couple's sexuality, nurses must be comfortable with their own sexuality so that they can better help couples understand why the private act of lovemaking needs to be shared with health care professionals. Nurses need up-to-date factual knowledge about human sexual practices and must be accepting of the preferences and activities of others without being judgmental. They must be skilled in interviewing and in therapeutic use of self, sensitive to the nonverbal cues of others, and knowledgeable regarding each couple's sociocultural and religious beliefs (see Critical Thinking Exercise).

The woman or couple facing infertility exhibit behaviors of the grieving process that are associated with other types of loss. The loss of one's genetic continuity with the generations to come can lead to a loss of self-esteem, a sense of inadequacy as a woman or a man, a loss of control over one's destiny, and a reduced sense of self. Infertile individuals can have impaired self-concept and greater dissatisfaction with their marriages. Not all people have all the reactions described, nor can it be predicted how long any reaction will last for an individual.

CRITICAL THINKING EXERCISE

Infertility Workup

Crista is 31 years old and is a registered nurse working in the operating room at a local hospital. Anthony is 34 years old and is a fireman. They have been trying to become pregnant for the past 8 years. They have come for an infertility workup and are wondering about the possibility of in vitro fertilization. The nurse will do the initial intake interview and some counseling. Crista and Anthony express discouragement, disillusionment, and anxiety. They have many questions about the probability of achieving pregnancy after this length of time.

1. Evidence—Is there sufficient evidence to draw conclusions about the probability of achieving pregnancy?
2. Assumptions—What assumptions can be made about a couple experiencing infertility?
3. What implications and priorities for nursing care can be drawn at this time?
4. Does the evidence objectively support your conclusion?
5. Are there alternative perspectives to your conclusion?

If the couple conceives, their concerns and problems concerning infertility may not be over. Many couples are overjoyed with the pregnancy; however, some are not. Some couples rearrange their lives, sense of self, and personal goals based on accepting their infertile state. The couple may think that those who worked with them to identify and treat impaired fertility expect them to be happy with the pregnancy. They may be shocked to find that they feel resentment because the pregnancy, once a cherished dream, now necessitates another change in goals, aspirations, and identities. The normal ambivalence toward pregnancy may be perceived as reneging on the original choice to become parents. The couple might choose to abort the pregnancy at this time. Other couples worry about miscarriage. If the couple wishes to continue with the pregnancy, they will need the care other expectant couples need.

If the couple does not conceive, they are assessed regarding their desire to be referred for help with adoption, therapeutic intrauterine insemination, other reproductive alternatives, or choosing a childfree state. The couple may find helpful a list of agencies, support groups, and other resources in their community such as ASRM *(www.asrm.org)* and RESOLVE *(www.resolve.org)*.

Nonmedical

Simple changes in lifestyle may be effective in the treatment of subfertile men. Only water-soluble lubricants should be used during intercourse because many commonly used lubricants contain spermicides or have spermicidal properties.

evolve Nursing Care Plan–Infertility

High scrotal temperatures may be caused by daily hot tub baths or saunas that keep the testes at temperatures too high for efficient spermatogenesis. These conditions lead to only lessened fertility and should not be used as a means of contraception.

Treatment is available for women who have immunologic reactions to sperm. The use of condoms during genital intercourse for 6 to 12 months will reduce female antibody production in most women who have elevated antisperm antibody titers. After the serum reaction subsides, condoms are used at all times except at the expected time of ovulation. Approximately one third of couples with this problem conceive by following this course of action.

Changes in nutrition and habits may increase fertility for both men and women. For example, a well-balanced diet, exercise, decreased alcohol intake, abstinence from smoking or abusing drugs, and stress management may be effective.

Herbal Alternative Measures

Most herbal remedies have not been proven clinically to promote fertility or to be safe in early pregnancy and should be taken by the woman only as prescribed by a physician or nurse-midwife who has expertise in herbology. Relaxation, osteopathy, stress management (e.g., aromatherapy, yoga), and nutritional and exercise counseling have been reported to increase pregnancy rates in some women. Herbal remedies that promote fertility in general include red clover flowers, nettle leaves, dong quai, and false unicorn root (Weed, 1986). Vitamin E, calcium, and magnesium may promote fertility and conception. Vitamins E and C, glutathione, and coenzyme Q10 are antioxidants that have proven beneficial effects for male infertility (Sheweita, Tilmisany, Al-Sawaf, 2005). Herbs to avoid while trying to conceive include licorice root, yarrow, wormwood, ephedra, fennel, goldenseal, lavender, juniper, flaxseed, pennyroyal, passionflower, wild cherry, cascara, sage, thyme, and periwinkle.

Medical

Pharmacologic therapy for female infertility is often directed at treating ovulatory dysfunction by either stimulating or enhancing ovulation so that more oocytes mature. These medications include clomiphene citrate, human menopausal gonadotropin (HMG), FSH, recombinant FSH (rFSH), and human chorionic gonadotropin. Gonadotropin-releasing hormone (GnRH) agonists, progesterone, and bromocriptine (Parlodel) also are used.

These medications are extremely potent and require daily monitoring with ovarian ultrasonography and monitoring of estradiol levels to prevent hyperstimulation. The incidence of multiple pregnancies with the use of these medications is greater than 25%. When failure to ovulate is caused by hypothalamic-pituitary dysfunction or failure to respond to clomiphene, GnRH may be used. Thyroid-stimulating hormone (Synthroid) is indicated if the woman has hypothyroidism.

The woman with low estrogen levels may be a candidate for conjugated estrogens and medroxyprogesterone. A hypoestrogenic condition may result from a high stress level or from a decreased percentage of body fat as a result of an eating disorder (e.g., anorexia nervosa) or excessive exercise. Hydroxyprogesterone supplementation with vaginal suppositories or intramuscular injection is used to treat luteal phase defects. In the presence of adrenal hyperplasia, prednisone, a glucocorticoid, is taken orally. Treatment of endometriosis may include danazol, progesterone, combined oral contraceptives, or GnRH agonists. Infections are treated with appropriate antimicrobial formulations.

Drug therapy may be indicated for male infertility. Problems with the thyroid or adrenal glands are corrected with appropriate medications. Infections are identified and treated with antimicrobials. FSH, HMG, and clomiphene may be used to stimulate spermatogenesis in men with hypogonadism.

The primary care provider is responsible for fully informing patients about the prescribed medications. However, the nurse must be ready to answer patients' questions and to confirm their understanding of the drug, its administration, potential side effects, and expected outcomes. Because information varies with each drug, the nurse must consult the medication package inserts, pharmacology references, the physician, and the pharmacist as necessary.

Surgical

A number of surgical procedures can be used for problems causing female infertility. Ovarian tumors must be excised. Whenever possible, functional ovarian tissue is left intact. Scar tissue adhesions caused by chronic infections may cover much or all of the ovary. These adhesions usually necessitate surgery to free and expose the ovary so that ovulation can occur.

Hysterosalpingography is useful for identification of tubal obstruction and also for the release of blockage (Fig. 7-2). During laparoscopy delicate adhesions may be divided and removed, and endometrial implants may be destroyed by electrocoagulation or laser (Fig. 7-3). Laparotomy and even microsurgery may be required for extensive repair of the damaged tube. Prognosis depends on the degree to which tubal patency and function can be restored.

Reconstructive surgery (e.g., the unification operation for bicornuate uterus) often improves a woman's ability to

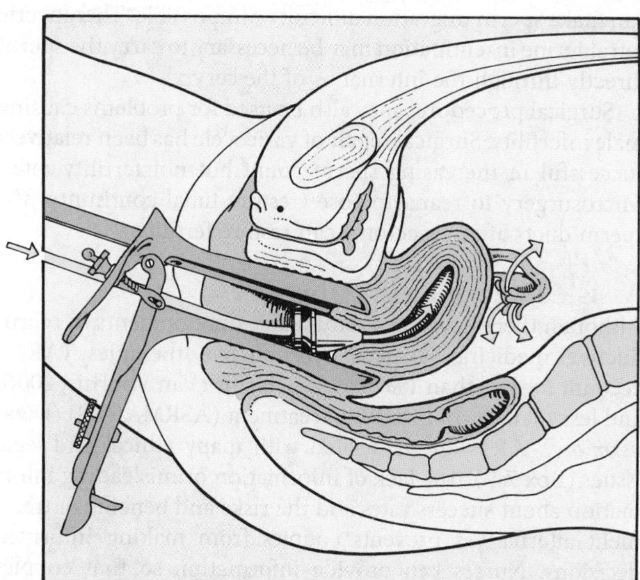

Fig. 7-2 Hysterosalpingography. Note that the contrast medium flows through the intrauterine cannula and out through the uterine tubes.

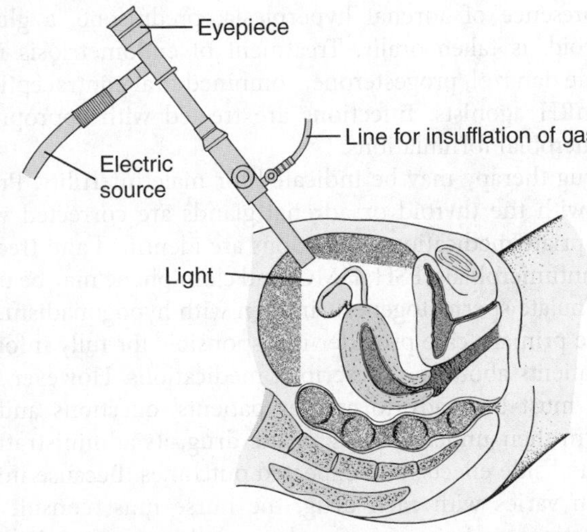

Fig. 7-3 Laparoscopy.

conceive and carry the fetus to term. Surgical removal of tumors or fibroids involving the endometrium or uterus often improves the woman's chance of conceiving and maintaining the pregnancy to viability. Surgical treatment of uterine tumors or maldevelopment that results in successful pregnancy usually requires birth by cesarean surgery near term gestation because the enlarging uterus may rupture as a result of weakness in the area of reconstructive surgery.

Chronic inflammation and infection can be eliminated by radial chemocautery (destruction of tissue with chemicals) or thermocautery (destruction of tissue with heat, usually electrical) of the cervix, cryosurgery (destruction of tissue by application of extreme cold, usually liquid nitrogen), or conization (excision of a cone-shaped piece of tissue from the endocervix). When the cervix has been deeply cauterized or frozen or when extensive conization has been performed, extreme limitation of mucus production by the cervix may result. Therefore the absence of a mucus bridge from the vagina to the uterus can make sperm migration difficult or impossible. Therapeutic intrauterine insemination may be necessary to carry the sperm directly through the internal os of the cervix.

Surgical procedures may also be used for problems causing male infertility. Surgical repair of varicocele has been relatively successful in increasing sperm count but not fertility rates. Microsurgery to reanastomose (restore tubal continuity) the sperm ducts after vasectomy can restore fertility.

Assisted Reproductive Therapies

Although there have been remarkable developments in reproductive medicine, assisted reproductive therapies (ARTs) account for less than 1% of all U.S. births (Van Voorhis, 2006) and less than 3% of infertility treatment (ASRM, 2008) *(www.asrm.org)*. ARTs are associated with many ethical and legal issues (Box 7-7). The lack of information or misleading information about success rates and the risks and benefits of treatment alternatives prevents couples from making informed decisions. Nurses can provide information so that couples have an accurate understanding of their chances for a successful pregnancy and live birth. Nurses also can provide anticipatory guidance about the moral and ethical dilemmas regarding the use of ARTs. Some of the ARTs for treatment of infertility include in vitro fertilization–embryo transfer (IVF-ET), gamete intrafallopian transfer (GIFT) (Fig. 7-4), zygote intrafallopian transfer (ZIFT), ovum transfer (oocyte donation), embryo adoption, embryo hosting and surrogate parenting, and therapeutic donor insemination (TDI). Table 7-2 describes these procedures and the possible indications for ARTs. Other options include intracytoplasmic sperm injection, assisted hatching, and adoption.

BOX 7-7 Issues to Be Addressed by Infertile Couples Before Treatment

- Risks of multiple gestation
- Possible need for multifetal reduction
- Possible need for donor oocytes, sperm, or embryos or for gestational carrier (surrogate mother)
- Whether to or how to disclose facts of conception to offspring
- Freezing embryos for later use
- Possible risks of long-term effects of medications and treatment on women, children, and families

LEGAL TIP Cryopreservation of Human Embryos Couples who have excess embryos frozen for later transfer must be fully informed before consenting to the procedure to make decisions regarding the disposal of embryos in the event of death, divorce, or the decision at a later time that the couple no longer wants the embryos.

Complications

Other than the established risks associated with laparoscopy and general anesthesia, few risks are associated with IVF-ET, GIFT, and ZIFT. The more common transvaginal needle aspiration requires only local or intravenous analgesia. Congenital anomalies occur no more frequently than among naturally conceived embryos. Multiple gestations are more likely and are associated with increased risks for both the mother and fetuses. However, ectopic pregnancies do occur more often, and these carry a significant maternal risk. There is no increase in maternal or perinatal complications with TDI; the same frequencies of anomalies (about 5%) and obstetric complications (between 5% and 10%) that accompany natural insemination (through sexual intercourse) also apply to TDI.

Preimplantation Genetic Diagnosis

Preimplantation genetic diagnosis (PGD) is a form of early genetic testing designed to eliminate embryos with serious genetic diseases before implantation through one of the ARTs and to avoid future termination of pregnancy for genetic reasons. Micromanipulation allows removal of a single cell from a multicellular embryo for genetic study (i.e., embryo biopsy) (Georgia Reproductive Specialists, 2007; Kearnes et al, 2005). PGD is used clinically in over 20 centers around the world. Couples must be counseled about their options and choices and the implications of their choices when genetic analysis is considered. For example, the transfer of only

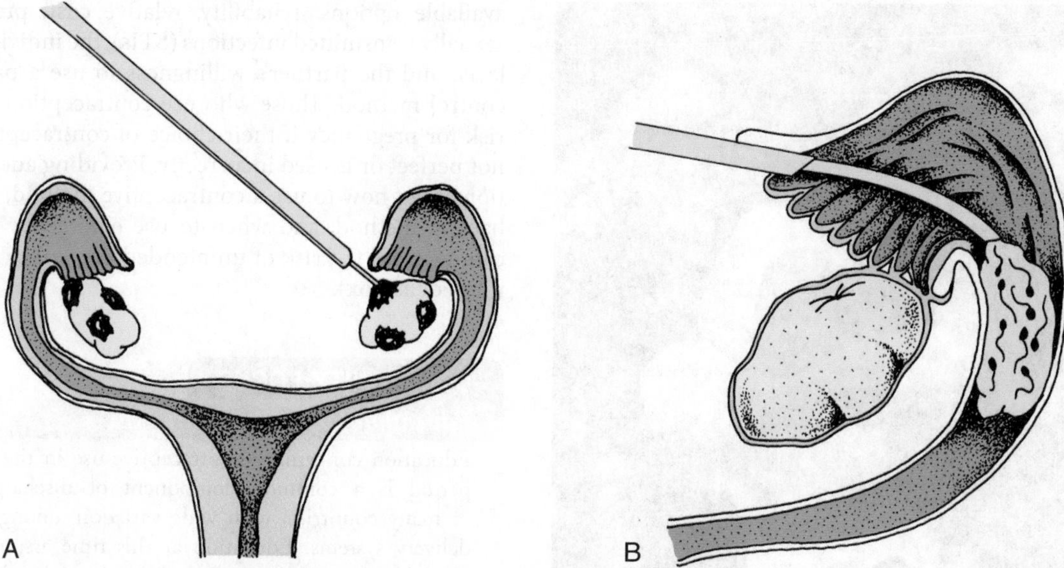

Fig. 7-4 Gamete intrafallopian transfer (GIFT). **A,** Through laparoscopy a ripe follicle is located, and fluid containing the egg is removed. **B,** The sperm and egg are placed separately in the uterine tube, where fertilization occurs.

Table 7-2 Assisted Reproductive Therapies

PROCEDURE	DEFINITION	INDICATIONS
In vitro fertilization–embryo transfer (IVF-ET)	A woman's eggs are collected from her ovaries, fertilized in the laboratory with sperm, and transferred to her uterus after normal embryo development has occurred.	Tubal disease or blockage; severe male infertility; endometriosis; unexplained infertility; cervical factor; immunologic infertility
Gamete intrafallopian transfer (GIFT)	Oocytes are retrieved from the ovary, placed in a catheter with washed motile sperm, and immediately transferred into the fimbriated end of the uterine tube. Fertilization occurs in the uterine tube.	Same as for IVF-ET, except there must be normal tubal anatomy, patency, and absence of previous tubal disease in at least one uterine tube
IVF-ET and GIFT with donor sperm	This process is the same as described previously except in cases where the husband's fertility is severely compromised and donor sperm can be used; if donor sperm are used, the wife must have indications for IVF and GIFT.	Severe male infertility; azoospermia; indications for IVF-ET or GIFT
Zygote intrafallopian transfer (ZIFT)	This process is similar to IVF-ET; after in vitro fertilization the ova are placed in one uterine tube during the zygote stage.	Same as for GIFT
Donor oocyte	Eggs are donated by an IVF procedure, and the donated eggs are inseminated. The embryos are transferred into the recipient's uterus, which is hormonally prepared with estrogen/progesterone therapy.	Early menopause; surgical removal of ovaries; congenitally absent ovaries; autosomal or sex-linked disorders; lack of fertilization in repeated IVF attempts because of subtle oocyte abnormalities or defects in oocyte-spermatozoa interaction
Donor embryo (embryo adoption)	A donated embryo is transferred to the uterus of an infertile woman at the appropriate time (normal or induced) of the menstrual cycle.	Infertility not resolved by less aggressive forms of therapy; absence of ovaries; male partner is azoospermic or severely compromised
Gestational carrier (embryo host); surrogate mother	A couple undertakes an IVF cycle, and the embryo(s) is transferred to another woman's uterus (the carrier), who has contracted with the couple to carry the baby to term. The carrier has no genetic investment in the child. Surrogate motherhood is a process by which a woman is inseminated with semen from the infertile woman's partner and then carries the baby until birth.	Congenital absence or surgical removal of uterus; a reproductively impaired uterus, myomas, uterine adhesions, or other congenital abnormalities; a medical condition that might be life threatening during pregnancy such as diabetes, immunologic problems, or severe heart, kidney, or liver disease
Therapeutic donor insemination (TDI)	Donor sperm are used to inseminate the female partner.	Male partner is azoospermic or has a very low sperm count; couple has a genetic defect; male partner has antisperm antibodies
Intracytoplasmic sperm injection	One sperm cell is selected to be injected directly into the egg to achieve fertilization. It is used with IVF.	Same as TDI
Assisted hatching	The zona pellucida is penetrated chemically or manually to create an opening for the dividing embryo to hatch and implant into the uterine wall.	Recurrent miscarriages; to improve implantation rate in women with previously unsuccessful IVF attempts; advanced age

Data from American Society for Reproductive Medicine: *Frequently asked questions about infertility,* 2008. Available at www.asrm.org (accessed February 21, 2009); Van Voorhis BJ: Outcomes from assisted reproductive technology, *Obstet Gynecol* 107 (1):183-200, 2006.

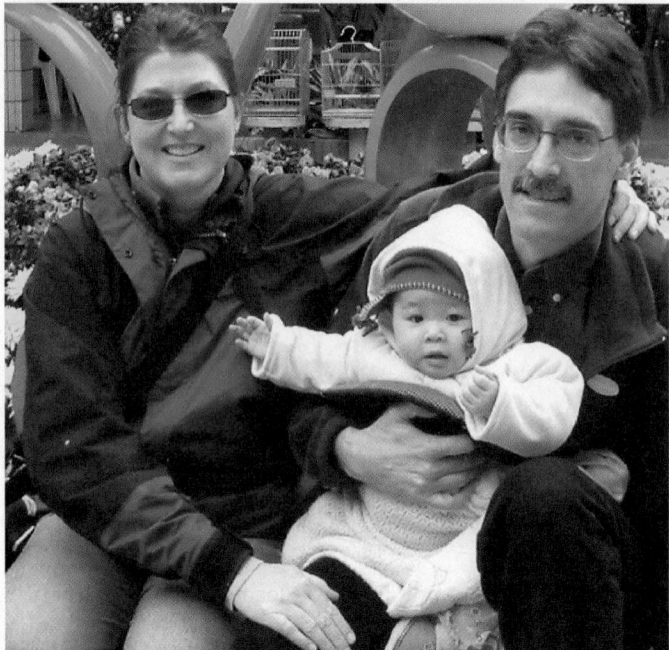

Fig. 7-5 After two miscarriages this couple chose foreign adoption. *(Courtesy Shannon Perry, Phoenix, AZ.)*

embryos that are free from abnormalities can increase the implantation rate and decrease the miscarriage rate and may increase the likelihood of the birth of a healthy infant (Kearnes et al, 2005).

Adoption

Couples may choose to build their family by adopting children who are not their own biologically. With increased availability of birth control and abortion and an increase in single mothers who choose to keep their babies, the availability of Caucasian infants for adoption is extremely limited. Minority infants, infants with special needs, older children, and foreign adoptions are other options (Fig. 7-5).

Couples who decide to adopt a child have decided that being a parent is more important than the actual process of birthing the child. The birth process is a very small aspect of having a baby and becoming a parent. So much emphasis is placed on being pregnant and having a child composed of one's own genetic makeup that the focus of the reason to have a child becomes cloudy. The question to be answered by couples who want to adopt is, "Do you want to give birth to a baby, or do you want to become parents?"

Contraception

Contraception is the intentional prevention of pregnancy during sexual intercourse. Birth control is the device and/or practice to decrease the risk of conceiving, or bearing, offspring. Family planning is the conscious decision on when to conceive or to avoid pregnancy throughout the reproductive years. With the wide assortment of birth control options available, it is possible for a woman to use several different contraceptive methods at various stages throughout her fertile years. Nurses interact with the woman to compare and contrast available options, reliability, relative cost, protection from sexually transmitted infections (STIs), the individual's comfort level, and the partner's willingness to use a particular birth control method. Those who use contraception can still be at risk for pregnancy if their choice of contraceptive method is not perfect or is used incorrectly. Providing adequate instruction about how to use a contraceptive method, when to use a backup method, and when to use emergency contraception can decrease the risk of unintended pregnancy (see Community Focus box).

COMMUNITY FOCUS

Education for Contraceptive Use

Education concerning contraceptive use in the postpartum period is a common component of discharge planning in many countries, with wide variation among health care delivery systems. Education at this time assumes women's receptiveness to information about contraception and that education or receptiveness to such information will be less at a later period. However, clinical trials have not demonstrated that education in the immediate postpartum period is effective. When assessing effectiveness of contraceptive education, attendance at family planning clinics, cessation of breastfeeding, knowledge about contraception, unplanned pregnancies, and satisfaction with care are factors that should be included. The content, timing, and organization of contraceptive education offered in the postpartum period needs to be addressed. Nurses provide discharge planning after childbirth; they commonly staff family planning clinics and provide contraceptive information. Evaluation of the effectiveness of their efforts must be implemented, and results used to make appropriate changes.

❀ Nursing Care Management

A multidisciplinary approach may assist a woman in choosing and correctly using an appropriate contraceptive method (see Nursing Process box). Nurses, nurse-midwives, nurse practitioners, and other advanced practice nurses and physicians have the knowledge and expertise to assist a woman in making decisions about contraception that will satisfy the woman's personal, social, cultural, and interpersonal needs. These needs include appropriate spacing of pregnancies (see Evidence-Based Practice box).

Unbiased patient teaching is fundamental to initiating and maintaining any form of contraception. The nurse counters myths with facts, clarifies misinformation, and fills in gaps of knowledge. The ideal contraceptive should be safe, easily available, economical, acceptable, simple to use, and promptly reversible. Although no method may ever achieve all of these objectives, significant advances in the development of new contraceptive technologies have occurred over the past 30 years.

Contraceptive failure rate refers to the percentage of contraceptive users expected to have an unplanned pregnancy during the first year even when they use a method consistently and correctly. Contraceptive effectiveness varies from couple

NURSING PROCESS: CONTRACEPTION

Assessment

Obtain a history (including menstrual, contraceptive, and obstetric).

Perform a physical examination (including pelvic examination).

Complete laboratory tests.

Determine woman's knowledge about contraception and her sexual partner's commitment to any particular method (Fig. 7-6).

Obtain data about the frequency of coitus, number of sexual partners, level of contraceptive involvement, and her or her partner's objections to any specific method(s).

Assess woman's level of comfort and willingness to touch her genitals and cervical mucus.

Identify myths and determine religious and cultural factors.

Carefully note the woman's verbal and nonverbal responses to hearing about the various available methods. An individual's reproductive life plan must be considered.

Nursing Diagnoses

Decisional conflict related to
- contraceptive alternatives
- partner's willingness to agree on a contraceptive method

Risk for infection related to
- unprotected sexual intercourse
- use of contraceptive method
- broken skin or mucous membrane secondary to surgery, intrauterine device insertion, or hormonal implant

Spiritual distress related to
- discrepancy between religious or cultural beliefs and choice of contraception

Planning

Expected outcomes are that the woman will do the following:
- Verbalize understanding about contraceptive methods
- State comfort and satisfaction with the method chosen
- Use the contraceptive method correctly and consistently
- Experience no adverse sequelae as a result of the chosen method of contraception
- Prevent unplanned pregnancy or plan a pregnancy

Interventions

Informed consent is a vital component in the education of the woman concerning contraception or sterilization.

The nurse has the responsibility of documenting information provided and the woman's understanding of that information.

Counter myths with facts, clarify misinformation, and fill in gaps of knowledge (see pp. 139-156).

Evaluation

The nurse can be reasonably assured that care was effective when the patient-centered expected outcomes have been achieved: the woman and her partner learn about the various methods of contraception, the couple achieves pregnancy only when planned, and they have no adverse sequelae as a result of the chosen method of contraception.

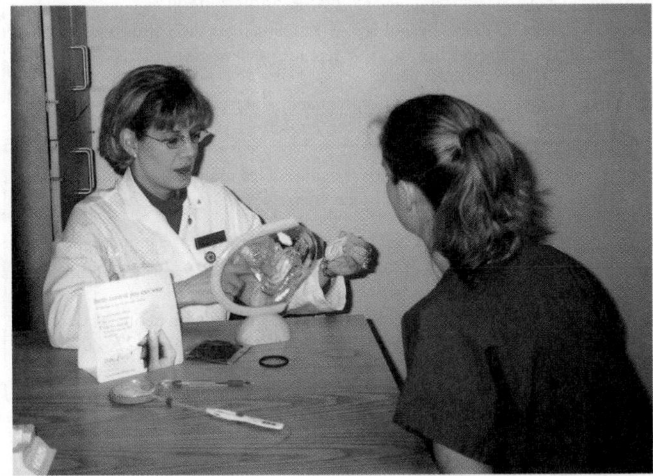

Fig. 7-6 Nurse counseling woman about contraceptive methods. *(Courtesy Dee Lowdermilk, Chapel Hill, NC.)*

to couple and depends on both the properties of the method and the characteristics of the user (Box 7-8). Failure rates decrease over time, either because a user gains experience with and uses a method more appropriately or because the less effective users stop using the method.

Safety of a method depends on the woman's medical history. Barrier methods offer some protection from STIs, and oral contraceptives may lower the incidence of ovarian and endometrial cancer but increase the risk of thromboembolic problems.

Methods of Contraception

The following discussion of contraceptive methods provides the nurse with information needed for patient teaching. After implementing the appropriate teaching for contraceptive use, the nurse supervises return demonstrations and practice to assess patient understanding (see Critical Thinking Exercise). The woman is given written instructions and telephone numbers for questions. If the woman has difficulty understanding written instructions, she (and her partner, if available) is offered graphic material and a telephone number to call as necessary or an opportunity to return for further instruction.

evolve Critical Thinking Exercise—Patient Teaching: Contraception

Coitus Interruptus

Coitus interruptus (withdrawal) involves the male partner withdrawing his penis from the woman's vagina before he ejaculates. Although coitus interruptus has been criticized as being an ineffective method of contraception, it is a good choice for couples who do not have another contraceptive available. Effectiveness is similar to barrier methods and depends on the man's ability to withdraw his penis before ejaculation. The percentage of women who will experience an

EVIDENCE-BASED PRACTICE Optimal Birth Spacing

—*Pat Gingrich*

Ask the Question

What interval between pregnancies is optimal for maternal and neonatal health?

Search for Evidence

Search Strategies

Professional organization guidelines, meta-analyses, systematic reviews, randomized controlled trials, nonrandomized prospective studies, and retrospective studies since 2006

Databases Searched

CINAHL, Cochrane, Medline, National Guideline Clearinghouse, TRIP Database Plus, and the websites for AWHONN, CDC, Family Health International, Planned Parenthood, and WHO

Critically Analyze the Evidence

In a systematic review of 22 eligible studies (Dewey & Cohen, 2007), the interpregnancy interval (IPI) was defined as the time between the end of one pregnancy and the beginning of the next. In some countries longer IPI was associated with a significantly lower risk of child malnutrition. The risk of stunting (height-for-age greater than 2 SD below the normal range) is decreased if the IPI is 36 months or more. In a Canadian cohort of 98,330 women, being unmarried increases the risk for small-for-gestational-age status in an IPI of less than 12 months (Auger et al, 2008).

Dewey and Cohen (2007) further speculated that breastfeeding may place additional nutritional pressure on the women. Eight studies showed no link between the recuperative interval (the time between weaning and subsequent pregnancy) and maternal weight or body mass index. Four studies they reviewed showed no relationship between IPI and maternal micronutrients, most notably anemia.

In another systematic review of 22 eligible studies (Conde-Agudelo, Rosas-Bermúdez, & Kafury-Goeta, 2007), a longer IPI is associated with an increased risk for preeclampsia, especially after 5 years. Some speculate that, as that much time passes, the woman's immune system becomes resensitized to foreign protein, much like that of a nulliparous woman. Similarly women who experienced labor dystocia showed a decreased risk of dystocia in subsequent labors, but that protective effect faded as the IPI lengthened. Short IPI (less than 18 months) was associated with bleeding (placenta previa and abruption), premature rupture of membranes, endometritis, and maternal mortality. Women attempting trial of labor after cesareans were more at risk for uterine rupture and blood transfusion with a short IPI, especially if the IPI was less than 6 months.

An Indian study of 80,164 women demonstrated that births spaced 36 to 59 months apart had fewer stillbirths and neonatal deaths than either shorter or longer birth intervals (Williams et al, 2008).

In a prospective comparative study of 562 births, Rodrigues and Barros (2008) demonstrated that an IPI of less than 6 months increased the risk for early preterm birth (less than 34 weeks of gestation) but had no effect on late preterm birth (34 to 37 weeks of gestation). Similarly, in a population-based cohort study of 156,330 women, DeFranco et al (2007) found an increasing risk of preterm birth as the IPI decreased.

Implications for Practice

There is strong evidence that avoiding pregnancy for at least a year after birth, especially after a cesarean birth, contributes to maternal and neonatal health. Single marital status, a marker for psychosocial stressors, may heighten the negative effects on fetal growth when the IPI is less than 12 months. Optimal interpregnancy interval will enable the woman's body to fully recover from the previous pregnancy and birth to provide adequate nutrition to herself and a subsequent fetus, while retaining the protective effects against recurrent dystocia and preeclampsia. An IPI of 18 to 36 months seems to meet these criteria.

Implications for Contraception

Such a window of time might comfortably include such highly effective methods as an intrauterine device, Depo-Provera for the first year, and combined hormonal contraceptives after weaning.

References

Auger N et al: The joint influence of marital status, interpregnancy interval, and neighborhood on small for gestational age birth: a retrospective cohort study, *BMC Pregnancy Childbirth* 28(8):7, 2008.

Conde-Agudelo A, Rosas-Bermúdez A, Kafury-Goeta AC: Effects of birth spacing on maternal health: a systematic review, *Am J Obstet Gynecol* 196(4):297-308, 2007.

DeFranco EA et al: A short interpregnancy interval is a risk factor for preterm birth and recurrence, *Am J Obstet Gynecol* 197(3):264.e1-6, 2007.

Dewey KG, Cohen RJ: Does birth spacing affect maternal or child nutritional status? A systematic literature review, *Matern Child Nutr* 3 (3):151-173, 2007.

Rodrigues T, Barros H: Short interpregnancy interval and risk of spontaneous preterm delivery, *Eur J Obstet Gynecol Reprod Biol* 136 (2):184-188, 2008.

Williams EK et al: Birth interval and risk of stillbirth or neonatal death: findings from rural north India, *J Trop Pediatr* 54(5):321-327, 2008.

BOX 7-8 Factors Affecting Contraceptive Method Effectiveness

- Frequency of intercourse
- Motivation to prevent pregnancy
- Understanding of how to use the method
- Adherence to the method
- Provision of short-term or long-term protection
- Likelihood of pregnancy for the individual woman
- Consistent use of the method

unintended pregnancy within the first year of typical use (failure rate) of withdrawal is about 27% (Trussell, 2007). Coitus interruptus does not protect against STIs or human immunodeficiency virus (HIV) infection.

Fertility Awareness Methods

Fertility awareness methods (FAMs) of contraception depend on identifying the beginning and end of the fertile period of the menstrual cycle. When women who want to use FAMs are educated about the menstrual cycle, three phases are identified:

CRITICAL THINKING EXERCISE

Contraception for Adolescents

Maria is a 16-year-old Hispanic female who comes to the family planning clinic seeking contraception. She has recently become sexually active and tells the nurse that she is concerned that her mother will find out. She also has many questions about the type of contraception to use. She seeks the nurse's advice to help in her decision making.

1. Evidence—Is there sufficient evidence to draw conclusions about what advice to give Maria?
2. Assumptions—What assumptions can be made about contraception for adolescents (types, legal issues, and implications of culture on choice)?
3. What implications and priorities for nursing care can be drawn at this time?
4. Does the evidence objectively support your conclusion?
5. Are there alternative perspectives to your conclusion?

1. Infertile phase: before ovulation
2. Fertile phase: about 5 to 7 days around the middle of the cycle, including several days before and during ovulation and the day afterward
3. Infertile phase: after ovulation

Although ovulation can be unpredictable in many women, teaching the woman about how she can directly observe her fertility patterns is an empowering tool. There are nearly a dozen categories of FAMs. To prevent pregnancy, each one uses a combination of charts, records, calculations, tools, observations, and either abstinence (natural family planning [NFP]) or barrier methods of birth control during the fertile period in the menstrual cycle. The charts and calculations associated with these methods can also be used to increase the likelihood of detecting the optimal timing of intercourse to achieve conception.

Advantages of these methods include low-to-no cost, absence of chemicals and hormones, and lack of alteration in the menstrual flow pattern. Disadvantages of FAMs include adherence to strict record keeping, unintentional interference from external influences that may alter the woman's core body temperature and vaginal secretions, decreased effectiveness in women with irregular cycles (particularly adolescents who have not established regular ovulatory patterns), decreased spontaneity of coitus, and attending possibly time-consuming training sessions by qualified instructors. The typical failure rate for most FAMs is 25% during the first year of use. FAMs do not protect against STIs or HIV infection. A systematic review of randomized controlled trials of FAMs concluded that the efficacy of these methods is unknown (Grimes et al, 2005).

FAMs involve several techniques to identify high risk, fertile days. The following discussion includes the most common techniques, as well as some promising techniques for the future.

Natural Family Planning (Periodic Abstinence)

NFP, or periodic abstinence, provides contraception by using methods that rely on avoidance of intercourse during fertile days. NFP methods are the only methods of contraception acceptable to the Roman Catholic Church. Signs and symptoms of fertility awareness most commonly used with abstinence are menstrual bleeding, cervical mucus, and BBT (see later discussions).

The human ovum can be fertilized no later than 16 to 24 hours after ovulation. Motile sperm have been recovered from the uterus and the oviducts as long as 7 days after coitus. However, their ability to fertilize the ovum probably lasts no longer than 24 to 48 hours. Pregnancy is unlikely to occur if a couple abstains from intercourse for 4 days before and 3 or 4 days after ovulation (fertile period). Unprotected intercourse on the other days of the cycle (safe period) should not result in pregnancy. However, the exact time of ovulation cannot be predicted accurately, and couples may find it difficult to abstain from sexual intercourse for several days before and after ovulation. Women with irregular menstrual periods have the greatest risk of failure with this form of contraception.

Calendar Rhythm Method

Practice of the calendar rhythm method is based on the number of days in each cycle, counting from the first day of menses. The fertile period is determined after accurately recording the lengths of menstrual cycles for 6 months. The beginning of the fertile period is estimated by subtracting 18 days from the length of the shortest cycle. The end of the fertile period is determined by subtracting 11 days from the length of the longest cycle. If the shortest cycle is 24 days and the longest is 30 days, application of the formula to calculate the fertile period is as follows:

$$\text{Shortest cycle, } 24-18=\text{day } 6$$

$$\text{Longest cycle, } 30-11=\text{day } 19$$

To avoid conception the couple would abstain during the fertile period, days 6 through 19.

If the woman has very regular cycles of 28 days each, the formula indicates the fertile days to be as follows:

$$\text{Shortest cycle, } 28-18=\text{day } 10$$

$$\text{Longest cycle, } 28-11=\text{day } 17$$

To avoid conception, the couple would abstain from day 10 through 17 because ovulation occurs on day 14 ± 2 days. A major drawback of the calendar method is that one is trying to predict future events with past data. The unpredictability of the menstrual cycle is also not taken into consideration. The calendar rhythm method is most useful as an adjunct to the BBT or cervical mucus method.

Standard Days Method

The Standard Days Method (SDM) is essentially a modified form of the calendar rhythm method that has a "fixed" number of days of fertility for each cycle (i.e., days 8 to 19). A CycleBeads necklace (i.e., a color-coded string of beads) can be purchased as a concrete tool to track fertility (Fig. 7-7). Day 1 of the menstrual flow is counted as the first day to begin the counting. Women who use this device are taught to avoid unprotected intercourse on days 8 to 19 (white beads on

evolve Spanish Guidelines—Contraception

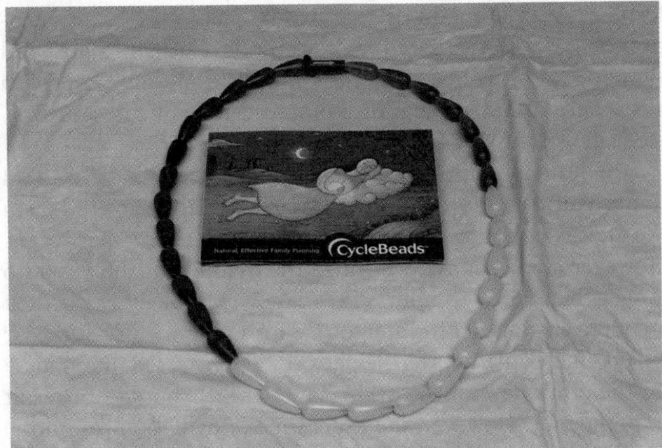

Fig. 7-7 Cyclebeads. *Red bead* marks the first day of the menstrual cycle. *White beads* mark days that are likely to be fertile days; therefore unprotected intercourse should be avoided. *Brown beads* are days when pregnancy is unlikely and unprotected intercourse is permitted. *(Courtesy Dee Lowdermilk, Chapel Hill, NC.)*

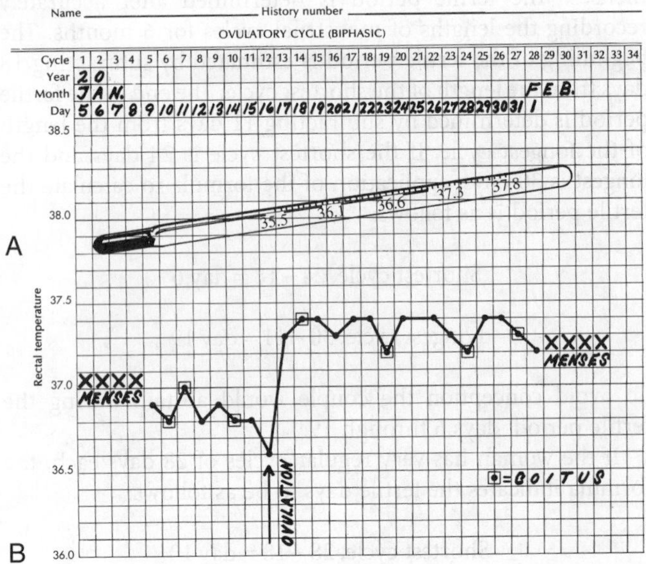

Fig. 7-8 **A**, Special thermometer for recording basal body temperature, marked in tenths to enable person to read more easily. **B**, Basal temperature record shows decrease and sharp increase at time of ovulation. Biphasic curve indicates ovulatory cycle.

CycleBeads necklace). Although this method is useful to women whose cycles are 26 to 32 days long, it is unreliable for those who have longer or shorter cycles (CycleBeads, 2007). The typical failure rate for the SDM is 12% during the first year of use (Sinai, Jennings, & Arevalo, 2004).

Basal Body Temperature Method

The BBT is the lowest body temperature of a healthy person, taken immediately after waking and before getting out of bed. The BBT usually varies from 36.2° to 36.3° C during menses and for approximately 5 to 7 days afterward (Fig. 7-8).

About the time of ovulation a slight drop in temperature (approximately 0.5° C) may occur in some women, but others may have no decrease at all. After ovulation, in concert with the increasing progesterone levels of the early luteal phase of the cycle, the BBT increases slightly (approximately 0.4° to 0.8° C). The temperature remains on an elevated plateau until 2 to 4 days before menstruation. Then it decreases to the low levels recorded during the previous cycle unless pregnancy has occurred. In that event the temperature remains elevated. If ovulation fails to occur, the pattern of lower body temperature continues throughout the cycle.

To use this method, the fertile period is defined as the day of first temperature drop, or first elevation, through 3 consecutive days of elevated temperature. Abstinence begins the first day of menstrual bleeding and lasts through 3 consecutive days of sustained temperature rise (at least 0.2° C). The decrease and subsequent increase in temperature are referred to as the thermal shift. When the entire month's temperatures are recorded on a graph, the pattern described is more apparent. It is more difficult to perceive day-to-day variations without the entire picture (see Guidelines box). Infection, fatigue, less than 3 hours of sleep per night, awakening late, and anxiety may cause temperature fluctuations and alter the expected pattern. If a new BBT thermometer is purchased, this fact is noted on the chart because the readings may vary slightly. Jet lag, alcohol taken the evening before, or sleeping in a heated waterbed must also be noted on the chart because each affects the BBT. Therefore the BBT alone is not a reliable method of predicting ovulation.

GUIDELINES Basal Body Temperature

- Discuss basal body temperature (BBT) with the woman.
- Show the woman a diagram depicting the phases of the menstrual cycle.
- Discuss the hormones in the woman's body that are responsible for her menstrual cycle and ovulation. Leave time for questions.
- Show the woman a sample BBT graph (see Fig. 7-8) and the biphasic line seen in ovulatory cycles.
- Show the woman the BBT thermometer and how it is calibrated.
- Provide a demonstration.
- Encourage the woman to demonstrate taking and reading the thermometer and graphing the temperature while the nurse watches.
- Encourage the woman to start a log to keep track of any other activity that might interfere with her true BBT.

Cervical Mucus Ovulation-Detection Method

The cervical mucus ovulation-detection method (Billings method; Creighton model ovulation method) requires that the woman recognize and interpret the cyclic changes in the amount and consistency of cervical mucus that characterize her own unique pattern of changes. The cervical mucus that accompanies ovulation is necessary for viability and motility of sperm. Without adequate cervical mucus, coitus does not result in conception. Women check quantity and character of mucus on the vulva or introitus with fingers or tissue paper each day for several months to learn the cycle. To ensure an accurate assessment of changes, the cervical mucus should be free from semen, contraceptive gels or foams, and blood or discharge from vaginal infections for at least one full cycle. Other factors that create difficulty in identifying mucus changes include douches and vaginal deodorants, being in the sexually aroused state (which thins the mucus), and taking medications such as antihistamines, which dry the mucus. Intercourse is considered safe without restriction beginning the fourth day after the last day of wet, clear, slippery mucus (postovulation).

Some women find this method unacceptable if they are uncomfortable touching their genitals. Whether or not a woman wants to use this method for contraception, it is to her advantage to learn to recognize mucus characteristics at ovulation (see Guidelines box). Self-evaluation of cervical mucus can be highly accurate and useful diagnostically for any of the following purposes:

- To alert the couple to the reestablishment of ovulation while breastfeeding and after discontinuation of oral contraception
- To note anovulatory cycles at any time and at the beginning of menopause
- To assist couples in planning a pregnancy

Symptothermal Method

The symptothermal method combines the BBT and cervical mucus methods with awareness of secondary, cycle phase–related symptoms. The woman gains fertility awareness as she learns the psychologic and physiologic symptoms that mark the phases of her cycle. Secondary symptoms include increased

GUIDELINES Cervical Mucus Characteristics

Setting the Stage

Show charts of menstrual cycle along with changes in the cervical mucus.

Have the woman practice with raw egg white.

Supply her with a basal body temperature (BBT) log and graph if she does not already have one.

Explain that the assessment of cervical mucus characteristics is best when mucus is not mixed with semen, contraceptive jellies or foams, or discharge from infections.

Content Related to Cervical Mucus

Explain to the woman (or couple) how cervical mucus changes throughout the menstrual cycle.

Right before ovulation the watery, thin, clear mucus becomes more abundant and thick. It feels like a lubricant and can be stretched approximately 5 cm between the thumb and forefinger; this is called ***spinnbarkeit.*** This characteristic indicates the period of maximum fertility. Sperm deposited in this type of mucus can survive until ovulation occurs.

Assessment Technique

Stress that good handwashing is imperative to begin and end all self-assessment.

Start observation from last day of menstrual flow.

Assess cervical mucus several times a day for several cycles. Mucus can be obtained from vaginal introitus; there is no need to reach into vagina to cervix.

Record findings on the same record on which her BBT is entered.

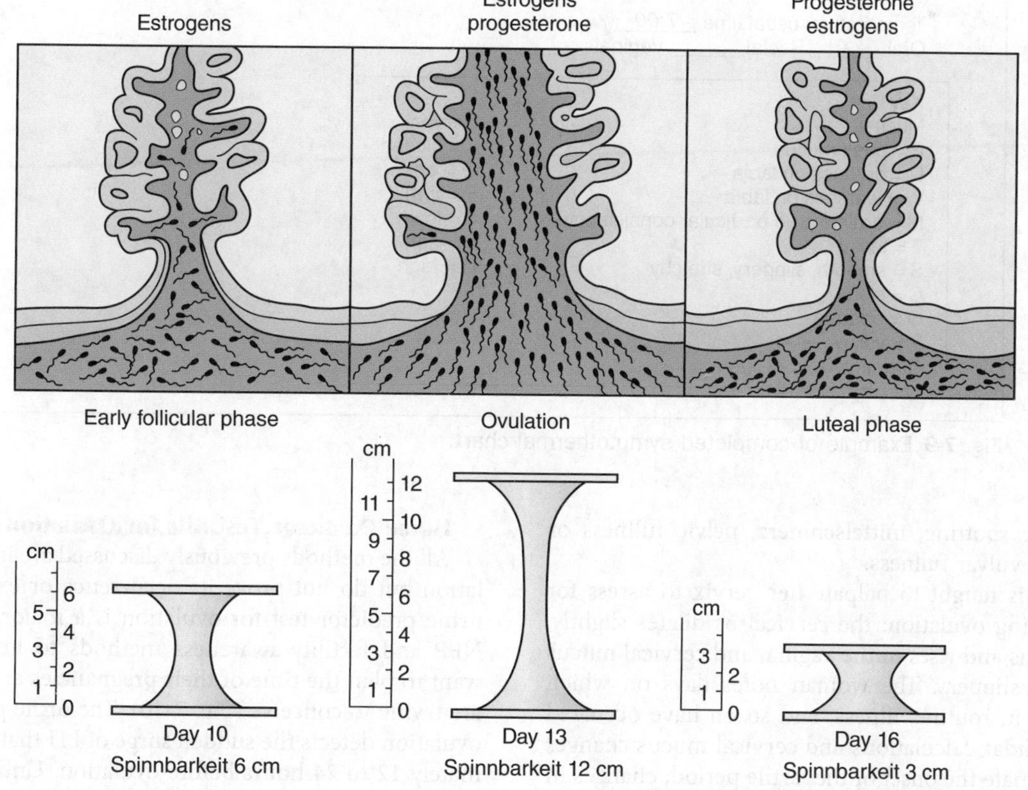

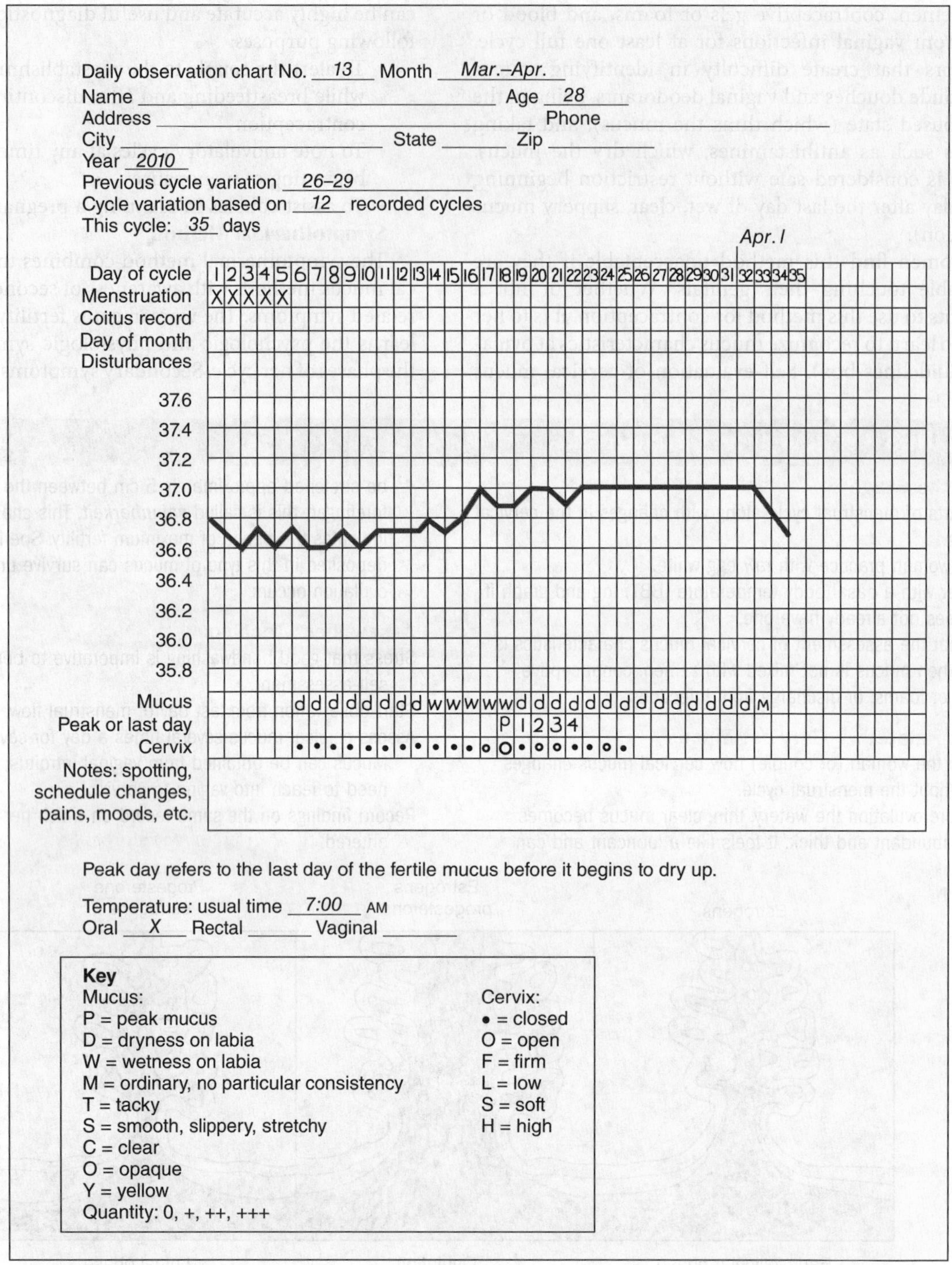

Fig. 7-9 Example of completed symptothermal chart.

libido, midcycle spotting, mittelschmerz, pelvic fullness or tenderness, and vulvar fullness.

The woman is taught to palpate her cervix to assess for changes indicating ovulation: the cervical os dilates slightly, the cervix softens and rises in the vagina, and cervical mucus is copious and slippery. The woman notes days on which coitus, changes in routine, illness, and so on have occurred (Fig. 7-9). Calendar calculations and cervical mucus changes are used to estimate the onset of the fertile period; changes in cervical mucus or the BBT are used to estimate its end.

Home Predictor Test Kits for Ovulation

All the methods previously discussed are indicative of ovulation but do not prove its occurrence or exact timing. The urine predictor test for ovulation is a major addition to the NFP and fertility-awareness methods to help women who want to plan the time of their pregnancies and for those who are trying to conceive (Fig. 7-10). The urine predictor test for ovulation detects the sudden surge of LH that occurs approximately 12 to 24 hours before ovulation. Unlike BBT, the test is not affected by illness, emotional upset, or physical activity.

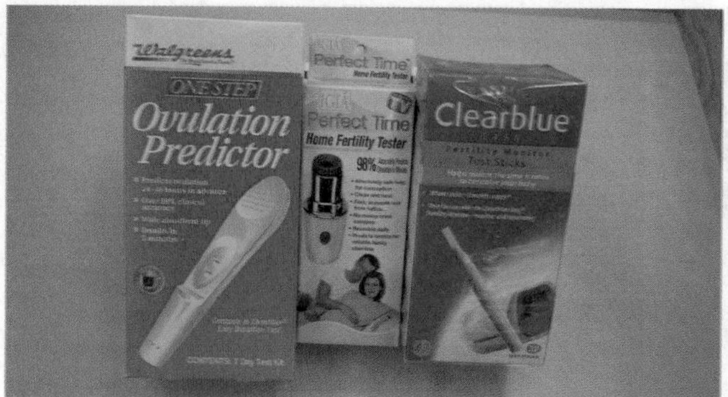

Fig. 7-10 Examples of ovulation predictor tests. *(Courtesy Shannon Perry, Phoenix, AZ.)*

For home use, a test kit contains sufficient material for several days' testing during each cycle. A positive response indicating an LH surge is noted by a color change that is easy to read. Directions for use of urine predictor test kits vary with the manufacturer. Saliva predictor tests for ovulation use dried, nonfoamy saliva as a tool to show fertility patterns. More research is needed to determine the efficacy of use of these tests for pregnancy prevention.

TwoDay Method of Family Planning

Based on monitoring and the recording of cervical secretions, a new algorithm for identifying the fertile window has been developed by the Institute for Reproductive Health at Georgetown University (Arevalo et al, 2004). The TwoDay algorithm appears to be simpler to teach, learn, and use than current natural methods. Results suggest that the algorithm can be an effective alternative for low literacy populations or for programs that find current NFP methods too time consuming or otherwise not feasible to incorporate into their services. Two questions are posed. Each day the woman is to ask herself, (1) "Did I note secretions today?" and (2) "Did I note secretions yesterday?" If the answer to either is yes, she should avoid coitus or use a backup method of birth control. If the answer to both questions is no, her probability of getting pregnant is very low. Further studies are needed to determine the efficacy of the TwoDay algorithm in avoiding pregnancy and to assess its acceptability to users and providers.

Breastfeeding: Lactational Amenorrhea Method

Lactational amenorrhea method (LAM) can be a highly effective, *temporary* method of birth control. It is more popular in underdeveloped countries and traditional societies where breastfeeding is used to prolong birth intervals. The method has seen limited use in the United States since only about half of new mothers initiate breastfeeding, and most American women do not establish breastfeeding patterns that provide maximum protection against pregnancy (Kennedy & Trussell, 2007).

When the infant suckles at the mother's breast, a surge of prolactin hormone is released, which inhibits estrogen production and suppresses ovulation and the return of menses. LAM works best if the mother is exclusively or almost exclusively breastfeeding, if the woman has not had a menstrual flow since giving birth, and if the infant is under 6 months of age. Effectiveness is enhanced by frequent feedings at intervals of less than 4 hours during the day and no more than 6 hours during the night, long duration of each feeding, and no bottle supplementation or limited supplementation by spoon or cup. The woman should be counseled that disruption of the breastfeeding pattern or supplementation can increase the risk of pregnancy. The typical failure rate is 2% (Kennedy & Trussell, 2007).

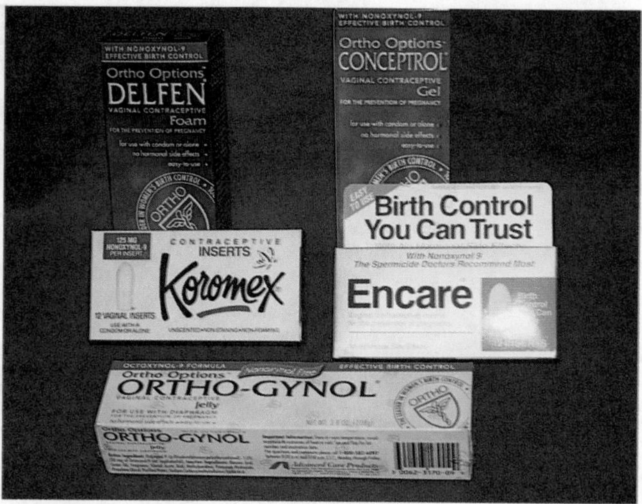

Fig. 7-11 Spermicides. *(Courtesy Marjorie Pyle, RNC, Life Circle, Costa Mesa, CA.)*

Barrier Methods

Barrier contraceptives have gained in popularity not only as a contraceptive method but also as protection against the spread of STIs such as human papilloma virus and herpes simplex virus (HSV). Some male condoms and female vaginal methods provide a physical barrier to several STIs, and some male condoms provide protection against HIV. Spermicides serve as chemical barriers against the sperm.

Spermicides

Spermicides such as nonoxynol-9 (N-9) work by reducing the sperm's mobility; the chemicals attack the sperm flagella and body, thereby preventing the sperm from reaching the cervical os. N-9, the most commonly used spermicidal chemical in the United States, is a surfactant that destroys the sperm cell membrane; however, data now suggest that frequent use (more than two times a day) of N-9 or use as a lubricant during anal intercourse may increase the transmission of HIV and can cause lesions (Cates & Raymond, 2007). Women with high risk behaviors that increase their likelihood of contracting HIV and other STIs are advised to avoid the use of spermicidal products containing N-9, including lubricated condoms, diaphragms, and cervical caps to which N-9 is added.

Intravaginal spermicides are marketed and sold without prescriptions as aerosol foams, tablets, suppositories, creams, films, and gels (Fig. 7-11). Preloaded, single-dose applicators small enough to be carried in a small purse are available. Effectiveness of spermicides depends on consistent and accurate use. Not more than 1 hour before sexual intercourse, the spermicide should be inserted high into the vagina so that it makes contact with the cervix. Spermicide must be reapplied for each additional act of intercourse, even if a barrier method

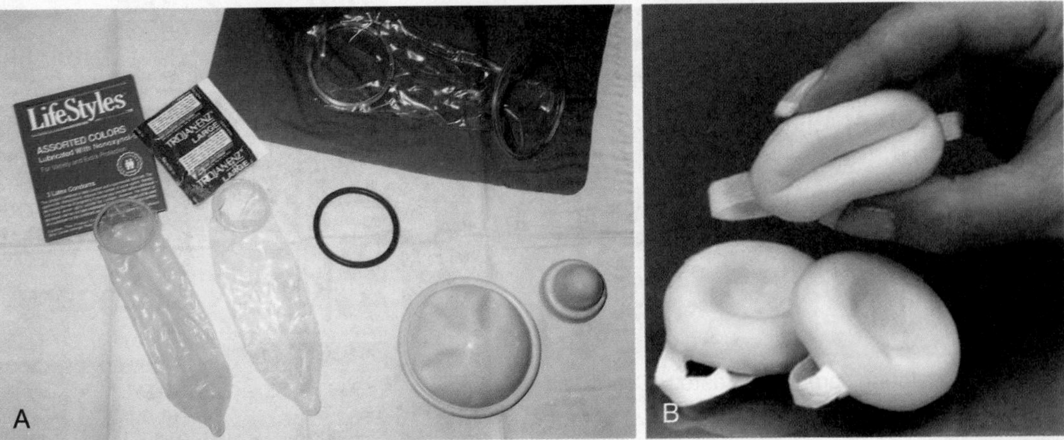

Fig. 7-12 A, Mechanical barriers. *Clockwise from top:* female condom, cervical cap, diaphragm, types of male condoms, vaginal ring (hormonal) *(center)*. B, Contraceptive sponge. *(A, Courtesy Donna Rowe, University of North Carolina Student Health, Chapel Hill, NC. B, Courtesy Allendale Pharmaceuticals, Inc., Allendale, NJ.).*

is used. Studies have shown varying effectiveness rates for spermicidal use alone. Typical failure rate in the first year of spermicidal use alone is 29% (Trussell, 2007).

Condoms

The male condom is a thin, stretchable sheath that covers the penis before genital, oral, or anal contact and is removed when the penis is withdrawn from the partner's orifice after ejaculation (Fig. 7-12). Condoms lubricated with N-9 are not recommended for preventing STIs or HIV (Centers for Disease Control and Prevention [CDC], Workowski, & Berman, 2006). Latex condoms break down with oil-based lubricants (e.g., petroleum jelly and suntan oil) and should be used only with water-based or silicone lubricants. Because of the growing number of people with latex allergies, condom manufacturers have begun using polyurethane, which is thinner and stronger than latex. Research is being conducted to determine the effectiveness of polyurethane condoms in protecting against STIs and HIV.

NURSING ALERT All patients should be questioned about the potential for latex allergy. Latex condom use is contraindicated for patients with latex sensitivity.

Condoms are made of latex rubber, which provides a barrier to sperm and STIs (including HIV); polyurethane (strong, thin plastic); or natural membranes (animal tissue). In addition to providing a physical barrier for sperm, nonspermicidal latex condoms also provide a barrier for STIs (particularly gonorrhea, chlamydia, and trichomonas) and HIV transmission. A small percentage of condoms are made from lamb cecum (natural skin). Natural skin condoms do not provide the same protection against STIs and HIV infection as latex condoms. Natural skin condoms contain small pores that could allow passage of viruses such as hepatitis B, HSV, and HIV.

A functional difference in condom shape is the presence or absence of a sperm reservoir tip. To enhance vaginal stimulation, some condoms are contoured and rippled or have ribbed or roughened surfaces. Thinner construction increases heat transmission and sensitivity; a variety of colors increases their acceptability and attractiveness. A wet jelly or dry powder lubricates some condoms. Spermicide is added to the interior or exterior surfaces of some condoms. Typical failure rate for the first year of use of the male condom is 15%.

NURSING ALERT It is a false assumption that everyone knows how to use condoms. To prevent unintended pregnancy and the spread of STIs, it is essential that condoms be used correctly. Proper instruction in use must be provided. The sheath is applied over the erect penis before insertion and before the loss of preejaculatory drops of semen (Box 7-9). All types of condoms must be discarded after each single use. They are available without prescription.

The female condom is a vaginal sheath made of polyurethane and has flexible rings at both ends (see Fig. 7-12, *A*). The closed end of the pouch is inserted into the vagina and anchored around the cervix; the open ring covers the labia. Women whose partner will not wear a male condom can use this as a protective mechanical barrier. Rewetting drops or oil- or water-based lubricants can be used to help decrease the distracting noise that is produced while penile thrusting occurs. The female condom is available in one size, is intended for single use only, and is sold over the counter. Male condoms should not be used concurrently because the friction from both sheaths can increase the likelihood of either or both tearing (Female Health Company, 2008). Typical failure rate in the first year of female condom use is 21% (Trussell, 2007).

Diaphragm

The contraceptive diaphragm is a shallow, dome-shaped, latex or silicone device with a flexible rim that covers the cervix (see Fig. 7-12, *A*). The diaphragm is a mechanical barrier to the meeting of sperm with the ovum. By holding spermicide in place against the cervix for the 6 hours it takes to destroy the sperm, the diaphragm also provides a chemical barrier to pregnancy. Diaphragms are available in a wide range of diameters (50 to 95 mm) and differ in the inner construction of the circular rim. The types of rims are coil

BOX 7-9 Male Condoms

Mechanism of Action

Sheath is applied over the erect penis before insertion or loss of preejaculatory drops of semen. Used correctly, condoms prevent sperm from entering the cervix. Spermicide-coated condoms cause ejaculated sperm to be immobilized rapidly, thus increasing contraceptive effectiveness.

Failure Rate

- Typical users, 15%
- Correct and consistent users, 2%

Advantages

- Safe
- No side effects
- Readily available
- Premalignant changes in cervix can be prevented or ameliorated in women whose partners use condoms
- Method of male nonsurgical contraception

Disadvantages

- Lovemaking must be interrupted to apply sheath.
- Sensation may be altered.
- If used improperly, spillage of sperm can result in pregnancy.
- Condoms occasionally may tear during intercourse.

STI Protection

If a condom is used throughout the act of intercourse and there is no unprotected contact with female genitals, a latex rubber condom, which is impermeable to viruses, can act as a protective measure against sexually transmitted infections.

Nursing Considerations

Teach man to do the following:

- Use a new condom (check expiration date) for each act of sexual intercourse or other acts between partners that involve contact with the penis.
- Place the condom after penis is erect and before intimate contact.
- Place the condom on the head of the penis (**A**) and unroll it all the way to the base (**B**).
- Leave an empty space at the tip (**A**); remove any air remaining in the tip by gently pressing air out toward the base of the penis.

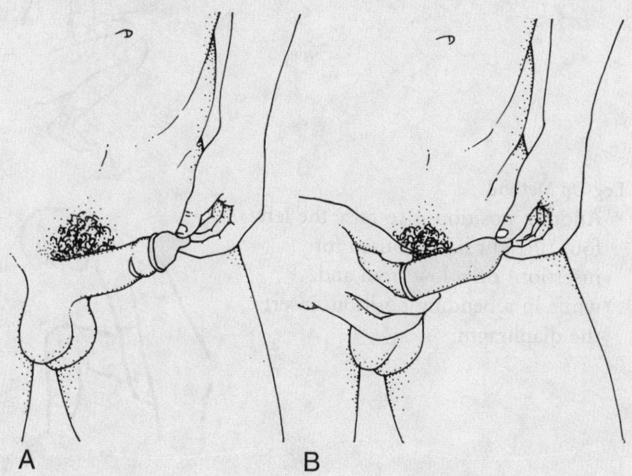

- If a lubricant is desired, use water-based products such as K-Y lubricating jelly. Do not use petroleum-based products because they can cause the condom to break.
- After ejaculation carefully withdraw the still-erect penis from the vagina, holding onto the condom rim; remove and discard the condom.
- Store unused condoms in a cool, dry place.
- Do not use condoms that are sticky, brittle, or obviously damaged.

spring, arcing spring, and wide-seal rim. The diaphragm should be the largest size the woman can wear without being aware of its presence. Typical failure rate of the diaphragm combined with spermicide is 16% in the first year of use (Trussell, 2007).

Nursing Considerations The woman using a diaphragm needs an annual gynecologic examination to assess the fit of the diaphragm. The device should be replaced every 2 years and may need to be refitted after a 20% weight loss or gain, term birth, or second-trimester miscarriage and after any abdominal or pelvic surgery (Planned Parenthood, 2008). Because various types of diaphragms are on the market, the nurse uses the package insert when teaching the woman how to use and care for the diaphragm (see Home Care box).

Disadvantages of diaphragm use include the reluctance of some women to insert and remove the diaphragm. Although it can be inserted up to 6 hours before intercourse, a cold diaphragm and a cold gel temporarily reduce vaginal response to sexual stimulation if insertion of the diaphragm occurs immediately before intercourse. Some women or couples object to the messiness of the spermicide. These annoyances of diaphragm use, along with failure to insert the device once foreplay has begun, are the most common reasons for failures of this method. Side effects may include irritation of tissues related to contact with spermicides. The diaphragm is not a good option for women with poor vaginal muscle tone or recurrent urinary tract infections. For proper placement, the diaphragm must rest behind the pubic symphysis and completely cover the cervix. To decrease the chance of exerting urethral pressure, the woman should be reminded to empty her bladder before diaphragm insertion and immediately after intercourse. Diaphragms are contraindicated for women with pelvic relaxation (uterine prolapse) or a large cystocele. Women with a latex allergy should not use latex diaphragms.

Toxic shock syndrome (TSS), although reported in very small numbers, can occur in association with the use of the contraceptive diaphragm and cervical caps. The nurse should instruct the woman about ways to reduce her risk for TSS. These measures include prompt removal 6 to 8 hours after

HOME CARE

Use and Care of the Diaphragm

Positions for Insertion of Diaphragm

Squatting

- Squatting is the most commonly used position, and most women find it satisfactory.

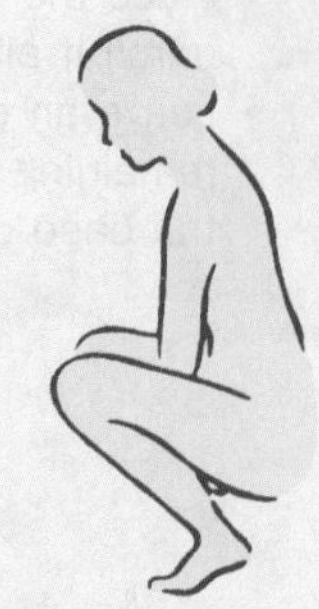

Leg-Up Method

- Another position is to raise the left foot (if right hand is used for insertion) on a low stool and, while in a bending position, insert the diaphragm.

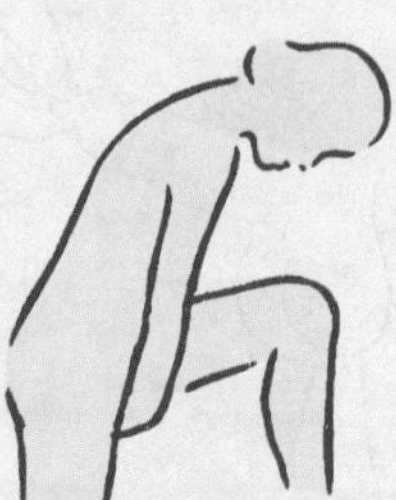

Chair Method

- Another practical method for diaphragm insertion is to sit far forward on the edge of a chair.

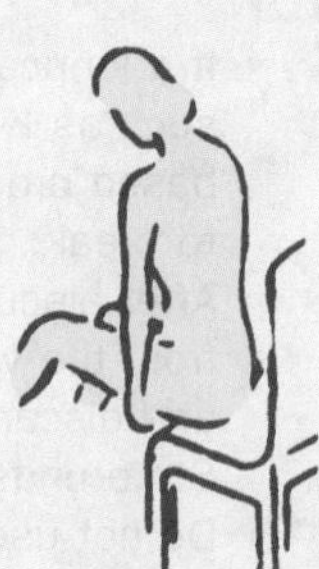

Reclining

- You may prefer to insert the diaphragm while in a semireclining position in bed.

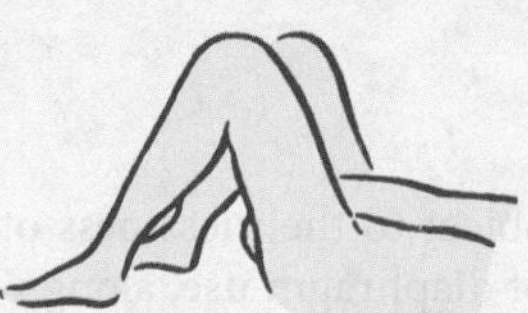

Inspection of Diaphragm

Your diaphragm must be inspected carefully before each use. The best way to do this is:

- Hold the diaphragm up to a light source. Carefully stretch the diaphragm at the area of the rim, on all sides, to make sure that there are no holes. Remember, it is possible to puncture the diaphragm with sharp fingernails.
- Another way to check for pinholes is to carefully fill the diaphragm with water. If there is any problem, it will be seen immediately.
- If your diaphragm is puckered, especially near the rim, this could mean thin spots.
- The diaphragm should not be used if you see any of these; consult your health care provider.

Preparation of Diaphragm

- Rinse off cornstarch. Your diaphragm must always be used with a spermicidal lubricant to be effective. Pregnancy cannot be prevented effectively by the diaphragm alone.
- Always empty your bladder before inserting the diaphragm. Place about 2 tsp of contraceptive jelly or contraceptive cream on the side of the diaphragm that will rest against the cervix (or whichever way you have been instructed). Spread it around to coat the surface and the rim. This aids in insertion and offers a more complete seal. Many women also spread some jelly or cream on the other side of the diaphragm.

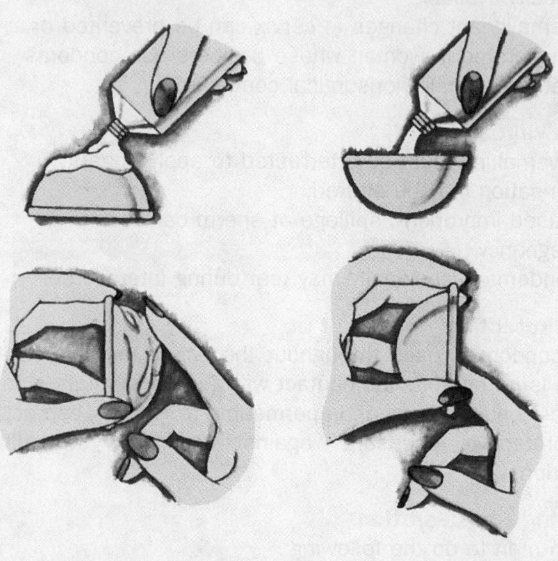

Insertion of Diaphragm

- The diaphragm can be inserted as long as 6 hours before intercourse. Hold the diaphragm between your thumb and fingers. The dome can either be up or down, as directed by your health care provider. Place your index finger on the outer rim of the compressed diaphragm.

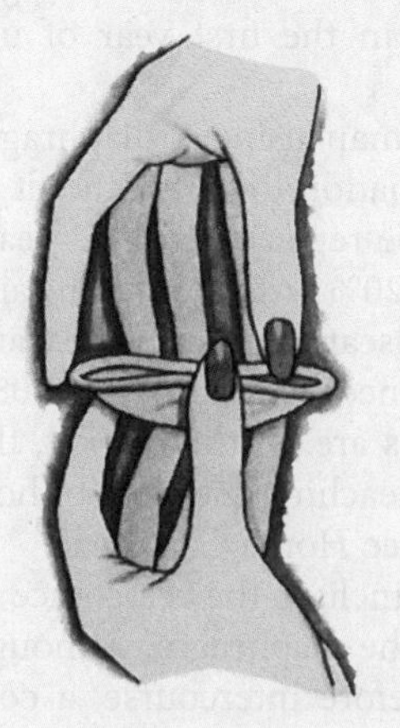

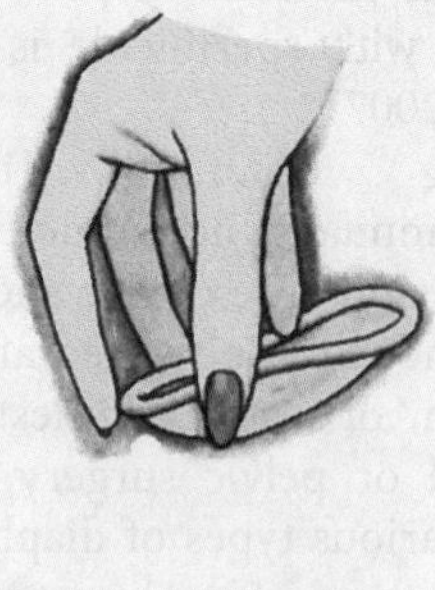

HOME CARE

Use and Care of the Diaphragm—cont'd

- Use the fingers of the other hand to spread the labia (lips of the vagina). This will assist in guiding the diaphragm into place.
- Insert the diaphragm into the vagina. Direct it inward and downward as far as it will go to the space behind and below the cervix.

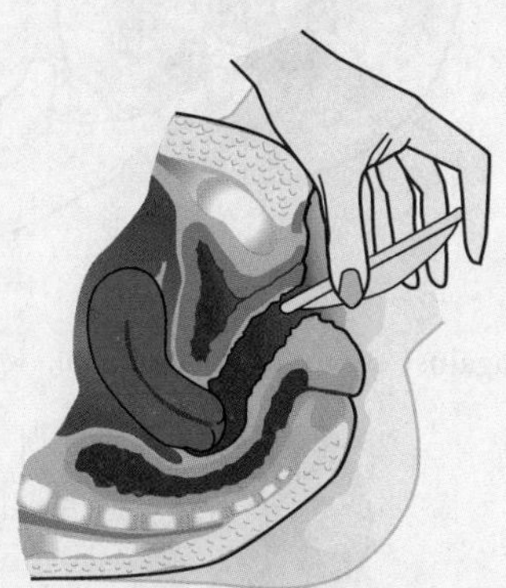

- Tuck the front of the rim of the diaphragm behind the pubic bone so that the rubber hugs the front wall of the vagina.

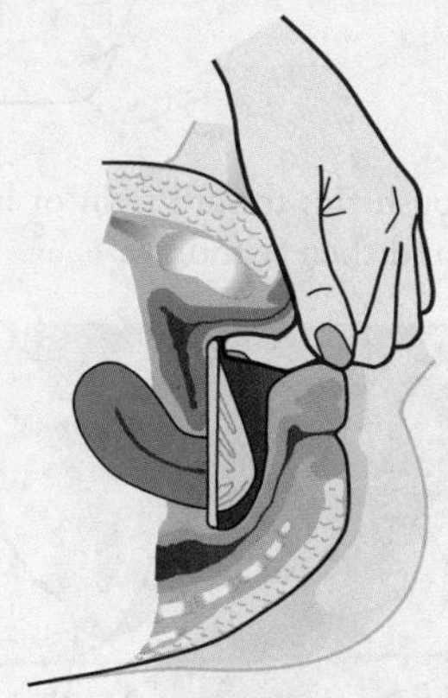

- Feel for your cervix through the diaphragm to be certain it is properly placed and securely covered by the rubber dome.

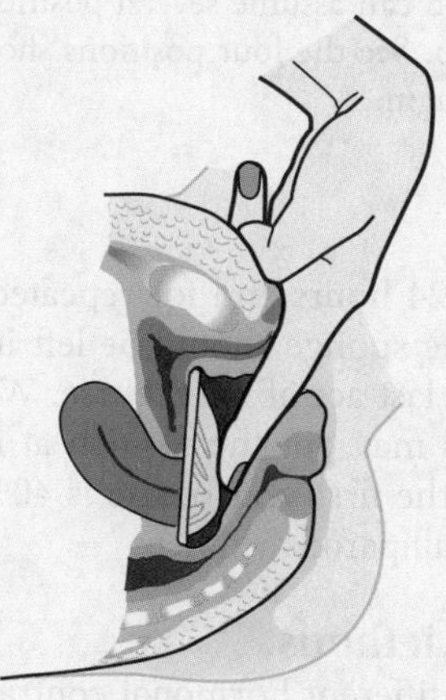

General Information

- Regardless of the time of the month, you must use your diaphragm every time intercourse takes place. Your diaphragm must be left in place for at least 6 hours after the last intercourse. If you remove your diaphragm before the 6-hour period, your chance of becoming pregnant could be greatly increased. If you have repeated acts of intercourse, you must add more spermicide for each act of intercourse.

Removal of Diaphragm

- The only proper way to remove the diaphragm is to insert your forefinger up and over the top side of the diaphragm and slightly to the side.
- Next turn the palm of your hand downward and backward, hooking the forefinger firmly on top of the inside of the upper rim of the diaphragm, breaking the suction.
- Pull the diaphragm down and out. This avoids the possibility of tearing it with the fingernails. You should not remove the diaphragm by trying to catch the rim from below the dome.

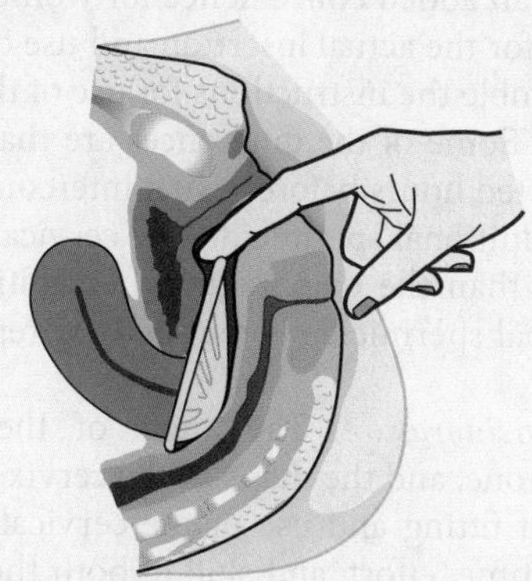

Care of Diaphragm

- When using a vaginal diaphragm, avoid using oil-based products such as certain body lubricants, mineral oil, baby oil, vaginal lubricants, or vaginitis preparations. These products can weaken the rubber.
- A little care means longer wear for your diaphragm. After each use wash the diaphragm in warm water and mild soap. Do not use detergent soaps, cold-cream soaps, deodorant soaps, and soaps containing oil products because they can weaken the rubber.
- After washing, dry the diaphragm thoroughly. All water and moisture should be removed with a towel. Dust the diaphragm with cornstarch. Scented talc, body powder, baby powder, and the like should not be used because they can weaken the rubber.
- To clean the introducer (if one is used), wash with mild soap and warm water, rinse, and dry thoroughly.
- Place the diaphragm back in the plastic case for storage. Do not store it near a radiator or heat source or exposed to light for an extended period.

intercourse, not using the diaphragm or cervical caps during menses, and learning and watching for danger signs of TSS.

NURSING ALERT The nurse should alert the woman who uses a diaphragm or cervical cap as a contraceptive method for signs of TSS. The most common signs include a sunburn type of rash, diarrhea, dizziness, faintness, weakness, sore throat, aching muscles and joints, sudden high fever, and vomiting.

Cervical Cap

Three types of cervical caps are available; two come in varying sizes, and one is one-size-fits-all. They are made of rubber or latex-free silicone and have soft domes and firm brims (see Fig. 7-12, *A*). The cap fits snugly around the base of the cervix close to the junction of the cervix and vaginal fornices. It is recommended that the cap remain in place no less than 6 hours and not more than 48 hours at a time. It is left in place at least 6 hours after the last act of intercourse. The seal provides a physical barrier to sperm: spermicide inside the cap adds a chemical barrier. The extended period of wear may be an added convenience for women.

Instructions for the actual insertion and use of the cervical cap closely resemble the instructions for use of the contraceptive diaphragm. Some of the differences are that the cervical cap can be inserted hours before sexual intercourse without a later need for additional spermicide, the cervical cap requires less spermicide than the diaphragm when initially inserted, and no additional spermicide is required for repeated acts of intercourse.

Nursing Considerations The angle of the uterus, the vaginal muscle tone, and the shape of the cervix may interfere with the ease of fitting and use of the cervical cap. Correct fitting requires time, effort, and skill of both the woman and the clinician (see Home Care box). The woman must check the position of the cap before and after each act of intercourse.

Because of the potential risk of TSS associated with the use of the cervical cap, another form of birth control is recommended for use during menstrual bleeding and up to at least 6 weeks postpartum. The cap should be refitted after any gynecologic surgery or birth and after major weight losses or gains. Otherwise the size should be checked at least once a year.

Women who are not good candidates for wearing the cervical cap include those with abnormal Pap test results, those who cannot be fitted properly with the existing cap sizes or who find the insertion and removal of the device too difficult, those with a history of TSS or with vaginal or cervical infections, and those who experience allergic responses to the cap or to spermicide. Failure rate with typical use for parous women is 32% and for nulliparous women, 16%.

Contraceptive Sponge

The vaginal sponge is a small, round, polyurethane sponge that contains N-9 spermicide (see Fig. 7-12, *B*). It is designed to fit over the cervix (one size fits all). The side that is placed next to the cervix is concave for better fit. The opposite side has a woven polyester loop to be used for removal of the sponge.

The sponge must be moistened with water before it is inserted into the vagina to cover the cervix. It provides protection for up to 24 hours and for repeated instances of sexual intercourse. The sponge should be left in place for at least 6 hours after the last act of intercourse. Wearing it longer than 24 to 30 hours may put the woman at risk for TSS. Typical failure rate in the first year of use is 40% for parous women and 20% for nulliparous women.

HOME CARE

Use of the Cervical Cap

- Push cap up into vagina until it covers cervix.

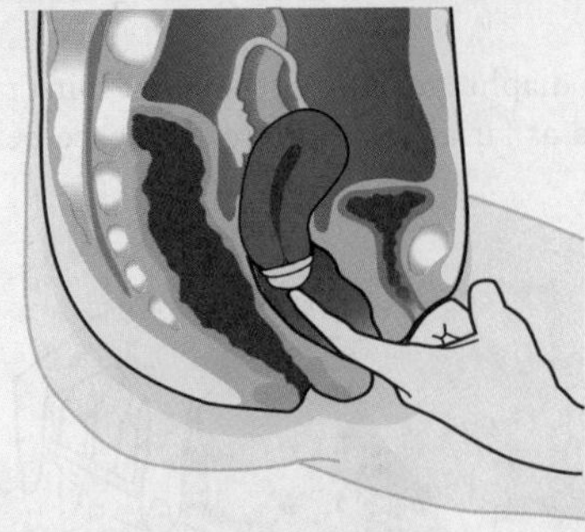

- Press rim against cervix to create a seal.

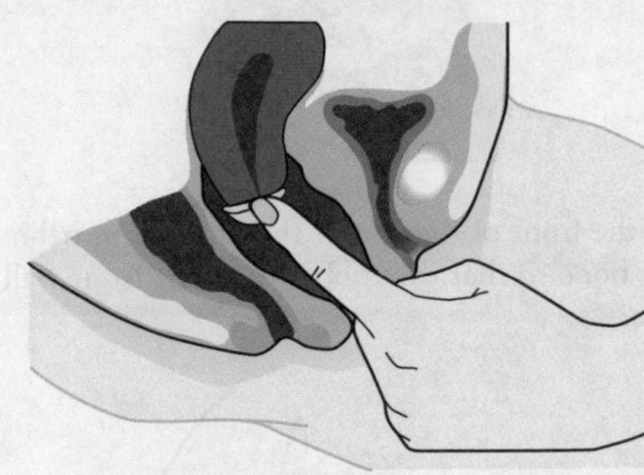

- To remove, push rim toward right or left hip to loosen from cervix and then withdraw.

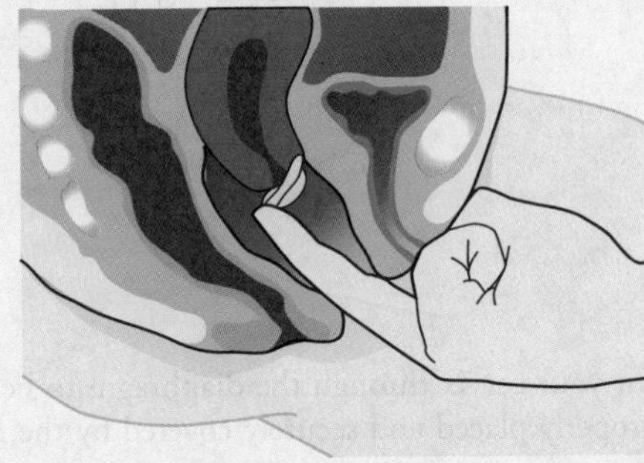

- The woman can assume several positions to insert the cervical cap. See the four positions shown for inserting the diaphragm.

Hormonal Methods

More than 30 different hormonal contraceptive formulations are available in the United States today. General classes are described in Table 7-3. Because of the wide variety of prepara-

Table 7-3 Hormonal Contraception

COMPOSITION	ROUTE OF ADMINISTRATION	DURATION OF EFFECT
Combination estrogen and progestin (synthetic estrogens and progestins in varying doses and formulations)	Oral Transdermal patch Vaginal ring insertion	24 hours; extended cycle—12 weeks 7 days 3 weeks
Progestin only		
Norethindrone, norgestrel	Oral	24 hours
Medroxyprogesterone acetate	Intramuscular or subcutaneous injection	3 months
Progestin etonogestrel	Subdermal implant	Up to 3 years
Levonorgestrel	Intrauterine device	1 year

tions available, the woman and nurse must read the package insert for information about specific products prescribed. Formulations include combined estrogen-progestin steroidal medications or progestational agents. The formulations are administered orally, transdermally, vaginally, by implantation, or by injection.

Combined Estrogen-Progestin Contraceptives

Oral Contraceptives The normal menstrual cycle is maintained by a feedback mechanism. FSH and LH are secreted in response to fluctuating levels of ovarian estrogen and progesterone. Regular ingestion of combined oral contraceptive pills (COCs) suppresses the action of the hypothalamus and anterior pituitary, leading to insufficient secretion of FSH and LH; therefore follicles do not mature, and ovulation is inhibited.

Other contraceptive effects are induced by the combined steroids. Maturation of the endometrium is altered, making it a less favorable site for implantation. COCs also have a direct effect on the endometrium so that, from 1 to 4 days after the last COC is taken, the endometrium sloughs and bleeds as a result of hormone withdrawal. The withdrawal bleeding is usually less profuse than that of normal menstruation and may last only 2 to 3 days. Some women have no bleeding at all. The cervical mucus remains thick from the effect of the progestin. Cervical mucus under the effect of progesterone does not provide as suitable an environment for sperm penetration as does the thin, watery mucus at ovulation.

Monophasic pills provide fixed dosages of estrogen and progestin. They alter the amount of progestin and sometimes the amount of estrogen within each cycle. These preparations reduce the total dosage of hormones in a single cycle without sacrificing contraceptive efficacy. To maintain adequate hormone levels for contraception and enhance compliance, COCs should be taken at the same time each day. Taken exactly as directed, COCs prevent ovulation, and pregnancy cannot occur. The overall effectiveness rate is almost 100%.

Because taking the pill does not relate directly to the sexual act, its acceptability may be increased. Improvement in sexual response may occur once the possibility of pregnancy is not an issue. For some women it is convenient to know when to expect the next menstrual flow.

Contraindications for COC use include a history of thromboembolic disorders, cerebrovascular or coronary artery disease, breast cancer, estrogen-dependent tumors, pregnancy, impaired liver function, liver tumor, lactation less than 6 weeks postpartum, smoking if older than 35 years (more than 15 cigarettes a day), headaches with focal neurologic symptoms, surgery with prolonged immobilization or any surgery on the legs, hypertension (160/100), and diabetes mellitus (of more than 20 years' duration) with vascular disease.

The effectiveness of oral contraceptives is decreased when the following medications are taken simultaneously:

- Anticonvulsants such as barbiturates, oxycarbazepine, phenytoin, phenobarbital, carbamazepine, primidone, and topiramate
- Systemic antifungals such as griseofulvin
- Antituberculosis drugs such as rifampicin and rifabutin
- Anti-HIV protease inhibitors such as nelfinavir and amprenavir

After discontinuing oral contraception, fertility usually returns quickly, but fertility rates are slightly lower the first 3 to 12 months after discontinuation.

Nursing Considerations Many different preparations of oral hormonal contraceptives are available. Because of the wide variations, each woman must be clear about the unique dosage regimen for the preparation prescribed for her and follow directions on the package insert. Directions for care after missing one or two tablets also vary (Fig. 7-13). Signs of potential complications associated with the use of oral contraceptives must be reviewed with the woman (Box 7-10). Oral

BOX 7-10 Signs of Potential Complications: Oral Contraceptives

Before oral contraceptives are prescribed and periodically throughout hormone therapy, the woman is alerted to stop taking the pill and report immediately any of the following symptoms to the health care provider. The word *aches* helps in remembering this list:

A—Abdominal pain: may indicate a problem with the liver or gallbladder
C—Chest pain or shortness of breath: may indicate possible clot problem within lungs or heart
H—Headaches (sudden or persistent): may be caused by cardiovascular accident or hypertension
E—Eye problems: may indicate vascular accident or hypertension
S—Severe leg pain: may indicate a thromboembolic process

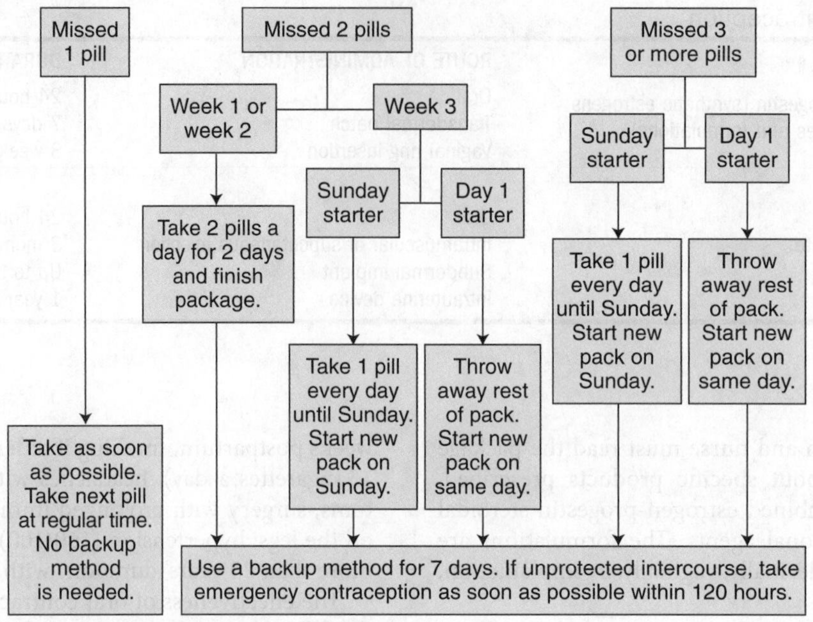

Fig. 7-13 Flowchart for missed contraceptive pills. *(Courtesy Patsy Huff, PharmD, Chapel Hill, NC.)*

contraceptives do not protect a woman against STIs. A barrier method such as condoms and spermicide should be used for protection.

Transdermal Contraceptive System The contraceptive patch delivers continuous levels of progesterone and ethynyl estradiol. The patch can be applied to the lower abdomen, upper outer arm, buttock, or upper torso (except the breasts). Application is on the same day once a week for 3 weeks, followed by a week without the patch. Withdrawal bleeding occurs during the "no patch" week. Mechanisms of action, contraindications, and side effects are similar to those of COCs. The typical failure rate during the first year of use is under 2% in women weighing less than 198 lb.

Vaginal Contraceptive Ring The vaginal ring (made of ethylene vinyl acetate copolymer) delivers continuous levels of progesterone and ethynyl estradiol. One vaginal ring is worn for 3 weeks, followed by a week without the ring. Withdrawal bleeding occurs during the "no ring" week. The ring can be inserted by the woman and does not have to be fitted. Some wearers may experience vaginitis, leukorrhea, and vaginal discomfort. Mechanisms of action, contraindications, and side effects are similar to those of COCs. The typical failure rate of the vaginal contraceptive ring is reportedly under 2% during the first year of use.

Progestin-Only Contraception

Progestin-only methods impair fertility by inhibiting ovulation, thickening and decreasing the amount of cervical mucus, thinning the endometrium, and altering cilia in the uterine tubes.

Oral Progestins (Minipill) Progestin-only pills are less effective than COCs. Failure rate for typical users is 8% in the first year of use. Effectiveness is increased if minipills are taken correctly. Because minipills contain such a low dose of progestin, the minipill must be taken at the same time every day. Users often complain of irregular vaginal bleeding.

Injectable Progestins Depot medroxyprogesterone acetate (DMPA; Depo-Provera) is given subcutaneously or intramuscularly in the deltoid or gluteus maximus muscle. DMPA should be initiated during the first 5 days of the menstrual cycle and administered every 11 to 13 weeks.

NURSING ALERT **When administering an injection of progestin (e.g., Depo-Provera), the site should not be massaged after the injection because this action can hasten the absorption and shorten the period of effectiveness.**

Advantages of DMPA include a contraceptive effectiveness comparable to that of combined oral contraceptives, long-lasting effects, requirement of injections only four times a year, and the unlikelihood of lactation being impaired. Side effects at the end of a year include decreased bone mineral density, weight gain, lipid changes, increased risk of venous thrombosis and thromboembolism, irregular vaginal spotting, decreased libido, and breast changes. Other disadvantages include no protection against STIs (including HIV). Return to fertility may be delayed as long as up to 18 months after discontinuing DMPA. Typical failure rate is 3% in the first year of use.

NURSING ALERT **Women who use DMPA may lose significant bone mineral density with increasing duration of use. It is unknown if this effect is reversible. It is unknown if use of DMPA during adolescence or early adulthood, a critical period of bone accretion, will reduce peak bone mass and increase the risk of osteoporotic fracture in later life. Women who receive DMPA should be counseled about calcium intake and exercise.**

Implantable Progestins Contraceptive implants consist of one or more nonbiodegradable flexible tubes or rods that are inserted under the skin of a woman's arm. These implants contain a progestin hormone and are effective for contraception for at least 3 years. They must be removed at the end of the recommended time.

Implanon is a single-rod implant that is FDA approved for use in the United States. Insertion and removal of the capsule are minor surgical procedures involving a local anesthetic, a small incision, and no sutures. The capsule is placed subdermally in the inner aspect of the nondominant upper arm. The progestin prevents some, but not all, ovulatory cycles and thickens cervical mucus. Other advantages include reversibility and long-term continuous contraception that is not related to frequency of coitus (Raymond, 2007). It can be implanted immediately postpartum in breastfeeding women without affecting lactation (Newberry, 2007). Irregular menstrual bleeding is the most common side effect. Less common side effects include headaches, nervousness, nausea, skin changes, and vertigo (Fischer, 2008). Implanon does not protect against STIs, so condoms should be used for protection. Typical failure rates for the first year of use are 0.05% (Trussell, 2007).

Emergency Contraception

Emergency contraception (EC) is available in over 100 countries, and in about one third of these countries it is available without a prescription. In the United States Plan B has been the only EC method available without a prescription and only in limited pharmacies and clinics in pharmacy access states (states where legislation has been passed to allow this practice)—Alaska, California, Hawaii, Maine, Massachusetts, New Hampshire, New Mexico, Vermont, and Washington. However, on August 24, 2006, the Food and Drug Administration (FDA) approved Plan B for over-the-counter sale to women ages 18 and older (FDA, 2006).

Plan B contains two doses of levonorgestrel. Other options that the FDA has determined to be safe for EC include high doses of oral estrogen or COCs (termed *emergency contractive pills [ECPs]*) and insertion of the copper intrauterine device (IUD). These options will continue to be available by prescription only. Plan B will be prescription only for women under the age of 18 except in the designated pharmacy access states (FDA, 2006).

EC should be taken by a woman as soon as possible but within 72 hours of unprotected intercourse or birth control mishap (e.g., broken condom, dislodged ring or cervical cap, missed oral contraceptive pills, late for injection) to prevent unintended pregnancy (American College of Obstetricians and Gynecologists [ACOG], 2009). If taken before ovulation, EC prevents ovulation by inhibiting follicular development. If taken after ovulation occurs, there is little effect on ovarian hormone production or the endometrium. To minimize the side effect of nausea that occurs with high doses of estrogen and progestin, the woman can be advised to take an over-the-counter antiemetic 1 hour before each dose. Women with contraindications for estrogen use should use progestin-only EC. No medical contraindications for EC exist, except pregnancy and undiagnosed abnormal vaginal bleeding (Stewart, Trussell, & Van Look, 2007). If the woman does not begin menstruation within 21 days after taking the pills, she should be evaluated for pregnancy (Stewart, Trussell, & Van Look, 2007). EC is ineffective if the woman is pregnant since the pills do not disturb an implanted pregnancy. Risk of pregnancy is reduced by as much as 75% and 89% if the woman takes ECPs (Stewart, Trussell, & Van Look, 2007).

NURSING ALERT EC will not protect the woman against pregnancy if she engages in unprotected intercourse in the days or weeks that follow treatment. Because ingestion of ECPs may delay ovulation, caution the woman that she needs to establish a reliable form of birth control to prevent unintended pregnancy (Stewart, Trussell, & Van Look, 2007). Information about EC method options and access to providers are available on the Internet at *www.NOT-2-LATE.com* or by calling 888-NOT-2-LATE.

IUDs containing copper (see later discussion) provide another EC option. The IUD should be inserted within 8 days of unprotected intercourse (Stewart, Trussell, & Van Look, 2007). This method is suggested only for women who wish to have the benefit of long-term contraception. The risk of pregnancy is reduced by as much as 99% with emergency insertion of the copper-releasing IUD.

Contraceptive counseling should be provided to all women requesting EC, including a discussion of modification of risky sexual behaviors to prevent STIs and unwanted pregnancy.

Intrauterine Devices

An IUD is a small T-shaped device with bendable arms for insertion through the cervix into the uterine cavity. Two strings hang from the base of the stem through the cervix and protrude into the vagina for the woman to feel for assurance that the device has not been dislodged (Fig. 7-14). There are two FDA-approved IUDs. The Copper T380A (Paragard) IUD is made of radiopaque polyethylene and fine solid copper and is approved for 10 years of use. The copper primarily serves as a spermicide and inflames the endometrium, preventing fertilization. Sometimes women experience an increase in bleeding and cramping within the first year after insertion, but nonsteroidal antiinflammatory drugs (NSAIDs) can provide pain relief. The typical failure rate in the first year of use of the copper IUD is 0.8% (Trussell, 2007).

The levonorgestrel intrauterine system (Mirena) releases levonorgestrel from its vertical reservoir. Effective for up to 5 years, it impairs sperm motility, irritates the lining of the uterus, and has some anovulatory effects (Grimes, 2007). Uterine cramping and uterine bleeding are usually decreased with this device, although irregular spotting is common in the first few months following insertion. The typical failure rate in the first year of use is 0.2% (Trussell, 2007).

The IUD offers constant contraception without the need to remember to take pills each day or engage in other manipulation before or between coital acts. If pregnancy can be excluded, an IUD can be placed at any time during the menstrual cycle. An IUD may be inserted immediately after childbirth or first-trimester abortion. Contraceptive effects are reversible. When pregnancy is desired, the IUD may be removed by the health care provider.

Disadvantages of IUD use include increased risk of pelvic inflammatory disease in the first 20 days after insertion and

evolve Nursing Care Plan—Sexual Activity/Contraception

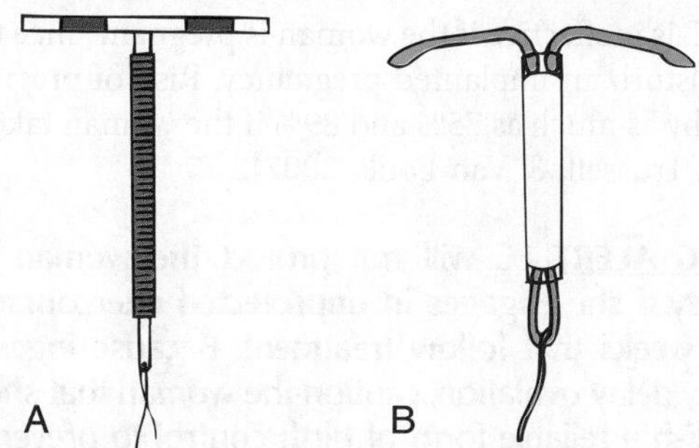

Fig. 7-14 Intrauterine devices. A, Copper T380A. B, Levonorgestrel-releasing intrauterine device.

BOX 7-11 Signs of Potential Complications: Intrauterine Devices

Signs of potential complications related to intrauterine devices can be remembered using the *pains* mnemonic:

P—Period late, abnormal spotting or bleeding
A—Abdominal pain, pain with intercourse
I—Infection exposure, abnormal vaginal discharge
N—Not feeling well, fever, or chills
S—String missing; shorter or longer

risk of bacterial vaginosis and uterine perforation. The IUD offers no protection against STIs or HIV.

Nursing Considerations

The woman should be taught to check for the presence of the IUD thread after menstruation to rule out expulsion of the device. If pregnancy occurs with the IUD in place, the IUD should be removed immediately in the first trimester if the strings are visible. Later in pregnancy ultrasound examination should be used to localize the IUD and to rule out placenta previa. Retention of the IUD during pregnancy increases the risk of septic miscarriage and ectopic pregnancy (Grimes, 2007). Some women allergic to copper develop a rash, necessitating removal of the copper-bearing IUD. Signs of potential complications are listed in Box 7-11.

Sterilization

Sterilization refers to surgical procedures intended to render the person infertile. Most procedures involve the occlusion of the passageways for the ova and sperm (Fig. 7-15, *A*). For the woman the oviducts (uterine tubes) are occluded; for the man the sperm ducts (vas deferens) are occluded. Only surgical removal of the ovaries (oophorectomy) or uterus (hysterectomy) or both result in absolute sterility for the woman. All other sterilization procedures have a small but definite failure rate (i.e., pregnancy may result).

Female Sterilization

Female sterilization (bilateral tubal ligation) may be done immediately after giving birth (within 24 to 48 hours), concomitantly with abortion, or as an interval procedure (during any phase of the menstrual cycle). Half of all female sterilization procedures are performed immediately after a pregnancy. Sterilization procedures can be done safely on an outpatient basis. Failure rate for methods of female sterilization vary by the method and the woman's age, but the average is 0.5% (Trussell, 2007).

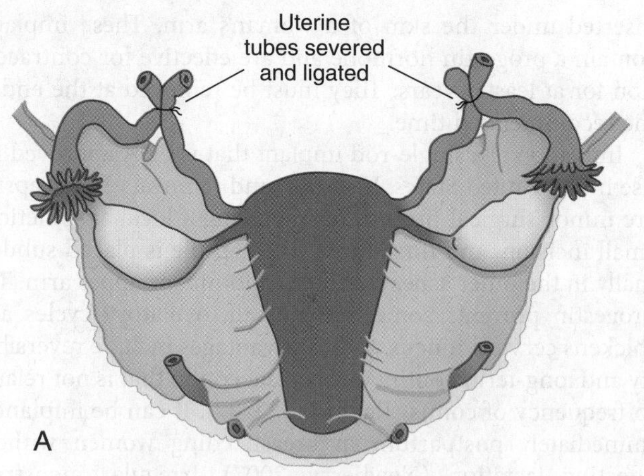

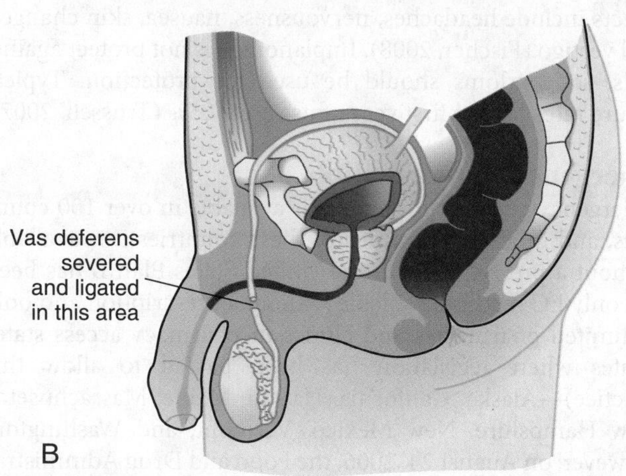

Fig. 7-15 Sterilization. A, Uterine tubes ligated and severed (tubal ligation). B, Sperm duct ligated and severed (vasectomy).

Tubal Occlusion A laparoscopic approach or a minilaparotomy may be used for tubal ligation (Fig. 7-16), tubal electrocoagulation, or the application of bands or clips. Electrocoagulation and ligation are considered to be permanent methods. Use of the bands or clips has the theoretic advantage of possible removal and return of tubal patency (see Patient Teaching box).

Tubal Reconstruction Restoration of tubal continuity (reanastomosis) and function is technically feasible except after laparoscopic tubal electrocoagulation. Sterilization reversal is costly, difficult (requiring microsurgery), and uncertain. The success rate varies with the extent of tubal destruction and removal. The risk of ectopic pregnancy after tubal reanastomosis is increased by 2% to 12.5%.

Male Sterilization

Vasectomy is the sealing, tying, or cutting of a man's vas deferens so that the sperm cannot travel from the testes to the penis. Vasectomy is the easiest and most commonly used operation for male sterilization. It can be done with local anesthesia on an outpatient basis. Pain, bleeding, infection,

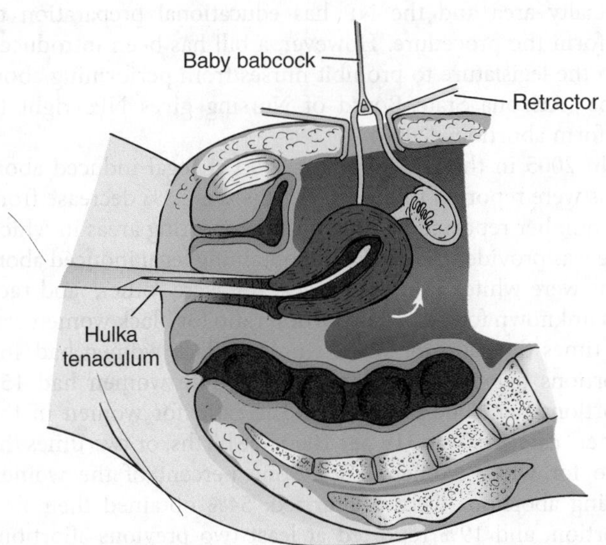

Fig. 7-16 Use of minilaparotomy to gain access to uterine tubes for occlusion procedures. Tenaculum is used to lift uterus upward *(arrow)* toward incision.

PATIENT TEACHING What to Expect After Tubal Ligation

- You should expect no change in hormones and their influence.
- Your menstrual period will be about the same as before the sterilization.
- You may feel pain at ovulation.
- The ovum disintegrates within the abdominal cavity.
- It is highly unlikely that you will become pregnant.
- You should not have a change in sexual functioning; you may enjoy sexual relations more because you will not be concerned about becoming pregnant.
- Sterilization offers no protection against sexually transmitted infections. Therefore you may need to use condoms.

and other postsurgical complications are considered the disadvantages to the surgical procedure.

Two methods are used for scrotal entry: conventional and no-scalpel vasectomy. The surgeon identifies and immobilizes the vas deferens through the scrotum. Then the vas is ligated or cauterized (see Fig. 7-15, *B*). Surgeons vary in their techniques to occlude the vas deferens: ligation with sutures, division, cautery, application of clips, excision of a segment of the vas, fascial interposition, or some combination of these methods.

Vasectomy has no effect on potency (ability to achieve and maintain erection) or volume of ejaculate. Endocrine production of testosterone continues so that secondary sex characteristics are not affected. Sperm production continues, but sperm are unable to leave the epididymis and are lysed by the immune system.

Complications after bilateral vasectomy are uncommon and usually not serious. They include bleeding (usually external), suture reaction, and reaction to the anesthetic agent. Men occasionally may develop a hematoma, infection, or epididymitis. Less common are painful granulomas from accumulation of sperm. The failure rate for male sterilization is 0.15% (Trussell, 2007).

Tubal Reconstruction Microsurgery to reanastomose (restore tubal continuity) the sperm ducts can be accomplished successfully (i.e., sperm in the ejaculate) in more than 90% of cases; however, the fertility rate is only about 50%. The rate of success decreases as the time since the procedure increases. The vasectomy may result in permanent changes in the testes that leave men unable to father children. The changes are those ordinarily seen only in the elderly (e.g., interstitial fibrosis [scar tissue between the seminiferous tubules]). Some men develop antibodies against their own sperm (autoimmunization).

Laws and Regulations

All states have strict regulations for informed consent. Many states permit voluntary sterilization of any mature, rational woman without reference to her marital or pregnancy status. Although the partner's consent is not required by law, the woman is encouraged to discuss the situation with her partner, and health care providers may request the partner's consent. Sterilization of minors or mentally incompetent individuals is restricted by most states and often requires the approval of a board of eugenicists or other court-appointed individuals.

LEGAL TIP Sterilization If federal funds are used for sterilization, the person must be at least 21 years old.

Informed consent must include an explanation of the risks, benefits, and alternatives; a statement that describes sterilization as a permanent, irreversible method of birth control; and a statement that mandates a 30-day waiting period between giving consent and the sterilization.

Informed consent must be in the person's native language, or an interpreter must be provided to read the consent form to the person.

Nursing Considerations

The nurse plays an important role in assisting people with decision making so that all requirements for informed consent are met. The nurse also provides information about alternatives to sterilization such as contraception.

Information must be given about what is entailed in the various procedures, how much discomfort or pain can be expected, and what type of care is needed. Many individuals fear sterilization procedures because of the imagined effect on their sexual life. They need reassurance concerning the hormonal and psychologic basis for sexual function and that uterine tube occlusion or vasectomy has no biologic sequelae in terms of sexual adequacy.

Preoperative care includes health assessment, which includes a psychologic assessment, physical examination, and laboratory tests. The nurse confirms the woman's understanding of printed instructions. Ambivalence and extreme fear of the procedure are reported to the physician.

Postoperative care depends on the procedure performed (e.g., laparoscopy, laparotomy for tubal occlusion, or vasectomy). General care includes recovery after anesthesia, vital signs, fluid-electrolyte balance (intake and output, laboratory values), prevention of or early identification and treatment of infection or hemorrhage, control of discomfort, and assessment of emotional response to the procedure and recovery.

Discharge planning depends on the type of procedure performed. In general, the patient is given written instructions about observing for and reporting symptoms and signs of complications, the type of recovery to be expected, and the date and time for a follow-up appointment.

Abortion

Induced abortion is the purposeful interruption of a pregnancy before 20 weeks of gestation. (Miscarriage is discussed in Chapter 14.) If the abortion is performed at the woman's request, the term *elective abortion* is usually used; if performed for reasons of maternal or fetal health or disease, the term *therapeutic abortion* applies. Many factors contribute to a woman's decision to have an abortion. Indications include (1) preservation of the life or health of the mother, (2) genetic disorders of the fetus, (3) rape or incest, and (4) the pregnant woman's request. The control of birth, dealing as it does with human sexuality and the question of life and death, is one of the most emotional components of health care. It has been the most controversial social issue in the last half of the twentieth century and the beginning of the twenty-first century. Regulations exist to protect the mother from the complications of abortion.

Abortion is regulated in most countries, including the United States. Before 1970 legal abortion was not widely available in the United States. However, in January 1973 the U.S. Supreme Court set aside previous antiabortion laws and legalized abortion. This decision established a trimester approach to abortion.

In the first trimester abortion is permissible, the decision is between the woman and her health care provider, and a state has little right to interfere (Paul & Stewart, 2007). In the second trimester abortion is left to the discretion of the individual states to regulate procedures as long as they are reasonably related to the woman's health. In the third trimester abortions may be limited or even prohibited by state regulation unless the restriction interferes with the life or health of the pregnant woman (Paul & Stewart, 2007). Hospitals maintained by Roman Catholics and some of those maintained by strict fundamentalists forbid abortion (and often sterilization) despite legal challenges.

In 1992 the U.S. Supreme Court made another landmark ruling, this time allowing states to restrict early abortion services as long as the restrictions did not place an "undue burden" on the woman's ability to choose abortion. Since then many bills have been introduced to limit access and funds for women seeking abortion. In 2006 several states introduced bills to ban most abortions; the U.S. Supreme Court will again play a major role in deciding the future of abortions.

In 2008 the Arizona State Board of Nursing became the first state to determine that it is within the scope of practice of registered nurse practitioners (NPs) to perform first-trimester aspiration abortion if the patient population is within the NP's specialty area and the NP has educational preparation to perform the procedure. However, a bill has been introduced into the legislature to prohibit nurses from performing abortions (Arizona State Board of Nursing gives NPs right to perform abortions, 2008).

In 2005 in the United States 820,151 legal induced abortions were reported to the CDC. This is a 2.3% decrease from the number reported in 2004. In the reporting areas in which race was provided, 53% of those obtaining legal induced abortions were white, 35% were black, 8% were "other," and race was unknown for 4%. The abortion ratio for black women was 2.9 times the ratio for white women. Black women had 467 abortions per 1000 live births, and white women had 158 abortions per 1000 live births. The ratio for women in the "other" category was 319 per 1000 live births, or two times the ratio for white women. Eighty-one percent of the women having abortions were unmarried; 54% obtained their first abortion, and 19% reported at least two previous abortions (Gamble et al, 2008).

The laws for abortion in Canada have also changed over the last 35 years, from being very restricted before 1969 to unrestricted in 1988. Today Canada is one of the only countries in the world without abortion regulation. Abortion is available throughout pregnancy, although more than 90% are performed in the first trimester and only 2% to 3% are performed after 16 weeks. In 2005 Canadian women had 96,815 abortions (AbortioninCanada.ca, 2008).

LEGAL TIP Induced Abortion It is important for nurses to know the laws regarding abortion in their state or province of practice before they offer abortion counseling or nursing care to a woman choosing an abortion. Many states enforce a mandatory delay or state-directed counseling before a woman may legally obtain an abortion.

Rates of biologic complications after abortions such as ectopic pregnancy, infection, or hemorrhage tend to be low if the woman aborts during the first trimester. Psychologic sequelae of induced abortion are uncommon and may be related to circumstances and support systems surrounding the pregnant woman such as the attitudes reflected by friends, family, and health care workers. The woman facing an abortion is pregnant and will exhibit the emotional responses shared by all pregnant women, including the possibility of postbirth depression.

Nurses and other health care providers often struggle with the same values and moral convictions as those of the pregnant woman. The conflicts and doubts of the nurse can be readily communicated to women who are already anxious. Regardless of personal views on abortion, nurses who provide care to women seeking abortion have an ethical responsibility to counsel women about their options and to make appropriate referrals.

The Association of Women's Health, Obstetric and Neonatal Nurses (AWHONN, 1999) continues to support a nurse's right to choose to participate or not in abortion procedures in keeping with his or her "personal, moral, ethical, or religious beliefs." AWHONN also advocates that "nurses have an obligation to inform their employers, at the time of employment, of any attitudes and beliefs that may interfere with essential job functions."

NURSING ALERT Nurses whose religious or moral beliefs do not support abortion have the right to refuse such an assignment. Reassignment is usually an option so that the abortion patient receives needed care.

LEGAL TIP Institutional Policies for Nurses' Rights and Responsibilities Related to Abortion Nurses' rights and responsibilities related to caring for abortion patients should be protected through policies that describe how the institution will accommodate the nurse's ethical or moral beliefs and what the nurse should do to avoid patient abandonment in such situations. Nurses should know what policies are in place in their institutions and encourage such policies to be written.

Counseling about abortion includes helping the woman identify how she perceives the pregnancy, providing information about the choices available (i.e., having an abortion or carrying the pregnancy to term and then either keeping the infant or placing the baby for adoption), and information about the types of abortion procedures (see Critical Thinking Exercise).

CRITICAL THINKING EXERCISE

Termination of Pregnancy

Angelica is a 19-year-old single woman whose contraceptive failed. She is 6 weeks pregnant and is seeking termination of the pregnancy. She has many questions for the nurse in the family planning clinic: What procedure is most likely to be chosen at this gestation? What are the risks associated with the procedure? Should her boyfriend be involved in the decision to terminate the pregnancy?

1. Evidence—Is there sufficient evidence to draw conclusions about what information the nurse should provide Tricia?
2. Assumptions—What assumptions can be made about Tricia's reaction to termination of the pregnancy?
   a. Psychologic/emotional reaction and sequelae
   b. Physical response
   c. Future childbearing
   d. Relationship with her boyfriend
3. What implications and priorities for nursing care can be drawn at this time?
4. Does the evidence objectively support your conclusion?
5. Are there alternative perspectives to your conclusion?

First-Trimester Abortion

Methods for performing early elective abortion (less than 9 weeks of gestation) include surgical (aspiration) and medical methods (mifepristone with prostaglandin and methotrexate with misoprostol).

Surgical (Aspiration) Abortion

Aspiration (vacuum or suction curettage) is the most common procedure in the first trimester, with almost 88% of all procedures being performed by this method (Gamble et al, 2008). Aspiration abortion is usually performed under local anesthesia in a physician's office, a clinic, or a hospital. The ideal time for performing this procedure is 8 to 12 weeks after the last menstrual period. The suction procedure for performing an early elective abortion usually requires less than 5 minutes.

A bimanual examination is done before the procedure to assess uterine size and position. A speculum is inserted, and the cervix is anesthetized with a local anesthetic agent. The cervix is dilated if necessary, and a cannula connected to suction is inserted into the uterine cavity. The products of conception are evacuated from the uterus.

During the procedure the woman is kept informed about what to expect next (e.g., menstrual-like cramping and sounds of the suction machine). The nurse assesses the woman's vital signs. The aspirated uterine contents must be carefully inspected to ascertain whether all fetal parts and adequate placental tissue have been evacuated. After the abortion the woman rests on the table until she is ready to stand. She then remains in the recovery area or waiting room for 1 to 3 hours for detection of excessive cramping or bleeding; then she is discharged.

Bleeding after the operation is normally about the equivalent of a heavy menstrual period, and cramps are rarely severe. Excessive vaginal bleeding and infection such as endometritis or salpingitis are the most common complications of induced abortion. Retained products of conception are the primary cause of vaginal bleeding. Evacuation of the uterus, uterine massage, and administration of oxytocin or methylergonovine (Methergine) may be necessary. Prophylactic antibiotics to decrease the risk of infection are commonly prescribed. Postabortion pain can be relieved with NSAIDs such as ibuprofen.

Nursing Interventions

Instructions following a surgical abortion differ among health care providers (e.g., tampons should not be used for at least 3 days or should be avoided for up to 3 weeks, and resumption of sexual intercourse may be permitted within 1 week or discouraged for 2 weeks). The woman may shower daily. Instruction is given to watch for excessive bleeding and other signs of complications (Box 7-12) and to avoid douches of any type. The woman may expect her menstrual period to resume 4 to 6 weeks after the day of the procedure. The nurse offers information about the birth control method the woman prefers if this has not been done during the counseling interview that usually precedes the decision to have an abortion. The woman must be strongly encouraged to return for her follow-up visit so that complications can be detected and an acceptable contraceptive method prescribed. A pregnancy test may also be performed to determine if the pregnancy has been terminated successfully.

Medical Abortion

Early medical abortion has been popular in Canada and Europe for more than 15 years, but it is a relatively new procedure in the United States. Medical abortions are available for use in the United States for up to 9 weeks after the last menstrual period. Methotrexate, misoprostol, and mifepristone are the drugs used in the current regimens to induce early

BOX 7-12 Induced Abortion Complications

Call your health care provider if you have any of the following signs:

- Fever greater than 38° C (100.4° F)
- Chills
- Bleeding greater than two saturated pads in 2 hours or heavy bleeding lasting a few days
- Foul-smelling vaginal discharge
- Severe abdominal pain, cramping, or backache
- Abdominal tenderness (when pressure applied)
- No return of menstrual period within 6 weeks

Reference: Paul M, Stewart F: Abortion. In Hatcher R et al (editors): *Contraceptive technology*, ed 19 rev, New York, 2007, Ardent Media.

abortion. About 10% of all reported abortion procedures in 2005 were medical procedures (Gamble et al, 2008).

Methotrexate is a cytotoxic drug that causes early abortion by blocking folic acid in fetal cells so they cannot divide. Misoprostol (Cytotec) is a prostaglandin analog that acts directly on the cervix to soften and dilate and on the uterine muscle to stimulate contractions. Mifepristone, formerly known as RU 486, was approved by the FDA in 2000. It works by binding to progesterone receptors and blocking the action of progesterone, which is necessary for maintaining pregnancy.

Methotrexate and Misoprostol

Methotrexate can be given intramuscularly or orally (usually mixed with orange juice). Vaginal placement of misoprostol follows in 3 to 7 days. Women commonly have nausea, vomiting, and cramping after the misoprostol insertion. The woman returns for a follow-up visit to confirm the abortion is complete. If abortion does not occur, misoprostol is repeated, or vacuum aspiration is performed.

Mifepristone and Misoprostol

Mifepristone can be taken up to 7 weeks after the last menstrual period. The FDA-approved regimen is that the woman takes 600 mg of mifepristone orally; 48 hours later she returns to the office and takes 400 mcg of misoprostol orally (unless abortion has already occurred and been confirmed). Two weeks after the administration of mifepristone, the woman must return to the office for a clinical examination or ultrasound to confirm that the pregnancy has been terminated. In 1% to 5% of cases the drugs do not work, and surgical abortion (aspiration) is needed.

With any medical abortion regimen, the woman usually will experience bleeding and cramping. Side effects of the medications include nausea, vomiting, diarrhea, headache, dizziness, fever, and chills. These are attributed to misoprostol and usually subside in a few hours after administration.

Second-Trimester Abortion

Second-trimester abortion is associated with more complications and costs than first-trimester abortions. Dilation and evacuation (D&E) accounts for almost all procedures performed in the United States. Induction of uterine contractions with hypertonic solutions (e.g., saline, urea) injected directly into the uterus and uterotonic agents (e.g., misoprostol, dinoprostone) accounts for only about 0.8% of all abortions (Gamble et al, 2008).

Dilation and Evacuation

D&E can be performed at any point up to 20 weeks of gestation, although it is more often performed between 13 and 16 weeks. The cervix requires more dilation because the products of conception are larger. Often laminaria are inserted several hours or several days before the procedure, or misoprostol can be applied to the cervix. The procedure is similar to that of vaginal aspiration, except that a larger cannula is used and other instruments may be needed to remove the fetus and placenta. Nursing care includes monitoring vital signs, providing emotional support, administering analgesics, and postoperative monitoring. Disadvantages of D&E include possible long-term harmful effects on the cervix.

Emotional Considerations

The woman considering an abortion will need help to explore the meaning of the various alternatives and consequences to herself and her significant others. It is often difficult for a woman to express her true feelings (e.g., what abortion means to her now and in the future and what support or regret her friends and peers may demonstrate). A calm, matter-of-fact approach on the part of the nurse can be helpful. Clarifying, restating, and reflecting statements; open-ended questions; and feedback are communication techniques that can be used to maintain a realistic focus on the situation and bring the woman's problems into the open. If family or friends cannot be involved, scheduling time for nursing personnel to give the necessary support is an essential component of the care plan.

Information about alternatives to abortion such as referral to adoption agencies or to support services if the woman chooses to keep her baby is provided. If a decision is made to have an abortion, the woman must be assured of continued support. Information about what is entailed in various procedures, how much discomfort or pain can be expected, and what type of care is needed must be given. A discussion of the various feelings, including depression, guilt, regret, and relief, that the woman might experience after the abortion is needed. Information about community resources for postabortion counseling may be needed.

After the abortion, studies have indicated that most women report relief, but some have temporary distress or mixed emotions. Evidence of long-term depression after elective abortion has been inconclusive. Guilt and anxiety may occur more with young women, women with poor social support, multiparous women, and women with a history of psychiatric illness. Women having second-trimester abortions may have more emotional distress than women having abortions in the first trimester. Because symptoms can vary among women who have had abortions, nurses must assess women for grief reactions and facilitate the grieving process through active listening and nonjudgmental support and care.

Key Points

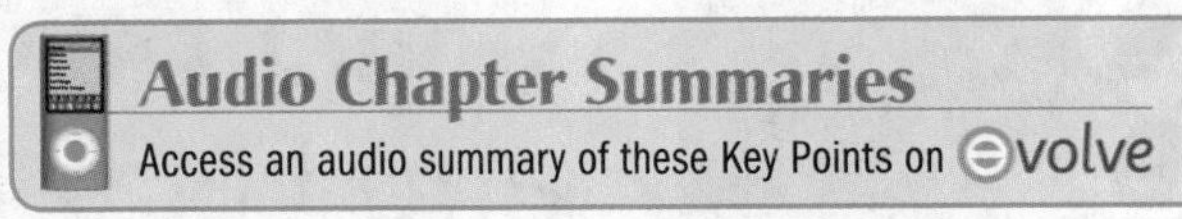
Audio Chapter Summaries
Access an audio summary of these Key Points on evolve

- Infertility is the inability to conceive and carry a fetus to term gestation at a time the couple has chosen to do so.
- Infertility affects about 10% of otherwise healthy adults. It increases in women older than 35 years.
- In the United States about one third of infertility is related to female causes, one third is related to male causes, and 20% of the causes are unexplained.
- Common etiologic factors of infertility include decreased sperm production, ovulation disorders, tubal occlusion, and endometriosis.
- Reproductive alternatives for family building include IVF-ET, GIFT, ZIFT, oocyte donation, embryo donation, TDI, surrogate motherhood, and adoption.
- A variety of contraceptive methods with various effectiveness rates, advantages, and disadvantages are available.
- Women and their partners should choose the contraceptive method(s) best suited to them.
- Effective contraceptives are available through both prescription and nonprescription sources.
- Proper concurrent use of spermicides and latex condoms provides protection against STIs.
- Tubal ligations and vasectomies are permanent sterilization methods used by increasing numbers of women and men.
- Induced abortion performed in the first trimester is safer and less complex than an abortion performed in the second trimester.
- The most common complications of induced abortion include infection, retained products of conception, and excessive vaginal bleeding.

References

AbortioninCanada.ca, 2008. Available at www.AbortioninCanada.ca (accessed February 21, 2009).

American College of Obstetricians and Gynecologists (ACOG): *Frequently asked questions about hormonal approaches to emergency contraception*, 2009. Available at www.acog.org/departments/dept_notice.cfm?recno=18&bulletin=1084 (accessed February 20, 2009).

American Society for Reproductive Medicine (ASRM): *Frequently asked questions about infertility*, 2008. Available at www.asrm.org (accessed February 21, 2009).

Arevalo M et al: Efficacy of the new TwoDay method of family planning, *Fertil Steril* 82(4):885-892, 2004.

Arizona State Board of Nursing gives NPs right to perform abortion, *Nurse Week*, June 2008, p 12.

Association of Women's Health, Obstetric and Neonatal Nurses (AWHONN): *Nurses' rights and responsibilities related to abortion and sterilization, Policy Position Statement*, 1999. Available at www.awhonn.org (accessed February 21, 2009).

Cates W, Raymond E: Vaginal barriers and spermicides. In Hatcher R et al (editors): *Contraceptive technology*, ed 19, New York, 2007, Ardent Media.

Centers for Disease Control and Prevention, Workowski KA, Berman SM: Sexually transmitted disease treatment guidelines 2006, *MMWR Morb Mortal Wkly Rep* 55(RR-11):1-100, 2006.

Cunningham FG et al: *Williams obstetrics*, ed 22, New York, 2005, McGraw-Hill.

CycleBeads: *Frequently asked questions*, 2007. Available at www.cyclebeads.com (accessed February 20, 2009).

D'Avanzo CE: *Pocket guide to cultural health assessment*, ed 4, St Louis, 2008, Mosby.

Female Health Company: *Female condom: the product*, 2008. Available at www.femalehealth.com/theproduct.html (accessed February 20, 2009).

Fischer M: Implanon: a new contraceptive implant, *J Obstet Gynecol Neonatal Nurs* 37(3):361-368, 2008.

Food and Drug Administration: *FDA approves over-the-counter access for Plan B for women 18 and older. Prescription remains required for those 17 and under*, Press release August 24, 2006. Available at www.fda.gov/bbs/topics/NEWS/2006/NEW01436.html (accessed February 21, 2009).

Gamble SB et al: Abortion surveillance—United States, 2005, *MMWR CDC Surveill Summ* 57(SS-13):1-36, 2008.

Georgia Reproductive Specialists: *Micromanipulation*, 2007. Available at www.ivf.com/icsi.html (accessed February 21, 2009).

Grimes D: Intrauterine devices (IUDs). In R Hatcher et al (editors): *Contraceptive technology*, ed 19, New York, 2007, Ardent Media.

Grimes D et al: Fertility awareness-based methods for contraception: systematic review of randomized controlled trials, *Contraception* 72(2):85-90, 2005.

Kearnes W et al: Preimplantation genetic diagnosis and screening, *Semin Reprod Med* 23(4):336-347, 2005.

Kennedy K, Trussell J: Postpartum contraception and lactation. In Hatcher R et al (editors): *Contraceptive technology*, ed 19, New York, 2007, Ardent Media.

Lobo R: Infertility: etiology, diagnostic evaluation, management, prognosis. In Katz VL et al: *Comprehensive gynecology*, ed 5, St Louis, 2007, Mosby.

Nelson A, Marshall J: Impaired fertility. In Hatcher R et al (editors): *Contraceptive technology*, ed 19, New York, 2007, Ardent Media.

Newberry Y: Implanon: a new implantable contraceptive, *Nurs Women's Health* 11(6):607-611, 2007.

Paul M, Stewart F: Abortion. In Hatcher R et al (editors): *Contraceptive technology*, ed 19, New York, 2007, Ardent Media.

Planned Parenthood: *Diaphragms*, updated May 15, 2008. Available at www.plannedparenthood.org (accessed February 20, 2009).

Raymond E: Progestin-only pills. In Hatcher R et al (editors): *Contraceptive technology*, ed 19, New York, 2007, Ardent Media.

RESOLVE: *Demystifying infertility*, 2008. Available at www.resolve.org/site/PageServer?pagename=cop_demis_home#myths (accessed February 21, 2009).

Sherrod RA: Understanding the emotional aspects of infertility: implications for nursing practice, *J Psychosoc Nurs Ment Health Serv* 42(3):40-49, 2004.

Sheweita S, Tilmisany A, Al-Sawaf H: Mechanisms of male infertility: role of antioxidants, *Curr Drug Metab* 6(5):495-501, 2005.

Sinai I, Jennings V, Arevalo M: The importance of screening and monitoring the standard day method and cycle regularity, *Contraception* 69(3):201-206, 2004.

Stewart F, Trussell J, Van Look P: Emergency contraception. In Hatcher R et al (editors): *Contraceptive technology*, ed 19, New York, 2007, Ardent Media.

Trussell J: The essentials of contraception: efficacy, safety, and personal considerations. In Hatcher R et al (editors): *Contraceptive technology*, ed 19, New York, 2007, Ardent Media.

Van Voorhis B: Outcomes from assisted reproductive technology, *Obstet Gynecol* 107(1):183-200, 2006.

Weed S: *Wise woman herbal for the childbearing year*, Woodstock, NY, 1986, Ash Tree Publishing.

Unit 3

8 Genetics, Conception, and Fetal Development

Learning Objectives

On completion of this chapter the reader will be able to:

- Explain the key concepts of basic human genetics.
- Discuss the purpose, key findings, and potential outcomes of the Human Genome Project.
- Describe expanded roles for nurses in genetics and genetic counseling.
- Examine ethical dimensions of genetic screening.
- Discuss the current status of gene therapy (gene transfer).
- Summarize the process of fertilization.
- Describe the development, structure, and functions of the placenta.
- Describe the composition and functions of the amniotic fluid.
- Identify three organs or tissues arising from each of the three primary germ layers.
- Summarize the significant changes in growth and development of the embryo and fetus.
- Identify the potential effects of teratogens during vulnerable periods of embryonic and fetal development.

Electronic Resources

Additional information related to the content in Chapter 8 can be found on

evolve the Companion Website at
http://evolve.elsevier.com/Perry/maternal/

- NCLEX Review Questions
- Animation: Fertilization and Implantation
- Animation: First Trimester, Fetal Development
- Animation: Male Accessory Sex Glands
- Animation: Male External Genitalia
- Animation: Male Reproductive Ducts
- Animation: Maternal and Fetal Circulation
- Animation: Oogenesis and Meiosis
- Animation: Pathway of Ovum
- Animation: Pathway of Sperm
- Animation: Second Trimester, Fetal Development
- Animation: Spermatogenesis
- Animation: Spermatozoa
- Animation: Testes
- Animation: Third Trimester, Fetal Development
- Critical Thinking Exercise—Genetic Counseling
- Nursing Care Plan—The Family with a Neonate with Down Syndrome

This chapter presents a brief discussion of genetics and the role of the nurse in genetics. It also provides an overview of the processes of fertilization and development of the normal embryo and fetus.

Genetics

Recent advances in molecular biology and genomics have revolutionized the field of health care by providing the tools needed to determine the hereditary component of many diseases and improve our ability to predict susceptibility to disease, onset and progression of disease, and response to medications (Guttmacher & Collins, 2005; Loescher & Merkle, 2005; Seo & Ginsburg, 2005). With this increase in genetic knowledge there has been a gradual shift from genetics (the study of single genes and their effects) to genomics (the study of the functions and interactions of all the genes in the genome) (Lea, 2008).

The demand for genetic services, especially genetic testing, has never been greater. Genetics is currently recognized as a contributing factor in virtually all human illnesses. In maternity care genetics issues occur before, during, and after pregnancy. With growing public interest in genetics, increasing commercial pressures, and Internet opportunities for individuals, families, and communities to participate in the direction and design of their genetic health care, genetic services are rapidly becoming an integral part of routine health care (Rubinstein & Roy, 2005).

For most genetic conditions therapeutic or preventive measures do not exist or are very limited. Consequently the most useful means of reducing the incidence of these disorders is by preventing their transmission. It is standard practice to assess all pregnant women for heritable disorders to identify potential problems. The incidence of chromosome aberrations is estimated to be 0.5% to 0.6% in newborns. Approximately 62% of miscarriages and 5% to 7% of stillbirths and perinatal deaths are caused by chromosome abnormalities (Hamilton & Wynshaw-Boris, 2009; Lashley, 2005).

Genetic disorders affect people of all ages, from all socioeconomic levels, and from all racial and ethnic backgrounds. They affect not only individuals, but also families, communities, and society. Advances in genetic testing and genetically based treatments have altered the care provided to affected individuals. Improvements in diagnostic capability have resulted in earlier diagnosis and enabled individuals who previously would have died in childhood to survive into adulthood (Lashley, 2005). The genetic aberrations that lead to a disorder are present at birth but may not be manifested for many years, or possibly never manifested.

Some disorders appear more often in ethnic groups. Examples include Tay-Sachs disease in Ashkenazi Jews, French Canadians of the Eastern St. Laurence River valley area of Quebec, Cajuns from Louisiana, and the Amish in Pennsylvania; β-thalassemia in Mediterranean, Middle Eastern, Transcaucasus, Central Asian, Indian, and Far Eastern groups, as well as those of African heritage; sickle cell anemia in African-Americans; α-thalassemia in those from Southeast Asia, South China, the Philippine Islands, Thailand, Greece, and Cyprus; lactase deficiency in adult Chinese and Thailanders; neural tube defects in Irish, Scots, and Welsh; phenylketonuria (PKU) in Irish, Scots, Scandinavians, Icelanders, and Polish; cystic fibrosis (CF) in Caucasians, Ashkenazi Jews, and Hispanics; and Niemann-Pick disease, type A, in Ashkenazi Jews (Hamilton & Wynshaw-Boris, 2009; Wapner, Jenkins, & Khalek, 2009).

Relevance of Genetics to Nursing

Genetic disorders span every clinical practice specialty and site, including school, clinic, office, hospital, mental health agency, and community health settings. Because the potential impact on families and the community is significant (Box 8-1), genetics must be integrated into nursing education and practice. Genetic information, technology, and testing must be incorporated in health care services.

BOX 8-1 Potential Impact of Genetic Disease on Family and Community

- Financial cost to family
- Decrease in planned family size
- Loss of geographic mobility
- Decreased opportunities for siblings
- Loss of family integrity
- Loss of career opportunities and job flexibility
- Social isolation
- Lifestyle alterations
- Reduction in contributions to their community by families
- Disruption of husband-wife or partner relationship
- Threatened family self-concept
- Coping with intolerant public attitudes
- Psychologic effects
- Stresses and uncertainty of treatment
- Physical health problems
- Loss of dreams and aspirations
- Cost to society of institutionalization or home or community care
- Cost to society because of additional problems and needs of other family members
- Cost of long-term care
- Housing and living arrangement changes

From Lashley F: *Clinical genetics in nursing practice*, ed 3, New York, 2005, Springer.

Expanded or new roles for nurses with expertise in genetics and genomics are developing in many areas of maternity and women's health nursing. These areas include but are not limited to preconception counseling and preimplantation diagnosis for patients at risk for the transmission of a genetic disorder, prenatal screening and testing, prenatal care for women with psychiatric disorders that have a genetic component such as bipolar disorder and schizophrenia, newborn screening and testing, the care of families who have lost a fetus or a child affected by a genetic condition, the identification and care of children with genetic conditions and their families, and the care of women with genetic conditions who require specialized care during pregnancy such as women with congenital heart disease, CF, Marfan syndrome *(www.marfan.org)*, and factor V Leiden.

In 2005 a panel of over 50 nursing leaders from clinical, research, and academic settings developed and came to consensus on a document, *Essential Nursing Competencies and Curricula Guidelines for Genetics and Genomics.* The competencies in the document reflect the minimal amount of genetic and genomic competency expected of all nurses. The competencies are not intended to replace or recreate current standards of practice. The document is available at *www.genome.gov/Pages/Careers/HealthProfessionalEducation/geneticscompetency.pdf.*

Genetics-related activities that all nurses should be able to provide are further delineated in the *Genetics/Genomics Nursing: Scope and Standards of Practice* (International Society of Nurses in Genetics [ISONG], 2007). This document includes standards and levels of practice for genetics nursing that were established cooperatively by ISONG and the American Nurses Association (ANA). ISONG has developed two credentials: one to recognize advanced practice nurses in genetics for their advanced knowledge, skills, and abilities; and another to recognize the special knowledge base and skills of genetics nurses who have a bachelor's degree. In addition, ISONG is working cooperatively with the American Nurses Credentialing Center to develop recognition of nurses in genetics.

Although diagnosis and treatment of genetic disorders requires medical skills, nurses with advanced preparation are assuming important roles in counseling people about genetically transmitted or genetically influenced conditions. Nurses are usually the ones who provide follow-up care and maintain contact with the patients. Community health nurses can identify groups within populations that are high risk for illness and provide care to individuals, families, and groups. They are a vital link in follow-up for newborns who may need newborn screening.

Referral to appropriate agencies is an essential part of the follow-up management. Many organizations and foundations (e.g., the Cystic Fibrosis Foundation and the Muscular Dystrophy Association) help provide services and equipment for affected children. There are also numerous parent groups in which the family can share experiences and derive mutual support from other families with similar problems.

Probably the most important of all nursing functions is providing emotional support to the family during all aspects of the counseling process. Feelings that are generated under the real or imagined threat posed by a genetic disorder are as varied as the people being counseled. Responses may include a variety of stress reactions such as apathy, denial, anger, hostility, fear, embarrassment, grief, and loss of self-esteem.

Genetic History Taking and Counseling Services

It is standard practice in obstetrics to determine whether a heritable disorder exists in a couple or in anyone in either of their families. The goal of screening is to detect or define risk for disease in low risk populations and identify those for whom diagnostic testing may be appropriate. A nurse can obtain a genetic history using a questionnaire or checklist such as the one in Fig. 8-1.

Genetic counseling that follows may occur in the office, or referral to a geneticist may be necessary. The most efficient counseling services are associated with the larger universities and major medical centers. This is also where support services are available (e.g., biochemistry and cytology laboratories), usually from a group of specialists under the leadership of a physician trained in medical genetics. Health professionals should become familiar with people who provide genetic counseling and the places that offer counseling services in their area of practice (see Community Focus box).

Individuals and families seek out or are referred for genetic counseling for a wide variety of reasons and at all stages of

evolve Critical Thinking Exercise—Genetic Counseling

Risk Factors for Genetic Disorders

Answer the following questions about risk factors. If you answer "yes" to any of them, you may be at increased risk for having a baby with a genetic disorder.

_____Will you be age 35 years or older when your baby is due?

_____Will the baby's father be age 50 years or older when your baby is due?

_____If you or the baby's father are of Mediterranean or Asian descent, do either of you or anyone in your families have thalassemia?

_____Is there a family history of neural tube defects?

_____Have you or the baby's father ever had a child with a neural tube defect?

_____Is there a family history of congenital heart defects?

_____Is there a family history of Down syndrome?

_____Have your or the baby's father ever had a child with Down syndrome?

_____If you or the baby's father are of Eastern European Jewish, French Canadian, or Cajun descent, is there a family history of Tay-Sachs disease?

_____If you or your partner are of Eastern European Jewish descent, is there a family history of Canavan disease or any other genetic disorders?

_____If you or your partner are African American, is there a family history of sickle cell disease or sickle cell trait?

_____Is there a family history of hemophilia?

_____Is there a family history of muscular dystrophy?

_____Is there a family history of cystic fibrosis?

_____Is there a family history of Huntington's disease?

_____Does anyone in your family or the family of the baby's father have cystic fibrosis?

_____Is anyone in your family or the baby's father's family mentally retarded?

_____If so, was that person tested for fragile X syndrome?

_____Do you, the baby's father, anyone in your families, or any of your children have any other genetic diseases, chromosomal disorders, or birth defects?

_____Do you have a metabolic disorder such as diabetes or phenylketonuria?

_____Do you have a history of pregnancy issues (miscarriage or stillbirth)?

Fig. 8-1 Questionnaire for identifying couples having increased risk for offspring with genetic disorders. (Courtesy American College of Obstetricians and Gynecologists [ACOG]: *Your pregnancy & birth*, ed 4, Washington, DC, 2005, ACOG.)

COMMUNITY FOCUS

Resources for Families with Children with Genetic Disorders

Select an organization that is specific to a genetic disorder (e.g., neurofibromatosis, Marfan syndrome, Down syndrome). Access the website for the organization. What services and resources are available for families? Are these services and resources free, or must the family pay for them? Is there a branch of the organization available in your city? If there is not branch of the organization available in your city, where could families go for information and assistance? For your selected genetic disorder, prepare a list of resources for families with a child with the disorder.

their lives. Some seek preconception or prenatal information; others are referred after the birth of a child with a birth defect or a suspected genetic condition; still others seek information because they have a family history of a genetic condition. Regardless of the setting or the individual and family's stage of life, genetic counseling should be offered and available to all individuals and families who have questions about genetics and their health.

Estimation of Risk

Most families with a history of genetic disease want an answer to the following question: What is the chance that our future children will have this disease? Because the answer to this question may have profound implications for individual family members and the family as a whole, health care professionals must be able to answer this question as accurately as they can in a timely manner.

If a couple has not yet had children but are known to be at risk for having children with a genetic disease, they will be given an *occurrence risk.* Once the mating of a couple has produced one or more children with a genetic disease, the couple will be given a *recurrence risk.* Both occurrence and recurrence risks are determined by the mode of inheritance for the genetic disease in question. For genetic diseases caused by a factor that segregates during cell division (genes and chromosomes), risk can be estimated with a high degree of accuracy by application of the Mendelian principles *(www.ncbi.nlm.nih.gov/entrez/query.fcgi?db=OMIM)* (see Community Focus box).

COMMUNITY FOCUS

Internet Resources on Genetics

Identify two websites for resources on genetics for parents from a search of the Internet. Access the sites.

- Compare and contrast the appearance, readability, and information contained in the sites.
- To whom would you recommend these sites?
- Is the information contained culturally relevant?
- What information would parents need?
- How could you as a nurse use this information?

In an autosomal dominant disorder, both the occurrence and recurrence risk is 50%, or one in two, that a subsequent offspring will be affected. The recurrence risk for autosomal recessive disorders is 25% or one-in-four. For X-linked disorders, recurrence is related to the sex of the child. Translocation chromosomes have a high risk of recurrence.

The risk of recurrence for multifactorial conditions can be estimated empirically. An empiric risk is based not on genetics theory but rather on experience and observation of the disorder in other families. Recurrence risks are determined by applying the frequency of a similar disorder in other families to the case under consideration.

Disorders in which a subsequent pregnancy would carry no more risk than there is for pregnancy alone (estimated at 1 in 30) include those resulting from isolated incidences not likely to be present in another pregnancy. These disorders include maternal infections (e.g., rubella and toxoplasmosis), maternal ingestion of drugs, most chromosomal abnormalities, and a disorder determined to be the result of a fresh mutation.

Interpretation of Risk

The guiding principle for genetics counselors has traditionally been the principle of nondirectiveness. According to the principle of nondirectiveness, the individual who is providing genetics counseling respects the right of the individual or family being counseled to make autonomous decisions. Counselors using a nondirective approach avoid making recommendations, and they try to communicate genetics information in an unbiased manner. The first step in providing nondirective counseling is becoming aware of one's own values and beliefs. Another important step is recognizing how one's values and beliefs can influence or interfere with the communication of genetics information.

The counselor provides appropriate information about the nature of the disorder, the extent of the risks in the specific case, the probable consequences, and (if appropriate) alternative options available; however, the final decision to become pregnant or to continue a pregnancy must be left to the family. An important nursing role is reinforcing the information the families are given and continuing to interpret this information on their level of understanding.

An important concept that must be emphasized to families is that *each pregnancy is an independent event.* For example, in monogenic disorders in which the risk factor is one in four that the child will be affected, the risk remains the same no matter how many affected children are already in the family. Families may make the erroneous assumption that the presence of one affected child ensures that the next three will be free of the disorder. However, "chance has no memory." The risk is one in four for each pregnancy. On the other hand, in a family with a child who has a disorder with multifactorial causes, the risk increases with each subsequent child born with the disorder.

The Human Genome Project

The Human Genome Project was a publicly funded international effort coordinated by the National Institutes of Health and the U.S. Department of Energy *(www.doegenomes.org).*

When the Human Genome Project was initiated in 1990, the ultimate goal of the project was to map the human genome (the complete set of genetic instructions in the nucleus of each human cell) by 2005. Considering that the human genome consists of approximately 3 billion base pairs of DNA, many people considered this to be an impossible task. However, on June 26, 2000, an announcement was made at the White House that a working draft of the Human Genome Project had been completed by two groups: scientists working on the Human Genome Project and scientists from Celera Genomics, a privately funded effort. Simultaneous publications describing the initial draft sequence and analysis of the human genome appeared in *Nature* (International Human Genome Sequencing Consortium, 2001) and *Science* (Venter et al, 2001) on February 12, 2001. A substantially complete version of the human genome was announced in April 2003 *(www.genome.gov/11006929).*

Two key findings from initial efforts to sequence and analyze the human genome are that (1) all humans are 99.9% identical at the DNA level, and (2) approximately 20,000 to 25,000 genes (pieces or sequences of DNA that contain information needed to make proteins) make up the human genome. This is a much smaller number than the 80,000 to 150,000 estimated by scientists. A new explanation for human complexity, given the relatively small number of genes, is that humans use their genes more efficiently. Humans are able to do much more with their genes than other species. Instead of producing only one protein per gene, most human genes produce at least three proteins.

Initial efforts to sequence and analyze the human genome have proven invaluable in the identification of genes involved in disease and in the development of genetic tests. Hundreds of genes involved in diseases such as Huntington's disease (HD), breast cancer, colon cancer, Alzheimer's disease, achondroplasia, and CF have been identified. The number of commercially available genetic tests continues to increase and can be found at GeneTests *(www.genetests.org).*

Genetic Testing

Genetic testing involves the analysis of human DNA, ribonucleic acid (RNA), chromosomes (threadlike packages of genes and other DNA in the nucleus of a cell), or proteins to detect abnormalities related to an inherited condition. Genetic tests can be used to examine directly the DNA and RNA that make up a gene (direct or molecular testing), look at markers that are coinherited with a gene that causes a genetic condition (linkage analysis), examine the protein products of genes (biochemical testing), or examine chromosomes (cytogenetic testing).

Most of the genetic tests now being offered in clinical practice are tests for single-gene disorders in patients with clinical symptoms or who have a family history of a genetic disease. Some of these genetic tests are prenatal tests or tests used to identify the genetic status of a pregnancy at risk for a genetic condition. Current prenatal testing options include maternal serum screening (a blood test used to see if a pregnant woman is at increased risk for carrying a fetus with a neural tube defect or a chromosome abnormality such as Down syndrome) and invasive procedures (amniocentesis and chorionic villus sampling). Other tests are carrier screening tests, which are used to identify individuals who have a gene mutation for a genetic condition but do not show symptoms of the condition because it is a condition that is inherited in an autosomal recessive form (e.g., CF, sickle cell disease, Tay-Sachs disease).

Another type of genetic testing is predictive testing, which is used to clarify the genetic status of asymptomatic family members. The two types of predictive testing are presymptomatic and predispositional. Mutation analysis for HD, a neurodegenerative disorder, is an example of presymptomatic testing. If the gene mutation for HD is present, symptoms of HD are certain to appear if the individual lives long enough. Testing for a BRCA1 gene mutation to determine breast cancer susceptibility is an example of predispositional testing. Predispositional testing differs from presymptomatic testing in that a positive result (indicating that a BRCA1 mutation is present) does not indicate a 100% risk of developing the condition (breast cancer).

In addition to using genetic tests to test for single-gene disorders, they are being used for population-based screening (e.g., state-mandated newborn screening for PKU and other inborn errors of metabolism [IEMs]) and to test for common complex diseases such as cancer and cardiovascular conditions. Genetic tests also are being used to determine paternity, identify victims of war and other tragedies, and profile criminals *(www.genetests.org).*

Factors Influencing the Decision to Undergo Genetic Testing

Decisions about genetic testing are shaped, and in many instances constrained, by factors such as social norms, where care is received, and socioeconomic status. Most pregnant women in the United States now have at least one ultrasound examination, many undergo some type of multiple-marker screening, and a growing number undergo other types of prenatal testing. The range of prenatal testing options available to a pregnant woman and her family may vary significantly, based on where the pregnant woman receives prenatal care and her socioeconomic status. Certain types of prenatal testing may not be available in smaller communities and rural settings (e.g., chorionic villus sampling and fluorescent in situ hybridization analysis. In addition, certain types of genetic testing may not be offered in conservative medical communities (e.g., preimplantation diagnosis). Some types of genetic testing are expensive and typically not covered by health insurance. Because of this, these tests may be available only to a relatively small number of individuals and families—those who can afford to pay for them.

Cultural and ethnic differences also have a significant impact on decisions about genetic testing. When prenatal diagnosis was first introduced, the principal constituency was a self-selected group of Caucasian, well-informed, middle- to upper-class women. Today the widespread use of genetic testing has introduced prenatal testing to new groups of women, women who had not previously considered genetics services. The fact that many of the women currently undergoing prenatal testing may not share mainstream United States views about the role of medicine and prenatal care, the meaning of disability, or how to respond to scientific risks and uncertainties further amplifies the complexity of ethical issues associated with prenatal testing.

There are ethical dimensions in the decision to be tested. The decision to undergo testing is seldom an autonomous decision based solely on the needs and preferences of the individual being tested. Instead it is often a decision based on feelings of responsibility and commitment to others (Van Riper, 2005; Van Riper & McKinnon, 2004). For example, a woman who is receiving treatment for breast cancer may undergo BRCA1/BRCA2 mutation testing not because she wants to find out if she carries a BRCA1 or BRCA2 mutation, but because her two unaffected sisters have asked her to be tested and she feels a sense of responsibility and commitment to them. A female airline pilot with a family history of HD who has no desire to find out if she has the gene mutation associated with HD may undergo mutation analysis for HD because she believes that she has an obligation to her family, her employer, and the people who fly with her.

Pharmacogenomics

One of the immediate clinical applications of the Human Genome Project may be pharmacogenomics, or the use of genetic information to individualize drug therapy. There has been speculation that pharmacogenomics may become part of standard practice for a large number of disorders and drugs by 2020 (Collins & McKusick, 2001). The expectation is that by identifying common variants in genes that are associated with the likelihood of a good or bad response to a specific drug, drug prescriptions can be individualized on the basis of the individual's unique genetic makeup. A primary benefit of pharmacogenomics is the potential to reduce adverse drug reactions.

Gene Therapy (Gene Transfer)

The aim of gene therapy is to correct defective genes that are responsible for disease development. The most common technique is to insert a normal gene in a location within the genome to replace a gene that is nonfunctional *(www.ornl.gov/sci/techresources/Human_Genome/medicine/genetherapy.shtml)*. In the early 1990s there was a great deal of optimism about the possibility of using genetic information to provide quick solutions to a long list of health problems. Although the early optimism about gene therapy was probably never fully justified, it is likely that the development of safer and more effective methods for gene delivery will ensure a significant role for gene therapy in the treatment of some diseases. Major challenges include targeting the right gene to the right location in the right cells, expressing the transferred gene at the right time, and minimizing adverse reactions. No human gene therapy product has yet been approved by the Food and Drug Administration for sale. Current research includes treatment for inherited blindness, lung cancer tumors, melanoma, myeloid disorders, deafness, sickle cell disease, and other blood disorders.

Ethical, Legal, and Social Implications

Because of widespread concern about misuse of the information gained through genetics research, 5% of the Human Genome Project budget was designated for the study of the Ethical, Legal, and Social Implications (ELSIs) of human genome research. Two large ELSI programs were created to identify, analyze, and address the ELSIs of human genome research at the same time that the basic science issues were being studied. The two ELSI programs are separate but complementary. During the past decade issues of high priority for these programs have been privacy and fairness in the use and interpretation of genetic information, clinical integration of new genetic technologies, issues surrounding genetics research such as possible discrimination and stigmatization, and education for professionals and the general public about genetics, genetics health care, and the ELSIs of human genome research. Both ELSI programs have excellent websites that include educational information, as well as links to other informative sites *(www.genome.gov/10001618; www.ornl.gov/sci/techresources/Human_Genome/elsi/elsi.shtml)*.

These programs address the potential that genetic information may be used to discriminate against individuals or for eugenic purposes. Informed consent is very difficult to ensure when some of the outcomes, benefits, and risks of genetic testing remain unknown. Continued awareness of and vigilance against such misuse of information is the collective responsibility of health care providers, ethicists, and society. Some ethical considerations include: What is normal or a disability and who decides? Are disabilities diseases that need to be prevented or cured? Who will have access to these expensive therapies; who will pay for them?

Clinical Genetics

Genetic Transmission

Human development is a complicated process that depends on the systematic unraveling of instructions found in the genetic material of the egg and the sperm. Development from conception to birth of a normal, healthy baby occurs without incident in most cases; however, occasionally some anomaly in the genetic code of the embryo creates a birth defect or disorder. The science of genetics seeks to explain the underlying causes of congenital disorders (disorders present at birth) and the patterns in which inherited disorders are passed from generation to generation.

Genes and Chromosomes

The hereditary material carried in the nucleus of each somatic (body) cell determines an individual's physical characteristics. This material, called *DNA*, forms threadlike strands known as chromosomes. Each chromosome is composed of many smaller segments of DNA referred to as genes. Genes or combinations of genes contain coded information that determines an individual's unique characteristics. The code consists of the specific linear order of the molecules that combine to form the strands of DNA. Genes control both the types of proteins that are made and the rate at which they are produced. Genes never act in isolation; they always interact with other genes and the environment.

All normal human somatic cells contain 46 chromosomes arranged as 23 pairs of homologous (matched) chromosomes; one chromosome of each pair is inherited from each parent. There are 22 pairs of autosomes, which control most traits in the body, and one pair of sex chromosomes, which determines sex and some other traits. The larger female chromosome is called the X; the smaller male chromosome is the Y. Generally the presence of a Y chromosome causes an embryo to develop as a male; in the absence of a Y chromosome, the individual develops as a female. Thus in a normal female the homologous pair of sex chromosomes are XX, and in a normal male the homologous pair are XY.

Homologous chromosomes (except the X and Y chromosomes in males) have the same number and arrangement of genes. In other words, if an autosome has a gene for hair color, its partner also has a gene for hair color—in the same location on the chromosome. Although both genes code for hair color, they may not code for the same hair color. Genes at corresponding loci on homologous chromosomes that code for different forms or variations of the same trait are called *alleles*. An individual with two copies of the same allele for a given trait is said to be homozygous for that trait. With two different alleles the person is heterozygous for the trait.

The term *genotype* typically is used to refer to the genetic makeup of an individual when discussing a specific gene pair, but at times genotype is used to refer to an individual's entire genetic makeup or all the genes that the individual can pass on to future generations. Phenotype refers to the observable expression of an individual's genotype such as physical features, a biochemical or molecular trait, and even a psychologic trait. A trait or disorder is considered dominant if it is expressed or phenotypically apparent when only one copy of the gene is present. It is considered recessive if it is expressed only when two copies of the gene are present.

As more is learned about genetics, the concepts of dominance and recessivity have become more complex, especially in X-linked disorders (Lashley, 2005). For example, traits considered to be recessive may be expressed even when only one copy of a gene located on the X chromosome is present. This occurs frequently in males because males have only one X chromosome; thus they have only one copy of the genes located on the X chromosome. Whichever gene is present on the one X chromosome determines which trait is expressed. Conversely, females have two X chromosomes; thus they have two copies of the genes located on the X chromosome. However, in any female somatic cell only one X chromosome is functioning (otherwise there would be inequality in gene dosage between males and females). This process, known as *X-inactivation* or the *Lyon hypothesis*, is generally a random occurrence (i.e., there is a 50:50 chance as to whether the maternal X or the paternal X is inactivated). Occasionally the percentage of cells that have the X with an abnormal or mutant gene is very high. This helps explain why hemophilia, an X-linked recessive disorder, can clinically manifest itself in a female known to be a heterozygous carrier (a female who has only one copy of the gene mutation). It also helps explain why traditional methods of carrier detection are less effective for X-linked recessive disorders; the possible range for enzyme activity values can vary greatly, depending on which X chromosome is inactivated.

Chromosome Abnormalities

Chromosome abnormalities are a major cause of reproductive loss, congenital problems, and gynecologic disorders and account for approximately 4% to 7% of perinatal deaths and 0.5% to 1% of infants born with multiple anomalies. Errors resulting in chromosome abnormalities can occur in mitosis or meiosis. These errors can occur in either the autosomes or the sex chromosomes. Even without the presence of obvious structural malformations, small deviations in chromosomes can cause problems in fetal development.

The pictorial analysis of the number, form, and size of an individual's chromosomes is known as a karyotype. Cells from any nucleated, replicating body tissue (not red blood cells, nerves, or muscles) can be used. The most commonly used tissues are white blood cells and fetal cells in amniotic fluid. The cells are grown in a culture and arrested when they are in metaphase and then dropped onto a slide. This breaks the cell membranes and spreads the chromosomes, making them easier to visualize. The cells are stained with special stains (e.g., Giemsa stain) that create striping or "banding" patterns. These patterns aid in the analysis because they are consistent from person to person. Once the chromosome spreads are photographed or scanned by a computer, they are cut out and arranged in a specific numeric order according to their length and shape. They are numbered from largest to smallest, 1 to 22, and the sex chromosomes are designated by the letter X or Y. Each chromosome is divided into two "arms" designated by *p* (short arm) and *q* (long arm). A female karyotype is designated as 46, XX, and a male karyotype is designated as 46, XY. Fig. 8-2 illustrates the chromosomes in a body cell and a karyotype. Karyotypes can be used to determine the sex of a child and the presence of any gross chromosomal abnormalities.

Autosome Abnormalities

Autosome abnormalities involve differences in the number or structure of autosome chromosomes (pairs 1 to 22) resulting from unequal distribution of the genetic material during gamete (egg and sperm) formation.

Abnormalities of Chromosome Number Euploidy is the term used to denote the correct number of chromosomes. Deviations from the correct number of chromosomes or the diploid number (2N, 46 chromosomes) can be one of two types: (1) polyploidy, in which the deviation is an exact multiple of the haploid number of chromosomes or one chromosome set (23 chromosomes); or (2) aneuploidy, in which the numeric deviation is not an exact multiple of the haploid set (Lashley, 2005). A triploid (3N) cell is an example of a polyploidy. It has 69 chromosomes. A tetraploid (4N) cell, also an example of a polyploidy, has 92 chromosomes.

Aneuploidy is the most commonly identified chromosome abnormality in humans. It occurs in at least 5% of all clinically recognized pregnancies, and it is the leading known cause of pregnancy loss. Aneuploidy also is the leading genetic cause of mental retardation. The two most common aneuploid conditions are monosomies and trisomies. A monosomy is the product of the union between a normal gamete and a gamete that is missing a chromosome. Monosomic individuals only have 45 chromosomes in each of their cells. The product of the union of a normal gamete with a gamete containing an extra chromosome is a trisomy. Trisomies are more common than monosomies. Trisomic individuals have 47 chromosomes in each of their cells.

Limited data are available concerning the origin of monosomies because, when an embryo is missing an autosomal chromosome, the embryo never survives. Although a great

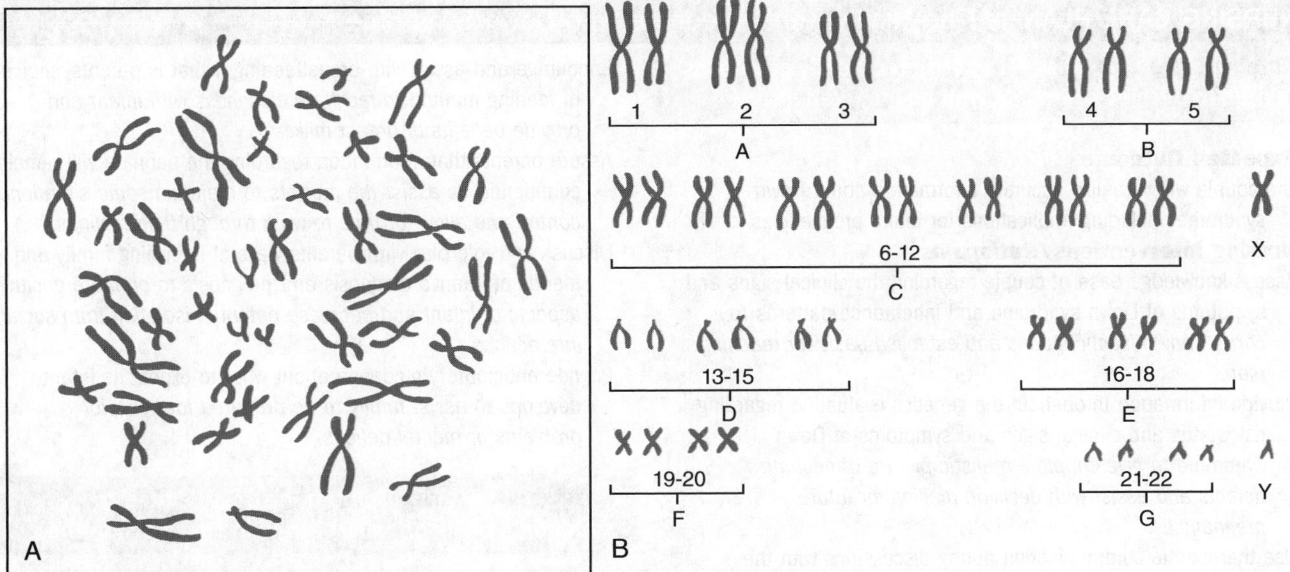

Fig. 8-2 Chromosomes during cell division. **A**, Example of photomicrograph. **B**, Chromosomes arranged in karyotype; female and male sex-determining chromosomes.

deal of variation exists among trisomies with regard to the parent and stage of origin of the extra chromosome, most trisomies are maternal meiosis I errors. This means that most trisomies are caused by nondisjunction during the first meiotic division (i.e., one pair of chromosomes fails to separate). One of the resulting cells contains two chromosomes, and the other contains none.

The most common trisomal abnormality is Down syndrome, or trisomy 21 (47,XX+21, female with Down syndrome; or 47,XY+21, male with Down syndrome). Although the risk of having a child with Down syndrome increases with maternal age (incidence is approximately 1 in 1200 for a 25-year-old woman; 1 in 350 for a 35-year-old woman; and 1 in 30 for a 45-year-old woman), children with Down syndrome can be born to mothers of any age. Eighty percent of children with Down syndrome are born to mothers younger than 35 years (National Down Syndrome Society, 2009a; National Down Syndrome Society, 2009b). The average age of mothers when they give birth to children with Down syndrome is about 27 years. The risk of a mother having a second child with Down syndrome is about 1% when the cause of the Down syndrome is trisomy 21 (see Nursing Care Plan) (see also Fig. 42-6 and discussion in Chapter 42).

Other autosomal trisomies that have been identified are trisomy 18 (Edwards' syndrome) and trisomy 13 (Patau's syndrome). Infants with trisomy 18 and trisomy 13 are usually severely to profoundly retarded. Although both conditions have a very poor prognosis, with the vast majority of affected infants dying within the first few days of life, a significant percentage of these infants survive the first 6 months to 1 year of life; some children with trisomy 18 and trisomy 13 have lived beyond 10 years of age.

Nondisjunction can also occur during mitosis. If this occurs early in development when cell lines are forming, the individual has a mixture of cells, some with a normal number of chromosomes and others either missing a chromosome or containing an extra chromosome. This condition is known as mosaicism. Mosaicism in autosomes is most commonly seen as another form of Down syndrome. Approximately 1% to 2% of individuals with Down syndrome have mosaic Down syndrome.

Abnormalities of Chromosome Structure Structural abnormalities can occur in any chromosome. Types of structural abnormalities include translocation, duplication, deletion, microdeletion, and inversion. Translocation occurs when there is an exchange of chromosome material between two chromosomes. Exposure to certain drugs, viruses, and radiation can cause translocations, but often they arise for no apparent reason. Thus, instead of two normal pairs of chromosomes, the individual has one normal chromosome of each pair and a third chromosome that is a fusion of the other two chromosomes. As long as all genetic material is retained in the cell, the individual is unaffected but is a carrier of a balanced translocation.

If a gamete receives the two normal chromosomes or the fused chromosome, the resulting offspring will be clinically normal. If the gamete receives one of the two normal chromosomes and the fused version, the resulting offspring will have an extra copy of one of the chromosomes. This condition is called an *unbalanced translocation* and often has serious clinical effects.

Whenever a portion of a chromosome is deleted from one chromosome and added to another, the gamete produced may have either extra copies of genes or too few copies. The clinical effects produced may be mild or severe, depending on the amount of genetic material involved. Two of the more common conditions are the deletion of the short arm of chromosome 5 (cri du chat syndrome) and the deletion of the long arm of chromosome 18.

Sex Chromosome Abnormalities

Several sex chromosome abnormalities are caused by nondisjunction during gametogenesis in either parent. The most common deviation in females is Turner's syndrome, or

NURSING CARE PLAN The Family with a Neonate with Down Syndrome

Nursing Diagnosis: Risk for interrupted family processes related to birth of a neonate with an inherited disorder

Expected Outcome

The couple will verbalize accurate information about Down syndrome, including implications for future pregnancies.

Nursing Interventions/*Rationales*

Assess knowledge base of couple regarding the clinical signs and symptoms of Down syndrome and inheritance patterns *to correct any misconceptions and establish basis for teaching plan.*

Provide information throughout the genetics evaluation regarding risk status and clinical signs and symptoms of Down syndrome *to give couple a realistic picture of neonate's defects and assist with decision making for future pregnancies.*

Use therapeutic communication during discussions with the couple *to provide opportunity for expression of concern.*

Refer to support groups, social services, or counseling *to assist with family cohesive actions and decision making.*

Refer to child development specialist *to provide family with realistic expectations regarding cognitive and behavioral differences of child with Down syndrome.*

Nursing Diagnosis: Situational low self-esteem related to diagnosis of inherited disorder as evidenced by parents' statements of guilt and shame

Expected Outcome

The parents will express an increased number of positive statements regarding the birth of a neonate with Down syndrome.

Nursing Interventions/*Rationales*

Assist parents to list strengths and coping strategies that have been helpful in past situations *to use appropriate strategies during this situational crisis.*

Encourage expression of feelings using therapeutic communication *to provide clarification and emotional support.*

Clarify and provide information regarding Down syndrome *to decrease feelings of guilt and gradually increase feelings of positive self-esteem.*

Refer for further counseling as needed *to provide more in-depth and ongoing support.*

Nursing Diagnosis: Risk for impaired parenting related to birth of neonate with Down syndrome

Expected Outcome

Parents demonstrate competent skills in parenting a child with Down syndrome and willingness to care for neonate.

Nursing Interventions/*Rationales*

Assist parents to see and describe normal aspects of infant *to promote bonding.*

Encourage and assist with breastfeeding if that is parents' choice of feeding method *to facilitate closeness with infant and provide benefits of breast milk.*

Assure parents that information regarding the neonate will remain confidential *to assist the parents to maintain some situational control and allow for time to work through their feelings.*

Discuss and role play with parents ways of informing family and friends of infant's diagnosis and prognosis *to promote positive aspects of infant and decrease potential isolation from social interactions.*

Provide anticipatory guidance about what to expect as infant develops *to assist family to be prepared for behavior problems or mental deficits.*

Nursing Diagnosis: Spiritual distress related to situational crisis of child born with Down syndrome

Expected Outcome

Parents seek appropriate support persons (e.g., family members, priest, minister, rabbi) for assistance.

Nursing Interventions/*Rationales*

Listen for cues indicative of parents' feelings ("Why did God do this to us?") *to identify messages indicating spiritual distress.*

Acknowledge parents' spiritual concerns and encourage expression of feelings *to help build a therapeutic relationship.*

Facilitate visits from clergy and provide privacy during visits *to demonstrate respect for parents' relationship with clergy.*

Encourage parents to discuss concerns with clergy *to use expert spiritual care resources to help the parents.*

Facilitate interaction with family members and other support persons *to encourage expressions of concern and seek comfort.*

Nursing Diagnosis: Risk for social isolation related to full-time caretaking responsibilities for a neonate with Down syndrome

Expected Outcome

Parents will describe a plan to use resources to prevent social isolation.

Nursing Interventions/*Rationales*

Provide opportunity for parents to express feelings about caring for a neonate with Down syndrome *to facilitate effective communication and trust.*

Discuss with parents their expectations about caring for the neonate *to identify potential areas of concern.*

Assist parents to identify potential caregiving resources *to permit parents to return to a routine at home.*

Identify appropriate referrals for home care *to provide continuity of care.*

Refer to support groups of parents of children with Down syndrome *to enlist support, understanding, and strategies for coping.*

evolve Nursing Care Plan–The Family with a Neonate with Down Syndrome

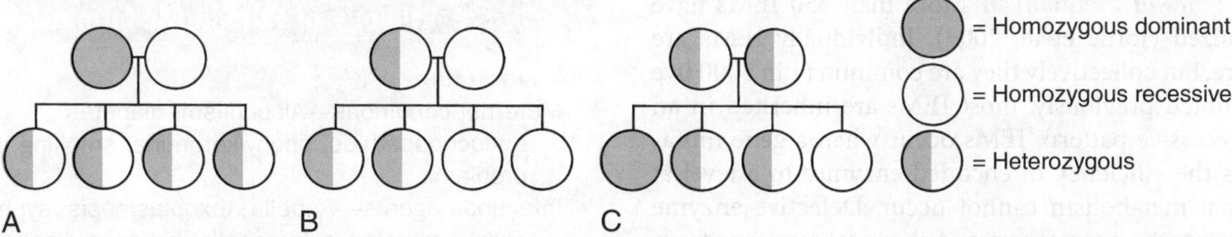

Fig. 8-3 Possible offspring in three types of matings. **A,** Homozygous-dominant parent and homozygous-recessive parent. Children: all heterozygous, displaying dominant trait. **B,** Heterozygous parent and homozygous-recessive parent. Children: 50% heterozygous, displaying dominant trait; 50% homozygous, displaying recessive trait. **C,** Both parents heterozygous. Children: 25% homozygous, displaying dominant trait; 25% homozygous, displaying recessive trait; 50% heterozygous, displaying dominant trait.

monosomy X (45,X). The affected female exhibits juvenile external genitalia with undeveloped ovaries. She is usually short in stature with webbing of the neck and lymphedema of her hands and feet. Intelligence may be impaired. Most affected embryos miscarry spontaneously.

The most common deviation in males is Klinefelter's syndrome, or trisomy XXY. The affected male has poorly developed secondary sexual characteristics and small testes. He is infertile, usually tall, and effeminate and may be slow to learn. Males who have mosaic Klinefelter's syndrome may be fertile.

Patterns of Genetic Transmission

Heritable characteristics are those that can be passed on to offspring. The patterns by which genetic material is transmitted to the next generation are affected by the number of genes involved in the expression of the trait. Many phenotypic characteristics result from two or more genes on different chromosomes acting together (referred to as multifactorial inheritance); others are controlled by a single gene (unifactorial inheritance). Specialists in genetics (e.g., geneticists, genetics counselors, and nurses with advanced expertise in genetics) predict the probability of the presence of an abnormal gene from the known occurrence of the trait in the individual's family and the known patterns by which the trait is inherited.

Multifactorial Inheritance

Most common congenital malformations result from multifactorial inheritance, a combination of genetic and environmental factors. Examples are cleft lip, cleft palate, congenital heart disease, neural tube defects, and pyloric stenosis. Each malformation may range from mild to severe, depending on the number of genes for the defect present or the amount of environmental influence. A neural tube defect may range from spina bifida, a bony defect in the lumbar region of the vertebrae with little or no neurologic impairment, to anencephaly, absence of brain development, which is always fatal. Some malformations occur more often in one sex. For example, pyloric stenosis and cleft lip are more common in males, and cleft palate is more common in females.

Unifactorial Inheritance

If a single gene controls a particular trait, disorder, or defect, its pattern of inheritance is referred to as unifactorial Mendelian or single-gene inheritance. The number of single-gene disorders far exceeds the number of chromosomal abnormalities. Potential patterns of inheritance for single-gene disorders include autosomal dominant, autosomal recessive, and X-linked dominant and recessive modes of inheritance (Fig. 8-3).

Autosomal Dominant Inheritance

Autosomal dominant inheritance disorders are those in which only one copy of a variant allele is needed for phenotypic expression. The variant allele may appear as a result of a mutation, a spontaneous and permanent change in the normal gene structure. In this case the disorder occurs for the first time in the family. Usually an affected individual comes from multiple generations having the disorder (see Fig. 8-3, *B* and *C*). There is a vertical pattern of inheritance (there is no skipping of generations; if an individual has an autosomal dominant disorder such as HD, so must one of his or her parents). Males and females are affected equally.

Autosomal dominant disorders are not always expressed with the same severity of symptoms. For example, a woman who has an autosomal dominant disorder may show few symptoms and may not become aware of her diagnosis until after she gives birth to a severely affected child. Predicting whether an offspring will have a minor or severe abnormality is not possible. Examples of autosomal dominant disorders are Marfan syndrome, neurofibromatosis, myotonic dystrophy, Stickler's syndrome, Treacher Collins syndrome, and achondroplasia (dwarfism).

Autosomal Recessive Inheritance

Autosomal recessive inheritance disorders are those in which both genes of a pair must be abnormal for the disorder to be expressed. Heterozygous individuals have only one variant allele and are unaffected clinically because their normal gene overshadows the variant allele. They are known as carriers of the recessive trait. Because these recessive traits are inherited by generations of the same family, an increased incidence of the disorder occurs in consanguineous matings (closely related parents). For the trait to be expressed, two carriers must each contribute a variant allele to the offspring (see Fig. 8-3, *C*). The chance of the trait occurring in each child is 25%. A clinically normal offspring may be a carrier of the gene. Autosomal recessive disorders have a horizontal pattern of inheritance rather than the vertical pattern seen with autosomal dominant disorders (i.e., autosomal recessive disorders are usually observed in one or more siblings but not in earlier generations). Males and females are equally affected. Most IEMs such as PKU, galactosemia, maple syrup urine disease, Tay-Sachs disease, sickle cell anemia, and CF are autosomal recessive inherited disorders.

Inborn Errors of Metabolism More than 350 IEMs have been recognized (Jorde et al, 2003). Individually IEMs are relatively rare, but collectively they are common (1 in 5000 live births). As noted previously, most IEMs are inherited in an autosomal recessive pattern. IEMs occur when a gene mutation reduces the efficiency of encoded enzymes to a level at which normal metabolism cannot occur. Defective enzyme action interrupts the normal series of chemical reactions from the affected point onward. The result may be an accumulation of a damaging product such as phenylalanine in PKU or the absence of a necessary product such as the lack of melanin in albinism caused by lack of tyrosinase. Diagnostic and carrier testing are available for a growing number of IEMs. In addition, many states in the United States have started screening for specific IEMs as part of their expanded newborn screening programs using tandem mass spectrometry. However, many of the deaths caused by IEMs are the result of enzyme variants not currently screened for in many of the newborn screening programs (Jorde et al, 2003). (See Table 25-3 for screening tests for IEMs.) (See discussion of IEMs in Chapter 25.)

X-Linked Dominant Inheritance

X-linked dominant inheritance disorders occur in males and heterozygous females; but because of X inactivation, affected females are usually less severely affected than affected males, and they are more likely to transmit the variant allele to their offspring (Lashley, 2005). Heterozygous females have a 50% chance of transmitting the variant allele to each offspring. The variant allele is often lethal in affected males since, unlike affected females, they have no normal gene. Mating of an affected male and an unaffected female is uncommon as a result of the tendency for the variant allele to be lethal in affected males. Relatively few X-linked dominant disorders have been identified. Two examples are vitamin D–resistant rickets and fragile X syndrome. (See discussion in Chapter 42.)

X-Linked Recessive Inheritance

Abnormal genes for X-linked recessive inheritance disorders are carried on the X chromosome. Females may be heterozygous or homozygous for traits carried on the X chromosome because they have two X chromosomes. Males are hemizygous because they have only one X chromosome carrying genes, with no alleles on the Y chromosome. Therefore X-linked recessive disorders are most often manifested in the male, with the abnormal gene on his single X chromosome. Hemophilia, color blindness, and Duchenne muscular dystrophy are all X-linked recessive disorders.

The male receives the disease-associated allele from his carrier mother on her affected X chromosome. Female carriers (those heterozygous for the trait) have a 50% probability of transmitting the disease-associated allele to each offspring. An affected male can pass the disease-associated allele to his daughters but not to his sons. The daughters will be carriers of the trait if they receive a normal gene on the X chromosome from their mother. They will be affected only if they receive a disease-associated allele on the X chromosome from both their mother and their father.

Nongenetic Factors Influencing Development

Not all congenital disorders are inherited. Congenital means that the condition was present at birth. Some congenital malformations may be the result of teratogens (i.e., environmental substances or exposures that result in functional or structural disability). In contrast to other forms of developmental disabilities, disabilities caused by teratogens are in theory totally preventable. Known human teratogens are drugs and chemicals, infections, exposure to radiation, and certain maternal conditions such as diabetes and PKU (Box 8-2). A teratogen has the greatest effect on the organs and parts of an embryo during its periods of rapid differentiation. This occurs during the embryonic period, specifically from days 15 to 60. During the first 2 weeks of development, teratogens either have no effect on the embryo or have effects so severe that they cause miscarriage. Brain growth and development continue during the fetal period, and teratogens can severely affect mental development throughout gestation (Fig. 8-4).

BOX 8-2 Etiology of Human Malformations

Environmental

Maternal conditions—Alcoholism, diabetes, endocrinopathies, phenylketonuria, smoking, nutritional problems

Infectious agents—Rubella, toxoplasmosis, syphilis, herpes simplex, cytomegalic inclusion disease, varicella, Venezuelan equine encephalitis

Mechanical problems (deformations)—Amniotic band constrictions, umbilical cord constraint, disparity in uterine size and uterine contents

Chemicals, drugs, radiation, hyperthermia

Genetic

Single-gene disorders

Chromosomal abnormalities

Unknown

Polygenic/multifactorial (gene-environment interactions)

"Spontaneous" errors of development

Other unknowns

Modified from Hudgins L, Cassidy SB: Congenital anomalies. In RJ Martin, AA Fanaroff, MC Walsh (editors): *Fanaroff and Martin's neonatal-perinatal medicine: diseases of the fetus and infant*, ed 8, St Louis, 2006, Mosby.

In addition to genetic makeup and the influence of teratogens, the adequacy of maternal nutrition influences development. The embryo and fetus must obtain the nutrients they need from the mother's diet; they cannot tap the maternal reserves. Malnutrition during pregnancy produces low-birth-weight newborns who are susceptible to infection. Malnutrition also affects brain development during the latter half of gestation and may result in learning disabilities in the child. Inadequate folic acid is associated with neural tube defects.

Behavioral Genetics

The field of human behavioral genetics seeks to understand genetic and environmental influences on variations in human behavior (McInerney, 2007). Behavior involves multiple genes. Study of behavior and genes requires analysis of families and populations to compare those who have the trait with those who do not. The result is an estimate of the amount of variation in the population attributable to genetic factors. The findings of this research have significant political and social

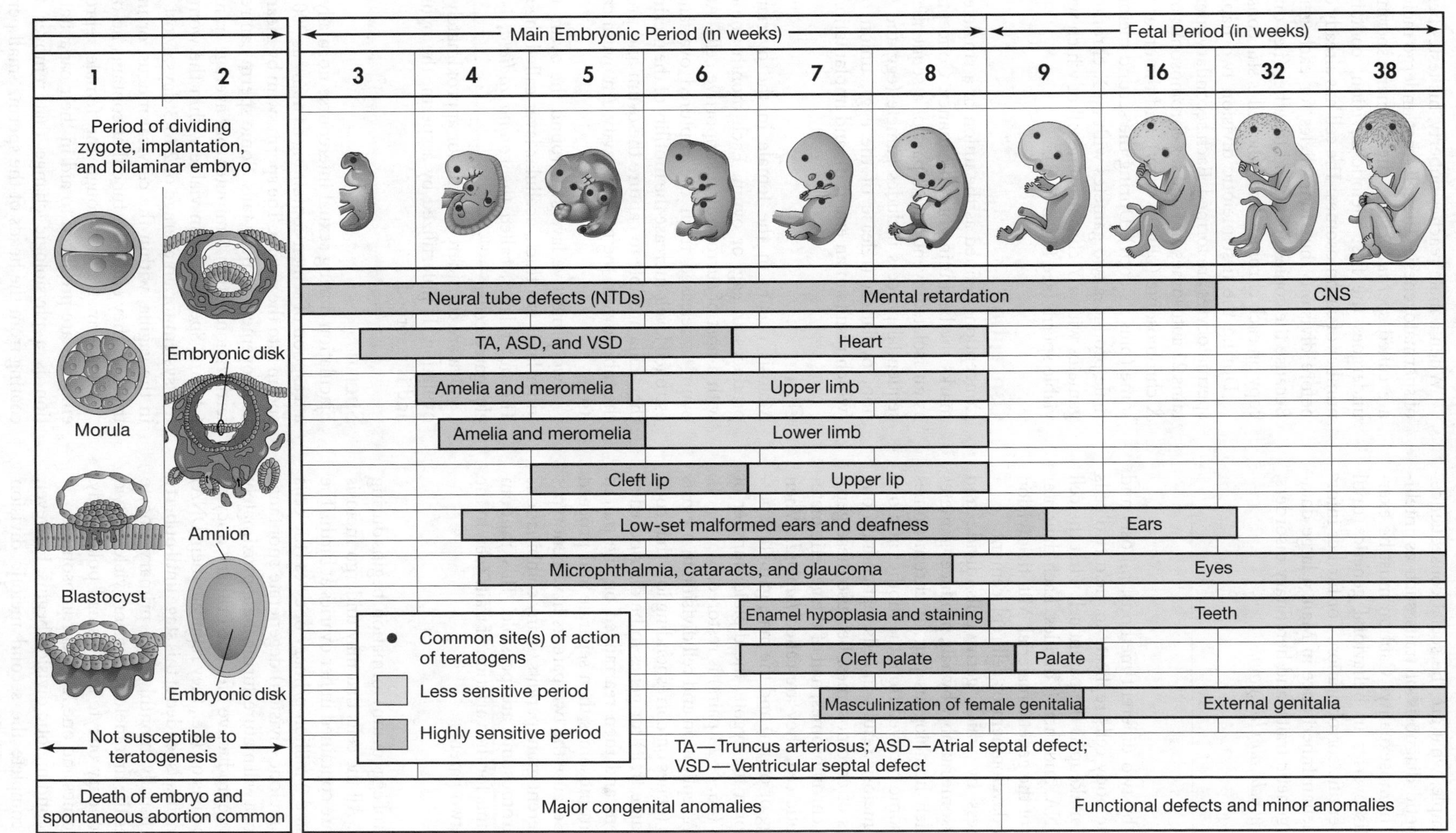

Fig. 8-4 Sensitive, or critical, periods in human development. *Dark color* denotes highly sensitive periods; *light color* indicates stages that are less sensitive to teratogens. (From Moore KL, Persaud TVN: *Before we are born: essentials of embryology and birth defects*, ed 7, Philadelphia, 2008, Saunders.)

implications. For example, what are the social consequences of determining a genetic diagnosis of traits such as intelligence, criminality, or homosexuality? Caution must be exercised in accepting discoveries in behavioral genetics until there is substantial scientific corroboration. For further information, Online Mendelian Inheritance in Man, a large database involving genes, genetic traits, and hereditary disorders, can be consulted *(www.ncbi.nlm.hih.gov).*

Conception

Cell Division

Cells are reproduced by two different methods: mitosis and meiosis. In mitosis the body cells replicate to yield two cells with the same genetic makeup as the parent cell. First the cell makes a copy of its DNA, and then it divides. Each daughter cell receives one copy of the genetic material. Mitotic division facilitates growth and development or cell replacement.

Meiosis, the process by which germ cells divide and decrease their chromosome number by half, produces gametes (eggs and sperm). Each homologous pair of chromosomes contains one chromosome received from the mother and one from the father; thus meiosis results in cells that contain one of each of the 23 pairs of chromosomes. Because these germ cells contain 23 single chromosomes, half of the genetic material of a normal somatic cell, they are called *haploid*. When the female gamete (egg or ovum) and the male gamete (spermatozoon) unite to form the zygote, the diploid number of human chromosomes (46, or 23 pairs) is restored.

The process of DNA replication and cell division in meiosis allows different alleles (genes on corresponding loci that code for variations of the same trait) for genes to be distributed at random by each parent and then rearranged on the paired chromosomes. The chromosomes then separate and proceed to different gametes. Because the two parents have genotypes derived from four different grandparents, many combinations of genes on each chromosome are possible. This random mixing of alleles accounts for the variation of traits seen in the offspring of the same two parents.

Gametogenesis

Oogenesis, the process of egg (ovum) formation, begins during fetal life of the female. All the cells that may undergo meiosis in a woman's lifetime are contained in her ovaries at birth. The majority of the estimated 2 million primary oocytes (the cells that undergo the first meiotic division) degenerate spontaneously. Only 400 to 500 ova will mature during the approximately 35 years of a woman's reproductive life. The primary oocytes begin the first meiotic division (i.e., they replicate their DNA) during fetal life but remain suspended at this stage until puberty (Fig. 8-5, *A*). Then, usually monthly, one primary oocyte matures and completes the first meiotic division, yielding two unequal cells: the secondary oocyte and a small polar body. Both contain 22 autosomes and one X sex chromosome.

At ovulation the second meiotic division begins. However, the ovum does not complete the second meiotic division unless fertilization occurs. At fertilization a second polar body and the zygote (the united egg and sperm) are produced (see Fig. 8-5, *C*). The three polar bodies degenerate. If fertilization does not occur, the ovum also degenerates.

evolve Animation: Pathway of Ovum

evolve Animation: Pathway of Sperm

evolve Animation: Spermatozoa

evolve Animation: Spermatogenesis

When a male reaches puberty, his testes begin the process of spermatogenesis. The cells that undergo meiosis in the male are called *spermatocytes*. The primary spermatocyte, which undergoes the first meiotic division, contains the diploid number of chromosomes. The cell has already copied its DNA before division; thus four alleles for each gene are present. Because the copies are bound together (i.e., one allele plus its copy on each chromosome), the cell is still considered diploid.

During the first meiotic division two haploid secondary spermatocytes are formed. Each secondary spermatocyte contains 22 autosomes and one sex chromosome; one contains the X chromosome (plus its copy), and the other the Y chromosome (plus its copy). During the second meiotic division the male produces two gametes with an X chromosome and two gametes with a Y chromosome, all of which will develop into viable sperm (see Fig. 8-5, *B*).

Conception

Conception, defined as the union of a single egg and sperm, marks the beginning of a pregnancy. Conception occurs not as an isolated event but as part of a sequential process. This sequential process includes gamete (egg and sperm) formation, ovulation (release of the egg), union of the gametes (which results in an embryo), and implantation in the uterus.

Ovum

Meiosis occurs in the female in the ovarian follicles and produces an egg, or ovum. Each month one ovum matures with a host of surrounding supportive cells. At ovulation the ovum is released from the ruptured ovarian follicle. High estrogen levels increase the motility of the uterine tubes so that their cilia are able to capture the ovum and propel it through the tube toward the uterine cavity. An ovum cannot move by itself.

Two protective layers surround the ovum (Fig. 8-6). The inner layer is a thick, acellular layer called the *zona pellucida*. The outer layer, called the *corona radiata*, is composed of elongated cells.

Ova are considered fertile for approximately 24 hours after ovulation. If unfertilized by a sperm, the ovum degenerates and is resorbed.

Sperm

Ejaculation during sexual intercourse normally propels about a teaspoon of semen containing as many as 200 to 500 million sperm into the vagina. The sperm swim by means of the flagellar movement of their tails. Some sperm can reach the site of fertilization within 5 minutes, but average transit time is 4 to 6 hours. Sperm remain viable within the woman's reproductive system for an average of 2 to 3 days. Most sperm are lost in the vagina, within the cervical mucus, or in the endometrium or they enter the tube that contains no ovum.

As sperm travel through the female reproductive tract, enzymes are produced to aid in their capacitation. Capacitation is a physiologic change that removes the protective coating from the heads of the sperm. Small perforations then form in the acrosome (a cap on the sperm) and allow enzymes (e.g., hyaluronidase) to escape (see Fig. 8-6). These enzymes are necessary for the sperm to penetrate the protective layers of the ovum before fertilization.

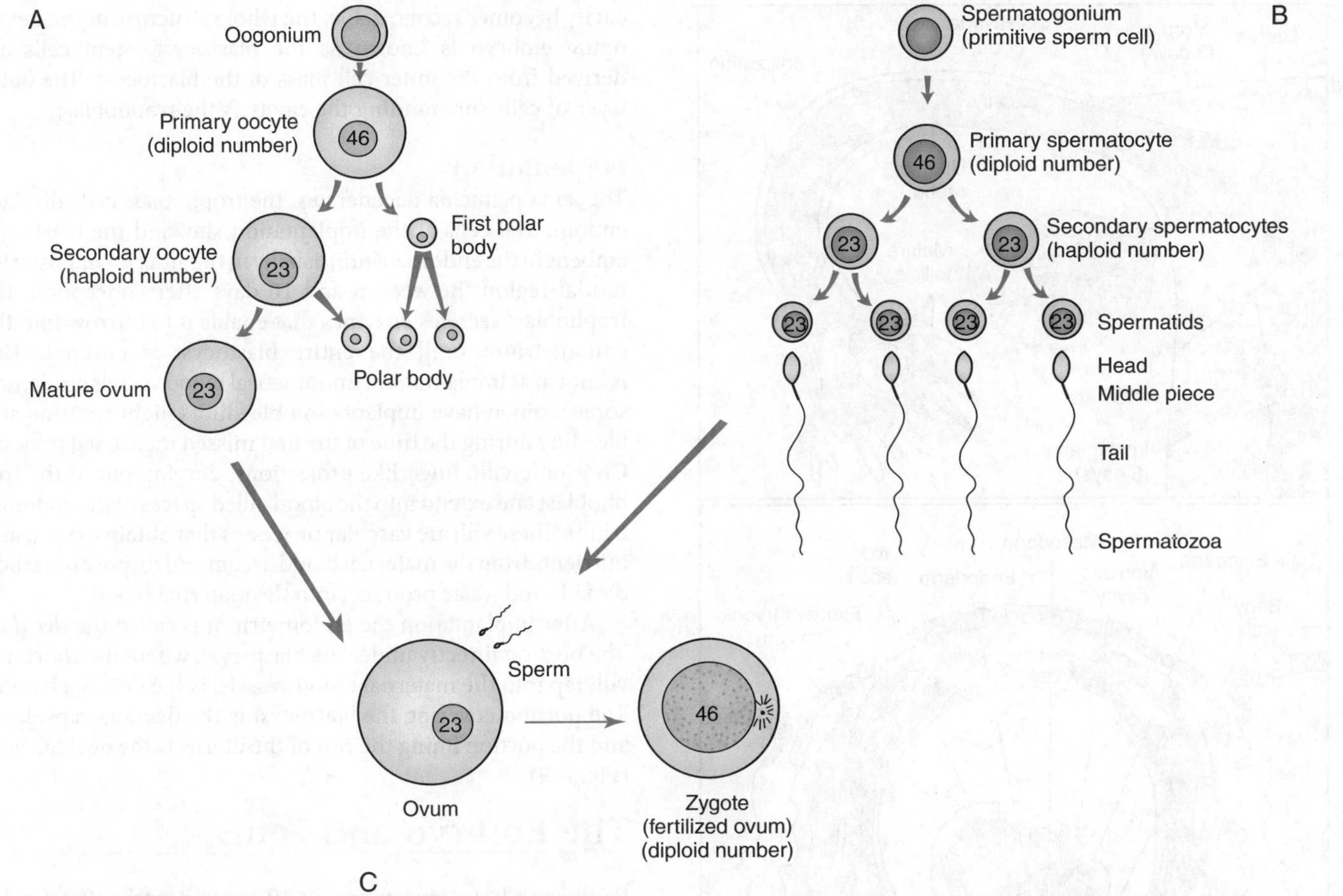

Fig. 8-5 Gametogenesis and fertilization. **A,** Oogenesis. Gametogenesis in the female produces one mature ovum and three polar bodies. Note relative difference in overall size between ovum and sperm. **B,** Spermatogenesis. Gametogenesis in the male produces four mature gametes, the sperm. **C,** Fertilization results in the single-cell zygote and restoration of the diploid number of chromosomes.

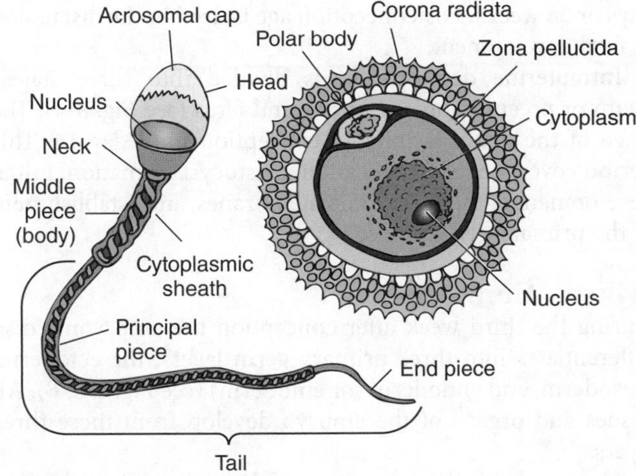

Fig. 8-6 Sperm and ovum.

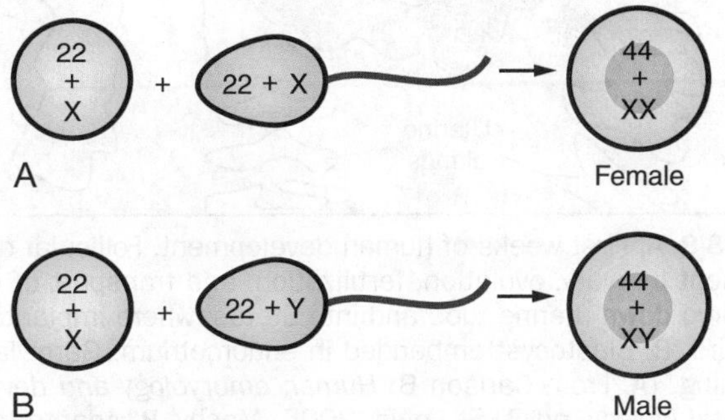

Fig. 8-7 Fertilization. **A,** Ovum fertilized by X-bearing sperm to form female zygote. **B,** Ovum fertilized by Y-bearing sperm to form male zygote.

Fertilization

Fertilization takes place in the ampulla (the outer third) of the uterine tube. When a sperm successfully penetrates the membrane surrounding the ovum, both sperm and ovum are enclosed within the membrane, and the membrane becomes impenetrable to other sperm; this process is termed the *zona reaction.* The second meiotic division of the secondary oocyte is then completed, and the ovum nucleus becomes the female pronucleus. The head of the sperm enlarges to become the male pronucleus, and the tail degenerates. The nuclei fuse, and the chromosomes combine, restoring the diploid number (46) (Fig. 8-7). Conception, the formation of the zygote (the first cell of the new individual), has been achieved.

Mitotic cellular replication, called *cleavage*, begins as the zygote travels the length of the uterine tube into the uterus. This voyage takes 3 to 4 days. Because the fertilized egg divides rapidly with no increase in size, successively smaller cells,

evolve Animation: Testes

evolve Animation: Oogenesis and Meiosis

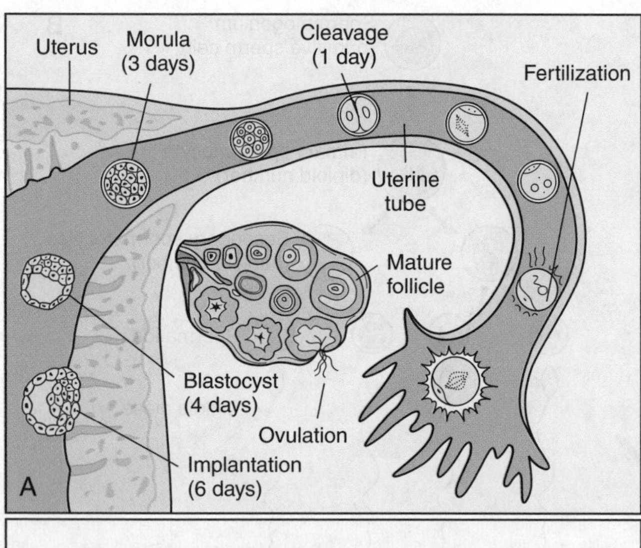

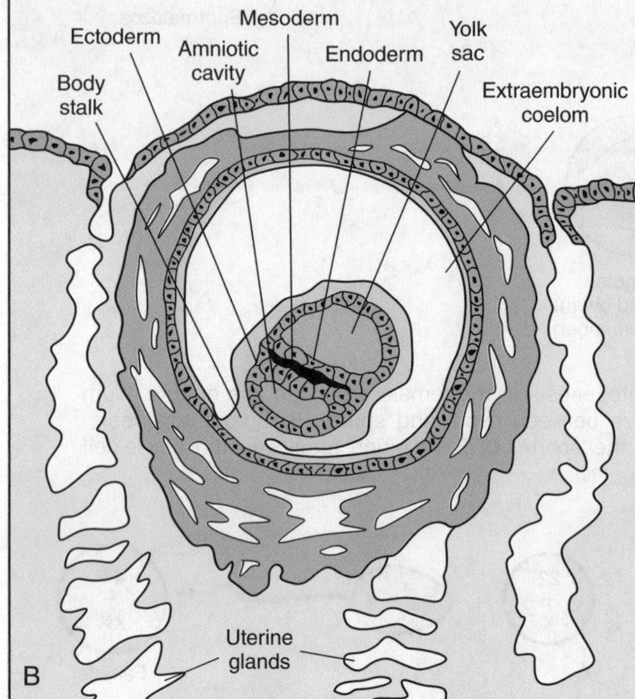

Fig. 8-8 A, First weeks of human development. Follicular development in ovary, ovulation, fertilization, and transport of early embryo down uterine tube and into uterus, where implantation occurs. **B,** Blastocyst embedded in endometrium. Germ layers forming. (**A,** From Carlson B: *Human embryology and developmental biology*, ed 3, St Louis, 2005, Mosby. **B,** Adapted from Langley L et al: *Dynamic human anatomy and physiology*, ed 5, New York, 1980, McGraw-Hill.)

called *blastomeres*, are formed with each division. A 16-cell morula, a solid ball of cells, is produced within 3 days and is still surrounded by the protective zona pellucida (Fig. 8-8, *A*). Further development occurs as the morula floats freely within the uterus. Fluid passes through the zona pellucida into the intercellular spaces between the blastomeres, separating them into two parts: the trophoblast (which gives rise to the placenta) and the embryoblast (which gives rise to the embryo). A cavity forms within the cell mass as the spaces come together, forming a structure called the *blastocyst cavity*. When the cavity becomes recognizable, the whole structure of the developing embryo is known as the blastocyst. Stem cells are derived from the inner cell mass of the blastocyst. The outer layer of cells surrounding the cavity is the trophoblast.

evolve Animation: Fertilization and Implantation
evolve Animation: Male Reproductive Ducts

Implantation

The zona pellucida degenerates; the trophoblast cells displace endometrial cells at the implantation site; and the blastocyst embeds in the endometrium, usually in the anterior or posterior fundal region. Between 6 and 10 days after conception, the trophoblast secretes enzymes that enable it to burrow into the endometrium until the entire blastocyst is covered. This is known as implantation. Endometrial blood vessels erode, and some women have implantation bleeding (slight spotting and bleeding during the time of the first missed menstrual period). Chorionic villi, fingerlike projections, develop out of the trophoblast and extend into the blood-filled spaces of the endometrium. These villi are vascular processes that obtain oxygen and nutrients from the maternal bloodstream and dispose of carbon dioxide and waste products into the maternal blood.

After implantation the endometrium is called the *decidua*. The portion directly under the blastocyst, where the chorionic villi tap into the maternal blood vessels, is the decidua basalis. The portion covering the blastocyst is the decidua capsularis, and the portion lining the rest of the uterus is the decidua vera (Fig. 8-9).

The Embryo and Fetus

Pregnancy lasts approximately 10 lunar months, 9 calendar months, 40 weeks, or 280 days. Length of pregnancy is computed from the first day of the last menstrual period (LMP) until the day of birth. However, conception occurs approximately 2 weeks after the first day of the LMP. Thus the postconception age of the fetus is 2 weeks less, for a total of 266 days or 38 weeks. Postconception age is used in the discussion of fetal development.

Intrauterine development is divided into three stages: ovum or preembryonic, embryo, and fetus (see Fig. 8-4). The stage of the ovum lasts from conception until day 14. This period covers cellular replication, blastocyst formation, initial development of the embryonic membranes, and establishment of the primary germ layers.

Primary Germ Layers

During the third week after conception the embryonic disk differentiates into three primary germ layers: the ectoderm, mesoderm, and endoderm (or entoderm) (see Fig. 8-8, *B*). All tissues and organs of the embryo develop from these three layers.

The ectoderm, the upper layer of the embryonic disk, gives rise to the epidermis, glands (anterior pituitary, cutaneous, and mammary), nails and hair, central and peripheral nervous systems, lens of the eye, tooth enamel, and floor of the amniotic cavity.

The mesoderm, the middle layer, develops into the bones and teeth, muscles (skeletal, smooth, and cardiac), dermis and connective tissue, cardiovascular system and spleen, and urogenital system.

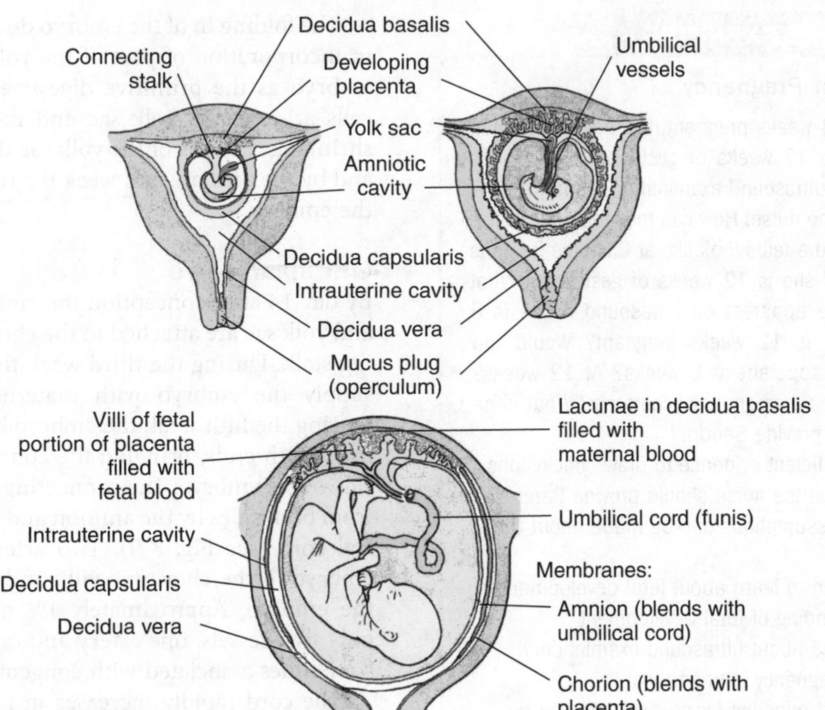

Fig. 8-9 Development of fetal membranes. Note gradual obliteration of intrauterine cavity as decidua capsularis and decidua vera meet. Also note thinning of uterine wall. Chorionic and amnionic membranes are in apposition to each other but may be peeled apart.

evolve Animation: Male External Genitalia

evolve Animation: Male Accessory Sex Glands

The endoderm, the lower layer, gives rise to the epithelium lining the respiratory and digestive tracts, including the oropharynx, liver and pancreas, urethra, bladder, and vagina. The endoderm forms the roof of the yolk sac.

Development of the Embryo

The stage of the embryo lasts from day 15 until approximately 8 weeks after conception, when the embryo measures approximately 3 cm from crown to rump. The embryonic stage is the most critical time in the development of the organ systems and the main external features. Developing areas with rapid cell division are the most vulnerable to malformation caused by environmental teratogens. At the end of the eighth week, all organ systems and external structures are present, and the embryo is unmistakably human (see Fig. 8-4 and Visible Embryo, *www.visembryo.com,* for a pictorial view of normal and abnormal development).

Membranes

At the time of implantation, two fetal membranes that will surround the developing embryo begin to form. The chorion develops from the trophoblast and contains the chorionic villi on its surface. The villi burrow into the decidua basalis and increase in size and complexity as the vascular processes develop into the placenta. The chorion becomes the covering of the fetal side of the placenta. It contains the major umbilical blood vessels that branch out over the surface of the placenta. As the embryo grows, the decidua capsularis stretches. The chorionic villi on this side atrophy and degenerate, leaving a smooth chorionic membrane.

The inner cell membrane, the amnion, develops from the interior cells of the blastocyst. The cavity that develops between this inner cell mass and the outer layer of cells (trophoblast) is the amniotic cavity (see Fig. 8-8, *B*). As it grows larger, the amnion forms on the side opposite the developing blastocyst (see Fig. 8-8, *B*, and Fig. 8-9). The developing embryo draws the amnion around itself to form a fluid-filled sac. The amnion becomes the covering of the umbilical cord and covers the chorion on the fetal surface of the placenta. As the embryo grows larger, the amnion enlarges to accommodate the embryo/fetus and the surrounding amniotic fluid. The amnion eventually comes in contact with the chorion surrounding the fetus (see Critical Thinking Exercise).

Amniotic Fluid

At first the amniotic cavity derives its fluid by diffusion from the maternal blood. The amount of fluid increases weekly, and 800 to 1200 ml of transparent liquid is normally present at term. The volume of amniotic fluid changes constantly. The fetus swallows fluid, and fluid flows into and out of the fetal lungs. The fetus urinates into the fluid, greatly increasing its volume.

The amniotic fluid serves many functions for the embryo/fetus. Amniotic fluid helps maintain a constant body temperature. It serves as a source of oral fluid and as a repository for waste. It cushions the fetus from trauma by blunting and dispersing outside forces. It allows freedom of movement for musculoskeletal development. The fluid keeps the embryo from tangling with the membranes, facilitating symmetric growth of the fetus. If the embryo does become tangled with

CRITICAL THINKING EXERCISE

Ultrasound Dating of Pregnancy

Sandra believes she is 8 weeks pregnant, but her obstetrician believes she is closer to 12 weeks of gestation. Sandra has come to the clinic for an ultrasound examination for dating. She has many questions for the nurse: How can they tell what gestation she is? What would the fetus look like at this time if she is 8 weeks of gestation? If she is 12 weeks of gestation? What fetal structures would be apparent on ultrasound if she is 8 weeks pregnant? If she is 12 weeks pregnant? Would any structural anomalies be apparent at 8 weeks? At 12 weeks? Why is it important to date a pregnancy accurately? What information should the nurse provide Sandra?

1. Evidence—Is there sufficient evidence to draw conclusions about what information the nurse should provide Sandra?
2. Assumptions—What assumptions can be made about the following factors?
   a. Sandra's motivation to learn about fetal development
   b. Sandra's understanding of fetal development
   c. Sandra's knowledge about ultrasound examinations
   d. Why dating the pregnancy is important
3. What implications and priorities for nursing care can be drawn at this time?
4. Does the evidence objectively support your conclusion?
5. Are there alternative perspectives to your conclusion?

the membranes, amputations of extremities or other deformities can occur from constricting amniotic bands.

The volume of amniotic fluid is an important factor in assessing fetal well-being. Having less than 300 ml of amniotic fluid (oligohydramnios) is associated with fetal renal abnormalities. Having more than 2 L of amniotic fluid (hydramnios) is associated with gastrointestinal and other malformations.

Amniotic fluid contains albumin, urea, uric acid, creatinine, lecithin, sphingomyelin, bilirubin, fructose, fat, leukocytes, proteins, epithelial cells, enzymes, and lanugo hair. Study of fetal cells in amniotic fluid through amniocentesis yields much information about the fetus. Genetic studies (karyotyping) provide knowledge about the sex and the number and structure of chromosomes. Other studies such as the lecithin/sphingomyelin (L/S) ratio determine the health or maturity of the fetus (see Chapter 9).

Yolk Sac

At the same time the amniotic cavity and amnion are forming, another blastocyst cavity forms on the other side of the developing embryonic disk (see Fig. 8-8, *B*). This cavity becomes surrounded by a membrane, forming the yolk sac. The yolk sac aids in transferring maternal nutrients and oxygen, which have diffused through the chorion, to the embryo. Blood vessels form to aid transport. Blood cells and plasma are manufactured in the yolk sac during the second and third weeks while uteroplacental circulation is being established and forming primitive blood cells until hematopoietic activity begins. At the end of the third week the primitive heart begins to beat and circulate the blood through the embryo, connecting stalk, chorion, and yolk sac.

The folding in of the embryo during the fourth week results in incorporation of part of the yolk sac into the body of the embryo as the primitive digestive system. Primordial germ cells arise in the yolk sac and move into the embryo. The shrinking remains of the yolk sac degenerate (see Fig. 8-8, *B*), and by the fifth or sixth week the remnant has separated from the embryo.

Umbilical Cord

By day 14 after conception the embryonic disk, amniotic sac, and yolk sac are attached to the chorionic villi by the connecting stalk. During the third week the blood vessels develop to supply the embryo with maternal nutrients and oxygen. During the fifth week the embryo has curved inward on itself from both ends, bringing the connecting stalk to the ventral side of the embryo. The connecting stalk becomes compressed from both sides by the amnion and forms the narrower umbilical cord (see Fig. 8-9). Two arteries carry blood from the embryo to the chorionic villi, and one vein returns blood to the embryo. Approximately 1% of umbilical cords contain only two vessels: one artery and one vein. This occurrence is sometimes associated with congenital malformations.

The cord rapidly increases in length. At term the cord is 2 cm in diameter and ranges from 30 to 90 cm in length (with an average of 55 cm). It twists spirally on itself and loops around the embryo/fetus. A true knot is rare, but false knots occur as folds or kinks in the cord and may jeopardize circulation to the fetus. Connective tissue called Wharton's jelly prevents compression of the blood vessels and ensures continued nourishment of the embryo/fetus. Compression can occur if the cord lies between the fetal head and the pelvis or is twisted around the fetal body. When the cord is wrapped around the fetal neck, it is called a nuchal cord.

Because the placenta develops from the chorionic villi, the umbilical cord is usually located centrally. The blood vessels are arrayed out from the center to all parts of the placenta (see Fig. 8-10, *B*). A peripheral location is less common and is known as a battledore placenta (see Fig. 14-15, *B*).

Placenta

Structure

The placenta begins to form at implantation. During the third week after conception the trophoblast cells of the chorionic villi continue to invade the decidua basalis. As the uterine capillaries are tapped, the endometrial spiral arteries fill with maternal blood. The chorionic villi grow into the spaces with two layers of cells: the outer syncytium and the inner cytotrophoblast. A third layer develops into anchoring septa, dividing the projecting decidua into separate areas called cotyledons. In each of the 15 to 20 cotyledons the chorionic villi branch out, and a complex system of fetal blood vessels forms. Each cotyledon is a functional unit. The whole structure is the placenta (Fig. 8-10).

The maternal-placental-embryonic circulation is in place by day 17, when the embryonic heart starts beating. By the end of the third week, embryonic blood is circulating between the embryo and the chorionic villi. In the intervillous spaces maternal blood supplies oxygen and nutrients to the embryonic capillaries in the villi (Fig. 8-11). Waste products and carbon dioxide diffuse into the maternal blood.

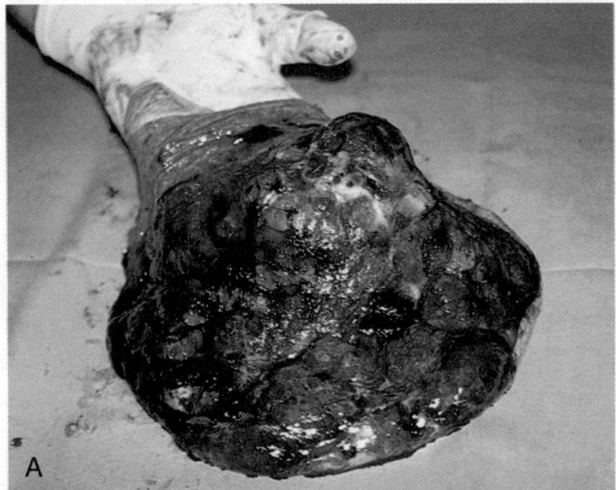

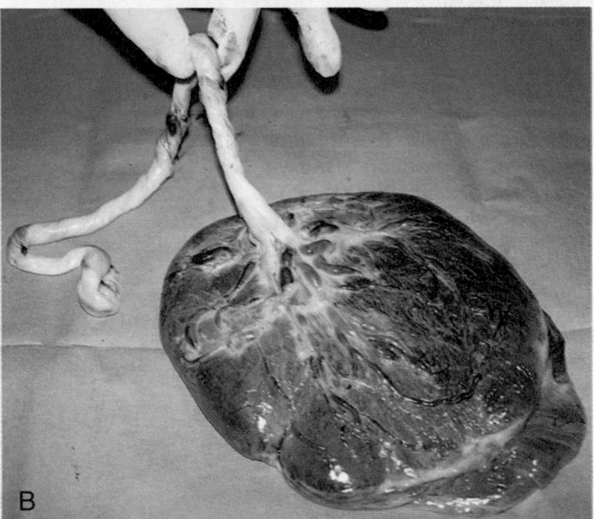

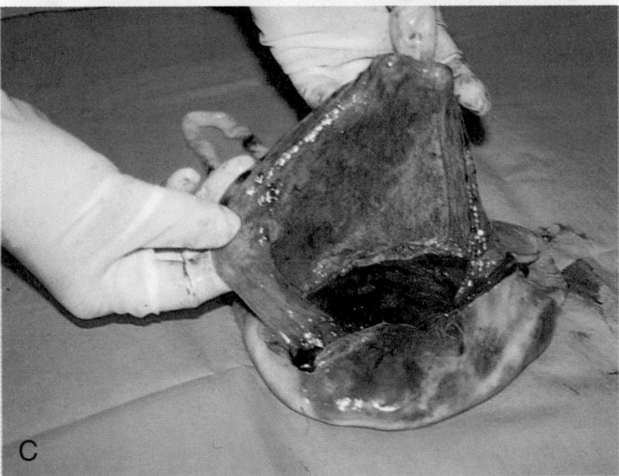

Fig. 8-10 Full-term placenta. **A,** Maternal (or uterine) surface, showing cotyledons and grooves. **B,** Fetal (or amniotic) surface, showing blood vessels running under amnion and converging to form umbilical vessels at attachment of umbilical cord. **C,** Amnion and smooth chorion are arranged to show that they are (1) fused and (2) continuous with margins of placenta. *(Courtesy Marjorie Pyle, RNC, Lifecircle, Costa Mesa, CA.)*

The placenta functions as a means of metabolic exchange. Exchange is minimal at this time because the two cell layers of the villous membrane are too thick. Permeability increases as the cytotrophoblast thins and disappears; by the fifth month only the single layer of syncytium is left between the maternal blood and the fetal capillaries. The syncytium is the functional layer of the placenta. By the eighth week genetic testing may be done on a sample of chorionic villi obtained by aspiration biopsy; however, limb defects have been associated with chorionic villi sampling done before 10 weeks. The structure of the placenta is complete by the twelfth week. The placenta continues to grow wider until 20 weeks, when it covers about half of the uterine surface. It then continues to grow thicker. The branching villi continue to develop within the body of the placenta, increasing the functional surface area.

Functions

One of the early functions of the placenta is as an endocrine gland that produces four hormones necessary to maintain the pregnancy and support the embryo/fetus. The hormones are produced in the syncytium.

The protein hormone human chorionic gonadotropin (hCG) can be detected in the maternal serum by 8 to 10 days after conception, shortly after implantation. This hormone is the basis for pregnancy tests. The hCG preserves the function of the ovarian corpus luteum, ensuring a continued supply of estrogen and progesterone needed to maintain the pregnancy. Miscarriage occurs if the corpus luteum stops functioning before the placenta can produce sufficient estrogen and progesterone. The hCG reaches its maximum level at 50 to 70 days and then begins to decrease.

The other protein hormone produced by the placenta is human chorionic somatomammotropin (hCS) or human placental lactogen (hPL). This substance is similar to a growth hormone and stimulates maternal metabolism to supply needed nutrients for fetal growth. This hormone increases the resistance to insulin, facilitates glucose transport across the placental membrane, and stimulates breast development to prepare for lactation.

The placenta eventually produces more of the steroid hormone progesterone than the corpus luteum does during the first few months of pregnancy. Progesterone maintains the endometrium, decreases the contractility of the uterus, and stimulates development of breast alveoli and maternal metabolism.

By 7 weeks after fertilization the placenta is producing most of the maternal estrogens, which are steroid hormones. The major estrogen secreted by the placenta is estriol, whereas the ovaries produce mostly estradiol. Measuring estriol levels is a clinical assay for placental functioning. Estrogen stimulates uterine growth and uteroplacental blood flow. It causes a proliferation of the breast glandular tissue and stimulates myometrial contractility. Placental estrogen production increases greatly toward the end of pregnancy. One theory for the cause of the onset of labor is the decrease in circulating levels of progesterone and the increased levels of estrogen.

The metabolic functions of the placenta are respiration, nutrition, excretion, and storage. Oxygen diffuses from the maternal blood across the placental membrane into the fetal

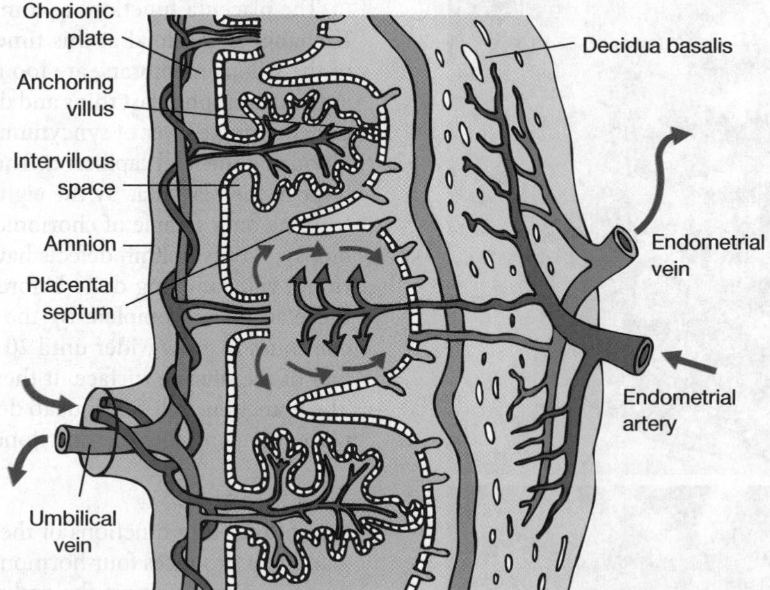

Fig. 8-11 Schematic drawing of placenta illustrating how it supplies oxygen and nutrition to embryo and removes its waste products. Deoxygenated blood leaves fetus through umbilical arteries and enters placenta, where it is oxygenated. Oxygenated blood leaves placenta through umbilical vein, which enters fetus via the umbilical cord.

blood, and carbon dioxide diffuses in the opposite direction. In this way the placenta functions as a lung for the fetus.

Carbohydrates, proteins, calcium, and iron are stored in the placenta for ready access to meet fetal needs. Water, inorganic salts, carbohydrates, proteins, fats, and vitamins pass from the maternal blood supply across the placental membrane into the fetal blood, supplying nutrition. Water and most electrolytes with a molecular weight less than 500 readily diffuse through the membrane. Hydrostatic and osmotic pressures aid in the flow of water and some solutions. Facilitated and active transport assist in the transfer of glucose, amino acids, calcium, iron, and substances with higher molecular weights. Amino acids and calcium are transported against the concentration gradient between the maternal blood and fetal blood.

The fetal concentration of glucose is lower than the glucose level in the maternal blood because of its rapid metabolism by the fetus. This fetal requirement demands larger concentrations of glucose than simple diffusion can provide. Therefore maternal glucose moves into the fetal circulation by active transport.

Pinocytosis is a mechanism used for transferring large molecules such as albumin and gamma (γ) globulins across the placental membrane. This mechanism conveys the maternal immunoglobulins that provide early passive immunity to the fetus.

Metabolic waste products of the fetus cross the placental membrane from the fetal blood into the maternal blood. The maternal kidneys then excrete them. Many viruses can cross the placental membrane and infect the fetus. Some bacteria and protozoa first infect the placenta and then infect the fetus. Drugs can also cross the placental membrane and may harm the fetus. Caffeine, alcohol, nicotine, carbon monoxide and other toxic substances in cigarette smoke, and prescription

BOX 8-3 Developmentally Toxic Exposures in Humans

- Aminopterin
- Androgens
- Angiotensin-converting enzyme inhibitors
- Carbamazepine
- Cigarette smoking
- Cocaine
- Coumarin anticoagulants
- Cytomegalovirus
- Diethylstilbestrol
- Ethanol (more than 1 drink/day)
- Etretinate
- Hyperthermia
- Iodides
- Ionizing radiation (more than 10 rads)
- Isotretinoin
- Lead
- Lithium
- Methimazole
- Methyl mercury
- Parvovirus B19
- Penicillamine
- Phenytoin
- Radioiodine
- Rubella
- Syphilis
- Tetracycline
- Thalidomide
- Toxoplasmosis
- Trimethadione
- Valproic acid
- Varicella

and recreational drugs (such as marijuana and cocaine) readily cross the placenta (Box 8-3).

Although no direct link exists between the fetal blood in the vessels of the chorionic villi and the maternal blood in the intervillous spaces, only one cell layer separates them. Breaks occasionally occur in the placental membrane. Fetal erythrocytes then leak into the maternal circulation, and the mother may develop antibodies to the fetal red blood cells. This is often the way the Rh-negative mother becomes sensitized to the erythrocytes of her Rh-positive fetus (see the discussion of isoimmunization in Chapter 28).

Although the placenta and fetus are analogous to living tissue transplants, they are not destroyed by the host mother. Either the placental hormones suppress the immunologic response, or the tissue evokes no response.

Placental function depends on the maternal blood pressure supplying the circulation. Maternal arterial blood, under pressure in the small uterine spiral arteries, spurts into the intervillous spaces (see Fig. 8-11). As long as rich arterial blood continues to be supplied, pressure is exerted on the blood already in the intervillous spaces, pushing it toward drainage by the low-pressure uterine veins. At term gestation 10% of the maternal cardiac output goes to the uterus.

If there is interference with the circulation to the placenta, the placenta cannot supply the embryo or fetus. Vasoconstriction such as that caused by hypertension or cocaine use diminishes uterine blood flow. Decreased maternal blood pressure or decreased cardiac output also diminishes uterine blood flow.

When a woman lies on her back with the pressure of the uterus compressing the vena cava, blood return to the right atrium is diminished (see Fig. 18-4 and the discussion of supine hypotension in Chapter 11). Excessive maternal exercise that diverts blood to the muscles away from the uterus compromises placental circulation. Optimal circulation is achieved when the woman is lying at rest on her side. Decreased uterine circulation may lead to intrauterine growth restriction of the fetus and infants who are small for gestational age.

Uterine contractions seem to enhance the movement of blood through the intervillous spaces, aiding placental circulation. However, prolonged contractions or too-short intervals between contractions during labor can reduce the blood flow to the placenta.

Fetal Maturation

The stage of the fetus lasts from 9 weeks (when the fetus becomes recognizable as a human being) until the pregnancy ends. Changes during the fetal period are not as dramatic because refinement of structure and function is taking place. The fetus is less vulnerable to teratogens, except for those that affect central nervous system functioning.

Viability refers to the capability of the fetus to survive outside the uterus. In the past the earliest age at which fetal survival could be expected was 28 weeks after conception. With modern technology and advances in maternal and neonatal care, viability is now possible at 20 weeks after conception (22 weeks since LMP; fetal weight of 500 g or more). The limitations on survival outside the uterus are based on central nervous system function and oxygenation capability of the lungs.

Respiratory System

The respiratory system begins development during embryonic life and continues through fetal life and into childhood. The development of the respiratory tract begins in week 4 and continues through week 17 with formation of the larynx, trachea, bronchi, and lung buds. Between 16 and 24 weeks the bronchi and terminal bronchioles enlarge, and vascular structures and primitive alveoli are formed. Between 24 weeks and term birth, more alveoli form. Specialized alveolar cells, type I and type II cells, secrete pulmonary surfactants to line the interior of the alveoli. After 32 weeks sufficient surfactant is present in developed alveoli to provide infants with a good chance of survival.

Pulmonary Surfactants

The detection of the presence of pulmonary surfactants, surface-active phospholipids, in amniotic fluid has been used to determine the degree of fetal lung maturity, or the ability of the lungs to function after birth. Lecithin (L) is the most critical alveolar surfactant required for postnatal lung expansion. It is detectable at approximately 21 weeks and increases in amount after week 24. Another pulmonary phospholipid, sphingomyelin (S), remains constant in amount. Thus the measure of lecithin in relation to sphingomyelin, or the L/S ratio, is used to determine fetal lung maturity. When the L/S ratio reaches 2:1, the infant's lungs are considered to be mature. This occurs at approximately 35 weeks of gestation.

Certain maternal conditions that cause decreased maternal placental blood flow such as maternal hypertension, placental dysfunction, infection, or corticosteroid use accelerate lung maturity. This apparently is caused by the resulting fetal hypoxia, which stresses the fetus and increases the blood levels of corticosteroids that accelerate alveolar and surfactant development.

Conditions such as gestational diabetes and chronic glomerulonephritis can retard fetal lung maturity. The use of intrabronchial synthetic surfactant in the treatment of respiratory distress syndrome in the newborn has greatly improved the chances of survival for preterm infants.

Fetal respiratory movements have been seen on ultrasound as early as week 11. These fetal respiratory movements may aid in development of the chest wall muscles and regulate lung fluid volume. The fetal lungs produce fluid that expands the air spaces in the lungs. The fluid drains into the amniotic fluid or is swallowed by the fetus.

Before birth secretion of lung fluid decreases. The normal birth process squeezes out approximately one third of the fluid. Infants of cesarean births do not benefit from this squeezing process; thus they may have more respiratory difficulty at birth. The fluid remaining in the lungs at birth is usually resorbed into the infant's bloodstream within 2 hours of birth.

Fetal Circulatory System

The cardiovascular system is the first organ system to function in the developing human. Blood vessel and blood cell formation begin in the third week and supply the embryo with oxygen and nutrients from the mother. By the end of the third week the tubular heart begins to beat, and the primitive cardiovascular system links the embryo, connecting stalk, chorion, and yolk sac. During the fourth and fifth weeks the heart develops into a four-chambered organ. By the end of the embryonic stage the heart is developmentally complete.

The fetal lungs do not function for respiratory gas exchange; thus a special circulatory pathway, the ductus arteriosus, bypasses the lungs. Oxygen-rich blood from the placenta flows rapidly through the umbilical vein into the fetal abdomen (Fig. 8-12). When the umbilical vein reaches the liver, it divides into two branches. One branch circulates some oxygenated blood through the liver. Most of the blood passes through the ductus venosus into the inferior vena cava. There it mixes with the deoxygenated blood from the fetal legs and abdomen on its way to the right atrium. Most of this blood passes straight through the right atrium and through the foramen ovale, an opening into the left atrium. There it mixes with the small amount of deoxygenated blood returning from the fetal lungs through the pulmonary veins.

The blood flows into the left ventricle and is squeezed out into the aorta, where the arteries supplying the heart, head, neck, and arms receive most of the oxygen-rich blood. This pattern of supplying the highest levels of oxygen and nutrients to the head, neck, and arms enhances the cephalocaudal (head-to-rump) development of the embryo/fetus.

Deoxygenated blood returning from the head and arms enters the right atrium through the superior vena cava. This blood is directed downward into the right ventricle, where it is squeezed into the pulmonary artery. A small amount of blood circulates through the resistant lung tissue, but the majority follows the path with less resistance through the ductus arteriosus into the aorta, distal to the point of exit of the arteries supplying the head and arms with oxygenated blood. The oxygen-poor blood flows through the abdominal aorta into the internal iliac arteries, where the umbilical arteries direct most of it back through the umbilical cord to the

evolve Animation: Maternal and Fetal Circulation

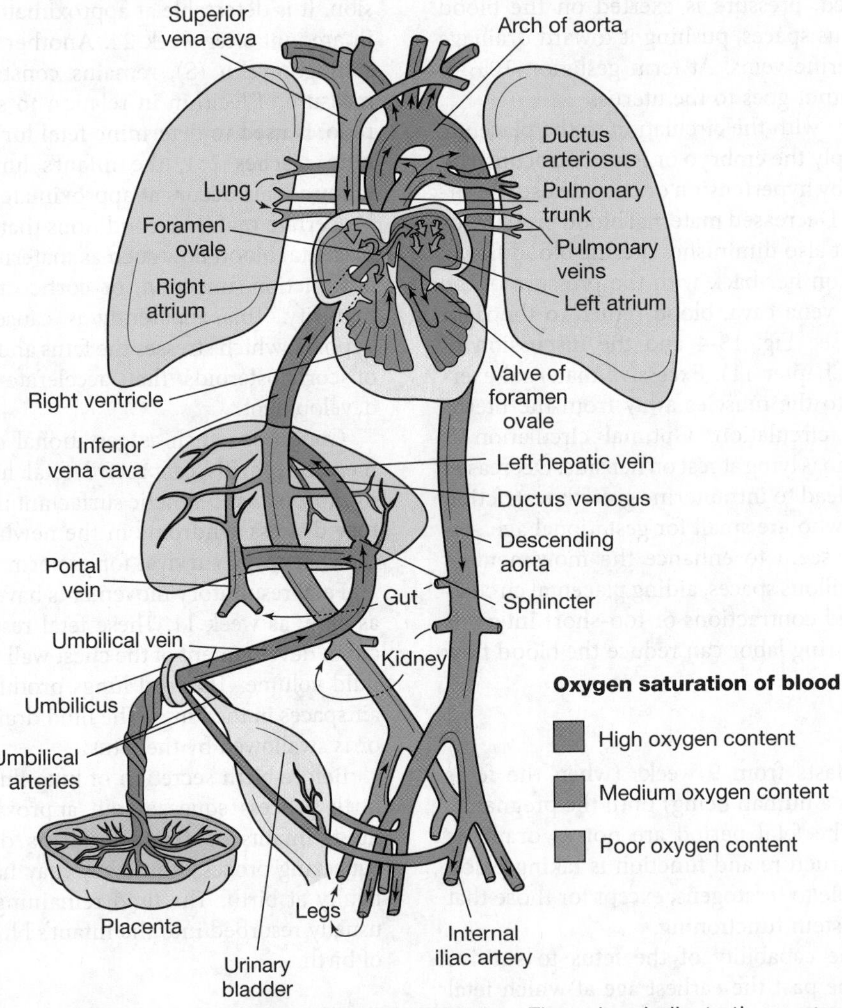

Fig. 8-12 Schematic illustration of fetal circulation. The colors indicate the oxygen saturation of the blood, and the arrows show the course of the blood from the placenta to the heart. The organs are not drawn to scale. Observe that three shunts permit most of the blood to bypass the liver and lungs: (1) ductus venosus, (2) foramen ovale, and (3) ductus arteriosus. The poorly oxygenated blood returns to the placenta for oxygen and nutrients through the umbilical arteries. (From Moore KL, Persaud TVN: *Before we are born: essentials of embryology and birth defects*, ed 7, Philadelphia, 2008, Saunders.)

placenta. There the blood gives up its wastes and carbon dioxide in exchange for nutrients and oxygen. The blood remaining in the iliac arteries flows through the fetal abdomen and legs, ultimately returning through the inferior vena cava to the heart.

The following three special characteristics enable the fetus to obtain sufficient oxygen from the maternal blood:

1. Fetal hemoglobin carries 20% to 30% more oxygen than maternal hemoglobin.
2. The hemoglobin concentration of the fetus is about 50% greater than that of the mother.
3. The fetal heart rate is 110 to 160 beats/min, making the cardiac output per unit of body weight higher than that of an adult.

Hematopoietic System

Hematopoiesis, the formation of blood, occurs in the yolk sac (see Fig. 8-8, *B*) beginning in the third week. Hematopoietic stem cells seed the fetal liver during the fifth week, and hematopoiesis begins there during the sixth week. This accounts for the relatively large size of the liver between the seventh and ninth weeks. Stem cells seed the fetal bone marrow, spleen and thymus, and lymph nodes between weeks 8 and 11 (for more information about stem cells see *http://stemcells.nih.gov/index.asp*).

The antigenic factors that determine blood type are present in the erythrocytes soon after the sixth week. For this reason the Rh-negative woman is at risk for isoimmunization in any pregnancy that lasts longer than 6 weeks after fertilization.

Hepatic System

The liver and biliary tract develop from the foregut during the fourth week of gestation. Hematopoiesis begins during the sixth week and requires that the liver be large. The embryonic liver is prominent, occupying most of the abdominal cavity. Bile, a constituent of meconium, begins to form in the twelfth week.

Glycogen is stored in the fetal liver beginning at week 9 or 10. At term glycogen stores are twice those of the adult. Glycogen is the major source of energy for the fetus and for the neonate stressed by in utero hypoxia, extrauterine loss of the maternal glucose supply, the work of breathing, or cold stress.

Iron is also stored in the fetal liver. If maternal intake is sufficient, the fetus can store enough iron to last for 5 months after birth.

During fetal life the liver does not have to conjugate bilirubin for excretion because the unconjugated bilirubin is cleared by the placenta. Therefore the glucuronyl transferase enzyme needed for conjugation is present in the fetal liver in amounts less than those required after birth. This predisposes the neonate, especially the preterm infant, to hyperbilirubinemia.

Coagulation factors II, VII, IX, and X cannot be synthesized in the fetal liver because of the lack of vitamin K synthesis in the sterile fetal gut. This coagulation deficiency persists after birth for several days and is the rationale for the prophylactic administration of vitamin K to the newborn.

Gastrointestinal System

During the fourth week the shape of the embryo changes from being almost straight to a C shape as both ends fold in toward the ventral surface. A portion of the yolk sac is incorporated into the body from head to tail as the primitive gut (digestive system).

The foregut produces the pharynx, part of the lower respiratory tract, the esophagus, the stomach, the first half of the duodenum, the liver, the pancreas, and the gallbladder. These structures evolve during the fifth and sixth weeks. Malformations that can occur in these areas include esophageal atresia, hypertrophic pyloric stenosis, duodenal stenosis or atresia, and biliary atresia.

The midgut becomes the distal half of the duodenum, the jejunum and ileum, the cecum and appendix, and the proximal half of the colon. The midgut loop projects into the umbilical cord between weeks 5 and 10. A malformation, omphalocele, results if the midgut fails to return to the abdominal cavity, causing the intestines to protrude from the umbilicus. Meckel diverticulum is the most common malformation of the midgut. It occurs when a remnant of the yolk stalk that has failed to degenerate attaches to the ileum, leaving a blind sac.

The hindgut develops into the distal half of the colon, the rectum and parts of the anal canal, the urinary bladder, and the urethra. Anorectal malformations are the most common abnormalities of the digestive system.

The fetus swallows amniotic fluid beginning in the fifth month. Gastric emptying and intestinal peristalsis occur. Fetal nutrition and elimination needs are taken care of by the placenta. As the fetus nears term, fetal waste products accumulate in the intestines as dark green–to-black, tarry meconium. Normally this substance is passed through the rectum within 24 hours of birth. Sometimes with a breech presentation or fetal hypoxia, meconium is passed in utero into the amniotic fluid. The failure to pass meconium after birth may indicate atresia somewhere in the digestive tract; an imperforate anus; or meconium ileus, in which a firm meconium plug blocks passage (seen in infants with CF).

The metabolic rate of the fetus is relatively low, but the infant has great growth and development needs. Beginning in week 9 the fetus synthesizes glycogen for storage in the liver. Between 26 and 30 weeks the fetus begins to lay down stores of brown fat in preparation for extrauterine cold stress. Thermoregulation in the neonate requires increased metabolism and adequate oxygenation.

The gastrointestinal system is mature by 36 weeks. Digestive enzymes (except pancreatic amylase and lipase) are present in sufficient quantity to facilitate digestion. The neonate cannot digest starches or fats efficiently. Little saliva is produced.

Renal System

The kidneys form during the fifth week and begin to function approximately 4 weeks later. Urine is excreted into the amniotic fluid and forms a major part of the amniotic fluid volume. Oligohydramnios is indicative of renal dysfunction. Because the placenta acts as the organ of excretion and maintains fetal water and electrolyte balance, the fetus does not need functioning kidneys while in utero. However, at birth the kidneys are required immediately for excretory and acid-base regulatory functions.

A fetal renal malformation can be diagnosed in utero. Corrective or palliative fetal surgery may treat the malformation successfully, or plans can be made for treatment immediately after birth.

At term the fetus has fully developed kidneys. However, the glomerular filtration rate is low, and the kidneys lack the ability to concentrate urine. This makes the newborn more susceptible to both overhydration and dehydration.

Most newborns void within 24 hours of birth. With the loss of the swallowed amniotic fluid and the metabolism of nutrients provided by the placenta, voidings for the first days of life are scant until fluid intake increases.

Neurologic System

The nervous system originates from the ectoderm during the third week after fertilization. The open neural tube forms during the fourth week. It initially closes at what will be the junction of the brain and spinal cord, leaving both ends open. The embryo folds in on itself lengthwise at this time, forming a head fold in the neural tube at this junction. The cranial end of the neural tube closes; then the caudal end closes. During week 5 different growth rates cause more flexures in the neural tube, delineating three brain areas: the forebrain, midbrain, and hindbrain.

The forebrain develops into the eyes (cranial nerve II) and cerebral hemispheres. The development of all areas of the cerebral cortex continues throughout fetal life and into childhood. The olfactory system (cranial nerve I) and thalamus also develop from the forebrain. Cranial nerves III and IV (oculomotor and trochlear) form from the midbrain. The hindbrain forms the medulla, the pons, the cerebellum, and the remainder of the cranial nerves. Brain waves can be recorded on an electroencephalogram by week 8.

The spinal cord develops from the long end of the neural tube. Another ectodermal structure, the neural crest, develops into the peripheral nervous system. By the eighth week nerve fibers traverse throughout the body. By week 11 or 12 the fetus makes respiratory movements, moves all extremities, and changes position in utero. The fetus can suck his or her thumb, swim in the amniotic fluid pool, and turn somersaults and sometimes ties a knot in the umbilical cord. Sometime between 16 and 20 weeks, when the movements are strong enough to be perceived by the mother as "the baby moving," quickening has occurred. The perception of movement occurs earlier in the multipara than in the primipara. The mother also becomes aware of the sleep and wake cycles of the fetus.

Sensory Awareness

Purposeful movements of the fetus have been demonstrated in response to a firm touch transmitted through the mother's abdomen. Because it can feel, the fetus requires anesthesia when invasive procedures are done.

Fetuses respond to sound by 24 weeks. Different types of music evoke different movements. The fetus can be soothed by the sound of the mother's voice. Acoustic stimulation can be used to evoke a fetal heart rate response. The fetus becomes accustomed (habituates) to noises heard repeatedly. Hearing is fully developed at birth.

The fetus is able to distinguish taste. By the fifth month, when the fetus is swallowing amniotic fluid, a sweetener added to the fluid causes the fetus to swallow faster. The fetus also reacts to temperature changes. A cold solution placed into the amniotic fluid can cause fetal hiccups.

The fetus can see. Eyes have both rods and cones in the retina by the seventh month. A bright light shone on the mother's abdomen in late pregnancy causes abrupt fetal movements. During sleep time rapid eye movements have been observed similar to those occurring in children and adults while dreaming.

At term the fetal brain is approximately one fourth the size of an adult brain. Neurologic development continues. Stressors on the fetus and neonate (e.g., chronic poor nutrition or hypoxia, drugs, environmental toxins, trauma, disease) cause damage to the central nervous system long after the vulnerable embryonic time for malformations in other organ systems. Neurologic insult can result in cerebral palsy, neuromuscular impairment, mental retardation, and learning disabilities.

Endocrine System

The thyroid gland develops along with structures in the head and neck during the third and fourth weeks. The secretion of thyroxine begins during the eighth week. Maternal thyroxine does not readily cross the placenta; therefore the fetus that does not produce thyroid hormones will be born with congenital hypothyroidism. If untreated, hypothyroidism can result in severe mental retardation. Screening for hypothyroidism is typically included in the testing when screening for PKU after birth.

The adrenal cortex is formed during the sixth week and produces hormones by the eighth or ninth week. As term approaches, the fetus produces more cortisol. This is believed to aid in initiation of labor by decreasing the maternal progesterone and stimulating production of prostaglandins.

The pancreas forms from the foregut during the fifth through eighth weeks. The islets of Langerhans develop during the twelfth week. Insulin is produced by week 20. In infants of mothers with uncontrolled diabetes, maternal hyperglycemia produces fetal hyperglycemia, stimulating hyperinsulinemia and islet cell hyperplasia. This results in a macrosomatic (large-size) fetus. The hyperinsulinemia also blocks lung maturation, placing the neonate at risk for respiratory distress and hypoglycemia when the maternal glucose source is lost at birth. Control of the maternal glucose level before and during pregnancy minimizes problems for the fetus and infant.

Reproductive System

Sex differentiation begins in the embryo during the seventh week. Female and male external genitalia are indistinguishable until after the ninth week. Distinguishing characteristics appear around the ninth week and are fully differentiated by the twelfth week. When a Y chromosome is present, testes are formed. By the end of the embryonic period testosterone is being secreted and causes formation of the male genitalia. By week 28 the testes begin descending into the scrotum. After birth low levels of testosterone continue to be secreted until the pubertal surge.

The female, with two X chromosomes, forms ovaries and female external genitalia. By the sixteenth week, oogenesis has been established. At birth the ovaries contain the female's lifetime supply of ova. Most female hormone production is delayed until puberty. However, the fetal endometrium responds to maternal hormones, and withdrawal bleeding or vaginal discharge (pseudomenstruation) may occur at birth when these hormones are lost. The high level of maternal estrogen also stimulates mammary engorgement and secretion of fluid ("witch's milk") in newborn infants of both sexes.

Musculoskeletal System

Bones and muscles develop from the mesoderm by the fourth week of embryonic development. At that time the cardiac muscle is already beating. The mesoderm next to the neural tube forms the vertebral column and ribs. The parts of the vertebral column grow toward each other to enclose the developing spinal cord. Ossification, or bone formation, begins. If there is a defect in the bony fusion, various forms of spina bifida may occur. A large defect affecting several vertebrae may allow the membranes and spinal cord to pouch out from the back, producing neurologic deficits and skeletal deformity.

The flat bones of the skull develop during the embryonic period, and ossification continues throughout childhood. At birth connective tissue sutures exist where the bones of the skull meet. The areas where more than two bones meet (called fontanels) are especially prominent. The sutures and fontanels allow the bones of the skull to mold, or move during birth, enabling the head to pass through the birth canal.

The bones of the shoulders, arms, hips, and legs appear in the sixth week as a continuous skeleton with no joints. Differentiation occurs, producing separate bones and joints. Ossification continues through childhood to allow growth. Beginning in the seventh week muscles contract spontaneously. Arm and leg movements are visible on ultrasound examination, although the mother does not perceive them until sometime between 16 and 20 weeks.

Integumentary System

The epidermis begins as a single layer of cells derived from the ectoderm at 4 weeks. By the seventh week there are two layers of cells. The cells of the superficial layer are sloughed and become mixed with the sebaceous gland secretions to form the white, cheesy vernix caseosa, the material that protects the skin of the fetus. The vernix is thick at 24 weeks but becomes scant by term.

The basal layer of the epidermis is the germinal layer, which replaces lost cells. Until 17 weeks the skin is thin and wrinkled, with blood vessels visible underneath. The skin thickens, and all layers are present at term. After 32 weeks, as subcutaneous fat is deposited under the dermis, the skin becomes less wrinkled and red in appearance.

By 16 weeks the epidermal ridges are present on the palms of the hands, the fingers, the bottom of the feet, and the toes. These handprints and footprints are unique to that infant.

Hairs form from hair bulbs in the epidermis that project into the dermis. Cells in the hair bulb keratinize to form the hair shaft. As the cells at the base of the hair shaft proliferate, the hair grows to the surface of the epithelium. Very fine hairs, called *lanugo,* appear first at 12 weeks on the eyebrows and upper lip. By week 20 they cover the entire body. At this time the eyelashes, eyebrows, and scalp hair are beginning to grow. By week 28 the scalp hair is longer than the lanugo, which thins and may disappear by term gestation.

Fingernails and toenails develop from thickened epidermis at the tips of the digits beginning during the tenth week. They grow slowly. Fingernails usually reach the fingertips by 32 weeks, and toenails reach toe tips by 36 weeks.

Immunologic System

During the third trimester albumin and globulin are present in the fetus. The only immunoglobulin that crosses the placenta, IgG, provides passive acquired immunity to specific bacterial toxins. The fetus produces IgM by the end of the first trimester. This is produced in response to blood group antigens, gram-negative enteric organisms, and some viruses. IgA is not produced by the fetus; however, colostrum, the precursor to breast milk, contains large amounts of IgA and can provide passive immunity to the neonate who is breastfed.

The normal term neonate can fight infection but not as effectively as an older child. The preterm infant is at much greater risk for infection.

Table 8-1 summarizes embryonic and fetal development.

Multifetal Pregnancy

Twins

The incidence of twinning is 1 in 43 pregnancies (Benirschke, 2009). There has been a steady rise in multiple births since 1973. This is partly attributed to delayed childbearing. The use of ovulation-enhancing drugs is also a factor.

Dizygotic Twins

When two mature ova are produced in one ovarian cycle, both have the potential to be fertilized by separate sperm. This results in two zygotes, or dizygotic twins (Fig. 8-13). There are always two amnions, two chorions, and two placentas that may be fused together. These dizygotic or fraternal twins may be the same sex or different sexes and are genetically no more alike than siblings born at different times. Dizygotic twinning occurs most often in families with a history of twinning, is more common among African-American women than Caucasian women, and is least common among Asian-American women. Dizygotic twinning increases in frequency with maternal age up to 35 years, with parity, and with the use of fertility drugs.

Monozygotic Twins

Identical or monozygotic twins develop from one fertilized ovum, which then divides (Fig. 8-14). They are the same sex and have the same genotype. If division occurs soon after fertilization, two embryos, two amnions, two chorions, and two placentas that may be fused will develop. Most often division occurs between 4 and 8 days after fertilization; there are

Table 8-1 Milestones in Human Development Before Birth Since Last Menstrual Period

4 wk	8 wk	12 wk
External Appearance		
Body flexed, C shaped; arm and leg buds present; head at right angles to body	Body fairly well formed; nose flat, eyes far apart; digits well formed; head elevating; tail almost disappeared; eyes, ears, nose, and mouth recognizable	Nails appearing; resembles a human; head erect but disproportionately large; skin pink, delicate
Crown-to-Rump Measurement; Weight		
0.4-0.5 cm; 0.4 g	2.5-3 cm; 2 g	6-9 cm; 19 g
Gastrointestinal System		
Stomach at midline and fusiform; conspicuous liver; esophagus short; intestine a short tube	Intestinal villi developing; small intestines coil within umbilical cord; palatal folds present; liver very large	Bile secreted; palatal fusion complete; intestines have withdrawn from cord and assume characteristic positions
Musculoskeletal System		
All somites present	First indication of ossification—occiput, mandible, and humerus; fetus capable of some movement; definitive muscles of trunk, limbs, and head well represented	Some bones well outlined, ossification spreading; upper cervical to lower sacral arches and bodies ossify; smooth muscle layers indicated in hollow viscera
Circulatory System		
Heart develops, double chambers visible, begins to beat; aortic arch and major veins completed	Main blood vessels assume final plan; enucleated red cells predominate in blood	Blood forming in marrow
Respiratory System		
Primary lung buds appear	Pleural and pericardial cavities forming; branching bronchioles; nostrils closed by epithelial plugs	Lungs acquire definite shape; vocal cords appear
Renal System		
Rudimentary ureteral buds appear	Earliest secretory tubules differentiating; bladder-urethra separates from rectum	Kidney able to secrete urine; bladder expands as a sac
Nervous System		
Well-marked midbrain flexure; no hindbrain or cervical flexures; neural groove closed	Cerebral cortex begins to acquire typical cells; differentiation of cerebral cortex, meninges, ventricular foramina, cerebrospinal fluid circulation; spinal cord extends entire length of spine	Brain structural configuration almost complete; cord shows cervical and lumbar enlargements; fourth ventricle foramina are developed; sucking present
Sensory Organs		
Eye and ear appearing as optic vessel and otocyst	Primordial choroid plexuses develop; ventricles large relative to cortex; development progressing; eyes converging rapidly; internal ear developing	Earliest taste buds indicated; characteristic organization of eye attained
Genital System		
Genital ridge appears (fifth week)	Testes and ovaries distinguishable; external genitalia sexless but begin to differentiate	Sex recognizable; internal and external sex organs specific

evolve Animation: First Trimester, Fetal Development

Table 8-1 Milestones in Human Development Before Birth Since Last Menstrual Period—cont'd

16 wk	20 wk	24 wk
External Appearance		
Head still dominant; face looks human; eyes, ears, and nose approach typical appearance on gross examination; arm/leg ratio proportionate; scalp hair appears	Vernix caseosa appears; lanugo appears; legs lengthen considerably; sebaceous glands appear	Body lean but fairly well proportioned; skin red and wrinkled; vernix caseosa present; sweat glands forming
Crown-to-Rump Measurement; Weight		
11.5-13.5 cm; 100 g	16-18.5 cm; 300 g	23 cm; 600 g
Gastrointestinal System		
Meconium in bowel; some enzyme secretion; anus open	Enamel and dentine depositing; ascending colon recognizable	
Musculoskeletal System		
Most bones distinctly indicated throughout body; joint cavities appear; muscular movements can be detected	Sternum ossifies; fetal movements strong enough for mother to feel	
Circulatory System		
Heart muscle well developed; blood formation active in spleen		Blood formation increases in bone marrow and decreases in liver
Respiratory System		
Elastic fibers appear in lungs; terminal and respiratory bronchioles appear	Nostrils reopen; primitive respiratory-like movements begin	Alveolar ducts and sacs present; lecithin begins to appear in amniotic fluid (wk 26-27)
Renal System		
Kidney in position; attains typical shape and plan		
Nervous System		
Cerebral lobes delineated; cerebellum assumes some prominence	Brain grossly formed; cord myelination begins; spinal cord ends at level of first sacral vertebra (S-1)	Cerebral cortex layered typically; neuronal proliferation in cerebral cortex ends
Sensory Organs		
General sense organs differentiated	Nose and ears ossify	Can hear
Genital System		
Testes in position for descent into scrotum; vagina open		Testes at inguinal ring in descent to scrotum

Continued

evolve Animation: Second Trimester, Fetal Development

Table 8-1 Milestones in Human Development Before Birth Since Last Menstrual Period—cont'd

28 wk	30-31 wk	36 AND 40 wk
External Appearance		
Lean body, less wrinkled and red; nails appear	Subcutaneous fat beginning to collect; more rounded appearance; skin pink and smooth; has assumed birth position	**36 wk**–Skin pink, body rounded; general lanugo disappearing; body usually plump **40 wk**–Skin smooth and pink; scant vernix caseosa; moderate-to-profuse hair; lanugo on shoulders and upper body only; nasal and alar cartilage apparent
Crown-to-Rump Measurement; Weight		
27 cm; 1100 g	31 cm; 1800-2100 g	**36 wk**–35 cm; 2200-2900 g **40 wk**–40 cm; 3200+ g
Musculoskeletal System		
Astragalus (talus, ankle bone) ossifies; weak, fleeting movements; minimum tone	Middle fourth phalanxes ossify; permanent teeth primordia seen; can turn head to side	**36 wk**–Distal femoral ossification centers present; sustained, definite movements; fair tone; can turn and elevate head **40 wk**–Active, sustained movement; good tone; may lift head
Respiratory System		
Lecithin forming on alveolar surfaces	L/S ratio = 1.2:1	**36 wk**–L/S ratio ≥2:1 **40 wk**–Pulmonary branching only two-thirds complete
Renal System		
		36 wk–Formation of new nephrons ceases
Nervous System		
Appearance of cerebral fissures, convolutions rapidly appearing; indefinite sleep-wake cycle; cry weak or absent; weak suck reflex		**36 wk**–End of spinal cord at level of third lumbar vertebra (L3); definite sleep-wake cycle **40 wk**–Myelination of brain begins; patterned sleep-wake cycle with alert periods; cries when hungry or uncomfortable; strong suck reflex
Sensory Organs		
Eyelids reopen; retinal layers completed, light receptive; pupils capable of reacting to light	Sense of taste present; aware of sounds outside mother's body	
Genital System		
	Testes descending to scrotum	**40 wk**–Testes in scrotum; labia majora well developed

L/S, Lecithin/sphingomyelin.

Animation: Third Trimester, Fetal Development

two embryos, two amnions, one chorion, and one placenta. Rarely division occurs after the eighth day following fertilization. In this case there are two embryos within a common amnion and a common chorion with one placenta. This often causes circulatory problems because the umbilical cords may tangle together, and one or both fetuses may die. If division occurs very late, cleavage may not be complete, and conjoined or "Siamese" twins could result (see Fig. 8-14,*C*). Monozygotic twinning occurs in approximately 1 of 250 births (Benirschke, 2009). There is no association with race, heredity, maternal age, or parity. Fertility drugs also increase the incidence of monozygotic twinning.

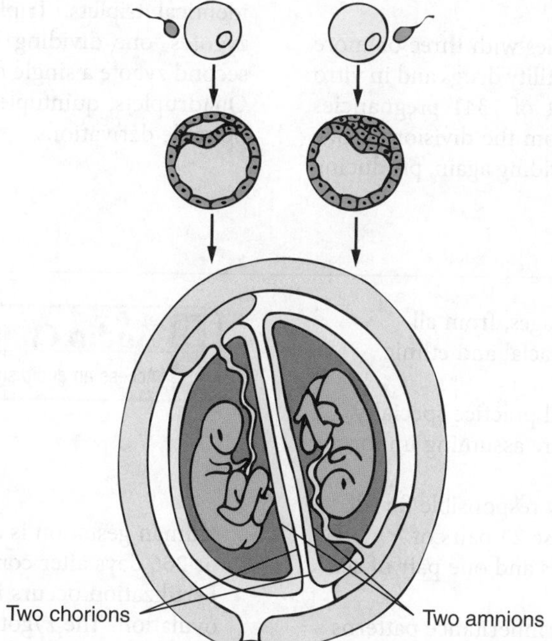

Fig. 8-13 Formation of dizygotic twins. There is fertilization of two ova, two implantations, two placentas, two chorions, and two amnions.

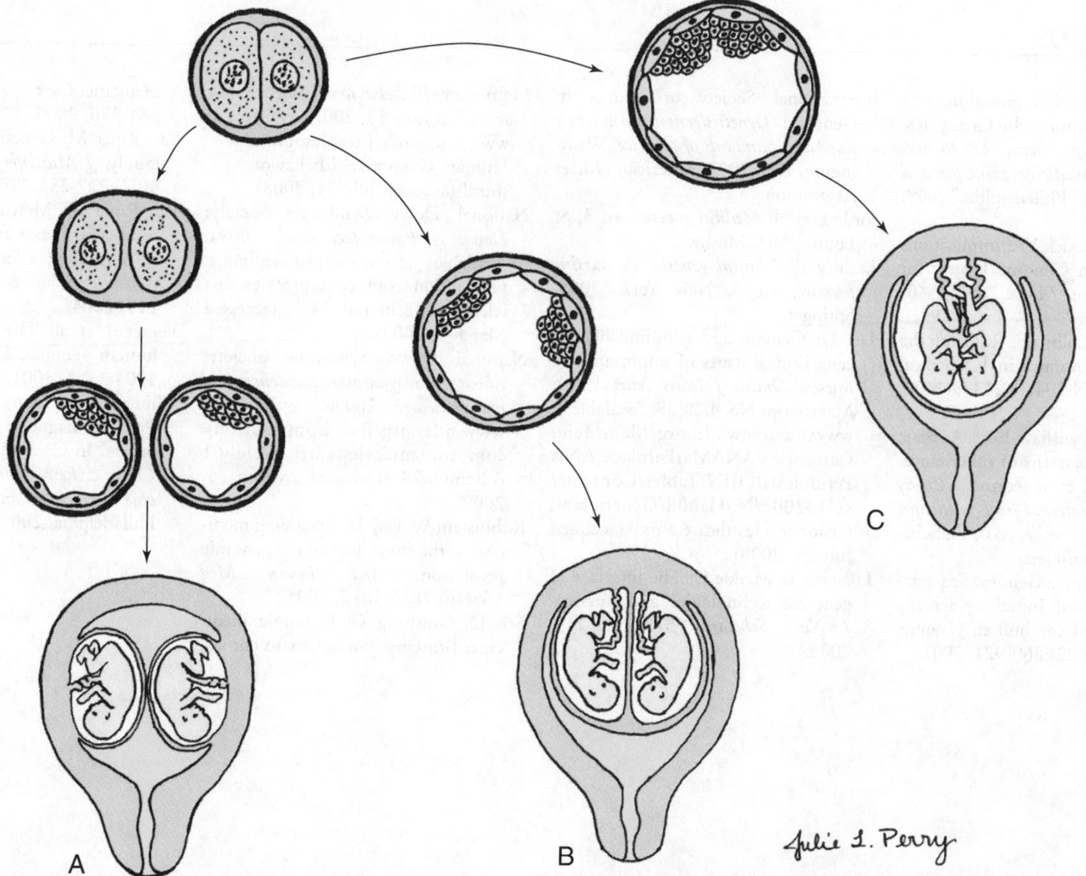

Fig. 8-14 Formation of monozygotic twins. **A**, One fertilization: blastomeres separate, resulting in two implantations, two placentas, and two sets of membranes. **B**, One blastomere with two inner cell masses, one fused placenta, one chorion, and separate amnions. **C**, One blastomere with incomplete separation of cell mass, resulting in conjoined twins.

Other Multifetal Pregnancies

The occurrence of multifetal pregnancies with three or more fetuses has increased with the use of fertility drugs and in vitro fertilization. Triplets occur in about 1 of 1341 pregnancies (Benirschke, 2009). They can occur from the division of one zygote into two, with one of the two dividing again, producing identical triplets. Triplets can also be produced from two zygotes, one dividing into a set of identical twins and the second zygote a single fraternal sibling, or from three zygotes. Quadruplets, quintuplets, sextuplets, and so on have similar possible derivations.

Key Points

- Genetic disease affects people of all ages, from all socioeconomic levels, and from all racial and ethnic backgrounds.
- Genetic disorders span every clinical practice specialty.
- Nurses with advanced preparation are assuming important roles in genetic counseling.
- Genes are the basic units of heredity responsible for all human characteristics. They comprise 23 pairs of chromosomes: 22 pairs of autosomes and one pair of sex chromosomes.
- Genetic disorders follow Mendelian inheritance patterns of dominance, segregation, and independent assortment of normal genetic transmission.
- Multifactorial inheritance includes both genetic and environmental contributions.

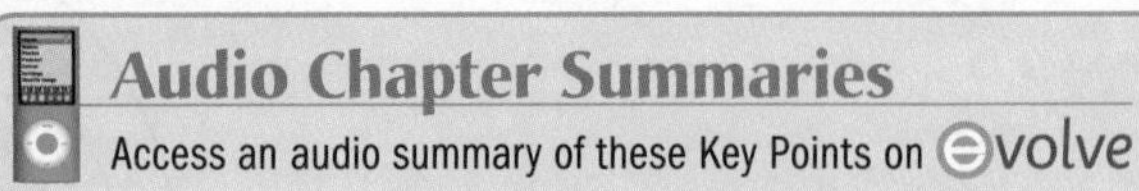
Audio Chapter Summaries
Access an audio summary of these Key Points on evolve

- Human gestation is approximately 280 days after the LMP or 266 days after conception.
- Fertilization occurs in the uterine tube within 24 hours of ovulation. The zygote undergoes mitotic divisions, creating a 16-cell morula.
- Critical periods occur in human development during which the embryo/fetus is vulnerable to environmental teratogens.

References

Benirschke K: Multiple gestation. The biology of twinning. In Creasy RK et al (editors): *Creasy & Resnik's maternal-fetal medicine: principles and practice*, ed 6, Philadelphia, 2009, Saunders.

Collins FS, McKusick VA: Implications of the Human Genome Project for medical science, *JAMA* 285(5):540-544, 2001.

Guttmacher A, Collins F: Realizing the promise of genomics in biomedical research, *JAMA* 294(11):1399-1402, 2005.

Hamilton BA, Wynshaw-Boris A: Basic genetics and patterns of inheritance. In Creasy RK et al (editors): *Creasy & Resnik's maternal-fetal medicine: principles and practice*, ed 6, Philadelphia, 2009, Saunders.

International Human Genome Sequencing Consortium: Initial sequencing and analysis of the human genome, *Nature* 409(6822):860-921, 2001.

International Society of Nurses in Genetics: *Genetics/genomics nursing: scope and standards of practice*, Washington, DC, 2007, American Nurses Association.

Jorde L et al: *Medical genetics*, ed 3, St Louis, 2003, Mosby.

Lashley F: *Clinical genetics in nursing practice*, ed 3, New York, 2005, Springer.

Lea D: Genetic and genomic healthcare: Ethical issues of importance to nurses, *Online J Issues Nurs* 13(1): Manuscript No. 4, 2008. Available at www.nursingworld.org/MainMenuCategories/ANAMarketplace?ANAPeridoicals/OJIN/Tables/Contents/vol132008/No1Jan08/GeneticsandGenomicsHealthcare.aspx (accessed July 24, 2008).

Loescher L, Merkle C: The interface of genomic technologies and nursing, *J Nurs Scholarsh* 37(2):111-119, 2005.

McInerney J: *Behavioral genetics*, last modified June 15, 2007. Available at www.ornl.gov/sci/techresources/Human_Genome/elsi/behavior.shtml (accessed July 24, 2008).

National Down Syndrome Society: *Down syndrome fact sheet*, 2009a. Available at www.ndss.org/index.php?option=com_content&view=article&id=54&Itemid=74 (accessed March 5, 2009).

National Down Syndrome Society: *About down syndrome. Incidences and maternal age*, 2009b. Available at www.ndss.org/index.php?option=com_content&view=article&id=61&Itemid=78 (accessed March 5, 2009).

Rubinstein W, Roy H: Practicing medicine at the front lines of the genomic revolution, *Arch Intern Med* 165(16):1815-1817, 2005.

Seo D, Ginsburg G: Genomic medicine: Bringing biomarkers to clinical medicine, *Curr Opin Chem Biol* 9(4): 381-386, 2005.

Van Riper M: Genetic testing and the family, *J Midwifery Womens Health* 50(3):227-233, 2005.

Van Riper M, McKinnon W: Genetic testing for breast and ovarian cancer susceptibility: a family experience, *J Midwifery Womens Health* 43(3):210-219, 2004.

Venter J et al: The sequence of the human genome, *Science* 291(5507): 1304-1351, 2001.

Wapner RJ, Jenkins TM, Khalek N: Prenatal diagnosis of congenital disorders. In Creasy RK et al (editors): *Creasy & Resnik's maternal-fetal medicine: principles and practice*, ed 6, Philadelphia, 2009, Saunders.

Unit 3

9 Assessment for Risk Factors

Learning Objectives

On completion of this chapter the reader will be able to:

- Explore the scope of high risk pregnancy.
- Examine risk factors identified through history, physical examination, and diagnostic techniques.
- Describe diagnostic techniques and implications of findings.
- Describe the nursing role in antepartal risk assessment.
- Discuss psychologic considerations associated with a high risk pregnancy diagnosis.

Electronic Resources

Additional information related to the content in Chapter 9 can be found on

evolve the Companion Website at http://evolve.elsevier.com/Perry/maternal/

- NCLEX Review Questions
- Spanish Guidelines—High Risk Factors

Approximately 500,000 of the 4 million births that occur in the United States each year are categorized as high risk because of maternal or fetal complications. Identification of the risks, together with appropriate and timely intervention during the perinatal period, can prevent morbidity and mortality among mothers and infants.

With the changing demographics in the United States, more women and families can be identified as at risk because of factors other than biophysical criteria. The increasing numbers of homeless, single, or uninsured pregnant women who have no access to prenatal care during any stage of pregnancy and the behaviors and lifestyles that pose a risk to the health of the mother and fetus contribute to the problem.

Care of these high risk patients requires the collaborative efforts of medical and nursing personnel. The high risk woman and the factors associated with a diagnosis of high risk are discussed in this chapter. Diagnostic techniques used to monitor the maternal-fetal unit are emphasized. Psychologic considerations of care of the woman experiencing a high risk pregnancy are addressed.

Definition and Scope of the Problem

A high risk pregnancy is one in which the life or health of the mother or infant is jeopardized by a disorder coincidental with or unique to pregnancy. For the mother the high risk status arbitrarily extends through the puerperium (4 to 6 weeks after childbirth). Postbirth maternal complications usually are resolved within 1 month of birth, but perinatal morbidity may continue for months or years.

High risk pregnancy is a critical problem for modern medical and nursing care. The current social emphasis on the quality of life and the wanted child has resulted in a reduction of family size and the number of unwanted pregnancies. At the same time technologic advances have facilitated pregnancies in previously infertile couples. As a consequence, emphasis is on the safe birth of normal infants who can develop to their potential. Scientific and technologic advances have allowed perinatal health care to reach a level far beyond that previously available.

The diagnosis of high risk imposes a situational crisis on the family. These crises include, for example, loss of pregnancy before the anticipated date; development of gestational diabetes mellitus with its potential complications; or birth of a neonate who does not meet cultural, societal, or familial norms and expectations.

Maternal Health Problems

The leading causes of maternal death attributable to pregnancy differ throughout the world. In general, three major causes have persisted for the last 50 years: hypertensive disorders, infection, and hemorrhage. In the United States today the three leading causes of maternal mortality are gestational hypertension, pulmonary embolism, and hemorrhage. Factors that are strongly related to maternal death include age (younger than 20 years or 35 years or older), lack of prenatal care, low educational attainment, unmarried status, and nonwhite race. African-American maternal mortality rates are more than three times higher than those for Caucasian women (Hoyert et al, 2006). Reaching the goal set by *Healthy People 2010* of no more than 3.3 maternal deaths per 100,000 live births (U.S. Department of Health and Human Services, 2000) presents a significant challenge.

Although the overall number of maternal deaths is small, maternal mortality remains a significant problem because a high proportion of these deaths are preventable, primarily through improving access to and use of prenatal care services. Nurses can be instrumental in educating the public about the importance of obtaining early and regular care during pregnancy.

Fetal and Neonatal Health Problems

The leading causes of death in the neonatal period are congenital anomalies (Hoyert et al, 2006). Other causes of neonatal death include disorders relating to short gestation and low birth weight, respiratory distress syndrome, the effects of maternal complications, and sudden infant death. Racial differences in the infant mortality rates continue to challenge public health experts. Increased rates of survival during the neonatal period have resulted largely from high-quality prenatal care and the improvement in perinatal services, including technologic advances in neonatal intensive care and obstetrics.

Reducing infant mortality rates requires the removal of financial, educational, sociocultural, and logistic barriers to care so that pregnant women can seek and receive health services. Commitment at national, state, and local levels is required. More research is needed to identify the extent to which financial, educational, sociocultural, and behavioral factors individually and collectively affect perinatal morbidity and mortality. Barriers to care must be removed, and perinatal services modified to meet contemporary health care needs.

Regionalization of Health Care Services

Early and ongoing risk assessment is a crucial component of perinatal care. Conditions associated with perinatal morbidity and mortality can be prevented, treated, or referred to more skilled health care providers. Factors to consider when determining a patient's risk status include resources available locally to treat the condition, availability of appropriate facilities for transport if needed, and determination of the best match for the patient's needs.

It is neither feasible nor reasonable for each hospital to develop and maintain the full spectrum of services required for high risk perinatal patients. As a consequence, regionalization of health care emerged. This system of coordinated care, in which facilities within a geographic region are organized to provide different levels of care, was also applied to preconception and ambulatory prenatal care services.

Assessment for Risk Factors

Pregnancies can be designated as high risk for any of several undesirable outcomes. Those considered to be at risk for uteroplacental insufficiency carry a serious threat for fetal growth restriction, intrauterine fetal death, intrapartum death, intrapartum fetal distress, and various types of neonatal morbidity.

When using a medical model perspective, a woman is at risk only from adverse medical, obstetric, or physiologic conditions. Today a more comprehensive approach to high risk pregnancy is used, and the factors associated with high risk childbearing are grouped into broad categories based on threats to health and pregnancy outcome. Categories of risk include genetic, demographic, and behavioral (Gilbert, 2007a) (Box 9-1).

Genetic risks include heritable factors that originate within the mother or fetus and affect the development or functioning of either or both.

Demographic risks result from geographic location (e.g., altitude, unsafe soil conditions), socioeconomic status (e.g., limited income, poor nutritional status), educational attainment, marital status (single status is associated with adverse perinatal outcome), maternal age (adverse perinatal outcome for mothers younger than 20 years or older than 34 years), racial and ethnic origins (significant racial disparities between Caucasians and other races and ethnicities) (Box 9-2), and occupational hazards.

Behavioral risks arise from the mother and her family and place the mother and fetus at risk. Examples include substance abuse, failure to seek prenatal care, inadequate nutritional status, poor dental hygiene, psychosocial stressors, abuse and violence, and multiple births (see Box 9-1).

Risk factors are interrelated and cumulative in their effects (see Community Focus box). Specific pregnancy problems and risk factors are listed in Box 9-3. Risk factors of the postpartum woman and the neonate are outlined in Box 9-4. A comprehensive database for pregnancy risk assessment can help generate appropriate nursing diagnoses (Box 9-5).

COMMUNITY FOCUS

Resources for Parents Experiencing a High Risk Pregnancy

Contact the nearest March of Dimes office to assess the resources available for parents (e.g., pamphlets, websites for high risk pregnancies) and to learn what screening is recommended during pregnancy to identify problems. For what problems is the screening conducted? How can pregnant women access March of Dimes information? What information or resources are available in your community for the problems identified?

Antepartum Testing and Biophysical Assessment

The major expected outcome of antepartum testing is the detection of potential fetal compromise. Ideally the technique used will identify fetal compromise before intrauterine asphyxia of the fetus occurs so that the health care provider can take measures to prevent or minimize adverse perinatal outcomes. No single test can provide this information. Assessment tests should be selected based on their effectiveness, and the results must be interpreted in light of the complete clinical picture. The most reliable evidence for effectiveness is provided by randomized controlled trials. Nurses can be informed about the most recent research on fetal assessment by using an up-to-date systematic review such as the Cochrane Database of Systematic Reviews (*www.cochrane.org.au/libraryguide/guide_data.asp*). Box 9-6 lists evidence for

BOX 9-1 High Risk Factors

Genetic Factors

Genetic considerations—Genetic factors may interfere with normal fetal or neonatal development, result in congenital anomalies, or create difficulties for the mother. These factors include defective genes, transmittable inherited disorders, chromosome anomalies, multiple pregnancy, large fetal size, and ABO incompatibility. A genetic risk assessment should be done to determine the family's heritable risk.

Demographic Characteristics

Geographic location—The availability and quality of prenatal care vary greatly with geographic region. Women in metropolitan areas have more prenatal visits than those in rural areas who have fewer opportunities for specialized care and consequently a higher incidence of maternal mortality. Health care in an inner city, where residents are usually poorer and begin childbearing earlier and continue for longer, may be of lower quality than in a more affluent neighborhood. There may be unsafe soil and water conditions and environmental exposure to pollutants.

Socioeconomic status—Poverty underlies many other risk factors and leads to inadequate financial resources for food and prenatal care; poor general health; increased risk for medical complications of pregnancy; and greater prevalence of adverse environmental influences such as substandard living conditions, poor hygiene, and inadequate nutrition.

Educational attainment—Risk for adverse perinatal outcomes decreases as educational level increases.

Marital status—The increased mortality and morbidity rates for unmarried women, including a greater risk for preeclampsia, are often related to inadequate prenatal care and a younger childbearing age.

Maternal age—Mothers younger than 20 years and older than 34 years have a slight increase in adverse perinatal outcomes

Racial and ethnic origins—Although race and ethnicity by themselves are not major risks, race is an indicator of other sociodemographic risk factors. Non-Caucasian women are more than three times as likely as Caucasian women to die of pregnancy-related causes. African-American babies have the highest rates of prematurity and low birth weight, with the infant mortality rates among African-Americans being more than double that among Caucasians.

Occupational hazards—Occupational hazards can be grouped into chemical, physical, biologic, and psychologic hazards. The risk to the fetus depends on the timing of exposure, the dose, and fetal and maternal susceptibility.

Behavioral Characteristics

Substance abuse—Smoking is associated with intrauterine growth restriction and low birth weight; alcohol exerts adverse effects on the fetus, resulting in fetal alcohol spectrum disorders, which include fetal alcohol syndrome, alcohol-related neurodevelopmental disorder, and alcohol-related birth defects; drugs can be teratogenic, cause metabolic disturbances, produce chemical effects, or cause depression or alteration of central nervous system function.

Failure to seek prenatal care—Failure to diagnose and treat complications early is a major risk factor arising from financial barriers or lack of access to care; depersonalization of the system, resulting in long waits, routine visits, variability in health care personnel, and unpleasant physical surroundings; lack of understanding of need for early and continued care or cultural beliefs that do not support the need; and fear of the health care system and its providers.

Nutritional status—Adequate nutrition, without which fetal growth and development cannot proceed normally, is one of the most important determinants of pregnancy outcome. Conditions that influence nutritional status include the following: young age; three pregnancies in the previous 2 years; tobacco, alcohol, or drug use; inadequate dietary intake because of chronic illness or food fads; inadequate or excessive weight gain; and hematocrit value less than 32%.

Dental hygiene—Periodontal disease increases the risk for preterm birth and low birth weight.

Psychosocial stressors—Childbearing triggers profound and complex physiologic, psychologic, and social changes, with evidence to suggest a relationship between emotional distress and birth complications. This risk factor includes conditions such as specific intrapsychic disturbances and addictive lifestyles; a history of child or spouse abuse; inadequate support systems; family disruption or dissolution; maternal role changes or conflicts; noncompliance with cultural norms; unsafe cultural, ethnic, or religious practices; and situational crises.

Abuse and violence—Domestic violence is a serious problem; the risk of violence increases during pregnancy. Abuse during pregnancy increases the risk for abruptio placenta, preterm birth, and low-birth-weight infants and infections from forced sex.

Modified from Gilbert ES: *Manual of high risk pregnancy & delivery*, ed 4, St Louis, 2007, Mosby.

recommending care for fetal assessment screening based on this database.

Daily Fetal Movement Count

Assessment of fetal activity by the mother is a simple yet valuable method for monitoring the condition of the fetus (see Critical Thinking Exercise). The daily fetal movement count (DFMC) (also called "kick counts") can be done at home, is simple to understand, is noninvasive, and usually does not interfere with a daily routine. The DFMC is frequently used to monitor the fetus in pregnancies complicated by conditions that may affect fetal oxygenation. These conditions include but are not limited to gestational hypertension or chronic hypertension and diabetes. The presence of movements is generally a reassuring sign of fetal health.

Women should be taught the significance of the presence and/or absence of FMs, the procedure to use for counting, how to record findings on a daily FM record, and when to notify their health care provider (Fig. 9-1, p. 195).

BOX 9-2 Antepartum Cultural Assessment

All cultures recognize pregnancy as a special transitional period and have particular customs and beliefs that dictate behavior during this time. In the antepartum period the nurse should assess the following:

- Beliefs of whether pregnancy is a state of illness or health
- Behavioral expectations of the mother and the health care provider
- Dietary prescriptions or restrictions (e.g., hot/cold balance theory, pica)
- Activity restrictions or prescriptions (e.g., use of massage)
- Availability of advice (e.g., from whom and at what time advice will be sought and when prenatal care will begin [if at all])
- Considerations of modesty

Several protocols are used for counting. One recommendation is to count all fetal movements in a 12-hour period each day until a minimum of 10 movements are counted. Another common recommendation is that mothers count fetal activity two or three times daily (e.g., after meals or before bedtime) for 2 hours or until 10 movements are counted. Except for noting a very low number of daily fetal movements (FMs) or a trend toward decreased motion, the clinical value of the absolute number of FMs has not been established. The only exception is if FMs cease entirely for 12 hours (the so-called fetal alarm signal). If fewer than 10 FMs are felt within the specified time or movement is perceived to be less than the previous day, the woman should notify her health care provider for further evaluation.

NURSING ALERT In assessing FMs it is important to remember that they are usually not present during the fetal sleep cycle; they may be temporarily reduced if the woman is taking depressant medication, drinking alcohol, or smoking a cigarette. They do not decrease as the woman nears term. Obesity decreases perception of FM and consequently, the ability of the mother to count FMs.

Ultrasonography

Sound is a form of wave energy that causes small particles in a medium to oscillate. The frequency of sound, which refers to the number of peaks or waves that move over a given point

BOX 9-3 Specific Pregnancy Problems and Related Risk Factors

Preterm Labor

Age younger than 16 or older than 35 years
Low socioeconomic status
Maternal weight below 50 kg (110 lb)
Poor nutrition
Previous preterm birth
Incompetent cervix
Uterine anomalies
Smoking
Drug addiction and alcohol abuse
Pyelonephritis, pneumonia
Multiple gestation
Anemia
Abnormal fetal presentation
Preterm rupture of membranes
Placental abnormalities
Infection

Polyhydramnios

Diabetes mellitus
Multiple gestation
Fetal congenital abnormalities
Isoimmunization (Rh or ABO)
Nonimmune hydrops
Abnormal fetal presentation

Intrauterine Growth Restriction

Multiple gestation
Poor nutrition
Maternal cyanotic heart disease
Prior pregnancy with intrauterine growth restriction
Maternal collagen diseases
Chronic hypertension
Gestational hypertension
Recurrent antepartum hemorrhage
Smoking
Maternal diabetes with vascular problems
Fetal infections
Fetal cardiovascular anomalies
Drug addiction and alcohol abuse
Fetal congenital anomalies
Hemoglobinopathies

Oligohydramnios

Renal agenesis (Potter's syndrome)
Prolonged rupture of membranes
Intrauterine growth restriction
Intrauterine fetal death

Postterm Pregnancy

Anencephaly
Placental sulfatase deficiency
Perinatal hypoxia, acidosis
Placental insufficiency

Chromosome Abnormalities

Maternal age 35 years or older at birth
Balanced translocation (maternal and paternal)

From Gillen-Goldstein J et al: Methods of assessment for pregnancy at risk. In DeCherney AH, Nathan L (editors): *Current obstetric and gynecologic diagnosis and treatment*, ed 9, New York, 2003, Lange Medical Books/McGraw-Hill.

BOX 9-4 Factors That Place the Postpartum Woman and Neonate at High Risk

Mother
Hemorrhage
Infection
Abnormal vital signs
Traumatic labor or birth
Psychosocial factors

Infant (for Admission to Neonatal Intensive Care Unit)

High Risk
Infants who continue with or develop signs of RDS or other respiratory distress
Asphyxiated infants (Apgar scores less than 6 at 5 minutes); resuscitation required at birth
Preterm infants; dysmature infants
Infants with cyanosis or suspected cardiovascular disease; persistent cyanosis
Infants with major congenital malformations requiring surgery; chromosome anomalies
Infants with convulsions, sepsis, hemorrhagic diathesis, or shock
Meconium aspiration syndrome
CNS depression for longer than 24 hours
Hypoglycemia
Hypocalcemia
Hyperbilirubinemia

Moderate Risk
Dysmaturity
Prematurity (weight between 2000 and 2500 g)
Apgar score less than 5 at 1 minute
Feeding problems
Multifetal birth
Transient tachypnea
Hypomagnesemia or hypermagnesemia
Hypoparathyroidism
Failure to gain weight
Jitteriness or hyperactivity
Cardiac anomalies not requiring immediate catheterization
Heart murmur
Anemia
CNS depression for less than 24 hours

CNS, Central nervous system; *RDS*, respiratory distress syndrome.

BOX 9-5 Pregnancy Risk Assessment Monitoring System

The Pregnancy Risk Assessment Monitoring System (PRAMS) is a surveillance project of the Centers for Disease Control and Prevention and state health departments. It was started in 1987 to improve the health of mothers and infants by reducing adverse outcomes. The sample in PRAMS is chosen from all women who recently had a live birth. Currently 37 states, New York City, and South Dakota (Yankton Sioux Tribe) participate in PRAMS. The PRAMS questionnaire contains questions asked by all states and some state-specific questions. Data are used to plan maternal and infant health programs and develop partnerships among agencies that have important contributions to make in developing programs.

Information from www.cdc.gov/PRAMS/ (accessed March 5, 2009).

per unit of time, is expressed in hertz (Hz). Sound with a frequency of 1 cycle, or one peak per second, has a frequency of 1 Hz. When directional beams of sound strike an object, an echo is returned. The time delay between the emission of the sound and the return of the echo and the direction of the echo are noted. From these data the distance and location of an object can be calculated. Ultrasound is sound frequency higher than that detectable by humans (greater than 20,000 Hz). Diagnostic ultrasound instruments operate within a frequency range of 2 to 10 million Hz (or 2 to 10 MHz), which is below the range used by sonar and radar equipment. Ultrasound images are a reflection of the strength of the sending beam, the strength of the returning echo, and the density of the medium (e.g., muscle [uterus], bone, tissue [placenta], fluid, or blood) through which the beam is sent and returned.

CRITICAL THINKING EXERCISE

Fetal Activity Monitoring

Barbra is an elementary school teacher. She is at 30 weeks of gestation with her first baby. This is a planned pregnancy, and Barbra and her husband are excited about becoming parents. They have read extensively about pregnancy and selected midwifery care after a careful review of the literature on childbirth and interviewing other patients of the midwife they selected to provide care. Barbra has kept all of her recommended appointments with the nurse-midwife. On the last two visits to her nurse-midwife, Barbra's blood pressure has been elevated. She has been advised to monitor fetal activity at home. As her nurse, you are responsible for developing a teaching plan that includes the following: the purpose of monitoring fetal activity; the significance of fetal activity; the times when monitoring is to take place; and instructing Barbra on the way to count movements, the best time of the day to complete the counts, how to record the counts, and when to notify you or her nurse-midwife with findings.

1. Evidence—Is there sufficient evidence to draw conclusions about the benefits of monitoring fetal activity?
2. Assumptions—Describe an underlying assumption about each of the following topics:
   a. Barbra's motivation for learning about fetal activity monitoring
   b. Barbra's motivation to perform fetal activity monitoring
   c. The best time of the day for Barbra to complete the counts
   d. Barbra's ability to comply with instructions
3. What implications and priorities for nursing care can be drawn at this time?
4. Does the evidence objectively support your conclusion?
5. Are there alternative perspectives to your conclusion?

BOX 9-6 Fetal Assessment Screening: Recommendations for Care

Beneficial Effects

Doppler ultrasound use in pregnancy at high risk for fetal compromise

Effects Likely to Be Beneficial

Ultrasound use to estimate gestational age in first and early second trimesters
Ultrasound use to confirm suspected multiple pregnancy
Ultrasound use for placental location in suspected placenta previa
Ultrasound use to assess amniotic fluid volume
Early second-trimester amniocentesis for identification of chromosome abnormalities
Transabdominal instead of transvaginal chorionic villus sampling

Trade-Off Between Beneficial and Adverse Effects

Formal systems of risk scoring
Routine use of early ultrasound
Chorionic villus sampling versus amniocentesis for diagnosing chromosome abnormalities
Serum alpha-fetoprotein screening for neural tube defects
Triple screen test for Down syndrome and neural tube defects

Effectiveness Unknown

Placental grading by ultrasound to improve perinatal outcome
Biophysical profile for fetal surveillance
Routine fetal movement counts to improve perinatal outcome

Effects Unlikely to Be Beneficial

Routine use of ultrasound for fetal anthropometry (body measurements) in late pregnancy
Use of Doppler ultrasound screening in all pregnancies
Measurement of placental hormones (estriol and human placental lactogen)

Effects Likely to Be Ineffective or Harmful

Nipple stimulation test to improve perinatal outcome
Nonselective nonstress test to improve perinatal outcome
Contraction stress test to improve perinatal outcome

Source: Enkin M et al: Effective care in pregnancy and childbirth: a synopsis, *Birth* 28(1):41-51, 2001.

Diagnostic ultrasonography is an important technique in antepartum fetal surveillance (Fig. 9-2). It provides critical information to health care providers regarding fetal activity and gestational age, normal versus abnormal fetal growth curves, visual assistance with which invasive tests may be performed more safely, fetal and placental anatomy, and fetal well-being. Ultrasound examination can be done abdominally or transvaginally during pregnancy. Both methods produce a three-dimensional view from which a pictorial image is obtained. Abdominal ultrasonography is more useful after the first trimester when the pregnant uterus becomes an abdominal organ.

For the procedure the woman is usually required to have a full bladder to push the uterus up to get a better image of the fetus. Transmission gel or paste is applied to the abdomen before a transducer is moved over the skin to enhance transmission and reception of the sound waves. She is positioned with small pillows under her head and knees. The display panel is positioned so that the woman and/or her partner can observe the images on the screen if they desire.

Transvaginal ultrasonography, in which the probe is inserted into the vagina, allows pelvic anatomy to be evaluated in greater detail and allows intrauterine pregnancy to be diagnosed earlier. Transvaginal ultrasonography is used in the first trimester to detect ectopic pregnancies, monitor the developing embryo, help identify abnormalities, and help establish gestational age. In some instances it may be used as an adjunct to abdominal scanning to evaluate preterm labor in second- and third-trimester pregnancies. A transvaginal ultrasound examination is well tolerated by most patients because it alleviates the need for a full bladder. It is especially useful in obese patients whose thick abdominal layers cannot be penetrated adequately with an abdominal approach.

A transvaginal ultrasound may be performed either with the woman in a lithotomy position or with her pelvis elevated by towels, cushions, or a folded pillow. This pelvic tilt is optimal to image the pelvic structures. A protective cover such as a condom, the finger of a clean rubber surgical glove, or a special cover provided by the manufacturer is used to cover the probe. The probe is lubricated with a water-soluble gel and placed in the vagina either by the examiner or by the woman herself. During the examination the position of the probe or the tilt of the examining table may be changed to view the complete pelvis. The procedure is not physically painful, although the woman will feel pressure as the probe is moved.

Levels of Ultrasonography

The American College of Obstetricians and Gynecologists (ACOG, 2004a) describes three levels of ultrasonography. The standard examination is used most frequently and can be performed by ultrasonographers or other health care professionals, including nurses, who have had special training. Indications for standard ultrasonography are described in detail in the next section; its primary purposes are to detect fetal viability, determine the presentation of the fetus, assess gestational age, locate the placenta, examine the fetal anatomy for malformations, and determine amniotic fluid volume (AFV). Limited examinations are performed for specific indications such as identifying fetal presentation during labor or evaluating fetal heart activity when it is not detected by other methods (ACOG, 2004a). Specialized or targeted examinations are performed if a woman is suspected of carrying an anatomically or a physiologically abnormal fetus. Indications for a comprehensive examination include abnormal findings on clinical examination, especially with polyhydramnios or oligohydramnios, elevated alpha-fetoprotein (AFP) levels, and a

FETAL MOVEMENT CHART

1. This chart will help us find out how your baby is doing.
2. Carefully count the number of baby movements during the same hour every evening. (Baby moves more during the evening hours.) Example: 8-9 PM every evening.
3. If the baby has not moved for 12 hours, it is important that you notify the clinic (555-1234). If the clinic is closed, a recorded message will give you further instructions for contacting a doctor who is on-call.
4. Bring this chart with you whenever you come to the clinic or hospital.

DAILY CHART OF BABY KICKS

DAYS OF WEEK	MON	TUES	WED	THURS	FRI	SAT	SUN
DATE							
KICKS							
DATE							
KICKS							
DATE							
KICKS							
DATE							
KICKS							
DATE							
KICKS							
DATE							
KICKS							
DATE							
KICKS							
DATE							
KICKS							
DATE							
KICKS							

X-IMR-2211 (03/C1) OTHER

Fig. 9-1 Fetal movement (kick count) chart. *(Courtesy St. Joseph Hospital and Medical Center, Phoenix, AZ.)*

history of offspring with anomalies that can be detected by ultrasound examination. Specialized ultrasonography is performed by highly trained and experienced personnel.

Indications for Use

Major indications for the use of obstetric sonography are shown by trimester in Box 9-7. Ultrasonography can lead to earlier diagnoses, allowing therapy to be instituted early in pregnancy. This decreases the severity and duration of morbidity, both physical and emotional, for the family. For example, early diagnosis of a fetal anomaly gives the family choices such as (1) preparation for the care of an infant with a disorder, (2) intrauterine surgery or other therapy for the fetus, or (3) termination of the pregnancy.

Fetal Heart Activity

Fetal heart activity can be demonstrated as early as 6 to 7 weeks by real-time echo scanners and at 10 to 12 weeks by Doppler mode. By 9 to 10 weeks gestational trophoblastic disease can be diagnosed. Fetal death can be confirmed by lack of heart motion; the presence of fetal scalp edema, and maceration; and overlap of the cranial bones.

Gestational Age

Gestational dating by ultrasonography is indicated for conditions such as the following: (1) uncertain dates for the last normal menstrual period, (2) recent discontinuation of oral contraceptives, (3) bleeding episode during the first trimester, (4) uterine size that does not agree with dates, and (5) other high risk conditions.

During the first 20 weeks of gestation, ultrasonography provides an accurate assessment of gestational age because most normal fetuses grow at the same rate. With increased fetal age the accuracy of gestational age estimates using ultrasound also increases because more variables are measured. Four methods of fetal age estimation are used: (1) determination of gestational sac dimensions (at about 8 weeks), (2)

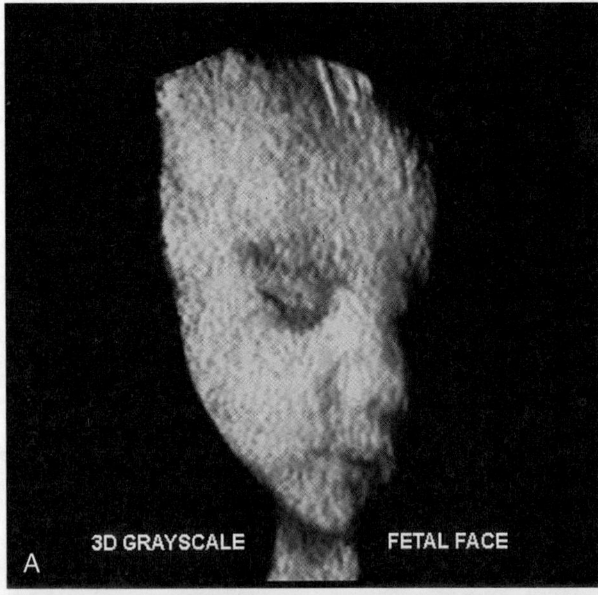

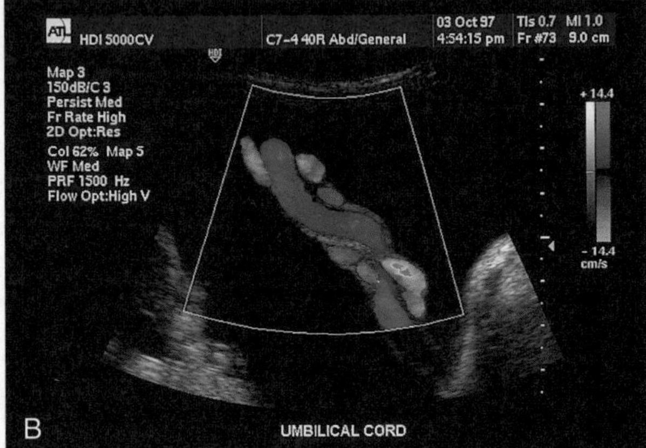

Fig. 9-2 Two views of the fetus during ultrasonography. **A,** Fetal face (20 weeks). **B,** Umbilical cord (26 weeks). *(Courtesy Advanced Technology Laboratories, Bothell, WA.)*

BOX 9-7 Major Uses of Ultrasonography During Pregnancy

First Trimester

- Confirm pregnancy
- Confirm viability
- Determine gestational age
- Rule out ectopic pregnancy
- Detect multiple gestation
- Visualization during chorionic villus sampling
- Detect maternal abnormalities such as bicornuate uterus, ovarian cysts, fibroids
- Detect presence and location of an intrauterine contraceptive device

Second Trimester

- Establish or confirm dates
- Confirm viability
- Detect polyhydramnios, oligohydramnios
- Detect congenital anomalies
- Detect intrauterine growth restriction (IUGR)
- Confirm placental placement
- Visualization during amniocentesis

Third Trimester

- Confirm gestational age
- Confirm viability
- Detect macrosomia
- Detect congenital anomalies
- Detect IUGR
- Determine fetal position
- Detect placenta previa or abruptio placentae
- Visualization during amniocentesis, external version
- Biophysical profile
- Assess amniotic fluid volume
- Doppler flow studies
- Detect placental maturity

measurement of crown-rump length (between 5 and 10 weeks), (3) measurement of the biparietal diameter (BPD) (after 12 weeks), and (4) measurement of femur length (after 12 weeks) (Richards, 2007). Fetal BPD at 36 weeks should be approximately 8.7 cm. Term pregnancy and fetal maturity can be diagnosed with some confidence if the biparietal measurement by ultrasound is greater than 9.8 cm (Fig. 9-3), especially when this is combined with appropriate femur length measurement.

Fetal Growth

Fetal growth is determined by intrinsic growth potential and the environmental factors that may enhance or inhibit that growth. Conditions that indicate the need for ultrasound assessment of fetal growth include the following: (1) poor maternal weight gain or pattern of weight gain, (2) previous pregnancy with intrauterine growth restriction (IUGR), (3) chronic infections, (4) ingestion of drugs (tobacco, alcohol, over-the-counter drugs, and street drugs), (5) maternal diabetes mellitus, (6) hypertension, (7) multifetal pregnancy, and (8) other medical or surgical complications.

Serial evaluations of BPD (see Fig. 9-3), head circumference (Fig. 9-4), limb length, and abdominal circumference (Fig. 9-5) can differentiate among size discrepancy resulting from inaccurate dates, true IUGR, and macrosomia. IUGR may be symmetric (the fetus is small in all parameters) or asymmetric (head and body growth vary). Symmetric IUGR implies a chronic or long-standing insult and may be caused by low genetic growth potential, intrauterine infection, undernutrition, heavy smoking, or chromosome aberration. Asymmetric growth reflects an acute or late-occurring deprivation such as placental insufficiency resulting from hypertension, renal disease, or cardiovascular disease. Reduced fetal growth is still one of the most frequent conditions associated with stillbirth.

Macrosomic infants (those weighing 4000 g or more) are at increased risk for dystocia, traumatic injury, and asphyxia during birth. Fetal macrosomia associated with maternal glucose intolerance or diabetes carries an increased risk of intrauterine fetal death. Macrosomia in the infant of a mother with diabetes is asymmetric and characterized by increases in

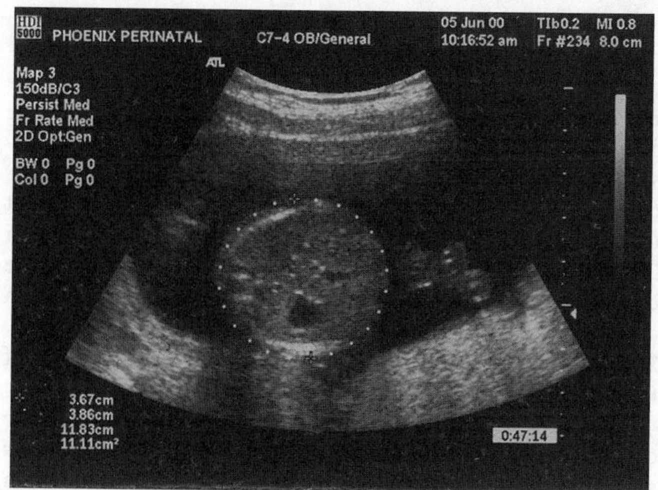

Fig. 9-3 Biparietal cephalometry by ultrasound. *(Courtesy Michael S. Clement, MD, Mesa, AZ.)*

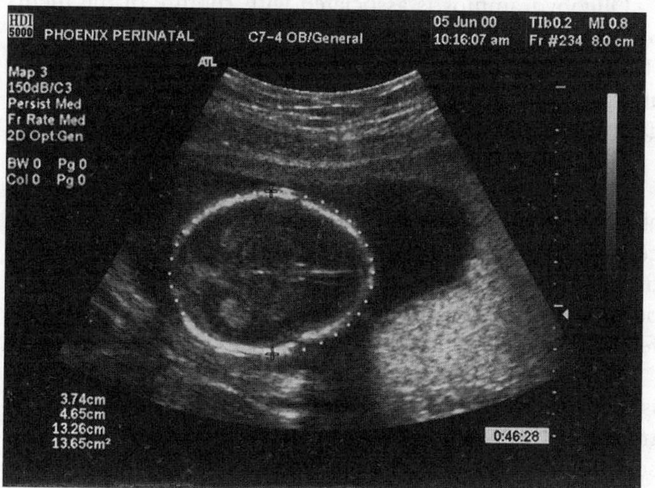

Fig. 9-4 Head circumference. *(Courtesy Michael S. Clement, MD, Mesa, AZ.)*

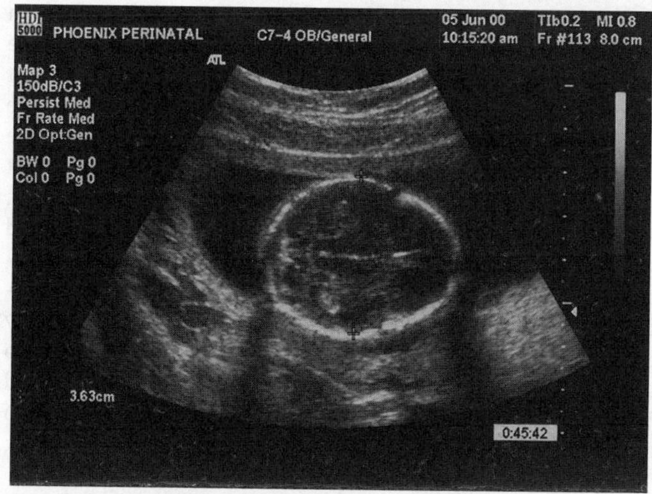

Fig. 9-5 Abdominal circumference. *(Courtesy Michael S. Clement, MD, Mesa, AZ.)*

fat and muscle in the abdomen and shoulders; head circumference remains normal. Macrosomia in an infant whose mother is obese without glucose intolerance results in symmetric changes (i.e., excessive growth of abdominal and head circumferences).

Fetal Anatomy

Depending on the gestational age, the following structures can be identified by ultrasonography: head (including ventricles and blood vessels), neck, spine, heart, stomach, small bowel, liver, kidneys, bladder, limbs, and umbilical cord. Ultrasonography permits the confirmation of normal anatomy and the detection of major fetal malformations. The presence of an anomaly may influence the birth location (e.g., delivery room instead of a labor-delivery-recovery room or a subspecialty center versus a basic care center) and the method of birth to optimize neonatal outcomes (vaginal versus cesarean).

The number of fetuses and their presentations also may be assessed by ultrasonography, allowing plans for therapy and mode of birth to be made in advance.

Fetal Genetic Disorders and Physical Anomalies

A prenatal screening technique called *fetal nuchal translucency (FNT)* screening uses ultrasound measurement of fluid in the nape of the fetal neck between 10 and 14 weeks of gestation to identify possible fetal abnormalities (Fig. 9-6). A finding of abnormal fluid collection that is greater than 2.5 mm is considered abnormal, whereas a measurement of 3 mm or greater is highly indicative of genetic disorders or physical anomalies. If the FNT is abnormal, diagnostic genetic testing is recommended (ACOG, 2004b).

Placental Position and Function

The pattern of uterine and placental growth and the fullness of the maternal bladder influence the apparent location of the placenta as viewed by ultrasonography. During the first trimester differentiation between the endometrium and small placenta is difficult. By 14 to 16 weeks the placenta is clearly defined, but its relationship to the internal cervical os can sometimes be altered dramatically by changing the degree of fullness of the maternal bladder. In approximately 15% to 20% of all pregnancies in which ultrasound scanning is performed during the second trimester, the placenta seems to be overlying the os, but at term the incidence of placenta previa at term is only 0.5%. Thus the diagnosis of placenta previa can seldom be confirmed before 27 weeks, primarily because of the elongation of the lower uterine segment as pregnancy advances.

Another use of ultrasonography is grading of placental maturation. Calcium deposits are of significance in postterm pregnancies because, as they increase, the available surface area that can be adequately bathed by maternal blood decreases. The point at which this results in fetal wastage and hypoxia cannot be determined precisely; however, effects usually are observable by 42 weeks and are progressive.

Adjunct to Amniocentesis, Percutaneous Umbilical Blood Sampling, and Chorionic Villus Sampling

The safety of amniocentesis is increased when the exact position of the fetus, placenta, and pockets of amniotic fluid can be identified accurately. Ultrasound scanning has reduced the risks previously associated with amniocentesis

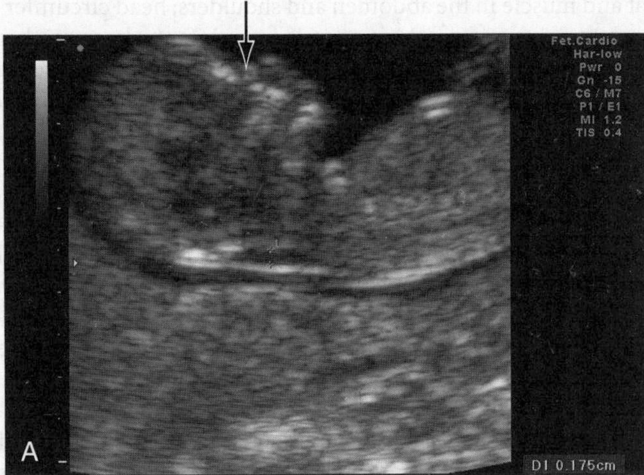

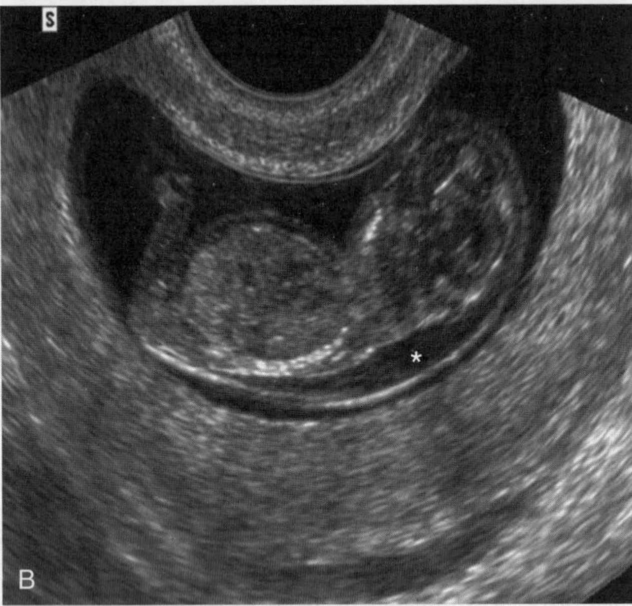

Fig. 9-6 Fetal nuchal translucency. **A,** Nuchal lucency (calipers) and nasal bone (*arrow*) in 12-week fetus. **B,** Increased nuchal translucency. Transvaginal ultrasound performed at 12 weeks demonstrates a sonolucent area (*asterisk*) over the posterior neck and upper thorax. (From Martin RJ, Fanaroff AA, Walsh MC: *Fanaroff and Martin's neonatal-perinatal medicine: diseases of the fetus and infant*, ed 8, Philadelphia, 2006, Mosby.)

such as fetomaternal hemorrhage from a pierced placenta. Percutaneous umbilical blood sampling (PUBS) and chorionic villus sampling (CVS) are also guided by ultrasonography to accurately identify the cord and chorion frondosum (see Fig. 9-2, *B*).

Fetal Well-Being

Physiologic parameters of the fetus that can be assessed with ultrasound scanning include amniotic fluid volume, vascular waveforms from the fetal circulation, heart motion, fetal breathing movements, fetal urine production, and fetal limb and head movements. Assessment of these parameters, singly or in combination, yields a fairly reliable picture of fetal well-being. The significance of these findings is discussed in the following sections.

Amniotic Fluid Volume

Abnormalities in amniotic fluid volume (AFV) are frequently associated with fetal disorders. Subjective determinants of oligohydramnios (decreased fluid) include the absence of fluid pockets in the uterine cavity and the impression of crowding of fetal small parts (arms and legs). An objective criterion of decreased AFV is met when the largest pocket of fluid measured in two perpendicular planes is less than 2 cm. In the case of polyhydramnios (increased fluid), the criteria include multiple large pockets of fluid, the impression of a floating fetus, and free movement of fetal limbs (Harman, 2009). The diagnosis may be made when the largest pocket of fluid exceeds 8 cm in one vertical pocket.

The total AFV can be evaluated by a method in which the depths (in centimeters) of amniotic fluid in all four quadrants surrounding the maternal umbilicus are totaled, resulting in an amniotic fluid index (AFI). An AFI of less than 5 cm indicates oligohydramnios; 5 to 19 cm is considered a normal measurement; and a measurement greater than 20 cm reflects polyhydramnios (Gilbert, 2007b).

Oligohydramnios is associated with rupture of the membranes and congenital anomalies (such as renal agenesis), IUGR, and fetal distress in labor. Polyhydramnios is associated with neural tube defects (NTDs), obstruction of the fetal gastrointestinal tract, multiple fetuses, and fetal hydrops.

Doppler Blood Flow Analysis

One of the major advances in perinatal medicine is the ability to study blood flow noninvasively in the fetus and placenta with ultrasonography. Doppler blood flow analysis is a useful adjunct in the management of pregnancies at risk because of hypertension, IUGR, diabetes mellitus, multiple fetuses, or preterm labor.

When a sound wave is reflected from a moving target, there is a change in frequency of the reflected wave relative to the transmitted wave. This is called the *Doppler effect.* An ultrasound beam scattered by a group of red blood cells (RBCs) is an example of this effect. The velocity of the RBCs can be determined by measuring the change in the frequency in the sound wave reflected off the cells.

The shifted frequencies can be displayed as a plot of velocity versus time, and the shape of these waveforms can be analyzed to give information about blood flow and resistance in a given circulation. Velocity waveforms from umbilical and uterine arteries, reported in systolic/diastolic (S/D) ratios, can be first detected at 15 weeks of pregnancy. Because of progressive decline in resistance in both the umbilical and the uterine arteries, this ratio decreases as pregnancy advances. Most fetuses achieve an S/D ratio of 3 or less by 30 weeks (Fig. 9-7). Persistent elevation of S/D ratios after 30 weeks is associated with IUGR, usually resulting from uteroplacental insufficiency. In postterm pregnancies evaluated by Doppler umbilical flow studies, an elevated S/D ratio indicates a poorly perfused placenta. Abnormal velocity study results are also seen with certain chromosome abnormalities (trisomy 13 and 18) and with lupus erythematosus in the mother. Exposure to nicotine from maternal smoking also increases the S/D ratio.

Biophysical Profile

Real-time ultrasound permits detailed assessment of the physical and physiologic characteristics of the developing

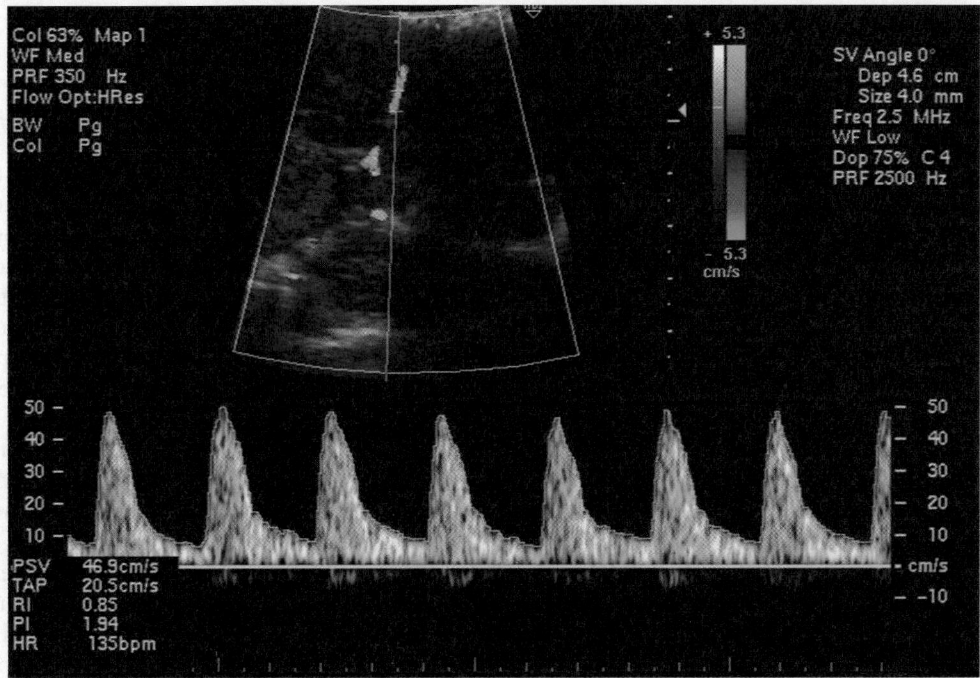

Fig. 9-7 Umbilical artery velocity waveform. (From Callen P: *Ultrasonography in obstetrics and gynecology*, ed 4, Philadelphia, 2000, Saunders.)

fetus to such an extent that it is possible to examine the fetus in detail and to catalog normal and abnormal biophysical responses to stimuli. The biophysical profile (BPP) is a noninvasive dynamic assessment of a fetus that is based on the assessment of acute and chronic markers of fetal disease. The BPP includes fetal breathing movements, FMs, fetal tone, fetal heart rate (FHR) patterns by means of a nonstress test (NST), and AFV.

The BPP may be considered as a physical examination of the fetus, including determination of vital signs. The fetus responds to central hypoxia by alteration in movement, muscle tone, breathing, and heart rate patterns. The presence of normal fetal biophysical activities indicates that the central nervous system is functional; therefore the fetus is not hypoxemic. BPP variables and scoring are detailed in Table 9-1.

The BPP is an accurate indicator of impending fetal death. Fetal acidosis can be diagnosed early with a nonreactive NST and absent fetal breathing movements. An abnormal score and oligohydramnios indicate labor should be induced. Fetal infection in women whose membranes rupture prematurely (at less than 37 weeks of gestation) can be diagnosed early by changes in biophysical activities that precede the clinical signs of infection and indicate the necessity for immediate birth. When the BPP score is normal and the risk of fetal death low, intervention is indicated only for obstetric or maternal factors.

Nursing Role

Although a growing number of nurses perform ultrasound scans and BPPs in certain centers, the main role of nurses is in counseling and educating women about the procedure. Providing accurate information regarding the procedure is imperative to allay the mother's anxiety. Although ultrasound

Table 9-1 Biophysical Profile

VARIABLES	NORMAL (SCORE = 2)	ABNORMAL (SCORE = 0)
Fetal breathing movements	One or more episodes in 30 min, each lasting ≥30 sec	Episodes absent or no episode ≥30 sec in 30 min
Fetal movements	At least three trunk or limb movements in 30 min	Fewer than three episodes of body or limb movements in 30 min
Fetal tone	At least one episode of active extension with return to flexion of fetal limb or trunk; opening and closing of hand is considered normal tone	Absence of movement or slow extension/ flexion
Amniotic fluid index	AFI >5 cm or at least one pocket >2 cm	AFI ≤5 cm and no single pocket >2 cm
Nonstress test	Reactive	Nonreactive
Score		
Normal	8-10 (if amniotic fluid index is adequate)	
Suspicious	6	Repeat testing next day
Abnormal	<6	Associated with increased perinatal morbidity and mortality; usually hospitalize for further evaluation or birth

Reference: Tucker SM, Miller LA, Miller DA: *Mosby's pocket guide to fetal monitoring; a multidisciplinary approach*, ed 6, St Louis, 2009, Mosby.
AFI, Amniotic fluid index.

scanning has become a widely used diagnostic tool, recommendations for the procedure are based on expectations of a fetal problem and therefore may cause concern. Women should be provided ample opportunity to ask questions and be reassured that the procedure is safe. In the 35+ years that diagnostic ultrasonography has been used, no conclusive evidence of any harmful effects on humans has emerged. Although the possibility of unidentified biologic effects exists, the benefits to the woman of prudent use of diagnostic ultrasonography appear to outweigh any possible risk.

LEGAL TIP Performance of Limited Ultrasound Examinations Nurses who have the training and competence may perform limited ultrasound examinations if it is within the scope of practice in their state or area and consistent with regulations of the agencies in which they practice. Limited ultrasound examinations include identification of fetal number, fetal presentation, fetal cardiac activity, location of the placenta, and BPP, including AFV assessment. Women should be informed about the limited information provided by these examinations. They are not meant to evaluate or identify fetal anomalies, assess fetal age, or estimate fetal weight. The obstetric health care provider is responsible for obtaining a more comprehensive ultrasound examination when complete patient assessment is necessary (Association of Women's Health, Obstetric and Neonatal Nurses, 1998).

Magnetic Resonance Imaging

Magnetic resonance imaging (MRI) is a noninvasive radiologic tool used for obstetric and gynecologic diagnosis. Like computed tomography (CT), MRI provides excellent pictures of soft tissue. Unlike CT, ionizing radiation is not used; therefore vascular structures within the body can be visualized and evaluated without injection of an iodinated contrast medium, thus eliminating any known biologic risk. Like sonography, MRI is noninvasive and can provide images in multiple planes; but there is no interference from skeletal, fatty, or gas-filled structures; and imaging of deep pelvic structures does not require a full bladder.

With MRI the examiner can evaluate (1) fetal structure (central nervous system, thorax, abdomen, genitourinary tract, and musculoskeletal system) and overall growth; (2) placenta (position, density, and presence of gestational trophoblastic disease); (3) amniotic fluid quantity; (4) maternal structures (uterus, cervix, adnexa, and pelvis); (5) biochemical status (pH, adenosine triphosphate content) of tissues and organs; and (6) soft tissue, metabolic, or functional malformations.

The woman is placed on a table in a supine position and slid into the bore of the main magnet, which is similar in appearance to a CT scanner. Depending on the reason for the study, the entire procedure may take from 20 to 60 minutes, during which time the woman must be perfectly still except for short respites. Because of the long time needed to produce MRIs, it is likely that the fetus will move and obscure anatomic details. The only way to ensure that this does not occur is to administer a sedative to the mother, but this approach should be reserved for selected cases in which visualization of fetal detail is critical.

MRI has little effect on the fetus; concerns that the FHR or FMs would decrease have not been supported.

Biochemical Assessment

Biochemical assessment involves biologic examination (e.g., chromosomes in exfoliated cells) and chemical determinations (e.g., lecithin/sphingomyelin (L/S) ratio and bilirubin level) (Table 9-2). Procedures used to obtain the specimens for

Table 9-2 Summary of Biochemical Monitoring Techniques

TEST	POSSIBLE FINDINGS	CLINICAL SIGNIFICANCE
Maternal Blood		
Coombs' test	Titer of 1:8 and rising	Significant Rh incompatibility
Alpha-fetoprotein (AFP)	See below	See below
Amniotic Fluid Analysis		
Color	Meconium	Possible hypoxia or asphyxia
Lung profile		
L/S ratio	>2:1	Fetal lung maturity
Phosphatidylglycerol	Present	Fetal lung maturity
Creatinine	>2 mg/dl	Gestational age >36 wk
Bilirubin (ΔOD 450 nm)*	<0.015	Gestational age >36 wk, normal pregnancy
	High levels	Fetal hemolytic disease in Rh-isoimmunized pregnancies
Lipid cells	>10%	Gestational age >35 wk
AFP	High levels after 15-wk gestation	Open neural tube or other defect
Osmolality	Decline after 20-wk gestation	Advancing nonspecific gestational age
Genetic disorders Sex-linked Chromosomal Metabolic	Dependent on cultured cells for karyotype and enzymatic activity	Counseling possibly required

*The presence of bilirubin changes the color of amniotic fluid. The change in optical density (ΔOD) is a measure of the amount of bilirubin in the amniotic fluid.

study include amniocentesis, PUBS, CVS, and maternal sampling (see Box 9-10).

Amniocentesis

Amniocentesis is performed to obtain amniotic fluid, which contains fetal cells. Under direct ultrasonographic visualization a needle is inserted transabdominally into the uterus, amniotic fluid is withdrawn into a syringe, and various assessments are performed (Fig. 9-8). Amniocentesis is possible after week 14 of pregnancy, when the uterus becomes an abdominal organ and sufficient amniotic fluid is available for testing (see Table 9-2). Indications for the procedure include prenatal diagnosis of genetic disorders or congenital anomalies (NTDs in particular), assessment of pulmonary maturity, and diagnosis of fetal hemolytic disease.

Complications in the mother and fetus occur in less than 1% of cases and include the following:

Maternal—Hemorrhage, fetomaternal hemorrhage with possible maternal Rh isoimmunization, infection, labor, abruptio placentae, inadvertent damage to the intestines or bladder, and amniotic fluid embolism. Due to the possibility of fetomaternal hemorrhage, it is standard practice after an amniocentesis to administer immune globulin D (e.g., RhoGAM) to the woman who is Rh negative.

Fetal—Death, hemorrhage, infection (amnionitis), direct injury from the needle, miscarriage or preterm labor, and leakage of amniotic fluid.

Many of the complications have been minimized or eliminated by using ultrasonography to direct the procedure.

Indications for Use

Genetic Concerns

Prenatal assessment of genetic disorders is indicated for women older than 35 years (Box 9-8), those with a previous child with a chromosome abnormality, or those with a family history of chromosome anomalies. Inherited inborn errors of metabolism and other disorders for which marker genes are known may also be detected.

Fetal cells are cultured for karyotyping of chromosomes (see Chapter 8). Karyotyping also permits determination of fetal sex, which is important if a sex-linked disorder (occurring almost always in a male fetus) is suspected.

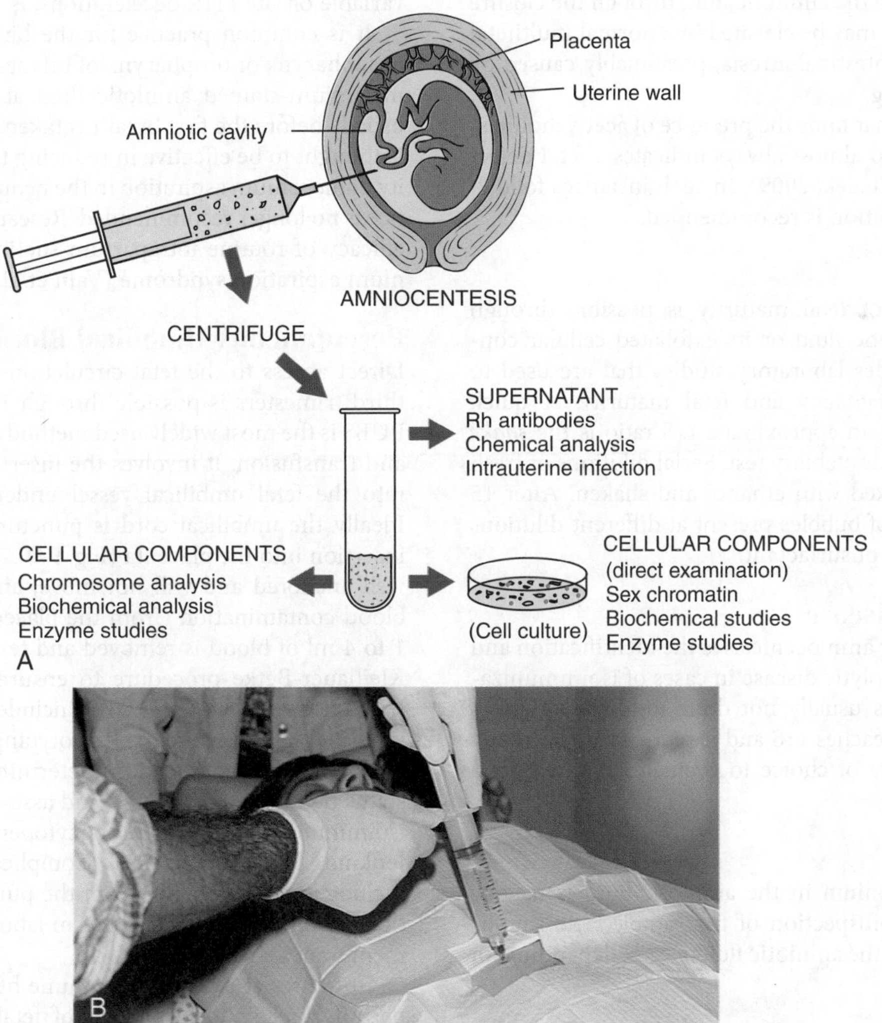

Fig. 9-8 A, Amniocentesis and laboratory use of amniotic fluid aspirant. B, Transabdominal amniocentesis. *(B, Courtesy Marjorie Pyle, RNC, Lifecircle, Costa Mesa, CA.)*

BOX 9-8 Elimination of Maternal Age as an Indication for Invasive Prenatal Diagnosis

Maternal age of 35 years and older has been a standard indication for invasive prenatal testing since 1979 despite a sensitivity of only 30%. The importance of age as a single indication for testing is being reevaluated as serum screening has evolved. The most effective use of resources involves screening the entire population of pregnant women. Presently many centers offer the option of screening before invasive testing for women over 35 years of age (March of Dimes, 2008; Wapner, Jenkins, & Khalek, 2009).

Biochemical analysis of enzymes in amniotic fluid can detect inborn errors of metabolism. For example, AFP levels in amniotic fluid are assessed as a follow-up for elevated levels in maternal serum. High AFP levels in amniotic fluid help confirm the diagnosis of an open NTD such as spina bifida or anencephaly or an open abdominal wall defect such as omphalocele. The elevation results from the increased leakage of cerebrospinal fluid into the amniotic fluid through the closure defect. AFP levels also may be elevated in a normal multifetal pregnancy and with intestinal atresia, presumably caused by lack of fetal swallowing.

A concurrent test that finds the presence of acetylcholinesterase in amniotic fluid almost always indicates a fetal defect (Wapner, Jenkins, & Khalek, 2009). In such instances follow-up ultrasound examination is recommended.

Fetal Maturity

Accurate assessment of fetal maturity is possible through examination of amniotic fluid or its exfoliated cellular contents. Table 9-2 includes laboratory studies that are used to demonstrate term pregnancy and fetal maturity. A quick means of determining an approximate L/S ratio is the *shake test,* foam test, or bubble stability test. Serial dilutions of fresh amniotic fluid are mixed with ethanol and shaken. After 15 minutes, the amount of bubbles present at different dilutions indicates the presence of surfactant.

Fetal Hemolytic Disease

Another indication for amniocentesis is the identification and follow-up of fetal hemolytic disease in cases of isoimmunization. The procedure is usually not done until the mother's serum antibody titer reaches 1:8 and is increasing. Currently PUBS is the procedure of choice to evaluate and treat fetal hemolytic disease.

Meconium

The presence of meconium in the amniotic fluid is usually determined by visual inspection of the sample. The significance of meconium in the amniotic fluid varies, depending on when it is found.

Antepartal Period

Meconium in the amniotic fluid before early labor begins is not usually associated with an adverse fetal outcome. The finding may be the result of an acute and subsequently corrected fetal stress, chronic ongoing stress, or simply the physiologic passage of meconium. Because there is some association between meconium in amniotic fluid in the third trimester and hypertensive conditions and postmaturity, the fetus should undergo further antepartum evaluation. Labor induction may be considered if the fetal status appears compromised (Resnik & Resnik, 2009).

Intrapartal Period

Intrapartal meconium-stained amniotic fluid is an indication for more careful evaluation by electronic fetal monitoring (EFM) and perhaps fetal scalp blood sampling. However, the presence of meconium should not be the sole indicator for intervention.

Three possible reasons exist for the passage of meconium during the intrapartal period: (1) it is a normal physiologic function that occurs with maturity (meconium passage is uncommon before weeks 23 to 24, but there is an increased incidence after 38 weeks); (2) it is the result of hypoxia-induced peristalsis and sphincter relaxation; and (3) it may be a sequel to umbilical cord compression–induced vagal stimulation in mature fetuses. Thick, fresh meconium passed for the first time in late labor, associated with nonremediable severe variable or late FHR decelerations, is an ominous sign.

It is common practice for the birth team to suction the nasopharynx or oropharynx of infants born in the presence of meconium-stained amniotic fluid at the time of the birth, usually before the first breath is taken. Suctioning at this time is thought to be effective in reducing the incidence and severity of meconium aspiration in the neonate. However, this practice is no longer recommended. Research does not support the efficacy of routine intrapartum suctioning to prevent meconium aspiration syndrome (Vain et al, 2004).

Percutaneous Umbilical Blood Sampling

Direct access to the fetal circulation during the second and third trimesters is possible through PUBS, or cordocentesis. PUBS is the most widely used method for fetal blood sampling and transfusion. It involves the insertion of a needle directly into the fetal umbilical vessel under ultrasound guidance. Ideally the umbilical cord is punctured 1 to 2 cm from its insertion into the placenta (Fig. 9-9). At this point the cord is well anchored and will not move, and the risk of maternal blood contamination (from the placenta) is slight. Generally 1 to 4 ml of blood is removed and tested immediately by the Kleihauer-Betke procedure to ensure that it is fetal blood. Indications for use of PUBS include prenatal diagnosis of inherited blood disorders, karyotyping of malformed fetuses, detection of fetal infection, determination of the acid-base status of fetuses with IUGR, and assessment and treatment of isoimmunization and thrombocytopenia in the fetus (Wapner, Jenkins, & Khalek, 2009). Complications that can occur include leaking of blood from the puncture site, cord laceration, thromboembolism, preterm labor, premature rupture of membranes, and infection.

In fetuses at risk for isoimmune hemolytic anemia, PUBS permits precise identification of fetal blood type and RBC count and may eliminate the need for further intervention. If the fetus is positive for the presence of maternal antibodies, a direct blood test can confirm the degree of anemia resulting

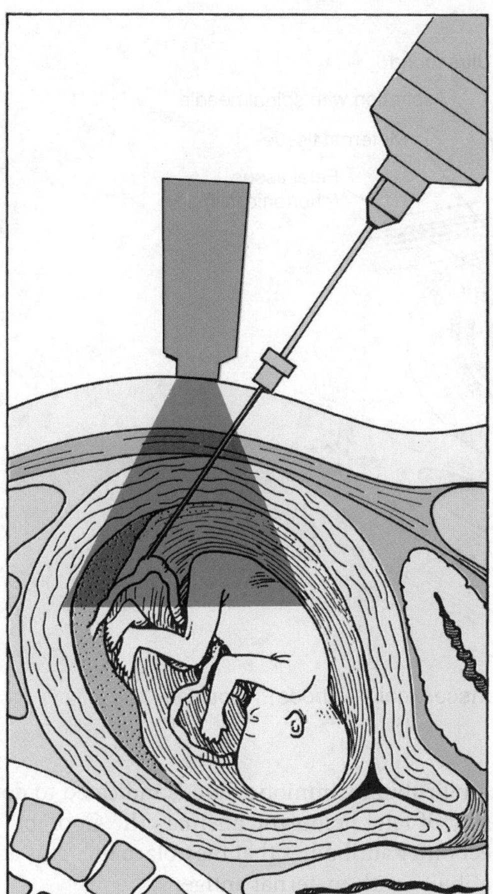

Fig. 9-9 Technique for percutaneous umbilical blood sampling guided by ultrasound.

from hemolysis. Intrauterine transfusion of severely anemic fetuses can be done 4 to 5 weeks earlier than through the intraperitoneal route.

Follow-up includes continuous FHR monitoring for several minutes to 1 hour and a repeat ultrasound examination 1 hour later to ensure that no bleeding or hematoma formation has occurred.

Chorionic Villus Sampling

The combined advantages of earlier diagnosis and rapid results have made chorionic villus sampling (CVS) a popular technique for genetic studies, although some risks to the fetus exist. Indications for CVS are similar to those for amniocentesis; however, second-trimester amniocentesis appears to be safer than CVS (Alfirevic, Sunberg, & Brigham, 2004). The benefits of earlier diagnosis must be weighed against the increased risk of pregnancy loss and risk of anomalies.

The procedure is performed between 10 and 12 weeks of gestation and involves the removal of a small tissue specimen from the fetal portion of the placenta. Because chorionic villi originate in the zygote, that tissue reflects the genetic makeup of the fetus.

CVS can be accomplished either transcervically or transabdominally. In transcervical sampling a sterile catheter is introduced into the cervix under continuous ultrasonographic guidance, and a small portion of the chorionic villi is aspirated with a syringe. The aspiration cannula and obturator must be placed at a suitable site, and rupture of the amniotic sac must be avoided.

If the abdominal approach is used, an 18-gauge spinal needle with stylet is inserted under sterile conditions through the abdominal wall into the chorion frondosum under ultrasound guidance. The stylet is then withdrawn, and the chorionic tissue is aspirated into a syringe (Fig. 9-10).

Complications of the procedure include vaginal spotting or bleeding immediately afterward (Box 9-9), miscarriage (0.3%), rupture of membranes (0.1%), and chorioamnionitis (0.5%). Because of the possibility of fetomaternal hemorrhage, women who are Rh negative should receive immune globulin to avoid isoimmunization. An increased risk of limb anomalies (transverse digital anomalies) has been noted when CVS is done before 10 weeks of gestation (Box 9-10).

Use of amniocentesis and CVS is declining because of advances in noninvasive screening techniques. These techniques include measurement of nuchal translucency, maternal serum screening tests in the first and second trimesters, and ultrasonography in the second trimester (Benn et al, 2004).

BOX 9-9 Apt Test for Differentiation of Maternal and Fetal Blood

The Apt test is used to differentiate maternal and fetal blood when vaginal bleeding occurs during pregnancy or labor. It may be performed quickly by the following method: Add 0.5 ml of bloody fluid to 4.5 ml of distilled water and shake. Add 1 ml of 1% sodium hydroxide. Fetal and cord blood remains pink for 1 to 2 minutes. Maternal blood turns brown in 30 seconds. A Kleihauer-Betke procedure can be done in the laboratory to confirm the presence of fetal blood.

BOX 9-10 Fetal Rights

Amniocentesis, percutaneous umbilical blood sampling, and chorionic villus sampling are prenatal tests used for diagnosing fetal defects in pregnancy. They are invasive and carry risks to the mother and fetus. A consideration of elective abortion is linked to the performance of these tests because there is no treatment for genetically affected fetuses. Thus the issue of fetal rights is a key ethical concern in prenatal testing for fetal defects.

Maternal Assays

Alpha-Fetoprotein

Maternal serum AFP (MSAFP) levels are used as a screening tool for NTDs in pregnancy. Through this technique approximately 80% to 85% of all open NTDs and open abdominal wall defects can be detected early in pregnancy. Screening is recommended for all pregnant women.

The cause of NTDs is not well understood, but 95% of all affected infants are born to women with no family history of similar anomalies (Wapner, Jenkins, & Khalek, 2009). The defect occurs in 1 to 2 per 1000 births in most parts of the

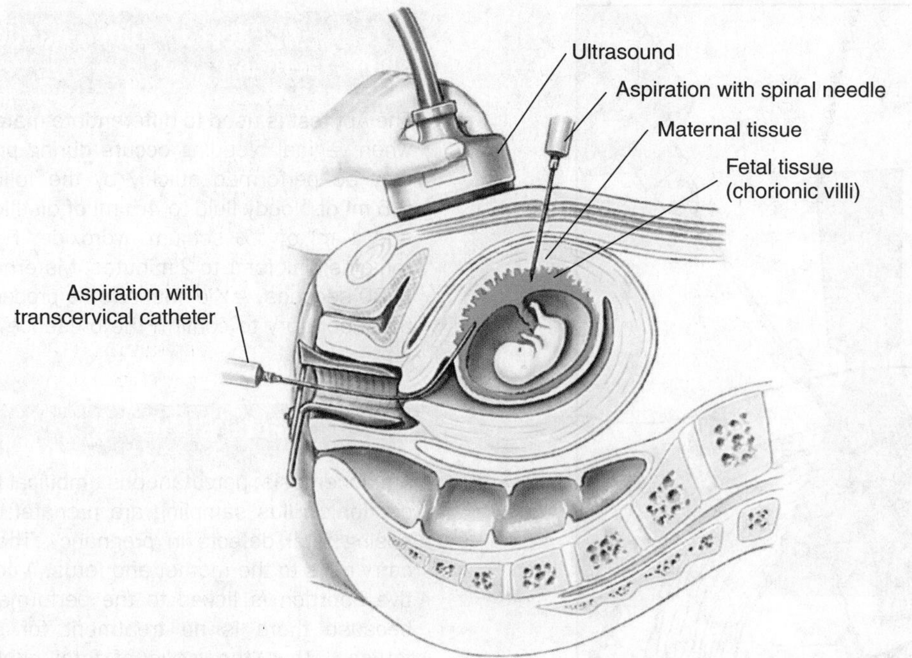

Fig. 9-10 Chorionic villi sampling (abdominal and transcervical methods). *(Courtesy Medical and Scientific Illustration, Crozet, VA.)*

United States. The birth of one affected child increases the risk of NTD recurrence in future pregnancies (Manning, 2009).

AFP is produced by the fetal liver and is detectable in increasing quantities in the serum of pregnant women from 14 to 34 weeks. Although amniotic fluid AFP is diagnostic for NTD, MSAFP is a screening tool only and identifies candidates for the more definitive procedures of amniocentesis and ultrasound examination. MSAFP screening can be done with reasonable reliability any time between 15 and 22 weeks of gestation (16 to 18 weeks being ideal) (Wapner, Jenkins, & Khalek, 2009).

Down syndrome—and probably other autosomal trisomies—is associated with lower-than-normal levels of MSAFP and amniotic fluid AFP. The triple-marker test is also performed at 16 to 18 weeks of gestation and uses the levels of three maternal serum markers: MSAFP, unconjugated estriol, and human chorionic gonadotropin (hCG), in combination with maternal age to calculate a new risk level. If a fetus has Down syndrome, the MSAFP and unconjugated estriol levels are low, and the hCG level is elevated. With these two additional screening tests, approximately 60% of fetuses with Down syndrome can be identified. Other maternal markers are being investigated as predictors of fetal abnormalities as well. Serum pregnancy-associated placental protein A is low in Down syndrome, whereas another substance, inhibin-A, is elevated in Down syndrome and other trisomies.

As with MSAFP, these tests are screening procedures only and are not diagnostic. A definitive examination of amniotic fluid for AFP and chromosome analysis, combined with ultrasound visualization of the fetus, is necessary for diagnosis.

Coombs' Test

The indirect Coombs' test is a screening test for Rh incompatibility and is discussed in Chapter 28. If the maternal titer for Rh antibodies is greater than 1 : 8, amniocentesis for determination of bilirubin in amniotic fluid is indicated to determine the severity of fetal hemolytic anemia. The Coombs' test can also detect other antibodies that may place the fetus at risk for incompatibility with maternal antigens.

Antepartal Assessment Using Electronic Fetal Monitoring

Indications

Assessment during the first and second trimesters is directed primarily at the diagnosis of fetal anomalies. The goal of third-trimester testing is to determine whether the intrauterine environment continues to be supportive to the fetus. The testing is often used to determine the timing of childbirth for patients at risk for uteroplacental insufficiency. Gradual loss of placental function results first in inadequate nutrient delivery to the fetus, leading to IUGR. Subsequently respiratory function is compromised, resulting in fetal hypoxia. Indications for the NST and the contraction stress test (CST) are listed in Box 9-11.

No clinical contraindications exist for the NST, but results may be inconclusive if gestation is 26 weeks or less. Absolute contraindications for the CST are rupture of membranes, previous classic incision for cesarean birth, preterm labor, placenta previa, and abruptio placentae. Multifetal pregnancy, previous preterm labor, hydramnios, more than 36 weeks of gestation, and incompetent cervix are relative contraindications for the CST. As a rule, reactive patterns with the NST or negative results with the CST are associated with favorable outcomes.

Fetal Responses to Hypoxia and Asphyxia

Observable fetal responses to hypoxia or asphyxia are the clinical basis for testing with EFM. Hypoxia or asphyxia elicits a number of responses in the fetus. There is a redistribution

BOX 9-11 Indications for the Nonstress Test and the Contraction Stress Test

- Maternal diabetes mellitus
- Chronic hypertension
- Hypertensive disorders in pregnancy
- Intrauterine growth restriction
- Sickle cell disease
- Maternal cyanotic heart disease
- Postmaturity
- History of previous stillbirth
- Decreased fetal movement
- Isoimmunization
- Meconium-stained amniotic fluid at third-trimester amniocentesis
- Hyperthyroidism
- Collagen disease
- Older pregnant woman
- Chronic renal disease

of blood flow to certain vital organs. This series of responses (redistribution of blood flow favoring vital organs, decreased total oxygen consumption, and a switch to anaerobic glycolysis) is a temporary mechanism that enables the fetus to survive up to 30 minutes with limited oxygen supply without decompensation of vital organs. However, during more severe asphyxia or sustained hypoxemia, these compensatory responses are no longer maintained; and a decrease in the cardiac output, arterial blood pressure, and blood flow to the brain and heart occurs (Nageotte & Gilstrap, 2009), with characteristic FHR patterns reflecting these changes.

Variability

Considerable evidence supports the clinical belief that FHR variability indicates an intact nervous pathway through the cerebral cortex, midbrain, vagus nerve, and cardiac conduction system. With 98% accuracy in predicting fetal well-being, the presence of normal FHR variability is a reassuring indicator. Input from various areas of the brain decreases after cerebral asphyxia, leading to a decrease in variability after failure of the fetal hemodynamic compensatory mechanisms to maintain cerebral oxygenation (Nageotte & Gilstrap, 2009).

Nonstress Test

The NST is the most widely applied technique for antepartum evaluation of the fetus. The basis for the NST is that the normal fetus produces characteristic heart rate patterns in response to FM. In the healthy fetus with an intact central nervous system, 90% of gross fetal body movements are associated with FHR accelerations. The acceleration with movement response may be blunted by hypoxia, acidosis, drugs (analgesics, barbiturates, and β-blockers), fetal sleep, and some congenital anomalies (Tucker, Miller, & Miller, 2009).

The NST can be performed easily and quickly in an outpatient setting because it is noninvasive, relatively inexpensive, and has no known contraindications. Disadvantages center around the high rate of false-positive results for nonreactivity as a result of fetal sleep cycles, chronic tobacco smoking, medications, and fetal immaturity. The test is slightly less sensitive in detecting fetal compromise than are the CST or BPP.

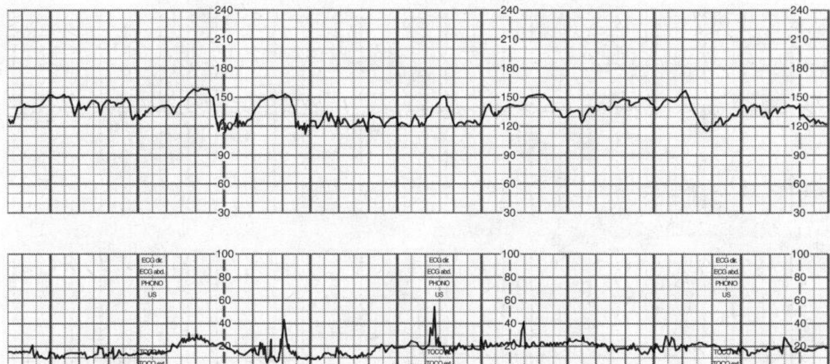

Fig. 9-11 Reactive nonstress test. Fetal heart rate accelerations with fetal movement. (From Tucker SM: *Pocket guide to fetal monitoring and assessment*, ed 5, St Louis, 2004, Mosby.)

Procedure

The woman is seated in a reclining chair (or in a semi-Fowler position) with a slight left tilt to optimize uterine perfusion and avoid supine hypotension. The FHR is recorded with a Doppler transducer, and a tocodynamometer is applied to detect uterine contractions or fetal movements. The tracing is observed for signs of fetal activity and a concurrent acceleration of FHR. If evidence of FM is not apparent on the strip, the woman may be asked to depress a button on a handheld event marker connected to the monitor when she feels FM. The movement is then noted on the tracing. Because almost all accelerations are accompanied by FMs, the movements need not be recorded for the test to be considered reactive. The test usually is completed in 20 to 30 minutes, but it may take longer if the fetus must be awakened from a sleep state.

It has been suggested that the woman drink orange juice or be given glucose to increase her blood sugar level and thereby stimulate FMs. This practice is common; however, research has not proven it to be effective (Tan & Sabapathy, 2004). Some sources suggest that FMs increase when maternal glucose levels are low. Other methods that have been used in an effort to stimulate fetal activity such as manipulating the woman's abdomen or using a transvaginal light are not very effective either. Only vibroacoustic stimulation has had some impact (Tan & Smyth, 2004).

Interpretation

Generally accepted criteria for a reactive tracing are as follows (Fig. 9-11):

- Two or more accelerations of 15 beats/min lasting for 15 seconds over a 20-minute period
- Normal baseline rate
- Moderate variability

If the test does not meet the criteria after 40 minutes, it is considered nonreactive (Fig. 9-12 and Table 9-3), in which case further assessments are needed with a CST or BPP. The current recommendation is that the NST be performed twice weekly (after 28 weeks of gestation) with patients who have diabetes or are at risk for fetal death.

Vibroacoustic Stimulation

Vibroacoustic stimulation (also called *fetal acoustic stimulation test*) is another method of testing antepartum FHR

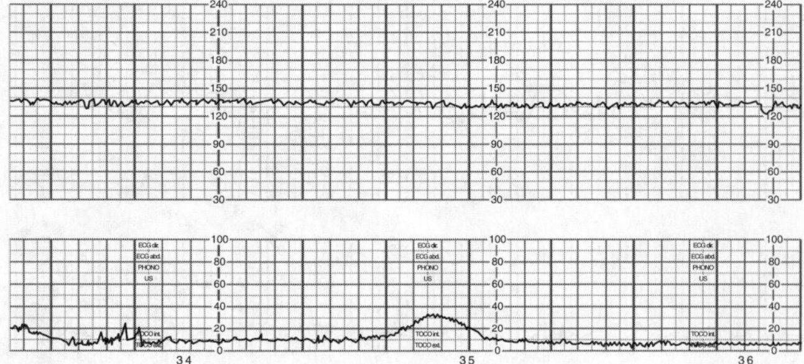

Fig. 9-12 Nonreactive nonstress test (no fetal heart rate accelerations). (From Tucker SM: *Pocket guide to fetal monitoring and assessment*, ed 5, St Louis, 2004, Mosby.)

Table 9-3 Interpretation of the Nonstress Test

RESULT	INTERPRETATION	CLINICAL SIGNIFICANCE
Reactive	Two accelerations of FHR of 15 beats/min lasting 15 sec or more, associated with each fetal movement in a 20-min period (see Fig. 9-11)	As long as twice-weekly NSTs remain reactive, most high risk pregnancies are allowed to continue.
Nonreactive	Any tracing with no FHR accelerations or accelerations <15 beats/min or lasting <15 sec throughout any FMs during testing period	Further indirect monitoring may be attempted with abdominal fetal electrocardiography in an effort to clarify FHR pattern and quantify variability; external monitoring should continue, and a CST or BPP should be done.
Unsatisfactory	Quality of FHR recording not adequate for interpretation	Test is repeated in 24 hr, or a CST is done, depending on the clinical situation.

Reference: Tucker SM, Miller LA, Miller DA: *Mosby's pocket guide to fetal monitoring; a multidisciplinary approach*, ed 6, St Louis, 2009, Mosby.
BPP, Biophysical profile; *CST,* contraction stress test; *FHR,* fetal heart rate; *FM,* fetal movement; *NST,* nonstress test.

response and is sometimes used in conjunction with the NST. The test takes approximately 15 minutes to complete, with the fetus monitored for 5 to 10 minutes before stimulation to obtain a baseline FHR. If the fetal baseline pattern is nonreactive, the sound source (usually a laryngeal stimulator) is then activated for 3 seconds on the maternal abdomen over the fetal head. Monitoring continues for another 5 minutes, after which the monitor tracing is assessed. A test is considered reactive if there is an immediate and sustained increase in variability and heart rate accelerations. The test may be repeated at 1-minute intervals up to three times when there is no response. Further evaluation is needed with BPP or CST if the pattern is still nonreactive.

Contraction Stress Test

The CST was one of the first electronic methods to be developed for assessment of fetal well-being. It was devised as a graded stress test of the fetus. Its purpose was to identify the jeopardized fetus that was stable at rest but showed evidence of compromise after stress. Uterine contractions decrease uterine blood flow and placental perfusion. If this decrease is sufficient to produce hypoxia in the fetus, a deceleration in FHR results, beginning at the peak of the contraction and persisting after its conclusion (late deceleration).

NURSING ALERT In a healthy fetoplacental unit, uterine contractions usually do not produce late decelerations; when there is underlying uteroplacental insufficiency, contractions produce late decelerations.

The CST provides a warning of fetal compromise earlier than the NST and with fewer false-positive tests. In addition to the contraindications described earlier, the CST is more time-consuming and expensive than an NST. It also is an invasive procedure if exogenous oxytocin stimulation is required.

Procedure

The woman is placed in semi-Fowler position or sits in a reclining chair with a slight lateral tilt to optimize uterine perfusion and avoid supine hypotension. She is monitored electronically with the fetal ultrasound transducer and uterine tocodynamometer. The tracing is observed for 10 to 20 minutes for baseline rate, long-term variability, and the possible occurrence of spontaneous contractions. Two methods of the CST are the nipple-stimulated contraction test and the oxytocin-stimulated contraction test.

Nipple-Stimulated Contraction Test

Several methods of nipple stimulation have been described. In one approach the woman applies warm, moist washcloths to both breasts for several minutes. She is then asked to massage one nipple for 10 minutes. Massaging the nipples causes a release of oxytocin from the posterior pituitary. An alternative approach is for her to massage the nipple for 2 minutes, rest for 5 minutes, and repeat the cycles of massage and rest as necessary to achieve adequate uterine activity. When adequate contractions or hyperstimulation occurs, stimulation should be stopped (Tucker, Miller, & Miller, 2009).

Oxytocin-Stimulated Contraction Test

Exogenous oxytocin can also be used to stimulate uterine contractions. An intravenous (IV) infusion is begun with a scalp needle. The oxytocin is diluted in an IV solution (usually 10 units in 1000 ml of fluid) and infused through a piggyback port into the tubing of the main IV device. An infusion pump is used to ensure accurate dosage. The oxytocin infusion usually is begun at 0.5 milliunits/min and increased by 0.5 milliunits/min at 15- to 30-minute intervals until three uterine contractions of good quality are observed within a 10-minute period. A rate of 10 milliunits/min is usually adequate to elicit uterine contractions.

Interpretation

If no late decelerations are observed with the contractions, the findings are considered to be negative (Fig. 9-13). Repetitive late decelerations render the test results positive (Fig. 9-14 and Table 9-4).

After interpretation of the FHR pattern, the oxytocin infusion is discontinued, and the maintenance IV solution is infused until the uterine activity has returned to the prestimulation level. If the CST is negative, the IV device is removed, and the fetal monitor disconnected. If the CST is positive, continued monitoring and further evaluation of fetal well-being are indicated.

Nursing Role in Antenatal Assessment for Risk

The nurse's role is that of educator and support person when the woman is undergoing examinations such as ultrasonography, MRI, CVS, PUBS, and amniocentesis. In some instances the nurse may assist the physician with the procedure. In many settings nurses perform NSTs, CSTs, BPPs, and basic ultrasonography; conduct an initial assessment; and begin necessary interventions for nonreassuring patterns. These nursing procedures are accomplished after additional education and training, under guidance of established protocols, and in collaboration with physicians. Patient teaching, which is an integral component of this role, involves preparing the woman for the procedure, interpreting the findings, and providing psychosocial support when needed.

Psychologic Considerations

All women who undergo antenatal assessments are at risk for real and potential problems and may be anxious. In most instances the tests are ordered because of suspected fetal compromise, deterioration of a maternal condition, or both. In the third trimester pregnant women are most concerned about protecting themselves and their fetuses and consider themselves most vulnerable to outside influences. The label of high risk increases this sense of vulnerability.

When a woman is diagnosed with a high risk pregnancy, she and her family will likely experience stress related to the diagnosis. The woman may exhibit various psychologic

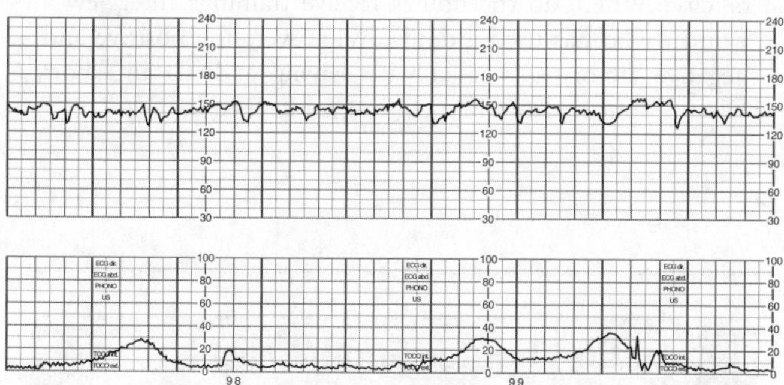

Fig. 9-13 Negative contraction stress test (reassuring external fetal heart rate tracing). (From Tucker SM: *Pocket guide to fetal monitoring and assessment*, ed 5, St Louis, 2004, Mosby.)

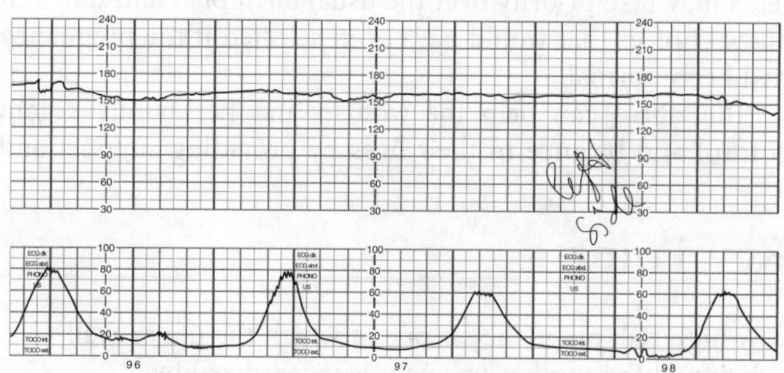

Fig. 9-14 Positive contraction stress test (nonreassuring late decelerations with uterine contractions). (From Tucker SM: *Pocket guide to fetal monitoring and assessment*, ed 5, St Louis, 2004, Mosby.)

Table 9-4 Interpretation of the Contraction Stress Test

INTERPRETATION	CLINICAL SIGNIFICANCE
Negative	
No late decelerations, with minimum of three uterine contractions within 10-min period (see Fig. 9-13)	Reassurance that the fetus is likely to survive labor should it occur within 1 wk; more frequent testing may be indicated by clinical situation
Positive	
Late decelerations occurring with at least half of contractions (see Fig. 9-14)	Management lies between use of other tools of fetal assessment such as BPP and termination of pregnancy; positive test result indicates that fetus is at increased risk for perinatal morbidity and mortality; physician may perform expeditious vaginal birth after successful induction or may proceed directly to cesarean birth; decision to intervene determined by fetal monitoring and presence of FHR reactivity
Suspicious or Equivocal	
Prolonged, variable, or late decelerations occurring with less then 50% of the contractions	NST and CST should be repeated within 24 hr; if interpretable data cannot be achieved, other methods of fetal assessment must be used*
Equivocal-Hyperstimulatory	
Decelerations that occur in the presence of contractions more frequent than every 2 min or lasting longer then 90 sec	Repeat test next day
Unsatisfactory	
Inadequate uterine contraction pattern or tracing too poor to interpret	Repeat test next day

Reference: Tucker SM, Miller LA, Miller DA: *Mosby's pocket guide to fetal monitoring; a multidisciplinary approach*, ed 6, St Louis, 2009, Mosby.
BPP, Biophysical profile; *FHR,* fetal heart rate; *NST,* nonstress test; *CST,* contraction stress test.
*Applies to results noted as suspicious, hyperstimulation, or unsatisfactory.

responses, including anxiety, low self-esteem, guilt, frustration, and inability to function. The development of a high risk pregnancy also can affect parental attachment, accomplishment of the tasks of pregnancy, and family adaptation to the pregnancy.

If the woman is fearful for her own well-being, she may continue to feel ambivalence about the pregnancy or not accept the reality of the pregnancy. She may not be able to complete preparations for the baby or go to childbirth classes if she is on bed rest or hospitalized. The family may become frustrated because they cannot engage in these activities that prepare them for parenthood.

Antepartal hospitalization is an added stressor for the high risk pregnant woman and her family. The woman may be lonely because she is separated from her home and family. She may feel powerless and unable to make decisions for herself because her care is out of her control. Likewise, preparation for the birth process may be out of control of the woman and her family. Unexpected procedures and care for the woman or fetus may take priority over the usual birth plan and may not allow choices that would have been selected if the pregnancy had been normal.

The nurse can help the woman and her family regain control and balance in their lives by providing support and encouragement, information about the pregnancy problem and its management, and opportunities to make as many choices as possible about the woman's care (see Community Focus box).

COMMUNITY FOCUS

Support for At-Risk Pregnant Women

At-risk pregnant women experience many stressors. Social support can relieve some of the stress, including during labor. Nurses, social workers, and midwives—as well as trained lay persons—have provided labor support. Investigate in your setting whether such support is available for low-income women. Is there a doula program at the hospital where you did your maternity clinical rotation or in your city? Does the program provide this service on a sliding scale for low-income women? What is the background of the doulas in your setting or city? Where do the doulas receive training? Interview a woman who has used a doula. What were the positive and negative factors associated with having a doula in labor? Discuss your findings in a clinical conference.

Key Points

- A high risk pregnancy is one in which the life or well-being of the mother or infant is jeopardized by a biophysical or psychosocial disorder coincidental with or unique to pregnancy.
- The pregnancy, fetus, or neonate can be placed at risk by biophysical, sociodemographic, psychosocial, and environmental factors.
- Psychosocial perinatal warning indicators include characteristics of the parents, the fetus, the neonate, their support systems, and family circumstances.
- There are racial and ethnic disparities in maternal and perinatal mortality rates in the United States.
- Mortality rate decreases when risks are identified early and intensive care is applied.

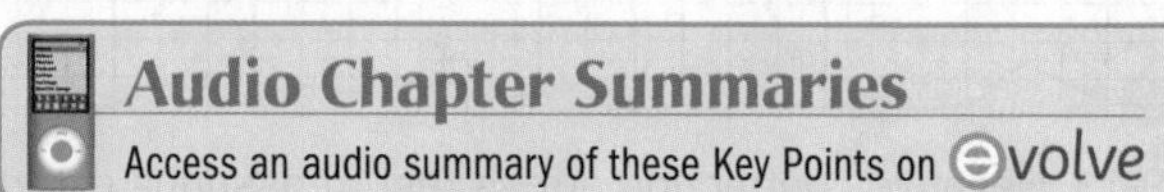
Audio Chapter Summaries
Access an audio summary of these Key Points on evolve

- Biophysical assessment techniques include FM counts, ultrasonography, and MRI.
- Biochemical monitoring techniques include amniocentesis, PUBS, CVS, and MSAFP.
- Reactive NSTs and negative CSTs suggest fetal well-being.
- Most assessment tests have some degree of risk for the mother and fetus and usually cause some anxiety for the woman and her family.

References

Alfirevic Z, Sunberg S, Brigham S: Amniocentesis and chorionic villi sampling for prenatal diagnosis (Cochrane Review). In *The Cochrane Library,* Issue 2, Chichester, UK, 2004, John Wiley & Sons.

American College of Obstetricians and Gynecologists: Ultrasonography in pregnancy. Practice Bulletin Number 58, *Obstet Gynecol* 104(6):1149-1158, 2004a.

American College of Obstetricians and Gynecologists: News release. *ACOG issues position on first-trimester screening methods,* 2004b. Available at www.acog.org/from_home/publications/press_releases/nr06-30-04.cfm (accessed March 5, 2009).

Association of Women's Health, Obstetric and Neonatal Nurses (AWHONN): *Nursing practice competencies and educational guidelines for limited ultrasound examination in obstetric and gynecology/infertility settings,* ed 2, Washington, DC, 1998, AWHONN.

Benn P et al: Changes in utilization of prenatal diagnosis, *Obstet Gynecol* 103(6):1255-1260, 2004.

Gilbert ES: *Manual of high risk pregnancy & delivery,* ed 4, St Louis, 2007a, Mosby.

Gilbert WM: Amniotic fluid disorders. In Gabbe SG, Niebyl JR, Simpson JL (editors): *Obstetrics: normal and problem pregnancies,* ed 5, Philadelphia, 2007b, Churchill Livingstone.

Harman CR: Assessment of fetal health. In Creasy RK et al (editors): *Creasy & Resnik's maternal-fetal medicine: principles and practice,* ed 6, Philadelphia, 2009, Saunders.

Hoyert D et al: *Deaths: final data for 2003,* Health E-Stats, Hyattsville, Md, released January 19, 2006, National Center for Health Statistics.

Manning F: Imaging in the diagnosis of fetal anomalies. In Creasy RK et al (editors): *Creasy & Resnik's maternal-fetal medicine: principles and practice,* ed 6, Philadelphia, 2009, Saunders.

March of Dimes: *Pregnancy after 35,* 2008. Available at www.marchofdimes.com/professionals/14332_1155.asp (accessed March 5, 2009).

Nageotte MP, Gilstrap LC: Intrapartum fetal surveillance. In Creasy RK et al (editors): *Creasy & Resnik's maternal-fetal medicine: principles and practice,* ed 6, Philadelphia, 2009, Saunders.

Resnik JL, Resnik R: Post-term pregnancy. In Creasy RK et al (editors): *Creasy & Resnik's maternal-fetal medicine: principles and practice*, ed 6, Philadelphia, 2009, Saunders.

Richards DS: Ultrasound for pregnancy dating, growth and diagnosis of fetal malformations. In Gabbe SG, Niebyl JR, Simpson JL (editors): *Obstetrics: normal and problem pregnancies*, ed 5, Philadelphia, 2007, Churchill Livingstone.

Tan KH, Sabapathy A: Maternal glucose administration for facilitating tests of fetal wellbeing (Cochrane Review), *The Cochrane Library*, Issue 3, Chichester, UK, 2004, John Wiley & Sons.

Tan KH, Smyth R: Fetal vibroacoustic stimulation for facilitation of tests of fetal wellbeing (Cochrane Review), *The Cochrane Library*, Issue 3, Chichester, UK, 2004, John Wiley & Sons.

Tucker SM, Miller LA, Miller DA: *Mosby's pocket guide to fetal monitoring: a multidisciplinary approach*, ed 6, St Louis, 2009, Mosby.

U.S. Department of Health and Human Services: *Healthy People 2010* (Conference Edition) (vols. 1-2), Washington, DC, 2000, US Government Printing Office.

Vain NE et al: Oropharyngeal and nasopharyngeal suctioning of meconium-stained neonates before delivery of their shoulders: multicentre, randomized controlled trial, *Lancet* 364(9434):597-602, 2004.

Wapner RJ, Jenkins TM, Khalek N: Prenatal diagnosis of congenital disorders. In Creasy RK et al (editors): *Creasy & Resnik's maternal-fetal medicine: principles and practice*, ed 6, Philadelphia, 2009, Saunders.

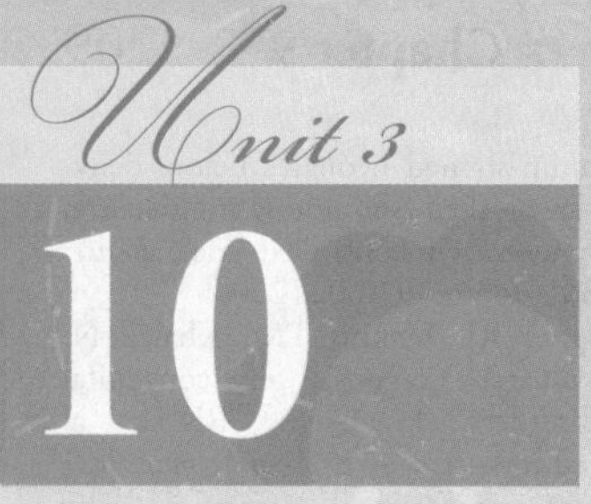

10 Anatomy and Physiology of Pregnancy

Learning Objectives

On completion of this chapter the reader will be able to:

- Determine gravidity and parity using the five- and two-digit systems.
- Describe the various types of pregnancy tests, including the timing of tests and interpretation of results.
- Explain the expected maternal anatomic and physiologic adaptations to pregnancy.
- Differentiate among presumptive, probable, and positive signs of pregnancy.
- Identify maternal hormones produced during pregnancy, their target organs, and their major effects on pregnancy.
- Compare the characteristics of the abdomen, vulva, and cervix of the nullipara and multipara.

Electronic Resources

Additional information related to the content in Chapter 10 can be found on

evolve the Companion Website at

http://evolve.elsevier.com/Perry/maternal/

- NCLEX Review Questions

The goal of maternity care is a healthy pregnancy with a physically safe and emotionally satisfying outcome for mother, infant, and family. Consistent health supervision and surveillance are of utmost importance. However, many maternal adaptations are unfamiliar to pregnant women and their families. Helping the pregnant woman recognize the relationship between her physical status and the plan for her care assists her in making decisions and encourages her to participate in her own care.

Gravidity and Parity

An understanding of the following terms used to describe pregnancy and the pregnant woman (Cunningham et al, 2005) is essential to the study of maternity care:

Gravida—A woman who is pregnant

Gravidity—Pregnancy

Multigravida—A woman who has had two or more pregnancies

Multipara—A woman who has completed two or more pregnancies to 20 weeks of gestation or more

Nulligravida—A woman who has never been pregnant

Nullipara—A woman who has not completed a pregnancy with a fetus or fetuses beyond 20 weeks of gestation

Parity—The number of pregnancies in which the fetus or fetuses have reached 20 weeks of gestation, not the number of fetuses (e.g., twins) born. Parity is not affected by whether the fetus is born alive or is stillborn (i.e., showing no signs of life at birth).

Postdate or postterm—Pregnancy that goes beyond 42 weeks of gestation

Preterm—A pregnancy that has reached 20 weeks of gestation but before completion of 37 weeks of gestation

Primigravida—A woman who is pregnant for the first time

Primipara—A woman who has completed one pregnancy with a fetus or fetuses who have reached 20 weeks of gestation

Term—A pregnancy from the beginning of week 38 of gestation to the end of week 42 of gestation

Viability—Capacity to live outside the uterus, occurring about 22 to 25 weeks of gestation

Gravidity and parity information is obtained during history-taking interviews. Obtaining and documenting this information accurately is important in planning care for the pregnant women. Information may be recorded in patient records in a variety of ways because there is no one standardized system. It is important that the nurse understand the documentation system used by the health care facility. Gravidity and parity can be described with only two digits: the first digit indicates the number of pregnancies the woman has had, including the present one, and parity the number of pregnancies that have reached 20 weeks of gestation. For example, the abbreviation gravida 1, para 0 (1/0) means that a woman is pregnant for the first time (primigravida) and has not carried a pregnancy to 20 weeks (nullipara). If a woman had twins at 36 weeks with her first pregnancy, she would also be gravida 1, para 1 (remember that para refers to pregnancies, not fetuses) (Cunningham et al, 2005).

Table 10-1 Gravidity and Parity Using Five-Digit (GTPAL) and Two-Digit Systems

	Five-Digit System					Two-Digit System
	G	T	P	A	L	G/P
CONDITION	GRAVIDITY	TERM BIRTH	PRETERM BIRTHS	ABORTIONS AND MISCARRIAGES	LIVING CHILDREN	GRAVIDITY/PARITY
Kathy is pregnant for the first time.	1	0	0	0	0	1/0
She carries the pregnancy to term, and the neonate survives.	1	1	0	0	1	1/1
She is pregnant again.	2	1	0	0	1	2/1
Her second pregnancy ends in miscarriage at 10 wk.	2	1	0	1	1	2/1
During her third pregnancy she gives birth at 36 wk to twins.	3	1	2	1	3	3/2

Another system, consisting of five digits separated by hyphens, is commonly used in maternity centers. This system provides more information about the woman's obstetric history, although it may not provide accurate information about parity since it provides information about births and not pregnancies reaching 20 weeks of gestation (Beebe, 2005). The first digit represents gravidity; the second digit represents the total number of term births; the third indicates the number of preterm births; the fourth identifies the number of abortions (miscarriage or elective termination of pregnancy); and the fifth is the number of children currently living. The acronym *GTPAL* (gravidity, term, preterm, abortions, living children) may be helpful in remembering this system of notation. For example, if a woman pregnant only once gives birth at week 35 and the infant survives, the abbreviation that represents this information is "1-0-1-0-1." During her next pregnancy the abbreviation is "2-0-1-0-1." Additional examples are in Table 10-1.

Pregnancy Tests

Early detection of pregnancy allows for early initiation of care. Human chorionic gonadotropin (hCG) is the earliest biologic marker for pregnancy. Pregnancy tests are based on the recognition of hCG or a beta (β) subunit of hCG. Production of β-hCG begins as early as the day of implantation and can be detected as early as 7 to 10 days after conception (Blackburn, 2007). The level of hCG rises until it peaks at about 60 to 70 days of gestation and then declines until about 80 days of gestation. It remains stable until about 30 weeks and then gradually increases until term. Higher than normal levels of hCG may indicate ectopic pregnancy, abnormal gestation (e.g., fetus with Down syndrome), or multiple gestation; abnormally slow increase or a decrease in hCG levels may indicate impending miscarriage (Cunningham et al, 2005).

Serum and urine pregnancy tests are performed in clinics, offices, women's health centers, and laboratory settings. Urine pregnancy tests may be performed at home (see Community Focus box). Both serum and urine tests can provide accurate results. A 7- to 10-ml sample of venous blood is collected for serum testing. Most urine tests require a first-voided morning urine specimen because it contains levels of hCG approximately the same as those in serum. Random urine samples usually have lower levels. Urine tests are less expensive and provide more immediate results than serum tests.

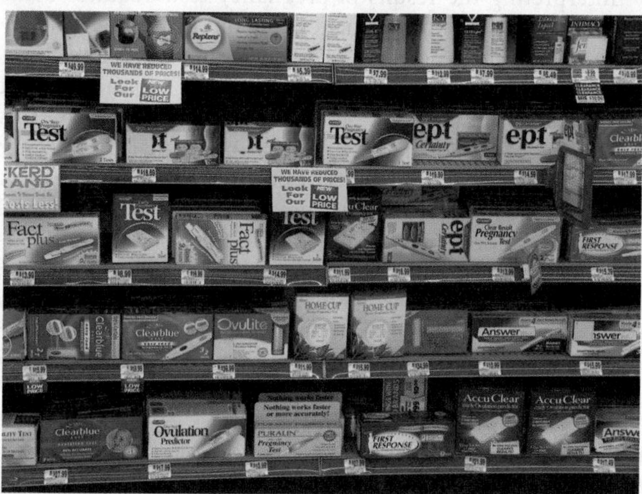

Fig. 10-1 Many pregnancy test products are available over the counter. *(Courtesy Dee Lowdermilk, Chapel Hill, NC.)*

COMMUNITY FOCUS

Home Pregnancy Test Kits

Visit a pharmacy in your neighborhood. How many different types of pregnancy home test kits are available in the pharmacy? Read the labels on three different types of pregnancy home test kits. Do the kits include material for more than one test? Are the directions printed in more than one language? After reading the directions, do you have questions about how to perform the test or how to interpret the results? If so, what does that say about the likelihood that the tests will be used correctly?

Many different pregnancy tests are available (Fig. 10-1). The wide variety of tests precludes discussion of each. The nurse should read the manufacturer's directions for the test that is used.

Enzyme-linked immunosorbent assay (ELISA) testing is the most popular method of testing for pregnancy. It uses a specific monoclonal antibody (anti-hCG) with enzymes that bond with hCG in urine. ELISA technology is the basis for most over-the-counter home pregnancy tests. With these one-step tests the woman usually applies urine to a strip or absorbent-tipped applicator and reads the results. The test kits come with directions for collection of the specimen, the testing procedure, and reading of results. A positive test result is indicated by a simple color change reaction or a digital reading. Most manufacturers of the kits provide a toll-free telephone number to call if users have concerns and questions about test procedures or results. The most common error in performing home pregnancy tests is doing the test too early in pregnancy (Pagana & Pagana, 2006).

Interpreting the results of pregnancy tests requires some judgment. The type of pregnancy test and its degree of sensitivity (the ability to detect low levels of a substance) and specificity (the ability to discern the absence of a substance) must be considered in conjunction with the woman's history. This includes the date of her last normal menstrual period, her usual cycle length, and results of previous pregnancy tests. It is important to know if the woman abuses substances and what medications she is taking. Medications such as anticonvulsants and tranquilizers can cause false-positive results, whereas diuretics and promethazine can cause false-negative results (Pagana & Pagana, 2006). Improper collection of the specimen, hormone-producing tumors, and laboratory errors can also cause inaccurate results.

Women who use a home pregnancy test should be advised about the variations in accuracy reporting and to use caution when interpreting results. Whenever there is any question, further evaluation or retesting may be appropriate.

Adaptations to Pregnancy

Maternal physiologic adaptations are attributed to the hormones of pregnancy and to mechanical pressures arising from the enlarging uterus and other tissues. These adaptations protect the woman's normal physiologic functioning, meet the metabolic demands that pregnancy imposes on her body, and provide a nurturing environment for fetal development and growth (see Critical Thinking Exercise). Although pregnancy is a normal phenomenon, problems can occur.

Signs of Pregnancy

Some physiologic adaptations are recognized as the signs and symptoms of pregnancy. Three commonly used categories of these signs and symptoms are (1) presumptive—those changes felt by the woman (e.g., amenorrhea, fatigue, breast changes); (2) probable—those changes observed by an examiner (e.g., Hegar sign, ballottement, pregnancy tests); and (3) positive—those signs attributed only to the presence of the fetus (e.g., hearing fetal heart tones, visualizing the fetus, palpating fetal movements). Table 10-2 summarizes these signs of pregnancy in relation to when they might occur and gives other possible causes for their occurrence.

CRITICAL THINKING EXERCISE

Awareness of Physiologic Changes of Pregnancy

Marlys is pregnant with her first child, and Janice is pregnant with her third child. They are both at approximately 18 weeks of gestation and have come to a prenatal appointment. While they are in the waiting room, you overhear Marlys asking Janice about some "old wives' tales" that she has heard:

- If she raises her arms above her head, the cord will wrap around the baby's neck.
- Putting a knife under the bed while she is laboring will "cut" the pain.
- If she dangles a needle in front of her abdomen, she will be able to tell if the baby is a boy or a girl.
- A rapid fetal heartbeat means that the baby will be a boy.

Marlys says that she has not felt her baby move yet, whereas Janice says that she has been feeling fetal movement for over 2 weeks. Marlys also has questions about some of the changes in her body that she has experienced or expects to experience. Janice bases her responses on her own experience. Based on the conversation you have overheard, you identify a need to spend some time with Marlys and Janice discussing physiologic changes of pregnancy.

1. Evidence—Is there sufficient evidence to draw conclusions about the normal physiologic changes in pregnancy in primigravidas and multiparas that the nurse should discuss with Marlys and Janice?
2. Assumptions—Describe an underlying assumption about each of the following topics:
   a. Differences in the normal physiologic changes in pregnancy between primigravidas and multiparas
   b. Reversibility of these physiologic changes in pregnancy
   c. Information provided by the health care provider
   d. Deviations from normal in the physiologic changes of pregnancy
3. What implications and priorities for nursing care can be drawn at this time?
4. Does the evidence objectively support your conclusion?
5. Are there alternative perspectives to your conclusion?

Reproductive System and Breasts

Uterus

Changes in Size, Shape, and Position

High levels of estrogen and progesterone stimulate phenomenal uterine growth in the first trimester. Early uterine enlargement results from increased vascularity and dilation of blood vessels, hyperplasia (production of new muscle fibers and fibroelastic tissue) and hypertrophy (enlargement of preexisting muscle fibers and fibroelastic tissue), and development of the decidua. By 7 weeks of gestation the uterus is the size of a large hen's egg; by 10 weeks it is the size of an orange (twice its nonpregnant size); and by 12 weeks it is the size of a grapefruit. After the third month uterine enlargement is primarily the result of mechanical pressure of the growing fetus.

As the uterus enlarges, it also changes in shape and position. At conception the uterus is shaped like an upside-down

Table 10-2 Signs of Pregnancy

TIME OF OCCURRENCE (GESTATIONAL AGE)	SIGN	OTHER POSSIBLE CAUSE
Presumptive		
3-4 wk	Breast changes	Premenstrual changes, oral contraceptives
4 wk	Amenorrhea	Stress, vigorous exercise, early menopause, endocrine problems, malnutrition
4-14 wk	Nausea, vomiting	Gastrointestinal virus, food poisoning
6-12 wk	Urinary frequency	Infection, pelvic tumors
12 wk	Fatigue	Stress, illness
16-20 wk	Quickening	Gas, peristalsis
Probable		
5 wk	Goodell sign	Pelvic congestion
6-8 wk	Chadwick sign	Pelvic congestion
6-12 wk	Hegar sign	Pelvic congestion
4-12 wk	Positive pregnancy test (serum)	Hydatidiform mole, choriocarcinoma
6-12 wk	Positive pregnancy test (urine)	False-positive result may be caused by pelvic infection, tumors
16 wk	Braxton Hicks contractions	Myomas, other tumors
16-28 wk	Ballottement	Tumors, cervical polyps
Positive		
5-6 wk	Visualization of fetus by real-time ultrasound examination	No other causes
6 wk	Fetal heart tones detected by ultrasound	No other causes
16 wk	Visualization of fetus by radiographic study	No other causes
8-17 wk	Fetal heart tones detected by Doppler ultrasound stethoscope	No other causes
17-19 wk	Fetal heart tones detected by fetal stethoscope	No other causes
19-22 wk	Fetal movements palpated	No other causes
Late pregnancy	Fetal movements visible	No other causes

pear. During the second trimester, as the muscular walls strengthen and become more elastic, the uterus becomes spherical or globular. Later, as the fetus lengthens, the uterus becomes larger and more ovoid and rises out of the pelvis into the abdominal cavity.

The pregnancy may "show" after the fourteenth week, although this depends to some degree on the woman's height and weight. Abdominal enlargement may be less apparent in the nullipara with good abdominal muscle tone (Fig. 10-2). Posture also influences the type and degree of abdominal enlargement that occurs. In normal pregnancies the uterus enlarges at a predictable rate.

As the uterus grows, it may be palpated above the symphysis pubis sometime between the twelfth and fourteenth weeks of pregnancy (Fig. 10-3). The uterus rises gradually to the level of the umbilicus at 22 to 24 weeks of gestation and nearly reaches the xiphoid process at term. Between weeks 38 and 40 fundal height decreases as the fetus begins to descend and engage in the pelvis (lightening) (see Fig. 10-3, *dashed line*). Generally lightening occurs in the nullipara about 2 weeks before the onset of labor and in the multipara at the start of labor.

Uterine enlargement is determined by measuring fundal height (see Fig. 11-7). This measurement is commonly used to estimate the duration of pregnancy. However, variation in the position of the fundus or the fetus, variations in the amount of amniotic fluid present, the presence of more than one fetus, maternal obesity, and variation in examiner technique can reduce the accuracy of this estimation.

Generally the uterus rotates to the right as it elevates, probably because of the presence of the rectosigmoid colon on the left side. However, the extensive hypertrophy (enlargement) of the round ligaments keeps the uterus in the midline. Eventually the growing uterus touches the anterior abdominal wall and displaces the intestines to either side of the abdomen (Fig. 10-4). When a pregnant woman is standing, most of her uterus rests against the anterior abdominal wall and contributes to altering her center of gravity.

At approximately 6 weeks of gestation softening and compressibility of the lower uterine segment (uterine isthmus) occurs (Hegar sign) (Fig. 10-5). This results in exaggerated uterine anteflexion during the first 3 months of pregnancy. In this position the uterine fundus presses on the urinary bladder, causing the woman to have urinary frequency.

Changes in Contractility

Soon after the fourth month of pregnancy uterine contractions can be felt through the abdominal wall. These contractions are referred to as Braxton Hicks contractions. Braxton

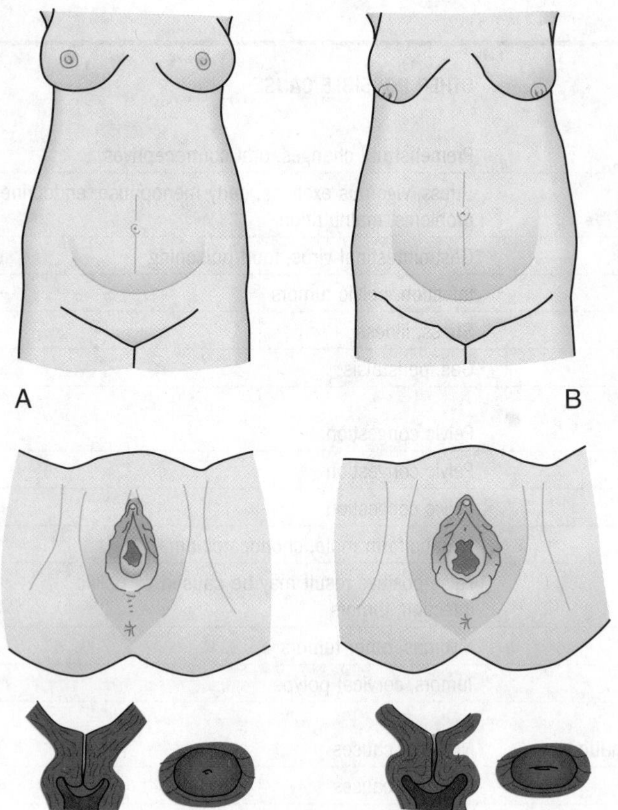

Fig. 10-2 Comparison of abdomen, vulva, and cervix in **A**, nullipara, and **B**, multipara, at the same stage of pregnancy.

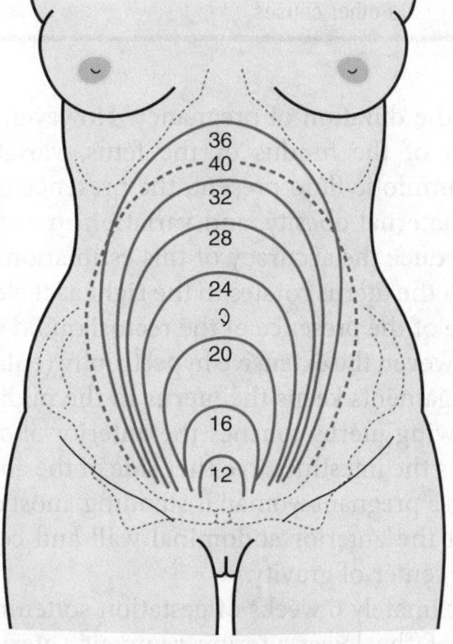

Fig. 10-3 Height of fundus by weeks of normal gestation with a single fetus. *Dashed line,* Height after lightening.

Hicks contractions are irregular and painless contractions that occur intermittently throughout pregnancy. These contractions facilitate uterine blood flow through the intervillous spaces of the placenta and promote oxygen delivery to the fetus. Although Braxton Hicks contractions are not painful, some women complain that they are annoying. After the twenty-eighth week, these contractions become more definite, but they usually cease with walking or exercise. Braxton Hicks contractions can be mistaken for true labor; however, they do not increase in intensity or duration or cause cervical dilation. Conversely premature labor contractions can be mistaken for Braxton Hicks contractions and lead to a delay in seeking treatment.

Uteroplacental Blood Flow

Placental perfusion depends on the maternal blood flow to the uterus. Blood flow increases rapidly as the uterus increases in size. Although uterine blood flow increases twentyfold, the fetoplacental unit grows even more rapidly. Consequently more oxygen is extracted from the uterine blood during the latter part of pregnancy (Cunningham et al, 2005). In a normal term pregnancy one sixth of the total maternal blood volume is within the uterine vascular system. The rate of blood flow through the uterus averages 500 ml/min, and oxygen consumption of the gravid uterus increases to meet fetal needs. Three factors known to decrease uterine blood flow are low maternal arterial pressure, contractions of the uterus, and maternal supine position. Estrogen stimulation may increase uterine blood flow. Doppler ultrasound examination can be used to measure uterine blood flow velocity, especially in pregnancies at risk because of conditions associated with decreased placental perfusion such as hypertension, intrauterine growth restriction, diabetes mellitus, and multiple gestation (Blackburn, 2007) (see Fig. 9-7).

Using an ultrasound device or a fetal stethoscope, the examiner may hear the uterine souffle or bruit, a rushing or blowing sound of maternal blood flowing through uterine arteries to the placenta that is synchronous with the maternal pulse. The funic souffle, which is synchronous with the fetal heart rate and is caused by fetal blood coursing through the umbilical cord, may also be heard, as well as the actual heartbeat of the fetus.

Cervical Changes

In a normal, unscarred cervix, a softening of the cervical tip may be observed about the beginning of the sixth week. This probable sign of pregnancy, Goodell sign, is brought about by increased vascularity, slight hypertrophy, and hyperplasia (increase in number of cells). The muscle and its collagen-rich connective tissue become loose, edematous, highly elastic, and increased in volume. The glands near the external os proliferate beneath the stratified squamous epithelium, giving the cervix the velvety appearance characteristic of pregnancy. Friability is increased and can result in slight bleeding after vaginal examination or after coitus with deep penetration.

Pregnancy can also cause the squamocolumnar junction, the site for obtaining cells for cervical cancer screening, to be located away from the cervix. Because of these changes, evaluation of abnormal Papanicolaou tests during pregnancy can be complicated. However, careful assessment of all pregnant women is important because approximately 3% of all cervical cancers are diagnosed during pregnancy (Copeland & Landon, 2007).

The cervix of the nullipara is rounded. Lacerations of the cervix almost always occur during the birth process. After

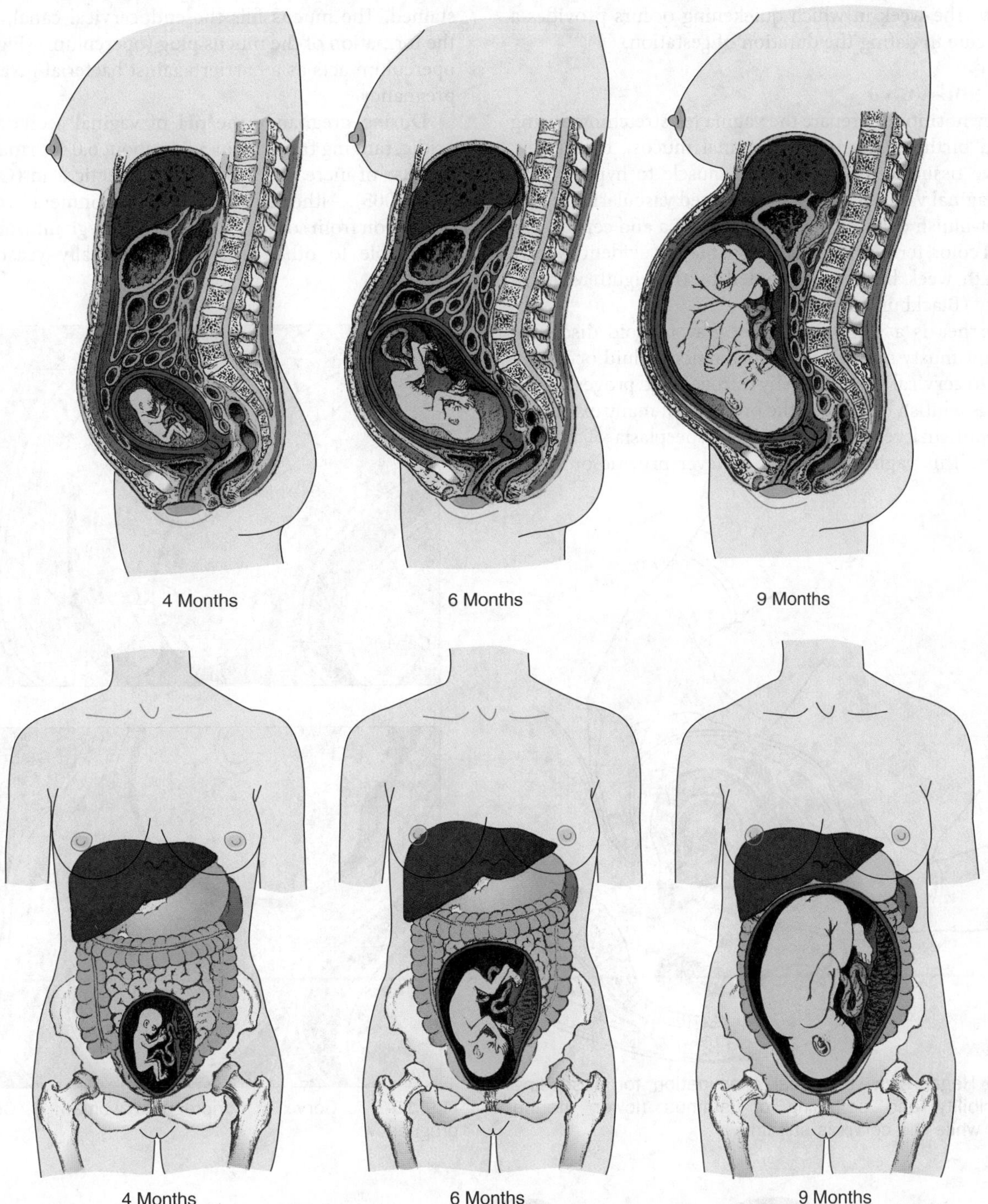

Fig. 10-4 Displacement of internal abdominal structures and diaphragm by the enlarging uterus at 4, 6, and 9 months of gestation.

childbirth, with or without lacerations, the cervix becomes more oval in the horizontal plane, and the external os appears as a transverse slit (see Fig. 10-2).

Changes Related to the Presence of the Fetus

Passive movement of the unengaged fetus is called *ballottement* and can be identified generally between the sixteenth and eighteenth week. Ballottement is a technique of palpating a floating structure by bouncing it gently and feeling it rebound. To palpate the fetus the examiner places a finger within the vagina and taps gently upward, causing the fetus to rise. The fetus then sinks, and a gentle tap is felt on the finger (Fig. 10-6).

The first recognition of fetal movements, or "feeling life," by the multiparous woman may occur as early as the sixteenth week. The nulliparous woman may not notice these sensations until the eighteenth week or later. Quickening is commonly described as a flutter and is difficult to distinguish from peristalsis. Fetal movements gradually increase in intensity and frequency. The week in which quickening occurs provides a tentative clue in dating the duration of gestation.

Vagina and Vulva

Pregnancy hormones prepare the vagina for stretching during labor and birth by causing the vaginal mucosa to thicken, connective tissue to loosen, smooth muscle to hypertrophy, and the vaginal vault to lengthen. Increased vascularity results in a violet-bluish color of the vaginal mucosa and cervix. The deepened color, termed *Chadwick sign,* may be evident as early as the sixth week but is easily noted by the eighth week of pregnancy (Blackburn, 2007).

Leukorrhea is a white or slightly gray mucoid discharge with a faint musty odor. This copious mucoid fluid occurs in response to cervical stimulation by estrogen and progesterone. The fluid is whitish because of the presence of many exfoliated vaginal epithelial cells caused by the hyperplasia of normal pregnancy. This vaginal discharge is never pruritic or blood stained. The mucus fills the endocervical canal, resulting in the formation of the mucus plug (operculum) (Fig. 10-7). The operculum acts as a barrier against bacterial invasion during pregnancy.

During pregnancy the pH of vaginal secretions is more acidic, ranging from about 3.5 to about 6.0 (normal 4.0 to 7.0), because of increased production of lactic acid (Cunningham et al, 2005). Although this acidic environment provides more protection from some organisms, the pregnant woman is more vulnerable to other infections, especially yeast infections,

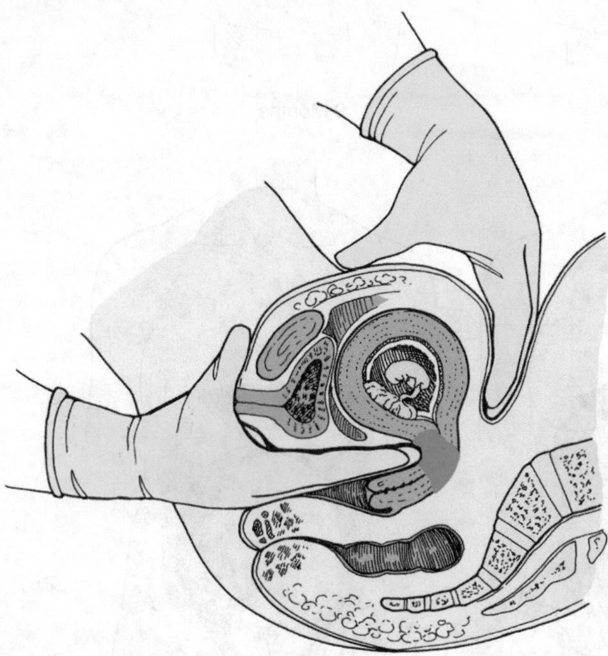

Fig. 10-5 Hegar sign. Bimanual examination for assessing compressibility and softening of isthmus (lower uterine segment) while the cervix is still firm.

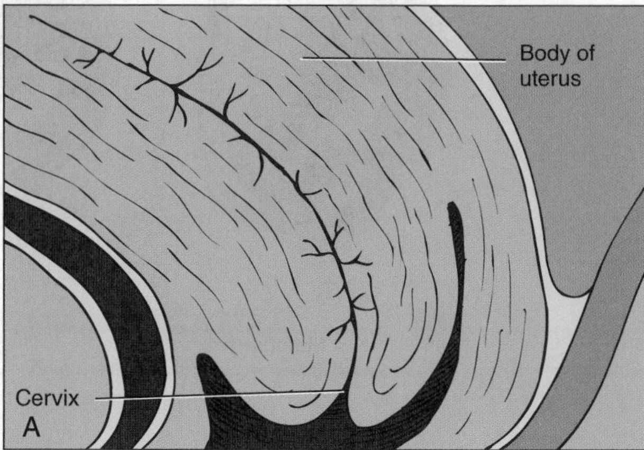

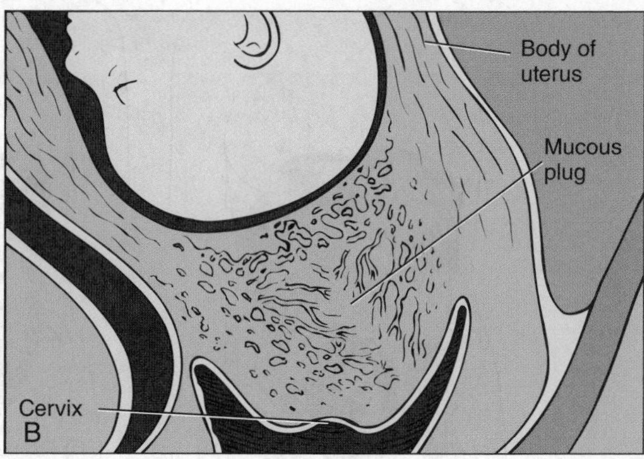

Fig. 10-7 A, Cervix in nonpregnant woman. **B,** Cervix during pregnancy.

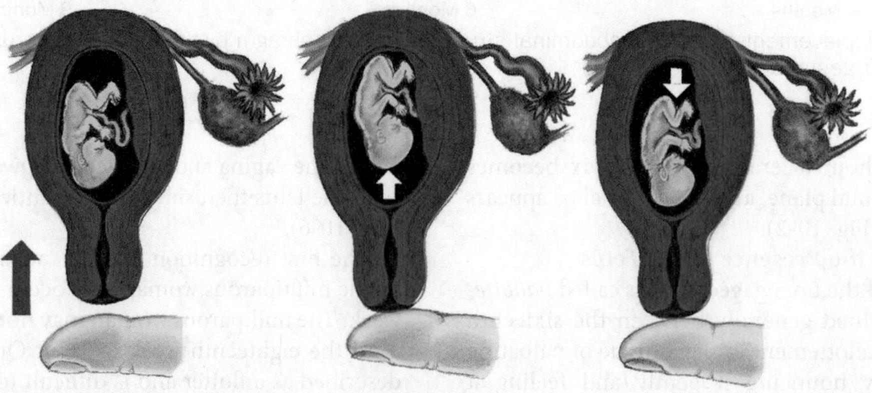

Fig. 10-6 Internal ballottement (18 weeks).

because the glycogen-rich environment of the vagina is more susceptible to *Candida albicans* (Duff, Sweet, & Edwards, 2009).

The increased vascularity of the vagina and other pelvic viscera results in a marked increase in sensitivity. The increased sensitivity may lead to a high degree of sexual interest and arousal, especially during the second trimester of pregnancy. The increased congestion, plus the relaxed walls of the blood vessels and the heavy uterus, may result in edema and varicosities of the vulva. The edema and varicosities usually resolve during the postpartum period.

External structures of the perineum are enlarged during pregnancy because of an increase in vasculature, hypertrophy of the perineal body, and deposition of fat (Fig. 10-8). The labia majora of nullipara women approximate (come together) and obscure the vaginal introitus; those of the parous woman separate and gape after childbirth and perineal or vaginal injury. See Fig. 10-2 for a comparison of the perineum of the nullipara and the multipara in relation to the pregnant abdomen, vulva, and cervix.

Breasts

Fullness, heightened sensitivity, tingling, and heaviness of the breasts begin in the early weeks of gestation in response to increased levels of estrogen and progesterone. Breast sensitivity varies from mild tingling to sharp pain. Nipples and areolae become more pigmented; secondary pinkish areolae develop, extending beyond the primary areolae; and nipples become more erectile. Hypertrophy of the sebaceous (oil) glands embedded in the primary areolae, called *Montgomery tubercles,* may be seen around the nipples. These sebaceous glands may have a protective role in that they keep the nipples lubricated for breastfeeding.

The richer blood supply causes the vessels beneath the skin to dilate. Once barely noticeable, the blood vessels become visible, often appearing in an intertwining blue network beneath the surface of the skin. Venous congestion in the breasts is more obvious in primigravidas. Striae gravidarum may appear at the outer aspects of the breasts.

During the second and third trimesters growth of the mammary glands accounts for the progressive breast enlargement (Fig. 10-9). The high levels of luteal and placental hormones in pregnancy promote proliferation of the lactiferous ducts and lobule-alveolar tissue so that palpation of the breasts reveals a generalized, coarse nodularity. Glandular tissue displaces connective tissue, and as a result the tissue becomes softer and looser.

Although development of the mammary glands is functionally complete by midpregnancy, lactation is inhibited until a decrease in estrogen level occurs after birth. A thin, clear, viscous secretory material (precolostrum) can be found in the acini cells by the third month of gestation. Colostrum, the creamy, white-to-yellowish-to-orange premilk fluid, may be expressed from the nipples as early as 16 weeks of gestation (Blackburn, 2007). See Chapter 26 for a discussion of lactation.

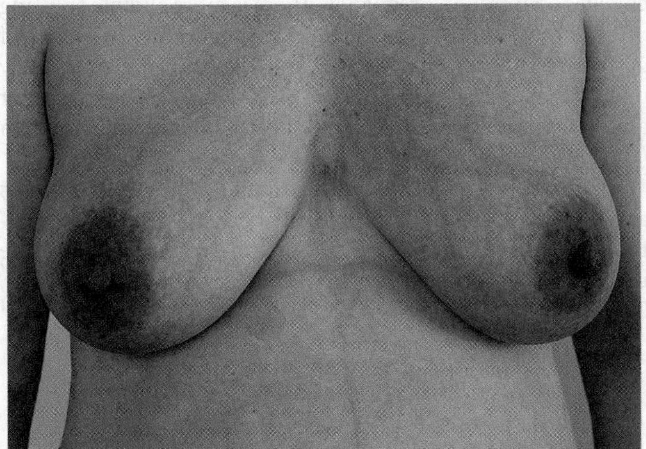

Fig. 10-9 Enlarged breasts in pregnancy with venous network and darkened areolae and nipples. (From Seidel HM et al: *Mosby's guide to physical examination*, ed 6, St. Louis, 2006, Mosby.)

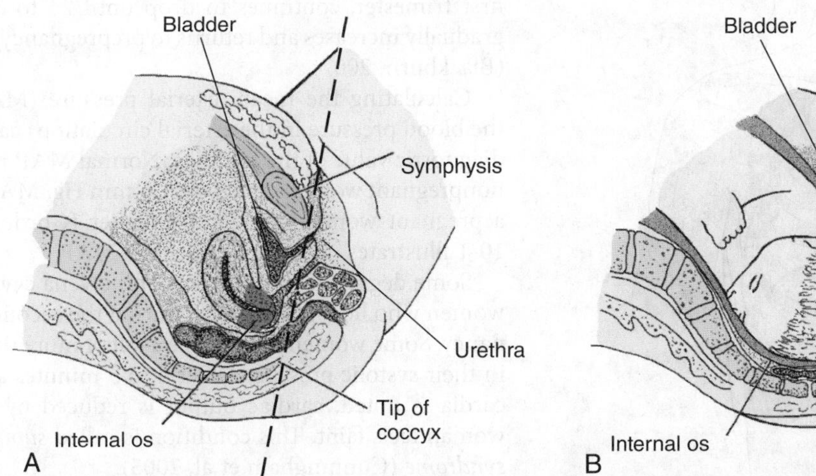

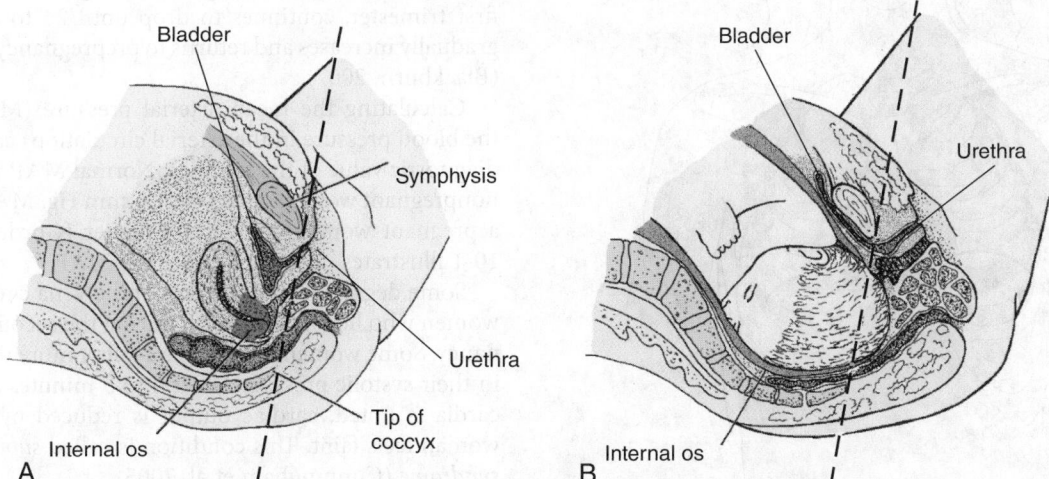

Fig. 10-8 A, Pelvic floor in nonpregnant woman. B, Pelvic floor at end of pregnancy. Note marked hypertrophy and hyperplasia below dotted line joining tip of coccyx and inferior margin of symphysis. Note elongation of bladder and urethra as a result of compression. Fat deposits are increased.

General Body Systems

Cardiovascular System

Maternal adjustments to pregnancy involve extensive anatomic and physiologic changes in the cardiovascular system. Cardiovascular adaptations protect the woman's normal physiologic functioning, meet the metabolic demands pregnancy imposes on her body, and provide for fetal developmental and growth needs.

Slight cardiac hypertrophy (enlargement) is probably secondary to increased blood volume and cardiac output that occurs in pregnancy. The heart returns to its normal size after childbirth. As the diaphragm is displaced upward by the enlarging uterus, the heart is elevated upward and rotated forward to the left (Fig. 10-10). The apical impulse, a point of maximal intensity, is shifted upward and laterally about 1 to 1.5 cm. The degree of shift depends on the duration of pregnancy and the size and position of the uterus.

The changes in heart size and position and the increases in blood volume and cardiac output contribute to auscultatory changes common in pregnancy. There is more audible splitting of S_1 and S_2, and S_3 may be readily heard after 20 weeks of gestation. In addition, systolic and diastolic murmurs may be heard over the pulmonic area. These changes are transient and disappear in most women shortly after they give birth (Cunningham et al, 2005).

Between 14 and 20 weeks of gestation, the pulse increases about 10 to 15 beats/min, and this persists to term. Palpitations may occur. In twin gestations the maternal heart rate increases significantly in the third trimester (Blackburn, 2007).

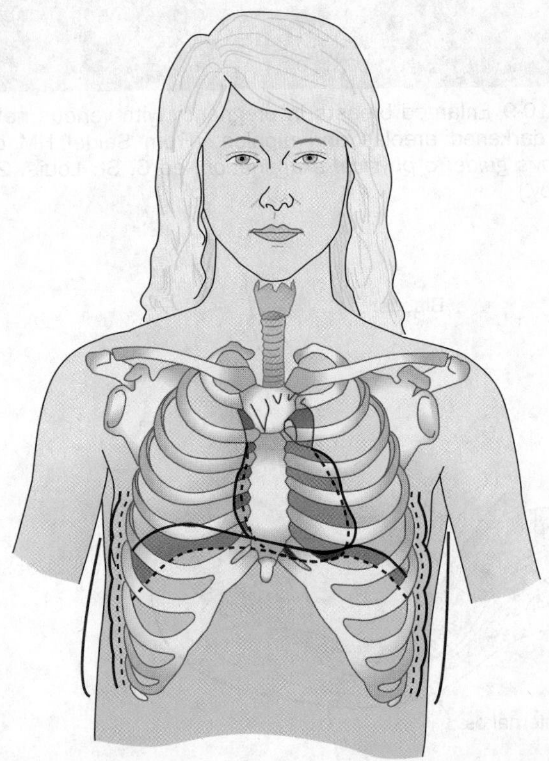

Fig. 10-10 Changes in position of heart, lungs, and thoracic cage in pregnancy. *Broken line,* Nonpregnant state; *solid line,* change that occurs in pregnancy.

The cardiac rhythm may be disturbed. The pregnant woman may experience sinus arrhythmia, premature atrial contractions, and premature ventricular systole. In the healthy woman with no underlying heart disease, no therapy is needed. Women with preexisting heart disease need close medical and obstetric supervision during pregnancy (see Chapter 13).

Blood Pressure

Arterial blood pressure (brachial artery) varies with age; activity level; presence of health problems; circadian rhythm; and use of alcohol, smoking, and pain. Additional factors to consider during pregnancy include maternal anxiety, maternal position, and type of blood pressure apparatus (Pickering et al, 2005).

Maternal anxiety can elevate readings. If an elevated reading is found, the woman is given time to rest, and the reading is repeated.

Maternal position affects readings. Brachial blood pressure is highest when the woman is sitting; lowest when she is lying in the lateral recumbent position; and intermediate when she is supine, except for some women who experience hypotensive syndrome (see later discussion). Therefore at each prenatal visit the reading should be obtained in the same arm and with the woman in a seated position with her back and arm supported and her upper arm at the level of the right atrium (Pickering et al, 2005; Sibai, 2007). The position and arm used should be recorded along with the reading.

The proper-size cuff is essential for accurate readings. The cuff should have a bladder length that is 80% and a width that is at least 40% of the arm circumference. For example, an adult-size cuff (16 cm × 30 cm) should be used for an arm circumference of 27 to 34 cm. A cuff that is too small yields a falsely high reading; a cuff that is too large yields a falsely low reading (Pickering et al, 2005).

Caution should be used when comparing auscultatory and oscillatory blood pressure readings because discrepancies can occur. Automated monitors may give inaccurate readings in women with hypertensive conditions (Gordon, 2007).

Systolic blood pressure usually remains the same as the prepregnancy level but may decrease slightly as pregnancy advances. Diastolic blood pressure begins to decrease in the first trimester, continues to drop until 24 to 32 weeks, and gradually increases and returns to prepregnancy levels by term (Blackburn, 2007).

Calculating the mean arterial pressure (MAP) (mean of the blood pressure in the arterial circulation) can increase the diagnostic value of the findings. Normal MAP readings in the nonpregnant woman are 86.4 ± 7.5 mm Hg. MAP readings for a pregnant woman are slightly higher (Gordon, 2007). Box 10-1 illustrates one way to calculate MAP.

Some degree of compression of the vena cava occurs in all women who lie on their backs during the second half of pregnancy. Some women experience a fall of more than 30 mm Hg in their systolic pressure. After 4 to 5 minutes a reflex bradycardia is noted, cardiac output is reduced by half, and the woman feels faint. This condition is called *supine hypotensive syndrome* (Cunningham et al, 2005).

Compression of the iliac veins and inferior vena cava by the uterus causes increased venous pressure and reduced blood flow in the legs, except when the woman is in the lateral

BOX 10-1 Calculation of Mean Arterial Pressure

Blood pressure: 106/70
Formula:
Systolic + 2(Diastolic)/3
106 + 2(70)/3
106 + 140/3
246/3 = 82 mm Hg

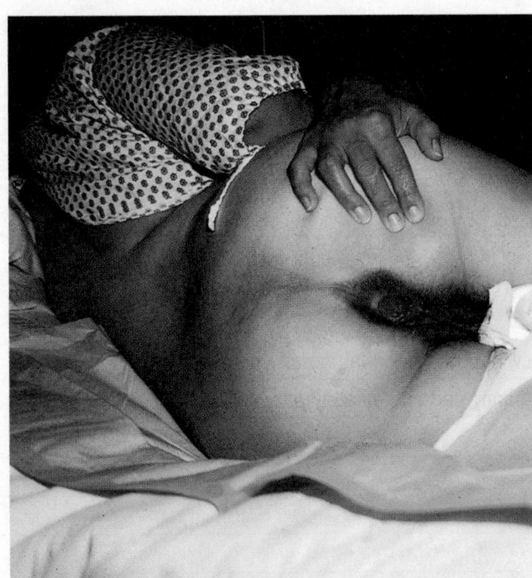

Fig. 10-11 Hemorrhoids. *(Courtesy Marjorie Pyle, RNC, Lifecircle, Costa Mesa, CA.)*

position. These alterations contribute to the dependent edema, varicose veins in the legs and vulva, and hemorrhoids that develop in the latter part of term pregnancy (Fig. 10-11).

Blood Volume and Composition

The degree of blood volume expansion varies considerably. Blood volume increases by approximately 1500 ml, or 40% to 50% above nonpregnancy levels (Cunningham et al, 2005). This increase consists of 1000 ml of plasma plus 450 ml of red blood cells (RBCs). The increase in volume starts at weeks 10 to 12, peaks at weeks 32 to 34, and decreases slightly at week 40. The volume in a multiple gestation increases above that for a single fetus (Blackburn, 2007). Increased blood volume is a protective mechanism. It is essential for meeting the blood volume needs of the hypertrophied vascular system of the enlarged uterus, for adequately hydrating fetal and maternal tissues when the woman assumes an erect or supine position, and for providing a fluid reserve to compensate for blood loss during birth and the puerperium. Peripheral vasodilation allows for a normal blood pressure despite the increased blood volume in pregnancy.

During pregnancy there is an accelerated production of RBCs (normal, 4.2 to 5.4 million/mm^3). The percentage of increase depends on the amount of iron available. The RBC mass increases by 20% to 30% (Blackburn, 2007).

Because the plasma increase is greater than the increase in RBC production, there is a decrease in normal hemoglobin values (12 to 16 g/dl blood) and hematocrit values (37% to 47%). This state of hemodilution is referred to as physiologic anemia. The decrease is more noticeable during the second trimester, when rapid expansion of blood volume occurs faster than RBC production. If the hemoglobin value drops to 11 g/dl or less or if the hematocrit decreases to 32% or less, the woman is considered anemic (Samuels, 2007).

The total white blood cell count increases during the second trimester and peaks during the third trimester. This increase is primarily in the granulocytes; the lymphocyte count stays about the same throughout pregnancy. See Table 10-3 for laboratory values during pregnancy.

Cardiac Output

Cardiac output increases from 30% to 50% over the nonpregnant rate by week 32 of pregnancy; it declines to about a 20% increase at 40 weeks of gestation. This elevated cardiac output is largely a result of increased stroke volume and heart rate and occurs in response to increased tissue demands for oxygen (Blackburn, 2007).

Cardiac output in late pregnancy is appreciably higher when the woman is in the lateral recumbent position than when she is supine. In the supine position the large, heavy uterus often impedes venous return to the heart and affects blood pressure. Cardiac output increases with any exertion such as labor and birth. Table 10-4 summarizes cardiovascular changes in pregnancy.

Circulation and Coagulation Times

The circulation time decreases slightly by week 32. It returns to near normal by term. There is a greater tendency for blood to coagulate (clot) during pregnancy because of increases in various clotting factors (i.e., factors VII, VIII, IX, X, and fibrinogen). This tendency, combined with the fact that fibrinolytic activity (the splitting up or dissolving of a clot) is depressed during pregnancy and the postpartum period, provides a protective function to decrease the chance of bleeding but also makes the woman more vulnerable to thrombosis, especially after cesarean birth.

Respiratory System

Structural and ventilatory adaptations occur during pregnancy to provide for maternal and fetal needs. Maternal oxygen requirements increase in response to the acceleration in metabolic rate and the need to add to the tissue mass in the uterus and breasts. In addition, the fetus requires oxygen and a way to eliminate carbon dioxide.

Elevated levels of estrogen cause the ligaments of the rib cage to relax, permitting increased chest expansion (see Fig. 10-10). The transverse diameter of the thoracic cage increases by about 2 cm, and the circumference by 6 cm (Cunningham et al, 2005). The costal angle increases, and the lower rib cage appears to flare out. The chest may not return to its prepregnant state after birth (Seidel et al, 2006).

The diaphragm is displaced by as much as 4 cm during pregnancy. With advancing pregnancy chest breathing replaces abdominal breathing, and it becomes less possible for the diaphragm to descend with inspiration. Thoracic breathing is primarily accomplished by the diaphragm rather than by the costal muscles (Blackburn, 2007).

The upper respiratory tract becomes more vascular in response to elevated levels of estrogen. As the capillaries

Table 10-3 Laboratory Values for Pregnant and Nonpregnant Women

VALUES	NONPREGNANT	PREGNANT
Hematologic		
Complete Blood Count		
Hemoglobin, g/dl	12-16*	>11*
Hematocrit, packed cell volume, %	37-47	>32*
RBC volume, per milliliter	1400	1650
Plasma volume, per milliliter	2400	40%-60% increase
RBC count, million/mm^3	4.2-5.4	5-6.25
White blood cells, total per mm^3	5000-10,000	5000-15,000
Neutrophils, %	55-70	60-85
Lymphocytes, %	20-40	15-40
Erythrocyte sedimentation rate, mm/hr	20	Elevated in second and third trimesters
Mean corpuscular hemoglobin concentration, g/dl packed RBCs	32-36	No change
Mean corpuscular hemoglobin, pg	27-31	No change
Mean corpuscular volume per mm^3	80-95	No change
Blood Coagulation and Fibrinolytic Activity†		
Factor VII	65-140	Increases in pregnancy, returns to normal in early puerperium
Factor VIII	55-145	Increases during pregnancy and immediately after birth
Factor IX	60-140	Same as factor VII
Factor X	45-155	Same as factor VII
Factor XI	65-135	Decreases in pregnancy
Factor XII	50-150	Same as factor VII
Prothrombin time, sec	11-12.5	Decreases slightly in pregnancy
Partial thromboplastin time, sec	60-70	Decreases slightly in pregnancy and decreases during second and third stage of labor (indicates clotting at placental site)
Bleeding time, min	1-9 (Ivy method)	No appreciable change
Coagulation time, min	6-10 (Lee-White method)	No appreciable change
Platelets, per mm^3	150,000-400,000	No significant change until 3-5 days after birth and then increases rapidly (may predispose woman to thrombosis) and gradually returns to normal
Fibrinolytic activity		Decreases in pregnancy and then abruptly returns to normal (protection against thromboembolism)
Fibrinogen, mg/dl	200-400	Levels increase late in pregnancy
Mineral/Vitamin Concentrations		
Vitamin B_{12}, folic acid, ascorbic acid	Normal	Moderate decrease
Serum Proteins		
Total, g/dl	6.4-8.3	5.5-7.5
Albumin, g/dl	3.5-5	Slight increase
Globulin, total, g/dl	2.3-3.4	3.0-4.0
Blood Glucose		
Fasting, mg/dl	70-105	Decreases
2-hr postprandial, mg/dl	<140	<140 after a 100-g carbohydrate meal is considered normal
Acid-Base Values in Arterial Blood		
Po_2, mm Hg	80-100	104-108 (increased)
Pco_2, mm Hg	35-45	27-32 (decreased)
Sodium bicarbonate (HCO_3), mEq/L	21-28	18-31 (decreased)
Blood pH	7.35-7.45	7.40-7.45 (slightly increased, more alkaline)

Table 10-3 Laboratory Values for Pregnant and Nonpregnant Women—cont'd

VALUES	NONPREGNANT	PREGNANT
Hepatic		
Bilirubin, total, mg/dl	≤1	Unchanged
Serum cholesterol, mg/dl	120-200	Increases from 16-32 wk of pregnancy; remains at this level until after birth
Serum alkaline phosphatase, units/L	30-120	Increases from wk 12 of pregnancy to 6 wk after birth
Serum albumin, g/dl	3.5-5	Increases slightly
Renal		
Bladder capacity, ml	1300	1500
Renal plasma flow, ml/min	490-700	Increases by 25%-30%
Glomerular filtration rate, ml/min	88-128	Increases by 30%-50%
Nonprotein nitrogen, mg/dl	25-40	Decreases
Blood urea nitrogen, mg/dl	10-20	Decreases
Serum creatinine, mg/dl	0.5-1.1	Decreases
Serum uric acid, mg/dl	2.7-7.3	Decreases but returns to prepregnancy level by end of pregnancy
Urine glucose	Negative	Present in 20% of pregnant women
Intravenous pyelogram	Normal	Slight-to-moderate hydroureter and hydronephrosis; right kidney larger than left kidney

References: Blackburn S: *Maternal, fetal, & neonatal physiology: a clinical perspective*, ed 3, St Louis, 2007, Saunders; Gordon M: Maternal physiology in pregnancy. In Gabbe SG, Niebyl JR, Simpson JL (editors): *Obstetrics: normal and problem pregnancies*, ed 5, New York, 2007, Churchill Livingstone; Pagana KD, Pagana TJ: *Mosby's manual of diagnostic and laboratory tests*, ed 3, St Louis, 2006, Mosby; Samuels P: Hematology complications of pregnancy. In Gabbe SG, Niebyl JR, Simpson JL (editors): *Obstetrics: normal and problem pregnancies*, ed 5, Philadelphia, 2007, Churchill Livingstone.
*At sea level. Permanent residents of higher levels (e.g., Denver) require higher levels of hemoglobin.
†Pregnancy represents a hypercoagulable state.
RBC, Red blood cell.
NOTE: Abbreviations should not be used in practice.

Table 10-4 Cardiovascular Changes in Pregnancy

PARAMETER	CHANGE
Heart rate	Increases 10-15 beats/min
Blood pressure	
Systolic	Slight or no decrease from prepregnancy levels
Diastolic	Slight decrease to midpregnancy (24-32 wk) and gradual return to prepregnancy levels by end of pregnancy
Blood volume	Increases by 1500 ml or 40%-50% above prepregnancy level
Red blood cell mass	Increases 17%
Hemoglobin	Decreases
Hematocrit	Decreases
White blood cell count	Increases in second and third trimesters
Cardiac output	Increases 30%-50%

become engorged, edema and hyperemia develop within the nose, pharynx, larynx, trachea, and bronchi. This congestion within the tissues of the respiratory tract gives rise to several conditions commonly seen during pregnancy, including nasal and sinus stuffiness, epistaxis (nosebleed), changes in the voice, and marked inflammatory response to even a mild upper respiratory infection.

Increased vascularity of the upper respiratory tract also can cause the tympanic membranes and eustachian tubes to swell, giving rise to symptoms of impaired hearing, earaches, or a sense of fullness in the ears.

Pulmonary Function

Respiratory changes in pregnancy are related to the elevation of the diaphragm and changes in the chest wall. Changes in the respiratory center result in a lowered threshold for carbon dioxide. The actions of progesterone and estrogen are presumed to be responsible for the increased sensitivity of the respiratory center to carbon dioxide. In addition, pregnant women become more aware of the need to breathe; many complain of nasal stuffiness, and some have epistaxis (Gordon, 2007) (see Table 10-5 for respiratory changes in pregnancy). Although pulmonary function is not impaired by pregnancy, diseases of the respiratory tract may be more serious during this time (Cunningham et al, 2005). One important factor responsible for this may be the increase in oxygen requirements.

Basal Metabolic Rate

The basal metabolic rate (BMR) increases during pregnancy. This increase varies considerably, depending on the prepregnancy nutritional status of the woman and fetal growth (Blackburn, 2007). The BMR returns to nonpregnant levels by 5 to 6 days after birth. The elevation in BMR reflects increased oxygen demands of the uterine-placental-fetal unit and greater oxygen consumption because of increased maternal cardiac work. Peripheral vasodilation and acceleration of sweat gland activity help dissipate the excess heat resulting from the

Table 10-5 Respiratory Changes in Pregnancy

PARAMETER	CHANGE
Respiratory rate	Unchanged or slightly increased
Tidal volume	Increased 30%-40%
Vital capacity	Unchanged
Inspiratory capacity	Increased
Expiratory volume	Decreased
Total lung capacity	Unchanged to slightly decreased
Oxygen consumption	Increased 20%-40%

Source: Gordon M: Maternal physiology. In Gabbe SG, Niebyl JR, Simpson JL (editors): *Obstetrics: normal and problem pregnancies*, ed 5, Philadelphia, 2007, Churchill Livingstone.

increased BMR during pregnancy. Pregnant women may experience heat intolerance. Lassitude and fatigability after only slight exertion are experienced by many women in early pregnancy. These feelings, along with a greater need for sleep, may persist and may be caused in part by the increased metabolic activity.

Acid-Base Balance

By about the tenth week of pregnancy there is a decrease of about 5 mm Hg in the partial pressure of carbon dioxide (Pco_2). Progesterone may be responsible for increasing the sensitivity of the respiratory center receptors so that tidal volume increases and Pco_2 decreases, the base excess (HCO_3, or bicarbonate) decreases, and pH increases slightly. These alterations in acid-base balance indicate that pregnancy is a state of respiratory alkalosis compensated by mild metabolic acidosis (Gordon, 2007). These changes also facilitate the transport of CO_2 from the fetus and O_2 release from the mother to the fetus (see Table 10-5).

Renal System

The kidneys are responsible for maintaining electrolyte and acid-base balance, regulating extracellular fluid volume, excreting waste products, and conserving essential nutrients.

Anatomic Changes

Changes in renal structure result from hormonal activity (estrogen and progesterone), pressure from an enlarging uterus, and an increase in blood volume. As early as the tenth week of pregnancy the renal pelves and the ureters dilate. Dilation of the ureters is more pronounced above the pelvic brim, in part because they are compressed between the uterus and the pelvic brim. In most women the ureters below the pelvic brim are of normal size. The smooth-muscle walls of the ureters undergo hyperplasia and hypertrophy and muscle tone relaxation. The ureters elongate, become tortuous, and form single or double curves. In the latter part of pregnancy the renal pelvis and ureter dilate more on the right side than on the left because the heavy uterus is displaced to the right by the sigmoid colon.

Because of these changes, a larger volume of urine is held in the pelves and ureters, and urine flow rate is slowed. Urinary stasis or stagnation has several consequences:

- There is a lag between the time urine is formed and when it reaches the bladder. Therefore clearance test results may reflect substances contained in glomerular filtrate several hours before.
- Stagnated urine is an excellent medium for the growth of microorganisms. In addition, the urine of pregnant women contains more nutrients, including glucose, that increase the pH (making the urine more alkaline). This makes pregnant women more susceptible to urinary tract infection.

Bladder irritability, nocturia, and urinary frequency and urgency (without dysuria) are commonly reported in early pregnancy. These bladder symptoms may return near term, especially after lightening occurs.

Urinary frequency results initially from increased bladder sensitivity and later from compression of the bladder (see Fig. 10-8). In the second trimester the bladder is pulled up out of the true pelvis into the abdomen. The urethra lengthens to 7.5 cm as the bladder is displaced upward. The pelvic congestion that occurs in pregnancy is reflected in hyperemia of the bladder and urethra. This increased vascularity causes the bladder mucosa to be traumatized and bleed easily. Bladder tone may decrease, which increases the bladder capacity to 1500 ml. At the same time the bladder is compressed by the enlarging uterus, resulting in the urge to void even if the bladder contains only a small amount of urine.

Functional Changes

In normal pregnancy renal function is altered considerably. Glomerular filtration rate (GFR) and renal plasma flow increase early in pregnancy (Cunningham et al, 2005). These changes are caused by pregnancy hormones; an increase in blood volume; and the woman's posture, physical activity, and nutritional intake. The woman's kidneys must manage the increased metabolic and circulatory demands of the maternal body and also the excretion of fetal waste products.

Renal function is most efficient when the woman lies in the lateral recumbent position and least efficient when the woman assumes a supine position. A side-lying position increases renal perfusion, which increases urine output and decreases edema. When the pregnant woman is lying supine, the heavy uterus compresses the vena cava and the aorta, and cardiac output decreases. As a result, blood flow to the brain and heart is continued at the expense of other organs, including the kidneys and uterus.

Fluid and Electrolyte Balance

Selective renal tubular resorption maintains sodium and water balance, regardless of changes in dietary intake and losses through sweat, vomitus, or diarrhea. From 500 to 900 mEq of sodium is normally retained during pregnancy to meet fetal needs. To prevent excessive sodium depletion, the maternal kidneys undergo a significant adaptation by increasing tubular resorption. Because of the need for increased maternal intravascular and extracellular fluid volume, additional sodium is needed to expand fluid volume and maintain an isotonic state. As efficient as the renal system is, it can be overstressed by excessive dietary sodium intake or restriction or by use of diuretics. Severe hypovolemia and reduced placental perfusion are two consequences of using diuretics during pregnancy.

The capacity of the kidneys to excrete water is more efficient during the early weeks than later in pregnancy. As a result, some women feel thirsty in early pregnancy because of the greater amount of water loss. The pooling of fluid in the legs in the latter part of pregnancy decreases renal blood flow and GFR. This pooling is sometimes referred to as physiologic or dependent edema and requires no treatment. The normal diuretic response to the water load is triggered when the woman lies down, preferably on her side, and the pooled fluid reenters general circulation.

Normally the kidney resorbs almost all the glucose and other nutrients from the plasma filtrate. However, in pregnant women tubular resorption of glucose is impaired so that glucosuria occurs at varying times and to varying degrees. Normal values range from 0 to 20 mg/dl, meaning that during any day the urine is sometimes positive and sometimes negative for glucose. In nonpregnant women blood glucose levels must be at 160 to 180 mg/dl before glucose is "spilled" into the urine (not resorbed). During pregnancy glucosuria occurs when maternal glucose levels are lower than 160 mg/dl. Why glucose, as well as other nutrients such as amino acids, is wasted during pregnancy is not understood, nor has the exact mechanism been discovered. Although glucosuria may be found in normal pregnancies (2+ levels may be seen with increased anxiety states), the possibility of diabetes mellitus and gestational diabetes must be kept in mind.

Proteinuria does not usually occur in normal pregnancy except during labor or after birth (Cunningham et al, 2005). However, the increased amounts of amino acids that must be filtered may exceed the capacity of the renal tubules to absorb them, and small amounts of protein may be lost in the urine. The amount of protein excreted is not an indication of the severity of renal disease, nor does an increase in protein excretion in a pregnant woman with known renal disease necessarily indicate a progression in her disease. However, a pregnant woman with hypertension and proteinuria must be evaluated carefully because she may be at greater risk for an adverse pregnancy outcome (Gordon, 2007) (Table 10-6).

Integumentary System

Alterations in hormone balance and mechanical stretching are responsible for several changes in the integumentary system during pregnancy. Hyperpigmentation is stimulated by the anterior pituitary hormone melanotropin, which is increased during pregnancy. Darkening of the nipples, areolae, axillae, and vulva occurs at about the sixteenth week of gestation. Facial melasma (also called *chloasma* or *mask of pregnancy*) is a blotchy, brownish hyperpigmentation of the skin over the cheeks, nose, and forehead, especially in pregnant women with dark complexions. Chloasma appears in 50% to 70% of pregnant women, beginning after the sixteenth week and increasing gradually until term. The sun intensifies this pigmentation in susceptible women. Chloasma caused by normal pregnancy usually fades after birth.

The linea nigra (Fig. 10-12) is a pigmented line extending from the symphysis pubis to the top of the fundus in the midline. This line is known as the linea alba before hormone-induced pigmentation. In primigravidas the extension of the linea nigra, beginning in the third month, keeps pace with the rising height of the fundus; in multigravidas the entire line often appears earlier than the third month. Not all pregnant women develop lineae nigra, and some women notice hair growth along the line with or without the change in pigmentation.

Striae gravidarum or stretch marks (seen over the lower abdomen in Fig. 10-12) appear in 50% to 90% of pregnant women during the second half of pregnancy. These may be caused by the action of adrenocorticosteroids. Striae reflect separation within the underlying connective (collagen) tissue of the skin. These slightly depressed streaks tend to occur over areas of maximum stretch (the abdomen, thighs, and breasts). The stretching sometimes causes a sensation that resembles itching. The tendency to develop striae may be familial. After birth they usually fade, although they never disappear completely. Color of striae varies, depending on the pregnant woman's skin color. The striae appear pinkish on a woman with light skin and are lighter than the surrounding skin in dark-skinned women. In the multipara, in addition to the striae of the present pregnancy, glistening silvery lines (in light-skinned women) or purplish lines (in dark-skinned women) are commonly seen. These represent the scars of striae from previous pregnancies.

Angiomas are commonly referred to as vascular spiders. These tiny, star-shaped or branched, slightly raised, and pulsating end-arterioles are usually found on the neck, thorax, face, and arms. They occur as a result of elevated levels of circulating estrogens. The spiders are bluish in color and do not blanch with pressure. Vascular spiders appear during the second to fifth month of pregnancy in about 65% of Caucasian

Table 10-6 Renal Changes in Pregnancy

PARAMETER	CHANGE
Bladder capacity	Increased
Glomerular filtration rate	Increased 30%-50%
Renal plasma flow	Increased 30%
Blood urea nitrogen	Decreased
Creatinine	Decreased
Glucose (in urine)	Present in 20% of pregnant women

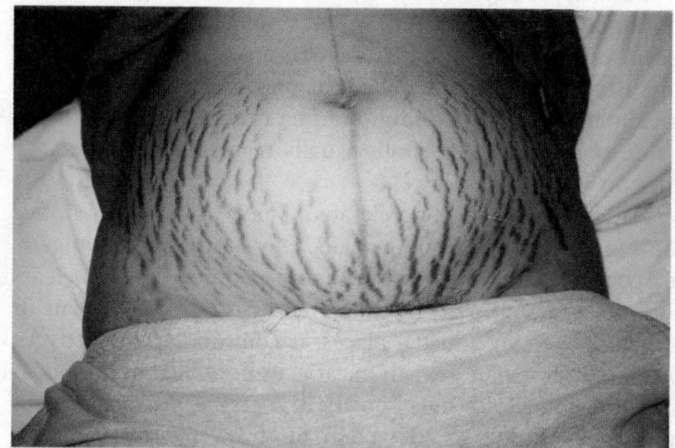

Fig. 10-12 Striae gravidarum and linea nigra in a dark-skinned person. *(Courtesy Shannon Perry, Phoenix, AZ.)*

BOX 10-2 Ethnic Considerations for Skin Assessment During Pregnancy

Integumentary system changes vary greatly among women of different racial backgrounds. For example, vascular spiders and palmar erythema are seen more often in Caucasian women than in African-American women. Areolar pigmentation varies by race: African-American women have the darkest areolae, Caucasian women have the lightest, and Asian and Native American women have intermediate pigmentation. When performing physical assessments, the color of the woman's skin should be noted, along with any changes that may be attributed to pregnancy.

BOX 10-3 Prevalence of Dermatologic Disorders of Pregnancy

Pruritic urticarial papules and plaques of pregnancy (PUPPP)—1:130 to 1:300
Prurigo of pregnancy (PP)—1:300 to 1:450
Herpes gestationis (HG)—1:50,000
Pruritic folliculitis of pregnancy (PFP)—Very rare; about 30 cases

Source: Papoutsis J, Kroupouzos G: Dermatologic disorders In Gabbe SG, Niebyl JR, Simpson JL (editors): *Obstetrics: normal and problem pregnancies*, ed 5, Philadelphia, 2007, Churchill Livingstone.

women and 10% of African-American women. The spiders usually disappear after birth (Blackburn, 2007).

Pinkish-red diffusely mottled or well-defined blotches are seen over the palmar surfaces of the hands in about 60% of Caucasian women and 35% of African-American women during pregnancy (Blackburn, 2007). These color changes, called *palmar erythema*, are related primarily to increased estrogen levels (Box 10-2).

Some dermatologic conditions have been identified as unique to pregnancy or as having an increased incidence during pregnancy. Mild pruritus (pruritus gravidarum) is a relatively common dermatologic symptom during pregnancy. The goal of management is to relieve the itching. Topical steroids and emollients are the usual treatment. The problem usually resolves during the postpartum period (Papoutsis & Kroupouzos, 2007). Systemic diseases can also cause pruritus, but these causes are uncommon or rare (Cappell, 2007) (Box 10-3). Preexisting skin diseases may complicate pregnancy or be improved.

NURSING ALERT Women with severe acne taking isotretinoin (Accutane) should avoid pregnancy while receiving the treatment because it is teratogenic and associated with major fetal malformations.

Gum hypertrophy may occur. An epulis (gingival granuloma gravidarum) is a red, raised nodule on the gums that bleeds easily. This lesion may develop around the third month and usually continues to enlarge as pregnancy progresses. It is usually managed by avoiding trauma to the gums (e.g., using a soft toothbrush). An epulis usually regresses spontaneously after birth.

Nail growth may be accelerated. Some women may notice thinning and softening of the nails. Oily skin and acne vulgaris may occur during pregnancy. In some women the skin clears and looks radiant. Hirsutism, the excessive growth of hair or growth of hair in unusual places, is commonly reported. An increase in fine hair growth may occur but tends to disappear after pregnancy. However, growth of coarse or bristly hair does not usually disappear after pregnancy. The rate of scalp hair loss slows during pregnancy; increased hair loss may be noted in the postpartum period.

Increased blood supply to the skin leads to increased perspiration. Women feel hotter during pregnancy, possibly related to a progesterone-induced increase in body temperature and the increased BMR.

Musculoskeletal System

The gradually changing body and increasing weight of the pregnant woman usually cause noticeable changes in her posture (Fig. 10-13) and in the way she walks. The great abdominal distention gives the pelvis a forward tilt, decreased abdominal muscle tone, and increased weight bearing. The woman's center of gravity shifts forward, requiring a realignment of the spinal curvatures. An increase in the normal lumbosacral curve (lordosis) develops, and a compensatory curvature in the cervicodorsal region (exaggerated anterior flexion of the head) develops to help her maintain balance. Aching, numbness, and weakness of the upper extremities may result. Large breasts and a stoop-shouldered stance further accentuate the lumbar and dorsal curves. Walking is more difficult, and the waddling gait of the pregnant woman, called "the proud walk of pregnancy" by Shakespeare, is well known. The ligamentous and muscular structures of the middle and lower spine may be severely stressed. These and related changes often cause musculoskeletal discomfort, especially in older women or those with a back disorder or a faulty sense of balance.

Slight relaxation and increased mobility of the pelvic joints are normal during pregnancy. This is secondary to the exaggerated elasticity and softening of connective and collagen tissue caused by increased circulating steroid sex hormones, especially estrogen. Relaxin, an ovarian hormone, assists in this relaxation and softening. These adaptations permit enlargement of pelvic dimensions to facilitate labor and birth. The degree of relaxation varies, but considerable separation of the symphysis pubis and the instability of the sacroiliac joints may cause pain and difficulty in walking. Obesity or multifetal pregnancy tends to increase the pelvic instability. Peripheral joint laxity also increases as pregnancy progresses, but the cause is not known (Cunningham et al, 2005).

The muscles of the abdominal wall stretch and ultimately lose some tone. During the third trimester the rectus abdominis muscles may separate (Fig. 10-14), allowing abdominal

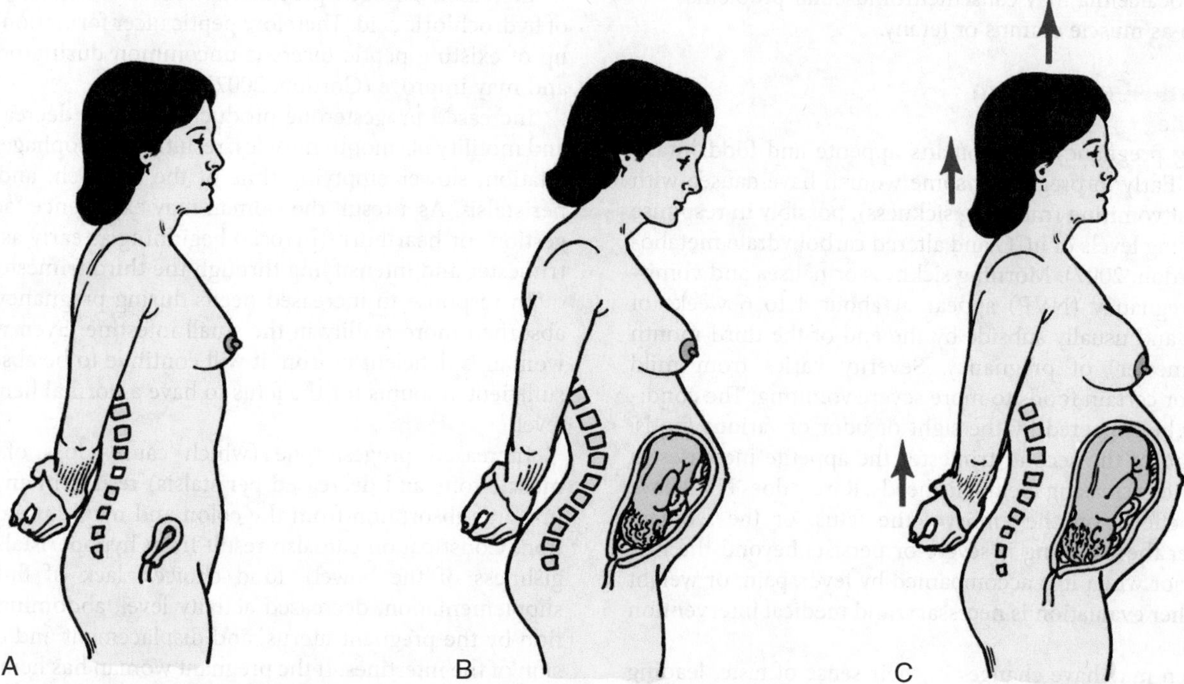

Fig. 10-13 Postural changes during pregnancy. A, Nonpregnant. B, Incorrect posture during pregnancy. C, Correct posture during pregnancy.

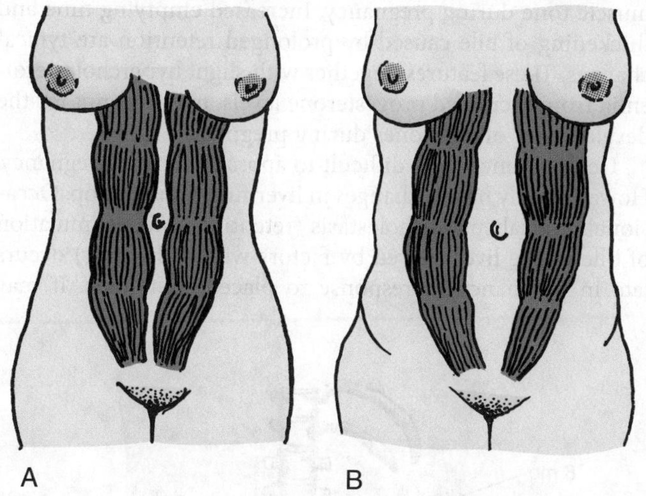

Fig. 10-14 Possible change in rectus abdominis muscles during pregnancy. A, Normal position in nonpregnant woman. B, Diastasis recti abdominis in pregnant women.

contents to protrude at the midline. The umbilicus flattens or protrudes. After birth the muscles gradually regain tone. However, separation of the muscles (diastasis recti abdominis) may persist.

Neurologic System

Little is known regarding specific alterations in function of the neurologic system during pregnancy, aside from hypothalamic-pituitary neurohormonal changes. Specific physiologic alterations resulting from pregnancy may cause the following neurologic or neuromuscular symptoms:

- Sensory changes in the legs as a result of compression of pelvic nerves or vascular stasis caused by enlargement of the uterus.
- Pain from dorsolumbar lordosis because of traction on nerves or compression of nerve roots.
- Carpal tunnel syndrome from edema of the peripheral nerves during the third trimester (Samuels & Niebyl, 2007). The edema compresses the median nerve beneath the carpal ligament of the wrist. Smoking and alcohol consumption can impair the microcirculation and may worsen the symptoms. The syndrome is characterized by paresthesia (abnormal sensation such as burning or tingling caused by a disorder of the sensory nervous system) and pain in the hand, radiating to the elbow. The dominant hand is usually affected most, although as many as 80% of women report symptoms in both hands. Symptoms usually regress after pregnancy. Some patients may require surgical treatment (Samuels & Niebyl, 2007).
- Acroesthesia (numbness and tingling of the hands) is caused by the stoop-shouldered stance (see Fig. 10-13, *B*) assumed by some women during pregnancy. The condition is associated with traction on segments of the brachial plexus.
- Tension headache is common when anxiety or uncertainty complicates gestation. However, vision problems such as refractive errors, sinusitis, or migraine may also be responsible for headaches.
- "Light-headedness," faintness, and even syncope (fainting) are common during early pregnancy. Vasomotor instability, postural hypotension, or hypoglycemia may be responsible.

- Hypocalcemia may cause neuromuscular problems such as muscle cramps or tetany.

Gastrointestinal System

Appetite

During pregnancy the woman's appetite and food intake fluctuate. Early in pregnancy some women have nausea with or without vomiting (morning sickness), possibly in response to increasing levels of hCG and altered carbohydrate metabolism (Gordon, 2007). Morning sickness or nausea and vomiting of pregnancy (NVP) appear at about 4 to 6 weeks of gestation and usually subside by the end of the third month (first trimester) of pregnancy. Severity varies from mild distaste for certain foods to more severe vomiting. The condition may be triggered by the sight or odor of various foods. By the end of the second trimester the appetite increases in response to increasing metabolic needs. Rarely does NVP have harmful effects on the embryo, the fetus, or the woman. Whenever the vomiting is severe or persists beyond the first trimester or when it is accompanied by fever, pain, or weight loss, further evaluation is necessary, and medical intervention is likely.

Women may have changes in their sense of taste, leading to cravings and changes in dietary intake. Some women have nonfood cravings (pica) such as for ice, clay, and laundry starch. Usually the subjects of these cravings, if consumed in moderation, are not harmful to the pregnancy if the woman has adequate nutrition with appropriate weight gain (Gordon, 2007).

Mouth

The gums become hyperemic, spongy, and swollen during pregnancy. They tend to bleed easily because the increasing levels of estrogen cause selective increased vascularity and connective tissue proliferation (a nonspecific gingivitis). Epulis (discussed in the section on the integumentary system) may develop at the gum line. Some pregnant women complain of ptyalism (excessive salivation), which may be caused by the decrease in unconscious swallowing by the woman when nauseated or from stimulation of salivary glands by eating starch (Cunningham et al, 2005).

Teeth

The pregnant woman requires about 1.2 g of calcium and approximately the same amount of phosphorus every day during pregnancy. This is an increase of about 0.4 g of each of these elements over nonpregnant needs. With a well-balanced diet these requirements are satisfied. Serious dietary deficiency may deplete the mother's bony stores of these elements but does not draw on calcium in her teeth. Demineralization of teeth does not occur during pregnancy; the old adage, "for every child a tooth" is untrue. Gingivitis and poor dental hygiene during pregnancy (or anytime) may contribute to dental caries, which can lead to the loss of a tooth.

Esophagus, Stomach, and Intestines

Herniation of the upper portion of the stomach (hiatal hernia) occurs in 15% to 20% of pregnant women after the seventh or eighth month. This condition results from upward displacement of the stomach, which causes a widening of the hiatus of the diaphragm. It occurs more often in multiparas and older or obese women.

Increased estrogen production causes decreased secretion of hydrochloric acid. Therefore peptic ulcer formation or flare-up of existing peptic ulcers is uncommon during pregnancy and may improve (Gordon, 2007).

Increased progesterone production causes decreased tone and motility of smooth muscles, resulting in esophageal regurgitation, slower emptying time of the stomach, and reverse peristalsis. As a result the woman may experience "acid indigestion" or heartburn (pyrosis) beginning as early as the first trimester and intensifying through the third trimester.

In response to increased needs during pregnancy, iron is absorbed more readily in the small intestine. Even when the woman is deficient in iron, it will continue to be absorbed in sufficient amounts for the fetus to have a normal hemoglobin level.

Increased progesterone (which causes loss of smooth muscle tone and decreased peristalsis) results in an increase in water absorption from the colon and may cause constipation. Constipation can also result from hypoperistalsis (sluggishness of the bowel), food choices, lack of fluids, iron supplementation, decreased activity level, abdominal distention by the pregnant uterus, and displacement and compression of the intestines. If the pregnant woman has hemorrhoids (see Fig. 10-11) and is constipated, the hemorrhoids can evert or bleed during straining at stool.

Gallbladder and Liver

The gallbladder is often distended because of its decreased muscle tone during pregnancy. Increased emptying time and thickening of bile caused by prolonged retention are typical changes. These features, together with slight hypercholesterolemia from increased progesterone levels, may account for the development of gallstones during pregnancy.

Hepatic function is difficult to appraise during pregnancy. However, only minor changes in liver function develop. Occasionally intrahepatic cholestasis (retention and accumulation of bile in the liver caused by factors within the liver) occurs late in pregnancy in response to placental steroids. It may

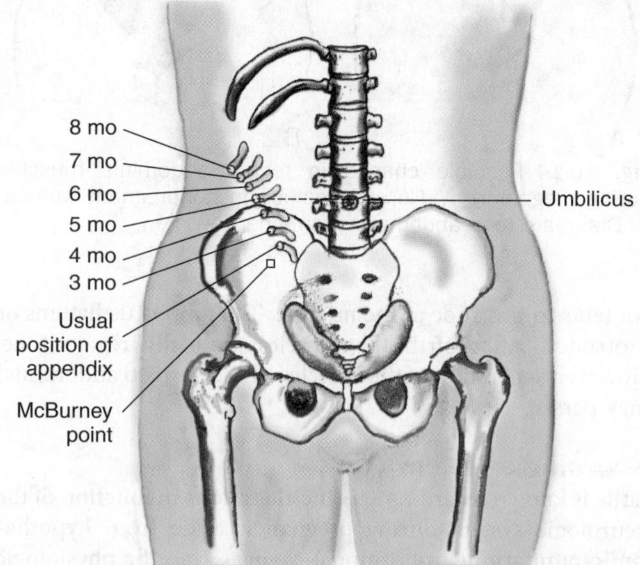

Fig. 10-15 Change in position of appendix in pregnancy. Note McBurney point.

Table 10-7 Hormones and Effects of Changes During Pregnancy

HORMONE	SOURCE	EFFECTS OF CHANGES DURING PREGNANCY
Human chorionic gonadotropin	Fertilized ovum and chorionic villi	Maintains corpus luteum production of estrogen and progesterone until placenta takes over the function
Progesterone	Corpus luteum until 14 wk of gestation, then the placenta	Suppresses secretion of FSH and LH by the anterior pituitary; maintains pregnancy by relaxing smooth muscles, decreasing uterine contractility; causes fat to deposit in subcutaneous tissues over the maternal abdomen, back, and upper thighs; decreases mother's ability to use insulin
Estrogen	Corpus luteum until 14 wk of gestation, then the placenta	Suppresses secretion of FSH and LH by the anterior pituitary; causes fat to deposit in subcutaneous tissues over the maternal abdomen, back, and upper thighs; promotes enlargement of genitals, uterus, and breasts; increases vascularity; relaxes pelvic ligaments and joints; interferes with folic acid metabolism; increases the level of total body proteins; promotes retention of sodium and water; decreases secretion of hydrochloric acid and pepsin; decreases mother's ability to use insulin
Serum prolactin	Anterior pituitary	Responsible for initial lactation
Oxytocin	Posterior pituitary	Stimulates uterine contractions; stimulates the let-down or milk-ejection reflex
Human chorionic somatomammotropin (previously called human placental lactogen)	Placenta	Acts as a growth hormone; contributes to breast development; decreases maternal metabolism of glucose; increases the amount of fatty acids for metabolic needs
Thyroxine-binding globulin, thyroxine, triiodothyronine	Thyroid	Causes moderate enlargement of the thyroid gland but woman remains euthyroid; possibly plays role in early neural development of the fetus
Parathyroid	Parathyroid	Controls calcium and magnesium metabolism
Insulin	Pancreas	Decreases production of insulin to protect fetus and its need for glucose
Cortisol	Adrenal glands	Stimulates production of insulin; increases peripheral resistance to insulin
Aldosterone	Adrenal glands	Stimulates resorption of excess sodium from the renal tubules

FSH, Follicle-stimulating hormone; *LH*, luteinizing hormone.

result in pruritus gravidarum (severe itching) with or without jaundice. These distressing symptoms are difficult to treat during pregnancy and may be associated with fetal risk. However, symptoms subside after birth (Cappell, 2007).

Abdominal Discomfort

Intraabdominal alterations that can cause discomfort include pelvic heaviness or pressure, round ligament tension, flatulence, distention and bowel cramping, and uterine contractions. In addition to displacement of intestines, pressure from the expanding uterus causes an increase in venous pressure in the pelvic organs. Although most abdominal discomfort is a consequence of normal maternal alterations, the health care provider must be constantly alert to the possibility of disorders such as bowel obstruction or an inflammatory process.

Appendicitis may be difficult to diagnose in pregnancy because the appendix is displaced upward and laterally, high and to the right, away from McBurney point (Fig. 10-15).

Endocrine System

Profound endocrine changes are essential for pregnancy maintenance, normal fetal growth, and postpartum recovery. Hormones, their sources, and their effects on the pregnancy are presented in Table 10-7.

Key Points

- The biochemical, physiologic, and anatomic adaptations that occur during pregnancy are profound and revert to the nonpregnant state after birth and lactation.
- Maternal adaptations are attributed to the hormones of pregnancy and to mechanical pressures arising from the enlarging uterus and other tissues.
- Adaptations to pregnancy protect the woman's normal physiologic functioning, meet the metabolic demands that

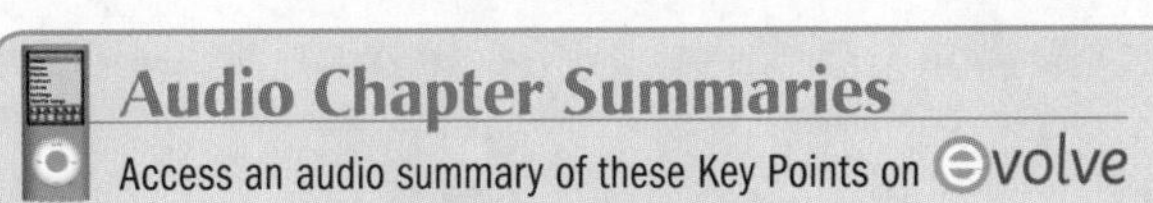
Audio Chapter Summaries
Access an audio summary of these Key Points on evolve

pregnancy imposes, and provide for fetal developmental and growth needs.
- ELISA testing, with monoclonal antibody technology, is the most popular method of pregnancy testing and

is the basis for most over-the-counter home pregnancy tests.

- Presumptive, probable, and positive signs of pregnancy aid in the diagnosis of pregnancy; only positive signs (identification of a fetal heart tone, verification of fetal movements, and visualization of the fetus) can establish the diagnosis of pregnancy.
- Although the pH of the pregnant woman's vaginal secretions is more acidic than in the nonpregnant state, she is more vulnerable to some vaginal infections, especially yeast infections.
- Increased vascularity and sensitivity of the vagina and other pelvic viscera may lead to a high degree of sexual interest and arousal.
- Some adaptations to pregnancy result in discomforts such as fatigue, urinary frequency, nausea, constipation, and breast sensitivity.
- Balance and coordination are affected by changes in joints and in the woman's center of gravity as pregnancy progresses.

References

Beebe K: The perplexing parity puzzle, *AWHONN Lifelines* 9(5):394-399, 2005.

Blackburn S: *Maternal, fetal, & neonatal physiology: a clinical perspective*, ed 3, St Louis, 2007, Saunders.

Cappell M: Hepatic and gastrointestinal diseases. In Gabbe SG, Niebyl JR, Simpson JL (editors): *Obstetrics: normal and problem pregnancies*, ed 5, Philadelphia, 2007, Churchill Livingstone.

Copeland L, Landon M: Malignant diseases and pregnancy. In Gabbe SG, Niebyl JR, Simpson JL (editors): *Obstetrics: normal and problem pregnancies*, ed 5, Philadelphia, 2007, Churchill Livingstone.

Cunningham F et al: *Williams obstetrics*, ed 22, New York, 2005, McGraw-Hill.

Duff W, Sweet R, Edwards RK: Maternal and fetal infections. In Creasy RK et al (editors): *Creasy & Resnik's maternal-fetal medicine: principles and practice*, ed 6, Philadelphia, 2009, Saunders.

Gordon M: Maternal physiology. In Gabbe SG, Niebyl JR, Simpson JL (editors): *Obstetrics: normal and problem pregnancies*, ed 5, Philadelphia, 2007, Churchill Livingstone.

Pagana KD, Pagana TJ: *Mosby's diagnostic and laboratory test reference*, ed 7, St Louis, 2006, Mosby.

Papoutsis J, Kroupouzos G: Dermatologic disorders. In Gabbe SG, Niebyl JR, Simpson JL (editors): *Obstetrics: normal and problem pregnancies*, ed 5, Philadelphia, 2007, Churchill Livingstone.

Pickering T et al: Recommendations for blood pressure measurement in humans and experimental animals. Part 1: Blood pressure measurement in humans: statement for professionals from the Subcommittee of Professional and Public Education of the American Heart Association Council on High Blood Pressure Research, *Hypertension* 45(1):142-161, 2005.

Samuels P: Hematology complications of pregnancy. In Gabbe SG, Niebyl JR, Simpson JL (editors): *Obstetrics: normal and problem pregnancies*, ed 5, Philadelphia, 2007, Churchill Livingstone.

Samuels P, Niebyl J: Neurologic disorders. In Gabbe SG, Niebyl JR, Simpson JL (editors): *Obstetrics: normal and problem pregnancies*, ed 5, Philadelphia, 2007, Churchill Livingstone.

Seidel H et al: *Mosby's guide to physical examination*, ed 6, St Louis, 2006, Mosby.

Sibai B: Hypertension. In Gabbe SG, Niebyl JR, Simpson JL (editors): *Obstetrics: normal and problem pregnancies*, Philadelphia, 2007, Churchill Livingstone.

11 Nursing Care During Pregnancy

Learning Objectives

On completion of this chapter the reader will be able to:

- Describe the processes of confirming pregnancy and estimating the date of birth.
- Summarize the physical, psychosocial, and behavioral changes that usually occur as the mother and other family members adapt to pregnancy.
- Discuss the benefits of prenatal care and problems of accessibility for some women.
- Outline the patterns of health care to assess maternal and fetal health status at the initial visit and follow-up visits during pregnancy.
- Identify the typical nursing assessments, diagnoses, interventions, and methods of evaluation in providing care for the pregnant woman.
- Discuss education needed by pregnant women to understand physical discomforts related to pregnancy and to recognize the signs and symptoms of potential complications.
- Explain the impact of culture, age, parity, and number of fetuses on the response of the family to the pregnancy and on the prenatal care provided.
- Determine the scope of childbirth and perinatal education in the community.
- Compare philosophies underlying maternal choices for childbirth.
- Compare the advantages and disadvantages of choosing different care providers.

Electronic Resources

Additional information related to the content in Chapter 11 can be found on

evolve the Companion Website at

http://evolve.elsevier.com/Perry/maternal/

- NCLEX Review Questions
- Assessment Video—Chest Wall, Breast, Abdomen/Fundal Height, Fetal Lie, Presentation, Position, Fetal Heart Rate
- Case Study—First Trimester
- Case Study—Second Trimester
- Case Study—Third Trimester
- Critical Thinking Exercise—Teenage Pregnancy
- Critical Thinking Exercise—Discomforts of Pregnancy
- Nursing Care Plan—Discomforts of Pregnancy and Warning Signs
- Nursing Care Plan—Adolescent Pregnancy
- Spanish Guidelines—Assessment of Respiratory Symptoms
- Spanish Guidelines—Prenatal Interview
- Spanish Guidelines—Prenatal Physical Examination

The prenatal period is a time of physical and psychologic preparation for birth and parenthood. Becoming a parent is one of the maturational milestones of adult life. It is a time of intense learning for parents and those close to them. The prenatal period provides a unique opportunity for nurses and other members of the health care team to influence family health. During this period essentially healthy women seek regular care and guidance. The nurse's health promotion interventions can affect the well-being of the woman, her unborn child, and the rest of her family for many years.

Regular prenatal visits, ideally beginning soon after the first missed menstrual period, offer opportunities to ensure the health of the expectant mother and her infant. Prenatal health care permits diagnosis and treatment of preexisting maternal disorders and those that may develop during the pregnancy. Care is designed to monitor the growth and development of the fetus and identify abnormalities that may interfere with the course of normal labor. The woman and her family can seek support to reduce stress and learn parenting skills.

Pregnancy lasts 9 calendar months. However, health care providers use the concept of lunar months, which last 28 days (or 4 weeks) to describe the duration of pregnancy or gestational age. Thus normal pregnancy lasts about 10 lunar months, that is, 40 weeks, or 280 days. Pregnancy is divided into three 3-month periods, or trimesters. The first trimester covers weeks 1 through 13; the second, weeks 14 through 26; and the third, weeks 27 through term gestation (38 to 40 weeks). The focus of this chapter is on meeting the health needs of the expectant family over the course of pregnancy, which is known as the prenatal period.

Diagnosis of Pregnancy

Women may suspect pregnancy when they miss a menstrual period. Many women come to the first visit after a positive home pregnancy test. However, the clinical diagnosis of pregnancy before the second missed period may be difficult in some women. Factors such as physical variations, lack of relaxation, obesity, or tumors may confound even the experienced examiner. However, accuracy is important because emotional, social, medical, or legal consequences related to an inaccurate diagnosis, either positive or negative, can be extremely serious. A correct date for the first day of the last (normal) menstrual period (LMP), the date of intercourse, and a basal body temperature record may be of great value in the accurate diagnosis of pregnancy (see Chapter 7).

Signs and Symptoms

Great variability is possible in the subjective and objective symptoms of pregnancy. Therefore the diagnosis of pregnancy may be uncertain for a time. It is based on signs and symptoms that are reported during history taking or found during physical examination. These signs and symptoms are classified as presumptive, probable, and positive (see Table 10-2).

Estimating Date of Birth

When pregnancy is confirmed, the woman's first question usually concerns when she will give birth. This date has traditionally been called the estimated date of confinement or estimated date of delivery. However, to promote a more positive perception of both pregnancy and birth, the term *estimated date of birth* (EDB) is now used. Because the exact date of conception is usually unknown, several formulas have been suggested for calculating the EDB. None of these guides is infallible, but Nägele's rule is reasonably accurate and is the method usually used.

Nägele's rule is as follows: after determining the first day of the LMP, subtract 3 months, add 7 days and 1 year; or alternatively, add 7 days to the LMP and count forward 9 months. For example, if the first day of the LMP was September 10, 2009, the EDB is June 17, 2010.

Nägele's rule assumes that the woman has a 28-day menstrual cycle and that the pregnancy occurred on the fourteenth day of the cycle. An adjustment is in order if the cycle is longer or shorter than 28 days. Only about 5% of pregnant women give birth spontaneously on the EDB as determined by Nägele's rule. Most women give birth during the period extending from 7 days before to 7 days after the EDB.

Adaptation to Pregnancy

Pregnancy affects all family members, and each family member must adapt to the pregnancy and interpret its meaning in light of his or her own needs. This process of family adaptation to pregnancy takes place within a cultural environment influenced by societal trends. Dramatic changes have occurred in Western society in recent years, and the nurse must be prepared to support not only traditional families but also single-parent families, reconstituted families, dual-career families, and alternative families.

Much of the investigation of family dynamics in pregnancy by scholars in the United States and Canada has been done with Caucasian, middle-class nuclear families; thus findings may not apply to families who do not fit the traditional North American model. For example, terms such as *spouse, husband,* and *wife* are used consistently in family literature but may not fit the configuration of a given family in the nurse's care. Adaptation of terms is appropriate to avoid offense to the family and embarrassment to the nurse.

Maternal Adaptation

Women of all ages use the months of pregnancy to adapt to the maternal role, a complex process of social and cognitive learning (see Family-Centered Care box).

Pregnancy can be stressful but also rewarding as the woman prepares for a new level of caring and responsibility. Her self-concept changes in readiness for parenthood as she prepares for her new role. She moves gradually from being self-contained and independent to being committed to a lifelong concern for another human being. This growth requires mastery of certain developmental tasks: accepting the pregnancy, identifying with the role of mother, reordering the relationships between herself and her mother and between herself and her partner, establishing a relationship with the unborn child, and preparing for the birth experience. The partner's emotional support is an important factor in the successful accomplishment of these developmental tasks. Single women with limited support may have difficulty making this adaptation.

Accepting the Pregnancy

The first step in adapting to the maternal role is accepting the idea of pregnancy and assimilating the pregnant state into the woman's way of life. Mercer (1995) described this process as cognitive restructuring and credited Reva Rubin (1984) as the nurse theorist who pioneered our understanding of maternal role attainment.

The degree of acceptance is reflected in the woman's emotional responses. Initially many women are dismayed at finding themselves pregnant, especially if the pregnancy is unplanned. Eventual acceptance of pregnancy parallels the growing acceptance of the reality of a child. Nonacceptance of the pregnancy should not be equated with rejection of the child. A woman may dislike being pregnant but feel love for the child to be born.

Women who are happy and pleased about their pregnancy have high self-esteem and tend to be confident about outcomes for themselves, their babies, and other family members. Despite a general feeling of well-being, many pregnant women are surprised to experience emotional lability (i.e., rapid and unpredictable changes in mood). These swings in emotions and increased sensitivity to others are disconcerting to the expectant mother and those around her. Increased irritability, explosions of tears and anger, and feelings of great joy and cheerfulness alternate, apparently with little or no provocation. Profound hormonal changes that are part of the maternal response to pregnancy may be responsible for mood changes.

Most women have ambivalent feelings during pregnancy, whether or not the pregnancy was intended. Ambivalence—

FAMILY-CENTERED CARE

Maternal Adaptation

Adaptation to the maternal role involves a complex social and cognitive learning process. Pregnancy functions as a rite of passage and indicates that maturity has been reached. Reva Rubin began studying maternal role adaptation in the 1960s. She described the developmental tasks of pregnancy as accepting the pregnancy, identifying the role of mother, reordering the relationships between her mother and herself and between herself and her partner, establishing a relationship with the unborn child, and preparing for the birth experience.

The partner's emotional support is an important factor in the successful accomplishment of these developmental tasks. Women who are prepared to accept a pregnancy seek medical validation early. When pregnancy is confirmed, a woman's emotional responses may range from delight to shock, disbelief, and despair. A general state of well-being predominates, but emotional lability is common. These rapid mood changes include increased irritability, explosions of tears and anger, and feelings of great joy and cheerfulness. Such changes are often attributed to hormonal changes.

Rubin described changes in pregnancy as follows. The subjective experience of time and space changes during pregnancy; early in pregnancy nothing seems to be happening, and the woman spends much time sleeping. With quickening (feelings of fetal movement) in the second trimester, there is a reduction of time and space, both geographic and social, as the woman turns her attention inward to her pregnancy. She examines or fosters relationships with her mother and other women who have been or are pregnant. With the third trimester there is a slower pace and a sense that time is running out as the woman's activities are curtailed. A mother's reaction to her daughter's pregnancy signifies her acceptance of the grandchild and of her daughter. If the mother is supportive, the daughter has an opportunity to discuss pregnancy and labor and her feelings of joy or ambivalence with a knowledgeable and accepting woman.

Women express two major needs within the partner relationship during pregnancy: feeling loved and valued and having the child accepted by the partner. The addition of a child changes forever the nature of the bond between partners. The partner can be a stabilizing influence, a good listener to expressions of doubts and fears, and a source of physical and emotional reassurance. The partner can also feel jealous of the unborn baby. Lesbian and unpartnered women have received little attention in the literature. Some suggest that a woman partner may be better able to understand and meet the needs of her partner for nurturing more effectively. An unpartnered woman may seek out her mother or other women friends to meet her dependence needs.

Data from Mercer R: *Becoming a mother*, New York, 1995, Springer.

having conflicting feelings at the same time—is considered a normal response for people preparing for a new role. For example, during pregnancy women may feel great pleasure that they are fulfilling a lifelong dream, but they also may feel great regret that life as they now know it is ending.

Even women who are pleased to be pregnant may experience feelings of hostility toward the pregnancy or the unborn child from time to time. Intense feelings of ambivalence that persist through the third trimester may indicate an unresolved conflict with the motherhood role (Mercer, 1995). After the birth of a healthy child, memories of these ambivalent feelings usually are dismissed. If the child is born with a defect, a woman may look back at the times when she did not want the pregnancy and feel intense guilt. She may believe that her ambivalence caused the birth defect. She will need reassurance that her feelings were not responsible for the problem.

Identifying with the Mother Role

The process of identifying with the mother role begins early in each woman's life when she is being mothered as a child. Her social group's perception of what constitutes the feminine role can subsequently influence her toward choosing between motherhood or a career, being married or single, being independent rather than interdependent, or being able to manage multiple roles. Practice roles such as playing with dolls, babysitting, and taking care of siblings may increase her understanding of what being a mother entails.

Many women have always wanted a baby; they like children, and look forward to motherhood. Their high motivation to become a parent promotes acceptance of pregnancy and eventual prenatal and parental adaptation. Other women apparently have not considered in any detail what motherhood means to them. During pregnancy conflicts such as not wanting the pregnancy and child-related or career-related decisions need to be resolved.

Reordering Personal Relationships

Close relationships held by the pregnant woman undergo change as she prepares emotionally for the new role of mother. As family members learn their new roles, periods of tension and conflict may occur. Promoting effective communication patterns between the expectant mother and her own mother and between the expectant mother and her partner are common nursing interventions provided during the prenatal visits.

The woman's relationship with her mother is significant in adapting to pregnancy and motherhood. Important components in the pregnant woman's relationship with her mother are the mother's availability (past and present), her reactions to the daughter's pregnancy, respect for her daughter's autonomy, and the willingness to reminisce (Mercer, 1995).

The mother's reaction to the daughter's pregnancy signifies her acceptance of the grandchild and of her daughter. If the mother is supportive, the daughter has an opportunity to discuss pregnancy and labor and her feelings of joy or ambivalence with a knowledgeable and accepting woman (Fig. 11-1). Reminiscing about the pregnant woman's early childhood and sharing the grandmother-to-be's account of her childbirth experience help the daughter anticipate and prepare for labor and birth.

Although the woman's relationship with her mother is significant in considering her adaptation in pregnancy, the most important person to the pregnant woman is usually the father of her child. A woman who is nurtured by her partner during

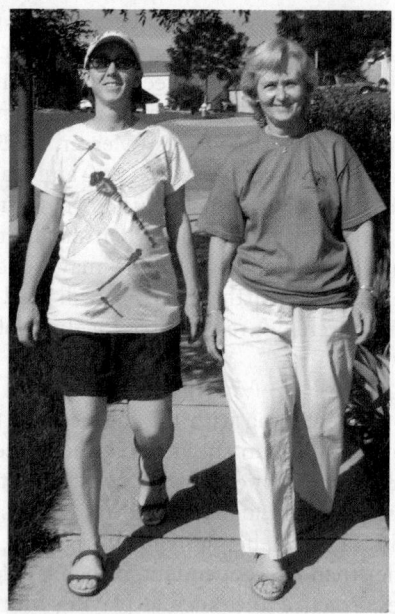

Fig. 11-1 A pregnant woman and her mother enjoy a walk together. *(Courtesy Shannon Perry, Phoenix, AZ.)*

pregnancy has fewer emotional and physical symptoms, fewer labor and childbirth complications, and an easier postpartum adjustment. Women express two major needs within this relationship during pregnancy: feeling loved and valued and having the child accepted by the partner.

The marital or committed relationship is not static but evolves over time. The addition of a child changes forever the nature of the bond between partners. This can be a time when couples grow closer and the pregnancy has a maturing effect on the partners' relationship as they assume new roles and discover new aspects of one another. Partners who trust and support each other are able to share mutual dependency needs (Mercer, 1995).

Sexual expression during pregnancy is highly individual. The sexual relationship is affected by physical, emotional, and interactional factors, including myths about sex during pregnancy, sexual dysfunction, and physical changes in the woman. Myths about body functions and fantasies about the influence of the fetus as a third party in lovemaking are commonly expressed. An individual may also inaccurately attribute anomalies, mental retardation, and other injuries to the fetus and mother to sexual relations during pregnancy. Some couples fear that the woman's genitals will be drastically changed by the birth process. Couples may not express their concerns to the health care provider because of embarrassment or because they do not want to appear foolish.

As pregnancy progresses, changes in body shape, body image, and levels of discomfort influence both partners' desire for sexual expression. During the first trimester the woman's sexual desire may decrease, especially if she has breast tenderness, nausea, fatigue, or sleepiness. As she progresses into the second trimester, her sense of well-being, combined with the increased pelvic congestion that occurs at this time, may increase her desire for sexual release. In the third trimester somatic complaints and physical bulkiness may increase her physical discomfort and diminish her interest in sex. As a woman's pregnancy progresses, her enlarging gravid abdomen may limit the use of the man-on-top position for intercourse. Therefore other positions (e.g., side to side or the woman on top) can allow intercourse while minimizing pressure on the woman's abdomen.

Establishing a Relationship with the Fetus

Emotional attachment—feelings of being tied by affection or love—begins during the prenatal period as women use fantasizing and daydreaming to prepare themselves for motherhood (Rubin, 1975). They think of themselves as mothers and imagine maternal qualities they would like to possess. Expectant parents desire to be warm, loving, and close to their child. They try to anticipate changes that the child will bring in their lives and wonder how they will react to noise, disorder, reduced freedom, and caregiving activities. The mother-child relationship progresses through pregnancy as a developmental process that unfolds in three phases.

In phase 1 the woman accepts the biologic fact of pregnancy. She needs to be able to state, "I am pregnant." In phase 2 the woman accepts the growing fetus as distinct from herself and as a person to nurture. She can now say, "I am going to have a baby." Attachment by a mother to her child is enhanced by experiencing a planned pregnancy, and it increases when ultrasound examination and quickening confirm the reality of the fetus. During phase 3 the woman prepares realistically for the birth and parenting of the child. She expresses the thought, "I am going to be a mother," and defines the nature and characteristics of the child. For example, she may speculate about the child's sex (if she has not had an ultrasound that confirms the sex) and personality traits based on patterns of fetal activity.

Although the mother alone experiences the child within, both parents and siblings believe the unborn child responds in a very individualized, personal manner. Family members may interact with the unborn child by talking to the fetus and stroking the mother's abdomen, especially when the fetus shifts position. They may sing to, play music for, or read to the fetus. The fetus may have a nickname used by family members.

Parents may occasionally show or voice disappointment over the sex of the child. The parents may experience grief and a sense of loss at birth as they release their fantasized image of the child and begin to accept the real child. However, these negative responses are usually temporary. Providing an accepting environment for parental reactions facilitates the parent's ability to move beyond disappointment to acceptance.

Preparing for Childbirth

Many women actively prepare for birth. They read books, view films, attend parenting classes, and talk to other women. They seek the best caregiver possible for advice, monitoring, and caring. The multipara has her own history of labor and birth, which influences her approach to preparation for this childbirth experience.

Anxiety can arise from concern about safe passage for herself and her child during the birth process (Mercer, 1995; Rubin, 1975). This concern may not be expressed overtly, but cues are given as the nurse listens to plans women make for care of the new baby and other children in case "anything should happen." These feelings persist despite statistical evidence about the safe outcome of pregnancy for mothers and their infants. Many women fear the pain of childbirth or mutilation because they do not understand anatomy and the birth process. Education by the nurse can alleviate many of these fears.

Toward the end of the third trimester breathing is difficult and fetal movements become vigorous enough to disturb the mother's sleep. Backaches, frequency and urgency of urination, constipation, and varicose veins can become troublesome. The bulkiness and awkwardness of her body interfere with the woman's ability to care for other children, perform routine work-related duties, and assume a comfortable position for sleep and rest. A strong desire to see the end of pregnancy, to be over and done with it, makes women at this stage ready to move on to childbirth.

Paternal Adaptation

The father's beliefs and feelings about the ideal mother and father and his cultural expectation of appropriate behavior during pregnancy affect his response to his partner's need for him. For most men, pregnancy can be a time of preparation for the parental role with intense learning (see Family-Centered Care box).

FAMILY-CENTERED CARE

Paternal Adaptation

A man's emotional responses to becoming a father, his concerns, and his informational needs change during the course of pregnancy. Three styles of involvement provide examples of different ways men can experience pregnancy (May, 1980, 1982). Men may be involved in pregnancy as an observer (i.e., avoiding direct involvement in activities such as parent education classes and decisions about breastfeeding). Others are more expressive and display a strong emotional response to pregnancy and a desire to be a full partner in the project. Some expectant fathers experience the couvade syndrome and have pregnancy-like symptoms such as nausea and other gastrointestinal complaints, fatigue, and other physical discomforts. Other fathers adopt the instrumental style, seeing tasks they can perform in their role as manager of the pregnancy. They feel responsible for the outcome of the pregnancy and are protective and supportive of their wives.

The father's beliefs and feelings about the ideal mother and father and his cultural expectation of appropriate behavior during pregnancy affect his response to his partner's need for him. One man may engage in nurturing behavior; another may feel lonely and alienated as the woman becomes physically and emotionally engrossed in the unborn child. The man may seek comfort and understanding outside the home or become interested in a new hobby or involved with his work. Some men view pregnancy as a proof of their masculinity and their dominant role. To others pregnancy has no meaning in terms of responsibility to either mother or child. However, for most men pregnancy is a time of preparation for the parental role, fantasy, great pleasure, and intense learning.

Accepting the Pregnancy

The ways in which fathers adjust to the parental role has been the subject of considerable research. In older societies the man enacted the ritual couvades; that is, he behaved in specific ways and respected taboos associated with pregnancy and giving birth. In this way the man's new status was recognized and endorsed. During the past 30 years changing cultural and professional attitudes have encouraged fathers' participation in the childbirth experience (Fig. 11-2).

Identifying with the Father Role

Each man brings to pregnancy attitudes that affect the way in which he adjusts to the pregnancy and parental role. His memories of the fathering he received from his own father, the experiences he has had with child care, and the perceptions of the male and father roles within his social group guide his selection of the tasks and responsibilities he will assume. Some men are highly motivated to nurture and love a child. They may be excited and pleased about the anticipated role of father. Others may be more detached or even hostile to the idea of fatherhood.

Reordering Personal Relationships

The partner's main role in pregnancy is to nurture and respond to the pregnant woman's feelings of vulnerability. The partner also must deal with the reality of the pregnancy. The partner's support indicates involvement in the pregnancy and preparation for attachment to the child.

Some aspects of a partner's behavior indicate rivalry. Direct rivalry with the fetus may be evident, especially during sexual activity. Men may protest that fetal movements prevent sexual gratification or that the fetus is watching them during sexual activity. Feelings of rivalry may be unconscious and not verbalized, but expressed in subtle behaviors.

The woman's increased introspection may cause her partner to feel uneasy as she becomes preoccupied with thoughts of the child and of motherhood, with her growing dependence

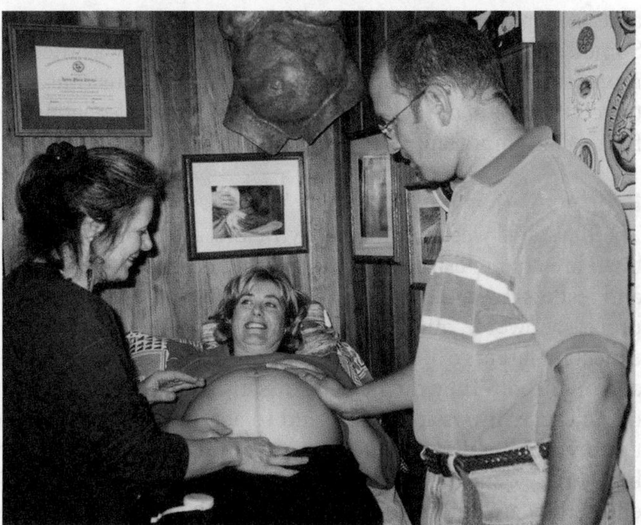

Fig. 11-2 Father participating in prenatal visit. Nurse-midwife instructs him in palpating fundus. *(Courtesy Shannon Perry, Phoenix, AZ.)*

on her physician or midwife, and with her reevaluation of the couple's relationship.

Establishing a Relationship with the Fetus

The father-child attachment can be as strong as the mother-child relationship, and fathers can be as competent as mothers in nurturing their infants. The father-child attachment also begins in pregnancy. A father may rub or kiss the maternal abdomen; try to listen, talk, or sing to the fetus; or play with the fetus as he notes fetal movement. Calling the unborn child by name or nickname helps to confirm the reality of pregnancy and promote attachment.

Men prepare for fatherhood in many of the same ways that women prepare for motherhood (i.e., by reading and fantasizing about the baby). Daydreaming about their role as father is common in the last weeks before the birth; men rarely describe their thoughts unless they are reassured that such daydreams are normal. They may adjust work commitments or plan vacations so that they can spend time with their new family.

Nurses can help fathers identify concerns and prepare for the reality of a baby by asking questions such as the following:

- What do you expect the baby to look and act like?
- What do you think being a father will be like?
- Have you thought about the baby's crying? Changing diapers? Burping the baby? Being awakened at night? Sharing your partner with the baby?

The father may not wish to answer such questions when he is asked but may need time to think them through or discuss them with his partner.

As the birth day approaches, fathers have more questions about fetal and newborn behaviors. Some fathers are shocked or amazed at the small size of the clothes and furniture for the baby. The nurse can tell the father about the unborn child's ability to respond to light, sound, and touch and encourage him to feel and talk to the fetus. A tour of a newborn nursery or discussions with new fathers, as in childbirth classes, may be welcomed.

Some men become involved by choosing the child's name and anticipating the child's sex, if it is not already known. Some couples select the name of the child as early as the first month of pregnancy. Family tradition, religious customs, and the continuation of the parent's name or names of relatives or friends are important in the selection process.

Preparing for Childbirth

The days and weeks immediately before the expected day of birth are characterized by anticipation and anxiety. Boredom and restlessness are common as the couple focuses on the birth process; however, during the last 2 months of pregnancy many expectant fathers experience a surge of creative energy at home and on the job. They can become dissatisfied with their present living space. If possible, they tend to act on the need to alter the environment (e.g., remodeling, painting). This activity can be overt evidence of their sharing in the childbearing experience. They are able to channel the anxiety and other feelings experienced during the final weeks before birth into productive activities. This behavior earns recognition and compliments from friends, relatives, and their partners.

The father's major concerns are getting the mother to a medical facility in time for the birth and not appearing ignorant. Many men want to be able to recognize labor and determine when it is appropriate to leave for the hospital or call the physician or midwife. They fantasize different situations and plan what they will do in response to them; they may rehearse taking various routes to the hospital, timing each route at different times of the day.

Some prospective fathers have questions about the labor suite's furniture, nursing staff, and location, as well as the availability of the physician and anesthesiologist. Others want to know what is expected of them when their partners are in labor. The man may have fears concerning safe passage of his partner and the mutilation or death of his partner or child. It is important he verbalize these fears; otherwise he cannot help his mate deal with her unspoken or overt apprehension.

With the exception of childbirth preparation classes, a man has few opportunities to learn ways to be an involved and active partner in this rite of passage into parenthood (see Family Centered Care box). The tensions and apprehensions of the unprepared, unsupportive father are readily transmitted to the mother and may increase her fears.

The same fears, questions, and concerns may affect birth partners who are not the biologic fathers. Birth partners need to be kept informed, supported, and included in all activities in which the mother desires their participation. The nurse can do much to promote pregnancy and birth as a family experience.

Sibling Adaptation

Sharing the spotlight with a new brother or sister may be the first major crisis for a child. The older child often experiences a sense of loss or feels jealous at being "replaced" by the new baby. Some of the factors that influence the child's response are age, the parents' attitudes, the father's role, the length of separation from the mother, the hospital's visitation policy, and how the child has been prepared for the change.

The mother with other children must devote time and energy to reorganizing her relationships with these children. She needs to prepare siblings for the birth of the baby (Box 11-1). She can begin the process of role transition in the family by including the children in the pregnancy and being sympathetic to older children's concerns about losing their places in the family hierarchy (Fig. 11-3). No child willingly gives up a familiar position.

Classes to prepare children for the birth of a new brother or sister are available in many communities (Fig. 11-4) (see Family Centered Care box).

Grandparent Adaptation

Expectant grandparenthood can represent a maturational milestone for the parent of an expectant parent. Some grandparents describe having a grandchild as the best thing that ever happened to them; they can enjoy the child without assuming responsibility for its care (Fig. 11-5). For other grandparents, when the mother is a young adolescent or for other reasons such as a substance-abusing mother, the grandchild may mean assuming care and raising another child when they thought childrearing was over.

FAMILY-CENTERED CARE

Maternal-Paternal-Fetal Relationship

Emotional attachment to the child begins during the prenatal period. Parents fantasize and daydream to prepare for parenthood. Early in pregnancy the woman accepts the biologic fact of pregnancy and incorporates the idea of a child into her body and self-image. When the fetus is viewed on ultrasound, it becomes more real. During the second trimester there is growing awareness of the child as a separate being. When she accepts the reality of the child, the woman becomes more introspective. She seems to withdraw and concentrate her interest on the unborn child. Her partner may feel left out, and other children in the family become more demanding in efforts to redirect the mother's attention to themselves.

The *fantasy child* may have familial characteristics and superior abilities; its appearance may be that of a 3- or 4-month-old infant. Both parents and siblings believe the unborn child responds in an individualized, personal manner. Some families become involved by choosing the child's name and anticipating the child's sex if it is not already known. Some families select the child's name as early as the first month of pregnancy. Family tradition, religious customs, and continuation of one's own name or names of relatives and friends are important in the selection process. Family members may interact a great deal with the unborn child by trying to listen to, talk to, and play with the fetus and stroking or kissing the mother's abdomen, especially when the fetus moves.

Nurses must continue to seek to understand and foster attitudes and behaviors that promote early attachment and reduce the risk of negative long-term effects such as child neglect and abuse. More research relating psychologic variables to prenatal attachment and maternal-paternal-fetal interaction with maternal-paternal-child interaction is needed, including research with lesbian couples and unpartnered women. Tools to measure maternal-fetal attachment are the Maternal-Fetal Attachment Scale* and the Prenatal Attachment Inventory.†

*Cranley MS: Development of a tool for the measurement of maternal attachment during pregnancy, *Nurs Res* 30(5):281-284, 1981.

†Müller ME: Development of the prenatal attachment inventory, *West J Nurs Res* 15(2):199-211, 1993.

BOX 11-1 Tips for Sibling Preparation

Prenatal

Adjust the timing and content of information about an anticipated infant to the age and understanding of the older child.

Take your child on a prenatal visit. Let the child listen to the fetal heartbeat and feel the baby move.

Involve the child in preparations for the baby such as helping to decorate the baby's room.

Move the child to a bed (if still sleeping in a crib) at least 2 months before the baby is due.

Read books, show videos, or take child to sibling preparation classes, including a hospital tour.

Answer your child's questions about the coming birth, what babies are like, and any other questions.

Take your child to the homes of friends who have babies so that the child has realistic expectations of what babies are like.

During the Hospital Stay

Have someone bring the child to the hospital to visit you and the baby (unless you plan to have the child attend the birth).

Don't force interactions between the child and the baby. Often the child will be more interested in seeing you and being reassured of your love.

Help the child explore the infant by showing how and where to touch the baby.

Give the child a gift (from you or from you, the father, and the baby).

Going Home

Leave the child at home with a relative or baby-sitter.

Have someone else carry the baby from the car so that you can hug the child first.

Adjustment After the Baby Is Home

Arrange for a special time with the child alone with each parent.

Don't exclude the child during infant feeding times. The child can sit with you and the baby and feed a doll or drink juice or milk with you or sit quietly with a game.

Prepare small gifts for the child so that, when the baby gets gifts, the sibling won't feel left out. The child can also help open the baby gifts.

Praise the child for acting age appropriately (so that being a baby does not seem better than being older).

To be truly family oriented, maternity care must include the grandparent in the implementation of the nursing process with the whole childbearing family. A class for grandparents is one method of incorporating the grandparents into the family system and encouraging communication between the generations (see Family-Centered Care box, p. 237).

Nursing Care Management

The purpose of prenatal care is to identify existing risk factors and other deviations from normal so that pregnancy outcomes can be enhanced (Johnson, Gregory, & Niebyl, 2007). Major emphasis is placed on preventive aspects of care, primarily to motivate the pregnant woman to practice optimal self-management and report unusual changes early so that problems can be minimized or prevented. In holistic care nurses provide information and guidance about not only the physical changes but also the psychosocial impact of pregnancy on the woman and members of her family. Therefore the goals of prenatal nursing care are to foster a safe birth for the infant and mother and to promote satisfaction of the mother and family with the pregnancy and birth experience (Box 11-2).

Advances have been made in the number of women in the United States who receive adequate prenatal care; in 2005 84% of pregnant women received care in the first trimester (Martin

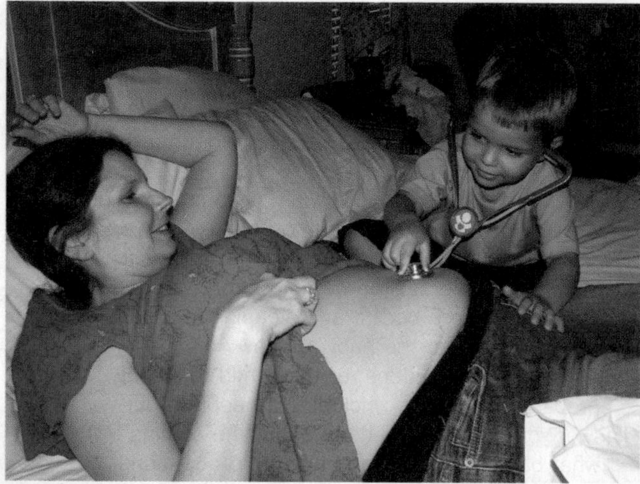

Fig. 11-3 Four-year-old likes to examine the pregnant abdomen of his mother. *(Courtesy Kara George, Phoenix, AZ.)*

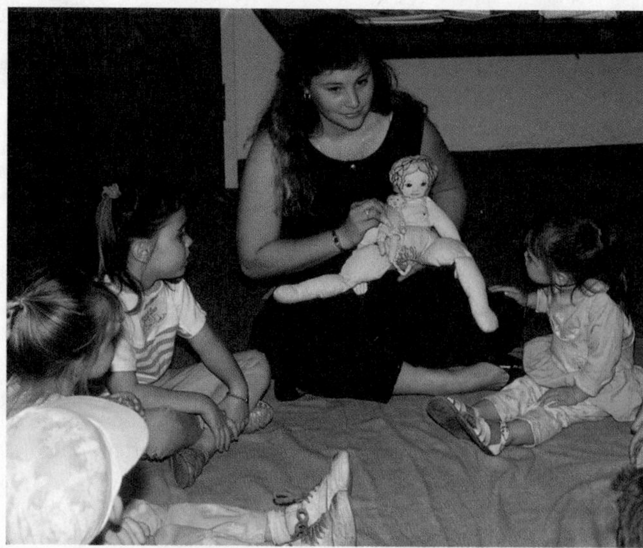

Fig. 11-4 A sibling class of preschoolers learns about childbirth and infant care using dolls. *(Courtesy Marjorie Pyle, RNC, Lifecircle, Costa Mesa, CA.)*

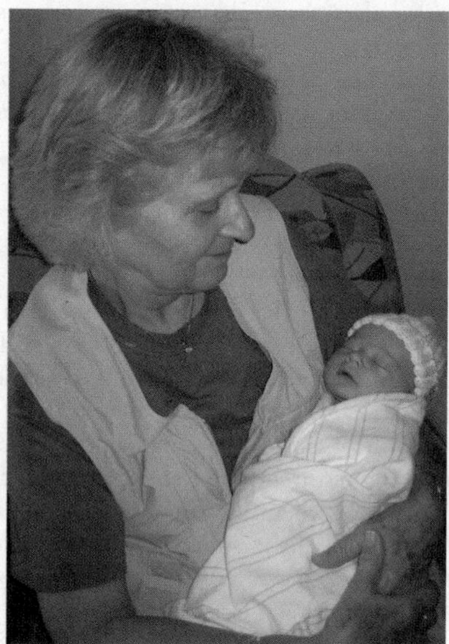

Fig. 11-5 A grandmother relaxes with her grandson. *(Courtesy Shannon Perry, Phoenix, AZ.)*

FAMILY-CENTERED CARE

Sibling Adaptation to Pregnancy and Birth

Sibling responses to pregnancy vary with age and dependency needs. The 1-year-old infant seems largely unaware of the process, but the 2-year-old child notices the change in the mother's appearance and may comment, "Mommy's fat." The 2-year-old child's need for sameness in the environment makes the child aware of any change. Toddlers may exhibit more clinging behavior and revert to dependent behaviors in toilet training or eating.

By age 3 or 4 years, children like to be told the story of their own beginning and accept its being compared to the present pregnancy. They like to listen to heartbeats and feel the baby moving in utero (see Fig. 11-3). Sometimes they worry about how the baby is being fed and what it wears.

School-age children take a more clinical interest in their mother's pregnancy. They may want to know in more detail, "How did the baby get in there?" and "How will it get out?" Children in this age group notice pregnant women in stores, churches, and schools and sometimes seem shy if they need to approach a pregnant woman directly. On the whole they look forward to the new baby, see themselves as "mothers" or "fathers," and enjoy buying baby supplies and readying a place for the baby. Because they still think in concrete terms and base judgments on the here and now, they respond positively to their mother's current good health.

Early and middle adolescents preoccupied with the establishment of their own sexual identity may have difficulty accepting the overwhelming evidence of the sexual activity of their parents. They reason that if they are too young for such activity, certainly their parents are too old. They seem to take on a critical parental role and may ask, "What will people think?" or "How can you let yourself get so fat?" Many pregnant women with teenage children confess that their teenagers are the most difficult factor in their current pregnancy.

Late adolescents do not appear to be unduly disturbed. They realize that they soon will be gone from home. Parents usually report that they are comforting and act more like other adults than children.

et al, 2008). Prenatal care is sought routinely by women of middle or high socioeconomic status. However, women living in poverty or who lack health insurance may not be able to use public medical services or gain access to private care. Lack of culturally sensitive care providers and barriers in communication caused by differences in language also interfere with access to care. Immigrant women from cultures in which prenatal care is not emphasized may not know to seek routine prenatal care. Thus birth outcomes in these populations are less positive, with higher rates of maternal and fetal or newborn complications. In particular, problems with low birth weight (LBW) (less than 2500 g) and infant mortality have been associated with inadequate prenatal care.

Barriers to obtaining health care during pregnancy include inadequate numbers of health care providers, unpleasant

FAMILY-CENTERED CARE

Grandparent Adaptation to Pregnancy and Birth

Every pregnancy affects all family relationships. For expectant grandparents a first pregnancy in a child is undeniable evidence that they are growing older. Many think of a grandparent as old, white haired, and becoming feeble of mind and body; however, some people face grandparenthood while still in their thirties or forties. A mother-to-be announcing her pregnancy to her mother may be greeted by a negative response that indicates she is not ready to be a grandmother. Both daughter and mother may be startled and hurt by the response.

Some expectant grandparents not only are nonsupportive but also use subtle means to decrease the self-esteem of the young parents-to-be. Mothers may talk about their terrible pregnancies; fathers may discuss the endless cost of rearing children; and mothers-in-law may complain that their sons are neglecting them because their concern is now directed toward the pregnant daughters-in-law.

However, most grandparents are delighted with the prospect of a new baby in the family. It reawakens their feelings of their own youth, the excitement of giving birth, and their delight in the behavior of the parents-to-be when they were infants. They set up a memory store of their child's first smiles, first words, and first steps that can be used later for "claiming" the newborn as a member of the family. Their satisfaction and that of the parents comes with the realization that continuity between past and present is guaranteed.

The grandparent is the historian who transmits the family history, a resource person who shares knowledge based on experience, a role model, and a support person. The grandparent's presence and support can strengthen family systems by widening the circle of support and nurturance (see Fig. 11-5). Other sources of information cannot replace the unique contribution that grandparents make *(www.grandparenting.org)*.

Many women report that their pregnancies bridged the final gap between them and their own mothers. The estrangement that began in adolescence disappears as the now-pregnant daughter experiences joys, concerns, and anxieties similar to those her mother felt before her.

BOX 11-2 Lamaze Philosophy of Pregnancy

- Pregnancy is a normal, natural life event.
- Women's bodies are perfectly designed to nourish and nurture their babies through pregnancy.
- The months of pregnancy are necessary for babies to develop and grow, for women's bodies to prepare for birth, and for women to become mothers.
- Pregnancy provides an opportunity for mothers and fathers to begin forming lifelong bonds with their babies.
- A good support system, a healthy lifestyle, and the ability to cope with the stresses of life promote a healthy pregnancy, a healthy birth, and a healthy baby.
- The health care system and care provider can increase or decrease a woman's confidence in the normality of pregnancy and in her ability to have a healthy baby.
- Lamaze education empowers women to gain confidence in their bodies, trust their inner wisdom, and make informed decisions about pregnancy, birth, breastfeeding, and parenting.

Source: www.lamaze.org/AboutLamaze/MissionandVision/LamazePhilosophyofPregnancy/tabid/379/Default.aspx (accessed July 31, 2008).

BOX 11-3 Sharing Care—Planning Safe Passage

Pamela, a 38-year-old professional, pregnant with her second child, planned a home birth. After successfully giving birth to her first child at home, she contracted with a home birth lay midwife for pregnancy care and birth for the second child. During pregnancy she scheduled three visits with an obstetrician to ensure that, in the case of problems, a skilled practitioner with access to high risk hospital care was familiar with her. She was able to give birth at home with family and friends in attendance and to fulfill her desire for a home birth, while at the same time ensuring expert care in the event of problems.

clinic facilities or procedures, inconvenient clinic hours, distance from health care facilities, lack of transportation, fragmentation of services, inadequate finances, and personal attitudes. The availability and accessibility of prenatal care may be improved by increasing the use of advanced practice nurses in collaborative practice with physicians or midwives (Box 11-3). The effectiveness of a regular schedule of home visiting by nurses during pregnancy also has been validated.

The current model for providing prenatal care has been used for more than a century. The initial visit usually occurs in the first trimester, with monthly visits through week 28 of pregnancy. Thereafter visits are scheduled every 2 weeks until week 36 and then every week until birth. This model is currently being questioned, and in some practices there is a growing tendency to have fewer visits with women who are at low risk for complications. Health care providers are challenged to create a system of prenatal care that has minimal barriers and a focus on individualized care (Box 11-4). A prenatal history form is the best way to document information obtained (see Nursing Process box and *www.acog.org/acb-custom/aa128.pdf* for a sample form available from the American College of Obstetricians and Gynecologists).

The therapeutic relationship between the nurse and the woman is established during the initial assessment interview (Fig. 11-6). It is a time for planned, purposeful communication that focuses on specific content. The data collected are of two types: the woman's subjective appraisal of her health status and the nurse's objective observations. The nurse observes the woman's affect, posture, body language, skin color, and other physical and emotional signs.

Often the pregnant woman is accompanied by one or more family members. The nurse needs to build a relationship with these people as part of the social context of the patient. With her permission, those accompanying the woman can be

NURSING PROCESS: NURSING CARE DURING PREGNANCY

Assessment

The assessment process begins at the initial prenatal visit and is continued throughout the pregnancy.

- History (comprehensive health history, obstetric and gynecologic history, family history; physical abuse)
- Interview (psychosocial profile; mental status; risk assessment; symptoms she is experiencing)
- Physical examination (review of body systems; vital signs, weight; pelvic examination; fetal heart rate)
- Review of laboratory tests

Nursing Diagnoses

Nursing diagnoses that may be appropriate in the prenatal period include the following:

Anxiety related to

- physical discomforts of pregnancy
- ambivalent and labile emotions
- changes in family dynamics
- fetal well-being
- ability to manage anticipated labor

Interrupted family processes related to

- changing roles and responsibilities
- inadequate understanding of physical and emotional changes in pregnancy
- increased concern about labor

Deficient knowledge regarding self-care measures for

- posture and body mechanics
- rest and relaxation
- personal hygiene
- activity and exercise
- safety

Disturbed sleep pattern related to

- discomforts of late pregnancy
- anxiety about approaching labor

Planning

Prenatal care ideally is a multidisciplinary activity in which nurses work with physicians or midwives, nutritionists, social workers, and others. Collaboration among these individuals is necessary to provide holistic care that meets the needs of individual women.

Examples of expected outcomes of prenatal care include that the pregnant woman will achieve the following:

- Indicate decreased anxiety about the health of her fetus and herself
- Describe improved family dynamics
- Show appropriate weight gain patterns
- Report signs and symptoms of complications
- Describe appropriate measures taken to relieve physical discomforts
- Develop a realistic birth plan

Interventions

The nurse-patient relationship is critical in setting the tone for further interaction.

- Listen with an attentive expression, use touch, and maintain eye contact.
- Recognize the woman's feelings and her right to express these feelings.
- Be perceptive in identifying unvoiced needs; ask for a patient-generated solution and a subsequent report of its effectiveness.
- Teach for self-management (see text).
- Supportive care involves developing, augmenting, or changing the mechanisms used by women and their families in coping with stress.
- The woman must be a willing partner in a purely voluntary relationship. The relationship can be refused or terminated at any time by the pregnant woman or her family.

Evaluation

Evaluation of the effectiveness of care of the woman during pregnancy is based on the previously stated outcomes.

BOX 11-4 Centering Pregnancy Approach

In response to the call of the United States Public Health Service (1989) to develop new models of prenatal care, Rising (1998), a certified nurse-midwife, developed an innovative approach that emphasizes the assessment of risk, education, and support in a group setting using a holistic and comprehensive focus. In this centering pregnancy (CP) approach, women have over 20 contact hours with a health care provider during pregnancy and after delivery. Eight to 12 women are placed in gestational age cohort groups; group sessions begin at 12 to 16 weeks of gestation and end with an early postpartum meeting (Carlson & Lowe, 2006).

Before groups begin, each woman has an individual assessment, physical examination, and history. At the beginning of the group meeting women measure their own blood pressure, weigh themselves, test their own urine with dipsticks, and record the results. Fundal height and the fetal heart rate are assessed individually and privately. Individual follow-up is scheduled as needed (Carlson & Lowe, 2006).

Results assessing the effectiveness of this approach have been promising; in a study of adolescents, the incidence of low birth weight was reduced, and rates of breastfeeding were increased (Grady & Bloom, 2004). Other studies of CP are ongoing.

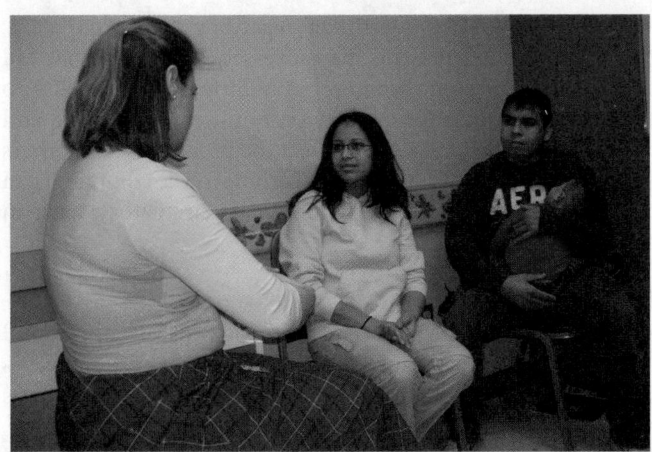

Fig. 11-6 Prenatal interview. *(Courtesy Dee Lowdermilk, Chapel Hill, NC.)*

included in the initial prenatal interview, and the observations and information about the woman's family form part of the database. For example, if the woman is accompanied by small children, the nurse can ask about her plans for child care during the time of labor and birth. Special needs are noted at this time (e.g., wheelchair access, assistance in getting on and off the examining table, and cognitive deficits).

Reason for Seeking Care

Although pregnant women are scheduled for "routine" prenatal visits, they often come to the health care provider seeking information or reassurance about a particular concern. When the woman is asked a broad, open-ended question such as "How have you been feeling?", she may reveal problems that could otherwise be overlooked. The woman's chief concerns should be recorded in her own words to alert other personnel to the priority of needs identified by her. At the initial visit a typical desire is for information about what is normal in the course of pregnancy.

Current Pregnancy

The presumptive signs of pregnancy may be of great concern to the woman. A review of symptoms she is experiencing and how she is coping with them helps establish a database to develop a plan of care. Some early teaching may be provided at this time.

Obstetric and Gynecologic History

Data are gathered on the woman's age at menarche; menstrual history; contraceptive history; the nature of any infertility or gynecologic conditions; history of any sexually transmitted infections (STIs); her sexual history; and a detailed history of all her pregnancies, including the present one, and their outcomes. The date of the last Papanicolaou test and the result are noted. The date of her LMP is obtained to establish the EDB.

Medical History

The medical history includes medical or surgical conditions that may affect the pregnancy or that may be affected by the pregnancy. For example, a pregnant woman who has diabetes or epilepsy requires special care. Because most women are anxious during the initial interview, the nurse's reference to cues such as a MedicAlert bracelet prompts the woman to explain allergies; chronic diseases; or medications being taken such as cortisone, insulin, or anticonvulsants.

The nature of previous surgical procedures should also be described. If a woman has had uterine surgery or extensive repair of the pelvic floor, a cesarean birth may be necessary; appendectomy rules out appendicitis as a cause of right lower quadrant pain in pregnancy; spinal surgery may contraindicate the use of spinal or epidural anesthesia; and breast augmentation or reduction procedures may influence the ability to breastfeed. Any injury involving the pelvis is noted.

Often women who have chronic or handicapping conditions forget to mention them during the initial assessment because they have adapted to them. Special shoes or a limp may indicate the existence of a pelvic structural defect, an important consideration in pregnant women. The nurse who observes these special characteristics and sensitively inquires about them can obtain individualized data that will provide the basis for a comprehensive nursing care plan. Observations are a vital component of the interview process because they prompt the nurse and the woman to focus on the specific needs of the woman and her family.

evolve Spanish Guidelines—Prenatal Interview

Nutritional History

The nutritional status of a pregnant woman has a direct effect on the growth and development of the fetus. A dietary assessment can reveal special diet practices, food allergies, eating behaviors, the practice of pica, and other factors related to her nutritional status (see Box 12-6). Pregnant women are usually motivated to learn about good nutrition and respond well to nutritional advice generated by this assessment. Cultural influences on diet and food selection should also be considered.

History of Use of Drugs and Herbal Preparations

A woman's past and present use of drugs, both legal (over-the-counter [OTC], prescription, and herbal drugs; caffeine; alcohol; nicotine) and illegal (marijuana, cocaine, heroin) must be assessed because many substances cross the placenta and can harm the developing fetus. Periodic urine toxicology screening tests are often recommended during pregnancy for women who have a history of illegal drug use. Results of such tests have been used for criminal prosecution, which results in a breach in the patient-provider relationship and in ethical responsibilities to the patient.

Nurses may have ethical concerns if pregnant women are not informed of the possibility of random urine testing for presence of drugs. The other side of this concern is the unborn child and whether the mother has a duty not to harm him or her. Today increased numbers of individuals are using herbal preparations, and this usage includes pregnant women. Therefore it is important for health care providers to question prenatal women regarding the use of herbal preparations and document the woman's responses.

LEGAL TIP Screening for Drug Use Hospitals must obtain informed consent from a pregnant woman before she can be tested for drug use (Kehringer, 2003).

Family History

The family history provides information about the woman's immediate family, including parents, siblings, and children. These data help identify familial or genetic disorders or conditions that could affect the present health status of the woman or her fetus.

Social, Experiential, and Occupational History

Situational factors such as the family's ethnic and cultural background and socioeconomic status are assessed while the history is obtained. The following information may be obtained over several encounters. The woman's perception of this pregnancy is explored by asking her such questions as the following: Is this pregnancy wanted or not, planned or not? Is the woman/couple pleased or displeased, accepting or nonaccepting? What problems related to finances, career, or living accommodations may arise as a result of the pregnancy? The family support system is determined by asking her such questions as the following: What primary support is available to her? Are changes needed to promote adequate support? What are the existing relationships among mother, father/partner, siblings, and in-laws? What preparations are being made for her care and that of dependent family members during labor and for the care of the infant after birth? Is financial, educational, or other support needed from the community? What are the woman's ideas about childbearing, her expectations of the infant's behavior, and her outlook on life and the female role?

Other questions that should be asked include the following: What does the woman think it will be like to have a baby in the home? How is her life going to change by having a baby? What plans are interrupted by having a baby at this time? During interviews throughout the pregnancy, the nurse should remain alert for the appearance of potential parenting problems such as depression, lack of family support, and inadequate living conditions. The nurse must assess the woman's attitude toward health care, particularly during childbearing; her expectations of health care providers; and her view of the relationship between herself and the nurse.

Coping mechanisms and patterns of interacting are identified. Early in the pregnancy the nurse should determine the woman's knowledge of pregnancy, maternal changes, fetal growth, self-management, and care of the newborn, including feeding. It is important to ask about attitudes toward unmedicated or medicated childbirth and about her knowledge of the availability of parenting skills classes. Before planning for nursing care, the nurse needs information about the woman's decision-making abilities and living habits (e.g., exercise, sleep, diet, diversional interests, personal hygiene, clothing). Common stressors during childbearing include the baby's welfare, the labor and birth process, the behaviors of the newborn, the relationship with the baby's father and her family, changes in body image, and physical symptoms.

Attitudes concerning the range of acceptable sexual behaviors during pregnancy are explored. Questions such as the following could be asked: What has your family (partner, friends) told you about sex during pregnancy? The woman's sexual self-concept is given emphasis by asking questions such as the following: How do you feel about the changes in your appearance? How does your partner feel about your body now? How do you feel about wearing maternity clothes?

Women should be questioned regarding their occupation, past and present, since this may adversely affect maternal and fetal health. For some women heavy lifting and exposure to chemicals and radiation may be part of their daily work, and these activities can negatively affect the pregnancy. For others long hours of sitting at a desk working on a computer can contribute to carpal tunnel syndrome or circulatory stasis in the legs.

History of Physical Abuse

All women should be assessed for a history or risk of physical abuse, particularly because the likelihood of abuse increases during pregnancy. Although visual cues from the woman's appearance or behavior may suggest the possibility of abuse, no one profile of the battered woman exists. Identification of abuse and immediate clinical intervention that includes information about safety can result in behavior that may prevent future abuse and increase the safety and well-being of the woman and her infant. During pregnancy the target body parts change during abusive episodes. Women report physical blows directed to the head, breasts, abdomen, and genitalia. Sexual assault is common.

Battering and pregnancy in teenagers constitutes a particularly difficult situation. Adolescents may be trapped in the abusive relationship because of their inexperience. Many professionals and the adolescents themselves ignore the violence because it may not be believable, because relationships are transient, and because the jealous and controlling behavior is interpreted as love and devotion. Routine screening for abuse and sexual assault is recommended for pregnant adolescents. Because pregnancy in young adolescent girls is commonly the result of sexual abuse, the nurse should assess the desire to maintain the pregnancy.

Review of Systems

During this portion of the interview the woman is asked to identify and describe preexisting or concurrent problems in any of the body systems, and her mental status is assessed. The woman is questioned about physical symptoms she has experienced such as shortness of breath or pain. Pregnancy affects and is affected by all body systems; therefore information on the present status of body systems is important in planning care. For each sign or symptom described, the following additional data should be obtained: body location, quality, quantity, chronology, aggravating or alleviating factors, and associated manifestations (onset, character, and course) (Seidel et al, 2006).

Physical Examination

The initial physical examination provides the baseline for assessing subsequent changes. The examiner should determine the woman's needs for basic information regarding reproductive anatomy and provide this information, along with a demonstration of the equipment that may be used during the examination and an explanation of the procedure itself. The interaction requires an unhurried, sensitive, and gentle approach with a matter-of-fact attitude.

The physical examination begins with assessment of vital signs, including blood pressure [BP], height, and weight (for calculation of body mass index [BMI]). The bladder should be

evolve Case Study—First Trimester

empty before pelvic examination. A urine specimen can be obtained to test for protein, glucose, or leukocytes or for other tests.

Each examiner develops a routine for proceeding with the physical examination; most choose the head-to-toe progression. Heart and lung sounds are evaluated, and extremities examined. The skin is assessed for changes in pigmentation, rashes, and edema. Distribution, amount, and quality of body hair are of particular importance because the findings reflect nutritional status, endocrine function, and attention to hygiene. The thyroid gland is assessed carefully, as are the breasts and abdomen. The height of the fundus is noted if the first examination occurs after the first trimester of pregnancy. During the examination the examiner must remain alert to the woman's cues that give direction to the remainder of the assessment and that indicate imminent untoward response such as supine hypotension (low BP that occurs while the woman is lying on her back, causing feelings of faintness). See Chapter 5 for a detailed description of the physical examination.

Whenever a pelvic examination is performed, the tone of the pelvic musculature and the woman's knowledge of Kegel exercises are assessed. Particular attention is paid to the size of the uterus because this is an indication of the duration of gestation. The nurse present during the examination can coach the woman at this time in breathing and relaxation techniques as needed. One vaginal examination during pregnancy is recommended; another is usually not done unless indicated for medical reasons.

Laboratory Tests

The data yielded by laboratory examination of specimens obtained during the examination add important information concerning the symptoms of pregnancy and the woman's health status.

Specimens are collected at the initial visit so that any abnormal findings can be treated. Blood is drawn for a variety of tests (Table 11-1). A sickle cell screen is recommended for women of African, Asian, or Middle Eastern descent. The folate level is measured when indicated. Testing for antibody to the human immunodeficiency virus (HIV) is strongly recommended for all pregnant women (Centers for Disease Control and Prevention, Workowski, & Berman, 2006) (Box 11-5). In addition, pregnant women and fathers with a family history of cystic fibrosis and of Caucasian ethnicity may elect to have blood drawn for testing to ascertain if they are a cystic fibrosis carrier (Fries, Bashford, & Nunes, 2006). Urine is tested for glucose (diabetes), protein (preeclampsia), and nitrites and leukocytes (urinary tract infection). Urine specimens are usually tested by dipstick. Culture and sensitivity tests are ordered as necessary. A purified protein derivative tuberculin test may be administered to assess exposure to tuberculosis. During the pelvic examination cervical and vaginal smears may be obtained for cytologic studies and diagnosis of infection (e.g., *Chlamydia*, gonorrhea, group B streptococcus).

The finding of risk factors during pregnancy may indicate the need to repeat some tests at other times. For example, exposure to tuberculosis or an STI would necessitate repeat testing. STIs are common in pregnancy and may have negative effects on mother and fetus. Careful assessment and thorough screening are essential.

Table 11-1 Laboratory Tests in Prenatal Period

LABORATORY TEST	PURPOSE
Hemoglobin, hematocrit/WBC, differential	Detects anemia/detects infection
Hemoglobin electrophoresis	Identifies women with hemoglobinopathies (e.g., sickle cell anemia, thalassemia)
Blood type, Rh, and irregular antibody	Identifies fetuses at risk for developing erythroblastosis fetalis or hyperbilirubinemia in neonatal period
Rubella titer	Determines immunity to rubella
Tuberculin skin testing; chest film after 20 wk of gestation in women with reactive tuberculin tests	Screens for exposure to tuberculosis
Urinalysis, including microscopic examination of urinary sediment; pH, specific gravity, color, glucose, albumin, protein, RBCs, WBCs, casts, acetone; hCG	Identifies women with unsuspected diabetes mellitus, renal disease, hypertensive disease of pregnancy; infection; occult hematuria
Urine culture	Identifies women with asymptomatic bacteriuria
Renal function tests: BUN, creatinine, electrolytes, creatinine clearance, total protein excretion	Evaluates level of possible renal compromise in women with a history of diabetes, hypertension, or renal disease
Papanicolaou test	Screens for cervical intraepithelial neoplasia, herpes simplex type 2, and HPV
Vaginal or rectal smear for *Neisseria gonorrhoeae*, *Chlamydia*, HPV, GBS	Screens high risk population for asymptomatic infection; GBS done at 35-37 wk
RPR/VDRL/FTA-ABS	Identifies women with untreated syphilis
HIV antibody,* hepatitis B surface antigen, toxoplasmosis	Screens for infection
1-hr glucose tolerance	Screens for gestational diabetes; done at initial visit for women with risk factors; done at 28 wk for all pregnant women
3-hr glucose tolerance	Screens for diabetes in women with elevated glucose level after 1-hr test; must have two elevated readings for diagnosis
Cardiac evaluation: ECG, chest x-ray film, and echocardiogram	Evaluates cardiac function in women with a history of hypertension or cardiac disease

BUN, Blood urea nitrogen; *ECG*, electrocardiogram; *FTA-ABS*, fluorescent treponemal antibody absorption test; *GBS*, group B streptococcus; *hCG*, human chorionic gonadotropin; *HIV*, human immunodeficiency virus; *HPV*, human papilloma virus; *RBC*, red blood cell; *RPR*, rapid plasma reagin; *VDRL*, Venereal Disease Research Laboratories; *WBC*, white blood cell.
*With patient permission.

evolve Spanish Guidelines—Prenatal Physical Examination

Follow-Up Visits

Monthly visits are scheduled routinely during the first and second trimesters, although additional appointments may be made as the need arises. However, during the third trimester the possibility for complications increases, and closer moni-

BOX 11-5 Human Immunodeficiency Virus Screening

Pregnant women are ethically obligated to seek reasonable care during pregnancy and to avoid causing harm to the fetus. Maternity nurses should be advocates for the fetus while accepting the pregnant woman's decision regarding testing and/or treatment for human immunodeficiency virus (HIV).

The incidence of perinatal transmission from an HIV-positive mother to her fetus ranges from 25% to 35%. Zidovudine decreases perinatal transmission and the risk of infant death. Elective cesarean birth significantly reduces the risk of transmission from the mother to child. Thus testing has the potential to identify HIV-positive women who can then be treated. Health care providers have an obligation to ensure that pregnant women are well informed about HIV symptoms, testing, and methods of decreasing maternal-fetal transmission. However, mandatory HIV screening involves ethical issues related to privacy invasion, discrimination, social stigma, and reproductive risks to the pregnant woman.

toring is warranted. Starting with week 28, visits are scheduled every 2 weeks until week 36 and then every week until birth unless the health care provider individualizes the schedule. Individual needs, complications, and risks of the pregnant woman may warrant visits more or less often. The pattern of interviewing the woman first and then assessing physical changes and performing laboratory tests is maintained.

Interview

Follow-up visits are less intensive than the initial prenatal visit. At each of these follow-up visits the woman is asked to summarize relevant events that have occurred since the previous visit. She is asked about her general emotional and physiologic well-being, complaints or problems, and questions she may have. Personal and family needs are identified and explored.

A woman's emotional state can affect her and her family's general well-being. Therefore the nurse asks whether the woman has had any mood swings, reactions to changes in her body image, bad dreams, or worries. Positive feelings (her own and those of her family) are also noted. The reactions of family members to the pregnancy and the woman's progression through the developmental tasks of pregnancy are also assessed and recorded.

During the third trimester current family situations and their effect on the woman are assessed (e.g., the response of partner, siblings, and grandparents to the pregnancy and the coming child). The nurse needs to assess the parents' understanding of the following: the warning signs that indicate emergencies such as bleeding and abdominal pain, the signs of preterm and term labor, the labor process and anxieties about labor, fetal development, and methods to assess fetal well-being. The nurse should ascertain whether the woman is planning to attend childbirth preparation classes and what she knows about the control of discomfort during labor. If she is having a home birth, she should be queried as to whether all the necessary supplies have been obtained.

A review of the woman's physical systems is appropriate at each visit, and any suggestive signs or symptoms are assessed in depth. Discomforts reflecting adaptations to pregnancy are identified. Special inquiries are made about possible infections (e.g., genitourinary tract, respiratory tract). The woman's knowledge of and success with self-management measures are assessed, as well as outcomes of prescribed therapy.

Physical Examination

Reevaluation is a constant aspect of a pregnant woman's care. Each woman reacts differently to pregnancy. As a result, careful monitoring of the pregnancy and her reactions to care is vital. Physiologic changes are documented as the pregnancy progresses and reviewed for possible deviations from normal progress.

At each visit physical parameters are measured. BP is taken at every visit using the same arm and with the woman seated. Her weight is measured, and the appropriateness of the weight gain is evaluated in relation to her BMI. Urine may be checked by dipstick. The presence and degree of edema are noted. For examination of the abdomen, the woman lies on her back with her arms by her side and head supported by a pillow. The bladder should be empty. Abdominal inspection is followed by measurement of the height of the fundus (Fig. 11-7). While the woman lies on her back, the nurse should be alert for the occurrence of supine hypotension (see Emergency box).

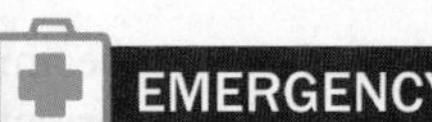

Supine Hypotension

Signs and Symptoms

Pallor
Dizziness, faintness, breathlessness
Tachycardia
Nausea
Clammy (damp, cool) skin; sweating

Intervention

Position woman on her side until her signs and symptoms subside and vital signs stabilize within normal limits.

The findings revealed during the interview and physical examination reflect the status of maternal adaptations. When any of the findings is suspicious, an in-depth examination is performed. For example, careful interpretation of BP is important in the risk factor analysis of all pregnant women. BP is evaluated on the basis of absolute values and the length of gestation and is interpreted in the light of modifying factors.

NURSING ALERT Individuals whose systolic BP (SBP) is 120 to 139 mm Hg or whose diastolic DBP (DBP) is 80 to 89 mm Hg should be viewed as prehypertensive. To prevent cardiovascular disease, they require health-promoting lifestyle modifications.

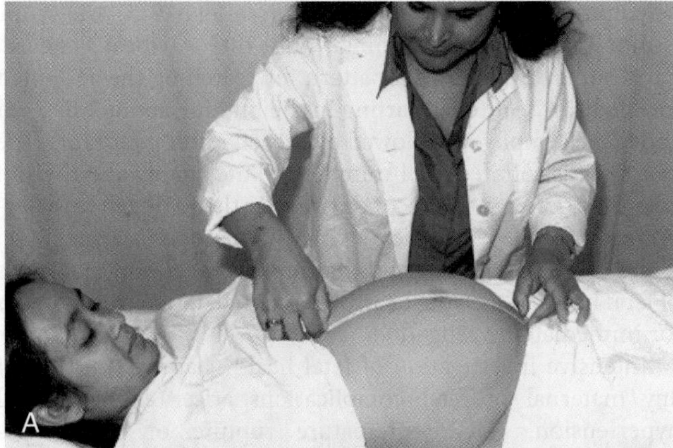

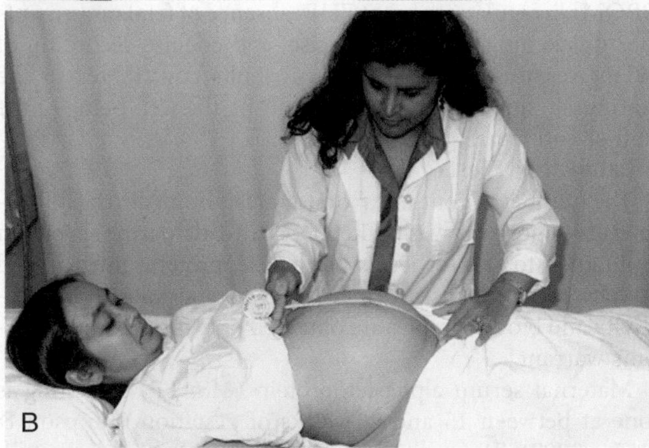

Fig. 11-7 Measurement of fundal height from symphysis that **A**, includes the upper curve of the fundus and **B**, does not include the upper curve of the fundus. Note position of hands and measuring tape. *(Courtesy Chris Rozales, San Francisco, CA.)*

An absolute SBP of 140 mm Hg or more and a DBP of 90 mm Hg or more suggest the presence of hypertension. An SBP of 125 mm Hg or more or a DBP of 75 mm Hg or more in midpregnancy or an SBP of 130 mm Hg or more or a DBP of 85 mm Hg or more in later pregnancy are indicative of problems and should be reported to the primary health care provider immediately.

A rise in SBP of 30 mm Hg or more over the baseline pressure or a rise in the DBP of 15 mm Hg over the baseline pressure is also a significant finding, regardless of the absolute values, and should be closely monitored. See Chapter 14 for an in-depth discussion of problems associated with hypertension.

The pregnant woman is monitored continuously for a range of signs and symptoms that indicate potential complications in addition to hypertension. For example, persistent and excessive vomiting and ketonuria may indicate the development of hyperemesis gravidarum. Uterine cramping and vaginal bleeding are signs of threatened miscarriage. Chills and fever are symptoms of infection. Discharge from the vagina may be amniotic fluid or associated with infection (Box 11-6).

BOX 11-6 Signs of Potential Complications During the First, Second, and Third Trimesters

First Trimester

Signs and Symptoms	Possible Causes
Severe vomiting	Hyperemesis gravidarum
Chills, fever	Infection
Burning on urination	Infection
Diarrhea	Infection
Abdominal cramping; vaginal bleeding	Miscarriage, ectopic pregnancy

Second and Third Trimesters

Signs and Symptoms	Possible Causes
Persistent, severe vomiting	Hyperemesis gravidarum, hypertension, preeclampsia
Sudden discharge of fluid from vagina before 37 weeks	Premature rupture of membranes
Vaginal bleeding, severe abdominal pain	Miscarriage, placenta previa, abruptio placentae
Chills, fever, burning on urination, diarrhea	Infection
Severe backache or flank pain	Kidney infection or stones; preterm labor
Change in fetal movements: absence of fetal movements after quickening, any unusual change in pattern or amount	Fetal jeopardy or intrauterine fetal death
Uterine contractions; pressure; cramping before 37 weeks	Preterm labor
Visual disturbances: blurring, double vision, or spots	Hypertensive conditions, preeclampsia
Swelling of face or fingers and over sacrum	Hypertensive conditions, preeclampsia
Headaches: severe, frequent, or continuous	Hypertensive conditions, preeclampsia
Muscular irritability or convulsions	Hypertensive conditions, preeclampsia
Epigastric or abdominal pain (perceived as severe stomachache)	Hypertensive conditions, preeclampsia, abruptio placentae
Glycosuria, positive glucose tolerance test reaction	Gestational diabetes mellitus

Fetal Assessment

Toward the end of the first trimester, before the uterus is an abdominal organ, the fetal heart tones (FHTs) can be heard with an ultrasound fetoscope or an ultrasound stethoscope. To hear the FHTs, place the instrument in the midline just above the symphysis pubis and apply firm pressure. The woman and her family should be offered the opportunity to listen to the FHTs. The health status of the fetus is assessed at each visit for the remainder of the pregnancy.

Fundal Height

During the second trimester the uterus becomes an abdominal organ. The fundal height, or measurement of the height of the uterus above the symphysis pubis, is used as one indicator of fetal growth. The measurement also provides a gross estimate of the duration of pregnancy. During the second and third trimesters (weeks 18 to 30) the height of the fundus in centimeters is approximately the same as the number of weeks of gestation if the woman's bladder is empty at the time of

evolve Assessment Video

measurement (Cunningham et al, 2005). Measurement of fundal height may aid in the identification of high risk factors. A stable or decreased fundal height may indicate the presence of intrauterine growth restriction (IUGR); an excessive increase could indicate the presence of multifetal gestation (more than one fetus) or hydramnios.

A paper tape is typically used to measure fundal height. To increase the reliability of the measurement, the same person examines the pregnant woman at each of her prenatal visits; often this is not possible. All clinicians who examine a particular pregnant woman should be consistent in their measurement technique. Ideally a protocol should be established for the setting in which the measurement technique is explicitly set forth; and the woman's position on the examining table, the measuring device, and method of measurement used are specified. Fig. 11-7 presents two methods of measuring fundal height.

Gestational Age

In an uncomplicated pregnancy fetal gestational age is estimated after the duration of pregnancy and the EDB are determined. Fetal gestational age is determined from the menstrual history, contraceptive history, pregnancy test results, and the following findings obtained from the clinical evaluation:

- First uterine evaluation: date, size
- Fetal heart first heard: date, method (Doppler stethoscope, fetoscope)
- Date of quickening
- Current fundal height, estimated fetal weight
- Current week of gestation by history of LMP or ultrasound examination (or both)
- Ultrasound examination: date, week of gestation, biparietal diameter
- Reliability of dates

Quickening ("feeling life") refers to the mother's first perception of fetal movement. It usually occurs between weeks 16 and 20 of gestation and is initially experienced as a fluttering sensation. The mother's report should be recorded. Multiparas often perceive fetal movement earlier than primigravidas.

Routine use of ultrasound examination (also called a sonogram) in early pregnancy has been recommended, and many health care providers have this equipment available in the office. This procedure may be used to establish the duration of pregnancy if the woman cannot give a precise date for her LMP or if the size of the uterus does not conform to the EDB as calculated by Nägele's rule. Ultrasound also provides information about the well-being of the fetus. However, the routine use of ultrasound has not been found to substantively improve fetal outcome.

Health Status

The assessment of fetal health status includes consideration of fetal movement. The mother is instructed to note the extent and timing of fetal movements and report immediately if the pattern changes or movement ceases. Regular movement has been found to be a reliable indicator of fetal health (Cunningham et al, 2005).

The fetal heart rate (FHR) is checked on routine visits once it has been heard (Fig. 11-8). Early in the second trimester the heartbeat may be heard with the Doppler stethoscope (see Fig. 11-8, *B*). To detect the heartbeat before the fetal position can be palpated by Leopold maneuvers (see Fig. 18-5), the scope is moved around the abdomen until the heartbeat is heard. Each nurse develops a set pattern for searching the abdomen for the heartbeat (e.g., starting in the midline about 2 to 3 cm above the symphysis, followed by the left lower quadrant). The heartbeat is counted for 1 minute, and the quality and rhythm are noted. Later in the second trimester the FHR can be determined with the fetoscope or Pinard fetoscope (see Fig. 11-8, *A* and *C*). A normal rate and rhythm are other good indicators of fetal health. Once the heartbeat is noted, its absence is cause for immediate investigation.

Intensive investigation of fetal health status is initiated if any maternal or fetal complications arise (e.g., maternal hypertension, IUGR, premature rupture of membranes [PROM], irregular or absent FHR, absence of fetal movements after quickening). Careful, precise, and concise recording of patient responses and laboratory results contributes to the continuous supervision vital to ensuring the well-being of the mother and fetus.

Laboratory Tests

The number of routine laboratory tests done during follow-up visits in pregnancy is limited. A clean-catch urine specimen is obtained to test for levels of glucose, protein, nitrites, and leukocytes at each visit. Urine specimens for culture and sensitivity and blood samples are obtained only if signs and symptoms warrant.

Maternal serum alpha-fetoprotein (MSAFP) screening is done at between 15 and 20 weeks of gestation (Simpson & Otaño, 2007). The multiple marker test, or triple screen test, is used to detect Down syndrome and other chromosome abnormalities. Done between 16 and 18 weeks of gestation, it measures MSAFP, human chorionic gonadotropin, and unconjugated estriol (Gilbert, 2007). Combining these three markers with maternal age allows a high detection rate for Down syndrome. High levels are associated with neural tube defects, and abnormally low levels may be associated with Down syndrome or other trisomies (Gilbert, 2007).

Other blood tests are repeated as necessary.

Other Tests

Other diagnostic tests are available to assess the health status of both the pregnant woman and the fetus. For example, ultrasonography may be performed to determine the status of the pregnancy and to confirm gestational age of the fetus. Fetal nuchal translucency screening uses ultrasound measurement of fluid in the nape of the fetal neck between 10 and 14 weeks of gestation to identify possible fetal abnormalities (see Fig. 9-6). Chorionic villus sampling or amniocentesis may be needed to evaluate the fetus for genetic disorders or gestational maturity. These and other tests used to determine health risks for the mother and infant are described in Chapters 9 and 17.

Nursing Care

Because of the large number of health care professionals involved in care of the expectant mother, unintentional gaps or overlaps in care may occur. To better coordinate prenatal care services for childbearing families, a care path can be used to improve consistency of care and reduce costs. It can also guide health care providers in carrying out the appropriate

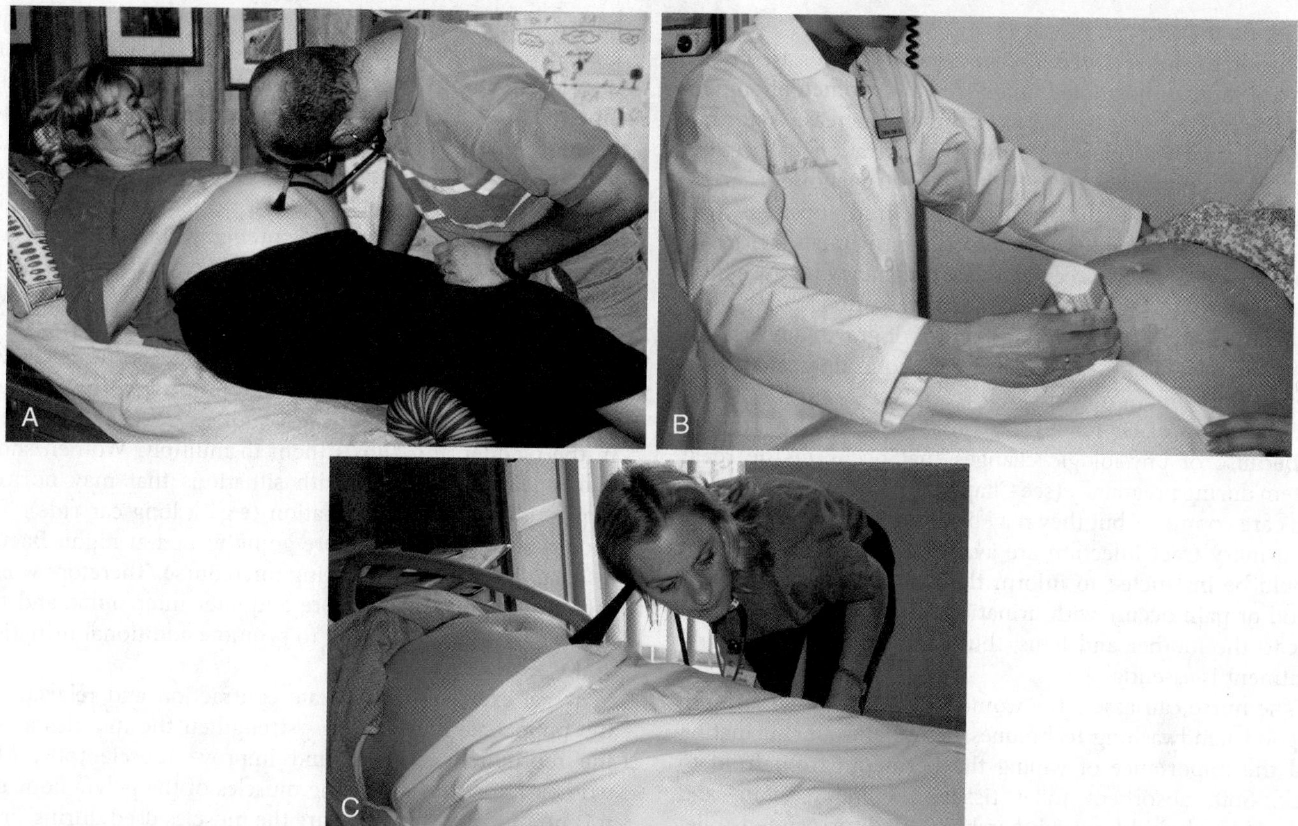

Fig. 11-8 Detecting fetal heartbeat. A, Father can listen to the fetal heart with a fetoscope (first detectable at 18 to 20 weeks with a fetoscope). B, Doppler ultrasound stethoscope (fetal heartbeat detectable at 12 weeks). C, Pinard's stethoscope. NOTE: Hands should not touch stethoscope while nurse is listening. *(A, Courtesy Shannon Perry, Phoenix, AZ. B, Courtesy Dee Lowdermilk, Chapel Hill, NC. C, Courtesy Julie Perry Nelson, Loveland, CO.)*

assessments and interventions in a timely way. Use of care paths also can contribute to improved satisfaction of families with the prenatal care provided, and members of the health care team may function more efficiently and effectively.

Education About Maternal and Fetal Changes

Expectant parents typically are curious about the growth and development of the fetus and the consequent changes that occur in the mother's body. Mothers may be more tolerant of the discomforts related to the continuing pregnancy if they understand the underlying causes. Educational literature (electronic and written materials) that describes fetal and maternal changes is available and can be used to explain changes as they occur. To be most effective the material must reflect the pregnant woman's or couple's ethnicity, culture, and literacy level and the agency's resources.

Education for Self-Management

The expectant mother needs information on many topics. The nurse who is observant, listens, and knows typical concerns of expectant parents can anticipate what questions will be asked and prompt mothers and their partners to discuss what is on their minds. Printed literature can be given to supplement the individualized teaching the nurse provides, and women often avidly read books and pamphlets related to their own experience. When nurses read the literature before they distribute it, they have an opportunity to point out areas that may not correspond with local health care practices. It is important to include family members in health education. As more individuals use the computer for information, the pregnant woman or couple may have questions from their Internet reviews. Nurses can share recommended electronic sites from reliable sources.

Patients who receive conflicting advice or instruction are likely to grow increasingly frustrated with members of the health care team and the care provided. Several topics that may cause concern in pregnant women are discussed in the following sections.

Nutrition

Good nutrition is important in the maintenance of maternal health during pregnancy and in the provision of adequate nutrients for embryonic and fetal development. Assessing a woman's nutritional status and weight gain and providing information on nutrition are part of the nurse's responsibilities in providing prenatal care. Teaching may include discussion about foods high in iron, encouragement to take prenatal vitamins, and recommendations to limit caffeine intake. In some settings a registered dietitian conducts classes for pregnant women on the topics of nutritional status and nutrition during pregnancy or interviews them to assess their knowledge of these topics. Nurses can refer women to a registered dietitian if a need is revealed during the nursing assessment. (For detailed information concerning maternal and fetal nutritional needs and related nursing care, see Chapter 12.)

Personal Hygiene

During pregnancy the sebaceous (sweat) glands are highly active because of hormonal influences, and women often perspire freely. They may be reassured that the increase is normal and that their previous patterns of perspiration will return after the postpartum period. Baths and warm showers can be therapeutic because they relax tense, tired muscles; help counter insomnia; and make the pregnant woman feel fresh. Tub bathing is permitted even in late pregnancy because little water enters the vagina unless under pressure. However, late in pregnancy, when the woman's center of gravity lowers, she is at risk for falling. Tub bathing is contraindicated after rupture of the membranes.

Prevention of Urinary Tract Infection

Because of physiologic changes that occur in the renal system during pregnancy (see Chapter 10), urinary tract infections are common, but they may be asymptomatic. OTC tests for urinary tract infection are available (Fig. 11-9). Women should be instructed to inform their health care provider if blood or pain occurs with urination. These infections pose a risk to the mother and fetus; thus their prevention or early treatment is essential.

The nurse can assess the woman's understanding and use of good handwashing techniques before and after urinating and the importance of wiping the perineum from front to back. Soft, absorbent toilet tissue, preferably white and unscented, should be used; harsh, scented, or printed toilet paper may cause irritation. Bubble bath or other bath oils should be avoided because these can irritate the urethra. Women should wear underpants and panty hose with a cotton crotch and avoid wearing tight-fitting slacks or jeans for long periods. Anything that allows a buildup of heat and moisture in the genital area can foster the growth of bacteria.

Some women do not consume enough fluid and food. After ascertaining the woman's food preferences, the nurse should advise the woman to drink at least 2 L (eight glasses) of liquid a day to maintain an adequate fluid intake that ensures frequent urination. Pregnant women should not limit fluids in an effort to reduce the frequency of urination. Women need to know that, if urine looks dark (concentrated), they must increase their fluid intake. The consumption of yogurt and acidophilus milk can help prevent urinary tract and vaginal infections. Although drinking cranberry juice is often recommended, there is conflicting evidence regarding its effectiveness and, in particular, the effective dose needed to prevent urinary tract infections.

The nurse should review healthy urination practices with the woman. Women should be told not to ignore the urge to urinate because holding urine lengthens the time bacteria are in the bladder and allows them to multiply. Women should plan ahead when faced with situations that may normally require them to delay urination (e.g., a long car ride). They should always urinate before going to bed at night. Bacteria also can be introduced during intercourse. Therefore women are advised to urinate before and after intercourse and then drink a large glass of water to promote additional urination.

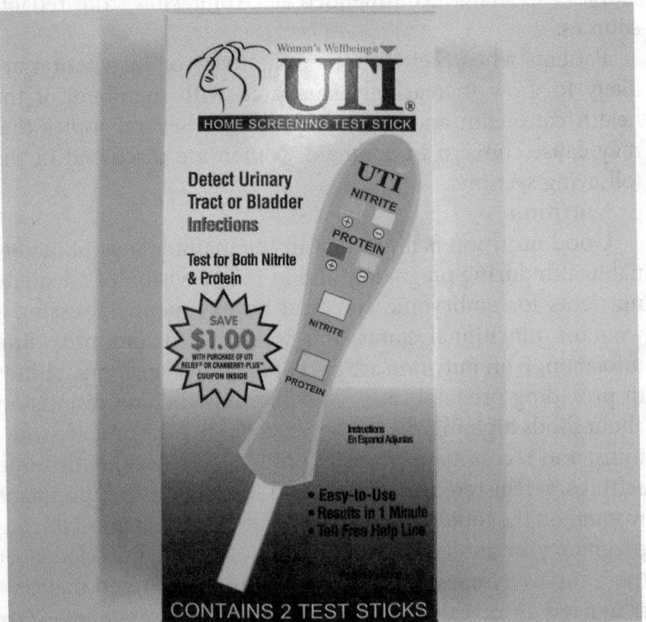

Fig. 11-9 Over-the-counter urinary tract infection detection kit. *(Courtesy Julie Perry Nelson, Loveland, CO.)*

Kegel Exercises

Kegel exercises—deliberate contraction and relaxation of the pubococcygeus muscle—strengthen the muscles around the reproductive organs and improve muscle tone. Many women are not aware of the muscles of the pelvic floor until it is pointed out that these are the muscles used during urination and sexual intercourse and that they can be consciously controlled. The pelvic floor muscles encircle the vaginal outlet, and they need to be exercised. An exercised muscle can stretch and contract readily at birth. Practice of pelvic muscle exercise during pregnancy also results in fewer complaints of urinary incontinence in late pregnancy and postpartum (see Patient Teaching box, p. 53).

Preparation for Breastfeeding the Newborn

Pregnant women are usually eager to discuss their plans for feeding the newborn. Breast milk is the food of choice, in part because breastfeeding is associated with a decreased incidence in perinatal morbidity and mortality. The American Academy of Pediatrics recommends breastfeeding for at least 1 year. However, a deep-seated aversion to breastfeeding by the mother or partner, the mother's need for certain medications, and certain medical complications such as active tuberculosis and newly diagnosed breast cancer are contraindications to breastfeeding. Although hepatitis B antigen has not been shown to be transmitted through breast milk, as an added precaution it is recommended that infants born to hepatitis B antigen–positive women receive hepatitis B vaccine and hepatitis B immune globulin immediately after birth. Nursing is discouraged in women who are HIV positive because of the risk of HIV transmission (Lawrence & Lawrence, 2005).

A woman's decision about the method of infant feeding is made before pregnancy; thus it is essential to educate women of childbearing age about the benefits of breastfeeding. The woman and her partner are encouraged to decide what method of feeding is suitable for them; however, the benefits of breastfeeding should be emphasized. Once the couple has been given information about the advantages and disadvantages of breastfeeding and bottle-feeding, they can make an informed

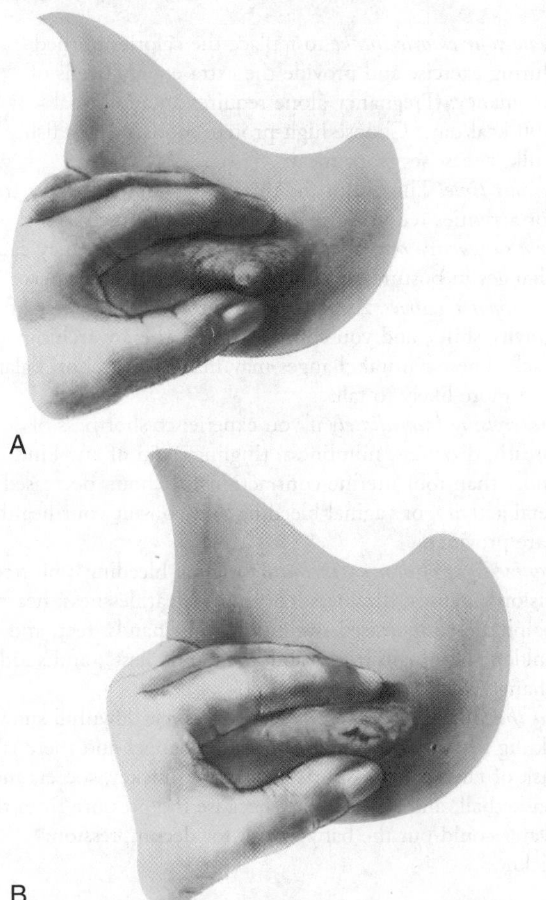

Fig. 11-10 Pinch test. **A,** Normal nipple everts with gentle pressure. **B,** Inverted nipple inverts with gentle pressure. (Modified from Lawrence RA, Lawrence RM: *Breastfeeding: a guide for the medical profession*, ed 5, St Louis, 2005, Mosby.)

choice. Health care providers support these decisions and provide any needed assistance.

Women with inverted nipples need special consideration if they are planning to breastfeed. The pinch test is done to determine whether the nipple is everted or inverted (Fig. 11-10). To perform the pinch test, the woman places her thumb and forefinger on her areola and presses inward gently. This action will cause her nipple either to stand erect or to invert. Most nipples will stand erect.

Exercises to break the adhesions that cause the nipple to invert do not work and may in fact cause uterine contractions (Lawrence & Lawrence, 2005). The use of breast shells, small plastic devices that fit over the nipple, by women with flat or inverted nipples is sometimes recommended (Fig. 11-11). Breast shells exert a continuous, gentle pressure around the areola that pushes the nipple through a central opening in the inner shield. Breast shells should be worn for 1 to 2 hours daily during the last trimester of pregnancy. Breast stimulation is contraindicated in women at risk for preterm labor; therefore the decision to suggest the use of breast shells to women with flat or inverted nipples must be made judiciously.

The woman is taught to cleanse the nipples with warm water to prevent blocking of the ducts with dried colostrum. Soap, ointments, alcohol, and tinctures should not be applied

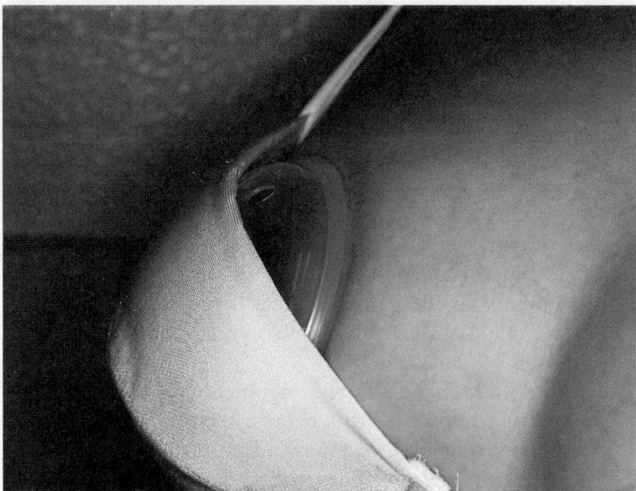

Fig. 11-11 Breast shell in place inside bra to evert nipple. *(Courtesy Michael S. Clement, MD, Mesa, AZ.)*

because they remove protective oils that keep nipples supple. The use of these substances may cause the nipple to crack during early lactation (Lawrence & Lawrence, 2005).

The woman who plans to breastfeed should purchase a nursing bra that will accommodate her increased breast size during the last few months of pregnancy and during lactation. If her breasts are very heavy or if the woman feels uncomfortable with the weight unsupported, the bra can be worn day and night.

Dental Health

Dental care during pregnancy is especially important because nausea during pregnancy may lead to poor oral hygiene and allow dental caries to develop. Fluoride toothpaste should be used daily. Inflammation and infection of the gingival and periodontal tissues may occur. There is some evidence linking periodontal infections and preterm birth, LBW (Lopez, 2005), and an increased risk for preeclampsia (Boggess et al, 2003).

Because calcium and phosphorus in the teeth are fixed in enamel, the old adage "for every child a tooth" is not true. There is no scientific evidence indicating that filling teeth or even dental extraction using local or nitrous oxide–oxygen anesthesia causes miscarriage or premature labor. However, antibacterial therapy should be considered for sepsis, especially in pregnant women who have had rheumatic heart disease or nephritis. Emergency dental surgery is not contraindicated during pregnancy; however, the risks and benefits of surgery need to be explained to the mother. If dental treatment is necessary, the woman will be most comfortable during the second trimester.

Physical Activity

Physical activity promotes a feeling of well-being in the pregnant woman. It improves circulation, promotes relaxation and rest, and counteracts boredom, as it does in the nonpregnant woman. Detailed exercise tips for pregnancy are presented in the Home Care box.

Exercises that help relieve the low back pain that often arises during the second trimester because of the increased weight of the fetus are demonstrated in Fig. 11-12.

HOME CARE

Exercise Tips for Pregnant Women

Consult your health care provider when you know or suspect that you are pregnant. Discuss your medical and obstetric history, your current exercise regimen, and the exercises you would like to continue throughout pregnancy.

Seek help in determining an exercise routine that is well within your limit of tolerance, especially if you have not been exercising regularly.

Consider decreasing weight-bearing exercises (jogging, running) and concentrating on non–weight bearing activities such as swimming, cycling, or stretching. If you are a runner, starting in your seventh month you may wish to walk instead.

Avoid risky activities such as surfing, mountain climbing, skydiving, and racquetball because such activities that require precise balance and coordination may be dangerous. Avoid activities that require holding your breath and bearing down (Valsalva maneuver). Jerky, bouncy motions also should be avoided.

Exercise regularly at least three times a week, as long as you are healthy, to improve muscle tone and increase or maintain your stamina. If you exercise sporadically, this may put undue strain on your muscles. Limit activity to shorter intervals. Exercise for 10 to 15 minutes, rest for 2 to 3 minutes, and then exercise for another 10 to 15 minutes.

Decrease your exercise level as your pregnancy progresses. The normal alterations of advancing pregnancy such as decreased cardiac reserve and increased respiratory effort may produce physiologic stress if you exercise strenuously for a long time.

Take your pulse every 10 to 15 minutes while you are exercising. If it is more than 140 beats/min, slow down until it returns to a maximum of 90 beats/min. You should be able to converse easily while exercising. If you cannot, you need to slow down.

Avoid becoming overheated for extended periods of time. It is best not to exercise for more than 35 minutes, especially in hot, humid weather. As your body temperature rises, the heat is transmitted to your fetus. Prolonged or repeated elevation of fetal temperature may result in birth defects, especially during the first 3 months. Your temperature should not exceed 38° C.

Do not use hot tubs and saunas.

Perform warm-up and stretching exercises to prepare your joints for more strenuous exercise and lessen the likelihood of strain or injury to your joints. After the fourth month of gestation you should not perform exercises flat on your back.

Include a cool-down period of mild activity involving your legs after an exercise period to help bring your respiration, heart, and metabolic rates back to normal and prevent the pooling of blood in the exercised muscles.

Rest for 10 minutes after exercising, lying on your side. As the uterus grows, it puts pressure on a major vein in your abdomen, which carries blood to your heart. Lying on your side removes the pressure and promotes return circulation from your extremities and muscles to your heart, thereby increasing blood flow to your placenta and fetus. You should rise gradually from the floor to prevent dizziness or fainting (orthostatic hypotension).

Drink two or three 8-oz glasses of water after you exercise to replace the body fluids lost through perspiration. While exercising, drink water whenever you feel the need.

Increase your caloric intake to replace the calories burned during exercise and provide the extra energy needs of pregnancy. (Pregnancy alone requires an additional 300 kcal/day.) Choose high-protein foods such as fish, milk, cheese, eggs, or meat.

Take your time. This is not the time to be competitive or train for activities requiring speed or long endurance.

Wear a supportive bra. Your increased breast weight may cause changes in posture and put pressure on the ulnar nerve.

Wear supportive shoes. As your uterus grows, your center of gravity shifts, and you compensate for this by arching your back. These natural changes may make you feel off balance and more likely to fall.

Stop exercising immediately if you experience shortness of breath, dizziness, numbness, tingling, pain of any kind, more than four uterine contractions per hour, decreased fetal activity, or vaginal bleeding and consult your health care provider.

Recognize signs of danger, including vaginal bleeding*; blurred vision*; nausea; dizziness; fainting*; breathlessness; heart palpitations; increased swelling in your hands, feet, and ankles; sharp pain in the abdomen and chest*; and sudden change in body temperature.

Avoid the following exercises during pregnancy: downhill snow skiing because the center of gravity changes and there is risk of falls; contact sports such as ice hockey, soccer, and basketball; and scuba diving because the pressure from the water could put the baby at risk for decompression sickness.

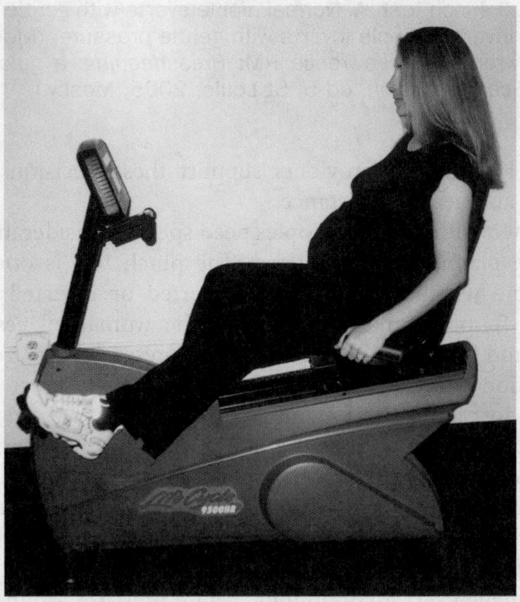

Riding a recumbent bicycle provides exercise while supplying back support. *(Courtesy Shannon Perry, Phoenix, AZ.)*

*If you experience any of these signs, contact your physician or midwife immediately.

Source: ACOG: *Exercise during pregnancy, ACOG Education Pamphlet*, 2003; *Exercises recommended throughout pregnancy*. Available at www.babycenter.com.au/pregnancy/fitness/recommendedexercises (accessed August 3, 2008); *Exercise during pregnancy: signs of danger*. Available at www.babycenter.com.au/pregnancy/fitnes/dangersigns (accessed August 3, 2008); *Fitness and exercise in pregnancy*. Available at www.babycenter.com.au/pregnancy/fitness (accessed August 3, 2008).

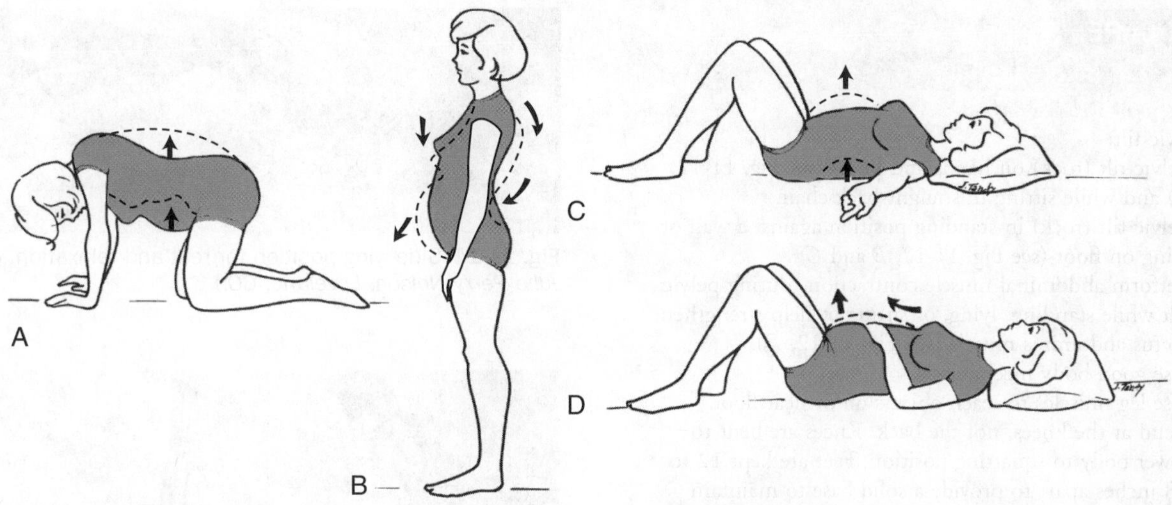

Fig. 11-12 Exercises. A to C, Pelvic rocking relieves low backache (excellent for relief of menstrual cramps as well); D, Abdominal breathing aids relaxation and lifts abdominal wall off uterus.

Posture and Body Mechanics

Skeletal, musculature, and hormonal changes (relaxin) in pregnancy can predispose the woman to backache and possible injury. As pregnancy progresses, the pregnant woman's center of gravity changes, pelvic joints soften and relax, and stress is placed on abdominal musculature. Poor posture and body mechanics contribute to the discomfort and potential for injury (see Patient Teaching box). To minimize these problems, women can learn good body posture and body mechanics (Fig. 11-13; see Fig. 10-13). The activities described in the Home Care box (p. 250) can also promote greater physical comfort.

PATIENT TEACHING Safety During Pregnancy

Changes in the body caused by pregnancy include relaxation of joints, alteration to center of gravity, faintness, and discomforts. Problems with coordination and balance are common. Therefore the woman should follow these guidelines:

- Use good body mechanics.
- Use safety features on tools/vehicles (safety seat belts, shoulder harnesses, headrests, goggles, helmets) as specified.
- Avoid activities requiring coordination, balance, and concentration.
- Take rest periods; reschedule daily activities to meet rest and relaxation needs.

Embryonic and fetal development are vulnerable to environmental teratogens. Many potentially dangerous chemicals are present in the home, yard, and workplace: cleaning agents, paints, sprays, herbicides, and pesticides. The soil and water supply may be unsafe. Therefore the woman should follow these guidelines:

- Read all labels for ingredients and proper use of product.
- Ensure adequate ventilation with clean air.
- Dispose of wastes appropriately.
- Wear gloves when handling chemicals.
- Change job assignments or workplace as necessary.
- Avoid high altitudes (not in pressurized aircraft), which could jeopardize oxygen intake.

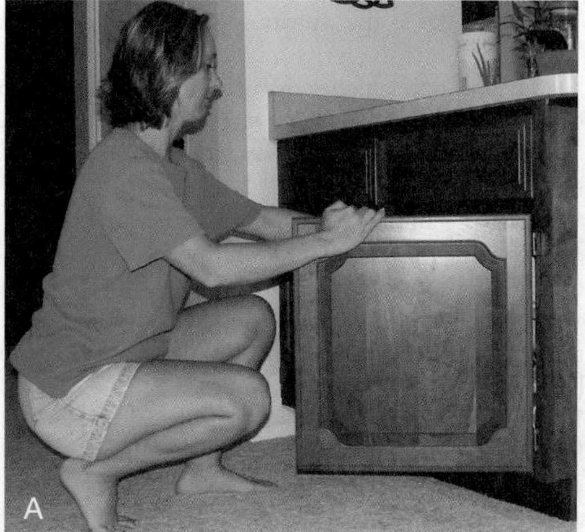

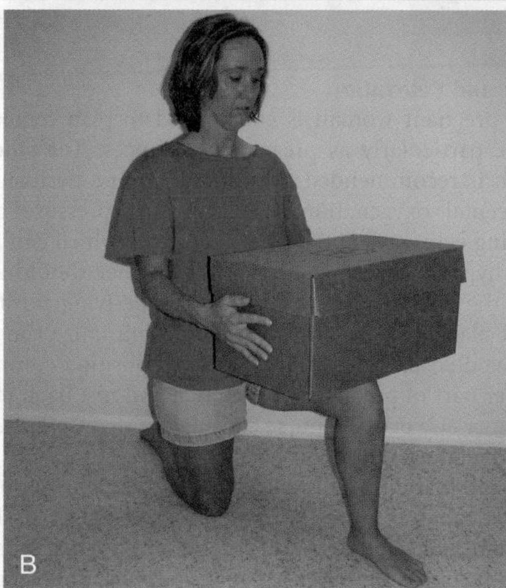

Fig. 11-13 Correct body mechanics. A, Squatting. B, Lifting. *(Courtesy Julie Perry Nelson, Loveland, CO.)*

HOME CARE

Posture and Body Mechanics

To Prevent or Relieve Backache

Do pelvic tilt:

- Pelvic tilt (rock) on hands and knees (see Fig. 11-12, *A*) and while sitting in straight-back chair.
- Pelvic tilt (rock) in standing position against a wall or lying on floor (see Fig. 11-12, *B* and *C*).
- Perform abdominal muscle contractions during pelvic tilt while standing, lying, or sitting to help strengthen rectus abdominis muscle (see Fig. 11-12, *D*).
- Use good body mechanics.
- Use leg muscles to reach objects on or near floor. Bend at the knees, not the back. Knees are bent to lower body to squatting position. Feet are kept 12 to 18 inches apart to provide a solid base to maintain balance (see Fig. 11-13, *A*).
- Lift with the legs. To lift a heavy object (e.g., young child), one foot is placed slightly in front of the other and kept flat as the woman lowers herself onto one knee. She lifts the weight, holding it close to her body and never higher than the chest. To stand up or sit down, one leg is placed slightly behind the other as she raises or lowers herself (see Fig. 11-13, *B*).

To Restrict the Lumbar Curve

For prolonged standing (e.g., ironing or because of employment), place one foot on low footstool or box; change positions often.

Move car seat forward so that knees are bent and higher than hips. If needed, use a small pillow to support low back area.

Sit in chairs low enough to allow both feet to be placed on floor, preferably with knees higher than hips.

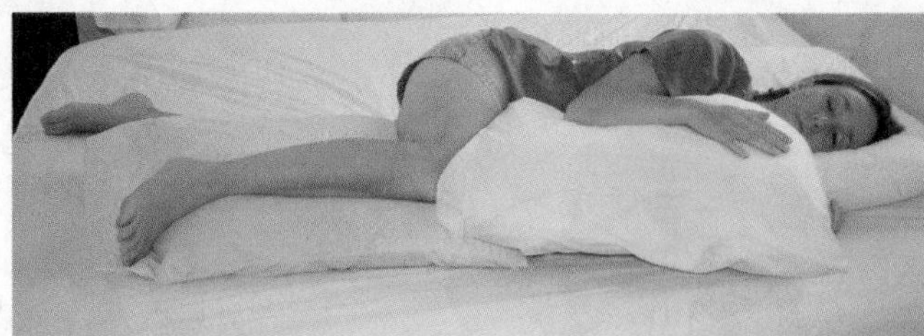

Fig. 11-14 Side-lying position for rest and relaxation. *(Courtesy Julie Perry Nelson, Loveland, CO.)*

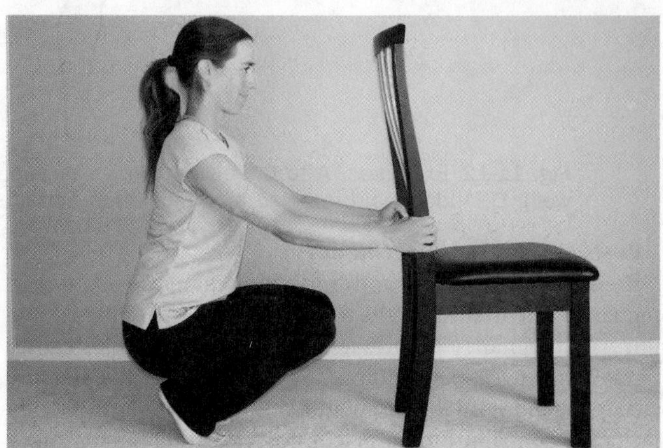

Fig. 11-15 Squatting for muscle relaxation and strengthening and for keeping leg and hip joints flexible. *(Courtesy Julie Perry Nelson, Loveland, CO.)*

Rest and Relaxation

The pregnant woman is encouraged to plan regular rest periods, particularly as pregnancy advances. The side-lying position is recommended to promote uterine perfusion and fetoplacental oxygenation by eliminating pressure on the ascending vena cava and descending aorta, which can lead to supine hypotension (Fig. 11-14). The mother should also be shown the way to rise slowly from a side-lying position to prevent placing strain on the back and minimize the orthostatic hypotension caused by changes in position common in the latter part of pregnancy. To stretch and rest back muscles at home or at work, the nurse can suggest that the woman do the following exercises:

- While standing behind a chair, the woman supports and balances herself using the back of the chair (Fig. 11-15). She squats for 30 seconds and then stands for 15 seconds. She should repeat six times, in several sets per day, as needed.
- While sitting in a chair, the woman lowers her head to her knees for 30 seconds and then raises her head. She should repeat six times, several times per day, as needed.

Conscious relaxation is the process of releasing tension from the mind and body through deliberate effort and practice. The ability to relax consciously and intentionally can be beneficial for the following reasons:

- To relieve the normal discomforts related to pregnancy
- To reduce stress and diminish pain perception during the childbearing cycle
- To heighten self-awareness and trust in one's own ability to control responses and functions
- To help cope with stress in everyday life situations, whether the woman is pregnant or not

The techniques for conscious relaxation are numerous and varied. The guidelines given in Box 11-7 can be used by anyone.

Employment

Employment of pregnant women usually has no adverse effects on pregnancy outcomes. Job discrimination that is based solely on pregnancy is illegal. However, some job environments pose potential risk to the fetus (e.g., dry cleaning plants, chemical laboratories, and parking garages). Excessive fatigue is usually the deciding factor in the termination of employment. Strategies to improve safety during pregnancy are described in the Patient Teaching box on p. 249.

Women in sedentary jobs need to walk around at intervals to counter the sluggish circulation in the legs. They should neither sit nor stand in one position for long periods. They should avoid crossing their legs at the knees because all of these activities can foster the development of varices and

BOX 11-7 Conscious Relaxation Tips

Preparation—Loosen clothing, assume a comfortable sitting or side-lying position with all parts of body well supported with pillows. The use of soothing music is optional.

Beginning—Allow self to feel warm and comfortable. Inhale and exhale slowly and imagine peaceful relaxation coming over each part of the body, starting with the neck and working down to the toes. People who learn conscious relaxation often speak of feeling relaxed even if some discomfort is present.

Maintenance—Use imagery (fantasy or daydream) to maintain the state of relaxation. Using *active imagery*, imagine yourself moving or doing some activity and experiencing its sensations. Using *passive imagery*, imagine yourself watching a scene such as a lovely sunset.

Awakening—Return to the wakeful state gradually. Slowly begin to take in stimuli from the surrounding environment.

Further retention and development of the skill—Practice regularly for some periods each day (e.g., at the same hour for 10 to 15 minutes each day to feel refreshed, revitalized, and invigorated).

thrombophlebitis. Standing for long periods also increases the risk of preterm labor. The pregnant woman's chair should provide adequate back support. Use of a footstool can prevent pressure on veins, relieve strain on varicosities, minimize swelling of feet, and prevent backache.

Clothing

Some women continue to wear their usual clothes during pregnancy as long as they fit and feel comfortable. If maternity clothing is needed, outfits may be purchased new or found in good condition at thrift shops or garage sales. Comfortable, loose clothing is best. Tight bras and belts, stretch pants, garters, tight-top knee socks, body shapers, and other constrictive clothing should be avoided because tight clothing over the perineum encourages vaginitis and miliaria (heat rash) and impaired circulation in the legs can cause varicosities.

Maternity bras are constructed to accommodate the increased breast weight, chest circumference, and size of breast tail tissue (under the arm). These bras have drop-flaps over the nipples to facilitate breastfeeding. A good bra can help prevent neck ache and backache.

Maternity support hose give considerable comfort and promote greater venous emptying in women with large varicose veins. Ideally support stockings should be put on before the woman gets out of bed in the morning. Figure 11-16 demonstrates a position to rest the legs and reduce swelling.

Comfortable shoes that provide firm support and promote good posture and balance are advisable. Very high heels and platform shoes are not recommended because of the woman's changed center of gravity, which can cause her to lose her balance. In addition, the woman's pelvis tilts forward in the third trimester, increasing her lumbar curve. The resulting leg aches and cramps will be aggravated by shoes that do not provide good support. Figure 11-17 shows exercises to relieve leg cramps.

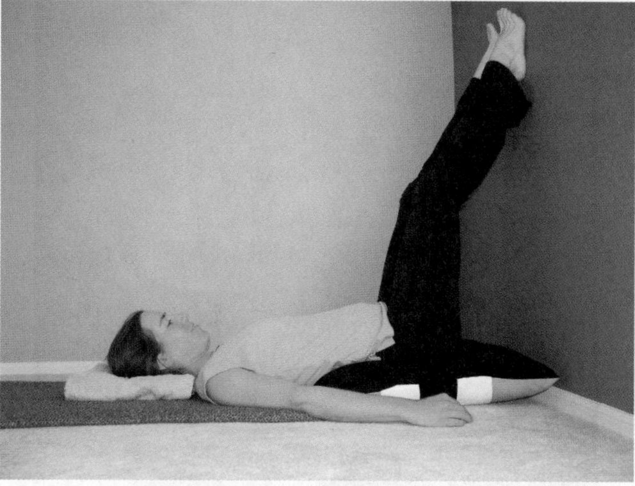

Fig. 11-16 Position for resting legs and reducing edema and varicosities. Encourage the woman with vulvar varicosities to include a pillow under her hips. *(Courtesy Julie Perry Nelson, Loveland, CO.)*

Travel

Travel is not contraindicated for low risk pregnant women. Women with high risk pregnancies are advised to avoid long-distance travel after fetal viability has been reached to avert the economic and psychologic consequences of giving birth to a preterm infant far from home. Travel to areas where medical care is poor, water is untreated, and malaria is prevalent should be avoided if possible. Women who contemplate foreign travel should be aware that many health insurance carriers do not cover birth in a foreign setting or even hospitalization for preterm labor. In addition, vaccinations for foreign travel may be contraindicated during pregnancy.

Pregnant women who travel for long distances should schedule periods of activity and rest. While sitting, the woman can practice deep breathing, foot circling, and alternately contracting and relaxing different muscle groups. She should avoid becoming fatigued. Although travel in itself is not a cause of adverse outcomes such as miscarriage or preterm labor, certain precautions are recommended when traveling in a car. For example, women riding in a car should wear automobile restraints and stop and walk every hour.

Maternal death as a result of injury is the most common cause of fetal death. The next most common cause is placental separation (abruptio placentae) that occurs because body contours change in reaction to the force of a collision. The uterus as a muscular organ can adapt its shape to that of the body, but the placenta is not resilient. At the impact of collision, placental separation can occur. A combination lap belt and shoulder harness is the most effective automobile restraint, and both should be used. The lap belt should be worn low across the hip bones and as snug as is comfortable (Fig. 11-18). The shoulder harness should be worn above the gravid uterus and below the neck to prevent chafing. The pregnant woman

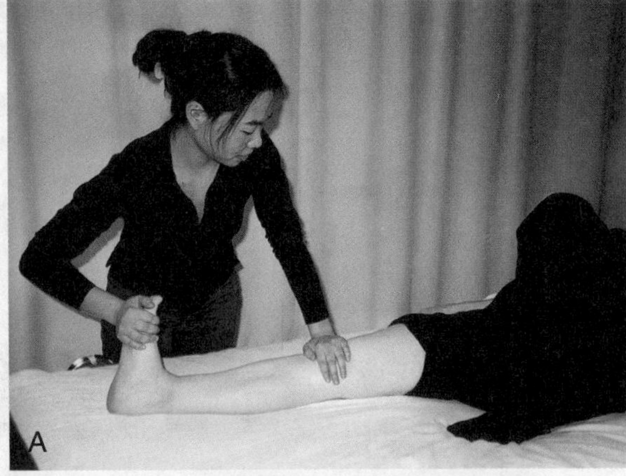

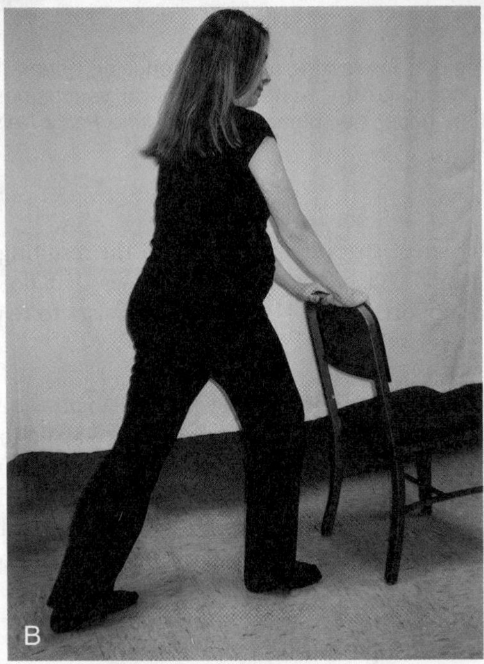

Fig. 11-17 Relief of muscle spasm (leg cramps). A, Another person dorsiflexes foot with knee extended. B, Woman stands and leans forward, thereby dorsiflexing foot of affected leg. *(Courtesy Shannon Perry, Phoenix, AZ.)*

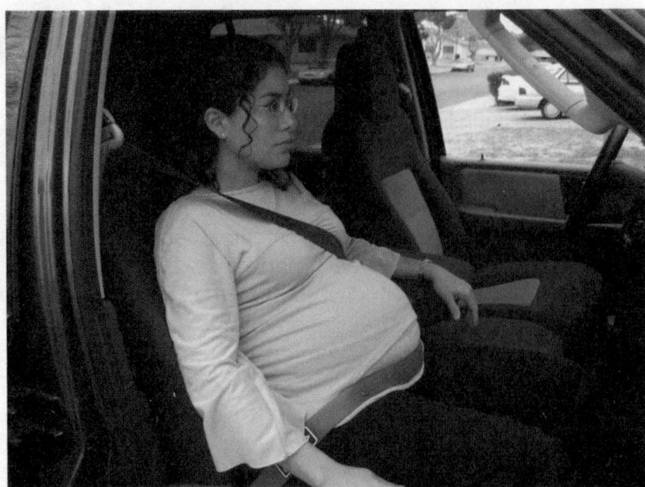

Fig. 11-18 Proper use of seat belt and headrest. *(Courtesy Brian and Mayannyn Sallee, Las Vegas, NV.)*

should sit upright. The headrest should be used to avoid whiplash injury.

Air travel in large commercial jets usually poses little risk to the pregnant woman, but policies vary from airline to airline. The pregnant woman is advised to inquire about restrictions or recommendations from her carrier. Most health care providers allow air travel up to 36 weeks of gestation in women without medical or pregnancy complications. Magnetometers (metal detectors) used at airport security checkpoints are not harmful to the fetus. The 8% humidity at which cabins are maintained in commercial airlines may result in some water loss; hydration (with water) should be maintained under these conditions. Sitting in the cramped seat of an airliner for prolonged periods may increase the risk of superficial and deep thrombophlebitis. A pregnant woman is encouraged to take a 15-minute walk around the aircraft during each hour of travel to minimize this risk (see the Patient Teaching box earlier in this chapter). However, women who are pilots, flight attendants, or frequent flyers expose themselves to in-flight radiation that exceeds recommended levels (Barish, 2004). Resources from the U.S. Federal Aviation Administration *(www.faa.gov)* will assist the health care provider in determining safe levels for women at high risk for radiation exposure.

Medications and Herbal Preparations

Although much has been learned in recent years about fetal drug toxicity, the possible teratogenicity of many drugs, both prescription and OTC, is still unknown. This is especially true for new medications and combinations of medications. Moreover, certain subclinical errors or deficiencies in intermediate metabolism in the fetus may cause an otherwise harmless drug to be converted into a hazardous one. The greatest danger of drug-caused developmental defects in the fetus extends from the time of fertilization through the first trimester, a time when the woman may not realize she is pregnant. Self-treatment must be discouraged. The use of all drugs, including OTC medications, herbs, and vitamins, should be limited; and a careful record kept of all therapeutic and nontherapeutic agents used.

Immunizations

Some concern has been raised over the safety of various immunization practices during pregnancy. Immunization with live or attenuated live viruses is contraindicated during pregnancy because of potential teratogenicity. Live virus vaccines include those for measles (rubeola and rubella), chickenpox, mumps, and the Sabin (oral) poliomyelitis vaccine (no longer used in the United States). Vaccines consisting of killed viruses that may be administered during pregnancy include tetanus, diphtheria, recombinant hepatitis B, and rabies vaccines.

Alcohol, Cigarette Smoke, Caffeine, and Drugs

A safe level of alcohol consumption during pregnancy has not yet been established. Although the consumption of occasional alcoholic beverages may not be harmful to the mother or her developing embryo or fetus, complete abstinence is strongly advised. Maternal alcoholism is associated with high rates of miscarriage and fetal alcohol syndrome; the risk for miscarriage in the first trimester is dose related (three or more drinks per day). Growing evidence indicates that the pattern of drinking (frequency, timing, and duration), especially in the first trimester, is more predictive of fetal damage than is the amount. Considerably less alcohol use is reported among pregnant women than in nonpregnant women, but a high prevalence of some alcohol use among pregnant women still exists. Such a finding underscores the need for more systematic public health efforts to educate women about the hazards of alcohol consumption during pregnancy.

Cigarette smoking or continued exposure to secondhand smoke (even if the mother does not smoke) is associated with IUGR and an increase in perinatal and infant morbidity and mortality. Smoking is associated with an increased frequency of preterm labor, PROM, abruptio placentae, placenta previa, and fetal death, possibly resulting from decreased placental perfusion (Niebyl & Simpson, 2007). Smoking cessation activities should be incorporated into routine prenatal care.

All women who smoke should be strongly encouraged to quit or at least reduce the number of cigarettes they smoke. Pregnant women need to be told about the negative effects of secondhand smoke on the fetus and encouraged to avoid such environments. Efforts focused on preventing girls and women from beginning to smoke should be intensified.

Most studies of human pregnancy have revealed no association between caffeine consumption and birth defects or LBW (Weng, Odouli, & Li, 2008). However, some studies have documented an increased risk for miscarriage with caffeine intake greater than 300 mg/day or fetal growth restriction with caffeine intake greater than 223 mg/day. Therefore, because other effects are unknown, pregnant women are advised to limit their caffeine intake to no more than 3 cups of coffee or cola per day (Resnik & Creasy, 2009).

Any drug or environmental agent that enters the pregnant woman's bloodstream has the potential to cross the placenta and harm the fetus. Marijuana, heroin, and cocaine are common examples of such substances. Although substance abuse in pregnancy is a major public health concern and comprehensive care of drug-addicted women improves maternal and neonatal outcomes, few facilities are available for treatment of these women (see Chapter 13).

Normal Discomforts

Pregnant women are confronted with symptoms that would be considered abnormal in the nonpregnant state. Women pregnant for the first time have an increased need for explanations of the causes of the discomforts and advice on ways to relieve the discomforts. The discomforts are fairly specific to each trimester of pregnancy. Table 11-2 provides information about the physiology, prevention, and self-management of discomforts experienced during the three trimesters. Box 11-8 lists alternative therapies used in pregnancy (see also Fig. 1-1). Nurses can do much to allay a first-time mother's anxiety about such symptoms by telling her about them in advance, using terminology that the woman (or couple) can understand. Understanding the rationale for treatment promotes their participation in their care. Interventions should be individualized, with attention given to the woman's lifestyle and culture.

BOX 11-8 Alternative Therapies Used in Pregnancy

Touch and Energetic Therapies

Massage
Acupressure
Therapeutic touch
Healing touch

Mind-Body Healing

Imagery
Meditation, prayer, reflection
Biofeedback
Other modalities that may fall outside of nurse practice guidelines unless the nurse has completed additional training or certification:

- Herbs
- Homeopathy
- Traditional Chinese medicine

NURSING ALERT Although complementary and alternative therapies may benefit the woman during pregnancy, some practices should be avoided because they may cause miscarriage or preterm labor. It is important to ask the woman what therapies she may be using.

Recognizing Potential Complications

One of the most important responsibilities of care providers is to alert the pregnant woman to signs and symptoms that indicate a potential complication of pregnancy. The woman needs to know how and to whom such warning signs should be reported (see Box 11-6). It is difficult to remember specifics when stressed by a disturbing symptom. Therefore the woman and her family can be reassured if they receive and use a printed form written at the appropriate literacy level listing the signs and symptoms that warrant an investigation and the phone numbers to call with questions or in an emergency.

The nurse must answer questions honestly as they arise during pregnancy. Pregnant women often have difficulty deciding when to report signs and symptoms. The mother is encouraged to refer to the printed list of potential complications and to listen to her body. If she senses that something is wrong, she should call her care provider immediately. Several signs and symptoms must be discussed more extensively. These include vaginal bleeding, alteration in fetal movements, symptoms of preeclampsia, rupture of membranes, and preterm labor.

Recognizing Preterm Labor

Teaching each expectant mother to recognize preterm labor is necessary for early diagnosis and treatment. Preterm labor occurs after the twentieth week but before the thirty-seventh week of pregnancy. It consists of uterine contractions that, if untreated, cause the cervix to open earlier than normal, resulting in preterm birth.

Although the exact etiology of preterm labor is unknown, it is assumed to have multiple causes. An increased incidence of preterm birth is associated with sociodemographic factors such as poverty, low educational level, lack of social support, smoking, domestic violence, and stress. Other risk factors

evolve Nursing Care Plan—Discomforts of Pregnancy and Warning Signs

Table 11-2 Discomforts Related to Pregnancy

DISCOMFORT	PHYSIOLOGY	EDUCATION FOR SELF-MANAGEMENT
First Trimester		
Breast changes, new sensation; pain, tingling, tenderness	Hypertrophy of mammary glandular tissue and increased vascularization, pigmentation, and size and prominence of nipples and areolae caused by hormonal stimulation	Wear supportive maternity bras with pads to absorb discharge (may be worn at night); wash with warm water and keep dry; breast tenderness may interfere with sexual expression/foreplay but is temporary
Urgency and frequency of urination	Vascular engorgement and altered bladder function caused by hormones; bladder capacity reduced by enlarging uterus and fetal presenting part	Empty bladder regularly; perform Kegel exercises; limit fluid intake before bedtime; wear perineal pad; report pain or burning sensation to primary health care provider
Languor and malaise; fatigue (early pregnancy, most commonly)	Unexplained; may be caused by increasing levels of estrogen, progesterone, and hCG or by elevated BBT; psychologic response to pregnancy and its required physical/psychologic adaptations	Rest as needed; eat well-balanced diet to prevent anemia
Nausea and vomiting, morning sickness—occurs in 50%-75% of pregnant women; starts between first and second missed periods and lasts until about fourth missed period; may occur any time during day; fathers also may have symptoms	Cause unknown; may result from hormonal changes, possibly hCG; may be partly emotional, reflecting pride in, ambivalence about, or rejection of pregnant state	Avoid empty or overloaded stomach; maintain good posture—give stomach ample room; stop smoking; eat dry carbohydrate on awakening; remain in bed until feeling subsides or alternate dry carbohydrate 1 hr with fluids such as hot herbal decaffeinated tea, milk, or clear coffee the next hour until feeling subsides; eat five to six small meals per day; avoid fried, odorous, spicy, greasy, or gas-forming foods; consult primary health care provider if intractable vomiting occurs
Ptyalism (excessive salivation) may occur starting 2-3 wk after first missed period	Possibly caused by elevated estrogen levels; may be related to reluctance to swallow because of nausea	Use astringent mouthwash, chew gum, eat hard candy as comfort measures
Gingivitis and epulis (hyperemia, hypertrophy, bleeding, tenderness); condition disappears spontaneously 1-2 mo after birth	Increased vascularity and proliferation of connective tissue from estrogen stimulation	Eat well-balanced diet, with adequate protein and fresh fruits and vegetables; brush teeth gently and observe good dental hygiene; avoid infection; see dentist
Nasal stuffiness; epistaxis (nosebleed)	Hyperemia of mucous membranes related to high estrogen levels	Use humidifier; avoid trauma; normal saline nose drops or spray may be used
Leukorrhea: often noted throughout pregnancy	Hormonally stimulated cervix becomes hypertrophic and hyperactive, producing abundant amount of mucus	Not preventable; do not douche; wear perineal pads; perform hygienic practices such as wiping front to back; report to primary health care provider if accompanied by pruritus, foul odor, or change in character or color
Psychosocial dynamics, mood swings, mixed feelings	Hormonal and metabolic adaptations; feelings about female role, sexuality, timing of pregnancy, and resultant changes in life and lifestyle	Participate in pregnancy support group; communicate concerns to partner, family, and others; request referral for supportive services if needed (financial assistance)
Second Trimester		
Pigmentation deepens, acne, oily skin	Melanocyte-stimulating hormone (from anterior pituitary)	Not preventable; it usually resolves during puerperium
Spider nevi (angiomas) appear over neck, thorax, face, and arms during second or third trimester	Focal networks of dilated arterioles (end-arteries) from increased concentration of estrogens	Not preventable; they fade slowly during late puerperium but rarely disappear completely
Palmar erythema occurs in 50% of pregnant women; may accompany spider nevi	Diffuse reddish mottling over palms and suffused skin over thenar eminences and fingertips; may be caused by genetic predisposition or hyperestrogenism	Not preventable; condition fades within 1 wk after giving birth
Pruritus (noninflammatory)	Unknown cause; various types as follows: nonpapular; closely aggregated pruritic papules Increased excretory function of skin and stretching of skin possible factors	Keep fingernails short and clean; contact primary health care provider for diagnosis of cause Not preventable; symptomatic; can be managed with Keri baths, mild sedation, distraction, tepid baths with sodium bicarbonate or oatmeal added to water, lotions and oils, change of soaps or reduction in use of soap, loose clothing

evolve Critical Thinking Exercise–Discomforts of Pregnancy

Table 11-2 Discomforts Related to Pregnancy—cont'd

DISCOMFORT	PHYSIOLOGY	EDUCATION FOR SELF-MANAGEMENT
Palpitations	Unknown; should not be accompanied by persistent cardiac irregularity	Not preventable; contact primary health care provider if accompanied by symptoms of cardiac decompensation
Supine hypotension (vena cava syndrome) and bradycardia	Induced by pressure of gravid uterus on ascending vena cava when woman is supine; reduces uteroplacental and renal perfusion	Assume side-lying position or semisitting posture, with knees slightly flexed (see also Emergency box, p. 242)
Faintness and, rarely, syncope (orthostatic hypotension): may persist throughout pregnancy	Vasomotor lability or postural hypotension from hormones; in late pregnancy may be caused by venous stasis in lower extremities	Exercise moderately (deep breathing, vigorous leg movements); avoid sudden changes in position* and warm crowded areas; move slowly and deliberately; keep environment cool; avoid hypoglycemia by eating five to six small meals per day; wear elastic hose; sit as necessary; if symptoms are serious, contact primary health care provider
Food cravings	Cause unknown; craving determined by culture or geographic area	Not preventable; satisfy craving unless it interferes with well-balanced diet; report unusual cravings to primary health care provider
Heartburn (pyrosis or acid indigestion): burning sensation, occasionally with burping and regurgitation of a little sour-tasting fluid	Progesterone slows GI tract motility and digestion, reverses peristalsis, relaxes cardiac sphincter, and delays emptying time of stomach; stomach displaced upward and compressed by enlarging uterus	Limit or avoid gas-producing or fatty foods and large meals; maintain good posture; sip milk for temporary relief; drink hot herbal tea; primary health care provider may prescribe antacid between meals; contact primary health care provider for persistent symptoms
Constipation	GI tract motility slowed because of progesterone, resulting in increased reabsorption of water and drying of stool; intestines compressed by enlarging uterus; predisposition to constipation because of oral iron supplementation	Drink six glasses of water per day; include roughage in diet; exercise moderately; maintain regular schedule for bowel movements; use relaxation techniques and deep breathing; do not take stool softener, laxatives, mineral oil, other drugs, or enemas without first consulting primary health care provider
Flatulence with bloating and belching	Reduced GI motility because of hormones, allowing time for bacterial action that produces gas; swallowing air	Chew foods slowly and thoroughly; avoid gas-producing foods, fatty foods, large meals; exercise, maintain regular bowel habits
Varicose veins (varicosities): may be associated with aching legs and tenderness; may be present in legs and vulva; hemorrhoids are varicosities in perianal area	Hereditary predisposition; relaxation of smooth muscle walls of veins because of hormones causing tortuous dilated veins in legs and pelvic vasocongestion; condition aggravated by enlarging uterus, gravity, and bearing down for bowel movements; thrombi from leg varices rare but may be produced by hemorrhoids	Avoid obesity, lengthy standing or sitting, constrictive clothing, and constipation and bearing down with bowel movements; exercise moderately; rest with legs and hips elevated (see Fig. 11-16); wear support stockings; thrombosed hemorrhoid may be evacuated; relieve swelling and pain with warm sitz baths; apply astringent compresses locally
Leukorrhea: often noted throughout pregnancy	Hormonally stimulated cervix becomes hypertrophic and hyperactive, producing abundant amount of mucus	Not preventable; do not douche; maintain good hygiene; wear perineal pads; report to primary health care provider if accompanied by pruritus, foul odor, or change in character or color
Headaches (through wk 26)	Emotional tension (more common than vascular migraine headache); eye strain (refractory errors); vascular engorgement and congestion of sinuses resulting from hormone stimulation	Conscious relaxation; contact primary health care provider for constant "splitting" headache to assess for preeclampsia
Carpal tunnel syndrome (involves thumb, second and third fingers, lateral side of little finger)	Compression of median nerve resulting from changes in surrounding tissues; pain, numbness, tingling, burning; loss of skilled movements (typing); dropping of objects	Not preventable; elevate affected arms; splinting of affected hand may help; regressive after pregnancy; surgery is curative
Periodic numbness, tingling of fingers (acrodysesthesia) occurs in 5% of pregnant women	Brachial plexus traction syndrome resulting from drooping of shoulders during pregnancy (occurs especially at night and early morning)	Maintain good posture; wear supportive maternity bra; condition will disappear if lifting and carrying baby does not aggravate it

Continued

Table 11-2 Discomforts Related to Pregnancy—cont'd

DISCOMFORT	PHYSIOLOGY	EDUCATION FOR SELF-MANAGEMENT
Round ligament pain (tenderness)	Stretching of ligament caused by enlarging uterus	Not preventable; rest, maintain good body mechanics to avoid overstretching ligament; relieve cramping by squatting or bringing knees to chest; sometimes heat helps
Joint pain, backache, and pelvic pressure; hypermobility of joints	Relaxation of symphyseal and sacroiliac joints because of hormones, resulting in unstable pelvis; exaggerated lumbar and cervicothoracic curves caused by change in center of gravity resulting from enlarging abdomen	Maintain good posture and body mechanics; avoid fatigue; wear low-heeled shoes; abdominal supports may be useful; practice conscious relaxation; sleep on firm mattress; apply local heat or ice; get back rubs; do pelvic rock exercise; rest; condition disappears 6-8 wk after birth
Third Trimester		
Shortness of breath and dyspnea: occur in 60% of pregnant women	Expansion of diaphragm limited by enlarging uterus; diaphragm elevated about 4 cm; some relief after lightening	Maintain good posture; sleep with extra pillows; avoid overloading stomach; stop smoking; contact health care provider if symptoms worsen to rule out anemia, emphysema, and asthma
Insomnia (later weeks of pregnancy)	Fetal movements, muscle cramping, urinary frequency, shortness of breath, or other discomforts	Reassurance, conscious relaxation, back massage or effleurage, support of body parts with pillows, and warm milk or warm shower before retiring are helpful
Psychosocial responses: mood swings, mixed feelings, increased anxiety	Hormonal and metabolic adaptations; feelings about impending labor, birth, and parenthood	Reassurance and support from significant other and nurse and improved communication with partner, family, and others are helpful
Gingivitis and epulis (hyperemia, hypertrophy, bleeding, tenderness): condition disappears spontaneously 1-2 mo after birth	Increased vascularity and proliferation of connective tissue from estrogen stimulation	Eat a well-balanced diet with adequate protein and fresh fruits and vegetables; gently brush teeth and practice good dental hygiene; avoid infection; see dentist for teeth cleaning
Urinary frequency and urgency return	Vascular engorgement and altered bladder function caused by hormones; bladder capacity reduced by enlarging uterus and fetal presenting part	Empty bladder regularly, do Kegel exercises; limit fluid intake before bedtime; reassurance is helpful; wear perineal pad; contact health care provider for pain or burning sensation
Perineal discomfort and pressure	Pressure from enlarging uterus, especially when standing or walking; multifetal gestation	Rest, conscious relaxation, and good posture are helpful; contact health care provider for assessment and treatment if pain is present
Leg cramps (gastrocnemius spasm), especially when reclining	Compression of nerves supplying lower extremities because of enlarging uterus; reduced level of diffusible serum calcium or elevation of serum phosphorus; aggravating factors: fatigue, poor peripheral circulation, pointing toes when stretching legs or when walking, drinking more than 1 L (1 qt) of milk per day	Check for Homans' sign; if negative, use massage and heat over affected muscle; dorsiflex foot until spasm relaxes (see Fig. 11-17, *A*); stand on cold surface; supplement orally with calcium carbonate or calcium lactate tablets; aluminum hydroxide gel, 30 ml, with each meal removes phosphorus by absorbing it
Ankle edema (nonpitting) to lower extremities	Edema aggravated by prolonged standing, sitting, poor posture, lack of exercise, constrictive clothing (e.g., garters), or hot weather	Intake ample fluid for natural diuretic effect; put on support stockings before arising; rest periodically with legs and hips elevated (see Fig. 11-16); exercise moderately; contact health care provider if generalized edema develops; *diuretics are contraindicated*

BBT, Basal body temperature; *GI*, gastrointestinal; *hCG*, human chorionic gonadotropin.
*Caution woman to rise slowly and sit on edge of bed or to assume hands-and-knees posture before rising and to get up slowly after sitting or squatting.

include a previous preterm labor (McPheeters et al, 2005), current multifetal gestation, and some uterine and cervical variations (March of Dimes Birth Defects Foundation, 2005). The rate of prematurity is almost twice as high in the African-American population as in Caucasians.

If a woman knows the warning signs and symptoms of preterm labor and seeks care early enough, prevention of preterm birth may be possible. Warning signs and symptoms of preterm labor are given in the Home Care box. Fig. 11-19 shows where in the body the signs and symptoms of preterm labor may be located.

Sex Counseling

Sex counseling of expectant couples includes countering misinformation, providing reassurance of normality, and suggesting alternative behaviors. The uniqueness of each couple is

HOME CARE
How to Recognize Preterm Labor

Because the onset of preterm labor is subtle and often hard to recognize, it is important to know how to feel your abdomen for uterine contractions. You can feel for contractions in the following way. While lying down, place your fingertips on the top of your uterus. A contraction is the periodic tightening or hardening of your uterus. If your uterus is contracting, you will actually feel your abdomen get tight or hard and then feel it relax or soften when the contraction is over.

If you think you are having any of the other signs and symptoms of preterm labor, empty your bladder, drink three to four glasses of water for hydration, lie down tilted toward your side, and place a pillow at your back for support.

Check for contractions for 1 hour. To tell how often contractions are occurring, check the minutes that elapse from the beginning of one contraction to the beginning of the next.

It is *not normal* to have frequent uterine contractions (every 10 minutes or more often for 1 hour).

Contractions of labor are regular, frequent, and hard. They also may be felt as a tightening of the abdomen or a backache. This type of contraction causes the cervix to efface and dilate.

Call your doctor, nurse-midwife, clinic, or labor and birth unit or go to the hospital if any of the following signs occur:

- You have uterine contractions every 10 minutes or more often for 1 hour *or*
- You have any of the other signs and symptoms for 1 hour *or*
- You have any bloody spotting or leaking of fluid from your vagina

It is often difficult to identify preterm labor. Accurate diagnosis requires assessment by the health care provider, usually in the hospital or clinic.

Post these instructions where they can be seen by everyone in the family.

considered within a biopsychosocial framework (see Home Care box). Nurses can initiate discussion about sexual adaptations that must be made during pregnancy. They need a sound knowledge base about the physical, social, and emotional responses to sex during pregnancy. Not all maternity nurses are comfortable dealing with the sexual concerns of their patients; nurses who are aware of their personal strengths and limitations in dealing with sexual content are better prepared to make referrals if necessary (Westheimer & Lopater, 2005).

Many women merely need "permission" to be sexually active during pregnancy. However, other women need information about the physiologic changes that occur during pregnancy and to dispel myths associated with sex during pregnancy. Discussions of positions for intercourse that decrease pressure on the gravid abdomen can be included (Westheimer & Lopater, 2005). Such tasks are within the purview of the maternity nurse and should be an integral component of the health care provided.

Some couples need to be referred for sex or family therapy. Couples whose long-standing problems with sexual dysfunction are intensified by pregnancy are good candidates for sex therapy. When a sexual problem is a symptom of a more serious relationship problem, the couple would benefit from family therapy.

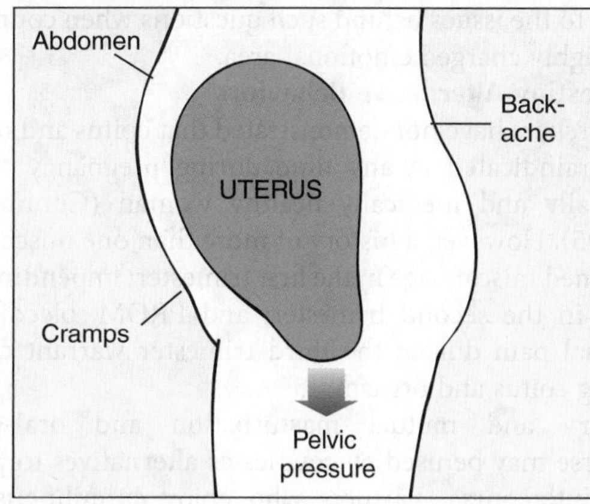

Fig. 11-19 Symptoms of preterm labor.

HOME CARE
Sexuality in Pregnancy

Be aware that maternal physiologic changes such as breast enlargement, nausea, fatigue, abdominal changes, perineal enlargement, leukorrhea, pelvic vasocongestion, and orgasmic responses may affect sexuality and sexual expression.

Discuss responses to pregnancy with your partner.

Keep in mind that cultural prescriptions (do's) and proscriptions (don'ts) may affect your responses.

Although your libido may be depressed during the first trimester, it often increases during the second and third trimesters.

Discuss and explore the following with your partner:

- Alternative behaviors (e.g., mutual masturbation, foot massage, cuddling).
- Alternative positions (e.g., female superior, side lying) for sexual intercourse.

Intercourse is safe as long as it is not uncomfortable. There is no correlation between intercourse and miscarriage, but observe the following precautions:

- Abstain from intercourse if you experience uterine cramping or vaginal bleeding; report event to your caregiver as soon as possible.
- Abstain from intercourse (or any activity that results in orgasm) if you have a history of premature dilation of the cervix until the problem is corrected.

Continue to use risk reduction behaviors. Women at risk for acquiring or conveying sexually transmitted infections are encouraged to use condoms during sexual intercourse throughout pregnancy.

Countering Misinformation

Many myths and much of the misinformation related to sex and pregnancy are masked by seemingly unrelated issues. For example, a discussion about the baby's ability to hear and see in utero may be prompted by questions about the baby being an observer of lovemaking. The counselor must be extremely sensitive to the issues behind such questions when counseling in this highly charged emotional area.

Suggesting Alternative Behaviors

Researchers have not demonstrated that coitus and orgasm are contraindicated at any time during pregnancy for the obstetrically and medically healthy woman (Cunningham et al, 2005). However, a history of more than one miscarriage; a threatened miscarriage in the first trimester; impending miscarriage in the second trimester; and PROM, bleeding, or abdominal pain during the third trimester warrant caution regarding coitus and orgasm.

Solitary and mutual masturbation and oral-genital intercourse may be used by couples as alternatives to penile-vaginal intercourse. Partners who enjoy cunnilingus (oral stimulation of the clitoris or vagina) may feel "turned off" by the normal increase in amount and odor of vaginal discharge during pregnancy. Couples who practice cunnilingus should be cautioned against the blowing of air into the vagina, particularly during the last few weeks of pregnancy, when the cervix may be slightly open. An air embolism can occur if air is forced between the uterine wall and fetal membranes and enters the maternal vascular system through the placenta.

Showing the woman or couple illustrations of the possible variations of coital position is helpful (Fig. 11-20). The female-superior, side-by-side, rear-entry, and facing-each-other positions are alternatives to the traditional male-superior position. The woman astride (superior position) allows her to control the angle and depth of penile penetration, as well as protect her breasts and abdomen. During the third trimester the side-by-side position or any position that places less pressure on the pregnant abdomen and requires less energy may be preferred.

Multiparous women sometimes have significant breast tenderness in the first trimester. A coital position that avoids direct pressure on the woman's breasts and decreased breast fondling during love play can be recommended to such couples. The woman should also be reassured that this condition is normal and temporary.

Some women complain of lower abdominal cramping and backache after orgasm during the first and third trimesters. A back rub can often relieve some of the discomfort and provide a pleasant experience. A tonic uterine contraction, often lasting up to a minute, replaces the rhythmic contractions of orgasm during the third trimester. Changes in FHR without fetal distress have also been reported.

The objective of risk reduction is to provide prophylaxis against the acquisition and transmission of STIs (e.g., herpes simplex virus, human papilloma virus, and HIV). Because these diseases may be transmitted to the woman and her fetus, the use of condoms is recommended throughout pregnancy if the woman is at risk for acquiring an STI.

Well-informed nurses who are comfortable with their own sexuality and the sex counseling needs of expectant couples can offer information and advice in this valuable but often neglected area. They can establish an open environment in which couples can feel free to introduce their concerns about sexual adjustment and seek support and guidance. This intervention is as important for lesbian women and their partners as it is for women partnered with men.

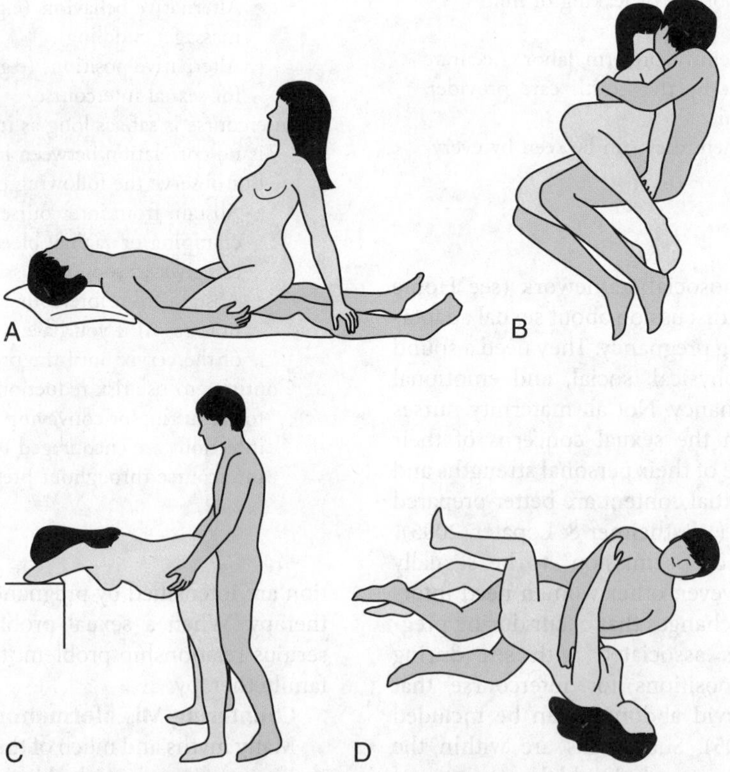

Fig. 11-20 Positions for sexual intercourse during pregnancy. A, Female superior. B, Side by side. C, Rear entry. D, Facing each other.

Psychosocial Support

Esteem, affection, trust, concern, consideration of cultural and religious responses, and listening are all components of the emotional support given to the pregnant woman and her family. The woman's satisfaction with her relationships and support, her feeling of competence, and her sense of being in control are important issues to be addressed in the third trimester. A discussion of fetal responses to stimuli such as sound, light, maternal posture, and tension, as well as patterns of sleeping and waking, can be helpful. Other issues of concern that can arise for the pregnant woman and couple include fear of pain, loss of control, and possible birth of the infant before reaching the hospital. Parental concerns about the responsibilities and tasks of parenthood; the safety of the mother and unborn child; siblings and their acceptance of the new baby; social and economic responsibilities; and possible conflicts in cultural, religious, or personal value systems are addressed.

The father's or partner's commitment to the pregnancy, the couple's relationship, and their concerns about sexuality and sexual expression can emerge as issues for many expectant parents.

Providing the prospective mother and father with opportunities to discuss their concerns and validating the normality of their responses can meet their needs to some degree. Nurses must also recognize that men feel more vulnerable during their partner's pregnancy. Female partners may also have these feelings. Anticipatory guidance and health promotion strategies can help partners cope with their concerns. Nursing intervention may help them to deal with such concerns either directly through counseling or indirectly through the education of the mothers. Health care providers can stimulate and encourage open dialogue between the couple.

Variations in Prenatal Care

The course of prenatal care described thus far can seem to suggest that the experiences of childbearing women are similar and that nursing interventions are uniform across all populations. Although typical patterns of response to pregnancy are easily recognized and many aspects of prenatal care indeed are consistent, pregnant women enter the health care system with individual concerns and needs. The nurse's ability to assess unique needs and tailor interventions to the individual is the hallmark of expertise in providing care. Variations that influence prenatal care include culture, age, and number of fetuses.

Cultural Influences

Prenatal care as we know it is a phenomenon of Western medicine. In the U.S. biomedical model of care, women are encouraged to seek prenatal care as early as possible in their pregnancy by visiting a physician, nurse-midwife, office, or clinic. Such visits are routine and follow a systematic sequence, with the initial visit followed by monthly, then semimonthly, then weekly visits. Monitoring weight and BP; testing blood and urine; teaching specific information about diet, rest, and activity; and preparing for childbirth are common components of prenatal care. This model is not only unfamiliar but may seem strange to many groups. Different models for providing prenatal care for women in other parts of the world are being explored.

Many cultural variations in prenatal care exist. Even if the prenatal care described is familiar to a woman, some practices may conflict with the beliefs and practices of a subculture group to which she belongs. Because of these and other factors such as lack of money, lack of transportation, and language barriers, women from diverse cultures may not keep prenatal appointments. The nurse may misinterpret their behavior as uncaring, lazy, or ignorant.

For many women concern for modesty is a deterrent for seeking prenatal care. Some women consider exposing body parts, especially to a man, a major violation of their modesty. For many women invasive procedures such as vaginal examination may be so threatening that they cannot be discussed even with their own husbands. Thus they prefer a female health care provider. Too often health care providers assume that women lose this modesty during pregnancy and labor, but most women value and appreciate efforts to maintain their modesty.

In many cultural groups a physician is deemed appropriate only in times of illness. Because pregnancy is considered a normal process and the woman is in a state of health, the services of a physician are considered inappropriate. Western medicine's view of problems in pregnancy may differ from that of members of other cultural groups.

Although pregnancy is considered normal by many, certain practices are expected of women of all cultures to ensure a good outcome. Cultural prescriptions tell women what to do, and cultural proscriptions establish taboos. The purposes of these practices are to prevent maternal illness caused by a pregnancy-induced imbalanced state and to protect the vulnerable fetus. Prescriptions and proscriptions regulate the woman's emotional response, clothing, physical activity and rest, sexual activity, and dietary practices. Exploration of the woman's beliefs, perceptions of the meaning of childbearing, and health care practices may help health care providers foster her self-actualization, promote attainment of the maternal role, and positively influence her relationship with her spouse.

To provide culturally sensitive care, the nurse must be knowledgeable about practices and customs, although it is not possible to know all there is to know about every culture and subculture or the many lifestyles that exist. It is important to learn about the varied cultures in the setting in which a nurse practices. When exploring cultural beliefs and practices related to childbearing, the nurse can support and nurture the beliefs that promote physical or emotional adaptation (Fig. 11-21). However, if potentially harmful beliefs or activities are identified, the nurse should sensitively provide education and propose modifications.

Emotional Response

Virtually all cultures emphasize the importance of maintaining a socially harmonious and agreeable environment for the pregnant woman (see Community Focus box). A lifestyle with minimal stress is important in ensuring a successful outcome for the mother and baby. Harmony with other people must be fostered, and visits from extended family members may be required to demonstrate pleasant and noncontroversial relationships. If discord exists in a relationship, it is usually dealt with in culturally prescribed ways.

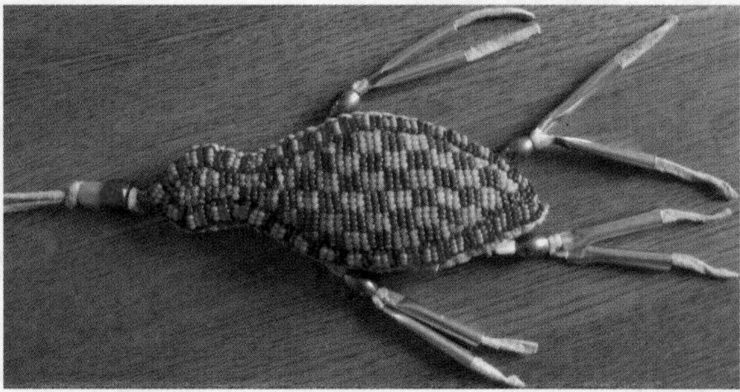

Fig. 11-21 Umbilical amulet. Northern plains tribes of Native Americans made amulets to hold the umbilical cord of a newborn child. The parents protected the child by ensuring that it was carried or worn by the child. *(Courtesy Shannon Perry, Phoenix, AZ.)*

COMMUNITY FOCUS

Culture and Childbirth Beliefs and Practices

Select an immigrant or other minority group in your community and identify childbirth-related beliefs and practices that are unique to that group. Are there stores in the area that sell items that meet the needs of that group? Does the community center have activities or classes that are directed toward that group? Are childbirth education programs available that provide essential information while incorporating cultural patterns? Are childbirth classes available in languages other then English? What could you, as a nurse, contribute to the community that would help meet the needs of that group?

Besides proscriptions regarding food, other proscriptions involve forms of magic. For example, some Mexicans believe pregnant women should not be allowed to witness an eclipse of the moon because it may cause a cleft palate in the infant. They also believe that exposure to an earthquake may precipitate preterm birth, miscarriage, or a breech presentation. In some cultures a pregnant woman must not ridicule someone with an affliction for fear her child might be born with the same handicap. A mother should not hate a person lest her child resemble that person. Dental work should not be done during pregnancy because it may cause a baby to have a "harelip." A folk belief widely held in many cultures is that the pregnant woman should refrain from raising her arms above her head and from tying knots because such movements tie knots in the umbilical cord and may cause it to wrap around the baby's neck. Another belief is that placing a knife under the bed of a laboring woman will "cut" her pain.

Clothing

Although most cultural groups do not prescribe specific clothing for pregnancy, modesty is an expectation for many. Some Mexican women of the Southwest wear a cord beneath the breasts and knotted over the umbilicus. This cord, called a *muñeco,* is thought to prevent morning sickness and ensure a safe birth. Amulets, medals, and beads also may be worn to ward off evil spirits.

Physical Activity and Rest

Norms that regulate physical activity of mothers during pregnancy vary tremendously. Many groups, including Native Americans and some Asian groups, encourage women to be active, to walk, and to engage in normal although not strenuous activities to ensure that the baby is healthy and not too large. Other groups such as Filipinos believe that any activity is dangerous, and others willingly take over the work of the pregnant woman. Some Filipinos believe that this inactivity protects the mother and child. The mother is encouraged simply to produce the succeeding generation. If health care providers do not know of this belief, they could misinterpret this behavior as laziness or noncompliance with the desired prenatal health care regimen. It is important for the nurse to find out the way each pregnant woman views activity and rest.

Sexual Activity

In most cultures sexual activity is not prohibited until the end of pregnancy. Some Latinos view sexual activity as necessary to keep the birth canal lubricated. Conversely some Vietnamese have definite proscriptions about sexual intercourse, requiring abstinence throughout the pregnancy because it is thought that sexual intercourse may harm the mother and the fetus.

Nutrition

Nutritional information given by Western health care providers may be a source of conflict for many cultural groups. Such a conflict commonly is not known by health care providers unless they understand the dietary beliefs and practices of the particular people for whom they are caring. For example, Muslims have strict regulations regarding preparation of food; and if meat cannot be prepared as prescribed, they may omit it from their diets. Many cultures permit pregnant women to eat only warm foods.

Age Differences

The age of the childbearing couple may have a significant influence on their physical and psychosocial adaptation to pregnancy. Normal developmental processes that occur in both very young and older mothers are interrupted by pregnancy and require a different type of adaptation to pregnancy than that of the woman of typical childbearing age. Although the individuality of each pregnant woman is recognized, special needs of expectant mothers 15 years of age or younger or those 35 years of age or older are summarized here.

Adolescents

Teenage pregnancy is a worldwide problem. About 1 million adolescent females in the United States, or 4 of every 10 girls, become pregnant each year. Most of the pregnancies are unintended. Adolescents are responsible for almost 450,000 births in the United States annually. Hispanic adolescents currently have the highest birth rate, although the rate for African-American adolescents also is high (Martin et al, 2008). Most of these young women are unmarried, and many are not ready for the emotional, psychosocial, and financial responsibilities of parenthood.

Despite these alarming statistics and the fact that the United States has the highest adolescent birth rate in the industrialized world, the birth rate for adolescents declined steadily from 1991 until 2006 when the rate rose 3% (Martin et al, 2008). Concentrated national efforts have spawned a host of adolescent pregnancy prevention programs that have had varying degrees of success. Characteristics of programs that make a difference are those that have sustained commitment to adolescents over a long period, involve the parents and other adults in the community, promote abstinence and personal responsibility, and assist adolescents to develop a clear strategy for reaching future goals such as a college education or a career.

When adolescents become pregnant and decide to give birth, they are much less likely than older women to receive adequate prenatal care, with many receiving no care at all. These young women also are more likely to smoke and less likely to gain adequate weight during pregnancy. As a result of these and other factors, babies born to adolescents are at greatly increased risk of LBW, serious and long-term disability, and dying during the first year of life.

Delayed entry into prenatal care may be the result of late recognition of pregnancy, denial of pregnancy, or confusion about the services that are available. Such a delay in care may leave inadequate time before birth to attend to correctable problems. The very young pregnant adolescent is at higher risk for each of the confounding variables associated with poor pregnancy outcomes (e.g., socioeconomic factors) and for the conditions associated with a first pregnancy, regardless of age (e.g., gestational hypertension). However, when prenatal care is initiated early and consistently and confounding variables are controlled, very young pregnant adolescents are at no greater risk (nor are their infants) for an adverse outcome than older pregnant women. Thus the role of the nurse in reducing the risks and consequences of adolescent pregnancy is twofold: first, to encourage early and continued prenatal care; and second, to refer the adolescent, if necessary, for appropriate social support services, which can help reverse the effects of a negative socioeconomic environment (Fig. 11-22; see Nursing Care Plan).

Women Older Than 35 Years of Age

Two groups of older parents have emerged in the population of women having a child late in their childbearing years. One group consists of women who have many children or who have an additional child during the menopausal period. The other group consists of women who have deliberately delayed childbearing until their late thirties or early forties.

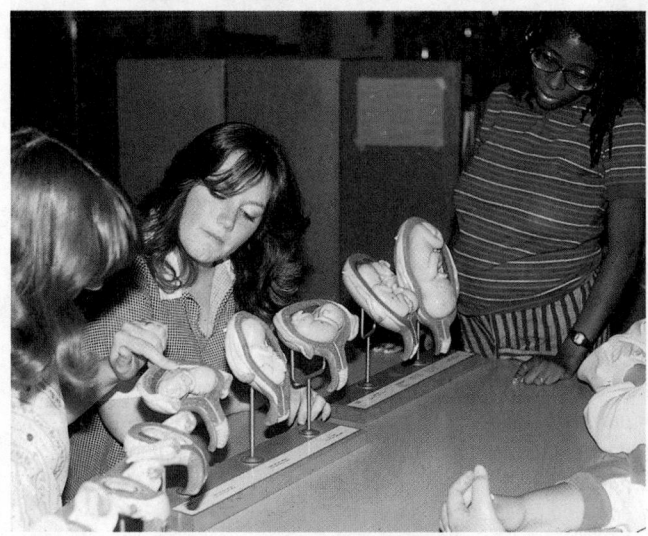

Fig. 11-22 Pregnant adolescents review fetal development. *(Courtesy Marjorie Pyle, RNC, Lifecircle, Costa Mesa, CA).*

Multiparous Women Multiparous women may have never used contraceptives because of personal choice or a lack of knowledge concerning contraceptives. They also may be women who have used contraceptives successfully during the childbearing years but, as menopause approaches, cease menstruating regularly or stop using contraception and subsequently become pregnant. The older multiparous woman may believe that pregnancy separates her from her peer group and that her age is a hindrance to close associations with young mothers. Other parents welcome the unexpected infant as evidence of continuing maternal and paternal roles.

Nulliparous Women The number of first-time pregnancies in women between ages 35 and 40 has increased significantly over the last three decades. Reasons for delaying pregnancy include advanced education, career priorities, better contraceptive measures, and infertility.

These women choose parenthood over a childfree lifestyle. They often are established in a career and a lifestyle with a partner that includes time for self-attention, the establishment of a home with accumulated possessions, and freedom to travel (Benzies et al, 2006). The dilemma of choice includes recognition that being a parent will have both positive and negative consequences. Couples need to discuss the consequences of childbearing and childrearing before committing themselves to this lifelong venture. Partners in this group seem to share the preparation for parenthood, the planning for a family-centered birth, and the desire to be loving and competent parents. However, the reality of child care may prove difficult for them.

During pregnancy parents explore the possibilities and responsibilities of changing identities and new roles. They must prepare a safe and nurturing environment during pregnancy and after birth. They must integrate the child into an established family system and negotiate new roles (parent, sibling, and grandparent roles) for family members.

Adverse perinatal outcomes are more common in older primiparas than in younger women, even when they receive good prenatal care. Women 35 years of age and older are more likely than younger primiparas to have LBW infants, premature birth, IUGR, abruptio placentae, and multiple births (Montan, 2007). The incidence of malpresentation also is more common in older primiparas, and they are more likely to have a cesarean birth. The occurrence of these complications is quite stressful for the new parents, and nursing interventions that provide information and psychosocial support in addition to care for physical needs are important.

Multifetal Pregnancy

A multifetal pregnancy, or pregnancy with more than one fetus, places the mother and fetuses at increased risk for adverse outcomes. The maternal blood volume is increased, resulting in an increased strain on the maternal cardiovascular system. Anemia often develops because of a greater demand for iron by the fetuses. Marked uterine distention, increased pressure on the adjacent viscera and pelvic vasculature, and diastasis of the two rectus abdominis muscles may occur (see Fig. 10-14). Placenta previa develops more commonly in multifetal pregnancies because of the large size or placement of the placentas. Premature separation of the placenta may occur before the second and any subsequent fetuses are born.

evolve Critical Thinking Exercise—Teenage Pregnancy

NURSING CARE PLAN Adolescent Pregnancy

Nursing Diagnosis: Imbalanced nutrition: less than body requirements related to intake insufficient to meet metabolic needs of fetus and adolescent patient

Expected Outcomes

Patient will gain weight as prescribed by age, take prenatal vitamins/iron as prescribed, and maintain normal hematocrit and hemoglobin.

Nursing Interventions/*Rationales*

Assess current diet history/intake *to determine prescriptions for additions or changes in present dietary pattern.*

Compare prepregnancy weight with current weight *to determine if pattern is consistent with appropriate fetal growth and development.*

Provide information concerning food prescriptions for appropriate weight gain, considering preferences for "fast food" and peer influences, *to correct any misconceptions and increase chances for compliance with diet.*

Include patient's immediate family or support system during instruction *to ensure that person preparing family meals receives information.*

Nursing Diagnosis: Risk for injury, maternal or fetal, related to inadequate prenatal care and screening

Expected Outcomes

Patient will experience uncomplicated pregnancy and give birth to a healthy fetus at term.

Nursing Interventions/*Rationales*

Provide information, using therapeutic communication and confidentiality, *to establish relationship and build trust.*

Discuss importance of ongoing prenatal care and possible risks to adolescent patient and fetus *to reinforce that ongoing assessment is crucial to health and well-being of patient and fetus, even if patient feels well.* The adolescent patient is more at risk for certain complications that may be avoided or managed early if prenatal visits are maintained.

Discuss risks of alcohol, tobacco, and recreational drug use during pregnancy *to minimize risks to patient and fetus because adolescent patients have a higher abuse rate than the rest of the pregnant population.*

Assess for evidence of sexually transmitted infection (STI) and provide information regarding safer sexual practices *to minimize risk to patient and fetus because adolescent is more at risk for STIs.*

Screen for preeclampsia on an ongoing basis *to minimize risk because adolescent population is more at risk for preeclampsia.*

Nursing Diagnosis: Social isolation related to body image changes of pregnant adolescent as evidenced by patient statements and concerns

Expected Outcomes

Patient will identify support systems and report decreased feelings of social isolation.

Nursing Interventions/*Rationales*

Establish a therapeutic relationship *to listen objectively and establish trust.*

Discuss with patient changes in relationships that have occurred as a result of the pregnancy *to determine extent of isolation from family, peers, and father of the baby.*

Provide referrals and resources appropriate for developmental stage of patient *to give information for patient support.*

Provide information regarding parenting classes, breastfeeding classes, and childbirth preparation classes *to give further information and group support, which lessens social isolation.*

Nursing Diagnosis: Interrupted family processes related to adolescent pregnancy

Expected Outcome

Patient will reestablish relationship with her mother and father of baby.

Nursing Interventions/*Rationales*

Encourage communication with mother *to clarify roles and relationships related to birth of infant.*

Encourage communication with father of baby (if she desires continued contact) *to ascertain level of support to be expected of father of baby.*

Refer to support group *to learn more effective problem-solving methods and reduce conflict within the family.*

Nursing Diagnosis: Disturbed body image related to situational crisis of pregnancy

Expected Outcome

Pregnant adolescent will verbalize positive comments regarding her body image during the pregnancy.

Nursing Interventions/*Rationales*

Assess pregnant adolescent's perception of self related to pregnancy *to provide basis for further interventions.*

Give information regarding expected body changes occurring during pregnancy *to provide a realistic view of these temporary changes.*

Provide opportunity to discuss personal feelings and concerns *to promote trust and support.*

Nursing Diagnosis: Risk for impaired parenting related to immaturity and lack of experience in new role of adolescent mother

Expected Outcome

Parents will demonstrate parenting roles with confidence.

Nursing Interventions/*Rationales*

Provide information on growth and development *to enhance knowledge so that adolescent mother can have basis for caring for her infant.*

Refer to parenting classes *to enhance knowledge and obtain support for providing appropriate care to newborn and infant.*

Initiate discussion of child care *to assist adolescent in problem solving for future needs.*

Assess parenting abilities of adolescent mother and father *to provide baseline for education.*

Provide information on parenting classes that are appropriate for parents' developmental stage *to give opportunity to share common feelings and concerns.*

Assist parents to identify pertinent support systems *to give assistance with parenting as needed.*

Twin pregnancies often end prematurely. Spontaneous rupture of membranes before term is common. Congenital malformations are twice as common in monozygotic twins as in singletons, although there is no increase in the incidence of congenital anomalies in dizygotic twins. Two-vessel cords (i.e., cords with a single umbilical artery) occur more often in twins than in singletons; this abnormality is most common in monozygotic twins. The most serious problem for the fetus is the local shunting of blood between placentas (twin-to-twin transfusion); this causes the recipient twin to be larger and the donor twin to be small, pallid, dehydrated, malnourished, and hypovolemic. However, the larger twin may develop congenital heart failure during the first 24 hours after birth.

The clinical diagnosis of multifetal pregnancy is accurate in about 90% of cases. The likelihood of a multifetal pregnancy is increased if any one or a combination of the following factors is noted during a careful assessment:

- History of dizygotic twins in the female lineage
- Use of fertility drugs
- More rapid uterine growth for the number of weeks of gestation
- Hydramnios
- Palpation of more than the expected number of small or large parts
- Asynchronous fetal heartbeats or more than one fetal electrocardiographic tracing
- Ultrasonographic evidence of more than one fetus

The diagnosis of multifetal pregnancy can come as a shock to many expectant parents, and they may need additional support and education to help them cope with the changes they face. The mother needs nutrition counseling so she gains more weight than that needed for a singleton birth. She should also be counseled that maternal adaptations will probably be more uncomfortable and provided with information about the possibility of a preterm birth.

If the presence of more than three fetuses is diagnosed, the parents may receive counseling regarding selective reduction of the fetuses to reduce the incidence of premature birth and improve the opportunities for the remaining fetuses to grow to term gestation (Cleary-Goldman, Chitkara, & Berkowitz, 2007). This situation poses an ethical dilemma for many couples, especially those who have worked hard to overcome problems with infertility and those who harbor strong values regarding the right to life. Nurse-initiated discussions to identify what resources could help the couple (e.g., a minister, priest, rabbi, or mental health counselor) can make the decision-making process somewhat less traumatic.

Prenatal care given to women with multifetal pregnancies includes changes in the pattern of care and modifications in other aspects such as the amount of weight gained and the nutritional intake necessary. The prenatal visits of these mothers are scheduled at least every 2 weeks in the second trimester and weekly thereafter. The recommended weight gain in twin gestations is 16 to 20 kg (Cleary-Goldman, Chitkara, & Berkowitz, 2007). Iron and vitamin supplements are desirable. Since preeclampsia and eclampsia occur more commonly during multifetal pregnancies, the health care team works aggressively to prevent, identify, and treat these complications of pregnancy.

The considerable uterine distention involved in a multifetal pregnancy can cause the backache commonly experienced by pregnant women to be even worse. Maternity support hose may be worn to control leg varicosities. Every multifetal pregnancy is at risk for preterm labor; thus the women receive frequent ultrasound examinations, FHR monitoring, and nonstress tests (Elliott, 2007). Some practitioners recommend bed rest beginning at 20 weeks in women carrying multiple fetuses to prevent preterm labor. Other practitioners question the value of prolonged bed rest. If bed rest is recommended, the mother needs to assume the lateral position to promote increased placental perfusion. If birth is delayed until after the thirty-sixth week, the risk of morbidity and mortality decreases for the neonates (see Home Care box).

HOME CARE

Example of How One Organization Uses Case Management to Keep Preterm Birth Rate Low

A regional health maintenance organization targets women at risk for preterm birth using a case management model. Women complete a risk assessment form when they enroll in the health plan. Once a woman has been identified as having high risk factors, a case manager (CM) makes an outreach call. The CM educates the women regarding what to expect, what they should watch for, and when to report findings to their physician. When a physician orders bed rest at home or for those women with small children or who need extra help, the health plan provides the services of a doula before and after childbirth. The CM follow-up and the doula ensure that the woman has the physical and emotional support that is needed for a healthy outcome of the pregnancy. Through this program the health plan has been able to reduce the preterm rate of their members (6.5% to 7.8%) to a rate well below the national rate (11.3% to 12.7%).

Data from: CM program keeps preterm delivery rate low, *Case Manag Advis* 18(6):51-52, 2007.

Multiple newborns will likely place a strain on finances, space, workload, and the mother's and family's coping abilities. Lifestyle changes may be necessary. Parents will need assistance in making realistic plans for the care of the babies (e.g., whether to breastfeed and whether to raise them as "alike" or as separate individuals). Parents can be referred to national organizations such as Mother of Twins *(www.nomotc.org)*, Parents of Twins and Triplets *(www.potatonet.org)*, and the La Leche League *(www.lalecheleague.org)* for further support.

Childbirth and Perinatal Education

A goal of childbirth and perinatal education is to assist individuals and their family members to make informed, safe decisions about pregnancy, birth, and early parenthood. A specific focus is to assist them to comprehend the long-lasting potential that empowering birth experiences have in the lives of women. It also aims to convey the impact that early experiences have on the development of children and the family. Perinatal education programs are an expansion of the earlier childbirth education movement that originally offered only a set of classes in the third trimester of pregnancy to prepare parents for birth.

Today perinatal education programs consist of a menu of class series and activities from preconception through pregnancy, childbirth, and the early months of parenting. It takes a well-informed, articulate childbirth educator to teach consumer-oriented childbirth classes. Optimally these classes help women trust their bodies and offer them a way to take full advantage of the opportunities presented by a prepared-for and well-supported childbirth experience.

For the new family, prior experience related to the pregnancy and birth of others or in the care of younger siblings or relatives is increasingly uncommon, given the small size of many North American families. As a result, many individuals facing parenthood may have little information about what to expect and thus do not have the important skills necessary to deal effectively with pregnancy, childbirth, or parenthood. Perinatal education classes can partially fill this void.

Preconception education and care are designed to foster conscious conception and health maintenance, promote healthy behaviors for the health of the woman and her potential fetus, and foster risk management as needed. Therefore preconception and early pregnancy education fosters behaviors in potential parents to do the following:

- Establish lifestyle behaviors to maintain optimal health (e.g., eating a healthy diet, including sources of folic acid; getting enough rest and exercise; and avoiding alcohol use, smoking, and other drugs)
- Prepare psychologically for pregnancy and the responsibilities that come with parenthood and build a support system to sustain the new family throughout the perinatal year
- Identify, minimize, or treat risk factors before conception (e.g., medical conditions such as diabetes mellitus, substance abuse, use of medications for chronic illness, or infections, including STIs)
- Screen for health hazards in the workplace or home
- Obtain, when warranted, genetic counseling to identify carriers of inherited diseases (e.g., Tay-Sachs disease, sickle cell disease, or thalassemia)
- Compare the quality and philosophic bases of the perinatal care options available

The components of general preconception education such as health promotion, risk assessment, and interventions are outlined in Box 11-9.

All health-promoting education should be provided in a context that emphasizes how well designed a healthy body is to adapt to the changes that accompany pregnancy. Without this context of health, routine care and testing for risks may contribute to a mindset of families that pregnancy is a pathologic as opposed to a healthy mind-body-spirit event.

Previous pregnancy and childbirth experiences are important elements that influence current learning needs. The woman's (and support person's) age, cultural background, personal philosophy in regard to childbirth, socioeconomic status, spiritual beliefs, and learning styles all need to be assessed to develop the best plan to help the woman meet her needs.

Most childbirth education classes are attended by the pregnant woman and her partner, although a friend, teenage daughter, or parent may be the designated support person. Classes may also be held for grandparents and siblings to prepare them for their attendance at birth or the arrival of the

BOX 11-9 Components of Preconception Care

Health Promotion: General Teaching

Nutrition
- Healthy diet, including folic acid
- Optimal weight

Exercise and rest
Avoidance of substance abuse (tobacco, alcohol, "recreational" drugs)
Use of sex practices that reduce risk
Attending to family and social needs

Risk Factor Assessment

Medical history
- Immune status (e.g., rubella)
- Family history (e.g., genetic disorders)
- Illnesses (e.g., infections)
- Current use of medication (prescription, nonprescription, herbal)

Reproductive history
- Contraceptive
- Obstetric

Psychosocial history
- Spouse/partner and family situation, including domestic violence
- Availability of family or other support systems
- Readiness for pregnancy (e.g., age, life goals, stress)

Financial resources
Environmental (home, workplace) conditions
- Safety hazards
- Toxic chemicals
- Radiation

Occupational
- Sitting or standing for long periods
- Heavy lifting
- Work requiring fine motor skills or repetitive activities

Interventions as Indicated

Anticipatory guidance/teaching
Treatment of medical conditions and results
- Medications
- Cessation/reduction in substance use/abuse
- Immunizations (e.g., rubella, hepatitis)

Nutrition, diet, and weight management
Exercise
Referral for genetic counseling
Referral to and use of:
- Family planning services
- Family and social needs management

baby (see Fig. 11-4). Siblings often see a film about birth and learn ways they can help welcome the baby. They also learn to cope with changes that include a reduction in parental time and attention. Grandparents learn about current child-care practices and how to help their adult children adapt to parenting in a supportive way.

Perinatal Care Choices

The environment in which a woman gives birth is equally as influential as education about how to listen to and work with her body during childbirth. The Coalition to Improve Maternity Services (CIMS), a group of more than 50 nursing and maternity care–oriented organizations, produced a document to assist women in selecting their perinatal care. After some explanation of choices, women are encouraged to ask potential care providers the following questions:

- Who can be with me during labor and birth?
- What happens during a normal labor and birth in your setting?
- How do you allow for differences in culture and beliefs?
- Can I walk and move around during labor? What position do you suggest for birth?
- How do you make sure everything goes smoothly when my nurse, doctor, midwife, or agency work with each other?
- What things do you normally do to a woman in labor?
- How do you help mothers stay as comfortable as they can be? Besides drugs, how do you help mothers relieve the pain of labor?
- What if my baby is born early or has special problems?
- Do you circumcise babies?
- How do you help mothers who want to breastfeed?

The entire document can be downloaded from *www.motherfriendly.org*. CIMS has also produced a Mother-Friendly Childbirth Initiative with guidelines for identifying and designating "mother-friendly" birth sites, including hospitals, birth centers, and home-birth services. This information is available at the same website. CIMS identified several principles for mother-friendly services. They should do the following:

- Promote birth as a normal, natural, and healthy process
- Empower a woman to develop confidence in her ability to give birth and care for her baby
- Give the woman autonomy to make informed choices about the care she and her baby receive
- Do no harm by applying only medically necessary interventions
- Take responsibility for the quality of care provided, based on the needs of the mother and child

Childbirth Education

When one is prepared and well supported, childbirth presents to women a unique and powerful opportunity to find their core strength in a manner that forever changes their self-perception. Expectant parents and their families have different interests and information needs as the pregnancy progresses.

Early pregnancy ("early bird") classes provide fundamental information. Classes are developed around the following areas: (1) early fetal development, (2) physiologic and emotional changes of pregnancy, (3) human sexuality, and (4) the nutritional needs of the mother and fetus. Environmental and workplace hazards may be addressed. Exercises, nutrition, warning signs, drugs, and self-medication are topics of interest and concern.

Midpregnancy classes emphasize the woman's participation in self-management. Classes provide information on preparation for breastfeeding and formula feeding; infant care; basic hygiene; common complaints and simple, safe remedies; infant health; parenting; and updating and refining the birth plans (see Evidence-Based Practice box).

Late pregnancy classes emphasize labor and birth. Different methods of coping with labor and birth have been developed and are often the basis for various prenatal classes. These include Lamaze, Bradley, and Dick-Read. A hospital tour is usually included.

Throughout the series of classes there is discussion of support systems that people can use during pregnancy and after birth. Such support systems help parents function independently and effectively. During all the classes the open expression of feelings and concerns about any aspect of pregnancy, birth, and parenting is welcomed.

Fathers or partners often worry about their role during childbirth classes and labor and birth, as well as the safety of their partner and baby during the birth. Many fathers elect to participate actively during labor and the birth of their child (see Fig. 1-2). However, as noted earlier, some men, through personal or cultural conception of the father role, neither want nor intend to participate. It is important that the partners agree on each other's roles.

Current Practices in Childbirth Education

A variety of approaches to childbirth education have evolved as childbirth educators attempt to meet learning needs. In addition to classes designed specifically for pregnant adolescents, their partners, or parents, classes exist for other groups with special learning needs. These include classes for first-time mothers over age 35, single women, adoptive parents, and parents of twins. Refresher classes for parents with children not only review coping techniques for labor and birth but also help couples prepare for sibling reactions and adjustments to a new baby. Cesarean birth classes are offered for couples who have this kind of birth scheduled because of breech position or other risk factors. Other classes focus on vaginal birth after cesarean (VBAC) because many women successfully give birth vaginally after previous cesarean birth.

Strategies for Childbirth Education

Because of the multicultural composition of the population in North America, there is great diversity in attitudes, expectations, and behaviors judged appropriate during pregnancy and early parenthood. No one approach can meet all needs. For example, classes for new immigrants are particularly effective when taught in their first language (e.g., Spanish, Tagalog, Cantonese). For classes to be meaningful, parent educators must understand the value systems in other cultures and their influence on issues such as nutrition, exercise, valuing of early prenatal care, maternal weight gain, and infant feeding prac-

EVIDENCE-BASED PRACTICE The Usefulness of Prenatal Breastfeeding Education

—*Pat Gingrich*

Ask the Questions

Does prenatal education about breastfeeding promote initiating breastfeeding and continuing exclusive breastfeeding for 3 and 6 months? If so, what prenatal education strategies are most effective?

Search for Evidence

Search Strategies

Professional organization guidelines, meta-analyses, systematic reviews, randomized controlled trials, nonrandomized prospective studies, and retrospective studies since 2006

Databases Searched

CINAHL; Cochrane; Medline; and the websites for AWHONN, CDC, NICE, and the Academy of Breastfeeding Medicine

Critically Analyze the Evidence

After reviewing scientific literature indicating that health care provider attitude and ongoing support have significant impact on initiation and duration of exclusive breastfeeding, the Academy of Breastfeeding Medicine published a protocol calling for health care providers to discuss the benefits of breastfeeding, beginning with the first visit in the first trimester (Academy of Breastfeeding Medicine Protocol Committee, 2006). The guidelines encourage an ongoing conversation with the patient and her family about feeding plans, attitudes, and previous experiences. Both parents are encouraged to attend prenatal breastfeeding classes before making a decision. Educational materials should include written, nonformula-advertising materials and may also include visual aids, books, and videos.

A Cochrane Systematic Review of nine prenatal education trials totaling 2284 women found that the benefits and strategies of prenatal education are difficult to compare because of greatly differing interventions and outcome measures (Gagnon & Sandall, 2007). One particular challenge of studying this topic is the difficulty of randomizing women to the interventions or control, when randomization may contradict a woman's choice. The reviewers were not able to determine benefits or best strategies for prenatal education.

However, a subsequent randomized, controlled trial (RCT) of 450 healthy women in Singapore who were over 34 weeks of gestation demonstrated that breastfeeding initiation and duration were significantly improved if the women were given either a prenatal education session (video, individual instruction, and written materials) or two postnatal support sessions (individual instruction in hospital and at 2 weeks, with written materials) when compared to women receiving usual care (Su et al, 2007).

Group prenatal education sessions may also be both effective and efficient for the health care provider. In a more recent RCT of 1047 pregnant women, the participants randomized to receive weekly group educational and facilitated support sessions with their gestational peers from 18 weeks until term had significantly increased breastfeeding initiation, more prenatal knowledge, more readiness for labor and delivery, and increased satisfaction compared to women receiving usual treatment. There were no differences in costs, and birth weights remained similar. Interestingly, the women in the support group also had significantly fewer preterm births (Ickovics et al, 2007).

Implications for Practice

On balance the literature and expert opinion confirm the value of prenatal education for initiation and duration of exclusive breastfeeding. Especially for the primipara or the woman lacking social support for breastfeeding, it makes sense for the health care provider to start the dialogue early in pregnancy or possibly before pregnancy and use each contact to further educate the expectant family on the many benefits of breastfeeding. There is enough information to recommend combinations of individual instruction and noncommercial written and multimedia material. Group education sessions may provide cost-effective use of the educator's time, along with added emotional and social support for participating families at similar gestational ages.

References

Academy of Breastfeeding Medicine Protocol Committee: ABM clinical protocol No. 14: Breastfeeding-friendly physician's office. Part 1: Optimizing care for infants and children, *Breastfeed Med* 1(2):115-119, 2006.

Gagnon AJ, Sandall J: Individual or group antenatal education for childbirth or parenthood, or both. In *The Cochrane Database of Systematic Reviews* 2007, Issue 3, Chichester, UK, 2007, John Wiley & Sons.

Ickovics J R et al: Group prenatal care and perinatal outcomes: a randomized, controlled trial, *Obstet Gynecol* 110(2 Pt 1):330-339, 2007.

Su L-L et al: Antenatal education and postnatal support strategies for improving rates of exclusive breastfeeding: randomized controlled trial, *BMJ* 335(7620):596, 2007.

tices. Parent educators must establish rapport, be understood, and build on cultural practices, reinforcing the positive and promoting change only if a practice such as pica is directly harmful.

Options for Care Providers

Maternity care providers are typically split into two ideologic groups, with the medical model more oriented toward intervention and the midwifery model inclined to be more holistic and natural. There are many gradations between the two models of care; however, the emphasis of the former is on the use of technology versus an emphasis on health promotion and problem prevention by the latter.

Physicians (obstetricians, family practice physicians) attended 92% of births in the United States and Canada in 2005 (Martin et al, 2007). Physicians see low risk and high risk patients. Care often includes pharmacologic and medical management of problems and the early use of technologic procedures such as ultrasonography and amniocentesis. Family practice physicians may need backup by obstetricians if a specialist is needed for a problem such as cesarean birth. Almost all physicians manage births in a hospital setting.

Nurse-Midwives

Certified nurse-midwives are registered nurses with education in the two disciplines of nursing and midwifery. Throughout history midwives have held a holistic view of childbirth. They provide care for about 8% of the births in the United States (Martin et al, 2007). Nurse-midwives may practice with physicians or independently with an arrangement for physician backup. They usually see low risk obstetric patients. Care is often noninterventionist, and the woman and her family are encouraged to be active participants in the care. Nurse-midwives refer patients with complications to physicians. Most births are managed in hospital settings or alternative birth centers; a few may be managed in a home setting.

Direct-Entry Midwives

Direct-entry midwives (also called certified professional midwives) are trained in midwifery schools or universities as a profession distinct from nursing. In the United States their certification process is administered by the American College of Nurse-Midwives. They also refer the patients in whom problems develop to physicians. Increasing numbers of midwives in the United Kingdom and Ireland are in this category.

Independent Midwives

Independent midwives, who also may be called lay midwives, are nonprofessional caregivers. Their training varies greatly, from self-teaching to formal training. They manage about 1% of births in the United States. Patients who develop problems are referred to a physician. A majority of births are managed in the home setting. In many international settings lay midwives are called traditional birth attendants. Births are in the home.

Doula

A doula is professionally trained to provide labor or postpartum support, including physical, emotional, and informational support to women and their partners during labor and birth and in the postpartum period. The doula does not become involved with clinical tasks (Doulas of North America, 2008). Although the doula role originally developed as an assistant during labor, some women need assistance during the postpartum period. There are small but growing numbers of postnatal doulas who provide assistance to the new mother as she develops competence with infant care, feeding, and other maternal tasks.

Some childbirth educators serve in the doula role for those who attend their classes. Today many couples, no matter which type of childbirth classes they take, also employ a doula for labor or postpartum support. A Cochrane synopsis of 15 trials involving 12,791 women found that "continuous labor support like that provided by doulas reduces a woman's likelihood of having pain medication, increases her satisfaction and chances for spontaneous birth, and has no known risks" (Hodnett et al, 2007).

A doula typically meets with the mother and her partner before labor to ascertain their expectations and desires for the birth experience. With this information as her guide during labor and birth, the doula focuses her efforts on assisting the woman to achieve her goals. Working collaboratively with other health care providers and the woman's supportive individuals, the doula focuses efforts on assisting the woman and the couple to achieve their goals. See *www.dona.org* for information on how to support the father's participation in the birth and during the postpartum period. Box 11-10 provides questions to ask when interviewing a prospective doula.

BOX 11-10 Questions to Ask When Choosing a Doula

To discover the specific training, experience, and services offered by anyone who provides labor support, potential patients, nursing supervisors, physicians, midwives, and others should ask the following questions of that person:

- What training have you had?
- Tell me about your experience with birth, personally and as a doula.
- What is your philosophy about childbirth and supporting women and their partners through labor?
- May we meet to discuss our birth plans and the role you will play in supporting me through childbirth?
- May we call you with questions or concerns before and after the birth?
- When do you try to join women in labor? Do you come to our home or meet us at the hospital?
- Do you meet with us after the birth to review the labor and answer questions?
- Do you work with one or more backup doulas for times when you are not available? May we meet them?
- What is your fee?

From Doulas of North America: *Doulas of North America position paper: the birth doula's contribution to modern maternity care*, 2008. Available at www.dona.org/pdfs/position_papers/BIRTH%20Paper--%204%20page.pdf (accessed March 8, 2009).

Birth Plans

The birth plan is a natural evolution of a contemporary wellness-oriented lifestyle in which patients assume a level of responsibility for their own health. The birth plan is a tool with which parents can explore their childbirth options and choose those that are most important to them. The plan must be viewed as tentative since the realities of what is feasible may change as the actual labor and birth unfold. It is understood to be a preference list based on a best-case scenario.

It is useful for the nurse in a prenatal practice setting to initiate a discussion of choices and birth planning during the first and second prenatal visits. Some maternity practices provide printed material describing available options and giving answers to commonly asked questions, and tours of the birth setting are offered by almost all birthing facilities. The nurse can provide couples with pertinent information and make them aware of the various options for care and the advantages and consequences of each so they can begin making informed decisions. Early plans can be modified as the couple learns more details in their childbirth class.

The birth plan can serve as a means of open communication between the pregnant woman and her partner and also between the couple and health care providers. An early introduction to the idea of a birth plan allows the couple time to think about events or situations that could make their childbearing experience more meaningful and those they would prefer to avoid.

Topics for birth plan discussion and decision making may include any or all of the following:

Partner's participation: Attend prenatal visits? Childbirth and parent education classes? Present during labor? During birth? During cesarean birth?

Birth setting: Hospital delivery room or birthing room (if available)? A birthing center? Home?

Labor management: Walk around during labor? Use a rocking chair? Use a shower? Use a Jacuzzi, if available? Intermittent versus continuous use of an electronic fetal monitor? Have music or dimmed lighting? Have older children or other people present? Is telemetry monitoring available? Consider stimulation of labor? Consider medication—what kind?

Birth: Positions—Side-lying? On hands and knees, kneeling, or squatting? Use a birthing bed or delivery table? Will you be photographing, videotaping, or recording any of the labor or birth? Who would you like to be present—partner, older siblings, other family members, or friends? What do you know about the use of forceps? Episiotomies? Will your partner want to cut the umbilical cord?

Immediately after birth: Do you want to hold the baby right away? Breastfeed immediately?

Postpartum care: What kind of care do you anticipate—labor, delivery, recovery, postpartum room; mother-baby coupling? How long does your insurance company provide coverage for you to stay? Would you like to attend self-management classes, or do you prefer to get such information from videotapes? On which subjects?

Birth Setting Choices

With careful thought the concept of natural, family, or woman-centered maternity care can be implemented in any setting. The three primary options for birth settings today are the hospital, birth center, and home. Women consider several factors in choosing a setting for childbirth, including the preference of their health care provider, characteristics of the birthing unit, and preference of their third-party payer. Approximately 99% of all births in the United States take place in a hospital setting (Martin et al, 2007). However, the types of labor and birth services vary greatly, from the traditional labor and delivery rooms with separate postpartum and newborn units to in-hospital birthing centers where all or almost all care takes place in a single unit.

Labor, Delivery, Recovery, Postpartum (Birthing) Rooms

Labor, delivery, and recovery (LDR) and labor, delivery, recovery, and postpartum (LDRP) rooms offer families a comfortable, private space for childbirth (Fig. 11-23). Women are admitted to LDR units, labor and give birth, and spend the first 1 to 2 hours postpartum there for immediate recovery and to have time with their families to bond with their newborns. After this period of recovery the mothers and newborns are transferred to a postpartum unit and nursery or mother-baby unit for the duration of their stay. Care is provided by different nursing staff (e.g., labor and delivery nurses, postpartum nurses, nursery nurses). In some hospitals the same nurse provides care for both mothers and newborns (mother-baby or couplet care).

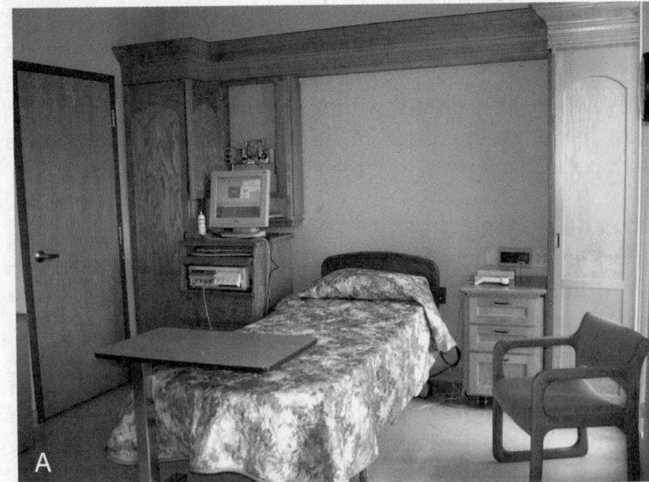

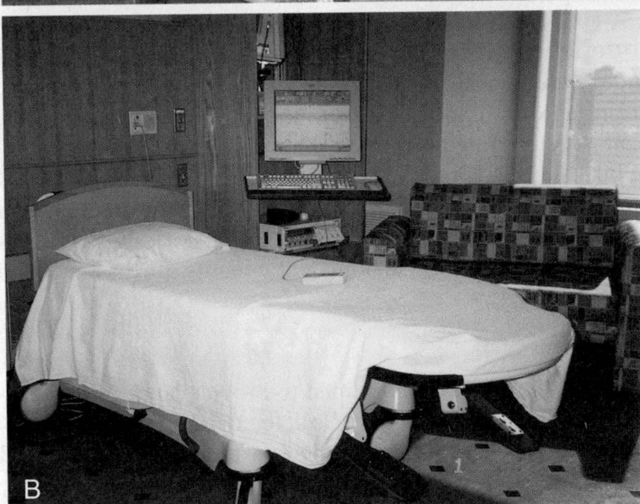

Fig. 11-23 A, Labor, delivery, and recovery unit. B, Labor, delivery, recovery, and postpartum unit. *(A, Courtesy Julie Perry Nelson, Loveland, CO. B, Courtesy Dee Lowdermilk, Chapel Hill, NC.)*

In LDRP units total care is provided from admission for labor through postpartum discharge in the same room and usually by the same nursing staff. The woman and her family may stay in this unit for 6 to 48 hours after giving birth. The units are furnished in a homelike atmosphere, similar to LDR units, but have accommodations for family members to stay overnight (see Fig. 11-23, *B*).

Both units are equipped with fetal monitors, emergency resuscitation equipment for both mother and newborn, and heated cribs or warming units for the newborn. Often this equipment is out of sight in cabinets or closets when it is not being used (see Fig. 11-23, *A*).

Birth Centers

Free-standing birth centers are usually built in locations separate from the hospital but may be located nearby in case transfer of the woman or newborn is needed. These birth centers are intended to offer families a safe and cost-effective alternative to hospital or home birth, providing a third choice that is a safe and cost-effective compromise. The centers are usually

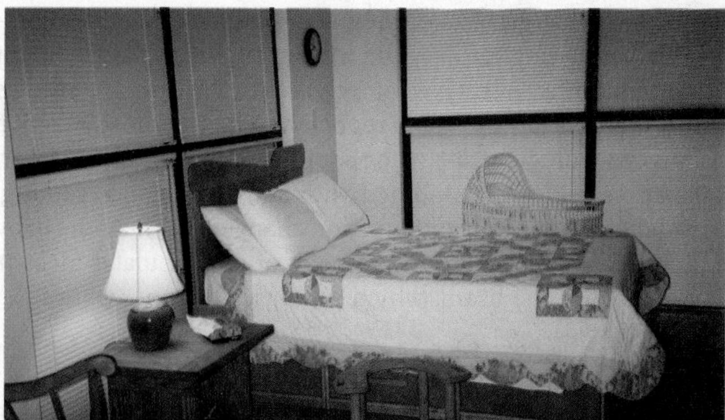

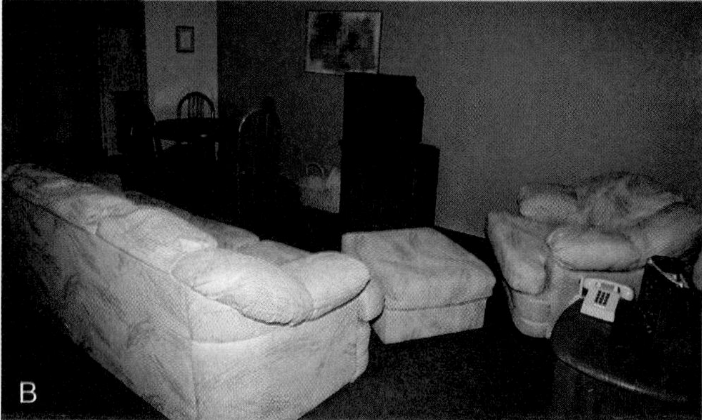

Fig. 11-24 Birth center. A, Note double bed, baby crib, and birthing stool. B, Lounge and kitchen. *(A, Courtesy Dee Lowdermilk, Chapel Hill, NC. B, Courtesy Michael S. Clement, MD, Mesa, AZ. Photo location: Bethany Birth Center, Phoenix, AZ.)*

staffed by nurse-midwives or physicians who also have privileges at the local hospital. Only women at low risk for complications are included for care.

Birth centers typically have homelike accommodations, including a double bed for the couple and a crib for the newborn (Fig. 11-24, *A*). Emergency equipment and drugs are available but stored out of view. Private bathroom facilities are incorporated into each birth unit. There may be an early labor lounge or a living room and small kitchen (see Fig. 11-24, *B*). The family is admitted to the birth center for labor and birth and will remain there until discharge, which often takes place within 6 hours of the birth.

Other services provided by the free-standing birth centers include those necessary for safe management during the childbearing cycle. Attendance at childbirth and parenting classes is required of all patients. Expectant families develop birth plans (i.e., the practices and procedures they would like to either include or exclude from their childbirth experience). Patients must understand that some situations require transfer to a hospital, and they must agree to abide by those guidelines.

Birth centers and hospitals with a comprehensive birthing program may have resources for parents such as a lending library that includes books and videotapes; reference files on related topics; recycled maternity clothes, baby clothes, and equipment; and supplies and reference materials for childbirth educators. The centers may also have referral files for community resources that offer services relating to childbirth and early parenting, including support groups (e.g., for single parents, postbirth support, and parents of twins), genetic counseling, women's issues, and consumer action.

When births occur in a birth center or a home setting, they should be located close to a major hospital so that quick transfer to that institution is possible when necessary. Ambulance service and emergency procedures must be readily available. Fees vary with the services provided but typically are less than or equal to those charged by local hospitals. Some base fees on the ability of the family to pay (a reduced-fee sliding scale). Several third-party payers, as well as Medicaid and the Civilian Health and Medical Programs of the Uniformed Services (TRICARE/CHAMPUS), recognize and reimburse these centers.

Home Birth

Home birth has always been popular in certain countries such as Sweden and The Netherlands. In developing countries hospitals or adequate lying-in facilities often are unavailable to most pregnant women, and home birth is a necessity. In North America home births account for less than 1% of births (Martin et al, 2005).

National groups supporting home birth are the Home-Oriented Maternity Experience and the National Association of Parents for Safe Alternatives in Childbirth *(www.napsac.org)*. These groups work to foster more humane childbearing practices at all levels, integrating the alternatives for childbirth to meet the needs of the total population.

With a home birth the family is in control of the experience, and the birth may be more physiologically natural in familiar surroundings (see Critical Thinking Exercise). The mother may be more relaxed than she would be in the hospital environment. The family can assist in and be a part of the birth, and the mother-father/partner-infant (and sibling-infant) contact is immediate and sustained. Home birth may be less expensive than a hospital confinement. Serious infection may be less likely (assuming strict aseptic principles are followed) because it is usual for people to be relatively immune to the bacteria in their own home.

Over time many studies have documented the safety of home births. Olsen and Jewell (1998) reported a metaanalysis of observational studies that found that planned home birth is safe, with fewer interventions than planned hospital births. Most recently the surveillance and risk assessment division in the Public Health Agency of Canada conducted a prospective cohort study involving certified professional midwives of 5418 births across the United Sates and Canada. Substantially lower rates of epidurals, episiotomies, forceps, vacuum extractions, and cesarean births occurred among them, including the 12% who were transferred to the hospital. No mothers died, and infant mortality was similar to rates of other low risk home and hospital births. Thus, although home births are considered countercultural by many in the United States, there is no evidence base to discourage low risk couples who desire a carefully planned out-of-the-hospital birth (Johnson & Daviss, 2005).

Components of Perinatal Education Programs

A variety of approaches to perinatal education beyond preparation for birth have evolved as educators attempt to meet

CRITICAL THINKING EXERCISE

Deciding About a Home Birth

Maxine, 37 years old and gravida 1, para 0, is interested in having a home birth. She has insulin-dependent diabetes. She is currently 14 weeks pregnant, and her pregnancy is progressing normally. According to an ultrasound examination she has one fetus of appropriate size for gestational age with no detectable anomalies. She asks a nurse on the obstetric clinic about how to find a midwife who will attend a home birth.

1. Evidence—Is there sufficient evidence to draw conclusions about the safety of a home birth for Maxine?
2. Assumptions—Describe an underlying assumption about each of the following issues:
   a. Assessments that are necessary to identify whether it is feasible and safe for Maxine to have a home birth
   b. Supports necessary for a home birth
   c. How to identify providers who are willing to attend a home birth
   d. Ethics of the nurse assisting Maxine to find a midwife who will attend a home birth
3. What implications and priorities for nursing care can be drawn at this time?
4. Does the evidence objectively support your conclusion?
5. Are there alternative perspectives to your conclusion?

learning and support needs of expectant parents and capitalize on the openness to learning they exhibit. For example, prenatal and new-mother weekly exercise classes can offer both physiologic and social support for a mixture of expectant and new mothers who may even elect to stay connected by e-mail for support between weekly classes. However, it is important that a focus on preparation for birth not become lost in all the topics that could be offered to expectant parents. Some of the additional topics mentioned below might fit well into a second-trimester class as part of an organized series for the perinatal year.

Pain Management

Fear of pain in labor is a key issue for pregnant women and the reason many give for attending childbirth education classes. Numerous studies show that women who have received childbirth preparation later report no less pain but do report greater ability to cope with the pain during labor and birth and increased birth satisfaction compared to unprepared women. Thus, although pain management strategies are an essential component of childbirth education, pain eradication is not the primary source of birth satisfaction. Control in childbirth (i.e., participation in decision making) has repeatedly been found to be the primary source of birth satisfaction. The advantages and disadvantages of pain medication for coping with labor are discussed in Chapter 16.

Relaxation

Relaxation or reduction of body tension is a technique suggested by virtually all childbirth education organizations. Learning relaxation in childbirth education classes can help couples with the stresses of pregnancy, childbirth, and adjustment to parenting and can be a form of stress management throughout life. A review of research across many studies found that relaxation skill is reported to be the most effective nonpharmacologic strategy for coping with the stress of labor. Relaxation is ideally combined with activity such as walking, slow dancing, rocking, and position changes that help the baby rotate through the pelvis. Rhythmic motion stimulates mechanoreceptors in the brain, which decreases pain perception.

Imagery and Visualization

Imagery and visualization also are taught in classes during preparation for birth. Although research on their use in childbirth is scant, clinical reports suggest that imagery and visualization can be used to produce a sense of well-being during pregnancy, assist with cervical dilation, and decrease the experience of pain and tension during labor. A variety of skills taught in childbirth classes augment relaxation during pregnancy and labor. All can be taught as lifetime skills useful to the couple and can be used to teach their children to cope with the stresses of life.

Conscious Breathing

Using conscious breathing patterns is a visible technique and thus is frequently used in the media to characterize childbirth preparation. Relaxed individuals automatically slow their breathing; conversely, slowing one's breathing serves to increase one's relaxation. During labor nursing support includes guiding couples in the application of breathing and relaxation methods and adapting methods to their particular needs.

Biofeedback

The use of observation in class (informal biofeedback) helps couples develop awareness of their bodies and learn strategies to change their responses to stress. During preparation for birth, formal biofeedback (which uses machines prenatally to detect skin temperature, blood flow, or muscle tension) can prepare women to perfect their relaxation response.

Energy Work, Massage, Music, and Acupressure

Energy work such as therapeutic touch or healing touch involves energy fields around the body and can be taught in class for use during labor to decrease anxiety and pain and increase relaxation. Certified practitioners in energy work are consulted throughout pregnancy and during childbirth by women who have access to such care.

Music promotes relaxation and has been known for centuries to be generally therapeutic. Acupressure, which consists of applying pressure to various pressure points, has been correlated with relief of dizziness, headaches, back pain, nausea, leg cramps, and labor pain. Massage has been shown in a randomized trial to decrease pain and anxiety during labor, and the husbands' participation in massage positively increases the experience for the woman.

Preparation for Cesarean Birth

Given that almost 30% of births in the United States are by cesarean surgery, this is an important topic for birth preparation education *(www.childbirth.org/section/ICAN)*. The expectant parents can be helped to know what they can do to avoid the necessity of a cesarean birth. Cesarean birth rates vary widely by care provider and care setting. They are more common in women who choose epidurals, in part because the powers of the mother's muscles do not effectively assist the infant in rotation through the pelvis; in part because, if given early, epidurals prolong labor; and in part because the mother has less urge to push. In a setting where nursing support during labor is low and care provider rate of cesarean birth is high, women should be aware that their chances of a cesarean birth are increased.

Effort can be directed to prevent the need for a subsequent cesarean or to prepare for it when it is inevitable or highly likely. Women with a prior cesarean birth can be encouraged to explore the availability of a vaginal birth, with the exception of those who have a history of classic vertical or unknown uterine incisions or those with medical contraindication. In many communities there are VBAC support groups, physicians who are known to be supportive, and special childbirth classes for those attempting a VBAC. Mothers can be prepared for the differences in postpartum recovery for women after a cesarean birth. Their hospital stay will be longer, their need for assistance at home will be greater, and they may need extra support to establish breastfeeding comfortably.

Childbirth Education Outcomes

The effects of childbirth education have consistently been shown to be in birth satisfaction, building confidence, and building relationships. Physiologic outcomes are not demonstrated to be strongly influenced by educating expectant parents. One reason for this finding may be that research has not focused on this. Many researchers treat childbirth education as a direct influence on the birth without considering the mediating influence of care providers' philosophy and their usual type of care. If considered, a more accurate evaluation of childbirth education influence on birth outcomes might be obtained.

Pregnancy is a time when expectant parents expect change in their lives and are open to many types of education. This education can enhance their health and coping skills in pregnancy, childbirth, and early parenting. It also can influence how they relate to health professionals over a lifetime, how they problem solve with each other, and how they launch their new family. It is an opportunity for nurses to engage in meaningful health promotion and the building of resilience and connection in families.

Key Points

- The prenatal period is a preparatory one, both physically and psychologically.
- Psychosocial aspects of care may affect pregnancy, childbirth, and the adjustment of the new family.
- The pregnant woman's readiness to learn is at a high level, making this an excellent time to help her expand her self-management skills.
- Maternal physical and familial adaptations to pregnancy generate needs that the nurse can anticipate and meet.
- Even with a normal pregnancy the nurse must remain alert to hazards such as supine hypotension, warning signs and symptoms, and signs of family maladaptations.
- Each pregnant woman needs to know how to recognize and report preterm labor.
- Parent-child, sibling-child, and grandparent-child relationships are affected by pregnancy.

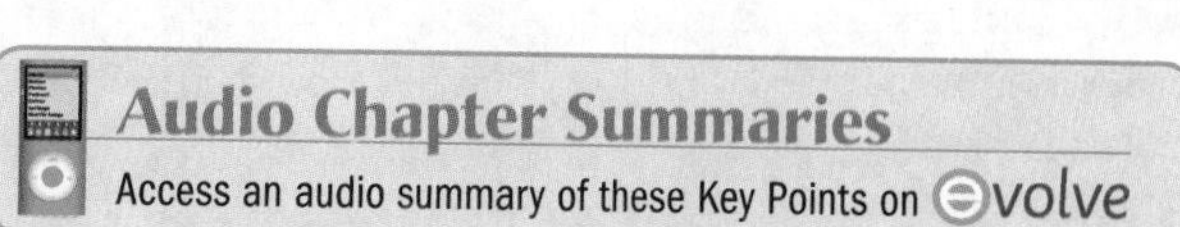
Audio Chapter Summaries
Access an audio summary of these Key Points on evolve

- Cultural prescriptions and proscriptions influence responses to pregnancy and to the health care delivery system.
- Childbirth education teaches tuning in to the body's inner wisdom and coping strategies that enhance women's ability to know how to give birth.
- Childbirth education is a process designed to help parents make the transition from the role of expectant parents to the role and responsibilities of parents of a new baby.

References

Barish R: In-flight radiation exposure during pregnancy, *Obstet Gynecol* 103(6):1326-1330, 2004.

Benzies K et al: Factors influencing women's decisions about timing of motherhood, *J Obstet Gynecol Neonatal Nurs* 35(5):625-633, 2006.

Boggess K et al: Maternal periodontal disease is associated with an increased risk for preeclampsia, *Obstet Gynecol* 101(2):227-231, 2003.

Carlson NS, Lowe NK: Centering pregnancy: a new approach to prenatal care, *MCN Am J Matern Child Nurs* 31(4):218-223, 2006.

Centers for Disease Control and Prevention, Workowski K, Berman S: Sexually transmitted diseases treatment guidelines, 2006, *MMWR Morb Mortal Wkly Rep* 55(RR-11):1-94, 2006.

Cleary-Goldman J, Chitkara U, & Berkowitz R: Multiple gestation. In Gabbe SG, Niebyl JR, Simpson JL: *Obstetrics: normal and problem pregnancies*, ed 5, Philadelphia, 2007, Churchill Livingstone.

Cunningham F et al: *Williams obstetrics*, ed 22, New York, 2005, McGraw Hill.

Doulas of North America: *Doulas of North America position paper: the birth doula's contribution to modern maternity care*, 2008. Available at www.dona.org/ (accessed March 8, 2009).

Elliott JP: Preterm labor in twins and high-order multiples, *Clin Perinatol* 34(4):599-609, 2007.

Fries M, Bashford M, Nunes M: Implementing prenatal screening for cystic fibrosis in routine obstetric practice, *Am J Obstet Gynecol* 192(2):527-534, 2006.

Gilbert ES: *Manual of high risk pregnancy & delivery*, ed 4, St Louis, 2007, Mosby.

Grady M, Bloom K: Pregnancy outcomes of adolescents enrolled in a Centering Pregnancy Program, *J Midwifery Womens Health* 49(5):412-420, 2004.

Hodnett E et al: Continuous support for women during childbirth, *The Cochrane Database of Systematic Reviews* 2007, Issue 3, CD003766.

Johnson K, Daviss B: Outcomes of planned home births and certified professional midwives: large prospective study in North America, *BMJ* 330(7505):1416, 2005.

Johnson TRB, Gregory KD, Niebyl JR: Preconception and prenatal care: part of the continuum. In Gabbe SG, Niebyl JR, Simpson JL: *Obstetrics: normal and problem pregnancies*, ed 5, Philadelphia, 2007, Churchill Livingstone.

Kehringer K: Informed consent: hospitals must obtain informed consent prior to drug testing pregnant patients, *J Law Med Ethics* 32(3):455-457, 2003.

Lawrence RA, Lawrence RM: *Breastfeeding: a guide for the medical profession*, ed 5, St Louis, 2005, Mosby.

Lopez R: Periodontal disease, preterm birth, and low birth weight, *Evid Based Dent* 6(4):90-91, 2005.

March of Dimes Birth Defects Foundation: *PeriStats: born too soon and too small in the United States*, 2005. Available at www.marchofdimes.com/peristats (accessed August 3, 2008).

Martin JA et al: Births: final data for 2003, *Natl Vital Stat Rep* 54(2):1-116, 2005.

Martin JA et al: Births: final data for 2005, *Natl Vital Stat Rep* 56(6):1-104, 2007.

Martin JA et al: Annual summary of vital statistics: 2006, *Pediatrics* 121(4):788-801, 2008.

May KA: A typology of detachment and involvement styles adopted during pregnancy by first-time expectant fathers, *West J Nurs Res* 2(2):444-461, 1980.

May KA: Three phases of father involvement in pregnancy, *Nurs Res* 31(6):337-342, 1982.

McPheeters M et al: The epidemiology of threatened preterm labor: a prospective cohort study, *Am J Obstet Gynecol* 192(4):1325-1330, 2005.

Mercer R: *Becoming a mother*, New York, 1995, Springer.

Montan S: Increased risk in the elderly parturient, *Curr Opin Obstet Gynecol* 19(2):110-112, 2007.

Niebyl JR, Simpson JL: Drugs and environmental agents in pregnancy and lactation: embryology, teratology, epidemiology. In Gabbe SG, Niebyl JR, Simpson JL (editors): *Obstetrics: normal and problem pregnancies*, ed 5, Philadelphia, 2007, Churchill Livingstone.

Olsen O, Jewell M: Home versus hospital birth, *The Cochrane Database of Systematic Reviews* 1998, Issue 3, CD000352.

Resnik R, Creasy RK: Intrauterine growth restriction. In Creasy RK et al (editors): *Creasy & Resnik's maternal-fetal medicine: principles and practice*, ed 6, Philadelphia, 2009, Saunders.

Rising S: Centering pregnancy: an interdisciplinary model of empowerment, *J Nurse-Midwifery* 43(1): 46-54, 1998.

Rubin R: Maternal tasks in pregnancy, *Matern Child Nurs J* 4(3):143-153, 1975.

Rubin R: *Maternity identity and the maternal experience*, New York, 1984, Springer.

Seidel HM et al: *Mosby's guide to physical examination*, ed 6, St Louis, 2006, Mosby.

Simpson JL, Otaño L: Prenatal genetic diagnosis. In Gabbe SG, Niebyl JR, Simpson JL, *Obstetrics: normal and problem pregnancies*, ed 5, Philadelphia, 2007, Churchill Livingstone Elsevier.

US Public Health Service: *Caring for our future: the content of prenatal care*, Washington, DC, 1989, Department of Health and Human Services.

Weng X, Odouli R, Li D: Maternal caffeine consumption during pregnancy and the risk of miscarriage: a prospective cohort study, *Am J Obstet Gynecol* 198(3):279.e1-8, 2008.

Westheimer R, Lopater S: *Human sexuality: a psychosocial perspective*, ed 2, Philadelphia, 2005, Lippincott Williams & Wilkins.

Unit 3

12 Maternal and Fetal Nutrition

Learning Objectives

On completion of this chapter the reader will be able to:

- Explain recommended maternal weight gain during pregnancy.
- Compare the recommended level of intake of energy sources, protein, and key vitamins and minerals during pregnancy and lactation.
- Give examples of the food sources that provide the nutrients required for optimal maternal nutrition during pregnancy and lactation.
- Examine the role of nutrition supplements during pregnancy.
- List five nutritional risk factors during pregnancy.
- Compare the dietary needs of adolescent and mature pregnant women.
- Analyze examples of eating patterns of women from two different ethnic or cultural backgrounds and identify potential dietary problems.
- Assess nutritional status during pregnancy.

Electronic Resources

Additional information related to the content in Chapter 12 can be found on

evolve the Companion Website at

http://evolve.elsevier.com/Perry/maternal/

- NCLEX Review Questions
- Critical Thinking Exercise—Nutrition Education
- Nursing Care Plan—Nutrition During Pregnancy
- Spanish Guidelines—Diet and Nutrition

Nutrition is one of the many factors that influence the outcome of pregnancy (Fig. 12-1). However, maternal nutritional status is an especially significant factor, both because it is potentially alterable and because good nutrition before and during pregnancy is an important preventive measure for a variety of problems. These problems include birth of low-birth-weight (LBW) (birth weight of 2500 g or less) and preterm infants. Neonatal and infant death rates for moderately LBW infants (1500 to 2499 g) are five times higher than that of infants born weighing more than 2500 g; the risk for very LBW (VLBW) infants (less than 1500 g) is more than 100 times that of infants born weighing 2500 g or more (Hoyert et al, 2006). Thus it is essential that the importance of good nutrition be emphasized to all women of childbearing potential. Nutrition assessment, intervention, and evaluation must be an integral part of the nursing care given to all pregnant women.

Nutrient Needs Before Conception

The first trimester of pregnancy is a crucial one for embryonic and fetal organ development. A healthful diet before conception is the best way to ensure that adequate nutrients are available for the developing fetus. Folate or folic acid intake is of particular concern in the periconceptual period. Folate is the form in which this vitamin is found naturally in foods, and folic acid is the form used in fortification of grain products and other foods and in vitamin supplements. Neural tube defects (failure in closure of the neural tube) are more common in infants of women with poor folic acid intake. Proper closure of the neural tube is required for normal formation of the spinal cord, and the neural tube begins to close within the first month of gestation, often before the woman realizes that she is pregnant. It is estimated that the incidence of neural tube defects could be decreased by as much as 70% if all women had an adequate folate intake during the periconceptual period (Cornel, Smit, & de Jong-van den Berg, 2005). All women capable of becoming pregnant are advised to consume 0.4 mg (400 mcg) of folic acid daily in fortified foods (ready-to-eat cereals and enriched grain products) or supplements and a diet rich in folate-containing foods such as green leafy vegetables, whole grains, and fruits (Box 12-1).

Both maternal and fetal risks in pregnancy are increased when the mother is significantly underweight or overweight when pregnancy begins. Ideally all women would achieve their desirable body weights before conception.

Nutrient Needs During Pregnancy

Nutrient needs are determined, at least in part, by the stage of gestation. The amount of fetal growth varies during the different stages of pregnancy. During the first trimester the synthesis of fetal tissues places relatively few demands on maternal nutrition. Therefore during the first trimester, when the embryo or fetus is very small, the needs are only slightly

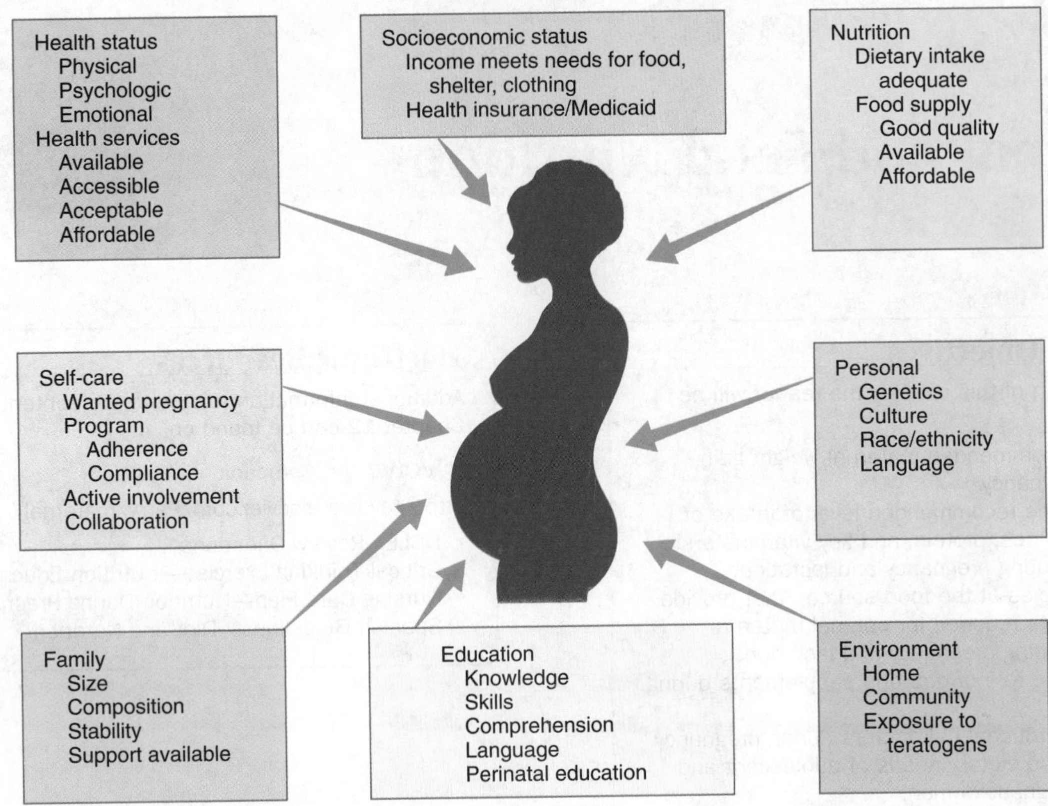

Fig. 12-1 Factors that influence the outcome of pregnancy.

BOX 12-1 Food Sources of Folate

Foods Providing 500 mcg or More per Serving

Liver: chicken, turkey, goose (3.5 oz)

Foods Providing 200 mcg or More per Serving

Liver: lamb, beef, veal (3.5 oz)

Foods Providing 100 mcg or More per Serving

Legumes, cooked (½ cup)
Peas: black-eye, chickpea (garbanzo)
Beans: black, kidney, pinto, red, navy
Lentils
Vegetables (½ cup)
Asparagus
Spinach, cooked
Papaya (1 medium)
Breakfast cereal, ready-to-eat (½ to 1 cup)
Wheat germ (¼ cup)

Foods Providing 50 mcg or More per Serving

Vegetables (½ cup)
Broccoli
Beans: lima beans, baked beans, or pork and beans
Greens: collards or mustard, cooked
Spinach, raw
Fruits (½ cup)
Avocado
Orange or orange juice
Pasta, cooked (1 cup)
Rice, cooked (1 cup)

Foods Providing 20 mcg or More per Serving

Bread (1 slice)
Egg (1 large)
Corn (½ cup)

increased over those before pregnancy. In contrast, the last trimester is a period of noticeable fetal growth when most of the fetal stores of energy sources and minerals are deposited. Thus, as fetal growth progresses during the second and third trimesters, the pregnant woman's need for some nutrients increases greatly.

The Food and Nutrition Board of the National Academy of Sciences publishes recommendations for the people of the United States, the Dietary Reference Intakes (DRIs) (*www.iom.edu*). The DRIs consist of Recommended Dietary Allowances (RDAs), Adequate Intakes (AIs), and Upper Limits (ULs) (i.e., guidelines for avoiding excessive intakes of nutrients that may be toxic if consumed in excess). RDAs for some nutrients have been available for many years, and they have been revised periodically. They are recommendations for daily nutritional intakes that meet the needs of almost all (97% to 98%) of the healthy members of the population. AIs are similar to the RDAs and are believed to cover the needs for virtually all healthy individuals in a group, except that they deal with nutrients for which there are not enough data to be certain of their requirements. The RDAs and AIs include a wide variety of nutrients and food components; they are divided into age, sex, and life-stage categories (e.g., infancy, pregnancy, and lactation). They can be used as goals in planning the diets of individuals (Table 12-1).

Energy Needs

Energy (kilocalories or kcal) needs are met by carbohydrate, fat, and protein in the diet. No specific recommendations exist for the amount of carbohydrate and fat in the diet of the pregnant women. However, intake of these nutrients should be

Table 12-1 Recommendations for Daily Intakes of Selected Nutrients During Pregnancy and Lactation

NUTRIENT (units)	RECOMMENDATION FOR NONPREGNANT WOMAN	RECOMMENDATION FOR PREGNANCY*	RECOMMENDATION FOR LACTATION*	ROLE IN RELATION TO PREGNANCY AND LACTATION	FOOD SOURCES
Energy (kilocalories [kcal] or kilojoules [kJ]†)	Variable	First trimester, same as nonpregnant; second trimester, nonpregnant needs + 81 kcal (340 kJ); third trimester, nonpregnant needs + 108 kcal (452 kJ)	First 6 mo, nonpregnant needs + 79 kcal (330 kJ); second 6 mo, nonpregnant needs + 55 kcal (230 kJ)	Growth of fetal and maternal tissues; milk production	Carbohydrate, fat, and protein
Protein (g)	46	First trimester, same as nonpregnant; second and third trimesters, nonpregnant needs + 25 g‡	Nonpregnant needs + 25 g	Synthesis of the products of conception; growth of maternal tissue and expansion of blood volume; secretion of milk protein during lactation	Meats, eggs, cheese, yogurt, legumes (dry beans and peas, peanuts), nuts, grains
Water (L)	2.7 total (2.2 in beverages)	3 total (2.3 in beverages)	3.8 total (3.1 in beverages)	Expansion of blood volume, excretion of wastes; milk secretion	Water and beverages made with water, milk, juices; all foods, especially frozen desserts, fruits, lettuce and other fresh vegetables
Fiber (g)	25	28	29	Promote regular bowel elimination; reduce long-term risk of heart disease, diverticulosis, and diabetes	Whole grains, bran, vegetables, fruits, nuts and seeds
Minerals					
Calcium (mg)	1300/1000	1300/1000	1300/1000	Fetal and infant skeleton and tooth formation; maintenance of maternal bone and tooth mineralization	Milk, cheese, yogurt, sardines or other fish eaten with bones left in; deep green leafy vegetables except spinach or Swiss chard; calcium-set tofu, baked beans, tortillas
Iron (mg)	15/18	30	10/9	Maternal hemoglobin formation; fetal liver iron storage	Liver, meats, whole grain or enriched breads and cereals, deep green leafy vegetables, legumes, dried fruits
Zinc (mg)	98	12/11	11/12	Component of numerous enzyme systems; possibly important in preventing congenital malformations	Liver, shellfish, meats, whole grains, milk
Iodine (mcg)	150	220	290	Increased maternal metabolic rate	Iodized salt, seafood, milk and milk products, commercial yeast breads, rolls, and donuts

Continued

Table 12-1 Recommendations for Daily Intakes of Selected Nutrients During Pregnancy and Lactation—cont'd

NUTRIENT (units)	RECOMMENDATION FOR NONPREGNANT WOMAN	RECOMMENDATION FOR PREGNANCY*	RECOMMENDATION FOR LACTATION*	ROLE IN RELATION TO PREGNANCY AND LACTATION	FOOD SOURCES
Magnesium (mg)	360/310-320	400/350-360	360/310-320	Involved in energy and protein metabolism, tissue growth, muscle action	Nuts, legumes, cocoa, meats, whole grains
Fat-Soluble Vitamins					
A (mcg)	700	750/770	1200/1300	Essential for cell development, tooth bud formation, bone growth	Deep green leafy vegetables, dark yellow vegetables, fruits, chili peppers, liver, fortified margarine and butter
D (mcg)	5	5	5	Involved in absorption of calcium and phosphorus; improves mineralization	Fortified milk and margarine, egg yolk, butter, liver, seafood
E (mg)	15	15	19	Antioxidant (protects cell membranes from damage), especially important for preventing breakdown of RBCs	Vegetable oils, green leafy vegetables, whole grains, liver, nuts and seeds, cheese, fish
K (mcg)	90	75 (14-18 yr old) 90 (19-50 yr old)	75 (14-18 yr old) 90 (19-50 yr old)	Involved in synthesis of protein, blood coagulation, and bone metabolism	Green leafy vegetables, plant oils, margarine, soybeans, lentils
Water-Soluble Vitamins					
C (mg)	65/75	80/85	115/120	Tissue formation and integrity, formation of connective tissue; enhancement of iron absorption	Citrus fruits, strawberries, melons, broccoli, tomatoes, peppers, raw deep green leafy vegetables
Folate (mcg)	400	600	500	Prevention of neural tube defects, support for increased maternal RBC formation	Fortified ready-to-eat cereals and other grain products, green leafy vegetables, oranges, broccoli, asparagus, artichokes, liver
B_6 or pyridoxine (mg)	1.2/1.3	1.9	2	Involved in protein metabolism	Meats, liver, deep green vegetables, whole grains
B_{12} (mcg)	2.4	2.6	2.8	Production of nucleic acids and proteins; especially important in formation of RBC and neural functioning	Milk and milk products, eggs, meats, liver, fortified soy milk

Sources: Institute of Medicine: *Dietary reference intakes for energy, carbohydrate, fiber, fat, fatty acids, cholesterol, protein, and amino acids*, Washington, DC, 2002, National Academies Press; Institute of Medicine: *Dietary reference intakes: applications in dietary planning*, Washington, DC, 2003, National Academies Press; and Institute of Medicine: *Dietary reference intakes for water, potassium, sodium, chloride, and sulfate*, Washington, DC, 2004, National Academies Press.

RBC, Red blood cell.

*When two values appear, separated by a diagonal slash, the first is for females younger than 19 years, and the second is for those 19 to 50 years of age.

†The international metric unit of energy measurement is the joule (J). 1 kcal = 4.184 kJ.

‡Add an additional 25 g in twin pregnancies.

adequate to support the recommended weight gain. Although protein can be used to supply energy, its primary role is to provide amino acids for the synthesis of new tissues (see discussion later in this chapter). The estimated energy expenditure for the first trimester is the same as in the prepregnant state; during the second trimester the RDA is 340 kcal greater than the prepregnancy needs, and during the third trimester it is 462 kcal more than the prepregnant needs (Institute of Medicine, 2003). Longitudinal assessment of weight gain during pregnancy is the best way to determine whether the kilocalorie intake is adequate; very underweight or active women may require more than the recommended increase in kilocalories to sustain the desired rate of weight gain.

Weight Gain

The optimal weight gain during pregnancy is not known precisely. However, it is known that the amount of weight gained by the mother during pregnancy has an important bearing on the course and outcome of pregnancy. Although adequate weight gain does not necessarily indicate that the diet is nutritionally adequate, it is associated with a reduced risk of giving birth to a small-for-gestational-age (SGA) or preterm infant.

The desirable weight gain during pregnancy varies among women. The primary factor to consider in making a weight gain recommendation is the appropriateness of the prepregnancy weight for the woman's height (see Box 12-3). Maternal and fetal risks in pregnancy are increased when the mother is either significantly underweight or overweight before pregnancy and when weight gain during pregnancy is either too low or too high. Severely underweight women are more likely to have preterm labor and to give birth to LBW infants. Women with inadequate weight gain have an increased risk of giving birth to an infant with intrauterine growth restriction (IUGR). Greater-than-expected weight gain during pregnancy may occur for many reasons, including multiple gestation, edema, preeclampsia, and overeating. When obesity is present (either preexisting or developed during pregnancy), there is an increased likelihood of macrosomia and fetopelvic disproportion; operative birth; emergency cesarean birth; postpartum hemorrhage; wound, genital tract, or urinary tract infection; birth trauma; and late fetal death. Obese women are more likely than normal-weight women to have preeclampsia and gestational diabetes.

A commonly used method of evaluating the appropriateness of weight for height is the body mass index (BMI), which is calculated by the following formula:

$$\text{BMI} = \text{Weight} \div \text{Height}^2$$

where the weight is in kilograms and height is in meters. Thus for a woman who weighed 51 kg before pregnancy and is 1.57 m tall:

$$\text{BMI} = 51\text{ kg} \div (1.57\text{ m})^2\text{, or } 20.7$$

Prepregnant BMI can be classified into the following categories: less than 18.5, underweight or low; 18.5 to 24.9, normal; 25 to 29.9, overweight or high; and greater than 30, obese *(www.nhlbisupport.com/bmi/)*. This website also contains a BMI table so that calculating the BMI is not necessary.

Pattern of Weight Gain

Weight gain should take place throughout pregnancy. The risk of delivering an SGA infant is greater when the weight gain early in pregnancy has been poor. The likelihood of preterm birth is greater when the gains during the last half of pregnancy have been inadequate. These risks exist even when the total gain for the pregnancy is in the recommended range.

The optimal rate of weight gain depends on the stage of pregnancy. During the first and second trimesters growth takes place primarily in maternal tissues; during the third trimester growth occurs primarily in fetal tissues (Fig. 12-2).

In multiple gestations weight gain during the first half of pregnancy appears to be especially important (Luke, 2005). For the first trimester of twin gestation, a gain of 0.3 to 0.8 kg a week has been associated with positive outcomes. This general goal should be adjusted for prepregnancy weight (i.e., 0.6 to 0.8 kg weekly for underweight women and 0.3 to 0.6 kg weekly for obese women). Similarly, during mid-pregnancy in twin gestation, recommended weekly weight gains are 0.45 to 0.9 kg, with the lower value for obese women and the higher for underweight women. During late pregnancy weekly gains of 0.3 to 0.6 kg are recommended for the woman pregnant with twins (Luke, 2005).

The recommended energy (kcal) intake corresponds to the recommended pattern of gain. For the first trimester there is no increment; an additional 340 kcal per day and 462 kcal per day over the prepregnant intake during the second and third trimester, respectively, are recommended. The amount of food providing the needed increase is not great. The 340 additional kcal needed during the second trimester can be provided by one additional serving from any one of the following groups: milk, yogurt, or cheese (all skim milk products); fruits; vegetables; and bread, cereal, rice, or pasta. In the third trimester, an additional one-third serving will provide the needed kilocalories.

The reasons for an inadequate weight gain (less than 1 kg per month for normal-weight women or less than 0.5 kg per month for obese women during the last two trimesters) or excessive weight gain (more than 3 kg per month) should be evaluated thoroughly. Possible reasons for deviations from the expected rate of weight gain, besides inadequate or excessive dietary intake, include measurement or recording errors, differences in weight of clothing, time of day, and accumulation of fluids. An exceptionally high gain is likely to be caused by an accumulation of fluids; and a gain of more than 3 kg in a month, especially after the twentieth week of gestation, often indicates the development of preeclampsia.

Hazards of Restricting Adequate Weight Gain

An obsession with thinness and dieting pervades the North American culture. Figure-conscious women may find it difficult to make the transition from guarding against weight gain before pregnancy to valuing weight gain during pregnancy. In counseling these women the nurse can emphasize both the positive effects of good nutrition and the adverse effects of

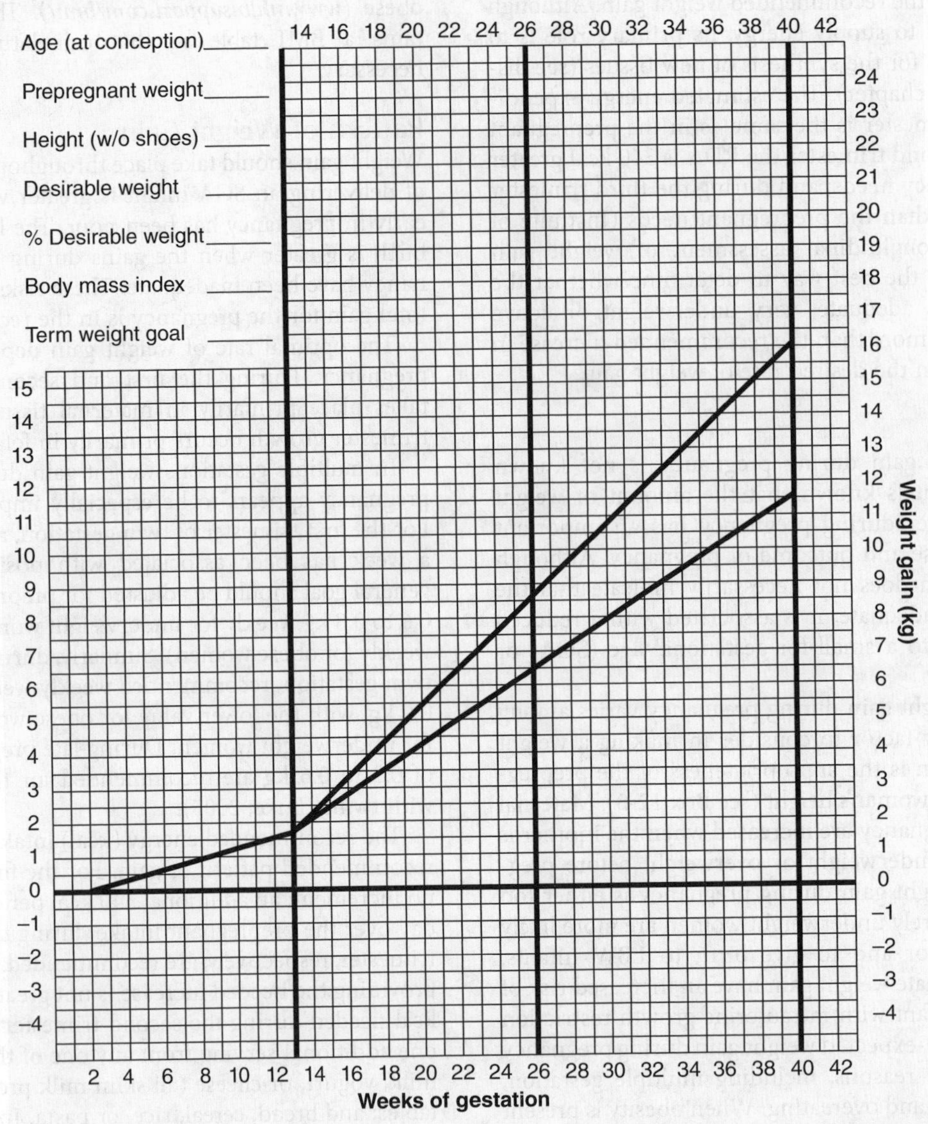

Fig. 12-2 Prenatal weight gain chart for plotting weight gain of normal-weight women. NOTE: Young adolescents, African-American women, and smokers should aim for the upper end of the recommended range; short women (less than 157 cm) should strive for gains at the lower end of the range.

maternal malnutrition (manifested by poor weight gain) on infant growth and development. This counseling includes information on the components of weight gain during pregnancy (Table 12-2) and the amount of this weight that will be lost at birth. Because lactation can help to reduce maternal energy stores gradually, this also provides an opportunity to promote breastfeeding.

In the United States 20% of women who give birth are obese (Paul, 2008). However, pregnancy is not a time for weight reduction. Even overweight or obese pregnant women need to gain at least enough weight to equal the weight of the products of conception (fetus, placenta, and amniotic fluid). If overweight women limit their energy intake to prevent weight gain, they may also excessively limit their intake of important nutrients. Moreover, dietary restriction results in

Table 12-2 Tissues Contributing to Maternal Weight Gain at 40 Weeks of Gestation

TISSUE	WEIGHT (lb)
Fetus	7-8.5
Placenta	2-2.5
Amniotic fluid	2
Increase in uterine tissue	2
Breast tissue	1-4
Increased blood volume	4-5
Increased tissue fluid	3-5
Increased stores (fat)	4-6

catabolism of fat stores, which in turn augments the production of ketones. The long-term effects of mild ketonemia during pregnancy are not known, but ketonuria has been found to be correlated with the occurrence of preterm labor. It should be stressed to obese women (and to all pregnant women) that the quality of the weight gain is important, with emphasis placed on the consumption of nutrient-dense foods and the avoidance of empty-calorie foods (see Critical Thinking Exercise).

CRITICAL THINKING EXERCISE

Nutrition and the Overweight Pregnant Woman

Tamara, age 27, of African-American and Asian heritage, is 3 months pregnant and comes to her initial appointment for diagnosis and care. She appears to be overweight for her height (5 foot 6 inches tall, 172 lb). To provide optimal care for her, you plan to calculate her prepregnancy body mass index. When her pregnancy is confirmed, you are asked to plan a diet with Tamara that meets the minimum daily requirements and allows for growth of the pregnancy. You know that it is important to include consideration of personal preferences and cultural factors in your plan. With Tamara, identify barriers to implementing the plan.

1. Evidence—Is there sufficient evidence to draw conclusions about an appropriate nutrition plan, taking into consideration personal preferences and cultural factors?
2. Assumptions—Describe underlying assumptions about each of the following issues:
   a. Dietary Reference Intakes for pregnancy and lactation
   b. Indicators of nutritional risk in pregnancy; possibility of lactose intolerance
   c. Daily food guide for pregnancy and lactation
   d. Sources of calcium for women who do not drink milk
3. What implications and priorities for nursing care can be drawn at this time?
4. Does the evidence objectively support your conclusion?
5. Are there alternative perspectives to your conclusion?

Weight gain is important, but pregnancy is not an excuse for uncontrolled dietary indulgence. The woman should place an emphasis on the quality of her food intake as she considers her needs and those of her fetus. Excessive weight gained during pregnancy may be difficult to lose after pregnancy, thus contributing to chronic overweight or obesity, an etiologic factor in a host of chronic diseases, including hypertension, diabetes mellitus, and arteriosclerotic heart disease. The woman who gains 18 kg or more during pregnancy is especially at risk. Food energy intake and particularly intake of fat is likely to be high among pregnant women, especially low-income women.

Protein

Protein, with its essential constituent nitrogen, is the nutrition element basic to growth. Adequate protein intake is essential to meet increasing demands in pregnancy. These demands arise from the rapid growth of the fetus; the enlargement of the uterus and its supporting structures, the mammary glands, and the placenta; an increase in maternal circulating blood volume and subsequent demand for increased amounts of plasma protein to maintain colloidal osmotic pressure; and the formation of amniotic fluid.

Milk, meat, eggs, and cheese are complete-protein foods with a high biologic value. Legumes (dried beans and peas), whole grains, and nuts are also valuable sources of protein. In addition, these protein-rich foods are a source of other nutrients such as calcium, iron, and B vitamins; plant sources of protein often provide needed dietary fiber. The recommended daily food plan (Table 12-3) is a guide to the amounts of these foods that would supply the quantities of protein needed. The recommendations provide for only a modest increase in protein intake over the prepregnant levels in adult women.

Protein intake in many people in the United States is relatively high; thus many women need not increase their protein intake at all during pregnancy. Three servings of milk, yogurt, or cheese (four for adolescents) and 5 to 6 oz (140 to 168 g) (two servings) of meat, poultry, or fish supply the recommended protein for the pregnant woman. Additional protein is provided by vegetables and breads, cereals, rice, and pasta. Pregnant adolescents, women from impoverished backgrounds, and women adhering to unusual diets such as a macrobiotic (highly restricted vegetarian) diet are those most likely to have inadequate protein intake. The use of high-protein supplements is not recommended because these have been associated with an increased incidence of preterm births.

When choosing fish, pregnant and nursing women should be especially careful to select those that are low in mercury.

NURSING ALERT High levels of mercury can harm the developing nervous system of the fetus or young child, and certain fish are especially high in mercury. Women who may become pregnant, women who are pregnant or nursing, and young children need to follow some precautions: (1) avoid eating shark, swordfish, king mackerel, and tilefish; (2) check local advisories about the safety of fish caught by family and friends in local bodies of water, but if no advisory is available, limit intake of these fish to 6 oz and eat no other fish that week; and (3) eat as much as 12 oz/wk of a variety of commercially caught fish and shellfish low in mercury such as shrimp, salmon, pollock, catfish, and canned light tuna (but limit intake of albacore or "white" tuna and tuna steaks, which contain more mercury, to 6 oz/wk). Additional information about mercury levels in a variety of commercial fish is available at *www.cfsan.fda.gov/~frf/sea-mehg.html*.

Fluids

Essential during the exchange of nutrients and waste products across cell membranes, water is the main substance of cells, blood, lymph, amniotic fluid, and other vital body fluids. It also aids in maintaining body temperature. A good fluid intake promotes regular bowel function; constipation is sometimes a problem during pregnancy. The recommended daily intake is about 8 glasses (2 L) of fluid. Water, milk, and juices are good sources. Foods in the diet should supply an

Table 12-3 Daily Food Guide for Pregnancy and Lactation

FOOD GROUP	SERVING SIZE	NONPREGNANT, NONLACTATING WOMAN	PREGNANT WOMAN	LACTATING WOMAN
		Suggested Number of Servings		
Grain Products Include whole-grain and enriched breads, cereals, pasta, and rice.	1 slice bread; ½ bun, bagel, or English muffin; 1 oz ready-to-eat cereal; ½ cup cooked grains	6-11	6-11	6-11
Vegetables Eat dark green leafy and deep yellow often. Eat dried beans and peas often; count ½ cup cooked dried beans or peas as a serving of vegetables or 1 oz from meat group.	1 cup raw leafy greens; ½ cup of others	3-5	3-5	3-5
Fruits Include citrus fruits, strawberries, or melons frequently.	1 medium apple, orange, banana, peach, etc; ½ cup small or diced fruit; ¾ cup juice	2-4	2-4	2-4
Milk and Milk Products	1 cup milk or yogurt; 1½ oz cheese	2-3	≥3	≥4
Meat, Poultry, Fish, Dry Beans, Nuts, and Eggs Eat peanut butter or nuts rarely to avoid excessive fat intake. Limit egg intake to reduce cholesterol intake; trim fat from meat, and remove skin from poultry.	½ cup cooked dried beans, 1 egg, or ½ tbsp peanut butter is equivalent to 1 oz of meat	Up to 6 oz total	≤6 oz total	≤6 oz total

additional 700 ml or more of fluid. Dehydration may increase the risk of cramping, contractions, and preterm labor.

Caffeine in moderate amounts has not been proven to cause adverse effects during pregnancy. However, women who consume more than 300 mg of caffeine daily (equivalent to about 3 cups of coffee) may be at increased risk of miscarriage and giving birth to infants with IUGR. The ill effects of caffeine have been proposed to result from vasoconstriction of the blood vessels supplying the uterus or from interference with cell division in the developing fetus. Consequently caffeine-containing products such as caffeinated coffee, tea, soft drinks, and cocoa beverages should be avoided or consumed only in limited quantities.

Aspartame (NutraSweet, Equal), acesulfame potassium (Sunett), and sucralose (Splenda), artificial sweeteners commonly used in low- or no-calorie beverages and low-calorie food products, have not been found to have adverse effects on the normal mother or fetus and therefore are approved by the U.S. Food and Drug Administration (FDA) for use during pregnancy. Aspartame, which contains phenylalanine, should be avoided by pregnant women with phenylketonuria (PKU) (Box 12-2). Stevia (stevioside) is a sweetener that has not been approved by the FDA.

Minerals, Vitamins, and Electrolytes

In general the nutrient needs of pregnant women, except perhaps the need for folate and iron, can be met through dietary sources. Counseling about the need for a varied diet rich in vitamins and minerals should be a part of every pregnant woman's early prenatal care and should be reinforced throughout pregnancy. Supplements of certain nutrients are recommended when the woman's diet is very poor or when significant nutritional risk factors are present. Nutritional risk factors in pregnancy are listed in Box 12-3 (see Evidence-Based Practice box).

Iron

Iron is needed both to allow transfer of adequate iron to the fetus and to permit expansion of the maternal red blood cell (RBC) mass. However, poor iron intake and absorption, which can result in iron deficiency anemia, is relatively common among women in the childbearing years. Iron deficiency (not necessarily anemia) is estimated to affect approximately 10% of nonpregnant women in the childbearing years in the United States. Anemic women are poorly prepared to tolerate hemorrhage at the time of birth. In addition, women who have iron deficiency anemia during early pregnancy are at increased risk of preterm birth. Iron deficiency during the third trimester apparently does not carry the same risk. In the United States anemia is most common among adolescents, African-American women, and women of lower socioeconomic status.

The RDA of iron during pregnancy is 27 mg per day (Office of Dietary Supplements, 2007). Pregnant women should receive a supplement of 30 mg of ferrous iron daily, starting by 12 weeks of gestation. (Iron supplements may be poorly tolerated during the nausea that is prevalent in the first trimester.) Iron supplementation of women with iron deficiency can improve maternal hematologic indices and appears to reduce LBW births. If maternal iron deficiency anemia is present (preferably diagnosed by measurement of serum ferritin, a storage form of iron), increased dosages (60 to 120 mg daily) are recommended. Certain foods taken with an iron supplement can promote or inhibit absorption of iron from the supplement. See the Patient Teaching box later in the chapter regarding iron supplementation. Even when a woman is taking an iron supplement, she should include good food sources of iron in her daily diet (see Table 12-1).

Calcium

There is no increase in the DRI of calcium during pregnancy and lactation compared to the recommendation for the non-

BOX 12-2 Use of Artificial Sweeteners During Pregnancy

All of the following sweeteners are approved for use in all age groups, including pregnant women, in the United States:

Acesulfame K

Brand names—Sunett, Sweet One
Primary uses—Baked goods, frozen desserts, candies, beverages
Sweetness—200 times sweeter than sugar
Shelf life—Long
Suitability for cooking—Good; does not break down when heated
Health concerns—None known

Aspartame

Brand names—Equal, NutraSweet, NatraTaste
Primary uses—Beverages, frozen desserts, dairy products, chewing gum, breakfast cereals, table-top sweetener
Sweetness—180 times sweeter than sugar
Shelf life—Relatively short (about 5 months in a soft drink)
Suitability for cooking—Breaks down and loses sweetness if cooked at high temperatures or for long periods
Health concerns—Contains phenylalanine, a consideration in the diets of people with phenylketonuria

Neotame

Brand names—None (not currently available)
Primary uses—Approved in the United States but not currently marketed; proposed use in beverages, frozen desserts, yogurt, chewing gum, toppings, fillings, fruit spreads, table-top sweetener
Sweetness—8000 times sweeter than sugar
Shelf life—Similar to aspartame (about 5 months in a soft drink)
Suitability for cooking—Good, but loses sweetness if cooked at high temperatures or for prolonged periods
Health concerns—None known; contains phenylalanine but not in a form that can be metabolized

Saccharin

Brand name—Sweet'n Low
Primary uses—Fountain drinks, chewable vitamins and medications, table-top sweetener
Sweetness—300 times sweeter than sugar
Shelf life—Long
Suitable for cooking—Good, does not lose sweetness during cooking
Health concerns—Linked to bladder cancer in rats

Sucralose

Brand name—Splenda
Primary uses—Baked goods, beverages, frozen desserts, gelatins, table-top sweetener
Sweetness—600 times sweeter than sugar
Shelf life—Long
Suitability for cooking—Very good; does not break down during cooking (maltodextrin is added to give products better bulk and texture)
Health concerns—None known

Sugar Alcohols (Not Technically Artificial Sweeteners; Contain Almost as Many Calories as Sugar)

Types—Sorbitol, xylitol, lactitol, mannitol, and maltitol
Primary uses—Sugar-free candy, cookies, and chewing gum
Sweetness—Most are about 70% as sweet as sugar; xylitol equals sugar in sweetness
Shelf life—Long
Suitability for cooking—Good
Advantages over sugar—Do not promote tooth decay; more slowly metabolized so that they do not create a rapid peak in blood glucose
Health concerns—Diarrhea can occur with large intakes

NOTE: Sugar is important for the volume and moisture of baked goods. Artificial sweeteners may produce a good-tasting product, but some sugar is necessary in many recipes to yield normal volume and texture.

BOX 12-3 Indicators of Nutritional Risk in Pregnancy

- Adolescence
- Frequent pregnancies: three within 2 years
- Poor fetal outcome in a previous pregnancy
- Poverty
- Poor diet habits with resistance to change
- Use of tobacco, alcohol, or drugs
- Weight at conception under or over normal weight
- Problems with weight gain
- Any weight loss
- Weight gain of less than 1 kg/mo after the first trimester
- Weight gain of more than 1 kg/wk after the first trimester
- Multifetal pregnancy
- Low hemoglobin or hematocrit values (or both)

pregnant woman (see Table 12-1). The DRI (1000 mg daily for women 19 years and older and 1300 mg for those younger than 19 years) appears to provide sufficient calcium for fetal bone and tooth development to proceed while maintaining maternal bone mass.

Milk and yogurt are especially rich sources of calcium, providing approximately 300 mg per cup (240 ml). Nevertheless, many women do not consume these foods or do not consume adequate amounts to provide the recommended intakes of calcium. One problem that can interfere with milk consumption is lactose intolerance, the inability to digest milk sugar (lactose) caused by the lack of the lactase enzyme in the small intestine. Lactose intolerance is relatively common in adults, particularly African-Americans, Asians, Native Americans, and Inuits (Alaska Natives). Milk consumption can cause abdominal cramping, bloating, and diarrhea in such people, although many lactose-intolerant individuals can tolerate small amounts of milk without symptoms. Yogurt, sweet acidophilus milk, buttermilk, cheese, chocolate milk, and cocoa

EVIDENCE-BASED PRACTICE Nutrition Supplements Other Than Folic Acid That Promote Optimal Health During Pregnancy

—Pat Gingrich

Ask the Question

In addition to folic acid, what nutrition supplements should be recommended to pregnant women?

Search for Evidence

Search Strategies

Professional organization guidelines, meta-analyses, systematic reviews, randomized controlled trials, nonrandomized prospective studies, and retrospective studies since 2006

Databases Searched

CINAHL; Cochrane; Medline; National Guideline Clearinghouse; and the websites for AWHONN, CDC, and NICE

Critically Analyze the Evidence

The National Institute of Health and Clinical Evidence clinical guidelines for prenatal care included the recommendation that all women be informed about the importance of vitamin D supplementation, especially for women with darker skin, low vitamin D diets, obesity, or low sun exposure (National Institute for Health and Clinical Excellence, 2008). By facilitating the absorption of calcium, vitamin D prevents rickets and may protect against preeclampsia. Calcium is known to decrease the risk of preeclampsia by half, especially for women with risk factors of low dietary calcium (Hofmeyr, Duley, & Atallah, 2007).

Norwegian women who were given vitamin A lowered their risk for delivering babies with cleft palate (Johansen et al, 2008).

Since preeclampsia is a result of oxidative stress, it has been suggested that antioxidants may be protective. However, a Cochrane systematic review of 10 trials involving 6533 women found that vitamins C and E, selenium, and lycopene supplements did not result in any improvement in preeclampsia, preterm birth, small-for-gestational-age status, or perinatal death (Rumbold et al, 2008).

Another Cochrane review of 17 trials involving more than 9000 women revealed that zinc supplementation in pregnancy may reduce preterm births in areas of high perinatal mortality, but there is no evidence of benefit in other settings (Mahomed, Bhutta, & Middleton, 2007). The reviewers recommend a more comprehensive approach to dietary nutrition in pregnancy rather than focusing on specific micronutrients.

Implications for Practice

Good nutrition is essential to good health, especially in pregnancy. Although certain micronutrients may go in and out of scientific favor, women from low-resource areas will most benefit themselves and their fetuses with comprehensive vitamin and mineral supplementation and dietary adequacy and variety. Women at risk for certain conditions can benefit from additional protective micronutrients such as vitamin D and calcium to decrease the risk of preeclampsia.

References

Hofmeyr GJ, Duley L, Atallah A: Dietary calcium supplementation for prevention of pre-eclampsia and related problems: a systematic review and commentary, *Br J Obstet Gynecol* 1114:933-943, 2007.

Johansen AM et al: Maternal dietary intake of vitamin A and risk of orofacial clefts: a population-based case-control study in Norway, *Am J Epidemiol* 167(10):1164-1170, 2008.

Mahomed K, Bhutta Z, Middleton P: Zinc supplementation for improving pregnancy and infant outcome. In *The Cochrane Database of Systematic Reviews* 2007, Issue 2, Chichester, UK, 2007, John Wiley & Sons.

National Institute for Health and Clinical Excellence: *Antenatal care: routine care for the healthy pregnant woman, NICE Clinical Guideline 62*, London, 2008, NICE. Available at www.nice.org.uk/nicemedia/pdf/CG062NICEguideline.pdf (accessed June 22, 2008).

Rumbold A et al: Antioxidants for preventing pre-eclampsia. In *The Cochrane Database of Systematic Reviews* 2007, Issue 3. Chichester, UK, 2008, John Wiley & Sons.

may be tolerated even when fresh fluid milk is not. Commercial lactase supplements (e.g., Lactaid) are widely available to consume with milk. Many supermarkets stock lactase-treated milk. The lactase in these products hydrolyzes, or digests, the lactose in milk, making it possible for lactose-intolerant people to drink milk.

In some cultures adults rarely drink milk. For example, Puerto Ricans and other Hispanic people may use milk only as an additive in coffee. Pregnant women from these cultures may need to consume nondairy sources of calcium (Box 12-4). Vegetarian diets may also be deficient in calcium. If calcium intake appears low and the woman does not change her dietary habits despite counseling, a daily supplement containing 600 mg of elemental calcium may be needed. Calcium supplements may also be recommended when a pregnant woman experiences leg cramps caused by an imbalance in the calcium-to-phosphorus ratio. Bone meal supplements are not recommended in pregnancy (Box 12-5).

Magnesium

Diets of women in the childbearing years are likely to be low in magnesium, and as many as half of pregnant and lactating women may have inadequate intakes (Institute of Medicine, 2004). Adolescents and low-income women are especially at risk. Dairy products, nuts, whole grains, and green leafy vegetables are good sources of magnesium.

Sodium

During pregnancy the need for sodium increases slightly, primarily because the body water is expanding (e.g., the expanding blood volume). Sodium is essential for maintaining body water balance. In the past dietary sodium was routinely restricted in an effort to control the peripheral edema that commonly occurs during pregnancy. It is now recognized that moderate peripheral edema is normal in pregnancy, occurring as a response to the fluid-retaining effects of elevated levels of estrogen. Severe sodium restriction may make it difficult for pregnant women to achieve an adequate diet. Grain, milk, and meat products, which are good sources of nutrients needed during pregnancy, are significant sources of sodium. In addition, sodium restriction may stress the adrenal glands and the kidney as they attempt to retain adequate sodium. In general, sodium restriction is necessary only if the woman has a medical condition such as

BOX 12-4 Calcium Sources for Women Who Do Not Drink Milk

Each of the following provides approximately the same amount of calcium as 1 cup of milk:

Fish
3 oz can of sardines
4½ oz can of salmon (if bones are eaten)

Beans and Legumes
3 cups of cooked dried beans
2½ cups of refried beans
2 cups of baked beans with molasses
1 cup of tofu (calcium is added in processing)

Greens
1 cup of collards
1½ cups of kale or turnip greens

Baked Products
3 pieces of cornbread
3 English muffins
4 slices of French toast
2 waffles (7 inches in diameter)

Fruits
11 dried figs
1⅛ cups of orange juice with calcium added

Sauces
3 oz of pesto sauce
5 oz of cheese sauce

BOX 12-5 Complementary and Alternative Therapies

Bone meal, which is sometimes used as a calcium source by pregnant women, is frequently found to be contaminated with lead. Lead freely crosses the placenta; thus regular maternal intake of bone meal may result in high levels of lead in the fetus.

Reference: Shannon M: Severe lead poisoning in pregnancy, *Ambul Pediatr* 3(1):37-39, 2003.

renal or liver failure or hypertension that warrants such a restriction.

Excessive intake of sodium is discouraged during pregnancy just as it is in nonpregnant women because it may contribute to development of hypertension in salt-sensitive individuals. An adequate sodium intake for pregnant and lactating women, as well as nonpregnant women in the childbearing years, is estimated to be 1.5 g/day, with a recommended upper limit of intake of 2.3 g/day (Institute of Medicine, 2003). Table salt (sodium chloride) is the richest source of sodium, with approximately 2.3 g of sodium contained in 1 tsp (6 g) of salt. Most canned foods contain added salt unless the label states otherwise. Large amounts of sodium are also found in many processed foods, including meats (e.g., smoked or cured meats, cold cuts, and corned beef), frozen entrees and meals, baked goods, mixes for casseroles or grain products, soups, and condiments. Products low in nutritive value and excessively high in sodium include pretzels, potato and other chips (except salt free), pickles, catsup, prepared mustard, steak and Worcestershire sauces, some soft drinks, and bouillon. A moderate sodium intake can usually be achieved by salting food lightly in cooking; adding no additional salt at the table; and avoiding low-nutrient, high-sodium foods.

Potassium

Diets including adequate intakes of potassium are associated with reduced risk of hypertension. Potassium has been identified as one of the nutrients most likely to be lacking in the diets of women of childbearing years (Institute of Medicine, 2004). A diet including 8 to 10 servings of unprocessed fruits and vegetables daily, along with moderate amounts of low-fat meats and dairy products, has been effective in reducing sodium intake while providing adequate amounts of potassium.

Zinc

Zinc is a constituent of numerous enzymes involved in major metabolic pathways. Zinc deficiency is associated with malformations of the central nervous system in infants. When large amounts of iron and folic acid are consumed, the absorption of zinc is inhibited, and serum zinc levels are reduced as a result. Because iron and folic acid supplements are commonly prescribed during pregnancy, pregnant women should be encouraged to consume recommended sources of zinc daily (see Table 12-1). Women with anemia who receive high-dose iron supplements also need supplements of zinc and copper.

Fluoride

There is no evidence that prenatal fluoride supplementation reduces the child's likelihood of tooth decay during the preschool years. No increase in fluoride intake over the nonpregnant DRI is currently recommended during pregnancy (Institute of Medicine, 2003).

Fat-Soluble Vitamins

Fat-soluble vitamins—A, D, E, and K—are stored in the body tissues. These are of special concern during pregnancy because vitamin E intake is among the nutrients most likely to be lacking in the diets of women of childbearing age and intake of vitamins A and D is also low in the diets of some women (Institute of Medicine, 2004). With chronic overdoses these vitamins can reach toxic levels. Because of the high potential for toxicity, pregnant women are advised to take fat-soluble vitamin supplements only as prescribed.

Adequate intake of vitamin A is needed so that sufficient amounts of the vitamin can be stored in the fetus. A well-chosen diet, including adequate amounts of deep yellow and deep green vegetables and fruits such as leafy greens, broccoli, carrots, cantaloupe, and apricots, provides sufficient amounts of carotenes that can be converted in the body to vitamin A. Congenital malformations have occurred in infants of mothers who took excessive amounts of preformed vitamin A (from supplements) during pregnancy; thus supplements are not recommended for pregnant women. Vitamin A analogs such as isotretinoin (Accutane), which are prescribed for the treatment of cystic acne, are a special concern. Isotretinoin use during early pregnancy has been associated with an increased incidence of heart malformations, facial abnormalities, cleft palate, hydrocephalus, and deafness and blindness in the infant, as well as an increased risk of miscarriage. Topical agents such as tretinoin (Retin-A) do not appear to enter the circulation in any substantial amounts, but their safety in pregnancy has not been confirmed.

Vitamin D plays an important role in absorption and metabolism of calcium. The main food sources of this vitamin are enriched or fortified foods such as milk and ready-to-eat cereals. Vitamin D is also produced in the skin by the action of ultraviolet light (in sunlight). Severe deficiency may lead to neonatal hypocalcemia and tetany, as well as to hypoplasia of the tooth enamel. Women with lactose intolerance and those who do not include milk in their diet for any reason are at risk for vitamin D deficiency. Other risk factors are dark skin; habitual use of clothing that covers most of the skin (e.g., Moslem women with extensive body covering); and living in northern latitudes where sunlight exposure is limited, especially during the winter. Use of recommended amounts of sunscreen with a sun protection factor (SPF) rating of 15 or greater reduces skin vitamin D production by as much as 99%, thus bringing about a need for regular intake of fortified foods or a supplement.

Vitamin E is needed for protection against oxidative stress, and pregnancy is associated with increased oxidative stress. Indeed, oxidative stress has been proposed as an explanation for the etiology of preeclampsia (Allen, 2005). Vegetable oils and nuts are especially good sources of vitamin E, and whole grains and green leafy vegetables are moderate sources.

Vitamin K is involved in the synthesis of proteins involved in blood coagulation and bone metabolism. The AI for men is 120 mcg/day and for women 90 mcg/day. The classic sign of vitamin K deficiency is an increase in prothrombin time; severe cases result in hemorrhage. Food sources are green leafy vegetables, plant oils and margarine, and soybeans and lentils.

Water-Soluble Vitamins

Body stores of water-soluble vitamins are much smaller than those of fat-soluble vitamins. In contrast to fat-soluble vitamins, water-soluble vitamins are readily excreted in the urine. Therefore recommended sources of these vitamins must be consumed frequently. Toxicity with overdose is less likely than with fat-soluble vitamins.

Folate or Folic Acid

Because of the increase in RBC production during pregnancy and the nutrition requirements of the rapidly growing cells in the fetus and placenta, pregnant women should consume about 50% more folic acid than nonpregnant women, between 0.4 mg (400 mcg) and 0.6 mg (600 mcg) daily. In the United States all enriched grain products (which includes most white breads, flour, and pasta) must contain folic acid at a level of 1.4 mg/kg of flour. This level of fortification is designed to supply approximately 0.1 mg of folic acid daily in the average American diet and has significantly increased folic acid consumption in the population as a whole. All women of childbearing potential need careful counseling about including good sources of folate in their diets (see Box 12-1). Supplemental folic acid is usually prescribed to ensure that intake is adequate. Women who have borne a child with a neural tube defect are advised to consume 4 mg (4000 mcg) of folic acid daily, and a supplement is required for them to achieve this level of intake.

Pyridoxine

Pyridoxine, or vitamin B_6, is involved in protein metabolism. Although levels of a pyridoxine-containing enzyme have been reported to be low in women with preeclampsia, there is no evidence that supplementation prevents or corrects the condition. No supplement is recommended routinely, but women with poor diets and those at nutritional risk (see Box 12-3) may need a supplement providing 2 mg/day. Pyridoxine has been effective in reducing the nausea and vomiting of early pregnancy in some trials.

Vitamin C

Vitamin C, or ascorbic acid, plays an important role in tissue formation and enhances the absorption of iron. The vitamin C needs of most women are readily met by a diet that includes at least one daily serving of citrus fruit or juice or another good source of the vitamin (see Table 12-1), but women who smoke need more. For women at nutritional risk, a supplement of 50 mg/day is recommended. However, if the mother takes excessive doses of this vitamin during pregnancy, a vitamin C deficiency may develop in the infant after birth.

Vitamin B_{12}

Vitamin B_{12} is involved in production of nucleic acids and proteins; it is especially important in formation of RBCs and neural functioning. It is found in milk and milk products, eggs, meats, liver, and fortified soy milk.

Multivitamin-Multimineral Supplements During Pregnancy

Food can and should be the normal vehicle to meet the additional needs imposed by pregnancy, except for iron. In addition, the recommended folate/folic acid intake may be difficult for some women to achieve. Some women habitually consume diets that are deficient in necessary nutrients and for whatever reason may be unable to change this intake. For these women a multivitamin-multimineral supplement should be considered to ensure that they consume the RDA for most known vitamins and minerals. It is important that the pregnant woman understand that the use of a vitamin-mineral supplement does not lessen the need to consume a nutritious, well-balanced diet.

Other Nutritional Issues During Pregnancy

Pica and Food Cravings

Pica, the practice of consuming nonfood substances (e.g., clay, dirt, and laundry starch) or excessive amounts of foodstuffs low in nutritional value (e.g., cornstarch, ice or freezer frost, baking powder, and baking soda), is often influenced by the woman's cultural background (Fig. 12-3). In the United States it appears to be most common among African-American women, women from rural areas, and women with a family history of pica. Regular and heavy consumption of low-

evolve Spanish Guidelines–Diet and Nutrition

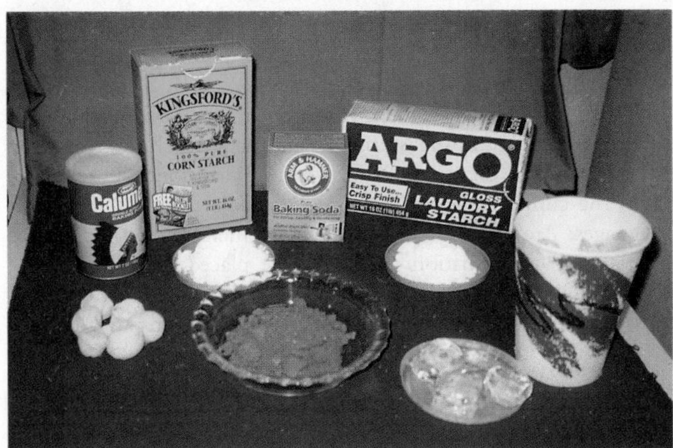

Fig. 12-3 Nonfood substances consumed in pica: red clay from Georgia, Nzu from Eastern Nigeria, baking powder, corn starch, baking soda, laundry starch, and ice. Some individuals practice poly-pica (consuming more than one of these substances). *(Courtesy Shannon Perry, Phoenix, AZ.)*

nutrient products may cause more nutritious foods to be displaced from the diet, and the items consumed may interfere with the absorption of nutrients, especially minerals. As an example, cornstarch ingestion is popular among African-American women. It is a source of "empty" calories; half a cup (64 g) provides 240 kcal (57 kJ) but almost no vitamins, minerals, or protein. Grotegut and colleagues (2006) reported a case of a 31-week gestation multigravida ingesting a box of baking soda (454 g of sodium bicarbonate) each day, which resulted in severe hypokalemic metabolic alkalosis and rhabdomyolysis. More than one substance may be ingested (Ngozi, 2008). Women with pica have lower hemoglobin levels than those without pica.

Moreover, there is a risk that nonfood items are contaminated with heavy metals or other toxic substances. Among Mexican-American women, consumption of "tierra" includes both soil and pulverized Mexican pottery (Klitzman et al, 2002; Shannon, 2003). Lead contamination of soils and soil-based products has caused high levels of lead in both pregnant women and their newborns. Regular household use of Mexican pottery in cooking or serving food or ingestion of ground pottery must be included in interviews or questionnaires regarding nutrition intake of pregnant women. The possibility of pica must be considered when pregnant women are found to be anemic, and the nurse should provide counseling about the health risks associated with pica (Corbett, Ryan, & Weinrich, 2003).

The existence of pica and details of the types and amounts of products ingested are likely to be discovered only by the sensitive interviewer who has developed a relationship of trust with the woman. It has been proposed that pica and food cravings (e.g., the urge to have ice cream, pickles, or pizza) during pregnancy are caused by an innate drive to consume nutrients missing from the diet. However, research has not supported this hypothesis.

Adolescent Pregnancy Needs

Many adolescent females have diets that provide less than the recommended intakes of key nutrients, including energy, calcium, and iron. Pregnant adolescents and their infants are at increased risk of complications during pregnancy and parturition. Growth of the pelvis is delayed in comparison with growth in stature, and this helps to explain why cephalopelvic disproportion and other mechanical problems associated with labor are common among young adolescents. Competition for nutrients between the growing adolescent and the fetus may also contribute to some of the poor outcomes apparent in teen pregnancies. Pregnant adolescents are encouraged to choose a weight gain goal at the upper end of the range for their BMI.

Efforts to improve the nutritional health of pregnant adolescents focus on improving the nutrition knowledge, meal planning, and selection and food preparation skills of young women; promoting access to prenatal care; developing nutrition interventions and educational programs that are effective with adolescents; and striving to understand the factors that create barriers to change in the adolescent population.

Preeclampsia

The cause of preeclampsia is not known. There has been speculation that the poor intake of several nutrients, including calcium, magnesium, vitamin B_6, and protein, might foster its development. There is no definite evidence that nutrition deficiencies are causes or that nutrition supplements can help prevent it. At present, a diet adequate in the recommended nutrients (see Table 12-1) appears to be the best means of reducing the risk of preeclampsia.

Physical Activity During Pregnancy

Moderate exercise during pregnancy yields numerous benefits, including improving muscle tone, potentially shortening the course of labor, and promoting a sense of well-being. If no medical or obstetric problems contraindicate physical activity, pregnant women should obtain 30 minutes of moderate physical exercise on most, if not all, days of the week. Two nutritional concepts are especially important for women who choose to exercise during pregnancy. First, a liberal amount of fluid should be consumed before, during, and after exercise because dehydration can trigger premature labor. Second, the calorie intake should be sufficient to meet the increased needs of pregnancy and the demands of exercise.

Nutrient Needs During Lactation

Nutrition needs during lactation are similar in many ways to those during pregnancy (see Table 12-1). Needs for energy (calories), protein, calcium, iodine, zinc, the B vitamins (thiamine, riboflavin, niacin, pyridoxine, and vitamin B_{12}), and vitamin C remain greater than nonpregnant needs. The recommendations for some of these (e.g., vitamin C, zinc, and protein) are slightly-to-moderately higher than during pregnancy (see Table 12-1). This allowance covers the amount of the nutrients released in the milk, as well as the needs of the mother for tissue maintenance. In the case of iron and folic acid, the recommendation during lactation is lower than during pregnancy. Both of these nutrients are essential for RBC formation and thus for maintaining the increase in the blood volume that occurs during pregnancy. With the decrease in maternal blood volume to nonpregnant levels after birth, maternal iron and folic acid needs also decrease. Many lactating women have a delay in the return of menses; this conserves blood cells and also reduces iron and folic acid needs. It is especially important that the calcium intake be adequate; if it is not and the woman does not respond to nutrition counseling, a supplement of 600 mg of calcium per day may be needed.

The recommended energy intake for the first 6 months is an increase of 330 kcal more than the woman's nonpregnant intake. It is difficult to obtain adequate nutrients for maintenance of lactation if total caloric intake is less than 1800 kcal. Because of the deposition of energy stores, the woman who has gained the optimal amount of weight during pregnancy is heavier after birth than at the beginning of pregnancy. However, as a result of the caloric demands of lactation, the lactating mother usually experiences a gradual but steady weight loss. Most women rapidly lose several pounds during the first month after birth, whether or not they breastfeed. After the first month the average loss during lactation is 0.5 to 1 kg a month. A woman who is overweight may be able to lose up to 2 kg without decreasing her milk supply.

Fluid intake must be adequate to maintain milk production, but the mother's level of thirst is the best guide to the right amount. There is no need to consume more fluids than those needed to satisfy thirst.

Smoking, alcohol intake, and excessive caffeine intake should be avoided during lactation. Smoking can impair milk production, and it exposes the infant to the risk of passive smoking. It is speculated that the infant's psychomotor development may be affected by maternal alcohol use, and alcoholic beverages (two drinks per day) may impair the milk ejection reflex. Caffeine intake can lead to a reduced iron concentration in milk and consequently contribute to the development of anemia in the infant. The caffeine concentration in milk is only approximately 1% of the mother's plasma level, but caffeine seems to accumulate in the infant. Breastfed infants of mothers who drink large amounts of coffee or caffeine-containing soft drinks may be unusually active and wakeful.

Nursing Care Management

During pregnancy nutrition plays a key role in achieving an optimal outcome for the mother and her unborn baby (see Nursing Process box). Motivation to learn about nutrition is usually higher during pregnancy as parents strive to "do what's right for the baby." Optimal nutrition cannot eliminate all problems that may arise during pregnancy, but it does establish a good foundation for supporting the needs of the mother and her unborn baby (see Community Focus box).

evolve Critical Thinking Exercise–Nutrition Education

Diet History

A diet history is a description of the woman's usual food and beverage intake and factors affecting her nutritional status. These include such factors as medications being taken and adequacy of income to allow her to purchase the necessary foods.

> **COMMUNITY FOCUS**
>
> *Nutrition Education in the Prenatal Clinic*
>
> Visit a prenatal clinic. Identify sources of nutrition education that are evident in the waiting room. Does the clinic employ a nutritionist/dietitian? Who provides nutrition counseling in the clinic? Are print materials available in multiple languages? Are interpreters available? Are there sources for free materials on nutrition that could be placed in the clinic? Identify strengths and weaknesses of nutrition education in that setting. Develop a feasible plan for improving nutrition education in the clinic.

Obstetric and Gynecologic Effects on Nutrition

Nutrition reserves may be depleted in the multiparous woman or one who has had frequent pregnancies (especially three pregnancies within 2 years). A history of preterm birth or the birth of an LBW or SGA infant may indicate inadequate dietary intake. Preeclampsia may also be a factor in poor maternal nutrition. Birth of a large-for-gestational-age infant may indicate the existence of maternal diabetes mellitus. Previous contraceptive methods also may affect reproductive health. Increased menstrual blood loss often occurs during the first 3 to 6 months after placement of an intrauterine contraceptive device. Consequently the user may have low iron stores or even iron deficiency anemia. Oral contraceptive agents are associated with decreased menstrual losses and increased iron stores. However, oral contraceptives may interfere with folic acid metabolism.

Medical History

Chronic maternal illnesses such as diabetes mellitus, renal disease, liver disease, cystic fibrosis or other malabsorptive disorders; seizure disorders and the use of anticonvulsant agents; hypertension; and PKU may affect a woman's nutritional status and dietary needs. In women with illnesses that have resulted in nutrition deficits or that require dietary treatment (e.g., diabetes mellitus, PKU), it is extremely important for nutritional care to be started and for the condition to be optimally controlled before conception. A registered dietitian can provide in-depth counseling for the woman who requires medical nutrition therapy during pregnancy and lactation.

Usual Maternal Diet

The woman's usual food and beverage intake, adequacy of income and other resources to meet her nutrition needs, any dietary modifications, food allergies and intolerances, all medications and nutrition supplements being taken, and pica and cultural dietary requirements should be ascertained. In addition, the presence and severity of nutrition-related discomforts of pregnancy such as morning sickness, constipation, and pyrosis (heartburn) should be determined. The nurse should be alert to any evidence of eating disorders such as anorexia nervosa, bulimia, or frequent and rigorous dieting before or during pregnancy.

The impact of food allergies and intolerances on nutritional status ranges from very important to almost nil. Lactose intolerance is of special concern in pregnant and lactating women

NURSING PROCESS: NUTRITION

Assessment

Assessment is based on a diet history obtained from an interview and review of the woman's health records, physical examination, and laboratory results (see discussion in text, pp. 286-288). Ideally a nutritional assessment is performed before conception so that any recommended changes in diet, lifestyle, and weight can be undertaken before the woman becomes pregnant.

Nursing Diagnoses

Imbalanced nutrition: less than body requirements related to

- inadequate information about nutrition needs and weight gain during pregnancy
- misperceptions regarding normal body changes during pregnancy and inappropriate fear of becoming fat
- inadequate income or skills in meal planning and preparation

Imbalanced nutrition: more than body requirements related to

- excessive intake of energy (calories) or decrease in activity during pregnancy
- use of unnecessary dietary supplements

Constipation related to

- decrease in gastrointestinal motility because of elevated progesterone levels
- compression of intestines by the enlarging uterus
- oral iron supplementation

Planning

Nutrition-related outcomes are that the woman will do the following:

- Achieve an appropriate weight gain during pregnancy, which takes into account such factors as prepregnancy weight, whether she is overweight/obese or underweight, and whether the pregnancy is single or multifetal
- Consume adequate nutrients from the diet and supplements to meet estimated needs
- Cope successfully with nutrition-related discomforts associated with pregnancy such as morning sickness, pyrosis (heartburn), and constipation
- Avoid or reduce potentially harmful practices such as smoking, alcohol consumption, and caffeine intake
- Return to prepregnancy weight (or an appropriate weight for height) within 6 months of giving birth

Interventions

- Acquaint the woman with nutrition needs during pregnancy and, if necessary, the characteristics of an adequate diet.
- Help her individualize her diet so that she achieves an adequate intake while conforming to her personal, cultural, financial, and health circumstances.
- Acquaint her with strategies for coping with the nutrition-related discomforts of pregnancy.
- Help her use nutrition supplements appropriately.
- Consult with and make referrals to other professionals or services as indicated.

See discussion in text on pp. 286-288.

Evaluation

- Compare the woman's weight gain with standardized grids showing recommended patterns.
- Compare the woman's diet with the plan in Table 12-3. It is essential that individual factors affecting nutrition needs and dietary intake be considered.
- Use data from physical examination and laboratory testing to confirm that nutritional status is adequate.

because no other food group equals milk and milk products in terms of calcium content. If a woman has lactose intolerance, the interviewer should explore her intake of other calcium sources (see Box 12-4).

The assessment must include an evaluation of the woman's financial status and her knowledge of sound dietary practices. The quality of the diet improves with increasing socioeconomic status and educational level. Poor women may not have access to adequate refrigeration and cooking facilities and may find it difficult to obtain adequate nutritious food. Pregnancy rates are high among homeless women, and many such women cannot or do not take advantage of services such as food stamps.

Box 12-6 provides a simple tool for obtaining diet history information. When potential problems are identified, they should be followed up with a careful interview.

Physical Examination

Anthropometric (body) measurements provide short- and long-term information on a woman's nutritional status and are thus essential to the assessment. At a minimum the woman's height and weight must be determined at the time of her first prenatal visit, and her weight should be measured at each subsequent visit (see earlier discussion of BMI).

A careful physical examination can reveal objective signs of malnutrition (Table 12-4). However, it is important to note that some of these signs are nonspecific and that the physiologic changes of pregnancy may complicate the interpretation of physical findings. For example, lower extremity edema often occurs in calorie and protein deficiency, but it may also be a normal finding in the third trimester of pregnancy. Interpretation of physical findings is made easier by a thorough health history and laboratory testing if indicated.

Laboratory Testing The only nutrition-related laboratory testing needed by most pregnant women is a hematocrit or hemoglobin measurement to screen for the presence of anemia. Because of the physiologic anemia of pregnancy, the reference values for hemoglobin and hematocrit must be adjusted during pregnancy. The lower limit of the normal range for hemoglobin during pregnancy is 11 g/dl (compared with 12 g/dl in the nonpregnant state). The lower limit of the normal range for hematocrit is 32% (compared with 37% in the nonpregnant state). Cutoff values for anemia are higher in

BOX 12-6 Food Intake Questionnaire

How many servings of the following did you eat or drink yesterday? If the way you ate yesterday wasn't the way you usually eat, choose a recent day that was typical for you.

Beer, wine, other alcoholic drinks ______
Tea ______
Coffee ______
Fruit drink ______
Water ______
Cheese ______
Macaroni and cheese ______
Other foods with cheese (such as lasagna, enchiladas, cheeseburgers) ______
Orange or grapefruit ______
Bananas ______
Peaches or apricots ______
Green salad ______
Spinach or greens ______
Green peas ______
Sweet potatoes ______
Carrots ______
Meat ______
Fish ______
Peanut butter ______
Dried beans or peas ______
Bacon or sausage ______
Bread ______

Rice ______
Spaghetti or other pasta ______
Tortillas ______
French fries ______
Cookie ______
Pie ______
Orange or grapefruit juice ______
Fruit juice other than orange or grapefruit ______
Soft drinks ______
Milk ______
Cereal with milk ______
Yogurt ______
Pizza ______
Melon (such as watermelon, cantaloupe, honeydew) ______
Berries (specify kind) ______
Apples ______
Other fruit ______
Broccoli ______
Green beans ______
Potatoes (other than fried) ______

Corn ______
Other vegetables ______
Chicken or turkey ______
Egg ______
Nuts ______
Hot dog ______
Cold cuts ______

Roll ______
Cereal ______
Noodles ______
Chips ______
Cake ______
Donut or pastry ______

Are you often bothered by any of the following? (Circle all that apply)
Nausea Vomiting Heartburn Constipation
Are you on a special diet? No ______ Yes ______ If yes, what kind? ______
Do you try to limit the amount or kind of food you eat to control your weight? No ______ Yes ______
Do you avoid any foods for health or religious reasons? No ______ Yes ______ If yes, what foods? ______
Do you take any prescribed drugs or medications? No ______ Yes ______ If yes, what are they? ______
Do you take any over-the-counter medications (such as aspirin, cold medicines, Tylenol)? No ______ Yes ______ If yes, what are they? ______
Do you ever have trouble affording the food you need? No ______ Yes ______
Do you have any help getting the food you need? No ______ Yes ______ (Circle all that apply)
Food stamps WIC School lunch or breakfast
Food from a food pantry, soup kitchen, or food bank

women who smoke or live at high altitudes because the decreased oxygen-carrying capacity of their RBCs causes them to produce more RBCs than other women.

A woman's history or physical findings may indicate the need for additional testing. These tests might include a complete blood cell count with a differential to identify megaloblastic or macrocytic anemia and measurement of levels of specific vitamins or minerals believed to be lacking in the diet.

For many women with uncomplicated pregnancies, the nurse can serve as the primary source of nutrition education during pregnancy. The registered dietitian who has specialized training in evaluating diets, planning nutrition needs during illness, ethnic and cultural food patterns, and translating nutrient needs into food patterns often serves as a consultant. Pregnant women with serious nutrition problems, those with intervening illnesses such as diabetes (either preexisting or gestational), and any others requiring in-depth dietary counseling should be referred to the dietitian.

Two programs that provide nutrition services are the food stamp program and the Special Supplemental Program for Women, Infants, and Children (WIC). These programs provide vouchers for selected foods to pregnant and lactating women and infants and children at nutritional risk. WIC foods include items such as eggs, cheese, milk, juice, and fortified cereals—foods chosen because they provide iron, protein, vitamin C, and other vitamins.

Adequate Dietary Intake

Nutrition teaching can take place in a one-on-one interview or in a group setting. In either case teaching should emphasize the importance of choosing a varied diet composed of readily available foods rather than specialized diet supplements. The importance of consuming adequate amounts from the milk, yogurt, and cheese group must be emphasized, especially for adolescents and women younger than 25 years of age who are still actively adding calcium to their skeletons; adolescents need at least 3 to 4 cups from the milk group daily. Good nutrition practices (and avoidance of poor practices such as smoking and alcohol or drug use) are essential content for prenatal classes designed for women in early pregnancy.

MyPyramid can be used as a guide to making daily food choices during pregnancy and lactation, just as it is during other stages of the life cycle. Additional individualized information and resources are available from the website *www.mypyramid.gov*. On the website is an option for MyPyramid for Moms. By selecting pregnancy or breastfeeding as appropriate, a women can fill in the requested information (age, due date, height, prepregnancy weight, amount of exercise), and the program will calculate a plan for calories and amounts of food to be consumed daily to promote an appropriate weight gain.

Pregnancy

The pregnant woman must understand what adequate weight gain during pregnancy means, recognize the reasons

Table 12-4 Physical Assessment of Nutritional Status

SIGNS OF GOOD NUTRITION	SIGNS OF POOR NUTRITION
General Appearance	
Alert, responsive, energetic, good endurance	Listless, apathetic, cachectic, easily fatigued, looks tired
Muscles	
Well developed, firm, good tone, some fat under skin	Flaccid, poor tone, undeveloped, tender, "wasted" appearance
Nervous Control	
Good attention span, not irritable or restless, normal reflexes, psychologic stability	Inattentive, irritable, confused, burning and tingling of hands and feet, loss of position and vibratory sense, weakness and tenderness of muscles, decrease or loss of ankle and knee reflexes
Gastrointestinal Function	
Good appetite and digestion, normal regular elimination, no palpable organs or masses	Anorexia, indigestion, constipation or diarrhea, liver or spleen enlargement
Cardiovascular Function	
Normal heart rate and rhythm, no murmurs, normal blood pressure for age	Rapid heart rate, enlarged heart, abnormal rhythm, elevated blood pressure
Hair	
Shiny, lustrous, firm, not easily plucked, healthy scalp	Stringy, dull, brittle, dry, thin and sparse, depigmented, can be easily plucked
Skin (General)	
Smooth, slightly moist, good color	Rough, dry, scaly, pale, pigmented, irritated, easily bruised, petechiae
Face and Neck	
Skin color uniform, smooth, pink, healthy appearance; no enlargement of thyroid gland; lips not chapped or swollen	Scaly, swollen, skin dark over cheeks and under eyes; lumpiness or flakiness of skin around nose and mouth; thyroid enlarged; lips swollen; angular lesions or fissures at corners of mouth
Oral Cavity	
Reddish pink mucous membranes and gums; no swelling or bleeding of gums; tongue healthy pink or deep red in appearance, not swollen or smooth, surface papillae present; teeth bright and clean, no cavities, no pain, no discoloration	Gums spongy, bleed easily, inflamed or receding; tongue swollen, scarlet and raw, magenta color, beefy, hyperemic and hypertrophic papillae, atrophic papillae; teeth with unfilled caries, absent teeth, worn surfaces, mottled
Eyes	
Bright, clear, shiny, no sores at corners of eyelids, membranes moist and healthy pink color, no prominent blood vessels or mound of tissue (Bitot's spots) on sclera, no fatigue circles beneath	Eye membranes pale, redness of membrane, dryness, signs of infection, Bitot's spots, redness and fissuring of eyelid corners, dryness of eye membrane, dull appearance of cornea, soft cornea, blue sclerae
Extremities	
No tenderness, weakness, or swelling; nails firm and pink	Edema, tender calves, tingling, weakness; nails spoon-shaped, brittle
Skeleton	
No malformations	Bowlegs, knock-knees, chest deformity at diaphragm, beaded ribs, prominent scapulas

for its importance, and be able to evaluate her own gain in terms of the desirable pattern. Many women, particularly those who have worked hard to control their weight before pregnancy, may find it difficult to understand why the weight gain goal is so high when a newborn infant is so small. The nurse can explain that maternal weight gain consists of increments in the weight of many tissues, not just the growing fetus (see Table 12-2).

Dietary overindulgence, which may result in excessive fat stores that persist after giving birth, should be discouraged. Nevertheless, it is best not to focus unduly on weight gain because this could result in feelings of stress and guilt in the woman who does not follow the preferred pattern of gain. Teaching regarding weight gain during pregnancy is summarized in Box 12-7.

Postpartum Period

The need for a varied diet with food from all food groups continues throughout lactation. As mentioned previously, the lactating woman should be advised to consume at least 1800 kcal daily, and she should receive counseling if her intake appears to be inadequate in any nutrients. Special attention should be given to her zinc, vitamin B_6, and folic acid intake because the recommendations for these remain higher than for nonpregnant women (see Table 12-1). Sufficient calcium is needed to allow for both milk formation and maintenance of maternal bone mass. It may be difficult for lactating women to consume enough of these nutrients without careful meal planning.

The woman who does not breastfeed loses weight gradually if she consumes a balanced diet that provides slightly less than her daily energy expenditure. A reasonable weight loss goal for nonlactating women is 0.5 to 1 kg per week; a loss of 1 kg per month is recommended for most lactating women who need to lose weight. On average, at 6 weeks after giving birth women retain 3 to 7 kg of the weight gained during pregnancy, and two thirds of them weigh more than they did before preg-

BOX 12-7 Weight Gain During Pregnancy

- Progressive weight gain during pregnancy is essential to ensure normal fetal growth and development and the deposition of maternal stores that promote successful lactation.
- Recommended weight gain during pregnancy for women with a single fetus is determined largely by prepregnancy weight for height: normal-weight women, 11.5 to 16 kg; underweight women, 12.5 to 18 kg; overweight women, 7 to 11.5 kg, and obese women should gain at least 7 kg.
- Adolescents are encouraged to strive for weight gains at the upper end of the recommended range for their BMI because it appears that the fetus and the still-growing mother compete for nutrients.
- In twin gestations the total weight gain at term should be 21 to 28 kg for women who are underweight before conception, 17 to 24.5 kg for normal-weight women, 16.4 to 20.4 kg for overweight women, and 12 to 17.7 kg for obese women (Luke, 2005).
- Weight gain should be achieved through a balanced diet of regular foods chosen from all the different food groups (see Table 12-3).
- The pattern of weight gain is important: approximately 0.4 kg per week during the second and third trimesters for normal-weight women; 0.5 kg per week for underweight women; and 0.3 kg per week for overweight women.

nancy (Walker, Sterling, & Timmerman, 2005). Those at risk for obesity and overweight need follow-up to ensure that they know how to make wise food choices, primarily from fruits, vegetables, whole grains, lean meats, and low-fat dairy products. An hour of moderately vigorous physical activity (e.g., walking, jogging, swimming, cycling, aerobic dance) most days of the week will improve the ability of the woman to lose weight gradually and maintain the weight loss.

Daily Food Guide and Menu Planning

The daily food plan (see Table 12-3) can be used as a guide for educating women about nutrition needs during pregnancy and lactation. This food plan is general enough to be used by women from a variety of cultures, including those following a vegetarian diet. One of the more helpful teaching strategies is to assist the woman to plan daily menus that follow the food plan and are affordable, have realistic preparation times, and are compatible with personal preferences and cultural practices. Information regarding cultural food patterns is provided later in this chapter.

Medical Nutrition Therapy

During pregnancy and lactation the food plan for women with special medical nutrition therapy may have to be modified. The registered dietitian can instruct these women about their diets and assist them in meal planning. However, the nurse should understand the basic principles of the diet and be able to reinforce the diet teaching.

The nurse should be especially aware of the dietary modifications necessary for women with diabetes mellitus (either gestational or preexisting). This disease is relatively common, and fetal morbidity and mortality occur more often in pregnancies complicated by hyperglycemia or hypoglycemia (see discussion of diabetes in Chapter 13). Every effort should be made to maintain blood glucose levels in the normal range throughout pregnancy. The food plan of the woman with diabetes usually includes four to six meals and snacks daily, with the daily carbohydrate intake distributed fairly evenly among the meals and snacks. The complex carbohydrates—fibers and starches—should be well represented in the diet. To maintain strict control of the blood glucose level, the pregnant woman with diabetes usually must monitor her own blood glucose daily.

Counseling About Iron Supplementation

As mentioned earlier, the nutrition supplement most commonly needed during pregnancy is iron. However, a variety of dietary factors can affect the completeness of absorption of an iron supplement. The Patient Teaching box summarizes important points regarding iron supplementation.

PATIENT TEACHING
Iron Supplementation

- Vitamin C (in citrus fruits, tomatoes, melons, and strawberries) and heme iron (in meats) increase the absorption of iron supplement; therefore include these in the diet often.
- Bran, tea, coffee, milk, oxalates (in spinach and Swiss chard), and egg yolk decrease iron absorption. Avoid consuming them at the same time as the supplement.
- Iron is absorbed best if it is taken when the stomach is empty (i.e., take it between meals with a beverage other than tea, coffee, or milk).
- Iron can be taken at bedtime if abdominal discomfort occurs when it is taken between meals.
- If an iron dose is missed, take it as soon as it is remembered if that is within 13 hours of the scheduled dose. Do not double up on the dose.
- Keep the supplement in a childproof container and out of the reach of any children in the household.
- The iron may cause stools to be black or dark green.
- Constipation is common with iron supplementation. A diet high in fiber with adequate fluid intake is recommended.

Coping with Nutrition-Related Discomforts of Pregnancy

The most common nutrition-related discomforts of pregnancy are nausea and vomiting (or "morning sickness"), constipation, and pyrosis.

Nausea and Vomiting

Nausea and vomiting are most common during the first trimester. Usually nausea and vomiting cause only mild-to-moderate nutrition problems, although they may be a source of substantial discomfort. Antiemetic medications, vitamin B_6, ginger, and pericardium 6 acupressure (Fig. 12-4) may be

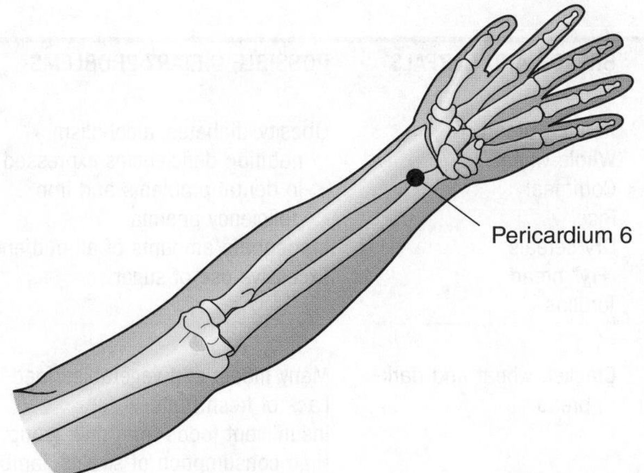

Fig. 12-4 Pericardium 6 (P6) acupressure/acupuncture point for nausea.

effective in reducing the severity of nausea (Borrelli et al, 2005; Jewell & Young, 2004). The pregnant woman may find the following suggestions helpful in alleviating the problems:

- Eat dry, starchy foods such as dry toast, Melba toast, or crackers on awakening in the morning and at other times when nausea occurs.
- Avoid consuming excessive amounts of fluids early in the day or when nauseated (but compensate by drinking fluids at other times).
- Eat small amounts frequently (every 2 to 3 hours) and avoid large meals that distend the stomach.
- Avoid skipping meals and thus becoming extremely hungry, which may worsen nausea. Have a snack such as cereal with milk, a small sandwich, or yogurt before bedtime.
- Avoid sudden movements. Get out of bed slowly.
- Decrease intake of fried and other fatty foods. Good choices are starches such as pastas, rice, and breads and low-fat, high-protein foods such as skinless broiled or baked poultry, cooked dry beans or peas, lean meats, and broiled or canned fish.
- Some women find that tart foods or drinks (e.g., lemonade) or salty foods (e.g., potato chips) are tolerated during periods of nausea.
- Breathe fresh air to help relieve nausea. Keep the environment well ventilated (e.g., open a window), go for a walk outside, or decrease cooking odors by using an exhaust fan.
- Eat foods served at cool temperatures and foods that give off little aroma.
- Try herbal teas such as those made with raspberry leaf or peppermint to decrease nausea.
- Avoid brushing teeth immediately after eating.

Hyperemesis gravidarum (severe and persistent vomiting causing weight loss, dehydration, and electrolyte abnormalities) occurs in up to 1% of pregnant women. Intravenous fluid and electrolyte replacement is usually necessary for women who lose 5% of their body weight. Often this is followed by improved tolerance of oral intake; therapy then consists of frequently consuming small amounts of low-fat foods. Enteral tube feeding using small-bore nasogastric tubes has been successful for some women. Because pulmonary aspiration of the feeding is a potential complication if vomiting occurs, antiemetic medications are sometimes used in conjunction with tube feedings. Tube feedings may be used to supplement oral intake, with the volume of the tube feeding gradually being decreased as oral intake improves. In some instances total parenteral nutrition (balanced intravenous feedings of amino acids, carbohydrate, lipid, vitamins, and minerals) is used to nourish women with hyperemesis gravidarum when their nutritional status has been severely impaired. None of the interventions already mentioned for morning sickness (i.e., antihistamines, vitamin B_6, ginger) have shown any benefit in hyperemesis gravidarum.

Constipation

Improved bowel function generally results from increasing the intake of fiber (e.g., wheat bran and whole-wheat products, popcorn, and raw or lightly steamed vegetables) in the diet. Fiber helps retain water within the stool, creating a bulky stool that stimulates intestinal peristalsis. The recommendation for pregnant women for fiber is 28 g per day. An adequate fluid intake (at least 50 ml/kg/day) helps hydrate the fiber and increase the bulk of the stool. Making a habit of regular exercise that uses large muscle groups (walking, swimming, cycling) also helps stimulate bowel motility.

Pyrosis

Pyrosis, or heartburn, is usually caused by reflux of gastric contents into the esophagus. This condition can be minimized by eating small, frequent meals rather than two or three larger meals daily. Because fluids increase the distention of the stomach, they should not be consumed with foods. The woman needs to be sure to drink adequate amounts between meals. Avoiding spicy foods may help alleviate the problem. Reflux can be exacerbated by lying down immediately after eating and wearing clothing that is tight across the abdomen.

Cultural Influences

Consideration of a woman's cultural food preferences enhances communication and provides a greater opportunity for following the agreed-on pattern of intake. Women in most cultures are encouraged to eat a diet typical for them. The nurse needs to be aware of what constitutes a typical diet for each cultural or ethnic group present in her patient population. However, several variations may occur within one cultural group. Thus a careful exploration of individual preferences is needed. Although ethnic and cultural food beliefs may seem at first glance to conflict with the dietary instruction provided by physicians, nurses, and dietitians, it is often possible for the empathic health care provider to identify cultural beliefs that are congruent with the modern understanding of pregnancy and fetal development. Many cultural food practices have some merit, or the culture would not have survived. Food cravings during pregnancy are considered normal by many cultures, but the kinds of cravings often are culturally specific. In most cultures women crave acceptable foods such as chicken, fish, and greens among African-Americans. Cultural influences on food intake usually lessen if the woman and her family become more integrated into the dominant culture. Nutrition beliefs and the practices of selected cultural groups are summarized in Table 12-5.

Table 12-5 Characteristic Food Patterns of Selected Cultures

MILK GROUP	PROTEIN GROUP	FRUITS AND VEGETABLES	BREADS AND CEREALS	POSSIBLE DIETARY PROBLEMS
Native American (Many Tribal Variations; Many "Americanized")				
Fresh milk Evaporated milk for cooking Ice cream Cream pie	Pork, beef, lamb, rabbit Fowl, fish, eggs Legumes Sunflower seeds Nuts: walnuts, acorn, pine, peanut butter Game meat	Green peas, beans Beets, turnips Green leafy and other vegetables Grapes, bananas, peaches, other fresh fruits Roots	Refined bread Whole wheat Cornmeal Rice Dry cereals "Fry" bread Tortillas	Obesity, diabetes, alcoholism, nutrition deficiencies expressed in dental problems and iron deficiency anemia Inadequate amounts of all nutrients Excessive use of sugar
Middle Eastern* (Armenian, Greek, Syrian, Turkish)				
Yogurt Little butter	Lamb Nuts Dried peas, beans, lentils Sesame seeds	Peppers, tomatoes, cabbage, grape leaves, cucumbers, squash Dried apricots, raisins, dates	Cracked wheat and dark bread	Many meats and vegetables fried Lack of fresh fruits Insufficient foods from milk group High consumption of sweets, lamb fat, and olive oil
African-American (Particularly Southern and Rural)				
Milk† Ice cream Cheese: longhorn, American	Pork: all cuts, plus organs, chitterlings Beef, lamb Chicken, giblets Eggs Nuts Legumes Fish, game	Leafy vegetables Green and yellow vegetables Potato: white, sweet Stewed fruit Bananas and other fresh fruit	Cornmeal and hominy grits Rice Biscuits, pancakes, white breads Puddings: bread, rice	Extensive use of frying, smothering in gravy, or simmering Fats: salt pork, bacon drippings, lard, and gravies High consumption of sweets Insufficient citrus Vegetables often boiled for long periods with pork fat and much salt Limited amounts from milk group†
Chinese (Cantonese Most Prevalent)				
Milk: water buffalo	Pork sausage‡ Eggs and pigeon eggs Fish Lamb, beef, goat Fowl: chicken, duck Nuts Legumes Soybean curd (tofu)	Many vegetables Radish leaves Bean, bamboo sprouts	Rice/rice flour products Cereals, noodles Wheat, corn, millet seed	Tendency of some immigrants to use large amounts of grease in cooking Limited use of milk and milk products Often low in protein, calories, or both Soy sauce (high sodium)
Filipino (Spanish-Chinese Influence)				
Flavored milk Milk in coffee Cheese: gouda, cheddar	Pork, beef, goat, rabbit Chicken Fish Eggs, nuts, legumes	Many vegetables and fruits	Rice, cooked cereals Noodles: rice, wheat	Limited use of milk and milk products Tendency to prewash rice Tendency to have only small portions of protein foods
Italian				
Cheese Some ice cream	Meat Eggs Dried beans	Leafy vegetables Potatoes Eggplant, tomatoes, peppers Fruits	Pasta White breads, some whole wheat Farina Cereals	Prefer expensive imported cheeses; reluctant to substitute less expensive domestic varieties Tendency to overcook vegetables Limited use of whole grains High consumption of sweets Extensive use of olive oil Insufficient servings from milk group
Japanese (Isei, More Japanese Influence; Nisei, More Westernized)				
Increasing amounts being used by younger generations	Pork, beef, chicken Fish Eggs Legumes: soy, red, lima beans Tofu Nuts	Many vegetables and fruits Seaweed	Rice, rice cakes Wheat noodles Refined bread, noodles	Excessive sodium: pickles, salty crisp seaweed, MSG, and soy sauce Insufficient servings from milk group May use prewashed rice

Table 12-5 Characteristic Food Patterns of Selected Cultures—cont'd

MILK GROUP	PROTEIN GROUP	FRUITS AND VEGETABLES	BREADS AND CEREALS	POSSIBLE DIETARY PROBLEMS
Hispanic, Mexican-American				
Milk Cheese Flan, ice cream	Beef, pork, lamb, chicken, tripe, hot sausage, beef intestines Fish Eggs Nuts Dry beans: pinto, chickpeas (often eaten more than once daily)	Spinach, wild greens, tomatoes, chilies, corn, cactus leaves, cabbage, avocado, potatoes Pumpkin, zapote, peaches, guava, papaya, citrus	Rice, cornmeal Sweet bread, pastries Tortilla: corn, flour Vermicelli *(fideo)*	Limited meats primarily because of cost Limited use of milk and milk products Large amounts of lard Abundant use of sugar Tendency to boil vegetables for long periods
Puerto Rican				
Limited use of milk products Coffee with milk *(café con leche)*	Pork Poultry Eggs (Fridays) Dried codfish Beans (habichuelas)	Avocado, okra Eggplant Sweet yams Starchy vegetables and fruits *(viandas)*	Rice Cornmeal	Small amounts of pork and poultry Extensive use of fat, lard, salt pork, and olive oil Lack of milk products
Scandinavian (Danish, Finnish, Norwegian, Swedish)				
Cream Butter Cheeses	Wild game Reindeer Fish (fresh or dried) Eggs	Berries Dried fruit Vegetables: cole slaw, roots	Whole wheat, rye, barley, sweets (cookies and sweet breads)	Insufficient fresh fruits and vegetables High consumption of sweets, pickled or salted meats, and fish
Southeast Asian (Vietnamese, Cambodian)				
Generally not taken Coffee with condensed cow's milk Plain yogurt Ice cream (rare) Soybean milk	Fish (daily): fresh, dried, salted Poultry/egg, duck, chicken Pork Beef (seldom) Dry beans Tofu	Seasonal variety: fresh or preserved Green leafy vegetables Yams Corn	Rice: grains, flour, noodles French bread "Cellophane" (bean starch) noodles	Fresh milk products generally not consumed Poultry/eggs may be limited Meat considered "unclean" avoided Preference for diet high in salt and pepper, as well as rice and pork High intake of MSG and soy sauce
Jewish: Orthodox*				
Milk† Cheese†	Meat (bloodless; Kosher prepared): beef, lamb, goat, deer, poultry (all types), no pork Fish with fins and scales only No crustaceans	Wide variety	Wide variety	High intake of sodium in meat products

MSG, Monosodium L-glutamate.
*Religious holidays may involve fasting, which is believed to increase the likelihood of preterm labor. Fasting requirement may be waived during pregnancy.
†Lactose intolerance relatively common in adults.
‡Lower in fat content than Western sausage.

Vegetarian Diets

Vegetarian diets represent another cultural effect on nutritional status. Foods basic to almost all vegetarian diets are vegetables, fruits, legumes, nuts, seeds, and grains, but with many variations. Semivegetarians, who are not true vegetarians, include fish, poultry, eggs, and dairy products in their diets but do not eat beef or pork. Such a diet can be completely adequate for pregnant women. Another type of vegetarians, ovolacto-vegetarians, consumes eggs and dairy products in addition to plant products. Iron and zinc intake may not be adequate in these women, but such diets can be otherwise nutritionally sound. Strict vegetarians, or vegans, consume only plant products. Because vitamin B_{12} is found only in foods of animal origin, this diet is deficient in vitamin B_{12}. As a result, strict vegetarians should take a supplement or regularly consume vitamin B_{12}–fortified foods (e.g., soy milk). Vitamin B_{12} deficiency can result in megaloblastic anemia, glossitis (inflamed red tongue), and neurologic deficits in the mother. Infants born to affected mothers are likely to have megaloblastic anemia and exhibit neurodevelopmental delays. Iron, calcium, zinc, and vitamin B_6 intake may also be low in women on this diet; and some strict vegetarians have excessively low caloric intakes. The protein intake should be assessed especially carefully because plant proteins tend to be incomplete in that they lack one or more amino acids required for growth and maintenance of body tissues. However, the daily consumption of a variety of different plant proteins—grains, dried beans and peas, nuts, and seeds—helps to provide all of the essential amino acids.

Key Points

- A woman's nutritional status before, during, and after pregnancy contributes significantly to her well-being and that of her infant.
- Many physiologic changes occurring during pregnancy influence the need for additional nutrients and the efficiency with which the body uses them.
- Both the total maternal weight gain and the pattern of weight gain are important determinants of the outcome of pregnancy.
- The appropriateness of the mother's prepregnancy weight for height (BMI) is a major determinant of her recommended weight gain during pregnancy.
- Nutritional risk factors include adolescent pregnancy, nicotine use, alcohol or drug use, bizarre or faddish food habits, a low weight for height, and frequent pregnancies.

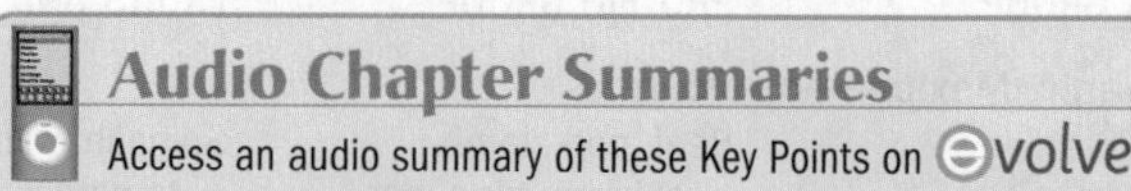
Audio Chapter Summaries
Access an audio summary of these Key Points on evolve

- Iron supplementation is usually routinely recommended during pregnancy. Other supplements may be warranted when nutritional risk factors are present.
- The nurse and the woman are influenced by cultural and personal values and beliefs during nutrition counseling.
- Pregnancy complications that may be nutrition related include anemia, gestational hypertension, gestational diabetes, and IUGR.
- Dietary adaptation can be an effective intervention for some of the common discomforts of pregnancy, including nausea and vomiting, constipation, and heartburn.

References

Allen L: Multiple micronutrients in pregnancy and lactation: an overview, *Am J Clin Nutr* 81(5):1206S-1212S, 2005.

Borrelli F et al: Effectiveness and safety of ginger in the treatment of pregnancy-induced nausea and vomiting, *Obstet Gynecol* 105(4):849-856, 2005.

Corbett R, Ryan C, Weinrich S: Pica in pregnancy: does it affect pregnancy outcomes? *MCN Am J Matern Child Nurs* 28(3):183-189, 2003.

Cornel M, Smit D, de Jong-van den Berg L: Folic acid—the scientific debate as a base for public health policy, *Reprod Toxicol* 20(3):411-415, 2005.

Grotegut CA et al: Baking soda pica: a case of hypokalemic metabolic alkalosis and rhabdomyolysis in pregnancy, *Obstet Gynecol* 107(2 pt 2):484-486, 2006.

Hoyert D et al: *Deaths: Final data for 2003*, Health E-Stats, Hyattsville, Md, released January 19, 2006, National Center for Health Statistics.

Institute of Medicine: *Dietary reference intakes: applications in dietary planning*, Washington, DC, 2003, National Academies Press.

Institute of Medicine: *Dietary reference intakes for water, potassium, sodium, chloride, and sulfate*, Washington, DC, 2004, National Academies Press.

Jewell D, Young G: Interventions for nausea and vomiting in early pregnancy (Cochrane Review), 2004. In *The Cochrane Library*, Issue 4, Chichester, UK, 2004, John Wiley & Sons.

Klitzman S et al: Lead poisoning among pregnant women in New York City: risk factors and screening practices, *J Urban Health* 79(2):225-237, 2002.

Luke B: Nutrition in multiple gestations, *Clin Perinatol* 32(2):403-429, vii, 2005.

Ngozi PO: Pica practices of pregnant women in Nairobi, Kenya, *East Afr Med J* 85(2):72-79, 2008.

Office of Dietary Supplements: *Dietary Supplement Fact Sheet: Iron*, National Institutes of Health, 2007. Available at www.dietary-supplements.info.nih.gov/factsheets/iron.asp (accessed August 7, 2008).

Paul AM: Too fat and pregnant, *New York Times*, July 13, 2008.

Shannon M: Severe lead poisoning in pregnancy, *Ambul Pediatr* 3(1):37-39, 2003.

Walker L, Sterling B, Timmerman G: Retention of pregnancy-related weight in the early postpartum period: Implications for women's health services, *J Obstet Gynecol Neonatal Nurs* 34(4):418-427, 2005.

Unit 3

13

Pregnancy at Risk: Preexisting Conditions

Learning Objectives

On completion of this chapter the reader will be able to:

- Differentiate the types of diabetes mellitus and their respective risk factors in pregnancy.
- Compare insulin requirements during pregnancy, the postpartum period, and lactation.
- Identify maternal and fetal risks or complications associated with diabetes in pregnancy.
- Develop a plan of care for the pregnant woman with pregestational or gestational diabetes.
- Compare the management of a pregnant woman with hyperthyroidism with one who has hypothyroidism.
- Differentiate the management of various cardiovascular disorders in pregnant women.
- Discuss the different types of anemia and their effects during pregnancy.
- Explain the care of pregnant women with pulmonary disorders.
- Describe the effects of gastrointestinal disorders on pregnancy.
- Review the effects of neurologic disorders on pregnancy.
- Describe the care of women whose pregnancies are complicated by autoimmune disorders.
- Explain the effects on and the management of pregnant women with human immunodeficiency virus.
- Discuss the care of pregnant women who use, abuse, or are dependent on alcohol or illicit or prescription drugs.

Electronic Resources

Additional information related to the content in Chapter 13 can be found on

evolve the Companion Website at http://evolve.elsevier.com/Perry/maternal/

- NCLEX Review Questions
- Case Study—Class III Cardiac Disorder
- Case Study—Pregestational Diabetes
- Critical Thinking Exercise—Gestational Diabetes
- Nursing Care Plan—Pregnancy Complicated by Pregestational Diabetes
- Nursing Care Plan—The Pregnant Woman with Heart Disease
- Nursing Care Plan—Substance Abuse During Pregnancy

For most women pregnancy represents a normal part of life. However, for some women pregnancy presents a significant risk because it is superimposed on a chronic illness. With well-motivated patients who actively participate in the treatment plan and with careful management from a multidisciplinary health care team, positive pregnancy outcomes are often possible.

Providing safe and effective care for women experiencing high risk pregnancy and their fetuses is a challenge. Although unique maternal and fetal needs prompted by these conditions exist, these women also experience many of the same pregnancy-related feelings, needs, and concerns as their "normal" counterparts. The primary objective of nursing care must be to guide and support the woman and her family in achieving optimal outcomes for both the pregnant woman and the fetus.

This chapter focuses on metabolic disorders, including diabetes mellitus and thyroid disorders; cardiovascular disorders; selected disorders of the respiratory, gastrointestinal, integumentary, and central nervous systems; and autoimmune disorders. Substance abuse and human immunodeficiency virus (HIV) infection are also discussed.

Metabolic Disorders

Diabetes Mellitus

Despite advances in care, the woman whose pregnancy is complicated by diabetes may still have poor outcomes. Diabetes during pregnancy is most successfully managed with a multidisciplinary approach involving the obstetrician, internist or diabetologist, neonatologist, nurse, nutritionist, and social worker. Favorable outcome of pregnancy requires commitment and active participation by the woman and her family. The woman must comply with a schedule of frequent prenatal visits, strict adherence to the dietary regimen, regular self-monitoring of blood glucose level, frequent laboratory evaluation, intensive fetal surveillance, and possible hospitalization.

The perinatal mortality rate for women with well-controlled diabetes, excluding major congenital malformations, is about the same as that for any other pregnancy (Landon, Catalano, & Gabbe, 2007). The incidence of major congenital malformations in infants born to women with diabetes has not changed significantly over time. Experts have concluded that the key to optimal pregnancy outcome is strict maternal glucose control before conception and throughout the pregnancy. Consequently much emphasis is placed on preconception counseling for women with diabetes.

Care of the pregnant woman who has diabetes requires that the nurse fully understand the normal physiologic responses to pregnancy, as well as the altered metabolism of diabetes. Furthermore, the nurse must understand the relationship between pregnancy and diabetes, including psychosocial implications, to accurately assess the woman, plan for her care, and intervene appropriately.

Pathogenesis

Diabetes mellitus is a group of metabolic diseases characterized by hyperglycemia resulting from defects in insulin secretion, insulin action, or both (Expert Committee on the Diagnosis and Classification of Diabetes Mellitus, 2003). Insulin, produced by β-cells in the islets of Langerhans of the pancreas, regulates blood glucose levels by enabling glucose to enter adipose and muscle cells, where it is used for energy. Insulin also stimulates protein synthesis and storage of free fatty acids. When insulin is insufficient or ineffective in promoting glucose uptake by the muscle and adipose cells, glucose accumulates in the bloodstream, resulting in hyperglycemia. Hyperglycemia causes hyperosmolarity of the blood, which attracts intracellular fluid into the vascular system, resulting in cellular dehydration and expanded blood volume. Consequently the kidneys function to excrete large volumes of urine (polyuria) in an attempt to regulate excess vascular volume and excrete the unused glucose (glycosuria). Polyuria and cellular dehydration cause excessive thirst (polydipsia).

The body compensates for its inability to convert carbohydrate (glucose) into energy by burning proteins (muscle) and fats. The end products of this metabolism are ketones and fatty acids, which in excess quantity produce ketoacidosis and acetonuria. Weight loss occurs because of the breakdown of fat and muscle tissue. This tissue breakdown causes a state of starvation that compels the individual to eat excessive amounts of food (polyphagia).

Over time diabetes causes significant changes in both the microvascular and macrovascular circulations. These structural changes affect a variety of organ systems, primarily the heart, eyes, kidneys, and nerves. Complications resulting from diabetes include premature atherosclerosis, retinopathy, nephropathy, and neuropathy.

Diabetes may be caused by either impaired insulin secretion when β-cells of the pancreas are destroyed by an autoimmune process or inadequate insulin action in target tissues at one or more points along the metabolic pathway. Both of these conditions are commonly present in the same person, and it is unclear which abnormality, if either, is the primary cause of the disease (Expert Committee on the Diagnosis and Classification of Diabetes Mellitus, 2003).

Classification

The current classification system includes four groups: type 1 diabetes, type 2 diabetes, other specific types (e.g., diabetes caused by infection, drug-induced diabetes), and gestational diabetes mellitus (GDM). A major change proposed by the Expert Committee was a move away from a system that classified the disease by its pharmacologic management to one based on disease etiology (Expert Committee on the Diagnosis and Classification of Diabetes Mellitus, 2003).

Type 1 diabetes includes cases that are primarily caused by pancreatic islet β-cell destruction and prone to ketoacidosis. People with type 1 diabetes usually have an absolute insulin deficiency. Type 1 diabetes includes cases currently thought to be caused by an autoimmune process, as well as those for which the cause is unknown (Expert Committee on the Diagnosis and Classification of Diabetes Mellitus, 2003).

Type 2 diabetes is the most prevalent form of the disease and includes individuals who have insulin resistance and usually relative (rather than absolute) insulin deficiency. Specific etiologies for type 2 diabetes are unknown at this time. It often goes undiagnosed for years because hyperglycemia develops gradually and often is not severe enough for the person to recognize the classic signs of polyuria, polydipsia, and polyphagia. Many people who develop type 2 diabetes are obese or have an increased amount of body fat distributed primarily in the abdominal area. Other risk factors include aging, a sedentary lifestyle, hypertension, and prior gestational diabetes. Type 2 diabetes often has a strong genetic predisposition (Expert Committee on the Diagnosis and Classification of Diabetes Mellitus, 2003).

Pregestational diabetes is the label sometimes given to type 1 or type 2 diabetes that existed before pregnancy.

GDM is any degree of glucose intolerance with its onset or first recognition during pregnancy. This definition is appropriate whether or not insulin is used for treatment or whether the diabetes persists after pregnancy. It does not exclude the possibility that the glucose intolerance preceded the pregnancy. Women experiencing gestational diabetes should be reclassified 6 weeks or more after the pregnancy ends (Expert Committee on the Diagnosis and Classification of Diabetes Mellitus, 2003).

An alternative classification used commonly in obstetrics is that of Priscilla White (Table 13-1). This classification is based on duration of disease and vascular damage to retinal, renal, and cardiovascular structures. The ADA classification is preferred today (Moore & Catalano, 2009).

Metabolic Changes Associated with Pregnancy

Normal pregnancy is characterized by complex alterations in maternal glucose metabolism, insulin production, and metabolic homeostasis. During normal pregnancy adjustments in maternal metabolism allow for adequate nutrition for both the mother and the developing fetus. Glucose, the primary fuel used by the fetus, is transported across the placenta through the process of carrier-mediated facilitated diffusion. This means that the glucose levels in the fetus are directly proportional to maternal levels. Although glucose crosses the placenta, insulin does not. By the tenth week of gestation the embryo or fetus secretes its own insulin at levels adequate to use the glucose obtained from the mother. Thus, as maternal glucose levels rise, fetal glucose levels are increased, resulting in increased fetal insulin secretion.

Table 13-1 The White Classification of Diabetes in Pregnancy

CLASS	AGE AT ONSET (yr)		DURATION (yr)	COMPLICATIONS
A	Any		Any	Diagnosed before pregnancy; no vascular disease
B	≥20	or	<10	No vascular disease
C	10-19	or	10-19	No vascular disease
D	<10	or	≥20	Background retinopathy only or hypertension
E				Calcification of pelvic arteries (no longer used)
F				Nephropathy (>500 mg of proteinuria per day)
H				Arteriosclerotic heart disease
R				Proliferative retinopathy or vitreous hemorrhage
T				After renal transplantation

Adapted from Hare JW, White P: Gestational diabetes and the White classification, *Diabetes Care* 3:394, 1980.

During the first trimester of pregnancy the pregnant woman's metabolic status is significantly influenced by the rising levels of estrogen and progesterone. These hormones stimulate the β-cells in the pancreas to increase insulin production, which promotes increased peripheral use of glucose and decreased blood glucose, with fasting levels being reduced by approximately 10% (Fig. 13-1, *A*). There is a concomitant increase in tissue glycogen stores and a decrease in hepatic glucose production, which further encourage lower fasting glucose levels. As a result of these normal metabolic changes of pregnancy, women with insulin-dependent diabetes are prone to hypoglycemia (low blood glucose) during the first trimester.

During the second and third trimesters pregnancy exerts a diabetogenic effect on the maternal metabolic status. Because of the major hormonal changes, there is decreased tolerance to glucose, increased insulin resistance, decreased hepatic glycogen stores, and increased hepatic production of glucose. Increasing levels of human chorionic somatomammotropin, estrogen, progesterone, prolactin, cortisol, and insulinase increase insulin resistance through their actions as insulin antagonists. Insulin resistance is a glucose-sparing mechanism that ensures an abundant supply of glucose for the fetus. Maternal insulin requirements gradually increase from about 18 to 24 weeks of gestation to about 36 weeks of gestation. At this time insulin requirements usually level off until labor begins (see Fig. 13-1, *B* and *C*).

At birth expulsion of the placenta prompts an abrupt decrease in levels of circulating placental hormones, cortisol, and insulinase (see Fig. 13-1, *D*). Maternal tissues quickly regain their prepregnancy sensitivity to insulin. For the nonbreastfeeding mother, the prepregnancy insulin-carbohydrate

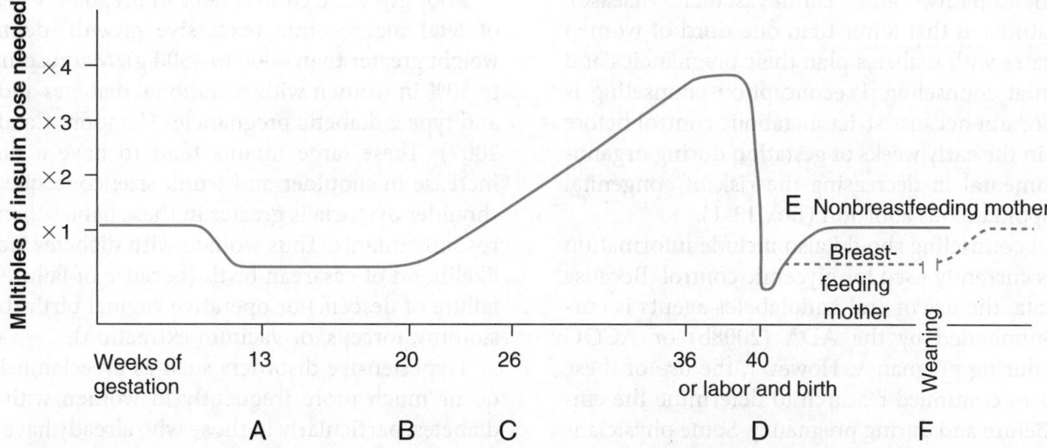

Fig. 13-1 Changing insulin needs during pregnancy. **A**, First trimester: Insulin need is reduced because of increased insulin production by the pancreas and increased peripheral sensitivity to insulin; nausea, vomiting, and decreased food intake by mother and glucose transfer to embryo/fetus contribute to hypoglycemia. **B**, Second trimester: Insulin need increases as placental hormones, cortisol, and insulinase act as insulin antagonists, decreasing the effectiveness of insulin. **C**, Third trimester: Insulin requirements gradually increase until about 36 weeks of gestation. **D**, Day of delivery: Maternal insulin requirements drop drastically to approach prepregnancy levels. **E**, Breastfeeding mother maintains lower insulin requirements, as much as 25% less than prepregnancy; insulin need of nonbreastfeeding mother returns to prepregnancy levels in 7 to 10 days. **F**, At weaning of breastfeeding infant, mother's insulin need returns to prepregnancy levels.

balance usually returns in about 7 to 10 days (see Fig. 13-1, *E*). Lactation uses maternal glucose; thus the breastfeeding mother's insulin requirements remain low as long as she is nursing (see Fig. 13-1, *E*). On completion of weaning the mother's prepregnancy insulin requirement is reestablished (see Fig. 13-1, *F*).

evolve Case Study—Pregestational Diabetes

Pregestational Diabetes Mellitus

Approximately 2 per 1000 pregnancies are complicated by preexisting diabetes. Women with pregestational diabetes may have either type 1 or type 2 diabetes, with type 1 now the more common diagnosis. As the incidence of type 2 diabetes increases in the general population, it may become the more prevalent form of the disease in childbearing-age women. Fetal risks for women with type 1 and type 2 diabetes are about the same. However, maternal risks tend to be greater in women with type 1 diabetes. Their blood sugar control is usually more erratic because of their absolute lack of insulin production. They also are more likely to have the vascular, retinal, or renal complications that often accompany the disease because their duration of illness is usually longer than that of women with type 2 diabetes. Almost all women with pregestational diabetes are insulin dependent during pregnancy.

Preconception Counseling

Preconception counseling, which is recommended by the American Diabetes Association (ADA) and the American College of Obstetricians and Gynecologists (ACOG) for all women of reproductive age with diabetes, is associated with improved pregnancy outcomes (ADA, 2008b; ACOG, 2005).

Under ideal circumstances the woman with pregestational diabetes is counseled before the time of conception to evaluate the mother's health status, plan the optimal time for pregnancy, establish glycemic control before conception, and diagnose any vascular complications of diabetes (retinopathy, nephropathy, neuropathy, and cardiovascular disease). However, it is estimated that fewer than one third of women in the United States with diabetes plan their pregnancies and seek preconceptual counseling. Preconception counseling is particularly important because strict metabolic control before conception and in the early weeks of gestation during organogenesis is instrumental in decreasing the risk of congenital anomalies and spontaneous abortion (Box 13-1).

Preconceptual counseling should also include information regarding agents currently used for glycemic control. Because of insufficient data, the use of oral antidiabetes agents is currently not recommended by the ADA (2008b) or ACOG (2001a) for use during pregnancy. However, the use of these agents is a focus of continued research to determine the efficacy and safety before and during pregnancy. Some physicians may recommend that oral hypoglycemic agents be discontinued in the preconception period in women with type 2 diabetes. These women are started on insulin before pregnancy when the pregnancy is planned or as soon as the pregnancy is diagnosed when it is unplanned (Cunningham et al, 2005).

The woman's partner should be included in the counseling to assess the couple's level of understanding related to the effects of pregnancy on the diabetic condition and the potential complications of pregnancy as a result of diabetes. The couple also should be informed of the anticipated alterations in management of diabetes during pregnancy and the need for a multidisciplinary team approach to health care. Financial implications of diabetic pregnancy and other demands related to frequent maternal and fetal surveillance should be discussed. Contraception is an important aspect of preconception counseling to assist the couple in planning effectively for pregnancy.

BOX 13-1 Goals for Self-Monitored Glucose Levels in Preconceptional Period

Before meals—Capillary plasma glucose: 80 to 110 mg/dl

2 hours after meals—Capillary plasma glucose: less than 155 mg/dl

Maternal Risks and Complications

Although maternal morbidity and mortality rates have improved significantly, the pregnant woman with diabetes remains at risk for the development of significant complications during pregnancy. Risk assessment is best done by evaluating the woman's blood glucose control, the length of time since diagnosis of the woman's diabetes, and the presence of vascular disease. Women with poor glycemic control, longer durations of diabetes, and vascular disease have inferior pregnancy outcomes.

Women with pregestational diabetes who have poor glycemic control (defined as a glycosylated hemoglobin value greater than 6 standard deviations above the mean) around the time of conception and in the early weeks of pregnancy have a twofold increased incidence of early pregnancy loss (28%). Women with good glycemic control before conception and in the first trimester are no more likely to have a miscarriage than women without diabetes.

Poor glycemic control later in pregnancy increases the rate of fetal macrosomia (excessive growth; defined as a birth weight greater than 4000 to 4500 g). Macrosomia occurs in up to 50% in women with gestational diabetes and 40% of type 1 and type 2 diabetic pregnancies (Landon, Catalano, & Gabbe, 2007). These large infants tend to have a disproportionate increase in shoulder and trunk size; consequently the risk of shoulder dystocia is greater in these babies than in other macrosomic infants. Thus women with diabetes face an increased likelihood of cesarean birth (because of failure to progress or failure of descent) or operative vaginal birth (birth using episiotomy, forceps, or vacuum extraction).

Hypertensive disorders such as preeclampsia or eclampsia occur much more frequently in women with pregestational diabetes, particularly in those who already have renal dysfunction. Preterm labor/birth also is more likely to occur, especially with more severe diabetes, elevated glucose levels, and genital or urinary tract infections. The risk for induced preterm birth also is greater in women with pregestational diabetes (Landon, Catalano, & Gabbe, 2007).

Hydramnios (polyhydramnios; amniotic fluid in excess of 2000 ml) occurs about 10 times more often in diabetic pregnancies than in nondiabetic pregnancies. The etiology for hydramnios has been theorized as increased amniotic glucose concentration or fetal hyperglycemia and polyuria; however, it is still unknown (Cunningham et al, 2005). Overdistention of the uterus caused by hydramnios increases the possibility of compression of maternal abdominal blood vessels (vena cava and aorta), causing supine hypotension. Premature rupture of the membranes, preterm labor, and postpartum hemorrhage are also associated with hydramnios.

Infections are more common and more serious in pregnant women with diabetes. Disorders of carbohydrate metabolism alter the body's normal resistance to infection. The inflammatory response, leukocyte function, and vaginal pH are all affected. Vaginal infections, particularly monilial vaginitis, are more common. Urinary tract infections also are more prevalent. Infection in the pregnant woman with diabetes may be critical, causing increased insulin resistance, which may result in ketoacidosis. Postpartum infection is also more common among women who are insulin dependent.

Ketoacidosis (accumulation of ketones in the blood resulting from hyperglycemia and leading to metabolic acidosis) occurs most often during the second and third trimesters when the diabetogenic effect of pregnancy is the greatest. When the maternal metabolism is stressed by illness or infection, the woman with diabetes is at increased risk for diabetic ketoacidosis (DKA). The use of tocolytic drugs such as terbutaline (Brethine) to treat premature labor may also contribute to the risk for hyperglycemia and subsequent DKA. DKA may also occur because of the woman's failure to take insulin appropriately. The onset of previously undiagnosed diabetes during pregnancy is another cause of DKA. It may occur with blood glucose levels barely exceeding 200 mg/dl compared with 300 to 350 mg/dl in the nonpregnant state. In response to stress factors such as infection or illness, hyperglycemia occurs as a result of increased hepatic glucose production and decreased peripheral glucose use. Stress hormones, which act to impair insulin action and further contribute to insulin deficiency, are released. Fatty acids are mobilized from fat stores into the circulation. As they are oxidized, ketone bodies are released into the peripheral circulation. The woman's buffering system is unable to compensate, and metabolic acidosis develops. The excessive blood glucose and ketone bodies result in osmotic diuresis, with subsequent loss of fluid and electrolytes, volume depletion, and cellular dehydration. Prompt treatment of DKA is necessary to avoid maternal coma or death. Ketoacidosis at any time during pregnancy can lead to intrauterine fetal death; it is also a cause of preterm labor. The fetal mortality rate is approximately 20% with maternal ketoacidosis (Cunningham et al, 2005).

The risk of hypoglycemia is also increased. Early in pregnancy, when hepatic production of glucose is diminished and peripheral use of glucose is enhanced, hypoglycemia occurs frequently, often during sleep. Later in pregnancy hypoglycemia may also result as insulin doses are adjusted to maintain euglycemia (a normal blood glucose level). Women with a prepregnancy history of severe hypoglycemia are at increased risk for severe hypoglycemia during gestation. Mild-to-moderate hypoglycemic episodes do not appear to have significant deleterious effects on fetal well-being. The long-term fetal effects of severe maternal hypoglycemia are as yet uncertain.

Fetal and Neonatal Risks and Complications

Despite the improvements in care of pregnant women with diabetes, sudden and unexplained stillbirth is still a significant risk (Landon, Catalano, & Gabbe, 2007). The other major cause of perinatal deaths in pregnancies complicated by diabetes is congenital anomalies. The incidence of congenital anomalies in infants born to women with diabetes is 6% to 10%, a twofold to fourfold increase over that of the general population (Reece & Homko, 2007). Central nervous system (CNS) defects (e.g., anencephaly, open spina bifida) are increased tenfold (Reece & Homko, 2007). Cardiac defects, especially ventricular septal defects (VSDs) and transposition of the great vessels, are increased fivefold (Landon, Catalano, & Gabbe, 2007). Caudal regression (also called caudal dysplasia or sacral agenesis) is a fetal anomaly found 200 to 400 times more often in pregnancies of mothers with diabetes (Landon, Catalano, & Gabbe, 2007).

Other problems that cause significant neonatal morbidity include macrosomia, hypoglycemia, respiratory distress syndrome, polycythemia, and hyperbilirubinemia (Cunningham et al, 2005; Landon, Catalano, & Gabbe, 2007). See Chapter 27 for further discussion of neonatal risks associated with maternal diabetes.

✱ Nursing Care Management

Effective management of diabetic pregnancy depends on the woman's adherence to a plan of care (see Nursing Process box). For the woman to care for her diabetes on a daily basis, she must have an adequate understanding of her disease and the prescribed regimen. Thus with the initial prenatal visit the woman's knowledge regarding diabetes and pregnancy, potential maternal and fetal complications, and the plan of care are assessed. With subsequent visits follow-up assessments are completed. Data from these assessments are used to identify the woman's specific learning needs. The support person's knowledge of diabetes is also assessed, and teaching needs are identified.

Assessment of Past Glycemic Control

For the woman with pregestational type 1 or type 2 diabetes, the glycosylated hemoglobin A_{1c} level may be measured. With prolonged hyperglycemia some of the hemoglobin remains saturated with glucose for the life of the red blood cell. Therefore a test for glycosylated hemoglobin provides a measurement of glycemic control over time, specifically over the previous 8 to 12 weeks. Regular measurements of glycosylated hemoglobin provide data for altering the treatment plan and lead to improvement of glycemic control. A hemoglobin A_{1c} of 5% to 6% is the desired goal, which correlates to an average glucose of 90 to 120 mg/dl (Gabbe, Carpenter, & Garrison, 2007).

Fasting blood glucose and random (1 to 2 hours after eating) glucose levels may be assessed during antepartum visits (Fig. 13-2). Blood glucose self-monitoring records should also be reviewed.

Antepartum

Because of her high risk status, the woman with diabetes is monitored more frequently than low risk pregnant women. In the past routine hospitalization for management of diabetes

evolve Nursing Care Plan—Pregnancy Complicated by Pregestational Diabetes

NURSING PROCESS: PREGESTATIONAL DIABETES

Assessment

When a pregnant woman with diabetes initiates prenatal care, a thorough evaluation of her health status is completed. The assessment includes:

History

Routine prenatal history
Onset and course of diabetes
Degree of glycemic control before pregnancy

Interview

Learning needs:

- Diabetes and pregnancy
- Potential fetal complications
- Plan of care

Emotional status:

- Coping with pregnancy superimposed on preexisting diabetes
- Dealing with "high risk" status
- Fear of maternal and fetal complications

Support system:

- Identifying significant persons and their roles
- Assessing reactions to the pregnancy and the management plan
- Assessing involvement in the treatment regimen
- Reviewing socioeconomic factors

Physical Examination

Current health status
Routine prenatal examination
Effects of diabetes on pregnancy

- Baseline electrocardiogram to assess cardiovascular status
- Evaluation for retinopathy with follow-up as needed by an ophthalmologist each trimester and more often if retinopathy is diagnosed
- Blood pressure: increased risk for preeclampsia
- Weight gain
- Fundal height: abnormal increase in size for dates may indicate hydramnios or fetal macrosomia

Laboratory Tests

Glycosylated hemoglobin (glycemic control over time)
Baseline renal function with a 24-hour urine collection for total protein excretion and creatinine clearance
Urinalysis and culture: initial prenatal visit and throughout the pregnancy (urinary tract infections are common in diabetic pregnancy)
Urine (ketones)
Thyroid function tests may be performed (see later discussion of thyroid disorders)

Nursing Diagnoses

Nursing diagnoses for the woman with pregestational diabetes include the following:

Deficient knowledge related to

– diabetic pregnancy, management, and potential effects on pregnant woman and fetus

Anxiety, fear, dysfunctional grieving, powerlessness, disturbed body image, situational low self-esteem, spiritual distress, ineffective role performance, interrupted family processes related to

– stigma of being labeled diabetic
– effects of diabetes and its potential sequelae on the pregnant woman and the fetus

Risk for injury to fetus related to

– uteroplacental insufficiency
– birth trauma

Risk for injury to mother related to

– improper insulin administration
– hypoglycemia and hyperglycemia
– cesarean or operative vaginal birth
– postpartum infection

Planning

A plan of care is developed with the woman in collaboration with the multidisciplinary care team.

Expected outcomes of care for the pregnant woman with pregestational diabetes include that she will do the following:

- Demonstrate or verbalize understanding of diabetic pregnancy, the plan of care, and the importance of glycemic control
- Achieve and maintain glycemic control
- Demonstrate effective coping
- Experience no complications (maternal morbidity or mortality)
- Give birth to a healthy infant at term

Interventions

Antepartum

Schedule routine prenatal visits every 1 to 2 weeks in first and second trimesters and one to two times per week in the third trimester.

Education:

- Home glucose monitoring
- Importance of a consistent daily schedule to maintain tight glucose control
- Importance of good foot care and general skin care
- Diet: Nutrition counseling by registered dietitian
- Insulin therapy

Exercise as prescribed by the primary health care provider
Fetal surveillance
Sonograms (to determine gestational age and fetal growth; estimate fetal weight; detect hydramnios, macrosomia, and anomalies)

- Maternal serum alpha-fetoprotein (to detect neural tube defects)
- Fetal echocardiography (to detect cardiac anomalies)
- Doppler studies of the umbilical artery (to detect placental compromise)
- Kick counts
- Nonstress tests (to evaluate fetal well-being)

Intrapartum

Monitor closely to prevent complications (dehydration, hypoglycemia, hyperglycemia).
Determine blood glucose hourly.
Monitor fetal heart rate continuously.
Observe for fetal dystocia.
Ensure that a neonatal care provider is present at birth.

NURSING PROCESS: PREGESTATIONAL DIABETES—cont'd

Interventions—cont'd

Postpartum

Monitor blood glucose levels and adjust insulin dosage as appropriate.
Observe for complications (preeclampsia, hemorrhage, infection).
Encourage breastfeeding.
Provide family planning education.

Evaluation

Evaluation of the effectiveness of care of the pregnant woman with pregestational diabetes is based on the previously stated outcomes, which are closely associated with the degree of maternal metabolic control during pregnancy.

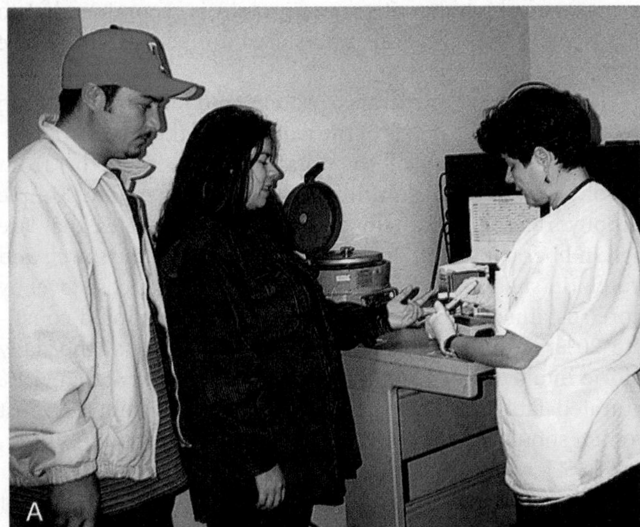

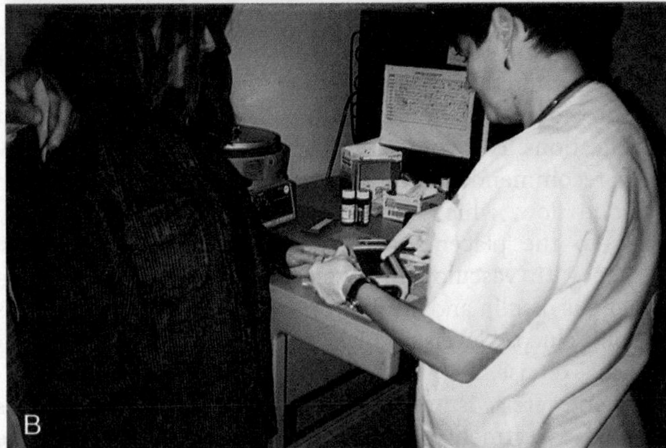

Fig. 13-2 A, Clinic nurse collects blood to determine glucose level. **B,** Nurse interprets glucose value displayed by monitor. *(Courtesy Dee Lowdermilk, UNC Ambulatory Care Clinics, Chapel Hill, NC.)*

such as insulin dose changes was common. With the availability of better home glucose monitoring and the growing reluctance of third-party payers to reimburse for hospitalization, pregnant women with diabetes are now generally managed as outpatients. Some patient and family education and maternal and fetal assessment may be done in the home, depending on the woman's insurance coverage and care provider preference.

Achieving and maintaining euglycemia (normal blood glucose level; also called *normogylcemia*) with blood glucose levels in the range of 60 to 120 mg/dl (Table 13-2) is the

Table 13-2 Target Blood Glucose Levels During Pregnancy

TIME OF MEASUREMENT	TARGET GLUCOSE LEVEL (mg/dl)*
Fasting	60-90
Premeal (lunch, dinner)	60-105
Bedtime	90-120
Postmeal	
1 hr	100-120
2 hr	90-120
2 AM to 4 AM	60-120

Source: American Diabetes Association: *Medical management of pregnancy complicated by diabetes,* ed 3, Alexandria, Va, 2000, The Association.
*Add 15% if plasma values are used.

primary goal of medical therapy for the pregnant woman with diabetes. Euglycemia is achieved through a combination of diet, insulin, exercise, and blood glucose determinations. Providing the woman with the knowledge, skill, and motivation she needs to achieve and maintain excellent blood glucose control is the primary nursing goal.

Achieving euglycemia requires commitment of the woman and her family to make the necessary lifestyle changes, which can sometimes seem overwhelming. Maintaining tight blood glucose control necessitates that the woman follow a consistent daily schedule. She must go to bed and get up, eat, exercise, and take insulin at the same time every day. Blood glucose is measured frequently to determine how well the major components of therapy (diet, insulin, and exercise) are working together to control blood glucose levels.

The woman should wear an identification bracelet at all times and carry insulin, syringes, and "glucose boosters" with her whenever she is away from home (see Community Focus box). She should be given written instructions for reporting the development of problems such as nausea, vomiting, and infections; and directions for reaching her health care provider by phone at night and on weekends and holidays (see Guidelines box).

Because the woman with diabetes is at risk for infections, eye problems, and neurologic changes, foot care and general skin care are important. A daily bath that includes good perineal and foot care is important. Lotions, creams, or oils can be applied to dry skin. Tight clothing should be avoided. Shoes or slippers that fit properly should be worn at all times and are best worn with socks or stockings. Feet should be inspected regularly, toenails should be cut straight across, and profes-

COMMUNITY FOCUS

Accessibility of Diabetes Supplies

Visit your local pharmacy and examine the diabetes equipment and supplies that are available. Locate glucose meters, urine test strips, insulin syringes, and insulin pens. How much does each of these items cost? Check to see which items are covered by most types of insurance and Medicaid. Read the directions for use of each item. How easily could you follow the instructions? Could a woman with low literacy skills read and understand them? Do the directions contain illustrations? Are the directions written in more than one language (e.g., in Spanish or French) in addition to English? Does the pharmacy have someone who can teach women? How can you use the information you have obtained in this exercise in your patient teaching?

GUIDELINES Treatment for Hypoglycemia

Be familiar with signs and symptoms of hypoglycemia (nervousness, headache, shaking, irritability, personality change, hunger, blurred vision, sweaty skin, tingling of mouth or extremities).

Check blood glucose level immediately when hypoglycemic symptoms occur.

If blood glucose is below 60 mg/dl, immediately eat or drink something that contains 10 to 15 g of simple carbohydrate. Examples:

- ½ cup (4 oz) unsweetened fruit juice
- ½ cup (4 oz) regular (not diet) soda
- 5 to 6 Life Savers candies
- 1 tbsp honey or corn (Karo) syrup
- 1 cup (8 oz) milk
- 2 to 3 glucose tablets

Rest for 15 minutes; then recheck blood glucose.

If glucose level is still below 60 mg/dl, eat or drink another serving of one of the "glucose boosters" listed here.

Wait 15 minutes; then recheck blood glucose. If it is still below 60 mg/dl, notify health care provider immediately.

Source: American Diabetes Association: *Medical management of pregnancy complicated by diabetes*, ed 3, Alexandria, Va, 2000, The Association; Becton Dickinson & Co: *Controlling low blood sugar reactions*, Franklin Lakes, NJ, 1997, Becton Dickinson.

sional help should be sought for any foot problems. Extremes of temperature should be avoided.

Diet The woman with pregestational diabetes has usually had nutrition counseling regarding the management of diabetes. Because pregnancy precipitates special nutrition concerns and needs, the woman should be educated to incorporate these changes into dietary planning. Nutrition counseling is usually provided by a registered dietitian.

Dietary management during diabetic pregnancy must be based on blood (not urine) glucose levels. The diet is individualized to allow for increased fetal and metabolic requirements, with consideration of such factors as prepregnancy weight and dietary habits, overall health, ethnic background, lifestyle, stage of pregnancy, knowledge of nutrition, and insulin therapy. The dietary goals are to provide weight gain consistent with a normal pregnancy, prevent ketoacidosis, and minimize wide fluctuation of blood glucose levels.

Energy needs are usually calculated on the basis of 30 to 35 calories per kilogram of ideal body weight, with the average diet including 2200 calories (first trimester) to 2500 calories (second and third trimesters). Total calories may be distributed among three meals and one evening snack or, more commonly, three meals and at least two snacks. Meals should be eaten on time and never skipped. Snacks must be carefully planned in accordance with insulin therapy to avoid fluctuations in blood glucose levels. A large bedtime snack of at least 25 g of carbohydrate with some protein is recommended to help prevent hypoglycemia and starvation ketosis during the night.

The ratio of carbohydrates, protein, and fat is important to meet the metabolic needs of the woman and the fetus. Approximately 40% to 50% of the total calories should be from carbohydrates, with a minimum of 250 g per day. Simple carbohydrates are limited; complex carbohydrates that are high in fiber content are recommended because the starch and protein in such foods help regulate the blood glucose level by more sustained glucose release. Protein intake should constitute 20% of the total kilocalories; 30% to 40% of the daily caloric intake should come from fat, with no more than 10% saturated fats (see Home Care box). Weight gain for most women should be about 12 kg during the pregnancy (Gilbert, 2007).

Exercise Although exercise enhances the utilization of glucose and decreases insulin need in nonpregnant women with diabetes, there are limited data regarding exercise during pregnancy. Any prescription of exercise during pregnancy for a woman with diabetes should be done by the primary health care provider and should be monitored closely to prevent complications. For women with vasculopathy only mild exercise is recommended because exercise causes a redistribution of blood flow, which increases the potential for ischemic injury to the placenta and already compromised organs. Women with vasculopathy typically depend completely on exogenous insulin and are at greater risk for wide fluctuations in blood glucose levels and ketoacidosis, which can be worsened by exercise.

When exercise is prescribed by the health care provider as part of the treatment plan, careful instructions are given. The exercise need not be vigorous to be beneficial: 15 to 30 minutes of walking four to six times a week is satisfactory for most pregnant women. Other exercises that may be recommended include non–weight-bearing activities such as arm ergometry or use of a recumbent bicycle. The best time for exercise is after meals when the blood glucose level is rising. To monitor the effect of insulin on blood glucose levels, the woman can measure blood glucose before, during, and after exercise (see also Home Care box: Exercise Tips for Pregnant Women in Chapter 11).

Insulin Therapy Adequate insulinization is the primary factor in the maintenance of euglycemia during pregnancy, thus ensuring proper glucose metabolism of the mother and fetus. Insulin requirements during pregnancy change dramatically as the pregnancy progresses, necessitating frequent adjustments in insulin dosage. In the first trimester, little or

HOME CARE

Dietary Management of Diabetic Pregnancy

- Follow the prescribed diet plan.
- Eat a well-balanced diet, including daily food requirements for a normal pregnancy.
- Divide daily food intake between three meals and two to four snacks, depending on individual needs.
- Eat a substantial bedtime snack to prevent a severe drop in blood glucose level during the night.
- Limit the intake of fats if weight gain occurs too rapidly.
- Take daily vitamins and iron as prescribed by the health care provider.
- Avoid foods high in refined sugar.
- Eat consistently each day; never skip meals or snacks.
- Reduce the intake of saturated fat and cholesterol.
- Eat foods high in dietary fiber.
- Avoid alcohol and caffeine.

no change occurs in prepregnancy insulin requirements; however, insulin dosage may need to be decreased because of hypoglycemia. During the second and third trimesters, because of insulin resistance, the dosage must be increased to maintain target glucose levels.

The goal of administration of exogenous insulin during pregnancy is to achieve diurnal glucose levels that are similar to those of a nondiabetic pregnant woman. The insulin regimen for a pregnant woman differs from that which is effective in the nonpregnant state in combinations and timing of insulin injections (Landon, Catalano, & Gabbe, 2007). Thus, for the woman with type 1 pregestational diabetes who has typically been accustomed to one injection per day of intermediate-acting insulin, multiple daily injections of mixed insulin are a new experience. The woman with type 2 diabetes previously treated with oral hypoglycemics is faced with the task of learning to self-administer injections of insulin. The nurse is instrumental in education and support with regard to insulin administration and the adjustment of insulin dosage to maintain euglycemia (see Patient Teaching box).

Many types of insulin are available today. Beef and pork insulin have largely been replaced by biosynthetic human insulin preparations (Humulin or Novolin), which are less likely to cause antibody formation. Patients with new onset of diabetes are almost always started on this type of insulin. Lispro (Humalog) is a rapid-acting insulin preparation that has an onset of action within 25 minutes of injection and peaks in 30 minutes to 1½ hours. Advantages of lispro include convenience; because it is injected immediately before mealtime, there is less hyperglycemia after meals and fewer hypoglycemic episodes. Lispro insulin has a total duration of action of 4 to 5 hours (Landon, Catalano, & Gabbe, 2007) (Table 13-3). Insulin-dependent diabetes is managed in most women with two to three injections per day. Usually two thirds of the daily insulin dose, with longer-acting (NPH) and short-acting (regular or Lispro) insulin combined in a 2 : 1 ratio, is given before breakfast. The remaining one third, again a combination of longer- and short-acting insulin, is administered in the evening before dinner. To reduce the risk of hypoglycemia during the night, separate injections often are administered, with short-acting insulin given before dinner, followed by longer-acting insulin at bedtime. An alternative insulin regimen that works well for some women is to administer short-acting insulin before each meal and longer-acting insulin at bedtime (Landon, Catalano, & Gabbe, 2007).

Although subcutaneous insulin injections are most commonly used, increasing numbers of pregnant women are using continuous insulin infusion systems. The insulin pump is designed to mimic more closely the function of the pancreas in secreting insulin (Fig. 13-3). This portable, battery-powered

PATIENT TEACHING Administration of Insulin

Procedure for Mixing Intermediate-Acting (NPH) and Short-Acting (Regular) Insulin

1. Wash hands thoroughly and gather supplies. Be sure that the insulin syringe corresponds to the concentration of insulin you are using.
2. Check insulin bottle to be certain that it is the appropriate type and check the expiration date.
3. Gently rotate (do not shake) the insulin vial to mix the insulin.
4. Wipe off rubber stopper of each vial with alcohol.
5. Draw into syringe the amount of air equal to total dose.
6. Inject air equal to NPH dose into NPH vial. Remove syringe from vial.
7. Inject air equal to regular insulin dose into regular insulin vial.
8. Invert regular insulin bottle and withdraw regular insulin dose.
9. Without adding more air to NPH vial, carefully withdraw NPH dose.

Procedure for Self-Injection of Insulin

1. Select proper injection site (remember to rotate sites).
2. Injection site should be clean. Use of alcohol is not necessary. If alcohol is used, let it dry before injecting.
3. Pinch the skin up to form a subcutaneous pocket and, holding the syringe like a pencil, puncture the skin at a 45- to 90-degree angle. If there is a great deal of fatty tissue at the site, spread the skin taut and inject the syringe at a 90-degree angle.
4. Slowly inject the insulin.
5. As you withdraw the needle, cover the injection site with sterile gauze and apply gentle pressure to prevent bleeding.
6. Record insulin dose and time of injection.

Table 13-3 Insulin Administration During Pregnancy: Expected Time of Action

TYPE OF INSULIN	ONSET	PEAK	DURATION
Lispro (rapid acting)	Within 15 min	2-3 hr	3-4 hr
Regular (short acting)	30 min	3-4 hr	6-8 hr
Intermediate acting	2-4 hr	4-12 hr	12-24 hr
Long acting	3-4 hr	14-24 hr	24-36 hr

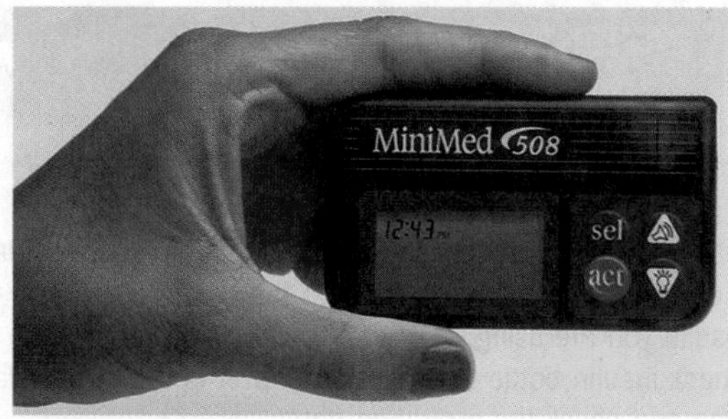

Fig. 13-3 Insulin pump shows basal rate for pregnant women with diabetes. *(Courtesy MiniMed, Inc., Sylmar, CA.)*

device is worn like a pager during most daily activities. The pump infuses regular insulin at a set basal rate and has the capacity to deliver up to four different basal rates in 24 hours. It also delivers bolus doses of insulin before meals to control postprandial blood glucose levels. A fine-gauge plastic catheter is inserted into subcutaneous tissue, usually in the abdomen, and attached to the pump syringe by connecting tubing. The subcutaneous catheter and connecting tubing are changed every 2 to 3 days. Although the insulin pump is convenient and generally provides good glycemic control, complications such as DKA, infection, or hypoglycemic coma can still develop. Use of the insulin pump requires a knowledgeable, motivated patient; skilled health care providers; and 24-hour availability of emergency assistance (Landon, Catalano, & Gabbe, 2007).

Monitoring Blood Glucose Levels Blood glucose testing at home is the commonly accepted method for monitoring blood glucose levels. It is the most important tool available to the woman to assess her degree of glycemic control. In addition, this monitoring provides motivation to continue the prescribed treatment plan. The data obtained facilitate interaction with the health care team in maintaining glycemic control and minimizing fetal risk (see Home Care box).

Women with pregestational diabetes are often familiar with self-monitoring of blood glucose levels because it is typically included in the management plan for type 1 and some cases of type 2 diabetes. However, a thorough assessment of the woman's knowledge and skill related to blood glucose testing is essential to ensure accurate monitoring of glucose levels during pregnancy. The nurse observes the woman performing blood glucose monitoring to determine her accuracy and comfort with the system. The family is included in the assessment and in subsequent instruction.

Glucometers incorporate memory to store a large number of readings; however, the woman is still encouraged to keep written records of glucose levels. She should bring her written records, her meter containing stored test results, or both with her to each appointment. It is important that the monitoring equipment be checked for accuracy at intervals by comparing the woman's results on her machine with the results of a laboratory test done at the same time on a capillary whole blood sample.

Blood glucose levels are routinely measured at various times throughout the day such as before breakfast, lunch, and dinner; 2 hours after meals; at bedtime; and in the middle of the night. The primary health care provider will determine for each individual woman the number and timing of routine blood glucose determinations. Because hyperglycemia is to be avoided, postprandial measurements are often performed.

HOME CARE

Testing Blood Glucose Level

1. Gather supplies, check expiration date, and read instructions on testing materials. Prepare glucose reflectance meter for use according to manufacturer's directions.
2. Wash hands in warm water (warmth increases circulation).
3. Select site on side of any finger (all fingers should be used in rotation).
4. Pierce site with lancet (may use automatic, spring-loaded, puncturing device). Cleaning the site with alcohol is not necessary.
5. Drop hand down to side; with other hand gently squeeze finger from hand to fingertip.
6. Allow blood to drop onto testing strip. Be sure to cover entire reagent area.
7. Determine blood glucose value using the glucose reflectance meter, following manufacturer's instructions.
8. Record results.
9. Repeat daily as instructed by health care provider and as needed for signs of hypoglycemia or hyperglycemia.

Source: American Diabetes Association: *Medical management of pregnancy complicated by diabetes*, ed 3, Alexandria, Va, 2000, The Association.

NURSING ALERT Hyperglycemia will most likely be identified in the 2-hour postprandial values because blood glucose levels peak about 2 hours after a meal.

Special circumstances may necessitate more frequent testing. Women are instructed to check glucose levels at any sign of hypoglycemia or hyperglycemia. When there is any readjustment in insulin dosage or diet, more frequent measurement of blood glucose is warranted. If nausea, vomiting, or diarrhea occurs or if any infection is present, the woman will probably be asked to monitor her blood glucose levels more closely.

Target levels of blood glucose during pregnancy are lower than nonpregnant values. Acceptable fasting levels are generally between 60 and 90 mg/dl, and 2-hour postprandial levels should be less than 120 mg/dl (see Table 13-2) (ADA, 2008b). The woman should be told to report episodes of hypoglycemia (less than 60 mg/dl) and hyperglycemia (greater than 200 mg/dl) to her health care provider immediately so that adjustments in diet or insulin therapy can be made.

Pregnant women with diabetes are much more likely to develop hypoglycemia than hyperglycemia because the goal of therapy is to maintain the blood glucose in a narrow, low-normal range of 60 to 120 mg/dl. Although a blood glucose level greater than 120 mg/dl is considered too high for a pregnant woman, it will not produce the classic signs and symptoms of hyperglycemia. However, many women will have signs and symptoms of hypoglycemia with blood glucose levels below 60 mg/dl.

Most episodes of mild or moderate hypoglycemia can be treated with oral intake of 10 to 15 g of simple carbohydrates (see Guidelines box, p. 302). If severe hypoglycemia occurs in which the woman experiences a decrease in or loss of consciousness or an inability to swallow, she will require a parenteral injection of glucagon or intravenous (IV) glucose. Because hypoglycemia can develop rapidly and impaired judgment can be associated with even moderate episodes, it is vital that family members, friends, and work colleagues be able to recognize signs and symptoms quickly and initiate proper treatment if necessary.

Although hyperglycemia is less likely to occur, it is still a dangerous complication. Hyperglycemia can rapidly progress to DKA. Women and their family members should be alert for signs and symptoms of hyperglycemia, especially when infections or other illnesses occur (see Home Care box).

HOME CARE

What to Do When Illness Occurs

Be sure to take insulin even though appetite and food intake may be less than normal. (Insulin needs are increased with illness or infection.)

Call the health care provider and relay the following information:

- Symptoms of illness (e.g., nausea, vomiting, diarrhea)
- Fever
- Most recent blood glucose level
- Urine ketones
- Time and amount of last insulin dose

Increase oral intake of fluids to prevent dehydration.

Rest as much as possible.

If unable to reach health care provider and blood glucose exceeds 200 mg/dl with urine ketones present, seek emergency treatment at the nearest health care facility. Do not attempt to self-treat.

Complications Requiring Hospitalization Occasionally hospitalization may be required to regulate insulin dosage and stabilize glucose levels. Hospitalization offers a controlled situation to initiate and regulate insulin therapy while providing opportunity for intensive education in self-administration of insulin and regulation of blood glucose. Infection, which can lead to hyperglycemia and DKA, is an indication for hospitalization, regardless of gestational age. Hospitalization during the third trimester for closer maternal and fetal observation may be indicated for women whose diabetes is poorly controlled or who also have hypertension.

Determination of Birth Date and Mode of Delivery Today the majority of diabetic pregnancies are allowed to progress to term (38 to 40 weeks of gestation), as long as good metabolic control is maintained and all parameters of antepartum fetal surveillance remain within normal limits. Reasons to proceed with delivery before term include poor metabolic control, worsening hypertensive disorders, fetal macrosomia, prior stillbirth, or fetal growth restriction (Landon, Catalano, & Gabbe, 2007).

Many practitioners plan labor induction between 38 and 40 weeks provided maternal glucose levels are well controlled. To confirm fetal lung maturity before birth, an amniocentesis may be performed in pregnancies of less than 39 weeks. For the pregnancy complicated by diabetes, fetal lung maturation is better predicted by the amniotic fluid phosphatidylglycerol than by the lecithin/sphingomyelin (L/S) ratio. If the fetal lungs are still immature, birth should be postponed as long as the results of fetal assessment remain reassuring. Induced labor and birth despite poor fetal lung maturity may be essential when testing suggests fetal compromise or if preeclampsia, deteriorating vision resulting from proliferative retinopathy, or worsening renal function develops.

The mode of birth for women with pregestational diabetes is a subject of controversy among practitioners. The rate of cesarean births for these women is high, around 45%. Cesarean birth is often performed when antepartum testing suggests a compromised fetal status or if the estimated fetal weight is 4000 to 4500 g. When induction of labor is desired and the cervix fails to respond, cesarean birth often is necessary (Landon, Catalano, & Gabbe, 2007).

Intrapartum

During the intrapartum period the woman with pregestational diabetes must be monitored closely to prevent complications related to dehydration, hypoglycemia, and hyperglycemia. Most women use large amounts of energy (calories) to accomplish the work and manage the stress of labor and birth; however, this calorie expenditure varies with the individual. Blood glucose levels and hydration must be controlled carefully during labor. An IV line is inserted for infusion of a maintenance fluid such as lactated Ringer's solution or 5% dextrose in lactated Ringer's solution. Insulin may be administered by continuous infusion or intermittent subcutaneous injection.

Determinations of blood glucose are made every hour, and fluids and insulin are adjusted to maintain blood glucose levels between 70 and 90 mg/dl or capillary whole blood glucose levels at 60 to 80 mg/dl. It is essential that these target glucose levels be maintained because hyperglycemia during labor can precipitate metabolic problems in the neonate, particularly hypoglycemia.

During labor continuous fetal heart monitoring is necessary. The mother should assume an upright or side-lying position during bed rest in labor to prevent supine hypotension because of a large fetus or polyhydramnios. Labor is allowed to progress without intervention, provided normal rates of cervical dilation, fetal descent, and fetal well-being are maintained. Failure to progress may indicate a macrosomic infant and cephalopelvic disproportion, necessitating cesarean birth. The woman is observed and treated during labor for diabetic complications such as hyperglycemia, ketosis, ketoacidosis, and glycosuria. During second-stage labor the nurse should be alert for the possibility of shoulder dystocia if delivery of a macrosomic infant is attempted and be prepared to assist with maneuvers to free the fetal shoulder that is lodged behind the symphysis pubis (see Chapter 19). A neonatologist, pediatrician, or neonatal nurse practitioner may be present at the birth to initiate assessment and neonatal care.

If a cesarean birth is planned, it should be scheduled in the early morning to facilitate glycemic control. The morning dose of insulin is withheld, and the woman is given nothing by mouth. Regional anesthesia (epidural or spinal) is recommended because hypoglycemia can be detected earlier if the woman is awake.

Postpartum

In the immediate postpartum period insulin requirements decrease substantially because the major source of insulin resistance, the placenta, has been removed. Women with type 1 diabetes may require only one half the prenatal insulin dose on the first postpartum day, provided that they are eating a full diet. It takes several days after birth to reestablish carbohydrate homeostasis. Blood glucose levels are monitored in the postpartum period, and insulin dosage is adjusted accordingly. Blood glucose levels do not require such a tight control after birth. Usually insulin is not given until the blood glucose level is greater than 200 mg/dl. The woman who is insulin dependent must eat on time even if the baby needs feeding or other pressing demands exist. Women with type 2 diabetes often require no insulin in the postpartum period and are able to maintain euglycemia through diet alone or with oral hypoglycemics.

Possible postpartum complications include preeclampsia-eclampsia, hemorrhage, and infection. Hemorrhage is a possibility if the mother's uterus was overdistended (by hydramnios or a macrosomic fetus) or overstimulated (by oxytocin induction). Postpartum infections such as endometritis are more likely to occur in a woman with diabetes.

Mothers are encouraged to breastfeed. In addition to the advantages of maternal satisfaction, breastfeeding has an antidiabetogenic effect. Insulin requirements may be half of prepregnancy levels because of the carbohydrate used in human milk production. Because glucose levels are lower, breastfeeding women are at increased risk for hypoglycemia, especially in the early postpartum period and after breastfeeding sessions.

The mother may have early breastfeeding difficulties. Poor metabolic control may delay lactogenesis and contribute to decreased milk production. Because many women give birth by cesarean, the effects of anesthesia and postoperative discomfort may delay maternal contact and make breastfeeding more difficult. Initial contact and opportunity to breastfeed the infant are often delayed because many institutions place infants of mothers with diabetes in neonatal intensive care units or special care nurseries for observation during the first few hours after birth. Support and assistance from nursing staff and lactation specialists can facilitate the mother's early experience with breastfeeding and encourage her to continue.

Infants who are exclusively breastfed are less likely to develop diabetes; exposure to cow's milk products before 8 days of age is an important risk factor for the disease.

Breastfeeding mothers with diabetes may be at increased risk for mastitis and yeast infections of the breast. Insulin dosage, which is decreased during lactation, must be recalculated at the time of weaning.

Family Planning and Contraception The new mother needs information about family planning and contraception. Family planning is important for all women, but it is essential for the woman with diabetes to safeguard her own health and to promote optimal outcomes in future pregnancies. Because excellent glucose control at conception is crucial for all women with diabetes, the importance of conscientiously using a reliable contraceptive method until another pregnancy is desired should be stressed. No one best form of contraception exists for women with diabetes. Instead emphasis should be placed on consistent use of a reliable and effective birth control method. The risks and benefits of contraceptive methods should be discussed with the mother and her partner before discharge from the hospital.

The barrier methods are often recommended as safe, inexpensive options that have no inherent risks for women with diabetes (Landon, Catalano, & Gabbe, 2007). However, barrier methods are not as effective or convenient as some other forms of contraception.

Use of oral contraceptives is controversial because of the risk of thromboembolic events and myocardial infarction and the effect on carbohydrate metabolism. In women without vascular disease or other risk factors, combination low-dose oral contraceptives may be prescribed. Close monitoring of blood pressure and lipid levels is necessary to detect complications (Landon, Catalano, & Gabbe, 2007). Progestin-only oral contraceptives can be used because they minimally affect carbohydrate metabolism (Cunningham et al, 2005).

Some health care providers are reluctant to use intrauterine devices (IUDs) in women with diabetes because of concerns about infection. However, these women have used this method successfully.

Opinion is divided about the use of long-acting parenteral or implantable progestins such as Depo-Provera. Some authorities recommend their use, especially in women who may not be compliant with daily dosing of oral contraceptives or appropriate follow-up care. Others believe that these methods may adversely affect diabetic control (Landon, Catalano, & Gabbe, 2007).

The woman and her partner should be informed that the risks associated with pregnancy increase with the duration and severity of the diabetic condition and that pregnancy may contribute to vascular changes associated with diabetes. Therefore sterilization should be discussed with the woman who has completed her family or who has significant vasculopathy (see Nursing Care Plan).

Gestational Diabetes Mellitus

GDM complicates approximately 4% of all pregnancies in the United States and accounts for 90% of all cases of diabetic pregnancy (ADA, 2008a). Prevalence varies by race and ethnicity. GDM is more likely to occur among Hispanic, Native American, Asian, and African-American populations than in Caucasians (Centers for Disease Control and Prevention [CDC], 2007a; Landon, Catalano, & Gabbe, 2007). Women with GDM are at significant risk of developing glucose intolerance later in life; about 50% will be diagnosed as having diabetes within 5 to 10 years. This is especially true of women whose GDM is diagnosed early in pregnancy and who also are obese. Classic risk factors for GDM include maternal age older than 30; obesity; family history of type 2 diabetes; and an obstetric history of an infant weighing more than 9 lb, hydramnios, unexplained stillbirth, miscarriage, or an infant with congenital anomalies. Other factors include hypertensive disorders, recurrent monilial vaginitis, and glucosuria on two consecutive visits to the clinic or office (ADA, 2008a).

evolve Critical Thinking Exercise—Gestational Diabetes

NURSING CARE PLAN Pregnancy Complicated by Pregestational Diabetes

Nursing Diagnosis: Deficient knowledge related to lack of recall of information as evidenced by patient questions and concerns

Expected Outcome

Patient will be able to verbalize important information regarding diabetes, its management, and potential effects on the pregnant woman and fetus.

Nursing Interventions/*Rationales*

Assess patient's current knowledge base regarding disease process, management, effects on pregnancy and fetus, and potential complications *to provide database for further teaching.*

Review the pathophysiology of diabetes, effects on pregnancy and fetus, and potential complications *to promote patient recall of information and compliance with treatment plan.*

Review procedure for insulin administration, demonstrate procedure for blood glucose monitoring and insulin measurement and administration, and obtain return demonstration *to establish patient comfort and competence with procedures.*

Discuss diet and exercise as *prescribed* by diabetologist *to promote self-management.*

Review signs and symptoms of complications of hypoglycemia and hyperglycemia and appropriate interventions *to promote prompt recognition of complications and self-management.*

Provide contact numbers for health care team for prompt interventions and answers to questions on an ongoing basis *to promote patient and health team collaboration.*

Nursing Diagnosis: Risk for fetal injury related to elevated maternal glucose levels

Expected Outcome

Fetus will remain free of injury and be born at term in a healthy state.

Nursing Interventions/*Rationales*

Assess patient's current control of diabetes *to identify risk for fetal death and congenital anomalies.*

Monitor fundal height during each prenatal visit *to identify appropriate fetal growth.*

Monitor for signs and symptoms of pregnancy-induced hypertension *to identify early manifestations because pregnant women with diabetes are more at risk.*

Assess fetal movement and heart rate during each prenatal visit and perform weekly nonstress tests during the last 4 weeks of pregnancy *to assess fetal well-being.*

Review procedure for blood glucose testing and insulin administration *to promote self-management.*

Nursing Diagnosis: Anxiety related to threat to maternal and fetal well-being as evidenced by patient verbal expressions of concern

Expected Outcome

Patient will identify sources of anxiety and report feeling less anxious.

Nursing Interventions/*Rationales*

Through therapeutic communication promote an open relationship with patient *to promote patient trust.*

Listen to patient's feelings and concerns *to assess for any misconception or misinformation that may be contributing to anxiety.*

Review potential dangers by providing factual information *to correct any misconceptions or misinformation.*

Encourage patient to share concerns with her health care team *to promote patient and team collaboration in her care.*

Nursing Diagnosis: Risk for imbalanced nutrition: less than body requirements related to inability to ingest nutrients that are needed for pregnancy complicated by diabetes

Expected Outcomes

Patient will verbalize understanding of dietary needs during pregnancy, gain weight that is consistent with a normal pregnancy, and maintain blood sugar levels between 60 and 120 mg/dl.

Nursing Interventions/*Rationales*

Assess caloric intake and dietary pattern using 24-hour recall *to evaluate patient understanding and adherence to dietary regimen.*

Review importance of regularity of meals and snacks *to promote compliance with treatment plan.*

Review blood glucose monitoring *to determine if patient is competent with procedure.*

Weigh patient at each prenatal visit *to assess appropriate weight gain.*

Refer to dietitian for individualized counseling if needed *to plan diet that assists the woman to maintain normoglycemia and gain the appropriate amount of weight.*

The diagnosis of gestational diabetes is usually made during the second half of pregnancy. As fetal nutrient demands rise during the late second and third trimesters, maternal nutrient ingestion induces greater and more sustained levels of blood glucose. At the same time maternal insulin resistance is also increasing as a result of the insulin antagonistic effects of the placental hormones, cortisol and insulinase. Consequently maternal insulin demands rise as much as threefold. Most pregnant women are capable of increasing insulin production to compensate for the insulin resistance and maintain euglycemia. When the pancreas is unable to produce sufficient insulin or the insulin is not used effectively, GDM can result.

Maternal and Fetal Risks

Women with GDM have twice the risk of developing hypertensive disorders compared with normal pregnant women. They also have increased risk for fetal macrosomia, which can

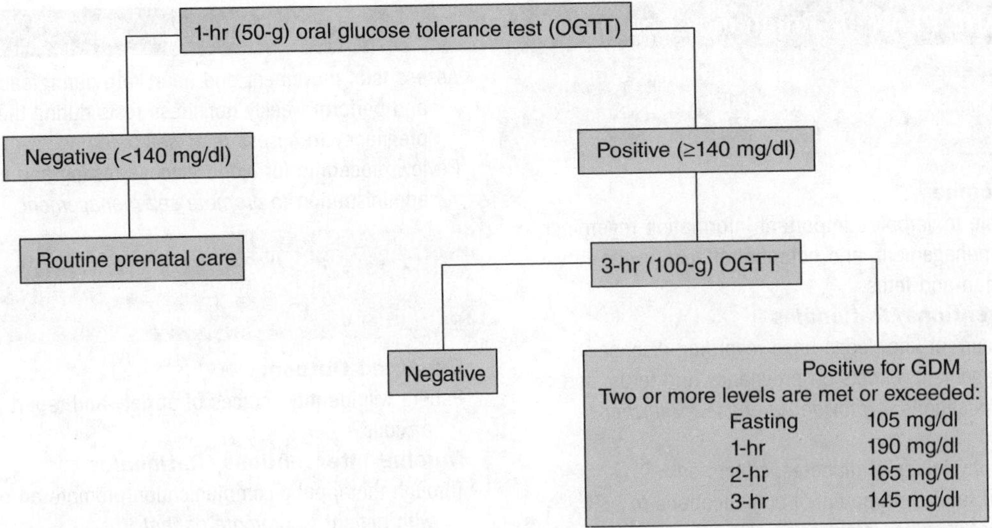

Fig. 13-4 Screening and diagnosis for gestational diabetes. (From American Diabetes Association: Position statement: gestational diabetes mellitus, *Diabetes Care* 27[suppl 1]:S88-S90, 2004.)

lead to increased rates of perineal lacerations, episiotomy, and cesarean birth. In addition, fetal macrosomia may be associated with shoulder dystocia and birth trauma. GDM also places the neonate at increased risk for hypoglycemia, hypocalcemia, hyperbilirubinemia, thrombocytopenia, polycythemia, and respiratory distress syndrome.

The overall incidence of congenital anomalies among infants of women with GDM approaches that of the general population because GDM usually develops after week 20 of pregnancy—after the critical period of organogenesis (first trimester) has passed.

Screening for Gestational Diabetes Mellitus

Nurses involved in prenatal care delivery can be instrumental in the identification of women with GDM. Although protocols regarding which women will undergo screening and exactly how the screening will be done vary among care providers, nurses are often responsible for ensuring that the screen is performed on the identified group of women at the proper gestational age. Careful adherence to screening protocols is crucial to correctly identify women with GDM.

ACOG (2001a) recommends that all pregnant women be screened for GDM, either by history, clinical risk factors, or laboratory screening of blood glucose levels (Fig. 13-4). Based on history and clinical risk factors, some women are at such low risk for the development of GDM that glucose testing is neither necessary nor cost-effective (Expert Committee on the Diagnosis and Classification of Diabetes Mellitus, 2003). This group at low risk includes normal-weight women younger than 25 years who have no family history of diabetes, are not members of an ethnic or a racial group known to have a high prevalence of the disease, and have no previous history of abnormal glucose tolerance or adverse obstetric outcomes usually associated with GDM (ACOG, 2001a; Expert Committee on the Diagnosis and Classification of Diabetes Mellitus, 2003). Women at high risk for developing GDM should be screened at the first prenatal visit and again at 24 to 28 weeks of gestation (ADA, 2008b).

Nursing diagnoses and expected outcomes of care for the woman with GDM are basically the same as those for women with pregestational diabetes; however, the time frame for planning may be shortened with GDM because the diagnosis is usually made later in pregnancy.

Interventions

Antepartum

When the diagnosis of gestational diabetes is made, treatment begins immediately, allowing little or no time for the woman and her family to adjust to the diagnosis before they are expected to participate in the treatment plan. This is in contrast to the woman with pregestational diabetes who may have had years to learn about the disease and adapt to dietary modifications, self-monitoring of glucose, and insulin administration. With each step of the treatment plan, the nurse and other health care providers should educate the woman and her family, providing detailed and comprehensive explanations to ensure understanding, participation, and adherence to the necessary interventions. Potential complications should be discussed, and the need for maintenance of euglycemia throughout the remainder of the pregnancy is reinforced. It may be reassuring for the woman and her family to know that GDM typically disappears when the pregnancy is over.

As with pregestational diabetes, the aim of therapy in women with GDM is meticulous blood glucose control. Fasting (preprandial) blood glucose levels should be less than or equal to 105 mg/dl; 1 hour after meals (postprandial) they should be less than or equal to 155; and 2-hour postprandial blood levels should be less than or equal to 130 mg/dl (ADA, 2008b).

Diet Dietary modification is the mainstay of treatment for GDM. The woman with GDM is placed on a standard diabetic diet immediately on diagnosis. Some authorities recommend fewer calories for overweight or morbidly obese women, believing that such a diet will cause less hyperglycemia and reduce the need for insulin (Landon, Catalano, & Gabbe, 2007). Dietary counseling by a nutritionist is recommended.

Exercise Exercise in women with GDM appears to be safe. It helps lower blood glucose levels and may be instrumental in eliminating the need for insulin.

Monitoring Blood Glucose Levels Regular blood glucose monitoring is necessary to determine if euglycemia can be maintained by diet and exercise. Women with GDM are encouraged to perform self-monitoring with reflectance meters to adjust the management plan to achieve near-normal glycemia. Testing may be done at fasting, preprandial, and postprandial times with values recorded in a log for review by the health care provider.

Insulin Therapy Up to 20% of women with GDM require insulin during the pregnancy to maintain adequate blood glucose levels, despite compliance with the prescribed diet. The nurse should never assume that increased blood glucose levels in the woman with GDM have been caused by dietary indiscretion alone without first taking a thorough history.

Women who repeatedly exceed glucose thresholds for fasting and 2-hour postprandial values are usually started on insulin therapy. The woman and her family should be taught the necessary skills to manage insulin administration. The use of oral hypoglycemic agents, commonly used in the treatment of nonpregnant patients, is currently being studied to determine safety for use during pregnancy and the long-term effects of in utero exposure. However, glyburide, a second-generation oral hypoglycemic agent, has been shown not to pass through the placenta. Langer and colleagues (2000) compared the use of glyburide and insulin in women with GDM. They found similar improvement in maternal glucose levels in both groups. Furthermore, the incidence of fetal macrosomia and neonatal hypoglycemia in the two study groups also was similar. Even though oral hypoglycemic agents are becoming more widely used, more studies are recommended before their endorsement for general use in all women with GDM

Fetal Surveillance There is no standard recommendation for fetal surveillance in pregnancies complicated by GDM. Women whose blood glucose levels are well controlled by diet are at low risk for fetal death. Many practitioners do not routinely perform antepartum fetal testing on them as long as their fasting and 2-hour postprandial blood glucose levels remain within normal limits and they have no other risk factors. Usually these women are allowed to progress to term and spontaneous labor without intervention. Once the woman reaches 40 weeks of gestation, fetal surveillance once or twice weekly is usually instituted (ACOG, 2001a).

Women with GDM whose blood glucose levels are not well controlled or who require insulin therapy, have hypertension, or have a history of previous stillbirth generally receive more intensive fetal biophysical monitoring. There is no standard recommendation regarding initiation of testing. Nonstress tests and biophysical profiles are often performed weekly, beginning from 32 to 36 weeks of gestation (ACOG, 2001a).

Intrapartum

During labor and birth blood glucose levels are monitored at least every 1 to 2 hours to maintain levels less than 110 mg/dl (ACOG, 2005). Glucose levels within this range will decrease the severity of neonatal hypoglycemia. Women whose GDM has been managed on insulin can be controlled by an infusion of regular insulin during labor. Even though IV fluids containing glucose may be given as maintenance fluids during birth, they should not be given as a bolus to the woman who has GDM. Routine uterine activity and fetal heart rate assessments are done. Although GDM is not an indication for cesarean birth, it may be necessary in the presence of problems such as preeclampsia or macrosomia.

Postpartum

Most women with GDM return to normal glucose levels after childbirth. However, GDM is likely to recur in future pregnancies, and women with GDM are at significant risk of developing glucose intolerance later in life. Assessment for carbohydrate intolerance can be initiated 6 to 12 weeks postpartum or after breastfeeding has stopped and should be repeated at regular intervals throughout the woman's life. Obesity is a major risk factor for the later development of diabetes. Thus women with a history of GDM, particularly those who are overweight, should be encouraged to make lifestyle changes that include weight loss and exercise to reduce this risk. Because offspring of women with GDM are at risk to develop obesity and diabetes in childhood or adolescence, regular health care for these children is essential.

Thyroid Disorders

Hyperthyroidism

Hyperthyroidism occurs in approximately 2 of every 1000 pregnancies (Mestman, 2007). In 90% to 95% of pregnant women it is caused by Graves' disease. Other rare but possible causes include toxic nodular goiter and thyroiditis (Mestman, 2007). Clinical manifestations of hyperthyroidism usually begin between 4 to 8 weeks of gestation and involve severe nausea and vomiting. Hyperemesis gravidarum may be diagnosed and is often associated with elevated thyroid hormone levels. Other symptoms are associated with an increased basal metabolic rate and increased sympathetic nervous system activity. Typical symptoms include fatigue, heat intolerance, warm skin, diaphoresis, emotional lability, tremulousness, tachycardia, and a wide pulse pressure. Many of these symptoms also occur with pregnancy; thus the disorder can be difficult to diagnose. Signs that may help differentiate hyperthyroidism from normal pregnancy include unplanned weight loss, onycholysis (loose nails), and a pulse rate greater than 100 beats/min that does not decrease with the Valsalva maneuver. Laboratory findings include an elevated free thyroxine (T_4) level and a suppressed serum thyroid-stimulating hormone (TSH) level. Hyperthyroidism is best treated before pregnancy. Moderate and severe hyperthyroidism must be treated during pregnancy; untreated or inadequately treated women may give birth to infants with low birth weight, intrauterine growth restriction (IUGR), hyperthyroidism, prematurity, stillbirth, and central hypothyroidism (Mestman, 2007). Women with hyperthyroidism are also at increased risk of developing severe preeclampsia, congestive heart failure, thyroid storm, miscarriage, placental abruption and infection. (Mestman, 2007).

The primary treatment of hyperthyroidism during pregnancy is drug therapy; the medication of choice is propylthiouracil (PTU). Patients generally show clinical improvement within 2 to 6 weeks of beginning therapy, but the medication requires 6 to 8 weeks to reach full effectiveness. During therapy the woman's free T_4 levels are measured monthly; the results are used to taper the drug to the smallest effective dosage to prevent unnecessary fetal hypothyroidism (Mestman, 2007; Nader, 2009). PTU is well tolerated by most patients. Rare side effects include pruritus, skin rash, a metallic taste, nausea, bronchospasm, oral ulcerations, hepatitis, and a lupuslike syndrome (Mestman, 2007; Nader, 2009). The most severe side effect is agranulocytosis, which is more common in women over 40 years of age and in those taking high doses of PTU. Symptoms of agranulocytosis are fever, malaise, gingivitis, and sore throat, which should be reported immediately to the health care provider; the woman should stop taking the PTU. Leukopenia of a transient and benign nature may occur as a result of PTU therapy. PTU readily crosses the placenta and may induce fetal hypothyroidism and goiter (Mestman, 2007; Nader, 2009).

β-Adrenergic blockers such as propranolol may be used in women with severe hyperthyroidism symptoms. Long-term use is not recommended because of the potential for IUGR and altered response to anoxic stress, postnatal bradycardia, and hypoglycemia.

Radioactive iodine must not be used in diagnosis or treatment of hyperthyroidism because it may compromise the fetal thyroid. If a mother taking hyperthyroid medication chooses to breastfeed, she needs to be aware that physiologically significant doses of the drug are passed to the infant through the breast milk. The infant's thyroid status should be monitored periodically so hypothyroidism can be prevented.

In severe cases hyperthyroidism may be treated surgically with subtotal thyroidectomy during the second or third trimester. Because of the increased risk of miscarriage and preterm labor associated with major surgery, this treatment is usually reserved for women with severe disease, those for whom drug therapy proves toxic, and those who are unable to adhere to the prescribed medical regimen. Postoperative hypothyroidism is common, occurring in at least 20% of women with hyperthyroidism.

NURSING ALERT A serious but uncommon complication of undiagnosed or partially treated hyperthyroidism is thyroid storm, which may occur in response to stresses such as infection, birth, or surgery. A woman experiencing this emergent condition may have fever, restlessness, tachycardia, vomiting, hypotension, or stupor. Congestive heart failure occurs frequently. Prompt treatment is essential; IV fluids and oxygen are administered along with high doses of PTU. Potassium iodide, antipyretics, glucocorticoids, and β-adrenergic blockers may also be given; sedation may be necessary for extreme restlessness (Mestman, 2007; Nader, 2009).

Hypothyroidism

Hypothyroidism during pregnancy is rare because women with this condition are often infertile. Hypothyroidism is usually the result of Hashimoto's disease (autoimmune thyroiditis), thyroid gland ablation by radiation, previous surgery, or antithyroid medications. Reduced thyroid function because of hypothalamic or pituitary failure is rare, with only a few reported cases. Iodine deficiency in the United States is also rare (Mestman, 2007; Nader, 2009).

Characteristic symptoms of hypothyroidism include fatigue, weight gain, cold intolerance, constipation, cool and dry skin, coarsened hair, and muscle weakness. Laboratory findings during pregnancy include low or low-normal T_3 and T_4 levels and elevated levels of TSH.

Pregnant women with untreated hypothyroidism are at risk for preeclampsia, placental abruption, and stillbirth. Infants born to mothers with hypothyroidism may be of low birth weight but for the most part are healthy, without evidence of thyroid dysfunction.

Thyroid hormone supplements are used to treat hypothyroidism. Levothyroxine (L-thyroxine [Synthroid]) is most often prescribed during pregnancy. As pregnancy progresses, the woman usually requires increased amounts of L-thyroxine. The aim of drug therapy is to maintain the woman's TSH level within the normal range for pregnant women. Dosage adjustments are made as necessary by measuring TSH levels periodically. Each dosage change should be followed 4 to 6 weeks later by determining the TSH level.

NURSING ALERT Pregnant women should be told to take L-thyroxine 2 hours before or after iron tablets because ferrous sulfate lowers the effectiveness of the medication (Cooper et al, 2007)).

The fetus depends on maternal thyroid hormones until 12 weeks of gestation, when fetal production begins. Thus maternal hypothyroidism does not cause fetal hypothyroidism. However, maternal treatment of hypothyroidism may result in increased fetal levels of thyroid hormones. Careful monitoring of the neonate's thyroid status is important to detect any abnormalities.

Nursing Care

Education of the pregnant woman with thyroid dysfunction is essential to promote compliance with the plan of treatment. The woman is instructed regarding the disorder and its potential impact on herself and her fetus, the medication regimen and possible side effects, the need for continuing medical supervision, and the importance of compliance. The family is incorporated into the plan of care to foster mutuality and support among the members.

The woman often needs assistance from the nurse in coping with the discomforts and frustrations associated with symptoms of the disorder. For example, the woman with hyperthyroidism who has nervousness and hyperactivity concomitant with weakness and fatigue may benefit from suggestions to channel excess energies into quiet diversional activities such as reading or crafts. Discomfort associated with hypersensitivity to heat (hyperthyroidism) or cold intolerance (hypothyroidism) can be minimized by wearing appropriate clothing, regulating environmental temperatures, and avoiding temperature extremes when possible.

Nutrition counseling with a registered dietitian can provide guidance in selecting a well-balanced diet. The woman with hyperthyroidism who has increased appetite and poor weight gain and the hypothyroid woman who has anorexia and lethargy need counseling to ensure adequate intake of nutritionally sound foods to meet both maternal and fetal needs.

Maternal Phenylketonuria

Phenylketonuria (PKU), a recognized cause of mental retardation, is an inborn error of metabolism caused by an autosomal recessive trait that creates a deficiency in the enzyme phenylalanine hydrolase. Absence of this enzyme impairs the ability of the body to metabolize the amino acid phenylalanine found in all protein foods. Consequently there is toxic accumulation of phenylalanine in the blood, which interferes with brain development and function. PKU affects approximately 1 of every 15,000 infants in the United States (Mayo Clinic Staff, 2007).

All newborns are tested for this disorder soon after birth; prompt diagnosis and therapy with a phenylalanine-restricted diet significantly decreases the incidence of mental retardation. Diet therapy for PKU is recommended to continue throughout life (Mayo Clinic Staff, 2007). Subtle but detrimental effects of elevated levels of phenylalanine on neurologic, behavioral, and intellectual function have been found in women who discontinued treatment in childhood.

The key to prevention of fetal anomalies caused by PKU is the identification of women in their reproductive years who have the disorder. Screening programs during the school years and in the premarital period may help identify individuals with PKU so dietary therapy can be instituted before conception occurs. Before conception these women and their families should be educated about the potential risks to the fetus if phenylalanine levels are not controlled.

Screening for undiagnosed maternal PKU at the first prenatal visit may be warranted, especially in individuals with a family history of the disorder, with low intelligence of uncertain etiology, or who have given birth to microcephalic infants. Although it may be too late to improve the current pregnancy outcome through diet therapy, the woman and her family will be aware of the problem and the necessary treatment should future pregnancies occur.

Normal pregnancy weight gain reduces the incidence of microcephaly and should be encouraged. Adequate protein and vitamin intake early in pregnancy may prevent congenital heart disease even when the blood phenylalanine level is elevated.

Women with PKU have been discouraged from breastfeeding because their milk contains a high concentration of phenylalanine. Infants diagnosed with PKU can be safely breastfed if the amount of breast milk ingested is monitored so that phenylalanine levels do not get too high. Mothers who choose to breastfeed must supplement the infant's diet with a special milk preparation that contains little or no phenylalanine.

Cardiovascular Disorders

During a normal pregnancy the maternal cardiovascular system undergoes many changes that put a physiologic strain on the heart. The major cardiovascular changes that occur during a normal pregnancy and affect the patient with cardiac disease are increased intravascular volume; decreased systemic vascular resistance; cardiac output changes occurring during pregnancy, labor, and birth; and the intravascular volume changes that occur just after childbirth. The strain is present during pregnancy and continues for a few weeks after birth. The normal heart can compensate for the increased workload; and pregnancy, labor, and birth are generally well tolerated; but the diseased heart is hemodynamically challenged.

If the cardiovascular changes are not well tolerated, cardiac failure can develop during pregnancy, labor, or the postpartum period. In addition, if myocardial disease develops, valvular disease exists, or a congenital heart defect is present, cardiac decompensation (inability of the heart to maintain a sufficient cardiac output) may occur.

From 0.4% to 4% of pregnancies are complicated by heart disease (Grewal, Biswas, & Perloff, 2003), the leading cause of nonobstetric maternal death. The two broad categories of cardiac disease are congenital and acquired. The incidence of acquired disease (e.g., rheumatic heart disease) is decreasing in developed countries. However, pregnancy in women with congenital cardiac disease is increasing because of advances in diagnosis, technology, and treatment, which has improved survival rates in these women (Arafeh & Baird, 2006). Cardiac disease ranks fourth overall as a cause of maternal death. A maternal mortality rate of up to 50% is anticipated in women with persistent cardiac decompensation (Arafeh & Baird, 2006). Box 13-2 lists maternal cardiac disease risk groups.

The New York Heart Association (NYHA) classification of functional capacity of patients with heart disease, a widely accepted standard, is as follows (Criteria Committee of the New York Heart Association, 1994):

Class I—Asymptomatic at normal levels of activity
Class II—Symptomatic with ordinary activity
Class III—Symptomatic with less than ordinary activity
Class IV—Symptomatic at rest

BOX 13-2 Maternal Cardiac Disease Risk Groups

Group I (Mortality Rate 1%)
Corrected tetralogy of Fallot
Pulmonic/tricuspid disease
Mitral stenosis (classes I and II)
Patent ductus arteriosus
Ventricular septal defect
Atrial septal defect
Porcine valve

Group II (Mortality Rate 5% to 15%)
Mitral stenosis with atrial fibrillation
Artificial heart valves
Mitral stenosis (classes III and IV)
Uncorrected tetralogy of Fallot
Aortic coarctation (uncomplicated)
Aortic stenosis
Marfan syndrome with normal aorta

Group III (Mortality Rate 25% to 50%)
Aortic coarctation (complicated)
Myocardial infarction (previous)
Marfan syndrome with aortic involvement
Pulmonary hypertension

From Foley MR: Cardiac disease. In Dildy GA et al (editors): *Critical care obstetrics*, ed 4, Malden, Mass, 2004, Blackwell Science.

evolve Case Study—Class III Cardiac Disorder

No classification of heart disease can be considered rigid or absolute, but the NYHA classification offers a basic practical guide for treatment, assuming that frequent prenatal visits, good patient cooperation, and appropriate obstetric care occur. Medical therapy is conducted by a team approach that includes the cardiologist, obstetrician, anesthesia care providers, and nurses. The functional classification may change over the course of the pregnancy because of the hemodynamic changes that occur in the cardiovascular system. There is a 45% to 50% increase in cardiac output compared with nonpregnancy resting values, with the majority of the increase in the first trimester and the peaks around 25 to 32 weeks of gestation (Blanchard & Shabetai, 2009). The functional classification of the disease is determined at 3 months and again at 7 or 8 months of gestation. Pregnant women may progress from class I or II to III or IV during pregnancy. Women with cyanotic congenital heart disease do not fit into the NYHA classification because their exercise-induced symptoms have causes not related to heart failure. An ability index was developed for assessment of these patients (Gei & Hankins, 2001).

Contraindications to pregnancy in women with heart disease are listed in Box 13-3. The incidence of miscarriage is increased, and preterm labor and birth are more prevalent in the pregnant woman with cardiac problems. In addition, IUGR is common, which may be the result of low oxygen pressure (Po_2) in the mother. The incidence of congenital heart lesions is increased in children of mothers with congenital heart disease; thus preconception counseling is important.

A diagnosis of cardiac disease depends on the history, physical examination, chest film findings, and, if indicated, sonogram results. The differential diagnosis of heart disease also involves ruling out respiratory problems and other potential causes of chest pain.

General intrapartum management for cardiac disease focuses on preventing hypotension and maternal tachycardia (heart rate greater than 110 beats/min) and optimizing cardiac output with volume and maternal position (e.g., left or right side to increase cardiac output) (Arafeh & Baird, 2006). Pulmonary artery catheter and arterial line placement, epidural anesthesia, and scheduled induction of labor should be strongly considered for women with moderate-to-high risk lesions or with symptoms in NYHA classes III and IV. Second stage should be managed with "laboring down" technique, preventing Valsalva maneuver (forced expiration against a closed airway, which when released causes blood to rush to the heart and overload the cardiac system), open glottis pushing, and consideration for operative vaginal delivery.

BOX 13-3 Contraindications to Pregnancy in a Woman with Heart Disease

- Dilated cardiomyopathy
- Primary pulmonary hypertension
- Eisenmenger's syndrome
- Marfan syndrome with aortic root dilation

Source: Blanchard DG, Shabetai R: Cardiac diseases. In Creasy RK et al (editors): *Creasy & Resnik's maternal-fetal medicine: principles and practice*, ed 6, Philadelphia, 2009, Saunders.

Cesarean birth is recommended only for obstetric issues (e.g., cephalopelvic disproportion). Bacterial endocarditis prophylaxis should be in accordance with the American Heart Association recommendations. During the immediate postpartum period, diuretic therapy may be required.

Peripartum Cardiomyopathy

The criteria for the diagnosis of peripartum cardiomyopathy (PPCM) include development of congestive heart failure in the last month of pregnancy or within the first 5 postpartum months, lack of another cause for heart failure, and absence of heart disease before the last month of pregnancy (Easterling & Stout, 2007). Some data suggest that this definition be expanded because the diagnosis of PPCM has been made at other times during gestation. The etiology of the disease is unknown; theories suggest genetic predisposition, autoimmunity, and viral infections.

PPCM is more common in African-American women, twin pregnancies, and women with preeclampsia (Grewal, Biswas, & Perloff, 2003). In the United States the incidence is 1 in 3000 to 4000 live births. Maternal mortality rate has been estimated in the range of 25% to 50%, whereas infant mortality rate is approximately 10% (Ramsey, Ramin, & Ramin, 2001). Maternal death is usually caused by thromboembolism, arrhythmia, or progressive heart failure. Symptoms include breathlessness, dyspnea, cough, orthopnea, tachydysrhythmias, and edema, with radiologic findings of cardiomegaly. The prognosis is good if cardiomegaly does not persist after 6 months postpartum. Women whose hearts remain enlarged after 6 months postpartum will have PPCM in future pregnancies (Blanchard & Shabetai, 2009). Pregnancy is contraindicated for women with persistent cardiomegaly or cardiac dysfunction.

Medical management of cardiomyopathy during pregnancy includes a regimen used for congestive heart failure and the potential for thromboembolism: diuretics, sodium restriction, afterload-reducing agents, anticoagulants, and digoxin. Angiotensin-converting enzyme inhibitors can be used only in the postpartum period because they are teratogenic agents. The nursing care of women with PPCM is essentially the same as that for women with other types of cardiac problems.

Rheumatic Heart Disease

Rheumatic fever is increasingly uncommon in the United States. When it occurs, it usually develops suddenly, often several symptom-free weeks after an inadequately treated group A β-hemolytic streptococcal throat infection. Episodes of rheumatic fever create an autoimmune reaction in the heart tissue that leads to permanent damage of heart valves (usually the mitral valve) and the chorda tendineae cordis. This damage is referred to as *rheumatic heart disease* (RHD). RHD may be evident during acute rheumatic fever or discovered years later. Recurrences of rheumatic fever are common; each has the potential to increase the severity of heart damage. The American Heart Association recommends prophylaxis to prevent infective endocarditis only in those patients who are at highest risk (Blanchard & Shabetai, 2009). Heart murmurs resulting from stenosis, valvular insufficiency, or thickening of the walls of the heart characterize RHD. Abnormal pulse rate and rhythm and congestive heart failure are common.

Mitral and Aortic Valve Stenosis

The concern regarding mitral and aortic valve lesions in the pregnant women is the need for cardiac output fluctuations during pregnancy, labor, and birth. With many of these lesions only allowing a "fixed" cardiac output, pregnant women and their fetuses may have hemodynamic decompensation if cardiac output cannot meet the needs for tissue perfusion and oxygen transport. Mitral valve stenosis (narrowing of the opening of the mitral valve caused by stiffening of valve leaflets, thereby obstructing blood flow from the atrium to the ventricles) is the characteristic lesion resulting from RHD. Even though a history of rheumatic fever may be absent, it remains the most likely cause of mitral stenosis. As the mitral valve narrows, cardiac output decreases, and dyspnea worsens, occurring first on exertion and eventually at rest. A tight stenosis plus the increase in blood volume and required cardiac output demands of normal pregnancy and birth may cause ventricular failure, pulmonary edema, and death (Blanchard & Shabetai, 2009).

Rheumatic fever can also affect the aortic valve. However, significant aortic stenosis in pregnant women is usually congenital. With this in mind, a fetal echocardiogram may be done. When the aortic valve orifice is less than one third of normal, limited cardiac output is possible, leading to increased left ventricular afterload, left ventricular hypertrophy, and failure. As with any left-sided heart lesion, the pregnant woman is very sensitive to changes in intravascular volume. Intravascular volume balance is essential to prevent hypotension caused by hypovolemia and pulmonary edema caused by hypervolemia (Easterling & Stout, 2007)

Antepartum care of the pregnant woman with mitral and/or aortic stenosis typically is managed by reducing her activity, restricting dietary sodium, diuretic therapy, β-blocking medications to lower heart rate, and increasing bed rest. She should be monitored frequently for clinical symptoms and with routine echocardiograms to monitor atrial and ventricular size and heart valve function. For patients with NYHA class III or IV symptoms, balloon valvuloplasty may be considered. This procedure should be considered only when symptoms cannot be controlled by standard medical treatments. Balloon valvuloplasty is optimally performed after 20 weeks of gestation to decrease radiation risks to the fetus.

Mitral Valve Prolapse

Mitral valve prolapse (MVP) is a common, usually benign, condition occurring in 1% of women (Blanchard & Shabetai, 2009). The mitral valve leaflets prolapse into the left atrium during ventricular systole, allowing some backflow of blood. Midsystolic click and late systolic murmur are hallmarks of this syndrome. Most cases are asymptomatic. A few women have atypical chest pain (sharp and located in the left side of the chest) that occurs at rest, is unrelated to exercise, and does not respond to nitrates. They may have anxiety, palpitations, dyspnea on exertion, and syncope. Specific treatment is usually not necessary except for symptomatic tachyarrhythmias. Pregnancy and its associated hemodynamic changes may change or alleviate the murmur and click of MVP, as well as its symptoms. Pregnancy is usually well tolerated; but, as with RHD, antibiotic prophylaxis may be given before invasive procedures for at-risk patients and for complicated vaginal births in patients with MVP.

Eisenmenger's Syndrome

Eisenmenger's syndrome is a right-to-left or bidirectional shunting that can be at the atrial or ventricular level and is combined with elevated pulmonary vascular resistance (Easterling & Stout, 2007). The syndrome is associated with a mortality rate of approximately 50% during pregnancy; thus pregnancy is contraindicated. If pregnancy occurs, termination may be recommended if the woman has significant pulmonary hypertension.

In women who continue pregnancy despite the risks, physical activity is strictly limited; prophylactic anticoagulation is considered (Easterling & Stout, 2007). Intensive care monitoring during labor and birth, guided by invasive hemodynamic parameters obtained with a pulmonary artery and arterial catheter, is essential to optimize outcomes for mother and fetus. A team approach involving a perinatologist, skilled critical care and obstetric nurses, and cardiology and anesthesia care providers is essential.

Atrial and Ventricular Septal Defects

Atrial septal defects (ASDs: an abnormal opening between the atria) and VSDs are causes of a left-to-right shunting that can lead to Eisenmenger's syndrome. These defects may go undetected because the woman usually is asymptomatic until pregnancy hemodynamic changes occur. The pregnant woman with an ASD or VSD will most likely have an uncomplicated pregnancy unless the defect causes significant shunting and increased pulmonary vascular resistance. As a result of the increased plasma volume, some women may have right-sided heart failure or tachyarrhythmias as the pregnancy progresses.

Tetralogy of Fallot

Tetralogy of Fallot includes several abnormalities caused by maldevelopment of the truncus arteriosus. The cardiac abnormalities include a VSD, pulmonary stenosis, overriding aorta, and right ventricular hypertrophy, leading to a right-to-left shunt. Surgical correction of tetralogy of Fallot includes correction of the VSD and possibly the pulmonary stenosis. Women with corrected tetralogy of Fallot have a low mortality rate; however, women with uncorrected tetralogy of Fallot have a high maternal risk and high rate of fetal loss (Blanchard & Shabetai, 2009). Medical management for women with uncorrected tetralogy of Fallot includes anticoagulant therapy, high-concentration oxygen administration, and hemodynamic monitoring during labor and birth as well as prophylactic antibiotics.

Marfan Syndrome

Marfan syndrome is an autosomal dominant genetic disorder characterized by generalized weakness of the connective tissue, resulting in joint deformities, ocular lens dislocation, and weakness of the aortic wall and root (Arafeh & Baird, 2006). About 90% of individuals with this syndrome have

MVP, and 25% have aortic insufficiency, with an increased risk of aortic dissection and rupture during pregnancy. Excruciating chest pain and sudden cardiac decompensation is the most common symptom of aortic dissection and rupture. Aortic dissection and/or rupture most often occurs in the third trimester or the postpartum period. Therapy includes limiting physical activity, preventing hypertensive or hypotensive complications, and administering β-blockers as needed. Aortic root measurements are taken early in pregnancy as a baseline and then at intervals to detect an increasing diameter. Preconception and genetic counseling are recommended to make women aware of the risks of pregnancy with this condition (i.e., a 50% risk of mortality and inheritance of the syndrome) (Easterling & Stout, 2007)

Heart Transplantation

Increasing numbers of heart recipients are successfully completing pregnancies but risk complications. Before conception the woman should be assessed for quality of ventricular function and potential rejection of the transplant. She should be stabilized on the immunosuppressant regimen. Conception should be postponed for at least 1 year after transplantation to avoid acute rejection episodes (Blanchard & Shabetai, 2009). Risks to the woman include hypertension, preeclampsia, preterm labor (50%), renal insufficiency, small-for-gestational-age (SGA) neonate, rejection, and infections. During labor β-blocking agents may be needed to prevent tachycardia caused by vagal denervation from the transplant surgery. Management of the intrapartal period requires the coordination of care among all health care providers involved in the care of the woman and her fetus.

After birth the neonate may exhibit immunosuppressive effects during the first week of life. Breastfeeding is not advised for infants of mothers taking cyclosporine.

Nursing Care Management

Nursing care of the woman with a cardiovascular disorder combines routine peripartum care with care specific for the cardiac diagnosis and function (see Nursing Process box). Care of these women at high risk requires a multidisciplinary approach. The multidisciplinary team includes a cardiologist who is familiar with expected cardiovascular changes in pregnancy; a perinatologist; an anesthesiologist; and nurses expert in labor, birth, and maternal hemodynamic monitoring.

Cardiac conditions vary in their impact on pregnancy because of acuteness or chronicity. The presence of cardiac disease makes the decision to become pregnant more difficult. Planned pregnancy requires that the woman understand the peripartum risks. If the pregnancy is unplanned, the nurse needs to explore the woman's desire to continue the pregnancy. The nurse should review with the woman options for pregnancy termination if her cardiac status is tenuous and abortion is an acceptable alternative. The woman's significant other and family should be included in the discussion. Teaching sessions for the woman and her support people should be offered as indicated by their learning needs. Table 13-4 lists the normal and abnormal cardiovascular signs and symptoms during pregnancy.

The pregnant woman with cardiovascular problems faces curtailment of her activities. Bed rest during pregnancy affects all of the organ systems, but especially the cardiovascular and musculoskeletal. In addition, psychologic side effects can be debilitating, especially stress (Cunningham et al, 2005; Maloni, Brezinski-Tomasi, & Johnson, 2001). The community health nurse, social worker, and physical or occupational therapist are some of the resource people whose services may be incorporated into the plan of care.

Table 13-4 Cardiovascular Signs and Symptoms During Pregnancy

NORMAL	ABNORMAL
Signs	
Neck vein pulsation	Neck vein distention
Diffuse/displaced apical	Cardiomegaly; heave pulse
Split S_1, accentuated S_2	Loud P_2; wide split of S_2
Third heart sound	Summation gallop
Systolic murmur (1-2/6)	Loud systolic murmur (4-6/6)
Venous hum	Diastolic murmur
Sinus dysrhythmia	Sustained dysrhythmia
Peripheral edema	Clubbing/cyanosis
Symptoms	
Fatigue	Symptoms at rest
Chest pain	Exertional chest pain
Dyspnea	Exertional, severe dyspnea
Orthopnea	Orthopnea (progressive)
Hyperpnea	Paroxysmal nocturnal dyspnea
Palpitations	Tachycardia (>120 beats/min); dysrhythmia
Syncope (vasovagal)	Exertional syncope

Adapted from Mendelson MA: Congenital cardiac disease and pregnancy, *Clin Perinatol* 24(2):467-482, 1997.

Symptoms of cardiac decompensation may appear abruptly or gradually. Medical intervention must be instituted immediately to maintain optimal cardiac status. Dyspnea, palpitations, syncope, and edema commonly occur in pregnant women and can mask the symptoms of a developing or worsening cardiovascular disorder. A woman's sudden inability to perform activities she previously was comfortable doing may indicate cardiovascular decompensation (Box 13-4).

The woman's cultural background may affect the amount of support that she is able to receive from significant others. Family size (number of children and extended family members in the home) and role expectations within the family may be dictated by cultural norms. For the woman with cardiac impairment, family expectations may be a cause of major stress if she is unable to bear the expected number of children or if it is unacceptable to receive help with domestic chores.

Plan of Care and Implementation

Therapy for the pregnant woman with heart disease is focused on minimizing stress on the heart. This stress is greatest between 28 and 32 weeks as the hemodynamic changes reach their maximum. The workload of the cardiovascular system is reduced by appropriate treatment of any coexisting emotional stress, hypertension, anemia, hyperthyroidism, or obesity.

NURSING PROCESS: CARDIAC DISEASE

Assessment

The pregnant woman with cardiac disease requires detailed assessment throughout the peripartum period to determine the potential for optimal maternal health, progression of symptoms, and a viable fetus. If she chooses to continue the pregnancy, the high risk pregnant woman's condition may be assessed as often as weekly.

Interview

The nurse elicits the following information from the woman:

Her personal medical history and that of her family

- Diseases of cardiovascular significance, including congenital heart disease, streptococcal infections, rheumatic fever, valvular disease, endocarditis, congestive heart failure, angina, or myocardial infarction

Factors that would increase stress on the heart (anemia, infection, and edema)

How the woman is adapting to the physiologic changes of pregnancy

- Review of the cardiovascular and pulmonary systems
- Whether the woman has experienced chest pain at rest or on exertion
- Edema of the face, hands, or feet; hypertension; heart murmurs; palpitations; paroxysmal nocturnal dyspnea; diaphoresis; and pallor or syncope
- Pulmonary symptoms such as cough, hemoptysis, shortness of breath, and orthopnea

Document all medications taken by the woman.

Assess for undue emotional stress that might further compromise cardiac status.

Physical Examination

Monitor the following:

- Amount and pattern of edema
- Vital signs
- Discomforts of pregnancy
- Amount and pattern of weight gain

Observe for signs of cardiac decompensation:

- Progressive generalized edema
- Crackles at base of lungs
- Pulse irregularity

Review results of laboratory tests:

- Routine urinalysis and blood work (complete blood count and blood chemistry)
- Baseline 12-lead electrocardiogram (ECG) at the beginning of the pregnancy, if not before pregnancy (permits vital diagnostic comparisons with subsequent ECGs)
- Echocardiograms and pulse oximetry studies as indicated

Chest films may be necessary during late pregnancy; the abdomen must be carefully shielded

- Fetal ultrasound, fetal movement studies, or fetal nonstress tests (to determine fetal well-being)

Nursing Diagnoses

The following examples are some nursing diagnoses that may be formulated. As always, individualizing diagnoses is vital.

Prenatal Period

Fear related to

– increased peripartum risk

Deficient knowledge related to

– cardiac condition
– pregnancy and how it affects cardiac condition
– requirements to alter self-management activities

Activity intolerance related to

– cardiac condition

Risk for self-care deficit (bathing, grooming, and dressing) related to

– fatigue or activity intolerance
– need for bed rest

Impaired home maintenance related to

– woman's confinement to bed or limited activity level

Postpartum Period

Anxiety related to

– fear for infant's safety

Fear of dying related to

– perceived physiologic inability to cope with stress of labor

Risk for impaired gas exchange related to

– cardiac condition

Risk for excess fluid volume related to

– extravascular fluid shifts

Ineffective breastfeeding related to

– fatigue from cardiac condition

Planning

Nursing care of the woman with a cardiovascular disorder combines routine peripartum care with care specific for the cardiac diagnosis and function. Care of these women at high risk requires a multidisciplinary approach.

Expected outcomes might include that the pregnant woman (and family, if appropriate) will do the following:

- Verbalize understanding of the disorder, management, and probable outcome
- Describe her role in management, including when and how to take medication, adjust diet, and prepare for and participate in treatment
- Cope with emotional reactions to pregnancy and an infant at risk
- Adapt to the physiologic stressors of pregnancy, labor, and birth
- Identify and use support systems
- Carry her fetus to viability or to term

Interventions

Review signs and symptoms of cardiac decompensation with the pregnant woman and her family.

Provide patient teaching.

The Woman with Class I or II Heart Disease

Woman requires 8 to 10 hours of sleep every day and should take 30-minute naps after meals.

Restrict activities (limit housework, shopping, and exercise) to the amount recommended for the functional classification of her heart disease.

The Woman with Class II Cardiac Disease

Avoid heavy exertion; stop any activity that causes even minor signs and symptoms of cardiac decompensation.

NURSING PROCESS: CARDIAC DISEASE–cont'd

Interventions—cont'd

The Woman with Class II Cardiac Disease—cont'd

She will be admitted to the hospital near term (or earlier if signs of cardiac overload or dysrhythmia develop) for evaluation and treatment.

The Pregnant Woman with Class III Cardiac Disease

Emphasize that bed rest for much of the day is necessary.

Treat infections promptly; administer prophylactic antibiotics against bacterial endocarditis as ordered.

Provide nutrition counseling. Refer to a registered dietitian as necessary.

Administer cardiac medications as prescribed.

Monitor drug levels.

Monitor the woman's blood work.

Review results of tests for fetal maturity and well-being and placental sufficiency.

Reinforce the need for close medical supervision.

Evaluation

The nurse uses the previously stated expected outcomes as criteria to evaluate the care of the woman with cardiac disease.

BOX 13-4 Signs of Potential Complications: Cardiac Decompensation

Pregnant Woman: Subjective Symptoms

Increasing fatigue or difficulty breathing or both with usual activities

Feeling of smothering

Frequent cough

Palpitations; feeling that her heart is racing

Swelling of face, feet, legs, fingers (e.g., rings do not fit anymore)

Nurse: Objective Signs

Irregular weak, rapid pulse (100 or more beats/min)

Progressive, generalized edema

Crackles at base of lungs after two inspirations and exhalations

Orthopnea; increasing dyspnea

Rapid respirations (25 or more breaths/min)

Moist, frequent cough

Increasing fatigue

Cyanosis of lips and nail beds

PATIENT TEACHING The Pregnant Woman at Risk for Cardiac Decompensation

- Assess lifestyle patterns, emotional status, and environment of woman.
- Arrange for consultations as needed (e.g., dietitian, home care, child care, social work).
- Determine woman's and her family's understanding of her heart disease and how the disease affects her pregnancy.
- Determine stressors in the woman's life. Assist woman in identifying effective coping strategies.
- Instruct woman to report signs of cardiac decompensation or congestive heart failure: generalized edema, distention of neck veins, dyspnea, pulmonary crackles, cough, palpitations, sudden weight gain.
- Instruct woman to be watchful for signs of thromboembolism such as redness, tenderness, pain, or swelling of the legs. Instruct woman to seek medical help immediately if such symptoms occur.
- Instruct woman to avoid constipation and thus straining with bowel movements (Valsalva maneuver) by taking in adequate fluids and fiber. A stool softener may be ordered.
- Explore with woman ways to obtain the needed rest throughout the day. Depending on the level of her cardiac disease, she may need to sleep 10 hours per night and rest for 30 minutes after meals (class I or II) or for most of the day (class III or IV).
- Help woman make use of community resources, including support groups, as indicated.
- Emphasize the importance of keeping her prenatal visits.

References: Gilbert ES: *Manual of high risk pregnancy and delivery*, ed 4, St Louis, 2007, Elsevier; Arafeh JM, Baird SM: Cardiac disease in pregnancy, *Crit Care Nurs Q* 29(1):32-52, 2006.

The woman needs a well-balanced diet with iron and folic acid supplementation, high protein, and adequate calories to gain weight. Iron supplements tend to cause constipation. She should increase her intake of fluids and fiber. A stool softener may be prescribed. It is important that the pregnant woman with cardiac disease avoid straining during defecation, thus causing the Valsalva maneuver (see Patient Teaching box). If sodium restriction is necessary, the amount should not be less than 2.5 g/day (Gilbert, 2007). The woman's intake of potassium is monitored to prevent hypokalemia, especially if she is taking diuretics. A referral to a registered dietitian may be necessary.

Cardiac medications are prescribed as needed for the pregnant woman, with attention to fetal well-being. The hemodynamic changes that occur during pregnancy such as increased plasma volume and increased renal clearance of drugs can alter the amount of medication needed to establish and maintain a therapeutic drug level (Blanchard & Shabetai, 2009). Monitoring of the drug levels during the pregnancy is crucial to maintain effective therapy for the woman while minimizing risk to the fetus. Research on the effects of cardiovascular drugs on the fetus and pregnant woman has been limited. The nurse should review current pharmacologic literature, especially when administering any medication to a pregnant woman (Table 13-5).

Table 13-5 Medications Used in Pregnancy for Cardiac Conditions

MEDICATION	SELECTED MATERNAL INDICATIONS	FDA PREGNANCY CATEGORY*	POSSIBLE ADVERSE FETAL EFFECTS
Cardiac Glycoside			
Digoxin, digitoxin	Arrhythmia	C	Maternal overdose can cause fetal toxicity and death
Anticoagulants			
Heparin	Thrombophlebitis Pulmonary hypertension	Does not cross the placenta	Heparin considered safe in pregnancy for the fetus
Warfarin	Same as heparin	X	Fetal anomalies, congenital malformations, hemorrhage; contraindicated in first trimester and at term
Diuretics			
Furosemide Thiazides	Hypertension	C	No known teratogenic effects; possible growth restriction; neonatal jaundice, thrombocytopenia, hemolytic anemia, hypoglycemia
β-Blockers			
Propranolol Metoprolol	Angina, hypertension, mitral valve prolapse, arrhythmia	C	During labor can cause bradycardia; after birth can cause hypoglycemia, hyperbilirubinemia
Vasodilators			
Hydralazine	Severe hypertension, pulmonary hypertension	C	Leukopenia and thrombocytopenia reported in newborns
Calcium Channel Blockers			
Nifedipine Verapamil	Angina, hypertension, arrhythmia (verapamil only)	C	Considered safe for use in pregnancy but no controlled human studies on fetal effects
Antiarrhythmias			
Quinidine Procainamide	Arrhythmia	C	Neonatal thrombocytopenia reported; quinidine preferred over procainamide

References: Blanchard DG, Shabetai T: Cardiac diseases. In Creasy RK et al (editors): *Creasy & Resnik's maternal-fetal medicine: principles and practice*, ed 6, Philadelphia, 2009, Saunders; Arafeh JM, Baird SM: Cardiac disease in pregnancy, *Crit Care Nurs Q* 29(1):32-52, 2006.

*U.S. Food and Drug Administration (FDA) pregnancy categories: *category A*, controlled studies have not demonstrated a risk to the fetus; *category C*, animal studies have shown no adverse effects on the fetus, but there are no adequate studies in humans; potential benefits may be acceptable despite potential risks; *category X*, studies demonstrate fetal risk or abnormalities; risks outweigh potential benefits.

If anticoagulant therapy is required during pregnancy for conditions such as recurrent venous thrombosis, pulmonary embolus, RHD, prosthetic valves, or cyanotic congenital heart defects, heparin may be used because this large-molecule drug does not cross the placenta (Blanchard & Shabetai, 2009). The nurse should closely monitor the woman's blood work, including clotting factors. The woman may need to learn to self-administer heparin. She also requires specific nutrition education to avoid foods high in vitamin K such as raw, dark green leafy vegetables, which counteract the effects of the heparin. In addition, she will require a folic acid supplement.

Tests for fetal maturity and well-being and placental sufficiency may be necessary. Other therapy is directly related to the functional classification of heart disease. The nurse may need to reinforce the need for close medical supervision.

LEGAL TIP Cardiac and Metabolic Emergencies The management of emergencies such as maternal cardiopulmonary distress or arrest or maternal metabolic crisis should be documented in policies, procedures, and protocols. Any independent nursing actions appropriate to the emergency should be clearly identified.

Heart Surgery During Pregnancy

Ideally a woman would have surgical correction of the cardiac lesion before pregnancy; however, cardiac disease may be diagnosed for the first time during pregnancy. When medical therapy for a pregnant woman fails, cardiac surgery may be performed. Early in the second trimester is the best time for surgery. The woman, fetus, and uterine activity must be monitored carefully during surgery. Closed cardiac surgery such as release of a stenotic mitral orifice can be accomplished with little risk to mother or fetus. Open heart surgery requires extracorporeal circulation, and under these circumstances hypoxia and fetal bradycardia may occur as a result of low blood-flow rates. Periods of hypoxemia for the fetus can lead to various kinds of neurologic insults. Increase in flow rates on cardiopulmonary bypass may correct fetal bradycardia. Uterine contractions also increase in frequency before and during cardiopulmonary bypass and can be alleviated by medication.

Intrapartum

For all pregnant women the intrapartum period evokes the most apprehension in patients and caregivers. The woman with impaired cardiac function has additional reasons to be anxious because labor and giving birth place an additional burden on her already compromised cardiovascular system.

Assessments include the routine assessments for all laboring women, as well as assessments for cardiac decompensation. In addition, arterial line placement and arterial blood gas evaluations may be needed to assess for adequate oxygenation. A pulmonary artery catheter (Swan-Ganz catheter) may be inserted to monitor hemodynamic status accurately during labor and birth. Electrocardiographic monitoring and continuous monitoring of blood pressure and pulse oximetry should be instituted for all women, and the fetus is continuously monitored electronically (Arafeh & Baird, 2006).

NURSING ALERT A pulse rate of 100 beats/min or greater or a respiratory rate of 25 breaths/min or greater is a concern. Respiratory status is checked frequently for developing dyspnea, coughing, or crackles at the base of the lungs. The color and temperature of the skin are noted. Pale, cool, clammy skin may indicate cardiac shock.

Nursing care during labor and birth focuses on the promotion of cardiac function. Anxiety is minimized by maintaining a calm atmosphere in the labor and birth rooms. The nurse provides anticipatory guidance by keeping the woman and her family informed of labor progress and events that will probably occur and answering any questions they have. The woman's childbirth preparation method should be supported to the degree it is feasible for her cardiac condition. Nursing techniques that promote comfort such as back massage are used.

Cardiac function is supported by keeping the woman's head and shoulders elevated and body parts resting on pillows. The side-lying position usually facilitates hemodynamics during labor. Discomfort is relieved with medication and supportive care. Epidural regional analgesia provides better pain relief than narcotics and causes fewer alterations in hemodynamics. Hypotension must be avoided.

The woman may require other types of medication (e.g., anticoagulants, prophylactic antibiotics). If evidence of cardiac decompensation appears, the physician may order deslanoside (Cedilanid-D) for rapid digitalization, furosemide (Lasix) for rapid diuresis, and oxygen by intermittent positive pressure to decrease the development of pulmonary edema.

β-Adrenergic agents (i.e., ritodrine and terbutaline) should not be used for tocolysis. These medications are associated with various cardiac side effects, including tachycardia and myocardial ischemia.

Labor and/or planned induction of labor is the preferred method of birth for women with cardiac disease. If there are no obstetric problems, vaginal birth can be accomplished with the woman in a side-lying position to facilitate uterine perfusion. To prevent compression of popliteal veins and an increase in blood volume in the chest and trunk as a result of the effects of gravity, stirrups are not used. The "laboring down" method or open-glottis pushing is recommended for the second stage of labor. Valsalva maneuver should be avoided during pushing in the second stage of labor because it reduces diastolic ventricular filling and obstructs left ventricular outflow. Supplemental oxygen is administered throughout labor to optimize maternal and fetal tissue perfusion.

Vacuum extraction or outlet forceps may be used to decrease the length and workload of the heart in second-stage labor. Cesarean birth is not routinely recommended for women who have cardiovascular disease because there is risk of dramatic fluid shifts, sustained hemodynamic changes, and increased blood loss.

Penicillin prophylaxis may be ordered for nonallergic pregnant women with class II or higher cardiac disease to protect against bacterial endocarditis in labor and during early puerperium. Dilute IV oxytocin immediately after birth may be used to prevent hemorrhage. Ergot products should not be used because they tend to increase blood pressure. Fluid balance should be maintained, and blood loss replaced. If tubal sterilization is desired, surgery is delayed at least several days to ensure homeostasis.

Postpartum

Monitoring for cardiac decompensation in the postpartum period is essential. The first 24 to 48 hours postpartum are the most hemodynamically difficult for the woman. Hemorrhage, infection, or both, may worsen the cardiac condition. The woman with a cardiac disorder may continue to require a pulmonary artery catheter and arterial catheter to monitor volume status, cardiac output, blood pressure, and arterial blood gases.

NURSING ALERT The immediate postbirth period is hazardous for a woman whose heart function is compromised. Cardiac output increases rapidly as extravascular fluid is remobilized into the vascular compartment. At the moment of birth intraabdominal pressure is reduced drastically; pressure on veins is removed, the splanchnic vessels engorge, and blood flow to the heart is increased. When blood flow increases to the heart, a reflex bradycardia may result.

Care in the postpartum period is tailored to the woman's functional capacity. Postpartum assessment of the woman with cardiac disease includes vital signs, oxygen saturation levels, lung and heart auscultation, edema, amount and character of bleeding, uterine tone and fundal height, urinary output, pain (especially chest pain), the activity-rest pattern, dietary intake, mother-infant interactions, and emotional state. The head of the bed is elevated, and the woman is encouraged to lie on her side. Bed rest may be ordered, with or without bathroom privileges. Progressive ambulation may be permitted as tolerated. The nurse may help the woman meet her grooming and hygiene needs and other activities. Bowel movements without stress or strain for the woman are promoted with stool softeners, diet, and fluids.

The woman may need a family member to help in the care of the infant. Breastfeeding is not contraindicated, but not all women with heart disease will be able to nurse their infants. The woman who chooses to breastfeed will need the support of her family and the nursing staff to be successful. She may need assistance in positioning herself or the infant for feeding. To conserve the woman's energy, the infant may need to be brought to the mother and taken from her after the feeding. Women who breastfeed may need less medication, especially fewer diuretics, for their cardiac condition. Because diuretics can cause neonatal diuresis that can lead to dehydration, lactating women must be monitored closely to determine if medication doses can be reduced and still be effective.

If the woman is unable to breastfeed and her energies do not allow her to bottle-feed the infant, the baby can be kept at the bedside so she can look at and touch her baby to establish an emotional bond with a low expenditure of energy. If the mother is unable to hold her infant, the nurse or a family member can hold the infant at the mother's eye level and close enough for her to touch.

Discharge is carefully planned with the woman and family. Provision of help for the woman in the home by relatives, friends, and others must be addressed. The family is referred to community resources (e.g., homemaking services) as appropriate. Rest and sleep periods, activity, and diet must be planned. The couple may need information about reestablishing sexual relations and contraception or sterilization. Potential hazards of a subsequent pregnancy need to be examined by the woman and her partner. If sterilization is selected as a method of contraception, the risks of surgery, especially for the woman with class III or IV heart disease, need to be explained. Oral contraceptives are often contraindicated because of the risk of thromboembolism. IUDs may put the woman at risk for infection, especially if she has a valve replacement. Injectable progestins are effective and safe (Easterling & Stout, 2007). Both the woman and her partner need to be involved in the decision-making process.

Monitoring for cardiac decompensation continues through the first few weeks after birth because of hormone shifts that affect hemodynamics. Maternal cardiac output is usually stabilized by 2 weeks postpartum (Easterling & Stout, 2007).

Cardiopulmonary Resuscitation of the Pregnant Woman

Cardiac arrest in a pregnant woman is most often related to events at the time of birth such as amniotic fluid embolism, eclampsia, and drug toxicity. It can also be related to congestive cardiomyopathy, aortic dissection, pulmonary embolism, or hemorrhage caused by a pregnancy-related pathologic condition. Other problems are motor vehicle accidents, falls, assault, suicide attempts, and trauma (stabbing, gunshot wounds) (American Heart Association [AHA], 2000). Preexisting disorders such as heart or pulmonary disease, hypertension, or autoimmune collagen vascular disease increase this risk.

Various protocols exist for cardiopulmonary resuscitation (CPR) during pregnancy. The most widely used guide is the AHA advanced cardiac life support (ACLS) protocol (AHA, 2005). This protocol recommends standard CPR with the uterus displaced laterally, fluid volume restoration, and defibrillation if indicated. The decision for cesarean birth should be made within 4 to 5 minutes of the mother's cardiac arrest. No matter what protocol is used, nurses and other health care providers must be prepared if CPR is to be successful.

In the event of cardiac arrest, standard resuscitative efforts with a few modifications are implemented. To prevent supine hypotension, the woman is placed on a flat, firm surface with the uterus displaced laterally either manually or with a wedge or rolled towel under her right hip or on her side supported by angled thighs of several rescuers or angled backs of several chairs (AHA, 2005). If defibrillation is needed, the paddles must be placed one rib interspace higher than usual because the heart is slightly displaced by the enlarged uterus. If possible, the fetus should be monitored during the cardiac arrest (see Emergency box).

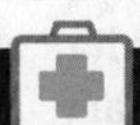

EMERGENCY

Cardiopulmonary Resuscitation of the Pregnant Woman

Airway

Determine unresponsiveness.

Activate emergency medical system and get the automated external defibrillator (AED) if available.

Position woman on flat, firm surface with uterus displaced laterally with a wedge (e.g., a rolled towel placed under her hip) or manually or place her in a lateral position.

Open airway with head tilt–chin lift maneuver.

Breathing

Determine breathlessness (look, listen, feel).

If the woman is not breathing, give two slow breaths; each breath over 1-second duration to make the chest rise.

Rescue breathing without chest compressions should be given at a rate of 10 to 12 breaths/min.

Circulation

Determine pulselessness by feeling carotid pulse.

If there is no pulse, begin chest compressions at rate of 100/min at a compression depth of 1½ to 2 inches. Allow the chest to completely recoil after compression. Chest compressions may be performed slightly higher on the sternum if the uterus is enlarged enough to displace the diaphragm into a higher position.

After four cycles of 30 compressions and two breaths, check her pulse. If pulse is not present, continue cardiopulmonary resuscitation.

Defibrillation

Use an AED according to standard protocol to analyze heart rhythm and deliver shock if indicated.

Delivery

Consider perimortem cesarean birth within 5 minutes if chest compressions are unsuccessful.

Relief of Foreign-Body Airway Obstruction

If the pregnant woman is unable to speak or cough, perform chest thrusts.

Stand behind the woman and place your arms under her armpits to encircle her chest. Press backward with quick thrusts until the foreign body is expelled (see Fig. 13-5).

If the woman becomes unresponsive, follow the steps for victims who become unresponsive, but use chest thrusts instead of abdominal thrusts.

Source: American Heart Association: *2005 Guidelines for cardiopulmonary resuscitation and emergency cardiovascular care*, November 2005, The Association.

Complications that may be associated with CPR of a pregnant woman include laceration of the liver, rupture of the uterus, hemothorax, and hemoperitoneum. Fetal complications that may occur include cardiac dysrhythmia or asystole related to maternal defibrillation and medications, CNS depression related to antidysrhythmic drugs and inadequate uteroplacental perfusion, and onset of preterm labor.

If resuscitation is successful, the woman and her fetus must receive careful monitoring. The woman remains at increased risk for recurrent pulmonary arrest and dysrhythmias (ventricular tachycardia, supraventricular tachycardia, and bradycardia). Therefore her cardiovascular, pulmonary, and neurologic status should be assessed continuously. Uterine activity and resting tone must be monitored. Fetal status and gestational age should be determined and used in decision making regarding continuation of the pregnancy or the timing and route of birth.

Clearing an airway obstruction in a woman in the second or third trimester of pregnancy also requires a modification of the Heimlich maneuver (Fig. 13-5) (see Nursing Care Plan).

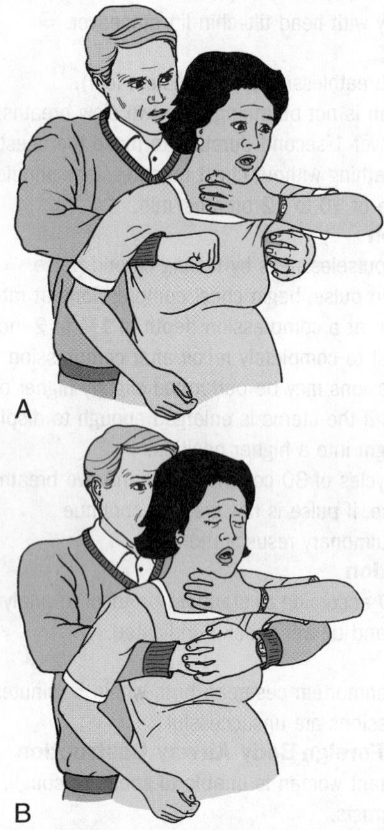

Fig. 13-5 Heimlich maneuver. Clearing airway obstruction in a woman in the late stages of pregnancy (can also be used in markedly obese person). **A,** Standing behind victim, place your arms under woman's armpits and across the chest. Place thumb side of your clenched fist against the middle of the sternum and place other hand over fist. **B,** Perform backward chest thrusts until foreign body is expelled or woman loses consciousness. If pregnant woman becomes unconscious because of foreign body airway obstruction, place her on her back and kneel close to her side. (Be sure that uterus is displaced laterally by using, for example, a rolled blanket under her hip.) Open her mouth with tongue-jaw lift, perform finger sweep, and attempt rescue breathing. If unable to ventilate, position hands as for chest compression. Deliver five chest thrusts firmly to remove the obstruction. Repeat the sequence of Heimlich maneuver, finger sweep, and attempt to ventilate. Continue sequence until pregnant woman's airway is clear of obstruction or help has arrived to relieve you. If woman is unconscious, give chest compressions as for woman without a pulse.

Anemia

Anemia is the most common medical disorder of pregnancy, affecting at least 20% of pregnant women. Anemia results in reduction of the oxygen-carrying capacity of the blood, and the heart tries to compensate by increasing the cardiac output. This effort increases the workload of the heart and stresses ventricular function. Therefore anemia that occurs with any other complication (e.g., preeclampsia) may result in congestive heart failure.

An indirect index of the oxygen-carrying capacity is the packed red blood cell volume, or hematocrit level. The normal hematocrit range in nonpregnant women is 37% to 47%. Normal values for pregnant women with adequate iron stores may be as low as 32%. This has been explained by the blood volume expansion by approximately 50% and total red blood cell mass expansion of approximately 25%. This hydremia (dilution of blood) is also called the *physiologic anemia of pregnancy.*

The CDC defines anemia in the pregnant woman as a hemoglobin level of less than 11 g/dl or a hematocrit of less than or equal to 32% (CDC, 1998). When a woman has anemia during pregnancy, the loss of blood at birth, even if minimal, is not well tolerated. She is at an increased risk for requiring blood transfusions. Women with anemia have a higher incidence of puerperal complications such as infection than do pregnant women with normal hematologic values (Box 13-5). Severe anemia, defined as a hemoglobin level of less than 6 g/dl, has been associated with decreased fetal oxygen levels that result in abnormal fetal heart rate patterns, decreased amniotic fluid volume, and fetal death.

Nursing care of the pregnant woman with anemia requires that the nurse be able to distinguish between the normal physiologic anemia of pregnancy and the disease states. About 90% of cases of anemia in pregnancy are of the iron deficiency type. The remaining 10% embrace a considerable variety of acquired and hereditary anemias, including folic acid deficiency, sickle cell anemia, and thalassemia.

During prenatal visits the nurse should take a diet history and provide dietary teaching as appropriate. Pregnancy may cause increased fatigue, stress, and financial difficulties for a

BOX 13-5 Restless Legs Syndrome

Restless legs syndrome (RLS) is a sensorimotor disorder characterized by discomfort of the legs and an urge to move them, usually during rest or inactivity. The discomfort is relieved by movement. RLS occurs mostly in the evening. It is generally idiopathic but is associated with anemia and pregnancy. Pregnant women have two to three times the risk of having RLS than the general population. Preexisting RLS worsens during pregnancy, having the highest degree of severity in the third trimester, and disappears at the time of birth.

Sources: Manconi M et al: Pregnancy as a risk factor for restless legs syndrome, *Sleep Med* 5(3):305-308, 2004; Zucconi M, Ferini-Strambi L: Epidemiology and clinical findings of restless legs syndrome, *Sleep Med* 5(3):293-299, 2004.

NURSING CARE PLAN The Pregnant Woman with Heart Disease

Nursing Diagnosis: Activity intolerance related to effects of pregnancy on the patient with rheumatic heart disease with mitral valve stenosis

Expected Outcome

Woman will verbalize a plan to change her lifestyle throughout pregnancy to avoid risk of cardiac decompensation.

Nursing Interventions/*Rationales*

Assist woman to identify factors that decrease activity tolerance and explore extent of limitations *to establish a baseline for evaluation.*

Help woman to develop an individualized program of activity and rest, taking into account the living and working environment, as well as support of family and friends, *to maintain sufficient cardiac output.*

Teach woman to monitor physiologic response to activity (i.e., pulse rate, respiratory rate) and reduce activity that causes fatigue or pain *to maintain sufficient cardiac output and prevent potential injury to fetus.*

Enlist family and friends to assist woman in pacing activities and provide support in performing role functions and self-management activities that are too strenuous *to increase chances of compliance with activity restrictions.*

Suggest that woman maintain an activity log that records activities, time, duration, intensity, and physiologic response *to evaluate effectiveness of and adherence to activity program.*

Discuss various quiet diversional activities that could be done by the woman *to decrease the potential for boredom during rest periods.*

Nursing Diagnosis: Risk for ineffective therapeutic regimen management related to woman's first pregnancy and perceived sense of wellness

Expected Outcome

Woman will participate in an effective therapeutic regimen for pregnancy complicated by heart disease.

Nursing Interventions/*Rationales*

Identify factors that could inhibit the woman from participating in a therapeutic regimen such as insufficient knowledge about the effect of cardiac disease on pregnancy *to promote early interventions such as teaching about the importance of rest.*

Teach woman and family about factors such as lack of rest or not taking prescribed medications that could adversely affect the pregnancy *to provide information and promote empowerment over the situation.*

Encourage expression of feelings about the disease and its potential effect on the pregnancy *to promote a sense of trust.*

Identify resources in the community *to provide a shared sense of common experiences.*

Encourage woman to verbalize her plan for carrying out the regimen of care *to evaluate the effects of teaching.*

Nursing Diagnosis: Decreased cardiac output related to increased circulatory volume secondary to pregnancy and cardiac disease

Expected Outcome

The woman will exhibit signs of adequate cardiac output (i.e., normal pulse and blood pressure; normal heart and breath sounds; normal skin color, tone, and turgor; normal capillary refill; normal urine output; and no evidence of edema).

Nursing Interventions/*Rationales*

Reinforce the importance of activity/rest cycles *to prevent cardiac complications.*

Plan with woman a frequent visit schedule to caregiver *to provide adequate surveillance of high risk pregnancy.*

Teach woman to lie in lateral position *to increase uteroplacental blood flow* and to elevate legs while sitting *to promote venous return.*

Monitor intake and output and check for edema *to assess for renal complications or venous return problems.*

Monitor fetal heart rate (FHR) and fetal activity and perform nonstress test (NST) as indicated *to assess fetal status and detect uteroplacental insufficiency.*

Nursing Diagnosis: Risk for ineffective tissue perfusion related to cardiac condition secondary to increased circulatory needs during pregnancy

Expected Outcomes

The woman will exhibit signs of hemodynamic stability (i.e., blood pressure, pulse, arterial blood gases [ABGs], and white blood cell [WBC] counts are within normal limits). The fetus will exhibit signs of well-being (i.e., fetal activity and FHR are within normal limits).

Nursing Interventions/*Rationales*

Monitor heart rate and rhythm, blood pressure, skin color and temperature, WBCs, hemoglobin and hematocrit, and ABGs *to detect early signs of cardiac failure/hypoxia.*

Monitor fetal activity and FHR and perform NST as indicated *to assess fetal status and detect uteroplacental insufficiency.*

Teach woman how to detect and report early signs of cardiac decompensation *to prevent maternal/fetal complications.*

woman with anemia as she copes with her activities of daily living. The nurse should assess the pregnant woman's needs and provide her with appropriate resources or referral.

Iron Deficiency Anemia

Pathologic anemia of pregnancy is mainly the result of iron deficiency. Without iron therapy even pregnant women who enjoy excellent nutrition conclude pregnancy with an iron deficit. Iron is actively transported across the placenta for fetal erythropoiesis. Ferritin levels are the primary screening tests to diagnose iron deficiency anemia. A ferritin level of less than 10 to 15 mcg/L confirms the diagnosis.

If iron deficiency anemia is diagnosed, increased iron dosages are recommended (elemental iron, 60 to 120 mg/day).

Diet alone cannot replace gestational iron losses. Inadequate nutrition without therapy will certainly mean iron deficiency anemia during late pregnancy and the puerperium. It is important to teach the pregnant woman the significance of iron therapy (see Table 12-1). In addition, the woman should be instructed to decrease the gastrointestinal side effects of iron therapy through diet. Some pregnant women cannot tolerate the prescribed oral iron because of nausea and vomiting. In such cases they should receive parenteral iron such as an iron-dextran complex (Imferon). Blood transfusions should be considered for the woman with severe anemia to prevent fetal and maternal complications of decreased oxygen delivery.

Folic Acid Deficiency Anemia

Folic acid deficiency during conception and early pregnancy increases the incidence of neural tube defects, cleft lip, and cleft palate. Even in well-nourished women it is common to have a folate deficiency. Poor diet, cooking with large volumes of water, or home canning of food (especially vegetables) may lead to folate deficiency. Malabsorption may play a part in the development of anemia caused by a lack of folic acid. Folic acid deficiency is common in multiple gestations. During pregnancy the recommended daily intake is 400 mcg per day of folic acid, although women who have a deficiency may need 1 mg or more per day (see Box 12-1).

Since 1998 the U.S. Food and Drug Administration has required the addition of folic acid to cereals, pasta, breads, and other food that are labeled "enriched." However, the amount added is small, and most pregnant women need a supplement.

Sickle Cell Hemoglobinopathy

Sickle cell hemoglobinopathy is a disease caused by the presence of abnormal hemoglobin in the blood. Sickle cell trait (SA hemoglobin pattern), sickling of the red blood cells but with a normal red blood cell life span, usually causes only mild clinical symptoms. Sickle cell anemia (sickle cell disease) is a recessive, hereditary, familial hemolytic anemia that affects those of African-American or Mediterranean ancestry. These individuals usually have abnormal hemoglobin types (SS or SC). People with sickle cell anemia have recurrent attacks (crises) of fever and pain in the abdomen or extremities. These attacks are attributed to vascular occlusion (from abnormal cells), tissue hypoxia, edema, and red blood cell destruction. Crises are associated with normochromic anemia, jaundice, reticulocytosis, a positive sickle cell test, and the demonstration of abnormal hemoglobin (usually SS or SC).

Almost 10% of African-Americans in North America have the sickle cell trait, but fewer than 1% have sickle cell anemia. The anemia often is complicated by iron and folic acid deficiency.

Women with sickle cell trait usually do well in pregnancy, although they are at increased risk for urinary tract infections and hematuria and may be deficient in iron (Kilpatrick, 2009). If the woman has sickle cell anemia, the anemia that occurs in normal pregnancies may aggravate the condition and bring on more crises. Fetal complications include being small for gestational age, IUGR, and skeletal changes. Pregnant women with sickle cell anemia are prone to pyelonephritis, leg ulcers, bone abnormalities, strokes, cardiopathy, congestive heart failure, and preeclampsia. An aplastic crisis may follow serious infection. Transfusions have been the usual treatment for symptomatic patients; however, partial exchange transfusions or prophylactic transfusions are common as well and significantly reduce the number of painful crises (Kilpatrick, 2009). Cesarean birth is warranted only for obstetric indications. Oral contraceptives are contraindicated.

Table 13-6 identifies some potential problems faced by the woman with sickle cell disease and some preventive and maintenance interventions.

Thalassemia

Thalassemia (Mediterranean or Cooley anemia) is a relatively common anemia in which an insufficient amount of globin is produced to fill the red blood cells. The condition eventually manifests itself in severe bone deformities caused by massive marrow tissue expansion. Thalassemia is a hereditary disorder that involves the abnormal synthesis of the alpha (α) or beta (β) chains of hemoglobin. β-Thalassemia is the more common variety in the United States and is more common in individuals of Mediterranean, Middle Eastern, and Asian descent (Kilpatrick, 2009). The unbalanced synthesis of hemoglobin leads to premature red blood cell death, resulting in severe anemia. Thalassemia major is the homozygous form of the disorder; thalassemia minor is the heterozygous form. Couples with the thalassemia trait should seek genetic counseling. Women with the thalassemia trait usually have an uncomplicated pregnancy.

Women with thalassemia major or minor have infertility problems; thus few pregnancies result. As many as 50% of these pregnancies have been complicated by stillbirth, IUGR, preeclampsia, and preterm birth. Medical management consists of ongoing monitoring and transfusion therapy.

Women with thalassemia minor have a mild, persistent anemia; but the red blood cell level may be normal or even elevated. However, no systemic problems are caused by the anemia. Thalassemia minor must be distinguished from iron deficiency anemia.

The anemia does not respond to iron therapy; and prolonged parenteral iron therapy can lead to harmful, excessive iron storage. People with thalassemia minor should have a normal life span despite a moderately reduced hemoglobin level.

Pulmonary Disorders

As pregnancy advances and the uterus impinges on the thoracic cavity, any pregnant woman may have increased respiratory difficulty. This difficulty is compounded by pulmonary disease.

A pregnant woman with a pulmonary disorder requires assessment, planning, and interventions specific to the disease process, in addition to the routine peripartum care. The nurse also must be alert to pulmonary complications precipitated by the pregnancy.

Asthma

Bronchial asthma is an acute respiratory illness caused by allergens, irritants, marked changes in ambient temperature, certain medications (e.g., aspirin and β-blockers) or exercise. In many cases the cause may be unknown. A history of posi-

Table 13-6 Sickle Cell Anemia: Potential Problems, Prevention, and Maintenance

POTENTIAL PROBLEM	PREVENTION AND MAINTENANCE
1. Inadequate oxygen to meet needs of labor and prevent sickling	1. a. Monitor Hb level and HCT to maintain Hb at ≥8 g and HCT at ≥20%. b. Have typed and crossmatched blood available. c. Assist with transfusions. d. Administer oxygen continuously during labor. e. Coach for relaxation and to lessen anxiety.
2. Infection: UTI, pyelonephritis, pneumonia	2. a. Continue actions as under No. 1. b. Maintain adequate hydration. c. Administer antibiotics as ordered. d. Maintain strict asepsis. e. Encourage frequent voiding to keep bladder empty.
3. Sequestration crisis caused by need for and destruction of RBCs	3. Administer folic acid supplement (1 mg/day) to decrease erythropoietic demands and reduce probability of capillary stasis.
4. Crisis caused by hypoxia, hypotension, acidosis, dehydration, exertion, sudden cooling, low-grade fever	4. a. Continue actions as under No. 1. b. Avoid supine hypotension. c. Maintain adequate hydration. d. Maintain comfortable room temperature: use warm blankets or cool cloths as needed. e. Assist with analgesia and anesthesia.
5. Hypertension, proteinuria, no large weight gain; often accompanying bone pain crisis	5. a. If true preeclampsia occurs, care is the same as for preeclampsia. b. Monitor blood pressure and urine.
6. Thromboembolism (from increased blood viscosity)	6. a. Monitor for positive Homans' sign. b. Initiate bed rest if Homans' sign is positive or if reddened, warm areas or lump appears in calf. c. Maintain adequate hydration. d. Administer heparin as ordered. e. Apply warm compresses. f. Apply antiembolism stockings.
7. Congestive heart failure	7. a. Assess pulse, respiratory rate. b. Place in semirecumbent position; lateral position for labor. c. Auscultate frequently for crackles in the lungs. d. Administer oxygen and medications (e.g., digitalis, antibiotics, diuretics, analgesics). e. Regional analgesia for pain relief in labor.
8. Pulmonary infarction (hemoptysis, cough, temperature to 38.9° C, friction rub)	8. Assess for this possible complication to facilitate early diagnosis.
9. Postpartum hemorrhage (resulting from heparin therapy)	9. Administer ordered oxytocic medication.

Hb, Hemoglobin; *HCT,* hematocrit; *RBC,* red blood cell; *UTI,* urinary tract infection.

tive allergen testing is common (75% to 85%) in people with asthma. In response to stimuli, there is widespread but reversible narrowing of the hyperreactive airways, making it difficult to breathe. The clinical manifestations are some or all of the following: expiratory wheezing, productive cough, thick sputum, and dyspnea.

Approximately 4% to 8% of pregnant women have diagnosed asthma, making it the most common pulmonary disease in pregnancy (Whitty & Dombrowski, 2009). To classify the severity of asthma and determine management guidelines, the National Asthma Education and Prevention Program (NAEPP) Working Group on Asthma and Pregnancy published guidelines for classification. Pregnant women are classified as having mild intermittent, mild persistent, moderate persistent, and severe persistent asthma based on exacerbation of symptoms, peak expiratory flow rate (PEFR), and forced expiratory volume in 1 second (FEV_1) (NAEPP, 2004) (Table 13-7). The effect of pregnancy on asthma is unpredictable. Approximately 23% improve, and 30% worsen (Whitty & Dombrowski, 2009). Maternal morbidity is 2.3% with mild, 19.3% with moderate, and 26.9% with severe symptoms that required hospitalization (Whitty & Dombrowski, 2009). Physiologic alterations induced by pregnancy do not make the pregnant woman more prone to asthmatic attacks. Women often have few symptoms of asthma in the first trimester and the last weeks of pregnancy. The severity of symptoms usually peaks between 29 and 36 weeks of gestation (Burton & Reyes, 2001).

The ultimate goal of therapy for asthma is to prevent hypoxic episodes in the mother and fetus. The therapy has four objectives: (1) relieve the bronchospasm, (2) limit irritant stimuli, (3) decrease the pulmonary response to allergen exposure, and (4) limit the inflammatory response in the airways. These goals can be achieved in pregnancy by eliminating environmental triggers (e.g., dust mites, animal dander, pollen), drug therapy (e.g., bronchodilators and anti-inflammatory agents), and patient education. Respiratory infections should be treated, and mist or steam inhalation should be used to aid expectoration of mucus. Acute episodes may require albuterol, steroids, aminophylline, β-adrenergic agents, and oxygen. Pharmacotherapy to control symptoms and treat airway inflammation is safer than exacerbations of symptoms during pregnancy. Patients should determine their PEFR before taking medications (Whitty & Dombrowski, 2009).

Table 13-7 Modified National Asthma Education and Prevention Program Asthma Severity Classification

CLASS	CRITERIA	TREATMENT
Mild intermittent	Symptoms ≤ twice/week Nocturnal symptoms ≤ twice/month PEFR or FEV_1 ≥80%, variability ≤20%	No daily medications needed
Mild persistent	Symptoms > twice/week but not daily Nocturnal symptoms > twice/month PEFR or FEV_1 ≥80%, variability 20%-30%	Preferred–Low-dose inhaled corticosteroid Alternative–Cromolyn, leukotriene receptor antagonist, *or* theophylline (serum level 5-12 mcg/ml)
Moderate persistent	Daily symptoms Nocturnal symptoms > once/week PEFR or FEV_1 >60%-80% predicted, variability >30% Regular medications necessary to control symptoms	Preferred–Low-to-medium inhaled corticosteroid and salmeterol *or* medium dose inhaled corticosteroid Alternative–Low-to-medium dose inhaled corticosteroid and leukotriene receptor antagonist *or* low-to-medium dose inhaled corticosteroid and theophylline (serum level 5-12 mcg/ml)
Severe	Continuous symptoms/frequent exacerbations Frequent nocturnal symptoms PEFR or FEV_1 ≤60% predicted, variability >30% Regular oral corticosteroids necessary to control symptoms	Preferred–High-dose inhaled corticosteroid and salmeterol *and* oral corticosteroid if needed Alternative–High-dose inhaled corticosteroid and theophylline (serum level 5-12 mcg/ml) *and* oral corticosteroid if needed Albuterol 2-4 puffs as needed for PEFR or FEV_1 <80%, asthma exacerbations, or exposure to exercise or allergens; oral corticosteroid burst if inadequate response to albuterol, regardless of asthma severity

NAEPP expert panel report managing asthma during pregnancy: *Recommendations for pharmacologic treatment–2004 update.* NHLBI, NIH Publication No. 05-3279. Available at www.med.umich.edu/obgyn/resdir/AsthmaGuidelines2004.pdf (accessed March 22, 2009).
FEV_1, Forced expiratory volume in 1 second; *PEFR,* peak expiratory flow rate.

Asthma attacks can occur in labor; thus medications for asthma are continued in labor and postpartum. Pulse oximetry should be instituted during labor. Epidural analgesia reduces oxygen consumption and minute ventilation during labor. Meperidine is a histamine-releasing narcotic but rarely causes bronchospasm (Whitty & Dombrowski, 2009).

During the postpartum period women who have asthma are at increased risk for hemorrhage. If excessive bleeding occurs, oxytocin is the recommended drug. Asthma medications are usually safe for administration during the postpartum period and lactation. The woman usually returns to her prepregnancy asthma status within 3 months after giving birth.

Cystic Fibrosis

Cystic fibrosis is a common autosomal recessive genetic disorder in which the exocrine glands produce excessive viscous secretions, causing problems with both respiratory and digestive functions. There is an increase in pulmonary capillary permeability, decrease of lung volume, and shunting, which results in arterial hypoxemia. Respiratory failure and early death (in the early twenties) may occur.

The gene for cystic fibrosis was identified in 1989. All infants born to mothers with cystic fibrosis are carriers of the gene. The disease occurs in 1 in 3300 Caucasian live births (Slack et al, 2006). Improvements in diagnosis and treatment have allowed an increasing number of women with cystic fibrosis to survive to adulthood. One of the genetic testing recommendations from ACOG is cystic fibrosis carrier screening to couples who are planning a pregnancy (ACOG, 2001b). Preconception counseling is essential for women with cystic fibrosis. Infertility appears to relate to changes in cervical mucus. As a result of the advances in diagnostic capabilities and treatment, the median survival has increased from 14 years of age to 30 to 35 years of age. The median age of survival for women with pancreatic insufficiency is 27 years (Whitty & Dombrowski, 2009).

In women with good nutritional status, mild obstructive lung disease, and minimal impairment of lung function, pregnancy is tolerated well. In those with severe disease the pregnancy is often complicated by chronic hypoxia and frequent pulmonary infections. Women with cystic fibrosis show a decrease in their residual lung volume during pregnancy, as do normal pregnant women, and are unable to maintain vital capacity. Presumably the pulmonary vasculature cannot accommodate the increased cardiac output of pregnancy. The results are decreased oxygen to the myocardium, decreased cardiac output, and increased hypoxia. A pregnant woman with less than 50% of expected vital capacity usually has a difficult pregnancy. Increased maternal and perinatal mortality rates are related to severe pulmonary infection. There is an increased incidence of preterm births, IUGR, and neonatal deaths in patients with cystic fibrosis. Predictors of adverse effects to the fetus and neonate are inadequate weight gain, dyspnea, and cyanosis.

In addition to the respiratory problems, pregnant women with cystic fibrosis have decreased insulin secretion and increased insulin resistance, resulting in a higher incidence for the development of GDM. Pancreatic insufficiency may also put the woman at risk for malnutrition because she cannot meet the increased nutrition requirements of pregnancy. Fat-soluble vitamins may not be utilized because of diminished absorption.

Weight and symptoms of malabsorption should be monitored at each prenatal visit, and pancreatic enzymes should be adjusted as necessary. Women with severe pancreatic insufficiency may require total parenteral nutrition. A glucose tolerance test should be done at 20 weeks of gestation. Routine respiratory management is continued throughout the pregnancy. Hospitalization and antibiotic therapy are recommended when a pulmonary infection has been identified. Because cystic fibrosis places the pregnant woman at risk, nonstress testing should be initiated at 32 weeks.

During labor, monitoring for fluid and electrolyte balance is required. The amount of sodium lost through sweat can be significant, and hypovolemia can occur. Conversely, if the woman has any degree of cor pulmonale, fluid overload is a concern. Oxygen is given freely during labor, and monitoring by pulse oximetry is recommended. Epidural or local anesthesia is the preferred analgesic for birth. Vaginal birth is preferable; cesarean birth should be reserved for the usual obstetric indications.

Breastfeeding appears to be safe as long as the sodium content of the mother's milk is not abnormal. The milk is pumped and discarded until the sodium content has been determined. Milk samples should be tested periodically for sodium, chloride, and total fat; and the infant's growth pattern should be followed (Lawrence & Lawrence, 2005).

Gastrointestinal Disorders

Compromise of gastrointestinal function during pregnancy is a concern. Obvious physiologic alterations such as the greatly enlarged uterus and less apparent changes such as hormonal differences and hypochlorhydria (deficiency of hydrochloric acid in the stomach's gastric juice) require understanding for proper diagnosis and treatment. Gallbladder disease and inflammatory bowel disease are two gastrointestinal disorders that may occur during pregnancy.

Cholelithiasis and Cholecystitis

Women are twice as likely to have cholelithiasis (presence of gallstones in the gallbladder) than are men, and pregnancy seems to make the woman more vulnerable to gallstone formation. Decreased muscle tone allows gallbladder distention and thickening of the bile and prolongs emptying time. Increased progesterone levels result in a slight hypercholesterolemia. Nutrition counseling is important (see Home Care box).

HOME CARE

Nutrition Counseling for the Pregnant Woman with Cholecystitis or Cholelithiasis

- Assess your diet for foods that cause discomfort and flatulence and omit foods that trigger episodes.
- Reduce dietary fat intake to 40 to 50 g/day.
- Limit protein to 10% to 12% of total calories.
- Choose foods so that most of the calories come from carbohydrates.
- Prepare food without adding fats or oils as much as possible.
- Avoid fried foods.

Cholecystitis (inflammation of the gallbladder) may also occur during pregnancy, probably because pressure of the enlarged uterus interferes with the normal circulation and drainage of the gallbladder. Acute cholecystitis occurs most often in older women who have been pregnant several times and who have a history of previous attacks.

Women with acute cholecystitis usually have fatty food intolerance along with colicky abdominal pain radiating to the back or shoulder, nausea, and vomiting. Fever and an increased leukocyte count may also be present. Ultrasound is often used to detect the presence of stones or dilation of the common bile duct.

Generally gallbladder surgery should be postponed until the puerperium. Usually the woman can be treated with medical therapy consisting of antibiotics, analgesics, IV fluids, bowel rest, and nasogastric suctioning. Total parenteral nutrition can be used in some cases as an alternative to surgery. Morphine should not be used as an analgesic because it may cause ductal spasm. The woman's condition should improve significantly within 48 hours of beginning treatment. Surgery may be necessary if the woman has repeated attacks of biliary colic, acute cholecystitis, obstructive jaundice, peritonitis, or pancreatitis. Laparoscopic cholecystectomy performed in the second trimester poses minimal risk to both mother and fetus. Other procedures performed may be endoscopic retrograde cholangiopancreatography or open cholecystectomy (Williamson & Mackillop, 2009).

Inflammatory Bowel Disease

Treatment of inflammatory bowel disease is the same for the pregnant woman as it is for the nonpregnant woman. Medications include prednisone and sulfasalazine. Vitamin and folic acid supplementation is especially important because of problems with malabsorption. Effects of inflammatory bowel disease on pregnancy are usually minimal. If the woman is severely debilitated, miscarriage, preterm birth, or fetal death can occur.

Integumentary Disorders

The skin surface may exhibit many physiologic and pathologic conditions during pregnancy. Dermatologic disorders induced by pregnancy include melasma (chloasma), vascular "spiders," palmar erythema, and striae gravidarum. Skin problems generally aggravated by pregnancy are acne vulgaris (in the first trimester), erythema multiforme, herpetiform dermatitis (fever blisters and genital herpes), granuloma inguinale (Donovan bodies), condylomata acuminata (genital warts), neurofibromatosis (von Recklinghausen's disease), and pemphigus. Dermatologic disorders usually improved by pregnancy include acne vulgaris (in the third trimester), seborrheic dermatitis (dandruff), and psoriasis. An unpredictable course during pregnancy may be expected in atopic dermatitis, lupus erythematosus, and herpes simplex. Disease processes during and soon after pregnancy may be extremely difficult to diagnose and treat.

NURSING ALERT Isotretinoin (Accutane), commonly prescribed for acne, is contraindicated in pregnancy because of its high teratogenicity. Fetuses exposed to this medication are at increased risk for craniofacial, cardiac, and CNS anomalies.

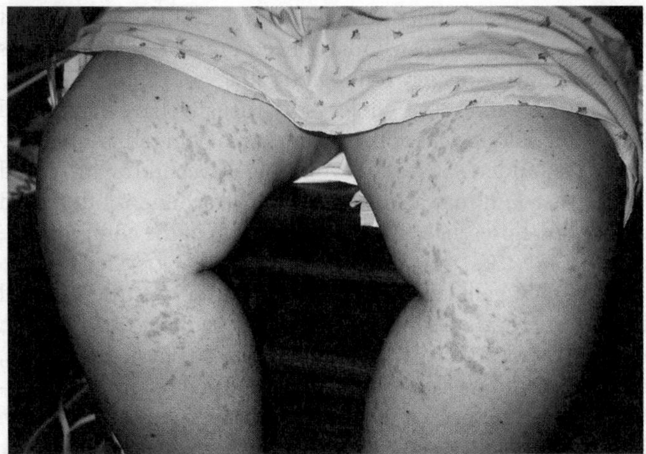

Fig. 13-6 Woman with pruritic urticarial papules and plaques of pregnancy. Lesions also are present on her arms, back, abdomen, and buttocks. *(Courtesy Shannon Perry, Phoenix, AZ.)*

Pruritus is a common symptom in pregnancy-specific inflammatory skin diseases. The most common pregnancy-specific causes of pruritus are polymorphic eruption of pregnancy (also known as pruritic urticarial papules and plaques of pregnancy [PUPPP]) (Fig. 13-6), prurigo gestationis, and cholestasis of pregnancy. Symptoms usually appear in the third trimester and usually subside in the postpartum period. The abdomen is usually affected; but lesions can spread to the arms, thighs, back, and buttocks. Topical steroid therapy usually provides relief, but some women may require systemic steroid therapy for severe symptoms (Papoutsis & Kroumpouzos, 2007).

Neurologic Disorders

The pregnant woman with a neurologic disorder needs to deal with the potential teratogenic effects of prescribed medications, changes of mobility during pregnancy, and impaired ability to care for the baby. The nurse should be aware of all drugs the pregnant woman is taking and the associated potential for producing congenital anomalies. As the pregnancy progresses, the woman's center of gravity shifts and causes balance and gait changes. The woman should be advised of these expected changes and suggest safety measures as appropriate. Family and community resources should be assessed to provide child care for the neurologically impaired woman.

Epilepsy

Epilepsy is a disorder of the brain causing recurrent seizures; it is the most common neurologic disorder accompanying pregnancy. Epilepsy may result from developmental abnormalities or injury or have no identified cause. Convulsive seizures may be more frequent or severe during complications of pregnancy such as edema, alkalosis, fluid-electrolyte imbalance, cerebral hypoxia, hypoglycemia, and hypocalcemia. They also may be related to hormonal changes, fatigue, or sleep deprivation.

NURSING ALERT Anticonvulsants and oral contraceptive agents may have interactions that decrease the effectiveness of the contraceptive, leading to unplanned pregnancy.

The effects of pregnancy on epilepsy are unpredictable. Most women have no change in seizure activity during pregnancy; some have an increase, whereas others have a decrease in seizures.

The differential diagnosis between epilepsy and eclampsia may pose a problem. Epilepsy and eclampsia can coexist. However, a history of seizures, a normal plasma uric acid level, and the absence of hypertension and generalized edema or proteinuria point to epilepsy.

During pregnancy risk of vaginal bleeding is doubled, and there is a threefold risk of abruptio placentae. Abnormal presentations are more common in labor and delivery. There is an increased possibility that the fetus will experience seizures in utero.

Metabolic changes in pregnancy usually alter pharmacokinetics. In addition, nausea and vomiting may interfere with ingestion and absorption of medication.

Teratogenicity of antiepileptic drugs (AEDs) has been described thoroughly. However, failure to take medications is a common factor leading to worsening of seizure activity during pregnancy. Babies born to mothers exposed to AEDs are at increased risk of congenital malformations, cognitive impairment, and fetal death. Congenital anomalies associated with AEDs include cleft lip or palate, congenital heart disease, urogenital defects, and neural tube defects. AEDs should be monotherapeutic and used in the smallest therapeutic dose. Daily folic acid supplementation is essential because of the depletion that occurs when taking AEDs.

A small risk of seizure activity exists during labor. If the woman cannot take oral AEDs, phenytoin can be administered intravenously. Serum levels of AEDs should be checked within 48 hours and at 1 to 2 weeks after birth because levels can change quickly and toxicity can develop.

During the neonatal period infants can have a hemorrhagic disorder associated with AED-induced vitamin K deficiency. Prophylaxis consists of administering vitamin K, 20 mg orally, daily during the last month of pregnancy and 1 mg intramuscularly to the newborn at birth. Neonates also should be monitored for drug withdrawal. All of the most prescribed AEDs cross into breast milk; however, their use is not contraindicated with breastfeeding. Some AEDs may have a sedative effect and cause possible withdrawal symptoms in the newborn (e.g., phenobarbital, primidone, benzodiazepines). Newborn weight loss has been associated with the use of topiramine and may not be an option for the breastfeeding mother (Samuels & Niebyl, 2007).

Multiple Sclerosis

Multiple sclerosis (MS), a patchy demyelinization of the spinal cord and CNS, may be a viral disorder. Women are affected twice as often as men, with the most common onset occurring during the childbearing years between ages 20 and 40. MS does not affect the normal course of pregnancy or birth (Aminoff, 2009).

Occasionally MS may complicate pregnancy, but exacerbations and remissions are unrelated to the pregnant state. Bed rest and steroids are commonly used to treat acute exacerbations. Nursing care of the pregnant woman with MS is similar to that of the pregnant woman with an uncomplicated pregnancy. Women with MS may have an almost painless labor, although the character of uterine contractions is unaffected by the disease.

Bell's Palsy

An association between Bell's palsy (idiopathic facial paralysis) and pregnancy was first cited by Bell in 1830. The incidence of Bell's palsy in pregnancy is about 57 per 100,000 per year. The clinical manifestations include the sudden development of a unilateral facial weakness, often discovered first thing in the morning. In addition, taste on the anterior two thirds of the tongue may be lost, depending on the location of the lesion. Pain may occur in and around the ear. The incidence usually peaks during the third trimester and the puerperium. There is no relationship between the appearance of Bell's palsy and any complications of pregnancy.

No effects of maternal Bell's palsy have been observed in infants. Maternal outcome is generally good unless there is a complete block in nerve conduction. Steroids sometimes are prescribed for the condition, but they do not hasten recovery. In most affected women 90% or more of facial function can be expected to return. Supportive care includes prevention of injury to the exposed cornea, facial muscle massage, careful chewing and manual removal of food from inside the affected cheek, and reassurance that return of total neurologic function is likely.

Autoimmune Disorders

Autoimmune disorders make up a large group of diseases that disrupt the function of the immune system of the body. In these types of disorders the body develops antibodies that attack its normally present antigens, causing tissue damage. Autoimmune disorders have a predilection for women in their reproductive years; therefore associations with pregnancy are not uncommon. Pregnancy may affect the disease process. Some disorders adversely affect the course of pregnancy or are detrimental to the fetus. Autoimmune disorders of concern in pregnancy include systemic lupus erythematosus, myasthenia gravis, and rheumatoid arthritis.

Systemic Lupus Erythematosus

One of the most common serious disorders in women of childbearing age, systemic lupus erythematosus (SLE), is a chronic multisystem inflammatory disease characterized by autoimmune antibody production that affects skin, joints, kidneys, lungs, CNS, liver, and other body organs. The exact cause is unknown, but viral infection and hormonal and genetic factors may be related. SLE is four times more common in African-American than in Caucasian women.

Early symptoms such as fatigue, fever, skin rashes, weight loss, and arthralgias may be overlooked. Pericarditis is often the initial symptom. Eventually all organs become involved. The condition is characterized by a series of exacerbations and remissions.

If the diagnosis has been established and the woman desires a child, she is advised to wait until she is in remission and cytotoxic drugs (e.g., azathioprine, methotrexate, cyclophosphamide) have been stopped (Holmgren & Branch, 2007). An exacerbation of SLE during pregnancy or postpartum occurs in 15% to 60% of women (Holmgren & Branch, 2007).

SLE during pregnancy is associated with increased rates of preterm deliveries, IUGR, stillbirth, postpartum hemorrhage, and perinatal death. Complications such as preeclampsia and HELLP syndrome are common.

Medical therapy is kept to a minimum in women who are in remission or who have a mild form of SLE. Antiinflammatory medications such as prednisone and aspirin may be used. Immunosuppressive medications are not recommended during pregnancy but may be used in some situations when there is more risk in not treating SLE. Nursing care focuses on early recognition of signs of SLE exacerbation and pregnancy complications, education and support of the woman and her family, and assessment of fetal well-being.

Vaginal birth is preferred, but cesarean birth is common because of maternal and fetal complications. During labor efforts are aimed at reducing the risk of infection, which is the leading cause of death in women with SLE.

During the postpartum period the mother should rest as much as possible to prevent an exacerbation of SLE. Breastfeeding is encouraged unless the mother is taking immunosuppressive agents. Women with SLE should limit their number of pregnancies because of increased adverse perinatal outcomes and the guarded maternal prognosis (Holmgren & Branch, 2007). Family planning is important. Oral contraceptives with synthetic estrogens should not be used in women with active lupus nephritis.

Myasthenia Gravis

Myasthenia gravis (MG), an autoimmune motor (muscle) end-plate disorder that involves acetylcholine use, affects the motor function at the myoneural junction. Muscle weakness results, particularly in the eyes, face, tongue, neck, limbs, and respiratory muscles. Symptoms include easy fatigability; intermittent double vision (diplopia); upper eyelid drooping; and difficulty speaking, swallowing, and clearing secretions. In more serious cases upper arm weakness and breathing difficulty are seen. The response of women with MG to pregnancy is unpredictable; remission, exacerbation, or remaining stable during pregnancy may occur.

NURSING ALERT If preterm labor occurs, magnesium sulfate, which interferes with neuromuscular transmission, is absolutely contraindicated.

Treatment is the same as that for a nonpregnant woman. Usual medications include immunosuppressive medications and acetylcholinesterase inhibitors. Monitoring blood glucose values is important because hyperglycemia may be the result of corticosteroid therapy. Thymectomy may result in remission of the disease but is best performed before or after pregnancy if at all possible. Plasmapheresis or IV immunoglobulin therapy may be needed for severe weakness.

Women with MG usually tolerate labor well, but vacuum or forceps assistance for birth may be required because of muscle weakness. Oxytocin may be given to stimulate contractions. Narcotic analgesia should be avoided because it may precipitate respiratory depression. Regional analgesia is preferred. After birth women must be carefully supervised because relapses often occur during the puerperium.

In approximately 10% to 15% of neonates neonatal myasthenia develops, with symptoms of feeble cry, respiratory distress, and weak suck. These neonates may require ventilatory support. With proper management, complete recovery of the neonate should occur within 6 weeks (Aminoff, 2009).

Human Immunodeficiency Virus and Acquired Immunodeficiency Syndrome

Infection with HIV and the resultant acquired immunodeficiency syndrome (AIDS) are increasingly occurring in women. Although HIV and AIDS have traditionally been associated with homosexual populations, women are now the fastest-growing population of individuals with HIV infection and AIDS. Women are more likely to have acquired the infection through heterosexual contact or IV drug use. Women of color are disproportionately affected; about 78% of HIV-infected women are African-American or Hispanic. This section addresses management of the pregnant woman who is HIV positive or who has developed full-blown AIDS. See Chapter 6 for more information about the diagnosis and management of nonpregnant women with HIV and Chapter 28 for a discussion of HIV/AIDS in infants.

CRITICAL THINKING EXERCISE

The Pregnant Woman Who Is Positive for Human Immunodeficiency Virus

Betsy is being seen in the prenatal clinic at 34 weeks of gestation. She is positive for immunodeficiency virus (HIV) and has a past history of intravenous cocaine and heroin use. She has been drug free for the last 18 months. She tells you she is taking "some AIDS drug" during pregnancy but does not seem to know much about it. As part of your care, you will be providing information regarding risk factors in her lifestyle and future planning for her own care and that of her infant.

1. Evidence—Is there sufficient evidence to draw conclusions about the necessity of continued treatment for Betsy and her infant? Can risk factors in Betsy's background be identified?
2. Assumptions—What assumptions can be made about the following issues?
   a. The drug Betsy has most likely been taking and the rationale for its use
   b. Continuation of the therapy during the intrapartum and postpartum periods
   c. Therapy for the infant
   d. Risk factors for acquiring HIV infection present in Betsy's background
   e. Precautions necessary to protect yourself as you provide care for Betsy
3. What implications and priorities for nursing care can be drawn at this time?
4. Does the evidence objectively support your conclusion?
5. Are there alternative perspectives to your conclusion?

AIDS, Acquired immunodeficiency syndrome.

Preconception Counseling

Pregnancy is discouraged in HIV-positive women; preconception counseling is recommended. Exposure to the virus has a significant impact on the pregnancy, the neonatal feeding method, and neonatal health status. HIV-positive women should be counseled extensively about the risk of perinatal transmission and possible obstetric complications. Pregnancy itself does not appear to significantly accelerate the progression of HIV infection. HIV-positive women should be encouraged to seek prenatal care immediately if they suspect pregnancy to maximize chances for a positive outcome.

Pregnancy Risks

Perinatal Transmission

Even though the number of AIDS cases from perinatal transmission has decreased dramatically, approximately 100 to 200 infants in the United States are still infected with HIV every year. Data show that almost all AIDS diagnoses in children are caused by mother-to-child transmission and were from minority races and ethnicities (CDC, 2007b). Perinatal transmission may occur to the fetus through the maternal circulation as early as the first trimester of pregnancy; to the infant during labor and birth by inoculation or ingestion of maternal blood and other infected fluids; or to the infant through breast milk. Factors that increase the likelihood of perinatal viral transmission are listed in Box 13-6.

Treatment of HIV-infected women with the antiviral drug zidovudine (AZT) during pregnancy and labor and birth and treatment of their infants for the first 6 weeks of life with zidovudine decreases the rate of viral transmission from 25.5% to 8.3%. In the United States 25% of women who do not undergo antiviral treatment will transmit the virus to their unborn child (CDC, 2007b). These women should also be given the option of having a scheduled cesarean birth at 38 weeks to decrease the risk of perinatal transmission. If a woman with HIV has a cesarean birth and receives antiviral treatment during pregnancy, labor, and birth and if her newborn is treated, the perinatal transmission rate is less than 2% (CDC, 2007b).

Obstetric Complications

It is difficult to determine obstetric risk in persons with HIV infection because so many confounding variables are often present. Many HIV-positive women also suffer from drug and alcohol addiction, poor nutrition, limited access to prenatal care, or concurrent sexually transmitted infections (STIs). HIV-positive women are probably at risk for preterm labor

BOX 13-6 Factors That Increase the Risk of Perinatal Human Immunodeficiency Virus Transmission

- Previous history of a child with HIV infection
- Acquired immunodeficiency syndrome
- Preterm birth
- Decreased maternal CD4 count
- High maternal viral load
- Firstborn twin
- Chorioamnionitis
- Intrapartum blood exposure
- Failure to treat mother and fetus with zidovudine during the perinatal period

Source: Berstein H: Maternal and perinatal infection: In Gabbe SG, Niebyl JR, Simpson JL (editors): *Obstetrics: normal and problem pregnancies*, ed 5, New York, 2007, Churchill Livingstone.

and birth, premature rupture of membranes, IUGR, perinatal death, and postpartum endometritis.

Nursing Care Management

HIV counseling and testing should be offered to all women when they initially enter prenatal care. Most states in the United States have enacted legislation to ensure that this is offered. If only those presumed to be at high risk are screened, about half of all HIV-positive women will not be detected. Identification of HIV-positive pregnant women is especially important because antepartum and intrapartum antiviral drug therapy has been shown to greatly decrease the risk of viral transmission to the fetus. To increase screening and provide earlier detection and treatment, the "Opt-out" approach is recommended by the CDC and some states. This approach includes the HIV testing in the standard group of prenatal tests given to all pregnant women early in pregnancy. Therefore, unless the woman declines the test, she will receive an HIV test (CDC, 2007b). Any woman or newborn whose HIV status is unknown at the time of labor and/or birth should be screened with a rapid HIV test unless she declines, using the opt-out method of screening (CDC, 2007b).

HIV-infected women should also be tested for other STIs such as gonorrhea; syphilis; chlamydial infection; hepatitis B, C, and D; and herpes. Cytomegalovirus and toxoplasmosis antibody testing should be done because both infections can cause significant maternal and fetal complications and can be successfully treated with antimicrobial agents. Any history of vaccination and immune status should be documented, and chickenpox (varicella) and rubella titers should be determined. Women who are HIV positive should also be vaccinated against hepatitis B, pneumococcal infection, hemophilus B influenza, and viral influenza. A tuberculin skin test should be performed; a positive test necessitates a chest x-ray film to identify active pulmonary disease. A Papanicolaou test should also be done.

All HIV-infected women should be treated with highly active anitretroviral therapy (HAART) during pregnancy, regardless of the CD4 counts. HAART should include three drugs from at least two classes of antiretroviral medications. The major side effect of these drugs is bone marrow suppression. Periodic hematocrit, white blood cell count, and platelet count assessments should be performed. Women with CD4 counts of less than 200 cells/mm^3 should receive prophylactic treatment for *Pneumocystis carinii* pneumonia with daily trimethoprim-sulfamethoxazole. Any other opportunistic infections should be treated with medications specific for the infection; often dosages must be higher for women with HIV infection or AIDS. If women are treated with HAART and have an undetectable viral load, the risk of perinatal transmission is 1% to 2% (Bernstein, 2007).

To support any pregnant woman's immune system, appropriate counseling is provided about optimal nutrition, sleep, rest, exercise, and stress reduction. The HIV-infected woman needs a greater amount of nutritional support and counseling about diet choices, food preparation, and food handling. Weight gain or maintenance in pregnancy is a challenge with the HIV-infected patient. The infected patient is counseled regarding risk reduction techniques. Use of condoms and a spermicide is encouraged to minimize further exposure to HIV if her partner is the source. Orogenital sex is discouraged.

The woman is referred for drug rehabilitation as necessary to discontinue substance abuse. Abuse of alcohol, methamphetamines ("speed," "ice"), marijuana, cocaine, nitrites ("poppers," "snappers"), or other drugs compromises the body's immune system and increases the risks of AIDS and associated conditions. It also interferes with many medical and alternative therapies for AIDS. In addition, alcohol and other drugs affect the judgment of abusers, who may be more likely to engage in high risk activities that increase their exposure to HIV.

IV zidovudine is administered to the HIV-positive woman during the intrapartum period. A loading dose is initiated on her admission in labor, followed by a continuous maintenance dosage throughout labor.

Every effort should be made during the birthing process to decrease the neonate's exposure to infected maternal blood and secretions if cesarean birth is not scheduled and the woman goes into labor. If feasible, the membranes should be left intact until the birth. Increased duration of ruptured amniotic membranes has been associated with increased perinatal transmission. However, research has not shown these data to be statistically significant (Bernstein, 2007). If rupture of membranes occurs before labor, induction of uterine contractions with oxytocin may be appropriate. Fetal scalp electrode and scalp pH sampling should be avoided because these procedures may result in inoculation of the virus into the fetus. Operative vaginal delivery (forceps and/or vacuum extractor) and episiotomy should also be avoided when possible (Bernstein, 2007).

The postpartum period for the woman infected with HIV may be notable for infection, hemorrhage, or both. Women without symptoms may have an unremarkable postpartum course; on the other hand, immunosuppressed women with symptoms may be at increased risk for postpartum urinary tract infections, vaginitis, postpartum endometritis, and poor wound healing. HIV-related thrombocytopenia may also increase the risk of hemorrhage.

Immediately after birth infants should be wiped free of all body fluids and then bathed as soon as they are in stable condition. All staff working with the mother or infant must adhere strictly to infection control techniques and observe Standard Universal Precautions for blood and other body fluids. The cleansed neonate can be with the mother after birth, but breastfeeding is discouraged because of the risk of transmission through breast milk. Oral zidovudine treatment for the infant is initiated before discharge. After discharge the woman and her infant are referred to physicians who are experienced in the treatment of AIDS and associated conditions.

Substance Abuse

evolve Nursing Care Plan–Substance Abuse During Pregnancy

The damaging effects of alcohol and illicit drugs on pregnant women and their unborn babies are well documented (Wisner et al, 2007). Alcohol and other drugs easily pass from a mother to her baby through the placenta. Smoking during pregnancy has serious health risks, including bleeding complications, miscarriage, stillbirth, prematurity, placenta previa, placental abruption, low birth weight, and sudden infant death syndrome (Wisner et al, 2007). Congenital abnormalities have occurred in infants of mothers who have taken drugs. The safest pregnancy is one in which the mother is totally drug and alcohol free, with one exception: for pregnant women addicted to heroin, methadone maintenance is safer for the fetus than acute opiate detoxification.

Substance abuse refers to the continued use of substances despite related problems in physical, social, or interpersonal areas. Recurrent abuse results in failure to fulfill major role obligations, and there may be substance-related legal problems.

Barriers to Treatment

Pregnant women often do not seek help because of the fear of losing custody of the child or of criminal prosecution. Pregnant women who abuse substances commonly have little understanding of the ways in which these substances affect them, their pregnancies, and their babies. They often delay seeking prenatal care until labor begins. Stigma, shame, and guilt lead to a high denial of drinking or drug problems both by the woman herself and by family members and friends who conceal the abuse from outsiders to protect the abuser (Wisner et al, 2007). Traditionally substance abuse treatment programs have not addressed issues that affect pregnant women such as concurrent need for obstetric care and child care for other children. Long waiting lists and lack of health insurance present further barriers to treatment.

Legal Considerations

Because of the risks to the unborn children, pregnant women who abuse substances may face criminal charges under expanded interpretations of child abuse and drug-trafficking statutes. At least 35 states have prosecuted pregnant women on a variety of charges for suspected harm to the fetus (Jos, Perlmutter, & Marshall, 2003). Some policymakers have proposed that pregnant women who abuse substances should be jailed, placed under house arrest, or committed to psychiatric hospitals for the remainder of their pregnancies. Nurses who screen for substance abuse in pregnancy and encourage prenatal care, counseling, and treatment will be of greater benefit to the mother and child than prosecution. A public health approach to substance abuse can inspire macrolevel policy that is designed to strengthen communities, as well as specific treatment and prevention programs embedded in the communities (Jos, Perlmutter, & Marshall, 2003).

LEGAL TIP Drug Testing During Pregnancy There is no state requirement for a health care provider to test either the mother or the newborn for the presence of drugs. However, nurses need to know the practices of the states in which they are working. In some states a woman whose urine drug screen test is positive at the time of labor and birth must be referred to child protective services. If the mother is not in a drug treatment program or is judged unable to provide care, the infant may be placed in foster care. In all states the U.S. Supreme Court has ruled that it is unlawful to test for drug use without the pregnant woman's permission (Harris & Paltrow, 2003).

Nursing Care Management

The care of the substance-dependent pregnant woman is based on historical data, symptoms, physical findings, and laboratory results. Screening questions for alcohol and drug abuse should be included in the overall assessment of the first prenatal visit of all women. Because women often deny or greatly underreport usage when asked directly about drug or alcohol consumption, it is crucial that the nurse display a nonjudgmental and matter-of-fact attitude while taking the history to gain the woman's trust and elicit a reasonably accurate estimate. Information about drug use should be obtained by first asking about the woman's intake of over-the-counter and prescribed medications. Next her use of "legal" drugs such as caffeine, nicotine, and alcohol should be ascertained. Finally, the woman should be questioned about her use of illicit drugs such as cocaine, heroin, and marijuana. The approximate frequency and amount should be documented for each drug used.

Alcohol screening questionnaires generally ask about consequences of heavy drinking, alcohol intake, or both. The Michigan Alcoholism Screening Test (MAST) and the CAGE test are two well-known screens that are used. The T-ACE (Hankin & Sokol, 1995) (Box 13-7) was developed to screen specifically for alcohol use during pregnancy. Urine screening is unreliable because alcohol is undetectable within a few hours after ingestion. Abnormal liver function studies can provide diagnostic data about the physical effects of alcohol abuse.

Urine toxicology testing is often performed to screen for illicit drug use. Drugs may be found in urine days to weeks after ingestion, depending on how quickly they are metabolized and excreted from the body. Meconium (from the neonate) and hair can also be analyzed to determine past drug use over a longer period of time. In addition to screening for alcohol and drug abuse, the nurse should also screen for physical and sexual abuse and history of psychiatric illness because these are risk factors in women who abuse substances.

Initial and serial ultrasound studies are usually performed to determine gestational age because the woman may have had

BOX 13-7 T-ACE Test

- How many drinks can you hold before getting sleepy or passing out? (TOLERANCE)
- Have people ANNOYED you by criticizing your drinking?
- Have you ever thought that you ought to CUT DOWN on your drinking?
- Have you ever had a drink first thing in the morning to steady your nerves or get rid of a hangover? (EYE-OPENER)

Scoring: Two points are given for the TOLERANCE question for the ability to hold at least a six-pack of beer or a bottle of wine. A "yes" answer to any of the other questions receives one point. An overall score of 2 or more indicates a high probability that the woman is a risk drinker.

From Hankin JR, Sokol RJ: Identification and care of problems associated with alcohol ingestion in pregnancy, *Semin Perinatol* 19(4):286-292, 1995.

amenorrhea as a result of her drug use or may not know when her last menstrual period occurred. Because of concerns about stillbirth, an increased frequency of the birth of SGA infants, and the potential for hypoxia, some experts recommend that nonstress testing be done in women who are known substance abusers.

Planning the care for a pregnant woman who is a substance abuser must take into consideration the woman's lifestyle and habits. Although the ideal long-term outcome is total abstinence, it is not likely that the woman will either desire or be able to stop alcohol and drug use suddenly. Indeed, it may be harmful to the fetus for her to do so. A realistic goal may be to decrease substance use, and short-term outcomes will be necessary.

An interdisciplinary model is essential when planning the care for women who abuse substances. Major issues that must be addressed in treatment for women that generally are not part of treatment for men are low self-esteem, stigmatization, high probability of sexual abuse and physical abuse, lack of social support, need for social services and child care, need for women's health services, and need for support and education in the mothering role. Drug-free public housing or residential communities may offer an ideal route to stabilization in a safe environment. Treatment must demonstrate cultural sensitivity and responsiveness to recognize ethnicity and culture as an important part of her identity. Other needs of many women include relationship counseling, coping skills training, and vocational and legal assistance (Jos, Perlmutter, & Marshall, 2003).

Intervention with the pregnant substance abuser begins with education about specific effects on pregnancy, the fetus, and the newborn for each drug used. Consequences of perinatal drug use should be clearly communicated, and abstinence recommended as the safest course of action. Women are often more receptive to making lifestyle changes during pregnancy than at any other time in their lives. The casual, experimental, or recreational drug user is often able to achieve and maintain sobriety when she receives education, support, and continued monitoring throughout pregnancy. Periodic screening during pregnancy of women who have admitted to drug use may help them continue abstinence. Pregnancy presents a window of opportunity for motivating women to stop their abuse of substances.

Treatment for substance abuse will be individualized for each woman, depending on the type of drug used and the frequency and amount of use. Detoxification, short-term inpatient or outpatient treatment, long-term residential treatment, aftercare services, and self-help support groups are all possible options. Neonatal outcomes are improved among infants whose mothers received an integration of substance abuse treatment with prenatal care.

Women for Sobriety may be a more helpful organization for women than Alcoholics Anonymous or Narcotics Anonymous, which are based on the 12-step program. The emphasis on powerlessness over addiction and avoidance of codependency found in 12-step programs may disempower and isolate women, particularly women of color. The confrontational techniques of the 12-step program, developed to break down denial in men, may be especially threatening to women, who often feel unworthy and full of shame and guilt.

In general, long-term treatment of any sort is becoming increasingly more difficult to obtain, particularly for women who lack insurance coverage. Although some programs allow a woman to keep her child with her at the treatment facility, far too few are available to meet the demand.

Methadone maintenance treatment for pregnant women dependent on opiates is the current standard (Wisner et al, 2007). Methadone therapy, along with behavioral counseling, has been shown to decrease the use of opiates and other drugs, reduce criminal activity, improve birth weight and decrease the rates of preeclampsia and HIV. Disadvantages of methadone therapy include fetal heart rate changes (e.g., fewer accelerations, decreased rate and variability), a decrease in fetal breathing episodes, and neonatal abstinence syndrome (Wisner et al, 2007).

Cocaine use during pregnancy has increased dramatically in the last few years. A number of maternal and fetal complications accompany cocaine use, including placental abruption and stillbirth, prematurity, and SGA infants. When it is determined that a pregnant woman is using cocaine, she should be advised to stop using immediately. She will need a great deal of assistance such as an alcohol and drug treatment program, individual or group counseling, and participation in self-help support groups to successfully accomplish this major lifestyle change.

Because of the lifestyle often associated with drug use, substance-abusing women are at risk for STIs, including HIV. Laboratory assessments will likely include screening for STIs such as gonorrhea and chlamydial infection and antibody determinations for hepatitis B and HIV. A chest x-ray film may be taken to assess for pulmonary problems such as hilar lymphadenopathy, pulmonary edema, bacterial pneumonia, and foreign-body emboli. A skin test to screen for tuberculosis may also be ordered.

Although substance abusers may be difficult to care for at any time, they are often particularly challenging during the intrapartum and postpartum periods because of manipulative and demanding behavior. Typically these women display poor control over their behavior and a low threshold for pain.

BOX 13-8 Dealing with Pregnant Substance Abusers

- Realize that the decision to become and remain sober can *only* be made by the substance abuser.
- Understand that nurses do not have the power to cure anyone. They are only cheerleaders and supporters!
- Educate yourself about the effects of drug use in general and its effect on pregnancy and the newborn specifically.
- Treat substance abusers with the same respect and consideration that you show other people.
- Become familiar with your local treatment centers. Learn which of them will accept pregnant women. Keep an up-to-date list of groups meeting in your community.
- Remember that there are no "hopeless cases." It is never too late to quit!
- Practice patience and persistence. It may take months or years to see the effects of your work.

Increased dependency needs and poor parenting skills may also be apparent.

Nurses must understand that substance abuse is an illness and that these women deserve to be treated with patience, kindness, consistency, and firmness when necessary (Box 13-8). Even women who are actively abusing drugs experience pain during labor and after giving birth. Withholding analgesia or anesthesia in an attempt to "punish" them for prenatal substance abuse is not helpful and should be avoided. It is helpful to develop a standardized plan of care so that patients have limited opportunities to play staff members against each other. Mother-infant attachment should be promoted by identifying the woman's strengths and reinforcing positive maternal feelings and behaviors. Staffing should be sufficient to ensure strict surveillance of visitors and prevent unsupervised drug use.

Advice regarding breastfeeding must be individualized. Although all abuse substances appear in breast milk, some in greater amounts than others, breastfeeding is definitely contraindicated in women who continue to use amphetamines, alcohol, cocaine, heroin, or marijuana. The baby's nutrition and safety needs are of primary importance in this consideration. For some women a desire to breastfeed may provide strong motivation to achieve and maintain sobriety.

Before a known substance abuser is discharged with her baby, the home situation must be assessed to determine that the environment is safe and that someone will be available to meet the infant's needs if the mother proves unable to do so. Usually the social services department of the hospital will be involved in interviewing the mother before discharge to ensure that the infant's needs will be met. Sometimes family members or friends will be asked to become actively involved with the mother before discharge. A home care or public health nurse may be asked to make home visits to assess the mother's ability to care for the baby and provide guidance and support. If serious questions about the infant's well-being exist, the case can be referred to the state's child protective services agency for further action.

Key Points

- Careful monitoring of blood glucose levels, insulin administration when necessary, and dietary counseling are used to create a normal intrauterine environment for fetal growth and development in the pregnancy complicated by diabetes mellitus.
- Poor maternal glycemic control before conception and in the first trimester of pregnancy may be responsible for fetal congenital malformations and maternal complications such as miscarriage, infection, preeclampsia, and dystocia (difficult labor) caused by macrosomia.
- Maternal insulin requirements increase as the pregnancy progresses and may quadruple by term as a result of insulin resistance created by placental hormones, insulinase, and cortisol.
- Thyroid dysfunction during pregnancy requires close monitoring of thyroid hormone levels to regulate therapy and prevent fetal insult.
- High levels of phenylalanine in the maternal bloodstream cross the placenta and are teratogenic to the fetus. Damage can be prevented or minimized by dietary restriction of phenylalanine.

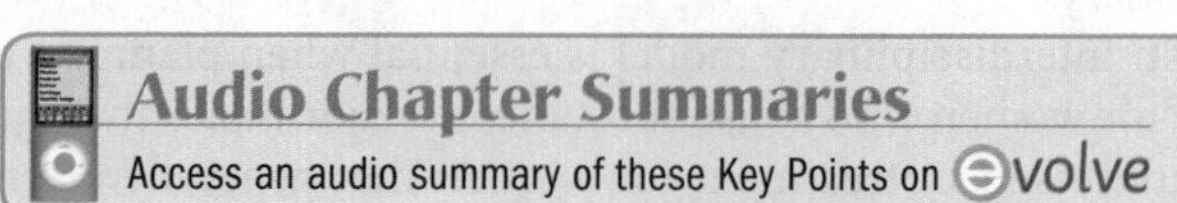
Audio Chapter Summaries
Access an audio summary of these Key Points on evolve

- The stress of the normal maternal adaptations to pregnancy on a heart whose functions are already taxed may cause cardiac decompensation.
- In the case of cardiac arrest in a pregnant woman, the ACLS guidelines should be implemented without modification.
- Anemia, the most common medical disorder of pregnancy, affects at least 20% of pregnant women.
- Women in their reproductive years show a predilection for autoimmune disorders (e.g., systemic lupus erythematosus and myasthenia gravis); therefore they may occur during pregnancy.
- Perinatal administration of HAART is recommended to decrease transmission of HIV from mother to fetus.
- Support from a variety of sources—including family and friends, health care providers, and the recovery community—is needed to help perinatal substance abusers achieve and maintain sobriety.

References

American College of Obstetricians and Gynecologists (ACOG): *Gestational diabetes, ACOG Practice Bulletin*, number 30, Washington, DC, 2001a, ACOG.

American College of Obstetricians and Gynecologists (ACOG), American College of Medical Genetics: *Preconception and prenatal carrier screening for cystic fibrosis: clinical and laboratory guidelines*, Washington, DC, 2001b, ACOG.

American College of Obstetricians and Gynecologists (ACOG): *Pregestational diabetes mellitus: ACOG Practice Bulletin*, No 60, Washington, DC, March 2005, ACOG.

American Diabetes Association: Position statement: diagnosis and classification of diabetes mellitus, *Diabetes Care* 31(suppl 1):S55-S60, 2008a.

American Diabetes Association: Standards of medical care in diabetes, *Diabetes Care* 31:S12-S54, 2008b.

American Heart Association: Part 8: Advanced challenges in resuscitation. Section 3: Special challenges in ECC. 3F: Cardiac arrest associated with pregnancy, *Resuscitation* 46:293-295, 2000.

American Heart Association: Guidelines for cardiopulmonary resuscitation and emergency cardiovascular care. Part 10.8. Cardiac arrest associated with pregnancy, *Circulation* 112:IV-150–IV-153, 2005.

Aminoff MJ: Neurologic disorders. In Creasy RK et al (editors): *Creasy & Resnik's maternal-fetal medicine: principles and practice*, ed 6, Philadelphia, 2009, Saunders.

Arafeh JM, Baird SM: Cardiac disease in pregnancy, *Crit Care Nurs Q* 29(1):32-52, 2006.

Bernstein H: Maternal and perinatal infection—viral: In Gabbe SG, Niebyl JR, Simpson JL (editors): *Obstetrics: normal and problem pregnancies*, ed 5, New York, 2007, Churchill Livingstone.

Blanchard DG, Shabetai R: Cardiac diseases. In Creasy RK et al (editors): *Creasy & Resnik's maternal-fetal medicine: principles and practice*, ed 6, Philadelphia, 2009, Saunders.

Burton J, Reyes J: Breathe in, breathe out, controlling asthma during pregnancy, *AWHONN Lifelines* 5(1):24-30, 2001.

Centers for Disease Control and Prevention: Recommendations to prevent and control iron deficiency in the United States, *MMWR Recomm Rep* 47(RR-3):1-29, 1998.

Centers for Disease Control and Prevention: *National diabetes fact sheet*, 2007a. Available at www.cdc.gov/diabetes/pubs/pdf/ndfs_2007.pdf (accessed March 22, 2009).

Centers for Disease Control and Prevention: Reducing HIV transmission from mother to child: an opt-out approach to HIV screening, 2007b. Available at www.cdc.gov/hiv/topics/perinatal/resources/factsheets/pdf/opt-out.pdf (accessed March 22, 2009).

Cooper DS et al: The thyroid gland. In Gardner DG, Shoback D (editors): *Greenspan's basic & clinical endocrinology*, ed 8, New York, 2007, McGraw-Hill.

Criteria Committee of the New York Heart Association: *Nomenclature and criteria for diagnosis of diseases of the heart and great vessels*, ed 9, Boston, 1994, Little, Brown.

Cunningham FG et al: *Williams obstetrics*, ed 22, New York, 2005, McGraw-Hill.

Easterling TR, Stout K: Heart disease. In Gabbe SG, Niebyl JR, Simpson JL (editors): *Obstetrics: normal and problem pregnancies*, ed 5, New York, 2007, Churchill Livingstone.

Expert Committee on the Diagnosis and Classification of Diabetes Mellitus: Report of the Expert Committee, *Diabetes Care* 26(suppl 1):S5-S20, 2003.

Gabbe SA, Carpenter LB, Garrison EA: New strategies for glucose control in patients with type 1 and type 2 diabetes mellitus in pregnancy, *Clin Obst Gynecol* 50(4):1014-1024, 2007.

Gei AF, Hankins GD: Cardiac disease and pregnancy, *Obstet Gynecol Clin North Am* 28(3):465-512, 2001.

Gilbert ES: *Manual of high risk pregnancy and delivery*, ed 4, St Louis, 2007, Mosby.

Grewal M, Biswas MK, Perloff D: Cardiac, hematologic, pulmonary, renal and urinary tract disorders in pregnancy. In DeCherney AH, Nathan L: *Current obstetric and gynecologic diagnosis and treatment*, ed 9, New York, 2003, Lange Medical Books/McGraw-Hill.

Hankin JR, Sokol RJ: Identification and care of problems associated with alcohol ingestion in pregnancy, *Semin Perinatol* 19(4):286-292, 1995.

Harris LH, Paltrow L: The status of pregnant women and fetuses in US criminal law, *JAMA* 289(13):1697-1699, 2003.

Holmgren C, Branch DW: Collagen vascular diseases. In Gabbe SG, Niebyl JR, Simpson JL (editors): *Obstetrics: normal and problem pregnancies*, ed 5, New York, 2007, Churchill Livingstone.

Jos PH, Perlmutter M, Marshall MF: Substance abuse during pregnancy: clinical and public health approaches, *J Law Med Ethics* 31(3):340-350, 2003.

Kilpatrick SJ: Anemia and pregnancy. In Creasy RK et al (editors): *Creasy & Resnik's maternal-fetal medicine: principles and practice*, ed 6, Philadelphia, 2009, Saunders.

Landon MB, Catalano PM, Gabbe SG: Diabetes mellitus. In Gabbe SG, Niebyl JR, Simpson JL (editors): *Obstetrics: normal and problem pregnancies*, ed 5, New York, 2007, Churchill Livingstone.

Langer O et al: A comparison of glyburide and insulin in women with gestational diabetes mellitus, *N Engl J Med* 343(16):1134-1138, 2000.

Lawrence RA, Lawrence RM: *Breastfeeding: a guide for the medical profession*, ed 6, St Louis, 2005, Mosby.

Maloni JA, Brezinski-Tomasi JE, Johnson LA: Antepartum bed rest: effect upon the family, *J Obstet Gynecol Neonatal Nurs* 30(2):67-77, 2001.

Mayo Clinic Staff: *Phenylketonuria*, December 20, 2007. Available at www.mayoclinic.com/invoke.cfm?id=DS00514&dsection=1 (accessed March 22, 2009).

Mestman JH: Endocrine diseases in pregnancy. In Gabbe SG, Niebyl JR, Simpson JL (editors): *Obstetrics: normal and problem pregnancies*, ed 5, New York, 2007, Churchill Livingstone.

Moore TR, Catalano P: Diabetes in pregnancy. In Creasy RK et al (editors): *Creasy & Resnik's maternal-fetal medicine: principles and practice*, ed 6, Philadelphia, 2009, Saunders.

Nader S: Thyroid disease and pregnancy. In Creasy RK et al (editors): *Creasy & Resnik's maternal-fetal medicine: principles and practice*, ed 6, Philadelphia, 2009, Saunders.

NAEPP expert panel report managing asthma during pregnancy: Recommendations for pharmacologic treatment—2004 update. NHLBI, NIH Publication No 05-3279. Available at www.nhlbi.nih.gov.proxy.library.vanderbilt.edu/health/prof/lung/asthma/astpreg.htm (accessed March 22, 2009).

Papoutsis J, Kroumpouzos G: Dermatologic disorders. In Gabbe SG, Niebyl JR, Simpson JL (editors): *Obstetrics: normal and problem pregnancies*, ed 5, New York, 2007, Churchill Livingstone.

Ramsey PS, Ramin KD, Ramin SM: Cardiac disease in pregnancy, *Am J Perinatol* 18(5):245-266, 2001.

Reece EA, Homko CJ: Prepregnancy care and the prevention of fetal malformations in the pregnancy complicated by diabetes, *Clin Obstet Gynecol* 50(4):990-997, 2007.

Samuels P, Niebyl JR: Neurologic disorders. In Gabbe SG, Niebyl JR, Simpson JL (editors): *Obstetrics: normal and problem pregnancies*, ed 5, New York, 2007, Churchill Livingstone.

Slack C et al: Prenatal genetics: The evolution and future directions of screening and diagnosis, *J Perinat Neonatal Nurs* 20(1):93-97, 2006.

Whitty JE, Dombrowski MP: Respiratory diseases in pregnancy. In Creasy RK et al (editors): *Creasy & Resnik's maternal-fetal medicine: principles and practice*, ed 6, Philadelphia, 2009, Saunders.

Williamson C, Mackillop L: Diseases of the liver, biliary system, and pancreas. In Creasy RK et al (editors): *Creasy & Resnik's maternal-fetal medicine: principles and practice*, ed 6, Philadelphia, 2009, Saunders.

Wisner KL et al: Psychiatric disorders. In Gabbe SG, Niebyl JR, Simpson JL (editors): *Obstetrics: normal and problem pregnancies*, ed 5, New York, 2007, Churchill Livingstone.

Unit 3

14 Pregnancy at Risk: Gestational Conditions

Learning Objectives

On completion of this chapter the reader will be able to:

- Differentiate among gestational hypertension, preeclampsia/eclampsia, and chronic hypertension.
- Describe the etiologic theories and pathophysiology of preeclampsia.
- Compare care management of women with mild preeclampsia vs. care management of women with severe preeclampsia.
- Describe HELLP syndrome, including appropriate nursing actions.
- Explain the effects of hyperemesis gravidarum on maternal and fetal well-being.
- Differentiate among causes, signs and symptoms, possible complications, and management of miscarriage, ectopic pregnancy, cervical insufficiency, and hydatidiform mole.
- Compare and contrast placenta previa and abruptio placentae in relation to signs and symptoms, complications, and management.
- Discuss the diagnosis and management of disseminated intravascular coagulation.
- Explain the basic principles of care for a pregnant woman undergoing abdominal surgery.
- Discuss implications of trauma on mother and fetus during pregnancy.
- Identify priorities in assessment and stabilization measures for the pregnant trauma victim.

Electronic Resources

Additional information related to the content in Chapter 14 can be found on

evolve the Companion Website at

http://evolve.elsevier.com/Perry/maternal/

- NCLEX Review Questions
- Case Study—Preeclampsia
- Critical Thinking Exercise—Preeclampsia
- Nursing Care Plan—Hyperemesis Gravidarum
- Nursing Care Plan—Mild Preeclampsia: Home Care
- Nursing Care Plan—Placenta Previa
- Nursing Care Plan—Severe Preeclampsia: Hospital Care
- Spanish Guidelines—Assessment of Bleeding in Early Pregnancy

Providing safe and effective care for the high risk patient requires a joint effort from all members of the health care team, with each member contributing unique skills and talents to provide optimum outcomes for mother and infant. This chapter discusses a wide range of disorders that did not exist before pregnancy, all of which have at least one thing in common: their occurrence in pregnancy puts the woman and fetus at risk. Hypertension in pregnancy, hyperemesis gravidarum, hemorrhagic complications of early and late pregnancy, surgery during pregnancy, and trauma are discussed.

Hypertension in Pregnancy

Significance and Incidence

Hypertensive disorders complicate 6% to 8% of all pregnancies and are the most common medical complications of pregnancy (Martin et al, 2005). The rate of pregnancy-related hypertension has risen steadily, by approximately 30% to 40%, since 1990 for all ages, races, and ethnic groups to the current rate of 39.9 per 1000 live births, the highest since the data were first reported (Martin et al, 2007). Rates for chronic hypertension have increased (10.4 per 1000 live births), whereas the rate for eclampsia has declined (4 per 1000 live births) (Martin et al, 2007). Age distribution remains U shaped, with women younger than age 20 and older than age 40 having the highest rates of occurrence for pregnancy-related hypertension. However, rates of chronic hypertension in mothers ages 40 and older are eight times higher than for those under age 20 (29.2 compared to 3.7 per 1000 live births). Maternal race also influences the rate of pregnancy-associated hypertension, with the highest rates seen in non-Hispanic black women and non-Hispanic white women. Hispanic women have an intermediate rate (Martin et al, 2007).

Morbidity and Mortality

"Preeclampsia is the second leading cause of maternal morbidity and mortality in the U.S." (Hawfield & Freedman, 2009). Maternal complications of preeclampsia include renal and liver failure, HELLP syndrome, and cerebral edema with seizures (Mutter & Karumanchi, 2008). Maternal deaths that are associated with preeclampsia primarily result from complications of hepatic rupture, abruptio placentae, and eclampsia (Roberts & Funai, 2009).

Preeclampsia usually occurs after the second trimester of pregnancy (earlier with hydatidiform mole and hydrops) and contributes to intrauterine fetal death and perinatal mortality. Causes of perinatal death related to preeclampsia are uteroplacental insufficiency and abruptio placentae, which lead to intrauterine death, preterm birth, and low birth weight.

Eclampsia (characterized by seizures) from profound cerebral effects of preeclampsia is the major maternal risk. As a rule, maternal and perinatal morbidity and mortality rates are highest when eclampsia is seen early in gestation (before 28 weeks), maternal age is greater than 25 years, the woman is a multigravida, and chronic hypertension or renal disease is present (Sibai, 2007). The fetus of the eclamptic woman is at increased risk from abruptio placentae, preterm birth, intrauterine growth restriction, and acute hypoxia.

Classification

The classification system most commonly used in the United States is based on reports from the American College of Obstetricians and Gynecologists (ACOG) (2002b) and the National High Blood Pressure Education Program (NHBPEP) Working Group on High Blood Pressure in Pregnancy (2000). This classification system is summarized in Table 14-1.

Gestational Hypertension

Gestational hypertension is the onset of hypertension during pregnancy or in the first 24 hours after birth without other signs or symptoms of preeclampsia and without preexisting hypertension. The blood pressure (BP) returns to normal within 6 weeks of birth (Sibai, 2007). *Gestational hypertension* is a nonspecific term that replaces the term *pregnancy-induced hypertension.* Gestational hypertension is a provisional diagnosis that includes women with preeclampsia who do not yet have proteinuria and women who do not have preeclampsia (Roberts & Funai, 2009).

Preeclampsia

Preeclampsia is a pregnancy-specific syndrome in which hypertension develops after 20 weeks of gestation in a previously normotensive woman. It is a multisystem, vasospastic disease process of reduced organ perfusion characterized by the presence of hypertension and proteinuria with a clinical continuum from mild to severe (Table 14-2). With mild preeclampsia, hypertension (systolic BP below 160 mm Hg and diastolic BP below 110 mm Hg) and proteinuria are present, and there is no evidence of organ dysfunction (Roberts & Funai, 2009; Sibai, 2007).

Hypertension, whether gestational or chronic, is defined as a systolic BP greater than 140 mm Hg, a diastolic BP greater than 90 mm Hg, or a mean arterial pressure greater than 105 mm Hg recorded on two separate occasions at least 4 hours apart (Sibai, 2007). Elevations over prepregnancy values are no longer considered diagnostic for preeclampsia. However, women who demonstrate an increase in BP of 30 mm Hg systolic or 15 mm Hg diastolic warrant close observation if the BP elevation occurs with proteinuria and hyperuricemia (uric acid of 6 mg/dl or more) (ACOG, 2002b; Roberts & Funai, 2009). Uric acid levels may be higher than 6 mg/dl in normotensive women with multifetal gestation; thus it is not diagnostic for preeclampsia (Sibai, 2007).

Proteinuria is defined as a concentration of 30 mg/dl or more in at least two random urine specimens collected at least 6 hours apart with no evidence of urinary tract infection. In a 24-hour specimen, proteinuria is defined as a concentration of 300 mg/L or greater per 24 hours (Box 14-1). The diagnosis of proteinuria should be based on a 24-hour urine collection or a timed collection corrected for creatinine excretion if a

Evolve Critical Thinking Exercise—Preeclampsia

Table 14-1 Classification of Hypertensive States of Pregnancy

TYPE	DESCRIPTION
Gestational hypertension	Blood pressure elevation detected first time after midpregnancy without proteinuria (previously known as pregnancy-induced hypertension)
Transient hypertension	Gestational hypertension with no signs of preeclampsia present at the time of birth and hypertension resolves by 12 weeks after birth; this is a retrospective diagnosis
Preeclampsia	Pregnancy-specific syndrome that usually occurs after 20 weeks of gestation and is determined by gestational hypertension plus proteinuria
Eclampsia	The occurrence of seizures in a woman with preeclampsia that cannot be attributed to other causes
Chronic hypertension	Hypertension that is present and observable before pregnancy or that is diagnosed before week 20 of gestation
Preeclampsia superimposed on chronic hypertension	Chronic hypertension with new proteinuria or an exacerbation of hypertension (previously well controlled) or proteinuria, thrombocytopenia, or increases in hepatocellular enzymes

Adapted from American College of Obstetricians and Gynecologists: *Diagnosis and management of preeclampsia and eclampsia: ACOG Practice Bulletin number 33,* Washington, DC, 2002b, ACOG; Blackburn ST: *Maternal, fetal, and neonatal physiology: a clinical perspective,* ed 3, St Louis, 2007, Saunders; National High Blood Pressure Education Program: *Working group report on high blood pressure in pregnancy:* NIH Pub No 00-3029, Bethesda, Md, 2000, National Institutes of Health, National Heart, Lung, and Blood Institute.

Table 14-2 Differentiation Between Mild and Severe Preeclampsia

	MILD PREECLAMPSIA	SEVERE PREECLAMPSIA
Maternal Effects		
Blood pressure (BP)	BP reading of 140/90 mm Hg ×2, >4-6 hr apart, no more than 1 wk apart	Rise to ≥160/110 mm Hg on two separate occasions
Mean arterial pressure	>105 mm Hg	>105 mm Hg
Proteinuria		
Quantitative 24-hr analysis	Proteinuria of >0.3 g in a 24-hr specimen	Proteinuria of >2 g in 24 hr
Qualitative dipstick	≥30 mg/dl on dipstick	2+ to 3+ protein on dipstick
Reflexes	May be normal	Hyperreflexia >3+, possible ankle clonus
Urine output	Output matching intake, ≥30 ml/hr or <650 ml/24 hr	20 ml/hr or <400 ml-500 ml/24 hr
Headache	Absent/transient	Severe
Visual problems	Absent	Blurred, photophobia, blind spots on funduscopy
Irritability/changes in affect	Transient	Severe
Epigastric pain	Absent	Present
Serum creatinine	Normal	Elevated
Thrombocytopenia	Absent	Present
AST elevation	Normal or minimal	Marked
Fetal Effects		
Placental perfusion	Reduced	Decreased perfusion expressing as IUGR in fetus; FHR: late decelerations
Premature placental aging	Not apparent	At birth placenta appearing smaller than normal for duration of pregnancy; premature aging apparent with numerous areas of broken syncytia, ischemic necroses (white infarcts); numerous, intervillous fibrin deposition (red infarcts)

Sources: American College of Obstetricians and Gynecologists: *Diagnosis and management of preeclampsia and eclampsia, ACOG Practice Bulletin number 33,* Washington, DC, 2002b, American College of Obstetricians and Gynecologists; Report of the National High Blood Pressure Education Program Working Group on High Blood Pressure in Pregnancy: Summary report, *Am J Obstet Gynecol* 183(1):S1-S22, 2002.
AST, Aspartate aminotransferase; *FHR,* fetal heart rate; *IUGR,* intrauterine growth restriction.

BOX 14-1 Urine Protein Values

Protein readings are designated as follows:
- 0—Negative
- Trace—Trace
- +1—30 mg/dl
- +2—100 mg/dl
- +3—300 mg/dl
- +4—more than 1000 mg (1 g)/dl

24-hour specimen is not feasible (ACOG, 2002b; Roberts & Funai, 2009).

Severe Preeclampsia

Severe preeclampsia is the presence of a systolic BP of greater than 160 mm Hg or diastolic BP of at least 110 mm Hg and proteinuria of 5 g or more per 24-hour specimen (Sibai, 2007). Other signs and symptoms associated with severe preeclampsia include the following: oliguria, cerebral disturbances such as altered level of consciousness, confusion, or headache; visual disturbances such as scotomata or blurred vision; hepatic involvement, including epigastric pain, right upper quadrant pain, impaired liver function or elevated liver enzymes; thrombocytopenia with a platelet count less than 100,000/mm^3; hemolytic anemia; pulmonary edema; and fetal growth restriction (ACOG, 2002b; Roberts & Funai, 2009; Sibai, 2007).

Eclampsia

Eclampsia is the onset of seizure activity or coma in the woman diagnosed with preeclampsia, with no history of preexisting pathology that can result in seizure activity (Roberts & Funai, 2009; Sibai, 2007). The initial presentation of eclampsia varies, with one third of the women developing eclampsia during the pregnancy, one third during labor, and one third within 72 hours after giving birth (Emery, 2005).

Chronic Hypertension

Chronic hypertension is defined as hypertension present before the pregnancy or diagnosed before 20 weeks of gestation (Roberts & Funai, 2009). Most women experience uncomplicated pregnancies; however, there is an increased risk of poor fetal growth and fetal demise. Preconception counseling is recommended for women with chronic hypertension (ACOG, 2002b).

evolve Nursing Care Plan–Severe Preeclampsia: Hospital Care

Chronic Hypertension with Superimposed Preeclampsia

Approximately 25% of women with chronic hypertension develop preeclampsia or eclampsia. This disorder is associated with severe maternal and fetal complications. Chronic hypertension with superimposed preeclampsia is defined in the presence of the following findings:

- Hypertension before 20 weeks of gestation, with new-onset proteinuria
- Both hypertension and proteinuria before 20 weeks of gestation
- Sudden increase in proteinuria
- A sudden increase in BP in a woman whose hypertension has previously been well controlled
- Thrombocytopenia
- Elevated liver enzymes

Preeclampsia

Etiology

Preeclampsia is a condition unique to human pregnancy; signs and symptoms develop only during pregnancy and disappear soon after birth of the fetus and placenta. The ultimate cause remains unknown. Preeclampsia is seen more frequently in primigravidas. Age distribution remains U shaped, with women younger than 20 years and older than 40 years having the highest rates of occurrence. Certain risk factors are associated with development of the condition such as nulliparity, family history of preeclampsia, multiple gestation, obesity, and chronic medical disorders (Box 14-2) (Sibai, 2007). Some studies have shown an increased risk for preeclampsia in multiparous women with new partners for subsequent pregnancies (Sibai, 2007). There appears to be a paternal factor involved (i.e., men who fathered one pregnancy complicated by preeclampsia were nearly twice as likely to father a preeclamptic pregnancy in a different woman) (Sibai, 2007).

BOX 14-2 Risk Factors for Preeclampsia

Nulliparity
Family history of preeclampsia
Obesity
Multifetal gestation
Preeclampsia in previous pregnancy
Poor outcome in previous pregnancy
- Intrauterine growth restriction, abruptio placentae, fetal death

Preexisting medical or genetic conditions
- Chronic hypertension
- Renal disease
- Type 1 diabetes mellitus
- Thrombophilias
- Antiphospholipid antibody syndrome
- Proteins C and S, antithrombin deficiency
- Factor V Leiden

From Sibai BM: Hypertension. In Gabbe SF, Niebyl JR, Simpson JL: *Obstetrics: normal and problem pregnancies*, ed 5, Philadelphia, 2007, Churchill Livingstone.

The etiology of preeclampsia is theorized to include various possibilities: abnormal prostaglandin action, endothelial cell dysfunction, coagulation abnormalities, vasoconstrictor tone, and dietary deficiencies or excesses (Fig. 14-1). Immunologic factors and genetic disposition may also play an important role (Sibai, 2007). Animal studies have suggested that abnormalities of the placenta are the cause of preeclampsia. The trophoblast cells of the placenta usually alter the spiral arteries in the uterus to accommodate increased blood flow. Instead the vessels seen in preeclampsia are abnormally thick walled and muscular and have higher resistance. The condition also results in a distinctive lesion called acute atherosis, and there are increased numbers of placental infarcts. Placental perfusion is decreased, resulting in hypoxia; this causes several pathophysiologic abnormalities, especially endothelial damage. Thus many of the pathophysiologic changes of preeclampsia occur before clinical symptoms develop (Sibai, 2007).

Since the etiology of preeclampsia is unknown, various clinical trials have attempted to correct theoretic abnormalities present in preeclampsia as a means of preventing preeclampsia. Some methods used to prevent preeclampsia are listed in Box 14-3.

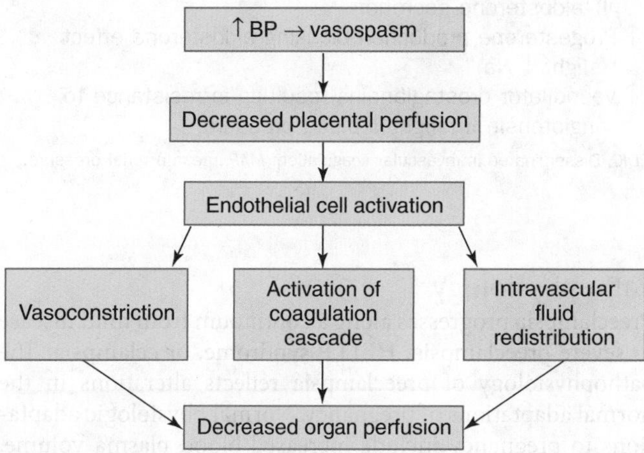

Fig. 14-1 Etiology of preeclampsia. *BP,* Blood pressure.

BOX 14-3 Methods Used to Prevent Preeclampsia

- High-protein and low-salt diet
- Nutrition supplementation (protein)
- Calcium
- Magnesium
- Zinc
- Fish and evening primrose oil
- Antihypertensive drugs, including diuretics
- Antithrombotic agents
- Low-dose aspirin
- Dipyridamole
- Heparin
- Vitamins E and C

From Sibai BM: Hypertension. In Gabbe SF, Niebyl JR, Simpson JL: *Obstetrics: normal and problem pregnancies*, ed 5, Philadelphia, 2007, Churchill Livingstone.

evolve Case Study—Preeclampsia

BOX 14-4 Normal Physiologic Adaptations to Pregnancy

Cardiovascular

↑ Blood volume; plasma volume expansion greater than red cell mass expansion, leading to physiologic anemia of pregnancy

↓ Total peripheral resistance, decreases in blood pressure readings, and MAP

↑ Cardiac output resulting from increased blood volume; slight increase in heart rate to compensate for peripheral relaxation

↑ Oxygen consumption

Physiologic edema related to ↓ plasma colloid osmotic pressure and ↑ venous capillary hydrostatic pressure

Hematologic

↑ Clotting factors, predisposing to DIC and clotting

↓ Serum albumin resulting in decreases in colloid osmotic pressure, predisposing to pulmonary edema

Renal

↑ Renal plasma flow and glomerular filtration rate

Endocrine

↑ Estrogen production resulting in ↑ renin–angiotensin II–aldosterone secretion

↑ Progesterone production blocking aldosterone effect (slight ↓ Na)

↑ Vasodilator prostaglandins resulting in resistance to angiotensin II (slight ↓ blood pressure)

DIC, Disseminated intravascular coagulation; *MAP*, mean arterial pressure.

COMMUNITY FOCUS

The Woman with Preeclampsia

Margie, a 25-year-old, G1 P0, single woman who is a school secretary, is seen in the clinic for her routine prenatal visit at 30 weeks of gestation. On examination you note that she has gained 8 lb since her last clinic visit 2 weeks ago, her blood pressure is 150/94, and on a urine dipstick she has 1+ proteinuria.

- What is the likely diagnosis for Margie? What other signs and symptoms of this condition might you find? Develop a nursing care plan for Margie. What teaching about diet, rest, signs and symptoms to observe, and fetal assessment should be included in the plan?
- Margie has no insurance. What community agencies or assistance is available to her? Develop a list of community resources for women in circumstances similar to Margie.

Pathophysiology

Preeclampsia progresses along a continuum from mild disease to severe preeclampsia, HELLP syndrome, or eclampsia. The pathophysiology of preeclampsia reflects alterations in the normal adaptations of pregnancy. Normal physiologic adaptations to pregnancy include increased blood plasma volume, vasodilation, decreased systemic vascular resistance, elevated cardiac output, and decreased colloid osmotic pressure (Box 14-4; see Community Focus box). The main pathogenic factor is not an increase in BP but poor perfusion as a result of vasospasm. Arteriolar vasospasm diminishes the diameter of blood vessels, which impedes blood flow to all organs and increases BP (Roberts et al & NHLBI Working Group on Research on Hypertension During Pregnancy, 2003; Roberts & Funai, 2009). Function in organs such as the placenta, kidneys, liver, and brain is depressed by as much as 40% to 60%. The pathophysiologic sequelae are shown in Fig. 14-2.

Preeclampsia contributes significantly to restrictions of fetal growth and incidence of placental abruption. Impaired placental perfusion leads to early degenerative aging of the placenta. The rate of fetal complications is directly related to the severity of the disease (Sibai, 2007).

HELLP Syndrome

HELLP syndrome is a laboratory diagnosis for a variant of severe preeclampsia that is characterized by hemolysis *(H),* elevated liver enzymes *(EL),* and low platelets *(LPs)* (ACOG, 2002b, Sibai, 2007). To have a diagnosis of HELLP syndrome, the platelet count must be less than 100,000/mm^3, and the liver enzyme levels (aspartate aminotransferase [AST] and alanine aminotransferase [ALT]) must be elevated. A unique form of coagulopathy (not DIC) occurs with HELLP syndrome. The platelet count is low, but coagulation factor assays, prothrombin time (PT), partial thromboplastin time (PTT), and bleeding time remain normal. In some instances hemolysis does not occur, and the condition is termed ELLP (Sibai, 2007; Sibai, Dekker, & Kupferminc, 2005).

HELLP syndrome appears in approximately 20% of women with severe preeclampsia (ACOG, 2002b; Emery, 2005). Most commonly HELLP syndrome is seen in older, Caucasian, multiparous women. About 90% of women report a history of malaise for several days. Many women (65%) experience epigastric or right upper quadrant abdominal pain (possibly related to hepatic ischemia), and approximately half develop nausea and vomiting. Many women with HELLP syndrome may not have signs and symptoms of severe preeclampsia; many are normotensive and have no proteinuria. As a result, women with HELLP syndrome are often misdiagnosed with a variety of other medical or surgical disorders (Sibai, 2007).

Recognition of the clinical and laboratory findings associated with HELLP syndrome is important if early, aggressive therapy is to be initiated to prevent maternal and neonatal death. Complications reported with HELLP syndrome include renal failure, pulmonary edema, ruptured liver hematoma, DIC, and abruptio placentae (Sibai, 2007).

Nursing Care Management

Hypertensive disorders of pregnancy can occur without warning or with the gradual development of symptoms (see Nursing Process box). The best prevention methods include early prenatal care for identification of women at risk and early detection of preeclampsia. The woman is assessed for risk factors at her first prenatal visit (see Box 14-2).

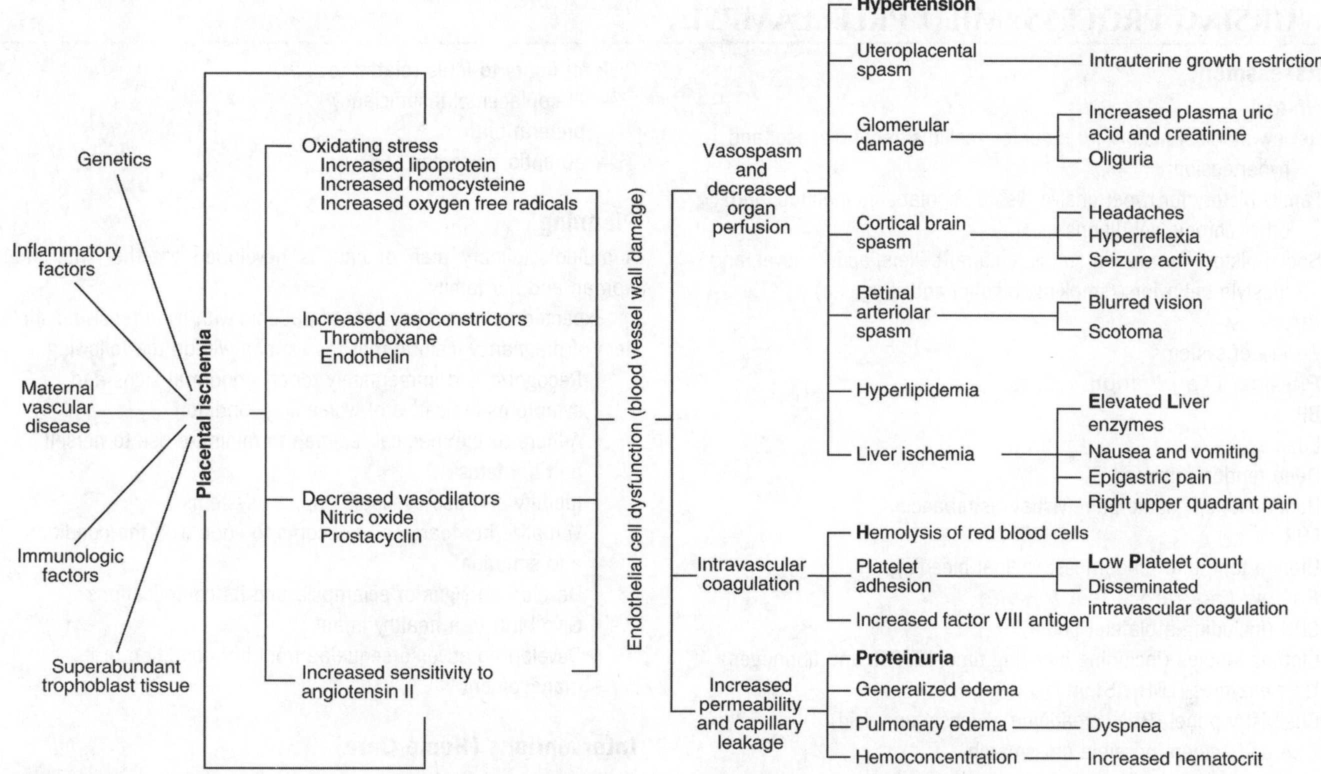

Fig. 14-2 Pathophysiology of preeclampsia. (Modified from Gilbert ES: *Manual of high risk pregnancy & delivery*, ed 4, St Louis, 2007, Mosby.)

BOX 14-5 Protocol for Blood Pressure Measurement

- Measure blood pressure in the same arm with the woman in the same position each time (e.g., seated or in a 30-degree tilt on her left side).
- After positioning, allow the woman 5 minutes of quiet rest before blood pressure measurement to encourage relaxation.
- If the woman is seated, her arm should be resting on a surface at the level of her heart.
- If the woman is in a lateral position, the lower arm should be positioned so the woman is not lying on the arm, and the blood pressure is then taken in the dependent arm. This more closely approximates the arterial pressure, whereas using the arm of the opposite side falsely reduces the measurement.
- Use the proper-size cuff (cuff should cover 80% of the upper arm).
- In women who have an upper arm too large for a standard-size cuff (cuff is too short), a more accurate measure is obtained by taking the blood pressure with the cuff placed on the forearm and recording Korotkoff phase V at the radial artery.
- Maintain a slow, steady deflation rate.
- Take the average of two readings 6 hours apart to minimize recorded blood pressure variations across time.
- Use Korotkoff phase V (disappearance of sound) for recording the diastolic value (some sources recommend recording both phase IV [the muffled sound] and phase V).
- Use accurate equipment.
- If interchanging manual and electronic devices, use caution in interpreting different blood pressure values.

Accurate and consistent BP assessment is important for establishing a baseline and monitoring subtle changes throughout the pregnancy. BP readings are affected by maternal position and measurement techniques. Consistency must be ensured. Normally the diastolic BP drops an average of 10 mm Hg below nonpregnant values by midgestation and then slowly reaches nonpregnant levels in the third trimester. Evaluation of BP focuses on trends, not on a single reading (ACOG, 2002b; Roberts & Funai, 2009). Box 14-5 presents recommendations for standardizing this procedure.

Observation of edema in addition to hypertension warrants additional investigation, although there is universal agreement that edema should not be considered in the diagnosis of preeclampsia (Sibai, 2007). Edema is assessed for distribution, degree, and pitting. It may be described as dependent or pitting.

Dependent edema is edema of the lowest or most dependent parts of the body where hydrostatic pressure is greatest. Many normotensive pregnant women have dependent edema. If a pregnant woman is ambulatory, this edema may first be

NURSING PROCESS: MILD PREECLAMPSIA

Assessment

History

Review medical history for diabetes mellitus, renal disease, and hypertension

Family history for hypertensive disorders, diabetes mellitus, and other chronic conditions

Social history for marital status, cultural beliefs, activity level, and lifestyle behaviors (smoking; alcohol and drug use)

Interview

Review of systems

Physical Examination

BP

Edema

Deep tendon reflexes

Headache, epigastric pain, visual disturbances

FHR

Uterine tone and tenderness; vaginal bleeding

Review Laboratory Test Results

CBC (including a platelet count)

Clotting studies (including bleeding time, PT, PTT, and fibrinogen)

Liver enzymes (LDH, AST, ALT)

Chemistry panel (BUN, creatinine, glucose, uric acid)

Type and screen, possible crossmatch

Nursing Diagnoses

Nursing diagnoses for the woman with hypertensive disorders in pregnancy include the following:

Anxiety related to
- preeclampsia and its effect on woman and infant

Ineffective individual/family coping related to
- the woman's restricted activity and concern over a complicated pregnancy
- the woman's inability to work outside the home
- the transfer of the woman to a tertiary center for more intensive management

Powerlessness related to
- inability to prevent or control condition and outcomes

Ineffective tissue perfusion related to
- hypertension
- cyclic vasospasms
- cerebral edema
- hemorrhage

Risk for injury to fetus related to
- uteroplacental insufficiency
- preterm birth
- abruptio placentae

Planning

A multidisciplinary plan of care is developed together with the woman and her family.

Expected outcomes for care of patients with hypertensive disorders of pregnancy include that the woman will do the following:

- Recognize and immediately report abnormal signs and symptoms indicative of worsening condition
- Adhere to the medical regimen to minimize risk to herself and her fetus
- Identify and use available support systems
- Verbalize her fears and concerns to cope with the condition and situation
- Develop no signs of eclampsia and its complications
- Give birth to a healthy infant
- Develop no adverse sequelae from her condition or its management

Interventions (Home Care)

Assess maternal-fetal unit two to three times/wk.

Evaluate fetal growth by ultrasound every 3 weeks.

Teach daily fetal movement counts.

Perform nonstress test one to two times/wk.

Recommend bed rest in lateral recumbent position.

Teach how to cope with bed rest.

Recommend diet as for normal pregnant women.

Review clinical signs to report.

Involve woman and family in plan of care.

Evaluate support systems.

Evaluation

Evaluation of the effectiveness of care of the woman with preeclampsia is based on the expected outcomes.

ALT, Alanine aminotransferase; *AST*, aspartate aminotransferase; *BP*, blood pressure; *BUN*, blood urea nitrogen; *CBC*, complete blood count; *FHR*, fetal heart rate; *LDH*, lactate dehydrogenase; *PT*, prothrombin time; *PTT*, partial thromboplastin time.

evident in the feet and ankles. If the woman is confined to bed, the edema is more likely to occur in the sacral region.

Pitting edema is edema that leaves a small depression or pit after finger pressure is applied to the swollen area (Fig. 14-3). The pit, caused by movement of fluid away from the point of pressure to adjacent tissues, normally disappears within 10 to 30 seconds. Although the amount of edema is difficult to quantify, the method shown in Fig. 14-4 may be used to record relative degrees of edema formation.

Although it is not a routine assessment during the prenatal period, evaluation of the fundus of the eye yields valuable data. An initial baseline finding of normal eye grounds assists in differentiating a preexisting from a new disease process.

Deep tendon reflexes (DTRs) are evaluated as a baseline and to detect any changes. The biceps and patellar reflexes and ankle clonus are assessed, and the findings recorded (Fig. 14-5 and Table 14-3). The evaluation of DTRs is especially important if the woman is being treated with magnesium sulfate. Absence of DTRs may be an indication of impending magnesium toxicity.

To elicit the biceps reflex a downward blow is struck over the thumb, which is placed over the biceps tendon. Normal response is flexion of the arm at the elbow, described as a 2+ response (see Fig. 14-5, *A*, and Table 14-3).

The patellar reflex is elicited with the woman's legs hanging freely over the end of the examining table or with the woman lying on her side with the knee slightly flexed. A blow with a percussion hammer is dealt directly to the patellar tendon, inferior to the patella. Normal response is the extension or kicking out of the leg, which is recorded as 2+ (see Fig. 14-5, *B*, and Table 14-3).

To assess for hyperactive reflexes (clonus) at the ankle joint, the examiner supports the leg with the knee flexed. With one hand the examiner sharply dorsiflexes the foot, maintains the position for a moment, and then releases the foot (see Fig. 14-5, *C*). Normal (negative clonus) response is elicited when no rhythmic oscillations (jerks) are felt while the foot is held

Table 14-3 Assessing Deep Tendon Reflexes

GRADE	DEEP TENDON REFLEX RESPONSE
0	No response
1+	Sluggish or diminished
2+	Active or expected response
3+	More brisk than expected; slightly hyperactive
4+	Brisk, hyperactive, with intermittent or transient clonus

From Seidel HM et al: *Mosby's guide to physical examination,* ed 6, St Louis, 2006, Mosby.

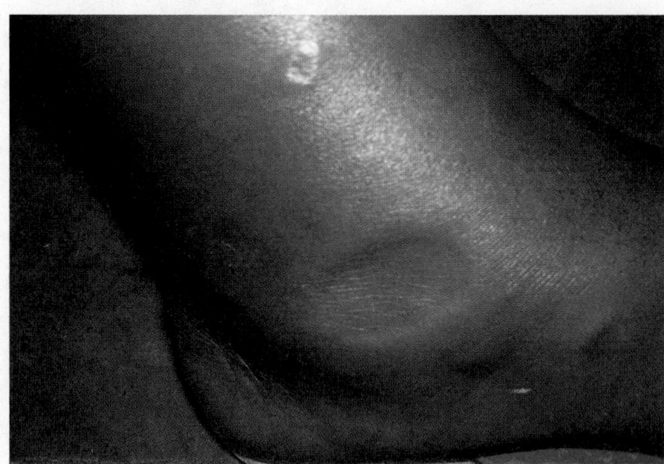

Fig. 14-3 Pitting edema. *(Courtesy Shannon Perry, Phoenix, AZ.)*

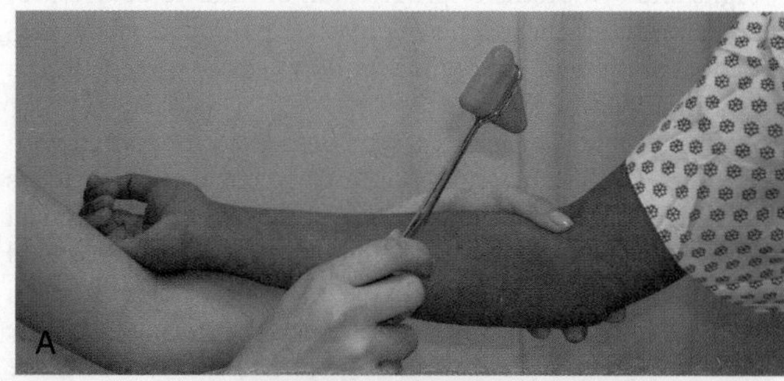

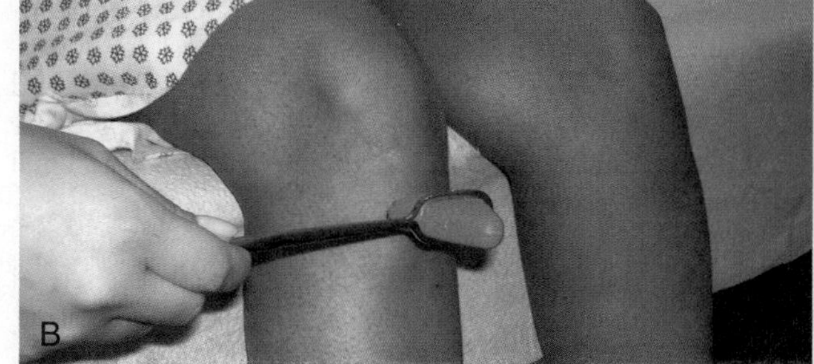

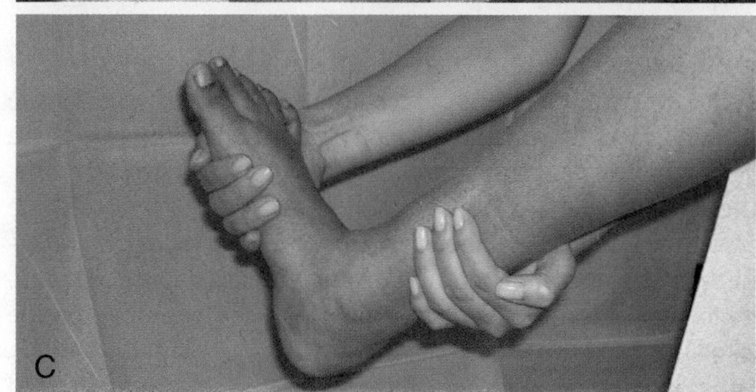

Fig. 14-5 Deep tendon reflexes. **A,** Biceps reflex. **B,** Patellar reflex with woman's legs hanging freely over end of examining table. **C,** Test for ankle clonus. *(Courtesy Shannon Perry, Phoenix, AZ.)*

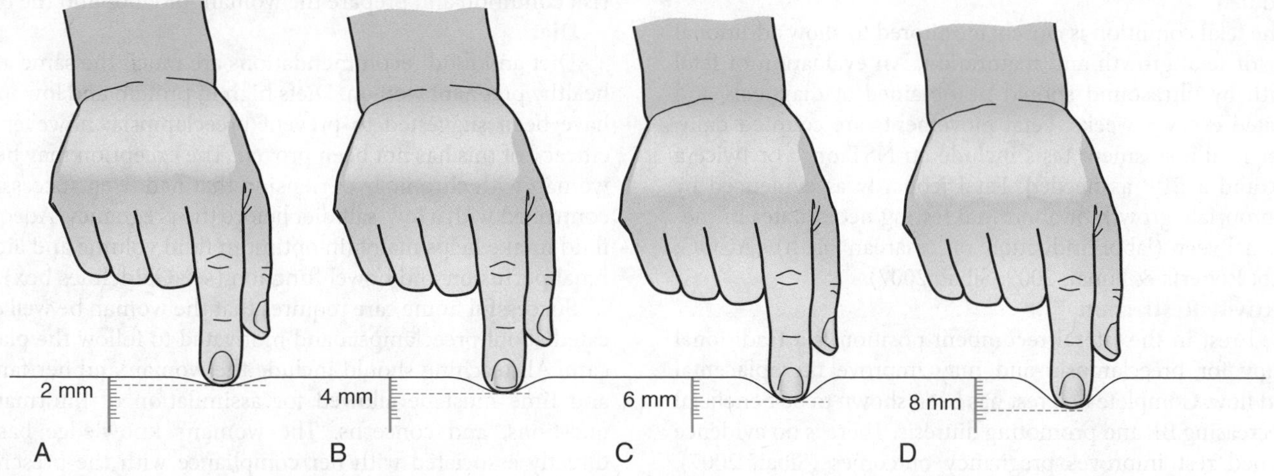

Fig. 14-4 Assessment of pitting edema. **A,** 1+; **B,** 2+; **C,** 3+; **D,** 4+.

in dorsiflexion. When the foot is released, no oscillations are seen as the foot drops to the plantar-flexed position. Abnormal (positive clonus) response is recognized by rhythmic oscillations of one or more beats felt when the foot is in dorsiflexion and seen as the foot drops to the plantar-flexed position.

Signs and symptoms of progression of mild-to-severe preeclampsia such as headaches, epigastric pain, and visual disturbances are noted. The signs of mild vs. severe preeclampsia are summarized in Table 14-2.

Uteroplacental perfusion can be decreased in women with preeclampsia. Biophysical monitoring such as nonstress testing (NST), contraction stress testing (CST), biophysical profile (BPP), and serial ultrasonography is used to assess fetal status. The fetal heart rate (FHR) is assessed for baseline rate, variability, and presence of accelerations. Abnormal baseline rate, decreased or absent variability, or late decelerations are indications of fetal intolerance to the intrauterine environment. Since the woman with preeclampsia is at risk for abruptio placentae, it is important to assess uterine tone and tenderness and the presence of vaginal bleeding. Doppler flow velocimetry studies can be used to evaluate uteroplacental perfusion (see Chapter 17).

NURSING ALERT Uterine tenderness in the presence of increasing tone may be the earliest finding of an abruption. Idiopathic preterm contractions also may be an early sign.

Mild Preeclampsia and Home Care

If the woman has mild preeclampsia (BP is stable, urine protein is less than 300 mg in a 24-hour collection, and there are no subjective complaints), she may be managed at home. The maternal-fetal condition should be assessed two to three times per week. Many agencies are able to provide this assessment in the home, depending on the woman's insurance coverage. If home nursing is not possible, the woman may be asked to perform self-assessment daily, including weight, urine dipstick, protein determinations, BP measurement, and fetal movement counting. She will be instructed to report immediately any subjective symptoms to her primary health care provider (see Home Care box) and to return to the high risk clinic or physician's office for all appointments as scheduled.

The fetal condition is closely monitored to allow additional time for fetal growth and maturation. An evaluation of fetal growth by ultrasound should be obtained at diagnosis and repeated every 3 weeks. Fetal movements are counted daily. Other fetal assessment tests include an NST once or twice a week and a BPP as needed. Fetal jeopardy as evidenced by inappropriate growth or abnormal testing necessitates immediate delivery (labor induction or cesarean birth) (ACOG, 2002b; Roberts & Funai, 2009; Sibai, 2007).

Activity Restriction

Bed rest in the lateral recumbent position is a traditional therapy for preeclampsia and may improve uteroplacental blood flow. Complete bed rest has been shown to be beneficial in decreasing BP and promoting diuresis. There is no evidence that bed rest improves pregnancy outcomes (Sibai, 2007). Adverse physiologic outcomes related to bed rest include cardiovascular deconditioning; diuresis with accompanying fluid, electrolyte, and weight loss; muscle atrophy; and psychologic stress. These changes begin on the first day of bed rest and continue for the duration of therapy. Thus modified bed rest with bathroom privileges may be ordered to help decrease negative effects (Maloni et al, 2004; Sibai, 2007).

Women with mild preeclampsia feel reasonably well; thus boredom from the restriction is common. Diversionary activities, visits from friends, telephone conversations, and creation of a comfortable and convenient environment are ways to cope with the boredom (see Home Care box on p. 343). Gentle exercise (e.g., range of motion, stretching, Kegel exercises, and pelvic tilts) is important in maintaining muscle tone, blood flow, regularity of bowel function, and a sense of well-being. Relaxation techniques can help reduce stress associated with the high risk condition and prepare the woman for labor and the birth.

Diet

Diet and fluid recommendations are much the same as for healthy pregnant women. Diets high in protein and low in salt have been suggested to prevent preeclampsia; however, the efficacy of this has not been proven. The exception may be the woman with chronic hypertension that had been successfully controlled with a low-salt diet before the pregnancy. Adequate fluid intake helps maintain optimum fluid volume and aids in renal perfusion and bowel function (see Guidelines box).

Successful home care requires that the woman be well educated about preeclampsia and motivated to follow the plan of care. All teaching should include the woman and her family; and time must be allowed for assimilation of information, questions, and concerns. The woman's knowledge base is directly associated with her compliance with the prescribed treatment program. Methods for enhancing learning include

HOME CARE

Assessing and Reporting Clinical Signs of Preeclampsia

Report immediately any increase in your blood pressure, protein in urine, weight gain, decreased fetal movement.*

Take your blood pressure on the same arm in a sitting position each time for consistent and accurate readings. Support arm on a table in a horizontal position at heart level.

Use the same scale, wearing the same clothes, at the same time each day, after voiding, and before breakfast for reliable daily weights.

Dipstick test your clean-catch urine sample to assess proteinuria; report frequency or burning on urination.

Assess your baby's activity daily. Decreased activity (three or fewer movements per hour) may indicate fetal compromise.

It is important to keep your scheduled prenatal appointments so that any changes in your or your baby's condition can be detected immediately.

Keep a daily log or diary of your assessments for your home health care nurse or bring it with you to your next prenatal visit.

*Thresholds for blood pressure, weight gain, fetal movement counts, and proteinuria are set by the physician or institutional protocol.

evolve Nursing Care Plan—Mild Preeclampsia: Home Care

HOME CARE

Coping with Bed Rest

In bed lie on your side. This allows more blood to get to your uterus (womb) and baby. The bed or sofa should be near a window and a bathroom.

Increase your fluid intake to eight glasses per day and add roughage (bran, fruits, leafy vegetables) to your diet to decrease constipation. Keep a bowl of fruit and a large container full of water close by.

Include diversionary activities such as puzzles, reading, and crafts to reduce boredom. Place a box or table within reach to store magazines, books, telephone, and other useful items.

Do gentle exercises such as circling your hands and feet or gently tensing and relaxing arm and leg muscles. This improves muscle tone, circulation, and sense of well-being.

Encourage family participation in your care.

Have significant others assist you with care of the house and children and any other duties.

Use relaxation to help cope with stress. Relax your body one muscle at a time or imagine some pleasant scene, word, or image. Soothing music can also help you relax.

GUIDELINES Nutrition

- Eat a nutritious, balanced diet (60 to 70 g protein; 1200 mg calcium; and adequate zinc, magnesium, and vitamins). Consult with registered dietitian on the diet best suited for you as an individual.
- There is no sodium restriction; however, consider limiting excessively salty foods (luncheon meats, pretzels, potato chips, pickles, sauerkraut).
- Eat foods with roughage (whole grains, raw fruits, and vegetables).
- Drink six to eight 8-oz glasses of water per day.
- Avoid alcohol and limit caffeine intake.

visual aids, videotapes, handouts, and demonstrations with return demonstrations. Furthermore the effects of illness, language, age, culture, beliefs, and support systems must be considered (see Nursing Care Plan).

Severe Preeclampsia or HELLP Syndrome

Hospital Care

The woman with severe preeclampsia or HELLP syndrome should receive appropriate management in a tertiary care center (see Nursing Care Plan). The woman may be admitted to an antepartum or a labor and birth unit, depending on the hospital. If the woman's condition is serious, she may be placed in an obstetric critical care unit or a medical intensive care unit for hemodynamic monitoring. If severe preeclampsia is diagnosed at less than 32 weeks, an initial observation period and conservative management may be attempted. With a gestational age of 32 to 36 weeks, labor is usually induced. Vaginal birth is considered safer than cesarean birth and should be attempted unless there are indications for a cesarean birth such as an unfavorable (uneffaced and undilated) cervix. In pregnancies of less than 34 weeks antenatal corticosteroids may be given to promote fetal lung maturation. If the birth can be delayed for 48 hours, steroids such as betamethasone (12 mg intramuscularly 24 hours apart) may be given to the woman (ACOG, 2002b; Cunningham et al, 2005; Sibai, Dekker, & Kupferminc, 2005).

Recognition of the clinical and laboratory findings of severe preeclampsia or HELLP syndrome is important to prevent maternal and perinatal mortality. The woman with severe preeclampsia or HELLP syndrome has multiple problems, and nursing care must focus on both the mother and fetus. Maternal and fetal surveillance, patient education regarding the disease process, and supportive measures directed toward the woman and her family are initiated. Assessments include review of the central nervous, cardiovascular, pulmonary, and renal systems. Weight is measured on admission and usually at the same time every day thereafter. Breath sounds are auscultated for crackles or diminished breath sounds, which may indicate pulmonary edema. An indwelling urinary catheter may be inserted to measure urinary output. Hemoglobin oxygen saturation can be assessed with a pulse oximeter. Baseline laboratory assessments include metabolic studies for liver enzyme (AST, ALT, lactate dehydrogenase [LDH]) determination, complete blood count (CBC) with platelets, coagulation profile to assess for DIC, and electrolyte studies to establish renal functioning (ACOG, 2002b; Roberts & Funai, 2009).

Weight should be measured on admission and every day thereafter. An indwelling urinary catheter facilitates monitoring of renal function and effectiveness of therapy; however, the risk of urinary tract infection should be considered in the stable antepartum woman. If appropriate, vaginal examination may be done to check for cervical changes. Abdominal palpation establishes uterine tonicity and fetal size, activity, and position. Assessments of fetal well-being (e.g., NST, BPP) are ordered because of the potential for hypoxia related to uteroplacental insufficiency. Electronic monitoring to determine fetal status is initiated at least once a day. The nurse's skill in implementing the techniques described here can be reassuring to the woman and her family. The woman's room should be close to staff and emergency drugs, supplies, and equipment. Seizure precautions are taken (Box 14-6). Because of the risk for thromboembolism for the woman on bed rest, she may wear TED (antiembolism) hose and SCD (intermittent compression device) boots while in bed.

Intrapartum nursing care of the woman with severe preeclampsia or HELLP syndrome involves continuous maternal and fetal assessments as labor progresses. Invasive hemodynamic monitoring with a pulmonary artery catheter (Swan-Ganz catheter) may be required for accurate intravascular fluid volume measurement in the presence of pulmonary edema or acute renal failure (ACOG, 2002b; Roberts & Funai, 2009).

Magnesium Sulfate

One of the important goals of care for the woman with preeclampsia is prevention or control of convulsions. Magnesium sulfate is the drug of choice in the prevention and treatment of convulsions caused by preeclampsia or eclampsia. It

NURSING CARE PLAN Mild Preeclampsia: Home Care

Nursing Diagnosis: Risk for injury related to signs of preeclampsia

Expected Outcomes

Patient will demonstrate ability to assess self and fetus for signs of worsening preeclampsia; no adverse sequelae will occur as result of preeclamptic condition.

Nursing Interventions/*Rationales*

Review warning signs/symptoms of preeclampsia *to ensure adequate knowledge base exists for decision making.*

Assess home environment, including woman's ability to assume self-management responsibilities, support systems, language, age, culture, beliefs, and effects of illness *to determine if home care is a viable option.*

Teach woman how to do a self-assessment for clinical signs of preeclampsia (take and record blood pressure, measure urine protein, maintain daily weight log, assess edema formation, assess fetal activity) *to provide immediate evidence of a worsening condition.*

Teach woman to report any increases in blood pressure, proteinuria of 2+ or more, weight gain, and decreased fetal activity to her health care provider immediately *to prevent worsening of preeclamptic condition.*

Teach woman about use of rest and relaxation as palliative treatment options *to decrease blood pressure and promote diuresis.*

Nursing Diagnosis: Fear/anxiety related to preeclampsia and its effect on the fetus

Expected Outcome

Patient's feelings and symptoms of fear/anxiety will decrease/ease.

Nursing Interventions/*Rationales*

Provide a calm, soothing atmosphere and teach family to provide emotional support *to facilitate coping.*

Encourage verbalization of fears *to decrease intensity of emotional response.*

Involve woman and family in the management of her preeclamptic condition *to promote a greater sense of control.*

Help woman identify and use appropriate coping strategies and support systems *to reduce fear/anxiety.*

Explore use of desensitization strategies such as progressive muscle relaxation, visual imagery, or thought stopping *to reduce fear-related emotions and related physical symptoms.*

Nursing Diagnosis: Deficient diversional activity related to imposed bed rest

Expected Outcome

Patient will verbalize diminished feelings of boredom.

Nursing Interventions/*Rationales*

Assist woman to creatively explore personally meaningful activities that can be pursued from the bed *to ensure activities that have meaning, purpose, and value to the individual.*

Maintain emphasis on personal choices of woman *to promote control and minimize imposition of routines by others.*

Evaluate what support and system resources are available in the environment *to assist in providing diversional activities.*

Explore ways for woman to remain an active participant in home management and decision making *to promote control.*

Engage support of family and friends in carrying out chosen activities and making necessary environmental alterations *to ensure success.*

Teach woman about stress-management and relaxation techniques *to help manage tension of confinement.*

BOX 14-6 Hospital Precautionary Measures

Environment
- Quiet
- Nonstimulating
- Lighting subdued

Seizure precautions
- Suction equipment tested and ready to use
- Oxygen administration equipment tested and ready to use

Call button within easy reach

Emergency medication tray immediately accessible
- Hydralazine or other antihypertensive medication and magnesium sulfate immediately available
- Calcium gluconate immediately available

Emergency birth pack accessible

is administered as a secondary infusion ("piggyback") to the main intravenous (IV) line by volumetric infusion pump. An initial loading dose of 4 to 6 g diluted in at least 100 ml of IV fluid per protocol or physician's order is infused over 15 to 30 minutes. This dose is followed by a maintenance dosage of magnesium sulfate diluted in an IV solution per physician's order (e.g., 40 g of magnesium sulfate in 1000 ml of lactated Ringer's solution) and administered by infusion pump at 2 g/hr (Gilbert, 2007). This dosage should maintain a therapeutic serum magnesium level of 4 to 7.5 mEq/L or 5 to 7 mg/dl (Gilbert, 2007). No data exist to support the routine drawing of serial serum magnesium levels, although levels are often checked daily (Gilbert, 2007). After the loading dose there may be a transient lowering of the arterial BP secondary to relaxation of smooth muscle.

NURSING ALERT The woman's BP, pulse, and respiratory status should be monitored closely while the loading dose is being administered intravenously and every 15 to 30 minutes at other times, depending on the stability of the woman's condition.

NURSING CARE PLAN Severe Preeclampsia: Hospital Care

Nursing Diagnosis: Risk for injury to mother and fetus related to CNS irritability

Expected Outcomes

Patient will show diminished signs of CNS irritability (e.g., DTRs 2+, absence of clonus) and have no convulsions.

Nursing Interventions/*Rationales*

Establish baseline data (e.g., DTRs, clonus) *to use as basis for evaluating effectiveness of treatment.*

Administer IV magnesium sulfate per physician's orders *to decrease hyperreflexia and minimize risk of convulsions.*

Monitor maternal vital signs, FHR, urine output, DTRs, IV flow rate, and serum levels of magnesium sulfate *to assess for and prevent magnesium sulfate toxicity* (e.g., depressed respirations, oliguria, sudden drop in blood pressure, hyporeflexia, fetal distress).

Have calcium gluconate available if needed *as antidote for magnesium sulfate toxicity.*

Maintain a quiet, darkened environment *to avoid stimuli that may precipitate seizure activity.*

Nursing Diagnosis: Ineffective tissue perfusion related to preeclampsia secondary to arteriolar vasospasm

Expected Outcome

Patient will exhibit signs of increased vasodilation (diuresis, decreased edema, weight loss).

Nursing Interventions/*Rationales*

Establish baseline data (weight, degree of edema) *to use as basis for evaluating effectiveness of treatment.*

Administer IV magnesium sulfate per physician order, *which serves to relax vasospasms and increase renal perfusion.*

Place woman on bed rest in a side-lying position *to maximize uteroplacental blood flow, reduce blood pressure, and promote diuresis.*

Monitor intake and output, edema, and weight *to assess for evidence of vasodilation and increased tissue perfusion.*

Nursing Diagnoses: Risk for excess fluid volume related to increased sodium retention secondary to administration of magnesium sulfate

Risk for impaired gas exchange related to pulmonary edema secondary to increased vascular resistance

Risk for decreased cardiac output related to use of antihypertensive drugs

Risk for injury to fetus related to uteroplacental insufficiency secondary to use of antihypertensive medications

Expected Outcomes

Patient will exhibit signs of normal fluid volume (balanced intake and output, normal serum creatinine levels, normal breath sounds), adequate oxygenation (normal respirations, fully oriented to person, time, and place), normal range of cardiac output (normal pulse rate and rhythm), and fetal well-being (adequate fetal movement, normal FHR).

Nursing Interventions/*Rationales*

Monitor woman for signs of third spacing of fluid volume (increased edema, decreased urine output, elevated serum creatinine level, weight gain, dyspnea, crackles) *to prevent complications.*

Monitor woman for signs of impaired gas exchange (increased respirations, dyspnea, altered blood gases, hypoxemia) *to prevent complications.*

Monitor woman for signs of decreased cardiac output (altered pulse rate and rhythm) *to prevent complications.*

Monitor fetus for signs of compromise (decreased fetal activity, abnormal EFM pattern) *to prevent complications.*

Record findings and report signs of increasing problems to physician *to enable timely interventions.*

CNS, Central nervous system; *DTRs*, deep tendon reflexes; *EFM*, electronic fetal monitoring; *FHR*, fetal heart rate; *IV*, intravenous.

Magnesium sulfate is rarely given intramuscularly because the absorption rate cannot be controlled, injections are painful, and tissue necrosis can occur. The intramuscular (IM) route may be used with some women who are being transported to a tertiary care center. The IM dose is 4 to 5 g given in each buttock, for a total of 10 g (1% procaine may be ordered to be added to the solution to reduce injection pain), and can be repeated at 4-hour intervals. Z-track technique should be used for the deep IM injection, followed by gentle massage at the site.

Magnesium sulfate interferes with the release of acetylcholine at the synapses, decreasing neuromuscular irritability, depressing cardiac conduction, and decreasing central nervous system (CNS) irritability. Because magnesium circulates free and unbound to protein and is excreted in the urine, accurate recordings of maternal urine output must be maintained.

Diuresis within 24 to 48 hours is an excellent prognostic sign. It is considered evidence that perfusion of the kidneys has improved as a result of relaxation of arteriolar spasm. With improved perfusion fluid moves from interstitial spaces to the intravascular bed, and edema is reduced. Diuresis results in weight loss. Although diuresis generally indicates improvement, in the presence of worsening clinical status it may indicate impending renal failure. As renal function declines and serum creatinine levels rise, renal filtration is compromised. The woman can excrete large volumes of urine (greater than 200 ml/hr) but does not excrete magnesium sulfate.

Because magnesium sulfate is a CNS depressant, the nurse assesses for signs and symptoms of magnesium toxicity. Serum magnesium levels are obtained on the basis of the woman's response and if any signs of toxicity are present. Early symptoms of toxicity include decreased DTRs, nausea, a feeling of warmth, flushing, muscle weakness, decreased reflexes, and slurred speech.

NURSING ALERT Loss of patellar reflexes, respiratory and muscular depression, oliguria, and decreased level of consciousness are signs of magnesium toxicity. If magnesium toxicity is suspected, the infusion should be discontinued immediately. Calcium gluconate, the antidote for magnesium sulfate, may also be ordered (10 ml of a 10% solution, or 1 g) and given by slow IV push (usually by the physician) over at least 3 minutes to avoid undesirable reactions such as dysrhythmias, bradycardia, and ventricular fibrillation.

Magnesium sulfate does not seem to affect FHR variability in a healthy term fetus. Neonatal serum magnesium levels approximate those of the mother. Doses of magnesium sulfate that prevent maternal seizures have been determined to be safe for the fetus. Toxic levels in the newborn can cause depressed respirations and hyporeflexia at birth. It is important that the neonatal team attend the birth to provide resuscitation measures as needed. In a 2-year follow-up study, magnesium administration was not found to result in an excess of disability or death in mothers (Magpie Trial Follow-Up Study Collaborative Group, 2007b). At the 18-month follow-up magnesium administration was not associated with a difference in disability or death in infants who had in utero exposure to magnesium sulfate when compared with infants who were exposed to a placebo (Magpie Trial Follow-Up Study Collaborative Group, 2007a).

NURSING ALERT Because magnesium sulfate is also a tocolytic agent, its use can increase the duration of labor. The labor of a woman with preeclampsia receiving magnesium sulfate may need augmentation with oxytocin. The amount of oxytocin needed to stimulate labor may be more than that needed for a woman who is not receiving magnesium sulfate.

Control of Blood Pressure

Antihypertensive medications may be ordered to lower the diastolic BP. Initiation of antihypertensive therapy reduces maternal morbidity and mortality rates associated with left ventricular failure and cerebral hemorrhage. Because a degree of maternal hypertension is necessary to maintain uteroplacental perfusion, antihypertensive therapy must not decrease the arterial pressure too much or too rapidly. Therefore the target range for the diastolic pressure is less than 110 mm Hg, and the systolic pressure less than 160 mm Hg (ACOG, 2002b; Cunningham et al, 2005).

IV hydralazine remains the antihypertensive agent of choice for the treatment of hypertension. Labetalol hydrochloride, nifedipine, verapamil, and oral methyldopa are also used (ACOG, 2002b; Chan & Winkle, 2006; Cunningham et al, 2005; Roberts & Funai, 2009; Sibai, 2007). The choice of agent used depends on the woman's response and physician preference. Table 14-4 compares antihypertensive agents used to treat hypertension in pregnancy.

NURSING ALERT When administering antihypertensive therapy, the nurse must remember that the drug effects depend on intravascular volume. Because preeclampsia is associated with contracted intravascular volume, initial doses should be given with caution, and maternal response monitored closely.

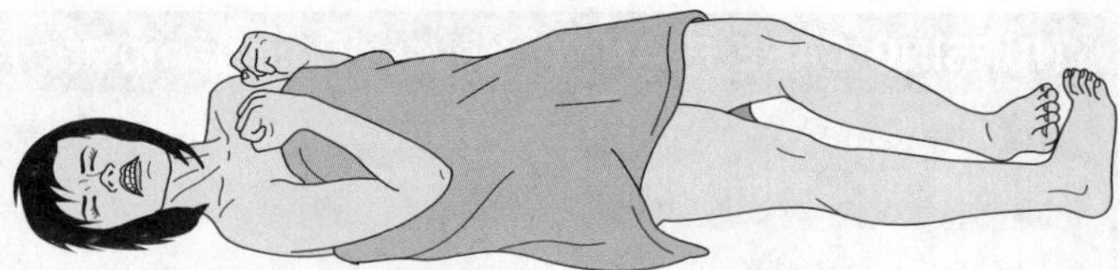

Fig. 14-6 Eclampsia (convulsion or seizure).

Eclampsia

Eclampsia is usually preceded by various premonitory symptoms and signs, including headache, severe epigastric pain, and hyperreflexia. However, convulsions can appear suddenly and without warning in a seemingly stable woman with only minimum BP elevations (Sibai, 2007). Increased hypertension and tonic contraction of all body muscles (seen as arms flexed, hands clenched, legs inverted) precede the convulsions (Fig. 14-6). During this stage muscles alternately relax and contract. Respirations are halted and then begin again with long, deep, stertorous inhalations.

Hypotension and then coma follow. Nystagmus and muscular twitching persist for a time. Disorientation and amnesia cloud the immediate recovery. Seizures may recur within minutes of the first convulsion, or the woman may never have another. During the convulsion the pregnant woman and fetus are not receiving oxygen; thus eclamptic seizures produce a marked metabolic insult to both the woman and the fetus (Cunningham et al, 2005).

Immediate Care

The immediate goal of care during a convulsion is to ensure a patent airway (see Emergency box). Time, duration, and a description of the convulsions are recorded; and any urinary or fecal incontinence is noted. If possible, the fetus is monitored for adverse effects; however, this task should not take precedence over other stabilizing care measures. Transient fetal bradycardia and decreased FHR variability are common.

A rapid assessment of uterine activity, cervical status, and fetal status is performed after a convulsion. During the convulsion membranes can rupture, and the cervix can dilate because the uterus becomes hypercontractile and hypertonic; birth may be imminent. If birth is not imminent, once a woman's seizure activity and BP are controlled, a decision should be made regarding whether birth should take place. Since delivery is the definitive cure for the disease, the more serious the condition of the woman, the greater the need to proceed to the birth following the cessation of seizure activity. The means of birth (i.e., induction of labor vs. cesarean birth) depends on maternal and fetal condition, fetal gestational age, presence of labor, and the cervical Bishop score. If fetal lungs are not mature and the birth can be delayed for 48 hours, steroids such as betamethasone can be given.

If the woman has been incontinent of urine and stool, or the membranes have ruptured during the convulsion, she will

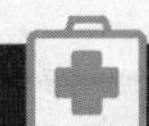

EMERGENCY

Eclampsia

Tonic-Clonic Convulsion Signs

Stage of invasion–2 to 3 seconds: eyes are fixed; twitching of facial muscles occurs

Stage of contraction–15 to 20 seconds: eyes protrude and are bloodshot; all body muscles are in tonic contraction

Stage of convulsion–Muscles relax and contract alternately (clonic); respirations are halted and then begin again with long, deep, stertorous inhalation; coma ensues

Intervention

Keep airway patent: turn head to one side, place pillow under one shoulder or back if possible.

Call for assistance.

Protect with side rails up.

Observe and record convulsion activity.

After Convulsion or Seizure

Do not leave unattended until fully alert.

Observe for postconvulsion coma, incontinence.

Use suction as needed.

Administer oxygen via face mask at 10 L/min.

Start intravenous fluids and monitor intake.

Give magnesium sulfate or anticonvulsant drug as ordered.

Insert indwelling urinary catheter and monitor output.

Monitor blood pressure.

Monitor fetal and uterine status.

Expedite laboratory work as ordered to monitor kidney function, liver function, coagulation system, and drug levels.

Provide hygiene and a quiet environment.

Support and keep woman and family informed.

Be prepared to assist with birth when woman is in stable condition.

need assistance with hygiene and a change of gown. Oral care with a soft toothbrush may be of comfort.

NURSING ALERT Immediately after a seizure, the woman may be very confused and can be combative. Pad the side rails to prevent injury and maintain a quiet, darkened environment. It may take several hours for the woman to regain her usual level of mental functioning. She should not be left alone. Provide emotional support to the family and discuss with them the management, its rationale, and the woman's progress.

Laboratory tests are ordered to assess for HELLP syndrome. Blood is typed and crossmatched for administration of packed red blood cells as needed. The eclamptic woman is at high risk for abruptio placentae, with accompanying hemorrhage and shock. Other tests include determination of electrolyte levels; liver function; and a complete hemogram and clotting profile, including platelet count and fibrin split product levels (to assess for DIC).

Aspiration is a leading cause of maternal morbidity and mortality after an eclamptic seizure. After initial stabilization and airway management, the nurse should anticipate orders for a chest x-ray film and possibly arterial blood gases to determine whether aspiration occurred.

Postpartum Nursing Care

After birth the symptoms of preeclampsia or eclampsia resolve quickly, usually within 48 hours. Resolution of the disease process is manifested by diuresis, which usually occurs within 24 hours after the birth. The hematopoietic and hepatic complications of HELLP syndrome may persist longer. Usually an abrupt decrease in platelet count occurs with a concomitant increase in LDH and AST levels after a trend toward normalization of values has begun. Generally the laboratory abnormalities seen with HELLP syndrome resolve in 72 to 96 hours.

The nursing care of the woman with hypertensive disease differs in a number of respects from that required in a normal postpartum period. These variations in the nursing process are described in the following paragraphs.

The woman will need careful assessment of her vital signs, intake and output, DTRs, level of consciousness, uterine tone, and lochia flow throughout the postpartum period. The magnesium sulfate infusion is continued 12 to 24 hours for seizure prophylaxis. Even if no convulsions occurred before the birth, they may occur during the postpartum period. The same assessments continue until the medication is discontinued.

NURSING ALERT The woman is at risk for a boggy uterus and a large lochia flow as a result of the tocolytic effects of magnesium sulfate therapy. Uterine tone and lochial flow must be monitored closely.

The preeclamptic woman is usually hemoconcentrated and unable to tolerate excessive postpartum blood loss. Oxytocin or prostaglandin products are used to control bleeding. Ergot products (e.g., ergonovine [Ergotrate] and methylergonovine [Methergine]) are contraindicated because they increase BP. The woman is asked to report symptoms such as headaches and blurred vision. The nurse assesses affect, level of consciousness, BP, pulse, and respiratory status before an analgesic is given for headache. Magnesium sulfate potentiates the action of narcotics, CNS depressants, and calcium channel blockers; these medications must be administered with caution. The woman may need to continue antihypertensive medication if her diastolic BP exceeds 100 mm Hg at discharge.

Postpartum recovery may be prolonged as a result of the physiologic consequences of prolonged bed rest. The nurse should accompany the woman when she ambulates after prolonged bed rest and assess for weakness, dizziness, shortness of breath, and muscle soreness. The woman will also need reassurance that the physiologic effects of bed rest will reverse over time when she resumes normal activity (Simpson & James, 2005).

The woman's and family's responses to labor, the birth, and the newborn are monitored. Interactions and involvement in the care of the newborn are encouraged as much as the woman

Table 14-4 Pharmacologic Control of Hypertension in Pregnancy

ACTION	TARGET TISSUE	Effects: MATERNAL	Effects: FETAL	NURSING ACTIONS
Hydralazine (Apresoline, Neopresol)				
Arteriolar vasodilator	Peripheral arterioles: to decrease muscle tone, decrease peripheral resistance; hypothalamus and medullary vasomotor center for minor decrease in sympathetic tone	Headache, flushing, palpitation, tachycardia, some decrease in uteroplacental blood flow, increase in heart rate and cardiac output, increase in oxygen consumption, nausea and vomiting	Tachycardia; late decelerations and bradycardia if maternal diastolic pressure <90 mm Hg	Assess for effects of medications, alert woman (family) to expected effects of medications, assess blood pressure frequently because precipitate decrease can lead to shock and perhaps abruptio placentae; assess urinary output; maintain bed rest in a lateral position with side rails up; use with caution in presence of maternal tachycardia
Labetalol Hydrochloride (Normodyne)				
β-Blocking agent causing vasodilation without significant change in cardiac output	Peripheral arterioles (see hydralazine)	Minimal: flushing, tremulousness; minimal change in pulse rate	Minimal, if any	See hydralazine; less likely to cause excessive hypotension and tachycardia; less rebound hypertension than hydralazine
Methyldopa (Aldomet)				
Maintenance therapy if needed: 250-500 mg orally every 8 hr (α_2-receptor agonist)	Postganglionic nerve endings: interferes with chemical neurotransmission to reduce peripheral vascular resistance, causes CNS sedation	Sleepiness, postural hypotension, constipation; rare: drug-induced fever in 1% of women and positive Coombs' test result in 20%	After 4 mo maternal therapy, positive Coombs' test result in infant	See hydralazine
Nifedipine (Procardia)				
Calcium channel blocker	Arterioles: to reduce systemic vascular resistance by relaxation of arterial smooth muscle	Headache, flushing; possible potentiation of effects on CNS if administered concurrent with magnesium sulfate, may interfere with labor	Minimal	See hydralazine; use caution if patient also getting magnesium sulfate

CNS, Central nervous system.

and her family desire. If the preeclampsia was severe, the infant may be premature and in a special care nursery. The woman and her family may be worried about their infant's survival, and the day-to-day fluctuations in the infant's status can be emotionally draining (Simpson & James, 2005). In addition, the woman and her family need opportunities to discuss their emotional response to complications. The nurse provides information concerning the prognosis. Preeclampsia and eclampsia do not necessarily recur in subsequent pregnancies (recurrence rate is approximately 30%), but prenatal care is essential for assessment and early intervention. If the outcome for the mother or baby is unfavorable, the family is assisted in coping with loss and grief.

Chronic Hypertension

Chronic hypertension occurs in 5% of pregnant women. Chronic hypertension in pregnancy is associated with increased incidence of abruptio placentae, superimposed preeclampsia, and increased perinatal mortality. Fetal effects include fetal growth restriction, small-for-gestational-age infants, and fetal death (Cunningham et al, 2005; Roberts & Funai, 2009; Sibai, 2007).

Women with chronic hypertension ideally should be screened before conception or at the first prenatal visit. Medications that could have adverse effects on the fetus should be discussed and can be discontinued or changed to another medication. Because of the antihypertensive effects of pregnancy, the antihypertensive medication may be discontinued or changed to another medication. Antihypertensive medications are reinstituted when the BP increases with gestational age, especially after 28 weeks (Sibai, 2007).

Based on the history and physical findings, women with chronic hypertension are identified as either at high or low risk for pregnancy complications (Sibai, 2007). Women who are high risk are usually managed with antihypertensive therapy and frequent assessments of maternal and fetal well-being. The goal of treatment is to maintain a BP below 150 to 160 mm Hg systolic and 100 to 110 mm Hg diastolic. Methyldopa (Aldomet) is the drug of choice for treating chronic hypertension in pregnancy. If methyldopa is ineffective in reducing BP, β-blockers or calcium channel blockers can be used (Chan & Winkle, 2006; Cunningham et al, 2005). The treatment of low risk women is controversial. Evidence has not shown improvement in maternal or fetal outcome or a decreased risk of developing superimposed preeclampsia with treatment (Sibai, 2007).

Lifestyle changes may be necessary (e.g., limiting sodium in the diet, limiting exercise during pregnancy, not smoking or using alcohol, limiting caffeine, and losing weight in the preconception period if overweight). The woman should be taught how to monitor her BP and count fetal movements and the importance of bed rest (Gilbert, 2007).

The time of birth is individualized, but a woman at low risk can usually wait until her cervix is favorable for induction at 37 weeks of gestation. The woman at high risk is followed closely, and the method and timing of the birth depends on maternal and fetal status. After giving birth women with chronic hypertension, especially if at high risk, should be monitored for signs of complications such as renal failure, pulmonary edema, heart failure, and encephalopathy (Sibai, 2007). Because all antihypertensive drugs are found in breast milk, the drugs of choice are methyldopa or hydralazine. Short-term studies have not found any adverse effects on infants, but no long-term human studies have examined the drug effects on infants.

The risks and benefits of contraception should be discussed with the mother and her family before discharge from the hospital. Provided that the woman is compliant and there is close follow-up, she can use all types of contraception. The risks of oral contraceptives must be discussed, including the risk of thromboembolic events. Estrogen has a negative effect on some clotting factors, angiotensinogen, total cholesterol, and triglycerides. Progesterone has a negative effect on lipoproteins and insulin resistance (Gilbert, 2007).

Hyperemesis Gravidarum

Nausea and vomiting complicate approximately 70% of all pregnancies and are usually confined to the first trimester (Gordon, 2007). Although these manifestations are distressing, they are typically benign, with no significant alterations or risks to the mother or fetus. Pregnancies complicated by nausea and vomiting have a more favorable outcome than pregnancies without such symptoms (Gordon, 2007).

When vomiting during pregnancy becomes excessive enough to cause weight loss of at least 5% of prepregnancy weight and is accompanied by dehydration, electrolyte imbalance, ketosis, and acetonuria, the disorder is termed *hyperemesis gravidarum.* The estimated incidence is 0.5% of all pregnancies (Kelly & Savides, 2009). Hyperemesis gravidarum usually begins during the first 10 weeks of pregnancy. It has been associated with women who are nulliparous, have increased body weight, have a history of migraines, or are pregnant with twins or hydatidiform mole (Kelly & Savides, 2009). In addition, an interrelated psychologic component has been associated with hyperemesis and must be assessed (Cunningham et al, 2005; Kelly & Savides, 2009). The effects of hyperemesis gravidarum on perinatal outcome vary with the severity of the disorder.

Etiology

The etiology of hyperemesis gravidarum remains obscure. Several theories have been proposed as to the cause, although none of them adequately explains the disorder. Hyperemesis gravidarum may be related to high levels of estrogen or human chorionic gonadotropin (hCG) and associated with transient hyperthyroidism during pregnancy. Some research has found that a woman who has severe nausea and vomiting has a 1.5-fold increased chance of carrying a female infant, supporting the association between increased estrogen exposure and hyperemesis gravidarum (Cunningham et al, 2005; Kelly & Savides, 2009). Esophageal reflux, reduced gastric motility, and decreased secretion of free hydrochloric acid may contribute to the disorder.

Psychologic and social factors can also play a part in the development of hyperemesis gravidarum. Ambivalence toward the pregnancy and increased stress may be associated with this condition (Cunningham et al, 2005; Kelly & Savides, 2009). Conflicting feelings regarding prospective motherhood, body changes, and lifestyle alterations—all normal reactions to pregnancy—may contribute to episodes of vomiting, particularly if these feelings are excessive or unresolved.

Clinical Manifestations

The woman with hyperemesis usually has significant weight loss and symptoms of dehydration such as decreased BP, increased pulse rate, and poor skin turgor (Kelly & Savides, 2009). She is almost always unable to keep down even clear liquids taken by mouth. Laboratory tests may reveal electrolyte imbalances.

Collaborative Care

Whenever a pregnant woman has nausea and vomiting, the first priority is a thorough assessment to determine the severity of the problem. In most cases the woman should be told to come to the health care provider's office or the emergency department immediately because the severity of illness is often difficult to determine by phone. The frequency, severity, and duration of episodes of nausea and vomiting should be assessed. Other symptoms such as diarrhea, indigestion, and abdominal pain or distention are also identified. Pharmacologic and nonpharmacologic treatments used should be recorded. Prepregnancy weight and documented weight gain or loss during pregnancy are important to note.

The woman's weight and vital signs are measured, and a complete physical examination is performed, with attention to signs of fluid and electrolyte imbalance and nutritional status. The most important initial laboratory test to be obtained is a dipstick determination of ketonuria. Other laboratory tests that may be ordered include a urinalysis, CBC, electrolytes, liver enzymes, and bilirubin levels. These tests help rule out the presence of underlying diseases such as pyelonephritis, pancreatitis, cholecystitis, and hepatitis. Because of the recognized association between hyperemesis gravidarum and hyperthyroidism, thyroid function may also be assessed (Kelly & Savides, 2009).

Psychosocial assessment includes asking the woman about anxiety, fears, and concerns related to her own health and the effects on pregnancy outcome. Family members should be

evolve Nursing Care Plan—Hyperemesis Gravidarum

assessed both for anxiety and in regard to their role in providing support for the woman.

Initial Care

Initially the woman who is unable to keep down clear liquids by mouth requires IV therapy for correction of fluid and electrolyte imbalances. She should receive nothing by mouth until dehydration has been resolved and for at least 48 hours after vomiting has stopped. In the past women requiring IV therapy were admitted to the hospital. Today they often are successfully managed at home even if on enteral therapy. Antiemetic medications may be used if nausea and vomiting are uncontrolled. Commonly used medications include pyridoxine (vitamin B_6) alone or in combination with doxylamine (Unisom), promethazine (Phenergan), and metoclopramide (Reglan) (ACOG, 2004; Cunningham et al, 2005; Kelly & Savides, 2009). Other less commonly used medications include meclizine (Antivert), dimenhydrinate (Dramamine), diphenhydramine (Benadryl), prochlorperazine (Compazine), and ondansetron (Zofran) (Cunningham et al, 2005). Corticosteroids (methylprednisolone [Medrol]) may also be used to treat refractory hyperemesis gravidarum. Some women also benefit from psychotherapy or stress reduction techniques.

Interventions may include initiating and monitoring IV therapy, administering drugs and nutrition supplements, and monitoring the woman's response to interventions. The nurse observes the woman for any signs of complications such as metabolic acidosis, jaundice, or hemorrhage and alerts the physician should these occur. Monitoring includes assessment of the woman's nausea, retching without vomiting, and vomiting since the two symptoms, although related, are separate. A standardized assessment tool such as the Pregnancy-Unique Quantification of Emesis allows quantification of the presence and severity of the nausea and vomiting and promotes accurate monitoring (Davis, 2004).

Accurate measurement of intake and output, including the amount of emesis, is an important aspect of nursing care. Oral hygiene while the woman is on nothing-by-mouth status and after episodes of vomiting helps allay associated discomforts. Assistance with positioning and providing a quiet, restful environment that is free from odors may increase the woman's comfort. When the woman begins responding to therapy, limited amounts of oral fluids and bland foods such as crackers, toast, or baked chicken are begun. The diet is progressed slowly as tolerated by the woman until she is able to consume a nutritionally sound diet. Because sleep disturbances may accompany hyperemesis gravidarum, promoting adequate rest is important. The nurse can assist in coordinating treatment measures and periods of visitation to provide opportunity for rest periods (see Nursing Care Plan).

Follow-Up Care

Most women are able to take nourishment by mouth after several days of treatment. They should be encouraged to eat small, frequent meals consisting of low-fat, high-protein foods; to avoid greasy and highly seasoned foods; and to increase dietary intake of potassium and magnesium. Herbal teas such as ginger, chamomile, and raspberry leaf may decrease nausea. Taking fluids between meals rather than with them sometimes helps decrease nausea. Many pregnant women find exposure to cooking odors nauseating; having other family members cook may decrease nausea. Dietary instructions include eating dry, bland foods; high-protein foods; small, frequent meals; cold foods; or a snack before bedtime; and drinking liquids from a cup with a lid, drinking tea or water with lemon slices, and avoiding high-fat or spicy foods (Davis, 2004). The woman is counseled to contact her health care provider immediately if the nausea and vomiting recur, especially if accompanied by abdominal pain, dehydration, or weight loss greater than 2.3 kg (5 lb) in 1 week.

A few women will continue to experience intractable nausea and vomiting throughout pregnancy. Rarely it may be necessary to maintain a woman on enteral, parenteral, or total parenteral nutrition to provide adequate nutrition for the mother and fetus. Many home health agencies are able to provide these services, and arrangements for service may be made, depending on the woman's insurance coverage.

The woman with hyperemesis gravidarum needs calm, compassionate, and sympathetic care, with recognition that the manifestations of hyperemesis can be physically and emotionally debilitating to the woman and stressful for her family. Irritability, tearfulness, and mood changes are often consistent with this disorder. Fetal well-being is a primary concern of the woman. The nurse can provide an environment conducive to discussion of concerns and assist the woman in identifying and mobilizing sources of support. The family should be included in the plan of care whenever possible. Their participation may help alleviate some of the emotional stress associated with this disorder.

Hemorrhagic Disorders

Bleeding in pregnancy may jeopardize maternal and fetal well-being. Maternal blood loss decreases oxygen-carrying capacity; predisposes the woman to increased risk for hypovolemia, anemia, infection, preterm labor, and preterm birth; and adversely affects oxygen delivery to the fetus. Fetal risks from maternal hemorrhage include blood loss or anemia, hypoxemia, hypoxia, anoxia, and preterm birth.

Hemorrhagic disorders in pregnancy are medical emergencies. The incidence and type of bleeding vary by trimester. In the first trimester most bleeding is a result of miscarriage and ectopic pregnancy. Approximately 50% of bleeding in the third trimester is caused by placenta previa and abruptio placentae. Antepartal hemorrhage is a leading cause of maternal death, with ectopic pregnancy rupture, uterine rupture, and abruptio placentae being responsible for most maternal deaths.

With approximately 750 ml/min to 1000 ml/min (15% of maternal cardiac output) of blood flow to the uterine vasculature and placenta, disruption of vascular integrity has the potential for maternal exsanguination within 8 to 10 minutes. Prompt, expert teamwork on the part of the health care providers is essential to save the lives of the mother and infant.

Early Pregnancy Bleeding

Bleeding during early pregnancy is alarming to the woman and of concern to health care providers. The common bleeding disorders of early pregnancy include miscarriage, prema-

Evolve Spanish Guidelines—Assessment of Bleeding in Early Pregnancy

NURSING CARE PLAN Hyperemesis Gravidarum

Nursing Diagnosis: Imbalanced nutrition: less than body requirements related to nausea and persistent vomiting as evidenced by weight decrease as compared with prepregnant weight

Expected Outcomes

Woman will exhibit no further weight losses, and weight will stabilize. Woman will tolerate regular diet with adequate nutrients for pregnancy with no further nausea and vomiting.

Nursing Interventions/*Rationales*

Ascertain woman's prepregnant weight and monitor woman's current weight and intake and output *to provide a database for care planning.*

Resume oral diet as tolerated and prescribed by caregiver *to provide oral nutrition at optimal time.*

Provide small, frequent bland meals as woman tolerates *to assess woman's response to limited oral intake.*

Administer antiemetic medications as prescribed *to decrease or eliminate episodes of vomiting.*

Provide a quiet, restful environment *to decrease associated discomforts.*

Teach woman the importance of a low-fat, high-protein diet with fluids between meals *to provide optimal nutrition for fetal growth and keep nausea to a minimum.*

Refer to dietitian to develop optimal diet plan individualized to woman's current preferences, culture, and lifestyle *to encourage ongoing compliance.*

Discuss with woman the importance of contacting health care provider if intractable nausea and vomiting recur *to provide prompt treatment and avoid complications.*

Nursing Diagnosis: Deficient fluid volume related to excessive vomiting as evidenced by fluid and electrolyte imbalance

Expected Outcome

Woman's fluid and electrolyte balance will be restored.

Nursing Interventions/*Rationales*

Assess and document skin turgor, condition of mucous membranes, vital signs, and urine specific gravity *to provide database for planning care.*

Obtain daily weight *to provide ongoing evaluation of care.*

Monitor laboratory values and report deviations from normal *to prevent complications.*

Maintain accurate intake and output record *to assess for evidence of fluid deficit.*

Initiate and maintain intravenous therapy carefully *to maintain fluid balance.*

Administer antiemetics as prescribed *to inhibit nausea and vomiting.*

Begin oral fluids slowly and carefully *to increase tolerance and restore fluid balance.*

Nursing Diagnosis: Anxiety related to effects of hyperemesis on fetal well-being as evidenced by woman's statements of concern

Expected Outcome

Woman will exhibit decreased anxiety.

Nursing Interventions/*Rationales*

Use therapeutic communication to listen to woman's concerns *to maintain a relationship and feeling of trust.*

Provide information regarding any potential risks to the fetus *to alleviate anxiety.*

Assist woman to identify personal strengths and previous coping mechanisms *to reinforce to woman the strengths and coping mechanisms that may be of assistance during this illness.*

Help woman identify sources of support and mobilize support person or group of her choice *to provide support as needed.*

Refer to social services as needed *for ongoing evaluation and assistance.*

ture dilation of the cervix, ectopic pregnancy, and hydatidiform mole (molar pregnancy). Women with advanced maternal age, smoking exposure, and prior preterm birth are more likely to experience intense vaginal bleeding during pregnancy (Yang et al, 2005).

Miscarriage (Spontaneous Abortion)

A pregnancy that ends without medical or surgical method before 20 weeks of gestation or 500-g birth weight is defined as a *miscarriage* or *spontaneous abortion* (Cunningham et al, 2005).

The term *miscarriage* is used throughout this discussion because it is a more appropriate term to use with patients; *abortion* may be an insensitive term to use with families who are grieving a pregnancy loss. Therapeutic and elective abortion is discussed in Chapter 7.

Incidence and Etiology

Approximately 10% to 12% of all confirmed pregnancies in the United States end in miscarriage (Simpson & Jauniaux, 2007). An early miscarriage is one that occurs before 12 weeks of gestation. At least 50% of all clinically recognized pregnancy losses result from chromosome abnormalities (Griebel et al, 2005). More than 90% of miscarriages occur early, before 8 weeks and only 2% to 3% occur after 8 weeks of gestation (Simpson & Jauniaux, 2007). Possible causes of early miscarriage include endocrine imbalance (as in women who have luteal phase defects or insulin-dependent diabetes mellitus with high blood-glucose levels in the first trimester), immunologic factors (e.g., antiphospholipid antibodies), infections (e.g., bacteriuria and *Chlamydia trachomatis*), systemic disorders (e.g., lupus erythematosus), and genetic factors (Gilbert, 2007; Simpson & Jauniaux, 2007).

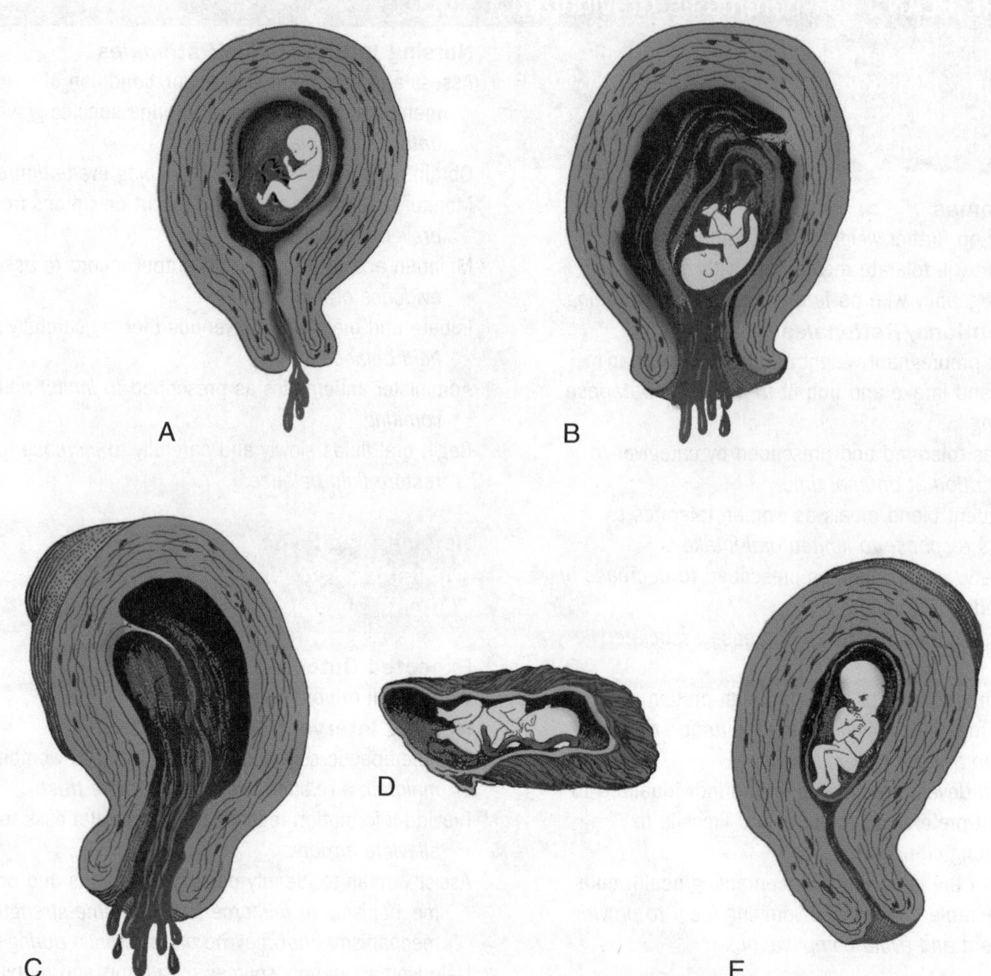

Fig. 14-7 Miscarriage. **A,** Threatened. **B,** Inevitable. **C,** Incomplete. **D,** Complete. **E,** Missed.

A late miscarriage occurs between 12 and 20 weeks of gestation. It usually results from maternal causes such as advancing maternal age and parity, chronic infections, premature dilation of the cervix and other anomalies of the reproductive tract, chronic debilitating diseases, inadequate nutrition, and recreational drug use (Cunningham et al, 2005). Little can be done to avoid genetic causes of pregnancy loss, but correction of maternal disorders, immunization against infectious diseases, adequate early prenatal care, and treatment of pregnancy complications can do much to prevent miscarriage.

Types

The types of miscarriage include threatened, inevitable, incomplete, complete, and missed (Fig. 14-7). All types of miscarriages can recur in subsequent pregnancies; all types but the threatened miscarriage can lead to infection.

Clinical Manifestations

Signs and symptoms of miscarriage depend on the duration of the pregnancy. The presence of uterine bleeding, uterine contractions, or uterine pain is an ominous sign in early pregnancy and must be considered a threatened miscarriage until proven otherwise.

If miscarriage occurs before the sixth week of pregnancy, the woman may report a heavy menstrual flow. Miscarriage that occurs between weeks 6 and 12 of pregnancy causes moderate discomfort and blood loss. After week 12 miscarriage is typified by more severe pain, similar to that of labor, because the fetus must be expelled. Diagnosis of the type of miscarriage is based on the signs and symptoms present (Table 14-5).

Symptoms of a threatened miscarriage (see Fig. 14-7, *A*) include spotting of blood with a closed cervical os. Mild uterine cramping may be present.

Inevitable (see Fig. 14-7, *B*) and incomplete (see Fig. 14-7, *C*) miscarriages involve a moderate-to-heavy amount of bleeding with an open cervical os. Tissue may be present with the bleeding. Mild-to-severe uterine cramping may be present. An inevitable miscarriage is often accompanied by rupture of membranes (ROM) and cervical dilation; passage of the products of conception occurs. An incomplete miscarriage involves the expulsion of the fetus with retention of the placenta (Cunningham et al, 2005).

In a complete miscarriage (see Fig. 14-7, *D*) all fetal tissue is passed, the cervix is closed, and there may be slight bleeding. Mild uterine cramping may be present.

Table 14-5 Types of Miscarriage and Usual Management

TYPE OF MISCARRIAGE	AMOUNT OF BLEEDING	UTERINE CRAMPING	PASSAGE OF TISSUE	CERVICAL DILATION	MANAGEMENT
Threatened	Slight, spotting	Mild	No	No	Bed rest, sedation, and avoidance of stress and orgasm usually recommended; further treatment depends on woman's response to treatment
Inevitable	Moderate	Mild to severe	No	Yes	Prompt termination of pregnancy accomplished, usually by dilation and curettage
Incomplete	Heavy, profuse	Severe	Yes	Yes, with tissue in cervix	Prompt termination of pregnancy accomplished, usually by dilation and curettage
Complete	Slight	Mild	Yes	No	May not need further intervention if uterine contractions adequate to prevent hemorrhage and there is no infection
Missed	None, spotting	None	No	No	If spontaneous evacuation of the uterus does not occur within 1 mo, pregnancy terminated by method appropriate to duration of pregnancy; blood clotting factors monitored until uterus is empty; possible DIC and incoagulability of blood with uncontrolled hemorrhage in cases of fetal death after the twelfth week if products of conception are retained for >5 wk
Septic	Varies, usually malodorous	Varies	Varies	Yes, usually	Immediate termination of pregnancy by method appropriate to duration of pregnancy; cervical culture and sensitivity studies done, and broad-spectrum antibiotic therapy (e.g., ampicillin) started; treatment for septic shock initiated if necessary
Recurrent	Varies	Varies	Yes	Yes, usually	Varies, depends on type; prophylactic cerclage may be done if premature cervical dilation is cause

Adapted from Gilbert ES: *Manual of high risk pregnancy & delivery*, ed 4, St Louis, 2007, Mosby.
DIC, Disseminated intravascular coagulation.

The term *missed miscarriage* (see Fig. 14-7, *E*) refers to a pregnancy in which the fetus has died but the products of conception are retained in utero for up to several weeks. It may be diagnosed by ultrasonic examination after the uterus stops increasing or even decreases in size. There may be no bleeding or cramping, and the cervical os remains closed. If the products of conception are retained after a missed miscarriage, they may calcify, forming a uterine lithopedion or "womb stone."

Habitual miscarriage or recurrent spontaneous abortion is three or more consecutive pregnancy losses before 20 weeks of gestation. The etiology is often unclear but is thought to be multifactorial in nature (Pandey, Rani, & Agrawal, 2005). Women with a history of habitual miscarriage are at increased risk for preterm birth, placenta previa, and fetal anomalies in subsequent pregnancies (Cunningham et al, 2005). Miscarriage can become septic, although this is not a common occurrence. Symptoms of sepsis include fever and abdominal tenderness. Vaginal bleeding, which may be slight to heavy, is usually malodorous. Surgical evacuation is required at this point.

Nursing Care Management

When a woman has vaginal bleeding early in pregnancy, a thorough assessment should be performed (Box 14-7). It is not uncommon for the woman and her family to be anxious and fearful regarding what may happen to her and to her pregnancy.

BOX 14-7 Assessment of Bleeding in Pregnancy

Initial Database

Chief complaint
Vital signs
Gravidity, parity
Last menstrual period/estimated date of birth
Pregnancy history (previous and current)
Allergies
Nausea and vomiting
Pain (onset, quality, precipitating event, location)
Bleeding or coagulation problems
Level of consciousness
Emotional status

Early Pregnancy

Confirmation of pregnancy
Bleeding (bright or dark, intermittent or continuous)
Pain (type, intensity, persistence)
Vaginal discharge

Late Pregnancy

Estimated date of birth
Bleeding (quantity, associated pain)
Vaginal discharge
Amniotic membrane status
Uterine activity
Abdominal pain
Fetal status/viability

Various laboratory findings are characteristic of miscarriage. Evaluation of the placental hormone hCG is used in the diagnosis of pregnancy and pregnancy loss. hCG is produced by the syncytiotrophoblast, and the β-subunit of hCG (β-hCG) can be detected in maternal plasma and urine 8 to 9 days after ovulation if the woman is pregnant. In early pregnancy the concentration of β-hCG should double every 1.4 to 2 days until about 60 or 70 days of gestation (Cunningham et al, 2005). Before 8 weeks of gestation, if miscarriage is suspected, two serum quantitative β-hCG levels are measured 48 hours apart. If a normal pregnancy is present, the β-hCG level doubles within that time. Ultrasonography can then be used to determine the presence of a viable gestational sac. With considerable or persistent blood loss anemia is likely (hemoglobin level less than 11 g/dl). If infection is present, the white blood cell count is greater than 12,000/mm^3. Sedimentation rate is not helpful for differential diagnostic purposes because an increased sedimentation rate occurs with pregnancy, anemia, or infection.

Medical-Surgical Management

Medical management of miscarriage (see Table 14-5) depends on the classification of the miscarriage and on signs and symptoms. Traditionally threatened miscarriages have been managed with bed rest and supportive care. Follow-up treatment depends on whether the threatened miscarriage progresses to actual miscarriage or symptoms subside and the pregnancy remains intact. Dilation and curettage (D&C) is a surgical procedure in which the cervix is dilated and a curette is inserted to scrape the uterine walls and remove uterine contents. A D&C is commonly used to treat inevitable and incomplete miscarriages. The nurse reinforces explanations, answers any questions or concerns, and prepares the woman for surgery.

Dilation and evacuation, performed after 16 weeks of gestation, consists of wide cervical dilation followed by instrumental removal of the uterine contents.

Before either surgical procedure is performed, a full history should be obtained, and general and pelvic examinations should be performed. General preoperative and postoperative care is appropriate for the woman requiring surgical intervention. Analgesia and anesthesia appropriate to the procedure are used.

Outpatient management of first-trimester pregnancy loss may be accomplished with the use of misoprostol (a synthetic prostaglandin E_1 analog) intravaginally for up to 2 days (Moodliar, Bagratee, & Moodley, 2005; Yang et al, 2005). There has been no difference in short-term psychologic outcomes between expectant and surgical management. If evidence of infection, unstable vital signs, or uncontrollable bleeding exists, a surgical evacuation is performed.

For late incomplete, inevitable, or missed miscarriages (16 to 20 weeks), misoprostol can be given orally or vaginally to induce labor and achieve vaginal delivery of the fetus(s). Prostaglandin (PGE_2) has been used for induction in this patient population; however, the extreme systemic side effects of this medication make it a less attractive option. IV oxytocin can also be used after 20 weeks gestation when myometrial oxytocin binding sites have developed.

Nursing Care

Nursing care is similar to care for any woman whose labor is being induced (see Chapter 19). Special care may be needed for management of side effects of PGE_2 suppositories such as nausea, vomiting, and diarrhea. If the fetus(es) and placenta are not passed in their entirety, the woman may be prepared for manual or surgical evacuation of the uterus.

After evacuation of the uterus, 10 to 20 units of oxytocin in 1000 ml of fluids can be given to prevent hemorrhage. For excessive bleeding ergot products such as ergonovine or a prostaglandin derivative such as carboprost tromethamine can be given to contract the uterus. Three or four doses of ergonovine (e.g., 0.2 mg orally or intramuscularly every 4 hours) can be given if the woman is normotensive. A 25-mg dose of carboprost can be given intramuscularly every 15 to 90 minutes for as many as eight doses (Cunningham et al, 2005). Antibiotics are given as necessary. Analgesics such as antiprostaglandin agents may decrease discomfort from cramping. Transfusion may be required for shock or anemia. The woman who is Rh negative and has not developed isoimmunization is given an IM injection of Rh_o(D) immune globulin within 72 hours of the miscarriage.

Psychosocial aspects of care focus on what the pregnancy loss means to the woman and her family. Grief from perinatal loss is complex and unique to each individual. Explanations of expected procedures, possible complications, and future implications for childbearing are provided. Culturally sensitive education regarding recognition of grief responses and how to manage these responses effectively may prevent adverse outcomes (Van & Meleis, 2003).

As with other fetal or neonatal loss, the woman should be offered the option of seeing the fetal remains. She may also want to know what the hospital does with the fetus or whether she needs to make a decision about final disposition of remains.

NURSING ALERT Procedures for disposition of the fetal remains vary from hospital to hospital and state to state. The nurse should know what the usual procedures are in his or her setting.

Home Care

The woman is usually discharged home after delivery or after a D&C when vital signs are stable, vaginal bleeding remains minimal, and she has recovered from anesthesia. Discharge teaching emphasizes the need for rest. If significant blood loss has occurred, iron supplementation may be ordered. Teaching includes information about normal physical findings such as cramping and type and amount of bleeding, resumption of sexual activity, and family planning. Follow-up care is needed to assess the woman's physical and emotional recovery. Referrals to local support groups or counseling are provided as necessary (see Patient Teaching box).

Follow-up phone calls after a loss are important. The woman may appreciate a phone call on what would have been her due date. These calls provide opportunities for the woman to ask questions, seek advice, and receive information to help process her grief.

PATIENT TEACHING Discharge Teaching for the Woman After Early Miscarriage

- Advise the woman to report any heavy, profuse, or bright red bleeding to health care provider.
- Reassure the woman that a scant, dark discharge may persist for 1 to 2 weeks.
- To reduce the risk of infection, remind the woman not to put anything into the vagina for 2 weeks or until bleeding has stopped (e.g., no tampons, no vaginal intercourse). She should take antibiotics as prescribed.
- Advise the woman to eat foods high in iron and protein.
- Acknowledge that the woman has experienced a loss and that time is required for recovery. She may have mood swings and depression.
- Refer the woman to support groups, clergy, or professional counseling as needed.
- Advise the woman that attempts at pregnancy should be postponed for at least 2 months to allow her body to recover.

From Gilbert ES: *Manual of high risk pregnancy & delivery*, ed 4, St Louis, 2007, Mosby.

Recurrent Premature Dilation of Cervix (Incompetent Cervix)

Passive and painless dilation of the cervical os without labor or contractions of the uterus (incompetent cervix) may occur in the second trimester or early in the third trimester of pregnancy; miscarriage or preterm birth may result. This description assumes an "all or nothing" role for the cervix; it is either "competent" or "incompetent." Current researchers contend that cervical competence is variable and exists as a continuum that is determined in part by cervical length. Other factors include composition of the cervical tissue and the individual circumstances associated with the pregnancy in terms of maternal stress and lifestyle. Iams (2009) refers to this condition as *cervical insufficiency.*

Etiology

Etiologic factors include a history of cervical trauma such as lacerations during childbirth, excessive cervical dilation for curettage or biopsy, and ingestion of diethylstilbestrol (DES) by the woman's mother while pregnant with the woman (see Community Focus box). Other causes are a congenitally short cervix and cervical or uterine anomalies. Reduced cervical competence is a clinical diagnosis based on history. Short labors and recurring loss of the pregnancy at progressively earlier gestational ages are characteristics of reduced cervical competence. Ultrasound examination is used to diagnose this condition objectively. A short cervix (less than 25 mm in length) is indicative of reduced cervical competence. Often, but not always, the short cervix is accompanied by cervical funneling (beaking), or effacement of the internal cervical os (Iams & Romero, 2007; Rust et al, 2005).

COMMUNITY FOCUS

Diethylstilbestrol Exposure

Diethylstilbestrol (DES), a synthetic nonsteroidal estrogen, was used in the United States between 1938 and 1971 to prevent miscarriage and other pregnancy complications. When a relationship was found between exposure to DES and clear cell adenocarcinoma of the vagina and cervix in young women whose mothers had taken DES while pregnant, the U.S. Food and Drug Administration issued a warning in 1971 about the use of DES. Although DES has not been given to pregnant women for more than 30 years, effects continue to be seen. Women who took it during pregnancy have a higher risk of breast cancer than other women. Women who were exposed to it in utero have a higher incidence of structural reproductive tract anomalies, increased infertility, and poorer pregnancy outcomes than women who were not exposed. They also have a higher rate of miscarriage, ectopic pregnancy, and preterm birth. Male offspring of women who took DES while pregnant have more genital abnormalities and a possible increased risk of prostate and testicular cancer. Women who took DES during pregnancy should be encouraged to have regular mammography. Women exposed to DES in utero should have vaginal and cervical digital palpation to assess for clear cell adenocarcinoma. Colposcopic examination may be indicated. Men exposed to DES in utero should have routine prostate cancer screening and perform testicular self-examination.

Source: Schrager S, Potter BE: Diethylstilbestrol exposure, *Am Fam Physician* 69(10):2395-2400, 2004.

Collaborative Care

Medical-Surgical Management

Conservative management consists of bed rest, hydration, and tocolysis (inhibition of uterine contractions). A cervical cerclage may be performed. During pregnancy a Shirodkar or McDonald procedure may be performed. In the Shirodkar maternal fascia lata is threaded submucosally in the cervix anteriorly and posteriorly and tied. In the McDonald cerclage nonabsorbable ribbon (Mersilene) is placed around the cervix beneath the mucosa to constrict the internal os of the cervix (Fig. 14-8). A cerclage procedure can be classified according to time or whether it is elective (prophylactic), urgent, or emergent (Rust & Roberts, 2005).

Prophylactic cerclage is placed at 11 to 15 weeks of gestation, after which the woman is told to refrain from intercourse, prolonged (i.e., more than 90 minutes) standing, and heavy lifting (Iams, 2009). She is monitored during the rest of her pregnancy with ultrasound scans to assess for cervical shortening and funneling. The cerclage is electively removed (usually an office or a clinic procedure) when the woman reaches 37 weeks of gestation, or it may be left in place, and a cesarean birth performed. Approximately 80% to 90% of pregnancies treated with cerclage result in live, viable births. If removed, the cerclage must be repeated with each successive pregnancy.

A woman whose reduced cervical competence is diagnosed during the current pregnancy may undergo emergency cer-

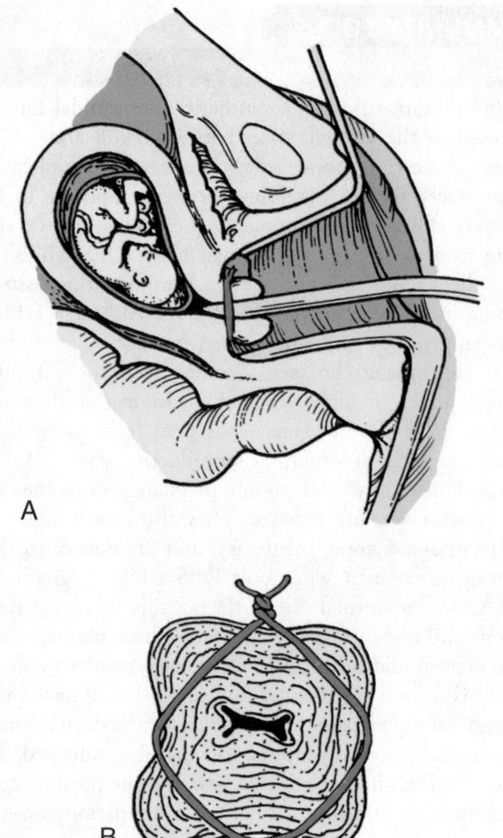

Fig. 14-8 A, Cerclage correction of recurrent premature dilation of cervix. B, Cross section of closed internal os.

clage placement. Risks of the procedure include premature rupture of membranes (PROM), preterm labor, and chorioamnionitis. Because of these risks and because bed rest and tocolytic therapy can be used to prolong the pregnancy, cerclage is rarely performed after 25 weeks of gestation (Iams, 2009).

Nursing Care

The nurse assesses the woman's feelings about her pregnancy and her understanding of reduced cervical competence. Because the diagnosis of reduced cervical competence is usually not made until the woman has lost one or two pregnancies, she may feel guilty or to blame for this impending loss. Therefore it is important to assess for previous reactions to stresses and appropriateness of coping responses and to evaluate the woman's support systems. She needs the support of her family, as well as that of health care providers.

If a cervical cerclage is performed, the nurse monitors the woman after surgery for contractions, ROM, and signs of infection. Discharge teaching focuses on continued monitoring of these aspects at home. Home uterine monitoring may be indicated with follow-up from a home health agency.

Home Care

The woman must understand the importance of activity restriction at home and the need for close observation and supervision. Tocolytics can be given to prevent uterine contractions and further dilation of the cervix. The woman must be instructed on the importance of taking oral tocolytic medication as prescribed, on the expected response, and about

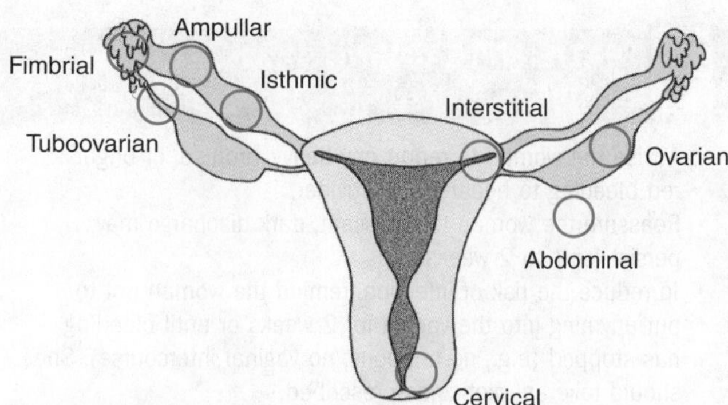

Fig. 14-9 Sites of implantation of ectopic pregnancies. Order of frequency of occurrence is ampullar, isthmic, interstitial, fimbrial, tuboovarian ligament, ovarian, abdominal cavity, and cervical (external os).

possible side effects. If home uterine monitoring is implemented, the woman is taught how to apply a uterine contraction monitor and transmit the monitor tracing by telephone to the monitoring center. Nurses at the monitoring center assess the tracing for contractions, answer questions, provide emotional support and education, and report information to the woman's physician or midwife. The woman should know the signs that warrant immediate transfer to the hospital, including strong contractions less than 5 minutes apart, ROM, severe perineal pressure, and an urge to push. If the fetus is born prematurely, appropriate anticipatory guidance and support are necessary. If management is unsuccessful and the fetus is born before viability, appropriate grief support should be provided.

Ectopic Pregnancy

Incidence and Etiology

An ectopic pregnancy is one in which the fertilized ovum is implanted outside the uterine cavity (Fig. 14-9). It accounts for 2% of all pregnancies in the United States (Sepilian, 2007). The frequency is consistent across maternal age ranges and ethnic origins (Murray et al, 2005).

Approximately 95% of ectopic pregnancies occur in the uterine (fallopian) tube, with most located on the ampullar or largest portion of the tube. Other sites include the ovary (0.5%), abdominal cavity (1.5%), and cervix (0.3%) (Gilbert, 2007). Ectopic pregnancy is classified according to the site of implantation (e.g., tubal, ovarian). The uterus is the only organ capable of containing and sustaining a term pregnancy. However, 5% to 25% of abdominal pregnancies with birth by laparotomy may result in a living infant (Fig. 14-10). The risk of deformity in these infants is as high as 40% (Gilbert, 2007).

Ectopic pregnancy is the leading pregnancy-related cause of first-trimester maternal death in the United States and is responsible for 9% of pregnancy-related deaths (Sepilian, 2007). Ectopic pregnancy is a leading cause of infertility. Women who have been treated surgically for ectopic pregnancy have a subsequent intrauterine pregnancy rate of 50% to 80%; recurrent ectopic pregnancy rate is up to 10% to 25%. Women treated with methotrexate have an intrauterine pregnancy rate of 64%; recurrent ectopic pregnancy rate is approximately 11% (Sepilian, 2007).

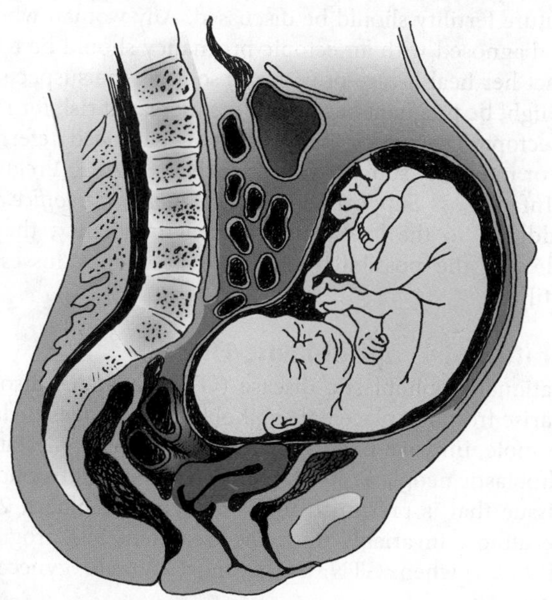

Fig. 14-10 Ectopic pregnancy, abdominal.

The reported incidence of ectopic pregnancy is rising as a result of improved diagnostic techniques such as more sensitive β-hCG assays and the availability of transvaginal ultrasound. An increased incidence of STIs, better treatment of pelvic inflammatory disease (which formerly would have caused sterility), increased numbers of tubal sterilizations, and surgical reversal of tubal sterilizations also have resulted in more ectopic pregnancies (Sepilian, 2007).

Clinical Manifestations

A missed menstrual period, adnexal fullness, and tenderness may suggest an unruptured tubal pregnancy. The tenderness can progress from a dull to a colicky pain when the tube stretches. Pain may be unilateral, bilateral, or diffuse over the abdomen. Dark red or brown abnormal vaginal bleeding occurs in 50% to 80% of women. If the ectopic pregnancy ruptures, pain increases. It may be generalized, unilateral, or acute deep lower quadrant pain caused by blood irritating the peritoneum. Referred shoulder pain can occur from diaphragmatic irritation caused by blood in the peritoneal cavity. The woman may exhibit signs of shock related to the amount of bleeding in the abdominal cavity and not necessarily to obvious vaginal bleeding. An ecchymotic blueness around the umbilicus (Cullen sign), indicating hematoperitoneum, may develop in an undiagnosed, ruptured intraabdominal ectopic pregnancy.

Collaborative Care

The differential diagnosis of ectopic pregnancy involves consideration of numerous disorders that share many signs and symptoms. Many of these women present to the emergency department experiencing first-trimester bleeding or pain. Miscarriage, ruptured corpus luteum cyst, appendicitis, salpingitis, ovarian cysts, torsion of the ovary, and urinary tract infection must be considered. The key to early detection of ectopic pregnancy is having a high index of suspicion for this condition. Any woman with complaints of abdominal pain, vaginal spotting or bleeding, and a positive pregnancy test should undergo screening for ectopic pregnancy.

Laboratory screening includes determination of serum progesterone and β-hCG levels. If either of these values is lower than would be expected for a normal pregnancy, the woman is asked to return within 48 hours for serial measurements. Transvaginal ultrasonography is done to confirm intrauterine or tubal pregnancy (Sepilian, 2007). Ultrasonographic identification of an intrauterine pregnancy (gestational sac plus yolk sac) rules out ectopic pregnancy in most women.

The woman should be assessed for the presence of active bleeding, which is associated with tubal rupture. If internal bleeding is present, the woman may have vertigo, shoulder pain, hypotension, and tachycardia. A vaginal examination should be performed only once, and then with great caution. Approximately half of women with tubal pregnancies have a palpable mass on examination. It is possible to rupture the mass during a bimanual examination; thus gentleness is critical.

Removal of the ectopic pregnancy by salpingostomy is possible before rupture. Residual tissue is dissolved with a dose of methotrexate after surgery. Methotrexate is an antimetabolite and folic acid antagonist that destroys rapidly dividing cells. It may be used in a single-dose IM injection to treat unruptured pregnancies. It has been shown to produce results similar to those of surgical therapy in terms of high success rate, low complication rate, and good reproductive potential (Sepilian, 2007) (see Medication Guide).

MEDICATION GUIDE

Methotrexate (Trexall)

Action

Decreases action of dihydrofolic acid reductase enzyme, which stops growth of actively proliferating tissue such as a tumor or fetus; immunosuppressant

Indication

Ectopic pregnancy, rheumatic conditions, psoriasis, chemotherapy

Dose

50 mg/m^2 intramuscularly ×1: may repeat in 1 week if β-hCG is increased

Adverse Reactions

Thrombocytopenia and other blood related disorders, neurotoxicity, nausea and vomiting, fever, dizziness, diarrhea, pruritus

Nursing Considerations

Provide grief support for loss of pregnancy. Counsel woman to report increased abdominal pain, which could indicate tubal rupture. Follow-up care is needed until β-hCG levels are nondetectable. If methotrexate treatment fails, surgical intervention may be necessary.

NURSING ALERT Women receiving methotrexate should refrain from taking any analgesic stronger than acetaminophen. Stronger analgesics can mask symptoms of tubal rupture.

Advanced ectopic abdominal pregnancy requires laparotomy as soon as the woman has been stabilized for surgery. If the placenta of a second- or third-trimester abdominal pregnancy is attached to a vital organ such as the liver, separation and removal are usually not attempted because of risk of hemorrhage. The cord is cut flush with the placenta, and the abdomen is closed, leaving the placenta in place. Degeneration and absorption of the placenta usually occur without complication, although infection and intestinal obstruction may occur. Methotrexate may be given to dissolve the residual tissue (Gilbert, 2007).

Hospital Care

If surgery is planned for the woman with an ectopic pregnancy, general preoperative and postoperative care is appropriate. Vital signs (pulse, respirations, and BP) are assessed before surgery every 15 minutes or as needed based on severity of the bleeding and the woman's condition. Preoperative laboratory tests include determination of blood type and Rh factor, CBC, and serum quantitative β-hCG assay. Ultrasonography is used to confirm an extrauterine pregnancy. Blood replacement may be necessary. The nurse verifies the woman's Rh and antibody status and administers Rh_o(D) immune globulin if appropriate. The woman should be encouraged to verbalize her feelings related to the loss. Referral to community resources may be appropriate.

Home Care

Some women can be treated on an outpatient basis if they meet certain criteria. Hemodynamically stable women with ectopic pregnancies are eligible for methotrexate therapy if the mass is unruptured and measures less than 3.5 cm in diameter by ultrasound, there is no fetal cardiac activity noted on ultrasound, the serum β-hCG level is less than 5000 IU/ml, there is no free fluid in the cul-de-sac (which indicates possible tubal rupture), and the woman is willing to comply with post-treatment monitoring (Sepilian, 2007). Methotrexate therapy avoids surgery and is a safe, effective, and cost-effective way of managing many cases of tubal pregnancy. The woman is informed about how the medication works, what adverse effects are possible, who to call if she has concerns or if problems develop, and the importance of follow-up care (see Patient Teaching box).

PATIENT TEACHING Methotrexate for Ectopic Pregnancy

- Keep all appointments (2 to 8 weeks).
- Report any vaginal bleeding or abdominal pain.
- Do not take any vitamins or folic acid.
- Do not drink any alcohol.
- Avoid prolonged sun exposure.
- Avoid gas-forming foods.
- Put nothing in the vagina (i.e., no tampons, douches, or intercourse).

NURSING ALERT The woman receiving methotrexate therapy who drinks alcohol and takes vitamins containing folic acid (e.g., prenatal vitamins) increases her risk of having drug side effects or exacerbating the ectopic rupture.

Future fertility should be discussed. Any woman who has been diagnosed with an ectopic pregnancy should be told to contact her health care provider as soon as she suspects that she might be pregnant because of the increased risk for recurrent ectopic pregnancy. These women may need referral to grief or infertility support groups such as SHARE: Pregnancy and Infant Loss Support Inc. (*www.nationalshareoffice.com*). In addition to the loss of the current pregnancy, they are faced with the possibility of future pregnancy losses and infertility.

Gestational Trophoblastic Disease

Gestational trophoblastic disease (GTD) includes disorders that arise from the placental trophoblast. It includes hydatidiform mole, invasive mole, and choriocarcinoma. Gestational trophoblastic neoplasia (GTN) refers to persistent trophoblastic tissue that is presumed to be malignant (Gilbert, 2007). Once almost invariably fatal, the treatment has progressed until today when GTN is the most curable gynecologic malignancy.

Hydatidiform Mole

Hydatidiform mole (molar pregnancy) is a GTD. There are two distinct types: complete (or classic) mole and partial mole.

Incidence and Etiology

Hydatidiform mole occurs in 1 in 1000 pregnancies in the United States (Cohn, Ramaswamy, & Blum, 2009). The etiology is unknown, although there may be an ovular defect or nutrition deficiency. Women at higher risk for hydatidiform mole are those in their early teens or over age 40 or who have undergone ovulation stimulation with clomiphene (Clomid). The risk of developing a second mole is 1% to 2%.

Types

The complete mole results from fertilization of an egg, the nucleus of which has been lost or inactivated. The nucleus of a sperm (23,X) duplicates itself (resulting in the diploid number, 46,XX) because the ovum has no genetic material or the material is inactive. The mole resembles a bunch of white grapes (Fig. 14-11). The hydropic (fluid-filled) vesicles grow rapidly, causing the uterus to be larger than expected for the duration of the pregnancy. Usually the complete mole contains no fetus, placenta, amniotic membranes, or fluid. Maternal blood has no placenta to receive it; therefore hemorrhage into the uterine cavity and vaginal bleeding occur. In about 20% of complete moles progression toward choriocarcinoma occurs.

For a partial mole, chromosome studies often show a karyotype of 69,XXY; 69,XXX; or 69,XYY. This occurs as a result of two sperm fertilizing an apparently normal ovum. Partial moles often have embryonic or fetal parts and an amniotic sac. Congenital anomalies are usually present. The potential for malignant transformation is less than 6% (Copeland & Landon, 2007).

Clinical Manifestations

In the early stages the clinical manifestations of a complete hydatidiform mole cannot be distinguished from normal pregnancy. Vaginal bleeding occurs in almost 95% of patients. The vaginal discharge may be dark brown (resembling prune juice) or bright red and either scant or profuse. It may continue for only a few days or intermittently for weeks. In early

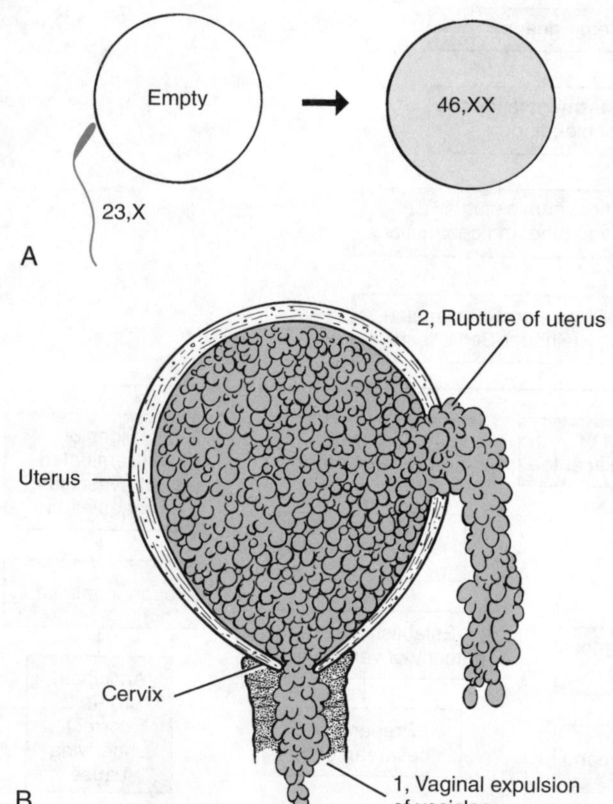

Fig. 14-11 A, Chromosome origin of complete mole. Single sperm (in color) fertilizes an "empty" ovum. Reduplication of sperm's 23,X set gives completely homozygous diploid 46,XX. Similar process follows fertilization of empty ovum by two sperm with two independently drawn sets of 23,X or 23,Y; both karyotypes of 46,XX and 46,YY can therefore result. **B,** Uterine rupture with hydatidiform mole. *1,* Evacuation of mole through cervix. *2,* Rupture of uterus and spillage of mole into peritoneal cavity (rare).

pregnancy in about half of affected women the uterus is significantly larger than expected from menstrual dates.

Anemia from blood loss, excessive nausea and vomiting (hyperemesis gravidarum), and abdominal cramps caused by uterine distention are relatively common findings. Preeclampsia occurs in about 15% of cases (usually between 9 and 12 weeks of gestation), but any symptoms of gestational hypertension before 24 weeks of gestation may suggest hydatidiform mole. Hyperthyroidism and pulmonary embolization of trophoblastic elements occur less commonly but are serious complications of hydatidiform mole. Partial mole causes few of these symptoms and may be mistaken for an incomplete or a missed miscarriage.

Collaborative Care

Medical-Surgical Management Although most moles pass spontaneously, suction curettage offers a safe, rapid, and effective method of evacuation of hydatidiform mole if necessary (Copeland & Landon, 2007). An alternative management plan for a woman who desires sterilization is hysterectomy. The use of oxytocic agents or prostaglandins is not recommended because of the increased risk of embolization of trophoblastic tissue (Copeland & Landon, 2007). Administration of Rh_o(D) immune globulin to women who are Rh negative is needed to prevent isoimmunization.

Nursing Care Nursing assessments during prenatal visits should include observation for signs of molar pregnancy during the first 24 weeks. If hydatidiform mole is suspected, ultrasonography and serial β-hCG immunoassays are used to confirm the diagnosis. The sonographic pattern of a molar pregnancy is characterized by a diffuse snowstorm appearance. The β-hCG titer remains high or rises above the normal peak after the time it normally drops (i.e., 70 to 100 days).

The nurse provides the woman and her family with information about the disease process, the necessity for a long course of follow-up, and the possible consequences of the disease. The nurse helps the woman understand and cope with pregnancy loss and recognize that the pregnancy was abnormal. The woman and her family are encouraged to express their feelings, and information is provided about support groups or counseling resources if needed (e.g., International Society for the Study of Trophoblastic Disease, *www.isstd.org*). Explanations about the importance of contraceptive counseling and the need to postpone a subsequent pregnancy are provided to emphasize the importance of consistent and reliable use of the method chosen.

NURSING ALERT To avoid confusing the signs of choriocarcinoma with the signs of pregnancy, pregnancy should be avoided for 1 year. Any contraceptive method except the intrauterine device is acceptable. Oral contraceptives are highly effective.

Home Care Follow-up management includes frequent physical and pelvic examinations along with measurement of serum β-hCG until the level drops to normal and remains normal for 3 weeks. Monthly measurements are usually taken for a year (Gilbert, 2007). A rising titer and an enlarging uterus may indicate choriocarcinoma. Women with a complete hydatidiform molar pregnancy are at a 15% to 28% risk of requiring further management with chemotherapy for persistent trophoblastic disease (Wolfberg et al, 2005).

Gestational Trophoblastic Neoplasia

These types of tumors are classified as nonmetastatic, metastatic low risk, and metastatic high risk. After the evacuation of a hydatidiform molar pregnancy, approximately 20% of women are treated for malignancy. Almost 50% of these tumors occur after a hydatidiform mole. Approximately 30% follow an ectopic pregnancy or miscarriage, and 20% occur after an apparently normal birth at term. There is an almost 100% cure rate after nonmetastatic and low risk metastatic GTN. Common sites of metastasis are the lungs, vagina, vulva/cervix, liver, and brain (Copeland & Landon, 2007). There is a 20% risk of maternal death after high risk metastatic GTN.

Continued bleeding after evacuation of a hydatidiform mole is usually the most suggestive symptom of GTN. Other clinical signs include abdominal pain and uterine and ovarian enlargement. Signs of metastasis include pulmonary symptoms (e.g., dyspnea, cough). The diagnosis is usually confirmed by increasing or plateauing hCG levels after evacuation

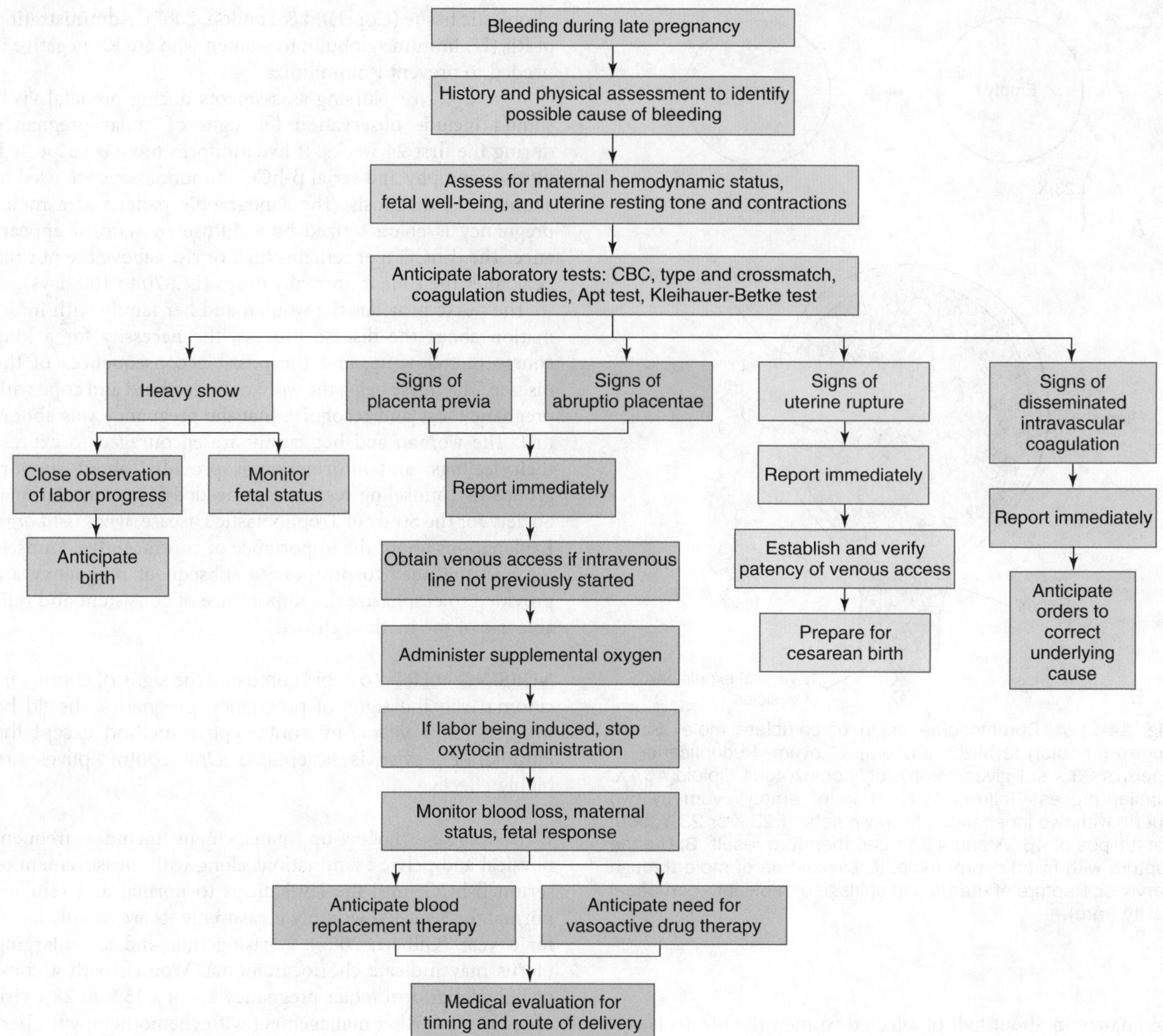

Fig. 14-12 Bleeding during late pregnancy.

of a molar pregnancy. Once diagnosis is confirmed, other clinical studies (e.g., computed tomography scan of lungs and brain, chest x-ray, pelvic ultrasound, and liver scan) are done to determine the extent of the disease.

Single-agent chemotherapy is usually effective. Methotrexate has been the treatment of choice for years. Dactinomycin also has been used with equally good results and is used for women with liver or renal disease, both of which are contraindications for methotrexate. Hysterectomy with adjuvant chemotherapy is often the choice of treatment for nonmetastatic tumors in women who have completed their childbearing.

Therapy is continued until negative hCG levels are obtained. Follow-up after successful chemotherapy is by serum hCG levels obtained every month for a year (Gilbert, 2007). Physical examinations are done at least annually, and chest x-rays are done if indicated. Contraception is needed until the woman has been in remission for at least 6 months. Oral contraceptives are preferred, but barrier methods are acceptable if oral contraceptives are contraindicated. During a subsequent pregnancy, pelvic ultrasonography is recommended because the woman is at higher risk to develop another molar pregnancy. Serum hCG levels should be obtained 6 weeks after the birth.

Late Pregnancy Bleeding

Late pregnancy bleeding disorders include placenta previa, premature separation of placenta (abruptio placentae), and variations in the insertion of the cord and the placenta (Fig. 14-12). Expedient assessment for and diagnosis of the cause of bleeding are essential to reduce the risk of maternal and perinatal morbidity and mortality.

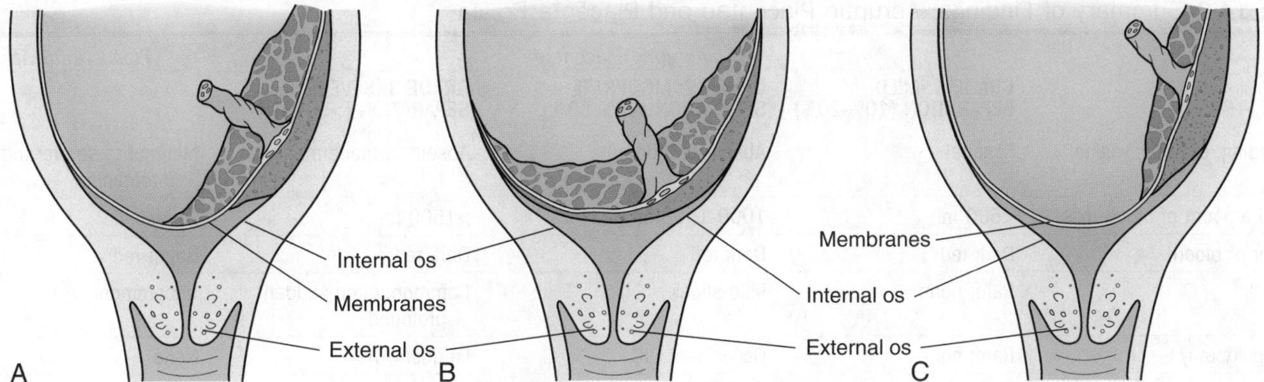

Fig. 14-13 Types of placenta previa. **A,** Low-lying placenta in second trimester. **B,** Placenta previa. **C,** Marginal placenta previa.

Placenta Previa

In placenta previa the placenta is implanted in the lower uterine segment near or over the internal cervical os. The degree to which the internal cervical os is covered by the placenta has traditionally been used to classify three types of placenta previa (Fig. 14-13). Placenta previa often is described as complete, total, or central if the internal os is entirely covered by the placenta when the cervix is fully dilated. Partial placenta previa implies incomplete coverage of the internal os. Marginal placenta previa indicates that only an edge of the placenta extends to the internal os, but it may extend onto the os during dilation of the cervix during labor. The term *low-lying placenta* is used when the placenta is implanted in the lower uterine segment but does not reach the os.

Recent advances in sonographic diagnosis and a better understanding of the changing relationship of the internal cervical os and the placenta as pregnancy progresses have made these traditional definitions and classifications obsolete. If the placenta implants in the lower uterine segment, a diagnosis of placenta previa may be made in the second trimester. However, as uterine growth continues throughout gestation, the placenta will usually grow away from the os toward the fundus, and the lower uterine segment will develop (placental migration) (Hull & Resnik, 2009). The presence of placenta previa during the second trimester is a risk factor for the development of vasa previa. A more descriptive classification is complete placenta previa (in the third trimester the placenta covers the internal os) and marginal placenta previa (the distance of the placenta is 2 to 3 cm from the internal os and does not cover it). When the exact relationship of the os to the placenta has not been determined or in cases of apparent placenta previa in the second trimester, the term *low-lying placenta* can be used (Hull & Resnik, 2009) (see Fig. 14-13).

Incidence and Etiology

The incidence of placenta previa is approximately 0.5% of births. The most important risk factors are previous placenta previa, previous cesarean birth, and suction curettage for miscarriage or induced abortion, possibly related to endometrial scarring (see Critical Thinking Exercise). The risk also increases with multiple gestation (because of the larger placental area), multiparity, maternal age over 35 years, African or Asian ethnicity, and smoking (Hull & Resnik, 2009).

> **CRITICAL THINKING EXERCISE**
>
> **Placenta Previa**
>
> Marta is a 26-year-old woman, G6, P4, Ab1 at 26 weeks of gestation, who is seen in the emergency department with bright red vaginal bleeding. She asks you what is wrong and whether this means she will lose the baby.
>
> 1. Evidence—Is there sufficient evidence to draw conclusions about her diagnosis and preferred treatment?
> 2. Assumptions—What assumptions can be made about the following items?
>   a. Possible diagnoses for Marta
>   b. Physical assessment, laboratory tests, and diagnostic procedures that will be done to make a diagnosis
>   c. The circumstances under which Marta would be transferred to the antepartum unit
>   d. The circumstances under which Marta would be discharged home
> 3. What implications and priorities for nursing care can be drawn at this time?
> 4. Does the evidence objectively support your conclusion?
> 5. Are there alternative perspectives to your conclusion?

evolve Nursing Care Plan—Placenta Previa

Clinical Manifestations

Approximately 70% of women with placenta previa have painless uterine bleeding; 20% have vaginal bleeding associated with uterine activity. Previa should be suspected whenever vaginal bleeding occurs after 20 weeks of gestation. The bleeding is associated with the stretching and thinning of the lower uterine segment that occurs during the third trimester. Placental attachment is gradually disrupted, and bleeding occurs when the uterus is not able to contract adequately and stop blood flow from open vessels. The initial bleeding is usually a small amount and stops as clots form; however, it can recur at any time (Table 14-6). It is bright red.

Vital signs may be normal even with heavy blood loss because a pregnant woman can lose up to 40% of blood volume without showing signs of shock. Clinical presentation and decreasing urinary output may be better indicators of acute blood loss than vital signs alone. FHR changes are unlikely

Table 14-6 Summary of Findings: Abruptio Placentae and Placenta Previa

	Abruptio Placentae			*Placenta Previa*
	GRADE 1: MILD SEPARATION (10%-20%)	**GRADE 2: MODERATE SEPARATION (20%-50%)**	**GRADE 3: SEVERE SEPARATION (>50%)**	
Bleeding, external, vaginal	Minimal	Absent or moderate	Absent to moderate	Minimal to severe and life threatening
Total amount of blood loss	<500 ml	1000-1500 ml	>1500 ml	Varies
Color of blood	Dark red	Dark red	Dark red	Bright red
Shock	Rare; none	Mild shock	Common, often sudden, profound	Uncommon
Coagulopathy	Rare; none	Occasional DIC	Frequent DIC	None
Uterine tonicity	Normal	Increased; may be localized to one region or diffuse over uterus; uterus fails to relax between contractions	Tetanic, persistent uterine contraction; boardlike uterus	Normal
Tenderness (pain)	Usually absent	Present	Agonizing, unremitting uterine pain	Absent
Ultrasonographic findings				
Location of placenta	Normal; upper uterine segment	Normal; upper uterine segment	Normal; upper uterine segment	Abnormal; lower uterine segment
Station of presenting part	Variable to engaged	Variable to engaged	Variable to engaged	High, not engaged
Fetal position	Usual distribution*	Usual distribution*	Usual distribution*	Commonly transverse, breech, or oblique
Gestational or chronic hypertension	Usual distribution*	Commonly present	Commonly present	Usual distribution*
Fetal effects	Normal fetal heart rate pattern	Nonreassuring fetal heart rate pattern	Nonreassuring fetal heart rate pattern; death can occur	Normal fetal heart rate pattern

*Usual distribution refers to the usual variations of incidence seen when there is no concurrent problem.
DIC, Disseminated intravascular coagulation.

unless there is a major detachment of the placenta (Gilbert, 2007).

Abdominal examination usually reveals a soft, relaxed, nontender uterus with normal tone. If the fetus is lying longitudinally, the fundal height is usually greater than expected for gestational age because the low placenta hinders descent of the presenting fetal part. Leopold's maneuvers may reveal a fetus in an oblique or breech position or lying transverse because of the abnormal site of placental implantation.

Maternal and Fetal Outcome

Complications associated with placenta previa include PROM, preterm labor and birth, surgery-related trauma to structures adjacent to the uterus, anesthesia complications, blood transfusion reactions, overinfusion of fluids, abnormal placental attachments (e.g., placenta accreta), vasa previa, postpartum hemorrhage, anemia, thrombophlebitis, and infection.

The greatest risk of fetal death is caused by preterm birth. Other fetal risks include malpresentation and congenital anomalies (Gilbert, 2007). Infants who are small for gestational age or have intrauterine growth restriction also have been associated with placenta previa. This association may be related to poor placental exchange or hypovolemia resulting from maternal blood loss and maternal anemia.

Nursing Care Management

The standard for the diagnosis of placenta previa is a transabdominal ultrasound examination (see Nursing Process box). It is accurate 93% to 97% of the time. Transvaginal ultrasound also is used for placental location, particularly when the exact relation of the lower placental margin to the internal os is not clearly seen with transabdominal examination (Hull & Resnik, 2009). If ultrasonographic scanning reveals a normally implanted placenta, a speculum examination is performed to rule out local causes of bleeding (e.g., cervicitis, polyps, or carcinoma of the cervix), and a coagulation profile is obtained to rule out other causes of bleeding.

If expectant management is to be implemented, a vaginal speculum examination is postponed until fetal viability is reached (preferably after 34 weeks of gestation). If a pelvic examination is needed before that time, anticipate the possibility that an immediate cesarean birth may be required. The woman is taken to a delivery room or an operating room set up for cesarean birth because profound hemorrhage can occur during the examination. This type of vaginal examination, known as the double-setup procedure, is not often performed.

NURSING PROCESS: PLACENTA PREVIA

Assessment

A woman with third-trimester vaginal bleeding requires immediate evaluation. The assessment includes:

History

Pregnancy (gravidity, parity, estimated date of birth)

Course of pregnancy

Interview

General status

Bleeding (quantity, precipitating event, associated pain)

Physical Examination

Vital signs

Fetal status

Presence of contractions or abdominal discomfort

Review Laboratory Test Results

Complete blood count

Blood type and Rh factor

Coagulation profile

Possible type and crossmatch

Planning

Once placenta previa has been diagnosed, a management plan is developed based on gestational age, amount of bleeding, and fetal condition. Expectant management (observation and bed rest) usually is implemented when the fetus is not mature.

Expected outcomes for the woman experiencing placenta previa may include that the woman will do the following:

- Verbalize understanding of her condition and its management
- Identify and use available support systems
- Demonstrate compliance with prescribed activity limitations
- Develop no complications related to bleeding
- Give birth to a healthy term infant

Nursing Diagnoses

Potential nursing diagnoses for the woman with a placenta previa include the following:

Decreased cardiac output related to

– excessive blood loss secondary to placenta previa

Deficient fluid volume related to

– excessive blood loss secondary to placenta previa

Ineffective peripheral tissue perfusion related to

– hypovolemia and shunting of blood to central circulation

Anxiety/fear related to

– maternal condition and pregnancy outcome

Anticipatory grieving related to

– actual/perceived threat to self, pregnancy, or infant

Interventions

Monitor

- Vital signs.
- Fetal status.
- Amount of bleeding.
- Urine output.
- Level of consciousness.

Provide emotional support to the woman and her family.

Explain all procedures.

Administer medications as ordered.

Be prepared for an emergency cesarean birth.

Notify hospital chaplain or other support services as desired by the woman.

Evaluation

The expected outcomes of care are used to evaluate the care for the woman with placenta previa (see Nursing Care Plan).

Hospital Care

Active Management

Acute care of a patient with a diagnosed placenta previa should be carried out in a labor and birth unit with continuous electronic fetal and uterine contraction monitoring. Maternal vital signs are assessed frequently for BP changes, increasing pulse rate, changes in level of consciousness, and oliguria. If the woman is at term (longer than or equal to 37 weeks of gestation) and in labor or bleeding persistently, immediate birth by cesarean is almost always indicated. The nurse should continuously assess maternal and fetal status while preparing the woman for surgery. In women with partial or marginal placenta previa (placental edge is 2 to 3 cm from the cervical os) who have minimal bleeding, vaginal birth may be attempted (Francois & Foley, 2007).

Blood loss may not cease with the infant's birth. The large vascular channels in the lower uterine segment may continue to bleed because of the diminished muscle content in that region. The natural mechanism to control bleeding (i.e., the interlacing muscle bundles contracting around open vessels [the "living ligature" characteristic of the upper part of the uterus]) is absent in the lower part of the uterus. Postpartum hemorrhage may occur even if the fundus is contracted firmly.

Emotional support for the woman and her family is extremely important. The actively bleeding woman is concerned not only for her own well-being but for the well-being of her fetus. All procedures should be explained, and a support person should be present. The woman should be encouraged to express her concerns and feelings. If the woman and her support person or family desire pastoral support, the nurse can notify the hospital chaplain service or provide information about other supportive resources.

Expectant Management

If the woman is less than 36 weeks of gestation, is not in labor, and the bleeding is mild or has stopped, expectant management (i.e., rest and close observation) is generally the treatment of choice to give the fetus time to mature in utero. The woman may remain in the hospital on bed rest with bathroom privileges and limited activity (up in a wheelchair for short periods of time). Bleeding is assessed by checking the amount of bleeding on perineal pads, bed pads, and linens. Weighing pads, although not often used, is one way to more accurately assess blood loss; 1 g is equal to 1 ml of blood.

Ultrasonographic examinations may be done every 2 to 3 weeks. Fetal surveillance may include NST or BPP once or twice weekly. Serial laboratory values are evaluated for decreasing hemoglobin and hematocrit levels and changes in coagulation values. Venous access with an IV infusion or heparin lock may be placed in case blood or blood component therapy is needed. Antepartum steroids (betamethasone) may be ordered to promote fetal lung maturity if the woman is at less than 34 weeks of gestation. No vaginal or rectal examinations are performed, and the woman is placed on pelvic rest (nothing in the vagina). Once she reaches 37 weeks of gestation and fetal lung maturity is documented, cesarean birth can be scheduled.

The woman with placenta previa should always be considered a potential emergency because massive blood loss with resulting hypovolemic shock can occur quickly if bleeding resumes. The possibility always exists that she may require an emergency cesarean for birth. Placenta previa in a preterm gestation may be an indication for admission to a tertiary perinatal center because many community hospitals are not equipped to perform emergency cesarean births 24 hours per day, 7 days per week, nor can they provide neonatal intensive care.

Home Care

Criteria for home care management vary among primary perinatal providers and home care agencies and are usually determined on a case-by-case basis. To be considered for home care referral, the woman must be in stable condition with no evidence of active bleeding and must have resources to be able to return to the hospital immediately if active bleeding resumes.

She must have close supervision by family or friends in the home. She should be taught how to assess fetal and uterine activity and bleeding and told to avoid intercourse, douching, and enemas. She should limit her activities according to the advice of her physician and be advised to keep all appointments for fetal testing, laboratory assessments, and prenatal care. Visits by a perinatal home care nurse may be arranged (see Nursing Care Plan).

NURSING CARE PLAN — Placenta Previa

Nursing Diagnosis: Decreased cardiac output related to bleeding secondary to placenta previa

Expected Outcome

Patient will exhibit signs of increased blood volume and restoration of cardiac output (i.e., normal pulse and blood pressure; normal heart and breath sounds; normal skin color, tone, and turgor; normal capillary refill).

Nursing Interventions/*Rationales*

Woman uterus for tenderness and tone; assess bleeding rate, amount, color, degree of bleeding, CBC values, and coagulation profile *to determine severity of situation.* Do not perform vaginal examination *because it may stimulate further bleeding.*

Establish baseline data for cardiac output (vital signs; heart and breath sounds; skin color, tone, turgor; capillary refill; level of consciousness; urinary output; pulse oximetry) *to use as a basis for evaluating effectiveness of treatment.*

Initiate intravenous therapy or blood transfusions and medications per physician order *to restore blood volume and prevent organ compromise to mother and fetus.*

Place woman on bed rest *to decrease oxygen demands.*

Monitor vital signs, intake and output, hemodynamic status, and laboratory values *to evaluate treatment response.*

Provide emotional support to woman and her family (e.g., explain procedures and their rationale; explain what is happening and what to expect; keep support person present) *to allay fears and provide the family with some sense of control.*

After stabilization, teach woman home management, including bed rest, watching for spotting/bleeding, close follow-up with her health care provider, and preparation for immediate return to hospital if needed *to prevent or stem further complications.*

Nursing Diagnosis: Risk for injury to fetus related to decreased uterine/placental perfusion secondary to bleeding

Expected Outcome

Woman will exhibit ongoing signs of fetal well-being (i.e., adequate fetal movement, normal fetal heart rate, reactive NST, normal BPP).

Nursing Interventions/*Rationales*

Monitor fetus daily for signs of tachycardia, decreased movement, loss of reactivity on NST *to identify and treat changes in fetal status early.*

Obtain BPP per physician order *to assess for signs of chronic asphyxia.*

Maintain maternal side-lying position *to prevent compression of aorta and vena cava.*

Nursing Diagnosis: Risk for infection related to anemia and bleeding secondary to placenta previa

Expected Outcome

Woman will show no signs of intrauterine infection.

Nursing Interventions/*Rationales*

Monitor vital signs for elevated temperature, pulse, and decreased blood pressure; monitor laboratory results for elevated white blood cell count, differential shift; check for uterine tenderness and malodorous vaginal discharge *to detect early signs of infection resulting from exposure of placental tissue.*

Provide/teach perineal hygiene *to decrease the risk of ascending infection.*

Discuss need to increase dietary iron and protein intake to treat anemia.

BPP, Biophysical profile; *CBC*, complete blood count; *NST*, nonstress test.

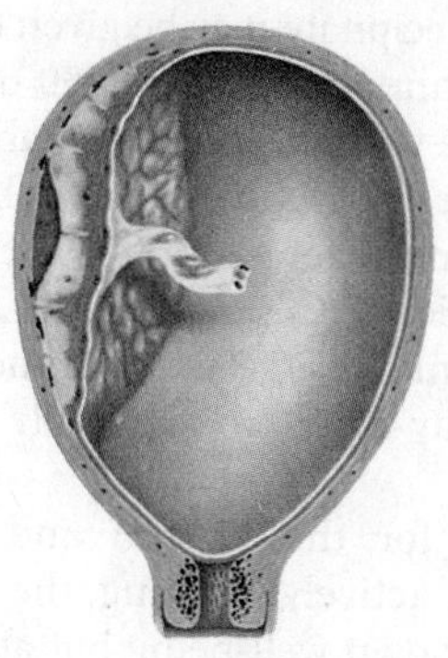

Partial separation (concealed hemorrhage)

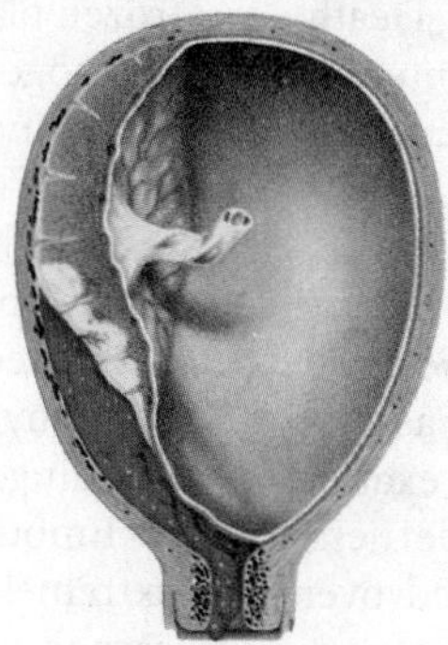

Partial separation (apparent hemorrhage)

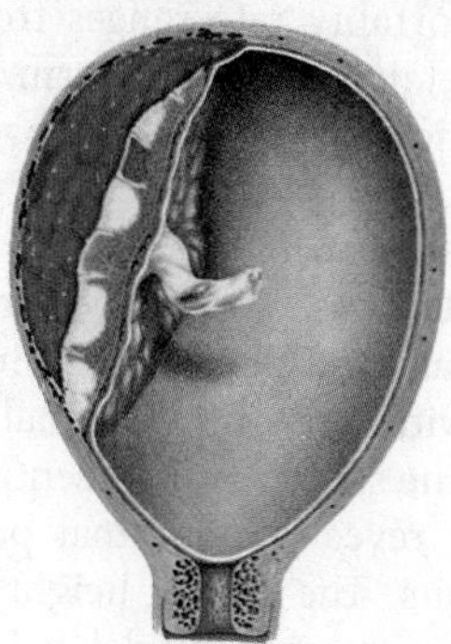

Complete separation (concealed hemorrhage)

Fig. 14-14 Abruptio placentae. Premature separation of normally implanted placenta.

Placental Abruption (Premature Separation of Placenta)

Premature separation of the placenta, or abruptio placentae, is the detachment of part or all of the placenta from its implantation site (Fig. 14-14). Separation occurs in the area of the decidua basalis after 20 weeks of pregnancy and before birth of the baby.

Incidence and Etiology

Premature separation of the placenta is a serious event that accounts for significant maternal and fetal morbidity and mortality. Maternal hypertension is probably the most consistently identified risk factor for abruption. Cocaine use also is a risk factor as a result of cocaine-induced vasospasm leading to placental ischemia, reflex vasodilation, and disruption in the placental vasculature (Francois & Foley, 2007). Blunt external abdominal trauma, most often the result of motor vehicle accidents or maternal battering, is an increasingly significant cause of placental abruption (Francois & Foley, 2007). Maternal smoking significantly increases the risk of placental abruption. In the past maternal age older than 35, parity, short umbilical cord, and folic acid deficiency were all thought to increase risk; however, more recent research has failed to confirm any of these (Francois & Foley, 2007). Abruption is more likely to occur with polyhydramnios and in multiple gestation after birth of the first infant because of rapid uterine decompression. There is a significant (5% to 17%) recurrence risk for placental abruption. A woman who has had two previous premature separations has a recurrence risk of 25% in the next pregnancy (Francois & Foley, 2007).

Classification Systems

The most common classification of placental abruption is according to type and severity. This classification is summarized in Table 14-6.

Clinical Manifestations

The separation may be partial or complete, or only the margin of the placenta may be involved. Bleeding from the placental site may dissect (separate) the membranes from the decidua basalis and flow out through the vagina; it may remain concealed (retroplacental hemorrhage); or it may do both (see Fig. 14-14). Clinical symptoms vary with the degree of separation (see Table 14-6).

Typically vaginal bleeding, abdominal pain, "port wine" stained amniotic fluid, uterine contractions or hypertonus, uterine tenderness, and abnormal FHR patterns or fetal death are seen with abruptio placentae. Although abdominal pain and uterine tenderness are characteristic of abruption, either finding may be absent in the presence of a silent abruption (Baird & Kennedy, 2008; Hull & Resnik, 2009). Bleeding may result in maternal hypovolemia (i.e., shock, oliguria, anuria) and coagulopathy. Mild-to-severe uterine hypertonicity is present. Pain is mild to severe and localized over one region of the uterus or diffuse over the uterus with a "boardlike" abdomen (Baird & Kennedy, 2008).

Extensive myometrial bleeding damages the uterine muscle. If blood accumulates between the separated placenta and the uterine wall, it may produce a Couvelaire uterus. The uterus appears purplish and copper colored, it is ecchymotic, and contractility is lost. Shock may occur and is out of proportion to blood loss. The Apt test result (for blood in amniotic fluid) is positive, hemoglobin and hematocrit levels decrease, and coagulation factor levels decrease. Clotting defects (e.g., DIC) develop in 10% to 30% of women, in most cases within 8 hours of hospital admission. A Kleihauer-Betke stain may be ordered to determine the presence of fetal-to-maternal bleeding (transplacental hemorrhage), although this test appears to be of no value in the general workup of patients with placental abruption (Hull & Resnik, 2009).

Maternal, Fetal, and Neonatal Outcomes

Maternal mortality rate approaches 1% in abruptio placentae; this condition remains one of the leading causes of maternal death. The mother's prognosis depends on the extent of placental detachment, overall blood loss, degree of DIC, and time between placental detachment and birth.

Maternal complications are associated with the abruption or its treatment. Hemorrhage, hypovolemic shock, hypofibrinogenemia, and thrombocytopenia are associated with severe abruption. Couvelaire uterus, DIC, and infection may occur. Renal failure and pituitary necrosis (Sheehan's syndrome) may result from ischemia. In rare cases women who are Rh negative can become sensitized if fetal-to-maternal hemorrhage occurs and the fetal blood type is Rh positive.

Perinatal mortality rate ranges from 20% to 30%. Death occurs from fetal hypoxia, preterm birth, and intrauterine growth restriction. Risks of neurologic deficits are increased (Hull & Resnik, 2009).

Collaborative Care

Abruptio placentae should be strongly suspected in the woman who has a sudden onset of intense, usually localized uterine pain, with or without vaginal bleeding. Initial assessment is much the same as for placenta previa. Physical examination usually reveals abdominal pain, uterine tenderness, and contractions. The fundal height may be measured over time, because increasing fundal height could indicate concealed bleeding. Approximately 60% of live fetuses exhibit abnormal signs on the electronic fetal heart monitor such as loss of variability and late decelerations; uterine hyperstimulation and increased resting tone may also be noted on the monitor tracing (Francois & Foley, 2007).

Many women demonstrate coagulopathy, as evidenced by abnormal clotting studies (fibrinogen, platelet count, PT, PTT, fibrin split products). Sonographic examination is used to rule out placenta previa; however, it is not always diagnostic for abruption. A retroplacental mass may be detected with ultrasonographic examination, but negative findings do not rule out a life-threatening abruption (Hull & Resnik, 2009).

Nursing diagnoses and expected outcomes are similar to those described for placenta previa.

Hospital Care Treatment depends on severity of blood loss and fetal maturity and status. If the abruption is mild, expectant management is implemented if the fetus is less than 36 weeks of gestation and not in distress. The woman is hospitalized and closely observed for signs of bleeding and labor. The fetal status is monitored with intermittent FHR monitoring and NST or BPP until fetal maturity is achieved. If the woman's condition deteriorates, immediate birth is indicated. Use of corticosteroids to accelerate fetal lung maturity is appropriately included in the plan of care for the woman managed expectantly (ACOG, 2002a; Hull & Resnik, 2009). Women who are Rh negative may be given $Rh_o(D)$ immune globulin if fetal-to-maternal hemorrhage occurs and the fetal blood is Rh positive.

If the mother is hemodynamically stable, a vaginal birth may be attempted if the fetus is alive and in no acute distress or if the fetus is dead. In the presence of fetal compromise, severe hemorrhage, coagulopathy, poor labor progress, or increasing uterine resting tone, a cesarean birth is performed. At least one large-bore (16-gauge) IV line should be started. Maternal vital signs are monitored frequently to observe for signs of declining hemodynamic status such as increasing pulse rate and decreasing BP. Serial laboratory studies include hematocrit or hemoglobin determinations and clotting studies. Continuous electronic fetal monitoring is mandatory. An indwelling Foley catheter can be inserted for continuous assessment of urine output, an excellent indirect measure of maternal organ perfusion.

Blood and fluid volume replacement will most likely be ordered, with the goals of maintaining the urine output at 30 ml/hr or more and the hematocrit at 30% or more. If these goals are not reached despite vigorous attempts at replacement, hemodynamic monitoring may be necessary. Fresh frozen plasma or cryoprecipitate may be given to maintain the fibrinogen level at a minimum of 100 to 150 mg/dl.

Vaginal birth may be feasible and is desirable especially in cases of fetal death. Cesarean birth should be reserved for cases of abnormal electronic fetal monitor (EFM) patterns or other obstetric indications. Cesarean birth should not be attempted when the woman has severe and uncorrected coagulopathy because it may result in surgically uncontrollable bleeding.

Emotional support for the woman and her family is extremely important. If actively bleeding, the woman is concerned not only for her own well-being but also for the well-being of her fetus. All procedures should be explained, and a support person should be present.

Home Care Women with abruptio placentae are usually not managed out of the hospital because the placenta can separate at any time and immediate intervention or birth may be necessary.

Cord Insertion and Placental Variations

Placenta accreta is a serious complication of placenta previa. In this condition, trophoblastic invasion extends beyond the normal endometrial barrier. If the invasion extends into the myometrium, it is called *placenta increta.* Placenta percreta exists when the placental invasion extends beyond the uterine serosa (Hull & Resnik, 2009). Massive hemorrhage can occur with these conditions. Cesarean birth through a fundal incision, followed by total abdominal hysterectomy, may be indicated (Hull & Resnik, 2009).

Velamentous insertion of the cord and vasa previa are rare placental anomalies with a higher incidence in multiple gestation. Velamentous insertion of the cord occurs when the umbilical vessels begin to branch at the membranes and then course onto the placenta (Fig. 14-15, *A*). When some of the umbilical vessels cross the cervical os below the presenting part, vasa previa is diagnosed. ROM or traction on the cord may tear one or more of the fetal vessels. As a result, the fetus may rapidly bleed to death. Battledore (marginal) insertion of the cord (see Fig. 14-15, *B*) increases the risk of fetal hemorrhage, especially after marginal separation of the placenta.

Rarely the placenta may be divided into two or more separate lobes, resulting in succenturiate placenta (see Fig. 14-15, *C*). Each lobe has a distinct circulation. The vessels collect at the periphery, and the main trunks eventually unite to form the vessels of the cord. Blood vessels joining the lobes may be supported only by the fetal membranes; therefore they are in danger of tearing during labor, birth, or expulsion of the placenta. During expulsion of the placenta one or more of the separate lobes may remain attached to the decidua basalis, preventing uterine contraction and increasing the risk of postpartum hemorrhage.

Clotting Disorders in Pregnancy

Normal Clotting

Normally a delicate balance (homeostasis) is maintained between the opposing hemostatic and fibrinolytic systems. The hemostatic system is involved in the lifesaving process by stopping the flow of blood from injured vessels, in part through the formation of insoluble fibrin, which acts as a hemostatic

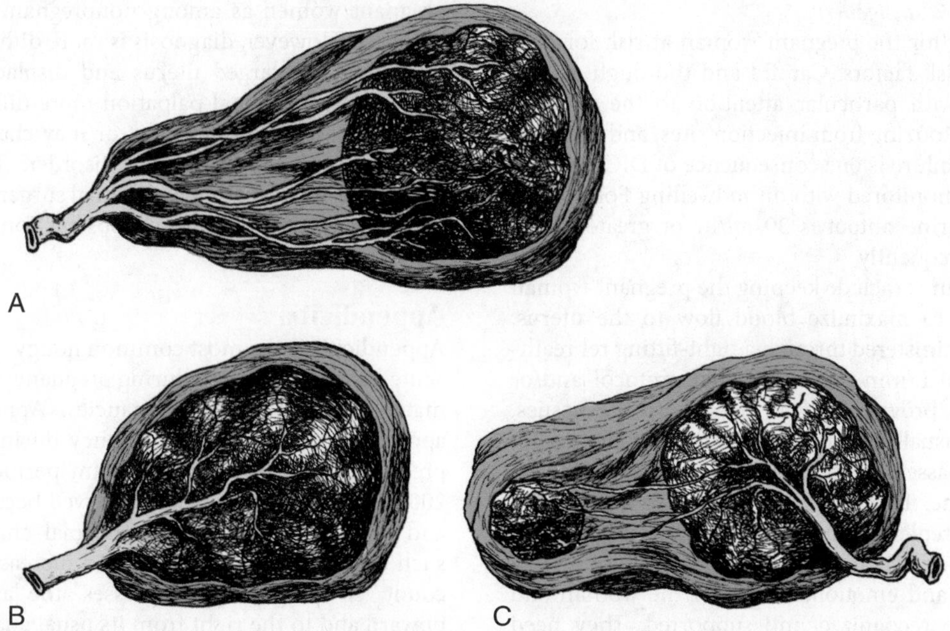

Fig. 14-15 Cord insertion and placental variations. A, Velamentous insertion of cord. B, Battledore placenta. C, Succenturiate placenta.

platelet plug. The coagulation process involves an interaction of the coagulation factors in which each factor sequentially activates the factor next in line, the "cascade effect" sequence. The fibrinolytic system is the process by which the fibrin is split into fibrin degradation products and circulation is restored.

Clotting Problems

A history of abnormal bleeding, inheritance of unusual bleeding tendencies, or a report of significant aberrations of laboratory findings indicates a bleeding or clotting problem. For the pregnant woman, bleeding disorders are suspected if the woman has gestational hypertension, HELLP syndrome, retained dead fetus syndrome, amniotic fluid embolism, sepsis, or hemorrhage. Determination of hemostasis is made by testing the usual mechanisms for the control of bleeding, the function of platelets, and the necessary clotting factors. Most clotting disorders are more a concern in the immediate postpartum period. Recognition in the antepartal period may decrease hemorrhagic problems.

Disseminated Intravascular Coagulation

DIC is a pathologic form of clotting that is diffuse and consumes large amounts of clotting factors, causing widespread external or internal bleeding or both. DIC is an overactivation of the clotting cascade and the fibrinolytic system, resulting in depletion of platelets and clotting factors. This results in the formation of multiple fibrin clots throughout the body's vasculature, even in the microcirculation. Blood cells are destroyed as they pass through these fibrin-choked vessels. Thus DIC results in a clinical picture of hemorrhage, anemia, and ischemia.

DIC is always a secondary diagnosis. In the obstetric population it is most often triggered by the release of large amounts of tissue thromboplastin; this occurs in abruptio placentae, retained dead fetus, and amniotic fluid embolus. Severe preeclampsia and sepsis are examples of conditions that can trigger DIC because of widespread damage to vascular integrity.

Medical Management The diagnosis of DIC is based on clinical findings and laboratory markers. Physical examination reveals unusual bleeding. Spontaneous bleeding from the woman's gums or nose may be noted. Petechiae may appear around the BP cuff placed on her arm. Excessive bleeding may occur from the site of a slight trauma (e.g., venipuncture sites, IM or subcutaneous injection sites, or injury from insertion of urinary catheter). Maternal symptoms may include tachycardia and diaphoresis.

Laboratory tests reveal decreased hematocrit, hemoglobin, platelets, fibrinogen, proaccelerin, antihemophilic factor, and prothrombin (the factors consumed during coagulation). Fibrinolysis is first increased but later severely depressed. Degradation of fibrin leads to the accumulation of fibrin split products in the blood. Fibrin split products have anticoagulant properties and thus prolong the PT. Bleeding time is normal, coagulation time shows no clot, clot retraction time shows no clot, and PTT is increased.

The primary management of DIC involves correction of the underlying cause, which may be treatment of existing infection, preeclampsia or eclampsia, or removal of a placental abruption. Concomitantly treatment is directed toward support of maternal physiologic functioning and replacing essential factors faster than the body can consume them. IV fluids are given to replace volume lost through severe bleeding. Packed red blood cells are administered to maintain enough circulating red blood cells to ensure tissue oxygenation. Fresh frozen plasma or cryoprecipitate is given to replace fibrinogen and coagulation factors. Platelets may also be administered. Warming fluids and blood prior to administration helps to keep the patient's body temperature within normal range, allowing oxygen use in the organs and tissues.

Nursing Care Management

The nurse caring for the pregnant woman at risk for DIC must be aware of risk factors. Careful and thorough assessment is required, with particular attention to the signs of bleeding (petechiae, oozing from injection sites, and hematuria). Because renal failure is one consequence of DIC, urinary output is carefully monitored with an indwelling Foley catheter. The goal for urine output is 30 ml/hr or greater. Vital signs are assessed frequently.

Supportive measures include keeping the pregnant woman in a side-lying tilt to maximize blood flow to the uterus. Oxygen may be administered through a tight-fitting rebreathing mask at 8 to 10 L/min or per hospital protocol and/or physician order. To provide oxygen delivery to the tissues, blood products are usually administered. If the woman has not yet given birth, fetal assessments by continuous electronic fetal monitoring are done. DIC is usually corrected with birth, blood and volume replacement, and resolution of the cause and as coagulation abnormalities resolve.

The educational and emotional needs of the woman and her family must be recognized and supported. They need information about her condition and explanations of unfamiliar equipment and procedures and will most likely be very anxious about the health of the mother and baby.

von Willebrand's Disease

von Willebrand's disease, a type of hemophilia, is probably the most common of all hereditary bleeding disorders. It results from a factor VIII deficiency and platelet dysfunction. It is transmitted as an incomplete autosomal dominant trait to both sexes. Although von Willebrand's disease is rare, it is one of the most common congenital clotting defects in American women of childbearing age. Symptoms include a familial bleeding tendency, previous bleeding episodes, prolonged bleeding time (the most important test), factor VIII deficiency (mild to moderate), and bleeding from mucous membranes. Factor VIII increases during pregnancy, and this increase may be sufficient to offset danger from hemorrhage during childbirth. von Willebrand's disease is variable in its clinical course, severity, and laboratory values; thus it is possible for this condition to go undetected throughout pregnancy until bleeding problems develop after birth. A primary treatment for many women is desmopressin, which increases levels of plasma factor VIII and vWF (Lockwood & Silver, 2009). If the woman is known to have von Willebrand's disease before labor, factor VIII levels should be monitored and factor VIII/vWF plasma concentrate given as needed to maintain activity at 50% of normal near-term gestation (Lockwood & Silver, 2009). Hemorrhage may occur 4 or 5 days after birth. The woman should remain in the hospital for several days after birth to monitor her for that complication.

Nonobstetric Surgery During Pregnancy

The incidence of surgery requiring anesthesia during pregnancy ranges from 1.5% to 2.0%, affecting an estimated 75,000 women in the United States each year (Kuczkowski, 2004). The need for abdominal surgery occurs as often among pregnant women as among nonpregnant women of comparable age. However, diagnosis is more difficult in the pregnant woman. An enlarged uterus and displaced internal organs may make abdominal palpation more difficult, may alter the position of an affected organ, or may change the usual signs associated with a particular disorder. The most common conditions necessitating abdominal surgery during pregnancy are appendicitis, intestinal obstruction, and gynecologic problems.

Appendicitis

Appendicitis is the most common nongynecologic cause of an acute surgical abdomen during pregnancy, occurring approximately once in 1500 pregnancies. Appendicitis occurs in approximately the same frequency during each trimester of pregnancy and in the postpartum period (Kelly & Savides, 2009). The diagnosis is often delayed because the usual signs and symptoms mimic some normal changes of pregnancy such as nausea and vomiting and increased white blood cell count. As pregnancy progresses, the appendix is pushed upward and to the right from its usual anatomic location (see Fig. 10-15). Because of these changes, appendiceal rupture and peritonitis occur two to three times more often in pregnant women than in nonpregnant women. The fetal loss rate associated with appendectomy is higher than with other surgical procedures (Kelly & Savides, 2009).

The woman with appendicitis most commonly has right lower quadrant pain, nausea and vomiting, and loss of appetite. Approximately half of these women will have muscle guarding. Moving the uterus tends to increase the pain. Temperature may be normal or mildly increased (to 38.3° C). Because of the physiologic increase in white blood cells that occurs in pregnancy, laboratory findings are not helpful in the diagnosis (Kelly & Savides, 2009).

The diagnosis of appendicitis requires a high level of suspicion because the typical signs and symptoms are similar to those found in many other conditions, including pyelonephritis, round ligament pain, placental abruption, torsion of an ovarian cyst, cholecystitis, and preterm labor (Kelly & Savides, 2009).

Appendectomy before rupture usually does not require either antibiotic or tocolytic therapy. If surgery is delayed until after rupture, multiple antibiotics are ordered. Rupture is likely to result in preterm labor and necessitate the use of tocolytic agents.

Intestinal Obstruction

The second most common nonobstetric abdominal emergency in pregnancy is intestinal obstruction. Any woman with a laparotomy scar is more likely to have an intestinal obstruction (adynamic ileus) during gestation. Adhesions as a result of previous surgery or pelvic inflammatory disease, an enlarging uterus, and displacement of the intestines are etiologic factors.

Constipation; persistent cramplike, abdominal pain; vomiting; auscultatory rushes within the abdomen; and "laddering" of the intestinal shadows on x-ray films aid in the diagnosis of intestinal obstruction. Immediate surgical intervention is required for release of the obstruction. Pregnancy is rarely affected by the surgery, assuming the absence of complications such as peritonitis.

Gynecologic Problems

Pregnancy predisposes a woman to ovarian problems, especially during the first trimester. Ovarian cysts and twisting of ovarian cysts or adnexal tissues may occur. Other problems include retained or enlarged cystic corpus luteum of pregnancy and bacterial invasion of reproductive or other intraperitoneal organs.

Laparotomy or laparoscopy may be required to discriminate between ovarian problems and early ectopic pregnancy, appendicitis, or an infectious process.

Nursing Care Management

Initial assessment of the pregnant woman requiring surgery focuses on her presenting signs and symptoms. A thorough history and physical examination are performed. Laboratory testing includes, at a minimum, a CBC with differential and a urinalysis. FHR and activity and uterine activity should be monitored; constant vigilance is maintained for symptoms of impending obstetric complications. The extent of preoperative assessment is determined by the immediacy of surgical intervention and the specific condition that requires surgery.

Hospital Care

When surgery becomes necessary during pregnancy, the woman and her family are concerned about the effects of the procedure and medication on fetal well-being and the course of pregnancy. An important part of preoperative nursing care is encouraging the woman to express her fears, concerns, and questions.

Preoperative care for a pregnant woman differs from that of a nonpregnant woman in one significant aspect: the presence of at least one other person—the fetus. Continuous FHR and uterine contraction monitoring may be performed if the fetus is considered viable. Procedures such as preparation of the operative site and time of insertion of IV lines and urinary retention catheters vary with the physician and the facility. However, in every instance there is total restriction of solid food and fluids or a clear specification of the type, amount, and time at which clear liquids may be taken before surgery. Some bowel preparation such as clear liquids and laxatives may be required before surgery. Food by mouth is restricted for several hours before a scheduled procedure. If the woman experiences a prolonged nothing-by-mouth status, IV fluids with dextrose should be given. Even if she has had nothing by mouth—but more important, if surgery is unexpected—the woman is in danger of vomiting and aspirating; and special precautions are taken before the anesthetic is administered (e.g., administering an antacid).

During surgery perinatal nurses may collaborate with the surgical staff to meet the special needs of pregnant women. To improve fetal oxygenation the woman should be positioned on the operating table with a lateral tilt to avoid maternal compression of the vena cava. Continuous fetal and uterine monitoring during the procedure may be ordered because the risk of preterm labor is great. Depending on the surgical procedure, monitoring can be accomplished using sterile Aquasonic gel and a sterile sleeve for the transducer. Uterine contractions may be palpated manually.

BOX 14-8 Discharge Teaching for Home Care

- Care of incision site
- Diet and elimination related to gastrointestinal function
- Signs and symptoms of developing complications (wound infection, thrombophlebitis, pneumonia)
- Equipment needed and technique for assessing temperature
- Recommended schedule for resumption of activities of daily living
- Treatments and medications ordered
- List of resource persons and their telephone numbers
- Schedule of follow-up visits
- If birth has not occurred:
  - Assessment of fetal activity (kick counts)
  - Signs of preterm labor

In the immediate recovery period general observations and care pertinent to postoperative recovery are initiated. Frequent assessments are carried out for several hours after surgery. Whether the woman is cared for in the surgical postanesthesia recovery area or in a labor and delivery unit, continuous fetal and uterine monitoring will likely be initiated or resumed because of the increased risk of preterm labor. Tocolysis may be necessary if preterm labor occurs.

Home Care

Plans for the woman's return home and for convalescent care should be completed as early as possible before discharge. Depending on her insurance coverage, nursing care may be provided through a home health agency. If not, the woman and other support persons must be taught necessary skills and procedures such as wound care. Provision should be made for supervised practice before discharge. Box 14-8 lists information that should be included in discharge teaching for the postoperative patient. The woman may also need referrals to various community agencies for evaluation of the home situation, child care, home health care, and financial or other assistance.

Trauma During Pregnancy

Trauma is a common complication during pregnancy because most pregnant women in the United States continue activities as usual. Thus pregnant women are at the same risk as others for vehicular crashes, falls, burns, industrial mishaps, violence, gunshot wounds, and other injuries in the home and community. Treatment of pregnant trauma victims is complicated because doctors and nurses who have expertise in the care of trauma victims rarely have similar expertise in the care of pregnant women.

Significance

Approximately 6% to 7% of pregnancies are complicated by physical trauma, which accounts for 46% of maternal mortality (Chames & Pearlman, 2008). As pregnancy progresses, the risk of trauma seems to increase, with more cases of trauma reported in the third trimester than earlier in gestation. Motor vehicle crashes are the most common cause of trauma in pregnancy, accounting for 49%. Other common causes are falls (25%), assaults (18%), gunshot wounds (4%), and burns (1%) (El-Kady et al, 2004). Approximately 50% of fetal deaths are associated with maternal trauma, and most of these are from motor vehicle crashes (Mattox & Goetzl, 2005). Maternal death caused by trauma is usually the result of head injury or hemorrhagic shock. Fetal death usually occurs as a sequela to maternal death or as a result of placental abruption.

Acts of violence are a significant health problem in the United States. The risk of trauma caused by battering and abuse is increased during pregnancy, and rates of recurrence are high. The reported incidence of physical abuse during pregnancy ranges from 4% to 8% (McFarlane, 2007). As many as 45% of women subject to intimate partner violence before pregnancy continue to be abused during the pregnancy. Women who are abused during pregnancy have a threefold risk of being murdered compared with their nonpregnant abused controls (McFarlane, 2007). African-American women have a threefold higher risk than Caucasian women in the same pregnancy group (McFarlane, 2007).

Trauma increases the incidence of miscarriage, preterm labor, abruptio placentae, and stillbirth (Mattox & Goetzl, 2005). The effect of trauma on pregnancy is influenced by the length of gestation, type and severity of the trauma, and degree of disruption of uterine and fetal physiologic features. Fetal death as a result of trauma is more common than the occurrence of both maternal and fetal death (Shah & Kilcline, 2003). Less serious trauma is associated with numerous complications for pregnancy, including fetomaternal hemorrhage, abruptio placentae, intrauterine fetal death, and preterm labor and birth. Careful evaluation of mother and fetus after all types of trauma is imperative.

Multisystem trauma during pregnancy is usually the result of a serious motor vehicle crash, especially if the woman is not wearing a seat belt with a shoulder harness and is ejected from the vehicle. To improve chances of survival for both mother and fetus, pregnant women should wear properly positioned restraints at all times when in a motor vehicle (see Fig. 11-18). Failure to wear restraining devices occurred in 66% of cases in one study (Ikossi et al, 2005). Other researchers found that 95% of pregnant women surveyed either maintained or increased their seat belt use during pregnancy, and a large majority (73%) demonstrated correct usage. The perception that wearing a seat belt would protect them and their baby positively influenced their decision to wear a seat belt, although only 37% of these women reported being given seat belt information during their pregnancy (McGwin et al, 2004).

Special considerations for the pregnant woman and her fetus are necessary when trauma occurs because of the physiologic alterations that accompany pregnancy and the presence of the fetus. Fetal survival depends on maternal survival; therefore the pregnant woman must receive immediate stabilization and appropriate care for optimal fetal outcome.

Maternal Physiologic Characteristics

Optimal care for the pregnant woman after trauma depends on understanding the physiologic state of pregnancy and its effects on trauma. The pregnant woman's body exhibits responses different from those of a nonpregnant person to the same traumatic insults. Because of the different responses to injury during pregnancy, management strategies must be adapted for appropriate resuscitation, fluid therapy, positioning, assessments, and most other interventions. Significant maternal adaptations and the relation to trauma are summarized in Table 14-7.

The uterus and bladder are confined to the bony pelvis during the first trimester of pregnancy and are at reduced risk for injury in cases of abdominal trauma. After pregnancy progresses beyond the fourteenth week, the uterus becomes an abdominal organ, and the risk for injury increases in cases of abdominal trauma. During the second and third trimesters the distended bladder becomes an abdominal organ and is at increased risk for injury and rupture. Bowel injuries occur less often during pregnancy because of the protection provided by the enlarged uterus.

The elevated levels of progesterone that accompany pregnancy relax smooth muscle and profoundly affect the gastrointestinal tract. Gastrointestinal motility decreases, with a resultant increased time required for gastric emptying; the production of hydrochloric acid increases in the last trimester, and the gastroesophageal sphincter relaxes. Airway management of the unconscious pregnant woman is of critical importance.

NURSING ALERT The unconscious pregnant woman is at increased risk for regurgitation of gastric contents and aspiration whenever her head is positioned lower than her stomach or if abdominal pressure is applied.

A pregnant woman has decreased tolerance for hypoxia and apnea because of her decreased functional residual capacity and increased renal loss of bicarbonate. Acidosis develops more quickly in the pregnant woman than in the nonpregnant state.

Cardiac output increases approximately 50% over prepregnancy values by 32 weeks of gestation and is positionally dependent in the third trimester. Because of compression of the inferior vena cava and descending aorta by the pregnant uterus, cardiac output decreases dramatically if the woman is placed in the supine position. The supine position must be avoided, even in women with cervical spine injuries. It is a primary priority that lateral uterine displacement be accomplished without any head movement. As soon as the neck is immobilized, the stretcher should be tilted laterally.

Circulating blood volume increases 50% during a singleton gestation, and pregnant women can tolerate a 1000-ml blood loss readily without demonstrating clinical signs. Hemodynamic instability that indicates the need for transfusion may not be apparent until blood loss nears 1200 to 1500 ml (Martin & Foley, 2009). Clinical signs of hemorrhage do not appear until after a 20% to 25% loss of circulating volume occurs. Although heart rate increases with pregnancy, a maternal heart rate greater than 100 beats/min should be considered abnormal.

Fetal Physiologic Characteristics

Perfusion of the uterine arteries, which provide the primary blood supply to the uteroplacental unit, depends on adequate

Table 14-7 Maternal Adaptations During Pregnancy and Relation to Trauma

SYSTEM	ALTERATION	CLINICAL RESPONSES
Respiratory	↑ Oxygen consumption ↑ Tidal volume ↓ Functional residual capacity Chronic compensated alkalosis ↓ $Paco_2$ ↓ Serum bicarbonate	↑ Risk of acidosis ↑ Risk of respiratory mismanagement ↓ Blood-buffering capacity
Cardiovascular	↑ Circulating volume, 1600 ml ↑ Cardiac output ↑ Heart rate ↓ Systemic vascular resistance ↓ Arterial blood pressure Heart displaced upward to left	Can lose 1000 ml blood No signs of shock until blood loss >30% total blood volume ↓ Placental perfusion in supine position Point of maximal impulse, fourth intercostal space
Renal	↑ Renal plasma flow Dilation of ureters and urethra Bladder displaced forward	 ↑ Risk of stasis, infection ↑ Risk of bladder trauma
Gastrointestinal	↓ Gastric motility ↑ Hydrochloric acid production ↓ Competency of gastroesophageal sphincter	↑ Risk of aspiration Passive regurgitation of stomach acids if head lower than stomach
Reproductive	↑ Blood flow to organs Uterine enlargement	Source of ↑ blood loss Vena caval compression in supine position
Musculoskeletal	Displacement of abdominal viscera Pelvic venous congestion Cartilage softened Fetal head in pelvis	↑ Risk of injury, altered rebound response Altered pain referral ↑ Risk of pelvic fracture Center of gravity changed ↑ Risk of fetal injury
Hematologic	↑ Clotting factors ↓ Fibrinolytic activity	↑ Risk of thrombus formation

maternal arterial pressure because these vessels lack autoregulation. Therefore maternal hypotension decreases uterine and fetal perfusion. Maternal shock results in splanchnic and uterine artery vasoconstriction, which decreases blood flow and oxygen transport to the fetus. EFM tracings can assist in the evaluation of maternal status after trauma. They reflect fetal cardiac responses to hypoxia and hypoperfusion, including tachycardia or bradycardia, decreased or absent baseline variability, and/or late decelerations.

Careful monitoring of fetal status assists greatly in maternal assessment because the fetal monitor tracing works as an "oximeter" of internal maternal well-being. Hypoperfusion can be present in the pregnant woman before the onset of clinical signs of shock. The EFM tracings may show the first signs of maternal compromise such as when maternal heart rate, BP, and color appear normal yet the EFM printout shows signs of fetal hypoxia (Tucker, Miller, & Miller, 2009).

Mechanisms of Trauma

Blunt Abdominal Trauma

Blunt abdominal trauma is most commonly the result of motor vehicle crashes but also may be the result of battering or falls. Maternal and fetal morbidity and mortality rates associated with motor vehicle crashes are directly correlated with whether the mother remains inside the vehicle or is ejected. Maternal death is usually the result of a head injury or exsanguination from a major vessel rupture. Serious retroperitoneal hemorrhage after lower abdominal and pelvic trauma is reported more frequently during pregnancy. Serious maternal abdominal injuries are usually the result of splenic rupture or liver and renal injury.

When maternal survival of trauma occurs, fetal death is usually the result of abruptio placentae. Placental separation is thought to be a result of deformation of the elastic myometrium around the relatively inelastic placenta. Shearing of the placental edge from the underlying decidua basalis results and is worsened by the increased intrauterine pressure caused by the impact. It is imperative that all pregnant victims be evaluated carefully for signs and symptoms of abruptio placentae after even minor blunt abdominal trauma.

NURSING ALERT Signs and symptoms of abruptio placentae include uterine tenderness or pain, uterine irritability and/or frequent uterine contractions, vaginal bleeding, blood-stained amniotic fluid, and a change in FHR characteristics.

Pelvic fracture can result from severe injury and produce bladder trauma or retroperitoneal bleeding with two-point displacement of pelvic bones. One point of displacement is common at the symphysis pubis, and the second point is posterior because of the structure of the pelvis. Careful evaluation for clinical signs of internal hemorrhage is indicated.

Direct fetal injury as a complication of blunt trauma during pregnancy most often involves the fetal skull and brain

(Chames & Pearlman, 2008). Most commonly this injury accompanies maternal pelvic fracture in late gestation after the fetal head becomes engaged. When the force of the impact is great enough to fracture the maternal pelvis, the fetus often sustains a skull fracture. Evaluation for fetal skull fracture or intracranial hemorrhage is indicated.

Uterine rupture as a result of trauma is rare, occurring in only 0.6% of all reported cases of trauma during pregnancy. Uterine rupture depends on numerous factors, including gestational age, the intensity of the impact, the presence of a predisposing factor such as a distended uterus caused by polyhydramnios or multiple gestation, or the presence of a uterine scar from previous uterine surgery (Cunningham et al, 2005). When uterine rupture occurs, the force responsible is usually a direct, high-energy blow. Fetal death is common with traumatic uterine rupture. However, maternal death occurs less than 10% of the time; when it occurs, it is usually the result of massive injuries sustained from an impact severe enough to rupture the uterus.

Penetrating Abdominal Trauma

Bullet wounds are the most frequent cause of penetrating abdominal injury, followed by stab wounds. In most cases of penetrating abdominal wounds the woman survives, but the fetus does not. The enlarged uterus may protect other maternal organs, but the fetus is more vulnerable.

Numerous factors determine the extent and severity of maternal and fetal injury from a bullet wound, including size and velocity of the bullet, anatomic region penetrated, angle of entry, path of the bullet, organs damaged, gestational age, and exit wound. Once the bullet enters the body, it may ricochet several times as it encounters organs or bone, or it may sever a large blood vessel. During the second half of pregnancy the fetus usually sustains a direct injury from the bullet. Gunshot wounds require surgical exploration to determine the extent of maternal injury and repair damage as needed.

Stab wounds are limited by the length and width of the penetrating object and are usually confined to the pathway of the weapon. Maternal and fetal injuries are less likely if the stab wound is located in the upper abdomen and if the angle of penetration is downward rather than upward. Stab wounds usually require surgical exploration to clean out debris, determine extent of injury, and repair damage.

Thoracic Trauma

Thoracic trauma is reported to produce 25% of all trauma deaths. Pulmonary contusion results from nearly 75% of blunt thoracic trauma and is a potentially life-threatening condition. Pulmonary contusion can be difficult to recognize, especially if flail chest is also present or if there is no evidence of thoracic injury. It should be suspected in cases of thoracic injury, especially after blunt acceleration or deceleration trauma such as that occurring when a rapidly moving vehicle crashes into an immovable object.

Penetrating wounds into the chest can result in pneumothorax or hemothorax. This type of injury is usually caused by a vehicular crash that results in impalement by the steering column or a loose article in the vehicle that became a projectile with the force of impact. Stab wounds in the chest also may occur as a result of violence.

❋ Nursing Care Management

Immediate Stabilization

Immediate priorities for stabilization of the pregnant woman after trauma should be identical to those of the nonpregnant trauma patient. Pregnancy should not result in any restriction of the usual diagnostic, pharmacologic, or resuscitative procedures or maneuvers. Fetal survival depends on maternal survival, and stabilization of the mother improves fetal chance of survival. The perinatal nurse is often called on to function collaboratively with emergency department or trauma unit staff members in providing care for the pregnant trauma victim.

NURSING ALERT Priorities of care for the pregnant woman after trauma must be to resuscitate the woman and stabilize her condition *first* and then consider fetal needs.

In cases of minor trauma, the woman is evaluated for vaginal bleeding, uterine irritability, abdominal tenderness, abdominal pain or cramps, and evidence of hypovolemia. A change in or absence of FHR or fetal activity, leakage of amniotic fluid, and presence of fetal cells in the maternal circulation are also included in the assessment.

Primary Survey

In cases of major trauma, the systematic evaluation begins with a primary survey and the initial ABCs of resuscitation:

Airway—Establish and maintain an airway.
Breathing—Ensure adequate breathing.
Circulation—Maintain an adequate circulatory volume.

Increased oxygen needs during gestation necessitate a rapid response. The presence of a cervical spine injury is always assumed.

NURSING ALERT Hyperextension of the neck is avoided; instead jaw thrust is used to establish an airway for the trauma victim.

Once an airway is established, assessment should focus on adequacy of oxygenation. The chest wall is observed for movement. If breathing is absent, ventilations and endotracheal intubation are initiated. Supplemental oxygen should be administered with a tight-fitting, nonrebreathing face mask at 10 to 12 L/min to attempt to normalize maternal arterial oxygen tension (Pao_2 104 to 108 mm Hg) and hemoglobin saturation greater than 95% to optimize maternal and fetal status. The chest wall is assessed for penetrating chest wound or flail chest. Breathing with a flail chest will be rapid and labored; chest wall movements will be uncoordinated and asymmetric; crepitus from bony fragments may be palpated.

Rapid placement of two large-bore (14- to 16-gauge) IV lines is necessary in most seriously injured patients. It is important to place the lines while veins are still distended. Cardiac arrest during the immediate stabilization period is usually the result of profound hypovolemia, necessitating massive fluid resuscitation. Infusion of crystalloids such as Ringer's solution or normal saline solution should be given as a 3 : 1 ratio (i.e., 3 ml of crystalloid replacement to 1 ml of the estimated blood loss is given over the first 30 to 60 minutes of acute resuscitation). Because of the 50% increase in blood volume during pregnancy, published formulas for nonpregnant adults used for estimating crystalloid and blood replacement to counter blood loss must be adjusted upward for pregnancy.

Replacement of red blood cells and other blood components is anticipated; and blood is drawn for type, crossmatch, CBC, and platelet count. Infusion of type-specific packed red blood cells is usually necessary to improve fetal oxygenation status and replace blood loss. During an extreme emergency type O Rh-negative blood may be administered without matching.

If possible, vasopressor drugs to restore maternal arterial BP should be avoided until volume replacement is administered. Although vasopressor agents result in decreased perfusion to the uterus, they should be given and not withheld if needed for successful resuscitation of the mother.

After 20 weeks of gestation, venous return to the heart is best accomplished by positioning the uterus to one side to eliminate the weight of the uterus compressing the inferior vena cava or the descending aorta. This facilitates efforts to establish the forward flow of blood through resuscitation and stabilization. If a lateral position is not possible because of resuscitative efforts or cervical spine immobilization, the uterus can be manually deflected to the left, or a wedge can be inserted underneath the right side of the backboard or stretcher.

Signs of bleeding may be more difficult to recognize in the pregnant woman because a 30% to 35% loss of maternal blood volume may produce only a minimal change in maternal mean arterial pressure. Hypovolemia can be detrimental for the fetus because the vascular bed of the uterus is a low-resistance system that depends on adequate maternal cardiac output and arterial pressure to maintain uterine and fetal perfusion. Maternal hypovolemia can be fatal for the fetus (Friese & Wojciehoski, 2005).

Establishing a baseline neurologic status (level of consciousness, pupil size, and reactivity) is essential. The Glasgow Coma Scale is commonly used at the scene of the accident to help determine the extent of the head injury.

Secondary Survey

After immediate resuscitation and successful stabilization measures, a more detailed secondary survey of the mother and fetus should be accomplished. A complete physical assessment to include all body systems is performed.

The maternal abdomen should be evaluated carefully because a large percentage of serious injuries involve the uterus, intraperitoneal structures, and retroperitoneum. The pregnant woman's stomach is assumed to be full. A nasogastric tube can be used to empty the stomach to help prevent acid aspiration syndrome. An empty stomach facilitates respiratory efforts. The uterus should be evaluated for evidence of gross deformity, tenderness, irritability, or contractions.

The greatest clinical concern after a vehicular crash is abruptio placentae because as many as 40% of these women will have an abruption (Mattox & Goetzl, 2005). Assessments should focus on recognition of this complication, with careful evaluation of fetal monitor tracings, uterine tenderness, labor, or vaginal bleeding. Ultrasound examination may be performed to determine gestational age, viability of fetus, and placental location. However, ultrasound studies cannot exclude abruptio placentae.

Peritoneal lavage for the pregnant woman after blunt abdominal trauma has proven to be a safe procedure and can be helpful in the early diagnosis of intraperitoneal injury or hemorrhage. Under direct visualization the peritoneum is incised, and a peritoneal dialysis catheter is positioned. If aspiration yields free-flowing blood, the test is considered positive, and a laparotomy should be performed. This procedure is not necessary before laparotomy if intraperitoneal bleeding is clinically apparent. Indications for peritoneal lavage include abdominal symptoms or signs suggestive of intraperitoneal bleeding, alteration in mental status, unexplained shock, and severe multiple injuries (Cunningham et al, 2005).

If trauma is the result of a penetrating wound, the woman should be completely undressed and carefully examined for all entrance and exit wounds. A bullet may be located on x-ray films. Exploratory laparotomy is necessary after a gunshot wound to explore the abdominal cavity for organ damage and repair any damage present, with careful examination of all organs, the entire bowel, and posterior vessels. If uterine injury is determined, the risks and benefits of cesarean birth are quickly evaluated. A cesarean birth is desirable if the fetus is alive and near term and may be necessary for the preterm fetus because of the high incidence of fetal injury in these cases. The fetus usually tolerates surgery and anesthesia if adequate uterine perfusion and oxygenation are maintained. Tetanus prophylaxis guidelines are not changed by pregnancy.

Electronic Fetal Monitoring

Continuous electronic fetal monitoring may show early signs of abruptio placentae, including a change in baseline rate, loss of accelerations, and/or the presence of late decelerations. If the estimated gestational age is 24 weeks or greater, fetal monitoring should be initiated soon after the woman is stable because abruptio placentae usually becomes apparent shortly after the injury. Fetal monitoring should be continued, and further evaluation initiated if any of the aforementioned signs occur. Palpation is required to evaluate the intensity of contractions and the uterine resting tone. It is important to palpate between contractions to verify that the uterus is well relaxed. If the uterus does not relax between contractions, abruptio placentae could be present.

Abruptio placentae occurring after trauma may be delayed up to 48 hours after the incident. Electronic fetal monitoring periods of 2 to 6 hours after minor trauma are adequate if there are no uterine contractions, uterine tenderness, or bleeding.

LEGAL TIP Care of the Pregnant Woman After Minor Trauma After minor trauma the pregnant woman may be discharged after an adequate period of electronic fetal monitoring that demonstrates fetal reassurance and absence of uterine contractions. However, clear instructions must be given for immediate return if vaginal bleeding, leaking of amniotic fluid, decreased fetal movement, or abdominal pain occurs.

In addition to helping to stabilize the woman, the nurse provides emotional support for her and her family. If the trauma is the result of a motor vehicle accident, other family members may also have been critically injured or killed. The nurse collaborates with other staff to make sure that questions are answered and consistent information given. Grief support may be necessary.

Discharge Planning

The woman may be discharged home after several hours of evaluation following minor trauma. Her vital signs should be stable, with no evidence of bleeding at the time of discharge. The fetal tracing should be reassuring before monitoring is discontinued and the woman discharged. Education for the woman and her family is very important. She should be instructed to contact her health care provider immediately if changes in fetal movement or signs and symptoms indicative of preterm labor, PROM, or placental abruption develop. If the trauma occurred as a result of a motor vehicle crash, the importance of wearing a seat belt should be reinforced, and she should be given directions for using it correctly during pregnancy (i.e., position the lap belt over hips and thighs rather than across the abdomen; see Fig. 11-18). If the trauma occurred as a result of domestic violence, the woman may need information about the abuse cycle; referral to a crisis center, law enforcement agency, or counseling center; and help in forming a safety plan.

Perimortem Cesarean Delivery

In the presence of multisystem trauma, perimortem cesarean birth may be indicated. Removal of the stressor of pregnancy early in the process of resuscitation can increase the chance for maternal survival. Fetal survival is unlikely if cesarean birth is accomplished more than 20 minutes after maternal death. Therefore, to facilitate resuscitative efforts, consideration may be given to cesarean birth for maternal benefit after 5 minutes of resuscitative efforts that produce no response in the mother (Martin & Foley, 2009).

Key Points

- Hypertensive disorders during pregnancy are a leading cause of maternal and perinatal morbidity and mortality worldwide.
- The cause of preeclampsia is unknown, and there are no known reliable tests for predicting women at risk for developing preeclampsia/eclampsia.
- Preeclampsia/eclampsia is a multisystem disease, and the pathologic changes are present long before clinical manifestations such as hypertension are evident.
- Once preeclampsia becomes clinically evident, therapeutic interventions are palliative (e.g., bed rest and diet) and may slow the progression of the disease, allowing the pregnancy to continue, but the underlying pathology continues.
- HELLP syndrome, which is a complication of preeclampsia/eclampsia, is considered life threatening.
- Magnesium sulfate, the anticonvulsant of choice for preventing or controlling eclampsic seizures, requires careful monitoring of reflexes, respirations, and renal function; its antidote, calcium gluconate, should be at the bedside.
- Intent of emergency interventions for eclampsia is to prevent self-injury, enhance oxygenation, reduce aspiration risk, and establish control with magnesium sulfate.

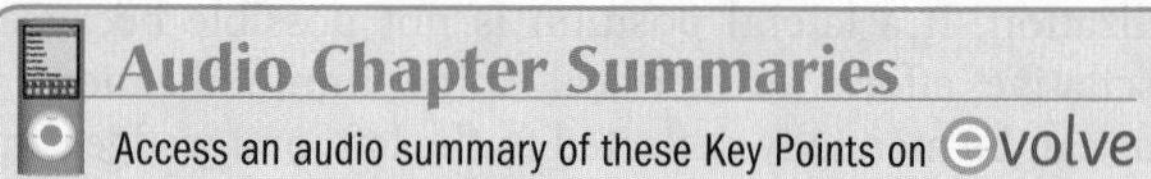
Audio Chapter Summaries
Access an audio summary of these Key Points on evolve

- Ectopic pregnancy is a significant cause of maternal morbidity and mortality even in developed countries.
- Abruptio placentae and placenta previa are differentiated by type of bleeding, uterine tonicity, and presence or absence of pain.
- Clotting disorders are associated with many obstetric complications.
- The physiologic adaptations of pregnancy mask warning signs and changes in vital signs during early shock state.
- Preoperative care for a pregnant woman differs from that for a nonpregnant woman in one significant aspect: the presence of at least one other person—the fetus.
- Trauma from accidents is the most common cause of death in women of childbearing age.
- Fetal survival depends on maternal survival. After trauma the first priority is resuscitation and stabilization of the mother before consideration of fetal concerns.
- Minor trauma is associated with major complications for the pregnancy, including abruptio placentae, fetomaternal hemorrhage, preterm labor and birth, and fetal death.

References

American College of Obstetricians and Gynecologists (ACOG): *Antenatal corticosteroid therapy for fetal maturation: ACOG Committee Opinion No. 210*, Washington, DC, 2002a, ACOG.

American College of Obstetricians and Gynecologists (ACOG): *Diagnosis and management of preeclampsia and eclampsia: ACOG Practice Bulletin number 33*, Washington, DC, 2002b, ACOG.

American College of Obstetricians and Gynecologists (ACOG): *Nausea and vomiting of pregnancy: ACOG Practice Bulletin No. 52*, Washington, DC, 2004, ACOG.

Baird SM, Kennedy, BB: Obstetric emergencies. In Kennedy BB, Ruth DJ, Martin EJ (editors): *Intrapartum management modules: a perinatal education program*, Philadelphia, 2008, Wolters-Kluwer.

Chames MC, Pearlman MD: Trauma during pregnancy: outcomes and clinical management, *Clin Obstet Gynecol* 51(2):398-408, 2008.

Chan P, Winkle C: *Gynecology and obstetrics: current clinical strategies*, Laguna Hills, Calif, 2006, CCS Publishing.

Cohn D, Ramaswamy B, Blum K: Malignancy and pregnancy. In

Creasy RK et al (editors): *Creasy & Resnik's maternal-fetal medicine: principles and practice*, ed 6, Philadelphia, 2009, Saunders.

Copeland L, Landon M: Malignant diseases in pregnancy. In Gabbe SG, Niebyl JR, Simpson JL (editors): *Obstetrics: normal and problem pregnancies*, ed 5, New York, 2007, Churchill Livingstone.

Cunningham F et al: *Williams obstetrics*, ed 22, New York, 2005, McGraw-Hill.

Davis M: Nausea and vomiting of pregnancy: an evidence-based review, *J Perinat Neonatal Nurs* 18(4):312-328, 2004.

El-Kady D et al: Trauma during pregnancy: an analysis of maternal and fetal outcomes in a large population, *Am J Obstet Gynecol* 190:1661-1668, 2004.

Emery S: Hypertensive disorders of pregnancy: over-diagnosis is appropriate, *Cleve Clin J Med* 72(4):345-352, 2005.

Francois KE, Foley MR: Antepartum and postpartum hemorrhage. In Gabbe SG, Niebyl JR, Simpson JL (editors): *Obstetrics: normal and problem pregnancies*, ed 5, New York, 2007, Churchill Livingstone.

Friese G, Wojciehoski R: Fetal trauma from motor vehicle collisions, *JEMS* 30(5):110-127, 2005.

Gilbert ES: *Manual of high risk pregnancy & delivery*, ed 4, St Louis, 2007, Mosby.

Gordon MC: Maternal physiology. In Gabbe S, Niebyl J, & Simpson J (editors): *Obstetrics: normal and problem pregnancies*, ed 5, New York, 2007, Churchill Livingstone.

Griebel C et al: Management of spontaneous abortion, *Am Fam Physician* 72(7):1243-1250, 2005.

Hawfield A, Freedman BI: Pre-eclampsia: the pivotal role of the placenta in its pathophysiology and markers for early detection, *Ther Adv Cardiovasc Dis* 3(1):65-73, 2009.

Hull AD, Resnik R: Placenta previa, placenta accrete, abruption placentae, and vasa previa. In Creasy RK et al (editors): *Creasy & Resnik's maternal-fetal medicine: principles and practice*, ed 6, Philadelphia, 2009, Saunders.

Iams JD: Cervical insufficiency. In Creasy RK et al (editors): *Creasy & Resnik's maternal-fetal medicine: principles and practice*, ed 6, Philadelphia, 2009, Saunders.

Iams JD, Romero R: Preterm birth. In Gabbe S, Niebyl J, & Simpson J (editors): *Obstetrics: normal and problem pregnancies*, ed 5, New York, 2007, Churchill Livingstone.

Ikossi D et al: Profile of mothers at risk: an analysis of injury and pregnancy loss in 1,195 trauma patients, *J Am Coll Surg* 200(1):49-56, 2005.

Kelly TF, Savides TJ: Gastrointestinal disease in pregnancy. In Creasy RK et al (editors): *Creasy & Resnik's maternal-fetal medicine: principles and practice*, ed 6, Philadelphia, 2009, Saunders.

Kuczkowski KM: Nonobstetric surgery during pregnancy: what are the risks of anesthesia? *Obstet Gynecol Surv* 59(1):52-56, 2004.

Lockwood CJ, Silver RM: Coagulation disorders in pregnancy. In Creasy RK et al (editors): *Creasy & Resnik's maternal-fetal medicine: principles and practice*, ed 6, Philadelphia, 2009, Saunders.

Magpie Trial Follow-Up Study Collaborative Group: The Magpie Trial: a randomised trial comparing magnesium sulphate with placebo for preeclampsia. Outcome for children at 18 months, *Br J Obstet Gynaecol* 114(3):289-299, 2007a.

Magpie Trial Follow-Up Study Collaborative Group: The Magpie Trial: a randomised trial comparing magnesium sulphate with placebo for preeclampsia. Outcome for women at 2 years, *Br J Obstet Gynaecol* 114(3):300-309, 2007b.

Maloni JA et al: Antepartum bed rest: maternal weight change and infant birth weight, *Biol Res Nurs* 5(3):177-186, 2004.

Martin J et al: Births: Final data for 2003, *Natl Vital Stat Rep* 54(2):1-116, 2005.

Martin J et al: Births: final data for 2005, *Natl Vital Stat Rep* 56(6):1-104, 2007.

Martin SR, Foley MR: Intensive care monitoring of the critically ill pregnant patient. In Creasy RK et al (editors): *Creasy & Resnik's maternal-fetal medicine: principles and practice*, ed 6, Philadelphia, 2009, Saunders.

Mattox K, Goetzl L: Trauma in pregnancy, *Crit Care Med* 33(10S):S385-S389, 2005.

McFarlane J: Pregnancy following partner rape. What we know and what we need to know, *Trauma Violence Abuse* 8(2):127-134, 2007.

McGwin G et al: Knowledge, beliefs, and practices concerning seat belt use during pregnancy, *J Trauma* 56(3):670-675, 2004.

Moodliar S, Bagratee J, Moodley J: Medical versus surgical evacuation of first-trimester spontaneous abortion, *Int J Gynaecol Obstet* 91(1):21-26, 2005.

Murray H et al: Diagnosis and treatment of ectopic pregnancy, *Can Med Assoc J* 173(8):905-912, 2005.

Mutter WP, Karumanchi SA: Molecular mechanisms of preeclampsia, *Microvasc Res* 75(1):1-8, 2008.

National High Blood Pressure Education Program: *Working group report on high blood pressure in pregnancy*, NIH Pub No 00-3029, Bethesda, Md, 2000, National Institutes of Health, National Heart, Lung, and Blood Institute.

Pandey M, Rani R, Agrawal S: An update in recurrent spontaneous abortion, *Arch Gynecol Obstet* 272(2):95-108, 2005.

Roberts J, Funai EF: Pregnancy-related hypertension. In Creasy RK et al (editors): *Creasy & Resnik's maternal-fetal medicine: principles and practice*, ed 6, Philadelphia, 2009, Saunders.

Roberts J et al, NHLBI Working Group on Research on Hypertension During Pregnancy: Summary of the NHLBI working group on research on hypertension during pregnancy, *Hypertension* 41(3):437-445, 2003.

Rust O, Roberts W: Does cerclage prevent preterm birth? *Obstet Gynecol Clin North Am* 32(3):441-456, 2005.

Rust O et al: Does the presence of a funnel increase the risk of adverse perinatal outcome in a patient with a short cervix? *Am J Obstet Gynecol* 192(4):1060-1066, 2005.

Sepilian VP: Ectopic pregnancy, *Emedicine*, August 17, 2007. Available at www.emedicine.com/med/topic3212.htm (accessed March 30, 2009).

Shah A, Kilcline B: Trauma in pregnancy, *Emerg Med Clin North Am* 21(3):615-629, 2003.

Sibai B: Hypertension in pregnancy. In Gabbe S, Niebyl J, Simpson J (editors), *Obstetrics: normal and problem pregnancies*, ed 5, New York, 2007, Churchill Livingstone.

Sibai B, Dekker G, Kupferminc M: Preeclampsia. *Lancet* 365(9461):785-799, 2005.

Simpson K, James D: *Postpartum care*, White Plains, NY, 2005, March of Dimes.

Simpson JL, Jauniaux, ERM: Pregnancy loss. In Gabbe S, Niebyl J, Simpson J (editors): *Obstetrics: normal and problem pregnancies*, ed 5, New York, 2007, Churchill Livingstone.

Tucker SM, Miller LA, Miller DA: *Pocket guide to fetal monitoring: a multidisciplinary approach*, ed 6, St Louis, 2009, Mosby.

Van P, Meleis AI: Coping with grief after involuntary pregnancy loss: perspectives of African American women, *J Obstet Gynecol Neonatal Nurs* 32(1):28-39, 2003.

Wolfberg A et al: Postevacuation hCG levels and risk of gestational trophoblastic neoplasia in women with complete molar pregnancy, *Obstet Gynecol* 106(3):548-552, 2005.

Yang J et al: Predictors of vaginal bleeding during the first two trimesters of pregnancy, *Paediatr Perinat Epidemiol* 19(4):276-283, 2005.

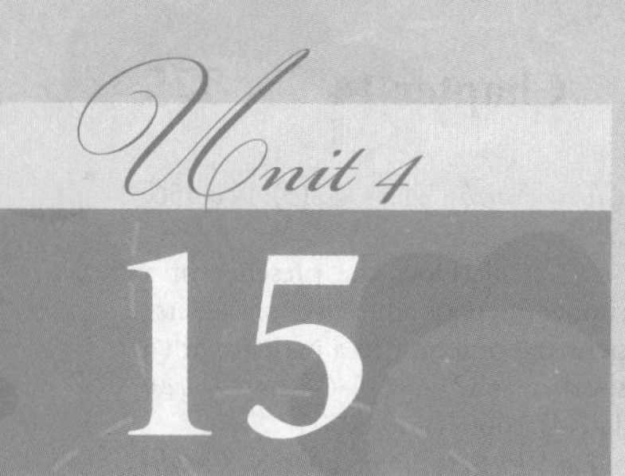

Unit 4

15 Labor and Birth Processes

Learning Objectives

On completion of this chapter the reader will be able to:

- Explain five factors that affect the labor process.
- Describe the anatomic structure of the bony pelvis.
- Recognize the normal measurements of the diameters of the pelvic inlet, cavity, and outlet.
- Explain the significance of the size and position of the fetal head during labor and birth.
- Summarize the cardinal movements of the mechanism of labor for a vertex presentation.
- Assess the maternal anatomic and physiologic adaptations to labor.
- Describe fetal adaptations to labor.

Electronic Resources

Additional information related to the content in Chapter 15 can be found on

evolve the Companion Website at
http://evolve.elsevier.com/Perry/maternal/

- NCLEX Review Questions
- Critical Thinking Exercise—Fetal Presentation

During late pregnancy the woman and fetus prepare for the labor process. The fetus has grown and developed in preparation for extrauterine life. The woman has undergone various physiologic adaptations during pregnancy that prepare her for birth and motherhood. Labor and birth represent the end of pregnancy, the beginning of extrauterine life for the newborn, and a change in the lives of the family. This chapter discusses the factors affecting labor, the processes involved, the normal progression of events, and the adaptations made by both the woman and fetus.

Factors Affecting Labor

At least five factors affect the process of labor and birth. These are easily remembered as the five *P's*: passenger (fetus and placenta), passageway (birth canal), powers (contractions), position of the mother, and psychologic response. The first four factors are presented here as the basis of understanding the physiologic process of labor. The fifth factor is discussed in Chapter 18. Other factors that may be a part of the woman's labor experience may be important as well. VandeVusse (1999) identified external forces, including place of birth, preparation, type of provider (especially nurses), and procedures. Physiology (sensations) was identified as an internal force. These factors are discussed generally in Chapter 18 as they relate to nursing care during labor. Further research investigating essential forces of labor is recommended.

Passenger

The movement of the passenger, or fetus, through the birth canal is determined by several interacting factors: the size of the fetal head, fetal presentation, fetal lie, fetal attitude, and fetal position. Because the placenta also must pass through the birth canal, it can be considered a passenger along with the fetus; however, the placenta rarely impedes the process of labor in normal vaginal birth. An exception is the case of placenta previa (see Chapter 14).

Size of the Fetal Head

Because of its size and relative rigidity, the fetal head has a major effect on the birth process. The fetal skull is composed of two parietal bones, two temporal bones, the frontal bone, and the occipital bone (Fig. 15-1, *A*). These bones are united by membranous sutures: the sagittal, lambdoidal, coronal, and frontal (see Fig. 15-1, *B*). Membrane-filled spaces called fontanels are located where the sutures intersect. During labor, after rupture of membranes, palpation of fontanels and sutures during vaginal examination reveals fetal presentation, position, and attitude.

The two most important fontanels are the anterior and posterior (see Fig. 15-1, *B*). The larger of these, the anterior fontanel, is diamond shaped, about 3 cm × 2 cm, and lies at the junction of the sagittal, coronal, and frontal sutures. It closes by 18 months after birth. The posterior fontanel lies at the junction of the sutures of the two parietal bones and the one occipital bone, is triangular, and is about 1 cm × 2 cm. It closes 6 to 8 weeks after birth.

Sutures and fontanels make the skull flexible to accommodate the infant brain, which continues to grow for some time after birth. However, because the bones are not firmly united, slight overlapping of the bones, or molding of the shape of the head, occurs during labor. This capacity of the bones to slide

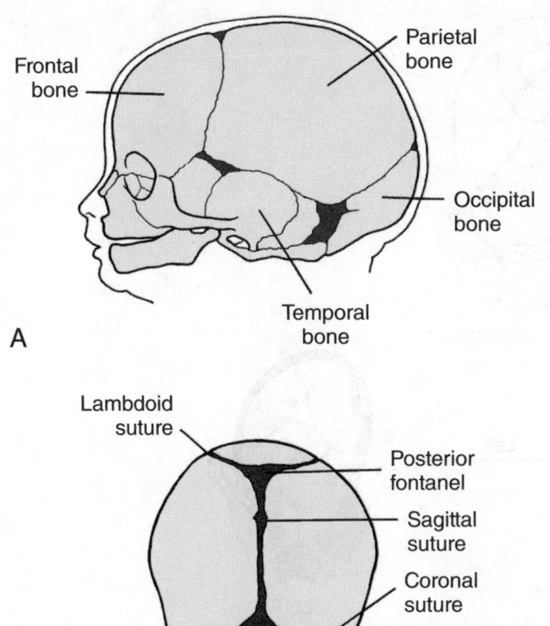

Fig. 15-1 Fetal head at term. **A,** Bones. **B,** Sutures and fontanels.

over one another also permits adaptation to the various diameters of the maternal pelvis. Molding can be extensive, but the heads of most newborns assume their normal shape within 3 days after birth.

Although the size of the fetal shoulders may affect passage, their position can be altered relatively easily during labor so that one shoulder may occupy a lower level than the other. This creates a shoulder diameter that is smaller than the skull, facilitating passage through the birth canal. The circumference of the fetal hips is usually small enough not to create problems.

Fetal Presentation

Presentation refers to the part of the fetus that enters the pelvic inlet first and leads through the birth canal during labor at term. The three main presentations are cephalic (head first), occurring in 96% of births (Fig. 15-2); breech (buttocks or feet first), occurring in 3% of births (Fig. 15-3, *A-C*); and shoulder, seen in 1% of births (see Fig. 15-3, *D*). Presenting part refers to that part of the fetal body first felt by the examining finger during a vaginal examination. In a cephalic presentation the presenting part is usually the occiput; in a breech presentation it is the sacrum; in the shoulder presentation it is the scapula. When the presenting part is the occiput, the presentation is noted as vertex (see Fig. 15-2). Factors that determine the presenting part include fetal lie, fetal attitude, and extension or flexion of the fetal head.

Fetal Lie

Lie is the relation of the long axis (spine) of the fetus to the long axis (spine) of the mother. The two primary lies are longitudinal, or vertical, in which the long axis of the fetus is parallel with the long axis of the mother (see Fig. 15-2); and transverse, horizontal, or oblique, in which the long axis of the fetus is at a right angle diagonal to the long axis of the mother (see Fig. 15-3, *D*). Longitudinal lies are either cephalic or breech presentations, depending on the fetal structure that first enters the mother's pelvis. Vaginal birth cannot occur when the fetus stays in a transverse lie. An oblique lie, one in which the long axis of the fetus is lying at an angle to the long axis of the mother, is less common and usually converts to a longitudinal or transverse lie during labor (Cunningham et al, 2005).

Fetal Attitude

Attitude is the relation of the fetal body parts to one another. The fetus assumes a characteristic posture (attitude) in utero partly because of the mode of fetal growth and partly because of the way the fetus conforms to the shape of the uterine cavity. Normally the back of the fetus is rounded so that the chin is flexed on the chest, the thighs are flexed on the abdomen, and the legs are flexed at the knees. The arms are crossed over the thorax, and the umbilical cord lies between the arms and the legs. This attitude is termed *general flexion* (see Fig. 15-2).

Deviations from the normal attitude may cause difficulties in childbirth. For example, in a cephalic presentation the fetal head may be extended or flexed in a manner that presents a head diameter that exceeds the limits of the maternal pelvis, leading to prolonged labor, forceps- or vacuum-assisted birth, or cesarean birth (see Fig. 15-5, *B* and *C*).

Certain critical diameters of the fetal head are usually measured. The biparietal diameter, which is about 9.25 cm at term, is the largest transverse diameter and an important indicator of fetal head size (Fig. 15-4, *B*). In a well-flexed cephalic presentation the biparietal diameter is the widest part of the head entering the pelvic inlet. Of the several anteroposterior diameters, the smallest and the most critical one is the suboccipitobregmatic diameter (about 9.5 cm at term). When the head is in complete flexion, this diameter allows the fetal head to pass through the true pelvis easily (Fig. 15-5, *A*). As the head is more extended, the anteroposterior diameter widens, and the head may not be able to enter the true pelvis (see Fig. 15-5, *B* and *C*).

Fetal Position

The presentation or presenting part indicates the portion of the fetus that overlies the pelvic inlet. Position is the relation of the presenting part (occiput, sacrum, mentum [chin], or sinciput [deflexed vertex]) to the four quadrants of the mother's pelvis (see Fig. 15-2). Position is denoted by a three-letter abbreviation. The first letter of the abbreviation denotes the location of the presenting part in the right (R) or left (L) side of the mother's pelvis. The middle letter stands for the specific presenting part of the fetus (O for occiput, S for sacrum, M for mentum [chin], and Sc for scapula [shoulder]). The third letter stands for the location of the presenting part in relation to the anterior (A), posterior (P), or transverse (T) portion of the maternal pelvis. For example, ROA means that the occiput is the presenting part and is located in the right anterior quadrant of the maternal pelvis (see Fig. 15-2). LSP

evolve Critical Thinking Exercise—Fetal Presentation

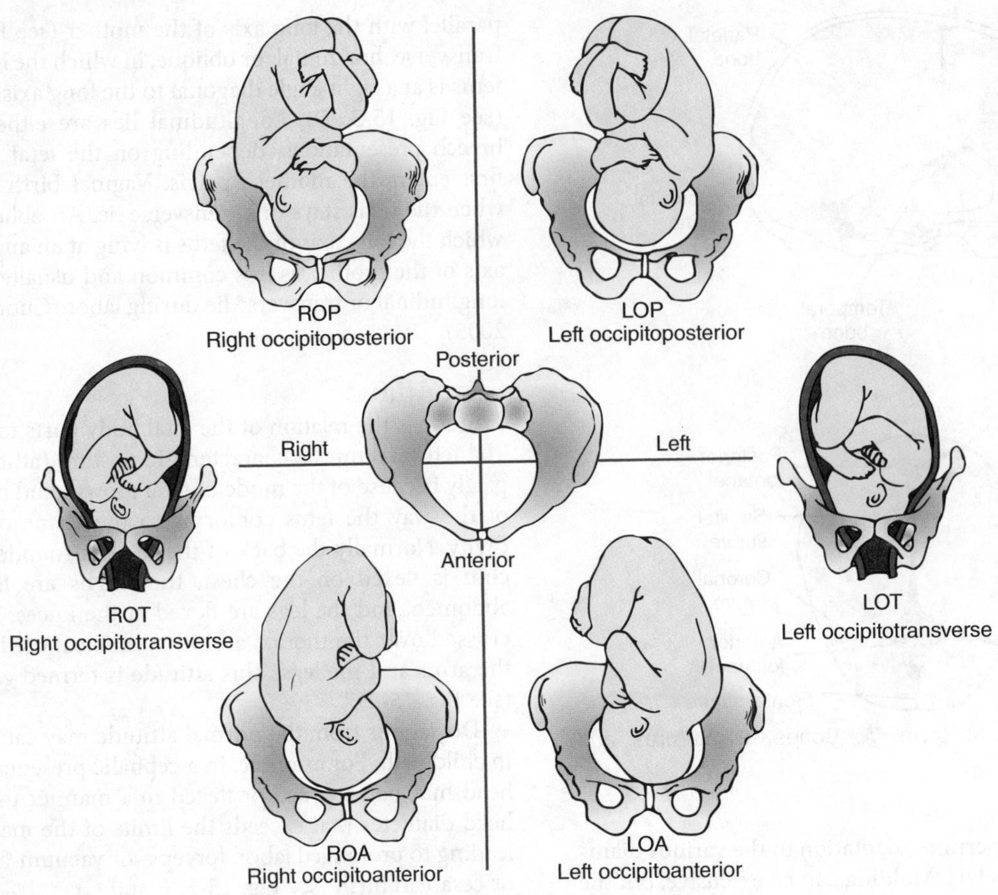

Fig. 15-2 Examples of fetal vertex (occiput) presentations in relation to front, back, or side of maternal pelvis.

means that the sacrum is the presenting part and is located in the left posterior quadrant of the maternal pelvis (see Fig. 15-3).

Station is the relation of the presenting part of the fetus to an imaginary line drawn between the maternal ischial spines and is a measure of the degree of descent of the presenting part of the fetus through the birth canal. The placement of the presenting part is measured in centimeters above or below the ischial spines (Fig. 15-6). For example, when the lowermost portion of the presenting part is 1 cm above the spines, it is noted as being minus (−) 1. At the level of the spines, the station is referred to as 0 (zero). When the presenting part is 1 cm below the spines, the station is said to be plus (+) 1. Birth is imminent when the presenting part is at +4 to +5 cm. The station of the presenting part should be determined when labor begins so that the rate of descent of the fetus during labor can be accurately determined.

Engagement is the term used to indicate that the largest transverse diameter of the presenting part (usually the biparietal diameter) has passed through the maternal pelvic brim or inlet into the true pelvis and usually corresponds to station 0. Engagement often occurs in the weeks just before labor begins in nulliparas and may occur before or during labor in multiparas. Engagement can be determined by abdominal or vaginal examination.

Passageway

The passageway, or birth canal, is composed of the mother's rigid bony pelvis and the soft tissues of the cervix, pelvic floor, vagina, and introitus (the external opening to the vagina). Although the soft tissues, particularly the muscular layers of the pelvic floor, contribute to vaginal birth of the fetus, the maternal pelvis plays a far greater role in the labor process because the fetus must successfully accommodate itself to this relatively rigid passageway. Therefore the size and shape of the pelvis must be determined before labor begins.

Bony Pelvis

The anatomy of the bony pelvis is described in Chapter 5. The following discussion focuses on the importance of pelvic configurations as they relate to the labor process. (It may be helpful to refer to Figs. 5-5 and 5-6.)

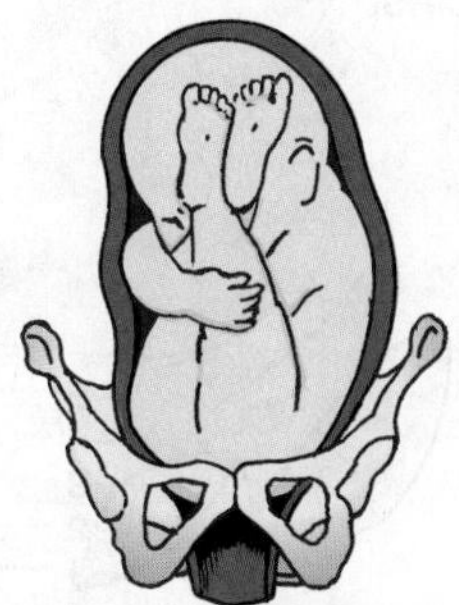

Frank breech

Lie: Longitudinal or vertical
Presentation: Breech (incomplete)
Presenting part: Sacrum
Attitude: Flexion, except for legs at knees

A

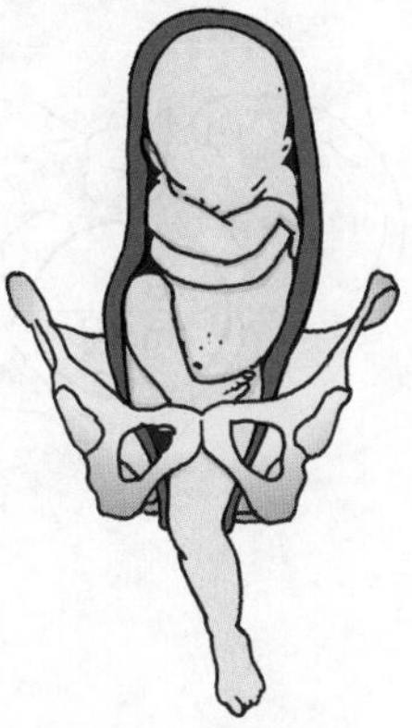

Single footling breech

Lie: Longitudinal or vertical
Presentation: Breech (incomplete)
Presenting part: Sacrum
Attitude: Flexion, except for one leg extended at hip and knee

B

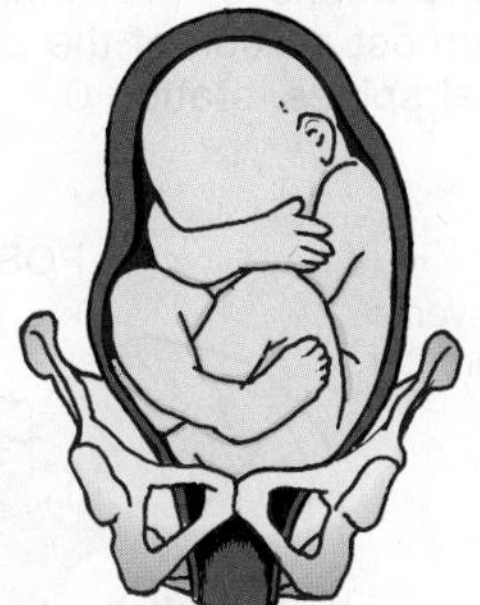

Complete breech

Lie: Longitudinal or vertical
Presentation: Breech (sacrum and feet presenting)
Presenting part: Sacrum (with feet)
Attitude: General flexion

C

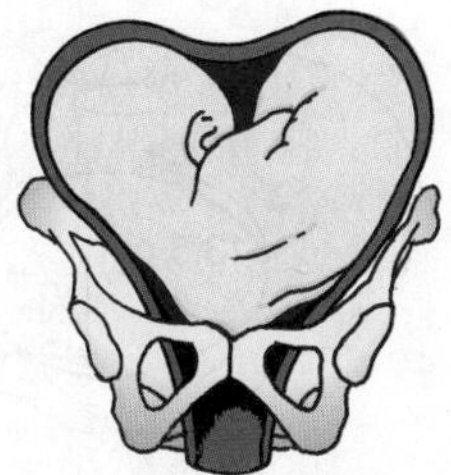

Shoulder presentation

Lie: Transverse or horizontal
Presentation: Shoulder
Presenting part: Scapula
Attitude: Flexion

D

Fig. 15-3 Fetal presentations. **A** to **C**, Breech (sacral) presentation. **D**, Shoulder presentation.

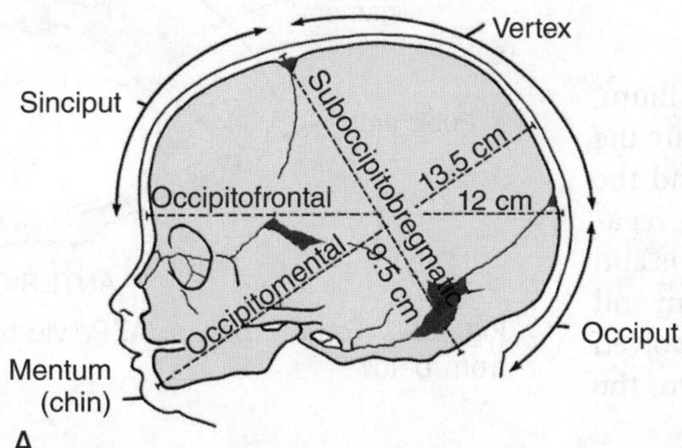

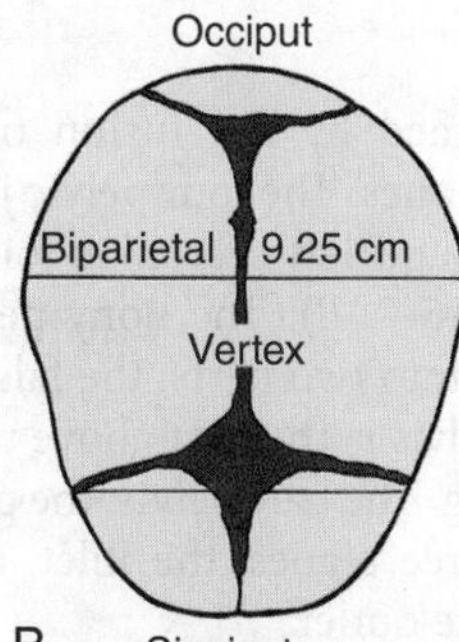

Fig. 15-4 Diameters of the fetal head at term. **A**, Cephalic presentations: occiput, vertex, and sinciput; and cephalic diameters: suboccipitobregmatic, occipitofrontal, and occipitomental. **B**, Biparietal diameter.

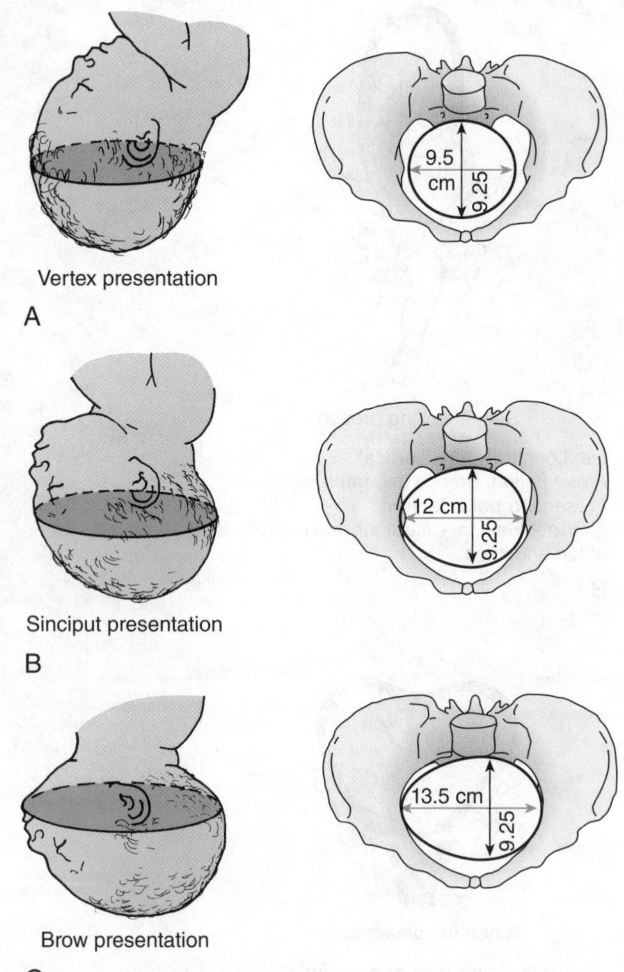

Fig. 15-5 Head entering pelvis. Biparietal diameter is indicated with shading (9.25 cm). A, Suboccipitobregmatic diameter: complete flexion of head on chest so that smallest diameter enters. B, Occipitofrontal diameter: moderate extension (military attitude) so that large diameter enters. C, Occipitomental diameter: marked extension (deflection) so that the largest diameter, which is too large to permit head to enter pelvis, is presenting.

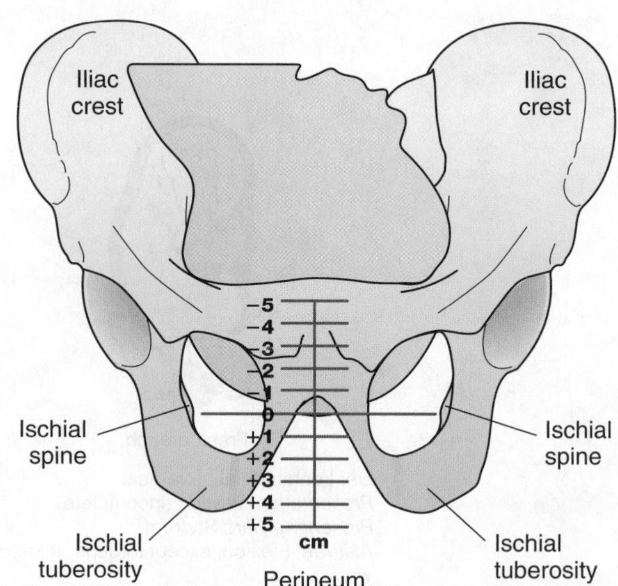

Fig. 15-6 Stations of presenting part, or degree of descent. The lowermost portion of the presenting part is at the level of the ischial spines, station 0.

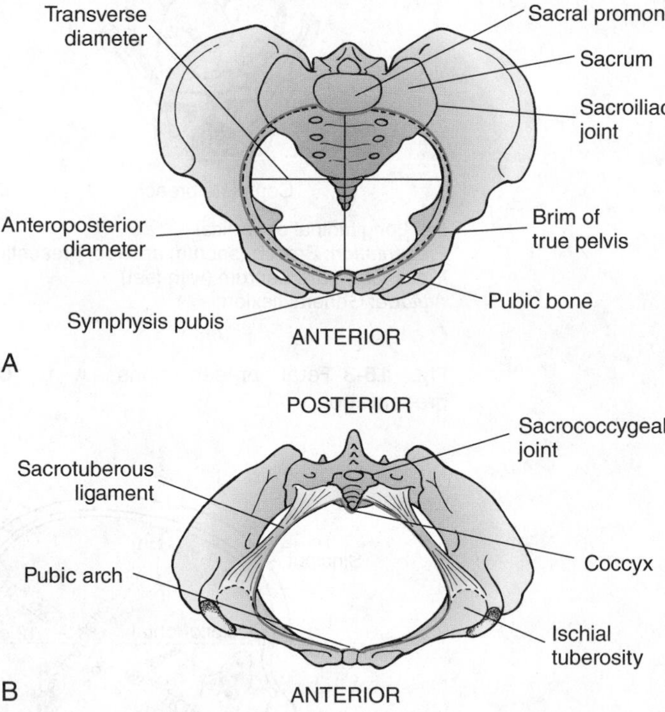

Fig. 15-7 Female pelvis. A, Pelvic brim above. B, Pelvic outlet from below.

The bony pelvis is formed by the fusion of the ilium, ischium, pubis, and sacral bones. The four pelvic joints are the symphysis pubis, the right and left sacroiliac joints, and the sacrococcygeal joint (Fig. 15-7, *B*). The bony pelvis is separated by the brim, or inlet, into two parts: the false pelvis and the true pelvis. The false pelvis is the part above the brim and plays no part in childbearing. The true pelvis, the part involved in birth, is divided into three planes: the inlet, or brim; the midpelvis, or cavity; and the outlet.

The pelvic inlet, which is the upper border of the true pelvis, is formed anteriorly by the upper margins of the pubic bone, laterally by the iliopectineal lines along the innominate bones, and posteriorly by the anterior, upper margin of the sacrum and the sacral promontory.

The pelvic cavity, or midpelvis, is a curved passage with a short anterior wall and a much longer concave posterior wall. It is bounded by the posterior aspect of the symphysis pubis, the ischium, a portion of the ilium, the sacrum, and the coccyx.

The pelvic outlet is the lower border of the true pelvis. Viewed from below, it is ovoid; somewhat diamond shaped; and bounded by the pubic arch anteriorly, the ischial tuberosities laterally, and the tip of the coccyx posteriorly (see Fig. 15-7, *B*). In the latter part of pregnancy the coccyx is movable (unless it has been broken in a fall during skiing or

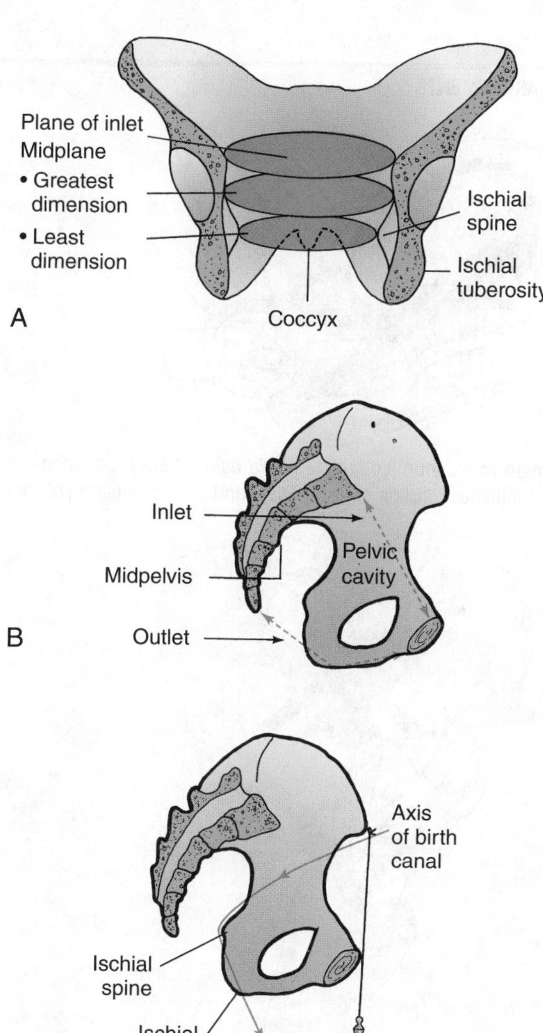

Fig. 15-8 Pelvic cavity. **A,** Inlet and midplane. Outlet not shown. **B,** Cavity of true pelvis. **C,** Note curve of sacrum and axis of birth canal.

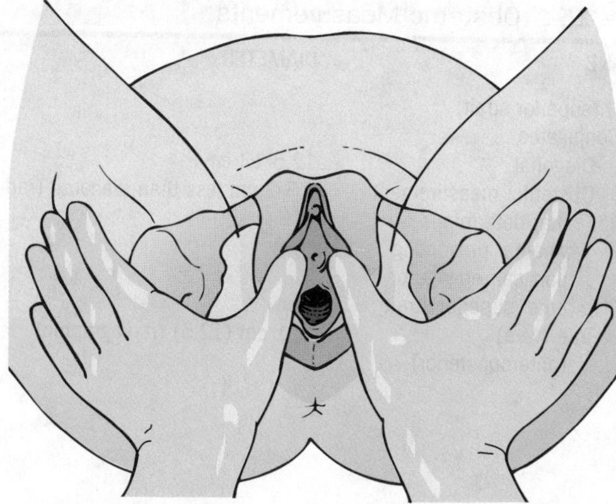

Fig. 15-9 Estimation of angle of subpubic arch. With both thumbs, examiner externally traces descending rami down to tuberosities. (From Barkauskas VH, Baumann LC, Darling-Fisher CS: *Health and physical assessment*, ed 3, St Louis, 2002, Mosby.)

skating, for example, and has fused to the sacrum during healing).

The pelvic canal varies in size and shape at various levels. The diameters at the plane of the pelvic inlet, midpelvis, and outlet, plus the axis of the birth canal (Fig. 15-8) determine whether vaginal birth is possible and the manner by which the fetus may pass down the birth canal.

The subpubic angle, which determines the type of pubic arch, together with the length of the pubic rami and the intertuberous diameter, is of great importance. Because the fetus must first pass beneath the pubic arch, a narrow subpubic angle is less accommodating than a rounded wide arch. The method of measurement of the subpubic arch is shown in Fig. 15-9. A summary of obstetric measurements is given in Table 15-1.

The four basic types of pelves are classified as follows:

1. Gynecoid (the classic female type)
2. Android (resembling the male pelvis)
3. Anthropoid (resembling the pelvis of anthropoid apes)
4. Platypelloid (the flat pelvis)

The gynecoid pelvis is the most common, with major gynecoid pelvic features present in 50% of all women. Anthropoid and android features are less common, and platypelloid pelvic features are the least common. Mixed types of pelves are more common than are pure types (Cunningham et al, 2005). Examples of pelvic variations and their effects on mode of birth are given in Table 15-2.

Assessment of the bony pelvis can be performed during the first prenatal evaluation and need not be repeated if the pelvis is of adequate size and suitable shape. In the third trimester of pregnancy the examination of the bony pelvis may be more thorough, and the results more accurate because there is relaxation and increased mobility of the pelvic joints and ligaments as a result of hormonal influences. Widening of the joint of the symphysis pubis and the resulting instability may cause pain in any or all of the pelvic joints.

Because the examiner does not have direct access to the bony structures and because the bones are covered with varying amounts of soft tissue, estimates of size and shape are approximate. Precise bony pelvis measurements can be determined by use of computed tomography, ultrasound, or x-ray films. However, radiographic examination is rarely done during pregnancy because the x-ray may damage the developing fetus.

Soft Tissues

The soft tissues of the passageway include the distensible lower uterine segment, cervix, pelvic floor muscles, vagina, and introitus. Before labor begins the uterus is composed of the uterine body (corpus) and cervix (neck). After labor has begun, uterine contractions cause the uterine body to have a thick and muscular upper segment and a thin-walled, passive, muscular lower segment. A physiologic retraction ring separates the two segments (Fig. 15-10). The lower uterine segment gradually distends to accommodate the intrauterine contents as the wall of the upper segment thickens and its accommo-

Table 15-1 Obstetric Measurements

PLANE	DIAMETER	MEASUREMENTS
Inlet (superior strait)		Length of diagonal conjugate *(solid colored line)*, obstetric conjugate *(broken colored line)*, and true conjugate *(black line)**
Conjugates		
Diagonal	12.5-13 cm	
Obstetric: measurement that determines whether presenting part can engage or enter superior strait	1.5-2 cm less than diagonal (radiographic)	
True (vera) (anteroposterior)	≥11 cm (12.5) (radiographic)	
Midplane		Measurement of interspinous diameter*
Transverse diameter (interspinous diameter)	10.5 cm	
The midplane of the pelvis normally is its largest plane and the one of greatest diameter.		
Outlet		Use of Thom's pelvimeter to measure intertuberous diameter*
Transverse diameter (intertuberous diameter) (biischial)	≥8 cm	
The outlet presents the smallest plane of the pelvic canal.		

*From Seidel HM et al: *Mosby's guide to physical examination*, ed 6, St Louis, 2006, Mosby.

dating capacity is reduced. The contractions of the uterine body thus exert downward pressure on the fetus, pushing it against the cervix.

The cervix effaces (thins) and dilates (opens) sufficiently to allow the first fetal portion to descend into the vagina. As the fetus descends, the cervix is actually drawn upward and over this first portion.

The pelvic floor is a muscular layer that separates the pelvic cavity above from the perineal space below. This structure helps the fetus rotate anteriorly as it passes through the birth

Table 15-2 Comparison of Pelvic Types

	GYNECOID (50% OF WOMEN)	ANDROID (23% OF WOMEN)	ANTHROPOID (24% OF WOMEN)	PLATYPELLOID (3% OF WOMEN)
Brim	Slightly ovoid or transversely rounded	Heart shaped, angulated	Oval, wider anteroposteriorly	Flattened anteroposteriorly, wide transversely
	Round	Heart	Oval	Flat
Depth	Moderate	Deep	Deep	Shallow
Side walls	Straight	Convergent	Straight	Straight
Ischial spines	Blunt, somewhat widely separated	Prominent, narrow interspinous diameter	Prominent, often with narrow interspinous diameter	Blunt, widely separated
Sacrum	Deep, curved	Slightly curved, terminal portion often beaked	Slightly curved	Slightly curved
Subpubic arch	Wide	Narrow	Narrow	Wide
Usual mode of birth	Vaginal Spontaneous Occipitoanterior position	Cesarean Vaginal Difficult with forceps	Forceps/spontaneous Occipitoposterior or occipitoanterior position	Vaginal Spontaneous

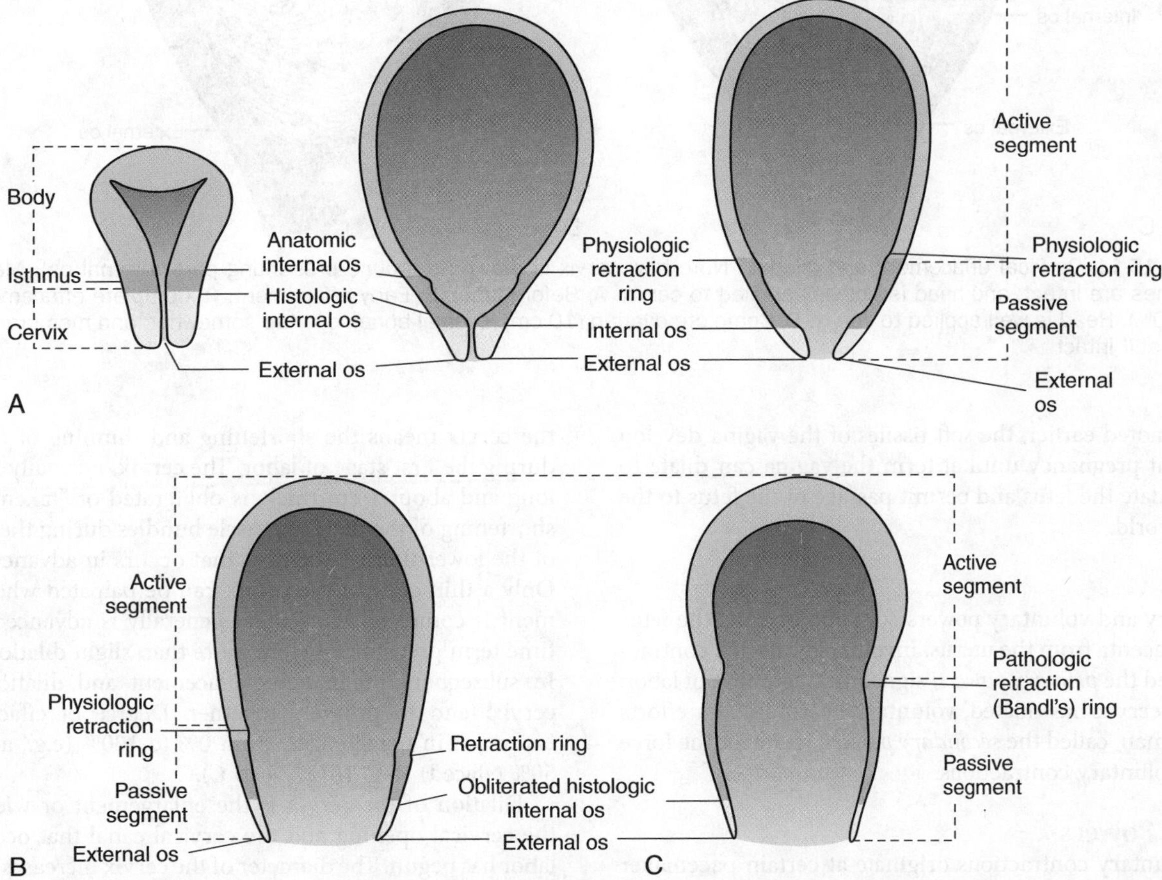

Fig. 15-10 Uterus in normal labor **A,** in early first stage; and **B,** in second stage. Passive segment is derived from lower uterine segment (isthmus) and cervix, and physiologic retraction ring is derived from anatomic internal os. **C,** Uterus in abnormal labor in second-stage dystocia. Pathologic retraction (Bandl's) ring that forms under abnormal conditions develops from the physiologic ring.

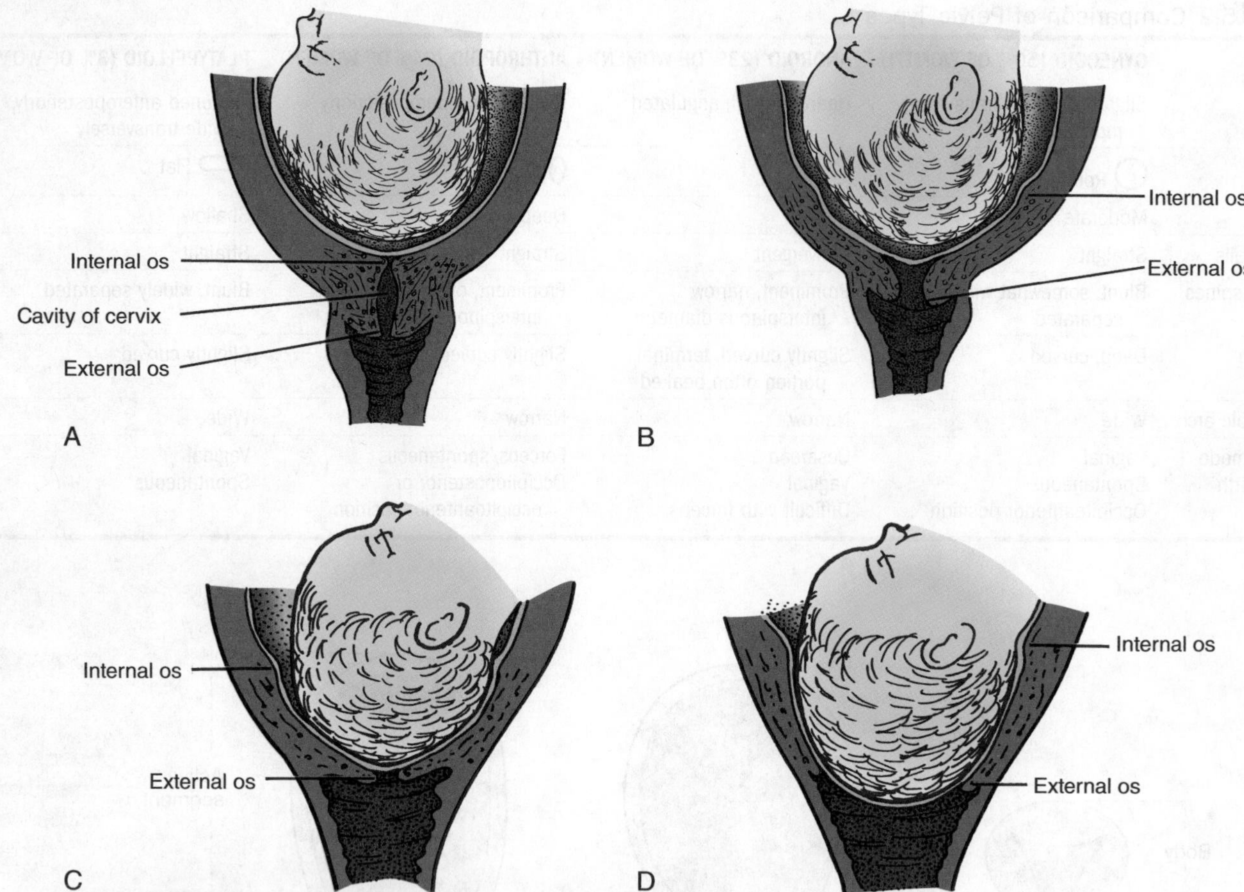

Fig. 15-11 Cervical effacement and dilation. Note how cervix is drawn up around presenting part (internal os). Membranes are intact, and head is not well applied to cervix. A, Before labor. B, Early effacement. C, Complete effacement (100%). Head is well applied to cervix. D, Complete dilation (10 cm). Cranial bones overlap somewhat, and membranes are still intact.

canal. As noted earlier, the soft tissues of the vagina develop throughout pregnancy until at term the vagina can dilate to accommodate the fetus and permit passage of the fetus to the external world.

Powers

Involuntary and voluntary powers combine to expel the fetus and the placenta from the uterus. Involuntary uterine contractions, called the *primary powers,* signal the beginning of labor. Once the cervix has dilated, voluntary bearing-down efforts by the woman, called the *secondary powers,* augment the force of the involuntary contractions.

Primary Powers

The involuntary contractions originate at certain pacemaker points in the thickened muscle layers of the upper uterine segment. From the pacemaker points contractions move downward over the uterus in waves, separated by short rest periods. Terms used to describe these involuntary contractions include *frequency* (the time from the beginning of one contraction to the beginning of the next), *duration* (length of contraction), and *intensity* (strength of contraction).

The primary powers are responsible for the effacement and dilation of the cervix and descent of the fetus. Effacement of the cervix means the shortening and thinning of the cervix during the first stage of labor. The cervix, normally 2 to 3 cm long and about 1 cm thick, is obliterated or "taken up" by a shortening of the uterine muscle bundles during the thinning of the lower uterine segment that occurs in advancing labor. Only a thin edge of the cervix can be palpated when effacement is complete. Effacement generally is advanced in first-time term pregnancy before more than slight dilation occurs. In subsequent pregnancies effacement and dilation of the cervix tend to progress together. Degree of effacement is expressed in percentages, from 0% to 100% (e.g., a cervix is 50% effaced) (Fig. 15-11, *A* to *C*).

Dilation of the cervix is the enlargement or widening of the cervical opening and the cervical canal that occurs once labor has begun. The diameter of the cervix increases from less than 1 cm to full dilation (approximately 10 cm) to allow birth of a term fetus. When the cervix is fully dilated (and completely retracted), it can no longer be palpated (see Fig. 15-11, *D*). Full cervical dilation marks the end of the first stage of labor.

Dilation of the cervix occurs by the drawing upward of the musculofibrous components of the cervix caused by strong uterine contractions. Pressure exerted by the amniotic fluid while the membranes are intact or by the force applied by the presenting part can promote cervical dilation. Scarring of the cervix as a result of prior infection or surgery may slow cervical dilation.

In the first and second stages of labor, increased intrauterine pressure caused by contractions exerts pressure on the descending fetus and the cervix. When the presenting part of the fetus reaches the perineal floor, mechanical stretching of the cervix occurs. Stretch receptors in the posterior vagina cause release of endogenous oxytocin that triggers the maternal urge to bear down, or the Ferguson reflex.

Uterine contractions are usually independent of external forces. For example, laboring women who are paralyzed because of spinal cord lesions above T-12 have normal but painless uterine contractions (Cunningham et al, 2005). However, uterine contractions may decrease temporarily in frequency and intensity if narcotic analgesic medication is given early in labor. Studies of effects of epidural analgesia have demonstrated prolonged length of labor for nulliparas both in the active phase of first-stage labor and in second-stage labor (Salim et al, 2005; Schiessl et al, 2005).

Secondary Powers

As soon as the presenting part reaches the pelvic floor, the contractions change in character and become expulsive. The laboring woman experiences an involuntary urge to push. She uses secondary powers (bearing-down efforts) to aid in expulsion of the fetus as she contracts her diaphragm and abdominal muscles and pushes. These bearing-down efforts result in increased intraabdominal pressure that compresses the uterus on all sides and adds to the power of the expulsive forces.

The secondary powers have no effect on cervical dilation, but they are of considerable importance in the expulsion of the infant from the uterus and vagina after the cervix is fully dilated. Studies have shown that pushing in the second stage is more effective and the woman is less fatigued when she begins to push only after she has the urge to do so rather than beginning to push when she is fully dilated without an urge to do so (Jacobson & Turner, 2008; Simpson & James, 2005; Yildirim & Beji, 2008).

When and how a woman pushes in the second stage is a much-debated topic. Studies have investigated the effects of spontaneous bearing-down efforts, directed pushing, delayed pushing, Valsalva maneuver (closed glottis and prolonged bearing down), and open glottis pushing (Gupta, Hofmeyr, & Smyth, 2004; Simpson & James, 2005). Although no significant differences have been found in the duration of second-stage labor, adverse effects of certain types of pushing techniques have been reported. Fetal hypoxia and subsequent acidosis have been associated with prolonged breath holding and forceful pushing efforts (Simpson & James, 2005). Perineal floor problems have been associated with directed pushing (Schaffer et al, 2005). Continued study is needed to determine the effectiveness and appropriateness of strategies used by nurses to teach pushing techniques, the suitability and effectiveness of various pushing techniques related to nonreassuring fetal heart patterns, and the standards for length of pushing in terms of maternal and fetal outcomes (Gennaro, Mayberry, & Kafulafula, 2007).

Position of the Laboring Woman

Position affects the woman's anatomic and physiologic adaptations to labor. Frequent changes in position relieve fatigue, increase comfort, and improve circulation. Therefore a laboring woman should be encouraged to find positions that are most comfortable to her (Fig. 15-12, *A*).

An upright position (walking, sitting, kneeling, or squatting) offers a number of advantages. Gravity can promote the descent of the fetus. Uterine contractions are generally stronger and more efficient in effacing and dilating the cervix, resulting in shorter labor (Gupta, Hofmeyr, & Smyth, 2004).

An upright position also is beneficial to the mother's cardiac output, which normally increases during labor as uterine contractions return blood to the vascular bed. The increased cardiac output improves blood flow to the uteroplacental unit and the maternal kidneys. Cardiac output is compromised if the descending aorta and ascending vena cava are compressed during labor. Compression of these major vessels may result in supine hypotension that decreases placental perfusion. With the woman in an upright position, pressure on the maternal vessels is reduced, and compression is prevented. If the woman wishes to lie down, a lateral position is suggested (Blackburn, 2007). Upright positions for women who have epidural analgesia are associated with a reduced duration of labor (Roberts et al, 2005).

The "all fours" position (hands and knees) may be used to relieve backache if the fetus is in an occipitoposterior position and may assist in anterior rotation of the fetus and in cases of shoulder dystocia (Hunter, Hofmeyr, & Kulier, 2007; Jevitt, Morse, & O'Donnell, 2008).

Positioning for second-stage labor (see Fig. 15-12, *B*) may be determined by the woman's preference, but it is constrained by the condition of the woman or fetus, the environment, and the health care provider's confidence in assisting in a birth in a specific position. The predominant position in the United States in physician-attended births is the lithotomy position. Alternative positions and position changes that result in more births over an intact perineum are more commonly practiced by nurse-midwives (Jacobson & Turner, 2008).

A woman who pushes in a semirecumbent position needs adequate body support to push effectively because her weight will be on her sacrum, moving the coccyx forward and causing a reduction in the pelvic outlet. In a sitting or squatting position abdominal muscles work in greater synchrony with uterine contractions during bearing-down efforts. Kneeling or squatting moves the uterus forward and aligns the fetus with the pelvic inlet and can facilitate the second stage of labor by increasing the pelvic outlet (Jacobson & Turner, 2008).

The lateral position can be used by the woman to help rotate a fetus that is in a posterior position. It also can be used when less force is needed for bearing down such as when there is a need to control the speed of a precipitate birth (Simkin & Ancheta, 2000).

No evidence exists that any of these positions suggested for second-stage labor increases the need for use of operative techniques (e.g., forceps- or vacuum-assisted birth, cesarean birth, episiotomy), causes perineal trauma, or adversely affects the newborn (Gupta, Hofmeyr, & Smyth, 2004; Roberts et al, 2005).

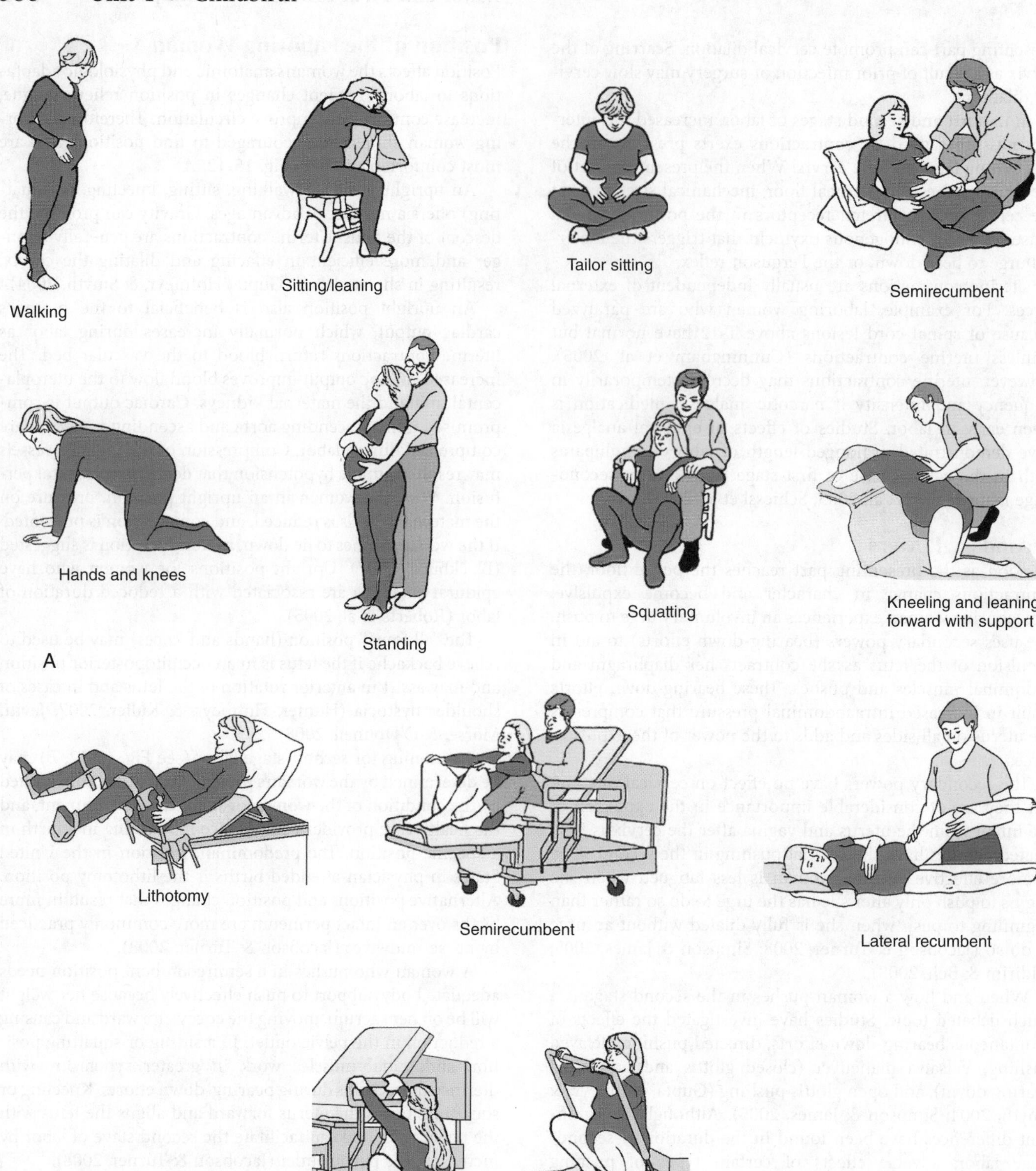

Fig. 15-12 Positions for labor and birth. A, Positions for labor. B, Positions for birth.

Process of Labor

The term *labor* refers to the process of moving the fetus, placenta, and membranes out of the uterus and through the birth canal. Various changes take place in the woman's reproductive system in the days and weeks before labor begins. Labor itself can be discussed in terms of the mechanisms involved in the process and the stages the woman moves through.

Signs Preceding Labor

In first-time pregnancies the uterus sinks downward and forward about 2 weeks before term, when the fetus's presenting part (usually the fetal head) descends into the true pelvis. This settling is called lightening, or "dropping," and usually happens gradually. After lightening women feel less congested and breathe more easily, but usually more bladder pressure results from this shift, and consequently there is a return of urinary frequency. In a multiparous pregnancy lightening may not take place until after uterine contractions are established and true labor is in progress.

The woman may complain of persistent low backache and sacroiliac distress as a result of relaxation of the pelvic joints. She may identify strong, frequent, but irregular uterine (Braxton Hicks) contractions.

The vaginal mucus becomes more profuse in response to the extreme congestion of the vaginal mucous membranes. Brownish or blood-tinged cervical mucus may be passed (bloody show). The cervix becomes soft (ripens) and partially effaced and may begin to dilate. The membranes may rupture spontaneously.

Other phenomena are common in the days preceding labor: (1) loss of 0.5 to 1.5 kg in weight, caused by water loss resulting from electrolyte shifts that in turn are produced by changes in estrogen and progesterone levels; and (2) a surge of energy. Women speak of having a burst of energy that they often use to clean the house and put everything in order. Less commonly some women have diarrhea, nausea, vomiting, and indigestion (see Community Focus box). Box 15-1 lists signs that may precede labor.

COMMUNITY FOCUS

The Processes of Childbirth: Class for Adolescents

You have been asked by your friend, a teacher in the local high school, to speak to the young people in her family life class about childbirth and what happens to the body during labor. The class has just learned that one of the young women is 4 months pregnant.

1. Identify essential content to be covered and describe how you would collect data about the group's knowledge and educational levels.
2. Plan a 25- to 30-minute class, including audiovisuals. Discuss the plan with your faculty.
3. Would you include mention of the young woman who is 4 months pregnant? Why or why not?
4. Present the class and ask the teacher to evaluate it in terms of level of content and appropriate cultural content.

BOX 15-1 Signs Preceding Labor

- Lightening
- Return of urinary frequency
- Backache
- Stronger Braxton Hicks contractions
- Weight loss of 0.5 to 1.5 kg
- Surge of energy
- Increased vaginal discharge; bloody show
- Cervical ripening
- Possible rupture of membranes

Onset of Labor

The onset of true labor cannot be ascribed to a single cause. Many factors, including changes in the maternal uterus, cervix, and pituitary gland, are involved. Hormones produced by the normal fetal hypothalamus, pituitary, and adrenal cortex probably contribute to the onset of labor. Progressive uterine distention, increasing intrauterine pressure, and aging of the placenta seem to be associated with increasing myometrial irritability. This is a result of increased concentrations of estrogen and prostaglandins, as well as decreasing progesterone levels. The mutually coordinated effects of these factors result in the occurrence of strong, regular, rhythmic uterine contractions. The outcome of these factors working together is normally the birth of the fetus and the expulsion of the placenta; however, how certain alterations trigger others and the ways in which proper checks and balances are maintained is not known.

Fetal fibronectin is a protein found in plasma and cervicovaginal secretions of pregnant women before the onset of labor. Assessment for the presence of fetal fibronectin is being used to predict the likelihood of preterm labor in women who are at increased risk for this complication, including those with twin gestation (Blackburn, 2007). The value of detection of fetal fibronectin in management of women with preterm labor continues to be investigated; therefore the test is not indicated for screening for preterm labor in low risk pregnant women (Pagana & Pagana, 2006).

Stages of Labor

Labor is considered "normal" when the woman is at or near term, no complications exist, a single fetus presents by vertex, and labor is completed within 18 hours. The course of normal labor, which is remarkably constant, consists of (1) regular progression of uterine contractions, (2) effacement and progressive dilation of the cervix, and (3) progress in descent of the presenting part. Four stages of labor are recognized. These stages are discussed in greater detail, along with nursing care for the laboring woman and family, in Chapter 18.

The first stage of labor is considered to last from the onset of regular uterine contractions to full dilation of the cervix. Commonly the onset of labor is difficult to establish because the woman may be admitted to the labor unit just before birth and the beginning of labor may be only an estimate. The first stage is much longer than the second and third combined. However, great variability is the rule, depending on the factors discussed previously in this chapter. Parity has a strong effect on the duration of first-stage labor (Gross, Drobnic, & Keirse, 2005). Full dilation may occur in less than 1 hour in some multiparous pregnancies. In first-time pregnancy complete dilation of the cervix can take 18 hours or longer. Variations may reflect differences in the patient population (e.g., risk status, age) or in clinical management of the labor and birth.

The first stage of labor is divided into three phases: a latent phase, an active phase, and a transition phase. During the latent phase there is more progress in effacement of the cervix and little increase in descent. During the active and transition phases there is more rapid dilation of the cervix and increased rate of descent of the presenting part. Maternal prepregnancy overweight and obesity can cause the active phase of labor to be longer than for women of normal weight (Liao, Buhimschi, & Norwitz, 2005).

The second stage of labor lasts from the time the cervix is fully dilated to the birth of the fetus. It takes an average of 20 minutes for a multiparous woman and 50 minutes for a nulliparous woman. Labor of up to 2 hours has been considered within the normal range for the second stage, but Cesaro (2004) found that a wider range of normal was still associated with no adverse effects on the mother or infant. Cheng, Hopkins, and Caughey (2004) found that a prolonged second stage was associated with increased rates of operative births and maternal morbidity. Epidural analgesia will likely prolong the second stage (Salim et al, 2005; Schiessl et al, 2005). Ethnicity may play a role in length of second-stage labor. Greenberg and associates (2006) found that nulliparous Asian women had a longer second stage than nulliparous white women, whereas African-American and Latino women had shorter second stages of labor.

Roberts (2002) described three phases of second-stage labor. The first phase is a period that begins about the time of complete dilation of the uterus, when the contractions are weak or not noticeable and the woman is not feeling the urge to push, is resting, or is exerting only small bearing-down efforts with contractions. The second phase is a period when contractions resume, the woman is making strong bearing-down efforts, and the fetal station is advancing. The third phase is a period lasting from the crowning until the birth.

The third stage of labor lasts from the birth of the fetus until the placenta is delivered. The placenta normally separates with the third or fourth strong uterine contraction after the infant has been born. After it has separated, the placenta can be delivered with the next uterine contraction. The duration of the third stage may be as short as 3 to 5 minutes, although up to 1 hour is considered within normal limits. The risk of hemorrhage increases as the length of the third stage increases (Cunningham et al, 2005).

The fourth stage of labor arbitrarily lasts about 2 hours after delivery of the placenta. It is the period of immediate recovery, when homeostasis is reestablished. It is an important period of observation for complications such as abnormal bleeding (see Chapter 23).

Mechanism of Labor

As already discussed, the female pelvis has varied contours and diameters at different levels, and the presenting part of the passenger is large in proportion to the passage. Therefore for vaginal birth to occur the fetus must adapt to the birth canal during the descent. The turns and other adjustments necessary in the human birth process are termed the *mechanism of labor* (Fig. 15-13). The seven cardinal movements of the mechanism of labor that occur in a vertex presentation are engagement, descent, flexion, internal rotation, extension, external rotation (restitution), and finally birth by expulsion. Although these movements are discussed separately, in actuality a combination of movements occurs simultaneously. For example, engagement involves both descent and flexion.

Engagement

When the biparietal diameter of the head passes the pelvic inlet, the head is said to be engaged in the pelvic inlet (see Fig. 15-13, *A*). In most nulliparous pregnancies this occurs before the onset of active labor because the firmer abdominal muscles direct the presenting part into the pelvis. In multiparous pregnancies in which the abdominal musculature is more relaxed, the head often remains freely movable above the pelvic brim until labor is established.

Asynclitism

The head usually engages in the pelvis in a synclitic position (i.e., one that is parallel to the anteroposterior plane of the pelvis). Frequently asynclitism occurs (the head is deflected anteriorly or posteriorly in the pelvis), which can facilitate descent because the head is being positioned to accommodate to the pelvic cavity (Fig. 15-14). Extreme asynclitism can cause cephalopelvic disproportion, even in a normal-size pelvis, because the head is positioned so that it cannot descend.

Descent

Descent refers to the progress of the presenting part through the pelvis. Descent depends on at least four forces: (1) pressure exerted by the amniotic fluid, (2) direct pressure exerted by the contracting fundus on the fetus, (3) force of the contraction of the maternal diaphragm and abdominal muscles in the second stage of labor, and (4) extension and straightening of the fetal body. The effects of these forces are modified by the size and shape of the maternal pelvic planes and the size of the fetal head and its capacity to mold.

The degree of descent is measured by the station of the presenting part (see Fig. 15-6). As mentioned, little descent occurs during the latent phase of the first stage of labor. Descent accelerates in the active phase when the cervix has dilated to 5 to 7 cm. It is especially apparent when the membranes have ruptured.

In a first-time pregnancy descent is usually slow but steady; in subsequent pregnancies descent may be rapid. Progress in descent of the presenting part is determined by abdominal palpation and vaginal examination until the presenting part can be seen at the introitus.

Flexion

As soon as the descending head meets resistance from the cervix, pelvic wall, or pelvic floor, it normally flexes so that the chin is brought into closer contact with the fetal chest (see Fig. 15-13, *B*). Flexion permits the smaller suboccipitobreg-

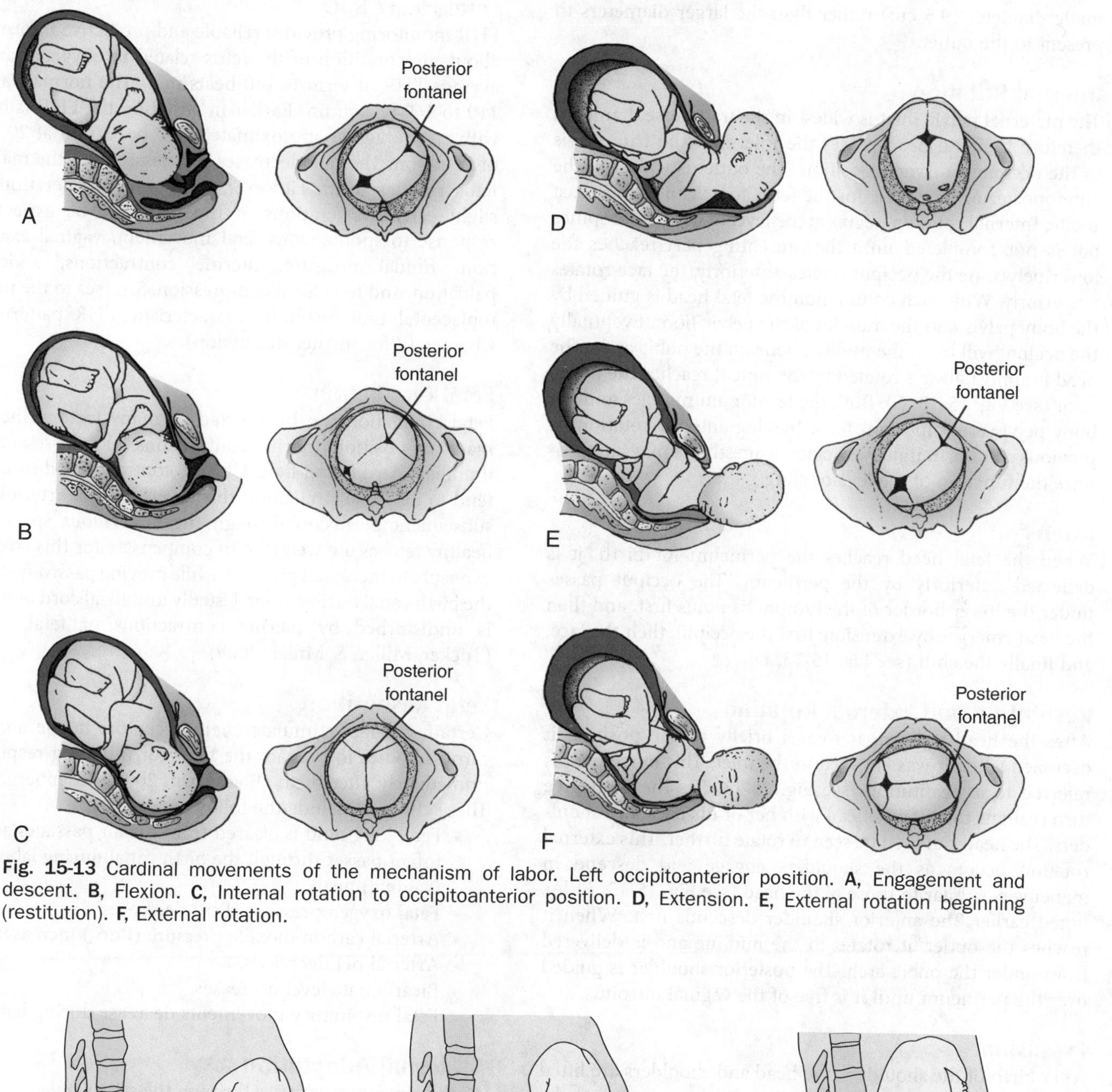

Posterior fontanel

A

D

Posterior fontanel

B

E

Posterior fontanel

C

F

Fig. 15-13 Cardinal movements of the mechanism of labor. Left occipitoanterior position. A, Engagement and descent. B, Flexion. C, Internal rotation to occipitoanterior position. D, Extension. E, External rotation beginning (restitution). F, External rotation.

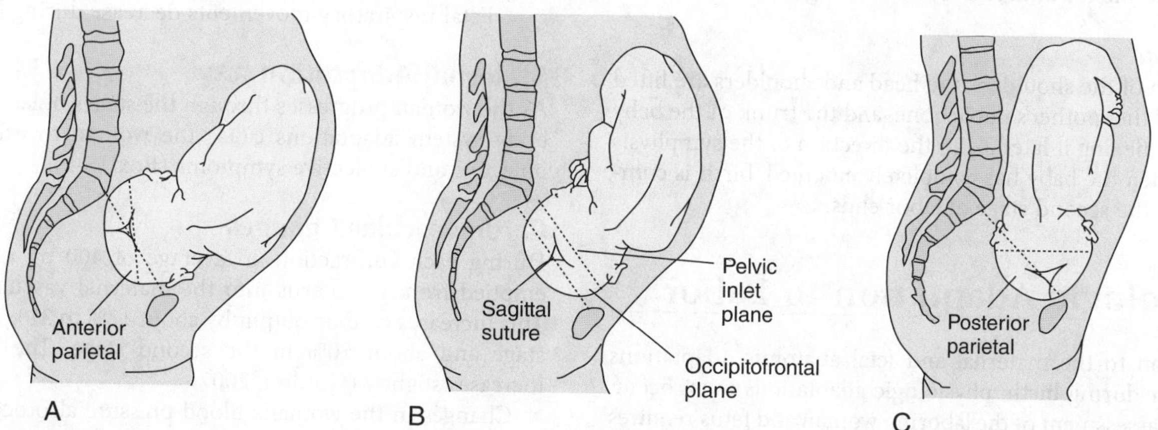

Fig. 15-14 Synclitism and asynclitism. A, Anterior asynclitism. B, Normal synclitism. C, Posterior asynclitism.

matic diameter (9.5 cm) rather than the larger diameters to present to the outlet.

Internal Rotation

The maternal pelvic inlet is widest in the transverse diameter; therefore the fetal head passes the inlet into the true pelvis in the occipitotransverse position. The outlet is widest in the anteroposterior diameter; for the fetus to exit the head must rotate. Internal rotation begins at the level of the ischial spines but is not completed until the presenting part reaches the lower pelvis. As the occiput rotates anteriorly, the face rotates posteriorly. With each contraction the fetal head is guided by the bony pelvis and the muscles of the pelvic floor. Eventually the occiput will be in the midline beneath the pubic arch. The head is almost always rotated by the time it reaches the pelvic floor (see Fig. 15-13, *C*). Both the levator ani muscles and the bony pelvis are important for achieving anterior rotation. A previous childbirth injury or regional anesthesia may compromise the function of the levator sling.

Extension

When the fetal head reaches the perineum for birth, it is deflected anteriorly by the perineum. The occiput passes under the lower border of the symphysis pubis first, and then the head emerges by extension: first the occiput, then the face, and finally the chin (see Fig. 15-13, *D*).

Restitution and External Rotation

After the head is born, it rotates briefly to the position it occupied when it was engaged in the inlet. This movement is referred to as restitution (see Fig. 15-13, *E*). The 45-degree turn realigns the infant's head with her or his back and shoulders. The head can then be seen to rotate further. This external rotation occurs as the shoulders engage and descend in maneuvers similar to those of the head (see Fig. 15-13, *F*). As noted earlier, the anterior shoulder descends first. When it reaches the outlet, it rotates to the midline and is delivered from under the pubic arch. The posterior shoulder is guided over the perineum until it is free of the vaginal introitus.

Expulsion

After birth of the shoulders, the head and shoulders are lifted up toward the mother's pubic bone, and the trunk of the baby is born by flexing it laterally in the direction of the symphysis pubis. When the baby has completely emerged, birth is complete, and the second stage of labor ends.

Physiologic Adaptation to Labor

In addition to the maternal and fetal anatomic adaptations that occur during birth, physiologic adaptations must occur. Accurate assessment of the laboring woman and fetus requires knowledge of these expected adaptations.

Fetal Adaptation

Several important physiologic adaptations occur in the fetus. These changes occur in fetal heart rate (FHR), fetal circulation, respiratory movements, and other behaviors.

Fetal Heart Rate

FHR monitoring provides reliable and predictive information about the condition of the fetus related to oxygenation. The average FHR at term is 140 beats/min. The normal range is 110 to 160 beats/min. Earlier in gestation the FHR is higher, with an average of approximately 160 beats/min at 20 weeks of gestation. The rate decreases progressively as the maturing fetus reaches term. However, temporary accelerations and slight early decelerations of the FHR can be expected in response to spontaneous fetal movement, vaginal examination, fundal pressure, uterine contractions, abdominal palpation, and fetal head compression. Stresses to the uterofetoplacental unit result in characteristic FHR patterns (see Chapter 17 for further discussion).

Fetal Circulation

Fetal circulation can be affected by many factors, including maternal position, uterine contractions, blood pressure, and umbilical cord blood flow. Uterine contractions during labor tend to decrease circulation through the spiral arterioles and subsequent perfusion through the intervillous space. Most healthy fetuses are well able to compensate for this stress and exposure to increased pressure while moving passively through the birth canal during labor. Usually umbilical cord blood flow is undisturbed by uterine contractions or fetal position (Tucker, Miller, & Miller, 2009).

Fetal Respiration

Certain changes stimulate chemoreceptors in the aorta and carotid bodies to prepare the fetus for initiating respirations immediately after birth (Blackburn, 2007; Rosenberg, 2007). These changes include the following:

- Fetal lung fluid is cleared from the air passages as the infant passes through the birth canal during labor and (vaginal) birth.
- Fetal oxygen pressure (Po_2) decreases.
- Arterial carbon dioxide pressure (Pco_2) increases.
- Arterial pH decreases.
- Bicarbonate level decreases.
- Fetal respiratory movements decrease during labor.

Maternal Adaptation

As the woman progresses through the stages of labor, various body system adaptations cause the woman to exhibit both objective and subjective symptoms (Box 15-2).

Cardiovascular Changes

During each contraction an average of 400 ml of blood is emptied from the uterus into the maternal vascular system. This increases cardiac output by about 12% to 31% in the first stage and about 50% in the second stage. The heart rate increases slightly (Gordon, 2007).

Changes in the woman's blood pressure also occur. Blood flow, which is reduced in the uterine artery by contractions, is redirected to peripheral vessels. As a result, peripheral resistance increases, and blood pressure increases (Gordon, 2007). During the first stage of labor uterine contractions cause systolic readings to increase by approximately 10 mm Hg; therefore assessing blood pressure between contractions provides

BOX 15-2 Maternal Physiologic Changes During Labor

- Cardiac output increases 10% to 15% in first stage; 30% to 50% in second stage.
- Heart rate increases slightly in first and second stages.
- Systolic blood pressure increases during uterine contractions in first stage; systolic and diastolic pressures increase during uterine contractions in second stage.
- White blood cell count increases.
- Respiratory rate increases.
- Temperature may be slightly elevated.
- Proteinuria (+1) may occur.
- Gastric motility and absorption of solid food is decreased; nausea and vomiting may occur during transition to second-stage labor.
- Blood glucose level decreases.

more accurate readings. During the second stage contractions may cause systolic pressures to increase by 30 mm Hg and diastolic readings to increase by 25 mm Hg, with both systolic and diastolic pressures remaining somewhat elevated even between contractions (Gordon, 2007). Therefore the woman already at risk for hypertension is at increased risk for complications such as cerebral hemorrhage.

CRITICAL THINKING EXERCISE

Anxiety in a Multipara in Active Labor

Jody was admitted in labor to an LDR room 2 hours ago. She is 39 weeks of gestation in her second pregnancy. She is noticeably anxious and tells you that her first pregnancy ended at term but that the labor was "terrible. It was 22 hours long. I had an epidural but had to push and push to get the baby out." What interventions are appropriate?

1. Evidence—Is there sufficient evidence to draw conclusions about what intervention is needed?
2. Assumptions—Describe underlying assumptions about the following issues:
   a. Effects of anxiety on progress in labor
   b. Effect of parity on labor
   c. Effect of epidural analgesia on ability to push
   d. Education needed by Jody
3. What implications and priorities for nursing care can be made at this time?
4. Does the evidence objectively support your conclusion?
5. Are there alternative perspectives to your conclusions?

LDR, Labor, delivery, and recovery.

Supine hypotension (see Fig. 18-4, p. 451) occurs when the ascending vena cava and descending aorta are compressed. The laboring woman is at greater risk for supine hypotension if the uterus is particularly large because of multifetal pregnancy, hydramnios, or obesity or if the woman is dehydrated or hypovolemic. In addition, anxiety and pain, as well as some medications, can cause hypotension.

The woman should be discouraged from using the Valsalva maneuver (holding one's breath and tightening abdominal muscles) for pushing during the second stage. This activity increases intrathoracic pressure, reduces venous return, and increases venous pressure. The cardiac output and blood pressure increase, and the pulse slows temporarily. During the Valsalva maneuver fetal hypoxia may occur. The process is reversed when the woman takes a breath.

The white blood cell (WBC) count can increase (Blackburn, 2007). Although the mechanism leading to this increase in WBCs is unknown, it may be secondary to physical or emotional stress or to tissue trauma. Labor is strenuous, and physical exercise alone can increase the WBC count.

Some peripheral vascular changes occur, perhaps in response to cervical dilation or compression of maternal vessels by the fetus passing through the birth canal. Flushed cheeks, hot or cold feet, and eversion of hemorrhoids may result.

Respiratory Changes

Increased physical activity with greater oxygen consumption is reflected in an increase in the respiratory rate. Hyperventilation may cause respiratory alkalosis (an increase in pH), hypoxia, and hypocapnia (decrease in carbon dioxide). In the unmedicated woman in the second stage, oxygen consumption almost doubles. Anxiety also increases oxygen consumption.

Renal Changes

During labor spontaneous voiding may be difficult for various reasons: tissue edema caused by pressure from the presenting part, discomfort, analgesia, and embarrassment. Proteinuria up to +1 is a normal finding because it can occur in response to the breakdown of muscle tissue from the physical work of labor.

Integumentary Changes

The integumentary system changes are evident, especially in the great distensibility (stretching) in the area of the vaginal introitus. The degree of distensibility varies with the individual. Despite this ability to stretch, even in the absence of episiotomy or lacerations, minute tears in the skin around the vaginal introitus occur.

Musculoskeletal Changes

The musculoskeletal system is stressed during labor. Diaphoresis, fatigue, proteinuria (+1), and possibly an increased temperature accompany the marked increase in muscle activity. Backache and joint ache (unrelated to fetal position) occur as a result of increased joint laxity at term. The labor process itself and the woman's pointing her toes can cause leg cramps.

Neurologic Changes

Sensorial changes occur as the woman moves through phases of the first stage of labor and from one stage to the next. Initially she may be euphoric. Euphoria gives way to increased seriousness, to amnesia between contractions during the second stage, and finally to elation or fatigue after giving birth. Endogenous endorphins (morphinelike chemicals produced naturally by the body) raise the pain threshold and produce sedation. In addition, physiologic anesthesia of perineal tissues, caused by pressure of the presenting part, decreases perception of pain.

Gastrointestinal Changes

During labor gastrointestinal motility and absorption of solid foods are decreased, and stomach-emptying time is slowed. Nausea and vomiting of undigested food eaten after onset of labor are common. Nausea and belching also occur as a reflex response to full cervical dilation. The woman may state that diarrhea accompanied the onset of labor, or the nurse may palpate the presence of hard or impacted stool in the rectum.

Endocrine Changes

The onset of labor may be triggered by decreasing levels of progesterone and increasing levels of estrogen, prostaglandins, and oxytocin. Metabolism increases, and blood glucose levels may decrease with the work of labor.

Accurate assessment of the mother and fetus during labor and birth depends on knowledge of these expected adaptations so that appropriate interventions can be implemented.

Key Points

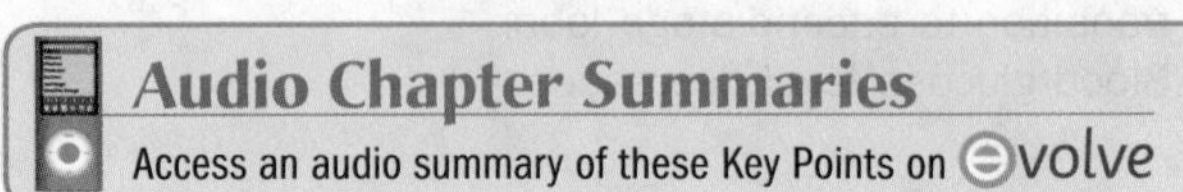
Audio Chapter Summaries
Access an audio summary of these Key Points on evolve

- Labor and birth are affected by the five *P's*: passenger, passageway, powers, position of the woman, and psychologic response.
- Because of its size and relative rigidity, the fetal head is a major factor in determining the course of birth.
- The diameters at the plane of the pelvic inlet, midpelvis, and outlet, plus the axis of the birth canal, determine whether vaginal birth is possible and the manner in which the fetus passes down the birth canal.
- Involuntary uterine contractions act to expel the fetus and placenta during the first stage of labor; these are augmented by voluntary bearing-down efforts during the second stage.
- The first stage of labor lasts from the time dilation begins to the time when the cervix is fully dilated. The second stage of labor lasts from the time of full dilation to the birth of the infant. The third stage of labor lasts from the infant's birth to the expulsion of the placenta. The fourth stage is the first 2 hours after birth.
- The cardinal movements of the mechanism of labor are engagement, descent, flexion, internal rotation, extension, restitution and external rotation, and expulsion of the infant.
- Although the events precipitating the onset of labor are unknown, many factors, including changes in the maternal uterus, cervix, and pituitary gland, are thought to be involved.
- A healthy fetus with an adequate uterofetoplacental circulation will be able to compensate for the stress of uterine contractions.
- As the woman progresses through labor, various body systems adapt to the birth process.
- When pushing, the woman should be encouraged to use the open-glottis method rather than the closed-glottis method.

References

Blackburn ST: *Maternal, fetal, and neonatal physiology: a clinical perspective*, ed 3, St Louis, 2007, Saunders.

Cesaro S: Reevaluation of Friedman's labor curve: a pilot study, *J Obstet Gynecol Neonatal Nurs* 33(6):713-722, 2004.

Cheng Y, Hopkins L, Caughey A: How long is too long: does a prolonged second stage of labor in nulliparous women affect maternal and neonatal outcomes? *Am J Obstet Gynecol* 191(3):933-938, 2004.

Cunningham F et al: *Williams obstetrics*, ed 22, New York, 2005, McGraw-Hill.

Gennaro S, Mayberry L, Kafulafula U: The evidence supporting nursing management of labor, *J Obstet Gynecol Neonatal Nurs* 36(6):598-604, 2007.

Gordon M: Maternal physiology. In Gabbe SG, Niebyl JR, Simpson JL (editors): *Obstetrics: normal and problem pregnancies*, ed 5, Philadelphia, 2007, Churchill Livingstone.

Greenberg M et al: Are there ethnic differences in the length of labor? *Am J Obstet Gynecol* 195(3):743-748, 2006.

Gross M, Drobnic S, Keirse M: Influence of fixed and time-dependent factors on duration of normal first stage labor, *Birth* 32(1): 27-33, 2005.

Gupta JK, Hofmeyr GJ, Smyth RMD: Position in the second stage of labour for women without epidural anaesthesia (Cochrane Review). *Cochrane Database of Systematic Reviews*, 2004, Issue 1, Art No CD002006. DOI: 10.1002/14651858.CD002006.pub2.

Hunter S, Hofmeyr GJ, Kulier R: Hands and knees posture in late pregnancy or labour for fetal malposition (lateral or posterior). *Cochrane Database of Systematic Reviews*, 2007, Issue 4, Art No CD001063. DOI: 10.1002/14651858.CD001063.pub3.

Jacobson P, Turner L: Management of the second stage of labor in women with epidural analgesia, *J Midwifery Women's Health* 53(1):82-85, 2008.

Jevitt CM, Morse S, O'Donnell YS: Shoulder dystocia: nursing prevention and posttrauma care, *J Perinat Neonatal Nurs* 22(1):14-20, 2008.

Liao J, Buhimschi D, Norwitz E: Normal labor: mechanism and duration, *Obstet Gynecol Clin North Am* 32(2):145-164, 2005.

Pagana KD, Pagana TJ: *Mosby's manual of diagnostic and laboratory tests*, ed 3, St Louis, 2006, Mosby.

Roberts C et al: A meta-analysis of upright positions in the second stage to reduce instrumental deliveries in women with epidural analgesia, *Acta Obstet Gynecol Scand* 84(8):794-798, 2005.

Roberts JE: The "push" for evidence: management of the second stage, *J Midwifery Womens Health* 47(1):2-15, 2002.

Rosenberg A: The neonate. In Gabbe SG, Niebyl JR, Simpson JL (editors): *Obstetrics: normal and problem pregnancies*, ed 5, New York, 2007, Churchill Livingstone.

Salim R et al: Continuous compared with intermittent epidural infusion on progress of labor and patient satisfaction, *Obstet Gynecol* 106(2): 301-306, 2005.

Schaffer J et al: A randomized trial of the effects of coached vs. uncoached maternal pushing during the second stage of labor on postpartum pelvic floor structure and function, *Am J Obstet Gynecol* 192(5):1692-1696, 2005.

Schiessl B et al: Obstetrical parameters influencing the duration of second stage labor, *Eur J Obstet Gynecol Reprod Biol* 118(1):17-20, 2005.

Simkin P, Ancheta R: *The labor progress handbook: early interventions to prevent and treat dystocia*, Oxford, 2000, Blackwell Science.

Simpson K, James D: Effects of immediate versus delayed pushing during second-stage labor on fetal well-being: a randomized clinical trial, *Nurs Res* 54(3):149-157, 2005.

Tucker S, Miller L, Miller D: *Mosby's pocket guide to fetal monitoring: a multidisciplinary approach*, ed 6, St Louis, 2009, Mosby.

VandeVusse L: The essential forces of labor revisited: 13 Ps reported in women's stories, *MCN Am J Matern Child Nurs* 24(4):176-184, 1999.

Yildirim G, Beji N: Effects of pushing techniques in birth on mother and fetus: randomized study, *Birth* 35(1):25-30, 2008.

Unit 4

16 Management of Discomfort

Learning Objectives

On completion of this chapter the reader will be able to:

- Compare various childbirth preparation methods.
- Describe breathing and relaxation techniques used for each stage of labor.
- Identify nonpharmacologic strategies to enhance relaxation and decrease discomfort during labor.
- Discuss types of analgesia and anesthesia used during labor.
- Compare pharmacologic methods of relief of discomfort in different stages of labor and for different methods of birth.
- Describe nursing responsibilities appropriate for a woman receiving analgesia and anesthesia during labor.

Electronic Resources

Additional information related to the content in Chapter 16 can be found on

evolve the Companion Website at

http://evolve.elsevier.com/Perry/maternal/

- NCLEX Review Questions
- Critical Thinking Exercise—Patient Receiving Epidural Block
- Nursing Care Plan—Epidural Block During Labor
- Nursing Care Plan—Nonpharmacologic Management of Discomfort
- Spanish Guidelines—Pain Management

Pain is an unpleasant, complex, highly individualized phenomenon with both sensory and emotional components. Pregnant women commonly worry about the pain they will experience during labor and birth and how they will react to and deal with that pain. Many physiologic, psychosocial, and environmental factors influence the nature and degree of pain of a woman in labor and the manner in which she will respond to and cope with the pain (Lowe, 2002). A variety of childbirth preparation methods are available to help the woman or couple cope with the discomfort of labor. The methods selected depend on the situation, availability, and the preferences of the woman and her primary health care provider.

The discomforts experienced during labor are discussed in this chapter, as are nonpharmacologic and pharmacologic interventions to relieve the discomforts during the different stages of labor. This information provides the basis for understanding the nurse's role in management of maternal discomfort during labor.

Discomfort During Labor and Birth

Neurologic Origins

The pain and discomfort experienced during labor has two origins: visceral and somatic (Lowe, 2002). During the first stage of labor uterine contractions cause cervical dilation and effacement. Uterine ischemia (decreased blood flow and therefore local oxygen deficit) results from compression of the arteries supplying the myometrium during uterine contractions. Pain impulses during the first stage of labor are transmitted through the T10 to T12 spinal nerve segment and accessory lower thoracic and upper lumbar sympathetic nerves. These nerves originate in the uterine body and cervix.

The pain from cervical changes, distention of the lower uterine segment, and uterine ischemia that predominates during the first stage of labor is visceral pain. It is located over the lower portion of the abdomen. Referred pain occurs when the pain that originates in the uterus radiates to the abdominal wall, lumbosacral area of the back, iliac crests, gluteal area, and down the thighs. The woman usually has discomfort only during contractions and is free of pain between contractions, although some women have continuous contraction-related low back pain, even in the interval between contractions (Lowe, 2002; Trout, 2004).

During the second stage of labor, the stage of expulsion of the baby, the woman experiences somatic pain. This pain is often described as intense, sharp, burning, and well localized. Pain results from stretching and distention of perineal tissues and the pelvic floor to allow passage of the fetus, from distention and traction on the peritoneum and uterocervical supports during contractions, and from lacerations of soft tissue (e.g., cervix, vagina, perineum). Discomfort also can be produced by expulsive forces or pressure exerted by the presenting part on the bladder, bowel, or other sensitive pelvic structures. Pain impulses during the second stage of labor are carried from perineal tissues via the S2 to S4 spinal nerve segments and the parasympathetic system (Lowe, 2002).

Pain during the third stage of labor and the afterpains of the early postpartum period are uterine, similar to that expe-

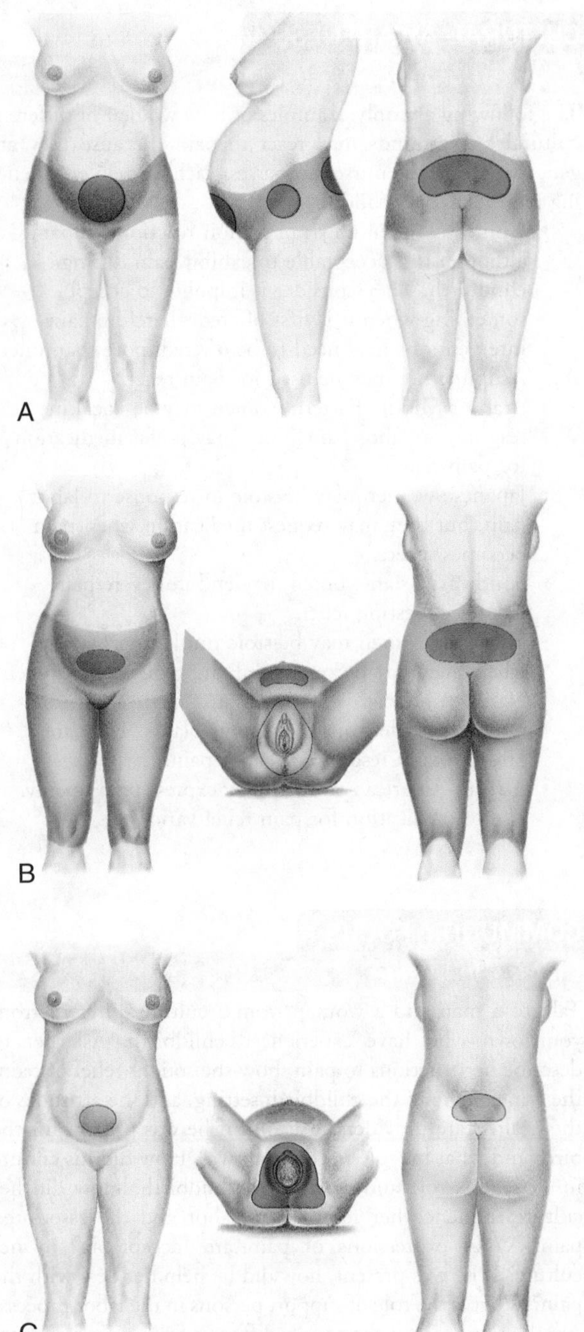

Fig. 16-1 Discomfort during labor. A, Distribution of labor pain during first stage. B, Distribution of labor pain during later phase of first stage and early phase of second stage. C, Distribution of labor pain during later phase of second stage and during birth. (*Gray shading* indicates areas of mild discomfort; *light-colored shading* indicates areas of moderate discomfort; *dark-colored shading* indicates areas of intense discomfort.)

rienced early in the first stage of labor. Areas of discomfort during labor are illustrated in Fig. 16-1.

Perception of Pain

Although the pain threshold is remarkably similar in all persons regardless of gender, social, ethnic, or cultural differences, these differences play a definite role in the person's perception of and behavioral responses to pain. The effects of factors such as culture, counterstimuli, and distraction in coping with pain are not fully understood. The meaning of pain and the verbal and nonverbal expressions given to pain are apparently learned from interactions within the primary social group. Cultural influences may impose unrealistic expectations. For instance, women from some cultural groups (e.g., Asian, Amish) believe it is shameful and counterproductive to scream or show pain and therefore avoid outward expressions when they are in pain (Trout, 2004).

Expression of Pain

Pain results in physiologic effects and sensory and emotional (affective) responses. During childbirth pain gives rise to identifiable physiologic effects. Sympathetic nervous system activity is stimulated in response to intensifying pain, resulting in increased catecholamine levels. Blood pressure and heart rate increase. Maternal respiratory patterns change in response to an increase in oxygen consumption. Hyperventilation, sometimes accompanied by respiratory alkalosis, can occur as pain intensifies. Pallor and diaphoresis may be seen. Gastric acidity increases, and nausea and vomiting are common in the active phase of labor. Placental perfusion may decrease, and uterine activity may diminish, potentially prolonging labor and affecting fetal well-being.

The sensory quality of visceral and somatic pain has been described as prickling, stabbing, burning, bursting, aching, heavy, pulling, throbbing, sharp, shooting, stinging, or cramping. The emotional (affective) quality of pain has been described as tiring, exhausting, annoying, sickening, and nauseating (Lowe, 2002).

Certain emotional (affective) expressions of suffering are often seen. Such changes include increasing anxiety with lessened perceptual field, writhing, crying, groaning, gesturing (hand clenching and wringing), and excessive muscular excitability throughout the body. Cultural expression of pain may vary. For example, Native American women may endure pain quietly, whereas Hispanic women may endure pain stoically because it is expected and esteemed but consider it acceptable to cry out. Chinese women often use soft voices and calm demeanors to cope with pain as a means of conserving energy during labor, whereas Mayan women may repeat a mantra and call out to the Lord to cope with pain and enhance the labor process (Callister et al, 2003).

Factors Influencing Pain Response

Pain during childbirth is unique to each woman. How she perceives or interprets that pain is influenced by a variety of physiologic, psychologic, emotional, social, cultural, and environmental factors (Trout, 2004). Women who approach pain as a challenge for which they have sufficient resources to cope effectively are unlikely to equate pain with suffering. In contrast, women without sufficient self-confidence and coping strategies may feel threatened and view their pain experience as suffering (Lowe, 2002; Simkin & Bolding, 2004).

Physiologic Factors

A variety of physiologic factors can affect the intensity of pain experienced by women during childbirth. Women with a history of dysmenorrhea may experience increased pain during childbirth as a result of higher prostaglandin levels. Back pain associated with menstruation also may increase the likelihood of contraction-related low back pain. When upright positions are assumed during labor, they seem to result in decreased pain and an overall increase in comfort when compared with the supine position. Women also report that being able to move freely to find a position of comfort is an important factor in reducing pain and muscle tension and maintaining control during labor. The relation of fetal size to the dimensions of the maternal pelvis may influence pain intensity (Lowe, 2002; Simkin & O'Hara, 2002).

Endorphins are endogenous opioids secreted by the pituitary gland that act on the central and peripheral nervous systems to reduce pain. β-Endorphin is the most potent of the endorphins. Although the physiologic role of endorphins is not completely understood, it is thought that endorphin levels increase during pregnancy and birth in humans. Higher endorphin levels may increase the ability of women in labor to tolerate acute pain and may reduce their irritability and anxiety. Levels of β-endorphins are higher when a woman experiences a spontaneous, natural childbirth.

Culture

The obstetric population reflects the increasingly multicultural nature of U.S. society. As nurses care for women and families from a variety of cultural backgrounds, they must have knowledge and understanding of how culture mediates pain. Although all women expect to experience at least some pain and discomfort during childbirth, it is their culture and religious belief system that determines how they will perceive, interpret, and respond to and manage the pain. For example, women with strong religious beliefs often accept pain as a necessary and inevitable part of bringing a new life into the world (Callister et al, 2003). An understanding of the beliefs, values, expectations, and practices of various cultures will narrow the cultural gap and help the nurse to assess the laboring woman's pain experience more accurately. This will enable the nurse to provide culturally sensitive care by using appropriate pain relief measures that preserve the woman's sense of control and self-confidence (see Cultural Awareness box) (see Table 18-1). It is important for the nurse to recognize that, although a woman's behavior in response to pain may vary according to her cultural background, it may not accurately reflect the intensity of the pain she is experiencing. The nurse must assess the woman for the physiologic effects of pain and listen to the words the woman uses to describe the sensory and affective qualities of her pain (Lowe, 2002) (see Community Focus box).

Anxiety and Fear

Anxiety and fear are commonly associated with increased pain during labor. Mild anxiety is considered normal for a woman during labor and birth. However, excessive anxiety and fear cause catecholamine secretion, resulting in more pelvic pain stimuli reaching the brain; this in turn magnifies pain perception (Lowe, 2002). As anxiety heightens, muscle tension increases, the effectiveness of the uterine contractions decreases, and discomfort intensifies; a cycle of increased fear and anxiety begins. Ultimately this cycle will slow the progress of labor. The woman's "self-efficacy" or confidence in her ability to cope with pain will be diminished, potentially resulting in reduced effectiveness of pain relief measures being used.

CULTURAL AWARENESS

Some Cultural Beliefs About Pain

The following are only examples of how women of different cultural backgrounds may react to pain. Because they are generalizations, the nurse must assess each woman experiencing pain related to childbirth.

- Chinese women may not exhibit reactions to pain, although it is acceptable to exhibit pain during childbirth. They consider it impolite to accept something when it is first offered; therefore pain interventions may need to be offered more than once. Acupuncture may be used for pain relief.
- Arab or Middle Eastern women may be vocal in response to labor pain. They may prefer medication for pain relief.
- Japanese women may be stoic in response to labor pain, but they may request medication when pain becomes severe.
- Southeast Asian women may endure severe pain before requesting relief.
- Hispanic women may be stoic until late in labor, when they may become vocal and request pain relief.
- Native American women may use medications or remedies made from indigenous plants. They are often stoic in response to labor pain.
- African-American women may express pain openly. Use of medication for pain relief varies.

COMMUNITY FOCUS

Culture and Pain

Talk to a man and a woman from a culture different from your own who have experienced childbirth. Ask her to describe her reactions to pain, how she sought relief of pain, the atmosphere of the childbirth setting, and the attitudes of the health care providers. Ask him if he was present for the birth and what his role in the birth was. How did his culture influence his role and reaction to childbirth? How did her culture influence her response to labor and the associated pain? What expressions of pain are "acceptable" in her culture? If he was present, how did he help her deal with the pain? What is the role of support persons in the labor process? Are the responses of the couple different from your responses to those same questions?

Previous Experience

Previous experience with pain and childbirth may affect a woman's description of her pain and her ability to cope with the pain. Childbirth may be a healthy young adult woman's first experience with significant pain, and as a result she may not have developed effective pain coping strategies. She may describe the intensity of even early labor pain as pain "as bad as it can be." The nature of previous childbirth experiences also may affect a woman's responses to pain. For women who have had a difficult and painful previous birth experience, anxiety and fear from the past experience may lead to an increased perception of pain. Conversely, a woman who has experienced a labor and birth in which the degree of pain matched her expectations and in which her coping skills were successful may experience decreased anxiety and a sense of pride in her accomplishment (Trout, 2004). However, anxiety will increase if previous successful coping skills are ineffective during a more difficult labor.

Sensory pain for nulliparous women is often greater than that for multiparous women during early labor (dilation less than 5 cm) because their reproductive tract structures are less supple. During the transition phase of the first stage of labor and during the second stage of labor, multiparous women may experience greater sensory pain than nulliparous women because their more supple tissue increases the speed of fetal descent and thereby intensifies pain. The firmer tissue of nulliparous women results in a slower, more gradual descent. Affective pain is usually greater for nulliparous women throughout the first stage of labor but decreases for both nulliparous and multiparous women during the second stage of labor (Lowe, 2002).

Fatigue and sleep deprivation magnify pain. Most women have a decrease in quality of sleep over the last few days of pregnancy, and the spontaneous onset of labor occurs most often during the night (Beebe & Lee, 2007). Thus many women have an increased perception of the intensity of pain during labor.

Gate-Control Theory of Pain

Even particularly intense pain can at times be ignored. This is possible because certain nerve cell groupings within the spinal cord, brainstem, and cerebral cortex have the ability to modulate the pain impulse through a blocking mechanism. The gate-control theory of pain helps explain the way hypnosis and the pain relief techniques taught in childbirth preparation classes work to relieve the pain of labor. According to this theory, pain sensations travel along sensory nerve pathways to the brain, but only a limited number of sensations, or messages, can travel through these nerve pathways at one time. By using distraction techniques such as massage or stroking, music, focal points, and imagery, the capacity of nerve pathways to transmit pain is reduced or completely blocked. These distractions are thought to work by closing down a hypothetic gate in the spinal cord, thus preventing pain signals from reaching the brain. Perception of pain stimuli is thereby diminished.

In addition, when the woman in labor engages in neuromuscular and motor activity, activity within the spinal cord itself further modifies the transmission of pain. Cognitive work involving concentration on breathing and relaxation requires selective and directed cortical activity that activates and closes the gating mechanism as well. As labor intensifies, more complex cognitive techniques are required to maintain effectiveness. Therefore the gate-control theory underscores the need for a supportive birth setting that allows the laboring woman to relax and use various higher mental activities.

Comfort

Although the predominant medical approach to labor is that it is painful and the pain must be removed, an alternative view is that labor is a natural process and women can experience comfort and transcend the discomfort or pain to reach the joyful outcome of birth. Having needs and desires met engenders a feeling of comfort. Comfort may be viewed as strengthening. The most helpful interventions in enhancing comfort are a caring nursing approach and supportive presence.

Support

A woman's satisfaction with her childbirth experience is primarily influenced by the attitudes and behaviors of her caregivers, including the caregivers' ability to communicate and be helpful, supportive, accepting, and kind. In addition, satisfaction is influenced by the degree to which she was able to stay in control of her labor and participate in decision making regarding it, including the pain relief measures to be used. However, decisions can be based on inadequate or anecdotal information. There is a discrepancy between the perceived and actual knowledge of the likely consequence of labor analgesia (Raynes-Greenow et al, 2007).

The continuous supportive presence of a person (e.g., women with or without special training, including doulas, childbirth educators, family members, friends, nurses) who provides physical comfort, emotional support, ease of communication, and information and guidance to the woman in labor is a beneficial form of care. Continuous support begun early in labor significantly relieves pain, improves outcomes, decreases interventions (e.g., use of pharmacologic pain relief measures) and complication rates (e.g., cesarean rates) associated with labor, and enhances overall maternal satisfaction. Interestingly, a more positive effect was achieved when the continuous support was provided by a woman who was not part of the staff of the hospital (Enkin et al, 2000; Hodnett et al, 2007; Simkin & O'Hara, 2002).

Environment

According to Lowe (2002), environment should be viewed in terms of the persons present (e.g., how they communicate, their philosophy of care, practice policies, and quality of support) and the physical space in which the labor occurs. The quality of the environment can influence a woman's ability to cope with the pain of labor. Women prefer to be cared for by familiar caregivers in a comfortable, homelike setting (Hodnett, 2002). An environment should be safe and private, allowing a woman to feel free to be herself as she tries out different comfort measures. Stimuli, including light, noise, and temperature, should be adjusted according to the woman's preferences. There should be space for movement, and equipment should be readily available for a variety of nonpharmacologic pain relief measures such as birth balls, comfortable chairs, tubs, and showers. The familiarity of the environment can be enhanced by bringing items from home such as pillows, objects for a focal point, music, and videos or DVDs.

Nonpharmacologic Management of Discomfort

The alleviation of pain is important. Commonly it is not the amount of pain the woman experiences but whether she meets her goals for herself in coping with the pain that influences her perception of the birth experience as "good" or "bad." The observant nurse looks for cues to identify the woman's desired level of control in the management of pain and its relief.

Nonpharmacologic measures are often simple, safe, and relatively inexpensive. They provide the woman with a sense of control over her childbirth as she makes choices about the measures that are best for her. During the prenatal period the woman should explore a variety of nonpharmacologic measures. Techniques she finds helpful in relieving stress and enhancing relaxation (e.g., music, meditation, massage, warm baths) also may be very effective as components of a plan for managing labor pain. The woman should be encouraged to communicate to her health care providers her preferences for relaxation and pain relief measures and to actively participate in their implementation. She can prepare a birth plan that includes her preferences for pain relief measures (Box 16-1). Using these measures requires the woman's active participation and support from her partner and caregivers.

Many of the nonpharmacologic methods for relief of discomfort are taught in different types of prenatal preparation classes, or the woman or couple may have read various books and magazine articles on the subject in advance (see Community Focus box). Many of these methods require practice for best results (e.g., hypnosis, patterned breathing and controlled relaxation techniques, biofeedback), although the nurse may use some of them successfully without the woman or couple having prior knowledge (e.g., slow-paced breathing, massage and touch, effleurage, counterpressure). Women should be encouraged to try a variety of methods and to seek alternatives, including pharmacologic methods, if the measure being used is no longer effective (Box 16-2).

COMMUNITY FOCUS

Resources for Alternative and Complementary Methods of Pain Relief

Survey your community for services that provide pregnant women with instruction in complementary or alternative nonpharmacologic methods (e.g., biofeedback, aromatherapy, yoga, transcutaneous electrical nerve stimulation, massage, hypnosis) to relieve and cope with discomforts in pregnancy and pain during labor. Create a booklet that describes each of the methods. Include the following information in the booklet:

- A description of the methods and how they work
- Evidence available to validate effectiveness of the methods
- Internet addresses for the methods
- Agencies providing instruction in the methods; include contact information (address, telephone number), cost of the classes or service, and credentials of persons providing instruction
- At what point in pregnancy instruction should begin and the level of preparation and practice necessary for effective use

The analgesic effect of many nonpharmacologic measures is comparable to or even superior to opioids that are administered parenterally. However, none of these measures is more effective than methods of epidural analgesia. Nonpharmacologic measures are relatively inexpensive and safe with few, if any, major adverse reactions, and they can be used throughout labor. There is limited scientific evidence regarding the effectiveness of nonpharmacologic measures in relieving the pain of childbirth (Simkin & Bolding, 2004; Smith et al, 2006).

BOX 16-1 Birth Plan

The birth plan is a tool with which parents can explore their childbirth options and choose those that are most important to them. It can serve as a means of open communication between the pregnant woman and her partner and between the couple and health care providers. The plan must be viewed as tentative and based on a best-case scenario since the realities of what is feasible may change as the actual labor and birth unfold. The options of women with a high risk pregnancy or those in whom complications develop during labor may be more limited.

Some health care providers provide birth plan templates, and there are numerous interactive programs on the Internet that will assist couples to create their birth plans. However, childbirth educators should screen any such programs before referring couples to them since some contain advertising that is contrary to promoting good health.

Topics for birth plan discussion and decision making may include any or all of the following:

Partner's participation—Attend prenatal visits? Childbirth and parent education classes? Present during labor? During birth? During cesarean birth?

Birth setting—Hospital delivery room or birthing room (if available)? A birthing center? Home?

Labor management—Walk around during labor? Use a rocking chair? Use a shower? Use a Jacuzzi if available? Intermittent vs. continuous use of an electronic fetal monitor? Have music or dimmed lighting? Have older children or other people present? Is telemetry monitoring available? Consider stimulation of labor? Consider medication—what kind?

Birth—Positions—Side-lying? On hands and knees, kneeling, or squatting? Use a birthing bed? Or delivery table? Will you be photographing, videotaping, or recording any of the labor or birth? Who would you like to be present—partner, older siblings, other family members, or friends? What do you know about the use of forceps? Episiotomies? Will your partner want to cut the umbilical cord?

Immediately after birth—Do you want to hold the baby right away? Breastfeed immediately?

Postpartum care—What kind of care do you anticipate—labor, delivery, recovery, postpartum room; mother-baby coupling? How long does your insurance company provide coverage for you to stay? Would you like to attend self-management classes, or do you prefer to get such information from videotapes/DVDs? On which subjects?

Childbirth Preparation Methods

Most health care providers recommend or offer childbirth preparation classes to expectant parents. Most proponents of

BOX 16-2 Nonpharmacologic Strategies to Encourage Relaxation and Relieve Pain

Cutaneous Stimulation Strategies
Counterpressure*
Effleurage (light massage)*
Therapeutic touch and massage*
Walking*
Rocking*
Changing positions*
Applying heat or cold*
Transcutaneous electrical nerve stimulation
Acupressure
Water therapy (hydrotherapy)
Intradermal water block

Sensory Stimulation Strategies
Aromatherapy
Breathing techniques*
Music*
Imagery*
Use of focal points*

Cognitive Strategies
Childbirth education*
Hypnosis
Biofeedback

*Forms of care likely to be beneficial (Enkin et al, 2000).

CRITICAL THINKING EXERCISE

Pain Management

You are assigned to a 17-year-old, single, nulliparous woman in active labor who is thrashing about in her bed and requesting something for "this terrible pain." She did not attend childbirth preparation classes. She has the prn orders for pain that are routine on your unit and has an intravenous line of lactated Ringer's solution in place infusing at 125 ml/hr. She can ambulate and has periodic electronic fetal monitor strips run to check on fetal status.

1. Evidence—Is there sufficient evidence to draw conclusions about what nonpharmacologic and pharmacologic pain relief techniques can be instituted?
2. Assumptions—What assumptions can be made about the following issues?
   a. Reactions to pain of young, single women who lack support in labor
   b. Degree of pain relief expected by the woman
   c. Degree of pain relief expected by the nurse
   d. Nonpharmacologic measures that are effective
3. What implications and priorities for nursing care can be drawn at this time?
4. Does the evidence objectively support your conclusion?
5. Are there alternative perspectives to your conclusion?

prepared childbirth agree that the major causes of pain in labor are fear and tension (see Critical Thinking Exercise). All childbirth methods attempt to reduce these two factors and eliminate pain by increasing the woman's knowledge of the labor and birth process, enhancing her self-confidence and sense of control, preparing a support person, and training the woman in physical conditioning and relaxation breathing.

There are a few fine differences in approach. For example, in the Lamaze method external focusing and distraction are stressed. In the Bradley method women are discouraged from using medication and encouraged to focus inwardly and take direction from their own body. In reality, few instructors adhere strictly to one particular method but instead incorporate a variety of strategies aimed at increasing the woman's ability to cope with labor and minimize her need for medication.

Early Methods of Childbirth Education

Dick-Read Method

An English physician, Grantly Dick-Read, published two books (*Natural Childbirth,* 1933; *Childbirth Without Fear,* 1944) in which he theorized that pain in childbirth is socially conditioned and caused by a fear-tension-pain syndrome. In 1960 those prepared through such programs established the International Childbirth Education Association (ICEA). The Grantly Dick-Read method, referred to as *Childbirth Without Fear,* initially recommended deep abdominal breathing during early first-stage contractions, shallow breathing for later first stage, and sustained pushing with breath holding (Dick-Read, 1987). Women were taught to relax different muscle groups through the entire body, consciously and progressively, until a high degree of skill at relaxation was achieved. Consequently a woman was taught to relax completely between contractions and keep all muscles except the uterus relaxed during contractions.

Lamaze Method

During the 1960s the Lamaze method, originally known as the psychoprophylactic method (PPM), was introduced in the United States by Marjorie Karmel in her book *Thank You, Dr. Lamaze,* published in 1959. The PPM offered new perspectives on preparation for childbirth by emphasizing control using the mind. The PPM combined controlled muscular relaxation and breathing techniques. Active relaxation has been an integral part of the Lamaze method. The woman was taught to contract specific muscle groups (neuromuscular control) while relaxing the remainder of her body. She thus learned to relax the uninvolved muscles in her body while her uterus contracted. Instead of tensing during uterine contractions, women were conditioned to respond with relaxation and breathing patterns.

In 1960 the American Society for Psychoprophylaxis in Obstetrics was formed in New York and became a national organization to promote use of the Lamaze method and prepare teachers of the method. It continues to be an active organization, known since 1998 as *Lamaze International* and dedicated to advancing normal birth. Lamaze's Institute of Normal Birth publishes reviews of research related to normal birth. In the official Lamaze *Guide to Giving Birth with Confidence,* the authors state that "Mothers do know how to give birth, simply; and doctors, hospitals, and technology have not made normal birth safer" (Lothian & Devries, 2005). They further state that women need to rediscover birth as a natural part of life based on research that confirms that interfering in the normal birth process is harmful unless there is clear evidence that interference provides benefits.

Bradley Method

A third early advocate of prepared childbirth was the Denver obstetrician, Robert Bradley, who published *Husband-Coached Childbirth* in 1965. He advocated what he called true "natural" childbirth, without any form of anesthesia or analgesia and with a husband-coach and breathing techniques for labor. The American Academy of Husband-Coached Childbirth was founded to make the Bradley method available and to prepare teachers *(www.bradleybirth.com)*. This method of partner-coached childbirth used breath control, abdominal breathing, and general body relaxation. Working in harmony with the body was emphasized (Bradley, 1981). Bradley's technique emphasized environmental variables such as darkness, solitude, and quiet to make childbirth a more natural experience. Women using the Bradley method may appear to be sleeping during labor because they are in such a deep state of mental relaxation. Medication is discouraged.

These three organizations continue to exist but are now less focused on a "method" approach. Rather women are assisted to develop their birth philosophy and inner knowledge and then offered many skills from which to choose. Many childbirth educators teach a plethora of techniques that originated in several different organizations or publications. Women are encouraged to choose the techniques that work for them. Other childbirth educator organizations include *BirthWorks, Association of Childbirth Educators and Labor Assistants, Birthing From Within, Childbirth and Postpartum Association (CAPPA)*, and *Hypnobirth.*

Newer Methods of Childbirth Education

The Coalition to Improve Maternity Services

The Coalition to Improve Maternity Services (CIMS) *(www.motherfriendly.org)* was founded in 1996 after a summit meeting of maternity organizations was held. The group drafted standards for normal birth entitled the Mother-Friendly Childbirth Initiative. This document was ratified by Lamaze International *(www.lamaze-childbirth.com)*; La Leche League *(www.lalecheleague.org)*; BirthWorks *(www.birthworks.org)*; the American Academy of Husband-Coached Childbirth *(http://aahhc.com)*; the American College of Nurse Midwives *(www.midwife.org)*; the Association of Women's Health, Obstetric, and Neonatal Nurses *(www.awhonn.org)*; ICEA *(www.icea.org)*; the Midwife Alliance of North America *(www.mana.org)*; and Physicians for Midwifery.

The CIMS adopted the Lamaze International philosophy of birth, which follows:

- Birth is normal, natural, and healthy.
- The experience of birth profoundly affects women and their families.
- Women's inner wisdom guides them through birth.
- Women's confidence and ability to give birth is either enhanced or diminished by the care provider and place of birth.
- Women have a right to give birth free from routine medical interventions.
- Birth can safely take place in birth centers and homes and hospitals.
- Childbirth education empowers women to make informed choices in health care, to assume responsibility for their health, and to trust their inner wisdom (Lothian & Devries, 2005).

This philosophy has become an ideal for many childbirth education organizations in the United States. It fits closely with the principles of perinatal care put forth by the World Health Organization (WHO, 1998), which states that care for normal pregnancy and birth should be removed from total control of doctors, based on the use of appropriate technology (as opposed to overuse), evidence based, regionalized, multidisciplinary, holistic, family centered, and culturally appropriate; should involve women in decision making; and should respect the privacy, dignity, and confidentiality of women.

A Guide to Effective Care in Pregnancy and Childbirth (Enkin et al, 2000) presents the evidence base for effective care in pregnancy and childbirth based on systematic reviews from the Cochrane Pregnancy and Childbirth Group. Free Internet access to this book is available *(www.maternitywise.org)*. How the childbirth educator uses this evidence in education programs depends on both the population who attend classes and the care-provider practices in the community. Expectant parents can ask their care providers if they are familiar with this database and if they use it to discontinue routines that have been found to be useless or harmful. In the role as advocate, the childbirth educator can let families know that items on the list of ineffective or harmful care routines might affect their choice of care provision.

The Maternity Center Association released a survey report in 2002 conducted by Harris Interactive from the Harris Poll group entitled *Listening to Mothers*, which is available at *www.maternitywise.org/listeningtomothers/*. This is the first national U.S. survey of women's childbearing experiences. A total of 136 mothers were interviewed by telephone, and 1447 completed a written survey. The results suggest that a large percentage of mothers giving birth receive interventions that are not evidence based. It takes skill, judgment, and tact for the childbirth educator to help consumers make choices about their desired care without undermining medical colleagues when local routine care frequently lacks an evidence base.

The Lamaze Institute for Normal Birth (LINB) is an evidence-based resource for new and expectant parents and childbirth professionals, whether they practice from a medical, nursing, or midwifery model of care. Its foundation comprises six care principles modified from the WHO recommendations:

1. Labor to begin on its own
2. Freedom of movement throughout labor
3. Continuous labor support
4. No routine interventions
5. Nonsupine (e.g., upright or side-lying) positions for birth
6. No separation of mother and baby after birth, with unlimited opportunity for breastfeeding

Brief papers documenting the research supporting each of these care principles is available at *www.lamaze.org*. In addition, the LINB produces a free Internet-based newsletter that reviews recent studies that address some aspect of normal birth. Thus all perinatal educators, perinatal care providers, and consumers can have ready access to current research on the subject of normal birth.

Three organizations that function with this or a similar philosophy are HypnoBirthing, Birthing From Within, and the CAPPA.

HypnoBirthing

HypnoBirthing, the Mongan Method, grew out of the work of Dr. Grantly Dick-Read, an English obstetrician, who taught that fear (of pain or birth) and tension (resulting from the fear) lead to pain (HypnoBirthing, 2004; Mottershead, 2006). In HypnoBirthing pregnant women (couples) learn how the birthing muscles work when the woman is in a state of relaxation. The woman will be relaxed and in control. She will experience surges (contractions) while calm and relaxed, free of fear and tension. Testimonials from birthing women and their attendants attest to the effectiveness of this technique, describing births as rapid and pain free (HypnoBirthing, 2004).

Birthing From Within

Birthing From Within mentors (teachers) believe that childbirth is not a medical event but a profound rite of passage. Parents are taught the power of birthing-in awareness. Mentors create a safe, nurturing class experience and assist parents to find their personal strength and wisdom. Birth is taught from four perspectives: mother, father, baby, and culture. Parents are assisted to develop a pain-coping mindset. Parents deserve support for whatever birth option they choose. Fathers provide most help as loving partners and birth guardians, not coaches (Birthing From Within, n.d.).

Childbirth and Postpartum Professional Association

The CAPPA is a nonprofit international organization, formed in 1998, that provides professional membership and training to antepartum doulas, childbirth educators, labor doulas, postpartum doulas, and lactation educators. They are proponents of evidence-based practice in childbirth education. Their childbirth educators teach parents that childbirth is painful but there are ways to deal with the pain. They generally recommend deep abdominal breathing in labor. Relaxation is vital to achieve their goals. Vocalization, position changes, walking, frequent urination, and hydrotherapy are useful techniques (CAPPA, 2008).

Childbirth Education Outcomes

Researchers studying childbirth education outcomes have not adopted a standard set of operational definitions of childbirth education or a theoretic framework that acknowledges that multiple factors, as opposed to childbirth education alone, impact the outcomes. Research on the influence of childbirth education on biologic birth outcomes has not accounted for the management mindset of those providing care during labor.

However, the research findings on positive childbirth education outcomes have been consistent over many decades. The effects of childbirth education have consistently been shown to be in birth satisfaction, building confidence, and building relationships. Physiologic outcomes are not demonstrated to be strongly influenced by educating expectant parents.

Pregnancy is a time when expectant parents expect change in their lives and are open to many types of education. This education can enhance their health and coping in pregnancy, childbirth, and early parenting. It also can influence how they relate to health professionals over a lifetime, problem solve with each other, and launch their new family. It is an opportunity for nurses to engage in meaningful health promotion and the building of resilience and connection in families.

Relaxation and Breathing Techniques

Relaxation

Relaxation or reduction of body tension is a technique suggested by virtually all childbirth education organizations. Learning relaxation in childbirth education classes can help couples with the stresses of pregnancy, childbirth, and adjustment to parenting and can be a form of stress management throughout life (Fig. 16-2). The research is clear that relaxation skill is the most effective nonpharmacologic strategy for coping with the stress of labor. Relaxation is ideally combined with activity such as walking, slow dancing, rocking, and position changes that help the baby rotate through the pelvis. Rhythmic motion stimulates mechanoreceptors in the brain, which decreases pain perception.

Imagery and Visualization

Imagery and visualization are useful techniques in preparation for birth. Although research on their use is scant, clinical reports suggest that imagery and visualization can be used to produce a sense of well-being during pregnancy, assist with cervical dilation, and decrease the experience of pain and tension during labor. Imagery involves techniques such as imagining a walk through a restful garden or breathing in light, energy, and healing color and breathing out worries and tension. A variety of skills taught in childbirth classes augment relaxation during pregnancy and labor. All can be taught as lifetime skills useful to the couple and can be used to teach their children to cope with the stresses of life.

Music

Music, taped or live, enhances relaxation during labor, thereby reducing stress, anxiety, and the perception of pain. Women can prepare their musical preferences in advance and bring their tape or compact disk player to the hospital or birthing center. Use of a headset or earphones may increase the effectiveness of the music because other sounds will be shut out.

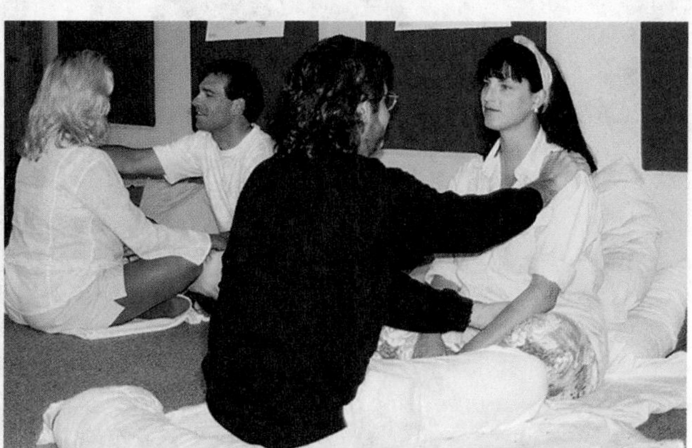

Fig. 16-2 Expectant parents learning relaxation techniques. *(Courtesy Marjorie Pyle, RNC, Lifecircle, Costa Mesa, CA.)*

Live music provided at the bedside by a support person may also be very helpful in transmitting energy that decreases tension and elevates mood. Ocean waves and Baroque and New Age music assist in relaxation.

Touch and Massage

Touch and massage have been an integral part of the traditional care process for women in labor. Touch can be as simple as holding the woman's hand, stroking her body, and embracing her. Head, hand, back, and foot massage may be very effective in reducing tension and enhancing comfort. Hand and foot massage may be especially relaxing in advanced labor when hyperesthesia limits a woman's tolerance for touch on other parts of her body.

Energy Work

Energy work such as therapeutic touch or healing touch involves manipulation of energy fields around the body and can be taught in class for use during labor to decrease anxiety and pain and increase relaxation. Certified practitioners in energy work are consulted throughout pregnancy and during childbirth by some women who have access to such care.

Conscious Breathing

Using conscious breathing patterns is a visible technique and thus is frequently used in the media to characterize childbirth preparation. Relaxed individuals automatically slow their breathing; conversely, slowing one's breathing serves to increase one's relaxation. Different approaches to childbirth preparation use varying breathing techniques to help the woman maintain control through contractions (Fig. 16-3 and Box 16-3). During labor, nursing support includes guiding couples in applying breathing and relaxation methods, adapting methods to their particular needs, and using pushing techniques for birth that avoid breath holding. Such techniques often involve moaning or other noises as the woman pushes without holding her breath.

The woman and her support person must be aware of and watch for symptoms of respiratory alkalosis when rapid shallow breathing results in hyperventilation: lightheadedness, dizziness, tingling of fingers, or circumoral numbness. Such alkalosis may be eliminated by having the woman breathe into a paper bag held tightly around the mouth and nose. This enables her to rebreathe carbon dioxide and replace the bicarbonate ion. She can also breathe into her cupped hands if no bag is available.

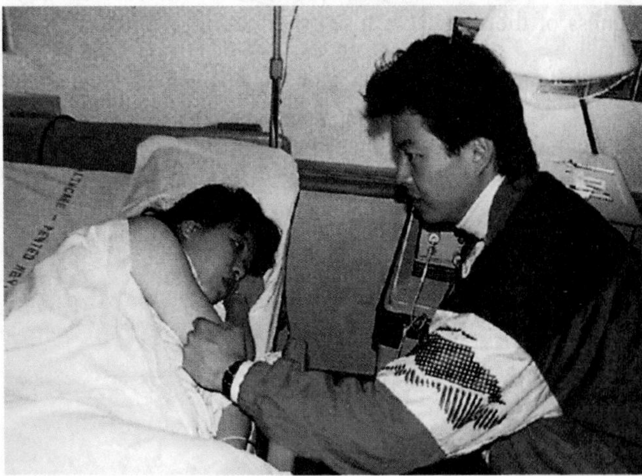

Fig. 16-3 Laboring woman using focusing and breathing techniques during contraction with coaching from her partner. *(Courtesy Marjorie Pyle, RNC, Lifecircle, Costa Mesa, CA.)*

Effleurage and Counterpressure

Effleurage (light massage) and counterpressure bring relief to many women during the first stage of labor. Effleurage is a

BOX 16-3 Paced Breathing Techniques

Cleansing Breath

Relaxed breath in through nose and out mouth, keeping shoulders relaxed

Used at the beginning and end of each contraction

Slow-Paced Breathing (Approximately 6 to 8 breaths/min)

Not less than half normal breathing rate (breaths/min ÷ 2)

IN-2-3-4/OUT-2-3-4/IN-2-3-4/OUT-2-3-4

Modified-Paced Breathing (Approximately 32 to 40 breaths/min)

Not more than twice normal breathing rate (breaths/min × 2)

IN-2-OUT-2/IN-2-OUT-2/IN-2-OUT-2

Patterned-Paced Breathing (Same Rate as Modified)

Enhances concentration

3:1 Patterned breathing IN-OUT/IN-OUT/IN-OUT/IN-BLOW (repeat through contractions)

4:1 Patterned breathing IN-OUT/IN-OUT/IN-OUT/IN-OUT/IN-BLOW (repeat through contractions)

Pant-Blow Breathing (Same Rate as Modified-Paced Breathing)

Not more than twice normal breathing rate (breaths/min × 2)

Upper chest, shallow breaths followed by relaxed exhales

The pant is an in breath and an out breath

Pattern may vary: PANT-2-3-4-BLOW, or PANT-2-3-BLOW

Keep facial muscles relaxed

Breathing During Second Stage—Pushing

Spontaneous Pushing

Urge to push is nearly involuntary. Many women hold their breath; remember to breathe.

Slow Exhalation Pushing (Open-Glottis Pushing)

Work with contraction; inhale and exhale slowly through pursed lips.

Grunting or making noise with exhalation keeps glottis open.

Directed Pushing (Closed-Glottis Pushing)

During contraction woman inhales and holds breath while support person counts to 10 (about 6 seconds). Exhale and inhale rapidly again, holding for another count of 10. Repeat until contraction is over.

Adapted from BirthSource: *Breathing*, Centerville, OH, 1999-2009, Perinatal Education Associates. Available at www.birthsource.com (accessed May 10, 2009).

light stroking, usually of the abdomen, in rhythm with breathing during contractions. It is used to distract the woman from contraction pain. Often the presence of monitor belts makes it difficult to perform effleurage on the abdomen; thus a thigh or the chest may be used.

Counterpressure is steady pressure in the sacral area with the fist or heel of the hand, which may help the woman cope with the sensations of internal pressure and pain in the lower back.

Water Therapy (Hydrotherapy)

Bathing, showering, or jet hydrotherapy (whirlpool baths) using warm water are nonpharmacologic measures that can be used to promote comfort and relaxation during labor, reduce fear of pain, and cope with pain (Maude & Foureur, 2007) (Fig. 16-4). Showers in early labor may provide relaxation and comfort. Sitting in a tub of water up to the shoulders for 1 to 2 hours has several immediate benefits. Buoyancy in the water results in general body relaxation and temporary relief from discomfort and pain. This reduces the woman's anxiety and enhances a feeling of well-being. Catecholamine production decreases. This triggers an increase in the levels of oxytocin (to stimulate uterine contractions) and endorphins (to reduce pain perception).

If the woman is experiencing "back labor" as a result of an occiput posterior or transverse position, she is encouraged to assume the hands-and-knees or the side-lying position in the tub. Because this position decreases pain and increases relaxation and the production of oxytocin, the fetus can rotate spontaneously to the occiput anterior position.

In some settings jet hydrotherapy may need to be approved by the woman's primary health care provider. The woman's vital signs must be within normal limits, and she should be in the active phase of the first stage of labor. If she is in the latent phase, her contractions may slow down. Fetal well-being must also be documented. Fetal heart rate (FHR) monitoring is done by Doppler device, fetoscope, or wireless external monitor device (see Fig. 16-4, *C*). Placement of internal electrodes is contraindicated for jet hydrotherapy. The woman's membranes may be intact or ruptured. If the membranes are ruptured, the fluid must be clear or only lightly stained with meconium.

There is no limit to the time women can stay in the bath, and often they are encouraged to stay in it as long as desired. Most women use jet hydrotherapy for 30 to 60 minutes at a time. Repeated baths with occasional breaks may be more effective in relieving pain in long labors than unlimited amounts of time in the water. Fluids to maintain hydration, ice chips, and a cool face cloth are offered during the bath.

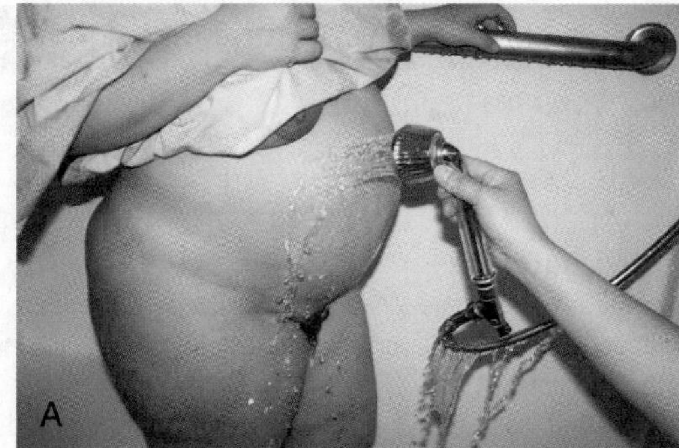

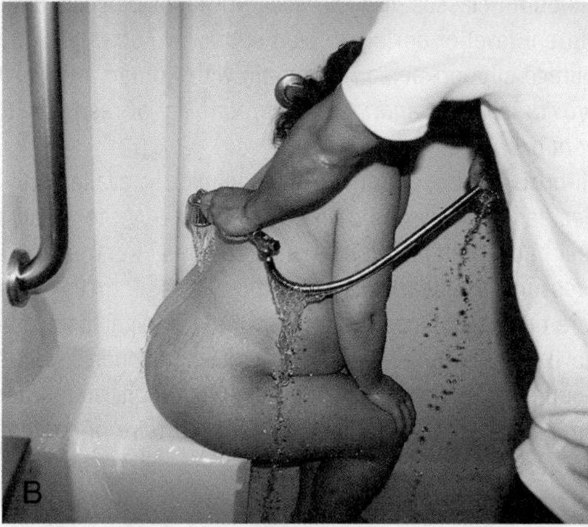

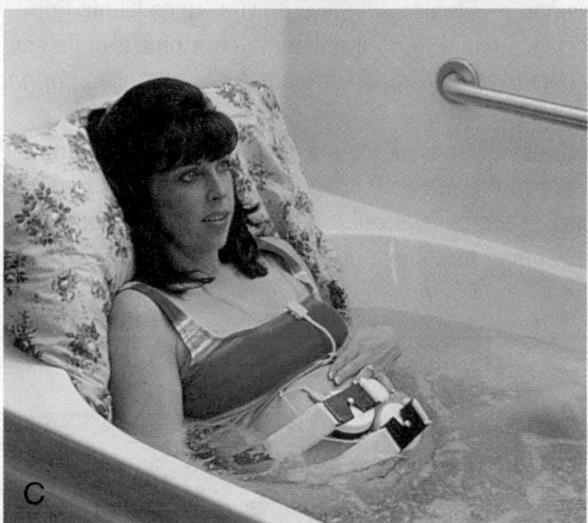

Fig. 16-4 Water therapy during labor. **A,** Use of shower during labor. **B,** Woman experiencing back labor relaxes as husband sprays warm water on her back. **C,** Woman relaxing in Jacuzzi. *(**A** and **B**, Courtesy Marjorie Pyle, RNC, Lifecircle, Costa Mesa, CA. **C**, Courtesy Spacelabs Medical, Redmond, WA.)*

Transcutaneous Electrical Nerve Stimulation

Transcutaneous electrical nerve stimulation (TENS) involves placing two pairs of electrodes on either side of the woman's thoracic and sacral spine (Fig. 16-5). These electrodes provide continuous mild electrical current from a battery-operated device. During a contraction the woman increases the stimulation from low to high intensity by turning control knobs on the device. High intensity should be maintained for at least 1 minute to facilitate release of endorphins. Women describe the resulting sensation as a tingling or buzzing and pain relief as good or very good. TENS is most useful for lower back pain during the early first stage of labor. It is now considered a form of care with insufficient quality data to recommend its use (Enkin et al, 2000). The nurse assists the woman in using TENS by explaining the device and its use, by carefully placing and securing the electrodes, and by closely evaluating its effectiveness (see Nursing Care Plan).

Acupressure and Acupuncture

Acupressure techniques can be used in pregnancy, labor, and postpartum to relieve pain and other discomforts. Pressure, heat, or cold is applied to acupuncture points termed *tsubos.*

NURSING CARE PLAN Nonpharmacologic Management of Discomfort

Nursing Diagnosis: Anxiety related to lack of confidence in ability to cope effectively with pain during labor

Expected Outcome

Woman will express decrease in anxiety and experience satisfaction with her labor and birth performance.

Nursing Interventions/*Rationales*

Assess whether woman and significant other have attended childbirth classes, her knowledge of labor process, and her current level of anxiety *to plan supportive strategies.*

Encourage support person to remain with woman in labor *to provide support and increase probability of response to comfort measures.*

Teach or review nonpharmacologic techniques available to decrease anxiety and pain during labor (e.g., focusing and feedback, breathing techniques, effleurage, and sacral pressure) *to enhance chances of success in using techniques.*

Explore other techniques that the woman or significant other may have learned in childbirth classes (e.g., hypnosis, yoga, acupressure, biofeedback, therapeutic touch, aromatherapy, imaging, music) *to provide largest repertoire of coping strategies.*

Explore use of jet hydrotherapy if ordered by physician and if woman meets use criteria (i.e., vital signs within normal limits, cervix 4 to 5 cm dilated, active phase of first-stage labor) *to aid relaxation and stimulate production of natural oxytocin.*

Explore use of transcutaneous nerve stimulation per physician order *to provide an increased perception of control over pain and an increase in release of endogenous opiates.*

Assist woman to change positions and to use pillows *to reduce stiffness, aid circulation, and promote comfort.*

Assess bladder for distention and encourage voiding often *to avoid bladder distention and subsequent discomfort.*

Encourage rest between contractions *to minimize fatigue.*

Keep woman and significant other informed about progress *to allay anxiety.*

Guide couple through the labor stages and phases, helping them use and modify comfort techniques that are appropriate to each phase, *to ensure greatest effectiveness of techniques used.*

Support couple if pharmacologic measures are required to increase pain relief, explaining safety and effectiveness, *to reduce anxiety and maintain self-esteem and sense of control over labor process.*

Nursing Diagnosis: Health-seeking behavior (labor) related to desire for a healthy outcome of labor and birth

Expected Outcome

Woman will participate in care planning for labor.

Nursing Interventions/*Rationales*

Discuss woman's birth plan and knowledge about the birth process *to collect data for plan of care.*

Provide information about the labor process *to correct any misconceptions.*

Inform woman about her labor status and fetus's well-being *to promote comfort and confidence.*

Discuss rationales for all interventions *to incorporate woman into plan of care.*

Incorporate nonpharmacologic interventions into plan of care *to increase woman's sense of control during labor.*

Provide emotional support and ongoing positive feedback *to enhance positive coping mechanisms.*

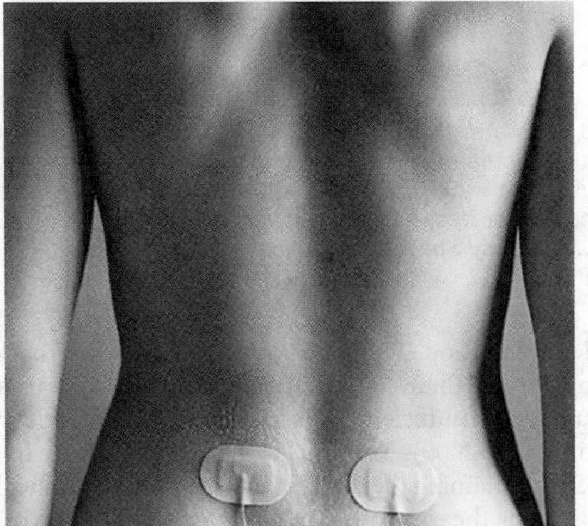

Fig. 16-5 Placement of TENS electrodes on back for relief of labor pain.

These points have an increased density of neuroreceptors and increased electrical conductivity. Acupressure is best applied over the skin without using lubricants. Pressure is usually applied with the heel of the hand, fist, or pads of the thumbs and fingers (Fig. 16-6). Synchronized breathing by the caregiver and the woman is suggested for greater effectiveness. Acupressure points are found on the neck; shoulders; wrists; lower back, including sacral points; hips; area below the kneecaps; ankles; nails on the small toes; and soles of the feet.

Acupuncture is the insertion of fine needles into specific areas of the body to restore the flow of *qi* (energy) and decrease pain, which is thought to be obstructing the flow of energy. It should be done by a trained certified therapist. Current evidence indicates that acupuncture may be beneficial for relief of labor pain; however, further study is indicated (Florence & Palmer, 2003; Smith et al, 2006).

Application of Heat and Cold

Warmed blankets, warm compresses, heated rice bags, a warm bath or shower, or a moist heating pad can enhance relaxation and reduce pain during labor. Heat relieves muscle ischemia

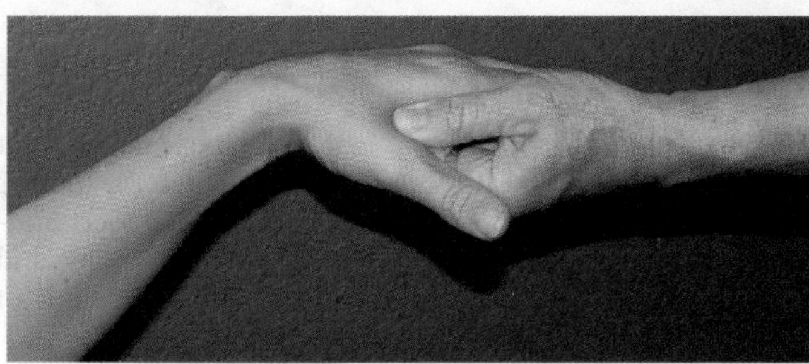

Fig. 16-6 Ho-Ku acupressure point (back of hand where thumb and index finger come together) used to enhance uterine contractions without increasing pain. *(Courtesy Julie Perry Nelson, Loveland, CO.)*

and increases blood flow to the area of discomfort. Heat application is effective for back pain caused by a posterior presentation or general backache from fatigue.

Cold application such as cool cloths or ice packs applied to the back, chest, and/or face during labor may be effective in increasing comfort when the woman feels warm. They may also be applied to areas of pain. Cooling relieves pain by lowering the muscle temperature and relieving muscle spasms. A woman's culture may make the use of cold during labor unacceptable (Simkin & Bolding, 2004).

Heat and cold may be used alternately for a greater effect. Neither heat nor cold should be applied over ischemic or anesthetized areas because tissues can be damaged. One or two layers of cloth should be placed between the skin and a hot or cold pack to prevent damage to the underlying integument (Simkin & Bolding, 2004).

Hypnosis

Although hypnosis is not commonly used for pain management in the United States, it is associated with shorter labors and less analgesia and in higher 1-minute Apgar scores (VandeVusse et al, 2007). Current evidence suggests that hypnosis may relieve pain, increase the likelihood of vaginal birth, reduce the use of oxytocin, and enhance maternal satisfaction. Further research is required to confirm these potentially promising outcomes (Simkin & Bolding, 2004; Smith et al, 2006). Hypnosis techniques used for labor and birth place an emphasis on relaxation and diminishing fear, anxiety, and perception of pain (see earlier discussion of HypnoBirthing). The woman may be given direct suggestions about pain relief or indirect suggestions that she is experiencing diminished sensations. The woman receives posthypnotic suggestions such as "you will be able to push the baby out easily," to increase her confidence. To be successful the woman must be educated regarding hypnosis and practice the techniques during the prenatal period.

Biofeedback

Biofeedback is a relaxation technique that can be used for labor. It is based on the theory that, if a person can recognize physical signals, certain internal physiologic events can be changed (i.e., whatever signs the woman has that are associated with her pain). For biofeedback to be effective, the woman must be educated during the prenatal period to become aware of her body and its responses and how to relax. The woman

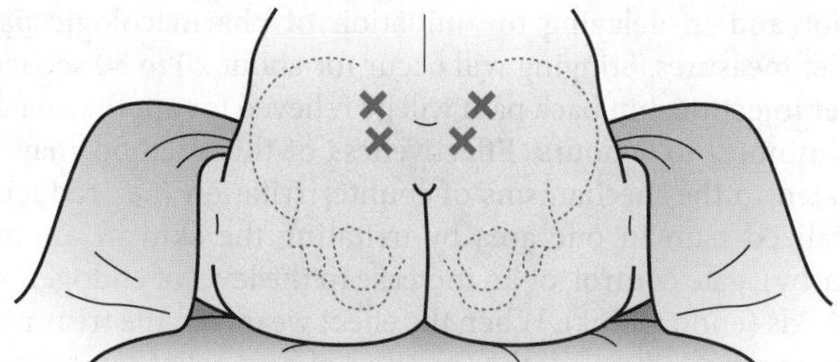

Fig. 16-7 Intradermal injections of 0.1 ml of sterile water in the treatment of women with back pain during labor. Sterile water is injected into four locations on the lower back, two over each posterior superior iliac spine (PSIS) and two 3 cm below and 1 cm medial to the PSIS. The injections should raise a bleb on the skin. Simultaneous injections administered by two clinicians decreases the pain of the injections. (Leeman L et al: The nature and management of labor pain. Part I: Nonpharmacologic pain relief, *Am Fam Physician* 68(6):1109-1112, 2003.)

must learn how to use thinking and mental processes (e.g., focusing) to control body responses and functions. Informal biofeedback helps couples develop awareness of their bodies and learn strategies to change their responses to stress. If the woman responds to pain during a contraction with tightening of muscles, frowning, moaning, and breath holding, her partner uses verbal and touch feedback to help her relax. Formal biofeedback, which uses machines to detect skin temperature, blood flow, or muscle tension, also can prepare women to intensify their relaxation responses.

Aromatherapy

Aromatherapy uses oils distilled from plants, flowers, herbs, and trees to promote health and well-being and to treat illnesses. The use of herbal teas and vapors is reported to have positive effects in pregnancy and labor for some women. Lavender, clary sage, and bergamot promote relaxation and can be used by adding a few drops to a warm bath, to warm water used for soaking compresses that can be applied to the body, to an aromatherapy lamp to vaporize a room, or to oil for a back massage. Drops of essential oils can also be put on a pillow or on a woman's brow or palms (Simkin & Bolding, 2004). Certain odors or scents can evoke pleasant memories and feelings of love and security. It would be helpful for a woman to choose the scents that she will use (Trout, 2004). Currently there is insufficient evidence to support the effectiveness of aromatherapy for pain relief in labor, although its use has elicited promising results (Smith et al, 2006).

NURSING ALERT Never apply the essential oils used for aromatherapy full strength directly to the skin. Most oils should be diluted in a vegetable oil base before use. Essential oils vary in terms of safe use during pregnancy. Inhaling vapors from the oils can lead to unpleasant side effects, including nausea or headaches.

Intradermal Water Block

An intradermal water block involves the injection of small amounts of sterile water (e.g., 0.05 to 0.1 ml) by using a fine needle (e.g., 25-gauge) into four locations on the lower back to relieve back pain (Fig. 16-7). It may be effective in early labor and in delaying the initiation of pharmacologic pain relief measures. Stinging will occur for about 20 to 30 seconds after injection, but back pain will be relieved for approximately 45 minutes to 2 hours. Effectiveness of this method may be related to the mechanisms of counterirritation (i.e., reducing localized pain in one area by irritating the skin in an area nearby), gate control, or an increase in the level of endogenous opioids (endorphins). When the effect wears off, the treatment can be repeated, or another method of pain relief can be used (Simkin & O'Hara, 2002).

Pharmacologic Management of Discomfort

evolve Spanish Guidelines—Pain Management

Pharmacologic measures for pain management should be implemented before pain becomes so severe that catecholamines increase and labor is prolonged. When pharmacologic and nonpharmacologic measures are used together, they increase the level of pain relief and create a more positive labor experience for the woman and her family. Nonpharmacologic measures can be used for relaxation and pain relief, especially in early labor. Pharmacologic measures can be implemented as labor becomes more active and discomfort and pain intensify; nonpharmacologic measures enhance relaxation and potentiate the effect of the analgesic. Since 1981 more women are taking advantage of pharmacologic measures and fewer opt for no pharmacologic support. The largest increase was noted in the use of epidural forms of analgesia (Bucklin et al, 2005).

Sedatives

Sedatives relieve anxiety and induce sleep. They can be given to a woman when she is having a prolonged latent phase of labor or when there is a need to decrease anxiety or promote sleep. They can also be given to augment analgesics and reduce nausea when an opioid is used. Barbiturates such as secobarbital sodium (Seconal) can cause undesirable side effects, including respiratory and vasomotor depression that affects the woman and newborn. These effects are increased if a barbiturate is administered with another central nervous system (CNS) depressant such as an opioid analgesic. However, pain will be magnified if a barbiturate is given without an analgesic to women experiencing pain. Because of these disadvantages, barbiturates are seldom used.

Phenothiazines (e.g., promethazine [Phenergan], hydroxyzine [Vistaril]) do not relieve pain but decrease anxiety and apprehension, increase sedation, and potentiate opioid analgesic effects. This potentiation effect causes the two drugs to work together more effectively so the opioid dose can be reduced. They can also be used to reduce the nausea and vomiting that often accompany opioid use. Metoclopramide (Reglan) is an antiemetic that also can be used for this purpose.

Benzodiazepines (e.g., diazepam [Valium], lorazepam [Ativan]), when given with an opioid analgesic, seem to enhance pain relief and reduce nausea and vomiting, although the increased sedation experienced may be unacceptable to women in labor (Lehne, 2007).

Analgesia and Anesthesia

The ideal obstetric analgesic or anesthetic provides adequate pain relief to women without increasing maternal or fetal risk or affecting the progress of labor. Nursing management of obstetric analgesia and anesthesia combines the nurse's expertise in maternity care with a knowledge and understanding of anatomy and physiology and of medications and their therapeutic effects, adverse reactions, and methods of administration.

Anesthesia encompasses analgesia, amnesia, relaxation, and reflex activity. Anesthesia abolishes pain perception by interrupting the nerve impulses to the brain. The loss of sensation may be partial or complete, sometimes with the loss of consciousness.

The term *analgesia* refers to the alleviation of the sensation of pain or the raising of the threshold for pain perception without loss of consciousness.

The type of analgesic or anesthetic chosen is determined in part by the stage of labor and the method of birth planned (Box 16-4).

Systemic Analgesia

Systemic analgesia remains the major method of analgesia for the woman in labor when personnel trained in regional analgesia (i.e., epidural analgesia) are not available. It is a form of

BOX 16-4 Pharmacologic Control of Discomfort by Stage of Labor and Method of Birth

First Stage
Systemic analgesia
- Opioid agonist analgesics
- Opioid agonist-antagonist analgesics, co-drugs

Epidural (block) analgesia
Combined spinal-epidural (CSE) analgesia
Paracervical block (rarely used)
Nitrous oxide

Second Stage
Nerve block analgesia/anesthesia
- Local infiltration anesthesia
- Pudendal block
- Spinal (block) anesthesia
- Epidural (block) analgesia
- CSE analgesia

Nitrous oxide

Vaginal Birth
Local infiltration anesthesia
Pudendal block
Epidural (block) analgesia/anesthesia
Spinal (block) anesthesia
CSE analgesia/anesthesia
Nitrous oxide

Cesarean Birth
Spinal (block) anesthesia
Epidural (block) anesthesia
General anesthesia

care with a trade-off between beneficial and adverse effects (Enkin et al, 2000). Systemic analgesics cross the blood-brain barrier to provide central analgesic effects. They also cross through the placenta. Once transferred to the fetus, analgesics cross the fetal blood-brain barrier more readily than the maternal blood-brain barrier. The duration of action will be longer in the fetus and newborn because the systemic analgesics used during labor have a significantly longer half-life in the fetus and newborn. Effects on the fetus and the newborn can be profound (e.g., respiratory depression, decreased alertness, delayed sucking), depending on the characteristics of the specific systemic analgesic used, the dosage given, and the route and timing of administration.

Intravenous (IV) administration is preferred to intramuscular (IM) administration because the onset of action of the medication is faster and more predictable; as a result a higher level of pain relief usually occurs. IV patient-controlled analgesia is available for use during labor. With this method the woman self-administers small doses of an opioid analgesic by using a pump programmed for dose and frequency. Overall a lower total amount of analgesic is used, and maternal satisfaction is high. Classifications of analgesic medications used to relieve the pain of childbirth include opioid (narcotic) agonists and opioid (narcotic) agonist-antagonist compounds.

Choice of which medication to use often depends on preferences of the primary health care provider and the characteristics of the laboring woman. Types of systemic analgesics used may also vary from one obstetric unit to another.

Opioid (Narcotic) Agonist Analgesics

Opioid agonist analgesics such as meperidine (Demerol), hydromorphone (Dilaudid), fentanyl (Sublimaze), and sufentanil citrate (Sufenta) are effective for the relief of severe, persistent, or recurrent pain. They have no amnesic effect but create a feeling of well-being or euphoria (Medication Guides). These analgesics decrease gastric emptying and increase nausea and vomiting. Bladder and bowel elimination can be inhibited.

NURSING ALERT Because heart rate (e.g., bradycardia, tachycardia), blood pressure (e.g., hypotension), and respiratory effort (e.g., depression) can be adversely affected, opioid analgesics should be used cautiously in women with respiratory and cardiovascular disorders. Safety precautions should be taken because sedation and dizziness can occur after administration, increasing the risk for injury.

Women who receive opioids for their labor pain have less effective pain relief and are less satisfied with their pain management method than women whose pain is managed by using epidural analgesia. However, opioid use is associated with shorter labors, less oxytocin augmentation, and fewer instrumental vaginal births (e.g., forceps- or vacuum-assisted birth) when compared with epidural analgesia.

Meperidine hydrochloride (also known as pethidine) used to be the most commonly used opioid agonist analgesic for women in labor, but it is no longer the preferred choice because other medications have fewer side effects. Its short half-life requires more frequent administration, increasing the risk for adverse reactions (e.g., dysphoria, irritability, seizures, tremors) related to the accumulation of a toxic metabolite (Lehne, 2007) (see Medication Guide).

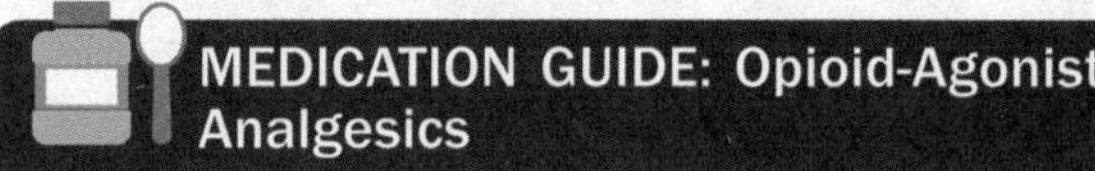

MEDICATION GUIDE: Opioid-Agonist Analgesics

Meperidine (Demerol)
Hydromorphone Hydrochloride (Dilaudid)

Action

Opioid agonist analgesics stimulate mu and kappa opioid receptors to decrease transmission of pain impulses

Indication

Moderate-to-severe labor pain; postoperative pain after cesarean birth

Dosage and Route

Meperidine hydrochloride—25 mg intravenously; 50 to 100 mg intramuscularly or subcutaneously; may repeat in 1 to 3 hours

Hydromorphone hydrochloride—1 mg IV every 3 hours as needed; 1 to 2 mg IM, may repeat in 3 to 6 hours if needed; or 3 to 4 mg, may repeat in 4 to 6 hours if needed.

Adverse Effects

Nausea and vomiting, sedation, confusion, drowsiness, tachycardia or bradycardia, hypotension, dry mouth, pruritus, urinary retention, respiratory depression (woman and newborn), decreased fetal heart rate (FHR) variability, decreased uterine activity if given in early labor

Nursing Considerations

Assess maternal vital signs, degree of pain, FHR and pattern, and uterine activity before and after administration; observe for respiratory depression, notifying primary health care provider if maternal respirations are 12 breaths/min or less; encourage voiding every 2 hours and palpate for bladder distention; administer with a phenothiazine or benzodiazepine, if ordered, to potentiate the analgesic effect, enhance sedation, and decrease nausea and vomiting; if birth occurs within 1 to 4 hours of dose, observe newborn for respiratory depression; have naloxone available as antidote; implement safety measures as appropriate, including use of side rails and assistance with ambulation; continue use of nonpharmacologic pain relief measures

Fentanyl citrate (Sublimaze) and sufentanil citrate (Sufenta) are potent, short-acting opioid agonist analgesics (see Medication Guide, p. 408). Sufentanil use is increasing since it is has a more potent analgesic action than fentanyl when given epidurally. In addition, less sufentanil crosses the placenta, resulting in reduced fetal exposure. Onset of action after IV injection of either fentanyl or sufentanil occurs within 2 to 5 minutes; the action peaks in 3 to 5 minutes, and the duration of action is 30 to 60 minutes. More frequent dosing is required with fentanyl and sufentanil because of their relatively short duration of action. As a result these opioids are most commonly administered intrathecally or epidurally, alone or in combination with a local anesthetic agent (e.g., bupivacaine) (Lehne, 2007).

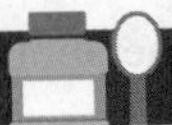

MEDICATION GUIDE

Fentanyl (Sublimaze) and Sufentanil (Sufenta)

Action

Opioid analgesics, rapid action with short duration (1 to 2 hours intramuscularly; 30 minutes to 1 hour intravenously)

Indication

For epidural or intrathecal analgesia, alone or in combination with a local anesthetic

Dosage and Route

Fentanyl—50 to 100 mcg intramuscularly; 25 to 50 mcg intravenously

Epidural—fentanyl, 1 to 2 mcg with 0.125% bupivacaine at a rate of 8 to 10 ml/hr; sufentanil, 1 mcg with 0.125% bupivacaine at rate of 10 ml/hr

Adverse Effects

Dizziness, drowsiness, allergic reactions, rash, pruritus, respiratory depression, nausea and vomiting, urinary retention

Nursing Considerations

Assess for respiratory depression; naloxone should be available as antidote

Opioid (Narcotic) Agonist-Antagonist Analgesics

An agonist is an agent that activates or stimulates a receptor to act; an antagonist is an agent that blocks a receptor or a medication designed to activate a receptor. Opioid agonist-antagonist compounds such as butorphanol (Stadol) and nalbuphine (Nubain) in the doses used during labor provide analgesia without causing respiratory depression in the mother or the neonate (see Medication Guide). They are less likely to cause nausea and vomiting when compared with meperidine, but sedation may be as great or greater when compared with pure opioid agonists. Both IM and IV routes are used for administration, but the IV route is preferred. These opioid analgesics, especially nalbuphine, are not suitable for women with an opioid dependence because the antagonist activity could precipitate withdrawal symptoms (abstinence syndrome) in both the mother and her newborn (Box 16-5).

BOX 16-5 Signs of Potential Complications—Maternal Opioid Abstinence Syndrome (Opioid/Narcotic Withdrawal)

- Yawning, rhinorrhea (runny nose), sweating, lacrimation (tearing), mydriasis (dilation of pupils)
- Anorexia
- Irritability, restlessness, generalized anxiety
- Tremor
- Chills and hot flashes
- Piloerection ("gooseflesh")
- Violent sneezing
- Weakness, fatigue, and drowsiness
- Nausea and vomiting
- Diarrhea, abdominal cramps
- Bone and muscle pain, muscle spasm, kicking movements

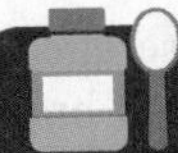

MEDICATION GUIDE: Opioid Agonist-Antagonist Analgesics

Butorphanol Tartrate (Stadol)

Action

Mixed agonist-antagonist analgesic; stimulates kappa opioid receptor and blocks mu opioid receptor

Indication

Labor pain; postoperative pain after cesarean birth

Dosage and Route

1 mg intravenously q3-4hr; 2 mg intramuscularly q3-4hr

Adverse Effects

Confusion, sedation, sweating; transient sinusoidal-like fetal heart rhythm; less respiratory depression, nausea and vomiting

Nursing Considerations

See meperidine; may precipitate withdrawal symptoms in opioid-dependent women and their newborns

Nalbuphine (Nubain)

Action

Mixed agonist-antagonist analgesic; stimulates kappa opioid receptor and blocks mu opioid receptor

Indication

Labor pain; postoperative pain after cesarean birth

Dosage and Route

10 mg intravenously; 10 to 20 mg intramuscularly q3-6hr

Adverse Effects

See butorphanol

Nursing Considerations

See butorphanol

Opioid (Narcotic) Antagonists

Opioids such as hydromorphone, meperidine, and fentanyl can cause excessive CNS depression in the mother and newborn. Current practice of giving lower doses of opioids intravenously has reduced the incidence and severity of opioid-induced CNS depression. Opioid antagonists such as naloxone (Narcan) can promptly reverse the CNS depressant effects, especially respiratory depression (see Medication Guide). In addition, the antagonist counters the effect of stress-induced levels of endorphins. An opioid antagonist is especially valuable if labor is more rapid than expected and birth is anticipated when the opioid is at its peak effect.

The antagonist may be given through the woman's IV line or it can be administered intramuscularly. The woman should be told the pain that was relieved with the use of the opioid analgesic will return with the administration of the opioid antagonist. Some authorities believe that unless maternal CNS depression is severe enough to affect her well-being and that of her fetus, the woman should not receive naloxone just before birth in an attempt to prevent neonatal CNS depression. Placental transfer of naloxone is unpredictable; the newborn may not require treatment with an opioid antagonist;

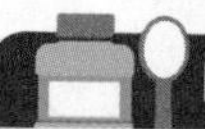

MEDICATION GUIDE: Opioid Antagonist

Naloxone Hydrochloride (Narcan)

Action

Opioid antagonist that blocks both mu and kappa opioid receptors from the effects of opioid agonists

Indication

Reverses opioid-induced respiratory depression in woman or newborn; may be used to reverse pruritus from epidural opioids

Dosage and Route

Adult: Opioid overdose—0.4 to 2 mg intravenously, may repeat IV at 2- to 3-minute intervals up to 10 mg; if IV route unavailable, IM or SC administration may be used

Adult: Postoperative opioid depression—Initial dose 0.1 to 0.2 mg IV at 2- to 3-minute intervals up to three doses to desired degree of reversal obtained; may repeat dose in 1 to 2 hours if needed.

Newborn: Opioid-induced depression—Initial dose is 0.1 mg/kg intravenously, intramuscularly, or subcutaneously; may be repeated at 2- to 3-minute intervals up to three doses until desired degree of reversal is obtained

Adverse Effects

Maternal hypotension and hypertension, tachycardia, hyperventilation, nausea and vomiting, sweating, and tremulousness

Nursing Considerations

Woman should delay breastfeeding until medication is out of system; do not give to mother or newborn if woman is opioid dependent—may cause abrupt withdrawal in woman and newborn if given to woman for reversal of respiratory depression caused by opioid analgesic; pain will return suddenly

and the sudden return of severe pain could have adverse physiologic and psychologic effects on the mother (Lehne, 2007).

NURSING ALERT An opioid antagonist is contraindicated for an infant of an opioid-dependent woman because it may precipitate abstinence syndrome (withdrawal symptoms) (see Box 16-5).

An opioid antagonist can be given to the newborn as one part of the treatment for neonatal narcosis, which is a state of CNS depression in the newborn caused by an opioid. Prophylactic administration of naloxone is controversial. Affected infants may exhibit respiratory depression, hypotonia, lethargy, and a delay in temperature regulation. Risk for hypoxia, hypercarbia, and acidosis increases if neonatal narcosis is not treated promptly. Treatment involves ventilation, administration of oxygen, and gentle stimulation. Naloxone is administered, if still required, to reverse CNS depression. More than one dose of naloxone may be required because its half-life is shorter than the half-life of opioids. Alterations in neurologic and behavioral responses may be evident for as long as 2 to 4 days after birth. Some depression of attention and social responsiveness can be evident for up to 6 weeks after birth. The significance of these neurobehavioral changes is unknown (Lehne, 2007).

Nerve Block Analgesia and Anesthesia

A variety of local anesthetic agents are used in obstetrics to produce regional analgesia (some pain relief and motor block) and anesthesia (complete pain relief and motor block). Most of these agents are related chemically to cocaine and end with the suffix *-caine*. This helps to identify a local anesthetic.

The principal pharmacologic effect of local anesthetics is the temporary interruption of the conduction of nerve impulses, notably pain. Examples of common agents are lidocaine (Xylocaine), bupivacaine (Marcaine), chloroprocaine (Nesacaine), tetracaine (Pontocaine), and mepivacaine (Carbocaine). The solution strength of the local anesthetic agent and the amount used depend on the type of nerve block being performed.

In rare instances people are sensitive (allergic) to one or more local anesthetics. Such a reaction may include respiratory depression, hypotension, and other serious adverse effects. Epinephrine, antihistamines, oxygen, and supportive measures should reverse these effects. Sensitivity may be identified by administering minute amounts of the medication to test for an allergic reaction.

Local Infiltration Anesthesia

Local infiltration anesthesia of perineal tissues is commonly used when an episiotomy is to be performed or when lacerations must be sutured after birth in a woman who does not have regional anesthesia. Rapid anesthesia is produced by injecting 10 to 20 ml of 1% lidocaine or 2% chloroprocaine into the skin and then subcutaneously into the region to be anesthetized. Epinephrine often is added to the solution to localize and intensify the anesthesia in a limited region and prevent excessive bleeding and systemic absorption by constricting local blood vessels. Repeated injections will prolong the anesthesia as long as needed.

Pudendal Nerve Block

Pudendal nerve block, administered late in the second stage of labor, is useful if an episiotomy is to be performed or if forceps or a vacuum extractor is to be used to facilitate birth. It can also be administered during the third stage of labor if an episiotomy or lacerations have to be repaired. Its use has declined as a result of the increased use of epidural anesthesia. Although it does not relieve pain from uterine contractions, it does relieve pain in the lower vagina, vulva, and perineum (Fig. 16-8, *A*). A pudendal nerve block must be administered 10 to 20 minutes before perineal anesthesia is needed.

The pudendal nerve traverses the sacrosciatic notch just medial to the tip of the ischial spine on each side. Injection of an anesthetic solution at or near these points anesthetizes the pudendal nerves peripherally (Fig. 16-9). The transvaginal approach is generally used because it is less painful for the woman, has a higher rate of success in blocking pain, and tends to cause fewer fetal complications. Pudendal block does not change maternal hemodynamic or respiratory functions, vital signs, or FHR. However, the bearing-down reflex is lessened or lost completely.

Spinal Anesthesia (Block)

In spinal anesthesia (block) an anesthetic solution containing a local anesthetic alone or in combination with fentanyl is injected through the third, fourth, or fifth lumbar interspace into the subarachnoid space (Fig. 16-10, *A* and *B*), where the

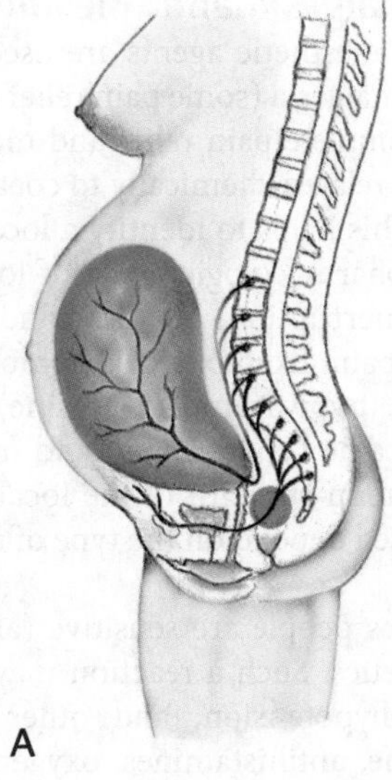

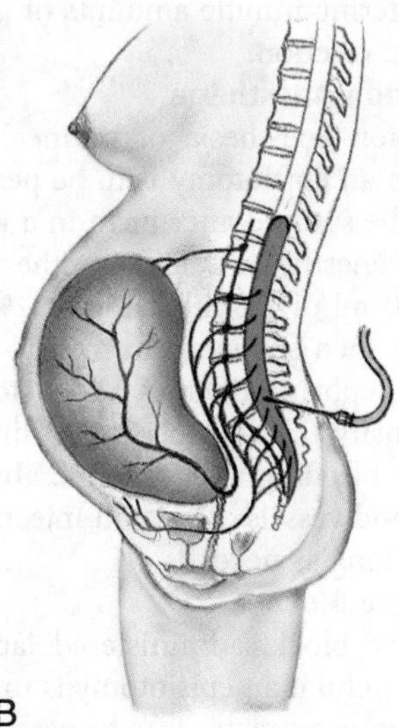

Fig. 16-8 Pain pathways and sites of pharmacologic nerve blocks. **A,** Pudendal block; suitable during second and third stages of labor and for repair of episiotomy. **B,** Epidural block; suitable during all stages of labor and for repair of episiotomy.

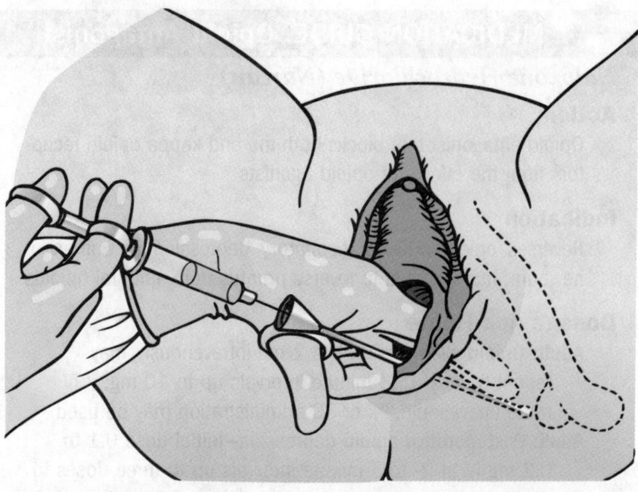

Fig. 16-9 Pudendal block. Use of needle guide ("Iowa trumpet") and Luer-Lok syringe to inject medication.

anesthetic solution mixes with cerebrospinal fluid (CSF). The use of this technique has increased for both elective and emergent cesarean births and is more common than epidural anesthesia for these types of births. Low spinal anesthesia (block) may be used for vaginal birth, but it is not suitable for labor. Spinal anesthesia (block) used for cesarean birth provides anesthesia from the nipple (T6) to the feet. If it is used for vaginal birth, the anesthesia level is from the hips (T10) to the feet (see Fig. 16-10, *C*).

To initiate spinal anesthesia (block), the woman is sitting or lying on her side (e.g., modified Sims position) with back curved to widen the intervertebral space to facilitate insertion of a small-gauge spinal needle and injection of the anesthetic solution. The nurse supports the woman because she must remain still during the placement of the spinal needle. The insertion is made between contractions. After the anesthetic solution has been injected, the woman may be positioned upright to allow the heavier (hyperbaric) anesthetic solution to flow downward to obtain the lower level of anesthesia suitable for a vaginal birth. She may be positioned supine with head and shoulders slightly elevated and the uterus displaced with a wedge under one of her hips to obtain the higher level of anesthesia desired for cesarean birth (see Fig. 16-10, *C*). The anesthetic effect usually begins 1 to 2 minutes after the anesthetic solution is injected and lasts 1 to 3 hours, depending on the type of agent used.

Marked hypotension, impaired placental perfusion, and an ineffective breathing pattern may occur during any spinal anesthesia. Before induction of the spinal anesthetic (block), the woman's fluid balance is assessed, and IV fluid is usually administered to decrease the potential for hypotension caused by sympathetic blockade (vasodilation with pooling of blood in the lower extremities decreases cardiac output). After induction of the anesthetic, maternal blood pressure, pulse, and respirations and FHR and pattern must be checked and documented every 5 to 10 minutes. If signs of serious maternal hypotension (e.g., a drop in the baseline blood pressure of more than 20%) or fetal distress (e.g., bradycardia, diminished variability, late decelerations) develop, emergency care must be given (see Emergency box).

Because the mother is not able to sense her contractions, she must be instructed when to bear down during a vaginal birth. Use of a combination of local anesthetic agent and an opioid reduces the degree of motor function loss, thereby enhancing a woman's ability to push effectively. If the birth occurs in a delivery room (rather than a labor-delivery-recovery room), the woman will need assistance in the transfer to a recovery bed after expulsion of the placenta.

Advantages of spinal anesthesia include ease of administration and absence of fetal hypoxia with maintenance of normotension. Maternal consciousness is maintained, excellent muscular relaxation is achieved, and blood loss is not excessive.

Disadvantages of spinal anesthesia include medication reactions (e.g., allergy), hypotension, and an ineffective breathing pattern; cardiopulmonary resuscitation may be

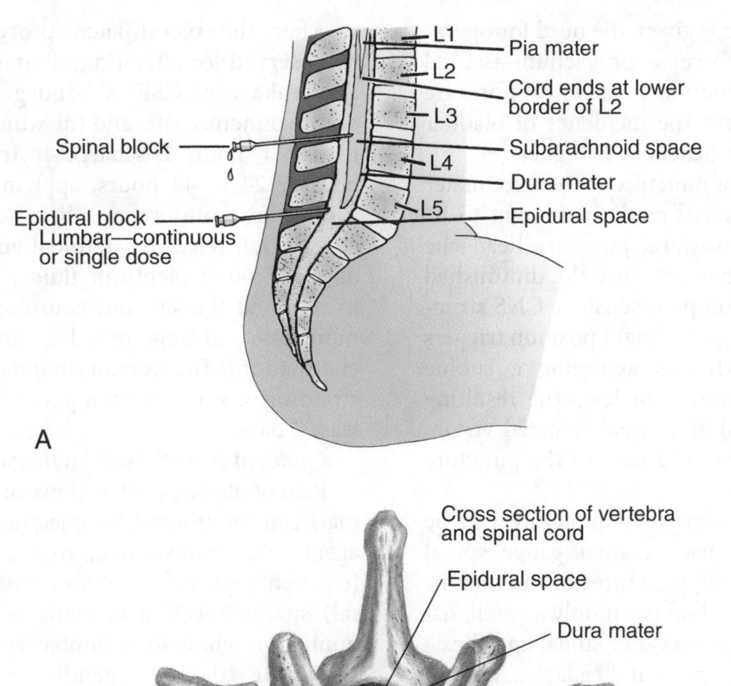

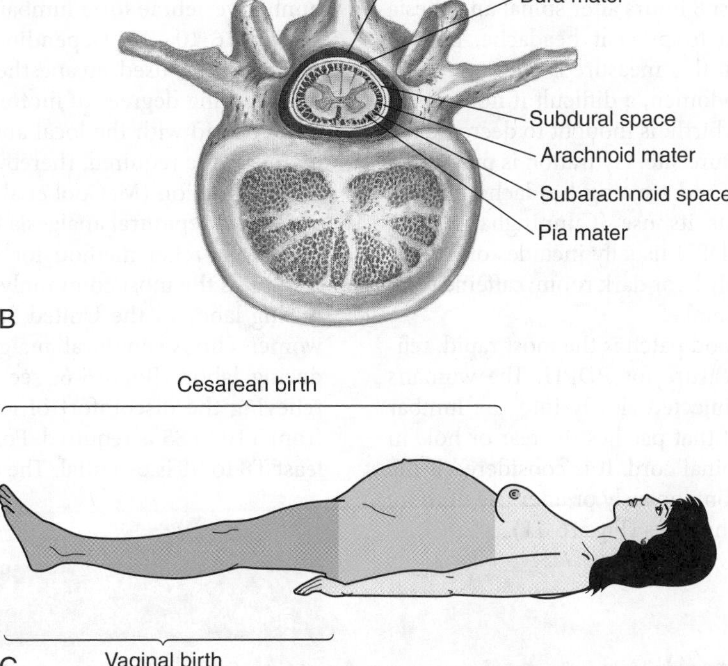

Cesarean birth

Vaginal birth

C

Fig. 16-10 **A,** Membranes and spaces of spinal cord and levels of sacral, lumbar, and thoracic nerves. **B,** Cross section of vertebra and spinal cord. **C,** Levels of anesthesia necessary for cesarean and vaginal births.

EMERGENCY

Maternal Hypotension with Decreased Placental Perfusion

Signs and Symptoms

Maternal hypotension (20% drop from preblock level or less than 100 mm Hg systolic)

Fetal bradycardia

Decreased beat-to-beat fetal heart rate variability

Interventions

Turn woman to lateral position or place pillow or wedge under hip (see Fig. 18-4, *D*) to deflect uterus.

Maintain intravenous infusion at rate specified, or increase prn per hospital protocol.

Administer oxygen by face mask at 10 to 12 L/min or per protocol.

Elevate woman's legs.

Notify physician/midwife/anesthesiologist/nurse anesthetist.

Administer intravenous vasopressor (e.g., ephedrine) per protocol.

Remain with woman; continue to monitor maternal blood pressure and fetal heart rate every 5 minutes until her condition is stable or per primary health care provider's order.

needed. When a spinal anesthetic is given, the need for operative delivery (i.e., episiotomy; forceps- or vacuum-assisted birth) tends to increase because voluntary expulsive efforts are reduced or eliminated. After birth the incidence of bladder and uterine atony and postspinal headache is higher.

Leakage of CSF from the site of puncture of the dura mater (membranous covering of the spinal cord) is thought to be the major causative factor in postdural puncture headache (PDPH). Presumably postural changes cause the diminished volume of CSF to exert traction on pain-sensitive CNS structures. Characteristically, assuming an upright position triggers or intensifies the headache, whereas assuming a supine position achieves relief in 30 minutes or less. The resulting headache and auditory (tinnitus) and visual (blurred vision, photophobia) problems begin within 2 days of the puncture and may persist for days or weeks.

The likelihood of headache after dural puncture can be reduced if the anesthesiologist uses a small-gauge spinal needle and avoids making multiple punctures of the meninges. Positioning the woman flat in bed (with only a small, flat pillow for her head) for at least 8 hours after spinal anesthesia also has been recommended to prevent headache, but no definitive evidence shows that this measure is effective. Positioning the woman on her abdomen, a difficult if not impossible position after a cesarean birth, is thought to decrease the loss of CSF through the puncture site. Hydration is purported to be of value in preventing and treating headache, but no compelling evidence supports its use (Cunningham et al, 2005). Initial treatment for PDPH usually includes oral analgesics; bed rest in a quiet, dimly lit or dark room; caffeine (oral liquids); and increased fluid intake.

An autologous epidural blood patch is the most rapid, reliable, and beneficial relief measure for PDPH. The woman's blood (i.e., 10 to 20 ml) is injected slowly into the lumbar epidural space, creating a clot that patches the tear or hole in the dura mater around the spinal cord. It is considered if the headache does not resolve spontaneously or after use of more conservative, noninvasive techniques (Fig. 16-11).

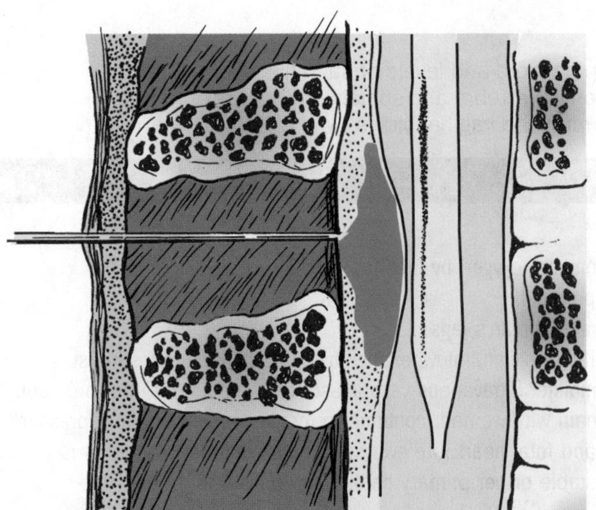

Fig. 16-11 Blood-patch therapy for spinal headache.

After the blood-patch procedure, the woman should be observed for alteration of vital signs, pallor, clammy skin, and leakage of CSF. A bandage and cold pack are placed on the puncture site, and the woman rests in bed for approximately 1 hour. Discharge instructions include resting in bed for 24 to 48 hours, applying cold packs to the site as needed for comfort, avoiding analgesics that affect platelet aggregation (e.g., nonsteroidal antiinflammatory drugs for 2 days, drinking plenty of fluids, and observing for signs of infection at the site and neurologic symptoms such as pain, numbness and tingling in legs, and difficulty with walking or elimination). The woman should be cautioned to avoid lifting, straining at stool, coughing, tub bathing, or swimming for at least 2 days.

Epidural Anesthesia/Analgesia (Block)

Pain of uterine contractions and birth (vaginal and abdominal) can be relieved by injecting a suitable local anesthetic agent (e.g., bupivacaine, ropivacaine), an opioid analgesic (e.g., fentanyl, sufentanil), or both into the epidural (peridural) space. Injection is made between the fourth and fifth lumbar vertebrae for a lumbar epidural block (see Figs. 16-8, *B,* and 16-10, *A*). Depending on the type and amount of medication(s) used, an anesthetic or analgesic effect will occur with varying degrees of motor impairment. The combination of an opioid with the local anesthetic agent reduces the dose of anesthetic required, thereby preserving a greater degree of motor function (McCool et al, 2004).

Lumbar epidural analgesia is the most effective pharmacologic pain relief method for labor currently available. As a result it is the most commonly used method for relieving pain during labor in the United States. Nearly two thirds of U.S. women choose epidural analgesia for their plan of pain care during labor (Box 16-6; see Cultural Awareness box). For relieving the discomfort of labor and vaginal birth, a block from T10 to S5 is required. For cesarean birth a block from at least T8 to S1 is essential. The diffusion of epidural anesthesia

BOX 16-6 Do Women Have a Choice for Labor Analgesia?

"A technologic birthing model that uses labor induction, epidural analgesia, continuous electronic fetal monitoring, and cesarean delivery increasingly dominates labor and delivery wards in the United States and other industrialized countries" (Leeman et al, 2003a). The American Society of Anesthesiologists has suggested that smaller hospitals that cannot support universal access to epidural analgesia should be closed. It is unknown whether the use of epidural analgesia by women in labor in the United States is a true preference or if it is selected because the only other choice is parenteral opioids. For example, nitrous oxide is rarely used in the United States. There is ample evidence of the benefits of the use of doulas and continuous support in labor, yet many women are not offered these options. Research is needed to discover which pain relief methods women would choose if they were offered a wide range of options (Leeman et al, 2003b).

depends on the location of the catheter tip, the dose and volume of the anesthetic agent used, and the woman's position (e.g., horizontal or head-up position).

CULTURAL AWARENESS

Access to Epidural Analgesia in Labor

Epidural analgesia is a highly effective, widely available method of providing pain relief in labor. However, Hispanic women and those on Medicaid are less likely than non-Hispanic women with private insurance or no insurance to receive epidurals (Atherton, Feeg, & el-Adham, 2004; Glance et al, 2007). When Medicaid was introduced in Tennessee, there was a significant decrease in the epidural rate (Johnson & Rosenfeld, 1995). It is not known whether provider preference for type of analgesia is influenced by racial or ethnic considerations. For health care providers to manage labor pain effectively, race, ethnicity, and insurance should not be determining factors.

Before placement of the epidural, an IV bolus of 500 to 1000 ml of crystalloids is usually given. The woman is positioned as for a spinal block (i.e., sitting) or in a modified Sims position. For the modified lateral Sims position, the woman is placed on her side with her shoulders parallel, legs slightly flexed, and back arched (Fig. 16-12). It is essential that the woman cooperate and maintain her position without moving during the insertion of the epidural catheter to prevent misplacement, neurologic injury, or hematoma formation. Administration of an opioid analgesic may be necessary to decrease pain and enhance her ability to remain still during the procedure (Cunningham et al, 2005).

After the epidural has been placed, the woman is preferably positioned on her side so that the uterus does not compress the ascending vena cava and descending aorta, which can impair venous return, reduce cardiac output, and decrease placental perfusion. Her position should be alternated from side to side every hour. Upright positions and ambulation may be encouraged, depending on the degree of motor impairment. Oxygen should be available to treat hypotension should it occur despite maintenance of hydration with IV fluid and displacement of the uterus to the side. Ephedrine (a vasopressor used to increase maternal blood pressure) and increased IV fluid infusion may be needed (see Emergency box). The FHR and pattern and progress in labor must be monitored carefully because the woman in labor may not be aware of changes in strength of uterine contractions or of descent of the presenting part.

Several methods can be used for an epidural block. The most commonly used method is the continuous block, achieved by using a pump to infuse the anesthetic solution through an indwelling plastic catheter. The least common method is an intermittent block, which is achieved by using repeated injections of anesthetic solution. Patient-controlled epidural analgesia, the newest method, uses an indwelling catheter and a programmed pump that allows the woman to control the dosing. This method enhances a woman's sense of

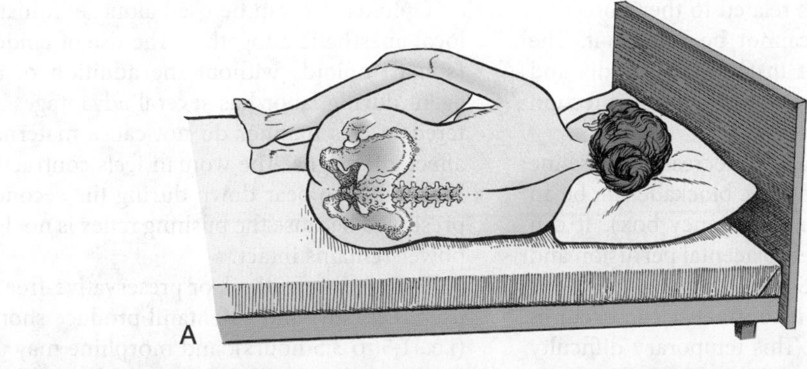

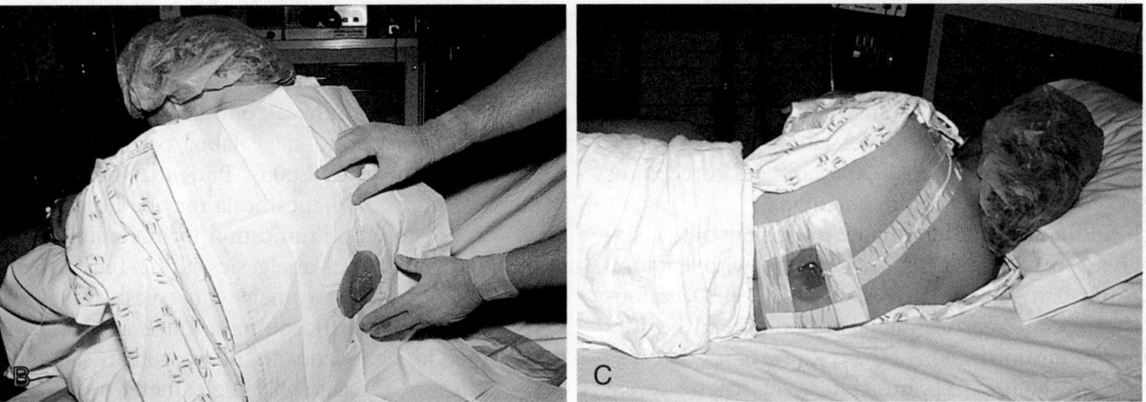

Fig. 16-12 Position for spinal and epidural blocks. A, Lateral position. B, Upright position. C, Catheter is taped to woman's back with port segment located near her shoulder. *(B and C, Courtesy Michael S. Clement, MD, Mesa, AZ.)*

control over her labor and has been found to decrease the total amount of medication used.

The advantages of an epidural block are numerous: the woman remains alert and is more comfortable and able to participate, good relaxation is achieved, airway reflexes remain intact, only partial motor paralysis develops, gastric emptying is not delayed, and blood loss is not excessive. Fetal complications are rare but may occur in the event of rapid absorption of the medication or marked maternal hypotension. The dose, volume, and type of medication(s) used can be modified to allow the woman to push; assume upright positions and walk; produce perineal anesthesia; and permit forceps-assisted, vacuum-assisted, or cesarean birth if required (Cunningham et al, 2005).

The disadvantages of an epidural block are also numerous. Length of labor is longer; there are increased requirements for oxygen and oxytocin (Kukulu & Demirok, 2008). The woman's ability to move freely and maintain control of her labor is limited, related to the use of numerous medical interventions (e.g., an IV infusion, electronic monitoring, Foley catheterization), the occurrence of orthostatic hypotension and dizziness, sedation, and weakness of the legs. CNS effects such as excitation, bizarre behavior, tinnitus, disorientation, paresthesia, and convulsions can occur if a solution containing a local anesthetic agent is accidentally injected into a blood vessel. Respiratory arrest can occur if the relatively high dosage used with an epidural block is accidentally injected into the subarachnoid space. Women who receive an epidural have a higher rate of fever (i.e., intrapartum temperature of 38° C or higher), especially when labor lasts longer that 12 hours. The temperature elevation most likely is related to thermoregulatory changes, although infection cannot be ruled out. The elevation in temperature can result in fetal tachycardia and neonatal workup for sepsis, whether or not signs of infection are present.

Severe hypotension (more than a 20% decrease in baseline blood pressure) as a result of sympathetic blockade can be an outcome of an epidural block (see Emergency box). It can result in a significant decrease in uteroplacental perfusion and oxygen delivery to the fetus (Anim-Somuah, Smyth, & Howell, 2005). Urinary retention and stress incontinence can occur in the immediate postpartum period. This temporary difficulty in urinary elimination could be related not only to the effects of the epidural block but also to the increased duration of labor and need for instrumental birth associated with the block. Pruritus (itching) is a side effect associated with the use of an opioid, including fentanyl and morphine. A relation between epidural analgesia and longer labor, increased incidence of fetal malposition, use of oxytocin, and forceps- or vacuum-assisted birth has been documented.

Research findings have been unable to demonstrate a significant increase in cesarean birth associated with epidural analgesia (Anim-Somuah, Smyth, & Howell, 2005). Occasionally a PDPH can occur after accidental perforation of the dura mater during the administration of the epidural block. Because a larger needle is used for an epidural block, the risk for severe headache is high as a result of greater CSF loss. For some women the epidural block is not effective, and a second form of analgesia is required to establish effective pain relief. When women progress rapidly in labor, pain relief may not be obtained before birth occurs.

Combined Spinal-Epidural Analgesia

Using opioids such as fentanyl and sufentanil to potentiate the effects of local anesthetic agents reduces the amount of the local anesthetic used, thereby reducing motor blockade. A combined spinal-epidural analgesia (CSEA) technique is an increasingly popular approach that can be used to block pain transmission without compromising motor ability (Kuczkowski, 2007). The opioid is injected into the subarachnoid space for rapid activation of the opioid receptors. A catheter is left in place in the epidural space to extend the duration of the analgesia by using a lower dose of a local anesthetic agent alone or in combination with an opioid agonist analgesic. Although women can walk (hence the term *walking epidural*), they often choose not to do so because of sedation and fatigue, abnormal sensations in and weakness of the legs, and a feeling of insecurity. Often health care providers are reluctant to encourage or assist women to ambulate for fear of injury. However, women can be assisted to change positions and use upright positions during labor and birth. Enhanced motor function facilitates more effective bearing-down efforts, thereby reducing the risk for forceps or vacuum-assisted birth (Mayberry et al, 2003; McCool et al, 2004).

CSEA may be associated with fetal bradycardia, necessitating close assessment of FHR and pattern. Since it involves both the puncture of the dura and the placement of a catheter in the epidural space, there is a higher risk for infection and PDPH.

Epidural and Intrathecal Opioids

Opioids also can be used alone, eliminating the effect of a local anesthetic altogether. The use of epidural or intrathecal (spinal) opioids without the addition of a local anesthetic agent during labor has several advantages. Opioids administered in this manner do not cause maternal hypotension or affect vital signs. The woman feels contractions but not pain. Her ability to bear down during the second stage of labor is preserved because the pushing reflex is not lost, and her motor power remains intact.

Fentanyl, sufentanil, or preservative-free morphine may be used. Fentanyl and sufentanil produce short-acting analgesia (i.e., 1.5 to 3.5 hours), and morphine may provide pain relief for 4 to 7 hours. Morphine may be combined with fentanyl or sufentanil. Short-acting opioids are often used with multiparous women, and morphine may be used with nulliparous women or women with a history of long labor. For most women intrathecal opioids do not provide adequate analgesia for second-stage labor pain, episiotomy, or birth (Cunningham et al, 2005). Pudendal nerve blocks or local perineal infiltration anesthesia may be necessary.

A more common indication for the administration of epidural or intrathecal analgesics is the relief of postoperative pain. For example, women who give birth by cesarean can receive fentanyl or morphine through a catheter. The catheter may then be removed, and the women are usually free of pain for 24 hours. Occasionally the catheter is left in place in the epidural space in case another dose is needed.

Women who receive epidurally administered morphine after cesarean birth are up soon after surgery with surprising ease and are able to care for their babies. Early ambulation and freedom from pain also facilitate bladder emptying, enhance peristalsis, and prevent clot formation in the lower extremities (e.g., thrombophlebitis). To those women who have had a previous cesarean birth and experienced the usual postoperative pain, the effects of this approach seem miraculous. However, the mother may not understand why she may have pain after the opioid effect wears off.

Side effects of opioids administered by the epidural and intrathecal routes include nausea, vomiting, pruritus (itching), urinary retention, and delayed respiratory depression. These side effects are more common when morphine or fentanyl is administered. Antiemetics, antipruritics, and opioid antagonists are used to relieve these symptoms. For example, naloxone (Narcan), promethazine (Phenergan), or metoclopramide (Reglan) may be administered. Hospital protocols should provide specific instructions for treatment of these side effects. Use of epidural opioids is not without risks. Respiratory depression is a serious concern; for this reason the woman's respiratory rate should be assessed and documented every hour for 24 hours or per hospital protocol. Naloxone should be readily available for use if the respiratory rate decreases to less than 10 breaths/min or if the oxygen saturation rate decreases to less than 89%. Administration of oxygen by face mask may also be initiated, and the anesthesia care provider should be notified.

Contraindications to Epidural Blocks Contraindications to epidural analgesia include the following:

- Acute antepartum hemorrhage—Acute hypovolemia leads to increased sympathetic tone to maintain the blood pressure; any anesthetic technique that blocks the sympathetic fibers can produce significant hypotension that can endanger the mother and the baby.
- Anticoagulant therapy or bleeding disorder—If a woman is receiving anticoagulant therapy or has a bleeding disorder, injury to a blood vessel may cause the formation of a hematoma that may compress the cauda equina or the spinal cord and lead to serious CNS complications.
- Infection at the injection site—Infection can be spread through the peridural or subarachnoid spaces if the needle traverses an infected area.
- Allergy to the anesthetic drug
- Maternal refusal or inability to cooperate
- Some types of maternal cardiac conditions

Effects of Epidural Block on Neonate Debate persists concerning the effects of epidural anesthesia and analgesia on the newborn's neurobehavioral responses. Findings from studies that examine associations between neurobehavioral outcome and epidural block are far from consistent. For example, studies comparing the neonatal neurobehavioral scores for infants born to mothers who did and mothers who did not receive epidural analgesia either have shown little or no difference in the scores or have shown that the infants of mothers who received epidural anesthesia did not score as well on neurobehavioral tests. In one research study infants exposed to an epidural block tended to have less muscle tone but were better able to orient and habituate to sound when compared with infants whose mothers received opioids during labor (Lieberman & O'Donoghue, 2002).

Paracervical (Uterosacral) Block

Paracervical block has been used during the first stage of labor to relieve pain from uterine contractions and cervical dilation. It is rarely used now for labor because of its association with fetal bradycardia. It may be used for anesthesia during abortion or other gynecologic procedures.

Nitrous Oxide for Analgesia

Nitrous oxide mixed with oxygen can be inhaled in a low concentration (50% or less) to reduce but not eliminate pain during the first and second stages of labor. At the lower doses used for analgesia, the woman remains awake, and the danger of aspiration is avoided because the laryngeal reflexes are unaffected. It can be used in combination with other nonpharmacologic and pharmacologic measures for pain relief.

A face mask or mouthpiece is used to self-administer the gas. The woman should place the mask over her mouth and nose or insert the mouthpiece 30 seconds before the onset of a contraction (if regular) or as soon as a contraction begins (if irregular). When she inhales, a valve opens, and the gas is released. She should continue to inhale the gas slowly and deeply until the contraction starts to subside. When inhalation stops, the valve closes. Onset of action is 50 seconds; therefore beginning the inhalation process 30 seconds before the onset of a contraction provides the best pain relief. During the interval between contractions the woman should remove the device and breathe normally.

Most women who use nitrous oxide obtain adequate pain relief and are satisfied with the method. The nurse should observe the woman for nausea and vomiting, drowsiness, dizziness, hazy memory, and loss of consciousness. Loss of consciousness is more likely to occur if opioids are used with the nitrous oxide. The use of nitrous oxide does not appear to depress uterine contractions or cause adverse reactions in the fetus and newborn.

Nitrous oxide for pain relief during labor is more readily available in Canada and European countries than in the United States.

General Anesthesia

General anesthesia is used rarely for uncomplicated vaginal birth and is used infrequently for elective cesarean birth. It may be necessary if there is a contraindication to spinal or epidural anesthesia or if indications necessitate a rapid birth (vaginal or emergent cesarean) without sufficient time to perform a block. In addition, being awake and aware during major surgery may be unacceptable for some women having a cesarean birth.

If general anesthesia is being considered, the nurse gives the woman nothing by mouth for 6 to 8 hours (per protocol) and sees that an IV infusion is in place. If time allows, the nurse premedicates the woman with a nonparticulate (clear) oral antacid (e.g., such as sodium citrate, Bicitra, Alka-Seltzer) to neutralize the acidic contents of the stomach. Aspiration of highly acidic gastric contents will damage lung tissue. Some anesthesia care providers and physicians also order the administration of a histamine blocker such as cimetidine (Tagamet) to decrease production of gastric acid and metoclopramide (Reglan) to increase gastric emptying. Before the anesthesia is given, a wedge should be placed under one of the woman's hips

evolve Critical Thinking Exercise—Patient Receiving Epidural Block

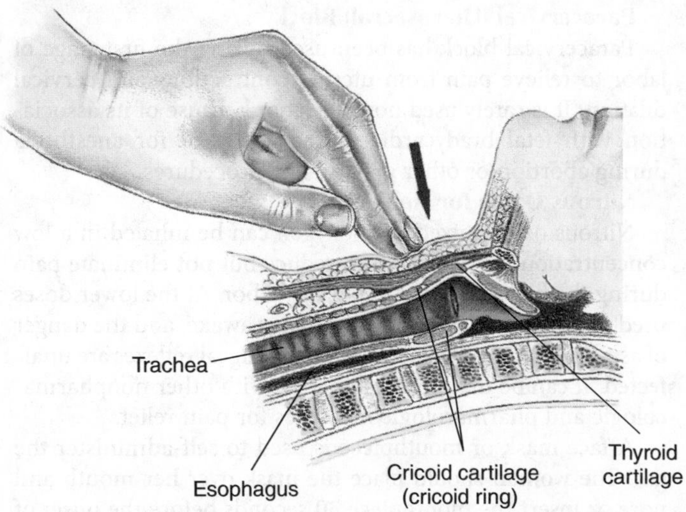

Fig. 16-13 Technique of applying pressure on cricoid cartilage to occlude esophagus to prevent pulmonary aspiration of gastric contents during induction of general anesthesia.

to displace the uterus. Uterine displacement prevents aortocaval compression, which interferes with placental perfusion.

Thiopental, a short-acting barbiturate, is administered intravenously to render the woman unconscious; succinylcholine, a muscle relaxer, is then administered to facilitate passage of an endotracheal tube. Sometimes the nurse is asked to assist with applying cricoid pressure before intubation as the woman begins to lose consciousness. This maneuver blocks the esophagus and prevents aspiration should the woman vomit or regurgitate (Fig. 16-13). Pressure is released once the endotracheal tube is securely in place.

After the woman is intubated, nitrous oxide and oxygen in a 50:50 mixture are administered. A low concentration of a volatile halogenated agent (e.g., isoflurane) also may be administered to increase pain relief and reduce maternal awareness and recall. In higher concentrations isoflurane or methoxyflurane relaxes the uterus quickly and facilitates intrauterine manipulation, version, and extraction. However, at higher concentrations these agents readily cross the placenta and can produce narcosis in the fetus and could reduce uterine tone after birth, increasing the risk for hemorrhage.

Priorities for recovery room care are to maintain an open airway and cardiopulmonary function and to prevent postpartum hemorrhage. Routine postpartum care is organized to facilitate parent-infant interaction as soon as possible and to answer the mother's questions. When appropriate the nurse assesses the mother's readiness to see the baby, as well as her response to the anesthesia and to the event that necessitated general anesthesia (e.g., emergency cesarean birth when vaginal birth was anticipated).

Nursing Care Management

The choice of pain relief depends on a combination of factors, including the woman's special needs and wishes, the availability of the desired method(s), the knowledge and expertise in nonpharmacologic and pharmacologic methods of the health care providers involved in the woman's care, and the phase and stage of labor (see Nursing Process box).

The needs of each woman are different, and many factors must be considered before deciding whether nonpharmacologic methods, pharmacologic methods, or a combination of both will be used to manage labor pain. Women often underestimate the amount of pain they will experience in labor (Lally et al, 2008). It is critical that the nurse take note of all pain characteristics, including location, intensity, quality, frequency, duration, and effectiveness of relief measures.

The nurse should never assume that, because a woman is in labor, her pain must be uterine in origin. Because pain is a subjective phenomenon, the nurse must listen to the woman's description of her pain. A self-assessment tool such as a visual analog scale allows the woman to indicate on a line how severe or intense she perceives her pain to be. Pain is rated from "no pain" to "pain as bad as it can possibly be." Self-assessment is recommended to ensure that pain management is based on the subjective nature of the woman's pain rather than just on the nurse's judgment. It is not unusual for a nurse to overestimate or underestimate the pain being experienced by a patient. When there are major cultural differences between the health care provider and the patient, inaccurate interpretation of pain intensity is more likely.

The woman's perception of her behavior during labor is of utmost importance. If she planned a nonmedicated birth but then needs and accepts medication, her self-esteem may falter. Verbal and nonverbal acceptance of her behavior is given as necessary by the nurse and reinforced by discussion and reassurance after birth. Providing explanations about the fetal response to maternal discomfort, the effects of maternal stress and fatigue on the progress of labor, and the medication itself is a supportive measure. The woman also may experience anxiety and stress related to anticipated or actual pain. Stress can cause increased maternal catecholamine production. Increased levels of catecholamines have been linked to dysfunctional labor and fetal and neonatal distress and illness. Nurses must be able to implement strategies aimed at reducing this stress.

Informed Consent

The primary health care provider and anesthesia care provider are responsible for informing women of the alternative methods of pharmacologic pain relief available in the hospital. Nurses play a part in the informed consent process by clarifying and describing procedures and acting as the woman's advocate by asking the primary health care provider for further explanations.

LEGAL TIP Informed Consent for Anesthesia The woman receives (in an understandable manner) all of the following:

- Explanation of the alternative methods of analgesia and anesthesia available
- Description of anesthetic and procedure for administration
- Description of the benefits, discomfort, risks, and consequences of the selected anesthetic for the mother and the fetus
- Explanation of how complications can be treated
- Information that the anesthetic is not always effective

NURSING PROCESS: DISCOMFORT IN LABOR

Assessment

The assessment of the woman, her fetus, and her labor is a joint effort of the nurse and the primary health care providers who consult with the woman regarding their findings and recommendations. The assessment includes the following.

History

Review prenatal record (parity, estimated date of birth, complications, medications)

Allergies

History of smoking; neurologic and spinal disorders

Interview (by a Member of the Anesthesia Care Team and the Nurse)

Time of woman's last meal; type of food and fluid consumed

Nature of existing respiratory condition (cold, allergy), allergies to medications, cleansing agents, or tape

Childbirth preparation, knowledge and preferences for management of discomfort

Type of analgesia or anesthesia preferred (see Box 16-4)

Herbal medications used

Relevant events that have occurred since last contact with her primary health care provider

If evidence of substance abuse, identify type of drug, last time drug taken, and method of administration; a urine drug screen may be ordered

Physical Examination

Character and status of labor and fetal response
- Maternal vital signs
- Fetal heart rate and pattern
- Uterine contractions
- Amniotic membranes and fluid
- Cervical effacement and dilation and station
- Length of labor and fatigue

Hydration status (intake and output, mucous membranes, skin turgor, urine concentration)

Bladder distention

Signs of apprehension (fist clenching; restlessness)

Review of Results of Laboratory Tests

Hemoglobin and hematocrit (anemia)

Prothrombin time and platelet count (coagulopathy or bleeding disorder) (if ordered)

White blood cell count and differential (infection)

Nursing Diagnoses

The following nursing diagnoses are relevant in the management of discomfort during labor and birth:

Acute pain related to
- processes of labor and birth

Risk for ineffective tissue perfusion related to
- effects of analgesia or anesthesia
- maternal position

Situational low self-esteem related to
- negative perception of the woman's (or her family's) behavior

Anxiety or fear related to deficient knowledge of
- procedure for nerve block analgesia
- expected sensation during nerve block analgesia

Risk for injury to fetus related to
- maternal hypotension
- maternal position (aortocaval compression)

Planning

A plan of care is developed for each woman to address her particular clinical and nursing problems. The nurse collaborates with the primary health care provider, the anesthesia care provider, and the laboring woman to select the aspects of care relevant to the woman and her family.

The expected outcomes for nursing care in the management of discomfort during labor and birth include the following:
- The woman will promptly report the characteristics of her pain and discomfort.
- The woman will verbalize understanding of her needs and rights with regard to pain relief management that uses a variety of nonpharmacologic and pharmacologic methods reflecting her preferences.
- The woman will experience adequate pain relief without adding to maternal risk (e.g., through the use of appropriate nonpharmacologic methods and appropriate medication, including the appropriate dose, timing, and route of administration).
- The fetus will maintain well-being, and the neonate will adjust to extrauterine life without problems related to the management of maternal pain.

Interventions

Assist woman in use of nonpharmacologic interventions.

Provide explanations of fetal response to maternal discomfort and effects of maternal stress and fatigue on the progress of labor.

Ensure informed consent to procedures and anesthesia.

Administer pharmacologic measures.

Prepare woman for procedures.

Monitor for sign of potential problems.

Protect from injury.

Monitor and record response to interventions.

Evaluation

Evaluation of the effectiveness of care of the woman needing management of discomfort during labor and birth is based on the previously stated outcomes.

- Indication that the woman may withdraw consent at any time
- Opportunity to have any questions answered
- Opportunity to explain in her own words components of the consent

The consent form will
- Be written or explained in the woman's primary language.
- Have the woman's signature.
- Have the date of consent.

- Carry the signature of anesthesia care provider, certifying that the woman has received and appears to understand the explanation.

Administration of Medication

Timing of Administration

Accurate monitoring of the progress of labor forms the basis for the nurse's judgment that a woman needs pharmacologic control of discomfort. It is usually the nurse who notifies the primary health care provider that the woman is in need of pharmacologic measures to relieve her discomfort. Knowledge of the medications used during childbirth is essential. The most effective route of administration is selected for each woman; then the medication is prepared and administered correctly.

Orders are often written for the administration of pain medication as needed by the woman and based on the nurse's clinical judgment. Generally pharmacologic measures for pain relief are not implemented until labor has advanced to the active phase of the first stage of labor and the cervix is dilated approximately 4 to 5 cm to avoid suppressing the progress of labor (see Box 16-4). Nonpharmacologic measures can be used to relieve pain in early labor while relieving stress and enhancing progress (see Box 16-2).

Preparation for Procedures

The nurse reviews the methods of pain relief available to the woman (or validates her choices) and clarifies information as necessary. The procedure and what will be asked of the woman (e.g., to maintain flexed position during insertion of epidural needle) must be explained. The woman can also benefit from knowing the route of administration of the medication, the degree of discomfort to expect from administration of the medication, the interval before the medication takes effect, and the expected pain relief from the medication. When an indwelling epidural catheter is to be threaded, the woman should be told that she may experience a momentary twinge down her leg, hip, or back and that this feeling is not a sign of injury.

A long needle is used for pudendal blocks (see Fig. 16-9). The sight of this needle may be frightening, and the woman can be reassured that only the tip of the needle will be inserted.

Intravenous Route The preferred route of administration of medications such as fentanyl and nalbuphine is through IV tubing administered into the port nearest the woman while the infusion of IV solution is stopped. The medication is given slowly in small doses at the beginning of a contraction and over three to five consecutive contractions. Because uterine blood vessels are constricted during contractions, the medication stays within the maternal vascular system for several seconds before the uterine blood vessels reopen. The IV infusion is then restarted slowly to prevent a bolus of medication from being administered. With this method of injection, the amount of medication crossing the placenta to the fetus is minimized. With decreased placental transfer, the mother's degree of pain relief is maximized. The IV route has the following advantages:

- Onset of pain relief is rapid and more predictable.
- Pain relief is obtained with small doses of the drug.
- Duration of effect is more predictable.

Intramuscular Route Although IM injections of analgesics are still used, they are not the preferred route of administration for the woman in labor. The advantages of using the IM route are quick administration and no need to site an IV line.

Disadvantages of the IM route include the following:

- Onset of pain relief is delayed.
- Higher doses of medication are required.
- Medication is released at an unpredictable rate from the muscle tissue and is available for transfer across the placenta to the fetus.

IM injections given in the upper portion of the arm (deltoid site) seem to result in more rapid absorption and higher blood levels of the medication than injections given in other sites. The deltoid is the preferred site if regional anesthesia is planned later in labor because the autonomic blockage from the regional (e.g., epidural) anesthesia causes blood flow to the gluteal region to be increased and accelerates absorption of the drug. The maternal plasma level of the drug necessary to bring pain relief usually is reached 45 minutes after IM injection, followed by a decline in plasma levels. The maternal drug levels (after IM injections) are unequal because of uneven distribution (maternal uptake) and metabolism.

Spinal Nerve Blocks An IV line is usually established before induction of nerve blocks such as epidural and spinal blocks. Anesthesia protocols often include the prophylactic administration of a bolus of IV fluid before epidural and spinal anesthesia for blood volume expansion to prevent maternal hypotension. However, routine preloading with IV fluids before epidural analgesia is a form of care with a trade-off between beneficial and adverse effects (Enkin et al, 2000).

Lactated Ringer's and normal saline solutions are commonly used infusion solutions. Infusion solutions without dextrose are preferred, especially when the solution must be infused rapidly (e.g., to treat dehydration or maintain blood pressure) because solutions containing dextrose rapidly raise maternal blood glucose levels. The fetus responds to high blood glucose levels by increasing insulin production; fetal or neonatal hypoglycemia may result as the glucose is metabolized. In addition, dextrose changes osmotic pressure so that fluid is excreted from the kidneys more rapidly.

Because spinal nerve blocks can reduce bladder sensation, resulting in difficulty in voiding, the woman should empty her bladder before the induction of the block and should be encouraged to void at least every 2 hours thereafter. The nurse should palpate for bladder distention and measure urinary output to ensure that the bladder is being emptied completely. A distended bladder can inhibit uterine contractions and fetal descent, resulting in a slowing of the progress of labor. The status of the maternal-fetal unit and the progress of labor must be established before the block is performed. The nurse or the woman's partner must assist the woman to assume and maintain the correct position for induction of epidural and spinal anesthesia (see Fig. 16-12).

Signs of Potential Problems

The woman should be questioned about the use of herbal medications. There is potential for alternations in maternal hemodynamics (e.g., tachycardia, hypertension) and increased bleeding tendencies with herbal self-therapy (Kuczkowski, 2006).

Any medication can cause an allergic reaction that may be minor or as severe as anaphylaxis. Minor reactions can consist of a rash, rhinitis, fever, asthma, or pruritus. Management of the less acute allergic response is not an emergency. As part of the assessment for such allergic reactions, the nurse should monitor the woman's vital signs, respiratory status, cardiovascular status, platelet count, and white blood cell count. The woman is observed for side effects of medications, especially drowsiness.

Severe allergic reactions may occur suddenly and lead to shock. The most dramatic form of anaphylaxis is sudden severe bronchospasm, vasospasm, severe hypotension, and death. Signs of anaphylaxis are largely caused by contraction of smooth muscles and may begin with irritability, extreme weakness, nausea, and vomiting. This may then lead to dyspnea, cyanosis, convulsions, and cardiac arrest. An acute allergic reaction—anaphylaxis—must be diagnosed and treated immediately. Treatment usually consists of 1:1000 epinephrine injected subcutaneously or intramuscularly, followed by parenteral administration of antihistamines. Supportive care is given to alleviate symptoms. The type of care is determined by the rapidly assessed cardiovascular and respiratory response of the woman to primary interventions. Cardiopulmonary resuscitation may be necessary. The nurse must also be alert to changes in fetal status: nonreassuring changes in FHR and pattern should be noted and reported to the primary health care provider.

Safety and General Care

After administration of a spinal nerve block, the woman is protected from injury by raising the side rails and placing a call bell within easy reach when the nurse is not in attendance. Oxygen and suction should be readily available at the bedside. The nurse must make sure that there is no prolonged pressure on an anesthetized part (e.g., lying on one side with weight on one leg; tight bed linen on feet). If stirrups are used for birth, the nurse should pad them, adjust both stirrups at the same level and angle, place both of the woman's legs into them while avoiding putting pressure to the popliteal angle, and apply restraints without restricting circulation.

Depending on the level of motor blockade, the woman should be assisted to remain as mobile as possible. When in bed, her position should be alternated from side to side every hour to ensure adequate distribution of the anesthetic solution and maintain circulation to the uterus and placenta. Assisting the woman to assume upright positions such as sitting (e.g., modified throne position in which the woman sits on the bed with the bottom part lowered to place her feet below her body) (Fig. 16-14), tug-of-war position (woman tugs on towel or sheet that is tied to the bar on the bed or held by the nurse), and squatting by using the head of the bed or a squatting bar for support (Fig. 16-15) will facilitate fetal descent and enhance bearing-down efforts (Gilder et al, 2002; Mayberry et al, 2003). Ambulation should be encouraged if the woman has received a "walking" epidural. Upright positions are important in the prevention of operative births (e.g., forceps- or vacuum-assisted birth). To prevent injury the nurse must assess the level of motor function (e.g., three unassisted steps with accompaniment; standing and closing eyes, noting the degree of unsteadiness; ability to flex legs or rise from a supine position), level of sensation in legs (e.g., degree of numbness), and level of sedation before the woman is assisted out of bed and periodically thereafter (Mayberry et al, 2003). The woman should sit on the side of the bed before standing to determine if orthostatic hypotension occurs. If she is not dizzy or light-headed, she can stand at the side of the bed and finally walk.

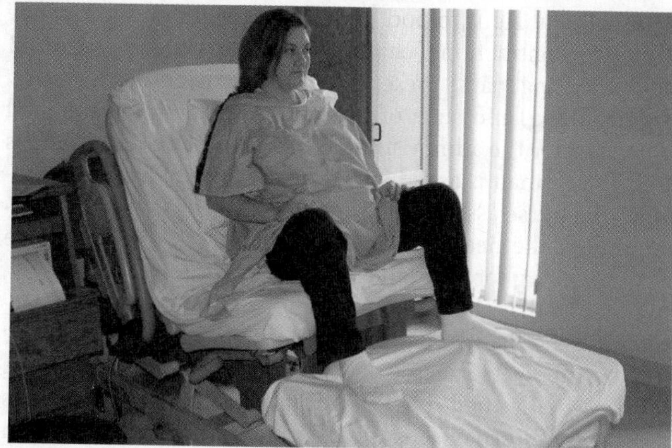

Fig. 16-14 Throne position. *(Courtesy Julie Perry Nelson, Loveland, CO.)*

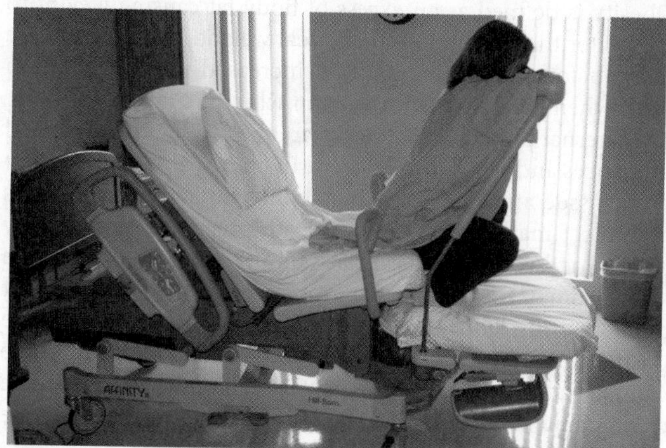

Fig. 16-15 Using squatting bar during labor. *(Courtesy Julie Perry Nelson, Loveland, CO.)*

The second stage of labor is often prolonged in women who use epidural analgesia for pain management. Research evidence indicates that as long as the well-being of the maternal-fetal unit is established, a period of "laboring down" to allow the fetus to descend and rotate with uterine contractions and the use of open-glottis pushing techniques when the fetus has reached a +1 station and is rotating to an anterior position are the best approaches to use for the management of second-stage labor (Mayberry, Clemmens, & De, 2002) (see Chapter 18 for a full discussion of second-stage labor management).

The nurse monitors and records the woman's response to nonpharmacologic pain relief methods and medication(s). This includes the degree of pain relief, the level of apprehension, the return of sensations and perception of pain, and allergic or untoward reactions (e.g., hypotension, respiratory depression, and hypothermia). The nurse continues to monitor maternal vital signs, blood pressure, strength and frequency of uterine contractions, changes in the cervix and station of the presenting part, presence of the bearing-down reflex, bladder filling, and state of hydration. Determining the fetal response after the administration of analgesia or anesthesia is vital. The woman is asked if she (or the family) has any questions. The nurse assesses the woman's and her family's understanding of the need to ensure her safety (e.g., keeping side rails up, calling for assistance as needed).

The time that elapses between the administration of a narcotic and the baby's birth is noted. Medication given to the newborn to reverse narcotic effects is recorded. After birth the woman who has had spinal, epidural, or general anesthesia is assessed for return of sensory and motor function, in addition to the usual postpartum assessments.

Anesthesia in the Obese Woman

Obesity is defined as an excess of body fat causing weight to be greater than 20% more than ideal weight. Women who are obese before pregnancy have an increased risk for cesarean birth when compared with women who are not obese.

Maternal physiologic changes are the product of hormonal influences and mechanical effects. In obese women the weight of fat tissue and the added metabolic demands this involves also affect maternal physiology. Both pregnancy and obesity cause blood volume and cardiac output to increase, and in the obese woman they expand in proportion to the amount of fat tissue. During labor and vaginal birth and in the immediate postpartum period, blood values and cardiac output in obese women can reach levels 80% greater than prelabor values. The enlarged uterus and abdominal fat mass also further increase the possibility of aortocaval compression.

The respiratory system also is stressed in obese pregnant women, and the pulmonary function of an obese laboring woman is in a precarious state. Therefore the woman's oxygenation must be monitored carefully during birth and the immediate postpartum period. Monitoring by pulse oximeter has been recommended.

The gastric emptying time is delayed, the tone of the cardiac sphincter is decreased, and the gastric contents are hyperacidic in all pregnant women. The obese woman also is more likely to have a hiatal hernia and a marked increase in intragastric pressure and volume; therefore these women are at great risk for regurgitation and aspiration.

Management of the obese woman during labor should focus on efforts to minimize oxygen consumption and maximize pulmonary function. Epidural analgesia administered during the first stage of labor can bring about a decreased demand on the metabolic and respiratory systems and improved oxygenation. This is because pain causes the catecholamine levels to increase, which in turn causes cardiac output to increase. Effective epidural analgesia retards this increase in catecholamine levels.

IV opioids may be used during the first stage of labor; however, the doses and the effects must be monitored carefully because obese women are extremely sensitive to the respiratory depressant effects of opioids. An epidural block during the second stage of labor provides complete pain relief and also supports cardiovascular function.

Combined spinal epidural anesthesia is an alternative to epidural anesthesia. This option is now available in the morbidly obese pregnant woman because there is an appropriate long needle manufactured for this purpose (Kuczkowski, 2005).

An epidural block is preferred to general anesthesia in the obese woman who must give birth by cesarean. Problems associated with general anesthesia in obese women include potential difficulties during intubation, a hypertensive effect of laryngoscopy and intubation, and aspiration and pulmonary complications. A spinal block may be used if there is insufficient time to induce an epidural block. Uterine displacement to prevent aortocaval compression is more difficult to achieve in the obese woman in the supine position needed for cesarean birth. If the woman is extremely obese, a wedge may not be able to elevate one hip enough to prevent compression. In this case it may be necessary to lift the abdominal fat pad off the abdomen manually until the peritoneal cavity has been entered.

Maternal Hypothermia After Analgesia and Anesthesia

Hypothermia is defined as a core body temperature of less than 35° C. During labor and immediately after the birth, women are predisposed to hypothermia because of the combination of the vasodilation that normally occurs during pregnancy and the effects of the analgesia and anesthesia.

Opioids, barbiturates, tranquilizers, and antiemetics are thought to affect thermoregulation by increasing vasodilation and radiant loss; general anesthetic agents are thought to do so by depressing thermoregulation; and epidural and spinal anesthesia are thought to do so by inducing peripheral dilation. During labor, during vaginal or cesarean birth, or immediately after birth, women may have shivering, hypotension, and respiratory distress. The hypothermia may result in cardiovascular, pulmonary, circulatory, hematologic, neurologic, or renal complications. The nurse can minimize these complications by making sure that the birthing areas are warm, wet drapes and towels are removed, women are covered with warm blankets after birth, and hypothermia is recognized early. Explaining these effects to the woman and her support people will help allay concerns.

Key Points

- The expected outcome of preparation for childbirth and parenting is "education for choice."
- Nonpharmacologic pain and stress management strategies are valuable for managing labor discomfort alone or in combination with pharmacologic methods.

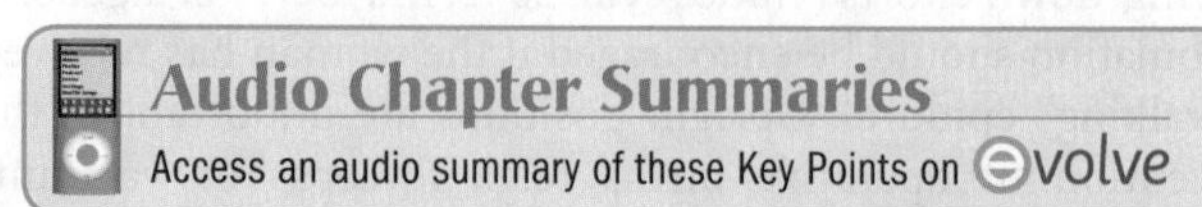
Audio Chapter Summaries
Access an audio summary of these Key Points on evolve

- The gate-control theory of pain and the stress response are the bases for many of the nonpharmacologic methods of pain relief.
- The type of analgesic or anesthetic to be used is determined by maternal and health care provider preference, the stage of labor, and the method of birth.
- Sedatives may be appropriate for women in prolonged early labor when there is a need to decrease anxiety or promote sleep or therapeutic rest.
- Phenothiazines and benzodiazepines can be used during labor to decrease anxiety and apprehension, increase sedation, potentiate opioid analgesic effects, and reduce nausea and vomiting.
- Naloxone (Narcan) is an opioid (narcotic) antagonist that can reverse narcotic effects, especially respiratory depression.
- Pharmacologic control of discomfort during labor requires collaboration among the health care providers and the woman in labor.
- The nurse must understand medications, their expected effects, potential side effects, and methods of administration.
- Maintenance of maternal fluid balance is essential during spinal and epidural nerve blocks.
- Maternal analgesia or anesthesia potentially affects neonatal neurobehavioral response.
- The use of opioid agonist-antagonist analgesics in women with preexisting opioid dependence may cause symptoms of abstinence syndrome (opioid withdrawal).
- General anesthesia is rarely used for vaginal birth but may be used for cesarean birth or whenever rapid anesthesia is needed in an emergency childbirth situation.

References

Anim-Somuah M, Smyth R, Howell C: Epidural versus no epidural or no analgesia in labor, *The Cochrane Database of Systematic Reviews*, 2005, Issue 4, Chichester, UK, 2005, John Wiley & Sons.

Atherton MJ, Feeg VD, el-Adham AF: Race, ethnicity, and insurance as determinants of epidural use: analysis of a national sample survey, *Nurs Econ* 22(1):6-13, 2004.

Beebe KR, Lee K: Sleep disturbance in late pregnancy and early labor, *J Perinat Neonatal Nurs* 21(2):103-108, 2007.

Birthing From Within, n.d. Available at www.birthingfromwithin.com (accessed March 31, 2009).

Bradley R: *Husband-coached childbirth*, ed 3, New York, 1981, Harper & Collins.

Bucklin B et al: Obstetric anesthesia workforce survey, *Anesthesiology* 103(3):645-653, 2005.

Callister LC et al: The pain of childbirth: perceptions of culturally diverse women, *Pain Manag Nurs* 4(4):145-154, 2003.

Childbirth and Postpartum Professional Association (CAPPA), 2008. Available at www.cappa.net (accessed March 31, 2009).

Cunningham FG et al: *Williams obstetrics*, ed 22, New York, 2005, McGraw-Hill.

Dick-Read G: *Childbirth without fear*, ed 5, New York, 1987, Harper & Collins.

Enkin M et al: *A guide to effective care in pregnancy and childbirth*, ed 3, Oxford, NY, 2000, Oxford University Press.

Florence DJ, Palmer DG: Therapeutic choices for the discomforts of labor, *J Perinat Neonatal Nurs* 17(4):238-249, 2003.

Gilder K et al: Maternal positions in labor with epidural analgesia: results from a multi-site survey, *AWHONN Lifelines* 6(1):40-45, 2002.

Glance LG et al: Racial differences in the use of epidural analgesia for labor, *Anesthesiology* 106(1):19-25, 2007.

Hodnett ED: Pain and women's satisfaction with the experience of childbirth: a systematic review, *Am J Obstet Gynecol* 186(5 suppl Nature): S160-S172, 2002.

Hodnett ED et al: Continuous support for women during childbirth, *The Cochrane Database of Systematic Reviews*, 2007, Issue 3, Chichester, UK, 2007, John Wiley & Sons.

HypnoBirthing: Available at www.hypnosisforawakening.com, 2004 (accessed March 31, 2009).

Johnson S, Rosenfeld JA: The effect of epidural anesthesia on the length of labor, *J Fam Pract* 40(3):244-247, 1995.

Karmel M: *Thank you, Dr. Lamaze*, New York, 1959, Dolphin Books.

Kuczkowski KM: Labor analgesia for the morbidly obese parturient: an old problem—new solution, *Arch Gynecol Obstet* 271(4):302-303, 2005.

Kuczkowski KM: Labor analgesia for the parturient with herbal medicine use: what does an obstetrician need to know? *Arch Gynecol Obstet* 274(4):233-239, 2006.

Kuczkowski KM: Labor pain and its management with the combined spinal-epidural analgesia: what does an obstetrician need to know? *Arch Gynecol Obstet* 275(3):183-185, 2007.

Kukulu K, Demirok H: Effects of epidural anesthesia on labor progress, *Pain Manag Nurs* 9(1):10-16, 2008.

Lally JE et al: More in hope than expectation: a systematic review of women's expectations and experience of pain relief in labour, *BMC Med* 6:7, 2008.

Leeman L et al: Editorial: management of labor pain: promoting patient choice, *Am Fam Physician* 68(6):1023-1026, 2003a.

Leeman L et al: The nature and management of labor pain. Part II. Pharmacologic pain relief, *Am Fam Physician* 68(6):1115-1120, 2003b.

Lehne RA: *Pharmacology for nursing care*, ed 6, Philadelphia, 2007, Saunders.

Lieberman E, O'Donoghue C: Unintended effects of epidural anesthesia during labor: a systematic review, *Am J Obstet Gynecol* 186(5 suppl Nature):S31-S68, 2002.

Lothian J, Devries C: *The official Lamaze guide: Giving birth with confidence*, New York, 2005, Meadowbrook Press.

Lowe NK: The nature of labor pain, *Am J Obstet Gynecol* 186(5 suppl Nature):S16-S24, 2002.

Maude RM, Foureur MJ: It's beyond water; stories of women's experience of using water for labour and birth, *Women Birth* 20(1):17-24, 2007.

Mayberry LJ, Clemmens D, De A: Epidural analgesia side effects, co-interventions, and care of women during childbirth: a systematic review, *Am J Obstet Gynecol* 186(5 suppl Nature):S81-S93, 2002.

Mayberry LJ et al: Use of upright positioning with epidural analgesia: findings from an observational study, *MCN Am J Matern Child Nurs* 28(3):152-159, 2003.

McCool WF et al: Obstetric anesthesia: Changes and choices, *J Midwifery Womens Health* 49(6):505-513, 2004.

Mottershead N: Hypnosis: removing the labour from birth, *Pract Midwife* 9(3):26-27, 2006.

Raynes-Greenow CH et al: Knowledge and decision-making for labour analgesia of Australian primiparous women, *Midwifery* 23(2):139-145, 2007.

Simkin P, Bolding A: Update on nonpharmacologic approaches to relieve labor pain and prevent suffering, *J Midwifery Womens Health* 49(6):489-504, 2004.

Simkin PP, O'Hara M: Nonpharmacologic relief of pain during labor: systematic reviews of five methods, *Am J Obstet Gynecol* 186(5 suppl Nature):S131-S159, 2002.

Smith C et al: Complementary and alternative therapies for pain management in labour, *The Cochrane Database of Systematic Reviews*, 2006, Issue 4, Chichester, UK, 2006, John Wiley & Sons.

Trout K: The neuromatrix theory of pain: Implications for selected nonpharmacologic methods of pain relief for labor. *J Midwifery Womens Health* 49(6):482-488, 2004.

VandeVusse L et al: Hypnosis for childbirth: a retrospective comparative analysis of outcomes in one obstetrician's practice, *J Midwifery Womens Health* 50(2):109-119, 2007.

World Health Organization (WHO): *Workshop on perinatal care proceedings*, Venice, April 16-18, Geneva, 1998, Author.

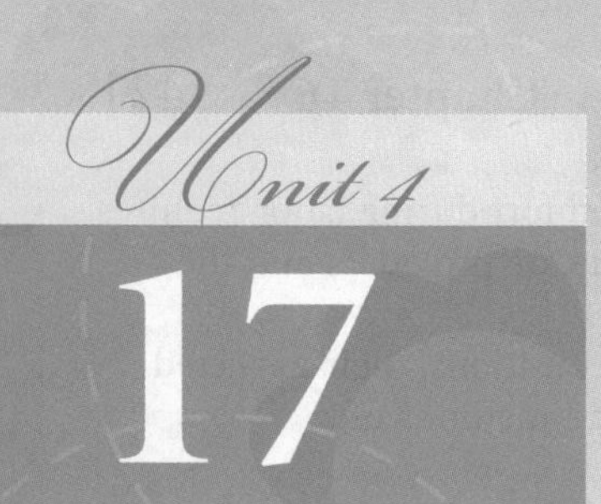

17 Fetal Assessment During Labor

Learning Objectives

On completion of this chapter the reader will be able to:

- Explain baseline fetal heart rate (FHR) and evaluate periodic changes.
- Identify typical signs of nonreassuring FHR patterns.
- Compare FHR monitoring done by intermittent auscultation with external and internal electronic methods.
- Describe nursing measures that can be used to maintain FHR patterns within normal limits.
- Differentiate among the nursing interventions used for managing specific FHR patterns, including tachycardia and bradycardia, increased and decreased variability, and late and variable decelerations.
- Review the documentation of the monitoring process necessary during labor.

Electronic Resources

Additional information related to the content in Chapter 17 can be found on

evolve the Companion Website at

http://evolve.elsevier.com/Perry/maternal/

- NCLEX Review Questions
- Critical Thinking Exercise—Fetal Monitoring
- Nursing Care Plan—Electronic Fetal Monitoring During Labor
- Spanish Guidelines—Fetal Monitoring

The ability to assess the fetus by auscultation of fetal heart tones was initially described more than 300 years ago. With the advent of the fetoscope and stethoscope after the turn of the twentieth century, the listener could hear clearly enough to count the fetal heart rate (FHR). When electronic fetal monitoring (EFM) was first used clinically in the early 1970s, it was anticipated that its use would effect a decrease in cerebral palsy and be more sensitive than stethoscopic auscultation in predicting and preventing fetal compromise (Garite, 2007). Consequently the use of EFM rapidly expanded. However, the rate of cerebral palsy has risen slightly since that time and is not likely to improve (Gilbert, 2007). The cesarean birth rate continues to rise markedly in the United States, with the incidence of cesarean births reported as 31.1% of live births in 2006 (Hamilton, Martin, & Ventura, 2007).

EFM is a useful tool for visualizing FHR patterns on a monitor screen or printed tracing and continues to be the primary mode of intrapartum fetal assessment. Currently in the United States about 85% of women have continuous EFM during labor (Tucker, Miller, & Miller, 2009). Pregnant women should be informed about the equipment and procedures used and the risks, benefits, and limitations of intermittent auscultation (IA) and EFM.

This chapter discusses the basis for fetal monitoring, the types of monitoring, and nursing assessment and management of nonreassuring fetal status. In clinical practice the patterns of the FHR are described as reassuring (progressing normally; no intervention needed) or nonreassuring (abnormal; needing intervention).

Basis for Monitoring

Fetal Response

Because labor is a period of physiologic stress for the fetus, frequent monitoring of fetal status is part of the nursing care during labor. The fetal oxygen supply must be maintained during labor to prevent fetal compromise and promote newborn health after birth. The fetal oxygen supply can decrease in a number of ways:

- Reduction of blood flow through the maternal vessels as a result of maternal hypertension (chronic hypertension or gestational hypertension), hypotension (caused by supine maternal position, hemorrhage, or epidural analgesia or anesthesia), or hypovolemia (caused by hemorrhage)
- Reduction of the oxygen content in the maternal blood as a result of hemorrhage or severe anemia
- Alterations in fetal circulation occurring with compression of the umbilical cord (transient, during uterine contractions [UCs]; or prolonged, resulting from cord prolapse), placental separation or complete abruption, or head compression (head compression causes increased intracranial pressure and vagal nerve stimulation with an accompanying decrease in the FHR)

- Reduction in blood flow to the intervillous space in the placenta secondary to uterine hypertonus (generally caused by excessive exogenous oxytocin) or deterioration of the placental vasculature associated with maternal disorders such as hypertension or diabetes mellitus

Uterine Activity

A normal uterine activity (UA) pattern in labor is characterized by contractions occurring every 2 to 5 minutes and lasting less than 90 seconds. Such contractions are moderate to strong in intensity as assessed by palpation, or intensity is less than 100 mm Hg as measured by an intrauterine pressure catheter (IUPC); 30 seconds or more should elapse between the end of one contraction and the beginning of the next. Between contractions uterine relaxation should be detected by palpation or by an average intrauterine pressure of 15 mm Hg or less.

UA can be described as:

Normal—5 or fewer contractions in 10 minutes averaged over a 30-minute window

Tachysystole—5 or more contractions in 10 minutes averaged over a 30-minute window

Characteristics of UCs:

- Tachysystole should always be qualified by presence or absence of associated FHR decelerations.
- Tachysystole applies to both spontaneous or stimulated labor.
- The terms *hyperstimulation* and *hypercontractility* are not defined and should be abandoned (Macones et al, 2008).

Fetal Compromise

The goals of intrapartum FHR monitoring are to identify and differentiate reassuring patterns from nonreassuring patterns, which can indicate fetal compromise.

Reassuring FHR includes the following:

- Normal baseline rate of 110 to 160 beats/min
- Moderate variability
- Presence of accelerations
- Absence of decelerations (Tucker, Miller, & Miller, 2009)

Nonreassuring FHR patterns are those associated with fetal hypoxemia, which is a deficiency of oxygen in the arterial blood. If uncorrected, hypoxemia can deteriorate to severe fetal hypoxia, which is an inadequate supply of oxygen at the cellular level. Nonreassuring FHR includes the following:

- A baseline FHR of less than 110 beats/min or more than 160 beats/min
- Absent or persistently minimal variability
- Recurrent late or variable decelerations
- Bradycardia (Tucker, Miller, & Miller, 2009)

Monitoring Techniques

The ideal method of fetal assessment during labor continues to be debated. Results from research studies indicate that IA of the FHR and EFM are associated with similar fetal outcomes in low risk intrapartum patients (Gilbert, 2007). The continued use of EFM in place of IA is thought to be caused by concerns about liability and the increased nurse-to-patient ratio required with IA (Tucker, Miller, & Miller, 2009).

Intermittent Auscultation

IA uses listening to fetal heart sounds at periodic intervals to assess the FHR. IA of the fetal heart can be performed with a Leff scope, a DeLee-Hillis fetoscope, a Pinard fetoscope (used commonly in countries outside the United States) (see Fig. 11-8, C), or an ultrasound device. If a Leff scope is used, the domed side should be opened to the connective tubing to the earpieces. The domed side is then applied to the maternal abdomen. The fetoscope is applied over the listener's head because bone conduction amplifies the fetal heart sounds for counting. The bell of the Pinard fetoscope is applied to the maternal abdomen while the nurse's ear is applied to the opposite end. The ultrasound device transmits ultrahigh-frequency sound waves reflecting movement of the fetal heart and converts these sounds into an electronic signal that can be counted (Fig. 17-1).

One procedure for performing auscultation is as follows:

1. Perform Leopold's maneuvers (see Fig. 18-5) by palpating the maternal abdomen to identify fetal presentation and position.
2. Place the listening device over the area of maximal intensity and clarity of the fetal heart sounds to obtain the clearest and loudest sound, which is easiest to count. Apply ultrasound gel to Doppler ultrasound device if used.
3. Palpate the abdomen for the absence of UA to be able to count the FHR between contractions.
4. Count the maternal radial pulse at the same time as listening to the FHR to differentiate it from the fetal rate.
5. Count the FHR for 30 to 60 seconds between contractions to identify the baseline rate. This rate can be assessed only during the absence of UA.
6. Auscultate the FHR during a contraction and for 30 seconds after the end of the contraction to identify any increases or decreases in FHR in response to the contraction.

IA is easy to use, inexpensive, and less invasive than EFM. It is often more comfortable for the woman and gives her more freedom of movement. However, IA may be difficult to perform in women who are obese. Because IA is intermittent, significant events may occur during a time when the FHR is not auscultated. In addition, IA does not provide a permanent

evolve Critical Thinking Exercise—Fetal Monitoring

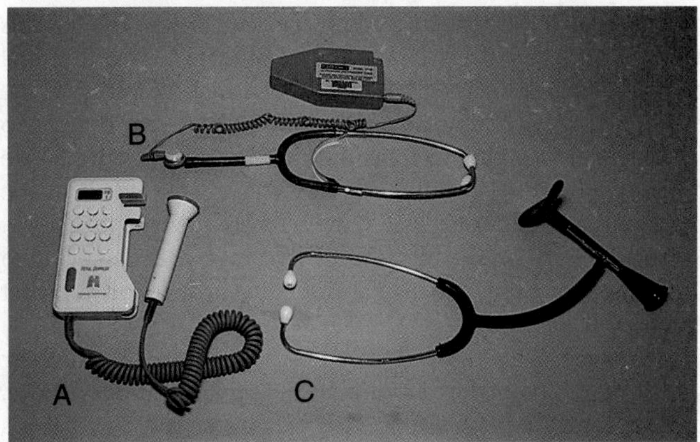

Fig. 17-1 **A**, Ultrasound fetoscope. **B**, Ultrasound stethoscope. **C**, DeLee-Hillis fetoscope. *(Courtesy Michael S. Clement, MD, Mesa, AZ.)*

documented visual record of the FHR and cannot be used to assess visual patterns of the FHR variability or periodic changes (Tucker, Miller, & Miller, 2009). By using IA, the nurse can assess the FHR baseline rate, rhythm, and increases and decreases from baseline. The method and frequency of fetal surveillance during labor will vary, depending on maternal-fetal risk factors and the preference of the facility.

There is no recommended practice for assessing the FHR in the latent phase of first-stage labor; however, the Association of Women's Health, Obstetric and Neonatal Nurses (AWHONN) suggests that the FHR be assessed as frequently as maternal vital signs. It is also assessed before and after ambulation, rupture of membranes, administration of medications and anesthesia, and more frequently when nonreassuring FHR patterns are heard (AWHONN, 2003). The National Institute of Health and Clinical Excellence (NICE) recommends IA at admission and during labor with a stethoscope or Doppler for the low risk laboring patient (NICE, 2008).

NURSING ALERT When the FHR is auscultated and documented, it is inappropriate to use the descriptive terms associated with EFM (e.g., moderate variability, variable deceleration) because most of the terms are visual descriptions of the patterns produced on the monitor tracing. However, terms that are numerically defined such as bradycardia and tachycardia can be used.

Every effort should be made to use the method of fetal assessment the woman desires. However, auscultation of the FHR in accordance with the frequency recommended may be difficult in today's busy labor and birth units. When used as the primary method of fetal assessment, auscultation requires a 1:1 nurse-to-patient staffing ratio. If acuity and census change so that auscultation standards are no longer met, the nurse must discuss this with the laboring woman and inform the woman and the physician or nurse-midwife that continuous EFM will be used until staffing can be arranged to meet the standards.

The woman can become anxious if the examiner cannot readily count the fetal heartbeats. It often takes time for the inexperienced listener to locate the heartbeat and find the area of maximal intensity. To allay the mother's concerns, she can be told that the nurse is "finding the spot where the sounds are loudest." If it takes considerable time to locate the fetal heartbeats, after locating them the examiner can reassure the mother by offering her an opportunity to listen to them, too (see Critical Thinking Exercise). If the examiner cannot locate the fetal heartbeat, assistance should be requested. In some cases ultrasound can be used to help locate the fetal heartbeat. Seeing the FHR on the ultrasound screen can be reassuring to the mother if there was initial difficulty in locating the best area for auscultation.

When using IA, UA is assessed by palpation. The examiner should keep his or her hand placed over the fundus before, during, and after contractions. The contraction intensity is usually described as mild, moderate, or strong. The contraction duration is measured in seconds, from the beginning to the end of the contraction. The frequency of contractions is measured in minutes, from the beginning of one contraction to the beginning of the next contraction. The examiner should keep his or her hand on the fundus after the contraction is over to evaluate uterine resting tone or relaxation between contractions. Normal resting tone between contractions is usually described as soft or relaxed.

Accurate and complete documentation of fetal status and UA is especially important when IA and palpation are being used because no paper tracing record of these assessments is provided as it is by continuous EFM. Labor flow records or computer charting systems that prompt notations of all assessments are useful for ensuring such comprehensive documentation.

CRITICAL THINKING EXERCISE

Fetal Heart Rate Recording

You are assigned to a woman who is in the first stage of labor. She wonders why the fetal heart rate (FHR) is sometimes not being recorded on the monitor paper. She asks if there is "something wrong with the baby" when the FHR is not recording continuously. Based on your knowledge of how the external monitor works, you explain the lack of continuous recording of the FHR and how you plan to improve the tracing and document your observations.

1. Evidence—Is there sufficient evidence to draw conclusions about what causes gaps in recording on the monitor paper and ways to improve the tracing?
2. Assumptions—What assumptions can be made about the following issues?
   a. Efficacy of FHR monitoring in improving pregnancy outcome
   b. Signs of nonreassuring FHR patterns
   c. Causes of periodic and episodic changes in the FHR
   d. Patient choice in fetal monitoring techniques
3. What implications and priorities for nursing care can be drawn at this time?
4. Does the evidence objectively support your conclusion?
5. Are there alternative perspectives to your conclusion?

Electronic Fetal Monitoring

The purpose of electronic FHR monitoring is the ongoing assessment of fetal oxygenation. The goal is to detect fetal hypoxia and metabolic acidosis during labor so that interventions to resolve the problem can be implemented in a timely manner before permanent damage or death occurs (Garite, 2007).

The FHR and UA tracings are evaluated regularly throughout labor. The *Guidelines for Perinatal Care,* jointly published by the American Academy of Pediatrics (AAP) and the American College of Obstetricians and Gynecologists (ACOG) (2007), recommend that the FHR tracing be evaluated at least every 30 minutes during the first stage of labor and every 15 minutes during the second stage of labor in low risk women. If risk factors are present, the FHR tracing should be evaluated more frequently, every 15 minutes in the first stage of labor and every 5 minutes in the second stage of labor.

The two modes of EFM are (1) the external mode, which uses external transducers placed on the maternal abdomen to assess FHR and UA; and (2) the internal mode, which uses a spiral electrode applied to the fetal presenting part to assess the FHR and an IUPC to assess UA and pressure. In some countries EFM is called cardiotocography or CTG (Tucker, Miller, & Miller, 2009) (see Evidence-Based Practice box). The differences between the external and internal modes of EFM are summarized in Table 17-1.

External Monitoring

Separate transducers are used to monitor the FHR and UCs (Fig. 17-2). The ultrasound transducer works by reflecting high-frequency sound waves off a moving interface: in this case the fetal heart and valves. It is sometimes difficult to reproduce a continuous and precise record of the FHR because of artifacts introduced by fetal and maternal movement. The FHR is printed on specially formatted monitor paper. The standard paper speed used in the United States is 3 cm/min. Once the area of maximal intensity of the FHR has been located, conductive gel is applied to the surface of the ultrasound transducer, and the transducer is then positioned over this area.

The tocotransducer (tocodynamometer) measures UA transabdominally. The device is placed over the fundus above the umbilicus. UCs or fetal movements depress a pressure-sensitive surface on the side next to the abdomen. The tocotransducer can measure and record the frequency, regularity, and approximate duration of UCs but not their intensity. This method is especially valuable for measuring UA during the first stage of labor in women with intact membranes or for antepartum testing. Because the tocotransducer of most electronic fetal monitors is designed for assessing UA in term pregnancy, it may not be sensitive enough to detect preterm UA. When monitoring the woman in preterm labor, remember that the fundus may be located below the level of the umbilicus. The nurse may need to rely on the woman to indicate when UA is occurring and to use palpation as an additional way of assessing contraction frequency and validating the monitor tracing.

The external transducer is easily applied by the nurse, but it must be repositioned as the woman or fetus changes posi-

EVIDENCE-BASED PRACTICE Fetal Monitoring and the Machine That Goes "Beep" —*Pat Gingrich*

Ask the Question

What are the optimal methods of assessing fetal well-being during labor?

Search for Evidence

Search Strategies

Professional organization guidelines, meta-analyses, systematic reviews, randomized controlled trials, nonrandomized prospective studies, and retrospective studies since 2006

Databases Searched

CINAHL, Cochrane, Medline, National Guideline Clearinghouse, TRIP Database Plus, and the websites for ACOG, AWHONN, and NICE

Critically Analyze the Evidence

Electronic fetal heart monitoring (EFM; also known as cardiotocography [CTG]) has become standard practice in the labor and birth setting for many decades, especially in the United States. It has been suggested that such monitoring is not necessary for the low risk labor patient and may even present a risk of false abnormal readings leading to high rates of cesarean births.

A meta-analysis of trials measuring fetal outcomes and use of EFM revealed that there was no significant change in APGAR scores for women who had EFM on admission for labor when compared to women who were not monitored at admission. However, there was a statistically increased risk for cesarean birth in the monitored women (Gourounti & Sandall, 2007).

The National Institute of Health and Clinical Excellence (NICE) issued professional guidelines for intrapartum care that do not recommend EFM for the low risk laboring patient (NICE, 2008). Instead, the guidelines recommend IA at admission and during labor with a stethoscope or Doppler. Use of continuous EFM should begin in the presence of meconium, bleeding, abnormal fetal heart rate (less than 110 beats/min or more than 160 beats/min), oxytocin use, or patient request. Similar clinical practice guidelines from the Society of Obstetricians and Gynaecologists of Canada also recommend IA in the absence of risk factors (Liston et al, 2007). EFM should be used for high risk women, with fetal scalp blood pH testing if abnormal patterns arise. The guidelines do not recommend the routine use of fetal pulse oximetry.

Implications for Practice

Electronic fetal monitoring is here to stay, but it is only a tool. Women and providers have come to expect the constant feedback, and busy nurses have come to rely on the remote screens as they move from room to room. However, the risks of false alarms and the legal vulnerability of ambiguous patterns may be contributing to the soaring cesarean rate, which carries its own risks. Continuous monitoring of low risk women restricts patient mobility, which may prolong labor and increase discomfort. In high risk situations EFM can be valuable for picking up some fetal stress early but also may be inaccurate and ambiguous and cause needless anxiety. Women who expect routine monitoring need explanations about the risks and benefits of continuous monitoring vs. IA and should be given informed choices. The health care team may also need to become more proficient and familiar with auscultation as an assessment tool.

References

Gourounti K, Sandall J: Admission cardiotocography versus intermittent auscultation of fetal heart rate: effects on neonatal Apgar score, on the rate of caesarean sections, and on the rate of instrumental delivery—a systematic review, *Int J Nurs Stud* 44(6):1029-1035, 2007.

Liston R et al: Fetal health surveillance: antepartum and intrapartum consensus guideline, *J Obstet Gynaecol Can* 29(9 suppl 4):s1-s56, 2007, Society of Obstetricians and Gynaecologists of Canada (SOGC) Clinical Practice Guideline 197, Ottawa, Ontario, Canada, SOGC. Available at www.sogc.org/guidelines/documents/gui197CPG0709.pdf (accessed April 1, 2009).

National Institute for Health and Clinical Excellence (NICE): *Intrapartal care: care for healthy women and their babies during childbirth*, NICE Clin Guideline 55, London, 2008, NICE. Available at www.nice.org.uk/nicemedia/pdf/IPCNICEGuidance.pdf (accessed April 1, 2009).

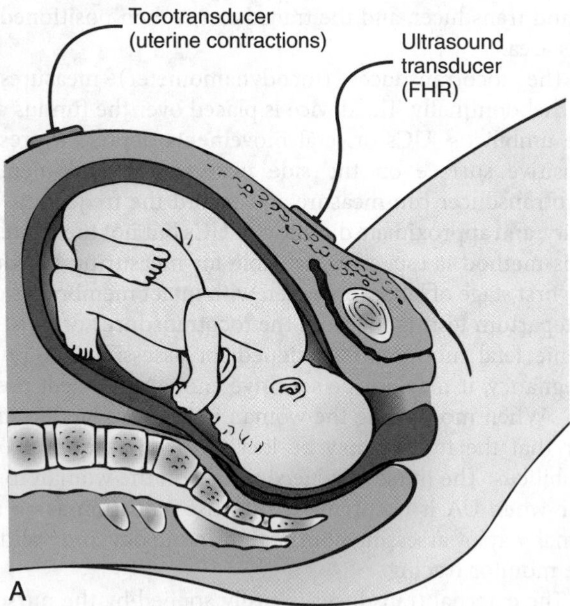

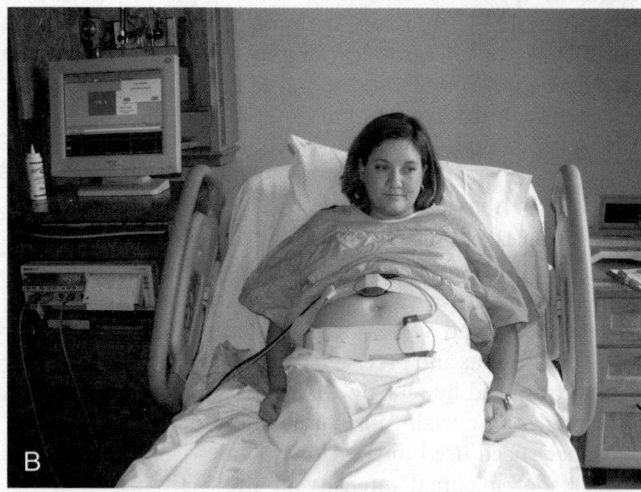

Fig. 17-2 A, External noninvasive fetal monitoring with tocotransducer and ultrasound transducer. *FHR,* Fetal heart rate. **B,** Ultrasound transducer is placed below umbilicus over the area where fetal heart rate is best heard, and tocotransducer is placed on uterine fundus. *(B, Courtesy Julie Perry Nelson, Loveland, CO.)*

Table 17-1 External and Internal Modes of Monitoring

EXTERNAL MODE	INTERNAL MODE
Fetal Heart Rate	
Ultrasound transducer: High-frequency sound waves reflect mechanical action of the fetal heart. It is noninvasive, does not require rupture of membranes or cervical dilation, and is used during both the antepartum and intrapartum periods.	*Spiral electrode:* This electrode converts the fetal ECG as obtained from the presenting part to the FHR via a cardiotachometer. This method can be used only when membranes are ruptured and the cervix is sufficiently dilated during the intrapartum period. The electrode penetrates into fetal presenting part by 1.5 mm and must be attached securely to ensure a good signal.
Uterine Activity	
Tocotransducer: This instrument monitors frequency and duration of contractions by means of a pressure-sensing device applied to the maternal abdomen. It is used during both the antepartum and intrapartum periods.	*Intrauterine pressure catheter (IUPC):* This instrument monitors the frequency, duration, and intensity of contractions. The two types of IUPCs are a fluid-filled system and a solid catheter. Both measure intrauterine pressure at the catheter tip and convert the pressure into millimeters of mercury on the uterine activity panel of the strip chart. Both can be used only when membranes are ruptured and the cervix is sufficiently dilated during the intrapartum period.

ECG, Electrocardiogram; *FHR,* fetal heart rate.

tion (see Fig. 17-2, *B*). The woman is asked to assume a semi-sitting or lateral position. Use of an external transducer confines the woman to bed or chair. Portable telemetry monitors allow observation of the FHR and UC patterns by means of centrally located electronic display stations. These portable units permit the woman to walk around during electronic monitoring.

Internal Monitoring

The technique of continuous internal monitoring provides a more accurate appraisal of fetal well-being during labor than external monitoring since it is not interrupted by fetal or maternal movement (Fig. 17-3). For this type of monitoring the membranes must be ruptured, and the cervix sufficiently dilated (2 to 3 cm) to allow placement of the spiral electrode and/or IUPC. Internal and external modes of monitoring may be combined (i.e., internal FHR with external UA or external FHR with internal UA) without difficulty.

Internal monitoring of the FHR is accomplished by attaching a small spiral electrode to the presenting part; a continuous FHR will be displayed on the fetal monitor strip. To monitor UA internally a solid or fluid-filled IUPC is introduced into the uterine cavity. A solid catheter has a pressure-sensitive tip that measures changes in intrauterine pressure. A fluid-filled (with sterile water) catheter detects pressure changes in the sterile water through a strain gauge. As the catheter is compressed during a contraction, pressure is placed on the pressure transducer or strain gauge; this pressure is then converted into a pressure reading in millimeters of mercury. The average pressure during a contraction ranges from 50 to 85 mm Hg. The IUPC can measure the frequency, duration, and intensity of UCs as well as uterine resting tone.

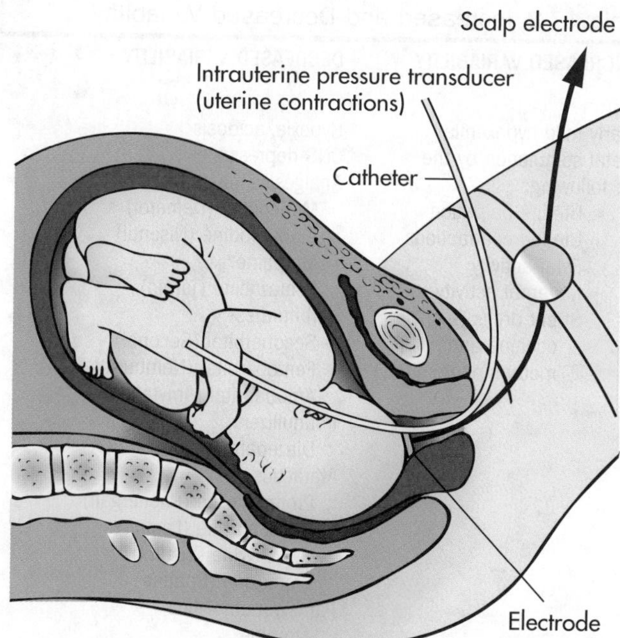

Fig. 17-3 Diagrammatic representation of internal invasive fetal monitoring with intrauterine pressure catheter and spiral electrode in place (membranes ruptured and cervix dilated).

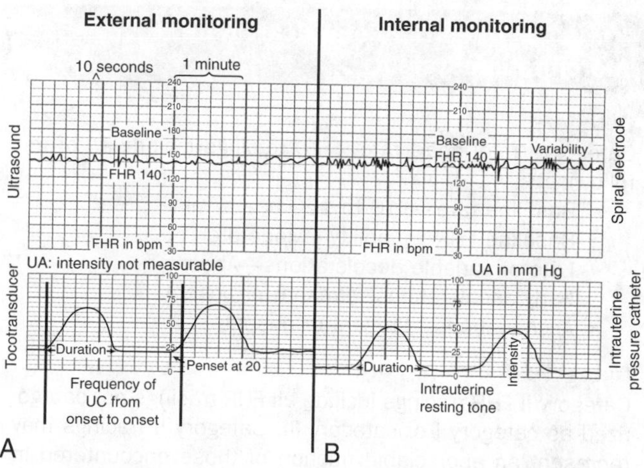

Fig. 17-4 Display of fetal heart rate and uterine activity on monitor paper. **A,** External mode with ultrasound and tocotransducer as signal source. *FHR,* Fetal heart rate; *UC,* uterine contractions. **B,** Internal mode with spiral electrode and intrauterine catheter as signal source. Frequency of contractions is measured from the beginning of one contraction to the beginning of the next. *FHR,* Fetal heart rate; *UA,* uterine activity. (From Tucker SM, Miller LA, Miller DA: *Mosby's pocket guide to fetal monitoring: a multidisciplinary approach,* ed 6, St Louis, 2009, Mosby.)

The FHR and UA are displayed on the monitor paper with the FHR in the upper section and UA in the lower section. Figure 17-4 contrasts the internal and external modes of electronic monitoring. Note that each small square represents 10 seconds; each larger box of six squares equals 1 minute (when paper is moving through the monitor at the rate of 3 cm/min).

Fetal Heart Rate Patterns

Characteristic FHR patterns are associated with fetal and maternal physiologic processes and have been identified for many years. However, because EFM was introduced into clinical practice before consensus was reached in regard to standardized terminology, there were often wide variations in the description and interpretation of common FHR patterns. In 1997 the National Institute of Child Health and Human Development (NICHD) published a proposed nomenclature system for electronic fetal monitor interpretation with standardized definitions for FHR monitoring (NICHD, 1997). These recommendations were incorporated into clinical practice after endorsement by the American College of Obstetricians and Gynecologists (ACOG) in 2005 and AWHONN and the American College of Nurse Midwives (ACNM) in 2006. In 2008 the NICHD updated the 1997 nomenclature system (Macones et al, 2008). ACOG, AWHONN, and ACNM adopted the 1997 NICHD terminology and participated in preparing the 2008 update (Macones et al, 2008).

In the Macones and colleagues' paper (2008), a three-tier system for categorization of FHR was recommended (Box 17-1). Category I tracings are normal (reassuring); category II tracings are indeterminate and require evaluation and continued surveillance; category III tracings are abnormal (nonreassuring) and need evaluation and intervention.

Baseline Fetal Heart Rate

The intrinsic rhythmicity of the fetal heart, the central nervous system (CNS), and the fetal autonomic nervous system control the FHR. An increase in sympathetic response results in acceleration of the FHR, whereas an augmentation in parasympathetic response produces a slowing of the FHR. Usually a balanced increase of sympathetic and parasympathetic response occurs during contractions, with no observable change in the baseline FHR.

Baseline FHR is the average rate during a 10-minute segment that excludes accelerations, decelerations, and periods of marked variability. There must be at least 2 minutes of baseline segments in a 10-minute segment (Macones et al, 2008). The normal range at term is 110 to 160 beats/min. The baseline rate is documented as a single number rather than a range (Tucker, Miller, & Miller, 2009).

Baseline variability of the FHR can be described as fluctuations in the baseline FHR that are irregular in amplitude and frequency (Macones et al, 2008). Variability is classified as follows:

- Absent or undetectable variability
- Minimal variability (> undetectable but ≤5 beats/min)
- Moderate variability (6 to 25 beats/min)
- Marked variability (>25 beats/min) (Fig. 17-5)

The interpretation of the FHR tracing should be within the context of the overall clinical picture. The presence of accelerations is reliable in predicting the absence of fetal metabolic acidemia. However, the converse is not true; the absence of variability does not predict fetal acidemia (Macones et al, 2008).

FHR accelerations can be stimulated by direct fetal scalp or vibroacoustic stimulation or with transabdominal halogen light (Macones et al, 2008). Diminished variability can result

BOX 17-1 Three-Tier Fetal Heart Rate Interpretation System

Category I

Category I fetal heart rate (FHR) tracings include *all* of the following:

- Baseline rate—110 to 160 beats/min
- Baseline FHR variability—Moderate
- Late or variable decelerations—Absent
- Early decelerations—Present or absent
- Accelerations—Present or absent

Category II

Category II FHR tracings include all FHR tracings not categorized as category I or category III. Category II tracings may represent an appreciable fraction of those encountered in clinical care. Examples of category II FHR tracings include any of the following:

Baseline rate

- Bradycardia not accompanied by absent baseline variability
- Tachycardia

Baseline FHR variability

- Minimal baseline variability
- Absent baseline variability not accompanied by recurrent decelerations
- Marked baseline variability

Accelerations

- Absence of induced accelerations after fetal stimulation

Periodic or episodic decelerations

- Recurrent variable decelerations accompanied by minimal or moderate baseline variability
- Prolonged deceleration of 2 minutes or more but less than 10 minutes
- Recurrent late decelerations with moderate baseline variability
- Variable decelerations with other characteristics such as slow return to baseline, "overshoots," or "shoulders"

Category III

Category III FHR tracings include:

Absent baseline FHR variability and any of the following:

- Recurrent late decelerations
- Recurrent variable decelerations
- Bradycardia

Sinusoidal pattern

Source: Macones GA et al: The 2008 National Institute of Child Health and Human Development Workshop Report on Electronic Fetal Monitoring: update on definitions, interpretation, and research guidelines, *J Obstet Gynecol Neonatal Nurs* 37(5):510-515, 2008.

Table 17-2 Increased and Decreased Variability

INCREASED VARIABILITY	DECREASED VARIABILITY
Cause	
Early mild hypoxemia Fetal stimulation by the following: Uterine palpation Uterine contractions Fetal activity Maternal activity Street drugs (e.g., cocaine and methamphetamines)	Hypoxia/acidosis CNS depressants Analgesics/narcotics Meperidine (Demerol) Alphaprodine (Nisentil) Morphine Pentazocine (Talwin) Barbiturates Secobarbital (Seconal) Pentobarbital (Nembutal) Amobarbital (Amytal) Tranquilizers Diazepam (Valium) Ataractics Promethazine (Phenergan) Propiomazine (Largon) Hydroxyzine (Vistaril) Promazine (Sparine) Parasympatholytics Atropine General anesthetics Prematurity–less than 24 wk Fetal sleep cycles Congenital abnormalities Fetal cardiac dysrhythmias
Clinical Significance	
Significance of marked variability not known; increased variability from a previous average variability is earliest FHR sign of mild hypoxemia	Benign when associated with periodic fetal sleep states, which last 20 to 30 min; if caused by drugs, variability usually increases as drugs are excreted; decreased variability is not reassuring and is considered a sign of fetal stress *unless* it has an identifiable temporary (e.g., fetal sleep) or correctable cause
Nursing Intervention	
Observe FHR tracing carefully for any nonreassuring patterns, including decreasing variability and late decelerations; if using external mode of monitoring, consider using internal mode (spiral electrode) for more accurate tracing	Dependent on cause; intervention not warranted if associated with fetal sleep states or temporarily associated with CNS depressants; consider performing external stimulation of scalp during a vaginal examination to elicit an acceleration of FHR or return to average variability; consider application of internal mode (spiral electrode); assist health care provider with fetal oxygen saturation monitoring if ordered; prepare for birth if so indicated by primary health care provider

CNS, Central nervous system; *FHR*, fetal heart rate.

from fetal hypoxemia and acidosis and from certain drugs that depress the CNS, including analgesics, opioids (morphine), barbiturates (secobarbital [Seconal] and pentobarbital [Nembutal]), tranquilizers (diazepam [Valium]), ataractics (promethazine [Phenergan]), and general anesthetics. In addition, a temporary decrease in variability can occur when the fetus is in a sleep state. These sleep states do not usually last longer than 30 minutes. Table 17-2 contrasts key differences between increased and decreased variability.

A sinusoidal FHR pattern has a visually apparent, smooth, undulating sine wavelike pattern in baseline FHR. The cycle frequency is 3 to 5/min, which persists for 20 minutes or more (Macones et al, 2008). This uncommon pattern occurs

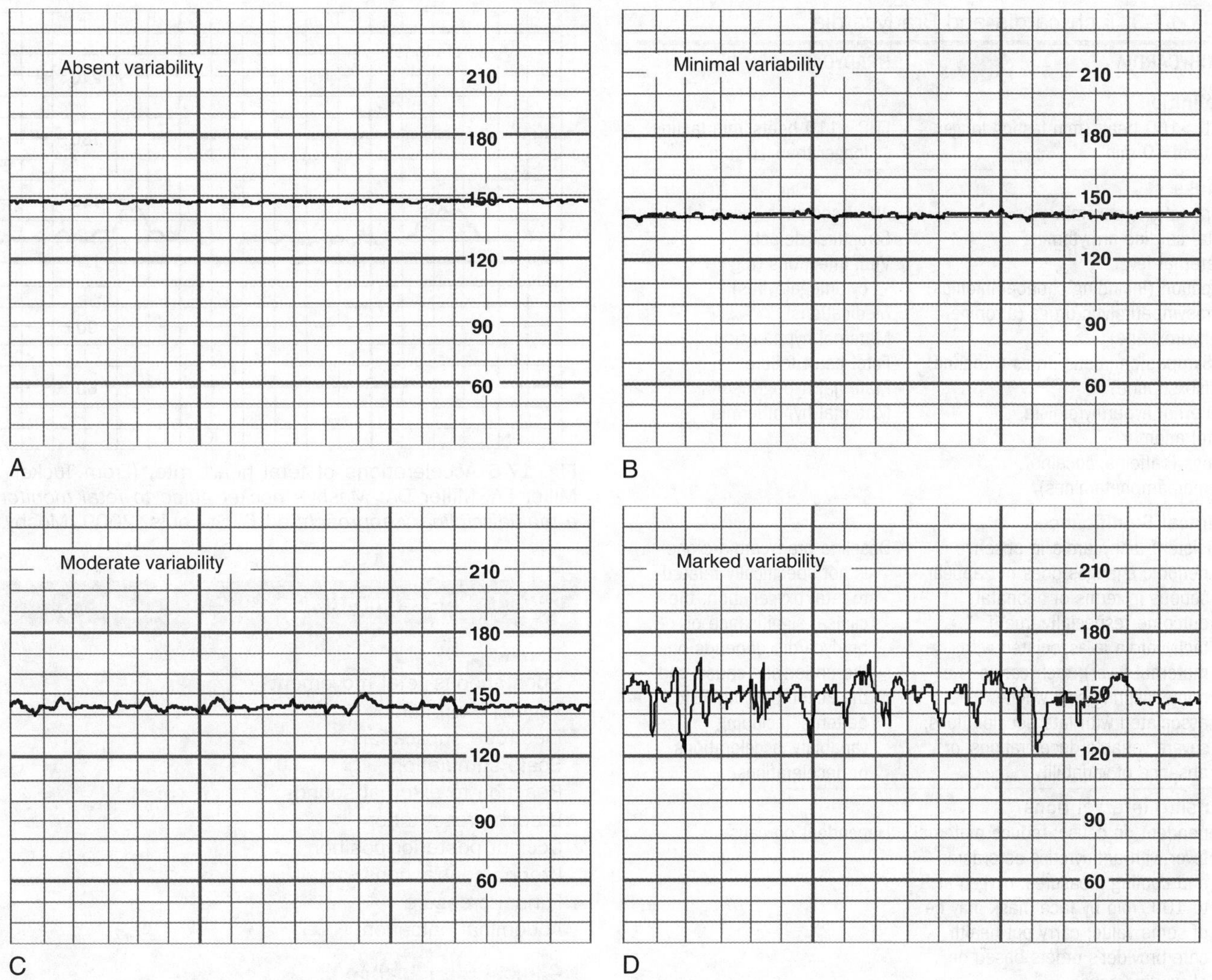

Fig. 17-5 Fetal heart rate variability. **A**, Absent or undetected. **B**, Minimal. **C**, Moderate. **D**, Marked. (Modified from Tucker SM, Miller LA, Miller DA: *Mosby's pocket guide to fetal monitoring: a multidisciplinary approach,* ed 6, St Louis, 2009, Mosby.)

when fetal hypoxia results from Rh isoimmunization or fetal anemia.

Tachycardia is a baseline FHR greater than 160 beats/min for a duration of 10 minutes or longer. It can be considered an early sign of fetal hypoxemia, especially when associated with late decelerations and minimal or absent variability. Fetal tachycardia can result from maternal or fetal infection such as prolonged rupture of membranes with amnionitis; from maternal hyperthyroidism or fetal anemia; or in response to drugs such as atropine, hydroxyzine (Vistaril), and terbutaline or illicit drugs such as cocaine or methamphetamines.

Bradycardia is a baseline FHR less than 110 beats/min for a duration of 10 minutes or longer. True bradycardia occurs rarely and is not specifically related to fetal oxygenation. It is critical to distinguish true bradycardia from a prolonged deceleration since the causes and management of these two conditions are very different. Bradycardia is often caused by some type of fetal cardiac problem such as structural defects involving the pacemakers or conduction system or fetal heart failure. Other causes of bradycardia include viral infections (cytomegalovirus), maternal hypoglycemia, and maternal hypothermia. The clinical significance of the bradycardia depends on the underlying cause and accompanying FHR patterns, including variability and the presence of accelerations or decelerations (Tucker, Miller, & Miller, 2009). Table 17-3 lists causes, clinical significance, and nursing interventions for bradycardia.

Periodic and Episodic Changes in Fetal Heart Rate

Changes in FHR from the baseline are categorized as periodic or episodic. Periodic changes are those that occur with UCs. Episodic changes are those that are not associated with UCs. These patterns include accelerations and decelerations (Macones et al, 2008).

Accelerations

Acceleration of the FHR is defined as a visually apparent, abrupt increase in FHR above the baseline rate. Abrupt is defined as an increase from onset to peak of acceleration in less than 30 seconds (Macones et al, 2008) (Fig. 17-6). To be classed as an acceleration, the increase must be 15 beats/min

Table 17-3 Tachycardia and Bradycardia

TACHYCARDIA	BRADYCARDIA
Definition	
FHR >160 beats/min lasting longer than 10 min	FHR <110 beats/min lasting longer than 10 min
Cause	
Early fetal hypoxemia Fetal cardiac arrhythmias Maternal fever Infection (including chorioamnionitis) Parasympatholytic drugs (atropine, hydroxyzine) β-Sympathomimetic drugs (ritodrine, isoxsuprine) Maternal hyperthyroidism Fetal anemia Drugs (caffeine, cocaine, methamphetamines)	AV dissociation (heart block) Structural defects Viral infections (e.g., cytomegalovirus) Medications Maternal hypotension Fetal heart failure Maternal hypoglycemia Maternal hypothermia
Clinical Significance	
Persistent tachycardia in absence of periodic changes does not appear serious in terms of neonatal outcome (especially true if tachycardia is associated with maternal fever); tachycardia is a nonreassuring sign when associated with late decelerations, severe variable decelerations, or absence of variability	Baseline bradycardia alone is not specifically related to fetal oxygenation; the clinical significance of bradycardia depends on the underlying cause and the accompanying FHR patterns, including variability, accelerations, or decelerations
Nursing Interventions	
Dependent on cause; reduce maternal fever with antipyretics as ordered and cooling measures; oxygen at 8 to 10 L/min by face mask may be of some value; carry out health care provider's orders based on alleviating cause	Dependent on cause

ECG, Electrocardiogram; *FHR*, fetal heart rate.

or greater and last 15 seconds or more, with the return to baseline less than 2 minutes from the beginning of the acceleration. A prolonged acceleration is 2 minutes or more but less than 10 minutes in length (Macones et al, 2008). Acceleration of the FHR for more than 10 minutes is considered a change in baseline rate. In preterm gestations the definition of an acceleration is a peak of 10 beats/min or more above baseline for at least 10 seconds.

Accelerations can be periodic or episodic. They may occur in association with fetal movement or spontaneously. If accelerations do not occur spontaneously, they can be elicited by fetal scalp stimulation or vibroacoustic stimulation. Accelerations are considered a sign of fetal well-being. Their presence is highly predictive of a normal fetal acid-base balance (absence of fetal metabolic acidemia) (Tucker, Miller, & Miller, 2009). Box 17-2 lists causes, clinical significance, and nursing interventions for accelerations.

Decelerations

Decelerations are classified as *early, late, prolonged,* and *variable.* FHR decelerations are described by their visual relation to the onset and end of a contraction and by their shape.

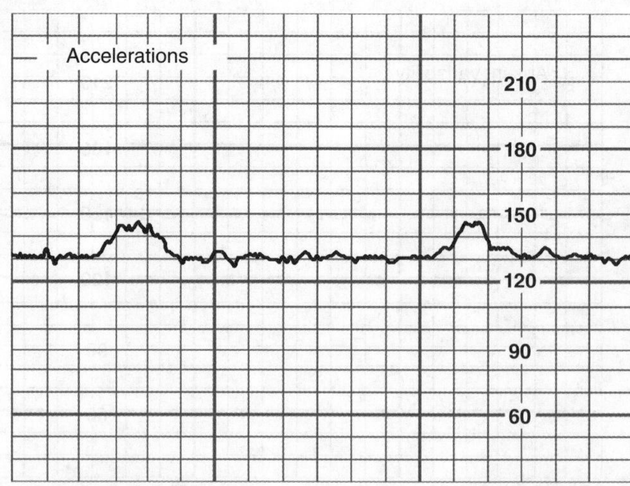

Fig. 17-6 Accelerations of fetal heart rate. (From Tucker SM, Miller LA, Miller DA: *Mosby's pocket guide to fetal monitoring: a multidisciplinary approach,* ed 6, St Louis, 2009, Mosby.)

BOX 17-2 Accelerations

Cause

Spontaneous fetal movement
Vaginal examination
Electrode application
Scalp stimulation
Reaction to external sounds
Breech presentation
Occiput posterior position
Uterine contractions
Fundal pressure
Abdominal palpation

Clinical Significance

Acceleration with fetal movement signifies fetal well-being, representing fetal alertness or arousal states.

Nursing Interventions

None required

Early Decelerations

Early deceleration of the FHR is a visually apparent gradual decrease and return to baseline FHR associated with UCs (Fig. 17-7, *A*) (Macones et al, 2008). Generally the onset, nadir, and recovery of the deceleration correspond to the beginning, peak, and end of the contraction. For this reason early decelerations are sometimes referred to as the "mirror image" of a contraction.

Early decelerations are thought to be caused by transient fetal head compression and are considered a benign finding. They may also occur during vaginal examinations, as a result of fundal pressure, and during placement of the internal mode of fetal monitoring. When present, they usually occur during the first stage of labor when the cervix is dilated 4 to 7 cm but can also be seen during the second stage when the woman is pushing.

Because early decelerations are considered to be benign, interventions are not necessary. Early decelerations should be

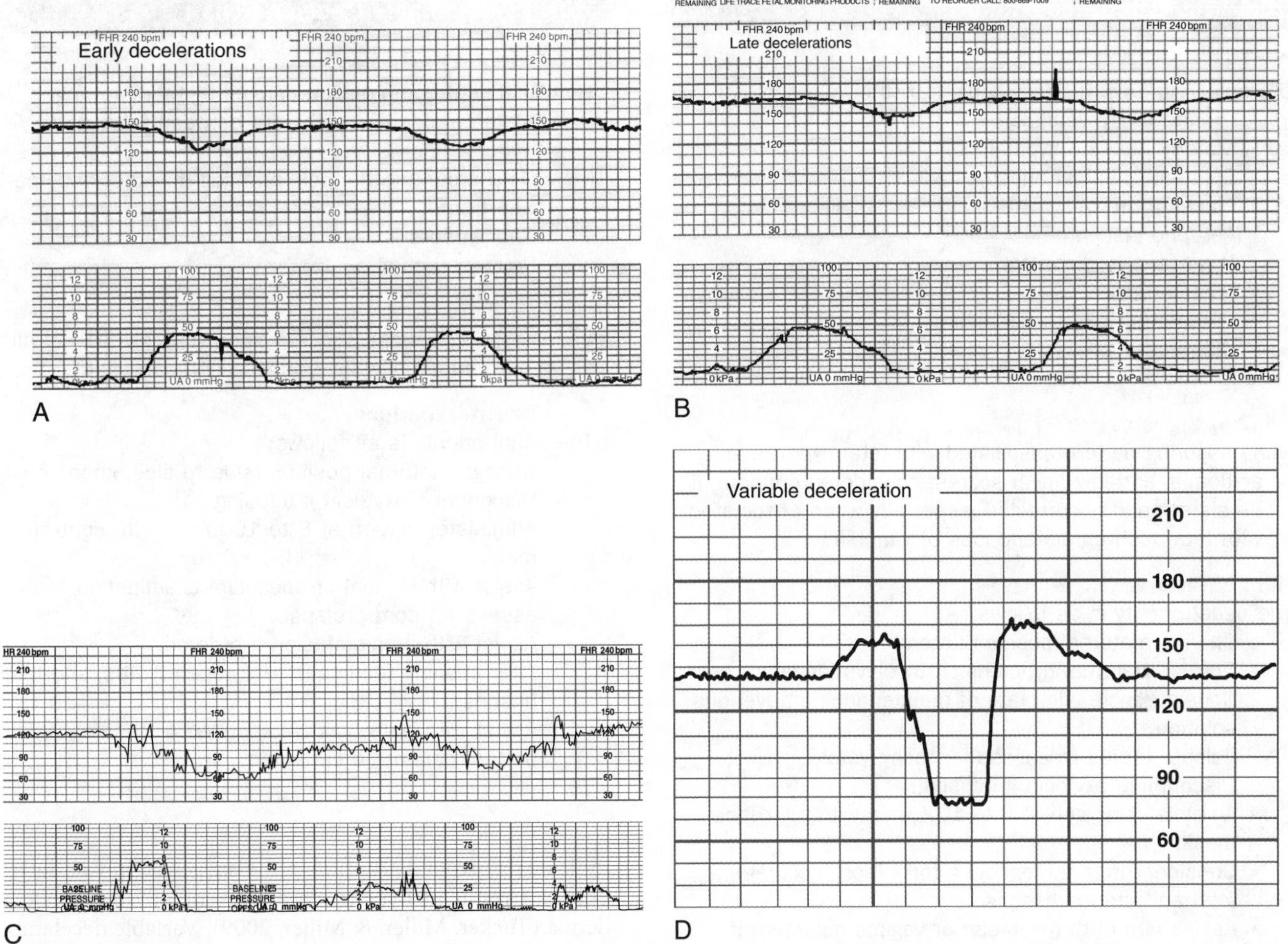

Fig. 17-7 Deceleration patterns. **A,** Early. **B,** Late. **C,** Prolonged, **D,** Variable. (From Tucker SM, Miller LA, Miller DA: *Mosby's pocket guide to fetal monitoring: a multidisciplinary approach,* ed 6, St Louis, 2009, Mosby.)

identified so that they can be distinguished from late or variable decelerations, which can be nonreassuring and for which interventions are appropriate. Box 17-3 lists cause, clinical significance, and nursing interventions for early decelerations.

Late Decelerations

Late deceleration of the FHR is a visually apparent gradual decrease in and return to baseline FHR associated with UCs (Macones et al, 2008). The deceleration begins after the contraction has started, and the lowest point of the deceleration occurs after the peak of the contraction. The deceleration usually does not return to baseline until after the contraction is over (see Fig. 17-7, *B*). Late decelerations reflect a transient disruption of oxygen transfer to the fetus, which results in transient fetal hypoxemia (Tucker, Miller, & Miller, 2009).

Persistent and repetitive late decelerations usually indicate the presence of fetal hypoxemia stemming from insufficient placental perfusion. They can be associated with fetal hypoxemia progressing to hypoxia and metabolic acidemia (Tucker, Miller, & Miller, 2009). They should be considered an ominous sign when they are uncorrectable, especially if they are associated with decreased variability and tachycardia. A number of things can disrupt oxygen transfer to the fetus. The causes, clinical significance, and nursing interventions for late decelerations are described in Box 17-4.

A prolonged deceleration is a decrease in FHR from the baseline that is greater than 15 beats/min lasting more than 2 minutes but less than 10 minutes (see Fig. 17-7, *C*). A decrease from the baseline in FHR that lasts more than 10 minutes is a baseline change (Macones et al, 2008).

BOX 17-3 Early Decelerations

Cause

Head compression resulting from the following:

- Uterine contractions
- Vaginal examination
- Fundal pressure
- Placement of internal mode of monitoring

Clinical Significance

Reassuring pattern is not associated with fetal hypoxemia, acidemia, or low Apgar scores.

Nursing Interventions

None required

BOX 17-4 Late Decelerations

Cause

Uteroplacental insufficiency caused by the following:

- Uterine tachysystole
- Maternal supine hypotension
- Epidural or spinal anesthesia
- Placenta previa
- Abruptio placentae
- Hypertensive disorders
- Postmaturity
- Intrauterine growth restriction
- Diabetes mellitus
- Intraamniotic infection

Clinical Significance

Nonreassuring pattern associated with fetal hypoxemia, acidemia, and low Apgar scores; considered ominous if persistent and uncorrected, especially when associated with fetal tachycardia and loss of variability.

Nursing Interventions

The usual priority is as follows:

- Change maternal position (lateral).
- Correct maternal hypotension by elevating legs.
- Consider increasing rate of maintenance intravenous solution.
- Palpate uterus to assess for tachysystole.
- Discontinue oxytocin if infusing.
- Administer oxygen at 8 to 10 L/min with tight face mask.
- Consider internal monitoring for a more accurate fetal and uterine assessment.
- Assist with birth (cesarean or vaginal assisted) if pattern cannot be corrected.

BOX 17-5 Variable Decelerations

Cause

Umbilical cord compression caused by the following:

- Maternal position with cord between fetus and maternal pelvis
- Cord around fetal neck, arm, leg, or other body part
- Short cord
- Knot in cord
- Prolapsed cord

Clinical Significance

Variable decelerations occur in approximately 50% of all labors and usually are transient and correctable.

Nursing Interventions

The usual priority is as follows:

- Change maternal position (side to side, knee chest).
- Discontinue oxytocin if infusing.
- Administer oxygen at 8 to 10 L/min with tight face mask.
- Assist with vaginal or speculum examination to assess for cord prolapse.
- Assist with amnioinfusion if ordered.
- Alter pushing technique (e.g., open glottis, shorter pushes).
- Assist with birth (vaginal assisted or cesarean) if pattern cannot be corrected.

Decelerations can be further defined as recurrent or intermittent. Recurrent decelerations occur with more than 50% of UCs. If the decelerations occur with less than 50% of UCs, they are labeled intermittent (Macones et al, 2008).

Variable Decelerations

Variable deceleration is defined as a visual abrupt decrease in FHR below the baseline. The decrease is 15 beats/min or more, lasts at least 15 seconds, and returns to baseline in less than 2 minutes from the time of onset (Macones et al, 2008). Variable decelerations occur any time during the uterine contracting phase and are caused by compression of the umbilical cord (Tucker, Miller, & Miller, 2009).

The appearance of variable decelerations differs from those of early and late decelerations, which closely approximate the shape of the corresponding UC. Instead variable decelerations often have a U, V, or W shape, characterized by a rapid descent and ascent to and from the nadir (or depth) of the deceleration (see Fig. 17-7, *D*). Some variable decelerations are preceded and followed by brief accelerations of the FHR, known as *shouldering,* which is an appropriate compensatory response to compression of the umbilical cord.

Occasional variable decelerations have little clinical significance. On the other hand, repetitive variable decelerations indicate recurrent disruption in the oxygen supply of the fetus. This can result in hypoxemia and eventually metabolic academia (Tucker, Miller, & Miller, 2009). Variable decelerations are most commonly found during the transition phase of the first stage of labor and during the second stage of labor as a result of umbilical cord compression and stretching during fetal descent (Garite, 2007). Box 17-5 lists causes, clinical significance, and nursing interventions for variable decelerations.

Prolonged Decelerations

A prolonged deceleration is a visually apparent decrease in FHR below the baseline 15 beats/min or more and lasting more than 2 minutes but less than 10 minutes. A deceleration lasting more than 10 minutes is considered a baseline change (Macones et al, 2008). Generally the benign causes are pelvic examination, application of a spiral electrode, rapid fetal descent, and sustained maternal Valsalva maneuver. Other less benign causes are progressive severe variable decelerations, sudden umbilical cord prolapse, hypotension produced by spinal or epidural analgesia or anesthesia, paracervical anesthesia, tetanic contraction, placental hemorrhage, uterine rupture, and maternal hypoxia, which may occur during a seizure.

When the deceleration lasts longer than 1 to 2 minutes, a loss of variability with rebound tachycardia usually occurs. Occasionally a period of late decelerations follows. Prolonged decelerations usually are isolated events that end spontaneously. However, when a prolonged deceleration is seen late in the course of severe variable decelerations or during a prolonged series of late decelerations, the prolonged deceleration may occur just before fetal death.

NURSING ALERT Nurses should notify the physician or nurse-midwife immediately and initiate appropriate treatment when they see a prolonged deceleration.

Nursing Care Management

The primary goals of nursing care are to have healthy fetal and maternal outcomes. Knowledge of fetal status and standards for care determine the interventions implemented. The planning process includes accommodating the wishes of the woman and family, answering questions, and explaining nursing interventions (see Nursing Process box).

Although the use of EFM can be reassuring to many parents, it can be a source of anxiety to some. Therefore the nurse must be particularly sensitive to and respond appropriately to the emotional, informational, and comfort needs of the woman in labor and those of her family (Fig. 17-8 and Box 17-6).

Electronic Fetal Monitoring Pattern Recognition

Nurses must evaluate five essential components of an FHR tracing to determine whether immediate intervention is needed or whether there are indications to expedite birth. These components are baseline rate, baseline variability, accelerations, decelerations, and changes or trends in the FHR pattern over time (Tucker, Miller, & Miller, 2009). Nurses evaluate these factors on the basis of other obstetric complications, progress in labor, and analgesia or anesthesia. They also must consider the estimated time interval until birth. Therefore interventions are based on clinical judgment of a complex, integrated process (Simpson & James, 2005).

NURSING PROCESS: FETAL MONITORING

Assessment

Maternal temperature, pulse, respiratory rate, blood pressure, position, comfort, voiding pattern, status of membranes, uterine contraction pattern, cervical effacement and dilation, and emotional status are assessed.

Fetal assessment includes fetal presentation, fetal position, fetal heart rate (FHR), and identification of both reassuring and nonreassuring FHR patterns.

A checklist can be used by the nurse to assess the FHR.

All of the assessment information must be documented in the woman's medical record.

The electronic fetal monitoring (EFM) equipment is evaluated to ensure that the equipment is working properly and to allow an accurate assessment of the woman and fetus.

A checklist for EFM equipment can be used to evaluate the equipment functions

Nursing Diagnoses

Possible nursing diagnoses include the following:

Decreased maternal cardiac output related to
- supine hypotension secondary to maternal position

Anxiety related to
- lack of knowledge concerning fetal monitoring during labor
- restriction of mobility or movement during monitoring

Impaired fetal gas exchange related to
- umbilical cord compression
- placental insufficiency

Acute pain related to
- use of belts to position transducers
- maternal position
- vaginal examinations associated with application of maternal or fetal internal monitoring equipment or fetal blood sampling

Risk for fetal injury related to
- unrecognized hypoxemia, hypoxia, or anoxia
- infection secondary to internal monitoring or scalp blood sampling

Planning

The care given to women being monitored by EFM or auscultation is the same as that given to the woman having a low risk labor. Care of the woman being monitored by internal methods may vary. FHR pattern recognition and intervention may require a nurse to have additional education and clinical experience.

Expected outcomes for the pregnant woman and family and the fetus include the following:

- The pregnant woman and family will verbalize their understanding of the need for monitoring.
- The pregnant woman and family will recognize and avoid situations that compromise maternal and fetal circulation.
- The fetus will not have any hypoxemic, hypoxic, or anoxic episodes.
- Should fetal compromise occur, it will be identified promptly, appropriate nursing interventions such as intrauterine resuscitation will be initiated, and the physician or nurse-midwife will be notified.

Interventions

Assess FHR patterns.

Implement independent nursing interventions.

Document observations and actions.

Observe established standards of care.

Report nonreassuring FHR patterns to the primary care provider.

Provide reassurance to woman and family.

Evaluation

Evaluation is a continuous process. The nurse can assume that care was effective when the outcomes for care have been achieved (see Nursing Care Plan).

NURSING CARE PLAN Electronic Fetal Monitoring During Labor

Nursing Diagnosis: Maternal anxiety related to lack of knowledge about use of electronic monitor

Expected Outcomes

The woman will exhibit increased understanding about fetal monitoring and signs of reduced anxiety (i.e., absence of physical indicators, absence of perceived threat, and absence of feelings of dread).

Nursing Interventions/*Rationales*

Explain and demonstrate to woman and labor support partner how the electronic fetal monitor (EFM) (internal or external) works in assessing fetal heart rate (FHR) and detecting and assessing quality of uterine contractions *to remove fear of unknown and ensure that woman can move with the monitor.*

When adjusting the monitor, explain to the couple what is being done and why *because information increases understanding and allays anxiety.*

Explain that, although a side-lying or Fowler's position provides for optimal monitoring, position changes decrease discomfort; therefore encourage frequent changes in position (other than supine) and explain any monitoring adjustments that are being made as a result *to reduce discomfort and allay anxiety.*

Nursing Diagnosis: Risk for fetal injury related to inaccurate placement of transducers/electrodes, misinterpretation of results, or failure to use other assessment techniques to monitor fetal well-being

Expected Outcomes

Fetal well-being is adequately assessed, and any fetal compromise is identified immediately.

Nursing Interventions/*Rationales*

Carefully follow guidelines and checklist for application and initiation of monitoring *to ensure proper placement of monitoring devices and production of accurate output from monitoring device.*

Check placement throughout monitoring process *to ensure that devices remain correctly placed.*

Regularly assess and record results of electronic fetal monitoring (FHR and variability, decelerations, accelerations, uterine activity, contractions, uterine resting tone) *to provide consistent and timely evaluation of fetal well-being and progress of labor.*

Auscultate FHR and palpate contractions on a regular basis *to provide a cross-check on the EFM output and ensure fetal well-being.*

Nursing Diagnosis: Risk for maternal injury related to incorrect placement of external or internal monitors or misinterpretation of contraction pattern

Expected Outcomes

Maternal well-being is assessed continuously, and any alterations are identified promptly.

Nursing Interventions/*Rationales*

Palpate uterine contractions *to correlate data with electronic monitoring results.*

Periodically recheck placement *to verify that all monitoring devices are accurately placed.*

Assess uterine activity, contraction pattern, and baseline *to provide ongoing evaluation and basis for further interventions.*

Use correct aseptic technique for insertion of internal monitors *to prevent infection.*

Monitor maternal temperature and color, odor, and amount of amniotic fluid *to determine indicators of infection.*

Nursing Diagnosis: Risk for impaired physical mobility related to restriction of movement with monitoring devices

Expected Outcome

Woman will be able to change positions and ambulate at intervals.

Nursing Interventions/*Rationales*

Discontinue continuous electronic monitoring at intervals *to change position and increase mobility.*

Encourage woman to change position and reposition monitor as needed *to decrease complications of immobility.*

Place external monitor manually at intervals *to collect data while woman is out of bed.*

evolve Nursing Care Plan—Electronic Fetal Monitoring During Labor

LEGAL TIP Fetal Monitoring Standards Nurses who care for women during childbirth are legally responsible for correctly interpreting FHR patterns, initiating appropriate nursing interventions based on those patterns, and documenting the outcomes of those interventions. Perinatal nurses are responsible for the timely notification of the physician or nurse-midwife in the event of nonreassuring FHR patterns (i.e., patterns that indicate the need for intervention or expedited birth). Perinatal nurses also are responsible for initiating the institutional chain of command should differences in opinion arise among health care providers concerning the interpretation of the FHR pattern and the intervention required.

Nursing Management of Nonreassuring Patterns

Whenever one of the five essential components of the FHR tracing is assessed as abnormal, corrective measures must immediately be taken. The purpose of these actions is to improve fetal oxygenation (Tucker, Miller, & Miller, 2009). The term *intrauterine resuscitation* is sometimes used to refer to the interventions initiated when a nonreassuring FHR pattern is noted. Basic corrective measures include providing supplemental oxygen, instituting maternal position changes, and increasing intravenous fluid administration. The purpose of these interventions is to improve uterine and intervillous space blood flow and increase maternal oxygenation and cardiac output (Simpson & James, 2005). Box 17-7 lists basic

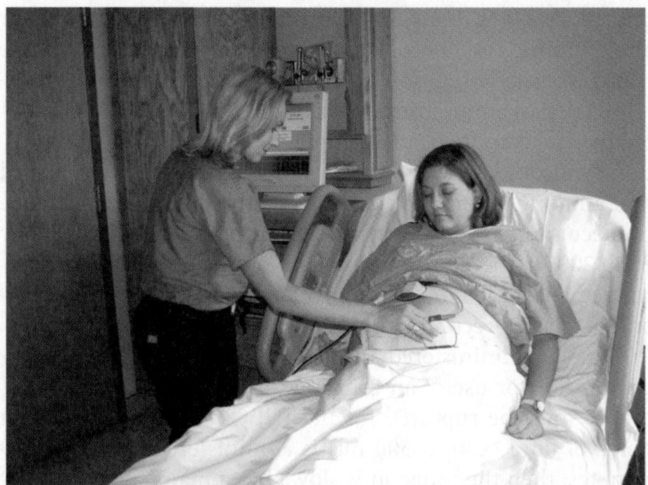

Fig. 17-8 Nurse explains electronic fetal monitoring as ultrasound transducer monitors the fetal heart rate. *(Courtesy Julie Perry Nelson, Loveland, CO.)*

BOX 17-6 Patient and Family Teaching When Electronic Fetal Monitor Is Used

The following guidelines relate to patient teaching and the functioning of the monitor:

- Explain the purpose of monitoring.
- Explain each procedure.
- Provide rationale for maternal position other than supine.
- Explain that fetal status can be continuously assessed by electronic fetal monitoring, even during contractions.
- Explain that the lower tracing on the monitor strip paper shows uterine activity; the upper tracing shows the fetal heart rate (FHR).
- Reassure woman and partner that prepared childbirth techniques can be implemented without difficulty.
- Explain that during external monitoring effleurage can be performed on sides of abdomen or upper portion of thighs.
- Explain that breathing patterns based on the time and intensity of contractions can be enhanced by the observation of uterine activity on the monitor strip paper, which shows the onset of contractions.
- Note peak of contraction; knowing that contraction will not get stronger and is half over is usually helpful.
- Note diminishing intensity.
- Coordinate with appropriate breathing and relaxation techniques.
- Reassure woman and partner that the use of internal monitoring does not restrict movement, although she is confined to bed.*
- Explain that use of external monitoring usually requires the woman's cooperation during positioning and movement.
- Reassure woman and partner that use of monitoring does not imply fetal jeopardy.

*Portable telemetry monitors allow the FHR and uterine contraction patterns to be observed on centrally located display stations. These portable units permit ambulation during electronic monitoring.

BOX 17-7 Management of Nonreassuring FHR Patterns

Basic Interventions

Administer oxygen by nonrebreather face mask at a rate of 10 L/min.

Assist the woman to a side-lying (lateral) position.

Increase maternal blood volume by increasing the rate of the primary intravenous (IV) infusion.

Interventions for Specific Problems

Maternal hypotension

- Increase the rate of the primary IV infusion.
- Change to lateral or Trendelenburg positioning.
- Administer ephedrine or phenylephrine if other measures are unsuccessful in increasing blood pressure.

Uterine tachysystole

- Reduce or discontinue the dose of any uterine stimulants in use (e.g., oxytocin [Pitocin]).
- Administer a uterine relaxant (tocolytic) (e.g., terbutaline [Brethine]).

Nonreassuring FHR tracing during second-stage labor

- Use open glottis, rather than Valsalva-style pushing.
- Use fewer pushing efforts during each contraction.
- Make individual pushing efforts shorter.
- Push only with every second or third contraction.
- Push only with a perceived urge to push (with use of regional anesthesia).

interventions to improve maternal and fetal oxygenation status.

Nurses must assign priorities to interventions to maximize the efficacy of the intrauterine resuscitation. The first priority is to open the maternal and fetal vascular systems; the second priority is to increase blood volume; and the third priority is to optimize oxygenation of the circulating blood volume.

Depending on the underlying cause of the nonreassuring FHR pattern, other interventions such as correcting maternal hypotension, reducing UA, and altering second-stage pushing techniques may also be instituted (Tucker, Miller, & Miller, 2009). Some interventions are specific to the FHR pattern. Nursing interventions appropriate for the management of tachycardia and bradycardia are given in Table 17-3, and those appropriate for the management of increased or decreased variability are given in Table 17-2. No specific nursing interventions are required for the management of FHR acceleration or early deceleration (see Boxes 17-2 and 17-3). However, late and some types of variable FHR decelerations require aggressive intervention (see Box 17-4). The primary health care provider decides whether medical intervention should be instituted, what intervention is indicated, or whether immediate vaginal or cesarean birth should be performed.

Additional Methods of Assessment and Intervention

Other methods of assessment and intervention are designed to be used in conjunction with EFM in an effort to identify and intervene in the presence of a nonreassuring FHR or pattern. These methods include FHR response to stimulation, fetal oxygen saturation monitoring, fetal blood sampling, amnioinfusion, and tocolysis. Umbilical cord acid-base determination is an assessment technique that is a useful adjunct to the Apgar score in assessing the immediate condition of the newborn.

Fetal Heart Rate Response to Stimulation

Stimulation of the fetus is done to elicit an acceleration of the FHR of 15 beats/min for at least 15 seconds and/or to improve FHR variability. The two methods of fetal stimulation currently in practice are scalp stimulation (using digital pressure during a vaginal examination) and vibroacoustic stimulation (using an artificial larynx or fetal acoustic stimulation device over the fetal head for 1 to 2 seconds). Fetal stimulation procedures should only be performed when the FHR is at baseline. Neither fetal scalp stimulation nor vibroacoustic stimulation should be instituted if FHR decelerations or bradycardia is present (Tucker, Miller, & Miller, 2009). FHR acceleration usually indicates fetal well-being. However, if the fetus does not have an acceleration, it does not necessarily indicate fetal compromise but rather that further evaluation of fetal well-being is needed.

Fetal Oxygen Saturation Monitoring

Continuous monitoring of fetal oxygen saturation ($FSpo_2$) or fetal pulse oximetry (FPO) is a method of fetal assessment that was approved for clinical use by the Food and Drug Administration in May 2000 (Dildy, 2004). FPO works in a way similar to the pulse oximetry used in children and adults. A specially designed sensor inserted next to the fetal cheek or temple area provides a continuous estimation of $FSpo_2$. After a number of randomized trials that indicated no consistent impact on newborn outcomes or overall cesarean rate, the manufacturer announced that it would no longer distribute the sensor, which effectively withdraws the product from the market (Tucker, Miller, & Miller, 2009).

Fetal Scalp Blood Sampling

A sample of fetal scalp blood is obtained through the dilated cervix after the membranes have ruptured. Many factors limit its use: the requirement for cervical dilation and membrane rupture, the technical difficulty of the procedure, the need for repeated pH determinations, and the uncertainty regarding interpretation and application of results. This procedure is now seldom used in the United States but remains a common practice in other countries (Tucker, Miller, & Miller, 2009).

Amnioinfusion

Amnioinfusion is infusion of room temperature isotonic fluid (usually normal saline or lactated Ringer's solution) into the uterine cavity through a double lumen IUPC when the volume of amniotic fluid is low. Without the buffer of amniotic fluid, the umbilical cord can easily become compressed during contractions or fetal movement, diminishing the flow of blood between the fetus and placenta and resulting in variable decelerations and transient fetal hypoxemia. The purpose of amnioinfusion is to relieve intermittent umbilical cord compression by restoring the amniotic fluid volume to a normal or near-normal level (Tucker, Miller, & Miller, 2009). Women with an abnormally small amount of amniotic fluid (oligohydramnios) or no amniotic fluid (anhydramnios) are candidates for this procedure. Conditions that can result in oligohydramnios or anhydramnios are uteroplacental insufficiency and premature rupture of membranes.

In the past amnioinfusion was also used to dilute moderate-to-thick meconium in an attempt to prevent meconium aspiration syndrome. However, a recent large research study found that amnioinfusion did not significantly reduce the incidence of meconium aspiration syndrome or perinatal death (Fraser et al, 2005). Therefore routine amnioinfusion for meconium-stained amniotic fluid without the presence of variable decelerations is not recommended by ACOG (2006).

Fluid is administered through a double-lumen IUPC by gravity flow or use of an infusion pump. The woman's membranes must be ruptured for the IUPC placement. Usually a bolus of fluid (250 to 500 ml) is administered over 20 to 30 minutes; then the infusion is slowed to a maintenance rate (2 to 3 ml/min; maximum 180 ml/hr). Only approximately a maximum of 1000 ml of fluid will need to be administered. The fluid can be warmed with a blood warmer before administration for the preterm or small-for-gestational-age fetus (Tucker, Miller, & Miller, 2009). It can be infused by bolus or continuous flow or a combination of these two methods. Risks of amnioinfusion are overdistention of the uterine cavity and increased uterine tone.

Intensity and frequency of UCs should be assessed continually during the procedure. The recorded uterine resting tone during amnioinfusion will appear higher than normal because of resistance to outflow and turbulence at the end of the catheter. The amount of fluid return should be estimated and documented during amnioinfusion to avoid overdistention of the uterus (Tucker, Miller, & Miller, 2009).

Tocolytic Therapy

Tocolysis (relaxation of the uterus) can be achieved through the administration of drugs that inhibit UCs. This therapy can be used as an adjunct to other interventions in the management of fetal stress when the fetus has nonreassuring FHR patterns associated with increased UA. Tocolysis improves blood flow through the placenta by inhibiting UCs. It may be considered by the primary health care provider and implemented when other interventions to reduce UA such as maternal position change and discontinuance of an oxytocin infusion have no effect on diminishing the UCs. Tocolytics are often administered when women are having excessive UCs spontaneously or after a decision for cesarean birth has been made while preparations for surgery are underway. The most commonly used tocolytic in these situations is terbutaline (Brethine) given subcutaneously. Terbutaline works quickly and has been demonstrated to improve Apgar scores and cord pH values without apparent complications (Garite, 2007). If the FHR and UC patterns improve, the woman may be allowed to continue labor; if there is no improvement, immediate surgical intervention for birth may be needed.

Umbilical Cord Acid-Base Determination

In assessing the immediate condition of the newborn after birth, a sample of cord blood is a useful adjunct to the Apgar score. Generally blood is withdrawn from the umbilical artery and tested for pH, Pco_2, and Po_2. Umbilical arterial values reflect fetal condition; umbilical venous blood values reflect placental function (Tucker, Miller, & Miller, 2009). Umbilical

Table 17-4 Approximate Normal Values for Cord Blood

CORD BLOOD	pH	PCO_2 (mm Hg)	PO_2 (mm Hg)	BASE DEFICIT (mmol/L)
Artery	7.2-7.3	45-55	15-25	<12
Vein	7.3-7.4	35-45	25-35	<12

From: Tucker SM, Miller LA, Miller DA: *Mosby's pocket guide to fetal monitoring: a multidisciplinary approach*, ed 6, St Louis, 2009, Mosby.

Table 17-5 Types of Acidemia

	RESPIRATORY	METABOLIC	MIXED
pH	<7.20	<7.20	<7.20
PCO_2 (mm Hg)	Elevated	Normal	Elevated
Base deficit	<12 mmol/L	<12 mmol/L	<12 mmol/L

From: Tucker SM, Miller LA, Miller DA: *Mosby's pocket guide to fetal monitoring: a multidisciplinary approach*, ed 6, St Louis, 2009, Mosby.

cord gas measurements reflect the acid-base status of the newborn at birth, a measurement not reflected in the Apgar score (Table 17-4). If acidemia is present, the type—respiratory, metabolic, or mixed—is determined by analyzing the blood gas values (Table 17-5).

Patient and Family Teaching

Part of the nurse's role includes acting as a partner with the woman to achieve a high-quality birthing experience (see Community Focus box). In addition to teaching and supporting the woman and her family with understanding of the laboring and birth process, breathing techniques, use of equipment, and pain management techniques, the nurse should provide information and support regarding two factors that have an effect on fetal status: pushing and positioning.

COMMUNITY FOCUS

Education About Electronic Fetal Monitoring

Interview childbirth educators from two different types of childbirth preparation classes (e.g., Lamaze, Bradley) regarding what they teach expectant parents about electronic fetal monitoring. Do the educators regard it to be "normal"? Do they discuss its advantages and disadvantages, or do they just describe it as a usual intervention? Do they discuss choice in labor (i.e., are parents able to select auscultation rather than electronic monitoring)? Intermittent rather than continuous monitoring? What implications does this information have for your practice as a labor and birth nurse?

Maternal Positioning

Maternal supine hypotensive syndrome is caused by the weight and pressure of the gravid uterus on the ascending vena cava when the woman is in a supine position. The supine position decreases venous return to the woman's heart and cardiac output and subsequently reduces her blood pressure. Low maternal blood pressure decreases intervillous space blood flow during UCs and results in fetal hypoxemia. This is reflected on the fetal monitor as a nonreassuring FHR pattern, usually as late decelerations. The nurse should solicit the woman's cooperation in avoiding the supine position. She should be encouraged to maintain a side-lying or semi-Fowler position with a lateral tilt to the uterus. Either the right or left lateral maternal position effectively enhances uteroplacental blood flow.

Discouraging the Valsalva Maneuver

The Valsalva maneuver can be described as the process of making a forceful bearing-down attempt while holding one's breath with a closed glottis and tightening the abdominal muscles. This process stimulates the parasympathetic division of the autonomic nervous system, producing a vagal response, and results in the decrease of the maternal heart rate and blood pressure. Prolonged pushing in this manner can decrease placental blood flow, alter maternal and fetal oxygenation, decrease the fetal pH and PO_2, increase the fetal PCO_2, and increase the likelihood of fetal hypoxemia, as reflected in FHR pattern changes.

During the second stage of labor, when the woman needs to push, an alternative to breath holding with a closed glottis is to perform the open-mouth and open-glottis breathing-pushing technique. The nurse can instruct the woman to keep her mouth and glottis open and let air escape from the lungs during the pushing process. This may result in an audible grunting sound and will prevent the Valsalva maneuver.

Some providers of care prefer the laboring-down process or delayed pushing, which is to refrain from pushing in the early second stage of labor. The natural forces of labor contractions are used to move the fetus down the birth canal; focused pushing is then used for a short period to expel the fetus from the birth canal.

Documentation

Clear and complete documentation in the woman's medical record is essential. Each FHR and UA assessment must be documented completely in the woman's medical record. Currently more and more hospitals are moving to use of the electronic medical record and computer charting. With computerized charting each required component usually appears on the screen so that it will be addressed routinely. Often computerized charting includes forced choices that greatly increase the use of standardized FHR terminology by all members of the health care team.

In the past nurses were often encouraged to chart both on the monitor strip and in the medical record. However, charting directly on the monitor strip is unnecessary when an electronic medical record is used (Fig. 17-9). Any information that is handwritten on the monitor strip will not be recorded in the computer record. Furthermore, since the electronic fetal monitor tracing is stored on computer, the paper strips are destroyed after the woman is discharged. No permanent record of the handwritten charting exists.

In institutions that still use a paper chart, documentation on the woman's monitor strip is started before the initiation of monitoring and consists of identifying information plus other relevant data. This documentation is continued and updated according to institutional protocol as monitoring progresses.

Fetal Monitor Integration

Quantitative Sentinel - PerinatalUser Split Stored Strip User: Quantitative Sentinel (OBU) (System Staff) 07/02/02 12:02
Security Roster Chalkboard Required Data Surveillance Help
(((Fetal Monitoring Strip))) - NID, OB (22332421)
11/19/94 20:42
240 180 120 60 100 50 0

Adm General Info - NID, OB (22332421)

Patient Name: DOE, JANE
Attending: Dr. W.
Pt. Age: 25
Height In: 64.0 Cm: 162.6
Prepreg Wt Lbs: 128 Kg: 58.18

PREGNANCY INFORMATION

Grav**	Para**	Term	Preterm	SAB	IAB	Living
3	2	0	2	0	0	2

LMP: 03/02/2002 EDC: 12/03/2002 EDC per U/S: MM/dd/yyyy
Exported data**

ALLERGIES

Medication	Y N U	Details...
Food	Y N U	Details...
Environmental	Y N U	Details...
Latex	Y N U	Details...
Potential Latex*	Y N U	Details...

*Sensitive to Nuts, Avocados, Kiwi, Balloons, Bananas, Condoms, etc.

COMMUNICATION
Primary Language: ENGLISH Prim. language, Other
-- If primary language is not English, enter ability with English language
No understanding, INTERPRETER needed
Understands verbal communication
Speaks English
Reads English
Communication Barriers identified:
None
Language barrier
Hearing deficit
Visual deficit
Mental retardation
Other
Communication Aids needed

Demographics | Patient Care | OB/Med/Surg Hx | Current Admission

Name: DOE, JANE Id: 22332421 Attend: Dr. W. Location: TEACHIN 168 GA: Allergies:

Adm/Disch | Interdisciplinary | Labor | Delivery | FM/Summary | MAR/I&O | Lab Results | Data Review | Full Screen | Split Screen
OB Triage | Adm INDEX | General Admit Info | Admit Assess | Problem List | Discharge | Select Beds | Active Beds
Help | F2-Home | F3-Select Pt | F4-Create Pt | F5-Transfer | F6-Discharge | F7-Select FMS | F8-Active Beds | F9-Stored Strip | F10-Chalkbd | F11-OnCall | F12-Logoff

Fig. 17-9 With integration of the fetal monitor tracing into the electronic medical record, the nurse can view the fetal tracing while charting. *(Courtesy General Electric Healthcare Technologies, Barrington, IL.)*

In some institutions observations noted and interventions implemented are recorded on the monitor strip to produce a comprehensive document that chronicles the course of labor and the care rendered. In other institutions this documentation is confined to the labor flow record. Advocates of documenting on both the medical record and the electronic fetal monitor strip cite as advantages of this approach the ease of writing directly on the strip while at the bedside and the improved accuracy in documenting critical events and the interventions implemented. Others believe that charting on the electronic fetal monitor strip constitutes duplicate documentation of the same information noted in the medical record and thus it is unnecessary additional paperwork for the nurse. This documentation is continued and updated according to institutional protocol as monitoring progresses.

A disadvantage of documenting on both the electronic fetal monitor strip and the medical record is that frequently the times noted for events and interventions on the electronic fetal monitor strip do not match what is later documented in the medical record. These differences can lead those involved in the retrospective review process carried out during litigation to infer that documentation errors have occurred. Therefore, if institutional policy mandates documentation on both the monitor strip and the medical record, it is critically important for the nurse to make sure that the times and notations of events and interventions recorded in each place agree.

Key Points

- Fetal well-being during labor is gauged by the response of the FHR to UCs.
- FHR characteristics include the baseline FHR and periodic/episodic changes in the FHR.
- The monitoring of fetal well-being includes FHR assessment, watching for meconium-stained amniotic fluid, and assessment of maternal vital signs and UA.
- It is the responsibility of the nurse to assess FHR and patterns, implement independent nursing interventions, and report nonreassuring patterns to the physician or nurse-midwife.

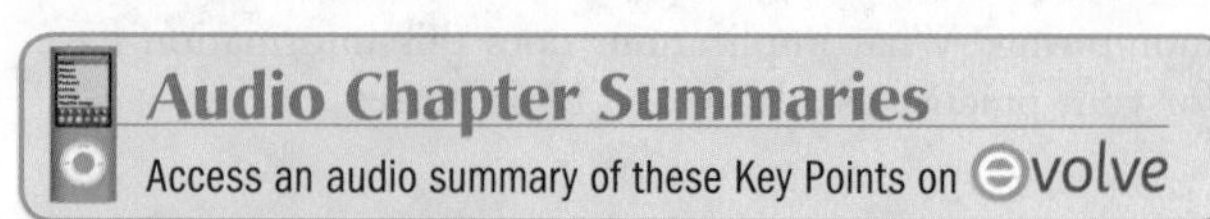
Audio Chapter Summaries
Access an audio summary of these Key Points on evolve

- AWHONN and ACOG established and published health care provider standards and guidelines for fetal heart monitoring.
- The emotional, informational, and comfort needs of the woman and her family must be addressed when the mother and her fetus are being monitored.
- Documentation is initiated and updated according to institutional protocol.

References

American Academy of Pediatrics (AAP), American College of Obstetricians and Gynecologists (ACOG): *Guidelines for perinatal care*, ed 6, Washington, DC, 2007, AAP and ACOG.

American College of Obstetricians and Gynecologists (ACOG): Amnioinfusion does not prevent meconium aspiration syndrome, ACOG Committee Opinion Number 346, Washington, DC, 2006, ACOG.

Association of Women's Health, Obstetric and Neonatal Nurses: *Fetal heart monitoring principles and practice*, ed 3, Dubuque, Ia, 2003, Kendall/Hunt.

Dildy G: Fetal pulse oximetry: a critical appraisal, *Best Pract Res Clin Obstet Gynaecol* 18(3):477-484, 2004.

Fraser WD et al: Amnioinfusion Trial Group: Amnioinfusion for the prevention of the meconium aspiration syndrome, *New Eng J Med* 353(9): 909-917, 2005.

Garite TJ: Intrapartum fetal evaluation. In Gabbe S, Niebyl J, Simpson J (editors): *Obstetrics: normal and problem pregnancies*, ed 5, Philadelphia, 2007, Churchill Livingstone.

Gilbert ES: *Manual of high risk pregnancy & delivery*, ed 4, St Louis, 2007, Mosby.

Hamilton BE, Martin JA, Ventura SJ: Births: preliminary data for 2006, *Natl Vital Stat Rep* 56(7):1-18, 2007.

Macones GA et al: The 2008 National Institute of Child Health and Human Development Workshop Report on Electronic Fetal Monitoring: update on definitions, interpretation, and research guidelines, *J Obstet Gynecol Neonatal Nurs* 37(5): 510-515, 2008.

National Institute of Child Health and Human Development Research Planning Workshop: Electronic fetal heart rate monitoring: research guidelines for interpretation, *Am J Obstet Gynecol* 177(6):1385-1390, 1997.

National Institute for Health and Clinical Excellence (NICE): *Intrapartal care: care for healthy women and their babies during childbirth*, NICE Clin Guideline 55, London, 2008, NICE. Available at www.nice.org.uk/nicemedia/pdf/IPCNICEGuidance.pdf (accessed April 1, 2009).

Simpson K, James D: Efficacy of intrauterine resuscitation techniques in improving fetal oxygen status during labor, *Obstet Gynecol* 105(6):1362-1368, 2005.

Tucker SM, Miller LA, Miller DA: *Mosby's pocket guide to fetal monitoring: a multidisciplinary approach*, ed 6, St Louis, 2009, Mosby.

Unit 4

18 Nursing Care During Labor and Birth

Learning Objectives

On completion of this chapter the reader will be able to:

- Review the factors included in the initial assessment of the woman in labor.
- Describe the ongoing assessment of maternal progress during the first, second, and third stages of labor.
- Recognize the physical and psychosocial findings that indicate maternal progress during labor.
- Describe fetal assessment during labor.
- Identify signs of developing complications during labor and birth.
- Develop a comprehensive plan of care for the woman and her significant others (support person[s], family) relevant to each stage of labor.
- Analyze the influence of cultural and religious beliefs and practices on the process of labor and birth.
- Evaluate research findings on the importance of support from family, partner, doula, and nurse in facilitating maternal progress during labor and birth.
- Describe the role and responsibilities of the nurse in an emergency childbirth situation.
- Evaluate the impact of perineal trauma on the woman's reproductive and sexual health.
- Discuss ways the nurse can use evidence-based practices to enhance the quality of care a woman receives during labor and birth.

Electronic Resources

Additional information related to the content in Chapter 18 can be found on

evolve the Companion Website at

http://evolve.elsevier.com/Perry/maternal/

- NCLEX Review Questions
- Animation—Vaginal Birth
- Assessment Video—Leopold's Maneuvers
- Case Study—First Stage of Labor
- Case Study—Second/Third Stages of Labor
- Critical Thinking Exercise—Positioning During Labor
- Nursing Care Plan—Labor and Birth
- Spanish Guidelines—Care During Labor
- Spanish Guidelines—Labor Assessment
- Video—Childbirth (Vaginal)

The labor process is an exciting and anxious time for the woman and her significant others (support people, family). In a relatively short period they experience one of the most profound changes in their lives.

For most women labor begins with the first uterine contraction, continues with hours of hard work during cervical dilation and birth, and ends as the woman and her family begin the attachment process with the newborn. Nursing care management focuses on assessment and support of the woman and her support people and family throughout labor and birth, with the goal of ensuring the best possible outcome for all involved.

First Stage of Labor

Nursing Care Management

The first stage of labor begins with the onset of regular uterine contractions and ends with complete cervical effacement and dilation (see Nursing Process box). The first stage of labor consists of three phases: the latent phase (up to 3 cm of dilation), the active phase (4 to 7 cm of dilation), and the transition phase (8 to 10 cm of dilation). Most nulliparous women seek admission to the hospital in the latent phase because they have not experienced labor before and are unsure of the "right" time to come in. Multiparous women usually do not come to the hospital until they are in the active phase. Even though no two labors are identical, women who have given birth before appear less anxious about the process unless their previous experience was negative.

A woman often has lingering impressions of her childbirth experiences. Satisfaction with childbirth depends on the woman's ability to maintain a sense of control. Caregivers who encourage a woman to be actively involved in decision making and who are respectful, supportive, available, protective, encouraging, kind, patient, professional, calm, and comforting help the woman to remember her childbirth experiences in positive terms. A satisfactory view of childbirth contributes to a woman's self-esteem and sense of accomplishment with her performance. Adaptation to her role as a mother can also be enhanced. Frustrations a woman feels regarding her childbirth experience stem from unmet expectations, poorly managed pain, loss of control, lack of knowledge, or the negative behaviors of some caregivers. A woman who perceives her childbirth

NURSING PROCESS: LABOR

Assessment

Assessment begins at the first contact with the woman, whether by telephone or in person.

- Review prenatal data from chart/patient.
- Perform physical examination including Leopold's maneuvers, uterine contractions, FHR, and status of cervix and membranes.
- Review laboratory data.
- Assess psychosocial factors.
- Assess cultural factors.

See text for discussion.

Nursing Diagnoses

Nursing diagnoses appropriate for the woman in first-stage labor include the following:

Anxiety related to
- negative experience with previous childbirth
- cultural differences

Impaired urinary elimination related to
- reduced intake of oral fluids
- diminished sensation of bladder fullness associated with epidural anesthesia/analgesia

Impaired fetal gas exchange related to
- maternal hypotension or hypertension
- intense uterine contractions
- compression of umbilical cord

Situational low self-esteem (maternal) related to
- inability to meet self-expectations concerning performance during childbirth
- loss of control during labor

Nursing diagnoses that represent potential areas for concern during the second stage of labor include the following:

Risk for injury to mother and fetus related to
- persistent use of Valsalva maneuver

Situational low self-esteem related to
- deficient knowledge of normal, beneficial effects of vocalization during bearing-down efforts
- inability to carry out plan for birth without medication

Ineffective coping related to
- coaching that contradicts woman's physiologic urge to push

Anxiety related to
- inability to control defecation with bearing-down efforts
- lack of knowledge of perineal sensations associated with the urge to bear down

Examples of nursing diagnoses relevant to the third stage of labor include the following:

Risk for deficient fluid volume related to
- blood loss occurring following placental separation and expulsion
- inadequate contraction of the uterus

Anxiety related to
- lack of knowledge regarding birth of the placenta
- occurrence of perineal trauma and the need for repair

Fatigue related to
- energy expenditure associated with childbirth and the bearing-down efforts of the second stage

Planning

The nurse and woman set and prioritize expected outcomes that focus on the woman, the fetus, and the woman's significant others.

Expected outcomes for the woman in labor are that the woman will accomplish the following:

- Continue normal progression of labor while the fetal heart rate and pattern remain reassuring and without signs of distress
- Maintain adequate hydration status through oral or intravenous intake (or both)
- Actively participate in the labor process
- Verbalize discomfort and indicate the need for measures that help reduce discomfort and promote relaxation
- Accept comfort and support measures from significant others and health care providers as needed
- Sustain no injury to herself or the fetus during labor
- Expel the placenta with maternal blood loss of less than 500 ml or less than 1% of body weight
- Initiate, along with the partner and family, the processes of bonding and attachment with the newborn
- Express satisfaction with her performance during labor

Interventions

Nursing care during first-stage labor includes both physical care and supportive care. Nursing interventions are described in the text (pp. 440-455) and in Table 18-4.

Evaluation

Evaluation is an ongoing process and is based on expected outcomes of care (see the Nursing Care Plan on pp. 458-459).

to be unsatisfactory or traumatic could be at risk for postpartum depression and cesarean birth for a subsequent pregnancy.

Certain factors are assessed initially to determine if the woman is in true labor and should come for further assessment or admission (see Patient Teaching box). The pregnant woman may call her primary health care provider or come to the hospital while in false labor or early in the latent phase of the first stage of labor. She may feel discouraged, angry, or confused on learning that the contractions that feel so strong and regular to her are not true contractions because they are not causing cervical dilation or are still not strong or frequent enough for admission.

PATIENT TEACHING How to Distinguish True Labor from False Labor

True Labor

Contractions

- Occur regularly, becoming stronger, lasting longer, and occurring closer together.
- Become more intense with walking.
- Usually felt in lower back, radiating to lower portion of abdomen.
- Continue despite use of comfort measures.

Cervix (by vaginal examination)

- Shows progressive change (softening, effacement, and dilation signaled by the appearance of bloody show).
- Moves to an increasingly anterior position.

Fetus

- Presenting part usually becomes engaged in the pelvis. This results in increased ease of breathing; at the same time the presenting part presses downward and compresses the bladder, resulting in urinary frequency.

False Labor

Contractions

- Occur irregularly or become regular only temporarily.
- Often stop with walking or position change.
- Can be felt in the back or abdomen above the navel.
- Often can be stopped through the use of comfort measures.

Cervix (by vaginal examination)

- May be soft, but there is no significant change in effacement or dilation or evidence of bloody show.
- Is often in a posterior position.

Fetus

- Presenting part is usually not engaged in the pelvis.

BOX 18-1 Telephone Interview with Woman in Latent Phase of Labor*

The perinatal nurse performs the following steps of the nursing process:

Assessment

Gathers data regarding the woman's status, including signs and symptoms indicative of true or false labor

Discusses instructions given by the woman's primary health care provider regarding when to come for admission

Planning and Implementation

Decides whether the woman will come for labor assessment and admission or be encouraged to stay at home until contractions increase in duration, frequency, and intensity

Assures the woman that she is welcome to call the perinatal unit at any time to discuss her labor status

Answers questions the woman and her family may have regarding labor or provides instruction as needed (e.g., which entrance of the hospital to enter)

Suggests a variety of positions she can assume to maximally enhance uteroplacental and renal blood flow (e.g., side-lying position) and enhance the progress of labor (e.g., upright positions and ambulation)

Suggests diversional activities such as walking, reading, watching television, talking to friends

Suggests measures to maintain comfort such as a warm shower or a back or foot massage

Discusses the oral intake of foods and fluids appropriate for early labor (light foods or fluids or clear liquids, depending on the preference of her primary health care provider)

Instructs the woman to come in immediately if membranes rupture, bleeding occurs, or fetal movements change

Evaluation

Evaluates whether instructions and information have been understood by the woman by asking her to verbalize her understanding

Documentation

Documents all advice given over the telephone in the woman's record

*In some settings, nurses are no longer allowed to provide advice over the telephone but must refer the caller to her primary health care provider.

During the third trimester of pregnancy women should be instructed regarding the stages of labor and the signs indicating its onset. They should be informed of the possibility that they will not be admitted if they are 3 cm or less dilated. Later admission (i.e., during the active phase of labor at 4 cm or greater dilation) for low risk women has been associated with an increased rate of spontaneous vaginal birth and fewer obstetric interventions.

If the woman lives near the hospital and has adequate support and transportation, she may be asked to stay home or return home to allow labor to progress (i.e., until the contractions are more frequent and intense). The ideal setting for low risk women in early labor is the familiar environment of her home. The nurse can use a telephone interview (Box 18-1) to assess the woman's status, give instructions regarding the optimal timing for admission, reinforce teaching of the signs that require immediate notification of the primary health care provider, and provide support and encouragement. The nurse should describe measures the woman and her significant others can use to enhance the progress of labor, reduce anxiety, and maintain comfort. The woman should be informed that she can call back at any time to report concerns she may have or to ask questions.

This is especially important for the primigravida who may be very anxious and lack confidence in her ability to cope with labor.

A warm shower can be relaxing for the woman in early labor; however, warm baths should be avoided until the cervix is approximately 4 to 5 cm dilated, because water immersion in early labor can prolong the labor process and increase the use of oxytocin to stimulate uterine contractions and epidural analgesia for pain reduction. Soothing back, foot, and hand massages or a warm drink of preferred liquids such as tea or milk can help the woman rest and even sleep, especially if false or early labor is occurring at night. Diversional activities such as walking, reading, watching television, doing needlework, or talking with friends can reduce the perception of early discomfort, help the time pass, and reduce anxiety.

The woman who lives at a considerable distance from the hospital or who lacks adequate support and transportation may be admitted in early labor. The same measures used by the woman at home should be offered to the hospitalized woman in early labor.

Admission to Labor Unit

When the woman arrives at the perinatal unit, assessment is the top priority (Fig. 18-1). The nurse first performs a screening assessment, using the techniques of interview and physical assessment, and reviews laboratory and diagnostic test findings to determine the health status of the woman and her fetus and the progress of her labor. The primary health care provider is notified; if the woman is admitted, a detailed systems assessment is done.

LEGAL TIP Obstetric Triage and Emergency Medical Treatment and Active Labor Act The Emergency Medical Treatment and Active Labor Act (EMTALA) is a federal regulation enacted to ensure that a woman gets emergency treatment or active labor care whenever such treatment is sought. According to the EMTALA, true labor is considered to be an emergency medical condition. Nurses working in labor and birth units must be familiar with their responsibilities according to the EMTALA regulations, which include providing services to pregnant women when they experience an urgent pregnancy problem (e.g., labor, decreased fetal movement, rupture of membranes [ROM], recent trauma) and fully documenting all relevant information (e.g., assessment findings, interventions implemented, client responses to care measures provided). A pregnant woman presenting in an obstetric triage is considered to be in "true" labor until a qualified health care provider certifies that she is not. Agencies need to have specific policies and procedures in place so that compliance with the EMTALA regulations is achieved while safe and efficient care is provided (Angelini & Mahlmeister, 2005; Caliendo et al, 2004).

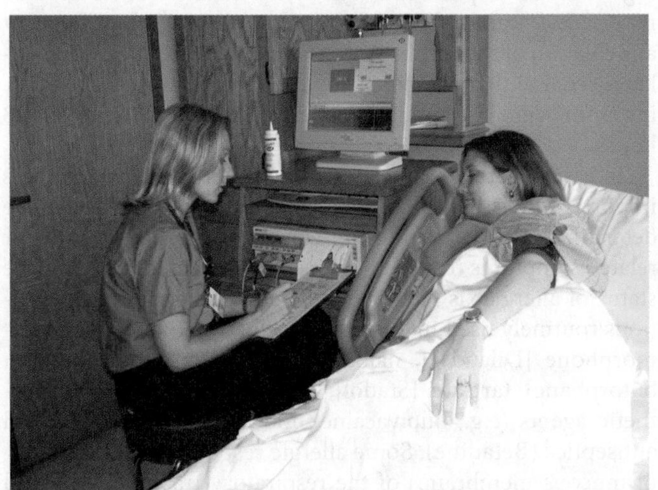

Fig. 18-1 Woman being admitted. *(Courtesy Julie Perry Nelson, Loveland, CO.)*

When the woman is admitted, she usually is moved from an observation area to the room where she will labor and give birth: the labor, delivery, and recovery (LDR) room or the labor, delivery, recovery, and postpartum (LDRP) room. Anyone coming in the room should be introduced; women often express concern regarding the number of people intruding on their labor experience, especially if the role of the person and purpose for his or her presence are not clearly identified.

Family-centered care is important in maternity today. This approach views labor as wellness and the woman and her support people as active participants in the process of labor and birth. LDR or LDRP rooms are essential components of family-centered care, and the woman is encouraged to have anyone she wishes present for her support. After birth the mother, baby, and support people are permitted to stay together to celebrate the arrival of a new family member.

The woman is asked to undress and put on her own gown or a hospital gown. An admissions band is placed on the woman's wrist and, when relevant, an allergy band (usually colored). Her personal belongings are put away safely or given to family members according to agency policy and her preference. Often women who participate in expectant parent classes bring a birth bag or Lamaze bag with them. Tennis balls or rolling pins for counterpressure, a pillow for comfort and reminder of home, an object for a focal point (e.g., meaningful picture, stuffed animal), and rice bags for warm packs may be included in her bag.

The nurse orients the woman and her partner to the layout and operation of the unit and room. This includes the use of the call light and telephone system, the location of personal storage areas in the bedside and over-the-bed tables, and how to adjust lighting in the room and positions of the bed.

The nurse reassures the woman that she is in competent, caring hands and that she and her partner can ask questions related to her care and the status of herself and her fetus at any time during labor. The woman's anxiety can be minimized by explaining terms commonly used during labor. Her interest, response, and prior experience guide the depth of these explanations.

Admission Data

Hospital admission forms in either paper format or, more commonly today, computerized can provide guidelines for the acquisition of important assessment information when a

evolve Case Study–First Stage of Labor

woman in labor is being evaluated or admitted. Additional sources of data include the following: (1) prenatal record, (2) initial interview, (3) physical examination to determine baseline physiologic parameters (e.g., vital signs), (4) laboratory and diagnostic test results, (5) expressed psychosocial and cultural factors, and (6) clinical evaluation of labor status.

Prenatal Data

The nurse reviews the prenatal record to identify the woman's individual needs and risks. Complete information regarding the woman's prenatal health status is essential to ensure the quality and safety of the care provided to her and her fetus or newborn during labor and birth and in the postpartum period.

If the woman has not had any prenatal care or her prenatal record is unavailable, certain baseline information must be obtained. If she is having discomfort, the nurse should ask questions between contractions when she can concentrate more fully on her responses. At times the partner or support person(s) may need to be secondary sources of essential information.

It is important to know the woman's age so that the plan of care can be tailored to the needs of her age group. For example, a 14-year-old and a 40-year-old have different but specific needs, and their ages place them at risk for different problems. Height and weight relations are important to determine because a weight gain greater than that recommended may place the woman at a higher risk for cephalopelvic disproportion and cesarean birth. This is especially true for women who are petite and have gained 16 kg or more. Other factors to consider are the woman's general health status, current medical conditions or allergies, respiratory status, and previous surgical procedures. Questioning about physical and substance abuse should form an integral part of the initial and ongoing assessment.

Her past and present pregnancy histories are carefully noted. These include gravidity; parity; and problems such as history of vaginal bleeding, gestational hypertension, anemia, pregestational or gestational diabetes, infections (e.g., bacterial or sexually transmitted), and immunodeficiency.

If this is not the woman's first labor and birth experience, it is important to note the characteristics of her previous experiences. This information includes the duration of previous labors, the type of anesthesia used, the kind of birth (e.g., spontaneous vaginal, forceps- or vacuum-assisted, or cesarean birth), and the condition of the newborn. The woman's perception of her previous labor and birth experiences should be explored because it may influence her attitude toward her current experience.

It is important to confirm the expected date of birth. Other data in the prenatal record include patterns of maternal weight gain, physiologic measurements such as maternal vital signs (blood pressure; temperature, pulse, respiration), fundal height, baseline fetal heart rate (FHR), and laboratory and diagnostic test results.

Laboratory tests include the woman's blood type and Rh factor, a complete or partial blood cell count (complete blood cell count [CBC], hemoglobin, and hematocrit), the 50-g blood glucose test, determination of the rubella titer, serologic tests (Venereal Disease Research Laboratories [VDRL] or rapid plasma reagin [RPR] test) for syphilis, hepatitis B surface antigen, culture for group B streptococci, and urinalysis. Additional tests may include a tuberculosis screen with purified protein derivative (PPD), screening for the human immunodeficiency virus, and a screen for sickle cell trait or other genetic disorders (e.g., maternal serum alpha-fetoprotein). Diagnostic tests include amniocentesis, nonstress test, contraction stress test, biophysical profile, and ultrasound examination.

Interview

The woman's primary reason for coming to the hospital is determined in the interview. Her primary reason may be that her bag of waters (i.e., amniotic membranes) ruptured, with or without contractions. The woman may have come in for an obstetric check, which is a period of observation reserved for women who are unsure whether they are in labor. This allows time on the unit for diagnosis of labor without official admission and minimizes or avoids cost to the woman when used by the hospital and approved by her health insurance plan.

Even the experienced mother may have difficulty determining the onset of labor. The woman is asked to recall the events of the previous days and to describe the following:

- Time of onset of contractions and progress in terms of intensity, frequency, and duration
- Location and character of discomfort from the contractions (e.g., back pain, suprapubic discomfort)
- Persistence of contractions despite changes in maternal position and activity (e.g., walking or lying down)
- Presence and character of vaginal discharge or "show"
- Status of amniotic membranes such as gush or seepage of fluid ([spontaneous] ROM [S][ROM])

If there has been a discharge that may be amniotic fluid, the woman is asked the date and time the fluid was first noted and the fluid's characteristics (e.g., amount, color, or unusual odor). In many instances a sterile speculum examination and a nitrazine (pH) or fern test can confirm that the membranes are ruptured (Box 18-2).

These descriptions help the nurse assess the degree of progress in labor. Bloody or pink show is distinguished from bleeding in that it is pink and feels sticky because of its mucoid nature. It is scant to begin with and increases with effacement and dilation of the cervix. A woman may report a scant brownish discharge that can be attributed to cervical trauma resulting from vaginal examination or coitus within the previous 48 hours.

In case general anesthesia is required in an emergency, it is important to assess the woman's respiratory status. The nurse determines this by asking the woman if she has a "cold" or related symptoms (e.g., stuffy nose, sore throat, or cough). The status of allergies is rechecked, including allergies to medications routinely used in obstetrics such as opioids (e.g., hydromorphone [Dilaudid], nalbuphine hydrochloride [Nubain], butorphanol tartrate [Stadol], fentanyl [Sublimaze]), anesthetic agents (e.g., bupivacaine, lidocaine, ropivacaine), and antiseptics (Betadine). Some allergic responses cause swelling of mucous membranes of the respiratory tract, which could interfere with breathing and the administration of inhalation anesthetics.

BOX 18-2 Procedure: Tests for Rupture of Membranes

Nitrazine Test for pH*

Explain procedure to woman/couple.

Procedure

Wash hands.

Use *nitrazine test* paper, a dye-impregnated test paper for determining pH (differentiates amniotic fluid, which is slightly alkaline, from urine and purulent material [pus], which are acidic).

Wearing a sterile glove lubricated with water, place a piece of test paper at the cervical os.

or

Use a sterile, cotton-tipped applicator to dip deep into vagina to pick up fluid; touch applicator to test paper. (Procedure may be done during speculum examination.)

or

Use *amniotic fluid indicator swabs* (which have been impregnated with nitrazine).

Read Results

Membranes probably intact—Identifies vaginal and most body fluids that are acidic:

Yellow	pH 5.0
Olive-yellow	pH 5.5
Olive-green	pH 6.0

Membranes probably ruptured—Identifies amniotic fluid that is alkaline:

Blue-green	pH 6.5
Blue-gray	pH 7.0
Deep blue	pH 7.5

Realize that false test results are possible because of presence of bloody show, insufficient amniotic fluid, or semen.

Remove gloves and wash hands.

Document Results

Positive or negative

Test for Ferning or Fern Pattern*

Explain procedure to woman/couple.

Wash hands, apply sterile gloves, obtain specimen of fluid (usually during sterile speculum examination).

Spread a drop of fluid from vagina on a clean glass slide with a sterile, cotton-tipped applicator.

Allow fluid to dry.

Examine slide under microscope. Observe for appearance of ferning (a frondlike crystalline pattern). (Do not confuse with cervical mucus test, when high levels of estrogen are responsible for causing the ferning.)

Observe for absence of ferning (alert staff to possibility that amount of specimen was inadequate or that specimen was urine, vaginal discharge, or blood).

Remove gloves and wash hands.

Document Results

Positive or negative

*In some settings the specimen is collected by the nurse or primary health care provider and sent to the laboratory for interpretation of results.

Because vomiting and subsequent aspiration into the respiratory tract can complicate an otherwise normal labor, the nurse records the type and time of the woman's last solid food and liquid intake.

Any information not found in the prenatal record is obtained during the admission assessment. Pertinent data include the birth plan (see Chapter 11; *www.childbirth.org*), the choice of infant feeding method, the type of pain management, and the name of the pediatric health care provider. A patient profile is obtained that identifies the woman's preparation for childbirth, the support person or family members desired during childbirth and their availability, and ethnic or cultural expectations and needs. The woman's use of alcohol, drugs, and tobacco before or during pregnancy should be determined. After birth the nurse assesses the neonate for signs indicating maternal substance use during pregnancy (e.g., abstinence syndrome, size, and appearance) (see Community Focus box). Screening of the neonate for substances abused by the mother may be required.

The nurse reviews the birth plan. If no written plan has been prepared, the nurse helps the woman formulate a birth plan by describing options available and finds out the woman's wishes and preferences. The nurse prepares the woman for the possibility that changes may be needed in her plan as labor progresses and assures her that information will be provided so that she can make informed decisions. The nurse uses the birth plan information to plan individualized care for the woman during labor.

The nurse should discuss with the woman and her partner their plans for preserving childbirth memories using photography and videotaping. The nurse should provide information about the agency's policies regarding these practices and

COMMUNITY FOCUS

Availability of Alternative Childbirth Options in the Community

Consult the yellow pages of the telephone directory and the Internet to explore options for childbearing families in your community. Are certified nurse-midwives available in your community? Are other types of licensed midwives available? Is there an option for a home birth? For a water birth? During your clinical rotation in maternity nursing, interview a staff nurse in labor and delivery (L&D) and ascertain his or her views of midwives and home births. Interview a childbirth educator and ascertain his or her views of midwives and home births. Contrast the views of the L&D nurse and the childbirth educator. Is there a difference in their views? Prepare a patient handout listing the options for childbearing families in your community. Discuss the findings from your interview with your clinical group.

under what circumstances they are allowed. Protection of privacy and safety and infection control (e.g., where the person who is recording the event should stand) are major concerns for the parents-to-be and the agency. The woman's record should reflect that the birth was recorded.

Psychosocial Factors

The woman's general appearance and behavior (and that of her partner) provide valuable clues to the type of supportive care she will need. However, the nurse should keep in mind that general appearance and behavior may vary, depending on the stage and phase of labor (Table 18-1). Psychosocial factors to assess include the following:

Verbal interactions—Does the woman ask questions? Can she ask for what she needs? Does she talk to her support person(s)? Does she talk freely with the nurse or respond only to questions?

Body language—Is she relaxed or tense? What is her anxiety level? How does she react to being touched by the nurse or support person? Does she change positions or lie rigidly still? Does she avoid eye contact? Does she look tired? How much rest has she had during the past 24 hours?

Perceptual ability—Does she understand what the nurse says? Is there a language barrier? Are repeated explanations necessary because her anxiety level interferes with her ability to comprehend? Can she repeat what she has been told or demonstrate her understanding?

Discomfort level—To what degree does the woman describe what she is experiencing? How does she react to a contraction? Are any nonverbal pain messages seen? Does she complain to the nurse or her partner? Can she ask for comfort measures?

Women with a History of Sexual Abuse

Memories of sexual abuse can be triggered during labor by intrusive procedures such as vaginal examination; loss of control; feeling helpless and isolated in a strange environment; being unable to move freely as a result of being confined to bed and "restrained" by monitors, intravenous (IV) lines, and epidural catheters; being watched by students; and having intense sensations in the uterus and genital area, especially at the time when she must push the baby out. Women who are survivors of abuse may fight the labor process by reacting in panic or anger toward care providers, take control of everyone and everything related to their childbirth, surrender by being submissive and dependent, or retreat by mentally dissociating themselves from the sensations of labor and birth (Hobbins, 2004; Simkin & Klaus, 2004).

The nurse can help these women to associate the sensations they are experiencing with the process of childbirth and not with their past abuse. The woman's sense of control should be maintained by explaining all procedures and why they are needed, validating her needs and paying close attention to her requests, proceeding at the woman's pace by waiting for her permission to touch her, accepting her often extreme reactions to labor, and protecting her privacy by limiting the exposure of her body and the number of people involved in her care. It

Table 18-1 Sociocultural Basis of Pain Experience

WOMAN IN LABOR	NURSE
Perception of Meaning	
Origin: Cultural concept of and personal experience with pain; for example: Pain in childbirth is inevitable, something to be endured. Pain in childbirth can be avoided completely. Pain in childbirth is punishment for sin. Pain in childbirth can be controlled.	Origin: Cultural concept of and personal experience with pain; in addition, nurse becomes accustomed to working with certain "expected" pain trajectories. For example, in obstetrics pain is expected to increase as labor progresses, be intermittent, and have an end point; relief can be derived from medications once labor is well established and fetus or newborn can cope with amount and elimination of medications; relief can also come from woman's knowledge, attitude, and support from family or friends.
Coping Mechanisms	
Woman may exhibit the following behaviors: She may be traditionally vocal or nonvocal; crying out or groaning or both may be part of her ritual response to pain. Use counterstimulation to minimize pain (e.g., rubbing, applying heat, or applying counterpressure). Use relaxation, distraction, or autosuggestion as pain-countering techniques. Resist any use of "needles" as modes of administering pain-relief agents.	Nurse may respond by: Using self effectively (e.g., using tone of voice, closeness in space, and touch as media for conveying message of interest and caring). Using avoidance, belittling, or other distracting actions as protective device for self. Using pharmacologic resources at hand judiciously. Using comfort measures. Assuming accountability for control and management of pain.
Expectations of Others	
Nurse may be seen as someone who will accept woman's statement of pain and act as her advocate. Medical personnel may be expected to relieve woman of all pain sensations. Nurse may be expected to be interested, gentle, kind, and accepting of behavior exhibited.	Only certain verbal or nonverbal responses to pain may be accepted as appropriate responses. Couple that is prepared for childbirth may be expected to refuse medication and wish to "do everything on their own." Woman's definition of pain may not be accepted (i.e., woman may wish to experience and participate in controlling pain or may not be able to accept any pain as reasonable).

is recommended that all laboring women be cared for in this manner because it is not unusual for a woman to choose not to reveal a history of sexual abuse (Hobbins, 2004; Simkin & Klaus, 2004).

Stress in Labor

The way in which women and their support person or family members approach labor is related to the manner in which they have been socialized to the childbearing process. Their reactions reflect their life experiences regarding childbirth—physical, social, cultural, and religious. Society communicates its expectations regarding acceptable and unacceptable maternal behaviors during labor and birth. These expectations may be used by some women as the basis for evaluating their own actions during childbirth. An idealized perception of labor and birth may be a source of guilt and a sense of failure if the woman finds the process less than joyous, especially when the pregnancy is unplanned or is the product of a shaky or terminated relationship. Often women have heard horror stories or seen friends or relatives going through labors that appear anything but easy. Multiparous women often base their expectations of the present labor on their previous childbirth experiences.

Feelings a woman has about her pregnancy and fears regarding childbirth should be discussed. This is especially important if the woman is a primigravida who has not attended childbirth classes or a multiparous woman who had a previous negative childbirth experience. Major fears and concerns relate to the process and effects of childbirth, maternal and fetal well-being, and the attitude and actions of the health care staff. Unresolved fears increase a woman's stress and can slow the process of labor as a result of the inhibiting effects of catecholamines associated with the stress response on uterine contractions.

Women in labor usually have a variety of concerns that they will voice if asked but rarely volunteer. It is important to ask the woman what she expects or to suggest that she ask her primary health care provider about an issue. The following are common concerns that women in labor have: Will my baby be all right? Will I be able to stand labor? Will my labor be long? How will I act? Will I need medication? Will it work for me? Will my partner or someone be there to support me?

The nurse's responsibility to the woman in labor with regard to these concerns is to answer her questions or find out the answers, provide support for her and her support person and family, take care of her in partnership with the people the woman wants as her support team, and serve as their advocate. Women can equate emotional support with information giving. Nurses are perceived as supportive when they explain things in detail by using positive terms and provide accurate information and specific directions. Women feel empowered when they are given information they can understand and that reflects support of their efforts. This feeling of empowerment contributes to a positive perception of the birth experience. In contrast, a woman's level of anxiety and fear may increase when she does not understand what is being said.

The nurse communicates to the woman that she is not expected to act in any particular way and that the process will end in the birth of her baby, which is the only expectation she should have. Women need to be able to behave in a manner that is natural for them. The woman's views and expectations regarding the nurse's role as caregiver should be determined. The nurse-patient relationship will become increasingly important as labor progresses. Women need to trust in their own innate ability to give birth; nurses need to support and protect each woman's efforts to achieve this outcome.

The father, coach, or significant other(s) also experience stress during labor. The nurse can assist and support these individuals by identifying their needs and expectations and helping to make sure these are met. The nurse can ascertain what role the support person intends to fulfill and whether he or she is prepared for that role by making observations and asking him or her questions such as the following: Has the couple attended childbirth classes? What role does this person expect to play? Is he or she nervous, anxious, aggressive, or hostile? Does he or she look hungry, tired, worried, or confused? Does he or she watch television, sleep, or stay out of the room instead of paying attention to the woman? Does he or she touch the woman? What is the character of the touch? The nurse should be sensitive to needs of support people and provide teaching and support as appropriate. Often the support this person is able to give the laboring woman is in direct proportion to the support he or she receives from nurses and other health care providers.

Cultural Factors

As the population of the United States and Canada becomes more diverse, it is increasingly important to recognize a pregnant woman's ethnic (cultural) and religious values, beliefs, and practices to anticipate nursing interventions that should be included in a mutually acceptable plan of care that facilitates a feeling of safety and control. Nurses should be committed to providing culturally sensitive care and to developing an appreciation and respect for cultural diversity (Callister, 2005). The woman should be encouraged to request caregiving behaviors and practices that are important to her. If a special request contradicts usual practices in that setting, the woman or nurse can ask the woman's primary health care provider to write an order to accommodate the special request. For example, in many cultures it is unacceptable to have a male caregiver examine a pregnant woman. In some cultures it is traditional to take the placenta home; in others the woman is given only certain nourishments during labor. Some women believe that cutting her body, as with an episiotomy, allows her spirit to leave her body and that rupturing the membranes prolongs, not shortens, labor. It is important that the rationale for required care measures be carefully explained (see Cultural Awareness box).

Cultural beliefs and values can influence a woman's reliance on her primary health care provider during labor and her desire to participate in making decisions about the care she receives (Callister, 2005). It may be noted that a Japanese woman in labor may assume the traditional role of a passive patient and may be reluctant to express her needs unless specifically asked to do so (Ito & Sharts-Hopko, 2002). Native American women who view childbirth as a natural event may find the high-technology environment of a hospital frightening and a disruption of the balance and harmony that are

CULTURAL AWARENESS

Cultural Variations in Birth Practices

South Korea—Stoic response to labor pain; fathers usually not present

Japan—Natural childbirth methods practiced; may labor silently; may eat during labor; father may be present

China—Stoic response to pain; fathers usually not present; side-lying position preferred for labor and birth because this position is thought to reduce infant trauma

India—Natural childbirth methods preferred; father usually not present; female relatives usually present

Iran—Father not present; prefers female support and female caregivers

Mexico—May be stoic about discomfort until second stage; then may request pain relief; fathers and female relatives may be present

Laos—May use squatting position for birth; fathers may or may not be present; prefers female attendants

Modified from D'Avanzo CE: *Mosby's pocket guide to cultural health assessment*, ed 4, St Louis, 2008, Mosby.

critical for a positive birth experience. They often prefer to be surrounded by a large number of family members, especially the grandparents, and become anxious in the presence of a large number of health care providers who come into the labor room and loudly discuss the progress of labor with each other (Molina, 2001). During contractions a Navajo woman may wish to pull on a rope or sash belt that is suspended from the ceiling (Fig. 18-2). As the woman pulls on the rope, a caring person chosen by the woman (e.g., her husband, mother, or other female companion) sits, kneels, or stands behind her and holds her tight under her breasts and over her pregnant abdomen to support her in an upright position and to provide warmth against her back (Begay, 2004). Chinese women who believe in the balance of *yin-yang* view childbirth as a source of heat loss from the body. Providing hot fluids and a warm shower to these women during labor would be measures they would accept as a means of restoring the heat that is being lost (Cioffi, 2004).

When assessing a woman's cultural and religious preferences, the nurse can ask questions regarding the following:

- The value and meaning placed on the childbirth experience
- The view of childbirth as a wellness or illness experience and as a private or social event
- Practices regarding diet, medications, activity, and emotional and physical support
- Appropriate maternal and paternal behaviors
- Birth companions—who they should be and what they should do
- Views regarding the newborn and newborn care immediately after birth

Within cultures women may learn the "right" way to behave in labor and react to the pain experienced in that way. These behaviors can range from total silence to moaning or screaming, but they are not in and of themselves a gauge of the degree of pain. A woman who moans with contractions may not be in as much physical pain as a woman who is silent but winces

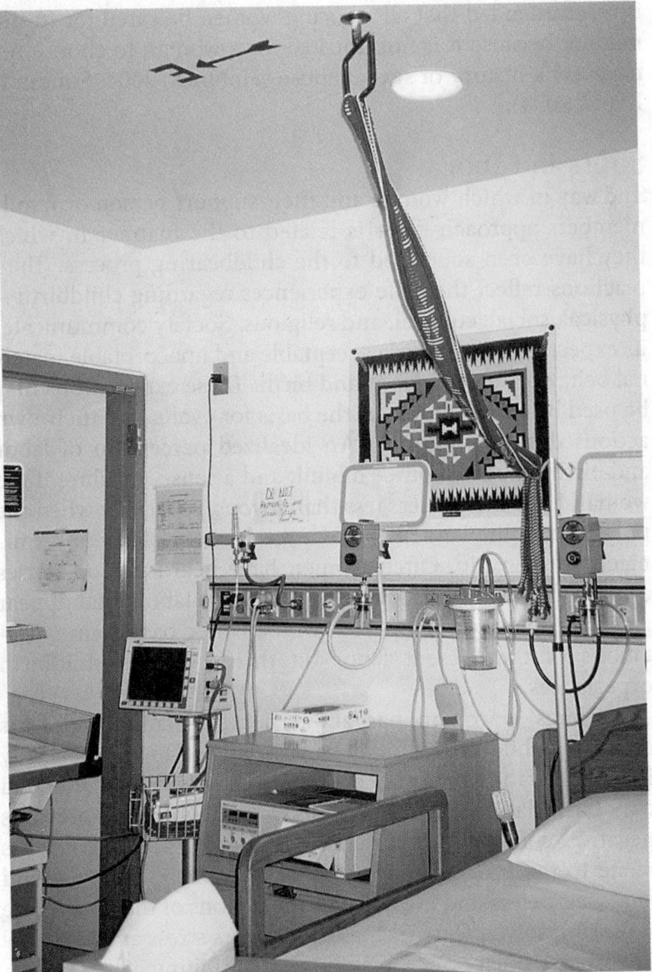

Fig. 18-2 Birthing room specific to a Native American population. Note the arrow pointing east, the rug on the wall, and the cord hanging from the ceiling. *(Chinle Comprehensive Health Care Center, Chinle, AZ; photo courtesy Patricia Hess, San Francisco, CA.)*

during contractions (see Table 18-1). For example, Chinese women may be stoic and quiet during labor and merely grimace during a contraction but not shout out. Rather than using pharmacologic measures for pain relief, they may prefer the support of family members and nonpharmacologic measures (Brathwaite & Williams, 2004; Cioffi, 2004). Some women believe that it is shameful to scream or cry out in pain if a man is present. If the woman's support person is her mother, she may perceive the need to "behave" more strongly than if her support person is the father of the baby. She will perceive herself as failing or succeeding on the basis of her ability to adhere to these "standards" of behavior. Conversely, a woman's behavior in response to pain may influence the support received from significant others. In some cultures women who lose control and cry out in pain may be scolded, whereas in other cultures support people will become more helpful.

Culture and Father Participation

A companion is an important source of support, encouragement, and comfort to women during childbirth. The choice of a birth companion is influenced by the woman's cultural and religious background and by trends in the society in which she lives. For example, in Western societies the father is viewed as the ideal birth companion. For European-American couples, attending childbirth classes together has become a traditional, expected activity. In some other cultures the father's presence in the labor and birth room is inappropriate (e.g., Mexican, Filipino, Chinese, Islamic, and Ethiopian) (D'Avanzo, 2008). However, among the Laotian (Hmong) the father plays an important role in the birth.

Mexican-American and Filipina women share an affectional bond with their female relatives when it comes to home-related activities such as childbearing. This also is true for the women of many other cultural groups. The presence of another woman or women is highly desired at such occasions. Women who come from some of these cultures and who give birth in the hospital like to have at least one woman present for assistance. Vietnamese, Chinese, Indian, Syrian, and Orthodox Jewish women prefer a female companion during childbirth and are very concerned about their modesty. In addition to feeling shy, they cite the belief that female caregivers are more respectful and would provide a higher degree of comfort and psychosocial support (Bashour & Abdulsalam, 2005; D'Avanzo, 2008). Islamic women also are very modest (i.e., need to keep hair and body covered) and would not accept the presence of a man during childbirth, not even the father. In India women are attended by other women and in rural areas by a local untrained midwife or *dai*. If couples from these cultures immigrate to the United States or Canada, their roles may change. The nurse will need to talk with the woman and her support people to determine the roles they wish to assume.

The Non–English-Speaking Woman in Labor

A woman's level of anxiety in labor rises when she does not understand what is happening to her or what is being said. Some misunderstanding may occur with English-speaking women and cause some stress; but the effect of misunderstanding on non–English-speaking women is much more dramatic. These women often feel a complete loss of control over their situation if there is no health care provider present who speaks their language. They can panic and withdraw or become physically abusive when someone tries to do something that they perceive might harm them or their babies. Sometimes a support person is able to serve as an interpreter. However, this must be done with caution because the interpreter may not be able to convey exactly what the nurse or others are saying or what the woman is saying, and this may raise the woman's stress level even more.

Ideally a bilingual nurse will care for the woman. Alternatively an employee or volunteer interpreter may be contacted for assistance. Preferably the interpreter is from the woman's culture. For some women a female interpreter may be more acceptable. If no one in the hospital is able to interpret, a translation service can be called so that an interpretation can take place over the telephone. Another alternative is for the labor and birth staff to prepare a set of cards with graphic depictions that illustrate common situations. These cards can be used to communicate with non–English-speaking women. Even when the nurse has limited ability to communicate orally with the woman, in most instances the nurse's efforts to communicate are meaningful and appreciated by the woman. Speaking slowly and avoiding complex words and medical terms can help a woman and her partner to understand.

Physical Examination

The initial physical examination includes a general systems assessment; performance of Leopold's maneuvers to determine fetal presentation, position, and point of maximal intensity (PMI) for auscultating the FHR; assessment of fetal status; assessment of uterine contractions; and vaginal examination to assess cervical effacement and dilation, fetal descent, and amniotic membranes and fluid. The findings of the admission physical examination serve as a baseline for assessing the woman's progress from that point.

It is important to obtain as many related pieces of information as possible before planning and implementing care. Women often focus on the nature of their contractions as the clearest indicator of how far advanced their labor is. However, the findings from the vaginal examination are more valid indicators of the phase of labor, especially for nulliparous women.

Expected maternal progress and minimum assessment guidelines during the first stage of labor are presented in Table 18-2. Standard Precautions should be used for all assessment and care measures (Box 18-3). Hand hygiene (e.g., washing hands with soap or application of an alcohol-based antibacterial solution) before and after assessing the woman and providing care is a critical step in the prevention of infection transmission. The assessment findings are explained to the woman whenever possible. Throughout labor accurate documentation, following agency policy, is done as soon as possible after a procedure has been performed (Fig. 18-3).

General Systems Assessment

A brief systems assessment is performed. This includes assessment of the heart, lungs, and skin; an examination to determine the presence and extent of edema of the legs, face, hands, and sacrum; and testing of deep tendon reflexes and for clonus.

Vital Signs

Vital signs (temperature, pulse, respirations, and blood pressure) are assessed on admission, and initial values are used for comparison with subsequent values. If blood pressure is elevated, it should be reassessed 30 minutes later, between

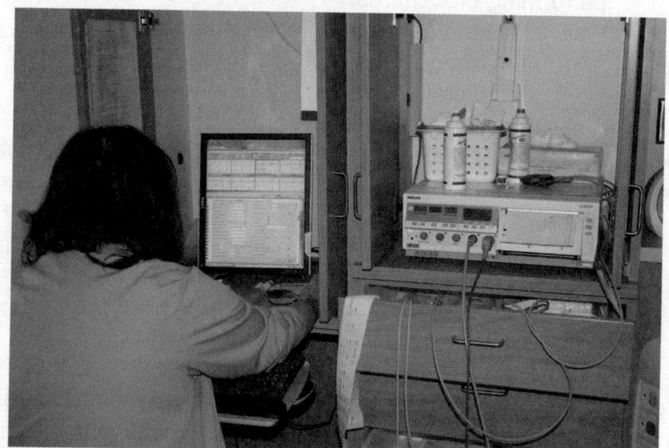

Fig. 18-3 Nurse documenting assessment findings on computer in a labor, delivery, recovery, postpartum room. *(Courtesy Shannon Perry, Phoenix, AZ.)*

Table 18-2 Expected Maternal Progress During First Stage of Labor

	Phases Marked by Cervical Dilation*		
CRITERION	0-3 cm (LATENT)	4-7 cm (ACTIVE)	8-10 cm (TRANSITION)
Duration†	About 6-8 hr	About 3-6 hr	About 20-40 min
Contractions			
Strength	Mild to moderate	Moderate to strong	Strong to very strong
Rhythm	Irregular	More regular	Regular
Frequency	5-30 min apart	3-5 min apart	2-3 min apart
Duration	30-45 sec	40-70 sec	45-90 sec
Descent			
Station of presenting part	Nulliparous: 0 Multiparous: 0 to −2 cm	Varies: +1 to +2 cm Varies: +1 to +2 cm	Varies: +2 to +3 cm Varies: +2 to +3 cm
Show			
Color	Brownish discharge, mucous plug, or pale pink mucus	Pink-to-bloody mucus	Bloody mucus
Amount	Scant	Scant to moderate	Copious
Behavior and appearance‡	Excited; thoughts center on self, labor, and baby; may be talkative or silent, calm or tense; some apprehension; pain controlled fairly well; alert, follows directions readily; open to instructions	Becomes more serious, doubtful of pain control, more apprehensive; desires companionship and encouragement; attention more inner directed; fatigue evidenced; malar (cheeks) flush; has some difficulty following directions	Pain described as severe; backache common; frustration, fear of loss of control, and irritability surface; vague in communications; amnesia between contractions; writhing with contractions; nausea and vomiting, especially if hyperventilating; hyperesthesia; circumoral pallor, perspiration of forehead and upper lips; shaking tremor of thighs; feeling of need to defecate, pressure on anus

*In the nullipara effacement is often complete before dilation begins; in the multipara it occurs simultaneous with dilation.
†Duration of each phase is influenced by such factors as parity, maternal emotions, position, level of activity, fetal size, and presentation position. For example, the labor of a nullipara tends to last longer, on average, than the labor of a multipara. Women who ambulate and assume upright positions or change positions frequently during labor tend to experience a shorter first stage. Descent is often prolonged in breech presentations and occiput posterior positions.
‡Women who have epidural analgesia for pain relief may not demonstrate some of these behaviors.

BOX 18-3 Standard Precautions During Childbirth

Birth is a time when nurses and other health care providers are exposed to a great deal of maternal and newborn blood and body fluids. Observation of Standard Precautions is necessary to prevent the transmission of infection. Perinatal infections most often are transmitted through contact with body fluids. The Standard Precautions applicable to childbirth include the following:

- Wash hands before and after putting on gloves and performing procedures.
- Wear gloves (clean or sterile, as appropriate) when performing procedures that require contact with the woman's genitalia and body fluids, including bloody show (e.g., during vaginal examination, amniotomy, hygienic care of the perineum, insertion of an internal scalp electrode and intrauterine pressure monitor, and catheterization).
- Wear cap, a mask that has a shield or protective eyewear, and shoe covers and cover gown during the birth. Gowns worn by the primary health care provider who is attending the birth should have a waterproof front and sleeves and should be sterile.
- Drape the woman with sterile towels and sheets as appropriate. Explain to the woman what can and cannot be touched.
- Help the woman's partner put on appropriate coverings for the birth such as cap, mask, gown, and shoe covers. Show the partner where to stand and what can and cannot be touched.
- Wear gloves and gown when handling the newborn immediately after birth.
- Use an appropriate method to suction the newborn's airway such as a bulb syringe, mechanical wall suction, or DeLee oral suction device that prevents the newborn's mucus from getting into the user's airway.

contractions, using a correct-size blood pressure cuff to obtain a reading after the woman has relaxed. To prevent supine hypotension and fetal distress, the woman should be encouraged to lie on her side and not supine (Fig. 18-4). Her temperature is monitored so that signs of infection or fluid deficit (e.g., dehydration associated with inadequate intake of fluids) can be identified. The woman's intake and output should be measured at least every 8 hours. When indicated, urinary protein and ketone levels may be determined by using a dipstick.

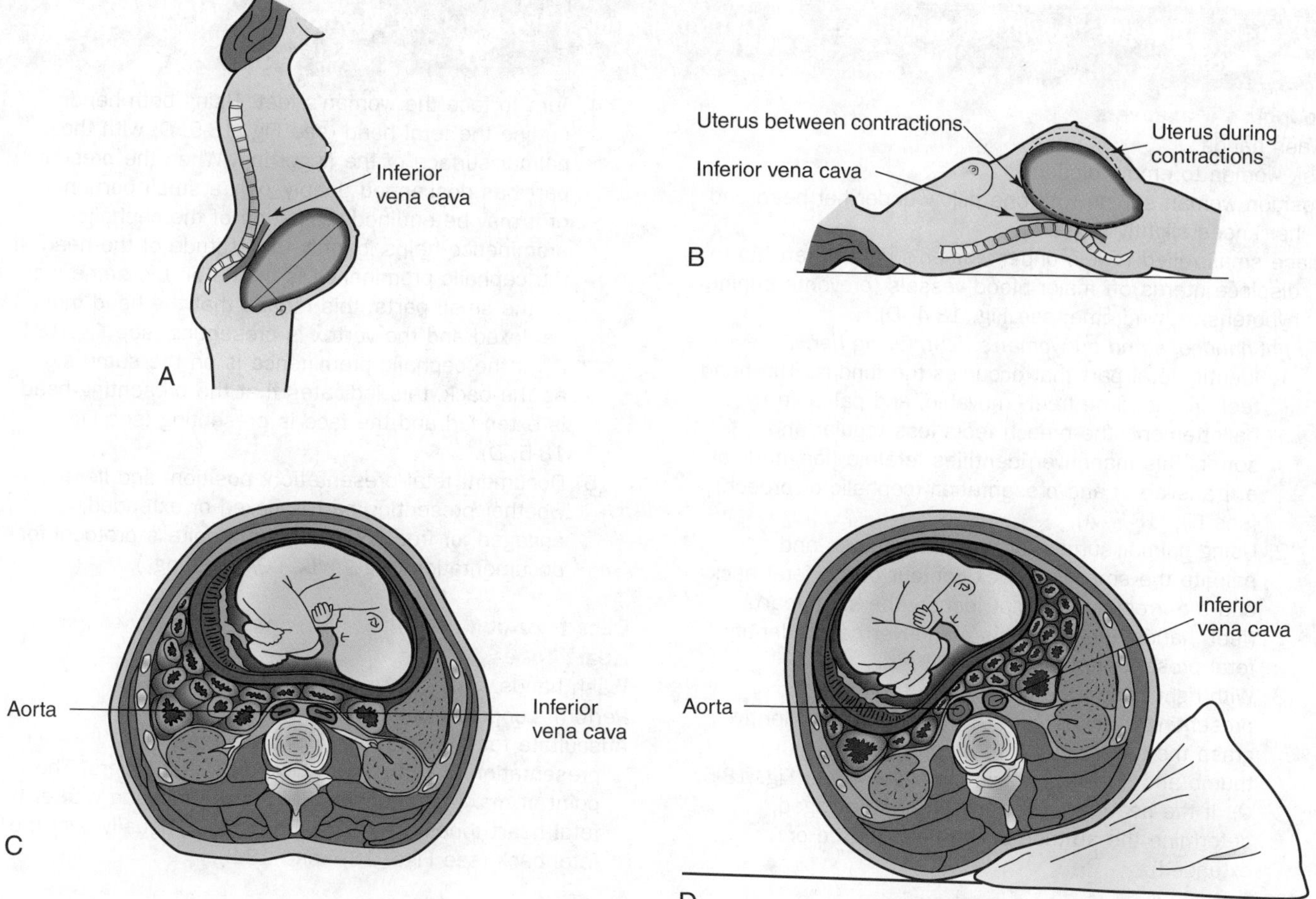

Fig. 18-4 Supine hypotension. Note relationship of gravid uterus to ascending vena cava in standing posture (**A**) and supine posture (**B**). **C**, Compression of aorta and inferior vena cava with woman in supine position. **D**, Relieved by use of a wedge pillow placed under woman's right side.

NURSING ALERT During labor blood pressure should be assessed with a sphygmomanometer and stethoscope for the most accurate results. Automatic devices that measure blood pressure have been found to overestimate the systolic pressure and underestimate the diastolic pressure. These devices further restrict freedom of movement and can also increase the discomfort of the woman as the cuff inflates and deflates on a regular basis. Maternal heart rate should be assessed by auscultation (i.e., apical rate) or palpation (i.e., radial pulse rate) rather than with a pulse oximeter (Simpson, 2005).

Leopold's Maneuvers (Abdominal Palpation)

Leopold's maneuvers are performed with the woman briefly lying on her back (Box 18-4 and Fig. 18-5). These maneuvers help to identify the following: (1) number of fetuses; (2) presenting part, fetal lie, and fetal attitude; (3) degree of descent of the presenting part into the pelvis; and (4) expected location of the PMI of the FHR on the woman's abdomen.

Assessment of Fetal Heart Rate and Pattern

It is important for the nurse to understand the relationship between the location of the PMI of the FHR and fetal presentation, lie, and position. A risk for childbirth complications may be revealed by variations in these findings. The PMI of the FHR is the location on the maternal abdomen where the FHR is heard the loudest. It is usually directly over the fetal back. The PMI is also an aid in determining the fetal presentation and position (Fig. 18-6). In a vertex presentation FHR is heard below the mother's umbilicus in either the right or left lower quadrant of the abdomen. In a breech presentation the FHR is heard above the mother's umbilicus (see Fig. 18-6, *A*, and Fig. 18-7, *C*). As the fetus descends and rotates internally, the FHR is heard lower and closer to the midline of the maternal abdomen. The PMI of the fetus in the right occipitoanterior position moves to the midline just over the symphysis pubis (see Fig. 18-7, *A* and *B*). Just before birth the fetal position is occipitoanterior, and the fetal back is directly above the symphysis pubis.

The FHR and pattern must also be assessed (1) immediately after ROM because this is the most common time for the umbilical cord to prolapse, (2) after any change in the contraction pattern or maternal status, and (3) before and after medicating the woman or performing a procedure.

Assessment of Uterine Contractions

A general characteristic of effective labor is regular uterine activity (i.e., contractions becoming more frequent and of increased duration); however, uterine activity is not directly related to labor progress. Uterine contractions are the primary powers that act involuntarily to expel the fetus and placenta

BOX 18-4 Procedure: Leopold's Maneuvers and Determination of the Points of Maximal Intensity of the Fetal Heart Rate

Leopold's Maneuvers

Wash hands.

Ask woman to empty bladder.

Position woman supine with one pillow under her head and her knees slightly flexed.

Place small rolled towels under woman's right or left hip to displace uterus off major blood vessels (prevents supine hypotensive syndrome; see Fig. 18-4, *D*).

If right-handed, stand on woman's right, facing her:

1. Identify fetal part that occupies the fundus. The head feels round, firm, freely movable, and palpable by ballottement; the breech feels less regular and softer. This maneuver identifies fetal lie (longitudinal or transverse) and presentation (cephalic or breech) (see Fig. 18-5, *A*).
2. Using palmar surface of one hand, locate and palpate the smooth convex contour of the fetal back and the irregularities that identify the small parts (feet, hands, elbows). This maneuver helps identify fetal presentation (see Fig. 18-5, *B*).
3. With right hand determine which fetal part is presenting over the inlet to the true pelvis. Gently grasp the lower pole of the uterus between the thumb and fingers, pressing in slightly (see Fig. 18-5, *C*). If the head is presenting and not engaged, determine the attitude of the head (flexed or extended).
4. Turn to face the woman's feet. Using both hands, outline the fetal head (see Fig. 18-5, *D*) with the palmar surface of the fingertips. When the presenting part has descended deeply, only a small portion of it may be outlined. Palpation of the cephalic prominence helps identify the attitude of the head. If the cephalic prominence is bound on the same side as the small parts, this means that the head must be flexed and the vertex is presenting (see Fig. 18-5, *D*). If the cephalic prominence is on the same side as the back, this indicates that the presenting head is extended and the face is presenting (see Fig. 18-5, *D*).
5. Document fetal presentation, position, and lie and whether presenting part is flexed or extended, engaged, or free floating. Use hospital's protocol for documentation (e.g., "Vtx, LOA, floating").

Determination of Point of Maximal Intensity of Fetal Heart Tones

Wash hands.

Perform Leopold's maneuvers.

Auscultate fetal heart rate (FHR) based on fetal presentation identified with Leopold's maneuvers. The point of maximal intensity (PMI) is the location where the fetal heart tones are heard the loudest, usually over the fetal back (see Figs. 18-7 and 18-8).

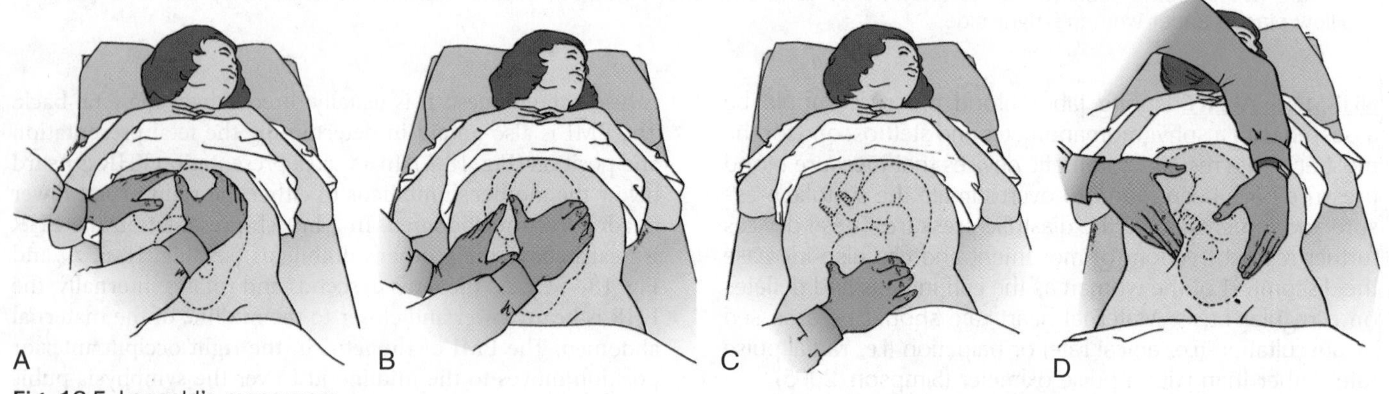

Fig. 18-5 Leopold's maneuvers.

evolve Assessment Video—Leopold's Maneuvers

from the uterus. Several methods are used to evaluate uterine contractions. These include the woman's subjective description, palpation and timing of the contraction by a health care provider, and internal electronic monitoring.

Each contraction exhibits a wavelike pattern. It begins with a slow increment (the "building up" of a contraction from its onset) gradually reaches an acme (the peak, with intrauterine pressure less than 80 mm Hg), and then diminishes rapidly (decrement, the "letting down" of the contraction). An interval of rest (intrauterine pressure less than 20 mm Hg) ends when the next contraction begins. The outward appearance of the woman's abdomen during and between contractions and the pattern of a typical uterine contraction are shown in Fig. 18-8.

The following characteristics are used to describe a uterine contraction:

Frequency—How often uterine contractions occur; the time that elapses from the beginning of one contraction to the beginning of the next

Intensity—The strength of a contraction at its peak

Duration—The time that elapses between the onset and the end of a contraction

Resting tone—The tension in the uterine muscle between contractions

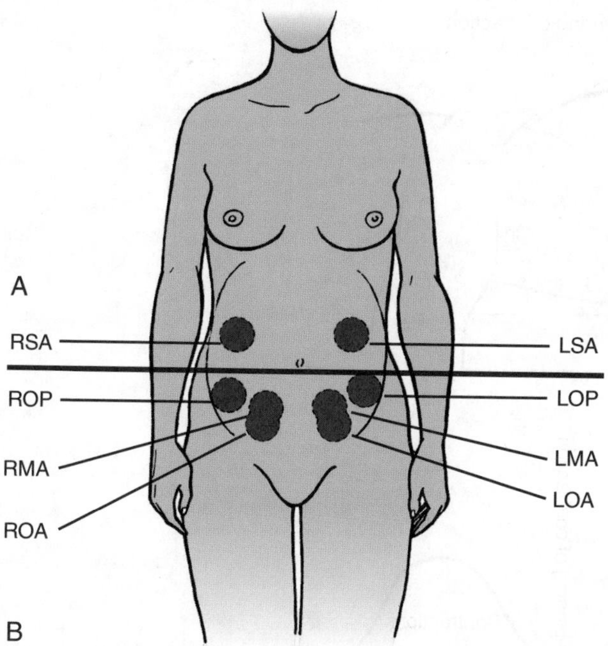

Fig. 18-6 Areas of maximal intensity of fetal heart rate for differing positions. *RSA*, Right sacrum anterior; *ROP*, right occipitoposterior; *RMA*, right mentum anterior; *ROA*, right occipitoanterior; *LSA*, left sacrum anterior; *LOP*, left occipitoposterior; *LMA*, left mentum anterior; and *LOA*, left occipitoanterior. **A**, Presentation is *breech* if fetal heart tones (FHTs) are heard *above* umbilicus. **B**, Presentation is *vertex* if FHTs are heard *below* umbilicus.

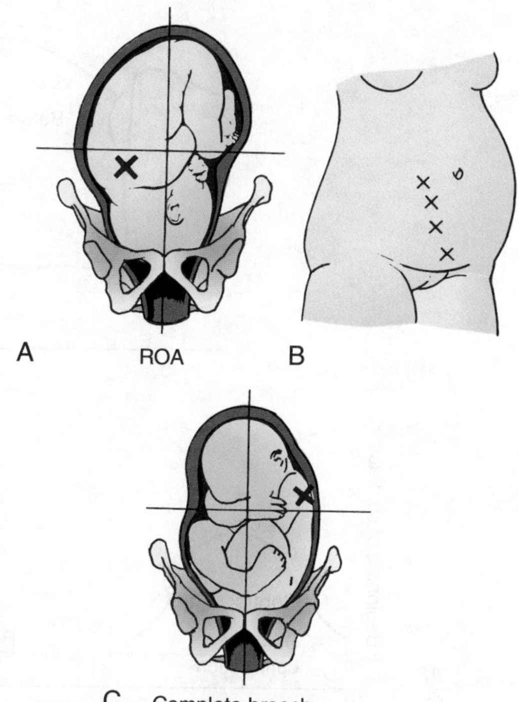

Fig. 18-7 Location of the fetal heart rate. **A**, With fetus in right occipitoanterior *(ROA)* position. **B**, Changes in location of point of maximal intensity of fetal heart tones as fetus undergoes internal rotation from ROA to OA for birth. **C**, With fetus in left sacrum posterior position. *(A and C, Courtesy Ross Laboratories, Columbus, OH.)*

Uterine contractions are assessed by palpation or by an external or internal electronic monitor. Frequency and duration can be measured by all three methods of uterine activity monitoring. The accuracy of determining intensity varies by the method used. Palpation is subjective and is a less precise way of determining the intensity of uterine contractions. The following terms are used to describe what is felt on palpation:

Mild—Slightly tense fundus that is easy to indent with fingertips (feels like touching finger to tip of nose)

Moderate—Firm fundus that is difficult to indent with fingertips (feels like touching finger to chin)

Strong—Rigid, boardlike fundus that is almost impossible to indent with fingertips (feels like touching finger to forehead)

Women in labor tend to describe the pain of contractions in terms of their sensations in the lower abdomen or the back, which may be unrelated to the firmness of the uterine fundus. Thus their assessment of the strength of their contractions can be less valid than that of an experienced health care provider, although the amount of discomfort reported is valid.

External electronic monitoring is not a valid measure of the intensity of uterine contractions. Internal electronic monitoring with an intrauterine pressure catheter is the most valid way of assessing the intensity of uterine contractions.

On admission a 20- to 30-minute baseline monitoring of uterine contractions and the FHR and pattern is usually done. The findings expected as labor progresses are summarized in Tables 18-2 and 18-6.

The nurse's responsibility in monitoring uterine contractions is to ascertain whether they are powerful and frequent enough to accomplish the work of expelling the fetus and the placenta.

NURSING ALERT If the characteristics of contractions are found to be abnormal, either exceeding or falling below what is considered acceptable in terms of the standard characteristics, the nurse should report this finding to the primary health care provider.

Cervical Effacement, Dilation, Fetal Descent Uterine activity must be considered in the context of its effect on cervical effacement and dilation and the degree of descent of the presenting part. The effect on the fetus must also be considered.

NURSING ALERT It is important for the nurse to recognize that active labor can last longer than the expected labor patterns. This finding should not be a cause for concern unless the maternal-fetal unit exhibits signs of distress (e.g., abnormal FHR and patterns, maternal fever).

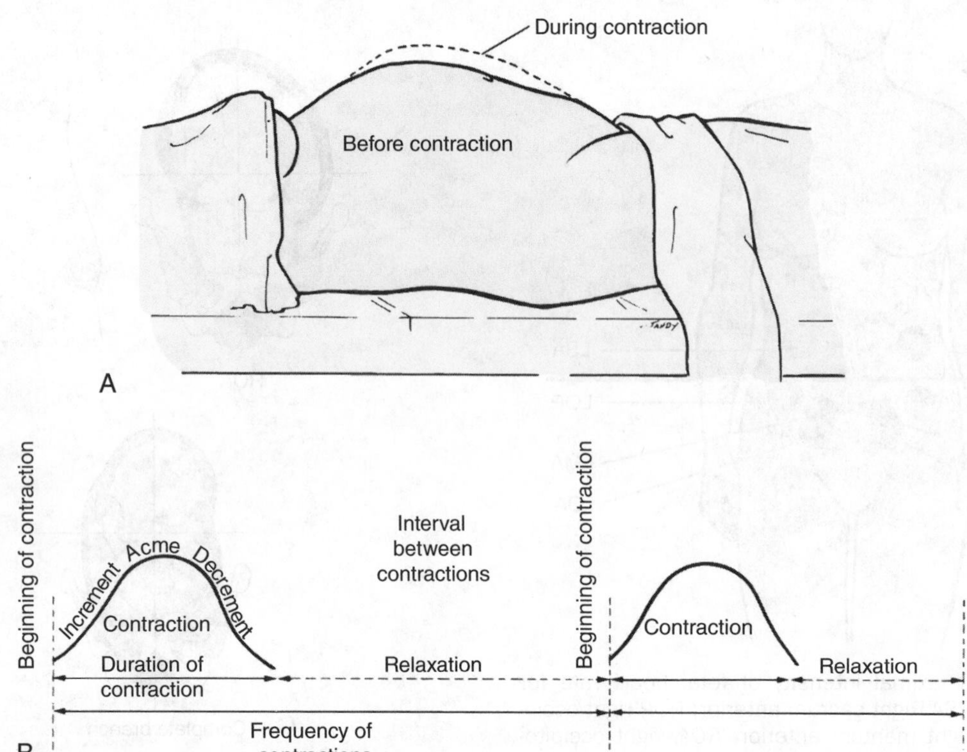

Fig. 18-8 Assessment of uterine contractions. **A**, Abdominal contour before and during uterine contractions. **B**, Wavelike pattern of contractile activity.

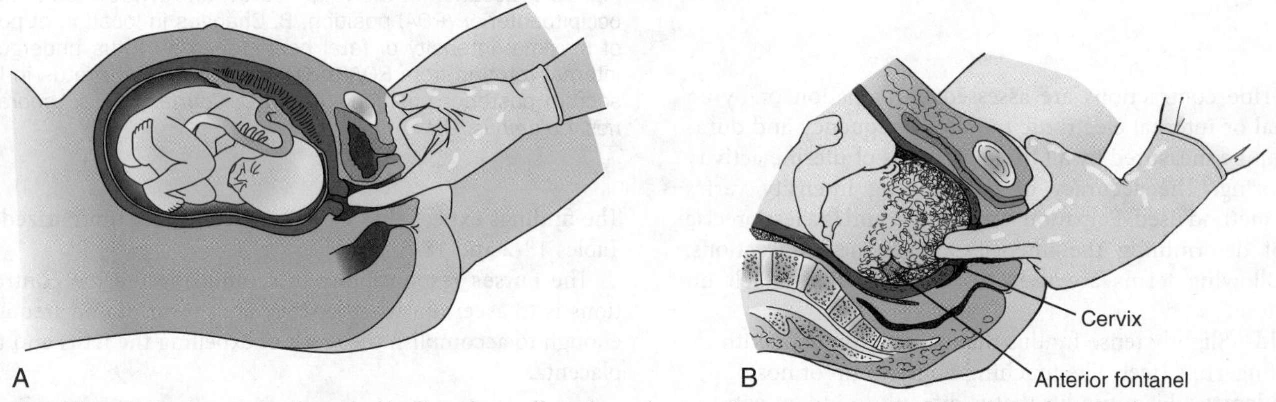

Fig. 18-9 Vaginal examination. **A**, Undilated, uneffaced cervix; membranes intact. **B**, Palpation of sagittal suture line. Cervix effaced and partially dilated.

Vaginal Examination

The vaginal examination reveals whether the woman is in true labor and enables the examiner to determine whether the membranes have ruptured (Fig. 18-9). Because this examination is often stressful and uncomfortable for the woman, it should be performed only when indicated by the status of the woman and her fetus. For example, a vaginal examination should be performed on admission, when significant change has occurred in uterine activity, on maternal perception of perineal pressure or the urge to bear down, when membranes rupture, or when variable decelerations of the FHR are noted. A full explanation of the examination and support of the woman are important factors in reducing the stress and discomfort associated with the examination.

Laboratory and Diagnostic Tests

Analysis of Urine Specimen

A clean-catch urine specimen may be obtained to gather more data about the pregnant woman's health. It is a convenient and simple procedure that can provide information about her hydration status (e.g., by specific gravity, color, and amount), nutritional status (e.g., ketones), infection (e.g., leukocytes), or the status of possible complications such as preeclampsia (shown by finding protein in the urine). The results can be obtained quickly and help the nurse to determine appropriate interventions to implement.

Blood Tests

Blood tests performed vary with hospital protocol and the woman's health status. An example of minimal assessment is a hematocrit determination, in which the specimen is centrifuged on the perinatal unit. Blood can be obtained by a finger stick or from the hub of a catheter used to start an IV line. More comprehensive assessments such as white blood cell count, red blood cell count, hemoglobin level, hematocrit, and platelet values are included in the CBC. A CBC may be ordered for women with a history of infection, anemia, gestational hypertension, or other disorders.

If the woman's blood type has not been verified, blood is drawn to determine the type and Rh factor. If blood typing has already been done, the primary health care provider may choose not to repeat the test. If obvious signs of immunocompromise or substance abuse are present, other blood tests may be ordered.

Assessment of Amniotic Membranes and Fluid

Labor is initiated at term by SROM in approximately 25% of pregnant women. A lag period, rarely exceeding 24 hours, may precede the onset of labor. Membranes (the bag of waters) can also rupture spontaneously at any time during labor but most commonly in the transition phase of the first stage of labor.

NURSING ALERT The umbilical cord may prolapse when the membranes rupture. The FHR and pattern should be monitored closely for several minutes immediately after ROM to ascertain fetal well-being, and the findings should be documented.

Artificial ROM or amniotomy may be done to augment or induce labor or facilitate placement of internal monitors when fetal status indicates the need for some form of direct assessment method (e.g., insertion of a fetal scalp electrode to the presenting part or an intrauterine pressure catheter). (For the tests used to assess ROM, see Box 18-2.) Assessment of amniotic fluid characteristics is described in Table 18-3.

Infection After membranes rupture, microorganisms from the vagina can ascend into the amniotic sac, causing chorioamnionitis and placentitis to develop. For this reason maternal temperature and vaginal discharge are assessed frequently (every 1 to 2 hours) so that an infection developing after ROM can be identified early. However, even when membranes are intact, microorganisms may ascend and cause premature ROM. Controversy exists regarding whether prophylactic antibiotic therapy can protect against infection (chorioamnionitis), which involves both the maternal and fetal sides of the membrane. The effectiveness of prophylactic antibiotics for prelabor ROM at term or preterm is unknown (Enkin et al, 2000).

The nurse's responsibility is to report findings promptly to the primary health care provider and document them in the labor record and on the monitor strip (if that is agency policy). If abnormal findings are noted, continuous electronic monitoring is usually initiated and maintained for the duration of labor. The presence of meconium-stained amniotic fluid alerts the nurse of the need to observe fetal status more closely. After birth the newborn may be at high risk for alteration in respiratory status if meconium is aspirated into the lungs with the first breath.

Assessment findings serve as a baseline for evaluating the woman's progress during labor. Although some problems of labor are anticipated, others may appear unexpectedly during the clinical course of labor (Box 18-5).

Plan of Care and Implementation

Standards of Care

Standards of care guide the nurse in preparing for and implementing procedures with the expectant mother. Protocols for care based on standards include the following tasks:

1. Check the primary health care provider's orders.
2. Assess the orders for appropriateness and correctness (e.g., the dosage and route of administration of the analgesic to be administered to relieve discomfort).

Table 18-3 Assessment of Amniotic Fluid

CHARACTERISTIC OF FLUID	NORMAL FINDING	DEVIATION FROM NORMAL FINDING	CAUSE OF DEVIATION FROM NORMAL
Color	Pale, straw colored; may contain white flecks of vernix caseosa, lanugo, scalp hair	Greenish-brown color	Hypoxic episode in fetus; meconium in fluid
		Yellow-stained fluid	May be normal finding in breech presentation as pressure is exerted on fetal abdominal wall during descent Fetal hypoxia ≥36 hr before ROM; fetal hemolytic disease; intrauterine infection
		Port wine–colored	Bleeding associated with abruptio placentae
Viscosity and odor	Watery; no strong odor	Thick, cloudy, foul-smelling	Intrauterine infection Large amount of meconium can make fluid thick
Amount (normally varies with gestational age)	400 ml (20 weeks of gestation) 1000 ml (36 to 38 weeks of gestation)	≥2000 ml (32 to 36 weeks of gestation)	Hydramnios; associated with congenital anomalies of the fetus when fetus cannot drink or fluid is trapped in the body (e.g., fetal gastrointestinal obstruction or atresias); increased risk with maternal pregestational or gestational diabetes mellitus
		≤500 ml (32 to 36 weeks of gestation)	Oligohydramnios; associated with incomplete or absent kidney; obstruction of urethra; infant cannot secrete or excrete urine

ROM, Rupture of membranes.

BOX 18-5 Signs of Potential Labor Complications

- Intrauterine pressure of more than 75 mm Hg (determined by intrauterine pressure catheter monitoring) or resting tone of more than 15 mm Hg
- Contractions consistently lasting 90 seconds or more
- Contractions consistently occurring 2 minutes or less apart
- Fetal bradycardia, tachycardia, or persistently decreased variability
- Irregular fetal heart rate; suspected fetal dysrhythmias
- Appearance of meconium-stained or bloody fluid from the vagina
- Arrest in progress of cervical dilation or effacement, descent of the fetus, or both
- Maternal temperature of 38° C or more
- Foul-smelling vaginal discharge
- Persistent bright-red or dark-red vaginal bleeding

3. Check labels on IV solutions, medications, and other materials used for nursing care.
4. Check the expiration date on any packs of supplies used for procedures.
5. Ensure that information on the woman's identification band is accurate (e.g., that the band is the appropriate color for allergies).
6. Use an empathic approach when giving care:
   - Establish rapport with the woman and her significant others.
   - Respect the woman's individual needs and behaviors.
   - Be kind, caring, and competent when performing necessary procedures.
   - When explaining procedures, use words the woman can understand; repeat as necessary.
   - Be aware that pain and discomfort are as the woman describes them.
   - Carry out appropriate comfort measures such as mouth and back care.
   - Include the support people in the care as desired by the woman and the support people.
   - Recognize that a woman's current childbirth experience and the actions of nurses and other health care providers can have a positive or negative effect on her future childbirth experiences.
7. Use Standard Precautions, including precautions for invasive procedures as needed (see Box 18-3).
8. Document care according to hospital guidelines and communicate information to the primary health care provider when indicated.

evolve Spanish Guidelines–Care During Labor

Physical Nursing Care During Labor

Physical nursing care of the woman in labor is an essential component of her care. The current emphasis on evidence-based practice supports the management of care by using this approach to enhance the safety, effectiveness, and acceptability of the physical care measures chosen to support the woman during labor and birth (Enkin et al, 2000). The various physical needs, the requisite nursing actions, and the rationale for care are presented in Table 18-4 and the Nursing Care Plan.

General Hygiene

Women in labor should be offered the use of showers or warm water baths, if they are available, to enhance the feeling of well-being and minimize the discomfort of contractions. Women should also be encouraged to wash their hands after voiding and to perform self-hygiene measures. Linen should be changed if it becomes wet or stained with blood, and linen savers (Chux) should be used and changed as needed.

Nutrient and Fluid Intake

Oral Intake Traditionally the laboring woman has been offered only clear liquids or ice chips or given nothing by mouth during the active phase of labor. This was to minimize the risk of anesthesia complications and their sequelae should general anesthesia be required in an emergency. These sequelae include aspiration of gastric contents and resultant compromise in oxygen perfusion, which may endanger the lives of the mother and fetus. This practice is being challenged today because regional anesthesia is used more often than general anesthesia, even for emergency cesarean births. Women are awake during regional anesthesia and are able to participate in their own care and protect their airway.

Although gastric emptying is slowed as a result of labor, stress, and the use of narcotics or sedatives, fasting does not cause gastric contents to be eliminated and may even cause them to be more acidic. In addition, fasting is identified by many laboring women as a stressor with which they must cope and a source of frustration during labor related to a loss of control with regard to meeting their own nourishment needs.

Adequate intake of fluids and calories is required to meet the energy demands and fluid losses associated with childbirth. The progress of labor slows, and ketosis develops if these demands are not met and fat is metabolized. Reduced energy for bearing-down efforts (pushing) increases the risk for a forceps- or vacuum-assisted birth. This is most likely to occur in women who begin to labor early in the morning after a night without caloric intake. Common practice is to allow clear liquids (e.g., water, tea, apple juice, clear sodas, gelatin, broth) during early labor, tapering off to ice chips and sips of water as labor progresses and becomes more active. However, when women are permitted to consume fluids and food freely, they typically regulate their own oral intake, eating light foods (e.g., eggs, yogurt, ice cream, dry toast and jelly, fruit) and drinking fluids during early labor and then tapering off to an intake of clear fluid and sips of water or ice chips as labor intensifies and the second stage approaches. Food and fluid consumed orally during labor can meet a laboring woman's hydration and energy demands and relieve stress (American College of Nurse-Midwives, 2008). Women who use nonpharmacologic pain-relief measures and labor at home or in birthing centers are more likely to eat and drink during labor. In addition, the woman's sense of control and level of comfort are enhanced.

Withholding food and drink from women in labor has been identified as a form of care unlikely to be beneficial; offering oral fluids is demonstrably useful and should be encouraged (Enkin et al, 2000; Hofmeyr, 2005). Nurses should follow the orders of the woman's primary health care provider when offering the woman food or fluids during labor. However,

Table 18-4 Physical Nursing Care During Labor

NEED	NURSING ACTIONS	RATIONALE
General Hygiene		
Showers/bed baths, Jacuzzi bath	Assess for progress in labor Supervise showers closely if woman is in true labor Suggest allowing warm water to flow over back	Determines appropriateness of activity Prevents injury from fall; labor may be accelerated Aids relaxation; increases comfort
Perineum	Cleanse frequently, especially after rupture of membranes and when show increases	Enhances comfort and reduces risk of infection
Oral hygiene	Offer toothbrush or mouthwash or wash the teeth with an ice-cold, wet washcloth as needed	Refreshes mouth; helps counteract dry, thirsty feeling
Hair	Brush, braid per woman's wishes	Improves morale; increases comfort
Handwashing	Offer washcloths before and after voiding and as needed	Maintains cleanliness; prevents infection
Face	Offer cool washcloth	Provides relief from diaphoresis; cools and refreshes
Gowns/linens	Change prn; fluff pillows	Improves comfort; enhances relaxation
Nutrient and Fluid Intake		
Oral	Offer fluids and solid foods, following orders of primary health care provider and desires of laboring woman	Provides hydration and calories; enhances positive emotional experience and maternal control
Intravenous (IV)	Establish and maintain IV as ordered	Maintains hydration; provides venous access for medications
Elimination		
Voiding	Encourage voiding at least every 2 hr	A full bladder may impede descent of presenting part; overdistention may cause bladder atony and injury and postpartum voiding difficulty
Ambulatory woman	Allow ambulation to bathroom according to orders of primary health care provider, if: The presenting part is engaged The membranes are not ruptured The woman is not medicated	 Reinforces normal process of urination Precautionary measure to protect against prolapse of umbilical cord Precautionary measure to protect against injury
Woman on bed rest	Offer bedpan Allow tap water to run; pour warm water over vulva; give positive suggestion Provide privacy Put up side rails on bed Place call bell within reach Offer washcloth for hands Wash vulvar area	Prevents complications of bladder distention and ambulation Encourages voiding Shows respect for woman Prevents injury from fall Maintains cleanliness; prevents infection Maintains cleanliness; enhances comfort; prevents infection
Catheterization	Catheterize according to orders of primary health care provider or hospital protocol if measures to facilitate voiding are ineffective Insert catheter between contractions Avoid force if obstacle to insertion is noted	Prevents complications of bladder distention Minimizes discomfort "Obstacle" may be caused by compression of urethra by presenting part
Bowel elimination—sensation of rectal pressure	Help woman ambulate to bathroom or offer bedpan after careful assessment Perform vaginal examination Cleanse perineum immediately after passage of stool	Prevents misinterpretation of rectal pressure from the presenting part as need to defecate Determines degree of descent of presenting part Reduces risk of infection and sense of embarrassment

as advocates nurses can facilitate change by informing others of the current research findings that support the safety and effectiveness of the oral intake of food and fluid during labor and by initiating such research themselves.

Intravenous Intake Fluids are administered intravenously to the laboring woman to maintain hydration, especially when labor is long and the woman is unable to ingest a sufficient amount of fluid orally or if she is receiving epidural or intrathecal analgesia. However, routine use of IV fluids during labor is a form of care that is unlikely to be beneficial and may be harmful (Enkin et al, 2000). In most cases an electrolyte solution without glucose is adequate and does not introduce excess glucose into the bloodstream, which results in fetal hyperglycemia and fetal hyperinsulinism. After birth the neonate's high level of insulin will then deplete his or her glucose stores, and hypoglycemia will result. If maternal ketosis occurs, the primary health care provider may order an IV solution containing a small amount of dextrose to provide the glucose needed to assist in fatty acid metabolism.

NURSING ALERT Nurses should carefully monitor the intake and output of laboring women receiving IV fluids because

NURSING CARE PLAN Labor and Birth

Nursing Diagnosis: Anxiety related to labor and the birthing process

Expected Outcome

Woman exhibits decreased signs of anxiety.

Nursing Interventions/*Rationales*

Orient woman and significant others to labor and birth unit and explain admission protocol *to allay initial feelings of anxiety.*

Assess woman's knowledge, experience, and expectations of labor; note any signs or expressions of anxiety, nervousness, or fear *to establish a baseline for intervention.*

Discuss the expected progression of labor and describe what to expect during the process *to allay anxiety associated with the unknown.*

Actively involve woman in care decisions during labor, interpret sights and sounds of environment (monitor sights and sounds, unit activities), and share information on progression of labor (vital signs, fetal heart rate, dilation, effacement) *to increase her sense of control and allay fears.*

Nursing Diagnosis: Acute pain related to increasing frequency and intensity of contractions

Expected Outcome

Woman exhibits signs of ability to cope with discomfort.

Nursing Interventions/*Rationales*

Assess woman's level of pain and strategies that she has used to cope with pain *to establish a baseline for intervention.*

Encourage significant other to remain as support person during labor process *to assist with support and comfort measures because measures are often more effective when delivered by a familiar person.*

Instruct woman and support person in use of specific techniques such as conscious relaxation, focused breathing, effleurage, massage, and application of sacral pressure *to increase relaxation, decrease intensity of contractions, and promote use of controlled thought and direction of energy.*

Provide comfort measures such as frequent mouth care *to prevent dry mouth;* application of damp cloth to forehead and changing of damp gown or bed covers *to relieve discomfort associated with diaphoresis;* and position changes *to reduce stiffness.*

Explain which analgesics and anesthetics are available for use during labor and birth *to provide knowledge to help woman make decisions about pain control.*

Nursing Diagnosis: Risk for impaired urinary elimination related to sensory impairment secondary to labor

Expected Outcome

Bladder does not show signs of distention.

Nursing Interventions/*Rationales*

Palpate the bladder superior to the symphysis on a frequent basis *to detect a full bladder that occurs from increased fluid intake and inability to feel urge to void.*

Encourage frequent voiding (at least every 2 hours) and catheterize if necessary to avoid bladder distention *because it impedes progress of fetus down birth canal and may result in trauma to the bladder.*

Assist to bathroom or commode to void if appropriate and provide privacy *to facilitate bladder emptying with an upright position (natural) and relaxation.*

Nursing Diagnosis: Risk for ineffective individual coping related to birthing process

Expected Outcome

Woman actively participates in the birth process with no evidence of injury to her or her fetus.

Nursing Interventions/*Rationales*

Constantly monitor events of second-stage labor and birth, including physiologic responses of woman and fetus and emotional responses of woman and partner *to ensure maternal, partner, and fetal well-being.*

Provide ongoing feedback to woman and partner *to allay anxiety and enhance participation.*

Continue to provide comfort measures and minimize distractions *to decrease discomfort and aid in focus on the birth process.*

Encourage woman to experiment with various positions *to assist downward movement of fetus.*

Ensure that woman takes deep cleansing breaths before and after each contraction *to enhance gas exchange and oxygen transport to the fetus.*

Encourage woman to push spontaneously when urge to bear down is perceived during a contraction *to aid descent and rotation of fetus.*

Encourage woman to exhale, holding breath for short periods while bearing down, *to avoid holding breath and triggering a Valsalva maneuver, increasing intrathoracic and cardiovascular pressure, and decreasing perfusion of placental oxygen, placing the fetus at risk.*

Have woman take deep breaths and relax between contractions *to reduce fatigue and increase effectiveness of pushing efforts.*

Have mother pant as fetal head crowns *to control birth of head.*

Explain to woman and labor partner what is expected in the third stage of labor *to enlist cooperation.*

Have woman maintain her position *to facilitate delivery of the placenta.*

Nursing Diagnosis: Fatigue related to energy expenditure required during labor and birth

Expected Outcome

Woman's energy levels are restored.

Nursing Interventions/*Rationales*

Educate woman and partner about need for rest and help them plan strategies (e.g., restricting visitors, increasing role of support systems in performing functions associated with daily routines) that allow specific times for rest and sleep *to ensure that woman can restore depleted energy levels in preparation for caring for a new infant.*

evolve Nursing Care Plan—Labor and Birth

NURSING CARE PLAN Labor and Birth—cont'd

Monitor woman's fatigue level and the amount of rest received *to ensure restoration of energy.*

Nursing Diagnosis: Risk for deficient fluid volume related to decreased fluid intake and increased fluid loss during labor and birth

Expected Outcomes

Fluid balance is maintained, and there are no signs of dehydration.

Nursing Interventions/*Rationales*

Monitor fluid loss (i.e., blood, urine, perspiration) and vital signs; inspect skin turgor and mucous membranes for dryness *to evaluate hydration status.*

Administer oral/parenteral fluid per physician/nurse-midwife orders *to maintain hydration.*

Monitor the fundus for firmness after placental separation *to ensure adequate contraction and prevent further blood loss.*

they also face an increased danger of hypervolemia as a result of the fluid retention that occurs during pregnancy.

Elimination

Voiding Voiding every 2 hours should be encouraged. A distended bladder may impede descent of the presenting part, inhibit uterine contractions, and lead to decreased bladder tone or atony after birth. Women who receive epidural analgesia or anesthesia are especially at risk for retention of urine, and the need to void should be assessed more frequently in them.

The woman should be assisted to the bathroom to void unless the primary health care provider has ordered bed rest, the woman is receiving epidural analgesia or anesthesia, or in the nurse's judgment ambulation would compromise the status of the laboring woman or her fetus. External monitoring can usually be interrupted for the woman to go to the bathroom.

Catheterization If the woman is unable to void and her bladder is distended, she may need to be catheterized. Most hospitals have protocols that rely on the nurse's judgment concerning the need for catheterization. Before performing the catheterization, the nurse should clean the vulva and perineum because vaginal show and amniotic fluid may be present. If there appears to be an obstacle that prevents advancement of the catheter, it is most likely the presenting part. If the catheter cannot be advanced, the nurse should stop the procedure and notify the primary health care provider of the difficulty.

Bowel Elimination Most women do not have bowel movements during labor because of decreased intestinal motility. Stool that has formed in the large intestine often is moved downward toward the anorectal area by the pressure exerted by the fetal presenting part as it descends. This stool is often expelled during second-stage pushing and birth. However, the passage of stool with bearing-down efforts increases the risk of infection and may embarrass the woman, thereby reducing the effectiveness of these efforts. To prevent these problems, the nurse should immediately cleanse the perineal area to remove any stool, while at the same time reassuring the woman that the passage of stool at this time is a normal and expected event because the same muscles used to expel the baby also expel stool. Routine use of an enema to empty the rectum is considered to be harmful or ineffective and should be eliminated (Enkin et al, 2000).

When the presenting part is deep in the pelvis, even in the absence of stool in the anorectal area, the woman may feel rectal pressure and think she needs to defecate. If the woman expresses the need to defecate, the nurse should perform a vaginal examination to assess cervical dilation and station. When a multiparous woman experiences the urge to defecate, this often means that birth will follow quickly.

Ambulation and Positioning

Freedom of maternal movement and choice of position through labor are forms of care likely to be beneficial for the laboring woman and should be encouraged (Enkin et al, 2000). The increased use of epidurals during childbirth accompanied by multiple medical interventions (e.g., monitors, IV infusions) and reduced motor control interfere with a woman's freedom of movement.

The potential advantages of ambulation include enhanced uterine activity, distraction from the discomfort of labor, enhanced maternal control, and an opportunity for close interaction with the woman's partner and care provider as they help her to walk. Ambulation is associated with a reduced rate of operative delivery (i.e., cesarean birth, forceps- and vacuum-assisted birth) and less frequent use of opioid analgesics.

Walking, sitting, or standing during early labor is more comfortable than lying down and facilitates the progress of labor. Ambulation should be encouraged if membranes are intact, if the fetal presenting part is engaged after ROM, and if the woman has not received medication for pain (Fig. 18-10). The woman may find it comfortable to stand and lean forward on her partner, doula, or nurse for support at times during labor (Fig. 18-11, *A*). At times, ambulation is contraindicated because of maternal or fetal status.

When the woman lies in bed she will usually change her position spontaneously as labor progresses. If she does not change position every 30 to 60 minutes, she should be assisted to do so. The side-lying (lateral) position promotes optimal uteroplacental and renal blood flow and increases oxygen saturation (see Fig. 18-11, *B*). If the woman wants to lie supine, the nurse may place a pillow under one hip as a wedge to prevent the uterus from compressing the aorta and vena cava. Sitting is not contraindicated unless it adversely affects fetal status, which can be determined by checking the FHR and pattern. If the fetus is in the occiput posterior position, it may be helpful to encourage the woman to squat during contractions because this position increases pelvic diameter, allowing

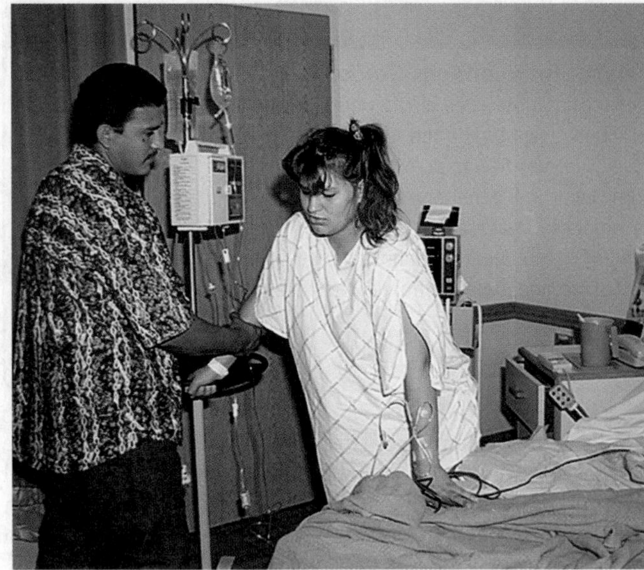

Fig. 18-10 Woman preparing to walk with partner. *(Courtesy Marjorie Pyle, RNC, Lifecircle, Costa Mesa, CA.)*

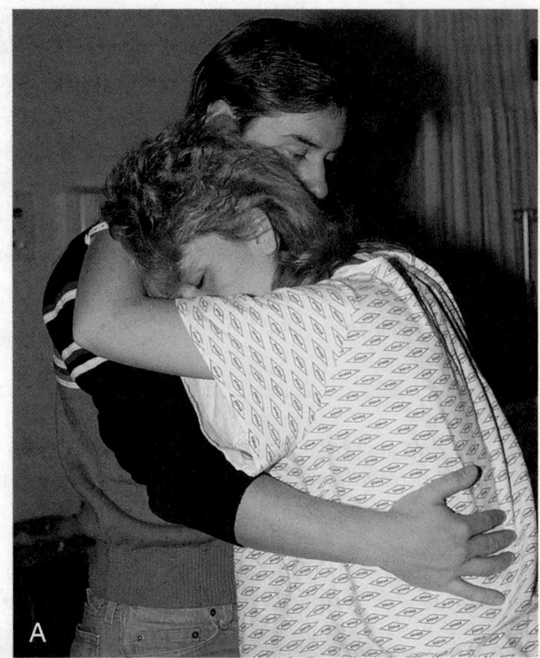

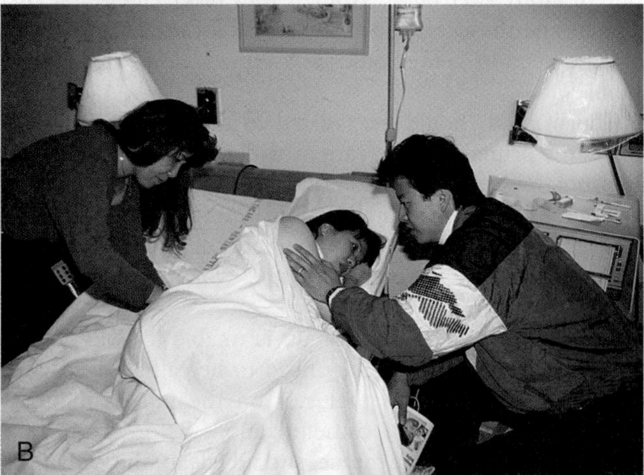

Fig. 18-11 A, Woman standing and leaning forward with support. B, Lateral position. Support person is applying sacral pressure while partner provides encouragement. *(Courtesy Marjorie Pyle, RNC, Lifecircle, Costa Mesa, CA.)*

the head to rotate to a more anterior position (Fig. 18-12, *A*). A hands-and-knees position during contractions is also recommended to facilitate the rotation of the fetal occiput from a posterior to an anterior position as gravity pulls the fetal back forward (see Fig. 18-12, *B*). A variety of positions recommended for the laboring woman are described in Box 18-6.

A birth ball (gymnastic ball, also used in physical therapy) can be used to support a woman's body as she assumes a variety of labor and birth positions (Fig. 18-13). The woman can sit on the ball while leaning over the bed, or she can lean over the ball to support her upper body and reduce stress on her arms and hands when she assumes a hands-and-knees position. The birth ball can encourage pelvic mobility and pelvic and perineal relaxation when the woman sits on the firm yet pliable ball and rocks in rhythmic movements. Warm compresses applied to the perineum can maximize this relaxation effect. The birth ball should be large enough so that, when the woman sits, her knees are bent at a 90-degree angle and her feet are flat on the floor and approximately 2 feet apart.

Supportive Care During Labor and Birth

Support during labor and birth involves emotional support, physical care and comfort measures, and provision of advice and information. Effective support provided to women during labor can result in shorter labors, reduced rates of complications and surgical or obstetric interventions (e.g., cesarean births, labor augmentations and inductions, episiotomies, and forceps- and vacuum-assisted births), and enhanced self-esteem and satisfaction. Physical, emotional, and psychologic support of the woman during labor and birth is a beneficial form of care demonstrated by clear research evidence (see Evidence-Based Practice box) (Enkin et al, 2000; MacKinnon, McIntyre, & Quance, 2005).

Labor rooms should be airy, clean, and homelike. The laboring woman should feel safe in this environment and free to be herself and use the comfort and relaxation measures she prefers. To enhance relaxation bright overhead lights should be turned off when not needed. Noise and intrusions should be kept to a minimum. The temperature is controlled to ensure the laboring woman's comfort. The room should be large enough to accommodate a comfortable chair for the woman's partner, the monitoring equipment, and hospital personnel. Couples can bring their own pillows to make the hospital surroundings more homelike and facilitate position changes. This type of an environment can help women to view their childbirth experience as normal and not related to illness. Environmental modifications should reflect the preferences of the woman, including the number of visitors and availability of a telephone, television, and music. Nurses should ensure that each woman labors in an optimal birth environment.

Labor Support by the Nurse

The nurse can alleviate a woman's anxiety by communicating clearly, explaining unfamiliar terms, providing information and explanations without her having to ask and at a level

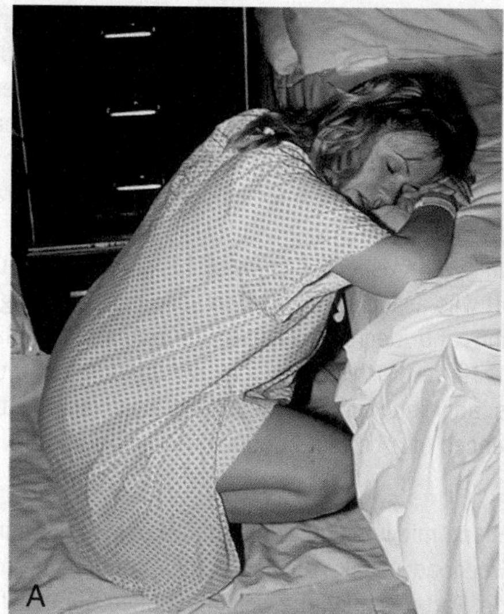

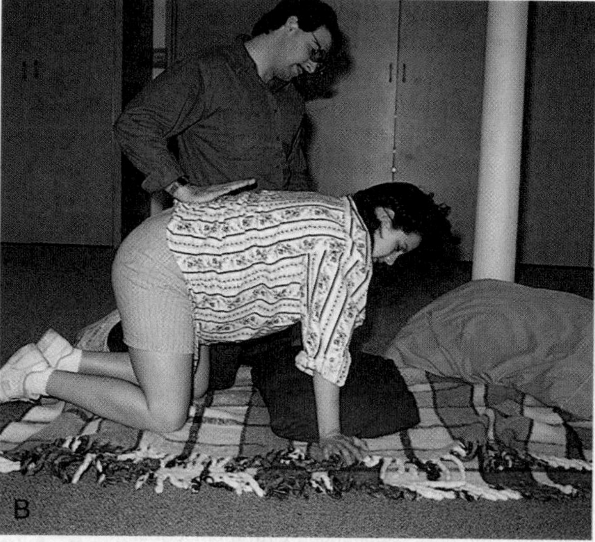

Fig. 18-12 Maternal positions for labor. **A,** Squatting. **B,** Woman in hands-and-knees position. *(Courtesy Marjorie Pyle, RNC, Lifecircle, Costa Mesa, CA.)*

BOX 18-6 Some Maternal Positions* During Labor and Birth

Semirecumbent Position

With woman sitting with her upper body elevated to at least a 30-degree angle, place wedge or small pillow under hip to prevent vena caval compression and reduce likelihood of supine hypotension (see Fig. 18-4, *B*).

- The greater the angle of elevation, the more gravity or pressure is exerted, which promotes fetal descent, the progress of contractions, and the widening of pelvic dimensions.
- It is convenient for rendering care measures and for external fetal monitoring.

Lateral Position (see Fig. 18-11, *B*)

Have woman alternate between left and right side-lying position and provide abdominal and back support as needed for comfort.

- Removes pressure from the vena cava and back; enhances uteroplacental perfusion and relieves backache
- Makes it easier to perform back massage or counterpressure
- Associated with less frequent but more intense contractions
- May make obtaining good external fetal monitor tracings more difficult
- May be used as a birthing position
- Takes pressure off perineum

Upright Position

The gravity effect enhances the contraction cycle and fetal descent: the weight of the fetus places increasing pressure on the cervix; the cervix is pulled upward, facilitating effacement and dilation; impulses from the cervix to the pituitary gland increase, causing more oxytocin to be secreted; and contractions are intensified, thereby applying more forceful downward pressure on the fetus, but they are less painful.

- Fetus is aligned with pelvis, and pelvic diameters are widened slightly.
- Effective upright positions include the following:
  - Ambulation (see Fig. 18-10)
  - Standing and leaning forward with support provided by coach, end of bed, back of chair, or birth ball; relieves backache and facilitates application of counterpressure or back massage (see Fig. 18-11 and Fig. 18-13)
  - Sitting up in bed, chair, birthing chair, on toilet or bedside commode
  - Squatting (see Fig. 18-12, *A*)

Hands-and-Knees Position—Ideal Position for Posterior Positions of the Presenting Part (see Fig. 18-12, *B*)

Assume an "all-fours" position in bed or on a covered floor; allows for pelvic rocking.

- Relieves backache characteristic of "back labor."
- Facilitates internal rotation of the fetus by increasing mobility of the coccyx, increasing the pelvic diameters, and using gravity to turn the fetal back and rotate the head.

*Assess the effect of each position on the laboring woman's comfort and anxiety level, progress of labor, and fetal heart rate and pattern. Alternate positions every 30 to 60 minutes.

she understands, and preparing her for sensations she will experience and procedures that will follow. By encouraging the woman or couple to ask questions and providing honest, understandable answers, the nurse can play a significant role in helping the woman achieve a satisfying birth experience.

Supportive, empathic nursing care for a woman in labor includes the following:

- Helping the woman maintain control and participate to the extent she wishes in the birth of her infant

EVIDENCE-BASED PRACTICE The Benefits of Continuous Labor Support

—Pat Gingrich

Ask the Question

How does continuous labor support benefit laboring patients? Who should provide this support? Is this a nursing role?

Search for Evidence

Search Strategies

Professional organization guidelines, meta-analyses, systematic reviews, randomized controlled trials, nonrandomized prospective studies, and retrospective studies since 2006

Databases Searched

CINAHL, Cochrane, Medline, National Guideline Clearinghouse, and the websites for AWHONN, National Practice Guidelines, Lamaze International, SGOC, and WHO

Critically Analyze the Evidence

For millennia women have labored in the company of other women—usually family or friends who have experienced birth themselves. In the last century Western women in labor became more isolated in institutional, high-technology settings. Loss of dedicated labor support coincided with increasing technology, pain management, and operative birth. Observers now question whether returning the human touch of birthing assistants could improve outcomes. Lamaze International defines labor support as a trusted friend or doula not employed by the facility who offers to the laboring women and her partner physical and emotional support, information, and advocacy but never medical advice. The Lamaze Practice Guideline recommends that all women should have access to doula care covered under insurance (Green, Amis, & Hotelling, 2007).

A Cochrane systematic analysis reviewed 16 randomized, controlled trials involving 13,391 women from 11 countries. Taken as a whole the studies demonstrated that continuous labor support leads to shorter labors, increased vaginal birth, decreased analgesia, and decreased dissatisfaction (Hodnett et al, 2007). These associations were especially true if the labor support was not an employee of the facility, the support was begun early in labor, and the setting did not typically use epidural analgesia.

In a randomized, controlled trial of 420 women, continuous labor support was associated with decreased cesarean and instrumental birth, decreased need for pain medication or regional analgesia, and 100% positive feelings about birth (McGrath & Kennell, 2008).

Finally, a retrospective study of 11,471 women found that doula support was associated with increased breastfeeding intention and initiation and decreased cesarean births (Motti-Santiago et al, 2008). However, this study did not randomize; thus the use of doulas and intention to breastfeed may represent prior related preferences of a certain population of women.

Implications for Practice

Nurses and midwives provide attentive care for laboring women, but their workload usually precludes their continuous presence at the bedside. Partners might be well intentioned but may find the powerful reality of birth to be overwhelming. An experienced doula or birth attendant can keep the laboring woman calm and comfortable, which not only improves the experience emotionally but also reduces pain, stress hormones, and muscular tension, thereby facilitating vaginal birth. Doulas are not there to replace the nurse or partner but to provide support as needs arise. Insurance companies and institutions that see the measurable benefits of doulas are wise to value and encourage their contribution.

References

Green J, Amis D, Hotelling BA: Care practice No 3: continuous labor support, *J Perinat Educ* 16 (3):25-28, 2007.

Hodnett ED et al: Continuous support for women during childbirth. In *The Cochrane Database of Systematic Reviews* 2007, Issue 3, Chichester, UK, 2007, John Wiley & Sons.

McGrath SK, Kennell JN: A randomized controlled trial of continuous labor support: effect on cesarean delivery rates, *Birth* 35(2):92-97, 2008.

Motti-Santiago J et al: A hospital-based doula program and childbirth outcomes in an urban, multicultural setting, *Matern Child Health J* 35(3):372-377, 2008.

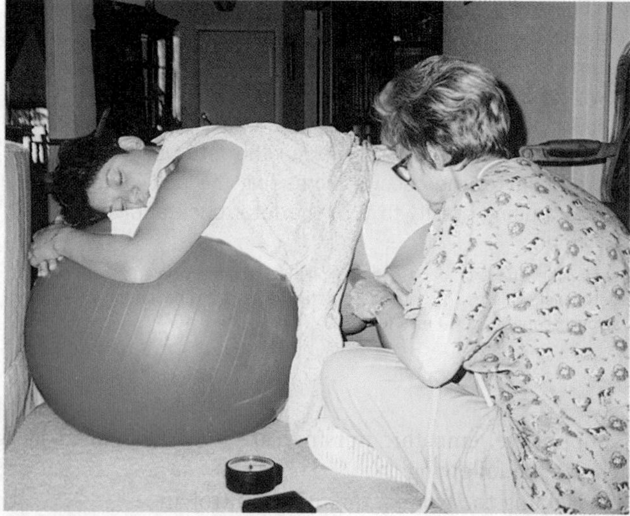

Fig. 18-13 Laboring woman using birth ball. *(Courtesy Polly Perez, Cutting Edge Press, Johnson, VT.)*

- Providing continuity of care that is nonjudgmental and respectful of her cultural and religious values and beliefs
- Meeting the woman's expected outcomes for her labor
- Listening to the woman's concerns and encouraging her to express her feelings
- Acting as the woman's advocate, supporting her decisions and respecting her choices as appropriate, and relating her wishes as needed to other health care providers
- Helping the woman conserve her energy and cope effectively with her pain and discomfort by using a variety of comfort measures that are acceptable to her
- Helping control the woman's discomfort
- Acknowledging the woman's efforts during labor, including her strength and courage, as well as those of her partner, and providing positive reinforcement
- Protecting the woman's privacy and modesty

Couples who have attended childbirth education programs will know something about the labor process, coaching techniques, and comfort measures. The nurse should play a supportive role and keep the couple informed of the progress. Breathing and relaxation techniques and comfort measures described in Chapter 16 can be implemented.

Even when expectant parents have not attended childbirth education classes, the nurse can teach them simple breathing and relaxation techniques during the early phase of labor. In this case the nurse may provide more of the coaching and supportive care until the support person feels ready to take on a more active coaching role.

Comfort measures vary with the situation (Figs. 18-14 and 18-15, *B*). The nurse can draw on the couple's repertoire of comfort measures and relaxation techniques learned during the pregnancy and through life experiences. Such measures include maintaining a comfortable, supportive atmosphere in the labor and birth area; using touch therapeutically (e.g., heat or cold applied to the lower back in the event of back labor, a cool cloth applied to the forehead); providing nonpharmacologic measures to relieve discomfort; administering analgesics when necessary; and most of all just being there (see Tables 18-1 and 18-5). See Chapter 16 for a full discussion of both pharmacologic and nonpharmacologic comfort measures.

Most women in labor respond positively to touch, but permission should be obtained before any measure involving touch. They appreciate gentle handling by staff members. Back rubs and counterpressure may be offered, especially if the woman is experiencing back labor. A support person may be taught to exert counterpressure against the woman's sacrum over the occiput of the head of a fetus in a posterior position (see Fig. 18-11, *B*). The back pain is caused by the occiput pressing on spinal nerves, and counterpressure lifts the occiput off these nerves, thereby providing some relief from pain. Once counterpressure is initiated, the woman usually asks her partner to continue doing this for each following contraction. However, the partner will need to be relieved after a while because exerting counterpressure is hard work. Hand and foot massage also can be soothing and relaxing.

Many women become more sensitive to touch (hyperesthesia) as labor progresses; this is a typical response during transition (see Table 18-2). They may tell their coach to leave them alone or not to touch them. The partner who is unprepared for this normal response may feel rejected and react by withdrawing active support. The nurse can reassure him or her that this response is a positive indication that the first stage is ending and the second stage is approaching. Women with increased sensitivity to touch may have a positive response when touched on surfaces of the body where hair does not grow such as the forehead, the palms of the hands, and the soles of the feet.

Labor Support by the Father or Partner

Although a woman or a man other than the father may be the woman's partner, the father of the baby is usually the support person during labor. He often is able to provide the comfort measures and touch that the laboring woman needs. When the woman becomes focused on her pain, sometimes the partner can persuade her to try nonpharmacologic variations of comfort measures. In addition, he usually is able to interpret the woman's needs and desires to staff members.

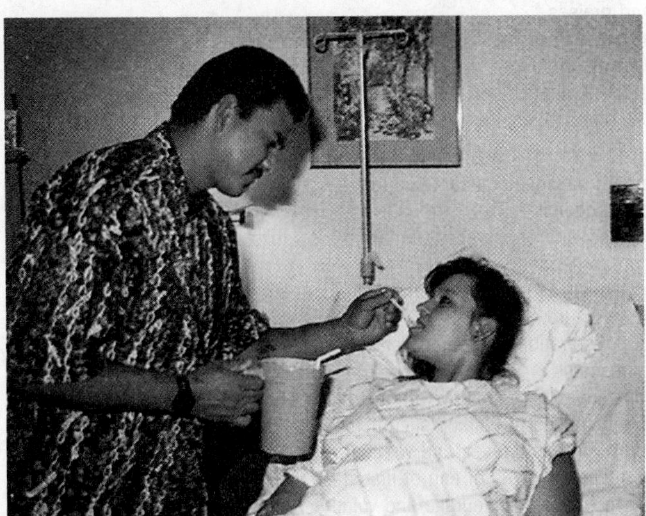

Fig. 18-14 Partner providing comfort measures. *(Courtesy Marjorie Pyle, RNC, Lifecircle, Costa Mesa, CA.)*

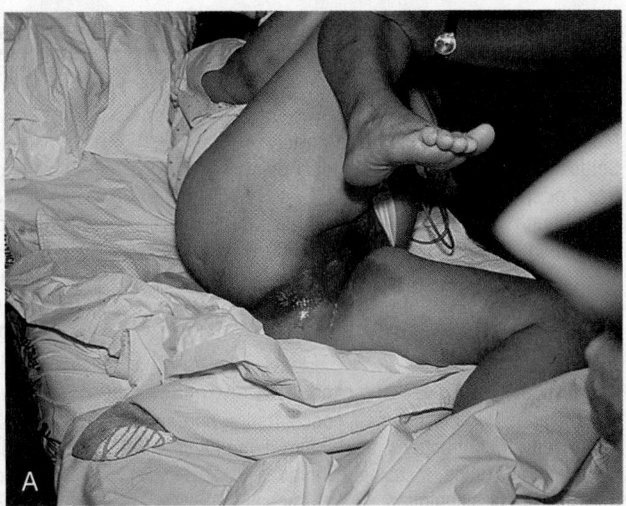

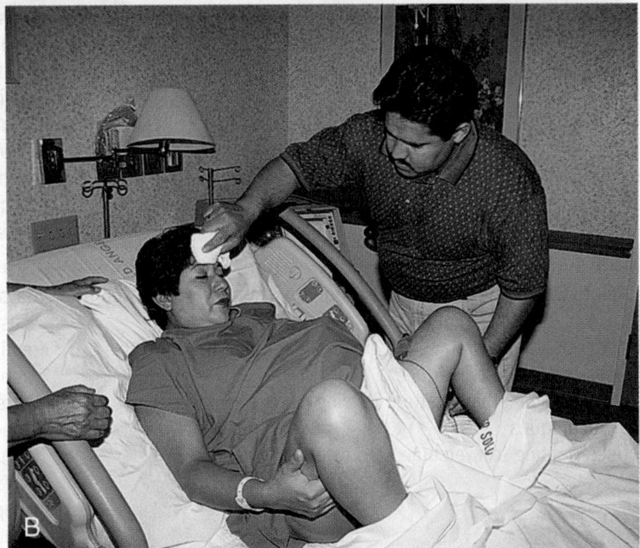

Fig. 18-15 A, Pushing, side-lying position, perineal bulging. **B,** Pushing, semisitting. Partner wiping woman's face with cool cloth between contractions. *(A, Courtesy Michael S. Clement, MD, Mesa, AZ. B, Courtesy Marjorie Pyle, RNC, Lifecircle, Costa Mesa, CA.)*

Throughout the past 30 years childbirth preparation education has been widely available. In the United States and Canada the father's ideal role was thought to be that of labor coach, and he was expected to actively help the woman cope with labor. However, this expectation may be unrealistic because some men have concerns about their labor-coaching abilities. Because the father can participate in labor and birth in different ways, the nurse should encourage him to adopt the role most comfortable for him and for the woman rather than to assume an unnatural role. Participation in the birth is ego building. The father can be of assistance; his presence is important.

The feelings of a first-time father change as labor progresses. Although he is often calm at the onset of labor, feelings of fear and helplessness begin to dominate as labor becomes more active and the father realizes that labor is more work than he anticipated. The first-time father may feel excluded as birth preparations begin during the transition phase. Once the second stage begins and birth nears, the father's focus changes from the woman to the baby who is about to be born (Table 18-5).

Ways in which the nurse can support the father-partner are detailed in Box 18-7. A well-informed father can make an important contribution to the health and well-being of the mother and child, their family interrelationship, and his self-esteem.

Labor Support by Doulas

Continuity of care has been cited by women as a critical component of a satisfying childbirth experience. This need can be met by a specially trained, experienced female labor attendant called a *doula.* The doula provides a continuous, one-on-one caring presence throughout the labor and birth process of the woman she is attending. This is a beneficial form of care (Enkin et al, 2000).

The primary role of the doula is to focus on the laboring woman and provide physical and emotional support by using soft, reassuring words; touching, stroking, and hugging; administering comfort measures to reduce pain and enhance

Table 18-5 Woman's Responses and Support Person's Actions During First Stage of Labor

WOMAN'S RESPONSES	NURSE/SUPPORT PERSON'S ACTIONS*
Dilation of Cervix 0-3 cm (Latent) (Contractions 10-30 sec Long, 5-30 min Apart, Mild to Moderate)	
Mood: alert, happy, excited, mild anxiety Settles into labor room; selects focal point Rests or sleeps if possible Uses breathing techniques Uses effleurage, focusing, and relaxation techniques	Provides encouragement, feedback for relaxation, companionship Helps to cope with contractions Encourages use of focusing techniques Helps to concentrate on breathing techniques Uses comfort measures Assists woman into comfortable position Informs woman of progress; explains procedures and routines Gives praise Offers fluids, ice chips as ordered
Dilation of Cervix 4-7 cm (Active) (Contractions 30-45 sec Long, 3-5 min Apart, Moderate to Strong)	
Mood: seriously labor oriented, concentration and energy needed for contractions, alert, more demanding Continues relaxation, focusing techniques Uses breathing techniques	Acts as buffer; limits assessment techniques to between contractions Assists with contractions Encourages woman as needed to help her maintain breathing techniques Uses comfort measures Assists with frequent position changes, emphasizing side-lying and upright positions Encourages voluntary relaxation of muscles of back, buttocks, thighs, and perineum; effleurage Applies counterpressure to sacrococcygeal area Encourages and praises Keeps woman aware of progress Offers analgesics as ordered Checks bladder; encourages her to void Gives oral care; offers fluids, ice chips as ordered
Dilation of Cervix 8-10 cm (Transition) (Contractions 45-90 sec Long, 2-3 min Apart, Strong)	
Mood: irritable, intense concentration, symptoms of transition (e.g., nausea, vomiting) Continues relaxation, needs greater concentration to do this Uses breathing techniques Uses 4:1 breathing pattern if using psychoprophylactic techniques Uses panting to overcome urge to push	Stays with woman; provides constant support Assists with contractions Reminds, reassures, and encourages woman to reestablish breathing pattern and concentration as needed Alerts woman to begin breathing pattern before contraction becomes too intense if she is sedated or drowsy Prompts panting respirations if woman begins to push prematurely Uses comfort measures Accepts woman's inability to comply with instructions Accepts irritable response to helping such as counterpressure Supports woman who has nausea and vomiting; gives oral care as needed; gives reassurance regarding signs of end of first stage Uses relaxation techniques (effleurage and voluntary relaxation) Keeps woman aware of progress

*Provided by nurses and support people in collaboration with primary nurse.

BOX 18-7 Guidelines for Supporting the Father

- Orient to the labor room and the unit; explain location of the cafeteria, toilet, waiting room, and nursery; visiting hours; names and functions of personnel present.
- Inform him of sights and smells he can expect to encounter; encourage him to leave the room if necessary.
- Respect his or the couple's decision about the degree of his involvement. Offer them freedom to make decisions.
- Tell him when his presence has been helpful and continue to reinforce this throughout labor.
- Offer to teach him comfort measures.
- Inform him frequently of the progress of the labor and the woman's needs. Keep him informed about procedures to be performed.
- Prepare him for changes in the woman's behavior and physical appearance.
- Remind him to eat; offer him snacks and fluids if possible.
- Relieve him of the job of support person as necessary. Offer him blankets if he is to sleep in a chair by the bedside.
- Acknowledge the stress experienced by each partner during labor and birth and identify normal responses.
- Attempt to modify or eliminate unsettling stimuli such as extra noise and extra light.

relaxation; and walking with the woman, helping her to change positions, and encouraging her spontaneous bearing-down efforts. Doulas provide information and explain procedures and events. They advocate for the woman's right to participate actively in the management of her labor. These forms of caring help to reduce a woman's level of anxiety and fear, make her more confident and calm, and reduce the stress response that could inhibit the progress of labor.

The doula also supports the woman's partner, who often feels unqualified to be the sole labor support and may find it difficult to watch the woman when she is experiencing pain. The doula can encourage and praise the partner's efforts, create a partnership as caregivers, and provide respite care. Doulas also facilitate communication between the laboring woman and her partner and between the couple and the health care team (Simkin & Way, 2008).

Continuous supportive care that begins early in labor significantly reduces the cesarean birth rate; duration of labor; use of oxytocin, analgesics, and forceps or vacuum-extractor; and requests for epidural anesthesia (McGrath & Kennell, 2008). Laboring women also reported a higher level of satisfaction with their childbirth experience and greater success with breastfeeding. Long-term benefits of doula care are reflected in more positive maternal feelings regarding their parenting ability and lower rates of postpartum depression.

The role of the nurse and the doula are complementary. They should work together as a team, recognizing and respecting the role each plays in supporting and caring for the woman and her partner during the childbirth process. The doula provides supportive nonmedical care measures; whereas the nurse focuses on monitoring the status of the maternal-fetal unit and implementing clinical care protocols, including pharmacologic interventions, and documenting assessment findings, actions, and responses (Simkin & Way, 2008).

Labor Support by the Grandparents

When grandparents act as labor coaches, it is important to support them and treat them with respect. They may have ways to deal with pain based on their experience. They should be encouraged to help as long as their actions do not compromise the status of the mother or the fetus. One example of an acceptable practice would be giving the woman herbal tea during labor. The nurse acts as a role model for parents by acknowledging the value of the grandparent's contributions to parental support and recognizing the difficulty parents have in witnessing their child's discomfort or crisis, regardless of the age of that child. If they have never witnessed a birth, the nurse may need to provide explanations about what is happening. Many of the activities used to support fathers also are appropriate for grandparents.

Other grandparents are health professionals, have knowledge and experience with the birthing process, and can provide effective labor support. However, if adverse events occur, their knowledge will cause additional stress.

When possible, the nurse offers the grandparents emotional support. A nurse can show such support by offering them liquid refreshment and initiating discussion with open-ended questions or statements such as, "It is sometimes hard to watch a daughter in labor." Nursing actions that provide support for the grandparents can have a therapeutic effect on all members of the family. In turn, a strong, supportive family unit is important for the optimal growth and development of its newest member.

Siblings During Labor and Birth

The preparation of siblings for acceptance of the new child helps promote the attachment process. Such preparation and participation during pregnancy and labor may help the older children accept this change. The older child or children who know that they are important to the family become active participants. Rehearsal for the event before labor is essential.

The age and developmental level of children influence their responses; therefore preparation for the children to be present during labor is adjusted to meet each child's needs. The child younger than 2 years shows little interest in pregnancy and labor; for the older child such preparation may reduce fears and misconceptions. Parents need to be prepared for labor and birth themselves and feel comfortable about the process and the presence of their children. Most parents have a "feel" for their children's maturational level and their physical and emotional ability to observe and cope with the events of the labor and birth process.

Preparation can include a description of the anticipated sights, events (e.g., ROM, monitors, IV infusions), smells, and sounds; a labor and birth demonstration; a tour of the birthing unit; and an opportunity to be around a real newborn. Children must learn that their mother will be working hard during labor and birth. She will not be able to talk to them during contractions. She may groan, scream, grunt, and pant at times and say things she would not say otherwise (e.g., "I can't take this anymore;" "Take this baby out of me;" or "This pain is killing me"). They can be told that labor is uncomfortable but that their mother's body is made for the job.

Storybooks about the birth process can be read to or by children to prepare them for the event. Films are available for preparing preschool and school-age children to participate in the labor and birth experience. Most agencies require that a specific person be designated to watch over the children who are participating in their mother's childbirth experience to provide them with support, explanations, diversions, and comfort as needed. Health care providers involved in attending women during birth must be comfortable with the presence of children and the unpredictability of their questions, comments, and behaviors.

Emergency Interventions

Emergency conditions that require immediate nursing intervention can arise with startling speed. Interventions for abnormal FHR, inadequate uterine relaxation, vaginal bleeding, infection, and prolapse of the cord are detailed in the Emergency box.

Second Stage of Labor

evolve Case Study—Second/Third Stages of Labor

The second stage of labor is the stage in which the infant is born. This stage begins with full cervical dilation (10 cm) and complete effacement (100%) and ends with the baby's birth. The force exerted by uterine contractions, gravity, and maternal bearing-down efforts facilitates achievement of the expected outcome of a spontaneous, uncomplicated, vaginal birth.

The second stage comprises three phases: latent, descent, and transition phases. These phases are characterized by maternal verbal and nonverbal behaviors, uterine activity, the urge to bear down, and fetal descent.

The latent phase is a period of rest and relative calm (i.e., "laboring down"). During this early phase the fetus continues to descend passively through the birth canal and rotate to an anterior position as a result of ongoing uterine contractions. The woman is quiet and often relaxes with her eyes closed between contractions. The urge to bear down is not well established and is experienced only during the acme of a contraction or may not be experienced at all. Allowing a woman to rest during this phase and waiting until the urge to push intensifies reduces maternal fatigue, conserves energy for bearing-down efforts, and provides optimal maternal and fetal outcomes. Coaching a woman to push before her body signals readiness can result in a prolonged period of active pushing with limited-to-no progress. The woman can become dependent on her coach or nurses to tell her when and how to push. Women who have epidural analgesia may not feel the urge to bear down and will need coaching.

The descent phase or phase of active pushing is characterized by strong urges to bear down as the Ferguson reflex is activated by pressure of the presenting part on the stretch receptors of the pelvic floor. At this point the fetal station is usually 1+, and the position is anterior. This stimulation causes the release of oxytocin from the posterior pituitary gland, which stimulates stronger, expulsive uterine contractions. The woman becomes more focused on bearing-down efforts, which become rhythmic. She changes positions frequently to find a more comfortable pushing position. The woman often announces the onset of contractions and becomes more vocal as she bears down. The urge to bear down intensifies as descent progresses.

In the transition phase the presenting part is on the perineum, and bearing-down efforts are most effective for promoting birth. The woman may be more verbal about the pain she is experiencing; she may scream or swear and act out of control.

The nurse encourages the woman to "listen" to and trust her body as she progresses through the phases of the second stage of labor. When a woman listens to her body to tell her when to bear down, her efforts become more effective, and she often feels more satisfied with her efforts to give birth to her baby.

If a woman is confined to bed, especially in a recumbent position, the rhythmic urge to bear down is delayed because gravity is not being used to press the presenting part against the pelvic floor. Being moved to another room and placed on a delivery table in the lithotomy position, as has been the custom in North America, also has an inhibiting effect on the urge to bear down. Today Western societies have adopted the birthing practice of most non-Western societies where labor and birth occur in the same room and women use various positions for bearing down such as side-lying, kneeling, squatting, sitting, or standing.

Duration of Second Stage

The duration of the second stage of labor is influenced by several factors such as the effectiveness of the primary and secondary powers of labor; the type and amount of analgesia or anesthesia used; the physical and emotional condition, position, activity level, parity, and pelvic adequacy of the laboring woman; the size, presentation, and position of the fetus; and the nature and source of support the woman receives.

For many multiparous women birth occurs within minutes of complete dilation, perhaps only one push later. Nulliparous women usually push for 1 to 2 hours before giving birth. If the woman has been given epidural analgesia, pushing can last more than 2 hours. Epidural analgesia blocks or reduces the urge to bear down and limits the woman's ability to attain an upright position to push. By adjusting dosages to the lowest effective level, allowing the epidural to wear off at full dilation or after 1 hour of pushing, or using mixtures containing an opioid-agonist analgesic and a local anesthetic, the woman is able to perceive more fully the urge to bear down, move more freely, and attain an upright position with assistance as a result of increased strength and sensation in her legs. This approach can enhance the ability to bear down effectively and achieve an uncomplicated vaginal birth. However, allowing the analgesia to wear off means that women will have an increase in distress and the severity of pain. This results in an increase in sympathetic activity and the release of catecholamines. Catecholamines inhibit uterine contractions, potentially prolonging the second stage of labor. Allowing these women a "laboring down" period for fetal descent and rotation may result in a more positive outcome.

Commonly a second stage of more than 2 hours may be considered prolonged in women without regional analgesia

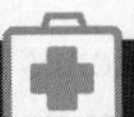

EMERGENCY

Interventions for Emergencies

Signs	Interventions*
Nonreassuring Fetal Heart Rate Pattern	
Fetal bradycardia (fetal heart rate [FHR] less than 110 beats/min for more than 10 minutes)†	Notify primary health care provider.‡
Fetal tachycardia (FHR above 160 beats/min for more than 10 minutes in term pregnancy)§	Change woman to side-lying position.
Irregular FHR; abnormal sinus rhythm shown by internal monitor	Discontinue oxytocin (Pitocin) infusion if being infused.
Persistent decrease in baseline FHR variability without any identified cause	Increase intravenous (IV) fluid rate if fluid is being infused per protocol order.
Late, severe variable, and prolonged deceleration patterns	Administer oxygen at 8 to 10 L/min by tight face mask.
Absence of FHR	Check maternal temperature for elevation.
	Start an IV line if one is not in place.
	Administer amnioinfusion if ordered.
Inadequate Uterine Relaxation	
Intrauterine pressure greater than 75 mm Hg (shown by intrauterine pressure catheter monitoring)	Notify primary health care provider.‡
Contractions consistently lasting more than 90 seconds	Discontinue oxytocin infusion if being infused.
Contraction interval less than 2 minutes	Change woman to side-lying position.
	Increase IV fluid rate if fluid is being infused.
	Administer oxygen at 8 to 10 L/min by tight face mask.
	Start an IV line if one is not in place.
	Palpate and evaluate contractions.
	Give tocolytics (terbutaline) as ordered.
Vaginal Bleeding	
Vaginal bleeding (bright red, dark red, or in amount in excess of that expected during normal cervical dilation)	Notify primary health care provider.‡
Continuous vaginal bleeding with FHR changes	Anticipate emergency (stat) cesarean birth.
Pain may or may not be present	Do NOT perform a vaginal examination.
Infection	
Foul-smelling amniotic fluid	Notify primary health care provider.‡
Maternal temperature above 38° C in presence of adequate hydration (straw-colored urine)	Institute cooling measures for laboring woman.
Fetal tachycardia greater than 160 beats/min for more than 10 minutes	Start an IV line if one is not in place.
	Assist with or perform collection of catheterized urine specimen and amniotic fluid sample and send to the laboratory for urinalysis and cultures.
Prolapse of Cord	
Fetal bradycardia with variable deceleration during uterine contraction	Call for assistance.
Woman reports feeling the cord after membranes rupture	Have someone notify the primary health care provider immediately.
Cord lies alongside or below the presenting part of the fetus; can be seen or felt in or protruding from the vagina	Glove the examining hand quickly and insert two fingers into the vagina to the cervix; with one finger on either side of the cord or both fingers to one side, exert upward pressure against the presenting part to relieve compression of the cord.
Major predisposing factors:	Place a rolled towel under the woman's hip.
• Rupture of membranes with a gush	Place woman in extreme Trendelenburg or modified Sims' position or knee-chest position.
• Loose fit of presenting part in lower uterine segment	Wrap the cord loosely in a sterile towel saturated with warm sterile normal saline if the cord is protruding from the vagina.
• Presenting part not yet engaged	Administer oxygen at 8 to 10 L/min by face mask until birth is accomplished.
	Start IV fluids or increase existing drip rate.
	Continue to monitor FHR by internal fetal scalp electrode if possible.
	Do not attempt to replace cord into cervix.
	Prepare for immediate birth (vaginal or cesarean).

*Because emergency situations are often frightening events, it is important for the nurse to explain to the woman and her support person what is happening and how it is being managed.

†Practice is to intervene within 2 to 30 minutes if FHR is less than 110 beats/min.

‡In most emergency situations nurses take immediate action, following a protocol and standards of nursing practice. Another person can notify the primary health care provider, or this can be done by the nurse as soon as possible.

§Nonreassuring sign when associated with late decelerations or absence of variability, especially if FHR is greater than 180 beats/min.

and is reported to the primary health care provider. By using assessment findings such as the FHR and pattern, the descent of the presenting part, the quality of the uterine contractions, and the status of the woman, premature intervention with episiotomy or forceps- or vacuum-assisted birth can be avoided. If the status of the maternal-fetal unit is reassuring and progress is continuing, interventions to end the second stage of labor are unwarranted. Less emphasis should be placed on a definite time limit for the second stage. The duration of active pushing has been found to be more relevant to the newborn's condition at birth than the duration of the second stage of labor itself.

Nursing Care Management

The only certain objective sign that the second stage of labor has begun is the inability to feel the cervix during vaginal examination, indicating that the cervix is fully dilated and effaced. The precise moment that this occurs is not easily determined because it depends on when a vaginal examination is performed to validate full dilation and effacement. This makes timing of the actual duration of the second stage difficult. Other signs that suggest the onset of the second stage include the following:

- Sudden appearance of sweat on upper lip
- An episode of vomiting
- Increased bloody show
- Shaking of extremities
- Increased restlessness; verbalization (e.g., "I can't go on")
- Involuntary bearing-down efforts

These signs commonly appear when the cervix reaches full dilation; however, women with an epidural block may not exhibit such signs. Other indicators for each phase of the second stage are given in Table 18-6.

Women can begin to experience an irresistible urge to bear down before full dilation. For some women this occurs as early as 5 cm dilation. This is most often related to the station of the presenting part below the level of the ischial spines of the maternal pelvis. This occurrence creates a conflict between the woman, whose body is telling her to push, and her health care providers, who believe that pushing the fetal presenting part against an incompletely dilated cervix will result in cervical edema and lacerations and a slowing down of labor progress. The premature urge to bear down must be evaluated as a phase of labor progress, possibly indicating the onset of the second stage of labor. The timing when a woman pushes in relation to whether or not her cervix is fully dilated should be based on research evidence rather than on tradition or routine practice. It may be safe and effective for a woman to push with the urge to bear down at the acme of a contraction if her cervix is soft, retracting, and 8 cm or more dilated and if the fetus is at a 1+ station and rotating to an anterior position.

Assessment is continuous during the second stage of labor. Professional standards and agency policy determine the specific type and timing of assessments and the way in which findings are documented. Signs and symptoms of impending birth (see Table 18-6) may appear unexpectedly, requiring immediate action by the nurse (see Box 18-8).

In the hospital birth may occur in an LDR, LDRP, or delivery room. If the mother is to be transferred to the delivery room

Table 18-6 Expected Maternal Progress During Second Stage of Labor

CRITERION	LATENT PHASE (AVERAGE DURATION, 10-30 min)	DESCENT PHASE (AVERAGE DURATION VARIES)*	TRANSITION PHASE (AVERAGE DURATION 5-15 min)
Contractions	Period of physiologic lull for all criteria; period of peace and rest		
Magnitude (intensity)		Significant increase	Overwhelmingly strong; expulsive
Frequency		2-2.5 min	1-2 min
Duration		90 sec	90 sec
Descent, station	0 to +2	Increases and Ferguson reflex† activated, +2 to +4	Rapid, +4 to birth Fetal head visible in introitus
Show: color and amount		Significant increase in dark-red bloody show	Bloody show accompanies birth of head
Spontaneous bearing-down efforts	Slight to absent, except during acme of strongest contractions	Increased urge to bear down	Greatly increased
Vocalization	Quiet; concern over progress	Grunting sounds or expiratory vocalization; announces contractions	Grunting sounds and expiratory vocalizations continue; may scream or swear
Maternal behavior	Experiences sense of relief that transition to second stage is finished Feels fatigued and sleepy Feels a sense of accomplishment and optimism, because the "worst is over" Feels in control	Senses increased urge to push Alters respiratory pattern: has short 4- to 5-sec breath holds with regular breaths in between five to seven times per contraction Makes grunting sounds or expiratory vocalizations Frequent repositioning	Describes extreme pain Expresses feelings of powerlessness Shows decreased ability to listen or concentrate on anything but giving birth Describes *ring of fire* (burning sensation of acute pain as vagina stretches and fetal head crowns) Often shows excitement immediately after birth of head

*Duration of descent phase can vary, depending on maternal parity, effectiveness of bearing-down effort, and presence of spinal or epidural analgesia.
†Pressure of presenting part on stretch receptors of pelvic floor stimulates release of oxytocin from posterior pituitary, resulting in more intense uterine contractions.

for birth, the nurse makes the transfer early enough to avoid rushing the woman. The birth area is readied for the birth.

Maternal Position

There is no single position for childbirth. Labor is a dynamic, interactive process involving the woman's uterus, pelvis, and voluntary muscles. In addition, angles between the woman's pelvis and the baby constantly change as the fetus turns and flexes down the birth canal. The woman may want to assume various positions for childbirth, and she should be encouraged and helped to attain and maintain her positions of choice. Supine, semi-recumbent, or lithotomy positions are still widely used in Western societies despite evidence that women prefer upright positions for their bearing-down efforts and birth.

Birth attendants play a major role in influencing a woman's choice of position for birth, with midwives tending to advocate the nonlithotomy positions for the second stage of labor. Upright positions for women with or without epidural anesthesia facilitate birth and fetal descent and reduce the duration of the second stage of labor and the need for episiotomy, forceps, or vacuum extractor in the following ways:

- Straighten the longitudinal axis of the birth canal and improve the alignment of the fetus for passage through the pelvis
- Use gravity to direct the fetal head toward the pelvic inlet, thereby facilitating descent
- Enlarge pelvic dimensions and restrict the encroachment of the sacrum and coccyx into the pelvic inlet
- Increase uteroplacental circulation, resulting in more intense, efficient uterine contractions
- Enhance the woman's ability to bear down effectively, thereby minimizing maternal exhaustion

However, the upright positions may slightly increase the risk for second-degree lacerations and a blood loss greater than 500 ml. Further investigation is needed to determine the exact mechanism for these outcomes.

Squatting is highly effective in facilitating the descent and birth of the fetus. It is considered to be one of the best and most natural positions for the second stage of labor. Women should assume a modified, supported squat until the fetal head is engaged, at which time a deep squat can be used. A firm surface is required for this position, and the woman will need side support (see Fig. 18-12, *A*). In a birthing bed a squatting bar is available that she can use to help support herself (see Fig. 16-15). A birth ball can help a woman maintain the squatting position. The fetus will be aligned with the birth canal, and pelvic and perineal relaxation are facilitated as she sits on the ball or holds it in front of her for support as she squats (see Fig. 18-13).

When a woman uses the supported standing position for bearing down, her weight is borne on both femoral heads, allowing the pressure in the acetabulum to increase the transverse diameter of the pelvic outlet by up to 1 cm. This can be helpful if descent of the head is delayed because the occiput has not rotated from the lateral (transverse diameter of pelvis) to the anterior position. Birthing or rocking chairs may be used to provide women with a good physiologic position to enhance bearing-down efforts during childbirth, although some women feel restricted by a chair. The upright position provides a potential psychologic advantage in that it allows the mother to see the birth as it occurs and maintain eye contact with the attendant. Most birthing chairs are designed so that, if an emergency occurs, the chair can be adjusted to the horizontal or the Trendelenburg position.

Oversized beanbag chairs and large floor pillows may be used for both labor and birth. They can mold around and support the mother in whatever position she selects. These chairs are of particular value for mothers who wish to be actively involved in the birth process. Birthing stools can be used to support the woman in an upright position similar to squatting. Women may want to sit on the toilet to push because they are concerned about stool incontinence during this stage. These women must be closely monitored and removed from the toilet before birth is imminent. Because sitting on chairs, stools, toilets, or commodes can increase perineal edema and blood loss, it is important to assist the woman to change her position frequently.

The side-lying position, with the upper part of the woman's leg held by the nurse or coach or placed on a pillow, is an effective position for the second stage of labor (see Fig. 18-15, *A*). Women using the lateral position have more control over their bearing-down efforts. In addition, a slower, more controlled descent of the fetus results in a reduced risk of perineal trauma. Some women prefer a semisitting (semirecumbent) position. To maintain good uteroplacental circulation and enhance the woman's bearing-down efforts in this position, the woman's back and shoulders should be elevated to at least a 30-degree angle, and a wedge should be placed under one hip (see Fig. 18-15, *B*). The episiotomy rate for nulliparas has been found to be highest in this position.

The hands-and-knees position, along with pelvic rocking and abdominal stroking, is an effective position for birth because it enhances placental perfusion, helps rotate the fetus from a posterior to an anterior position, and may facilitate the birth of the shoulders, especially if the fetus is large (see Fig. 18-12, *B*). Perineal trauma may also be reduced.

The birthing bed is commonly used today and can be set for different positions according to the woman's needs (Fig. 18-16). The woman can squat, kneel, sit, recline, or lie on her side, choosing the position most comfortable for her without having to climb into bed for the birth. At the same time there is excellent exposure for examination, electrode placement, and birth. Squatting bars, over-the-bed tables, birth balls, and pillows can be used for support. The bed can be positioned for the administration of anesthesia and is ideal to help women receiving an epidural to assume different positions to facilitate birth. The bed can be used to transport the woman to the operating room if a cesarean birth is necessary.

Bearing-Down Efforts

As the fetal head reaches the pelvic floor, most women experience the urge to bear down. Reflexively the woman will begin to exert downward pressure by contracting her abdominal muscles while relaxing her pelvic floor. This bearing down is an involuntary response to the Ferguson reflex.

A strong expiratory grunt or groan (vocalization) often accompanies pushing when the woman exhales as she pushes. This natural vocalization by women during open-glottis bearing-down efforts should not be discouraged by nurses.

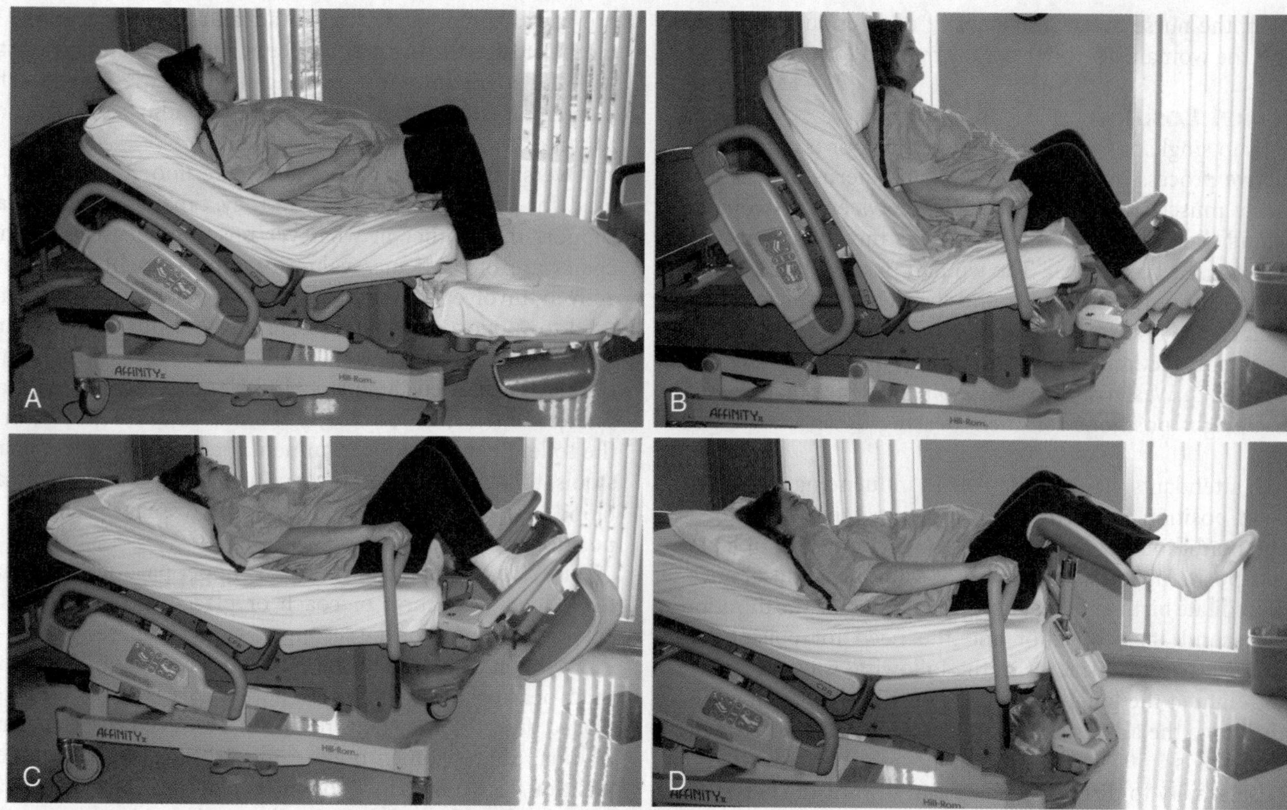

Fig. 18-16 The versatility of today's birthing bed makes it practical in many settings. NOTE: OB table used for lithotomy position. A, Labor bed. B, Birth chair. C, Birth bed. D, OB table. *(Courtesy Julie Perry Nelson, Loveland, CO.)*

When assisting a woman to push, the nurse should encourage her to push as she feels like pushing (instinctive, spontaneous pushing) rather than to give a prolonged push on command (Yildirim & Beji, 2008). A woman can become confused and anxious when she is being told to do something in conflict with what her body is telling her. Using phrases such as "you are doing so well," "you are moving the baby down," and "follow what your body is telling you," rather than "Push, push, push," encourages a woman to feel confident in her body and what she is feeling (Sampselle et al, 2005).

Women usually begin to push naturally as the contractions increase in intensity and the Ferguson reflex strengthens. The nurse should monitor the woman's breathing so that she does not hold her breath for more than 5 to 7 seconds at a time and should remind her to ventilate her lungs fully by taking deep cleansing breaths before and after each contraction. Bearing down while exhaling (open-glottis pushing) and taking breaths between bearing-down efforts help to maintain adequate oxygen levels for the mother and fetus, thereby enhancing fetal well-being. Approximately five pushes occur during a contraction, with each push lasting about 5 seconds. Maternal benefits associated with spontaneous pushing include less perineal trauma, less maternal fatigue, and fewer forceps- or vacuum-assisted births. In addition, evidence is indicating that the integrity of the pelvic floor is preserved, reducing the risk for future incontinence and pelvic organ prolapse (Sampselle et al, 2005; Simpson & James, 2005).

Prolonged breath holding or sustained, directed bearing down is still a common practice often beginning at 10 cm dilation and before the urge to bear down is perceived. The woman is coached to hold her breath, closing her glottis, and to push while the nurse or partner counts to 10. This method of bearing down triggers the Valsalva maneuver when the woman closes her glottis (closed-glottis pushing), thereby increasing intrathoracic and cardiovascular pressure, reducing cardiac output, and inhibiting perfusion of the uterus and the placenta. Breath holding for more than 5 to 7 seconds causes the perfusion of oxygen across the placenta to be diminished, resulting in fetal hypoxia (Simpson, 2005; Yildirim & Beji, 2008). This approach to bearing down is harmful or ineffective and should be discouraged (Enkin et al, 2000) (see Critical Thinking Exercise).

A woman may reach the second stage of labor and then experience a lack of readiness to complete the process and give birth to her child. She may have doubts about her readiness to be a mother or desire to wait for her support person or primary health care provider to arrive. Fear, anxiety, or embarrassment regarding the unfamiliar or painful sensations and behaviors during pushing (e.g., sounds made, passage of stool) may be other inhibiting factors. Fear that the baby will be in danger once it emerges from the protective intrauterine environment may also be present.

By recognizing that a woman may experience a need to hold back the birth of her baby, the nurse can address her concerns and effectively coach her through this stage of labor.

To ensure slow birth of the fetal head, the nurse encourages the woman to control the urge to bear down by coaching her to take panting breaths or exhale slowly through pursed lips

CRITICAL THINKING EXERCISE

Spontaneous vs. Directed Bearing-Down Efforts

A controversy has arisen on the labor unit where you have your maternal-newborn clinical rotation. Some of the nurses and midwives and most of the obstetricians believe that women must be coached to begin pushing as soon as full dilation occurs to ensure that the second stage is not prolonged. The rest of the nurses and midwives and a few obstetricians believe that women know best when and how to push and encourage women in labor to follow what their bodies tell them. The nurse manager of the labor unit has encouraged those believing in spontaneous pushing to present a unit in-service to provide evidence to show that spontaneous pushing enhances the well-being of the maternal-fetal unit without a significant effect on the progress of the second stage of labor. What should the proponents of spontaneous pushing present at the unit in-service?

1. Evidence—Is there evidence that supports the benefits of spontaneous pushing?
2. Assumptions—What assumptions can be made about the following issues related to spontaneous pushing during the second stage of labor?
   a. Benefits of spontaneous pushing
   b. Risks associated with directed pushing
   c. Impact of timing for the onset of pushing during the second stage of labor
3. What influence does a woman's position have on the effectiveness of the pushing technique she uses?
4. Does the evidence support a recommended position to enhance the woman's bearing-down efforts?
5. Are there alternative perspectives to your conclusion?

as the baby's head crowns. At this point the woman needs simple, clear directions from one person.

Amnesia between contractions is often pronounced in the second stage, and the woman may have to be roused to cooperate in the bearing-down process. Parents who have attended childbirth education classes may have devised a set of verbal cues for the laboring woman to follow. It is helpful for them to have these cues printed on a card that can be attached to the head of the bed so that the nurse can better substitute as coach if the partner has to leave the room for a short period of time.

Fetal Heart Rate and Pattern

As noted previously, the FHR must be checked. If the baseline rate begins to slow, if there is a loss of variability, or if deceleration patterns develop (e.g., late, variable), prompt treatment must be initiated. The woman can be turned on her side to reduce the pressure of the uterus against the ascending vena cava and descending aorta (see Fig. 18-4), and oxygen can be administered by nonrebreather face mask at 10 L/min (Tucker, Miller, & Miller, 2009). Often this is all that is required to restore a reassuring pattern. If the FHR and pattern do not become reassuring immediately, the primary health care provider should be notified quickly because medical intervention to hasten birth may be indicated.

Support of the Father or Partner

During the second stage of labor the woman needs continuous support and coaching (Table 18-7). Because the coaching process can be physically and emotionally tiring for support people, the nurse offers them nourishment and fluids and encourages them to take short breaks. If birth occurs in an LDR or LDRP room, the partner may be allowed to wear street clothes or required to wear a clean scrub outfit, cap, and mask (for the birth). The support person who attends the birth in a delivery room is instructed to put on a cover gown or scrub clothes, mask, hat, and shoe covers as required by agency policy. The nurse also specifies support measures that can be used for the laboring woman and points out areas of the room in which the partner can move freely.

LEGAL TIP Documentation All observations (e.g., maternal vital signs, FHR and pattern, progress of labor) and nursing interventions, including patient response, should be documented concurrently with care. The course of labor and maternal-fetal response may change without warning. It is important that all documentation be accurate, complete, timely, and according to agency policy.

Supplies, Instruments, and Equipment

To prepare for birth in any setting, the birthing table is usually set up during the transition phase for nulliparous women and during the active phase for multiparous women.

The birthing supplies and instruments are arranged on a table or cart (Fig. 18-17). Standard procedures are followed for gloving, identifying and opening sterile packages, adding sterile supplies to the table, unwrapping sterile instruments, and handing them to the primary health care provider. The crib or radiant warmer and equipment are readied for the support and stabilization of the infant (Fig. 18-18).

The items used for birth may vary among different facilities; therefore the procedure manual of each facility should be consulted to determine the protocols specific to that facility.

The nurse estimates the time until the birth will occur and notifies the primary health care provider if he or she is not in the patient's room. Even the most experienced nurse can miscalculate the time left before birth occurs; thus every nurse who attends a woman in labor must be prepared to assist with a birth if the primary health care provider is not present (see Box 18-8).

Birth in a Delivery Room or Birthing Room

The woman will need assistance if she must move from the labor bed to the delivery table (Fig. 18-19). The various

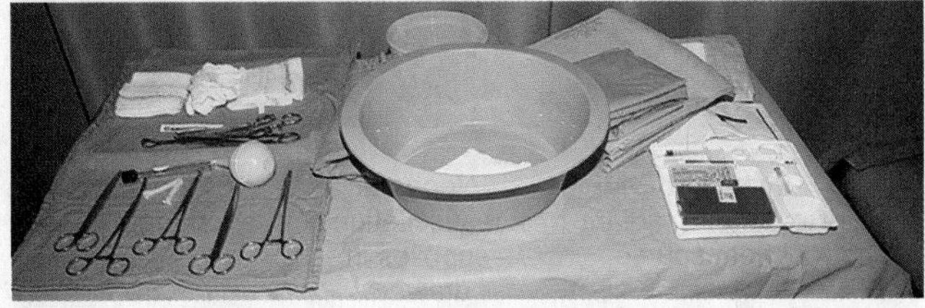

Fig. 18-17 Instrument table. *(Courtesy Marjorie Pyle, RNC, Lifecircle, Costa Mesa, CA.)*

Table 18-7 Woman's Responses and Support Person's Action During Second Stage of Labor

WOMAN'S RESPONSES	NURSE OR SUPPORT PERSON'S ACTIONS*
Latent Phase	
Experiences a short period of peace and rest	Encourages woman to "listen" to her body Continues support measures Suggests an upright position to encourage progression of descent if descent phase does not begin after 20 min
Descent Phase	
Senses increased urgency to bear down as Ferguson reflex is activated Notes increase in intensity of uterine contractions—alters respiratory pattern: short 4- to 5-sec breath holds five to seven times per contraction Makes grunting sounds or expiratory vocalizations	Encourages respiratory pattern of short breath holds Stresses normality and benefits of grunting sounds and expiratory vocalizations Encourages bearing-down efforts with urge to push Encourages/suggests maternal movement and position changes (upright, if descent is not occurring) Encourages woman to "listen" to her body regarding movement and position change if descent is occurring Discourages long breath holds If birth is to occur in a delivery room, transfers woman to delivery room early to avoid rushing or, if permitted, offers her option of walking to delivery room Places woman in lateral recumbent position to slow descent if descent is too fast
Transitional Phase	
Behaves in manner similar to behavior during transition in first stage (8-10 cm) Experiences a sense of severe pain and powerlessness Shows decreased ability to listen Concentrates on birth of baby until head is born Experiences contractions as overwhelming in intensity Reports feeling ring of fire as head crowns Maintains respiratory pattern of three to five 7-sec breath holds per contraction, followed by forced expiration Eases head out with short expirations Responds with excitement and relief after head is born	Encourages slow, gentle pushing Explains that "blowing away the contraction" facilitates a slower birth of the head Provides mirror to help woman see or touch the emerging fetal head (best to extend over two to three contractions) to help her understand the perinatal sensations Coaches woman to relax mouth, throat, and neck to promote relaxation of pelvic floor Applies warm compress to perineum to promote relaxation

*Provided by nurses and support people in collaboration with the primary nurse.

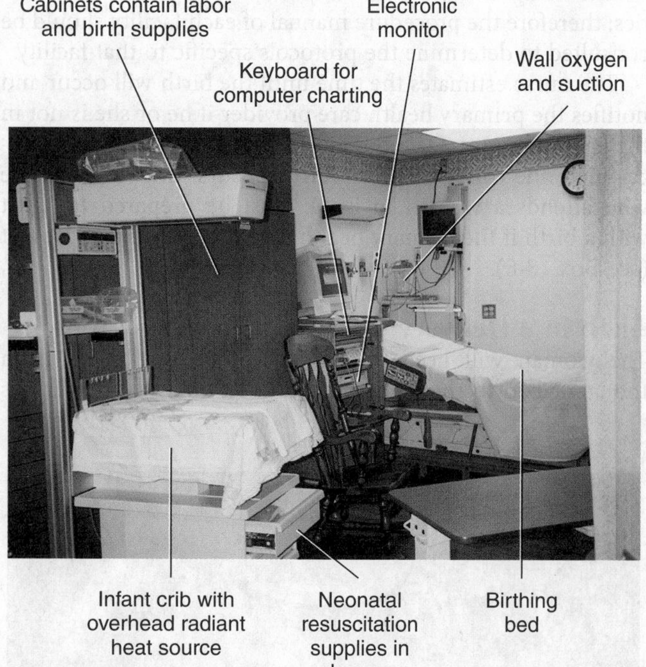

Fig. 18-18 Birthing room. *(Courtesy Dee Lowdermilk, Chapel Hill, NC.)*

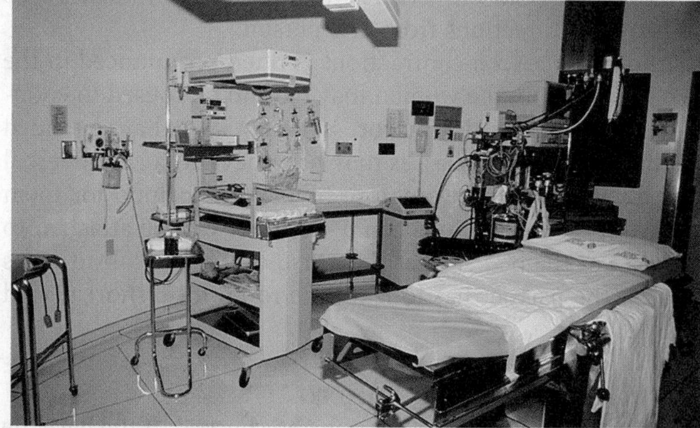

Fig. 18-19 Delivery room. *(Courtesy Michael S. Clement, MD, Mesa, AZ.)*

positions assumed for birth in a delivery room are the Sims' or lateral position in which the attendant supports the upper part of the woman's leg, the dorsal position (supine position with one hip elevated), and the lithotomy position.

The lithotomy position has been the position most commonly used for birth in Western cultures, although this practice is changing slowly. The lithotomy position makes it more convenient for the primary health care provider to deal with complications that arise. To place the woman in this position, her buttocks are brought to the edge of the table, and her legs are placed in stirrups. Care must be taken to pad the stirrups, raise and place both legs simultaneously, and adjust the shanks of the stirrups so that the calves of the legs are supported. There should be no pressure on the popliteal space. If the stirrups are not the same height, ligaments in the woman's back can be strained as she bears down, leading to considerable discomfort in the postpartum period. The lower portion of the table may be dropped down and rolled back under the table.

It should be noted that the routine use of a supine or lithotomy position for labor and birth has been identified as a clearly harmful or ineffective practice and should be discouraged (Enkin et al, 2000).

Birth in a Labor, Delivery, Recovery or Labor, Delivery, Recovery, Postpartum Room

The maternal position for birth varies from a lithotomy position with the woman's legs in stirrups to one in which her feet rest on footrests while she holds onto a squatting bar to a side-lying position with the woman's upper leg supported by the coach, nurse, or squatting bar. The foot of the bed can be removed so that the primary health care provider attending the birth can gain better perineal access for performing an episiotomy, delivering a large baby, using forceps or vacuum extractor, or gaining access to the emerging head to facilitate suctioning. Otherwise the foot of the bed is left in place and lowered slightly to form a ledge that allows access for birth and also serves as a place to lay the newborn (see Fig. 18-16, *A*).

Once the woman is positioned for birth, the vulva and perineum are cleansed. Hospital protocols and preferences of the primary health care provider for cleansing may vary.

The nurse continues to coach and encourage the woman. She auscultates the FHR or evaluates the electronic monitor tracing every 5 to 15 minutes, depending on whether the woman is at low or high risk for problems or per protocol of the birthing facility. She keeps the primary health care provider informed of the rate and pattern of the fetal heart. An oxytocic medication such as oxytocin (Pitocin) can be prepared so that it is ready to administer after expulsion of the placenta.

In the delivery room the primary health care provider puts on a cap, a mask that has a shield or protective eyewear, and shoe covers. Hands are scrubbed, a sterile gown (with waterproof front and sleeves) is donned, and gloves are put on. Nurses attending the birth may also need to wear caps, protective eyewear, masks, gowns, and gloves. The woman may then be draped with sterile drapes. In the birthing room Standard Precautions are observed, but the amount and types of protective coverings worn by those in attendance may vary (see Box 18-3).

Nursing contact with the parents is maintained by touching, verbal comforting, explaining the reasons for care, and sharing in the parents' joy at the birth of their child.

Water Birth

There is evidence that immersion in water during first-stage labor can reduce pain and anxiety and does not appear to affect neonatal outcomes adversely. However, the effects of immersion during birth and in the third stage have not been determined by randomized, controlled trials that have a large enough sample to make a determination about maternal and neonatal outcomes.

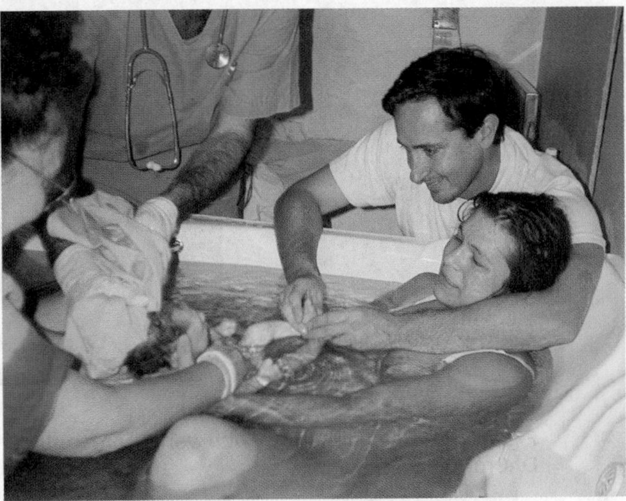

Fig. 18-20 Waterbirth. *(Courtesy Global Maternal/Child Health Association, Inc., Wilsonville, OR.)*

If a woman wishes to have a water birth (Fig. 18-20) in the United States, the newborn will usually be removed from the water immediately after birth (Waterbirth International, 2007). The infant can be placed in the mother's arms until the cord is cut. The woman usually is assisted from the tub to the bed to deliver the placenta.

Mechanism of Birth: Vertex Presentation

The three phases of spontaneous birth of a fetus in a vertex presentation are (1) birth of the head, (2) birth of the shoulders, and (3) birth of the body and extremities (see Chapter 15).

With voluntary bearing-down efforts, the head appears at the introitus (Fig. 18-21). Crowning occurs when the widest part of the head (the biparietal diameter) distends the vulva just before birth. The birth attendant may apply mineral oil to the perineum and stretch it as the head is crowning. Immediately before birth the perineal musculature becomes greatly distended. If an episiotomy (incision into the perineum to enlarge the vaginal outlet) is necessary, it is done at this time to minimize soft tissue damage. Local anesthetic is administered before the episiotomy.

The primary health care provider may use a hands-on approach to control the birth of the head, believing that guarding the perineum results in a gradual birth that will prevent fetal intracranial injury, protect maternal tissues, and reduce postpartum perineal pain. This approach involves (1) applying pressure against the rectum, drawing it downward to aid in flexing the head as the back of the neck catches under the symphysis pubis; (2) applying upward pressure from the coccygeal region (modified Ritgen maneuver) (Fig. 18-22) to extend the head during the actual birth, thereby protecting the musculature of the perineum; and (3) assisting the mother with voluntary control of the bearing-down efforts by coaching her to pant while letting uterine forces expel the fetus.

Some health care providers use a hands-poised (hands-off) approach when attending a birth. In this approach hands are prepared to place light pressure on the fetal head to prevent

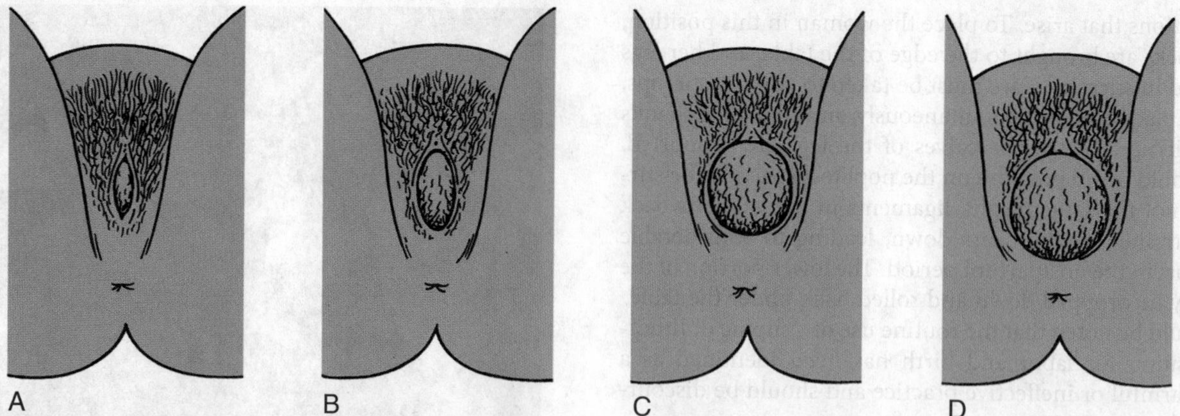

Fig. 18-21 Beginning birth with vertex presenting. A, Anteroposterior slit. B, Oval opening. C, Circular shape. D, Crowning.

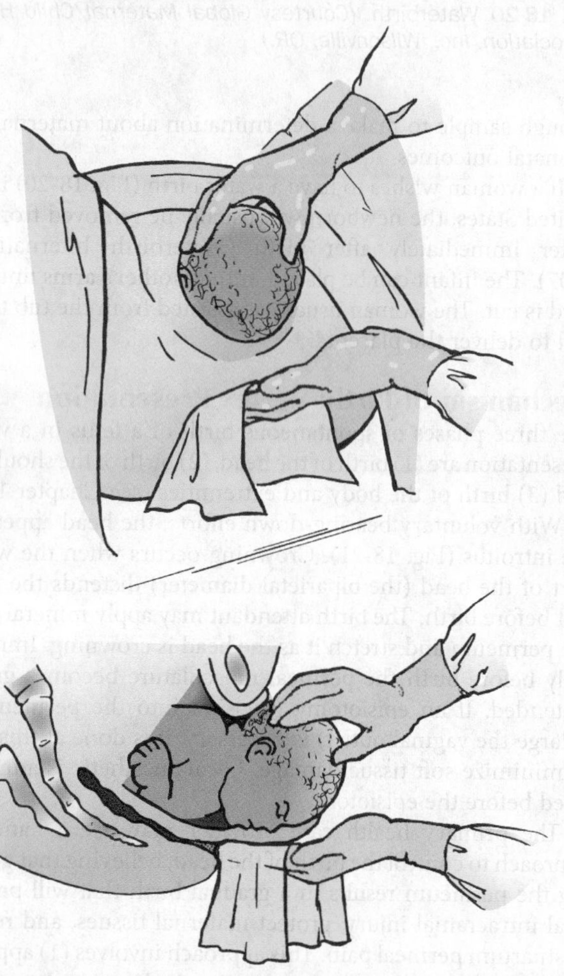

Fig. 18-22 Birth of head with modified Ritgen maneuver. Note control to prevent too rapid birth of head.

rapid expulsion. They are not placed on the perineum or used to assist with birth of the shoulders and body.

The hands-on and hands-poised approaches have similar results in terms of perineal trauma and condition of the newborn. However, perineal pain is slightly less 10 days after birth when the hands-on approach is used. Guarding the perineum is a form of care likely to be beneficial (Enkin et al, 2000).

The umbilical cord often encircles the neck (nuchal cord) but rarely so tightly as to cause hypoxia. After the head is born, gentle palpation is used to feel for the cord. If present, the cord should be slipped gently over the head. If the loop is tight or if there is a second loop, the cord is clamped twice, cut between the clamps, and unwound from around the neck before the birth is allowed to continue. Mucus, blood, or meconium in the nasal or oral passages may prevent the newborn from breathing. To eliminate this problem, moist gauze sponges are used to wipe the nose and mouth. The tip of a bulb syringe is inserted into the mouth and then the oropharynx to aspirate contents. The nares are cleared in the same fashion while the head is supported.

Management of Infant Born in Meconium-Stained Fluid

Meconium staining of the amniotic fluid occurs when the fetus passes meconium at some time before birth. Meconium-stained fluid is green in color. The consistency of the fluid is described as either thin (light) or thick (heavy), depending on the amount of meconium present. Meconium-stained fluid can indicate a nonreassuring fetal status. However, many infants with meconium staining exhibit no signs of depression at birth. The major risk with meconium-stained fluid is the development of meconium aspiration syndrome (see Chapter 27).

The International Liaison Committee on Resuscitation (ILCOR) (2006) and the American Heart Association (2006) have published treatment recommendations for initial resuscitation of the newborn that include peripartum management of meconium. The widely used practice of routinely suctioning meconium from the infant's airway after the head is born but before the shoulders are born is no longer recommended. This recommendation is based on studies that have yielded conflicting results about the value of this practice and the results of a large multicenter randomized trial that found that intrapartum suctioning of meconium does not decrease the incidence of meconium aspiration syndrome (Vain et al, 2004). ILCOR continues to recommend tracheal suctioning immediately after birth for meconium-stained depressed infants but not for meconium-stained infants who are at term gestation and vigorous.

NURSING ALERT Personnel skilled in neonatal resuscitation should be present for the birth of a meconium-stained infant (Miller, Fanaroff, & Martin, 2006).

Use of Fundal Pressure

Fundal pressure is the application of gentle, steady pressure against the fundus of the uterus to facilitate vaginal birth. Historically it has been used when the administration of analgesia and anesthesia decreased the woman's ability to push during the birth, for maternal exhaustion, or when second-stage fetal bradycardia or other nonreassuring FHR patterns were present. Use of fundal pressure by nurses is not advised because there is no standard technique available for this maneuver and no current legal, professional, or regulatory standards exist for its use. Fundal pressure is contraindicated in shoulder dystocia (see Critical Thinking Exercise). The all-fours position (the Gaskin maneuver), suprapubic pressure, and maternal position changes are among the recommended interventions.

CRITICAL THINKING EXERCISE

Applying Fundal Pressure

Myra is a gravida 1, para 0 who has been in labor for 18 hours; her cervix has been completely effaced and 10 cm dilated for 2½ hours; the station has been at +1 for 45 minutes. She has been pushing for 2 hours and is exhausted. To assist in descent of the fetus, the primary health care provider has asked you to apply fundal pressure while he stretches the vaginal orifice and perineum. What should be your response to this request?

1. Evidence—Is there sufficient evidence to draw conclusions about what your proper action should be?
2. Assumptions—What assumptions can be made about the following issues?
   a. Benefits of fundal pressure
   b. Risks of fundal pressure
   c. Contraindications to fundal pressure
   d. Alternative approaches to the use of fundal pressure
3. What implications and priorities for nursing care can be drawn at this time?
4. Does the evidence objectively support your conclusion?
5. Are there alternative perspectives to your conclusion?

Reference: Simpson KR, Knox GE: Fundal pressure during the second stage of labor: clinical perspectives and risk management issues, *MCN Am J Matern Child Nurs* 26(2):64-71, 2001.

Immediate Assessment and Care of the Newborn

The time of birth is the precise time when the entire body is out of the mother. This time must be noted on the record. If the condition of the newborn is not compromised, he or she may be placed on the mother's abdomen immediately after birth and covered with a warm, dry blanket. The cord can be clamped at this time, and the primary health care provider may ask if the woman's partner would like to cut the cord. If so, the partner is given a sterile pair of scissors and instructed to cut the cord 1 inch (2.5 cm) above the clamp.

Care given immediately after the birth focuses on assessing and stabilizing the newborn. The nurse's primary responsibility at this time is the infant because the primary health care provider is involved with the delivery of the placenta and care of the mother. The nurse must watch the infant for signs of distress and initiate appropriate interventions should any appear.

A brief assessment can be performed while the mother is holding the infant. This includes checking the infant's airway and obtaining the Apgar score. Maintaining a patent airway; supporting respiratory effort; and preventing cold stress by drying and placing the infant skin-to-skin on the mother's chest, covering the newborn with a warm blanket, or placing him or her under a radiant warmer are the major priorities for the newborn's immediate care. Further examination, identification procedures, and care can be postponed until later in the third stage of labor or early in the fourth stage.

Perineal Trauma Related to Childbirth

Lacerations

Most acute injuries and lacerations of the perineum, vagina, uterus, and their support tissues occur during childbirth. Some injuries to the supporting tissues, whether they were acute or nonacute and whether they were repaired or not, may lead to genitourinary and sexual problems later in life (e.g., pelvic relaxation, fistulas, uterine prolapse, cystocele, rectocele, dyspareunia, or urinary and bowel dysfunction).

During every birth some damage occurs to the soft tissues of the birth canal and adjacent structures. The tendency to sustain lacerations varies with each woman because the soft tissue in some women may be less distensible. Damage usually is more pronounced in nulliparous women because the tissues are firmer and more resistant than those in multiparous women. Heredity may also be a factor. For example, the tissue of light-skinned women, especially those with reddish hair, is not as readily distensible as that of darker-skinned women, and healing may be less efficient. The perineal skin and vaginal mucosa may appear intact, but numerous small lacerations in underlying muscle and its fascia may be obscured. Damage to pelvic supports usually is readily apparent and is repaired after birth.

Immediate repair promotes healing, limits residual damage, and decreases the possibility of infection. Immediately after birth the cervix, vagina, and perineum are inspected to look for damage. In addition, during the early postpartum period the nurse and primary health care provider continue to inspect the perineum carefully and evaluate lochia and symptoms to identify any previously missed damage.

Perineal Lacerations

If perineal lacerations are present, they usually occur when the fetal head is being born. The extent of the laceration is defined in terms of its depth:

First degree—Laceration extends through the skin and structures superficial to muscles.

Second degree—Laceration extends through muscles of perineal body.

Third degree—Laceration continues through anal sphincter muscle.

Fourth degree—Laceration also involves the anterior rectal wall.

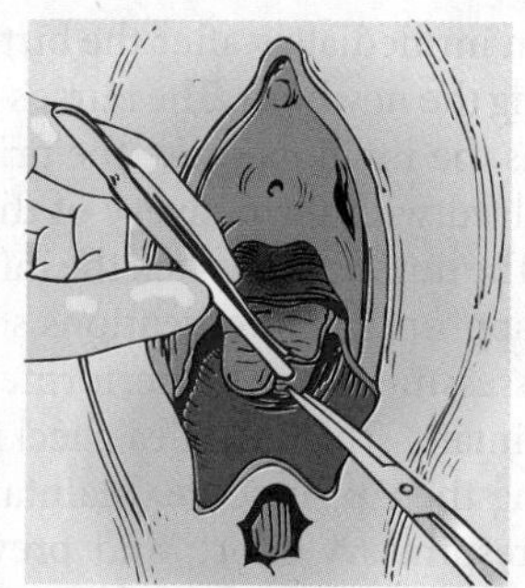

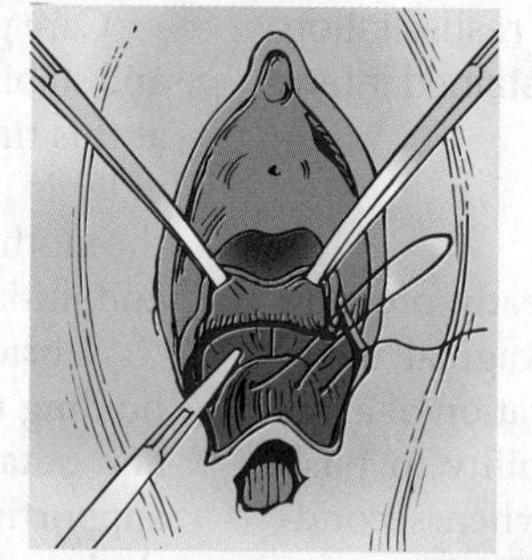

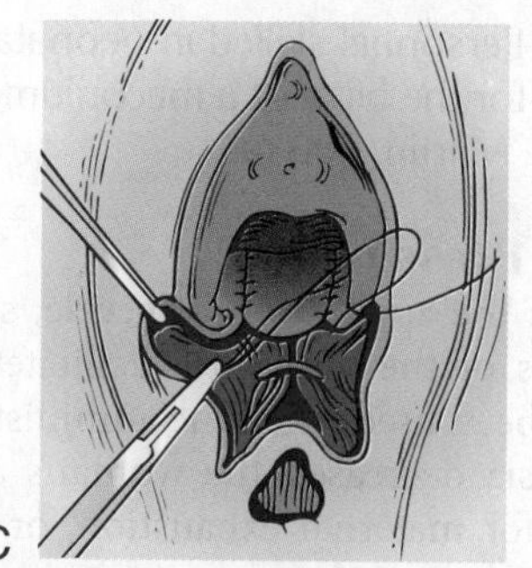

Fig. 18-23 Perineal lacerations. **A,** Bilateral sulcus tears, periurethral tear, and separation of anal sphincter. **B,** Exposure and approximation of levator ani structures. **C,** Approximation of torn bulbocavernous muscle.

Perineal injury is often accompanied by small lacerations on the medial surfaces of the labia minora below the pubic rami and to the sides of the urethra (periurethral) and clitoris. Lacerations in this highly vascular area often result in profuse bleeding. Such lacerations must be repaired with absorbable suture (Fig. 18-23).

Special attention must be paid to third- and fourth-degree lacerations so that the woman retains fecal continence. Measures are taken to promote soft stools (e.g., roughage, fluid, activity, and stool softeners) to increase the woman's comfort and foster healing. Antimicrobial therapy may be used in some cases. Enemas and suppositories are contraindicated for these women. Simple perineal injuries usually heal without permanent disability, regardless of whether they were repaired. However, it is easier to repair a new perineal injury to prevent sequelae than it is to correct long-term damage.

Vaginal and Urethral Lacerations

Vaginal lacerations often occur in conjunction with perineal lacerations. Vaginal lacerations tend to extend up the lateral walls (sulci) and, if deep enough, involve the levator ani. Additional injury may occur high in the vaginal vault near the level of the ischial spines. Vaginal vault lacerations may be circular and may result from use of forceps to rotate the fetal head or from rapid fetal descent or precipitous birth.

Cervical Injuries

Cervical injuries occur when the cervix retracts over the advancing fetal head. These cervical lacerations occur at the lateral angles of the external os; most are shallow, and bleeding is minimal. More extensive lacerations may extend to the vaginal vault or beyond it into the lower uterine segment; serious bleeding may occur. Extensive lacerations may follow hasty attempts to enlarge the cervical opening artificially or to deliver the fetus before full cervical dilation is achieved. Injuries to the cervix can have adverse effects on future pregnancies and childbirths.

Episiotomy

An episiotomy is an incision made in the perineum to enlarge the vaginal outlet. It is performed more commonly in the United States and Canada than in Europe. The side-lying position for birth causes less tension on the perineum, making possible a gradual stretching of the perineum with fewer indications for episiotomies. There is clear evidence that routine or liberal performance of an episiotomy for birth is a form of care that is likely to be harmful or ineffective (Enkin et al, 2000; Hofmeyr, 2005).

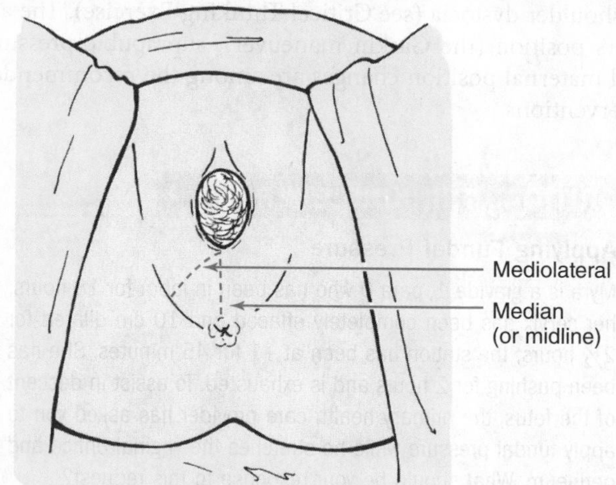

Fig. 18-24 Types of episiotomies.

Currently the practice in many settings is to manually support the perineum during birth and allow it to tear rather than perform an episiotomy. Tears are often smaller than an episiotomy, are repaired easily or not at all, and heal quickly. The pain and discomfort resulting from episiotomies can interfere with mother-infant interaction, breastfeeding, reestablishment of sexual relationship with partner, and even emotional recovery after birth. The rate of episiotomies is lower when nurse-midwives rather than obstetricians attend births.

The type of episiotomy is designated by the site and direction of the incision (Fig. 18-24). Midline (median) episiotomy is used most commonly in the United States. It is effective, easily repaired, and generally the least painful. However, it is associated with a higher incidence of third- and fourth-degree lacerations. Sphincter tone is usually restored following primary healing and a good repair.

Mediolateral episiotomy is used in operative births when the need for posterior extension is likely. Although a fourth-degree laceration may be prevented, a third-degree laceration may occur. The blood loss is greater, and the repair more difficult and painful than with midline episiotomies. It is more painful in the postpartum period, and the pain lasts longer.

Alternative measures for perineal management such as warm compresses and massage with a lubricant (e.g., prenatal and intrapartum) have limited effectiveness in reducing perineal trauma, although they may lessen the degree of perineal lacerations. Use of Kegel exercises in the prenatal and postpartum periods improves and restores the tone and strength of the perineal muscles. Health practices, including good nutrition and appropriate hygienic measures, help to maintain the integrity and suppleness of the perineal tissue, enhance healing, and prevent infection.

Emergency Childbirth

Even under the best of circumstances there probably will come a time when the perinatal nurse will be required to assist with the birth of an infant without medical assistance. Because it is neither possible nor desirable to prevent an impending birth, the perinatal nurse must be able to function independently and be skilled in the safe birth of a vertex fetus (Box 18-8).

A lateral Sims' position may be the position of choice for birth when (1) the birth is progressing rapidly and there is insufficient time for slow distention of the perineum; (2) the fetal head seems too large to pass through the introitus without laceration, and episiotomy is not possible; or (3) the apparent size of the fetus is consistent with possible shoulder dystocia. In the lateral Sims position less stress is placed on the perineum, and better visualization of the perineum is possible as the upper leg is supported by the woman's partner or the nurse (see Fig. 18-15, *A*). In the event of shoulder dystocia, the lateral Sims' position increases the space needed for birth.

Third Stage of Labor

The third stage of labor lasts from the birth of the baby until the placenta is expelled. The goal in the management of the third stage of labor is the prompt separation and expulsion of the placenta in the easiest, safest manner.

The placenta is attached to the decidual layer of the thin endometrium of the basal plate by numerous fibrous anchor villi. After the birth of the fetus, strong uterine contractions cause the placental site to shrink markedly. This causes the anchor villi to break and the placenta to separate from its attachments. Normally the first few strong contractions 5 to 7 minutes after the baby's birth cause the placenta to be sheared from the basal plate. A placenta cannot detach itself from a flaccid (relaxed) uterus because the placental site is not reduced in size.

Placental separation is indicated by the following signs (Fig. 18-25):

- A firmly contracting fundus
- A change in the uterus from a discoid to a globular ovoid shape as the placenta moves into the lower uterine segment
- A sudden gush of dark blood from the introitus

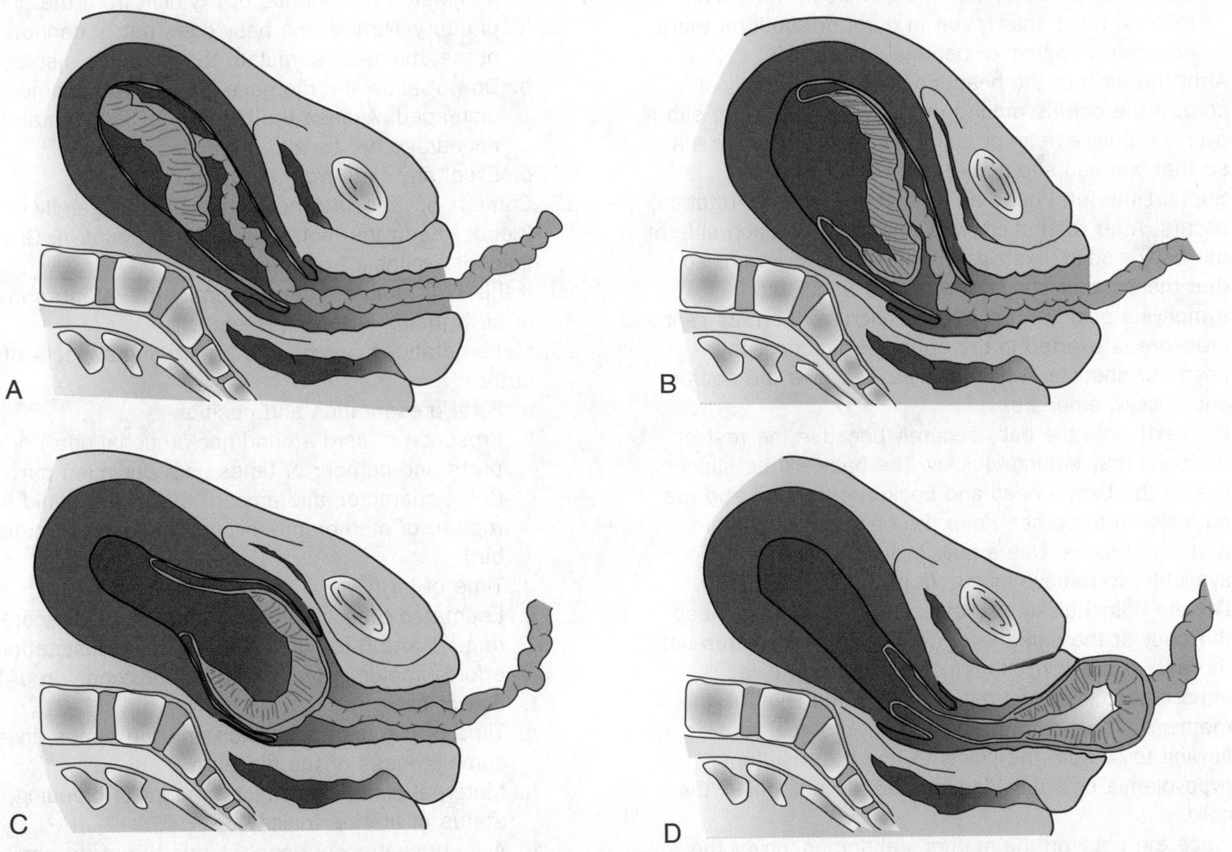

Fig. 18-25 Third stage of labor. **A,** Placenta begins the separation process in central portion with retroplacental bleeding. Uterus changes from discoid to globular shape. **B,** Placenta completes separation and enters lower uterine segment. Uterus is globular in shape. **C,** Placenta enters vagina, cord is seen to lengthen, and there may be increased bleeding. **D,** Expulsion (birth) of placenta and completion of third stage.

BOX 18-8 Guidelines for Assistance at the Emergency Birth of a Fetus in the Vertex Presentation

1. The woman usually assumes the position most comfortable for her. A lateral position is often recommended.
2. Reassure the woman that birth is usually uncomplicated and easy in these situations. Use eye-to-eye contact and a calm, relaxed manner. If someone else is available such as the partner, that person could help support the woman in the position, assist with coaching, and compliment her on her efforts.
3. Wash your hands and put on gloves if available.
4. Place under woman's buttocks whatever clean material is available.
5. Avoid touching the vaginal area to decrease the possibility of infection.
6. As the head begins to crown, you should do the following:
   a. Tear the amniotic membrane if it is still intact.
   b. Instruct the woman to pant or pant-blow, thus minimizing the urge to push.
   c. Place the flat side of your hand on the exposed fetal head and apply *gentle* pressure toward the vagina to prevent the head from "popping out." The mother may participate by placing her hand under yours on the emerging head. NOTE: Rapid delivery of the fetal head must be prevented because a rapid change of pressure within the molded fetal skull follows, which may result in dural or subdural tears and cause vaginal or perineal lacerations.
7. After the birth of the head, check for the umbilical cord. If the cord is around the baby's neck, try to slip it over the baby's head or pull it *gently* to get some slack so that you can slip it over the shoulders.
8. Support the fetal head as restitution (external rotation) occurs. After restitution, with one hand on each side of the baby's head, exert *gentle* pressure downward so that the anterior shoulder emerges under the symphysis pubis and acts as a fulcrum; then, as *gentle* pressure is exerted in the opposite direction, the posterior shoulder, which has passed over the sacrum and coccyx, emerges.
9. Be alert! Hold the baby securely because the rest of the body may emerge quickly. The baby will be slippery!
10. Cradle the baby's head and back in one hand and the buttocks in the other. Keep the head down to drain away the mucus. Use a bulb syringe, if one is available, to remove mucus from the baby's mouth.
11. Dry the baby quickly to prevent rapid heat loss. Keep the baby at the same level as the mother's uterus until the end of the cord stops pulsating. Note: It is important to keep the baby at the same level as the mother's uterus to prevent the baby's blood from flowing to or from the placenta and the resultant hypovolemia or hypervolemia. Also, do not "milk" the cord.
12. Place the baby on the mother's abdomen, cover the baby (remember to keep the head warm, too) with the mother's clothing, and have her cuddle the baby. Compliment her (them) on a job well done and on the baby, if appropriate.
13. *Wait* for the placenta to separate; do *not* tug on the cord. NOTE: Injudicious traction may tear the cord, separate the placenta, or invert the uterus. Signs of placental separation include a slight gush of dark blood from the introitus, lengthening of the cord, and change in the uterine contour from a discoid to globular shape.
14. Instruct the mother to push to deliver the separated placenta. Gently ease out the placental membranes using an up-and-down motion until the membranes are removed. If birth occurs outside a hospital setting, to minimize complications do not cut the cord without proper clamps and a sterile cutting tool. Inspect the placenta for intactness. Place the baby on the placenta and wrap the two together for additional warmth.
15. Check the firmness of the uterus. Gently massage the fundus and demonstrate to the mother how she can massage her own fundus properly.
16. If supplies are available, clean the mother's perineal area and apply a peripad.
17. In addition to gentle massage of the fundus, the following measures can be taken to prevent or minimize hemorrhage:
    a. Put the baby to the mother's breast as soon as possible. Sucking or nuzzling and licking the nipple stimulates the release of oxytocin from the posterior pituitary. NOTE: If the baby does not or cannot nurse, manually stimulate the mother's nipples.
    b. Do not allow the mother's bladder to become distended. Assess the bladder for fullness and encourage her to void if fullness is found.
    c. Expel any clots from the mother's uterus.
18. Comfort or reassure the mother and her family or friends. Keep the mother and the baby warm. Give her fluids if available and tolerated.
19. If this is a multifetal birth, identify the infants in order of birth (using letters *A, B,* etc.).
20. Make notations regarding the following aspects of the birth:
    a. Fetal presentation and position
    b. Presence of cord around neck (nuchal cord) or other parts and number of times cord encircled part
    c. Color, character, and amount of amniotic fluid if rupture of membranes occurs immediately before birth
    d. Time of birth
    e. Estimated time of determination of Apgar score (e.g., 1 and 5 minutes after birth), resuscitation efforts implemented, and ultimate condition of baby
    f. Sex of baby
    g. Time of placental expulsion and the appearance and completeness of the placenta
    h. Maternal condition: affect, amount of bleeding, and status of uterine tonicity
    i. Any unusual occurrences during the birth (e.g., maternal or paternal response, verbalizations, or gestures in response to birth of baby)

- Apparent lengthening of the umbilical cord as the placenta descends to the introitus
- The finding of vaginal fullness (the placenta) on vaginal or rectal examination or of fetal membranes at the introitus

Depending on the preferences of the primary health care provider, an expectant or active approach may be used to manage the third stage of labor. Expectant management (watchful waiting) involves the natural, spontaneous separation and expulsion of the placenta by efforts of the mother with clamping and cutting of the cord after pulsation ceases. It may involve the use of gravity or nipple stimulation to facilitate separation and expulsion, but no oxytocic (uterotonic) medications are given. A quiet, relaxed environment that supports close skin-to-skin contact between mother and newborn also promotes the release of endogenous oxytocin.

Active management facilitates placental separation and expulsion with administration of one or more oxytocic (uterotonic) medications after the birth of the anterior shoulder of the fetus, clamping and cutting of the umbilical cord immediately, and delivery of the placenta by application of controlled cord traction when signs of separation are noted. Research findings support the superiority of active management in terms of less blood loss and reduced risk of hemorrhage and other complications of the third stage of labor. Active management of the third stage of labor is a beneficial form of care (Enkin et al, 2000).

To assist in the delivery of the placenta, the woman is instructed to push when signs of separation have occurred. If possible, the placenta should be expelled by maternal effort during a uterine contraction. Alternate compression and elevation of the fundus plus minimal controlled traction on the umbilical cord may be used to facilitate delivery of the placenta and amniotic membranes. Oxytocics may be administered after the placenta is removed because they stimulate the uterus to contract, thereby helping to prevent hemorrhage.

Whether the placenta first appears by its shiny fetal surface (Schultze mechanism) or turns to show its dark roughened maternal surface (Duncan mechanism) is of no clinical importance. After the placenta and the amniotic membranes emerge, the primary health care provider examines them for intactness to ensure that no portion remains in the uterine cavity (i.e., no fragments of the placenta or membranes are retained) (Fig. 18-26).

Some women and their families may have culturally based beliefs regarding the care of the placenta and the manner of its disposal after birth, viewing the care and disposal of the placenta as a way of protecting the newborn from bad luck and illness. Requests by the woman to take the placenta home and dispose of it according to her customs may be at odds with health care agency policies, especially those related to infection control and the disposal of biologic wastes. Many cultures follow specific rules regarding the disposal of the placenta in terms of method (burning, drying, burying, or eating); site for disposal (in or near the home); and timing of disposal (immediately after birth, time of day, or by astrologic signs). Disposal rituals may vary according to the gender of the child and the length of time before another child is desired. If eaten, the placenta can be a means of restoring a woman's well-being after birth or ensuring quality breast milk. Health care providers can provide culturally sensitive health care by encouraging women and their families to express their wishes regarding the care and disposal of the placenta and establishing a policy to fulfill these requests (D'Avanzo, 2008).

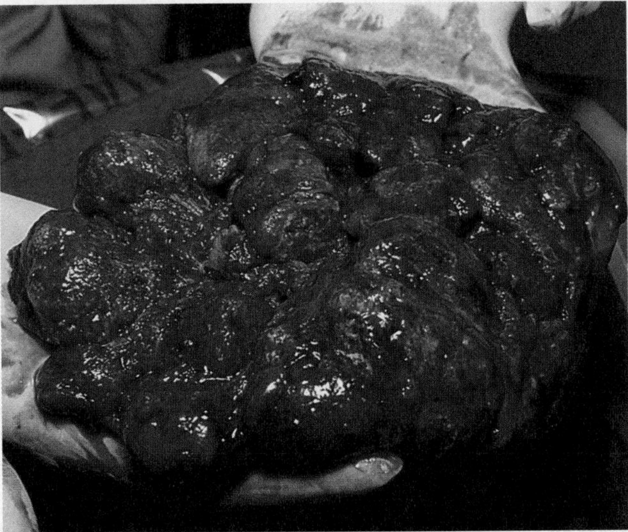

Fig. 18-26 Examination of the placenta. *(Courtesy Michael S. Clement, MD, Mesa, AZ.)*

Maternal Physical Status

Physiologic changes after birth are profound. The cardiac output increases rapidly as maternal circulation to the placenta ceases and the pooled blood from the lower extremities is mobilized. The pulse rate slows in response to the change in cardiac output and tends to remain slightly slower than before pregnancy for about 1 week.

Soon after the birth the woman's blood pressure usually returns to prepregnancy levels. Several factors contribute to an elevated blood pressure at this time: the excitement of the second stage, certain medications, and the time of day (blood pressure is highest during the late afternoon). Analgesics and anesthetics may also cause hypotension to develop in the hour after birth.

Signs of Potential Problems

The major risk for women during the third stage of labor is postpartum hemorrhage. While the primary health care provider completes the delivery of the placenta, the nurse observes the mother for signs of excessive blood loss, including alteration in vital signs, pallor, light-headedness, restlessness, decreased urinary output, and alteration in level of consciousness and orientation.

Because of the rapid cardiovascular changes taking place (e.g., the increased intracranial pressure during pushing and the rapid increase in cardiac output), the risks of rupture of a preexisting cerebral aneurysm and formation of pulmonary emboli are greater than usual during this period. Another dangerous, unpredictable problem is amniotic fluid embolism (see Chapter 19).

Women with a history of cardiac disorders are at increased risk for cardiac decompensation and pulmonary edema as a result of circulatory changes associated with the birth of the fetus and expulsion of the placenta. The nurse should carefully assess the woman's respiratory pattern and effort, especially in the early postpartum period.

Care After Placental Delivery

The woman may feel some discomfort when the placenta is delivered and while the primary health care provider carries out the postbirth vaginal examination. The nurse can encourage her to use breathing and relaxation or distraction techniques to help her cope with the discomfort.

While the mother is being examined, the nurse has an opportunity to complete an assessment of the newborn's physical condition. The baby can be weighed and measured; given a vitamin K injection; given an identification bracelet that corresponds to the mother's identification bracelet; wrapped in clean, warm blankets; and then given to the partner or back to the mother to hold when she is ready. In some agencies the father of the baby (or another person designated by the mother) is also given a corresponding identification bracelet. Administration of eye prophylaxis can be delayed to promote parent-newborn attachment.

When the third stage is complete and any lacerations are repaired or an episiotomy is sutured; the vulvar area is gently cleansed with warm, sterile water or normal saline solution; and a perineal pad or an ice pack is applied to the perineum (some agencies or primary health care providers may require the use of sterile technique for perineal care immediately after birth). The birthing table or bed is repositioned, and the woman's legs are lowered simultaneously if she gave birth in the lithotomy position. Drapes are removed, and dry linen is placed under the woman's buttocks; she is provided with a clean gown and a warm blanket. She is assisted into her bed if she is to be transferred from the birthing area to the recovery area. The side rails are raised during transfer. She may be given the baby to hold during the transfer, or the father or partner may carry the baby or transport it in a crib, either to the recovery area or to the nursery. If the woman labors, gives birth, and recovers in the same bed and room, she is refreshed following the protocol already described. Maternal and neonatal assessments for the fourth stage of labor are instituted. Box 18-9 summarizes normal vaginal childbirth.

Fourth Stage of Labor

The first 1 to 2 hours after birth, sometimes called the fourth stage of labor, is a crucial time for mother and newborn. Both not only are recovering from the physical process of birth but also are becoming acquainted with each other and additional family members. During this time maternal organs undergo their initial readjustment to the nonpregnant state, and the functions of body systems begin to stabilize. Meanwhile the newborn continues the transition from intrauterine to extrauterine existence.

The fourth stage of labor is an excellent time to begin breastfeeding because the infant is in an alert state and ready to nurse. Breastfeeding at this time also aids in the contraction of the uterus and the prevention of maternal hemorrhage. In most centers the mother remains in the labor and birth area during this recovery time. In an institution in which LDR rooms are used, the woman stays in the same room where she gave birth. In traditional settings women are taken from the delivery room to a separate recovery area for observation. Arrangements for care of the newborn vary during the fourth stage of labor. In many settings the baby remains at the mother's bedside, and the labor or birth nurse cares for both of them. In other institutions the baby is taken to the nursery for several hours of observation after an initial bonding period with the parents (see Fig. 21-6).

If the recovery nurse has not previously cared for the new mother, her assessment begins with an oral report from the nurse who attended the woman during labor and birth and a review of the prenatal, labor, and birth records. Of primary importance are conditions that could predispose the mother to hemorrhage such as precipitous labor, large baby, grand multiparity (having given birth many times), or induced labor. For healthy women hemorrhage is probably the most dangerous potential complication.

During the first hour in the recovery room, physical assessments of the mother are frequent. All factors except temperature are assessed every 15 minutes for 1 hour. Temperature is assessed at the beginning and end of the recovery period. After the fourth 15-minute assessment, if all parameters have stabilized within the normal range, assessments are continued every 30 minutes in the second hour. Box 18-10 describes the physical assessment of the mother during the fourth stage of labor.

During the fourth stage of labor many women experience intense tremors that resemble shivering from a chill. They are commonly seen and are not related to infection. Several theories have been offered to explain these tremors or shivering such as their being the result of a sudden release of pressure on pelvic nerves after birth, a response to a fetus-to-mother transfusion that occurred during placental separation, a reaction to maternal adrenaline production during labor and birth, or a reaction to epidural anesthesia. Warm blankets and reassurance that the chills or tremors are common and self-limiting and last only a short while are useful interventions.

The nutritional status of the woman is assessed. Restriction of food and fluid intake and the loss of fluids (blood, perspiration, or emesis) during labor cause many women to express a strong desire to eat or drink soon after birth. In the absence of complications, a woman who has given birth vaginally; has recovered from the effects of the anesthetic; and has stable vital signs, a firm uterus, and small-to-moderate lochial flow may have fluids and a regular diet as desired.

Postanesthesia Recovery

The woman who has given birth by cesarean or who has received regional anesthesia for a vaginal birth requires special attention during the recovery period. Obstetric recovery areas are held to the same standard of care that would be expected of any other postanesthesia recovery room. A recovery from anesthesia requires the nurse to have available cardiopulmo-

BOX 18-9 Normal Vaginal Childbirth

First Stage

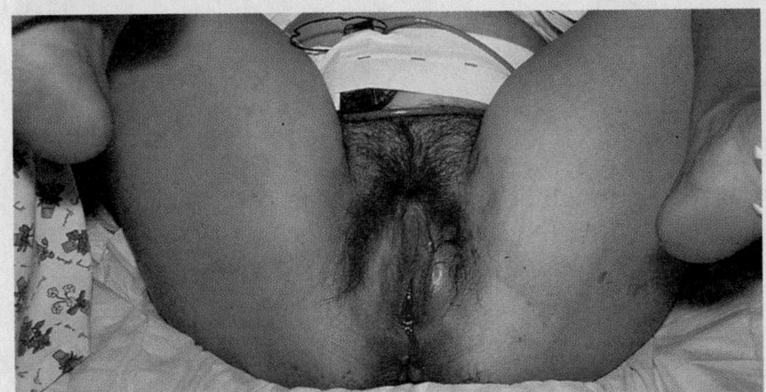

Anteroposterior slit; vertex visible during contraction.

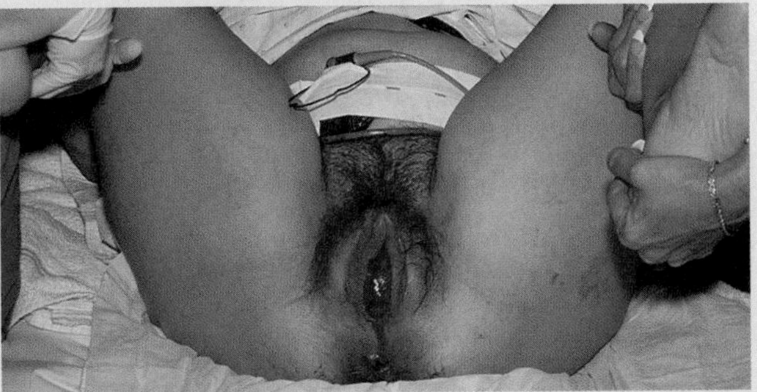

Oval opening; vertex presenting; NOTE: nurse *(on left)* is wearing gloves but support person *(on right)* is not.

Second Stage

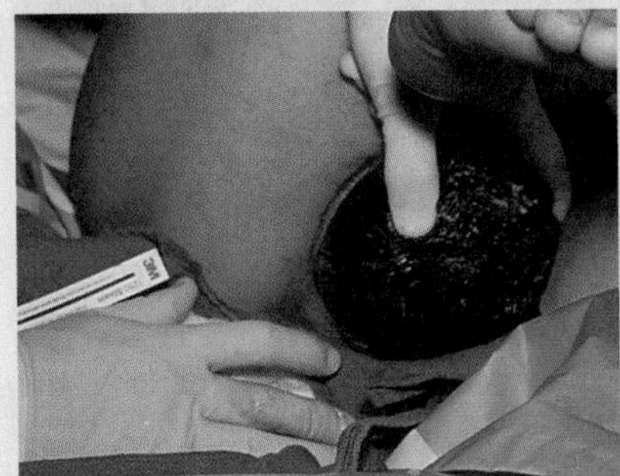

Crowning.

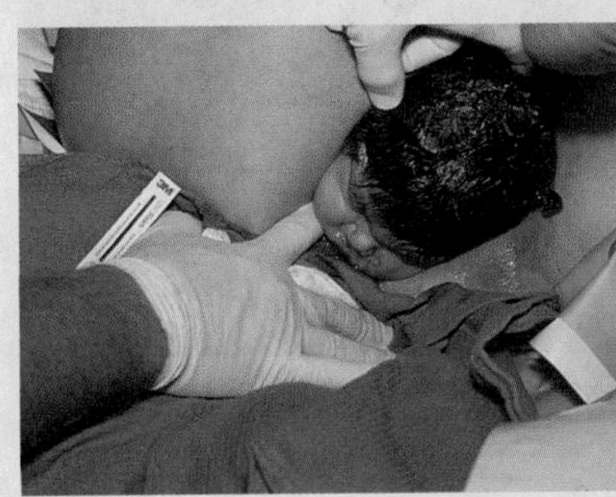

Nurse-midwife using Ritgen maneuver as head is born by extension.

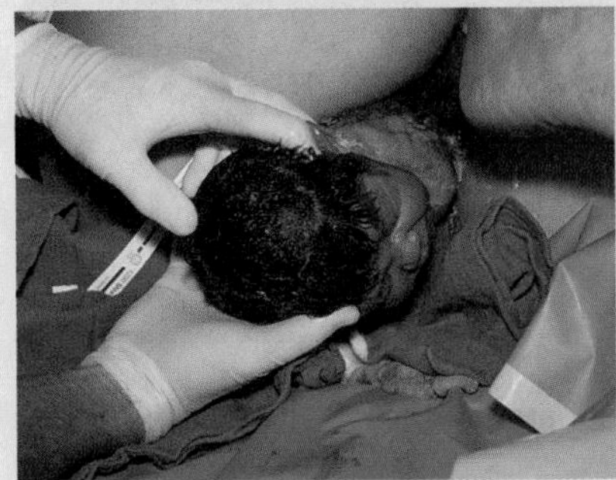

After nurse-midwife checks for nuchal cord, she supports head during external rotation and restitution.

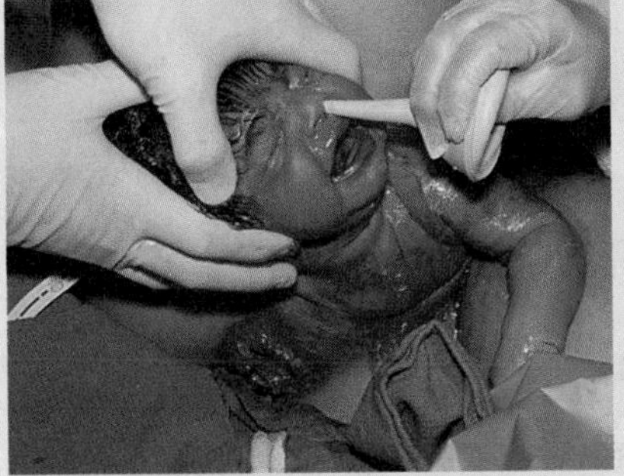

Use of bulb syringe to suction mucus.

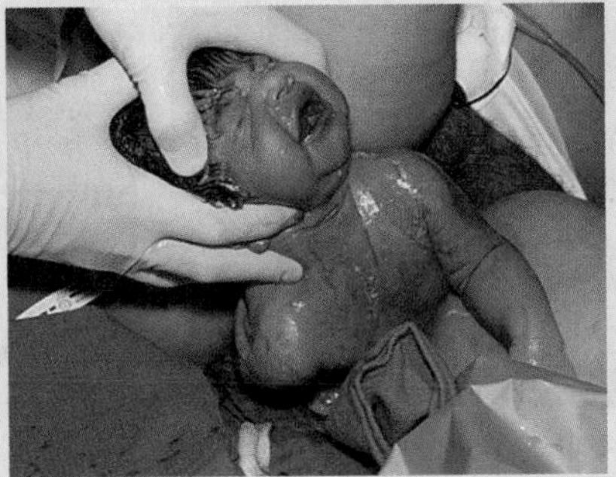

Birth of posterior shoulder.

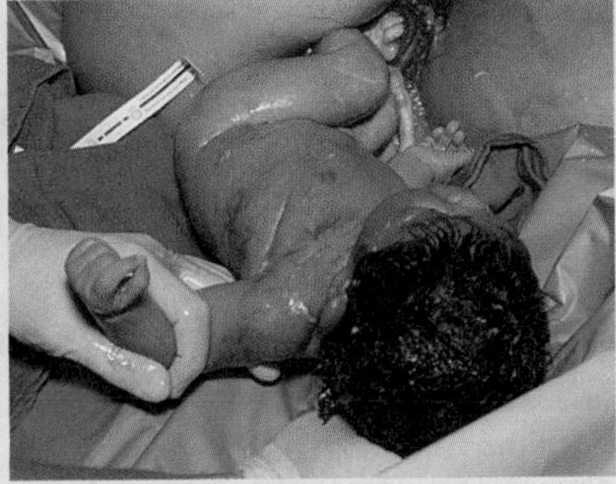

Birth of newborn by slow expulsion.

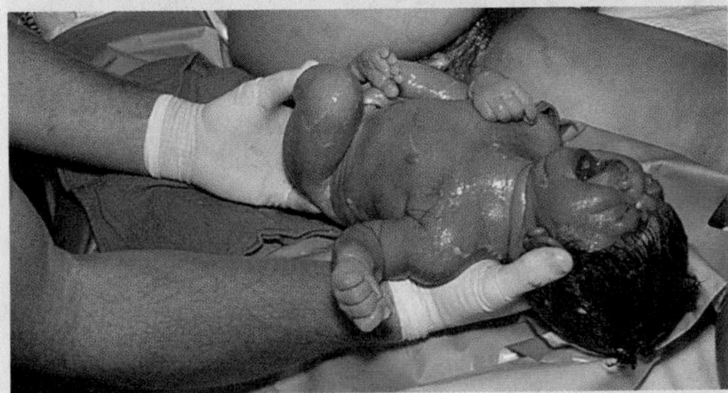

Second stage complete; note that newborn is not completely pink yet.

Continued

evolve Video—Childbirth (Vaginal)

BOX 18-9 Normal Vaginal Childbirth—cont'd

Third Stage

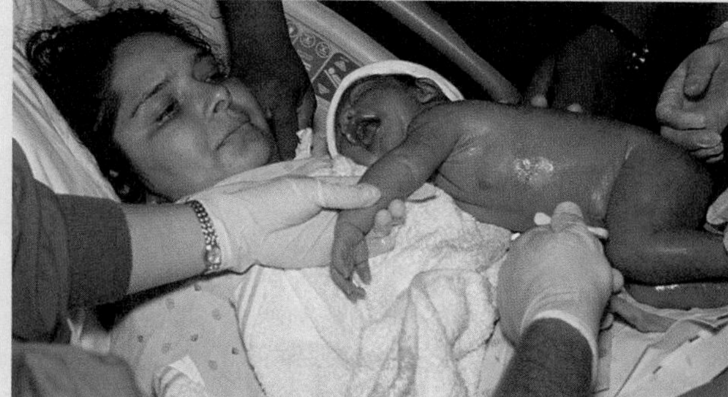

Newborn placed on mother's abdomen while cord is clamped and cut.

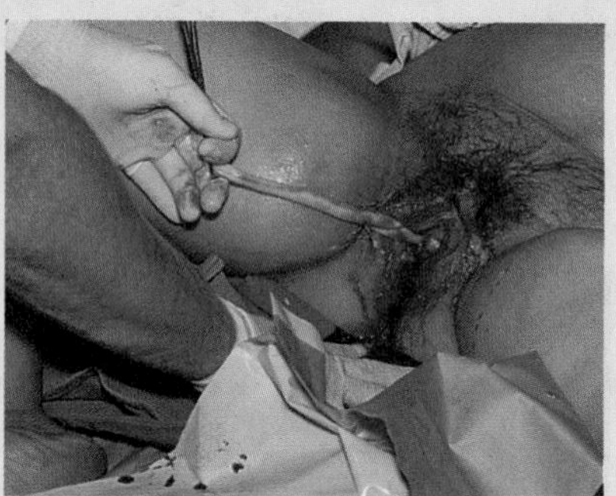

Note increased bleeding as placenta separates.

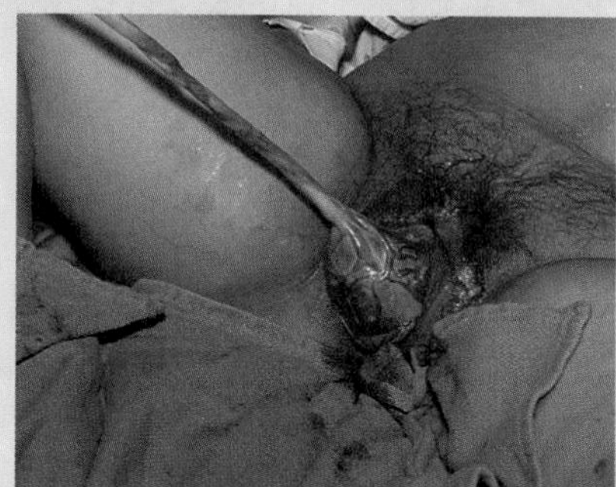

Expulsion of placenta.

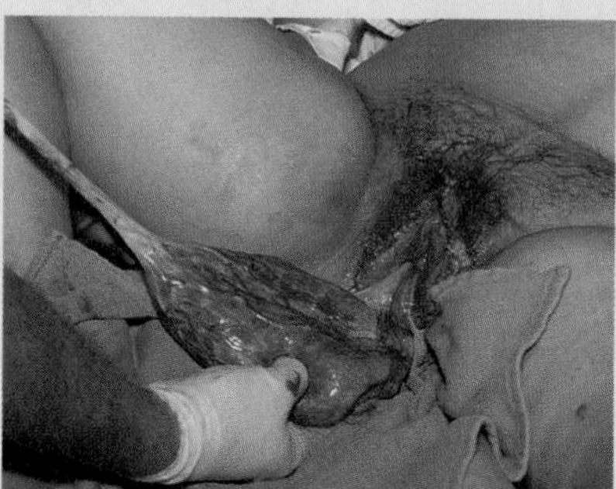

Expulsion is complete, marking the end of the third stage.

The Newborn

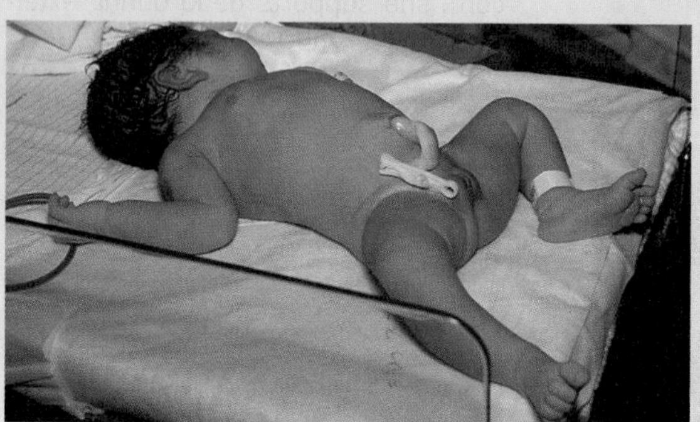

Newborn awaiting assessment; note that color is almost completely pink.

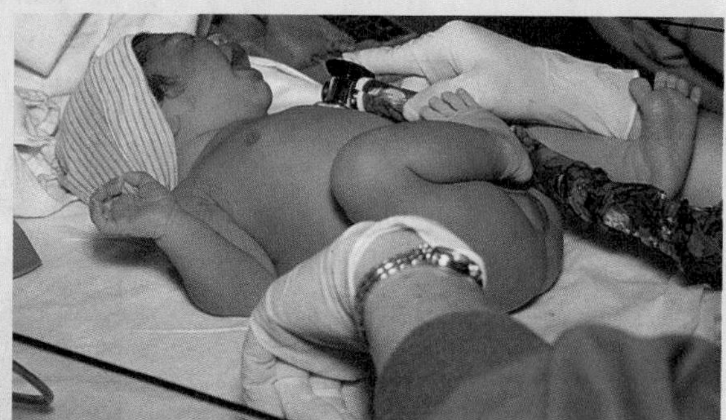

Newborn assessment under radiant warmer.

Parents admiring their newborn.

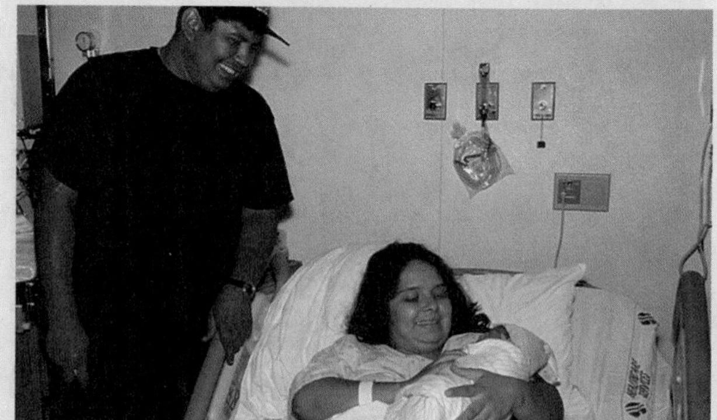

Courtesy Michael S. Clement, MD, Mesa, AZ.

evolve Animation–Vaginal Birth

BOX 18-10 Assessment During Fourth Stage of Labor

Before beginning the assessment, wash hands thoroughly, assemble necessary equipment, and explain the procedure to the patient.

Blood Pressure

Measure blood pressure per assessment schedule.

Pulse

Assess rate and regularity.

Temperature

Determine temperature.

Fundus

Put on clean examination gloves.
Position woman with knees flexed and head flat.
Just below umbilicus, cup hand and press firmly into abdomen. At the same time stabilize uterus at symphysis with the opposite hand.
If fundus is firm (and bladder is empty), with uterus in midline, measure its position relative to woman's umbilicus. Lay fingers flat on abdomen under umbilicus; measure how many fingerbreadths (fb) or centimeters (cm) fit between umbilicus and top of fundus. If the fundus is above umbilicus, this is recorded as plus fb or cm; if below, as minus fb or cm.
If fundus is not firm, massage it gently to contract and expel any clots before measuring distance from umbilicus.
Place hands appropriately; massage gently only until firm.
Expel clots while keeping hands placed as in Fig. 21-3.
With upper hand firmly apply pressure downward toward vagina; observe perineum for amount and size of expelled clots.

Bladder

Assess distention by noting location and firmness of uterine fundus and observing and palpating bladder. Distended bladder is seen as a suprapubic rounded bulge that is dull to percussion and fluctuates like a water-filled balloon. When bladder is distended, uterus is usually boggy in consistency, well above umbilicus and to woman's right side.
Assist woman to void spontaneously. Measure amount of urine voided.
Catheterize as necessary.
Reassess after voiding or catheterization to make sure that bladder is not palpable and fundus is firm and in the midline.

Lochia

Observe lochia on perineal pads and on linen under mother's buttocks. Determine amount and color; note size and number of clots; note odor.
Observe perineum for source of bleeding (e.g., episiotomy, lacerations).

Perineum

Ask or assist woman to turn on her side and flex upper leg on hip.
Lift upper buttock.
Observe perineum in good lighting.
Assess episiotomy site or laceration repair for intactness, hematoma, edema, bruising, redness, and drainage.
Assess for presence of hemorrhoids.

nary support and emergency supplies. A postanesthesia recovery (PAR) score is determined for each patient on her arrival and is updated as part of every 15-minute assessment. Components of the PAR score include activity, respirations, blood pressure, level of consciousness, and color.

NURSING ALERT Regardless of her obstetric status, no woman should be discharged from the recovery area until she has completely recovered from the effects of anesthesia.

If the woman received general anesthesia, she should be awake and alert and oriented to time, place, and person. Her respiratory rate should be within normal limits, and her oxygen saturation levels at least 95% as measured by a pulse oximeter. If the woman received epidural or spinal anesthesia, she should be able to raise her legs, extended at the knees, off the bed; or to flex her knees, place her feet flat on the bed, and raise her buttocks well off the bed. The numb or tingling, prickly sensation should be entirely gone from her legs. Women vary greatly in regard to length of time required to recover from regional anesthesia. Often it takes several hours for these anesthetic effects to disappear.

When fourth-stage recovery is complete, the woman will remain in her room if she is in an LDRP unit or transferred via wheelchair to a room on the postpartum unit if she gave birth in an LDR or delivery room.

Interactions with the Newborn

Most parents enjoy being able to handle, hold, explore, and examine the baby immediately after birth. Both parents can assist with the thorough drying of the infant. The infant may be wrapped in a receiving blanket and placed on the woman's abdomen. If skin-to-skin contact is desired, the unwrapped infant may be placed on the woman's abdomen and then covered with a warm blanket. Holding the newborn next to her skin helps the mother maintain the baby's body heat and provides skin-to-skin contact; care must be taken to keep the head warm as well. Stockinette caps are sometimes used to cover the newborn's head.

Many women wish to begin breastfeeding their newborns at this time to take advantage of the infant's alert state (first period of reactivity) and to stimulate the production of oxytocin, which promotes contraction of the uterus. Others prefer to wait until the newborn, parents, and older siblings are together in the recovery area. In some cultures breastfeeding is not considered acceptable until the milk comes in. In baby-friendly hospitals and many other hospitals, the baby is put to breast within the first hour after birth.

Family-Newborn Relationships

The woman's reaction to the sight of her newborn may range from excited outbursts of laughing, talking, and even crying to apparent apathy. A polite smile and nod may be her only acknowledgment of the comments of nurses and the primary health care provider. Occasionally the reaction is one of anger or indifference; the woman turns away from the baby, concentrates on her own pain, and may make hostile comments. These varied reactions can arise from pleasure, exhaustion, or deep disappointment. When evaluating parent-newborn interactions after birth, the nurse should also consider the cultural characteristics of the woman and her family and the expected behaviors of that culture. In some cultures the birth of a male child is preferred, and women may grieve when a female child is born (D'Avanzo, 2008).

Whatever the reaction and its cause may be, the woman needs continuing acceptance and support from all staff. Notation regarding the parents' reaction to the newborn can be made in the recovery record. Nurses can assess this reaction by asking themselves questions such as the following: How do the parents look? What do they say? What do they do? Further assessment of the parent-newborn relationship can be conducted as care is given during the period of recovery. This is especially important if warning signs (e.g., passive or hostile reactions to newborn, disappointment with sex or appearance of newborn, absence of eye contact, or limited interaction of parents with each other) were noted immediately after birth. The nurse may find it helpful to discuss with the woman's primary health care provider any warning signs that may have been noted.

Siblings who may have appeared only remotely interested in the final phases of the second stage tend to experience renewed interest and excitement when the newborn appears. They can then be encouraged to touch or hold the baby (Fig. 18-27).

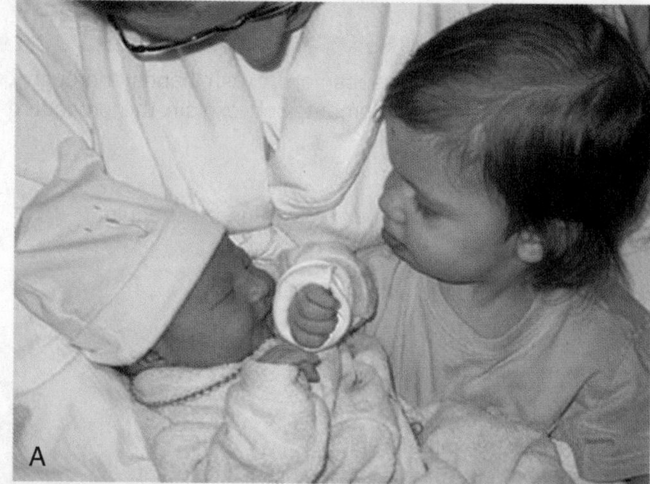
A

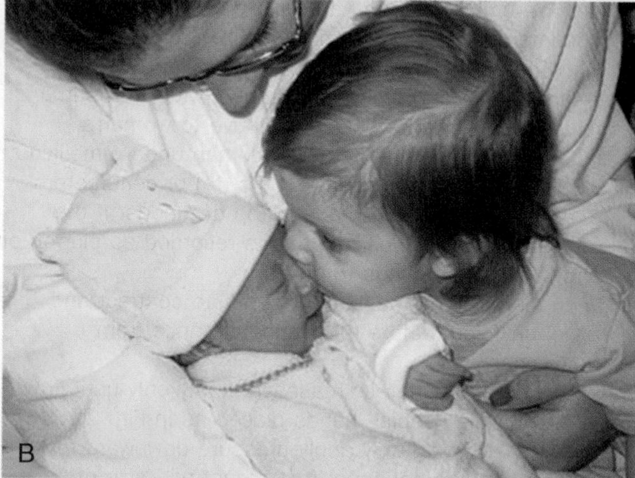
B

Fig. 18-27 Big sister being introduced to baby brother. **A,** Not sure who this new person is. **B,** A kiss says he is OK. *(Courtesy Rebekah Vogel, Ft. Collins, CO.)*

Parents usually respond to praise of their newborn. Many need to be reassured that the dusky appearance of the baby's extremities immediately after birth is normal until circulation is well established. If appropriate, the nurse should explain the reason for the molding of the newborn's head. Information about hospital routine can be communicated. However, it is important for nurses to recognize that the cultural background of the parents may influence expectations regarding care and handling of their newborn immediately after birth. For example, some traditional Southeast Asians believe that the head should not be touched because it is the most sacred part of a person's body. They also believe that praise of the baby is dangerous because jealous spirits may cause the baby harm or take it away (D'Avanzo, 2008). Hospital staff members, by their interest and concern, can provide an environment for making this time a satisfying experience for parents, family, and significant others.

Determining a woman's satisfaction with and impressions of her childbirth experience is a critical component in the provision of high-quality maternal-newborn health care that meets the individual needs of women and families using these services. Reviewing the childbirth experience with someone who will listen, support, and explain has been found to reduce the degree of postpartum depression experienced by many women during the first week or so after birth.

Key Points

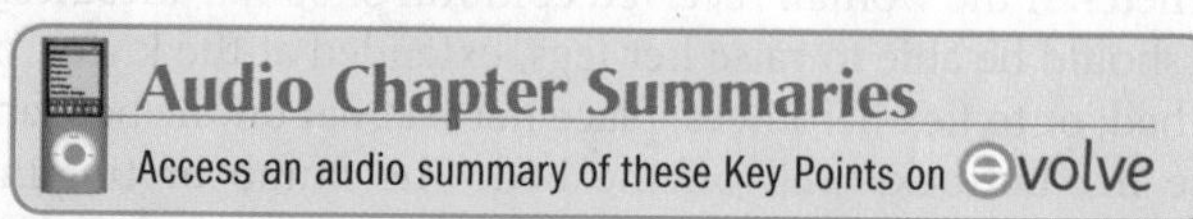
Audio Chapter Summaries
Access an audio summary of these Key Points on evolve

- The onset of labor may be difficult to determine for both nulliparous and multiparous women.
- The familiar environment of her home is most often the ideal place for a woman during the latent phase of the first stage of labor.
- The nurse assumes much of the responsibility for assessing the progress of labor and keeping the primary health care provider informed about progress in labor and deviations from expected findings.
- The FHR and pattern reveal the fetal response to the stress of the labor process.
- Regardless of the actual labor and birth experience, the woman's or couple's perception of the birth experience is most likely to be positive when events and performances

are consistent with expectations, especially in terms of maintaining control and adequacy of pain relief.

- The woman's level of anxiety may rise when she does not understand what is being said to her about her labor because of the medical terminology used or because of a language barrier.
- Coaching, emotional support, and comfort measures assist the woman to use her energy constructively in relaxing and working with the contractions.
- The progress of labor is enhanced when a woman changes her position frequently during the first stage of labor.
- Doulas provide a continuous supportive presence during labor that can have a positive effect on the process of childbirth and its outcome.
- The cultural beliefs and practices of a woman and her significant others, including her partner, can have a profound influence on their approach to labor and birth.
- The quality of the nurse-patient relationship is a factor in the woman's ability to cope with the stressors of the labor process.
- Women with a history of sexual abuse often experience profound stress and anxiety during childbirth.
- Inability to palpate the cervix during vaginal examination indicates that complete effacement and full dilation have occurred and is the only certain, objective sign that the second stage has begun.
- When allowed to respond to the rhythmic nature of the second stage of labor, the woman normally changes body position, bears down spontaneously, and vocalizes (open-glottis pushing) when she perceives the urge to push (Ferguson reflex).
- Women should bear down several times during a contraction using the open-glottis pushing method; sustained closed-glottis pushing should be avoided because oxygen transport to the fetus will be inhibited.
- Objective signs indicate that the placenta has separated and is ready to be expelled; excessive traction (pulling) on the umbilical cord, before the placenta has separated, can result in maternal injury.
- Siblings present for labor and birth need preparation and support for the event.
- Most parents/families enjoy being able to handle, hold, explore, and examine the baby immediately after birth.
- Nurses should observe progress in the development of parent-child relationships and be alert for warning signs that may appear during the immediate postpartum period.
- After an emergency childbirth out of the hospital, stimulation of the mothers' nipple manually or by the infant's suckling stimulates the release of oxytocin from the maternal posterior pituitary gland; oxytocin stimulates the uterus to contract and thereby prevents hemorrhage.
- A woman benefits from reviewing her childbirth experience with the nurse who managed her care during the process of labor and birth.

References

American College of Nurse-Midwives: Providing oral nutrition to women in labor, *J Midwifery Womens Health* 53(3):276-283, 2008.

American Heart Association: 2005 American Heart Association (AHA) guidelines for cardiopulmonary resuscitation (CPR) and emergency cardiovascular care (ECC) of pediatric and neonatal patient: pediatric basic life support, *Pediatrics* 117(5):e989-e1004, 2006.

Angelini D, Mahlmeister L: Liability in triage: Management of EMTALA regulations and common obstetric risks, *J Midwifery Womens Health* 50 (6):472-478, 2005.

Bashour H, Abdulsalam A: Syrian women's preferences for birth attendant and birth place, *Birth* 32(1):20-25, 2005.

Begay R: Changes in childbirth knowledge, *Am Indian Q* 28(3 & 4):550-565, 2004.

Brathwaite A, Williams C: Childbirth experiences of professional Chinese Canadian women, *J Obstet Gynecol Neonatal Nurs* 33(6):748-755, 2004.

Caliendo C et al: Obstetric triage and EMTALA: practice strategies for labor and delivery nursing units, *AWHONN Lifelines* 8(5):442-448, 2004.

Callister LC: What has the literature taught us about culturally competent care of women and children? *MCN Am J Matern Child Nurs* 30(6):380-388, 2005.

Cioffi J: Caring for women from culturally diverse backgrounds: midwives' experiences, *J Midwifery Womens Health* 49(5):437-442, 2004.

D'Avanzo CE: *Mosby's pocket guide to cultural health assessment*, ed 4, St Louis, 2008, Mosby.

Enkin M et al: *A guide to effective care in pregnancy and childbirth*, ed 3, Oxford, NY, 2000, Oxford University Press.

Hobbins D: Survivors of childhood sexual abuse: implications for perinatal nursing, *J Obstet Gynecol Neonatal Nurs* 33(4):485-497, 2004.

Hofmeyr G: Evidence-based intrapartum care, *Best Pract Res Clin Obstet Gynaecol* 19(1):103-115, 2005.

International Liaison Committee on Resuscitation (ILCOR): The International Liaison Committee on Resuscitation (ILCOR) consensus on science with treatment recommendations for pediatric and neonatal patients: neonatal resuscitation, *Pediatrics* 117(5):e978-e988, 2006.

Ito M, Sharts-Hopko N: Japanese women's experience of childbirth in the United States, *Health Care Women Int* 23 (6-7):666-677, 2002.

MacKinnon K, McIntyre M, Quance M: The meaning of the nurse's presence during childbirth, *J Obstet Gynecol Neonatal Nurs* 34(1):28-36, 2005.

McGrath SK, Kennell JH: A randomized controlled trial of continuous labor support for middle-class couples: effect on cesarean delivery rates, *Birth* 35(2):92-97, 2008.

Miller M, Fanaroff A, Martin R: Respiratory disorders: preterm and term infants. In Martin R, Fanaroff A, Walsh M (editors): *Fanaroff and Martin's neonatal-perinatal medicine: diseases of the fetus and infant*, ed 8, Philadelphia, 2006, Mosby.

Molina JW: Traditional Native American practices in obstetrics, *Clin Obstet Gynecol* 44(4):661-670, 2001.

Sampselle C et al: Provider support of spontaneous pushing during the second stage of labor, *J Obstet Gynecol Neonatal Nurs* 34(6):695-702, 2005.

Simkin P, Klaus P: *When survivors give birth*, Seattle, Wash, 2004, Classic Day.

Simkin P, Way K: *Doulas of North America (DONA) International Position Paper: the birth doula's contribution to modern maternity care*, 2008. Available at www.DONA.org (accessed October 6, 2008).

Simpson K: The context and clinical evidence for common nursing practices during labor, *MCN Am J Matern Child Nurs* 30(6):356-363, 2005.

Simpson K, James D: Effects of immediate versus delayed pushing during second-stage labor on fetal well-being: a randomized clinical trial, *Nurs Res* 54(3):149-157, 2005.

Tucker SM, Miller LA, Miller DA: *Pocket guide to fetal monitoring and assessment*, ed 6, St Louis, 2009, Mosby.

Vain N et al: Oropharyngeal and nasopharyngeal suctioning of meconium-stained neonates before delivery of their shoulders: multicentre, randomized controlled trial, *Lancet* 364 (9434):597-602, 2004.

Waterbirth International: *Frequently asked questions: how long is the baby in the water?* 2007. Available at www.waterbirth.org (accessed October 7, 2008).

Yildirim G, Beji NK: Effects of pushing techniques in birth on mother and fetus: a randomized study, *Birth* 35(1):31-32, 2008.

Unit 4

19 Labor and Birth at Risk

Learning Objectives

On completion of this chapter the reader will be able to:

- Differentiate between preterm birth and low birth weight.
- Identify risk factors for preterm labor and birth.
- Discuss current interventions to prevent preterm labor and birth.
- Discuss the use of tocolytics and antenatal glucocorticoids in preterm labor and birth.
- Evaluate the effects of prescribed bed rest on pregnant women and their families.
- Design a nursing care management plan for women with preterm premature rupture of the membranes.
- Summarize the nursing care management for a trial of labor, induction and augmentation of labor, forceps- and vacuum-assisted birth, cesarean birth, and vaginal birth after a cesarean birth.
- Describe the care of a woman experiencing postterm pregnancy.
- Discuss obstetric emergencies and their appropriate management.

Electronic Resources

Additional information related to the content in Chapter 19 can be found on

evolve the Companion Website at
http://evolve.elsevier.com/Perry/maternal/

- NCLEX Review Questions
- Animation—Breech Birth
- Animation—Breech Examination
- Animation—Cord Prolapse
- Animation—Shoulder Dystocia
- Case Study—Postdate Pregnancy
- Case Study—Preterm Labor
- Nursing Care Plan—Dysfunctional Labor: Hypotonic Uterine Dysfunction with Protracted Active Phase
- Nursing Care Plan—Preterm Labor
- Spanish Guidelines—Cesarean Birth
- Spanish Guidelines—Induction of Labor
- Video—Childbirth (Cesarean)

When complications arise during labor and birth, perinatal morbidity and mortality risks increase. Some complications may be anticipated, especially if the woman is identified as high risk during the antepartum period; others are unexpected or unforeseen. The woman, her family, and the health care team can feel devastated when things go wrong. Nurses must recognize these feelings if they are to provide effective support. It is crucial for nurses to understand the normal birth process to prevent and detect deviations from normal labor and birth and implement nursing measures when complications arise. Optimum care of the laboring woman, the fetus, and the family with complications is possible only when the nurse and other members of the obstetric team use their knowledge and skills in a concerted effort to provide care. This chapter focuses on the problems of preterm labor and birth, dystocia, postterm pregnancy, and obstetric emergencies.

Preterm Labor and Birth

Preterm labor is defined as cervical changes and uterine contractions occurring between 20 and 37 weeks of pregnancy. *Preterm birth* is any birth that occurs before the completion of 37 weeks of pregnancy. Preterm labor and preterm birth are the most serious complications of pregnancy because they lead to about 90% of all neonatal deaths, with more than 75% of these deaths occurring in infants born at fewer than 32 weeks of gestation. Preterm birth is second only to congenital anomalies as a cause of infant death. In 2005 the overall preterm birth rate for all races in the United States was 12.7%. The very low preterm birth rate (birth that occurs before the completion of 32 weeks of pregnancy) was 2.03% in 2005 (Martin et al, 2007).

Preterm Birth vs. Low Birth Weight

Although they have distinctly different meanings, the terms *preterm birth* or *prematurity* and *low birth weight* are often used interchangeably. Preterm birth describes length of gestation (i.e., less than 37 weeks regardless of the weight of the infant), whereas low birth weight describes only weight at the time of birth (i.e., 2500 g or less). Low birth weight is far easier to measure than preterm birth; thus in many settings and publications low birth weight has been used as a substitute term for preterm birth. However, preterm birth is a more dangerous health condition for an infant because length of time in the uterus correlates with immaturity of body systems. Low-birth-weight babies can be but are not necessarily preterm. Pregnant women who are poorly nourished or have various complications of pregnancy that interfere with uteroplacental perfusion such as gestational hypertension may give birth to a baby at term who is low birth weight because of intrauterine growth restriction (IUGR).

The incidence of preterm birth in the United States is increasing and varies according to race; the 2005 rate for non-Hispanic black women (18.4%) was considerable higher than that for Hispanics (12.1%) and non-Hispanic white women (11.7%) (Martin et al, 2007). The increase in rates is attributed largely to the increase in multiple births.

Sociodemographics may play a part in the race-based differences in preterm birth. Preterm birth rates are higher among socially disadvantaged populations, including minorities, women with low levels of education, and women who receive late or no prenatal care (Martin et al, 2007; Maupin et al, 2004). The preterm birth rate is higher among women younger than 15 years of age or older than 45 years (Martin et al, 2007). Multifetal pregnancy from in vitro fertilization also is associated with an increase in preterm births.

Predicting Preterm Labor and Birth

The known risk factors for preterm birth are shown in Box 19-1. The risk factors most commonly associated with preterm labor and birth are a history of preterm birth, race (i.e., non-Hispanic black women), and multiple gestation (Martin et al, 2007) (see Critical Thinking Exercise). Using these risk factors, researchers have tried to determine which women might go into labor prematurely. However, no risk-scoring system has resulted in lowering the preterm birth rate in the United States because at least 50% of all women who ultimately give birth prematurely have no identifiable risk factors (Martin et al, 2007). In 2005 The March of Dimes began a 5-year, $75 million campaign to address the problems of prematurity. The Association of Women's Health, Obstetric and Neonatal Nurses (AWHONN), the American College of Obstetrics and Gynecologists (ACOG), and the American Academy of Pediatrics (AAP) are professional organizations that have partnered in this project. AWHONN helped to increase screening for known risk factors and to teach women the signs and symptoms of preterm labor.

Biochemical Markers

The two most common biochemical markers used in an effort to predict who might experience preterm labor are fetal fibronectin and salivary estriol.

Fetal fibronectins are glycoproteins found in plasma and produced during fetal life. They appear in the cervical canal early in pregnancy and again in late pregnancy. Their appearance between 24 and 34 weeks of gestation predicts labor. The test is done during a vaginal examination.

Endocervical Length

Another possible predictor of imminent preterm labor is endocervical length. Some studies have suggested that a shortened cervix precedes preterm labor and can be determined by ultrasound measurement. Women whose cervical length is more than 30 mm before 34 weeks of gestation are less likely to have a preterm birth than women whose cervical length is less than 30 mm (Iams, Romero, & Creasy, 2009). When a woman has a short cervix combined with a positive fetal fibronectin result, her risk for spontaneous preterm birth is substantially higher than that for women positive for only one marker or none at all (Iams, Romero, & Creasy, 2009).

BOX 19-1 Risk Factors for Preterm Labor

Demographic Risks
Nonwhite race
Age (less than 15 years or more than 35 years)
Low socioeconomic status
Unmarried
Less than high school education

Biophysical Risks
Previous preterm labor or birth
Second-trimester abortion (more than two spontaneous or therapeutic); stillbirths
Grand multiparity; short interval between pregnancies (1 year or less since last birth); family history of preterm labor and birth
Progesterone deficiency
Uterine anomalies or fibroids; uterine irritability
Cervical insufficiency, trauma, shortened length
Exposure to diethylstilbestrol or other toxic substances
Medical diseases (e.g., diabetes, hypertension, anemia)
Small stature (less than 119 cm in height; less than 45.5 kg or underweight for height)
Current pregnancy risks:
- Multifetal pregnancy
- Hydramnios
- Bleeding
- Placental problems (e.g., placenta previa, abruptio placentae)
- Infections (e.g., pyelonephritis, recurrent urinary tract infections, asymptomatic bacteriuria, bacterial vaginosis, chorioamnionitis)
- Gestational hypertension
- Premature rupture of the membranes
- Fetal anomalies
- Inadequate plasma volume expansion; anemia

Behavioral-Psychosocial Risks
Poor nutrition; weight loss or low weight gain
Smoking (more than 10 cigarettes a day)
Substance abuse (e.g., alcohol; illicit drugs, especially cocaine)
Inadequate prenatal care
Commutes of more than 1½ hours each way
Excessive physical activity (heavy physical work, prolonged standing, heavy lifting, young child care)
Excessive lifestyle stressors

From Gilbert ES: *Manual of high risk pregnancy & delivery,* ed 4, St Louis, 2007, Mosby; Iams JD, Romero R: Preterm birth. In Gabbe SG, Niebyl JR, Simpson JL (editors): *Obstetrics: normal and problem pregnancies,* ed 5, New York, 2007, Churchill Livingstone; Varney H: *Varney's textbook for midwives,* ed 4, Sudbury, Mass, 2004, Jones & Bartlett.

evolve Case Study–Preterm Labor

Causes of Preterm Labor and Birth

The cause of preterm labor may be unknown and is assumed to be multifactorial (Cunningham et al, 2005) (Box 19-2).

CRITICAL THINKING EXERCISE

Preterm Labor

You are assigned to Yolanda, who is experiencing preterm labor at 28 weeks of gestation. She has a 2-year-old son at home. This is her third admission for preterm labor during this pregnancy. Her primary health care provider had told her she must remain hospitalized on bed rest until she reaches 37 weeks of gestation or until birth of the baby, whichever comes first. She tearfully asks you why she can't be at home on bed rest, who will help care for her son, and how she will manage to keep from going crazy staying in bed that long. How will you respond to her concerns?

1. Evidence—Is there sufficient evidence to draw conclusions about the benefits of bed rest to prevent preterm birth?
2. Assumptions—What assumptions can be made about the following issues?
   a. The impact her history might have on the medical and nursing care she receives during this pregnancy
   b. The pros and cons of home management vs. hospital management for the prevention of preterm birth for this woman
   c. Ways to reduce the frustration and boredom that the woman will experience if she is restricted to bed rest for the next several weeks
   d. Resources available to assist with care of her 2-year-old son
3. What implications and priorities for nursing care can be drawn at this time?
4. Does the evidence objectively support your conclusion?
5. Are there alternative perspectives to your conclusion?

BOX 19-2 Multifactorial Etiology of Preterm Labor and Birth

Maternal Behaviors
- Smoking
- Substance use (alcohol or illegal drugs)
- Poor nutrition
- Work/fatigue
- Short interpregnancy interval
- Sexual activity

Maternal Characteristics
- Young or older age
- Previous preterm birth
- Short stature
- Short cervix
- Uterine anomalies
- Diethylstilbestrol exposure
- Prematurely dilated cervix
- Low prepregnancy weight
- Race (e.g., African-American, Hispanic)
- Unmarried
- Low socioeconomic status
- Victim of domestic violence

Other Factors
- Inadequate support systems
- Stress
- Uterine irritability
- Multiple gestation
- Late or no prenatal care
- Preterm premature rupture of membranes
- Anemia
- Infection
- Catecholamine release
- Decreased progesterone production
- Decidual cell disruption
- Prostaglandin synthesis
- Cytokine release

Infection is thought to be a major etiologic factor in some preterm labors, but trials of antibiotic therapy for all women at risk have not resulted in statistically significant reductions in preterm births (Iams, Romero, & Creasy, 2009). When cervical, bacterial, or urinary tract infections are present, the risk of preterm birth is increased. Thus early continuous and comprehensive prenatal care, which can detect and treat infection, is essential in dealing with this aspect of preterm birth prevention.

Recent evidence has demonstrated a link between periodontal infection and preterm labor and birth as a result of increased levels of prostaglandins released by the causative pathogens. Although research is ongoing, recommendations for all pregnant women include regular dental care before and during pregnancy, oral assessment as part of prenatal health care, and strict oral hygiene measures (e.g., brushing teeth, using dental floss, rinsing with baking soda and water after vomiting) (Wener & Lavigne, 2004).

Not all preterm births can or even should be prevented. About 25% of all preterm births are indicated (i.e., babies are intentionally delivered prematurely because of pregnancy complications that put the life or health of the fetus or the mother in danger and not because of preterm labor). Another 25% are preceded by spontaneous rupture of membranes (preterm premature rupture of membranes [PPROM]) followed by labor and are not known to be preventable. Therefore only about 50% of preterm births can possibly be prevented and are considered idiopathic preterm births (Iams, Romero, & Creasy, 2009).

Sociodemographic factors such as poverty, low educational level, lack of social support, smoking, little or no prenatal care, domestic violence, and stress are thought to contribute to the 50% of the preterm births that may be preventable (Iams, Romero, & Creasy, 2009). If prenatal care programs are to be effective in reducing the rate of preterm labor and birth, they must address these sociodemographic factors and develop strategies to attract all women to participate, including those at high risk for preterm labor.

Nursing Care Management

Preconception and prenatal care should be made available to all women. This care should focus on performing ongoing holistic risk assessment, encouraging women to participate in health-promoting activity (e.g., good nutrition, exercise, stress

NURSING PROCESS: PRETERM LABOR

Assessment

Nursing assessment begins at the time of entry to prenatal care. It is essential that nurses teach pregnant women how to detect the early symptoms of preterm labor.

History

Review prenatal record (parity, estimated date of birth, previous preterm pregnancies/births)

Dental health

Cervical, bacterial, or urinary tract infections

Domestic violence

Interview

Symptoms of preterm labor

Activities that trigger symptoms (e.g., sexual activity, carrying heavy loads, heavy housework)

Psychosocial and emotional status of the woman

Impact of treatment on woman and her family

Physical Examination

Ultrasound examination of cervical length

Cervical status

Evidence of rupture of membranes

Uterine activity

Fetal heart rate

Review of Results of Laboratory Tests

Fetal fibronectin (if done)

Salivary estriol (if done)

Nursing Diagnoses

Nursing diagnoses relevant for women at risk for preterm birth include the following:

Deficient knowledge related to
– recognition of preterm labor symptoms

Risk for excess maternal fluid volume related to
– administration of tocolytics to suppress preterm labor

Impaired mobility related to
– prescribed bed rest

Risk for complicated grieving related to
– potential for birth of preterm infant

Planning

A plan of care is developed for each woman to address her particular clinical and nursing problems. The nurse collaborates with the primary health care provider and the woman to provide home or hospital care as appropriate.

Expected outcomes include that the woman will do the following:

- Learn the symptoms of preterm labor and be able to assess herself and her need for intervention
- Follow teaching suggestions and call her primary health care provider if symptoms occur
- Not experience preterm symptoms or, if she does, take appropriate action
- Maintain her pregnancy for at least 37 completed weeks
- Give birth to a healthy, full-term infant

Interventions

Teach woman early recognition of preterm labor symptoms.

Teach woman what to do if symptoms of preterm labor occur.

Support woman at home on bed rest.

Modify home environment for woman's convenience.

Monitor uterine activity.

Provide telephone support.

Administer tocolytics and antenatal glucocorticoids as prescribed.

If preterm birth in inevitable, transfer woman to tertiary care center.

Evaluation

Evaluation of the nursing care provided a woman at risk for preterm labor is based on the expected outcomes of care (see Nursing Care Plan).

management), and implementing appropriate medical and psychosocial interventions (see Nursing Process box).

Prevention

Prevention strategies that address risk factors associated with preterm labor and birth are less costly in human and financial terms than the high-tech and often lifelong care required by preterm infants and their families (Box 19-3). Programs aimed at health promotion and disease prevention that encourage healthy lifestyles for the population in general and women of childbearing age in particular should be developed to prevent preterm labor and birth. One of the most important nursing interventions aimed at preventing preterm birth is the education of pregnant women about the early symptoms of preterm labor so that, if symptoms occur, the woman can be referred promptly to her care provider for more intensive care (Fritz & Smith, 2008) (Box 19-4). Patient education regarding any symptoms of regular contractions or cramping between 20 and 37 weeks of gestation should be directed toward telling the woman that these symptoms are not normal discomforts of pregnancy and that contractions or cramping that does not go away, that becomes regular in timing, and/or that increases in intensity should prompt the woman to contact her primary health care provider. Because no one can discriminate between Braxton Hicks contractions and the contractions of early preterm labor, Freda and Patterson (2001) suggest that the term *Braxton Hicks contractions* be eliminated from teaching about pregnancy expectations (Fig. 19-1).

Some women wait hours or days before contacting a health care provider after preterm labor symptoms have begun. Women may ignore the symptoms because of ignorance regarding their significance or a belief that the symptoms are expected during pregnancy. The symptoms may be attributed to other factors such as the flu, incontinence of urine, or working too hard. Some women become more vigilant, waiting to see if the symptoms subside, go away, or become worse.

NURSING CARE PLAN — Preterm Labor

Nursing Diagnosis: Deficient knowledge related to recognition of preterm labor

Expected Outcome

Woman and partner (if applicable) delineate the signs and symptoms of preterm labor.

Nursing Interventions/*Rationales*

Assess what the woman and partner know about abnormal signs and symptoms during pregnancy *to identify areas of deficit.*

Discuss signs and symptoms that serve as warning signs of preterm labor *so that the woman or her partner has adequate information to identify problems early.*

Provide written supplemental materials that include a list of warning signs and instructions regarding what to do if any of the listed signs occur *so that the couple can reinforce and review learning and act swiftly and appropriately should a sign occur.*

Discuss and demonstrate how to assess and time the contractions *to provide needed skills to assess the signs of labor.*

Nursing Diagnosis: Risk for maternal/fetal injury related to recurrence of preterm labor

Expected Outcome

Woman demonstrates ability to assess self and fetus for signs of recurring labor; maternal-fetal well-being is maintained.

Nursing Interventions/*Rationales*

Teach woman/partner how to monitor fetal and uterine contraction activity daily *to provide immediate evidence of a worsening condition.*

Have woman/partner report rupture of membranes, vaginal bleeding, cramping, pelvic pressure, or low backache to appropriate health care resource immediately *because such symptoms are signs of labor.*

If home uterine activity monitoring is to be used, teach woman/partner how to use the monitoring device and how to transmit the data to the health care provider via telephone *to enhance correct use of monitoring device and increase the accuracy of detection of early labor.*

Have woman monitor her weight, diet, fluid intake, and vital signs on a daily basis *to evaluate for potential problems.*

Use a side-lying position *to enhance placental perfusion.*

Teach woman signs and symptoms of thrombophlebitis and encourage gentle exercise of lower extremities *because pregnancy and limited activity increase risk for clot formation.*

Abstain from sexual intercourse and nipple stimulation *because such activities may stimulate uterine contractions.*

Practice relaxation techniques *to decrease uterine tone and anxiety and stress.*

Take tocolytic or other medications per physician's orders *to inhibit uterine contractions.*

Teach woman/partner about and have them report any medication side effects immediately *to prevent medication-induced complications.*

Have family arrange for alternative strategies in carrying out the woman's usual roles and functions *to decrease stress and limit temptations to increase activity.*

If small children are part of the household, encourage family to make alternative arrangements for child care *to enhance woman's adherence to bed rest protocol.*

Nursing Diagnosis: Anxiety related to preterm labor and potentially premature neonate

Expected Outcome

Feeling and symptoms of anxiety are reduced.

Nursing Interventions/*Rationales*

Provide a calm, soothing atmosphere and teach family to provide emotional support *to facilitate coping.*

Encourage verbalization of fears *to decrease intensity of emotional response.*

Involve woman and family in the home management of her condition *to promote a greater sense of control.*

Help the woman identify and use appropriate coping strategies and support systems *to reduce fear/anxiety.*

Explore the use of desensitization strategies such as progressive muscle relaxation, visual imagery, or thought stopping *to reduce fear-related emotions and related physical symptoms.*

Nursing Diagnosis: Deficient diversional activity related to imposed bed rest

Expected Outcome

The woman will verbalize diminished feelings of boredom.

Nursing Interventions/*Rationales*

Assist woman to creatively explore personally meaningful activities that can be pursued from the bed *to ensure activities that have meaning, purpose, and value to the individual.*

Maintain emphasis on personal choices of the woman *to promote control and minimize imposition of routines by others.*

Evaluate what support and system resources are available in the environment *to assist in providing diversional activities.*

Explore ways for the woman to remain an active participant in home management and decision making *to promote control.*

Engage support of family and friends in carrying out chosen activities and making necessary environmental alterations *to ensure success.*

Encourage woman to use the Internet to communicate with other women on bed rest *to obtain support and share feelings.*

Teach woman about stress management and relaxation techniques *to help manage tension of confinement.*

They may take action by seeking advice about what to do from family or friends, resting more, increasing fluid intake, taking a bath, or rubbing the back or abdomen. Persistence of symptoms and increasing severity finally compel women to seek health care. Waiting too long to see a health care provider could result in inevitable preterm birth without the benefit of the administration of antenatal glucocorticoids (i.e., medication given to accelerate fetal lung maturity). In this event the neonate is born at higher risk for respiratory distress syndrome and intraventricular hemorrhage.

BOX 19-3 Progesterone Supplementation to Prevent Preterm Labor

In 2003 the American College of Obstetricians and Gynecologists (2003a) issued a committee opinion that a weekly injection of progesterone can be used to help prevent preterm birth. The use of progesterone for this purpose should be restricted to pregnant women who have a history of preterm birth before 37 weeks. The treatment must be administered before the occurrence of symptoms of labor. The treatment is not effective for women at risk for preterm birth because of multiple gestation.

References: Farino D et al: The use of progesterone for prevention of preterm birth, *J Obstet Gynaecol Can* 30(1):67-77, 2008; Meis PJ, Aleman A: Progesterone treatment to prevent preterm birth, *Drugs* 64(21):2463-2474, 2004; Spong CY: Prediction and prevention of recurrent spontaneous preterm birth, *Obstet Gynecol* 110(2pt1):405-415, 2007.

BOX 19-4 Signs and Symptoms of Preterm Labor

Uterine Activity

Uterine contractions more frequent than every 10 minutes, persisting for 1 hour or more

Uterine contractions painful or painless

Discomfort

Lower abdominal cramping similar to gas pains; may be accompanied by diarrhea

Dull, intermittent low back pain (below the waist)

Painful, menstrual-like cramps

Suprapubic pain or pressure

Pelvic pressure or heaviness

Urinary frequency

Vaginal Discharge

Change in character and amount of usual discharge: thicker (mucoid) or thinner (watery), bloody, brown or colorless, increased amount, odor

Rupture of amniotic membranes

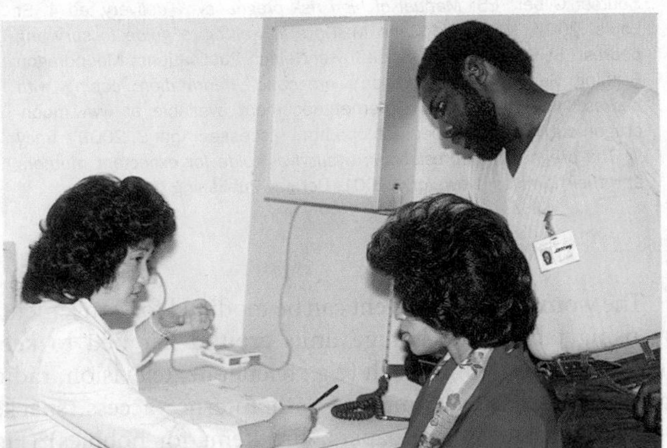

Fig. 19-1 Nurse teaching woman signs and symptoms of preterm labor. *(Courtesy Marjorie Pyle, RNC, Lifecircle, Costa Mesa, CA.)*

Early Recognition and Diagnosis

Early recognition of preterm labor is essential to successfully implement interventions such as tocolytic therapy and administration of antenatal glucocorticoids. The diagnosis of preterm labor is based on three major diagnostic criteria:

1. Gestational age between 20 and 37 weeks
2. Uterine activity (contractions)
3. Progressive cervical change (e.g., cervical effacement of 80% or cervical dilation of 2 cm or greater)

If the presence of fetal fibronectin is used as another diagnostic criterion, a sample of cervical mucus for testing should be obtained before an examination for cervical changes because the lubricant used to examine the cervix can reduce the accuracy of the test for fetal fibronectin.

The pregnant woman at 30 weeks of gestation with an irritable uterus but no documented cervical change is not in preterm labor. Misdiagnosis of preterm labor can lead to inappropriate use of pharmacologic agents that can be dangerous to the health of the woman, the fetus, or both (Iams & Romero, 2007).

Lifestyle Modifications

Nurses caring for women with symptoms of preterm labor should question the women about whether they have symptoms when engaged in any of the following activities:

- Sexual activity
- Riding long distances in automobiles, trains, or buses
- Carrying heavy loads such as laundry, groceries, or a small child
- Standing more than 50% of the time
- Heavy housework
- Climbing stairs
- Hard physical work
- Being unable to stop and rest when tired

If symptoms occur when the woman is engaged in any of these activities, the woman should consider what she was doing when the symptoms began and consider stopping those activities until 37 weeks of pregnancy when preterm birth is no longer a risk. Counseling about lifestyle modifications should be individualized; only women who have symptoms of preterm labor when they are engaged in certain activities need to alter their lifestyles. There are no specific rules for which activities are safe for pregnant women and which are not. For example, sexual activity is not contraindicated during pregnancy. However, if symptoms of preterm labor occur after sexual activity, such activity may need to be curtailed until 37 weeks of gestation.

Bed Rest

Bed rest is a commonly used intervention for the prevention of preterm labor. Although frequently prescribed, bed rest is not a benign intervention, and there is no evidence in the literature to support the efficacy of this intervention in reducing preterm birth rates. It is a form of care of unknown effectiveness (Enkin et al, 2000; Sosa et al, 2004; Sprague et al, 2008). The deleterious effects of bed rest on women are well known (Box 19-5). Symptoms often are not resolved by 6 weeks postpartum (Maloni & Park, 2005).

The father's constant worry about his partner and baby and increased stress with the assumption of new roles and responsibilities when bed rest is prescribed for his partner

BOX 19-5 Adverse Effects of Bed Rest

Maternal Effects (Physical)

Weight loss; indigestion; loss of appetite
Muscle wasting, weakness; aching muscles
Potential for thrombus formation and thromboembolism
Bone demineralization and calcium loss
Decreased plasma volume and cardiac output
Increased clotting tendency; risk for thrombophlebitis
Alteration in bowel function
Sleep disturbance, fatigue
Prolonged postpartum recovery

Maternal Effects (Psychosocial)

Loss of control associated with role reversals
Dysphoria—anxiety, depression, hostility, and anger
Guilt associated with difficulty complying with activity restriction and inability to meet role responsibilities
Boredom, loneliness
Emotional lability (mood swings); difficulty concentrating
Increased stress

Effects on Support System

Stress associated with role reversals, increased responsibilities, and disruption of family routines
Financial strain associated with loss of maternal income and cost of treatment
Fear and anxiety regarding well-being of the mother and fetus

have also been documented. Bed rest is costly for society; the estimated economic costs are based on lost wages, household help and child care expenses, and hospital costs. Prolongation of pregnancy does not necessarily occur despite the increased costs incurred.

Women on bed rest need support and encouragement whether they are at home or hospitalized. Nurses can create support groups of hospitalized women on bed rest. Family, friends, and Internet resources (e.g., *www.pregnancybedrest.com* and *www.sidelines.com*), including chat rooms for women on bed rest at home, can be important sources of support for women and reduce the sense of isolation they can feel. Interacting with other women experiencing preterm labor and bed rest has been found to be highly therapeutic.

Health care providers must recognize the difficulty that women face when placed on bed rest. When these women try to do too much, nurses can explore with them the realities of their daily lives and work with them to set realistic guidelines for activity limitations that they will follow, thereby avoiding feelings of cheating and its associated guilt. This approach can help to communicate to women that the nurses empathize with the impact that bed rest has on their lives and the lives of their families (Sprague, 2004).

Home Care

The home care of the woman at risk for preterm birth is a challenge for the nurse, who must help the woman and her family deal with the many difficulties faced by families in which one member is incapacitated. The scope of care given to women in their homes ranges from occasional visits to monitor the maternal and fetal condition to daily telephone consultation and reading of uterine monitoring strips.

Regardless of the frequency of the visits, nursing care for the woman and family in the home demands organization and a sense of just how this family's life has been disrupted by the loss of activity of this essential family member. Families who are often anxious regarding the health status of the mother and baby may need help in learning how to organize time and space or restructure family routines so that the pregnant woman can remain a part of family activity while still maintaining bed rest. The nurse should also assist the family members to explore their feelings regarding the anxieties of preterm labor and help them share their feelings with each other. The Home Care and Family-Centered Care boxes detail activities for women on bed rest and for their children.

HOME CARE

Suggested Activities for Women on Bed Rest

- Set a routine for daily activities (e.g., getting dressed, moving from the bedroom to a "day bed rest place," having social time, eating meals, self-monitoring fetal and uterine activity).
- Do passive exercises as allowed.
- Review childbirth education information or have a childbirth class at home if this can be arranged.
- Plan menus and make up grocery shopping lists.
- Shop by phone or Internet.
- Read books about high risk pregnancy or other topics.
- Keep a journal of the pregnancy.
- Keep a calendar of your progress.
- Reorganize files, recipes, household budget.
- Update address book.
- Do mending, sewing.
- Listen to audiotapes, watch videos or television.
- Do crossword puzzles, jigsaw puzzles, Sudoku, etc.
- Do craft projects; make something for the baby.
- Put pictures in photo albums.
- Call or email a friend, family member, or support person each day.
- Treat yourself to a facial, manicure, neck massage, or other special treat when you need a lift.

Source: Gilbert ES: *Manual of high risk pregnancy & delivery,* ed 4, St Louis, 2007, Mosby; McCann M: *Days in waiting: a guide to surviving bedrest,* St Paul, MN, 2003, deRuyter-Nelson Publications; Moondragon Birthing Services: *Moondragon's pregnancy information: coping with bedrest during pregnancy.* Internet document available at www.moondragon.org/pregnancy/bedrestcope.html (accessed April 3, 2009); Tracy A: *The pregnancy bedrest book: a survival guide for expectant mothers and their families,* New York, 2001, Berkley Publishing Group.

The woman's environment can be modified for convenience by using tables and storage units around her bed to keep essential items within reach (e.g., telephone, television, radio, tape or CD player, computer with Internet access, snacks, books, magazines, newspapers, and items for hobbies) (Fig. 19-2). Ensuring that the bed or couch is near a window and the bathroom is also helpful. Covering the bed with an egg

FAMILY-CENTERED CARE

Activities for Children of Women on Bed Rest

- Schedule brief play periods throughout the day.
- Keep a few favorite toys in a box or basket close to the bed or couch.
- Read to the child or children.
- Put puzzles together.
- Watch videos, play video games (remote control for television is ideal).
- Play cards or board games.
- Color in coloring books.
- Cut out pictures from magazines and paste on cardboard.
- Play bed basketball with a soft (sponge) ball or rolled up sock and a trash can or empty laundry basket.

Source: McCann M: *Days in waiting: a guide to surviving bedrest*, St Paul, MN, 2003, deRuyter-Nelson Publications; Tracy A: *The pregnancy bedrest book: a survival guide for expectant mothers and their families*, New York, 2001, Berkley Publishing Group.

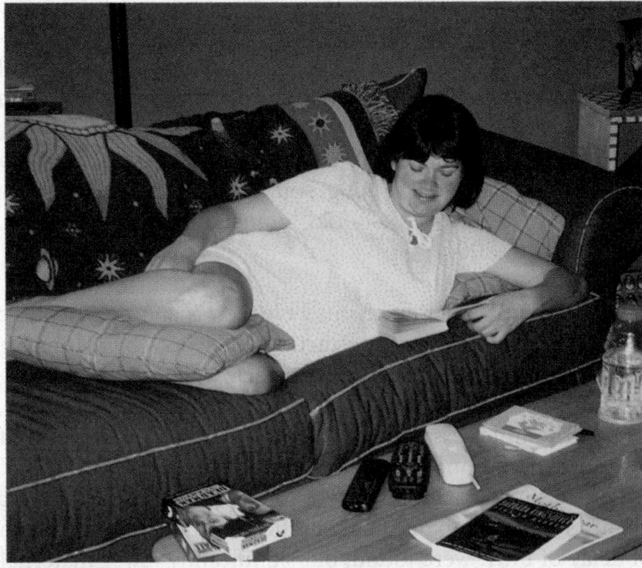

Fig. 19-2 Woman at home on restricted activity for preterm labor prevention. Note how she has arranged her daytime resting area so that needed items are close at hand. *(Courtesy Amy Turner, Cary, NC.)*

crate mattress can relieve discomfort. Women often find that preparing a daily schedule of meals, activities, and hygiene and grooming (e.g., shower, dressing in street clothes, applying makeup) reduces boredom and helps them maintain control and normalcy. Limiting naps, eating smaller but more frequent meals, and performing gentle range-of-motion exercises can help reduce some of the detrimental effects of bed rest. It is essential that a woman and her family recognize that postpartum recovery will be slower as she works to regain strength and stamina.

Home Uterine Activity Monitoring

Home uterine monitoring systems were developed to provide uterine monitoring services in the home for women diagnosed with preterm labor. Nurses are usually an integral part of the systems developed by companies to educate the patients they serve. The use and effectiveness of home uterine activity monitoring (HUAM) continues to be controversial. Research evidence indicates that HUAM is a form of care unlikely to be beneficial in preventing preterm birth (ACOG, 2001; Enkin et al, 2000). Palpation of the uterus is more effective than a monitor for detecting uterine contractions when a woman is obese (e.g., excessive abdominal adipose tissue) or the gestational age is less than 26 weeks. However, a comprehensive evidence-based review of clinical data suggests that, if used correctly (e.g., twice daily monitoring of uterine activity and daily nursing care) in patients at risk for preterm birth, HUAM increases the incidence of early diagnosis of preterm labor and prolongation of pregnancy, with fewer preterm births and reduced neonatal morbidity, when study groups are compared to control groups of women receiving standard prenatal care in the United States (Morrison & Chauhan, 2003).

Suppression of Uterine Activity

Tocolytics

Should preterm labor occur, women are usually admitted to the hospital for assessment; fetal monitoring; cervical and/or vaginal cultures; and assessment of cervical status, amniotic fluid leakage, and maternal temperature (an early sign of chorioamnionitis). The initiation of tocolytic therapy might be considered at this time. Once the pregnancy has progressed beyond 34 weeks of gestation, the benefits of prolonging the pregnancy do not justify its risk to the woman.

Tocolytic therapy, the administration of pharmaceutical agents that suppress uterine activity, has been studied since the late 1970s. At first it was thought that tocolytic therapy could prolong a threatened pregnancy indefinitely; research has demonstrated that a gain of 48 hours to several days is the best outcome that can be expected if the woman's cervix is less than 6 cm dilated. Once uterine contractions are suppressed, maintenance therapy may be implemented in an attempt to continue the suppression, or tocolytic treatment can be discontinued and resumed only if uterine contractions begin again. Research findings are complicated by selection of participants, some of whom may not be in preterm labor and would have delivered at term without treatment (Iams, Romero, & Creasy, 2009).

It is now thought that the best reason to use tocolytics is that they afford the opportunity to begin administering antenatal glucocorticoids to accelerate fetal lung maturity and reduce the severity of sequelae in infants born preterm (Iams & Romero, 2007). Time also is provided for maternal transport to a facility with a neonatal intensive care unit.

The medications most commonly used for this purpose are ritodrine (Yutopar), terbutaline (Brethine), magnesium sulfate, indomethacin (Indocin), and nifedipine (Procardia). Ritodrine, approved in 1980, is the only medication approved by the Food and Drug Administration specifically for the purpose of cessation of uterine contractions. Because of serious side effects associated with its use, ritodrine is no longer marketed (Iams, Romero, & Creasy, 2009); however, magnesium sulfate, terbutaline, and nifedipine are more commonly used in U.S. hospitals, although there is no clear first-line tocolytic drug. These medications are used on an

BOX 19-6 Contraindications to Tocolysis

Maternal
Severe preeclampsia or eclampsia
Active vaginal bleeding
Intrauterine infection (chorioamnionitis)
Cardiac disease
Medical or obstetric condition that contraindicates continuation of pregnancy
Dilation greater than 6 cm

Fetal
Estimated gestational age greater than 34 weeks
Fetal death
Lethal fetal anomaly
Acute fetal distress
Chronic intrauterine growth restriction

BOX 19-7 Nursing Care for Women Receiving Tocolytic Therapy

- Explain the purpose and side effects of tocolytic therapy to woman and her family.
- Position woman on her side to enhance placental perfusion and reduce pressure on the cervix.
- Monitor maternal vital signs, including lung sounds and respiratory effort, fetal heart rate and pattern, and labor status according to hospital protocol and professional standards.
- Assess mother and fetus for signs of adverse reactions related to the tocolytic being administered.
- Determine maternal fluid balance by measuring daily weight and intake and output.
- Limit fluid intake to 1500 to 2500 ml/day, especially if a β-adrenergic agonist or magnesium sulfate is being administered.
- Provide psychosocial support and opportunities for women and family to express feelings and concerns.
- Offer comfort measures as required.
- Encourage diversional activities and relaxation techniques.

"unlabeled" basis (i.e., medications known to be effective for a specific purpose although not specifically developed and tested for this purpose) (see Medication Guide). There are important contraindications to the use of all tocolytics (Box 19-6). Because these medications have the potential for serious adverse reactions for mother and fetus, close nursing supervision during treatment is critical (Lehne, 2007) (Box 19-7) (see Box 19-6).

Magnesium sulfate is the most commonly used tocolytic agent because maternal and fetal/neonatal adverse reactions are less common than with the β-adrenergic agonists. Although its exact mechanism of action on uterine muscle is unclear, magnesium sulfate does promote relaxation of smooth muscles (Iams & Romero, 2007). At the onset of preterm labor, magnesium sulfate is administered via an intravenous infusion.

Terbutaline, a β-adrenergic agonist medication for tocolysis, works by relaxing uterine smooth muscle as a result of stimulation of β_2-receptors on uterine smooth muscle. Terbutaline is most commonly administered by a subcutaneous injection of 0.25 mg to suppress uterine hyperactivity or a subcutaneous pump in the home setting. Continuous subcutaneous infusion has fewer side effects at lower doses than does oral administration (Iams, Romero, & Creasy, 2009). β_2-Adrenergic agonists have many maternal and fetal cardiopulmonary and metabolic adverse reactions, in part related to β_1-stimulation, and must always be used with extreme caution and careful, conscientious nursing care. Fewer neonatal adverse reactions occur if the administration of the β-adrenergic agonist is discontinued at least 4 hours before birth. Medication administration and nursing care are aimed at maintaining a therapeutic level of medication and avoiding the most serious side effects while maintaining optimal health of the fetus.

NURSING ALERT Caution must be used when administering intravenous fluids to women in preterm labor because this practice can increase the risk for tocolytic-induced pulmonary edema, especially when a β-adrenergic agonist or magnesium sulfate is used. It is recommended that the total oral and intravenous fluid intake in 24 hours should be restricted to 1500 to 2500 ml. Strict intake and output measurement, daily weight determination, and assessment of pulmonary function (e.g., auscultate lung sounds for crackles; observe for signs of orthopnea) should be instituted (Fritz & Smith, 2008; Gilbert, 2007).

Nifedipine, a calcium channel blocker, is another tocolytic agent that can suppress contractions. It works by inhibiting calcium from entering smooth muscle cells, thus reducing uterine contractions (Fritz & Smith, 2008; Iams & Romero, 2007). The mildness of maternal side effects and the ease of oral administration have increased its use. When the tocolytic effects and maternal tolerance of nifedipine and β-adrenergic agonists were compared, no significant differences in length of delay of birth were found, but significantly fewer maternal side effects occurred with nifedipine. Maternal side effects relate primarily to hypotension that occurs with administration. Concerns regarding adverse fetal effects have been reduced. Safety is achieved by following recommended dosages and maintaining maternal blood pressure, thereby preserving effective uteroplacental perfusion (Fritz & Smith, 2008; Iams & Romero, 2007).

Indomethacin, a nonsteroidal antiinflammatory drug (NSAID), has been shown in some trials to suppress preterm labor by blocking the production of prostaglandins. Two prostaglandins are affected, prostacyclin and thromboxane. The decrease in prostacyclin suppresses uterine contractions, and the decrease in thromboxane suppresses platelet aggregation. However, both of these actions increase the risk for postpartum hemorrhage. Although NSAIDs pose the lowest risk for maternal adverse reactions, the severity of fetal side effects associated with their use for tocolysis makes them less common than other classes of tocolytic drugs. Risk for premature closure of the ductus arteriosus increases if treatment goes

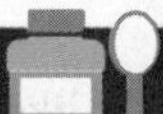

MEDICATION GUIDE: Tocolytic Therapy for Preterm Labor

*Terbutaline (Brethine)**

Action

β_2-Adrenergic agonist; relaxes smooth muscles, inhibiting uterine activity and causing bronchodilation

Dosage and Route†

Subcutaneous injection: 0.25 mg q20-30min for up to 3 hours (hold for heart rate greater than 120 beats/min)

Adverse Reactions

Maternal reactions include shortness of breath, coughing, nasal stuffiness, tachypnea, pulmonary edema, tachycardia, palpitations, skipped beats, myocardial ischemia, chest pain, hypotension, fluid retention and decreased urine production, tremors, dizziness, nervousness, muscle cramps and weakness, headache, hyperinsulinemia, hyperglycemia, hypokalemia, hypocalcemia, metabolic acidosis, nausea and vomiting, fever, and altered thyroid function.

Fetal reactions include hyperinsulinemia, hyperglycemia, and tachycardia.

Neonatal reactions include hypoglycemia, hypocalcemia, hyperbilirubinemia, hypotension, and ileus.

Nursing Considerations

Teach woman and family assessment measures (pulse, BP, respiratory effort, insertion site for infection, signs of PTL, and adverse reactions of terbutaline), whom to call if problems or concerns arise, site care and pump maintenance, activity restrictions, and how to arrange for follow-up and home care.

*Magnesium Sulfate**

Action

Central nervous system depressant; relaxes smooth muscles, including uterus

Dosage and Route†

Mix 40 g in 1000 ml intravenous solution, piggyback to primary infusion, and administer using controller pump:

- Loading dose of 4 to 6 g over 20 minutes
- Maintenance dosage: gradually increase from 2 g/hr to 4 g/hr as needed to suppress contractions; continue until contractions stop (or one contraction or less in 10 to 15 minutes) or intolerable adverse reactions develop

Adverse Reactions

Maternal adverse reactions include hot flushes, sweating, nausea and vomiting, drowsiness, blurred vision, diplopia, headache, ileus, generalized muscle weakness, dizziness, hypocalcemia, SOB, and transient hypotension. Some may subside when loading dose is completed.

Fetal and newborn reactions are uncommon and include decreased breathing movement, reduced FHR variability, nonreactive NST, hypocalcemia, lethargy, hypotonia, and respiratory depression.

Intolerable adverse reactions include respiratory rate less than 12, pulmonary edema, absent DTRs, chest pain, severe hypotension, altered level of consciousness, extreme muscle weakness, urine output less than 25 to 30 ml/hr or less than 100 ml/4 hr, and serum magnesium level of 10 mEq/L (9 mg/dl) or greater.

Nursing Considerations

Assess woman and fetus to obtain baseline before beginning therapy and then before and after each increment; follow frequency of agency protocol. Monitor serum magnesium levels with higher doses; therapeutic range is between 4 and 7.5 mEq/L or 5 and 8 mg/dl. Discontinue infusion and notify physician if intolerable adverse reactions occur. Ensure that calcium gluconate (1 g = 10 ml of 10% solution) is available for emergency administration to reverse magnesium sulfate toxicity.

*Nifedipine (Procardia; Adalat)**

Action

Calcium channel blocker; relaxes smooth muscles, including the uterus by blocking calcium entry

Dosage and Route†

Loading dose: 30 mg PO

Maintenance dosage: 10 to 20 mg PO q4-6h

Adverse Reactions

Maternal reactions include transient tachycardia, palpitations, hypotension, dizziness, headache, nervousness, peripheral edema, fatigue, nausea, and facial flushing. Fetal and newborn reactions are rare and are related to maternal hypotension, which would affect uteroplacental perfusion.

Nursing Considerations

Do not use sublingual route. Avoid use or use cautiously with magnesium sulfate because severe hypotension can result. Assess woman and fetus according to agency protocol, being alert for adverse reactions.

*Indomethacin**

Action

Prostaglandin synthetase inhibitor; relaxes uterine smooth muscle

Dosage and Route†

Loading dose: 50 mg rectally or 50 to 100 mg orally; then 25 to 50 mg orally q6h for 48 hours

Adverse Reactions

Maternal reactions include nausea and vomiting, dyspepsia, pyrosis, dizziness, oligohydramnios, and reduced platelet aggregation increasing risk for hemorrhage. Fetal reactions involve constriction of ductus arteriosus progressing to premature closure. Neonatal reactions include bronchopulmonary dysplasia, respiratory distress syndrome, intracranial hemorrhage, necrotizing enterocolitis, and hyperbilirubinemia.

Nursing Considerations

Used if gestational age is less than 32 weeks. Administer for 48 hours or less. Do not use for women with bleeding potential (coagulopathy), peptic ulcer disease, or oligohydramnios. Assess woman and fetus according to agency policy, being alert for adverse reactions. Determine amniotic fluid volume and function of ductus arteriosus before initiating therapy and within 48 hours of discontinuing therapy; assessment is critical if therapy continues for more than 48 hours. Administer with food or use rectal route to decrease GI distress. Monitor for signs of postpartum hemorrhage

BP, Blood pressure; *DTRs,* deep tendon reflexes; *ECG,* electrocardiogram; *FHR,* fetal heart rate; *GI,* gastrointestinal; *NST,* nonstress test; *PTL,* preterm labor; *SOB,* shortness of breath.

*NOTE: For variations in recommended administration protocols, always consult agency protocols, which should be evidence based.

†Caution: Not approved by Food and Drug Administration for PTL (unlabeled use).

beyond 48 hours or if the gestational age of the fetus is 32 or more weeks. Therefore limiting the use of indomethacin to a short duration of treatment (e.g., 2 to 3 days) or to women at less than 32 weeks of gestation is recommended (Fritz & Smith, 2008; Iams & Romero, 2007)

Promotion of Fetal Lung Maturity

Antenatal Glucocorticoids

Antenatal glucocorticoids given as intramuscular injections to the mother accelerate fetal lung maturity. In addition, corticosteroid administration has been associated with a decrease in the incidence of neonatal intraventricular hemorrhage and necrotizing enterocolitis. It is viewed as a form of

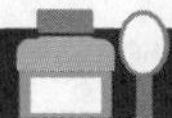

care likely to be beneficial (Enkin et al, 2000). All women between 24 and 34 weeks of gestation should be given antenatal glucocorticoids when preterm birth is a threat unless there is a medical indication for immediate delivery such as cord prolapse, chorioamnionitis, or abruptio placentae (National Institutes of Health, 2000). The regimen for administration of antenatal glucocorticoids is given in the Medication Guide.

> **MEDICATION GUIDE**
>
> ***Antenatal Glucocorticoid Therapy with Betamethasone, Dexamethasone***
>
> **Action**
>
> Stimulates fetal lung maturation by promoting release of enzymes that induce production or release of lung surfactant
>
> NOTE: The Food and Drug Administration has not approved these medications for this use (i.e., this is an unlabeled use for obstetrics).
>
> **Indication**
>
> To prevent or reduce the severity of respiratory distress syndrome in preterm infants between 24 and 34 weeks of gestation
>
> **Dosage and Route**
>
> Betamethasone: 12 mg IM × 2 doses 24 hours apart
> Dexamethasone: 6 mg IM × 4 doses 12 hours apart
>
> **Adverse Reactions**
>
> Possible maternal infection, pulmonary edema (if given with β-adrenergic medications), may worsen maternal condition (diabetes, hypertension)
>
> **Nursing Considerations**
>
> Give deep intramuscular injection. Teach signs of pulmonary edema. Assess blood glucose levels and lung sounds. Do not give if woman has infection. Use in women with PPROM not universally recommended.
>
> *IM*, Intramuscularly; *PPROM*, preterm premature rupture of membranes.

NURSING ALERT Nurses need to know that any woman who is admitted to the hospital 24 to 34 weeks pregnant should receive antenatal glucocorticoids unless she has chorioamnionitis. These drugs require a 24-hour period to become effective; thus timely administration is essential.

Management of Inevitable Preterm Birth

Labor that has progressed to a cervical dilation of 4 cm is likely to lead to inevitable preterm birth. Preterm births that occur in tertiary care centers lead to better neonatal and maternal outcomes. Therefore women considered at risk for inevitable preterm birth should be transferred quickly to such a facility to ensure the best possible outcome. The first dose of antenatal corticosteroids should be given before transfer.

Although maternal transport may help to ensure a better health outcome for the mother and the baby, it may have a negative psychosocial impact. Women may be transported to tertiary centers far from home, making visits by the family difficult and increasing the anxiety levels of both the woman and her family. Attention to the needs of the woman and her family before, during, and after the transport is essential to comprehensive nursing care for these families (see Family-Centered Care box).

> **FAMILY-CENTERED CARE**
>
> ***Impact of Preterm Birth***
>
> Parental concern for the well-being of the infant is apparent during labor. Parents need to be aware of the interest and support of staff members. However, false assurance of fetal health must be avoided. For some parents the reality of the situation is not appreciated until they see their daughter or son in the intensive care unit. For those who experience fetal or neonatal death, the loss intensifies once the stress of labor and childbirth is over.
>
> During the postpartum period physical care of the mother is similar to that required after any vaginal birth. However, the family will be very anxious concerning the health and prognosis of the infant. Care of the preterm infant involves not only medical and nursing personnel but also parent participation. The nurse must be aware of the impact that a preterm birth may have on family dynamics. Parents must accept that the infant has special needs, and they must learn to meet those needs before discharge so that they have more realistic expectations when they are at home.

Preterm Premature Rupture of Membranes

Premature rupture of membranes (PROM) is the rupture of the amniotic sac and leakage of amniotic fluid beginning at least 1 hour before the onset of labor at any gestational age. PPROM (i.e., membranes rupture before 37 weeks of gestation) occurs in up to 25% of all cases of preterm labor. Infection often precedes it, but its etiology remains unknown. Symptoms suggestive of PPROM are complaints of either a sudden gush of fluid or a slow leak of fluid from the vagina.

Infection and umbilical cord compression are serious side effects of PPROM, making the diagnosis a major complication of pregnancy. Chorioamnionitis is an intraamniotic infection of the chorion and amnion that is potentially life-threatening for the fetus and the woman. Most cases of intrauterine infection respond well to antibiotics, but sepsis can occur and can lead to maternal death. Fetal and neonatal complications from chorioamnionitis include congenital pneumonia, sepsis, and meningitis (Mercer, 2007). Even in the absence of infection, PPROM can precipitate cord prolapse or cause oligohydramnios, leading to cord compression, potentially life-threatening complications for the fetus.

Nursing Care Management: Home vs. Hospital

Since digital cervical examination before birth has been associated with neonatal infection and mortality, examinations should be avoided unless there is suspicion that birth is imminent. If cervical examination is required to determine dilation, a sterile speculum examination is recommended (Mercer, 2007). A visual pool of fluid in the posterior vaginal fornix, fluid passing from the cervical os, vaginal pH of greater than 6.0 to 6.5 (tested with nitrazine paper), or a positive "fern" test (microscopic arborized crystals) is used to determine if the discharge is amniotic fluid or urine (see Box 18-2). A woman with this diagnosis may be cared for at home (see Fig. 3-3), with more frequent visits to her primary health care provider (see Home Care box). Expectant management will continue as long as there are no signs of infection or fetal distress. Nursing support of the woman and her family is critical at this time. The nurse should encourage expression of feelings and concerns, provide information, and make referrals as needed.

HOME CARE

The Woman with Preterm Premature Rupture of Membranes

- Take your temperature and assess pulse q4h when awake.
- Report temperature of more than 38° C.
- Remain on modified bed rest.
- Insert nothing in the vagina.
- Do not engage in sexual activity.
- Assess for uterine contractions.
- Do fetal movement counts daily.
- Do not take tub baths.
- Watch for foul-smelling vaginal discharge.
- Wipe front to back after urinating or having a bowel movement.
- Take antibiotics if prescribed.
- See primary health care provider as scheduled.

Frequent biophysical profiles are performed to determine fetal health status and estimate amniotic fluid volume (AFV). The woman with PPROM also should be taught how to count fetal movements daily because a slowing of fetal movement has been shown to be a precursor to severe fetal compromise. Several methods are commonly used to count fetal movements; one method for fetal movement counting is described in the Guidelines box. Antenatal glucocorticoids may be administered if chorioamnionitis is absent (Mercer, 2007).

Vigilance for signs of infection is a major part of the nursing care and patient education after PPROM. The woman must be taught how to keep her genital area clean and that nothing should be introduced into her vagina. Signs of infection (e.g., fever, foul-smelling vaginal discharge, maternal and fetal tachycardia) should be reported to the primary health care provider immediately. Prophylactic antibiotic therapy may be ordered in an effort to improve perinatal outcome by preventing infection (Mercer, 2007). However, in the absence of a positive group B streptococcus culture or signs of chorioamnionitis, the use of prophylactic antibiotics for PROM before labor at term or preterm is not recommended because of the possibility of resistant organisms if neonatal sepsis occurs (Mercer, 2007).

GUIDELINES Counting Fetal Movements (Kick Counts)

Choose a time of day when you can sit or lie quietly.
Choices for counting strategies (see Fig. 9-1):

- Starting at 9 AM count the baby's movements until you have counted 10. If you have not counted 10 movements in 12 hours, notify your primary health care provider immediately.
- Count movements three times a day after meals. Most people count four movements in 1 hour. If you don't, count for 1 more hour. If, at the end of 2 hours, you still have not felt four movements, call your primary health care provider immediately.

Dystocia

Dystocia is defined as long, difficult, or abnormal labor; it is caused by various conditions associated with the five factors affecting labor. It is estimated that dystocia occurs in approximately 8% to 11% of women during the first stage of labor and is the primary cause for cesarean birth (Gilbert, 2007). Dystocia can be caused by any of the following:

- Dysfunctional labor, resulting in ineffective uterine contractions or maternal bearing-down efforts (the powers); the most common cause of dystocia
- Alterations in the pelvic structure (the passage)
- Fetal causes, including abnormal presentation or position, anomalies, excessive size, and number of fetuses (the passenger)
- Maternal position during labor and birth
- Psychologic responses of the mother to labor related to past experiences, preparation, culture and heritage, and support system

These five factors are interdependent. In assessing the woman for an abnormal labor pattern, the nurse must consider the way in which they interact and influence labor progress. Dystocia is suspected when there is an alteration in the characteristics of uterine contractions, a lack of progress in the rate of cervical dilation, or a lack of progress in fetal descent and expulsion.

Dysfunctional Labor

Dysfunctional labor is described as abnormal uterine contractions that prevent the normal progress of cervical dilation, effacement (primary powers), or descent (secondary powers). Gilbert (2007) lists several factors that are suspected to increase a woman's risk for uterine dystocia, including the following:

- Body build (e.g., 30 lb or more overweight; short stature)
- Uterine abnormalities (e.g., congenital malformations; overdistention, as with multiple gestation or hydramnios)
- Malpresentations and positions of the fetus
- Cephalopelvic disproportion (CPD)
- Overstimulation with oxytocin
- Maternal fatigue, dehydration and electrolyte imbalance, and fear
- Inappropriate timing of analgesic or anesthetic administration

Dysfunction of uterine contractions can be further described as being hypertonic or hypotonic.

Hypertonic Uterine Dysfunction

The woman experiencing hypertonic uterine dysfunction, or primary dysfunctional labor, is often an anxious first-time mother who is having painful and frequent contractions that are ineffective in causing cervical dilation or effacement to progress. These contractions usually occur in the latent stage (cervical dilation of less than 4 cm) and are usually uncoordinated. The force of the contraction may be in the midsection of the uterus rather than in the fundus; therefore the uterus is unable to apply downward pressure to push the presenting part against the cervix. The uterus may not relax completely between contractions (Gilbert, 2007).

Therapeutic rest, which is achieved with a warm bath or shower and the administration of analgesics such as morphine, butorphanol (Stadol), or nalbuphine (Nubain) to inhibit uterine contractions, reduce pain, and encourage sleep, is usually prescribed for the management of hypertonic uterine dysfunction (Gilbert, 2007). After a 4 to 6-hour rest these women are likely to awaken in active labor with a normal uterine contraction pattern.

Hypotonic Uterine Dysfunction

The second and more common type of uterine dysfunction is hypotonic uterine dysfunction, or secondary uterine inertia. The woman initially makes normal progress into the active stage of labor; then the contractions become weak and inefficient or stop altogether (see Fig. 19-4, *B*). The uterus is easily indented, even at the peak of contractions. Intrauterine pressure during the contraction (usually less than 25 mm Hg) is insufficient for progress of cervical effacement and dilation (Gilbert, 2007). CPD and malpositions are common causes of this type of uterine dysfunction.

Management usually consists of performing an ultrasound examination to determine fetal positioning and assessing the fetal heart rate (FHR) and pattern, characteristics of amniotic fluid if membranes are ruptured, and maternal well-being. If findings are normal, measures such as ambulation, hydrotherapy, enema, stripping or rupture of membranes, nipple stimulation, and oxytocin infusion can be used to augment labor (see Nursing Care Plan).

Alterations in Pelvic Structure

Pelvic Dystocia Pelvic dystocia can occur whenever there are contractures of the pelvic diameters that reduce the capacity of the bony pelvis, including the inlet, midpelvis, outlet, or any combination of these planes.

Disproportion of the pelvis is the least common cause of dystocia. Pelvic contractures may be caused by congenital abnormalities, maternal malnutrition, neoplasms, or lower spinal disorders. An immature pelvic size predisposes some adolescent mothers to pelvic dystocia. Pelvic deformities may also be the result of automobile or other accidents or trauma.

An inlet contracture is diagnosed when the diagonal conjugate is less than 11.5 cm. The incidence of face and shoulder presentation is increased. Because these presentations interfere with engagement and fetal descent, the risk of prolapse of the umbilical cord is increased. Inlet contracture is associated with maternal rickets and a flat pelvis. Weak uterine contractions may be noted during the first stage of labor in affected women.

Midplane contracture, the most common cause of pelvic dystocia, is diagnosed when the sum of the interischial spinous and posterior sagittal diameters of the midpelvis is 13.5 cm or less. Fetal descent is arrested (transverse arrest of the fetal head) because the head cannot rotate internally. These infants are usually born by cesarean, but vacuum-assisted birth has been used safely when the cervix is fully dilated. Midforceps-assisted birth usually is not recommended because of the increased perinatal morbidity associated with this intervention.

Outlet contracture exists when the interischial diameter is 8 cm or less. It rarely occurs in the absence of midplane contracture. Women with outlet contracture have a long, narrow pubic arch and an android pelvis, which causes fetal descent to be arrested. Maternal complications include extensive perineal lacerations during vaginal birth because the fetal head is pushed posteriorly.

Soft-Tissue Dystocia Soft-tissue dystocia results from obstruction of the birth passage by an anatomic abnormality other than that involving the bony pelvis. The obstruction may result from placenta previa that partially or completely obstructs the internal os of the cervix. Other causes such as leiomyomas (uterine fibroids) in the lower uterine segment, ovarian tumors, and a full bladder or rectum may prevent the fetus from entering the pelvis. Occasionally cervical edema occurs during labor when the cervix is caught between the presenting part and the symphysis pubis or when the woman begins bearing-down efforts prematurely, inhibiting complete dilation. Sexually transmitted infections (e.g., human papillomavirus) can alter cervical tissue integrity and thus interfere with adequate effacement and dilation.

Bandl's ring, a pathologic retraction ring that forms between the upper and lower uterine segments (see Fig. 15-10, *C*), is associated with prolonged rupture of membranes, protracted labor, and increased risk of uterine rupture (Cunningham et al, 2005).

Fetal Causes

Dystocia of fetal origin may be caused by anomalies, excessive fetal size and malpresentation, malposition, or multifetal pregnancy. Complications associated with dystocia of fetal origin include neonatal asphyxia, fetal injuries or fractures, and maternal vaginal lacerations. Although spontaneous vaginal birth is possible in these instances, a low-forceps or vacuum-assisted or cesarean birth often is necessary.

Anomalies

Gross ascites, large tumors, and open neural tube defects such as myelomeningocele and hydrocephalus are fetal anomalies that can cause dystocia. The anomalies affect the relationship of the fetal anatomy to the maternal pelvic capacity, with

NURSING CARE PLAN Dysfunctional Labor: Hypotonic Uterine Dysfunction with Protracted Active Phase

Nursing Diagnosis: Risk for injury to mother or fetus (or both) related to oxytocin augmentation secondary to dysfunctional labor

Expected Outcomes

Maternal-fetal well-being is maintained; labor progresses, and birth occurs.

Nursing Interventions/*Rationales*

Explain oxytocin protocol to woman and her labor partner *to allay apprehension and enhance participation.*

Encourage woman to void before beginning protocol *to prevent discomfort and remove a barrier to labor progress.*

Apply the electronic fetal monitor per hospital protocol and obtain a 15- to 20-minute baseline strip *to ensure adequate assessment of fetal heart rate (FHR) and contractions.*

Position woman in a side-lying position and administer the oxytocin per physician order using an (IV) infusion pump *to stimulate uterine activity and provide adequate control of the flow rate.*

Regulate the oxytocin per protocol (e.g., advancing the dosage in increments of 1 to 2 mU/min every 30 to 60 minutes) *to allow adequate evaluation of the woman's response to stimulation and prevent hyperstimulation and fetal hypoxia.*

Maintain oxytocin dosage and rate when contractions occur every 2 to 3 minutes with a duration of 40 to 90 seconds and intrauterine pressures are 60 to 90 mm Hg (if internal monitoring is used) *to produce effective uterine stimulation without risk of hyperstimulation.*

Monitor maternal vital signs every 30 to 60 minutes *to assess for oxytocin-induced hypertension.*

Monitor contractility pattern and FHR and pattern every 15 minutes *to assess uterine activity for possible hypertonicity or ineffective uterine response to oxytocin and to detect evidence of fetal distress.*

Monitor intake, output, and specific gravity (limit intake to 1000 ml/8 hr; output should be at least 120 ml/4 hr) *to assess for urinary retention and prevent water intoxication.*

Monitor cervical dilation, effacement, and station *to assess progress of labor.*

If hypertonicity or signs of a nonreassuring fetal status is detected, discontinue oxytocin immediately *to arrest the progress of hypertonicity;* turn woman on her side *to increase placental blood flow;* increase primary IV rate to 200 ml/hr (unless signs of water toxicity are present); administer oxygen via nonrebreather face mask *to enhance placental perfusion;* notify primary health care provider; and continuously monitor maternal vital signs and FHR *to provide ongoing assessment of maternal/fetal status.*

Maintain Standard Precautions and use scrupulous handwashing techniques when providing care *to prevent the spread of infection.*

Nursing Diagnosis: Acute pain related to increasing frequency, regularity, intensity, and prolonged peak of contractions

Expected Outcome

The woman exhibits signs of decreased discomfort and increased coping with pain.

Nursing Interventions/*Rationales*

Prepare woman and labor partner for the change in the nature of the contractions once the oxytocin drip is initiated *to prepare them and allow for more effective coping.*

Review the use of specific techniques such as conscious relaxation, focused breathing, effleurage, massage, and application of sacral pressure *to increase relaxation, decrease intensity of pain of contractions, and promote use of controlled thought and direction of energy.*

Provide comfort measures such as frequent mouth care *to prevent dry mouth,* application of damp cloth to forehead and changing of damp gown or bed covers *to relieve discomfort of diaphoresis,* and positioning *to reduce stiffness.*

Encourage conscious relaxation between contractions to prevent fatigue, *which contributes to increased pain perceptions.*

Remind woman and labor partner that analgesics are available for use during labor *to provide knowledge to help them make decisions about pain control.*

Nursing Diagnosis: Anxiety related to prolonged labor, increased pain, and fatigue

Expected Outcomes

Woman's anxiety is reduced; woman actively participates in the labor process.

Nursing Interventions/*Rationales*

Provide ongoing feedback to woman and partner *to allay anxiety and enhance participation.*

Present care options when possible *to increase feelings of control.*

Continue to provide comfort measures *to maintain a posture of support and caring and help woman to focus on the labor process.*

Encourage woman and partner to continue to use the mechanisms that promote effective labor (e.g., breathing, activity, positioning) *to keep woman and partner actively involved in process.*

the result that the fetus is unable to descend through the birth canal.

Cephalopelvic Disproportion

CPD, also called *fetopelvic disproportion*, is often related to excessive fetal size (i.e., 4000 g or more). When CPD is present, the fetus cannot fit through the maternal pelvis to be born vaginally. Excessive fetal size, or macrosomia, is associated with maternal diabetes mellitus, obesity, multiparity, or the large size of one or both parents. If the maternal pelvis is too small, abnormally shaped, or deformed, CPD may be of maternal origin. In this case the fetus may be of average size or even smaller.

BOX 19-8 Back Labor—Occiput Posterior Position

Measures to Reduce Back Pain During a Contraction

Counterpressure—Apply fist or heel of hand to sacral area

Heat or cold applications—Apply to sacral area

Double hip squeeze:

- Woman assumes a position with hip joints flexed such as knee-chest position.
- Partner, nurse, or doula places hands over gluteal muscles and presses with palms of hands up and inward toward center of pelvis.

Knee press:

- Woman assumes a sitting position with knees a few inches apart and feet flat on the floor or on a stool.
- Partner, nurse, or doula cups a knee in each hand with heels of hands on top of tibia and then presses the knees straight back toward the woman's hips while leaning forward toward the woman.

Measures to Facilitate Rotation of Fetal Head (May Also Relieve Back Pain)

Lateral abdominal stroking—Stroke abdomen in direction that fetal head should rotate

Hands-and-knees position (all-fours)—Can also be accomplished by kneeling while leaning forward over a birth ball, padded chair seat, bed, or over-the-bed table

Squatting

Pelvic rocking

Stair climbing

Lateral position—Lie on side toward which the fetus should turn

Lunges—Widen pelvis on side toward which woman lunges

- Woman stands, facing forward, next to/alongside a chair so that she can lunge toward the side the fetal back is on or in the direction of the fetal occiput.
- Woman places foot on seat of chair with toes pointed toward the back of the chair and then lunges.
- Alternative position for lunge is kneeling.

evolve Animation–Breech Birth

evolve Animation–Breech Examination

Malposition

The most common fetal malposition is persistent occipitoposterior position (i.e., right occipitoposterior or left occipitoposterior) (see Fig. 15-2), occurring in about 25% of all labors. Labor, especially the second stage, is prolonged; the woman typically complains of severe back pain from the pressure of the fetal head (occiput) pressing against her sacrum. Box 19-8 identifies suggested measures to relieve back pain and facilitate rotation of the fetal occiput to an anterior position, which will facilitate birth (Gilbert, 2007).

Malpresentation

Malpresentation occurred at a rate of 47.1 per 1000 live births in 2005, with the highest rate (71/1000) among women 40 to 54 years of age (Martin et al, 2007). Breech presentation is the most common form of malpresentation. The four main types of breech presentation are frank breech (thighs flexed, knees extended); complete breech (thighs and knees flexed); and two types of incomplete breech, one in which the knee extends below the buttocks and the other in which the foot extends below the buttocks (Fig. 19-3). Breech presentations are associated with multifetal gestation, preterm birth, fetal and maternal anomalies, hydramnios, and oligohydramnios. Diagnosis is made by abdominal palpation (e.g., Leopold's maneuvers) and vaginal examination and usually is confirmed by ultrasound scan (Lanni & Seeds, 2007).

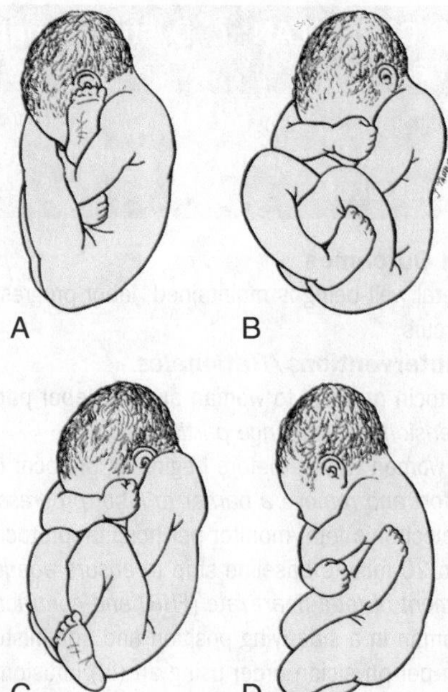

Fig. 19-3 Types of breech presentation. **A,** Frank breech: thighs are flexed on hips; knees are extended. **B,** Complete breech: thighs and knees are flexed. **C,** Incomplete breech: foot extends below the buttocks. **D,** Incomplete breech: knee extends below the buttocks.

During labor fetal descent may be slow because the breech is not as good a dilating wedge as the fetal head; the labor itself is usually not prolonged. There is risk of prolapse of the umbilical cord if the membranes rupture in early labor. The aftercoming head can be trapped by an incompletely dilated cervix. The presence of meconium in amniotic fluid is not necessarily a sign of fetal compromise because it results from pressure on the fetal abdominal wall as it traverses the birth canal. The fetal heart tones of infants in a breech position are best heard at or above the maternal umbilicus.

Vaginal birth is accomplished by mechanisms of labor that manipulate the buttocks and lower extremities as they emerge from the birth canal. Piper forceps sometimes are used to deliver the head (see Fig. 19-8). Late in pregnancy external cephalic version (ECV) may be tried to turn the fetus to a vertex presentation. When ECV is performed, the success rate is approximately 60% to 70% (Lanni & Seeds, 2007).

Although opinions vary, a cesarean birth is commonly performed when the fetus is estimated to be larger than 3800 g or smaller than 1500 g if this is a first pregnancy, if labor is ineffective, or if complications occur. Although cesarean birth reduces the risks to the fetus, the maternal risks are increased. ECV also poses risks of abruption, nonreassuring FHR patterns, rupture of membranes, and cord prolapse and is not always successful. Women whose breech presentation occurs late in pregnancy need to be informed about the options for birth, including the risks associated with each option.

Face and brow presentations are uncommon and are associated with fetal anomalies, pelvic contractures, and CPD. Vaginal birth is possible if the fetus flexes to a vertex presentation, although forceps often are used. Cesarean birth is indicated if the presentation persists, if there is an abnormal FHR and pattern, or if labor stops progressing.

Cesarean birth is usually necessary for a fetus in a shoulder presentation (i.e., the fetus is in a transverse lie), although ECV may be attempted after 36 to 37 weeks of gestation in patients with intact membranes, no CPD, and no placenta previa (Thorp, 2009).

Multifetal Pregnancy

Multifetal pregnancy is the gestation of twins, triplets, quadruplets, or more infants. The twin birth rate was 32.2 per 1000 live births in 2005. The higher-order multiple birth rate (i.e., triplet and more) was 161.8 per 100,000 live births in 2005 (Martin et al, 2007). The incidence of twin births has been increasing since 1980; however, there is a decreasing trend in triplet and higher-order multiple births since 1999. It is likely that the increased trend in twins is related to the use of fertility-enhancing medications and procedures and the older age of childbearing women (Malone & D'Alton, 2009). The decrease in higher order multiple births is likely due to voluntary limits imposed in assisted reproduction centers in the number of embryos transferred and to multifetal pregnancy reduction (Malone & D'Alton, 2009). When compared with younger women, women age 35 years and older are more likely to have a multifetal pregnancy with or without fertility-enhancing drugs.

Multiple births are associated with more complications, including dysfunctional labor, than are single births. The high incidence of fetal/newborn complications and higher risk of perinatal death primarily stems from the birth of low-birth-weight infants resulting from preterm birth and IUGR. Fetuses may experience hypoxia leading to asphyxia during birth as a result of cord prolapse and the onset of placental separation with the birth of the first fetus (Malone & D'Alton, 2009). As a result, the risk for long-term problems such as cerebral palsy is higher among multiple births.

In addition, fetal complications such as congenital anomalies and abnormal presentations can lead to dystocia and an increased incidence of cesarean birth. For example, in only half of all twin pregnancies do both fetuses present in the vertex presentation, the most favorable for vaginal birth; in one third of pregnancies one twin may present in the vertex presentation and one in the breech.

The health status of the mother may be compromised by an increased risk for hypertension, anemia, and hemorrhage associated with uterine atony, abruptio placentae, and multiple or adherent placentas (Malone & D'Alton, 2009). Duration of the phases and stages of labor may vary from that experienced with singleton births.

Teamwork and planning are essential in the management of childbirth in multiple pregnancies, especially those of the higher-order multiples. The nurse plays a key role in coordinating the activities of many highly skilled health care professionals. Early detection and effective care of maternal, fetal, and newborn complications associated with multiple births are essential to achieve a positive outcome for mothers and babies. Maternal positioning and active support are used to enhance labor progress and placental perfusion. Stimulation of labor with oxytocin, epidural anesthesia, forceps and vacuum assistance, and internal or ECV may be used to accomplish the vaginal birth of twins. Cesarean birth is most likely with higher-order multiple births. Each infant may have its own team of health care providers present at the birth. Emotional support that includes expression of feelings and full explanations of events as they occur and of the status of the mother and the fetuses/newborns is important to reduce the anxiety and stress the mother and her family experience. Websites such as *www.nomotc.org* and *www.tripletconnection.org* may be helpful for families having a multiple birth.

Position of the Woman

The functional relationships among the uterine contractions, the fetus, and the mother's pelvis are altered by the maternal position. The position can provide a mechanical advantage or disadvantage to the mechanisms of labor by altering the effects of gravity and the body part relations important to the progress of labor. For example, the hands-and-knees position facilitates rotation from a posterior occiput position more effectively than does the lateral position. Upright positions such as sitting and squatting facilitate fetal descent during pushing and shorten the second stage of labor (Terry et al, 2006). Discouraging maternal movement or restricting labor to the recumbent or lithotomy position may compromise progress. The incidence of dystocia in women confined to these positions is increased, resulting in increased need for augmentation of labor, the use of forceps, and vacuum-assisted or cesarean birth.

Psychologic Responses

Hormones and neurotransmitters released in response to stress (e.g., catecholamines) can cause dystocia. Sources of stress vary for each woman, but pain and the absence of a support person are two recognized factors. Confinement to bed and restriction of maternal movement can be a source of psychologic stress that compounds the physiologic stress caused by immobility in the unmedicated laboring woman. When anxiety is excessive, it can inhibit normal cervical dilation and result in prolonged labor and increased pain perception. Anxiety also causes increased levels of stress-related hormones (e.g., β-endorphin, adrenocorticotropic hormone, cortisol, and epinephrine). These hormones act on the smooth muscles of the uterus; increased levels can cause dystocia by reducing uterine contractility.

Abnormal Labor Patterns

Six abnormal labor patterns were identified and classified by Friedman (1989) according to the nature of cervical dilation and fetal descent. The labor patterns seen in normal and abnormal labor are described in Table 19-1.

These abnormal patterns may result from a variety of causes that include ineffective uterine contractions, pelvic contractures, CPD, abnormal fetal presentation or position, early use of analgesics, nerve block analgesia/anesthesia, and anxiety

Table 19-1 Labor Patterns in Normal and Abnormal Labor

Normal Labor

1. Dilation: continues
   a. Latent phase: <4 cm and low slope
   b. Active phase: >5 cm or high slope
   c. Deceleration phase: ≥9 cm
2. Descent: active at ≥9 cm dilation

Abnormal Labor

PATTERN	NULLIPARAS	MULTIPARAS
Prolonged latent phase	>20 hr	>14 hr
Protracted active phase dilation	<1.2 cm/hr	<1.5 cm/hr
Secondary arrest: no change	≥2 hr	≥2 hr
Protracted descent	<1 cm/hr	<2 cm/hr
Arrest of descent	≥1 hr	≥½ hr
Failure of descent	No change during deceleration phase and second stage	
Precipitous labor	>5 cm/hr	10 cm/hr

and stress. Progress in either the first or second stage of labor can be protracted (prolonged) or arrested (stopped).

Abnormal progress can be identified by plotting cervical dilation and fetal descent on a labor graph (partogram) at various intervals after the onset of labor and comparing the resulting curve with the expected labor curve for a nulliparous or multiparous labor. Fig. 19-4, *A*, is a labor graph illustrating progress in a normal labor for a primigravida. Fig. 19-4, *B*, illustrates major types of deviation from the normal progress of labor. If a woman exhibits an abnormal labor pattern, the primary health care provider should be notified.

Health care providers must be careful when diagnosing a labor pattern as prolonged and when intervening based on this diagnosis. Criteria defining the differences between false, latent, and active labor should be established. Using hospital or unit admission areas to evaluate a woman's labor status is helpful in preventing the premature implementation of labor interventions such as administration of systemic opioid analgesics or induction of epidural analgesia/anesthesia. If a woman is found to be in false or latent (early) labor, she can be sent home or remain in the admission area until labor becomes active. Women in active labor are admitted to the labor and birth unit.

Maternal morbidity and death may occur as a result of uterine rupture, infection, severe dehydration, and postpartum hemorrhage. The fetus is at increased risk for hypoxia. A long, difficult labor also can have an adverse psychologic effect on the mother, father, and family.

Precipitous Labor

Precipitous labor is defined as labor that lasts less than 3 hours from the onset of contractions to the time of birth. This abnormal labor pattern occurred at a rate of 20 per 1000 live births in 2005. Precipitous labor occurred at the highest rate (23.1/1000) among women age 35 to 39 and at the lowest rate (13.7/1000) among women younger than 20 years (Martin et al, 2007).

Precipitous labor may result from hypertonic uterine contractions that are tetanic in intensity. Maternal and fetal complications can occur as a result. Maternal complications can include uterine rupture, lacerations of the birth canal, and postpartum hemorrhage. Fetal complications can include hypoxia caused by decreased periods of uterine relaxation between contractions and intracranial hemorrhage related to rapid birth (Cunningham et al, 2005).

Women who have experienced precipitate labor often describe feelings of disbelief that their labor began so quickly, alarm that their labor progressed so rapidly, panic about the possibility that they would not make it to the hospital on time to give birth, and finally relief when they arrived at the hospital. In addition, women have expressed frustration when nurses would not believe them when they reported their readiness to push.

Nursing Care Management

Fetal scalp or acoustic stimulation can be used to assess the fetal acid-base status. Any acceleration is a reassuring assessment finding that indicates the absence of fetal acidosis. Ultrasound scanning can identify potential dysfunctional labor problems related to the fetus (e.g., abnormal fetal position) or maternal pelvis. All of these assessments contribute to accurate identification of potential and actual nursing diagnoses related to dystocia and maternal-fetal compromise (see Nursing Process box).

Version

Version is the turning of the fetus artificially from one presentation to another by the physician. Version may be done externally or internally.

External Cephalic Version

ECV is used to attempt to turn the fetus from a breech or shoulder presentation to a vertex presentation for birth. It may be attempted in a labor and birth setting after 37 weeks of gestation. ECV is accomplished by the exertion of gentle, constant pressure on the abdomen (Fig. 19-5). Before it is attempted, ultrasound scanning is done to determine the fetal position; locate the umbilical cord; rule out placenta previa; evaluate the adequacy of the maternal pelvis; and assess the amount of amniotic fluid, fetal age, and presence of any anomalies (Thorp, 2009). A nonstress test (NST) is performed to confirm fetal well-being, or the FHR and pattern are monitored for a period of time (usually 10 to 20 minutes). Informed consent is obtained. Contraindications to ECV include uterine anomalies, previous cesarean birth, CPD, placenta previa, multifetal gestation, and oligohydramnios (Cunningham et al, 2005; Lanni & Seeds, 2007). A tocolytic agent such as terbutaline often is given to relax the uterus and facilitate the maneuver. ECV performed at term to avoid breech birth is a beneficial form of care (Enkin et al, 2000).

Before and during an attempted ECV, the nurse and/or physician monitors the FHR and pattern either with the external fetal monitor or by ultrasound especially for bradycardia and variable decelerations; checks maternal vital signs; and assesses the woman's level of comfort because the procedure may cause discomfort. After the procedure is completed, the nurse continues to monitor maternal vital signs, uterine activ-

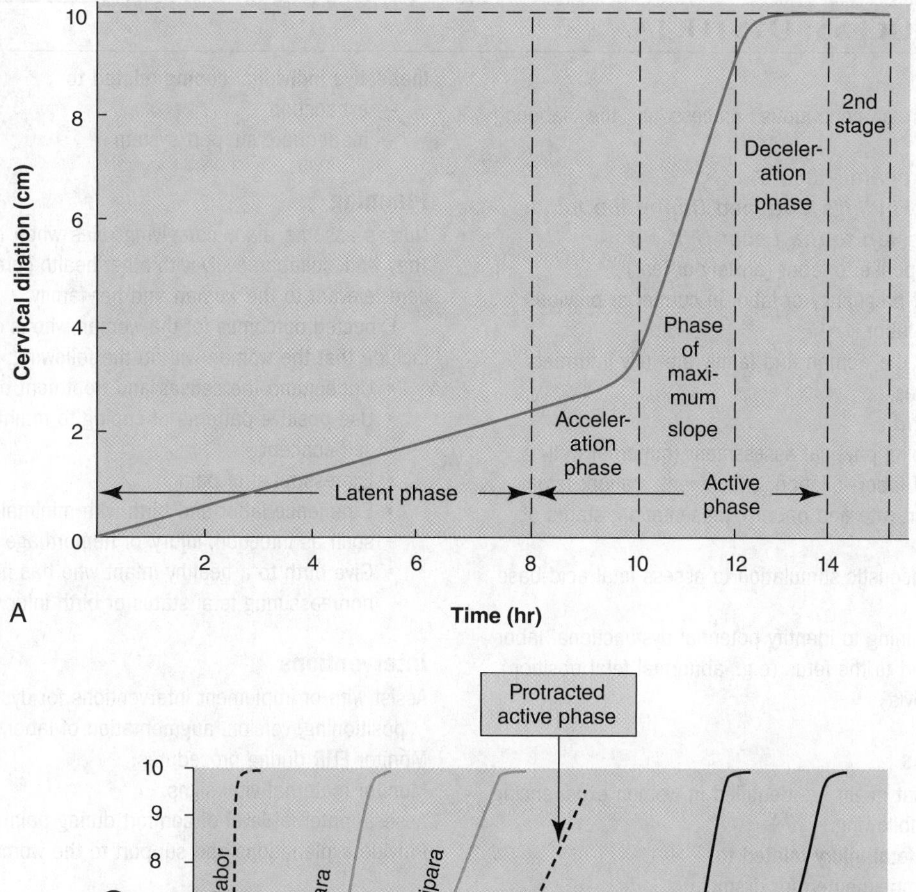

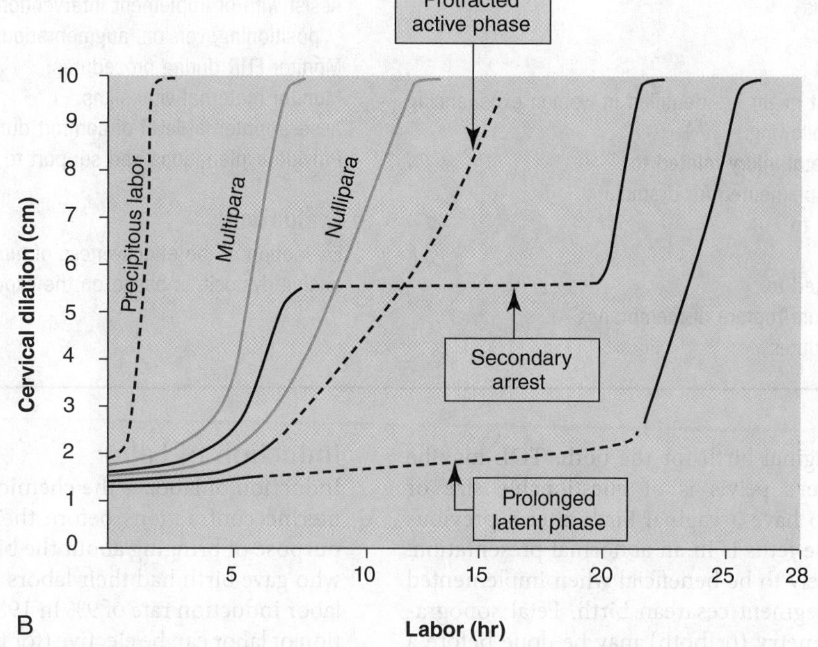

Fig. 19-4 Progress in labor. **A,** Depiction of a normal labor for a primigravida. **B,** Major types of deviation from normal progress of labor may be detected by noting dilation of cervix at various intervals after labor begins. If a woman exhibits an abnormal labor pattern, as depicted by *broken lines,* the primary health care provider should be notified.

ity, and FHR and pattern and assess for vaginal bleeding until the woman's condition is stable. Women who are Rh-negative should receive Rh immune globulin because the manipulation can cause fetomaternal bleeding (Cunningham et al, 2005).

Internal Version

With internal version the fetus is turned by the physician, who inserts a hand into the uterus and changes the presentation to cephalic (head) or podalic (foot). Internal version may be used in multifetal pregnancies to deliver the second fetus. The safety of this procedure has not been documented; maternal and fetal injury are possible. Cesarean birth is the usual method for managing malpresentation in multifetal pregnancies. The nurse's role is to monitor the status of the fetus and support the woman.

Trial of Labor

A trial of labor (TOL) is the observance of a woman and her fetus for a reasonable period of spontaneous active labor to

NURSING PROCESS: DYSTOCIA

Assessment

Risk assessment is a continuous process in the laboring woman.

History (Review Prenatal Record)

Interview (Review Findings Obtained During the Initial Interview at Admission to the Labor Unit)

- Psychologic response to labor (anxiety or fear)
- Complication of pregnancy or labor in current or previous pregnancy and labor
- Assess whether the woman and family are fully informed about procedures

Physical Examination

- Initial and ongoing physical assessment (maternal well-being; status of labor–dilation, effacement, station; fetal well-being–heart rate and pattern, presentation; status of membranes)
- Fetal scalp or acoustic stimulation to assess fetal acid-base status
- Ultrasound scanning to identify potential dysfunctional labor problems related to the fetus (e.g., abnormal fetal position) or maternal pelvis

Nursing Diagnoses

Nursing diagnoses that might be identified in women experiencing dystocia include the following:

Risk for maternal or fetal injury related to

– interventions implemented for dystocia

Powerlessness related to

– loss of control

Risk for infection related to

– preterm premature rupture of membranes

– operative procedures

Ineffective individual coping related to

– exhaustion

– inadequate support system

Planning

Nurses assume many caregiving roles when labor is complicated. They work collaboratively with other health care providers to provide care relevant to the woman and her family.

Expected outcomes for the woman who is experiencing dystocia include that the woman will do the following:

- Understand the causes and treatment of dysfunctional labor
- Use positive patterns of coping to maintain a positive self-concept
- Express relief of pain
- Experience labor and birth with minimal or no complications such as infection, injury, or hemorrhage
- Give birth to a healthy infant who has not experienced a nonreassuring fetal status or birth injury

Interventions

Assist with or implement interventions for dystocia (e.g., positioning, version, augmentation of labor, cervical ripening)

Monitor FHR during procedures.

Monitor maternal vital signs.

Assess maternal level of comfort during painful procedures.

Provide explanations and support to the woman and her family

Evaluation

Evaluation of the effectiveness of nursing care for a woman experiencing dystocia is based on the expected outcomes.

evolve Spanish Guidelines—Induction of Labor

assess the safety of vaginal birth for the both. TOL may be initiated if the mother's pelvis is of questionable size or shape, if she wishes to have a vaginal birth after a previous cesarean birth, or if the fetus is in an abnormal presentation. It is a form of care likely to be beneficial when implemented after a previous low-segment cesarean birth. Fetal sonography or maternal pelvimetry (or both) may be done before a TOL to estimate fetal weight and maternal pelvic measurements. The cervix must be ripe (soft and dilatable). During a TOL the woman is evaluated for the occurrence of active labor, including adequate contractions, engagement and descent of the presenting part, and effacement and dilation of the cervix.

The nurse assesses maternal vital signs and FHR and pattern and is alert for signs of potential complications. If complications develop, the nurse is responsible for initiating appropriate actions, including notifying the primary health care provider, and for evaluating and documenting the maternal and fetal responses to the interventions. Supporting and encouraging the woman and her partner and providing information regarding progress can reduce stress, enhance the labor process, and facilitate a successful outcome.

Induction of Labor

Induction of labor is the chemical or mechanical initiation of uterine contractions before their spontaneous onset for the purpose of bringing about the birth. In 2005 22.8% of women who gave birth had their labors induced, more than twice the labor induction rate of 9% in 1989 (Martin et al, 2007). Induction of labor can be elective (for the convenience of the woman or staff) or indicated for medical, obstetric, or fetal reasons. Medical and obstetric reasons include hypertensive disorders, diabetes mellitus, chorioamnionitis, and other maternal medical problems; PROM; postdate gestation; suspected fetal jeopardy (e.g., IUGR, oligohydramnios); logistic factors such as history of previous rapid birth or distance of the woman's home from the hospital; and fetal death. Under such conditions the risk to the mother or fetus is less than the risk of continuing the pregnancy. There is evidence that elective induction increases the risk for cesarean birth, especially for nulliparous women (Battista & Wing, 2007).

Success rates for induction of labor are higher when the cervix is favorable, or inducible. A rating system such as the Bishop score (Table 19-2) can be used to evaluate inducibility. For example, a score of 9 or more on this 13-point scale

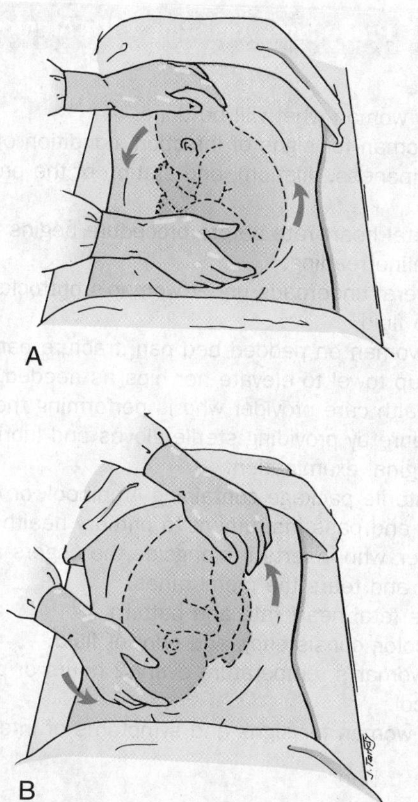

Fig. 19-5 External version of fetus from breech to vertex presentation. This must be achieved without force. **A,** Breech is pushed up out of pelvic inlet while head is pulled toward inlet. **B,** Head is pushed toward inlet while breech is pulled upward.

Table 19-2 Bishop Score

	Score			
	0	1	2	3
Dilation (cm)	Closed	1-2	3-4	≥5
Effacement (%)	0-30	40-50	60-70	≥80
Station (cm)	−3	−2	−1, 0	+1, +2
Cervical consistency	Firm	Medium	Soft	
Cervix position	Posterior	Midposition	Anterior	

indicates that the cervix is soft, anterior, 50% or more effaced, and dilated 2 cm or more and that the presenting part is engaged. Induction of labor is likely to be more successful if the score is 8 or more (Gilbert, 2007).

Cervical Ripening Methods

Both chemical and mechanical methods are used to induce labor. Intravenous oxytocin and amniotomy are the most common methods used in the United States. Prostaglandins are increasingly used for inducing labor. The most effective protocol (e.g., dosage, frequency) to follow when using prostaglandins continues to be investigated.

Less commonly used methods include nipple stimulation (manual or with a breast pump), the ingestion of castor oil or herbal preparations, a soapsuds enema, stripping of membranes, and acupuncture (Thorp, 2009). Many folk beliefs exist regarding methods to induce labor. These methods include activity (e.g., walking, exercise, strenuous work, sexual intercourse), fasting, and increasing stress (e.g., frightening the woman). It is important for the nurse to know the practices a woman may believe in and follow because some of these methods can be harmful (e.g., strenuous activity).

Chemical Agents

Preparations of prostaglandin E_1 and prostaglandin E_2 can be used before induction to "ripen" (soften and thin) the cervix (see Medication Guides). This treatment usually results in a higher success rate for the induction of labor, the need for lower dosages of oxytocin during the induction, and shorter induction times. In some cases women will go into labor after the application of prostaglandin, thereby eliminating the need to administer oxytocin to induce labor. Although prostaglandin E_1 is less expensive and more effective than oxytocin or prostaglandin E_2 for inducing labor and birth, it is associated with a higher risk for hyperstimulation of the uterus (Thorp, 2009).

Mechanical Methods

Mechanical dilators ripen the cervix by stimulating the release of endogenous prostaglandins from the fetal membranes and maternal decidua. Their use is a form of care with a trade-off between beneficial and adverse effects (Enkin et al, 2000). Balloon catheters (e.g., Foley catheter) can be inserted into the intracervical canal to ripen and dilate the cervix. Hygroscopic dilators (substances that absorb fluid from surrounding tissues and enlarge) also can be used for cervical ripening. Laminaria tents (natural cervical dilators made from desiccated seaweed) and synthetic dilators containing magnesium sulfate (Lamicel) are inserted into the endocervix without rupturing the membranes. As they absorb fluid, they expand and cause cervical dilation. These dilators are left in place for 6 to 12 hours before being removed to assess cervical dilation. Fresh dilators are inserted if further cervical dilation is necessary. Synthetic dilators swell faster than natural dilators and become larger with less discomfort (Simpson, 2008). Nursing responsibilities for women who have dilators inserted include documenting the number of dilators and sponges inserted during the procedure and the number removed and assessing for urinary retention, rupture of membranes, uterine tenderness/pain, contractions, vaginal bleeding, and fetal distress (Gilbert, 2007; Simpson, 2008).

Amniotomy

Amniotomy (i.e., artificial rupture of membranes) can be used to induce labor when the condition of the cervix is favorable (ripe) or to augment labor if progress begins to slow. Labor usually begins within 12 hours of the rupture; the duration of labor is decreased by up to 2 hours, especially if combined with oxytocin administration. If amniotomy does not stimulate labor, the resulting prolonged rupture may lead to infection. Other potential risks include umbilical cord prolapse and fetal injury. Once an amniotomy is performed, the woman is committed to giving birth. For this reason amniotomy often is used in combination with oxytocin induction. Evidence from controlled trials clearly demonstrates that amniotomy combined with oxytocin for induction is more effective than either amniotomy or oxytocin alone and is a beneficial form of care (Enkin et al, 2000).

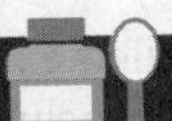

MEDICATION GUIDE

Cervical Ripening Using Prostaglandin E_1: Misoprostol (Cytotec)

Action

Prostaglandin E_1 (PGE_1) ripens the cervix, making it softer and causing it to begin to dilate and efface; it stimulates uterine contractions.

Indications

PGE_1 is used for preinduction cervical ripening (ripens cervix before oxytocin induction of labor when the Bishop score is 4 or less) and to induce labor or abortion (abortifacient agent).

Dosage

Insert 25 to 50 mcg (¼ to ½ of a 100-mcg tablet) intravaginally into the posterior fornix using the tips of index and middle fingers without the use of a lubricant. Repeat every 3 to 6 hours as needed to a maximum of 300 to 400 mcg in a 24-hour period or until an effective contraction pattern is established (three or more uterine contractions in 10 minutes), cervix ripens (Bishop score of 8 or higher), or significant adverse reactions occur. Administer 50 to 100 mcg PO q4-6h (gastrointestinal effects are increased; there are insufficient data to support effectiveness; therefore oral administration is generally not recommended).

Adverse Reactions

Higher dosages are more likely to result in adverse reactions such as nausea and vomiting, diarrhea, fever, tachysystole (12 or more uterine contractions in 20 minutes without alteration of fetal heart rate or pattern), hyperstimulation of the uterus (tachysystole with nonreassuring fetal heart patterns), or fetal passage of meconium. Risk for adverse reactions is reduced with lower dosages (i.e., 25 mcg) and longer intervals between doses (i.e., q6h).

Nursing Considerations

Explain procedure to woman and her family. Ensure that an informed consent has been obtained per agency policy. Assess maternal-fetal unit before each insertion and during treatment, following agency protocol for frequency. Assess maternal vital signs and health status, fetal heart rate and pattern, and status of pregnancy, including indications for cervical ripening or induction of labor, signs of labor or impending labor, and the Bishop score. Recognize that a nonreassuring fetal heart rate or pattern; maternal fever, infection, vaginal bleeding, or hypersensitivity; and regular, progressive uterine contractions and history of cesarean birth or uterine scar contraindicate the use of misoprostol. Use caution if the woman has a history of asthma; glaucoma; or renal, hepatic, or cardiovascular disorders. Have woman void before procedure. Assist woman to maintain a supine position with lateral tilt or a side-lying position for 30 to 40 minutes after insertion. Prepare to swab vagina to remove unabsorbed medication using saline-soaked gauze wrapped around fingers and to administer terbutaline 0.25 mg subcutaneously or intravenously if significant adverse reactions occur. Initiate oxytocin for induction of labor at least 4 hours after last dose of misoprostol was administered, following agency protocol, if ripening has occurred and labor has not begun. Document all assessment findings and administration procedures. A nonscored 100-mcg tablet must be cut in the pharmacy to ensure dosage accuracy.

BOX 19-9 Procedure: Assisting with Amniotomy

Procedure

Explain to woman what will be done.
Assess woman for signs of infection, condition of cervix (e.g., ripeness, dilation), and station of the presenting part.
Assess fetal heart rate before procedure begins to obtain a baseline reading.
Place several underpads under woman's buttocks to absorb fluid.
Position woman on padded bed pan, fracture pan, or rolled-up towel to elevate her hips as needed.
Assist health care provider who is performing the procedure by providing sterile gloves and lubricant for the vaginal examination.
Unwrap sterile package containing Amnihook or Allis clamp and pass instrument to primary health care provider, who inserts it alongside the fingers and then hooks and tears the membranes.
Reassess fetal heart rate and pattern.
Assess color, consistency, and odor of fluid.
Assess woman's temperature every 2 hours or per protocol.
Evaluate woman for signs and symptoms of infection.

Documentation

Record the following:

- Indication for amniotomy
- Time of rupture
- Color, odor, consistency and clarity of fluid
- Fetal heart rate and pattern before and after procedure
- Maternal status and how well procedure was tolerated

NURSING ALERT An amniotomy is performed by the primary health care provider (physician or midwife), never a nurse.

Before the procedure the woman should be told what to expect; she should also be assured that the actual rupture of membranes is painless for her and the fetus, although she may experience some discomfort when the Amnihook or other sharp instrument is inserted through the vagina and cervix (Box 19-9).

The presenting part of the fetus should be engaged and well applied to the cervix to reduce the risk of cord prolapse. The woman should be free of active infection of the genital tract (e.g., herpes) and human immunodeficiency virus (HIV) infection. The membranes are ruptured with an Amnihook or other sharp instrument, and the amniotic fluid is allowed to drain slowly. The fluid is assessed for color, odor, and consistency (i.e., for the presence or absence of meconium or blood). The time of rupture is recorded.

NURSING ALERT The FHR is assessed before and immediately after the amniotomy to detect any changes (transient tachycardia is common, but bradycardia and variable

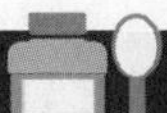

MEDICATION GUIDE

Cervical Ripening Using Prostaglandin E_2: Dinoprostone (Cervidil Insert; Prepidil Gel)

Action

Prostaglandin E_2 (PGE_2) ripens the cervix, making it softer and causing it to begin to dilate and efface; it stimulates uterine contractions.

Indications

PGE_2 is used for preinduction cervical ripening (to ripen cervix before oxytocin induction of labor when the Bishop score is 4 or less) and to induce labor or abortion (abortifacient agent).

Dosage and Route

Place Cervidil insert (10 mg dinoprostone gradually released over 12 hours) intravaginally into the posterior fornix. Remove after 12 hours or the onset of labor. Keep insert frozen until ready to use (no rewarming is needed). Uterine contractions usually begin in 5 to 7 hours. Induction may be initiated, if needed, 30 to 60 minutes after placement of the insert.

Insert Prepidil gel (2.5-ml syringe containing 0.5 mg of dinoprostone) into cervical canal just below internal cervical os or into posterior fornix; a shield can be used to prevent insertion past internal os. Repeat gel insertion in 6 hours as needed to a maximum of 1.5 mg in a 24-hour period. Bring gel to room temperature before administration. Do not force the warming process by using a warm water bath or other source of external heat such as microwave. Continue treatment until maximum dosage is administered or until an effective contraction pattern is established (three or more uterine contractions in 10 minutes), cervix ripens (Bishop score of 8 or more), or significant adverse reactions occur. Initiate oxytocin for induction of labor, if needed, within 6 to 12 hours after the last instillation of the gel.

Adverse Reactions

Potential adverse reactions include headache, nausea and vomiting, diarrhea, fever, hypotension, tachysystole (12 or more uterine contractions in 20 minutes without alteration of fetal heart rate or pattern), hyperstimulation of the uterus (tachysystole with nonreassuring fetal heart rate or patterns), or fetal passage of meconium. Adverse reactions are more common with intracervical administration.

Nursing Considerations

Explain procedure to woman and her family. Ensure that an informed consent has been obtained per agency policy. Assess maternal-fetal unit before each insertion and during treatment, following agency protocol for frequency. Assess maternal vital signs and health status, fetal heart rate and pattern, and status of pregnancy, including indications for cervical ripening or induction of labor, signs of labor or impending labor, and the Bishop score. Recognize that a nonreassuring fetal heart rate or pattern; maternal fever, infection, vaginal bleeding, or hypersensitivity; and regular, progressive uterine contractions and history of cesarean birth or uterine scar contraindicate the use of dinoprostone. Use caution if the woman has a history of asthma; glaucoma; or renal, hepatic, or cardiovascular disorders. Have woman void before insertion. Assist woman to maintain a supine position with lateral tilt or a side-lying position for 30 to 60 minutes after insertion of gel or for 2 hours after placement of insert. Allow woman to ambulate after recommended period of bed rest and observation. Prepare to swab vagina to remove remaining gel using saline-soaked gauze wrapped around fingers or pull string to remove insert and administer terbutaline, 0.25 mg subcutaneously or intravenously, if significant adverse reactions occur. Initiate oxytocin for induction of labor within 6 to 12 hours after last instillation of gel or at least 30 to 60 minutes after removal of the insert. Follow agency protocol for induction if ripening has occurred and labor has not begun. Document all assessment findings and administration procedures. Dinoprostone is the only FDA-approved medication for cervical ripening or labor induction.

FDA, Food and Drug Administration.

decelerations are not), which may indicate cord compression or prolapse.

The woman's temperature should be checked at least every 2 hours to rule out possible infection. If her temperature is 38° C or greater, the primary health care provider is notified. The nurse assesses for other signs and symptoms of infection such as maternal chills, fetal tachycardia, uterine tenderness on palpation, and foul-smelling vaginal drainage (Simpson, 2008). Comfort measures such as frequently changing the woman's underpads and perineal cleansing are implemented.

Oxytocin

Oxytocin is a hormone normally produced by the posterior pituitary gland; it stimulates uterine contractions. It may be used to either induce labor or augment a labor that is progressing slowly because of inadequate uterine contractions. See Box 19-10 for indications and contraindications for oxytocin induction or augmentation.

Although certain maternal and fetal conditions are not contraindications to the use of oxytocin to stimulate labor, they do require special caution during its administration. These conditions include the following:

- Multifetal presentation
- Breech presentation
- Presenting part above the pelvic inlet
- Abnormal FHR and pattern not requiring emergency birth
- Polyhydramnios
- Grand multiparity
- Maternal cardiac disease; hypertension

Oxytocin use can present hazards to the mother and the fetus. These hazards are primarily dose related; most problems are caused by high doses given rapidly. Maternal hazards include water intoxication and tumultuous labor with tetanic contractions, which may cause premature separation of the placenta, rupture of the uterus, lacerations of the cervix, or postpartum hemorrhage. These complications can lead to infection, hemorrhage, disseminated intravascular coagulation, or fetal compromise. Women may become anxious or fearful if the induction is not successful because they can then have concerns about the method of birth.

BOX 19-10 Indications and Contraindications for Use of Oxytocin for Induction or Augmentation of Labor

The indications for oxytocin induction or augmentation of labor may include but are not limited to the following:

- Suspected fetal jeopardy (e.g., intrauterine growth restriction)
- Inadequate uterine contractions; dystocia
- Premature rupture of membranes
- Postterm pregnancy
- Chorioamnionitis
- Maternal medical problems (e.g., woman with severe Rh isoimmunization, inadequately controlled diabetes, chronic renal disease, or chronic pulmonary disease)
- Gestational hypertension (e.g., preeclampsia, eclampsia)
- Fetal death
- Multiparous women with history of precipitous labor or who live far from the hospital

The management of stimulation of labor is the same, regardless of indication. Because of the potential dangers associated with the injection of oxytocin in the prenatal and perinatal periods, the Food and Drug Administration has issued restrictions on its use.

Contraindications to oxytocic stimulation of labor include but are not limited to the following:

- Cephalopelvic disproportion, prolapsed cord, transverse lie
- Abnormal fetal heart rate
- Placenta previa or vasa previa
- Prior classic uterine incision or uterine surgery
- Active genital herpes infection
- Invasive cancer of the cervix

Tachysystole (more than 5 uterine contractions in a 10-minute period) may reduce the blood flow through the placenta and result in FHR changes (bradycardia, tachycardia, decreased or absent baseline variability, late decelerations) and fetal asphyxia, which may lead to neonatal hypoxia. If the estimated date of birth is inaccurate, physical injury, neonatal hyperbilirubinemia, and prematurity are other hazards.

Informed consent to begin induction or augmentation of labor with oxytocin is the responsibility of the primary health care provider. Oxytocin is administered through a secondary intravenous line according to agency protocol and professional standards (Fig. 19-6 and Box 19-11). The nurse titrates the oxytocin dose to achieve a regular uterine contraction pattern that causes cervical change. In the past the aim of induction was to achieve a contraction pattern that simulates the active phase of labor as quickly as possible. However, research on uterine tolerance to oxytocin has now shown that lower physiologic doses (e.g., initial dose of 0.5 to 1 mU/min with increments of 1 to 2 mU/min) given over a longer time are as effective as previous protocols. A recommended dosage increment frequency is every 30 to 60 minutes because 30 to 40 minutes is required for a steady state of oxytocin to be reached and for the full effect of a dosage increment to be reflected in more intense, frequent, and longer contractions. Such an approach reduces the amount of oxytocin required to achieve a spontaneous vaginal birth and decreases the risk for tachysystole, dysfunctional labor, operative vaginal birth, cesarean birth, abnormal FHR patterns, and other adverse reactions such as water intoxication (Battista & Wing, 2007; Simpson, 2008).

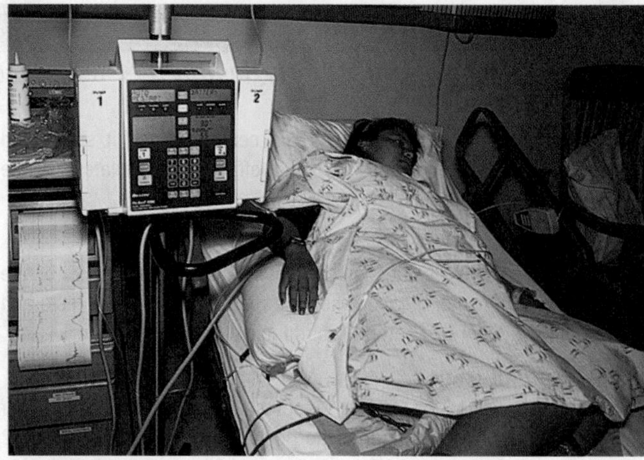

Fig. 19-6 Woman in side-lying position receiving oxytocin. *(Courtesy Michael S. Clement, MD, Mesa, AZ.)*

Nursing Considerations

An evidence-based written protocol for the preparation and administration of oxytocin should be established by the obstetric department (physicians, midwives, nurses) in each institution. One procedure recommended for a woman who is eligible for induction of labor is discussed in Box 19-11.

NURSING ALERT Oxytocin is decreased and/or discontinued and the health care provider notified, if tachysystole that results in an abnormal FHR and/or pattern occurs. Other nursing interventions such as administering 10 L oxygen by nonrebreather mask, positioning the woman on her side, and administering an intravenous fluid bolus, are independent nursing interventions and are implemented immediately (see Emergency box). Based on the status of the maternal-fetal unit, the primary health care provider may order that the infusion be restarted once the FHR and uterine activity return to acceptable levels. Depending on the FHR and pattern assessment and the length of time the infusion was discontinued, the oxytocin may be restarted at half the rate that resulted in tachysystole (e.g., discontinued for 10 to 20 minutes) or at the same rate as the initial rate (e.g., discontinued for more than 30 to 40 minutes) (Simpson, 2008) (see Nursing Care Plan: Dysfunctional Labor).

Augmentation of Labor

Augmentation of labor is the stimulation of uterine contractions after labor has started spontaneously but progress has been unsatisfactory. Augmentation is usually implemented for the management of hypotonic uterine dysfunction resulting in a slowing of labor (protracted active phase). Common augmentation methods include oxytocin infusion, amniotomy, and nipple stimulation. Noninvasive methods such as emptying the bladder, ambulation, position changes, relaxation measures, nourishment, hydration, and hydrotherapy can be attempted before invasive interventions are initiated. The procedures and nursing assessments are similar to those used for oxytocin induction of labor. Protocols for dosage and fre-

BOX 19-11 Protocol: Induction of Labor with Oxytocin

Patient/Family Teaching

Explain technique, rationale, and reactions to expect.

- Route and rate for administration of medication
- What "piggyback" is for
- Reasons for use—Induce labor, improve labor
- Reactions to expect concerning the nature of contractions—Intensity of contraction increases more rapidly, holds peak longer, and ends more quickly; contractions will come regularly and more often
- Monitoring to anticipate:
  Maternal—Blood pressure, pulse, uterine contractions, uterine tone
  Fetal—Heart rate, activity/movements
- Success to expect—Favorable outcome will depend on inducibility of cervix (e.g., Bishop score of 9)

Keep woman and support person informed of progress.

Administration

Verify that primary health care provider has discussed the indication and risks and benefits with the pregnant woman.

Verify that the indication for induction is documented.

Assess status of maternal-fetal unit (contractions, cervical status; monitor fetal heart rate [FHR] for at least 15 minutes before initiation of oxytocin infusion).

Position woman in side-lying or upright position.

Prepare solution and administer with pump delivery system according to prescribed orders.

- Infusion pump and solution are set up (e.g., 30 units/500 ml lactated Ringer's solution).
- Piggyback solution is connected to intravenous line at proximal port (port nearest point of venous insertion).
- Solution with oxytocin is flagged with medication label.
- Begin induction at 0.5 to 1 mU/min.
- Increase dosage 1 to 2 mU/min at intervals of 30 to 60 minutes until an adequate contraction pattern is established.
- Once labor is established, maintain or decrease oxytocin to a rate adequate for continued labor progress.
- Dosage may be increased up to 20 mU/min.

Maternal/Fetal Assessments

Monitor blood pressure, pulse, and respirations at least every 4 hours.

Monitor contraction pattern and uterine resting tone each time the FHR is evaluated and before every increment in dosage.

Assess intake and output; limit intravenous intake to 1000 ml/8 hr; output should be 120 ml or more every 4 hours.

Perform vaginal examination for effacement, dilation, and station as indicated.

Monitor amniotic fluid for character and amount.

Monitor character and amount of bloody show/vaginal bleeding.

Monitor for nausea, vomiting, headache, hypotension.

Assess fetal status using electronic fetal monitoring; evaluate tracing every 30 minutes during the active phase of labor, every 15 minutes during active pushing, and with each increment in dose.

Assess level of maternal discomfort/pain and effectiveness of pain management.

Observe emotional responses of woman and her partner.

Reportable Conditions

Uterine tachysystole

Abnormal FHR and pattern

Suspected uterine rupture

Inadequate uterine response at 20 mU/min

Emergency Measures

Discontinue use of oxytocin per hospital protocol:

- Turn woman on her side.
- Give intravenous bolus of at least 500 ml lactated Ringer's solution.
- If indeterminate or abnormal FHR pattern, consider giving woman oxygen by nonrebreather face mask at 8 to 10 units/min or per protocol or primary health care provider's order.

Documentation

Medication—Kind, amount, time of beginning, increasing dosage, maintaining dosage, and discontinuing medication

Reactions of mother and fetus:

- Uterine activity
- Progress of labor
- FHR and pattern
- Maternal vital signs
- Nursing interventions and woman's response

Communication with physician or nurse-midwife

From American College of Obstetricians and Gynecologists: *Induction of labor,* ACOG Practice Bulletin No 20, Washington, DC, 1999/2006, ACOG; Simpson KR: *Cervical ripening and induction and augmentation of labor,* ed 3, Washington, DC, 2008, Association of Women's Health, Obstetric and Neonatal Nurses.

quency of increments may vary (e.g., lower dosages may be needed to achieve spontaneous vaginal birth) (Gilbert, 2007; Simpson, 2008).

Some physicians advocate active management of labor in a primigravid woman (i.e., the augmentation of labor to establish efficient labor with aggressive use of oxytocin so that the woman gives birth within 12 hours of admission to the labor unit). The woman should be admitted only when labor is established (i.e., painful contractions, spontaneous rupture of membranes, complete effacement) (Kilpatrick & Garrison, 2007). Advocates of active management believe that intervening early (as soon as a nulliparous labor is not progressing at least 1 cm/hr) with amniotomy and the use of higher pharmacologic oxytocin doses administered at frequent increment intervals (e.g., a starting dose of 6 mU/min with increases of 6 mU/min every 15 minutes to a maximum dosage of 40 mU/min) shortens labor and is associated with a lower incidence of cesarean birth (Battista & Wing, 2007; Simpson, 2008). Active management of labor continues to be under study in the United States to determine effectiveness and impact on perinatal morbidity and

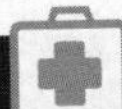

EMERGENCY

Uterine Hyperstimulation with Oxytocin

Signs

Greater than five uterine contractions in 10 minutes, averaged over a 30-minute window

Abnormal fetal heart rate and pattern:

- Absent baseline variability and any of the following: (1) recurrent late decelerations, (2) recurrent variable decelerations, and (3) bradycardia
- Sinusoidal pattern

Interventions

Maintain woman in side-lying position.

Turn off oxytocin infusion; keep maintenance intravenous line open; increase rate.

Start administering oxygen by nonrebreather face mask per protocol or physician's order.

Notify primary health care provider.

Prepare to administer terbutaline (Brethine), 0.25 mg subcutaneously, if ordered to decrease uterine activity.

Continue monitoring fetal heart rate and pattern and uterine activity.

Document responses to actions.

mortality rates. Thus far results have been disappointing, especially in terms of reducing the rate of cesarean births. The disappointing results have been attributed in part to a greater than one-to-one nurse/patient ratio and the high rate of epidural anesthesia. It is considered to be a form of care of unknown effectiveness (Enkin et al, 2000; Gilbert, 2007).

Forceps-Assisted Birth

A forceps-assisted vaginal birth is one in which an instrument with two curved blades is used to assist in the birth of the fetal head. The cephalic-like curve of the forceps commonly used is similar to the shape of the fetal head, with a pelvic curve to the blades conforming to the curve of the pelvic axis. The blades are joined by a groove arrangement and prevent the forceps from compressing the fetal skull. Maternal indications for forceps-assisted birth include a maternal disease state that inhibits pushing efforts (e.g., cardiac disease) or the need to shorten the second stage.

Fetal indications include certain abnormal presentations, arrest of rotation, an abnormal FHR and/or pattern that necessitates birth, and delivery of an aftercoming head in a breech presentation. The use of forceps during childbirth has been decreasing. In 2005 forceps or vacuum was used to assist 4.8% of births (Martin et al, 2007).

There are various definitions of forceps applications. Outlet forceps are used when the fetal scalp is visible on the perineum without manually separating the labia. Outlet forceps are used to shorten the second stage of labor (Fig. 19-7). Low forceps refers to the application of forceps to a fetal head that is at least at a +2 cm station. Midforceps is the application of forceps to the fetal head that is engaged (no higher than station 0) but above the +2 cm station. In no instances should the forceps be applied to an unengaged presenting part.

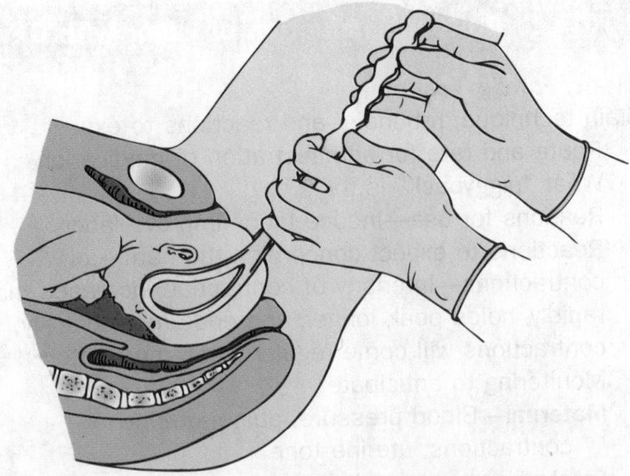

Fig. 19-7 Outlet forceps-assisted extraction of the head.

BOX 19-12 Prerequisites for Successful Forceps- or Vacuum-Assisted Birth

- Informed consent should be obtained by the physician before the procedure.
- The woman's cervix must be fully dilated to avoid lacerations and hemorrhage.
- The bladder should be empty.
- The vertex presenting part must be engaged and descended into a low station.
- Membranes must be ruptured so that the position of the fetal head can be determined and the forceps can firmly grasp the head during birth.
- Adequate maternal analgesia and appropriate support personnel need to be available.
- The maternal pelvis should be assessed, and fetal weight estimated by the physician to determine adequacy for delivery.

Nursing Considerations

Prerequisites for use must be met for the use of forceps to be successful (Box 19-12). The nurse obtains the type of forceps requested by the physician (Fig. 19-8). The nurse may explain to the mother that the forceps blades fit like two tablespoons around an egg, with the blades coming over the baby's ears.

NURSING ALERT Because compression of the cord between the fetal head and the forceps causes a drop in FHR, the FHR and pattern are checked, reported, and recorded before and after forceps are applied. If a decrease in FHR occurs, the physician can remove and reapply the forceps. Ordinarily traction is applied during contractions.

After birth the mother is assessed for vaginal and cervical lacerations (e.g., bleeding that occurs even with a contracted uterus); urine retention, which may result from bladder injuries or urethral injuries; and hematoma formation in the pelvic soft tissues, which may result from blood vessel damage. The infant should be assessed for bruising or abrasions at the site of the blade applications, facial palsy resulting from pressure of the blades on the facial nerve (cranial nerve VII), and subdural hematoma. Newborn and postpartum caregivers should be told that the birth was forceps assisted.

Vacuum-Assisted Birth

Vacuum-assisted birth, or vacuum extraction, is a birth method involving the attachment of a vacuum cup to the fetal head, using negative pressure to assist in the birth of the head.

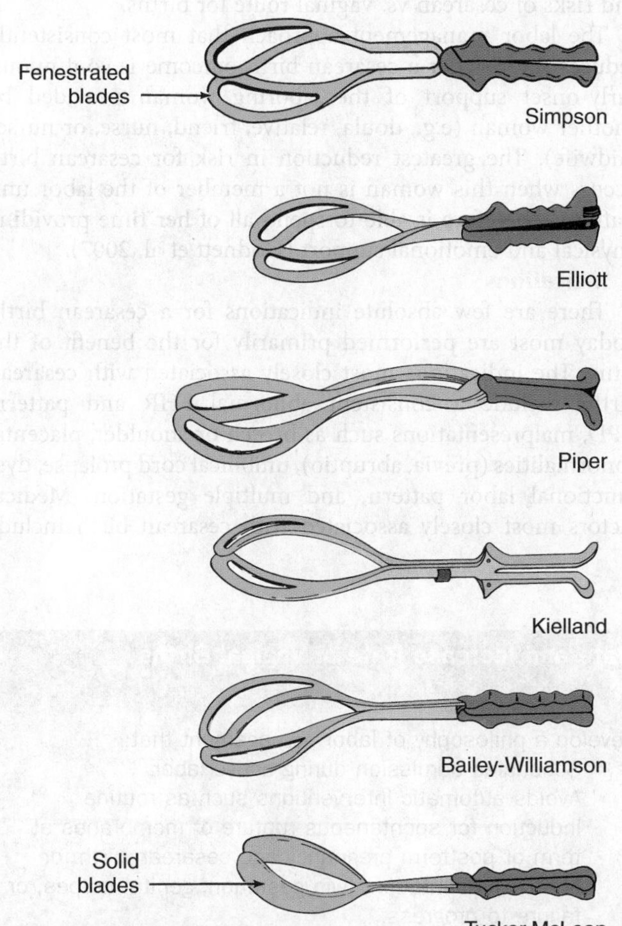

Fig. 19-8 Types of forceps. Piper forceps are used to assist delivery of the head in a breech birth.

Indications for use are similar to those for outlet forceps. When an operative vaginal birth is required, vacuum assistance is preferred as a beneficial form of care when compared with forceps assistance (Cunningham et al, 2005).

When the birth is to be vacuum assisted, the woman is prepared for a vaginal birth in the lithotomy position to allow for sufficient traction. The cup is applied to the fetal head, and a caput develops inside the cup as the pressure is initiated (Fig. 19-9). Traction is applied by the physician to facilitate descent of the fetal head, and the woman is encouraged to push as suction is applied. The vacuum cup is released and removed after birth of the head. If vacuum extraction is not successful, a forceps-assisted or cesarean birth is performed.

Risks to the newborn include cephalhematoma, scalp lacerations, and subdural hematoma. Fetal complications can be reduced by strict adherence to the manufacturer's recommendations for method of application, degree of suction, and duration of application. Maternal complications are uncommon but can include perineal, vaginal, and cervical lacerations and soft-tissue hematomas.

Nursing Considerations

The nurse's role for the woman who has a vacuum-assisted birth is one of support person and educator. The nurse can prepare the woman for birth and encourage her to remain active in the birth process by pushing during contractions. The FHR should be assessed frequently during the procedure. After birth the newborn should be observed for signs of trauma at the application site and cerebral irritation (e.g., poor sucking or listlessness). Documentation includes the number of applications, any "pop-offs," the number of pulls, and the maximum amount of suction used.

The newborn may be at risk for infection at the application site, hyperbilirubinemia and neonatal jaundice as bruising, a cephalhematoma, or subdural hematoma resolves. The parents may need to be reassured that the caput succedaneum will begin to disappear in a few hours. Neonatal caregivers should be told that the birth was vacuum assisted.

Cesarean Birth

Cesarean birth is the birth of a fetus through a transabdominal incision of the uterus (see Fig. 19-11). The purpose of cesarean birth is to preserve the life or health of the mother and/or her

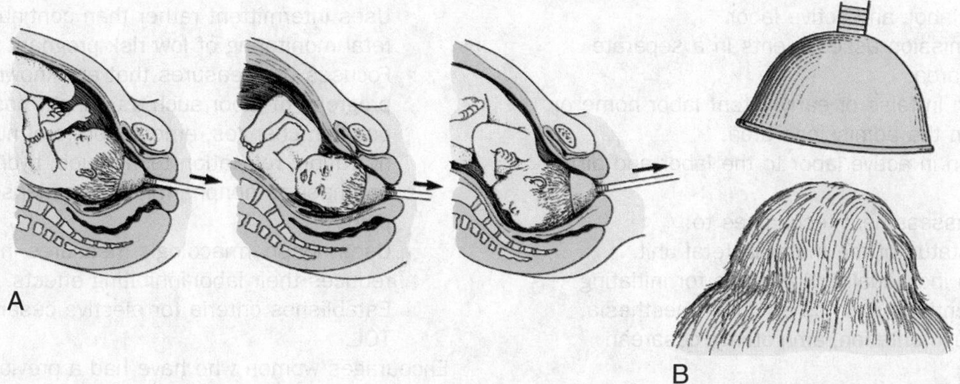

Fig. 19-9 Use of vacuum extraction to rotate fetal head and assist with descent. **A,** *Arrow* indicates direction of traction on the vacuum cup. **B,** Caput succedaneum formed by the vacuum cup.

fetus; it may be the best choice when there is evidence of maternal or fetal complications. Incisions are made into the lower uterine segment rather than into the muscular body of the uterus and thus promote more effective healing. Since the advent of modern surgical methods and care and the use of antibiotics, maternal and fetal morbidity and mortality rates have decreased. Despite these advances, cesarean birth still poses threats to the health of both mother and infant.

The incidence of cesarean births increased to 31.1% in 2006, the highest rate ever reported in the United States (Martin et al, 2007). Factors cited in this increase include the increase of primary elective cesarean births and the decline in the rate of vaginal birth after cesarean (VBAC) (Martin et al, 2007). Cesarean rates were highest for non-Hispanic black women (33.1%) compared with non-Hispanic white (31.3%) and Hispanic women (29.7%) (Martin et al, 2007). Women who have private insurance, who are of a higher socioeconomic status, or who deliver in a private hospital are more likely to experience cesarean birth than are women who are poor, have no insurance, are receiving public assistance (e.g., Medicaid), or give birth in a public hospital (Gilbert, 2007).

Approaches for the management of labor and birth to reduce the rate of cesarean births while increasing the rate of VBACs are presented in Box 19-13. These management approaches involve the combined efforts of health care professionals and pregnant women and their families. The type of nursing care given also may influence the rate of cesarean births. A labor management approach that uses one-to-one support and emphasizes ambulation, maternal position changes, relaxation measures, oral fluids and nutrition, hydrotherapy, and nonpharmacologic pain relief facilitates the progress of labor and reduces the incidence of dystocia. The rate of VBACs is decreasing. This decline may be the result of risks of VBAC (e.g., uterine rupture), legal pressures, conservative practice guidelines, and debate regarding the relative benefits and risks of cesarean vs. vaginal route for births.

The labor management approach that most consistently reduces the risk for a cesarean birth outcome is continuous, early-onset support of the laboring woman provided by another woman (e.g., doula, relative, friend, nurse, or nurse-midwife). The greatest reduction in risk for cesarean birth occurs when this woman is not a member of the labor unit staff and therefore is able to spend all of her time providing physical and emotional support (Hodnett et al, 2007).

Indications

There are few absolute indications for a cesarean birth. Today most are performed primarily for the benefit of the fetus. The indications most closely associated with cesarean births include a consistent abnormal FHR and pattern, CPD, malpresentations such as breech or shoulder, placental abnormalities (previa, abruptio), umbilical cord prolapse, dysfunctional labor pattern, and multiple gestation. Medical factors most closely associated with cesarean birth include

BOX 19-13 Selected Measures to Reduce Cesarean Birth Rate and Increase Rate of Vaginal Births After Cesarean

Educate women regarding:
- Advantages and safety of the home environment for early or latent labor.
- Indicators for hospital admission.
- Management techniques to use during labor to enhance progress.
- Nonpharmacologic measures to reduce pain and discomfort and enhance relaxation.
- Safety and effectiveness of TOL and VBAC.

Establish admission criteria for women in labor to:
- Distinguish clinical manifestations for false labor, latent/early labor, and active labor.
- Conduct admission assessments in a separate admissions area.
- Send women in false or early/latent labor home or keep them in the admissions area.
- Admit women in active labor to the labor and birth unit.

Use appropriate assessment techniques to:
- Determine status of the maternal-fetal unit.
- Establish an individualized rationale for initiating labor interventions such as epidural anesthesia, induction/augmentation, amniotomy, cesarean birth.

Initiate a doula program that:
- Provides one-to-one support for women in labor.

Develop a philosophy of labor management that:
- Schedules admission during active labor.
- Avoids automatic interventions such as routine induction for spontaneous rupture of membranes at term or postterm pregnancy and cesarean birth for breech presentation, twin gestation, genital herpes, or failure to progress.
- Relies on assessment findings reflective of the status of the maternal-fetal unit rather than strict adherence to set ranges for the duration of the stages and phases of labor.
- Uses intermittent rather than continuous electronic fetal monitoring of low risk pregnant women.
- Focuses on measures that are known to enhance the progress of labor such as upright positions, frequent position changes, ambulation, oral nutrition and hydration, relaxation techniques, hydrotherapy.
- Emphasizes nonpharmacologic measures to relieve pain.
- Uses nonpharmacologic measures in a manner that reduces their labor-inhibiting effects.
- Establishes criteria for elective cesarean birth and TOL.

Encourages women who have had a previous cesarean birth to participate in TOL to attempt a vaginal birth.

TOL, Trial of labor; *VBAC*, vaginal birth after cesarean.

hypertensive disorders, active genital herpes, positive HIV status, and diabetes (Martin et al, 2007).

Surgical Techniques

The two main types of cesarean operation are the classic and the lower-segment cesarean incisions. Classic cesarean birth is rarely performed today, although it may be used when rapid birth is necessary and in some cases of shoulder presentation, multiple gestation, and placenta previa. The incision is made vertically into the upper body of the uterus (Fig. 19-10, *A*). Because the procedure is associated with a higher incidence of blood loss, infection, and uterine rupture in subsequent pregnancies than is lower-segment cesarean birth, labor and vaginal birth after a classic cesarean are contraindicated.

Lower-segment cesarean birth can be achieved through a vertical or transverse incision into the uterus (see Fig. 19-10, *B* and *C*). The transverse incision is more popular because it is easier to perform, associated with less blood loss and fewer postoperative infections, and less likely to rupture in subsequent pregnancies (Cunningham et al, 2005).

Complications and Risks

Cesarean births are not without risk of complications for both the mother and fetus. Maternal complications include aspiration; pulmonary embolism; wound infection; wound dehiscence; thrombophlebitis; hemorrhage; urinary tract infection; injuries to bladder, ureters, or bowel; and complications related to anesthesia. The fetus may be born prematurely if gestational age has not been accurately determined; fetal injuries can occur during the surgery (Landon, 2007). Besides

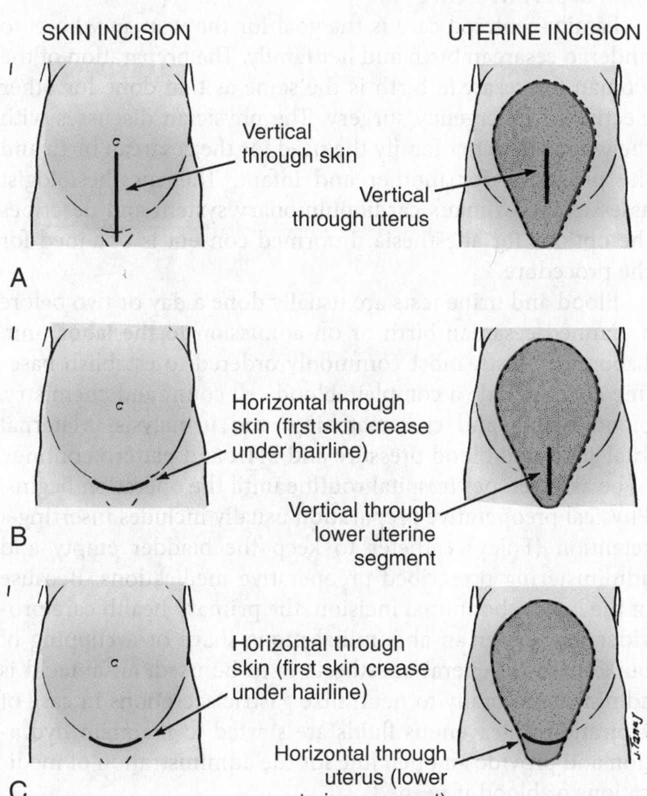

Fig. 19-10 Cesarean birth: skin and uterine incisions. **A**, Classic: vertical incisions of skin and uterus. **B**, Low cervical: horizontal incision of skin; vertical incision of uterus. **C**, Low cervical: horizontal incisions of skin and uterus.

these risks, the woman is at economic risk because the cost of a cesarean birth is higher than that of a vaginal birth and a longer recovery period may require additional expenditures.

Cesarean on Demand

The decrease in VBACs becomes more complex as women are requesting cesarean births for reasons other than medical, obstetric, or fetal indications. These reasons include the belief that the surgery will prevent future problems with pelvic support or sexual dysfunction and the convenience of planning a date when the father of the baby or support person is available. Some multiparous women may request a cesarean after a previous traumatic vaginal birth caused by physical injury or psychologic trauma (Gardner, 2003). In a committee opinion ACOG (2003b) notes that the right of patients to refuse surgery is well known. It is less clear if they have the right to ask for surgery. The Society of Obstetricians and Gynaecologists of Canada (SOGC) does not promote cesarean on demand and promotes natural childbirth but believes that the final decision as to the safest route for childbirth rests with the woman and her health care provider (SOGC, 2004). It is essential that women are fully informed about the risks and benefits of cesarean birth when they consider requesting elective cesarean birth.

Forced Cesarean Birth

A woman's refusal to undergo cesarean birth for fetal reasons is often described as a maternal-fetal conflict. Health care providers are ethically obliged to protect the well-being of both the mother and the fetus; a decision for one affects the other. If a woman refuses a cesarean birth that is recommended because of fetal jeopardy, health care providers must make every effort to find out why she is refusing and provide information that may persuade her to change her mind. If the woman continues to refuse surgery, the health care providers must decide if it is ethical to get a court order for the surgery; however, every effort should be made to avoid this legal step.

Anesthesia

Spinal, epidural, and general anesthetics are used for cesarean births. Regional blocks (epidural and spinal) are popular because women want to be awake for and aware of the birth experience. However, the choice of anesthetic depends on several factors. The mother's medical history or present condition such as a spinal injury, hemorrhage, or coagulopathy may rule out the use of regional anesthesia. Time is another factor, especially if there is an emergency and the life of the mother or infant is at risk. In such a case general anesthesia will most likely be used unless an epidural is already in place. The woman herself is a factor. She may not know all the options or may have fears about "a needle in her back" or of being awake and feeling pain. She needs to be fully informed about the risks and benefits of the different types of anesthesia so that she can participate in the decision whenever there is a choice.

Scheduled Cesarean Birth

Cesarean birth is scheduled or planned if labor and vaginal birth is contraindicated (e.g., complete placenta previa, active genital herpes, positive HIV status), if birth is necessary but labor is not inducible (e.g., hypertensive states that cause a poor intrauterine environment that threatens the fetus), or if this has been decided on by the physician and the woman (e.g., a repeat or elective cesarean birth).

Women who are scheduled to have a cesarean birth have time to prepare for it psychologically. However, the psychologic responses of these women may vary. Those having a repeat cesarean birth can have disturbing memories of the conditions preceding the initial surgical birth and their experiences in the postoperative recovery period. They can be concerned about the added burden of caring for an infant and perhaps other children while recovering from a surgical operation. Others can feel glad to have been relieved of the uncertainty about the date and time of birth and to be free from the pain of labor.

Unplanned Cesarean Birth

The psychosocial outcomes of unplanned or emergency cesarean birth are usually more pronounced and negative in nature when compared with the outcomes associated with a scheduled or planned cesarean birth. Women and their families experience abrupt changes in their expectations for birth, postpartum care, and the care of the new baby at home. This may be an extremely traumatic experience for all.

The woman usually approaches the procedure tired and discouraged after an ineffective and difficult labor. Fear predominates as she worries about her own safety and well-being and that of her fetus. Because preoperative procedures must be done quickly and competently, the time available for explanation of the procedures and operation is often short. Because maternal and family anxiety levels are high at this time, much of what is said may be forgotten or misunderstood. These women need much supportive care.

Therefore after surgery time must be spent reviewing the events preceding the operation and the operation itself to ensure that the woman understands what has happened and that gaps in her recollections are filled. This approach will help create more realistic memories of the childbirth experience, thereby having a more positive influence on future pregnancies and labors.

Prenatal Preparation

Whether a cesarean birth is planned (scheduled) or unplanned (emergency or determined to be necessary during labor), the loss of the experience of giving birth to an infant in the traditional manner may have a negative effect on a woman's self-concept. She may feel frustration at losing control, disappointment, anger, and loss of self-esteem. These feelings are related to a change in body image and perceived inability to give birth as she had expected and hoped. Often women experience a delay in the ability to interact with their newborn after a cesarean birth. They are less likely to breastfeed and may even have difficulty expressing positive feelings about their newborns for some time after birth. They often are less satisfied with their childbirth experience and report more fatigue and poor physical functioning during the first few weeks after discharge.

Success at mothering and in the recovery process can do much to restore the self-esteem of these women. Some women see the scar as mutilating, and worries concerning sexual attractiveness may surface. Some men are fearful of resuming intercourse because of the fear of hurting their partner. Parents may wonder if a cesarean birth was absolutely necessary, and such feelings may surface even years later. A clear explanation should be given to the woman and her family regarding why the cesarean birth was necessary. Opportunities should also be provided to discuss the childbirth in an effort to resolve concerns that may arise after the birth.

Concerned professionals and lay groups in the community have established councils for cesarean birth to meet the needs of these women and their families. Such groups advocate that a discussion of cesarean birth be included in all parenthood preparation classes. No woman can be guaranteed a vaginal birth, even if she is in good health and there is no indication of danger to the fetus before the onset of labor. For this reason every woman needs to be aware of and prepared for this eventuality.

Childbirth educators stress the importance of emphasizing the similarities and differences between a cesarean and vaginal birth. In support of the philosophy of family-centered birth, many hospitals have instituted policies that permit fathers and other partners and family members to share in these births as they do in vaginal ones. Women who have undergone cesarean birth agree that the continued presence and support of their partners helped them respond positively to the entire experience.

In addition to preparing women for the possibility of cesarean birth, childbirth educators should empower women to believe in their ability to give birth vaginally and to seek care measures during labor that will enhance the progress of their labors and reduce their risk for cesarean birth.

Preoperative Care

Family-centered care is the goal for the woman who is to undergo cesarean birth and her family. The preparation of the woman for cesarean birth is the same as that done for other elective or emergency surgery. The physician discusses with the woman and her family the need for the cesarean birth and the prognosis for mother and infant. The anesthesiologist assesses the woman's cardiopulmonary system and describes the options for anesthesia. Informed consent is obtained for the procedure.

Blood and urine tests are usually done a day or two before a planned cesarean birth or on admission to the labor unit. Laboratory tests, most commonly ordered to establish baseline data, include a complete blood cell count and chemistry, blood typing and crossmatching, and urinalysis. Maternal vital signs and blood pressure and FHR and pattern continue to be assessed per hospital routine until the operation begins. Physical preoperative preparation usually includes inserting a retention (Foley) catheter to keep the bladder empty and administering prescribed preoperative medications. Because of the lower abdominal incision, the primary health care provider may order an abdominal-mons shave or a clipping of pubic hair. If general anesthesia is to be used, an antacid is administered orally to neutralize gastric secretions in case of aspiration. Intravenous fluids are started to maintain hydration and provide an open line for the administration of medications or blood if needed.

Removal of dentures, nail polish, and jewelry may be optional, depending on hospital policies and type of anesthesia used. If the woman wears glasses and is going to be awake, the nurse should make sure that her glasses accompany her to the operating room so she can see her infant. If the woman wears contact lenses, the nurse can find out whether they can be worn for the birth.

During preoperative preparation the support person is encouraged to remain with the woman as much as possible to provide continuing emotional support (if this is culturally acceptable to the woman and support person). The nurse provides essential information about the preoperative procedures during this time. Although the nursing actions may be carried out quickly if a cesarean birth is unplanned, verbal communication, particularly explanations, is important. Silence can be frightening to the woman and her support person. The nurse's use of touch can communicate feelings of care and concern for the woman. The nurse can assess the woman's and her partner's perceptions about cesarean birth. As the woman expresses her feelings, the nurse may identify a potential for a disturbance in self-concept during the postpartum period that may need to be addressed. If there is time before the birth, the nurse can teach the woman about postoperative expectations and pain relief, turning, coughing, and deep-breathing measures.

Intraoperative Care

Cesarean births occur in operating rooms in the surgical suite or in the labor and birth unit. Once the woman has been taken to the operating room, her care becomes the responsibility of the obstetric team, surgeon, anesthesiologist, pediatrician, and surgical nursing staff (Fig. 19-11). If possible, the partner, who is gowned appropriately, accompanies the mother to the surgical unit and remains close to her so that continued support and comfort can be provided. In unplanned cesarean birth the nurse who cared for the woman during labor should be part of the nursing care team in the operating room if possible.

The nurse who is circulating can assist with positioning the woman on the birth (surgical) table. It is important to position her so that the uterus is displaced laterally to prevent compressing the inferior vena cava, which causes decreased placental perfusion. This is usually accomplished by placing a wedge under the hip. A Foley catheter is inserted into the bladder at this time if one is not already in place.

If the partner either is not allowed or chooses not to be present in the operative suite, the nurse can stay in communication with him or her and give progress reports whenever possible. If the mother is awake during the birth, the nurse or anesthesiologist can tell her what is happening and provide support. The mother may be anxious about the sensations she is experiencing such as the coldness of solutions used to prepare the abdomen and pressure or pulling during the actual birth of the infant. She also may be apprehensive because of the bright lights or the presence of unfamiliar equipment and masked and gowned personnel in the room. Explanations by the nurse can help decrease the woman's anxiety.

Care of the infant usually is delegated to a pediatrician or a nurse team skilled in neonatal resuscitation because these infants are considered to be at risk until there is evidence of physiologic stability after the birth. A crib with resuscitation equipment is readied before surgery. Those responsible for care are expert not only in resuscitative techniques but also in their ability to detect normal and abnormal infant responses. After birth, if the infant's condition permits and the mother is awake, the baby may be placed skin-to-skin on the mother or can be given to the woman's partner to hold (Fig. 19-12). The infant whose condition is compromised is transported after initial stabilization to the nursery for observation and the implementation of appropriate interventions. In some institutions the partner may accompany the infant; if not, personnel

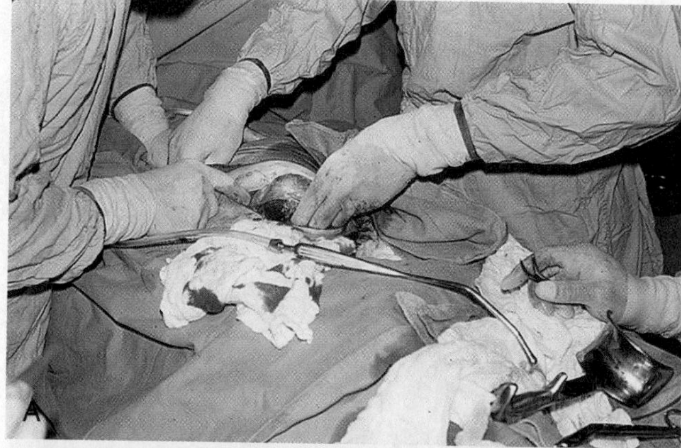

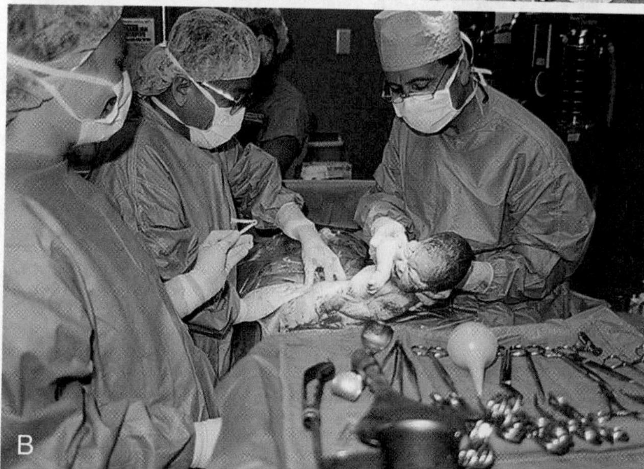

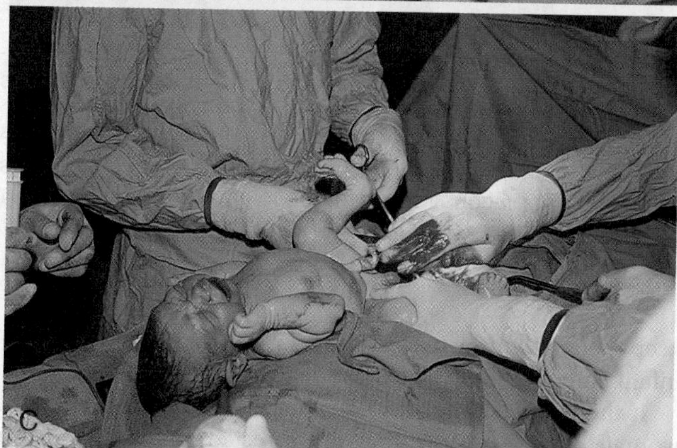

Fig. 19-11 Cesarean birth. **A**, "Bikini" incision has been made, the muscle layer is separated, the abdomen is entered, the uterus has been exposed and incised; suctioning of amniotic fluid continues as head is brought up through the incision. Note small amount of bleeding. **B**, The neonate's birth through the uterine incision is nearly complete. **C**, A quick assessment is performed; note significant molding of head resulting from cephalopelvic disproportion. *(Courtesy Marjorie Pyle, RNC, Lifecircle, Costa Mesa, CA.)*

evolve Video—Childbirth (Cesarean)

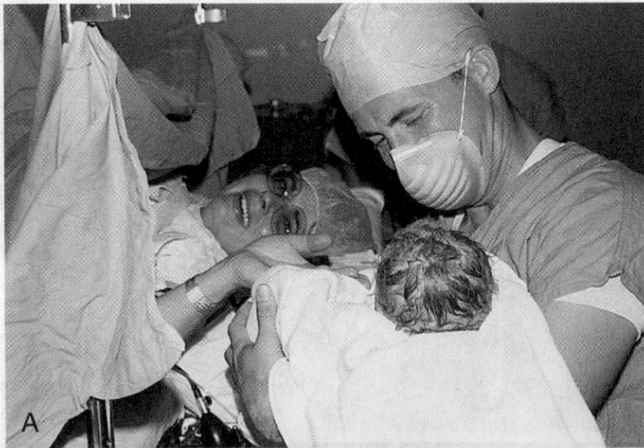

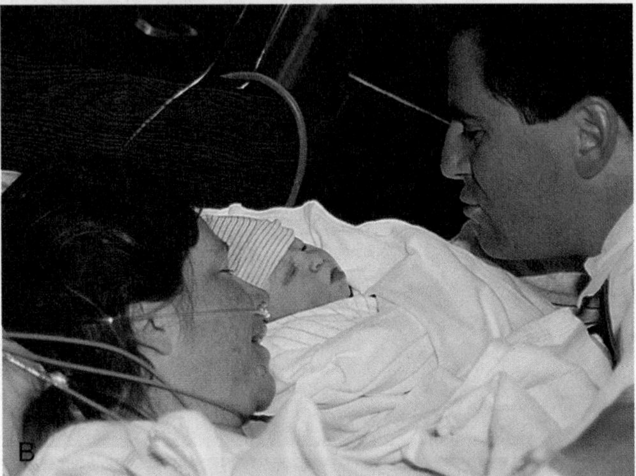

Fig. 19-12 A, Parents and their newborn. The physician manually removes the placenta; suctions the remaining amniotic fluid and blood from the uterine cavity; and closes the uterine incision, peritoneum, muscle layer, fatty tissue, and finally the skin while the new family shares some private time. B, Parents become better acquainted with their newborn while mother rests after surgery. *(Courtesy Marjorie Pyle, RNC, Lifecircle, Costa Mesa, CA.)*

keep the family informed of the infant's progress, and parent-infant contacts are initiated as soon as possible.

If the family cannot (or does not want to) accompany the woman during surgery, they are directed to the surgical or obstetric waiting room. The physician then reports on the condition of the mother and child to family members after the birth is completed. Family members may accompany the infant as he or she is transferred to the nursery, giving them an opportunity to see and admire the new baby.

NURSING ALERT Some mothers/parents want the privilege of informing family and friends of the sex of the infant (if it was not known before birth). Before responding to requests for such information from people waiting outside the birthing area, the nurse should check to see if the mother has given consent for such information to be released and to whom.

Immediate Postoperative Care

Once surgery is completed, the mother is transferred to a recovery room or back to her labor room. After a cesarean birth women have both postoperative and postpartum needs that must be addressed. They are surgical patients, as well as new mothers. Nursing assessments in this immediate postbirth period follow agency protocol and include degree of recovery from the effects of anesthesia, postoperative and postbirth status, and degree of pain. If general anesthesia was administered, it is essential that a patent airway be maintained, and the woman is positioned to prevent possible aspiration until she is fully alert and responsive. Vital signs are taken every 15 minutes for 1 to 2 hours or until stable. The condition of the incisional dressing, the fundus, and the amount of lochia are assessed, as well as intravenous intake and urine output through the Foley catheter. The woman is helped to turn and do coughing, deep-breathing, and leg exercises. Medications to relieve pain can be administered as ordered.

If the baby is present, the mother and her partner are given some time alone with him or her to facilitate bonding and attachment. Breastfeeding can be initiated when the mother feels like trying, preferably within the first 30 to 60 minutes. If the woman is in a recovery area or her labor room, she usually is transferred to the postpartum unit after 1 to 2 hours or once her condition is stable and the effects of anesthesia have worn off (i.e., she is alert, oriented, and able to feel and move extremities).

Postoperative or Postpartum Care

The attitude of the nurse and other health team members can influence the woman's perception of herself after a cesarean birth. The caregivers should stress that the woman is a new mother first and a surgical patient second. This attitude helps the woman perceive herself as having the same problems and needs as other new mothers while at the same time requiring supportive postoperative care.

The woman's physiologic concerns for the first few days may be dominated by pain at the incision site and pain resulting from intestinal gas; thus the need for pain relief. If epidural anesthesia was used for the surgery, epidural opioids can be given in the immediate postoperative period to provide pain relief for approximately 24 hours. Otherwise pain medications usually are given parenterally every 3 to 4 hours, or patient-controlled analgesia may be ordered. The most commonly used analgesics include opioids (e.g., hydromorphone, nalbuphine) and NSAIDs (e.g., ketorolac [Toradol]). If opioids are used, an antiemetic (e.g., promethazine [Phenergan], metoclopramide, ondansetron [Zofran]) is often ordered to be administered either as needed by the woman or around the clock as long as the opioid is used. Other comfort measures such as position changes, splinting the incision with pillows, and relaxation and breathing techniques may be implemented.

Ambulation and rocking in a rocking chair may relieve gas pains, and avoiding consumption of gas-forming foods and carbonated beverages may help minimize them (see Patient Teaching box).

Nurses must be alert to a woman's physiologic needs, managing care to ensure adequate rest and pain relief. Mother-baby care (couplet care) for a cesarean birth mother can be modified according to her physiologic limitations as a surgical patient.

PATIENT TEACHING Postpartum Pain Relief After Cesarean Birth

Incisional Pain

Splint incision with a pillow when moving or coughing.

Use relaxation techniques such as music, breathing, and dim lights.

Intestinal Gas

Walk as often as you can.

Do not eat or drink gas-forming foods, carbonated beverages, or whole milk.

Do not use straws for drinking fluids.

Take antiflatulence medication if prescribed.

Lie on your left side to expel gas.

Rock in a rocking chair.

Daily care includes perineal care, breast care, and routine hygienic care, including showering after the dressing has been removed (if showering is acceptable according to the woman's cultural beliefs and practices). The nurse assesses the woman's vital signs, incision, fundus, and lochia according to hospital policies, procedures, or protocols. Breath sounds, bowel sounds, circulatory status of lower extremities, and urinary and bowel elimination also are assessed. It is important to note maternal emotional status.

During the postpartum period the nurse can provide care that meets the psychologic and learning needs of mothers who have had cesarean births. The nurse can explain postpartum procedures to help the woman participate in her recovery from surgery. She can help the woman plan care and visits from family and friends that allow for adequate rest periods. Information and assistance with infant care can facilitate adjustment to her role as a mother. The woman is supported as she breastfeeds her baby by receiving individualized assistance to comfortably hold and position the baby at her breast. The side-lying position or football hold and the use of pillows to support the newborn can enhance comfort and facilitate successful breastfeeding.

Discharge after cesarean birth is usually by the third postoperative day. This time is often determined by criteria established by the woman's insurance carrier or the federal government (e.g., diagnosis-related groups). The Newborn's and Mother's Health Protection Act of 1996 provides for a length of stay of up to 96 hours for cesarean births. These criteria may not coincide with the woman's physical or psychosocial readiness for discharge. Some states have added home care provisions for mothers who meet appropriate criteria for discharge and choose to leave sooner than the allowed length of stay. This policy recognizes that home care is less costly than hospital care and in most cases is more beneficial for recovery.

The predominant needs at home for a woman who experienced cesarean birth are for rest and sleep; relief of pain and discomfort; and assistance with household chores, infant care and feeding, and self-management. The nurse must provide discharge teaching to prepare the woman for self-management and newborn care in a limited time, while trying to ensure that the woman is comfortable and able to rest. The nurse must assess the woman's information needs and coordinate the health care team's efforts to meet them.

Discharge teaching and planning should include information about nutrition; measures to relieve pain and discomfort (see Patient Teaching box); exercise and specific activity restrictions; time management that includes periods of uninterrupted rest and sleep; hygiene, breast, and incision care; timing for resumption of sexual activity and contraception; signs of complications (see Home Care box); and infant care. The nurse assesses the woman's need for continued support or counseling to facilitate her emotional recovery from the birth. Her family and friends should be educated regarding her needs during the recovery process, and their assistance should be coordinated before discharge. Referrals to support groups (e.g., *www.birthrites.org*) or community agencies may be indicated to further promote the recovery process. A postdischarge program of telephone follow-up and home visits can facilitate the woman's full recovery after cesarean birth.

HOME CARE

Signs of Postoperative Complications After Discharge

Report the following signs to your health care provider:

- Temperature exceeding 38° C
- Painful urination
- Lochia heavier than a normal period
- Foul-smelling lochia
- Wound separation
- Redness or oozing at the incision site
- Severe abdominal pain

Vaginal Birth After Cesarean

Indications for primary cesarean birth such as dystocia, breech presentation, or consistent abnormal FHR and patterns often are nonrecurring. Therefore a woman who has had a cesarean birth may subsequently become pregnant and not have any contraindications to labor and vaginal birth in that pregnancy and may attempt a VBAC.

Women who have had one previous cesarean birth by low transverse incision, who have an adequate pelvis, and who have no other uterine scars or previous ruptures may attempt a TOL and VBAC. A physician must be available throughout active labor and capable of performing an emergency cesarean birth. TOL after cesarean is relatively safe, but there is risk of uterine rupture through a lower uterine segment scar. Increased reports of uterine rupture in the United States and Canada raised concerns about the safety of VBAC. The incidence of uterine rupture appears to be related to the method of the second labor and birth (Thorp, 2009). The rate of uterine rupture was lowest with spontaneous vaginal birth and highest when labor was induced, especially if prostaglandins were used to ripen the cervix. Other risk factors include prior classic uterine incision extending into the fundus, single-layer rather than double-layer uterine closure, two or more previous cesarean births, an interdelivery interval of 18 to 24 months or less, maternal age of 30 years or older, postpartum fever, and CPD. Women are most often the primary decision makers with regard to choice of birth method. During the antepartal period the woman should be given information about VBAC and encouraged to choose it as an alternative to a repeat cesarean as long as no contraindications exist. VBAC support groups (e.g., *www.vbac.com*) and prenatal classes can help prepare the woman psychologically for labor and vaginal birth.

TOL should occur in a hospital facility that has the equipment and personnel available to begin surgery within 30 minutes from the time a decision is made for cesarean birth. Ideally the woman is admitted to the labor and birth unit at the onset of spontaneous labor. In the active phase of labor FHR and uterine activity are continuously monitored electronically, and intravenous access is established. Abnormal FHR patterns (e.g., prolonged decelerations, variable or late decelerations, and absent baseline variability) often precede rupture or signal its occurrence. The woman may also complain of abdominal, shoulder, or back pain even with an epidural and may exhibit signs of excessive blood loss. The physician should be immediately available during active labor.

There is conflicting evidence that administering oxytocin to induce or augment labor increases the risk of uterine rupture. If oxytocin is used for the TOL, caution and close monitoring of the laboring woman are urged. However, use of prostaglandins, especially misoprostol (prostaglandin E_1), to ripen the cervix or induce labor is not recommended because they have been associated with an increased risk for uterine rupture (Landon, 2007).

Attention should be given to the woman's psychologic and physical needs during the TOL. Anxiety increases the release of catecholamines and can inhibit the release of oxytocin, delaying the progress of labor and possibly leading to a repeat cesarean birth. To alleviate anxiety the nurse can encourage the woman to use breathing and relaxation techniques and change position to promote labor progress. The woman's partner can be encouraged to provide comfort measures and emotional support. Collaboration among the woman in labor, her partner, the nurse, and other health care providers often results in a successful VBAC. If a TOL does not proceed to vaginal birth, the woman will need support and encouragement to express her feelings about having another cesarean birth. It is very important that this outcome not be labeled a failed VBAC.

Postterm Pregnancy, Labor, and Birth

A postterm or postdate pregnancy is one that extends beyond the end of week 42 of gestation, or more than 294 days from the first day of the last menstrual period. The incidence of postterm pregnancy is estimated to be between 4% and 19% (Divon, 2007). Many pregnancies are misdiagnosed as prolonged. This can occur because (1) the pregnancy is inaccurately dated because the woman had an irregular menstrual cycle pattern, (2) an accurate date of the last menstrual period is unknown, or (3) entry into prenatal care was delayed or did not occur. Although the exact cause of postterm pregnancy is still unknown, a possible cause may be deficiency of placental estrogen and continued secretion of progesterone. Low levels of estrogen may result in a decrease in prostaglandin precursors and reduced formation of oxytocin receptors in the myometrium (Gilbert, 2007). A woman who experiences one postterm pregnancy is 50% more likely to experience it again in subsequent pregnancies (Divon, 2007).

Clinical manifestations of postterm pregnancy include maternal weight loss, decreased uterine size (because of decreased amniotic fluid), meconium in the amniotic fluid, and advanced bone maturation of the fetal skeleton with an exceptionally hard fetal skull (Gilbert, 2007).

Maternal and Fetal Risks

Maternal risks are often related to the birth of an excessively large infant. The woman is at increased risk for dysfunctional labor; birth canal trauma, including perineal lacerations and extension of episiotomy during vaginal birth; postpartum hemorrhage; and infection. Interventions such as induction of labor with prostaglandins or oxytocin, vacuum- or forceps-assisted birth, and cesarean birth are more likely to be necessary. The woman also may experience fatigue and psychologic reactions such as depression, frustration, and feelings of inadequacy as she passes her estimated date of birth (Gilbert, 2007).

Fetal risks appear to be twofold. The first is the possibility of prolonged labor, shoulder dystocia, birth trauma, and asphyxia from macrosomia, which is estimated to occur in approximately 25% of prolonged pregnancies (Divon, 2007). The second risk is the compromising effects on the fetus of an "aging" placenta. Placental function gradually decreases after 37 weeks of gestation. AFV declines to approximately 800 ml by 40 weeks of gestation and to about 400 ml by 42 weeks of gestation. The resulting oligohydramnios can lead to fetal hypoxia related to cord compression. If placental insufficiency is present, there is a high likelihood of an abnormal FHR pattern occurring during labor. Neonatal problems may include asphyxia, meconium aspiration syndrome, dysmaturity syndrome, hypoglycemia, polycythemia, and respiratory distress (Gilbert, 2007). Whether an infant born after a postterm pregnancy has neurologic, behavioral, intellectual, or developmental problems must be further investigated.

✱ Nursing Care Management

The management of postterm pregnancy is still controversial. The induction of labor at 41 to 42 weeks is suggested by some authorities as a means of reducing the rate of cesarean birth and stillbirth or neonatal death. Others follow a more individualized approach, allowing the pregnancy to proceed to 43 weeks as long as assessment of fetal well-being using a combination of tests is performed and the results of the tests are normal. Tests are usually performed on a weekly or twice-weekly basis (Divon, 2007).

Antepartum assessments for postterm pregnancy may include daily fetal movement counts, NSTs, AFV assessments, contraction stress tests, biophysical profiles (BPPs), and Doppler flow measurements. The woman and her family should be fully informed regarding the tests, including why they are performed and the meaning of the results obtained in terms of the health of the mother and fetus.

An amniotic fluid index (AFI) less than 5 has been associated with an increased risk of cesarean birth for a nonreassuring fetal status and an Apgar score of less than 7 at 5 minutes. Ideally amniotic fluid should be present throughout the uterine cavity (Gilbert, 2007). The BPP may be the best way of gauging fetal well-being because it combines nonstress testing with real-time ultrasound scanning to assess fetal movements, fetal breathing movements, and AFV. Determining the AFV is critical in women with a postterm pregnancy because decreased AFV has been associated with fetal stress. The AFI should be greater than 8, with at least one pocket of amniotic fluid greater than 2 cm, and amniotic fluid should be present throughout the uterine cavity (Gilbert, 2007).

Cervical checks usually are performed weekly after 40 weeks of gestation to determine whether the condition of the cervix is favorable for induction. Vaginal secretions may be assessed for the amount of fetal fibronectin; a low concentration may predict increased risk for prolonged pregnancy, but results of studies have thus far been inconclusive (Divon, 2007; Gilbert, 2007). Amniocentesis or amnioscopy may be performed to detect meconium in the amniotic fluid.

During the postterm period the woman is encouraged to assess fetal activity daily, assess for signs of labor, and keep appointments with her primary health care provider (see Home Care box). The woman and her family should be encouraged to express their feelings about the prolonged pregnancy. They should be helped to realize that feelings of frustration, anger, impatience, and fear are normal. At times the emotional and physical strain of a postterm pregnancy may seem insurmountable. Referral to a support group or other supportive resource may be needed.

HOME CARE

Postterm Pregnancy

- Perform daily fetal movement counts.
- Assess for signs of labor.
- Call your primary health care provider if your membranes rupture or if you perceive a decrease in or no fetal movement.
- Keep appointments for fetal assessment tests or cervical checks.
- Come to the hospital soon after labor begins.

If the woman's cervix is favorable, expectant management can be followed, but labor is usually induced with oxytocin. If the cervix is not favorable, fetal surveillance is continued, and a cervical ripening agent (e.g., prostaglandin insert, misoprostol) may be administered followed by oxytocin induction (Gilbert, 2007).

The fetus of a woman with a postterm pregnancy should be monitored electronically for a more accurate assessment of the FHR and pattern. Inadequate fluid volume leads to compression of the cord, which results in a transient fetal hypoxia that is reflected in variable or prolonged deceleration patterns. If oligohydramnios is present, amnioinfusion may be performed to restore AFV to maintain a cushioning of the cord. However, performing an amnioinfusion prophylactically is likely to be ineffective or harmful (Enkin et al, 2000). Although maternal-fetal risks related to amnioinfusion are rare, they can result from infection and overdistention of the uterine cavity with infused fluid and postpartum hemorrhage (Gilbert, 2007).

Emotional support is essential for the woman with a postterm pregnancy and her family. A vaginal birth is anticipated, but the couple should be prepared for a forceps- or vacuum-assisted birth or cesarean birth if complications arise.

Obstetric Emergencies

Shoulder Dystocia

evolve Animation—Shoulder Dystocia

Shoulder dystocia is an uncommon obstetric emergency that increases the risk for fetal/neonatal and maternal morbidity and mortality during the attempt to deliver the fetus vaginally. It is estimated that 0.24% to 2% of all vaginal births are complicated by shoulder dystocia (Thorp, 2009). Shoulder dystocia is not predictable; many women who have risk factors will not develop the problem, whereas others with no apparent risk factors experience it.

Shoulder dystocia is a condition in which the head is born but the anterior shoulder cannot pass under the pubic arch. Fetopelvic disproportion caused by excessive fetal size (greater than 4000 g) or maternal pelvic abnormalities may be a cause of shoulder dystocia, although it can occur in the absence of any known risk factors.

The nurse should be observant for risk factors that could indicate the possibility for shoulder dystocia, including maternal obesity, previous birth of an infant weighing more than 4000 g, estimated fetal weight of more than 4000 g, diabetes mellitus, prolonged second stage of labor, prolonged transition phase of labor, previous instrumental midpelvic delivery, and previous shoulder dystocia. When the head emerges, it retracts against the perineum (turtle sign), and external rotation does not occur (Lanni & Seeds, 2007; Baird & Kennedy, 2008).

Risks to the fetus/newborn include birth injuries, asphyxia, brachial plexus damage, and fracture, especially of the humerus or clavicle. The mother's primary risk stems from excessive blood loss as a result of uterine atony or rupture, lacerations, extension of the episiotomy, or endometritis.

Nursing Care Management

Many maneuvers such as suprapubic pressure and maternal position changes have been suggested and tried to free the anterior shoulder, although no one particular maneuver has been found to be most effective (Lanni & Seeds, 2007). Suprapubic pressure can be applied to the anterior shoulder using the Mazzanti or Rubin technique (Fig. 19-13) in an attempt to push the shoulder under the symphysis pubis.

In the McRoberts maneuver (Fig. 19-14) the woman's legs are flexed apart with her knees on her abdomen. This maneuver causes the sacrum to straighten, and the symphysis pubis rotates toward the mother's head; the angle of pelvic inclination is decreased, freeing the shoulder. Suprapubic pressure can be applied at this time. Having the woman move to a hands-and-knees position (the Gaskin maneuver), a squatting position, or a lateral recumbent position also has been used to resolve cases of shoulder dystocia (Baird & Kennedy, 2008;

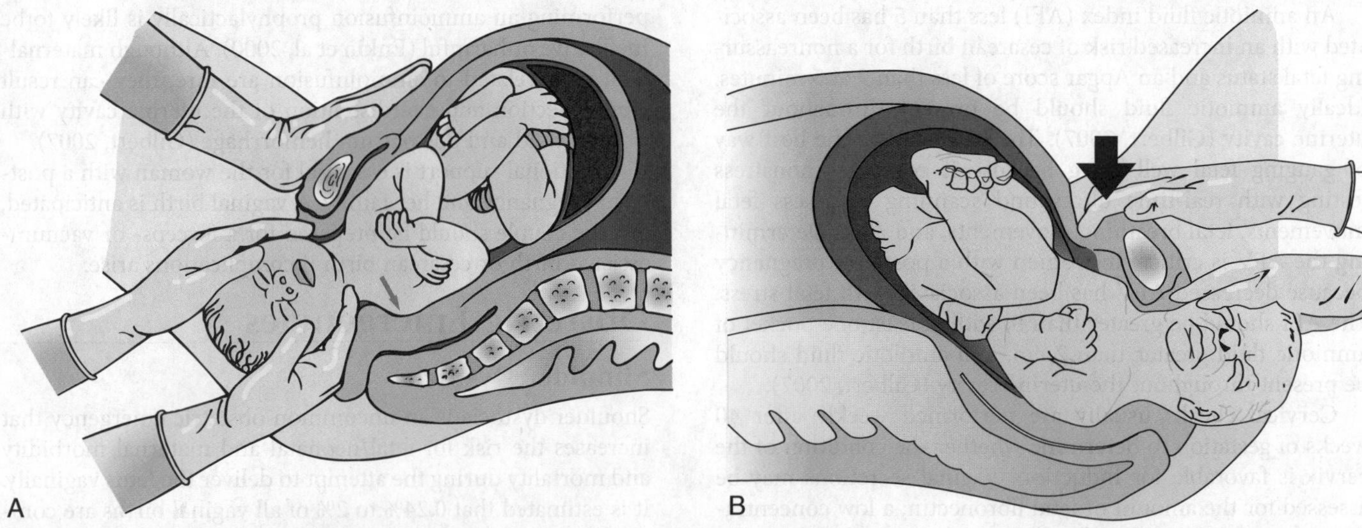

Fig. 19-13 Application of suprapubic pressure. A, Mazzanti technique: pressure is applied directly posteriorly and laterally above the symphysis pubis. B, Rubin technique: pressure is applied obliquely posteriorly against the anterior shoulder.

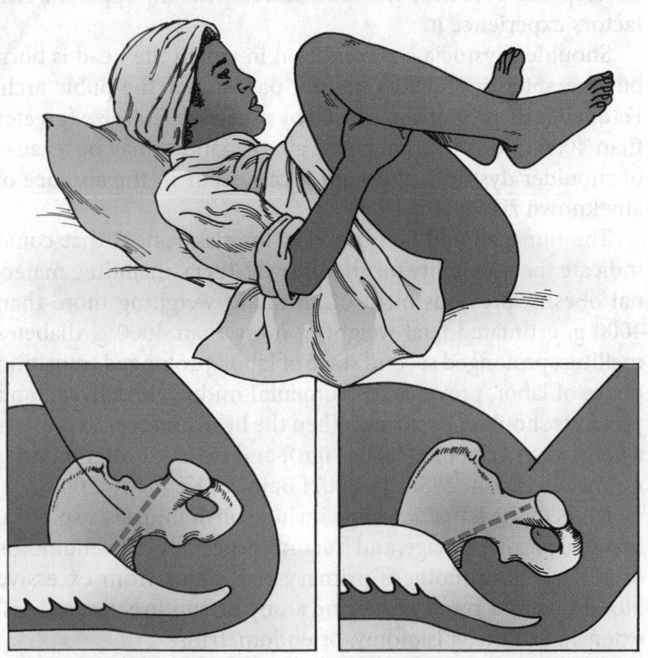

Fig. 19-14 McRoberts maneuver. (Modified from Lanni SM, Seeds JW: Malpresentations. In Gabbe SG, Niebyl JR, Simpson JL: *Obstetrics: normal and problem pregnancies*, ed 5, New York, 2007, Churchill Livingstone.)

Jevitt, 2005; Thorp, 2009). Fundal pressure is contraindicated as a method of relieving shoulder dystocia.

When shoulder dystocia is diagnosed, the nurse helps the woman assume the position(s) that may facilitate birth of the shoulders, assists the primary health care provider with these maneuvers, and monitors the fetal response. The nurse should also provide encouragement and support to reduce anxiety and fear.

Newborn assessment should include examination for fracture of the clavicle or humerus, brachial plexus injuries, and asphyxia. Maternal assessment should focus on early detection of hemorrhage and trauma to the soft tissue of the birth canal.

evolve Animation–Cord Prolapse

Prolapsed Umbilical Cord

Prolapse of the umbilical cord occurs when the cord lies below the presenting part of the fetus. Umbilical cord prolapse may be occult (hidden, not visible) at any time during labor whether or not membranes are ruptured (Fig. 19-15, *A* and *B*). It is most common to see frank (visible) prolapse directly after rupture of membranes, when gravity washes the cord in front of the presenting part (see Fig. 19-15, *C* and *D*). Frank prolapse occurs in 0.1% to 0.6% of all births (Lin, 2006). Contributing factors are a long cord (longer than 100 cm), malpresentation (footling breech), transverse lie, or unengaged presenting part.

If the presenting part does not fit snugly into the lower uterine segment, as in polyhydramnios, when the membranes rupture a sudden gush of amniotic fluid may cause the cord to be displaced downward. Similarly the cord may prolapse during amniotomy if the presenting part is high. A small or preterm fetus may not fit snugly into the lower uterine segment; as a result, cord prolapse is more likely to occur.

Nursing Care Management

Prompt recognition of a prolapsed cord is important because fetal hypoxia resulting from prolonged cord compression (i.e., occlusion of blood flow to and from the fetus for more than 5 minutes) can occur and potentially lead to fetal hypoxia, newborn asphyxia, neurologic brain injury, or death of the fetus. Pressure on the cord may be relieved by the examiner putting a sterile gloved hand into the vagina and holding the presenting part off of the umbilical cord (Fig. 19-16, *A* and *B*). The woman is assisted into a position such as a modified Sims' (see Fig. 19-16, *C*), Trendelenburg, or knee-chest (see Fig. 19-16, *D*) position, in which gravity keeps the presenting part off the cord. If the cervix is fully dilated, a forceps- or vacuum-assisted birth can be performed for the fetus in a cephalic presentation; otherwise emergent cesarean surgery is likely to be performed. Indications for immediate interventions are presented in the Emergency box. Ongoing assessment of the woman and her fetus is critical. The woman and her family are often aware of the seriousness of the situation; therefore the

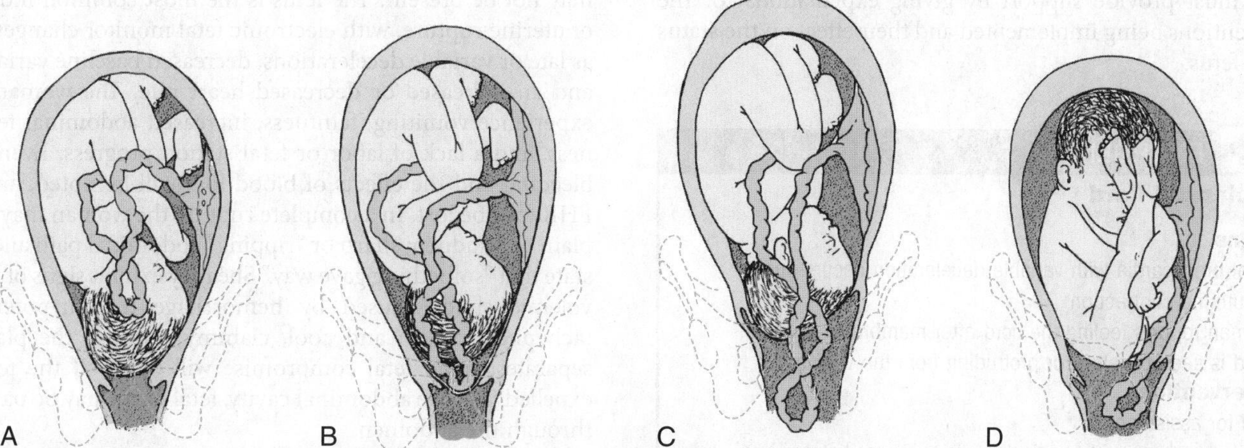

Fig. 19-15 Prolapse of umbilical cord. Note pressure of presenting part on umbilical cord, which endangers fetal circulation. **A**, Occult (hidden) prolapse of cord. **B**, Complete prolapse of cord. Note that membranes are intact. **C**, Cord presenting in front of fetal head may be seen in vagina. **D**, Frank breech presentation with prolapsed cord.

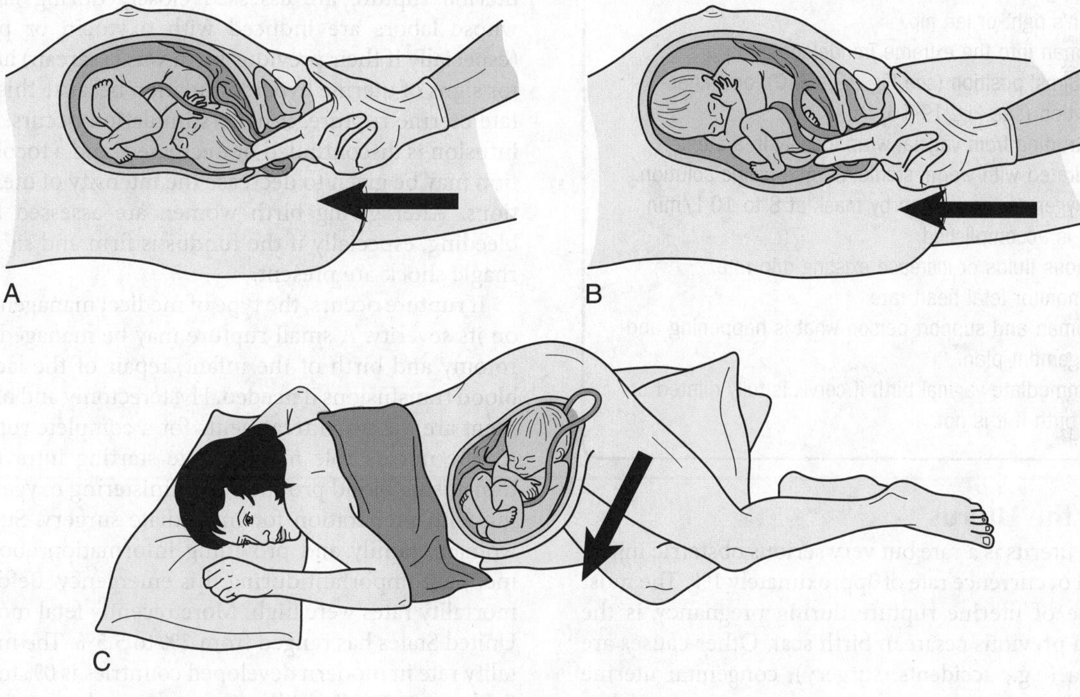

Fig. 19-16 *Arrows* indicate direction of pressure against presenting part to relieve compression of prolapsed umbilical cord. Pressure exerted by examiner's fingers in **A**, vertex presentation, and **B**, breech presentation. **C**, Gravity relieves pressure when woman is in modified Sims' position with hips elevated as high as possible with pillows. **D**, Knee-chest position.

nurse must provide support by giving explanations for the interventions being implemented and their effect on the status of the fetus.

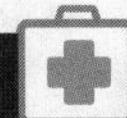

EMERGENCY

Prolapsed Cord

Signs

Fetal bradycardia with variable deceleration occurs during uterine contraction.

Woman reports feeling the cord after membranes rupture.

Cord is seen or felt in or protruding from the vagina.

Interventions

Call for assistance.

Notify physician with surgical privileges immediately.

Glove the examining hand quickly and insert two fingers into the vagina to the cervix. With one finger on either side of the cord or both fingers to one side, exert upward pressure against the presenting part to relieve compression of the cord (see Fig. 19-16, *A* and *B*). Place a rolled towel under the woman's right or left hip.

Place the woman into the extreme Trendelenburg or a modified Sims' position (see Fig. 19-16, *C*), or a knee-chest position (see Fig. 19-16, *D*).

If cord is protruding from vagina, wrap loosely in a sterile towel saturated with warm, sterile, normal saline solution.

Administer oxygen to the woman by mask at 8 to 10 L/min until birth is accomplished.

Start intravenous fluids or increase existing drip rate.

Continue to monitor fetal heart rate.

Explain to woman and support person what is happening and the management plan.

Prepare for immediate vaginal birth if cervix is fully dilated or cesarean birth if it is not.

Rupture of the Uterus

Rupture of the uterus is a rare but very serious obstetric injury with an overall occurrence rate of approximately 1%. The most common cause of uterine rupture during pregnancy is the separation of a previous cesarean birth scar. Other causes are uterine trauma (e.g., accidents, surgery), congenital uterine anomaly, intense spontaneous uterine contractions, labor stimulation (e.g., oxytocin, prostaglandin), an overdistended uterus (e.g., multifetal gestation), malpresentation, external or internal version, or a difficult forceps-assisted birth. It occurs more commonly in multigravidas than primigravidas.

A uterine rupture may be classified as complete or incomplete. A complete rupture extends through the entire uterine wall into the peritoneal cavity or broad ligament. An incomplete rupture extends into the peritoneum but not into the peritoneal cavity or broad ligament. Bleeding is usually internal. An incomplete rupture may also be a partial separation of an old cesarean scar and may go unnoticed unless the woman has a subsequent cesarean birth or other uterine surgery.

Signs and symptoms vary with the extent of the rupture and may be silent or dramatic. In an incomplete rupture, pain may not be present. The fetus is the most common indicator of uterine rupture, with electronic fetal monitor changes such as late or variable decelerations, decreased baseline variability, and an increased or decreased heart rate. The woman may experience vomiting, faintness, increased abdominal tenderness, and a lack of labor or fetal station progress. Eventually bleeding and the effects of blood loss will be noted, and the FHR may be lost. In a complete rupture the woman may complain of a sudden, sharp or "ripping" abdominal pain and may state that "something gave way." She may exhibit signs of hypovolemic shock caused by hemorrhage (i.e., hypotension; tachypnea; pallor; and cool, clammy skin). If the placenta separates, rapid fetal compromise will occur. If the fetus is expelled into the abdominal cavity, fetal parts may be palpable through the abdomen.

Nursing Care Management

Prevention is the best treatment. Women who have had a previous classic cesarean birth are advised not to attempt vaginal birth in subsequent pregnancies. Women at risk for uterine rupture are assessed closely during labor. Women whose labors are induced with oxytocin or prostaglandin (especially if their previous birth was cesarean) are monitored for signs of uterine hyperstimulation because this can precipitate uterine rupture. If hyperstimulation occurs, the oxytocin infusion is discontinued or decreased, and a tocolytic medication may be given to decrease the intensity of uterine contractions. After giving birth women are assessed for excessive bleeding, especially if the fundus is firm and signs of hemorrhagic shock are present.

If rupture occurs, the type of medical management depends on its severity. A small rupture may be managed with a laparotomy and birth of the infant, repair of the laceration, and blood transfusions if needed. Hysterectomy and blood replacement are the usual treatments for a complete rupture.

The nurse's role may include starting intravenous fluids, transfusing blood products, administering oxygen, and assisting with preparation for immediate surgery. Supporting the woman's family and providing information about the treatment are important during this emergency. Before 1978 fetal mortality rates were high. More recently fetal mortality in the United States has ranged from 2% to 5.5%. The maternal mortality rate in modern developed countries is 0% to 1% (Nahum & Pham, 2008). Providing information about spiritual support services or suggesting that the family contact their own support system may be warranted.

Amniotic Fluid Embolism (Anaphylactoid Syndrome of Pregnancy)

Amniotic fluid embolism (AFE) occurs when amniotic fluid, fetal cells, hair or other debris enter the maternal circulation, triggering a rapid, complex series of pathophysiologic events that lead to life-threatening maternal symptoms (Baird & Kennedy, 2008; Gilbert, 2007). This can occur because fluid can enter the maternal circulation any time there is an opening in the amniotic sac or maternal uterine veins accompanied by enough intrauterine pressure to force the amniotic fluid into the veins (e.g., if the placenta separates). Although uncommon (1 in 8000 to 30,000 pregnancies), this complication is estimated to be the cause of 5% to 10% of maternal deaths in the United States (Moore, 2008). The maternal mortality rate is approximately 61%, and fetal mortality rate is 79% in the United States (Moore, 2008). A common first symptom is acute dyspnea, followed by severe hypotension (Moore, 2008; Schoening, 2006).

AFE cannot be predicted or prevented, and the cause for the reaction is unknown. A history of allergies is present in 41% of women with exposure to amniotic fluid (Moore, 2008). The condition is similar but not identical to anaphylactic shock; hence a new diagnostic title, *anaphylactoid syndrome of pregnancy,* has been proposed.

Nursing Care Management

The immediate interventions for AFE are summarized in the Emergency box. Such medical management must be instituted immediately. Cardiopulmonary resuscitation is often needed. The woman is usually placed on mechanical ventilation, and rapid blood and volume replacement is initiated; coagulation defects are treated.

The nurse's immediate responsibility is to assist with the resuscitation efforts. The nurse should continuously monitor the fetus if the mother is undelivered and anticipate emergency cesarean birth and neonatal resuscitation (Baird & Kennedy, 2008). If the woman survives, she is usually moved to a critical care unit where hemodynamic monitoring, blood replacement, and coagulopathy treatment are implemented. If cardiopulmonary arrest occurs, for optimal fetal survival a perimortem cesarean birth should occur within 5 minutes.

Support of the woman's partner and family is needed; they will be anxious and distressed. Brief explanations of what is happening are important during the emergency and can be reinforced after the immediate crisis is over. If the woman dies and the infant survives, grieving, anger and blame may interfere with parent-infant attachment (Perozzi & Englert, 2004). When both the mother and infant die, it is important that the family has the opportunity to spend time with them. Emotional support and involvement of the perinatal loss support team or other resource for grief counseling, including the pastoral care team (if desired by the family), are needed. Referral to grief and loss support groups is appropriate. The nursing staff also may need help in coping with feelings and emotions that result from a maternal death.

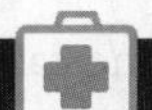

EMERGENCY

Amniotic Fluid Embolism (Anaphylactoid Syndrome of Pregnancy)

Signs

Respiratory distress
- Restlessness
- Dyspnea
- Cyanosis
- Pulmonary edema
- Respiratory arrest

Circulatory collapse
- Hypotension
- Tachycardia
- Shock
- Cardiac arrest

Hemorrhage
- Coagulation failure: bleeding from incisions, venipuncture sites, trauma (lacerations); petechiae, ecchymoses, purpura
- Uterine atony

Tonic-clonic seizure activity

Interventions

Oxygenate.
- Administer oxygen by nonrebreather face mask (10 L/min) or resuscitation bag delivering 100% oxygen.
- Prepare for intubation and mechanical ventilation.
- Initiate or assist with cardiopulmonary resuscitation. Tilt pregnant woman 30 degrees to side to displace uterus.

Maintain cardiac output and replace fluid losses.
- Position woman on her side.
- Administer intravenous fluids.
- Administer blood: packed cells, fresh frozen plasma.
- Insert indwelling catheter and measure hourly urine output.

Correct coagulation failure.

Monitor fetal and maternal status.

Prepare for emergency birth.

Anticipate pulmonary artery and arterial catheter placement.

Prepare mother and family for transfer to an intensive care environment or tertiary care center following stabilization.

Provide emotional support to woman, her partner, and her family.

Key Points

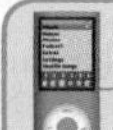

Audio Chapter Summaries

Access an audio summary of these Key Points on evolve

- Preterm labor is defined as uterine contractions leading to cervical change occurring between 20 and 37 completed weeks of pregnancy; preterm birth is any birth that occurs before the completion of 37 weeks of pregnancy.
- The incidence of preterm birth in the United States varies considerably by race.
- The cause of preterm labor is unknown and is assumed to be multifactorial.
- β-Mimetics are a class of medications that have many maternal and fetal side effects and must always be used with extreme caution.
- Bed rest, a commonly prescribed intervention for preterm labor, has many deleterious side effects and has never been shown to decrease preterm birth rates.
- Preterm birth that occurs in a tertiary care center leads to better neonatal and maternal outcomes.

- Vigilance for signs of infection is a major part of the care for women with PPROM.
- Dystocia results from differences in the normal relationships among any of the five factors affecting labor.
- Dysfunctional labor occurs as a result of hypertonic uterine dysfunction, hypotonic uterine dysfunction, or inadequate voluntary expulsive forces.
- The functional relationships among the uterine contractions, the fetus, and the mother's pelvis are altered by maternal positioning.
- Uterine contractility is increased by oxytocin and prostaglandin and decreased by tocolytic agents.
- Cervical ripening using chemical or mechanical measures can increase the success of labor induction.
- Expectant parents benefit from learning about operative obstetrics (e.g., forceps- or vacuum-assisted or cesarean birth) during the prenatal period.
- The basic purpose of cesarean birth is to preserve the life and health of the mother and her fetus.
- Unless contraindicated, a vaginal birth may be possible after a previous cesarean birth.
- Labor management that emphasizes one-to-one support of the laboring woman by another woman (doula, nurse, or nurse-midwife) can reduce the rate of cesarean birth and increase the rate of VBACs.
- Postterm pregnancy poses a risk to both the mother and the fetus.
- Obstetric emergencies (e.g., shoulder dystocia, prolapsed cord, rupture of the uterus, and amniotic fluid embolism) occur rarely but require immediate intervention.
- The perinatal loss support team or other resource for grief counseling, including the pastoral care team, provides support for families experiencing death of the mother and/or infant.

References

American College of Obstetricians and Gynecologists (ACOG): *Assessment of risk factors for preterm birth*, ACOG Practice Bulletin No 31, Washington, DC, 2001, Author.

American College of Obstetricians and Gynecologists (ACOG): *Management of preterm labor*, ACOG Practice Bulletin No 43, Washington, DC, 2003a, Author.

American College of Obstetricians and Gynecologists: *New ACOG opinion addresses elective cesarean controversy*, ACOG news release, Washington, DC, 2003b, Author.

Baird SM, Kennedy BB: Intrapartum emergencies. In Kennedy BB, Ruth DJ, Martin EJ (editors): *Intrapartum management modules: a perinatal education program*, ed 4, Philadelphia, 2008, Wolters Kluwer.

Battista LR, Wing DA: Abnormal labor and induction of labor. In Gabbe SG, Niebyl JR, Simpson JL (editors): *Obstetrics: normal and problem pregnancies*, ed 5, New York, 2007, Churchill Livingstone

Cunningham F et al: *Williams obstetrics*, ed 22, Stamford, Conn, 2005, Appleton & Lange.

Divon MY: Prolonged pregnancy. In Gabbe SG, Niebyl JR, Simpson JL (editors): *Obstetrics: normal and problem pregnancies*, ed 5, New York, 2007, Churchill Livingstone.

Enkin M et al: *A guide to effective care in pregnancy and childbirth*, ed 3, Oxford, NY, 2000, Oxford University Press.

Freda MC, Patterson E: *Preterm birth: prevention and nursing management*, ed 2, March of Dimes Nursing Module, New York, 2001, March of Dimes.

Friedman E: Normal and dysfunctional labor. In Cohen W et al (editors): *Management of labor*, ed 2, Rockville, Md, 1989, Aspen.

Fritz EA, Smith NW: Caring for the woman at risk for preterm labor or with premature rupture of membranes. In Kennedy BB, Ruth DJ, Martin EJ (editors): *Intrapartum management modules: a perinatal education program*, ed 4, Philadelphia, 2008, Wolters Kluwer.

Gardner PS: Previous traumatic birth: an impetus for requested cesarean birth, *J Perinatal Educ* 12(1):1-5, 2003.

Gilbert ES: *Manual of high risk pregnancy and delivery*, ed 3, St Louis, 2007, Mosby.

Hodnett E et al: Continuous support for women during childbirth. *The Cochrane Database of Systematic Reviews*, 2007, Issue 3, Chichester, UK, 2007, John Wiley & Sons.

Iams JD, Romero R, Creasy RK: Preterm labor and birth. In Creasy RK et al (editors): *Creasy & Resnik's maternal-fetal medicine: principles and practice*, ed 6, Philadelphia, 2009, Saunders.

Iams JD, Romero R: Preterm birth. In Gabbe SG, Niebyl JR, Simpson JL (editors): *Obstetrics: normal and problem pregnancies*, ed 5, New York, 2007, Churchill Livingstone.

Jevitt C: Shoulder dystocia: Etiology, common risk factors, and management, *J Midwifery Womens Health* 50(6):485-497, 2005.

Kilpatrick S, Garrison E: Normal labor and delivery. In Gabbe SG, Niebyl JR, Simpson JL (editors): *Obstetrics: normal and problem pregnancies*, ed 5, New York, 2007, Churchill Livingstone.

Landon MB: Cesarean delivery. In Gabbe SG, Niebyl JR, Simpson JL (editors): *Obstetrics: normal and problem pregnancies*, ed 5, New York, 2007, Churchill Livingstone.

Lanni SM, Seeds JW: Malpresentations. In Gabbe SG, Niebyl JR, Simpson JL (editors): *Obstetrics: normal and problem pregnancies*, ed 5, New York, 2007, Churchill Livingstone.

Lehne R: *Pharmacology for nursing care*, ed 6, Philadelphia, 2007, Saunders.

Lin MG: Umbilical cord prolapse, *Obstet Gynecol Surv* 61(4):269-277, 2006.

Malone FD, D'Alton ME: Multiple gestation. Clinical characteristics and management. In Creasy RK et al (editors): *Creasy & Resnik's maternal-fetal medicine: principles and practice*, ed 6, Philadelphia, 2009, Saunders.

Maloni J, Park S: Postpartum symptoms after antepartum bedrest, *J Obstet Gynecol Neonatal Nurs* 34(2):163-171, 2005.

Martin JA et al: Births: final data for 2005, *Natl Vital Stat Rep* 56(6):1-104, 2007.

Maupin RM et al: Characteristics of women who deliver with no prenatal care, *J Matern Fetal Neonatal Med* 16(1):45-50, 2004.

Mercer BM: Premature rupture of membranes. In Gabbe SG, Niebyl JR, Simpson JL (editors): *Obstetrics: normal and problem pregnancies*, ed 5, New York, 2007, Churchill Livingstone.

Moore LE: Amniotic fluid embolism, *eMedicine*, 2008. Available at www.emedicine.com/med/topic122.htm (accessed October 3, 2008).

Morrison JC, Chauhan SP: Current status of home uterine activity monitoring, *Clin Perinatol* 30(4):757-801, 2003.

Nahum GG, Pham KQ: Uterine rupture in pregnancy, *eMedicine*, 2008. Available at www.emedicine.com/med/topic3746.htm (accessed October 3, 2008).

National Institutes of Health: *Antenatal corticosteroids revisited: Consensus Development Conference Statement*, Bethesda, Md, 2000, National Institutes of Health. Available at http://consensus.nih.gov (accessed February 7, 2005).

Perozzi KJ, Englert NC: Amniotic fluid embolism: an obstetric emergency, *Crit Care Nurse* 24(4):54-61, 2004.

Schoening A: Amniotic fluid embolism: historical perspectives and new possibilities, *MCN Am J Matern Child Nurs* 31(2):78-83, 2006.

Simpson KR: *Cervical ripening and induction and augmentation of labor*, ed 3, Washington, DC, 2008, Association of Women's Health, Obstetric, and Neonatal Nurses.

Society of Obstetricians and Gynaecologists of Canada: News: C-sections on demand—SOGC's position, *Birth* 31(2):154, 2004.

Sosa C et al: Bed rest in singleton pregnancies for preventing preterm birth, *Cochrane Database Syst Rev* 1:CD003581, 2004.

Sprague A: The evolution of bed rest as a clinical intervention, *J Obstet Gynecol Neonatal Nurs* 33(5):542-549, 2004.

Sprague AE et al: Bed rest and activity restriction for women at risk for preterm birth: a survey of Canadian prenatal care providers, *J Obstet Gynaecol Can* 30(4):317-326, 2008.

Terry RR et al: Postpartum outcomes in supine delivery by physicians vs nonsupine delivery by midwives, *J Am Osteopath Assoc* 106(4):199-202, 2006.

Thorp JM: Clinical aspects of normal and abnormal labor. In Creasy RK et al (editors): *Creasy & Resnik's maternal-fetal medicine: principles and practice*, ed 6, Philadelphia, 2009, Saunders.

Wener M, Lavigne S: Can periodontal disease lead to premature delivery? *AWHONN Lifelines* 8(5):422-431, 2004.

Unit 5

20 Maternal Physiologic Changes

Learning Objectives

On completion of this chapter the reader will be able to:

- Describe the anatomic and physiologic changes that occur during the postpartum period.
- Identify characteristics of uterine involution and lochial flow and describe ways to measure them.
- List expected values for vital signs and blood pressure, deviations from normal findings, and probable causes of the deviations.

Electronic Resources

Additional information related to the content in Chapter 20 can be found on

evolve the Companion Website at

http://evolve.elsevier.com/Perry/maternal/

- NCLEX Review Questions
- Spanish Guidelines—Postpartum Physical Examination

The postpartum period is the interval between the birth of the newborn and the return of the reproductive organs to their normal nonpregnant state. This period is sometimes referred to as the *puerperium,* or fourth trimester of pregnancy. Although the puerperium has traditionally been considered to last 6 weeks, this time frame varies among women. The physiologic changes that occur during the reversal of the processes of pregnancy are distinctive, but they are normal. To provide care during the recovery period that is beneficial to the mother, her infant, and her family, the nurse must synthesize knowledge of maternal anatomy and physiology of the recovery period, the newborn's physical and behavioral characteristics, infant care activities, and the family response to the birth of the infant. This chapter focuses on anatomic and physiologic changes that occur in the mother during the postpartum period.

Reproductive System and Associated Structures

Uterus

Involution Process

The return of the uterus to a nonpregnant state following birth is called *involution.* This process begins immediately after expulsion of the placenta with contraction of the uterine smooth muscle.

At the end of the third stage of labor the uterus is in the midline, approximately 2 cm below the level of the umbilicus, with the fundus resting on the sacral promontory. At this time the uterus weighs approximately 1000 g.

Within 12 hours the fundus may rise to approximately 1 cm above the umbilicus (Fig. 20-1). By 24 hours after birth the uterus is about the same size as it was at 20 weeks of gestation. Involution progresses rapidly during the next few days. The fundus descends 1 to 2 cm every 24 hours. By the sixth postpartum day the fundus is normally located halfway between the umbilicus and the symphysis pubis. The uterus should not be palpable abdominally after 2 weeks.

The uterus, which at full term weighs approximately 11 times its prepregnancy weight, involutes to approximately 500 g by 1 week after birth and to 350 g by 2 weeks after birth. At 6 weeks postpartum it weighs 50 to 60 g (see Fig. 20-1).

Increased estrogen and progesterone levels are responsible for stimulating the massive growth of the uterus during pregnancy. Prenatal uterine growth results from both hyperplasia, an increase in the number of muscle cells, and hypertrophy, an enlargement of the existing cells. After birth the decrease in these hormones causes autolysis, the self-destruction of excess hypertrophied tissue. The additional cells laid down during pregnancy remain and account for the slight increase in uterine size after each pregnancy.

Subinvolution is the failure of the uterus to return to a nonpregnant state. The most common causes of subinvolution are retained placental fragments and infection.

Contractions

Postpartum hemostasis is achieved primarily by compression of intramyometrial blood vessels as the uterine muscle contracts rather than by platelet aggregation and clot formation. The hormone oxytocin, released from the pituitary gland, strengthens and coordinates these uterine contractions, which compress blood vessels and promote hemostasis. During the first 1 to 2 postpartum hours, uterine contractions may decrease in intensity and become uncoordinated. Because it is vital that the uterus remain firm and well contracted, exogenous oxytocin (Pitocin) is usually administered intravenously or intramuscularly immediately after expulsion of the placenta. Women who plan to breastfeed may be encouraged to put the baby to breast immediately after birth because suckling stimulates oxytocin release.

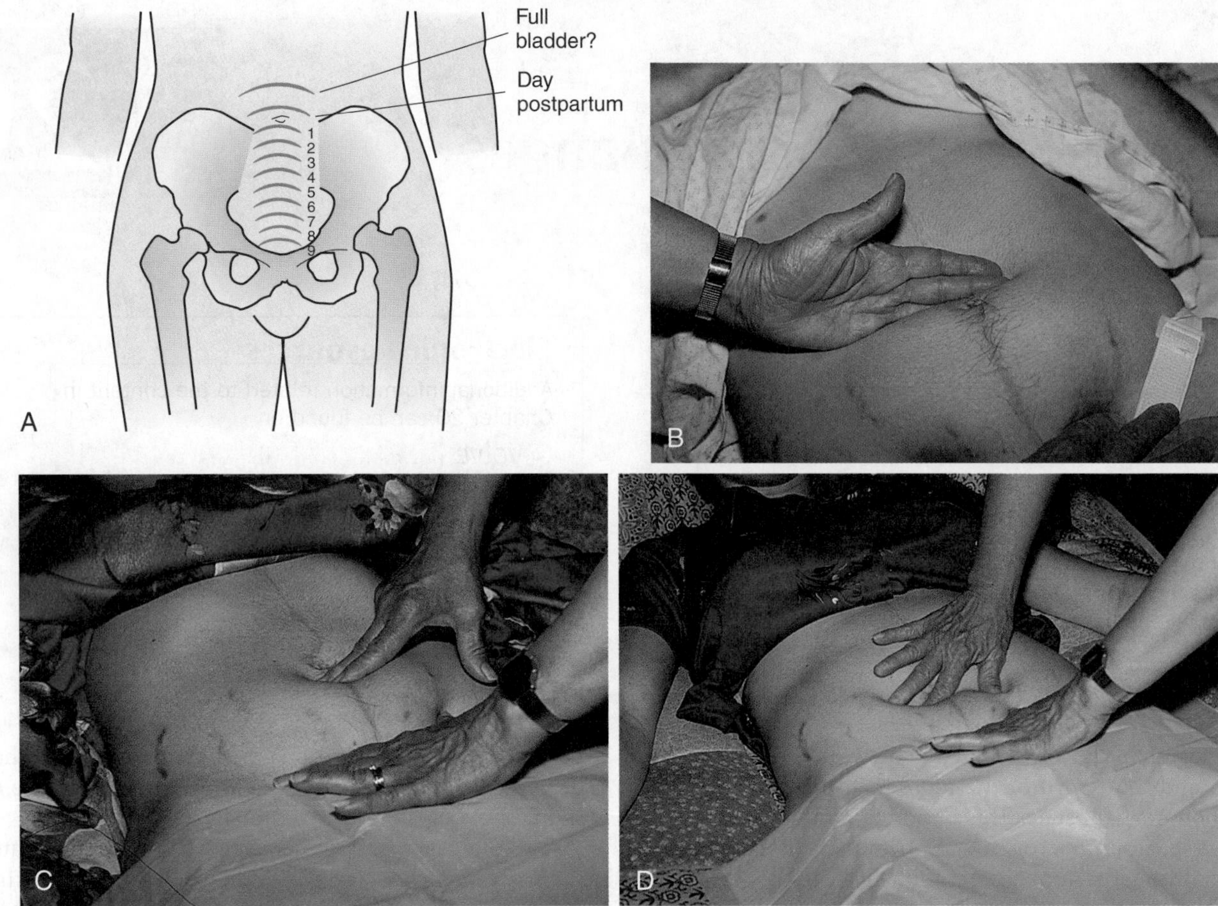

Fig. 20-1 Assessment of involution of uterus after childbirth. A, Normal progress, days 1 through 9. B, Size and position of uterus 2 hours after childbirth. C, Two days after childbirth. D, Four days after childbirth. *(B through D, Courtesy Marjorie Pyle, RNC, Lifecircle, Costa Mesa, CA.)*

Afterpains

In first-time mothers uterine tone is good, the fundus generally remains firm, and the woman usually perceives only mild uterine cramping. Periodic relaxation and vigorous contractions are more common in subsequent pregnancies and may cause uncomfortable cramping called *afterpains* (afterbirth pains), which persist throughout the early puerperium. Afterpains are more noticeable after births in which the uterus was overdistended (e.g., large baby, multifetal gestation, polyhydramnios). Breastfeeding and exogenous oxytocic medication usually intensify these afterpains because both stimulate uterine contractions.

Placental Site

Immediately after the placenta and membranes are expelled, vascular constriction and thromboses reduce the placental site to an irregular nodular and elevated area. Upward growth of the endometrium causes sloughing of necrotic tissue and prevents the scar formation characteristic of normal wound healing. This unique healing process enables the endometrium to resume its usual cycle of changes and permit implantation and placentation in future pregnancies. Endometrial regeneration is completed by postpartum day 16, except at the placental site. Regeneration at the placental site usually is not complete until 6 weeks after birth.

Lochia

Postbirth uterine discharge, commonly called *lochia,* initially is bright red (lochia rubra) and may contain small clots. For the first 2 hours after birth the amount of uterine discharge should be about that of a heavy menstrual period. After that time the lochia flow should steadily decrease.

Lochia rubra consists mainly of blood and decidual and trophoblastic debris. The flow pales, becoming pink or brown (lochia serosa) after 3 to 4 days. Lochia serosa consists of old blood, serum, leukocytes, and tissue debris. The median duration of lochia serosa discharge is 22 to 27 days (Katz, 2007). In most women about 10 days after childbirth the drainage becomes yellow to white (lochia alba). Lochia alba consists of leukocytes, decidua, epithelial cells, mucus, serum, and bacteria. It may continue for 2 to 6 weeks after the birth but may last longer and still be normal.

If the woman receives an oxytocic medication, regardless of the route of administration, the flow of lochia is often scant until the effects of the medication wear off. The amount of lochia is usually less after cesarean births. Flow of lochia usually increases with ambulation and breastfeeding. Lochia tends to pool in the vagina when the woman is lying in bed; the woman then may experience a gush of blood when she stands. This gush should not be confused with hemorrhage.

BOX 20-1 Lochial and Nonlochial Bleeding

Lochial Bleeding

Lochia usually trickles from the vaginal opening. The steady flow is greater as the uterus contracts.

A gush of lochia may result as the uterus is massaged. If it is dark in color, it has been pooled in the relaxed vagina, and the amount soon lessens to a trickle of bright red lochia (in the early puerperium).

Nonlochial Bleeding

If the bloody discharge spurts from the vagina, there may be cervical or vaginal tears in addition to the normal lochia.

If the amount of bleeding continues to be excessive and bright red, a tear may be the source.

Persistence of lochia rubra early in the postpartum period suggests continued bleeding as a result of retained fragments of the placenta or membranes. Recurrence of bleeding 7 to 14 days after birth is from the healing placental site. About 10% to 15% of women will still be having normal lochia serosa discharge at their 6-week postpartum examination (Katz, 2007). However, in most women the continued flow of lochia serosa or lochia alba by 3 to 4 weeks after birth can indicate endometritis, particularly if fever, pain, or abdominal tenderness is associated with the discharge. Lochia should smell like normal menstrual flow; an offensive odor usually indicates infection.

Not all postpartal vaginal bleeding is lochia; vaginal bleeding after birth may be caused by unrepaired vaginal or cervical lacerations. Box 20-1 distinguishes between lochial and nonlochial bleeding.

Cervix

The cervix is soft immediately after birth. However, within 2 to 3 postpartum days it has shortened, become firm, and regained its form. The cervix up to the lower uterine segment remains edematous, thin, and fragile for several days after birth. The ectocervix (part of the cervix that protrudes into the vagina) appears bruised and has some small lacerations—optimal conditions for the development of infection. The cervical os, which dilated to 10 cm during labor, closes gradually. Two fingers may still be introduced into the cervical os for the first 4 to 6 days after birth; however, only the smallest curette can be introduced by the end of 2 weeks. The external cervical os never regains its prepregnant appearance; it is no longer shaped like a circle but appears as a jagged slit that is often described as a "fish mouth." Lactation delays the production of cervical and other estrogen-influenced mucus and mucosal characteristics.

Vagina and Perineum

Postpartum estrogen deprivation is responsible for the thinness of the vaginal mucosa and the absence of rugae. The greatly distended, smooth-walled vagina gradually returns to its prepregnancy size by 6 to 10 weeks after childbirth. Rugae reappear within 3 weeks, but they are never as prominent as they are in the nulliparous woman. Most rugae are permanently flattened. The mucosa remains atrophic in the lactating woman, at least until menstruation resumes. Thickening of the vaginal mucosa occurs with the return of ovarian function. Reduced estrogen levels are also responsible for a decreased amount of vaginal lubrication. Localized dryness and coital discomfort (dyspareunia) may persist until ovarian function returns and menstruation resumes. The use of a water-soluble lubricant to reduce discomfort during sexual intercourse is usually recommended.

Initially the introitus is erythematous and edematous, especially in the area of the episiotomy or laceration repair. It is barely distinguishable from that of a nulliparous woman if lacerations and an episiotomy have been carefully repaired, hematomas are prevented or treated early, and the woman practices good hygiene during the first 2 weeks after birth.

Most episiotomies are visible only if the woman is lying on her side with her upper buttock raised or if she is placed in the lithotomy position. A good light source is essential for visualization of some episiotomies. An episiotomy heals the same way as any surgical incision. Signs of infection (pain, redness, warmth, swelling, or discharge) or loss of approximation (separation of the edges of the incision) may occur. Healing should occur within 2 to 3 weeks.

Hemorrhoids (anal varicosities) are commonly seen. Internal hemorrhoids may evert while the woman is pushing during birth. Women often experience associated symptoms such as itching, discomfort, and bright red bleeding upon defecation. Hemorrhoids usually decrease in size within 6 weeks of childbirth.

Pelvic Muscular Support

The supporting structure of the uterus and vagina may be injured during childbirth and may contribute to later gynecologic problems. Supportive tissues of the pelvic floor that are torn or stretched during childbirth may require up to 6 months to regain tone. Kegel exercises, which help strengthen perineal muscles and encourage healing, are recommended after childbirth (see Patient Teaching box, p. 53). Pelvic relaxation refers to the lengthening and weakening of the fascial supports of pelvic structures. These structures include the uterus, upper posterior vaginal wall, urethra, bladder, and rectum. Although relaxation can occur in any woman, it is commonly a direct but delayed complication of childbirth.

Abdomen

When the woman stands during the first days after birth, her abdomen protrudes and gives her a still-pregnant appearance. During the first 2 weeks after birth the abdominal wall is relaxed (see Fig. 20-1). It takes about 6 weeks for the abdominal wall to return almost to its prepregnancy state (Fig. 20-2). The skin regains most of its previous elasticity, but some striae may persist. The return of muscle tone depends on previous tone, proper exercise, and the amount of adipose tissue. Occasionally, with or without overdistention because of a large fetus or multiple fetuses, the abdominal wall muscles separate, a condition termed *diastasis recti abdominis* (see Fig. 10-14, *B*). Persistence of this separation may be disturbing to the woman, but surgical correction rarely is necessary. With time the separation becomes less apparent.

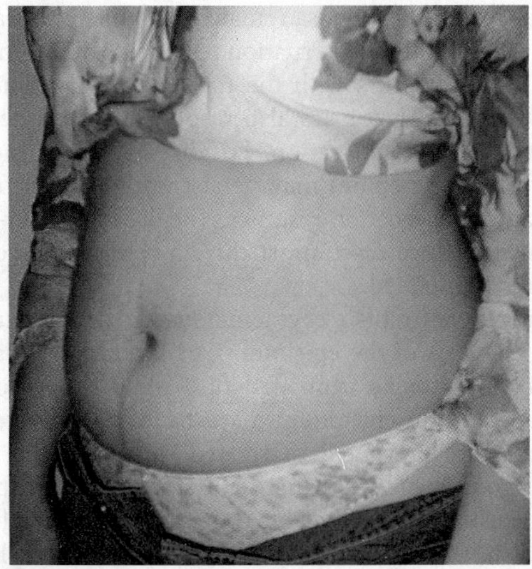

Fig. 20-2 Abdominal wall 6 weeks after vaginal birth is almost back to prepregnancy appearance. Note that the linea nigra is still visible. *(Courtesy Jodi Brackett, Phoenix, AZ.)*

Endocrine System

Placental Hormones

Significant hormonal changes occur during the postpartal period. Expulsion of the placenta results in dramatic decreases of the hormones produced by that organ. Decreases in human chorionic somatomammotropin (also called human placental lactogen), estrogens, cortisol, and the placental enzyme insulinase reverse the diabetogenic effects of pregnancy, resulting in significantly lower blood sugar levels in the immediate puerperium. Mothers with type 1 diabetes will likely require much less insulin for several days after birth. Because these normal hormonal changes make the puerperium a transitional period for carbohydrate metabolism, it is more difficult to interpret glucose tolerance tests at this time.

Estrogen and progesterone levels drop markedly after expulsion of the placenta and reach their lowest levels 1 week after birth. Decreased estrogen levels are associated with breast engorgement and the diuresis of excess extracellular fluid accumulated during pregnancy. In nonlactating women estrogen levels begin to increase by 2 weeks after birth and by postpartum day 17 are higher than in women who breastfeed (Katz, 2007).

Human chorionic gonadotropin disappears from maternal circulation in 14 days.

Pituitary Hormones and Ovarian Function

Prolactin levels in blood rise progressively throughout pregnancy. In women who breastfeed prolactin levels remain elevated and increase with each breastfeeding (Liu, 2009). Serum prolactin levels are influenced by the frequency of breastfeeding, the duration of each feeding, and the degree to which supplementary feedings are used. Individual differences in the strength of an infant's sucking stimulus probably also affect prolactin levels. In nonlactating women prolactin levels decline after birth and reach the prepregnant range in 3 to 4 weeks (Liu, 2009).

Lactating and nonlactating women differ considerably in the timing of their first ovulation and when menstruation resumes. The persistence of elevated serum prolactin levels in breastfeeding women appears to be responsible for suppressing ovulation (Liu, 2009).

Ovulation occurs as early as 27 days after birth in nonlactating women, with a mean time of about 10 weeks. About 70% of nonbreastfeeding women resume menstruating by 12 weeks after birth. The mean time to ovulation in women who breastfeed is about 6 months (Katz, 2007). In lactating women both the resumption of ovulation and the return of menses are determined in large part by breastfeeding patterns. Discussion of contraceptive options early in the puerperium is necessary.

The first menstrual flow after childbirth is usually heavier than normal. Within three or four cycles the amount of menstrual flow returns to the woman's prepregnancy volume.

Urinary System

The hormonal changes of pregnancy (i.e., high steroid levels) contribute to an increase in renal function; diminishing steroid levels after childbirth may partly explain the reduced renal function that occurs during the puerperium. Kidney function returns to normal within 1 month after birth. About 6 weeks are required for the pregnancy-induced hypotonia and dilation of the ureters and renal pelves to return to the nonpregnant state (Katz, 2007). In a small percentage of women dilation of the urinary tract may persist for 3 months or longer, increasing the chances of developing a urinary tract infection.

Urine Components

The renal glycosuria induced by pregnancy disappears, but lactosuria may occur in lactating women. The blood urea nitrogen increases during the puerperium as autolysis of the involuting uterus occurs. This breakdown of excess protein in the uterine muscle cells also results in a mild (+1) proteinuria for 1 to 2 days after childbirth in approximately 50% of women. Ketonuria may occur in women with an uncomplicated birth or after a prolonged labor with dehydration.

Postpartal Diuresis

Within 12 hours of birth women begin to lose excess tissue fluid accumulated during pregnancy. Profuse diaphoresis often occurs, especially at night, for the first 2 or 3 days after childbirth. Postpartal diuresis, caused by decreased estrogen levels, removal of increased venous pressure in the lower extremities, and loss of the remaining pregnancy-induced increase in blood volume, also aids the body in ridding itself of excess fluid. Fluid loss through perspiration and increased urinary output accounts for a weight loss of approximately 2.25 kg during the puerperium.

Urethra and Bladder

Birth-induced trauma, increased bladder capacity following childbirth, and the effects of conduction anesthesia combine to cause a decreased urge to void. In addition, pelvic soreness caused by the forces of labor, vaginal lacerations, or the episiotomy reduces or alters the voiding reflex. Decreased voiding combined with postpartal diuresis may result in bladder distention.

Immediately after birth excessive bleeding can occur if the bladder becomes distended because it pushes the uterus up and to the side and prevents it from contracting firmly. Later in the puerperium overdistention can make the bladder more susceptible to infection and impede the resumption of normal voiding (Cunningham et al, 2005). With adequate emptying of the bladder, bladder tone is usually restored by 5 to 7 days after childbirth.

Gastrointestinal System

Appetite

The mother usually is hungry shortly after birth and can tolerate a light diet. Most new mothers are very hungry after full recovery from analgesia, anesthesia, and fatigue. Requests for extra portions of food and frequent snacks are not uncommon.

Bowel Evacuation

A spontaneous bowel evacuation may not occur for 2 to 3 days after childbirth. This delay can be explained by decreased muscle tone in the intestines during labor and the immediate puerperium, prelabor diarrhea, lack of food, or dehydration. The mother often anticipates discomfort during the bowel movement because of perineal tenderness as a result of episiotomy, lacerations, or hemorrhoids and resists the urge to defecate. Regular bowel habits should be reestablished when bowel tone returns.

Operative vaginal birth (forceps or vacuum use) and anal sphincter lacerations are associated with an increased risk of postpartum anal incontinence. If it occurs, anal incontinence is often temporary and may resolve within 6 months (Katz, 2007). Women should be taught during pregnancy about episiotomy and its possible sequelae. Pelvic floor (Kegel) exercises should be encouraged.

Breasts

Promptly after birth there is a decrease in the concentrations of hormones (i.e., estrogen, progesterone, human chorionic gonadotropin, prolactin, cortisol, and insulin) that stimulated breast development during pregnancy. The time it takes for these hormones to return to prepregnancy levels is determined in part by whether the mother breastfeeds her infant.

Breastfeeding Mothers

During the first 24 hours after birth there is little, if any, change in the breast tissue. Colostrum, a clear, yellow fluid, may be expressed from the breasts. The breasts gradually become fuller and heavier as the colostrum transitions to milk by about 72 to 96 hours after birth; this is often referred to as the "milk coming in." The breasts may feel warm, firm, and somewhat tender. Bluish-white milk with a skim-milk appearance (true milk) can be expressed from the nipples. As milk glands and milk ducts fill with milk, breast tissue may feel somewhat nodular or lumpy. Unlike the lumps associated with fibrocystic breast disease or cancer (which can be palpated consistently in the same location), the nodularity associated with milk production tends to shift in position. Some women experience engorgement, but with frequent breastfeeding and proper care this is a temporary condition that typically lasts only 24 to 48 hours (see Chapter 26).

Nonbreastfeeding Mothers

The breasts generally feel nodular in contrast to the granular feel of breasts in nonpregnant women. The nodularity is bilateral and diffuse. Prolactin levels drop rapidly. Colostrum is present for the first few days after childbirth. Palpation of the breast on the second or third day as milk production begins may reveal tissue tenderness in some women. On the third or fourth postpartum day engorgement may occur. The breasts are distended (swollen), firm, tender, and warm to the touch (because of vasocongestion). Breast distention is caused primarily by the temporary congestion of veins and lymphatics rather than by an accumulation of milk. Milk is present but should not be expressed. Axillary breast tissue (the tail of Spence) and any accessory breast or nipple tissue along the milk line can be involved. Engorgement resolves spontaneously, and discomfort decreases usually within 24 to 36 hours. A breast binder or well-fitted supportive bra, ice packs, fresh cabbage leaves, and/or mild analgesics may be used to relieve discomfort. Nipple stimulation is avoided. If suckling is never begun (or is discontinued), lactation ceases within a few days to a week.

Cardiovascular System

Blood Volume

Changes in blood volume after birth depend on several factors such as blood loss during childbirth and the amount of extravascular water (physiologic edema) mobilized and excreted. Blood loss results in an immediate but limited decrease in total blood volume. Thereafter most of the blood volume increase during pregnancy (1000 to 1500 ml) is eliminated within the first 2 weeks after birth.

Pregnancy-induced hypervolemia (an increase in blood volume of at least 35% over prepregnancy values near term) (Katz, 2007) allows most women to tolerate considerable blood loss during childbirth. Many women lose approximately 500 ml of blood during vaginal birth of a single fetus and about twice this much during cesarean birth (Monga, 2009) (see Critical Thinking Exercise).

Readjustments in the maternal vasculature after childbirth are dramatic and rapid. The woman's response to blood loss during the early puerperium differs from that in a nonpregnant woman. Three postpartum physiologic changes protect the woman from excessive blood loss: (1) elimination of uteroplacental circulation reduces the size of the maternal vascular bed by 10% to 15%; (2) loss of placental endocrine function removes the stimulus for vasodilation; and (3) mobilization of extravascular water stored during pregnancy increases blood volume. Thus hypovolemic shock usually does not occur in women who experience a normal blood loss during the puerperium.

Cardiac Output

Pulse rate, stroke volume, and cardiac output increase throughout pregnancy. Cardiac output remains increased for at least 48 hours after birth because of an increase in stroke volume. This increased stroke volume is caused by the return of blood to the maternal systemic venous circulation, a result of rapid decrease in uterine blood flow and mobilization of extravascular fluid (Monga, 2009). Stroke volume, cardiac output, end-diastolic volume, and systemic vascular resistance remain elevated over nonpregnant values for 12 weeks after birth and may not stabilize until 24 weeks after birth (Monga, 2009).

CRITICAL THINKING EXERCISE

Maternal Postpartum Blood Loss and Fatigue

You are caring for four women on the postpartum unit, two of whom had vaginal births and two who had cesarean births. Each of the women has complained about feeling tired and has expressed concern about the amount of blood she lost during birth. Before providing patient education related to fatigue after birth and blood loss, you review the nurses' notes, the intake and output records, and patient records for estimated blood loss and hemoglobin and hematocrit values.

1. Evidence—Is there sufficient evidence to draw conclusions about the relation between tiredness (fatigue) after birth and blood loss?
2. Assumptions—What assumptions can be made about the following factors?
   a. Comparison of amount of blood loss between women who give birth vaginally and by cesarean
   b. Postpartum norms for hematocrit and hemoglobin for women who give birth vaginally and by cesarean
   c. Causes of fatigue after birth
   d. Interventions to alleviate fatigue and replace blood lost at birth
3. What implications and priorities for nursing care can be drawn at this time?
4. Does the evidence objectively support your conclusion?
5. Are there alternative perspectives to your conclusion?

Vital Signs

Few alterations in vital signs are seen under normal circumstances. Heart rate and blood pressure return to nonpregnant levels within a few days (Katz, 2007) (Table 20-1). Respiratory function returns to nonpregnant levels by 6 to 8 weeks after birth. After the uterus is emptied the diaphragm descends, the normal cardiac axis is restored, and the point of maximal impulse and the electrocardiogram are normalized.

Blood Components

Hematocrit and Hemoglobin

During the first 72 hours after childbirth there is a greater reduction of plasma volume than in the number of blood cells. This results in a rise in hematocrit and hemoglobin levels by the seventh day after birth. There is no increased red blood cell (RBC) destruction during the puerperium, but any excess will disappear gradually in accordance with the life span of the RBC. The exact time at which RBC volume returns to prepregnancy values is not known, but it is within normal limits when measured 8 weeks after childbirth (Katz, 2007).

White Blood Cell Count

Normal leukocytosis of pregnancy averages approximately 12,000/mm^3. During the first 10 to 12 days after childbirth values between 20,000 and 25,000/mm^3 are common. Neutrophils are the most numerous white blood cells. Leukocytosis, coupled with the normal increase in erythrocyte sedimentation rate that occurs, may obscure the diagnosis of acute infections at this time.

Table 20-1 Vital Signs After Childbirth

NORMAL FINDINGS	DEVIATIONS FROM NORMAL FINDINGS AND PROBABLE CAUSES
Temperature	
During first 24 hours temperature may increase to 38° C as a result of dehydrating effects of labor. After 24 hours the woman should be afebrile.	A diagnosis of puerperal sepsis is suggested if an increase in maternal temperature to 38° C is noted after the first 24 hours after childbirth and recurs or persists for 2 days. Other possibilities are mastitis, endometritis, urinary tract infections, and other systemic infections.
Pulse	
Pulse, along with stroke volume and cardiac output, remains elevated for the first hour or so after childbirth. It then begins to decrease at an unknown rate to a nonpregnant rate.	A rapid pulse rate or one that is increasing may indicate hypovolemia as a result of hemorrhage.
Respirations	
The respiratory rate should decrease to within the woman's normal prebirth range by 6-8 weeks after childbirth.	Hypoventilation may occur after an unusually high subarachnoid (spinal) block or epidural narcotic after a cesarean birth.
Blood Pressure	
Blood pressure is altered slightly if at all. Orthostatic hypotension, as indicated by feelings of faintness or dizziness immediately after standing up, can develop in the first 48 hours as a result of the splanchnic engorgement that may occur after birth.	A low or decreasing blood pressure may indicate the existence of hypovolemia secondary to hemorrhage; however, it is a late sign, and other symptoms of hemorrhage usually alert the staff. An increased reading may result from excessive use of vasopressor or oxytocic medications. Because gestational hypertension can persist into or occur first in the postpartum period, routine evaluation of blood pressure is needed. If a woman complains of headache, hypertension must be ruled out as a cause before analgesics are administered.

Coagulation Factors

Clotting factors and fibrinogen are normally increased during pregnancy and remain elevated in the immediate puerperium. When combined with vessel damage and immobility, this hypercoagulable state causes an increased risk of thromboembolism, especially after a cesarean birth. Fibrinolytic activity also increases during the first few days after childbirth (Katz, 2007). Factors I, II, VIII, IX, and X decrease to nonpregnant levels within a few days. Fibrin split products, probably released from the placental site, can also be found in maternal blood.

Varicosities

Varicosities (varices) of the legs and around the anus (hemorrhoids) are common during pregnancy. All varices, even the less common vulvar varices, regress (empty) rapidly immediately after childbirth. Total or nearly total regression of varicosities is expected after childbirth.

Neurologic System

Neurologic changes during the puerperium are those that result from a reversal of maternal adaptations to pregnancy and those resulting from trauma during labor and childbirth.

Pregnancy-induced neurologic discomforts disappear after birth. Elimination of physiologic edema through the diuresis that follows childbirth relieves carpal tunnel syndrome by easing compression of the median nerve. The periodic numbness and tingling of fingers that afflict 5% of pregnant women usually disappear after the birth, unless lifting and carrying the baby aggravates the condition. Headache requires careful assessment. Postpartum headaches may be caused by various conditions, including gestational hypertension, stress, and leakage of cerebrospinal fluid into the extradural space during placement of the needle for administration of epidural or spinal anesthesia. Depending on the cause and effectiveness of treatment, headaches last from 1 to 3 days to several weeks.

Musculoskeletal System

Adaptations of the mother's musculoskeletal system that occur during pregnancy are reversed in the puerperium. These adaptations include the relaxation and subsequent hypermobility of the joints and the change in the mother's center of gravity in response to the enlarging uterus. The joints are completely stabilized by 6 to 8 weeks after birth. Although all other joints return to their normal prepregnancy state, those in the parous woman's feet do not. The new mother may notice a permanent increase in her shoe size.

Integumentary System

Chloasma of pregnancy usually disappears at the end of pregnancy. Hyperpigmentation of the areolae and linea nigra may not regress completely after childbirth. Some women will have permanent darker pigmentation of those areas. Striae gravidarum (stretch marks) on the breasts, abdomen, and thighs may fade but usually do not disappear.

Vascular abnormalities such as spider angiomas (nevi), palmar erythema, and epulis generally regress in response to the rapid decline in estrogens after the end of pregnancy. For some women spider nevi persist indefinitely.

Hair growth slows during the postpartum period. Some women may experience hair loss because the amount of hair lost is temporarily more than the amount regrown. The abundance of fine hair seen during pregnancy usually disappears after giving birth; however, any coarse or bristly hair that appears during pregnancy usually remains. Fingernails return to their prepregnancy consistency and strength.

Profuse diaphoresis that occurs in the immediate postpartum period is the most noticeable change in the integumentary system.

Immune System

No significant changes in the maternal immune system occur during the postpartum period. The mother's need for a rubella vaccination or for $Rh_o(D)$ immune globulin for prevention of Rh isoimmunization is determined.

Key Points

- The uterus involutes rapidly after birth and returns to the true pelvis within 2 weeks.
- The rapid decrease in estrogen and progesterone levels after expulsion of the placenta is responsible for triggering many of the anatomic and physiologic changes in the puerperium.
- Assessment of lochia and fundal height is essential to monitor the progress of normal involution and to identify potential problems.
- The return of ovulation and menses is determined in part by whether the woman breastfeeds her infant.
- Few alterations in vital signs are seen after birth under normal circumstances.

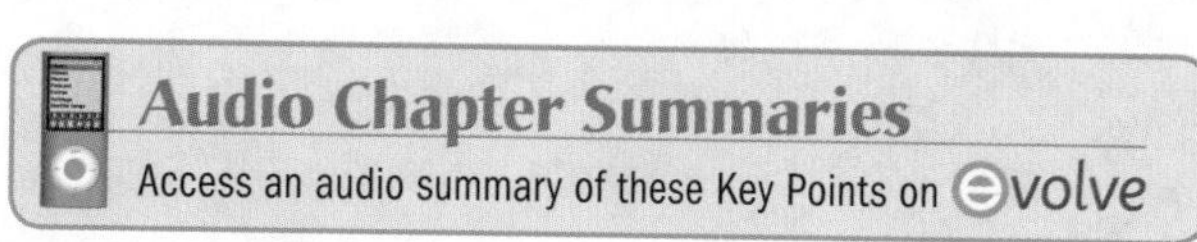
Audio Chapter Summaries
Access an audio summary of these Key Points on evolve

- Hypercoagulability, vessel damage, and immobility predispose the woman to thromboembolism.
- Marked diuresis, decreased bladder sensitivity, and overdistention of the bladder can lead to problems with urinary elimination.
- Pregnancy-induced hypervolemia, combined with several postpartum physiologic changes, allows the woman to tolerate considerable blood loss at birth.

References

Cunningham F et al: *Williams obstetrics*, ed 22, New York, 2005, McGraw Hill.

Katz V: Postpartum care. In Gabbe SG, Niebyl JR, Simpson JL (editors): *Obstetrics: normal and problem pregnancies*, ed 5, New York, 2007, Churchill Livingstone.

Liu JH: Endocrinology of pregnancy. In Creasy RK et al (editors): *Creasy & Resnik's maternal-fetal medicine: principles and practice*, ed 6, Philadelphia, 2009, Saunders.

Monga M: Maternal cardiovascular, respiratory, and renal adaptation to pregnancy. In Creasy RK et al (editors): *Creasy & Resnik's maternal-fetal medicine: principles and practice*, ed 6, Philadelphia, 2009, Saunders.

Unit 5

21

Nursing Care During the Fourth Trimester

Learning Objectives

On completion of this chapter the reader will be able to:

- Discuss postpartum care and discharge teaching.
- Summarize nursing interventions to prevent infection and excessive bleeding, promote normal bladder and bowel patterns, and care for the breasts of women who are breastfeeding or bottle-feeding.
- Identify common selection criteria for safe early postpartum discharge.
- Explain the influence of cultural expectations on postpartum adjustment.
- Describe the nurse's role in these postpartum follow-up strategies: home visits, telephone follow-up, warm lines and help lines, support groups, and referrals to community resources.

Electronic Resources

Additional information related to the content in Chapter 21 can be found on

evolve the Companion Website at
http://evolve.elsevier.com/Perry/maternal/

- NCLEX Review Questions
- Case Study—Fourth Trimester
- Critical Thinking Exercise—Postpartum Complications
- Critical Thinking Exercise—Priority Nursing Care: Postpartum Unit
- Nursing Care Plan—Postpartum Care: Vaginal Birth
- Spanish Guidelines—Assessing for Hemorrhage
- Spanish Guidelines—Assessing for Infection
- Spanish Guidelines—Discharge Teaching
- Spanish Guidelines—Postpartum Adjustment

The goal of nursing care in the immediate postpartum period is to assist women and their partners during their initial transition to parenting. The approach to the care of women after birth is wellness oriented. Consequently in the United States most women remain hospitalized no more than 1 or 2 days after giving birth, and some for as few as 6 hours. Because there is so much important information to be shared with these women in a very short time, it is vital that their care be thoughtfully planned and provided. Care is focused on the woman's physiologic recovery, her psychologic well-being, and her ability to care for herself and her new baby. In addition, the nurse considers the needs of other family members and includes strategies in the plan of care to assist the family in adjusting to the new baby.

Transfer from the Recovery Area

After the initial recovery period has been completed, the woman may be transferred to a postpartum room in the same or another nursing unit. In facilities with labor, delivery, recovery, postpartum rooms, the woman stays in the same room, and the nurse who provides care during the recovery period usually continues caring for the woman. Women who have received general or regional anesthesia must be cleared for transfer from the recovery area by a member of the anesthesia care team.

In preparing the transfer report, the recovery nurse uses information from the records of admission, birth record, and recovery. Information communicated to the postpartum nurse includes identity of the health care provider; gravidity and parity; age; anesthetic used; any medications given; duration of labor and time of rupture of membranes; whether labor was induced or augmented; type of birth and repair; blood type and Rh status; group B streptococcus status; status of rubella immunity; syphilis and hepatitis serology test results (if positive); intravenous infusion of any fluids; physiologic status since birth; description of fundus, lochia, bladder, and perineum; sex and weight of infant; time of birth; name of pediatric care provider; chosen method of feeding; any abnormalities noted; and assessment of initial parent-infant interaction.

Most of this information is also documented for the nursing staff in the newborn nursery if the infant is transferred to that unit. In addition, specific information should be provided regarding the infant's Apgar scores (see Chapter 25), weight, voiding, stooling, and whether fed since birth. Nursing interventions that have been completed (e.g., eye prophylaxis and vitamin K injection) also must be recorded. Table 21-1 gives examples for documenting this information before the transfer of the woman from the recovery area.

Women who give birth in birthing centers may go home within a few hours, after the woman's and infant's conditions are stable.

Table 21-1 Recovery Nurse's Report

ITEM	EXAMPLE OF DOCUMENTATION OF MOTHER	EXAMPLE OF DOCUMENTATION OF NEWBORN
Type of labor and birth; unusual observations, if any, of the placenta	Spontaneous or assisted (forceps, vacuum extraction) vaginal birth; vertex presentation; time of ROM	Spontaneous or assisted (forceps) vaginal birth; vertex presentation; time of ROM
Gravidity and parity, age	G1, P1, age 22 yr; 39 wk of gestation	G1, P1, age 22 yr; 39 wk of gestation
Anesthesia and analgesia used	None; epidural, low spinal, local	None; epidural, low spinal, local
Condition of perineum	Episiotomy; repair of lacerations; intact	
Events since birth	Vital signs, BP, fundus, lochia, intake and output, medications (dosage, time of administration, and results); response to newborn; observation of family interactions, including siblings, if present	Vital signs, blood glucose level (if assessed), nursed at breast for ____ min Voided ×1; meconium stool ×1 Eye prophylaxis given Vitamin K injection given Held by siblings who are happy (or have other response to newborn)
Condition and sex of newborn; other information	Time of birth; weight; whether breastfeeding or bottle-feeding; sex of the baby	Time of birth; Apgar at 1 and 5 min; Sex; weight; name of pediatrician; breastfeeding or bottle feeding; mother's hepatitis B status and GBS status; whether mother received magnesium sulfate; time of last systemic analgesia
Relevant information from prenatal record	Need for rubella vaccination; presence of infections; hepatitis B status; HIV status; blood type; Rh status; GBS status and treatment if positive	Unremarkable pregnancy
Miscellaneous information: IV drip	If IV drip is infusing, rate of infusion, medications added (e.g., oxytocin [Pitocin]), whether to keep open or discontinue after completion of bag that is hung	
Social factors	If woman is releasing baby for adoption, whether she wants to see baby, breastfeed, allow visitors, or other preferences she may have	Baby up for adoption; to stay in NBN until discharge

BP, Blood pressure; *GBS*, group B streptococcus; *HIV*, human immune deficiency virus; *IV*, intravenous; *NBN*, newborn nursery; *ROM*, rupture of membranes.

Discharge—Before 24 Hours and After 48 Hours

Early postpartum discharge, shortened hospital stay, and 1-day maternity stay are all terms for the decreasing length of hospital stays of mothers and their babies after a low risk birth. The trend of shortened hospital stays is based largely on efforts to reduce health care costs, coupled with consumer demands to have less medical intervention and more family-focused experiences (Box 21-1).

Laws Relating to Discharge

Health care providers expressed concern with shortened stays because some medical problems do not show up in the first 24 hours after birth. In this short time new mothers have not had sufficient time to learn to care for their newborns and identify newborn health problems such as jaundice and dehydration related to limited intake the first hours after birth.

The concern for the potential increase in adverse maternal-infant outcomes from hospital early discharge practices led the American College of Obstetricians and Gynecologists, the American Academy of Pediatrics (AAP), and other professional health care organizations to promote the enactment of federal and state maternity length-of-stay bills to ensure adequate care for both the mother and the newborn. The passage of the Newborns' and Mothers' Health Protection Act of 1996 provided minimum federal standards for health plan coverage for mothers and their newborns (AAP Committee on Fetus and Newborn, 2004). Under this Act all health plans are required to allow the new mother and newborn to remain in the hospital for a minimum of 48 hours after a normal vaginal birth and for 96 hours after a cesarean birth, unless the attending provider, in consultation with the mother, decides on early discharge.

Criteria for Discharge

Early discharge with postpartum home care can be a safe and satisfying option for women and their families when it is comprehensive and based on individual needs (AAP Committee on Fetus and Newborn, 2004). Hospital stays need to be long enough to identify problems and ensure that the woman is sufficiently recovered and prepared to care for herself and the baby at home.

It is essential that nurses consider the medical needs of the woman and her baby and provide care that is coordinated to meet those needs to provide timely physiologic interventions and treatment to prevent morbidity and hospital readmission. With predetermined criteria for identifying low risk in the mothers and newborns (Box 21-2), the length of hospitaliza-

BOX 21-1 Advantages and Disadvantages of Early Postpartum Discharge

Advantages

Reinforces the concept of childbirth as a normal physiologic event

Allows shorter separations between mothers and other children

Extends a couple's sense of control and participation beyond the birth itself

Capitalizes on the security of the home environment during the stressors of early parenting

Decreases unnecessary exposure to the pathogens in the hospital environment

Allows beds on the maternity service to be used more effectively (i.e., quick turnover in patients or greater availability for patients with a complication)

Allows more time for mother/father/partner/infant and other family members to bond

Creates less disruption in the daily life of the family

Promotes active involvement of family and support persons in assisting the mother and newborn

Disadvantages

Complications (maternal or newborn) may go unrecognized.

Families may be or feel unprepared for the reality they face once the baby is at home.

The mother is fatigued from the labor and childbirth process.

The mother is experiencing postpartum pain or discomfort.

The length of time for learning after the birth in the hospital setting is decreased.

A vulnerability and crisis potential exists for both women and families.

tion can be based on medical need for care in an acute care setting or in consideration of the ongoing care needed in the home environment (see Evidence-Based Practice box). Early follow-up visits are key to reducing readmission of newborns.

Hospital-based maternity nurses continue to play invaluable roles as caregivers, teachers, and patient and family advocates in developing and implementing effective home care strategies. Postpartum order sets and maternal-newborn teaching checklists (Fig. 21-1) can be used to accomplish patient care and educational outcomes. With coordination, clinical care and education can be planned and provided throughout pregnancy, during the hospital stay, and in the home after discharge to ensure the family's continued well-being.

LEGAL TIP Early Discharge Whether or not the woman and her family have chosen early discharge, the nurse and the primary health care provider are held responsible if the woman is discharged before her condition has stabilized within normal limits. If complications occur, the medical and nursing staff could be sued for abandonment.

BOX 21-2 Criteria for Early Discharge

Mother

Uncomplicated pregnancy, labor, vaginal birth, and postpartum course

No evidence of premature rupture of membranes

Blood pressure, temperature stable and within normal limits

Ambulating unassisted

Voiding adequate amounts without difficulty

Hemoglobin greater than 10 g

No significant vaginal bleeding; perineum intact or no more than second-degree episiotomy or laceration repair; uterus firm

Received instructions on postpartum self-management

Infant

Term infant (38 to 42 weeks) with weight appropriate for gestational age

Normal findings on physical assessment

Temperature, respirations, and heart rate within normal limits and stable for the 12 hours preceding discharge

At least two successful feedings completed (normal sucking and swallowing)

Urination and stooling have occurred at least once

No evidence of significant jaundice in the first 24 hours after the birth

No excessive bleeding at the circumcision site for at least 2 hours

Screening tests performed according to state regulations; tests to be repeated at follow-up visit if done before the infant is 24 hours old

Initial hepatitis B vaccine given or scheduled for first follow-up visit

Laboratory data reviewed: maternal syphilis and hepatitis B status; infant or cord blood type and Coombs' test results if indicated

General

No social, family, or environmental risk factors identified

Family or support person available to assist mother and infant at home

Follow-up scheduled within 1 week if discharged before 48 hours after the birth

Documentation of skill of mother in feeding (breast or bottle), cord care, skin care, perineal care, infant safety (use of car seat, sleeping positions), and recognizing signs of illness and common infant problems

Sources: American Academy of Pediatrics (AAP) Committee on Fetus and Newborn: Hospital stay for healthy term infants, *Pediatrics* 113(5):1434-1436, 2004.

Nursing Care Management—Physical Needs

The nursing plan of care includes both the postpartum woman and her infant, even if the nursery nurse retains primary responsibility for the infant (see Nursing Process box). In many hospitals couplet care (also called *mother-baby care* or *single-room maternity care*) is practiced. Nurses in these settings have been educated in both mother and infant care and

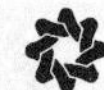

Abbott Northwestern Hospital
A HealthSpan™ Organization

SELF/FAMILY LEARNING CHECKLIST

Patient Name, Social Security #, Date of Birth

I learn best by: ☐ *Group classes* ☐ *Individual instruction* ☐ *Video instruction* ☐ *Reading it myself*

Please indicate your desired learning needs by placing a check in one of the columns next to each topic.

KEY *1 = Most important to learn before I go home*
2 = I already know

(Please DATE when learning need is met.)

CARING FOR YOURSELF	1	2	DATE	CARING FOR BABY	1	2	DATE
Episiotomy and perineal care				*Diapering*			
Vaginal discharge				*Baby bath, skin and cord care*			
Hemorrhoids/Constipation				*Circumcised/uncircumcised care*			
Breast care				*Burping*			
Nutrition				*Bowel movements/wet diapers*			
Activity				*Sleeping habits*			
Post partal exercises				*Newborn behavior*			
Return of menstruation				*Jaundice*			
Family planning				*Signs of illness*			
Blood clots				*Car seat safety*			
Post partum emotions				*General infant safety/poison control*			
Post partum warning signs				*Signs/symptoms of dehydration*			
				Bulb syringe			
Cesarean Birth							
Incisional care				**BREAST FEEDING**			
				Sore nipples			
				Positioning			
				Frequency of feedings			
AFTER DISCHARGE				*Expressing/storing milk*			
When to call health care provider				*Engorgement*			
				Feeding water			
				Nursing while working			
OTHER				*Weaning*			
Working mothers							
Day care							
Sibling adjustment				**BOTTLE FEEDING**			
Single parent support				*Types of formula*			
Time out for parents				*Preparing formula*			
Infant safety and security				*Frequency of feedings*			
Infant As A Person Class							
New Parent Connection							

MEDICATIONS AT HOME

MEDICATIONS	STRENGTH	DOSAGE	FREQUENCY	PURPOSE/SPECIAL INSTRUCTIONS
			times per day	
			times per day	
			times per day	

RESOURCES REFERRALS
☐ *Physician Discharge Instructions*
☐ *Home Care Agency* ______
☐ *Other Referrals* ______

VALUABLES: ☐ *Returned* ☐ *None* **MEDICATIONS:** ☐ *Returned* ☐ *None* ☐ *Room checked for belongings*

Patient verbalized understanding of discharge information received.

PATIENT OR SUPPORT PERSON ______ NURSE'S SIGNATURE ______ DATE ______

SELF/FAMILY LEARNING CHECKLIST

SELF/FAMILY LEARNING CHECKLIST

Fig. 21-1 Self/Family Learning Checklist. *(Copyright Abbott Northwestern Hospital of Allina Health System, Minneapolis and St Paul, MN.)*

EVIDENCE-BASED PRACTICE How Soon Is Too Soon? Early Discharge After Birth —*Pat Gingrich*

Ask the Question

What are the risks and benefits of early postpartum discharge for mother and baby? What do women want from their postpartum hospital experience?

Search for Evidence

Search Strategies

Professional organization guidelines, meta-analyses, systematic reviews, randomized controlled trials, nonrandomized prospective studies, and retrospective studies since 2006.

Databases Searched

CINAHL; Cochrane; Medline; National Guideline Clearinghouse; TRIP Database Plus; and the websites for AWHONN, SOGC, and NICE

Critically Analyze the Evidence

The optimum length of postpartum hospitalization has been debated for decades. After a period of shortened stays in the early 1990s, which critics dubbed "drive-through deliveries," research demonstrated an increase in infant problems and readmissions. New laws required insurance and Medicaid to cover 48 hours for vaginal birth and 72 hours for cesarean birth, which has decreased readmission rates.

Length of hospital stay after giving birth depends on many factors: the physical condition of the mother and baby, social support at home, patient education needs for self-care and infant care, mental and emotional status of the mother, and financial constraints.

Women who greatly prefer to go home will probably do better there. The professional recommendation by the National Institute for Health and Clinical Excellence (2004) is to allow early discharge at 24 hours after vaginal or cesarean birth as long as there is neither fever nor complications and there will be close follow-up. According to a survey of 2583 Canadian women, effective follow-up such as office or home visit or telephone contact with a health care provider within 72 hours of discharge can significantly decrease infant readmissions and maternal postpartum depression (Goulet, D'Amour, & Pineault, 2007).

According to the professional guidelines published by the Society of Obstetricians and Gynaecologists of Canada (SOGC), the risk with early discharge is mainly to the infant, who may develop jaundice, infection, unrecognized heart or respiratory problems, or feeding problems (Cargill, Martel, & SOGC, 2007). The rate of emergency department visits and readmissions was especially high for infants with young, primiparous, unmarried mothers.

Implications for Practice

In an ongoing population-based survey of 16,000 U.S. women, a qualitative analysis found six major themes for postpartum concerns of the women 2 to 9 months after birth: the need for social support, breastfeeding issues, newborn care, postpartum depression, perceived need to extend hospital stay, and need for insurance beyond birth (Kanotra et al, 2007). Nurses have the most opportunity to assess the physical, psychologic, and social well-being of their patients. Postpartum women deserve individualized patient education that includes comprehensive information and resources about infant care, breastfeeding, and postpartum depression. Educational information should be offered in many formats and include hand-on demonstrations. Written material should include 24-hour numbers to call for problems with infant care and breastfeeding and contact information for community parenting groups. All patients should go home with a realistic expectation of the social and financial support they will need. Finally, nurses can advocate for policies that support flexible lengths of hospital stays and programs recommended by the SOGC (i.e., early home visits, outpatient breastfeeding clinics, and early physician visits) (Cargill, Martel, & SOGC, 2007).

References

Cargill Y, Martel M J, Society of Obstetricians and Gynaecologists of Canada: SGOC policy statement No 190: postpartum maternal and newborn discharge, *J Obstet Gynaecol Can* 29(4):357-363, 2007.

Goulet L, D'Amour D, Pineault R: Type and timing of services following postnatal discharge: do they make a difference? *Womens Health* 45(4):19-39, 2007.

Kanotra S et al: Challenges faced by new mothers in the early postpartum period: an analysis of comment data from the 2000 Pregnancy Risk Assessment Monitoring System (PRAMS) survey, *Matern Child Health J* 11(6):549-558, 2007.

National Institute for Health and Clinical Excellence: *Caesarean section,* NICE Clinical Guideline 13, London, 2004, NICE. Available from www.nice.org.uk/CG013NICEguideline (accessed April 4, 2009).

function as primary nurses for both mother and infant, even if the infant is kept in the nursery. This approach is a variation of rooming-in, in which the mother and infant room together and mother and nurse share the care of the infant.

Plan of Care and Implementation

Once the nursing diagnoses are formulated, the nurse plans with the woman what nursing measures are appropriate and which are to be given priority. The nursing plan of care includes periodic assessments to detect deviations from normal physical changes, measures to relieve discomfort or pain, safety measures to prevent injury or infection, and teaching and counseling measures designed to promote the woman's feelings of competence in self-management and baby care. Family members are included in the teaching. The nurse evaluates continuously and is ready to change the plan if indicated. Almost all hospitals use standardized care plans as a base. The nurse's adaptation of the standardized plan to meet specific medical and nursing diagnoses results in individualized patient care (see Nursing Care Plan). Signs of potential problems that may be identified during the assessment process are listed in Box 21-3.

Nurses assume many roles while implementing the nursing plan of care. They provide direct physical care, teach mother and baby care, and provide anticipatory guidance and counseling. Perhaps most important of all, they nurture the woman by providing encouragement and support as she begins to assume the many tasks of motherhood. Nurses who take the time to "mother the mother" do much to increase feelings of self-confidence in new mothers.

The first step in providing individualized care is to confirm the woman's identity by checking her wristband. At the same

NURSING PROCESS: PHYSICAL NEEDS

Assessment

A focused physical assessment is performed on admission to the postpartum unit. If vital signs are within normal limits, assessment continues every 4 to 8 hours.

Interview (by Postpartum Nurse)

Mother's emotional status and energy level
Degree of physical discomfort, hunger, and thirst
Knowledge level concerning self-care and infant care

Physical Examination

Breasts (firmness)
Uterine fundus (location; consistency)
Lochia (amount; color)
Perineum (discomfort; condition of repair [if done])
Bladder and bowel function (amount; frequency)
Legs (edema; Homans' sign)
Intake and output if an intravenous infusion or a urinary catheter is in place
Incisional dressing if birth by cesarean

Review of Results of Laboratory Tests

Postpartum hemoglobin and hematocrit (if ordered)
Clean-catch or catheterized urine (in some settings)
Rubella and Rh (if status is unknown)

Nursing Diagnoses

Examples of nursing diagnoses commonly established for the postpartum patient include the following:

Risk for deficient fluid volume (hemorrhage) related to
- uterine atony after childbirth

Urinary retention or constipation related to
- postchildbirth discomfort
- childbirth trauma to tissues

Acute pain related to
- uterine involution
- episiotomy or lacerations
- hemorrhoids
- engorged breasts

Disturbed sleep pattern related to
- discomforts of postpartum period
- long labor process
- infant care and hospital routine

Ineffective breastfeeding related to
- maternal discomfort
- infant positioning

Planning

The nursing plan of care includes both the postpartum woman and her infant, even if the nursery nurse retains primary responsibility for the infant. The organization of the mother's care must take the newborn into consideration. The day actually revolves around the baby's feeding and care times.

Expected outcomes for the postpartum period are based on the nursing diagnoses identified for the individual patient. Examples of common expected outcomes for physiologic needs are that the woman will do the following:

- Remain free from infection
- Demonstrate normal involution and lochial characteristics
- Remain comfortable and injury free
- Demonstrate normal bladder and bowel patterns
- Demonstrate knowledge of breast care, whether breastfeeding or bottle-feeding
- Integrate the newborn into the family

Interventions

Provide direct care (e.g., administer analgesics, assist with ambulation, administer intravenous fluids, assist with personal hygiene, provide perineal care, change dressing).
Teach mother-baby care.
Provide anticipatory guidance and counseling.
Provide encouragement and support.
Teach mother to check identity of anyone who cares for the baby.
Additional interventions are discussed in the text.

Evaluation

The nurse can be reasonably assured that care was effective when the expected outcomes of care for physical needs have been achieved.

BOX 21-3 Signs of Potential Physiologic Complications

Temperature—More than 38° C after the first 24 hours
Pulse—Tachycardia or marked bradycardia
Blood Pressure—Hypotension or hypertension
Energy Level—Lethargy; extreme fatigue
Uterus—Deviated from the midline; boggy consistency; remains above the umbilicus after 24 hours
Lochia—Heavy, foul odor; bright red bleeding that is not lochia
Perineum—Pronounced edema; not intact; signs of infection; marked discomfort
Legs—Homans' sign positive; painful, reddened area; warmth on posterior aspect of calf
Breasts—Redness, heat, pain; cracked and fissured nipples; inverted nipples; palpable mass
Appetite—Lack of appetite
Elimination—Urine: inability to void, urgency, frequency, dysuria; bowel: constipation, diarrhea
Rest—Inability to rest or sleep

NURSING CARE PLAN Postpartum Care—Vaginal Birth

Nursing Diagnosis: Risk for deficient fluid volume related to uterine atony/hemorrhage

Expected Outcomes

Fundus is firm, lochia is moderate, and there is no evidence of hemorrhage.

Nursing Interventions/*Rationales*

Monitor lochia (color, amount, consistency) and count sanitary pads if lochia is heavy *to evaluate amount of bleeding.*

Monitor and palpate fundus for location and tone to determine status of uterus and dictate further interventions *because atonic uterus is the most common cause of postpartum hemorrhage.*

Monitor intake and output, assess for bladder fullness, and encourage voiding *because a full bladder interferes with involution of the uterus.*

Monitor vital signs (increased pulse and respirations, decreased blood pressure) and skin temperature and color *to detect signs of hemorrhage/shock.*

Monitor postpartum hematology studies *to assess effects of blood loss.*

If fundus is boggy, apply gentle massage and assess tone response *to promote uterine contractions and increase uterine tone.* (Do not overstimulate because doing so can cause fundal relaxation.)

Express uterine clots *to promote uterine contraction.*

Explain to the woman the process of involution and teach her to assess and massage the fundus and report any persistent bogginess *to involve her in self-management and increase sense of self-control.*

Administer oxytocic agents per physician/nurse-midwife order and evaluate effectiveness *to promote continuing uterine contraction.*

Administer fluids, blood, blood products, or plasma expanders as ordered *to replace lost fluid and lost blood volume.*

Nursing Diagnosis: Acute pain related to postpartum physiologic changes (hemorrhoids, episiotomy, breast engorgement, cracked/sore nipples)

Expected Outcome

Woman exhibits signs of decreased discomfort.

Nursing Interventions/*Rationales*

Assess location, type, and quality of pain *to direct intervention.*

Explain to the woman the source and reasons for the pain, its expected duration, and treatments *to decrease anxiety and increase sense of control.*

Administer prescribed pain medications *to provide pain relief.*

If pain is perineal (episiotomy, hemorrhoids), apply ice packs in the first 24 hours *to reduce edema and vulvar irritation and reduce discomfort;* encourage sitz baths using cool water the first 24 hours *to reduce edema* and warm water thereafter *to promote circulation;* apply witch hazel compresses *to reduce edema;* teach woman to use prescribed perineal creams, sprays, or ointments *to depress response of peripheral nerves;* teach woman to tighten buttocks before sitting and to sit on flat, hard surfaces *to compress buttocks and reduce pressure on the perineum.* (Avoid donuts and soft pillows because they separate the buttocks and decrease venous blood flow, increasing pain.)

If pain is from breasts and woman is breastfeeding, encourage use of a supportive bra *to increase comfort;* ascertain that infant has latched on correctly *to prevent sore nipples;* vary infant position during feeding *to prevent sore nipples.*

If breasts are engorged, have woman use warm compresses or take a warm shower before breastfeeding *to stimulate milk flow and relieve stasis.*

If nipples are sore, have woman air-dry nipples after feeding *to toughen nipples;* apply breast creams as prescribed *to soften nipples and relieve irritation;* and wear breast shields in her bra *to relieve irritation.*

If pain is from breast and woman is not breastfeeding, encourage use of a tight supportive bra or breast binder, as well as application of ice packs or cold cabbage leaves *to reduce lactation and decrease heaviness.*

Nursing Diagnosis: Disturbed sleep pattern related to excitement, discomfort, and environmental interruptions

Expected Outcome

Woman sleeps for uninterrupted periods of time and feels rested after waking.

Nursing Interventions/*Rationales*

Establish woman's routine sleep patterns and compare with current sleep pattern, exploring things that interfere with sleep, *to determine scope of problem and direct interventions.*

Individualize nursing routines to fit woman's natural body rhythms (i.e., wake/sleep cycles), provide a sleep-promoting environment (i.e., darkness, quiet, adequate ventilation, appropriate room temperature); prepare for sleep using woman's usual routines (i.e., back rub, soothing music, warm milk); teach use of guided imagery and relaxation techniques *to promote optimum conditions for sleep.*

Avoid things or routines (i.e., caffeine, foods that induce heartburn, fluids, strenuous mental/physical activity) *that may interfere with sleep.*

Administer sedation or pain medication as prescribed *to enhance quality of sleep.*

Advise woman/partner to limit visitors and activities *to avoid further taxation and fatigue.*

Teach woman to use infant nap time as a time for her also *to nap and replenish energy and decrease fatigue.*

Nursing Diagnosis: Risk for impaired urinary elimination related to perineal trauma and effects of anesthesia

Expected Outcomes

Woman will void within 6 to 8 hours after birth and empty bladder completely.

Continued

evolve Nursing Care Plan—Postpartum Care: Vaginal Birth

NURSING CARE PLAN Postpartum Care—Vaginal Birth—cont'd

Nursing Interventions/*Rationales*

Assess position and character of uterine fundus and bladder *to ascertain if any further interventions are indicated because of displacement of the fundus or distention of the bladder.*

Measure intake and output *to assess any evidence of dehydration and subsequent decreased anticipated urine output.*

Encourage voiding by walking woman to bathroom, running water over perineum, running water in sink, and providing privacy *to encourage voiding.*

Encourage oral intake *to replace any fluids lost during birth and prevent dehydration.*

Catheterize as necessary with indwelling or straight method *to ensure bladder emptying and allow uterine involution.*

time the infant's identification number is matched with the corresponding band on the mother's wrist and in some instances the father's wrist. The nurse determines how the mother wishes to be addressed and notes her preference in her record and in her nursing care plan.

The woman and her family are oriented to their surroundings. Familiarity with the unit, routines, resources, and personnel reduces one potential source of anxiety—the unknown. The mother is reassured through knowing whom and how she can call for assistance and what she can expect in the way of supplies and services. If the woman's usual daily routine before admission differs from the routine of the facility, the nurse works with the woman to develop a mutually acceptable routine.

Infant abduction from hospitals in the United States has increased over the past few years. The mother should be taught to check the identity of any person who comes to remove the baby from her room. Hospital personnel usually wear picture identification badges. On some units all staff members wear matching scrubs or special badges. Other units use closed-circuit television, computer monitoring systems, or fingerprint identification pads. As a rule the baby is never carried in a staff member's arms between the mother's room and the nursery but rather is always wheeled in a bassinet, which also contains baby care supplies. Patients and nurses must work together to ensure the safety of newborns in the hospital environment.

Prevention of Infection

One important means of preventing infection is maintenance of a clean environment. Bed linens should be changed as needed. Disposable pads should be changed frequently. Women should wear slippers when walking about to avoid contaminating the linens when they return to bed. A sitz bath or heat lamp used by more than one patient must be scrubbed after each woman's use. Personnel must be conscientious about their hand hygiene to prevent cross infection. Standard Precautions must be practiced. Staff members with colds, coughs, or skin infections (e.g., a cold sore on the lips [herpes simplex virus type I]) must follow hospital protocol when in contact with postpartum patients. In many hospitals staff with open herpetic lesions, strep throat, conjunctivitis, upper respiratory infections, or diarrhea are encouraged to avoid contact with mothers and infants by staying home until the condition is no longer contagious.

Proper care of the episiotomy site and any perineal lacerations prevents infection in the genitourinary area and aids the healing process. Educating the woman to wipe from front to back (urethra to anus) after voiding or defecating is a simple first step. In many hospitals a squeeze bottle filled with warm water or an antiseptic solution is used after each voiding to cleanse the perineal area (Box 21-4). The woman should change her perineal pad from front to back each time she voids or defecates and wash her hands thoroughly before and after doing so.

Prevention of Excessive Bleeding

The most frequent cause of excessive bleeding after childbirth is uterine atony, or failure of the uterine muscle to contract firmly. The two most important interventions for preventing excessive bleeding are maintaining good uterine tone and preventing bladder distention. If uterine atony occurs, the relaxed uterus distends with blood and clots, blood vessels in the placental site are not clamped off, and excessive bleeding results.

Excessive blood loss after childbirth can also be caused by vaginal or vulvar hematomas, unrepaired lacerations of the vagina or cervix, and retained placental fragments.

NURSING ALERT A perineal pad saturated in 15 minutes or less or pooling of blood under the buttocks is an indication of excessive blood loss requiring immediate assessment, intervention, and notification of the primary health care provider.

Accurate visual estimation of blood loss is an important nursing responsibility. Blood loss is usually described subjectively as scant, light, moderate, or heavy (profuse). Fig. 21-2 shows examples of perineal pad saturation corresponding to each of these descriptions.

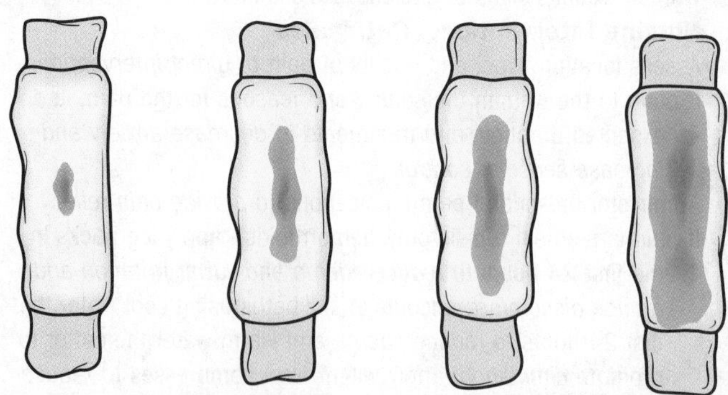

Fig. 21-2 Blood loss after birth is assessed by the extent of perineal pad saturation as *(from left to right)* scant (less than 2.5 cm); light (less than 10 cm); moderate (10 cm or more); or heavy (one pad saturated within 2 hours).

BOX 21-4 Interventions for Episiotomy, Lacerations, and Hemorrhoids

Explain both procedure and rationale before implementation.

Cleansing

Wash hands before and after cleansing perineum and changing pads.
Wash perineum with mild soap and warm water at least once daily.
Cleanse from symphysis pubis to anal area.
Apply peripad from front to back, protecting inner surface of pad from contamination.
Wrap soiled pad and place in covered waste container.
Change pad with each void or defecation or at least four times per day.
Assess amount and character of lochia with each pad change.

Ice Pack

Apply a covered ice pack to perineum from front to back:

- During first 2 hours to decrease edema formation and increase comfort
- After the first 2 hours following the birth to provide anesthetic effect

Squeeze Bottle

Demonstrate for and assist woman; explain rationale.
Fill bottle with tap water warmed to approximately 38° C (comfortably warm on the wrist).
Instruct woman to position nozzle between her legs so that squirts of water reach perineum as she sits on toilet seat. Explain that it will take whole bottle of water to cleanse perineum.
Remind her to blot dry with toilet paper or clean wipes.
Remind her to avoid contamination from anal area.
Apply clean pad.

Sitz Bath

Built-In Type

Prepare bath by thoroughly scrubbing with cleaning agent and rinsing.
Pad with towel before filling.
Fill one-third to one-half full with water of correct temperature 38° to 40.6° C. Some women prefer cool sitz baths. Ice is added to water to lower the temperature to the level comfortable for the woman.
Encourage woman to use at least twice a day for 20 minutes.
Place call bell within easy reach.
Teach woman to enter bath by tightening gluteal muscles and keeping them tightened and then relaxing them after she is in the bath.
Place dry towels within reach.
Ensure privacy.
Check woman in 15 minutes.

Disposable Type

Clamp tubing and fill bag with warm water.
Raise toilet seat, place bath in bowl with overflow opening directed toward back of toilet.
Place container above toilet bowl.
Attach tube into groove at front of bath.
Loosen tube clamp to regulate rate of flow; fill bath to about one-half full; continue as for built-in sitz bath.

Surgi-Gator

Assemble Surgi-Gator.
Instruct woman regarding use and rationale.
Follow package directions.
Instruct woman to sit on toilet with legs apart and put nozzle so tip is just past the perineum, adjusting placement as needed. Remind her to return her applicator to her bedside stand.

Topical Applications

Apply anesthetic cream or spray: use sparingly three to four times per day.
Offer witch hazel pads (Tucks) after voiding or defecating; woman pats perineum dry from front to back and then applies witch hazel pads.

Although postpartal blood loss may be estimated by observing the amount of staining on a perineal pad, it is difficult to judge the amount of lochial flow based only on observation of perineal pads. More objective estimates of blood loss include measuring serial hemoglobin or hematocrit values, weighing blood clots and items saturated with blood (1 g equals 1 ml), and establishing the milliliters it takes to saturate perineal pads being used.

Any estimation of lochial flow is inaccurate and incomplete without consideration of the time factor. The woman who saturates a perineal pad in 1 hour or less is bleeding much more heavily than the woman who saturates a perineal pad in 8 hours.

Nurses in general tend to overestimate rather than underestimate blood loss. Different brands of perineal pads vary in their saturation volume and soaking appearance. For example, blood placed on some brands tends to soak down into the pad, whereas on other brands it tends to spread outward. Nurses should determine saturation volume and soaking appearance for the perineal pad brands used in their institution to improve accuracy of blood loss estimation.

NURSING ALERT The nurse always checks under the mother's buttocks as well as on the perineal pad. Blood may flow between the buttocks onto the linens under the mother, although the amount on the perineal pad is slight; thus excessive bleeding goes undetected.

Blood pressure is not a reliable indicator of impending shock from early hemorrhage. More sensitive means of identifying shock are provided by respirations, pulse, skin condition, and urinary output. The frequent physical assessments performed during the fourth stage of labor are designed to provide prompt identification of excessive bleeding (see Emergency box).

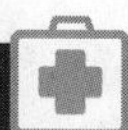

EMERGENCY

Hypovolemic Shock

Signs and Symptoms

Persistent significant bleeding—Perineal pad is soaked within 15 minutes; may not be accompanied by a change in vital signs or maternal color or behavior.

Woman states she feels weak, light-headed, "funny," "sick to my stomach," or "sees stars."

Woman begins to act anxious or exhibits air hunger.

Woman's skin turns ashen or grayish.

Skin feels cool and clammy.

Pulse rate increases.

Blood pressure declines.

Interventions

Notify primary health care provider.

If uterus is atonic, massage gently and expel clots to cause uterus to contract; compress uterus manually as needed, using two hands. Add oxytocic agent to IV drip as ordered.

Give oxygen by nonrebreather face mask or nasal prongs at 10 L/min.

Tilt the woman to her side or elevate the right hip; elevate her legs to at least a 30-degree angle.

Provide additional or maintain existing IV infusion of lactated Ringer's solution or normal saline solution to restore circulatory volume.

Administer blood or blood products as ordered.

Monitor vital signs.

Insert an indwelling urinary catheter to monitor perfusion of kidneys.

Administer emergency drugs as ordered.

Prepare for possible surgery or other emergency treatments or procedures.

Chart incident, medical and nursing interventions instituted, and results of treatments.

IV, Intravenous.

Maintenance of Uterine Tone

A major intervention to restore good tone is stimulation by gently massaging the uterine fundus until firm (Fig. 21-3). Fundal massage can cause a temporary increase in the amount of vaginal bleeding seen as pooled blood leaves the uterus. Clots can be expelled. The uterus may remain boggy even after massage and expulsion of clots.

Fundal massage is a very uncomfortable procedure. Understanding the causes and dangers of uterine atony and the purpose of fundal massage can help the woman cooperate. Teaching the woman to massage her own fundus enables her to maintain some control and decreases her anxiety.

Additional interventions likely to be used are administration of intravenous fluids and oxytocic medications (drugs that stimulate contraction of the uterine smooth muscle). See Medication Guide (p. 581) for information about common oxytocic medications.

Prevention of Bladder Distention

A full bladder causes the uterus to be displaced above the umbilicus and well to one side of the midline in the abdomen.

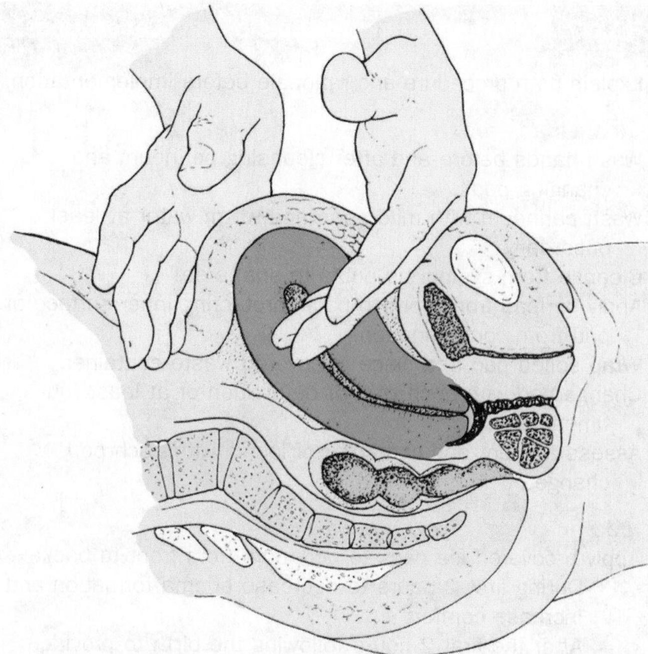

Fig. 21-3 Palpating fundus of uterus during fourth stage of labor. Note that upper hand is cupped over fundus; lower hand dips in above symphysis pubis and supports uterus while it is massaged gently.

It also prevents the uterus from contracting normally. Nursing interventions focus on helping the woman empty her bladder spontaneously as soon as possible. The first priority is to assist the woman to the bathroom or onto a bedpan if she is unable to ambulate. Having the woman listen to running water, placing her hands in warm water, or pouring water from a squeeze bottle over her perineum may stimulate voiding. Assisting the woman into the shower or sitz bath and encouraging her to void can be effective. Administering analgesics, if ordered, may be indicated because some women can anticipate pain and fear voiding. If these measures are unsuccessful, a sterile catheter can be inserted to drain the urine.

Promotion of Comfort

Most women experience some degree of discomfort during the postpartum period. Common causes of discomfort include afterbirth pains (afterpains), episiotomy or perineal lacerations, hemorrhoids, and breast engorgement. The woman's description of the type and severity of her pain is the best guide in choosing an appropriate intervention. To confirm the location and extent of discomfort, the nurse inspects and palpates areas of pain as appropriate for redness, swelling, discharge, and heat and observes for body tension, guarded movements, and facial tension. Blood pressure, pulse, and respirations may be elevated in response to acute pain. Diaphoresis may accompany severe pain. A lack of objective signs does not necessarily mean there is no pain because there may also be a cultural component to the expression of pain. Nursing interventions are intended to eliminate the pain sensation entirely or reduce it to a tolerable level that allows the woman to care for herself and her baby. Nurses may use both nonpharmacologic and pharmacologic interventions to promote comfort. Pain relief is enhanced by using more than one method or route.

Nonpharmacologic Interventions

Warmth, distraction, deep breathing, imagery, therapeutic touch, relaxation, and interaction with the infant may decrease the discomfort associated with afterbirth pains. Simple interventions that can decrease the discomfort associated with an episiotomy or perineal lacerations include encouraging the woman to lie on her side whenever possible and use a pillow when sitting. Other interventions include application of an ice pack; topical application (if ordered); dry heat; cleansing with a squeeze bottle; and a cleansing shower, tub bath, or sitz bath. Many of these interventions, especially ice packs, sitz baths, and topical applications (such as witch hazel pads), are also effective for hemorrhoids. Box 21-4 gives more specific information about these interventions.

The discomfort associated with engorged breasts may be lessened by applying ice, heat, or cold cabbage leaves to the breasts and wearing a well-fitted support bra. Decisions about specific interventions for relieving engorgement are based on whether the woman chooses breastfeeding or bottle-feeding (see Chapter 26).

Pharmacologic Interventions

Most health care providers routinely order a variety of analgesics to be administered as needed. These include both opioid (narcotic) and nonopioid (nonnarcotic) (e.g., nonsteroidal antiinflammatory drugs [NSAIDs]) choices, with their dosage and time frequency ranges. Topical application of antiseptic or anesthetic ointments or sprays is a common pharmacologic intervention for perineal pain. Patient-controlled analgesia pumps and epidural analgesia are technologies commonly used to provide pain relief after cesarean birth.

NURSING ALERT The nurse should carefully monitor all women receiving opioids because respiratory depression and decreased intestinal motility are side effects.

Many women want to participate in decisions about analgesia. However, severe pain may interfere with active participation in choosing pain relief measures. If an analgesic is to be given, the nurse must make a clinical judgment of the type, dosage, and frequency from the medications ordered. The woman is informed of the prescribed analgesic and its common side effects; this teaching is documented.

Breastfeeding mothers often have concerns about the effects of an analgesic on the infant. Although nearly all medications present in maternal circulation are also found in breast milk, many analgesics commonly used during the postpartum period are considered relatively safe for breastfeeding mothers. Often the timing of medications can be adjusted to minimize infant exposure. A mother may be given pain medication immediately after breastfeeding so that the interval between medication administration and the next nursing period is as long as possible. The decision to administer medications of any type to a breastfeeding mother must always be made by carefully weighing the woman's need against actual or potential risks to the infant.

If acceptable pain relief has not been obtained in 1 hour and there has been no change in the initial assessment, the nurse can contact the primary care provider for additional pain relief orders or further directions. Unrelieved pain results in fatigue, anxiety, and a worsening perception of the pain. It can also indicate the presence of a previously unidentified or untreated problem.

Promotion of Rest

The excitement and exhilaration experienced after the birth of the infant can make rest difficult. The new mother who is often anxious about her ability to care for her infant or is uncomfortable may also have difficulty sleeping. The demands of the infant, the hospital environment and routines, and the frequent presence of visitors contribute to alterations in her sleep pattern.

Fatigue is common in the postpartum period (Troy, 2003; Groër et al, 2005) and involves both physiologic components associated with long labors, cesarean birth, anemia, and breastfeeding; psychologic components related to depression and anxiety; and neuroendocrine and immune components. It is associated with symptoms of infection, postpartum stress, and depression. Lower serum prolactin levels are associated with depression and fatigue (Groër et al, 2005). Infant behavior can contribute to fatigue, particularly for mothers of more difficult infants. Conversely maternal fatigue can affect infant well-being. There can be an association with milk prolactin and melatonin and stress and fatigue in mothers who breastfeed. Prolactin and melatonin can be transferred to the infant. It is unknown what effect this might have on the infant (Groër et al, 2005).

CRITICAL THINKING EXERCISE

Fatigue and Rest After Childbirth

Patricia gave birth to her third baby; she has two children at home, ages 3 years and 18 months. Her husband travels frequently with his job. She is breastfeeding the baby without difficulty but is concerned about how she will care for all three of her children, stating "I remember how tired I was after my last baby. I'm not sure I can manage with three children since my husband is gone so much. Do you have any suggestions to help me?"

1. Evidence—Is there sufficient evidence to draw conclusions about whether support would be helpful for Patricia?
2. Assumptions—What assumptions can be made about the following factors?
    a. The relation of breastfeeding and fatigue
    b. Support in the postpartum period
    c. The role of sleep and rest in relation to fatigue and depression
    d. Spacing of pregnancies and fatigue
3. What implications and priorities for nursing care can be drawn at this time?
4. Does the evidence objectively support your conclusion?
5. Are there alternative perspectives to your conclusion?

evolve Case Study–Fourth Trimester

Interventions must be planned to meet the woman's individual needs for sleep and rest. Backrubs, other comfort measures, and medication for sleep for the first few nights may be necessary. The side-lying position for breastfeeding minimizes fatigue in nursing mothers (Troy, 2003). Support and encouragement in mothering behaviors help reduce anxiety. Hospital and nursing routines can be adjusted to meet individual needs. In addition, the nurse can help the family limit visitors and provide a comfortable chair or bed for the partner. Because milk contains high levels of melatonin (which induces sleep) at night and is not detectable during the day, fatigued mothers, who pump their milk might use morning milk to feed in the morning and evening milk to feed in the evening (Arendt, 2005; Groër et al, 2005).

Promotion of Ambulation

Early ambulation is successful in reducing the incidence of thromboembolism and promoting the woman's more rapid recovery of strength. Free movement is encouraged once anesthesia wears off unless an analgesic has been administered. After the initial recovery period is over, the mother is encouraged to ambulate frequently.

The rapid decrease in intraabdominal pressure after birth results in a dilation of blood vessels supplying the intestines (splanchnic engorgement) and causes blood to pool in the viscera. This condition contributes to the development of orthostatic hypotension and can occur when the woman who has recently given birth sits or stands, first ambulates, or takes a warm shower or sitz bath. The nurse must consider the baseline blood pressure; amount of blood loss; and type, amount, and timing of analgesic or anesthetic medications administered when assisting a woman to ambulate.

NURSING ALERT Having a hospital staff or family member present the first time the woman gets out of bed after birth is wise because she can feel weak, dizzy, faint, or light-headed.

Prevention of clot formation is important. Women who must remain in bed after giving birth are at increased risk for the development of a thrombus. They may have antiembolic stockings (TED hose) and/or a sequential compression device (SCD boots) ordered prophylactically. If a woman remains in bed longer than 8 hours (e.g., for postpartum magnesium sulfate therapy for preeclampsia), exercise to promote circulation in the legs is indicated using the following routine:

- Alternate flexion and extension of feet.
- Rotate ankles in circular motion.
- Alternate flexion and extension of legs.
- Press back of knee to bed surface; relax.

If the woman is susceptible to thromboembolism, she is encouraged to walk about actively and is discouraged from sitting immobile in a chair.

Women with varicosities are advised to wear support hose. If a thrombus is suspected, as evidenced by a positive Homans' sign (complaint of pain in calf muscles when the foot is dorsiflexed) or warmth, redness, or tenderness in the suspected leg, the primary health care provider should be notified immediately; meanwhile the woman should be confined to bed with the affected limb elevated on pillows.

Promotion of Exercise

Most women who have just given birth are interested in regaining their nonpregnant figures. Postpartum exercise can begin soon after birth, although the woman should be encouraged to start with simple exercises and gradually progress to more strenuous ones. Fig. 21-4 illustrates a number of exercises appropriate for the new mother. Abdominal exercises are postponed until about 4 weeks after cesarean birth.

Kegel exercises to strengthen muscle tone are extremely important, particularly after vaginal birth. Kegel exercises help women regain the muscle tone that is often lost as pelvic tissues are stretched and torn during pregnancy and birth. Women who maintain muscle strength may benefit years later by maintaining urinary continence.

It is essential that women learn to perform Kegel exercises correctly (see Patient Teaching box on p. 53). Approximately one fourth of all women who learn Kegel exercises do them incorrectly and may increase their risk of incontinence. This may occur when women inadvertently bear down on the pelvic floor muscles, thrusting the perineum outward. The woman's technique can be assessed during the pelvic examination at her checkup by inserting two fingers intravaginally and checking whether the pelvic floor muscles correctly contract and relax.

Promotion of Nutrition

During the hospital stay most women display a good appetite and eat well; nutritious snacks are usually welcomed. Women may request that family members bring to the hospital favorite or culturally appropriate foods (Fig. 21-5). Cultural dietary preferences must be respected. This interest in food presents an ideal opportunity for nutrition counseling on dietary needs after pregnancy such as for breastfeeding, preventing constipation and anemia, promoting weight loss, and promoting healing and well-being (see Chapter 12). Prenatal vitamins and iron supplements are often continued until 6 weeks after birth or until the ordered supply has been used.

Promotion of Normal Bladder Function

After giving birth the mother should void spontaneously within 6 to 8 hours. The first several voidings should be measured to document adequate emptying of the bladder. A volume of at least 150 ml is expected for each voiding. Some women experience difficulty in emptying the bladder, possibly as a result of diminished bladder tone, edema from trauma, or fear of discomfort. Nursing interventions for inability to void and bladder distention are discussed on p. 542.

Promotion of Normal Bowel Function

Nursing interventions to promote normal bowel elimination include educating the woman about measures to avoid constipation. These interventions include ensuring adequate roughage and fluid intake and promoting exercise. Alerting the woman to side effects of medications such as opioid analgesics (decreased gastrointestinal tract motility) may encourage her to implement measures to reduce the risk of constipation. Stool softeners or laxatives may be necessary during the early postpartum period. With early discharge a new mother may be home before having a bowel movement.

Some mothers experience gas pains. Antigas medications may be ordered. Ambulation or rocking in a rocking chair may stimulate passage of flatus and relief of discomfort.

evolve Critical Thinking Exercise—Postpartum Complications

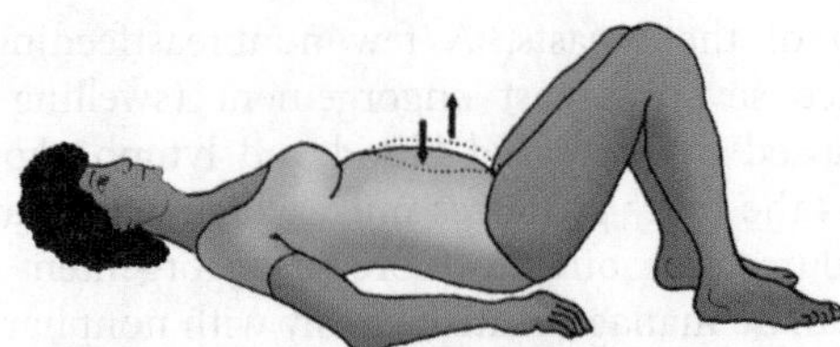

Abdominal Breathing. Lie on back with knees bent. Inhale deeply through nose. Keep ribs stationary and allow abdomen to expand upward. Exhale slowly but forcefully while contracting the abdominal muscles; hold for 3 to 5 seconds while exhaling. Relax.

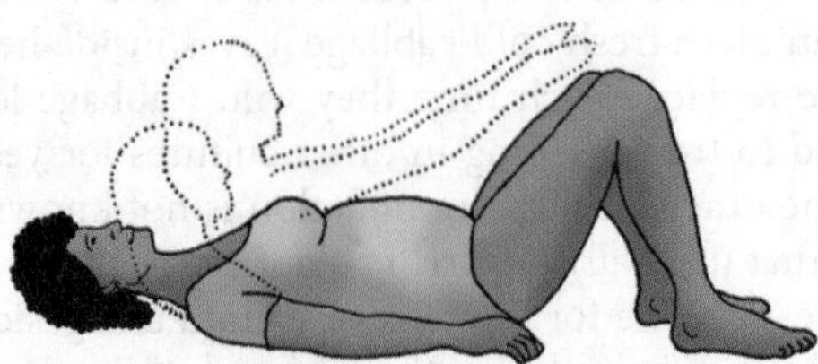

Reach for the Knees. Lie on back with knees bent. While inhaling, deeply lower chin onto chest. While exhaling, raise head and shoulders slowly and smoothly and reach for knees with arms outstretched. The body should rise only as far as the back will naturally bend while waist remains on floor or bed (about 6 to 8 inches). Slowly and smoothly lower head and shoulders back to starting position. Relax.

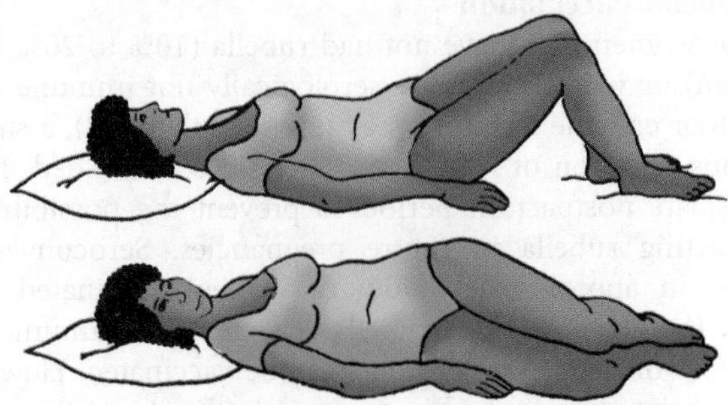

Double Knee Roll. Lie on back with knees bent. Keeping shoulders flat and feet stationary, slowly and smoothly roll knees over to the left to touch floor or bed. Maintaining a smooth motion, roll knees back over to the right until they touch floor or bed. Return to starting position and relax.

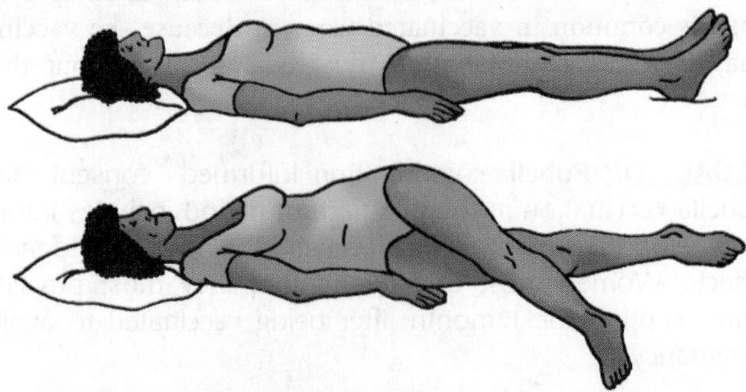

Leg Roll. Lie on back with legs straight. Keeping shoulders flat and legs straight, slowly and smoothly lift left leg and roll it over to touch the right side of floor or bed and return to starting position. Repeat, rolling right leg over to touch left side of floor or bed. Relax.

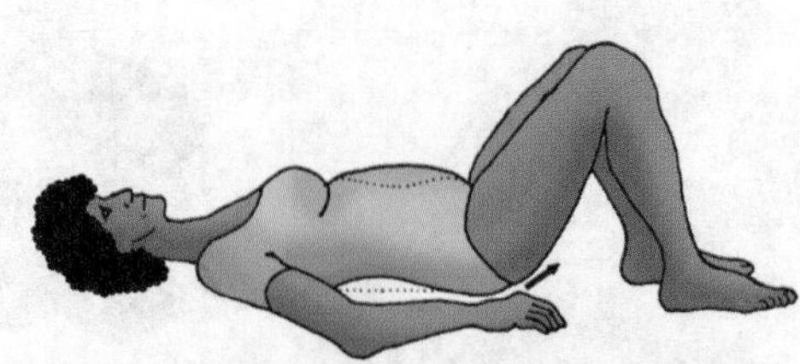

Combined Abdominal Breathing and Supine Pelvic Tilt (Pelvic Rock). Lie on back with knees bent. While inhaling deeply, roll pelvis back by flattening lower back on floor or bed. Exhale slowly but forcefully while contracting abdominal muscles and tightening buttocks. Hold for 3 to 5 seconds while exhaling. Relax.

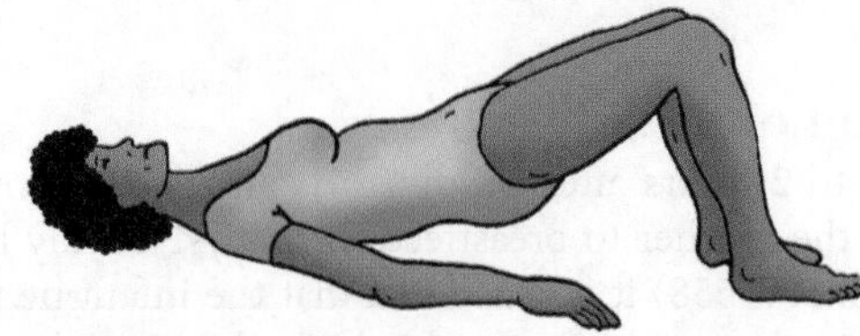

Buttocks Lift. Lie on back with arms at sides, knees bent, and feet flat. Slowly raise buttocks and arch back. Return slowly to starting position.

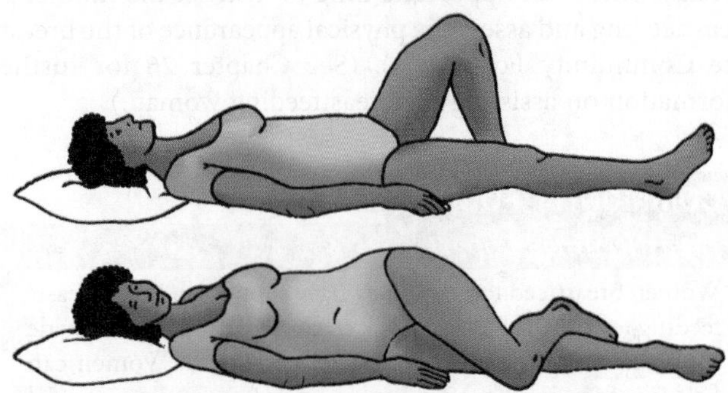

Single Knee Roll. Lie on back with right leg straight and left leg bent at the knee. Keeping shoulders flat, slowly and smoothly roll left knee over to the right to touch floor or bed and then back to starting position. Reverse position of legs. Roll right knee over to the left to touch floor or bed and return to starting position. Relax.

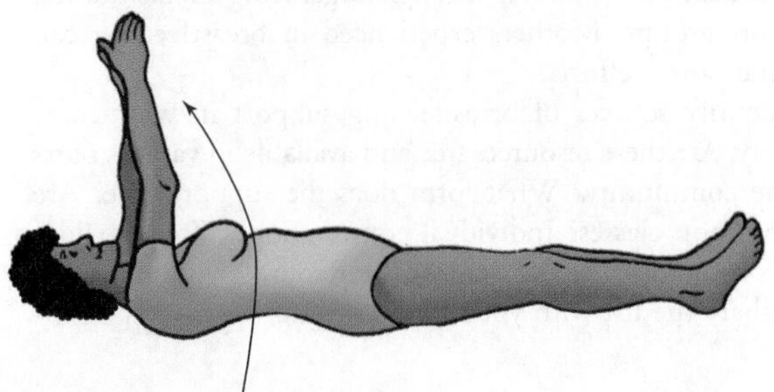

Arm Raises. Lie on back with arms extended at 90-degree angle from body. Raise arms so they are perpendicular and hands touch. Lower slowly.

Fig. 21-4 Postpartum exercise should begin as soon as possible. The woman should start with simple exercises and gradually progress to more strenuous ones.

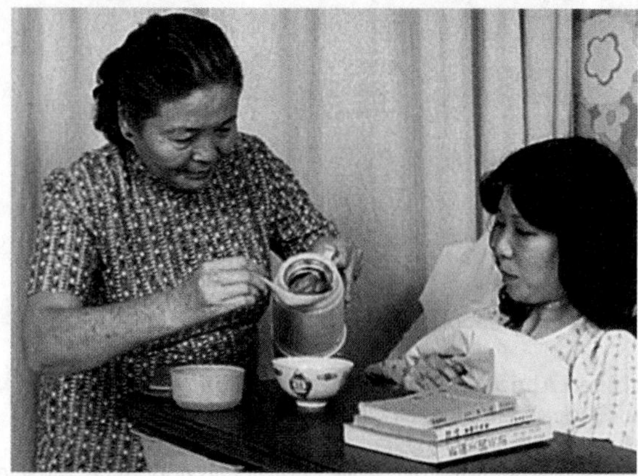

Fig. 21-5 Special foods are considered essential for recovery in the Asian culture. *(Courtesy Concept Media, Irvine, CA.)*

Promotion of Breastfeeding

The first 1 to 2 hours after childbirth is an excellent time to encourage the mother to breastfeed. In Baby-Friendly hospitals (see pp. 557-558) it is mandated that the infant be put to breast within the first hour after birth. At this time the infant is in an alert state and ready to nurse. Breastfeeding aids in the contraction of the uterus and prevention of maternal hemorrhage. This is an opportune time to instruct the mother in breastfeeding and assess the physical appearance of the breasts (see Community Focus box). (See Chapter 26 for further information on assisting the breastfeeding woman.)

COMMUNITY FOCUS

Breastfeeding Support

Women breastfeed longer if they have support in their breastfeeding efforts. Nurses and lactation consultants provide support during inpatient stays after childbirth. Women can find support in the community in various groups. Social support interventions that include peer support are successful in increasing the duration of exclusive breastfeeding and satisfaction with breastfeeding. In their discharge planning nurses can refer breastfeeding mothers to community groups for support. Community and home health nurses can facilitate breastfeeding efforts through organizing or facilitating support groups. Mothers experienced in breastfeeding can facilitate these efforts.

Identify sources of breastfeeding support in your community. Are these resources free and available in various parts of the community? What form does the support take? Are there group classes? Individual consultation? Who provides the consultation? Make a list of the resources you identified and share the list with your clinical group.

Suppression of Lactation

Suppression of lactation is necessary when the woman has decided not to breastfeed or in the case of neonatal death. Wearing a well-fitted support bra or breast binder continuously for at least the first 72 hours after giving birth is important. Women should avoid breast stimulation, including running warm water over the breasts, newborn suckling, or pumping of the breasts. A few nonbreastfeeding mothers experience severe breast engorgement (swelling of breast tissue caused by increased blood and lymph supply to the breasts as the body produces milk, which occurs at about 72 to 96 hours after birth). If breast engorgement occurs, it usually can be managed satisfactorily with nonpharmacologic interventions.

Ice packs to the breasts are helpful in decreasing the discomfort associated with engorgement. The woman should use a 15-minutes-on, 45-minutes-off schedule (to prevent the rebound swelling that can occur if ice is used continuously), or she can place fresh cold cabbage leaves inside her bra. The leaves are replaced each time they wilt. Cabbage leaves have been used to treat swelling in other cultures for years (Mass, 2004). The exact mechanism of action is not known, but it is thought that naturally occurring plant estrogens or salicylates may be responsible for the effects. A mild analgesic may also be necessary to help the mother through this uncomfortable time. Medications that were once prescribed for lactation suppression (estrogen, estrogen and testosterone, and bromocriptine) are no longer used.

Health Promotion for Planning Future Pregnancies and Children

Rubella Vaccination

For women who have not had rubella (10% to 20% of all women) or women who are serologically not immune (titer of 1:8 or enzyme immunoassay level less than 0.8), a subcutaneous injection of rubella vaccine is recommended in the immediate postpartum period to prevent the possibility of contracting rubella in future pregnancies. Seroconversion occurs in approximately 90% of women vaccinated after birth. The live attenuated rubella virus is not communicable; therefore breastfeeding mothers can be vaccinated. However, because the virus is shed in urine and other body fluids, the vaccine should not be given if the mother or other household members are immunocompromised. Rubella vaccine is made from duck eggs; thus women who have allergies to these eggs may develop a hypersensitivity reaction to the vaccine, for which they will need adrenaline. A transient arthralgia or rash is common in vaccinated women. Because the vaccine may be teratogenic, women must be informed about this fact.

LEGAL TIP **Rubella Vaccination** Informed consent for rubella vaccination in the postpartum period includes information about possible side effects and the risk of teratogenic effects. Women must understand that they must practice contraception for 1 month after being vaccinated to avoid pregnancy.

Prevention of Rh Isoimmunization

Injection of Rh immune globulin (a solution of γ-globulin that contains Rh antibodies) within 72 hours after birth prevents sensitization in the Rh-negative woman who has had a fetomaternal transfusion of Rh-positive fetal red blood cells (RBCs) (see Medication Guide). Rh immune globulin promotes lysis of fetal Rh-positive blood cells before the mother forms her own antibodies against them.

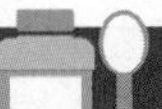

MEDICATION GUIDE

Rh Immune Globulin, RhoGAM, Gamulin Rh, HypRho-D, Rhophylac

Action

Suppression of immune response in nonsensitized women with Rh-negative blood who receive Rh-positive blood cells because of fetomaternal hemorrhage, transfusion, or accident

Indications

Routine antepartum prevention at 26 to 28 weeks of gestation in women with Rh-negative blood; suppression of antibody formation after birth, miscarriage/pregnancy termination, abdominal trauma, ectopic pregnancy, amniocentesis, version, or chorionic villi sampling

Dosage/Route

Standard dose: 1 vial (300 mcg) IM in deltoid or gluteal muscle; microdose: 1 vial (50 mcg) IM in deltoid muscle; Rho(D) immune globulin (Rhophylac) can be given IM or IV (available in prefilled syringes)

Adverse Effects

Myalgia, lethargy, localized tenderness and stiffness at injection site, mild and transient fever, malaise, headache, rarely nausea, vomiting, hypotension, tachycardia, and allergic response

Nursing Considerations

Give standard dose to mother at 28 weeks of gestation as prophylaxis or after an incident or exposure risk that occurs after 28 weeks of gestation (e.g., amniocentesis, second-trimester miscarriage or abortion, afterversion) and within 72 hours after birth if baby is Rh positive.

Give microdose for first-trimester miscarriage or abortion, ectopic pregnancy, chorionic villi sampling.

Verify that the woman is Rh negative and has not been sensitized, and if postpartum, that Coombs' test is negative, and that baby is Rh positive. Provide explanation to the woman about the procedure, including the purpose, possible side effects, and effect on future pregnancies. Have the woman sign a consent form if required by agency. Verify correct dosage and confirm lot number and woman's identity before giving injection (verify with another registered nurse or by other procedure per agency policy); document administration per agency policy. Observe patient for at least 20 minutes after administration for allergic response.

The medication is made from human plasma (a consideration if woman is a Jehovah's Witness). The risk of transmitting infectious agents, including viruses, cannot be completely eliminated.

IM, Intramuscularly; *IV,* intravenously.

NURSING ALERT After birth Rh immune globulin is administered to all Rh-negative, antibody (Coombs' test)–negative women who give birth to Rh-positive infants. Rh immune globulin is administered to the mother intramuscularly (RhoGAM, Gamulin RH, HypRho-D, Rhophylac) or intravenously (Rhophylac). It should never be given to an infant.

The administration of 300 mcg (1 vial) of Rh immune globulin is usually sufficient to prevent maternal sensitization. However, if a large fetomaternal transfusion is suspected, the dosage needed should be determined by performing a Kleihauer-Betke test, which detects the amount of fetal blood in the maternal circulation. If more than 15 ml of fetal blood is present in maternal circulation, the dosage of Rh immune globulin must be increased.

A 1:1000 dilution of Rh immune globulin is crossmatched to the mother's RBCs to ensure compatibility. Because Rh immune globulin is usually considered a blood product, precautions similar to those used for transfusing blood are necessary when it is given. The identification number on the woman's hospital wristband should correspond to the identification number found on the laboratory slip. The nurse must also check to see that the lot number of the laboratory slip corresponds to the lot number on the vial. Finally, the expiration date on the vial should be checked to ensure that it is a usable product.

Rh immune globulin suppresses the immune response. Therefore the woman who receives both Rh immune globulin and rubella vaccine must be tested in 3 months to see if she has developed rubella immunity. If not, the woman will need another dose of rubella vaccine.

There is some disagreement about whether Rh immune globulin should be considered a blood product. Health care providers need to discuss the most current information about this issue with women whose religious beliefs conflict with having blood products administered to them (e.g., Jehovah Witnesses).

Nursing Care Management—Psychosocial Needs

Meeting the psychosocial needs of new mothers involves assessing the parents' reactions to the birth experience, their feelings about themselves, and their interactions with the new baby (Fig. 21-6) and other family members. Specific interventions are then planned to increase the parents' knowledge and self-confidence as they assume the care and responsibility of the new baby and integrate this new member into their existing family structure in a way that meets their cultural expectations (see Nursing Process box and Chapter 22).

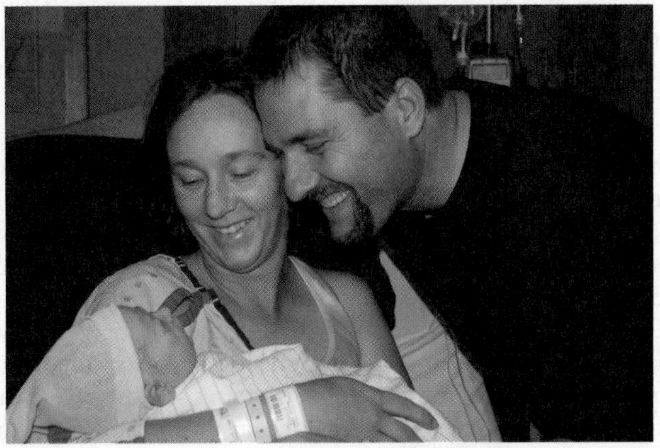

Fig. 21-6 Parents getting acquainted with their new son. *(Courtesy Julie and Darren Nelson, Loveland, CO.)*

evolve Spanish Guidelines—Postpartum Adjustment

NURSING PROCESS: PSYCHOSOCIAL NEEDS

Assessment

Assessment includes impact of birth experience, maternal self-image, and parent-infant interactions.

Nursing Diagnoses

Nursing diagnoses related to psychosocial issues that are often established for the postpartum patient include the following:

Interrupted family processes related to
- unexpected birth of twins

Impaired verbal communication related to
- patient's hearing impairment
- nurse's language not the same as patient's

Impaired parenting related to
- long, difficult labor
- unmet expectations of labor and birth

Anxiety related to
- newness of parenting role, sibling rivalry, or response of grandparent

Risk for situational low self-esteem related to
- body image changes

Planning

The nursing plan of care includes the family and observations of relationships among family members.

Examples of common expected outcomes include that the woman (family) will do the following:

- Identify measures that promote a healthy personal adjustment in the postpartum period
- Maintain healthy family functioning based on cultural norms and personal expectations

Interventions

Promote parenting skills.

Provide encouragement and support.

See text discussion for additional interventions.

Evaluation

The nurse can be reasonably assured that care was effective if expected outcomes of care for psychosocial needs have been met.

Impact of the Birth Experience

Many women indicate a need to examine the birth process itself and look at their own intrapartal behavior in retrospect. Their partners may express similar desires. If their birth experience was quite different from that planned (e.g., induction, epidural anesthesia, cesarean birth), both partners may need to mourn the loss of their expectations before they can adjust to the reality of their actual birth experience. Inviting them to review the events and describe how they feel helps the nurse assess how well they understand what happened and how well they have been able to put their childbirth experience into perspective.

Maternal Self-Image

An important assessment concerns the woman's self-concept, body image, and sexuality. How this new mother feels about herself and her body during the puerperium may affect her behavior and adaptation to parenting. The woman's self-concept and body image may also affect her sexuality. Overweight women can experience symptoms of depression and anxiety for several months postpartum.

Feelings related to sexual adjustment after childbirth are often a cause of concern for new parents. Women who have recently given birth may be reluctant to resume sexual intercourse for fear of pain or worry that coitus could damage healing perineal tissue. Because many new parents are anxious for information but reluctant to bring up the subject, postpartum nurses should matter-of-factly include the topic of postpartum sexuality during their routine physical assessment. For example, while examining the episiotomy site the nurse can say, "I know you're sore right now, but it probably won't be long until you (or you and your partner) are ready to make love again. Do you have any questions about resuming sex?" This approach assures the woman and her partner that resuming sexual activity is a legitimate concern for new parents and indicates the nurse's willingness to answer questions and share information.

Adaptation to Parenthood and Parent-Infant Interactions

The psychosocial assessment includes evaluating adaptation to parenthood as evidenced by the mother's and father's reactions to and interactions with the new baby. Clues indicating successful adaptation begin to appear early in the postbirth period as parents react positively to the newborn infant and continue the process of establishing a relationship with their child.

Parents are adapting well to their new roles when they exhibit a realistic perception and acceptance of their newborn's needs and his or her limited abilities, immature social responses, and helplessness. Examples of positive parent-infant interactions include taking pleasure in the infant and the tasks done for and with him or her; understanding the infant's emotional states and providing comfort; and reading the infant's cues for new experiences and sensing his or her fatigue level (see Chapter 22).

Should these indicators be missing, the nurse must investigate further what is hindering the normal adaptation process. The nurse can ask several questions such as "Do you feel sad often?" or "Do you have concerns about being a good parent?" that will help to determine if the woman is experiencing the normal "baby blues" or if there is a more serious underlying condition (i.e., postpartum depression) *(www.depressionafterdelivery.com)* (Jesse & Graham, 2005). See Chapter 23 for further discussion of postpartum depression.

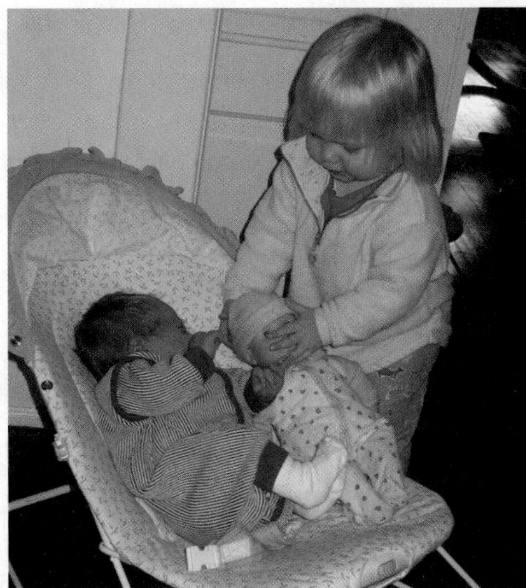

Fig. 21-7 Older sibling sharing her "baby" with brother. *(Courtesy Wendy and Marwood Larson-Harris, Roanoke, VA.)*

Family Structure and Functioning

A woman's adjustment to her role as mother is affected greatly by her relationships with her partner, her mother and other relatives, and any other children (Fig. 21-7). Nurses can help ease the new mother's return home by identifying possible conflicts among family members and helping the woman plan strategies for dealing with these problems before discharge. Such a conflict could arise when couples have very different ideas about parenting. Dealing with the stresses of sibling rivalry and unsolicited grandparent advice can also affect the woman's transition to motherhood. Only by asking about other nuclear and extended family members can the nurse discover potential problems in such relationships and help plan workable solutions for them.

Impact of Cultural Diversity

The final component of a complete psychosocial assessment is the woman's cultural beliefs and values. Much of a woman's behavior during the postpartum period is strongly influenced by her cultural background. Nurses are likely to come into contact with women from many different countries and cultures. All cultures have developed safe and satisfying methods of caring for new mothers and babies. Only by understanding and respecting the values and beliefs of each woman can the nurse design a plan of care to meet individual needs (see Cultural Awareness box).

Sometimes the findings of the psychosocial assessment indicate serious actual or potential problems that must be addressed. Box 21-5 lists several psychosocial needs that, at a minimum, warrant ongoing evaluation following hospital discharge. Women exhibiting these needs should be referred to appropriate community resources for assessment and management.

CULTURAL AWARENESS

A Clash of Cultures

A Vietnamese woman who had been in the United States for 4 years requested rooming-in facilities after childbirth. Instead of participating in the care of her infant, she refused to do so, remained in bed, wore a woolen cap, and appeared distressed and angry. The staff were puzzled and upset by her behavior. One nurse decided to put into effect her newly learned concepts concerning cross-cultural nursing. She began by praising the woman's ability to speak English and, after eliciting a smile, remarked, "Every country has developed good ways to look after mothers and babies. Would you tell me about the care in Vietnam?" There was an immediate response. The woman explained that in her country women remained in bed for at least 10 days after birth and the biggest danger to their health was getting a cold. The baby was kept in the room with his mother, but either a grandmother or nurse took complete charge of the care.

With this information the nurse was able to modify her plan of care to make it culturally relevant and therefore more satisfying for the woman.

BOX 21-5 Signs of Potential Psychosocial Complications

- Unable or unwilling to discuss labor and birth experience
- Refers to self as ugly and useless
- Excessively preoccupied with self (body image)
- Markedly depressed
- Lacks a support system
- Partner and/or other family members react negatively to baby
- Refuses to interact with or care for baby (e.g., does not name baby, does not want to hold or feed baby, is upset by vomiting and wet or dirty diapers) (cultural appropriateness of actions must be considered)
- Expresses disappointment over baby's sex
- Sees baby as messy or unattractive
- Baby reminds mother of family member or friend she doesn't like

✱ Nursing Care Management

The nurse functions in the roles of teacher, encourager, and supporter rather than doer while implementing the psychosocial plan of care for a postpartum woman. Implementation of the psychosocial care plan involves carrying out specific activities to achieve the expected outcome of care planned for each individual woman. Topics that should be included in the psychosocial plan of care include promotion of parenting skills and family member adjustment to the newborn infant (see Chapter 22).

Cultural issues must also be considered when planning care. Many traditional health beliefs and practices exist among the different cultures within the North American population. Traditional health practices that are used to maintain health or avoid illnesses deal with the whole person (body, mind, and spirit) and tend to be culturally based.

Women from various cultures may view health as a balance between opposing forces (e.g., cold vs. hot, yin vs. yang), being in harmony with nature, or just "feeling good." Traditional practices may include the observance of certain dietary restrictions, wearing certain clothing, or taboos for balancing the body; participation in certain activities such as sports and art for maintaining mental health; and use of silence, prayer, or meditation for developing spiritually. Some practices (e.g., using religious objects or eating garlic) are used to protect oneself from illness and may involve avoiding people who are believed to create hexes and spells or who have an "evil eye." Restoration of health may involve a person taking folk medicines (e.g., herbs, animal substances) or using a traditional healer.

Childbirth occurs within this sociocultural context. Rest, seclusion, dietary restraints, and ceremonies honoring the mother are all common traditional practices that are followed for the promotion of the health and well-being of the mother and baby.

Several common traditional health practices are used, and various beliefs are practiced during the postpartum period. For example, in Southeast Asia pregnancy is considered to be a "hot" state, and childbirth results in a sudden loss of this state. Therefore balance needs to be restored by increasing the return of the hot state, which is present physically or symbolically in hot food, hot water, and warm air.

Another common belief is that the mother and baby remain in a weak and vulnerable state for a period of several weeks following birth. During this time the mother may remain in a passive role, take no baths or showers, and stay in bed to prevent cold air from entering her body.

Women who have immigrated to the United States or other Western nations without their extended families may not have much help at home, making it difficult for them to observe these activity restrictions. Box 21-6 lists some common cultural beliefs about the postpartum period and family planning.

It is important that nurses consider all cultural aspects when planning care and not use their own cultural beliefs as the framework for that care. Although the beliefs and behaviors of other cultures may seem different or strange, they should be encouraged as long as the mother wants to conform to them and she and the baby have no ill effects. The nurse must determine whether a woman is using any folk medicine during the postpartum period because active ingredients in folk medicine can have adverse physiologic effects on the woman when ingested with prescribed medicines. Many young women who are first- or second-generation Americans follow their cultural traditions only when older family members are present or not at all.

BOX 21-6 Some Cultural Beliefs About the Postpartum Period and Family Planning

Postpartum Care

Chinese, Mexican, Korean, and *Southeast Asian women* may wish to eat only warm foods and drink hot drinks to replace blood loss and restore the balance of hot and cold in their bodies. These women may also wish to stay warm and avoid bathing, exercising, and hair washing for 7 to 30 days after childbirth. Self-management may not be a priority; care by family members is preferred. The woman has respect for elders and authority. These women may wear abdominal binders. They may prefer not to give their babies colostrum.

Haitian women may request to take the placenta home to bury or burn.

Muslim women follow strict religious laws on modesty and diet. A Muslim woman must keep her hair, body, arms to the wrist, and legs covered to the ankles at all times. She cannot be alone in the presence of a man other than her husband or a male relative. Observant Muslims do not eat pork or pork products and are obligated to eat meat slaughtered according to Islamic laws (halal meat). If halal meat is not available, kosher meat, seafood, or a vegetarian diet is usually accepted.

Family Planning

Birth control is government mandated in mainland *China.* Most *Chinese women* will have an intrauterine device inserted after the birth of their first child. Women do not want hormonal methods of contraception because they fear putting these medications in their bodies.

Saudi Arabian and *Hispanic women* will likely choose the rhythm method because most are Catholic.

(East) Indian men are encouraged to have voluntary sterilization by vasectomy.

Muslim couples may practice contraception by mutual consent as long as its use is not harmful to the woman. Acceptable contraceptive methods include foam and condoms, the diaphragm, and natural family planning.

Hmong women highly value and desire large families, which limits birth control practices.

Discharge Teaching

Self-Management and Signs of Complications

Discharge planning begins at the time of admission to the unit and should be reflected in the plan of care developed for each woman. Because of the limited time available for teaching, nurses must target their teaching on expressed needs of the woman. Giving the woman a list of topics and asking her to indicate her teaching needs will help the nurse maximize teaching efforts and can increase retention of information by the woman.

evolve Spanish Guidelines—Discharge Teaching

Just before the time of discharge, the nurse reviews the woman's chart to see that laboratory reports, medications, signatures, and other items are in order. Some hospitals use a checklist before the woman's discharge. The nurse verifies that medications, if ordered, have arrived on the unit; that any valuables kept secured during the woman's stay have been returned to her and that she has signed a receipt for them; and that the infant is ready to be discharged.

No medication that would make the mother sleepy should be administered if she is the one who will be holding the baby on the way out of the hospital. In most instances the woman is seated in a wheelchair and given the baby to hold. Some families leave unescorted and ambulatory, depending on hospital protocol. The woman's possessions are gathered and taken out with her and her family. The woman's and the baby's identification bands are carefully checked. The baby must be secured in a car seat for the drive home (see Fig. 25-18).

NURSING ALERT Prepackaged formula should not be given to mothers who are breastfeeding. Such "gifts" are associated with earlier cessation of breastfeeding.

Sexual Activity and Contraception

Many couples resume sexual activity before the traditional postpartum checkup 6 weeks after childbirth. Risk of hemorrhage and infection are minimal by approximately 2 weeks after birth. Couples may be anxious about the topic but uncomfortable and unwilling to bring it up. It is important that the nurse discuss the physical and psychologic effects that giving birth can have on sexual activity (see Home Care box). Contraceptive options should be discussed with women (and their partners if present) before discharge so that they can make informed decisions about fertility management before resuming sexual activity. Waiting to discuss contraception at the 6-week checkup may be too late. It is possible, particularly in women who bottle-feed, for ovulation to occur as soon as 1 month after birth. A woman who engages in unprotected sex risks becoming pregnant. Current contraceptive options are discussed in detail in Chapter 7. Women who are undecided about contraception at the time of discharge need information about using condoms with foam or creams until the first postpartum checkup.

Prescribed Medications

Women routinely continue to take their prenatal vitamins and iron during the postpartum period. It is especially important that women who are breastfeeding or discharged with a lower-than-normal hematocrit take these medications as prescribed. Women with vaginal lacerations (third or fourth degree) or extensive episiotomies are usually prescribed stool softeners to take at home. Pain relief medications (analgesics or NSAIDs) may be prescribed, especially for women who had cesarean birth. The nurse should make certain that the woman knows the route, dosage, frequency, and common side effects of all ordered medications.

Routine Mother and Baby Checkups

Women who have experienced uncomplicated vaginal births are still commonly scheduled for the traditional 6-week postpartum examination. Women who have had a cesarean birth are often seen in the health care provider's office or clinic within 2 weeks after hospital discharge. The date and time for the follow-up appointment should be included in the discharge instructions. If an appointment is not made before the woman leaves the hospital, she should be encouraged to call the health care provider's office or clinic to schedule one.

Parents who have not already done so need to make plans for newborn follow-up at the time of discharge. Most offices and clinics like to see newborns for an initial examination within the first week or by 2 weeks of age. If an appointment for a specific date and time was not made for the infant before leaving the hospital, the parents should be encouraged to call the office or clinic right away.

Dealing with Visitors

A newborn in the family or neighborhood draws visitors. The nurse can help the parents explore ways in which they can assert their needs in such situations. When family or friends ask what they can do to help, the family can respond with "Please bring us a casserole or a meal" or "Could you please pick up some items at the grocery store?" The couple can work out a signal for alerting the partner that the new mother is becoming tired or uncomfortable and needs to have the partner invite the visitors into another part of the house. Some new mothers have found that if they remain in their robes and do not appear ready for company, visitors stay for a shorter time. A "Please Do Not Disturb" sign on the front door may be useful when the mother is resting.

HOME CARE

Resumption of Sexual Intercourse

You can safely resume sexual intercourse by the second to fourth week after birth, when bleeding has stopped and the perineum is healed. For the first 6 weeks to 6 months the vagina does not lubricate well.

Your physiologic reactions to sexual stimulation for the first 3 months after birth will be slower and less intense. The strength of the orgasm is reduced.

A water-soluble gel, cocoa butter, or a contraceptive cream or jelly might be recommended for lubrication. If some vaginal tenderness is present, your partner can be instructed to insert one or more clean, lubricated fingers into the vagina and rotate them to help the vagina relax and identify possible areas of discomfort. A position in which you have control of the depth of the insertion of the penis also is useful. The side-by-side or female-on-top position may be more comfortable.

The presence of the baby influences postbirth lovemaking. Parents hear every sound made by the baby; conversely you may be concerned that the baby hears every sound you make. In either case any phase of the sexual response cycle may be interrupted by hearing the baby cry or move, leaving both of you frustrated and unsatisfied. In addition, the amount of psychologic energy expended by you in child care activities may lead to fatigue. Newborns require a great deal of attention and time.

Some women have reported feeling sexual stimulation and orgasms when breastfeeding their babies. Breastfeeding mothers often are interested in returning to sexual activity before non-breastfeeding mothers.

You should be instructed to correctly perform the Kegel exercises to strengthen your pubococcygeal muscle. This muscle is associated with bowel and bladder function and vaginal feeling during intercourse.

Follow-Up After Discharge

Home Visits

Home visits to new mothers and babies within a few days of discharge can help bridge the gap between hospital care and routine visits to health care providers. Nurses are able to assess the mother, infant, and home environment; answer questions and provide education; and make referrals to community resources if necessary. Home visits reduce the need for more expensive health care such as emergency department visits and rehospitalization. They can also help to improve the overall quality of care provided to infants and their parents. Ideally immediate follow-up contact and home visits are available 7 days a week.

Home nursing care may not be available, even if needed, because no agencies provide the service or insurance does not cover home care. If care is available, a referral form containing information about both mother and baby should be completed at hospital discharge and sent to the home care agency immediately.

The home visit is most commonly scheduled on the woman's second day home from the hospital, but it can be scheduled on any of the first 4 days at home, depending on the individual family's situation and needs. Additional visits are planned throughout the first week, as needed. The home visits can be extended beyond that time if the family's needs warrant it and if a home visit is the most appropriate option for carrying out the follow-up care required to meet the specific needs identified.

During the home visit the nurse conducts a systematic assessment of mother and newborn to determine physiologic adjustment, identify any existing complications, and answer any questions the mother has about herself or newborn care. Conducting the assessment in a separate room provides private time for the mother to ask questions on topics such as breast care, family planning, and constipation. The assessment also includes the mother's emotional adjustment and her knowledge of self- and infant care.

During the newborn assessment the nurse can demonstrate and explain normal newborn behavior and capabilities and encourage the mother and/or family to ask questions or express concerns they have. The home care nurse must verify if the newborn screen for phenylketonuria and other inborn errors of metabolism has been drawn. If the baby was discharged from the hospital before 24 hours of age, the specimen for the newborn screen can be done by the home care nurse, or the family will need to take the infant to the clinic or the physician's office.

Telephone Follow-Up

In addition to or instead of a home visit, many providers are implementing one or more postpartum telephone follow-up calls to their patients for assessment, health teaching, and identification of complications to effect timely intervention and referrals. Telephone follow-up can be among the services offered by the hospital, the private physician or clinic, or a private agency; it can be either a separate service or combined with other strategies for extending postpartum care. Telephonic nursing assessments are frequently used after a postpartum home care visit to reassess a woman's knowledge about the signs and symptoms of adequate intake by the breastfeeding infant or, after initiating home phototherapy, to assess the caregiver's knowledge regarding equipment complications.

Warm Lines

The warm line is another type of telephone link between the new family and concerned caregivers or experienced parent volunteers. A warm line is a helpline or consultation service, not a crisis intervention line. The warm line is appropriately used for dealing with less extreme concerns that can seem urgent at the time the call is placed but are not actual emergencies. Calls to warm lines commonly relate to infant feeding, prolonged crying, or sibling rivalry. Warm line services can extend beyond the fourth trimester. Families need to call when concerns arise and should be given telephone numbers for easy access to answers to their questions.

Support Groups

The woman adjusting to motherhood sometimes seeks a special group experience. Postpartum women who have met earlier in prenatal clinics or on the hospital unit can begin to associate for mutual support. Members of childbirth preparation classes who attend a postpartum reunion can decide to extend their relationship during the fourth trimester.

A postpartum support group enables mothers and fathers to share with and support each other as they adjust to parenting. Many new parents find it reassuring to discover that they are not alone in their feelings of confusion and uncertainty. An experienced parent can often impart concrete information to other members. Inexperienced parents can find themselves imitating the behavior of others in the group whom they perceive as particularly capable.

Referral to Community Resources

To develop an effective referral system, it is important that the nurse have a clear understanding of the needs of the woman and family and of the organization and community resources available for meeting those needs. Locating and compiling information about available community services contributes to the development of a referral system. It is important for the nurse to develop his or her own resource file of local and national services that are frequently useful to postpartum families.

Key Points

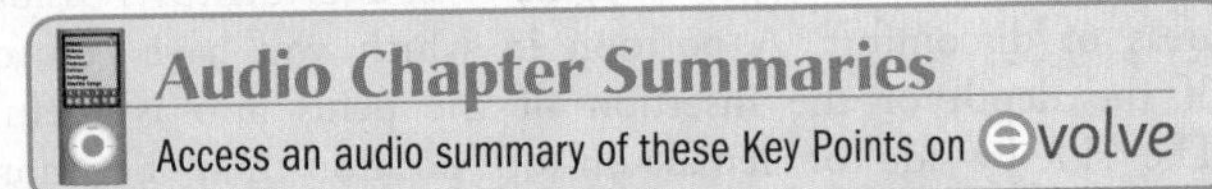
Audio Chapter Summaries
Access an audio summary of these Key Points on evolve

- Postpartum care is modeled on the concept of health.
- Cultural beliefs and practices affect the patient's response to the puerperium.
- The nursing care plan includes assessments to detect deviations from normal, comfort measures to relieve

discomfort or pain, and safety measures to prevent injury or infection.

- Teaching and counseling measures are designed to promote the woman's feelings of competence in self-management and baby care.
- Common nursing interventions in the postpartum period include evaluating and treating the boggy uterus and the full urinary bladder; providing for nonpharmacologic and pharmacologic relief of pain and discomfort associated with the episiotomy, lacerations, afterbirth pains, or breastfeeding; and instituting measures to promote or suppress lactation.
- Meeting the psychosocial needs of new mothers involves taking into consideration the composition and functioning of the entire family.
- Early postpartum discharge will continue as a result of consumer demand, medical necessity, discharge criteria for low risk childbirth, and cost-containment measures.
- Early discharge classes, telephone follow-up, home visits, warm lines, and support groups are effective means of facilitating physiologic and psychologic adjustments in the postpartum period.

References

American Academy of Pediatrics (AAP) Committee on Fetus and Newborn: Hospital stay for healthy term infants, *Pediatrics* 113(5):1434-1436, 2004.

Arendt J: Melatonin: characteristics, concerns, and prospect, *J Biol Rhythms* 20(4):291-303, 2005.

Groër M et al: Neuroendocrine and immune relationships in postpartum fatigue, *MCN Am J Matern Child Nurs* 30(2):133-138, 2005.

Jesse D, Graham M: Are you often sad and depressed? Brief measure to identify women at risk for depression in pregnancy, *MCN Am J Matern Child Nurs* 30(1):40-45, 2005.

Mass S: Breast pain: Engorgement, nipple pain and mastitis, *Clin Obstet Gynecol* 47(3):676-682, 2004.

Troy N: Is the significance of postpartum fatigue being overlooked in the lives of women? *MCN Am J Matern Child Nurs* 28(4):252-257, 2003.

Unit 5

22 Transition to Parenthood

Learning Objectives

On completion of this chapter the reader will be able to:

- Identify parental and infant behaviors that facilitate and those that inhibit parental attachment.
- Describe sensual responses that strengthen attachment.
- Examine the process of becoming a mother.
- Compare maternal and paternal adjustments to parenthood.
- Describe ways to facilitate parent-infant adjustment.
- Examine the effects of the following on parental response: parental age (i.e., adolescence and older than 35 years), social support, culture, socioeconomic conditions, personal aspirations, and sensory impairment.
- Describe sibling adjustment.
- Describe grandparent adaptation.

Electronic Resources

Additional information related to the content in Chapter 22 can be found on

evolve the Companion Website at

http://evolve.elsevier.com/Perry/maternal/

- NCLEX Review Questions
- Critical Thinking Exercise—Postpartum Home Care
- Nursing Care Plan—Home Care Follow-Up: Transition to Parenthood
- Nursing Care Plan—The Multiparous Woman and Family
- Skill—Swaddling

Becoming a parent creates a period of change and instability for all men and women, whether they made a conscious decision to have children or the pregnancy was unplanned. This holds true whether parenthood is biologic or adoptive and whether the parents are married husband-wife couples, cohabiting couples, single mothers, single fathers, lesbian couples with one woman as biologic mother, or gay male couples who adopt a child. Parenting can be described as a process of role transition that begins during pregnancy or while awaiting adoption. The transition is an ongoing process as the parents and infant develop and change.

A thorough understanding of the process parents go through during their transition to parenthood guides the nurse in helping family members adapt. The parenting process requires cognitive and affective skills and knowledge, as well as motor skills. The infant's well-being and development depend on these components. This chapter reviews the transition to parenthood, including the parenting process and the adjustment of parents, siblings, and grandparents.

Parental Attachment, Bonding, and Acquaintance

The process by which a parent comes to love and accept a child and a child comes to love and accept a parent is referred to as *attachment*. Using the terms *attachment* and *bonding*, Klaus and Kennell (1976) originally proposed that the period shortly after birth is important to mother-to-infant attachment. They defined the phenomenon of bonding as a sensitive period in the first minutes and hours after birth, when mothers and fathers must have close contact with their infants for optimal later development. In 1982 they revised their theory of parent-infant bonding, modifying their claim of the critical nature of immediate contact with the infant after birth. They acknowledged the adaptability of human parents, stating that it took longer than minutes or hours for parents to form an emotional relationship with their infants. The terms attachment and bonding continue to be used interchangeably.

Mothers become attached to their fetus. Factors that influence maternal-fetal attachment include family support, psychologic well-being, and having an ultrasound. Depression, substance abuse, and higher anxiety are associated with lower levels of attachment (Alhusen, 2008).

Attachment is developed and maintained by proximity and interaction with the infant; through it the parent becomes acquainted with the infant, identifies the infant as an individual, and claims the infant as a member of the family. Attachment is facilitated by positive feedback (i.e., social, verbal, and nonverbal responses, whether real or perceived, that indicate acceptance of one partner by the other). Attachment occurs through a mutually satisfying experience. A mother commented on her son's grasp reflex, "I put my finger in his hand, and he grabbed right on. It's just a reflex, I know, but it felt good anyway."

The concept of attachment has been extended to include mutuality (i.e., the infant's behaviors and characteristics call forth a corresponding set of maternal behaviors and characteristics). The infant displays signaling behaviors such as crying, smiling, and cooing that initiate the contact and bring the caregiver to the child. These behaviors are followed by executive behaviors such as rooting, grasping, and postural adjustments that maintain the contact. The caregiver is attracted to an alert, responsive, cuddly infant and repelled by an irritable, apparently disinterested infant. Attachment occurs more readily with the infant whose temperament, social capabilities, appearance, and sex fit the parent's expectations. If the child does not meet these expectations, resolution of the parent's disappointment can delay the attachment process. A list of infant behaviors affecting parental attachment that continues to be a classic comprehensive reference is presented in Table 22-1. A corresponding list of parental behaviors that affect infant attachment is presented in Table 22-2.

An important part of attachment is acquaintance. Parents use eye contact, touching, talking, and exploring to become acquainted with their infant during the immediate postpartum period. Adoptive parents undergo the same process when they first meet their new child. During this period families engage in the claiming process, which is the identification of the new baby. The child is first identified in terms of likeness to other family members, then in terms of differences, and finally in terms of uniqueness. The unique newcomer is thus incorporated into the family. Mother and father scrutinize their infant carefully and point out characteristics that the child shares with other family members and that are indicative of a relationship between them. The claiming process is revealed by maternal comments such as the following: "David held him close and said, 'He's the image of his father,' but I found one part like me—his toes are shaped like mine."

Conversely, some mothers react negatively. They "claim" the infant in terms of the discomfort or pain the baby causes.

Table 22-1 Infant Behaviors Affecting Parental Attachment

FACILITATING BEHAVIORS	INHIBITING BEHAVIORS
Visually alert; eye-to-eye contact; tracking or following of parent's face	Sleepy; eyes closed most of the time; gaze averted
Appealing facial appearance; randomness of body movements reflecting helplessness	Resemblance to person parent dislikes; hyperirritability or jerky body movements when touched
Smiles	Bland facial expression; infrequent smiles
Vocalization; crying only when hungry or wet	Crying for hours on end; colicky
Grasp reflex	Exaggerated motor reflex
Anticipatory approach behaviors for feedings; sucks well; feeds easily	Feeds poorly; regurgitates; vomits often
Enjoys being cuddled, held	Resists holding and cuddling by crying, stiffening body
Easily consolable	Inconsolable; unresponsive to parenting, caretaking tasks
Activity and regularity somewhat predictable	Unpredictable feeding and sleeping schedule
Attention span sufficient to focus on parents	Inability to attend to parent's face or offered stimulation
Differential crying, smiling, and vocalizing; recognizes and prefers parents	Shows no preference for parents over others
Approaches through locomotion	Unresponsive to parent's approaches
Clings to parent; puts arms around parent's neck	Seeks attention from any adult in room
Lifts arms to parents in greeting	Ignores parents

From Gerson E: *Infant behavior in the first year of life,* New York, 1973, Raven Press.

Table 22-2 Parental Behaviors Affecting Infant Attachment

FACILITATING BEHAVIORS	INHIBITING BEHAVIORS
Looks; gazes; takes in physical characteristics of infant; assumes en face position; eye contact	Turns away from infant; ignores infant's presence
Hovers; maintains proximity; directs attention to, points to infant	Avoids infant; does not seek proximity; refuses to hold infant when given opportunity
Identifies infant as unique individual	Identifies infant with someone parent dislikes; fails to discern any of infant's unique features
Claims infant as family member; names infant	Fails to place infant in family context or identify infant with family member; has difficulty naming
Touches; progresses from fingertip to fingers to palms to encompassing contact	Fails to move from fingertip touch to palmar contact and holding
Smiles at infant	Maintains bland countenance or frowns at infant
Talks to, coos, or sings to infant	Wakes infant when infant is sleeping; handles roughly; hurries feeding by moving nipple continuously
Expresses pride in infant	Expresses disappointment, displeasure in infant
Relates infant's behavior to familiar events	Does not incorporate infant into life
Assigns meaning to infant's actions and sensitively interprets infant's needs	Makes no effort to interpret infant's actions or needs
Views infant's behaviors and appearance in positive light	Views infant's behavior as exploiting, deliberately uncooperative; views appearance as distasteful, ugly

From Mercer R: Parent-infant attachment. In Sonstegard L, Kowalski K, Jennings B (editors): *Women's health.* Vol 2: *Childbearing,* New York, 1983, Grune & Stratton.

Table 22-3 Examples of Parent-Infant Attachment Interventions

INTERVENTION LABEL/DEFINITION	ACTIVITIES
Attachment Promotion	
Facilitation of development of parent-infant relationship	Provide opportunity for parent(s) to see, hold, and examine newborn immediately after birth. Encourage parent(s) to hold infant close to body. Help parent(s) participate in infant care. Provide rooming-in in hospitals.
Environmental Management: Attachment Process	
Manipulation of patient's surroundings to facilitate development of parent-infant relationship	Create environment that fosters privacy. Individualize daily routine to meet parent's needs. Permit father/significant other to sleep in room with mother. Develop policies that permit presence of significant others as much as desired.
Family Integrity Promotion: Childbearing Family	
Facilitation of growth of individuals or families who are adding infant to family unit	Prepare parent(s) for expected role changes involved in becoming a parent. Prepare parent(s) for responsibilities of parenthood. Monitor effects of newborn on family structure. Reinforce positive parenting behaviors.
Lactation Counseling	
Use of interactive helping process to assist in maintenance of successful breastfeeding	Correct misconceptions, misinformation, and inaccuracies about breastfeeding. Evaluate parent's understanding of infant's feeding cues (e.g., rooting, sucking, alertness). Determine frequency of feedings in relation to infant's needs. Demonstrate breast massage and discuss its advantages to increasing milk supply.
Parent Education: Infant	
Instruction on nurturing and physical care needed during first year of life	Determine parent(s) knowledge, readiness, and ability to learn about infant care. Provide anticipatory guidance about developmental changes during first year of life. Teach parent(s) skills to care for newborn. Demonstrate ways in which parent(s) can stimulate infant's development. Discuss infant's capabilities for interaction. Demonstrate quieting techniques.
Risk Identification: Childbearing Family	
Identification of individual or family likely to experience difficulties in parenting and assigning priorities to strategies to prevent parenting problems	Determine developmental stage of parent(s). Review prenatal history for factors that predispose patient to complications. Ascertain understanding of English or other language used in community. Monitor behavior that may indicate problem with attachment. Plan for risk-reduction activities in collaboration with individual or family.

Modified from Bulechek GM, Butcher, HK, Dochterman JM: *Nursing interventions classification (NIC)*, ed 5, St Louis, 2008, Mosby.

The mother interprets the infant's normal responses as being negative toward her and reacts to her child with dislike or indifference. She does not hold the child close or touch the child to be comforting; for example, "The nurse put the baby into Marie's arms. She promptly laid him across her knees and glanced up at the television. 'Stay still until I finish watching—you've been enough trouble already.' "

Nurses play an important role in facilitating parental attachment. They can enhance positive parent-infant contacts by heightening parental awareness of an infant's responses and ability to communicate. As the parent attempts to become competent and loving in that role, nurses can bolster his or her self-confidence and ego. Nurses are in prime positions to identify actual and potential problems and collaborate with other health care professionals who will provide care for the parents after discharge. Nursing interventions related to the promotion of parent-infant attachment are numerous and varied (Table 22-3).

Assessment of Attachment Behaviors

One of the most important areas of assessment is careful observation of behaviors thought to indicate the formation of emotional bonds between the newborn and family, especially the mother. Unlike physical assessment of the neonate, which has concrete guidelines to follow, assessment of parent-infant attachment requires much more skill in terms of observation and interviewing. Rooming-in of mother and infant and liberal visiting privileges for father, siblings, and grandparents facilitate recognition of behaviors that demonstrate positive or negative attachment. An excellent opportunity exists during feeding. Guidelines for assessment of attachment behaviors are presented in Box 22-1.

During pregnancy and often even before conception occurs, parents develop an image of the "ideal" or "fantasy" infant. At birth the fantasy infant becomes real. How closely the dream child resembles the real child influences the bonding process. Assessing such expectations during pregnancy and at the time of the infant's birth allows identification of discrepancies in the parents' view of the fantasy child and the real child.

The labor process significantly affects the immediate attachment of mothers to their newborn infants. Factors such as a long labor (Nystedt, Högberg, & Lundman, 2008), feeling tired or "drugged" after birth, and problems with breastfeeding can delay the development of initial positive feelings toward the

BOX 22-1 Assessing Attachment Behaviors

- When the infant is brought to the parents, do they reach out for the infant and call him or her by name? (Recognize that in some cultures parents may not name the infant in the early newborn period.)
- Do the parents speak about the infant in terms of identification? For example, do they surmise whom the infant looks like or identify what appears special about their infant in comparison with other infants?
- When parents are holding the infant, what kind of body contact is there? Do parents feel at ease in changing the infant's position? Are fingertips or whole hands used? Do they avoid touching parts of the body or do they investigate and scrutinize body parts?
- When the infant is awake, what kinds of stimulation do the parents provide? Do they talk to the infant, to each other, or to no one? How do they look at the infant? Do they use direct visual contact, avoid eye contact, or look at other people or objects?
- How comfortable do the parents appear in terms of caring for the infant? Do they express any concern regarding their ability or disgust for certain activities such as changing diapers?
- What type of affection do they demonstrate to the newborn (e.g., smiling, stroking, kissing, or rocking)?
- If the infant is fussy, what kinds of comforting techniques do the parents use (e.g., rocking, swaddling, talking, or stroking)?

newborn. Referral to groups such as La Leche League International *(www.llli.org)* or Postpartum Support International *(http://postpartum.net)* can be useful.

Parent-Infant Contact

Early Contact

Early close contact may facilitate the attachment process between parent and child. This does not mean that a delay will inhibit this process (humans are too resilient for that), but additional psychologic energy may be needed to achieve the same effect. No scientific evidence has demonstrated that immediate contact after birth is essential for the human parent-child relationship.

Parents who desire but are unable to have early contact with their newborn (e.g., the infant was transferred to the neonatal intensive care nursery) can be reassured that such contact is not essential for optimal parent-infant interactions. Otherwise adopted infants would not form the usual affectional ties with their parents. Nurses need to stress that the parent-infant relationship is a process that occurs over time.

Skin-to-Skin Contact

In a Cochrane review, early skin-to-skin contact (SSC) had a positive effect on breastfeeding, breastfeeding duration, maternal affectionate love/touch during observed breastfeeding, and maternal attachment behavior (Moore, Anderson, & Bergman, 2007). Better cardiorespiratory stability was observed in late-preterm infants with early SSC; no negative short- or long-term effects were observed (Moore, Anderson, & Bergman, 2007).

In a study examining the effects of kangaroo mother care (KMC) (SSC) on mother-baby attachment in low-birth-weight infants, Gathwaia, Singh, and Balhara (2008) found that attachment scores were higher in the KMC group and that mothers were more involved in the caretaking of the baby.

When fathers held their newborns skin-to-skin after a cesarean birth, the infants cried less, were calmer, and became drowsy sooner than babies cared for in a cot (Erlandsson et al, 2007).

Several and varied benefits of SSC have been observed. Nurses can facilitate this contact in most birth settings whether the infant is preterm or term, birthed vaginally or by cesarean, and with fathers and mothers.

evolve Skill–Swaddling

Extended Contact

Providing rooming-in facilities for the mother and her baby is common in family-centered care. The infant is transferred to the area from the transitional nursery (if the facility uses one) after showing satisfactory extrauterine adjustment. The father is encouraged to participate in the care of the infant, and siblings and grandparents are also encouraged to visit and become acquainted with the infant. Whether the method of family-centered care is rooming-in or a family birth unit, mothers and their partners are considered equal and integral parts of the developing family. Partners are encouraged to take as active a role as they wish (Fig. 22-1).

Extended contact with the infant should be available for all parents but especially for those at risk for parenting inadequacies such as adolescents and low-income women. Any activity that optimizes family-centered care is worthy of serious consideration by postpartum nurses. Baby-Friendly status for a hospital is one means to promote family-centered care.

The Baby Friendly Hospital Initiative, sponsored by the World Health Organization and the United Nations Children's Fund (UNICEF), was founded to encourage institutions to offer optimal levels of care for lactating mothers. When a hospital achieves *The Ten Steps to Successful Breastfeeding for Hospitals,* it is recognized as a Baby-Friendly hospital. The

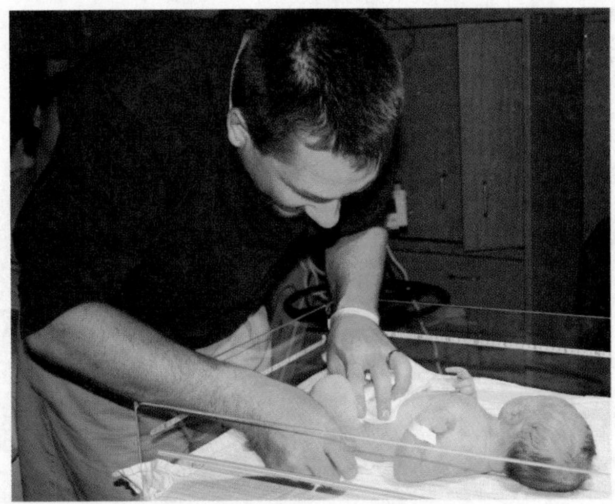

Fig. 22-1 Father changes diaper of his newborn son. *(Courtesy Darren Nelson, Loveland, CO.)*

steps include the following: having a written breastfeeding policy, training staff, informing pregnant women about the benefits of breastfeeding, initiating breastfeeding within 1 hour of birth, helping mothers maintain lactation even when separated from their infants, giving newborns only breast milk to drink, rooming-in 24 hours a day, breastfeeding on demand, avoiding pacifiers, and promoting the establishment of breastfeeding support groups and referring mothers to them.

Communication Between Parent and Infant

The parent-infant relationship is strengthened through the use of sensual responses and abilities by both partners in the interaction. The nurse should keep in mind that there may be cultural variations in these interactive behaviors.

The Senses

Touch

Touch, or the tactile sense, is used extensively by parents and other caregivers as a means of becoming acquainted with the newborn. Many mothers reach out for their infants as soon as they are born and the cord is cut. They lift them to their breasts, enfold them in their arms, and cradle them. Once the infant is close to them, they begin the exploration process with their fingertips, one of the most touch-sensitive areas of the body (Fig. 22-2). Within a short time the caregiver uses the palm to caress the baby's trunk and eventually enfolds the infant. Gentle stroking motions are used to soothe and quiet the infant. Patting or gently rubbing the infant's back is a comfort after feedings. Infants also pat the mother's breast as they nurse. Both seem to enjoy sharing each other's body warmth. There is a desire in parents to touch, pick up, and hold the infant. They comment on the softness of the baby's skin and are aware of milia and rashes. As parents become increasingly sensitive to the infant's like or dislike of different types of touch, they draw closer to their baby.

Variations in touching behaviors have been noted in mothers from different cultural groups. For example, minimal touching and cuddling is a traditional Southeast Asian practice thought to protect the infant from evil spirits. Because of traditions and spiritual beliefs, women in India and Bali have practiced infant massage since ancient times.

Eye Contact

Interest in having eye contact with the baby has been demonstrated repeatedly by parents. Some mothers remark that, once their babies have looked at them, they feel much closer to them. Parents spend much time getting their babies to open their eyes and look at them. In North American culture eye contact appears to cement the development of a trusting relationship and is an important factor in human relationships at all ages (Fig. 22-3). In other cultures eye-to-eye contact may be perceived differently (see Cultural Awareness box). For example, in Mexican culture sustained direct eye contact is considered to be rude, immodest, and dangerous for some. This danger may arise from the *mal ojo* (evil eye), resulting from excessive admiration. Women and children are thought to be more susceptible to the mal ojo (D'Avanzo, 2008).

As newborns become functionally able to sustain eye contact with their parents, time is spent in mutual gazing, often in the *en face* position. In this position the parent's face and the infant's face are approximately 8 inches apart and on the same plane.

Nursing and medical practices that encourage this interaction should be implemented. For example, immediately after birth the infant can be positioned on the mother's abdomen or breasts with the mother's and the infant's faces on the same plane so that they can easily make eye contact. Lights can be dimmed so that the infant's eyes will open. Instillation of prophylactic antibiotic ointment in the infant's eyes can be delayed until the infant and parents have had some time together in the first hour after birth.

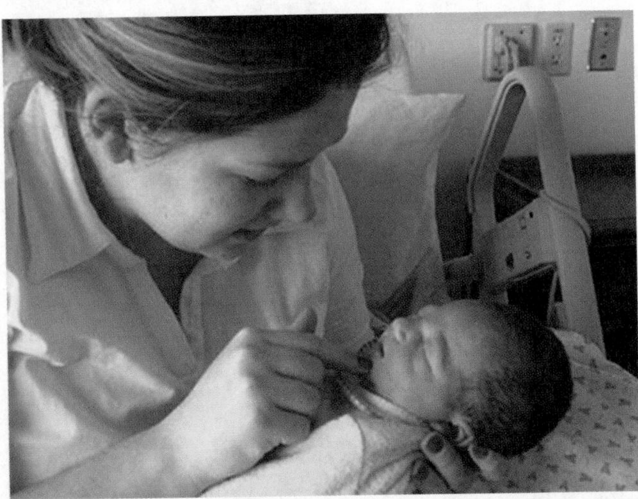

Fig. 22-2 Mother uses fingertip to explore infant. *(Courtesy Rebekah Vogel, Ft. Collins, CO.)*

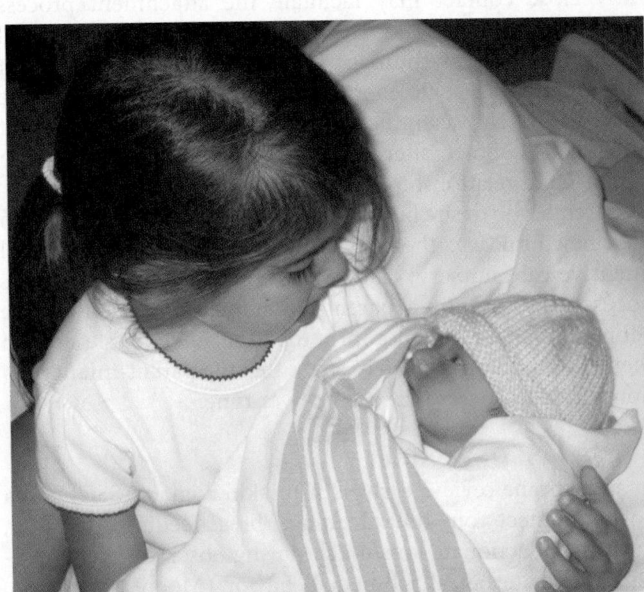

Fig. 22-3 Big sister in eye-to-eye contact with newborn brother. *(Courtesy Brian and Mayannyn Sallee, Las Vegas, NV.)*

CULTURAL AWARENESS

Fostering Bonding: Women of Varying Ethnic and Cultural Groups

Childbearing practices and rituals of other cultures may not be congruent with standard practices associated with bonding in the Anglo-American culture. For example, Chinese families traditionally use extended family members to care for the newborn so that the mother can rest and recover, especially after a cesarean birth. Some Native American, Asian, and Hispanic women do not initiate breastfeeding until their breast milk comes in. Haitian families do not name their babies until after the confinement month. Amount of eye contact varies among cultures, too. Yup'ik Eskimo mothers almost always position their babies so that eye contact can be made.

Nurses should become knowledgeable about the childbearing beliefs and practices of diverse cultural and ethnic groups. Because individual cultural variations exist within groups, nurses need to clarify with the patient and family members or friends what cultural norms the patient follows. Incorrect judgments may be made about mother-infant bonding if nurses do not practice culturally sensitive care.

Modified from D'Avanzo C: *Mosby's pocket guide to cultural health assessment*, ed 4, St Louis, 2008, Mosby.

Voice

The shared response of parents and infants to each other's voices is also remarkable. Parents wait tensely for the first cry. Once that cry has reassured them of the baby's health, they begin comforting behaviors. As the parents talk in high-pitched voices, the infant is alerted and turns toward them.

The infant responds to higher-pitched voices and can distinguish the mother's voice from others soon after birth. Infants use their cries to signal hunger, pain, boredom, and fatigue. With experience parents learn to distinguish such cries.

Odor

Another behavior shared by parents and infants is a response to each other's odor. Mothers comment on the smell of their babies when first born and have noted that each infant has a unique odor. Infants learn rapidly to distinguish the odor of their mother's breast milk.

Entrainment

Newborns move in time with the structure of adult speech. They wave their arms, lift their heads, and kick their legs, seemingly "dancing in tune" to a parent's voice. Culturally determined rhythms of speech are ingrained in the infant long before spoken language is used to communicate. This shared rhythm also gives the parent positive feedback and establishes a positive setting for effective communication.

Biorhythmicity

The fetus is in tune with the mother's natural rhythms such as heartbeats. After birth a crying infant may be soothed by being held in a position where the mother's heartbeat can be heard or by hearing a recording of a heartbeat. One of the newborn's tasks is to establish a personal biorhythm or to achieve biorhythmicity. Parents can help in this process by giving consistent loving care and using their infant's alert state to develop responsive behavior and thereby increase social interactions and opportunities for learning (Fig. 22-4). The more quickly parents become competent in child care activities, the more quickly their psychologic energy can be directed toward observing the communication cues the infant gives them.

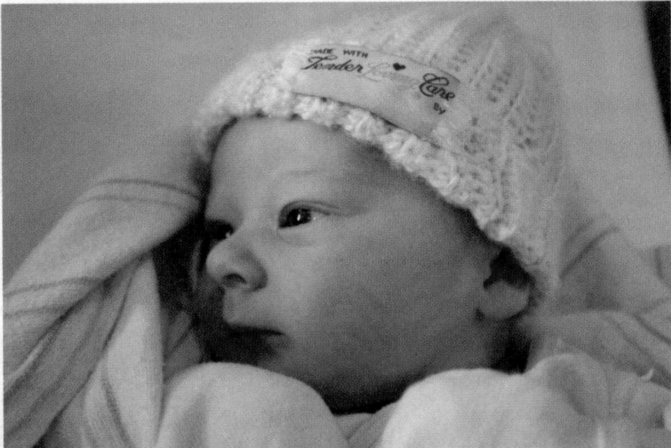

Fig. 22-4 Infant in alert state. *(Courtesy Julie and Darren Nelson, Loveland, CO.)*

Reciprocity and Synchrony

Reciprocity is a type of body movement or behavior that provides the observer with cues. The observer or receiver interprets the cues and responds to them. Reciprocity often takes several weeks to develop with a new baby. For example, when the newborn fusses and cries, the mother responds by picking up and cradling the infant; the baby becomes quiet and alert and establishes eye contact; the mother verbalizes, sings, and coos while the baby maintains eye contact. The baby then averts the eyes and yawns; the mother decreases her active response (Fig. 22-5). If the parent continues to stimulate the infant, the baby may become fussy.

Synchrony refers to the fit between the infant's cues and the parent's response. When parent and infant have a synchronous interaction, it is mutually rewarding. Parents need time to interpret the infant's cues correctly. For example, after a certain time the infant develops a specific cry in response to different situations such as boredom, loneliness, hunger, and discomfort. The parent may need assistance in deciphering these cries, along with trial and error interventions, before synchrony develops.

Parental Role After Childbirth

Adaptation involves stabilizing tasks and coming to terms with commitments. Parents demonstrate growing competence in child care activities and are more attuned to their infant's behavior. Typically the period from the decision to conceive through the first months of having a child is termed the *transition to parenthood.*

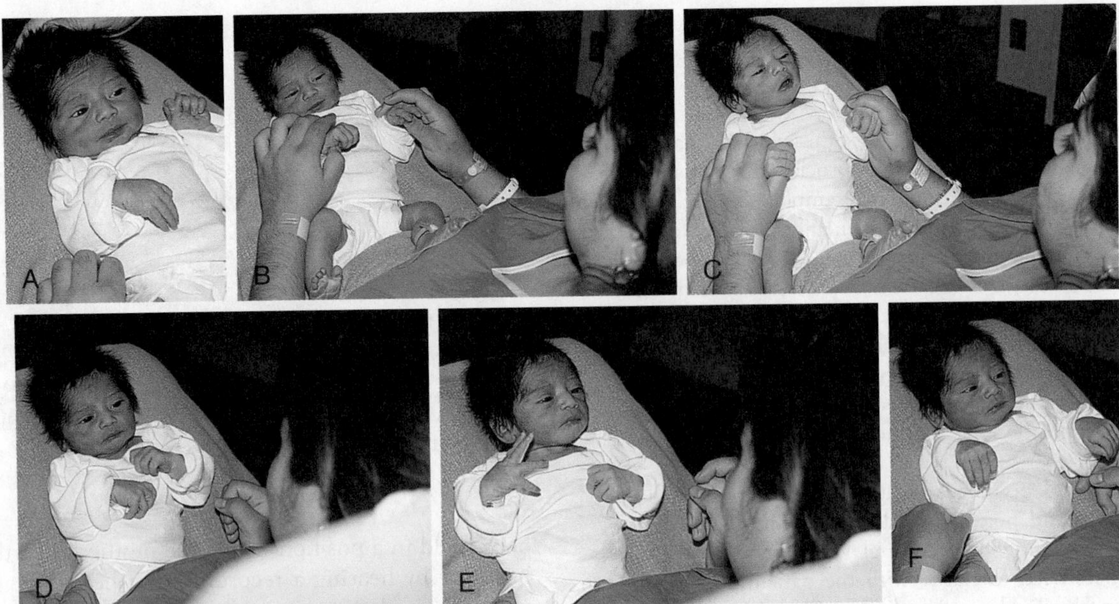

Fig. 22-5 Holding newborn in *en face* position, mother works to alert her daughter, 6 hours old. **A,** Infant is quiet and alert. **B,** Mother begins talking to daughter. **C,** Infant responds, opens mouth like her mother. **D,** Infant gazes at her mother. **E,** Infant waves hand. **F,** Infant glances away, resting. Hand relaxes. *(Courtesy Marjorie Pyle, RNC, Lifecircle, Costa Mesa, CA.)*

Transition to Parenthood

Historically the transition to parenthood was viewed as a crisis. The current perspective is that for the majority of families parenthood is a developmental transition rather than a major life crisis. The transition to parenthood is described as a time of disorder and disequilibrium, as well as satisfaction, for mothers and their partners. Usual methods of coping often seem ineffective. Some parents can be so distressed that they are unable to be supportive of each other. Since men typically identify their spouses as their primary or only source of support, the transition can be harder for the fathers, who feel deprived when the mothers, who are also experiencing stress, cannot provide their usual level of support. Strong emotions such as the helplessness, inadequacy, and anger that arise when dealing with a crying infant catch many parents unprepared. On the other hand, parenthood allows adults to develop and display a selfless, warm, and caring side of themselves that may not be expressed in other adult roles.

For most mothers and their partners the transition to parenthood is viewed as an opportunity rather than a time of danger. Parents are stimulated to try new coping strategies as they work to master their new roles and reach new developmental levels. As they work through the transition, personal strength and resourcefulness are revealed.

Some parents have limited knowledge of what being a parent entails. These parents can benefit from more information on child care, changes in relationships, and differing views of parenting held by partners. Women have more support from female relatives and postnatal groups, whereas men often lack support mechanisms and have only health professionals and work colleagues for information and support (Deave & Johnson, 2008; Deave, Johnson, & Ingram, 2008).

Parental Tasks and Responsibilities

Parents need to reconcile the actual child with the fantasy and dream child. This means coming to terms with the infant's physical appearance, sex, innate temperament, and physical status. If the real child differs greatly from the fantasy child, parents may delay acceptance of the child. In some instances they may never accept the child.

Some parents are startled by the normal appearance of the neonate—the size, color, molding of the head, Mongolian spots, or bowed appearance of the legs. Many fathers have commented that they thought the odd shape of the infant's head (molding) meant that the infant would be mentally retarded.

Parents may know the sex of the infant before birth because of ultrasound assessments; for those who do not have this information, disappointment over the sex can take time to resolve. The parents can provide adequate physical care but find it difficult to be sincerely involved with the infant until this internal conflict has been resolved. As one mother remarked,

"I really wanted a boy. I know it is silly and irrational, but when they said, 'She's a lovely little girl,' I was so disappointed and angry—yes, angry—that I could hardly look at her. Oh, I looked after her okay, her feedings and baths and things, but I couldn't feel excited. To tell the truth, I felt like a monster not liking my child. Then one day she was lying there and she turned her head and looked right at me. I felt a flooding of love for her come over me, and we looked at each other a long time. It's okay now. I wouldn't change her for all the boys in the world."

Parents need to become adept in the care of the infant, including caregiving activities, noting the communication cues the infant gives to indicate needs and responding appropriately to those needs. Self-esteem grows with competence. Breastfeeding makes mothers feel they are contributing in a unique way to the welfare of the infant. The infant's response to parental care and attention can be interpreted as a comment on the quality of that care. Infant behaviors that parents interpret as positive responses to their care include being consoled easily, enjoying being cuddled, and making eye contact. Spitting up frequently after feedings, crying, and being unpredictable may be perceived as negative responses to parental care. Continuation of these infant responses that are viewed as negative can result in alienation of parent and infant to the detriment of the infant.

Assistance, including advice by husbands, partners, wives, mothers, mothers-in-law, and professional workers, can be seen either as supportive or an indication of how inept these others judge the new parents to be. Criticism, real or imagined, of the new parents' ability to provide adequate physical care, nutrition, or social stimulation for the infant can prove to be devastating. By providing encouragement and praise for parenting efforts, nurses can bolster the new parents' confidence.

Parents must establish a place for the newborn within the family group. Whether the infant is the firstborn or the last born, all family members must adjust their roles to accommodate the newcomer. The firstborn child needs support to accept a rival for parental affections. An older child needs help dealing with losing a favored position in the family hierarchy. The parents are expected to negotiate these changes.

Becoming a Mother

Rubin (1961) identified three phases as the mother adjusts to her parental role. These phases are characterized by dependent behavior, dependent-independent behavior, and interdependent behavior. The phases extend over the first several weeks (Table 22-4). Rubin's research was conducted when the length of stay in the hospital was for a longer period of time (3 to 5 or more days). With today's early discharge women seem to move through the phases faster.

Mercer (2004) has suggested that the concept of maternal role attainment introduced by Rubin in 1967 be replaced with *becoming a mother* to signify the transformation and growth of the mother identity. Becoming a mother implies more than attaining a role. It includes learning new skills and increasing her confidence in herself as she meets new challenges in caring for her child(ren).

The transition to motherhood requires adjustment for the mother and her family. There is disruption inherent in that adjustment, and some circumstances, such as problems in postpartum recovery or giving birth to a high risk infant, add to the disruption (Nelson, 2003). Providing social support and enhancing maternal identity improve the ability of the mother to perceive and accurately interpret the signals of her infant and respond appropriately (Shin, Park, & Kim, 2006).

Nelson (2003) identified two social processes in maternal transition. The primary process is engagement (i.e., making a commitment to being a mother, actively caring for her child, and experiencing his or her presence). The secondary process is experiencing herself as a mother, which leads to growth and

Table 22-4 Phases of Maternal Postpartum Adjustment

PHASE	CHARACTERISTICS
Dependent: taking in*	First 24 hr (range of 1-2 days) Focus–Self and meeting of basic needs Reliance on others to meet needs for comfort, rest, closeness, and nourishment Excited and talkative Desire to review birth experience
Dependent-independent: taking hold*	Starts second or third day; lasts 10 days to several weeks Focus–Care of baby and competent mothering Desire to take charge Nurturing and acceptance by others still important Eagerness to learn and practice–Optimal period for teaching by nurses Handling of physical discomforts and emotional changes Possible experience with blues
Interdependent letting go*:	Focus–Forward movement of family as unit with interacting members Reassertion of relationship with partner Resumption of sexual intimacy Resolution of individual roles

*From Rubin R: Basic maternal behavior, *Nurs Outlook* 9:683-686, 1961.

transformation. During this process she must learn how to mother and adapt to a changed relationship with her partner, family, and friends; she must examine herself in relation to the past and present and come to view herself as a mother; and she must make decisions whether to and when to return to work.

Not all mothers experience the transition to motherhood in the same way. For some women becoming a mother entails multiple losses. For example, for some single women there may be a loss of the family of origin when they do not accept her decision to have the child and loss of a relationship with the father of the baby, with friends, and with their own sense of self. Women describe a loss of dreams, including loss of job, financial security, and a future profession (Keating-Lefler & Wilson, 2004). Accompanying these losses is a loss of support.

Mercer (2004) provides new names for the stages in the process of establishing a maternal identity while becoming a mother. These include "(a) commitment, attachment, and preparation (pregnancy); (b) acquaintance, learning, and physical restoration (first 2 to 6 weeks following birth); (c) moving toward a new normal (2 weeks to 4 months); and (d) achievement of the maternal identity (around 4 months)." The time of achievement of the stages varies, and the stages may overlap. Achievement is influenced by mother and infant variables and the social environment (Mercer, 2004).

Nurses must individualize their assessments and interventions. More reality-based perinatal education programs are necessary to prepare mothers better and decrease their anxiety. Mothers need to know that it is common to feel overwhelmed and insecure and to experience physical and mental fatigue in the first months of parenthood. Empathic listening and interactive dialogue are effective approaches to enhance mother-infant interactions and assist the parents in the transition (Mercer, 2006; Mercer & Walker, 2006). They need to be assured that this situation is temporary and that it will take 3 to 6 months to become comfortable in caregiving and in being a mother (Nelson, 2003). Maternal support by professionals should not end with hospital discharge but extend over the next 4 to 6 months. Nurses can advocate for the extension of such support services well into the postpartum period.

Nurses can discuss, before and after birth, the usual postpartum concerns that mothers experience and can provide anticipatory guidance on coping strategies such as resting when the infant sleeps and planning with an extended family member or friend to do the housework for the first week or two after the baby is born. Once a mother is home, periodic phone calls from a nurse who cared for her in the birth setting can provide her with an opportunity to vent her concerns and get support and advice from "her nurse." Nurses should plan additional supportive counseling for first-time mothers inexperienced in child care, women whose careers had provided outside stimulation, women who lack friends or family members with whom to share delights and concerns, and adolescent mothers. When possible, postpartum home visits are included in the plan of care.

Postpartum Blues

The "pink" period surrounding the first day or two after birth, characterized by heightened joy and feelings of well-being, is often followed by a "blue" period. Approximately 50% to 80% of women of all ethnic and racial groups experience the postpartum blues or baby blues. During the blues women are emotionally labile and often cry easily for no apparent reason. This lability seems to peak around the fifth day and subside by the tenth day. Other symptoms of postpartum blues include depression, a let-down feeling, restlessness, fatigue, insomnia, headache, anxiety, sadness, and anger. Biochemical, psychologic, social, and cultural factors have been explored as possible causes of the postpartum depressive state; however, the etiology remains unknown.

Whatever the cause, the early postpartum period appears to be one of emotional and physical vulnerability for new mothers who may be psychologically overwhelmed by the reality of parental responsibilities. The mother may feel deprived of the supportive care she received from family members and friends during pregnancy. Some mothers regret the loss of the mother-unborn child relationship and mourn its passing. Still others have a let-down feeling when labor and birth are complete. Most women experience fatigue after childbirth, which is compounded by the around-the-clock demands of the new baby and can accentuate the feelings of depression. Postpartum depressive symptoms can have a negative effect on maternal role attainment. To help mothers cope with postpartum blues, nurses can suggest various strategies (see Patient Teaching box).

A few questions on a discharge checklist can help mothers assess their level of blues and decide when to seek advice from their nurse, nurse-midwife, or physician (Fig. 22-6). Home visits and telephone follow-up calls by a nurse are important to assess the mother's pattern of blue feelings and behavior over time.

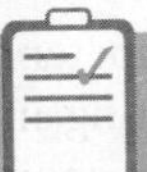

PATIENT TEACHING Coping with Postpartum Blues

- Remember that the blues are normal.
- Get plenty of rest; nap when the baby does if possible. Go to bed early and let friends know when to visit.
- Use relaxation techniques learned in childbirth classes (or ask the nurse to teach you and your partner some techniques).
- Do something for yourself. Take advantage of the time your partner or family members care for the baby—soak in the tub or go for a walk.
- Plan a day out of the house—go to the mall with the baby, being sure to take a stroller or carriage, or go out to eat with friends without the baby. Many communities have churches or other agencies that provide child care programs such as Mothers' Morning Out.
- Share your feelings with your partner. For example, talk about feeling tied down, how the birth met your expectations, and things that will help you.
- If you are breastfeeding, give yourself and your baby time to learn.
- Seek out and use community resources such as La Leche League or community mental health centers. One nationally recognized resource is:
  Postpartum Support International
  927 North Kellogg Avenue
  Santa Barbara, CA 93111
  Phone: 805-967-7636

Although the postpartum blues are usually mild and short lived, approximately 10% to 15% of women experience a more severe syndrome called postpartum depression (PPD) (see Chapter 23). PPD symptoms can range from mild to severe, with women having good and bad days. PPD may also occur in fathers (Goodman, 2004). Both mothers and fathers should be screened for PPD. It can go undetected because new parents generally do not voluntarily admit to this kind of emotional distress out of embarrassment, guilt, or fear. Nurses must include teaching about how to differentiate symptoms of the blues and PPD and urge parents to report depressive symptoms promptly if they occur (see Box 23-4).

Resuming Sexual Intimacy

The couple may begin to engage in sexual intercourse during the second to fourth week after the baby is born. Some couples begin earlier, as soon as it can be accomplished without discomfort, depending on factors such as timing, amount of vaginal dryness, and breastfeeding status. Sexual intimacy enhances the adult aspect of the family, and the adult pair shares a closeness denied to other family members. Changes in a woman's sexuality after childbirth are related to hormonal shifts, increased breast size, uneasiness with a body that has yet to return to a prepregnant size, chronic fatigue related to sleep deprivation, and physical exhaustion. Many new fathers speak of the alienation experienced when they observe the intimate mother-infant relationship, and some are frank in expressing feelings of jealousy toward the infant. The resumption of sexual intimacy seems to bring the parents' relationship

Am I Blue?

Many new mothers feel anxious, sad, or angry about the changes in their lives after the birth of their new baby. It is perfectly normal to feel this way, but sometimes the feelings grow so strong that they make life difficult. This quiz lists many feelings and experiences of "blue" or depressed mothers. Mark how strong each of these feelings or experiences is for you, compared with what is normal for you. For example: Do you feel no anger [0]; mild (very little) anger [1]; moderate (some) anger [2]; or severe (very strong) anger [3] compared with the way you usually feel? Add up your total score when you are finished, and discuss the results with your health care provider.

0 = Not there at all 1 = Mild 2 = Moderate 3 = Severe	0	1	2	3
Anger				
Anxiety attacks: periods of very strong fear, shortness of breath, rapid heartbeat				
Increased or decreased appetite and/or weight gain or loss that doesn't seem normal				
Strong feeling that you need to get away, need more time for your own interests				
Problems in a relationship with a family member, lover, close friend, etc.				
Crying spells				
Less interest in your personal appearance				
Less motivation—less energy or interest in accomplishing goals				
Depression				
Fatigue—feeling tired or exhausted				
Fear of harming yourself or your baby				
Loss of your sense of humor				
Nervousness, feeling tense or edgy				
Feelings of guilt				
Feelings of panic				
Feeling alone or lonely; without the support of others				
Feeling no love, or not enough love, for your baby				
Feeling forgetful, distracted, absent-minded—having trouble concentrating				
Frustration				
Hopelessness				
Insomnia				
Feeling irritable, bad-tempered				
Loss of sexual desire and/or pleasure in sex				
Loss of self-respect or confidence—feeling like you don't count or can't do anything right				
Feeling confused, uncertain				
Mood swings—your moods and emotions change all the time				
Obsessive thoughts—ideas or feelings you can't stop from repeating in your mind				
Odd or frightening thoughts—thoughts or images that scare you or that you can't control				
Thoughts of suicide, feeling like you want to die				
Feeling sad, unhappy				
TOTAL				

SCORE:

0 – 31 = MILD BLUES
This will probably pass, but pay attention to your feelings and needs.

32 – 64 = MODERATE BLUES
You may want to ask for help from a close friend or family member, or ask the advice of your health care provider.

65 – 98 = SEVERE BLUES
You could be depressed; see your health care provider for a check-up and advice as soon as possible.

If you are afraid you might harm yourself or your baby—ask a health care provider you trust for help—you don't have to be alone!

Fig. 22-6 Am I Blue? (Courtesy Johnson & Johnson: *Compendium of postpartum care*, Skillman, NJ, 1996, Johnson & Johnson Consumer Products.)

back into focus. Before and after birth nurses should review with new parents their plans for other pregnancies and their preferences for contraception.

Postpartum Adjustment in the Lesbian Couple

Little is known about postpartum maternal adjustment in the lesbian couple. Relationship satisfaction in first-time lesbian parent couples appears related to egalitarianism, commitment, sexual compatibility, communication skills, and the birth mother's decision for insemination by an anonymous sperm donor. Similar to heterosexual parent couples, most lesbian parent couples voice concern about less time and energy for their relationship after the arrival of the baby. Both partners consider themselves to be equal parents of the baby who share actively in childrearing. A primary concern of co-mothers is the legal vulnerability of lesbian families confounded by their social invisibility.

Lesbian couples face strong social sanctions regarding pregnancy and parenting. Their families may not have resolved the initial dismay and guilt over learning of their daughters' homosexuality, or they may disagree with the lesbian couple's decision to conceive and be parents. Lesbian parents deal with public ignorance, social and legal invisibility, and the lack of biologic connection to the child by using various techniques. These techniques include carefully planning and accomplishing their transition to parenthood, displaying public acts of equal mothering, sharing parenting at home, establishing a distinct parenting role within the family, and supporting each partner's sense of identity as a mother. In situations in which family support is limited or absent, the nurse can help lesbian couples locate more supportive social groups, lesbian or heterosexual.

Becoming a Father

Research on paternal adjustment to parenthood indicates that fathers go through predictable phases during their transition to parenthood (St. John, Cameron, & McVeigh, 2005). During this period fathers experience intense emotions. Many fathers acknowledge that their expectations were of limited value once they were immersed in the reality of parenthood. Feelings that often accompany this reality are sadness, ambivalence, jealousy, frustration at not being able to participate in breastfeeding, and an overwhelming desire to be more involved; most of which are different from the feelings mothers report. On the other hand, some fathers are pleasantly surprised at the ease and fun of parenting. In their transition to mastery, fathers take control and become more actively involved in the infant's life (Table 22-5).

First-time fathers perceive the first 4 to 10 weeks of parenthood in much the same way that mothers do (i.e., as a period characterized by uncertainty, increased responsibility, disruption of sleep, and inability to control time needed to care for the infant and reestablish the marital dyad). Fathers express concerns about decreased attention from their partners relative to their personal relationship, the mother's lack of recognition of the father's desire to participate in decision making for the infant, and limited time available to establish a relationship with their infants. These concerns can precipitate feelings of jealousy of the infant. To help alleviate these feelings the father should discuss his individual concerns/needs with the mother/partner and become more involved with the infant.

Table 22-5 Development of a Father-Infant Relationship: Process Components

COMPONENT	CHARACTERISTICS
Making a commitment	Is willing to invest in and take responsibility for nurturing the relationship despite difficulties in parenting and other life demands Feels reality of commitment—At confirmation of pregnancy; during pregnancy and birth; when providing infant care; when infant responds to them Feels duty to nurture and protect because of helpless nature of infant Desires to get to know and be psychologically involved Is rewarded by infant smile, increased self-esteem, gaining a new dimension in life, finding the child within self
Becoming connected	First meeting with infant—Feels joy, elation, awe, and wonderment Has sense of bond with the infant—May feel this at first meeting, when first touching/holding infant, or gradually during the first 2 mo Turning point—Perceives infant as more responsive, predictable, and familiar
Making room for baby	Makes changes in work and social/personal time, in relationship with wife/partner, and within self so he is more physically and emotionally available to infant

Concerns of fathers are often not addressed adequately in prenatal or postnatal education. The father's relationship with the child is fostered by time alone with the child. Health professionals must address the fathers' needs to assist in his transition to parenthood (Premberg, Hellström, & Berg, 2008).

Father-Infant Relationship

In North American culture neonates have a powerful impact on their fathers, who become intensely involved with their babies (Fig. 22-7). The term used for the father's absorption, preoccupation, and interest in the infant is *engrossment*. Characteristics of engrossment include some of the sensual responses relating to touch and eye-to-eye contact that were discussed earlier and also the father's keen awareness of features both unique and similar to himself that validate his claim to the infant. An outstanding response is one of strong attraction to the newborn. Fathers spend considerable time "communicating" with the infant and taking delight in the infant's response to them (Fig. 22-8). They experience increased self-esteem and a sense of being proud, larger, more mature, and older after seeing their baby for the first time.

Fathers spend less time than mothers with infants, and their interactions with their infants tend to be characterized by stimulating social play rather than caretaking. The subtle and more obvious differences in stimulation from two sources, mother and father, provide a wider social experience for the infant.

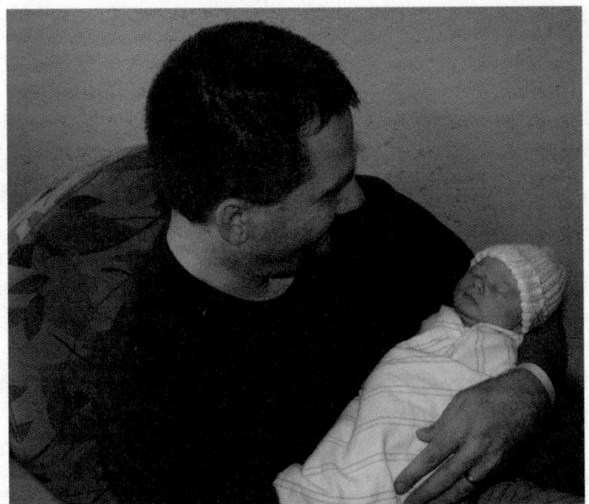

Fig. 22-7 Engrossment. Father absorbed in looking at his newborn son. *(Courtesy Darren Nelson, Loveland, CO.)*

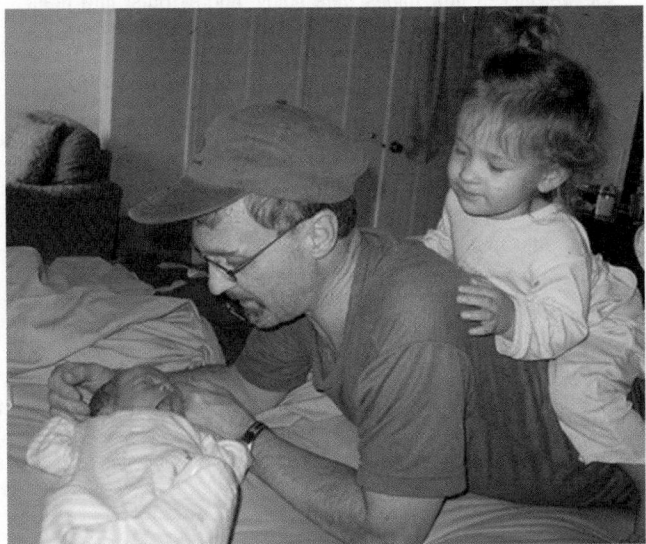

Fig. 22-8 Father interacting with newborn while sibling observes with interest. *(Courtesy Christine Brockett, Boulder, CO.)*

Fathers can benefit from nursing interventions during the postpartum period just as mothers can. Nurses can arrange to teach infant care when the father is present and provide anticipatory guidance for fathers about the transition to parenthood. Separate prenatal and parenting classes and parenting support groups for fathers can provide them with an opportunity to discuss their concerns and have some of their needs met. Postpartum phone calls and home visits by a nurse should include time for assessment of the father's adjustment and needs.

Infant-Parent Adjustment

Newborns participate actively in shaping their parents' reaction to them. Behavioral characteristics of the infant influence parenting behaviors. The infant and parent each have unique rhythms, behaviors, and response styles that are brought to every interaction. Infant-parent interactions can be facilitated in at least three ways: (1) modulation of rhythm, (2) modification of behavioral repertoires, and (3) mutual responsivity. Nurses can teach parents about these three aspects of infant-parent interaction through discussions, written materials, and videotapes on infant capabilities. A creative approach is to videotape the parent-infant pair during an interaction and then use the individualized tape to discuss the pair's rhythm, behavioral repertoire, and responsivity.

Rhythm

To modulate rhythm, both parent and infant must be able to interact. Therefore the infant must be in the alert state, one of the most difficult of the sleep-wake states to maintain. The alert state (see Fig. 22-4) occurs most often during a feeding or in face-to-face play. The parent must work hard to help the infant maintain the alert state long enough and often enough for interactions to take place. The *en face* position is usually assumed (see Fig. 22-5, *D*). Multiparous mothers in particular are very sensitive and responsive to the infant's feeding rhythms. Mothers learn to reserve stimulation for pauses in sucking activity and not to talk or smile excessively while the infant is sucking because the baby will stop feeding to interact with her. With maturity the infant can sustain longer interactions by modulating activity rhythms (i.e., limb movement, sucking, gaze alternation, and habituation). Meanwhile the parent becomes more attuned to the infant's rhythms and learns to modulate the rhythms, facilitating a rhythmic turn-taking interaction.

Behavioral Repertoires

Both the infant and the parent have a repertoire of behaviors they can use to facilitate interactions. Fathers and mothers engage in these behaviors, depending on the extent of contact and caregiving of the infant.

The infant's behavioral repertoire includes gazing, vocalizing, and facial expressions. The infant is able to focus and follow the human face from birth and also to alternate the gaze voluntarily, looking away from the parent's face when understimulated or overstimulated (see Fig. 22-5, *F*). One of the key responses for the parents to learn is to be sensitive to the infant's capacity for attention and inattention. Developing this sensitivity is especially important when interacting with preterm infants.

Body gestures form a part of the infant's early language. Babies greet parents with waving hands (see Fig. 22-5, *E*) or a reaching out of hands. They can raise an eyebrow or soften their expression to elicit loving attention. Game playing can stimulate them to smile or laugh. Pouting or crying, arching of the back, and general squirming usually signal the end of an interaction.

The parents' repertoire includes various types of interactive behaviors such as constantly looking at the infant and noting the infant's response. New parents often remark that they are exhausted from looking at the baby and smiling. Adults also "infantilize" their speech to help the infant listen. They do this by slowing the tempo, speaking loudly and rhythmically, and emphasizing key words. Phrases are repeated frequently. Infantilizing does not mean using baby talk, which involves distortion of sounds.

To communicate emotions to the infant, parents often use facial expressions such as slow and exaggerated looks of surprise, happiness, and confusion. Games such as "peek-a-boo" and imitation of the infant's behaviors are other means of interaction. For example, if the baby smiles, so does the parent; if the baby frowns, the parent responds in kind.

Responsivity

Contingent responses (responsivity) are those that occur within a specific time and are similar in form to a stimulus behavior. The adult has the feeling of having an influence on the interaction. Infant behaviors such as smiling, cooing, and sustained eye contact, usually in *en face* position, are viewed as contingent responses. The infant's responses act as rewards to the initiator and encourage the adult to continue with the game when the infant responds positively. When the adult imitates the infant, the infant appears to enjoy it. A progression occurs in the types of behaviors that parents present for the baby to imitate; for example, in early interactions the parent will grimace rather than laugh, which is in keeping with the infant's developmental level. Such behaviors sustain interactions and promote harmony in the relationship.

Diversity in Transitions to Parenthood

How parents respond to the birth of their child is influenced by various factors, including age, social networks, culture, socioeconomic conditions, and personal aspirations for the future.

Age

Maternal age has a definite effect on the outcome of pregnancy. The mother and fetus are at highest risk when the mother is an adolescent or is more than 35 years old (see Critical Thinking Exercise).

The Adolescent Mother

Although it is biologically possible for the adolescent female to become a parent, her egocentricity and concrete thinking interfere with her ability to parent effectively. The very young adolescent mother is inexperienced and unprepared to recognize the early signs of illness, potential danger, or household hazards. She may inadvertently neglect her child. The higher mortality rates among infants of adolescent mothers are attributed to the inexperience, lack of knowledge, and immaturity of the mothers, causing them to be unable to recognize a problem and obtain the necessary resources to rectify the situation. Nevertheless, in most instances, with adequate support and developmentally appropriate teaching, adolescents can learn effective parenting skills (Maputie, 2006).

The transition to parenthood may be difficult for adolescent parents. Coping with the developmental tasks of parenthood is often complicated by the unmet developmental needs and tasks of adolescence. Some young parents may experience difficulty accepting a changing self-image and adjusting to new roles related to the responsibilities of infant care. On the other hand, some adolescent parents may have higher self-concepts than their nonparenting peers.

CRITICAL THINKING EXERCISE

Postpartum Adjustment for the Adolescent and the Older Mother

You are a home care nurse and have had two patients referred to you. Carol is a 15-year-old first-time mother of a 5-day-old girl; she lives with her mother. The father of the baby, Robert, is 17 years old and attended childbirth classes with Carol. She is breastfeeding the baby but says that the baby sucks too slowly and takes too much time to eat. She said she thinks the baby should know enough to sleep longer at night. Robert would like to feed the baby some cereal since he heard that solid food will make a baby sleep longer at night.

Audrey is a 36-year-old attorney who has been practicing law for 7 years. She just gave birth to her first baby; she and her husband delayed parenting by choice until their careers were well established. She had an uneventful pregnancy, labor, and birth. During a telephone call 48 hours after discharge, when she was asked how things were going, Audrey burst into tears and said, "I didn't expect it to be like this! Nothing is going right."

1. Evidence—Is there sufficient evidence to draw conclusions about what teaching and care these new parents need?
2. Assumptions—What assumptions can be made about the following factors:
   a. The relationship of maternal age and postpartum adjustment
   b. The need for social support in the postnatal period
   c. The need for perinatal education
   d. Long-term prognosis for positive outcomes
3. What implications and priorities for nursing care can be drawn at this time?
4. Does the evidence objectively support your conclusion?
5. Are there alternative perspectives to your conclusion?

As adolescent parents move through the transition to parenthood, they may feel "different" from their peers, excluded from "fun" activities, and prematurely forced to enter an adult social role. The conflict between their own desires and the infant's demands, in addition to the low tolerance for frustration that is typical of adolescence, further contribute to the normal psychosocial stress of childbirth. Maintaining a relationship with the baby's father is beneficial for the teen mother and her infant.

Adolescent mothers provide warm and attentive physical care; however, they use less verbal interaction than do older parents, and adolescents tend to be less responsive and to interact less positively with their infants than do older mothers. Interventions emphasizing verbal and nonverbal communication skills between mother and infant are important. Such intervention strategies must be concrete and specific because of the cognitive level of adolescents. Although some observers suggest that some adolescents may use more aggressive behaviors, a higher incidence of child abuse by adolescent mothers has not been documented. In comparison with adult mothers, teenage mothers have a limited knowledge of child development. They tend to expect too much of their children too soon and often characterize their infants as being fussy. This limited knowledge may cause teenagers to respond to their infants inappropriately.

Many young mothers pattern their maternal role on what they themselves experienced. Therefore nurses need to determine the kind of support that people close to the young mother are able and prepared to give and the kinds of community aid available to supplement this support. Many teen mothers can identify a source of social support, with the predominant source being their own mothers.

The need for continued assessment of the new mother's parenting abilities during this postbirth period is essential. Continued support should be provided by involving the grandparents and other family members and through home visits and group sessions for discussion of infant care and parenting concerns. Outreach programs addressing self-management, parent-child interactions, child injuries, and failure to thrive, in addition to programs that provide prompt and effective community intervention, prevent serious problems from occurring. As the adolescent performs her mothering role within the framework of her family, she may need to address dependence vs. independence issues. The adolescent's family members also may need help adapting to their new roles.

The Adolescent Father

The adolescent father and mother face immediate developmental crises, which include completing the developmental tasks of adolescence, making a transition to parenthood, and sometimes adapting to marriage. These transitions can be stressful. The nurse may initiate interaction with the adolescent father by asking him to be present when postpartum home visits are made and to accompany the mother and the baby to well-baby checks at the clinic or pediatrician's office. With the adolescent mother's agreement, the nurse may contact the father directly. Adolescent fathers need support to discuss their emotional responses to the pregnancy. The father's feelings of guilt, powerlessness, or bravado should be recognized because of their negative consequences for both the parents and the child. Counseling of adolescent fathers needs to be reality oriented. Topics such as finances, child care, parenting skills, and the father's role in the birth experience must be discussed. Teenage fathers also need to know about reproductive physiology, birth control options, and risk-reducing sex practices.

The adolescent father may continue to be involved in an ongoing relationship with the young mother and his baby. In many instances he also plays an important role in the decisions about child care and raising the child. He may need help to develop realistic perceptions of his role as father to a child. He is encouraged to use coping mechanisms that are not detrimental to his own, his partner's, or his child's well-being. The nurse enlists support systems, parents, and professional agencies on his behalf.

Maternal Age Greater Than 35 Years

Women older than 35 years have always continued their childbearing either by choice or because of a lack of or failure of contraception during the perimenopausal years. Added to this group are women who have postponed pregnancy because of careers or other reasons and women of infertile couples who finally become pregnant with the aid of technologic advances (see Evidence-Based Practice box).

Adjustment of older mothers to changes involved in becoming a parent and seeing themselves as competent is aided by support from their partners. Support from other family members and friends is also important for positive self-evaluation of parenting, a sense of well-being and satisfaction, and help in dealing with stress.

Changes in the sexual aspect of a relationship can create a stressor for new midlife parents. Mothers report that finding time and energy for a romantic rendezvous is more difficult. They attribute much of this to the reality of caring for an infant and the decreasing libido that normally accompanies getting older.

Work, career issues, and child care are major sources of conflict and stress for older mothers. Conflicts emerge over being disinterested in work, worrying about giving enough attention to work with the distractions of a new baby, and anticipating what it will be like to return to work.

Another major issue for older mothers with careers is the perception of loss of control. Mothers older than 35 are at a different stage in their careers than younger mothers, having attained high levels of education, career, and income. The loss of control experienced when going from the consistency of a work role to the inconsistency of the parent role comes as a surprise to many. Helping the older mother have realistic expectations of herself and parenthood is essential.

New mothers who are also perimenopausal may find it hard to distinguish fatigue, loss of sleep, decreased libido, or other physiologic symptoms as the causes of the change in their sex lives. Although many women view menopause as a natural stage of life, for midlife mothers this cessation of menstruation coincides with the state of parenthood. The changes of midlife and menopause can add more emotional and physical stress to older mothers' lives because of the time- and energy-consuming aspects of raising a young child.

Paternal Age Greater Than 35 Years

Older fathers describe their experience of midlife parenting as wonderful but not without drawbacks. What they see as positive aspects of parenthood in older years include increased love and commitment between the spouses, a reinforcement of why one married in the first place, a feeling of being complete, experiencing "the child" in oneself again, more financial stability than in younger years, and more freedom to focus on parenting rather than on career. A common theme expressed is sharing: sharing joy, sharing in raising the child, sharing as a family. The main drawback of midlife parenting is the change that it makes in the relationships with their partners.

Social Support

Social support is strongly related to positive adaptation by new parents, including adolescent parents, during the transition to parenthood. Social support is multidimensional and includes the number of members in a person's social network, types of support, perceived general support, actual support received, and satisfaction with support available and received. The type

EVIDENCE-BASED PRACTICE Having a Baby Later in Life —*Pat Gingrich*

Ask the Question

What are the unique risks for advanced maternal age? Are there differences in expectations and nursing care for older primiparas than for younger new mothers?

Search for Evidence

Search Strategies

Professional organization guidelines, meta-analyses, systematic reviews, randomized controlled trials, nonrandomized prospective studies, and retrospective studies since 2006

Databases Searched

CINAHL, Cochrane, Medline, National Guideline Clearinghouse, TRIP Database Plus, and the websites for AWHONN and CDC

Critically Analyze the Evidence

The childbearing years can span four decades of life. Many women are delaying childbirth well into their thirties or forties. Older mothers are more likely to be educated and have a higher socioeconomic status but may lack some of the robust physical resilience of youth.

Advanced maternal age is a risk factor for not only trisomy 21 (Down syndrome) but also increased stillbirths, preterm births, small-for-gestational-age and low-birth-weight infants, particularly in primigravidas over 40 (Delpisheh et al, 2008). A systematic review of 37 studies confirms that the risk of stillbirth increases significantly over age 35 (Huang et al, 2007).

Interestingly, even advanced age in the father may affect the offspring. A Danish study of 102,879 couples who gave birth between 1980 and 1996 demonstrated a significantly increased risk of mortality in offspring of fathers over age 45. The risk for mortality persisted into adulthood (Zhu et al, 2008).

Implications for Practice

Most older mothers have healthy and normal births. The nurse can ask open-ended questions about the baby and pregnancy to assess the psychosocial and emotional status of the patient. According to Suplee, Dawley, & Bloch (2007), older first-time mothers may have spent many years seeking pregnancy and therefore may bring a "last-chance" focus on this new role. It is important for the nurse to facilitate realistic expectations in the parent regarding life changes. Some older women expect a trouble-free, controlled, "no-risk" birth and a quick return to normal. They may need reminders of the need for flexibility about the birth process and the realities of postpartum adjustment. Others may be insecure about their physical and mental abilities and may see themselves as "high-risk," requiring much care. The nurse can help her anxious mother focus on the normal and positive and encourage her to start envisioning holding her baby in her arms soon. Because they may live far from family and have aging parents and their partners may work long hours, many older first-time mothers may not have an extensive social support system or even realize how isolated they will feel. Even after birth the nurse can provide the mother at home with resources about support groups and services and encourage networking among new mothers and play groups (Suplee, Dawley, & Bloch, 2007).

References

Delpisheh A et al: Pregnancy late in life: a hospital-based study of birth outcomes, *J Womens Health* 17(6):1-6, 2008 [Epub ahead of print]. Available at www.liebertonline.com/doi/abs/10.1089/jwh.2008.0514 (accessed June 29, 2008).

Huang L et al: Maternal age and risk of stillbirth: a systematic review, *Can Med Assoc J* 178(2):165-172, 2007.

Suplee PD, Dawley K, Bloch JR: Tailoring peripartum nursing care for women of advanced maternal age, *J Obstet Gynecol Neonatal Nurs* 36(6):616-623, 2007.

Zhu JL et al: Paternal age and mortality in children, *Eur J Epidemiol* 23(7):443-447, 2008.

and satisfaction of support seem to be more important than the total number of support network members.

Across cultural groups, families and friends of new parents form an important dimension of the parent's social network. Through seeking help within the social network, new mothers learn culturally valued practices and develop role competency.

Social networks provide a support system on which parents can rely for assistance, but they also can be a source of conflict. Sometimes a large network can cause problems because it results in conflicting advice coming from numerous people. Grandparents or in-laws are most appreciated when they assist with household responsibilities and do not intrude into the parents' privacy or judge them critically.

Because of the extent of restructuring and reorganization that occurs in a family with the birth of another child, the mothers' moods and fatigue in the postpartum period can be helped more by situation-specific support from family and friends than by general support. General support addresses feeling loved, respected, and valued. Situation-specific support relates to practical concerns such as physical needs and child care. For example, the practical support of a grandparent bathing the infant can help lessen a second-time mother's feelings of loss by providing her time to be with her firstborn child.

Culture

Cultural beliefs and practices are important determinants of parenting behaviors. Culture defines what is socially acceptable in terms of eye contact, touch, and space. Culture influences the interactions with the baby and the parent's or family's caregiving style. For example, providing for a period of rest and recuperation for the mother after birth is prominent in several cultures. Asian mothers must remain at home with the baby at least 30 days after birth and are not supposed to engage in household chores, including care of the baby. Many times the grandmother takes over the baby's care immediately, even before discharge from the hospital (D'Avanzo, 2008). An example is the traditional Taiwanese ritual, *Tso-Yueh-Tzu* (translated "doing, within the first month postpartum"). Jordanian mothers have a 40-day lying-in after birth during which their mothers or sisters care for the baby (D'Avanzo, 2008). Japanese mothers rest for the first 2 months after childbirth. Hispanics practice an intergenerational family ritual, *la cuarentena.* For 40 days after birth the mother is expected to recuperate and get acquainted with her infant. Traditionally this involves many restrictions concerning food (spicy or cold foods, fish, pork, and citrus are avoided; tortillas and chicken soup are encouraged); exercise; and activities, including sexual intercourse. Many women avoid bathing and washing their hair. Traditional Hispanic husbands do not expect to see their wives or infants until both have been cleaned and dressed after birth. *La cuarentena* incorporates individuals into the family, instills parental responsibility, and integrates the family during a critical life event (D'Avanzo, 2008).

Desire for and valuing children is salient in all cultures. In Asian families children are valued as a source of family strength and stability, are perceived as wealth, and are objects of parental love and affection. Infants almost always are given an affectionate cradle name that is used during the first years of life (e.g., a Filipino girl might be called "Bong-Bong" and a boy "Ling-Ling"). See Table 2-2 for examples of some traditional cultural beliefs that may be important to parents from Hispanic, African-American, Asian-American, European American, and Native American cultures.

Differing cultural values can influence parents' interactions with health care professionals. For example, Asians are taught to be humble and obedient; it is frowned on to be outspoken. They are brought up to not question authority figures (such as a nurse), to avoid confrontation, and to respect the yin/yang balance in nature. Because of these learned values, an Asian mother might not confront the nurse about the length of time it has taken to receive the medication requested for her pain due to perineal laceration repair or a cesarean incision. A mother may nod and say, "Yes," in response to the nurse's directions for using an iced sitz bath but then will not use the sitz bath. The "yes" in this case is a gesture of courtesy, meaning, "I'm listening"; it is not an indication of agreement to comply. The mother does not use the iced sitz bath because of her traditional avoidance of bathing and cold in the puerperium. Because all members of a cultural group do not necessarily adhere to traditional practices, validating which cultural practices are important to individual parents is important.

Knowledge of cultural beliefs can help the nurse make more accurate assessments and diagnoses of observed parenting behaviors. For example, nurses may become concerned when they observe cultural practices that appear to reflect poor maternal-infant bonding. Algerian mothers may not unwrap and explore their infants as part of the acquaintance process because in Algeria babies are wrapped tightly in swaddling clothes to protect them physically and psychologically (D'Avanzo, 2008). The nurse may observe a Vietnamese woman who gives minimal care to her infant but refuses to cuddle or further interact with her baby. This apparent lack of interest in the newborn is this cultural group's attempt to ward off evil spirits and actually reflects an intense love and concern for the infant (Galanti, 2003). An Asian mother might be criticized for almost immediately relinquishing the care of the infant to the grandmother and not even attempting to hold her baby when it is brought to her room. However, in Asian extended families members show their support for a new mother's rest and recuperation by assisting with the care of the baby. Contrary to the guidance given to mothers in the United States about "nipple confusion," a mix of breastfeeding and bottle-feeding is standard practice for Japanese mothers. This is out of concern for the mother's rest during the first 2 to 3 months and does not lead to any problems with lactation; breastfeeding is widespread and successful among Japanese women.

Cultural beliefs and values give perspective to the meaning of childbirth for a new mother. Nurses can provide an opportunity for a new mother to talk about her perception of the meaning of childbearing. In helping new families adjust to parenthood, nurses must provide culturally sensitive care by following principles that facilitate nursing practice within transcultural situations.

Socioeconomic Conditions

Socioeconomic conditions often determine access to available resources. Parents whose economic condition is made worse with the birth of each child and who are unable to use an effective method of fertility management may find childbirth complicated by concern for their own health and a sense of helplessness. Mothers who are single; separated or divorced from their husbands; or without a partner, family, and friends for whatever reason may view the birth of a child with dread. Serious financial problems may override any desire for mothering the infant.

Personal Aspirations

Parenthood interferes with or blocks the plans of some women for personal freedom or advancement in their careers. Resentment concerning this loss may not have been resolved during the prenatal period; if it remains unresolved, it will spill over into caregiving activities. This may result in indifference and neglect of the infant or excessive concern and the setting of impossibly high standards for her own behavior or the child's performance.

Nursing intervention includes providing opportunities for mothers to express their feelings freely to an objective listener, discuss measures to permit personal growth, and learn about the care of their infant. Referring the woman to a support group of other mothers in the same situation may also be helpful.

Nurses also can be proactive in influencing changes in work policies related to maternity and paternity leaves, varying models of work sharing, and family-friendly work environments. Some corporations already structure their work sites to support new mothers (e.g., by providing on-site day care facilities and breastfeeding rooms).

Parental Sensory Impairment

In the early dialogue between the parent and child, each uses all senses—sight, hearing, touch, taste, and smell—to initiate and sustain the attachment process. A parent who has an impairment of one of the senses needs to maximize use of the remaining senses. Although these parents may need the assistance and support of a sighted or hearing person and other accommodations to their disability, they can become skilled parents. It is important for nurses and other health care professionals to remember that these people are parents living with a disability and not disabled parents.

Visually Impaired Parent

Visual impairment alone does not seem to have a negative effect on mothers' early parenting experiences. These mothers, just as sighted mothers, express the wonders of parenthood and encourage other visually impaired persons to become parents. Mothers with disabilities tend to value the importance of performing parenting tasks in the perceived culturally usual way.

Although visually impaired mothers initially feel a pressure to conform to traditional, sighted ways of parenting, they soon adapt these ways and develop methods better suited to themselves. Examples of activities that visually impaired mothers do differently include preparation of the infant's nursery, clothes, and supplies. Mothers may put an entire clothing outfit together and hang it in the closet rather than keeping the items separately in drawers. They might develop a labeling system for the infant's clothing and put diapering, bathing, and other care supplies where these will be easy to locate with minimal searching. A strength that visually impaired parents have is a heightened sensitivity to other sensory outputs. A blind mother can tell when her infant is facing her because she can feel the baby's breath on her face.

One of the major difficulties that visually impaired parents experience is the skepticism, open or hidden, of health care professionals. Visually impaired people sense reluctance on the part of others to acknowledge that they have a right to be parents. All too often nurses and doctors lack the experience to deal with the childbearing and childrearing needs of visually impaired mothers and mothers with other disabilities (such as the hearing impaired, physically impaired, and mentally challenged). The nurse's best approach is to assess the mother's capabilities. From that basis the nurse can make plans to assist the woman, often in much the same way as for a mother with sight. Visually impaired mothers have made suggestions for providing care for women such as themselves during childbearing (Box 22-2). Such approaches by the nurse can help avoid a sense of increased vulnerability on the mother's part. Childbirth education and other materials are available in Braille (*www.loc.gov/nls*).

Eye contact is considered important in North American culture. With a parent who is visually impaired, this critical factor in the parent-child attachment process is obviously missing. However, the visually impaired parent who may never have experienced this method of strengthening relationships does not miss it. The infant will need other sensory input from that parent. An infant looking into the eyes of a mother who is visually impaired may not be aware that the eyes are unseeing. Other people in the newborn's environment can participate in active eye contact to supply this need. However, a problem may arise if the visually impaired parent has an impassive facial expression. When her infant makes repeated unsuccessful attempts to engage in face play with the mother, he or she will abandon the behavior with her and intensify it with the father or other persons in the household. Nurses can provide anticipatory guidance regarding this situation and help the mother learn to nod and smile while talking and cooing to the infant.

BOX 22-2 Nursing Approaches for Working with Blind and Visually Impaired Parents

Parents who are blind need:
- Verbal teaching by health care providers because printed maternity information is not accessible to blind people.
- Explanations of routines.
- To feel devices (e.g., monitors, pelvic models) and hear descriptions of the devices.

Visually impaired parents need:
- An orientation to the hospital room that allows the parent to move about the room independently. For example, "Go to the left of the bed and trail the wall until you feel the first door. That is the bathroom."
- A chance to ask questions.
- The opportunity to hold and touch the baby after birth.

Nurses need:
- To demonstrate baby care by touch and follow with, "Now let me see you do it."
- To give instructions such as, "I'm going to give you the baby. The head is to your left side."

Hearing-Impaired Parent

The parent who has a hearing impairment faces another set of problems, particularly if the deafness dates from birth or early childhood. The mother and her partner are likely to have established an independent household. A number of devices that transform sound into light flashes are now marketed and can be fitted into the infant's room to permit immediate detection of crying. Even if the parent is not speech trained, vocalizing can serve as both a stimulus and a response to the infant's early vocalizing. Deaf parents can provide additional vocal training by use of recordings and television so that from birth the child is aware of the full range of the human voice. Young children acquire sign language readily, and the first sign used is as varied as the first word.

Section 504 of the Rehabilitation Act of 1973 requires that hospitals and other institutions receiving funds from the U.S. Department of Health and Human Services use various communication techniques and resources with the deaf, including having staff members or certified interpreters who are proficient in sign language. For example, providing written materials with demonstrations and having nurses stand where the parent can read their lips (if the parent practices lipreading) are two techniques that can be used. A creative approach is for the nursing unit to develop videotapes in which information on postpartum care, infant care, and parenting issues is signed by an interpreter and spoken by a nurse. A videotape in which a nurse signs while speaking would be ideal. With the advent of the Internet, many resources are available to the deaf parent.

Sibling Adaptation

Because the family is an interactive, open unit, the addition of a new family member affects everyone in the family. Siblings have to assume new positions within the family hierarchy. The older child's goal is to maintain the lead position. Parents are

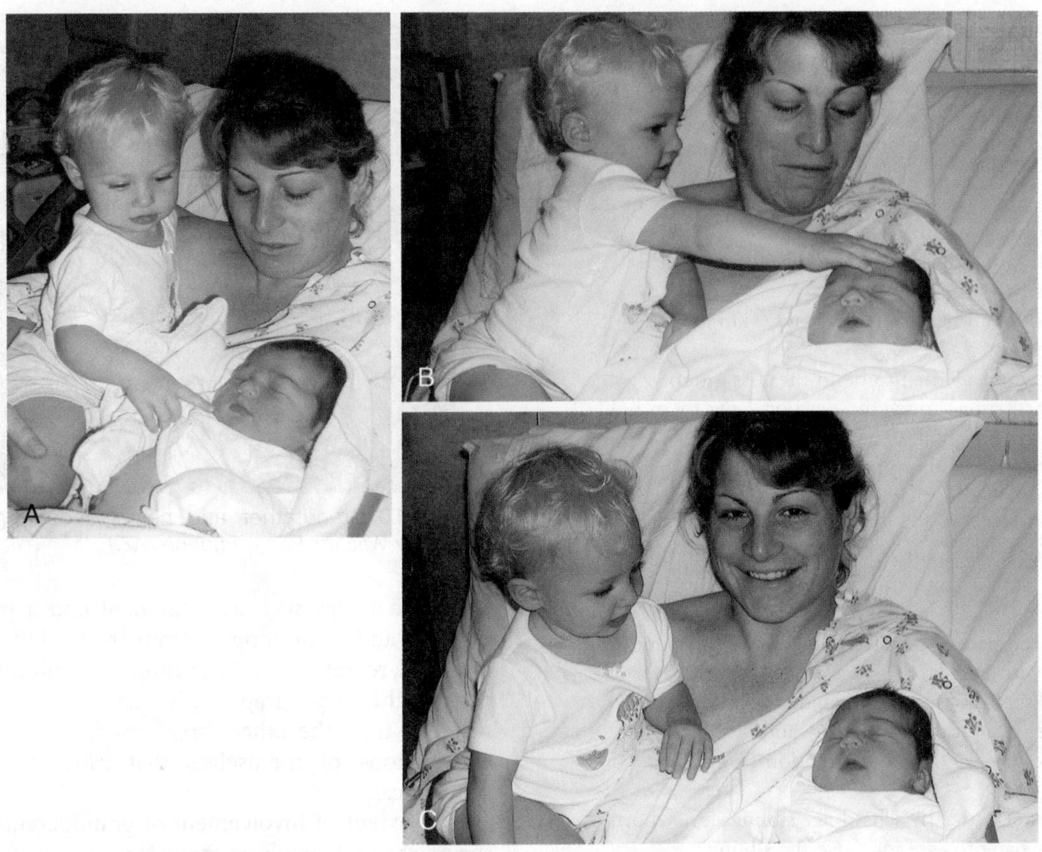

Fig. 22-9 First meeting. **A**, Sister touching new sibling with fingertip. **B**, Touching with whole hand. **C**, Smiles indicate acceptance. *(Courtesy Sara Kossuth, Los Angeles, CA.)*

faced with the task of caring for a new child while not neglecting the others. They need to distribute their attention in an equitable manner. When the newborn is born prematurely or has special needs, this can be difficult.

Reactions of siblings may result from temporary separation from the mother or changes in the mother's or father's behavior. Positive behavioral changes of siblings include interest in and concern for the baby (see Figs. 22-3 and 22-9) and increased independence. Regression in toileting and sleep habits, aggression toward the baby, and increased seeking of attention and whining are examples of negative behaviors.

The parents' attitudes toward the arrival of the baby can set the stage for the other children's reactions (Fig. 22-9). Because the baby absorbs the time and attention of the important people in the other children's lives, jealousy (sibling rivalry) is to be expected once the initial excitement of having a new baby in the home is over. However, sibling rivalry or negative behaviors in siblings may have been overemphasized in the past. Developmentally appropriate behaviors in siblings are similar before and after the baby arrives. Firstborn children seem to continue their usual routines and are more pleased with the newborns and more understanding of the baby's need for care than the parents predict.

Parents, especially mothers, spend much time and energy promoting sibling acceptance of a new baby. Participating in sibling preparation classes makes a difference in the ability of parents to cope with their behavior. Older children are actively involved in preparing for the infant, and this involvement intensifies after the birth of the child. Parents have to manage their feelings of guilt that the older children are being deprived of parental time and attention. They have to monitor the behavior of older children toward the more vulnerable infant and divert aggressive behavior. Strategies that parents have used to facilitate siblings' acceptance of a new baby are presented in the Family-Centered Care box.

Siblings demonstrate acquaintance behaviors with the newborn. The acquaintance process depends on the information given to the child before the baby is born and on the child's cognitive development level. The initial behaviors of siblings with the newborn include looking at the infant and touching the head (see Fig. 22-9). The adjustment of older children to a newborn takes time, and children should be allowed to interact at their own pace rather than be forced to do so. To expect a young child to accept and love a rival for the parents' affection assumes an unrealistic level of maturity. Sibling love grows as does other love (i.e., by being with another person and sharing experiences). This bond between siblings involves a secure base in which one child provides support for the other, is missed when absent, and is looked to for comfort and security.

evolve Nursing Care Plan–The Multiparous Woman and Family

Grandparent Adaptation

Grandparents experience a transition to grandparenthood. Intergenerational relationships shift, and grandparents must deal with changes in practices and attitudes toward childbirth, childrearing, and men's and women's roles at home and in the workplace (see Community Focus box). The degree to which

FAMILY-CENTERED CARE

Strategies for Facilitating Sibling Acceptance of a New Baby

- Take your firstborn child on a tour of your hospital room and point out similarities to his or her birth. "This is like the room I was in with you, and the baby is in the same kind of bassinet that you were in."
- Have a small gift from the baby to give to your older child each day.
- Give the older child a T-shirt that says, "I'm a big brother" (or "sister").
- Arrange for your children to be in the first group (grandparents, sister) to see the newborn. Let them hold the baby in the hospital. One mother and father arranged for their firstborn son to be present at the births of his three brothers and to be the first one to hold them.
- Plan time for both children. "When I get home, I'll arrange my day so that I can finish the baby's care in the morning while Sam (first child) is at school. Maybe the baby will sleep part of the afternoon and I can spend some time with Sam."
- Fathers can spend time with the older sibling while mothers are taking care of the baby and vice versa. Siblings like to have time and attention from both parents.
- Give preschool and early school-age siblings a newborn doll as their baby to care for. Give the sibling a photograph of the new baby to take to school to show off his or her baby. Older siblings may enjoy the responsibility of helping care for the newborn such as learning how to give the baby a bottle or change a diaper. One mother let her preschooler help burp the new baby by patting on the baby's back. She figured her son could pat the baby fairly firmly without harming him and at the same time let out some pent-up aggressive feelings.

grandparents understand and accept current practices can influence how supportive they are perceived to be by their adult children.

COMMUNITY FOCUS

Helping Grandparents Bridge the Generation Gap

Interview a grandfather and grandmother about their experiences with childbirth and infant care. Prepare a "letter to new parents" (written from the grandparents' perspective), which can be included in prenatal kits distributed in childbirth preparation classes and made available to all family members on the postpartum unit. Include how the birth of their adult child occurred, how things are different now, what role the grandparent can play in helping the new parents adjust to home and child care, and what the grandparent might contribute to the family in memories.

While they are adjusting to grandparenthood, most grandparents are experiencing normative middle- and old-age life transition issues such as retirement and a move to smaller housing and need support from their adult children. Some may feel regret about their limited involvement because of poor health or geographic distance. Maternal grandmothers, more so than the other three grandparents, may have high expectations of themselves that cause them to be very self-critical.

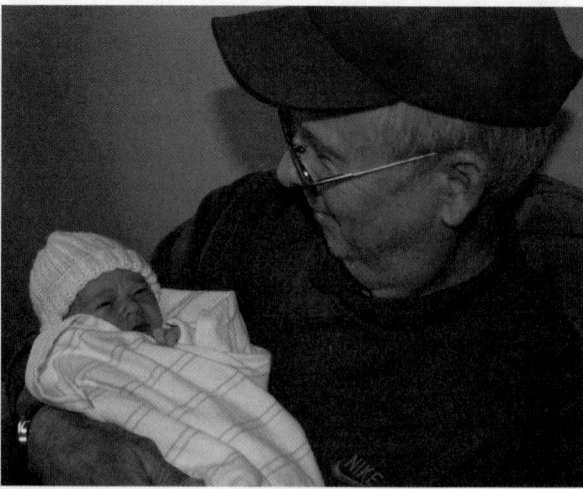

Fig. 22-10 Grandfather and new grandson get acquainted. *(Courtesy William Perry, Phoenix, AZ.)*

The extent of involvement of grandparents in the care of the newborn depends on many factors (e.g., the willingness of the grandparents to become involved, their proximity, and ethnic and cultural expectations of their role) (Fig. 22-10). If the new parents live in the United States, Asian grandparents typically are asked to come to the United States to care for the baby and mother after birth and to care for the children once the parents return to work. In the United States paternal grandparents, in contrast to those in other cultures, frequently consider themselves secondary to the maternal grandparents. Less seems expected of them, and they are initially less involved. Nevertheless these grandparents are eager to help and express great pleasure in their son's fatherhood and his involvement with the baby (Fig. 22-11).

For first-time parents pregnancy and parenthood can reawaken old issues related to dependence vs. independence. Some expectant parents may not plan on their parents' help immediately after the baby arrives. They want time "to be a family," inferring a couple-baby unit, not the intergenerational family network. Intergenerational help may be perceived as interference. However, contrary to their expectations, new parents do call on their parents for help, especially the maternal grandmother. Many grandparents are aware of their adult children's wishes for autonomy, respect these wishes, and remain available to help when asked.

Grandparents' classes can be used to bridge the generation gap and to help the grandparents understand their adult children's parenting concepts. The classes include information on up-to-date childbearing practices; family-centered care; infant care, feeding, and safety (car seats); and exploration of roles that grandparents play in the family unit.

Increasing numbers of grandparents are providing permanent care to their grandchildren as a result of divorce,

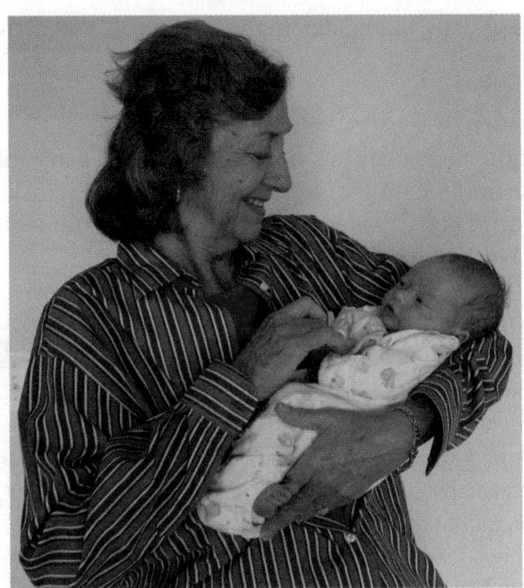

Fig. 22-11 Grandmother becoming acquainted with new grandson. *(Courtesy Diane Nelson, Las Vegas, NV.)*

substance abuse, child abuse and/or neglect, abandonment, teenage pregnancy, death, human immune deficiency virus and acquired immunodeficiency syndrome, unemployment, incarceration, and/or mental health problems. This emerging trend requires the nurse to evaluate the role of the grandparent in parenting the infant. Educational and financial considerations must be addressed, and available support systems identified for these families.

Nursing Care Management

Numerous changes occur during the first weeks of parenthood. Nursing care management should be directed toward helping parents cope with infant care, role changes, altered lifestyle, and change in family structure resulting from the addition of a new baby (see Nursing Process box). Developing skill and confidence in caring for an infant can be anxiety provoking. Anticipatory guidance can help prevent a shock of reality in the transition from hospital or birthing center to home that might negate the parents' joy or cause them undue

NURSING PROCESS: TRANSITION TO PARENTHOOD

Assessment

Assessment should include a psychosocial assessment focusing on the following:

- Parent-infant attachment
- Adjustment to the parental role
- Sibling adjustment
- Social support
- Education needs
- Mother's and baby's physical adaptation

Early home visits are an excellent opportunity for the nurse to assess beginnings of positive or negative parenting behaviors and provide positive reinforcement for loving and nurturing behaviors with the infant.

Parents who interact in inappropriate or abusive ways with their infants should be followed more closely, and an appropriate mental health practitioner or professional social worker should be notified.

Nursing Diagnoses

Readiness for enhanced family coping related to

- positive attitude and realistic expectations for newborn and adapting to parenthood
- nurturing behaviors with newborn
- verbalizing positive factors in lifestyle change

Risk for impaired parenting related to

- lack of knowledge in infant care
- feelings of incompetence and/or lack of confidence
- unrealistic expectations of newborn/infant
- fatigue from interrupted sleep

Ineffective parental role performance related to

- role transition and role attainment
- unwanted pregnancy
- lack of resources to support parenting (e.g., no paid leave)

Risk for impaired parent-infant attachment related to

- difficult labor and birth
- postpartum complications
- neonatal complications/anomalies

Planning

A plan of care is formulated in collaboration with the family that incorporates their priorities and preferences to meet their specific needs.

Expected outcomes for effective transition to parenthood include that the parents will do the following:

- Demonstrate behaviors that reflect appreciation of sensory and behavioral capacities of the infant
- Verbalize increasing confidence and competence in feeding, diapering, dressing, and sensory stimulation of the infant
- Identify deviations from normal in the infant that should be brought to the immediate attention of the primary health care provider
- Relate effectively to the newborn's siblings and grandparents

Interventions

Provide anticipatory guidance on what to expect as newborn grows and develops:

- Infant developmental milestones
- Sensory enrichment/infant stimulation

Provide interventions for promoting parent-infant attachment (see Table 22-3)

Provide suggestions for incorporating grandparents and siblings into interactions with newborn.

Evaluation

Evaluation is based on the expected outcomes of care. The plan is revised as necessary.

evolve Critical Thinking Exercise—Postpartum Home Care

stress. For example, the nurse can teach parents a number of strategies that help quiet a fussy baby, prevent crying, and induce quiet attention or sleep (see also Chapter 36).

Written information reinforcing education topics is helpful to provide to parents, as is a list of available community resources, both local and national. Classes in the prenatal period or during the postpartum stay are helpful. Instructions for the first days at home should include at a minimum activities of daily living, dealing with visitors, and activity and rest.

Recognizing Signs of Illness

In addition to explaining the need for well-baby follow-up visits, the nurse should discuss with parents the signs of illness in newborns. See Chapter 25 for specifics regarding this teaching (see Nursing Care Plan).

evolve Nursing Care Plan—Home Care Follow-Up: Transition to Parenthood

NURSING CARE PLAN Home Care Follow-Up: Transition to Parenthood

Nursing Diagnosis: Disturbed sleep pattern related to infant demands and environmental interruptions

Expected Outcomes

Woman sleeps for uninterrupted periods and feels rested on waking.

Nursing Interventions/*Rationales*

Discuss woman's routine and specify things that interfere with sleep *to determine scope of problem and direct interventions.*

Explore ways woman and significant others can make environment more conducive to sleep (e.g., privacy, darkness, quiet, back rubs, soothing music, warm milk); teach use of guided imagery and relaxation techniques *to promote optimal conditions for sleep.*

Eliminate things or routines (e.g., caffeine, foods that induce heartburn, strenuous mental/physical activity) *that may interfere with sleep.*

Advise family to limit visitors and activities *to avoid further taxation and fatigue.*

Have family plan specific times to care for the newborn *to allow mother time to sleep*; have mother learn to use infant nap time as a time for her to nap as well as *to replenish energy and decrease fatigue.*

Nursing Diagnosis: Risk for impaired home maintenance related to addition of new family member/inadequate resources/inadequate support systems

Expected Outcome

Home exhibits signs of safe and functional environment.

Nursing Interventions/*Rationales*

Observe the home environment (e.g., available living space and sleeping arrangements; adequacy of facilities for food preparation and storage, hygiene, and toileting; overall state of repair; cleanliness; presence of safety hazards) *to determine adequacy and effective use of resources.*

Observe arrangements for the newborn such as sleeping space, care equipment, and supplies (bathing, changing, feeding, transportation) *to determine adequacy of resources.*

Explore who is responsible for cooking, cleaning, child care, and newborn care and determine whether the mother seems adequately rested *to determine adequacy of support systems.*

Identify and arrange referrals to needed social agencies (e.g., Aid to Families with Dependent Children, Women, Infants, and Children program, food pantries) *to address resource deficits (finances, supplies, equipment).*

Nursing Diagnosis: Risk for interrupted family processes related to inclusion of new family member

Expected Outcome

Infant is successfully assimilated into family structure.

Nursing Interventions/*Rationales*

Explore with family the ways that the birth and neonate have changed family structure and function *to evaluate functional and role adjustment.*

Observe family interaction with the newborn and note degree of bonding, evidence of sibling rivalry, and involvement in newborn care *to evaluate acceptance of newest family member.*

Clarify identified misinformation and misperceptions *to promote clear communication.*

Assist family to explore options for solutions to identified problems *to promote effective problem resolution.*

Support family efforts as they move toward adjusting and incorporating the new member *to reinforce new functions and roles.*

If needed, make referrals to appropriate social services or community agencies *to ensure ongoing support and care.*

Key Points

- The birth of a child necessitates changes in the existing interactional structure of a family.
- Attachment is the process by which the parent and infant come to love and accept each other.
- Attachment is strengthened through the use of sensual responses or interactions by both partners in the parent-infant interaction.

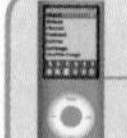

Audio Chapter Summaries

Access an audio summary of these Key Points on evolve

- In adjusting to the parental role, the mother moves from a dependent state (taking in) to an interdependent state (letting go).

- Mothers may exhibit signs of postpartum blues (baby blues) or PPD.
- Fathers experience emotions and adjustments during the transition to parenthood that are similar to and also distinctly different from those of mothers.
- Modulation of rhythm, modification of behavioral repertoires, and mutual responsivity facilitate infant-parent adjustment.
- Many factors (e.g., age, culture, socioeconomic level, and expectations of what the child will be like) influence adaptation to parenthood.
- Parents face a number of tasks related to sibling adjustment that require creative parental interventions.
- Grandparents can have a positive influence on the postpartum family.

References

Alhusen JL: A literature update on maternal-fetal attachment, *J Obstet Gynecol Neonatal Nurs* 37(5):315-328, 2008.

D'Avanzo C: *Mosby's pocket guide to cultural health assessment*, ed 4, St Louis, 2008, Mosby.

Deave T, Johnson D: The transition to parenthood: what does it mean for fathers? *J Adv Nurs* 63(6):626-633, 2008.

Deave T, Johnson D, Ingram J: Transition to parenthood: the needs of parents in pregnancy and early parenthood, *BMC Pregnancy Childbirth* 8:30, 2008. Available at www.biomedcentral.com/1471-2393/8/30 (accessed April 5, 2009).

Erlandsson K et al: Skin-to-skin care with the father after cesarean birth and its effect on newborn crying and prefeeding behavior, *Birth* 34(2):105-114, 2007.

Galanti G: *Caring for patients from different cultures*, ed 3, Philadelphia, 2003, University of Pennsylvania Press.

Gathwaia G, Singh B, Balhara B: KMC facilitates mother baby attachment in low birth weight infants, *Indian J Pediatr* 75(1):43-47, 2008.

Goodman JH: Paternal postpartum depression, its relationship to maternal postpartum depression, and implications for family health, *J Adv Nurs* 45(1):26-35, 2004.

Keating-Lefler R, Wilson M: The experience of becoming a mother for single, unpartnered, Medicaid-eligible, first-time mothers, *J Nurs Sch* 36(1):23-29, 2004.

Klaus M, Kennell J: *Maternal-infant bonding*, St Louis, 1976, Mosby.

Klaus M, Kennell J: *Parent-infant bonding*, ed 2, St Louis, 1982, Mosby.

Maputie MS: Becoming a mother: teenage mothers' experiences of first pregnancy, *Curationis* 29(2):87-95, 2006.

Mercer RT: Becoming a mother versus maternal role attainment, *J Nurs Sch* 36(3):226-232, 2004.

Mercer RT: Nursing support of the process of becoming a mother, *J Obstet Gynecol Neonatal Nurs* 35(5):649-651, 2006.

Mercer RT, Walker LO: A review of nursing interventions to foster becoming a mother, *J Obstet Gynecol Neonatal Nurs* 35(5):568-582, 2006.

Moore ER, Anderson GC, Bergman N: Early skin-to-skin contact for mothers and their healthy newborn infants, *Cochrane Database Syst Rev* 18(3):CD003519, 2007.

Nelson A: Transition to motherhood, *J Obstet Gynecol Neonatal Nurs* 32(4):465-477, 2003.

Nystedt A, Högberg U, Lundman B: Women's experiences of becoming a mother after prolonged labour, *J Adv Nurs* 63(3):250-258, 2008.

Premberg A, Hellström AL, Berg H: Experiences of the first year as father, *Scand J Caring Sci* 22(1):56-63, 2008.

Rubin R: Basic maternal behavior, *Nurs Outlook* 9:683-686, 1961.

Rubin R: Attainment of the maternal role. Part 1: Processes, *Nurs Res* 16(4):237-245, 1967.

Shin H, Park YJ, Kim MJ: Predictors of maternal sensitivity during the early postpartum period, *J Adv Nurs* 55(4):425-434, 2006.

St. John W, Cameron C, McVeigh C: Meeting the challenges of new fatherhood during the early weeks, *J Obstet Gynecol Neonatal Nurs* 34(2):180-190, 2005.

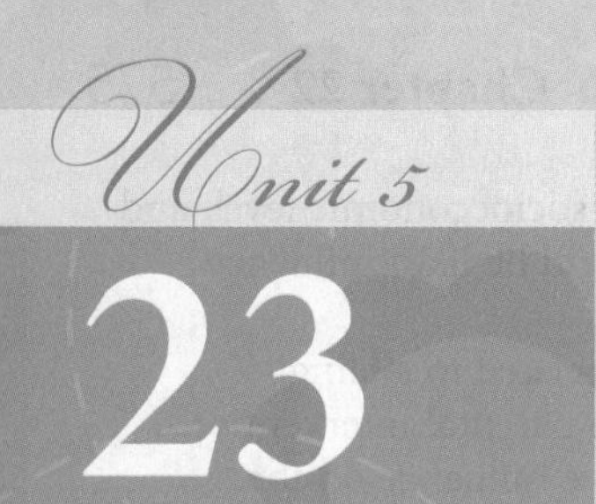

Postpartum Complications

Learning Objectives

On completion of this chapter the reader will be able to:

- Identify causes, signs and symptoms, possible complications, and medical and nursing management of postpartum hemorrhage.
- Describe hemorrhagic shock as a complication of postpartum hemorrhage, including management and hazards of therapy.
- Identify causes, signs and symptoms, possible complications, and medical and nursing management of postpartum infection.
- Describe thromboembolic disorders, including incidence, etiology, signs and symptoms, and management.
- Summarize the role of the nurse in the home setting in assessing potential problems and managing care of women with postpartum complications.
- Discuss emotional complications of pregnancy, including management of mood disorders.
- Differentiate among postpartum emotional complications, including incidence, risk factors, signs and symptoms, severity, and management.
- Describe emotional, behavioral, cognitive, and physical responses commonly experienced during the grieving process associated with perinatal loss.
- Identify specific nursing interventions to meet the special needs of parents and their families related to perinatal loss and grief.
- Differentiate among helpful and unhelpful responses in caring for parents experiencing loss and grief.

Electronic Resources

Additional information related to the content in Chapter 23 can be found on

evolve the Companion Website at http://evolve.elsevier.com/Perry/maternal/

- NCLEX Review Questions
- Critical Thinking Exercise—Postpartum Depression
- Nursing Care Plan—Fetal Death: 24 Weeks of Gestation
- Nursing Care Plan—Postpartum Depression
- Nursing Care Plan—Postpartum Hemorrhage

Providing safe and effective care of the woman and family experiencing postpartum physical and psychologic complications, sequelae of childbirth trauma, or grief related to perinatal loss requires a collaborative effort from all members of the health care team. This chapter focuses on the postpartum complications of hemorrhage and infection, sequelae of childbirth trauma, psychologic complications, and loss and grief.

Postpartum Hemorrhage

Definition and Incidence

Postpartum hemorrhage (PPH) is a leading cause of maternal morbidity and mortality in the United States and worldwide today. It is a life-threatening event that can occur with little warning and is often unrecognized until the mother has profound symptoms. PPH traditionally has been defined as the loss of 500 ml or more of blood after vaginal birth and 1000 ml or more after cesarean birth. Either a 10% change in hematocrit between admission for labor and postpartum or the need for erythrocyte transfusion has also been used to define PPH (Francois & Foley, 2007). It has been classified as early or late with respect to the birth. Early, acute, or primary PPH occurs within 24 hours of the birth. Late or secondary PPH occurs more than 24 hours but less than 6 weeks after the birth (Francois & Foley, 2007). Today's health care environment encourages shortened hospital stays after birth, which increases the potential for acute episodes of PPH to occur outside the traditional hospital or birth center setting.

Etiology and Risk Factors

Excessive bleeding can be considered with reference to the stages of labor. From birth of the fetus until separation of the placenta the character and quantity of blood passed may suggest excessive bleeding. For example, dark blood is probably of venous origin, perhaps from varices or superficial lacerations of the birth canal. Bright blood is arterial and may indicate deep lacerations of the cervix. Spurts of blood with clots may indicate partial placental separation. Failure of blood to clot or remain clotted indicates a pathologic condition or coagulopathy such as disseminated intravascular coagulation (DIC) (see later discussion).

Excessive bleeding may occur during the period from the separation of the placenta to its expulsion or removal. Commonly such bleeding is the result of incomplete placental separation, undue manipulation of the fundus, or excessive traction on the cord. After the placenta has been expelled or removed, persistent or excessive blood loss most commonly is a result of atony of the uterus (i.e., failure to contract well or maintain contraction) or prolapse of the uterus into the vagina. Late PPH most commonly is the result of infection, subinvolution of the placental site, retained placental tissue, or coagulopathy (Francois & Foley, 2007). Risk factors for and causes of PPH are listed in Box 23-1.

Uterine Atony

Uterine atony is marked hypotonia of the uterus. Normally placental separation and expulsion are facilitated by contraction of the uterus, which also prevents hemorrhage from the placental site. The uterine corpus is in essence a basket weave of strong, interlacing smooth-muscle bundles through which many large maternal blood vessels pass (see Fig. 5-3). If the uterus is flaccid after detachment of all or part of the placenta, brisk venous bleeding occurs, and normal coagulation of the open vasculature is impaired and continues until the uterine muscle is contracted.

BOX 23-1 Risk Factors and Causes of Postpartum Hemorrhage

Uterine atony
- Overdistended uterus—Large fetus, multiple fetuses, hydramnios, distention with clots
- Anesthesia and analgesia—Conduction anesthesia
- Previous history of uterine atony
- High parity
- Prolonged labor, oxytocin-induced labor
- Trauma during labor and birth—Forceps-assisted birth, vacuum-assisted birth, cesarean birth

Lacerations of the birth canal
Retained placental fragments
Ruptured uterus
Inversion of the uterus
Placenta accreta, increta, percreta
Coagulation disorders
Placental abruption
Placenta previa
Manual removal of a retained placenta
Magnesium sulfate administration during labor or postpartum period
Chorioamnionitis
Uterine subinvolution

Uterine atony is the leading cause of early PPH, complicating approximately 1 in 20 births (Francois & Foley, 2007). It is associated with high parity, hydramnios, a macrosomic fetus, and multifetal gestation. In such conditions the uterus is "overstretched" and contracts poorly after birth. Other causes of atony include traumatic birth, use of halogenated anesthesia (e.g., halothane) or magnesium sulfate, rapid or prolonged labor, chorioamnionitis, use of oxytocin for labor induction or augmentation, and uterine atony in a previous pregnancy (Francois & Foley, 2007).

Lacerations of the Genital Tract

Lacerations of the cervix, vagina, and perineum are also causes of PPH. Hemorrhage related to lacerations should be suspected if bleeding continues despite a firm, contracted uterine fundus. This bleeding can be a slow trickle, an oozing, or frank hemorrhage.

Factors that influence the causes and incidence of obstetric lacerations of the lower genital tract include operative birth, precipitous birth, congenital abnormalities of the maternal soft parts, and contracted pelvis. Size, abnormal presentation, and position of the fetus; relative size of the presenting part and the birth canal; previous scarring from infection, injury, or surgery; and vulvar, perineal, and vaginal varicosities can also cause lacerations.

Extreme vascularity in the labia and periclitoral areas often results in profuse bleeding if laceration occurs. Hematomas may also be present.

Lacerations of the perineum are the most common of all injuries in the lower portion of the genital tract. These are classified as first, second, third, and fourth degree (see Chapter 18). An episiotomy may extend to become either a third- or fourth-degree laceration.

Prolonged pressure of the fetal head on the vaginal mucosa ultimately interferes with the circulation and may produce ischemic or pressure necrosis. The state of the tissues in combination with the type of birth may result in deep vaginal lacerations, with consequent predisposition to vaginal hematomas.

After the bleeding has been controlled, the care of the woman with lacerations of the perineum is similar to that for women with episiotomies (i.e., analgesia as needed for pain and hot or cold applications as necessary). The need for increased roughage in the diet and increased intake of fluids is emphasized. Stool softeners may be used to assist the woman in reestablishing bowel habits without straining and putting stress on the suture lines.

NURSING ALERT To avoid injury to the suture line, a woman with third- or fourth-degree lacerations is not given rectal suppositories or enemas.

Hematomas

Pelvic hematomas (i.e., a collection of blood in the connective tissue) may be vulvar, vaginal, or retroperitoneal in origin.

Vulvar hematomas are the most common. Pain is the most common symptom, and most vulvar hematomas are visible. Vaginal hematomas occur more commonly in association with a forceps-assisted birth, an episiotomy, or primigravidity (Francois & Foley, 2007).

Retroperitoneal hematomas are the least common but are life threatening. They are caused by laceration of one of the vessels attached to the hypogastric artery, usually associated with rupture of a cesarean scar during labor. During the postpartum period, if the woman reports a persistent perineal or rectal pain or a feeling of pressure in the vagina, a careful examination is made. However, a retroperitoneal hematoma may cause minimal pain, and the initial symptoms may be signs of shock (Francois & Foley, 2007).

Cervical lacerations usually occur at the lateral angles of the external os. Most are shallow, and bleeding is minimal. More extensive lacerations may extend into the vaginal vault or the lower uterine segment.

Hematomas are usually surgically evacuated. Once the bleeding has been controlled, usual postpartum care is provided with attention to pain relief, monitoring amount of bleeding, replacing fluids, and reviewing laboratory results (hemoglobin and hematocrit).

Retained Placenta

Nonadherent Retained Placenta

Nonadherent retained placenta may result from partial separation of a normal placenta, entrapment of the partially or completely separated placenta by an hourglass constriction ring of the uterus, mismanagement of the third stage of labor, or abnormal adherence of the entire placenta or a portion of the placenta to the uterine wall. Placental retention because of poor separation is common in very preterm births (20 to 24 weeks of gestation).

Management of nonadherent retained placenta is by manual separation and removal by the primary health care provider. Supplementary anesthesia is usually not needed for women who have had regional anesthesia for birth. For other women administration of light nitrous oxide and oxygen inhalation anesthesia or intravenous (IV) thiopental facilitates intrauterine exploration and placental separation. After this removal the woman is at continued risk for PPH and infection.

Adherent Retained Placenta

Abnormal adherence of the placenta occurs for unknown reasons, but it is thought to result from zygote implantation in an area of defective endometrium so that no zone of separation exists between the placenta and the decidua. The incidence of placenta accreta is increasing as a result of the rise in cesarean birth rates (Oyelese & Smulian, 2006). Attempts to remove the placenta in the usual manner are unsuccessful, and laceration or perforation of the uterine wall may result, putting the woman at great risk for severe PPH and infection (Francois & Foley, 2007).

Unusual placental adherence may be partial or complete. The following degrees of attachment are recognized:

Placenta accreta—Slight penetration of myometrium by placental trophoblast

Placenta increta—Deep penetration of myometrium by placenta

Placenta percreta—Perforation of uterus by placenta

Bleeding with complete or total placenta accreta may not occur unless separation of the placenta is attempted. With more extensive involvement bleeding becomes profuse when delivery of the placenta is attempted. There is less blood loss if the diagnosis is made antenatally and no attempt is made to remove the placenta (Wong et al, 2008). Treatment includes blood component replacement therapy; hysterectomy may be indicated (Francois & Foley, 2007).

Inversion of the Uterus

Inversion (turning inside out) of the uterus after birth is a potentially life-threatening complication. The incidence of uterine inversion is approximately 1 in 2500 births (Francois & Foley, 2007) and may recur with a subsequent birth. Uterine inversion may be incomplete, complete, or prolapsed. Incomplete inversion cannot be seen but must be felt; a smooth mass can be palpated through the dilated cervix. In complete inversion the lining of the fundus crosses through the cervical os and forms a mass in the vagina. Prolapsed inversion of the uterus is obvious; a large, red, rounded mass (perhaps with the placenta attached) protrudes 20 to 30 cm outside the introitus.

Contributing factors to uterine inversion include fundal implantation of the placenta, vigorous fundal pressure, excessive traction applied to the cord, fetal macrosomia, tocolysis, prolonged labor, uterine atony, and abnormally adherent placental tissue (Francois & Foley, 2007). Uterine inversion occurs most often in multiparous women and with placenta accreta or increta. The primary presenting signs of uterine inversion are hemorrhage, shock, and pain. The uterus must be replaced into its proper position.

Prevention—always the easiest, cheapest, and most effective therapy—is especially appropriate for uterine inversion. The umbilical cord should not be pulled on unless the placenta has definitely separated.

Uterine inversion is an emergency situation requiring immediate recognition, maternal fluid resuscitation, replacement of the uterus within the pelvic cavity, and correction of associated clinical conditions. Tocolytics or halogenated anesthetics may be given to relax the uterus before attempting replacement (Francois & Foley, 2007). Oxytocic agents are given after the uterus is repositioned; broad-spectrum antibiotics are initiated. The woman's response to treatment is observed closely to prevent shock or fluid overload. If the uterus has been repositioned manually, care must be taken to avoid aggressive fundal massage.

Subinvolution of the Uterus

Late postpartum bleeding may occur as a result of subinvolution of the uterus (delayed return of the enlarged uterus to normal size and function). Recognized causes of subinvolution include retained placental fragments and pelvic infection. Signs and symptoms include prolonged lochial discharge, irregular or excessive bleeding, and sometimes hemorrhage. A pelvic examination usually reveals a larger-than-normal uterus that may be boggy.

Treatment of subinvolution depends on the cause. Ergonovine 0.2 mg every 4 hours for 2 or 3 days and antibiotic therapy are the most common medications used. Dilation and curettage (D&C) may be needed to remove retained placental fragments or to debride the placental site.

BOX 23-2 Noninvasive Assessments of Cardiac Output in Postpartum Patients Who Are Bleeding

Palpation of pulses (rate, quality, equality)
- Arterial
- Blood pressure

Auscultation
- Heart sounds/murmurs
- Breath sounds

Inspection
- Skin color, temperature, turgor
- Level of consciousness
- Capillary refill
- Urinary output
- Neck veins
- Pulse oximetry
- Mucous membranes

Presence or absence of anxiety, apprehension, restlessness, disorientation

Nursing Care Management

PPH may be sudden and even exsanguinating (see Nursing Process box). The nurse must be alert to the symptoms of hemorrhage and hypovolemic shock and be prepared to act quickly to minimize blood loss (Box 23-2).

Late PPH develops at least 24 hours after birth or later in the postpartum period. The woman may be at home when the symptoms occur. Discharge teaching should emphasize the signs of both normal involution and potential complications.

NURSING PROCESS: POSTPARTUM HEMORRHAGE

Assessment

Review history for factors that predispose woman to postpartum hemorrhage (PPH)

Assess the following:
- Fundus for consistency and height
- Bleeding for color and amount
- Perineum for signs of lacerations or hematomas
- Vital signs (VSs) (VSs may not be reliable indicator of shock because of physiologic adaptations of this period)
- Frequent VS checks may identify trends related to blood loss (tachycardia, tachypnea, decreasing blood pressure)
- Bladder for distention (distended bladder can displace uterus and prevent uterine contraction)
- Skin for warmth and dryness; nail beds for color and capillary refill

Laboratory studies (hemoglobin and hematocrit)

Nursing Diagnoses

Nursing diagnoses for women experiencing PPH include the following:

Deficient fluid volume related to
- excessive blood loss secondary to uterine atony, lacerations, or uterine inversion

Risk for injury (maternal) related to
- attempted manual removal of retained placenta
- administration of blood products
- operative procedures

Risk for impaired parenting related to
- separation from infant secondary to treatment regimen

Ineffective peripheral tissue perfusion related to
- excessive blood loss and shunting of blood to central circulation

Planning

Early recognition and diagnosis of PPH is critical to care management. Care is planned in collaboration with the primary health care provider.

Expected outcomes for the woman experiencing PPH include that she will do the following:
- Maintain normal vital signs and laboratory values
- Develop no complications related to excessive bleeding
- Verbalize understanding of her condition, its management, and discharge instructions
- Identify and use available support systems

Interventions

Massage fundus.

Empty bladder; monitor urinary output.

Ensure intravenous access.

Administer oxytocin or other drugs to stimulate uterine contraction per standing orders or protocols (see Medication Guide).

Notify primary health care provider.

Implement interventions to monitor or improve tissue perfusion (see Nursing Care Plan).

Provide fluid/blood replacement therapy as ordered.

Provide explanations to woman and family about interventions being performed and the need to act quickly.

Provide discharge instructions:
- Woman may feel fatigue and exhaustion because of blood loss.
- Limit activities to conserve strength.
- Increase dietary iron and protein intake; iron supplements may be ordered.

Observe for delayed or insufficient lactation and postpartum depression.

Refer for home care or to community resources.

Evaluation

The nurse can be reasonably assured that care was effective to the extent that the expected outcomes have been achieved (see Nursing Care Plan).

NURSING CARE PLAN Postpartum Hemorrhage

Nursing Diagnosis: Deficient fluid volume related to postpartum hemorrhage

Expected Outcome

Woman will demonstrate fluid balance as evidenced by stable vital signs, prompt capillary refill time, and balanced intake and output.

Nursing Interventions/*Rationales*

Monitor vital signs, oxygen saturation, urine specific gravity, and capillary refill *to provide baseline data.*

Measure and record amount and type of bleeding by weighing and counting saturated pads. If woman is at home, teach her to count pads and save any clots or tissue. If woman is admitted to hospital, save any clots and tissue for further examination *to estimate type and amount of blood loss for fluid replacement.*

Provide quiet environment *to promote rest and decrease metabolic demands.*

Give explanation of all procedures *to reduce anxiety.*

Begin intravenous access with 18-gauge or larger needle for infusion of isotonic solution as ordered *to provide fluid or blood replacement.*

Administer medications as ordered such as oxytocin, methylergonovine (Methergine), or prostaglandin $F_{2\alpha}$ (Prostin) as ordered *to increase contractility of the uterus.*

Insert indwelling urinary catheter *to provide most accurate assessment of renal function and hypovolemia.*

Prepare for surgical intervention as needed *to stop the source of bleeding.*

Nursing Diagnosis: Ineffective tissue perfusion related to hypovolemia

Expected Outcome

Woman will have stable vital signs, oxygen saturation, arterial blood gases, and adequate hematocrit and hemoglobin.

Nursing Interventions/*Rationales*

Monitor vital signs, oxygen saturation, arterial blood gases, and hematocrit and hemoglobin *to assess for hypovolemic shock and decreased tissue perfusion.*

Assess for any changes in level of consciousness *to assess for evidence of hypoxia.*

Assess capillary refill, mucous membranes, and skin temperature *to note indicators of vasoconstriction.*

Give supplementary oxygen as ordered *to provide additional oxygenation to tissues.*

Suction as needed, insert oral airway *to maintain clear, open airway for oxygenation.*

Monitor arterial blood gases *to provide information about acidosis or hypoxia.*

Administer sodium bicarbonate if ordered *to reverse metabolic acidosis.*

Nursing Diagnosis: Anxiety related to sudden change in health status

Expected Outcome

Woman will verbalize that anxious feelings are diminished.

Nursing Interventions/*Rationales*

Using therapeutic communication, evaluate woman's understanding of events *to provide clarification of any misconceptions.*

Provide calm, competent attitude and environment *to aid in decreasing anxiety.*

Explain all procedures *to decrease anxiety about the unknown.*

Allow woman to verbalize feelings *to permit clarification of information and promote trust.*

Continue to assess vital signs or other clinical indicators of hypovolemic shock *to evaluate if psychologic response of anxiety intensifies physiologic indicators.*

Keep family informed of condition *to enable them to provide support.*

Early recognition and diagnosis of PPH is critical to care management. The first step is to evaluate the contractility of the uterus. If the uterus is hypotonic, management is directed toward increasing contractility and minimizing blood loss.

The initial management of excessive postpartum bleeding is firm massage of the uterine fundus, expression of any clots in the uterus, eliminating bladder distention, and continuous IV infusion of 10 to 40 units of oxytocin in 1000 ml of Ringer's lactate or normal saline solution. If the uterus fails to respond to oxytocin, a dose of 0.2 mg ergonovine (Ergotrate) or methylergonovine (Methergine) may be given intramuscularly to produce sustained uterine contractions. However, it is more common to administer a 0.25-mg dose of a derivative of prostaglandin $F_{2\alpha}$ (carboprost tromethamine) intramuscularly. It also can be given intramyometrially at cesarean birth or intraabdominally after vaginal birth. Oral (400 to 800 mcg) and rectal (1000 mcg) misoprostol has also been administered, but there is no consensus about efficacy for management of PPH (Gülmezoglu et al, 2009; Magann & Lanneau, 2005). Recombinant factor VIIa may also be useful in managing PPH but requires testing in clinical trials (McLintock, 2005). See Medication Guide for a comparison of medications used to manage PPH. In addition to the medications used to contract the uterus, rapid administration of crystalloid solutions and/or blood or blood products are needed to restore the woman's intravascular volume (Francois & Foley, 2007).

NURSING ALERT Use of ergonovine or methylergonovine is contraindicated in the presence of hypertension or cardiovascular disease. Prostaglandin $F_{2\alpha}$ should be used cautiously in women with cardiovascular disease or asthma.

Hypotonic Uterus

Oxygen can be given to enhance oxygen delivery to the cells. A urinary catheter is usually inserted to monitor urine output as a measure of intravascular volume. Laboratory studies

MEDICATION GUIDE: Medications Used to Manage Postpartum Hemorrhage

Oxytocin (Pitocin)

Drug Action
Contraction of uterus; decreases bleeding

Side Effects
Infrequent: water intoxication; nausea and vomiting

Contraindications
None for postpartum hemorrhage

Dosage and Route
10 to 40 units/L diluted in lactated Ringer's solution or normal saline at 125 to 200 mU/min IV or 10 to 20 units IM

Nursing Considerations
Continue to monitor vaginal bleeding and uterine tone.

*Methylergonovine (Methergine)**

Drug Action
Contraction of uterus

Side Effects
Hypertension, nausea, vomiting, headache

Contraindications
Hypertension, cardiac disease

Dosage and Route
0.2 mg IM every 2 to 4 hours up to five doses; 0.2 mg IV only for emergency

Nursing Considerations
Check blood pressure before giving and do not give if more than 140/90 mm Hg; continue monitoring vaginal bleeding and uterine tone.

Prostaglandin $F_{2\alpha}$ (Prostin/15M; Hemabate)

Drug Action
Contraction of uterus

Side Effects
Headache, nausea and vomiting, fever, tachycardia, hypertension, diarrhea

Contraindications
Asthma, hypersensitivity

Dosage and Route
0.25 mg IM or intramyometrially every 15 to 90 minutes up to eight doses

Nursing Considerations
Continue to monitor vaginal bleeding and uterine tone.

Misoprostol (Cytotec)†

Drug Action
Contraction of uterus

Side Effects
Headache, nausea and vomiting, diarrhea

Contraindications
History of allergy to prostaglandins

Dosage and Route
400 mcg orally (range 200 to 800 mcg) or 600 to 1000 mcg rectally

Nursing Considerations
Continue to monitor vaginal bleeding and uterine tone.

IM, Intramuscularly; *IV*, intravenously.
*Information about methylergonovine may also be used to describe ergonovine (Ergotrate).
†Off-label use; research reports vary in conclusions about dosage and efficacy of use in comparison to other drugs used to manage postpartum hemorrhage.

usually include a complete blood count with platelet count, fibrinogen, fibrin split products, prothrombin time, and partial thromboplastin time. Blood type and antibody screen are done if not previously performed.

If bleeding persists, the obstetrician or nurse-midwife may consider bimanual compression. This procedure involves inserting a fist into the vagina and pressing the knuckles against the anterior side of the uterus while placing the other hand on the abdomen and massaging the posterior uterus. If the uterus still does not become firm, the uterine cavity is explored manually for retained placental fragments. If the preceding procedures are ineffective, surgical management may be the only alternative. Surgical management options include vessel ligation (i.e., uteroovarian, uterine, and hypogastric), selective arterial embolization, and hysterectomy (Francois & Foley, 2007).

Bleeding with a Contracted Uterus

If the uterus is firmly contracted and bleeding continues, the source of bleeding still needs to be identified and treated. Assessment may include visual or manual inspection of the perineum, vagina, cervix, or rectum and laboratory studies (e.g., hemoglobin, hematocrit, coagulation studies, and platelet count). Treatment depends on the source of the bleeding.

Herbal Remedies

Herbal remedies to control PPH have been used with some success in some settings. Some herbs have homeostatic actions, whereas others work as oxytocic agents to contract the uterus. Table 23-1 lists herbs that have been used and their actions. However, published evidence of the safety and efficacy of herbal therapy is lacking. Evidence from well-controlled studies is needed before recommendation for practice should be made (Skidmore-Roth, 2006).

Hemorrhagic (Hypovolemic) Shock

Hemorrhage may result in hemorrhagic (hypovolemic) shock. Shock is an emergency situation in which the perfusion of

Table 23-1 Herbal Remedies for Postpartum Hemorrhage

HERBS	ACTION
Witch hazel	Homeostatic
Lady's mantle	Homeostatic
Blue cohosh	Oxytocic
Cotton root bark	Oxytocic
Motherwort	Promotes uterine contraction; vasoconstrictive
Shepherd's purse	Promotes uterine contraction
Alfalfa leaf	Increases availability of vitamin K; increases hemoglobin
Nettle	Increases availability of vitamin K; increases hemoglobin
Red raspberry leaves	Homeostatic; promotes uterine contraction

Source: Schirmer G: *Herbal medicine*, Bedford, TX, 1998, MED2000; and Weed S: *Wise woman herbal for the childbearing years*, Woodstock, NY, 1986, Ash Tree.

EMERGENCY

Hemorrhagic Shock

Assessments	**Characteristics**
Respirations	Rapid and shallow
Pulse	Rapid, weak, irregular
Blood pressure	Decreasing (late sign)
Skin	Cool, pale, clammy
Urinary output	Decreasing
Level of consciousness	Lethargy → coma
Mental status	Anxiety → coma
Central venous pressure	Decreased

Intervention

Summon assistance and equipment

Start IV infusion per standing orders

Ensure patent airway; administer oxygen

Continue to monitor status

body organs may become severely compromised; death may occur. Physiologic compensatory mechanisms are activated in response to hemorrhage. The adrenal glands release catecholamines, causing arterioles and venules in the skin, lungs, gastrointestinal tract, liver, and kidneys to constrict. The available blood flow is diverted to the brain and heart and away from other organs, including the uterus. If shock is prolonged, the continued reduction in cellular oxygenation results in an accumulation of lactic acid and acidosis (from anaerobic glucose metabolism). Acidosis (lowered serum pH) causes arteriolar vasodilation; venule vasoconstriction persists. A circular pattern is established (i.e., decreased perfusion, increased tissue anoxia and acidosis, edema formation, and pooling of blood further decrease the perfusion). Cellular death occurs. See the Emergency box for assessments and interventions for hemorrhagic shock.

Medical Management

Vigorous treatment is necessary to prevent adverse sequelae. Management of hypovolemic shock involves restoring circulating blood volume and eliminating the cause of the hemorrhage (e.g., lacerations, uterine atony, or inversion). To restore circulating blood volume, a rapid IV infusion of crystalloid solution is given at a rate of 3 ml infused for every 1 ml of estimated blood loss (e.g., 3000 ml infused for 1000 ml of blood loss). Packed red blood cells (RBCs) are usually infused if the woman is still actively bleeding and no improvement in her condition is noted after the initial crystalloid infusion. Infusion of fresh frozen plasma may be needed if clotting factors and platelet counts are below normal values (Cunningham et al, 2005).

Nursing Interventions

Hemorrhagic shock can occur rapidly, but the classic signs of shock may not appear until the postpartum woman has lost 30% to 40% of blood volume. The nurse must continue to reassess the woman's condition as evidenced by the degree of measurable and anticipated blood loss and mobilize appropriate resources.

Most interventions are instituted to improve or monitor tissue perfusion. The nurse continues to monitor the woman's pulse and blood pressure. If invasive hemodynamic monitoring is ordered, the nurse may assist with placement of a central venous pressure (CVP) or pulmonary artery (Swan-Ganz) catheter. The nurse would then monitor CVP, pulmonary artery pressure, or pulmonary artery wedge pressure as ordered.

Additional assessments to be made include evaluation of skin temperature, color, and turgor and assessment of the woman's mucous membranes. If possible, breath sounds should be auscultated before fluid volume replacement to provide a baseline for future assessment. Inspection for oozing at the sites of incisions or injections and assessment of the presence of petechiae or ecchymosis in areas not associated with surgery or trauma are critical in the evaluation for DIC (see later discussion).

Oxygen is administered, preferably by a nonrebreathing face mask, at 10 to 12 L/min to maintain oxygen saturation. Oxygen saturation should be monitored with a pulse oximeter, although measurements may not always be accurate in a patient with hypovolemia or decreased perfusion. Level of consciousness is assessed frequently and provides additional indications of blood volume and oxygen saturation. In early stages of decreased blood flow, the woman may report "seeing stars" or feeling dizzy or nauseated. She may become restless and orthopneic. As cerebral hypoxia increases, she may become confused and react slowly to stimuli or not at all. Some women complain of headaches. An improved sensorium is an indicator of improved perfusion.

Continuous electrocardiographic monitoring may be indicated for the woman who is hypotensive or tachycardic, continues to bleed profusely, or is in shock. A Foley catheter with a urometer is inserted to allow hourly assessment of urine output. The most objective and least invasive assessment of adequate organ perfusion and oxygenation is a urine output of at least 30 ml/hr. Blood may be drawn and sent to the laboratory for studies that include hemoglobin and hematocrit levels, platelet count, and coagulation profile.

Fluid or Blood Replacement Therapy

Critical to successful management of the woman with a hemorrhagic complication is establishment of venous access, preferably with a large-bore IV catheter. The establishment of two IV lines facilitates fluid resuscitation. Vigorous fluid resuscitation includes the administration of crystalloids (lactated Ringer's, normal saline solution), colloids (albumin), blood, and blood components. Fluid resuscitation must be monitored carefully because fluid overload can occur. Intravascular fluid overload occurs most often with colloid therapy.

Transfusion reactions may follow administration of blood or blood components, including cryoprecipitates. Even in an emergency, each unit of fluid should be checked per hospital protocol. Complications of fluid or blood replacement therapy include hemolytic reactions, febrile reactions, allergic reactions, circulatory overloading, and air embolism.

LEGAL TIP Standard of Care for Bleeding Emergencies The standard of care for obstetric emergency situations such as PPH or hypovolemic shock is that provision should be made for the nurse to implement nursing actions independently. Policies, procedures, standing orders or protocols, and clinical guidelines should be established by each health care facility in which births occur and should be agreed on by health care providers involved in the care of obstetric patients.

Coagulopathies

When bleeding is continuous and there is no identifiable source, a coagulopathy may be the cause. The woman's coagulation status must be assessed quickly and continuously. The nurse may draw and send blood to the laboratory for studies. Abnormal results depend on the cause and may include increased prothrombin time, increased partial thromboplastin time, decreased platelets, decreased fibrinogen level, increased fibrin degradation products, and prolonged bleeding time. Causes of coagulopathies may be pregnancy complications such as idiopathic or immune thrombocytopenic purpura (ITP), von Willebrand (vW) disease, or DIC.

Idiopathic Thrombocytopenic Purpura

ITP is an autoimmune disorder in which antiplatelet antibodies decrease the life span of the platelets. Thrombocytopenia, capillary fragility, and increased bleeding time are diagnostic findings. ITP may cause severe hemorrhage after cesarean birth or from cervical or vaginal lacerations. The incidence of postpartum uterine bleeding and vaginal hematomas is also increased.

Medical management focuses on control of platelet stability. If ITP was diagnosed during pregnancy, the woman likely was treated with corticosteroids or IV immune globulin. Platelet transfusions are usually given when there is significant bleeding. A splenectomy may be needed if the ITP does not respond to medical management.

von Willebrand Disease

vW disease, a type of hemophilia, is probably the most common of all hereditary bleeding disorders. Although vW disease is rare, it is among the most common congenital clotting defects in North American women of childbearing age. It results from a factor VIII deficiency and platelet dysfunction that is transmitted as an incomplete autosomal dominant trait to both sexes. Symptoms include a familial bleeding tendency, previous bleeding episodes, prolonged bleeding time (the most important test), factor VIII deficiency (mild to moderate), and bleeding from mucous membranes. Although factor VIII increases during pregnancy, there is still a risk for PPH as levels of vW factor begin to decrease (Lockwood & Silver, 2009).

The woman may be at risk for bleeding for up to 4 weeks after birth. The treatment of choice is administration of desmopressin, which promotes the release of vW factor and factor VIII. It can be given nasally, intravenously, or orally. Transfusion therapy with plasma products that have been treated for viruses and contain factor VIII and vW factor also may be used. Concentrates of antihemophiliac factor (Humate-P or Alphanate) may also be used (Lockwood & Silver, 2009; Samuels, 2007).

Disseminated Intravascular Coagulation

DIC is a pathologic form of clotting that is diffuse and consumes large amounts of clotting factors, including platelets, fibrinogen, prothrombin, and factors V and VII. Widespread external bleeding, internal bleeding, or both can result. DIC also causes vascular occlusion of small vessels resulting from small clots forming in the microcirculation. In the obstetric population DIC may occur as a result of acute antepartum or PPH, abruptio placentae, amniotic fluid embolism, dead fetus syndrome (i.e., fetus dies but is retained in utero for at least 6 weeks), severe preeclampsia, sepsis, saline abortion, and acute fatty liver of pregnancy (Francois & Foley, 2007).

The diagnosis of DIC is made according to clinical findings and laboratory markers. Physical examination reveals unusual bleeding; spontaneous bleeding from the woman's gums or nose may be noted. Petechiae may appear around a blood pressure cuff placed on the woman's arm. Excessive bleeding may occur from the site of a slight trauma (e.g., venipuncture sites, intramuscular or subcutaneous injection sites, nicks from shaving of perineum or abdomen, and injury from insertion of a urinary catheter). Symptoms also may include tachycardia and diaphoresis. Laboratory tests reveal decreased levels of platelets, fibrinogen, proaccelerin, antihemophiliac factor, and prothrombin (the factors consumed during coagulation). Fibrinolysis is increased at first but is later severely depressed. Degradation of fibrin leads to the accumulation of fibrin split products in the blood; these have anticoagulant properties and prolong the prothrombin time. Bleeding time is normal, coagulation time shows no clot, clot-retraction time shows no clot, and partial thromboplastin time is increased.

DIC must be distinguished from other clotting disorders before therapy is initiated.

Primary medical management in all cases of DIC involves correction of the underlying cause (e.g., removal of the dead fetus, treatment of existing infection or of preeclampsia or eclampsia, or removal of a placental abruption). Volume replacement, blood component therapy, optimization of oxygenation and perfusion status, and continued reassessment of laboratory parameters are the usual forms of treatment (Francois & Foley, 2007). Resolution of DIC usually begins with the birth of the neonate (Francois & Foley, 2007).

Nursing interventions include assessing for signs of bleeding, administering fluid or blood replacement as ordered, observing for signs of complications from the administration of blood and blood products, and protecting from injury. Because renal failure is one consequence of DIC, urinary output is monitored, usually by insertion of an indwelling urinary catheter. Urinary output must be maintained at more than 30 ml/hr.

The woman and her family will be anxious or concerned about her condition and prognosis. The nurse offers explanations about care and provides emotional support to them through this critical time.

Thromboembolic Disease

A thrombosis results from the formation of a blood clot or clots inside a blood vessel and is caused by inflammation (thrombophlebitis) or partial obstruction of the vessel. Three thromboembolic conditions are of concern in the postpartum period:

Superficial venous thrombosis—Involvement of the superficial saphenous venous system

Deep venous thrombosis—Involvement varies but can extend from the foot to the iliofemoral region

Pulmonary embolism—Complication of deep venous thrombosis occurring when part of a blood clot dislodges and is carried to the pulmonary artery, where it occludes the vessel and obstructs blood flow to the lungs

Incidence and Etiology

The incidence of venous thromboembolism (VTE) varies from about 1 in 1000 to 1 in 2000 pregnancies (Pettker & Lockwood, 2007). VTE occurs in each trimester of pregnancy and in the postpartum period. The incidence of VTE in the postpartum period has declined in the last 30 years because early ambulation after childbirth has become standard practice. The major causes of thromboembolic disease are venous stasis and hypercoagulation, both of which are present in pregnancy and continue into the postpartum period. Other risk factors include cesarean birth, operative vaginal birth, history of venous thrombosis or varicosities, obesity, maternal age over 35, multiparity, and smoking (Pettker & Lockwood, 2007).

Clinical Manifestations

Superficial venous thrombosis is the most common form of postpartum thrombophlebitis. It is characterized by pain and tenderness in the lower extremity. Physical examination may reveal warmth; redness; and an enlarged, hardened vein over the site of the thrombosis. Deep vein thrombosis is more common in pregnancy and is characterized by unilateral leg pain, calf tenderness, and swelling. Physical examination may reveal redness and warmth, but women may also have a large clot with few symptoms. A positive Homans' sign may be present, but further evaluation is needed because the calf pain may be attributed to other causes such as a strained muscle resulting from the birthing position. Other signs and symptoms commonly seen include apprehension, cough, tachycardia, hemoptysis, elevated temperature, and pleuritic chest pain. Pulmonary embolism is characterized by dyspnea and tachypnea.

Physical examination is not a sensitive diagnostic indicator for thrombosis. Venography is the most accurate method for diagnosing deep venous thrombosis; however, it is an invasive procedure that exposes the woman and fetus to ionizing radiation and is associated with serious complications. Noninvasive diagnostic methods such as venous ultrasonography with or without color Doppler are the most commonly used. Magnetic resonance imaging and D-dimer assays may also be used (Pettker & Lockwood, 2007). Tachypnea and tachycardia are present with pulmonary embolism, and murmurs may be heard on cardiac auscultation. Echocardiographic abnormalities may be seen in right ventricular size or function (Pettker & Lockwood, 2007). Pregnancy limits the usefulness of arterial blood gases and oxygen saturation in diagnosis. A ventilation-perfusion scan, spiral computed tomography scan, magnetic resonance angiography, and pulmonary arteriogram may be used for diagnosis (Pettker & Lockwood, 2007).

Medical Management

Superficial venous thrombosis is treated with analgesia (nonsteroidal antiinflammatory agents), rest with elevation of the affected leg, and graduated elastic compression stockings or pneumatic compression devices (Pettker & Lockwood, 2007). Heat may also be applied locally. Deep venous thrombosis is initially treated with anticoagulant therapy (usually continuous IV heparin), bed rest with the affected leg elevated, and analgesia. After the symptoms have decreased, the woman may be fitted with graduated elastic compression stockings to use when she is allowed to ambulate. IV heparin therapy continues for 5 to 7 days. Oral anticoagulant therapy (warfarin [Coumadin]) is started during this time and will be continued for about 3 months. It is safe to use during lactation (see Medication Guide). Continuous IV heparin therapy is used for pulmonary embolism until symptoms have resolved. Intermittent subcutaneous heparin or oral anticoagulant therapy is usually continued for 6 months (Pettker & Lockwood, 2007).

In the hospital nursing care of the woman with a thrombosis consists of continued assessments: inspection and palpation of the affected area; palpation of peripheral pulses; checking Homans' sign; measurement and comparison of leg circumferences; inspection for signs of bleeding; monitoring for signs of pulmonary embolism, including chest pain, coughing, dyspnea, and tachypnea; and checking respiratory status for presence of crackles. Laboratory reports are monitored for prothrombin or partial thromboplastin times. The woman and her family are assessed for their level of under-

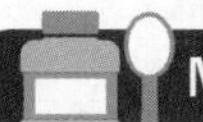

MEDICATION GUIDE

Warfarin Sodium (Coumadin)

Action

Blocks synthesis of clotting factors

Indications

For anticoagulation to prevent or treat blood clots

Dosage

Oral dosing dependent on blood tests

Adverse Reactions

Excessive bleeding, hemorrhage, rash, gastrointestinal upset

Nursing Considerations

It is contraindicated in pregnancy (can cause fetal death or birth defects). It is usually compatible with breastfeeding (APA, 2000). Blood levels of mother should be monitored. Inform woman to avoid alcohol, avoid cranberry products and large amounts of leafy green vegetables, and watch for bruising as it may be a sign of bleeding. Avoid aspirin and nonsteroidal agents such as naproxen or ibuprofen. It may be taken with food or on empty stomach. Dose compliance is very important!

standing about the diagnosis and their ability to cope during the unexpected extended period of recovery.

Interventions include explanations and education about the diagnosis and treatment. The woman will need assistance with personal care as long as she is on bed rest. The family should be encouraged to participate in the care if she and they wish. While the woman is on bed rest, she should be encouraged to change positions frequently but not to place the knees in a sharply flexed position that could cause pooling of blood in the lower extremities. She should also be cautioned not to rub the affected areas because rubbing could cause the clot to dislodge. Once the woman is allowed to ambulate, she is taught how to prevent venous congestion by putting on the elastic stockings before getting out of bed.

Heparin and warfarin are administered as ordered. The physician is notified if clotting times are outside the therapeutic level. If the woman is breastfeeding, she is assured that neither heparin nor warfarin is excreted in significant quantities in breast milk. If the infant has been discharged, the family is encouraged to bring the infant for feedings as permitted by hospital policy; the mother can also express milk to be sent home.

Pain can be managed with a variety of measures. Changing positions, elevating the leg, and applying moist heat may decrease discomfort. It may be necessary to administer analgesics and antiinflammatory medications.

NURSING ALERT Medications containing aspirin are not given to women on anticoagulant therapy because aspirin inhibits synthesis of clotting factors and can lead to prolonged clotting time and increased risk of bleeding.

The woman is usually discharged home on oral anticoagulants and will need an explanation of the treatment schedule and possible side effects. If subcutaneous injections are to be given, the woman and family are taught how to administer the medication and about site rotation. They should also be given information about safe care practices to prevent bleeding and injury while she is on anticoagulant therapy such as using a soft toothbrush and an electric razor. She will need information about follow-up with her health care provider to monitor clotting times and make sure that the correct dosage of anticoagulant therapy is maintained. The woman should also use a reliable form of contraception if taking warfarin because this medication is considered teratogenic (Pettker & Lockwood, 2007).

Postpartum Infections

Postpartum or puerperal infection is any clinical infection of the genital canal that occurs within 28 days after miscarriage, induced abortion, or childbirth. The definition in the United States continues to be the presence of a fever of 38° C or more on 2 successive days of the first 10 postpartum days (not counting the first 24 hours after birth) (Katz, 2007). Puerperal infection is one of the major causes of morbidity and mortality throughout the world; however, in the United States the incidence is 1% to 3% after vaginal births, 5% to 15% with planned cesarean birth, and 30% to 35% with cesarean birth after prolonged labor and ruptured membranes (Duff, 2007). Common postpartum infections include endometritis, wound infections, mastitis, urinary tract infections (UTIs), and respiratory tract infections.

The most common infecting organisms are the numerous streptococcal and anaerobic organisms. *Staphylococcus aureus,* gonococci, coliform bacteria, and clostridia are less common but serious pathogenic organisms that can cause puerperal infection. Postpartum infections are more common in women who have concurrent medical or immunosuppressive conditions or who had a cesarean or other operative birth. Intrapartal factors such as prolonged rupture of membranes, prolonged labor, and internal maternal or fetal monitoring also increase the risk of infection (Duff, 2007). Factors that predispose the woman to postpartum infection are listed in Box 23-3.

Endometritis

Endometritis (infection of the lining of the uterus) is the most common postpartum infection. It usually begins as a localized infection at the placental site but can spread to the entire endometrium. Incidence is higher after cesarean birth. Signs of endometritis include fever (usually greater than 38° C); increased pulse; chills; anorexia; nausea; fatigue and lethargy; pelvic pain; uterine tenderness; and foul-smelling, profuse lochia (Duff, 2007). Leukocytosis and a markedly increased RBC sedimentation rate are typical laboratory findings of postpartum infections. Anemia may also be present. Blood cultures or intracervical or intrauterine bacterial cultures (aerobic and anaerobic) should reveal the offending pathogens within 36 to 48 hours.

Wound Infections

Wound infections are common postpartum infections that often develop after the woman is at home. Sites of infection

BOX 23-3 Predisposing Factors for Postpartum Infection

Preconception or Antepartal Factors
History of previous venous thrombosis, urinary tract infection, mastitis, pneumonia
Diabetes mellitus
Alcoholism
Drug abuse
Immunosuppression
Anemia
Malnutrition

Intrapartal Factors
Cesarean birth
Prolonged rupture of membranes
Chorioamnionitis
Prolonged labor
Bladder catheterization
Internal fetal/uterine pressure monitoring
Multiple vaginal examinations after rupture of membranes
Epidural anesthesia
Retained placental fragments
Postpartum hemorrhage
Episiotomy or lacerations
Hematomas

include the cesarean incision and repaired laceration or episiotomy site. Predisposing factors are similar to those for endometritis (see Box 23-3). Signs of wound infection include erythema, edema, warmth, tenderness, seropurulent drainage, and wound separation. Fever and pain may also be present.

Urinary Tract Infections

UTIs occur in 2% to 4% of postpartum women. Risk factors include urinary catheterization, frequent pelvic examinations, epidural anesthesia, genital tract injury, history of UTI, and cesarean birth. Signs and symptoms include dysuria, frequency and urgency, low-grade fever, urinary retention, hematuria, and pyuria. Costovertebral angle tenderness or flank pain may indicate upper UTI. The most common infecting organism is *Escherichia coli,* although other gram-negative aerobic bacilli also may cause UTIs (Duff, 2007).

Mastitis

Mastitis, or breast infection, affects 2% to 10% of women soon after childbirth, most of whom are first-time mothers who are breastfeeding. It occurs in fewer than 1% of nonbreastfeeding mothers (Newton, 2007). Mastitis is almost always unilateral and develops well after the flow of milk has been established (Fig. 23-1). The infecting organism generally is the hemolytic *S. aureus.* An infected nipple fissure usually is the initial lesion, followed by ductal system involvement. Inflammatory edema and engorgement of the breast soon obstruct the flow of milk in a lobe; regional, then generalized, mastitis follows. If treatment is not prompt, mastitis may progress to a breast abscess.

Symptoms rarely appear before the end of the first postpartum week and are more common in the second to fourth weeks. Chills, fever, malaise, and local breast tenderness are noted first. Localized breast tenderness, pain, swelling, redness, and axillary adenopathy may also occur. Antibiotics are prescribed. Lactation can be maintained by emptying the breasts every 2 to 4 hours by breastfeeding, manual expression, or a breast pump.

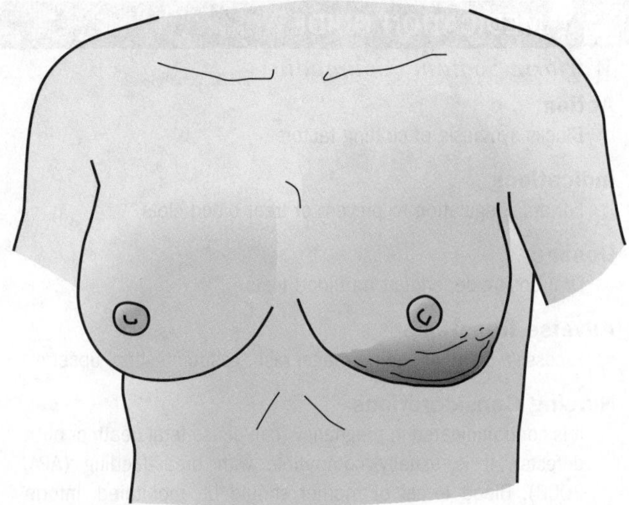

Fig. 23-1 Mastitis.

Nursing Care Management

Women with factors that predispose her to postpartum infection (see Box 23-3) should be assessed carefully. Signs and symptoms associated with postpartum infection were discussed with each infection. Elevation of temperature, redness, and swelling are common signs. The woman may also complain of chills, fever, localized tenderness, or pain. Laboratory tests usually performed include a complete blood count, venous blood cultures, and uterine tissue cultures. Review of the woman's history and the laboratory results should be included in the assessment.

Nursing diagnoses for women experiencing postpartum infection include the following:

- Deficient knowledge related to
  - — etiology, management, course of infection
  - — transmission and prevention of infection
- Impaired tissue integrity related to
  - — effects of infection process
- Acute pain related to
  - — mastitis
  - — puerperal infection
  - — UTI
- Interrupted family processes related to
  - — unexpected complication to expected postpartum recovery
  - — possible separation from newborn
  - — interruption in process of realigning relationships after the addition of the new family member
- Risk for impaired parenting related to
  - — fear of spread of infection to newborn

The most effective and least expensive treatment of postpartum infection is prevention. Preventive measures include good prenatal nutrition to control anemia and intrapartal hemorrhage. Good maternal perineal hygiene with thorough hand hygiene is emphasized. Strict adherence to aseptic techniques by all health care personnel during childbirth and the postpartum period is very important.

Management of endometritis consists of IV broad-spectrum antibiotic therapy (cephalosporins, penicillins, or clindamycin and gentamicin) and supportive care, including hydration, rest, and pain relief. Antibiotic therapy is usually discontinued 24 hours after the woman is asymptomatic. Assessments of lochia, vital signs, and changes in the woman's condition continue during treatment. Comfort measures depend on the symptoms and may include cool compresses, warm blankets, perineal care, and sitz baths. Teaching should include side effects of therapy, prevention of spread of infection, signs and symptoms of worsening condition, adherence to the treatment plan, and the need for follow-up care. Women may need to be encouraged or assisted to maintain mother-infant interactions and breastfeeding (if allowed during treatment).

Treatment of wound infections may combine antibiotic therapy with wound debridement. Wounds may be opened and drained. Nursing care includes frequent assessments of the wound and vital signs and wound care. Comfort measures include sitz baths, warm compresses, and perineal care. Teaching includes good hygiene techniques (e.g., changing perineal pads front to back, handwashing before and after perineal care), self-care measures, and signs of worsening conditions to report to the primary health care provider. The woman is usually discharged to home for self-care or home nursing care after treatment is initiated in the inpatient setting.

Medical management for UTIs consists of antibiotic therapy, analgesia, and hydration. Postpartum women are usually treated on an outpatient basis; therefore teaching should include instructions on how to monitor temperature, bladder function, and appearance of urine. The woman should also be taught about signs of potential complications and the importance of taking all antibiotics as prescribed. Other suggestions for prevention of UTIs include proper perineal care, wiping from front to back after urinating or having a bowel movement, and increasing fluid intake.

Because mastitis rarely occurs before the postpartum woman is discharged, teaching should include its warning signs and counseling about prevention of cracked nipples. Management includes intensive antibiotic therapy (e.g., cephalosporins and vancomycin, which are particularly useful in staphylococcal infections), support of breasts, local heat or cold, adequate hydration, and analgesics.

Almost all instances of acute mastitis can be avoided by using proper breastfeeding technique to prevent cracked nipples. Missed feedings, waiting too long between feedings, and abrupt weaning may lead to clogged nipples and mastitis. Cleanliness practiced by all who have contact with the newborn and new mother also reduces the incidence of mastitis. See also Chapter 26.

Postpartum women are usually discharged to home by 48 hours after birth. This is often before signs of infection are evident. Nurses in birth centers and hospital settings must be able to identify women at risk for postpartum infection and provide anticipatory teaching and counseling before discharge (see Community Focus box). After discharge, telephone follow-up, hot lines, support groups, lactation counselors, home visits by nurses, and teaching materials (videos, written materials) are all interventions that can be implemented to decrease the risk of postpartum infections. Home care nurses must be able to recognize signs and symptoms of postpartum infection so the woman can contact her primary health care provider. These nurses must also be able to provide the appropriate nursing care for women who need follow-up home care.

COMMUNITY FOCUS

Prevention of Postpartum Infection

After giving birth, many women are discharged home before an infection can develop. Prepare a "Fact Sheet About Postpartum Infection" that could be distributed to postpartum women on discharge from the hospitals or birth centers in your community. Include signs and symptoms and phone numbers and addresses of health care providers who could be contacted. If your community has a large population who do not speak English, consider a fact sheet in Spanish or other language as appropriate.

Sequelae of Childbirth Trauma

Women are at risk for problems related to the reproductive system from the age of menarche through menopause and the older years. These problems, which include structural disorders of the uterus and vagina related to pelvic relaxation and urinary incontinence (UI), are often the delayed but direct result of childbearing.

With fetopelvic disproportion, prolonged labor, or a precipitous birth, structures of the vesical and vaginal walls are stretched and may be injured. The bladder neck and urethra may be compressed between the presenting part and the pubic bones or forced downward ahead of the presenting part. Since soft-tissue damage usually occurs behind an intact vaginal epithelium, there is nothing visible to repair. However, defects may also occur in women who have never been pregnant.

Structural disorders can have far-reaching effects for the woman and her family. Beyond the obvious physiologic alterations, the woman also experiences threats to her self-concept and her ability to cope. A woman's concept of herself as a sexual being can be affected by the condition and its treatments. Her family is also challenged in the way it responds to her diagnosis.

Uterine Displacement and Prolapse

Normally the round ligaments hold the uterus in anteversion, and the uterosacral ligaments pull the cervix backward and upward. Uterine displacement is a variation of this normal placement. The most common type of displacement is posterior displacement, or retroversion, in which the uterus is tilted posteriorly and the cervix rotates anteriorly. Other variations include retroflexion and anteflexion (Fig. 23-2).

By 2 months postpartum the ligaments should return to normal length, but in about one third of women the uterus remains retroverted. This condition is rarely symptomatic, but

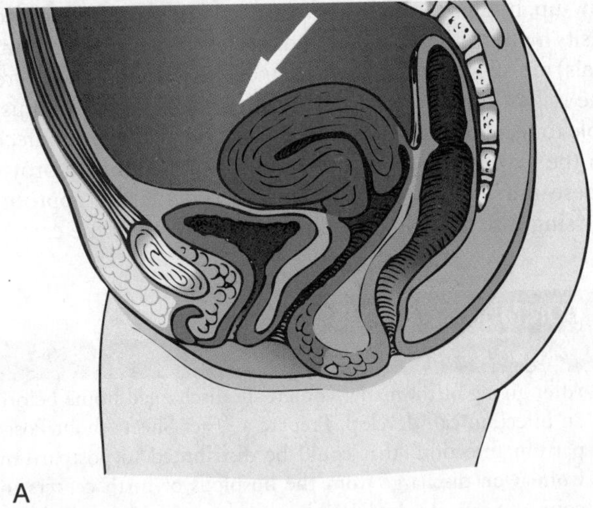

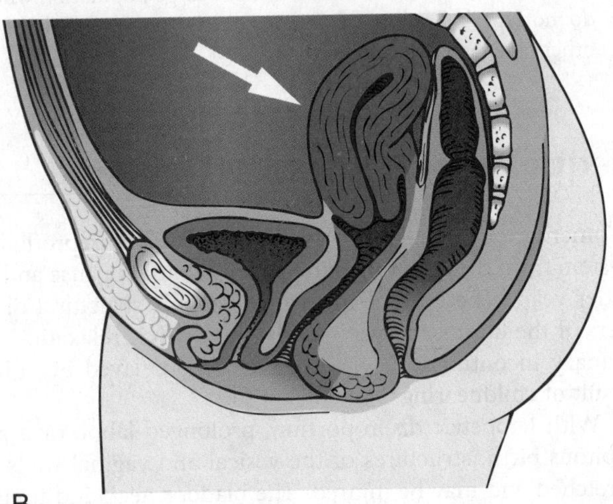

Fig. 23-2 Types of uterine displacement. **A,** Anterior displacement. **B,** Retroversion (backward displacement).

conception may be difficult because the cervix points toward the anterior vaginal wall and away from the posterior fornix, where seminal fluid pools after coitus. If symptoms occur, they may include pelvic and low back pain, exaggeration of premenstrual tension, and dyspareunia.

Uterine prolapse is a more serious type of displacement. Degrees of prolapse can vary from mild to complete. In complete prolapse the cervix and body of the uterus protrude through the vagina, and the vagina is inverted (Fig. 23-3).

Uterine displacement and prolapse can be caused by congenital or acquired weakness of the pelvic support structures (often referred to as pelvic relaxation). In many cases problems can be a delayed but direct result of childbearing. Although extensive damage may be noted and repaired shortly after birth, symptoms related to pelvic relaxation most often appear during the perimenopausal period, when the effects of ovarian hormones on pelvic tissues are lost and atrophic changes begin. Pelvic trauma, stress and strain, and the aging process are contributing causes. Other causes of pelvic relaxation include reproductive surgery and pelvic radiation.

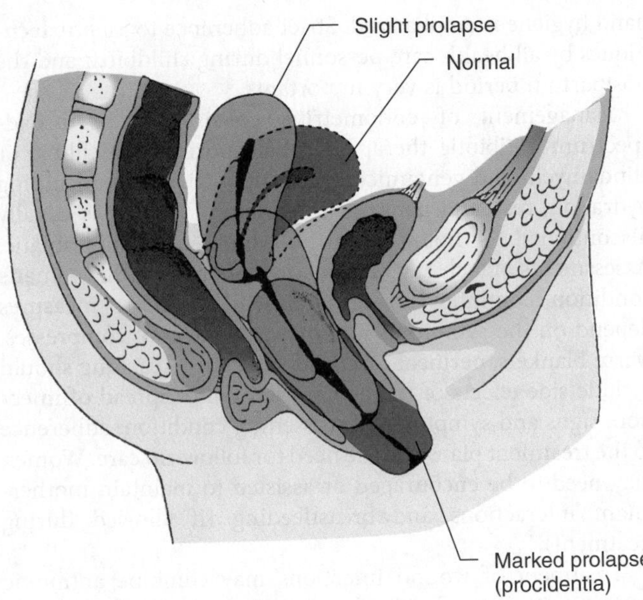

Fig. 23-3 Prolapse of uterus.

Clinical Manifestations

Generally symptoms of pelvic relaxation relate to the structure involved: urethra, bladder, uterus, vagina, cul-de-sac, or rectum. The most common complaints are pulling and dragging sensations, pressure, protrusions, fatigue, and low backache. Symptoms may be worse after prolonged standing or deep penile penetration during intercourse. Urinary incontinence may be present.

Cystocele and Rectocele

Cystocele and rectocele often occur with uterine prolapse (although they can occur independently), causing the uterus to sag even further backward and downward into the vagina. Cystocele (Fig. 23-4, *A*) is the protrusion of the bladder downward into the vagina that develops when supporting structures in the vesicovaginal septum are injured. Anterior wall relaxation develops gradually over time as a result of congenital defects of support structures, childbearing, obesity, or advanced age. When the woman stands, the weakened anterior vaginal wall cannot support the weight of the urine in the bladder; the vesicovaginal septum is forced downward, the bladder is stretched, and its capacity is increased. With time the cystocele enlarges until it protrudes into the vagina. Complete emptying of the bladder is difficult because the cystocele sags below the bladder neck. Rectocele is the herniation of the anterior rectal wall through the relaxed or ruptured vaginal fascia and rectovaginal septum; it appears as a large bulge that may be seen through the relaxed introitus (see Fig. 23-4, *B*).

Clinical Manifestations

Cystoceles and rectoceles often are asymptomatic. If symptoms of cystocele are present, they may include complaints of a bearing-down sensation or that "something is in my vagina." Other symptoms include urinary frequency, retention, incontinence, and possible recurrent cystitis and UTIs. On pelvic examination there is a bulging of the anterior wall of the vagina when the woman is asked to bear down. Unless the

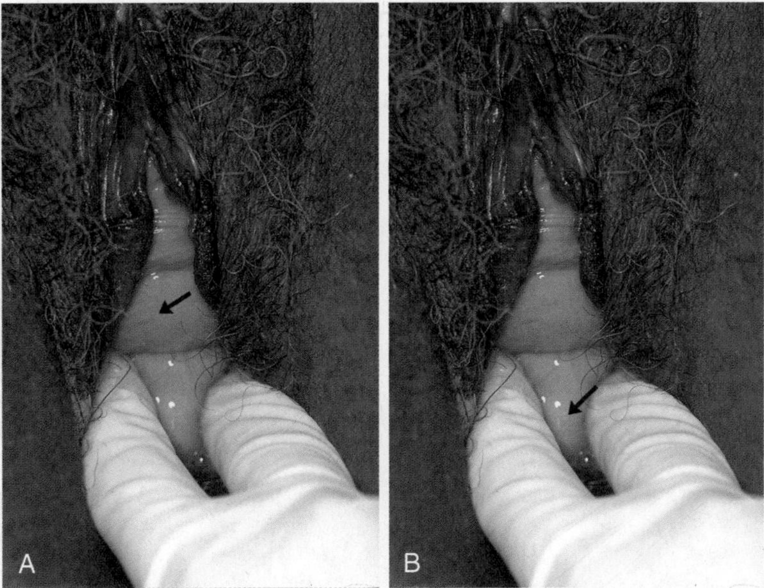

Fig. 23-4 Views of **A**, Cystocele. **B**, Rectocele. (From Seidel HM et al: *Mosby's guide to physical examination*, ed 6, St Louis, 2006, Mosby.)

bladder neck and urethra are damaged, urinary continence is unaffected. Women with large cystoceles complain of having to push upward on the sagging anterior vaginal wall to be able to void.

Rectoceles may be small and produce few symptoms, but some are so large that they protrude outside of the vagina when the woman stands. Symptoms are absent when the woman is lying down. A rectocele causes a disturbance in bowel function, a sensation of bearing down, or a sensation that the pelvic organs are falling out. With a very large rectocele it may be difficult to have a bowel movement. Each time the woman strains during bowel evacuation, the feces are forced against the thinned rectovaginal wall, stretching it even more. Some women facilitate evacuation by applying digital pressure vaginally to hold up the rectal pouch.

Urinary Incontinence

UI (uncontrollable leakage of urine) affects young and middle-age women; the prevalence increases as the woman ages. More than one third of women over the age of 60 have some form of UI (Mallett, 2005). Although nulliparous women can have UI, the incidence is higher in women who have given birth and also increases with parity. Conditions that disturb urinary control include stress UI, which is caused by sudden increases in intraabdominal pressure such as those caused by sneezing or coughing; urge incontinence, caused by disorders of the bladder and urethra such as urethritis and urethral stricture, trigonitis, and cystitis; neuropathies such as multiple sclerosis, diabetic neuritis, and pathologic conditions of the spinal cord; and congenital and acquired urinary tract abnormalities.

Stress UI may follow injury to bladder neck structures. A sphincter mechanism at the bladder neck compresses the upper urethra, pulls it upward behind the symphysis, and forms an acute angle at the junction of the posterior urethral wall and the base of the bladder (Fig. 23-5). To empty the bladder, the sphincter complex relaxes, and the trigone contracts to open the internal urethral orifice and pull the contracting bladder wall upward, forcing urine out. The angle between the urethra and the base of the bladder is lost or increased if the supporting pubococcygeus muscle is injured; this change, coupled with a urethrocele, causes incontinence. Urine spurts out when the woman is asked to bear down or cough while she is in the lithotomy position.

Clinical Manifestations

Involuntary leaking of urine is the main sign. Episodes of leaking are common during coughing, laughing, and exercise.

Genital Fistulas

Genital fistulas are perforations between genital tract organs. Most occur between the bladder and the genital tract (e.g., vesicovaginal); between the urethra and the vagina (urethrovaginal); and between the rectum or sigmoid colon and the vagina (rectovaginal) (Fig. 23-6). Genital fistulas may also be a result of a congenital anomaly, gynecologic surgery, obstetric trauma, cancer, radiation therapy, gynecologic trauma, or infection (e.g., in the episiotomy).

Clinical Manifestations

Signs and symptoms of vaginal fistulas depend on the site but may include the presence of urine, flatus, or feces in the vagina; odors of urine or feces in the vagina; and irritation of vaginal tissues.

Nursing Care Management

In general nurses working with these women can provide information and self-care education to prevent problems before they occur, manage or reduce symptoms and promote comfort and hygiene if symptoms are already present, and recognize when further intervention is needed (see Nursing

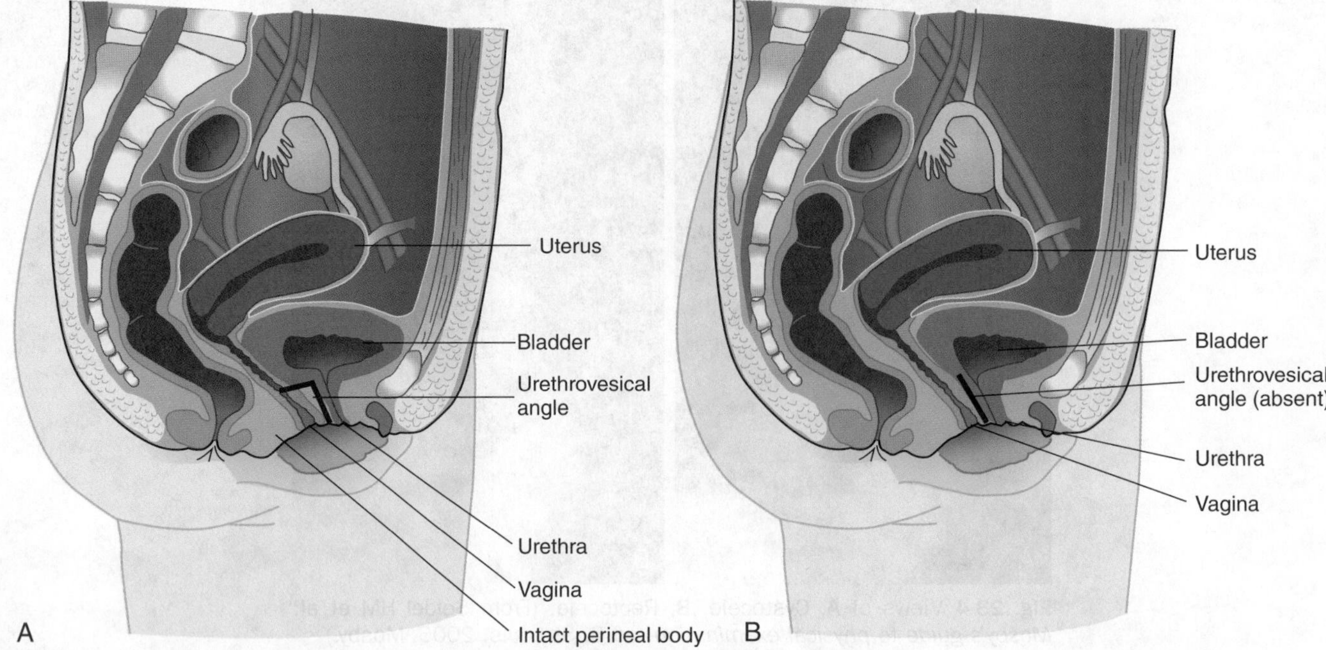

Fig. 23-5 Urethrovesical angle. **A**, Normal angle. **B**, Widening (absence) of angle.

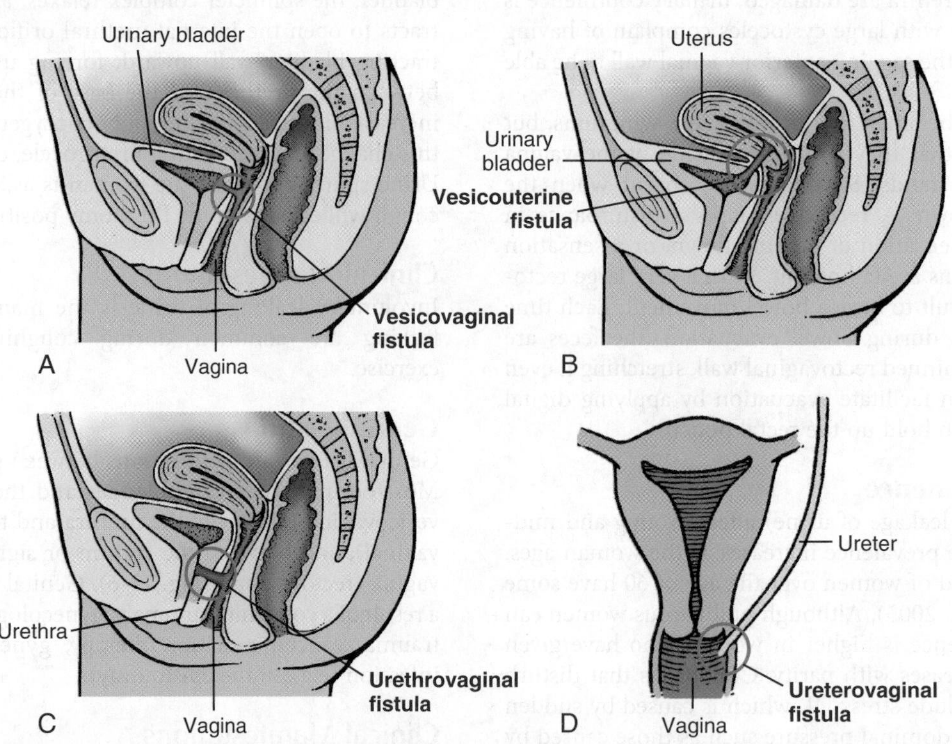

Fig. 23-6 Types of genitourinary fistulas. **A**, Vesicovaginal (bladder to vagina). **B**, Vesicouterine (bladder to uterus). **C**, Urethrovaginal (urethra to vagina). **D**, Ureterovaginal (ureter to vagina). Fistulas range in size from tiny and difficult to locate to large, disfiguring the base of the bladder. (From Monahan FD et al: *Phipps' medical-surgical nursing: health and illness perspectives*, ed 8, St Louis, 2007, Mosby.)

Process box). This information can be part of all postpartum discharge teaching or provided at postpartum follow-up visits in clinics or physician or nurse-midwife offices, during postpartum home visits, or during gynecologic health examinations. Information on how to prevent or recognize problems can be a topic for workshops for women or health fairs in community settings.

Interventions for specific problems depend on the problem and the severity of the symptoms. If discomfort related to uterine displacement is a problem, several interventions can

NURSING PROCESS: STRUCTURAL DISORDERS OF THE UTERUS AND VAGINA

Assessment

Assessment focuses primarily on the genitourinary tract, the reproductive organs, bowel elimination, and psychosocial and sexual factors. To support the appropriate medical diagnosis:

- Health history is taken.
- Physical examination is performed.
- Laboratory tests are done.
- Woman's knowledge of the disorder, its management, and the possible prognosis is assessed.

Nursing Diagnoses

Possible nursing diagnoses for the patient with a structural disorder of the uterus or vagina include the following:

Constipation or diarrhea related to
- anatomic changes

Ineffective coping related to
- changes in body image

Dysfunctional family processes related to
- the woman's anatomic and functional changes

Social isolation, spiritual distress, disturbed body image, or situational low self-esteem related to
- changes in anatomy and function

Anxiety related to
- surgical procedure
- prognosis

Planning

The health care team works together to treat the disorders related to alterations in pelvic support and to help the woman manage her symptoms.

Expected outcomes for the woman with structural abnormalities of the uterus and vagina include that she will do the following:

- Regain/maintain urinary and or fecal continence
- Cope with changes in body image
- Have satisfactory interpersonal relationships with her family and friends
- Have a reduction in anxiety related to her prognosis

Interventions

Various interventions are described in the text.

Evaluation

The nurse can be reasonably assured that care was effective to the extent that the expected outcomes have been achieved.

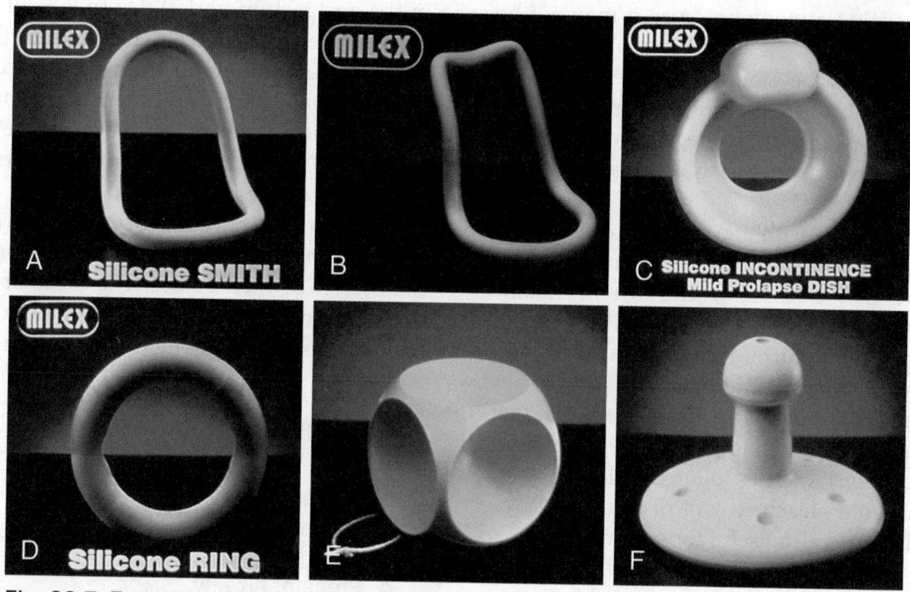

Fig. 23-7 Examples of pessaries. **A,** Smith. **B,** Hodge without support. **C,** Incontinence dish with support. **D,** Ring without support. **E,** Cube. **F,** Gellhorn. *(Courtesy Milex Products, Inc., a division of CooperSurgical, Trumbull, CT.)*

be implemented to treat uterine displacement. Kegel exercises can be performed several times a day to increase muscular strength. A knee-chest position performed for a few minutes several times a day can correct a mildly retroverted uterus. A pessary to support the uterus and hold it in the correct position may be inserted in the vagina (Fig. 23-7). Usually a pessary is used for only a short time because it can lead to pressure necrosis and vaginitis. Good hygiene is important; some women are taught to remove the pessary at night, cleanse it, and replace it in the morning. If the pessary is always left in place, regular douching with commercially prepared solutions or weak vinegar solutions (e.g., 1 tbsp to 1 qt of water) to remove increased secretions and keep the vaginal pH at 4.0 to 4.5 is suggested. After a period of treatment, most women are free of symptoms and do not require the pessary. Surgical correction is rarely indicated.

Treatment for uterine prolapse depends on the degree of prolapse. Pessaries may be useful in mild prolapse. Estrogen therapy also may be used in the older woman to improve tissue tone. If these conservative treatments do not correct the problem or there is a significant degree of prolapse, abdominal or vaginal hysterectomy is usually recommended.

Treatment for a cystocele includes use of a vaginal pessary or surgical repair. Pessaries may not be effective. Anterior repair (colporrhaphy) is the usual surgical procedure and is usually done for large symptomatic cystoceles. This involves a surgical shortening of pelvic muscles to provide better support for the bladder. An anterior repair is often combined with a vaginal hysterectomy.

Small rectoceles may not need treatment. The woman with mild symptoms may get relief from a high-fiber diet and adequate fluid intake, stool softeners, or mild laxatives. Vaginal pessaries usually are not effective. Large rectoceles that are causing significant symptoms are usually repaired surgically. A posterior repair (colporrhaphy) is the usual procedure. This surgery is performed vaginally and involves shortening the pelvic muscles to provide better support for the rectum. Anterior and posterior repairs may be performed at the same time and with vaginal hysterectomy.

Management of genital fistulas depends on the location. Surgical repair is the usual treatment; however, it may not be successful.

Mild-to-moderate UI can be significantly decreased or relieved in many women by bladder training and pelvic muscle (Kegel) exercises. Other management strategies include insertion of a bladder neck support prosthesis, estrogen therapy, and surgery.

Nursing care of the woman with a cystocele, rectocele, or fistula requires great sensitivity because the woman's reactions are often intense. She may become withdrawn or hostile because of embarrassment about odors and soiling of her clothing that are beyond her control. Her sexuality is threatened; her partner may refuse sexual intimacy.

The nurse may tactfully suggest hygiene practices that reduce odor. Commercial deodorizing douches are available, or noncommercial solutions such as diluted chlorine (e.g., 1 tsp of chlorine household bleach to 1 qt of water) may be used. The chlorine solution is also useful for external perineal irrigation. Sitz baths and thorough washing of the genitalia with unscented, mild soap and warm water help. Sparse dusting with deodorizing powders can be useful.

If a rectovaginal fistula is present, enemas given before leaving the house may provide temporary relief from oozing of fecal material until corrective surgery is performed. Irritated skin and tissues may benefit from use of a heat lamp or application of an emollient. Hygienic care is time consuming and may need to be repeated frequently throughout the day; protective pads or pants may need to be worn. All of these activities can be demoralizing to the woman and frustrating to her and her family.

Many of the nurse's efforts with these problems are directed toward participating in a team effort to prepare the woman for surgery. Preoperative teaching involves the primary nurse, operating room nurse, surgeon, and anesthesiologist. Postoperative nursing care focuses on preventing infection and helping the woman avoid putting stress on the surgical site.

The nurse in the health-promotion setting is usually most aware of the woman's living circumstances, physical limitations, and social problems and therefore may be best suited to coordinate continuity of care after discharge.

Postpartum Psychologic Complications

Mental health disorders in the postpartum period have implications for the mother, the newborn, and the entire family. Such conditions can interfere with attachment to the newborn and family integration, and some may threaten the safety and well-being of the mother, newborn, and other children. Fewer than 33% of women with substantial postpartum depression (PPD) or anxiety symptoms are detected by routine care (Coates, Schaefer, & Alexander, 2004). Because birth is usually thought to be a happy event, a new mother's emotional distress may puzzle and immobilize family and friends. When she most needs the caring attention of loved ones, they may either criticize or withdraw because of their own anxiety.

Mood Disorders

Mood disorders are the predominant mental health disorder in the postpartum period. Up to 70% of women experience a mild depression or baby blues after the birth of a child, although functioning of the woman is usually not impaired. However, baby blues and prepartum depression are predictors of depression (Kim et al, 2008; Reck et al, 2009; Watanabe et al, 2008). Box 23-4 lists 13 risk factors for PPD, with those having the greater effect listed first.

Some women have more serious depressions that can eventually incapacitate them to the point of being unable to care for themselves or their babies. The cause of PPD can be biologic, psychologic, situational, or multifactorial. It occurs in a variety of countries, although the manifestations may vary by culture;

BOX 23-4 Risk Factors for Postpartum Depression

1. Prenatal depression
2. Low self-esteem
3. Stress of child care
4. Prenatal anxiety
5. Life stress
6. Lack of social support
7. Marital relationship problems
8. History of depression
9. "Difficult" infant temperament
10. Postpartum blues
11. Single status
12. Low socioeconomic status
13. Unplanned/unwanted pregnancy

Source: Beck C: Predictors of postpartum depression: an update, *Nurs Res* 50(5):275-282, 2001; Beck C: Revision of the Postpartum Depression Predictors Inventory, *J Obstet Gynecol Neonatal Nurs* 31(4):394-402, 2002.

cultures have varying beliefs and rituals that can affect the severity of PPD (Bina, 2008; Goldbort, 2006). A study among postpartum Hispanic women in three U.S. cities revealed that 42.6% of participants were depressed (Kuo et al, 2004).

Depressive symptoms may also be evident in fathers; 10% of fathers exhibit such symptoms. This depression interferes with positive enrichment activities with their children (Paulson, Dauber, & Leiferman, 2006).

PPD exerts a moderate-to-large effect on the interaction of mothers and infants. Although a study in Taiwan showed that PPD had no significant effect on their infants' development (Wang et al, 2005), a study in the United Kingdom reported that infants of depressed mothers had significantly poorer weight gain (O'Brien et al, 2004). Nurses are strategically positioned to offer anticipatory guidance, assess the mental health of new mothers, offer therapeutic interventions, and make referrals when necessary. Failure to do so may result in tragic consequences. In the rarest of cases a disturbed mother may kill her infant, other family members, and/or herself (Lehmann, 2004).

The Diagnostic and Statistical Manual (DSM) of Mental Disorders contains the official guidelines for the assessment and diagnosis of psychiatric illness (APA, 2000). However, specific criteria for PPD are not listed. Instead, postpartum onset can be specified for any mood disorder either without psychotic features (i.e., PPD) or with psychotic features (i.e., postpartum psychosis) if the onset occurs within 4 weeks of childbirth (APA, 2000).

Postpartum Depression Without Psychotic Features

PPD is an intense and pervasive sadness with severe and labile mood swings and is more serious and persistent than postpartum blues. Intense fears, anger, anxiety, and despondency that persist past the baby's first few weeks are not a normal part of postpartum blues. Occurring in approximately 10% to 15% of new mothers, these symptoms rarely disappear without outside help (CDC, 2008; Paulson, Dauber, & Leiferman, 2006). Most of these mothers seek help only after reaching a "crisis point" (McCarthy & McMahon, 2008). The occurrence of PPD is higher among younger women, those with lower educational attainment, and those receiving Medicaid (CDC, 2008). African-American mothers were twice as likely as Caucasian mothers to experience PPD. Mothers who had no one to talk to about their problems after giving birth had a high rate of PPD and a low rate of seeking help. Having established

EVIDENCE-BASED PRACTICE Assessing for Postpartum Depression

—Pat Gingrich

Ask the Question

What is the best way to assess for postpartum depression?

Search for Evidence

Search Strategies

Professional organization guidelines, meta-analyses, systematic reviews, randomized controlled trials, nonrandomized prospective studies, and retrospective studies since 2006

Databases Searched

CINAHL, Cochrane, Medline, National Guideline Clearinghouse, TRIP Database Plus, and the websites for AWHONN and SOGC

Critically Analyze the Evidence

Postpartum depression (PPD) is a serious and insidious disease that can rob a new family of valuable nurturing time. Using data on U.S. women from the Pregnancy Risk Assessment Monitoring System (PRAMS), the Centers for Disease Control and Prevention (CDC) reported a prevalence of PPD in the first year after birth ranging from 11.7% to 20.4% (CDC, 2008). Risk factors for PPD included young age, low socioeconomic status, and use of Medicaid benefits. The CDC recommends incorporating PPD information into existing programs for high-risk women such as intimate partner violence services.

A large prospective study of 40,000 Australian women found that risk factors for PPD included previous history of depression, especially current/antenatal anxiety or depression, and low partner support (Milgrom et al, 2008). The authors recommend interventions targeted to women with current depression/anxiety and low social support.

Implications for Practice

In an update on the evidence-based guidelines of the Registered Nurses' Association of Ontario, nurses are encouraged to give individualized, flexible care; assess early and often, offering the Edinburgh Postnatal Depression Score (EPDS) as the most well-tested screening tool for patient self-test; intervene swiftly for a score greater than 12 on EPDS or if any evidence of self-harm ideation on score item No. 10 or in clinical judgment; and encourage peer support group participation (McQueen et al, 2008).

The Postpartum Social Support Questionnaire shows preliminary promise as a valid and reliable screening tool (Hopkins & Campbell, 2008).

A systematic review of telephone support revealed that proactive telephone support decreases the symptoms of PPD. Other postpartum benefits included preventing smoking relapse and promoting breastfeeding (Dennis & Kingston, 2008).

Nurses can also help by teaching women self-care, especially symptoms and risk factors for PPD; helping them to feel safe and empowered in discussing their mental and social health; and facilitating adequate social and partner support. Women and their families should be given written resources in their native language and emergency numbers to call. Last but not least, follow-up is a powerful tool for detection and deterrence of PPD.

References

Centers for Disease Control and Prevention: Prevalence of self-reported postpartum depression symptoms—17 states, 2004-2005, *MMWR Morb Mortal Wkly* 57(14):361-366, 2008.

Dennis CL, Kingston D: A systematic review of telephone support for women during pregnancy and the early postpartum period, *J Obstet Gynecol Neonatal Nurs* 37(3):301-314, 2008.

Hopkins J, Campbell SB: Development and validation of a scale to assess social support in the postpartum period, *Arch Womens Ment Health* 11(1):57-65, 2008.

McQueen K et al: Evidence-based recommendations for depressive symptoms in postpartum women, *J Obstet Gynecol Neonatal Nurs* 37(2):127-136, 2008.

Milgrom J et al: Antenatal risk factors for postnatal depression: a large prospective study, *J Affect Disord* 108(1-2):147-157, 2008.

evolve Nursing Care Plan—Postpartum Depression

and supportive relationships facilitates seeking care, as does outreach and follow-up (Sword et al, 2008).

The symptoms of postpartum major depression do not differ from those of nonpostpartum mood disorders except that the mother's ruminations of guilt and inadequacy feed her worries about being an incompetent and inadequate parent. In PPD there may be odd food cravings (often sweet desserts) and binges with abnormal appetite and weight gain. New mothers report an increased yearning for sleep, sleeping heavily but awakening instantly with any infant noise, and an inability to go back to sleep after infant feedings. Determining difficulty falling asleep is a relevant screening question to ascertain risk for PPD (Goyal, Gay, & Lee, 2007).

A distinguishing feature of PPD is irritability. These episodes of irritability may flare up with little provocation, and they may sometimes escalate to violent outbursts or dissolve into uncontrollable sobbing. Many of these outbursts are directed against significant others ("He never helps me.") or the baby ("She cries all the time, and I feel like hitting her."). Women with postpartum major depressive episodes often have severe anxiety, panic attacks, and spontaneous crying long after the usual duration of baby blues.

Many women feel especially guilty about having depressive feelings at a time when they believe they should be happy. They may be reluctant to discuss their symptoms or their negative feelings toward the infant. A prominent feature of PPD is rejection of the infant, often caused by abnormal jealousy. The mother may be obsessed by the notion that the baby may take her place in her partner's affections. Attitudes toward the infant may include disinterest, annoyance with care demands, and blaming because of her lack of maternal feeling. When observed, she may appear awkward in her responses to the baby. Obsessive thoughts about harming the infant are very frightening to her. Often she does not share these thoughts because of embarrassment; when she does, other family members become very frightened.

Medical Management

The natural course is one of gradual improvement over the 6 months after birth. However, supportive treatment alone is not efficacious for major PPD. Pharmacologic intervention is needed in most instances. Treatment options include antidepressants, antianxiety agents, and electroconvulsive therapy. Alternative therapies such as herbs, dietary supplements, massage, aromatherapy, and acupuncture may be helpful. Psychotherapy focuses on her fears and concerns regarding her new responsibilities and roles and monitoring for suicidal or homicidal thoughts. For some women hospitalization is necessary.

Postpartum Depression with Psychotic Features

Postpartum psychosis is a syndrome most often characterized by depression (as described previously), delusions, and thoughts by the mother of harming either the infant or herself (Kaplan & Sadock, 2005).

A postpartum mood disorder with psychotic features occurs in 1 to 2 per 1000 births (Kaplan & Sadock, 2005). Once a woman has had one postpartum episode with psychotic features, there is a 30% to 50% likelihood of recurrence with each subsequent birth (APA, 2000).

Symptoms often begin within days after the birth, although the mean time to onset is 2 to 3 weeks and almost always within 8 weeks of birth (Kaplan & Sadock, 2005). Characteristically the woman begins to complain of fatigue, insomnia, and restlessness and may have episodes of tearfulness and emotional lability. Complaints regarding the inability to move, stand, or work are also common. Suspiciousness, confusion, incoherence, irrational statements, and obsessive concerns about the baby's health and welfare may be present later (Kaplan & Sadock, 2005). Delusions may be present in 50% of all women, and hallucinations in about 25%. Auditory hallucinations that command the mother to kill the infant can also occur in severe cases. When delusions are present, they are often related to the infant. The mother may think the infant is possessed by the devil, has special powers, or is destined for a terrible fate (APA, 2000). Grossly disorganized behavior may be manifested as a disinterest in the infant or an inability to provide care. Some insist that something is wrong with the baby or accuse nurses or family of hurting or poisoning their child. Nurses are advised to be alert for mothers who are agitated, overactive, confused, complaining, or suspicious.

A specific illness included in depression with psychotic features is bipolar disorder (formerly called manic depressive illness). This mood disorder is preceded or accompanied by manic episodes characterized by elevated, expansive, or irritable moods. Clinical manifestations of a manic episode include at least three of the following symptoms that have been significantly present for at least 1 week: grandiosity, decreased need for sleep, pressured speech, flight of ideas, distractibility, psychomotor agitation, and excessive involvement in pleasurable activities without regard for negative consequences (APA, 2000). Because these women are hyperactive, they may not take the time to eat or sleep, which leads to inadequate nutrition, dehydration, and sleep deprivation. While in a manic state, mothers need constant supervision when caring for their infant. In most instances they are too preoccupied to provide child care.

Medical Management

A favorable outcome is associated with a positive premorbid adjustment (before the onset of the disorder) and a supportive family network (Kaplan & Sadock, 2005). Because mood disorders are usually episodic, women may experience another episode of symptoms within a year or two of the birth. Postpartum psychosis is a psychiatric emergency, and the mother will probably need psychiatric hospitalization. Antipsychotics and mood stabilizers such as lithium are the treatments of choice (see Tables 23-2 and 23-3 for Food and Drug Administration categories of risk during pregnancy). If the mother is breastfeeding, some sources recommend that no pharmacologic agents should be prescribed (Kaplan & Sadock, 2005), but other sources advise caution while prescribing some agents (Schatzberg & Nemeroff, 2004). It is usually advantageous for the mother to have contact with her baby if she so desires, but visits must be closely supervised. Psychotherapy is indicated after the period of acute psychosis is past.

Nursing Care Management

Even though the prevalence of PPD is fairly well established, women are unlikely to seek help from a mental health care provider (see Nursing Process box). Primary health care providers can usually recognize severe PPD or postpartum psychosis but may miss milder forms; even if it is recognized, the woman may be treated inappropriately or subtherapeutically. Identification and treatment of maternal depression must be continued beyond the immediate postbirth period to prevent negative effects of maternal depression on the children of these mothers (Horwitz et al, 2007).

To recognize symptoms of PPD as early as possible, the nurse should be an active listener and demonstrate a caring attitude. Nurses cannot depend on women to volunteer unsolicited information about their depression or ask for help. Examples of ways to initiate conversation include the following: "Now that you've had your baby, how are things going for you? Have you had to change many things in your life since having the baby?" and "How much time do you spend crying?" If the nurse assesses that the new mother is depressed, she or he must ask if the mother has thought about hurting herself or the baby. The woman may be more willing to answer honestly if the nurse says, "Lots of women feel depressed after having a baby, and some feel so badly that they think about hurting themselves or the baby. Have you had these thoughts?"

NURSING ALERT Because mothers with PPD with psychotic features may harm their infants, extra precaution is needed in assessment and intervention. The nurse needs to ask specifically if the mother has had thoughts about harming her baby.

On the Postpartum Unit

Nurses must discuss PPD to prepare new parents for potential problems in the postpartum period (see Patient Teaching box). Mothers are often discharged before the blues or depression occurs. The family must be able to recognize the symptoms and know where to go for help. Written materials that explain what the woman can do to prevent depression are useful.

NURSING PROCESS: POSTPARTUM DEPRESSION

Assessment

Observe for signs of depression.

Ask appropriate questions to determine moods, appetite, sleep, energy and fatigue levels, and ability to concentrate (see text for examples of questions to ask).

Use screening tools such as the Postpartum Depression Predictors Inventory–Revised (PDPI-R) (Beck, 2002) and the Edinburgh Postnatal Depression Scale (Cox, Holden, & Sagovsky, 1987) *(www.wellmother.com)*.

If initial screening indicates woman may be depressed, refer for formal screening to determine the urgency of referral and type of provider.

Assess the woman's family for information and the need to express how they have been affected by the woman's emotional disorder.

Nursing Diagnoses

Possible nursing diagnoses for the woman experiencing postpartum depression include the following:

Risk for violence toward self (mother) or children related to
- postpartum depression

Ineffective family coping related to
- increased care needs of mother and infant

Risk for impaired parenting related to
- inability of depressed mother to attach to and care for infant

Situational low self-esteem in the mother related to
- stresses associated with role changes

Risk for injury to newborn related to
- mother's depression (inattention to infant's needs for hygiene, nutrition, safety) and psychotropic medications via breast milk

Planning

Planning is focused on meeting the individualized needs of the family to ensure safety, especially for the mother and infant and any other children, and facilitate functional family coping.

Specific measurable criteria can be developed based on the following general outcomes:

- The mother will no longer be depressed.
- The mother's and infant's physical well-being will be maintained.
- The family will cope effectively.
- Family members will demonstrate continued healthy growth and development.
- The infant will be fully integrated into the family

Interventions

Observe mother carefully for signs of tearfulness; conduct further assessments as necessary.

Discuss postpartum depression to prepare new parents for potential problems in the postpartum period.

If postpartum nurse is concerned about the mother, request a mental health consult.

Provide routine instructions regarding postpartum depression to whoever takes the woman home (i.e., "If you notice that your wife (or daughter) is upset or crying a lot, please call the postpartum care provider immediately. Don't wait for the routine postpartum appointment.").

Provide information about community resources for support.

Evaluation

The nurse can be assured that care has been effective if the physical well-being of the mother and infant is maintained, the mother and family are able to cope effectively, and each family member continues to show a healthy adaptation to the presence of the new member of the family.

evolve Critical Thinking Exercise—Postpartum Depression

PATIENT TEACHING Activities to Prevent Postpartum Depression

- Share knowledge about postpartum emotional problems with close family and friends.
- Take care of yourself: eat a balanced diet, exercise on a regular basis, and get enough sleep. Ask someone to take care of the baby so you can get a full night's sleep.
- Share your feelings with someone close to you; don't isolate yourself at home with the TV.
- Don't overcommit yourself or feel like you need to be a superwoman.
- Don't place unrealistic expectations on yourself.
- Don't be ashamed of having emotional problems after your baby is born. It happens to approximately 15% of women.

NURSING ALERT Because the newborn may be scheduled for a checkup before the mother's 6-week checkup, nurses in well-baby clinics or pediatrician offices should be alert for signs of PPD in new mothers and be knowledgeable about community referral resources.

In the Home and Community

Postpartum home visits can reduce the incidence of or complications from depression. A brief home visit or phone call at least once a week until the new mother returns for her postpartum visit may save the life of a mother and her infant; however, home visits may not be feasible or available. Supervision of the mother with emotional complications may become a prime concern. Because depression can greatly interfere with her mothering functions, family and friends may need to participate in the infant's care. This is a time for the extended family and friends to determine what they can do to help; the nurse can work with them to ensure adequate supervision and their understanding of the woman's mental illness (Linter & Gray, 2006).

When the woman has PPD, a partner often reacts with confusion, shock, denial, and anger and feels neglected and blamed. The nurse can talk with the woman about how her condition is also hard for him and that he is probably very worried about her. Men often withdraw or criticize when they are deeply worried about their significant others. The nurse can provide nonjudgmental opportunities for the partner to verbalize feelings and concerns, help the partner identify positive coping strategies, and be a source of encouragement for the partner to continue supporting the woman. Suggestions for partners of women with PPD include helping around the house, setting limits with family and friends, going with her to doctor's appointments, educating himself or herself, writing down concerns and questions to take to the doctor or therapist, and just being with her—sitting quietly, hugging her, and telling her that you love her. Both the woman and her partner need an opportunity to express their needs, fears, thoughts, and feelings in a nonjudgmental environment.

Even if the woman is severely depressed, hospitalization can be avoided if adequate resources can be mobilized to ensure safety for both mother and infant. The nurse in home health care will need to make frequent phone calls or home visits for assessment and counseling. Community resources that may be helpful are temporary child care or foster care, homemaker service, meals on wheels, parenting guidance centers, mother's-day-out programs, and telephone support groups such as Postpartum Support International *(http://postpartum.net)* and Depression After Delivery *(www.depressionafterdelivery.com)*.

Referral

Women with moderate-to-severe cases of PPD should be referred to a mental health therapist such as an advanced practice psychiatric nurse or psychiatrist for evaluation and therapy. Inpatient psychiatric hospitalization may be necessary. This decision is made when the safety of the mother or children is threatened.

Providing Safety

When depression is suspected, the nurse asks, "Have you thought about hurting yourself?" If delusional thinking about the baby is suspected, the nurse asks, "Have you thought about hurting your baby?" Four criteria measure the seriousness of a suicidal plan: method, availability, specificity, and lethality. Has the woman specified a method? Is the method of choice available? How specific is the plan? If the method is concrete and detailed, with access to it right at hand, the suicide risk increases. How lethal is the method? The most lethal method is shooting, with hanging a close second. The least lethal is slashing one's wrists. Medication overdose with tricyclic antidepressants (TCAs) causes death. Avoid TCAs in suicidal women because of the danger of overdose.

NURSING ALERT Suicidal thoughts or attempts are among the most serious symptoms of PPD and require immediate assessment and intervention.

Psychiatric Hospitalization

Women with postpartum psychosis have a psychiatric emergency and must be referred immediately to a psychiatrist who is experienced in working with women with PPD, can prescribe medication and other forms of therapy, and can assess the need for hospitalization.

LEGAL TIP Commitment for Psychiatric Care If a woman with PPD is experiencing active suicidal ideation or harmful delusions about the baby and is unwilling to seek treatment, legal intervention may be necessary to commit the woman to an inpatient setting for treatment.

Within the hospital setting the reintroduction of the baby to the mother can occur at the mother's own pace. A schedule is set for increasing the number of hours the mother cares for the baby over several days, culminating in the infant staying overnight in the mother's room. This allows the mother to experience meeting the infant's needs and giving up sleep for the baby, a situation difficult for new mothers even under ideal conditions. The mother's readiness for discharge and caring for the baby is assessed. Her interactions with her baby also are carefully supervised and guided.

Nurses also should observe the mother for signs of bonding with the baby. Attachment behaviors are defined as eye-to-eye contact; physical contact that involves holding, touching, cuddling, and talking to the baby and calling the baby by name; and the initiation of appropriate care. A staff member is assigned to keep the baby in sight at all times. Indirect teaching, praise, and encouragement are designed to bolster the mother's self-esteem and self-confidence.

Psychotropic Medications

PPD is usually treated with antidepressant medications. If the woman with PPD is not breastfeeding, antidepressants can be prescribed without special precautions. In addition to tricyclic antidepressants, selective serotonin reuptake inhibitors and serotonin-norepinephrine reuptake inhibitors, monoamine oxidative inhibitors, and mood stabilizers, antipsychotic medications may be prescribed for nonbreastfeeding women.

Women taking mood stabilizers (Table 23-2) must be taught about their many side effects, and those on lithium especially need to be told to have serum lithium levels drawn every 6 months. Women with severe psychiatric syndromes such as schizophrenia, bipolar disorder, or psychotic depression will probably require antipsychotic medications (Table 23-3).

Patient education is important for those taking antipsychotic medications because most of these medications can cause sedation and orthostatic hypotension, both of which could interfere with the mother being able to safely care for her baby. The medications can also cause parasympathetic nervous system effects such as constipation, dry mouth, blurred vision, tachycardia, urinary retention, weight gain, and agranulocytosis. Central nervous system effects may include akathisia, dystonias, Parkinsonism-like symptoms, tardive dyskinesia (irreversible), and neuroleptic malignant syndrome (potentially fatal).

The newer, atypical antipsychotic medications such as aripiprazole, olanzapine, quetiapine, risperidone, and ziprasidone are usually safer and have fewer side effects than the older, more traditional antipsychotics; however, their safety in breastfeeding women has not been established.

Table 23-2 Mood Stabilizers

MOOD STABILIZERS	PREGNANCY RISK CATEGORY*	LACTATION RISK CATEGORY*
Carbamazepine (Tegretol XR)	C	L2
Clonazepam (Klonopin)	C	L3
Gabapentin (Neurontin)	C	L3
Lamotrigine (Lamictal)	C	L3
Lithium carbonate (Eskalith)	D	L4
Topiramate (Topamax)	C	L3
Valproic acid (Depakene, Depakote, and Depakote ER)	D	L2

*Source: Hale T: *Medications and mother's milk,* ed 11, Amarillo, Tex, 2004, Pharmasoft.

ER, XR, Extended release; *C,* animal studies show adverse effects on fetus but no controlled studies in pregnant women, *or* no studies available; *D,* positive evidence of human fetal risk; *L2,* drug studied in limited number of breastfeeding women with no adverse effects in infant, *or* evidence is remote; *L3,* no controlled studies, *or* studies show minimal nonthreatening effects; *L4,* possibly hazardous.

Psychotropic Medications and Lactation

A major clinical dilemma is the psychopharmacologic treatment of women with PPD who want to breastfeed their infants. In the past women were told to discontinue lactation. Current beliefs are that, although most drugs will diffuse into breast milk, there are very few instances in which breastfeeding has to be discontinued (Pigarelli, Kraus, & Potter, 2005). Several factors influence the amount of drug an infant will receive through breastfeeding: the amount of milk produced, the composition of the milk (mature milk vs. colostrum), the concentration of the medication, and the extent to which the breast was emptied during a previous feeding (Pigarelli, Kraus, & Potter, 2005). Infants also vary in their ability to absorb, metabolize, and excrete ingested medication. Premature infants may not have optimal liver function, and kidney function doesn't reach maturity until 2 to 4 months of age. Because all psychotropic medications pass through breast milk to the infant, the risks associated with the use of such medication must be weighed against the benefits associated with breastfeeding for both mother and infant. None of these medications has been proven to be safe during lactation.

When breastfeeding women have emotional complications and need psychotropic medications, referral to a mental health provider who specializes in postpartum disorders is preferred. Depressed women need the nurse to reinforce the need to take antidepressants as ordered. Because antidepressants do not exert any effect for about 2 weeks and usually do not reach full

Table 23-3 Antipsychotic Medications

ANTIPSYCHOTIC MEDICATIONS	PREGNANCY RISK CATEGORY*	LACTATION RISK CATEGORY*
Traditional Antipsychotics		
Chlorpromazine (Thorazine)	C	L3
Fluphenazine (Prolixin)	C	L3
Haloperidol (Haldol)	C	L2
Perphenazine (Trilafon)	C	L3
Thioridazine (Mellaril)	C	L4
Thiothixene (Navane)	C	L4
Trifluoperazine (Stelazine)	Unknown	Unknown
Atypical Antipsychotics		
Aripiprazole (Abilify)	C	L3
Clozapine (Clozaril)	C	L3
Loxapine (Loxitane)	C	L4
Olanzapine (Zyprexa)	C	L2
Quetiapine (Seroquel)	C	L4
Risperidone (Risperdal)	C	L3
Ziprasidone (Geodon)	C	L4

*Source: Hale T: *Medications and mother's milk,* ed 11, Amarillo, Tex, 2004, Pharmasoft.

C, Animal studies show adverse effects on fetus but no controlled studies in pregnant women, *or* no studies available; *L2,* drug studied in limited number of breastfeeding women with no adverse effects in infant, *or* evidence is remote; *L3,* no controlled studies, *or* studies show minimal nonthreatening effects; *L4,* possibly hazardous.

BOX 23-5 Possible Alternative and Complementary Therapies for Postpartum Depression

Acupuncture
Acupressure
Aromatherapy
- Jasmine
- Ylang Ylang
- Rose

Herbal
- Lavender tea

Healing touch/therapeutic touch
Massage
Relaxation techniques
Reflexology
Yoga

Source: Weier K, Beal M: Complementary therapies and adjuncts in the treatment of postpartum depression, *J Midwifery Womens Health* 49(2):96-104, 2004.

effect for 4 to 6 weeks, many women discontinue taking the medication on their own. Patient and family teaching should reinforce the schedule for taking medications in conjunction with the infant's feeding schedule and the necessity to continue to take the medication until therapeutic effects occur.

Other Treatments for PPD

Other treatments for PPD include complementary and alternative therapies such as those listed in Box 23-5, electroconvulsive therapy, and psychotherapy (group or individual). Alternative therapies may be used alone but often are used with other treatments for PPD. Safety and efficacy studies of these alternative therapies are needed to ensure that care and advice is based on evidence.

NURSING ALERT St. John's wort is often used to treat depression. It has not been proven safe for women who are breastfeeding.

Loss and Grief

Situational life crises can be superimposed on the experiences of childbearing. These may include infertility, premature labor/premature birth, a cesarean birth, any perception of loss of control during the birthing experience, the birth of a boy when the parents wanted a girl, the birth of a child with a handicap, a maternal death, and/or fetal or neonatal death (see Community Focus box). All of these situations have a common denominator: they are losses of what was hoped for, dreamed about, and/or planned.

From the perspective of health care providers, these crises vary in degree. However, from the perspective of the parents the perceived loss may be the most terrible thing that has ever happened to them. At the birth they are mourning instead of celebrating life.

The statistics on perinatal loss and death of an infant are grim. Each year approximately 7 of every 1000 births end in stillbirth or fetal death. Newborn death accounts for almost 28,500 deaths per year in the United States (Martin et al, 2008); 18,000 infants die in the early postpartum period from prematurity, birth defects, and other acute illnesses. Thus parents can experience grief before or during the childbearing experience. In addition, 15.1 women per 100,000 die in the United States of childbirth-related causes each year (Kung et al, 2008).

COMMUNITY FOCUS

Community Resources for Loss and Grief

Investigate what resources and support groups exist in your community to assist parents who have experienced a maternal death; birth of a "less-than-perfect" child; a cesarean birth; or the death of a baby through miscarriage, stillbirth, or newborn death. Are resources available? Are there groups available for people with languages other than English? Are there enough of these resources to assist parents? How difficult was it for you to identify these resources? What could you do to make resources more known to bereaved parents and families?

The focus of this section is to prepare the nurse to provide sensitive, supportive, and therapeutic interventions to parents and families experiencing perinatal loss in a variety of settings. An overview of the grief process is presented as a guide for assessing and understanding the responses of bereaved women, men, and their families. Guidelines for intervention are given, and specific intervention approaches are discussed.

Grief Responses

Grief or bereavement has been described as a cluster of painful responses experienced by individuals coping with the death of someone with whom they had a close relationship, generally a relative or close friend (Lindemann, 1944). Many authors believe that there are overlapping phases in the grief process, but most do not believe that grief is experienced in "stages." Based on years of clinical work with bereaved parents and building on the conceptualization of others regarding grief following the death of a spouse, Miles (1984) developed a model of parental grief. Parental grief responses occur in three overlapping phases. There is an early period of acute distress and shock followed by a period of intense grief that includes emotional, cognitive, behavioral, and physical responses. The phase of reorganization is reached when parents return to their usual level of functioning in society, although the pain associated with the death remains. The duration of grief varies with the individual, but there is general agreement that grief is a long-term process that can extend for months and years. With a very close relationship such as with one's baby, some aspects of grief never truly end.

Acute Distress

The loss of a pregnancy or death of an infant is an acute and distressing experience for mothers and fathers who planned for and expected a normal healthy infant as the outcome. The loss encompasses a loss of their identity as a mother or father and of their many dreams related to parenthood. The immediate reaction to news of a perinatal loss or infant death is a period of acute distress. Parents generally are in a state of shock and numbness. They may feel a sense of unreality, loss of innocence, and powerlessness as though they were in a bad dream or in a fog or trancelike state. Disbelief and denial can occur. Sadness, devastation, depression, and intense outbursts of emotion and crying are common. On the other hand, lack of affect, euphoria, and calmness may occur and may reflect numbness, denial, or a personal way of coping with stress.

Much of the attention during the time of a loss is on the mother; the father is expected to be her main support. The response of fathers may vary more than that of mothers and depends on the level of identification with the pregnancy. Many fathers are profoundly affected and grieve deeply for a perinatal loss, but their feelings are often ignored.

Fathers are distressed by the grief of the mother and often feel helpless as to how to help her with the intense pain. Some fathers appear stoic and unemotional to maintain the societal expectation that they be "strong" for the mother and other family members. Because many fathers do not easily share feelings or ask for help, special efforts are needed to help them acknowledge these feelings and realize that they too have a right to support from others in their pain.

During this time of acute distress parents face the first task of grief: accepting the reality of the loss. The pregnancy has ended, or the baby has died, and their lives have changed. Although parents are often required to make many decisions such as having an autopsy, naming the infant, and making funeral arrangements, normal functioning is impeded, and decisions are difficult to make. Grandparents, friends, clergy, or other relatives may be available to help the couple cope. However, it is important that the mother and father ultimately make the decisions that are right for them.

Intense Grief

The phase of intense grief encompasses many difficult emotions as the parents work through their pain and adjust to life without the wished-for child. In the early months after the loss parents often experience feelings of loneliness, emptiness, and yearning. The mother may report that her arms ache to hold or nurse her baby and that she wakes to the sound of a baby crying. Both mothers and fathers may be preoccupied with thoughts about the wished-for child. Some parents cope with these feelings by avoiding memories and not talking about the baby, whereas others want to reminisce and discuss their loss over and over.

Deciding what to do about the nursery and baby clothes is particularly difficult during this period. Some women want the room taken down before they go home, whereas others want the room left intact until they have had time to grieve their loss. It is not unusual for a grandparent or other family member to want to rush home to take down the nursery with the thought that they would be sparing additional painful grief. In fact, their actions might only complicate the grief if parents were not involved in the decision. The bereaved parents must go through these types of experiences in their own time frame so that healing can take place.

During this phase of intense grief, guilt may emerge from the deep feelings of helplessness in not somehow preventing the pregnancy loss or the death of the infant. Mothers are particularly vulnerable to guilt feelings because of their sense of responsibility for the well-being of the fetus and baby. With many perinatal losses there is no clear cause of the event, leaving the woman to speculate about what she might have done or not done to cause the loss. Guilt may be intense if the mother thinks she is being punished for some unrelated event such as having had a prior induced abortion. Such self-blame is torture for mothers, and they need repeated emotional reassurance that they were not at fault.

Other common responses during this phase are anger, resentment, bitterness, and irritability. Anger may be focused on the health care team who failed to save the pregnancy or infant; toward a God who allowed the loss to occur; or toward family, friends, or peers when they do not provide the support the bereaved parents need and want. Some parents focus their resentment on parents who do not appreciate their children or neglect and abuse them. A sense of bitterness or generalized irritability rather than frank anger may be another response.

Fear and anxiety can occur during the grief process as a profound worry that something else bad might happen to another. Some parents, especially mothers, are almost obsessed with the desire to become pregnant again; others struggle with whether they can cope with the possibility of another loss.

Deep sadness and depression occur when the parent is faced with the full awareness of the reality of the loss. This often occurs several months after a perinatal loss and can continue for some time. Sadness and depression can be accompanied by disorganization and problems with cognitive processing, leading to behavioral changes such as difficulty in getting things done, an inability to concentrate, restlessness, confused thought processes, difficulty solving problems, and poor decision making. Disorganization and depression often cause difficulties in keeping up with work and family expectations. In addition, parents returning to work face issues such as handling well-meaning but painful comments or the silence of co-workers.

Physical symptoms of grief include fatigue, headaches, dizziness, and backaches. Parents are at risk for developing health problems such as colds or hypertension. It may be difficult to sleep; the appetite may be depressed or voracious. Lack of sleep and inadequate nutrition and fluids can complicate other grief responses.

Grief responses are very personal, ongoing, and difficult to handle. Some parents may suppress or deny their feelings because of societal indifference toward pregnancy loss and infant death. On the surface, suppression of feelings may be more socially acceptable. However, denying the pain of grief may lead to eventual physical and emotional distress or illness. Although bereaved parents have many ups and downs for many months and even years after a child's death, few parents actually become mentally ill or commit suicide. Knowing that these feelings are normal and that others have felt the same is helpful. The grief process during this phase is often difficult for fathers. Some may continue to have difficulty sharing their feelings. A rift can occur if one parent, usually the mother, wants to talk about the loss and pain, and the other parent, often but not always the father, withdraws. Other signs of problems include reliance on alcohol and drugs, extramarital affairs, prolonged hours at work, and overinvolvement in activities outside the home as an escape.

Reorganization

From the time of the pregnancy loss or infant death, parents attempt to understand "why?" This leads to a long and intense search for meaning. At first the "why" is focused on the cause of death. Finding few good answers, parents next focus on "why me, why mine?" These questions lead some parents into an existential search about the meaning of life and death. This search continues into the phase of reorganization and may lead to profound changes in the parents' view of the fragility of life.

Time helps to slowly ease the painful feelings of grief. Reorganization occurs when the parent is better able to function at home and work, experiences a return of self-esteem and confidence, can cope with new challenges, and has placed the loss in perspective. Reorganization begins to peak sometime after the first year as parents begin to achieve the task of moving on with their lives. Enjoying the simple pleasures of life without feeling guilty, nurturing self and others, developing new interests, and reestablishing relationships are all signs of moving on. For some women and families another pregnancy and the birth of a subsequent child are important steps to be able to move on with their lives; however, the term *recovery* is used because the grief related to perinatal loss can continue in varying degrees for life.

Parents have shared that they will never forget the baby who died and they are not the same people as before the loss. The term *bittersweet grief* refers to the grief response that occurs with reminders of the loss. This typically happens on birthdays, death days, and anniversaries; at school events; during changes in the seasons; and during the time of the year when the loss occurred (Box 23-6). Grief feelings also can be triggered during subsequent pregnancies and after birth.

Resuming the sexual relationship is an important aspect of recovery but can be very complicated. Many parents are comforted by the belief that their babies were conceived in love, lived in love, and died in love. Their love and intimacy created this child, and parents may believe that they may never experience joy and closeness again. Some couples may have an increased need for sexual activity in an attempt for closeness and healing, whereas others have a decreased desire for sexual intimacy.

Sexuality also brings with it decisions about a future pregnancy. Some are eager to have another child, although one child cannot replace the one who died and the grief will continue despite being pregnant. Other parents have a deep fear of experiencing the pain of loss again, which can make the resumption of sexual activity difficult. These ambivalent feelings are normal, and couples find themselves moving back and forth between the emotions of exhilaration and fear. The excitement that many others experience with a pregnancy is very different for previously bereaved parents. For some this emotional distress can affect maternal attachment to the new baby. Mothers who became pregnant again within 6 months after a stillbirth had fewer depressive symptoms at a 3-year follow-up than those who did not have a subsequent pregnancy (Surkan et al, 2008).

BOX 23-6 Bittersweet Grief

To Jessica Mayo—on her eleventh birthday
Sunday, November 18, 1990
"The child who is born on the Sabbath day,
Is bonny and blithe and good and gay."
Sundays are special days,
...a day of rest, a day to play,
...a day to reflect on days past,
...a day to thank God for all that we bless.
I bless your memory.
I wish you were here.
On your eleventh birthday I still want to share,
...Your dreams of the future,
...Our memories past,
My baby's first cry,
My daughter's first laugh.
I was told you were an angel in heaven above.
Eleven years later, I'm an expert ...
At long-distance love.
On your third birthday I wrote my first poem
to you.
Eight years later, it's still true,
"... no birthday cake,
no presents unwrapped ...
no pictures of you in your party hat.
But the candles are lit,
Never to go out.
For they burn forever in my heart.
Love, Mom
Kathie Rataj Mayo
1990

Couples often mark the progress of the pregnancy in terms of fetal development, waiting anxiously until the number of weeks of the previous loss is passed. In some cases the fear of repeated loss, especially after a stillbirth, is so great that induction of labor is considered if lung maturity studies can confirm that the baby is mature. Support groups are important in helping women through pregnancies after loss.

Family Aspects of Grief

Grandparents and Siblings

It is extremely important for the nurse taking care of these patients to keep in mind that they have an entire family to whom to minister, especially grandparents and siblings. Grandparents have hopes and dreams for a grandchild; these have been shattered. The grief of grandparents is often complicated by the fact that they are experiencing intense emotional pain by witnessing and feeling the immense grief of their own child. It is extremely difficult to watch their son or daughter experience unimaginable emotional trauma with very few ways to comfort and end their pain. As a result, the grief response may be complicated or delayed for grandparents. On occasions some grandparents experience immense survivor guilt because they are alive and their grandchild has died.

The siblings of the expected infant also experience a profound loss. Most children have been prepared for having another child in the family once the pregnancy is confirmed. These children come in all ages and stages of development, and this must be considered in understanding how they view the event and their loss experience. A young child responds more to the response of his or her parents, picking up on the fact that they are behaving differently and are extremely sad. This can cause clinging, altered eating and sleeping patterns, or acting out behaviors; and it is a time when parents have limited patience for responding to and meeting the needs of the child. Older children have a more complete understanding of the loss. School-age children may be frightened by the entire event, whereas teens may understand fully but feel awkward in responding.

Older siblings need to be included in grieving rituals to the extent the parents and the child feel comfortable. They may need to see the baby to actualize the loss. Nurses need to have a basic understanding about how children view death and grief to reach out to siblings in an appropriate and sensitive manner. Nurses also need to help parents recognize and be sensitive to the grief of siblings, include them in family rituals, and keep the baby alive in the family memory.

Nursing Care Management

Nursing care of mothers and fathers experiencing a perinatal loss begins the first time they are faced with the potential loss of their pregnancy or death of their infant. Assessment is as important for families experiencing a miscarriage or ectopic pregnancy as it is for those experiencing stillbirth or neonatal loss. Supportive interventions are important both at the time of the loss and after the parents have returned home.

Parents often cannot recall details of their experiences at the time of death, but they may recall vividly a minor event that was perceived as particularly painful or particularly helpful. The interventions provided below are general ideas about what may be helpful to parents. However, care must be individualized to each parent and family. Cultural and spiritual beliefs and practices of individual parents and families must be considered.

Communicating and Caring Techniques

Mothers, fathers, and extended families look to the medical and nursing staff for support and understanding during the time of loss. Therapeutic communication and counseling techniques help the mother, father, and other family members express their feelings and emotions, understand their responses to the loss, and make decisions.

The nurse should listen patiently while people tell their story of loss and grief. It may be necessary to ask questions that help people talk about their grief and the experiences surrounding the loss. However, grief responses in the initial days of crisis make it difficult for individuals to concentrate on what is being asked, think about what the question means, and respond to the question. The use of silence often gives the bereaved person the opportunity to collect thoughts and respond to questions. The nurse should resist the temptation to give advice or use clichés in offering support (Box 23-7).

BOX 23-7 What to Say and What Not to Say to Bereaved Parents

What to Say

"I'm sad for you."
"How are you doing with all of this?"
"This must be hard for you."
"What can I do for you?"
"I'm sorry."
"I'm here, and I want to listen."

What Not to Say

"God had a purpose for her."
"Be thankful you have another child."
"The living must go on."
"I know how you feel."
"It's God's will."
"You have to keep on going for her sake."
"You're young; you can have others."
"We'll see you back here next year, and you'll be happier."
"Now you have an angel in heaven."
"This happened for the best."
"Better for this to happen now, before you knew the baby."
"There was something wrong with the baby anyway."

Nurses need to become comfortable with their own feelings of grief and loss to effectively support and care for the bereaved. It is appropriate to express feelings with the bereaved families and share the moment with them. The nurse might use the following techniques in helping the family share and express their grief.

Help Mother, Father, and Other Family Members Actualize the Loss

When a loss or death occurs, the nurse should be sure that parents have been honestly told about the situation by their physician or others on the health care team. It is important for their nurse to be with them during this time. With early pregnancy loss it is recommended that the term *miscarriage* be used consistently. With infant death caregivers should use the words "dead" and "died," rather than "lost" or "gone" to assist the bereaved in accepting this reality. One way of actualizing the loss is to tell the parents the sex of the baby and give them the option of naming the fetus or help them name an infant who has died. Choosing a name helps make the baby a member of their family so that the baby can be remembered in a special way.

NURSING ALERT A caution about naming is important. Naming is an individual decision that should never be imposed on parents. Beliefs and needs vary widely across individuals, cultures, and religions. Cultural taboos and rules in some religious faiths prohibit the naming of an infant who has died.

On the basis of vast clinical experiences with parents, many professionals believe that seeing the fetus/baby helps parents face the reality of the loss, reduces painful fantasies, and offers an opportunity for closure. However, parents should never be made to feel that they should see or hold their baby when this is something that they do not really want. It is a good policy for the nurse to first tell them about this option and then give them time to think about it. A question such as, "Some parents have found it helpful to see their baby. Would you like time to consider this?" is useful. Later the nurse can return and ask each parent individually what he or she decided. Because the need or willingness to see the child also may vary between the mother and father, it is extremely important to determine what each parent really wants. This should not be a joint decision made by one person or a decision made for the parents by grandparents or others.

In preparation for the visit with the baby, parents appreciate explanations about what to expect. A description of how their baby looks is important. For example, babies may have red, peeling skin like a bad sunburn, dark discoloration similar to bruises, molding of the head that makes the head look soft and swollen, or birth defects. The nurse should make the baby look as normal as possible and remember that parents see their baby with different eyes from health care professionals. Bathing the baby, applying lotion to the baby's skin, combing hair, placing identification bracelets on the arm and leg, dressing the baby in a diaper and special outfit, sprinkling powder in the baby's blanket, and wrapping the baby in a pretty blanket conveys to the parents that their baby has been cared for in a special way. If the baby has been in the morgue, he or she can be placed underneath a warmer for 20 to 30 minutes and wrapped in a warm blanket before being brought to the parents. Cold cream rubbed over stiffened joints can help in positioning the baby. The use of powder and lotion stimulates the parent's senses and provides pleasant memories of their baby.

When bringing the baby to the parents, it is important to treat the baby as one would a live baby. Holding the baby close, touching a hand or cheek, using the baby's name, and talking with the parents about the special features of their baby convey that it is all right for them to do likewise. If a baby has a congenital anomaly, the nurse can desensitize the family by pointing out aspects of the baby that are normal. Nurses can help parents explore the baby's body as they desire. Parents often seek to identify family resemblance. A good question might be: "Who in your family does Michael resemble?"

Some families may like to have the opportunity to bathe and dress their baby. Although the skin may be fragile, parents can still apply lotion with cotton balls; sprinkle powder; tie ribbons; fasten the diaper; and place amulets, medallions, rosaries, or special toys or mementos in their baby's hands or next to their baby. Volunteer women in communities across the country make special burial clothes to give parents at this difficult time. Parents may want to perform other parenting activities such as combing the hair, dressing the baby in a special outfit, wrapping the baby in a blanket, or placing the baby in a crib.

evolve Nursing Care Plan—Fetal Death: 24 Weeks of Gestation

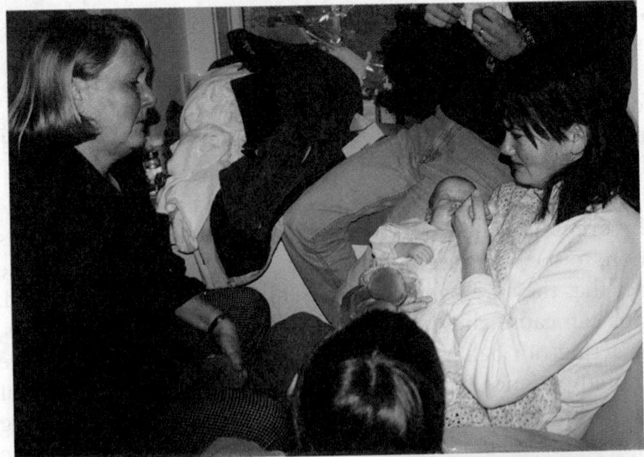

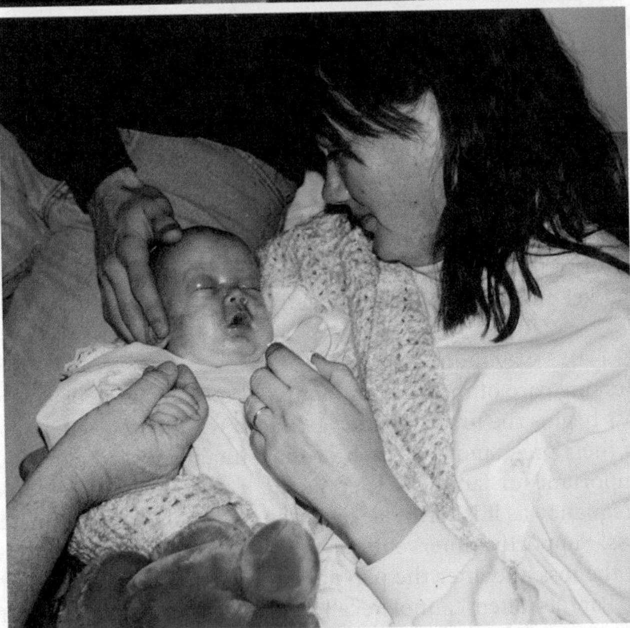

Fig. 23-8 Laura's family members say a special good-bye. *(Courtesy Amy and Ken Turner, Cary, NC.)*

Parents need to be offered time alone with their baby if they wish. They also need to know when the nurse will return and how to call if they should need anything. If at all possible, the family should be placed in a private room and, when possible, the room should have a rocking chair for the parents to sit in when holding their baby. This offers the mother and father special time together with their baby and other family members (Fig. 23-8). Marking the door to the room with a special card can be helpful in reminding the staff that this family has experienced a loss (Fig. 23-9).

Sensitivity to parental needs in actualizing the loss and coping with the reality of the death is essential for their healing. Grandparents should be offered the same opportunities to hold, rock, swaddle, and love their grandchildren so that their grief is started in a healthy way.

Help Parents with Decision Making

At a time when they are experiencing the great distress of a perinatal loss, and especially if the loss was of an infant, parents have many decisions to make. Mothers, fathers, and

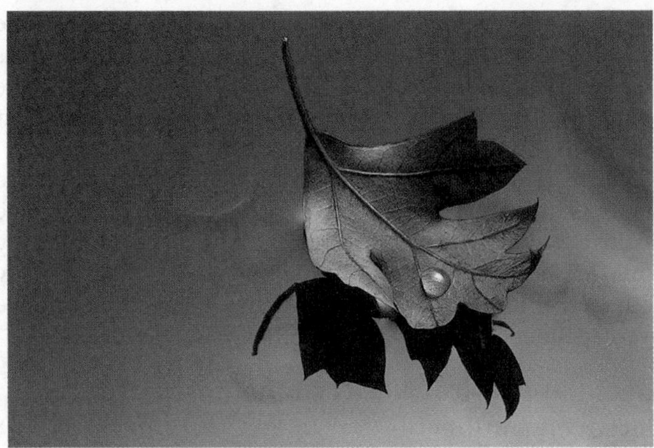

Fig. 23-9 Door card for room of mother who has experienced perinatal loss. *(Used with permission of Bereavement Services. Copyright Lutheran Hospital—La Crosse, Inc., a Gundersen Lutheran Affiliate, La Crosse, WI.)*

extended families look to the medical and nursing staff for guidance in knowing what decisions they must and can make and in understanding the options related to those decisions. Thus it is a primary responsibility of the nurse to help them and advocate for them because decisions made during the time of their loss will provide their memories for a lifetime.

One decision might be related to conducting an autopsy. An autopsy can be very important in answering the question "why" if there is a chance that the cause of death can be determined. This information can be helpful in processing grief and perhaps preventing another loss. However, the cost of an autopsy must be considered. Autopsies are not covered by insurance and are expensive. Some parents may believe that their baby has been through enough and prefer not to have further information about the cause of death. Some religions prohibit autopsy or limit the choice to times when it may help prevent another loss. Options for the type of autopsy such as excluding the head are available to parents. Parents may need time to make this decision. There is no need to rush them unless there was evidence of contagious disease or maternal infection at the time of death.

Organ donation can be an aid to grieving and an opportunity for the family to see something positive associated with their experience. The federal Gift of Life Act and HCFA-3005-F, enacted in 1998, shifted the responsibility for determining organ donation potential from the hospital staff to the state's organ procurement organization (OPO). States and hospitals have clear procedures for how and when to call the OPO. Generally, if a death certificate is issued, a call must be made to the OPO. Once contacted, they will decide whether to talk to the family, and either an OPO representative or a designated requester will contact them. This allows requests to be made by trained personnel in a consistent and compassionate manner. The most common donation is of cornea; donation of cornea from a baby can occur if the baby was born alive at 36 weeks of gestation or later.

Another important decision relates to spiritual rituals that may be helpful and important to parents. Support from the clergy is an option that should be offered to all parents. Parents may wish to have their own pastor, priest, rabbi, or spiritual leader contacted; or they may wish to see the hospital's chaplain. They may choose to do neither. Members from the clergy may offer the parents the opportunity for baptism when appropriate. Other rituals that may be important include a blessing, a naming ceremony, anointing, ritual of the sick, memorial service, or prayer.

One of the major decisions parents must make has to do with disposition of the body. Final disposition of all identifiable babies, regardless of gestational age, includes burial or cremation. Parents should be given information about the choices for the final disposition of their baby, regardless of gestational age. However, the nurses must be aware of cultural and spiritual beliefs that may dictate the choices of parents, issues related to the cost of burial, alternatives to burial, and state laws related to burial. A baby younger than 20 weeks of gestation is considered a product of conception; whereas embryos, uterine tubes removed with an ectopic pregnancy, and tissue from a pregnancy obtained during a D&C are all considered tissue. Many hospitals will make arrangements for the cremation of these infants or tissue. The nurse should know the hospital's policies and procedures and answer the parents' questions honestly. In most states, if a fetus is at least 20 weeks and 1 day of gestational age or is born alive, it is the parents' responsibility to make the final arrangements for their baby, although some hospitals will offer free cremation. In this case the family would not get the ashes.

LEGAL TIP Laws Regarding Live Birth Laws in all states govern what constitutes a live birth. In most states a live birth is considered to be any products of conception expelled from a woman that show any signs of life. Signs of life are considered to be any muscle irritability, respiratory effort, or heart rate, regardless of gestational age. All nurses should be knowledgeable about their state laws regarding what constitutes a live birth and what forms must be completed and filed in the case of fetal death, stillbirth, or newborn death.

In making final arrangements for their baby, parents may want a special service. They may choose to have a service in the hospital chapel, visitation at a funeral home or their own home, a funeral service, or a graveside service. Parents can make any of these services as special, personal, and memorable as they like. They can choose special music, poetry, or prose written by themselves or others.

The timing for actions such as naming the baby, seeing and holding the baby, disposition of the body, and funeral arrangements should never be rushed. In some cases the mother may be discharged home before these decisions are made. Then the family can think about them in the comfort of their home and contact the hospital in the following days to give their answers.

Help Bereaved to Acknowledge and Express Their Feelings

One of the most important goals of the nurse is to validate the experience and feelings of the parents by encouraging them to tell their stories and listening with care. Because nurses tend to be very focused on the physical and emotional needs of the mother, it is especially important to ask the father directly about his views of what happened and his feelings of loss.

Bereaved parents have many questions surrounding the event of their loss that can leave them feeling guilty. This is particularly true for mothers. Such questions include "What did I do?" "What caused this to happen?" "What do you think I should have, could have done?" Part of the grief process for bereaved parents is figuring out what happened, their role in the loss, why it happened to them, and why it happened to their baby. The nurse should recognize that these questions must be answered by the bereaved themselves; it is part of their healing. For example, a bereaved mother might ask, "Do you think that this was caused by painting the baby's room?" An appropriate response might be, "I understand you need to find an answer for why your baby died, but we really don't know why she died. What are some of the other things you have been thinking about?" Trying to give bereaved parents answers when there are no clear answers or trying to squelch their guilt feelings by telling them they should not feel guilty does not help them process their grief. In reality, many times there are no definite answers to the question of why this terrible thing has happened to them. However, factual information such as data about the frequency of miscarriages in pregnant women or the fact that there usually is no clear cause of a stillbirth can be helpful.

Feelings of anger, guilt, and sadness can occur immediately but often become more problematic in the early days and months after a loss. When a bereaved person expresses feelings of anger, it can be helpful to identify the feeling by simply saying, "You sound angry," or "You look angry." The nurse's willingness to sit down and listen to these surface feelings of anger can help the bereaved move past them into the underlying feelings of powerlessness and helplessness in not being able to control the many aspects of the situation.

Normalize the Grief Process and Facilitate Positive Coping

While helping parents share their feelings of pain, it is critical to help them understand their grief responses and know they are not alone in these painful responses. Most parents are not prepared for the raw feelings that they experience or the fact that these painful, complex feelings and related behavioral reactions continue for many weeks or months. Thus reassuring them of the normality of their responses and preparing them for the length of their grief is important.

The nurse can help the parent be prepared for the emptiness, loneliness, and yearning; for the feelings of helplessness that can lead to anger, guilt, and fear; and for the cognitive processing problems, disorganization, difficulty making decisions, and sadness and depression that are part of the grief process. Books and pamphlets about grief, if short and sensitive, can be given to parents to take home.

In the initial days after a loss, other useful strategies include follow-up phone calls, referrals to a perinatal grief support group, or providing a list of publications or websites intended for helping parents who have experienced a perinatal loss (e.g., *www.compassionatefriends.org, www.griefnet.org, www.growthhouse.org, www.nationalshareoffice.com*). However, as with any referral, the nurse should first read the materials or check out the websites.

To reduce relationship problems that can occur in grieving couples, it is particularly important to help them understand that they may respond and grieve in very different ways. The differences in grieving can lead to serious marital problems and be a risk factor for complicated bereavement. Remind the couple of the importance of being understanding and patient with each other.

Nurses can reinforce positive coping efforts and encourage attempts to resume normal activities; reinforce and encourage positive ways to hold onto memories of the pregnancy or baby while letting go; and help the parent organize a plan for daily activities, if needed. In particular, nurses should discourage overdependence on drugs and alcohol.

Meet the Physical Needs of the Postpartum Bereaved Mother

Coping with loss and grief after childbirth can be an overwhelming experience for the woman and her family. One particularly difficult aspect of the loss is the sound of crying babies and the happiness of other families on the unit who have given birth to healthy infants. The mother should be given the opportunity to decide if she wants to remain on the maternity unit or be moved to another hospital unit. She also should be helped to understand the pluses and minuses of each choice. Postpartum care and grief support may not be as good on another hospital unit where the staff are not experienced in postpartum and bereavement care.

The physical needs of a bereaved mother are the same as those of any woman who has given birth. The cruel reality for many bereaved mothers is that their milk can come in with no baby to nurse, their afterpains remind them of their emptiness, and gas pains feel as though a baby is still moving inside. The nurse should ensure that the mother receives appropriate medications to reduce these physical symptoms. Adequate rest, diet, and fluids must be offered to replenish her physical strength.

Mothers need postpartum care instructions on discharge. They also need ideas about how to cope with sleep problems such as decreasing food or fluids that contain caffeine, limiting alcohol and nicotine consumption, exercising regularly, using strategies for rest, taking a warm bath or drinking warm milk before bedtime, relaxation exercises, restful music, or a massage. Furthermore, the couple needs to be encouraged and supported in maintaining their relationship and keeping open channels of communication. They also need to be prepared for some of the issues related to resuming sexual relations after perinatal loss.

Create Memories for Parents to Take Home

Parents may want tangible mementos of their baby to allow them to actualize the loss. Some may want to bring in a previously purchased baby book. Special memory books, cards, and information on grief and mourning are available for purchase by parents, hospitals, or clinics through national perinatal bereavement organizations (Fig. 23-10).

The nurse can provide information about the baby's weight, length, and head circumference to the family. Footprints and handprints can be taken and placed with the other information on a special card or in a memory or baby book. Sometimes it is difficult to obtain good handprints or footprints. Application of alcohol or acetone on the palms or soles can help the ink adhere to make the prints clearer, especially for

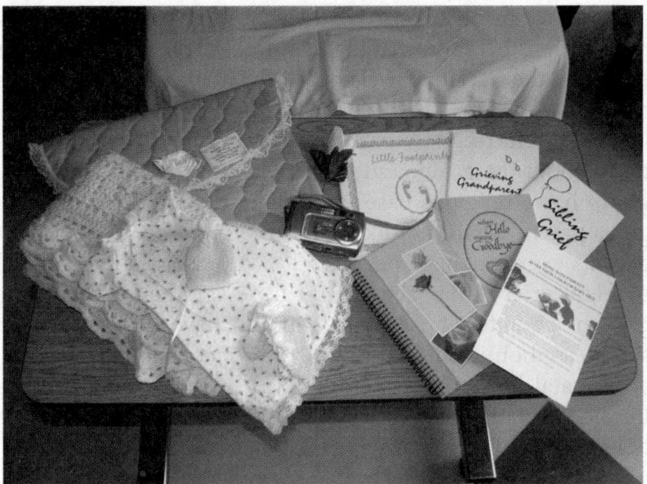

Fig. 23-10 Memory kit assembled at John C. Lincoln Hospital, Phoenix, AZ. Memory kits may include pictures of the infant, clothing, death certificate, footprints, ID bands, fetal monitor printout, and ultrasound picture. *(Courtesy Julie Perry Nelson, Loveland, CO.)*

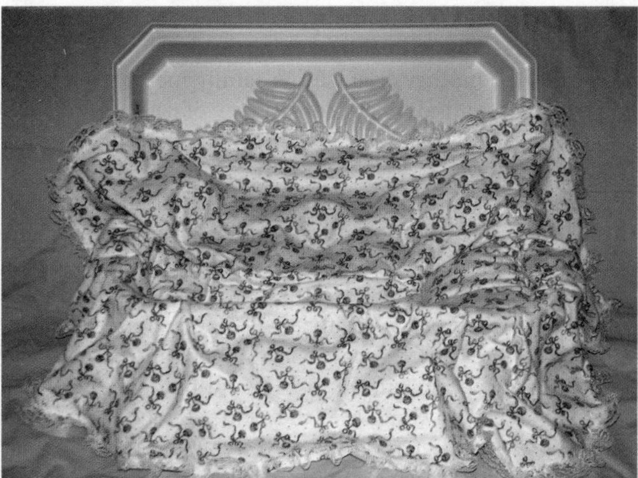

Fig. 23-11 Burial cradle (casket) for newborn infant. *(Courtesy Shannon Perry, Phoenix, AZ.)*

small babies. When making prints, have a hard surface underneath the paper to be printed. Place the baby's heel or palm down first and roll the foot or hand forward, keeping the toes or fingers extended. It may be helpful to have assistance in this procedure. If the print does not turn out, the nurse can trace around the baby's hands and feet, although this distorts the actual size. A form of plaster of paris can also be used to make an imprint of the baby's hand or foot.

Parents often appreciate articles that were in contact with or used in caring for the baby. This might include the tape measure used to measure the baby, baby lotions, combs, clothing, hats, blankets, crib cards, and identification bands. The identification band helps the parents remember the size of the baby and personalizes the mementos. The nurse should ask parents if they wish to have these articles. A lock of hair may be another important keepsake. Parents must be asked for permission before cutting a lock of hair, which can be removed from the nape of the neck where it is not noticeable.

For some, pictures are the most important memento. Photographs are generally taken whenever there is an identifiable baby and when it is culturally acceptable to the family. It does not matter how tiny the baby is, what the baby looks like, or how long the baby has been dead. Pictures should include close-ups of the baby's face, hands, and feet and photos of the baby clothed and wrapped in a blanket and unclothed. If there are any congenital anomalies, close-ups of these also should be taken. Flowers, blocks, stuffed animals, or toys can be placed in the background to make the picture more special. Parents may want their pictures taken holding the baby. Keeping a camera nearby and taking pictures when parents are spending special time with their baby can provide special memories. Some parents may have their own camera or video camera and ask the nurse to record them as they bathe, dress, hold, or diaper their baby.

Cultural and Spiritual Needs of Parents

Many of the responses to perinatal loss and suggested interventions described in this section are based on middle-class European-American views. Although there may be no particular differences in individual, intrapersonal experiences of grief based on culture, ethnicity, or religions, there are complex differences in the meaning of children and parenthood, the role of women and men, the beliefs and knowledge about modern medicine, views about death, mourning rituals and traditions, and behavioral expressions of grief. Thus the nurse must be sensitive to the responses and needs of parents from various cultural backgrounds and religious groups. To do this the nurse needs to be aware of her own values and beliefs and acknowledge the importance of understanding and accepting the values and beliefs of others that are different or even in conflict with hers. Further, it is critical to understand that the individual and unique responses of parents to a perinatal loss cannot be entirely predicted by their cultural or spiritual backgrounds. Each mother and father must be approached first as an individual needing support during a profoundly difficult and distressing life experience.

Provide Postmortem Care

Preparation of the baby's body and transport to the morgue depends on the procedures and protocols developed by individual hospitals. A sensitive and respectful approach for taking the fetus or infant to the morgue is the use of a burial cradle, which makes the process more dignified for parents and the nursing staff. These Styrofoam miniature coffins have a quilted lining and can be obtained from Zerbell's Bay Memorials (321 South 15th Street, Escanaba, MI; 906-786-2609) (Fig. 23-11). Postmortem care can be an emotional and sometimes difficult task for the nurse. However, nurses may find that providing postmortem care helps them find closure in their own grief related to a perinatal loss. This is particularly true for neonatal intensive care nurses who have cared for an infant for several hours, days, or weeks.

Documentation

Many hospitals have a checklist that is used in providing care, mobilizing members of the multidisciplinary health care team, communicating options the family has chosen, and keeping track of all the details in meeting the needs of bereaved parents. The checklists may or may not be a permanent part of the chart. Documentation in the nursing notes of primary concerns, grief responses, health teaching, health care advice, and referrals of the mother or any other family members is essential to ensure continuity and consistency of care.

Provide Sensitive Care at and After Discharge

When leaving the hospital, mothers are often taken out in a wheelchair. This can be a devastating experience for the mother who has experienced a pregnancy loss. Leaving the hospital without a baby in her arms is a very empty and painful experience. It is especially difficult if others are seen leaving with babies; thus the discharge of mothers and fathers who have experienced a perinatal loss should be done with great sensitivity to their feelings (i.e., they should not be discharged at a time when other mothers with live babies are leaving). Giving the mother a special flower to carry in her arms can be a thoughtful gesture.

The grief of the mother and her family does not end with discharge; rather it really begins once they return home, attend the funeral, and start to live their lives without their baby. There are numerous models for providing follow-up care to parents after discharge and, although there is no solid evidence from sound clinical trials regarding the benefit of these programs, nonexperimental studies and clinical evaluations suggest that these programs are helpful. Programs include hospital-based bereavement teams who provide support during hospitalization and follow-up contacts.

Phone calls after a loss may be helpful to some parents; however, it must be determined which parents do not want them. Follow-up calls let the parents know that someone still thinks and cares about them. The calls are made at predictably difficult times such as the first week at home, 1 month to 6 weeks later, 4 to 6 months after the loss, and at the anniversary of the death. Families who experienced a miscarriage, ectopic pregnancy, or death of a preterm baby may appreciate a phone call on the estimated date of birth. The calls provide an opportunity for parents to ask questions, share their feelings, seek advice, and receive information to help them process their grief.

A grief conference can be planned when parents return for an appointment with their doctor, nurses, and other health care providers. At the conference the loss or death of the infant is discussed in detail, parents are given information about the baby's autopsy report and genetic studies, and they have opportunities to ask the questions that have arisen since their baby's death. Parents appreciate the opportunity to review the events of hospitalization, go over the baby's and/or mother's chart with their primary health care provider, and talk with those who cared for them and their baby during hospitalization. This is an important time to help parents understand the cause of the loss or accept the fact that the cause will forever be unknown. This gives health care professionals the opportunity to assess how the family is coping with their loss and provide additional information and education on grief.

Some parents are very interested in finding a perinatal or parent grief support group. The opportunity to talk with others who have been through similar experiences, share memories of the pregnancy and the baby, and gain an understanding of the normality of the grief process generally have been found to be supportive. Over time it may be the only place where bereaved parents can talk about the wished-for child and their grief. However, not all parents find such groups helpful.

When referring to a group, it is important to know something about the group and how it operates. For example, if a group has a religious base for their interventions, a nonreligious parent would not likely find the group to be helpful. If parents experiencing a perinatal loss are referred to a general parental grief group, they might feel overwhelmed with the grief of parents whose older children have died of cancer, suicide, or homicide. In addition, the grief of parents following a perinatal loss might be minimized by other parents. Thus the needs of the parents must be matched with the focus of the group.

Maternal Death

It is rare for a woman to die in childbirth; the incidence of maternal deaths was 15.1 per 100,000 in 2005 (Kung et al, 2008) (see Critical Thinking Exercise). The father and extended family who are faced with not only mourning the death of a wife and mother but also the death of the baby have a particularly difficult time. On the other hand, the father may be faced with parenting a baby without a surviving mother. Death of a mother disrupts the family structure and leaves the father with the care of a baby at a time when he is greatly distressed. Thus the father and extended family, especially other children and grandparents, need supportive grief counseling at the time of death and following discharge to be able to heal after such a devastating loss.

The nursing care of families at this time is similar to that already described. Options need to be offered, memories made, and mementos obtained and held for the family until

CRITICAL THINKING EXERCISE

Reducing Maternal Mortality

One of the *Healthy People 2010* objectives is to reduce the maternal mortality rate to no more than 3.3 per 100,000 live births. The maternal mortality rate in the United States was 15.1 in 2005. What is the maternal mortality rate in your community? What efforts are being made in your community to reduce the maternal mortality rate? What efforts are being made to reduce disparities in mortality rates related to race and ethnicity?

1. Evidence—Is there sufficient evidence to draw conclusions about how to reduce the maternal mortality rate?
2. Assumptions—What assumptions can be made about the following factors:
   a. Causes of maternal mortality
   b. Factors associated with increased maternal mortality
   c. Access to prenatal care
   d. Racial disparities in mortality rates
3. What implications and priorities for nursing care can be drawn at this time?
4. Does the evidence objectively support your conclusion?
5. Are there alternative perspectives to your conclusion?

they are ready for them. These families are at risk for developing complicated bereavement and altered parenting of the surviving baby and other children in the family. Referral to social services to help the family mobilize support systems and for counseling can help combat potential problems before they develop and can be beneficial not only at the time of the loss but also in the future.

The emotional toll that a maternal death can take on the nursing and medical staff must also be addressed. Guilt, anger, fear, sadness, and depression are all common responses to a maternal death. The staff may want to review the situation surrounding the events, the medical record, and their responses in the forum of a mortality/morbidity review and a critical incident debriefing to help in coping with the feelings and emotions that result from a maternal death. Attending memorial or funeral services may benefit staff and family. Follow-up conferences with a social worker or grief counselor may be necessary.

Key Points

- PPH is the most common and most serious type of excessive obstetric blood loss.
- Hemorrhagic (hypovolemic) shock is an emergency situation in which the perfusion of body organs may become severely compromised and death may ensue.
- The potential hazards of therapeutic interventions may further compromise the woman with hemorrhagic disorders.
- Postpartum infection is a major cause of maternal morbidity and mortality throughout the world.
- Postpartum UTIs are common because of trauma experienced during labor.
- Breast infection affects about 1% of women soon after childbirth.
- Structural disorders of the uterus and vagina related to pelvic relaxation are often the delayed but direct result of childbearing.

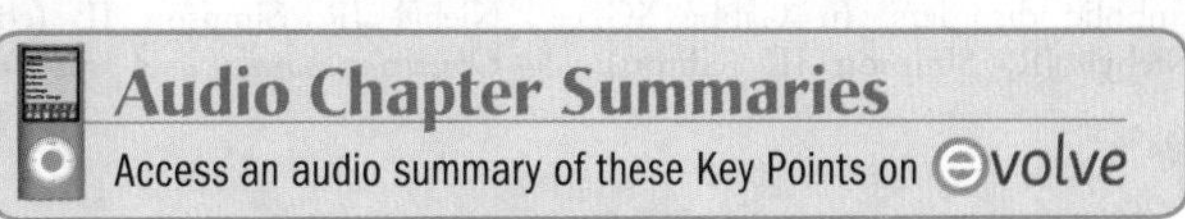
Audio Chapter Summaries
Access an audio summary of these Key Points on evolve

- An understanding of grief responses and the bereavement process is fundamental in the implementation of the nursing process.
- Therapeutic communication and counseling techniques can help families identify their feelings and feel comfortable in expressing their grief.
- Follow-up after discharge is an essential component in providing care to families who have experienced a loss.
- Nurses need to be aware of their own feelings of grief and loss to provide a nonjudgmental environment of care and support for bereaved families.

References

American Psychiatric Association (APA): *Diagnostic and statistical manual of mental disorders*, ed 4, revised, Washington, DC, 2000, APA Press.

Beck C: Revision of the Postpartum Depression Predictors Inventory, *J Obstet Gynecol Neonatal Nurs* 31(4):394-402, 2002.

Bina, R: The impact of cultural factors upon postpartum depression: a literature review, *Health Care Women Int* 29(6): 568-592, 2008.

Centers for Disease Control and Prevention: Prevalence of self-reported postpartum depressive symptoms —17 states, 2004-2005, *MMWR Morb Mortal Wkly Rep* 57(14):361-366, 2008.

Coates A, Schaefer C, Alexander J: Detection of postpartum depression and anxiety in a large health plan, *J Behav Health Serv Res* 31(2):117-133, 2004.

Cox JL, Holden JM, Sagovsky R: Detection of postnatal depression: development of the 10-item Edinburgh Postnatal Depression Scale, *Br J Psychiatry* 150:782-786, 1987.

Cunningham FG et al: *Williams obstetrics*, ed 22, Stamford, Conn, 2005, Appleton & Lange.

Duff P: Maternal and perinatal infection—bacterial. In Gabbe SG, Niebyl JR, Simpson JL (editors): *Obstetrics: normal and problem pregnancies*, ed 5, New York, 2007, Churchill Livingstone.

Francois KE, Foley MR: Antepartum and postpartum hemorrhage. In Gabbe SG, Niebyl JR, Simpson JL (editors): *Obstetrics: normal and problem pregnancies*, ed 5, New York, 2007, Churchill Livingstone.

Goldbort J: Transcultural analysis of postpartum depression, *MCN Am J Matern Child Nurs* 31(2):121-126, 2006.

Goyal D, Gay CL, Lee KA: Patterns of sleep disruption and depressive symptoms in new mothers, *J Perinat Neonatal Nurs* 21(2):323-329, 2007.

Gülmezoglu A et al: Prostaglandins for prevention of postpartum haemorrhage. In *The Cochrane Database of Systematic Reviews* 2007, Issue 3, Chichester, UK, 2009, John Wiley & Sons.

Horwitz SM et al: Prevalence, correlates, and persistence of maternal depression, *J Womens Health (Larchmt)* 16(5):678-691, 2007.

Kaplan H, Sadock B: *Synopsis of psychiatry*, ed 9, Baltimore, 2005, Williams & Wilkins.

Katz V: Postpartum care. In Gabbe SG, Niebyl JR, Simpson JL (editors): *Obstetrics: normal and problem pregnancies*, ed 5, New York, 2007, Churchill Livingstone.

Kim YK et al: Prediction of postpartum depression by sociodemographic, obstetric and psychological factors: a prospective study, *Psychiatry Clin Neurosci* 62(3):331-340, 2008.

Kung H-C et al: Deaths: final data for 2005, *Natl Vital Stat Rep* 56(10):1-120, 2008.

Kuo W et al: Depressive symptoms in the immediate postpartum period among Hispanic women in three US cities, *J Immigr Health* 6(4):145-153, 2004.

Lehmann C: House committee briefed on postpartum MH issues, *Psychiatr News* 39(21):26, 2004.

Lindemann E: Symptomatology and management of acute grief, *Am J Psychiatry* 101:141-148, 1944.

Linter N, Gray B: Childbearing and depression: what nurses need to know, *AWHONN Lifelines* 10(1):50-57, 2006.

Lockwood CJ, Silver RM: Coagulation disorders in pregnancy. In Creasy RK et al (editors): *Creasy & Resnik's maternal-fetal medicine: principles and practice*, ed 6, Philadelphia, 2009, Saunders.

Magann E, Lanneau G: Third stage of labor, *Obstet Gynecol Clin North Am* 32(2):323-332, 2005.

Mallett VT: Female urinary incontinence: what the epidemiologic data tell us, *Int J Fertil Womens Med* 50(1):12-17, 2005.

Martin JA et al: Annual summary of vital statistics: 2006, *Pediatrics* 121(4):788-801, 2008.

McCarthy M, McMahon C: Acceptance and experience of treatment for postnatal depression in a community mental health setting, *Health Care Women Int* 29(6):618-637, 2008.

McLintock C: Postpartum haemorrhage, *Thromb Res* 115(suppl 1):65-68, 2005.

Miles M: Helping adults mourn the death of a child. In Wass H, Corr C (editors): *Children and death*, Washington, DC, 1984, Hemisphere Publishing.

Newton ER: Breast-feeding. In Gabbe SG, Niebyl JR, Simpson JL (editors):

Obstetrics: normal and problem pregnancies, ed 5, New York, 2007, Churchill Livingstone.

O'Brien L et al: Postnatal depression and faltering growth: a community study, *Pediatrics* 113(5):1242-1247, 2004.

Oyelese Y, Smulian JC: Placenta previa, placenta accreta, and vasa previa, *Obstet Gynecol* 107(4):927-941, 2006.

Paulson JF, Dauber S, Leiferman JA: Individual and combined effects of postpartum depression in mothers and fathers on parenting behavior, *Pediatrics* 118(2):659-668, 2006.

Pettker CM, Lockwood CJ: Thromboembolic disorders. In Gabbe SG, Niebyl JR, Simpson JL (editors): *Obstetrics: normal and problem pregnancies*, ed 5, New York, 2007, Churchill Livingstone.

Pigarelli D, Kraus C, Potter B: Pregnancy and lactation: therapeutic considerations. In DiPiro J et al (editors), *Pharmacotherapy: a pathophysiologic approach*, ed 6, New York, 2005, McGraw-Hill.

Reck C et al: Maternity blues as a predictor of DSM-IV depression and anxiety disorders in the first three months' postpartum, *J Affect Disord* 113(1-2):77-87, 2009.

Samuels P: Hematologic complications of pregnancy. In Gabbe SG, Niebyl JR, Simpson JL (editors): *Obstetrics: normal and problem pregnancies*, ed 5, New York, 2007, Churchill Livingstone.

Schatzberg A, Nemeroff C (editors): *The American Psychiatric Publishing textbook of psychopharmacology*, ed 3, Washington, DC, 2004, American Psychiatric Publishing.

Skidmore-Roth L: *Mosby's handbook of herbs and natural supplements*, ed 2, St Louis, 2006, Mosby.

Surkan PJ et al: Events after stillbirth in relation to maternal depressive symptoms: a brief report, *Birth* 35(2):153-157, 2008.

Sword W et al: Women's care-seeking experiences after referral for postpartum depression, *Qual Health Res* 18(9):1161-1173, 2008.

Wang S et al: Impact of postpartum depression on the mother-infant couple, *Birth* 32(1):39-44, 2005.

Watanabe M et al: Maternity blues as a predictor of postpartum depression: a prospective cohort study among Japanese women, *J Psychosom Obstet Gynaecol* 29(3):211-217, 2008.

Wong HS et al: The maternal outcome in placenta accreta: the significance of antenatal diagnosis and non-separation of placenta at delivery, *NZ Med J* 121(1277):30-38, 2008.

Unit 6

24

Physiologic Adaptations of the Newborn

Learning Objectives

On completion of this chapter the reader will be able to:

- Describe the changes in the biologic system of the neonate during the transition to extrauterine life.
- Describe the sequence to follow in assessment of the newborn.
- Recognize deviations from normal physiologic findings during examination of the newborn.
- Compare and contrast the four types of heat loss in a neonate and describe how to prevent heat loss.
- Describe the behavioral adaptations of the newborn, including periods of reactivity and sleep-wake states.
- Describe the sensory and perceptual functioning of the neonate.

Electronic Resources

Additional information related to the content in Chapter 24 can be found on

evolve the Companion Website at http://evolve.elsevier.com/Perry/maternal/

- NCLEX Review Questions
- Anatomy Review—Sutures and Fontanels
- Case Study—Newborn Health Problems
- Nursing Care Plan—Immediate Care of the Newborn
- Skill—Thermoregulation
- Video—Buttocks
- Video—Cremasteric Reflex
- Video—Legs (Symmetry, Length)
- Video—Male Breasts (Supine Position)
- Video—Moro Reflex
- Video—Neck (Posterior)
- Video—Plantar Grasp
- Video—Rooting and Sucking
- Video—Upper Extremities

The neonatal period includes the time from birth through the twenty-eighth day of life. By term gestation, the fetus's various anatomic and physiologic systems have reached a level of development and functioning that permits a separate existence from the mother. At birth the newborn infant manifests behavioral competencies and a readiness for social interaction. These adaptations set the stage for future growth and development.

Transition to Extrauterine Life

Newborns undergo phases of relative instability during the first 6 to 8 hours after birth. These phases collectively are termed the *transition period* between intrauterine and extrauterine existence. The first phase of the transition period lasts up to 30 minutes after birth and is called the *first period of reactivity.* The newborn's heart rate increases rapidly to 160 to 180 beats/min but gradually falls by 30 minutes to a baseline rate between 100 and 120 beats/min. Respirations are irregular, with a rate between 60 and 80 breaths/min. Fine crackles may be present on auscultation; audible grunting, nasal flaring, and retractions of the chest may also be noted, but these should cease within the first hour of birth. The infant is alert and may have spontaneous startles, tremors, crying, and movement of the head from side to side. Bowel sounds are audible, and meconium may be passed.

After the first period of reactivity, the newborn either sleeps or has a marked decrease in motor activity. This period of unresponsiveness lasts from 60 to 100 minutes and is followed by a second period of reactivity.

The second period of reactivity occurs roughly between 4 and 8 hours after birth and lasts from 10 minutes to several hours. Brief periods of tachycardia and tachypnea occur, associated with increased muscle tone, skin color changes, and mucus production. Meconium is commonly passed at this time. Most healthy newborns experience this transition regardless of type of birth; extremely and very preterm infants do not because of physiologic immaturity.

Physiologic Adjustments

Respiratory System

With the cutting of the umbilical cord, the infant undergoes rapid and complex physiologic changes. The most critical and immediate adjustment is the establishment of respirations. With a vaginal birth some lung fluid is squeezed from the newborn's trachea and lungs; in infants who are born by cesarean birth some lung fluid may be retained within the alveoli. With the first breath of air, the newborn begins a dynamic sequence of cardiopulmonary changes.

Initial breathing is probably the result of a reflex triggered by pressure changes, cool air temperature, noise, light, and other sensations related to the birth process. In addition, the chemoreceptors in the aorta and carotid bodies initiate neurologic reflexes when arterial oxygen pressure (Po_2) falls, arterial carbon dioxide pressure (Pco_2) rises, and arterial pH falls. In most cases an exaggerated respiratory reaction follows within 1 minute of birth, and the infant takes the first gasping breath and cries.

Once respirations are established, they are shallow and irregular, ranging from 30 to 60 breaths/min, with periods of periodic breathing that include pauses in respirations lasting less than 20 seconds. These episodes of periodic breathing occur most often during the active REM sleep cycle and decrease in frequency and duration with age. Apneic periods lasting 20 seconds or longer are an indication of a pathologic process and should be carefully evaluated.

Signs of Respiratory Distress

Most term infants breathe spontaneously and continue to have normal respiratory patterns. Signs of respiratory distress may include nasal flaring, intercostal or subcostal retractions (i.e., drawing in of tissue between the ribs, or below the rib cage), or grunting with respirations. Suprasternal or subclavicular retractions with stridor or gasping most often represent an upper airway obstruction (Askin, 2003). Seesaw or paradoxical respirations (exaggerated rise in abdomen, with respiration, as chest falls) instead of abdominal respirations are abnormal and should be reported. A respiratory rate less than 30 or greater than 60 breaths/min with the infant at rest must be carefully evaluated. The respiratory rate can be negatively influenced (slowed, depressed, or absent) by analgesics or anesthetics administered to the mother during birth. Apneic episodes may be related to a number of events (rapid increase in body temperature, hypothermia, hypoglycemia, and sepsis) that require careful evaluation. Tachypnea may result from inadequate clearance of lung fluid, or it may be an indication of newborn respiratory distress syndrome.

Maintaining Adequate Oxygen Supply

During the first hour of life the pulmonary lymphatics continue to remove large amounts of fluid. Removal of fluid is also a result of the pressure gradient from alveoli to interstitial tissue to blood capillary. Reduced vascular resistance accommodates this flow of lung fluid. Retention of lung fluid may interfere with the infant's ability to maintain adequate oxygenation, especially if other factors (meconium aspiration, congenital diaphragmatic hernia, esophageal atresia with fistula, choanal atresia, congenital cardiac defect, immature alveoli [absent or decreased]) compromise respiration.

The newborn's chest circumference is approximately 30 to 33 cm at birth. Auscultation of the chest of a newborn infant reveals loud, clear breath sounds that seem very near because there is less chest wall musculature. The ribs of the infant articulate with the spine at a horizontal rather than a downward slope; consequently, the rib cage cannot expand with inspiration as readily as an adult's. Because neonatal respiratory function is largely a matter of diaphragmatic contraction, abdominal breathing is characteristic of newborns. That is, the newborn infant's chest and abdomen rise simultaneously with inspiration, but because of the large size of the abdomen, chest movement is not as visible.

The outer walls of the alveoli are lined with surfactant, a protein manufactured in type II cells of the lungs. Lung expansion is largely dependent on chest wall contraction and adequate presence and secretion of surfactant. Surfactant lowers surface tension, thereby requiring less inspiratory pressure to keep the alveoli open with inspiration, and prevents total alveolar collapse on exhalation, thus maintaining alveolar stability. With absent or decreased surfactant, more pressure must be generated for inspiration, which may soon tire or exhaust preterm or sick term infants. Surfactant may be compared with soapy water on the surface of a group of inflated latex balloons: as air is let out of the balloons (exhalation phase), the soapy water prevents total collapse of the balloons, and, conversely, inflation of the balloons occurs readily because of decreased tension (friction) on their surfaces.

Cardiovascular System

The cardiovascular system changes significantly after birth. The infant's first breaths, combined with increased alveolar capillary distention, inflate the lungs and reduce pulmonary vascular resistance to pulmonary blood flow from the pulmonary arteries. Pulmonary artery pressure drops, and pressure in the right atrium declines. Increased pulmonary blood flow from the left side of the heart increases pressure in the left atrium, which causes a functional closure of the foramen ovale. During the first few days of life, crying may temporarily reverse the flow through the foramen ovale and lead to mild cyanosis.

In utero, fetal Po_2 is 27 mm Hg. After birth, when the Po_2 level in the arterial blood approximates 50 mm Hg, the ductus arteriosus constricts in response to increased oxygenation. Circulating hormone prostaglandin (PGE_2) levels also have an important role in closure of the ductus arteriosus. Later, the ductus arteriosus closes completely and becomes a ligament. With the clamping of the cord, the umbilical arteries, umbilical vein, and ductus venosus close and are converted into ligaments. The hypogastric arteries also occlude and become ligaments.

Heart Rate and Sounds

The heart rate averages 120 to 140 beats/min at birth, with variations noted during sleeping and waking states. Shortly after the first cry, the infant's heart rate may be as high as 175 to 180 beats/min. The range of the heart rate in the full-term newborn is 80 to 90 beats/min during sleep and up to 170+ beats/min while awake. It is not unusual to find a heart rate of 180 beats/min when the infant cries. A heart rate that is either consistently high (more than 170 beats/min) or low (fewer than 80 beats/min) with the newborn at rest should be reevaluated within an hour or when the infant's activity changes.

The apical impulse (point of maximal impulse [PMI]) in the newborn is at the fourth intercostal space and to the left of the midclavicular line. The PMI is often visible and easily palpable because of the thin chest wall; this is also called *precordial activity.*

Apical pulse rates should be obtained on all infants. Auscultation should be for a full minute, preferably when the infant is asleep. An irregular heart rate in newborns is not uncommon in the first few hours of life. After this time an irregular heart rate not attributed to changes in activity or respiratory pattern should be further evaluated.

Heart sounds during the neonatal period are of higher pitch, shorter duration, and greater intensity than during adult life. The first sound (S_1) is typically louder and duller than the second sound (S_2), which is sharp. The third and fourth heart sounds are not auscultated in newborns. Most heart murmurs heard during the neonatal period have no pathologic significance, and more than half of the murmurs disappear by 6 months. However, the presence of a murmur and accompanying signs such as poor feeding, apnea, cyanosis, or pallor is considered abnormal and should be further investigated.

Blood Pressure

The newborn infant's average systolic blood pressure (BP) is 60 to 80 mm Hg and average diastolic BP is 40 to 50 mm Hg. The BP increases by the second day of life with minor variations noted during the first month of life. A drop in systolic BP (about 15 mm Hg) in the first hour of life is common. Crying and movement usually cause increases in the systolic BP. The measurement of BP is best accomplished with an oscillometric device while the infant is at rest. A correctly sized cuff must be used for accurate measurement of an infant's BP. Unless there is a specific indication, BP is not routinely measured in the newborn except as a baseline. The practice of obtaining four extremity pressures in the early newborn period to detect coarctation of the aorta (COA) has been recently questioned (Razmus & Lewis, 2006) in light of evidence that COA defects do not manifest in the immediate postpartum period but more typically at approximately 12 to 14 days of age, a time when the ductus arteriosus closes (Taylor, 2005).

Blood Volume

Blood volume in the newborn is about 80 to 85 ml/kg of body weight. Immediately after birth the total blood volume averages 300 ml, but this volume can increase by as much as 100 ml, depending on the length of time to cord clamping and cutting. The infant born prematurely has a relatively greater blood volume than the term newborn. This occurs because the preterm infant has a proportionately greater plasma volume, not a greater red blood cell (RBC) mass.

Early or late clamping of the cord changes circulatory dynamics of the newborn. Late clamping expands the blood volume from the so-called placental transfusion of blood to the newborn. Delayed cord clamping (more than 2 minutes after birth) has been reported to result in polycythemia with subsequent clinical signs of hyperviscosity (hematocrit 65% or greater, plethoric or ruddy red appearance, sluggish circulation leading to possible emboli in the microvasculature and organ damage, respiratory distress, and possibly hyperbilirubinemia as a result of red cell breakdown) (Armentrout & Huseby, 2003). However, recent data showed delayed cord clamping (no longer than 2 minutes after birth) in full-term neonates was beneficial in regards to improved hematocrit, improved iron status, and a decrease in anemia; such benefits were observed over ages 2 to 6 months (Hutton & Hassan, 2007). In this study polycythemia occurred with delayed clamping but was not harmful.

Hematopoietic System

The hematopoietic system of the newborn exhibits certain variations from that of the adult. Levels of RBCs and leukocytes differ, but platelets levels are relatively the same.

Red Blood Cells and Hemoglobin

At birth the average levels of RBCs and hemoglobin (fetal hemoglobin is predominant) are higher than those in the adult. Cord blood of the term newborn may have a hemoglobin concentration from 14 to 24 g/dl (mean 17 g/dl). The hematocrit ranges from 44% to 64% (mean 55%). The RBC count is correspondingly elevated, ranging from 4.8 to 7.1/mm^3. These values fall and reach the average levels of 11 to 17 g/dl (hemoglobin), 4.2 to 5.2/mm^3 (RBC), and 28% to 42% (hematocrit), by the end of the first month. The blood values may be affected by delayed clamping of the cord, which results in a rise in hemoglobin, RBCs, and hematocrit. The source of the sample is a significant factor because capillary blood yields higher values than venous blood. The timing of the neonate's blood sample is also significant; the slight rise in RBCs after birth is followed by a substantial drop. At birth the infant's blood contains an average of 70% fetal hemoglobin, but because of the shorter life span of the cells containing fetal hemoglobin, the percentage falls to 55% by 5 weeks and to 5% by 20 weeks. Iron stores generally are sufficient to sustain normal RBC production for 4 to 5 months in the term infant, at which time a physiologic anemia that is usually transient may occur.

Leukocytes

Leukocytosis, with a white blood cell (WBC) count of approximately 18,000/mm^3 (range 9000 to 30,000/mm^3), is normal at birth. The number of WBCs increases to 23,000 to 24,000/mm^3 during the first day after birth. The initial high WBC count of the newborn decreases rapidly, and a stable level of 11,500/mm^3 is normally maintained during the neonatal period. Serious infection is not well tolerated by the newborn; leukocytes are slow to recognize foreign protein and to localize and fight infection early in life. Sepsis may be accompanied by a concomitant rise in granulocytes (neutrophilia); however, some infants may initially be seen with clinical signs of sepsis without a significant elevation in WBCs. In addition, events other than infection—prolonged crying, maternal hypertension, asymptomatic hypoglycemia, hemolytic disease, meconium aspiration syndrome, labor induction with oxytocin, surgery, difficult labor, high altitude, and maternal fever—may cause neutrophilia in the newborn (Weinberg & Powell, 2001).

Platelets

Platelet count ranges between 200,000 and 300,000/mm^3 and is essentially the same in newborns as in adults. The levels of factors II, VII, IX, and X, found in the liver, are decreased during the first few days of life because the newborn cannot synthesize vitamin K. However, bleeding tendencies in the newborn are uncommon, and unless the vitamin K deficiency is great, clotting is sufficient to prevent hemorrhage.

Blood Groups

The infant's blood group is genetically determined and established early in fetal life. However, during the neonatal period there is a gradual increase in the strength of the agglutinogens present in the RBC membrane. Cord blood samples may be used to identify the infant's blood type and Rh status.

Thermogenic System

Next to establishing respiration and adequate circulation, heat regulation is most critical to the newborn's survival. Thermoregulation is the maintenance of balance between heat loss and heat production. Newborns attempt to stabilize their core body temperatures within a narrow range. Hypothermia from excessive heat loss is a common and dangerous problem in neonates. The newborn's ability to produce heat (thermogenesis) often approaches that of the adult; however, the tendency toward rapid heat loss in a cold environment is increased in the newborn and poses a significant hazard to the infant during transition to extrauterine life.

Thermogenesis

The shivering mechanism of heat production is rarely operable in the newborn. Nonshivering thermogenesis is accomplished primarily by brown fat, which is unique to the newborn, and secondarily by increased metabolic activity in the brain, heart, and liver. Brown fat is located in superficial deposits in the interscapular region and axillae, as well as in deep deposits at the thoracic inlet, along the vertebral column, and around the kidneys. Brown fat has a richer vascular and nerve supply than ordinary fat. Heat produced by intense lipid metabolic activity in brown fat can warm the neonate by increasing heat production as much as 100%. Reserves of brown fat, usually present for several weeks after birth, are rapidly depleted with cold stress. The less mature the infant, the less reserve of this essential fat is available at birth.

Heat Loss

Heat loss in the newborn occurs by four modes:

1. **Convection** is the flow of heat from the body surface to cooler ambient air. Because of heat loss by convection, the ambient temperature in the nursery is kept at approximately 24° C and newborns in open bassinets are wrapped to protect them from the cold. A cap may be worn to decrease heat loss from the infant's head.
2. **Radiation** is the loss of heat from the body surface to a cooler solid surface not in direct contact but in relative proximity. To prevent this type of loss, cribs and examining tables are placed away from outside windows and care is taken to avoid direct air drafts.
3. **Evaporation** is the loss of heat that occurs when a liquid is converted to a vapor. In the newborn, heat loss by evaporation occurs as a result of vaporization of moisture from the skin. This heat loss is intensified by failing to dry the newborn directly after birth or by drying the infant too slowly after a bath. The less mature the newborn, the more severe the evaporative heat loss. Evaporative heat loss, as a component of insensible water loss, is the most significant cause of heat loss in the first few days of life.
4. **Conduction** is the loss of heat from the body surface to cooler surfaces in direct contact. When admitted to the nursery, the newborn is placed in a warmed crib to minimize heat loss. The scales used for weighing the newborn should have a protective cover to minimize conductive heat loss as well.

Loss of heat must be controlled to protect the infant. Control of such modes of heat loss is the basis of caregiving policies and techniques. One method for promoting maternal-newborn interaction is to place the naked healthy newborn next to the mother's skin and cover both with a blanket. This skin-to-skin contact enhances newborn temperature control and interaction.

evolve Skill—Thermoregulation

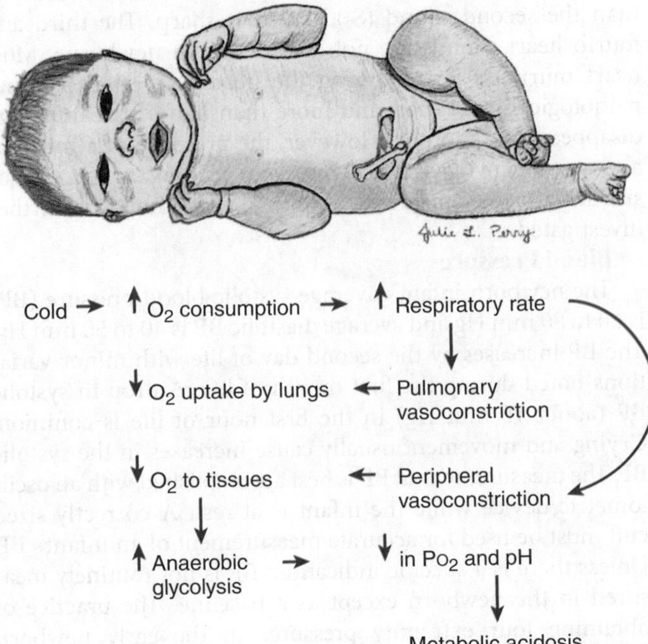

Fig. 24-1 Effects of cold stress. When an infant is stressed by cold, oxygen consumption increases and pulmonary and peripheral vasoconstriction occur, thereby decreasing oxygen uptake by the lungs and oxygen to the tissues; anaerobic glycolysis increases; and there is a decrease in Po_2 and pH, leading to metabolic acidosis.

Temperature Regulation

Anatomic and physiologic differences among the newborn, child, and adult are notable. The newborn's ability to produce heat initially is less than that of an adult. Newborns have larger body surface to body weight (mass) ratios than children and adults. The newborn's flexed position helps guard against heat loss because it diminishes the amount of body surface exposed to the environment. Infants can also reduce the loss of internal heat through the body surface by constricting peripheral blood vessels.

Cold stress imposes metabolic and physiologic problems on all infants, regardless of gestational age and condition. The respiratory rate increases in response to the increased need for oxygen. In the cold-stressed infant, oxygen consumption and energy are diverted from maintaining normal brain cell and cardiac function and growth to thermogenesis for survival. If the infant cannot maintain an adequate oxygen tension, vasoconstriction follows and jeopardizes pulmonary perfusion. As a consequence, the partial pressure of arterial oxygen (Pao_2) is decreased, and the blood pH drops. These changes may prompt a transient respiratory distress or may aggravate existing respiratory distress syndrome. Moreover, decreased pulmonary perfusion and oxygen tension may maintain or reopen the right-to-left shunt across the patent ductus arteriosus.

The basal metabolic rate increases with cold stress (Fig. 24-1). If cold stress is protracted, anaerobic glycolysis occurs, resulting in increased production of acids. Metabolic acidosis develops, and if a defect in respiratory function is present, respiratory acidosis also develops. Excessive fatty acids may displace the bilirubin from the albumin-binding sites and exacerbate hyperbilirubinemia. Another metabolic consequence of cold stress is hypoglycemia. The process of anaerobic glycolysis utilizes approximately three to four times the amount of blood glucose, thereby depleting existing stores; if the infant is sufficiently stressed and low glucose stores are not replaced, hypoglycemia, which can be asymptomatic in the newborn, may ensue.

Hyperthermia develops more rapidly in the newborn than in the adult because of decreased ability to increase evaporative skin water losses. Although newborn infants have six times as many sweat glands per unit area as adults, in most newborns these glands do not function sufficiently to allow the infant to sweat. Serious overheating of the newborn can cause cerebral damage from dehydration or heat stroke and death.

Renal System

At term the kidneys occupy a large portion of the posterior abdominal wall. The bladder lies close to the anterior abdominal wall and is an abdominal as well as a pelvic organ. In the newborn almost all palpable masses in the abdomen are renal in origin.

At birth a small quantity (approximately 40 ml) of urine is usually present in the bladder of a full-term infant. The frequency of voiding varies from two to six times per day during the first and second days of life and from 5 to 25 times during the subsequent 24 hours. About six to eight voidings per day of pale straw-colored urine are indicative of adequate fluid intake. Generally, term infants void 15 to 60 ml of urine per kilogram per day.

Full-term newborns have limited capacity to concentrate urine; therefore the specific gravity ranges from 1.001 to 1.020. The ability to concentrate urine fully is attained by about 3 months of age. After the first voiding the infant's urine may appear cloudy (because of mucus content) and have a much higher specific gravity. This decreases as fluid intake increases. Normal urine during early infancy is usually straw colored and almost odorless. Sometimes pink-tinged uric acid crystal stains appear on the diaper; these stains are normal.

Loss of fluid through urine, feces, lungs, increased metabolic rate, and limited fluid intake results in a 5% to 10% loss of the birth weight. This usually occurs over the first 3 to 5 days of life. If the mother is breastfeeding and her milk supply has not come in yet (which occurs by the third or fourth day after birth), the neonate is somewhat protected from dehydration by its increased extracellular fluid volume. The neonate should regain the birth weight within 10 to 14 days depending on the feeding method (breast or bottle).

Because renal thresholds are low in the infant, bicarbonate concentration and buffering capacity are decreased. This may lead to acidosis and electrolyte imbalance.

Fluid and Electrolyte Balance

About 40% of the body weight of the newborn is extracellular fluid. Each day the newborn takes in and excretes roughly 600 to 700 ml of water, which is 20% of the total body fluid or 50% of the extracellular fluid. The glomerular filtration rate of a newborn is about 30% to 50% that of an adult. This results in a decreased ability to remove nitrogenous and other waste products from the blood. However, the newborn's ingested protein is almost totally metabolized for growth.

Sodium reabsorption is decreased as a result of a lowered sodium and potassium-activated adenosine triphosphate activity. The decreased ability to excrete excessive sodium results in hypotonic urine compared with plasma. There is a higher concentration of sodium, phosphates, chloride, and organic acids and a lower concentration of bicarbonate ions. The infant has a higher renal threshold for glucose.

Gastrointestinal System

The full-term newborn is capable of swallowing, digesting, metabolizing, absorbing proteins and simple carbohydrates, and emulsifying fats. With the exception of pancreatic amylase, the characteristic enzymes and digestive juices are present even in low-birth-weight neonates.

In the adequately hydrated infant, the mucous membrane of the mouth is moist and pink; the hard and soft palates are intact. The presence of moderate to large amounts of mucus is common in the first few hours after birth. Small whitish areas (Epstein pearls) may be found on the gum margins and at the juncture of the hard and soft palate. The cheeks are full because of well-developed sucking pads. These, like the labial tubercles (sucking calluses) on the upper lip, disappear around the age of 12 months, when the sucking period is over.

Even though in utero sucking motions have been recorded by ultrasound, these motions are not coordinated with swallowing in any infant born before 32 to 33 weeks of gestation. Sucking behavior is influenced by neuromuscular maturity, maternal medications received during labor and birth, and the type of initial feeding.

A special mechanism present in healthy term newborns coordinates the breathing, sucking, and swallowing reflexes necessary for oral feeding. Sucking in the newborn takes place in small bursts of three or four sucks at a time. The infant is unable to move food from the lips to the pharynx; therefore placing the nipple (breast or bottle) well inside the baby's mouth is necessary. Peristaltic activity in the esophagus is uncoordinated in the first few days of life. It quickly becomes a coordinated pattern in healthy full-term infants, and they swallow easily.

Teeth begin developing in utero, with enamel formation continuing until about 10 years of age. Tooth development is influenced by neonatal or infant illnesses and medications, and by illnesses of or medications taken by the mother during pregnancy. The fluoride level in the water supply also influences tooth development. Occasionally an infant may be born with one or more teeth.

Bacteria are not present in the infant's gastrointestinal tract at birth. Soon after birth, oral and anal orifices permit entrance of bacteria and air. Generally the highest bacterial concentration is found in the lower portion of the intestine, particularly in the large intestine. Normal colonic bacteria are established within the first week after birth, and normal intestinal flora help synthesize vitamin K, folate, and biotin. Bowel sounds can usually be heard shortly after birth.

evolve Case Study—Newborn Health Problems

Stomach capacity varies from 30 to 90 ml, depending on the infant's size. Emptying time for the stomach is highly variable. Several factors, such as time and volume of feedings or type and temperature of food, may affect the emptying time. The cardiac sphincter and nervous control of the stomach are immature, so some regurgitation may occur. Regurgitation during the first day or two of life can be decreased by avoiding overfeeding, by burping the infant, and by positioning the infant with the head slightly elevated.

Digestion

The infant's ability to digest carbohydrates, fats, and proteins is regulated by the presence of certain enzymes. Most of these are functional at birth. One exception is amylase, produced by the salivary glands after about 3 months and by the pancreas at about 6 months of age. This enzyme is necessary to convert starch into maltose and occurs in high amounts in colostrum. The other exception is lipase, which is also secreted by the pancreas; it is necessary for the digestion of fat. Thus the normal newborn is capable of digesting simple carbohydrates and proteins but has a limited ability to digest fats.

Further digestion and absorption of nutrients occurs in the small intestine in the presence of pancreatic secretions, secretions from the liver through the common bile duct, and secretions from the duodenal portion of the small intestine.

Stools

At birth the lower intestine is filled with meconium. Meconium is formed during fetal life from the amniotic fluid and its constituents, intestinal secretions (including bilirubin), and cells (shed from the mucosa). Meconium is greenish black and viscous and contains occult blood. The first meconium passed is usually sterile, but within hours all meconium passed contains bacteria. The majority of healthy term infants pass meconium within 12 to 24 hours of life, and almost all do so by 48 hours (Blackburn, 2007). The number of stools passed varies during the first week, being most numerous between the third and sixth days. Newborns fed early pass stools sooner. Progressive changes in the stooling pattern indicate a properly functioning gastrointestinal tract (Box 24-1).

BOX 24-1 Changes in Stooling Patterns of Newborns

Meconium

Meconium is the infant's first stool, composed of amniotic fluid and its constituents, intestinal secretions, shed mucosal cells, and possibly blood (ingested maternal blood or minor bleeding of alimentary tract vessels).

Passage of meconium should occur within the first 24 to 48 hours, although it may be delayed up to 7 days in very-low-birth-weight infants.

Transitional Stools

These usually appear by third day after initiation of feeding.

They are greenish brown to yellowish brown; are thin and less sticky than meconium; and may contain some milk curds.

Milk Stool

Milk stool usually appears by the fourth day.

In *breastfed infants,* stools are yellow to golden, are pasty in consistency, and have an odor similar to that of sour milk.

In *formula-fed infants,* stools are pale yellow to light brown, are firmer in consistency, and have a more offensive odor.

Hepatic System

The liver and gallbladder are formed by the fourth week of gestation. In the newborn the liver can be palpated about 1 cm below the right costal margin because it is enlarged and occupies about 40% of the abdominal cavity. The infant's liver plays an important role in iron storage, carbohydrate metabolism, conjugation of bilirubin, and coagulation.

Iron Storage

The fetal liver, which serves as the site for production of hemoglobin after birth, begins storing iron in utero. The infant's iron store is proportional to total body hemoglobin content and length of gestation. At birth the term neonate has an iron store sufficient to last 4 to 6 months; the preterm infant's iron stores are often lower and are depleted sooner.

Carbohydrate Metabolism

At birth the newborn is cut off from its maternal glucose supply and, as a result, experiences an initial decrease in serum glucose levels. The newborn's increased energy needs, decreased hepatic release of glucose from glycogen stores, increased RBC volume, and increased brain size may initially contribute to the rapid depletion of stored glycogen within the first 24 hours after birth. In most healthy term newborns, blood glucose levels stabilize at 50 to 60 mg/dl during the first several hours after birth; by the third day of life, the blood glucose levels should be approximately 60 to 70 mg/dl. The initiation of feedings assists in the stabilization of the newborn's blood glucose levels. Colostrum contains high amounts of glucose, thus also assisting in the stabilization of blood glucose levels in breastfed neonates (see Evidence-Based Practice box).

Jaundice

Jaundice is the manifestation of the pigment bilirubin in the tissues of the body. Jaundice usually does not appear until the bilirubin level reaches 5 mg/dl. Any visible jaundice within the first 24 hours of life or persistence of jaundice beyond 7 to 10 days requires further investigation into the cause, since this may represent an underlying pathologic process (Fig. 24-2). See Chapter 25 for a further discussion of bilirubin metabolism and hyperbilirubinemia.

Coagulation

Coagulation factors, which are synthesized in the liver, are activated by vitamin K. The lack of intestinal bacteria needed to synthesize vitamin K results in transient blood coagulation deficiency between the second and fifth days of life. The administration of intramuscular vitamin K shortly after birth helps prevent clotting problems.

Immune System

The cells that provide the infant with immunity are developed early in fetal life; however, they are not activated for weeks to months. For the first 3 months of life, the healthy term infant

EVIDENCE-BASED PRACTICE Monitoring for Hypoglycemia

—*Pat Gingrich*

Ask the Question

What are the current recommendations for monitoring and treating neonatal hypoglycemia?

Search for Evidence

Search Strategies

Professional organization guidelines, meta-analyses, systematic reviews, randomized controlled trials, nonrandomized prospective studies, and retrospective studies since 2006

Databases Searched

CINAHL; Cochrane; Medline; National Guideline Clearinghouse; TRIP Database Plus; and websites for APA, AWHONN, CDC, and WHO

Critically Analyze the Evidence

Hypoglycemia affects less than 1% of healthy newborns. Risk factors for hypoglycemia included weight below 2 kg or above 4 kg, small or large for gestational age, intrauterine growth restriction, less than 37 weeks of gestation, maternal diabetes or glucose imbalance, or sepsis. Hypoglycemia of the newborn is infrequently a symptom of underlying disease. Signs of hypoglycemia include irritability, jitteriness, high-pitched cry, pallor, sweating, lethargy, poor feeding, seizures, and respiratory difficulties.

A Best Practice Guideline from the Joanna Briggs Institute (2006) concluded that breastfeeding early and often, with thermoregulation through skin-to-skin contact, will normalize the glucose levels of most term, normal-weight infants during their first 48 hours. The guidelines recommended against any supplemental glucose or water feedings or routine glucose monitoring, except in the case of obvious physical signs of hypoglycemia.

This emphasis on breastfeeding early (first hour) and often (10 to 12 feedings in first 24 hours) concurs with guidelines for breastfeeding by the Association of Women's Health, Obstetric and Neonatal Nurses (2007) and the Academy of Breastfeeding Medicine (Wight & Marinelli, 2006). The academy's guidelines recommend breastfeeding every 1 to 2 hours and monitoring blood glucose level. If the blood glucose does not reach the goal of more than 45 mg/dl, consider administering glucose intravenously.

Implications for Practice

As noted in the Evidence-Based Practice box for Chapter 27, skin-to-skin contact and early breastfeeding have proven benefits for early temperature and glucose stabilization of the newborn, as well as bonding during the newborn's first awake, interactive period. All nonessential tasks, such as administration of eye medications and vitamin K, should be delayed to facilitate this enriching time together. The nurse should be alert to the signs of hypoglycemia, which can appear late. For most infants without underlying pathologic conditions, monitoring the glucose levels and encouraging breastfeeding, rather than using supplemental formula or dextrose water, and skin-to-skin contact will correct the hypoglycemia within minutes or hours. Finally, the nurse can remember that every baby has his or her own normal range of glucose, which may run high or low in the normal range.

References

Association of Women's Health, Obstetric and Neonatal Nurses: *Breastfeeding support: prenatal care through the first year*, ed 2, Evidence-Based Clinical Practice Guideline, Washington, DC, 2007, The Association.

Joanna Briggs Institute of Evidence Based Nursing: Management of asymptomatic hypoglycemia in healthy term neonates for nurses and midwives, *Best Practice* 10(1):1-4, 2006.

Wight N, Marinelli KA: Academy of Breastfeeding Medicine Protocol Committee: ABM clinical protocol #1: guidelines for glucose monitoring and treatment of hypoglycemia in breastfed neonates, *Breastfeed Med* 1:178-184, 2006.

is somewhat protected by passive immunity received from the mother; however, this is dependent on the mother's previous exposure to antigens and her immunologic response. The membrane-protective IgA is missing from the respiratory and urinary tracts and, unless the newborn is breastfed, is also absent from the gastrointestinal tract. The infant begins to synthesize IgG, and levels reach about 40% of adult levels by 1 year of age. Significant amounts of IgM are produced at birth, and adult levels are reached by 9 months of age. The production of IgA, IgD, and IgE is much more gradual, and maximum levels are not attained until early childhood. The infant who is breastfed receives significant passive immunity through the colostrum and breast milk.

Integumentary System

All skin structures are present at birth. The epidermis and dermis are bound loosely and are very thin. Vernix caseosa (a cheeselike whitish substance) is fused with the epidermis and serves as a protective covering. The infant's skin is sensitive and can be easily damaged. The term infant has erythematous (red) skin for a few hours after birth, after which it fades to its normal color. The skin often appears blotchy or mottled, especially over the extremities. The hands and feet appear slightly cyanotic (acrocyanosis); this is caused by vasomotor instability and capillary stasis. Acrocyanosis is normal and appears intermittently over the first 7 to 10 days, especially with exposure to cold.

The healthy term infant usually has a plump appearance because of large amounts of subcutaneous tissue and extracellular water content. Subcutaneous fat accumulated during the last trimester acts as insulation. Fine lanugo hair may be noted over the face, shoulders, and back. Edema of the face and ecchymosis (bruising) may be noted as a result of face presentation, forceps-assisted birth, or vacuum extraction (see Family-Centered Care box).

Creases can be found on the palms of the hands. The simian line, a single palmar crease, is often found in Asian infants or in infants with Down syndrome.

Caput Succedaneum

Caput succedaneum is a generalized, easily identifiable edematous area of the scalp, most commonly found on the occiput (Fig. 24-3, *A*). The sustained pressure of the presenting vertex against the cervix results in compression of local vessels, thereby slowing venous return. The slower venous return causes an increase in tissue fluids within the skin of the scalp, and an edematous swelling develops. This edematous swelling,

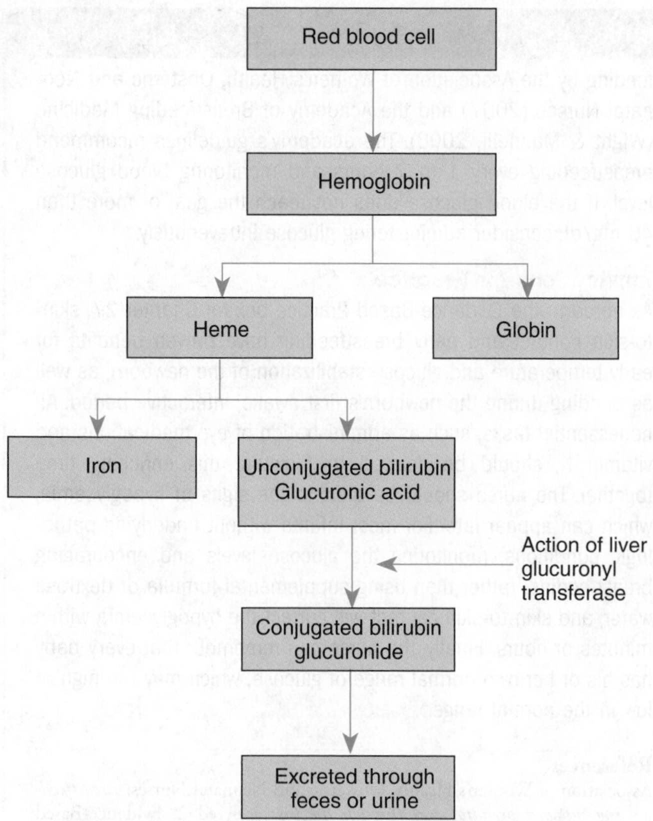

Fig. 24-2 Formation and excretion of bilirubin.

FAMILY-CENTERED CARE

Newborn Skin

A young couple with a healthy newborn girl calls the nurse because they are concerned about the small raised red dots on the baby's face and arms and that her skin is dry and flaky in certain places. The nurse assesses the newborn and concludes that the spots are not mosquito bites, as the family stated, but erythema toxicum. What further anticipatory guidance about normal newborn skin appearance could the nurse give the parents to reassure them that the newborn is healthy and "normal"?

present at birth, extends across the suture lines of the skull and disappears spontaneously within 3 to 4 days. Infants who are born with the assistance of vacuum extraction usually have a caput in the area where the cup was applied.

Cephalhematoma

Cephalhematoma is a collection of blood between a skull bone and its periosteum. Therefore a cephalhematoma does not cross a cranial suture line (see Fig. 24-3, *C*). Often caput succedaneum and cephalhematoma occur simultaneously.

Bleeding may occur with spontaneous birth from pressure against the maternal bony pelvis. Low forceps birth and difficult forceps rotation and extraction may also cause bleeding. This soft, fluctuating, irreducible fullness does not pulsate or bulge when the infant cries. It appears several hours or the day after birth and may not become apparent until a caput succedaneum is absorbed. A cephalhematoma is usually largest on the second or third day, by which time the bleeding stops (see Family-Centered Care box). The fullness of a cephalhematoma spontaneously resolves in 3 to 6 weeks. It is not aspirated because infection may develop if the skin is punctured. As the hematoma resolves, hemolysis of RBCs occurs and jaundice may result. Hyperbilirubinemia and jaundice may occur from a cephalhematoma after the newborn is discharged home.

FAMILY-CENTERED CARE

Swelling on the Scalp

A 2-day-old healthy newborn has a "bump" on the left side of the head. The mother is concerned that the baby may have somehow fallen out of the crib and injured the head. Nursing assessment reveals that the scalp swelling is raised and soft to the touch but does not cross cranial suture lines; there is no apparent bruising or discoloration. The neurologic assessment reveals no significant findings, and the newborn's behavior appears to be that of a healthy term infant. How could the nurse explain the condition and reassure the mother that her newborn has a common finding rather than an abnormal condition requiring immediate medical attention?

Subgaleal Hemorrhage

Subgaleal hemorrhage is bleeding into the subgaleal compartment (see Fig. 24-3, *B*). The subgaleal compartment is a potential space that contains loosely arranged connective tissue; it is located beneath the galea aponeurosis, the tendinous sheath that connects the frontal and occipital muscles and forms the inner surface of the scalp. The injury occurs as a result of forces that compress and then drag the head through the pelvic outlet (Paige & Moe, 2006). There have been reports of concern regarding the increased use of the vacuum extractor at birth and an association with cases of subgaleal hemorrhage, neonatal morbidity, and deaths (Boo et al, 2005; Uchil & Arulkumaran, 2003). The bleeding extends beyond bone, often posteriorly into the neck, and continues after birth, with the potential for serious complications such as anemia or hypovolemic shock.

Early detection of the hemorrhage is vital; serial head circumference measurements and inspection of the back of the neck for increasing edema and a firm mass are essential. A boggy scalp, pallor, tachycardia, and increasing head circumference may also be early signs of a subgaleal hemorrhage (Doumouchtsis & Arulkumaran, 2006). Computed tomography or magnetic resonance imaging is useful in confirming the diagnosis. Replacement of lost blood and clotting factors is required in acute cases of hemorrhage. Another possible early sign of subgaleal hemorrhage is a forward and lateral positioning of the newborn's ears because the hematoma extends posteriorly. Monitoring the infant for changes in level of consciousness and decreases in hematocrit is also key to early recognition and management. An increase in serum

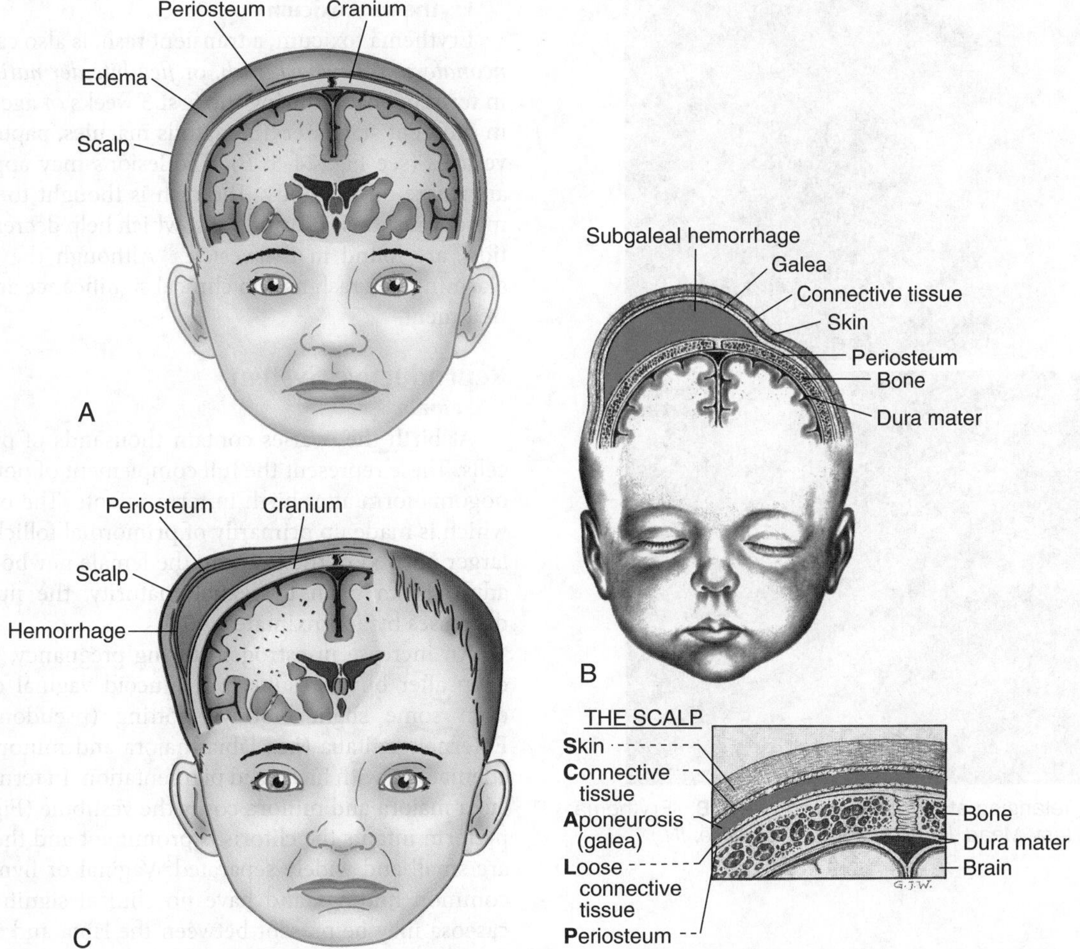

Fig. 24-3 A, Caput succedaneum. **B,** Subgaleal hemorrhage. **C,** Cephalhematoma. (**A** and **B,** From Seidel HM et al: *Mosby's guide to physical examination*, ed 6, St Louis, 2006, Mosby.)

bilirubin levels may be seen as a result of the degradation of blood cells within the hematoma.

Sweat Glands

Sweat glands are present at birth but do not respond to increases in ambient or body temperature. Some fetal sebaceous gland hyperplasia and secretion of sebum result from the hormonal influences of pregnancy. Vernix caseosa is a product of the sebaceous glands. Removal of the vernix is followed by desquamation of the epidermis in most infants. Vernix has been shown to be an epidermal barrier with positive benefits for neonatal skin such as decreasing the skin pH, decreasing skin erythema, and improving skin hydration (Visscher et al, 2005). Distended, small, white sebaceous glands, noticeable on the newborn face, are known as *milia.*

Desquamation

Desquamation (peeling) of the skin of the term infant does not occur until a few days after birth. Large generalized areas of skin desquamation present at birth may be an indication of postmaturity.

Mongolian Spots

Mongolian spots, bluish black areas of pigmentation, may appear over any part of the exterior surface of the body, including the extremities. They are more commonly noted on the back and buttocks (Fig. 24-4). These pigmented areas are most frequently noted in newborns whose ethnic origins are in the Mediterranean area, Latin America, Asia, or Africa. They are more common in dark-skinned individuals but may occur in 5% to 13% of Caucasians as well (Blackburn, 2007). They fade gradually over months or years.

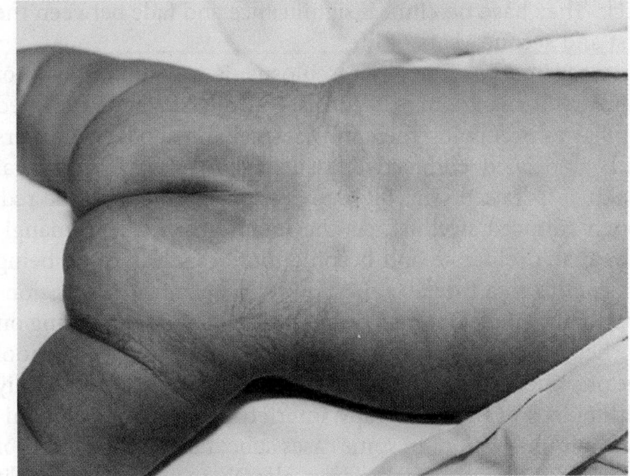

Fig. 24-4 Mongolian spot.

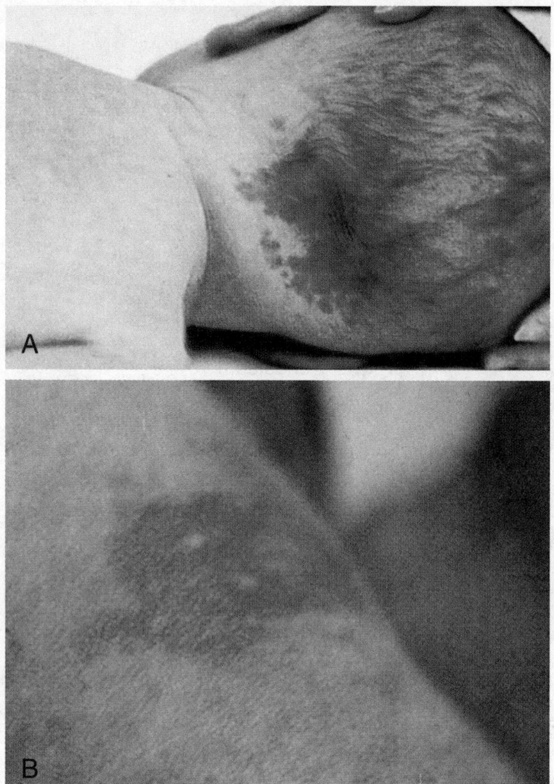

Fig. 24-5 A, Telangiectatic nevi (stork bite). B, Erythema toxicum. *(Courtesy Mead Johnson & Co., Evansville, IN.)*

Nevi

Known as "stork bites," telangiectatic nevi are pink and easily blanched (Fig. 24-5, *A*). They appear on the upper eyelids, nose, upper lip, lower occiput bone, and nape of the neck. They have no clinical significance and fade between the first and second years of life.

A red mark, or nevus vasculosus, is a common type of capillary hemangioma. It consists of dilated, newly formed capillaries occupying the entire dermal and subdermal layers with associated connective tissue hypertrophy. The typical lesion is a raised, sharply demarcated, bright or dark red, rough-surfaced swelling. As the infant grows, the hemangioma may proliferate and become more vascular, often being referred to as a *capillary* or *strawberry hemangioma.* Lesions are usually single but may be multiple, with 75% occurring on the head. These lesions can remain until the child is of school age or sometimes even longer but can be removed successfully with pulsed dye laser therapy, interferon therapy, and prednisone administration. In some cases subcutaneous injections of interferon alfa-2a or interferon alfa-2b may be required if prednisone therapy and the pulsed dye laser fail to control a problematic hemangioma.

A port-wine stain, or nevus flammeus, is usually observed at birth and is composed of a plexus of newly formed capillaries in the papillary layer of the corium. It is red to purple; varies in size, shape, and location; and is not elevated. True port-wine stains do not blanch on pressure or disappear. They are most commonly found on the face and neck.

Erythema Toxicum

Erythema toxicum, a transient rash, is also called *erythema neonatorum, newborn rash,* or *flea bite dermatitis.* It is found in term neonates during the first 3 weeks of age. It has lesions in different stages: erythematous macules, papules, and small vesicles (see Fig. 24-5, *B*). The lesions may appear suddenly anywhere on the body. The rash is thought to be an inflammatory response. Eosinophils, which help decrease inflammation, are found in the vesicles. Although the appearance is alarming, the rash has no clinical significance and requires no treatment.

Reproductive System

Female

At birth the ovaries contain thousands of primitive germ cells. These represent the full complement of potential ova; no oogonia form after birth in term infants. The ovarian cortex, which is made up primarily of primordial follicles, occupies a larger portion of the ovary in the female newborn than in the adult. From birth to sexual maturity, the number of ova decreases by approximately 90%.

An increase in estrogen during pregnancy, followed by a drop after birth, results in a mucoid vaginal discharge and even some slight bloody spotting (pseudomenstruation). External genitalia (i.e., labia majora and minora) are usually edematous, with increased pigmentation. In term neonates the labia majora and minora cover the vestibule (Fig. 24-6, *A*). In preterm infants the clitoris is prominent and the labia majora are small and widely separated. Vaginal or hymenal tags are common findings and have no clinical significance. Vernix caseosa may be present between the labia and should not be forcibly removed during bathing.

If the girl was born in the breech position, the labia may be edematous and bruised. The edema and bruising resolve in a few days; no treatment is necessary.

Male

The testes (see Fig. 24-6, *B*) descend into the scrotum by birth in 90% of newborn boys. Although this percentage drops with preterm birth, by 1 year of age the incidence of undescended testes in all boys is less than 1%.

A tight prepuce (foreskin) is common in newborns. The urethral opening may be completely covered by the prepuce, which may not be retractable for 3 to 4 years. Smegma, a white cheesy substance, is commonly found under the foreskin. Small, white, firm cysts called *epithelial pearls* may be seen at the tip of the prepuce. In the preterm boy of less than 28 weeks of gestation, the testes remain within the abdominal cavity and the scrotum appears high and close to the body. By 28 to 36 weeks of gestation, the testes can be palpated in the inguinal canal and a few rugae appear on the scrotum. At 36 to 40 weeks of gestation, the testes are palpable in the upper scrotum and rugae appear on the anterior portion. After 40 weeks, the testes can be palpated in the scrotum and rugae cover the scrotal sac. The postterm neonate has deep rugae and a pendulous scrotum. The scrotum is usually more deeply pigmented than the rest of the skin, a difference that is especially apparent in darker-skinned infants. This pigmentation is a response to maternal estrogen. A hydrocele, caused by an accumulation of fluid around the testes, may be found. This

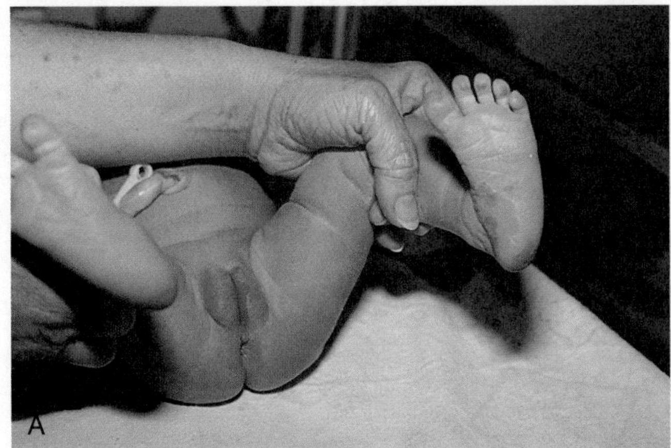

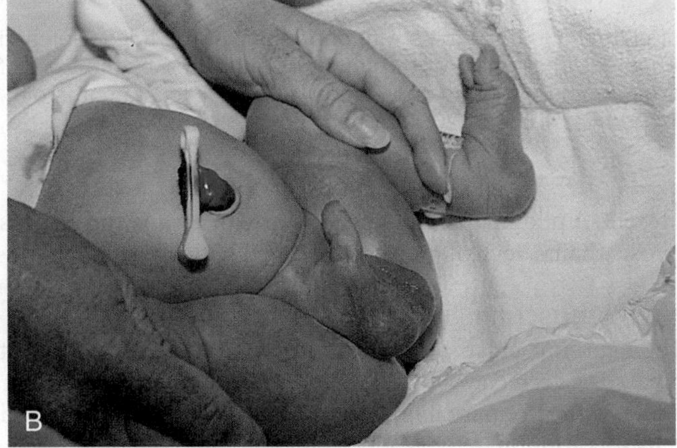

Fig. 24-6 External genitalia. **A,** Genitalia in female term infant. **B,** Genitalia in uncircumcised male infant. Rugae cover scrotum, indicating term gestation. Cord has been swabbed with ethylene blue to prevent infection. *(Courtesy Marjorie Pyle, RNC, Lifecircle, Costa Mesa, CA.)*

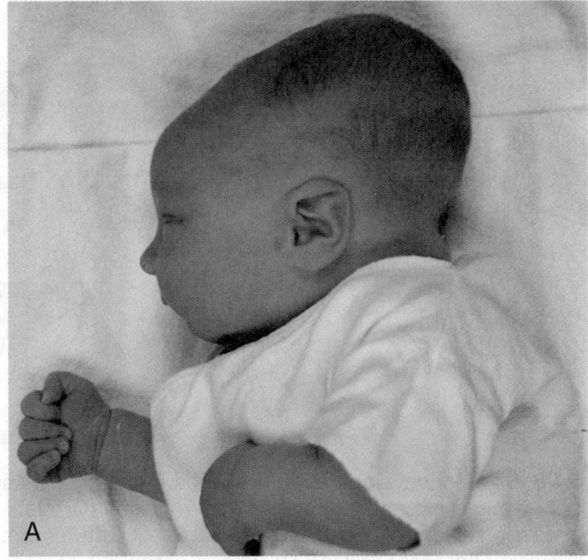

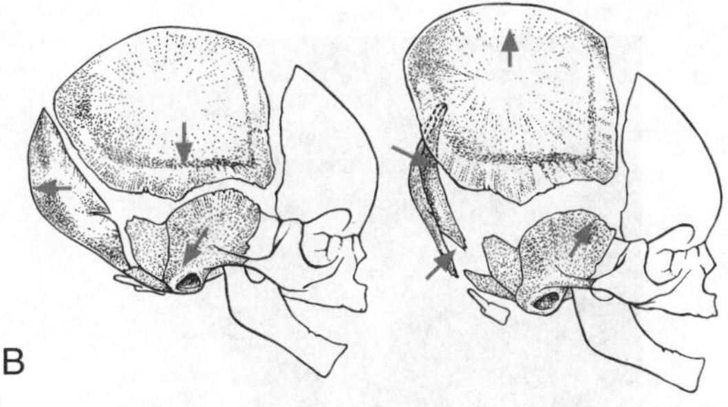

Fig. 24-7 Molding. **A,** Significant molding after vaginal birth. **B,** Schematic of bones of skull when molding is present. *(A, Courtesy Kim Molloy, Knoxville, IA.)*

can be transilluminated with a light and usually decreases in size without treatment.

If the male infant is born in a breech presentation, the scrotum is edematous and may be bruised (see Fig. 25-6). The swelling and discoloration subside within a few days.

Swelling of Breast Tissue

Swelling of the breast tissue in term infants of both sexes is caused by the hyperestrogenism of pregnancy. In a few infants a thin discharge (witch's milk) can be seen. This finding has no clinical significance, requires no treatment, and subsides within a few days as the maternal hormones are eliminated from the infant's body.

The nipples should be symmetric on the chest. Breast tissue and areola size increase with gestation. The areola appears slightly elevated at 34 weeks of gestation. By 36 weeks a breast bud of 1 to 2 mm is palpable; this increases to 12 mm by 42 weeks.

Skeletal System

The infant's skeletal system undergoes rapid development during the first year of life. At birth, more cartilage is present than ossified bone. Because of cephalocaudal (head-to-rump) development, the newborn looks somewhat out of proportion.

The head at term is one fourth of the total body length. The arms are slightly longer than the legs. In the newborn the legs are one third of the total body length but only 15% of the total body weight. As growth proceeds, the midpoint in head-to-toe measurements gradually descends from the level of the umbilicus at birth to the level of the symphysis pubis at maturity.

The face appears small in relation to the skull. The skull appears large and heavy. Cranial size and shape can be distorted by molding (the shaping of the fetal head by overlapping of the cranial bones to facilitate movement through the birth canal during labor) (Fig. 24-7).

The bones in the vertebral column of the newborn form two primary curvatures, one in the thoracic region and one in the sacral region. Both are forward, concave curvatures. As the infant gains head control, at approximately 3 months of age, a secondary curvature appears in the cervical region.

In some newborn infants, there is a significant separation of the knees when the ankles are held together, resulting in an appearance of bowlegs. At birth, there is no apparent arch to the foot. The extremities should be symmetric and of equal length. Skin folds should be equal and symmetric. The hips are checked for dysplasia by a trained clinician using Ortolani maneuver (Fig. 24-8). Fingers and toes should be equal in number and have nails. Extra digits (polydactyly) are some-

evolve Video—Male Breasts (Supine Position)
evolve Anatomy Review—Sutures and Fontanels

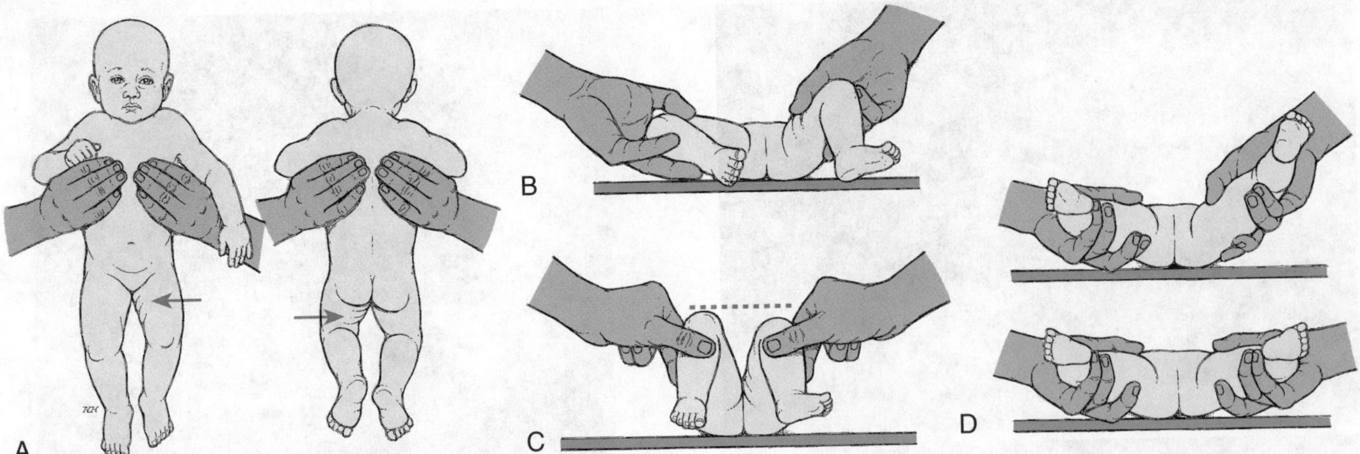

Fig. 24-8 Signs of developmental dysplasia of the hip. **A,** Asymmetry of gluteal and thigh folds with shortening of the thigh (Galeazzi sign). **B,** Limited hip abduction, as seen in flexion (Ortolani test). **C,** Apparent shortening of the femur, as indicated by the level of the knees in flexion (Allis sign). **D,** Ortolani test with femoral head moving in and out of acetabulum (in infants 1 to 2 months old). (From Hockenberry MJ, Wilson D: *Wong's essentials of pediatric nursing*, ed 8, St Louis, 2009, Mosby.)

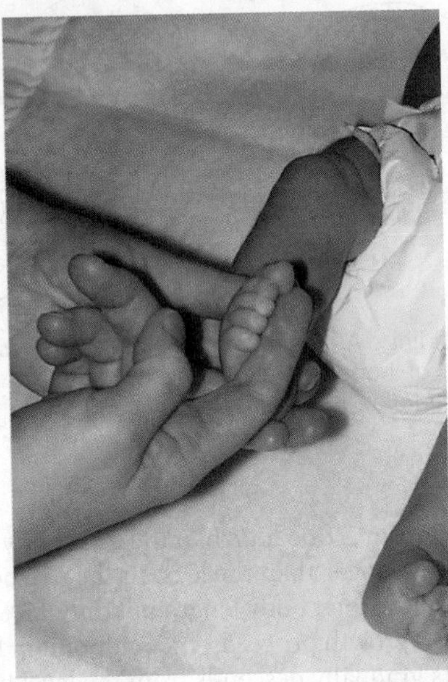

Fig. 24-9 Plantar grasp reflex. (From Zitelli BJ, Davis HW: *Atlas of pediatric physical diagnosis*, ed 5, St Louis, 2007, Mosby.)

evolve Video–Plantar Grasp

times found on the hands and feet. Fingers or toes may be fused (syndactyly). Creases can be found on the palms of the hands and cover the soles of the term newborn's feet. If the infant's presentation was breech, the knees may remain extended and the infant will maintain the in utero position for several weeks.

Two reflexes are elicited, the grasp and the Babinski. To elicit the grasp reflex, touch the palms of the hands or soles of the feet near the base of the digits, causing flexion or grasping (Fig. 24-9). To elicit the Babinski reflex, stroke the outer sole of the foot upward from the heel across the ball of the foot, causing the big toe to dorsiflex and the other toes to hyperextend (Table 24-1, p. 621).

The newborn's spine appears straight and can be flexed easily. The vertebrae should appear straight and flat. The base of the spine should be free from a dimple. If a dimple is noted, further inspection is required to determine whether a sinus is present. A pilonidal dimple, especially with a sinus and a nevus pilosis (hairy nevus), may be associated with spina bifida.

Neuromuscular System

The neuromuscular system is almost completely developed at birth. The term newborn is a vital, responsive, and reactive being with a remarkable capacity for social interaction and self-organization.

Growth of the brain after birth follows a predictable pattern of rapid growth during infancy and early childhood; growth becomes more gradual during the remainder of the first decade and minimal during adolescence. The cerebellum ends its growth spurt, which began at about 30 gestational weeks, by the end of the first year.

The brain requires glucose, as a source of energy, and a relatively large supply of oxygen for adequate metabolism. Such requirements signal a need for careful assessment of the infant's respiratory status. The necessity for glucose requires attentiveness to those neonates who are at risk for hypoglycemia (e.g., infants of diabetic mothers; infants who are macrosomic or small for gestational age; and newborns experiencing prolonged birth, hypoxia, or preterm birth).

Spontaneous motor activity may be seen as transient tremors of the mouth and chin, especially during crying episodes, and of the extremities, notably the arms and hands. Transient tremors are normal and can be observed in nearly every newborn. These tremors should not be present when the infant is quiet and should not persist beyond 1 month of age. Persistent tremors or tremors involving the entire body may indicate pathologic conditions. Normal tremors, tremors of hypoglycemia, and central nervous system (CNS) disorders need to be differentiated so corrective care can be instituted as necessary.

Neuromuscular control in the newborn, although limited, can be noted. If newborns are placed face down on a firm surface, they will turn their heads to the side. They attempt to hold their heads in line with their bodies if they are raised by

Text continued on p. 625

Table 24-1 Assessment of Newborn Reflexes

REFLEX	ELICITING THE REFLEX	CHARACTERISTIC RESPONSE	COMMENTS
Rooting	Touch infant's lip, cheek, or corner of mouth with nipple or finger.	Infant turns head toward stimulus and opens mouth. State dependent (e.g., if infant is in deep sleep, reflex may not be elicited)	Response is difficult if not impossible to elicit after infant has been fed; if response is weak or absent, consider preterm birth or neurologic defect. Parental guidance: Avoid trying to turn head toward breast or nipple; allow infant to root; response disappears after 3-4* mo but may persist up to 1 yr.
Sucking	Elicit rooting reflex as above. May also be elicited by gently stroking tongue with nipple.	Infant opens mouth and begins to suck on nipple. A gloved finger may be used to elicit and evaluate suck. State dependent (e.g., if infant is in deep sleep, reflex may not be elicited).	See above.
Swallowing	Feed infant; swallowing usually follows sucking and obtaining fluids.	Swallowing is usually coordinated with sucking and breathing and usually occurs without gagging, coughing, apnea, or vomiting.	If response is weak or absent, this may indicate preterm birth, effects of maternal analgesics, or illness that needs investigation. Sucking, swallowing, and breathing are often uncoordinated in preterm infant.
Grasp			
Palmar	Place finger in palm of hand.	Infant's fingers curl around examiner's fingers.	Palmar response lessens by 3-4 mo; parents enjoy this contact with infant.
Plantar (see Fig. 24-9)	Place finger at base of toes.	Toes curl downward.	Plantar response lessens by 8 mo.
Extrusion	Touch or depress tip of tongue.	Newborn forces tongue outward.	Response disappears about fourth to fifth month.
Glabellar (Myerson)	Tap over forehead, bridge of nose, or maxilla of newborn whose eyes are open.	Newborn blinks for first four or five taps.	Continued blinking with repeated taps is consistent with extrapyramidal signs.
Tonic neck or "fencing"	With infant in a supine neutral position, turn head to one side.	With infant facing left side, arm and leg on that side extend; opposite arm and leg flex (turn head to right, and extremities assume opposite postures).	Responses in leg are more consistent. Complete response disappears by 3-4 mo; incomplete response may be seen until third or fourth year. After 6 wk, persistent response is sign of an abnormality.

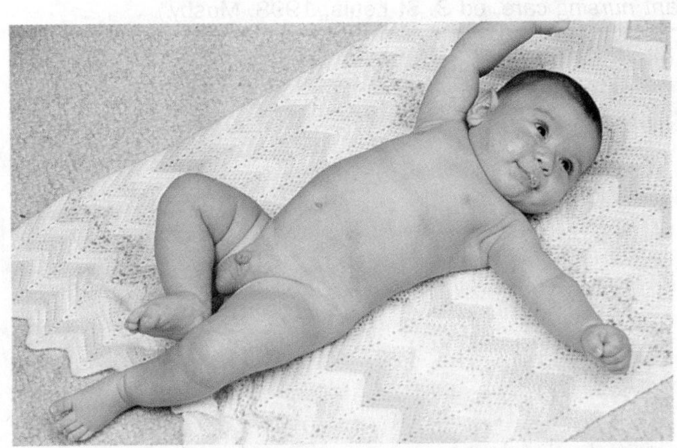

Classic pose in tonic neck reflex. *(Courtesy Marjorie Pyle, RNC, Lifecircle, Costa Mesa, CA.)*

*All durations for persistence of reflexes are based on time elapsed after 40 wk of gestation; that is, if newborn was born at 36 wk of gestation, add 1 mo to all time limits given.

Continued

evolve Video—Rooting and Sucking

evolve Video—Moro Reflex

Table 24-1 Assessment of Newborn Reflexes—cont'd

REFLEX	ELICITING THE REFLEX	CHARACTERISTIC RESPONSE	COMMENTS
Moro (or startle)	Hold infant in semisitting position, allowing head and trunk to fall backward (with support). Place infant supine on flat surface; make a loud abrupt noise. State dependent.	Symmetric abduction and extension of arms are seen; fingers fan out and form a C with thumb and forefinger; slight tremor may be noted; arms are adducted in embracing motion and return to relaxed flexion and movement. A cry may accompany or follow motor movement. Legs may follow similar pattern of response. Preterm infant does not complete "embrace"; instead, arms fall backward because of weakness.	Response is present at birth; complete response may be seen until 8 wk; body jerk only is seen between 8 and 18 wk; response is absent by 6 mo if neurologic maturation is not delayed; response may be incomplete if infant is in deep sleep state; give parental guidance about normal response. Asymmetric response may connote injury to brachial plexus, clavicle, or humerus. Persistent response after 6 mo indicates possible neurologic abnormality such as cerebral palsy.
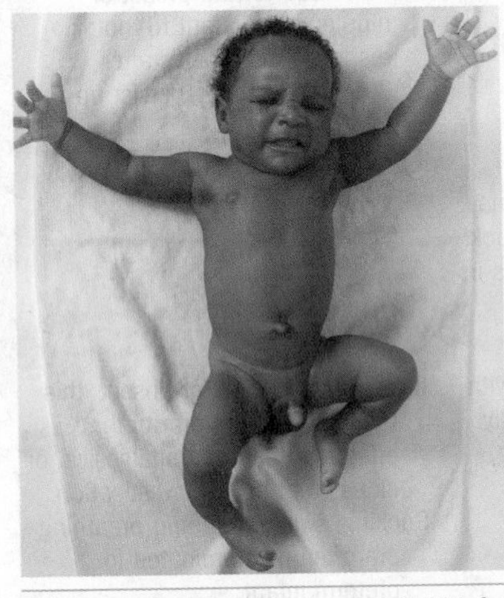 Moro reflex. *(Courtesy Paul Vincent Kuntz, Texas Children's Hospital, Houston.)*			
Stepping or "walking"	Hold infant vertically under arms or on trunk, allowing one foot to touch table surface.	Infant will simulate walking, alternating flexion and extension of feet; term infants walk on soles of their feet, and preterm infants walk on their toes.	Response is normally present for 3-4 wk.
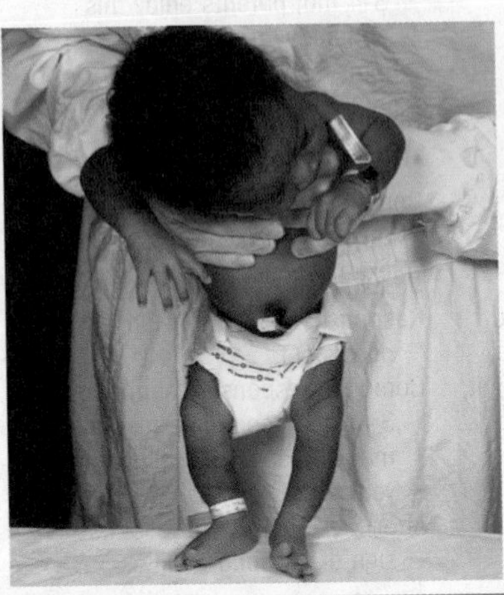 Stepping reflex. (From Dickason EJ, Silverman BL, Kaplan JA: *Maternal-infant nursing care*, ed 3, St Louis, 1998, Mosby.)			

Table 24-1 Assessment of Newborn Reflexes—cont'd

REFLEX	ELICITING THE REFLEX	CHARACTERISTIC RESPONSE	COMMENTS
Crawling	Place newborn on abdomen.	Newborn makes crawling movements with arms and legs.	Response should disappear about 6 wk of age.
	Crawling reflex. *(Courtesy Paul Vincent Kuntz, Texas Children's Hospital.)*		
Deep tendon	Use finger instead of percussion hammer to elicit patellar, or knee jerk, reflex; newborn must be relaxed.	Reflex jerk is present; even with newborn relaxed, nonselective overall reaction may occur.	
Crossed extension	With infant in supine position, examiner extends one leg of infant and presses down knee. Stimulation of sole of foot of fixated limb should cause free leg to flex, adduct, and extend as if attempting to push away stimulating agent.	Opposite leg flexes, adducts, and then extends.	This reflex should be present during newborn period.
	Crossed extension reflex. *(Courtesy Marjorie Pyle, RNC, Lifecircle, Costa Mesa, CA.)*		

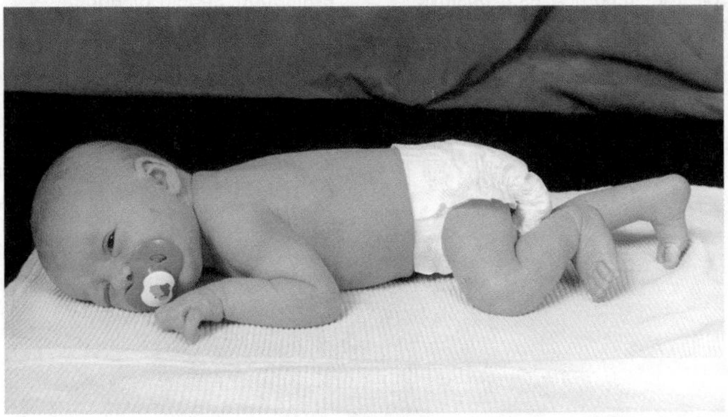

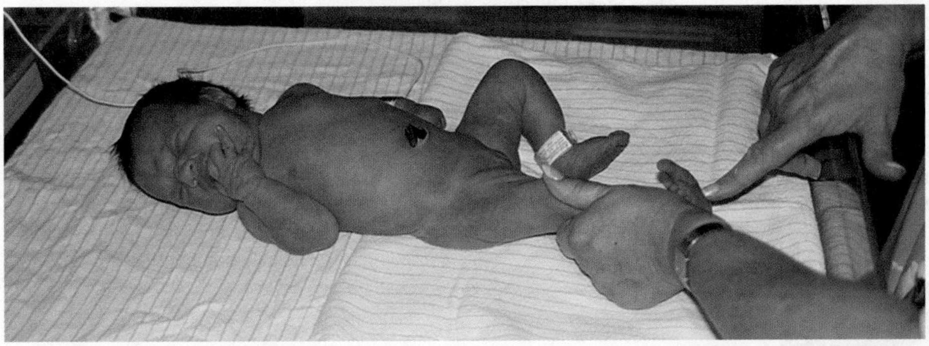

Continued

Table 24-1 Assessment of Newborn Reflexes—cont'd

REFLEX	ELICITING THE REFLEX	CHARACTERISTIC RESPONSE	COMMENTS
Babinski (plantar)	On sole of foot, beginning at heel, stroke upward along lateral aspect of sole, then move finger across ball of foot.	All toes hyperextend, with dorsiflexion of big toe—recorded as a positive sign.	Absence requires neurologic evaluation, should disappear after 1 yr of age. Response depends on infant's general muscle tone, maturity, and condition.
Pull-to-sit (traction response); postural tone	Pull infant up by wrists from supine position with head in midline.	Head comes forward with body with minimal lag; head falls forward when placed in sitting position.	Response disappears by fourth week.
Truncal incurvation (Galant)	Place infant prone on flat surface; run finger down back about 4-5 cm lateral to spine, first on one side and then down other. Correct response involves infant flexing trunk and swinging pelvis toward stimulus.	Trunk is flexed and pelvis is swung toward stimulated side.	Absence suggests general depression of nervous system. With transverse lesions of cord, no response below the level of lesion is present. Response may vary but should be obtainable in all infants, including the preterm. If not seen in first few days, it is usually apparent by 5-6 days.

Babinski reflex. **A**, Direction of stroke. **B**, Dorsiflexion of big toe. **C**, Fanning of toes. (From Hockenberry MJ, Wilson D: *Wong's nursing care of infants and children*, ed 8, St Louis, 2007, Mosby.)

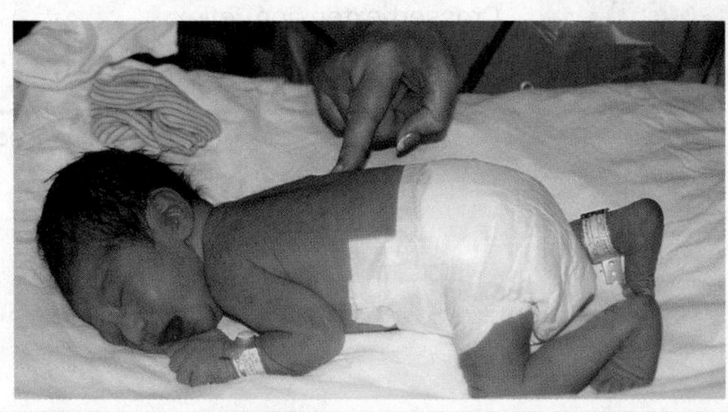

Trunk incurvation reflex. *(Courtesy Marjorie Pyle, RNC, Lifecircle, Costa Mesa, CA.)*

Table 24-1 Assessment of Newborn Reflexes—cont'd

REFLEX	ELICITING THE REFLEX	CHARACTERISTIC RESPONSE	COMMENTS
Magnet	Place infant in supine position, partially flex both lower extremities, and apply light pressure with fingers to soles of feet. Normally, while examiner's fingers maintain contact with soles of feet, lower limbs extend.	Both lower limbs should extend against examiner's pressure.	Absence suggests damage to central nervous system. Weak reflex may be seen after breech presentation *without* extended legs or may indicate sciatic nerve stretch syndrome. Breech presentation *with* extended legs may evoke exaggerated response.
Additional newborn responses: yawn, stretch, burp, hiccup, sneeze	These are spontaneous behaviors.	May be slightly depressed temporarily because of maternal analgesia or anesthesia, fetal hypoxia, or infection.	Parental guidance: Most of these behaviors are pleasurable to parents. Parents need to be assured that behaviors are normal. Sneeze is usually response to mucus in nose and not an indicator of a cold (upper respiratory tract infection). No treatment is needed for hiccups; sucking may help. In the preterm infant these are signs of neurodevelopmental immaturity and physiologic stress.

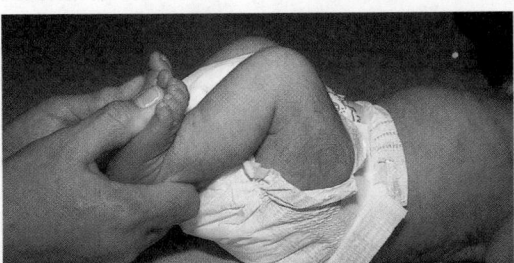

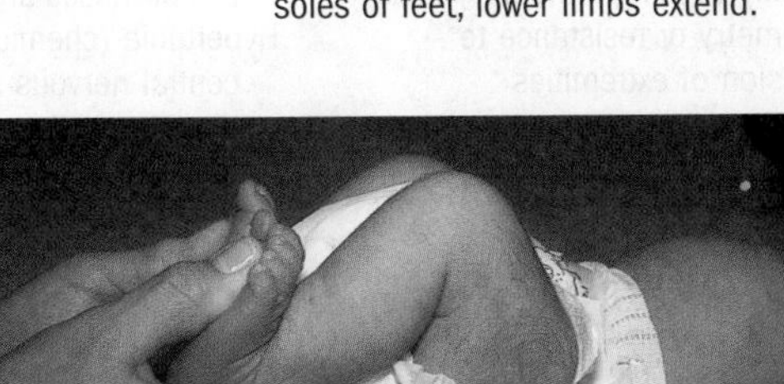

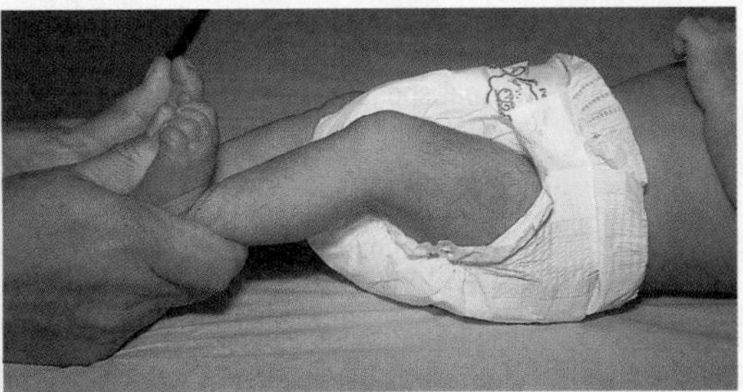

Magnet reflex. *(Courtesy Michael S. Clement, MD, Mesa, AZ.)*

their arms. Various reflexes serve to promote safety and adequate food intake.

Newborn Reflexes

The newborn infant has many primitive reflexes. The times at which these reflexes appear and disappear reflect the maturity and intactness of the developing nervous system. The most common reflexes found in the normal newborn are described in Table 24-1.

Physical Assessment

The assessment of the newborn should progress in a systematic manner, with evaluation and assessment of each system (e.g., respiratory and cardiovascular). It is recommended that assessment of features (e.g., observing general color and posture, auscultating heart tones and breath sounds), which least disturbs the newborn, be conducted first and then proceed in a head-to-toe manner once the newborn is awake and active. The findings provide a database for implementing the nursing process with newborns, and for providing anticipatory guidance for the parents.

An immediate assessment of the newborn is carried out to evaluate the infant's transition to extrauterine life. The Apgar score (see Chapter 25), determined at 1 and 5 minutes, provides information that must be considered in the context of data from the total assessment.

A complete physical examination should be done within 24 hours after birth, after the newborn's temperature stabilizes or under a radiant warmer. The area used for examination should be well lighted, warm, and free from drafts. The infant is undressed as needed and placed on a firm, warmed, flat surface. The physical assessment should begin with a review of the maternal history and prenatal and intrapartum records. This provides a background for the recognition of any potential problems. This assessment also includes general appearance, behavior, vital signs measurements, and maternal-infant interactions. Descriptions of any variations from normal and all abnormal findings are included (Table 24-2). Ideally the assessment should take place in the presence of the parents; this provides the parents an opportunity to learn about the unique characteristics of their infant. Ongoing assessments of

Text continued on p. 636

Table 24-2 Physical Assessment of Newborn Normal Findings

AREA ASSESSED AND APPRAISAL PROCEDURE	AVERAGE FINDINGS	NORMAL VARIATIONS	DEVIATIONS FROM NORMAL RANGE—POSSIBLE PROBLEMS (ETIOLOGY)
Posture			
Inspect newborn before disturbing for assessment. Refer to maternal chart for fetal presentation, position, and type of birth (vaginal, surgical), since newborn readily assumes in utero position.	Vertex: arms, legs in moderate flexion; fists clenched Resistance to having extremities extended for examination or measurement, crying possible when attempted Cessation of crying when allowed to resume curled-up fetal position (lateral) Normal spontaneous movement bilaterally asynchronous (legs flex and extend in alternating fashion) but equal extension in all extremities	Frank breech: legs straighter and stiff, newborn assuming intrauterine position in repose for a few days Prenatal pressure on limb or shoulder possibly causing temporary facial asymmetry or resistance to extension of extremities	Hypotonia, relaxed posture while awake (preterm or hypoxia in utero, maternal medications, neuromuscular disorder such as spinal muscular atrophy) Hypertonia (chemical dependence, central nervous system [CNS] disorder) Limitation of motion in any of extremities (see Skeletal System, p. 619)
Vital Signs			
Check heart rate and pulses: Thorax (chest): Inspection Palpation Auscultation Apex: mitral valve Second interspace, left of sternum: pulmonic valve Second interspace, right of sternum: aortic valve Junction of xiphoid process and sternum: tricuspid valve	Visible pulsations in left midclavicular line, fifth intercostal space Apical pulse, fourth intercostal space 120-140 beats/min Quality: *first sound* (closure of mitral and tricuspid valves) and *second sound* (closure of aortic and pulmonic valves) sharp and clear	80-100 beats/min (sleeping) to 180 beats/min (crying); possibly irregular for brief periods, especially after crying Murmur, especially over base or at left sternal border in interspace 3-4 (foramen ovale anatomically closing at about 1 yr)	Tachycardia: persistent, ≥180 beats/min (respiratory distress syndrome [RDS]; pneumonia) Bradycardia: persistent, ≤80 beats/min (congenital heart block, maternal lupus) Murmur (possibly functional) Arrhythmias: irregular rate Sounds: Distant (pneumopericardium) Poor quality Extra (S_3, S_4) Heart on right side of chest (dextrocardia), often accompanied by reversal of intestines
Peripheral pulses: femoral, brachial, popliteal, posterior tibial	Peripheral pulses equal and strong		Weak or absent peripheral pulses (decreased cardiac output, thrombus, possible coarctation of aorta if weak on left and strong on right) Bounding
Obtain temperature: Axillary: method of choice until 3 yr of age Temporal and intraauricular thermometers: not proved effective in measuring newborn temperature	Axillary: 37° C Temperature stabilized by 8-10 hr of age	36.5°-37.2° C Heat loss from evaporation, conduction, convection, radiation	Subnormal (preterm birth, infection, low environmental temperature, inadequate clothing, dehydration) Increased (infection, high environmental temperature, excessive clothing, proximity to heating unit or in direct sunshine, chemical dependence, diarrhea and dehydration) Temperature not stabilized by 6-8 hr after birth (if mother received magnesium sulfate, newborn less able to conserve heat by vasoconstriction; maternal analgesics possibly reducing thermal stability in newborn)

Table 24-2 Physical Assessment of Newborn Normal Findings—cont'd

AREA ASSESSED AND APPRAISAL PROCEDURE	AVERAGE FINDINGS	NORMAL VARIATIONS	DEVIATIONS FROM NORMAL RANGE—POSSIBLE PROBLEMS (ETIOLOGY)
Vital Signs—cont'd			
Observe and monitor respiratory rate and effort: Observe respirations when infant is at rest Count respirations for full minute Listen for sounds audible without stethoscope Observe respiratory effort	40 breaths/min Tendency to be shallow and irregular in rate, rhythm, and depth when infant is awake Crackles may be heard after birth No adventitious sounds audible on inspiration and expiration Breath sounds: bronchial: loud, clear	30-60 breaths/min Short periodic breathing episodes and no evidence of respiratory distress or apnea (>20 seconds); periodic breathing First period (reactivity): 50-60 breaths/min Second period: 50-70 breaths/min Stabilization (1-2 days): 30-40 breaths/min Crackles (fine)	Apneic episodes: >20 sec (preterm infant: rapid warming or cooling of infant; CNS or blood glucose instability) Bradypnea: <25 breaths/min (maternal narcosis from analgesics or anesthetics, birth trauma) Tachypnea: >60 breaths/min (RDS, transient tachypnea of the newborn, congenital diaphragmatic hernia) Breath sounds: Crackles (coarse), rhonchi, wheezing Expiratory grunt (narrowing of bronchi) Distress evidenced by nasal flaring, grunting, retractions, labored breathing Stridor (upper airway occlusion)
Obtain blood pressure (BP) Check oscillometric monitor BP cuff: BP cuff width affects readings; use appropriately sized cuff and palpate brachial, popliteal, or posterior tibial pulse (depending on measurement site)	80s-90s/40s-50s (approximate ranges) At birth: Systolic: 60-80 mm Hg Diastolic: 40-50 mm Hg At 10 days: Systolic: 95-100 mm Hg Diastolic: 45-75 mm Hg	Variation with change in activity level: awake, crying, sleeping	Difference between upper and lower extremity pressures (coarctation of aorta) Hypotension (sepsis, hypovolemia) Hypertension (coarctation of aorta, renal involvement, thrombus)
Weight			
Put protective liner cloth or paper in place and adjust scale to 0 g (or pounds/ounces) Weigh at same time each day Protect newborn from heat loss	Female: 3400 g Male: 3500 g Regaining of birth weight within first 2 wk	2500-4000 g Acceptable weight loss: 5% to 10% in first 3-5 days Second baby weighing more than first (on average)	Weight ≤2500 g (preterm, small for gestational age, rubella syndrome) Weight ≥4000 g (large for gestational age, maternal diabetes, heredity—normal for these parents) Weight loss 10%-15% (growth failure, dehydration); assess breastfeeding success, latch-on

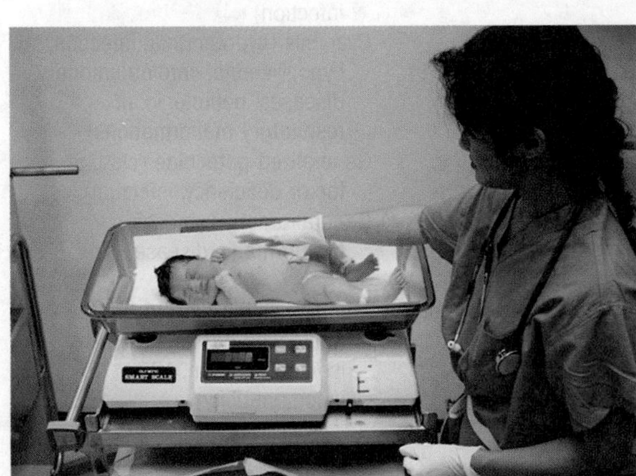

Weighing the infant. Note that a hand is held over infant as a safety measure. Scale is covered to protect against cross infection and heat loss. *(Courtesy Kim Molloy, Knoxville, IA.)*

NOTE: Weight, length, and head circumference should all be close to the same percentile for any child.

Continued

Table 24-2 Physical Assessment of Newborn Normal Findings—cont'd

AREA ASSESSED AND APPRAISAL PROCEDURE	AVERAGE FINDINGS	NORMAL VARIATIONS	DEVIATIONS FROM NORMAL RANGE—POSSIBLE PROBLEMS (ETIOLOGY)
Length			
Measure length from top of head to heel Measuring is difficult in term infant because of molding, incomplete extension of knees	50 cm	45-55 cm	<45 cm or >55 cm (chromosomal abnormality, heredity–normal for these parents); some syndromes result in shorter than average limb length (skeletal dysplasias, achondroplasia)

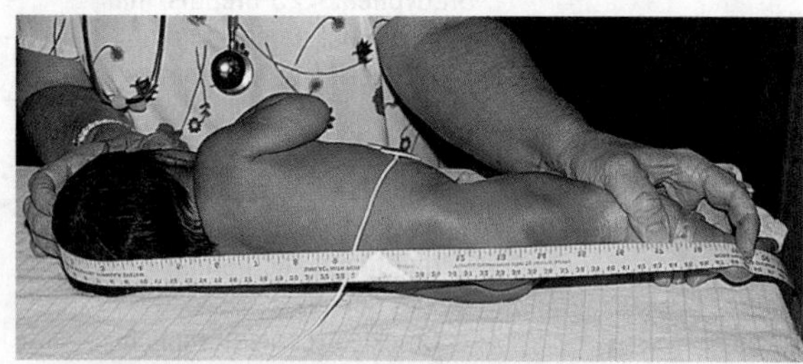

Length, crown to heel. To determine total length, include length of legs. If measurements are taken before the infant's initial bath, wear gloves. *(Courtesy Marjorie Pyle, RNC, Lifecircle, Costa Mesa, CA.)*

AREA ASSESSED AND APPRAISAL PROCEDURE	AVERAGE FINDINGS	NORMAL VARIATIONS	DEVIATIONS FROM NORMAL RANGE—POSSIBLE PROBLEMS (ETIOLOGY)
Head Circumference			
Measure head at greatest diameter: occipitofrontal circumference May need to remeasure on second or third day after resolution of molding and caput succedaneum	33-35 cm Circumference of head and chest approximately the same for first 1 or 2 days after birth; chest rarely measured on routine basis	32-36.8 cm	Microcephaly: head ≤32 cm (maternal rubella, toxoplasmosis, cytomegalovirus, fused cranial sutures [craniosynostosis]) Hydrocephaly: sutures widely separated, circumference ≥4 cm more than chest circumference (infection) Increased intracranial pressure (hemorrhage, space-occupying lesion)

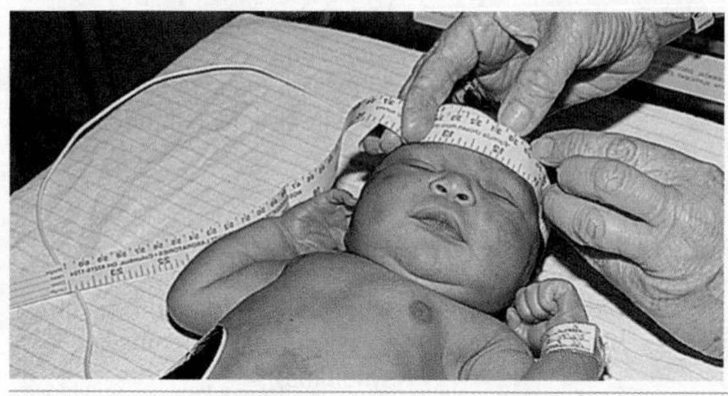

Circumference of head. *(Courtesy Marjorie Pyle, RNC, Lifecircle, Costa Mesa, CA.)*

AREA ASSESSED AND APPRAISAL PROCEDURE	AVERAGE FINDINGS	NORMAL VARIATIONS	DEVIATIONS FROM NORMAL RANGE—POSSIBLE PROBLEMS (ETIOLOGY)
Skin			
Check color Inspect and palpate: Inspect seminaked newborn in well-lit, warm area without drafts; natural daylight best Inspect newborn when quiet and alert	Generally pink Varying with ethnic origin; skin pigmentation beginning to deepen right after birth in basal layer of epidermis Acrocyanosis common after birth	Mottling Harlequin sign Plethora Telangiectases ("stork bites" or capillary hemangiomas) (see Fig. 24-5, *A*) Erythema toxicum neonatorum ("newborn rash") (see Fig. 24-5, *B*) Milia	Dark red (preterm, polycythemia) Gray (hypotension, poor perfusion) Pallor (cardiovascular problem, CNS damage, blood dyscrasia, blood loss, twin-to-twin transfusion, infection) Cyanosis (hypothermia, infection, hypoglycemia, cardiopulmonary diseases, neurologic, or respiratory malformations)
		Petechiae over presenting part	Generalized petechiae (clotting factor deficiency, infection)
		Ecchymoses from forceps in vertex births or over buttocks, genitalia, and legs in breech births	Generalized ecchymoses (hemorrhagic disease)
Observe for jaundice	None at birth	Physiologic jaundice in up to 60% of term infants in first week of life	Jaundice within first 24 hr (increased hemolysis, Rh isoimmunization, ABO incompatibility)

NOTE: Weight, length, and head circumference should all be close to the same percentile for any child.

Table 24-2 Physical Assessment of Newborn Normal Findings—cont'd

AREA ASSESSED AND APPRAISAL PROCEDURE	AVERAGE FINDINGS	NORMAL VARIATIONS	DEVIATIONS FROM NORMAL RANGE—POSSIBLE PROBLEMS (ETIOLOGY)
Skin—cont'd			
Observe for birthmarks or bruises: Inspect and palpate for location, size, distribution, characteristics, color, if obstructing airway or oral cavity		Mongolian spot (see Fig. 24-4) in infants of African-American, Asian, and Native American origin	Capillary hemangiomas Nevus flammeus: port-wine stain Nevus vasculosus: strawberry hemangioma Cavernous hemangioma
Check skin condition: Inspect and palpate for intactness, smoothness, texture, edema, pressure points if ill or immobilized	Confined to eyelid edema (result of eye prophylaxis) Opacity: few large blood vessels visible indistinctly over abdomen	Slightly thick; superficial cracking, peeling, especially of hands, feet No visible blood vessels, a few large vessels clearly visible over abdomen Some fingernail scratches	Edema on hands, feet; pitting over tibia; periorbital (overhydration; hydrops) Texture thin, smooth, or of medium thickness; rash or superficial peeling visible (preterm, postterm) Numerous vessels very visible over abdomen (preterm) Texture thick, parchmentlike; cracking, peeling (postterm) Skin tags, webbing Papules, pustules, vesicles, ulcers, maceration (impetigo, candidiasis, herpes, diaper rash)
Weigh infant routinely Inspect and palpate: Gently pinch skin between thumb and forefinger over abdomen and inner thigh to check for turgor Note presence of subcutaneous fat deposits (adipose pads) over cheeks, buttocks	After pinch released, skin returns to original state immediately	Normal weight loss after birth: up to 10% of birth weight Dehydration: loss of weight is best indicator Possibly puffy Variation in amount of subcutaneous fat	Loose, wrinkled skin (prematurity, postmaturity, dehydration: fold of skin persisting after release of pinch) Tense, tight, shiny skin (edema, extreme cold, shock, infection) Lack of subcutaneous fat, prominence of clavicle or ribs (preterm, malnutrition)
Check voiding	Voiding within 24 hr of birth Voiding 6-10 times/day by day 5-6		No void in first 24 hr Renal agenesis: Potter syndrome
Observe vernix caseosa: Observe color and odor before bath or removing	Whitish, cheesy, odorless	Usually more found in creases, folds	Absent or minimal (postterm) Abundant (preterm) Green color (possible in utero release of meconium or presence of bilirubin) Odor (possible intrauterine infection)
Assess lanugo: Inspect for this fine, downy hair, amount and distribution	Over shoulders, pinnae of ears, forehead	Variation in amount	Absent (postterm) Abundant (preterm, especially if lanugo abundant, long, and thick over back)
Head			
Palpate skin	See Skin	Caput succedaneum, possibly showing some ecchymosis (see Fig. 24-3, *A*)	Cephalhematoma (see Fig. 24-3, *C*)
Inspect shape, size	Making up one fourth of body length Molding (see Fig. 24-7)	Slight asymmetry from intrauterine position Lack of molding (preterm, breech presentation, cesarean birth)	Severe molding (birth trauma) Indentation (fracture from trauma)

Continued

Table 24-2 Physical Assessment of Newborn Normal Findings—cont'd

AREA ASSESSED AND APPRAISAL PROCEDURE	AVERAGE FINDINGS	NORMAL VARIATIONS	DEVIATIONS FROM NORMAL RANGE—POSSIBLE PROBLEMS (ETIOLOGY)
Head—cont'd			
Palpate, inspect, and note status of fontanels (open vs. closed)	Anterior fontanel 5-cm diamond, increasing as molding resolves Posterior fontanel triangle, smaller than anterior	Variation in fontanel size with degree of molding Difficulty in feeling fontanels possible because of molding	Fontanels: Full, bulging (tumor, hemorrhage, infection) Large, flat, soft (malnutrition, hydrocephaly, delayed bone age, hypothyroidism) Depressed (dehydration)
Palpate sutures	Palpable and separated sutures	Possible overlap of sutures with molding	Sutures: Widely spaced (hydrocephaly) Premature closure (fused) (craniosynostosis)
Inspect pattern, distribution, amount of hair; feel texture	Silky, single strands lying flat; growth pattern toward face and neck	Variation in amount	Fine, wooly (preterm) Unusual swirls, patterns, or hairline; or coarse, brittle (endocrine or genetic disorders)
Eyes			
Check placement on face	Eyes and space between eyes each one third the distance from outer-to-outer canthus	Epicanthal folds: characteristic in some ethnicities	Epicanthal folds when present with other signs (chromosomal disorders such as Down, cri-du-chat syndromes)

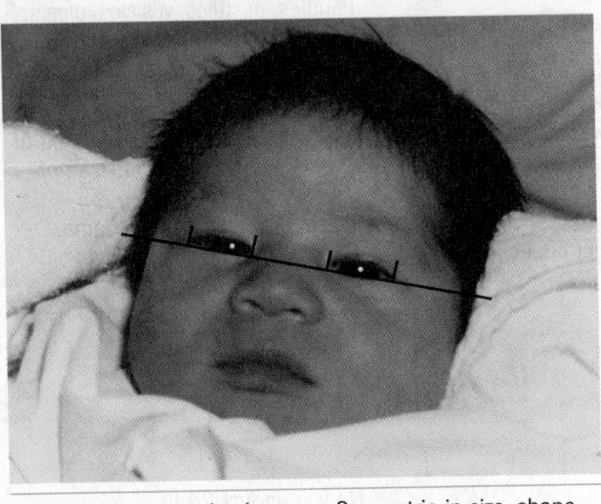

Eyes. In pseudostrabismus, inner epicanthal folds cause the eyes to appear misaligned; however, corneal light reflexes are perfectly symmetric. Eyes are symmetric in size and shape and are well placed.

AREA ASSESSED AND APPRAISAL PROCEDURE	AVERAGE FINDINGS	NORMAL VARIATIONS	DEVIATIONS FROM NORMAL RANGE—POSSIBLE PROBLEMS (ETIOLOGY)
Check for symmetry in size, shape	Symmetric in size, shape		
Check eyelids for size, movement, blink	Blink reflex	Edema if eye prophylaxis drops or ointment instilled	
Assess for discharge	None No tears	Some discharge if silver nitrate used Occasional presence of some tears	Discharge: purulent (infection) Chemical conjunctivitis from eye medication is common—requires no treatment
Evaluate eyeballs for presence, size, shape	Both present and of equal size, both round, firm	Subconjunctival hemorrhage	Agenesis or absence of one or both eyeballs Lens opacity or absence of red reflex (congenital cataracts, possibly from rubella, retinoblastoma [cat's eye reflex]) Lesions: coloboma, absence of part of iris (congenital) Pink color of iris (albinism) Jaundiced sclera (hyperbilirubinemia)

Table 24-2 Physical Assessment of Newborn Normal Findings—cont'd

AREA ASSESSED AND APPRAISAL PROCEDURE	AVERAGE FINDINGS	NORMAL VARIATIONS	DEVIATIONS FROM NORMAL RANGE—POSSIBLE PROBLEMS (ETIOLOGY)
Eyes—cont'd			
Check pupils	Present, equal in size, reactive to light		Pupils: unequal, constricted, dilated, fixed (intracranial pressure, medications, tumor)
Evaluate eyeball movement	Random, jerky, uneven, focus possible briefly, following to midline	Transient strabismus or nystagmus until third or fourth month	Persistent strabismus Doll's eyes (increased intracranial pressure) Sunset (increased intracranial pressure)
Assess eyebrows: amount of hair, pattern	Distinct (not connected in midline)		Connection in midline (Cornelia de Lange syndrome)
Nose			
Observe shape, placement, patency, configuration	Midline Some mucus but no drainage Preferential nose breather Sneezing to clear nose	Slight deformity (flat or deviated to one side) from passage through birth canal	Copious drainage (rarely, congenital syphilis) Blockage—membranous or bone with cyanosis at rest and return of pink color with crying (choanal atresia) Malformed (congenital syphilis, chromosomal disorder) Flaring of nares (respiratory distress)
Ears			
Observe size, placement on head, amount of cartilage, open auditory canal	Correct placement: line drawn through inner and outer canthi of eyes reaching to top notch of ears (at junction with scalp) Well-formed, firm cartilage	Size: small, large, floppy Darwin's tubercle (nodule on posterior helix)	Agenesis Lack of cartilage (preterm) Low placement (chromosomal disorder, cognitive impairment, kidney disorder) Preauricular tag or sinus Size: possibly overly prominent or protruding ears
Assess hearing	Responds to voice and other sounds	State (e.g., alert, asleep) influencing response	Perform universal newborn hearing screening to identify deficits Lack of response to loud noise *should not* imply deafness
Facies			
Observe overall appearance and symmetry of face	Rounded and symmetric; influenced by birth type or any molding	Positional deformities associated with intrauterine positioning, cranial molding	Asymmetric facial features may be accompanied by other characteristics such as low-set ears, absence of outer ear, or other structural disorders (hereditary, chromosomal aberration)

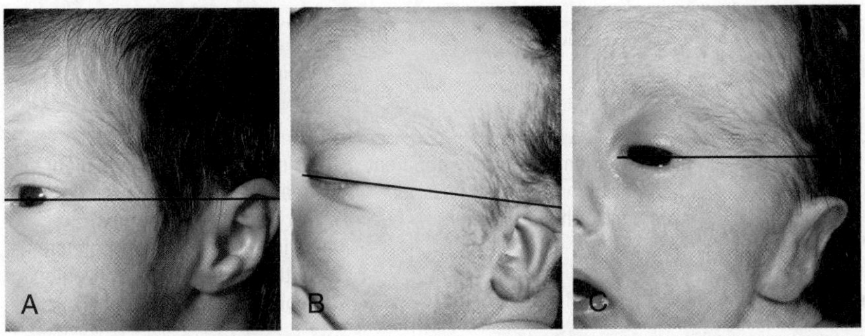

Placement of ears on the head in relation to a line drawn from the inner to the outer canthus of the eye. **A,** Normal position. **B,** Abnormally angled ear. **C,** True low-set ear. *(Courtesy Mead Johnson Nutritionals, Evansville, IN.)*

Continued

Table 24-2 Physical Assessment of Newborn Normal Findings—cont'd

AREA ASSESSED AND APPRAISAL PROCEDURE	AVERAGE FINDINGS	NORMAL VARIATIONS	DEVIATIONS FROM NORMAL RANGE—POSSIBLE PROBLEMS (ETIOLOGY)
Mouth			
Inspect and palpate Assess buccal mucosa: Dry or moist Pink Status intact Assess lips for color, configuration, movement	Symmetry of lip movement	Transient circumoral cyanosis	Apparent anomalies in placement, size, shape (cleft lip and/or palate, gums) Cyanosis, circumoral pallor (respiratory distress, hypothermia) Asymmetry in movement of lips (seventh cranial nerve paralysis)
Check gums	Pink gums	Inclusion cysts (Epstein pearls—Bohn nodules, whitish, hard nodules on gums or roof of mouth)	Teeth: predeciduous or deciduous (hereditary)
Assess tongue for color, mobility, movement, size	Tongue not protruding; freely movable; symmetric in shape, movement Sucking pads inside cheeks	Short lingual frenulum	Macroglossia (preterm, chromosomal disorder) Thrush: white plaques on cheeks or tongue that bleed if touched *(Candida albicans)*
Assess palate (soft, hard): Arch Uvula	Soft and hard palates intact Uvula in midline	Anatomic groove in palate to accommodate nipple, disappearance by 3-4 yr of age Epstein pearls	Cleft hard or soft palate
Assess chin	Distinct chin		Micrognathia—recessed chin with prominent overbite (Pierre Robin sequence or other syndrome)
Evaluate saliva for amount, character	Mouth moist, pink		Excessive salivation and choking or turning blue (esophageal atresia, tracheoesophageal fistula)
Check reflexes: Rooting Sucking Extrusion	Reflexes present	Reflex response dependent on state of wakefulness and hunger	Absent (preterm)
Neck			
Inspect and palpate for movement, flexibility, masses, bruising	Short, thick, surrounded by skin folds; no webbing		Webbing (Turner syndrome)
Check sternocleidomastoid muscles, movement and position of head	Head held in midline (sternocleidomastoid muscles equal), no masses Freedom of movement from side to side and flexion and extension; no movement of chin past shoulder	Transient positional deformity apparent when newborn is at rest; passive movement of head possible	Restricted movement, holding of head at angle (torticollis [wryneck], opisthotonos) Absence of head control (preterm birth, Down syndrome, hypotonia [spinal muscular atrophy])
Assess trachea for position and thyroid gland	Thyroid not palpable		Mass (enlarged thyroid, cystic hygroma) Distended veins (cardiopulmonary disorder) Skin tags
Chest			
Inspect and palpate: Shape	Almost circular, barrel shaped	Tip of sternum possibly prominent	Bulging of chest, unequal movement (pneumothorax, pneumomediastinum) Malformation (funnel chest—pectus excavatum)
Observe respiratory movements	Symmetric chest movements, chest and abdominal movements synchronized during respirations	Occasional retractions, especially when crying	Retractions with or without respiratory distress (preterm, RDS) Paradoxical breathing
Evaluate clavicles	Clavicles intact		Fracture of clavicle (trauma); crepitus

evolve Video–Neck (Posterior)

Table 24-2 Physical Assessment of Newborn Normal Findings—cont'd

AREA ASSESSED AND APPRAISAL PROCEDURE	AVERAGE FINDINGS	NORMAL VARIATIONS	DEVIATIONS FROM NORMAL RANGE—POSSIBLE PROBLEMS (ETIOLOGY)
Chest—cont'd			
Assess ribs	Rib cage symmetric, intact; moves with respirations		Poor development of rib cage and musculature (preterm)
Assess nipples for size, placement, number	Nipples prominent, well formed, symmetrically placed		Nipples: Supernumerary, along nipple line Malpositioned or widely spaced
Observe breast tissue	Breast nodule: approximately 6 mm in term infant	Breast nodule: 3-10 mm Secretion of witch's milk	Lack of breast tissue (preterm) Sounds: bowel sounds (see Abdomen)
Auscultate heart sounds and rate and breath sounds (see Vital Signs)			
Abdomen			
Inspect and palpate umbilical cord	Two arteries, one vein Whitish gray Definite demarcation between cord and skin; no intestinal structures within cord Dry around base, drying Odorless Cord clamp in place for 24 hr	Reducible umbilical hernia	One artery (renal anomaly) Meconium stained (intrauterine distress) Bleeding or oozing around cord (hemorrhagic disease) Redness or drainage around cord (infection, possible persistence of urachus) Hernia: herniation of abdominal contents through cord opening (e.g., omphalocele); defect covered with thin, friable membrane, possibly extensive
Inspect size of abdomen and palpate contour	Rounded, prominent, dome shaped because abdominal musculature not fully developed Liver possibly palpable 1-2 cm below right costal margin No other masses palpable No distention Few visible veins on abdominal surface	Some diastasis recti (separation) of abdominal musculature	Gastroschisis: herniation of abdominal contents to the side or above the cord; contents not covered by membranous tissue and may include liver Distention at birth (ruptured viscus, genitourinary masses or malformations: hydronephrosis, teratomas, abdominal tumors): Mild (overfeeding, high gastrointestinal tract obstruction) Marked (lower gastrointestinal tract obstruction, anorectal malformation, anal stenosis), often with bilious emesis Intermittent or transient (overfeeding) Partial intestinal obstruction (stenosis of bowel) Visible peristalsis (obstruction) Malrotation of bowel or adhesions Sepsis (infection)
Auscultate bowel sounds and note number, amount, and character of stools	Sounds present within minutes after birth in healthy term infant Meconium stool passing within 24-48 hr after birth		Scaphoid, with bowel sounds in chest and severe respiratory distress (congenital diaphragmatic hernia)
Assess color		Linea nigra possibly apparent and caused by hormone influence during pregnancy	
Observe movement with respiration	Respirations primarily diaphragmatic, abdominal and chest movement synchronous		Decreased or absent abdominal movement with breathing (phrenic nerve palsy, congenital diaphragmatic hernia)

Continued

Table 24-2 Physical Assessment of Newborn Normal Findings—cont'd

AREA ASSESSED AND APPRAISAL PROCEDURE	AVERAGE FINDINGS	NORMAL VARIATIONS	DEVIATIONS FROM NORMAL RANGE—POSSIBLE PROBLEMS (ETIOLOGY)
Genitalia			
Female (see Fig. 24-6, A)			
Inspect and palpate:			
General appearance	Female genitalia	Increased pigmentation caused by pregnancy hormones	Ambiguous genitalia—wide variation (small phallus not well distinguished from enlarged clitoris)
Clitoris	Usually edematous		
Labia majora	Usually edematous, covering labia minora in term newborns	Edema and ecchymosis after breech birth	Virilized female—extremely large clitoris (congenital adrenal hyperplasia)
Labia minora	Possible protrusion over labia majora	Blood-tinged discharge from pseudomenstruation caused by pregnancy hormones	Enlarged clitoris with urinary meatus on tip, absent scrotum, micropenis, fused labia
Discharge	Smegma	Some vernix caseosa between labia possible	Stenosed meatus Labia majora widely separated and labia minora prominent (preterm)
Vagina	Open orifice Mucoid discharge Hymenal/vaginal tag		Absence of vaginal orifice
Urinary meatus	Beneath clitoris, difficult to see	Rust-stained urine (uric acid crystals)	Fecal discharge (fistula) Bladder exstrophy (bladder outside abdominal cavity and turned inside out)
Male (see Fig. 24-6, B)			
Inspect and palpate:			
General appearance	Male genitalia	Increased size and pigmentation caused by pregnancy hormones Wide variation in size of genitalia	Ambiguous genitalia
Penis:			Micropenis
Urinary meatus appearance—should be at tip of penile shaft	Foreskin covers glans (if uncircumcised), meatus at tip of penis		Urinary meatus not on tip of glans penis (hypospadias, epispadias, foreskin may be retracted or absent); chordee (ventral curvature)
Prepuce (foreskin)—do not forcibly retract foreskin if uncircumcised	Prepuce covering glans penis and not retractable	Prepuce removed if circumcised	Round meatal opening
Scrotum Rugae (wrinkles)	Large, edematous, pendulous in term infant; covered with rugae	Scrotal edema and ecchymosis if breech birth Hydrocele, small, noncommunicating	Scrotum smooth and testes undescended (preterm, cryptorchidism) Bifid scrotum Hydrocele Inguinal hernia
Testes	Palpable on each side	Bulge palpable in inguinal canal	Undescended (preterm)
Check urination	Voiding within 24 hr, stream adequate, amount adequate	Rust-stained urine (uric acid crystals)	
Check reflexes: Cremasteric	Testes retracted, especially when newborn is chilled		
Extremities			
Make a general check: Inspect and palpate: Degree of flexion Range of motion Symmetry of motion Muscle tone	Assuming of position maintained in utero Attitude of general flexion Full range of motion, spontaneous movements	Transient (positional) deformities	Limited motion (malformations) Poor muscle tone (preterm, maternal medications, CNS anomalies)

evolve Video–Cremasteric Reflex

Table 24-2 Physical Assessment of Newborn Normal Findings—cont'd

AREA ASSESSED AND APPRAISAL PROCEDURE	AVERAGE FINDINGS	NORMAL VARIATIONS	DEVIATIONS FROM NORMAL RANGE–POSSIBLE PROBLEMS (ETIOLOGY)
Extremities—cont'd			
Observe arms and hands: Inspect and palpate: Color Intactness Appropriate placement	Longer than legs in newborn period Contours and movements symmetric	Slight tremors sometimes apparent Some acrocyanosis	Asymmetry of movement (fracture or crepitus, brachial nerve trauma, malformations) Asymmetry of contour (malformations, fracture) Amelia or phocomelia (teratogens) Palmar creases Simian line with short, incurved little fingers (Down syndrome)
Number of fingers	Five on each hand Fist often clenched with thumb under fingers		Webbing of fingers: syndactyly Absence or excess of fingers Strong, rigid flexion; persistent fists; positioning of fists in front of mouth constantly (CNS disorder) Yellowed nail beds (meconium staining)
Evaluate joints: Shoulder Elbow Wrist Fingers	Full range of motion, symmetric contour		Increased tonicity, clonus, prolonged tremors (CNS disorder)
Check reflex: grasp (palmar and plantar)			
Observe legs and feet: Inspect and palpate: Color Intactness Length in relation to arms and body and to each other	Appearance of bowing because lateral muscles more developed than medial muscles	Feet appearing to turn in but can be easily rotated externally, positional defects tending to correct while infant is crying Acrocyanosis	Amelia, phocomelia (chromosomal defect, teratogenic effect) Temperature of one leg differing from that of the other (circulatory deficiency, CNS disorder)
Number of toes	Five on each foot		Webbing, syndactyly (chromosomal defect) Absence or excess of digits (chromosomal defect, familial trait)
Femur	Intact femur		Femoral fracture (difficult breech birth)
Head of femur as legs are flexed and abducted, placement in acetabulum (see Fig. 24-8)			Developmental dysplasia of the hip
Major gluteal folds	Major gluteal folds even		Hip dysplasia
Soles of feet	Soles well lined (or wrinkled) over two thirds of foot in term infants Plantar fat pad giving flat-footed effect		Soles of feet: Few creases (preterm) Covered with creases (postterm) Congenital clubfoot
Evaluate joints: Hip Knee Ankle Toes	Full range of motion, symmetric contour		Hypermobility of joints (Down syndrome)
Check reflexes (see Table 24-1)			Asymmetric movement (trauma, CNS disorder)

Continued

evolve Video–Upper Extremities

evolve Video–Legs (Symmetry, Length)

Table 24-2 Physical Assessment of Newborn Normal Findings—cont'd

AREA ASSESSED AND APPRAISAL PROCEDURE	AVERAGE FINDINGS	NORMAL VARIATIONS	DEVIATIONS FROM NORMAL RANGE—POSSIBLE PROBLEMS (ETIOLOGY)
Back			
Assess anatomy: Inspect and palpate: Spine, shoulders, scapulae, iliac crests	Spine straight and easily flexed Infant able to raise and support head momentarily when prone	Temporary minor positional deformities; correction with passive manipulation	Limitation of movement (fusion or deformity of vertebra)
Base of spine—pilonidal dimple or sinus	Shoulders, scapulae, and iliac crests lining up in same plane		Meningocele, myelomeningocele (spina bifida cystica) Pigmented nevus with tuft of hair, located anywhere along the spine, often associated with spina bifida occulta Sinus (opening to spinal cord)
Check reflexes (spinal related): Test trunk incurvation reflex	Trunk flexed and pelvis swings to stimulated side	May not be apparent in first few days but is usually present in 5-6 days	If transverse lesion is present, no response below lesion; absence of response: CNS abnormality or CNS depression
Test magnet reflex	Lower limbs extend as pressure applied to feet with legs in semiflexed position	Weak or exaggerated response with breech presentation	Absence suggestive of CNS damage or malformation
Anus			
Inspect and palpate: Placement Patency Test for sphincter response (active "wink" reflex) Observe for the following: Abdominal distention Passage of meconium from anal opening Fecal drainage from perineum, penis, vagina	One anus with good sphincter tone Passage of meconium within 24 hr after birth Anal "wink" present, anal opening patent	Passage of meconium within 48 hr after birth	Imperforate anus without fistula Rectal atresia and stenosis Absence of anal opening; drainage of fecal material from vagina in female or urinary meatus in male (rectal fistula) or along perineal raphe (midline area between base of penis and anus) (anorectal malformation)
Stools			
Observe frequency, color, consistency	Meconium followed by transitional and soft yellow stool		No stool (obstruction) Frequent watery stools (infection, phototherapy)

evolve Video–Buttocks

the newborn are made, and an evaluation is performed before discharge.

General Appearance

The neonate's maturity level can be gauged by assessment of general appearance. Features to assess in the general survey include posture, activity, any overt signs of anomalies that may cause initial distress, presence of bruising or other consequences of birth, and state of alertness. The normal resting position of the neonate is one of general flexion (Fig. 24-10).

Vital Signs

The temperature, heart rate, and respiratory rate are always obtained. BP is assessed as a baseline unless cardiac problems are suspect. An irregular, very slow, or very fast heart rate may indicate a need for further evaluation of circulatory status, including BP measurement.

Axillary temperature is a safe, accurate substitute for rectal temperature. Electronic thermometers have expedited this task and provide a reading within 1 minute. Temporal artery, tympanic, and oral routes for measuring temperature in the newborn are not considered accurate (Asher & Northington, 2008). Taking an infant's temperature may cause the infant to cry and struggle against the placement of the thermometer in the axilla. Before taking the temperature, the examiner may determine the apical heart rate and respiratory rate while the infant is quiet and at rest. The normal axillary temperature averages 37° C with a range from 36.5° to 37.2° C.

The respiratory rate varies with the state of alertness and activity after birth. Respirations are abdominal and can be counted by observing or by lightly feeling the rise and fall of the abdomen. Neonatal respirations are shallow and irregular. It is important to count the respirations for a full minute to obtain an accurate count because of episodes of periodic breathing wherein respirations may cease for seconds (less than 20) and resume again. The examiner should also observe for symmetry of chest movement. The average respiratory rate is 40 breaths/min but will vary between 30 and 60 breaths/min or may be higher than 60 breaths/min if the newborn is very active or crying (see Table 24-2).

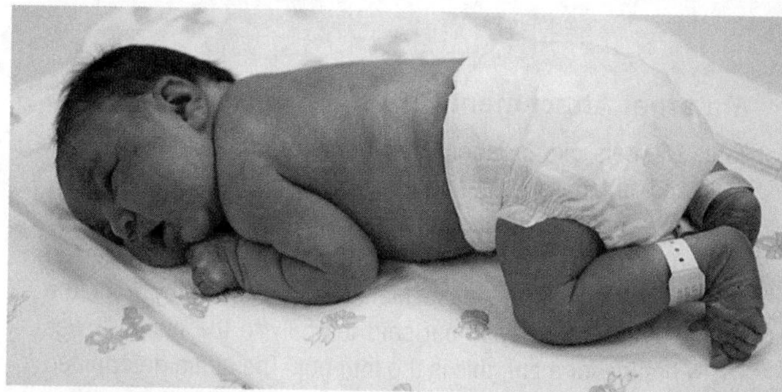

Fig. 24-10 Newborn in position of flexion in prone position while awake. (From Hockenberry MJ et al: *Wong's nursing care of infants and children*, ed 8, St Louis, 2007, Mosby.)

An apical pulse rate should be obtained on all newborns. Auscultation should be for a full minute, preferably when the infant is asleep or in a quiet alert state. The infant may need to be held and comforted during assessment. Heart rate may range from 80 to 170+ beats/min shortly after birth and, when the infant's condition has stabilized, from 120 to 140 beats/min. Brachial and femoral pulses are assessed for equality and strength.

If BP is measured, an oscillometric monitor calibrated for neonatal pressures is preferred. An appropriate sized cuff (width-to-arm or calf ratio of 0.45 to 0.70, or approximately ½ to ¾) is essential for accuracy. Neonatal BP usually is highest immediately after birth and falls to a minimum by 3 hours after birth. It then begins to rise steadily and reaches a plateau between 4 and 6 days after birth. This measurement is usually equal to that of the immediate postbirth BP. The BP varies with the neonate's activity; accurate measurement is best obtained while the newborn is at rest. In an Australian study of 406 infants born at term (without maternal diabetes or hypertension; birth weight range 2425 to 4990 g), median systolic and diastolic oscillometric BPs on the second day of life were 68 mm Hg (range 46 to 91 mm Hg) and 43 mm Hg (range 27 to 58 mm Hg), respectively (Kent et al, 2007). Median oscillometric BP increased slightly on the third and fourth days of life.

A baseline pulse oximetry measurement may be obtained along with palpation of peripheral pulses (brachial, femoral, pedal) before the infant's discharge from the birth institution, especially if there is concern for a congenital cardiac defect.

Baseline Measurements of Physical Growth

Baseline measurements are taken and recorded to help assess the progress and determine the growth patterns of the neonate. These may be recorded on growth charts. The following measurements are made when the neonate is assessed.

Weight

The newborn is usually weighed shortly after birth. This may be done in the labor and birthing area, in the mother's room, or on admission to the nursery. Care must be taken to ensure the scales are balanced. The totally unclothed neonate is placed in the center of the scale, which is usually covered with a disposable pad or cloth to prevent heat loss via conduction and cross infection. The nurse should place one hand over (but not touching) the neonate to prevent the infant from falling off the scales (p. 627). It is common to weigh the infant at the same time every day during the hospital stay. Birth weight of a term infant typically ranges from 2500 to 4000 g.

Head Circumference and Length

The head is measured at the widest part, which is the occipitofrontal diameter (p. 628). The tape measure is placed around the head just above the infant's eyebrows. The term neonate's head circumference ranges from 32 to 36.8 cm.

The length may be difficult to obtain because of the flexed posture of the newborn (p. 628). The examiner places the newborn on a flat surface and extends the leg until the knee is flat against the surface. Placing the head against a perpendicular surface and extending the leg may assist with this measurement. In the term neonate, head-to-heel length ranges from 45 to 55 cm.

Neurologic Assessment

The physical assessment includes a neurologic assessment of newborn reflexes (see Table 24-1). This provides useful information about the infant's nervous system and state of neurologic maturation. Many reflex behaviors (e.g., sucking and rooting) are important for proper development. Other reflexes such as gagging and sneezing act as primitive safety mechanisms. The assessment needs to be carried out as early as possible because abnormal signs present in the early neonatal period may require further investigation before the newborn is discharged home.

Behavioral Characteristics

The healthy newborn must accomplish behavioral and biologic tasks to develop normally. Behavioral characteristics form the basis of the infant's social capabilities. Normal newborns differ in their activity levels, feeding and sleeping patterns, and responsiveness. Parents' reactions to their newborns are often determined by these differences. Showing parents the unique characteristics of their infant helps parents develop a more positive perception of the infant, with increased interaction between infant and parent.

Behavioral responses, as well as physical characteristics, change during the period of transition. The Brazelton Neonatal Behavioral Assessment Scale (BNBAS) can be used to systematically assess the infant's behavior (Brazelton & Nugent, 1996). The BNBAS is an interactive examination that assesses the infant's response to 28 areas organized according to the clusters in Box 24-2. It is generally used as a research or diagnostic tool and requires special training.

In addition to its use as an initial and ongoing tool to assess neurologic and behavioral responses, the BNBAS can be used to assess initial parent-infant relationships and as a guide for parents to help them focus on their infant's individuality and to develop a deeper attachment to their child. See Chapter 22 for further discussion of attachment.

Sleep-Wake States

Variations in the state of consciousness of infants are called *sleep-wake states*. The six states form a continuum from deep sleep to crying (Fig. 24-11). There are two sleep states (i.e., deep sleep and light sleep) and four wake states (i.e., drowsy, quiet alert, active alert, and crying) (Blackburn, 2007). Each state has specific characteristics and state-related behaviors. The optimum state of arousal is the quiet alert state. During this state infants smile, vocalize, move in synchrony with speech, watch their parents' faces, and respond to people talking to them (see Family-Centered Care box). Infants respond to internal and external environmental factors by controlling sensory input and regulating the sleep-wake states; the ability to make smooth transitions between states is called *state modulation*. The ability to regulate sleep-wake states is

BOX 24-2 Clusters of Neonatal Behaviors in Brazelton Neonatal Behavioral Assessment Scale

Habituation—Ability to respond to and then inhibit responding to discrete stimulus (e.g., light, rattle, bell, pinprick) while asleep

Orientation—Quality of alert states and ability to attend to visual and auditory stimuli while alert

Motor performance—Quality of movement and tone

Range of state—Measure of general arousal level or arousability of infant

Regulation of state—How infant responds when aroused

Autonomic stability—Signs of stress (e.g., tremors, startles, skin color) related to homeostatic (self-regulator) adjustment of the nervous system

Reflexes—Assessment of several neonatal reflexes

CRITICAL THINKING EXERCISE

Maternal Attachment

Tara, 16 years old, in labor with her first baby, and Melanie, 38 years old, in labor with her fifth baby, gave birth at approximately the same time. Tara responded excitedly when her baby was placed in her arms but said, "Ugh!" when the nurse suggested placing the infant to breast. Melanie took the baby from the nurse, put him to breast, but said tearfully to the nurse, "I was really hoping for a girl; this is the fifth boy." The nurse determined there was a need to discuss infant feeding with Tara and to promote mother-infant attachment for Melanie. What suggestions would you have for the nurse?

1. Evidence—Is there sufficient evidence to draw conclusions about factors interfering with mother-infant attachment? About appropriate teaching related to breastfeeding and mother-infant attachment? Is age a risk factor in attachment?
2. Assumptions—What assumptions can be made about the following issues?
   a. Method of infant feeding used by adolescent mothers
   b. Attachment in adolescent mothers
   c. Attachment in experienced mothers
   d. Disappointment with the sex of an infant
3. What implications and priorities for nursing care can be drawn at this time?
4. Does the evidence objectively support your conclusion?
5. Are there alternative perspectives to your conclusion?

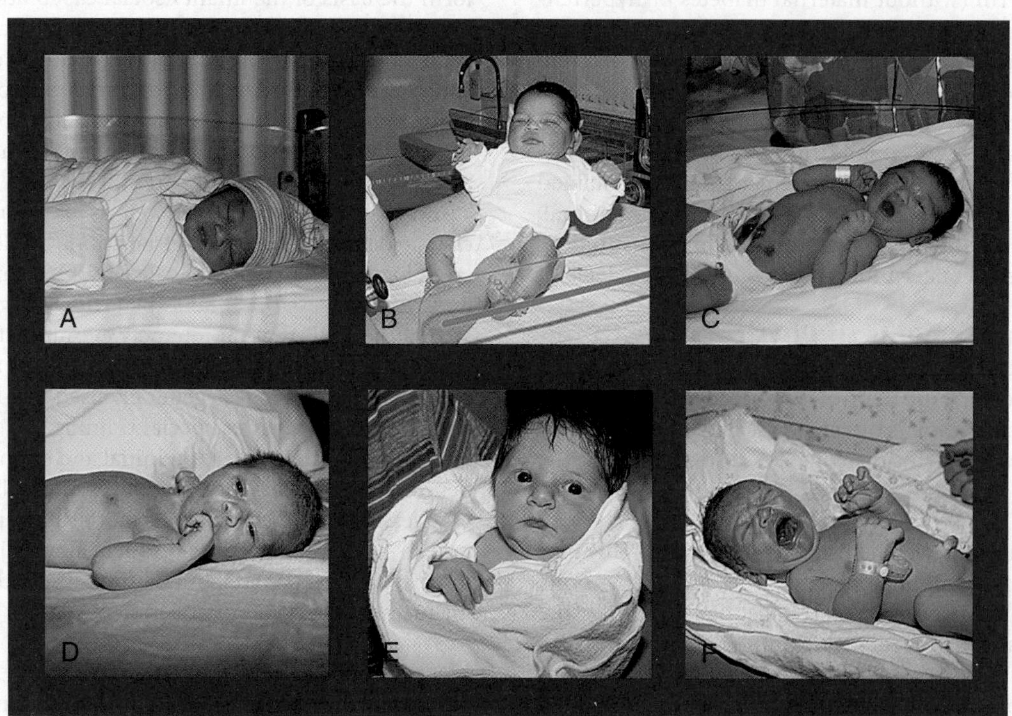

Fig. 24-11 Newborn sleep-wake states. A, Deep sleep. B, Light sleep; C, Drowsy. D, Quiet alert. E, Active alert. F, Crying. *(Courtesy Marjorie Pyle, RNC, Lifecircle, Costa Mesa, CA.)*

essential in the infant's neurobehavioral development. The more immature the infant, the less he or she is able to cope with factors, external or internal, that affect the sleep-wake patterns.

FAMILY-CENTERED CARE

Newborn Behavior

A first-time single mother asks the nurse about her newborn's activity. She voices concern that the newborn cries when she changes his diaper. "He sleeps a lot and only wakes up to eat or when I change his diaper. Is that normal?" Develop a short parent teaching lesson to present newborn behavior and care in relation to the following: sleep-wake states, newborn activities and relationship to crying behaviors in the first few days of life, and how to comfort and console the newborn.

Infants use purposeful behavior to maintain the optimum arousal state as follows: (1) actively withdrawing by increasing physical distance; (2) rejecting by pushing away with hands and feet; (3) decreasing sensitivity by falling asleep or breaking eye contact by turning head; or (4) using signaling behaviors, such as fussing and crying. These behaviors permit infants to quiet themselves and reinstate readiness to interact.

The first 6 weeks of life involve a steady decrease in the proportion of active REM sleep to total sleep. A steady increase in the proportion of quiet sleep to total sleep also occurs. Periods of wakefulness increase. For the first few weeks the wakeful periods seem dictated by hunger, but soon a need for socializing appears as well. The newborn sleeps approximately 16 to 18 hours a day, with periods of wakefulness gradually increasing. By the fourth week of life, some infants stay awake from one feeding to the next.

Other Factors Influencing Behavior of Newborns

Gestational Age

The gestational age of the infant and level of CNS maturity affect the observed behavior. In an infant with an immature CNS (preterm), the entire body responds to a pinprick of the foot, although the response may not be observed by an untrained observer; the mature infant withdraws only the foot. CNS immaturity is reflected in reflex development, sleep-wake states, and ability (or inability) to regulate or modulate a smooth transition between different states. Preterm infants have brief periods of alertness but have difficulty maintaining the state without becoming overstimulated, which leads to autonomic instability unless intervention is implemented. Preterm or sick infants show signs of fatigue or physiologic stress sooner than full-term healthy infants.

Time

The time elapsed since labor and birth affects infants' behavior as they attempt to become organized initially. Time elapsed since the previous feeding and time of day may also influence infants' responses.

Stimuli

Environmental events and stimuli affect infants' behavioral responses. The newborn responds to animate and inanimate stimuli. Nurses in intensive care nurseries observe that infants respond to loud noises, bright lights, monitor alarms, and tension in the unit. If a mother is tense and is nervous or uncomfortable while feeding her infant, the infant may sense her tension and demonstrate difficulty feeding.

Medication

Controversy surrounds the effects on infant behavior of maternal medication (e.g., analgesia and anesthesia) during labor. Some researchers note that infants of mothers given certain analgesic medications may continue to demonstrate poor state organization after the fifth day; medication effects have been noted as long as 30 days after birth. Other researchers maintain that the effect can be beneficial or nonexistent.

Sensory Behaviors

From birth, infants possess sensory capabilities that indicate a state of readiness for social interaction. Infants effectively use behavioral responses in establishing their first dialogues. These responses, coupled with the newborns' "baby appearance" (e.g., facial proportions of forehead and eyes larger than the lower part of the face) and their small size and helplessness, evoke feelings of wanting to hold, protect, and interact with them.

Vision

At birth the eye is structurally incomplete and the muscles are immature. The process of accommodation is not present at birth but improves over the first 3 months of life. The pupils react to light, the blink reflex is easily stimulated, and the corneal reflex is activated by light touch. Term newborns can see objects as far away as 2½ feet. The clearest visual distance is 20.3 to 30.4 cm (8 to 12 inches), which is about the distance the infant's face is from the mother's face as she breastfeeds or cuddles. Infants are sensitive to light; they will frown if a bright light is flashed in their eyes and will turn toward a soft, red light. If the room is darkened, they will open their eyes wide and look about. By 2 months of age, they can detect color; but at 5 days of age and younger, they seem more attracted by black-and-white patterns.

Response to movement is noticeable. If a bright light is shown to newborns (even at 15 minutes of age), they will follow it visually; some will even turn their heads to do so. Because human eyes are bright, shiny objects, newborns will track their parents' eyes. Parents often comment on how exciting this behavior is. The development of eye-to-eye contact is important for parent-infant attachment. Children of blind parents, and parents who have blind children, must circumvent this obstacle to form a relationship.

Visual acuity is surprising; even at 2 weeks of age, infants can distinguish patterns with stripes 3 mm apart. By 6 months their vision is as acute as that of an adult. They prefer to look at patterns rather than plain surfaces, even if the latter are brightly colored. Infants prefer more complex patterns to simple ones. They prefer novelty (changes in pattern) by 2 months of age. The infant of a few weeks of age

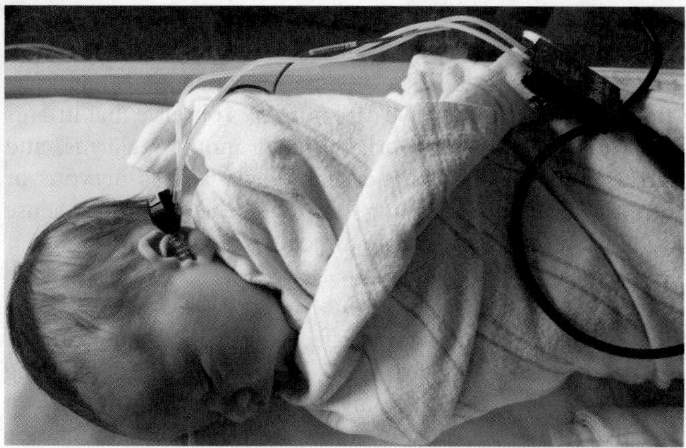

Fig. 24-12 Hearing screening in the newborn nursery. *(Courtesy Cheryl Briggs, RN, Annapolis, MD.)*

is therefore capable of responding actively to an enriched environment.

Hearing

As soon as the amniotic fluid drains from the ears, the infant's hearing is similar to that of an adult. Loud sounds of about 90 decibels cause the infant to react with a startle reflex. The newborn responds to low-frequency sounds such as a heartbeat or lullaby by decreasing motor activity or stopping crying. High-frequency sound elicits an alerting response.

The infant responds readily to the mother's voice. Studies indicate a selective listening to maternal voice sounds and rhythms during intrauterine life that prepares newborns for recognition and interaction with their primary caregivers—their mothers. Newborns are accustomed to hearing the regular rhythm of the mother's heartbeat. As a result, they respond by relaxing and ceasing to fuss and cry if a regular heartbeat simulator is placed in their cribs.

Hearing loss is a common major abnormality at birth; approximately one to three in 1000 normal term infants have bilateral hearing loss (American Academy of Pediatrics, 2000). To identify affected infants, the hearing of all infants is screened before discharge from the birth institution (Fig. 24-12).

Smell

Newborns react to strong odors such as alcohol or vinegar by turning their heads away. Breastfed infants are able to smell breast milk and can differentiate their mother from other lactating women by the smell (Lawrence & Lawrence, 2005).

Taste

The newborn can distinguish between tastes, and various types of solutions elicit differing facial expressions. A tasteless solution produces no response, a sweet solution elicits eager sucking, a sour solution causes puckering of the lips, and a bitter liquid produces a grimace.

Young infants are particularly oriented toward the use of their mouths, both for meeting their nutritional needs for rapid growth and for releasing tension through sucking. The early development of circumoral sensation, muscle activity, and taste would seem to be preparation for survival in the extrauterine environment.

Touch

The newborn is responsive to touch on all parts of the body. The face (especially the mouth), hands, and soles of the feet seem to be the most sensitive. Reflexes can be elicited by stroking the infant. The newborn's responses to touch suggest this sensory system is well prepared to receive and process tactile messages. Touch and motion are essential to normal growth and development. However, each infant is unique, and variations can be seen in newborns' responses to touch. Birth trauma or stress and depressant drugs taken by the mother decrease the infant's sensitivity to touch or painful stimuli.

Response to Environmental Stimuli

Temperament

Classic studies have identified individual variations in the primary reaction pattern of newborns and described them as *temperament.* Their style of behavioral response to stimuli is guided by the temperament, affecting newborns' sensory threshold, ability to habituate, and response to maternal behaviors. Newborns possess individual characteristics that affect selective responses to various stimuli present in the internal and external environments.

The three major patterns of behavioral style or temperament are as follows (Chess, 1969; Chess & Thomas, 1977):

1. The *easy child,* who demonstrates regularity in bodily functions, readily adapts to change, has a predominantly positive mood and moderate sensory threshold, and approaches new situations or objects with a moderate response
2. The *slow-to-warm-up child,* who has a low activity level, withdraws on first exposure to new stimuli, is slow to adapt and low in intensity of response, and is somewhat negative in mood
3. The *difficult child,* who is irregular in bodily functions, intense in reactions, generally negative in mood, and resistant to change or new stimuli and often cries loudly for long periods

Habituation

Habituation is a protective mechanism that allows the infant to become accustomed to environmental stimuli. Habituation is a psychologic and physiologic phenomenon in which the response to a constant or repetitive stimulus is decreased. In the term newborn, this can be demonstrated in several ways. Shining a bright light into a newborn's eyes will cause a startle or squinting the first two or three times. The third or fourth flash will elicit a diminished response, and by the fifth or sixth flash, the infant ceases to respond (Brazelton & Nugent, 1996). The same response pattern holds true for the sounds of a rattle or stroking the bottom of the foot.

The ability to habituate allows the healthy term newborn to select stimuli that promote continued learning about the social world, thus avoiding overload. The intrauterine environment seems to have programmed the newborn to be especially responsive to human voices, soft lights, soft sounds, and sweet tastes.

The newborn quickly learns the sounds in the home environment and is able to sleep in their midst. The selective responses of the newborn indicate cerebral organization capable of memory and making choices. The ability to habituate depends on the state of consciousness, hunger, fatigue, and temperament. These factors also affect consolability, cuddliness, irritability, and crying.

Consolability

Barr (1990) described variations in newborns' ability to console themselves or to be consoled. In the crying state, most newborns initiate one of several ways to reduce their distress. Hand-to-mouth movements are common, with or without sucking, as well as alerting to voices, noises, or visual stimuli.

Cuddliness

Cuddliness is especially important to parents because they often gauge their ability to care for the child by the child's responses to their actions. The degree to which newborns mold into the contours of the person holding them varies. Barr (1990) tested the effect of body contact and vestibular stimulation in both soothing babies and creating alertness. The vestibular stimulation of being picked up and moved had the greater effect.

Irritability

Some newborns cry longer and harder than others. For some the sensory threshold seems low. They are readily upset by unusual noises, hunger, wetness, or new experiences, and thus respond intensely. Others with a high sensory threshold require a great deal more stimulation and variation to reach the active, alert state.

Crying

Crying in an infant may signal hunger, discomfort, pain, desire for attention, or fussiness. Some mothers state that they learn to distinguish among the cries. The duration of crying is also highly variable in each infant; newborns may cry for as little as 5 minutes or as much as 2 hours or more per day. The amount of crying peaks in the second month and then decreases. There is a diurnal rhythm of crying, with more crying occurring in the evening hours. Crying does not seem to differ with different caretakers.

Key Points

- By full term the newborn's various anatomic and physiologic systems have reached a level of development and functioning that permits a physical existence apart from the mother.
- The appearance of jaundice during the first day of life or persistence of jaundice beyond 7 to 10 days may indicate a pathologic process that requires further investigation.
- Heat loss in the healthy term newborn may exceed the capacity to produce heat; this can lead to metabolic and respiratory complications that threaten the newborn's well-being.
- Assessment of the newborn requires data from the prenatal, intrapartum, and postpartum periods.
- The newborn assessment should proceed systematically so that each system is thoroughly evaluated.

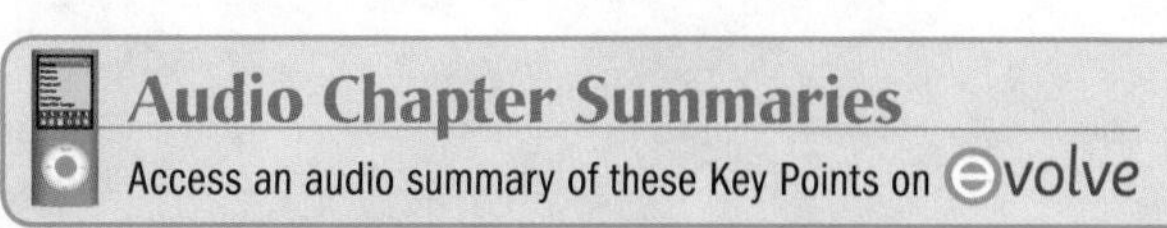
Audio Chapter Summaries
Access an audio summary of these Key Points on evolve

- Some reflex behaviors are important for the newborn's survival.
- Individual personalities and behavioral characteristics of infants play a major role in the ultimate relationship between infants and their parents.
- Each full-term newborn has a predisposed capacity to handle the multitude of stimuli in the external world.

References

American Academy of Pediatrics, Joint Committee on Infant Hearing: Year 2000 position statement: principle and guidelines for early hearing detection and intervention, *Pediatrics* 106(4):798-824, 2000.

Armentrout DC, Huseby V: Polycythemia in the newborn, *MCN Am J Matern Child Nurs* 28(4):234-239, 2003.

Asher C, Northington LK: Position statement for measurement of temperature/fever in children, *J Pediatr Nurs* 23(3):234-235, 2008.

Askin DF: Chest and lungs assessment. In Tappero EP, Honeyfield ME (editors): *Physical assessment of the newborn*, ed 3, Petaluma, CA, 2003, NICU Ink.

Barr RG: The normal crying curve: what do we really know? *Dev Med Child Neurol* 32(4):356-362, 1990.

Blackburn ST: *Maternal, fetal, and neonatal physiology: a clinical perspective*, ed 3, St Louis, 2007, Saunders.

Boo NY et al: Risk factors associated with subaponeurotic haemorrhage in full-term infants exposed to vacuum extraction, *Br J Obstet Gynaecol* 112:1516-1521, 2005.

Brazelton T, Nugent J: *Neonatal behavioural assessment scale*, ed 3, London, 1996, MacKeith.

Chess S: Individuality and baby care, *Dev Med Neurol* 11(6):749-754, 1969.

Chess S, Thomas A: Temperament and the parent-child interaction, *Pediatr Ann* 6(9):574-582, 1977.

Doumouchtsis SK, Arulkumaran S: Head injuries after instrumental vaginal deliveries, *Curr Opin Obstet Gynecol* 18(2):129-134, 2006.

Hutton EK, Hassan ES: Late vs early clamping of the umbilical cord in full-term neonates: systematic review and meta-analysis of controlled trials, *JAMA* 297(11):1241-1252, 2007.

Kent AL et al: Blood pressure in the first year of life in healthy infants born at term, *Pediatr Nephrol* 22(10):1743-1749, 2007.

Lawrence RA, Lawrence RM: *Breastfeeding: a guide for the medical profession*, ed 6, St Louis, 2005, Mosby.

Paige PL, Moe PC: Neurologic disorders. In Merenstein GB, Gardner SL (editors): *Handbook of neonatal intensive care*, ed 6, St Louis, 2006, Mosby.

Razmus IJ, Lewis L: Using four limb blood pressures as a screening tool in normal newborns, *Soc Pediatr Nurs News* 15(6):5-7, 2006.

Taylor ML: Coarctation of the aorta: critical catch for newborn well-being, *Nurse Pract* 30(12):34-43, 2005.

Uchil D, Arulkumaran S: Neonatal subgaleal hemorrhage and its relationship to delivery by vacuum extraction, *Obstet Gynecol Survey* 58(10):687-693, 2003.

Visscher MO et al: Vernix caseosa in neonatal adaptation, *J Perinatol* 25(7):440-446, 2005.

Weinberg JA, Powell KR: Laboratory aids for diagnosis of neonatal sepsis. In Remington JS, Klein JO (editors): *Infectious diseases of the fetus and newborn infant*, ed 5, Philadelphia, 2001, Saunders.

Unit 6

25

Nursing Care of the Newborn

Learning Objectives

On completion of this chapter the reader will be able to:

- Identify the purpose and components of the Apgar score.
- Compare and contrast the characteristics of preterm, late preterm, term, and postterm neonates.
- Perform a gestational age assessment on a newborn.
- Explain what is meant by a safe environment.
- Discuss phototherapy and the guidelines for teaching parents about this treatment.
- Explain purposes and methods of circumcision, the postoperative care of the circumcised infant, and parent teaching information regarding circumcision.
- Review procedures for performing a heel stick, collecting urine specimens, and assisting with venipuncture.
- Evaluate pain in the newborn based on physiologic changes and behavioral observations.
- Review anticipatory guidance nurses provide parents before discharge.

Electronic Resources

Additional information related to the content in Chapter 25 can be found on

evolve the Companion Website at
http://evolve.elsevier.com/Perry/maternal/

- NCLEX Review Questions
- Case Study—The Normal Newborn
- Critical Thinking Exercise—Circumcision
- Critical Thinking Exercise—Jaundice
- Nursing Care Plan—Home Care Follow-Up: Transition to Parenthood
- Nursing Care Plan—The Normal Newborn and Family
- Skill—Changing a Diaper
- Skill—Infant Bathing
- Skill—Pain Assessment
- Spanish Guidelines—Daily Care
- Spanish Guidelines—General Advice
- Spanish Guidelines—Infant Quieting Techniques
- Video—Circumcision
- Video—Crying Female Neonate

Although most infants make the necessary biopsychosocial adjustment to extrauterine existence without undue difficulty, their well-being depends on the care they receive from others. This chapter describes the assessment and care of the infant from immediately after birth until discharge.

Birth Through the First 2 Hours

Nursing Care Management

Care begins immediately after birth and focuses on assessing and stabilizing the newborn's condition. The nurse has primary responsibility for the infant during this period, since the physician or midwife is involved with the care of the mother. The nurse must be alert for any signs of distress and initiate appropriate interventions.

With the possibility of transmission of viruses such as hepatitis B virus and human immunodeficiency virus via maternal blood and blood-stained amniotic fluid, the newborn must be considered a potential contamination source until proved otherwise. As part of Standard Precautions, nurses should wear gloves when handling the newborn until blood and amniotic fluid are removed by bathing; gloves should be worn for all diaper changes as well.

Assessment

Initial Assessment and Apgar Scoring

The first assessment of the newborn is performed immediately after birth using the Apgar score (Table 25-1) and a brief physical examination (Box 25-1). A gestational age assessment is completed within the first hours of birth in the stable newborn (Fig. 25-1). A more comprehensive physical examination may be completed within 24 hours of birth (see Table 24-2).

Apgar Score

The Apgar score permits a rapid assessment of the newborn's transition to extrauterine existence based on five signs that indicate his or her physiologic state: (1) heart rate based on auscultation with a stethoscope or palpation of the umbilical cord; (2) respiratory rate based on observed movement of respiratory efforts; (3) muscle tone based on degree of flexion and movement of the extremities; (4) reflex irritability based on response to bulb or catheter inserted in nasopharynx; and

Table 25-1 Apgar Score

SIGN	Score 0	1	2
Heart rate	Absent	Slow (<100 beats/min)	>100 beats/min
Respiratory rate	Absent	Slow, weak cry	Good cry
Muscle tone	Flaccid	Some flexion of extremities	Well flexed
Reflex irritability	No response	Grimace	Cry
Color	Blue, pale	Body pink, extremities blue	Completely pink

BOX 25-1 Initial Physical Assessment by Body System

Central Nervous System
- ☐ Moves all four extremities, flexion, muscle tone good
- ☐ Symmetric features, movement
- ☐ Moro, suck, rooting, and grasp reflexes present
- ☐ Anterior fontanel soft and flat

Cardiovascular System
- ☐ Heart auscultation, regular in rate and rhythm
- ☐ Transient acrocyanosis, otherwise pink in color
- ☐ Pulses strong, equal bilaterally
- ☐ Capillary refill less than 3 seconds centrally and in peripheral tissues (not nail beds)

Respiratory System
- ☐ Lungs auscultated, clear bilaterally with minimal fine crackles shortly after birth
- ☐ Respiratory rate less than 60 breaths/min
- ☐ Respiratory effort nonlabored
- ☐ Absence of nasal flaring, grunting, retractions

Genitourinary System
- ☐ Male: urethral opening at tip of penis; testes descended bilaterally; female: labia minora and majora intact; hymenal tag may be visible

Gastrointestinal System
- ☐ Abdomen soft, no visible distention
- ☐ Cord attached and clamped
- ☐ Anus patent

Eyes, Ears, Nose, and Throat
- ☐ Eyes clear
- ☐ Palates intact
- ☐ Nares patent
- ☐ Ears in place; correct alignment

Skin

Color ☐ pink ☐ acrocyanotic
- ☐ Skin lesions or abrasions documented
- ☐ Birthmarks documented
- ☐ Caput/molding
- ☐ Other

(5) generalized skin color described as pallid, cyanotic, or pink (see Table 25-1). Evaluations are made at 1 and 5 minutes after birth and can be done by the nurse or birth attendant. Scores of 0 to 3 indicate severe distress, scores of 4 to 6 indicate moderate difficulty, and scores of 7 to 10 indicate that the infant is having minimal or no difficulty adjusting to extrauterine life. Apgar scores do not predict future neurologic outcome but are useful for describing the newborn's transition to the extrauterine environment (see Family-Centered Care box). Should resuscitation be required, it should be initiated before the 1-minute Apgar score (American Academy of Pediatrics & American College of Obstetricians and Gynecologists, 2007).

FAMILY-CENTERED CARE

Significance of the Apgar Score

The Apgar score was developed to provide a systematic method of assessing an infant's condition at birth. Researchers have tried to correlate Apgar scores with various outcomes such as development, intelligence, and neurologic development. In some instances, researchers have attempted to attribute causality to the Apgar score, that is, to suggest that the low Apgar score caused or predicted later problems. This is an inappropriate use of the Apgar score. Instead the score should be used to ensure that infants are systematically observed at birth to ascertain the need for immediate care. Either a physician or a nurse may assign the score; however, to avoid the real or perceived appearance of bias, the person assisting with the birth should not assign the score. Lack of consistency in the assigned scores limits studies of the Apgar's long-term predictive value. Prospective parents and the public need education on the significance of the Apgar, as well as its limits. *Because infants often do not receive the maximum score of 10, parents need to know that scores of 7 to 10 are within normal limits.* Attorneys involved in litigation related to injury of an infant at birth or negative outcomes, either short term or long term, also need education about the Apgar scoring system, its significance, and its limits. This useful tool needs to be used appropriately; health care providers, parents, and the public may need education to ensure appropriate use of the score.

Data from Montgomery K: Apgar scores: examining the long-term significance, *J Perinat Educ* 9(3):5-9, 2000.

ESTIMATION OF GESTATIONAL AGE BY MATURITY RATING

NEUROMUSCULAR MATURITY

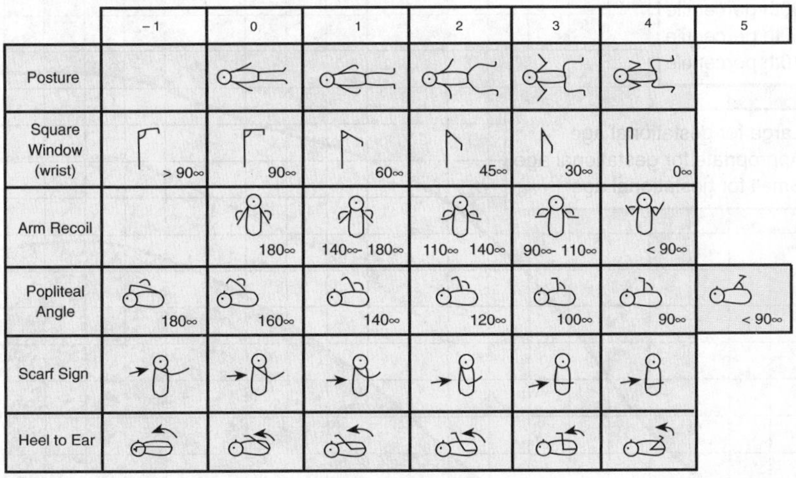

	−1	0	1	2	3	4	5
Posture							
Square Window (wrist)	> 90°	90°	60°	45°	30°	0°	
Arm Recoil		180°	140°- 180°	110° 140°	90°- 110°	< 90°	
Popliteal Angle	180°	160°	140°	120°	100°	90°	< 90°
Scarf Sign							
Heel to Ear							

PHYSICAL MATURITY

Skin	sticky friable transparent	gelatinous red, translucent	smooth pink, visible veins	superficial peeling &/or rash, few veins	cracking pale areas rare veins	parchment deep cracking no vessels	leathery cracked wrinkled
Lanugo	none	sparse	abundant	thinning	bald areas	mostly bald	
Plantar Surface	heel-toe 40-50 mm: -1 <40 mm: -2	>50 mm no crease	faint red marks	anterior transverse crease only	creases ant. 2/3	creases over entire sole	
Breast	imperceptible	barely perceptible	flat areola no bud	stippled areola 1-2 mm bud	raised areola 3-4 mm bud	full areola 5-10 mm bud	
Eye/Ear	lids fused loosely: -1 tightly: -2	lids open pinna flat stays folded	slightly curved pinna; soft; slow recoil	well-curved pinna; soft but ready recoil	formed & firm instant recoil	thick cartilage ear stiff	
Genitals (male)	scrotum flat, smooth	scrotum empty faint rugae	testes in upper canal rare rugae	testes descending few rugae	testes down good rugae	testes pendulous deep rugae	
Genitals (female)	clitoris prominent labia flat	prominent clitoris small labia minora	prominent clitoris enlarging minora	majora & minora equally prominent	majora large minora small	majora cover clitoris & minora	

MATURITY RATING

score	weeks
-10	20
-5	22
0	24
5	26
10	28
15	30
20	32
25	34
30	36
35	38
40	40
45	42
50	44

A

Fig. 25-1 Estimation of gestational age. **A,** New Ballard scale for newborn maturity rating. Expanded scale includes extremely preterm infants and has been refined to improve accuracy in more mature infants. (**A,** From Ballard J et al: New Ballard score, expanded to include extremely premature infants, *J Pediatr* 119(3):417, 1991.)

Continued

Initial Physical Assessment

The initial physical assessment includes a brief review of systems (see Box 25-1):

External—Note skin color, general activity, muscle tone, position; assess nasal patency by closing one nostril at a time while observing respirations; assess skin: peeling, lack of subcutaneous fat (preterm or postterm), temperature; note meconium staining of cord, skin, fingernails, or amniotic fluid (staining may indicate fetal release of meconium); note length of nails and development of creases on soles of feet.

Chest—Auscultate apical heart for rate and rhythm, heart tones, and presence of abnormal sounds; note character of respirations and presence of crackles or other adventitious sounds; note quality of breath sounds by auscultation and observation.

Abdomen—Verify characteristics of abdomen (rounded, flat, concave) and absence of anomalies; auscultate bowel sounds; note number of vessels in cord and general status of cord (e.g., thin, emaciated; thick, tortuous, presence of hematoma).

Neurologic—Check muscle tone and assess Moro and suck reflexes; palpate anterior fontanel; note by palpation the presence and size of the fontanels and sutures.

Genitourinary—Note external sex characteristics and any abnormality of same; check anal patency, presence of meconium; note passage of urine.

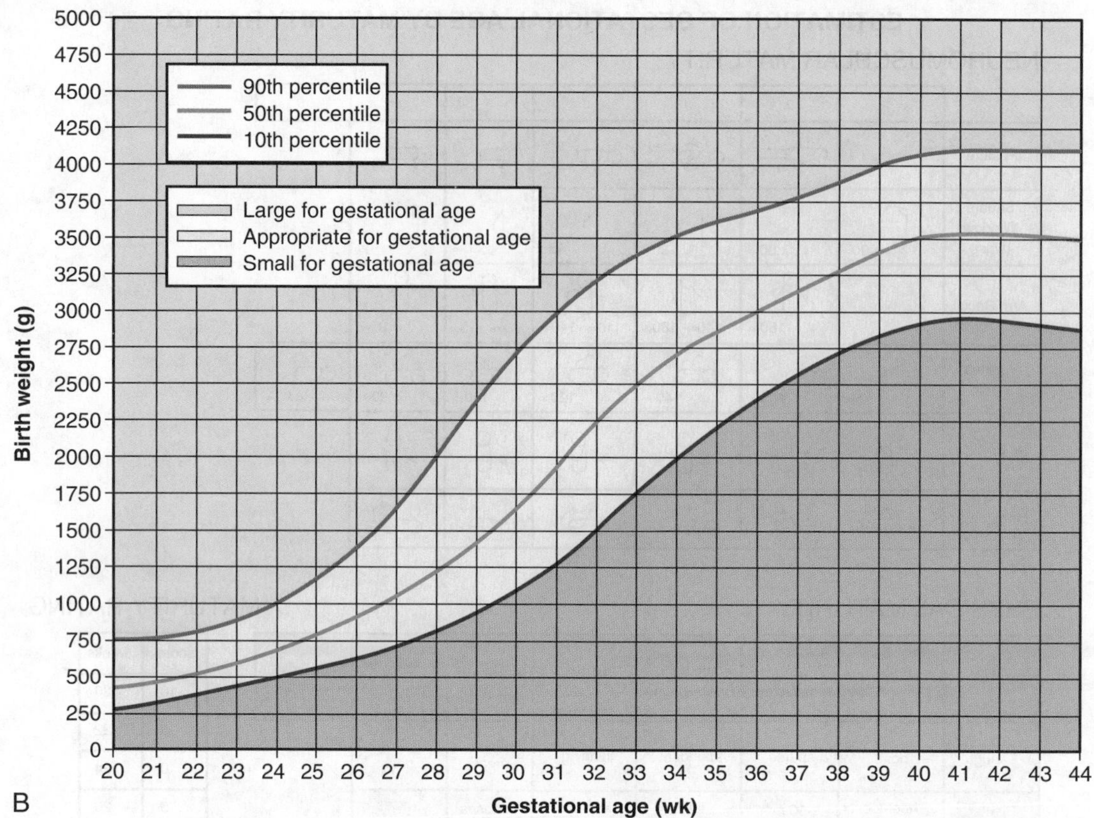

Fig. 25-1, cont'd B, Intrauterine growth: birth weight percentiles based on live single births at gestational ages 20 to 44 weeks. (**B,** Data from Alexander GR et al: A United States national reference for fetal growth, *Obstet Gynecol* 87(2):163-168, 1996.)

Other observations—Note gross structural malformation obvious at birth that may require immediate medical attention (e.g., omphalocele, meningocele).

The nurse responsible for the care of the newborn immediately after birth verifies that respirations have been established, dries the infant thoroughly, assesses temperature, and places identical identification bracelets on the infant and the mother. In some settings, the father or partner also wears an identification bracelet. The infant may be wrapped in a warm blanket and placed in the mother's arms, given to the partner to hold, or kept partially undressed under a radiant warmer. In many settings, immediately after birth the infant is placed on the mother's abdomen to allow skin-to-skin contact. This helps maintain the infant's optimum temperature and promotes parental bonding. The newborn may be placed to mom's breast within the first half hour to hour of life to begin the breastfeeding process or simply allowed to suckle at the mother's breast. The infant may be admitted to a nursery or remain with the parents throughout the hospital stay.

The initial examination of the newborn can occur while the nurse is drying and wrapping the infant, or observations can be made while the infant is lying on the mother's abdomen or in her arms immediately after birth. Efforts should be directed toward minimizing interference in the initial parent-infant acquaintance process. If the infant is breathing effectively, is pink, and has no apparent life-threatening anomalies or risk factors requiring immediate attention (e.g., infant of diabetic mother), further examination can be delayed until after the parents have had an opportunity to interact with the infant. Routine procedures and the admission process can be carried out in the mother's room or in a separate nursery.

The nursing process in the immediate care of the newborn and family is outlined in the Nursing Process box.

Implementation

Changes can occur rapidly in the newborn immediately after birth. Assessment must be followed by implementation of appropriate care.

Airway Maintenance

Generally, the normal term infant born vaginally has little difficulty clearing the airway. Most secretions are moved by gravity and brought by the cough reflex to the oropharynx to be drained or swallowed. The infant may initially be placed in a side-lying position (head stabilized, not in Trendelenburg position) until secretions are cleared and then placed supine.

If the infant has excess mucus in the respiratory tract, the mouth and nasal passages may be gently suctioned with a bulb syringe (Fig. 25-2). Routine chest percussion and suctioning of healthy term and near-term infants are avoided; there is insufficient evidence to support anything other than gentle nasopharyngeal and oropharyngeal suctioning to clear secretions (Hagedorn, 2006). The infant who is choking on

NURSING PROCESS: NEWBORN CARE

Assessment

A brief initial assessment is performed to detect any problems that may impair an effective newborn transition. Once the infant has stabilized and maternal-infant contact has occurred, a more thorough examination may take place, including the gestational age assessment.

Nursing Diagnoses

Nursing diagnoses are established after analysis of the findings of the physical assessment. Nursing diagnoses for the newborn include the following:

Ineffective airway clearance related to
- airway obstruction with mucus, blood, and amniotic fluid
- inability to clear mucus by cough and expectoration

Risk for imbalanced body temperature related to
- imbalance between body heat loss and heat production

Pain Related to
- heel stick, circumcision, venipuncture

Readiness for enhanced parenting related to
- knowledge of newborn's social capabilities
- knowledge of newborn's dependency needs
- knowledge of biologic characteristics of the newborn

Ineffective role performance related to
- misinterpretation of newborn's behavioral cues
- inadequate knowledge about newborn's basic care needs (feeding, bathing, sleep-wake patterns, stooling and voiding patterns)

Risk for unstable blood glucose related to
- increased glucose utilization at birth
- decreased endogenous glucose supply

Neonatal jaundice related to
- increasing serum bilirubin levels
- inability to metabolize and excrete bilirubin
- increased hemolysis

Implementation and Interventions

A number of intervention strategies for the newborn infant are discussed on pp. 643-649.

Planning

Expected outcomes can apply both to the infant and the parents. Expected outcomes for the newborn during the immediate recovery period include that the infant will do the following:

- Maintain effective breathing pattern
- Maintain effective thermoregulation
- Maintain adequate cardiac output, circulation, and tissue perfusion
- Remain free from infection
- Receive necessary nutrition for growth
- Receive bilirubin assessment and screening within the first week of life to determine risk for increasing levels of serum bilirubin

Expected outcomes for the parents include that they will do the following:

- Attain knowledge, skill, and confidence relevant to infant care activities
- State understanding of biologic and behavioral characteristics of the newborn
- Begin to integrate the newborn into the family

Evaluation

The nurse can be reasonably assured that care was effective to the extent that the expected outcomes for care have been achieved.

evolve Case Study—The Normal Newborn

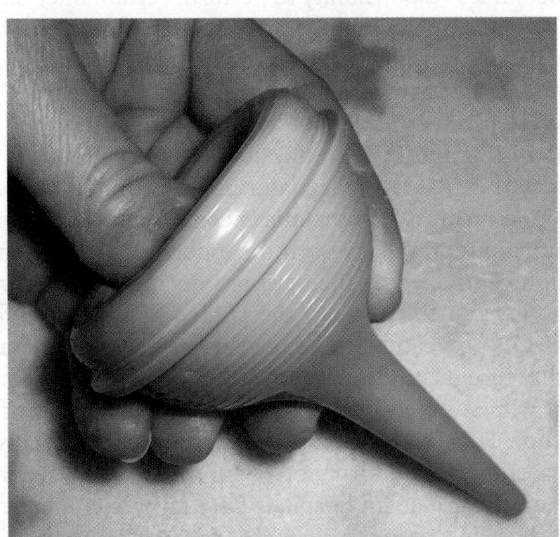

Fig. 25-2 Bulb syringe. Bulb must be compressed before insertion. *(Courtesy Cheryl Briggs, RN, Annapolis, MD.)*

secretions should be supported with his or her head to the side. The mouth is suctioned first to prevent the infant from inhaling pharyngeal secretions by gasping as the nares are touched. The bulb is compressed and inserted into one side of the mouth. The center of the infant's mouth is avoided because this could stimulate the gag reflex. The nasal passages are suctioned one nostril at a time. The bulb syringe should always be kept in the infant's crib. The parents should be shown how to use the bulb syringe and asked to perform a return demonstration. The nurse should also listen to the infant's respirations and lung sounds with a stethoscope to determine whether there are crackles, rhonchi, or inspiratory stridor. Fine crackles may be auscultated for several hours after birth. If air movement is adequate, the bulb syringe may be used to clear the mouth and nose. If the bulb syringe does not clear mucus interfering with respiratory effort, mechanical suction can be used. If the newborn has an obstruction that is not cleared with suctioning, further investigation is necessary to determine whether there is a mechanical defect (e.g., tracheoesoph-

BOX 25-2 Newborn Breathing: Signs of Distress

Bradypnea—Respirations (less than 30 breaths/min)
Tachypnea—Respirations (60 breaths/min or more)
Abnormal breath sounds—Crackles (fine crackles may be heard in first few hours after birth), wheezing, rhonchi, expiratory grunting, stridor, diminished or absent air movement
Respiratory distress—Nasal flaring, retractions, labored breathing, apnea lasting 20 seconds or longer

ageal fistula, choanal atresia [see Chapter 28]) causing the obstruction.

Deeper suctioning may be necessary to remove mucus from the infant's nasopharynx or posterior oropharynx; however, this should be performed only after an assessment of the risks involved. Proper catheter insertion and suctioning for 5 seconds or less per catheter insertion help prevent vagal stimulation and hypoxia. If wall suction is used, the pressure should be adjusted to less than 80 mm Hg. After the catheter is properly placed, suction is created by placing one's thumb over the control as the catheter is carefully rotated and gently withdrawn. This procedure may need to be repeated until the infant has a clear airway.

Maintaining an Adequate Oxygen Supply

Four conditions are essential for maintaining an adequate oxygen supply:

1. A clear airway
2. Effective establishment of respirations
3. Adequate circulation, adequate perfusion, and effective cardiac function
4. Adequate thermoregulation (Exposure to cold stress increases oxygen and glucose needs.)

Signs of potential complications related to abnormal newborn breathing are listed in Box 25-2.

Body Temperature Maintenance

Effective neonatal care includes maintenance of an optimal thermal environment (see Chapter 24). Cold stress increases the need for oxygen and may deplete glucose stores. The infant may react to exposure to cold by increasing the respiratory rate and may become cyanotic. Ways to stabilize the newborn's body temperature include placing the infant directly on the mother's abdomen and covering with a warm blanket (skin-to-skin contact), drying and wrapping the newborn in warmed blankets immediately after birth, keeping the head well covered, and keeping the ambient temperature at 22° to 26° C (American Academy of Pediatrics & American College of Obstetricians and Gynecologists, 2007). Allowing vernix caseosa to remain on the infant's skin has not been associated with a decrease in axillary temperature in the first hour after birth (Visscher et al, 2005).

If the infant does not remain with the mother during the first 1 to 2 hours after birth, the nurse places the thoroughly dried newborn under a radiant warmer or in a warm incubator unit until the body temperature stabilizes. The infant's skin temperature is used as the point of control when using a warmer with a servocontrolled mechanism. The control panel usually is maintained between 36° and 37° C. This setting should maintain the healthy term infant's skin temperature around 36.5° to 37° C. A thermistor probe (automatic sensor) is usually placed on the upper quadrant of the abdomen immediately below the right or left costal margin (never over a bone); a reflector adhesive patch may be used over the probe to provide adequate warming. This will ensure detection of minor temperature changes resulting from external environmental factors or neonatal factors (peripheral vasoconstriction, vasodilation, or increased metabolism) before a dramatic change in core body temperature develops; the servocontroller adjusts the warmer temperature to maintain the infant's skin temperature within the preset range. The sensor needs to be checked periodically to ensure that it is securely attached to the infant's skin. The newborn's axillary temperature is checked every hour (or more often as needed) until his or her temperature stabilizes. The time required to stabilize and maintain body temperature varies; each newborn should therefore be allowed to achieve thermal regulation as necessary, and care should be individualized.

During all procedures, heat loss must be avoided or minimized for the newborn; examinations and activities are performed with the newborn under a heat panel. The initial bath is postponed until the newborn's skin temperature is stable and can adjust to heat loss from a bath. The exact and optimal timing of the bath for every infant remains unknown and should be individualized according to the infant's ability to maintain a stable body temperature.

Even a healthy term infant can become hypothermic. Birth in a car on the way to the hospital, a cold birthing room, or inadequate drying and wrapping immediately after birth may cause the infant's temperature to fall below normal range (hypothermia). Warming the hypothermic newborn is accomplished with care. Rapid warming may cause apnea and acidosis in an infant. The warming process is therefore monitored to progress slowly over a period of 2 to 4 hours.

Immediate Interventions

It is the nurse's responsibility to perform certain interventions fairly soon after birth to provide for the safety of the newborn. Such interventions may be delayed for an hour or two in order for uninterrupted maternal-infant bonding to occur.

Eye Prophylaxis

The instillation of a prophylactic agent in the eyes of all neonates (Fig. 25-3) is mandatory in the United States as a precaution against ophthalmia neonatorum, which is an inflammation of the eyes from gonorrheal or chlamydial infection contracted by the newborn during passage through the mother's birth canal. In the United States, if the family objects to this treatment, the primary care provider may ask that the parents sign an informed refusal form, and their refusal will be noted in the neonate's record. The agent used for prophylaxis varies according to hospital protocols, but usual agents include forms of erythromycin, tetracycline, or silver nitrate. Canadian hospitals have not recommended the use of silver nitrate since 1986. It is rarely used in the United States because silver nitrate does not protect against chlamydial infection and can cause chemical conjunctivitis. Instil-

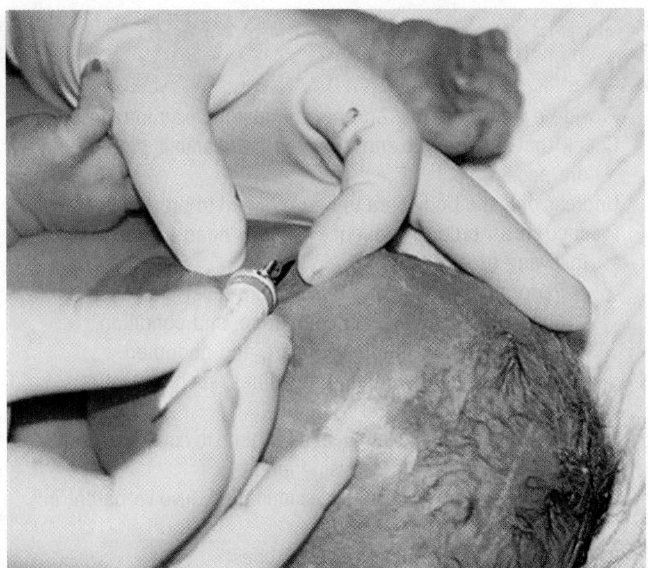

Fig. 25-3 Instillation of medication into eye of newborn. Thumb and forefinger are used to open the eye; medication is placed in the lower conjunctiva from the inner to the outer canthus. *(Courtesy Marjorie Pyle, RNC, Lifecircle, Costa Mesa, CA.)*

lation of eye prophylaxis may be delayed until an hour or so after birth (American Academy of Pediatrics & American College of Obstetricians and Gynecologists, 2007) (up to 2 hours in Canada) to facilitate eye contact and parent-infant attachment and bonding.

Topical antibiotics such as tetracycline and erythromycin, silver nitrate, and a 2.5% povidone-iodine solution (currently unavailable in commercial form in the United States) have not proved to be effective in the treatment of chlamydial conjunctivitis. A 14-day course of oral erythromycin or an oral sulfonamide may be given for chlamydial conjunctivitis (American Academy of Pediatrics, Committee on Infectious Diseases, 2006) (see Medication Guide).

Vitamin K Prophylaxis

Administering vitamin K intramuscularly is routine in the newborn period in the United States. A single injection of 0.5 to 1 mg of vitamin K is given soon after birth to prevent hemorrhagic disease of the newborn; administration may be delayed until after the first breastfeeding in the delivery room (American Academy of Pediatrics & American College of Obstetricians and Gynecologists, 2007). Vitamin K is produced in the gastrointestinal tract by bacteria, starting soon after microorganisms are introduced. By day 8, normal newborns are able to produce their own vitamin K (see Medication Guide).

NURSING ALERT Vitamin K is never administered via the intravenous route for prevention of hemorrhagic disease of the newborn except in some cases of a preterm infant who has no muscle mass. In such cases, the medication should be diluted and given over 10 to 15 minutes with the infant being closely monitored with a cardiorespiratory monitor. Rapid bolus administration of vitamin K may cause cardiac arrest.

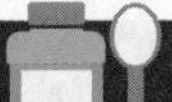

MEDICATION GUIDE

Eye Prophylaxis with Erythromycin Ophthalmic Ointment 0.5% and Tetracycline Ophthalmic Ointment 1%

Action

Erythromycin and tetracycline antibiotic ointments are both bacteriostatic and bactericidal. They provide prophylaxis against *Neisseria gonorrhoeae.* Topical treatment of neonatal conjunctivitis caused by *Chlamydia trachomatis* is not indicated; instead the infant should be treated with a 14-day course of either oral erythromycin or ethylsuccinate (American Academy of Pediatrics, Committee on Infectious Diseases, 2006).

Indication

These medications are used for the prevention of ophthalmia neonatorum in newborns of mothers who are infected with gonorrhea.

Neonatal Dosage

Apply a 1 to 2 cm ribbon of ointment to the lower conjunctival sac of each eye; the medicines may also be used in drop form.

Adverse Reactions

They may cause chemical conjunctivitis that lasts 24 to 48 hours; vision may be blurred temporarily.

Nursing Considerations

Administer within 1 to 2 hours of birth. Wear gloves. Cleanse eyes if necessary before administration. Open eyes by putting a thumb and finger at the corner of each lid and gently pressing on the periorbital ridges. Squeeze the tube and spread the ointment from the inner canthus of the eye to the outer canthus. Do not touch the tube to the eye. After 1 minute, excess ointment may be wiped off. Observe eyes for irritation. Explain treatment to parents.

Eye prophylaxis for ophthalmia neonatorum is required by law in all states of the United States.

Promoting Parent-Infant Bonding

Today's childbirth practices strive to promote the family as the focus of care. Parents generally desire to share in the birth process and to have early contact with their infants. Early contact between mother and newborn can be important in developing future relationships. It also has a positive effect on the duration of breastfeeding. There are physiologic benefits of early mother-infant contact. Oxytocin and prolactin levels rise in the mother, and suckling activity is activated in the infant. The process of developing active immunity begins as the infant ingests flora from the mother's colostrum.

From 2 Hours After Birth Until Discharge

Nursing Care Management

Many hospitals have adopted variations of single-room maternity care (SRMC) or mother-baby (couplet) care. One nurse

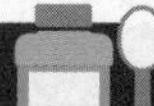

MEDICATION GUIDE

Vitamin K: Phytonadione (AquaMEPHYTON, Konakion)

Action

This intervention provides vitamin K because the newborn does not have the intestinal flora to produce this vitamin in the first week after birth. Vitamin K promotes formation of clotting factors (II, VII, IX, and X) in the liver.

Indication

Vitamin K is used for prevention and treatment of hemorrhagic disease in the newborn.

Neonatal Dosage

Administer a 0.5 to 1 mg (0.25 to 0.5 ml) dose intramuscularly within 2 hours of birth; the dose may be repeated if newborn shows bleeding tendencies.

Adverse Reactions

Edema, erythema, and pain at injection site may occur rarely; hemolysis, jaundice, and hyperbilirubinemia have been reported, particularly in preterm infants.

Nursing Considerations

Wear gloves. Administer in the middle third of the vastus lateralis muscle using a 25-gauge, ⅝-inch (16-mm) to ⅞-inch (22-mm) needle. Inject into skin that has been cleaned, or allow alcohol (or other skin antiseptic) to dry on puncture site for 1 minute to remove organisms and prevent infection. Stabilize leg firmly and grasp muscle between the thumb and fingers. Insert the needle at a 90-degree angle; aspirate and inject medication slowly if there is no blood return. After removing needle, rub gently on the injection site with a dry gauze square to decrease the pain. Observe for signs of bleeding from the site.

provides care for both the mother and the newborn. SRMC allows the infant to remain with the parents after the birth. Many of the procedures, such as assessment of weight and measurement, instillation of eye medication, administration of vitamin K, and physical assessment, may be carried out in the labor and birth unit. Nurses who work in an SRMC unit; a labor, delivery, and recovery (LDR) room; or a labor, delivery, recovery, and postpartum (LDRP) room must be educated in intrapartum, neonatal, and postpartum nursing care and be competent in providing it. If the infant is transferred to the nursery, the infant's identification is verified by the nurse receiving the infant, who places the baby in a warm environment and begins the admission process.

Assessment

Physical Assessment

A complete physical examination is performed within 24 hours, after the infant's condition has stabilized (see Guidelines box). See Chapter 24 for a detailed description of this examination.

GUIDELINES Physical Examination of the Newborn

Provide a normothermic and nonstimulating examination area.
Check that equipment and supplies are working properly and are accessible.
Undress only the body area to be examined to prevent heat loss.
Proceed in an orderly sequence (usually head to toe) with the following exceptions:
- Perform all procedures that require quiet first, such as observing position, skin color, tone, and condition.
- Next auscultate the lungs, heart, and abdomen.
- Perform more disturbing procedures, such as testing reflexes, last.
- Measure head and length at same time to compare results.

Proceed quickly to avoid stressing infant.
Comfort infant during and after examination; involve parent in:
- Talking softly
- Holding infant's hands against chest
- Swaddling and holding
- Giving pacifier or gloved finger to suck

Assessment of Gestational Age

Assessment of gestational age is important because perinatal morbidity and mortality rates are related to gestational age and birth weight. A frequently used method of determining gestational age is the simplified Assessment of Gestational Age scale by Ballard, Novak, and Driver (1979) (see Fig. 25-1, *A*). This scale, an abbreviated version of the Dubowitz scale, can be used to measure gestational ages of infants between 35 and 42 weeks. The Ballard scale assesses six external physical and six neuromuscular signs. Each sign has a number score, and the cumulative score correlates with a maturity rating of from 20 to 44 weeks of gestation.

The new simplified Ballard scale, a revision of the original scale, can be used with newborns as young as 20 weeks of gestation. The tool has the same physical and neuromuscular sections but includes −1 scores that reflect signs of extremely preterm infants, such as fused eyelids; imperceptible breast tissue; sticky, friable, transparent skin; no lanugo; and square-window (flexion of wrist) angle of greater than 90 degrees (see Fig. 25-1, *A*). The examination of infants with a gestational age of 26 weeks or less should be performed at a postnatal age of less than 12 hours. For infants with a gestational age of at least 26 weeks, the examination can be performed up to 96 hours after birth; however, to ensure accuracy, it is recommended that the initial examination be performed within the first 48 hours of life. Neuromuscular adjustments after birth in extremely immature neonates require that a follow-up examination be performed to further validate neuromuscular criteria. The new Ballard scale overestimates gestational age by 2 to 4 days in infants younger than 37 weeks of gestation, especially at gestational ages of 32 to 37 weeks (Ballard et al, 1991). See Box 25-3 for specific tests used in gestational age assessment.

BOX 25-3 Techniques Used in Assessing Gestational Age

Posture

With infant quiet and in a supine position, observe degree of flexion in arms and legs. Muscle tone and degree of flexion increase with maturity. Full flexion of the arms and legs = score 4.*

Square Window

With thumb supporting back of arm below wrist, apply gentle pressure with index and third fingers on dorsum of hand without rotating infant's wrist. Measure angle between base of thumb and forearm. Full flexion (hand lies flat on ventral surface of forearm) = score 4.

Arm Recoil

With infant supine, fully flex both forearms on upper arms and hold for 5 seconds; pull down on hands to fully extend and rapidly release arms. Observe rapidity and intensity of recoil to a state of flexion. A brisk return to full flexion = score 4.

Popliteal Angle

With infant supine and pelvis flat on a firm surface, flex lower leg on thigh and then flex thigh on abdomen. While holding knee with thumb and index finger, extend lower leg with index finger of other hand. Measure degree of angle behind knee (popliteal angle). An angle of less than 90 degrees = score 5.

Scarf Sign

With infant supine, support head in midline with one hand; use other hand to pull infant's arm across the shoulder so that infant's hand touches shoulder. Determine location of elbow in relation to midline. Elbow does not reach midline = score 4.

Heel to Ear

With infant supine and pelvis flat on a firm surface, pull foot as far as possible up toward ear on same side. Measure distance of foot from ear and degree of knee flexion (same as popliteal angle). Knees flexed with a popliteal angle of less than 10 degrees = score 4.

Source: Hockenberry MJ, Wilson D: *Wong's nursing care of infants and children*, ed 8, St Louis, 2007, Mosby.

*See Fig. 25-1 for scale and interpretation of scores.

Classification of Newborns by Gestational Age and Birth Weight

Classification of infants at birth by both birth weight and gestational age provides a more satisfactory method for predicting mortality risks and providing guidelines for management of the neonate than estimating gestational age or birth weight alone. The infant's birth weight, length, and head circumference are plotted on standardized graphs that identify normal values for gestational age (see Fig. 25-1, *B*, for weight chart and Box 27-1).

Intrauterine growth curves developed by Battaglia and Lubchenco (1967) have been used to classify infants according to birth weight and gestational age. Since that time, other intrauterine growth charts have emerged to reflect a more heterogeneous sample population than previously described (Cunningham et al, 2005). The primary intrauterine growth charts that provide national reference data include the work of Alexander and colleagues (1996), which represents more than 3.1 million live births in the United States; the work of Thomas and colleagues (2000); and the works of Arbuckle, Wilkins, and Sherman (1993) and Kramer and colleagues (2001), which represent intrauterine growth among the Canadian population. Thomas and colleagues (2000) concluded that intrauterine growth measured by head circumference, birth weight, and length varies according to race and gender. These researchers also found that altitude did not seem to significantly affect birth weight, as has been suggested by other authors. In one study, Asian and Hispanic newborns had lower mean birth weights, shorter mean lengths, and smaller mean head circumferences than Caucasian newborns (Madan et al, 2002). It is recommended that the reader access and use the most current intrauterine growth chart specific to the population being evaluated, especially when considering multiples such as twins.

The infant whose weight is appropriate for gestational age (AGA) (between the 10th and 90th percentiles) can be presumed to have grown at a normal rate regardless of the length of gestation—preterm, term, or postterm. The infant who is large for gestational age (LGA) (above the 90th percentile) can be presumed to have grown at an accelerated rate during fetal life; the small-for-gestational-age (SGA) infant (below the 10th percentile) can be presumed to have grown at a restricted rate during intrauterine life. When gestational age is determined according to the Ballard scale, the newborn will fall into one of the following nine possible categories for birth weight and gestational age: AGA—term, preterm, postterm; SGA—term, preterm, postterm; or LGA—term, preterm, postterm. Birth weight influences mortality: the lower the birth weight, the higher the mortality. The same is true for gestational age: the lower the gestational age, the higher the mortality (Stoll, 2007).

Late Preterm Infant

Much attention has recently been focused on infants who are considered "late preterm"; they are often the size and weight of term infants and may be admitted to the healthy newborn nursery and treated as healthy newborns. Late preterm infants, born at 34 to 36$\frac{6}{7}$ weeks of gestation, have risk factors due to their physiologic immaturity that require close attention by nurses working with them (Bakewell-Sachs, 2007; Engle et al, 2007). These risk factors include the tendency to develop respiratory distress, temperature instability, hypoglycemia, apnea, feeding difficulties, jaundice, and hyperbilirubinemia. Nurses must be cognizant of the risk factors for late preterm infants and be continually vigilant for the development of problems related to the infant's immaturity. The late preterm infant's care is further addressed in Chapter 27.

Umbilical Cord Care

Care of the umbilical cord is an important aspect of nursing care and parent teaching. The goal of care is prevention and early detection of hemorrhage or infection. The umbilical cord stump is an excellent medium for bacterial growth and can easily become infected.

Hospital protocol determines the technique for routine cord care. Common methods include the use of an antimicrobial agent such as bacitracin or triple dye, although some experts advocate the use of alcohol alone, soap and water, sterile water, povidone-iodine, or no treatment (natural healing). The use of antiseptic agents has been shown to prolong cord drying and separation (Zupan, Garner, & Omari, 2004). Studies regarding bacterial growth and colonization according to the cleansing method used have produced varied results (Janssen et al, 2003; Golombek, Brill, & Salice, 2002). A Cochrane Review of 21 studies found no significant difference between cords treated with antiseptics compared with dry cord care or placebo; there were no reported systemic infections or deaths, and a trend toward reduced colonization was found in cords treated with antiseptics (Zupan, Garner, & Omari, 2004). Recommendations for cord care by the Association of Women's Health, Obstetric and Neonatal Nurses (2007) include cleaning the cord initially with sterile water and subsequently cleaning the cord with water. A one-time application of triple dye has been shown to be superior to alcohol, povidone-iodine, or topical antibiotics in reducing colonization or infection; the use of alcohol is associated with prolonged cord drying and separation (McConnell et al, 2004).

The stump and base of the cord should be assessed for edema, erythema, and drainage with each diaper change. The nurse cleanses the cord and skin area around the base of the cord with the prescribed preparation (e.g., sterile water, erythromycin solution, or triple-blue dye). The stump deteriorates through the process of dry gangrene; therefore odor alone is not a positive indicator of omphalitis (infection of the umbilical stump). Cord separation time is influenced by a number of factors, including type of cord care, type of delivery, and other perinatal events. The average cord separation time is 10 to 14 days.

The cord clamp is removed once the stump has started drying and is no longer bleeding (Fig. 25-4), typically within 24 hours and prior to discharge from the hospital.

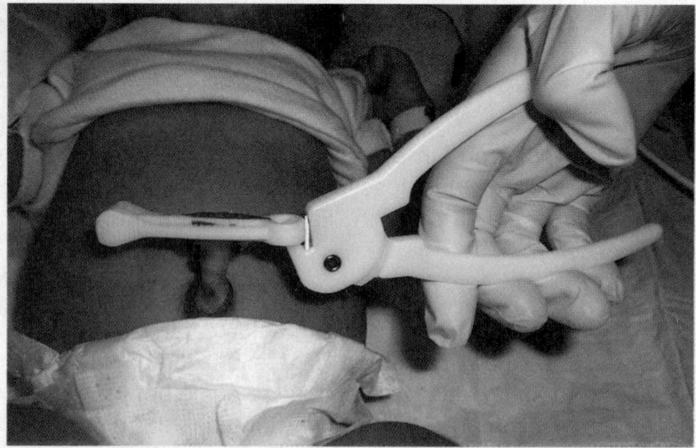

Fig. 25-4 Using special scissors, remove clamp after cord begins drying (about 24 hours). *(Courtesy Cheryl Briggs, RN, Annapolis, MD.)*

Common Newborn Problems

Physical Injuries

Birth trauma includes any physical injury sustained by a newborn during labor and birth. Many injuries are minor and readily resolve in the neonatal period without treatment. Other types of trauma require some form of intervention. A few are serious enough to be fatal.

Several factors predispose an infant to birth trauma. Maternal factors include uterine dysfunction that leads to prolonged or precipitous labor, preterm or postterm labor, and cephalopelvic disproportion. Injury may result from dystocia caused by fetal macrosomia, multifetal gestation, abnormal or difficult presentation, and congenital anomalies. Intrapartum events that can result in scalp injury include the use of intrapartum monitoring of the fetal heart rate and fetal scalp blood sampling. Obstetric birth techniques can also cause injury. These include forceps birth, vacuum extraction, external version and extraction, and cesarean birth (see Skeletal Injuries, and Peripheral Nervous System Injuries, Chapter 28). Caput succedaneum and cephalhematoma are described in Chapter 24 (see Fig. 24-3).

Soft-Tissue Injuries

Subconjunctival and retinal hemorrhages result from rupture of capillaries caused by increased pressure during birth. The hemorrhages clear within 5 days after birth and usually present no further problems. Parents need explanation and reassurance that these injuries are harmless.

Erythema, ecchymoses, petechiae, abrasions, lacerations, or edema of buttocks and extremities may be present. Localized discoloration may appear over presenting parts and may result from application of forceps or the vacuum extractor. Ecchymoses and edema may appear anywhere on the body. Petechiae, or pinpoint hemorrhagic areas, acquired during birth may extend over the upper trunk and face. These lesions are benign if they disappear within 2 or 3 days of birth and no new lesions appear. Ecchymoses and petechiae may be signs of a more serious disorder, such as thrombocytopenic purpura. To differentiate hemorrhagic areas from a skin rash or discoloration, apply pressure to the skin with two fingers. Petechiae and ecchymoses do not blanch because extravasated blood remains within the tissues, whereas skin rashes and discolorations do blanch.

Trauma secondary to dystocia occurs to the presenting fetal part. Forceps injury and bruising from the vacuum cup occur at the site of application of the instruments. In a forceps injury there is commonly a linear mark across both sides of the face that is in the shape of the blades of the forceps. The affected areas are kept clean to minimize risk of infection. These injuries usually resolve spontaneously within several days with no specific therapy. With the increased use of the vacuum extractor and use of padded forceps blades, the incidence of these lesions may be significantly reduced.

Bruises over the face may be the result of face presentation (Fig. 25-5). In a breech presentation, bruising and swelling may be seen over the buttocks or genitalia (Fig. 25-6). The skin

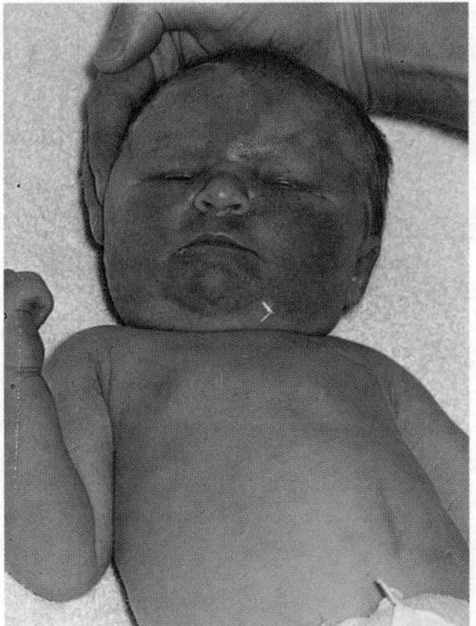

Fig. 25-5 Marked bruising on the entire face of an infant born vaginally after face presentation. Less severe ecchymoses were present on the extremities. Phototherapy was required for treatment of jaundice resulting from the breakdown of accumulated blood. (From O'Doherty N: *Neonatology: micro atlas of the newborn*, Nutley, NJ, 1986, Hoffmann–La Roche.)

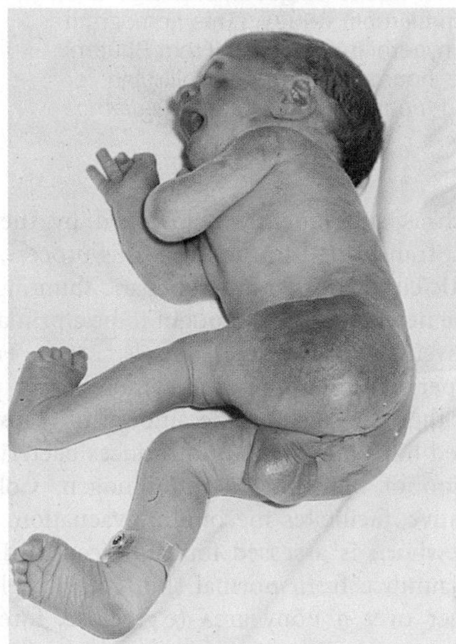

Fig. 25-6 Swelling of genitalia and bruising of the buttocks after a breech birth. (From O'Doherty N: *Neonatology: micro atlas of the newborn*, Nutley, NJ, 1986, Hoffmann–La Roche.)

over the entire head may be ecchymotic and covered with petechiae caused by a tight nuchal cord.

Accidental lacerations may be inflicted with a scalpel during cesarean birth. These cuts may occur on any part of the body but are most often found on the scalp, buttocks, and thighs. Usually they are superficial and only need to be kept clean. Butterfly adhesive strips will hold together the edges of more serious lacerations. Rarely sutures are needed.

Physiologic Problems

Conjugation of Bilirubin

Bilirubin is one of the products derived from the hemoglobin released with the breakdown of red blood cells (RBCs) and the myoglobin in muscle cells. The hemoglobin is broken down by the reticuloendothelial cells, converted to bilirubin, and released in an unconjugated form. Unconjugated (indirect) bilirubin is relatively insoluble and almost entirely bound to circulating albumin, a plasma protein. The unbound bilirubin can leave the vascular system and permeate other extravascular tissues (e.g., skin, sclera, and oral mucous membranes). The resulting yellow coloring is termed *jaundice.*

In the liver the unbound bilirubin is conjugated with glucuronide in the presence of the enzyme glucuronyl transferase. The conjugated form of bilirubin (direct bilirubin) is soluble and is excreted from liver cells as a constituent of bile. Along with other components of bile, direct bilirubin is excreted into the biliary tract system that carries the bile into the duodenum. Bilirubin is converted to urobilinogen and stercobilinogen within the duodenum through the action of the bacterial flora. Urobilinogen is excreted in urine and feces; stercobilinogen is excreted in the feces (see Fig. 24-2). The total serum bilirubin level is the sum of the levels of both conjugated and unconjugated bilirubin.

Physiologic Jaundice

evolve Critical Thinking Exercise—Jaundice

Approximately 50% to 60% of all full-term newborns are visibly jaundiced (yellow) by the second through fifth day of life. Serum bilirubin levels less than 5 mg/dl usually are not reflected in visible skin jaundice. Although the neonate has the functional capacity to convert bilirubin, physiologic hyperbilirubinemia commonly occurs in infants. Physiologic jaundice or neonatal hyperbilirubinemia occurs in 80% of preterm newborns. The incidence of physiologic jaundice is increased in Asian, Native-American, and Alaska Native infants. Although neonatal jaundice is considered benign, bilirubin may accumulate to hazardous levels and lead to a pathologic condition. Neonatal jaundice occurs because the newborn has a higher rate of bilirubin production than does an adult and the reabsorption of bilirubin from the neonatal small intestine is considerable.

Two phases of physiologic jaundice have been identified in full-term infants. In the first phase, bilirubin levels of formula-fed Caucasian and African-American infants gradually increase to approximately 5 to 6 mg/dl by 60 to 72 hours of life, then decrease to a plateau of 2 to 3 mg/dl by the fifth day (Blackburn, 2007). In Asian and Asian-American infants, levels reach a peak of 10 to 14 mg/dl around the third to fifth day of life; the levels gradually fall to 2 to 3 mg/dl by the seventh to tenth day. Bilirubin levels maintain a steady plateau state in the second phase without increasing or decreasing until approximately 12 to 14 days, at which time levels decrease to the normal value of 1 mg/dl (Blackburn, 2007). This pattern varies according to racial group, method of feeding (breast vs. bottle), and gestational age. In preterm formula-fed infants, serum bilirubin levels may peak as high as 10 to 12 mg/dl at 5 to 6 days of life and decrease slowly over a period of 2 to 4 weeks.

Some characteristics of physiologic jaundice include the following:

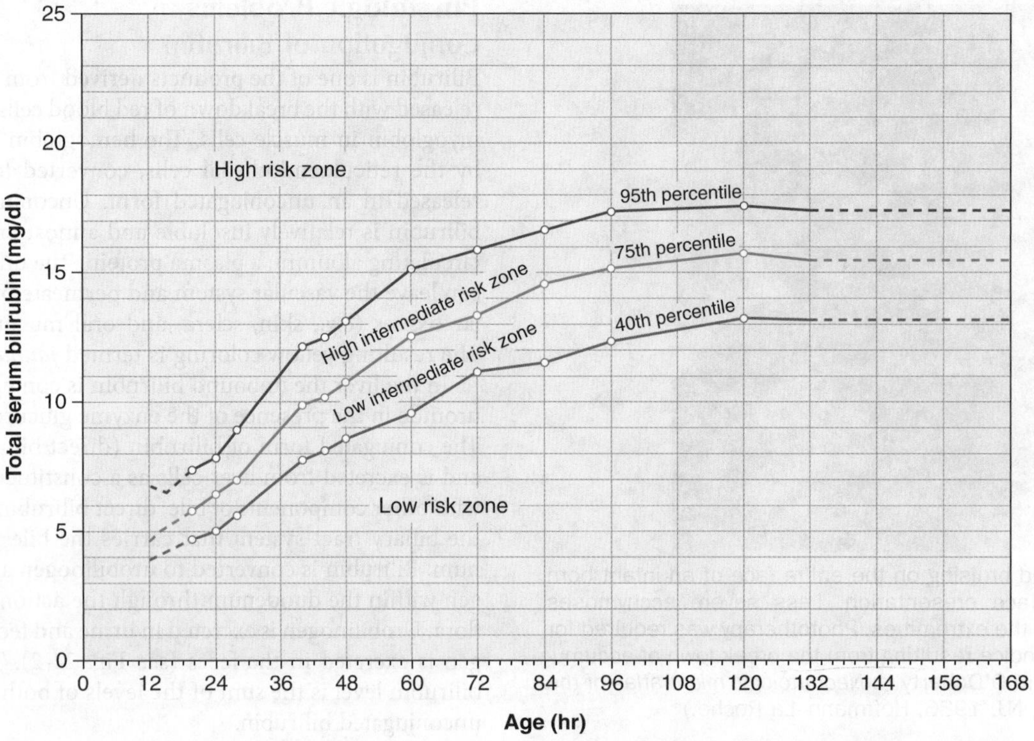

Fig. 25-7 Nomogram for designation of risk in 2840 well newborns at 36 or more weeks of gestational age with birth weight of 2000 g or more, or 35 or more weeks of gestational age and birth weight of 2500 g or more, based on the hour-specific serum bilirubin values. (This nomogram should not be used to represent the natural history of neonatal hyperbilirubinemia.) (From Bhutani VK, Johnson L, Sivieri EM: Predictive ability of a predischarge hour-specific serum bilirubin for subsequent significant hyperbilirubinemia in healthy term and near-term newborns, *Pediatrics* 103(1):6-14, 1999.)

- The infant is otherwise well in relation to cardiorespiratory status, neurologic status, carbohydrate metabolism, feeding pattern, and elimination.
- In term infants, jaundice first appears *after* 24 hours and disappears by the end of the seventh day.
- In preterm infants, jaundice is first evident after 48 hours and disappears by the ninth or tenth day.
- The infant's predischarge total serum bilirubin falls below the high risk category (below 95th percentile) on the hour-specific nomogram (Fig. 25-7).
- The serum concentration of unconjugated bilirubin usually does not exceed 12 mg/dl in term infants and 15 mg/dl in preterm infants.
- Direct bilirubin does not exceed 1 to 1.5 mg/dl.
- Indirect or unconjugated bilirubin concentration does not increase by more than 5 mg/dl/day.

See Table 25-2 for the varying causes of neonatal indirect hyperbilirubinemia.

NURSING ALERT The appearance of jaundice during the first 24 hours of life or persistence beyond the ages previously delineated usually indicates a potential pathologic process that requires further investigation.

In the newborn intestine the enzyme β-glucuronidase is able to convert conjugated bilirubin into the unconjugated form, which is subsequently reabsorbed by the intestinal mucosa and transported to the liver. This process, known as enterohepatic circulation or enterohepatic shunting, is accentuated in the newborn and is thought to be a primary mechanism in physiologic jaundice (Maisels, 2005). Feeding (1) stimulates peristalsis and produces more rapid passage of meconium, thus diminishing the amount of reabsorption of unconjugated bilirubin; and (2) introduces bacteria to aid in the reduction of bilirubin to urobilinogen. Colostrum, a natural laxative, facilitates meconium evacuation.

Every newborn is assessed for jaundice. To differentiate cutaneous jaundice from normal skin color, apply pressure with a finger over a bony area (e.g., nose, forehead, and sternum) for several seconds to empty all the capillaries in that spot. If jaundice is present, the blanched area will look yellow before the capillaries refill. The conjunctiva and buccal mucosa are also assessed, especially in darker-skinned infants. It is better to assess for jaundice in natural light because artificial lighting and the reflection from nursery walls can distort the actual skin color. Visual assessment of jaundice does not, however, provide an accurate assessment of the level of serum bilirubin.

Jaundice is generally first noticed in the head, especially the sclera and mucous membranes, and then progresses gradually to the thorax, abdomen, and extremities. The most common therapy used to treat a high serum bilirubin level or a rapidly increasing level is phototherapy. The degree of jaundice is

Table 25-2 Causes of Neonatal Indirect Hyperbilirubinemia

BASIS	CAUSES
Increased Production of Bilirubin	
Increased hemoglobin destruction	Fetomaternal blood group incompatibility (Rh, ABO) Congenital red blood cell abnormalities Congenital enzyme deficiencies (G6PD, galactosemia) Sepsis Enclosed hemorrhage (cephalhematoma, bruising)
Increased amount of hemoglobin	Polycythemia (maternal-fetal or twin-twin transfusion, SGA) Delayed cord clamping
Increased enterohepatic circulation	Delayed passage of meconium, meconium ileus, or plug Fasting or delayed initiation of feeding Intestinal atresia or stenosis
Altered Hepatic Clearance of Bilirubin	
Alteration in uridine diphosphoglucuronyl transferase production or activity	Immaturity Metabolic or endocrine disorders (e.g., Criglar-Najjar syndrome, hypothyroidism, disorders of amino acid metabolism)
Alteration in hepatic function and perfusion (and thus conjugating ability)	Sepsis (also causes inflammation) Asphyxia, hypoxia, hypothermia, hypoglycemia Drugs and hormones (e.g., novobiocin, pregnanediol)
Hepatic obstruction (associated with direct hyperbilirubinemia)	Congenital anomalies (biliary atresia, cystic fibrosis) Biliary stasis (hepatitis, sepsis) Excessive bilirubin load (often seen with severe hemolysis)

From Blackburn ST: *Maternal, fetal, and neonatal physiology: a clinical perspective*, ed 3, St Louis, 2007, Saunders.
G6PD, Glucose-6-phosphate dehydrogenase; *SGA*, small for gestational age.

determined by serum bilirubin measurements. Normal values of unconjugated bilirubin are 0.2 to 1.4 mg/dl.

It is important to note that the evaluation of jaundice is not based solely on serum bilirubin and transcutaneous bilirubin levels, but also on the timing of the appearance of clinical jaundice; gestational age at birth; age in hours since birth; family history, including maternal Rh factor; evidence of hemolysis; feeding method; infant's physiologic status; and the progression of serial serum bilirubin levels.

Pathologic jaundice is that level of serum bilirubin which, if left untreated, can result in sensorineural hearing loss; mild cognitive delays; and kernicterus, which is the deposition of bilirubin in the brain. With ever-changing medical terminology in the literature, there is less emphasis on pathologic jaundice more by omission than anything else. Nonetheless, one might consider any newborn jaundice as being physiologic (see preceding discussion) unless proven otherwise, in which case the condition may be considered pathologic.

Kernicterus describes the yellow staining of the brain cells that may result in bilirubin encephalopathy. The damage occurs when the serum concentration reaches toxic levels, regardless of cause. There is evidence that a fraction of unconjugated bilirubin crosses the blood-brain barrier in neonates with physiologic hyperbilirubinemia. When certain pathologic conditions exist in addition to elevated bilirubin levels, the blood-brain barrier has increased permeability to unconjugated bilirubin, creating the potential for irreversible damage. The exact level of serum bilirubin required to cause damage is not known. The signs of bilirubin encephalopathy are those of central nervous system depression or excitation. Prodromal symptoms consist of decreased activity, lethargy, irritability, hypotonia, and seizures. Those who survive may eventually show evidence of neurologic damage, such as cognitive impairment, cerebral palsy, attention-deficit/hyperactivity disorder, delayed or abnormal motor movement (especially ataxia or athetosis), behavior disorders, perceptual problems, or sensorineural hearing loss.

Noninvasive monitoring of bilirubin via cutaneous reflectance measurements (transcutaneous bilirubinometry [TcB]) allows for repetitive estimations of bilirubin. These devices work well on dark- and light-skinned infants and demonstrate linear correlation with serum determinations of bilirubin levels in full-term infants. TcB monitors may be used to screen clinically significant jaundice and decrease the need for serum bilirubin measurements (Ip et al, 2004). With shorter maternity stays, the value of transcutaneous bilirubin measurements as an assessment tool in follow-up home care has been demonstrated in a homogeneous population. However, because transcutaneous bilirubin measurements are affected by race, gestational age, and birth weight, their use in heterogeneous populations remains limited for diagnostic purposes (Engle et al, 2002). In addition, the intensity of jaundice is not always related to the degree of hyperbilirubinemia. The new TcB monitors provide accurate measurements within 2 to 3 mg/dl in most neonatal populations at serum levels below 15 mg/dl (American Academy of Pediatrics, Subcommittee on Hyperbilirubinemia, 2004). After phototherapy has been initiated, TcB is no longer useful as a screening tool.

The use of hour-specific serum bilirubin levels to predict term newborns at risk for rapidly rising levels has now become an official recommendation by the American Academy of Pediatrics, Subcommittee on Hyperbilirubinemia (2004), for monitoring healthy neonates at 35 weeks of gestation or greater before discharge from the hospital. Using a nomogram (see Fig. 25-7) with three levels (high, intermediate, or low risk) of rising total serum bilirubin values assists in the determination of which newborns might need further evaluation after discharge. Universal bilirubin screening based on hour-specific total serum bilirubin may be done at the same time as the routine newborn profile (phenylketonuria [PKU], galactosemia, and others) (American Academy of Pediatrics, Subcommittee on Hyperbilirubinemia, 2004; Bhutani, Johnson, & Sivieri, 1999). The hour-specific bilirubin risk nomogram is used to determine the infant's risk for development of hyperbilirubinemia requiring medical treatment or closer screening. Subsequent studies have demonstrated the accuracy of the nomogram in predicting infants with rapidly rising bilirubin levels requiring evaluation or treatment (Keren et al, 2008). Risk factors recognized to place infants in the high risk category include gestational age less than 38 weeks, breastfeeding, a sibling who had significant jaundice, and jaundice appearing before discharge (American Academy of Pediatrics, Subcommittee on Hyperbilirubinemia, 2004). It is recommended that healthy infants (35 weeks or greater) receive follow-up care and assessment of bilirubin within 3 days of discharge if discharged at less than 24 hours and a risk assessment with tools such as the hour-specific nomogram; likewise, newborns discharged at 24 to 47.9 hours should receive follow-up evaluation within 4 days (96 hours), and those discharged between 48 and 72 hours should receive follow-up within 5 days (American Academy of Pediatrics, Subcommittee on Hyperbilirubinemia, 2004). The guidelines for monitoring and treating neonatal hyperbilirubinemia are published extensively elsewhere (see Resources on this book's website). (See Community Focus box.)

COMMUNITY FOCUS

Neonatal Jaundice

Prepare a poster presentation for community health care workers that addresses the American Academy of Pediatrics, Subcommittee on Hyperbilirubinemia (2004), guidelines for monitoring jaundiced newborns in the first week of life according to the hour-specific risk nomogram. In the poster address the issue of monitoring breastfeeding progress and elimination in relation to neonatal jaundice.

One technology that is being investigated for noninvasive bilirubin monitoring includes measuring carbon monoxide indices (ETCOc) in exhaled breath (carbon monoxide is produced when RBCs are broken down; thus the extent of hemolysis may be appreciated). This technology is currently not being used significantly in the clinical setting because of its expense and lack of predictability in determining neonatal hemolysis (Mincey & Gonzaba, 2007).

Jaundice Associated with Breastfeeding

Breastfeeding is associated with an increased incidence of jaundice. Two types have been identified; however, nomenclature may vary among experts. In addition, these types may overlap and may not be easily differentiated from each other (Blackburn, 2007). Breastfeeding-associated jaundice (early-onset jaundice) begins at 2 to 4 days of age and occurs in approximately 10% to 25% of breastfed newborns. The jaundice is related to the process of breastfeeding and probably results from decreased caloric and fluid intake by breastfed infants before the milk supply is well established, since fasting is associated with decreased hepatic clearance of bilirubin (Blackburn, 2007; Porter & Dennis, 2002). The presence of decreased caloric intake (less milk), weight loss of more than 5% to 7% in the first 5 days of life, increasing serum bilirubin (unconjugated) levels, decreased stooling, and increased jaundice is also sometimes referred to as *starvation jaundice* or *nonbreastfeeding jaundice.* To prevent this pattern, the following measures are suggested: initiation of breastfeeding within the first few hours of life, continuous rooming-in with the mother, breastfeeding 10 to 12 times per day, no supplements, and recognition of and response to hunger cues (Gartner & Herschel, 2001). This set of newborns is at greater risk for developing high bilirubin levels in the first week of life and must be closely monitored.

Breast milk jaundice (late-onset jaundice) may initially begin as the early-onset variety or may begin at age 4 to 6 days and occurs in 2% to 3% of breastfed infants. Rising levels of bilirubin peak during the second week and gradually diminish. Despite high levels of bilirubin that may persist for 3 to 12 weeks, these infants are well and have no signs of hemolysis or liver dysfunction. The jaundice may be caused by factors in the breast milk (pregnanediol, fatty acids, and β-glucuronidase) that either inhibit the conjugation or decrease the excretion of bilirubin. Less frequent stooling by breastfed infants may allow extended time for reabsorption of bilirubin from stools (Blackburn, 2007) (see Chapter 26 for a discussion of these conditions in relation to nutrition).

Hypoglycemia

Hypoglycemia during the early newborn period of a term infant is often defined as a blood glucose concentration less than adequate to support adequate neurologic, organ, and tissue function; however, the precise level at which this occurs in every neonate is not known. At birth the maternal source of glucose is cut off with the clamping of the umbilical cord. Most healthy term newborns experience a transient decrease in glucose levels, with a subsequent mobilization of free fatty acids and ketones to help maintain adequate glucose levels (Blackburn, 2007). Insulin does not cross the placental barrier, thus predisposing some infants to low glucose levels as a result of increased insulin activity. Infants who are asphyxiated or have other physiologic stress may experience hypoglycemia as a result of a decreased glycogen supply, inadequate gluconeogenesis, or overutilization of glycogen stored during fetal life.

Cornblath and colleagues (2000) have suggested an operational threshold at which interventions to increase serum glucose levels should be instituted to prevent serious effects. For the healthy full-term infant, born after an uneventful pregnancy and delivery, recommendations are to monitor glucose levels only in the presence of risk factors (see following) or clinical manifestations of hypoglycemia; in these infants a plasma glucose of less than 45 mg/dl (2.5 mmol/L) requires intervention. Healthy full-term, breastfed newborns may not fit into this category because human milk appears to provide adequate substrate (Cornblath et al, 2000). Hoseth and colleagues (2000) evaluated blood glucose levels in healthy full-term, breastfed infants and found significant hypoglycemia in only two of the 223 infants during the first 4 days of life.

In infants who are at risk for altered metabolism as a result of maternal illness factors (diabetes, gestational hypertension, terbutaline administration) or newborn factors (perinatal hypoxia, infection, hypothermia, polycythemia, congenital malformations, hyperinsulinism, SGA, fetal hydrops), close observation and monitoring of blood glucose levels within 2 to 3 hours of birth are recommended. If the newborn has a blood glucose level below 36 mg/dl (2.0 mmol/L), intervention such as breastfeeding or bottle-feeding should be instituted. If levels remain low despite feeding, intravenous dextrose is warranted. In such infants the treatment should be aimed at maintaining the blood glucose levels above 45 mg/dl (2.5 mmol/L) (Cornblath et al, 2000). Blood glucose levels for infants with severe hyperinsulinism may need to be higher (60 mg/dl [3.3 mmol/L]) to prevent serious effects. Hypoglycemia in preterm infants requires further study, but it has been suggested that values be maintained above 47 mg/dl (2.6 mmol/L) (Cornblath et al, 2000).

Researchers further recommend that emphasis be placed less on an absolute glucose value and more on promoting normoglycemia with interventions for less optimal values (Blackburn, 2007). Monitoring blood glucose in the asymptomatic healthy term neonate (not at risk) on a routine basis is not recommended (Cornblath et al, 2000).

Signs of hypoglycemia include jitteriness; irregular respiratory effort; cyanosis; apnea; weak, high-pitched cry; feeding difficulty; lethargy; twitching; eye rolling; and seizures. The signs may be transient but recurrent.

Hypoglycemia in the low-risk term infant is usually eliminated by feeding the infant a source of carbohydrate (i.e., human milk or formula). Occasionally the intravenous administration of glucose is required for infants with persistently high insulin levels or in those with depleted stores of glycogen.

Hypocalcemia

Hypocalcemia in infants is defined as serum calcium levels less than 7.8 to 8 mg/dl in term infant, and slightly lower (7 mg/dl) in the preterm infant; ideally, ionized fraction levels reflect the biologically active form and levels range from 3 to 4.4 mg/dl depending on the measurement method (Blackburn, 2007). Hypocalcemia may occur in newborns of diabetic mothers, in those who experienced perinatal asphyxia or trauma, and in preterm infants. Early-onset hypocalcemia usually occurs within the first 24 to 48 hours after birth. Signs of hypocalcemia include jitteriness, tremors, twitching, high-pitched cry, irritability, apnea, and laryngospasm, although some infants may be asymptomatic (Blackburn, 2007).

Treatment for the condition includes early feeding of an appropriate sources of calcium such as fortified human milk or a preterm infant formula. In some cases (e.g., the medically unstable, extremely-low-birth-weight infant) the administration of intravenous elemental calcium and phosphorus may be necessary.

Because jitteriness is a symptom of both hypoglycemia and hypocalcemia, the latter must be considered if therapy for hypoglycemia is ineffective.

Laboratory and Diagnostic Tests

Because newborns experience many transitional events in the first 28 days of life, laboratory samples are often gathered to determine adequate physiologic adaptation and to identify disorders that may adversely affect the child's life beyond the neonatal period. Most laboratory tests for newborn screening may be obtained from the neonate with a heel puncture. Tests that may be performed include bilirubin levels, blood glucose, newborn screening tests (e.g., PKU, hypothyroidism [T4], sickle cell disease, and galactosemia), and drug serum levels. Box 25-4 lists standard laboratory values in a term newborn.

Tandem mass spectrometry has the potential for identifying as many as 40 inborn errors of metabolism (IEMs). With tandem mass spectrometry, earlier identification of IEMs may prevent further developmental delays and morbidities in affected children (MMWR Weekly, 2008; Schultze et al, 2003).

All states have programs for newborn screening, but such programs vary by state. With the increased mobility of the population, newborns at high risk for certain metabolic diseases may not be appropriately screened. It is therefore important that families be educated regarding the availability of metabolic tests routinely performed in their state of residence. Information about which tests are required in a state can be obtained from state health departments (see Resources on this book's website). Some of the major disorders for which infants are screened are described in Table 25-3.

Collection of Specimens

Ongoing evaluation and screening of the newborn often require obtaining blood by heel stick or venipuncture.

BOX 25-4 Standard Laboratory Values in a Term Newborn*

Hemoglobin	14-24 g/dl
Hematocrit	44%-64%
Glucose	45-65 mg/dl
Leukocytes (white blood cells)	9000-30,000/mm^3
Bilirubin, total serum	<2.0 mg/dl
Blood gases	
Arterial	pH 7.32-7.48
	P_{CO_2} 26-42 mm Hg
	P_{O_2} 60-70 mm Hg
Base excess	−10 to −2 mEq/L (whole blood)
Bicarbonate, serum	21-28 mmol/L(arterial)
Anion gap	7-16 mEq/L
Venous	pH 7.31-7.41
	P_{CO_2} 40-50 mm Hg
	P_{O_2} 40-50 mm Hg

*These values may change significantly in the first week of life.

Table 25-3 Newborn Screening Summary

DISORDER AND EVIDENCE	SYMPTOMS	SCREENING INCIDENCE	TREATMENT
PKU (classic) Elevated phenylalanine plasma concentrations (20 mg/dl)	Severe cognitive impairment if early detection and treatment not started, eczema, seizures, behavior disorders, decreased pigmentation, distinctive musty or mouselike odor	1:13,500 to 1:20,000 More common in Caucasians and Native Americans	Lifelong dietary management with low-phenylalanine diet; possible tyrosine supplementation
Congenital hypothyroidism (primary) Low T_4, elevated TSH	Asymptomatic at birth; mental and motor delays (although neonatal detection and treatment has decreased incidence of cognitive impairment); short stature; coarse, dry skin and hair; hoarse cry; constipation	1:3600 to 1:5000 live births with some ethnic variation 1:32,000 African-American 1:2000 Hispanic and Native American	Maintain L-thyroxine levels in upper half of normal range; periodic bone age testing to monitor growth
Galactosemia (transferase deficiency) Elevated galactose; low or absent fluorescence	Hypotonia, lethargy, vomiting, diarrhea, metabolic acidosis, *Escherichia coli* sepsis, liver dysfunction, cognitive impairment, jaundice, blindness, cataracts, long-term behavioral problems, neurologic impairment	1:60,000 to 1:250,000	Eliminate galactose and lactose from the diet; soy formulas in infancy; lactose-free solid foods
Maple syrup urine disease Elevated leucine	Poor feeding; lethargy; hypotonia; vomiting; ketoacidosis; seizures; sweet maple syrup odor in urine, cerumen, or sweat	1:90,000 to 1:100,000 Higher in certain Mennonite (Older Order) populations: 1:176 to 1:358	Branched-chain amino acid–free formula with added protein-based formula; thiamine supplement in some individuals; lifelong treatment and monitoring necessary
Homocystinuria Elevated methionine and homocysteine	Infancy: nonspecific growth failure; developmental delay; more commonly diagnosed around 3 yr Cognitive impairment, seizures, behavioral disorders, early-onset thromboses, dislocated lenses, tall lanky body habitus	1:150,000 to 1:200,000; more prevalent in Ireland and New South Wales, Australia (1:60,000)	Methionine-restricted diet; cysteine supplement; vitamin B_6 supplement if responsive
Congenital adrenal hyperplasia Elevated 17-hydroxyprogesterone; abnormal electrolytes	Hyponatremia, hyperkalemia, hypoglycemia, dehydration; weight loss; hypotension; shock in "salt wasting" type; female virilization; progressive virilization in both sexes	1:10,000 to 1:20,000 Higher in Native Eskimos: 1:300	Reduce excessive corticotropins; replace glucocorticoids and mineralocorticoids; corrective surgery for ambiguous genitalia (intersex assignment is controversial)
Sickle cell/hemoglobin SC (thalassemias)	Repeated infections, growth failure, pallor, hemolytic anemia; sickle cell crisis	Sickle cell anemia: 1:2647 in non–African-Americans; 1:375 in African-Americans; 1:36,000 in Hispanics	Preventive care: treatment of meningococcal and pneumococcal infections; hydroxyurea (antisickling agent); prevent human parvovirus B19 infection (limits production of reticulocytes)
Biotinidase deficiency Deficient or absent activity of biotinidase on colorimetric assay	Myoclonic seizures, hypotonia, feeding difficulties, organic aciduria, fungal infections, ataxia, skin rash, hearing loss, alopecia, optic nerve atrophy, developmental delay, coma, and death	1:60,000 to 1:137,000	5-20 mg biotin daily; less with partial deficiency

Data from Lashley FR: Newborn screening: new opportunities and new challenges, *Newborn Infant Nurs Rev* 2(4):228-242, 2002; DeBaun MR, Vichinsky E: Hemoglobinopathies. In Kliegman RM et al (editors): *Nelson textbook of pediatrics*, ed 18, Philadelphia, 2007, Saunders; Rezvani I: Metabolic diseases. In Kliegman RM et al (editors): *Nelson textbook of pediatrics*, ed 18, Philadelphia, 2007, Saunders; LaFranchini S: Disorders of the thyroid gland. In Kliegman RM et al (editors): *Nelson textbook of pediatrics*, ed 18, Philadelphia, 2007, Saunders.

PKU, Phenylketonuria; *TSH,* thyroid-stimulating hormone.

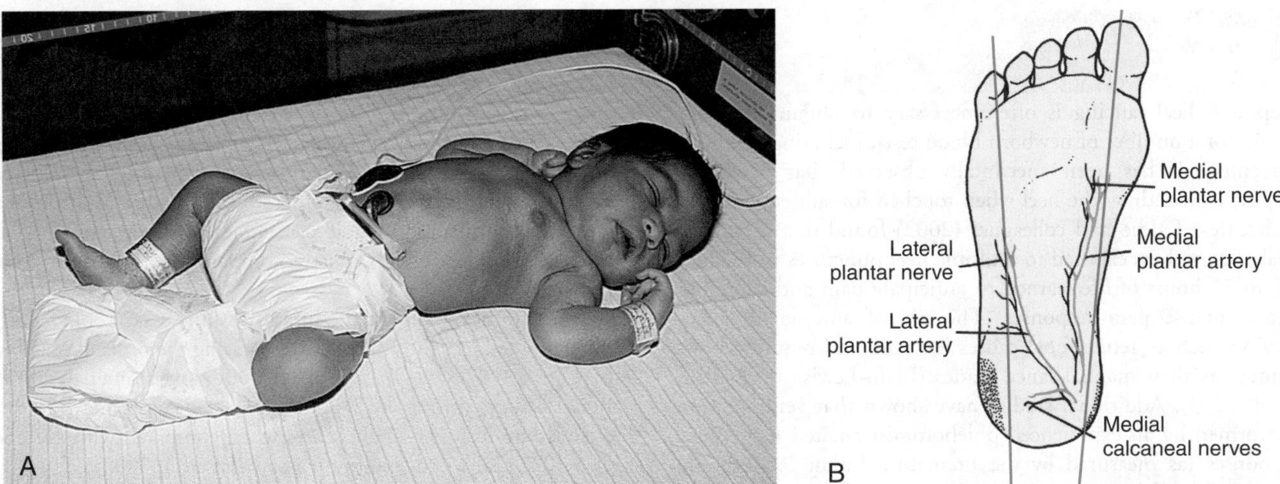

Fig. 25-8 Heel stick. **A**,Newborn with foot wrapped for warmth to increase blood flow to extremity before heel stick. **B**, Heel stick sites *(shaded areas)* on infant's foot for obtaining samples of capillary blood. *(A, Courtesy Marjorie Pyle, RNC, Lifecircle, Costa Mesa, CA.)*

Heel Stick

Most blood specimens are drawn by laboratory technicians. However, nurses may be required to perform heel sticks to obtain blood for glucose monitoring or newborn screening. The same technique is needed to complete the metabolic screening form on Guthrie paper or to test for galactosemia and hypothyroidism or other IEMs (see Table 25-3).

It is often helpful to warm the heel before the sample is taken; application of heat for 5 to 10 minutes helps dilate the blood vessels in the area. A cloth soaked with warm water and wrapped loosely around the foot provides effective warming (Fig. 25-8, *A*). Disposable heel warmers are available from a variety of companies; they should be used with care to prevent burns. Nurses should wear gloves when collecting any specimen. The nurse cleanses the area with an appropriate skin antiseptic, restrains the infant's foot with a free hand, and then punctures the site. A spring-loaded automatic puncture device causes less pain and requires fewer punctures than a manual lance blade; therefore manual lance blades should not be used on neonates. It is important to fill all of the circles on the metabolic screening form with blood.

The most serious complication of infant heel stick is necrotizing osteochondritis from lancet penetration of the bone (Meehan, 1998). To prevent this, the penetration should be made at the outer aspect of the heel and should be no deeper than 2.4 mm. To identify the appropriate puncture site, the nurse should draw an imaginary line running from between the fourth and fifth toes and parallel to the lateral aspect of the foot to the heel where the stick should be made; a second line can also be drawn from the great toe to the medial aspect of the heel (see Fig. 25-8, *B*). Repeated trauma to the walking surface of the heel can cause fibrosis and scarring that may lead to problems with walking later in life. After the specimen has been collected, pressure is applied with a dry gauze square. No further skin cleanser should be applied because this will cause the site to continue to bleed. The site is then covered with an adhesive bandage. The nurse ensures proper disposal of equipment used, reviews the laboratory requisition for correct identification, and checks the specimen for adequate labeling and routing.

A heel stick is traumatic for the infant and causes pain. After several heel sticks, infants have been observed to withdraw their feet when they are touched. To reassure the infant and to promote feelings of safety, the neonate should be cuddled and comforted when the procedure is complete, and appropriate pain management measures should be taken to minimize the pain (see Atraumatic Care box).

Venipuncture

Venous blood samples can be drawn from the antecubital, saphenous, superficial wrist, and, rarely, scalp veins. If an existing intravenous site is used to obtain a blood specimen, it is important to consider the type of infusion fluid; contamination of the blood with the fluid can alter results.

When venipuncture is required, positioning of the needle is extremely important. Although regular venipuncture needles may be used, some individuals prefer butterfly needles. A 25-gauge needle is adequate for blood sampling in neonates, with minimal hemolysis being observed when the proper procedure is followed. It is necessary to be patient during the procedure because the blood return from small veins is slow, and consequently the small needle must remain in place longer. A tourniquet is optional but may help increase blood flow with venipuncture. The mummy restraint commonly is used to help secure the infant (see Fig. 45-7).

For blood gas studies, the blood sample container is packed in ice (to reduce blood cell metabolism) and taken immediately to the laboratory for analysis.

Pressure must be maintained over an arterial puncture with a dry gauze square for at least 3 to 5 minutes to prevent bleeding from the site. The nurse should observe the infant frequently for evidence of bleeding or hematoma at the puncture site for at least an hour after any venipuncture. The infant's tolerance of the procedure should be noted and recorded. The infant should be cuddled and comforted (e.g., rocked, given a

ATRAUMATIC CARE

Heel Punctures

Repeated heel lancing is often necessary to obtain sufficient blood for a number of newborn blood tests, including newborn screening. It has been anecdotally observed that newborns appear to withdraw the heel when touched for subsequent heel punctures. Taddio and colleagues (2002) found that infants of diabetic mothers exposed to multiple heel punctures in the first 24 to 36 hours of life learned to anticipate pain and exhibited more intense pain responses. The use of automated lancet devices such as Tenderfoot* causes less pain and requires fewer punctures than manual lance blades (Blain-Lewis, 1992; Paes et al, 1993). Additional studies have shown that venipuncture performed by an experienced phlebotomist elicited fewer pain responses (as measured by the Premature Infant Pain Profile [PIPP]) from full-term newborns than did heel punctures (Shah & Ohlsson, 2001). The need for additional skin punctures was reduced with venipuncture. Although maternal anxiety was initially higher in the venipuncture group, mothers who observed the venipuncture reported observing less pain response than mothers who observed heel punctures.

Oral sucrose and nonnutritive sucking have proved effective in decreasing the pain associated with heel punctures in preterm and full-term infants during the first week of life (Stevens, Yamada, & Ohlsson, 2004; Gibbins et al, 2002; Harrison, Johnston, & Loughnan, 2003); however, the exact dose range that proves effective varies among several studies (Stevens, Yamada, & Ohlsson, 2004). In one study, infants experiencing venipuncture were given either oral sucrose (30%) and a skin placebo or the eutectic mixture of local anesthetic (EMLA). Pain scores were measured with the PIPP, and infants receiving the oral sucrose solution exhibited fewer pain signs than those in the EMLA group (Gradin et al, 2002). Giving newborns 2 ml of oral sucrose solution (25% and 50%) significantly reduced crying time and heart rate after 3 minutes in comparison with controls (sterile water) during heel stick sampling for serum bilirubin concentrations (Haouari et al, 1995). Newborns given 2 ml of concentrated oral sucrose solution showed a significant reduction in crying time and heart rate in comparison with controls (given sterile water) during heel stick sampling and other painful stimuli (Stevens, Yamada, & Ohlsson, 2004).

Evidence indicates that as little as 2 ml of a 24% oral sucrose solution is effective in decreasing pain in full-term and preterm infants. In addition, the best analgesic effect is achieved when sucrose is administered 2 minutes before the painful procedure with a pacifier or syringe. In one study protocol where oral sucrose was effective, 0.5 ml of 24% oral sucrose solution was administered 2 minutes before the heel puncture, during, and 5 minutes after the heel puncture (Gibbins et al, 2002). Eriksson and Finnstrom (2004) found that repeated administration of a 30% sucrose solution before heel lance in healthy full-term infants did not decrease the pain-relieving effect of the glucose solution; the study's aim was to determine whether multiple oral glucose administration would cause tolerance to glucose. Monitoring for adverse effects must accompany each administration (Noerr, 2001).

The mother's holding the infant in skin-to-skin contact significantly reduces the child's distress during the procedure (Blass & Watt, 1999; Gray, Watt, & Blass, 2000; Johnston et al, 2003). Breastfeeding during heel puncture in full-term newborns is effective in decreasing pain scores when compared with placebo or a 30% oral sucrose solution (Carbajal et al, 2003).

Applying the topical anesthetic EMLA to reduce the pain of heel lance has produced mixed results in full-term and preterm infants (Fitzgerald, Millard, & McIntosh, 1989; Taddio et al, 1998; Stevens et al, 1999). Grunau and colleagues (2004) noted that placing preterm infants in a prone (vs. supine) position for heel stick did not decrease the pain response and that additional pain-relieving measures for this population are necessary.

Music was found to decrease the pain response to heel stick in a small group of preterm infants (Butt & Kisilevsky, 2000). A study comparing the effects of swaddling and containment on preterm infants undergoing heel stick failed to demonstrate significant differences between the two interventions (Huang et al, 2004).

These studies provide evidence of a number of effective ways to decrease the pain associated with heel puncture in full-term and preterm newborns. It is essential that nurses use all available resources to advocate for the prevention and management of neonatal pain during such procedures as heel puncture. Because the overall goal is to decrease the effect on infants of painful interventions such as heel stick, a combination of pharmacologic and nonpharmacologic interventions is recommended. (See also Atraumatic Care box, p. 670.)

A number of commercially available oral sucrose solutions now exist, including Ora-Sweet† (54% solution), which can be diluted 1 : 1 to produce a 27% solution; and Sweet-Ease‡ (24% solution). When these are not available, the pharmacy can mix an oral sucrose solution to ensure a clean product. An approximate 25% sucrose solution is made by mixing 1 tsp of granulated (table) sugar with 4 tsp of sterile water; however, this method is the least desirable to prevent contamination of the solution and subsequent problems.

*International Technidyne Corporation, Edison, NJ.
†Paddock Laboratories, Minneapolis.
‡Children's Medical Ventures, Norwell, MA.

pacifier) when the procedure is completed, and appropriate pain management measures should be taken to minimize the pain.

NURSING ALERT Only venous or capillary blood samples may be used for newborn screening and genetic studies; cord blood is not used for such samples.

Obtaining a Urine Specimen

Examination of urine is a valuable laboratory tool for infant assessment, but the way in which the specimen is collected may influence the results. The urine sample should be fresh and examined within 1 hour of collection.

A variety of urine collection bags are available (Fig. 25-9) (see also Fig. 45-10). These are clear plastic, single-use bags

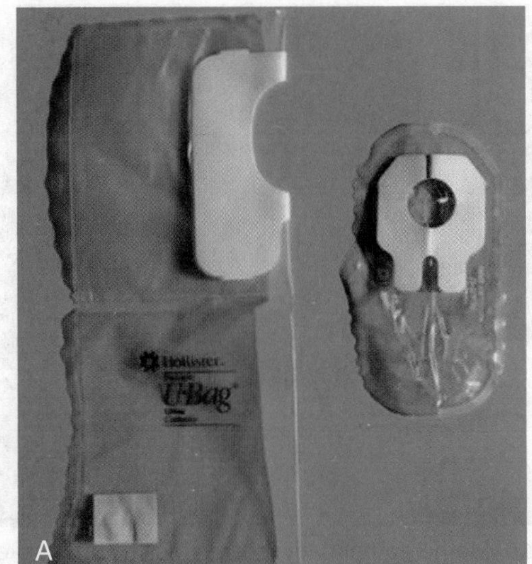

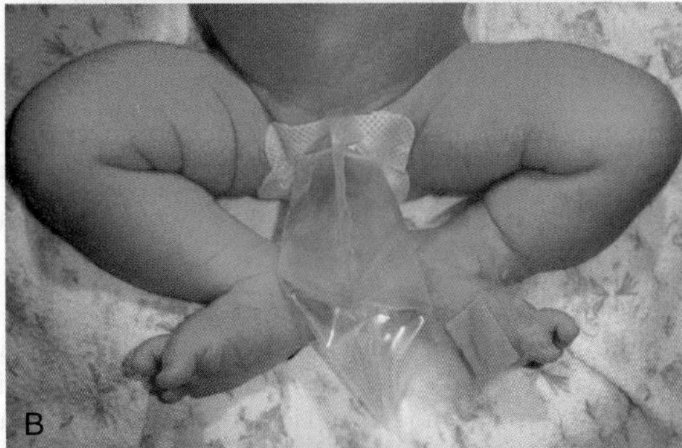

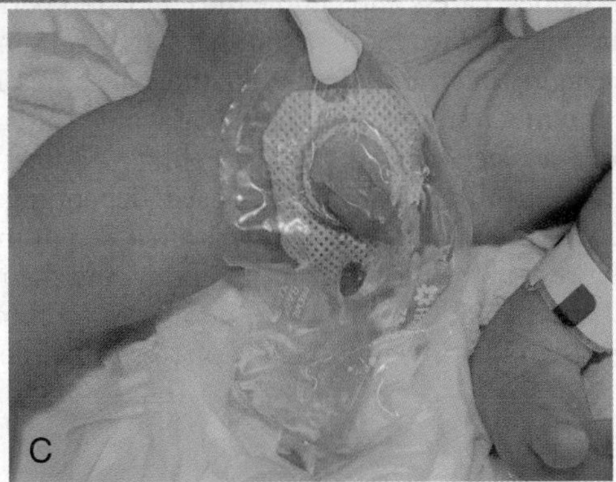

Fig. 25-9 Collection of urine specimen. **A**, Protective paper is removed from the adhesive surface. **B**, Applied to females. **C**, Applied to males. *(Courtesy Cheryl Briggs, RN, Annapolis, MD.)*

with adhesive material around the opening at the point of attachment.

To prepare the infant, the nurse removes the diaper and places the infant in a supine position. The genitalia, perineum, and surrounding skin are washed and thoroughly dried because the adhesive of the bag will not stick to moist, powdered, or oily skin surfaces. The protective paper is removed to expose the adhesive (see Fig. 25-9, *A*). In female infants, the perineum is stretched to flatten skin folds; then the adhesive area is pressed firmly to the skin all around the urinary meatus and vagina. (NOTE: Start with the narrow portion of the butterfly-shaped adhesive patch.) The nurse must be certain to start at the bridge of skin separating the rectum from the vagina and work upward (see Fig. 25-9, *B*). In male infants the penis (and scrotum, depending on the size of the collection device) is tucked through the opening of the collector before the nurse removes the protective paper from the adhesive; then the protective paper is removed, and the flaps are pressed firmly to the perineum, making certain the entire adhesive coating is firmly attached to skin and the edges of the opening do not pucker (see Fig. 25-9, *C*). This helps ensure a leak-proof seal and decreases the chance of contamination from stool. Cutting a slit in the diaper and pulling the bag through the slit may also help prevent leaking.

The diaper is carefully replaced and the bag is checked frequently. When a sufficient amount of urine (this amount varies according to the test done) has been obtained, the bag is removed. The infant's skin is observed for signs of irritation while the bag is in place. The specimen can be aspirated with a syringe or drained directly from the bag.

Collection of a 24-hour specimen from an infant can be a challenge, sometimes requiring need light restraint with elbow restraints. The 24-hour urine bag is applied in the manner just described, and the urine is placed in an appropriate receptacle. The infant's skin is watched closely for signs of irritation and for lack of a proper seal.

For some types of urine testing, urine can be aspirated directly from the diaper by means of a syringe without a needle. If the diaper has absorbent gelling material that traps urine, a small gauze pad or cotton balls are placed inside the diaper and the urine is aspirated from the cotton or gauze.

Implementation

In the inpatient setting, priorities of care must be established and a systematic teaching plan for infant care devised. One way to achieve this is to use critical path case management. A care path may be developed that covers the changes expected in the infant during the first few days of life. With early discharge (usually within 24 to 48 hours of birth), modifications in the care path to individualize newborn care will be necessary. The existing care path may also be used by nursing staff following the care of the mother-newborn dyad at home in the first few weeks of life to ensure that the infant receives appropriate care and screening, which was once provided in the acute care setting. When variations from the care path occur, further assessment and intervention may be necessary.

Protective Environment

The provision of a protective environment is basic to the care of the newborn. The construction, maintenance, and operation of nurseries in accredited hospitals is monitored by national professional organizations, such as the American Academy of Pediatrics, The Joint Commission, Occupational Health and Safety Administration, and local or state governing bodies. In addition, hospital personnel develop their own policies and procedures for protecting the newborns under their care. Prescribed standards cover areas such as environmental factors, measures to control infection, and safety factors.

Environmental Factors

Environmental factors that must be maintained include adequate lighting, elimination of potential fire hazards, safety of electric appliances, adequate ventilation, and controlled temperature (i.e., warm and free of drafts) and humidity (i.e., 40% to 60%) (American Academy of Pediatrics & American College of Obstetricians and Gynecologists, 2007).

Measures to Control Infection

Measures to control infection include adequate floor space to permit positioning bassinets at least 3 feet apart in all directions, handwashing facilities, and areas for cleaning and storing equipment and supplies. Only those personnel directly involved in the care of mothers and infants are allowed in these areas, thereby reducing the opportunities for the introduction of pathogenic organisms.

NURSING ALERT Personnel are instructed to use good handwashing techniques. The most important single measure in the prevention of neonatal infection is handwashing between handling different infants and after contact with potentially contaminated objects (e.g., computer keyboards, telephone, countertops). Inanimate objects should be cleaned with an appropriate bactericidal solution.

Health care workers must wear gloves when handling the infant before blood and amniotic fluid have been removed from the infant's skin; when drawing blood (e.g., heel stick); when caring for a fresh wound (e.g., circumcision); and during diaper changes.

Visitors and health care providers, including nurses, physicians, parents, siblings, and grandparents, are expected to wash their hands before having contact with infants or equipment. Individuals with infectious conditions are excluded from contact with newborns, or must take special precautions when working with infants. This includes persons with upper respiratory tract infections, gastrointestinal tract infections, and infectious skin conditions.

Safety Factors

Health care institutions must be proactive in protecting newborns from abduction. Measures taken include placing matching identification bracelets on newborns and their parents; using identification bands with radiofrequency transmitters that set off an alarm if the bracelet is removed or if a certain threshold is crossed (doorway to exit building or floor); and taking footprints or identification pictures after birth, before the infant leaves the mother's side. In addition, agencies must conduct periodic unit- and hospital-wide drills aimed at preventing newborn abductions. Personnel caring for newborns must be clearly identified by photo identification, and parents must be educated regarding measures to prevent abduction from the mother's room. Parents are also educated before discharge regarding measures to minimize and prevent abduction from the home setting.

evolve Spanish Guidelines—General Advice

Supporting Parents in the Care of Their Infant

The caregiver's sensitivity to the infant's social responses is basic to the development of a mutually satisfying parent-child relationship (Leitch, 1999). Sensitivity increases over time as parents become more aware of their infant's social capabilities.

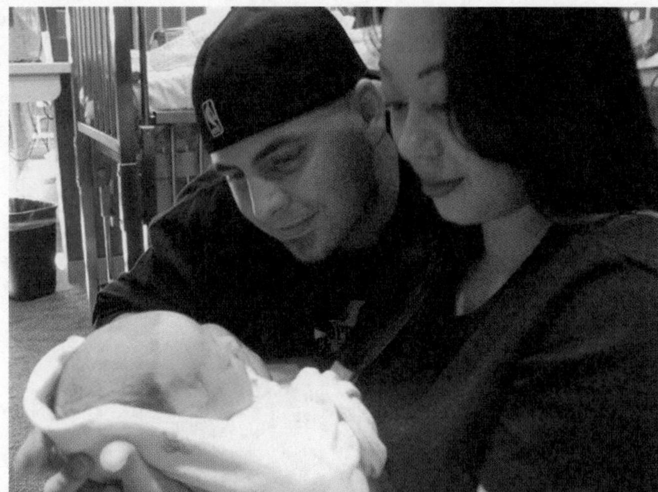

Fig. 25-10 Mother-father-baby interaction. (From Hockenberry MJ, Wilson D: *Wong's nursing care of infants and children*, ed 8, St Louis, 2007, Mosby.)

Social Interactions

The activities of daily care during the neonatal period present the best times for infant and family interactions (see Family-Centered Care box and Cultural Awareness box). While caring for their newborn, the mother and father can talk to the infant, play baby games, caress and cuddle the child, and perhaps use infant massage. In Fig. 25-10, a mother, father, and infant are shown engaging in arousal, imitation of facial expression, and smiling. Too much stimulation should be avoided after feeding and before a sleep period. Older siblings' contact with a newborn is encouraged and supervised depending on the child's developmental level. Parents often keep memento books that record the birth, the hospital stay, and their infant's progress; a personal blog may also be used to communicate with friends and family and to show photos of the newborn.

FAMILY-CENTERED CARE

Family Relationships and Social Support

The family's ethnic and cultural background is important in determining the health status, genetic or familial risk factors, and social support available to the woman throughout pregnancy and in the postpartum period. Family relationships, including husband-wife roles, vary among individuals and groups. The husband may be the decision maker, and his consent may be necessary before the woman agrees to prenatal treatment. Female rather than male family members may be involved in the pregnancy and birth. Mothers and mothers-in-law may be present and supportive during pregnancy, birth, and the early postnatal period to provide advice and care. In such instances, they need to be included in teaching sessions. Community and church support may be available. Assessment of family and community resources is an essential component of care.

CULTURAL AWARENESS

Cultural Beliefs and Practices

Nurses working with childbearing families from other cultures and ethnic groups must be aware of cultural beliefs and practices that are important to individual families. People with a strong sense of heritage may hold on to traditional health beliefs long after adopting other American lifestyle practices. These health beliefs may involve practices regarding the newborn. For example, some Asians, Hispanics, Eastern Europeans, and Native Americans delay breastfeeding because they believe that colostrum is "bad." Some Hispanics and African-Americans place a belly band over the infant's navel. The birth of a male child is generally preferred by Asians and Indians, and some Asians and Haitians delay naming their infant.

Source: D'Avanzo C: *Pocket guide to cultural health assessment,* ed 4, St Louis, 2008, Mosby.

Infant Feeding

The infant may be put to breast ideally within the first hour after birth, or at least within 4 hours of birth. Newborns are placed on demand feeding schedules and are allowed to feed when they awaken and demonstrate typical hunger cues, regardless of the time lapsed from the previous feeding. Ordinarily mothers are encouraged to breastfeed their infants at least every 2 to 3 hours (bottle-feed every 3 to 4 hours, or on demand) during the day and only when the infant awakens during the night in the first few days after birth. However, the newborn should not be allowed to sleep longer than 4 to 5 hours during the night to ensure adequate fluid intake and weight gain. Breastfed babies nurse more often than bottle-fed babies because breast milk is digested faster than formulas made from cow's milk and the stomach empties sooner as a result. Water and dextrose water supplements are not recommended in the newborn period, since these have the tendency to decrease breastfeeding. There is no evidence to support dextrose or water feedings in newborns (see Evidence-Based Practice box). For a thorough discussion of infant feeding, see Chapter 26.

Therapeutic and Surgical Procedures

Intramuscular Injection

As discussed previously, it is routine to administer a single dose of 0.5 to 1 mg of vitamin K intramuscularly (see Medication Guide earlier in this chapter).

Hepatitis B vaccination is recommended for all infants. Infants at highest risk of contracting hepatitis B are those born to women who have hepatitis B or whose hepatitis B status is unknown. If the infant is born to an infected mother or to a mother who is a chronic carrier, hepatitis B vaccine and hepatitis B immune globulin (HBIG) should be given within 12 hours of birth (see Medication Guides). The hepatitis B vaccine is given in one site and the HBIG in another. For infants born to a hepatitis B–negative woman, the first dose of the vaccine may be given at birth or at 1 month of age. Parental consent must be obtained before administering these medications.

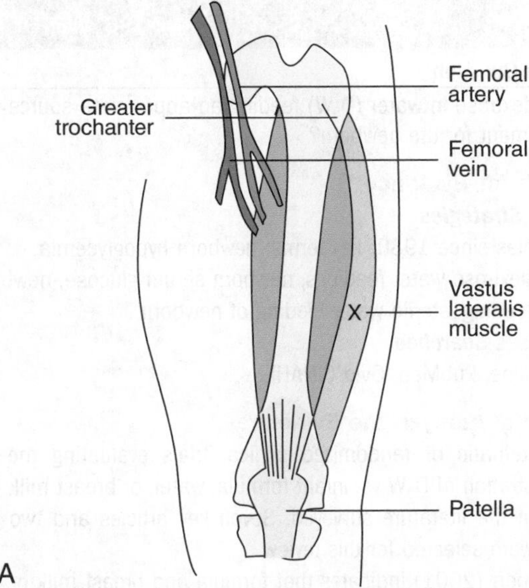

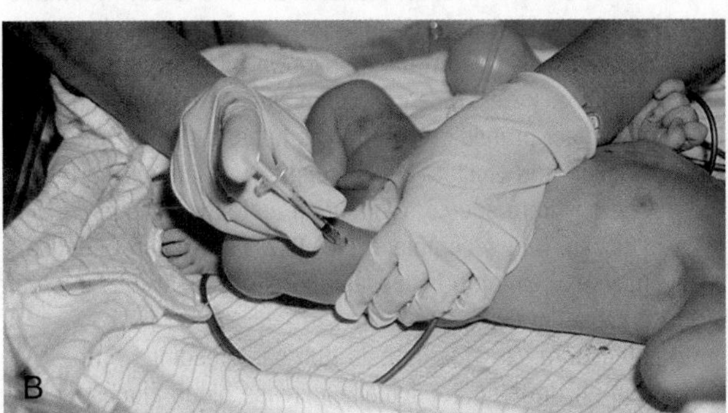

Fig. 25-11 Intramuscular injection. **A,** Acceptable intramuscular injection site *(X)* for newborn infant. **B,** Infant's leg stabilized for intramuscular injection. Nurse is wearing gloves to give injection. *(B, Courtesy Marjorie Pyle, RNC, Lifecircle, Costa Mesa, CA.)*

In most cases a 25-gauge, ⅝-inch (16-mm) to ⅞-inch (22-mm) needle should be used for the vitamin K and hepatitis B vaccine injections. Selection of the site for injection is important. Injections must be given in muscles large enough to accommodate the medication, and major nerves and blood vessels must be avoided. The muscles of newborns may not tolerate more than 0.5 ml per intramuscular injection. The preferred injection site for newborns is the vastus lateralis (Fig. 25-11). The dorsogluteal muscle is very small, poorly developed, and dangerously close to the sciatic nerve, which occupies a larger proportion of space in infants than in older children. Therefore it is not recommended as an injection site in small children. The newborn's deltoid muscle has an inadequate amount of muscle for intramuscular administration. An important factor in preventing and minimizing local reaction to intramuscular injections is adequate deposition of the fluid (medication) deep within the muscle; therefore muscle size, needle length, and amount of medication injected should be carefully considered.

EVIDENCE-BASED PRACTICE Glucose Water Feedings in the Newborn Period —*David Wilson*

Ask the Question

Is 5% dextrose in water (D_5W) feeding an appropriate source of nourishment for the newborn?

Search for Evidence

Search Strategies

Articles since 1980; key terms: newborn hypoglycemia, dextrose water feedings, newborn serum glucose, newborn feeding, sterile water feeding of newborn

Databases Searched

Medline, PubMed, Ovid CINAHL

Critically Analyze the Evidence

No systematic or randomized clinical trials evaluating the oral administration of D_5W vs. infant formula, water, or breast milk were found in the literature surveyed. Seven key articles and two textbooks were selected for this review.

- Noerr (2001) indicates that formula and breast milk or colostrum are ideal for the newborn who is asymptomatic (for hypoglycemia) and able to tolerate oral feedings; the free fatty acids from the breakdown of fat in formula or breast milk decrease peripheral glucose use and decrease the effect of insulin to suppress hepatic glucose production.
- Hashim and Guillet (2002) suggest that infants be fed a carbohydrate source to maintain a steady-state rise in glucose. They recommend that D_5W be avoided because it may lead to rapid increases and subsequent falls in serum glucose levels.
- Blackburn (2007) suggests that early feedings with a carbohydrate source initially increase blood glucose levels; this increase is accompanied by a subsequent increase in plasma insulin levels and the development of cyclic changes in insulin and blood glucose levels in full-term infants. Animal studies suggest that D_5W, if aspirated, is just as dangerous as formula.
- The American Academy of Pediatrics and American College of Obstetricians and Gynecologists (2007) do not recommend routine supplementation with D_5W for infants receiving phototherapy.
- Eidelman (2001) recommends the initiation of breastfeeding within the first 30 to 60 minutes of birth for the healthy term infant and suggests that feedings with water or dextrose water are unnecessary and counterproductive.
- Initial feedings of sterile water or glucose water in newborns were historically recommended by physicians on the premise that the infant's propensity to spit up and possibly aspirate the feeding source into the lungs was less likely to compromise the infant's respiratory status if the aspirate was water (or dextrose water) instead of formula, breast milk, or colostrum. Wakayama, Wilkins, and Kimura (1988) suggested that initial feedings of infant formula after surgical repair for inguinal hernia did not significantly increase the incidence of aspiration.
- Sperling and Menon (2004) indicate that the initiation of milk feedings in the full-term infant induces ketogenesis, thus sparing glucose for brain consumption and facilitating gluconeogenesis.
- Hoseth and colleagues (2000) found that healthy, appropriate-for-gestational-age (AGA), full-term, breastfed infants (n = 223) were not at risk for developing hypoglycemia. Diwakar and Sasidhar (2002) had similar findings in 200 exclusively breastfed healthy full-term, AGA infants. Blackburn (2007) suggests that healthy breastfed infants have a higher number of ketone bodies than formula-fed infants; this alternate source of energy (ketone bodies) enables the healthy full-term infant to maintain a steady-state serum glucose level while breastfeeding is being established.
- The physiologic effects of early milk intake (breast milk or formula) in the healthy newborn include the stimulation of gut maturation, promotion of intestinal mucosa integrity, and release of intestinal enzymes that enhance motility and perfusion (Blackburn, 2007). There is evidence that sterile water and dextrose water feedings do not promote intestinal maturation; these are primarily from studies in newborns who are jaundiced.

Implications for Practice

Currently no evidence exists to support the practice of oral dextrose water feedings in healthy AGA newborns as a substitute for breast milk or formula, even to treat mild, asymptomatic, transient hypoglycemia. Likewise, only physiologic evidence supports the practice of early oral feedings of breast milk, formula, or colostrum in healthy newborns.

References

American Academy of Pediatrics, American College of Obstetricians and Gynecologists: *Guidelines for perinatal care*, Elk Grove Village, Ill, 2007, The Academy.

Blackburn ST: *Maternal, fetal, and neonatal physiology: a clinical perspective*, ed 3, St Louis, 2007, Saunders.

Diwakar KK, Sasidhar MV: Plasma glucose levels in term infants who are appropriate size for gestation and exclusively breast fed, *Arch Dis Child Fetal Neonatal Educ* 87(1):F46-F48, 2002.

Eidelman AI: Hypoglycemia and the breastfed neonate, *Pediatr Clin North Am* 48(2):377-387, 2001.

Hashim MJ, Guillet R: Common issues in the care of sick neonates, *Am Fam Physician* 66(9):1685-1692, 2002.

Hoseth E et al: Blood glucose levels in a population of healthy, breast fed, term infants of appropriate size for gestational age, *Arch Dis Child Fetal Neonatal Educ* 83(2):F117-F119, 2000.

Noerr B: State of the science: neonatal hypoglycemia, *Adv Neonatal Care* 1(1):4-21, 2001.

Sperling MA, Menon RK: Differential diagnosis and management of neonatal hypoglycemia, *Pediatr Clin North Am* 51(3):703-723, 2004.

Wakayama Y, Wilkins S, Kimura K: Is 5% dextrose in water a proper choice for initial postoperative feeding in infants? *J Pediatr Surg* 23(7):644-666, 1988.

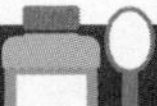

MEDICATION GUIDE

*Hepatitis B Vaccine (Recombivax HB, Engerix-B)**

Action

Hepatitis B vaccine induces protective anti–hepatitis B antibodies in 95% to 99% of healthy infants who receive the recommended three doses. The duration of protection of the vaccine is unknown.

Indication

Hepatitis B vaccine provides immunization against infection caused by all known subtypes of hepatitis B virus.

Neonatal Dosage

The usual dosage is Recombivax HB 5 mcg/0.5 ml or Engerix-B 10 mcg/0.5 ml at birth, 1 month, and 6 months. An alternative dosing schedule of birth, 1 month, 2 months, and 12 months is usually for newborns whose mothers were hepatitis B surface antigen (HBsAg) positive. (See also Immunizations, Chapter 36.)

Adverse Reactions

Common adverse reactions are rash, fever, erythema, swelling, and pain at injection site.

Nursing Considerations

Parental consent must be obtained before administration. Wear gloves. Administer in the middle third of the vastus lateralis muscle using a 25-gauge, ⅝-inch (16-mm) to ⅞-inch (22-mm) needle. Inject into skin that has been cleaned, or allow alcohol to dry on puncture site for 1 minute to remove organisms and prevent infection. Stabilize leg firmly and grasp muscle between the thumb and fingers. Insert the needle at a 90-degree angle; aspirate and inject medication slowly if there is no blood return. After removing needle, rub gently on the site with a dry gauze square to decrease pain sensation. If the infant was born to an HBsAg-positive mother, hepatitis B immune globulin (HBIG) should be given within 12 hours of birth in addition to the hepatitis B vaccine. Separate sites must be used. Document immunization administration on a vaccination card for parent(s) to have a record.

*Note: The combination vaccines containing hepatitis B are not recommended for the birth (first) dose.

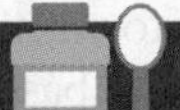

MEDICATION GUIDE

Hepatitis B Immune Globulin

Action

Hepatitis B immune globulin (HBIG) provides a high titer of antibody to hepatitis B surface antigen (HBsAg).

Indication

The HBIG vaccine provides prophylaxis against infection in infants born to HBsAg-positive mothers.

Neonatal Dosage

Administer one 0.5 ml dose intramuscularly within 12 hours of birth.

Adverse Reactions

Hypersensitivity may occur.

Nursing Considerations

The vaccine must be given within 12 hours of birth. Wear gloves. Administer in the middle third of the vastus lateralis muscle using a 25-gauge, ⅝-inch (16-mm) to ⅞-inch (22-mm) needle. Inject into skin that has been cleaned, or allow alcohol to dry on puncture site for 1 minute to remove organisms and prevent infection. Stabilize leg firmly and grasp muscle between the thumb and fingers. Insert the needle at a 90-degree angle; aspirate and inject medication slowly if there is no blood return. After removing needle, rub gently on the site with a dry gauze square to decrease pain sensation. HBIG may be given at same time as hepatitis B vaccine, but in a separate syringe and at a different site. Document immunization administration on a vaccination card for parent(s) to have a record.

For an injection, the neonate's leg should be stabilized (see Figure 45-8 for containment method). The nurse wears gloves and cleanses the injection site with an appropriate skin antiseptic. The needle is inserted into the vastus lateralis at a 90-degree angle. The plunger of the syringe is gently withdrawn, and if no blood is aspirated, the medication is injected. If blood is aspirated, the needle is withdrawn and the injection is given in another site. The needle is withdrawn quickly and pressure is maintained at the site to minimize the pain.

The nurse should always remember to comfort the infant after an injection. Needles should never be recapped but should be properly discarded in an appropriate safety container. It is important to record medication, date and time, amount, route, and site of injection on the newborn's medical record.

Therapy for Hyperbilirubinemia

The best therapy for hyperbilirubinemia is prevention. Because bilirubin is excreted in meconium, prevention can be facilitated by early feeding, which stimulates passage of meconium. However, despite early passage of meconium, the term infant may have trouble conjugating the increased amount of bilirubin derived from disintegrating fetal RBCs. As a result, the serum levels of unconjugated bilirubin may rise beyond normal limits, causing hyperbilirubinemia. The goal of treatment of hyperbilirubinemia is to help reduce the newborn's serum levels of unconjugated bilirubin. There are two ways to reduce unconjugated bilirubin levels: phototherapy and exchange blood transfusion. Exchange transfusion is used to treat those infants whose levels of serum bilirubin are rising rapidly despite the use of intensive phototherapy (see discussion on p. 767).

Phototherapy

During phototherapy the infant is placed, seminude, approximately 45 to 50 cm on or under special phototherapy lights. The distance may vary based on unit protocol and type of light used. The most effective therapy is achieved with lights at 400 to 550 nanometers, and a blue-green light spectrum is the most efficient (Steffensrud, 2004). The lamp energy output should be monitored routinely during treatment with a photometer to ensure efficacy of therapy. Phototherapy is carried out until the infant's serum bilirubin level decreases to within acceptable range. The decision to discontinue therapy is based on a definite downward trend in the serum bilirubin values.

Several precautions must be taken while the infant is undergoing phototherapy. The infant's eyes must be protected by an opaque mask to prevent overexposure to the light. The eye shield should cover the eyes completely but not occlude the nares. Before the mask is applied, the infant's eyes should be closed gently to prevent excoriation of the corneas. The mask should be removed periodically and during infant feedings so that the eyes can be checked and cleansed with water and the parents can have visual contact with the infant (Fig. 25-12, *A* and *B*, and Family-Centered Care box).

FAMILY-CENTERED CARE

Phototherapy and Parent-Infant Interaction

The traditional use of phototherapy has evoked concerns regarding a number of psychobehavioral issues, including parent-infant separation, potential social isolation, decreased sensorineural stimulation, altered biologic rhythms, altered feeding patterns, and activity changes. Parental anxiety is greatly increased, particularly at the sight of the newborn blindfolded and under special lights. The interruption of breastfeeding for phototherapy is a potential deterrent to successful maternal-infant attachment and interaction. Because research has demonstrated that bilirubin catabolism occurs primarily within the first few hours of the initiation of phototherapy, there is increased support for the removal of the infant from treatment for feeding and holding. Intermittent phototherapy may be just as effective as continuous therapy when used correctly. The benefits of stopping phototherapy for short periods so parents can feed and hold the newborn should be carefully weighed by the health care team and the parents.

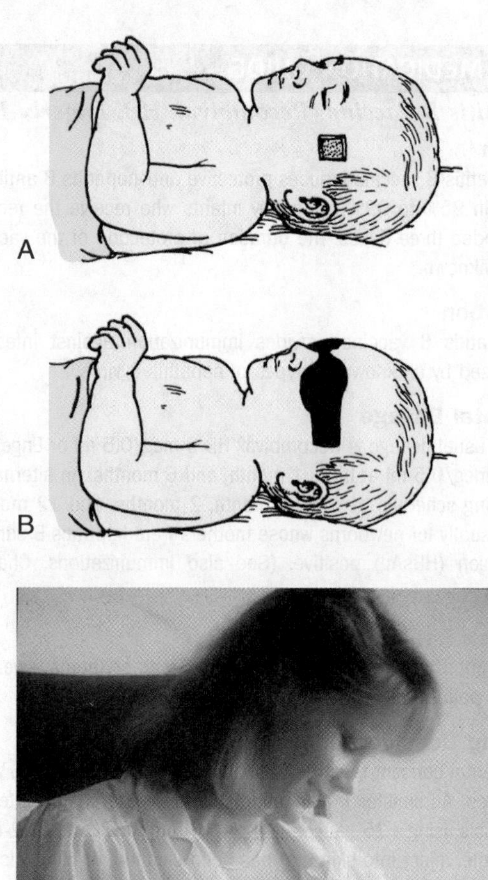

Fig. 25-12 Eye patches for newborns receiving phototherapy. **A,** Small Velcro patch stuck to both sides of head. **B,** Eye cover sticks to Velcro patch, which reduces movement of eye cover and facilitates removal for feedings. **C,** A mother can breastfeed her newborn without interrupting phototherapy when a fiberoptic blanket is used. *(**C**, Courtesy Respironics, Inc., Pittsburgh, PA.)*

Often a "string bikini" made from a disposable face mask is used instead of a diaper. This allows optimal skin exposure, yet provides sufficient protection to the genitalia and bedding. Before its application, the metal strip must be removed from the mask to avoid burning the infant. Lotions and ointments should not be used during phototherapy because they absorb heat and can cause burns.

Phototherapy may cause changes in the infant's temperature depending partially on the bed used: bassinet, incubator, or radiant warmer. The infant's temperature should be closely monitored. Phototherapy lights may increase the rate of insensible water loss, making it possible for fluid loss and dehydration to occur. Therefore it is important that the infant be adequately hydrated. Hydration maintenance in the healthy newborn is carried out with human milk or infant formula; there is no advantage or benefit to administering oral glucose or plain water because these do not promote excretion of bilirubin in stools and may in fact perpetuate enterohepatic circulation, thus delaying bilirubin excretion. Urine output may be decreased or unaltered; the urine may appear dark gold or brown.

The number and consistency of stools are monitored. Bilirubin breakdown increases gastric motility, which results in loose stools that can cause skin excoriation and breakdown. The infant's buttocks must be cleaned after each stool to help maintain skin integrity. A fine maculopapular rash may appear during phototherapy, but this is transient. Because visualization of the infant's skin color is difficult with blue light, appropriate cardiorespiratory monitoring should be implemented based on the infant's overall condition.

A number of newer phototherapy products including the Bilibed use fluorescent light for phototherapy. With such systems the infant may be kept in the mother's room to minimize separation and maximize therapy. Alternative devices for phototherapy include a fluorescent bank of lights, halogen spotlights, LED (light-emitting diode) units, and a fiberoptic pad. When a fiberoptic pad is used, the newborn can remain in the mother's room in an open crib or in her arms during treatment (see Fig. 25-12, C). Follow unit protocol for the use of eye patches. In certain situations the infant's bilirubin levels may be increasing rapidly and require intensive phototherapy; this involves the use of a combination of intensive conventional lights and fiberoptic or halogen lights to maximize bilirubin reduction. All aspects of phototherapy should be accurately recorded in the infant's medical record.

Parent Education

Serum levels of bilirubin in the newborn continue to rise until the fifth day of life. Many parents leave the hospital within 24 hours of birth, and some as early as 6 hours after birth. Therefore parents must receive education regarding jaundice and its treatment. They should have written instructions for assessing the infant's condition and the name of a contact person to whom they should report their findings and concerns. Some institutions or third-party payers cover a home visit to evaluate the infant's condition and to monitor the mother's health as well. If it proves necessary to measure serum bilirubin levels after discharge from the hospital, a health care technician or nurse may draw the blood for the specimen, or the parents may take the baby to a laboratory to have blood drawn for a serum bilirubin. In some cases parents may take the newborn to an outpatient clinic or physician's office to be evaluated.

Circumcision

Circumcision of male infants has traditionally been performed in the United States before discharge from the birth institution. The American Academy of Pediatrics, Task Force on Circumcision (1999), noted that, despite scientific evidence of potential medical benefits of circumcision, the data are not sufficient to recommend routine circumcision. The Task Force on Circumcision further recommended that if circumcision is performed, analgesia should be used; this policy statement was reaffirmed in 2005 (American Academy of Pediatrics, 2005).

Circumcision is a matter of personal parental choice. Parents usually decide to have their newborn circumcised based on one or more of the following factors: hygiene, religious conviction, tradition, culture, or social norms. Regardless of the reason for the decision, parents should be given unbiased information and the opportunity to discuss the benefits and risks (see Community Focus box).

Expectant parents need to begin learning about circumcision during the prenatal period, but circumcision often is not discussed with the parents before labor. In many instances, it is only when the mother is being admitted to the hospital or birth unit that she is first confronted with the decision regarding circumcision. Because the stress of the intrapartum period makes this a difficult time for parental decision making, this is not an ideal time to broach the topic of circumcision and expect a well-thought-out decision. Circumcision requires a signed consent form in addition to the safety measures that precede any surgical procedure (e.g., proper identification).

COMMUNITY FOCUS

Newborn Circumcision

Prepare a poster presentation to provide parents information on newborn circumcision. Because circumcision is considered an optional surgical procedure, it may not be performed until after the infant is discharged home. Include in your display the advantages and disadvantages of circumcision, as well as the care of the uncircumcised penis in infants and young children.

Procedure

Circumcision involves removing the prepuce (foreskin) of the glans. The procedure is not usually done immediately after birth because of the danger of cold stress and decreased clotting factors, but it is often performed in the hospital before the infant's discharge. The circumcision of a Jewish boy is performed on the eighth day after birth and is done at home in a ceremony called a *bris,* unless the infant is ill. The timing is logical from a physiologic standpoint because clotting factors drop somewhat immediately after birth and do not return to prebirth levels until the end of the first week.

evolve Critical Thinking Exercise—Circumcision

Feedings are usually withheld up to 2 to 3 hours before the circumcision to prevent vomiting and aspiration. To prepare the infant for the circumcision, he is positioned on a plastic restraint form (Fig. 25-13) or held by a staff member, and the penis is cleansed with soap and water or other prep solution such as povidone-iodine. The infant is draped to provide warmth and a sterile field, and the sterile equipment is readied for use.

Although some circumcision procedures require no special equipment or appliances (Fig. 25-14), numerous instruments have been designed for this purpose. Use of the Gomco clamp (Fig. 25-15) may make this an almost bloodless operation. The procedure itself takes only a few minutes to perform. After it is completed, a small petrolatum gauze dressing or a generous amount of petrolatum or A&D ointment may be applied to the penis for the first few days to prevent the diaper from

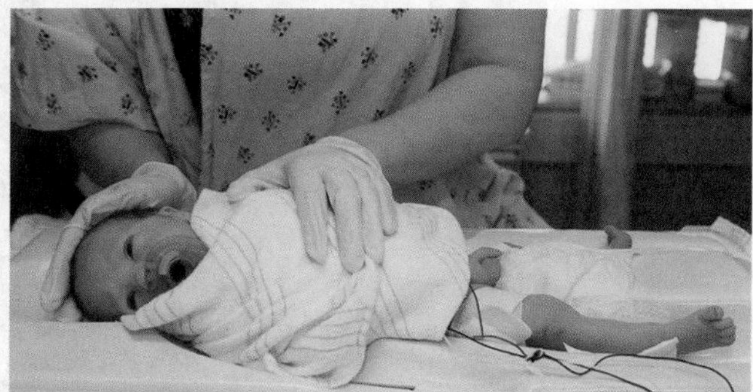

Fig. 25-13 Proper positioning of infant in Circumstraint. *(Courtesy Paul Vincent Kuntz, Texas Children's Hospital, Houston, TX.)*

adhering to the site. A PlastiBell is another method used for the circumcision. The advantages are that it applies constant direct pressure to prevent hemorrhage during the procedure and afterward protects against infection, keeps the site from sticking to the diaper, and prevents pain with urination. When using the plastic bell for circumcision, it is first fitted over the glans; the suture is tied around the rim of the bell; and excess prepuce is cut away. The plastic rim remains in place for about a week; it falls off after healing has taken place, usually within 5 to 7 days (Fig. 25-16). Petrolatum is not usually needed when the bell is used.

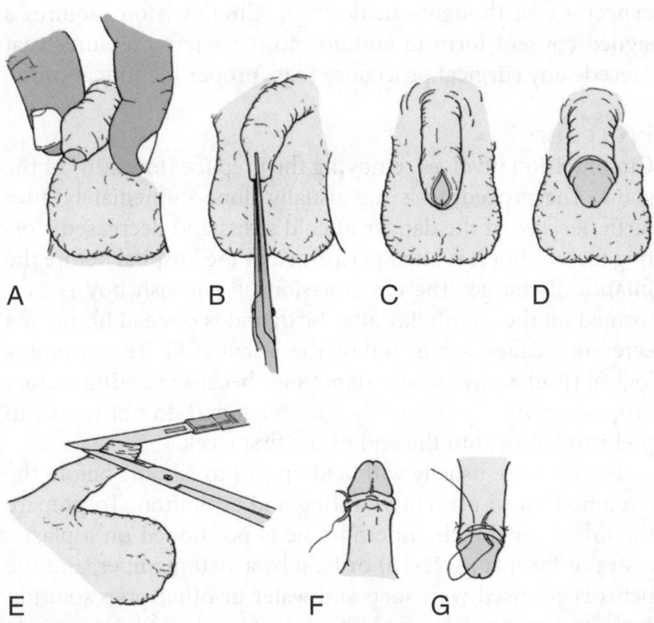

Fig. 25-14 Technique of circumcision. **A** to **D**, Prepuce is stripped and slit to facilitate its retraction behind glans penis. **E**, Prepuce is now clamped and excessive prepuce cut off. **F** and **G**, A very small needle with plain 2-0 or 3-0 catgut is used for suturing; some physicians prefer silk.

Procedural Pain Management

Circumcision is painful. The pain is manifested by both physiologic and behavioral changes in the infant (see discussion that follows). Four types of anesthesia and analgesia are used in newborns undergoing circumcision: ring block, dorsal penile nerve block (DPNB), topical anesthetic such as EMLA (prilocaine-lidocaine) or LMX4 (4% lidocaine), and concentrated oral sucrose. Nonpharmacologic methods such as nonnutritive sucking, containment, and swaddling may be used to enhance pain management. The Cochrane Group exploring pain relief for neonatal circumcision found that DPNB was the most effective intervention for decreasing pain (Brady-Fryer, Wiebe, & Lander, 2004). Studies exploring the use of several strategies concurrently, such as that conducted by Razmus, Dalton, and Wilson (2004), which included groups receiving both concentrated oral sucrose and ring block compared with

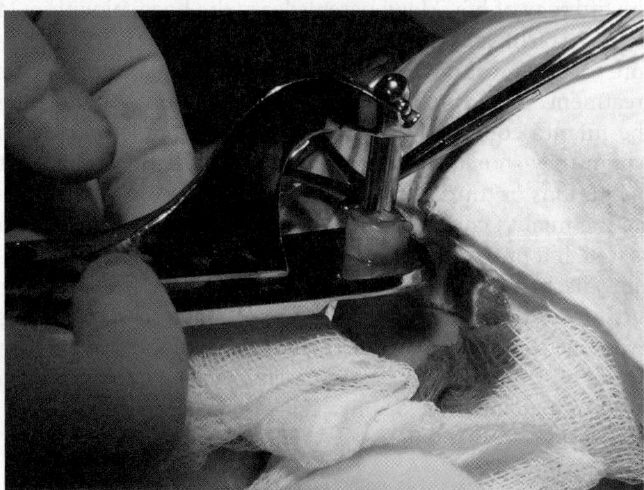

Fig. 25-15 Circumcision with Gomco clamp. Prepuce is drawn over cone and clamp is applied; hemostasis occurs, and then prepuce (over cone) is cut away. *(Courtesy Cheryl Briggs, RN, Annapolis, MD.)*

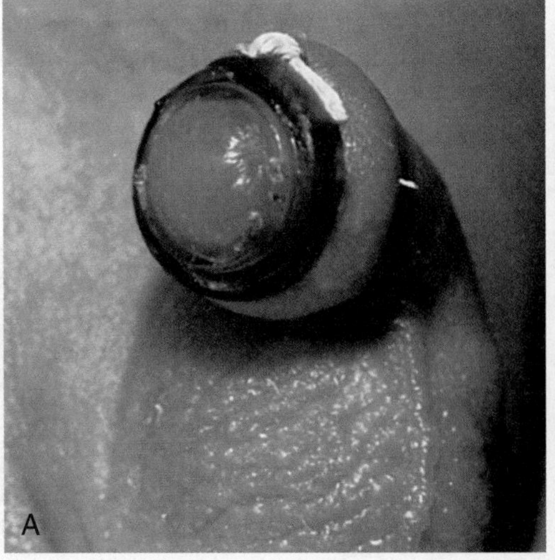

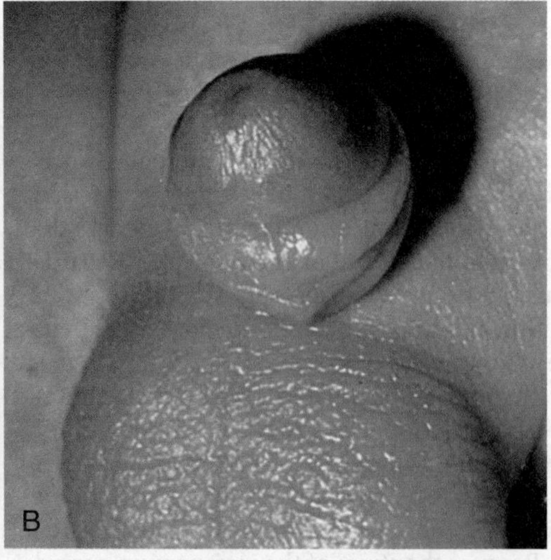

Fig. 25-16 Circumcision using Hollister PlastiBell. **A**, Suture around rim of PlastiBell controls bleeding. **B**, Plastic rim and suture drop off in 7 to 10 days. *(Permission to use and/or reproduce this copyrighted material has been granted by the owner, Hollister, Inc., Libertyville, IL.)*

evolve Video—Circumcision

ring block alone, have the most potential to clarify optimum strategies.

A ring block is the injection of buffered lidocaine administered subcutaneously on each side of the penile shaft. A DPNB includes subcutaneous injections of buffered lidocaine at the 2 o'clock and 10 o'clock positions at the base of the penis. The circumcision should not be done for at least 5 minutes after these injections.

A topical cream containing prilocaine-lidocaine such as eutectic mixture of local anesthetic (EMLA) can be applied to the base of the penis at least 1 hour before the circumcision. The area where the prepuce attaches to the glans is well coated with 1 g of the cream and then covered with a transparent occlusive dressing or finger cot. The cream is removed just before the procedure. Blanching or redness of the skin may occur.

After the circumcision, the infant is comforted until he is quieted. If the parents were not present during the procedure, the infant is returned to them. The infant may be fussy for several hours and may have disturbed sleep-wake states and disorganized feeding behaviors. Oral acetaminophen may be administered before the procedure and every 4 hours thereafter (as ordered by the practitioner) for a maximum of five doses in 24 hours or a maximum of 75 mg/kg/day (see Atraumatic Care box). For additional discussion of neonatal pain, see Chapter 35.

PATIENT TEACHING Care of the Circumcised Newborn at Home

Wash hands before touching the newly circumcised penis.

Check for Bleeding

Check circumcision for bleeding with each diaper change.

If bleeding occurs, apply gentle pressure with a folded sterile gauze square. If bleeding does not stop with pressure, notify primary health care provider.

Observe for Urination

Check to see that the infant urinates after being circumcised.

Infant should have a wet diaper 4 to 6 times per 24 hours.

Keep Area Clean

Change diaper and inspect circumcision at least every 4 hours.

Wash penis gently with warm water to remove urine and feces. Apply petrolatum liberally to the glans with each diaper change (omit petrolatum if PlastiBell was used).

Use soap only after circumcision is healed (5 to 6 days).

Fanfold diaper to prevent pressure on the circumcised area.

Check for Infection

Glans penis is dark red after circumcision, then becomes covered with yellow exudate in 24 hours. This is normal and will persist for 2 to 3 days. Do not attempt to remove it.

Redness, swelling, or discharge indicates infection. Notify primary health care provider if you think the circumcision area is infected.

Provide Comfort

Circumcision is painful. Handle the area gently.

Provide extra holding, feeding, and opportunities for nonnutritive sucking for a day or two.

Care of the Newly Circumcised Infant

The nurse checks the infant hourly for the next 4 to 6 hours to make certain that no bleeding is occurring and that voiding is normal. If bleeding is noted from the circumcision, the nurse applies gentle pressure to the site of bleeding with a folded sterile gauze pad or sprinkles powdered gel foam on it. If bleeding is not easily controlled, a blood vessel may need to be ligated. In this event, one nurse notifies the physician and prepares the necessary equipment (i.e., circumcision tray and suture materials) while another nurse maintains intermittent pressure until the physician arrives. If the parents take the baby home before the end of the observation period, they must be taught the proper home care (see Patient Teaching box). Nursing actions are planned and implemented to prevent infection. Prepackaged commercial wipes for cleaning the diaper area should not be used because they contain alcohol, which delays healing and causes discomfort. Instead, the nurse washes the penis gently with water to remove urine and feces and, if necessary, applies fresh petrolatum around the glans after each diaper change.

The glans penis, normally dark red during healing, becomes covered with a yellow exudate in 24 hours. This is part of normal healing, not an infective process. No attempt should be made to remove the exudate, which persists for 2 to 3 days. Parents should be taught to fanfold the diaper so that it does not press on the circumcised area. They should be encouraged to change the diaper at least every 4 hours to prevent it from sticking to the penis.

Discharge Planning and Teaching

Infant care activities can cause much anxiety for the new parent. Support from nursing staff members can be an important factor in determining whether new mothers seek and accept help in the future. Whether the couple is having their first newborn, the mother is an adolescent whose own mother will be the primary caregiver, or the couple attended parenthood preparation classes, parents appreciate anticipatory guidance in the care of their infant. The nurse should not try to cover all the content at one time because the parents can be overwhelmed by too much information and become anxious. However, because early discharge of new mothers is currently common practice, it may be a problem for the nurse to teach all the content that is necessary. As a result, many institutions have developed home visitation programs that take the necessary teaching to the new parents, although the hospital nurse still provides most of the essential information for newborn care.

To set priorities for teaching, the nurse follows parental cues. Deficient knowledge should be identified before beginning to teach. Normal growth and development and the infant's changing needs (e.g., for personal interaction and stimulation, growth milestones, exercise, injury prevention, and social contacts), as well as the topics that follow, should be included during discharge planning with parents.

evolve Nursing Care Plan—Home Care Follow-Up: Transition to Parenthood

ATRAUMATIC CARE

*Guidelines for Pain Management During Neonatal Circumcision**

Pharmacologic Interventions

Use of Topical Anesthetic Only

One hour before the procedure, administer acetaminophen (e.g., Tylenol, 15 mg/kg) as ordered by the practitioner.

Place a thick layer (1 g) of an eutectic mixture of lidocaine and prilocaine (EMLA)† or lidocaine 4% (LMX4)‡ cream around the penis where the prepuce (foreskin) attaches to the glans. Avoid placing cream on the tip of the penis where it may come in contact with the urethral opening.

Cover the penis with a "finger cot" that is cut from a vinyl or latex glove, or a piece of plastic wrap, and secure the bottom of the covering with tape. Avoid using Tegaderm or large amounts of tape on the skin because removing the adhesive causes pain and can irritate the fragile skin.

If the infant urinates during the time EMLA is applied (1 hour) and a significant amount of EMLA is removed, reapply the cream and covering. The total application of EMLA should not exceed a surface area of 10 cm^2 (1¼ × 1¼ inches).

Remove cream with clean cloth or tissue. Blanching of skin is an expected reaction to EMLA's application under an occlusive dressing; erythema and some edema may occur also.

Two minutes before starting the procedure, give the infant a sucrose solution; 24% (weight/volume) sucrose solution is available commercially. Use this solution to coat the pacifier (recoat several times before and during the procedure).

After the procedure, apply petrolatum or A&D ointment on a 2 × 2 inch dressing before diapering infant to prevent the wound from adhering to the dressing or diaper.

Administer acetaminophen as ordered by the practitioner 4 hours after the initial dose; give additional doses as needed but not to exceed five doses in 24 hours or a maximum dosage of 75 mg/kg/day.

Use of Dorsal Penile Nerve Block or Ring Block

One hour before the procedure administer acetaminophen as ordered by the practitioner.

One hour before procedure, apply EMLA. For the dorsal penile nerve block (DPNB) apply EMLA to the prepuce as described previously and at the penile base. For the ring block apply EMLA to the prepuce as described previously and to the shaft of the penis. Use a topical anesthetic in conjunction with the DPNB or ring block to avoid the pain of injecting the anesthetic.

Use a 30-gauge needle to administer the lidocaine.§ For the DPNB, 0.4 ml of the lidocaine is infiltrated at the 10:30 and 1:30 o'clock positions in Buck's fascia at the penile base. For the ring block, 0.4 ml of lidocaine is infiltrated subcutaneously on each side of the shaft of the penis below the prepuce.

For maximum anesthesia, wait 5 minutes after injection of lidocaine. An alternative anesthetic agent is chloroprocaine, which is as effective as lidocaine after 3 minutes.

Approximately 2 minutes before the circumcision, administer concentrated oral sucrose solution as described previously.

After the procedure, apply A&D ointment or petrolatum and administer acetaminophen as described previously.

Nonpharmacologic Interventions

In addition to the preceding pharmacologic interventions:

- If a Circumstraint board is used, pad with blankets or other thick, soft material such as lamb's wool. A more comfortable, padded, and physiologic restraint that places the infant semireclining can also decrease distress (Stang et al, 1997).‖
- Provide the parents, caregiver, or another staff member with the option of holding the infant during the procedure or being present during the circumcision.
- Swaddle the upper body and legs to provide warmth and containment and to reduce movement.
- If the baby is not swaddled and is unclothed, use a radiant warmer to prevent hypothermia. Shield infant's eyes from overhead lights.
- Prewarm any topical solutions to be used in sterile preparation of the surgical site by placing in a warm blanket or towel.
- Play infant relaxation music¶ before, during, and after procedure; allow parents or other caregiver the option of choosing the music.
- After the procedure, remove restraints and swaddle. Immediately have the parent, other caregiver, or nursing staff hold the infant. Continue to have the infant suck on pacifier or offer feeding.

Data from Broadman LM et al: Post-circumcision analgesia: a prospective evaluation of subcutaneous ring block of the penis, *Anesthesiology* 67:339-402, 1987; Howard CR, Howard FM, Weitzman ML: Acetaminophen analgesia in neonatal circumcision: the effect on pain, *Pediatrics* 93(4):641-646, 1994; Lander J et al: Comparison of ring block, dorsal penile nerve block, and topical anesthesia for neonatal circumcision, *JAMA* 278:2157-2162, 1997; Mintz MR, Grillo R: Dorsal penile nerve block for circumcision, *Clin Pediatr* 28:590-591, 1989; Serour F, Mandelberg A, Mori J: Slow injection of local anesthetic will decrease pain during dorsal penile nerve block, *Acta Anaesthesiol Scand* 42:926-928, 1998; Spencer DM et al: Dorsal penile nerve block in neonatal circumcision: chloroprocaine versus lidocaine, *Am J Perinatol* 9(3):214-218, 1992; Stang H et al: Beyond dorsal penile nerve block: a more humane circumcision, *Pediatrics* 100(2):e3, 1997. Stevens B et al: The efficacy of sucrose for relieving procedural pain in neonates—a systematic review and meta-analysis, *Acta Paediatr* 86:837-842, 1997; Taddio A et al: Efficacy and safety of lidocaine-prilocaine cream (EMLA) for pain during circumcision, *N Engl J Med* 336(17):1197-1201, 1997.

*There is sufficient evidence and support for use of a combination of pharmacologic and nonpharmacologic interventions to holistically manage neonatal circumcision pain. Combined analgesia, nonpharmacologic interventions (such as swaddling), and local anesthesia may be used during the procedure to provide holistic pain management (Taddio et al, 2000; Anand & International Evidence-Based Group for Neonatal Pain, 2001; Geyer et al, 2002; Razmus, Dalton, & Wilson, 2004).

†On March 11, 1999, the U.S. Food and Drug Administration approved use of EMLA in infants age 37 weeks of gestation. Although the package insert warns that patients taking acetaminophen are at greater risk for developing methemoglobinemia, there have been no reported cases of this complication in children taking acetaminophen and using EMLA. In fact, there is no evidence that acetaminophen induces methemoglobinemia in humans (Prescott, 1996). The only reported cases of methemoglobinemia from acetaminophen have been in cats and dogs (Hjelle & Grauer, 1986).

‡LMX4 (previously Ela-Max) is a 4% lidocaine cream reported to be effective within 30 minutes of application for venipuncture. There is no need to apply an occlusive dressing over LMX4 cream as recommended for EMLA (Wong, 2003). Use of LMX4 for pain relief of pediatric meatotomy has been reported previously (Smith & Gjellum, 2004). Despite anecdotal reports of its use in neonatal circumcision, at this time no studies are available regarding the use or effectiveness of LMX4 for neonatal circumcision analgesia.

§In one study the use of buffered lidocaine, which normally reduces stinging sensation of lidocaine, did not provide effective anesthesia for DPNB (Stang et al, 1997). The study on slow injection of the anesthetics lidocaine and bupivacaine compared 40 vs. 80 seconds in patients ages 15 to 53 years (Serour, Mandelberg, & Mori, 1998).

‖For information on Stang Circ Chair, contact Pedicraft, 4134 Saint Augustine Road, Jacksonville, FL 32247-5969, 800-223-7649; e-mail: info@pedicraft.com; www.pedicraft.com.

¶Suggested infant relaxation music: Heartbeat Lullabies by Terry Woodford. Available from Baby-Go-To-Sleep Center, Audio-Therapy Innovations, Inc., PO Box 550, Colorado Springs, CO 80901, 800-537-7748; www.babygotosleep.com.

Temperature

The nurse should review the following topics:

- The causes of elevation in body temperature (e.g., overwrapping, cold stress with resultant vasoconstriction, or response to infection) and the body's response to extremes in environmental temperature
- Signs to be reported, such as high or low temperatures with accompanying fussiness, lethargy, irritability, poor feeding, and crying
- Ways to promote normal body temperature, such as dressing the infant appropriately for the environmental air temperature and protecting the infant from exposure to direct sunlight
- Use of warm wraps or extra blankets in cold weather
- Technique for taking the newborn's axillary temperature

Respirations

The nurse should review the following points:

- Normal variations in the rate and rhythm
- Reflexes such as sneezing to clear the airway
- Need to protect the infant from (1) exposure to people with upper respiratory tract infections and respiratory syncytial virus (see Chapter 46); (2) exposure to secondhand tobacco smoke; and (3) suffocation from loose bedding, water beds, and beanbag chairs; drowning (in bath water); entrapment under excessive bedding or in soft bedding; anything tied around the infant's neck; and poorly constructed playpens, bassinets, or cribs
- Sleep position—on back when put to sleep
- Symptoms of the common cold

A commonly aspirated substance is baby powder, which usually is a mixture of talc (hydrous magnesium silicate) and other silicates. Parents are advised to substitute a cornstarch preparation if they prefer to use a powder. The powder should be placed in the caregiver's hand and then applied to the skin, never sprinkled directly onto the skin.

Symptoms of the common cold include nasal congestion and excessive drainage of mucus, coughing, sneezing, difficulty swallowing or breathing, decreased vigor in feeding, and low-grade fever. Advise the parents on measures to help the infant, such as the following:

- Feeding smaller amounts more often to prevent overtiring the infant
- Holding the baby in an upright position to feed
- For sleeping, raising the infant's head and chest by raising the mattress 30 degrees (do not use pillow)
- Avoiding drafts; not overdressing the baby
- Using only medications prescribed by a physician (Over-the-counter "cold" remedy medications are not appropriate for use in infants and should be avoided [Sharfstein et al, 2007].)
- Using nasal saline drops in each nostril and suctioning well with bulb syringe to remove secretions

Feeding Schedules

Feeding practices and schedules for newborns are discussed in Chapter 26.

Elimination

A review includes the following reminders:

- Color of normal urine and number of voidings to expect each day
- Changes to be expected in the color of the stool (i.e., meconium to transitional to soft yellow or golden yellow) and the number of bowel evacuations, plus the odor of stools for breastfed or bottle-fed infants (see Chapter 26)
- Expected pattern of stools in formula-fed infants (i.e., as few as one stool every other day after first few weeks of life)

Positioning and Holding

The Task Force on Sudden Infant Death Syndrome of the American Academy of Pediatrics (2005) continues to recommend placing the infant to sleep in the supine position to prevent sudden infant death syndrome (SIDS). The prone position has been associated with an increased incidence of SIDS. Death rates from SIDS have decreased by more than 40% in the United States since the original sleep position statement recommending supine sleeping for all newborns was made in 1992 (see Critical Thinking Exercise).

Anatomically, the infant's shape—a barrel chest and flat, curveless spine—makes it easy for the infant to roll from the side to the prone position; therefore the side-lying position for sleep is not recommended. When the infant is awake,

CRITICAL THINKING EXERCISE

Late Preterm Infant, Sudden Infant Death Syndrome, and Infant Sleep Position

Mary gave birth to a 35-week, 2250-g female infant. This is her third baby; the other children are 18 and 20 years old. Mary and Delilah are being discharged today. The nurse has given her instructions about feeding, stooling patterns, and jaundice but said nothing about sleeping position. Mary said that she has noticed that some of the nurses placed Delilah on her side in the nursery; the mother further indicates that she worked in the nursery during college and, if babies were placed on their backs, they tended to spit up and turn blue. Mary has voiced concerns to the nurse about placing her new baby on her back to sleep at home. How should the nurse respond to Mary's concerns?

1. Evidence–Is there sufficient evidence to draw conclusions about the safety and efficacy of the supine position for sleep for the late preterm infant in reducing the incidence of sudden infant death syndrome (SIDS)?
2. Assumptions–What assumptions can be made about the following factors related to infant positioning?
   a. Role modeling by nurses
   b. Sleep position in the nursery vs. sleep position at home
   c. Sleep position for late preterm vs. term infants
3. What implications and priorities for nursing care can be drawn at this time?
4. Does the evidence objectively support your conclusion?
5. Are there alternative perspectives to your conclusion?

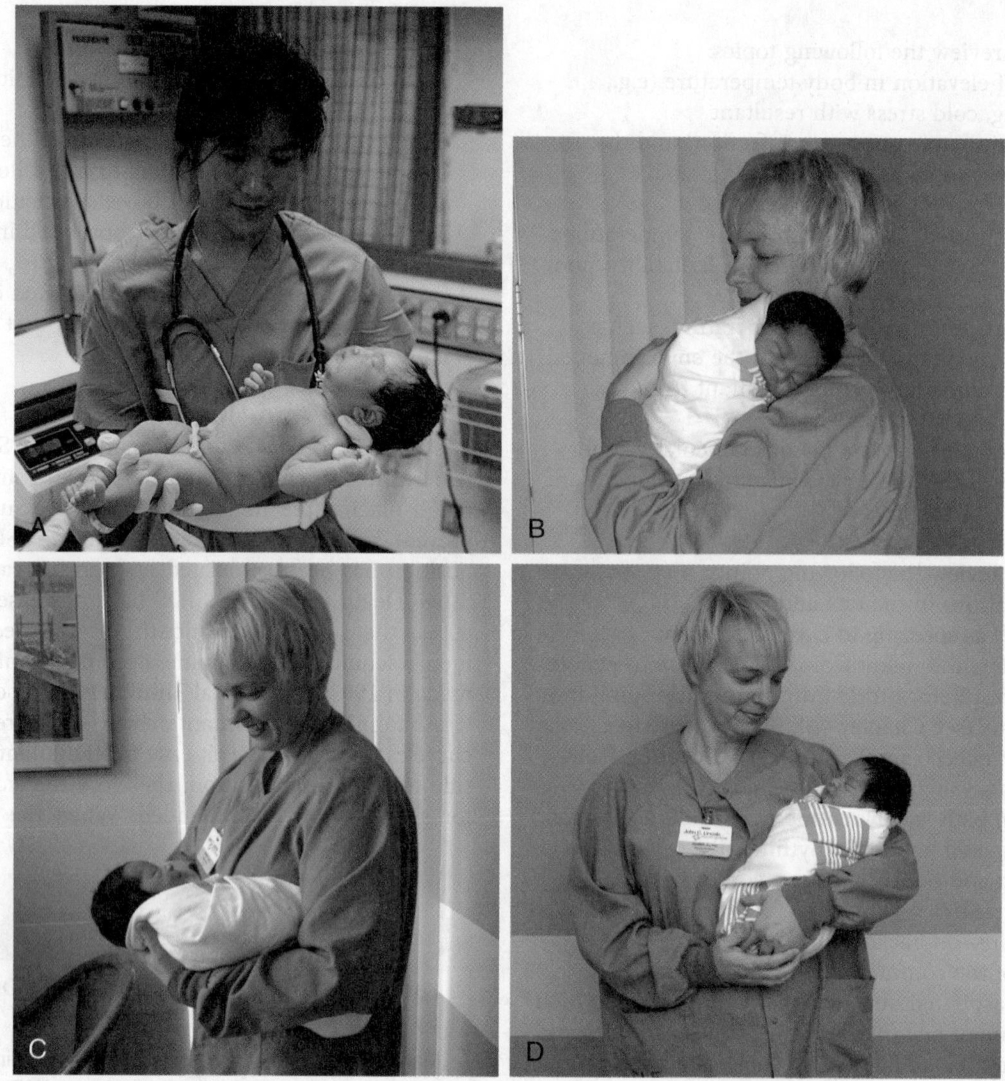

Fig. 25-17 Holding baby securely with support for head. **A,** Holding infant while moving from one place to another. Baby is undressed to show posture. **B,** Holding baby upright in "burping" position. **C,** "Football" hold. **D,** Cradling hold. *(A, Courtesy Kim Molloy, Knoxville, IA. B, C, and D, Courtesy Julie Perry Nelson, Loveland, CO.)*

tummy time can be provided under parental supervision so the infant may begin to develop appropriate muscle tone for eventual crawling; this tummy time is also effective in the prevention of a misshaped head (positional plagiocephaly).

Care must also be taken to prevent the infant from rolling off flat, unguarded surfaces. When an infant is on such a surface, the parent or nurse who must turn away from the infant even for a moment should always keep one hand placed securely on the infant. The infant is always held securely with his or her head supported because newborns are unable to maintain an erect head posture for more than a few moments. Fig. 25-17 illustrates various positions for holding an infant with adequate support.

All personnel working with infants must have current infant cardiopulmonary resuscitation (CPR) certification. Many institutions offer infant CPR courses to parents before discharge (see also Figs. 46-14 and 46-15).

evolve Skill—Changing a Diaper

Rashes

Diaper Rash

The warm, moist atmosphere in the diaper area provides an optimal environment for *Candida albicans* growth; dermatitis appears in the perianal area, inguinal folds, and lower abdomen. The affected area is intensely erythematous with a sharply demarcated, scalloped edge, often with numerous satellite lesions that extend beyond the larger lesion. The usual source of infection is from handling by persons who do not practice adequate handwashing. It may also appear 2 to 3 days after an oral infection (thrush).

Therapy consists of applications of an anticandidal ointment, such as clotrimazole or miconazole, with each diaper change. Sometimes the infant also is given an oral antifungal preparation such as nystatin or fluconazole to eliminate any gastrointestinal source of infection.

Washing and drying the wet and soiled area and changing the diaper immediately after voiding or stooling will prevent and help treat diaper rash. Parents can be taught to expose the buttocks to air to help dry up diaper rash. Because bacteria thrive in moist dark areas, exposing the skin to dry air decreases bacterial proliferation. A skin barrier ointment such as zinc oxide may be effective in preventing further excoriation, especially in the presence of loose stools or systemic gastrointestinal candidiasis; the latter will require treatment with a systemic antifungal drug.

Other Rashes

A rash on the cheeks may result from the infant's scratching with long unclipped fingernails or from rubbing the face against the crib sheets, particularly if regurgitated stomach contents are not washed off promptly. The newborn's skin begins a natural process of peeling and sloughing after birth. Dry skin may be treated with a neutral pH lotion, but this should be used sparingly. Newborn rash, erythema toxicum, is a common finding (see Fig. 24-5, *B*, p. 618) and needs no treatment.

Clothing

Parents commonly ask how warmly they should dress their infant. A simple rule of thumb is to dress the child as they dress themselves, adding or subtracting clothes and wraps for the child as necessary. A cotton shirt and diaper may be sufficient clothing for the young infant. A cap or bonnet is needed to protect the scalp and minimize heat loss if the weather is cool, or to protect against sunburn and shade the eyes if it is sunny and hot. Wrapping the infant snugly in a blanket maintains body temperature and promotes a feeling of security. Overdressing in warm temperatures can cause discomfort, as can underdressing in cold weather. Overdressing the infant has also been associated with SIDS. Parents are encouraged to dress the infant at all times in flame-retardant clothing. Infant sunglasses are available to protect the eyes when outdoors.

Safety: Use of Car Seat

Infants should travel only in federally approved, rear-facing safety seats secured in the rear seat (Fig. 25-18). The safest area of the car is the back seat. A car seat that faces the rear gives the best protection for the infant's disproportionately weak neck and heavy head. In this position, the force of a frontal crash is spread over the head, neck, and back; the back of the car seat supports the spine.

NURSING ALERT Infants should use a rear-facing car seat from birth to 9 kg (20 lb) and to 1 year of age. If the infant reaches the weight limit before the first birthday, the rear-facing position should still be used.

The car seat is secured using the vehicle seat belt; the infant is secured using the harness system in the car seat. If the infant must ride in the front seat, the air bag must be turned off to prevent injury from the air bag.*

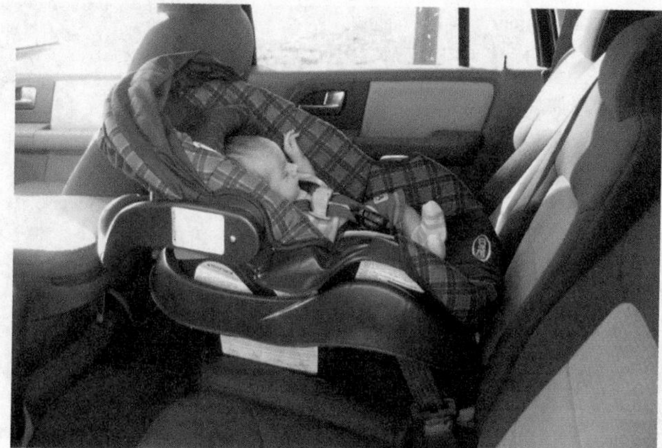

Fig. 25-18 Rear-facing infant seat in rear seat of car. Infant is placed in seat when going home from the hospital. *(Courtesy Brian and Mayannyn Sallee, Las Vegas, NV.)*

NURSING ALERT In cars equipped with air bags, rear-facing infant seats should not be placed in the front seat unless the air bag has been deactivated. Serious injury can occur if the air bag inflates because these types of infant seats fit closer to the dashboard than a passenger does.

Infants born at less than 37 weeks of gestation and with birth weight less than 2500 g should be observed in a car seat for a period (a minimum of 90 to 120 minutes is recommended by the American Academy of Pediatrics [Bull, Engle, & American Academy of Pediatrics, 2009]) before discharge. The infant is monitored for apnea, bradycardia, and a decrease in oxygen saturation. It may be necessary to place blanket rolls on either side of the infant for support of the head and trunk. To prevent slumping, the back-to-crotch strap distance should be 14 cm (see Motor Vehicle Injuries, Chapter 36, for additional car restraint information). If the preterm infant fails the car seat test, a car bed may used to provide safe transportation.

Nonnutritive Sucking

Sucking is the infant's chief pleasure. However, sucking needs may not be satisfied by breastfeeding or bottle-feeding alone. In fact, sucking is such a strong need that infants who are deprived of sucking, such as those with a cleft lip, will suck on their tongues. Some newborns are born with sucking pads on their fingers that developed during in utero sucking. Several benefits of nonnutritive sucking have been demonstrated, such as an increased weight gain in preterm infants,

Air bag safety sheets are available from the American Academy of Pediatrics, 141 Northwest Point Blvd., Elk Grove Village, IL 60007; 847-434-4000; fax: 847-434-8000; or access the website at www.aap.org for the latest guidelines for infant car seat restraints.

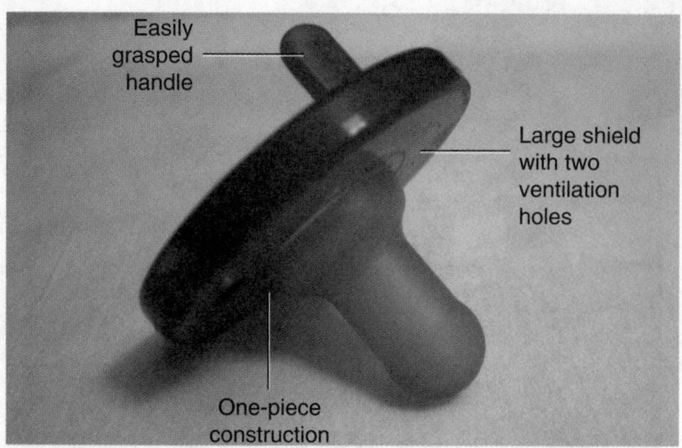

Fig. 25-19 Design of a safe pacifier. *(Courtesy Julie Perry Nelson, Loveland, CO.)*

increased ability to maintain an organized state, and decreased crying.

Problems arise when parents are concerned about the sucking of fingers, thumb, or pacifier and try to restrain this natural tendency. Before giving advice, nurses should investigate the parents' feelings and base the guidance they give on the information solicited. For example, some parents may see no problem with the use of a finger but may find the use of a pacifier objectionable. In general, there is no need to restrain either practice, unless thumb sucking persists past 4 years of age or past the time when the permanent teeth erupt. Parents are advised to consult with their pediatrician, pediatric dentist, or pediatric nurse practitioner on this topic.

A parent's excessive use of the pacifier to calm the child should also be explored, however. It is not unusual for parents to place a pacifier in the infant's mouth as soon as he or she begins to cry, thus reinforcing a pattern of distress-relief.

If parents choose to let their child use a pacifier, they need to be aware of certain safety considerations before purchasing one. A homemade or poorly designed pacifier can be dangerous because the entire object may be aspirated, if it is small, or a portion may become lodged in the pharynx. Improvised pacifiers, such as those commonly made in hospitals from a padded nipple, also pose dangers because the nipple may separate from the plastic collar and be aspirated. Safe pacifiers are made of one piece that includes a shield or flange large enough to prevent entry into the mouth and a handle that can be grasped (Fig. 25-19).

Bathing, Cord Care, and Skin Care

Bathing serves a number of purposes. It provides opportunities for (1) completely cleansing the infant, (2) observing the infant's condition, (3) promoting comfort, and (4) parent-child-family socializing.

An important consideration in skin cleansing is preservation of the skin's acid mantle, which is formed from the uppermost horny layer of the epidermis, sweat, superficial fat, metabolic products, and external substances such as amniotic fluid and microorganisms. At birth, the skin has a pH of 6.4. Within 4 days, the pH of the newborn's skin surface falls to within the bacteriostatic range (pH less than 5) (Krebs, 1998). Consequently, only plain, warm water should be used for the bath during that 4-day period. Alkaline soaps (such as Ivory) and oils, powders, and lotions should not be used during this time because they alter the acid mantle, thus providing a medium for bacterial growth.

Although the sponging technique is generally used, bathing the newborn by immersion has been found to allow less heat loss and provoke less crying. Immersion bathing is now considered a safe alternative to sponge bathing provided the infant's condition is stable (no temperature instability, respiratory or cardiac illness) and he or she is dried off immediately thereafter and kept warm (Association of Women's Health, Obstetric and Neonatal Nurses, 2007). A daily bath is not necessary for achieving cleanliness and may do more harm by disrupting the integrity of the newborn's skin; cleansing the perineum after a soiled diaper and daily cleansing of the face may suffice.

Until the initial bath is completed, personnel must wear gloves to handle the newborn.

The umbilical cord begins to dry, shrivel, and blacken by the second or third day of life depending in part on the cleansing method used. The umbilicus should be inspected often for signs of infection (e.g., foul odor, redness, and purulent discharge), granuloma (i.e., small, red, raw-appearing polyp where the umbilical cord separates), bleeding, and discharge. The cord clamp is removed when the cord is dry, in about 24 to 36 hours (see Fig. 25-4). The cord normally falls off 10 to 14 days after birth but may remain attached for as long as 3 weeks in some cases. Parents are instructed in appropriate home cord care (per practitioner or institution protocol) and the expected time of cord separation.

The Home Care box contains information regarding bathing, skin care, cord care, cutting nails, and dressing the infant.

Infant Follow-Up Care

With shorter hospital stays, the focus and site of infant care are changing. Home care may be provided either by a nurse as part of the routine follow-up care of patients, or through a visiting nurse or community health nurse referral service. For infants discharged early, newborn home care is essential (see Home Care box; see also Chapter 3).

Parents should plan for their child's follow-up health care at the following ages: within 2 or 3 days if early discharge to check for status of jaundice, feeding, and elimination (see also Physiologic Jaundice, p. 653, for follow-up guidelines); at 2 to 4 weeks of age; then every 2 months until 6 to 7 months of age; then every 3 months until 18 months; at 2 years; at 3 years; at preschool; and every 2 years thereafter.

Immunizations

The schedule for immunizations should be reviewed with the parents. Hepatitis B vaccine is currently administered to newborns before hospital discharge (depending on maternal hepatitis B status) or within 1 month of birth. See Chapter 36 for a complete discussion of infant immunizations.

HOME CARE

Newborn Bath

Fit Baths into the Family Schedule

Give a bath at any time convenient to you, but not immediately after a feeding period because the increased handling may cause regurgitation.

Prevent Heat Loss

The temperature of the room should be no cooler than 24° C (75.2 ° F), and the bathing area should be free of drafts.

Control heat loss during the bath to conserve the infant's energy. Bathing the infant quickly, exposing only a portion of the body at a time, and thoroughly drying the infant are all important parts of the bathing technique.

Gather Supplies and Clothing Before Starting

Clothing suitable for wearing indoors: diaper, shirt; stretch suit or nightgown optional

Towels for drying infant and a clean washcloth

Receiving blanket

Tub for water (Fill with only 3 to 4 inches of water.)

Bathe the Baby

Bring infant to bathing area when all supplies are ready.

***Never* leave the infant alone on bath table or in bath water, not even for a second! If you have to leave, take the infant with you or put back into crib.**

Test temperature of the water. It should feel pleasantly warm to the inner wrist (36.6° to 37.2° C [97.8° to 98.9° F]).

Do not hold infant under running water—water temperature may change, and infant may be scalded or chilled rapidly.

Use a mild, unscented, pH-neutral (5.5 to 7.0) soap or cleanser.

Wash infant's hair after body to prevent heat loss from prolonged exposure to cold (scalp loses heat rapidly due to size). You may wash face, neck, and ears first.

Cleanse the eyes from the inner canthus outward, using separate parts of a clean washcloth for each eye. For the first 2 or 3 days, there may be a discharge resulting from the reaction of the conjunctiva to the ointment (erythromycin) used as a prophylactic measure against infection. Any discharge should be considered abnormal and reported to the health care provider.

Wash the scalp with warm water and mild soap; dry thoroughly. Scalp desquamation, called *cradle cap,* often can be prevented by removing any scales with a fine-toothed comb or brush after washing. If condition persists, notify the health care provider.

Creases under the chin and arms and in the groin may need daily cleansing. The crease under the chin may be exposed by elevating the infant's shoulders 5 cm and letting the head drop back.

Cleanse ears and nose with twists of moistened cotton or a corner of the washcloth. Do not use cotton-tipped swabs because they may cause injury.

Undress baby and wash body, arms, and legs. Pat dry gently.

Prevent Skin Trauma

The fragile skin can be injured by too vigorous cleansing.

If stool or other debris has dried and caked on the skin, soak the area to remove it. Do not attempt to rub it off, since abrasion may result.

Being gentle, patting dry rather than rubbing, and using a mild soap without perfumes or coloring are recommended. Chemicals in the coloring and perfume can cause rashes on sensitive skin.

Care of the Cord

With a washcloth cleanse around base of the cord where it joins the skin. Notify the health care provider of any discharge or skin inflammation around the cord.

Because the cord skin essentially necroses (dies), there will be a slight odor until the cord falls off; however, any discharge or redness should be reported to the practitioner.

The clamp is usually removed before the newborn is discharged from the birth center (approximately 24 hours).

The diaper should not cover the cord because a wet or soiled diaper will slow or prevent drying of the cord and foster infection.

When the cord drops off after 10 to 15 days, small drops of blood may be seen when the baby cries. This will heal by itself. It is not dangerous.

Care of Hands and Feet

Wash and dry between the fingers and toes.

Use caution cutting the nails—use blunt scissors. The nails have to grow out far enough from the skin so that the skin is not cut by mistake. If the baby scratches himself or herself, you may apply loosely fitted mitts (or baby socks) over each of the baby's hands. Nails should be kept short.

Cleanse Genitalia

Cleanse the infant's genitalia daily and after voiding or defecating.

For girls, the genitalia may be cleansed by separating the labia and gently washing from the pubic area to the anus.

For uncircumcised boys, do not force (retract) the foreskin. Stop when resistance is felt. Wash and rinse the tip (glans) with soap and warm water and replace the foreskin. The foreskin must be returned to its original position to prevent constriction and swelling. In most newborns, the inner layer of the foreskin adheres to the glans and the foreskin cannot be retracted. By age 3 years in 90% of boys, the foreskin can be retracted easily without causing pain or trauma. For others, the foreskin is not retractable until adolescence. As soon as the foreskin is partly retractable and the child is old enough, he can be taught self-care.

Once healed, the circumcised penis does not require any special care other than cleansing with diaper changes.

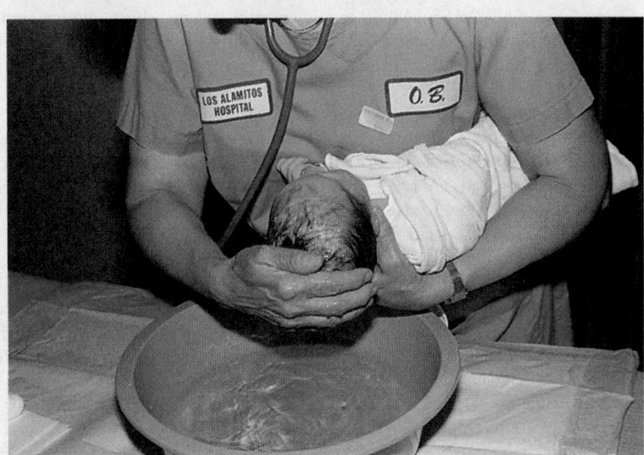

Wash hair with baby wrapped to prevent heat loss from wet scalp. *(Courtesy Marjorie Pyle, RNC, Lifecircle, Costa Mesa, CA.)*

evolve Skill—Infant Bathing

HOME CARE

*Newborn Home Care After Early Discharge**

Wet diapers—One wet diaper for each day of life until fifth to sixth day; then 6 to 10 per day.

Breastfeeding—Successful latch-on and feeding 10 to 12 times a day (24-hour period). Audible swallowing should be evident.

Formula feeding—Successfully, voiding as above, taking 2 to 3 oz (approximately) on demand or at least every 4 hours.

Circumcision—Wash with warm water only; yellow exudate forming, nonbleeding.

Stools—At least one soft stool every 48 to 72 hours (bottle-feeding), or two or three per day (breastfeeding).

Color—Pink to ruddy when crying; pink centrally when at rest or asleep.

Activity—Four or five wakeful periods per day; alerts to environmental sounds and voices.

Jaundice—Physiologic jaundice (not appearing in first 24 hours), feeding, voiding, and stooling as noted above. Notify practitioner of suspicion of pathologic jaundice (appears within 24 hours of birth; ABO/Rh problem suspected), decreased activity, poor feeding, or dark orange skin color persisting after the fifth day in light-skinned newborn. Obtain transcutaneous bilirubin levels before discharge and identify risk per hour-specific risk nomogram (see Fig. 25-7).

Cord—Kept above diaper line; nonodorous; drying.

Vital signs—Heart rate 120 to 140 beats/min at rest; respiratory rate 30 to 55 breath/min at rest without evidence of sternal retractions, grunting, or nasal flaring; temperature 36.5° to 37.2° C (97.7° to 99° F) axillary.

Position of sleep—On back.

From Hockenberry MJ, Wilson D: *Wong's nursing care of infants and children*, ed 8, St Louis, 2007, Mosby.

*Any deviation from the above or suspicion of poor newborn adaptation should be reported to the practitioner at once.

Key Points

- Assessment of the newborn requires data from the prenatal, intrapartum, and postnatal periods.
- Knowledge of biologic and behavioral characteristics is essential for guiding assessment and interpreting data.
- Providing a protective environment is a key responsibility of the nurse and includes such measures as careful identification procedures, protection from abduction, support of physiologic functions, and measures to prevent infection.
- Maintenance of adequate ventilation includes ensuring an open airway and body temperature within the normal range.

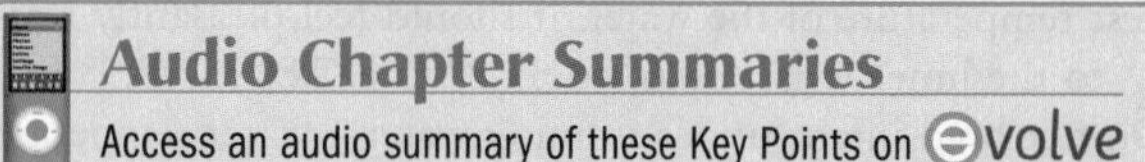
Audio Chapter Summaries
Access an audio summary of these Key Points on evolve

- Parent education is a major responsibility of the nurse and includes involvement of parents in all phases of the nursing process.
- The newborn has social as well as physical needs.
- Circumcision is an elective surgical procedure.
- Parents appreciate anticipatory guidance in the care of the newborn.

References

Alexander GR et al: A United States national reference for fetal growth, *Obstet Gynecol* 87(2):163-168, 1996.

American Academy of Pediatrics: AAP publications retired and reaffirmed, *Pediatrics* 116(3):796, 2005.

American Academy of Pediatrics, Committee on Infectious Diseases: *Red book: 2006 report of the Committee on Infectious Diseases*, ed 27, Elk Grove Village, IL, 2006, The Academy.

American Academy of Pediatrics, Subcommittee on Hyperbilirubinemia: Clinical practice guideline: management of hyperbilirubinemia in the newborn infant 35 or more weeks of gestation, *Pediatrics* 114(1):297-316, 2004.

American Academy of Pediatrics, Task Force on Circumcision: Circumcision policy statement, *Pediatrics* 103(3):686-693, 1999.

American Academy of Pediatrics, Task Force on Sudden Infant Death Syndrome: The changing concept of sudden infant death syndrome: diagnostic coding shifts, controversies regarding the sleeping environment, and new variables to consider in reducing risk, *Pediatrics* 116(5):1245-1255, 2005.

American Academy of Pediatrics, American College of Obstetricians and Gynecologists: *Guidelines for perinatal care*, ed 6, Elk Grove Village, IL, 2007, The Academy.

Anand KJS, International Evidence-Based Group for Neonatal Pain: Consensus statement for the prevention and management of pain in the newborn, *Arch Pediatr Adolesc Med* 155(2):173-179, 2001.

Arbuckle T, Wilkins R, Sherman G: Birth weight percentiles by gestational age in Canada, *Obstet Gynecol* 81(1):39-48, 1993.

Association of Women's Health, Obstetric and Neonatal Nurses: *Neonatal skin care: evidence-based clinical practice guideline*, ed 2, Washington, DC, 2007, The Association.

Bakewell-Sachs S: Near-term/late preterm infants, *Newborn Infant Nurs Rev* 7(2):67-71, 2007.

Ballard J, Novak K, Driver M: A simplified score for assessment of fetal maturity of newly born infants, *J Pediatr* 95(5 Pt 1):769-774, 1979.

Ballard J et al: New Ballard score, expanded to include extremely premature infants, *J Pediatr* 119(3):417-423, 1991.

Battaglia FC, Lubchenco LO: A practical classification of newborn infants by weight and gestational age, *J Pediatr* 71(2):159-161, 1967.

Bhutani VK, Johnson L, Sivieri EM: Predictive ability of a predischarge hour-specific serum bilirubin for subsequent significant hyperbilirubinemia in healthy term and near-term newborns, *Pediatrics* 103(1):6-14, 1999.

Blackburn ST: *Maternal, fetal, and neonatal physiology: a clinical perspective*, ed 3, St Louis, 2007, Saunders.

Blain-Lewis N: Comparative studies of bruising and healing after heelstick, *Neonatal Intensive Care* 5(5):18-21, 1992.

Blass EM, Watt LB: Suckling- and sucrose-induced analgesia in human newborns, *Pain* 83(3):611-623, 1999.

Brady-Fryer B, Wiebe N, Lander JA: Pain relief for newborn circumcision, *Cochrane Database Syst Rev* (4):CD004217, 2004.

Bull M, Engle WA, Committee on Injury, Violence, and Poison Prevention and Committee on Fetus and Newborn, American Academy of Pediatrics: Safe transportation of preterm and low birth weight infants at hospital discharge, *Pediatrics* 123(5):1424-1429, 2009.

Butt ML, Kisilevsky BS: Music modulates behaviour of premature infants following heel lance, *Can J Nurs Res* 31(4):17-39, 2000.

Carbajal R et al: Analgesic effect of breast feeding in term neonates: randomized controlled trial, *BMJ* 326(7379):13, 2003.

Cornblath M et al: Controversies regarding operational definition of neonatal hypoglycemia: suggested thresholds, *Pediatrics* 105(5):1141-1145, 2000.

Cunningham FG et al (editors): *Williams obstetrics*, ed 22, New York, 2005, McGraw-Hill.

Engle WA et al: "Late-preterm" infants: a population at risk, *Pediatrics* 120(6):1390-1401, 2007.

Engle WD et al: Assessment of a transcutaneous device in the evaluation of neonatal hyperbilirubinemia in a primarily Hispanic population, *Pediatrics* 110(1 Pt 1):61-67, 2002.

Eriksson M, Finnstrom O: Can daily repeated doses of orally administered glucose induce tolerance when given for neonatal pain relief? *Acta Paediatr* 93(2):246-249, 2004.

Fitzgerald M, Millard C, McIntosh N: Cutaneous hypersensitivity following peripheral tissue damage in newborn infants and its reversal with topical anaesthesia, *Pain* 3(1):31-36, 1989.

Gartner LM, Herschel M: The management of breastfeeding, part 2: Jaundice and breastfeeding, *Pediatr Clin North Am* 48(2):389-400, 2001.

Geyer J et al: An evidence-based multidisciplinary protocol for neonatal circumcision pain management, *J Obstet Gynecol Neonatal Nurs* 31(4):403-410, 2002.

Gibbins S et al: Efficacy and safety of sucrose for procedural pain relief in preterm and term neonates, *Nurs Res* 51(6):375-382, 2002.

Golombek SG, Brill PE, Salice AL: Randomized trial of alcohol versus triple dye for umbilical cord care, *Clin Pediatr* 41(6):419-423, 2002.

Gradin M et al: Pain reduction at venipuncture in newborns: oral glucose compared with local anesthetic cream, *Pediatrics* 110(6):1053-1057, 2002.

Gray L, Watt L, Blass EM: Skin-to-skin contact is analgesic in healthy newborns, *Pediatrics* 105(1):110-111, 2000. Available at www.pediatrics.org/cgi/content/full/105/1/e14 (accessed August 22, 2004).

Grunau RE et al: Does prone or supine position influence pain responses in preterm infants at 32 weeks gestational age? *Clin J Pain* 20(2):76-82, 2004.

Hagedorn ME: Respiratory distress. In Merenstein GB, Gardner SL (editors): *Handbook of neonatal intensive care*, ed 6, St Louis, 2006, Mosby.

Haouari N et al: The analgesic effect of sucrose in full-term infants: a randomised controlled trial, *BMJ* 310(6993):1498-1500, 1995.

Harrison D, Johnston L, Loughnan P: Oral sucrose for procedural pain in sick hospitalized infants: a randomized-controlled trial, *J Paediatr Child Health* 39(8):591-597, 2003.

Hjelle JJ, Grauer GF: Acetaminophen-induced toxicosis in dogs and cats, *J Am Vet Med Assoc* 188(7):742-749, 1986.

Hoseth E et al: Blood glucose levels in a population of healthy, breast fed, term infants of appropriate size for gestational age, *Arch Dis Child Fetal Neonatal Educ* 83(2):F117-F119, 2000.

Huang CM et al: Comparison of pain responses of premature infants to the heelstick between containment and swaddling, *J Nurs Res* 12(1):31-40, 2004.

Ip S et al: An evidence-based review on important issues concerning neonatal hyperbilirubinemia, *Pediatrics* 114 (1):e130-e153, 2004.

Janssen PA et al: To dye or not to dye: a randomized, clinical trial of a triple dye/alcohol regimen versus dry cord care, *Pediatrics* 111(1):15-20, 2003.

Johnston CC et al: Kangaroo care is effective in diminishing pain response in preterm neonates, *Arch Pediatr Adolesc Med* 157(11):1084-1088, 2003.

Keren R et al: A comparison of alternative risk-assessment strategies for predicting significant neonatal hyperbilirubinemia in term and near-term infants, *Pediatrics* 121(1):e170-e179, 2008.

Kramer MS et al: A new and improved population-based Canadian reference for birth weight for gestational age, *Pediatrics* 108(2):e35, 462, 2001.

Krebs T: Cord care: is it necessary? *Mother Baby J* 3(2):5-12, 18-20, 1998.

Leitch D: Mother-infant interaction: achieving synchrony, *Nurs Res* 48(1):55-58, 1999.

Madan A et al: Racial differences in birth weight of term infants in a northern California population, *J Perinatol* 22(3):230-235, 2002.

Maisels MJ: Jaundice. In MacDonald MG, Mullett MD, Seshia MM (editors): *Neonatology: pathophysiology and management of the newborn*, ed 6, Philadelphia, 2005, Lippincott.

McConnell TP et al: Trends in umbilical cord care: scientific evidence for practice, *Newborn Infant Nurs Rev* 4(4):211-222, 2004.

Meehan R: Heelsticks in neonates for capillary blood sampling, *Neonatal Netw* 17(1):17-24, 1998.

Mincey H, Gonzaba G: End tidal carbon monoxide: a new method to detect hyperbilirubinemia in newborns, *Newborn Infant Nurs Rev* 7(2):122-128, 2007.

MMWR Weekly: Impact of expanded newborn screening—United States, 2006, *MMWR Weekly* 57(37):1012-1015, 2008.

Noerr B: Sucrose for neonatal procedural pain, *Neonatal Netw* 20(7):63-67, 2001.

Paes B et al: A comparative study of heel-stick devices for infant blood collection, *Am J Dis Child* 147(3):346-348, 1993.

Porter ML, Dennis BL: Hyperbilirubinemia in the term newborn, *Am Fam Physician* 65(4):599-606, 613-614, 2002.

Prescott LF: *Paracetamol (acetaminophen): a critical bibliographic review*, Bristol, UK, 1996, Taylor & Francis.

Razmus IS, Dalton ME, Wilson D: Pain management for newborn circumcision, *Pediatr Nurs* 30(5):414-417, 427, 2004.

Schultze A et al: Expanded newborn screening for inborn errors of metabolism by electrospray ionization–tandem mass spectrometer: results, outcomes, and implications, *Pediatrics* 111(6):1399-1406, 2003.

Serour F, Mandelberg A, Mori J: Slow injection of local anesthetic will decrease pain during dorsal penile nerve block, *Acta Anaesthesiol Scand* 42(8):926-928, 1998.

Shah V, Ohlsson A: Venepuncture versus heel lance for blood sampling in term neonates, *Cochrane Database Syst Rev* (2):CD001452, 2001.

Sharfstein JM et al: Over the counter but no longer under the radar: pediatric cough and cold medications, *N Engl J Med* 357(23):2321-2324, 2007.

Smith DP, Gjellum M: The efficacy of LMX versus EMLA for pain relief in boys undergoing office meatotomy, *J Urol* 172(4 Pt 2):1760-1761, 2004.

Stang HJ et al: Beyond dorsal penile nerve block: a more humane circumcision, *Pediatrics* 100(2):E3, 1997.

Steffensrud S: Hyperbilirubinemia in term and near-term infants: kernicterus on the rise? *Newborn Infant Nurs Rev* 4(4):191-200, 2004.

Stevens B, Yamada J, Ohlsson A: Sucrose for analgesia in newborn infants undergoing painful procedures, *Cochrane Database Syst Rev* (3):CD001069, 2004.

Stevens B et al: Management of pain from heel lance with lidocaine-prilocaine (EMLA) cream: is it safe and efficacious in preterm infants? *J Dev Behav Pediatr* 20(4):216-221, 1999.

Stoll BJ: The fetus and the neonatal infant. In Kliegman RM et al (editors): *Nelson textbook of pediatrics*, ed 18, Philadelphia, 2007, Saunders.

Taddio A et al: Conditioning and hyperalgesia in newborns exposed to repeated heel lances, *JAMA* 288(7):857-861, 2002.

Taddio A et al: Combined analgesia and local anesthesia to minimize pain during circumcision, *Arch Pediatr Adolesc Med* 154(5):620-623, 2000.

Taddio A et al: A systematic review of lidocaine-prilocaine cream (EMLA) in the treatment of acute pain in neonates, *Pediatrics* 101(2):e1, 1998. Available at www.pediatrics.org/cgi/content/full/101/2/e1 (accessed August 22, 2004).

Thomas P et al: A new look at intrauterine growth and the impact of race, altitude, and gender, *Pediatrics* 106(2):e21, 2000.

Visscher MO et al: Vernix caseosa in neonatal adaptation, *J Perinatol* 25(7):440-446, 2005.

Wong D: Topical local anesthetics: two products for pain relief during minor procedures, *AJN* 103(6):42-45, 2003.

Zupan J, Garner P, Omari AA: Topical umbilical cord care at birth, *Cochrane Database Syst Rev* (3):CD001057, 2004.

Unit 6

26 Newborn Nutrition and Feeding

Learning Objectives

On completion of this chapter the reader will be able to:

- Describe current recommendations for infant feeding.
- Discuss benefits of breastfeeding for infants, mothers, families, and society.
- Describe the nutritional needs of newborns.
- List newborn feeding readiness cues.
- Describe the anatomy and physiology of breastfeeding.
- Identify nursing interventions to facilitate and promote successful breastfeeding.
- List signs of adequate intake in the breastfed infant.
- Identify common problems associated with breastfeeding and nursing interventions to help resolve them.
- Discuss patient teaching for the family who is formula-feeding their newborn.

Electronic Resources

Additional information related to the content in Chapter 26 can be found on

evolve the Companion Website at

http://evolve.elsevier.com/Perry/maternal/

- NCLEX Review Questions
- Case Study—Breastfeeding
- Critical Thinking Exercise—Breastfeeding
- Critical Thinking Exercise—Formula Preparation
- Nursing Care Plan—Breastfeeding and Infant Nutrition
- Nursing Care Plan—The Newborn with Insufficient Intake of Nutrients
- Skill—Infant Feeding
- Spanish Guidelines—Breastfeeding: Latching On
- Spanish Guidelines—Burping

Good nutrition in infancy fosters optimal growth and development. Infant feeding is more than the provision of nutrition; it represents an opportunity for social and psychologic interaction between parent and infant. It can also establish a basis for development of good eating habits and influence lifelong health habits. The health supervision of infants requires knowledge of their nutritional needs. This chapter primarily focuses on meeting nutritional needs for normal growth and development from birth to 6 months of age, with an emphasis on the neonatal period, when feeding practices and patterns are established. Both breastfeeding and formula-feeding are addressed.

Recommended Infant Nutrition

The American Academy of Pediatrics, Section on Breastfeeding (2005), recommends that infants be breastfed exclusively for the first 6 months of life and that breastfeeding continue for at least 12 months. If infants are weaned before 12 months, they should receive iron-fortified infant formula. *Healthy People 2010* goals include that 75% of women will breastfeed at birth, 50% will breastfeed for 6 months, and 25% will continue to breastfeed to 1 year of age (Department of Health and Human Services, 2000). Data from the 2003 Ross Mothers Survey indicate that the overall rate of breastfeeding in the hospital was 66%, down four points from 2002 (70.1%); breastfeeding at 6 months of age in 2003 was reported to be 32.8%, down slightly from the previous year (33.2%) (Ross Mothers Survey, 2003). The Centers for Disease Control and Prevention (2007) analyzed data from the National Immunization Survey and found that, among infants born in 2004, 30.5% and 11.3% were exclusively breastfeeding at 3 and 6 months, respectively. Both surveys found similar disparities in breastfeeding rates: lower breastfeeding rates at 6 months occurred in African-American women and in women without a college degree. Full-time employment at 6 months was a strong contributing factor to the decrease in breastfeeding, and enrollment in the Women, Infants, and Children (WIC) program was also found to have a negative impact on the initiation of breastfeeding in the hospital (55.2% for non-WIC vs. 32.3% for WIC participants) (Ross Mothers Survey, 2003).

Benefits of Breastfeeding

Human milk is designed specifically for human infants and is nutritionally superior to any alternative. Breast milk is considered a living tissue because it contains almost as many live cells as blood. It is bacteriologically safe and is always fresh. The nutrients in breast milk are more easily absorbed than those in formula.

Benefits of breastfeeding for the infant include the following:

- Breast milk enhances maturation of the gastrointestinal tract and contains immune factors that contribute to a lower incidence of gastroenteritis, neonatal necrotizing enterocolitis, lymphoma, childhood obesity, Crohn's disease, and celiac disease (Barnard, 1997; Grummer-Strawn, Mei, & Centers for Disease Control and Prevention Pediatric Nutrition Surveillance System, 2004; Scariati, Grummer-Strawn, & Fein, 1997).
- Breastfed infants receive specific antibodies and cell-mediated immunologic factors that help protect against otitis media, respiratory illnesses such as respiratory syncytial virus and pneumonia, urinary tract infections, bacteremia, and bacterial meningitis (Bachrach, Schwarz, & Bachrach, 2003; Cushing et al, 1998; Hanson & Korotkova, 2002).
- There is a lower incidence of certain allergies among breastfed infants from families at high risk. Atopic dermatitis is reduced by 42% among infants breastfed for at least 3 months (in children with a family history of atopy). Allergic manifestations occur at a greater rate and are more severe in formula-fed infants (Halken & Host, 1996; Ip et al, 2007).
- Breastfed infants are less likely to die from sudden infant death syndrome (SIDS) (Ford et al, 1993).
- Breast milk may have a protective effect against childhood lymphoma and type 1 and type 2 diabetes mellitus (Davis, 1998; Gerstein, 1994; Ip et al, 2007).
- Breast milk may enhance cognitive development for term and preterm infants (Anderson, Johnstone, & Remley, 1999; Horwood & Fergusson, 1998; Kramer et al, 2008; Vohr et al, 2006).
- Breastfeeding appears to have an analgesic effect for infants undergoing painful procedures such as venipuncture and heel stick (Carbajal et al, 2003; Gray et al, 2002).

Maternal benefits include the following:

- Women who have breastfed have a decreased risk of ovarian cancer, uterine cancer, rheumatoid arthritis, and breast cancer (Enger et al, 1998; Pikwer et al, 2009; Rosenblatt & Thomas, 1995).
- Breastfeeding promotes uterine involution and is associated with a decreased risk of postpartum hemorrhage (Lawrence & Lawrence, 2005).
- Mothers who are breastfeeding tend to return to their prepregnancy weight more quickly (Dewey, Heinig, & Nommsen, 1993).
- Breastfeeding may provide some protection against the development of osteoporosis and risk for hip fractures (Eisman, 1998).
- Breastfeeding provides a unique bonding experience, increases maternal role attainment (Lawrence & Lawrence, 2005), and may provide protection against postpartum depression when breastfeeding difficulties are appropriately addressed (Kendall-Tackett, 2007).

Benefits to families and society include the following:

- Breastfeeding is convenient; there are no bottles or other equipment to purchase, clean, or dispose of (benefit to community by not having to dispose of formula bottles and equipment used in manufacture).
- Breastfed babies are portable; when traveling, there are fewer supplies to take along.
- Parental absenteeism from work is decreased.
- Breastfeeding saves money. The cost of formula far exceeds the cost of extra food for the lactating mother. Breastfeeding families who are eligible for the Special Supplemental Nutrition Program for WIC represent a cost savings to the government. Because breastfed babies have a lower incidence of illness and infection, health care costs are lower for families and federal, state, and local governments.

Contraindications to Breastfeeding

Contraindications to breastfeeding include the following (American Academy of Pediatrics, Section on Breastfeeding, 2005):

- Maternal cancer therapy or diagnostic and therapeutic radioactive isotopes
- Active tuberculosis not under treatment in mother
- Human immunodeficiency virus (HIV) infection in mother
- Maternal herpes simplex lesion on a breast
- Galactosemia (classic) in infant
- Cytomegalovirus (CMV)—a primary risk to preterm infants receiving CMV-infected donor milk, not to infected mother's infant, who already has CMV
- Maternal substance abuse (e.g., cocaine, methamphetamines, marijuana)
- Maternal human T-cell leukemia virus type 1
- Some medications that may exert an untoward effect on the breastfeeding infant; require consultation of the practitioner and available references such as Hale (2008) or American Academy of Pediatrics, Committee on Drugs (2001)

Conditions that are not considered contraindications to breastfeeding include maternal infection with hepatitis C, hepatitis B surface antigen (HBsAg)–positive status, maternal fever and mothers who are CMV positive (American Academy of Pediatrics, Section on Breastfeeding, 2005).

Choosing an Infant Feeding Method

Women who elect to breastfeed usually do so because they are aware of the benefits to the infant. Many seek the unique bonding experience between mother and infant that is characteristic of breastfeeding. The support of her partner and family is a major factor in a mother's decision to breastfeed and in her ability to do so successfully. Prenatal preparation ideally includes the woman' s partner, providing information about the benefits of breastfeeding and how he or she can participate in infant care and nurturing.

Prenatal breastfeeding classes are an excellent vehicle to relay important information to expectant parents. Each encounter with an expectant mother is an opportunity to dispel myths, clarify misinformation, and address personal concerns. Connecting expectant mothers with women who are breastfeeding or who have successfully breastfed and are from similar backgrounds may be helpful. Peer counseling programs, such as those instituted by WIC and La Leche League, are beneficial, particularly in low socioeconomic

BOX 26-1 Guidelines for Breastfeeding Support

During pregnancy, a breast assessment is performed that includes a breastfeeding history, a breast examination, and a medication use history.

A prenatal care plan is developed to prepare the woman for lactation.

Immediately after birth, the newborn is kept with the mother when possible so that breastfeeding can be initiated when the newborn is most receptive.

After birth, the nurse:

- Assists with latch-on and positioning as needed
- Reinforces the need for frequent feedings
- Gives discharge instructions for recognizing signs of successful breastfeeding
- Provides information about community resources for breastfeeding
- Encourages breastfeeding, especially for preterm and low-birth-weight infants

Adapted from Association of Women's Health, Obstetric and Neonatal Nurses: *Standards and guidelines for professional nursing practice in the care of women and newborns*, ed 6, Washington, DC, 2003, The Association.

groups where bottle-feeding is common. To provide effective support for the mother, health care professionals must be knowledgeable about the benefits of breastfeeding, the basic process of breastfeeding, breastfeeding management, and interventions for common problems (Box 26-1).

Cultural Influences on Infant Feeding

Cultural beliefs and practices are significant influences on infant feeding methods. As many as 50 of 120 cultures studied typically do not give colostrum to newborns and only begin breastfeeding after the milk has "come in." These groups include some Filipinos, Hispanics, Vietnamese, Hmong, Koreans, and Nigerians. When breastfeeding is delayed until the milk is in, babies are given prelacteal food. In India, infants may be fed liquids such as honey, tea, water, or sugar water before the initiation of breastfeeding (Choudhry, 1997). Other cultures begin breastfeeding immediately and offer the breast each time the infant cries. Cultural attitudes regarding modesty and breastfeeding are important considerations. Language barriers may also prevent successful breastfeeding and counseling in some situations. Even among Hispanic Spanish-speaking people, terminology used in one country for the act of breastfeeding or describing the breasts may be offensive in another Spanish-speaking country.

Hernandez (2006) suggests that knowledge of the Hispanic woman's immigration status is important when discussing breastfeeding; U.S.-born Hispanic women are less likely to initiate breastfeeding, whereas those recently immigrated are more likely to continue the social norm of breastfeeding. Breastfeeding classes in Spanish for the new mother and grandmother may enhance discussion of practices related to exclusive breastfeeding in the first few months (Hernandez, 2006). Mexican women have a custom called *la cuarentena*, which means the woman has 40 days of rest after giving birth; during this time the mother is relieved of housekeeping duties and may focus on the new infant. The maternal grandmother traditionally assists the mother during this time. Other Hispanic customs related to infant feeding include the belief in herbal teas consumed by the breastfeeding mother to settle the infant's stomach; commonly given teas include *manzanilla* (chamomile) and anise. In Hispanic families the practice of the breastfeeding mother consuming traditional cultural foods to acculturate the infant to such foods is common (Hernandez, 2006).

The Muslim and Jewish cultures value breastfeeding of infants. Muslim women also have the tradition of the 40-day rest period in which the woman is relieved of housekeeping duties and other women help care for her. During this time the mother may exclusively breastfeed; however, Muslim women typically terminate exclusive breastfeeding early in infancy (Chertok, Shoham-Vardi, & Hallak, 2004). Breastfeeding for Jewish women is perceived as being important but is highly influenced by maternal education level, assimilated cultural values depending on geographic region of origin, and previous breastfeeding experience (Chertok, Shoham-Vardi, & Hallak, 2004).

With the large percentage of immigrants in the United States, it is incumbent on nurses to discuss cultural values related to breastfeeding and the benefits of breastfeeding so the mother can make an informed decision based on this knowledge. Hernandez (2006) relates the story of a young Mexican woman who delivered an infant in the United States but started bottle-feeding instead of breastfeeding. When asked about this, she told the nurse that since there was a packet of formula in the infant's crib at discharge, she interpreted this as the cultural norm in the United States and did not breastfeed. The nursing implications are clear: clarify with the mother what her expectations are regarding infant feeding and assist her in meeting those goals.

Sociocultural values may preclude the mother receiving adequate information regarding breastfeeding; for example, if the family is strongly patriarchal and the father is the only English-speaking person in the family, the necessary information being conveyed to the mother by the health care provider may not be correctly translated. Persons immigrating to the United States often tend to acquire the local customs, and, although breastfeeding may have been common in their own country, they may abandon the practice in the United States, considering it "outdated" (Riordan & Gill-Hopple, 2001).

Nutrient Needs

Energy

Infants require adequate caloric intake to provide energy for growth, digestion, physical activity, and maintenance of organ metabolic function. It is estimated that the average energy intake in a breastfeeding infant is 500 kcal/day (based on average milk intake of 0.78 L/day) (Institute of Medicine, 2005). For the first 3 months, the infant needs approximately 110 kcal/kg/day. From 3 months to 6 months, the requirement decreases to approximately 100 kcal/kg/day. This decreases slightly to 95 kcal/kg/day from 6 to 9 months, and increases to 100 kcal/kg/day from 9 months to 1 year.

Human milk provides approximately 67 kcal/dl or 20 kcal/oz; the greatest amount of energy is provided by the fat content of breast milk. Infant formulas are made to simulate the caloric content of human milk; standard formulas for healthy term infants contain 20 kcal/oz.

Carbohydrate

Because newborns have only small hepatic glycogen stores, carbohydrates should provide at least 40% to 45% of the total calories in the diet. Moreover, newborns may have limited ability for gluconeogenesis (formation of glucose from amino acids and other substrates) and ketogenesis (formation of ketone bodies from fat), which are mechanisms that provide alternative energy sources.

As the primary carbohydrate in human milk (approximately 75 g/L), lactose is the most abundant carbohydrate in the diet of infants up to 6 months of age. Lactose provides calories in an easily available form; its slow breakdown and absorption probably also increase calcium absorption. Corn syrup solids or glucose polymers are added to infant formulas to supplement the lactose in cow's milk and provide sufficient carbohydrates.

The Dietary Reference Intake Adequate Intake (DRI AI) for carbohydrate is 60 g/day in the first 6 months of life and 95 g/day for the next 6 months (Institute of Medicine, 2005).

Fat

For infants to acquire adequate calories from the limited amount of human milk or formula they are able to consume, at least 15% of the calories provided must come from fat (triglycerides). Fat is the major source of energy in the diet of the infant fed human milk. The fat must be easily digestible. Fat in human milk is easier to digest and absorb than that in cow's milk because of the arrangement of the fatty acids on the glycerol molecule and because of the presence of the enzyme lipase. The DRI AI for fat is 31 g/day, which reflects those infants fed human milk in the first 6 months of life (Institute of Medicine, 2005).

Modified cow's milk is used to make most infant formulas, but the milk fat is removed and replaced by another fat source, such as corn oil, that can be easily digested and absorbed by the infant. If whole milk or evaporated milk without added carbohydrate is fed to infants, the resulting fecal loss of fat (and therefore loss of energy) may be excessive because the milk moves through the infant's intestines too quickly for adequate absorption to take place. This can lead to poor weight gain. There is evidence that whole milk may also increase the infant's chances for developing allergies from cow's milk protein exposure.

In addition to its energy contributions, fat also furnishes essential fatty acids (EFAs), which are required for growth and tissue maintenance. EFAs are components of cell membranes and precursors of some hormones. Inadequate intake of EFAs results in eczema and growth failure. The lack of EFAs in skim and low-fat milk is another reason infants should not be fed these products.

In recent years the discovery of long-chain polyunsaturated fatty acids (LCPUFA) in human milk has led to the addition of arachidonic acid (ARA) and docosahexaenoic acid (DHA) to formula, both of which are considered important in the infant's growth, neurodevelopment, and visual function (Fleith & Clandinin, 2005; Morin, 2004). Studies in full-term infants receiving supplements with DHA and ARA have produced mixed results regarding cognitive function and visual acuity (Heird, 2007; Simmer, Patole, & Rao, 2008). LCPUFAs are available from a variety of sources, including egg yolk lipid, phospholipids, and triglyceride. The evidence for supplementation of formula for preterm infants with LCPUFAs, however, has been more convincing, producing some transient improvement in visual acuity and general development (American Academy of Pediatrics, 2009).

Protein

The protein requirement per unit of body weight is greater in the newborn than at any other time of life. The protein content of human milk, which is lower than that of unmodified cow's milk, is ideal for the newborn. Human milk contains far more lactalbumin (or whey protein) in relation to casein than does cow's milk, and lactalbumin is more easily digested than casein. In addition, the amino acid composition of human milk is suited to the newborn's metabolic capabilities. For example, phenylalanine and methionine levels are low, and cystine and taurine levels are high. The protein in some commercial formulas is modified to increase the amount of lactalbumin and to decrease the relative proportion of casein to more closely approximate human milk. The concentration of protein in infant formula is 1.45 to 1.6 g/dl (American Academy of Pediatrics, 2009). The DRI AI for protein is 1.52 g/kg/day (Institute of Medicine, 2005).

Water

The water requirement for healthy term infants is about 75 to 100 ml/kg/24 hr (Heird, 2007). The DRI for water intake for the 0- to 6-month-old infant is 700 ml/24 hr; for the 7- to 12-month-old, the DRI requirement is 800 ml/24 hr. Neither breastfed nor formula-fed infants, even those living in hot climates, need to be fed supplemental water. Breast milk contains 87% water, which easily meets fluid requirements. Feeding water to infants may cause water toxicity with resulting hyponatremia and seizures. Infants have little room for fluctuation in fluid balance and should be monitored closely for fluid intake and water loss if certain illness factors exist. Infants lose water through excretion of urine and through insensible losses such as respiration. Most healthy infants take in an adequate amount of fluid daily in either breast milk or commercial formula. Conditions that may lead to a decrease in oral intake and subsequent fluid deficit include gastroenteritis (vomiting and diarrhea), poor intake due to illness (congestive heart failure), or conditions affecting the mechanical process of eating (e.g., thrush, viral stomatitis, ankyloglossia [tight lingual frenulum], or poor latch-on early in breastfeeding). Juices are not necessary for proper nutrient intake. There is no evidence that juice intake provides better nutrients than human milk or fortified formula, but there are data indicating that excess juice consumption may replace essential elements, leading to nutritional deficits (American Academy of Pediatrics, Committee on Nutrition, 2001). Juices may also cause significant dental decay, especially when consumed from a bottle.

Vitamins

Human milk contains all the vitamins required for infant nutrition, with individual variations based on maternal diet and genetic differences. Vitamins are added to cow's milk formulas to approximate the levels in breast milk. Cow's milk contains adequate amounts of vitamin A and vitamin B complex; vitamin C (ascorbic acid) and vitamin E must be added.

Vitamin D is also added to commercial infant formulas. Because human milk is somewhat deficient in vitamin D (depending on maternal intake and metabolism) and to prevent vitamin D deficiency rickets, the American Academy of Pediatrics, Section on Breastfeeding and Committee on Nutrition (see Wagner et al, 2008) recommends that infants who are exclusively breastfed, who are breastfed and consuming less than 1000 ml of vitamin D–fortified formula or milk per day, or who are ingesting less than 1000 ml of vitamin D–fortified formula or milk per day be orally supplemented with 400 International Units of vitamin D per day; these supplements should be initiated in the first few days of life.

Vitamin K, required for blood coagulation, is produced by intestinal bacteria. However, the gut is relatively sterile at birth, and a few days are needed for intestinal flora to become established and produce vitamin K. To prevent hemorrhagic problems in the newborn, an injection of vitamin K is routinely given at birth. Oral vitamin K may not provide adequate stores necessary to prevent hemorrhage and is not recommended unless doses are repeatedly given during the first 4 months of life (American Academy of Pediatrics, Section on Breastfeeding, 2005).

Minerals

The mineral content of commercial infant formula is designed to reflect that of breast milk. Whole cow's milk is much higher in mineral content than human milk, which makes it unsuitable for infants in the first year of life. Minerals are typically highest in human milk during the first few days after birth and decrease slightly throughout lactation.

The ratio of calcium to phosphorus in human milk is 2:1, a proportion optimal for bone mineralization. Although cow's milk is high in calcium, the calcium-to-phosphorus ratio is low, resulting in decreased resorption. Consequently, young infants (less than 12 months) fed whole cow's milk are at risk for hypocalcemia, tetany, and seizures. The calcium-to-phosphorus ratio in commercial infant formulas is between the ratios of human and cow's milk.

Milk of all types is low in iron; however, iron from human milk is better absorbed than that from cow's milk, iron-fortified formula, or infant cereals. Breastfed infants benefit from the high lactose and vitamin C levels in human milk, which facilitate iron absorption. The infant who is totally breastfed normally maintains adequate hemoglobin levels for at least the first 6 months of life. After that time, iron-fortified cereals and other iron-rich foods may be added to the diet. Infants weaned from the breast before 6 months of age and all formula-fed infants should receive an iron-fortified commercial infant formula until 12 months of age. Infants should not be given low-iron formula (American Academy of Pediatrics, 2009).

The fluoride levels in human milk and in commercial formulas are low. This mineral, which is important in the prevention of dental caries, may cause staining of the permanent teeth (fluorosis) in excess amounts. Fluoride supplementation should be considered for any child over age 6 months whose drinking water is deficient in fluoride. Supplementation based on a fluoride concentration in the water supply of less than 0.3 parts per million is 0.25 mg for a child age 6 months to 3 years (American Academy of Pediatrics, Section on Pediatric Dentistry, 2003).

Overview of Lactation

Milk Production

Each female breast is composed of 15 to 20 segments (lobes) embedded in fat and connective tissue and well supplied with blood vessels, lymphatic tissue, and nerves (Fig. 26-1). Within each lobe are alveoli (the milk-producing cells) surrounded by myoepithelial cells, which contract to send the milk forward into the ductules. Each ductule enlarges into lactiferous ducts, where the milk is stored until the let-down reflex triggers the myoepithelial cells to contract and eject the milk out though the nipple pores (Riordan & Wambach, 2009). Each nipple has 5 to 19 pores through which milk is transferred to the suckling infant. The ducts do not widen into sinuses behind the nipple as previously thought.

Although nearly every woman can lactate, some mothers have insufficient glandular development to exclusively breastfeed their infants. Typically these women experienced few breast changes during either puberty or early pregnancy. In some cases, women may still be able to breastfeed and offer supplemental nutrition to support optimal infant growth. Devices are available that allow mothers to offer supplements while the baby is at the breast (Fig. 26-2).

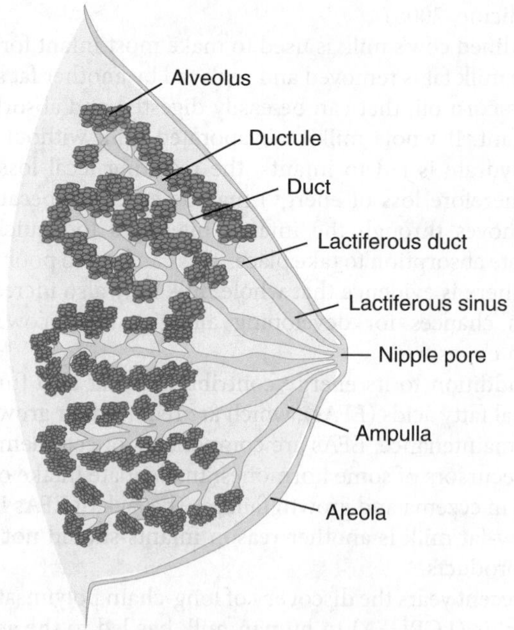

Fig. 26-1 Detailed structural features of human mammary gland.

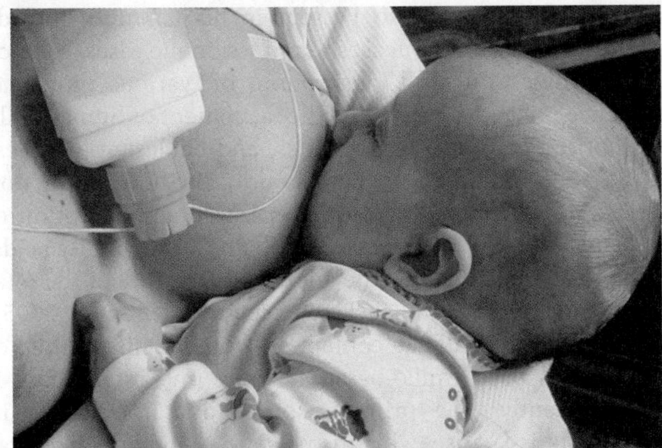

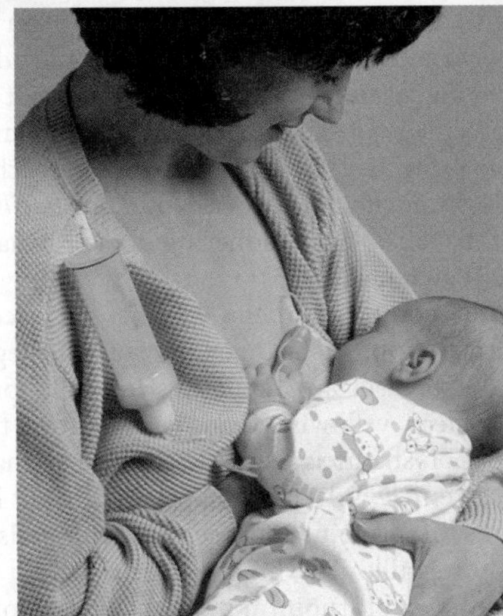

Fig. 26-2 Supplemental nursing system. *(Courtesy Medela, Inc., McHenry, IL.)*

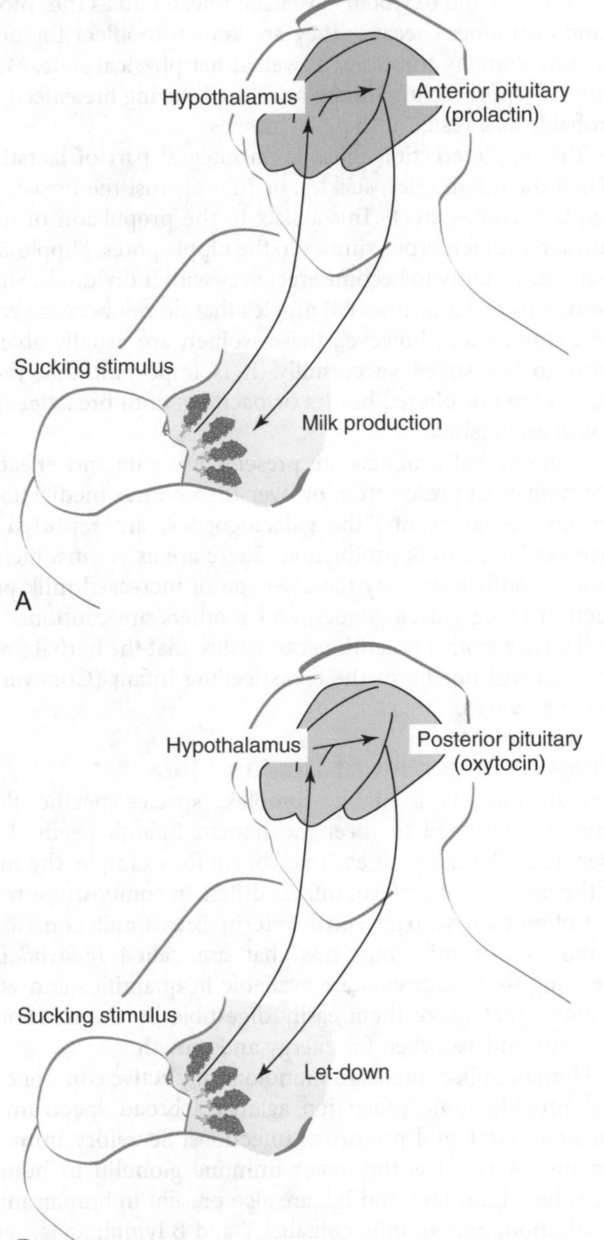

Fig. 26-3 Maternal breastfeeding reflexes. A, Milk production. B, Let-down.

After the mother gives birth, there is a precipitous fall in her estrogen and progesterone levels, which triggers release of prolactin from the anterior pituitary. Prolactin prepares the breasts to secrete milk during pregnancy and to synthesize and secrete milk during lactation. Prolactin levels are highest during the first 10 days after birth; they gradually decline over time, but remain above baseline levels for the duration of lactation. Prolactin is produced in response to infant suckling and emptying the breasts (lactating breasts are never completely empty; milk is constantly being produced by the alveoli as the infant feeds) (Fig. 26-3, *A*). Milk production is a supply-meets-demand system; that is, as milk is removed from the breast, more is produced. Incomplete emptying of the breasts with feedings can lead to a decrease in milk production.

Oxytocin is another hormone essential to lactation. As the nipple is stimulated by the suckling infant, the posterior pituitary is prompted by the hypothalamus to produce oxytocin. This hormone is responsible for the milk ejection reflex (MER), or let-down reflex (see Fig. 26-3, *B*). The myoepithelial cells surrounding the alveoli respond to oxytocin by contracting and sending the milk forward through the ducts to the nipple. Two to three "let-downs" can occur with each feeding session. The MER can be triggered by thoughts, sights, sounds, or odors that the mother associates with her baby (or other babies), such as hearing the baby cry. Many women report a tingling "pins and needles" sensation in the breasts as let-down occurs, although some mothers can detect milk ejection only by observing the infant's sucking and swallowing. Let-down may also occur during sexual activity because oxytocin is released during orgasm.

Oxytocin is the same hormone that stimulates uterine contractions during labor. Oxytocin contracts the mother's uterus after birth to control postpartum bleeding and to promote uterine involution. Thus mothers who breastfeed are at decreased risk for postpartum hemorrhage. The uterine contractions that occur with breastfeeding can be painful during and after the feeding, particularly in multiparas, for 3 to 5 days after giving birth.

evolve Case Study–Breastfeeding

Prolactin and oxytocin have been referred to as the "mothering hormones" because they are known to affect the postpartum woman's emotions, as well as her physical state. Many women report feeling thirsty or relaxed during breastfeeding, probably as a result of these hormones.

The nipple erection reflex is an integral part of lactation. When the infant cries, suckles, or rubs against the breast, the nipple becomes erect. This assists in the propulsion of milk through the lactiferous sinuses to the nipple pores. Nipple size, shape, and ability to become erect vary with individuals. Some women have flat or inverted nipples that do not become erect with stimulation; however, these women are usually able to learn to breastfeed successfully. It is important that these infants are not offered bottles or pacifiers until breastfeeding is well established.

Some herbal products are presented as safe and effective alternatives to prescription or over-the-counter medications; certain herbal agents, the galactogogues, are reported to increase breast milk production. There are as yet insufficient data to confirm or deny the assertion of increased milk production using galactogogues, and mothers are cautioned to seek advice from a practitioner to ensure that the herbal preparations will not harm the breastfeeding infant (Conover & Buehler, 2004).

Unique Properties of Human Milk

Human milk is a highly complex, species-specific fluid uniquely designed to meet the human infant's needs. It is specific to the needs of each newborn; for example, the milk of the mothers of preterm infants differs in composition from that of mothers who give birth at term. Breast milk consists of a number of micronutrients that are called *bioavailable,* meaning these nutrients are available in quantities and with qualities that make them easily digestible by the newborn's intestine and absorbed for energy and growth.

Human milk contains immunologically active components that provide some protection against a broad spectrum of bacterial, viral, and protozoan infections. Secretory immune globulin A (IgA) is the major immune globulin in human milk; IgG, IgM, IgD, and IgE are also present in human milk. In addition, human milk contains T and B lymphocytes, epidermal growth factor, cytokines, chemokines, interleukins, bifidus factor, complement (C3 and C4), and lactoferrin, all of which have specific roles in preventing localized and systemic bacterial and viral infections (Lawrence & Lawrence, 2005).

Human milk contains the two proteins, whey (lactalbumin) and casein (curd), in a ratio of approximately 60 : 40 (vs. 80 : 20 in most cow's milk–based formula). This ratio in human milk makes it more digestible and produces the soft stools seen in infants who breastfeed. Thus human milk has a laxative effect, and constipation is uncommon in breastfed infants. The whey protein, lactoferrin, in human milk has iron-binding characteristics with bacteriostatic capabilities, particularly against gram-positive and gram-negative aerobes, anaerobes, and yeasts (Lawrence & Lawrence, 2005). Casein in human milk greatly enhances the absorption of iron, thus preventing iron-dependent bacteria from proliferating in the gastrointestinal tract (Biancuzzo, 2003).

Digestive enzymes also present in human milk include amylases, lipases, proteases, and ribonucleases, which enhance digestion and absorption of various nutrients (Lawrence & Lawrence, 2005). The fat content of human milk is composed of lipids, triglycerides, and cholesterol; cholesterol is an essential element for brain growth. The function of these lipids is to allow optimum intestinal absorption of fatty acids and provide EFAs and polyunsaturated fatty acids. Furthermore lipids contribute approximately 50% of the total calories in human milk (Lawrence & Lawrence, 2005). Although the overall fat content in human milk is higher than that of cow's milk–based formula, the infant uses it more efficiently. The primary source of carbohydrate in human milk is lactose, which is present in higher concentrations (6.8 g/dl) than in cow's milk–based formula (4.9 g/dl). Other carbohydrates found in human milk include glucose, galactose, and glucosamine. The carbohydrates not only serve as a large percentage of the total calories in human milk, but also have a protective function; the oligosaccharides in human milk stimulate the growth of *Lactobacillus bifidus* and prevent bacteria from adhering to epithelial surfaces (Lawrence & Lawrence, 2005).

Human milk composition and volumes vary according to the stage of lactation. In lactogenesis stage I, beginning in pregnancy, the breasts are preparing for milk production. Colostrum, a clear, yellowish fluid, is present in the breasts at this time. Colostrum is more concentrated than mature milk and is extremely rich in immune globulins. It has higher concentrations of protein, glucose, and minerals, but less fat, than mature milk. The high protein level of colostrum facilitates binding of bilirubin, and the laxative action of colostrum promotes early passage of meconium. Colostrum gradually changes to mature milk; this is referred to as "the milk coming in," or lactogenesis stage II. By the third to fifth day after birth, most women have experienced this onset of copious milk secretion. Breast milk continues to change in composition for approximately 10 days, when the mature milk is established in stage III of lactogenesis (Lawrence & Lawrence, 2005).

Composition of mature milk changes during each feeding. As the infant nurses, the fat content of breast milk increases. Initially there is a release of bluish white foremilk that is part skim milk (about 60% of the volume) and part whole milk (about 35% of the volume). It provides primarily lactose, protein, and water-soluble vitamins. The hindmilk, or cream (about 5%), is usually let down 10 to 20 minutes into the feeding, although it may occur sooner. It contains the denser calories from fat necessary for optimal growth and contentment between feedings. Because of this changing composition of human milk during each feeding, it is important to breastfeed the infant long enough to supply a balanced feeding. Milk production gradually increases, so that by the time her infant is 2 weeks old, the mother produces 720 to 900 ml of milk every 24 hours. Babies experience fairly predictable growth spurts (i.e., at about 10 days, 3 weeks, 6 weeks, 3 months, and 4 to 6 months), when more frequent feedings stimulate increased milk production. These more frequent feedings usually last 24 to 48 hours, and then the infants resume their usual feeding pattern.

Nursing Care Management: The Breastfeeding Mother and Infant

Assessment

Infant

Before the initiation of breastfeeding, the nurse must consider several factors to effectively assist the breastfeeding infant. Maturity level, experience during labor and birth, any birth trauma or maternal risk factors, congenital defects or physical instability, and state of alertness all affect the infant's readiness and ability to breastfeed.

During feeding, the infant is assessed by direct observation for latch-on, position and alignment, and suckling and swallowing. After the feeding, the infant is observed for behavior such as contentment or sleepiness. Elimination patterns are noted: within 24 hours after birth, at least one wet diaper and one stool; by day 3, three or four wet diapers and one or two stools that are beginning to change from meconium to yellow; after day 4 (and mother's milk has "come in"), six to eight wet diapers and at least three stools per 24 hours. Other factors to assess include the presence of jaundice, weight loss greater than 7%, and a regain of birth weight by 10 to 14 days of age (see Critical Thinking Exercise).

> **CRITICAL THINKING EXERCISE**
>
> **Neonatal Breastfeeding**
>
> Neide is a 27-year-old married woman from Costa Rica currently living in the United States on a student visa who has a 5-day-old, 3288 g (7 lb, 4 oz) male infant. She is being seen in the clinic for a follow-up consultation on breastfeeding and jaundice; the baby's 2-year-old sister is at daycare. On examination the infant is alert, fussy, and visibly jaundiced. Neide admits that breastfeeding has not been going as well as planned and she is not certain the infant is receiving enough milk. She states, in tears, that all the baby does is cry and fuss when she places him to breast, and she wants to try formula. The baby has been having one or two stools per day and three or four wet diapers.
>
> 1. Evidence–Is there sufficient evidence to draw conclusions about the infant's breastfeeding pattern?
> 2. Assumptions–What assumptions can be made about the following factors?
>   a. The infant's ability to latch-on.
>   b. Adequacy of breast milk intake
>   c. Additional infant assessments
>   d. The mother's desire to give the infant formula.
> 3. What implications and priorities for nursing care can be drawn at this time?
> 4. Does the evidence objectively support your conclusion?
> 5. Are there alternative perspectives to your conclusion?

Mother

Before breastfeeding is begun, the nurse should carefully assess the mother's knowledge of breastfeeding and her physical and psychologic readiness to breastfeed. Factors to include are her previous experience with breastfeeding, knowledge about breastfeeding, cultural factors, physical features of the breasts or nipples or other physical limitations, psychologic readiness (time since birth, mood and energy level), and support of the newborn's father or other family members.

During the time in the hospital, the nurse can help the mother view each breastfeeding session as a "feeding lesson" or "practice session" that will foster maternal confidence and a satisfying breastfeeding experience for mother and infant. Assessment includes condition of nipples, transition to mature milk, breasts feeling lighter or softer after feeding, mother feeling relaxed or sleepy after feeding, uterine cramping or increased lochia flow during and after a feeding, and mother's appearance of comfort with breastfeeding techniques.

The nursing process in the care of the breastfeeding mother-infant pair is outlined in the Nursing Process box.

Implementation

In the early days after birth, interventions focus on helping the mother and the newborn initiate breastfeeding and achieve some degree of success and satisfaction before discharge from the hospital. Interventions to promote breastfeeding progress from basics such as latch-on and positioning to signs of adequate feeding and self-care measures such as prevention of engorgement. With early discharge from the hospital it is increasingly important to assess the mother-infant dyad in relation to feeding ability. In some cases either a home visit or return to primary practitioner visit is appropriate within 48 to 72 hours after discharge to ensure that adequate latch-on is taking place and that the infant is progressing in feeding, elimination, and jaundice patterns. The visit is also an excellent opportunity to evaluate the mother's status, answer any questions about self-care or newborn care, and reinforce positive parenting and child care abilities.

evolve Skill—Infant Feeding

The ideal time to begin breastfeeding is within the first hour after birth when the infant is in the quiet, alert state.

Positioning

There are four basic positions for breastfeeding: football hold; cradle; cross cradle, or across-the-lap; and side-lying position (Fig. 26-4). Initially it is best to use the position that most easily facilitates latch-on while allowing maximum comfort for the mother. The football hold is usually preferred by mothers who gave birth by cesarean. The cross cradle, or across-the-lap, hold also works well for early feedings. The side-lying position allows the mother to rest while breastfeeding and is often preferred by women experiencing perineal pain and swelling. Cradling is the most common breastfeeding position for infants who have learned to latch on easily and feed effectively. Before discharge from the hospital, the mother should be assisted in trying all of the positions so that she will feel confident in her ability to vary positions at home.

The mother should be comfortable in the position, with pillows used as needed to provide support for her back and arms. The infant is placed at the level of the breast, supported by pillows or folded blankets; turned completely on his or her side; and facing the mother so that the infant is "belly to belly" with the arms "hugging" the breast. The newborn's nose is directly in front of the nipple. It is important that the mother support the newborn's neck and shoulders with her hand and not push on the occiput. The infant's body is held in correct

NURSING PROCESS: BREASTFEEDING MOTHER-INFANT PAIR

Assessment

The assessment of the breastfeeding mother-newborn pair must include an assessment of infant feeding cues and the mother's physical and psychologic readiness to breastfeed. Additional assessment guidelines are discussed on p. 685.

Nursing Diagnoses

Nursing diagnoses for the breastfeeding woman and infant may include the following:

Effective breastfeeding related to
- mother's knowledge of breastfeeding techniques
- mother's appropriate response to infant's feeding readiness cues
- mother's ability to facilitate efficient breastfeeding

Risk for ineffective breastfeeding related to
- insufficient knowledge regarding newborn's reflexes and breastfeeding techniques
- lack of support by infant's father, family, friends
- lack of maternal self-confidence; presence of anxiety, fear of failure
- poor infant suckling reflex
- difficulty waking sleepy newborn

Risk for imbalanced nutrition: less than body requirements related to
- increased caloric and nutrient needs for breastfeeding (mother)
- incorrect latch-on and inability to transfer milk (infant)

Risk for deficient fluid volume related to
- ineffective suckling (infant)

Planning and Implementation

The expected outcomes include that the infant will do the following:

- Latch on and feed effectively at least 8 to 10 times per day
- Gain weight appropriately
- Remain well hydrated (have one wet diaper per day of life until the fifth day then six to eight wet diapers and at least three to four bowel movements every 24 hours)
- Sleep or seem contented between feedings

Examples of expected outcomes for the mother include that she will do the following:

- Verbalize and demonstrate understanding of breastfeeding techniques, including positioning and latch-on, signs of adequate feeding, and self-care
- Report no nipple discomfort with breastfeeding
- Express satisfaction with the breastfeeding experience
- Consume a nutritionally balanced diet with appropriate caloric and fluid intake to support breastfeeding

Nursing interventions for the breastfeeding mother-infant pair are discussed on pp. 685-700.

Evaluation

Evaluation is based on the expected outcomes, and the care plan is revised as needed based on the evaluation.

alignment (i.e., ears, shoulders, and hips are in a straight line) during latch-on and feeding (Fig. 26-5).

Latch-On

In preparation for latch-on, it may be helpful for the mother to manually express a few drops of colostrum or milk and spread it over the nipple. This lubricates the nipple and may entice the baby to open the mouth as the milk is tasted.

To facilitate latch-on, the mother supports her breast in one hand with the thumb on top and the fingers underneath at the back edge of the areola; this is called the C hold. She compresses the breast slightly so that an adequate amount of breast tissue is taken into the mouth with latch-on. Most mothers need to support the breast during feeding for at least the first few weeks until the infant can stay latched on easily.

The mother lightly touches the infant's lower lip with her nipple, stimulating the mouth to open (rooting reflex). When the mouth is open wide and the tongue is down, the mother positions her nipple upward and quickly pulls the infant onto the nipple. She brings the infant to the breast, not the breast to the infant. If the breast is pushed into the infant's mouth, the infant often closes the mouth too soon and does not latch on.

The amount of the areola in the newborn's mouth with latch-on depends on the size of the newborn's mouth and the size of the areola and nipple. In general, the infant's mouth should cover the nipple and an areolar radius of approximately 2 to 3 cm all around the nipple.

When the newborn is latched on correctly, the nose, cheeks, and chin should all be touching the breast (Fig. 26-6). The mother should not pull the nipple out of the mouth when trying to create a breathing space for the newborn's nose. Depressing the breast tissue around the newborn's nose is not necessary. If the mother is worried about the infant's breathing, she can raise the newborn's hips slightly to change the angle of the infant's head at the breast. If the newborn cannot breathe, reflexes will prompt the newborn to move the head and pull back to breathe.

Suckling creates a vacuum in the intraoral cavity as the breast is compressed between the tongue and the palate. If the mother experiences pinching or pain after the first few sucks, or does not feel a firm tugging on the nipple, the latch-on and positioning should be evaluated.

If each suck is painful, the infant may be having difficulty keeping the tongue out over the lower gum ridge. Clicking or smacking may be audible when this occurs. The nurse can place a finger on the side of the newborn's lower jaw, pulling down gently but firmly as the infant sucks, to help stabilize the jaw so that the tongue stays in place.

Any time the signs of adequate latch-on and sucking are not present, the newborn should be taken off the breast and

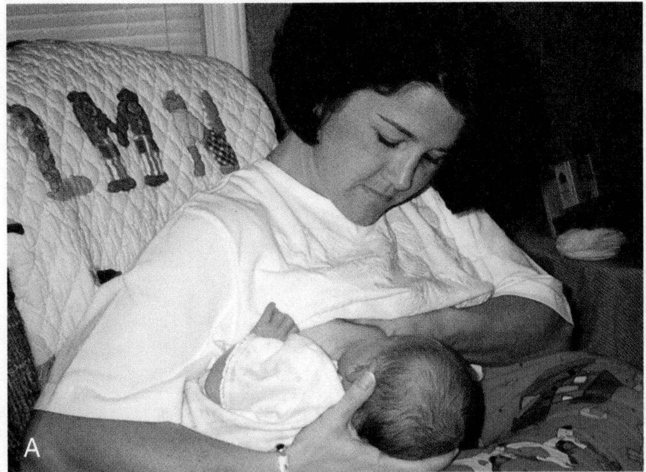

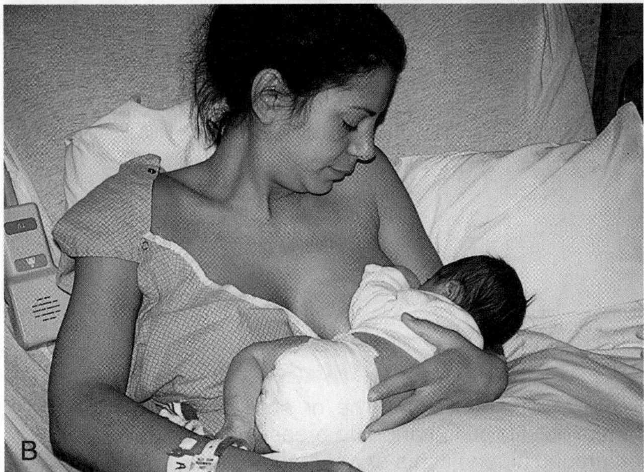

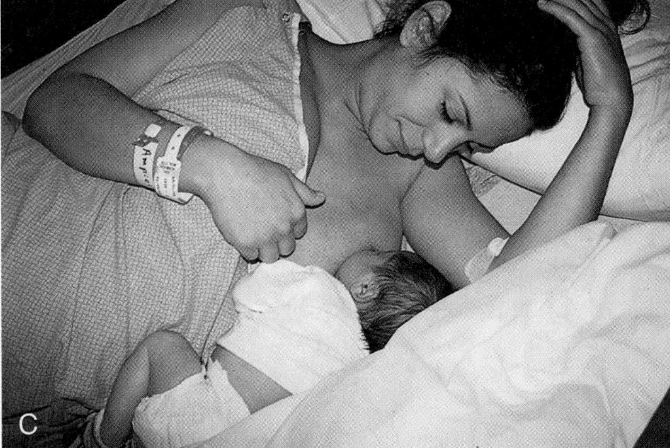

Fig. 26-4 Breastfeeding positions. **A**, Football hold. **B**, Cradling. **C**, Side-lying position. *(**B** and **C**, Courtesy Marjorie Pyle, RNC, Lifecircle, Costa Mesa, CA.)*

latch-on attempted again. To prevent nipple trauma as the newborn is taken off the breast, the mother is instructed to break the suction by inserting her finger in the side of the infant's mouth between the gums and keeping it there until the nipple is completely out of the newborn's mouth (Fig. 26-7).

When the newborn is latched on correctly and is sucking appropriately, (1) the mother reports a firm tug on her nipple, but no pinching or pain; (2) the newborn sucks with cheeks rounded, not dimpled; (3) the infant's jaw glides smoothly with sucking; and (4) swallowing is audible.

Milk Ejection, or Let-Down

As the newborn begins suckling on the nipple, the let-down, or milk ejection, reflex is stimulated. The hormone oxytocin causes milk to be sent forward from the milk ducts to the nipple. The following signs indicate that let-down has occurred:

- The mother may feel a tingling sensation in the nipples, although some women do not feel their milk let down.
- The newborn's suck changes from quick, shallow sucks to a slower, deeper, and stronger sucking pattern.
- Swallowing is audible after the newborn sucks.
- The mother feels relaxed, even sleepy, during feedings.
- The mother experiences uterine cramping and increased lochia flow during or after the feeding.
- The opposite breast may leak milk.

Frequency of Feedings

Newborns usually require 8 to 12 feedings in a 24-hour period. During the first 24 to 48 hours after birth, many newborns may not awaken this often to feed. On the other hand, some infants may nurse "nonstop" during this period to stimulate milk production. It is important that parents understand that they should awaken the infant to feed at least every 3 hours during the day and at least every 4 hours at night during the first few weeks of life. (Feeding frequency is determined by counting from the beginning of one feeding to the beginning of the next.) Once the newborn is feeding well and gaining weight appropriately, he or she can determine the timing of feedings through demand feedings.

Parents should be cautioned about attempting to place newborn infants on strict feeding schedules. Infants should be fed whenever they exhibit feeding cues such as hand-to-mouth movements, rooting, and mouth and tongue movements. Crying is a late sign of hunger, and infants may become frantic when they have to wait too long to feed. Some infants will shut down or go into a deep sleep when their needs are not met. Keeping the newborn close is the best way to observe and respond to infant feeding cues. One recommendation is that mother and breastfeeding infant sleep in close proximity to promote breastfeeding (American Academy of Pediatrics, Section on Breastfeeding, 2005). The issue of bed-sharing (cobedding) has raised concerns because of the association between a higher incidence of SIDS and bed-sharing with an adult. It is recommended that the breastfeeding infant be paced in a bassinet in close proximity to the mother, which would then allow for more convenient breastfeeding and at the same time prevent continuous bed-sharing (American Academy of Pediatrics, Task Force on Sudden Infant Death Syndrome, 2005).

evolve Critical Thinking Exercise—Breastfeeding

Duration of Feedings

The duration of breastfeeding sessions is highly variable, since the timing of milk transfer differs for each mother-infant pair. Whereas some infants may complete a feeding in 5 or 10 minutes, others may require 45 minutes or longer. The average time for feeding is 20 to 30 minutes, or approximately 15 minutes per breast. Instructing mothers to feed for a set

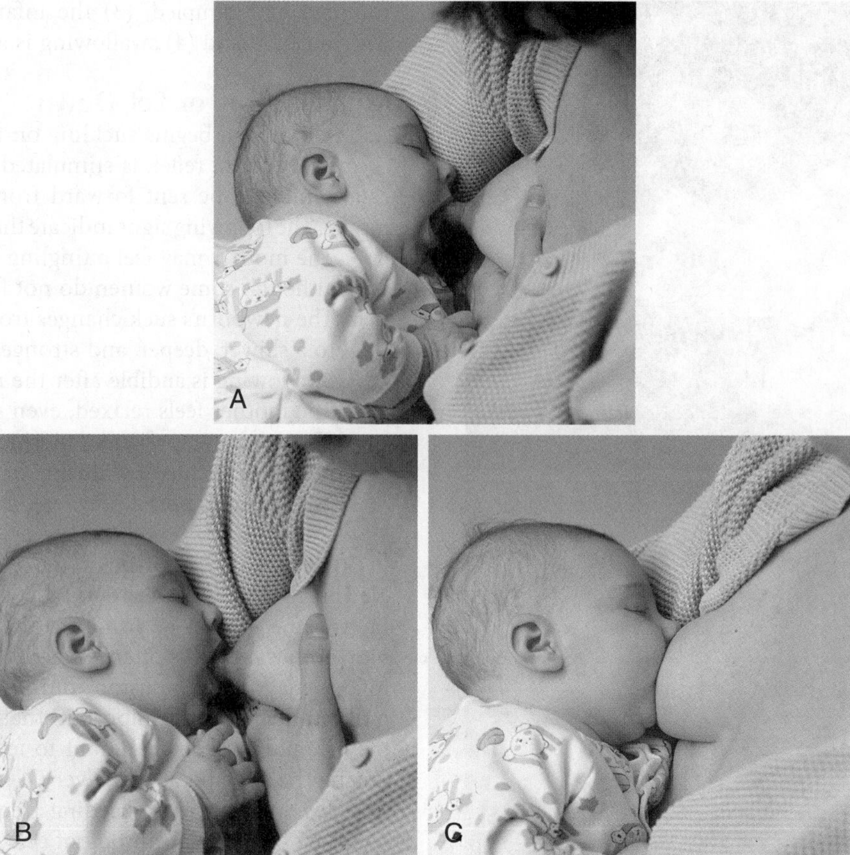

Fig. 26-5 Latching on. A, Tickle newborn's lip with your nipple until he or she opens wide. B, Once infant's mouth is opened wide, quickly pull infant onto breast. C, Infant should have as much areola (dark area around nipple) in his or her mouth as possible, not just the nipple. *(Courtesy Medela, Inc., McHenry, IL.)*

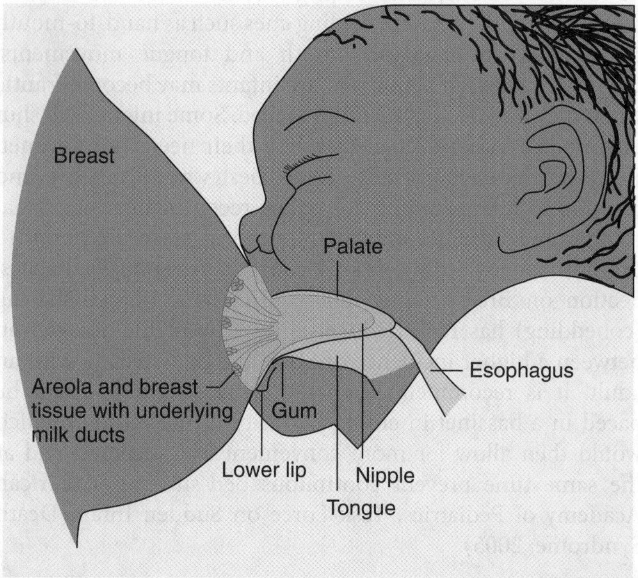

Fig. 26-6 Correct attachment (latch-on) of infant at breast.

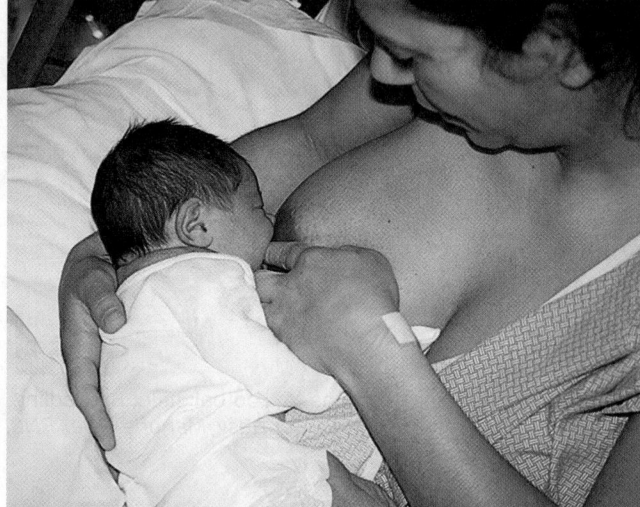

Fig. 26-7 Removing infant from the breast. *(Courtesy Marjorie Pyle, RNC, Lifecircle, Costa Mesa, CA.)*

number of minutes is inappropriate. It is better to teach mothers how to determine when an infant has finished a feeding: the infant's suck-swallow pattern has slowed, the breast is softened, and the newborn appears content and may fall asleep or release the nipple.

If a newborn seems to be feeding effectively and is having adequate urine output but not gaining weight well, the mother may be switching to the second breast too soon. The high lactose content in foremilk may cause the newborn to have explosive stools, gas pains, and inconsolable crying. Keeping the infant on the first breast until it is soft ensures that he or she receives the more calorie-dense, high-fat hindmilk, which usually results in increased weight gain.

Supplements, Bottles, and Pacifiers

The American Academy of Pediatrics, Section on Breastfeeding (2005), recommends that, unless a medical indication exists, *no supplements* be given to breastfeeding infants. Situations related to the infant that may necessitate supplemental feedings include low birth weight, hypoglycemia, or an inborn error of metabolism. Mothers may be unable to feed because of severe illness, or they may be taking medications incompatible with breastfeeding.

Offering a bottle after breastfeeding "just to make sure the baby is getting enough" is normally unnecessary and should be avoided. This can contribute to nipple confusion (i.e., difficulty knowing how to latch on to the breast) and to low milk supply because the baby becomes overly full and does not breastfeed often enough. Supplementation interferes with the supply-meets-demand cycle of milk production. The parents may interpret the newborn's willingness to take a bottle to mean that the mother's milk supply is inadequate. They need to know that a newborn will automatically suck from a bottle as the nipple triggers the suck-swallow reflex.

Newborns may become confused going from breast to bottle or bottle to breast when breastfeeding is first initiated. Although there is no research-based evidence to support this idea, there are anecdotal reports of infants who refused the breast once fed formula or even started on a pacifier. Breastfeeding and bottle-feeding require different oral motor skills. The ways newborns use their tongues, jaw, and lips, as well as the swallowing patterns, are very different. Some newborns can transition easily between breast and bottle, but others experience considerable difficulty. It is impossible to predict which infants will adapt well and which ones will not. Therefore many practitioners recommend avoiding bottles until breastfeeding is well established, usually after 3 to 4 weeks. If supplementation is needed, mechanisms such as supplemental nursing systems allow the infant to breastfeed while being supplemented (see Fig. 26-2). Although some parents combine breastfeeding and bottle-feeding, some infants never take a bottle and go directly from the breast to a cup as they grow.

Because a correlation has been identified between pacifier use at bedtime and a decreased incidence of SIDS, it is recommended that the caregiver consider offering the infant a pacifier at nap time or regular bedtime; in the breastfeeding infant, the pacifier may not be offered until after 1 month, which would ideally ensure that successful breastfeeding is occurring on a regular basis and the pacifier would not become a distraction from breastfeeding (American Academy of Pediatrics, Task Force on Sudden Infant Death Syndrome, 2005). This recommendation does not preclude pacifier use when the infant is demonstrating hunger cues. Biancuzzo (2003) suggests that health care workers maintain a commonsense approach to pacifier usage and breastfeeding. Parents should be informed of the relationship between pacifier use and early termination of breastfeeding so that they can make an informed decision. Furthermore, pacifier use should not replace actual feeding or suckling. Prohibiting pacifier use will not ensure an increase in the length of breastfeeding. The emphasis should be on allowing the infant to control the pace, frequency, and termination of feeding rather than allowing the pacifier (or anything else) to become the focus of the interaction (see Evidence-Based Practice box).

The use of a pacifier in infants has also been suggested as a causative factor in the increase in episodes of acute otitis media (Niemela, Uhari, & Mottonen, 1995). However, a later study showed a significant decrease in the incidence of acute otitis media when a pacifier was used only at bedtime (Niemela et al, 2000). Dental malocclusion has been found in some children using a pacifier, but the evidence supporting dental problems is lacking; however, pacifier use should not extend past 4 to 5 years of age (American Academy of Pediatrics, Task Force on Sudden Infant Death Syndrome, 2005; Early childhood pacifier use, 2005). The effect of continual pacifier use on early speech and language development is unknown, but the pacifier may decrease the infant's desire to imitate sounds and affect intelligibility. Parents need to be alerted that continual dependency on a pacifier may influence social and speech development.

If the infant uses a pacifier, safety considerations in purchasing one must be stressed. Parents should be cautioned against altering a pacifier, thus making it more dangerous.

At the time of this writing, there is no evidence that pacifier use and nonnutritive sucking in preterm infants have any effect on the initiation and length of breastfeeding. Nonnutritive sucking should not be withheld from preterm infants, especially in conjunction with the use of concentrated sucrose for pain management.

Special Considerations

Sleepy Newborn

During the first few days of life, some newborns need to be awakened for feedings. If the infant is awakened from a sound sleep, attempts at feeding are more likely to be unsuccessful. Unwrapping the newborn, changing the diaper, sitting the infant upright, talking to the newborn with variable pitch, gently massaging the infant's chest or back, and stroking the palms or soles may bring the newborn to an alert state.

Fussy Newborn

Infants sometimes awaken from sleep crying frantically. Although they may be hungry, they cannot focus on feeding until they are calmed. Calming techniques include swaddling, skin-to-skin contact and holding closely, talking soothingly, and allowing the infant to suck on a clean finger.

Some infants cry as soon as they are positioned for feeding. This may be due to a bruised head or previously undetected fractured clavicle. Changing the feeding position may solve the problem.

Fussiness may be related to gastrointestinal distress (i.e., cramping and gas pains). This may occur in response to an occasional feeding of infant formula, or it may be related to something the mother ingested. Although most mothers can consume their normal diet without affecting the infant, foods such as cabbage, broccoli, or onions may irritate some infants' stomachs. Others may react to cow's milk products ingested by the mother. There are no standard foods that all mothers should avoid when breastfeeding; each mother-newborn

EVIDENCE-BASED PRACTICE Pacifier Use in the Newborn

—*Pat Gingrich*

Ask the Question

What are the current recommendations regarding the use of pacifiers for breastfeeding neonates?

Search for Evidence

Search Strategies

Professional organization guidelines, meta-analyses, systematic reviews, randomized controlled trials, nonrandomized prospective studies, and retrospective studies since 2006

Databases Searched

CINAHL; Cochrane; Medline; TRIP Database Plus; and websites for AAP, ABM, AWHONN, and WHO

Critically Analyze the Evidence

The 10 points from the UNICEF and World Health Organization (2006) Baby-Friendly Hospital Initiative are designed to promote exclusive breastfeeding, skin-to-skin contact, and rooming-in. One of the 10 guidelines discourages pacifier use. There is a consensus among professional breastfeeding advocacy organizations that pacifier use during the first month of life can be detrimental to establishing exclusive breastfeeding. The Association of Women's Health, Obstetric and Neonatal Nurses (2007) suggests in its clinical protocol that parents consider introducing the pacifier after the first month, reflecting current research showing that pacifiers may have some protective effect against sudden infant death syndrome (SIDS). The Academy of Breastfeeding Medicine (2007) recommends that full-term, breastfed babies be offered pacifiers only in case of painful procedures, and that the pacifier be removed from the crib before returning the infant to the parents.

Researchers have shown that pacifier use can be effective as analgesia for painful procedures. They found in a randomized, controlled trial of 84 infants that this pain relief, as measured by the FLACC Scale (face, legs, activity, crying, and consolability), was enhanced with addition of sucrose (Curtis et al, 2007). Sucrose alone did not have any benefit as an analgesic.

Implications for Practice

Institutional pacifier use is a difficult habit to break. Nurses who bring babies into the nursery want to settle fussy babies, soothe them for necessary procedures, and avoid disturbing the other babies. Parents are accustomed to pacifiers and may have used them with their older children. It can be a real challenge to make pacifiers unavailable for breastfed babies. Newborns who are rooming in with their mothers and breastfed every 1 to 2 hours, at the first signs of hunger, are less likely to need nonnutritive sucking. Nurses must educate parents on the benefits of exclusive breastfeeding, emphasizing the importance of delaying the introduction of the pacifier until breastfeeding is firmly established, around 1 month of age.

The protective effect of pacifiers against SIDS outweighs the possible interruption of exclusive breastfeeding after the first month of life. The nurse needs to teach parents to wash the pacifier with soap and rinse thoroughly, but boiling the pacifier is not necessary. Except for painful procedures, the pacifier should not be coated with sucrose. Parents should actively wean the child from pacifier use by age 4 years to allow normal teeth and jaw development.

References

Academy of Breastfeeding Medicine Protocol Committee: ABM clinical protocol #7: model breastfeeding policy, *Breastfeed Med* 2(1):50-55, 2007.

Association of Women's Health, Obstetric and Neonatal Nurses: *Breastfeeding support: prenatal care through the first year, ed 2, Evidence-based clinical practice guideline*, Washington, DC, 2007, The Association.

Curtis SJ et al: A randomized, controlled trial of sucrose and/or pacifier use for analgesia for infants receiving venipuncture in a pediatric emergency department, *BMC Pediatr* 7(July 18):27, 2007.

UNICEF, World Health Organization: *Baby-Friendly Hospital Initiative, revised, updated and expanded for integrated care 2006*, Geneva, Switzerland, 2006, World Health Organization. Available at www.who.int/nutrition/topics/bfhi/en/index.html (accessed July 5, 2008).

couple responds individually. One rule of thumb is that if the food causes bloating and gas in the mother, there is a strong probability it will do the same for the infant. If gas is a problem, giving the newborn liquid simethicone drops before a feeding may help.

Persistent crying or refusing to breastfeed can indicate illness, and the health care provider should be notified. Ear infections, sore throat, or oral thrush may cause the infant to be fussy and not breastfeed well.

Slow Weight Gain

Commonly newborns lose 7% to 10% of their birth weight during the first 3 to 5 days after birth, which is mostly water weight acquired in utero. Thereafter, they should begin to gain weight at the rate of 110 to 200 g/wk, or 20 to 28 g/day. The infant who continues to lose weight after 5 days, who does not regain birth weight by 2 weeks, or whose weight is below the 10th percentile by 1 month should be evaluated and closely monitored by a health care provider.

At times, slow weight gain is related to inadequate breastfeeding. Feedings may be short or infrequent, or the infant may be latching on incorrectly or sucking ineffectively or inefficiently. Other causes are illness; infection; malabsorption; or circumstances that increase the newborn's energy needs, such as congenital heart disease, cystic fibrosis, or being small for gestational age. However, newborns gain weight in differing patterns, and one should not assume that the newborn is ill just because weight gain is not the same as that of another breastfed or bottle-fed infant.

Maternal factors may contribute to slow weight gain. There may be inadequate emptying of the breasts, pain with feeding, or inappropriate timing of feedings. Inadequate glandular breast tissue or previous breast surgery may affect milk supply. Severe intrapartum or postpartum hemorrhage, illness, or medications may decrease milk supply. Postpartum stress and fatigue may also negatively affect milk production.

Usually the solution to slow weight gain is to improve the feeding technique. Positioning and latch-on are evaluated and adjustments made. It may help to add a feeding or two in a 24-hour period. Massaging alternate breasts during feedings may help increase the amount of milk going to the infant. With this technique, the mother massages her breast from the chest wall to the nipple whenever the baby has sucking pauses. Some think that this technique may also increase the fat content of the milk, which aids in weight gain.

When newborns are calorie deprived and need supplementation, the extra breast milk or formula can be given with a spoon or cup, a nursing supplementer, or a bottle. If there are latch-on problems, it is best to avoid bottles and pacifiers. In most cases, supplementation is needed only for a short time until the newborn gains weight and is feeding adequately. Most breastfeeding problems require simple solutions; a lactation consultant can help solve problems by modifying feeding patterns.

Jaundice

Jaundice and hyperbilirubinemia in the newborn are discussed in detail in Chapter 25. Colostrum has a natural laxative effect and promotes early passage of meconium. Bilirubin is excreted from the body primarily (98%) through the intestines. Infrequent stooling allows bilirubin in the stool to be reabsorbed into the infant's system (enterohepatic shunting), thus promoting hyperbilirubinemia. Infants who receive water or glucose water supplements are more likely to have hyperbilirubinemia because these do not prevent enterohepatic shunting and only 2% of bilirubin is excreted through the kidneys (see also Evidence-Based Practice box, Chapter 25, p. 664). Breastfeeding-associated, or early breastfeeding, jaundice is reported to be related to an increased pattern of enterohepatic shunting, decreased caloric and fluid intake, less frequent stooling, and increased β-glucuronidase in human milk (Blackburn, 2007). This jaundice typically appears around the fourth or fifth day of life and may last as long as 2 weeks. The cause of late-onset breastfeeding jaundice, which may last as long as 12 weeks, is hypothesized to be related to substances in breast milk that interfere with bilirubin conjugation and excretion. These two phases may overlap and be indistinguishable from each other (Blackburn, 2007). Infants with either of these conditions are typically thriving, gaining weight, and stooling normally, and all pathologic causes of jaundice have been ruled out. The critical element in breastfeeding jaundice is to encourage early and frequent breastfeeding, often as frequently as every 2 hours in the first week of life, which will enhance stooling and decrease the chance for enterohepatic circulation. Achieving a successful latch-on in the first few days of life and a continuation of this pattern will probably do more to decrease jaundice than other medical therapies. The use of oral supplementation of glucose water or water is strongly discouraged.

The breastfeeding infant who becomes jaundiced should be carefully evaluated for weight loss over 7% of birth weight, decreased milk intake, infrequent stooling (less than three or four stools by day 4), decreased urine output (fewer than four to six wet diapers per day), and serum bilirubin levels or transcutaneous monitoring (Blackburn, 2007; American Academy of Pediatrics, Section on Breastfeeding, 2005). The 2004 American Academy of Pediatrics Subcommittee on Hyperbilirubinemia recommendations include monitoring the infant according to an hour-specific risk nomogram (see Chapter 25).

Preterm Infants

Human milk is the ideal food for preterm infants, with benefits that are unique to the individual preterm infant in addition to those received by healthy term infants. Initially, preterm human milk contains higher concentrations of energy, fat, sodium, and protein; however, by the second or third week of life, human milk protein content is less than adequate for preterm infant growth, and supplementation with human milk fortifier is recommended (Askin & Diehl-Jones, 2005). Human milk fortifier contains the protein, minerals (zinc, manganese, calcium, magnesium, phosphorus, sodium, potassium and copper), and vitamins (folic acid and vitamins B_2, B_6, C, D, E, and K) necessary to support growth and metabolism in the preterm infant (American Academy of Pediatrics, 2009). Human milk fortifiers are available in both liquid and powder form.

Mothers of preterm infants who are unable to breastfeed their infant due to either maternal or neonatal illness should begin pumping their breasts as soon as possible after birth with a hospital-grade electric pump. To establish an optimal milk supply, the mother should use a dual collection kit and pump 8 to 10 times daily for 10 to 15 minutes or until the milk flow has ceased for a few minutes (Meier, 1997). These women are taught proper handling and storage of breast milk to minimize bacterial contamination and growth.

See also Chapter 27 for additional information regarding discharge and nutrition of the preterm infant.

Breastfeeding Twins

Caring for twins takes some planning, but breastfeeding means that feedings are always ready instantly; no one has to wash bottles and fix formula; and some mothers can feed both babies at once. The mother with twins will need extra nourishment (200 to 500 kcal/day for each infant).

Each newborn feeds from one breast per feeding, usually for about 20 to 30 minutes. Some mothers assign each newborn a breast; others switch infants from one breast to the other, either on a schedule or randomly. The mother may find it easiest to use a modified demand feeding schedule; that is, feeding the first infant who wakes up and then waking the second infant for feeding.

During the early weeks, parents may find it helpful to keep a record of feeding times and which breast was used first by which infant. If one twin nurses more vigorously than the other, that infant should be alternated between breasts to equalize breast stimulation.

If the mother wants to feed the newborns simultaneously, she may wish to experiment with positions. For example, one newborn can be held in the football hold and the other in the cradle hold, or the newborns can each be held in a cradling position. Each infant can be supported on firm pillows while in the football hold. At first, some mothers using this position (Fig. 26-8) may require assistance to get the infants off the breasts.

Expressing and Storing Breast Milk

In some situations expression of breast milk is necessary or desirable, such as when engorgement occurs, the mother and infant are separated (e.g., preterm or sick infant is in neonatal intensive care), the mother is employed outside the home and

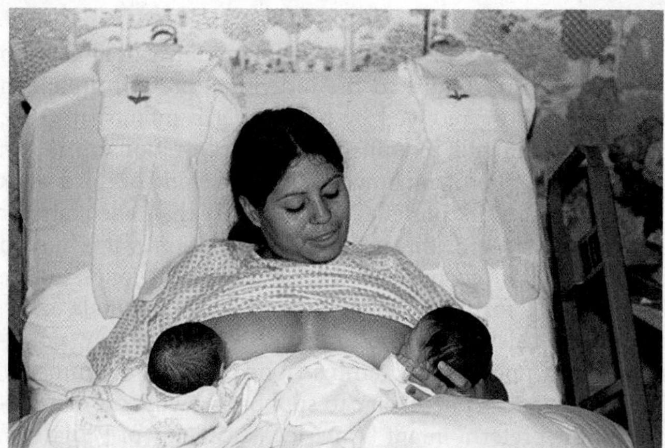

Fig. 26-8 Breastfeeding twins. *(Courtesy Marjorie Pyle, RNC, Lifecircle, Costa Mesa, CA.)*

wants to maintain her milk supply, the nipples are severely sore or cracked, or the mother leaves the infant with a caregiver and will not be present for feeding.

Because pumping and hand expression are rarely as effective as an infant in removing milk from the breast, the milk supply should never be judged based on the volume expressed.

Hand Expression

To manually express milk, after thoroughly washing her hands, the mother places one hand on her breast at the edge of the areola. With her thumb above and fingers below, she presses in toward her chest wall and gently compresses the breast while rolling her thumb and fingers forward. These motions are repeated rhythmically until the milk begins to flow. While the milk is flowing easily, the mother maintains a steady, light pressure. The thumb and fingers should not pinch the breast or slip down to the nipple. The hand should be rotated to reach all sections of each breast. After expressing milk from the second breast, she should return to the first breast and then repeat until all readily available milk is expressed.

Pumping

There are numerous ways to approach pumping. Some women pump when they first wake up in the morning or when the baby has fed but did not completely empty the breast. Others prefer to pump just before going to sleep. Some pump one breast while the infant is feeding from the other. Double pumping (pumping both breasts at the same time) saves time (Fig. 26-9).

The amount of milk obtained when pumping depends on the type of pump being used, the time of day, how long it has been since the infant breastfed, the mother's milk supply, how practiced she is at pumping, and her comfort level (pumping is uncomfortable for some women). Breast milk may vary in color and consistency, depending on the time of day, the infant's age, and foods the mother has eaten (e.g., the milk may appear green after the mother eats spinach).

Types of Pumps

There are many types of breast pumps (Fig. 26-10). Some are more effective than others, and they vary in price. Manual pumps are the least expensive and may be the most appropriate where portability and quietness of operation are critical, or when a mother is pumping only for an occasional bottle (see Fig. 26-10, *B*).

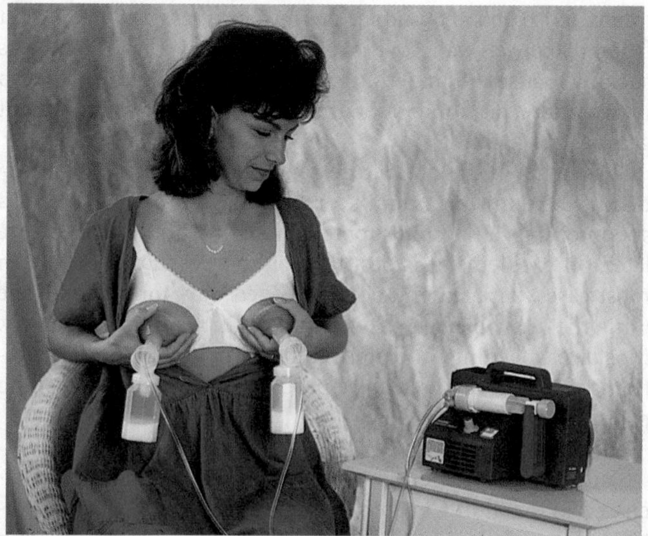

Fig. 26-9 Bilateral breast pumping. *(Courtesy Medela, Inc., McHenry, IL.)*

Full-service electric pumps, or hospital-grade pumps, are similar to the sucking action and pressure of the breastfeeding infant. These are expensive and therefore are usually rented. When breastfeeding is delayed after birth (e.g., the infant is preterm or ill), or when mother and baby are separated for lengthy periods, these pumps are most appropriate (see Fig. 26-10, *A*). Electric, self-cycling double pumps are efficient and easy to use. Some of these pumps come with carry bags containing coolers to store pumped milk (see Fig. 26-9).

Smaller battery-operated or electric pumps are also available. Some have automatic suck-release cycling, and others require use of a finger to regulate strength and speed of suction. These are typically used when pumping is done occasionally, but some models are satisfactory for working mothers or others who pump on a regular basis.

Storage of Breast Milk

Breast milk can be stored safely in any clean glass or plastic container (bisphenol A [BPA] free); some suggest plastic containers because cells in breast milk adhere to glass (Lawrence & Lawrence, 2005). Disposable bottle liners are easy and inexpensive to use when storing milk. When using bottle liners, double bagging is recommended to protect the milk most effectively.

Breast milk may be safely kept at room temperature for 6 to 8 hours as long as environmental temperatures do not exceed 77° F. Breast milk can be refrigerated safely for up to 5 days (39° F or 4° C) after it is expressed. If it is not used within that time, it can be frozen (at 0° C) for up to 6 months in a refrigerator/freezer with a separate freezer door; it should be kept in the middle or toward the back of the freezer to avoid variations in temperature. Milk can be stored for 1 year in a freezer at −18° C (Lawrence & Lawrence, 2005). When breast milk is stored, the container should be dated and the oldest milk used first.

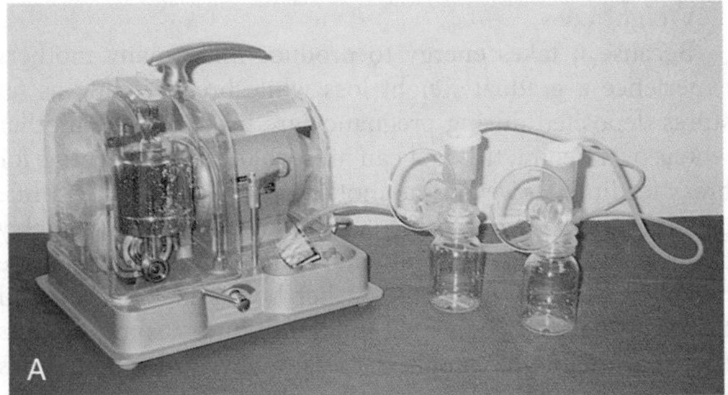

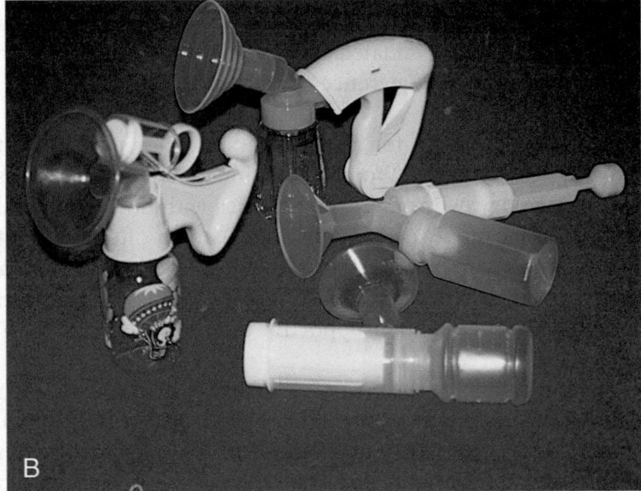

Fig. 26-10 **A,** Hospital-grade electric breast pump. **B,** Manual breast pumps. *(B, Courtesy Marjorie Pyle, RNC, Lifecircle, Costa Mesa, CA.)*

Frozen milk is thawed by placing the container in warm water or in the refrigerator. It should not be refrozen and should be used within 24 hours. After thawing, the container should be shaken gently to mix the layers that have separated.

NURSING ALERT Do not use a microwave to defrost frozen human milk. High-temperature microwaving (72° to 98° C) significantly destroys the antiinfective factors and vitamin C content. The safety of low-temperature microwaving (20° to 53° C) remains questionable. Microwaving does not heat evenly and can cause encapsulated boiling bubbles to form in the center of the liquid. Infants have sustained severe burns to the mouth, throat, and upper gastrointestinal tract as a result of microwaved milk (Lawrence & Lawrence, 2005). One of the best ways to thaw frozen human milk is to place under a warm flow of tap water. Another option is to let the frozen milk thaw overnight in the refrigerator to maintain high levels of secretory IgA (Biancuzzo, 2003). Test the temperature of the milk before feeding.

Being Away from the Infant (Maternal Employment)

Many women successfully combine breastfeeding with employment, school, or other commitments. If feedings are missed, the milk supply may be affected. Some women's bodies adjust the milk supply to the times she is with the infant for feedings. Other mothers must pump while away or their supply diminishes rapidly. Employed mothers can continue breastfeeding with guidance and encouragement. Mothers are encouraged to set realistic goals for employment and breastfeeding, with accurate information regarding the costs, risks, and benefits of available feeding options. Many mothers may find that a program of breast pumping when away from home and bottle-feeding the infant the expressed milk with or without formula supplementation is successful. Expressed breast milk may be stored in the refrigerator (4° C) without danger of bacterial contamination for up to 5 days (Lawrence & Lawrence, 2005). Although feeding the infant at home may occur on a demand basis, pumping milk away from home may be needed every 3 to 4 hours to maintain adequate supply. Breast milk may be expressed by hand or pump (manual or electric) and stored in an appropriate air-tight glass or plastic container (BPA free). Businesses are increasingly making available rooms where mothers can nurse their infants or use breast pumps.

In addition to efficient breast pumping, mothers also need child care by a trusted individual or agency and support and assistance from significant others. As with all breastfeeding mothers, these women must have proper nutrition and rest for adequate lactation. Maternal fatigue is considered the biggest threat to successful breastfeeding in employed mothers (Corbett-Dick & Bezek, 1997).

Weaning

Typically, weaning is initiated at a time chosen by the mother or the infant. Weaning can be accomplished with little effort and no discomfort when it is done gradually. Abrupt weaning is likely to be distressing for both mother and infant, as well as physically uncomfortable for the mother.

Infant-led weaning means that the infant moves at his or her own pace in omitting feedings. Drinking from a cup and increasing the amount of solid foods substitute for breastfeeding.

Mother-led weaning means that the mother decides which feedings to drop. This is most easily done by omitting the feeding of least interest to the infant or the one the infant is most likely to sleep through. It can also be the feeding most convenient for the mother to omit. After a week or more, another feeding is dropped, and so on, until the infant is weaned from the breast. Allowing time for the milk supply to adjust before omitting another feeding prevents discomfort for the mother as her supply gradually decreases.

Infants can be weaned directly from the breast to a cup. Bottles are usually offered to infants less than 6 months of age. If the infant is weaned before 1 year of age, formula should be offered instead of whole cow's milk.

If abrupt weaning is necessary, breast engorgement often occurs. The mother is instructed to take mild analgesics, wear a supportive bra, apply ice packs or cabbage leaves to the breasts, and pump if needed to increase comfort. The pump should not be used to empty the breasts, since they should remain full enough to promote a decrease in milk production.

Milk Banking

For those infants who cannot be breastfed but who also cannot survive except on human milk, banked donor milk is critically important. Because of the antiinfective and growth-promoting properties of human milk, as well as its superior nutrition, donor milk is used in some neonatal intensive care units for preterm or sick infants when the mother's own milk is not available. Donor milk is also used therapeutically for medical purposes, such as in transplant recipients who are immunocompromised.

The Human Milk Banking Association of North America (HMBANA) *(www.hmbana.org)* has established guidelines for the operation of donor human milk banks (Lawrence & Lawrence, 2005). Donor milk banks collect, screen, process, and distribute milk donated by breastfeeding mothers who are feeding their own infants and pumping a few extra ounces each day for the milk bank. All donors are screened both by interview and serologically for communicable diseases. Donor milk is stored frozen until it is heat processed to kill potential pathogens (bacteria and viruses), and then it is refrozen for storage until it is dispensed for use. The heat processing adds a level of protection for the recipient that is not possible with any other donor tissue or organ. Milk is dispensed only by prescription. A per-ounce fee is charged by the bank for processing, but the HMBANA guidelines prohibit payment to donors.

Care of the Mother

Diet

The composition of human milk varies slightly among women, regardless of their diets. The mother's milk automatically contains everything the baby needs, except in rare cases of maternal nutrient deficiencies. For most women, only 200 to 500 extra calories per day need to be added to the diet to provide adequate nutrients for the infant while also protecting the mother's body stores. The Institute of Medicine (2005) DRIs provide a guide for energy intake that is adjusted for lactating women. The Estimated Energy Requirement for a lactating woman during the first 6 months is approximately 2700 kcal/day; this amount increases to 2768 kcal/day in the second 6 months. Additional intake recommendations include micronutrients, vitamins, and minerals. For example, the Institute of Medicine recommends that a 19- to 30-year-old lactating woman consume 3.8 L of water, 210 g of carbohydrate, and 71 g of protein per day. The DRI tables may be accessed at *www.nap.edu.*

There are no specific foods or drinks that all breastfeeding mothers must either consume or avoid. Lactating mothers should ideally consume a balanced diet of nutrient-dense foods that includes a wide variety of breads and cereal grains, fruits and vegetables, and three or more servings of milk products daily. Diets or medications that promote rapid weight loss should be avoided, and caffeinated beverages should be consumed in moderation. Adequate amounts of calcium, minerals, and fat-soluble vitamins are important.

If the breastfeeding mother is drinking enough fluids to quench her thirst, she is likely drinking enough to support lactation. Because of her increased need for fluids, the breastfeeding mother may wish to keep a drink within reach during breastfeeding.

Weight Loss

Because it takes energy to produce milk, many mothers experience a gradual weight loss while breastfeeding as fat stores deposited during pregnancy are used. For the mother who is overweight, this fact can present an added incentive for breastfeeding. However, the mother who wants to diet while lactating should avoid losing large amounts of weight quickly because fat-soluble environmental contaminants to which she has been exposed are stored in her body's fat reserves, and these may be released into her milk. In addition, some mothers find that their milk supply decreases when caloric intake is severely restricted. A weight loss of 1 to 2 kg/mo reportedly will not affect milk production; however, more than that should be carefully evaluated in regards to infant weight gain and feeding pattern (Lawrence & Lawrence, 2005).

Exercise

There is no reason for a breastfeeding woman to restrict her physical activity. Women continue activities such as hiking, jogging, swimming, and aerobics with no detrimental effect on milk supply or composition. Women often find that they are more comfortable if they engage in exercise soon after breastfeeding when their breasts are as empty as possible. Wearing a well-designed, supportive bra may also help.

Rest

It is important for the breastfeeding mother to rest as much as possible, especially in the first 1 to 2 weeks after birth. Fatigue, stress, and worry may interfere with milk production and let-down. The nurse can encourage the mother to sleep when the baby sleeps. Household chores and care for other children can be done by the father, grandparents or other relatives, and friends.

Breast Care

The breastfeeding mother's normal bathing routine is all that is required to keep her breasts clean. Soap can have a drying effect on nipples, so she should be instructed to avoid washing the nipples with soap. The small amount of soap that runs down her breasts while washing her face and neck or shampooing her hair is of no concern.

Breast creams should not be used routinely because they may block the natural oil secreted by Montgomery's glands on the areola. Some breast creams contain alcohol, which may dry the nipples. Vitamin E oil or cream is not recommended for use on nipples because it is a fat-soluble vitamin and a breastfeeding infant might consume enough vitamin E from the nipple to reach toxic levels. In addition, some people are allergic to vitamin E oil.

Modified lanolin with reduced allergens can be used safely on dry or sore nipples. Because lanolin is made from sheep's wool, the nurse should ask the mother if she is allergic to wool before applying the ointment. Lanolin is not recommended if it is suspected that nipple soreness may be due to a monilial infection. Antifungal creams are used to treat yeast infections on nipples. Antiseptic sprays and premoistened towelettes containing alcohol are not recommended.

The mother with flat or inverted nipples is sometimes advised to wear breast shells in her bra. These hard plastic devices exert mild pressure around the base of the nipple to encourage nipple eversion; however, current information shows that little correction of the nipple actually takes place

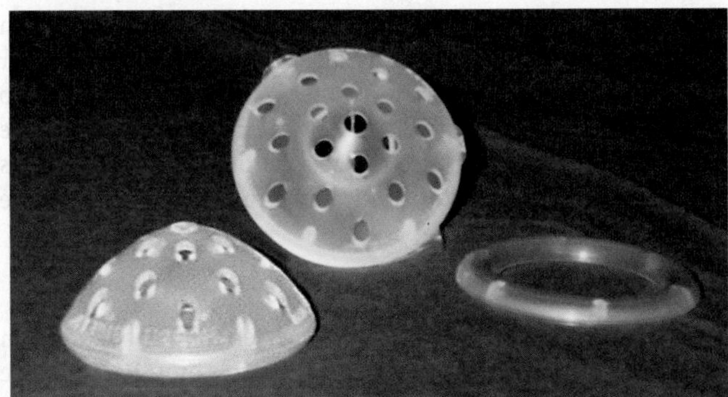

Fig. 26-11 Breast shells.

prenatally (Riordan & Wambach, 2009). Postnatally they are useful for sore nipples to keep the mother's bra or clothing from touching the nipples (Fig. 26-11).

If a mother needs breast support, she will be more comfortable wearing a bra, since the ligament that supports the breast (Cooper's ligament) will otherwise stretch and be painful. If she is comfortable without a bra, there is no reason for her to wear one. If a woman prefers to wear a bra, it should fit well, offer nonbinding support, and feel comfortable. Underwire bras or improperly fitting bras may contribute to clogged milk ducts. Mothers should be encouraged to breastfeed at least once daily without a bra on so that all milk ducts can empty well.

Leakage of milk between feedings is a problem for some women. Using breast pads (washable or disposable) inside a bra and wearing layered or printed tops can help camouflage the leakage. Plastic-lined pads are not recommended because they trap moisture and may lead to sore nipples. To stop leakage, the mother can be alert to any sensation, such as tingling, that her milk is letting down. If this happens, she can usually stop the let-down by pressing straight back on her nipples. In public the mother can fold her arms across her chest to apply pressure unobtrusively.

Breast Self-Examination

Although only 1% to 2% of cases of breast cancer are diagnosed during pregnancy or lactation, the breastfeeding woman should perform breast self-examination (BSE) (see Chapter 5). The woman who is not menstruating should choose a convenient date on which to do her BSE every month. She needs to become familiar with the normal nodularity of her lactating breasts so that she can detect anything unusual on examination. Nodules that match in location in both breasts are almost always breast tissue. Nodules that increase and decrease in size are probably milk glands or ducts. Because lactating breasts are very dense, mammography is of limited diagnostic value. Should a suspicious nodule be discovered, a biopsy can usually be done without interrupting breastfeeding.

Effect of Menstruation

The return of menstrual periods varies among lactating women. The majority will resume menstruation by 6 months postpartum. Menstruation has no effect on breastfeeding. There are no hormonal effects on the infant, although some babies may seem fussy for the first day. The quality of milk is not affected (Lawrence & Lawrence, 2005).

Sexual Sensations

Some women experience rhythmic uterine contractions during breastfeeding. Such sensations are not unusual because uterine contractions and milk ejection are both triggered by oxytocin, but they may be disturbing to some mothers who perceive them to be similar to orgasm.

Breastfeeding and Contraception

Although breastfeeding confers a period of infertility, it is not considered an effective method of contraception. Breastfeeding delays the return of ovulation and menstruation; however, ovulation may occur before the first menstrual period after birth. Thus the breastfeeding woman who is relying on the lactational amenorrhea method of birth control needs to be knowledgeable about ways to determine when ovulation occurs (i.e., basal body temperature, presence of cervical mucus, and cervical position). Hormonal contraceptives, including pills, injectables, and implants, may cause a decrease in the milk supply and decreased neonatal growth and are best avoided during the first 6 weeks postpartum. Oral contraceptives have historically not been recommended because of the tendency to decrease milk supply. Lawrence and Lawrence (2005), however, indicate that a number of studies show that low-dose contraceptives containing estrogen can be safely taken by the lactating woman. Progestin-only birth control pills are less likely to interfere with the milk supply. The etonogestrel implant Implanon is reported to be safe for use during lactation (Hohmann & Creinin, 2007). Contraceptives such as the progestin-only injection (Depo-Provera) have not been found to interfere with milk production. Nonhormonal contraceptive methods (e.g., foam, condom, nonhormonal intrauterine device, natural family planning, sterilization) are appropriate and have no detrimental effect on breastfeeding.

Recommendations from the World Health Organization are to avoid using combined oral contraceptives from 6 weeks to 6 months postpartum unless appropriate alternative methods are not available. The La Leche League International recommends avoiding combined oral contraceptives in breastfeeding women, and the American College of Obstetricians and Gynecologists recommends avoiding combined oral contraceptives until after 6 weeks postpartum and then only if lactation is well established and the infant's nutritional status is appropriately evaluated (Guthmann, Bang, & Nashelsky, 2005).

Breastfeeding During Pregnancy

It is possible for a breastfeeding woman to conceive and continue breastfeeding throughout the subsequent pregnancy if there are no medical contraindications (e.g., risk of preterm labor). When the second baby is born, colostrum is produced. The practice of breastfeeding a newborn and an older child is called *tandem nursing.* The nurse should remind the mother to always feed the newborn first to ensure that the newborn is receiving adequate nutrition. The supply-meets-demand principle works just as with breastfeeding multiple babies.

Diabetic Mother

The mother with type 2 diabetes is encouraged to breastfeed. In addition to benefits for the infant and maternal satisfaction, breastfeeding has an antidiabetogenic effect. Blood glucose levels and insulin requirements are lower because of the carbohydrate used in milk production. During lactation, the diabetic woman may be able to eat more food and still take less insulin. However, insulin dosage must be adjusted as the infant is weaned. Some diabetic women are at increased risk for sore nipples caused by monilial infections and may have an increased risk for mastitis (Lawrence & Lawrence, 2005).

Breastfeeding and Drugs

Despite much concern about the compatibility of drugs and breastfeeding, in fact few drugs are contraindicated during lactation (see Appendix A). Considerations in evaluating the safety of a specific medication during breastfeeding include the pharmacokinetics of the drug in the maternal system and the absorption, metabolism, distribution, storage, and excretion in the infant. The infant's gestational and chronologic age, body weight, and breastfeeding pattern are also considered (Lawrence & Lawrence, 2005). Most medications do not cause problems for the infant, but breastfeeding mothers should be cautioned about taking any but essential ones. In certain instances (e.g., radioactive diagnostic agents) the mother is instructed to pump her breasts and discard the pumped milk until the drug has cleared her body.

Smoking may impair milk production; it also exposes the infant to the risks of secondhand smoke. Mothers who continue to smoke tobacco when lactating should be advised not to smoke within 2 hours before breastfeeding and to never smoke in the same room with the infant. If a mother chooses to consume alcohol, she should be advised to minimize its effects by having only one drink and consuming it immediately after a feeding or waiting for 2 hours after drinking to breastfeed. Alcoholic beverages may impair the MER (milk ejection reflex). The mother who is pumping for a preterm or sick infant should avoid alcohol until her baby is healthy.

The caffeine concentration in milk is only about 1% of the level in the mother's plasma. The infant's immature renal system limits the ability to excrete the caffeine; caffeine accumulates in the infant's system and can cause irritability and poor sleeping patterns. Some infants are sensitive to even small amounts of caffeine; mothers of such infants should limit caffeine intake. Caffeine is found in coffee, tea, chocolate, and many soft drinks (Lawrence & Lawrence, 2005).

Herbs and herbal teas are becoming more widely used during lactation. Although some are considered safe, others contain pharmacologically active compounds that may have detrimental effects, particularly on the neonate. A thorough history should include the composition of any herbal remedies. Each remedy should then be evaluated for its compatibility with breastfeeding. Herbal teas that are considered safe during lactation include rose hips, orange spice, chicory, peppermint, raspberry, and red bush tea (Lawrence & Lawrence, 2005). A regional poison control center may provide information on the active properties of herbs. Consult resources online and Appendix A for more information about drugs in breast milk.

Environmental Contaminants

Except under unusual circumstances, breastfeeding is not contraindicated because of exposure to environmental contaminants such as DDT (an insecticide) and tetrachloroethylene (used in dry cleaning) (Lawrence & Lawrence, 2005). It is recommended that breastfeeding mothers not expose their infant to secondhand smoke; this often leads to an increase in the incidence of reactive airway disease, wheezing, and upper respiratory tract infections. Mothers who do not give up smoking should change clothes before breastfeeding because tobacco residue may adhere to most clothes and the infant is thus exposed to the effects of nicotine and smoke even in the absence of active smoking.

Special Considerations

The breastfeeding mother may experience some common problems. In the majority of cases these complications are preventable if the mother receives appropriate education about breastfeeding. Early recognition and resolution of these problems are important to prevent interruption of breastfeeding and to promote the mother's comfort and sense of well-being. Emotional support provided by the nurse or lactation consultant is essential to help allay the mother's frustration and anxiety and to prevent early cessation of breastfeeding.

Engorgement

Engorgement is a common response of the breasts to the sudden change in hormones and the increased volume of milk. It usually occurs on the third to fifth day postpartum when the milk comes in, and it lasts about 24 hours. Blood supply to the breasts increases and causes swelling of tissues surrounding the milk ducts. The ducts may be pinched shut, so that the milk does not flow. The breasts are firm, tender, swollen, and hot, and they may appear shiny and red. The tenderness and swelling extend into the axilla. The areolae are firm and the nipples may flatten, making it difficult for the newborn to latch on. Back pressure on full milk glands inhibits milk production if the milk is not removed from the breasts, and the milk supply may diminish.

When engorgement occurs, the nurse should assure the mother that this is a temporary condition usually resolved within 24 hours. The mother is instructed to feed every 2 hours, softening at least one breast, and pumping the other breast to soften. Pumping during engorgement will not cause a problematic increase in milk supply.

Because of the swelling of breast tissue surrounding the milk glands' ducts, ice packs are recommended in a 15 to 20 minutes on, 45 minutes off rotation between feedings. The ice packs should cover both breasts. Large bags of frozen peas or corn make easy packs and can be refrozen between uses. Standing in a warm shower and manually expressing some milk is an alternative treatment (Lawrence & Lawrence, 2005).

Fresh raw cabbage leaves placed over the breasts in between feedings may help reduce the swelling (Roberts, 1995). The mother washes the cabbage leaves and places them in her freezer until they are cold; she then places them over her breasts, leaving just the nipples exposed to air. The leaves are replaced when they begin to wilt. Although the exact mechanism of action of cabbage leaves in treatment of engorgement is not understood, it is thought that continuous application might decrease milk supply. Raw cabbage leaves are often effective for formula-feeding mothers who want their milk to "dry up."

Antiinflammatory medications such as ibuprofen may help reduce pain and swelling associated with engorgement. Mothers often have an elevated temperature and experience achiness in their breasts; ibuprofen can help remedy this.

Because heat increases blood flow, application of heat to an already congested breast is usually counterproductive. Occasionally, however, standing in a warm shower will start the milk leaking, or the mother may be able to manually express enough milk to soften the areola so the baby can latch on and feed.

Sore Nipples

Mild nipple discomfort at the beginning of feedings or mild nipple tenderness during the first few days of breastfeeding is common. Severe soreness and abraded, cracked, or bleeding nipples are not normal and most often result from poor positioning, incorrect latch-on, improper suck, or a monilial infection. Many women expect breastfeeding to be painful based on stories they have heard from family and friends; however, breastfeeding is not supposed to be painful.

For the first few days after birth, the nursing mother may experience some nipple tenderness with suckling. This should quickly dissipate as the milk begins to flow and acts as a lubricant. To minimize the initial suckling pain, the mother can express a few drops of milk to moisten the nipple and areola before latch-on. The mother should ensure that the newborn is well supported, is in straight body alignment, and has no pressure on the back of her or his head. The newborn's nose, cheeks, and chin should touch the breast, and the mother should support the breast with her hand during the early feedings. The nurse helps to reposition as necessary to try to resolve the nipple discomfort.

If the mother reports a pinching sensation of the nipple as the infant sucks, it may be helpful to gently pull down on the side of the newborn's jaw while he or she is sucking to increase the amount of breast tissue in the infant's mouth. If the nipple pain continues, the mother needs to remove the infant from the breast, breaking suction with her finger in the infant's mouth. She then attempts latch-on again, making certain the infant's mouth is open wide before the infant is pulled quickly to the breast (see Fig. 26-5).

The infant's suck can be assessed by the nurse or lactation consultant by inserting a clean gloved finger in the newborn's mouth and stimulating the newborn to suck. If the newborn is not extruding his or her tongue over the lower gum and the mother reports pain or pinching with sucking, the newborn may have a short frenulum (commonly referred to as being "tongue-tied"). In some cases ankyloglossia is corrected surgically to free the tongue for less painful, more effective breastfeeding (Dollberg et al, 2006).

The treatment for sore nipples is first to correct the cause. Once the problem is assessed, identified, and corrected, sore nipples should heal within a few days, even though the baby continues to breastfeed regularly. A common cause for sore nipples is positioning; the infant's ability to latch on to the areola should be carefully evaluated (Lawrence & Lawrence, 2005).

When sore nipples occur, it is more comfortable to start the feeding on the least sore nipple. A few drops of milk can be expressed, rubbed into the sore area, and allowed to air dry. Warm water compresses may also be comforting.

If nipples are extremely sore or damaged and the mother cannot tolerate breastfeeding, she may be advised to use an electric breast pump for 24 to 48 hours to allow the nipples to begin healing before resuming breastfeeding. It is important that the mother use a pump that will effectively empty the breasts.

Sore nipples should be open to air as much as possible. Breast shells worn inside the bra allow air to circulate while keeping clothing off sore nipples.

Silicone (flexible) nipple shields are helpful for a mother with flat or inverted nipples, for preterm babies who have trouble latching and maintaining suction, and for babies who develop a preference for a bottle nipple and refuse the breast (Riordan & Wambach, 2009). Nipple shields also help protect abraded, sore nipples. They should be applied on the nipple areola area just before putting the baby on the breast. Flip up the brim of the shield (like that of a sombrero), place the shield directly over the nipple, and gently pat down the brim. Nipple shields should be used for a short time only, or the baby may become so accustomed to them that he or she refuses the breast. In addition, lactation consultants should closely monitor the infant's growth and intake of milk (see Family-Centered Care box).

FAMILY-CENTERED CARE

Sore Nipples in Breastfeeding Mother

Role play how you could determine whether a mother's telephone call for help with sore nipples requires teaching about positioning and latch-on or whether she might have a monilial infection on her nipples. What specific questions would you ask? To whom might you refer her?

Monilial Infections

Sore nipples that occur after the newborn period are often due to a monilial (yeast) infection. The mother usually reports severe nipple pain and tenderness, burning, or stinging, and she may have sharp, shooting, burning pains in the breasts during and after feedings. The nipples appear somewhat pink and shiny or may be scaly or flaky; there may be a visible rash, small blisters, or thrush. Most often, the pain is out of proportion to the appearance of the nipple. Yeast infections of the nipples and breast can be excruciatingly painful and can lead to early cessation of breastfeeding if not recognized and treated promptly.

Infants may or may not exhibit symptoms of monilial infection. Oral thrush and a red, raised diaper rash are common indications of a yeast infection. An affected infant is often fussy and gassy. When feeding, the infant is likely to pull off the breast soon after starting to feed, crying with apparent pain. The infant may be biting or gumming at the breast.

The most common predisposing factors for yeast infections of the breast include previous antibiotic use, vaginal yeast infections, and nipple damage.

Mothers and infants must be treated simultaneously, even if the infant has no visible signs of infection. Treatment for mother is typically an antifungal cream applied to the nipples after feedings and, in some cases, a systemic antifungal medication such as fluconazole. Most pediatricians prescribe an oral antifungal medication, such as nystatin or fluconazole, for infants. Treatment should continue for at least 14 days even after symptoms begin to improve in 1 to 2 days (Lawrence & Lawrence, 2005). Careful handwashing is essential to prevent the spread of yeast.

Plugged Milk Ducts

A milk duct may become plugged or clogged, causing an area of the breast to become swollen and tender. This area typically does not empty or soften with feeding or pumping. There may also be a small white pearl on the tip of the nipple; this is the curd of milk blocking the flow. The mother is afebrile and has no generalized symptoms.

Plugged ducts are most often the result of inadequate emptying of the breast. This may be due to clothing that is too tight, a poorly fitting or underwire bra, or constant use of the same position for feeding. Application of warm compresses to the affected area and to the nipple before feeding helps promote emptying of the breast and release of the plug. (A disposable diaper filled with warm water makes an easy compress.)

Frequent feeding is recommended, with the infant beginning the feeding on the affected side to foster more complete emptying. The mother is advised to massage the affected area while the infant nurses or while she is pumping. Varying feeding positions and feeding without wearing a bra may be useful in resolving a plugged duct.

If the mother develops fever or flu-like symptoms, she may have developed mastitis and should notify her health care provider. Plugged milk ducts do not necessarily cause mastitis, but milk stasis may increase susceptibility to breast infection.

Mastitis

A breast infection, or mastitis, is characterized by the sudden onset of flu-like symptoms, including fever, chills, body aches, and headache. (Flu-like symptoms in a breastfeeding mother should be considered indicative of mastitis until proven otherwise.) There is localized breast pain and tenderness and a hot, reddened area on the breast, often resembling the shape of a pie wedge. Mastitis most commonly occurs in the upper outer quadrant of the breast; it may affect one or both breasts.

Certain factors may predispose a woman to mastitis. Inadequate emptying of the breasts is common, related to engorgement, plugged ducts, a sudden decrease in the number of feedings, abrupt weaning, or underwire bras. Sore, cracked nipples may lead to mastitis by providing a portal of entry for the causative organism (staphylococci, streptococci, and *Escherichia coli* are most common). Stress and fatigue, ill family members, breast trauma, and poor maternal nutrition are also predisposing factors for mastitis (Fetherston, 1998).

Breastfeeding mothers should be taught the signs of mastitis before they are discharged from the hospital, and they need to know to call the health care provider promptly if the symptoms occur. Treatment includes antibiotics such as cephalexin or dicloxacillin and analgesic-antipyretic medications such as ibuprofen. Rest is extremely important; the mother is advised to sleep whenever the baby sleeps. The mother should feed the baby or pump frequently, striving to adequately empty the affected side. Warm compresses to the breast before feeding or pumping may be useful; cool compresses may be applied to the breast after feeding. Adequate fluid intake and a balanced diet are important for the mother with mastitis.

Complications of mastitis include breast abscess, chronic mastitis, and fungal infections of the breast. Most complications can be prevented by early recognition and treatment.

Hepatitis B and C

The risk of perinatal transmission of hepatitis C is approximately 5% to 6%; transmission is believed to occur primarily at delivery and only in women who are hepatitis C virus ribonucleic acid (HCV RNA) positive at delivery. There is no evidence that HCV is transmitted in breast milk and therefore the Centers for Disease Control and Prevention guidelines maintain there is no increased risk of transmission with breastfeeding as long as the mother is also HIV negative and her nipples are not cracked or bleeding; breastfeeding by an HBsAg-positive mother is also reported to pose no additional risk of acquisition to the infant (American Academy of Pediatrics, Committee on Infectious Diseases, 2006) (see Contraindications to Breastfeeding, p. 679).

Role of the Nurse in Promoting Successful Lactation

Nurses play a major role in breastfeeding education and support for new parents. Nurses often work with lactation consultants in hospitals, physicians' offices, or community settings. Although the vast majority are registered nurses, lactation consultants come from a variety of educational backgrounds such as nutrition, physical and occupational therapy, home economics, psychology, social work, education, or the basic sciences. Lactation consultants have had specialized postbaccalaureate education, training, and clinical experience working with breastfeeding mothers, and they have passed a certifying examination that requires meeting defined academic and clinical experience criteria.

Nurses in prenatal settings can educate the mother and her partner about the advantages of breastfeeding and explore reasons why they may prefer bottle-feeding. They can provide expectant parents with current reading materials and information about prenatal classes. At each encounter, the nurse can answer questions and provide additional information as needed.

Assessment of the mother's breasts and nipples during pregnancy is important. Flat or inverted nipples are identified. The mother may be offered breast shells (see Fig. 26-11) to wear during the last trimester of pregnancy to encourage eversion of the nipples, although antepartum use may be ineffective. These breast shells can also be worn postpartum between feedings.

The nurse should determine whether the woman has had any breast surgery. Breast reduction or augmentation may interfere with the ability to produce milk and transfer it successfully to the baby.

No special nipple preparation is necessary during pregnancy. Efforts to "toughen" the nipples by pulling on them or rubbing them with a rough towel are to be avoided. Such stimulation can cause release of oxytocin and result in preterm labor, or damage the outer layer of protective skin cells, which may increase the risk of sore nipples.

In the immediate postpartum period, the nurse is instrumental in helping the mother initiate breastfeeding as soon as possible after birth. Encouraging parents to keep the baby in

NURSING CARE PLAN The Newborn with Insufficient Intake of Nutrients

Nursing Diagnosis: Ineffective breastfeeding related to deficient knowledge of mother as evidenced by ongoing incorrect latch-on technique

Expected Outcomes

Mother will express increased satisfaction with breastfeeding, and neonate will exhibit satisfaction of hunger and sucking needs.

Nursing Interventions/*Rationales*

Assess mother's knowledge and motivation for breastfeeding *to acknowledge mother's desire for effective outcome and provide starting point for teaching.*

Observe a breastfeeding session *to provide a database for positive reinforcement and problem identification.*

Describe and demonstrate ways to stimulate the sucking reflex, various positions for breastfeeding, and the use of pillows during a session *to promote maternal and neonatal comfort and effective latch-on.*

Monitor neonatal position of mouth on areola and position of head and body *to give positive reinforcement for correct latch-on position or to correct poor latch-on position.*

Teach mother ways to stimulate neonate to maintain an awake state by diapering, unwrapping, massaging, or burping *to complete a breastfeeding thoroughly and satisfactorily.*

Give mother information regarding lactation diet, expression of milk by hand or pump, and storage of expressed breast milk *to provide basic information.*

Make certain mother has written information on all aspects of breastfeeding *to reinforce verbal instructions and demonstrations.*

Refer to support group and lactation consultant if needed *to provide further information and group support.*

the mother's room (rooming-in) allows the opportunity for the mother to learn to recognize feeding cues and to feed the baby when these cues are present. The nurse provides help with positioning and latch-on until the mother can accomplish this independently. Explanations are given early regarding frequency and duration of feedings, how to wake a sleepy baby, and how to determine whether the baby is getting enough milk. Information about the transition to mature milk (milk coming in) and how to prevent or deal with engorgement is needed. The mother is informed about the prevention and treatment of sore nipples and about signs of mastitis (including the importance of contacting the primary health care provider if these occur). (See Nursing Care Plan.)

Parents often expect that because breastfeeding is "natural," it will come naturally for both mother and baby. This misconception needs to be clarified early so that parents may view breastfeeding as a learning process and not have unrealistic expectations. All health care providers who are knowledgeable about breastfeeding can offer needed support and encouragement to parents, helping to instill a sense of confidence.

The Baby-Friendly Hospital Initiative (BFHI) is a joint effort of the World Health Organization and the United Nations Children's Fund (UNICEF) to encourage, promote, and support breastfeeding as the model for optimum infant nutrition. BFHI developed 10 research-supported practices as a guideline for maternity facilities worldwide to promote breastfeeding (Kyenkya-Isabirye, 1992; Wright, Rice, & Wells, 1996) (Box 26-2). Research indicates that Baby-Friendly designated hospitals in the United States have higher rates for breastfeeding initiation and exclusivity than hospitals that are not Baby-Friendly designates (Merewood et al, 2005). In addition, BFHI implementation in birth facilities has increased breastfeeding rates among African-American women and other populations with lower breastfeeding rates. According to recent Centers for Disease Control and Prevention survey data (DiGirolamo et al, 2008), 24% of birth facilities (n = 2687 facilities) continue to offer supplements other than breast milk to approximately half of healthy term newborns; of those

BOX 26-2 Ten Steps to Successful Breastfeeding

Every facility providing maternity services and care for newborns should:

1. Have a written breastfeeding policy that is routinely communicated to all health care staff.
2. Train all health care staff in skills necessary to implement this policy.
3. Inform all pregnant women about the benefits and management of breastfeeding.
4. Help mothers initiate breastfeeding within a half hour of birth.
5. Show mothers how to breastfeed and how to maintain lactation, even if they are separated from their newborns.
6. Give newborns no food or drink other than breast milk, unless medically indicated.
7. Practice rooming-in—allow mothers and newborns to remain together—24 hours a day.
8. Encourage breastfeeding on demand.
9. Give no artificial teats or pacifiers (also called dummies or soothers) to breastfeeding newborns.
10. Foster the establishment of breastfeeding support groups and refer mothers to them on discharge from the hospital or clinic.

From Kyenkya-Isabirye M: UNICEF launches the Baby-Friendly Hospital Initiative, *MCN Am J Matern Child Nurs* 17(4):177-179, 1992; Wright A, Rice S, Wells C: Changing hospital practices to increase the duration of breastfeeding, *Pediatrics* 97(5):669-675, 1996.

facilities offering supplements, 30% reportedly gave the newborn glucose water, and 15% gave the newborn water. Of the birth facilities surveyed, 70% reported giving mothers gift bags containing formula. A population-based study indicates that mothers were more likely to continue breastfeeding when the birth facility supported all five practices recommended by BFHI: breastfeeding within the first hour after birth, no pacifiers, infant rooming-in, no supplements given, and a telephone number for consults after discharge (Murray, Ricketts, & Dellaport, 2007).

A survey of breastfeeding mothers indicated that the determining factors for changing to bottle-feeding included the mother's perception of the father's attitude toward breastfeeding and the mother's uncertainty regarding the amount of milk the infant would receive (Arora et al, 2000). These findings have important implications for involving fathers in education and discussion regarding breastfeeding before and during the pregnancy. Fathers may express concerns of feeling left out during the newborn period if they have little involvement other than diapering and holding the infant. Encouraging fathers regarding their positive role in supporting the mothers' breastfeeding may help decrease feelings of helplessness and isolation and may benefit mother-infant interaction.

Follow-Up After Hospital Discharge

Problems with sore nipples, engorgement, and jaundice are likely to occur after discharge. Thus it is the hospital nurse's role to educate and prepare the mother for problems she may encounter once she is home. It is critical that the mother be given a list of resources for help with breastfeeding concerns, and that she realizes when to call for assistance. Community resources for breastfeeding mothers include lactation consultants in hospitals, physicians' offices, or private practice; nurses in pediatric or obstetric offices; support groups such as La Leche League International; and peer counseling programs (such as those offered through WIC).

Telephone follow-up by hospital or office nurses within the first day or two after discharge can provide a means to identify any problems and offer needed advice and support. The American Academy of Pediatrics, Subcommittee on Hyperbilirubinemia (2004), recommends that infants discharged before 48 hours of age be seen by a health care provider within 48 hours. In some settings and circumstances, home care follow-up is available for mothers after hospital discharge.

Formula Feeding

Rationale for Formula Feeding

The decision to feed a baby infant formula may be the result of the mother's or partner's personal preference, the influence of other significant family members, or simply a lack of education and familiarity with breastfeeding. Occasionally no other option is available: the mother may have extensive breast scarring or may have had a bilateral mastectomy; the mother may be taking medications that preclude breastfeeding; or the baby may be adopted. Breast augmentation or reduction mammoplasty may interfere with the ability to produce an adequate milk supply and successful transfer to the baby. Some mothers are able to induce lactation for an adopted baby by using a supplemental nursing device during breastfeeding. Infants diagnosed with classic galactosemia must be fed a lactose-free formula; this excludes breastfeeding.

Infant formula may be used to supplement breastfeeding if the mother's milk supply is inadequate. It may also be fed to the baby if the mother will be away from home and wishes to leave a bottle of formula instead of expressed breast milk.

Formula-feeding is also recommended for mothers who are HIV positive or who are using recreational drugs (e.g., cocaine, methamphetamine, heroin).

Parent Education

Inexperienced mothers and fathers who are formula-feeding their infants usually need teaching, counseling, and support. They may need assistance with the feeding process and with any problems they may experience. Some parents who are formula-feeding may express concern that the baby will suffer as a result of their decision. Emphasis on the beneficial use of feeding times for close contact and socializing with the infant can help relieve some of this concern.

Readiness for Feeding

The first feeding of formula is ideally given after the initial transition to extrauterine life. Feeding readiness cues include stability of vital signs, bowel sounds, an active sucking reflex, an effective breathing pattern, and those cues described earlier for breastfed babies.

Feeding Patterns

Typically a newborn initially will take 10 to 15 ml of formula per feeding. Intake gradually increases during the first week of life. Most newborns are drinking 90 to 150 ml per feeding by the end of the second week, or sooner. The newborn infant should be fed at least every 3 to 4 hours, even if that requires waking the newborn for the feedings; rigid feeding schedules, however, are not recommended. The infant showing an adequate weight gain can be allowed to sleep at night and be fed only on awakening. Most newborns need six to eight feedings in 24 hours, and the number of feedings decreases as the infant matures. Usually by 3 to 4 weeks after birth a fairly predictable feeding pattern has developed. Scheduling feedings arbitrarily at predetermined intervals may not meet a newborn's needs, but initiating feedings at convenient times often moves the newborn's feedings to times that work for the family.

Mothers will usually notice an increase in the infant's appetite at ages 7 to 10 days, 3 weeks, 6 weeks, 3 months, and 6 months. These appetite spurts correspond to growth spurts. The amount of formula per feeding should be increased by about 30 ml at these times to meet the baby's needs.

Feeding Techniques

Parents who choose formula-feeding often need education regarding feeding techniques. Formula can be fed at room temperature or warmed. Formula should never be heated in a microwave oven. Microwaving does not heat evenly and can cause encapsulated boiling bubbles to form in the center of the liquid. This may not be detected when checking drops of milk for temperature. Babies have sustained severe burns to the mouth, throat, and upper gastrointestinal tract as a result of microwaved milk (Lawrence & Lawrence, 2005). If the formula is warmed, its temperature should be tested before it is given to the infant.

During feedings parents should be encouraged to sit comfortably, holding the infant closely in a semiupright position. Feedings provide an opportunity to bond with the infant through touching, talking, singing, or reading aloud. Parents

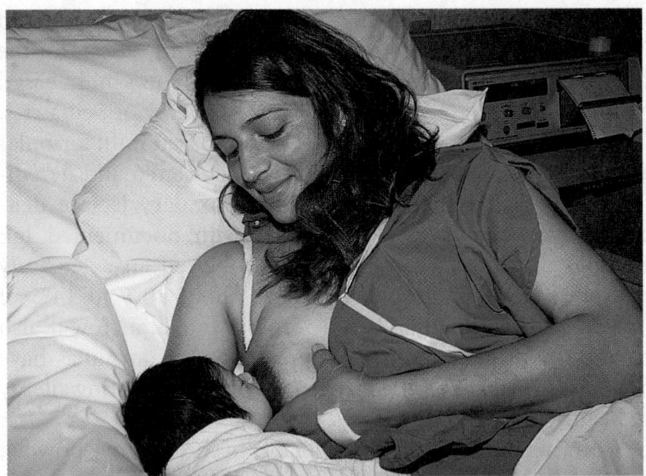

Fig. 26-12 Mother and infant enjoying breastfeeding. *(Courtesy Marjorie Pyle, RNC, Lifecircle, Costa Mesa, CA.)*

should consider feedings, whether breast or bottle, as a time of peaceful relaxation with their newborn (Fig. 26-12).

The bottle should never be propped with a pillow or other inanimate object and left with the infant. Likewise, small children should not be given charge of bottle-feeding the infant unless there is close adult supervision. This practice may result in choking, and it deprives the infant of important interaction during feeding. Moreover, propping the bottle has been implicated in causing nursing bottle caries, or decay of the first teeth, resulting from continuous bathing of the teeth with carbohydrate-containing fluid as the infant sporadically sucks the nipple.

The bottle should be held so that fluid fills the nipple and none of the air in the bottle is allowed to enter the nipple (Fig. 26-13). After the newborn period the infant who falls asleep, turns aside the head, or ceases to suck usually is signaling that enough formula has been taken. Parents should be taught to look for these cues and avoid overfeeding, which could contribute to obesity.

Once a bottle of formula has been prepared, it should be discarded to prevent contamination of the formula with bacteria from the baby's mouth. It is best to prepare only the amount the infant usually takes at each feeding to prevent discarding large portions of formula.

Most infants swallow air when fed from a bottle and should be given a chance to burp several times during a feeding (Fig. 26-14).

Bottles and Nipples

Various brands and styles of bottles and nipples are available. Most babies will feed well with any bottle and nipple. It is important that the bottles and nipples be washed in warm, soapy water using a bottle and nipple brush to facilitate thorough cleansing. Most household dishwashers use hot water and are safe for cleaning bottles and nipples. Boiling of bottles and nipples is not needed unless there is some question about the safety of the water supply or the infant has oral thrush. An angled bottle is preferable to a straight bottle, since it encourages more physiologic positioning of the infant, improves the infant's comfort level, and decreases the need for burping.

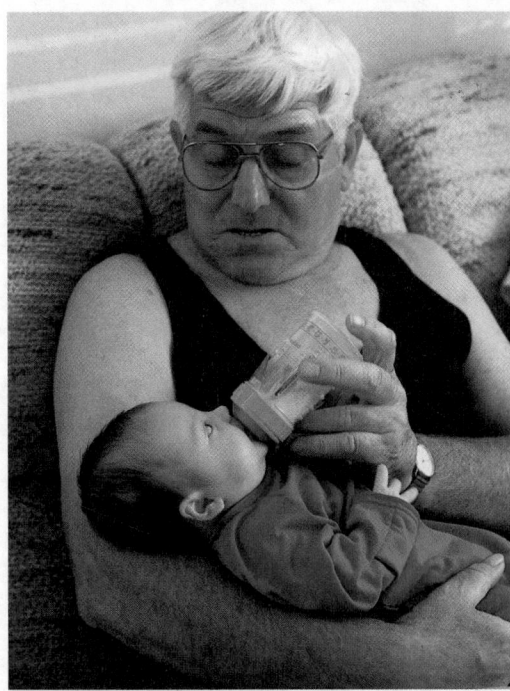

Fig. 26-13 Grandfather feeding infant granddaughter. Note angle of bottle, which ensures milk covers nipple area. *(Courtesy Kim Molloy, Knoxville, IA.)*

Infant Formulas

Commercial Formulas

Because human milk is species specific to meet the needs of the human infant, it is used as the standard for all infant formulas. Commercial infant formulas are designed to resemble human milk as closely as possible, although none has ever duplicated it.

Infants who are not breastfed should be given commercial iron-fortified formulas. If this is too expensive, the family may be eligible for services through the WIC program, which provides iron-fortified infant formula.

Commercially prepared formulas are cow's milk–based formulas that have been modified to closely resemble the nutritional content of human milk. These formulas are altered from cow's milk by removing butterfat, decreasing the protein content, and adding vegetable oil and carbohydrate. Some cow's milk–based formulas have demineralized whey added to yield a whey/casein ratio of 60:40. The standard cow's milk–based formulas, regardless of the commercial brand, have essentially the same compositions of vitamins, minerals, protein, carbohydrates, and essential amino acids, with minor variations such as the source of carbohydrate; nucleotides to enhance immune function; and LCPFUA, DHA, and ARA, which are thought to improve central nervous system, visual, and cognitive function (Georgieff, 2001; Gil, Ramirez, & Gil, 2003). Furthermore, the U.S. Food and Drug Administration regulates the manufacture of infant formula in the United States to ensure product safety. Standard cow's milk–based formulas are sold as low-iron and iron-fortified formulas; however, only the iron-fortified formulas meet the requirements of infants. There is no evidence that iron-fortified formula causes constipation in infants (Singhal et al, 2000).

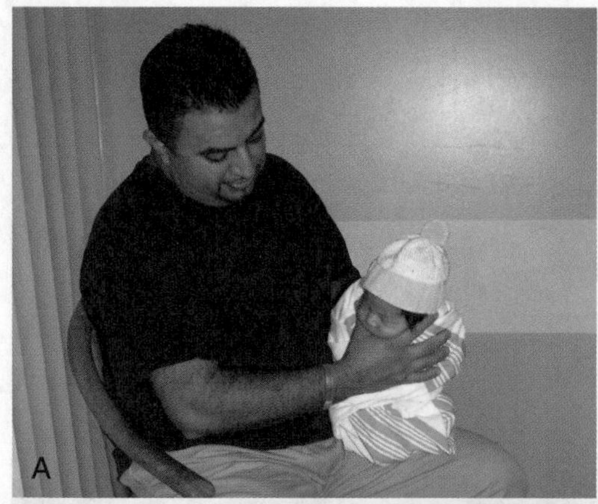

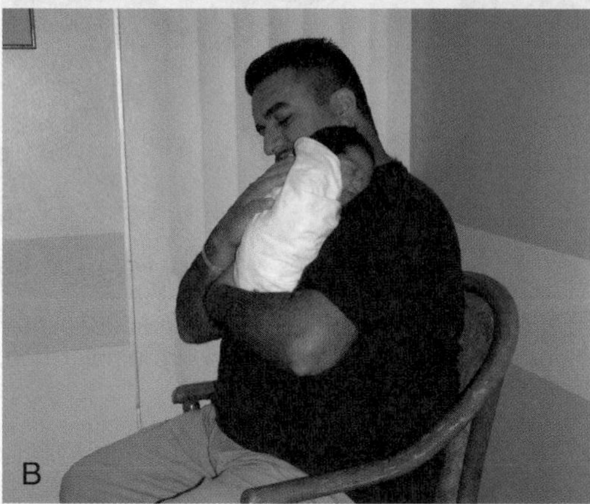

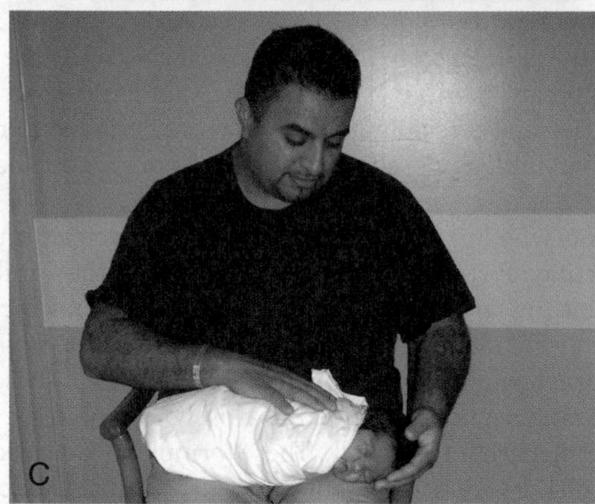

Fig. 26-14 Positions for burping an infant. **A,** Sitting. **B,** On the shoulder. **C,** Across the lap. *(Courtesy Julie Perry Nelson, Loveland, CO.)*

evolve Spanish Guidelines–Burping

Commercially prepared infant formulas come in four main categories: (1) *cow's milk–based formulas,* available in 20 kcal/fl oz as liquid (ready to feed), as powder (requires dilution with water), or as a concentrated liquid (requires dilution with water); (2) *soy-based formulas,* available commercially in ready-to-feed 20 kcal/fl oz powder and concentrated liquid forms, commonly used for children who are lactose or cow's milk protein intolerant; (3) *casein-* or *whey-hydrolysate formulas,* commercially available in ready-to-feed and powder forms and used primarily for children who cannot tolerate or digest cow's milk or soy-based formulas; and (4) *amino acid formulas.*

The American Academy of Pediatrics, Committee on Nutrition, indicates that there are few solid indications for the use of soy protein–based formulas instead of cow's milk–based formulas (Bhatia, Greer, & American Academy of Pediatrics, Committee on Nutrition, 2008). The soy-based milk formulas are recommended for infants with galactosemia and hereditary lactase deficiency; infants with secondary lactase deficiency may benefit as well. Infants with documented IgE allergies caused by cow's milk should be fed an extensively hydrolyzed protein formula because about 10% to 14% of infants with cow's milk–based formula intolerance will also have a soy protein allergy. Soy protein–based formulas have not been proved to be effective in colic or in preventing allergy in healthy or high risk infants.

Commercial formulas are available in three forms: powder, concentrate, and ready-to-feed. All are equivalent in nutritional content, but they vary considerably in price. Powdered formulas are least expensive and are convenient because they are lightweight and require no refrigeration before mixing with water. Concentrated liquid formula is more expensive than powder. It is diluted with water and can be stored in the refrigerator for 24 hours after opening. Ready-to-feed formula is most expensive but easiest to use. The desired amount is poured into the bottle. The opened can is safely refrigerated for 24 hours. This type of formula can also be purchased in individual disposable bottles for the most convenient feeding.

Alternate milk sources such as goat's milk; skim or low-fat milk; condensed milk; or raw, unpasteurized milk from any animal source should not be fed to infants, since these are inadequate to support growth and may contain excessive protein or an inadequate calcium/phosphorus ratio, which may cause seizures.

Formula Preparation

The commercial infant formula must include label directions for preparation and use of the formula with pictures and symbols for the benefit of individuals who cannot read. Some manufacturers translate the directions into languages such as Spanish, French, Vietnamese, Chinese, and Arabic to prevent misunderstanding and errors in formula preparation. It is important to impress on families that the proportions must not be altered—that is, neither diluted to extend the amount of formula nor concentrated to provide more calories.

Although manufacturers of commercial formulas include directions for preparing their products, the nurse should review formula preparation with the mother or primary caretaker. It is especially important that formula be mixed properly. The newborn's kidneys are immature; giving the infant overly concentrated formula may provide protein and minerals in amounts that exceed the kidneys' excretory ability. In contrast, if the formula is diluted too much (sometimes done to save money), the infant does not consume sufficient calories and does not grow appropriately. The water used to mix either powdered or concentrated liquid formula need not contain any fluoride, especially in the first 6 months of life; excess fluoride can permanently stain the teeth once they do appear.

Sterilization of formula is rarely recommended when families have access to a safe public water supply. Instead, formula is prepared with attention to cleanliness. When water from a private well is used in formula preparation, parents should be

HOME CARE

Formula Preparation and Feeding

Your newborn will be hungry about every 2½ to 3 hours, but sometimes may go 3 to 4 hours between feedings. The newborn should not go longer than 4 hours between feedings until a weight gain pattern is established—usually in about 2 weeks. Your newborn needs to be awake before being fed. If your newborn is sleepy, massage the newborn's back and chest and talk to him or her.

Your infant's feedings will change a lot in the first week after birth. The first day, most newborns drink only 15 to 25 ml (roughly 3 to 5 tsp) of formula at a feeding. By the time they are 1 week old, most infants drink 30 to 60 ml (1 to 2 oz) at a feeding and then gradually increase their intake as they grow. If you do not use all of the formula at a feeding, throw away what is left because it spoils once it has mixed with the infant's saliva.

You may want to write down how many ounces your infant drinks each day. When you take the infant in for a checkup, the physician or nurse will ask you about how much formula the infant drinks. By 1 to 2 weeks of age, most infants who weigh 3 to 4.0 kg (7 to 9 lb) are drinking about 840 ml in 24 hours (roughly 28 oz, or 3 to 3½ oz per feeding, based on eight feedings per day). Smaller infants may drink a little less because their stomach capacity is less. These figures, however, are approximations only, and infants will consume the amount necessary for growth, provided they are healthy. Do not force feed an infant if a smaller amount is consumed unless directed by the primary care practitioner.

To feed your newborn, place the nipple in the newborn's mouth on the tongue. It should touch the top of the tongue to stimulate the infant's sucking reflex. Hold the bottle like a pencil. Keep the bottle tipped so that the nipple stays filled with milk and the newborn does not suck in air. With most bottles you will notice air bubbles in the bottle as the infant sucks on the nipple; this means the infant is getting formula from the bottle. The plastic bag bottles will not have as many air bubbles as hard plastic or glass bottles. A curved bottle decreases the amount of air being swallowed during a feeding.

Hold your newborn close for feedings. This should be a pleasant time for social interaction and cuddling. Some newborns take longer to feed than others; be patient. It may be necessary to keep the infant awake and encourage continued sucking. Moving the nipple gently in the infant's mouth may stimulate more sucking.

Some newborns swallow air when sucking. Give your infant a chance to burp several times during early feedings. As your infant gets older and you get more experienced, you will know when to stop for burping.

If your infant fusses or cries between feedings, check the diaper to see if he or she needs to be changed and see if the infant needs to be picked up and cuddled. If the child continues to cry and acts hungry, he or she needs to be fed. Infants do not get hungry on a schedule.

Place your baby on his or her back to sleep. Do not use the side-lying position for sleep because the infant may roll forward onto his or her face and stomach. In the event that the infant does not usually sleep after a feeding, he or she may be placed on the tummy provided there is adult supervision; this does not occur until the infant is older because most infants sleep approximately 18 hours per day.

The stools (bowel movements) of a formula-fed newborn are yellow and soft but formed. The newborn will probably have a stool during or after each feeding in the first 2 weeks, but this will then gradually decrease to one or two stools each day.

Safety Tips

Infants should be held and never left alone while feeding. Do not prop the bottle: the infant could inhale formula or choke on any that was spit up.

Know how to use the bulb syringe in case your infant should choke.

Drinking bottles of formula or juice while falling asleep can cause tooth decay (nursing bottle caries) in young children.

Juice is not recommended in infants for nutritional purposes.

Formula Preparation

Wash your hands and clean the bottle, nipple, and can opener carefully before preparing formula.

If new nipples seem too hard, they can be softened by boiling them in water for 5 minutes before use.

Read the label on the container of formula and mix it exactly according to the directions.

Use tap water to mix concentrated or powdered formula unless directed otherwise by your infant's physician or nurse. Some manufacturers sell bottles of distilled or fluoridated water for formula preparation; however, neither of these is necessary for preparation of infant formulas unless prescribed by the primary care practitioner.

Test the size of the nipple hole by holding a prepared bottle upside down. The formula should drip slowly from the nipple. If it runs in a stream, the hole is too big and the nipple should not be used. If it has to be shaken for the formula to come out, the hole is too small. You can either buy a new nipple or enlarge the hole by boiling the nipple for 5 minutes with a sewing needle inserted in the hole.

If a nipple collapses when your infant sucks, loosen the nipple ring a little to let in air.

Opened cans of ready-to-feed or concentrated formula should be covered and refrigerated. Any unused portions must be discarded after 48 hours.

Unopened (sealed) bottles or cans of formula can be stored at room temperature.

Once a bottle of formula is prepared and fed to the infant, it must be discarded within 4 hours.

If the formula is refrigerated, warm it by placing the bottle in a pan of hot water. Never use a microwave to warm any food to be given to a baby. Test the temperature of the formula by letting a few drops fall on the inside of your wrist. If the formula feels comfortably warm to you, it is the correct temperature.

evolve Critical Thinking Exercise—Formula Preparation

advised to first contact the health department for a chemical and bacteriologic analysis of the water. The presence of nitrates, excess fluoride, or bacteria may be harmful to the infant.

If the sanitary conditions in the home appear unsafe, it would be better to recommend the use of ready-to-feed formula or to teach the mother to sterilize the formula. The two traditional methods for sterilization are terminal heating and the aseptic method. In the terminal heating method, the prepared formula is placed in the bottles, which are topped with the nipples placed upside down and covered with the caps, and then sealed loosely with the rings. The bottles are then boiled together in a water bath for 25 minutes. In the aseptic method, the bottles, rings, caps, nipples, and any other necessary equipment, such as a funnel, are boiled separately, after which the formula is poured into the bottles. Any formula left in the bottle after the feeding should be discarded because the infant's saliva has mixed with it. (Instructions for formula preparation and feeding are provided in the Home Care box.)

Vitamin and Mineral Supplementation

Commercial iron-fortified formula contains all the nutrients needed by the infant for the first 6 months of life. After 6 months, fluoride supplementation of 0.25 mg/day is required if the local water supply is not fluoridated. Vitamin D supplementation is discussed earlier in this chapter.

Weaning

The bottle-fed infant will gradually learn to use a cup, and the parents will find that they are preparing fewer bottles. Commonly the feeding before bedtime is the last one to remain. Infants have a strong need to suck, and the infant who has had the bottle taken away too early or abruptly will compensate with nonnutritive sucking on the fingers or thumb, a pacifier, or even the tongue. Weaning from a bottle should therefore be done gradually because the infant has learned to rely on the comfort that sucking provides.

Key Points

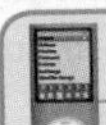

Audio Chapter Summaries

Access an audio summary of these Key Points on evolve

- Human milk is species specific and is the recommended form of nutrition for infants. It provides immunologic protection against many infections and diseases.
- Breast milk changes in composition with each stage of lactation, during each feeding, and as the infant grows.
- During the prenatal period, parents should be informed of the benefits of breastfeeding for infants, mothers, families, and society.
- Infants should be breastfed as soon as possible after birth and at least 8 to 12 times per day thereafter.
- There are objective, measurable indicators that the infant is breastfeeding effectively.
- Breast milk production is based on a supply-meets-demand principle; the more the infant nurses, the greater the milk supply.
- Commercial infant formulas provide satisfactory nutrition for most infants.
- Infants should be held for feedings.
- Parents should be instructed about the types of commercial infant formulas, proper preparation for feeding, and correct feeding technique.
- Unmodified (whole) cow's milk is not appropriate for feeding the infant during the first year of life.

References

American Academy of Pediatrics: *Pediatric nutrition handbook*, ed 6, Elk Grove Village, IL, 2009, The Academy.

American Academy of Pediatrics, Committee on Drugs: The transfer of drugs and other chemicals into milk, *Pediatrics* 108(3):776-789, 2001.

American Academy of Pediatrics, Committee on Infectious Diseases: *Red book: 2006 report of the Committee on Infectious Diseases*, ed 27, Elk Grove Village, IL, 2006, The Academy.

American Academy of Pediatrics, Committee on Nutrition: The use and misuse of fruit juices in pediatrics, *Pediatrics* 107(5):1210-1213, 2001. (Statement reaffirmed in 2007.)

American Academy of Pediatrics, Section on Breastfeeding: Breastfeeding and the use of human milk, *Pediatrics* 115(2):496-506, 2005.

American Academy of Pediatrics, Section on Pediatric Dentistry: Oral health risk assessment timing and establishment of the dental home, *Pediatrics* 111(5):1113-1116, 2003.

American Academy of Pediatrics, Subcommittee on Hyperbilirubinemia: Clinical practice guideline: management of hyperbilirubinemia in the newborn infant 35 or more weeks of gestation, *Pediatrics* 114(1):297-316, 2004.

American Academy of Pediatrics, Task Force on Sudden Infant Death Syndrome: The changing concept of sudden infant death syndrome: diagnostic coding shifts, controversies regarding the sleeping environment, and new variables to consider in reducing risk, *Pediatrics* 116(5):1245-1255, 2005.

Anderson JW, Johnstone BM, Remley DT: Breastfeeding and cognitive development: a meta-analysis, *Am J Clin Nutr* 70(4):525-535, 1999.

Arora S et al: Major factors influencing breastfeeding rates: mother's perception of father's attitude and milk supply, *Pediatrics* 106(5):E67, 2000.

Askin DF, Diehl-Jones WL: Improving on perfection: breast milk and breast-milk additives for preterm neonates, *Newborn Infant Nurs Rev* 5(1):10-18, 2005.

Bachrach VR, Schwarz E, Bachrach LR: Breastfeeding and the risk of hospitalization for respiratory disease in infancy, *Arch Pediatr Adolesc Med* 157(3):237-243, 2003.

Barnard J: Gastrointestinal disorders due to cow's milk consumption, *Pediatr Ann* 26(4):244-250, 1997.

Bhatia J, Greer F, & American Academy of Pediatrics, Committee on Nutrition: Use of soy protein–based formulas in infant feeding, *Pediatrics* 121(5):1062-1068, 2008.

Biancuzzo M: *Breastfeeding the newborn: clinical strategies for nurses*, ed 2, St Louis, 2003, Mosby.

Blackburn ST: *Maternal, fetal, and neonatal physiology: a clinical perspective*, ed 3, St Louis, 2007, Saunders.

Carbajal R et al: Analgesic effect of breast feeding in term neonates: randomized controlled trial, *BMJ* 326(7379):13, 2003.

Centers for Disease Control and Prevention: Breastfeeding trends and updated national health objectives for exclusive breastfeeding—United States, birth years 2000-2004, *Morb Mortal Wkly Rep* 56(30):760-763, 2007.

Chertok IR, Shoham-Vardi I, Hallak M: Four-month breastfeeding duration in postcesarean women of different cultures in the Israeli Negev, *J Perinat Neonatal Nurs* 18(2):145-160, 2004.

Choudhry UK: Traditional practices of women from India: pregnancy, childbirth, and newborn care, *J Obstet Gynecol Neonatal Nurs* 26(5):533-539, 1997.

Conover E, Buehler BA: Use of herbal agents by breastfeeding women may affect infants, *Pediatr Ann* 33(4):235-240, 2004.

Corbett-Dick P, Bezek SK: Breastfeeding promotion for the employed mother, *J Pediatr Health Care* 11(1):12-19, 1997.

Cushing AH et al: Breastfeeding reduces risk of respiratory illness in infants, *Am J Epidemiol* 147(9):863-870, 1998.

Davis M: Review of the evidence for an association between infant feeding and childhood cancer, *Int J Cancer Suppl* 11:29-33, 1998.

Department of Health and Human Services: Healthy people 2010, conference ed, vol 2, *Objectives for improving health,* Washington, DC, 2000, The Department. Available at www.health.gov/healthypeople/document/default.htm (accessed February 18, 2005).

Dewey KG, Heinig MJ, Nommsen LA: Maternal weight-loss patterns during prolonged lactation, *Am J Clin Nutr* 58:162-166, 1993.

DiGirolamo AM et al: Breastfeeding-related maternity practices at hospitals and birth centers—United States, 2007, *Morb Mortal Wkly Rep* 57(23):621-625, 2008.

Dollberg S et al: Immediate nipple pain relief after frenotomy in breast-fed infants with ankyloglossia: a randomized, prospective study, *J Pediatr Surg* 41(9):1598-1600, 2006.

Early childhood pacifier use in relation to breastfeeding, SIDS, infection, and dental occlusion, *Best Practice* 9(3):1-6, 2005.

Eisman J: Relevance of pregnancy and lactation to osteoporosis, *Clin Perinatol* 25(2):303-326, 1998.

Enger S et al: Breastfeeding experience and breast cancer risk among postmenopausal women, *Cancer Epidemiol Biomarkers Prev* 7(5):365-369, 1998.

Fetherston C: Risk factors for lactational mastitis, *J Hum Lact* 14(2):101-109, 1998.

Fleith M, Clandinin MT: Dietary PUFA for term and preterm infants: review of clinical studies, *Crit Rev Food Sci Nutr* 45(3):205-229, 2005.

Ford R et al: Breastfeeding and the risk of sudden infant death syndrome, *Int J Epidemiol* 22(5):885-890, 1993.

Georgieff MK: Taking a rational approach to the choice of formula, *Contemp Pediatr* 18(8):112-130, 2001.

Gerstein HC: Cow's milk exposure and type I diabetes mellitus, *Diabetes Care* 17:13-19, 1994.

Gil A, Ramirez M, Gil M: Role of long-chain polyunsaturated fatty acids in infant nutrition, *Eur J Clin Nutr* 57(Suppl 1):S31-S34, 2003.

Gray L et al: Breastfeeding is analgesic in healthy newborns, *Pediatrics* 109(4):590-593, 2002.

Grummer-Strawn LM, Mei Z, Centers for Disease Control and Prevention Pediatric Nutrition Surveillance System: Does breastfeeding protect against pediatric overweight? Analysis of longitudinal data from the Centers for Disease Control and Prevention Pediatric Nutrition Surveillance System, *Pediatrics* 113(2):E81-E86, 2004.

Guthmann RA, Bang J, Nashelsky J: FPIN's clinical inquiries: combined oral contraceptives for mothers who are breastfeeding, *Am Fam Physician* 72(7):1303-1304, 2005.

Hale TW: *Medications and mothers' milk*, ed 13, Amarillo, TX, 2008, Hale.

Halken S, Host A: Prevention of allergic disease: exposure to food allergens and dietetic intervention, *Pediatr Allergy Immunol* 7(9 Suppl):102-107, 1996.

Hanson LA, Korotkova M: The role of breastfeeding in prevention of neonatal infection, *Semin Neonatol* 7(4):275-281, 2002.

Heird WC: The feeding of infants and children. In Kliegman RM et al, editors: *Nelson textbook of pediatrics*, ed 18, Philadelphia, 2007, Saunders.

Hernandez IF: Promoting exclusive breastfeeding for Hispanic women, *MCN* 31(5):318-324, 2006.

Hohmann H, Creinin MD: The contraceptive implant, *Clin Obstet Gynecol* 50(4):907-917, 2007.

Horwood L, Fergusson D: Breastfeeding and later cognitive and academic outcomes, *Pediatrics* 101(1):E9, 1998.

Institute of Medicine: *Dietary Reference Intakes for energy, carbohydrate, fiber, fatty acids, cholesterol, protein, and amino acids*, Washington, DC, 2005, Food and Nutrition Board, Institute of Medicine, National Academies Press.

Ip S et al: *Breastfeeding and maternal and infant health outcomes in developed countries,* Pub. No. 07-E007, Rockville, MD, April 2007, Agency for Healthcare Research and Quality.

Kendall-Tackett K: A new paradigm for depression in new mothers: the central role of inflammation and how breastfeeding and anti-inflammatory treatments protect maternal health, *Int Breastfeed J* 2(March 30):2-6, 2007.

Kramer MS et al: Breastfeeding and child cognitive development: new evidence from a large randomized trial, *Arch Gen Psychiatry* 65(5):578-584, 2008.

Kyenkya-Isabirye M: UNICEF launches the Baby-Friendly Hospital Initiative, *MCN Am J Matern Child Nurs* 17(4):177-179, 1992.

Lawrence RA, Lawrence RM: *Breastfeeding: a guide for the medical profession*, ed 6, St Louis, 2005, Mosby.

Meier P: *Professional guide to breastfeeding premature infants*, Columbus, OH, 1997, Ross Products Division, Abbott Laboratories.

Merewood A et al: Breastfeeding rates in US Baby-Friendly hospitals: results of a national survey, *Pediatrics* 116(3):628-634, 2005.

Morin KH: Current thoughts on healthy term infant nutrition: the first 12 months, *MCN* 29(1):312-317, 2004.

Murray EK, Ricketts S, Dellaport J: Hospital practices that increase breastfeeding duration: results from a population-based study, *Birth* 34(3):202-211, 2007.

Niemela M, Uhari M, Mottonen M: A pacifier increases the risk of recurrent acute otitis media in children in day care centers, *Pediatrics* 96(5 Pt 1):884-888, 1995.

Niemela M et al: Pacifier as a risk factor for acute otitis media: a randomized, controlled trial of parental counseling, *Pediatrics* 106(3):483-488, 2000.

Pikwer M et al: Breast-feeding, but not oral contraceptives, is associated with a reduced risk of rheumatoid arthritis, *Ann Rheum Dis* 68(4):526-530, 2009 (Epub May 13, 2008).

Riordan J, Gill-Hopple K: Breastfeeding care in multicultural populations, *J Obstet Gynecol Neonatal Nurs* 30(2):216-223, 2001.

Riordan J, Wambach K: *Breastfeeding and human lactation*, ed 4, Sudbury, MA, 2009, Jones & Bartlett Publishers.

Roberts KL: A comparison of chilled cabbage leaves and chilled gelpaks in reducing breast engorgement, *J Hum Lact* 11(1):17-20, 1995.

Rosenblatt KA, Thomas DB: Prolonged lactation and endometrial cancer: WHO collaborative study of neoplasia and steroid contraceptives, *Int J Epidemiol* 24:499-503, 1995.

Ross Mothers Survey: *Breastfeeding trends—2003*, Columbus, OH, 2003, Ross Products Division, Abbott Laboratories. Available at http://abbottnutrition.com/resources/en_US/home/breastfeeding/BF_Trends_2003.pdf (accessed June 16, 2008).

Scariati PD, Grummer-Strawn LM, Fein SB: A longitudinal analysis of infant morbidity and the extent of breastfeeding in the United States, *Pediatrics* 99(6):E5, 1997.

Simmer K, Patole SK, Rao SC: Long-chain polyunsaturated fatty acid supplementation in infants born at term, *Cochrane Database Syst Rev* (1):CD000376, 2008.

Singhal A et al: Clinical safety of iron-fortified formulas, *Pediatrics* 105(3):e38, 2000.

Vohr BR et al: Beneficial effects of breast milk in the neonatal intensive care unit on the developmental outcome of extremely low birth weight infants at 18 months of age, *Pediatrics* 118(1):e115-e123, 2006.

Wagner CL et al: Prevention of rickets and vitamin D deficiency in infants, children, and adolescents, *Pediatrics* 122(5):1142-1150, 2008.

Wright A, Rice S, Wells S: Changing hospital practices to increase the duration of breastfeeding, *Pediatrics* 97(5):669-675, 1996.

Unit 6

27 Infants with Gestational Age–Related Problems

Learning Objectives

On completion of this chapter the reader will be able to:

- Compare and contrast the physical characteristics of preterm, term, and postterm neonates.
- Discuss respiratory distress syndrome and the approach to treatment.
- Compare methods of oxygen therapy for the high risk infant.
- Describe nursing interventions for nutritional care of the preterm infant.
- Discuss the pathophysiology of retinopathy of prematurity and bronchopulmonary dysplasia (chronic lung disease), and identify the predisposing risk factors.
- Describe the treatment of the infant with meconium aspiration.
- Describe risk factors associated with the birth and transition of an infant of a diabetic mother.
- Plan developmentally appropriate care for the high risk infant.
- Develop a plan to address the unique needs of parents of high risk infants.

Electronic Resources

Additional information related to the content in Chapter 27 can be found on

evolve the Companion Website at
http://evolve.elsevier.com/Perry/maternal/

- NCLEX Review Questions
- Critical Thinking Exercise—Patent Ductus Arteriosus
- Nursing Care Plan—The High Risk Preterm Newborn
- Nursing Care Plan—The Infant of Mother with Diabetes Mellitus
- Spanish Guidelines—Intensive Care Nursery: Parent Teaching on First Visit

Modern technology and expert nursing care have made important contributions to improving the health and overall survival of high risk infants. However, infants who are born considerably before term and survive are particularly susceptible to the development of sequelae related to their preterm birth. These conditions include necrotizing enterocolitis (NEC), growth failure, bronchopulmonary dysplasia (BPD), intraventricular and periventricular hemorrhage, and retinopathy of prematurity (ROP). This chapter focuses on care of the preterm infant, but care of other high risk infants with gestational age–related problems is also discussed. Infants born of mothers with diabetes are included because they may experience problems that place them at risk for improper function and development.

High risk infants are most often classified according to birth weight, gestational age, and predominant pathophysiologic problems (Box 27-1). Intrauterine growth rates are not the same for all infants, and other factors (e.g., heredity, placental insufficiency, and maternal disease) influence intrauterine growth and birth weight. The classification system in the box encompasses birth weight and gestational age.

The Preterm Infant

Preterm infants, those born before 37 weeks of gestation, are at risk because their organ systems are immature and they lack adequate physiologic reserves to function in an extrauterine environment. The range of birth weight and physiologic problems varies widely among preterm infants due to increased survival rates among those who weigh less than 1000 g. However, one general concept is that the lower the weight and the gestational age, the lower the chances of survival among infants born preterm. Preterm birth is responsible for almost two thirds of infant deaths. The cause of preterm birth is largely unknown; however, the incidence of preterm birth is highest among low socioeconomic groups. This is likely a result of the lack of comprehensive prenatal health care. Other factors found to be associated with preterm birth include gestational hypertension; maternal infection; multifetal pregnancy; HELLP syndrome (*h*emolysis, *e*levated *l*iver enzymes, and *l*ow *p*latelet count occurring in association with preeclampsia); premature dilation of the cervix; and placental or umbilical cord conditions that affect the fetus's reception of nutrients.

BOX 27-1 Classification of High Risk Infants

Classification According to Size

Low-birth-weight (LBW) infant—An infant whose birth weight is less than 2500 g, regardless of gestational age

Very-low-birth-weight (VLBW) infant—An infant whose birth weight is less than 1500 g

Extremely-low-birth-weight (ELBW) infant—An infant whose birth weight is less than 1000 g

Appropriate-for-gestational-age (AGA) infant—An infant whose birth weight falls between the 10th and 90th percentiles on intrauterine growth curves

Small-for-gestational-age (SGA) or small-for-date (SFD) infant—An infant whose rate of intrauterine growth was restricted and whose birth weight falls below the 10th percentile on intrauterine growth curves

Large-for-gestational-age (LGA) infant—An infant whose birth weight falls above the 90th percentile on intrauterine growth curves

Intrauterine growth restriction (IUGR)—Found in infants whose intrauterine growth is restricted (sometimes used as a more descriptive term for the *SGA infant*)

Symmetric IUGR—Growth restriction in which the weight, length, and head circumference are all affected

Asymmetric IUGR—Growth restriction in which the head circumference remains within normal parameters while the birth weight falls below the 10th percentile

Classification According to Gestational Age

Preterm infant—An infant born before completion of 37 weeks of gestation, regardless of birth weight

Late preterm (near-term) infant—An infant born between 34 0/7 and 36 6/7 weeks of gestation, regardless of birth weight*

Full-term infant—An infant born between the beginning of 38 weeks and the completion of 42 weeks of gestation, regardless of birth weight

Postterm infant—An infant born after 42 weeks of gestational age, regardless of birth weight

Classification According to Mortality

Live birth—Birth in which the neonate manifests any heartbeat, breathes, or displays voluntary movement, regardless of gestational age

Fetal death—Death of the fetus after 20 weeks of gestation and before delivery, with absence of any signs of life after birth

Neonatal death—Death that occurs in the first 27 days of life; early neonatal death occurs in the first week of life; late neonatal death occurs at 7 to 27 days

Perinatal mortality—Total number of fetal and early neonatal deaths per 1000 live births

*NOTE: Definitions of late preterm vary among experts, but Engle (2006) suggests the above (which corresponds to 239th to 259th day from first day of last menstrual period).

The potential problems and care needs of the preterm infant weighing 2000 g differ from those of the term or postterm infant of equal weight. The presence of physiologic disorders and anomalies affects the infant's response to treatment.

Opinions vary about the practical and ethical dimensions of resuscitation of extremely-low-birth-weight (ELBW) infants (those infants whose birth weight is 1000 g or less). Ethical issues associated with resuscitation of these infants include whether to resuscitate; who should make that decision; whether the cost of resuscitation is justified; and whether the benefits of technology outweigh the burdens on the infant, family, and society in relation to the infant's quality of life.

Late Preterm Infant

Within the last two decades, several significant changes have occurred in neonatal care. Early postpartum discharge for term and preterm infants gained popularity as health care institutions attempted to cut health care costs. Another change was in the arena of newborn care, as infants who appeared to be "near" term began to be treated much like term infants, thus avoiding the costs of neonatal intensive care for infants who appeared to be healthy. Recently it has been recommended that infants born between 34 and 36 6/7 weeks of gestation be referred to as *late preterm infants* rather than *near-term infants* (Engle, 2006; Engle et al, 2007). Late preterm infants may be able to make an effective transition to extrauterine life; however, such infants, by nature of their limited gestation, remain at risk for problems related to feeding, neurodevelopment, thermoregulation, hypoglycemia, hyperbilirubinemia, sepsis, and respiratory function (Bakewell-Sachs, 2007; Darcy, 2009). In one study children born at 34 to 36 weeks were more than three times as likely as children born at term to be diagnosed with cerebral palsy (Petrini et al, 2009). It is now estimated that late preterm infants represent 70% of the total preterm infant population and that the mortality rate for this group is significantly higher than that of term infants (7.9 vs. 2.4 per 1000 live births, respectively) (Tomashek et al, 2007). Because late preterm infants' birth weights often range from 2000 to 2500 g and they appear relatively mature in comparison to smaller preterm infants, they may be cared for in the same manner as healthy term infants, where risk factors for late preterm infants may be overlooked. Late preterm infants are often discharged early from the birth institution and have a significantly higher rate of rehospitalization than term infants (Escobar, Clark, & Greene, 2006). The Association of Women's Health, Obstetric and Neonatal Nurses has published the *Late Preterm Infant Assessment Guide* (Askin et al, 2007) for the education of perinatal nurses regarding the late preterm infant's risk factors and appropriate care and follow-up care (Table 27-1).

Nursing Care Management

Assessment

For the high risk infant, an accurate assessment of gestational age (see Chapter 25) is critical in helping the nurse identify the potential problems the newborn is likely to experience.

Table 27-1 Late Preterm Infant Assessment and Interventions

RISK FACTORS	ASSESSMENT	INTERVENTIONS*
Respiratory distress	Assess for cardinal signs of respiratory distress (nasal flaring, grunting, tachypnea, central cyanosis, retractions) and presence of apnea, especially during feedings. Assess for hypothermia, hypoglycemia.	Perform gestational age assessment. Observe for signs of respiratory distress; monitor oxygenation by pulse oximetry; provide supplemental oxygen judiciously.
Thermal instability	Monitor axillary temperature every 30 min immediately postpartum until stable; thereafter every 1-4 hr depending on gestational age and ability to maintain thermal stability.	Provide skin-to-skin care in immediate postpartum period for stable infant. Implement measures to avoid excess heat loss (adjust environmental temperature, avoid drafts). Bathe only after thermal stability has been maintained for 1 hr.
Hypoglycemia	Monitor for signs and symptoms of hypoglycemia. Assess feeding ability (latch-on, nipple feeding). Assess thermal stability and signs and symptoms of respiratory distress. Monitor bedside glucose in infants with additional risk factors (IDM, prolonged labor, respiratory distress, poor feeding).	Initiate early feedings of human milk or formula. Avoid dextrose water or water feedings. Provide IV dextrose as necessary for hypoglycemia.
Jaundice	Observe for jaundice in first 24 hr. Evaluate maternal-fetal history for additional risk factors that may cause increased hemolysis and circulating levels of unconjugated bilirubin (Rh, ABO, spherocytosis, bruising). Assess feeding method, voiding and stooling patterns.	Monitor transcutaneous bilirubin and note risk zone on hour-specific nomogram (see Fig. 25-7).
Feeding problems	Assess suck-swallow and breathing. Assess for respiratory distress, hypoglycemia, thermal stability. Assess latch-on, maternal comfort with feeding method. Determine weight loss (should be ≤10% of birth weight).	Initiate early feedings (human milk or formula). Ensure maternal knowledge of feeding method and signs of inadequate feeding (sleepiness, lethargy, color changes during feeding, apnea during feeding, decreased or absent urine output).
Neurodevelopmental problems	Assess for respiratory distress, neonatal jaundice, hypoglycemia, and thermal instability. Assess neurodevelopmental status. Assess for seizure activity.	Perform newborn screening, including hearing test. Implement individualized developmental care. Encourage parents to keep follow-up appointments with primary care physician for evaluation of growth and development (including cognitive function and achievement of appropriate milestones).
Infection	Evaluate maternal-fetal history for risk factors that may contribute to neonatal septicemia. Assess for signs and symptoms of neonatal infection (see Box 27-2 and Table 28-3).	Use Standard Precautions, especially handwashing between infants and after contact with surfaces that may harbor bacteria (e.g., keyboards, telephones). Maintain thermal stability. Administer hepatitis B vaccine. Encourage breastfeeding and assist mother-baby pair with breastfeeding. Encourage parents to decrease infant exposure to respiratory viruses after discharge and to obtain vaccines as appropriate to prevent development of respiratory viruses (e.g., influenza).

Portions adapted from Askin DF et al: *Late preterm infant assessment guide*, Washington, DC, 2007, Association of Women's Health, Obstetric and Neonatal Nurses.
IDM, Infant of diabetic mother; *IV*, intravenous.
*This is not an exhaustive list of nursing interventions; additional interventions include those discussed under the care of the high risk infant in this chapter.

The response of the preterm, late preterm, or postterm infant to extrauterine life is different from that of the term infant. By understanding the physiologic basis of these differences, the nurse can assess these infants; determine the response of the preterm, late preterm, or postterm infant; and discern which potential problems are most likely to occur.

Respiratory Function

An effective respiratory pattern is usually quickly established in nonstressed newborns as evidenced by vigorous activity, adequate tissue perfusion, and pink or acrocyanotic color. However, infants with a potential for respiratory depression at birth because of asphyxia, maternal analgesia or illness, pulmonary immaturity, or congenital malformations may exhibit cyanosis, gasping or ineffective respirations, decreased tissue perfusion, retractions, nasal flaring, tachypnea, decreased muscle tone, or a combination of these problems.

The preterm infant is likely to have difficulty making the pulmonary transition from intrauterine to extrauterine life.

Numerous problems may affect the respiratory system of preterm infants, including:
- Decreased number of functional alveoli
- Deficient surfactant levels
- Smaller airway lumen
- Decreased tracheal cartilage
- Obstruction of respiratory passages
- Insufficient calcification of the bony thorax
- Circulating hormones (prostaglandins) that may affect cardiovascular function
- Immature and fragile pulmonary vasculature
- Greater distance between functional alveoli and capillary bed, especially in ELBW infants

In combination, these deficits severely hinder the infant's respiratory efforts and can produce respiratory distress or respiratory failure. Early signs of respiratory distress include tachypnea, nasal flaring, and expiratory grunting. Depending on the severity of respiratory distress and its cause, retractions may begin as subcostal, intercostal, or suprasternal. Increasing respiratory effort (e.g., paradoxic breathing patterns, retractions, nasal flaring, expiratory grunting, tachypnea, or apnea) indicates increasing distress. As a result of pulmonary immaturity and residual function, very-low-birth-weight (VLBW) and ELBW infants may progress rapidly from respiratory distress to complete respiratory failure. Initially, a compromised infant's color may be cyanotic centrally or pale. Acrocyanosis is a normal finding in the neonate; however, central cyanosis indicates poor oxygenation.

Periodic breathing is a respiratory pattern commonly seen in preterm infants. Such infants exhibit 5- to 10-second respiratory pauses followed by 10 to 15 seconds of compensatory rapid respirations. Such periodic breathing should not be confused with apnea, which is a cessation of respirations of 20 seconds or more. The nurse must be prepared to provide supplemental oxygen and artificial ventilation as necessary when the newborn demonstrates an inability to initiate or maintain adequate respiratory function.

Cardiovascular Function

Evaluation of heart rate and rhythm, color, blood pressure, perfusion, pulses, oxygen saturation, and acid-base status provides information on cardiovascular status. The nurse must be prepared to intervene if symptoms of hypovolemia, shock, or both are found. These symptoms include prolonged capillary refill (longer than 3 seconds); pale color; poor muscle tone; lethargy; tachycardia initially, then bradycardia; and continued respiratory distress despite the provision of adequate oxygen and ventilation. Hypotension may initially be present or may occur in some infants as a late sign of shock.

Blood pressure is monitored routinely in the sick neonate by either internal or external means. Direct recording with arterial catheters is often used but carries the risks inherent in any procedure in which a catheter is introduced into an artery. An umbilical venous catheter may also be used to monitor the neonate's central venous pressure. Oscillometry (Dinamap) is a noninvasive, effective means for detecting alterations in systemic blood pressure (hypotension or hypertension) and implementing appropriate therapy to maintain cardiovascular function.

Body Temperature

Preterm infants are susceptible to temperature instability as a result of numerous factors, including:
- Large surface area in relation to body weight
- Minimal insulating subcutaneous fat
- Limited stores of brown fat (an internal source for the generation of heat present in normal term infants)
- Decreased or absent reflex control of skin capillaries (vasoconstriction)
- Inadequate muscle mass activity (leaving the preterm infant unable to produce his or her own heat)
- Poor muscle tone, resulting in more body surface area being exposed to the cooling effects of the environment
- An immature temperature regulation center in the brain
- Increased insensible water losses
- Decreased ability to increase oxygen consumption
- Decreased caloric intake

The goal of thermoregulation is a neutral thermal environment (NTE), which is the environmental temperature at which oxygen consumption and metabolic rate are minimal but adequate to maintain the body temperature (Blackburn, 2007). The NTE for preterm infants weighing less than 1000 g is very narrow, and the prediction of NTE for each infant is impossible. Extremely immature infants may require environmental temperatures equal to skin and core temperature or possibly higher to achieve thermoneutrality (Blackburn, 2007). With knowledge of the four mechanisms of heat transfer (i.e., convection, conduction, radiation, and evaporation), the nurse can create an environment for the preterm infant that prevents temperature instability (see Chapter 24). Since overheating produces an increase in oxygen and calorie consumption, the infant is also jeopardized if he or she becomes hyperthermic (apnea and flushed color may indicate hyperthermia). Unlike older children, the preterm infant is not able to sweat and thus dissipate heat.

Central Nervous System Function

The preterm infant's central nervous system (CNS) is susceptible to injury as a result of the following problems:
- Birth trauma with damage to immature intracranial structures
- Bleeding from fragile capillaries
- Impaired coagulation process, including prolonged prothrombin time
- Recurrent hypoxic and hyperoxic episodes
- Predisposition to hypoglycemia
- Fluctuating systemic blood pressure with concomitant variation in cerebral blood flow and pressure

In the preterm neonate neurologic function depends on gestational age; associated illness factors; and predisposing factors such as intrauterine asphyxia, which may have caused neurologic damage. Clinical signs of neurologic dysfunction may be subtle, nonspecific, or specific. Five categories of clinical manifestations should be carefully evaluated in the preterm infant: seizure activity, hyperirritability, CNS depression, elevated intracranial pressure, and abnormal movements such as decorticate posturing (Blackburn, 1998). Primary and tendon reflexes are generally present in preterm infants by 28 weeks of gestation and should be part of the neurologic examination.

Ongoing assessment and documentation of these neurologic signs are needed both for the purposes of discharge teaching and making follow-up recommendations, as well as for their predictive value.

Nutritional Status

The initial goal of neonatal nutrition in the preterm infant is to prevent catabolism and excess fluid losses. Once the infant has been stabilized in regard to respiratory and cardiac function, the goal of nutrition is to promote optimal growth and development. However, the maintenance of adequate nutrition in the preterm infant is complicated by problems with intake and metabolism of nutrients adequate to promote physical growth, including brain growth. The preterm infant has the following disadvantages with regard to intake of adequate nutrients: weak or absent suck, swallow, and gag reflexes; small stomach capacity; and immature digestive capacity. The preterm infant's metabolic functions are compromised by a limited store of nutrients, a decreased ability to digest proteins and absorb nutrients, and immature enzyme systems.

The nurse must continually assess the infant's nutritional status. Preterm infants often require gavage or intravenous (IV) feedings instead of oral feedings, depending on the gestational age and birth weight and existing illness factors such as respiratory distress.

Renal Function

The preterm infant's immature renal system is unable to (1) adequately excrete metabolites and drugs; (2) concentrate urine; or (3) maintain acid-base, fluid, or electrolyte balance. Therefore intake and output, as well as specific gravity, must be assessed. Laboratory tests must be performed to assess acid-base and electrolyte balance. Medication levels are also monitored in preterm infants because metabolism via renal and hepatic routes is often hindered. Because of great variability in drug metabolism, serum levels are obtained to ensure adequate therapeutic range for treatment and to prevent toxicity.

Hematologic Status

The preterm infant is predisposed to hematologic problems because of the following conditions:

- Increased capillary fragility
- Increased tendency to bleed (prolonged prothrombin time and partial thromboplastin time)
- Decreased production of red blood cells (RBCs) resulting from physiologic rapid decrease in erythropoiesis after birth
- Large amount of fetal hemoglobin (up to 80% of total volume)
- Loss of blood attributable to frequent blood sampling for laboratory tests
- Decreased RBC survival related to the increased size of the RBC and its increased permeability to sodium and potassium
- Decreased levels of circulating albumin

The nurse assesses such infants for any evidence of bleeding from puncture sites, the gastrointestinal (GI) tract, and pulmonary system. Infants are also examined for signs of anemia (e.g., decreased hemoglobin and hematocrit levels, pale skin, apnea, lethargy, tachycardia, and poor weight gain). In high risk infants the amount of blood withdrawn for laboratory testing is monitored.

Infection Prevention

Protection from infection is an integral part of all newborn care, but preterm and sick infants are particularly susceptible to infectious organisms. As with all aspects of care, strict handwashing is the single most important measure to prevent nosocomial infections. Personnel with known infectious disorders are barred from the unit until they are no longer infectious. Standard Precautions are instituted in all nursery areas as a method of infection control to protect the infants and staff.

Neonates are highly susceptible to infection as a result of diminished nonspecific (inflammatory) and specific (humoral) immunity, such as impaired phagocytosis, delayed chemotactic response, minimal or absent immune globulin A and immune globulin M, and decreased complement levels. Because of the infant's poor response to pathogenic agents, there is usually no local inflammatory reaction at the portal of entry to signal an infection, and the resulting symptoms tend to be vague and nonspecific. Consequently, diagnosis and treatment may be delayed. Preterm and term infants exhibit various nonspecific signs and symptoms of infection (Box 27-2). Early identification and treatment of sepsis are essential.

Parental Adaptation to Preterm Infant

Parents who experience the preterm birth of their infant have a much different experience from parents giving birth to a full-term infant. Because of this difference, parental attachment and adaptation to the parental role may differ as well.

Parental Tasks

Parents must accomplish a number of psychologic tasks before effective relationships and parenting patterns can evolve. These tasks include:

- Experiencing anticipatory grief over the potential loss of the infant. The parent grieves in preparation for the infant's possible death, although the parent clings to the hope that the infant will survive. This may begin during labor and often lasts until the infant dies or shows evidence of surviving.
- The mother accepting her failure to give birth to a healthy, full-term infant. Grief and depression typify this phase, which persists until the infant is out of danger and is expected to survive.
- Resuming the process of relating to the infant. As the infant's condition begins to improve and the infant gains weight, feeds by nipple, and is weaned from the incubator, the parent can begin the process of developing an attachment to the infant that was interrupted by the infant's critical condition at birth.
- Learning how this infant differs in special needs and growth patterns, caregiving needs, and growth and development expectations.
- Adjusting the home environment to the needs of the new infant. Visitors may be limited to reduce the risk

BOX 27-2 Signs and Symptoms of Neonatal Infection

Signs and symptoms that are subtle and nonspecific
- Temperature instability
- Hypothermia—most common
- Hyperthermia—rarely

Central nervous system changes
- Lethargy
- Irritability
- Altered level of consciousness

Changes in color
- Cyanosis, pallor
- Mottling (marbling)
- Jaundice

Cardiovascular instability
- Poor perfusion
- Hypotension
- Bradycardia or tachycardia
- Prolonged capillary refill (longer than 3 seconds)

Respiratory distress
- Tachypnea or bradypnea
- Apnea
- Retractions, nasal flaring, grunting

Gastrointestinal problems
- Feeding intolerance, increased residuals (when gavage fed)
- Vomiting
- Diarrhea
- Bloody stools (frank or occult positive)
- Abdominal distention

Metabolic instability
- Glucose instability
- Metabolic acidosis

Other
- Electrolyte imbalance
- Decreased urine output

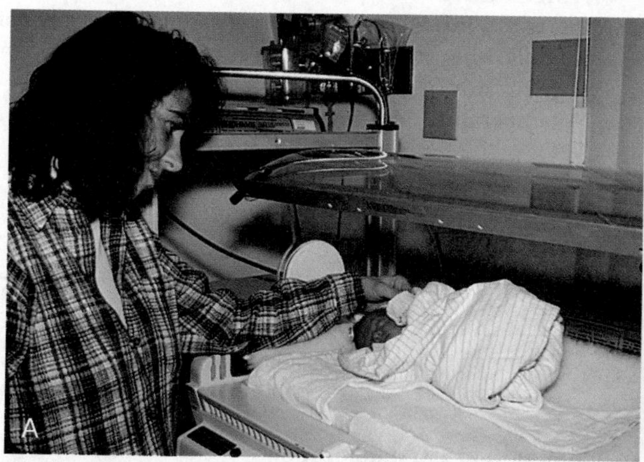

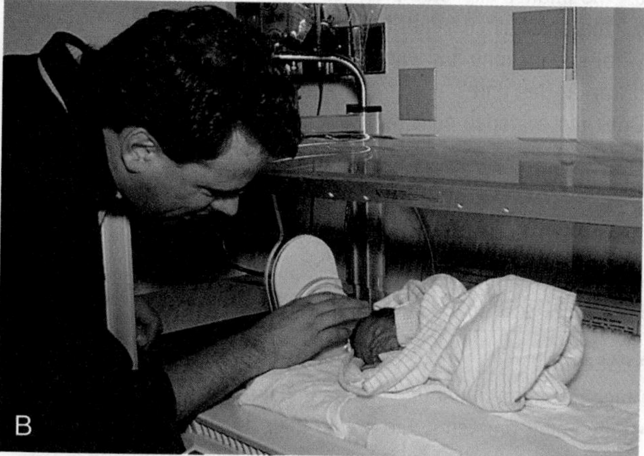

Fig. 27-1 A, Mother interacts with her preterm infant by touch. **B,** Father interacts with his newborn by stroking and touching infant with fingertips. *(Courtesy Michael S. Clement, MD, Mesa, AZ.)*

of exposure to pathogens, and the environmental temperature may be altered to optimize conditions for the infant.

Grandparents and siblings also react to the birth of the preterm infant. Parents must deal with the grief of grandparents and the bewilderment and anger of the infant's siblings at the apparent disproportionate amount of parental time spent with the newborn.

Parental Responses

Parents progress through stages as they interact with their infants, from maintaining an *en face* position and stroking and touching their infant (Fig. 27-1) to assuming some child care activities such as feeding, bathing, and diapering the infant.

Parental Maladaptation

The incidence of physical and emotional abuse is greater in infants who, because of preterm birth or high risk condition, are separated from their parents for a time after birth. Physical abuse includes varying degrees of poor nutrition, poor hygiene, and bodily harm. Emotional abuse ranges from subtle lack of interest to outright dislike of the infant. Appropriate resources should be made available to assess the parents' feelings regarding the preterm infant's birth. In addition, proper guidance and counseling are made available, including after hospital discharge, to help families adjust to and care for the preterm infant. The ultimate goal is for the family to incorporate the infant as a regular family member (see Critical Thinking Exercise).

Factors surrounding the birth may predispose parents to subconsciously or overtly reject the infant. These factors might include parental anxiety, unmet personal expectations surrounding the birth experience, a heavy financial burden because of the cost of the infant's care, unresolved anticipatory grief, threat to self-esteem, the infant being the product of an unwanted pregnancy, or discord in the relationship with the partner. The goal of health professionals is early identification of inadequate coping skills and potentially dysfunctional parenting to prevent further problems and enable early intervention.

evolve Spanish Guidelines—Intensive Care Nursery; Parent Teaching on First Visit

CRITICAL THINKING EXERCISE

Late Preterm Infant

A 2013 g (4 lb, 7 oz) male infant is born at an estimated gestational age of 35 weeks. The parents are excited about this birth because they have been trying to become pregnant for 6 years. The baby is placed on the mother's (Patti) abdomen after delivery for skin contact but does not breastfeed. The nurse assessing the baby notes that he has some mild grunting, nasal flaring and intercostal retractions; he is taken to the transitional nursery for further evaluation and treatment. Jorge, the father, speaks little English but asks when they will be able to hold their son again; Patti is crying and asks to have her baby brought back to her as soon as his condition is stable because she really wants to breastfeed him.

1. Evidence—Is there sufficient evidence to draw conclusions about what to tell Patti and Jorge about their infant son?
2. Assumptions—What assumptions can be made about the following?
   a. The mother's and father's reaction to their son's birth
   b. The infant's expected progress
   c. The possibility of Patti breastfeeding the baby
3. What implications and priorities for nursing care can be drawn at this time?
4. Does the evidence objectively support your conclusion?
5. Are there alternative perspectives to your conclusion?

The nursing process in the care of the late preterm and preterm infant is outlined in the Nursing Process box.

Implementation

The best environment for fetal growth and development is in the uterus of a healthy, well-nourished woman. The goal of care for the preterm infant is to provide an extrauterine environment that approximates a healthy intrauterine environment to promote normal growth and development. Medical and nursing personnel, respiratory therapists, occupational and physical therapists, dietitians, social workers, care managers, and pharmacists work as a team to provide the intensive care needed.

The admission of a preterm newborn to the intensive care nursery is usually an emergency situation. When required, resuscitation is started in the birthing unit, and warmth and oxygen are provided during transport to the nursery. A rapid initial assessment is performed to determine the infant's need for lifesaving treatment.

Physical Care

The preterm infant's environmental support typically consists of the following equipment and procedures:

- Incubator or radiant warmer to control body temperature and maintain NTE
- Oxygen administration, depending on infant's pulmonary and circulatory status

NURSING PROCESS: LATE PRETERM AND PRETERM INFANT CARE

Assessment

The high risk infant must undergo an initial physical assessment for life-threatening problems. The stable high risk infant may undergo a cursory gestational age assessment to identify potential risk factors.

Nursing Diagnoses

After assessment the following nursing diagnoses for high risk infants and their parents may include the following:

Ineffective breathing pattern related to
- decreased number of functional alveoli
- surfactant deficiency
- immature respiratory control
- increased pulmonary vascular resistance

Ineffective thermoregulation related to
- immature central nervous system thermoregulatory control
- increased heat loss to environment and inability to produce heat due to decreased brown fat reserves
- greater body surface exposed to environment

Risk for infection related to
- invasive procedures
- decreased immune response
- ineffective skin barrier

Anxiety (parental) related to
- lack of knowledge about infant's condition and prognosis (uncertain outcome)
- inability to perform expected caregiving activities
- neonatal intensive care unit environment noise and high-tech care

Planning and Implementation

Expected outcomes can apply both to the high risk infant and the parents. Expected outcomes are presented in patient-centered terms and include that the infant will do the following:

- Maintain adequate physiologic functioning (airway, breathing, circulation)
- Receive adequate nutrition for growth
- Maintain stable body temperature
- Remain free of infection
- Experience appropriate parent-infant interactions

Expected outcomes for the parents include that they will do the following:

- Perceive the infant as a family member
- Provide infant care comfortably
- Experience pride and satisfaction in the care of the infant
- Organize their time and energies to meet the love, attention, and care needs of the other members of the family as well as their own needs.

Numerous nursing implementation strategies are discussed on pp. 707-733.

Evaluation

The nurse can be reasonably assured that care was effective to the extent that the expected outcomes for care have been achieved.

- Electronic monitoring of respiratory and cardiac function
- Assistive devices for positioning the infant
- Clustering of care and minimization of stimulation and handling

Various metabolic support measures that may be instituted consist of the following:

- Parenteral fluids to support nutrition, hydration, and fluid and electrolyte balance
- IV access for fluids, parenteral nutrition, and medication administration
- Blood work to monitor arterial blood gases (ABGs), blood glucose level, electrolytes, and other diagnostic studies (C-reactive protein, white cell count with differential, hemoglobin and hematocrit) as indicated

Maintain Body Temperature

The high risk infant is susceptible to heat loss and its complications (see Fig. 24-1). In addition, low-birth-weight (LBW) infants may be unable to increase their metabolic rate because of impaired gas exchange, caloric intake restrictions in relation to high expenditure, or poor thermoregulation. Transepidermal water loss (TEWL) is greater because of skin immaturity in ELBW and VLBW infants and can contribute to temperature instability. The high risk infant should be transferred from the delivery room in a prewarmed incubator; ELBW infants may be placed in a polyethylene bag to decrease heat and water loss. Skin-to-skin (kangaroo) contact between the stable preterm infant and parent is also a viable option for interaction because it helps the infant maintain appropriate body temperature.

High risk infants are cared for in the NTE created by use of an external heat source. A probe applied to the infant is attached to an external heat source supplied by a radiant warmer or a servocontrolled incubator. Studies indicate that optimum thermoneutrality cannot be predicted for every high risk infant's needs. Guidelines for providing an optimum thermal environment for the VLBW infant suggest maintaining the infant's core temperature at rest within a range of 36.7° to 37.3° C, with core and mean temperatures changing less than 0.2° and 0.3° C an hour (Sauer, Dane, & Visser, 1984). Standard guidelines for maintaining NTE in the LBW infant are published (Blake & Murray, 2006). Further research is needed to define an NTE for the ELBW infant.

Care of the Hypothermic Infant

Rapid changes in body temperature may cause apnea and acidosis in the neonate. Therefore the warming of a hypothermic infant should occur over a period of hours. Rapid rewarming may cause apnea, and too slow rewarming increases metabolic distress and oxygen consumption. Rewarming must therefore be individualized for each infant according to illness and ability to produce heat. To accomplish this, the infant is placed either under a radiant warmer or in an incubator with a servocontrol mechanism. It has been suggested that rewarming proceed at a rate of 1° to 2° C per hour. Appropriate guidelines for rewarming the hypothermic infant should be consulted for further information.

Transition to the Incubator

To effectively wean the infant from the incubator, the incubator heat is decreased slowly over several hours to days. On average, infants who are medically stable, gaining weight, and tolerating enteral feedings and weigh 1300 to 1500 g may be weaned (depending on institution protocol). The following general guidelines may be followed to wean the infant from the incubator:

- Disconnect the servocontrol probe (if still in use).
- Dress the infant in a diaper, shirt, and cap.
- Lower the incubator temperature by no more than 0.5° C per each 2-hour period.
- Record the temperature of the infant, the air, and the incubator.
- Assess the infant's responses to the changes every hour until four stable readings are obtained.
- Monitor the infant's temperature and other vital signs.

This procedure is repeated until the incubator temperature is the same as the room temperature and the infant's body temperature consistently remains in the range of 36° to 37° C. The infant is placed in an open bassinet (away from any drafts) when the body temperature is stable, after which he or she is reassessed in conjunction with the delivery of routine care. If necessary, the infant may be returned to the incubator and weaning repeated once the infant is able to regulate his or her temperature. A pattern of steady daily weight gain and absence of any clinical signs such as poor feeding, respiratory distress, or temperature instability are appropriate measures of the effectiveness of weaning to an open bassinet.

Oxygen Therapy

The goals of oxygen therapy are to provide adequate oxygen to the tissues, prevent lactic acid accumulation resulting from hypoxia, and at the same time avoid the potentially negative effects of hyperoxemia and free radicals. Numerous methods have been devised to improve oxygenation. All require that the gas be warmed and humidified before entering the respiratory tract. If the infant does not require mechanical ventilation, oxygen can be supplied by plastic hood placed over the infant's head, by nasal cannula, or by nasal continuous positive airway pressure (CPAP) to supply variable concentrations of humidified oxygen. Because oxygen therapy has inherent hazards, each infant must be carefully monitored to prevent hyperoxemia and hypoxemia.

Infants who require oxygen should have frequent assessments of respiratory status and oxygenation; the time interval of assessments is based in part on the infant's status. Oxygenation assessment includes continuous pulse oximetry and, as warranted, ABG measurement. Vital signs, including heart rate, respiratory rate, and blood pressure, are monitored to ensure not only adequate respiratory function but also adequate circulation and perfusion of tissues.

Interest in the resuscitation of asphyxiated newborns with 21% oxygen rather than 100% oxygen has increased; preliminary studies demonstrate no significant neurologic morbidities at 18 to 24 months in newborns resuscitated with 21% oxygen (Saugstad et al, 2003). Proponents for room air resuscitation suggest fewer complications are associated with oxidative stress and hyperoxemia when room air is administered (Vento et al, 2003). The 2005 American Heart Association resuscitation standards for neonatal resuscitation stress that resuscitation may begin with no supplemental oxygen (i.e.,

21% oxygen or room air) but that, if the infant's condition does not improve within 90 seconds, supplemental oxygen should be available for use. The stated goal is to minimize oxygen free radicals by avoiding hyperoxia using supplemental oxygen at levels less than 100% (American Heart Association, 2005). A review of several studies indicates that neonatal mortality is reduced by 30% to 40% when room air is used instead of 100% oxygen for neonatal resuscitation; rates of ROP and BPD are lower in infants whose Sao_2 (saturation) is kept between 93% and 95%. Fluctuations in oxygen saturation are also deemed harmful. It is recommended that for ELBW infants, oxygen saturations be maintained between 85% and 93%, but definitely not exceeding 95% (Saugstad, 2007).

Oxygen Hood

Oxygen in a specified concentration can be administered by hood to infants who do not require positive pressure mechanical support. The hood is a clear plastic cover that is sized to fit over the head and neck of the infant (Fig. 27-2, *A*). Continuous pulse oximetry allows for monitoring oxygenation and making adjustments according to the infant's condition.

Nasal Cannula

Low-flow amounts of oxygen can be administered by nasal cannula (see Fig. 27-2, *B*). A nasal cannula is used for infants who require low concentrations of supplemental oxygen; this is often used for home oxygen administration. The infant receives an adequate, continuous flow of oxygen while allowing optimal vision, positioning, and parental holding. Infants can also breastfeed or bottle-feed while receiving oxygen by this method. The nasal prongs must be inspected often to ensure that they are not partially obstructed by milk or secretions.

Continuous Distending Pressure

Infants who are unable to maintain an adequate Pao_2 despite the administration of oxygen by hood or nasal cannula may require the delivery of oxygen using continuous distending airway pressure via CPAP or continuous negative pressure. CPAP delivers oxygen at a preset pressure (Fig. 27-3, *A*) by means of nasal prongs, nasopharyngeal tubes, endotracheal tube, or face mask. Nasal prongs are the most common method of CPAP delivery. An orogastric tube may be necessary for decompression of the stomach during use of nasal prongs.

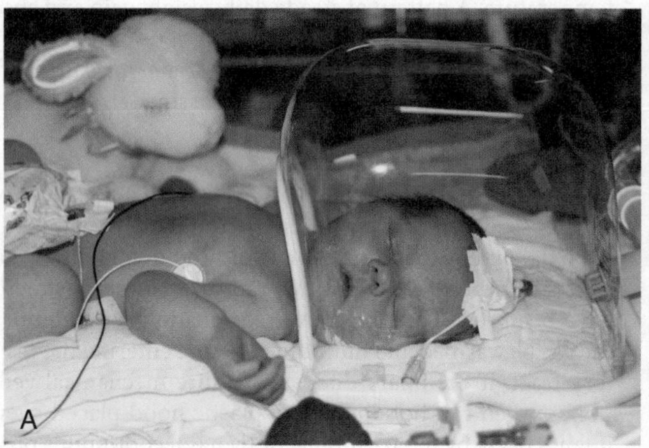

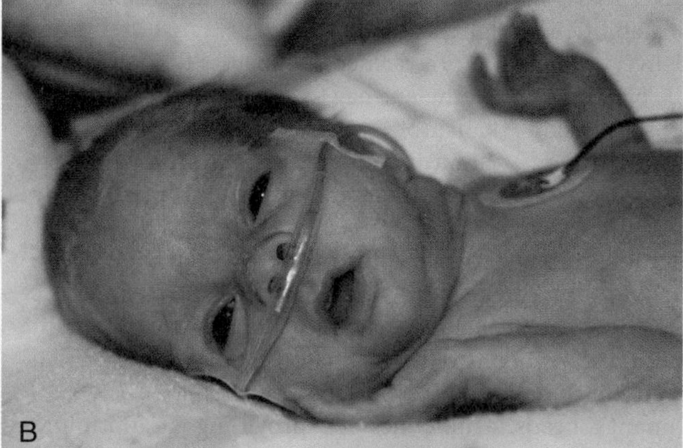

Fig. 27-2 A, Infant under hood. **B,** Infant with nasal cannula. (Courtesy Victoria Langer, RNC, MSN, NNP. From Dickason E, Silverman B, Kaplan J: *Maternal-infant nursing care*, ed 3, St Louis, 1998, Mosby.)

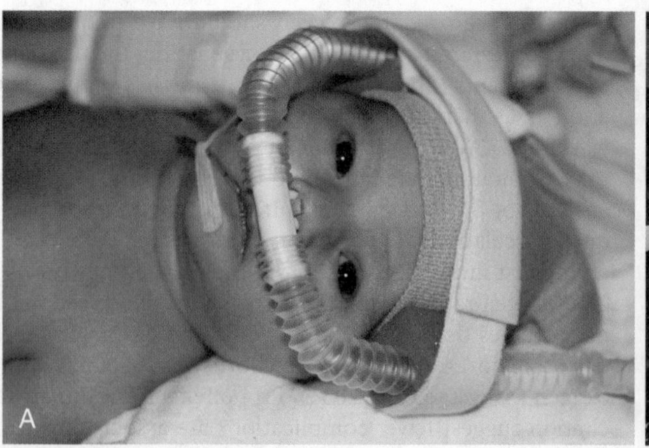

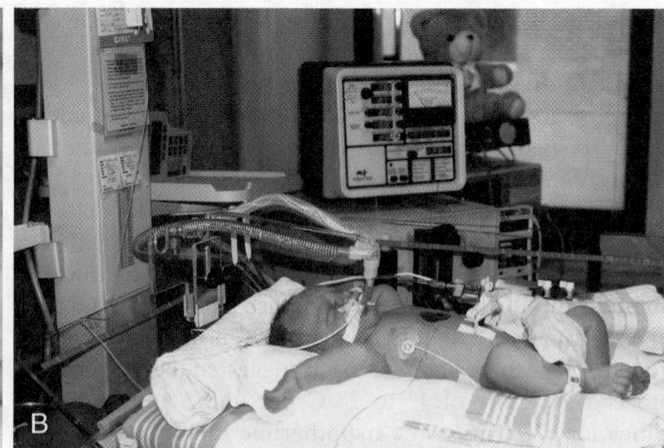

Fig. 27-3 A, Infant receiving ventilatory assistance with nasal continuous positive airway pressure. **B,** Infant intubated and on ventilator. (Courtesy Victoria Langer, RNC, MSN, NNP. From Dickason E, Silverman B, Kaplan J: *Maternal-infant nursing care*, ed 3, St Louis, 1998, Mosby.)

CPAP increases the functional residual capacity; improves the diffusion time of pulmonary gases, including oxygen; and can decrease pulmonary vascular resistance (PVR) and intrapulmonary shunting. If implemented early enough, CPAP may preclude the need for mechanical ventilation. CPAP is the preferred mode for infants who require minor distending pressure, and it avoids the trauma associated with endotracheal intubation and its inherent complications (Hagedorn et al, 2006). The infant with a nasal CPAP device must be monitored closely for signs of nasal damage and skin breakdown (Squires & Hyndman, 2009).

Mechanical Ventilation

Mechanical ventilation must be implemented if other methods of therapy cannot correct abnormalities in oxygenation. Its use is indicated whenever blood gas values reveal the existence of severe hypoxemia or severe hypercapnia (see Fig. 27-3, *B*). The condition of the infant experiencing apnea with bradycardia, ineffective respiratory effort, shock, asphyxia, infection, meconium aspiration syndrome (MAS), respiratory distress syndrome (RDS), or congenital defects that affect ventilation may also deteriorate and require intubation to reverse the process. Ventilator settings are determined by the infant's particular needs. The ventilator is set to provide a predetermined amount of oxygen during spontaneous respirations and also to provide mechanical ventilation in the absence of spontaneous respirations. Newer technologies in ventilation allow oxygen to be delivered at lower pressures and in assist modes, thereby preventing the overriding of the infant's spontaneous breathing and providing distending pressures within a physiologic range, decreasing barotrauma and associated complications such as pneumothorax and pulmonary interstitial emphysema. See Table 27-2 for an explanation of types of mechanical ventilation used in newborns.

Surfactant Replacement Therapy

Surfactant is a surface-active phospholipid secreted by the alveolar epithelium. Acting much like a detergent, this substance reduces the surface tension of fluids that line the alveoli and respiratory passages, resulting in uniform expansion and maintenance of lung expansion at low intraalveolar pressure. Immature development of these functions produces consequences that seriously compromise respiratory efficiency. Deficient surfactant production causes unequal inflation of alveoli on inspiration and the collapse of alveoli on end-expiration. Without surfactant, infants are unable to keep their lungs inflated and therefore exert a great deal of effort to reexpand the alveoli with each breath. With increasing exhaustion, infants are able to open fewer and fewer alveoli. This inability to maintain lung expansion produces widespread atelectasis.

In the absence of alveolar stability (normal functional residual capacity) and with progressive atelectasis, PVR increases, whereas with normal lung expansion PVR decreases. Consequently there is hypoperfusion to the lung tissue, with a decrease in effective pulmonary blood flow. The increase in PVR causes partial reversion to the fetal circulation, with a right-to-left shunting of blood through the persisting fetal communications—the ductus arteriosus and foramen ovale. Inadequate pulmonary perfusion and ventilation produce

Table 27-2 Common Methods for Assisted Ventilation in Neonatal Respiratory Distress*

METHOD	DESCRIPTION	HOW PROVIDED
Continuous distending pressure–continuous positive airway pressure (CPAP)	Provides constant distending pressure to airway in spontaneously breathing infant	Nasal prongs Endotracheal tube Face mask Nasal cannula or nasopharyngeal tubes Bubble CPAP using water resistance
Intermittent mandatory ventilation (IMV)	Allows infant to breathe spontaneously at own rate but provides mechanical cycled respirations and pressure at regular preset intervals; infant may maintain asynchronous ventilation efforts, which diminishes effective gas exchange, air leaks, and air trapping; uses positive end-expiratory pressure (PEEP)	Endotracheal intubation
Synchronized intermittent mandatory ventilation (SIMV)	Mechanically delivered breaths are synchronized to the onset of spontaneous patient breaths; assist/control (A/C) mode facilitates full inspiratory synchrony; involves signal detection of onset of spontaneous respiration from abdominal movement, thoracic impedance, and airway pressure or flow changes; *pressure support ventilation* provides an inspiratory pressure assist when spontaneous breathing is detected to decrease infant's work of breathing	Patient-triggered infant ventilator with signal detector and A/C mode; endotracheal tube; SIMV, A/C, and pressure support are also referred to as *patient-triggered ventilation*
Volume guarantee ventilation	Delivers a predetermined volume of gas using an inspiratory pressure that varies according to the infant's lung compliance (often used in conjunction with SIMV)	Volume guarantee ventilator with flow sensor; endotracheal tube
High-frequency oscillation (HFO)	Application of high-frequency, low-volume, sine-wave flow oscillations to airway at rates between 480 and 1200 breaths/min	Variable-speed piston pump (or loudspeaker, fluidic oscillator); endotracheal tube
High-frequency jet ventilation (HFJV)	Uses a separate, parallel, low-compliant circuit and injector port to deliver small pulses or jets of fresh gas deep into airway at rates between 250 and 900 breaths/min	May be used alone or with low-rate IMV; endotracheal tube

*This is not a comprehensive list of available ventilation modes. For more information, consult specific references on mechanical ventilation such as Donn and Sinha (2003).

hypoxemia and hypercapnia. Pulmonary arterioles, with their thick muscular layer, are markedly reactive to diminished oxygen concentration. Thus a decrease in oxygen tension causes vasoconstriction in the pulmonary arterioles that is further enhanced by a decrease in blood pH. This vasoconstriction contributes to a significant increase in PVR. In normal ventilation with increased oxygen concentration, the ductus arteriosus constricts, and the pulmonary vessels dilate to decrease PVR.

Surfactant can be administered as an adjunct to oxygen and ventilation therapy. Generally, infants born before 32 weeks of gestation do not have adequate amounts of pulmonary surfactant to survive extrauterine life. In many centers the use of prophylactic surfactant is reserved for infants younger than 29 weeks who will likely have RDS (Hagedorn et al, 2006). Exogenous surfactant is manufactured synthetically or extracted from bovine, porcine, or calf lung extract and is given as one or more doses through an endotracheal tube. The infant must be monitored for potential side effects such as patent ductus arteriosus (PDA) and pulmonary hemorrhage. Although the use of surfactant has been associated with a significantly reduced length of time on mechanical ventilation and oxygen therapy and an increased survival rate in preterm infants, it has not significantly decreased the incidence of BPD, intraventricular hemorrhage, or PDA in extremely immature infants. Studies have shown rapid improvement of respiratory status, less ROP and BPD, lower mortality, and decreased incidence of pneumothorax in infants who received natural surfactant in comparison with those who received synthetic (Hagedorn et al, 2006). However, other experts indicate that the newer synthetic surfactant products are equally effective (Engle & American Academy of Pediatrics, Committee on Fetus and Newborn, 2008). The American Academy of Pediatrics, Committee on Fetus and Newborn (Engle & American Academy of Pediatrics, Committee on Fetus and Newborn, 2008), recommends the use of surfactant in infants with RDS as soon as possible after delivery, especially ELBW infants and those not exposed to maternal antenatal steroids. The administration of antenatal steroids to the mother and surfactant replacement has decreased the incidence of RDS and concomitant morbidities.

Inhaled nitric oxide (INO) and extracorporeal membrane oxygenation (ECMO) are additional therapies used in the treatment of respiratory distress and respiratory failure in neonates. INO is used in term and late preterm infants with conditions such as persistent pulmonary hypertension of the newborn (PPHN), MAS, pneumonia, sepsis, and congenital diaphragmatic hernia to decrease or reverse pulmonary hypertension, pulmonary vasoconstriction, acidosis, and hypoxemia. Nitric oxide is a colorless, highly diffusible gas that can be administered through the ventilator circuit blended with oxygen. INO therapy may be used in conjunction with surfactant replacement therapy, high-frequency ventilation, or ECMO. INO has not proved to be significantly effective in decreasing RDS or in improved survival rates in preterm infants, although clinical trials are still ongoing (Barrington & Finer, 2007). Clinical trials have demonstrated, however, that the use of INO improved ventilatory status in infants with pulmonary hypertension, decreased requirements for ventilatory support (Sadiq et al, 2003), and decreased the need for ECMO (Field et al, 2007).

ECMO may be used in the management of term infants with acute severe respiratory failure for the same conditions as those mentioned for INO. This therapy involves a modified heart-lung machine, although in ECMO the heart is not stopped, and blood does not entirely bypass the lungs. Blood is shunted from a catheter in the right atrium or right internal jugular vein by gravity to a servo-regulated roller pump, pumped through a membrane lung where it is oxygenated, through a small heat exchanger where it is warmed, and then returned to the systemic circulation via a major artery such as the carotid artery to the aortic arch. ECMO provides oxygen to the circulation, allowing the lungs to "rest," and decreases pulmonary hypertension and hypoxemia in such conditions as PPHN, congenital diaphragmatic hernia, sepsis, meconium aspiration, and severe pneumonia. ECMO is not used in preterm infants younger than 34 weeks of gestation because the anticoagulant therapy required in the pump and circuits may increase the potential for intraventricular hemorrhage in such infants. In some centers the success of high-frequency ventilation and INO has greatly decreased the demand for ECMO.

High-Frequency Ventilation

Other modes of ventilator therapy include high-frequency oscillator ventilation and jet ventilation (see Table 27-2). These methods of high-frequency ventilation work by providing smaller volumes of oxygen at a significantly more rapid rate (more than 300 breaths/min) than traditional mechanical ventilators. As a result, the intrathoracic pressure and the risk of barotrauma are decreased.

Weaning from Respiratory Assistance

The infant is ready to be weaned from respiratory assistance when the ABG and oxygen saturation levels are maintained within normal limits and he or she is able to establish spontaneous ventilation sufficient to maintain acid-base balance. A spontaneous, adequate respiratory effort must be present, and the infant must show improved muscle tone during increased activity. Weaning is done in a stepwise and gradual manner. This may consist of the infant being extubated, placed on nasal CPAP, and then weaned to oxygen by means of a hood or nasal cannula. Throughout the weaning process the infant's oxygen levels are monitored by pulse oximetry, $tcPo_2$ monitoring, and blood gas levels.

Some infants are not able to be weaned from all oxygen support by the time of discharge from the hospital and may require home oxygen therapy for several months. BPD or congenital anomalies such as repaired congenital diaphragmatic hernia or tracheal defect, or a neurologic insult with resultant dysfunction, may prevent weaning.

The parents need to be given consistent information and be reassured about the infant's respiratory progress. Decisions regarding the nature of continued interventions should be included in a multidisciplinary care plan, and the therapy should be explained frequently to the family.

Frequent skin care assessments are essential when the infant is receiving supplemental oxygen with any of the methods described herein but particularly in infants with poor perfusion and in those requiring equipment that comes in continuous contact with the infant's skin (e.g., nasal CPAP, nasal cannula, pulse oximetry probes). A greater incidence of skin breakdown is noted in infants and children who use medical devices (e.g., nasal prongs, pulse oximetry probes) (Noonan, Quigley, & Curley, 2006).

Nutritional Care

Optimum nutrition is critical in the management of LBW and preterm infants, but providing for their nutritional needs is difficult. The various mechanisms for ingestion and digestion of foods are not fully developed; the more immature the infant, the greater the problem. In addition, the nutritional requirements for this group of infants are not known with certainty. It is known that all preterm infants are at risk because of poor nutritional stores and several physical and developmental characteristics.

An infant's need for rapid growth and daily maintenance must be met in the presence of several anatomic and physiologic disabilities. Although some sucking and swallowing activities are demonstrated before birth and in preterm infants, coordination of these mechanisms does not occur until approximately 32 to 34 weeks of gestation, and they are not fully synchronized until 36 to 37 weeks. Initial sucking is not accompanied by swallowing, and esophageal contractions are uncoordinated. The gag reflex may not be developed until 36 weeks of gestation. Consequently, infants are highly prone to aspiration and its attendant dangers. As infants mature, the suck-swallow pattern develops but is slow and ineffectual, and these reflexes may also become easily exhausted.

The amount and method of feeding are determined by the infant's size and condition. Nutrition can be provided by either the parenteral or enteral route or by a combination of the two. ELBW, VLBW, or critically ill infants are often initially fed exclusively by the parenteral route because of their inability to digest and absorb enteral nutrition. Illness factors resulting in hypoxia and major organ immaturity further preclude the use of enteral feeding until the infant's condition has stabilized. NEC has previously been associated with enteral feedings in acutely ill or distressed infants (see Necrotizing Enterocolitis, p. 731). Total parenteral nutrition (TPN) support of acutely ill infants may be accomplished successfully with commercially available IV solutions specifically designed to meet the infant's nutritional needs, including protein, amino acids, trace minerals, vitamins, carbohydrates (dextrose), and fat (lipid emulsion). There is evidence to support early (within hours of birth) introduction of parenteral nutrition, in particular amino acids, lipids, and protein, and the introduction of minimal enteral feedings within the first 5 days of life. These interventions improve neurodevelopmental outcome and prevent the growth failure often witnessed in ELBW infants (Anderson et al, 2006; Ehrenkranz, 2007).

Studies have shown that the early introduction of small amounts of enteral feedings in metabolically stable preterm infants is beneficial (American Academy of Pediatrics, 2009). These minimal enteral or trophic feedings have been shown to stimulate the infant's GI tract, preventing mucosal atrophy and subsequent enteral feeding difficulties. Minimal enteral feedings with as little as 0.1 to 4 ml/kg preterm formula or breast milk may be given by gavage as early as the first or second postnatal day. Parenteral hydration and nutrition are continued until the infant is able to tolerate an amount of enteral feeding sufficient to sustain growth. An increased incidence of NEC in those VLBW infants fed with minimal enteral feedings has not been substantiated (Mosqueda et al, 2008). Support for initiating minimal enteral feedings includes increased mineral absorption, increased serum calcium and alkaline phosphatase activity, and substantial decrease in the incidence of bilious gastric residuals and feeding intolerance in preterm infants (Schanler et al, 1999).

Type of Nourishment

The types of formulas used, the mode and volume of feeding, and the infant's feeding schedule are based on the findings yielded by assessment of the following variables:

- Weight of the infant
- Pattern of weight gain or loss (Infants weighing less than 1500 g require more energy for growth and thermoregulation.)
- Presence or absence of suck and swallow reflexes
- Behavioral readiness to take oral feedings
- Physical condition, including presence or absence of bowel sounds, abdominal distention, bloody stools, presence and degree of respiratory distress, and apneic episodes
- Residual from previous feeding, if being gavage fed
- Malformations (especially GI defects)
- Renal function, including urine output and laboratory values (e.g., nitrogen balance, electrolyte balance, and glucose level)

Sufficient evidence now indicates that human milk is the best source of nutrition for term and preterm infants. Studies indicate that even small preterm infants are able to breastfeed, if they have adequate sucking and swallowing reflexes and no other contraindications, such as respiratory complications, or concurrent illness are present (Morton, 2002). Mothers who wish to breastfeed their preterm infants are encouraged to pump their breasts until their infants are stable enough to tolerate breastfeeding. Appropriate guidelines for the storage of expressed mother's milk should be followed to decrease the risk of milk contamination and destruction of its beneficial properties (see Chapter 26).

Preterm infants may be able to successfully breastfeed earlier than previously believed (28 to 36 weeks); in addition, preterm infants who are breastfed rather than bottle-fed demonstrate fewer oxygen desaturations; absence of bradycardia; warmer skin temperature; and better coordination of breathing, sucking, and swallowing (Gardner, Snell, & Lawrence, 2006).

Commercially available preterm formulas are cow's milk based; are whey predominant; and have a higher concentration of protein, calcium, and phosphorus than term formulas to meet the unique needs of the preterm infant (American Academy of Pediatrics, 2009). Most preterm formulas are either 22 or 24 cal/oz. The preparation of powdered formula for preterm infants should be carefully performed under strict aseptic technique, preferably in a pharmacy, and the formula properly refrigerated to prevent infection (American Academy of Pediatrics, 2009). Preterm infants fed human milk with fortifier (protein, phosphorus, and calcium) experienced increased weight gain compared with nonfortified human milk intake and had improved bone mineralization; thus a human milk fortifier is recommended for LBW preterm infants (Lawrence & Lawrence, 2005). Supplementation with iron, vitamin D, and multivitamins may be considered in exclusively breastfed LBW infants.

NURSING ALERT Contamination of powdered infant formula in hospitals by *Enterobacter sakazakii* has been associated with serious neonatal infections, NEC, and death (*Enterobacter sakazakii* infections associated with the use of powdered infant formula, 2002; van Acker et al, 2001). When possible, alternatives to powdered formula should be chosen; otherwise, such formula should be carefully mixed in a pharmacy or designated formula preparation room using aseptic technique. Continuous infusion of powdered formula should not exceed 4 hours (*Enterobacter sakazakii* infections associated with the use of powdered infant formula, 2002).

BOX 27-3 Calculation of a Weight Loss or Gain

Example 1

Day 1 = 1750 g (birth weight)
Day 3 = −1680 g
70 g *loss*

$$\frac{70\text{ g}}{1750\text{ g}} = \frac{x}{100\%}$$

$$1750x = 7000\%$$

$$x = 7000\% \div 1750$$

$$x = 4.0\%\text{ weight loss}$$

Example 2

Day 3 = 1680 g
Day 4 = −1720 g
−40 g = 40 g *gain*

$$\frac{40\text{ g}}{1680\text{ g}} = \frac{x}{100\%}$$

$$1680x = 4000\%$$

$$x = 4000\% \div 1680$$

$$x = 2.4\%\text{ weight gain}$$

Hydration

High risk infants often receive supplemental parenteral fluids to supply additional calories, electrolytes, or water. Adequate hydration is particularly important in preterm infants because their extracellular water content is higher (70% in full-term infants and up to 90% in preterm infants), their body surface is larger, the skin barrier is immature and unable to prevent TEWL losses, and glomerular immaturity decreases the ability to concentrate urine. Therefore preterm infants are highly vulnerable to fluid depletion, fluid volume overload, and subsequent electrolyte abnormalities.

Infants who are ELBW, tachypneic, being given phototherapy, or in a radiant warmer have increased insensible water losses that require appropriate fluid adjustments. Methods to decrease insensitive fluid losses include placement of the infant in a highly humidified (40% to 60%) microenvironment (in an incubator) and use of plastic wrap covering, polyethylene bag, or emollient to decrease TEWL. Nurses must monitor fluid status by daily (or more frequent) weights and accurate intake and output of all fluids, including medications and blood products. Urine specific gravity and dipstick measurements are monitored per unit protocol, and serum electrolytes are obtained as warranted by the infant's condition. ELBW infants often require more frequent monitoring of these parameters because of their inordinate transepidermal fluid loss, immature renal function, and propensity for dehydration or overhydration. Intolerance of even dextrose 5% is not uncommon in the ELBW infant, with subsequent glycosuria and osmotic diuresis. Alterations in behavior, alertness, or activity level in these infants receiving IV fluids may signal an electrolyte imbalance, hypoglycemia, or hyperglycemia. The nurse is also observant for tremors or seizures in the VLBW or ELBW infant, since these may be a sign of hyponatremia or hypernatremia. Weight gain from fluid overload in the sick preterm infant may occur as a result of fluid retention (renal failure), inappropriate fluid administration (parenteral), or congestive heart failure. An increased fluid gain may result in the opening of a previously closed PDA, thus exacerbating associated illness. Growing preterm infants, especially those with BPD and those on oral electrolyte supplements, should be carefully monitored for rapid weight gain that may result in pulmonary congestion, PDA, and electrolyte imbalance. See Box 27-3 for calculation of a weight loss or gain.

Elimination Patterns

Frequency of urination, as well as the amount, color, pH, and specific gravity of the urine, is assessed. The assessment of bowel movements includes frequency of stooling; character of the stool; and presence of constipation, diarrhea, or loss of fats (steatorrhea). Infants with unexplained abdominal distention are assessed carefully to rule out NEC, ileus, or obstruction of the GI tract.

Oral Feeding

Nourishment by the oral route is preferred for the infant who has adequate strength and GI function. The best milk for an infant is human milk. Breast milk may be fed by breast, bottle, or gavage. Formula may be fed by bottle or gavage.

Many high risk infants cannot suck well enough to breastfeed or bottle-feed until they have recovered from their initial illness or matured physically. Preterm infants may be put to breast for practice feeds and nonnutritive suckling as soon as medically stable. Mothers of high risk infants are encouraged to continue pumping breast milk. Because of the significant breastfeeding attrition rates among these mothers, they need support and frequent encouragement to continue pumping while their infant is not yet able to nurse.

Gavage Feeding

Gavage feeding is a method of providing breast milk or formula through a nasogastric or orogastric tube (Fig. 27-4). Gavage feeding can be accomplished either with a tube inserted at each feeding (bolus) or continuously through an indwelling feeding tube. Breast milk or formula can be supplied intermittently using a syringe with gravity-controlled flow, or can be given continuously using an infusion pump. The type of fluid instilled is recorded with every syringe change. The volume of the continuous feedings is recorded hourly, and the residual gastric aspirate is measured before each feeding. Residuals of less than a fourth of a feeding can be refed to the infant, depending largely on unit protocol. Feeding may be stopped if the residual is greater than 2 to 4 ml/kg or a 1-hour volume and is not resumed until the infant can be assessed for a possible feeding intolerance (Anderson et al, 2006).

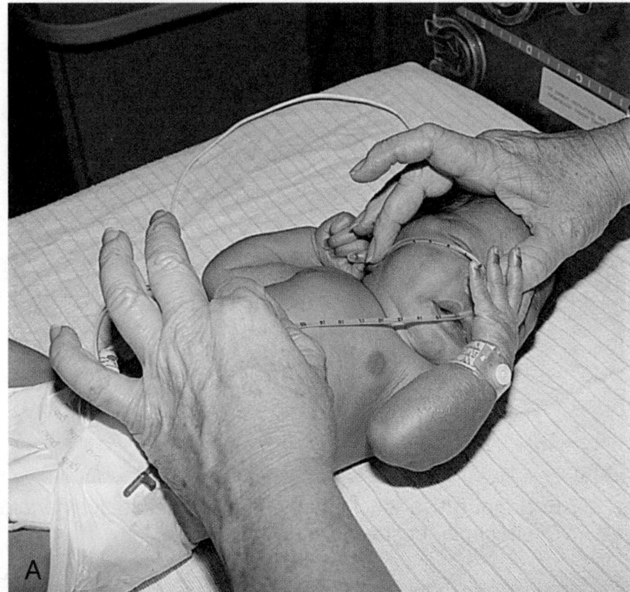

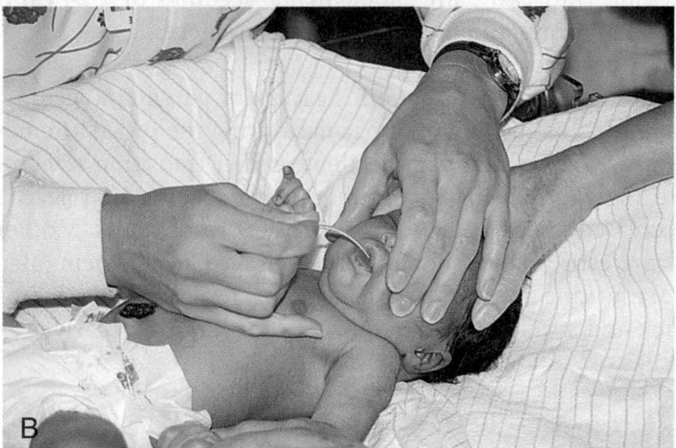

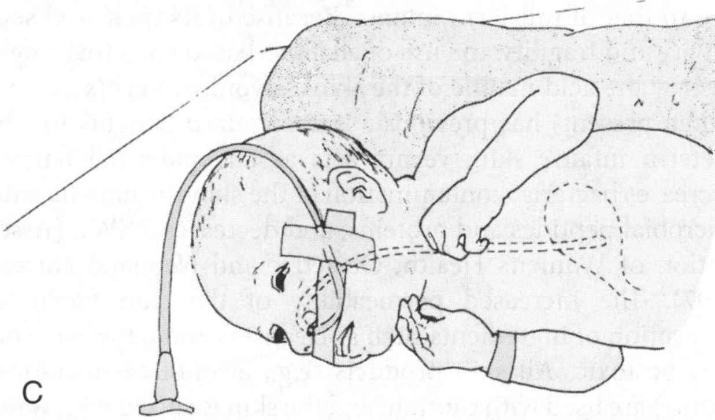

Fig. 27-4 Gavage feeding. **A,** Measurement of gavage feeding tube from tip of nose to earlobe and to midpoint between end of xiphoid process and umbilicus. Tape may be used to mark correct length on tube. **B,** Insertion of gavage tube using orogastric route. **C,** Indwelling gavage tube, nasogastric route. After feeding by orogastric or nasogastric tube, infant is propped on right side or placed prone (preterm infant) for 1 hour to facilitate emptying of stomach into small intestine. Note rolled towel for support. *(A and B, Courtesy Marjorie Pyle, RNC, Lifecircle, Costa Mesa, CA.)*

BOX 27-4 Procedure: Inserting a Gavage Feeding Tube

1. Measure the length of the gavage tube from the tip of the nose to the lobe of the ear to the midpoint between the xiphoid process and the umbilicus (see Fig. 27-4, *A*). Mark the tube with a piece of tape.
2. Lubricate the tip of the tube with sterile water and insert gently through the nose or mouth (see Fig. 27-4, *B*) until the predetermined mark is reached. Placement of the tube in the trachea will cause the infant to gag, cough, or become cyanotic.
3. Check correct placement of the tube by:
   a. Pulling back on the plunger to aspirate stomach contents. Lack of stomach aspirate or fluid is not necessarily evidence of improper placement. Aspirate consisting of respiratory secretions may be mistaken for stomach contents; however, the pH of the stomach contents is much lower (more acidic) than the pH of respiratory secretions.
   b. Injecting a small amount of air (1 to 3 ml) into the tube while listening for gurgling by using a stethoscope placed over the stomach. Ensure that the tube is inserted to the mark; it is possible to hear air entering the stomach even if the tube is positioned above the gastroesophageal (cardiac) sphincter.
   c. Performing abdominal radiography, which is 100% accurate in determining proper feeding tube placement in infants. In a small pilot study, carbon dioxide measurements of 0 (by capnography) indicated proper feeding tube placement in preterm infants (Ellett, Woodruff, & Stewart, 2007). Proper verification of feeding tube placement in neonates by assessing the pH of the aspirate has yet to be properly established; further studies are needed (Ellett et al, 2005).
4. Tape the tube in place and also tape it to the cheek to prevent accidental dislodgement and incorrect positioning (see Fig. 27-4, *C*).
   a. Assess the infant's skin integrity before taping the tube.
   b. Edematous or very preterm infants should have a pectin barrier placed under the tape to prevent abrasions, or use a hydrocolloid adhesive to prevent epidermal stripping (Lund & Durand, 2006).
5. Tube placement *must* be assessed before each feeding.

The orogastric route of gavage feedings may be preferred because most infants are preferential nose breathers. However, some infants do not tolerate oral tube placement. Smaller flexible feeding tubes (e.g., 3.5, 5, or 6 Fr) may be inserted via the nasal route without interfering with breathing. The procedure for inserting a gavage feeding tube is described in Box 27-4.

To begin the feeding, the nurse connects the barrel of a syringe to the gavage tube. While clamping (or pinching) the feeding tube, the nurse pours the specified amount of breast milk or formula into the syringe. The clamp in the tube is then released and the feeding allowed to flow by gravity at a rate that approximates that of an oral feeding (about 1 ml/min). The infant can be held or swaddled to help him or her associate the feeding with positive interactions.

Once the prescribed volume has been delivered, the tube is clamped or pinched and the syringe either removed or left in place. The gavage tube is capped (or the nurse continues to pinch it) while removing it in one steady motion. Capping or pinching the tube prevents breast milk or formula from leaking from the tube and being aspirated during removal of the tube.

After the feeding, the infant is positioned to prevent aspiration. Documentation of the procedure includes the size of the feeding tube, the amount and quality of the residual from the previous feeding, the type and quantity of fluid instilled, and the infant's response to the procedure.

Gastrostomy Feeding

Gastrostomy feeding involves the surgical placement of a tube through the skin of the abdomen into the stomach. With percutaneous gastrostomy insertion, feedings are often started within hours of insertion. Feedings by gravity are done slowly over 20 to 30 minutes, depending on the volume. Special care must be taken to avoid administering a rapid bolus of the fluid because this may lead to abdominal distention, GI reflux into the esophagus, diarrhea with malabsorption, or respiratory compromise. Meticulous skin care at the tube insertion site is necessary to prevent skin breakdown or infection. Intake and output are carefully monitored to ensure adequate fluid and calorie intake and adequate renal function.

Advancing Infant Feedings

Feedings are advanced from passive (parenteral and gavage) to active (nipple and breastfeeding) as assessment data and the infant's ability to tolerate feedings warrant. The infant's sucking patterns and demonstration of a quiet alert state can also be used to determine readiness to nipple feed.

The infant receiving nutrition parenterally is gradually weaned off this type of nutrition. The nourishment given by gavage feedings is increased as parenteral fluids are decreased, depending on the infant's tolerance of enteral feeding. Feedings are advanced slowly and cautiously; if feedings are advanced too rapidly, vomiting, diarrhea, abdominal distention, and apneic episodes may result.

The infant receiving gavage feedings progresses to nipple feeding or breast milk feedings. Gavage feedings are decreased as the infant's ability to suckle breast milk or formula improves. Often the infant is fed by both nipple or breast feeding and gavage feeding during this transition; this ensures intake of the prescribed volumes of both fluid and nutrients. The parents should be encouraged to interact by talking and making eye contact with the infant during feedings.

Because preterm infants are often being discharged at weights of 1500 g, the need to continue nutritional intake and growth to match intrauterine growth remains. A concern in recent years has been the delayed growth of preterm infants discharged home after neonatal intensive care. To address these growth needs, it has been recommended that formerly preterm infants receive either human breast milk with a preterm human milk fortifier or a 22 cal/oz formula until the postnatal age of 9 months. A suggested feeding regimen to meet the needs of the growing LBW infant includes breastfeeding with two daily supplemental feedings of a 24 cal/oz preterm formula to meet growth requirements.

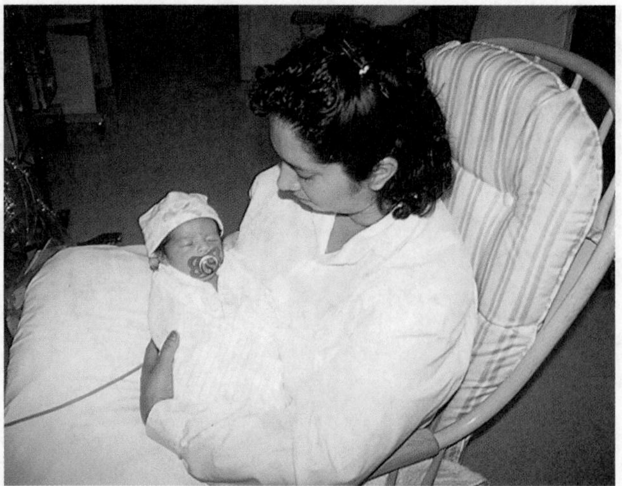

Fig. 27-5 Nonnutritive sucking by infant. *(Courtesy Marjorie Pyle, RNC, Lifecircle, Costa Mesa, CA.)*

Nonnutritive Sucking

For the infant who requires gavage or parenteral feedings, nonnutritive sucking on a pacifier during the procedure may improve oxygenation and facilitate earlier transition to nipple feeding (Fig. 27-5). Such nonnutritive sucking may lead to decreased energy expenditure with less restlessness. Mothers of preterm infants should be encouraged to let their infant start sucking at the breast during kangaroo care; some infant's suck and swallow reflexes may be coordinated as early as 32 weeks of gestation.

Skin Care

The skin of preterm infants is characteristically immature relative to that of full-term infants. Because of its increased sensitivity and fragility, the use of alkaline-based soap that might destroy the acid mantle of the skin is avoided. Vernix caseosa (when present) has previously unrecognized benefits for the preterm infant's skin; vernix acts as an epidermal barrier, decreases bacterial contamination of the skin through its antimicrobial peptides and proteins, and decreases TEWL (Association of Women's Health, Obstetric and Neonatal Nurses, 2007). The increased permeability of the skin facilitates absorption of ingredients such as cleansers and adhesives that may be toxic. All skin products (e.g., alcohol or povidone-iodine) are used with caution, and the skin is rinsed with water afterward because these substances may cause severe irritation and chemical burns in LBW infants.

Adhesives used after heel sticks or to secure monitoring equipment and IV infusions may excoriate the skin or adhere to the skin surface so firmly that the epidermis can be separated from understructures and pulled away with the adhesive. The use of pectin barriers and hydrocolloid adhesives may be useful because these products mold well to skin contours and adhere in moist conditions. Recommendations for protecting the integrity of preterm infant skin include using minimal adhesive tape, backing the tape with cotton, and delaying adhesive and pectin barrier removal until adherence is reduced (Lund & Kuller, 2007). Solvents used to remove tape are avoided because they tend to dry and burn the delicate skin.

An emollient such as Eucerin or Aquaphor may also be used to promote skin integrity and prevent dry, cracking, and peeling skin in infants at risk for skin breakdown. However, the use of an emollient in infants less than 750 g has been associated with *Staphylococcus epidermidis,* and its use in such infants must be carefully weighed against the risk of infection (Edwards, Conner, & Soll, 2004). In one small study, emollient application to the skin of infants born at less than 27 weeks of gestation decreased fluid loss during the first 2 weeks of life (Beeram et al, 2006).

Guidelines for skin care are listed in the Guidelines box. It is recommended that a validated skin assessment tool such as the Braden Q Scale or Neonatal Skin Condition Score be used once daily to evaluate the high risk infant's skin condition in order to implement interventions aimed at minimizing skin breakdown (Curley et al, 2003; Lund & Osborne, 2004).

GUIDELINES Neonatal Skin Care

General Skin Care

Assessment

Assess skin every day or more often as needed for redness, dryness, flaking, scaling, rashes, lesions, excoriation, or breakdown.

Identify risk factors for skin injury: gestational age less than 30 weeks, adhesive use, high-frequency ventilation, extracorporeal membrane oxygenation, nasal CPAP, hypotension requiring vasopressors.

Use a valid assessment tool to provide reliable and objective measurement of skin condition.

Evaluate and report abnormal skin findings and analyze for possible causes.

Intervene according to interpretation of findings or physician order.

Bathing

Initial Bath

Assess for stable temperature a minimum of 2 to 4 hours before first bath.

Use cleansing agents with neutral pH and minimal dyes or perfume in water.

Use Standard Precautions; wear gloves.

Do not completely remove vernix; allow vernix to wear off with normal care and handling.

Bathe preterm infant younger than 32 weeks only in warm sterile water for the first week.

Routine

Decrease frequency of baths to every second or third day by daily cleansing of eyes, oral and diaper areas, and pressure points.

Use cleanser or soaps no more than two or three times a week.

Avoid rubbing skin during bathing or drying.

Immerse stable infants fully (except head) in an appropriate-size tub.

Use swaddled immersion bathing technique: slow unwrapping after gently lowering into water for sensitive, but stable, infants needing assistance with motor system reactivity.

Emollients

Apply sparingly to dry, flaking, fissured areas as needed.

Choose petrolatum-based products that are free of preservatives, dyes, and perfume.

Observe neonates weighing less than 750 g receiving emollient therapy for increased risk of coagulase-negative staphylococcal infections.

Consider dispensing emollients from hospital pharmacy in a unit dose or patient-specific container. Follow hospital protocol or consider applying emollient as needed to infants older than 32 weeks for dry, flaking skin.

Adhesives

Decrease use as much as possible.

Use semipermeable transparent adhesive dressings to secure intravenous lines (IVs), nasogastric or orogastric tubes, silicone catheters, and central lines.

Use hydrogel or limb electrodes.

Consider pectin barriers (HolliHesive, DuoDERM) beneath adhesives to protect skin.

Secure pulse oximeter probe or electrodes with elasticized dressing material (carefully avoid restricting blood flow).

Do not use adhesive remover, solvents, or bonding agents.

Avoid removing adhesives for at least 24 hours after application.

Facilitate adhesive removal using water, mineral oil, or petrolatum.

Remove adhesives or skin barriers slowly, supporting the skin underneath with one hand and gently peeling away the product from the skin with the other hand.*

Antiseptic Agents

Apply before invasive procedures.

Consider the potential for skin breakdown or irritation with disinfectant.

No specific disinfectant is recommended for all neonates; remove completely with water or saline after use.

Apply povidone-iodine two times, air dry for 30 seconds; remove completely with sterile water or sterile saline solution immediately after procedure.

Avoid use of isopropyl alcohol for skin preparation or removal of other disinfectants.

Transepidermal Water Loss

Minimize transepidermal water loss and heat loss in small preterm infants at less than 30 weeks of gestation by:

- Measuring ambient humidity during first weeks of life
- Applying occlusive polyethylene body bag immediately at delivery and removing after infant is stabilized in the neonatal intensive care unit
- Considering an increase in humidity of more than 70% to 90% by using transparent dressings and/or a servocontrolled humidifying incubator for first 7 days; decreasing to 50% until 28 days of age; or following hospital guidelines
- Using supplemental conductive heat and reduce radiant heat source.
- Applying semipermeable transparent dressings to skin surfaces on infant's chest, abdomen, and back

*CAUTION: Scissors are not to be used for tape or dressing removal because of hazard of cutting skin or amputating tiny digits.

Continued

GUIDELINES Neonatal Skin Care—cont'd

Skin Breakdown

Prevention

Decrease pressure from externally applied forces using water, air, or gel mattresses; sheepskin; or cotton bedding.

Provide adequate nutrition, including protein, fat, and zinc.

Apply transparent adhesive dressings to protect arms, elbows, and knees from friction injury.

Use tracheostomy and gastrostomy dressings (Hydrasorb, Mepilex Lite, or Lyofoam) for drainage and relief of pressure from tracheostomy or gastrostomy tube.

Use emollient in the diaper area (groin and thighs) to reduce urine irritation.

Treating Skin Breakdown

Irrigate wound every 4 to 8 hours with warm half-strength normal saline using a 320-ml or larger syringe and 20-gauge Teflon catheter.

Culture wound and treat if signs of infection are present (excessive redness, swelling, pain on touch, heat, or resistance to healing).

Use transparent adhesive dressing for uninfected wounds.

Apply hydrogel with or without antibacterial or antifungal ointments (as ordered) for infected wounds (may need to moisten before removal).

Use hydrocolloid for deep, uninfected wounds (leave in place for 5 to 7 days) or as an ostomy barrier and to improve appliance adhesion; warm barrier in hand for several minutes to soften before applying to skin.

Avoid use of antiseptic solutions for wound cleansing (use for intact skin only).

Treating Diaper Dermatitis

Maintain clean, dry skin; use absorbent diapers and change often.

If mild irritation occurs, use petrolatum barrier.

For developing dermatitis, apply a generous quantity of zinc-oxide barrier.

For severe dermatitis, identify cause and treat (e.g., frequent stooling from spina bifida, severe opiate withdrawal, malabsorption syndrome).

Treat *Candida albicans* with antifungal ointment or cream.

Avoid powders and antibiotic ointments. (See Umbilical Cord Care and Care of the Newly Circumcised Infant, Chapter 25.)

Other Skin Care Concerns

Use of Substances on Skin

Evaluate all substances that come in contact with infant's skin.

Before using any topical agent, analyze components of preparation and:

- Use sparingly and only when necessary.
- Confine use to smallest possible area.
- Whenever possible and appropriate, wash off with water.
- Monitor infant carefully for signs of toxicity and systemic effects.

Use of Thermal Devices

Avoid heat lamps because of increased potential for burns. If needed, measure actual temperature of exposed skin every 15 minutes.

When using heating pads (Aqua K pads):

- Change infant's position every 15 minutes initially and then every 1 to 2 hours.
- Preset temperature of heating pads to less than 40° C (104° F).

When using preheated transcutaneous electrodes:

- Avoid use on infants.
- Set at lowest possible temperature.
- Use pulse oximetry rather than transcutaneous monitoring whenever possible.

When prewarming heels before phlebotomy, avoid temperatures over 40° C.

Provide warm ambient humidity, directed away from infant; use aerosolized sterile water and maintain ambient temperature so as to not exceed 40° C.

Document use of all heating devices.

Use of Fluid Therapy and Hemodynamic Monitoring

Be certain fingers or toes are visible whenever extremity is used for peripheral IV or arterial line.

Secure catheter or needle with transparent dressing and tape to promote easy visualization of site.

Assess site hourly for signs of ischemia, infiltration, and inadequate perfusion (check capillary refill, pulses, color).

Avoid use of restraints (e.g., arm boards); if used, check that they are secured safely and not restricting circulation or movement (check for pressure areas).

Use commercial IV protector (e.g., I.V. House) with minimal tape.

Data from Kuller JM: Skin breakdown: risk factors, prevention, and treatment, *NINR* 1(1):33-42, 2001; *Neonatal skin care: evidence-based clinical practice guideline,* ed 2, Washington, DC, 2007, Association of Women's Health, Obstetric and Neonatal Nurses; Johnson FE, Maikler VE: Nurses' adoption of the AWHONN/NANN Neonatal Skin Care Project, *NINR* 1(1):59-67, 2001; Lund CH, Kuller J, Lott JW: Neonatal skin care: clinical outcomes of the AWHONN/NANN evidence-based clinical practice guideline, *J Obstet Gynecol Neonatal Nurs* 30(1):41-51, 2001; Taquino LT: Promoting wound healing in the neonatal setting: process versus protocol, *J Perinat Neonatal Nurs* 14(1):108-118, 2000; Lund C, Lane A, Raines DA: Neonatal skin care: the scientific basis for practice, *J Obstet Gynecol Neonatal Nurs* 28(3):241-254, 1999; Malloy MB, Perez-Woods R: Neonatal skin care: prevention of skin breakdown, *Pediatr Nurs* 17(1):41-48, 1991.

Environmental Concerns

Infants in neonatal intensive care units (NICUs) are exposed to high levels of auditory input from the various machine alarms, and this can have adverse effects (Fig. 27-6). Continuous noise levels of 45 to 85 db are common in NICUs. An incubator produces a constant noise level of 60 to 80 db (Haubrich, 1998), and each new piece of life-support equipment used adds another 20 db to the background noise. The infant's hearing may be damaged if it is exposed to a constant decibel level of 90 db or frequent decibel swings higher than 110 db.

The noise level that results from monitoring equipment, alarms, and general unit activity has been correlated with the incidence of intracranial hemorrhage, especially in the ELBW or VLBW infant. Personnel should reduce noise-generating activities, such as closing doors (including incubator portholes), listening to loud radios, talking loudly, and handling equipment (e.g., trash containers). Byers, Waugh, and Lowman

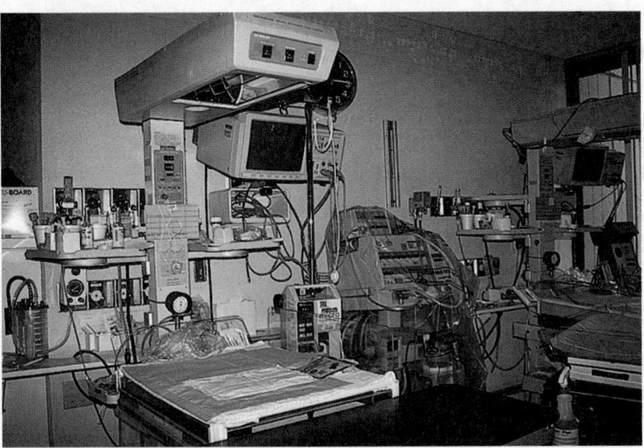

Fig. 27-6 Neonatal intensive care unit equipment, which, although necessary, may contribute to significant environmental stimulation. Note bed, wall oxygen attachments, monitor, ventilator, incubator, and pumps, all of which have alarm systems. *(Courtesy Marjorie Pyle, RNC, Lifecircle, Costa Mesa, CA.)*

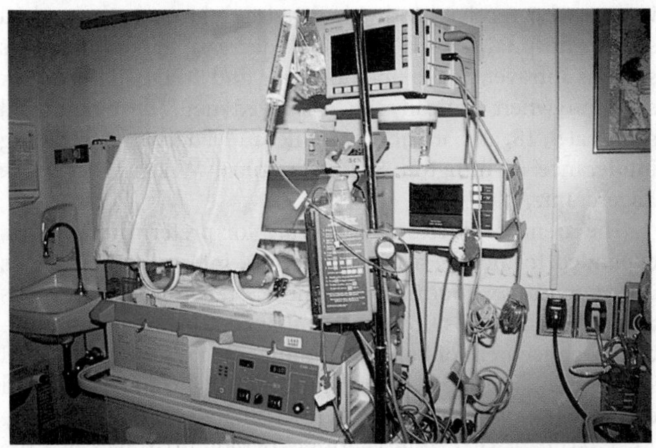

Fig. 27-7 Infant in double-walled incubator with a blanket for a light shield. *(Courtesy Marjorie Pyle, RNC, Lifecircle, Costa Mesa, CA.)*

(2006) suggest monitoring sound levels in the nursery to address problem areas.

Twenty-four-hour surveillance of sick infants implies maximum visibility and often bright lights. Units should establish a night-day sleep pattern by either darkening the room, covering cribs with blankets, or placing eye patches over the infants' eyes at night. Infants need scheduled rest periods during which the lights are dimmed, the incubators are covered with blankets, and the infants are not disturbed for handling of any kind (Fig. 27-7) (Holditch-Davis, Blackburn, & VandenBerg, 2007). Sleep periods should be undisturbed for at least 50 minutes to allow complete sleep cycles. Infants' eyes should be shielded from bright procedure lights to prevent potential harm. Many experts suggest that the human face, especially the parent's, is the best visual stimulus and that visual stimuli be kept to a minimum early in development.

Effects of environmental hazards can be potentiated by some drugs used for infant therapy. Diuretics (especially furosemide [Lasix]), ototoxic antibiotics such as gentamicin and kanamycin, and antimalarial agents can potentiate noise-induced hearing loss. Routine hearing screening should be performed on all infants before discharge.

Nurses can modify the environment to provide a neurodevelopmentally supportive milieu. In that way, the infant's neurobehavioral and physiologic needs can be better met, the infant's developing organization can be supported, and growth and development can be fostered.

Developmental Outcome

Much attention has been focused on the effects of early developmental intervention on both normal and preterm infants. Infants respond to a great variety of stimuli, and the atmosphere and activities of the NICU are overstimulating. Consequently, infants in the NICU are subjected to *inappropriate* stimulation that can be harmful. Nursing care activities, such as taking vital signs, changing the infant's position, weighing, and changing diapers, are associated with frequent periods of hypoxia, oxygen desaturation, and elevated intracranial pressure. The more immature the infant, the less able he or she is to habituate to a single procedure, such as taking an oscillometric blood pressure, without becoming overstimulated. The caregiver uses the infant's own behavior and physiologic functioning as the basis for planning care and providing interventions. Through observation, caregivers can identify the infant's strengths, thresholds for disorganization, and areas of vulnerability (Als, 1998).

Developmental care, accentuating the infant's unique ability to achieve behavioral state organization, is tailored to each infant's developmental level and tolerance based on a comprehensive behavioral assessment. During the early stages of development (especially before 33 weeks of gestation), external stimulation produces uncoordinated, random activity, such as jerky limb extension, hyperflexion, and irregular vital signs. At this stage infants need to have *minimum* environmental stimulation. Using the developmental model of supportive care, the nurse closely monitors physiologic and behavioral signs to promote organization and well-being of the high risk infant during handling. Softly calling the infant by name and then gently placing a hand on the body signal care is beginning and alleviate the abrupt interruption that precedes caregiving. Infants are handled with slow, controlled movements (some infants are unstable if moved abruptly), and their random movements are controlled with limbs held flexed close to their bodies during turning or other position changes. This *containment* or *facilitated tucking* may also be used before invasive procedures such as heel stick to alleviate distress. *Blanket swaddling* and *nesting* or containment has been shown to decrease physiologic and behavioral stress during routine care procedures such as bathing, weighing, and heel stick. A nest constructed by placing blanket rolls underneath the bed sheet helps infants maintain an attitude of flexion when prone or side lying.

Although it must be individually adjusted, *skin-to-skin contact (kangaroo care)* and short periods of gentle massage can help reduce stress in preterm infants. Regular passive skin-to-skin contact between parents (mother or father) and LBW infants has been shown to alleviate stress. The undressed (except for diaper) infant is placed in a vertical position on the parent's bare chest, which permits direct eye contact, skin-to-skin sensations, and close proximity. Skin-to-skin contact between parent and infant, in addition to being a safe and effective method for VLBW infant–parent acquaintance, can have a positive healing effect for the mother with a high risk pregnancy. Mothers may experience psychologic healing related to preterm delivery and regain the mothering role through early skin-to-skin contact with their VLBW infants. Additional benefits of skin-to-skin care include earlier contact with mechanically ventilated infants, maintenance of neonatal thermal stability and oxygen saturation, increased feeding vigor, maintenance of organized state, decreased pain perception during painful heel sticks, and minimal untoward effects of being held (Conde-Agudelo, Diaz-Rossello, & Belizan, 2008; Anderson, 1999; Dodd, 2005). In full-term and preterm newborns, skin-to-skin contact has a strong analgesic effect during procedures such as heel lance (Ludington-Hoe, Hosseini, & Torowicz, 2005; Johnston et al, 2008; Kostandy et al, 2008). LBW infants receiving skin-to-skin contact with breastfeeding mothers maintained higher oxygen saturation and were less likely to have desaturations below 90%, and their mothers were more likely to continue breastfeeding both in the hospital and for 1 month after discharge. Kangaroo care of preterm infants fosters appropriate neurobehavioral development by promoting stability of heart and respiratory function, minimizes purposeless movements, offers maternal proximity for attention, improves the infant's behavioral state, and permits self-regulating behaviors (McCain et al, 2005) (Fig. 27-8). The National Association of Neonatal Nurses has developed a clinical practice guideline for the stable healthy preterm infant age 30 weeks of gestation or older (Ludington-Hoe, Morgan, & Abouelfettoh, 2008) (see Evidence-Based Practice box).

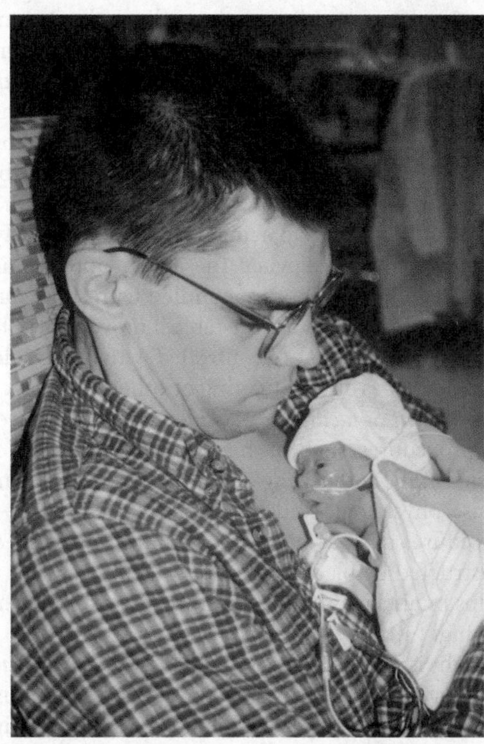

Fig. 27-8 Father providing kangaroo care. *(Courtesy Judy Meyr, St Louis, MO.)*

Cobedding of twins (or multiples) is another developmental intervention that has been implemented in neonatal intensive care and newborn nurseries to provide a better environment for neonatal growth and development (Altimier & Lutes, 2001; DellaPorta, Aforismo, & Butler-O'Hara, 1998). Cobedding involves placing twins or other multiples together in the same crib or incubator. Preliminary data from a multicenter study indicate that twins who are cobedding have improved thermoregulation, have significantly fewer apnea and bradycardia episodes, gain weight more quickly than their single counterparts, and have decreased length of stay. Parental satisfaction is also significantly greater with cobedded newborns. One major concern with cobedding is cross-transmission of infection between the neonates, but increased infection rates have not occurred with cobedding (LaMar & Dowling, 2006).

Additional research studies have confirmed the beneficial effects of developmental care with preterm infants. In addition to requiring fewer days of mechanical ventilation, preterm infants who received individualized developmental care had shorter hospital stays; a significant decrease in complications such as intraventricular hemorrhage and BPD; less need for sedation when critically ill; improved neurodevelopmental scores at 9, 18, and 36 months of life; and a decrease in feeding intolerance (Symington & Pinelli, 2006; Westrup, Sizun, & Lagercrantz, 2007).

The arena of developmental care for preterm infants has expanded to include a wide variety of interventions such as infant massage, soothing soft music, recordings of parents reading stories, positioning to enhance self-regulatory abilities, enhancement of hand-to-mouth activities, uninterrupted sleep periods, decreased environmental light and noise, and even the use of stuffed animals to facilitate infant positioning. As a result of such interventions, parents may perceive the NICU environment as less threatening. Active participation in providing such an environment for their special infant also involves the parents in the provision of daily care when the newborn is critically ill and cannot be fed or held.

When infants have reached sufficient developmental organization and stability, interventions are designed and implemented to support their growing abilities. Nurses and parents become adept at learning to read infants' behavioral cues and supplying appropriate interventions. Clues include both approach and avoidance behaviors. *Approach behaviors* that are supported and enhanced include tongue extension, hand clasp, hand-to-mouth movements, sucking, looking, and cooing. Signs of stress or fatigue that signal the infant's need for time-out include mottled, flushed, dusky, pale or gray skin; tachypnea; pauses; gasping; sighing; tremors; startles; twitches; hiccups; gagging or choking; spitting up; grunting and straining as if having a bowel movement; coughing; sneezing; yawning; arm or leg extensions; arm(s) outstretched with fingers splayed in salute gesture; and oxygen desaturations.

When infants are recovering and are free of support systems, medically stable, and on room air or minimal amounts of oxygen, they are assessed to document behavioral state organization and ability to self-regulate. When the infant is

EVIDENCE-BASED PRACTICE Skin-to-Skin Contact (Kangaroo Care) for Term and Preterm Infants

—*Pat Gingrich*

Ask the Question

What are the benefits of kangaroo care (skin-to-skin contact)?

Search for Evidence

Search Strategies

Professional organization guidelines, meta-analyses, systematic reviews, randomized controlled trials, nonrandomized prospective studies, and retrospective studies since 2006

Databases Searched

CINAHL; Cochrane; Medline; National Guideline Clearinghouse; TRIP Database Plus; and websites for ABM, AWHONN, CDC, and Lamaze International

Critically Analyze the Evidence

Kangaroo care (skin-to-skin contact) has proved to be so significantly beneficial to the infant and the mother (and/or father) that it is now promoted by most maternal-newborn professional organizations (American Academy of Pediatrics; Academy of Breastfeeding Medicine; Association of Women's Health, Obstetric and Neonatal Nurses; Lamaze International; National Institute for Health and Clinical Excellence; Joanna Briggs Institute). A Cochrane systematic review found that placing the dried newborn on the mother's bare abdomen at birth, covered with a warm towel, and early, frequent breastfeeding regulate newborn temperature, decrease stress hormones and crying, promote bonding, and encourage exclusive breastfeeding for a longer period (Moore, Anderson, & Bergman, 2007). As noted in Chapter 24, a program of skin-to-skin contact and frequent breastfeeding (10 to 12 times in 24 hours) regulates blood glucose for most term infants within minutes or hours.

For vulnerable preterm infants, these benefits may be even more protective. A randomized, controlled trial (RCT) comparing kangaroo care to typical care for preterm infants born at 32 to 36 weeks of gestation showed significant exclusive breastfeeding outcomes for as long as 6 months (Hake-Brooks & Anderson, 2008). In addition to breastfeeding and thermoregulation, another RCT concluded that regular skin-to-skin contact helps preterm infants better organize their sleep-awake states into more mature patterns (Ludington-Hoe et al, 2006).

Painful procedures can add to the stress hormones of the already fragile preterm neonate. A single-blind randomized crossover trial of 61 very preterm infants (gestational ages 28 to 32 weeks) compared the Premature Infant Pain Profile (PIPP) (heart rate, facial actions, and oxygen saturation) of infants being held in skin-to-skin contact during heel stick with those swaddled in incubators. The very preterm infants in kangaroo care had significantly lower PIPP scores than the controls (Johnston et al, 2008).

Implications for Practice

Skin-to-skin contact between parents and newborns, even preterm infants, is now an accepted way to promote well-being, foster bonding, encourage breastfeeding, and facilitate maturation. The parents feel "needed" and "more comfortable" participating in this highly beneficial intervention (Johnson, 2007). Preterm babies who receive pumped breast milk are not receiving the natural skin-to-skin contact, so nurses can advocate for a trial of kangaroo care, as tolerated. Although very preterm infants cannot tolerate the stimulation, late preterm infants can benefit very much from a policy of kangaroo care.

Mother-infant pairs should never be left alone during kangaroo care, especially in the first few hours of life, and will need frequent nursing assessment for signs of instability.

References

Hake-Brooks SJ, Anderson GC: Kangaroo care and breastfeeding of mother-preterm infant dyads 0-18 months: a randomized, controlled trial, *Neonatal Netw* 27(3):151-159, 2008.

Johnson AN: The maternal experience of kangaroo holding, *J Obstet Gynecol Neonatal Nurs* 36(6):568-573, 2007.

Johnston CC et al: Kangaroo mother care diminishes pain from heel lance in very preterm neonates: a crossover trial, *BMC Pediatr* 8:13, 2008. Available at www.pubmedcentral.nih.gov, doi: 10.1186/1471-2431-8-13 (accessed July 4, 2008).

Ludington-Hoe SM et al: Neurophysiological assessment of neonatal sleep organization: preliminary results of a randomized, controlled trial of skin contact with preterm infants, *Pediatrics* 117(5):e909-e923, 2006. Available at http://pediatrics.aappublications.org, DOI: 10.1542/peds.2004-1422 (accessed July 3, 2008).

Moore ER, Anderson GC, Bergman N: Early skin-to-skin contact for mothers and their healthy newborn infants, *Cochrane Database Syst Rev* (3):CD003519, 2007.

stable and mature enough to begin developmental intervention, activities are individualized according to each infant's cues, temperament, state, behavioral organization, and particular needs. Intervention periods are short (e.g., 2 to 3 minutes of voices, 5 minutes of quiet music). Hearing and vestibular interventions are initiated earlier than visual stimulation. One type of intervention at a time is applied to document the infant's tolerance and response. An intervention program for convalescing infants includes parents and siblings early in the infant's hospitalization; teaching parents to be responsive to the infant's individual cues is an important function of the NICU nurse. Parents, siblings, and health care providers are encouraged to adhere to the established developmental care plan to avoid disruption in sleep-wake cycles and minimize inappropriate stimuli.

Developmental care of the preterm neonate is an ongoing process in the NICU and is incorporated into the daily care given to each infant. The nurse is cognizant of the preterm infant's developmental needs, temperament, and newborn state, as well as environmental conditions that adversely affect the infant; nursing care is planned accordingly to enhance optimum physical, psychosocial, and neurologic development. This task is often difficult to accomplish when invasive treatments or interventions are required to stabilize the critically ill neonate.

One tool that may be used to evaluate the infant's neurodevelopmental status and adaptation to the environment is the NICU Network Neurobehavioral Scale (NNNS), which was developed by the National Institutes of Health and provides an assessment of neurologic, behavioral, and stress-abstinence function in the neonate. The test combines items from other tests such as the Neonatal Behavioral Assessment Scale; stress-abstinence items developed by Finnegan (1985); and a complete neurologic examination, which includes primitive reflexes and active and passive tone (Law et al, 2003).

Growth and Development Potential

Although it is impossible to predict with complete accuracy the growth and development potential of each preterm newborn, some findings support an anticipated favorable outcome in the absence of ongoing medical sequelae that can affect growth, such as BPD, NEC, and CNS problems. The lower the birth weight, the greater the likelihood of negative sequelae. The growth and development milestones (e.g., motor milestones, vocalization, and body growth) are corrected for gestational age until the child is approximately 3 years of age.

The age of a preterm newborn is calculated by subtracting the number of weeks born before 40 weeks of gestation from the chronologic age. For example, a 6-month-old (chronologic age) infant born at 32 weeks of gestation would have a corrected age of 4 months. The infant's responses are accordingly evaluated against the norm expected for a 4-month-old infant. Therefore, in the infant born preterm, chronologic age is not equal to corrected age (American Academy of Pediatrics, Committee on Fetus and Newborn, 2004).

An effective discharge plan should include frequent outpatient follow-up visits with a primary care practitioner and developmental specialist for monitoring growth and achievement of appropriate developmental milestones.

Parental Support

The nurse as support person and teacher shapes the environment and makes caregiving more responsive to the needs of parents and infant. Nurses help parents learn who their infant is and recognize behavioral cues in his or her development.

If a high risk birth is anticipated, the family can be given a tour of the NICU or shown a video to prepare them for the sights and activities of the unit. After the birth, the parents can be given a booklet, be shown a video, or have someone describe what they will see when they go to the unit to see their infant. As soon as possible, the parents should see and touch their infant so that they can begin to acknowledge the reality of the birth and the infant's true appearance and condition (Fig. 27-9). They need encouragement to begin to accomplish the psychologic tasks imposed by the preterm birth. A nurse and primary health care provider should be present during the parent's first visit to the infant for the following reasons:

- To help them "see" the infant rather than focus on equipment. The nurse and care provider should explain the significance and function of the apparatus that surrounds the infant.
- To explain the characteristics normal for an infant of their baby's gestational age. In this way, parents do not compare their infant with a full-term healthy baby.
- To encourage the parent to express feelings about the pregnancy, labor, and birth and the experience of having a preterm infant.

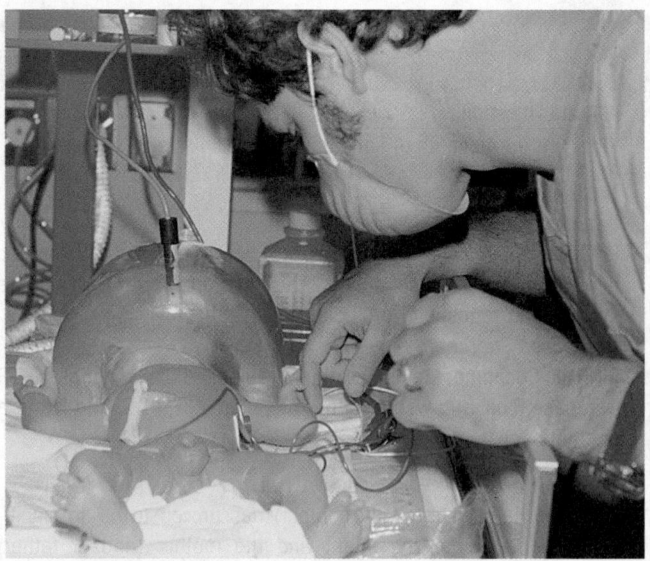

Fig. 27-9 A father caresses his tiny preterm infant receiving oxygen by hood in the neonatal intensive care unit. *(Courtesy Marjorie Pyle, RNC, Lifecircle, Costa Mesa, CA.)*

- To assess the parents' perceptions of the infant and determine the appropriate time for them to become actively involved in care.

Both parents, but especially the mother, are encouraged to visit the nursery as desired and to help with the infant's care. When the family cannot be present physically, staff members devise appropriate methods to keep the family in frequent touch with the newborn, such as daily phone calls, notes written as if from the infant, and video or photographs of the baby (see Family-Centered Care box).

FAMILY-CENTERED CARE

Preterm Infant

A multiparous, single woman has a preterm infant who was born at 28 weeks of gestation and subsequently transported to a special care nursery in a city 45 miles away from her home town. The mother is to be discharged tomorrow. It is anticipated that the infant will require a stay in the neonatal intensive care unit for at least 6 weeks. What information should the transport team provide the mother? What methods of assistance will this mother need now? Identify resources in the community with services that may be beneficial for the woman. Use your community or town as a guide to such resources.

Support groups for parents of infants in intensive care nurseries are often a source of comfort and support for parents who may feel isolated from peers because of the birth of the preterm infant. These groups encourage parents experiencing anxiety and grief to share their feelings. A parent with NICU experience often makes contact with a new member and provides additional support. These parents support the new NICU parent through hospital visits, phone contact, and home visits.

Parents of infants in NICU have identified the following four central themes for NICU staff to consider when caring for the family: (1) nurturing the parents, (2) providing accurate and consistent information, (3) clarifying NICU policies for neonatal treatment and family interaction, and (4) helping parents connect with other parents who have neonates in the NICU and graduates of NICU care (Woodwell, 2002). Ward (2001) developed a 20-item NICU Family Needs Inventory to help identify parents' particular needs. Perceived needs identified in the initial study included providing information about the infant's condition and treatment plan, answering parents' questions honestly, actively listening to parents' fears and concerns, assisting parents in understanding the infant's responses, and providing reassurance about the infant's progress.

Some high risk infants can be discharged earlier than expected. Criteria for early discharge require the infant to be physiologically stable, receive adequate nutrition and gain weight daily, and have a stable body temperature in an open bassinet. In addition, screening for hyperbilirubinemia, newborn metabolic and hematologic conditions, safe transportation (car seat testing), and hearing should occur before the preterm infant's discharge. An evaluation of the home environment and resources and arrangements for appropriate medical follow-up are essential. The parents or other caregivers must exhibit physical, emotional, and educational readiness to assume care of the infant. Ideally, the home environment is adequate for meeting the infant's needs. The parents need to show that they know the way to take the infant's temperature, signs and symptoms to report, and that they understand the infant's dietary needs.

Parent Education

Cardiopulmonary Resuscitation

Sudden infant death syndrome (SIDS) is more likely to occur in preterm infants than in term infants; infants discharged from an NICU are about twice as likely to die unexpectedly during the first year of life as infants in the general population. Instruction in cardiopulmonary resuscitation (CPR) is essential for parents of all infants but especially for parents of infants at risk for life-threatening events. Risk factors include preterm birth, apnea or bradycardia spells, neurologic immaturity, and the tendency to choke. Before taking the infant home, parents must be able to administer infant CPR. All parents should be encouraged to obtain instruction in CPR at the hospital, local Red Cross, or other community agency. It should be emphasized that CPR knowledge does not preclude the need for proper positioning of the infant in the crib (i.e., supine) when put to sleep, unless otherwise directed by the primary care physician. In addition the bed should have a firm mattress and be free of extra blankets, stuffed animals, or toys, which may cause the infant to become entangled and subsequently smothered.

Evaluation

The nurse uses the previously stated outcomes of care to evaluate the effectiveness of the physical and psychosocial aspects of care (see Nursing Care Plan).

Complications of Prematurity

Respiratory Distress Syndrome

RDS is a lung disorder usually affecting preterm infants, although a small percentage of term or late preterm infants may also be affected. Maternal and fetal conditions associated with a decreased incidence and severity of RDS include female infant; African-American race; maternal steroid (betamethasone) therapy; and stressors such as maternal gestational hypertension, maternal drug abuse, chronic retroplacental abruption, prolonged rupture of membranes, and intrauterine growth restriction (IUGR). The incidence and severity of RDS increase with a decrease in gestational age. Perinatal asphyxia, hypovolemia, male infant, Caucasian race, maternal diabetes, second-born twin, familial predisposition, maternal hypotension, cesarean birth without labor, hydrops fetalis, and third trimester bleeding are all factors that place an infant at increased risk for RDS (Hagedorn et al, 2006).

RDS is caused by a lack of pulmonary surfactant, which leads to progressive atelectasis, loss of functional residual capacity, and ventilation-perfusion imbalance with an uneven distribution of ventilation. Surfactant deficiency may be caused by insufficient surfactant production, abnormal composition and function, disruption of surfactant production, or a combination of these factors. The sequence of events is further compromised by weak respiratory muscles and an overly compliant chest wall, which are common in preterm infants. Lung capacity is compromised by proteinaceous material and epithelial debris in the airways. The resulting decreased oxygenation, cyanosis, and metabolic or respiratory acidosis can increase PVR. This increased PVR can lead to right-to-left shunting and a reopening of the ductus arteriosus and foramen ovale (Hagedorn et al, 2006).

Clinical symptoms of RDS include tachypnea, grunting, nasal flaring, intercostal or subcostal retractions, hypercapnia, respiratory or mixed acidosis, hypotension, and shock. These respiratory symptoms usually appear immediately after birth or within 6 hours of birth. Physical examination reveals crackles, poor air exchange, pallor, use of accessory muscles (retractions), and occasionally apnea. Radiographic findings include uniform reticulogranular appearance and air bronchograms. The infant's clinical course is variable. There is usually an increased oxygen requirement and increased respiratory effort as atelectasis, loss of functional residual capacity, and ventilation-perfusion imbalance worsen.

Severe RDS is often associated with a shocklike state, as manifested by diminished cardiac inflow and low arterial blood pressure. The ELBW or VLBW infant, as a result of extreme pulmonary immaturity, decreased glycogen stores, and lack of accessory muscles, may have severe RDS at birth.

RDS is a self-limiting disease with respiratory symptoms abating after 72 hours. The disappearance of respiratory symptoms coincides with the production of surfactant in type II cells of the alveoli.

The treatment for RDS is supportive. Adequate ventilation and oxygenation must be established and maintained in an attempt to prevent ventilation-perfusion mismatch and atelectasis. Exogenous surfactant, which alters the typical course of RDS, may be administered at or shortly after birth. Positive-pressure ventilation, CPAP, and oxygen therapy may be needed

NURSING CARE PLAN The High Risk Infant

Nursing Diagnosis: Ineffective breathing pattern related to pulmonary, cardiovascular, and neuromuscular immaturity; decreased energy reserves as evidenced by assessment findings (e.g., nasal flaring, tachypnea, grunting)

Expected Outcome

Infant exhibits adequate oxygenation (i.e., arterial blood gas [ABG] levels and acid-base balance within normal limits (WNL) for age; oxygen saturations 90% or greater; respiratory rate and pattern WNL for age; breath sounds clear; absence of grunting, nasal flaring; minimal retractions, skin color appropriate).

Nursing Interventions/*Rationales*

Position neonate prone or supine, avoiding neck hyperextension *to promote optimum air exchange.* Use a side-lying position to assist in draining excess mucus *to avoid aspiration.* Avoid Trendelenburg's position *because it can cause increased intracranial pressure (ICP) and reduce lung capacity. Once neonate's respiratory status is stable, use supine position.*

Suction nasopharynx, trachea, and endotracheal tube (if intubated) only as necessary *to remove mucus and secretions.* Avoid oversuctioning because it can cause bronchospasm, bradycardia, and hypoxia and can predispose the neonate to intraventricular hemorrhage.

Administer percussion, vibration, and postural drainage only as necessary *to facilitate drainage of secretions.*

Administer supplemental oxygen carefully and monitor neonatal response *to maintain oxygen saturation.*

Maintain a neutral thermal environment *to conserve oxygen and glucose use.*

Monitor ABG levels, acid-base balance, oxygen saturation, respiratory rate and pattern, breath sounds, and airway patency; observe for grunting, nasal flaring, retractions, and cyanosis *to detect signs of respiratory distress.*

Nursing Diagnosis: Ineffective thermoregulation related to immature central nervous system (CNS) temperature regulation, decreased brown fat, inability to effectively produce body heat, and minimal subcutaneous fat stores as evidenced by assessment findings (e.g., absent or decreased subcutaneous tissue, body temperature less than 36.5° C)

Expected Outcome

Infant exhibits maintenance of stable body temperature within normal range for postconceptional age (36.5° to 37.2° C).

Nursing Interventions/*Rationales*

Place neonate in a prewarmed radiant warmer *to maintain stable temperature.*

Place extremely-low-birth-weight infant's body in polyethylene bag or under plastic wrap immediately after delivery *to decrease body heat loss and transepidermal water loss (TEWL).*

Place temperature probe over tissue (not bone) such as abdomen *to control heat levels delivered by radiant warmer.*

Take axillary temperature periodically *to monitor temperature and cross-check functioning of warmer unit.*

Avoid exposing infant to cool air and drafts, cold scales, cold stethoscopes, cold examination tables, and prolonged bathing *to avoid heat loss.*

Use microenvironment (plastic wrap), double-walled incubator, and increased humidity to 60% *to prevent further heat loss from exposure to drafts and air currents and minimize insensible water loss.*

Monitor temperature sensor probe function (when used) and status frequently *because detachment can cause overheating or warmer-induced hyperthermia.*

Nursing Diagnosis: Risk for infection related to immature immune system and exposure to multiple sources of infection (invasive procedures) as evidenced by assessment findings (e.g., feeding intolerance, apnea, temperature instability)

Expected Outcome

Infant exhibits no evidence of infection.

Nursing Interventions/*Rationales*

Implement scrupulous handwashing techniques before and after handling neonate, ensure all supplies and equipment are clean before use, and ensure strict aseptic technique with invasive procedures *to minimize exposure to infective organisms.*

Prevent contact with persons who have communicable infections and instruct parents in infection control procedures *to minimize infection risk.*

Administer prescribed antibiotics *to provide coverage for infection during sepsis workup.*

Continually monitor vital signs for stability *because instability, hypothermia, or prolonged temperature elevations serve as indicators of infection.*

Nursing Diagnosis: Imbalanced nutrition: less than body requirements related to low birth weight, inability to ingest adequate nutrients for growth secondary to gastrointestinal (GI) immaturity, decreased stomach capacity, and associated illness factors as evidenced by inadequate weight gain

Expected Outcomes

Infant receives adequate amount of nutrients with sufficient caloric intake to maintain positive nitrogen balance; demonstrates steady weight gain (as appropriate to acuity).

Nursing Interventions/*Rationales*

Administer parenteral fluid or total parenteral nutrition (TPN) (protein, amino acids, lipids) *to provide adequate nutrition and fluid intake.*

Monitor for signs of intolerance to TPN, *which can interfere with effective replenishment of nutrients.*

Periodically assess readiness to orally feed (i.e., strong suck, swallow and gag reflexes) *to provide appropriate transition from gavage to oral feeding as soon as neonate is ready.*

evolve Nursing Care Plan–The High Risk Preterm Newborn

NURSING CARE PLAN The High Risk Infant—cont'd

Advance volume and concentration of formula per unit protocol *to avoid overfeeding and feeding intolerance.*

Provide expressed breast milk (including colostrum) when stable *to enhance GI development, provide natural immunity, and provide other benefits of human milk (digestive enzymes).*

If mother desires to breastfeed when neonate is stable, demonstrate how to express milk *to establish and maintain lactation until infant can breastfeed.*

Nursing Diagnosis: Risk for imbalanced (specify if deficient or excess) fluid volume related to large extracellular fluid volume, decreased ability to regulate fluid shifts, renal immaturity, permeable skin, and insensible water loss and TEWL as evidenced by excessive weight gain or loss

Expected Outcome

Infant exhibits evidence of fluid homeostasis.

Nursing Interventions/*Rationales*

Administer parenteral fluids as prescribed and regulate carefully *to maintain fluid balance.*

Avoid hypertonic fluids such as undiluted medications and concentrated glucose *to avoid excess solute load on immature kidneys.*

Implement strategies such as use of plastic covers and increase of ambient humidity *to minimize insensible water loss.*

Monitor hydration status (i.e., skin turgor, blood pressure, edema, weight, mucous membranes, fontanels, urine specific gravity, and electrolytes) and intake and output *to evaluate for evidence of dehydration or overhydration.*

Nursing Diagnosis: Risk for impaired skin integrity related to immature skin structure; poor perfusion; immobility; and invasive procedures as evidenced by epidermal stripping with adhesive removal or placement and translucent skin, erythema, abrasions

Expected Outcome

Infant's skin remains intact with no evidence of irritation or injury.

Nursing Interventions/*Rationales*

Cleanse skin as needed with warm water only and apply barrier or emollient to skin (as appropriate) *to prevent dryness and reduce friction across skin surface.*

When performing procedures, minimize use of tape and apply a skin barrier between tape and skin; use transparent elastic film for securing central and peripheral lines; use limb electrodes for monitoring or attach with hydrogel and rotate electrodes often; remove adhesives with water rather than alcohol or acetone-based adhesive removers *to minimize skin damage.*

Promptly remove skin cleansers such as povidone-iodine with water *to decrease absorption and potential toxicity.*

Monitor carefully use of thermal devices such as pulse oximeter probes, biliblankets, or thermal heating pads *to prevent burns.*

Monitor skin closely for evidence of redness, rash, irritation, bruising, breakdown, ischemia, and infiltration *to detect and treat potential complications early.*

Use a validated neonatal skin assessment tool *to objectively monitor infant's skin status.*

Nursing Diagnosis: Risk for (CNS) injury related to fluctuating systemic and intracranial pressures; immature CNS vascular bed; immature state regulatory ability; environmental stimuli; and episodes of hyperoxia and hypoxia as evidenced by episodes of hypoxia associated with handling, fluctuating blood pressure readings

Expected Outcome

Infant will exhibit normal ICP with no evidence of intraventricular hemorrhage.

Nursing Interventions/*Rationales*

Institute minimum stimulation protocol (e.g., minimal handling, clustering care techniques, avoidance of sudden head movements to one side, undisturbed sleep periods, light variations to simulate day and night, limitations on personnel and equipment noise in environment) *to decrease stress responses, which can increase ICP.*

Institute ordered pharmacologic and nonpharmacologic pain control methods *to manage pain and reduce physical stress.*

Avoid hypertonic solutions and medications *because they increase cerebral blood flow.*

Elevate head of bed 15 to 20 degrees *to decrease ICP.*

Monitor vital signs *for evidence of increased ICP.*

Recognize signs of overstimulation (e.g., flaccidity, yawning, irritability, crying, staring, and active averting) *so stimulation can be stopped to allow rest.*

Nursing Diagnosis: Risk for impaired parenting related to separation and interruption of parent-infant attachment secondary to preterm birth, severity of infant's illness, high-tech neonatal intensive care unit (NICU) environment, and anticipatory grieving over loss of perfect newborn as evidenced by physical separation from parents, verbalization of shock and disbelief at appearance of infant, lack of contact between infant and parent

Expected Outcomes

Parents establish contact with neonate and demonstrate competent parenting skills and willingness to care for neonate.

Nursing Interventions/*Rationales*

Before parents' first visit to the NICU, prepare them by explaining what the neonate will look like, what the equipment will look like, and its function *to diminish fear and decrease sense of shock.*

Keep parents informed about infant's condition (e.g., improvements and setbacks) and important aspects of infant's care; encourage and answer parental questions; actively listen to parent concerns *to establish trust, open communication, and caring atmosphere to aid in coping.*

Encourage parents to contact NICU staff any time, day or night, for concerns regarding the infant's condition *to maintain open*

Continued

NURSING CARE PLAN The High Risk Infant—cont'd

channels of communication regarding infant's status and decrease parents' fear of unknown.

Encourage parents to visit the NICU often; to name infant; to touch, hold, or caress infant as physical condition permits; to be actively involved in infant's care; to bring personal items (e.g., clothing, stuffed animals, or pictures of family) *to allow formation of emotional bond.*

Reinforce parent involvement and praise care endeavors *to increase self-confidence in their contribution.*

Encourage parents to bring other siblings to visit preterm infant as age-appropriate; explain to siblings what they are seeing; encourage siblings to draw pictures or write letters for infant and place in or near infant's crib *to promote family involvement, help ease sibling fears, and let them contribute to infant's care.*

Refer parents to social services as needed *to ensure comprehensive care.*

Provide consistent and frequent information regarding infant's condition through multidisciplinary conferences *to promote parent trust in caregivers and provide consistent information.*

Table 27-3 Normal Arterial Blood Gas Values for Neonates

VALUE	RANGE
pH	7.35-7.45
Arterial oxygen pressure (Pao_2)	60-80 mm Hg
Carbon dioxide pressure ($Paco_2$)	35-45 mm Hg
Bicarbonate (HCO_3^-)	22-26 mEq/L
Base excess	(−4) to (+4)
Oxygen saturation	92%-94%

From Parry WH, Zimmer J: Acid-base homeostasis and oxygenation. In Merenstein GB, Gardner SL (editors): *Handbook of neonatal intensive care*, ed 6, St Louis, 2006, Mosby.

during the respiratory illness. Prevention of complications associated with mechanical ventilation is critical. These complications include pulmonary interstitial emphysema, pneumothorax, pneumomediastinum, and pneumopericardium.

Acid-base balance is evaluated by monitoring ABG values (Table 27-3). Frequent blood sampling requires arterial access either by umbilical artery catheter or by a peripheral arterial line. Pulse oximetry and transcutaneous carbon dioxide and oxygen monitors document trends in ventilation and oxygenation. Capillary blood gas values may be used to evaluate pH and Pco_2 in infants whose condition is more stable.

The maintenance of a neutral thermal environment (NTE) continues to be of critical importance in infants with RDS; infants with hypoxemia are unable to increase their metabolic rate when cold stressed.

The clinical and radiographic presentation of neonatal pneumonia may be similar to that of RDS. Therefore sepsis evaluation, including blood culture, complete blood count with differential, and sometimes a lumbar puncture, is done in infants with RDS to rule out a concomitant systemic infection. Laboratory and radiographic tests rarely confirm the diagnosis of neonatal pneumonia; rather, the clinical history and presenting clinical signs provide a basis for the diagnosis and treatment (Stoll, 2007). Broad-spectrum antibiotics are initiated while the results of cultures are awaited.

Fluid and nutrition must be maintained for the infant critically ill with RDS. Parenteral nutrition can provide protein and fat to promote a positive nitrogen balance. Daily monitoring of electrolytes, urine output, specific gravity, and weight assists in the evaluation of hydration status.

Respiratory distress of a nonpulmonary origin in neonates may also be caused by sepsis, cardiac defects (structural or functional), exposure to cold, airway obstruction (atresia), intraventricular hemorrhage, hypoglycemia, metabolic acidosis, acute blood loss, and certain drugs. Pneumonia in the neonatal period may manifest as respiratory distress caused by bacterial or viral agents and may occur alone or as a complication of RDS.

Patent Ductus Arteriosus

The ductus arteriosus is a muscular contractile structure in the fetus connecting the left pulmonary artery and the dorsal aorta. The ductus constricts after birth as oxygenation, the levels of circulating prostaglandins, and the muscle mass increase. Other factors that promote ductal closure include catecholamines, low pH, bradykinin, and acetylcholine. When the fetal ductus arteriosus fails to close after birth, PDA occurs. Ductal closure usually occurs within hours or days in the term infant but may be delayed in preterm infants as a result of oxygenation and circulating hormones (prostaglandins).

The clinical presentation of an infant with a PDA includes systolic murmur, active precordium, bounding peripheral pulses, tachycardia, tachypnea, crackles, and hepatomegaly. The systolic murmur is heard best at the second or third intercostal space at the upper left sternal border. An active precordium is caused by an increased left ventricular stroke volume. A widened pulse pressure may result in bounding peripheral pulses.

Radiographic studies of infants with a large shunting PDA typically show cardiac enlargement and pulmonary edema; with a smaller PDA, the radiograph may appear normal for the infant's age (Knight & Washington, 2006). ABG findings reveal hypercarbia and metabolic acidosis. A color flow Doppler echocardiograph can demonstrate a PDA, identify the direction of the shunting (left to right, right to left, or both), and quantitate the amount of blood shunting across the PDA.

The PDA can be managed medically or surgically. Medical management consists of ventilatory support, fluid restriction, and the administration of diuretics and indomethacin or ibuprofen. Indomethacin is a prostaglandin synthetase inhibitor that blocks the effect of the arachidonic acid products on the ductus and causes the PDA to constrict. Ventilatory support is adjusted based on ABG levels. Fluid restriction is implemented to decrease cardiovascular volume overload in association with the diuretic therapy. Surgical ligation is performed when PDA is clinically significant and medical management has failed. The nonsteroidal antiinflammatory drug ibuprofen and indomethacin have been used in the medical closure of PDA in preterm infants. Ibuprofen administered orally reportedly has fewer side effects than indomethacin, yet a recent Cochrane review reports they are equally effective (Cherif, Jabnoun, & Khrouf, 2007; Ohlsson, Walia, & Shah, 2008).

Nursing care of the infant with PDA focuses on supportive care. The infant needs an NTE, adequate oxygenation, and meticulous fluid balance; parental support is imperative.

Periventricular-Intraventricular Hemorrhage

Periventricular-intraventricular hemorrhage (PV-IVH) is one of the most common types of neurologic injuries that occurs in neonates and is among the most severe in both short- and long-term outcomes. The true incidence of PV-IVH is unknown, but a general estimate is 15% in infants less than 32 weeks of gestation or under 1501 g (Volpe, 2008). PV-IVH occurs in approximately 3.5% to 5% of term infants, with 50% of those cases caused by asphyxia or trauma. In recent years research has shown that contributing events may occur antenatally and postnatally (Adams-Chapman & Stoll, 2007). In term infants the symptoms appear within 48 hours of birth (Paige & Moe, 2006).

The pathogenesis of PV-IVH includes intravascular factors (e.g., fluctuating or increasing cerebral blood flow, increases in cerebral venous pressure, and coagulopathy), vascular factors, extravascular factors (hypoglycemia, acidosis), and routine medical care (rapid volume expansion, blood transfusion). The developing preterm infant has highly vascularized areas of the brain with fragile blood vessels that are prone to bleeding when homeostasis is not maintained; the most common area affected is in and around the subependymal germinal matrix. PV-IVH events typically occur within the first 72 hours of birth. PV-IVH is classified according to severity, which determines long-term neurodevelopmental outcomes.

Nursing care focuses on recognition of factors that increase the risk of PV-IVH, interventions to decrease the risk of bleeding, and supportive care to infants who have bleeding episodes. The infant is positioned with the head in midline and the head of the bed elevated slightly to prevent or minimize fluctuations in intracranial blood pressure. NTE is maintained, as well as oxygenation. Rapid infusions of fluids should be avoided. Blood pressure is monitored closely for fluctuations. The infant is monitored for signs of pneumothorax because it often precedes PV-IVH.

Necrotizing Enterocolitis

NEC is an acute inflammatory disease of the GI mucosa, commonly complicated by perforation. This often fatal disease occurs in about 1% to 5% of newborns in NICUs. Three factors appear to play an important role in the development of NEC: intestinal ischemia, colonization by pathogenic bacteria, and substrate (formula feeding) in the intestinal lumen. The precise cause of NEC is still uncertain, but it appears to occur in infants whose GI tract has suffered vascular compromise. Intestinal ischemia of unknown cause, immature GI host defenses, bacterial proliferation, and feeding substrate are now believed to play multifactorial roles in the etiology of NEC. Preterm birth remains the most prominent risk factor in the development of NEC.

The onset of NEC in the full-term infant usually occurs between 4 and 10 days after birth. In the preterm infant the onset may be delayed for up to 30 days. Signs of developing NEC are nonspecific, which is characteristic of many neonatal disease processes. Some generalized signs include decreased activity, hypotonia, pallor, recurrent apnea and bradycardia, decreased oxygen saturation, respiratory distress, metabolic acidosis, oliguria, hypotension, decreased perfusion, temperature instability, and cyanosis. GI symptoms include abdominal distention, increasing or bile-stained residual gastric aspirates, vomiting (bile or blood), grossly bloody stools, abdominal tenderness, and erythema of the abdominal wall (Roaten, Bensard, & Price, 2006).

Diagnosis of NEC is confirmed by radiographic examination that reveals bowel loop distention, pneumatosis intestinalis, pneumoperitoneum, portal air, or a combination of these findings. The abnormal radiographic findings are caused by the bacterial colonization of the GI tract associated with NEC, resulting in an ileus. Pneumatosis intestinalis, pneumoperitoneum, and portal air are caused by gas produced by the bacteria that invade the wall of the intestines and escape into the peritoneum and portal system when perforation occurs. Laboratory evaluation includes a complete blood cell count with differential, coagulation studies, ABG analysis, serum electrolyte levels, and blood culture. The white blood cell count may be either increased or decreased. The platelet count and coagulation studies may be abnormal, with thrombocytopenia and disseminated intravascular coagulation. Electrolyte levels may be abnormal, with leaking capillary beds and fluid shifts with the infection.

Treatment of infants with NEC is supportive and preventive for bowel perforation. Oral or tube feedings are discontinued to rest the GI tract. A nasogastric tube is inserted and placed to low suction to provide gastric decompression. Parenteral therapy (often by TPN) is begun. NEC is an infectious disease; control of infection is imperative, with an emphasis on careful handwashing before and after infant contact. Systemic antibiotic therapy is instituted, and surgical resection may be performed if perforation or clinical deterioration occurs.

With early recognition and treatment, medical management is increasingly successful. If there is progressive deterioration under medical management or evidence of perforation, surgical resection and anastomosis are performed. Extensive involvement may necessitate surgical intervention and establishment of an ileostomy, jejunostomy, or colostomy. Sequelae in surviving infants include short-bowel syndrome, colonic stricture with obstruction, fat malabsorption, and failure to thrive secondary to intestinal dysfunction. Various surgical interventions for NEC are available and depend on the extent of bowel necrosis, associated illness factors, and infant stability. Intestinal transplantation has been successful in some former preterm infants with NEC-associated short-bowel syndrome who had already developed life-threatening TPN-related complications. Bowel-lengthening procedures and intestinal transplantation may be lifesaving options for infants who previously faced high morbidity and mortality (Nucci et al, 2008; Vennarecci et al, 2000). Therapy may be prolonged and recovery may be delayed by adhesions, complications of bowel resection, short-bowel syndrome (especially if the ileocecal valve is removed), and intolerance of oral feedings.

NURSING ALERT Observe for indications of early development of NEC by checking the appearance of the abdomen for distention (measuring abdominal girth, measuring residual gastric contents before feedings, and listening for bowel sounds) and performing all routine assessments for high risk neonates.

Minimal enteral feedings (trophic feeding, GI priming) have gained acceptance with no evidence of increased incidence of NEC. Early experience indicates such feedings may in fact be protective against NEC in nonasphyxiated preterm infants, in addition to providing other potential benefits. An increased incidence of NEC in those VLBW infants receiving minimal enteral nutrition has not been substantiated (Reynolds & Thureen, 2007). There is evidence that human milk may have a protective effect against the development of NEC (Diehl-Jones & Askin, 2004; Sisk et al, 2007). The role of probiotics such as *Lactobacillus acidophilus* and *Bifidobacterium infantis* administered with enteral feedings for the prevention of NEC has yet to be explored fully enough to advocate widespread use in all VLBW infants. In some studies probiotics decreased the incidence of NEC (Alfaleh & Bassler, 2008; Bin-Nun et al, 2005).

Retinopathy of Prematurity

ROP is a complex, multicausal disorder that affects the developing retinal vessels of preterm infants. The normal retinal vessels begin to form in utero at approximately 16 weeks of gestation in response to an unknown stimulus. The retinal vessels continue to develop until they reach maturity approximately 42 to 43 weeks after conception. Once the retina is completely vascularized, the retinal vessels are not susceptible to ROP.

The mechanism of injury in ROP is unclear. Oxygen tensions that are too high for the level of retinal maturity initially result in vasoconstriction. After oxygen therapy is discontinued, neovascularization occurs in the retina and vitreous, with capillary hemorrhages, fibrotic resolution, and possible retinal detachment. Scar tissue formation and consequent visual impairment may be mild or severe. The entire disease process in severe cases may take as long as 5 months to evolve. Examination by an ophthalmologist before discharge and a schedule for repeat examinations thereafter are recommended for the parents' guidance.

Studies have demonstrated an association between the development of ROP and high arterial oxygen saturations in ELBW and VLBW infants. Fluctuations in arterial oxygen saturation in the first few weeks of life have also been implicated in the development of ROP. Although there is no consensus as to what the ideal arterial oxygen saturation is in preterm infants—to prevent either hypoxemia or hyperoxemia—there is mounting evidence that oxygen saturations of 100% are undesirable and may have a significant role in the development of ROP in preterm infants. Further studies are needed to clarify optimal arterial oxygen saturation (Pollan, 2009).

Although exposure to bright light has not proven to contribute to ROP, such exposure is nevertheless undesirable from a neurobehavioral developmental perspective. All caregivers should use supplemental oxygen judiciously, monitor oxygen blood levels carefully, promptly attend to saturation monitor alarms, and prevent wide fluctuations in oxygen blood levels (hyperoxemia and hypoxemia).

Circumferential cryopexy, laser photocoagulation, vitamin E therapy, and decreased intensity of ambient light are used in the treatment of ROP with varying results. Early screening and detection should be provided in infants who are born at less than 32 weeks of gestation and who weigh less than 1500 g, and in infants weighing between 1500 and 2000 g who were born at more than 32 weeks of gestation, believed to be at high risk for development of ROP (American Academy of Pediatrics, Section on Ophthalmology, 2006). The Early Treatment for Retinopathy of Prematurity study found that early treatment of prethreshold ROP improved retinal and visual outcomes at 9 months corrected age (Jones et al, 2005).

Bronchopulmonary Dysplasia (Chronic Lung Disease)

BPD, or newborn chronic lung disease, is a result of lung injury in infants who require mechanical ventilation and supplemental oxygen (Dudell & Stoll, 2007). The etiology of BPD is multifactorial and includes pulmonary immaturity, surfactant deficiency, lung injury and stretch, barotrauma, inflammation caused by oxygen exposure, fluid overload, ligation of a PDA, and genetic predisposition (Hagedorn et al, 2006). The type of BPD witnessed has changed over the past decade, with the "classic" form observed less frequently; these changes are primarily morphologic rather than etiologic, and BPD remains a disease primarily seen in infants weighing less than 1000 g who are born at less than 28 weeks of gestation (Dudell & Stoll, 2007). The incidence of BPD in infants weighing less than 1500 g who require mechanical ventilation for RDS ranges from 23% to 80% (Berger et al, 2004; Gracey et al, 2002).

Clinical symptoms of BPD include tachypnea, retractions, nasal flaring, increased work of breathing, exercise intolerance (to handling and feeding), and tachycardia (Hagedorn et al, 2006). Auscultation of lung fields in affected infants reveals crackles, decreased air movement, and occasionally expiratory wheezing.

Treatment for BPD includes oxygen therapy, nutrition, fluid restriction, and medications (e.g., diuretics, corticosteroids, and bronchodilators). The use of corticosteroids to prevent or treat BPD is controversial because of the side effects and varied results in clinical trials; however, corticosteroids are used in many centers to treat or prevent BPD (American Academy of Pediatrics, Committee on Fetus and Newborn, 2002).The key to the management of BPD is prevention by reducing the incidence of preterm births and RDS and by using surfactant, giving antenatal steroids, and minimizing lung trauma from mechanical ventilation and high oxygen concentrations.

The prognosis for infants with BPD depends on the degree of pulmonary dysfunction. Most deaths occur within the first year of life as a result of cardiorespiratory failure, sepsis, or respiratory tract infection; in some infants the deaths are sudden and unexplained.

The Postterm Infant

Postterm (or postmature) infants are those whose gestation is prolonged beyond 42 weeks, regardless of birth weight. These infants may be large for gestational age (LGA) or small for gestational age (SGA), but most often their weight is appropriate for gestational age (AGA). It is important to determine whether the pregnancy is actually prolonged and also whether there is any evidence of fetal jeopardy as a result. The cause of prolonged pregnancy is unknown. Postmaturity can be associated with placental insufficiency, resulting in a newborn who has a thin, emaciated appearance (dysmature) at birth because of loss of subcutaneous fat and muscle mass. There may be meconium staining of the fingernails, the hair and nails may be long, and vernix may be absent. The skin may peel off. Not all postterm infants show signs of dysmaturity; some continue to grow in utero and are large at birth.

Perinatal mortality is significantly higher in the postterm fetus and neonate than in an infant born at term. During labor and birth, increased oxygen demands of the postterm fetus may not be met. Insufficient gas exchange in the postterm placenta increases the likelihood of intrauterine hypoxia, which may result in the passage of meconium in utero, thereby increasing the risk for MAS. In one study postterm infants were found to have a mortality rate almost three times higher than that of a control group of term infants (Stoll & Adams-Chapman, 2007).

Meconium Aspiration Syndrome

Meconium staining of the amniotic fluid can be indicative of nonreassuring fetal status, especially in a vertex presentation. It appears in 10% to 15% of all births and occurs primarily in term and postterm births. Many infants with meconium staining exhibit no signs of depression at birth; however, the presence of meconium in the amniotic fluid necessitates careful supervision of labor and close monitoring of fetal well-being. The presence of a team skilled in neonatal resuscitation is required at the birth of any infant with meconium-stained amniotic fluid (Fig. 27-10). The infant's mouth and nares are no longer routinely suctioned on the perineum before the infant's first breath (American Heart Association, 2005). In a multicentered, randomized, controlled trial, Vain and colleagues (2005) found no difference in outcomes between those infants who were suctioned and those who were not. For infants with meconium staining who are not vigorous, endotracheal suctioning should be performed immediately (American Heart Association, 2005).

If meconium is not removed from the airway at birth, it can migrate down to the terminal airways, causing mechanical

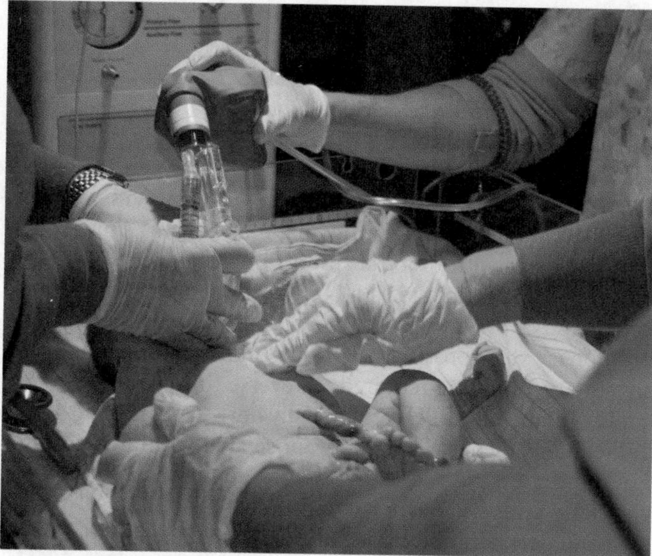

Fig. 27-10 Infant being resuscitated at birth. Note presence of meconium on abdomen, umbilical cord, and overbed warmer. *(Courtesy Shannon Perry, Phoenix, AZ.)*

obstruction and leading to MAS. The fetus may aspirate meconium in utero, which can cause a chemical pneumonitis. These infants may develop persistent pulmonary hypertension of the newborn (PPHN), further complicating their management. Infants with MAS who received surfactant had improved oxygenation and decreases in the severity of respiratory failure, need for ECMO, and air leaks (Engle & American Academy of Pediatrics, Committee on Fetus and Newborn, 2008).

Persistent Pulmonary Hypertension of the Newborn

PPHN is a term applied to the combined findings of pulmonary hypertension, right-to-left shunting, and a structurally normal heart. PPHN may manifest as either a single entity or the main component of MAS, congenital diaphragmatic hernia, RDS, hyperviscosity syndrome, or neonatal pneumonia or sepsis. PPHN is also called *persistent fetal circulation* because the syndrome includes reversion to fetal pathways for blood flow.

A brief review of fetal blood flow can help in the visualization of the problems with PPHN (see Fig. 8-12). In utero, oxygen-rich blood leaves the placenta via the umbilical vein, goes through the ductus venosus, and enters the inferior vena cava. From there, it empties into the right atrium and is mostly shunted across the foramen ovale to the left atrium, effectively bypassing the lungs. This blood enters the left ventricle, leaves through the aorta, and preferentially perfuses the carotid and coronary arteries. Thus the heart and brain receive the most oxygenated blood. Blood drains from the brain into the superior vena cava, reenters the right atrium, proceeds to the right ventricle, and exits through the main pulmonary artery. The lungs are a high-pressure circuit, needing only enough perfusion for growth and nutrition. The ductus arteriosus (connecting the main pulmonary artery and the aorta) is the path of least resistance for the blood leaving the right side of the fetal heart, shunting most of the cardiac output away from the lungs and toward the systemic system. This right-to-left shunting is the key to fetal circulation.

After birth, both the foramen ovale and the ductus arteriosus close in response to various biochemical processes, pressure changes within the heart, and dilation of the pulmonary vessels. This dilation allows virtually all of the cardiac output to enter the lungs, become oxygenated, and provide oxygen-rich blood to the tissues for normal metabolism. Any process that interferes with this transition from fetal to neonatal circulation may precipitate PPHN. PPHN characteristically proceeds into a downward spiral of exacerbating hypoxia and pulmonary vasoconstriction. Prompt recognition and aggressive intervention are required to reverse this process.

The infant with PPHN is typically born at term or postterm and exhibits tachycardia and cyanosis that within minutes or hours progress to severe respiratory compromise with concomitant acidosis, further compromising pulmonary perfusion and deteriorating oxygenation. Management depends on the underlying cause of the persistent pulmonary hypertension. The use of INO and ECMO (see previous discussion) has improved the chances of survival of these infants.

Another mode of treatment for PPHN and other respiratory disorders of the newborn is high-frequency ventilation, an assisted-ventilation method that delivers small volumes of gas at high frequencies and limits the development of high airway pressure, thus theoretically reducing barotrauma.

Other Problems Related to Gestation

Small-for-Gestational-Age Infants and Intrauterine Growth Restriction

Infants who are SGA (i.e., weight is below the 10th percentile expected at term) or infants who have IUGR (i.e., rate of growth does not meet expected growth pattern) are considered high risk, with the perimortality rate 5 to 20 times greater than that for the normal term infant (Kliegman, 2006).

Various conditions can affect and impede growth in the developing fetus. Conditions occurring in the first trimester (e.g., infections, teratogens, and chromosomal abnormalities) can affect all aspects of fetal growth, whereas extrinsic conditions early in pregnancy can result in symmetric IUGR (i.e., head circumference, length, and weight are all less than the 10th percentile). Conditions causing symmetric growth restriction result in an SGA infant, usually with a smaller head circumference and reduced brain capacity. Growth restriction in later stages of pregnancy, as a result of maternal or placental factors, results in asymmetric growth restriction (with respect to gestational age, weight will be less than the 10th percentile, whereas length and head circumference will be greater than the 10th percentile). Infants with asymmetric IUGR have the potential for normal growth and development. Abnormal fetal size may indicate an adaptive response, with diminished fetal weight-sparing brain growth.

Care of the SGA infant is based on the clinical problems present and is the same given to preterm infants with similar problems. Gas exchange is supported by maintaining a clear airway and preventing cold stress. Hypoglycemia is treated with oral feedings (e.g., breast, formula) or IV dextrose as the infant's condition warrants. An external heat source (radiant warmer or incubator) is used until the infant is able to maintain an adequate body temperature. Nursing support of parents is the same as that given to parents of preterm infants.

Common problems that affect SGA (IUGR) infants are perinatal asphyxia, meconium aspiration (discussed previously), immunodeficiency, hypoglycemia, polycythemia, and temperature instability.

Perinatal Asphyxia

Commonly, IUGR infants have been exposed to chronic hypoxia for varying periods before labor and birth. Labor is a stressor to the normal fetus; it is an even greater stressor for the growth-restricted fetus. The chronically hypoxic infant is severely compromised by a normal labor and has difficulty compensating after birth. The alert, wide-eyed appearance of the newborn is attributed to prolonged fetal hypoxia. Appropriate management and resuscitation are essential for the depressed infant.

The birth of the SGA newborn with perinatal asphyxia may be associated with a maternal history of heavy cigarette smoking; gestational hypertension; low socioeconomic status; multifetal gestation; gestational infections such as rubella, cytomegalovirus, and toxoplasmosis; advanced diabetes mellitus; and cardiac problems. Sequelae to perinatal asphyxia include MAS and hypoglycemia.

Hypoglycemia and Hyperglycemia

All high risk infants are at risk for hypoglycemia. Infants who experience physiologic stress may experience hypoglycemia as a result of a decreased glycogen supply, inadequate gluconeogenesis, or overutilization of glycogen stored during fetal and postnatal life. Preterm infants may also become hypoglycemic as a result of inadequate intake and increased metabolic demands as a result of illness factors (Blackburn, 2007). There is insufficient evidence to support the concept that the preterm or high risk infant can tolerate lower levels of serum glucose any better than healthy term infants (Blackburn, 2007) (see Chapter 25, p. 656, for discussion of hypoglycemia). The SGA infant, not unlike the preterm infant, is at higher risk for hypoglycemia as a result of decreased fetal stores and decreased rate of gluconeogenesis.

Hyperglycemia is defined as a blood glucose level greater than 125 mg/dl (whole blood) or a plasma glucose of 145 to 150 mg/dl (Blackburn, 2007). This condition is seen primarily in ELBW and VLBW infants receiving parenteral nutrition with dextrose concentrations of 5% or higher. Hyperglycemia may be just as harmful to the preterm infant as hypoglycemia. Increased circulating levels of glucose may lead to osmotic changes, increased urine output, and fluid shifts in the already compromised CNS of the preterm infant. The net result of hyperglycemia may be cellular dehydration and intraventricular hemorrhage. Preterm infants undergoing stress such as surgical intervention may also become hyperglycemic with increased catecholamine release, which inhibits insulin release and glucose utilization (Blackburn, 2007). In summary, ELBW and VLBW infants should be monitored closely for both hypoglycemia and hyperglycemia while receiving parenteral nutrition, both during the acute phase of illness and perioperatively.

Heat Loss

SGA infants are particularly susceptible to temperature instability as a result of decreased brown fat deposit; decreased adipose tissue; large body surface exposure and, often, poor flexion; and decreased glycogen storage in major organs such as the liver and heart. Therefore close attention must be given to maintain a thermoneutral environment. Nursing considerations focus on maintenance of thermoneutrality to promote recovery from perinatal asphyxia, since cold stress jeopardizes such recovery.

Large-for-Gestational-Age Infants

The LGA infant is defined as an infant weighing 4000 g or more at birth. An infant is considered LGA despite gestational age when the weight is above the 90th percentile on growth charts or two standard deviations above the mean weight for gestational age. The LGA infant is at greater risk for morbidity than the SGA and preterm infant; such infants have a higher incidence of birth injuries, asphyxia, and congenital anomalies such as heart defects (Stoll & Adams-Chapman, 2007).

All pregnancies of longer than 42 weeks of gestation must be carefully evaluated. All large fetuses are monitored during a trial of labor, and preparation is made for a cesarean birth if nonreassuring fetal status or poor progress of labor occurs. LGA newborns may be preterm, term, or postterm; they may be infants of diabetic mothers (IDMs). Each of these problems carries special concerns. Regardless of coexisting potential problems, the LGA infant is at risk by virtue of size alone.

The nurse assesses the LGA infant for hypoglycemia and trauma resulting from vaginal or cesarean birth. Any specific birth injuries are identified and treated appropriately.

Infants of Diabetic Mothers

All infants born to mothers with diabetes are at some risk for complications. The degree of risk is influenced by the severity and duration of maternal disease. Problems seen in IDMs include congenital anomalies (especially cardiac), macrosomia, birth trauma and perinatal asphyxia, RDS, hypoglycemia, hypocalcemia and hypomagnesemia, cardiomyopathy, hyperbilirubinemia, and polycythemia. Because some of these problems are also seen in infants with gestational age–related problems, discussion of IDMs is included here.

Pathophysiology

The mechanisms responsible for the problems seen in IDMs are not fully understood. Congenital anomalies are believed to be caused by fluctuations in blood glucose levels and episodes of ketoacidosis in early pregnancy. Later in pregnancy, when the mother's pancreas cannot release sufficient insulin to meet increased demands, maternal hyperglycemia results. The high levels of glucose cross the placenta and stimulate the fetal pancreas to release more insulin. The combination of the increased supply of maternal glucose and other nutrients, the inability of maternal insulin to cross the placenta, and increased fetal insulin results in excessive fetal growth called *macrosomia* (see the discussion that follows).

Hyperinsulinemia accounts for many of the problems the fetus or infant develops. In addition to fluctuating glucose levels, maternal vascular involvement or superimposed maternal infection adversely affects the fetus. Normally, maternal blood has a more alkaline pH than does carbon dioxide–rich fetal blood. This phenomenon encourages the exchange of oxygen and carbon dioxide across the placental membrane. When the maternal blood is more acidotic than the fetal blood, such as during ketoacidosis, little carbon dioxide or oxygen exchange occurs at the level of the placenta. The mortality for the unborn infant resulting from an episode of maternal ketoacidosis may be as high as 50% or more (Kalhan & Parimi, 2006).

The single most important factor influencing fetal well-being is the mother's glycemic status. There are indications that some neonatal conditions (e.g., macrosomia, hypoglycemia, polyhydramnios, preterm birth, and perhaps fetal lung immaturity) may be eliminated, or the incidence decreased, by maintaining tight control over maternal glucose levels within narrow limits (Reece et al, 1998). Tight glucose control is defined as maintenance of maternal blood glucose levels between 100 and 120 mg/dl.

Congenital Anomalies

Congenital anomalies occur in about 7% to 10% of IDMs. Their incidence is two to four times that for infants born to mothers without diabetes. The incidence is greatest among SGA newborns. IUGR leading to SGA infants is seen in IDMs with severe vascular disease. The most commonly occurring anomalies involve the cardiac, musculoskeletal, and central nervous systems. In most defects associated with diabetic pregnancies, the structural abnormality occurs before the eighth week after conception. This reinforces the importance of control of blood glucose both before conception and in the early stages of pregnancy.

The incidence of congenital heart lesions in these infants is five times higher than that in the general population. Coarctation of the aorta, transposition of the great vessels, and atrial or ventricular septal defects are the most common lesions encountered in the IDM. Maternal diabetic control is correlated with the incidence of defects; that is, the better the control, the lower the risk of defects.

CNS anomalies include anencephaly, encephalocele, meningomyelocele, and hydrocephalus. The musculoskeletal system may be affected by caudal regression syndrome (i.e., sacral agenesis, with weakness or deformities of the lower extremities, malformation and fixation of the hip joints, and shortening or deformity of the femurs). Hypertrichosis on the pinnae (excessive hair growth on the external ear) has been added to the list of characteristic clinical features. Other defects noted in this population include GI atresia and urinary tract malformations.

Macrosomia

Despite improvements in the control of maternal blood glucose levels, the incidence of macrosomia in infants of insulin-dependent diabetic is higher than in infants born of mothers who are not diabetic. At birth the typical LGA infant has a round, cherubic ("tomato" or cushingoid) face, chubby

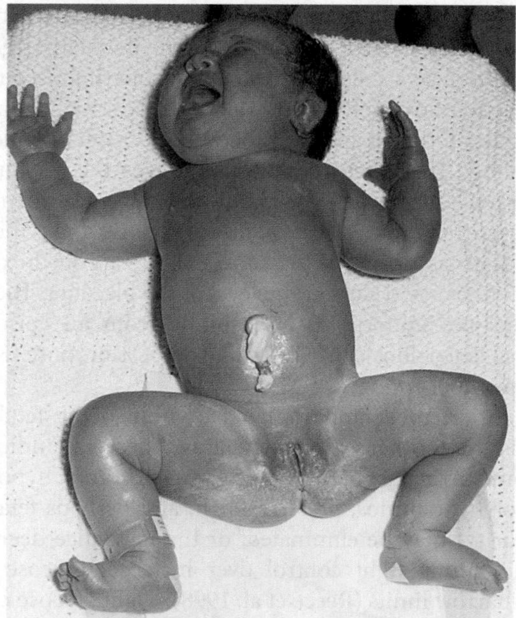

Fig. 27-11 Macrosomic newborn. (From O'Doherty N: *Neonatology: micro atlas of the newborn*, Nutley, NJ, 1986, Hoffmann–La Roche.)

body, and a plethoric or flushed complexion (Fig. 27-11). The infant has enlarged internal organs (i.e., hepatosplenomegaly, splanchnomegaly, and cardiomegaly) and increased body fat, especially around the shoulders. The placenta and umbilical cord are larger than average. The brain is the only organ that is not enlarged. IDMs may be LGA but physiologically immature.

The macrosomic infant is at risk for hypoglycemia, hypocalcemia, hyperviscosity, and hyperbilirubinemia. The excessive shoulder size in these infants often leads to dystocia, particularly because the head may be smaller in proportion to the shoulders than in a nonmacrosomic infant. Macrosomic infants born vaginally or by cesarean birth after a trial of labor may incur birth trauma.

Birth Trauma and Perinatal Asphyxia

Birth injury (resulting from macrosomia or method of birth) and perinatal asphyxia occur in 20% of infants of gestational diabetic mothers and 35% of IDMs. Examples of birth trauma include cephalhematoma; paralysis of the facial nerve (seventh cranial nerve) (see Fig. 28-3); fracture of the clavicle or humerus; brachial plexus paralysis, usually Erb-Duchenne (right upper arm) palsy (see Figs. 28-1 and 28-2); and phrenic nerve paralysis, invariably associated with diaphragmatic paralysis.

Respiratory Distress Syndrome

IDMs are four to six times more likely than normal infants to develop RDS. With improved maternal glucose control, this risk has been substantially reduced. In the fetus exposed to high levels of maternal glucose, synthesis of surfactant may be delayed because of the high fetal serum level of insulin. Before delivery, fetal lung maturation tests via amniocentesis are carried out, including lecithin/sphingomyelin ratio, phosphatidylglycerol, and disaturated phosphatidylcholine measurements. In the IDM, the presence of phosphatidylglycerol in the amniotic fluid is the best predictor of normal neonatal respiratory function.

Hypoglycemia

Hypoglycemia affects many IDMs. After constant exposure to high circulating levels of glucose, the fetal pancreas undergoes hyperplasia, resulting in hyperinsulinemia. Disruption of the fetal glucose supply occurs with the clamping of the umbilical cord, and the neonate's blood glucose level falls rapidly in the presence of fetal hyperinsulinism. Hypoglycemia is most common in the macrosomic or SGA infant, but blood glucose levels should be monitored in all infants of known or suspected diabetic mothers.

Asymptomatic or symptomatic hypoglycemia most commonly manifests within the first 1 to 3 hours after birth. Signs of hypoglycemia include jitteriness, apnea, tachypnea, and cyanosis. Significant hypoglycemia may result in seizures. Hypoglycemia is worsened by the presence of hypothermia or respiratory distress.

Studies confirm the importance of maintaining serum glucose levels above 50 mg/dl (2.8 mmol/L) in hyperinsulinemic infants with hypoglycemia to prevent serious neurologic sequelae (Cowett & Loughead, 2002; Schwartz, 1997).

Hypocalcemia and Hypomagnesemia

Hypocalcemia occurs in as many as 50% of IDMs. A number of these cases are related to hypoxia or prematurity; however, the overall incidence of hypocalcemia is higher than in nondiabetic pregnancies. Hypomagnesemia is believed to develop because of maternal renal losses that occur in diabetes. Hypocalcemia is associated with preterm birth, birth trauma, and perinatal asphyxia. Signs of hypocalcemia are similar to those of hypoglycemia, but they occur within the first 24 hours of age.

Cardiomyopathy

All IDMs need careful observation for cardiomegaly and heart failure, which are often found among these infants. Two types of cardiomyopathy can occur. Clinicians must be alert to identify correctly the type of lesion so that appropriate therapy is instituted. Both types of lesions are associated with respiratory symptoms and congestive heart failure.

Hypertrophic cardiomyopathy (HCM) is characterized by a hypercontractile and thickened myocardium. The ventricular walls are thickened, as is the septum, which in severe cases results in outflow tract obstructions. The mitral valve is poorly functioning. In nonhypertrophic cardiomyopathy (non-HCM) the myocardium is poorly contractile and overstretched. The ventricles are increased in size, but there is no outflow obstruction. Most infants are asymptomatic, but severe outflow obstruction may cause left ventricular heart failure. HCM may be treated with a beta-adrenergic blocker (such as propranolol to decrease contractility and heart rate). A cardiotonic agent is used to treat non-HCM (such as digoxin to increase contractility and decrease heart rate). The abnormality usually resolves in 3 to 12 months.

Hyperbilirubinemia and Polycythemia

IDMs are at increased risk of developing hyperbilirubinemia. Many IDMs are also polycythemic. Polycythemia increases blood viscosity, thereby impairing circulation. In addition, this increased number of RBCs to be hemolyzed increases the potential bilirubin load that the neonate must clear. The excessive RBCs are produced in extramedullary foci (liver and spleen) in addition to the usual sites in bone marrow. Therefore both liver function and bilirubin clearance may be adversely affected. Bruising associated with birth of a macrosomic infant will contribute further to high bilirubin levels.

Nursing Care

Ideally, planning for the IDM begins during the antenatal period. Pediatric staff members are present at the birth. Implementation of care depends on the neonate's particular problems. If the maternal blood glucose level was well controlled throughout the pregnancy, the infant may require only monitoring. Because euglycemia is not always possible, the nurse must promptly recognize and treat any consequences of maternal diabetes that arise (see Nursing Care Plan).

Discharge Planning

Discharge planning for the high risk newborn begins early in the hospitalization. Throughout the infant's hospitalization, the nurse gathers information from the health care team members and the family. This information is used to determine the infant's and family's readiness for discharge.

As the nurse assesses home care needs of the infant's parents, he or she takes steps to eliminate any knowledge deficits. Discharge teaching for the high risk newborn family is extensive, requires time and planning, and cannot be adequately accomplished on the day of discharge. Information is provided about infant care, especially as it pertains to the particular infant's home needs (e.g., supplemental oxygen, gastrostomy feedings, follow-up medical visits). Parent education includes having them give return demonstrations of their infant care skills to show whether they are becoming increasingly independent in the provision of this care. Parents of infants who have special needs or who were born at less than 34 weeks of gestation should be given the opportunity to spend a night or two in a predischarge room providing care

NURSING CARE PLAN The Infant of Mother with Diabetes Mellitus

Nursing Diagnosis: Risk for unstable blood glucose related to hypoglycemia secondary to hyperinsulinemia and maternal diabetes

Expected Outcome

Infant will exhibit serum blood glucose levels that are within normal limits.

Nursing Interventions/*Rationales*

Monitor blood glucose levels in infants at known risk for hypoglycemia (e.g., small for gestational age, preterm [extremely low birth weight, very low birth weight], infant of diabetic mother) *to assess and detect early onset to prevent complications.*

Observe for signs of hypoglycemia (e.g., jitteriness, twitching, lethargy, apathy, seizures, cyanosis, sweating, eye rolling, and refusal to eat) *to assess and detect signs of onset to prevent complications.*

Institute early feeding of breast milk or infant formula *to prevent or treat early hypoglycemia.*

Reduce adverse environmental factors (e.g., cold stress, hypoxia, and respiratory distress) *that can predispose infant to hypoglycemia.*

Nursing Diagnosis: Ineffective breathing pattern related to lung immaturity secondary to maternal gestational diabetes

Expected Outcome

Infant will exhibit breathing pattern adequate to maintain oxygenation (i.e., respiratory rate, rhythm, and characteristics).

Nursing Interventions/*Rationales*

Monitor infant vital signs and patency of airway *to evaluate pulmonary and circulatory status.*

Avoid activities that may lower body temperature and lead to cold stress, *which can induce respiratory distress.*

Suction as needed *to keep airway patent and prevent aspiration.*

Position infant on side initially *to facilitate mucus drainage.*

Have resuscitation equipment and oxygen available *for quick treatment of respiratory distress.*

Nursing Diagnosis: Risk for imbalanced body temperature related to physiologic immaturity

See the Nursing Process box for the term newborn in Chapter 25.

Nursing Diagnosis: Anxiety (maternal [risk for powerlessness, situational low self-esteem, ineffective coping]) related to neonate's condition, management, and prognosis

Expected Outcome

Parents demonstrate understanding of prognosis and therapy for infant.

Nursing Interventions/*Rationales*

Explain potential effects of maternal diabetic condition on newborn *to relieve fear of unknown and support ability to cope.*

Encourage open communication (e.g., inform parents of ongoing condition, procedures, and treatment; answer questions; correct misperceptions; actively listen to parental concerns) *to provide support and help provide sense of control.*

Encourage parents to interact with infant and to become involved in care routines *to foster emotional connection.*

Arrange for return demonstration of care by parents *to assess competence, provide positive reinforcement, and decrease their anxiety.*

for the infant away from the NICU to become better acquainted with the necessary care and to have a time of transition in which to ask questions regarding home care. Additional parent teaching should include bathing and skin care; requirements for meeting nutritional needs after discharge; safety in the home, including supine sleep position and prevention of infection (e.g., respiratory syncytial virus); and medication administration.

Durable medical equipment and supplies required for the care of the infant in the home should be delivered to the home before discharge; parents and care providers should have ample practice and education in the use of the equipment. Parents of infants being discharged with special needs such as gavage or gastrostomy feedings, nasal cannula oxygen, tracheostomy, or colostomy should receive several days of carefully planned education in the procedure before discharge.

Parents should obtain an age-appropriate car seat before discharge and demonstrate its use with the infant. Car seat safety is an essential aspect of discharge planning, and infants at less than 37 weeks of gestation should have a period of observation in an appropriate car seat to monitor for possible apnea, bradycardia, and decreased Sao_2.

Preterm infants have a high rate of readmission to acute care centers and emergency room visits. It is imperative that the family have a health professional they can contact for questions regarding infant care and behavior once they are home.

Before discharge all high risk or preterm infants should receive the appropriate immunizations, metabolic screening, hematology assessment (bilirubin risk as appropriate), and evaluation of hearing. Successful discharge of high risk infants to their homes requires a multidisciplinary approach. Medical, nursing, social services, and other professionals (physical therapy, occupational therapy, developmental follow-up specialist) are crucial to the smooth transition of these infants and their families to the community and home. If the infant is transported back to the community hospital that referred either the mother before birth or the infant after birth, interfacility communication is essential to continuity of care.

Discharge to home for high risk infants does not mean they can be treated like healthy term newborns. Follow-up by a specialized practitioner familiar with the complications common to the high risk newborn is essential. Further follow-up of specific complications by qualified specialists and referral to centers for developmental interventions can help ensure the best outcome possible for these infants.

Referrals for appropriate community resources also need to be made for infants with developmental disabilities, or those infants who may be at risk for further problems (e.g., preterm infants). Social service involvement is especially important for young or psychosocially high risk parents (e.g., parents with a history of substance abuse or child maltreatment).

For the family of the child who is technology dependent, special education needs are discussed before discharge. For further discussion of home care, see Chapter 43.

COMMUNITY FOCUS

Preterm and Near-Term Infant Car Seat Evaluation

The American Academy of Pediatrics recommends that infants born before 37 weeks of gestation be evaluated for apnea, bradycardia, and oxygen desaturation episodes before hospital discharge. The academy suggests that facilities develop policies for implementing an evaluation program; however, few evidence-based practice recommendations have been published to date delineating specific requirements for such a program. Based on the available literature, suggestions for providing a car seat evaluation of infants born before 37 weeks of gestation include:

- Use the parents' car seat for the evaluation.
- Perform the evaluation 1 to 7 days before the infant's anticipated discharge.
- Secure infant in car seat per guidelines using blanket rolls on side.
- Set pulse oximeter low alarm at 88% (arbitrary).
- Set heart rate low alarm limit at 80 beats/min and apnea alarm at 20 seconds (cardiorespiratory monitor).
- Leave the infant undisturbed in car seat for 90 to 120 minutes *or* for the time parents state it takes to arrive at their home (if more than the 90 minutes).
- Document infant's tolerance to car seat evaluation.
- An episode of desaturation, bradycardia, or apnea (20 seconds or more) constitutes a failure, and evaluation by the practitioner must occur before discharge.
- Repeat the test once modifications are made to the car seat, car bed, or infant's position in either restraint system (supplemental oxygen may be required).
- It is recommended that a certified car seat technician place the infant in the car seat (or bed) if a failure occurs (see National Highway Traffic Safety Administration website* for car seat inspection station).
- The technician will demonstrate appropriate positioning of the infant in the restraint device to the parents and have the parents do a return demonstration.
- Document the interventions, the infant's tolerance, and the parents' return demonstration.

Modified from American Academy of Pediatrics: Safe transportation of preterm and low birth weight infants at hospital discharge, *Pediatrics* 123(5):1424-1429, 2009; American Academy of Pediatrics: Transporting children with special health care needs, *Pediatrics* 104(4):988-992, 1999.

*www.nhtsa.dot.gov.

Transport to a Regional Center

If a hospital is not equipped to care for a high risk mother and fetus or a high risk infant, transfer to a specialized perinatal or regional tertiary care center is arranged. Maternal transport ideally occurs with the fetus in utero because this has two distinct advantages: (1) neonatal morbidity and mortality are decreased, and (2) the mother and infant are not separated at birth.

For a variety of reasons, it is not always possible to transport the mother before the birth. Therefore physicians and nurses in all facilities must have the skills and equipment necessary for making an accurate diagnosis and implementing emergency interventions to stabilize the infant's condition until transport can occur (Pettett, Pallotto, & Merenstein,

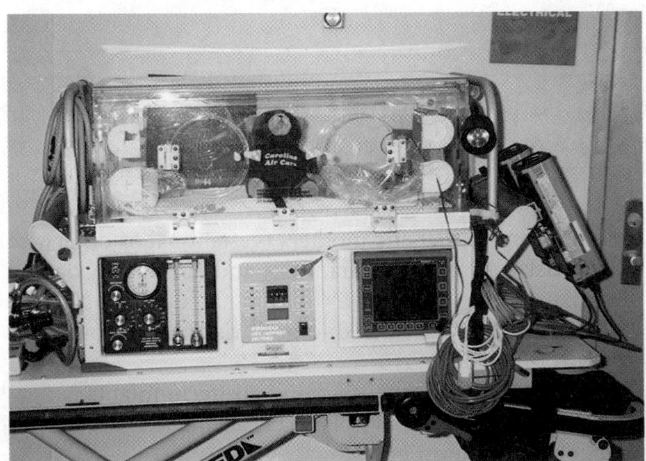

Fig. 27-12 Total life support system for transport of high risk newborns. *(Courtesy UNC Hospitals, Carolina Air Care, Chapel Hill, NC.)*

BOX 27-5 Information for Parents About the Tertiary Center

- Exact location of the unit—address, map, waiting area for relatives and friends
- Visiting hours and hospital rules
- Telephone numbers
- Names of individuals likely to be involved with the newborn's care (e.g., primary nurse, neonatologist, clinical manager)
- Information about the special care unit—what it is, what it does
- Location of parking facilities, nearby lodging, and rules regarding visitation by young children (siblings)
- Any particular rules or regulations regarding the special care unit

From Pettett G, Pallotto EK, Merenstein GB: Regionalization and transport in perinatal care. In Merenstein GB, Gardner SL (editors): *Handbook of neonatal intensive care,* ed 6, St Louis, 2006, Mosby.

2006). The goal of these interventions is to maintain the infant's condition within the normal physiologic range. Specific attention is given to vital signs, oxygenation and ventilation, thermoregulation, acid-base balance, fluid and electrolyte status, blood glucose, and developmental interventions.

Arrangements for transport to an intensive care facility are made as soon as the high risk infant is identified (see Community Focus box). The infant must be kept warm and adequately oxygenated (including intubation and surfactant replacement as indicated); have vital signs and oxygen saturation monitored; and, when indicated, receive an IV infusion. The infant is transported in a specially designed incubator unit containing a complete life support system and other emergency equipment that can be carried by ambulance, helicopter, or even a fixed-wing aircraft (Fig. 27-12).

COMMUNITY FOCUS

Neonatal Transport

During a scheduled clinical experience in the neonatal intensive care unit (NICU) or a special care nursery, observe a transport team leaving to pick up an infant from a referring hospital. Who are the transport team members? What are their job responsibilities when not transporting patients? What equipment are they taking on the transport? How was the referral made? What communication links are there between the special care nursery and the community hospitals in the surrounding area? What communication links exist between the NICU and the transport team when they are transporting the sick infant? How are parents kept informed of the infant's condition?

The transport team may consist of physicians, nurse practitioners, nurses, and respiratory therapists. The team must have experience in resuscitation, stabilization, and provision of critical care during the transport. Teams provide information for the parents about the tertiary center (Box 27-5).

The birth of any high risk infant can cause profound parental stress. Parents can grieve the loss of the ideal infant and fear the possible eventual outcomes. They must also deal with the technologic world surrounding their infant. Amid all the equipment, it is sometimes difficult for them to perceive the infant and respond to his or her needs. Parents of high risk infants who have been transported to regional centers therefore need special support.

Transport from a Regional Center

Infants may need to be transferred back (back transport) to the referring facility; however, in most cases the infant is discharged home from the tertiary center. Preterm infants who require thermoregulation and gavage feedings may be cared for in community hospitals closer to the parents' home. This allows parents to visit their infant more easily and to work with their personal health care provider on the long-range expected outcomes for the infant. Specialized incubators make these trips possible (see Fig. 27-12). However, parents may express mixed feelings about such return transports and may be reluctant to adapt to a different facility and group of caregivers. To minimize some of these concerns, it is important to give the parents clear information about return transports during the initial discharge planning.

Although at the time of discharge parents may not recognize the need for information on the various resources available to help them in the care of their infant, they can be given lists of agencies and telephone numbers for later use. Providing them with a patient-specific directory covering special programs, social support, community, and funding resources can help them make the transition to home care of their infants. As the nurse continually reinforces the idea that the infant will go home, this prompts the parents to plan for the days ahead and therefore be ready to take their infant home when the time comes.

Key Points

- Preterm infants are at risk for problems related to the immaturity of their organ systems.
- Late preterm infants are at higher risk for feeding problems, respiratory distress, jaundice, poor neurodevelopment, hypoglycemia, infection, and thermoregulation than their term counterparts.
- RDS, ROP, and chronic lung disease (BPD) are associated with preterm birth.
- High risk infants must be observed for respiratory distress and other early signs of physiologic distress.
- The adaptation of parents to preterm or high risk infants differs from that of parents of full-term infants.
- Parents need special instruction (e.g., CPR, oxygen therapy, suctioning, developmental care) before they take a high risk infant home.

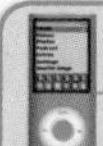

Audio Chapter Summaries

Access an audio summary of these Key Points on evolve

- Infants born to diabetic mothers (gestational or otherwise) are at risk for hypoglycemia, RDS, and birth asphyxia and trauma.
- SGA infants are considered to be at risk because of fetal growth restriction.
- Nonreassuring fetal status among postterm infants is related to the progressive placental insufficiency that can occur in a postterm pregnancy.
- Specially trained nurses may transport high risk infants to and from special care units.

References

Adams-Chapman I, Stoll B: Nervous system disorders. In Kliegman RM et al (editors): *Nelson textbook of pediatrics*, ed 18, Philadelphia, 2007, Saunders.

Alfaleh K, Bassler D: Probiotics for prevention of necrotizing enterocolitis in preterm infants, *Cochrane Database Syst Rev* (1):CD005496, 2008.

Als H: Developmental care in the newborn intensive care unit, *Curr Opin Pediatr* 10(2):138-142, 1998.

Altimier L, Lutes L: Cobedding multiples, *Newborn Infant Nurs Rev* 1(4):205-206, 2001.

American Academy of Pediatrics, Committee on Fetus and Newborn: Age terminology during the perinatal period, *Pediatrics* 114(5):1362-1364, 2004.

American Academy of Pediatrics, Committee on Fetus and Newborn: Postnatal corticosteroids to treat or prevent chronic lung disease in preterm infants, *Pediatrics* 109(2):330-337, 2002.

American Academy of Pediatrics: *Pediatric nutrition handbook*, ed 6, Elk Grove Village, IL, 2009, The Academy.

American Academy of Pediatrics, Section on Ophthalmology: Screening examination of premature infants for retinopathy of prematurity, *Pediatrics* 117(2):572-576, 2006.

American Heart Association: 2005 American Heart Association (AHA) guidelines for cardiopulmonary resuscitation (CPR) and emergency cardiovascular care (ECC) of pediatric and neonatal patients: pediatric basic life support, *Circulation* 112(24 Suppl):1-203, 2005.

Anderson GC: Kangaroo care of the premature infant. In Goldson E (editor): *Nurturing the premature infant: developmental interventions in the neonatal intensive care nursery*, New York, 1999, Oxford University Press.

Anderson MS et al: Enteral nutrition. In Merenstein GB, Gardner SL (editors): *Handbook of neonatal intensive care*, ed 6, St Louis, 2006, Mosby.

Askin DF et al: *Late preterm infant assessment guide*, Washington, DC, 2007, Association of Women's Health, Obstetric and Neonatal Nurses.

Association of Women's Health, Obstetric and Neonatal Nurses: *Neonatal skin care: evidence-based clinical practice guideline*, ed 2, Washington, DC, 2007, The Association.

Bakewell-Sachs S: Near-term/late preterm infants, *Newborn Infant Nurs Rev* 7(2):67-71, 2007.

Barrington KJ, Finer NN: Inhaled nitric oxide for respiratory failure in preterm infants: a systematic review, *Pediatrics* 120(5):1088-1099, 2007.

Beeram M et al: Effects of topical emollient therapy on infants at or less than 27 weeks' gestation, *J Natl Med Assoc* 98(2):261-264, 2006.

Berger TM et al: Impact of improved survival of very low–birth-weight infants on incidence and severity of bronchopulmonary dysplasia, *Biol Neonate* 86(2):124-130, 2004.

Bin-Nun A et al: Oral probiotics prevent necrotizing enterocolitis in very low birth weight neonates, *J Pediatr* 147(2):143-146, 2005.

Blackburn ST: *Maternal, fetal, and neonatal physiology: a clinical perspective*, ed 3, St. Louis, 2007, Saunders.

Blackburn ST: Environmental impact of the NICU on developmental outcomes, *J Pediatr Nurs* 13(5):279-289, 1998.

Blake WW, Murray JA: Heat balance. In Merenstein GB, Gardner SL: *Handbook of neonatal intensive care*, ed 6, St Louis, 2006, Mosby.

Byers JF, Waugh WR, Lowman LB: Sound level exposure of high-risk infants in different environmental conditions, *Neonatal Netw* 25(1):25-32, 2006.

Cherif A, Jabnoun S, Khrouf N: Oral ibuprofen in early curative closure of patent ductus arteriosus in very premature infants, *Am J Perinatol* 24(6):339-345, 2007.

Conde-Agudelo A, Diaz-Rossello JL, Belizan JM: Kangaroo mother care to reduce morbidity and mortality in low birthweight infants, *Cochrane Neonatal Rev* (2):CD 002771, 2008. Available at www.cochrane.org/reviews/en/ab002771.html (accessed June 9, 2008).

Cowett RM, Loughead JL: Neonatal glucose metabolism: differential diagnoses, evaluation, and treatment of hypoglycemia, *Neonat Netw* 21(4):9-19, 2002.

Curley MAQ et al: Predicting pressure ulcer risk in pediatric patients: the Braden Q scale, *Nurs Res* 52(1):22-33, 2003.

Darcy AE: Complications of the late preterm infant, *J Perinatal Neonatal Nurs* 23(1):78-86, 2009.

DellaPorta K, Aforismo D, Butler-O'Hara M: Co-bedding of twins in the neonatal intensive care, *Pediatr Nurs* 24(6):529-531, 1998.

Diehl-Jones WL, Askin DF: Nutritional modulation of neonatal outcomes, *AACN Clin Issues* 15(1):83-96, 2004.

Dodd VL: Implications of kangaroo care for growth and development in preterm infants, *J Obstet Gynecol Neonatal Nurs* 34(2):218-232, 2005.

Donn SM, Sinha SK: Invasive and noninvasive neonatal mechanical ventilation, *Respir Care* 48(4):426-441, 2003.

Dudell GG, Stoll BJ: Respiratory tract disorders. In Kliegman RM et al (editors): *Nelson textbook of pediatrics*, ed 18, Philadelphia, 2007, Saunders.

Edwards W, Conner J, Soll R: The effect of prophylactic ointment therapy on nosocomial sepsis rates and skin integrity in infants with birth weights of 501-1000g, *Pediatrics* 113(5):1195-1203, 2004.

Ehrenkranz RA: Early, aggressive nutritional management for very low birth weight infants: what is the evidence? *Semin Perinatol* 31(2):48-55, 2007.

Ellett M, Woodruff K, Stewart D: The use of carbon dioxide monitoring to determine orogastric tube placement in premature infants: a pilot study, *Gastroenterol Nurs* 30(6):414-417, 2007.

Ellett ML et al: Gastric tube placement in young children, *Clin Nurs Res* 14(3):238-252, 2005.

Engle WA: A recommendation for the definition of "late preterm" (near-term) and the birth weight–gestational age classification system, *Semin Perinatol* 30(1):2-7, 2006.

Engle WA, American Academy of Pediatrics, Committee on Fetus and Newborn: Surfactant replacement therapy for respiratory distress in the preterm and term neonate, *Pediatrics* 121(2):419-432, 2008.

Engle WA et al: Late-preterm infants: a population at risk, *Pediatrics* 120(6):1390-1401, 2007.

Enterobacter sakazakii infections associated with the use of powdered infant formula—Tennessee, 2001, *Morbid Mortal Wkly Rep* 51(14):297-300, 2002.

Escobar GJ, Clark RH, Greene JD: Short-term outcomes of infants born at 35 and 36 weeks gestation: we need to ask more questions, *Semin Perinatol* 30(1):28-33, 2006.

Field D et al: Neonatal ventilation with inhaled nitric oxide vs. ventilatory support without inhaled nitric oxide for infants with severe respiratory failure born at or neat term: the INNOVO multicenter randomised controlled trial. *Neonatology* 91(2):73-82, 2007.

Finnegan LP: Neonatal abstinence. In Nelson N, editor: *Current therapy in neonatal perinatal medicine 1985-1986*, Toronto, 1985, BC Decker.

Gardner SL, Snell BJ, Lawrence RA: Breastfeeding the neonate with special needs. In Merenstein GB, Gardner SL (editors): *Handbook of neonatal intensive care*, ed 6, St Louis, 2006, Mosby.

Gracey K et al: The changing face of bronchopulmonary dysplasia, part 1, *Adv Neonatal Care* 2(6):327-338, 2002.

Hagedorn MIE et al: Respiratory diseases. In Merenstein GB, Gardner SL (editors): *Handbook of neonatal intensive care*, ed 6, St Louis, 2006, Mosby.

Haubrich K: Assessment and management of auditory dysfunction. In Kenner C, Lott JW, Flandermyer A (editors): *Comprehensive neonatal nursing: a physiologic perspective*, ed 2, Philadelphia, 1998, Saunders.

Holditch-Davis D, Blackburn ST, VandenBerg K: Newborn and infant neurobehavioral development. In Kenner C, Lott J (editors): *Comprehensive neonatal care: an interdisciplinary approach*, ed 4, St Louis, 2007, Saunders.

Johnston CC et al: Kangaroo mother care diminishes pain from heel lance in very preterm neonates: a crossover trial, *BMC Pediatr* 8:13, 2008.

Jones JG et al: The Early Treatment for ROP (ETROP) randomized trial: study results and nursing care adaptations, *Insight* 30(2):7-13, 2005.

Kalhan SC, Parimi PS: Disorders of carbohydrate metabolism. In Martin RJ, Fanaroff AA, Walsh MC (editors): *Fanaroff and Martin's neonatal-perinatal medicine: diseases of the fetus and infant*, ed 8, Philadelphia, 2006, Mosby.

Kliegman RM: Intrauterine growth restriction. In Martin RJ, Fanaroff AA, Walsh MC (editors): *Fanaroff and Martin's neonatal-perinatal medicine: diseases of the fetus and infant*, ed 8, Philadelphia, 2006, Mosby.

Knight SE, Washington RL: Cardiovascular diseases and surgical interventions. In Merenstein GB, Gardner SL (editors): *Handbook of neonatal intensive care*, ed 6, St Louis, 2006, Mosby.

Kostandy RR et al: Kangaroo care (skin contact) reduces crying response to pain in preterm neonates: pilot results, *Pain Manage Nurs* 9(2):55-65, 2008.

LaMar K, Dowling DA: Incidence of infection for preterm twins cared for in cobedding in the neonatal intensive-care unit, *J Obstet Gynecol Neonatal Nurs* 35(2):193-198, 2006.

Law KL et al: Smoking during pregnancy and newborn neurobehavior, *Pediatrics* 111(6):1318-1323, 2003.

Lawrence RA, Lawrence RM: *Breastfeeding: a guide for the medical profession*, ed 6, Philadelphia, 2005, Mosby.

Ludington-Hoe SM, Hosseini R, Torowicz DL: Skin-to-skin contact (kangaroo care) analgesia for preterm infant heel stick, *AACN Clin Issues* 16(3):373-387, 2005.

Ludington-Hoe SM, Morgan K, Abouelfettoh A: A clinical guideline for implementation of kangaroo care with premature infants of 30 or more weeks' postmenstrual age, *Adv Neonatal Care* 8(3 Suppl):S3-S23, 2008.

Lund CH, Durand DJ: Skin and skin care. In Merenstein GB, Gardner SL (editors): *Handbook of neonatal intensive care*, ed 6, St Louis, 2006, Mosby.

Lund CH, Kuller JM: Assessment and management of the integumentary system. In Kenner C, Lott JW (editors): *Comprehensive neonatal care: an interdisciplinary approach*, ed 4, St Louis, 2007, Saunders.

Lund CH, Osborne JW: Validity and reliability of the Neonatal Skin Condition Score, *J Obstet Gynecol Neonatal Nurs* 33(3):320-327, 2004.

McCain GC et al: Heart rate variability responses of a preterm infant to kangaroo care, *J Obstet Gynecol Neonatal Nurs* 34(6):689-694, 2005.

Morton JA: Strategies to support extended breastfeeding of the premature infant, *Adv Neonatal Care*, 2(5): 267-282, 2002.

Mosqueda E et al: The early use of minimal enteral nutrition in extremely low birth weight newborns, *J Perinatol* 28(4):264-269, 2008.

Noonan C, Quigley S, Curley MAQ: Skin integrity in hospitalized infants and children, *J Pediatr Nurs* 21(6):445-453, 2006.

Nucci A et al: Interdisciplinary management of pediatric intestinal failure: a 10-year review of rehabilitation and transplantation, *J Gastrointest Surg* 12(3):429-435, 2008.

Ohlsson A, Walia R, Shah S: Ibuprofen for the treatment of patent ductus arteriosus in preterm and/or low birth weight infants, *Cochrane Database Syst Rev* (1):CD003481, 2008.

Paige PL, Moe PC: Neurologic disorders. In Merenstein GB, Gardner SL (editors): *Handbook of neonatal intensive care*, ed 6, St Louis, 2006, Mosby.

Petrini JR et al: Increased risk of adverse neurological development for late preterm infants, *J Pediatr* 154(2):169-176, 2009.

Pettett G, Pallotto EK, Merenstein GB: Regionalization and transport in perinatal care. In Merenstein GB, Gardner SL (editors): *Handbook of neonatal intensive care*, ed 6, St Louis, 2006, Mosby.

Pollan C: Retinopathy of prematurity: an eye toward better outcomes, *Neonatal Network* 28(2):93-101, 2009.

Reece EA et al: Pregnancy outcomes among women with and without diabetic microvascular disease (White's classes B to FR) versus nondiabetic controls, *Am J Perinatol* 15(9):549-555, 1998.

Reynolds RM, Thureen PJ: Special circumstances: trophic feeds, necrotizing enterocolitis and bronchopulmonary dysplasia, *Semin Fetal Neonatal Med* 12(1):64-70, 2007.

Roaten JB, Bensard DD, Price FN: Neonatal surgery. In Merenstein GB, Gardner SL (editors): *Handbook of neonatal intensive care*, ed 6, St Louis, 2006, Mosby.

Sadiq HF et al: Inhaled nitric oxide in the treatment of moderate persistent pulmonary hypertension of the newborn: a randomized controlled, multicenter trial, *J Perinatol* 23(2):98-103, 2003.

Sauer PJ, Dane HJ, Visser HK: New standards for neutral thermal environment of healthy very low birthweight infants in one week of life, *Arch Dis Child* 59(1):18-22, 1984.

Saugstad OD: Optimal oxygenation at birth and in the neonatal period, *Neonatology* 91(4):319-322, 2007.

Saugstad OD et al: Resuscitation of newborn infants with 21% or 100% oxygen: follow-up at 18 and 24 months, *Pediatrics* 112(2):296-300, 2003.

Schanler RJ et al: Feeding strategies for premature infants: randomized trial of gastrointestinal priming and tube-feeding method, *Pediatrics* 103(2): 434-439, 1999.

Schwartz RP: Neonatal hypoglycemia: how low is too low? *J Pediatr* 131(2):171-173, 1997.

Sisk PM et al: Early human milk feeding is associated with a lower risk of necrotizing enterocolitis in very low birth weight infants, *J Perinatol* 27(7):428-433, 2007.

Squires AJ, Hyndman M: Prevention of nasal injuries secondary to NCPAP application in the ELBW infant, *Neonatal Network* 28(1): 13-27, 2009.

Stoll BJ: Infections in the neonatal infant. In Kliegman RM et al (editors): *Nelson textbook of pediatrics*, ed 18, Philadelphia, 2007, Saunders.

Stoll BJ, Adams-Chapman I: The high-risk infant. In Kliegman RM et al (editors): *Nelson textbook of pediatrics*, ed 18, Philadelphia, 2007, Saunders.

Symington A, Pinelli J: Developmental care for promoting development and preventing morbidity in preterm infants, *Cochrane Database Syst Rev* (2):CD001814, 2006.

Tomashek KM et al: Differences in mortality between late-preterm and term singleton infants in the United States, 1995-2002, *J Pediatr* 151(5): 450-456, 2007.

Vain NE et al: Oropharyngeal and nasopharyngeal suctioning of meconium-stained neonates before delivery of their shoulders: multicenter, randomized, controlled trial, *Obstet Gynecol Surv* 60(2):88-89, 2005.

van Acker J et al: Outbreak of necrotizing enterocolitis associated with *Enterobacter sakazakii* in powdered milk formula, *J Clin Microbiol* 39(1):293-297, 2001.

Vennarecci G at al: Intestinal transplantation for short gut syndrome attributable to necrotizing enterocolitis, *Pediatrics* 105(2):1-5, 2000.

Vento M et al: Oxidative stress in asphyxiated term infants resuscitated with 100% oxygen, *J Pediatr* 142(3):240-246, 2003.

Volpe JJ: *Neurology of the newborn*, ed 5, Philadelphia, 2008, Saunders.

Ward K: Perceived needs of parents of critically ill infants in a neonatal intensive care unit (NICU), *Pediatr Nurs* 27(3):281-286, 2001.

Westrup B, Sizun J, Lagercrantz H: Family-centered developmental supportive care: a holistic and humane approach to reduce stress and pain in neonates, *J Perinatol* 27(Suppl 1):S12-S18, 2007.

Woodwell WH: The long road home: perspectives on parenting in the NICU, *Adv Neonatal Care* 2(3):161-169, 2002.

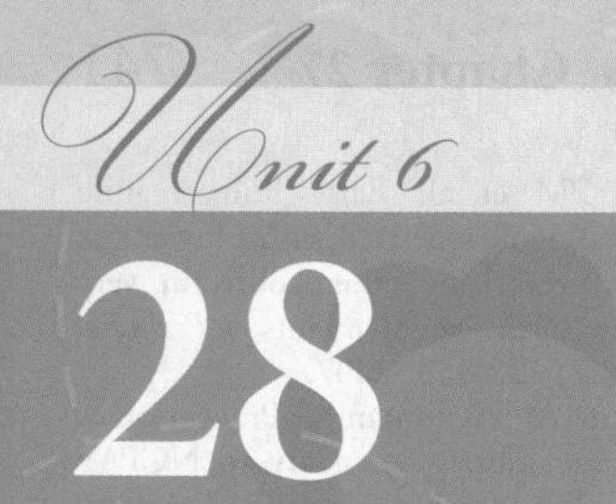

28 The Newborn at Risk: Acquired and Congenital Problems

Learning Objectives

On completion of this chapter the reader will be able to:

- Summarize assessment and care of the newborn with soft tissue, skeletal, and nervous system injuries due to birth trauma.
- Identify maternal conditions that place the newborn at risk for infection.
- Describe methods used to identify infection in the newborn.
- Identify the effects of maternal use of alcohol, heroin, methadone, marijuana, methamphetamine, cocaine, and tobacco on the fetus and newborn.
- Describe the assessment of a newborn exposed to recreational drugs in utero.
- Identify clinical signs of infection in the newborn.
- Describe the nurse's role in the diagnosis of neonatal sepsis.
- Compare characteristics of neonatal Rh and ABO incompatibility.
- Describe preoperative and postoperative nursing care of the newborn.
- Describe congenital disorders presented in this chapter and identify the priority of nursing care for each.

Electronic Resources

Additional information related to the content in Chapter 28 can be found on

evolve the Companion Website at

http://evolve.elsevier.com/Perry/maternal/

- NCLEX Review Questions
- Critical Thinking Exercise—Fetal Alcohol Syndrome
- Nursing Care Plan—The Drug-Exposed Newborn

A challenge for the nurse is the birth of an infant at risk because of conditions or circumstances that are superimposed on the normal course of events associated with birth and the adjustment to extrauterine existence. The infant may be considered high risk because of birth trauma, maternal substance abuse, infection, or congenital anomalies. Birth trauma includes physical injuries a neonate sustains during labor and birth. Congenital anomalies include such conditions as gastrointestinal (GI) malformations, neural tube defects, abdominal wall defects, and cardiac defects.

At times the nurse is able to anticipate problems, such as when a woman is admitted in premature labor or a congenital anomaly is diagnosed by ultrasound before birth. At other times the birth of a high risk infant is unanticipated. In either case, the personnel and equipment necessary for immediate care of the infant must be available.

Birth Trauma

Birth trauma (injury) is physical injury sustained by a neonate during labor and birth. It remains an important source of neonatal morbidity. Most birth injuries are avoidable, especially with careful assessment of risk factors and appropriate planning of the birth. The use of fetal ultrasonography allows antepartum diagnosis of certain fetal conditions that may be treated in utero or shortly after birth. Elective cesarean birth can be chosen for some pregnancies to prevent significant birth injury. A small percentage of significant birth injuries are unavoidable despite skilled and competent obstetric care, such as in especially difficult or prolonged labor or an abnormal fetal presentation. Some injuries cannot be anticipated until the specific circumstances are encountered during childbirth. Emergency cesarean birth may provide a last-minute salvage, but in these circumstances the injury may be truly unavoidable. The same injury might be caused in several ways; for example, a cephalhematoma could result from an obstetric technique such as forceps birth or vacuum extraction or from pressure of the fetal skull against the maternal pelvis.

Many injuries are minor and resolve readily in the neonatal period without treatment. Other trauma requires some degree of intervention; few are serious enough to be fatal. The nurse's contributions to the newborn's welfare begin with early

Table 28-1 Types of Birth Injuries

SITE OF INJURY	TYPE OF INJURY
Scalp	Caput succedaneum Subgaleal hemorrhage Cephalhematoma
Skull	Linear fracture Depressed fracture Occipital osteodiastasis
Intracranial	Epidural hematoma Subdural hematoma (laceration of falx, tentorium, or superficial veins) Subarachnoid hemorrhage Cerebral contusion Cerebellar contusion Intracerebellar hematoma
Spinal cord (cervical)	Vertebral artery injury Intraspinal hemorrhage Spinal cord transection or injury
Plexus	Erb's palsy Klumpke's paralysis Total (mixed) brachial plexus injury Horner's syndrome Diaphragmatic paralysis Lumbosacral plexus injury
Cranial and peripheral nerve	Radial nerve palsy Medial nerve palsy Sciatic nerve palsy Laryngeal nerve palsy Diaphragmatic paralysis Facial nerve palsy

From Paige PL, Moe PC: Neurologic disorders. In Merenstein GB, Gardner SL (editors): *Handbook of neonatal intensive care,* ed 6, St Louis, 2006, Mosby.

observation of his or her transition. The prompt reporting of signs that indicate deviations from normal permits early initiation of appropriate therapy. Table 28-1 provides an overview of neurologic birth injuries and the sites in which they occur.

Nursing Care Management

When the newborn is born, the nurse makes a rapid inspection and physical assessment to determine whether there are any life-threatening conditions requiring immediate medical or surgical attention. A comprehensive physical assessment of the newborn is performed after the parents have had the opportunity to interact with their new baby. Because evidence of some birth injuries may not be apparent at the initial examination, assessment continues during each contact with the neonate.

Soft-tissue injuries that commonly occur at birth are discussed at length in Chapter 25. Caput succedaneum and cephalhematoma are discussed in Chapter 24.

Skeletal Injuries

The newborn's immature, flexible skull can withstand a great degree of deformation (molding) before fracture results. Considerable force is required to fracture the newborn's skull. Two types of skull fractures typically identified in the newborn are linear fractures and depressed fractures. The location of the fracture and involvement of underlying structures determine its significance.

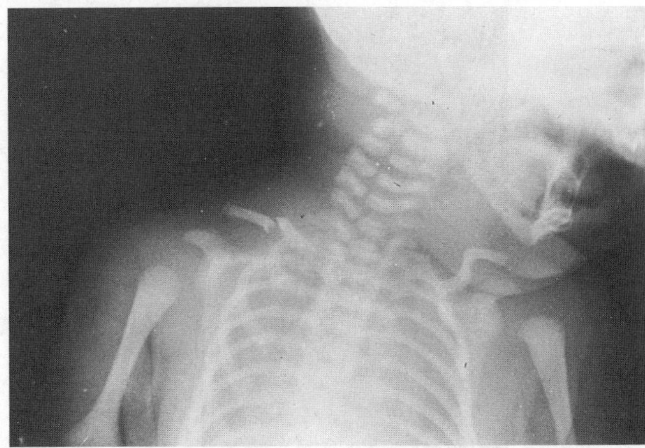

Fig. 28-1 Fractured clavicle after shoulder dystocia. (From O'Doherty N: *Neonatology: micro atlas of the newborn*, Nutley, NJ, 1986, Hoffmann–La Roche.)

If an artery lying in a groove on the undersurface of the skull is torn as a result of the fracture, increased intracranial pressure (ICP) will follow. Unless a blood vessel is involved, linear fractures, which account for 70% of all fractures for this age group, heal without special treatment. The soft skull may become indented without laceration of either the skin or the dural membrane. These depressed fractures, or ping-pong ball indentations, may occur during difficult births from pressure of the head on the bony pelvis. They also can occur as a result of injudicious application of forceps.

The clavicle is the bone most often fractured during birth. Generally the break is in the middle third of the bone (Fig. 28-1). Dystocia, particularly shoulder impaction, may be the predisposing problem. Limitation of motion of the arm, crepitus over the bone, and absence of the Moro reflex on the affected side are often present. Except for use of gentle rather than vigorous handling and containment of the limb against the chest, no accepted treatment for fractured clavicle of the newborn exists, and the prognosis is good. The humerus and femur are other bones that may be fractured during a difficult birth. Fractures in newborns generally heal rapidly. Immobilization is accomplished with slings, splints, swaddling, and other immobilization devices.

The parents need support in handling these infants because they often are fearful of hurting them. Parents are encouraged to practice handling, changing, and feeding the affected neonate under the guidance of nursery personnel. This increases their confidence and knowledge and facilitates attachment. A plan for follow-up therapy is developed with the parents so that the times and arrangements for therapy are acceptable to them.

Peripheral Nervous System Injuries

Plexus injury results from forces that alter the normal position and relationship of the arm, shoulder, and neck. Erb palsy (Erb-Duchenne paralysis) is caused by damage to the upper plexus and usually results from a stretching or pulling away of the shoulder from the head such as might occur with shoulder dystocia or with a difficult vertex or breech delivery. The less common lower plexus palsy, or Klumpke palsy, results from

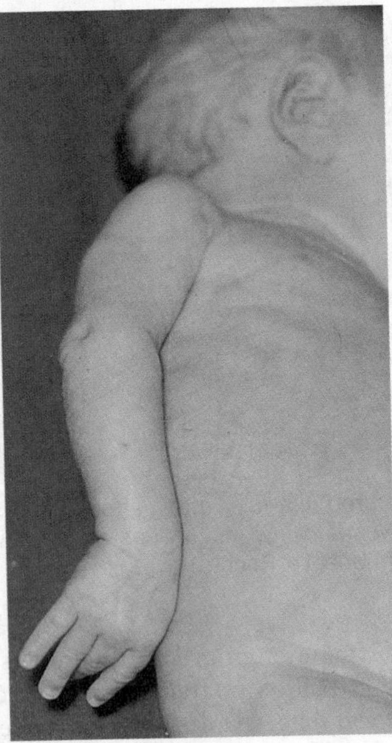

Fig. 28-2 Erb-Duchenne paralysis in newborn infant. Moro reflex is absent in right upper extremity. Recovery was complete. (From O'Doherty N: *Neonatology: micro atlas of the newborn*, Nutley, NJ, 1986, Hoffmann–La Roche.)

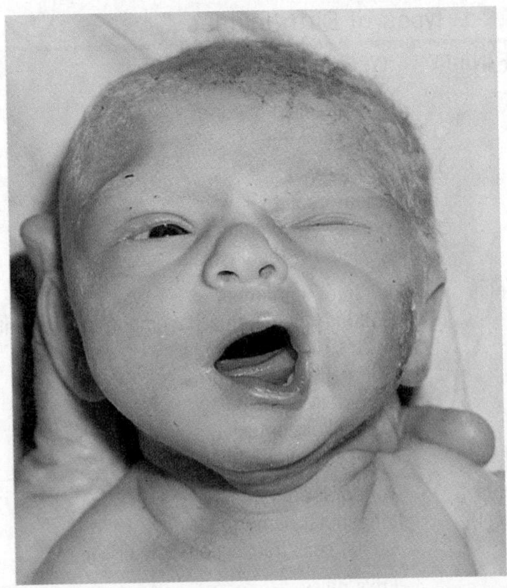

Fig. 28-3 Facial paralysis 15 minutes after forceps birth. Absence of movement on affected side is especially noticeable when infant cries. (From O'Doherty N: *Neonatology: micro atlas of the newborn*, Nutley, NJ, 1986, Hoffmann–La Roche.)

severe stretching of the upper extremity while the trunk is relatively less mobile.

The clinical manifestations of Erb palsy are related to the paralysis of the affected extremity and muscles. The arm hangs limp alongside the body. The shoulder and arm are adducted and internally rotated. The elbow is extended, and the forearm is pronated, with the wrist and fingers flexed; a grasp reflex may be present because finger and wrist movement remains normal (Adams-Chapman & Stoll, 2007) (Fig. 28-2). In lower plexus palsy, the muscles of the hand are paralyzed, with consequent wrist drop and relaxed fingers. In a third and more severe form of brachial palsy, the entire arm is paralyzed and hangs limp and motionless at the side. The Moro reflex is absent on the affected side for all of the forms of brachial palsy. Total plexus is the second most common type of plexus injury (Dunham, 2003).

Treatment of the affected arm is aimed at preventing contractures of the paralyzed muscles and maintaining correct placement of the humeral head within the glenoid fossa of the scapula. Complete recovery from stretched nerves usually takes 3 to 6 months. However, avulsion of the nerves (complete disconnection of the ganglia from the spinal cord that involves both anterior and posterior roots) results in permanent damage. For those injuries that do not improve by 3 to 6 months, surgical intervention may be needed to relieve pressure on the nerves or to repair the nerves with grafting (Adams-Chapman & Stoll, 2007).

Nursing care of the newborn with brachial palsy is concerned primarily with proper positioning of the affected arm. The affected arm should be abducted 90 degrees with external shoulder rotation, forearm supination, and extension at the wrist with the palm facing the infant's face (Adams-Chapman & Stoll, 2007). Passive range-of-motion exercises of the shoulder, wrist, elbow, and fingers are initiated in the latter part of the first week. Wrist flexion contractures may be prevented with the use of a wrist splint with padding in the fist. In dressing the infant, preference is given to the affected arm. Undressing begins with the unaffected arm, and redressing begins with the affected arm to prevent unnecessary manipulation and stress on the paralyzed muscles. Parents are taught to use the football position when holding the infant and to avoid picking the child up from under the axillae or by pulling on the arms.

Pressure on the facial nerve (cranial nerve VII) during delivery may result in injury to it. The primary clinical manifestations are loss of movement on the affected side, such as an inability to completely close the eye, drooping of the corner of the mouth, and absence of wrinkling of the forehead and nasolabial fold (Fig. 28-3). Facial palsy or paralysis is most noticeable when the infant cries. The mouth is drawn to the unaffected side, the wrinkles are deeper on the normal side, and the eye on the involved side remains open. Often the condition is temporary, resolving within hours or days of birth. Permanent paralysis is rare unless the nerve fibers were torn, in which case surgical intervention may be necessary.

Nursing care of the infant with facial nerve paralysis involves aiding the infant in sucking and helping the mother with feeding techniques. The infant may require gavage feeding to prevent aspiration. Breastfeeding is not contraindicated, but the mother will need additional assistance in helping the infant grasp and compress the areolar area.

If the lid of the eye on the affected side does not close completely, artificial tears can be instilled daily to prevent drying of the conjunctiva, sclera, and cornea. The lid is often taped shut to prevent accidental injury. If eye care is needed at home, the parents are taught the procedure for administering eyedrops before the infant is discharged.

Phrenic nerve paralysis results in diaphragmatic paralysis as demonstrated by ultrasonography, which shows paradoxic chest movement and an elevated diaphragm. Initially, radiography may not demonstrate an elevated diaphragm if the neonate is receiving positive pressure ventilation (Volpe, 2008). The injury sometimes occurs in conjunction with brachial palsy. Respiratory distress is the most common and important sign of injury. Because injury to the phrenic nerve is usually unilateral, the lung on the affected side does not expand, and respiratory efforts are ineffectual. The infant is positioned on the affected side to facilitate maximum expansion of the uninvolved lung. Breathing is primarily thoracic, and cyanosis, tachypnea, or complete respiratory failure may be seen. Pneumonia and atelectasis on the affected side may also occur.

The infant with phrenic nerve paralysis requires the same nursing care as any infant with respiratory distress. As with other birth injuries, the family's emotional needs are similar to those discussed for soft-tissue injury (see Chapter 25). Follow-up is also essential because of the extended length of recovery.

Central Nervous System Injuries

All types of intracranial hemorrhage (ICH) occur in newborns. ICH as a result of birth trauma is more likely to occur in the full-term, large infant. The frequency and degree of severity of ICH are different in the newborn than in older children or adults. In the newborn, more than one type of hemorrhage can and does commonly occur.

A subdural hematoma, or life-threatening collection of blood in the subdural space, most often is produced by the stretching and tearing of the large veins in the tentorium of the cerebellum, the dural membrane that separates the cerebrum from the cerebellum. When this type of bleeding occurs, the typical history includes a primiparous mother, with the total labor and birth occurring in less than 2 or 3 hours; a difficult birth involving high or midforceps application; or a large-for-gestational-age infant. Subdural hematoma occurs infrequently because of improvements in obstetric care. However, it is especially serious because of its inaccessibility to aspiration by subdural tap.

Subarachnoid hemorrhage occurs rarely and often without clinical manifestations. Small hemorrhages are the most common. Bleeding is of venous origin, and underlying contusion also may occur.

The clinical presentation of hemorrhage in the full-term infant can vary considerably. In many infants, signs are absent, and hemorrhaging is diagnosed only because of abnormal findings on lumbar puncture, for example, red blood cells (RBCs) in the cerebrospinal fluid (CSF) or a hemorrhage is seen on a computed tomography scan. The initial clinical manifestations of neonatal subarachnoid hemorrhage may be the early onset of alternating central nervous system (CNS) depression and irritability, with refractory seizure. Poor feeding, apnea, and unequal pupils may suggest an intracranial insult. Occasionally the infant appears normal initially then has seizures on the second day of life, followed by no apparent sequelae.

In general, nursing care of an infant with ICH is supportive and includes monitoring neurologic signs and intravenous therapy, observation and management of seizures, and prevention of increased ICP.

Spinal cord injuries almost always result from complicated breech births, especially difficult ones in which version and extraction are used. Clinical manifestations include respiratory failure and flaccid extremities; stillbirth is not uncommon.

Neonatal Infections

Sepsis

Sepsis (the presence of microorganisms or their toxins in the blood or other tissues) continues to be one of the most significant causes of neonatal morbidity and mortality. Maternal immune globulin M (IgM) does not cross the placenta. IgG levels in term infants are equal to maternal levels; however, in preterm infants the amount of IgG is directly proportional to gestational age (Stoll, 2007). IgA and IgM require time to reach optimum levels after birth. Neonatal neutrophils are present in term infants but have decreased functional capabilities; response to infections is sluggish. Phagocytosis is less efficient. Serum complement levels are low in term infants and even lower in the preterm infant; serum complement (C1 through C6) is involved in immunologic reactions, some of which kill or lyse bacteria and enhance phagocytosis. The gut mucosal barrier is initially immature in both term and preterm infants; this barrier is enhanced by the ingestion of human colostrum, which contains antiinfective properties. Dysmaturity seen with intrauterine growth restriction (IUGR) and preterm and postdate birth further compromises the neonate's immune system.

Table 28-2 outlines risk factors for neonatal sepsis. Special precautions for preventing infection, as well as prompt recognition when it occurs, are necessary for optimum newborn care. Neonatal infections may be acquired in utero, at birth or shortly thereafter, and nosocomially.

Table 28-2 Risk Factors for Neonatal Sepsis

SOURCE	RISK FACTORS
Maternal	Low socioeconomic status Poor prenatal care Poor nutrition Substance abuse
Intrapartum	Premature rupture of fetal membranes Maternal fever Chorioamnionitis Prolonged labor Rupture of membranes >18 hr Premature labor Maternal urinary tract infection
Neonatal	Twin or multiple gestation Male Birth asphyxia Meconium aspiration Congenital anomalies of skin or mucous membranes Galactosemia Absence of spleen Low birth weight or prematurity Malnourishment Prolonged hospitalization

Neonatal bacterial infection is classified into two patterns according to the time of presentation. Early-onset or congenital sepsis usually manifests within 24 to 48 hours of birth, progresses more rapidly than later-onset infection, and carries a mortality rate as high as 50%. Early-onset sepsis is acquired in the perinatal period; infection can occur from direct contact with organisms from the maternal GI and genitourinary tracts. The most common infecting organism is *Escherichia coli*, whereas group B streptococci (GBS) rates remain low (Stoll et al, 2005). *E. coli*, which may be present in the vagina, accounts for approximately half of all cases of sepsis caused by gram-negative organisms. GBS is an extremely virulent organism in neonates, with a high (50%) death rate in affected infants. Other bacteria noted to cause early-onset infection include *Haemophilus influenzae, Citrobacter* and *Enterobacter* organisms, coagulase-negative staphylococci, and *Streptococcus viridans* (Stoll et al, 2005). Other pathogens that are harbored in the vagina and may infect the infant include gonococci, *Candida albicans*, herpes simplex virus (HSV type 2), and chlamydia. Early-onset sepsis is associated with a history of obstetric events such as preterm labor, prolonged rupture of membranes (more than 18 hours), maternal fever during labor, and chorioamnionitis (Venkatesh et al, 2006).

Late-onset sepsis, occurring approximately at 7 to 30 days of age, may include maternally derived infection or nosocomial infection; the offending organisms are usually staphylococci, *Klebsiella* organisms, enterococci, *E. coli*, and *Pseudomonas* or *Candida* species (Stoll, 2007). Coagulase-negative staphylococci, considered to be primarily a contaminant in older children and adults, are commonly found to be the cause of septicemia in extremely-low-birth-weight (ELBW) and very-low-birth-weight (VLBW) infants. Additional infections of concern include methicillin-resistant *Staphylococcus aureus*, vancomycin-resistant enterococci, and multidrug-resistant gram-negative pathogens (Stoll, 2007). Bacterial invasion can occur through sites such as the umbilical stump; the skin; mucous membranes of the eye, nose, pharynx, and ear; and internal systems such as the respiratory, nervous, urinary, and GI systems.

Perinatally acquired infections may cause miscarriage, stillbirth, intrauterine infection, congenital malformations, and acute neonatal disease. Other viral infections such as respiratory syncytial virus (RSV), rotavirus, herpes, influenza, and varicella may occur in the neonatal intensive care unit (NICU). These pathogens also may cause chronic infection, with subtle manifestations that may be recognized only after a prolonged period. It is important to recognize the manifestations of infections in the neonatal period to be able to treat the acute infection, to prevent nosocomial infections in other infants, and to anticipate effects on the infant's subsequent growth and development.

Fungal infections are of greatest concern in the immunocompromised or preterm infant. Occasionally, fungal infections such as thrush are found in otherwise healthy term infants.

Septicemia refers to a generalized infection in the bloodstream. Pneumonia, the most common form of neonatal infection, is one of the leading causes of perinatal death. Bacterial meningitis occurs in approximately 0.2 to 0.4 cases per 1000 live births, with a higher rate in preterm infants. Gastroenteritis is sporadic, depending on epidemic outbreaks. Local infections such as conjunctivitis and omphalitis occur commonly. Infection continues to be a significant factor in fetal and neonatal morbidity and mortality.

Nursing Care Management

Assessment

The prenatal record is reviewed for risk factors associated with infection and the signs and symptoms suggestive of infection. Maternal vaginal or perineal infection may be transmitted directly to the infant during passage through the birth canal. Psychosocial history and history of sexually transmitted infections (STIs) may indicate possible human immunodeficiency virus (HIV), hepatitis B virus (HBV), herpes (type 2), or cytomegalovirus (CMV) infection.

Perinatal events also are reviewed. Premature rupture of membranes (PROM) may be caused by maternal or intrauterine infection. Ascending infection may occur after prolonged PROM, prolonged labor, or intrauterine fetal monitoring. In some cases infection may occur with intact membranes or contribute to early rupture. A maternal history of fever during labor or the presence of foul-smelling amniotic fluid may also indicate infection. Antibiotic therapy initiated during labor should be noted. The neonate's gestational age, maturity, birth weight, and gender all affect the incidence of infection. Sepsis occurs about twice as often and results in a higher mortality in male than in female infants. The neonate is assessed for respiratory distress, skin abscesses, rashes, and other indications of infection.

During the postnatal period, the time of onset of suspicious signs is noted. Onset within the first 48 hours of life is more often associated with prenatal or perinatal predisposing factors; onset after 2 or 3 days more often reflects a nosocomial infection.

The earliest clinical signs of neonatal sepsis are characterized by a lack of specificity. The nonspecific signs include lethargy, poor feeding, poor weight gain, and irritability. The nurse or parent may simply note that the infant is not doing as well as before. Differential diagnosis may be difficult because signs of sepsis are similar to signs of noninfectious neonatal problems such as hypoglycemia and respiratory distress. Additional clinical and laboratory information, including cultures, supplement the findings described. Table 28-3 outlines the clinical signs associated with neonatal sepsis.

Laboratory studies are important. Specimens for cultures include blood, CSF, stool, and urine. Fluids such as urine and CSF may be evaluated by counterimmune electrophoresis or latex agglutination to assist in the identification of the bacteria. A complete blood cell count with differential is performed to determine the presence of bacterial infection or increased or decreased white blood cell count (the latter is an ominous sign). The total neutrophil count, immature to total neutrophil (I/T) ratio, absolute neutrophil count, and C-reactive protein may be used to determine the presence of sepsis. Detection of viral deoxyribonucleic acid (DNA) or antibodies by polymerase chain reaction (PCR) amplification in fluids is also an important diagnostic tool (Frenkel, 2005). Antepartum infection can now be successfully treated with a number of antiviral medications to decrease viral replication and fetal transmis-

Table 28-3 Signs of Sepsis*

SYSTEM	SIGNS
Respiratory	Apnea, bradycardia Tachypnea Grunting, nasal flaring Retractions Decreased oxygen saturation Metabolic acidosis
Cardiovascular	Decreased cardiac output Tachycardia Hypotension Decreased perfusion
Central nervous	Temperature instability Lethargy Hypotonia Irritability, seizures
Gastrointestinal	Feeding intolerance (decreased suck strength and intake; increasing residuals) Abdominal distention Vomiting, diarrhea
Integumentary	Jaundice Pallor Petechiae Mottling

Modified from Askin DF: Bacterial and fungal sepsis in the neonate, *J Obstet Gynecol Neonatal Nurs* 24(7):635-643, 1995.

*Laboratory findings include neutropenia, increased bands, hypoglycemia or hyperglycemia, metabolic acidosis, and thrombocytopenia.

sion of disease; neonates may also be treated with antiviral medications such as acyclovir and ganciclovir. Treatment with antibiotics is initiated after blood cultures are obtained in neonates; in high risk infants with significant illness, antiviral or antibiotic treatment may begin once cultures are obtained. Once the pathogen is identified, antibiotic, antiviral, or antifungal therapy may be modified.

Vigilant assessment continues during and after treatment. The newborn continues to be assessed for sequelae to septicemia, which include meningitis, disseminated intravascular coagulation (DIC), necrotizing enterocolitis, pneumonia, and septic shock. Septic shock results from the toxins released into the bloodstream. The most common signs include decreasing oxygen saturation, poor perfusion (prolonged capillary refill, cool extremities, mottling), tachycardia, respiratory distress, and hypotension.

The nursing process in the care of the infant with suspected or confirmed infection (sepsis), or with risk factors that predispose to sepsis, is outlined in the Nursing Process box.

Plan of Care and Implementation

Prevention

Virtually all controlled clinical trials have demonstrated that effective handwashing is responsible for the prevention of nosocomial infection in nursery units. Nursing is directly or indirectly responsible for minimizing or eliminating environmental sources of infectious agents in the nursery. Measures to be taken include Standard Precautions, careful and thorough cleaning of contaminated equipment, frequent replacement of used equipment (e.g., changing intravenous and nasogastric tubing per hospital protocol, and cleaning resuscitation and ventilation equipment, intravenous pumps, and incubators), and appropriate disposal of contaminated linens and diapers. Overcrowding must be avoided in nurseries. Guidelines for space, visitation, and general infection control in areas where newborns receive care have been established and published (American Academy of Pediatrics & American College of Obstetricians and Gynecologists, 2007).

Infants cared for in NICUs are at high risk for infection. In a study of infants in the National Institute for Child Health and Human Development's Neonatal Research Network, of those who survived beyond 3 days, 25% had one or more instances of blood culture–proven sepsis. Of those infants with sepsis, 17% died. Infection rates vary from center to center, from 11.5% to 34% (Buus-Frank, 2004). Handwashing is the single most effective measure to reduce nosocomial infection. However, the rate of compliance with standards for hand hygiene is only 22%. The combined use of alcohol, hand hygiene, and gloves is effective in reducing the incidence of systemic infection (Buus-Frank, 2004). It is incumbent on caregivers to strictly adhere to recommended guidelines for hand hygiene.

Antibiotic is instilled into newborn's eyes 1 to 2 hours after birth to prevent infection (see Fig. 25-3). The skin, its secretions, and normal flora are natural defenses that protect against invading pathogens. Warm water may be used to remove blood and meconium from the neonate's face, head, and body. A mild nonmedicated soap (in single-use container) can be used with careful water rinsing. Vernix caseosa is not scrubbed vigorously for removal, since this further disrupts the skin barrier properties (see Guidelines box, p. 721). No single method of cord care has been shown to be more effective in the promotion of drying, separation, and prevention of colonization. Current recommendations for cord care by the Association of Women's Health, Obstetric and Neonatal Nurses (2007) include cleaning the cord with sterile water or a neutral pH cleanser; subsequent care entails cleansing the cord with water. Nurses must follow agency protocols for cord care, but they can recommend revision of protocols based on research (see also Umbilical Cord Care, Chapter 25, p. 651).

NURSING ALERT Artificial and long natural fingernails worn by nurses have been associated with serious neonatal infection and morbidity from *Pseudomonas aeruginosa* (Moolenaar et al, 2000) and *Klebsiella* organisms in the NICU (Gupta et al, 2004).

Care Management

Breastfeeding or feeding the newborn breast milk from the mother is encouraged. Breast milk provides protective mechanisms. Colostrum contains IgA, which offers protection against infection in the GI tract. Human milk contains iron-binding protein that exerts a bacteriostatic effect on *E. coli.* Human milk also contains macrophages and lymphocytes. The vulnerability of infants to common mucosal pathogens such as RSV may be reduced by passive transfer of maternal immunity in the colostrum and breast milk. Some evidence indicates that early enteral feedings with human milk (trophic or minimal enteral feedings) may be beneficial in establishing

NURSING PROCESS: NEWBORN WITH SUSPECTED SEPSIS

Assessment

The prenatal history, delivery history, and newborn's physical and gestational age assessment are reviewed for infection risk factors. Individual assessment findings are used to plan care for each newborn.

Nursing Diagnoses

Various nursing diagnoses are possible, depending on the type of infection, the newborn's gestational age and birth weight, and clinical manifestations. Examples of nursing diagnoses related to neonatal infections include the following:

Neonate

Risk for infection related to
- maternal infection (diagnosed or otherwise; e.g., chorioamnionitis)
- indwelling umbilical catheters, parenteral fluids (invasive procedures)
- intrauterine electronic fetal monitoring
- fetal dysmaturity, intrauterine growth restriction, low gestational age

Ineffective thermoregulation related to
- systemic infection

Impaired skin integrity related to
- use of multiple supportive invasive measures (e.g., physiologic monitoring, parenteral fluid therapy, inhalation therapy)

Pain (acute) related to
- multiple supportive invasive measures

Parents and Family

Anxiety, fear, or anticipatory grieving related to
- uncertainty about infant's prognosis
- therapy (invasive)

Risk for impaired parent-infant attachment related to
- separation of parent and newborn
- feelings of inadequacy in caring for infant

Powerlessness or spiritual distress related to
- perinatal events or newborn's condition beyond parents' control

Planning and Implementation

Parents and family are encouraged to participate in planning. Expected outcomes include the following:
- The newborn will remain free of infection.
- The newborn's clinical manifestations or suspicion of sepsis will be recognized and reported, and appropriate diagnosis and therapy will be instituted.
- If therapy is necessary, the newborn will suffer no harmful sequelae.
- Parents will begin interacting and caring for the newborn and be involved in his or her care.
- Parents will maintain self-esteem by understanding that their role as parents is important to the newborn's well-being.

A number of implementation strategies are discussed on pp. 746-748.

Evaluation

The nurse can be reasonably assured that care was effective if the outcomes established for care are met.

a natural barrier to infection in ELBW and VLBW infants (Anderson et al, 2006). Human milk is thought to provide some degree of protection from necrotizing enterocolitis (Diehl-Jones & Askin, 2004).

Administering medications, taking precautions when performing treatments, and following isolation procedures are also interventions to consider in the prevention and treatment of neonatal sepsis.

Monitoring the intravenous infusion rate and administering antibiotics are nursing responsibilities. It is important to administer the prescribed dose of antibiotic within 1 hour after it is prepared to avoid loss of drug stability. If the intravenous fluid the infant is receiving contains electrolytes, vitamins, or other medications, the nurse should check with the hospital pharmacy before adding antibiotics. The antibiotic (or other medication) may be deactivated or may form a precipitate when combined with other medications.

Care must be taken in suctioning secretions from any newborn's oropharynx or trachea. Routine suctioning is not recommended and may further compromise the infant's immune status, cause hypoxia, and increase ICP. Isolation procedures are implemented as indicated according to hospital policy. Isolation protocols change rapidly, and the nurse is urged to participate in continuing education and in-service programs to remain up to date.

Perinatally Acquired Infections

The occurrence of certain maternal infections during early pregnancy is known to be associated with various congenital malformations and disorders. An acronym that is often used in clinical practice is TORCH, which stands for *t*oxoplasmosis, *o*ther (gonorrhea, hepatitis B, syphilis, varicella-zoster virus, parvovirus B19, and HIV), *r*ubella, *c*ytomegalovirus, and *h*erpes simplex virus) (Box 28-1). Additional diagnostic studies specific to perinatal infectious agents are also considered. One of the problems with these viral infections is the lack of maternal symptomatology, resulting in lack of treatment and thus often producing an affected newborn at birth. With the advent of newer diagnostic methods, these viral infections may be diagnosed in utero and interventions planned based on the availability of intrauterine treatments.

HSV may result in a severe, often fatal systemic illness in neonates. Survivors of herpetic infection may have residual

BOX 28-1 TORCH Infections Affecting Newborns

T—Toxoplasmosis
O—Other: gonorrhea, syphilis, varicella, hepatitis B virus, human parvovirus B19, human immunodeficiency virus
R—Rubella
C—Cytomegalovirus
H—Herpes simplex virus

CNS damage (encephalitis) and chorioretinitis. The other congenital infections also may result in encephalopathy with various anomalies, including microcephaly, chorioretinitis, intracranial calcifications, microphthalmos, and cataracts. To a certain extent, the varied clinical manifestations of these infections overlap, but a specific diagnosis can be made by the clustering of clinical findings and specific antibody studies.

Toxoplasmosis

Toxoplasmosis is a multisystem disease caused by the protozoan *Toxoplasma gondii.* Cats that hunt infected birds and mice harbor the parasite and excrete the infective oocysts in their feces. Human infection follows hand-to-mouth contact, such as after disposing of cat litter or after handling or ingesting raw meat from cattle or sheep that grazed in contaminated fields, or from eating unwashed or unpeeled fruits or vegetables. First-trimester exposure to the protozoan is more serious for the fetus than third-trimester or perinatal transmission. Intrauterine detection of the condition may occur as early as 18 weeks using PCR of the gene (B1) of the protozoa in amniotic fluid. The detection of intrauterine infection and subsequent maternal treatment with spiramycin may prevent fetal infection (Boyer & Boyer, 2004).

More than 70% of affected infants are free of symptoms. The clinical features of toxoplasmosis resemble those of cytomegalic inclusion disease in the infant. Both diseases are responsible for serious perinatal mortality and morbidity: 10% to 15% die, 85% have severe psychomotor problems or cognitive impairment by age 2 to 4 years, and 50% have visual problems by age 1 year.

Severe toxoplasmosis is associated with preterm birth, growth restriction, microcephaly or hydrocephaly, microphthalmos, chorioretinitis, CNS calcification, thrombocytopenia, jaundice, and fever. Petechiae or a maculopapular rash may also be evident. Some clinical manifestations do not develop until later in life. The affected infant may be treated with pyrimethamine and oral sulfadiazine, but folic acid supplement will be required to prevent anemia.

Gonorrhea

The incidence of gonococcal infection in pregnant women ranges from 2.5% to 7.3%. Many women with gonorrhea often have a concurrent *Chlamydia trachomatis* infection (American Academy of Pediatrics, Committee on Infectious Diseases, 2006). After rupture of membranes, ascending *Neisseria gonorrhoeae* infection can result in orogastric contamination of the fetus. The organism also may invade mucosal surfaces such as the conjunctiva (ophthalmia neonatorum), rectal mucosa, and pharynx. Contamination may occur as the infant passes through the birth canal, or it may occur postnatally from an infected adult. Neonatal conjunctivitis usually appears 2 to 5 days after delivery. Neonatal gonococcal arthritis, septicemia, meningitis, vaginitis, and scalp abscesses can also develop.

Eye prophylaxis (e.g., with 0.5% erythromycin ointment) is administered within the first hour after birth to prevent ophthalmia neonatorum (American Academy of Pediatrics & American College of Obstetricians and Gynecologists, 2007). The infant with a mild infection often recovers completely with appropriate treatment (e.g., single dose of intramuscular or intravenous ceftriaxone). Occasionally, infants die of overwhelming infection in the early neonatal period. The newborn with clinical disease should be admitted to a hospital for treatment (American Academy of Pediatrics & American College of Obstetricians and Gynecologists, 2007).

Syphilis

Congenital and neonatal syphilis have reemerged in recent years as significant health problems. It is estimated that for every 100 women diagnosed with primary or secondary disease, two to five infants will contract congenital syphilis. If syphilis during pregnancy is untreated, 40% to 50% of neonates born to these women will have symptomatic congenital syphilis. Treatment failure can occur, particularly when treatment is given in the third trimester; therefore infants born to women treated after 20 weeks of gestation should be investigated for congenital syphilis.

Fetal infestation with the spirochete *Treponema pallidum* is blocked by Langhans' layer in the chorion until this layer begins to atrophy between 16 and 18 weeks of gestation. If spirochetemia is untreated, it will result in fetal death by midtrimester, miscarriage, or stillbirth (in one in four cases). All neonates in whom the infection occurs before 7 months of gestation are affected. Only 60% are affected if the infection occurs late in pregnancy. If maternal infection is treated adequately before the eighteenth week, neonates seldom demonstrate signs of the disease. Although treatment after the eighteenth week may cure fetal spirochetemia, pathologic changes may not be prevented completely.

Because the fetus becomes infected after the period of organogenesis (first trimester), organs develop normally. Congenital syphilis may stimulate preterm labor, but no evidence indicates that it causes IUGR. Organs affected later by congenital syphilis may include the liver, spleen, kidneys, adrenal glands, and bone covering and marrow. Disorders of the CNS, teeth, and cornea may not become evident until several months after birth.

The most severely affected infants have untreated mothers, and the newborn may be hydropic (edematous) and anemic, with enlarged liver and spleen. Hepatosplenomegaly probably results from extramedullary hematopoietic activity stimulated by the severe anemia. In some infants, signs of congenital syphilis do not appear until late in the neonatal period. In these newborns, early signs such as poor feeding, slight hyperthermia, and snuffles may be nonspecific. The term *snuffles* refers to the copious, clear, serosanguineous mucus discharge from the neonate's nose. A mucopurulent discharge indicates secondary infection, usually by streptococci or staphylococci.

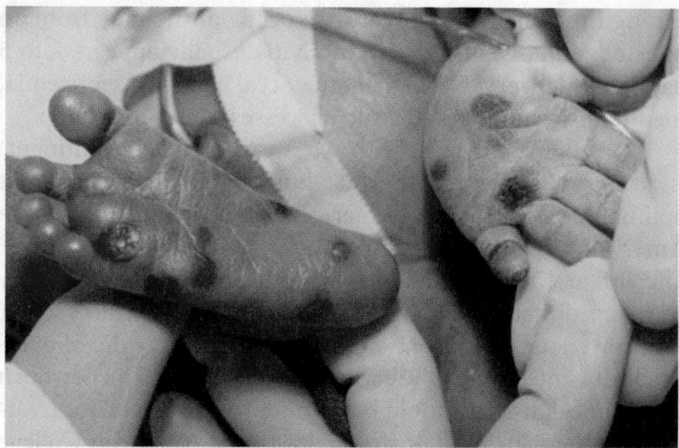

Fig. 28-4 Neonatal syphilis lesions on hands and feet. *(Courtesy Mahesh Kotwal, MD, Phoenix, AZ.)*

By the end of the first week of life, a copper-colored maculopapular dermal rash appears in untreated newborns. The rash is characteristically first noticeable on the palms of the hands, on the soles of the feet (Fig. 28-4), in the diaper area, and around the mouth and anus. The maculopapular lesions may become vesicular and confluent and extend over the trunk and extremities. Condylomata (elevated, wartlike lesions) may be seen around the anus. Rough, cracked, mucocutaneous lesions of the lips heal to form circumoral radiating scars known as *rhagades.*

If the mother was adequately treated before giving birth and serologic testing of the infant does not reveal syphilis, generally the infant is not treated with antibiotics. The infant is checked for antibody titer (received from the mother via the placenta) every 2 weeks for 3 months, at which time the test result should be negative. Some physicians recommend antibiotic therapy for asymptomatic or inconclusive cases.

A 10-day course of aqueous penicillin G or procaine penicillin G (consult drug references for dosage and administration route for each) is the usual treatment for congenital syphilis (Boyer & Boyer, 2004). Erythromycin is the substitute antibiotic of choice for infants sensitive to penicillin.

NURSING ALERT The infant with congenital syphilis may be entirely asymptomatic until after discharge from the birth hospital. It is therefore imperative that caregivers use Standard Precautions with all newborns.

In general, treatment of syphilis is more effective if it is begun early rather than later in the course of the disease. However, a recurrence rate of 5% can be expected. Even adequate treatment of congenital syphilis after birth does not always prevent late complication (e.g., 5 to 15 years after initial infection). Potential complications include neurosyphilis, deafness, Hutchinson's teeth (notched incisors), saber shins, joint involvement, saddle nose (depressed bridge), gummas (soft, gummy tumors) over the skin and other organs, and interstitial keratitis (inflammation of the cornea).

Varicella Zoster

The varicella zoster virus responsible for chickenpox and shingles is a member of the herpes family. About 90% of women in their childbearing years are immune; therefore risk of infection in pregnancy is low, 0.7 to 3 per 1000 bir (Birthistle & Carrington, 1998; Chapman, 1998).

Varicella transmission to the fetus may occur across placenta when the disease is contracted in the first half pregnancy, but this is relatively infrequent. When transm sion to the fetus does occur in the early part of pregnancy, effects on the fetus include limb atrophy, neurologic abn malities, eye abnormalities, and IUGR.

When maternal infection occurs in the last few days pregnancy, 20% of infants born to these mothers develop cli cal varicella (Boyer & Boyer, 2004). The severity of the infa illness increases greatly if maternal infection occurred wit 5 days before or 2 days after birth. The neonatal mortality severe illness is 30% (Chapman, 1998; Sauerbrei & Wutz 2007).

Infants born to mothers who develop chickenpox betwe 5 days before birth and 2 days after birth should be giv varicella zoster immune globulin (VariZIG) at birth becau of the risk of severe disease. Acyclovir can be used to tr infants with generalized involvement and pneumonia (Mye Seward, & LaRussa, 2007).

Term infants exposed to chickenpox after birth will ha either a mild infection or no infection if they are born immune mothers. Those born to nonimmune mothers m develop chickenpox, but the course is not usually severe. hospitalized preterm infants (28 or more weeks of gestatio whose mother lacks a reliable history of varicella or no e dence of protection, and hospitalized preterm infants less th 28 weeks of gestation or less than 1000 g at birth, are at r regardless of their mother's status and should receive eith acyclovir or VariZIG if exposed to chickenpox (Americ Academy of Pediatrics, Committee on Infectious Diseas 2006).

Hepatitis B Virus

HBV infection during pregnancy is not associated with increase in malformations, stillbirths, or IUGR; however, t risk for preterm birth increases about 32%. The transmissi rate of HBV to the newborn ranges from 70% to 90% wh the mother is seropositive for both hepatitis B surface an gen (HbsAg) and hepatitis B e antigen (HbeAg) (Americ Academy of Pediatrics, Committee on Infectious Diseas 2006). More than 90% of infants infected in the perina period will develop chronic HBV infection. Transmissi occurs infrequently (less than 2%) and occurs transplace tally; serum to serum; and by contact with contaminat blood, urine, feces, saliva, semen, or vaginal secretions duri birth. Infants are most commonly infected during birth or the first few days of life. The rate of transmission is high when the mother contracts the virus immediately before bir These mothers will be positive for HBsAg. Transmission m occur through breast milk, but antigens also develop formula-fed infants at the same or higher rate. Diagnosis made by viral culture of amniotic fluid and by the presence HBsAg and IgM in the cord blood or newborn's serum.

Neonatal and fetal effects are serious. Infants may symptom free at birth or show evidence of acute hepatitis wi changes in liver function. The mortality for severe cases hepatitis is 75%. Infants who become carriers are at high risk for chronic hepatitis, cirrhosis of the liver, or liver cancer even years later (Yudin & Gonik, 2006).

Infants whose mothers have antibodies for HBsAg or who have developed hepatitis during pregnancy or the postpartum period should be treated with hepatitis B immune globulin, 0.5 ml IM, as soon as possible after birth or within the first 12 hours of life. The hepatitis B vaccine should be given concurrently, but at a different site (American Academy of Pediatrics, Committee on Infectious Diseases, 2006). The second dose of vaccine is given at 1 month and the third dose at 6 months. The vaccine should protect the child for up to 9 years. After the infant has been cleansed thoroughly and has received the vaccine, breastfeeding may be initiated. Vaccination for infants not exposed to maternal HBV is recommended before discharge from the birth hospital; breastfeeding for these infants may begin before the vaccine is given.

Human Immunodeficiency Virus (Type 1)

It is estimated that, at the end of 2004, 2.2 million children under the age of 15 years were infected with HIV; more than 90% of those children lived in developing countries. The total number of children with active viral infection in the United States decreased by almost 95% by the year 2003 to less than 100 cases annually (Yogev & Chadwick, 2007). The decline is reportedly due to decreased perinatal transmission of the virus as a result of decreased maternal-to-infant transmission and potent antiretroviral drug therapy (American Academy of Pediatrics, Committee on Infectious Diseases, 2006). The majority of cases of pediatric acquired immunodeficiency syndrome (AIDS) (90% or more) result from maternal-to-fetal transmission. Universal counseling and screening of pregnant women is recommended in the United States and Canada.

Transmission of HIV from the mother to the infant may occur transplacentally at various gestational ages. The risk of infection in an infant born to an HIV-positive mother (not treated) is approximately 13% to 39% (American Academy of Pediatrics, Committee on Infectious Diseases, 2006). Globally the rate of maternal transmission of the virus is estimated to be 25%. With antepartum, intrapartum, and neonatal zidovudine treatment, the incidence of neonatal HIV infection is decreased to 5% to 8%, and compliance with highly active antiretroviral therapy (HAART) is said to further reduce newborn infection rates to 1% to 2% (American Academy of Pediatrics, Committee on Pediatric AIDS, 2008; Cooper et al, 2002; Kriebs, 2002). An elective cesarean section is said to further decrease perinatal transmission by 87% when zidovudine therapy is administered to both the mother and newborn. A critical factor in perinatal transmission is the maternal viral load; a high viral load (especially more than 100,000 copies/ml) creates a greater chance (up to 40%) for perinatal transmission of the virus. Postpartum transmission may also occur, with an additional risk of 14% attributed to breast milk contact (American Academy of Pediatrics, Committee on Infectious Diseases, 2006).

Diagnosis of HIV infection in the neonate is complicated by the presence of maternal IgG antibodies, which cross the placenta after 32 weeks of gestation. The most accurate test for newborns and infants younger than 18 months is the HIV-1 DNA PCR assay, which is performed on neonatal blood, not cord blood (American Academy of Pediatrics, Committee on Infectious Diseases, 2006). Follow-up testing for infants born to HIV-positive mothers is recommended at several intervals within the first year of life.

Typically the HIV-infected neonate is asymptomatic at birth. Early-onset illness (i.e., virus detected within 48 hours of birth) is attributed to prenatal infection and occurs in 10% to 15% of infected infants. These infants develop opportunistic infections (*Candida* and *pneumocystis carinii* pneumonia [PCP]) and rapid progression of immunodeficiency, which progresses to death in the first 1 to 2 years of life.

The remainder of infants seroconvert over a period of months to years. By 1 year of life, 80% to 90% of perinatally infected infants show signs of infection. Some children infected at birth show no signs of disease 8 to 10 years later. The age of onset of symptoms predicts the length of survival.

The presenting signs and symptoms of HIV infection vary from severe immunodeficiency to nonspecific findings such as growth failure, parotitis, and recurrent or persistent upper respiratory tract infections. In the first year of life, lymphadenopathy and hepatosplenomegaly are common. The infant may have fever, chronic diarrhea, chronic dermatitis, interstitial pneumonitis, persistent thrush, and AIDS-defining opportunistic infections. Common secondary opportunistic infections include PCP, candidiasis, CMV, cryptosporidiosis, herpes simplex or herpes zoster, and disseminated varicella.

Nursing Care Management

Although it is rare for an infant to be born with symptoms of HIV infection, all infants born to seropositive mothers should be presumed to be HIV positive until proven otherwise. Management begins by implementing Standard Precautions. Measures should also be taken to protect the infant from further exposure to maternal blood and body fluids. Breastfeeding is avoided completely if the mother is HIV positive. Regimens for the prevention of HIV transmission include antepartum, intrapartum, and neonatal treatment with HAART. Children who are HIV positive may be treated with a combination of three antiretroviral drugs: two nucleoside reverse transcriptase inhibitors, such as zidovudine and stavudine, plus either a protease inhibitor such as nelfinavir, lopinavir, or saquinavir, or a nonnucleoside reverse transcriptase such as nevirapine (American Academy of Pediatrics, Committee on Infectious Diseases, 2006; Yogev & Chadwick, 2007). Some children may not require treatment if viral load is low and risk for disease progression is minimal. In either case a consultation with a pediatric HIV specialist is recommended. If the infant is diagnosed with HIV infection, the family should be counseled about conventional and investigational treatment options.

The goal in the administration of antivirals is the suppression of the virus to undetectable concentrations; the available antiviral drugs do not, however, cure the child's disease (American Academy of Pediatrics, Committee on Infectious Diseases, 2006). HIV diagnosis in the neonatal period combined with aggressive antibiotic treatment of opportunistic infections such as PCP has the potential to prolong survival in children (American Academy of Pediatrics, Committee on Infectious Diseases, 2006). Studies of HIV symptoms in children treated in the era of HAART show a significant decrease in the incidence of secondary opportunistic infections (Nesheim et al, 2007). Long-term outcomes (18 and 36 months) in children treated with HAART show that children exposed to therapy had lower developmental scores and adaptive behavior scores than children who had not been exposed to HAART; however, the researchers attributed the lower scores to a high incidence and subsequent effect of maternal substance abuse (Alimenti et al, 2006).

Counseling regarding the care of the mothers themselves, the family's care of the infant, and future pregnancies should be provided. The risk for transmission among members of the same household is minimal. Social services are required in these cases. If the parent chooses to keep the infant, home health care may be arranged. For more information and updated information, parents are referred to the National AIDS Hotline, 1-800-342-AIDS.

In the United States, breastfeeding by the HIV-positive mother is contraindicated; however, in developing countries, the risks vs. benefits in relation to number of infant deaths attributed to poor sanitary conditions and availability of an appropriate food supply for infants are considered. The World Health Organization (2008) recommends exclusive breastfeeding for 6 months in infants with HIV-positive mothers in developing countries where the infant food supply is not readily available or has a greater chance of contamination (poor sanitary conditions, water supply). Studies in developing countries show that interrupting breastfeeding at 3 to 4 months, even if the mother is HIV positive, increases infant mortality rates from diarrhea and other illnesses (Ogundele & Coulter, 2003).

The family must be counseled about vaccinations. Children with symptomatic or asymptomatic HIV infection should receive all routine vaccines. Although data regarding children with HIV and varicella vaccine are limited, the American Academy of Pediatrics, Committee on Infectious Diseases (2006), recommends that children with no or mild symptoms be immunized for varicella.

Rubella Infection

Since rubella vaccination was begun in 1969, cases of congenital rubella have been reduced dramatically; however, it is still seen occasionally in the newborn. Vaccination failures, lack of compliance, and the immigration of unimmunized persons result in periodic outbreaks of rubella, also known as *German* or *3-day measles*.

The risk for congenital anomalies varies with the fetus's gestational age at the time maternal infection occurs. Abnormalities are most severe if the mother contracts the virus during the first trimester (occurrence of congenital defects as high as 85% in first 12 weeks of gestation, 54% in first 13 to 16 weeks of gestation, and 25% during the end of the second trimester [American Academy of Pediatrics, Committee on Infectious Diseases, 2006]).

More than two thirds of infected infants have no symptoms apparent at birth, but sequelae may develop years later. Hearing loss, the most common result, appears to be progressive after birth. Initially the newborn may be seen with hepatosplenomegaly, lymphedema, IUGR, jaundice, hepatitis, thrombocytopenic purpura with petechiae, and the characteristic blueberry muffin lesions (dermal erythropoiesis). Congenital rubella syndrome often includes chronic problems such as cataracts or glaucoma, sensorineural hearing impairment, hypogammaglobulinemia, peripheral pulmonary stenosis, and diabetes mellitus type 1 (Boyer & Boyer, 2004). The rubella virus has been cultured in infants for up to 18 months after their birth. These infants are a serious source of infection to susceptible individuals, particularly women in the childbearing years. Extended pediatric isolation is mandatory until the noncontagious stage of rubella has been reached (i.e., the infant should be isolated until pharyngeal mucus and the urine are free of virus).

Cytomegalovirus Infection

CMV infection during pregnancy may result in miscarriage, stillbirth, or congenital illness. It is the most common cause of congenital viral infections in the United States (Michaels, 2007; Boyer & Boyer, 2004). Most (90% to 95%) of the infected infants are asymptomatic at birth; however, sensorineural hearing impairment and learning disabilities have been reported in previously asymptomatic infants.

Only approximately 10% of infants with congenital CMV will display severe involvement and may have IUGR and microcephaly. The neonate may also have a rash, jaundice, and hepatosplenomegaly (Fig. 28-5). Anemia, thrombocytopenia, and hyperbilirubinemia are common in the early stages of the illness. Intracranial, periventricular calcification often is noted on radiography. Inclusion bodies ("owl's eye" figures) in cells sedimented from freshly voided urine or in liver biopsy specimens are typical.

The virus may be isolated from urine or saliva of the newborn using the PCR assay. Differential diagnosis includes other causes of jaundice, syphilis (positive Venereal Disease Research Laboratories findings), toxoplasmosis (positive Sabin-Feldman dye test result), hemolytic disease of the newborn (positive Coombs' test reaction), or coxsackievirus infection (positive culture).

Milder forms of the disease often result when the fetus is infected late in pregnancy. CMV can be transmitted through

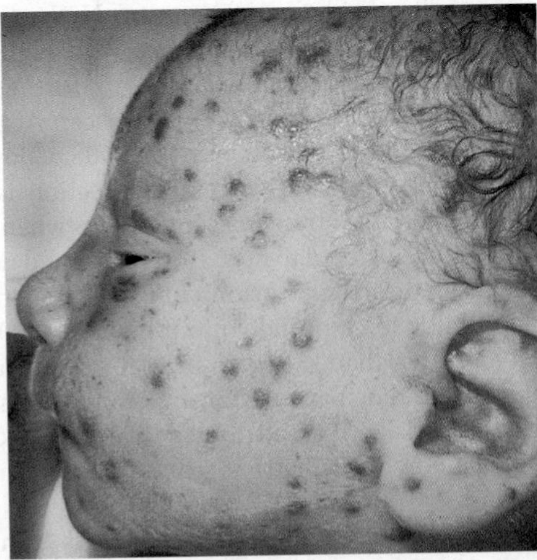

Fig. 28-5 Neonatal cytomegalovirus infection. Typical rash seen in a severely affected infant. *(Courtesy David A. Clarke, Philadelphia, PA.)*

breast milk while the mother is experiencing acute CMV syndrome. CMV infections acquired after birth are often asymptomatic and have no sequelae. Exceptions to this occur in preterm infants, in whom postnatal acquisition of CMV can result in pneumonia, hepatitis, thrombocytopenia, and long-term neurologic sequelae.

Antenatally infected infants who are asymptomatic at birth are at risk for late sequelae. Hearing loss may not be apparent until after the first year of life. Chorioretinitis, microcephaly, cognitive impairment, and neuromuscular deficits may occur by 2 years of age. Some children are at risk for a defect in tooth enamel, resulting in severe caries.

Treatment of the infected newborn with ganciclovir has proved effective in decreasing neurologic sequelae, in particular sensorineural hearing loss (Schleiss, 2008).

Herpes Simplex Virus

HSV infections among newborns are being diagnosed more frequently and are estimated to occur in as many as 1 in 3000 to 1 in 20,000 births. HSV type 2 is the most common cause of HSV illness in neonates (75%) (American Academy of Pediatrics, Committee on Infectious Diseases, 2006).

The neonate may acquire the virus by any of four modes of transmission:

1. Transplacental infection
2. Ascending infection by way of the birth canal
3. Direct contamination during passage through an infected birth canal
4. Direct transmission from infected personnel or family

Congenital infection is rare and is characterized by in utero destruction of normally formed organs. Affected infants are growth restricted and are more likely to be born preterm. They have severe psychomotor restriction, with intracranial calcifications, microcephaly, hypertonicity, and seizures. They suffer eye involvement, including microphthalmos, cataracts, chorioretinitis, blindness, and retinal dysplasia. Some infants have patent ductus arteriosus, limb anomalies, and recurrent skin vesicles, with a short life expectancy.

Most infants are infected directly during passage through the birth canal. The risk of infection during vaginal birth in the presence of genital herpes is estimated to be 33% to 50%, with active primary infection at term. The transmission rate of chronic vaginal herpes from the pregnant woman to her newborn is low. Passive intrauterine immunity to herpes may be responsible. In a recent study, clinical and laboratory features associated with neonatal herpes included maternal primary HSV infection, vaginal delivery, preterm birth, neonatal seizures, elevated liver enzymes, vesicular rash, and elevated CSF counts (Caviness, Demmler, & Selwyn, 2008).

Postnatal acquisition of the virus and spread within a nursery have been documented by DNA analysis. Both mother and father (including maternal breast lesions) have been implicated in neonatal infections. There also is concern regarding symptomatic and asymptomatic shedding among hospital personnel. Nursery personnel with cold sores should practice strict handwashing and wear a mask, but no evidence indicates they should be removed from the nursery unless they have a herpetic whitlow (primary HSV infection of the terminal segment of a finger).

Clinically, neonatal HSV infections are classified as disseminated infection; localized CNS disease; or localized infection of the skin, eye, or mouth. Disseminated infections may involve virtually every organ system, but those primarily involved are the liver, adrenal glands, and lungs. Affected infants exhibit initial symptoms usually in the first week of life but sometimes in the second week, with signs of bacterial sepsis or shock. Clinical manifestations include skin vesicles in about 33% of infants. Death results from progression of CNS involvement, respiratory distress and pneumonitis, shock, DIC, and bleeding; the mortality rate without antiviral therapy is approximately 25% (American Academy of Pediatrics, Committee on Infectious Diseases, 2006).

Nursing Care Management

Standard Precautions should be observed when caregivers have contact with these infants. The neonate's eyes, oral cavity, and skin are inspected carefully for the presence of any lesions (Fig. 28-6). Cultures are obtained from the mouth, eyes, and any lesions. Circumcision, if performed, is delayed until the infant is ready to be discharged. The infant may be discharged with the mother if the infant's cultures are negative for the virus. As long as no suspicious lesions are on the mother's breasts, breastfeeding is allowed. For the infant at risk, a prophylactic topical eye ointment (vidarabine, iododeoxyuridine, or trifluridine) is administered for 5 days to prevent keratoconjunctivitis. Parenteral acyclovir is recommended as standard therapy for neonatal herpes; neonates with ocular manifestations should receive acyclovir as well as the eye ointment. Blood, urine, and CSF specimens should be cultured when indicated clinically. If herpetic lesions first occur after 6 weeks of life, the risk of dissemination and severe illness is very low (Baley & Toltzis, 2006).

Parvovirus B19

Parvovirus B19 is well known in older children as fifth disease or "slapped cheek illness" because of the characteristic facial appearance of the affected child. During pregnancy, infection may result in fetal miscarriage or the development of fetal hydrops and IUGR. The estimated risk of transplacental

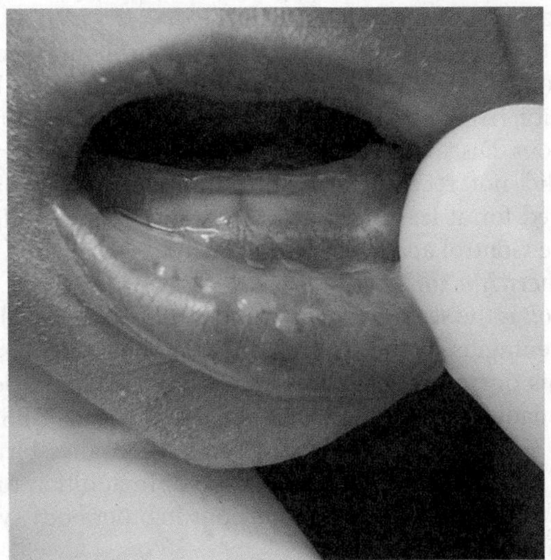

Fig. 28-6 Herpes simplex virus oral lesions. *(Courtesy David A. Clarke, Philadelphia, PA.)*

transmission is approximately 30%, and fetal death may occur in about 9% of those affected (Boyer & Boyer, 2004). Protocols for intrauterine management have not been well developed, but intrauterine transfusion to treat anemia is the only currently accepted therapy (de Jong et al, 2006). Serial ultrasounds to detect fetal hydrops are possible. The virus may be isolated from amniotic fluid, fetal blood, or tissues using DNA PCR assay (Boyer & Boyer, 2004). Pericardial, pleural, and peritoneal effusions are common and fatal if not treated immediately, with cardiac failure from anemia being the most common cause of death.

Bacterial Infections

Group B Streptococcus

Historically GBS was one of the most common causes of neonatal sepsis and meningitis in the United States; however, antepartum maternal screening and administration of penicillin have significantly decreased the incidence of GBS. The Centers for Disease Control and Prevention (2002b) reported that, as a result of screening and treatment of maternal GBS in the 1990s, the incidence of GBS decreased by 70% to a low of 0.5 cases per 1000 live births in 1999. Early-onset GBS rates decreased to 0.31 cases per 1000 live births from 2000 to 2003 and increased slightly to 0.40 cases per live births from 2003 to 2006 (Centers for Disease Control and Prevention, 2009b). Early-onset GBS infection in the neonate occurs in the first 7 days of life but most commonly manifests in the first 24 hours after birth. Risk factors for the development of early-onset GBS include low birth weight, preterm birth, rupture of membranes of more than 18 hours, maternal fever, previous GBS infant, maternal GBS bacteriuria, and multiple gestation. Usually resulting from vertical transmission from the birth canal, early-onset disease results in a respiratory illness that mimics the symptoms of severe respiratory distress syndrome. The infant may rapidly develop septic shock, which has a significant mortality rate.

Late-onset GBS infection manifests between 1 week and 3 months of age with an average age of onset of 24 days. Eighty-five percent of infants with late-onset GBS have meningitis; this population has a mortality rate of 5%. Fifty percent of the survivors develop neurologic damage.

In the newborn with presumptive or confirmed GBS infection, penicillin and an aminoglycoside are the therapy of choice (American Academy of Pediatrics, Committee on Infectious Diseases, 2006). The newborn born to a mother who did not receive complete intrapartum prophylaxis is observed for at least 48 hours before discharge (Centers for Disease Control and Prevention, 2002b).

Escherichia coli

E. coli is the second most common cause of neonatal sepsis and meningitis in the United States, although some suggest that this organism has increased in the VLBW and possibly term infant as a result of maternal prophylaxis for GBS (Stoll, 2007). *E. coli* is found in the GI tract soon after birth and makes up the bulk of human fecal flora. In addition to meningitis, *E. coli* can also cause infections in other body systems, including the urinary tract.

Tuberculosis

The incidence of tuberculosis (TB), which is caused by *Mycobacterium tuberculosis*, is increasing in Canada and the United States; most cases observed in children under 14 are in international adoptees and foreign-born immigrants (American Academy of Pediatrics, Committee on Infectious Diseases, 2006). Congenitally acquired TB, although rare, can cause otitis media, pneumonia, hepatosplenomegaly, enlarged lymph glands, or disseminated disease. After birth, exposed infants contract TB through droplets expelled by infected individuals, which results in pneumonia and necrosis of lung tissue. Untreated neonatal tuberculosis is almost always fatal.

Chlamydia Infection

Chlamydia trachomatis is an intracellular bacterium that causes neonatal conjunctivitis and pneumonia. Chlamydia infection is the most commonly reported notifiable disease in the United States and is one of the most common STIs (Centers for Disease Control and Prevention, 2008). The conjunctivitis, with minimal watery discharge, develops 5 days to 2 weeks after birth. Inclusion conjunctivitis is usually self-limiting, but if it is untreated, chronic follicular conjunctivitis (trachoma) with conjunctival scarring and corneal microgranulations has been reported. The organism may spread to the lungs from nasal secretions if left untreated, causing chlamydia pneumonia in about 33% of infected infants, with symptoms of a repetitive staccato cough, tachypnea, rales, hyperinflation, and bilateral diffuse infiltrates on radiographic examination (Popovich & McAlhany, 2004).

Ophthalmic silver nitrate, 0.5% erythromycin, and 1% tetracycline are not effective against *C. trachomatis;* therefore it is recommended that infants born to mothers who are positive for chlamydia be monitored closely for the development of symptoms. The neonate with positive cultures should be treated with oral erythromycin (American Academy of Pediatrics, Committee on Infectious Diseases, 2006) or oral sulfonamide for 2 to 3 weeks. Erythromycin administration in infants younger than 6 weeks has been associated with an increased risk of infantile hypertrophic pyloric stenosis; therefore parents should be educated regarding the symptoms of the condition (feeding intolerance, projectile vomiting, and abdominal distention).

Fungal Infections

Candidiasis

Candida infections, formerly known as *moniliasis,* may occur in the newborn. *C. albicans,* the organism usually responsible, may cause disease in any organ system. It is a yeastlike fungus (producing yeast cells and spores) that can be acquired from a maternal vaginal infection during birth; by person-to-person transmission; or from contaminated hands, bottles, nipples, or other articles. It usually is a benign disorder in the neonate, often confined to the oral and diaper regions. Diaper dermatitis caused by *Candida* organisms manifests as a moist, erythematous eruption with small white or yellow pebbly pustules. Small areas of skin erosion may also be seen.

Candidal diaper dermatitis appears on the perianal area, inguinal folds, and lower portion of the abdomen. The affected area is intensely erythematous, with a sharply demarcated, scalloped edge, often with numerous satellite lesions that extend beyond the larger lesion. The source of the infection can be through the GI tract or caretakers' hands. Topical application of 1 ml nystatin (Mycostatin) over the surfaces of the oral cavity four times a day, or every 6 hours, is usually suffi-

CRITICAL THINKING EXERCISE

Neonate with Chlamydia

An 8-day-old male infant is brought to the pediatric urgent care center on a Sunday morning by Maggie, an 18-year-old single mother, with a complaint of eye drainage for 2 days. Maggie is breastfeeding and states she was diagnosed and partially treated for a couple of sexually transmitted infections in late gestation; she does not remember the name but says one started with a "C." The medications made her stomach sick, so she quit taking them after 2 days. The practitioner examines the infant, who has a purulent yellowish discharge from both eyes but otherwise appears healthy; she suspects chlamydial conjunctivitis and orders cultures of the eye drainage. The retrieved medical record from the infant's birth indicates eye prophylaxis with erythromycin ophthalmic ointment was administered.

1. Evidence—Is there sufficient evidence to draw conclusions about the cause of the infant's eye drainage?
2. Assumptions—What assumptions can be made about the following factors:
   a. Treatment for neonatal chlamydia infection.
   b. Neonatal sequelae of inadequate chlamydia treatment in newborn.
   c. The mother's health status and possible treatment (she is not allergic to penicillin).
3. What implications and priorities for nursing care can be drawn at this time?
4. Does the evidence objectively support your conclusion?
5. Are there alternative perspectives to your conclusion?

cient to prevent spread of the disease or prolongation of its course. Several other drugs may be used, including amphotericin B (Fungizone), clotrimazole (Lotrimin, Mycelex), fluconazole (Diflucan), or miconazole (Monistat, Micatin) given intravenously, orally, or topically. To prevent relapse, therapy should be continued for at least 2 days after the lesions disappear (Lawrence & Lawrence, 2005). Gentian violet solution may be used in addition to one of the antifungal drugs in chronic cases of oral thrush; however, the former does not treat GI candida and may irritate the oral mucosa.

NURSING ALERT Nystatin is best absorbed when given either 1 hour before feeding or after a feeding. Using a needleless syringe or medicine dropper, apply the medication to each side of the infant's mouth for optimal absorption.

Oral candidiasis (thrush or mycotic stomatitis) is characterized by white plaques on the oral mucosa, gums, and tongue. The white patches are easily differentiated from milk curds; the patches cannot be removed and tend to bleed when touched. In most cases the infant does not seem to be in discomfort from the infection; however, some will pull away from the breast or bottle and cry. The child may be brought to the primary care provider with a complaint of poor oral intake.

Infants who are sick, debilitated, or receiving prolonged antibiotic therapy are more susceptible to thrush. Those with conditions such as cleft lip or palate, neoplasms, and hyperparathyroidism seem to be more vulnerable to mycotic infection.

Nursing Care Management

The objectives of management are to eradicate the causative organism and to control exposure to *C. albicans*. Interventions include maintenance of scrupulous cleanliness (by nursing personnel, parents, and others) to prevent reinfection. Good handwashing technique is always essential. Clean surfaces should be provided for changing neonates' diapers. Diaper dermatitis is treated with a topical fungicide at each diaper change. For the infant who is prone to diaper dermatitis, a barrier cream such as zinc oxide may be helpful, provided there is not already an infection. Diaper dermatitis that is not caused by *Candida* organisms may require treatment with a mild topical hydrocortisone ointment. When possible, exposing the perineal area to dry air is recommended because yeast prefers a moist environment. Other measures to control thrush include rinsing the infant's mouth with plain water after each feeding before applying the medication and boiling reusable nipples and bottles for at least 20 minutes after a thorough washing (spores are heat resistant). Pacifiers should be boiled for at least 20 minutes once daily, and the nipples of breastfeeding mothers should be treated with an antifungal to prevent reinfection.

Infants who are breastfed may acquire thrush from the mother. If the mother is colonized, treatment for mother and infant is recommended. There is no need to stop breastfeeding even if the mother is receiving systemic antifungal medications (Lawrence & Lawrence, 2005).

Substance Abuse

Certain maternal behaviors result in perinatal risk. Maternal habits hazardous to the fetus and neonate include recreational drug abuse, tobacco smoking, and alcohol consumption. Other than alcohol and tobacco use, cocaine and marijuana are the most commonly used substances by pregnant women. Physiologic signs of withdrawal have been reported in neonates of mothers who use to excess such drugs as barbiturates, alcohol, opioids, or amphetamines. Prescription opioids such as oxycodone (Percodan, OxyContin) have been identified as increasingly popular drugs of abuse, which may cause withdrawal symptoms in neonates (Sander & Hays, 2005; Rao & Desai, 2002). Serious withdrawal reactions may be seen in neonates whose mothers abuse psychoactive drugs. Mothers in substance abuse treatment receiving methadone may give birth to an infant who exhibits withdrawal symptoms requiring treatment. Almost 50% of pregnancies of women addicted to opioids result in low-birth-weight (LBW) infants who are not necessarily preterm. Alcohol is a teratogen that produces CNS effects that may not be evident for years. Maternal ethanol use during gestation can lead to a readily identifiable fetal alcohol syndrome (FAS, or ARBD [alcohol-related birth defect]) or a constellation of neurobehavioral and cognitive problems that may be identified only by maternal history and behavioral characteristics.

Historically the focus of maternal substance abuse has been on identifying the affected neonate and treating the withdrawal. However, such infants are often not easily identifiable in the perinatal period, and withdrawal may or may not occur. Perhaps of equal concern are issues related to birth of LBW infants, a population that continues to have the second highest infant mortality rate, and the long-term behavioral and neurodevelopmental effects that substance use by the pregnant mother has on the child.

It is important to note that the term *addiction* is often associated with behaviors whereby the person seeks the drug(s) to experience a high, achieve euphoria, escape from reality, or satisfy a personal need. Newborns who have been exposed to drugs in utero are not addicted in a behavioral sense, yet they may experience mild to strong physiologic signs as a result of the exposure. Therefore to say that an infant born to a mother who uses substances is addicted is incorrect; *drug-exposed newborn,* which implies intrauterine drug exposure, is a better term.

The adverse effects of exposure of the fetus to drugs are varied; many of these effects may not be identified until the child enters school. They include transient behavioral changes such as fetal breathing movements and irreversible effects such as fetal death, IUGR, structural malformations, cognitive and motor delay, and behavioral problems. Critical determinants of the drug's effect on the fetus include the specific drug, the dosage, the route of administration, the genotype of the mother or fetus, and the timing of the drug exposure. Fig. 28-7 shows critical periods in human embryogenesis and the teratogenic effects of drugs. Table 28-4 summarizes the effects of commonly abused substances on the fetus and neonate.

Alcohol

The incidence of FAS in the United States is about 0.2 to 1.5 per 1000 live births (Centers for Disease Control and Prevention, 2005). The term *fetal alcohol spectrum disorder* (FASD) has been suggested to encompass children with ARBD, FAS, or alcohol-related neurodevelopment disorder (ARND), all of which occur as a result of fetal exposure to alcohol (Centers

Table 28-4 Summary of Neonatal Effects of Commonly Abused Substances

SUBSTANCE	NEONATAL EFFECTS
Alcohol	*Fetal alcohol syndrome* (FAS)—Craniofacial features varied and may include short eyelid opening, flat midface, flat upper lip groove, thin upper lip; also may involve microcephaly, hyperactivity, developmental delays, attention deficits *Alcohol-related neurodevelopmental disorder* (ARND)—Varying forms of FAS; cognitive, behavioral, and psychosocial problems without typical physical features
Cocaine	Preterm birth, small for gestational age, microcephaly, poor feeding, irregular sleep patterns, diarrhea, visual attention problems, hyperactivity, difficulty being consoled, hypersensitivity to noise and external stimuli, irritability, developmental delays, congenital anomalies such as prune belly syndrome (i.e., distended, flabby, wrinkled abdomen caused by lack of abdominal muscles)
Heroin	Low birth weight, small for gestational age, irritability, tachypnea, feeding difficulties, vomiting, high-pitched cry, seizures
Methamphetamine	Small for gestational age, preterm birth, poor weight gain, lethargy, behavioral problems later in childhood
Tobacco	Preterm birth; low birth weight; increased risk for sudden infant death syndrome; increased risk for bronchitis, pneumonia, developmental delays, orofacial clefts
Marijuana	Possible neonatal tremors, low birth weight, growth restriction

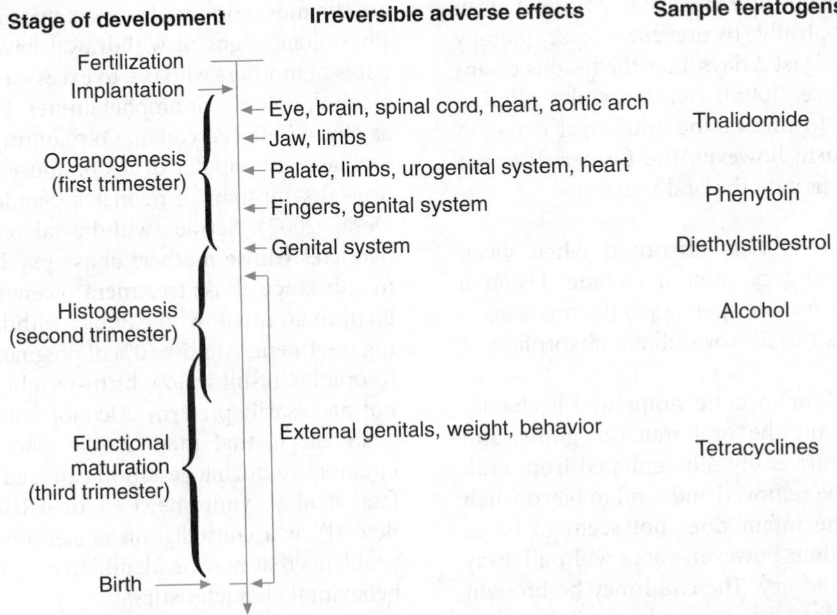

Fig. 28-7 Critical periods in human embryogenesis. (From Reed MD, Aranda JV, Hales BF: Developmental pharmacology. In Martin RJ, Fanaroff AA, Walsh MC (editors): *Fanaroff and Martin's neonatal-perinatal medicine: diseases of the fetus and infant*, ed 8, St Louis, 2006, Mosby.)

for Disease Control and Prevention, 2005). The three Centers for Disease Control and Prevention (2005) categories for diagnosis of FAS are (1) growth restriction, both prenatal and postnatal; (2) midfacial dysmorphic facial features; and (3) CNS involvement (structural, neurologic, or functional abnormality). Any single or multiple combinations of these may be present in addition to confirmed or unknown history of maternal alcohol consumption. The diagnosis of FAS is complicated by the absence of a specific single biologic marker and by manifestations that are often seen in other childhood conditions.

FAS is recognized as the leading cause of cognitive impairment (American Academy of Pediatrics, 2000). The incidence of FAS is on the rise in the United States despite public warnings, including the U.S. surgeon general's warning that consumption of alcohol during pregnancy may cause cognitive impairment and other defects. The reported incidence of maternal alcohol consumption during pregnancy also rose dramatically during the 1991 to 1995 period despite widespread education and information regarding periconceptional and gestational effects of drinking; recent surveillance indicates these rates have not decreased. The overall rates of alcohol consumption during pregnancy decreased from 1995 to 1999, but the incidence of binge drinking and frequent drinking during pregnancy did not decrease (Centers for Disease Control and Prevention, 2002a).

Alcohol (ethanol and ethyl alcohol) interferes with normal fetal development; the effects on the fetal brain are permanent, and even moderate use of alcohol during pregnancy may cause long-term postnatal difficulties, including impaired maternal-infant attachment. Because there is no known safe level of alcohol consumption in pregnancy, women should stop consuming alcohol at least 3 months before they plan to conceive.

Fetal abnormalities are not related to the amount of the mother's alcohol intake per se, but to the amount consumed in excess of the liver's ability to detoxify it. The liver's capacity to detoxify alcohol is limited and inflexible; when the liver receives more alcohol than it is able to handle, the excess is continually recirculated until the organ is able to reduce it to carbon dioxide and water. This circulating alcohol has a special affinity for brain tissue. Other factors that contribute to the teratogenic effects include toxic acetyl aldehyde (a degradation by-product of ethanol) and other substances that may be added to the alcohol. Poor nutritional state, smoking, polydrug intake, and infrequent or lack of prenatal care may compound the problem of alcohol abuse (Jones & Bass, 2003).

The effects on the fetal brain are reflected in CNS manifestations of FAS (Box 28-2). Cognitive and motor delays, hearing disorders, and a variety of defects in craniofacial development are prominent features (Fig. 28-8). Magnetic resonance imaging studies of children with diagnosed FAS revealed a high incidence of midbrain anomalies, particularly micrencephaly (Swayze et al, 1997). Some affected infants display physical features of the syndrome; behaviors, however, are nonspecific in newborns and may therefore pass undetected. These features include difficulty in establishing respiration, irritability, lethargy, poor suck reflex, and abdominal distention.

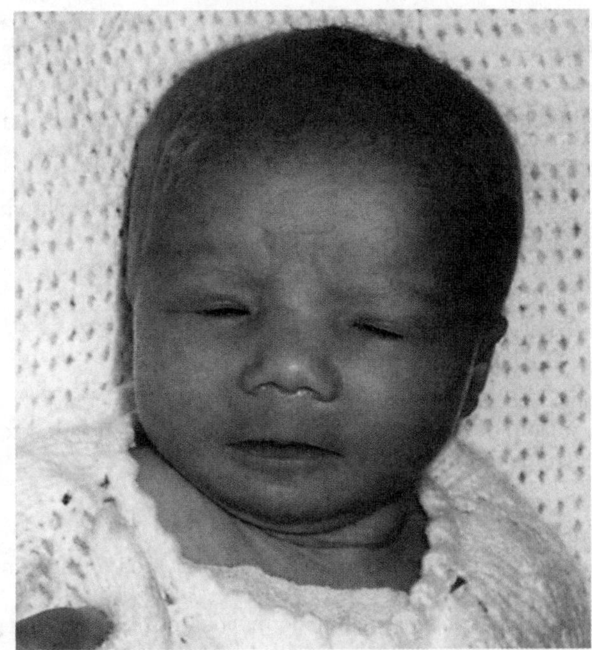

Fig. 28-8 Infant with fetal alcohol syndrome. (From Markiewicz M, Abrahamson E: *Diagnosis in color: neonatology*, St Louis, 1999, Mosby.)

The effects of FAS have been identified in adolescents and young adults, primarily in relation to growth deficiencies, delayed motor development, and cognitive impairment. In one study children who were exposed to only small amounts of alcohol prenatally showed more aggressiveness, delinquent behavior, and attention problems at 6 to 7 years of age compared with unexposed controls (Sood et al, 2001). Another study found that young adult offspring prenatally exposed to alcohol had significant alcohol-related problems by age 21 (Baer et al, 2003). Facial characteristics in adults tend to be more subtle than in infants and children.

evolve Critical Thinking Exercise—Fetal Alcohol Syndrome

The major goal of nursing care is prevention of these disorders through provision of adequate prenatal care for the expectant mother and precautions regarding exposure to potentially harmful infections. Nursing care of affected infants involves the same assessment and observations that are employed for any high risk infant. Poor feeding is characteristic of infants with FAS and can be a significant problem throughout infancy. Strategies to provide individualized developmental care are aimed at reducing noxious environmental stimuli and helping the infant achieve self-regulation. Special emphasis is placed on monitoring weight gain, analyzing feeding behaviors, and devising strategies to promote nutritional intake.

Early diagnosis and intervention are reported to be beneficial for reducing the effects of alcohol exposure on the growing child (Stoler & Holmes, 2004); therefore nurses should be actively involved in identifying and referring children exposed to alcohol prenatally.

When possible, long-term disabilities are prevented by early evaluation and implementation of therapy. The family is taught any special handling techniques needed for the care of their infant and signs of complications or possible sequelae. When sequelae are inevitable, the family will need assistance

BOX 28-2 Characteristics for Diagnosing Fetal Alcohol Syndrome

Facial Dysmorphia

On the basis of racial norms (i.e., those appropriate for a person's race), the person exhibits all three of the following characteristic facial features:

1. Smooth philtrum (University of Washington Lip-Philtrum Guide* rank 4 or 5*),
2. Thin vermillion border (University of Washington Lip-Philtrum Guide rank 4 or 5)
3. Small palpebral fissures (≤10th percentile).

Growth Problems

Confirmed, documented prenatal or postnatal height, weight, or both ≤10th percentile, adjusted for age, sex, gestational age, and race or ethnicity

Central Nervous System Abnormalities

Structural

Head circumference ≤10th percentile, adjusted for age and sex

Clinically meaningful brain abnormalities observable through imaging (e.g., reduction in size or change in shape of the corpus callosum, cerebellum, or basal ganglia)

Neurologic

Neurologic problems (e.g., motor problems or seizures) not resulting from a postnatal insult or fever, or other soft neurologic signs outside normal limits

Functional

Test performance substantially below that expected for a person's age, schooling, or circumstances, as evidenced by either:

1. Global cognitive or intellectual deficits representing multiple domains of deficit (or substantial developmental delay in younger children) with performance below the third percentile (i.e., 2 standard deviations below the mean for standardized testing); or
2. Functional deficits <16th percentile (i.e., 1 standard deviation below the mean for standardized testing) in at least three of the following domains:
   - Cognitive or developmental deficits or discrepancies
   - Executive functioning deficits
   - Motor functioning delays
   - Problems with attention or hyperactivity
   - Social skills
   - Other (e.g., sensory problems, pragmatic language problems, or memory deficits)

Maternal Alcohol Exposure

Confirmed prenatal exposure to alcohol

Unknown prenatal exposure to alcohol

Criteria for FAS Diagnosis

Diagnosis requires all three of the following findings:

1. Documentation of all three facial abnormalities listed above
2. Documentation of growth problems
3. Documentation of CNS abnormality

Source: Bertrand J et al: *Fetal alcohol syndrome: guidelines for referral and diagnosis*, Atlanta, 2004, US Department of Health and Human Services, Centers for Disease Control and Prevention. Available at www.cdc.gov/ncbddd/fas/documents/FAS_guidelines_accessible.pdf (accessed March 20, 2009).

*Astley SJ: *Diagnostic guide for fetal alcohol spectrum disorders: the four-digit diagnostic code*, ed 3, Seattle, 2004, University of Washington.

in determining how to best cope with the problems, such as with home care assistance, referral to appropriate agencies, or placement in an institution for care.

The dangers of heavy drinking are known, and *all* women should be counseled regarding the risks to the fetus. The nurse should emphasize to women of all ages that there is no known "safe" amount of alcohol intake during pregnancy that will preclude FAS, ARBD, ARND, or fetal alcohol effects. Furthermore, FAS is a totally preventable birth defect. A change in drinking habits even as late as the third trimester (when brain growth in the fetus is greatest) is associated with improved fetal outcome.

Tobacco

Cigarette smoking in pregnancy is associated with birth weight deficits of up to 250 g for a full-term neonate (Reed, Aranda, & Hales, 2006). Maternal cigarette smoking is implicated in 21% to 39% of LBW infants. Passive exposure to secondhand smoke by a pregnant woman may also result in the birth of an LBW infant. The rate of miscarriage and preterm birth is increased in the smoking population. Nicotine and cotinine, the two pharmacologically active substances in tobacco, are found in higher concentrations in infants whose mothers smoke. These substances can be secreted in breast milk for up to 2 hours after the mother has smoked. Cigarette smoke contains more than 2000 compounds, including carbon monoxide, dioxin, cyanide, and cadmium. Deficits in growth and intellectual and emotional development, poor auditory responsiveness, increased fine motor tremors, hypertonicity, and decreased verbal comprehension have been observed in infants exposed to smoke. There is also a positive dose-response relationship between the amount of tobacco exposure and newborn neurobehavior; increased tobacco exposure in utero is related to increasing negative neurobehavioral effects (Law et al, 2003). In addition, it is now recognized that neonates may experience withdrawal symptoms following exposure to nicotine.

Pregnant women must be informed about the harmful effects of smoking on their unborn baby's health. These include IUGR, miscarriage, PROM, placenta previa, perinatal death, LBW, deficits in learning and behavior, and sudden infant death syndrome (SIDS). The positive association between maternal smoking and SIDS (Lee, 1998; Milerad et al, 1998; Fleming & Blair, 2007; Mitchell & Milerad, 2006) reflects in utero exposure and passive exposure postnatally. Additional congenital defects or childhood problems associated with maternal tobacco use include congenital heart defects such as septal defects (Malik et al, 2008), orofacial clefts (cleft lip, cleft palate) (Honein et al, 2007), and increased incidence of childhood otitis media. Mothers and all others should refrain from smoking near the infant. Smoking cessation during pregnancy greatly decreases the chance of fetal complications; therefore women should be counseled regarding smoking cessation programs (see Family-Centered Care box).

FAMILY-CENTERED CARE

Smoking Cessation

You are the nurse working in a general family medicine clinic; you observe that many of the young mothers with newborns seen in the clinic smoke cigarettes. One young mother said, "I know it's bad for me but I can't quit. At least I don't smoke around the baby." What advice could you provide for the young mothers about the effect of tobacco smoke on young infants, especially those under 6 months of age? Prepare a short presentation that can be presented to the young mothers about the effects of tobacco on the infant's long-term health. Discuss options and resources for smoking cessation that are available from local community agencies.

Marijuana

Marijuana has replaced cocaine as the most common illicit drug used by women ages 18 to 44 years (nonpregnant and pregnant) in the United States (Ebrahim & Gfoerer, 2003). Marijuana crosses the placenta. Its use during pregnancy may result in a shortened gestation and a higher incidence of IUGR (Wagner et al, 1998). A strong association has been reported between the use of marijuana and a decrease in fetal growth and infant birth weight and length (Hurd et al, 2005). Other investigators have found a higher incidence of meconium staining (Bandstra & Accornero, 2006). Compounding the issue of the effects of marijuana, especially among women ages 18 to 30 years (Ebrahim & Gfoerer, 2003), is multidrug use, which combines the harmful effects of marijuana, tobacco, alcohol, opiates, and cocaine. Long-term follow-up studies on exposed infants are needed.

Cocaine

Cocaine, a common illicit drug used in the United States, has multiple modes of use. However, use of the relatively inexpensive and easily administered "crack" form is increasingly common, especially among women of childbearing age (Campbell, 2003; Eyler & Behnke, 1999). Because crack vaporizes at relatively low temperatures, it is smoked and absorbed in large quantities through pulmonary vasculature. The drug readily crosses the placenta, placing the fetus at risk (Malanga & Kosofsy, 1999).

Cocaine is a CNS stimulant and peripheral sympathomimetic. Legally it is classified as a narcotic, but it is not an opioid. The effects on the fetus are secondary to maternal effects—increased blood pressure, decreased uterine blood flow, and increased vascular resistance. Consequently, the fetus suffers decreased blood flow and oxygenation because of placental and fetal vasoconstriction. The difficulties encountered by cocaine-exposed infants are compounded when the mother is taking the drug in conjunction with other illicit drugs (Askin & Diehl-Jones, 2001). Researchers have concluded that variables such as the mother's lack of prenatal care; poor nutrition; and use of tobacco, alcohol, and other drugs during pregnancy compound the effects of cocaine exposure in the infant (Askin & Diehl-Jones, 2001; Tronick & Beeghly, 1999).

Infants may appear normal, or they may show neurologic problems at birth that may continue during the neonatal period. Fortunately, these findings are transient, and there has been little evidence of permanent sequelae. Either of two types of behavior may emerge as a result of cocaine effects on fetal development: neurobehavioral depression or excitability. The behaviors of the depressed infant include lethargy, poor suck, hypotonia, weak cry, and difficulty in arousing. The behaviors of the excitable neonate may include a high-pitched cry, hypertonicity, rigidity, irritability, inability to be consoled, and intolerance to a change in routine (Chiriboga et al, 1999; Richardson, Hamel, & Goldschmidt, 1996). Other behaviors may include frequent startling, poor awake state, sleeping difficulties, and persistent primitive reflexes. Some infants develop late onset of symptoms (2 to 8 weeks). They may become irritable and hypertonic, experience sleep-awake disruptions, and demonstrate an inability to tolerate change; they may also be slightly febrile. However, these findings have been refuted in other studies (Eyler & Behnke, 1999; Tronick & Beeghly, 1999).

The adverse effects on the cocaine-exposed neonate have a dose-response relationship. The higher the dose, the more effects such as IUGR, hypertonia, and decreased fetal head growth are noted (Chiriboga et al, 1999).

Sequelae of prenatal cocaine exposure include a smaller head circumference, decreased birth length, and decreased weight. Head growth may be one of the best predictors of long-term development (Bateman & Chiriboga, 2000). Other neonatal effects of cocaine exposure include increased incidence of gastroschisis, genitourinary anomalies, and periventricular and intraventricular hemorrhage. Some studies found that long-term sequelae for newborns exposed to cocaine include lower language, motor, and cognitive scores and an increased risk for learning disabilities (Singer et al, 2002; Koren et al, 1998; Morrow et al, 2006); however, one study revealed no significant differences in the total or verbal IQ scores but did note an increased risk of specific cognitive impairments (Singer et al, 2004). Arendt and colleagues (1999) noted that the fine and gross motor development indices in 2-year-old children who were exposed to cocaine prenatally were lower than in the control group. Some researchers noted that the exposed children may be affected emotionally rather than intellectually. In a study of first-grade students, Delaney-Black and colleagues (1998) concluded that the children who were exposed to cocaine prenatally were rated by their teachers as having more behavior problems than the control group. A more recent study, however, seems to refute these findings. In a large controlled study of children exposed to cocaine and opiates in utero, only subtle deficiencies in mental and psychomotor functioning were noted at 3 years of age (Messinger et al, 2004). Others suggest that the effects of cocaine in the

evolve Nursing Care Plan—The Drug-Exposed Newborn

newborn period are transient; cognitive function is reportedly only affected in relation to restriction of head growth (Chiriboga, 2003). No significant differences were noted in mental, psychomotor, or behavioral functioning. The environmental factors to which these children were exposed were perceived as an important factor in their development. Further long-term studies of exposed infants were recommended (Messinger et al, 2004).

Scores on the Brazelton Neonatal Behavioral Assessment Scale have shown cocaine-affected infants to be low in responding appropriately to arousal, auditory, and visual stimuli (Eyler, Behnke, & Conlon, 1998). However, other studies have not found significant differences (Frank et al, 1998; Richardson, Hamel, & Goldschmidt, 1996; Tronick et al, 1996).

Nursing care of cocaine-exposed infants is the same as that for other drug-exposed infants. Because they have increased flexor tone, these infants respond to swaddling in a semiflexed position (Askin & Diehl-Jones, 2001). Positioning, infant massage, and limited tactile stimulation have been shown to be effective interventions. Effects of the drug from breast milk have been reported (Kandall, 1999); therefore mothers should be cautioned about this hazard to their infants.

Referral to early intervention programs, including child health care, parental drug treatment, individualized developmental care, and parenting education, is essential in promoting the optimum outcome for these children. Many studies indicate that there is little or no significant difference between the cocaine-exposed and nonexposed groups. However, both groups (cocaine exposed and nonexposed) score significantly lower than published norms. Because cocaine-exposed children often live in an impoverished environment, they are at high risk for cognitive delays, lack of child health care, and inadequate nutrition and would benefit from an early intervention program (Tronick & Beeghly, 1999). A "one-stop shopping" model affords comprehensive care for mothers and children at one location, not only for drug treatment, but also for social and medical problems (Tanney & Lowenstein, 1997).

Phencyclidine ("Angel Dust")

Phencyclidine (PCP) increases the risk of injury to the pregnant woman and therefore also to her fetus. The user may be unaware that she is ingesting PCP because it often is misrepresented as another drug of abuse or is mixed with other drugs.

PCP crosses the placenta and is found in breast milk. Literature about the effects on infants is limited. Infants exposed to PCP may exhibit abnormal motor behavior such as irritability, jitteriness, and hypertonicity (D'Apolito, 1999).

Heroin

Heroin crosses the placenta and often results in IUGR. Heroin may have a direct growth-inhibiting effect on the fetus, but the exact mechanisms of growth inhibition are not clear. There is an increased rate of stillbirths but not of congenital anomalies. Additional neonatal effects include meconium aspiration, increased neonatal death, microcephaly, neurobehavioral problems, and a 74-fold increase in SIDS (Minozzi et al, 2008).

Many of the medical complications attributed to heroin ingestion result from preterm birth. Other risks include physical dependence in the fetus and the increased risk of exposure to infections, including hepatitis B and C virus and HIV.

Drug withdrawal in the expectant mother is accompanied by fetal withdrawal, which can lead to fetal death (Kaltenbach, Berghella, & Finnegan, 1998; Wagner et al, 1998). Maternal detoxification in the first trimester carries an increased risk of miscarriage. Detoxification is not recommended after the thirty-second week because of possible withdrawal-induced fetal distress (Kaltenbach, Berghella, & Finnegan, 1998).

Heroin withdrawal occurs in 50% to 80% of infants born to addicted mothers, usually within the first 24 to 72 hours of life (Wagner et al, 1998). The signs depend on the length of maternal addiction, the amount of drug taken, and the time of injection before birth. The infant whose mother is taking methadone may not demonstrate signs of withdrawal until a week or so after birth. The symptoms of infants whose mothers used heroin or methadone are similar. Initially the infant may be depressed. The withdrawal syndrome may manifest as a combination of any of the following signs:

- Infant may be jittery and hyperactive.
- Cry is shrill and persistent.
- Infant may yawn or sneeze frequently.
- Tendon reflexes are increased, but the Moro reflex is decreased.
- Neonate may exhibit poor feeding and sucking, tachypnea, vomiting, diarrhea, hypothermia or hyperthermia, and sweating.
- Infant may exhibit abnormal sleep cycle, with absence of quiet sleep and disturbance of active sleep.

The risk of SIDS is 5 to 10 times higher for infants with significant withdrawal problems than for infants in the general population. If withdrawal is not treated, vomiting, diarrhea, dehydration, apnea, and seizures may develop. Death may follow.

Therapy is individualized. Dehydration and electrolyte imbalance are prevented or treated. Usually the following drugs are given, singly or in combination: phenobarbital, diluted tincture of opium (paregoric), methadone, and morphine.

NURSING ALERT The use of naloxone (Narcan) is contraindicated in infants born to narcotic addicts because it may exacerbate neonatal abstinence syndrome (NAS) and cause seizures.

Methadone

Methadone, a synthetic opiate, has been the therapy of choice for heroin addiction since 1965. Methadone crosses the placenta. An increasing number of infants have been born to methadone-maintained mothers, who seem to have better prenatal care and a somewhat better lifestyle than those taking heroin.

Some question exists concerning the benefits of methadone therapy during pregnancy because of its effect on the fetus. Methadone withdrawal resembles heroin withdrawal but tends to be more severe and prolonged. Signs of methadone withdrawal include tremors, irritability, state lability, hypertonicity, hypersensitivity, vomiting, mottling, and nasal stuffiness (Jansson, Velez, & Harrow, 2004). These infants exhibit a disturbed sleep pattern similar to that seen in heroin withdrawal. They have a higher birth weight than those infants in heroin withdrawal and usually are appropriate for gestational age. No increased incidence of congenital anomalies is seen. The American Academy of Pediatrics, Committee on Drugs (2001), has revised its statement regarding breastfeeding for mothers who are in a methadone treatment program, suggesting such mothers be allowed to breastfeed regardless of the methadone treatment dosage. Follow-up counseling and monitoring of the mother and infant are recommended. The few available follow-up studies of these infants reveal a high incidence of hyperactivity, learning and behavior disorders, and poor social adjustment.

Late-onset withdrawal occurs at age 2 to 4 weeks and may continue for weeks or months. A higher incidence of SIDS also has been reported in these infants (Wagner et al, 1998). This factor is important for perinatal nurses who coordinate follow-up care for the infant and education for the mother or other caregiver. Community health nurses must know about the potential for withdrawal symptoms.

Therapy for methadone withdrawal is similar to that for heroin withdrawal. Buprenorphine, an opioid analgesic, has gained acceptance and Food and Drug Administration licensing in the treatment of opioid addiction. Preliminary studies indicate that this drug may have advantages over methadone in relation to neonatal outcomes. Offspring of mothers treated with buprenorphine had higher birth weights than those exposed to methadone, had shorter hospital stays, and had lower NAS scores (Jones et al, 2005; Kakko, Heilig, & Sarman, 2008).

Methamphetamine

The fetal and neonatal effects of maternal use of methamphetamines in pregnancy are not well known but appear to be dose related (Smith et al, 2003). LBW, preterm birth, and perinatal mortality may be consequences of higher doses used throughout pregnancy. In addition, a higher incidence of cleft lip and palate and cardiac defects has been reported in infants exposed to methamphetamines in utero (Plessinger, 1998).

Methamphetamine use has increased significantly during the past 10 years in certain regions of the United States. In Smith and colleagues' 2003 study, 63% of pregnant women who reported methamphetamine use reported using it throughout the pregnancy. A higher incidence of preterm delivery and placental abruption was associated with methamphetamine use. In addition, fetal growth restriction (being small for gestational age [SGA]) was slightly higher in methamphetamine-exposed offspring; however, 80% of these neonates' mothers also had significant intake of alcohol and tobacco use (Smith et al, 2003; Smith et al, 2006).

Study reports vary in the time of clinical manifestations of withdrawal from this drug; one study did not identify any signs of withdrawal in the first 3 days after birth, but long-term data were not collected (Smith et al, 2003). After birth, infants may experience bradycardia or tachycardia that resolves as the drug is cleared from the infant's system. Lethargy may continue for several months, along with frequent infections and poor weight gain. Emotional disturbances and delays in gross and fine motor coordination may be seen during early childhood.

One study found that prenatal methamphetamine users were also likely to smoke tobacco (25%), drink alcohol (22.8%), use marijuana (6%), and take barbiturates (1.3%) prenatally (Arria et al, 2006). Prenatal methamphetamine use was strongly associated with greater incidence of substance use among family and friends, lower maternal perception of quality of life, increased risk of legal difficulties, and increased likelihood of developing a substance abuse disorder (Derauf et al, 2007).

The long-term effects of methamphetamine exposure on children living in households where the product is manufactured are not known, but there are early reports of burns in exposed children and concerns regarding the effects of the toxic by-products of methamphetamine production on small children. Skin rashes and respiratory illnesses are common problems seen in methamphetamine-exposed children; physical neglect and speech and language developmental delays are of significant concern as well (Crocker, 2005).

Phenobarbital

Phenobarbital crosses the placenta readily and is subsequently found in high levels in the fetal liver and brain. Because of its slow metabolic rate, withdrawal onset is generally 2 to 14 days after birth and duration is about 2 to 4 months. Irritability, crying, hiccups, and sleepiness mark the initial response. During the second stage, the infant is extremely hungry; regurgitates and gags frequently; and demonstrates episodic irritability, sweating, and disturbed sleep pattern.

Caffeine

Caffeine has not been implicated as a teratogen in humans. Fernandes and colleagues (1998) reported that caffeine consumption greater than 150 mg/day was associated with IUGR and LBW. Santos and colleagues (1998) reported no adverse effects in the fetus with consumption of less than 300 mg of caffeine a day. Bracken and colleagues (2003) reported a slight decrease in birth weight in offspring of women consuming coffee during pregnancy; the authors indicated that caffeine intake of less than 600 mg/day is unlikely to have a significant impact on fetal growth. The American Dietetic Association (Kaiser, Allen, & American Dietetic Association, 2008) recommends that caffeine intake in pregnant women not exceed 300 mg/day. Caffeine is found in many beverages, including chocolate, colas, guarana, and mate (a tea consumed primarily in South America). High quantities of caffeine are in energy drinks as well.

Nursing Care Management

Assessment

Assessment of the newborn requires a review of the mother's prenatal record. A medical and social history of substance abuse, methadone treatment, or STIs is noted. The infant may have IUGR or be preterm and LBW. The woman who is using chemical substances may have infections that compound the risk to the infant, including hepatitis B; septicemia; and STIs, including HIV-positive status.

Table 28-5 Signs of Neonatal Abstinence Syndrome

SYSTEM	SIGNS
Gastrointestinal	Poor feeding, vomiting, regurgitation, diarrhea, excessive sucking
Central nervous	Irritability, tremors, shrill cry, incessant crying, hyperactivity, little sleep, excoriations on face, convulsions
Metabolic, vasomotor, respiratory	Nasal congestion, tachypnea, sweating, frequent yawning, increased respiratory rate >60 breaths/min, fever >37.2° C

The nurse often is the first to observe the signs of drug withdrawal in the infant; however, in many cases the newborn may be discharged before the appearance of any manifestations of withdrawal. The infant is assessed according to the guidelines discussed in Chapter 25. The infant's gestational age and maturity are noted. In utero exposure to some teratogens results in observable malformations or dysmorphism. Neonatal behavior may arouse suspicion. *Neonatal abstinence syndrome (NAS)* is the term used to describe the set of behaviors exhibited by the infant exposed to chemical substances in utero (Table 28-5). Fig. 28-9 provides an example of an NAS scoring system for assessing withdrawal symptoms. Because many women are multidrug users, the newborn initially may exhibit a variety of withdrawal manifestations.

Another scoring tool has been recently developed specifically aimed at measuring neurologic behavior and resultant effects on the neonate when substances are used during pregnancy. The NICU Network Neurobehavioral Scale (NNNS) was developed by the National Institutes of Health and provides an assessment of neurologic, behavioral, and stress-abstinence function in the neonate. The test combines items from other tests such as the Neonatal Behavioral Assessment Scale; stress-abstinence items developed by Finnegan (see Fig. 28-9); and a complete neurologic examination, which includes primitive reflexes and active and passive tone (Law et al, 2003; Lester & Tronick, 2004).

Newborn urine, hair, or meconium sampling may be required to identify drug exposure and implement appropriate early interventional therapies aimed at minimizing the consequences of intrauterine drug exposure. Methamphetamine may be found in fetal hair samples when intrauterine exposure occurs. Meconium sampling for fetal drug exposure is reported to provide more screening accuracy than urine, since drug metabolites accumulate in meconium (Ostrea, 2001). Urine toxicology screening has less accuracy because it reflects only recent substance intake by the mother (Huestis & Choo, 2002). Meconium testing for drug metabolites has the advantage of being easy to collect, noninvasive, and more accurate.

The nursing process in the care of the drug-exposed neonate is outlined in the Nursing Process box.

Plan of Care and Implementation

Caring for the infant born to a substance-abusing mother presents a challenge to the health care team. The parent, who is often single and unwed, is included in planning for the newborn's care and also encouraged to plan for her own care. A multidisciplinary approach is needed that includes home health or community resource personnel (e.g., regulatory agencies such as child protective services). Education and social support to prevent abuse of drugs provides the ideal approach. However, given the scope of the drug abuse problem, total prevention is unrealistic.

D'Apolito and Hepworth (2001) studied a small group (14) of infants exposed to multiple drugs in utero; these included opioids, stimulants, depressants, and sedatives. The most common symptoms observed were increased tone, increased respiratory rate, disturbed sleep, fever, frantic and increased sucking, and loose or watery stools. These findings are significant for nurses working in neonatal and obstetric areas; the presence of such findings may alert the nurse so documentation of events (per NAS scoring tool or other objective measure) may take place and therapy promptly implemented. Initial nursing interventions such as providing a quiet environment and offering a pacifier for frantic and excessive sucking may be implemented independently. It is important not to overfeed infants who demand frequent sucking as part of the withdrawal process.

Nursing care of the drug-exposed neonate involves supportive therapy for fluid and electrolyte balance, nutrition, infection control, individualized developmental care, and respiratory care. Swaddling, holding, reducing environmental stimuli, and feeding as necessary may be helpful in easing withdrawal (see Nursing Care Plan). Specific suggestions for providing care to infants experiencing withdrawal are listed in the Patient Teaching box.

PATIENT TEACHING Care of the Infant Experiencing Withdrawal

- Place the awake infant in a side-lying position with the spine and legs flexed.
- Position the infant's hands in midline with the arms at the side.
- Carry the infant in a flexed position.
- When interacting with the infant, introduce one stimulus at a time when the infant is in a quiet, alert state. Watch for time-out or distress signals (e.g., gaze aversion, yawning, sneezing, hiccups, arching, mottled color).
- When the infant is distressed, swaddle in a flexed position and rock in a slow, rhythmic fashion.
- Put the infant in a sitting position with chin tucked down for feeding.

Pharmacologic treatment is usually based on the severity of withdrawal symptoms, as determined by an assessment tool (see Fig. 28-9). Drug therapies to decrease withdrawal side effects include administration of phenobarbital, morphine, diluted tincture of opium (paregoric), or methadone (Coyle et al, 2002; Johnson, Gerada, & Greenough, 2003). A combination of these drugs may be necessary to treat infants exposed to multiple drugs in utero, and careful attention should be given to possible adverse effects of the treatment drugs (Johnson, Gerada, & Greenough, 2003).

NEONATAL ABSTINENCE SCORING SYSTEM

System	Signs and Symptoms	Score	AM	PM	Comments
Central Nervous System Disturbances	Excessive high-pitched (or other) cry	2			Daily weight:
	Continuous high-pitched (or other) cry	3			
	Sleeps <1 hour after feeding	3			
	Sleeps <2 hours after feeding	2			
	Sleeps <3 hours after feeding	1			
	Hyperactive Moro reflex	2			
	Markedly hyperactive Moro reflex	3			
	Mild tremors disturbed	1			
	Moderate-severe tremors disturbed	2			
	Mild tremors undisturbed	3			
	Moderate-severe tremors undisturbed	4			
	Increased muscle tone	2			
	Excoriation (specific area)	1			
	Myoclonic jerks	3			
	Generalized convulsions	5			
Metabolic/Vasomotor/Respiratory Disturbances	Sweating	1			
	Fever <101° (99–100.8° F/37.2–38.2° C)	1			
	Fever >101° (38.4° C and higher)	2			
	Frequent yawning (>3 or 4 times/interval)	1			
	Mottling	1			
	Nasal stuffiness	1			
	Sneezing (>3 or 4 times/interval)	1			
	Nasal flaring	2			
	Respiratory rate >60/min	1			
	Respiratory rate >60/min with retractions	2			
Gastrointestinal Disturbances	Excessive sucking	1			
	Poor feeding	2			
	Regurgitation	2			
	Projectile vomiting	3			
	Loose stools	2			
	Watery stools	3			
	Total Score				
	Initials of Scorer				

Fig. 28-9 Neonatal Abstinence Scoring (NAS) system, developed by L. Finnegan. (From Nelson N: *Current therapy in neonatal-perinatal medicine*, ed 2, St Louis, 1990, Mosby.)

NURSING PROCESS: DRUG-EXPOSED NEWBORN

Assessment

A comprehensive review of the maternal history and assessment of the neonate, including gestational age assessment, are performed on admission.

Nursing Diagnoses

Nursing diagnoses that may be derived from the neonatal assessment findings include the following:

Neonate

Risk for infection related to

- maternal risk behaviors that include promiscuous sexual activity
- prolonged rupture of membranes
- intrauterine growth restriction, preterm birth

Risk for disorganized infant behavior related to

- chemical effects of maternal substance abuse
- caregiver cue misreading
- caregiver cue knowledge deficit
- sensory overstimulation

Disturbed sleep pattern related to

- drug, chemical withdrawal

Risk for injury related to

- effects of drug exposure on growing fetal tissues

Parents

Risk for impaired parenting related to

- continuation of substance abuse or detoxification program
- guilt about infant's condition
- inability to cope with care needs of a special infant

Anxiety related to deficient knowledge regarding

- care needs of an affected infant

Violence: self-directed or directed toward infant related to

- drug-dependent lifestyle

Planning and Implementation

Examples of expected outcomes for neonates and parents are as follows:

Neonate

- The neonate will remain free of infection.
- Early manifestations of infection (viral or bacterial) will be recognized and appropriate therapy to minimize effects of disease will be implemented.
- Newborn manifestation of withdrawal (neonatal abstinence syndrome) will be recognized and appropriate therapy implemented to provide newborn state regulation.
- Newborn will receive appropriate physical and emotional care to minimize effects of maternal chemical substance use.
- Neonate will have steady patterns of uninterrupted sleep throughout the day.
- Neonate will demonstrate appropriate growth and development.

Parents

- Parent(s) will demonstrate ability to consistently meet basic caregiving needs of neonate.
- Parent(s) will continue to participate in substance abuse program to enhance ability to cope with life and effectively parent the newborn.
- Parent(s) will receive counseling and information from health care staff regarding newborn behavior, cues requiring comfort and feeding, signs of withdrawal, and general baby care.
- Parent(s) will recognize pattern of self-destructive behavior (substance abuse) and seek intervention.

A number of nursing interventions for the drug-exposed neonate are discussed on pp. 761-766.

Evaluation

Evaluation is based on the expected outcomes of care. The plan is revised as needed based on evaluation findings.

Pharmacologic treatment is based on assessment findings and validation of NAS. A suggested evaluation of NAS is recommended within 2 hours of the newborn's admission to the nursery and every 4 hours thereafter. A score of 8 or more requires more frequent assessment. With three consecutive scores of 8 or more, pharmacologic interventions are recommended (Weiner & Finnegan, 2006).

After the presence of NAS is identified in an infant, nursing care is directed toward treating the presenting signs, decreasing stimuli that may precipitate hyperactivity and irritability (e.g., dimming the lights, decreasing noise levels), providing adequate nutrition and hydration, and promoting positive maternal-infant relationships. Appropriate individualized developmental care is implemented to facilitate self-consoling and self-regulating behaviors. Irritable and hyperactive infants have been found to respond to physical comforting, movement, and close contact. Wrapping infants snugly and rocking and holding them tightly limits their ability to self-stimulate. The infant's arms should remain flexed with hands in close proximity of the mouth for sucking; sucking on fingers or hands is a form of self-control and comfort. Arranging nursing activities to reduce the amount of disturbance helps decrease exogenous stimulation. Rocking infants with signs of drug withdrawal in a bed designed to mimic the soothing intrauterine environment did not prove to be effective in decreasing withdrawal symptoms; the rocking bed was thought to be too stimulating for the infants studied (D'Apolito, 1999).

Loose stools, poor intake, and regurgitation after feeding predispose these infants to malnutrition, dehydration, and electrolyte imbalance. Daily weights to detect fluid losses or caloric intake, careful monitoring of intake and output, electrolytes, and additional caloric supplementation may be necessary. In addition, these infants burn up energy with continuous activity and increase oxygen consumption at the cellular level. It takes considerable time and patience to ensure that they receive a sufficient caloric and fluid intake.

Hyperactive infants must be protected from skin abrasions on the knees, toes, and cheeks that are caused by rubbing on

NURSING CARE PLAN The Drug-Exposed Newborn

Nursing Diagnosis: Risk for injury related to hyperactivity, irritability, and disorganized state

Expected Outcome

Infant exhibits age-appropriate state modulation regulation and stability (i.e., quiet alert state, deep sleep state, drowsy) with minimal irritability and inability to modulate state.

Nursing Interventions/*Rationales*

Use an objective measure or tool such as the Neonatal Abstinence Scoring system *to verify and document behaviors associated with withdrawal.*

Perform a comprehensive neurobehavioral assessment of the infant *to gather individual assessment data to assist in planning individualized care appropriate for the infant experiencing withdrawal as a result of intrauterine drug exposure.*

NOTE: These first two interventions take precedence over all others because manifestations of withdrawal may vary from one infant to another.

Administer medications *to decrease CNS irritability.*

Decrease environmental stimuli *that may trigger irritability and hyperactive behaviors.*

Plan care activities carefully *to allow for appropriate interaction as per infant's behavioral clues.*

Wrap infant snugly and hold infant tightly *to reduce self-stimulating behaviors.*

Monitor activity level, note the relationship between activity level and external stimulation, and stop external stimulation *if it causes activity increase.*

Provide scheduled periods of rest, decreased overhead lighting, and no physical care *to allow time for recovery of quiet state after periods of care.*

Help mother understand that infant behavioral cues are not a sign of rejection of her caretaking abilities, *to facilitate long-lasting maternal-infant interaction, decrease maternal guilt, and enhance environment conducive to infant growth (promote infant's sense of trust).*

Nursing Diagnosis: Imbalanced nutrition: less than body requirements related to central nervous system irritability; disorganized sucking pattern; vomiting; and loose, watery stools

Expected Outcome

Infant exhibits appropriate weight gain.

Nursing Interventions/*Rationales*

Observe for feeding cues indicating readiness for interaction (quiet alert, rooting) and feed frequent small amounts and burp well *to diminish vomiting and aspiration.*

Monitor weight daily and maintain strict intake and output *to evaluate success of feeding.*

If intake is insufficient, feed by gavage *to ensure ingestion of needed nutrients.*

Modify environment of feeding area as necessary *to decrease stimuli that detract from feeding process and interaction with caregiver.*

Nursing Diagnosis: Risk for impaired skin integrity related to hyperactivity; elbows and ankles rubbing against linen; and loose, watery stools

Expected Outcome

Infant exhibits evidence of intact skin.

Nursing Interventions/*Rationales*

Position infant supine with knees and arms flexed and place a blanket roll at front and back *to promote containment and comfort and minimize frantic, irritable activity.*

Monitor hydration and nutritional status (i.e., skin turgor, weight, mucous membranes, fontanels, urine specific gravity, electrolytes) *to decrease risk for skin breakdown.*

Administer medications intended to decrease hyperactivity, irritability, and frantic posturing, *to decrease exposure of skin to surfaces that may cause skin breakdown.*

Cleanse face and diaper area promptly after regurgitation or stooling *to prevent skin breakdown.*

Wrap infant snugly in blanket and place hands in midline next to face *to promote self-comforting and decrease frantic activity.*

Cuddle infant *to promote quiet and relaxation.*

Nursing Diagnosis: Ineffective maternal coping, anxiety, and powerlessness related to drug dependence, infant distress during withdrawal, and poor social support

Expected Outcome

Mother will accept newborn's condition and participate in care activities, showing evidence of maternal-infant bonding process.

Nursing Interventions/*Rationales*

Explain effects of maternal drug use on newborn and the withdrawal process *to provide understanding and information concerning effects of drug use.*

Encourage open communication (e.g., inform mother of ongoing condition, procedures, and treatment; answer questions; correct misperceptions; actively listen to her concerns) *to provide a sense of respect, provide support, and encourage a sense of control.*

Encourage mother to interact with infant and to become involved in care routines *to foster emotional connection.*

Explain how to do care procedures, how to avoid excess stimulation, and how to hold and comfort infant *to enhance mother's care abilities and her sense of confidence and control.*

If the infant demonstrates signs of withdrawal, explain to mother the infant's inability to interact, gaze aversion, arching back, and lack of response to cuddling *to enhance understanding of infant behaviors.*

Make appropriate referrals to community and social agencies for treatment of maternal substance abuse, infant development programs, and other needed support services *to ensure adequate resources for care of self and infant.*

Encourage maternal participation in a substance abuse counseling (and methadone maintenance, as appropriate) program *to enhance maternal coping skills for effective caretaking of affected newborn.*

bed linens while in a prone position while awake. The incidence of SIDS in such children is high, and parents should be reminded that the supine position for sleep is preferred. Monitoring and recording the activity level and its relationship to other activities, such as feeding and preventing complications, are important nursing functions.

Breastfeeding is encouraged for mothers who are not using illicit substances, are negative for HIV infection, and are compliant with a methadone program. Breastfeeding promotes maternal-infant bonding, and the small amount of methadone passed through breast milk has not proved to be harmful to the neonate (Berghella et al, 2003; Hale, 2002; Philipp, Merewood, & O'Brien, 2003). Lawrence and Lawrence (2005), however, suggest that maternal methadone regimens of 100 mg/day or more may cause increased withdrawal in infants, requiring paregoric for 6 to 8 weeks. Because many new drugs are being manufactured, the reader is advised to consult with updated references regarding the safety of medications for breastfeeding infants (see also Lawrence & Lawrence [2005] for a complete list of drugs that should be avoided with breastfeeding). It is reasonable to expect the pregnant mother to abstain from the so-called recreational drugs mentioned above because none of these is safe in any given quantity for any given fetus.

Hemolytic Disorders

Hyperbilirubinemia, physiologic jaundice, pathologic jaundice, and kernicterus are discussed in Chapter 25.

Hemolytic Disease of the Newborn

Hemolytic disease occurs when the blood groups of the mother and newborn are different; the most common of these are RhD factor and ABO incompatibilities. Hemolytic disorders occur when maternal antibodies are present naturally or form in response to an antigen from the fetal blood crossing the placenta and entering the maternal circulation. The maternal antibodies of the IgG class cross the placenta, causing hemolysis of the fetal RBCs, resulting in fetal anemia and often neonatal jaundice and hyperbilirubinemia.

Rh Incompatibility

Rh incompatibility, or isoimmunization, occurs when an RhD-negative mother has an RhD-positive fetus who inherits the dominant Rh-positive gene from the father. The Rh blood group consists of several antigens (since D is the most prevalent Rh antigen, the following discussion focuses on RhD isoimmunization). If the mother is Rh negative and the father is Rh positive and homozygous for the Rh factor, all the offspring will be Rh positive. If the father is heterozygous for the factor, there is a 50% chance that each infant born of the union will be Rh positive and a 50% chance that each will be Rh negative. An Rh-negative fetus is in no danger because he or she has the same Rh factor as the mother. An Rh-negative fetus with an Rh-positive mother is also in no danger. Only the Rh-positive offspring of an Rh-negative mother is at risk. From 10% to 15% of all Caucasian couples and about 5% of African-American couples have Rh incompatibility. Incompatibility is rare in Asian couples. The incidence of Rh sensitization and resulting hemolytic disease of the newborn have decreased dramatically since the development of Rh_o(D) immune globulin in 1968.

The pathogenesis of Rh incompatibility is as follows: hematopoiesis in the fetus, or the formation of blood cells, begins as early as the eighth week of gestation; in up to 40% of pregnancies, these cells pass through the placenta into the maternal circulation. When the fetus is Rh positive and the mother Rh negative, the mother forms antibodies against the fetal blood cells: first IgM antibodies that are too large to pass through the placenta and then IgG antibodies that can cross the placenta. The process of antibody formation is called *maternal sensitization.* Sensitization may occur during pregnancy, birth, induced abortion or miscarriage, or amniocentesis. Usually women become sensitized in their first pregnancy with an Rh-positive fetus but do not produce enough antibodies to cause lysis (destruction) of the fetal blood cells. In subsequent pregnancies, antibodies form in response to repeated contact with the antigen from the fetal blood, and lysis results. In approximately 10% to 15% of sensitized mothers, there is no hemolytic reaction in the newborn. In addition, some Rh-negative women, even though exposed to Rh-positive fetal blood, are immunologically unable to produce antibodies to the foreign antigen (Neal, 2001). Multiple gestations, abruptio placentae, placenta previa, manual removal of the placenta, and cesarean delivery increase the incidence of transplacental hemorrhage and subsequent isoimmunization (Moise, 2002).

Severe Rh incompatibility results in marked fetal hemolytic anemia because the fetal erythrocytes are destroyed by maternal Rh-positive antibodies. Although the placenta usually clears the bilirubin generated by the RBC breakdown, in extreme cases fetal bilirubin levels increase. The fetus compensates for the anemia by producing large numbers of immature erythrocytes to replace those hemolyzed—thus the name for this condition: *erythroblastosis fetalis.* In hydrops fetalis, the most severe form of this disease, the fetus has marked anemia, cardiac decompensation, cardiomegaly, and hepatosplenomegaly. Hypoxia results from the severe anemia. In addition, because of the decreased intravascular oncotic pressure involved, fluid leaks out of the intravascular space, resulting in generalized edema and effusions into the peritoneal (ascites), pericardial, and pleural (hydrothorax) spaces. The placenta is often edematous, which, along with the edematous fetus, can cause the uterus to rupture.

Intrauterine or early neonatal death may occur as a result of hydrops fetalis, although intrauterine transfusions and early delivery of the fetus may avert this. Intrauterine transfusion involves the infusion of Rh-negative, type O blood into the umbilical vein. The frequency of intrauterine transfusions may vary according to institution and fetal hydropic status, but it may be as often as every 2 weeks until the fetus reaches pulmonary maturity at approximately 37 to 38 weeks of gestation (Moise, 2002).

ABO Incompatibility

ABO incompatibility is more common than Rh incompatibility, but causes less severe problems in the affected infant. It occurs if the fetal blood type is A, B, or AB and the maternal type is O. It occurs rarely in infants with type B blood born to mothers with type A blood. The incompatibility arises because naturally occurring anti-A and anti-B antibodies are transferred across the placenta to the fetus. Unlike the situation that pertains to Rh incompatibility, first-born infants may be affected because mothers with type O blood already have anti-A and anti-B antibodies in their blood. Such a newborn may have a weakly positive direct Coombs' test (also referred to as a *direct antiglobulin test*). The cord bilirubin level usually is less than 4 mg/dl, and any resulting hyperbilirubinemia usually can be treated with phototherapy. Exchange transfusions are required only occasionally. Although ABO incompatibility is a common cause of hyperbilirubinemia, it rarely precipitates significant anemia resulting from the hemolysis of RBCs.

Other Hemolytic Disorders

It is not within the scope of this text to discuss the many potential causes of hemolytic jaundice in childhood. However, in some populations there is a high incidence of glucose-6-phosphate dehydrogenase deficiency (G6PD), which may cause an exaggerated jaundice in a newborn within 24 to 48 hours of birth. G6PD red cells hemolyze at a greater rate than healthy red cells, thus overwhelming the immature neonatal liver's ability to conjugate the indirect bilirubin. Some of the triggers that potentiate hemolysis include vitamin K, acetaminophen, aspirin, sepsis, and exposure to certain chemicals (Reiser, 2004). Hereditary spherocytosis may also cause serious neonatal hemolytic anemia as a result of high quantities of fetal hemoglobin; jaundice may develop rapidly and require phototherapy (Segel, 2007). Treatment is the same as for any newborn with rapidly rising serum bilirubin levels.

Other metabolic and inherited conditions that increase hemolysis and may cause jaundice in the infant include galactosemia, Crigler-Najjar disease, and hypothyroidism.

Nursing Care Management

At the first prenatal visit of an Rh-negative woman with a fetus who may be Rh positive, an indirect Coombs' test should be done to determine whether she has antibodies to the Rh antigen. In this test the maternal blood serum is mixed with Rh-positive RBCs. If the Rh-positive RBCs agglutinate or clump, this indicates that maternal antibodies are present or that the mother has been sensitized. The dilution of the specimen of blood at which clumping occurs determines the titer, or level, of maternal antibodies. This titer indicates the degree of maternal sensitization. A level of 1:8 rarely results in fetal jeopardy. If the titer reaches 1:16, amniocentesis is performed to determine the delta optical density (ΔOD) of the amniotic fluid to estimate fetal hemolytic process. Rising bilirubin levels may indicate the need for an intrauterine transfusion. Genetic testing allows early identification of paternal zygosity at the RhD gene locus, thus allowing earlier detection of the potential for isoimmunization and precluding further maternal or fetal testing (Moise, 2002).

The indirect Coombs' test is repeated at 28 weeks. If the result remains negative, indicating that sensitization has not occurred, the woman is given an intramuscular injection of $Rh_o(D)$ immune globulin. If the test result is positive, showing that sensitization has occurred, the test is repeated at 4- to 6-week intervals to monitor the maternal antibody titer as just described.

At birth, the neonate's cord blood is sent to the laboratory to determine the infant's blood type and Rh status. A direct Coombs' test is performed on cord blood to determine whether maternal antibodies are present in the fetal blood. If antibodies are present, the titer, which indicates the degree of maternal sensitization, is measured. The prevention of or prompt therapy for perinatal asphyxia, acidosis, cold stress, sepsis, and hypoglycemia will decrease the newborn's risk for severe hemolytic disease and his or her susceptibility to kernicterus. Early feeding in the stable newborn is also initiated to stimulate stooling and thus facilitate the removal of bilirubin.

If jaundice is present, the cause is determined and therapeutic management is begun. Phototherapy is used to reduce rapidly increasing serum bilirubin levels. See Chapter 25 for a discussion of phototherapy.

Exchange transfusions are needed infrequently because of the decrease in the incidence of severe hemolytic disease in newborns resulting from isoimmunization. Other factors must always be considered as well, particularly the infant's clinical condition, because it is a procedure with potential complications. Guidelines for the initiation of exchange transfusion in relation to serum bilirubin levels in infants at 35 weeks of gestation or greater may be found in the 2004 American Academy of Pediatrics, Subcommittee on Hyperbilirubinemia Clinical Practice Guideline.

Exchange transfusion is accomplished by alternately removing a small amount of the infant's blood and replacing it with an equal amount of donor blood. If the infant has Rh incompatibility, type O Rh-negative blood is used for transfusion, so the maternal antibodies still present in the infant do not hemolyze the transfused blood. Depending on the infant's size, maturity, and condition, 5 to 20 ml of the infant's blood are removed at one time and replaced with warmed donor blood. The total amount of blood exchanged approximates 170 ml/kg of body weight, or 75% to 85% of the infant's total blood volume. Preservatives in donor blood lower the infant's serum calcium level; therefore calcium gluconate is often given during the exchange transfusion. The neonate is monitored closely for signs of a blood transfusion reaction as well as hypotension, temperature instability, and cardiorespiratory compromise.

Congenital Anomalies

Congenital defects are reported to occur in 2% to 3% of all live births (Bay, Steele, & Davis, 2007), but this number increases to about 6% by 5 years, when more anomalies are diagnosed. In addition, the incidence of congenital malformations in fetuses that are aborted is higher than that in infants who are born alive, thus also adding to the overall incidence. Major congenital defects are the leading cause of death in infants younger than 1 year of age in the United States and account for 20% of neonatal deaths. Although the incidences of other causes of neonatal mortality have decreased, the death rate associated with most congenital anomalies has essentially remained stable since 1932.

The most common major congenital anomalies that cause serious problems in the neonate are congenital heart disease, abdominal wall defects, imperforate anus, neural tube defects (NTDs), cleft lip or palate, clubfoot, and developmental dysplasia of the hip. These are thought to result from the interaction of multiple genetic and environmental factors.

Ways of detecting and preventing some of these anomalies are being improved continuously, as are some surgical techniques for the care of the fetus with certain anomalies. Promoting the availability of these services to populations at risk challenges community health care systems. An interdisciplinary team approach is vital for providing holistic care: the surgical treatment, rehabilitation, and education of the child, as well as psychosocial and financial assistance for the parents. Parental disappointment and disillusion add to the complexity of the nursing care needed for these infants.

Central Nervous System Anomalies

Most congenital anomalies of the CNS result from defects in the closure of the neural tube during fetal development. Although the cause of NTDs is unknown, they are thought to stem from the interaction of many genes that may be influenced by factors in the fetal environment. Environmental influences such as treatment with valproic acid (an anticonvulsant), treatment with methotrexate (a chemotherapeutic agent), and alcohol and tobacco consumption have been implicated. Maternal folic acid deficit has a direct bearing on failure of the neural tube to close; therefore folic acid supplementation is recommended for women of childbearing age. In the United States, rates of NTDs declined by as much as 23% in the time beginning in 1995 to 1996 and ending in the year 2000; NTD rates have decreased an additional 6.9% between 2000 and 2005, primarily among African-American mothers. One concern is that NTD rates have not decreased among Hispanic and non-Hispanic Caucasian mothers since 1999 (Centers for Disease Control and Prevention, 2009a). The decline in NTDs in the late 1990s has been attributed in large part to the addition of folic acid to cereal grain products (Honein, 2001). Increased use of prenatal diagnostic techniques and termination of pregnancies have also affected the overall incidence of NTDs.

Although an NTD is usually an isolated defect, it can occur with some chromosomal abnormalities and syndromes and also with other defects such as cleft palate, ventricular septal defect, tracheoesophageal fistula (TEF), congenital diaphragmatic hernia (CDH), imperforate anus, and renal anomalies.

Encephalocele and Anencephaly

Encephalocele and anencephaly are abnormalities resulting from failure of the anterior end of the neural tube to close. An encephalocele is a herniation of the brain and meninges through a skull defect, usually at the base of the neck. The defect may be associated with hydrocephalus; the resulting sequelae depend on the amount of neural tissue within the protruding sac and associated neurologic defects. Treatment consists of surgical repair and shunting to relieve hydrocephalus, unless a major brain malformation is present. Anencephaly is the absence of both cerebral hemispheres and of the overlying skull. It is a condition that is incompatible with life; many of the infants are stillborn or die within a few days of birth. Comfort measures are provided until the infant eventually dies of temperature instability and respiratory failure.

Spina Bifida

Spina bifida, the most common defect of the CNS, results from failure of the neural tube to close at some point. There are two categories of spina bifida: spina bifida occulta and spina bifida cystica. Spina bifida occulta is a malformation in which the posterior portion of the laminae fails to close but the spinal cord or meninges do not herniate or protrude through the defect. It is usually asymptomatic and may not be diagnosed unless there are associated problems. Spina bifida cystica includes meningocele and myelomeningocele. A meningocele is an external sac that contains meninges and CSF and that protrudes through a defect in the vertebral column. A myelomeningocele is similar, except that it also contains nerves; therefore the infant has motor and sensory deficits below the lesion. A myelomeningocele is visible at birth, most often in the lumbosacral area. It is usually covered by a fragile, thin membrane (Fig. 28-10). The sac can tear easily, allowing CSF to leak out and providing an entry for infectious agents into the CNS (see Fig. 28-10, *B*). Myelomeningocele may be associ-

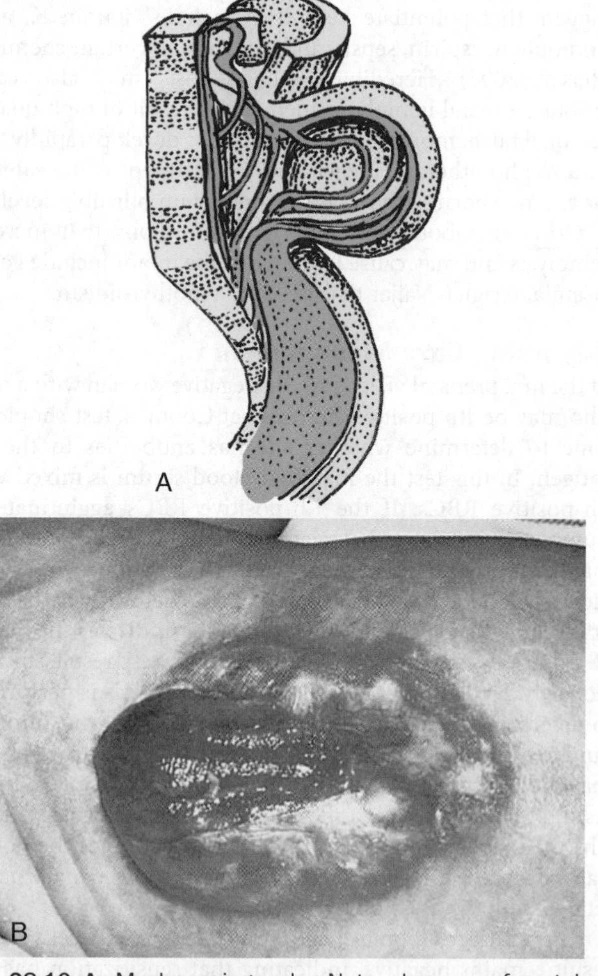

Fig. 28-10 **A**, Myelomeningocele. Note absence of vertebral arches. **B**, Myelomeningocele (ruptured sac exposing defect). (From Zitelli BJ, Davis HW: *Atlas of pediatric physical diagnosis*, ed 4, St Louis, 2002, Mosby.)

ated with an Arnold-Chiari malformation (70%), which results from the improper development and downward displacement of part of the brain into the cervical spinal canal. This in turn results in the development of hydrocephalus, which affects about 90% of children with myelomeningocele, although it is usually not present at birth.

The long-term prognosis in an affected infant can be determined to a large extent at birth, with the degree of neurologic dysfunction related to the level of the lesion, which determines the nerves involved. Most neurosurgeons recommend that treatment be instituted regardless of the level of the lesion unless there is a severe CNS anomaly, advanced hydrocephalus at birth, severe anoxic brain damage, active CNS infection, or a malformation or syndrome incompatible with long-term survival. Prenatal diagnosis makes possible a scheduled cesarean birth, allowing for more careful delivery of the infant's back to prevent rupture of the meningeal sac.

A major preoperative nursing intervention for a neonate with a myelomeningocele is to protect the protruding sac from injury, rupture, and resultant risk of CNS infection. Such infants should be positioned in a side-lying or prone position to prevent pressure on the sac until surgical repair is done. If the infant is able to be held, the nurse or parent must be careful to keep the defect from being injured. The sac should be covered with a sterile, moist, nonadherent dressing and cared for using sterile technique. The skin around the defect must be cleansed and dried carefully to prevent breakdown, which would establish a portal of entry for infectious agents. An important nursing intervention is providing support and needed information to parents as they learn to cope with an infant who has immediate needs for intensive care and who probably will have long-term needs as well. Surgical repair is performed in the neonatal period, often within the first 24 to 48 hours. Very early closure can prevent CNS infection and trauma to the exposed nerves. It can also prevent stretching of other nerve roots, which can occur as the sac continues to enlarge after birth. Surgical shunt procedures to prevent increasing hydrocephalus may be needed. Other problems, such as infection, are treated as they occur.

Hydrocephalus

Hydrocephalus is a condition in which the ventricles of the brain are enlarged as a result of an imbalance between the production and absorption of the CSF. Congenital hydrocephalus usually arises as a result of a malformation in the brain or an intrauterine infection. About one third of all cases of congenital hydrocephalus result from stenosis of the aqueduct of Sylvius in the brain. Hydrocephalus often occurs in conjunction with a myelomeningocele, which blocks the flow of CSF.

An infant with congenital hydrocephalus initially has a bulging anterior fontanel and a head circumference that increases at an abnormal rate, resulting from the increase in CSF pressure. Enlargement of the forehead with depressed eyes that are rotated downward, causing a "setting sun" sign, occurs as the condition worsens. If the surgical shunting of excess CSF from the brain is not done soon after birth, the resulting increasing ICP will lead to irreversible neurologic damage, as evidenced by palpably widening sutures and fontanels; distended scalp veins; lethargy; poor feeding; vomiting; irritability; opisthotonic positioning; and a high-pitched, shrill cry. Fetal ultrasound is helpful in the detection of hydrocephalus.

Nursing actions appropriate to the needs of a newborn with hydrocephalus include care similar to that for any high risk newborn. Measurement of the head circumference and neurologic assessments are done frequently. If the infant's head is large, a special pressure-sensitive mattress and frequent position changes are necessary to prevent skin breakdown. Chapter 51 contains a more detailed description of the evaluation and management of the child with hydrocephalus.

Microcephaly

Microcephaly refers to a head circumference that measures more than 3 standard deviations below the mean for age and sex. Brain growth is usually restricted and thus cognitive impairment is common. Microcephaly can be the result of an autosomal-dominant disorder; a chromosomal abnormality; fetal exposure to teratogens such as radiation; maternal substance abuse; and congenital infections such as rubella, toxoplasmosis, or CMV. Infants with microcephaly require supportive nursing care and medical observation to determine the extent of the psychomotor delay that almost always accompanies this abnormality. There is no treatment. Parents need support to learn to care for a child with cognitive impairment.

Cardiovascular System Anomalies

Congenital heart defects (CHDs) are anatomic abnormalities of the heart that are present at birth, although they may not be diagnosed immediately. Some type of congenital heart disease occurs in approximately 0.5% to 0.8% of live births, and about 2 to 3 in 1000 newborns will be symptomatic with heart disease in the first year of life (Bernstein, 2007). Ventricular septal defects, constituting more than 20% to 25% of all CHDs, are the most common type of acyanotic lesion. Tetralogy of Fallot, constituting 5% to 7% of all CHDs, is the most common type resulting in cyanosis. CHDs, often in association with other congenital anomalies, are the second major cause of death in the first year of life (the first being preterm births).

The cause of CHDs is unknown in many cases. Approximately 8% have a clear genetic cause, and most are associated with a chromosomal anomaly such as Down syndrome (40%) (Blackburn, 2007). Maternal factors associated with a higher incidence of CHD include diabetes mellitus, rubella, alcohol intake, systemic lupus erythematosus, phenylketonuria (PKU), poor nutrition, or antiepileptic medication use.

As a rule, CHDs are thought to be multifactorial in origin, involving both genetic and environmental influences; however, a familial occurrence of virtually all forms of CHD has been noted. See Chapter 48 for a discussion of classifications of CHDs.

Some CHDs are often evident immediately after birth, especially those defects that cause central cyanosis (e.g., transposition of the great vessels) despite 100% oxygen administration. Infants with these anomalies are transferred directly to an intensive care nursery or pediatric intensive care unit.

Affected newborns may have cyanosis that is unrelieved by oxygen treatment, with the cyanosis increasing whenever the child cries. Pulse oximetry readings that remain low (below 89%) despite oxygen administration are not unusual, and respiratory distress may or may not be present. In many cases the infant's color is unrelated to the severity of the defect. Other infants may be acyanotic and pale, with or without mottling on exertion, such as crying, feeding, or stooling.

The affected newborn's activity level varies from restlessness to lethargy and possible unresponsiveness, except to pain. Persistent bradycardia (i.e., resting heart rate of less than 80 to 100 beats/min) or tachycardia (i.e., rate exceeding 160 to 180 beats/min) may be noted. The infant born to a mother with systemic lupus may exhibit bradycardia with normal sinus rhythm and good perfusion; eventually cardioversion may be required if the rhythm persists. The cardiac rhythm may be abnormal, and a murmur may or may not be heard. In many cases, however, ductal (ductus arteriosus) dependent defects or large shunts will not be seen with a murmur. Signs of congestive heart failure, diminished cardiac output, and poor tissue perfusion may be occur within several days of birth.

Because the cardiac and respiratory systems function together, cardiac disease may also be manifested by respiratory signs and symptoms. The respiratory rate should be determined when the newborn is in a resting state. Abnormal findings may include tachypnea, which is a rate of 60 breaths/min or more; retractions with nasal flaring; grunting occurring with or without exertion; and dyspnea, which may worsen with crying and activity.

A major role of the nurse is to assess infants for abnormal findings such as central cyanosis and poor perfusion, which are an indication of decreased cardiac output. Newborns exhibiting these symptoms require prompt attention and appropriate therapy in a neonatal or pediatric intensive care unit. Interventions planned when a nursing diagnosis of decreased cardiac output is made include administering oxygen, although oxygen content is usually decreased once the defect is identified; administering cardiotonic medications to increase cardiac output, medications (prostaglandin) designed to prevent closure of the ductus arteriosus, and diuretic agents as needed for congestive heart failure; decreasing the work load of the heart by maintaining a thermoneutral environment; and feeding using the least strenuous method necessary. Various diagnostic tests such as echocardiography and cardiac catheterization are performed to obtain specific information about the defect and the need for surgical intervention.

Respiratory System Anomalies

Screening for congenital anomalies of the respiratory system is necessary even in infants who are apparently normal at birth. Respiratory distress at birth or shortly thereafter may be the result of lung immaturity or anomalous development. Respiratory distress caused by CDH and TEF may appear immediately or be delayed, depending on the severity of the defect.

Choanal Atresia

Choanal atresia, the most common congenital anomaly of the nose, is a bony or membranous septum located between the nose and the pharynx (Fig. 28-11). The atresia may be unilateral or bilateral. Because most infants are preferential nasal breathers, bilateral choanal atresia may be associated with apnea and cyanosis when the infant is at rest. When the infant cries, he or she breathes in through the mouth and pinks up. Unilateral choanal atresia may not be associated with apnea. Inability to pass a suction catheter through the nose into the pharynx or cyanosis without obvious respiratory distress usually leads to its detection. Nearly half of the infants with choanal atresia have other anomalies.

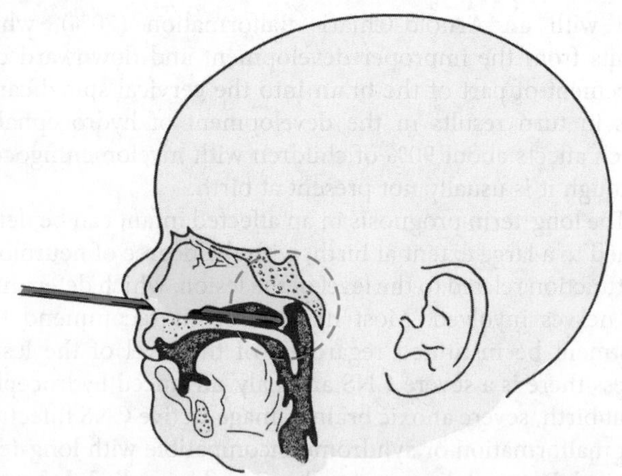

Fig. 28-11 Choanal atresia. Posterior nares are obstructed by membrane or bone, either bilaterally or unilaterally. Infant becomes cyanotic at rest. With crying, newborn's color improves. Nasal discharge is present. Snorting respirations often are observed with increased respiratory effort. Newborn may be unable to breathe and eat at the same time. Diagnosis is made by noting inability to pass small feeding tube through one or both nares. *(Used with permission of Ross Products Division, Abbott Laboratories, Inc., Columbus, OH 43216. From Clinical Education Aid No. 6, Copyright 1963, Ross Products Division, Abbott Laboratories, Inc.)*

Congenital Diaphragmatic Hernia

CDH results from a defect in the formation of the diaphragm, allowing the abdominal organs to be displaced into the thoracic cavity. It occurs in approximately 1 in 2000 to 1 in 5000 live births (Ehrlich & Coran, 2007). Herniation of the abdominal viscera into the thoracic cavity may cause severe respiratory distress and represent a neonatal emergency (Fig. 28-12). The defect and herniation may be minimal and easily repaired, or the defect may be so extensive that the viscera present in the thoracic cavity during embryonic life have prevented the normal development of pulmonary tissue. The defect is usually on the left (85%) because that is the side of the diaphragm that fuses last.

Most CDHs are discovered prenatally on ultrasound. Hernias may be repaired by fetal surgery in some research institutions. Intrauterine surgical correction of CDH has met with poor neonatal outcomes in many cases, primarily as a result of tocolysis failure and early delivery. At birth, most affected infants have severe respiratory distress, and respiratory assessment reveals worsening distress as the bowel fills with air. Typically the breath sounds are diminished and bowel sounds are heard in the chest. Heart sounds may be heard on the right side of the chest because the heart has been displaced there by the abdominal contents. Physical examination reveals a flat or scaphoid abdomen and a prominent ipsilateral chest.

Diagnosis can be made on the basis of the x-ray finding of loops of intestine in the thoracic cavity and the absence of intestine in the abdominal cavity.

Preoperative nursing interventions include helping stabilize the infant's condition until surgical repair can be performed. High-frequency oscillatory ventilation, conventional mechanical ventilation, and extracorporeal membrane oxygenation (ECMO) are used as respiratory support. Permissive hypercapnia may be allowed as long as the pH is maintained above or equal to 7.30 (Ehrlich & Coran, 2007). Inhaled nitric oxide to relieve pulmonary hypertension of CDH has also been used in some cases with mixed results. Gastric contents are aspirated and suction applied to decompress the GI tract and prevent further cardiothoracic compromise. Oxygen therapy, mechanical ventilation, and the correction of acidosis are necessary in infants with early clinical respiratory distress from CDH. ECMO may be used in infants with severe circulatory and respiratory complications. Traditional management has been early surgical repair of the defect. However, increased survival rates have been reported with surgery after a period of preoperative stabilization and resolution of pulmonary hypertension.

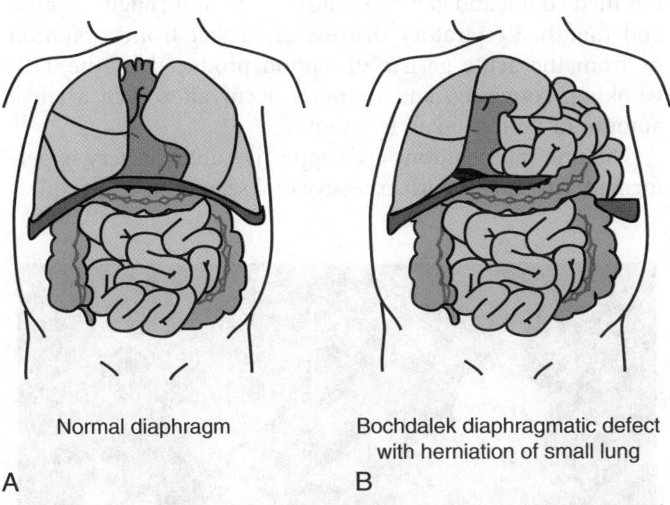

Fig. 28-12 **A,** Normal diaphragm separating the abdominal and thoracic cavities. **B,** Diaphragmatic hernia with a small lung and abdominal contents in the thoracic cavity. (From Ehrlich PF, Coran AG: Diaphragmatic hernia. In Kliegman RM et al (editors): *Nelson textbook of pediatrics*, ed 18, Philadelphia, 2007, Saunders.)

The prognosis depends largely on the degree of fetal pulmonary development, but the prognosis in severe cases is often poor. The overall survival rate for live-born infants is 67% (Ehrlich & Coran, 2007). The incidence of gastroesophageal reflux disease in survivors is approximately 50%, and a significant number will have neurocognitive deficits.

Gastrointestinal System Anomalies

Anomalies in the GI system can occur anywhere along the GI tract, from the mouth to the anus. Some anomalies, such as cleft lip, omphalocele, and gastroschisis, are apparent at birth. Others, including cleft palate, esophageal atresia (EA), intestinal obstruction, and imperforate anus, become apparent as the infant is further assessed or becomes symptomatic.

Cleft Lip and Palate

Cleft lip or palate is a commonly occurring congenital midline fissure, or opening, in the lip or palate resulting from failure of the primary palate to fuse (Fig. 28-13). One or both defor-

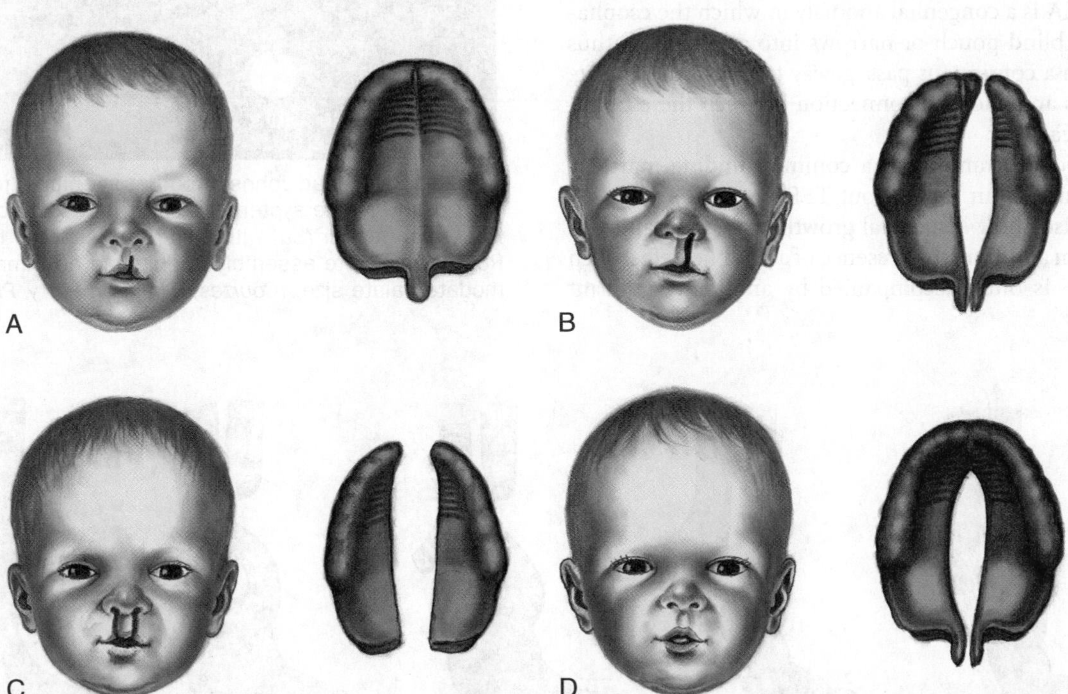

Fig. 28-13 Variations in clefts of lip and palate at birth. **A,** Notch in vermilion border. **B,** Unilateral cleft lip and cleft palate. **C,** Bilateral cleft lip and cleft palate. **D,** Cleft palate. (From Hockenberry MJ, Wilson D: *Wong's essentials of pediatric nursing*, ed 8, St. Louis, 2009, Mosby.)

mities may occur. Multiple genetic and, to a lesser extent, environmental factors (e.g., maternal infection; tobacco exposure; radiation exposure; alcohol ingestion; and treatment with medications such as corticosteroids, some tranquilizers, and antiepileptics) appear to be involved in their development. Pathophysiology, evaluation, and treatment are addressed in Chapter 47.

Feeding is difficult because the cleft lip renders the newborn unable to maintain a seal around a nipple; the cleft palate renders the infant unable to form a vacuum to maintain suction when feeding. In addition, the inability to suck and swallow normally allows milk to pool in the nasopharynx, which increases the likelihood of aspiration. Furthermore, as the infant attempts to suck, milk often comes out through the cleft and out of the nares. Although the degree of difficulty depends on the size of the cleft, feeding problems are greater in infants with a cleft palate than in those with a cleft lip alone (see Fig. 28-13). Breastfeeding can be successful in some infants. Special nipples, bottles, and appliances are available to aid in feeding (Fig. 28-14).

In general, parents of infants with these defects need a great deal of education and support as they learn to feed their baby, to prevent what should be a normal part of infant care from becoming a frustrating experience. Parents of infants with a cleft lip or palate need much support, particularly in the case of a cleft lip because this is both a cosmetic and functional defect. Recognizing that this may interfere with normal parent-infant bonding in the neonatal period, the nurse must assess for this and intervene appropriately.

Esophageal Atresia and Tracheoesophageal Fistula

EA and TEF often occur together, although they can also occur singly. EA is a congenital anomaly in which the esophagus ends in a blind pouch or narrows into a thin cord, thus failing to form a continuous passageway to the stomach (Fig. 28-15). TEF is an abnormal connection between the esophagus and trachea.

Maternal polyhydramnios is a common finding, particularly if the fetus has an EA without TEF. The infant with EA or TEF may also show some fetal growth restriction and will thus be SGA. In addition, the presence of a midline defect such as EA or TEF is often accompanied by another significant embryonic defect such as a cardiac anomaly; cleft lip and/or palate; or vertebral, genitourinary, or abdominal wall defect (Roaten, Bensard, & Price, 2006). Variations of the anomalies are possible, depending on the presence or absence of a TEF, the site of the fistula, and the location and degree of esophageal obstruction (see Fig. 28-15).

Infants with EA and TEF may demonstrate limited respiratory difficulty immediately after birth. EA with or without TEF results in excessive oral secretions, choking, and spitting up mucus through the nose. When fed, the infant may swallow, but then cough and gag and return the fluid through the nose and mouth. Respiratory distress can result from aspiration or from the acute gastric distention produced by the TEF. Choking, coughing, and cyanosis occur after even a small amount of fluid is taken by mouth.

Nursing interventions are supportive until surgery is performed. Any infant with excessive oral secretions and respira-

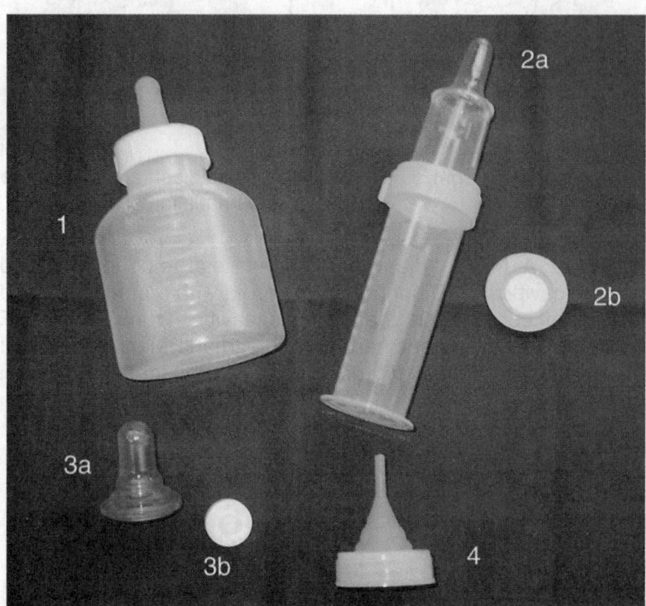

Fig. 28-14 *1,* Mead Johnson bottle and nipple for cleft palate. Cleft palate nipple system *(2a)* with valve *(2b)* to regulate flow. Haberman feeder *(3a)* with disc *(3b)* to control flow of milk. *4,* Ross cleft palate assembly. Nipple can be trimmed to accommodate palate size. *(Courtesy Shannon Perry, Phoenix, AZ.)*

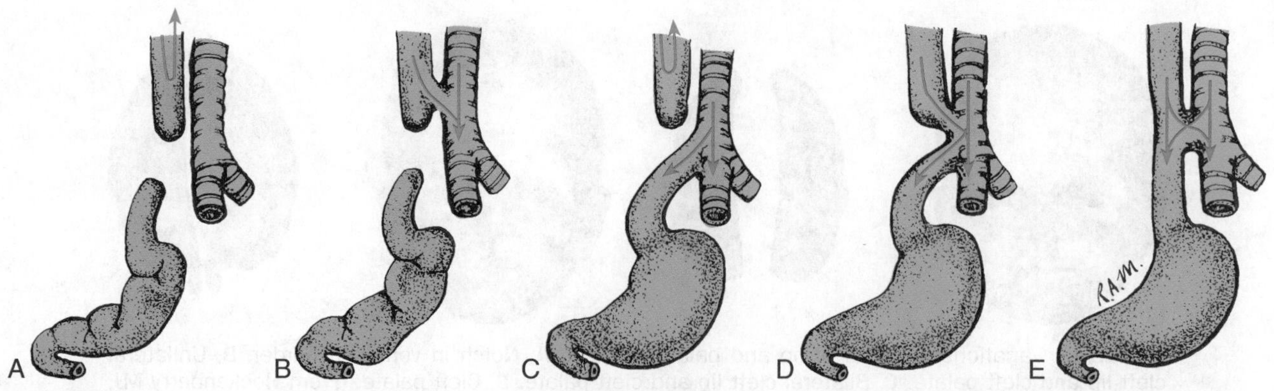

Fig. 28-15 **A** through **E**, Five most common types of esophageal atresia and tracheoesophageal fistula.

tory distress should not be fed orally until further evaluation is carried out. The infant is placed in the position least likely to cause aspiration of either mouth or stomach secretions. A double-lumen catheter is placed in the proximal esophageal pouch for drainage of swallowed secretions; this may minimize the possibility of aspiration. Other supportive measures include maintaining thermoregulation, fluid and electrolyte balance intravenously, and acid-base balance and preventing any further complications as a result of an associated defect. Surgical correction, often performed in one stage, consists of ligating the fistula and anastomosing the two segments of the esophagus. The chances for survival in those infants in a good-risk category exceed 95% depending on the presence of associated defects and the infant's birth weight. Many EA and TEF infants will have postoperative issues related to feeding difficulties such as gastroesophageal reflux (GER) and esophageal strictures requiring periodic dilation. (See Chapter 47 for further discussion of surgical treatment and nursing care.)

Omphalocele and Gastroschisis

Omphalocele and gastroschisis are two of the more common congenital defects that occur in the abdominal wall. They are rare, however, with omphalocele occurring in approximately 1 in 3000 to 10,000 live births, whereas the incidence of gastroschisis is 1 in 6000 live births (Blackburn, 2007).

An omphalocele is a covered defect of the umbilical ring into which varying amounts of the abdominal organs may herniate (Fig. 28-16). Although it is covered with a thin, often translucent peritoneal sac, the sac may rupture during or after birth. Many infants born with an omphalocele are preterm, and more than half have other defects involving the GI, cardiac, genitourinary, musculoskeletal, and nervous systems.

Gastroschisis is the herniation of the bowel through a defect in the abdominal wall to the right of the umbilical cord. No membrane covers the contents, as occurs with an omphalocele. Unlike infants with omphalocele, these infants have less than a 10% to 15% likelihood of associated anomalies, including intestinal atresia and cardiac anomalies.

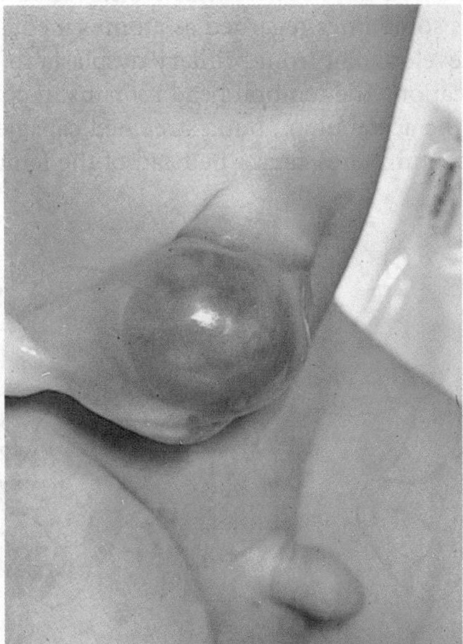

Fig. 28-16 Omphalocele. (From O'Doherty N: *Neonatology: micro atlas of the newborn*, Nutley, NJ, 1986, Hoffmann–La Roche.)

The preoperative nursing care is similar for infants with either defect. Exposure of the viscera causes problems with thermoregulation and fluid and electrolyte balance. Before closure is performed, the exposed viscera are covered with moistened saline gauze and plastic wrap. In some cases the infant may be placed in an impermeable, clear plastic bowel bag to decrease insensible water losses, maintain thermoregulation, and prevent contamination of the exposed viscera (Roaten, Bensard, & Price, 2006). Antibiotics, fluid and electrolyte replacement, gastric decompression, and thermoregulation are needed for physiologic support. If complete closure is impossible because of the small size of the abdominal cavity and the large amount of viscera to be replaced, a Silastic silo pouch is created and sewn to the fascia of the abdominal defect. The defect is closed surgically after the reduction of contents is complete, which usually takes 7 to 10 days. Gastric decompression is necessary preoperatively to prevent aspiration pneumonia and to allow as much bowel as possible to be placed into the abdomen during surgery. Surgery is usually performed soon after birth. With surgical treatment, nutritional support, and medical management, the prognosis has improved for infants born with an abdominal wall defect. It is estimated that more than 80% of infants born with omphalocele survive, as do more than 90% of those born with gastroschisis, although residual feeding difficulties such as GER are not uncommon.

Intestinal Obstruction

Congenital intestinal obstruction can occur anywhere in the GI tract and takes one of the following forms: atresia, which is a complete obliteration of the passage; partial obstruction, in which the symptoms may vary in severity and sometimes not be detected in the neonatal period; or malrotation of the intestine, which leads to twisting of the intestine (volvulus) and obstruction. EA, discussed previously, is a type of GI obstruction. Meconium ileus is an obstruction caused by impacted meconium and is the earliest symptom of cystic fibrosis, a life-threatening chronic illness. Infants with this type of obstruction should be tested for cystic fibrosis because 95% of infants with meconium ileus have cystic fibrosis. In addition to a history of maternal polyhydramnios, the infant with an ileus shows the following cardinal signs and symptoms: bilious vomiting, abdominal distention, and failure to pass normal amounts of meconium in the first 24 hours.

Nursing care is aimed at supporting the infant until surgical intervention can be carried out to eliminate the obstruction. Oral feedings are withheld, a nasogastric tube is placed for suction, and intravenous therapy is initiated to provide needed fluids and electrolytes. In infants with an intestinal obstruction, surgery consists of resecting the obstructed area of bowel and anastomosing the unaffected bowel. In recent years the survival rate for these infants has risen to 90% to 95% as a result of better treatments, improved neonatal intensive care, and an increased understanding of the total problem.

Anorectal Malformation

Anorectal malformation is a term used to describe a wide range of congenital disorders involving the anus and rectum and, in many cases, genitourinary system. These anomalies have an incidence of approximately 1 in 5000 to 1 in 15,000 live births (Blackburn, 2007). Occurring more in male than in female infants, they result from the failure of anorectal development in weeks 7 and 8 of gestational life. Such infants have no anal opening (Fig. 28-17), and commonly there is also a fistula from the rectum to the perineum or genitourinary system. Types of anorectal malformations include the typical cloaca in females, which involves the vagina, colon, and urethra forming a single common passage in the perineum. Others include the low rectovaginal fistula (female) and rectourethral bulbar fistula (male). Extensive surgical repair is often required in stages for the more complex types of anorectal malformations. In some cases the anomaly may involve stenotic areas, or there may be a thin translucent membrane covering the anal opening. Treatment for such a membrane is excision followed by daily dilation, which parents are taught to do. (See Chapter 47 for further discussion of surgical treatment.)

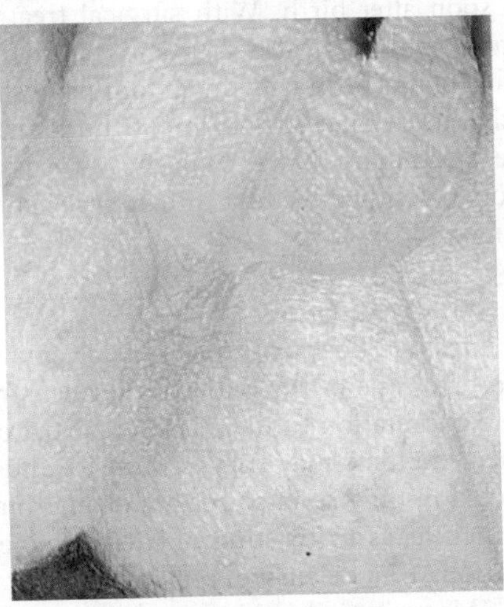

Fig. 28-17 Anorectal malformation (imperforate anus). (From Chessell G et al: *Diagnostic picture tests in clinical medicine*, vol 2, St Louis, 1984, Mosby.)

Musculoskeletal System Anomalies

Developmental Dysplasia of the Hip

The broad term *developmental dysplasia of the hip* (DDH) describes a spectrum of disorders related to abnormal development of the hip that may appear at any time during fetal life, infancy, or childhood. A change in terminology from *congenital hip dysplasia* and *congenital dislocation of the hip* to *DDH* more properly reflects a variety of hip abnormalities in which there is a shallow acetabulum, subluxation, or dislocation.

The incidence of hip instability of some kind is approximately 10 per 1000 live births. The incidence of frank dislocation or a dislocatable hip is 1 to 1.5 per 1000 live births (Hosalkar et al, 2007).

The cause of DDH is unknown, but certain factors such as sex, birth order, family history, intrauterine position, birth type, joint laxity, and postnatal positioning are believed to affect the risk of DDH. Predisposing factors associated with DDH may be divided into three broad categories: (1) physiologic factors, which include maternal hormone secretion and intrauterine positioning; (2) mechanical factors, which involve breech presentation, multiple fetuses, oligohydramnios, and large infant size; other mechanical factors may include continued maintenance of the hips in adduction and extension that will in time cause a dislocation; and (3) genetic factors, which entail a higher incidence (6%) of DDH in siblings of affected infants, and an even greater incidence (36%) of occurrence if a sibling and one parent were affected.

Three degrees of DDH are as follows (Fig. 28-18):

1. *Acetabular dysplasia (or preluxation)*—This is the mildest form of DDH in which there is neither subluxation nor dislocation. There is a delay in acetabular development evidenced by osseous hypoplasia of the acetabular roof that is oblique and shallow, although the cartilaginous roof is comparatively intact. The femoral head remains in the acetabulum.
2. *Subluxation*—The largest percentage of DDH, subluxation implies incomplete dislocation of the hip and is sometimes regarded as an intermediate stage in the development from primary dysplasia to complete dislocation. The femoral head remains in contact with the acetabulum, but a stretched capsule and ligamentum teres cause the head of the femur to be

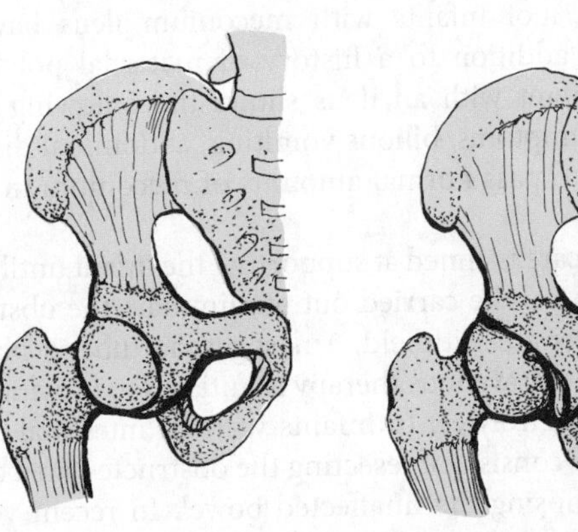

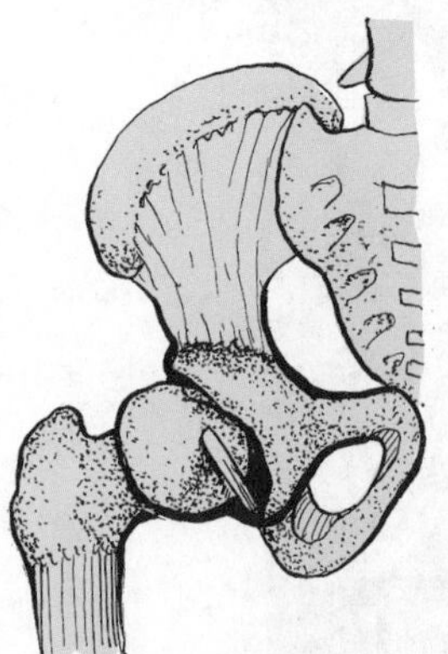

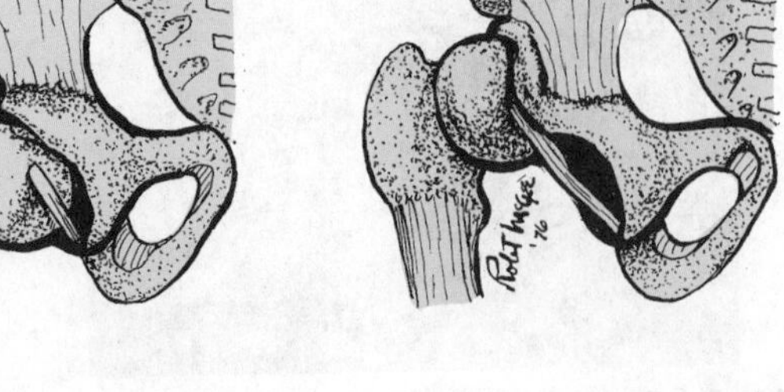

Fig. 28-18 Configuration and relationship of structures in developmental dysplasia of the hip.

partially displaced. Pressure on the cartilaginous roof inhibits ossification and produces a flattening of the socket.
3. *Dislocation*—The femoral head loses contact with the acetabulum and is displaced posteriorly and superiorly over the fibrocartilaginous rim. The ligamentum teres is elongated and taut.

DDH is often not detected at the initial examination after birth; thus all infants should be carefully monitored for hip dysplasia at follow-up visits throughout the first year of life. In the newborn period dysplasia usually appears as hip joint laxity rather than as outright dislocation. Subluxation and the tendency to dislocate can be demonstrated by the Ortolani or Barlow tests. The Ortolani and Barlow tests are most reliable from birth to 2 or 3 months of age. Other signs of DDH are shortening of the limb on the affected side (Galeazzi sign, Allis sign), asymmetric thigh and gluteal folds, and broadening of the perineum (in bilateral dislocation) (see also Fig. 24-8).

NURSING ALERT The Ortolani and Barlow tests must be performed by an experienced clinician to prevent fracture or further damage to the hip. If these tests are performed too vigorously in the first 2 days of life, when the hip subluxates freely, persistent dislocation may occur.

Treatment is initiated as soon as the condition is recognized, since early intervention is more favorable to the restoration of normal bony architecture and function. The longer treatment is delayed, the more severe the deformity, the more difficult the treatment, and the less favorable the prognosis. The treatment varies with the child's age and the extent of the dysplasia. The goal of treatment is to obtain and maintain a safe, congruent position of the hip joint to promote normal hip joint development and ambulation.

The hip joint is maintained by dynamic splinting in a safe position with the proximal femur centered in the acetabulum in an attitude of flexion. Of the numerous devices available, the Pavlik harness is the most widely used, and with time, motion, and gravity, the hip works into a more abducted, reduced position (Fig. 28-19). The harness is worn continuously until the hip is proved stable on clinical and radiographic examination, usually in about 3 to 5 months.

NURSING ALERT The former practice of double- or triple-diapering for DDH is not recommended because it promotes hip extension, thus worsening proper hip development.

See Chapter 54 for more detailed discussion of DDH.

Clubfoot

Congenital clubfoot is a complex deformity of the ankle and foot that includes forefoot adduction, midfoot supination, hindfoot varus, and ankle equinus. Deformities of the foot and ankle are described according to the position of the ankle and foot. The more common positions involve the following variations:

Talipes varus—An inversion, or a bending inward
Talipes valgus—An eversion, or bending outward
Talipes equinus—Plantar flexion, in which the toes are lower than the heel

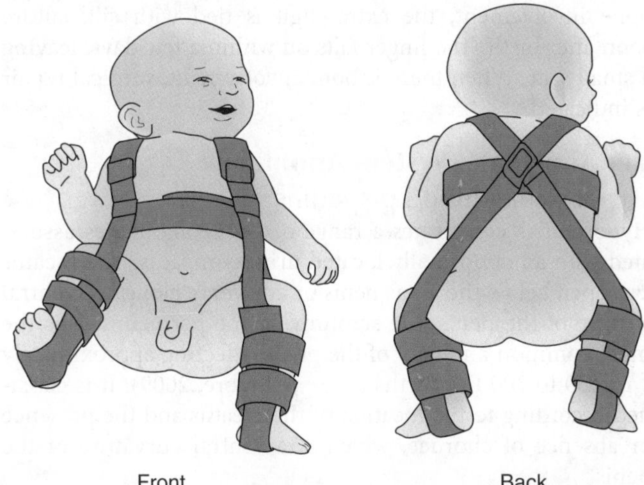

Fig. 28-19 Treatment for developmental hip dysplasia with Pavlik harness. (From Ball J: *Mosby's pediatric patient teaching guides*, St Louis, 1998, Mosby.)

Talipes calcaneus—Dorsiflexion, in which the toes are higher than the heel

Most cases of clubfoot are a combination of these positions, and the most frequently occurring type of clubfoot (approximately 95%) is the composite deformity talipes equinovarus, in which the foot is pointed downward and inward in varying degrees of severity (see Fig. 54-9, p. 1694). Unilateral clubfoot is somewhat more common than bilateral clubfoot and may occur as an isolated defect or in association with other disorders or syndromes, such as chromosomal aberrations, arthrogryposis (a generalized immobility of the joints), cerebral palsy, or spina bifida.

The goal of treatment for clubfoot is to achieve a painless, plantigrade (able to walk on the sole of the foot with the heel on the ground), and stable foot. Treatment of clubfoot involves three stages: (1) correction of the deformity, (2) maintenance of the correction until normal muscle balance is regained, and (3) follow-up observation to avert possible recurrence of the deformity. Some feet respond to treatment readily; some respond only to prolonged, vigorous, and sustained efforts; and improvement in others remains disappointing even with maximum effort on the part of all concerned.

Serial casting is begun shortly after birth, before discharge from the nursery. Successive casts allow for gradual stretching of skin and tight structures on the medial side of the foot. Manipulation and casting are repeated frequently (every week) to accommodate the rapid growth of early infancy. In some cases daily manipulation and stretching of tissues are accomplished with taping and splinting of the affected extremity. A continuous passive motion machine may be used several hours daily to stretch and strengthen muscle groups involved (Faulks & Luther, 2005). The extremity or extremities are often casted or splinted until maximum correction is achieved, usually within 8 to 12 weeks. A Denis Browne splint may be used to manage feet that correct with casting and manipulation.

Polydactyly

Occasionally hands or feet are seen with extra digits. In some instances, polydactyly is hereditary. If there is little or no bone involvement, the extra digit is tied with silk suture soon after birth. The finger falls off within a few days, leaving a small scar. When there is bone involvement, surgical repair is indicated.

Genitourinary System Anomalies

Hypospadias and Epispadias

Hypospadias constitutes a range of penile anomalies associated with an abnormally located urinary meatus. The meatus can open below the glans penis or anywhere along the ventral surface of the penis, the scrotum, or the perineum. It is the most common anomaly of the penis, affecting approximately 1 in 250 to 300 live births (Gray & Moore, 2009). It is classified according to the location of the meatus and the presence or absence of chordee, which is a ventral curvature of the penis.

Mild cases of hypospadias (Fig. 28-20) are often repaired for cosmetic reasons and involve a single surgical procedure. The goals are to improve the appearance of the genitalia and make it possible for the child to urinate in a standing position and have a sexually adequate organ. Historically these infants were not circumcised because the foreskin was used during surgical repair; the urologist should be consulted before circumcision. Repair is done early, often during or soon after the first year of life.

Epispadias results from failure of urethral canalization. About 55% of the affected infants are boys who have a widened pubic symphysis and a broad spadelike penis with the urethra opened on its dorsal surface. Girls have a wide urethra and a bifid clitoris. Severity ranges from mild anomaly to a severe one that is associated with exstrophy of the bladder. Surgical correction is necessary, and affected male infants should not be circumcised.

Exstrophy of the Bladder

The most common bladder anomaly is exstrophy (Fig. 28-21), which often occurs in conjunction with epispadias. It is rare, occurring only in about 1 in 35,000 to 40,000 live births (Elder, 2007). It results from abnormal development of the bladder, abdominal wall, and symphysis pubis that causes the bladder, urethra, and ureteral orifices to all be exposed. The bladder is visible in the suprapubic area as a red mass with numerous folds, with urine draining from it onto the infant's skin.

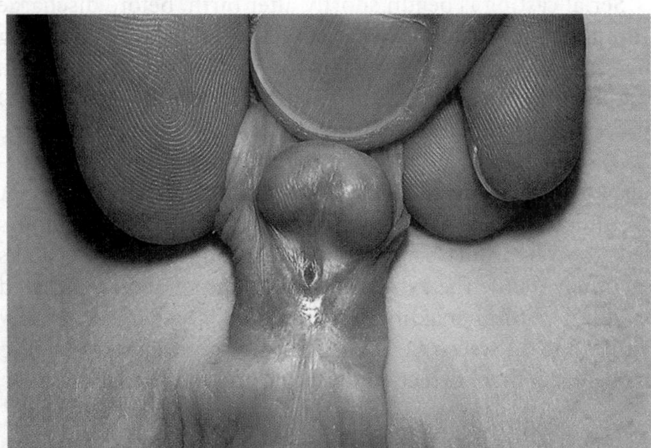

Fig. 28-20 Hypospadias. *(Courtesy H. Gil Rushton, MD, Children's National Medical Center, Washington, DC.)*

Immediately after birth the exposed bladder is covered with a sterile, nonadherent dressing to protect it until closure can be performed. It is recommended that reconstructive surgery be started in the neonatal period, preferably with the bladder being closed during the first or second day of life.

Disorders of Sex Development

A disorder of sex development (DSD) in the newborn (Fig. 28-22) often is discovered by the nurse during a physical assessment. Erroneous or abnormal sexual differentiation may be a genetic defect, such as congenital adrenal hypoplasia, which can be life threatening because it involves deficiency of all adrenocortical hormones. Other possible causes of DSD include chromosomal abnormalities, defective sex hormone synthesis in males, and the placental transfer of masculinizing

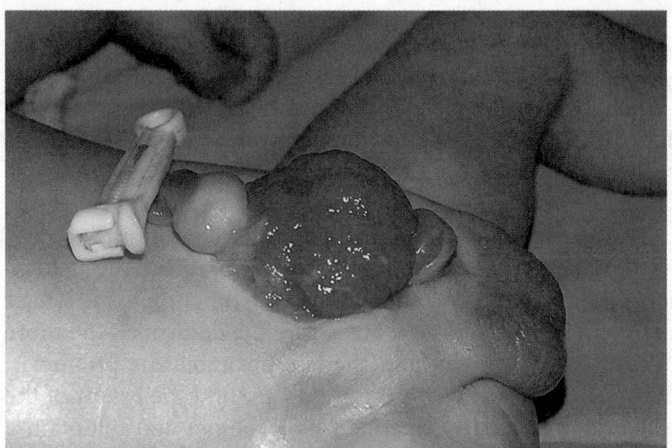

Fig. 28-21 Exstrophy of bladder. *(Courtesy H. Gil Rushton, MD, Children's National Medical Center, Washington, DC.)*

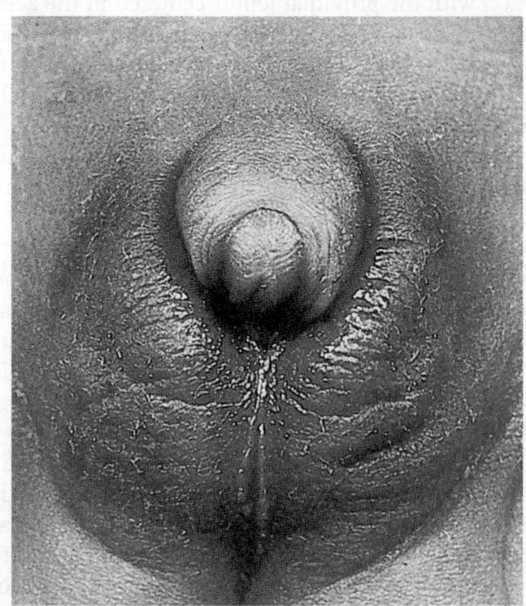

Fig. 28-22 Ambiguous external genitalia (i.e., structure may be enlarged clitoral hood and clitoris or micropenis and bifid scrotum). *(Courtesy Edward S. Tank, MD, Division of Urology, Oregon Health Sciences University, Portland, OR.)*

agents to female fetuses. Gender assignment should be based on data gathered from the following sources: maternal and family history, including the ingestion of steroids during pregnancy and relatives who had DSD or who died during the neonatal period; physical examination; chromosomal analysis (results are available in 2 or 3 days); endoscopy, ultrasonography, and radiographic contrast studies; biochemical tests, such as analysis of urinary steroid excretion, which helps detect several of the adrenocortical syndromes; and, in some instances, laparotomy or gonad biopsy.

Therapeutic intervention, including any counseling and surgery, should be started as soon as possible. Any child born with DSD should not receive gender assignment until a proper assessment has been done. An appropriate gender assignment should be based on age at presentation, potential for mature sexual function, potential fertility, and the long-term psychologic and intellectual impact on the child and family. Parents need much support as they learn to deal with this challenging situation.

Teratoma

A teratoma is an embryonal tumor that may be solid, cystic, or mixed. It is composed of at least two and usually three types of embryonal tissue: ectoderm, mesoderm, and endoderm. A teratoma in the newborn may occur in the skull, mediastinum, abdomen, or sacral area; more than half are located in the sacrococcygeal area. The treatment of choice for such neonates is complete surgical resection of the teratoma. Approximately 80% of all teratomas are benign, and no additional therapy is needed after complete resection done in the neonatal period. If the tumor is not surgically resected before the infant is 1 to 2 months old, the likelihood of the teratoma becoming malignant increases rapidly.

Nursing Care Management

Any deviations from normal are reported to the primary health care provider immediately. A thorough assessment of all body systems follows, with identification of both visible anomalies and those that might not be visible.

Some infants have multiple congenital anomalies. A recognized pattern of malformations is referred to as a *syndrome.* The most common is Down syndrome, with the diagnosis confirmed early in the neonatal period.

Genetic Diagnosis

Diagnostic procedures for the detection of genetic disorders are performed after birth at any time from the postnatal period through adulthood. Many tests are available for various disorders; only the most commonly used ones are discussed here.

Newborn Screening

The most widespread use of postnatal testing for genetic disease is the routine screening of newborns for inborn errors of metabolism (IEMs) such as PKU, galactosemia, hemoglobinopathy (sickle cell disease and thalassemias), and hypothyroidism. These are the minimum mandatory newborn screening tests in most states in the United States. An *IEM* is the term applied to a large group of disorders caused by a metabolic defect that results from the absence of or change in a protein, usually an enzyme, and mediated by the action of a certain gene. These defects can involve any substrate produced from protein, carbohydrate, or fat metabolism. IEMs are recessive disorders, and a person must receive a defective gene from each parent for them to occur. The parents usually are unaffected because their normal dominant gene directs the synthesis of sufficient protein to meet their metabolic needs under normal circumstances. With the advent of new biochemical techniques, it is now possible to detect the abnormal gene responsible for causing an increasing number of these disorders early in the neonatal period so appropriate therapies to prevent further morbidity may be implemented. Tandem mass spectrometry has the potential for identifying up to as many as 40 IEMs. With tandem mass spectrometry, earlier identification of IEMs may prevent further developmental delays and morbidities in affected children.

Phenylketonuria

PKU results from a deficiency of the enzyme phenylalanine dehydrogenase. The test for PKU is not reliable until the newborn has ingested an ample amount of the amino acid phenylalanine, a constituent of both human and cow's milk. The nurse must document the initial ingestion of milk and perform the test at least 24 hours after that time. The current trend toward early infant discharge from the hospital has the potential to cause neonates with a disorder such as PKU not to be adequately screened. The American Academy of Pediatrics, Committee on Genetics (1996), has made the following recommendations:

- Obtain a subsequent sample before 2 weeks of age if the initial specimen is collected before the newborn is 24 hours old.
- Designate a primary care provider for all newborns before discharge for adequate newborn screening follow-up.
- Collect the initial specimen as close as possible to discharge and no later than 7 days after birth.

If the infant is found to have PKU, a diet low in phenylalanine is begun soon after birth. A new drug, sapropterin dihydrochloride, has been recently approved for use in persons with PKU; the drug acts to decrease blood phenylalanine levels in persons with hyperphenylalaninemia (Stokowski, 2008). Breastfeeding or partial breastfeeding may be possible for some infants if the phenylalanine levels are monitored carefully and remain within acceptable limits (Lawrence & Lawrence, 2005). Many affected children have some intellectual impairment. Successful management and outcome are largely dependent on early identification of the condition, modification of the diet, and compliance with the treatment regimen throughout the entire life.

Galactosemia

Galactosemia, caused by a deficiency of the enzyme galactose-1-phosphate uridyltransferase, results in the inability to convert galactose to glucose. Galactosemia can be detected by measuring the blood levels of galactose in newborns suspected of having the disease who have ingested human milk (which contains galactose) or formula containing galactose. Infants with galactosemia appear normal at birth, but on ingestion of milk (which has a high lactose content), they begin to show progressive symptoms, including vomiting, diarrhea, and weight loss (Askin & Diehl-Jones, 2003). *E. coli* sepsis is another common initial clinical sign. If the disorder goes untreated, the galactose levels will continue to increase and the affected infant will show growth failure, cognitive impairment, cataracts, jaundice, hepatomegaly, and cirrhosis of the liver, with death possibly occurring in the first month of life. Therapy consists of eliminating lactose from the diet. This condition precludes breastfeeding, since lactose is present in breast milk.

Hypothyroidism

Congenital hypothyroidism results from a deficiency of thyroid hormones; it affects approximately 1 of every 3000 to 4000 newborns (Kaye & American Academy of Pediatrics, Committee on Genetics, 2006). All states in the United States routinely screen for hypothyroidism. Although a heel stick blood sample for the test is best obtained between 2 and 6 days of age, specimens are usually taken within the first 24 to 48 hours or before discharge as part of a concurrent screening for other metabolic defects. At this time the normally expected increase in thyroxine (T_4) would be lacking in newborns with hypothyroidism. Neonatal screening consists of an initial filter paper blood spot T_4 measurement followed by measurement of thyroid-stimulating hormone (TSH) in specimens with low T_4 values. Early screening may have false-positive results. In the newborn, thyroid function studies are elevated in comparison with values in older children; therefore it is important to document the timing of the tests. In preterm and sick full-term infants thyroid function tests are usually lower than in the healthy full-term infant. A repeat T_4 and TSH may be evaluated after 30 weeks (corrected age) in newborns born before that time and after resolution of the acute illness in the sick full-term infant.

Treatment involves lifelong thyroid hormone replacement therapy that begins as soon as possible after diagnosis to abolish all signs of hypothyroidism and to reestablish normal physical and mental development. The drug of choice is synthetic levothyroxine sodium (Synthroid, Levothroid).

Genetic Evaluation and Counseling

Genetic counseling is a communication process concerned with the human problems associated with the occurrence, or risk of occurrence, of a genetic disorder in a family. It involves relaying information about the diagnosis, treatment options, recurrence risk, and availability of prenatal diagnosis. With the completion of the Human Genome Project, the international project to determine the total genetic information in humans, a new era of human genetics is unfolding (International Human Genome Sequencing Consortium, 2004), and it will lead to a better understanding of specifically how genetic variation contributes to health and disease. It is essential that nurses master the basic principles of heredity, understand how heredity contributes to disorders, and be aware of the types of genetic testing available.

Nurses frequently encounter children with a genetic disorder, including an IEM, and families in which there is a risk that a disorder may be transmitted to or occur in an offspring. It is the nurse's responsibility to be alert to situations in which persons could benefit from a genetic evaluation and counseling to be aware of the local genetic resources, to aid the family in finding services, and to offer support and care for children and families affected by genetic conditions. Local genetic clinics can be located through several sites, such as GeneTests (*www.genetests.org*), a publicly funded medical genetics information resource developed for physicians and other health care providers, which is available at no cost to all interested persons.

Nursing Care

Newborn

A collaborative health team approach that includes specialists and community service representatives is needed in the care of the infant with a congenital anomaly. Surgical intervention in the neonatal period may be necessary for the infant requiring either immediate correction or a palliative procedure to relieve the symptoms of the anomaly until definitive correction can be done. There is also a higher morbidity and mortality in neonates than in older children or adults undergoing similar procedures. However, despite these problems unique to neonates, advances in surgical techniques, fluid and electrolyte management, anesthesia, pain management, and the nursing care given in intensive care nurseries have together been responsible for decreasing the risk of surgery in neonates.

The health care team must be highly skilled to meet these infants' needs. These needs are similar to those of other high risk infants. In addition to stabilization of the infant's condition (oxygenation and perfusion of tissues), other preoperative interventions, such as nasogastric tube placement for abdominal decompression, pain management, and the maintenance of fluid and electrolyte balance, are implemented to manage specific problems.

Postoperatively, the infant is often returned to the intensive care nursery, where he or she is closely monitored. The infant's respiratory efforts are supported; this often requires mechanical ventilation. Constant surveillance is necessary to detect any respiratory complications resulting from the anesthesia. A pulse oximeter is attached to measure the oxygen saturation, and oxygen is provided as needed. An indwelling gastric catheter may be placed to remove gastric secretions, thereby preventing aspiration and distention of the abdomen. The infant's fluid, electrolyte, and acid-base balances are monitored and adjusted as needed. Urine output is monitored and should equal 1 to 2 ml/kg/hr. Other nursing interventions are focused on caring for the surgical site, maintaining thermoregulation, managing pain, and promoting comfort.

Parents and Family

While the infant is receiving optimal care, the parents also have needs that must be met as they deal with the crisis of having an infant with an abnormal condition. Their reactions are carefully assessed and are likely to be those typical of a grief response. Facilitating their understanding of the information given them about their infant's condition is a vital nursing intervention. A newly diagnosed disorder often implies the need for the implementation of a therapeutic regimen. For example, the disorder may be an IEM, such as PKU, which requires consistent and rigid adherence to a diet. The family may need help with securing the required formula and receiving counseling from a clinical dietitian. The importance of maintaining the diet, keeping an adequate supply of special preparations, and avoiding the use of unauthorized substitutions must be impressed on the family. These conditions often require a drastic change in family lifestyle and functioning; families often depend on others for assistance, and family coping skills and resources may be stretched thin with a diagnosis such as PKU or galactosemia.

Referral to appropriate agencies is another essential component of the follow-up management, and the nurse should make the parents aware of all possible sources of aid, including pertinent literature, parent groups, and national organizations. Many organizations and foundations, such as the March of Dimes, provide services and counseling for families of affected children. Numerous parent support groups are also available, where they can share experiences and derive mutual support in coping with problems similar to those of other group members. Nurses must be familiar with the services available in their community that provide assistance and education to families with these special problems.

A major nursing function is providing emotional support to the family during all aspects of the care of the child born with an anomaly or disorder. The feelings stemming from the real or imagined threat posed by a congenital anomaly are as varied as the people being counseled. Responses may include apathy, denial, anger, hostility, fear, embarrassment, grief, and loss of self-esteem.

Parents may benefit from seeing before-and-after pictures of other babies born with the same defect. Coupled with other verbal and nonverbal supportive care, this visual reassurance may be effective in allaying their concerns.

Families need much information, guidance, and support as they make decisions regarding their infant's care. Once they have been given the facts and possible consequences and all the assistance they need in problem solving, the final decision regarding a course of action must be their own. It is then incumbent on health care providers to support the family's decision.

Key Points

- The identification of maternal and fetal risk factors in the antepartum and intrapartum periods is vital for planning adequate care of high risk infants.
- A small percentage of significant birth injuries may occur despite skilled and competent obstetric care.
- Metabolic abnormalities of diabetes mellitus in pregnancy adversely affect embryonic and fetal development.
- Infection in the newborn may be acquired in utero, at birth, in breast milk, or from within the nursery.
- The most common maternal infections during early pregnancy that are associated with various congenital malformations include toxoplasmosis, herpes, CMV, rubella, parvovirus B19, and varicella.
- HIV transmission from mother to infant occurs transplacentally at various gestational ages, perinatally by maternal blood and secretions, and by breast milk.
- Preterm infants are at risk for problems related to the immaturity of organ systems.
- Maternal-fetal Rh and ABO incompatibility may cause significant hemolysis and jaundice in the neonatal period.
- The injection of $Rh_o(D)$ immune globulin in Rh-negative and Coombs' test–negative women minimizes the possibility of isoimmunization.

Audio Chapter Summaries

Access an audio summary of these Key Points on evolve

- The nurse often first observes signs of newborn drug withdrawal (NAS) and acquires information from the maternal history.
- Congenital defects are now the leading cause of death in the first year of life.
- The curative and rehabilitative problems of a child with a congenital disorder are often complex, requiring a multidisciplinary approach to care.
- Parents often need special instruction (e.g., cardiopulmonary resuscitation, oxygen therapy, or nutrition requirements) before they take a high risk infant home.
- The supportive care given to the parents of infants with a congenital anomaly or IEM must begin at birth or at the time of diagnosis and continue for years.

References

Adams-Chapman I, Stoll B: Nervous system disorders. In Kliegman RM et al (editors): *Nelson textbook of pediatrics*, ed 18, Philadelphia, 2007, Saunders.

Alimenti A et al: A prospective controlled study of neurodevelopment in HIV-uninfected children exposed to combination retroviral drugs in pregnancy, *Pediatrics* 118(4):e1139-e1145, 2006.

American Academy of Pediatrics: Fetal alcohol syndrome and alcohol-related neurodevelopmental disorders, *Pediatrics* 106(2):358-361, 2000.

American Academy of Pediatrics, American College of Obstetricians and Gynecologists: *Guidelines for perinatal care*, ed 6, Elk Grove Village, IL, 2007, The Academy.

American Academy of Pediatrics, Committee on Drugs: The transfer of drugs and other chemicals into human milk, *Pediatrics* 108(3):776-789, 2001.

American Academy of Pediatrics, Committee on Genetics: Newborn screening fact sheet, *Pediatrics* 98(3 Pt 1):473-501, 1996.

American Academy of Pediatrics, Committee on Infectious Diseases: *Red book: 2006 report of the committee on infectious diseases*, ed 27, Elk Grove Village, IL, 2006, The Academy.

American Academy of Pediatrics, Committee on Pediatric AIDS: HIV testing and prophylaxis to prevent mother-to-child transmission in the United States, *Pediatrics* 122(5):1127-1134, 2008.

American Academy of Pediatrics, Subcommittee on Hyperbilirubinemia: Clinical practice guideline: management of hyperbilirubinemia in the newborn infant 35 or more weeks of gestation, *Pediatrics* 114(1):297-316, 2004.

Anderson MS et al: Enteral nutrition. In Merenstein GB, Gardner SL (editors): *Handbook of neonatal intensive care,* ed 6, St Louis, 2006, Mosby.

Arendt R et al: Motor development of cocaine-exposed children at age two years, *Pediatrics* 103(1):86-92, 1999.

Arria AM et al: Methamphetamine and other substance use during pregnancy: preliminary estimates from the Infant Development, Environment, and Lifestyle (IDEAL) study, *Matern Child Health* 10(3):293-302, 2006.

Askin DF, Diehl-Jones B: Liver, part 3, Pathophysiology of liver dysfunction, *Neonat Netw* 22(3):5-15, 2003.

Askin DF, Diehl-Jones B: Cocaine: effects of in utero exposure on the fetus and newborn, *J Perinat Neonatal Nurs* 14(4):83-102, 2001.

Association of Women's Health, Obstetric and Neonatal Nurses: *Evidence-based clinical practice guideline: neonatal skin care,* ed 2, Washington, DC, 2007, The Association.

Baer JS et al: A 21-year longitudinal analysis of the effects of prenatal alcohol exposure on young adult drinking, *Arch Gen Psychiatry* 60(4): 377-385, 2003.

Baley JE, Toltzis P: Viral infections. In Martin RJ, Fanaroff AA, Walsh MC (editors): *Fanaroff and Martin's neonatal-perinatal medicine: diseases of the fetus and infant,* ed 8, St Louis, 2006, Mosby.

Bandstra ES, Accornero VH: Infants of substance abusing mothers. In Martin RJ, Fanaroff AA, Walsh MC (editors): *Fanaroff and Martin's neonatal-perinatal medicine: diseases of the fetus and infant,* ed 8, St Louis, 2006, Mosby.

Bateman DA, Chiriboga CA: Dose-response effect of cocaine on newborn head circumference, *Pediatrics* 106(3):e33, 2000.

Bay CA, Steele MW, Davis H: Genetic disorders and dysmorphic conditions. In Zitelli B, Davis H (editors): *Atlas of pediatric physical diagnosis,* ed 5, St Louis, 2007, Mosby.

Berghella V et al: Maternal methadone dose and neonatal withdrawal, *Am J Obstet Gynecol* 189(2):312-317, 2003.

Bernstein D: Congenital heart disease. In Behrman RE et al (editors): *Nelson textbook of pediatrics,* ed 18, St Louis, 2007, Mosby.

Birthistle K, Carrington D: Fetal varicella syndrome: a reappraisal of the literature, *J Infect* 36(Suppl 1):25-29, 1998.

Blackburn S: *Maternal, fetal, and neonatal physiology: a clinical perspective,* ed 3, St Louis, 2007, Saunders.

Boyer SG, Boyer KM: Update on TORCH infections in the newborn infant, *Newborn Infant Nurs Rev* 4(1):70-80, 2004.

Bracken MB et al: Association of maternal caffeine consumption with decrements in fetal growth, *Am J Epidemiol* 157(5):456-466, 2003.

Buus-Frank M: Hands that heal—hands that harm, *Adv Neonatal Care* 4(5):251-255, 2004.

Campbell S: Prenatal cocaine exposure and neonatal/infant outcomes, *Neonatal Netw* 22(1):19-21, 2003.

Caviness AC, Demmler GJ, Selwyn BJ: Clinical and laboratory features of neonatal herpes simplex infection: a case-control study, *Pediatr Infect Dis J* 27(5):425-430, 2008.

Centers for Disease Control and Prevention: Racial/ethnic differences in the birth prevalence of spina bifida—United States, 1995-2005, *Morb Mortal Wkly Rep* 57(53):1409-1413, 2009a.

Centers for Disease Control and Prevention: Trends in perinatal group B streptococcal disease—United States, 2000-2006, *Morb Mortal Wkly Rep* 58(5):109-112, 2009b.

Centers for Disease Control and Prevention: *STD surveillance 2006, national profile,* January 2008. Available at www.cdc.gov/std/stats/chlamydia.htm (accessed on June 12, 2008).

Centers for Disease Control and Prevention: Guidelines for identifying and referring persons with fetal alcohol syndrome, *Morb Mortal Wkly Rep* 54(RR-11):1-15, 2005.

Centers for Disease Control and Prevention: Alcohol use among women of childbearing age—United States, 1991-1999, *Morb Mortal Wkly Rep* 51(13):273-276, 2002a.

Centers for Disease Control and Prevention: Prevention of perinatal group B streptococcal disease, *Morb Mortal Wkly Rep* 51(RR-11):1-231, 2002b.

Chapman SJ: Varicella in pregnancy, *Semin Perinatol* 22(4):339-346, 1998.

Chiriboga C et al: Dose-response of fetal cocaine exposure on newborn neurologic function, *Pediatrics* 103(6):79-85, 1999.

Chiriboga CA: Fetal alcohol and drug effects, *Neurologist* 9(6):267-279, 2003.

Cooper ER et al: Combination antiretroviral strategies for the treatment of pregnant HIV-1 infected women and prevention of perinatal HIV-1 transmission, *J AIDS* 29:484-494, 2002.

Coyle MG et al: Diluted tincture of opium (DTO) and phenobarbital versus DTO alone for neonatal opiate withdrawal in term infants, *J Pediatr* 140(5):561-564, 2002.

Crocker E: Meth's burning issues, *Nurse Week, Heartland Ed* 6(8):22-23, 2005.

D'Apolito K: Comparison of a rocking bed and standard bed for decreasing withdrawal symptoms in drug-exposed infants, *MCN Am J Matern Child Nurs* 24(3):138-144, 1999.

D'Apolito K, Hepworth JT: Prominence of withdrawal symptoms in polydrug-exposed infants, *J Perinat Neonatal Nurs* 14(4):46-60, 2001.

de Jong EP et al: Parvovirus B19 infection in pregnancy, *J Clin Virol* 36(1):1-7, 2006.

Delaney-Black V et al: Prenatal cocaine exposure and child behavior, *Pediatrics* 102(4 Pt 1):945-950, 1998.

Derauf C et al: Demographic and psychosocial characteristics of mothers using methamphetamine during pregnancy: preliminary results of the Infant Development, Environment and Lifestyle (IDEAL) study, *Am J Drug Alcohol Abuse* 33(2):281-289, 2007.

Diehl-Jones W, Askin DF: Nutritional modulation of neonatal outcomes, *AACN Clin Issues* 15(1):83-96, 2004.

Dunham EA: Obstetrical brachial plexus palsy, *Orthop Nurs* 22(2):106-116, 2003.

Ebrahim SH, Gfoerer J: Pregnancy-related substance use in the United States during 1996-1998, *Obstet Gynecol* 101(2):374-379, 2003.

Ehrlich PJ, Coran AG: Diaphragmatic hernia. In Kliegman RM et al (editors): *Nelson textbook of pediatrics,* ed 18, St Louis, 2007, Mosby.

Elder JS: Urologic disorders in infants and children: anomalies of the bladder. In Kliegman RM et al (editors): *Nelson textbook of pediatrics,* ed 18, St Louis, 2007, Mosby.

Eyler FD, Behnke M: Early development of infants exposed to drugs prenatally, *Clin Perinatol* 26(1):107-150, 1999.

Eyler FD, Behnke M, Conlon M: Birth outcome from a prospective, matched study of prenatal crack/cocaine use, part II, Interactive and dose effects on neurobehavioral assessment, *Pediatrics* 101(2):237-241, 1998.

Faulks S, Luther B: Changing paradigm for the treatment of clubfeet, *Orthop Nurs* 24(1):25-30, 2005.

Fernandes O et al: Moderate to heavy caffeine consumption during pregnancy and relationship to spontaneous abortion and abnormal fetal growth: a meta-analysis, *Reprod Toxicol* 12(4):435-444, 1998.

Fleming P, Blair PS: Sudden infant death syndrome and parental smoking, *Early Human Dev* 83(11): 721-725, 2007.

Frank DA et al: Heavily cocaine exposed children show positive effects of early intervention on Bayley Scales of Infant Development (abstract), *Pediatr Res* 43:214A, 1998.

Frenkel L: Challenges in the diagnosis and management of neonatal herpes simplex virus encephalitis, *Pediatrics* 115(3):795-797, 2005.

Gray M, Moore KN: *Urologic disorders: adult and pediatric care,* St Louis, 2009, Mosby.

Gupta A et al: Outbreak of extended-spectrum beta-lactamase-producing *Klebsiella pneumoniae* in a neonatal intensive care unit linked to artificial nails, *Infect Control Hosp Epidemiol* 25(3):210-215, 2004.

Hale TW: *Medications and mothers' milk,* Amarillo, TX, 2002, Pharmasoft Medical.

Honein MA: Impact of folic acid fortification of the US food supply and occurrence of neural tube defects, *JAMA* 285(23):2981-2986, 2001.

Honein MA et al: Maternal smoking and environmental tobacco smoke exposure and the risk of orofacial clefts, *Epidemiology* 18(2):226-233, 2007.

Hosalkar HS et al: The hip. In Kliegman RM et al (editors): *Nelson textbook of pediatrics,* ed 18, Philadelphia, 2007, Saunders.

Huestis MA, Choo RE: Drug abuse's smallest victims: in utero drug exposure, *Forensic Sci Int* 128(1-2):20-30, 2002.

Hurd YL et al: Marijuana impairs growth in mid-gestation fetuses, *Neurotoxicol Teratol* 27(2):221-229, 2005.

International Human Genome Sequencing Consortium: Finishing the euchromatic sequence of the human genome, *Nature* 431:931-945, 2004.

Jansson LM, Velez M, Harrow C: Methadone maintenance and lactation: a review of the literature and current management guidelines, *J Hum Lact* 20(1):62-71, 2004.

Johnson K, Gerada C, Greenough A: Treatment of neonatal abstinence syndrome, *Arch Dis Child Fetal Neonatal Ed* 88(1):F2-F5, 2003.

Jones HE et al: Buprenorphine versus methadone in the treatment of pregnant opioid-dependent patients: effects on the neonatal abstinence syndrome, *Drug Alcohol Depend* 79(1):1-10, 2005.

Jones MW, Bass WT: Fetal alcohol syndrome, *Neonatal Netw* 22(3):63-70, 2003.

Kaiser L, Allen LH, American Dietetic Association: Position of the American Dietetic Association: nutrition and lifestyle for a healthy pregnancy outcome, *J Am Diet Assoc* 108(3):553-561, 2008.

Kakko J, Heilig M, Sarman I: Buprenorphine and methadone treatment of opiate dependence during pregnancy: comparison of fetal growth and neonatal outcomes in two consecutive case series, *Drug Alcohol Depend* 96(1-2):69-78, 2008.

Kaltenbach K, Berghella V, Finnegan L: Opioid dependence during pregnancy: effects and management, *Obstet Gynecol Clin North Am* 25(1): 139-151, 1998.

Kandall SR: Treatment strategies for drug-exposed neonates, *Clin Perinatol* 26(1):231-243, 1999.

Kaye CI, American Academy of Pediatrics, Committee on Genetics:

Newborn screening fact sheets, *Pediatrics* 118(3):e934-e963, 2006.

Koren G et al: Long-term neurodevelopmental risks in children exposed in utero to cocaine: the Toronto adoption study, *Ann NY Acad Sci* 846:306-312, 1998.

Kriebs JM: The global reach of HIV: preventing mother-to-child transmission, *J Perinat Neonatal Nurs* 16(3):1-10, 2002.

Law KL et al: Smoking during pregnancy and newborn neurobehavior, *Pediatrics* 111(6):1318-1323, 2003.

Lawrence RA, Lawrence RM: *Breastfeeding: a guide for the medical profession*, ed 6, St Louis, 2005, Mosby.

Lee M: Marihuana and tobacco use in pregnancy, *Obstet Gynecol Clin North Am* 25(1):65-83, 1998.

Lester BM, Tronick EZ: History and description of the Neonatal Intensive Care Unit Network Neurobehavioral Scale, *Pediatrics* 113(3 Pt 2):634-640, 2004.

Malanga CJ, Kosofsy BE: Mechanism of action of drugs of abuse on the developing fetal brain, *Clin Perinatol* 26(1):17-37, 1999.

Malik S et al: Maternal smoking and congenital heart defects, *Pediatrics* 121(4):e810-e816, 2008.

Messinger DS et al: The maternal lifestyle study: cognitive, motor, and behavioral outcomes of cocaine-exposed and opiate-exposed infants through 3 years of age, *Pediatrics* 113(6):1677-1685, 2004.

Michaels MG: Treatment of congenital cytomegalovirus: where are we now? *Expert Rev Anti Infect Ther* 5(3):441-448, 2007.

Milerad J et al: Objective measurements of nicotine exposure in victims of sudden infant death syndrome and in other unexpected child deaths, *J Pediatr* 133(2):232-236, 1998.

Minozzi S et al: Maintenance agonist treatments for opiate dependent pregnant women, *Cochrane Database Syst Rev* (2):CD006318, 2008.

Mitchell EA, Milerad J: Smoking and the sudden infant death syndrome, *Rev Environ Health* 21(2):81-103, 2006.

Moise KJ: Management of rhesus alloimmunization in pregnancy, *Obstet Gynecol* 100(3):600-611, 2002.

Moolenaar RL et al: A prolonged outbreak of *Pseudomonas aeruginosa* in a neonatal intensive care unit: did staff fingernails play a role in disease transmission? *Infect Control Hosp Epidemiol* 21(2):80-85, 2000.

Morrow CE et al: Learning disabilities and intellectual functioning in school-aged children with prenatal cocaine exposure, *Dev Neuropsychol* 30(3):905-931, 2006.

Myers MG, Seward JF, LaRussa PS: Varicella-zoster virus. In Kliegman RM et al (editors): *Nelson textbook of pediatrics*, ed 18, Philadelphia, 2007, Saunders.

Neal JL: RhD isoimmunization and current management modalities, *J Obstet Gynecol Neonatal Nurs* 30(6):589-607, 2001.

Nesheim SR et al: Trends in opportunistic infections in the pre- and post-highly active antitretroviral therapy eras among HIV-infected children in the Perinatal AIDS Collaborative Transmission Study, 1986-2004, *Pediatrics* 120(1):100-109, 2007.

Ogundele MO, Coulter JB: HIV transmission through breastfeeding: problems and prevention, *Ann Trop Paediatr* 23(2):91-106, 2003.

Ostrea E: Understanding drug testing in the neonate and the role of meconium analysis, *J Perinat Neonatal Nurs* 14(4):61-82, 2001.

Philipp BL, Merewood A, O'Brien S: Commentary: methadone and breastfeeding: new horizons, *Pediatrics* 111(6 Pt 1):1429-1430, 2003.

Plessinger M: Prenatal exposure to amphetamines, *Obstet Gynecol Clin North Am* 25(1):119-138, 1998.

Popovich DM, McAlhany A: Practitioner care and screening guidelines for infants born to *Chlamydia*-positive mothers, *Newborn Infant Nurs Rev* 4(1):51-55, 2004.

Rao R, Desai NS: OxyContin and neonatal abstinence syndrome, *J Perinatol* 22(4):324-325, 2002.

Reed MD, Aranda JV, Hales BF: Developmental pharmacology. In Martin RJ, Fanaroff AA, Walsh MC (editors): *Fanaroff and Martin's neonatal-perinatal medicine: diseases of the fetus and infant*, ed 8, St Louis, 2006, Mosby.

Reiser DJ: Neonatal jaundice: physiologic variation or pathologic process, *Crit Care Nurs Clin North Am* 16: 257-269, 2004.

Richardson GA, Hamel SC, Goldschmidt L: The effects of cocaine use on neonatal neurobehavioral status, *Neurotoxicol Teratol* 18(5):519-528, 1996.

Roaten JB, Bensard DD, Price FN: Neonatal surgery. In Merenstein GB, Gardner SL (editors): *Handbook of neonatal intensive care*, ed 6, St Louis, 2006, Mosby.

Sander SC, Hays LR: Prescription opioid dependence and treatment with methadone in pregnancy, *J Opioid Manage* 1(2):91-97, 2005.

Santos I et al: Caffeine intake and low birth weight: a population-based case-control study, *Am J Epidemiol* 147(7):620-627, 1998.

Sauerbrei A, Wutzler P: Herpes simplex and varicella-zoster virus infections during pregnancy: current concepts of prevention, diagnosis and therapy, part 2, Varicella-zoster virus, *Med Microbiol Immunol* 196(2):95-102, 2007.

Schleiss MR: Congenital cytomegalovirus infection: update on management strategies, *Curr Treat Options Neurol* 10(3):186-192, 2008.

Segel GB: Hereditary spherocytosis. In Kliegman RM et al (editors): *Nelson textbook of pediatrics*, ed 18, Philadelphia, 2007, Saunders.

Singer LT et al: Cognitive outcomes of preschool children with prenatal cocaine exposure, *JAMA* 291(20): 2448-2456, 2004.

Singer LT et al: Cognitive and motor outcomes of cocaine-exposed infants, *JAMA* 287(15):1952-1960, 2002.

Smith L et al: Effects of prenatal methamphetamine exposure on fetal growth and drug withdrawal symptoms in infants born at term, *J Devel Behav Pediatr* 24(1):17-23, 2003.

Smith LM et al: The infant development, environment, and lifestyle study: effects of prenatal methamphetamine exposure, polydrug exposure, and poverty on intrauterine growth, *Pediatrics* 118(3):1149-1156, 2006.

Sood B et al: Prenatal alcohol exposure and childhood behavior at age 6 to 7 years, part I, Dose-response effect, *Pediatrics* 108(2):e34, 2001.

Stokowski LA: Noteworthy professional news: drug to treat phenylketonuria approved, *Adv Neonatal Care* 8(3):139-140, 2008.

Stoler JM, Holmes LB: Recognition of facial features of fetal alcohol syndrome in the newborn, *Am J Med Genet C Semin Med Genet* 127(1):21-27, 2004.

Stoll BJ: Infections in the neonatal infant. In Kliegman RM et al (editors): *Nelson textbook of pediatrics*, ed 18, Philadelphia, 2007, Saunders.

Stoll BJ et al: Very low birth weight preterm infants with early onset neonatal sepsis: the predominance of gram-negative infections continues in the National Institute of Child Health and Human Development Neonatal Research Network, 2002-2003, *Pediatr Infect Dis J* 24(7):635-639, 2005.

Swayze VW et al: Magnetic resonance imaging of brain anomalies in fetal alcohol syndrome, *Pediatrics* 99(2):232-240, 1997.

Tanney MR, Lowenstein V: One-stop shopping: description of a model program to provide primary care to substance-abusing women and their children, *J Pediatr Health Care* 11(1):20-25, 1997.

Tronick EZ, Beeghly M: Prenatal cocaine exposure, child development, and the compromising effects of cumulative risk, *Clin Perinatol* 26(1):151-171, 1999.

Tronick EZ et al: Late dose-response effects of prenatal cocaine exposure on neurobehavioral performance, *Pediatrics* 98(1):78-83, 1996.

Venkatesh M et al: Infection in the neonate. In Merenstein GB, Gardner SL (editors): *Handbook of neonatal intensive care*, ed 6, St Louis, 2006, Mosby.

Volpe JJ: *Neurology of the newborn*, ed 5, Philadelphia, 2008, Saunders.

Wagner C et al: The impact of prenatal drug exposure on the neonate, *Obstet Gynecol Clin North Am* 25(1):169-194, 1998.

Weiner SM, Finnegan LP: Drug withdrawal in the neonate. In Merenstein GB, Gardner SL (editors): *Handbook of neonatal intensive care*, ed 6, St Louis, 2006, Mosby.

World Health Organization: *Consensus statement: WHO HIV and infant feeding*, 2008, Geneva, Switzerland, The Organization. Available at www.who.int/child_adolescent_health/topics/prevention_care/child/nutrition/hivif/en/print.html. Accessed March 21, 2009).

Yogev R, Chadwick EG: Acquired immunodeficiency syndrome (human immmunodeficiency virus). In Kliegman RM et al (editors): *Nelson textbook of pediatrics*, ed 18, Philadelphia, 2007, Saunders.

Yudin MH, Gonik B: Perinatal infections. In Martin RJ, Fanaroff AA, Walsh MC (editors): *Fanaroff and Martin's neonatal-perinatal medicine: diseases of the fetus and infant*, ed 8, St Louis, 2006, Mosby.

Part 2

Pediatric Nursing

Unit 7 Children, Their Families, and the Nurse

Unit 8 Assessment of the Child and Family

Unit 9 Health Promotion and Special Health Problems

Unit 10 Special Needs, Illness, and Hospitalization

Unit 11 Health Problems of Children

Unit 7

29

Contemporary Pediatric Nursing

Learning Objectives

On completion of this chapter the reader will be able to:

- Define the terms *mortality* and *morbidity.*
- Identify two ways that knowledge of mortality and morbidity can improve child health.
- List three major causes of death during infancy, early childhood, later childhood, and adolescence.
- List two major causes of illness during childhood.
- Describe five broad functions of the pediatric nurse in promoting the health of children.
- Define the term *critical thinking.*
- Identify the five steps of the nursing process.
- Define the term *nursing diagnosis.*
- Define *evidence-based practice.*

Electronic Resources

Additional information related to the content in Chapter 29 can be found on

evolve the Companion Website at
http://evolve.elsevier.com/Perry/maternal/

- NCLEX Review Questions

Health Care for Children

The major goal for pediatric nursing is to improve the quality of health care for children. There are 73 million children 0 to 18 years of age in the United States, making up 25% of the population (Dougherty et al, 2005). The health of children living in the United States has improved in numerous areas, including vaccination coverage, adolescent birth rates, and child mortality. Although child mortality rates have declined dramatically, millions of families have no child health insurance, resulting in lack of access to care and health promotion services. And although most American children are healthy, disparities related to race, ethnicity, socioeconomic status, and geography prevail. Patterns of child health are shaped by medical progress and societal trends (Dougherty et al, 2005; Wise, 2004, 2005). The *Healthy People 2010* Leading Health Indicators provide a framework for identifying essential components for child health promotion programs designed to prevent future health problems in our nation's children.

The National Children's Study is the largest long-term study of children's health and development conducted in the United States. The study is designed to follow 100,000 children and their families from birth to age 21 to understand the link between children's environments and their physical and emotional health and development (National Children's Study, 2008). It is hoped that a study of this magnitude will provide innovative interventions for families, children, and health care providers to eradicate unhealthy diets, dental caries, and childhood obesity and bring a significant reduction in violence, injury, substance abuse, and mental health disorders among the nation's children. This study supports the *Healthy People 2010* primary goals to increase the quality and years of healthy life and eliminate health disparities related to race, ethnicity, and socioeconomic status (US Department of Health and Human Services, 2007).

Health Promotion

Many of tomorrow's leading causes of death, disease, and disability—including cardiovascular disease, cancer, chronic lung diseases, depression, violence, substance abuse, injuries, nutritional deficiencies, and human immunodeficiency virus/acquired immunodeficiency syndrome (HIV/AIDS)—can be significantly reduced in children and adolescents by preventing six categories of behavior (World Health Organization, 2007):

1. Tobacco use
2. Behavior that results in injury and violence
3. Alcohol and substance use
4. Dietary and hygienic practices that cause disease
5. Sedentary lifestyle
6. Sexual behavior that causes unintended pregnancy and disease

Child health promotion provides opportunities to reduce differences in current health status among members of different groups and ensure equal opportunities and resources to enable all children to achieve their fullest health potential.

Nutrition

Nutrition is an essential component for healthy growth and development, and its promotion begins at birth. Human milk is the preferred form of nutrition for all infants. *Breastfeeding* provides the infant with micronutrients, immunologic properties, and several enzymes that enhance digestion and absorption of these nutrients. Many working mothers tend to wean their infants early to avoid the hassle of breast pumping during the workday. However, there has been resurgence in breastfeeding due to the education of mothers and fathers regarding its benefits.

Young children tend to establish eating habits during the first 2 to 3 years of life, and the nurse is instrumental in guiding parents in the selection nutritious foods. During childhood, the eating preferences and attitudes related to food habits are established by family influences and culture. During adolescence, parental influence diminishes as the adolescent makes food choices related to peer acceptability and sociability; these choices may be detrimental for the chronically ill child with diabetes, hypertension, or heart or renal disease.

Unhealthy diets are common among lower income families, often because of the lack of nutritious fresh fruits and vegetables and adequate milk and protein intake. In addition, the lifestyles of homeless and migrant children place these populations at risk for inadequate food, causing nutrient deficiencies, developmental and growth delays, depression, hunger, and behavior problems.

Dental Care

The *Healthy People 2010* project reports that nearly one in five children between the ages of 2 and 4 years, particularly Latino children, has visible cavities (Edelstein, 2005). *Dental caries* is the single most common chronic disease of childhood (Heuer, 2007). The most common form of early dental disease is early childhood caries, which may begin at the first birthday and progress to pain and infection within the first 2 years of life (Edelstein, 2005). Preschoolers of low-income families are twice as likely to develop tooth decay and only half as likely to visit the dentist as other children (Edelstein, 2005). Since this is a preventable disease, nursing plays an essential role in promoting early tooth care by instructing the children and parents on practicing dental hygiene beginning with the first tooth eruption; drinking fluoridated water, including bottled water; and instituting early dental preventive care.

Immunizations

The two public health interventions that have had the greatest impact on world health are clean drinking water and vaccines. Differences in *immunizations rates* exist among children of different races and ethnicities, family incomes, states, and ages and also according to the type of vaccination (Dougherty et al, 2005). A child's immunization record should be reviewed at each clinic visit, and parents should be instructed to keep immunizations current, reinforcing the *Healthy People 2010* goal of vaccinating 90% of 2-year-olds (US Department of Health and Human Services, 2007).

Childhood Health Problems

The health of the nation's children continues to improve in many areas, such as lower pregnancy rates for adolescents and expanded vaccine coverage. However, changes in modern society, including disruptive influences on the family, the explosion of technology, and the proliferation of information systems, are influencing the emergence of significant medical problems that affect the health of children (Lichter, 2005). Recent concern has focused on groups of children who have increased morbidity: homeless and immigrant children, children living in poverty, low-birth-weight (LBW) children, children with chronic illnesses, foreign-born adopted children, and children in day care centers. A number of factors place these groups at risk for poor health. A major cause is barriers to health care, especially for the homeless, the poverty stricken, and those with chronic health problems. Other factors include improved survival of children with chronic health problems, particularly infants of very low birth weight (VLBW).

In addition to disease and injury, children face behavioral, social (family), and educational problems that are referred to as the *new morbidity* or *pediatric social illness*. These problems (e.g., poverty, violence, aggression, noncompliance, school failure, and adjustment to divorce or bereavement) interfere with children's social and academic development. *Mental health issues* also affect our children and adolescents. One out of five has mental health problems, and 1 out of 10 has serious emotional problems that affect daily functioning (Coury, 2006). Examples of increasing pediatric problems include obesity, type 2 diabetes, injuries, violence, substance abuse, and emotional and mental health problems during adolescence.

Obesity and Type 2 Diabetes

Childhood obesity is the most common nutritional problem among American children and is increasing in epidemic proportions, along with type 2 diabetes (Yensel, Preud'Homme, & Curry, 2004). *Obesity* in children and adolescents is defined as a body mass index at or greater than the 95th percentile for youth of the same age and gender (Dietz, 2005; Covington et al, 2001). The National Health and Nutrition Examination Survey reported that the prevalence of overweight children doubled and the prevalence of overweight adolescents tripled between 1980 and 2000 (Dietz, 2005).

Advancements in entertainment and technology such as television, computers, and video games have contributed to the growing childhood obesity problem in the United States. Approximately 63% of 8- to 18-years-olds have a television in their bedrooms and watch television an average of 4 hours a day (Robinson & Sargent, 2005). Minority populations, especially African-American and Hispanic children from families of low socioeconomic status, watch more than 4 hours of television daily, exacerbating the effects of sedentary activity with intake of high-caloric, fatty foods (Fitzgibbon & Stolley, 2004).

Lack of outside physical activity because of unsafe environments and inconvenient facilities for physical activities, combined with easy access to video games and television within the home, tend to promote obesity among low-income

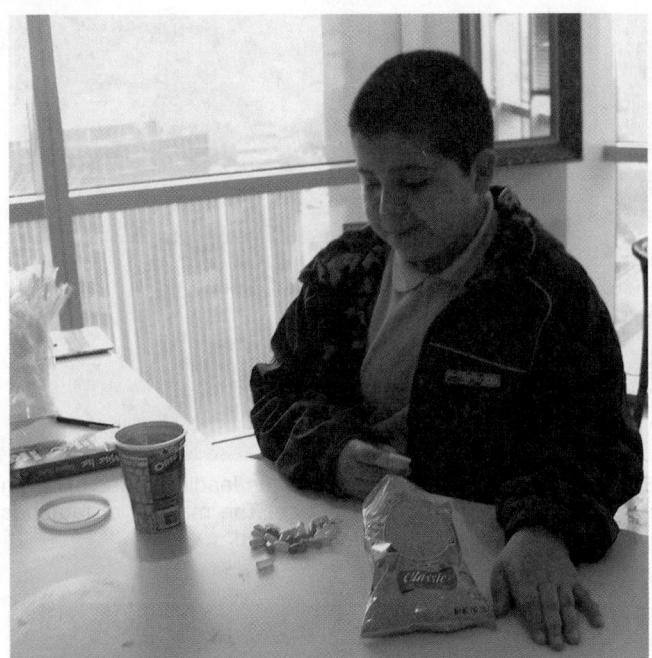

Fig. 29-1 The American cultural tendency toward excessive intake of high-caloric, fatty foods contributes to obesity in children.

minority children. Overweight youth, especially of Hispanic, African-American, and Native American descent, have increased risk for developing diabetes, insulin resistance, hypertension, and heart disease (Jackson, 2001; Yensel, Preud'Homme, & Curry, 2004) (Fig. 29-1). A major nursing health prevention focus, consistent with the *Healthy People 2010* primary goals, is the reduction of overweight children, ages 6 to 19 years, from the current 20% in all ethnic groups, to less than 6% (Duderstadt, 2004; US Department of Health and Human Services, 2007).

Childhood Injuries

Injuries are the most common cause of death and disability to children in the United States (Schnitzer, 2006). *Unintentional injuries* among children ages 19 and under have dropped to 39%, and the violent death rate has dropped 36% in the same age bracket; however, the trend has now plateaued (Rivara, 2005). Despite the decrease in injuries to children, motor vehicle (MV)–related accidents continue as the most common cause of death in children older than 1 year of age. As children grow older, the percentage of deaths from injuries increases. The most common types of unintentional injuries, in addition to MV accidents, include drowning, burns, and firearm accidents. Many childhood injury fatalities could be avoided. For example, the majority of bicycling deaths are from head injuries. Although helmets reduce the risk of head injury by 85%, few children wear them (National Safety Council, 2000).

The type of injury and the circumstances surrounding it are closely related to normal growth and developmental behavior. As children develop, their innate curiosity impels them to investigate activities and to mimic the behavior of others. This is essential to acquire competency as an adult, but it predisposes children to numerous hazards.

The child's *developmental stage* partially determines the types of injuries that are most likely to occur at a specific age and helps provide clues to preventive measures. For example, small infants are helpless in any environment. When they begin to roll over or propel themselves, they can fall from unprotected surfaces. The crawling infant, who has a natural tendency to place objects in the mouth, is at risk for aspiration or poisoning. The mobile toddler, with the instinct to explore and investigate and the ability to run and climb, may experience falls, burns, and collisions with objects. As children grow older, their absorption with play makes them oblivious to environmental hazards such as street traffic or water. The need to conform and gain acceptance compels older children and adolescents to accept challenges and dares. Although the rate of injuries is high in children less than 9 years of age, most fatal injuries occur in later childhood and adolescence.

The pattern of deaths caused by unintentional injuries, especially from MVs, drowning, and burns, is remarkably consistent in most Western societies. However, the United States far exceeds other countries in the number of *violent deaths*. The leading causes of death from injuries for each age group according to sex are presented in Table 29-1. Although the incidence of violence is increasing in the United States, it is important to note that accidents continue to account for more than three times as many teen deaths as any other cause (Annie E Casey Foundation, 2008). Fortunately, prevention strategies such as the use of car restraints, bicycle helmets, and smoke detectors have resulted in a significant decrease in fatalities for children. Currently, all states have enacted legislation requiring young children to be properly restrained in MVs. Despite safety efforts, the overwhelming cause of death in children is MV-related fatalities, including occupant, pedestrian, bicycle, and motorcycle deaths. In fact, MV-related accidents now account for more than half of all injury deaths (Hoyert, Kung, & Smith, 2005; National Center for Injury Prevention and Control, 2001). The majority of deaths from injuries occur in males. Even though the percentage of infants dying from MV injuries is small compared with the total number of deaths in that age group, children under 1 year of age still have a high death rate from MV accidents, primarily from a failure to use proper restraints (Fig. 29-2).

Pedestrian injuries in children account for significant numbers of MV-related deaths. Most pedestrian injuries occur at midblock, at intersections, in driveways, and in parking lots. Driveway injuries typically involve small children and large vehicles backing up. Parents may not be alert to the dangers leading to such injuries and consequently fail to protect their children.

Bicycle injuries are another important cause of childhood deaths. Children ages 5 to 9 years are at greatest risk of bicycling fatalities. The majority of bicycling deaths are from head injuries. Helmets reduce the risk of head injury by 85%, but few children wear helmets (National Safety Council, 2000). Community-wide bicycle helmet campaigns and mandatory use laws have resulted in significant increases in helmet use. Still, issues such as stylishness, comfort, and social acceptability remain important factors in compliance. Nurses can educate children and families about pedestrian and bicycle

Table 29-1 Mortality from Leading Types of Unintentional Injuries, United States, 1997 (Rate Per 100,000 Population in Each Age Group)

TYPE OF ACCIDENT	Age (yr) <1	1-4	5-14	15-24
Males				
All causes	818.0	39.8	24.0	124.4
Unintentional injuries (all types)	22.3	15.2	10.6	52.3
Motor vehicle	4.4 (2)	5.3 (1)	5.8 (1)	38.3 (1)
Drowning	1.8 (4)	3.9 (2)	1.6 (2)	3.2 (2)
Fires and burns	1.5 (5)	2.5 (3)	0.8 (3)	–
Firearms	–	–	0.5 (4)	1.5 (4)
Ingestion of food/object	2.5 (3)	0.5 (5)	–	–
Falls	–	–	–	1.2 (5)
Mechanical suffocation	9.1 (1)	0.6 (4)	0.4 (5)	–
Poisoning	–	–	–	2.8 (3)
All other unintentional injuries	3.1	2.3	1.4	5.3
Accidents as a percent of all deaths	2.7%	38.2%	44.3%	42.0%
Females				
All causes	662.9	31.8	17.4	46.0
Unintentional injuries (all types)	18.1	10.9	6.7	20.0
Motor vehicle	4.4 (2)	4.7 (1)	4.3 (1)	17.1 (1)
Drowning	1.4 (4)	2.0 (2)	0.6 (3)	0.4 (3)
Fires and burns	1.2 (5)	2.0 (2)	0.7 (2)	–
Firearms	–	–	0.1 (4)	0.1 (5)
Ingestion of food/object	1.5 (3)	0.4 (4)	–	–
Falls	–	–	–	0.2 (4)
Mechanical suffocation	6.9 (1)	0.3 (5)	0.1 (4)	–
Poisoning	–	–	–	0.8 (2)
All other unintentional injuries	2.7	1.5	0.9	1.5
Accidents as a percent of all deaths	2.7%	34.2%	38.2%	43.4%

Modified from National Safety Council: *Injury facts*, Itaska, IL, 2000, The Council. Data from National Center for Health Statistics.

safety. In particular, school nurses can promote helmet wearing and encourage peer leaders to act as role models.

Drowning and *burns* are among the top three leading causes of deaths for males and females throughout childhood (Fig. 29-3). In addition, improper use of firearms is a major cause of death among males. During infancy, more males succumb to death from aspiration or suffocation than do females (Fig. 29-4). More than half of all *poisonings* reported in 1999 occurred in children under 6 years of age (National Center for Injury Prevention and Control, 2001) (Fig. 29-5). By ages 4 to 5 years, unintentional poisonings are uncommon. Another increase occurs in the 15- to 24-year age group, where poisoning is the third leading cause of death in males and second in females. Poisoning in this age group is typically intentional and usually represents death from suicide (especially among females) or drug abuse.

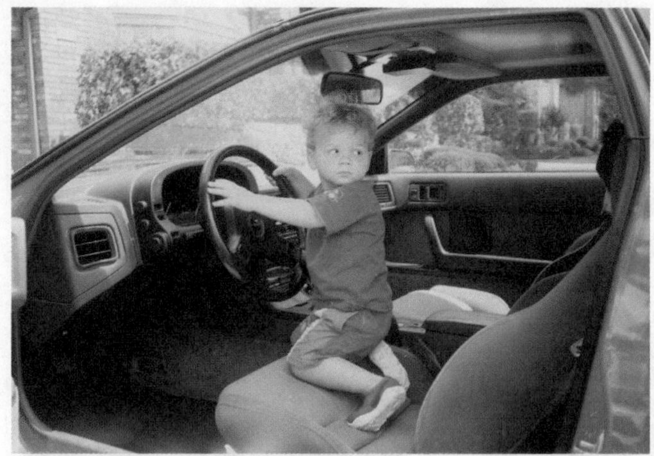

Fig. 29-2 Motor vehicle injuries are the leading cause of death in children older than 1 year of age. The majority of fatalities involve occupants who are unrestrained.

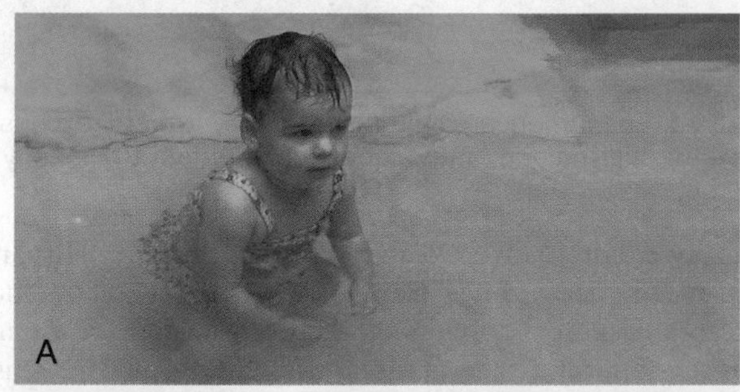

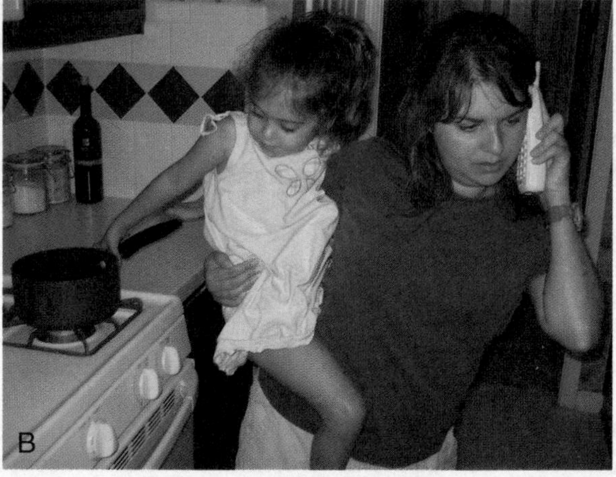

Fig. 29-3 A, Drowning is one of the leading causes of death. Children left unattended are unsafe even in shallow water. **B,** Burns are among the top three leading cause of death from injury in children ages 1 to 14 years.

Violence

Each day, 10 children in the United States are murdered by gunfire, equivalent to approximately one child every 2½ hours (Groves, 2005). Strikingly higher homicide rates are found among minority populations, especially African-American children. Violence permeates American households through

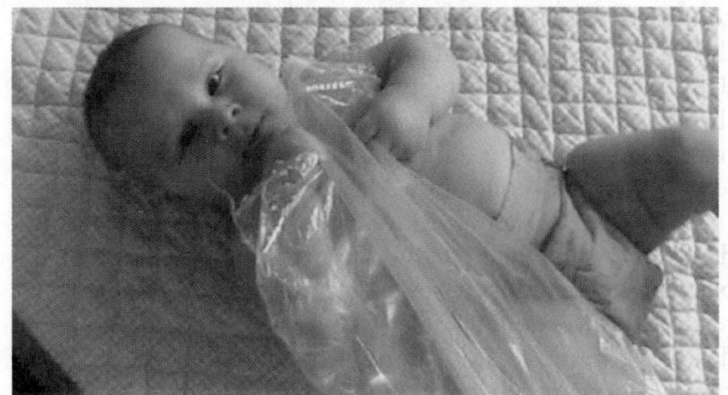

Fig. 29-4 Mechanical suffocation is the leading cause of death from injury in infants.

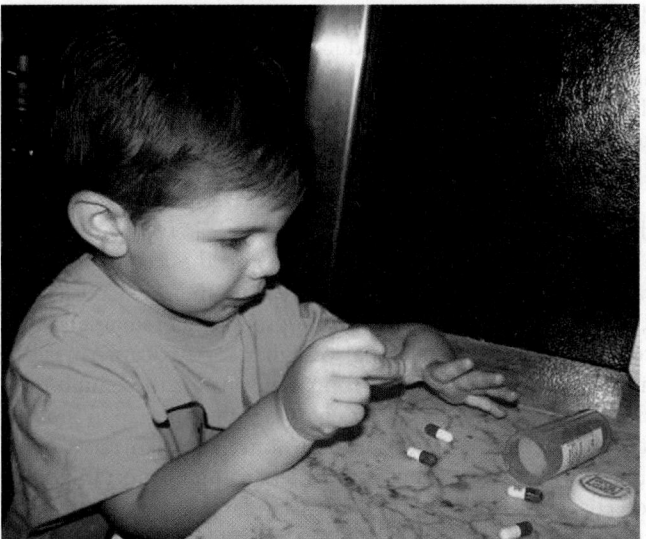

Fig. 29-5 Poisoning causes a considerable number of injuries in children under 4 years of age. Prescription drugs should never be left where young children can reach them.

television programs, commercials, video games, and movies that tend to desensitize the child toward violence. Between the time of preschool and graduation from high school, children will have viewed more than 200,000 violent acts on television (Groves, 2005). Violence also permeates the schools with the availability of guns and illicit drugs and the presence of gangs (Fisher & Kettl, 2003). Although declines from peak levels in 1993 have been observed in serious violent crimes with children as victims or as offenders (ages 12 to 17) (Federal Interagency Forum on Child and Family Statistics, 2007), assessment of high risk behaviors in our youth must continue to be a major focus of health promotion.

The causes of increased violence against children and self-inflicted violence are not fully understood. In young children the increase in homicide may represent a more accurate identification of child abuse. In all cases the problem of child homicide is extremely complex and involves numerous social, economic, and other influences. Prevention lies in better understanding of the social and psychologic factors that lead to the high rates of homicide and suicide. Nurses need to be especially aware of young people who are depressed, repeatedly in trouble with the criminal justice system, or associated with groups known to be violent. Prevention requires identification of these young people and therapeutic intervention by qualified professionals.

Pediatric nurses can assess children and adolescents for risk factors related to violence. Families that own firearms must be educated about their safe use and storage. The presence of a gun in a household increases the risk of suicide by about five-fold and the risk of homicide by about threefold. Legislative efforts may focus on preventing specific groups, such as felons and children, from having access to firearms. Technologic changes such as childproof safety devices and loading indicators could improve the safety of firearms.

Substance Abuse

Risk-taking behaviors, particularly in males, tends to begin in the first decade of life and continue into adolescence with drinking alcohol while driving, speeding, carrying a weapon, or using illicit drugs. In children, alcohol and illicit drug use occurs most commonly between ages 12 and 17 years and is associated with violence and injury (Jackson, 2001). About 10.9 million youths between the ages of 12 and 20 (primarily males) report drinking alcohol, with nearly 19.2% reported as being binge drinkers and 6.1% as being heavy drinkers (Substance Abuse and Mental Health Services Administration, 2004). Sixty-six percent of youths who drank alcohol heavily, and 52% of youths from 12 to 17 years of age who smoked cigarettes daily, were also users of illicit drugs (Substance Abuse and Mental Health Services Administration, 2004). An estimated 2.6 million new marijuana users emerged in 2002, with 69% under age 18 years. Use of marijuana, the most commonly used illicit drug, declined slightly from 20.6% in 2002 to 19.6% in 2003 (National Center for Health Statistics, 2007). During the same period, decreases were also seen in use of lysergic acid diethylamide (LSD) (1.3% to 0.6%), 3,4-methylenedioxymethamphetamine (MDMA, or ecstasy) (2.2% to 1.3%), and methamphetamine (0.9% to 0.7%) (National Center for Health Statistics, 2007). The slight decline in American youth's illicit drug use is attributed to education regarding the adverse effects of illicit drugs, parental disapproval, decreased availability of drugs, and consistent participation in church and organized activities such as scouts and sports.

Mental Health Problems

Mental health problems affect one out of five school-age children in the United States. Children and adolescents with mental health problems are more likely to drop out of school than those with other disabilities (Kelleher, 2005). One of the most common mental health problems is attention-deficit/hyperactivity disorder (ADHD) (Kelleher, 2005). ADHD is characterized by inattentiveness, impulsivity, and at times hyperactivity occurring in children as early as 3 years of age (Medd, 2003). ADHD affects every aspect of the child's life, but is most obvious in the classroom. Family education, counseling, medication, proper classroom placement, environmental manipulation, and behavior therapy are important management strategies for these children.

Suicide is defined as a self-chosen death and is the third leading cause of death in children ages 10 to 19 (Doucette, 2005). The American Association of Suicidology (2008) estimates that in a typical high school classroom, three students (one boy and two girls) have likely made a suicide attempt in the past year. Suicide is a preventable occurrence, placing a heavy burden on the nurse's ability to identify the at-risk child or adolescent, who may display mental health and emotional problems. There is a need for more completely integrated medical and mental health services for children and adolescents (Coury, 2006).

Mortality

Figures describing rates of occurrence for events such as death in children are referred to as *vital statistics. Mortality statistics* describe the incidence, or number of individuals who have died over a specific period. These statistics are usually presented as rates per 100,000 and are calculated from a sample of death certificates. In the United States the National Center for Health Statistics, under the Department of Health and Human Services, Public Health Service, is responsible for the collection, analysis, and dissemination of data on the health of the American people (Federal Interagency Forum on Child and Family Statistics, 2007).

The tabulation of race for live births (the denominator of infant mortality rates) has changed from race of child to race of mother. Formerly, to determine the child's race in mixed parentage in which one parent was Caucasian, the child was assigned the race of the non-Caucasian parent. In general, this change in assignment of race from child to mother has resulted in more Caucasian births and fewer non-Caucasian births. However, infant deaths are recorded by the decedent's race, resulting in a lower infant mortality rate for Caucasians than non-Caucasians. As a result of these changes in the early 1990s, figures for births, deaths, and infant mortality rates by race are not comparable to statistics reported before these changes were made.

Infant Mortality

The *infant mortality rate* is the number of deaths during the first year of life per 1000 live births. Infant mortality is divided into *neonatal mortality* (less than 28 days of life) and *postneonatal mortality* (28 days to 11 months). In the United States infant mortality has decreased dramatically. At the beginning of the twentieth century, the rate was approximately 200 infant deaths per 1000 live births. In 2003, the infant mortality rate was 6.85 per 1000 live births (Hoyert et al, 2006).

From a worldwide perspective, however, the United States lags behind other nations in reducing infant mortality. In 2001 the United States ranked last among 27 nations that have a population of at least 2.5 million and had infant mortality rates equal to or lower than that of the United States in 2000. Singapore, Hong Kong, and Japan have the three lowest rates, with the United States ranked last behind New Zealand and Cuba (Martin et al, 2005).

Birth weight is considered the major determinant of neonatal death in technologically developed countries. There is a definite relationship between birth weight and infant morbidity and mortality (Martin et al, 2005). The high incidence of LBW (under 2500 g) in the United States is a key factor in its higher neonatal mortality rates when compared with other countries. Access to and use of high-quality prenatal care is the single most important preventive strategy to decrease early delivery and infant mortality rates. Other factors that increase the risk of infant mortality include African-American race, male gender, short or long gestation, maternal age, and a low level of maternal education (Martin et al, 2005).

As Table 29-2 demonstrates, many of the leading causes of death during infancy continue to occur during the perinatal period. The first four causes—congenital anomalies, disorders relating to short gestation and unspecified LBW, sudden infant death syndrome (SIDS), and newborn affected by maternal complications of pregnancy—accounted for about half (53%) of all deaths of infants under 1 year of age (Martin et al, 2005). LBW is a major indicator of infant health and a significant predictor of infant mortality (Martin et al, 2005). Many birth defects are associated with LBW, and reducing the incidence of LBW can potentially reduce the incidence of congenital anomalies. Infant mortality resulting from HIV infection decreased significantly during the 1990s. In 2003 HIV/AIDS accounted for less than 0.2% of all infant deaths (Hoyert et al, 2006).

When infant death rates are categorized according to race, the infant mortality rate for Caucasians is lower than that for all other races in the United States, and the infant mortality rate for African-Americans is twice the rate for Caucasians. The gap between these two racial groups has remained fairly constant. The LBW rate is also higher for African-American infants than for any other group. Reasons for these high rates are unknown. One encouraging note is that the gap in mortality rates between Caucasian and non-Caucasian races other than African-Americans is narrowing. Infant mortality rates for Hispanics and Asian/Pacific Islanders decreased dramatically during the past 2 decades (Martin et al, 2005).

Table 29-2 Infant Mortality Rate and Percentage of Total Deaths for 10 Leading Causes of Infant Death in 2001 (Rate Per 1000 Live Births)

RANK	CAUSE OF DEATH (Based on 10th Revision, International Classification of Diseases)	PERCENT	RATE
	All races, all causes	100.00%	697.1
1	Congenital anomalies	20.1	139.8
2	Disorders relating to short gestation and unspecified low birth weight	16.5	115.3
3	Sudden infant death syndrome	8.2	57.1
4	Newborn affected by maternal complications of pregnancy	6.1	42.5
5	Newborn affected by complications of placenta, cord, and membranes	3.7	25.6
6	Accidents (unintentional injuries)	3.4	23.5
7	Respiratory distress of newborn	3.4	23.4
8	Bacterial sepsis of newborn	2.7	18.6
9	Diseases of circulatory system	2.4	18.6
10	Intrauterine hypoxia and birth asphyxia	2.1	14.5

Modified from Anderson RN, Smith BL: Deaths: leading causes for 2001, *Natl Vital Stat Rep* 52(9):1-85, 2003.

Table 29-3 Five Leading Causes of Death in Children in the United States: Selected Age Intervals, 2002 (Rate Per 100,000 Population)

	Ages 1-4 yr		Ages 5-9 yr		Ages 10-14 yr		Ages 15-19 yr	
RANK	CAUSE	RATE	CAUSE	RATE	CAUSE	RATE	CAUSE	RATE
	All causes	31.2	All causes	15.2	All causes	19.5	All causes	67.8
1	Accidents	10.5	Accidents	5.9	Accidents	7.3	Accidents	35.0
2	Congenital anomalies	3.4	Cancer	2.7	Cancer	2.5	Homicide	9.3
3	Homicide	2.7	Congenital anomalies	1.0	Suicide	1.2	Suicide	7.4
4	Cancer	2.6	Homicide	0.7	Congenital anomalies	1.0	Cancer	3.5
5	Heart disease	1.1	Heart disease	0.5	Homicide	1.0	Heart disease	2.0

Modified from Martin JA: Annual summary of vital statistics–2003, *Pediatrics* 115(3):632, 2005.

Childhood Mortality

Death rates for children older than 1 year of age have always been less than the rate for infants. Children ages 5 to 14 years have the lowest rate of death (Table 29-3). However, a sharp rise occurs during later adolescence, primarily from injuries, homicide, and suicide. In 2000 these conditions were responsible for approximately 73% of deaths in teenagers 15 to 19 years old (Hoyert et al, 2006). The trend in racial differences that occurs in infant mortality is also seen in childhood deaths for all ages and for both sexes. Caucasians have fewer deaths for all ages, and male deaths outnumber female deaths.

After 1 year of age there is a dramatic change in the cause of death. Unintentional injuries (accidents) are the leading cause of death from the youngest ages through the adolescent years. In addition, *violent deaths* are increasing among young people ages 10 through 25 years, especially among African-American males. Homicide is the second leading cause of death in the 15- to 19-year-old age group (see Table 29-3). Children 12 years of age and older are more likely to be killed by non–family members (acquaintances and gangs, typically of the same race) and most frequently by firearms. In 2004 African-American adolescent males were twice as likely to die as a result of a firearm injury as an MV injury (Federal Interagency Forum on Child and Family Statistics, 2007).

Morbidity

Measurements of the prevalence of specific illnesses in the population at a particular time are known as *morbidity statistics.* Morbidity statistics are generally presented as rates per 1000 population because of their frequency of occurrence. Unlike mortality, morbidity is difficult to define and may denote acute illness, chronic disease, or disability. Sources of data for morbidity statistics include reasons for visits to physicians, diagnoses for hospital admission, and household interviews. Unlike death rates, which are updated annually, morbidity statistics are revised less frequently and may not represent the general population.

Childhood Morbidity

Acute illness is defined as symptoms severe enough to limit activity or require medical attention. Respiratory illness accounts for about 50% of all acute conditions; infections and parasitic disease cause 11%, and injuries cause 15%. The chief illness of childhood is the common cold.

The types of diseases that children contract during childhood vary according to age. For example, upper respiratory tract infections and diarrhea decrease with age, but other disorders such as acne and headaches increase. Children who have had a particular type of problem are more likely to have that problem again. Morbidity is not distributed randomly in children. Children from poor families do not fare as well on health indicators as children from nonpoor families (Federal Interagency Forum on Child and Family Statistics, 2007). This finding suggests a need for heightened efforts to improve access to health care for low-income children.

Recent concern has focused on specific groups of children who have increased morbidity: homeless children, children living in poverty, LBW children, children with chronic illnesses, foreign-born adopted children, and children in day care centers. A number of factors place these groups at risk for poor health. A major cause is barriers to health care, especially for the homeless, the poverty stricken, and those with chronic health problems. Other factors include improved survival of children with chronic health problems, particularly VLBW infants.

The Art of Pediatric Nursing

Philosophy of Care

Nursing of infants and children is consistent with the *definition of nursing* as "the diagnosis and treatment of human responses to actual or potential health problems." This definition incorporates the four essential features of contemporary nursing practice (American Nurses Association, 2003):

1. Attention to the full range of human experiences and responses to health and illness without restriction to a problem-focused orientation
2. Integration of objective data with knowledge gained from an understanding of the patient's or group's subjective experience
3. Application of scientific knowledge to the processes of diagnosis and treatment
4. Provision of a caring relationship that facilitates health and healing

Family-Centered Care

The philosophy of *family-centered care* recognizes the family as the one constant in a child's life. Service systems and personnel must support, respect, encourage, and enhance the family's strength and competence by developing a partnership with parents (Newton, 2000). Nurses support families in their natural caregiving and decision-making roles by building on their unique strengths and acknowledging their expertise in caring for their child both within and outside the hospital setting (Newton, 2000). The needs of all family members, not just the child's, are considered (Box 29-1). The philosophy of family-centered care acknowledges diversity among family structures and backgrounds; family goals, dreams, strategies, and actions; and family support, service, and information needs.

Two basic concepts in family-centered care are enabling and empowerment. Professionals *enable* families by creating opportunities for all family members to display their current abilities and competencies and to acquire new ones that are necessary to meet the needs of the child and family. *Empowerment* describes the interaction of professionals with families in such a way that families maintain or acquire a sense of control over their lives and make positive changes that result from helping behaviors that foster their own strengths, abilities, and actions.

BOX 29-1 Key Elements of Family-Centered Care

- Incorporating into policy and practice the recognition that the *family is the constant* in a child's life while the service systems and support personnel within those systems fluctuate
- Facilitating *family-professional collaboration* at all levels of hospital, home, and community care:
  - Care of an individual child
  - Program development, implementation, and evaluation
  - Policy formation
- *Exchanging complete and unbiased information* between family members and professionals in a supportive manner at all times
- Incorporating into policy and practice the recognition and honoring of cultural diversity, strengths, and individuality within and across all families, including ethnic, racial, spiritual, social, economic, educational, and geographic diversity
- Recognizing and respecting *different methods of coping* and implementing comprehensive policies and programs that provide *developmental, educational, emotional, environmental, and financial support* to meet the diverse needs of families
- Encouraging and facilitating *family-to-family support* and networking
- Ensuring that *home, hospital,* and *community service* and *support systems* for children needing specialized health and developmental care and their families are *flexible, accessible,* and *comprehensive* in responding to diverse family-identified needs
- *Appreciating families as families* and children as children, recognizing that they possess a wide range of strengths, concerns, emotions, and aspirations beyond their need for specialized health and developmental services and support

From Shelton TL, Stepanek JS: *Family-centered care for children needing specialized health and developmental services,* Bethesda, MD, 1994, Association for the Care of Children's Health.

Atraumatic Care

Although tremendous advances have been made in pediatric care, many changes that have cured illnesses and prolonged life are traumatic, painful, upsetting, and frightening. Unfortunately, minimizing the trauma of medical interventions has not kept pace with the technologic advances. With knowledge of the stressors imposed on ill children and their families and armed with interventions that are safe and effective in eliminating or reducing the stressors, health professionals must direct their attention to providing atraumatic care.

Atraumatic care is the provision of therapeutic care in settings, by personnel, and through the use of interventions that eliminate or minimize the psychologic and physical distress experienced by children and their families in the health care system. *Therapeutic care* encompasses the prevention, diagnosis, treatment, or palliation of chronic or acute conditions. *Setting* refers to whatever place that care is given—the home, the hospital, or any other health care setting. *Personnel* include anyone directly involved in providing therapeutic care. *Interventions* range from psychologic approaches, such as preparing children for procedures, to physical interventions, such as providing space for a parent to room in with a child. *Psychologic distress* may include anxiety, fear, anger, disappointment, sadness, shame, or guilt. *Physical distress* may range from sleeplessness and immobilization to disturbing sensory stimuli such as pain, temperature extremes, loud noises, bright lights, or darkness. Thus atraumatic care is concerned with the who, what, when, where, why, and how of any procedure performed on a child for the purpose of preventing or minimizing psychologic and physical stress (Wong, 1989).

The overriding goal in providing atraumatic care is *first, do no harm.* Three principles provide the framework for achieving this goal: (1) prevent or minimize the child's separation from the family; (2) promote a sense of control; and (3) prevent or minimize bodily injury and pain. Examples of atraumatic care include fostering the parent-child relationship during hospitalization, preparing the child before any unfamiliar treatment or procedure, controlling pain, allowing the child privacy, providing play activities for expression of fear and aggression, providing choices to children, and respecting cultural differences.

Role of the Pediatric Nurse

Pediatric nurses are involved in every aspect of a child's and family's growth and development. Nursing functions vary according to regional job structures, individual education and experience, and personal career goals. Just as patients (children and their families) have unique backgrounds, each nurse brings an individual set of variables that affects the nurse-patient relationship. No matter where pediatric nurses practice, their primary concern is the welfare of the child and family.

Therapeutic Relationship

The establishment of a therapeutic relationship is the essential foundation for providing high-quality nursing care. Pediatric nurses need to have meaningful relationships with children and their families and yet remain separate enough to distinguish their own feelings and needs. In a *therapeutic relationship,* caring, well-defined boundaries separate the nurse from the child and family. These boundaries are positive and professional and promote the family's control over the child's health care. Effective family advocacy demands that these boundaries be established and promote therapeutic relationships (Jacobson, 2002). Both the nurse and the family are empowered, and open communication is maintained. In a *nontherapeutic relationship* these boundaries are blurred, and many of the nurse's actions may serve personal needs, such as a need to feel wanted and involved, rather than the family's needs.

Exploring whether relationships with patients are therapeutic or nontherapeutic helps nurses identify problem areas early in their interactions with children and families. Although questions for exploring types of involvement can be labeled negative or positive, no one action makes a relationship therapeutic or nontherapeutic. For example, nurses may spend additional time with the family but still recognize their own needs and maintain professional separateness. An important clue to nontherapeutic relationships is the staff's concerns about their peer's actions with the family.

Family Advocacy and Caring

Although nurses are responsible to themselves, the profession, and the institution of employment, their primary responsibility is to the consumer of nursing services—the child and the family. The nurse must work with family members, identify *their* goals and needs, and plan interventions that meet the defined problems. As an advocate, the nurse assists children and their families in making informed choices and acting in the child's best interest. Advocacy involves ensuring that families are aware of all available health services, informed of treatments and procedures, involved in the child's care, and encouraged to change or support existing health care practices. The United Nations Declaration of the Rights of the Child (Box 29-2) provides guidelines for nursing practice to ensure that every child receives optimum care. The nurse uses this knowledge to adapt care for the child's optimum physical and emotional well-being.

As nurses care for children and families, they must demonstrate *caring,* compassion, and empathy for others. Aspects of caring embody the concepts of atraumatic care and the development of a therapeutic relationship with patients. Parents perceive caring as a sign of high-quality nursing care, which is often focused on the nontechnical needs of the child and family. Parents describe "personable" care as actions by the nurse that include acknowledging the parents' presence, listening, making the parents feel comfortable, involving both the parents and the child in care, showing interest and concern for their welfare, showing affection and sensitivity to the parent and child, communicating with them, and individualizing the nursing care. Parents perceive "personable" nursing care as an integral part of a positive relationship.

BOX 29-2 United Nations Declaration of the Rights of the Child

All children need:

- To be free from discrimination
- To develop physically and mentally in freedom and dignity
- To have a name and nationality
- To have adequate nutrition, housing, recreation, and medical services
- To receive special treatment if handicapped
- To receive love, understanding, and material security
- To receive an education and develop their abilities
- To be the first to receive protection in disaster
- To be protected from neglect, cruelty, and exploitation
- To be brought up in a spirit of friendship among people

Disease Prevention and Health Promotion

Every nurse involved with child care must practice preventive health care. Regardless of the identified problem, the nurse's role is to plan care that fosters every aspect of growth and development. Based on a thorough assessment process, problems related to nutrition, immunizations, safety, dental care, development, socialization, discipline, or schooling often become obvious. Once the problem is identified, the nurse acts to intervene directly or to refer the family to other health care providers or agencies.

The best approach to prevention is *education* and *anticipatory guidance.* An appreciation of the hazards or conflicts of each developmental period enables the nurse to guide parents regarding childrearing practices aimed at preventing potential problems. One of the most significant examples is safety. Because each age group is at risk for special types of injuries, preventive teaching can significantly reduce injuries, lowering permanent disability and mortality rates.

Prevention also involves less obvious aspects of care. In addition to preventing physical disease or injury, the nurse also promotes mental health. For example, it is not sufficient to administer immunizations without regard to the psychologic trauma associated with the procedure. Optimum health care involves providing care with a humane approach; the nurse and all other health care professionals must ensure that *humane care* is provided.

Health Teaching

Health teaching is inseparable from family advocacy and prevention. Health teaching may be direct, as during parenting classes, or indirect, as when nurses help parents and children understand a diagnosis or treatment, encourage children to ask questions about their bodies, refer families to health-related professional or lay groups, supply appropriate literature, and provide anticipatory guidance. Health teaching is one area in which nurses often need preparation and practice with competent role models, since it involves transmitting information at the child's and family's level of understanding and desire for information. As an effective educator, the nurse focuses on providing the appropriate health teaching with generous feedback and evaluation to promote learning.

Support and Counseling

Attention to emotional needs requires support and sometimes counseling. The role of child advocate or health teacher is supportive because this role requires an individualized approach. Support can be offered by listening, by touching, and through physical presence. Touching and physical presence are helpful with children because these interventions facilitate nonverbal communication.

Counseling involves a mutual exchange of ideas and opinions that provides the basis for mutual problem solving. It involves supporting, teaching, fostering expression of feelings or thoughts, and helping families cope with stress. Optimally, counseling not only helps resolve a crisis or problem but also enables the family to attain a higher level of functioning, greater self-esteem, and closer relationships. Although advanced practice nurses frequently do most of the formal counseling of parents and children, counseling techniques are discussed in this text to help students and nurses cope with immediate crises and refer families for additional professional assistance.

Coordination and Collaboration

The nurse, as a member of the health team, collaborates and coordinates nursing services with the activities of other professionals. Working in isolation does not serve the child's best interest. The concept of holistic care can only be realized through a unified interdisciplinary approach. Being aware of individual contributions and limitations to the child's care, the nurse collaborates with other specialists to provide high-quality health services. Failure to recognize limitations can be nontherapeutic and perhaps destructive. For example, the nurse who feels competent in counseling but who is really inadequate in this area may not only prevent the child from dealing with a crisis but may also impede future success with a qualified professional.

Even nurses who practice in isolated geographic areas separated from other health professionals cannot be considered independent. Every nurse works interdependently with the child and family, collaborating on needs and interventions so the final care plan is one that truly meets the child's needs. Unfortunately, collaboration and coordination with the child and the family are sometimes not included in health care planning. Numerous disciplines often work together to formulate a comprehensive approach without consulting the child and the family regarding their preferences. The nurse is in a vital position to include the child and family members in their care, either directly or indirectly, by communicating their thoughts to the health care team.

Ethical Decision Making

Ethical dilemmas arise when competing moral considerations underlie various alternatives. Parents, nurses, physicians, and other health care team members may reach different but morally defensible decisions by assigning different weight to the competing moral values. These competing moral values may include *autonomy,* the patient's right to be self-governing; *nonmaleficence,* the obligation to minimize or prevent harm; *beneficence,* the obligation to promote the patient's well-being; and *justice,* the concept of fairness. Nurses are important role models for demonstrating how to create an environment of mutual respect and understanding for patients and their families. Respect for the individuals they care for is the affirmation that other persons matter in the same way as the nurses themselves (Milton, 2005).

Nurses must prepare themselves systematically for collaborative ethical decision making. This can be accomplished through formal course work, continuing education, contemporary literature, and work to establish an environment conducive to ethical discourse. Moreover, nurses must be educated on the mechanisms for dispute resolution, case review by ethics committees, procedural safeguards, state statutes, and case law (Woods, 2005).

The nurse also uses the professional code of ethics for guidance and as a means for professional self-regulation. The Code of Ethics for Nurses by the American Nurses Association focuses on the nurse's accountability and responsibility to the patient and emphasizes the nursing role as an independent professional, one that upholds its own legal liability (Box 29-3).

Nurses may face ethical issues regarding patient care, such as the use of lifesaving measures for VLBW newborns or the terminally ill child's right to refuse treatment. They may struggle with questions regarding truthfulness, balancing their rights and responsibilities in caring for children with AIDS, whistle-blowing, or allocating resources.

Research

Practicing nurses should contribute to research because they are the individuals observing human responses to health and illness. The current emphasis on measurable outcomes to determine the efficacy of interventions (often in relation to the cost) demands that nurses know whether clinical interventions result in positive outcomes for their patients. This demand has influenced the current trend toward *evidence-based practice* (EBP), which implies questioning why something is effective and whether a better approach exists. The concept of EBP also involves analyzing and translating published clinical research into the everyday practice of nursing. When nurses base their clinical practice on science and research and document their clinical outcomes, they will be able to validate their contributions to health, wellness, and cure, not only to their patients, third-party payers, and institutions but also to the nursing profession. Evaluation is essential to the nursing process, and research is one of the best ways to accomplish this.

Critical Thinking and the Process of Nursing Children and Families

Critical Thinking

A systematic thought process is essential to a profession. It assists the professional in meeting the patient's needs. *Critical thinking* is purposeful, goal-directed thinking that assists indi-

BOX 29-3 Standard 12: American Nurses Association: Ethics

The registered nurse integrates ethical provisions in all areas of practice.

Measurement Criteria

The registered nurse:

1. Uses the Code of Ethics for Nurses with Interpretive Statements to guide practice
2. Delivers care in a manner that preserves and protects patient autonomy, dignity, and rights
3. Maintains patient confidentiality within legal and regulatory parameters
4. Serves as a patient advocate, assisting patients in developing skills for self-advocacy
5. Maintains a therapeutic and professional patient-nurse relationship with appropriate professional role boundaries
6. Demonstrates a commitment to practicing self-care, managing stress, and connecting with self and others
7. Contributes to resolving ethical issues of patients, colleagues, or systems as evidenced in such activities as participating on ethics committees
8. Reports illegal, incompetent, or impaired practices

The advanced practice registered nurse:

1. Informs the patient of the risks, benefits, and outcomes of health care regimens
2. Participates in interdisciplinary teams that address ethical risks, benefits, and outcomes

The registered nurse in a nursing role specialty:

1. Participates on multidisciplinary and interdisciplinary teams that address ethical risks, benefits, and outcomes
2. Informs administrators or others of the risks, benefits, and outcomes of programs and decisions that affect health care delivery

From American Nurses Association: *Nursing: scope and standards of practice,* Silver Spring, MD, 2004, Nursesbooks.org.

viduals in making judgments based on evidence rather than guesswork (Alfaro-LeFevre, 2005). It is based on the scientific method of inquiry, which is also the root of the nursing process. Critical thinking and the nursing process are considered crucial to professional nursing in that they constitute a holistic approach to problem solving.

Critical thinking is a complex developmental process based on rational and deliberate thought. Becoming a critical thinker provides a common denominator for knowledge that exemplifies disciplined and self-directed thinking. The knowledge is acquired, assessed, and organized by thinking through the clinical situation and developing an outcome focused on optimum patient care. The cognitive skills used in high-quality thinking include intellectual discipline, self-evaluation, creativity, persistence, risk taking, and intuition (Ignatavicius, 2001). Critical thinking transforms the way in which individuals view themselves, understand the world, and make decisions.

Evidence-Based Practice

EBP is the collection, interpretation, and integration of valid, important, and applicable patient-reported, nurse-observed, and research-derived information (Simpson, 2004). Evidence-based nursing practice combines knowledge with clinical experience and intuition. It provides a rational approach to decision making that facilitates best practice (Newhouse et al, 2005). EBP is an important tool that complements the nursing process by using critical thinking skills to make decisions based on existing knowledge. The traditional nursing process approach to patient care can be used to conceptualize the essential components of EBP nursing (Table 29-4).

During the assessment and diagnostic phases of the nursing process, the nurse establishes important clinical questions and completes a critical review of existing knowledge. EBP also begins with identification of the problem. The nurse asks clinical questions in a concise, organized way that allows for clear answers. Once the specific questions are identified, extensive searching for the best information to answer the question begins. The nurse evaluates clinically relevant research, analyzes findings from the history and physical examinations, and reviews the specific pathophysiology of the defined problem. The third step in the nursing process is to develop a care plan. In evidence-based nursing practice, the care plan is established after a critical appraisal of what is known and not known about the defined problem. Next, in the traditional nursing process, the nurse implements the care plan. By integrating evidence with clinical expertise, the nurse focuses care on the patient's unique needs. The final step in EBP is consistent with the final phase of the nursing process: to evaluate the effectiveness of the care plan.

Searching for evidence in this modern era of technology can be overwhelming. Appropriate *resources* must be available for nurses to implement EBP. Resources include online search engines and journal access to the most recent information. In many institutions computer terminals are available on patient care units, with the Internet and online journals easily accessible. Another important resource for the implementation of EBP is *time.* The nursing shortage and ongoing changes that many institutions face have compounded the issue of nursing time allocation for patient care, education, and training. In some institutions nurses are given paid time away from performing patient care to participate in activities that promote EBP. This requires an organizational environment that values EBP and its potential impact on patient care. As knowledge is generated regarding the significant impact of EBP on patient care outcomes, it is hoped that the organizational culture will change to support the staff nurse's participation in EBP. As the amount of available evidence increases, so does our need to critically evaluate the evidence.

Nursing Process

The nursing process is a method of problem identification and problem solving that describes what the nurse actually does (Alfaro-LeFevre, 2005). The five-step model that is accepted as the nursing process is assessment, diagnosis (problem identification), planning (with outcome development), implementation, and evaluation. The second step of the nursing process, nursing diagnosis, involves naming the

Table 29-4 The Nursing Process and Evidence-Based Practice

NURSING PROCESS	ACTIONS	EVIDENCE-BASED PRACTICE	ACTIONS
Assessment	Collects patient data	Ask the question	Clearly identifies specific patient problems and needs
Diagnosis	Analyzes assessment data and determines diagnosis	Search for evidence	Collects information relevant to patient's identified problems and needs
Planning	Develops care plan	Analyze evidence	Critically appraises published literature
Implementation	Initiates interventions identified in care plan	Apply evidence to practice	Integrates evidence with clinical expertise and patient's unique needs
Evaluation	Evaluates patient's progress toward attainment of outcomes	Evaluate effectiveness	Evaluates effectiveness of integration of evidence

child's or family's problem in standardized nursing language. In the American Nurses Association (2003) Standards of Practice, the nursing diagnosis phase of the nursing process is separated into two steps: nursing diagnosis and outcome identification.

The nursing diagnosis is the naming of the cue clusters that are obtained during the assessment phase. According to NANDA International (formerly the North American Nursing Diagnosis Association), the currently accepted definition of the term *nursing diagnosis* is that it is a clinical judgment about individual, family, or community responses to actual and potential health problems and life processes. Nursing diagnoses provide the basis for selecting nursing interventions to achieve outcomes for which the nurse is accountable (Johnson et al, 2006). The Nursing Interventions Classification (NIC) consists of a standardized list of more than 400 examples of care provided by nurses in clinical practice. The Nursing Outcomes Classification (NOC) is a comprehensive, standardized system of patient outcomes that can be used to evaluate the results of specific nursing interventions. Not all children have actual health problems; some have a potential health problem, which is a risk state that requires nursing intervention to prevent the development of an actual problem. Potential health problems may be indicated by the presence of *risk factors*, or signs, that predispose a child and family to a dysfunctional health pattern and are limited to individuals at greater risk than the population as a whole. Nursing interventions are directed toward reducing risk factors. To differentiate actual from potential health problems, the word *risk* is included in the nursing diagnosis statement (e.g., risk for infection).

Signs and symptoms refer to a cluster of cues and defining characteristics that are derived from patient assessment and indicate actual health problems. When a defining characteristic is essential for the diagnosis to be made, it is considered critical. These critical defining characteristics help differentiate between diagnostic categories. For example, in deciding between the diagnostic categories related to family function and coping, the defining characteristics are critical in choosing the most appropriate nursing diagnosis.

Documentation

Although documentation is not one of the five steps of the nursing process, it is essential for evaluation. The nurse can assess, diagnose and identify problems, plan, and implement without documentation; however, evaluation is best performed with written evidence of progress toward outcomes.

Currently attention in health care is also focused on patient outcomes. The patient's care is evaluated not only at discharge but thereafter as well to ensure that the outcomes are met and there is adequate care for assisting the patient in resolving existing or potential health problems.

One federal agency that has developed clinical guidelines is the Agency for Healthcare Research and Quality.*

Health Care Planning

Today, the nurse's role has expanded beyond the nucleus of the family to include the community-based health-driven system. Traditionally, nurses were involved in public health either on a continuous or an episodic basis. Nurses were less frequently involved in health care planning on a political or legislative level. Future nurses will need to incorporate a political component into their professional identity and attempt to influence the decision-making body of government.†

As the largest health care profession, nursing has a valuable voice, especially as family and consumer advocate. Nurses must become aware of community needs, interested in the formulation of bills, and supportive of politicians to ensure passage (or rejection) of significant legislation. Nurses also need to become actively involved with groups that are dedicated to the welfare of children (e.g., professional nursing societies, parent-teacher organizations, parent support groups, and volunteer organizations).

Health care planning involves not only providing new services to children and their families but also promoting the highest quality in existing services. In addition to following the Code of Ethics for Nurses, nurses ensure excellence in their profession by following standards of practice. A *standard of practice* is the level of performance that is expected of a professional. In the past, pediatric nursing has not had national or international standards of care or education. Most pediatric

**540 Gaither Road, Suite 2000, Rockville, MD 20850; 301-427-1364; info@ahrq.gov;* www.ahrq.gov.

† The following are sources of information on government issues: White House Comment Line: 202-456-1111; White House fax: 202-456-2461; White House e-mail: president@whitehouse.gov.

nurses often merged with other specialties within nursing and followed the Standards of Maternal-Child Health Nursing or the standards of several of the pediatric specialties, such as pediatric oncology nursing or school nursing.* However, as the theoretic, practice, and research bases for pediatric nursing mature, the need for standards of practice for all basic pediatric nurses and for advanced practice registered nurses has become more evident. In 2003, the Society of Pediatric Nurses and the American Nurses Association published the *Scope and Standards of Pediatric Nursing.* This document identifies standards of practice that are congruent with current professional policy for both the nurse generalist and the advanced pediatric nurse.†

The highest standards of nursing practice are reflected in the emphasis on thorough assessment, the focus on scientific rationale as the basis for care, the summary of nursing care goals and responsibilities, and the comprehensive discussion of growth and development.

Future Trends

The present shift from treatment of disease to promotion of health has expanded nurses' roles in ambulatory care and highlighted the prevention and health teaching aspects of nursing practice. Prospective payment and the need for home care and community health services require nurses to be more independent and to acquire skills that are useful in settings beyond the hospital. As changing social policy shapes the expanding health care arena, the focus of nursing care is no longer on what we do *for* families, but what we do *in partnership with* them. The philosophy of family-centered care is no longer an option, but a mandate.

**Available from Association of Pediatric Hematology/Oncology Nurses, 4700 W. Lake Ave, Glenview, IL 60025-1485; 847-375-4724; fax: 877-734-6478;* www.apon.org *and National Association of School Nurses, 8484 Georgia Ave., Suite 420, Silver Spring, MD 29010; 866-627-6767 or 240-821-1130;* www.nasn.org.

†For more information on the Scope and Standards of Pediatric Nursing, *contact the Society of Pediatric Nurses, 7794 Grow Drive, Pensacola, FL 32514-7172; 800-723-2902; fax: 850-484-8762;* www.pedsnurses.org.

Today, technologic advances and the demand for computer knowledge in the work setting are obvious. The current shortage of nurses will persist into the future, and the pressure to create positions in the health care system that do not require a nursing background will intensify. As new categories of workers enter the health care field, nurses must continue to update their knowledge of technology and prove their unique contribution to health care. Nurses must use technology and learn to work collaboratively with unlicensed assistive personnel. *Unlicensed assistive personnel* "are individuals who are trained to function in an assistive role to the registered professional nurse in the provision of care activities as delegated by and under the supervision of the registered professional nurse" (American Nurses Association, 1994).

NURSING ALERT When the registered nurse determines that someone who is not licensed to practice nursing can safely provide a selected nursing activity or task for a patient and delegates that activity to the individual, the registered nurse remains responsible and legally accountable for the care provided.

Changing demographics will also influence pediatric nursing. Although the actual number of children under age 18 years will increase to an estimated 78 million in 2020, their relative importance in terms of the proportion of the total population will decrease from 26% to 24%. In the future, the adult population will grow faster than the pediatric population. Racial composition of the population will also change. The number of Caucasians in the population will decrease, whereas the number of individuals in minority groups will increase. The largest increases will occur in the number of Hispanic and Asian births. The impact of these changes will be an increase in the problems of adolescents and minority groups. Because the elderly will make up a larger percentage of the population, health care dollars will be split between the youngest and oldest groups, with shrinking resources to meet the needs of both. Nurses will need to be aware of developments in adolescent medicine and to continually adapt their care to the cultural milieu in which they practice. Finally, cost containment will present an ever-present challenge to providing high-quality care.

Key Points

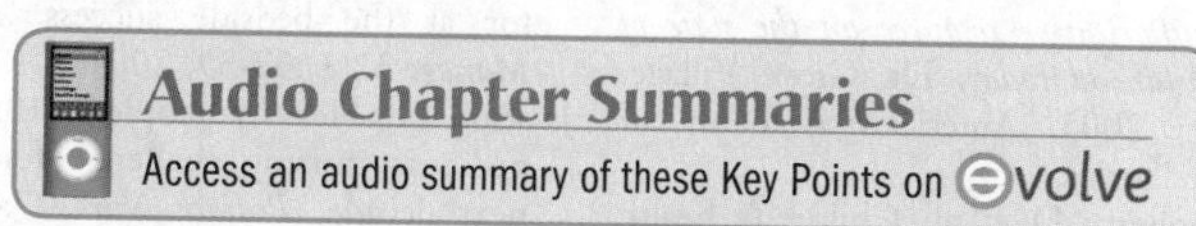
Audio Chapter Summaries
Access an audio summary of these Key Points on evolve

- *Healthy People 2010* broadened the health care objectives of the past and focuses on prevention as the method to accomplish health goals.
- Infant mortality rate in the United States is at an all-time low, but the nation continues to lag behind other major countries.
- LBW, which is closely related to early gestational age, is the leading cause of neonatal death in the United States.
- Injuries are the leading cause of death in children over age 1 year, with the majority being MV injuries.
- Childhood morbidity encompasses acute illness, chronic disease, and disability.
- Eighty percent of childhood illness is attributable to infections, with respiratory tract infections occurring two or three times more often than all other illnesses combined.
- The "new morbidity" refers to behavioral, social, and educational problems that can significantly alter a child's health.

- Developmental stage and environment are important factors in the prevalence of injuries at every age and should guide injury prevention measures.
- The philosophy of family-centered care recognizes the family as the constant in a child's life and that service systems and personnel must support, respect, encourage, and enhance the family's strength and competence.
- Atraumatic care is the provision of therapeutic care in settings, by personnel, and through the use of interventions that eliminate or minimize the psychologic and physical distress experienced by children and their families in the health care system.
- Roles of the pediatric nurse include establishing a therapeutic relationship, advocating for families, preventing disease and promoting health, health teaching, providing support and counseling, coordinating and collaborating on care, ethical decision making, and researching.
- With the shift in focus from treatment of disease to promotion of health, nurses' roles are expanding beyond traditional health care facilities into ambulatory care centers, schools, the family's home, and the community.
- EBP is the collection, interpretation, and integration of valid, important, and applicable patient-reported, nurse-observed, and research-derived information.
- The process of nursing for children and families includes accurate and complete *assessment*, analysis of assessment data to arrive at a *nursing diagnosis, planning* of care, *implementation* of the plan, and *evaluation* of interventions.

References

Alfaro-LeFevre R: *Applying nursing process: a tool for critical thinking*, ed 6, Philadelphia, 2005, Lippincott.

American Association of Suicidology: Youth suicide fact sheet, 2008. Available from www.suicidology.org/web/guest/stats-and-tools/fact-sheets (accessed March 11, 2009).

American Nurses Association: *Nursing: scope and standards of practice*, Washington, DC, 2003, The Association.

American Nurses Association: *Registered professional nurses and unlicensed assistive personnel*, Washington, DC, 1994, The Association.

Annie E Casey Foundation: *Kids count data book: state profiles of child well-being*, Baltimore, 2008, The Foundation.

Coury DL: Over the rainbow: advancing child health in the new millennium, *Ambul Pediatr* 6(3):134-137, 2006.

Covington CY et al: Kids on the move: preventing obesity among urban children, *Am J Nurs* 101(3):73-77, 79, 81-82, 2001.

Dietz WH: Overweight: an epidemic. In Cosby AG et al (editors): *About children: an authoritative resource on the state of childhood today*, Elk Grove Village, IL, 2005, American Academy of Pediatrics.

Doucette A: Youth suicide. In Cosby AG et al (editors): *About children: an authoritative resource on the state of childhood today*, Elk Grove Village, IL, 2005, American Academy of Pediatrics.

Dougherty D et al: Children's health care in the First National Healthcare Quality Report and National Healthcare Disparities Report, *Med Care* 43(3 Suppl):I58-I63, 2005.

Duderstadt KG: Advocacy for reducing childhood obesity, *J Pediatr Health Care* 18:103-105, 2004.

Edelstein BL: Tooth decay: the best of times, the worst of times. In Cosby AG et al (editors): *About children: an authoritative resource on the state of childhood today*, Elk Grove Village, IL, 2005, American Academy of Pediatrics.

Federal Interagency Forum on Child and Family Statistics: *America's children: key national indicators of well-being*, Washington, DC, 2007, US Government Printing Office.

Fisher K, Kettl P: Teachers' perceptions of school violence, *J Pediatr Health Care* 17:79-83, 2003.

Fitzgibbon ML, Stolley MR: Environmental changes may be needed for prevention of overweight in minority children, *Pediatr Ann* 33:45-49, 2004.

Groves BM: Violence in the lives of children. In Cosby AG et al (editors): *About children: an authoritative resource on the state of childhood today*, Elk Grove Village, IL, 2005, American Academy of Pediatrics.

Heuer S: Family-centered care, *J Spec Pediatr Nurs* 12(1):61-65, 2007.

Hoyert DL, Kung HC, Smith BL: Deaths: preliminary data for 2003, *Natl Vital Stat Rep* 53(15):1-48, 2005.

Hoyert DL et al: *Deaths: final data for 2003*, Washington, DC, 2006, National Center for Health Statistics. Available at www.cdc.gov/nchs/products/pubs/pubd/hestats/finaldeaths03/finaldeaths03.htm (accessed January 20, 2006).

Ignatavicius D: Critical thinking skills for at the bedside success, *Nurs Manage* 32(1):37-39, 2001.

Jackson PL: Healthy people 2010: the pediatric nursing challenge for the next decade, *Pediatr Nurs* 27:498-502, 2001.

Jacobson GA: Maintaining professional boundaries: preparing nursing students for the challenge, *J Nurs Educ* 41(6):279-281, 2002.

Johnson M et al: *NANDA, NOC, and NIC linkages: nursing diagnoses, outcomes and interventions*, ed 2, St Louis, 2006, Mosby.

Kelleher K: Mental health. In Cosby AG et al (editors): *About children: an authoritative resource on the state of childhood today*, Elk Grove Village, IL, 2005, American Academy of Pediatrics.

Lichter DT: Families: diversity and change. In Cosby AG et al (editors): *About children: an authoritative resource on the state of childhood today*, Elk Grove Village, IL, 2005, American Academy of Pediatrics.

Martin JA et al: Annual summary of vital statistics: 2003, *Pediatrics* 115(3):619-634, 2005.

Medd SE: Children with ADHD need our advocacy, *J Pediatr Health Care* 17:102-104, 2003.

Milton CL: The ethics of respect in nursing, *Nurs Sci Q* 18(1):20-23, 2005.

National Center for Health Statistics: *About Healthy People 2010*, 2007. Available at www.cdc.gov/nchs/about/otheract/hpdata2010/abouthp.htm (accessed February, 2, 2007).

National Center for Injury Prevention and Control: *Injury fact book 2001-2002*, Atlanta, 2001, Centers for Disease Control and Prevention.

National Children's Study: *What is the National Children's Study?* 2008. Available at www.nationalchildrensstudy.gov (accessed March 11, 2009).

National Safety Council: *Injury facts*, Itaska, IL, 2000, The Council.

Newhouse R et al: Evidence-based practice: a practical approach to implementation, *JONA* 35(1):35-40, 2005.

Newton MS: Family-centered care: current realities in parent participation, *Pediatr Nurs* 26(2):164-168, 2000.

Rivara FP: Impact of injury. In Cosby AG et al (editors): *About children: an authoritative resource on the state of childhood today*, Elk Grove Village, IL, 2005, American Academy of Pediatrics.

Robinson TN, Sargent JD: Children and media. In Cosby AG et al (editors): *About children: an authoritative resource on the state of childhood today*, Elk Grove Village, IL, 2005, American Academy of Pediatrics.

Schnitzer PG: Prevention of unintentional childhood injuries, *Am Fam Physician* 74(11):1864-1869, 2006.

Simpson R: Evidence-based nursing offers certainty in the uncertain world of healthcare, *Nurs Manage* 35(10):10-12, 2004.

Substance Abuse and Mental Health Services Administration, Office of Applied Studies: *2003 national survey on drug use and health: results*, 2004. Available at www.drugabusestatistics.samhsa.gov/NHSDA/2k3NSDUH/2k3results.htm (accessed February 2, 2007).

US Department of Health and Human Services: *Healthy people 2010*, 2007. Available at www.healthypeople.gov/default.htm (accessed January 8, 2008).

Wise PH: Medical progress and inequalities in child health. In Cosby AG et al (editors): *About children: an authoritative resource on the state of childhood today*, Elk Grove Village, IL, 2005, American Academy of Pediatrics.

Wise PH: The transformation of child health in the United States, *Health Affairs* 23(5):9-25, 2004.

Wong D: Principles of atraumatic care. In Feeg V (editor): *Pediatric nursing: forum on the future: looking toward the 21st century*, Pitman, NJ, 1989, Anthony J Jannetti.

Woods M: Nursing ethics education: are we really delivering the good(s)? *Nurs Ethics* 12(1):5-18, 2005.

World Health Organization: *School health and youth health promotion*, 2007. Available at www.who.int/school_youth_health/en (accessed January 26, 2007).

Yensel CS, Preud'Homme D, Curry DM: Childhood obesity and insulin-resistant syndrome, *J Pediatr Nurs* 19:238-246, 2004.

Community-Based Nursing Care of the Child and Family

30

Learning Objectives

On completion of this chapter the reader will be able to:

- Define community nursing.
- Describe community health nursing.
- Identify the roles and functions of the community health nurse.
- Discuss selected aspects of the epidemiologic process.
- Explain the purpose of an economic evaluation.
- Discuss the components of the community nursing process.

Electronic Resources

Additional information related to the content in Chapter 30 can be found on

evolve the Companion Website at
http://evolve.elsevier.com/Perry/maternal/

- NCLEX Review Questions

Nursing in the Community

The health of children and their families is greatly influenced by their community, and nurses can make a significant contribution by working with the community to promote children's heath. Nurses working with pediatric populations in the community need an understanding of the concepts and processes critical to address pediatric concerns from a community health perspective. Healthy communities not only provide excellent medical care; they also provide children a nurturing, safe place in which to live and grow. Healthy communities address concerns through collaboration between and among citizens, health care providers, businesses, and governmental and private agencies (Flynn & Ivanov, 2004).

This chapter discusses community health nursing as it relates to children. First it identifies and defines the concepts and principles that serve as the basis of community health nursing. Then it describes the community health nursing process, step by step. It includes a box that demonstrates use of the process to address a very real child health concern: obesity.

Community Concepts

Community

There are several ways to define a community. A *community* is a group of individuals with shared characteristics or interests who interact with each other (Allender & Spradley, 2005). A community is a system that includes children and families, the physical environment, educational facilities, safety and transportation resources, political and governmental agencies, health and social services, communication resources, economic resources, and recreational facilities. The community is also the client of the community health nurse (Anderson, 2008). Community health initiatives are directed at either the general health of the community as a whole or at specific populations within the community that have unique needs. In this context, *populations* can be described as groups of people who live in a community, for example, school-age children. *Target populations* or *subpopulations* are more narrowly defined groups (e.g., unimmunized preschoolers, or obese middle school children) toward whom nurses direct activities to improve the health status of individuals in the group. Common values often guide behaviors of populations and subpopulations in relation to health promotion and disease prevention (McEwen & Nies, 2007; Williams, 2004).

Community-oriented care involves a collaboration of individuals and groups, including health care providers, advocates, government, managed care organizations, businesses, children, and families within a specific community. The goal of the collaborative effort is to provide services that promote the child health initiatives of *Healthy People 2010* (see the *Healthy People 2010* website at *www.healthypeople.gov*). Community care is "without walls" in that the services of the health care system are frequently redesigned to meet the community's changing needs. Those involved in community care partner with community members to identify, plan, intervene, and evaluate activities that improve the community's health (Anderson & McFarlane, 2008).

Community Health Nursing

Community health nursing focuses on promoting and maintaining the health of individuals, families, and groups in the community setting. Community health nursing is a synthesis of nursing and public health. It involves nurses collaborating with other disciplines to assess, plan, and implement care that emphasizes personal responsibility for health and self-care by community members (Allender & Spradley, 2005; Williams,

2004). Community health nursing, at its best, empowers communities by enabling community members to gain the knowledge and skills needed to fulfill their own needs.

Although community health concepts can be used to address health concerns in any setting, traditional community health settings include the following: home health agencies, schools, physicians' offices, ambulatory health clinics, emergency rooms, triage call centers, insurance agencies, health departments, international relief agencies, health education agencies, juvenile detention facilities, camps, day care centers, foster care facilities, and rehabilitation agencies. The American Nurses Association (1986) has established nine standards for community health nursing to guide practice across settings. They include the following categories: theory, data collection, diagnosis, planning, intervention, evaluation, quality assurance and professional development, interdisciplinary collaboration, and research. The revised scope and standards of public health nursing describe the major components and measurement criteria for each standard (American Nurses Association, 2007).

Roles and Functions

The *roles and functions* of the community health nurse continue to evolve. In the future, many pediatric nurses will be working in community settings. The Health Resources and Services Administration (2004) reported that 14.9% of the total registered nurse workforce was employed in a community or public health setting, and 11.5% was employed in ambulatory care. Only 56.2% of registered nurses were employed in hospital settings.

Traditionally, the roles and functions of community health nurses included caregiver, advocate, case manager, case finder, counselor, educator, epidemiologist, group process leader, health planner, and manager. For example, the nurse employed in a pediatric outpatient clinic functions in a number of roles to provide care to a child with type 2 diabetes. The nurse provides case management by coordinating care between the disciplines, provides counseling by supporting the child and family through developmental crises, and acts as a case finder by identifying risk factors in the child's siblings.

The Institute of Medicine (1988) developed a list of *core functions* to guide the work of public health professionals, including nurses. The core functions are directed to population-wide services and to personal and home services for people at risk. The population-wide service is based on assessment of health status monitoring and disease *surveillance, policy development,* and *assurance* that policies are translated into service. The Council on Linkages Between Academia and Public Health Practice (2001), a group of university educators and public health professionals, further delineated the core functions and developed a list of skills to improve the ability of all public health workers, including nurses, to implement them. The eight categories of skills include analytic/assessment, policy development/program planning, communication, cultural competency, community dimensions of practice, basic public health sciences, financial planning and management, and leadership and systems thinking. Thus the pediatric nurse employed in a managed care environment may be asked to develop a creative approach to teaching children with asthma about peak flow meters during an emergency department visit. Included in the request may be a mechanism for evaluating the cost of the approach and the occurrence of repeated emergency department visits.

NURSING ALERT Nurses must be able to communicate and work with professionals from other disciplines. This includes being able to understand the terms used by demographers, epidemiologists, and economists.

Demography

Demography is the study of population characteristics. *Demographic characteristics* include age, gender, race/ethnicity, socioeconomic status, and education. Individuals, families, and communities may have demographic characteristics that affect their health risks (Cashaw, 2007). *Risk* is an increased probability of developing a disease, injury, or illness. Age is one of the most important risk factors for disease prevention and certain health conditions. For example, infants are most likely to die as a result of congenital malformations, children and adolescents as a result of accidents, and middle-age adults as a result of cancer (National Center for Health Statistics, 2006). Gender also plays an important role. Males are at much greater risk of having hemophilia A and B than females. Race and ethnicity have long been associated with increased risk for disease and disability, but it is now thought that, aside from genetic predisposition, there is a complicated relationship between minority status and socioeconomic status that increases the risk for disease and disability (Smith, 2000). Low socioeconomic status predisposes children to a variety of problems. Poor children are more likely to be obese and to have untreated dental problems. They are more likely to have no regular site for medical care and to be treated in emergency departments (National Center for Health Statistics, 2006).

Epidemiology

Epidemiology is the science of population health applied to the detection of morbidity and mortality in a population. The epidemiologic process identifies the distribution and causes of disease or injury across a population (Cashaw, 2007). It also serves as an important component in developing health programs. For example, *Healthy People 2010* incorporated the process to develop a set of health objectives for the United States. Health professionals in community, state, and national health care organizations use the objectives as a guide to develop programs that have the greatest impact on children's health.

Distribution of Disease, Injury, or Illness

Morbidity rates are used to measure disease and injury, and, along with *natality and mortality rates,* they present an objective picture of a community's health status. There are two types of morbidity rates: incidence and prevalence. *Incidence* measures the occurrence of new events in a population during a period of time. *Prevalence* measures existing events in a population during a period of time (Hennekens & Buring, 1987). For example, the incidence of type 1 diabetes in a community is estimated by counting the new cases of type 1 diabetes in a population and dividing that figure by the population at risk.

BOX 30-1 Frequently Used Mortality and Morbidity Rates

Crude Birth Rate

$$\frac{\text{Number of births in a population}}{\text{Total population}} \text{ within a time period} \times 1000$$

Crude Death Rate

$$\frac{\text{Number of deaths in a population}}{\text{Total population}} \text{ within a time period} \times 1000$$

Cause-Specific Death Rate

$$\frac{\text{Number of deaths in a population due to a certain disease}}{\text{Total population}} \text{ within a time period} \times 1000$$

Age-Specific Death Rate

$$\frac{\text{Number of deaths in a population in a certain age-group}}{\text{Total population in that age-group}} \text{ within a time period} \times 1000$$

Incidence of Disease

$$\frac{\text{Number of new events in a population}}{\text{Total at-risk population}} \text{ within a time period} \times 1000$$

Prevalence of Disease

$$\frac{\text{Number of existing events in a population}}{\text{Total at-risk population}} \text{ within a time period} \times 1000$$

The prevalence of type 1 diabetes is estimated by counting the existing cases of type 1 diabetes in a population and dividing that figure by the population at risk. Both incidence and prevalence are usually given as rates per 1000, 10,000, or 100,000 population, depending on their frequency. Box 30-1 presents frequently used mortality and morbidity rates.

Epidemiologic Triangle

Three factors form the epidemiologic triangle, and their interrelationship alters the risk of acquiring a disease or condition (McKeown & Hilfinger, 2004). These factors are agent, host, and environment (Fig. 30-1).

An *agent* is responsible for causing a disease and may be an infectious agent, such as *Mycobacterium tuberculosis;* a chemical agent, such as lead in paint; or a physical agent, such as fire. *Host factors* are those that are specific to an individual or group. These may be genetic factors, which cannot be controlled, or they may be lifestyle factors, such as food selections or exercise patterns. *Environmental factors* provide a setting for the host and include the climatic conditions in which the host lives and factors related to the home, neighborhood, and school.

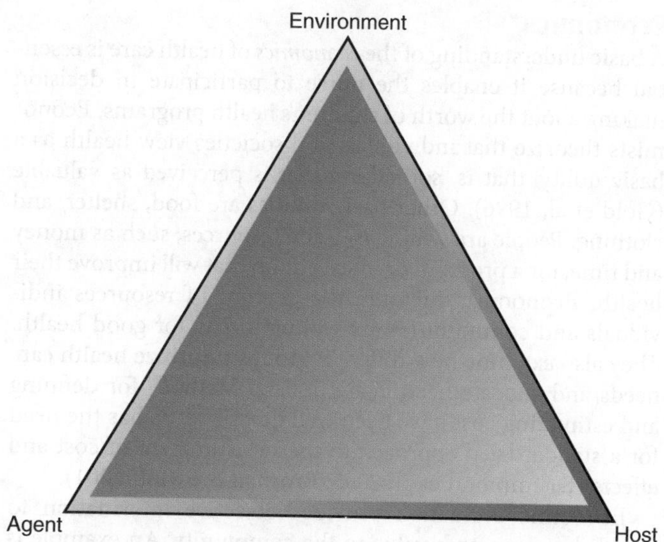

Fig. 30-1 The epidemiologic triangle.

Levels of Prevention

Community health programs are based on three classic levels of prevention (Leavell & Clark, 1965). *Primary prevention* focuses on health promotion and prevention of disease or injury. Examples of primary prevention activities include well-child care clinics, immunization programs, safety programs (bike helmets, car seats, seat belts, child-proof containers), nutrition programs, environmental efforts (clean air programs), sanitation measures (chlorinated water, garbage removal, sewage treatment), and community parenting classes. *Secondary prevention* focuses on screening and early diagnosis of disease. Examples of secondary interventions include tuberculosis and lead screening programs and mental health counseling for stressful events such as separation, divorce, death, or community natural disasters (e.g., earthquakes, floods, and hurricanes). *Tertiary prevention* focuses on optimizing function for children with a disability or chronic disease. Tertiary interventions include rehabilitation and disease management programs for asthma, sickle cell disease, cancer, and anorexia and special education programs for children.

Screening

Community health nurses are frequently involved in *screening,* a secondary prevention activity. The purpose of screening is to detect and treat disease early in the period of pathogenesis to prevent the spread and progression of the disease (Wilson & Jungner, 1968). However, screening is not appropriate for every condition. Although screening may bring benefits, a certain amount of risk is associated with any intervention. It is essential to determine the evidence for a proposed screening program before beginning it so that the benefits of screening exceed the risks and cost. For example, acanthosis nigricans (AN) is a thickening and darkening of the skin that is commonly found on the neck and is associated with insulin resistance (Centers for Disease Control and Prevention, 2005). Some school health officials have recommended screening for AN as a way to identify early type 2 diabetes in children, but others have argued that screening may not be effective. Because of this controversy, AN is a good example of the need to determine the evidence before establishing a screening program.

Economics

A basic understanding of the *economics* of health care is essential because it enables the nurse to participate in decision making about the worth of children's health programs. Economists theorize that individuals and societies view health as a basic utility, that is, something that is perceived as valuable (Gold et al, 1996). Other basic utilities are food, shelter, and clothing. People are willing to trade resources, such as money and time, for a program or intervention that will improve their health. Economists measure the amount of resources individuals and communities are willing to pay for good health. They also examine how different groups prioritize health care needs and allocate health care dollars. Methods for defining and estimating cost have been well described, as has the need for a standardized approach to the measurement of cost and effects (Drummond et al, 2005; Brosnan & Swint, 2001).

Economic evaluation provides objective information to establish a program's value to the community. An example is the evaluation of a school-based hepatitis B vaccination program by Wilson (2000). He concluded that the percentage of vaccinated sixth graders increased from 8% without the program to 82% with the program. The higher vaccination rate potentially saved money that might have eventually been spent to treat these children for hepatitis, cirrhosis, or cancer. The program resulted in potential cost savings of $24 million when compared with the no-program alternative.

Community Nursing Process

In community nursing the nursing process shifts its focus from the individual child and family to the community or target population (Box 30-2). The stages of the process (assessment, diagnosis, planning, implementation, and evaluation) are similar whether the client is one child or a population of children; only the type of interventions and indicators of wellness and illness differ (Anderson, 2008). *Assessment* is focused on collecting subjective and objective information about the target population in order to *diagnose* problems based on community needs. *Planning* involves the development of community-centered goals. During the *implementation* stage the nurse works with the community to implement a program that enables members to reach their goals. Finally, the nurse *evaluates* whether the goals were met.

BOX 30-2 The Community Nursing Process

Assessment and diagnosis—The nurse collects subjective and objective information about a community and develops a diagnosis based on community needs and problems.
Planning—The nurse develops community-centered goals to address the identified needs and problems.
Intervention—The nurse implements a program that enables community members to reach their goals.
Evaluation—The nurse conducts a systematic evaluation to determine that goals and program objectives were met.

Community nursing is collaborative, and the nurse is one member of a community team that includes other health professionals, educators, politicians, religious leaders, members of public and voluntary organizations, and consumers. The nurse's role depends on the project's scope, the target population, and the expertise of team members.

Students may be introduced to community collaboration through service learning. The community partnership model is an example of a model that enables nursing students to become part of a collaborative team and to directly contribute to a community's well-being. In this model the missions of nursing education, research, and practice are linked through three processes: evidence-based practice, service learning, and scholarly teaching (Brosnan et al, 2005).

Community Needs Assessment and Diagnosis

The assessment phase of the community nursing process is called a *community needs assessment.* Assessment involves the collection of *subjective and objective information* about a community. Subjective information indicates what community members say are their most important needs and can be determined in a number of ways. One way is to distribute questionnaires to a sample of people living in the community. Another way is to interview community members directly, phoning or meeting with individuals (such as community leaders) who represent the group or who have a special role in the group.

Objective information is data that the nurse collects either by direct observation or through written sources. A "windshield tour" is one method of direct observation. Nurses drive through a neighborhood and take notes about the environment, including the appearance of houses, the presence of sidewalks and gutters, the number of public areas, and so on. Objective information about the community's health status can also be obtained from such sources as the local chamber of commerce, the U.S. Census Bureau, libraries, state health departments, and the Internet sites of voluntary health organizations or government agencies. Information about service agencies can be found in resource directories, including the local telephone book, community resource directories compiled by such organizations as the United Way, and population-specific books provided by public and voluntary agencies.

One way to organize an assessment is to use a guide that lists community systems that need to be examined. This process is similar to using a physical assessment guide to examine the different body systems in an individual patient. Anderson and McFarlane (2008) described eight community systems that the nurse should examine: health and social services, communication, recreation, physical environment, education, safety and transportation, politics and government, and economics. During the assessment the nurse studies how well each component in the community functions and interacts to meet children's health needs, identifies the community's strengths, and determines whether any barriers disrupt the components and prevent access to care for children and their families.

After the assessment is completed, the community nurse collaborates with team members to analyze the results of surveys and questionnaires, determine whether the needs described by community members can be met by existing community agencies, and identify individuals at highest risk. During the analysis the community's demographic characteristics, morbidity rates, and mortality rates are compared with a standard. Comparisons can be made on the basis of time or place. In time comparisons, the nurse contrasts the rates in the current year with the rates during an earlier period. In comparisons of place, the nurse contrasts the rates in the community with those of a standard population. Standard rates may come from another community or from city, state, or national data. For example, the rate of tuberculosis in a group of preschool children in the community in 2002 could be compared with the rate of tuberculosis in preschool children in the state in 2002.

A *community health diagnosis* is the reflection of health status, risks, or needs as determined by a causative agent. The format of a community diagnosis is similar to that of an individual nursing diagnosis with a problem (need) and an etiology related to that problem (causative agent). An example of a community nursing diagnosis is "Child abuse related to a violent environment" (Visiting Nurse Association of Omaha, 1986).

NURSING ALERT All communities have strengths and limitations. The community health nurse draws on the community's strengths to solve problems.

Community Planning

The nurse collaborates with community members in developing a plan that addresses the target population's needs and problems. To maximize the use of community resources, problems should first be prioritized on the basis of their severity, the community's felt needs, and the community nurse's ability to bring about change. After prioritizing the problems, the nurse works with community members to develop at least one goal for each problem the members will address. *Goals* are outcomes that give direction to interventions and provide a measure of the change the interventions produced. Community interventions frequently take the form of *health programs* for improving the target population's health status. Community health programs are based on the three levels of prevention: primary, secondary, and tertiary. For example, a goal for preventing bicycle injuries is, "Within 1 year all students in the first grade will wear bicycle helmets." The nurse and community members then plan a program that includes health education about bicycle safety for students and their parents (primary prevention).

The planning group considers the resources that are already available in the community and resources that will be needed for implementing a health program, including personnel, supplies and equipment, office space, phones, and computers. Decisions are made about the program's timeline, the budget, and strategies to obtain funding. The nurse may also contact health professionals who have implemented successful programs in other communities; they can provide valuable, time-saving tips and suggestions. Program descriptions are found through professional contacts, online resources, and a review of the literature. An example of a community assessment and planning project is presented in Box 30-3.

BOX 30-3 An Example of Community Assessment and Planning

Sabine is an elementary school with 500 prekindergarten to sixth-grade children. The school nurse has been asked to conduct an assessment of the school community and to develop a care plan. The schoolchildren and their families are the target population.

Community Needs Assessment and Diagnosis

The school nurse formed a team of community members that included parents of students who attend Sabine Elementary School, faculty and staff, health care professionals, local religious leaders, and politicians. The group met at regularly scheduled intervals. Their first task was to complete the community assessment. Team members mailed questionnaires to a random sample of families who had children attending Sabine. They held focus groups with community members to obtain subjective information about the needs of the school community. Team members obtained objective data from the local health department, school records, and the U.S. Census Bureau. The nurse also conducted a windshield tour of the neighborhood surrounding the school. The following information was collected:

People—Sabine is located in an ethnically diverse area composed of 30% Hispanics, 30% African-Americans, 30% non-Hispanic Caucasians, and 10% Asians. The ethnicity of students in the school is representative of the surrounding area. Sabine is located in a large southwestern city.

Safety and transportation—School bus service was rated very good to excellent by a majority of those surveyed. Transportation records indicated that the last school bus accident occurred 1 year ago. There were no fatalities, but a number of children were injured. Other accidents occurred 2 years and 10 years prior to the most recent accident.

Economics—Although 94% of families had at least one fully employed member, 25% of the families lived below the poverty level. The number below poverty level had not changed in 10 years.

Education—Sixty percent of the adult population had a high school diploma, and 10% of this group had completed at least 1 year of college. School attendance at Sabine was higher than overall state attendance rates.

Communication—Ninety-five percent of homes had telephones, compared with 85% 10 years ago. An estimated 10% of the target population did not speak English, and Spanish was the primary language spoken in this group.

Recreation—Few places were available for small children to play. The focus groups recommended more parks and playgrounds.

Continued

BOX 30-3 An Example of Community Assessment and Planning—cont'd

Community Needs Assessment and Diagnosis—cont'd

Politics and government—The school system was strongly centralized and headed by a school superintendent. The city had a mayor and city council.

Social—Of those families living below the poverty level, 60% received some type of welfare assistance, including food stamps. The school lunch program served 95% of the children attending the school.

Health—The childhood immunization rate for all diseases among children in the community who were between 19 and 35 months of age was 90%, which compared favorably with the national level of 82% in 2005 (National Center for Health Statistics, 2006). The immunization rate for children attending Sabine Elementary School was 100%. Vision and hearing screening programs at Sabine resulted in the referral of 5% of the students for vision problems and 2% of the students for hearing problems. Review of student records indicated that all those children referred received diagnostic follow-up and treatment when indicated. Heights and weights were obtained on all students annually, and the body mass index (BMI) was determined for each student. BMI is calculated by dividing the weight in kilograms by the square of the height in meters (Flegal et al, 1998). Results indicated that 30% of students were above the 95th percentile for age and sex, compared with 19% nationally (National Center for Health Statistics, 2006). In focus groups, students and teachers noted that school breakfasts and lunches were high in carbohydrates and fats. They also observed that decreased recess time resulted in decreased student activity during school hours.

On the basis of these assessments, the following community diagnoses were made:

1. Increase in injuries related to school bus accidents.
2. Increase in obesity among students compared with the national standard related to high intake of calories and sedentary lifestyle.

Planning

Team members agreed that the number of school bus accidents should be closely monitored over the next 5 years. However, there was a consensus that increased obesity among students was the priority problem, and the team developed the following two goals:

1. Within 2 years the percentage of students with BMIs above the 95th percentile for age and sex will be 20%.
2. Within 5 years that percentage will be 10%.

Team members reviewed the literature for examples of communities that had experienced similar problems, contacted school and health department officials in other areas of the country, examined the results of successful programs, and planned a health program that addressed the unique needs of the target population. The program was titled "Sabine Excels in Health." Program activities were:

- Each September the nurse will address the school's parent association about the program and will discuss the importance of a healthy diet and exercise for all family members.
- Every month teachers will set aside 1 hour to talk with their students about healthy food choices and about the importance of limiting television viewing time.
- Within 6 months school administrators and community members will petition the city to provide a neighborhood park.
- Within 1 year the school dietitian will assess the nutritional value of the current school meals and, if indicated, revise the meal plan to ensure a healthy diet.
- Within 1 year the school will develop a plan to allow a minimum of 30 minutes of unrestricted play during the school day.

Team members determined the resources needed to implement the program, including personnel, supplies, and equipment. They estimated the total cost of setting up the program and maintaining it for 5 years and applied for funding to the school district and to the city and state health departments.

Implementation and Evaluation

The school nurse and other team members assumed responsibility for the timely implementation and evaluation of the Sabine Excels in Health program.

Community Intervention

During program implementation the nurse and community members carry out the intervention. Whether the program is simple or complex, oversight is needed to ensure that everyone involved is communicating with one another, following the plan's guidelines, keeping within the timeline, and documenting daily activities and expenses. The documentation will prove invaluable during the evaluation phase of the process.

Community Evaluation

Evaluation identifies whether the goals and program objectives were met. There are various models of program evaluation. Health care organizations commonly use the structure, process, and outcomes method. Donabedian (1980) described this approach as follows:

Structure—Where and by whom is the care delivered in a program?

Process—Was the care delivered using operational standards and within the program's financial guidelines?

Outcomes—What was the impact on health status? Was there any improvement?

Structure focuses on the qualifications of personnel; the adequacy of buildings and offices, supplies, and equipment; and the target population's characteristics. Process focuses on the interaction of patients and providers. Process indicators include the number of people who attended a health education program, the number of pamphlets distributed, and the program's efficiency. Outcome focuses on whether program objectives and community goals were met. Program evaluation should be ongoing so that performance improvement initiatives are monitored and so that an improvement in the way health care is delivered will affect the target population's health status.

Key Points

- Caring for children within a community requires a multidisciplinary approach.
- Healthy communities provide children with high-quality medical care and a nurturing, safe place to live and grow.
- Community health nursing focuses on promoting and maintaining the health of individuals, families, and groups in the community setting.
- Individual families and communities may have demographic characteristics that affect their risk for disease or injury.
- Epidemiology is the science of population health applied to the detection of morbidity and mortality in a population.
- Community health programs are based on three levels of intervention: primary, secondary, and tertiary.
- Economic evaluations provide objective information to establish a program's value to society.

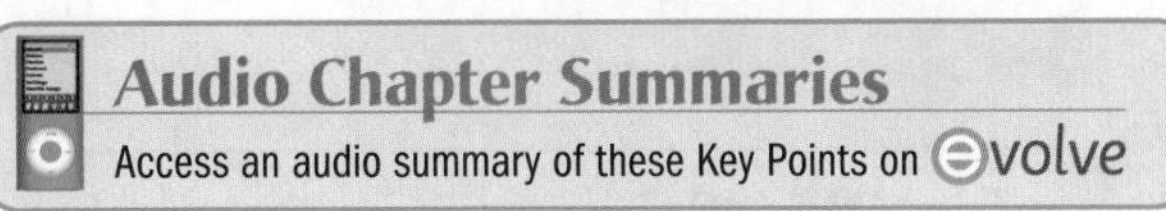
Audio Chapter Summaries
Access an audio summary of these Key Points on evolve

- A community needs assessment involves collection of subjective and objective information about the community.
- A community health diagnosis is a problem with a defined cause related to a community problem.
- Program planning and implementation in the community require collaboration between the nurse and community members who are in positions to promote change.
- Evaluation of effective community programs includes consideration of the structure, process, and outcomes related to the program.

References

Allender JA, Spradley BW: Opportunities and challenges of community health nursing. In Allender JA, Spradley BW (editors): *Community health nursing: promoting and protecting the public's health*, Philadelphia, 2005, Lippincott Williams & Wilkins.

American Nurses Association: *Public health nursing scope and standards*, Washington, DC, 2007, The Association.

American Nurses Association: *Standards of community health nursing practice*, Kansas City, MO, 1986, The Association.

Anderson ET: A model to guide practice. In Anderson ET, McFarlane J (editors): *Community as partner: theory and practice in nursing*, Philadelphia, 2008, Lippincott Williams & Wilkins.

Anderson ET, McFarlane J: Community assessment. In Anderson ET, McFarlane J (editors): *Community as partner: theory and practice in nursing*, Philadelphia, 2008, Lippincott Williams & Wilkins.

Brosnan CA, Swint JM: Cost analysis: concepts and application, *Public Health Nurs* 18(1):13-18, 2001.

Brosnan CA et al: Student nurses participate in public health research and practice through a school-based screening program, *Public Health Nurs* 22(3):260-266, 2005.

Cashaw SA: Epidemiology, demography and community health. In Anderson ET, McFarlane J (editors): *Community as partner*, ed 5, Philadelphia, 2007, Lippincott Williams & Wilkins.

Centers for Disease Control and Prevention: *CDC statement on screening children for acanthosis nigricans in schools and communities*, 2005. Available at www.cdc.gov/diabetes/news/docs/an.htm (accessed January 4, 2008).

Council on Linkages Between Academia and Public Health Practice: *Core competencies for public health professionals*, 2001. Available at www.phf.org/competencies.htm (accessed January 4, 2008).

Donabedian A: *The definition of quality and approaches to its assessment*, Ann Arbor, MI, 1980, Health Administration Press.

Drummond MF et al: *Methods for the economic evaluation of health care programmes*, ed 3, New York, 2005, Oxford University Press.

Flegal KM et al: Overweight and obesity in the United States: prevalence and trends, *Int J Obes Relat Metab Disord* 22(1):39-47, 1998.

Flynn BC, Ivanov LL: Health promotion through healthy communities and cities. In Stanhope M, Lancaster J: *Community and public health nursing*, St Louis, 2004, Mosby.

Gold MR et al: Identifying and valuing outcomes. In Gold MR et al (editors): *Cost-effectiveness in health and medicine*, New York, 1996, Oxford University Press.

Health Resources and Services Administration: *The registered nurse population*, Rockville, MD, 2004, US Department of Health and Human Services.

Hennekens CH, Buring JE: *Epidemiology in medicine*, Boston, 1987, Little, Brown.

Institute of Medicine: *The future of public health*, Washington, DC, 1988, National Academy Press.

Leavell HR, Clark EG: *Preventive medicine for the doctor in his community: an epidemiologic approach*, New York, 1965, McGraw-Hill.

McEwen M, Nies MA: Health: a community view. In Nies MA, McEwen M (editors): *Community/public health: promoting the health of populations*, Philadelphia, 2007, Saunders.

McKeown RE, Hilfinger DK: Epidemiology. In Stanhope M, Lancaster J (editors): *Community and public health nursing*, St Louis, 2004, Mosby.

National Center for Health Statistics: *Health, United States, 2006: with chartbook on trends in the health of Americans*, DHS Pub No 2006-1232, Hyattsville, MD, 2006, US Department of Health and Human Services. Available at www.cdc.gov/nchs/data/hus/hus06.pdf (accessed January 4, 2008).

Smith GD: Learning to live with complexity: ethnicity, socioeconomic position, and health in Britain and the United States, *Am J Public Health* 90:1694-1698, 2000.

Visiting Nurse Association of Omaha: *Client management information system for community health nursing agencies*, Rockville, MD, 1986, US Department of Health and Human Services.

Williams CA: Community-oriented populations-focused practice: the foundation of specialization in public health practice. In Stanhope M, Lancaster J (editors): *Community and public health nursing*, St Louis, 2004, Mosby.

Wilson JMG, Jungner G: Principles and practice of screening for disease, *Public Health Papers*, no. 34, Geneva, 1968, World Health Organization.

Wilson T: Economic evaluation of a metropolitan-wide, school-based hepatitis B vaccination program, *Public Health Nurs* 17(3):222-227, 2000.

Unit 7

31 Family Influences on Child Health Promotion

Learning Objectives

On completion of this chapter the reader will be able to:

- Discuss definitions of *family*.
- Describe three major family theories.
- Identify different family structures found in the United States.
- Discuss the effect of family size and configuration on personality development.
- Discuss the role transition experienced by new parents.
- Explain various parenting behaviors such as parenting styles, disciplinary patterns, and communication skills.
- Demonstrate an understanding of special parenting situations such as adoption, divorce, single parenting, parenting in reconstituted families, and dual-earner families.

Electronic Resources

Additional information related to the content in Chapter 31 can be found on

evolve **the Companion Website at**
http://evolve.elsevier.com/Perry/maternal/

- NCLEX Review Questions
- Case Study—Family Functioning

General Concepts

Definition of Family

The term *family* has been defined in many different ways according to the individual's own frame of reference, value judgment, or discipline. There is no universal definition of family; a family is what an individual considers it to be. Biology describes the family as fulfilling the biologic function of perpetuation of the species. Psychology emphasizes the interpersonal aspects of the family and its responsibility for personality development. Economics views the family as a productive unit providing for material needs. Sociology depicts the family as a social unit interacting with the larger society, creating the context within which cultural values and identity are formed. Others define family in terms of the relationships of the persons who make up the family unit. The most common type of relationships are *consanguineous* (blood relationships), *affinal* (marital relationships), and *family of origin* (family unit a person is born into).

Earlier definitions of family emphasized that family members were related by legal ties or genetic relationships and lived in the same household with specific roles. Later definitions have been broadened to reflect both structural and functional changes. A family can be defined as an institution where individuals, related through biology or enduring commitments, and representing similar or different generations and genders, participate in roles involving mutual socialization, nurturance, and emotional commitment (Lerner, Sparks, & McCubbin, 1999).

Considerable controversy has been generated about the newer concepts of family, such as communal families, single-parent families, and homosexual families. To accommodate these and other varieties of family styles, the descriptive term *household* is frequently used.

NURSING ALERT The nurse's knowledge and the sensitivity with which he or she assesses a household will help determine the types of interventions that are appropriate to support family members.

Nursing of infants and children is intimately involved with care of the child *and* the family. Consequently, nurses must be aware of the functions of the family, various types of family structures, and theories that provide a foundation for understanding the changes within a family and for directing family-oriented interventions.

Family Nursing Interventions

In working with children, the nurse must include family members in their care plan. To discover family dynamics, strengths, and weaknesses, a thorough family assessment is necessary (see Chapter 34). When working with families, the

BOX 31-1 Family Nursing Interventions

- Behavior modification
- Case management and coordination
- Collaborative strategies
- Contracting
- Counseling, including support, cognitive reappraisal, and reframing
- Empowering families through active participation
- Environmental modification
- Family advocacy
- Family crisis intervention
- Networking, including use of self-help groups and social support
- Providing information and technical expertise
- Role modeling
- Role supplementation
- Teaching strategies, including stress management, lifestyle modifications, and anticipatory guidance

From Friedman MM, Bowden VR, Jones EG: *Family nursing: research theory and practice*, ed 5, Upper Saddle River, NJ, 2003, Pearson Education.

nurse's choice of interventions depends on the theoretic family model that is used (Box 31-1). For example, in family systems theory, the focus is on the interaction of family members within the larger environment. In this case, using group dynamics to involve all members in the intervention process and being a skillful communicator are essential. Systems theory also presents excellent opportunities for anticipatory guidance. Because each family member reacts to every stress experienced by that system, nurses can intervene to help the family prepare for and cope with changes. Each stress point represents an opportunity for change and learning because families are more open to interventions at this time (Brazelton, 1995). In the family stress theory, crisis intervention strategies are employed to help family members cope with the challenging event. In the developmental theory, the nurse provides anticipatory guidance to prepare members for transition to the next family stage.

Family Roles, Relationships, and Strengths

Each individual has a position, or status, in the family structure and plays culturally and socially defined roles in interactions within the family. Each family also has its own traditions and values and sets its own standards for interaction within and outside the group. Each determines the experiences the children should have, those they are to be shielded from, and how each of these experiences meets the needs of family members. When family ties are strong, social control is highly effective, and most members conform to their roles willingly and with commitment. Conflicts arise when people do not fulfill their roles in ways that meet other family members' expectations, either because they are unaware of the expectations, they choose not to meet them, or they are incapable of meeting them.

Parental Roles

In all family groups the socially recognized status of father and mother exists with socially sanctioned roles that prescribe appropriate sexual behavior and childrearing responsibilities. The guides for behavior in these roles serve to control sexual conflict in society and provide for prolonged care of children. The degree to which parents are committed and the way they play their roles are influenced by a number of variables and by the parents' unique socialization experience.

Parental role definitions are changing as a result of the changing economy and increased opportunities for women. Women are achieving equality with men in education, more of them have entered the workforce, and the number of women who choose to have fewer children or none at all is increasing. As the role of the woman has changed, the complementary role of the man has also changed. Many fathers are taking a more active role in childrearing and household tasks. As the redefinition of sex roles continues in American families, there may be role conflicts in many families because of a cultural lag of the persisting traditional role definitions.

Role Learning

Roles are learned through the socialization process. During all stages of development children learn and practice, through interaction with others and in their play, a set of social roles and the characteristics of other roles. They behave in patterned and more or less predictable ways because they learn roles that define mutual expectations in typical social relationships. Although role definitions are changing, the basic determinants of parenting remain the same. Several determinants of parenting infants and young children are parental personality and mental well-being, systems of support, and child characteristics. These determinants have been used as consistent measurements to determine a person's success in fulfilling the parental role.

Parents, peers, authority figures, and other socializing agents who use positive and negative sanctions to ensure conformity to their norms transmit role conceptions. Role behaviors positively reinforced by rewards such as love, affection, friendship, and honors are strengthened. Negative reinforcement takes the form of ridicule, withdrawal of love, expressions of disapproval, or banishment.

In some cultures the role behavior expected of children conflicts with desirable adult behavior. For example, in the United States, children are expected to be submissive in childhood but dominant as adults. This conflict of expectations is known as *role discontinuity*. Other cultures value the same behaviors, such as courage and aggression, in both children and adults; this provides *role continuity*.

One responsibility of the family is to develop culturally appropriate role behavior in children. Children learn to perform in expected ways consistent with their position in the family and culture. The observed behavior of each child is a single manifestation—a combination of social influences and individual psychologic processes. In this way the uniting of the child's intrapersonal system (the self) with the interpersonal system (the family) is simultaneously understood as the child's conduct.

Role structuring initially takes place within the family unit, in which children fulfill a set of roles and respond to the roles of their parents and other family members. The children's roles are shaped primarily by the parents, who apply direct or indirect pressures to induce or force children into the desired patterns of behavior or direct their efforts toward modification of the child's role responses on a mutually acceptable basis. Parents have their own techniques and determine the course that the process of socialization follows.

Children respond to life situations according to behaviors learned in reciprocal transactions. As they acquire important role-taking skills, their relationships with others change. For instance, when a teenager is also the mother but lives in a household with the grandmother, the teenager may be viewed more as an adolescent than as a mother. Children become proficient at understanding others as they acquire the ability to discriminate their own perspectives from those of others. Children who get along well with others and attain status in the peer group have well-developed role-taking skills.

Family Size and Configuration

Parenting practices differ between small and large families. In small families, more emphasis is placed on the individual development of the children. Parenting is intensive rather than extensive, and there is constant pressure to measure up to family expectations. Children's development and achievement are measured against those of other children in the neighborhood and social class. In small families, there is more democratic participation by the children than in larger families. Adolescents in small families identify more strongly with their parents and rely more on their parents for advice. They have well-developed, autonomous inner controls as contrasted with adolescents from larger families, who rely more on adult authority.

evolve Case Study—Family Functioning

Children in a large family are able to adjust to a variety of changes and crises. There is more emphasis on the group and less on the individual (Fig. 31-1). Cooperation is essential, often because of economic necessity. The large number of people sharing a limited amount of space requires a greater degree of organization, administration, and authoritarian control. A dominant family member (a parent or older child) wields control. The number of children reduces the intimate, one-to-one contact between the parent and any individual child. Consequently, children turn to each other for what they cannot get from their parents. The reduced parent-child contact encourages individual children to adopt specialized roles to gain recognition in the family. Older siblings in large families often administer discipline. Siblings are usually attuned to what constitutes misbehavior. Sibling disapproval or ostracism is frequently a more meaningful disciplinary measure than parental interventions. In situations such as death or illness of a parent, an older sibling often assumes responsibility for the family at considerable personal sacrifice. Large families generate a sense of security in the children that is fostered by sibling support and cooperation. However, adolescents from a large family are more peer oriented than family oriented.

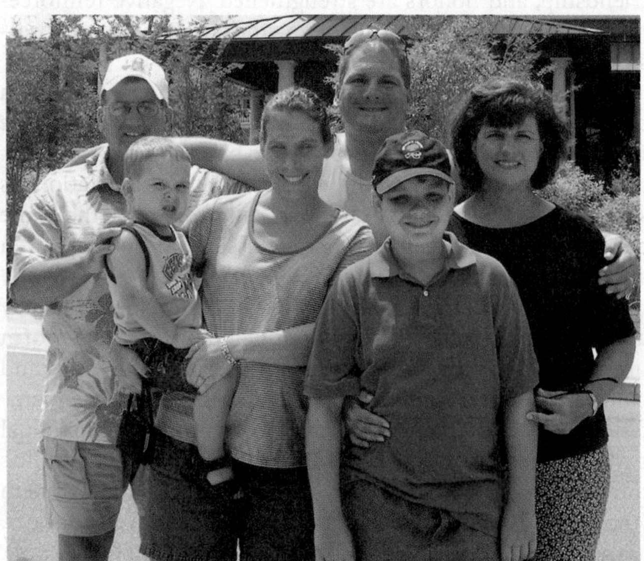

Fig. 31-1 Family structure promotes strong relationships among its members.

Sibling Interactions

Spacing of Children

Age differences between siblings affect the childhood environment, but to a lesser extent than does the sex of the sibling. The arrival of a sibling is difficult for toddlers and preschool children, especially between the ages of 2 and 3 years old. At this age, they are still attached to their parents and do not understand the concept of sharing. An older child is able to understand the situation and is less likely to see the newcomer as a threat, although the child does feel the loss of the only-child status. In general, the narrower the spacing between siblings, the more the children influence one another, especially in emotional characteristics. The wider the spacing, the greater the influence of the parents.

Traditionally, sibling relationships were viewed from a Freudian perspective that emphasized the concept of sibling rivalry. Recently, researchers have viewed siblings through developmental or ecologic frameworks that focus on interactions within family systems (Friedman, Bowden, & Jones, 2003). The results of these broader perspectives provide a picture of rich and varied sibling interactions (Fig. 31-2).

Sibling Functions

The sibling relationship's most unique feature is its duration. The longest relationship one will share with another human being is the sibling relationship, which lasts through a lifetime (often 50 to 80 years), compared with the child-parent relationship of approximately 30 to 50 years. Siblings spend long periods together and get to know each other at their best and worst.

Siblings exert power, exchange services, and express feelings in reciprocal ways that are often not revealed in the presence of the parents. They see themselves in their brother or sister, experience life vicariously through their sibling's behavior, and begin to expand on their own possibilities. Siblings can also be touchstones for what the other would *not* like to be, and they use each other as yardsticks for comparison. They provide a sounding board for each other and offer a safe forum for experimenting with new behaviors and roles. Brothers and sisters provide each other with tangible services (e.g., lending money, clothing, toys, or sports equipment; teaching a skill), help each other with childhood problems, provide support in dealing with parents or others outside the family, and provide introductions to new friendship groups. Children learn to

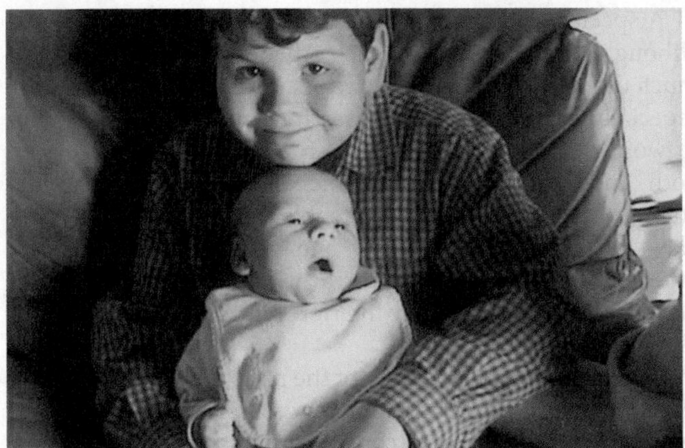

Fig. 31-2 Older school-age children often enjoy taking responsibility for the care of a younger sibling.

negotiate and bargain, and sometimes to manipulate, from their siblings. Their interactions with each other provide opportunities for conflict and conflict resolution. They protect one another from parental-executive abuse of power and can form a coalition to deal with the issues of authority, power, and emotional support. Negotiating with parents is stronger when siblings act together rather than singly.

Siblings interpret the outside world for each other and perform educative functions for the parents. A related function is *pioneering,* in which one sibling initiates a process, thereby giving the others permission to follow. These patterns include breaking explicit family rules, taking new pathways (such as leaving the family), or adopting different moral or political codes and lifestyles.

Tattling can be an important lever in sibling interactions. On the other hand, there is often a conspiracy of silence among siblings, leaving the parents feeling isolated and excluded. A willingness to maintain each other's privacy often serves as a powerful bond of loyalty that distinguishes the relationship between siblings from that between friends.

More Active Sibling Relationships

Sibling relationships vary among cultures. Some factors may be giving the sibling relationship greater significance in American families than in the past. Shrinking family size, longer life spans, divorce and remarriage, geographic mobility, maternal employment, alternative sources of child care, competitive pressures, stress, and parental insufficiency may be propelling siblings into greater contact and emotional interdependence than ever before. Siblings often join forces to confront the trauma of divorce, and they frequently rely on each other for support when parents remarry. The large number of working mothers means that young siblings today have significant amounts of time when a personally committed adult does not monitor their relationship. Often an older sibling is required to baby-sit, resulting in children spending more and more time together unsupervised. In a worried, mobile, small-family, high-stress, fast-paced, parent-absent society, children often turn to a brother or sister to meet their needs for contact, constancy, and permanency.

Ordinal Position

Researchers have observed that the birth position of children affects their personalities. Parents treat children differently, and sibling interactions are different, depending on the child's position within the family. Power is unequally distributed among siblings. Older siblings attempt to dominate younger ones. Therefore younger siblings develop interpersonal skills, the ability to negotiate, and an ability to accept unfavorable outcomes to a greater extent than older siblings. Later-born children are obliged to interact with other siblings from birth and seem to be more outgoing and make friends more easily than firstborns. Children vary tremendously, and generalizations do not always apply to the individual. General characteristics of children in the various ordinal positions are presented in Box 31-2.

BOX 31-2 Influence of Ordinal Position on Children

Firstborn Children
- Are more achievement oriented
- Are more dominant
- Receive more physical punishment
- Have stronger consciences; are more self-disciplined and inner directed
- Are more socially anxious
- Are prone to feelings of guilt
- Identify more with parents than with peers
- Are more conservative
- Are subject to greater parental expectations
- Begin to speak earlier in life
- Demonstrate higher intellectual achievement
- Plan better and experience fewer frustrations

Middle Children
- Have more demands made on them for household help
- Are praised less often
- Receive less of the parents' time
- Learn to compromise and be adaptable
- Are less stimulated toward achievement
- Are more difficult to characterize because of a variety of positions in the family

Youngest Children
- Are less dependent than firstborn children
- Are less tense, more affectionate, and more good-natured
- Tend to identify more with peer group than with parents
- Are more flexible in their thinking
- Have fewer demands placed on them for household help

Only Children
- Resemble firstborn children
- Are more mature and cultivated
- Experience greater parental pressure for mature behavior and achievement
- Demonstrate superiority in language facility
- Rarely develop into the stereotype of a spoiled, selfish child
- Often enjoy a rich fantasy life as a result of isolation

The Only Child

Being the only child in a family has traditionally been considered a disadvantage. Only children have been described as selfish, spoiled, dependent, and lonely. However, they do not demonstrate more evidence of maladjustment or self-centeredness than other children and tend to strongly resemble firstborn children in respects such as higher educational goals. Only children perform better on cognitive tests, are more mature, are more socially sensitive, and demonstrate superiority in language facility compared with other children.

Only children enjoy the advantage of having parents who can devote more time to them, talk to them, and stimulate them in intellectual activities. However, parents also exert greater pressure for mature behavior at an early age and for achievement. Relative isolation from peers contributes to intellectual pursuits and encourages a rich fantasy life, independence, and originality.

Multiple Births

A deviation in early development that occurs with variable frequency is multiple births. Twins are not uncommon in the population, but triplets are rare and quadruplets or quintuplets are extremely unusual. In any of these situations, the offspring can be of the like or unlike sex (i.e., derived from a single ovum; from multiple ova; or from a combination of the two, which can involve one or more cell divisions). The cause of twinning is unknown, but the increase in the number of larger multiples (quintuplets, sextuplets) during recent years has been associated with fertility treatments such as ovulation-inducing drugs or in vitro fertilization. Because women in their thirties are almost 2.5 times as likely as women in their twenties to have higher-order plural births, the rise in the multiple-birth ratio has been associated with increased childbearing among older women and the expanded use of fertility drugs (Hamilton et al, 2007).

Twins are of two distinct types: *identical*, or *monozygotic (MZ)*, and *fraternal*, or *dizygotic (DZ)* (Box 31-3). In 2004 in the United States the overall rate of twin birth was 32.2 per 1000 births, a record high (Hamilton et al, 2007); one third are MZ twins, and two thirds are DZ twins.

BOX 31-3 Characteristics of Twins

Monozygotic (Identical) Twins	Dizygotic (Fraternal) Twins
Result of one fertilized ovum that became separated early in development	Result of fertilization of two ova
Alike physically and genetically	Differ physically and genetically
Same sex	May be same or opposite sex
Frequency—Occurs uniformly in all populations	Frequency—Varies among races (highest in African-Americans; lowest in Asians; intermediate in Caucasians)
Unaffected by maternal age	More common with advancing maternal age (maximum at age 35 to 39 years, then decreases rapidly)
Tendency unaffected by heredity	Marked familial tendency
	Expressed only in the female
	Fathers appear to transmit disposition toward double ovulation to daughters
Similar behavior	Dissimilar behavior; more sibling rivalry

A special kind of sibling relationship is observed in twins, although getting along with each other and quarreling are not much different from these behaviors in any other two siblings, especially if they are different-sex fraternal twins. Twins tend to work out a relationship that is reasonably satisfactory to both and demonstrate early independence from parental attention. They develop a remarkable capacity for cooperative play and considerable loyalty and generosity toward each other. It is not uncommon for a private language to evolve between the twins that may interfere with the development of the family language.

In a twinship, one member of the pair, to a greater or lesser extent, is more dominant, outgoing, and assertive than the other, often to the parents' consternation. However, the seemingly more passive twin is able to accomplish as much and get his or her way as frequently as the more assertive twin.

Researchers have also observed a difference in behavior between identical and fraternal twins. There is near-unison in the actions of identical twins (although they alternate in assuming the leadership), but fraternal twins, even of the same sex, do not display this quality. Sibling rivalry can be pronounced in fraternal twins, especially in different-sex twins.

Identical twins also differ in their response to the tendency of some parents to treat twins exactly alike. The present philosophy is to determine the degree to which the children demonstrate an inclination toward togetherness. Some twins thrive best when they are constantly in each other's company; others prefer more individuality and separateness. The conservative approach is to allow the children to follow their natural inclinations. Early years of togetherness are often the basis of the children's security, and separating them too early may produce unnecessary stress. Fostering individual differences as they become evident could ease the process of separation when it becomes advisable.

Parental Adjustment

The entrance of any new member into a household creates stress, but with multiple births two or more new members must be incorporated into the family at the same time. The problems are obvious. Two infants must be provided with physical care, including feeding and diapering, and all of the purchasing and preparation that accompanies the care of any infant. Scheduling becomes crucial, and advancement in development brings new problems and adjustments (e.g., space and sleeping arrangements, selection of a stroller and other equipment). Care must be observed in selecting toys. As play becomes a serious business, some toys that would be safe and appropriate for a single child become weapons when two infants share a playpen. It is a good idea to select different toys for each child as they grow older and encourage sharing.

Parenting

Motivation for Parenthood

A dominant characteristic in all societies is that adults are expected to become parents and to be gratified by the experience. Pressures of tradition, sentiment regarding the state of parenthood, and religious beliefs influence decision making because conformity to social-role expectations is a strong influence in family planning.

Factors that influence family size are social class, religion, race, financial stability, type of conjugal-role relationships, and the social-psychologic aspects of sexual relations. In the case of divorce and remarriage, an individual may decide to have more children with the new spouse.

Preparation for Parenthood

The basic goals of parenting are to promote the children's physical survival and health, to foster the skills and abilities necessary to be a self-sustaining adult, and to foster behavioral capabilities for optimizing cultural values and beliefs. However, new parents often approach parenthood with limited experience and knowledge. Parents learn by trial and error, committing the same mistakes that have been committed by countless other parents, but they somehow manage to accomplish the task, becoming more skilled with each additional child. Tradition, rather than rational planning, furnishes the chief norms for childrearing. Experience in having been nurtured as a child is an essential component of successful parenting.

Their own parents are probably the only persons whom parents observe intimately in the parental role. This results in a *generational continuity*—parents rear their own children in much the same way as they themselves were reared. Other essential skills that parents need to feel comfortable in the parenting role include a basic understanding of childhood growth and development, bathing, feeding, use of play, and interpersonal communication skills.

Transition to Parenthood

Although experts disagree as to whether the birth of the first child should be labeled a *crisis,* the early weeks of an infant's life call for parents to make drastic adjustments. Even though the parents have anticipated and prepared for the child's arrival, the birth presents the challenge of providing total care 24 hours a day for a new member of the family. A crisis may occur if the event is perceived as disturbing old habits and relationships and eliciting new responses. The birth requires role changes or significantly modifies former relationships. In addition to the roles of husband and wife, the couple must assume the roles of father and mother.

The advent of a new family member requires that the family cope with greater financial responsibilities, a possible loss of income, changes in sleeping habits, and less time for the parents to spend with each other (especially if it is a firstborn) and with other children. If these events are perceived as adverse, it can disrupt the couple's bond and reduce the couple's intimacy and affection.

Other factors influencing the transition to the parental role include the following:

- Parents with previous experience, such as another child, appear to be more relaxed, have less conflict in disciplinary relationships, and are more aware of normal growth and development.
- The amount of stress experienced by one or both parents may interfere with their ability to exhibit patience and understanding and to cope with their children's behavior.
- Special characteristics of the infant, such as being temperamentally difficult, can cause the parents to lose confidence and doubt their abilities. Infants with special care needs (such as those associated with a disability) can be a significant source of added stress.
- Fathers who are highly involved with their child often feel more comfortable in the parenting role (Fig. 31-3).
- Stressed marital relationships can have a negative effect on parental transition because marital tension can alter caregiving routines and interfere with enjoyment of the infant. Conversely, parents' support and encouragement of one another serve as positive influences on establishment of a satisfying parental role.

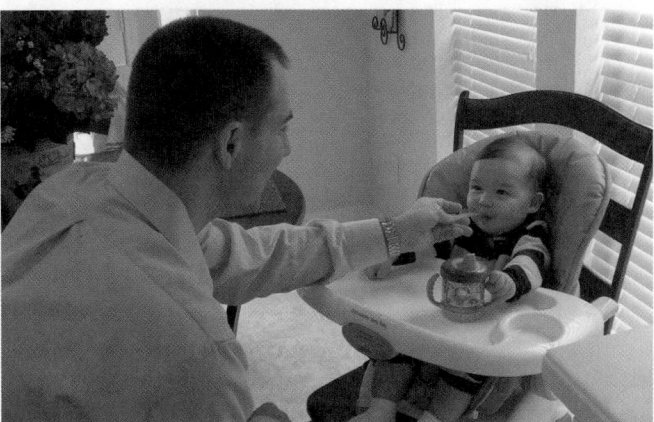

Fig. 31-3 Fathers who assume care of their children may feel more comfortable and successful in their parenting role.

Support Systems

Successful adaptation to the stress of transition to parenthood involves at least two types of family resources (McCubbin & McCubbin, 1994). *Internal resources* such as adaptability and integration are the first type. Changing from an orderly, predictable life to a relatively disordered, unpredictable one is a universal adaptation that families must make. Rigid schedules are impossible to maintain, and former activities must be curtailed or abandoned. Spending quality time with a child can promote health and a successful transition (Fig. 31-4). *Adaptation* is reflected in learning to be patient, becoming better organized, and becoming more flexible. *Integration* refers to the couple's attempt to continue some activities they engaged in before they became parents. In this way couples are able to maintain a sense of continuity and appreciate the importance of the husband-wife relationship.

The second resource for dealing with stress is the use of *coping strategies* that strengthen the family's organization and functioning. These include the use of social support systems and community resources and the adoption of a future orientation. Interpersonal supports that provide information, advice, and caretaking can be derived from friends, relatives, and neighbors. Relationships with family, friends, and community are essential. For parents, positive, supportive work relationships are important. Equally important is time spent with friends. Arranging for time away from the child or children is also beneficial. One parent can assume care of the family to allow the other parent some time to himself or herself. Adoption of a future orientation reassures parents that things will get better, that they will cope, and that it is realistic

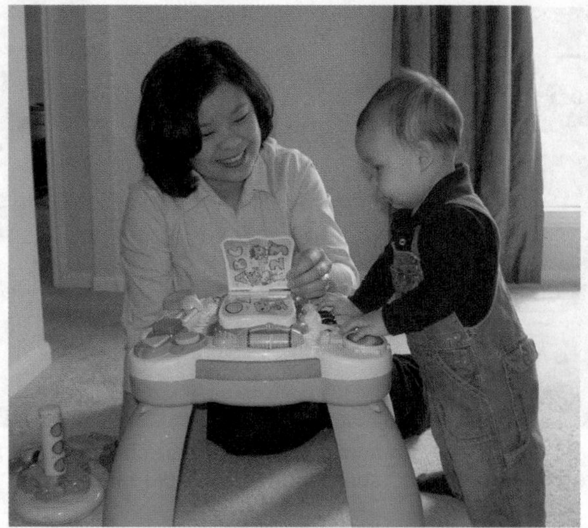

Fig. 31-4 Quality time spent with a child is essential to a family's health and well-being.

to plan for the time when they will be able to engage in self-fulfilling activities.

It is also reassuring to know that others experience ambivalent feelings toward parenthood and share the same difficulties and frustrations. Exchanging ideas and experiences with other parents and with one's partner provides an opportunity to voice concerns and to learn new ways to cope with multiple childrearing problems.

Parenting Behaviors

Parental Styles of Control

Parenting styles can be described as authoritarian, permissive, or authoritative. *Authoritarian* or *dictatorial* parents try to control their children's behavior and attitudes through unquestioned mandates. They establish rules and regulations or standards of conduct that they expect to be followed rigidly and unquestioningly. They value and reward absolute obedience, mute acceptance of their word, and unfailing respect for the family's principles and beliefs. They forcefully punish any behavior that is contrary to parental standards. Parental authority is exercised with little explanation and little involvement of the child in decision making. The message is: "Do it because I say so." Punishment need not be corporal but may be stern withdrawal of love and approval.

Careful training often results in rigidly conforming behavior in the children, who tend to be sensitive, shy, self-conscious, retiring, and submissive. They are more apt to be courteous, loyal, honest, and dependable but docile. These behaviors are more typically observed when close supervision and affection accompany parental authority. If not, this style of parenting may be associated with both defiant and antisocial behavior.

Permissive or *laissez-faire* parents exert little or no control over their children's actions. They avoid imposing their own standards of conduct and allow their children to regulate their own activity as much as possible. These parents consider themselves to be resources for the children, not role models. If rules do exist, the parents explain the underlying reason, elicit the children's opinions, and consult them in decision-making processes. They employ lax, inconsistent discipline; do not set sensible limits; and do not prevent the children from upsetting the home routine. These parents rarely punish the children. Consequently, the children control the parents and are often disobedient, disrespectful, and generally defiant of authority.

Authoritative or *democratic* parents combine practices from both of the previously described parenting styles. They direct their children's behavior and attitudes by emphasizing the reason for rules and negatively reinforcing deviations. They respect each child's individuality and allow him or her to voice objections to family standards or regulations. Parental control is firm and consistent but tempered with encouragement, understanding, and security. Control is focused on the issue, not on withdrawal of love or fear of punishment. These parents foster "inner-directedness," a conscience that regulates behavior based on feelings of guilt or shame for wrongdoing, not on fear of being caught or punished. Parents' realistic standards and reasonable expectations produce children with high self-esteem who are self-reliant, assertive, inquisitive, content, and highly interactive with other children.

Limit Setting and Discipline

In its broadest sense, *discipline* means *to teach* or refers to a set of rules governing conduct. In a narrower sense, it refers to the action taken to enforce the rules after noncompliance. *Limit setting* refers to establishing the rules or guidelines for behavior. For example, parents can place limits on the amount of time children spend watching television or chatting online. The clearer the limits that are set and the more consistently they are enforced, the less need there is for disciplinary action.

Nurses can help parents establish realistic and concrete "rules." Limit setting and discipline are positive, necessary components of childrearing and serve several useful functions as they help children:

- Test their limits of control
- Achieve in areas appropriate for mastery at their level
- Channel undesirable feelings into constructive activity
- Protect themselves from danger
- Learn socially acceptable behavior

Children want and need limits. Unrestricted freedom is a threat to their security and safety. Through testing the limits imposed on them, children learn the extent to which they can manipulate their environment and gain reassurance from knowing that others are there to protect them from potential harm.

Minimizing Misbehavior

The reasons for misbehavior may include attention, power, defiance, and a display of inadequacy (e.g., the child misses classes because of a fear that he or she is unable to do the work). Children may also misbehave because the rules are not clear or consistently applied. Acting-out behavior, such as a temper tantrum, may represent uncontrolled frustration, anger, depression, or pain. The best approach is to structure interactions with children so that unacceptable behavior is prevented or minimized (see Family-Centered Care box).

FAMILY-CENTERED CARE

Minimizing Misbehavior

- Set realistic goals for acceptable behavior and expected achievements.
- Structure opportunities for small successes to lessen feelings of inadequacy.
- Praise children for desirable behavior with attention and verbal approval.
- Structure the environment to prevent unnecessary difficulties (e.g., place fragile objects in inaccessible area).
- Set clear and reasonable rules; expect the same behavior regardless of the circumstances; if exceptions are made, clarify that the change is for one time only.
- Teach desirable behavior through own example, such as using a quiet, calm voice rather than screaming.
- Review expected behavior before special or unusual events, such as visiting a relative or having dinner in a restaurant.
- Phrase requests for appropriate behavior positively, such as "Put the book down," rather than "Don't touch the book."
- Call attention to unacceptable behavior as soon as it begins; use distraction to change the behavior or offer alternatives to annoying actions, such as a quiet toy for one that is excessively noisy.
- Give advance notice or "friendly reminders," such as "When the TV program is over, it is time for dinner" or "I'll give you to the count of three and then we have to go."
- Be attentive to situations that increase the likelihood of misbehaving, such as overexcitement or fatigue, or to decreased personal tolerance to minor infractions.
- Offer sympathetic explanations for not granting a request, such as "I am sorry I can't read you a story now, but I have to finish dinner. Then we can spend time together."
- Keep any promises made to children.
- Avoid outright conflicts; temper discussions with statements such as "Let's talk about it and see what we can decide together" or "I have to think about it first."
- Provide children with opportunities for power and control.

General Guidelines for Implementing Discipline

Regardless of the type of discipline used, certain principles are essential to ensure the efficacy of the approach (see Family-Centered Care box). Many strategies, such as behavior modification, can only be implemented effectively when principles of consistency and timing are followed. A pattern of intermittent or occasional enforcement of limits actually prolongs the undesired behavior because children learn that if they are persistent, the behavior is permitted eventually. Delaying punishment weakens its intent, and practices such as telling the child, "Wait until your father comes home," are not only ineffectual, but also convey negative messages about the other parent.*

**For parenting of kindergarten through sixth grade children, see* http://childparenting.about.com, *or see* www.kidshealth.org *for information about younger children and teens.*

FAMILY-CENTERED CARE

Implementing Discipline

Consistency—Implement disciplinary action exactly as agreed on and for each infraction.

Timing—Initiate discipline as soon as child misbehaves; if delays are necessary, such as to avoid embarrassment, verbally disapprove of the behavior and state that disciplinary action will be implemented.

Commitment—Follow through with the details of the discipline, such as timing of minutes; avoid distractions that may interfere with the plan, such as telephone calls.

Unity—Make certain that all caregivers agree on the plan and are familiar with the details to prevent confusion and alliances between child and one parent.

Flexibility—Choose disciplinary strategies that are appropriate to child's age and temperament and the severity of the misbehavior.

Planning—Plan disciplinary strategies in advance and prepare child if feasible (e.g., explain use of time-out); for unexpected misbehavior, try to discipline when you are calm.

Behavior orientation—Always disapprove of the behavior, not the child, with such statements as "That was a wrong thing to do. I am unhappy when I see behavior like that."

Privacy—Administer discipline in private, especially with older children, who may feel ashamed in front of others.

Termination—After the discipline is administered, consider child as having a "clean slate," and avoid bringing up the incident or lecturing.

Types of Discipline

To deal with misbehavior, parents need to implement appropriate disciplinary action. Many approaches are available. *Reasoning* involves explaining why an act is wrong and is usually appropriate for older children, especially when moral issues are involved. However, young children cannot be expected to "see the other side" because of their egocentrism. Children in the preoperative stage of cognitive development (toddlers and preschoolers) have a limited ability to distinguish between their point of view and those of others. Sometimes children use "reasoning" as a way of gaining attention. For example, they may misbehave thinking the parents will give them a lengthy explanation of the wrongdoing and knowing that negative attention is better than no attention. When children use this technique, parents should end the explanation by stating, "This is the rule, and this is how I expect you to behave. I won't explain it any further."

Unfortunately, reasoning is often combined with *scolding*, which sometimes takes the form of shame or criticism. For example, the parent may state, "You are a bad boy for hitting your brother." Children take such remarks seriously and personally, believing that they *are* bad.

NURSING ALERT When reprimanding children, focus only on the misbehavior, not on the child. Use of "I" messages rather than "you" messages expresses personal feelings without accusation or ridicule. For example, an "I" message attacks the behavior–"I am upset when Johnny is punched; I don't like to see him hurt"–not the child.

Positive and negative reinforcement is the basis of *behavior modification* theory—behavior that is rewarded will be repeated; behavior that is not rewarded will be extinguished. Using *rewards* is a positive approach. By encouraging children to behave in specified ways, the parents can decrease the tendency to misbehave. With young children, using star stickers is an effective method. For older children, the "token system" is appropriate, especially if a certain number of stars or tokens yields a special reward, such as a trip to the movies or a new book. In planning a reward system, the parents must explain expected behaviors to the child and establish rewards that are reinforcing. A chart should be used to record the stars or tokens, and an earned reward should be given promptly. Verbal approval should always accompany extrinsic rewards.

Consistently *ignoring* behavior will eventually extinguish or minimize the act. Although this approach sounds simple, it is often difficult to implement consistently. Parents frequently "give in" and resort to previous patterns of discipline. Consequently, the behavior is actually reinforced because the child learns that persistence gains parental attention. For ignoring to be effective, parents should (1) understand the process, (2) record the undesired behavior before using ignoring to determine whether a problem exists and to compare results after ignoring is begun, (3) determine whether parental attention acts as a reinforcer, and (4) be aware of "response burst." Response burst is a phenomenon that occurs when the undesired behavior increases after ignoring is initiated because the child is testing the parents to see if they are serious about the plan.

The strategy of *consequences* involves allowing children to experience the results of their misbehavior. It includes three types:

Natural—Those that occur without any intervention, such as being late and missing dinner

Logical—Those that are directly related to the rule, such as not being allowed to play with another toy until the used ones are put away

Unrelated—Those that are imposed deliberately, such as no playing until homework is completed or the use of time-out

Natural or logical consequences are preferred and effective if they are meaningful to children. For example, the natural consequence of living in a messy room may do little to encourage cleaning up, but allowing no friends over until the room is neat can be motivating! Withdrawing privileges is often an unrelated consequence. After the child experiences the consequence, the parent should refrain from any comment, since the usual tendency is for the child to try to place blame for imposing the rule.

Time-out is actually a refinement of the common practice of sending the child to his or her room and is a type of unrelated consequence. It is based on the premise of removing the reinforcer (i.e., the satisfaction or attention the child is receiving from the activity). When placed in an unstimulating and isolated place, children become bored and consequently agree to behave in order to reenter the family group. Time-out avoids many of the problems of other disciplinary approaches. No physical punishment is involved; no reasoning or scolding is given; and the parent does not need to be present for all of the time-out, thus facilitating his or her ability to consistently apply this type of discipline. Time-out offers both the child and the parent a "cooling off" time. To be effective, however, time-out must be planned in advance (see Family-Centered Care box).

FAMILY-CENTERED CARE

Using Time-Out

Select an area for time-out that is safe, convenient, and unstimulating, but where the child can be monitored, such as the bathroom, hallway, or laundry room.

Determine what behaviors warrant a time-out.

Make certain children understand the "rules" and how they are expected to behave.

Explain to children the process of time-out:

- When they misbehave, they will be given *one* warning.
- If they do not obey, they will be sent to the place designated for time-out.
- They are to sit there for a specified period.
- If they cry, refuse, or display any disruptive behavior, the time-out period will begin *after* they quiet down.
- When they are quiet for the duration of the time, they can then leave the room.

A rule for the length of time-out is *1 minute per year of age;* use a kitchen timer with an audible bell to record the time rather than a watch.

Implement time-out in a public place by selecting a suitable area, or explain to children that time-out will be spent immediately on returning home.

Corporal or *physical punishment* most often takes the form of spanking. Based on the principles of aversive therapy, inflicting pain through spanking causes a dramatic short-term decrease in the behavior. However, this approach has serious flaws: (1) it teaches children that violence is acceptable; (2) it may physically harm the child if it is the result of parental rage; and (3) children become accustomed to spanking, requiring more severe corporal punishment each time. Spanking can result in severe physical and psychologic injury, and it interferes with effective parent-child interaction. In addition, when the parent is not around, the misbehavior is likely to occur, since children have not learned to behave well for their own sake. Parental use of corporal punishment may also interfere with the child's development of moral reasoning.

Special Parenting Situations

Parenting is a demanding task under ideal circumstances, but when parents and children are faced with situations that deviate from what is considered the norm, the potential for family disruption is increased. Situations that are commonly encountered are divorce, single parenthood, blended families, adoption, and dual-career families. In addition, as cultural diversity increases in our communities, many immigrants are making the transition to parenthood and a new country, culture, and language simultaneously. Other situations that create unique parenting challenges are parental alcoholism, homelessness, and incarceration. Although these topics are not addressed here, the reader may wish to investigate them further.

Parenting the Adopted Child

Adoption establishes a legal relationship between a child and parents who are not related by birth, but who have the same rights and obligations that exist between children and their biologic parents. In the past the biologic mother alone made the decision to relinquish the rights to her child. In recent years the courts have acknowledged the legal rights of the biologic father regarding this decision. Concerned child advocates have questioned whether decisions that honor the father's rights are in the child's best interests. As the rights of the child have become recognized, older children have successfully dissolved their legal bond with their biologic parents to pursue adoption by adults of their choice. Furthermore, there is a growing interest and demand within the gay and lesbian community to adopt.

Unlike biologic parents, who prepare for their child's birth with prenatal classes and the support of friends and relatives, adoptive parents have few sources of support and preparation for the new addition to their family. Nurses can provide the information, support, and reassurance needed to reduce parental anxiety regarding the adoptive process and refer adoptive parents to state parental support groups. Such sources can be contacted through a state or county welfare office.

Most problems faced by adoptive parents are not different from those encountered by natural parents, but the desire to be a good parent is often intensified in adoptive parents. Adoptive parents have been portrayed as more apprehensive, insecure, and in need of assistance than biologic parents. However, some adoptive parents may actually need less assistance than biologic parents. This situation may be related to the adoptive parents' completely voluntary decision to become parents, the relatively long time they have to prepare for parenting, and the maturity associated with adoption.

The sooner infants enter their adoptive home, the better the chances of parent-infant attachment. However, the more caregivers the infant had before adoption, the greater the risk for attachment problems. The infant must break the bond with the previous caregiver and form a new bond with the adoptive parents. Difficulties in forming an attachment depend on the amount of time the infant has spent with earlier caregivers (e.g., the birth mother, nurse, adoption agency personnel).

Siblings, adopted or biologic, who are old enough to understand should be included in decisions regarding the commitment to adopt, with reassurance that they are not being replaced. Ways that the siblings can interact with the adopted child should be stressed (Fig. 31-5).

Issues of Origin

The task of telling children that they are adopted can be a cause of deep concern and anxiety. There are no clear-cut guidelines for parents to follow in determining when and at what age children are ready for the information. Parents are naturally reluctant to present the children with such potentially unsettling news. However, it is important that parents not withhold the adoption from the child, since it is an essential component of the child's identity (see Critical Thinking Exercise).

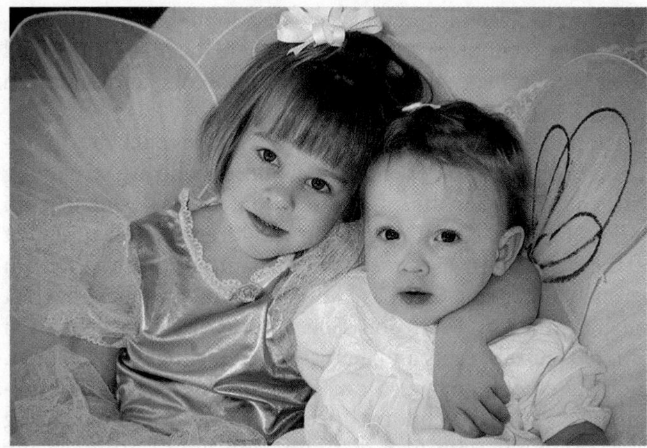

Fig. 31-5 An older sister lovingly embraces her adopted sister.

> **CRITICAL THINKING EXERCISE**
>
> **Parenting the Adopted Child**
>
> Twelve-month-old Justin was adopted at birth. His parents tell you that they wonder when they should tell Justin that he is adopted. As the nurse, what counseling and advice should you give Justin's parents?
>
> 1. Evidence—Is there sufficient information to draw any conclusions about this situation?
> 2. Assumptions—Describe some underlying assumptions about the following:
>   a. The best time to tell children that they are adopted
>   b. The manner in which parents should tell their child about adoption
>   c. Children's reactions to being told they are adopted
> 3. What implications for nursing care can be drawn at this time?
> 4. Does the evidence support your conclusion?
> 5. Are there alternative perspectives to consider?

The timing arises naturally, as parents become aware of the child's readiness. Most authorities believe that children should be informed at an age young enough so that, as they grow older, they do not remember a time when they did not know they were adopted. The time is highly individual, but must be right for both the parents and the child. It may be when children ask where babies come from, at which time children can also be told the facts of their adoption. If they are told in a way that conveys the idea that they were active participants in the selection process, they will be less likely to feel that they were abandoned, helpless victims. For example, parents can tell children that their personal qualities drew the parents to them. It is wise for parents who have not previously discussed adoption to tell children that they are adopted before the children enter school to avoid having them hear it from third parties. Complete honesty between parents and children strengthens the relationship.

Parents should anticipate behavior changes after the disclosure, especially in older children. Children who are struggling with the revelation that they are adopted may benefit from individual and family counseling. Children may use the fact of their adoption as a weapon to manipulate and threaten parents. Statements such as "My real mother would not treat me like this" or "You don't love me as much because I'm adopted" hurt parents and increase their feelings of insecurity. Such statements may also cause parents to become overpermissive. Adopted children need the same undemanding love, combined with firm discipline and limit setting, as any other child.

Adolescence

Adolescence may be an especially trying time for parents of adopted children. The normal confrontations of adolescents and parents assume more painful aspects in adoptive families. Adolescents may use their adoption to defy parental authority or as a justification for aberrant behavior. As they attempt to master the task of identity formation, the feeling of abandonment by their biologic parents comes into awareness and may be intensified.

Adopted children fantasize about their biologic parents and may feel the need to discover their parents' identity to define themselves and their own identity. It is important for parents to keep the lines of communication open and to reassure their child that they understand the need to search for their identity. In some states, birth certificates are made legally available to adopted children when they come of age. It is important for parents to be honest with questioning adolescents and to tell them of this possibility (the parents themselves are unable to obtain the birth certificate; it is the children's responsibility if they desire it).

Cross-Racial and International Adoption

Adoption of children from racial backgrounds different from that of the family is commonplace. In addition to the problems faced by adopted children in general, children of a cross-racial adoption must deal with physical and sometimes cultural differences. It is advised that parents who adopt such children do everything to preserve the adopted children's racial heritage.

NURSING ALERT As a health care provider, it is important not to ask the wrong questions, such as "Is she yours, or is she adopted?" "What do you know about the 'real' mother?" "Do they have the same father?" or "How much did it cost to adopt him?"

Although the children are full-fledged members of an adopting family and citizens of the adopted country, if they have a strikingly different appearance from other family members or exhibit distinct racial or ethnic characteristics, challenges may be encountered outside the family. Bigotry may appear among relatives and friends. Strangers may make thoughtless comments and talk about the children as though they were not members of the family. It is vital that family members declare to others that this is their child and a cherished member of the family.

In international adoptions the medical information the parents receive may be incomplete or sketchy; weight, height, and head circumference are often the only objective information present in the child's medical record. Many internationally adopted children were born prematurely, and common health problems such as infant diarrhea and malnutrition delay growth and development. Some children have serious or multiple health problems that can be stressful for the parents.

Parenting and Divorce

Since the mid-1960s, a marked change in the stability of families has been reflected in increased rates of divorce, single parenthood, and remarriage. In 2005 the divorce rate for the United States was 3.8 per 1000 total population (Munson & Sutton, 2006). The divorce rate has changed little since 1987. In the previous decade, the rate increased yearly, with a peak in 1979. Although almost half of all divorcing couples are childless, it is estimated that more than 1 million children experience divorce each year.

The process of divorce begins with a period of marital conflict of varying length and intensity, followed by a separation, the actual legal divorce, and the reestablishment of different living arrangements. Because a function of parenthood is to provide for the security and emotional welfare of children, disruption of the family structure often engenders strong feelings of guilt in the divorcing parents.

During a divorce, parents' coping abilities may be compromised. The parents may be preoccupied with their own feelings, needs, and life changes and unable to be available and supportive to their children. Newly employed parents, usually mothers, are likely to leave children with new caregivers, in strange settings, or alone after school. The parent may also spend more time away from home, searching for or establishing new relationships. Sometimes, however, the adult feels frightened and alone and begins to depend on the child as a substitute for the absent parent. This dependence places an enormous burden on the child.

Common characteristics in the custodial household after separation and divorce include disorder, coercive types of control, inflammable tempers in both parents and children, reduced parental competence, a greater sense of parental helplessness, poorly enforced discipline, and diminished regularity in enforcing household routines. Noncustodial parents are seldom prepared for the role of visitor, may assume the role of recreational and "fun" parent, and may not have a residence suitable for children's visits. They may also be concerned about maintaining the arrangement over the years to follow.

Impact of Divorce on Children

Numerous studies indicate that divorce has a profound effect on children. Many youngsters suffer for years from psychologic and social difficulties associated with continuing or new stresses in the postdivorce family. Even when a divorce is amicable and open, children recall parental separation with the same emotions felt by victims of a natural disaster: loss, grief, and vulnerability to forces beyond their control.

The impact of divorce on children depends on several factors, including the children's age and sex, parental interaction or conflict, and the quality of the parent-child relationship and parental care during the years following the divorce. Family characteristics are more crucial to the child's well-being than specific child characteristics, such as age or sex. High levels of ongoing family conflict are related to problems of social development, emotional stability, and cognitive skills for the child.

Complications associated with divorce include efforts on the part of one parent to subvert the child's loyalties to the other, abandonment to other caregivers, and adjustment to a stepparent. A major problem occurs when children are "caught in the middle" between the divorced parents. They become the message bearer between the parents, are often quizzed about the activities of the other parent, and have to listen to one parent criticize the other. A nurse may be able to intercede by helping the child get out of the middle by stating "I messages" based on the formula of "I feel . . . (state the feeling) when you . . . (state the source). I would like it if you . . . ." This approach enables the child to feel in control. An example of an "I message" is: "I do not feel comfortable when you ask me questions about Mom; maybe you could ask her yourself."

Feelings of children toward divorce vary with age (Box 31-4). Some children feel a sense of shame and embarrassment concerning the family situation. Some feelings cause children to see themselves as different, inferior, or unworthy of love, especially if they feel responsible for the family dissolution. Although the social stigma attached to divorce no longer produces the emotions it did in the past, such feelings may still exist in small towns or in some cultural groups and can reinforce children's negative self-image. The lasting effects of divorce depend on the children's and the parents' adjustment to the transition from an intact family to a single-parent family and, often, to a reconstituted family.

Although most studies have concentrated on the negative effects of divorce on youngsters, some positive outcomes of divorce have been reported. A successful postdivorce family, either a single-parent or a reconstituted family, can improve the quality of life for both adults and children. If conflict is

BOX 31-4 Feelings and Behaviors of Children Related to Divorce

Infants
- Effects of reduced mothering or lack of mothering
- Increased irritability
- Disturbance in eating, sleeping, and elimination
- Interference with attachment process

Early Preschool Children (Ages 2 to 3 Years)
- Frightened and confused
- Blame themselves for the divorce
- Fear of abandonment
- Increased irritability, whining, tantrums
- Regressive behaviors (e.g., thumb sucking, loss of elimination control)
- Separation anxiety

Later Preschool Children (Ages 3 to 5 Years)
- Fear of abandonment
- Blame themselves for the divorce; decreased self-esteem
- Bewilderment regarding all human relationships
- Become more aggressive in relationships with others (e.g., siblings, peers)
- Engage in fantasy to seek understanding of the divorce

Early School-Age Children (Ages 5 to 6 Years)
- Depression and immature behavior
- Loss of appetite and sleep disorders
- May be able to verbalize some feelings and understand some divorce-related changes
- Increased anxiety and aggression
- Feelings of abandonment by departing parent

Middle School-Age Children (Ages 6 to 8 Years)
- Panic reactions
- Feelings of deprivation—loss of parent, attention, money, and secure future
- Profound sadness, depression, fear, and insecurity
- Feelings of abandonment and rejection
- Fear regarding the future
- Difficulty expressing anger at parents
- Intense desire for reconciliation of parents
- Impaired capacity to play and enjoy outside activities
- Decline in school performance
- Altered peer relationships—become bossy, irritable, demanding, and manipulative
- Frequent crying, loss of appetite, sleep disorders
- Disturbed routine, forgetfulness

Later School-Age Children (Ages 9 to 12 Years)
- More realistic understanding of divorce
- Intense anger directed at one or both parents
- Divided loyalties
- Ability to express feelings of anger
- Ashamed of parental behavior
- Desire for revenge; may wish to punish the parent they hold responsible
- Feelings of loneliness, rejection, and abandonment
- Altered peer relationships
- Decline in school performance
- May develop somatic complaints
- May engage in aberrant behavior such as lying, stealing
- Temper tantrums
- Dictatorial attitude

Adolescents (Ages 12 to 18 Years)
- Able to disengage themselves from parental conflict
- Feelings of a profound sense of loss—of family, childhood
- Feelings of anxiety
- Worry about themselves, parents, siblings
- Expression of anger, sadness, shame, embarrassment
- May withdraw from family and friends
- Disturbed concept of sexuality
- May engage in acting-out behaviors

resolved, a better relationship with one or both parents may result, and some children may have less contact with a disturbed parent. Greater stability in the home setting and the removal of arguing parents can be a positive outcome for the child's long term well-being.

Age- and Sex-Related Responses to Divorce

Previously, it was believed that divorce had a greater impact on younger children, but recent observations indicate that divorce constitutes a major disruption for children of all ages. The feelings and behaviors of children may be different for various ages and gender, but all children suffer stress second only to the stress produced by the death of a parent. Although considerable research has looked at sex differences in children's adjustments to divorce, the findings are not conclusive.

Telling the Children

Parents are understandably hesitant to tell children about their decision to divorce. Most parents neglect to discuss either the divorce or its inevitable changes with their preschool child. Without preparation, even children who remain in the family home are confused by the parental separation. Frequently, children are already experiencing vague, uneasy feelings that are more difficult to cope with than being told the truth about the situation. If possible, the initial disclosure should include both parents and siblings, followed by individual discussions with each child. Sufficient time should be set aside for these discussions, and they should take place during a period of calm, not after an argument. The discussions should include the reason for the divorce (if age appropriate) and reassurance that the divorce is not the children's fault.

Parents should not fear crying in front of the children because their crying gives the children permission to cry also. Children may feel guilt, a sense of failure, or that they are being punished for misbehavior. They normally feel anger and resentment and should be allowed to communicate these feelings without punishment. They need consistency and order in their lives. They want to know where they will live, who will take care of them, if they will be with their siblings, and if there will be enough money to live on. Children fear that if their parents stopped loving each other, they could stop loving them. Their need for love and reassurance is tremendous at this time. Children may also wonder what will happen on special days such as birthdays and holidays, whether both parents will come to school events, and whether the child will still have the same friends.

Custody and Parenting Partnerships

In the past, when parents separated, the mother was given custody of the children with visitation agreements for the father. Now both parents and the courts are seeking alternatives. Current belief is that neither fathers nor mothers should be awarded custody automatically. Custody should be awarded to the parent who is best able to provide for the children's welfare. In some cases, children experience severe stress when living or spending time with a parent.

Two other types of custody arrangements are divided custody and joint custody. *Divided*, or *split*, *custody* means that each parent is awarded custody of one or more of the children, thereby separating siblings. For example, sons might live with the father and daughters with the mother.

Joint custody takes one of two forms. In *joint physical custody*, the parents alternate the physical care and control of the children on an equitable basis while maintaining shared parenting responsibilities legally. This custody arrangement works well for families who live close to each other and whose occupations permit an active role in the care and rearing of the children. In *joint legal custody*, the children reside with one parent but both parents are the children's legal guardians, and both participate in childrearing.

Co-parenting offers substantial benefits for the family: children can be close to both parents, and life with each parent can be more normal (as opposed to having a disciplinarian mother and a recreational father). To be successful, parents in these arrangements must place high value on the commitment to provide normal parenting and to separate their marital conflicts from their parenting roles. No matter what type of custody arrangement is awarded, the primary consideration is the welfare of the children.

Single Parenting

An individual may acquire single-parent status as a result of divorce, separation, death of a spouse, or birth or adoption of a child. Although divorce rates have stabilized, the number of single-parent households continues to rise. In 2005, 32% of children younger than 18 years of age lived in single-parent families, and the majority of single parents are women (US Census Bureau, 2003; Annie E Casey Foundation, 2007). It is estimated that at least half of the children born during the 1990s will spend part of their life in a family headed by a divorced, separated, widowed, or never-married mother. Although some women are single parents by choice, most of these women never planned on being single parents, and many feel pressure to marry or remarry.

Managing shortages of money, time, and energy is a major concern for single parents. Studies repeatedly confirm the financial difficulties of single-parent families, particularly single mothers. In 2004 only one third of mother-headed households received any child support or alimony (Annie E Casey Foundation, 2007). The stigma of poverty may be more keenly felt than the discrimination associated with being a single parent. These families are often forced by their financial status to live in communities with inadequate housing and personal safety concerns. Single parents often feel guilty about the time spent away from their children.

Being a teenage parent adds to the financial burden of being a single parent and can have long-term consequences for the mother and child. Poverty is a well-known predictor of adverse effects on a child's health and well-being. Approximately 78% of children born to a teenage mother who did not marry or graduate high school live in poverty. In contrast, only 9% of children born to women over 20 who marry and finish high school live in poverty (Annie E Casey Foundation, 2007).

Single Fathers

Fathers who have custody of their children have many of the same problems as divorced mothers. They feel overburdened by the responsibility, depressed, and concerned about their ability to cope with the emotional needs of the children, especially girls. Some fathers lack home-making skills. They find it difficult at first to coordinate household tasks, school visits, and other activities associated with managing a household alone. Fathers often demand more assistance with household tasks and more independence from their children than custodial mothers do, and they are likely to make use of alternative caregiving and support systems.

Parenting in Reconstituted Families

In the United States, many of the children living in homes where parents have divorced will experience another major change in their lives such as the addition of a stepparent or new siblings. The entry of a stepparent into an existing family requires adjustments for all family members. Some obstacles to the role adjustments and family problem solving include disruption of previous lifestyles and interaction patterns, complexity in the formation of new ones, and lack of social supports. Despite these problems, most children from divorced families want to live in a two-parent home.

Cooperative parenting relationships can allow more time for each set of parents to be alone to establish their own relationship with the children. Under ideal circumstances, power conflicts between the two households can be reduced, and tension and anxiety can be lessened for all family members. In addition, the children's self-esteem can be increased, and there is a greater likelihood of continued contact with grandparents. Flexibility, mutual support, and open communication are critical in successful relationships in stepfamilies and stepparenting situations. Unfortunately, stepfamilies usually do not seek help to prevent problems. Typically, information and counseling are sought only when problems have surfaced and can no longer be ignored. A preventive rather than remedial approach is needed.

Parenting in Dual-Earner Families

No change in family lifestyle has had more impact than the large numbers of women entering the workplace. As women moved away from the traditional homemaker role, the numbers of dual-earner families increased dramatically. This trend is unlikely to diminish significantly. As a result, the family is subjected to considerable stress as members attempt to meet the often competing demands of occupational needs and those regarded as necessary for a rich family life.

Role definitions are frequently altered to arrange an equitable division of time and labor, as well as to resolve conflict, especially conflict related to the traditional norms of the culture. Overload is a common source of stress in a dual-earner family, and social activities are significantly curtailed. Time demands and scheduling are major problems for all individuals who work. When the individuals are parents, the demands can be even more intense. Dual-earner couples may increase the strain on themselves to avoid creating stress for their children. Although there is no evidence to indicate that the dual-earner lifestyle is stressful to children, the stress experienced by the parents may affect the children indirectly.

Working Mothers

Working mothers have become the norm in the United States. Child care is critical to the working mother's sense of well-being. The quality of child care is a persistent concern for all working parents (see Evidence-Based Practice box). Determinants of child care quality are based on health and safety requirements, responsive and warm interaction between staff and children, developmentally appropriate activities, trained staff, limited group size, age-appropriate caregivers, adequate staff-to-child ratios, and adequate indoor and outdoor space. Nurses play an important role in helping families to find suitable sources of child care and to prepare children for this experience.

Foster Parenting

The term *foster care* is defined as placement in an approved living situation away from the family of origin. The living situation may be an approved foster home, possibly with other children, or a preadoptive home. Each state provides a standard for the role of foster parent and a process by which to become one. Most states require about 27 hours of training before being on contract and at least 12 hours of continuing education a year. Each state has guidelines regarding the relative health of the prospective foster parents and their families, background checks regarding legal issues for the adults, personal interviews, and a safety inspection of the residence and surroundings.

Nurses should be aware that nearly 700,000 children will spend time living in foster care in a given year, many of them facing developmental concerns (Annie E Casey Foundation, 2007; American Academy of Pediatrics, Committee on Early Childhood, Adoption, and Dependent Care, 2000). Children in foster care tend to have a higher than normal incidence of acute and chronic health problems and may experience feelings of isolation or confusion (Annie E Casey Foundation, 2007). Nurses should strive to implement strategies that will improve the health care for this group of children.

Accommodating Contemporary Parenting Situations

During recent years, both the private and government sectors have identified specific problems of contemporary families. Many of these issues involve working parents. One significant stressor for the working single parent or for dual-earner families is when a child becomes ill. The frequency of childhood illness, exclusion practices of most licensed child care programs, and employer's limited sick-leave policies are other contributing factors. Some employers have become more family focused and provide time off for parents to be with sick children. Flexible work schedules and family-oriented legislation can ease the burden of managing family and work responsibilities. The Family Medical Leave Act allows eligible employees to take up to 12 weeks of unpaid leave each year to care for newborn or newly adopted children, parents, or spouses who have serious health conditions, or to recover from their own serious health condition.

EVIDENCE-BASED PRACTICE Day Care for Preschool Children

Ask the Question

Does day care have an effect on preschool education, health, and welfare?

Search for Evidence

Search Strategies

Randomized controlled trials of day care for preschool children identified using electronic databases, hand searches of relevant literature, and contact with authors

Databases Searched

MEDLINE, EMBASE, Cochrane Controlled Trials Register, Social Science Citation Index, PsycLIT, Eric, and BIRD (French)

Critically Analyze the Evidence

Seven randomized control trials and one quasi-randomized study were identified after examining 920 abstracts and 19 books (Zortich, Roberts, & Oakley, 2000). In these eight studies, all conducted in the United States, a total of 2203 children were randomized to day care or a control group. All subjects were less than 4 years old at enrollment. Day care ranged from 2 hours a week for 8 months to 7 hours a day, 5 days a week for 7 years. All studies examined cognitive development, six studies examined school performance, four studies evaluated behavior, and one study assessed children's health.

- Brooks-Gunn et al (1994)—Two-year follow-up study of 985 preterm subjects of varying socioeconomic background. *Outcomes:* Developmental quotient and intelligence quotient (IQ), behavior, health status, health care usage, weight gain, maternal employment, public assistance, health insurance, and mother-child interactions.
- Campbell, Breitmayer, and Ramey (1994)—Follow-up study over 12 to 15 years of 111 children of disadvantaged families, age 6 weeks at enrollment. *Outcomes:* IQ, school achievement, mother-child interaction, maternal employment and education, child's psychologic well-being.
- Deutsch (1966)—Thirteen-year follow up of 504 children from disadvantaged families, 4 years old at enrollment. High attrition led to unbalanced groups. *Outcomes:* School competence, developed abilities, child's attitude, and impact on family.
- Garber (1988)—Quasi-randomized study, with 7-year follow up, of 40 children from disadvantaged background and low maternal IQ; age at enrollment 3 years. *Outcomes:* Developmental quotient, IQ, school achievement.
- Gray and Klaus (1970)—Twelve-year study of 65 subjects from varying social backgrounds, 3 years old at enrollment. *Outcomes:* IQ, achievement and language, follow up of school competence, developed abilities, child's attitude, and impact on family.
- Palmer and Siegel (1977)—Nine-year follow-up study of 310 subjects of mixed socioeconomic status, boys only, 2 years old at enrollment. *Outcomes:* IQ, language, developmental outcomes, school competence, developed abilities, child's attitude, and impact on family.
- Schweinhart, Barnes, and Wiekart (1993)—Twenty-four-year follow up of 128 disadvantaged children, 3 years old at enrollment. *Outcomes:* IQ, special education placement, grade retention, social development, parental satisfaction, delinquent behavior, employment, self-confidence, relationship with parents.
- Wasik et al (1990)—Six-month follow up of 65 children from disadvantaged families, 6 weeks old at enrollment. *Outcomes:* Developmental index, IQ, home environment, childrearing attitudes; home-based group performed worse than control.

Apply the Evidence: Nursing Implications

Studies revealed out-of-home day care has beneficial effects for children, enhancing cognitive development and preventing later school failures.

Observational studies have reported that day care can negatively affect child development. The studies reviewed show that preschool education has a beneficial effect on a child's behavior.

Center-based day care increases maternal employment and education, which could lead to improved socioeconomic status.

Mother-child interaction can be improved by day care, with studies showing improved communication between mother and child when compared with children who receive no day care.

Evidence suggests that out-of-home day care can have a positive effect on social outcomes for children and their families.

References

Brooks-Gunn J et al: Early intervention in low-birth-weight premature infants: results through age 5 years from the Infant Health and Development Program, *JAMA* 272(16):1257-1262, 1994.

Campbell FA, Breitmayer B, Ramey CT: Effects of early intervention on intellectual and academic achievement: a follow-up study of children from low-income families, *Child Devel* 65:684-698, 1994.

Deutsch M: Facilitating development in pre-school child: social and psychological perspectives. In Hechinger FM (editor): *Pre-school education today*, vol 73-97, Garden City, NJ, 1966, Doubleday.

Garber HL: *The Milwaukee project: preventing mental retardation in children at risk*, Washington, DC, 1988, American Association on Mental Retardation.

Gray SW, Klaus RA: The early training project: a seventh year report, *Child Devel* 41:909-924, 1970.

Palmer FH, Siegel RJ: Minimal intervention at ages 2 and 3 and subsequent intellectual changes. In Day MC, Parker RK (editors): *The pre-school in action: exploring early childhood programs*, ed 2, Boston, 1977, Allyn & Bacon.

Schweinhart LJ, Barnes HV, Wiekart DP: *Significant benefits: the High/Scope Perry Preschool Study through age 27*, Ypsilanti, MI, 1993, High/Scope Press.

Wasik BH et al: A longitudinal study of two early intervention strategies: Project CARE, *Child Devel* 61:1682-1696, 1990.

Zortich B, Roberts I, Oakley A: Day care for pre-school children, *Cochrane Database Syst Rev* (2):CD000564, 2000. In *The Cochrane Library*, Issue 3, 2005.

Key Points

- Because there is no agreement about the definition of family, a family is what an individual considers it to be.
- Three theories that have significant relevance and application to pediatric nursing are family systems theory, family stress theory, and developmental theory.
- Although the traditional family structure was nuclear or extended, in recent years other forms, such as the single-parent family, have emerged.
- Family size and position within the family structure have a strong impact on a child's development.
- Interpersonal skills and a basic understanding of childhood growth and development are two essential areas of focus for parents.
- Parental control tends to be predominantly one of three types: authoritarian, permissive, or authoritative.
- Three areas of special concern to adoptive families include the initial attachment process, the task of telling the children they are adopted, and identity formation during adolescence.
- Marital factors within the home significantly influence a child's development. The impact of divorce on a child depends on the child's age, the outcome, and the quality of the parent-child relationship and parental care following the divorce.
- Single parenting and stepparenting create adjustment difficulties and add stress to the already demanding parental role. Significant numbers of children will live in a single-parent or reconstituted family at some point.

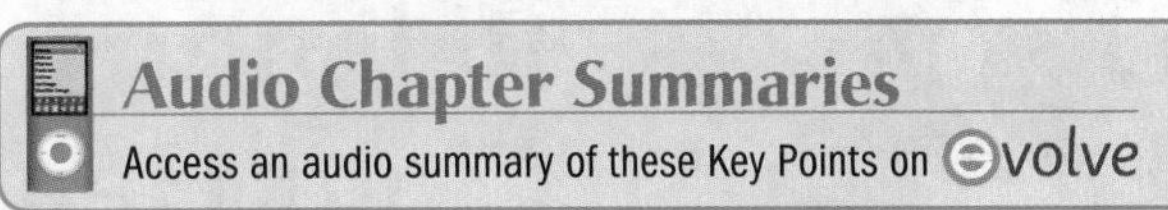
Audio Chapter Summaries
Access an audio summary of these Key Points on evolve

References

American Academy of Pediatrics, Committee on Early Childhood, Adoption, and Dependent Care: Development issues for young children in foster care (RE0012), *Pediatrics* 106(5):1145-1150, 2000.

Annie E Casey Foundation: *2007 Kids count data book: state profiles of child well-being*, Baltimore, 2007, The Foundation.

Brazelton TB: Working with families: opportunities for early intervention, *Pediatr Clin North Am* 42(1):1-10, 1995.

Friedman MM, Bowden VR, Jones EG: *Family nursing: research theory and practice*, ed 5, Upper Saddle River, NJ, 2003, Prentice Hall.

Hamilton BE et al: Annual summary of vital statistics: 2005, *Pediatrics* 119(2):345-360, 2007.

Lerner RM, Sparks EE, McCubbin LD: *Family diversity and family policy: strengthening families for America's children*, Boston, 1999, Kluwer.

McCubbin MA, McCubbin HI: Families coping with illness: the resiliency model of family stress, adjustment, and adaptation. In Danielson CB, Bissel BH, Winstead-Fry P (editors): *Families, health, and illness*, St Louis, 1994, Mosby.

Munson ML, Sutton PD: Births, marriages, divorces, and deaths: provisional data for 2005, *Natl Vital Stat Rep* 54(20):1-7, 2006.

US Census Bureau: *Two married parents the norm*, Washington DC, 2003, Department of Commerce News. Available at www.census.gov/Press-Release/www/2003/cb03-97.html (accessed January 8, 2008).

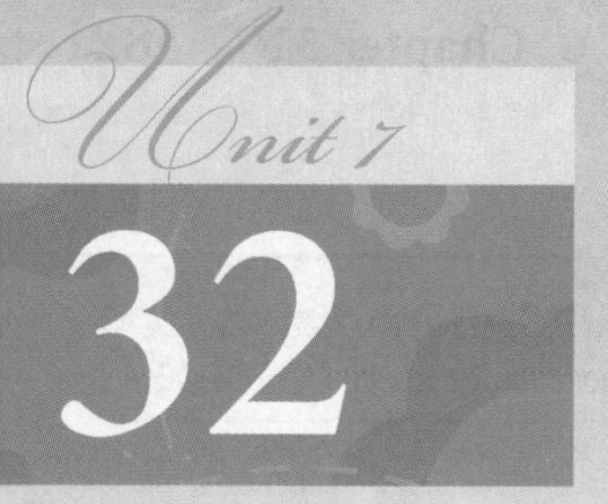

Unit 7

32

Social, Cultural, and Religious Influences on Child Health Promotion

Learning Objectives

On completion of this chapter the reader will be able to:

- Define culture, cultural competence, ethnocentrism, and cultural relativism.
- Describe the subcultural influences on child development in the areas of socioeconomic class, poverty, religion, and schools.
- Discuss the population shifts in number of minority children in the United States.
- Identify four common diseases or disorders that affect certain ethnic or cultural groups.
- Identify areas of potential conflict of values and customs for a nurse interacting with a family from a different cultural or ethnic group.
- Describe three religious groups whose beliefs significantly affect their health practices.

Electronic Resources

Additional information related to the content in Chapter 32 can be found on

evolve the Companion Website at http://evolve.elsevier.com/Perry/maternal/

- NCLEX Review Questions
- Case Study—Cultural Considerations
- Skill—Providing Culturally Sensitive Care

Culture

The future of any society depends on its children; therefore society must provide for their care, nurturing, and socialization. Culture plays a critical role in the parenting behaviors that facilitate children's development (Meléndez, 2005). The culture's customs and values help to organize a society's childrearing system and are transmitted from one generation to the next through the medium of the family. A holistic view of any child requires that nurses develop some understanding of the ways that culture contributes to the development of social and emotional relationships and influences childrearing practices and attitudes toward health.

As the ethnic, racial, and cultural diversity in the U.S. population increases, is it imperative that nurses become competent in transcultural nursing knowledge (Muñoz & Luckmann, 2005). This orientation to transcultural nursing includes an awareness of the nurse's own culture. The nurse who is becoming culturally competent learns about other cultures, becomes able to assess the perspectives of others, and shares his or her own culture with others (Dunn, 2002).

Culture is a pattern of learned beliefs, values, and practices that are shared within a group; it includes practices; customs; views on roles and relationships, including parenting; and communication patterns and language (Betancourt, 2004). Culture differs from both race and ethnicity. *Race* is defined as a division of humans possessing traits that are transmissible by descent and that are sufficient to characterize it as a distinct human type. One classification of race, based on skin color, is Caucasian (white), Negroid (African-American), and Mongoloid (yellow). *Ethnicity* is the affiliation of a set of persons who share a unique cultural, social, and linguistic heritage (Fig. 32-1). *Socialization* is the process by which society imparts its competencies, values, and expectations to children (Trawick-Smith, 2006).

Culture is a complex whole in which each part is interrelated. It provides the lens through which all facets of human behavior can be interpreted (Spector, 2004). Culture is not a surface veneer that covers a basic outlook shared by all human beings; rather, it is an ingrained orientation to life that serves as a frame of reference for individual perception and judgment. People from one culture differ from those in other cultures in the ways they think, solve problems, and perceive and structure the world. Culture is, essentially, the way of life of a group of people that incorporates experiences of the past, influences thought and action in the present, and transmits these traditions to future group members. Adaptation is necessary, however, for the culture to survive in an ever-changing world. Consciously and unconsciously, the members abandon, modify, or assume new patterns to meet the group's needs.

The cultural setting in which children are raised can influence many aspects of their life, from the food they eat to the way they behave in a social setting. To be acceptable members of the culture, children must learn how the culture expects them to behave toward others in the group. In turn, they learn how they can expect others to behave toward them.

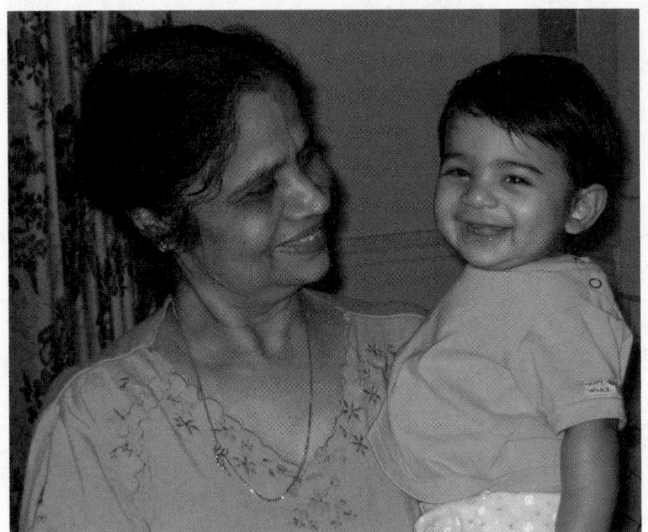

Fig. 32-1 Ethnicity is an individual's association with shared cultural, social, and linguistic heritage.

Cultures and subcultures contribute to the uniqueness of child members in such a subtle way and at such an early age that children grow up to think that their beliefs, attitudes, values, and practices are the "correct" or "normal" ones. By age 5, children can identify persons who belong to their own race or cultural background. During later primary years, children are able to identify people from different cultures (Trawick-Smith, 2006). A set of values learned in childhood is likely to characterize children's attitudes and behavior for life, guiding their long-range strivings and informing their short-range, impulsive inclinations. Thus every ongoing society socializes each succeeding generation to its cultural heritage.

The manner and sequence of the growth and development phenomenon are universal and fundamental features of all children; however, the variations in behavioral responses that children display to similar events are believed to be determined by their culture. Children acquire the skills, knowledge, beliefs, and values important to their own family and culture. The pace of acquisition of cognitive and motor skills can differ by cultural background as well as the child's social and emotional development (Trawick-Smith, 2006).

Cultures may also differ in whether status in the group is based on age or on skill. Even children's play and their types of games are culturally determined. In some cultures children play in groups composed of members of the same sex; in others, they play in mixed-sex groups. In some cultures team games predominate; in others, most play is limited to individual games.

Standards and norms vary from culture to culture and from location to location; a practice that is accepted in one area may meet with disapproval or create tension in another. The extent to which cultures tolerate divergence from the established norm also varies among cultures and subcultural groups. Although conformity provides a degree of security, it is often a deterrent to change.

Social Roles

Much of children's self-concept is derived from their ideas about their social roles. Roles are cultural creations; therefore the culture prescribes patterns of behavior for persons in a variety of social positions. All persons who hold similar social positions have an obligation to behave in a particular manner. A role prohibits some behaviors and allows others. Because it delineates and clarifies roles, the culture is a significant influence on the development of children's self-concept (i.e., attitudes and beliefs they have about themselves).

A social group consists of a system of roles carried out in both primary and secondary groups. A *primary group* is characterized by intimate, continued, face-to-face contact; mutual support of members; and the ability to order or constrain a considerable proportion of individual members' behavior. Two such groups are the family and the peer group, both of which exert a great deal of influence on the child.

Secondary groups are groups that have limited, intermittent contact and in which there is generally less concern for members' behavior. These groups offer little in terms of support or pressure toward conformity except in rigidly limited areas. Examples of secondary groups are professional associations and church organizations (also considered in relation to subgroups). The childrearing orientation in a secondary group environment, such as urban communities, differs considerably from that of a primary group community. An urban community is dynamic and rapidly changing; therefore many of the traditional behaviors and values do not meet its needs. Consequently, parents are often uncertain about what to teach their children. They may wish to rear their children with values consistent with their own, but the differences in experience between the generations are too great. As a result, they often grant their children autonomy in some areas of decision making early in the developmental process, and other secondary groups assume a greater influence. The children are exposed to an assortment of social groups with diverse sets of values and expectations. None of the groups is highly dominant in its influence; therefore the children are exposed to an eclectic set of values, some in agreement and some in conflict with the others. From these they must ultimately select those that they determine to be best for them and adopt them to form a consistent set of roles and behaviors to be incorporated into the self-concept.

Self-Esteem and Culture

A child's sense of self-esteem is influenced by his or her culture (Trawick-Smith, 2006). Some cultures are more collective in thought and action. A child from a collective culture will hold an inclusive view of self. Self-evaluation is related to the accomplishments or competencies of the entire family or community. School experiences that focus on personal achievement may promote positive self-esteem in some children but not in others, who are more dependent on the success of a whole family or peer group. A child's sense of control may not come from individual self-reliance but rather from a feeling of worth in his or her family or community (Trawick-Smith, 2006).

Families and culture also influence the criteria children use to evaluate their own abilities. Additionally, cultures vary in whether they instill an internal locus of control (a belief in the ability to regulate one's own life). Effects on self-esteem are minimal if these beliefs are directed by parents and are in accordance with cultural customs (Trawick-Smith, 2006). What is damaging to emotional health is helplessness that stems from prejudice. Ethnic pride is a factor that has helped maintain positive self-image and protect against the damage that prejudice can cause (Trawick-Smith, 2006).

Subcultural Influences

Except in rare situations, children grow and develop in a blend of cultures and subcultures. In a large, complex society such as that of the United States, different groups have their own set of standards, values, and expectations within the collective ways of the large culture. Although many cultural differences are related to geographic boundaries, subcultures are not always restricted by location.

Children's membership in a cultural subgroup is, for the most part, involuntary. They are born into a family with a specific ethnic or racial heritage, socioeconomic level, and religious beliefs. Although in the complex North American society there are countless subcultures and considerable variations in the way of life, those subcultures that seem to exert the greatest influence on childrearing are ethnicity, social class, and occupational role. In addition, schools and peer-group subcultures are strong influences in the socialization of the child.

evolve Case Study—Cultural Considerations

Ethnicity

Ethnicity is the classification of or affiliation with any of the basic groups or divisions of humans or any heterogeneous population differentiated by customs, characteristics, language, or similar distinguishing factors. Ethnic differences extend to many areas and include such manifestations as family structure, language, food preferences, moral codes, and expression of emotion. Some standards of behavior result from the cultural heritage of the specific ethnic group. The term *ethnic* has aroused strong negative feelings and is often rejected by the general population (Spector, 2004).

To establish their place in the group, children learn how to adhere to a mode of behavior that is in accordance with standards distinctive to the group and learn how they can expect others to behave toward them. They take their cues by observing and imitating those to whom they are exposed. For example, children of a racial minority form a perception of their role as a group member by observing the manner in which role models within the subgroup respond to treatment by people outside the subgroup. When they see group members display an attitude of inferiority, they assume this to be the appropriate behavior and incorporate these perceptions into their own self-concept.

In the United States the cross-cultural lines are becoming blurred as subcultures are assimilated and blend into the larger culture (Fig. 32-2). It is particularly difficult for persons to attempt to maintain an identity with a subculture while living and conforming to the requirements of the dominant culture. Universal customs and language used in commercial and educational systems are different from those of the minority culture. Consequently, children reared in this environment are confused about roles and values, and they usually adopt those of the more influential or higher status culture. Youths, in particular, are influenced by the locally dominant group.

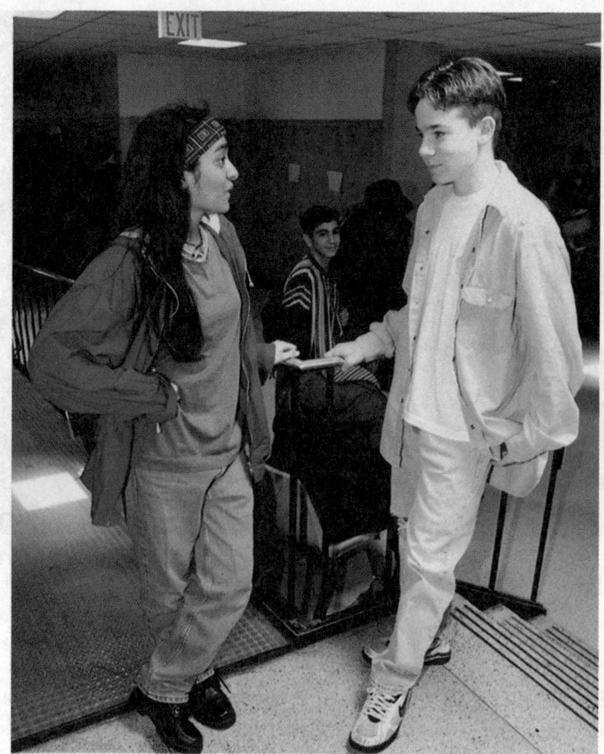

Fig. 32-2 Teenagers from different cultural backgrounds interact within the larger culture.

Ethnocentrism is the concept that one's own culture proves the right and natural way to do things while all other ways are unnatural and inferior (Galanti, 2004). *Ethnic stereotyping* or labeling stems from ethnocentric views of people. Ethnocentrism implies that all other groups are inferior and that their ways are not in the best interests of the group. It is a common attitude among a dominant ethnic group and strongly influences the ability of one person to objectively evaluate the beliefs and behaviors of others. This inherent viewpoint of individuals tends to bias their interpretation and understanding of the behavior of others. The culturally competent nurse should be empathetic and aware of his or her own views and that they may differ from another's based on culture or ethnicity. The nurse should be willing to ask questions that will provide a better understanding of patient or family views when appropriate.

Socioeconomic Class

It is important to recognize that family relationships may be stronger among some ethnic or cultural groups than others. However, the influence of socioeconomic class cannot be overlooked. Socioeconomic class relates to the family's economic and education levels. Strong family relationships exist among those of lower socioeconomic class who have few resources and must rely on the support of a family network to meet physical and emotional needs. Middle- and upper-class people often have resources that reach beyond the extended family. They are able to access physical and emotional support in the community (Giger & Davidhizar, 2008).

The term *socioeconomic class* should not be confused with cultural or ethnic diversity. Children of a specific race are not necessarily of low socioeconomic status. Additionally, children of poverty do not automatically have developmental delays (Trawick-Smith, 2006).

Poverty

A subcultural influence closely related to, but different from, social class is the condition known as poverty. It is a relative concept and is usually associated with the general standards of a population. The term *poverty* implies both visible and invisible impoverishment. It is a condition in which families live without adequate resources (Trawick-Smith, 2006). *Visible poverty* refers to lack of money or material resources, which includes insufficient clothing, poor sanitation, and deteriorating housing. *Invisible poverty* refers to social and cultural deprivation, such as limited employment opportunities, inferior educational opportunities, lack of or inferior medical services and health care facilities, and an absence of public services.

An *absolute standard* of poverty attempts to delimit some basic set of resources needed for adequate existence. *Relative poverty* reflects the median income and median standard of living in a society or country and is the term used in referring to childhood poverty in the United States (Scruggs & Allan, 2006); that is, what appears to be substandard living conditions in one area may be a standard or norm in another.

The number of children living in poverty has continued to increase during the twenty-first century. The child poverty rate in the United States is among the highest in the developed world (American Academy of Pediatrics, Committee on Community Health Services, 2005). In 2006, 18% of children were living in poverty, a 6% increase since the year 2000. In 2005, nearly 29 million U.S. children lived in low-income families. *Low income* is defined as having a family income (for a family of four) that is less than twice the federal poverty threshold with at least one parent working 50 or more weeks during the year. The majority of these children, or nearly 15 million, had at least one parent who worked regularly but were living on the economic edge and struggling to make ends meet (Annie E Casey Foundation, 2006). Poverty is a strong predictor of a child health and is closely associated with poorer physical, developmental, and mental health outcomes (American Academy of Pediatrics, Committee on Community Health Services, 2005).

Homelessness

One of the most pressing problems in the United States is the growing number of homeless families. Homeless individuals are those who lack resources and community ties necessary to provide for their own adequate shelter. Homeless children have increased in numbers as poverty has become feminized, minorities have become poorer, and low-income housing has become less accessible. Estimates of the number of homeless children in the United States are at 1.6 million children each year, with the number growing (American Academy of Pediatrics, Committee on Community Health Services, 2005). The majority of children are younger than 5 years of age and predominantly from minority groups.

Most homelessness is a direct result of increasing numbers of people in poverty combined with a lack of decent, affordable housing. Government housing subsidies have decreased, whereas the number of working poor has increased (Tropello, 2000). Other reasons include job layoffs, low income, parental mental illness, domestic conflict, and unexpected family or economic crises. Many families move into homelessness gradually after family members and friends are no longer willing to provide housing. Another group of homeless children are the "runaway" and "throwaway" adolescents. Many runaways are victims of physical and sexual abuse and leave home because of long-term family or school problems.

Migrant Farmworker Families

One of the most disadvantaged groups is migrant farm workers and their children. Indications suggest that in the United States there are between 3 million and 5 million migrant and seasonal workers and their dependents, whose average yearly income is well below the poverty level. In addition, most of these families have no health insurance.

The low position of these families on the economic scale and their rootless, mobile existence subject them to inadequate sanitation, substandard housing, social isolation, and lack of educational and medical facilities (American Academy of Pediatrics, Committee on Community Health Services, 2005). This lifestyle is especially deleterious to the children. Schooling and health care are inadequate. Children are likely to live in a number of localities and attend a variety of schools over the course of a year, with no continuity in either education or health care. Because both parents work in the fields, children receive little adult supervision; therefore injury rates are high and meals are erratic.

Immigrant Children

The 2000 U.S. Census informed us that a growing number of immigrants currently are living in the United States (US Census Bureau, 2001). In 2005 it is estimated that 21% of children (15.7 million) lived in immigrant families; the children were either born outside the United States or had at least one foreign-born parent (Annie E Casey Foundation, 2007). These children and families face unique stressors, including depression, grief, and anxiety related to migration and acculturation; separation from extended family and supports; language barriers; disparities in socioeconomic status compared with their country of origin; and possibly traumatic events that necessitated their immigration (American Academy of Pediatrics, 2005). Current laws restrict health benefits under government programs for immigrants who lawfully entered the United States after 1996; they must wait for 5 years to become eligible for comprehensive health benefits (American Academy of Pediatrics, 2005). Immigrant issues continue to require the attention of policymakers and child advocates.

Religion

An influential factor shaping the culture of the United States is the Judeo-Christian faith. Many immigrants came to the United States for religious freedom and established a religious and moral atmosphere that persists today. However, individual differences are part of the general culture.

The family's religious orientation dictates a code of morality and influences the family's attitudes toward education,

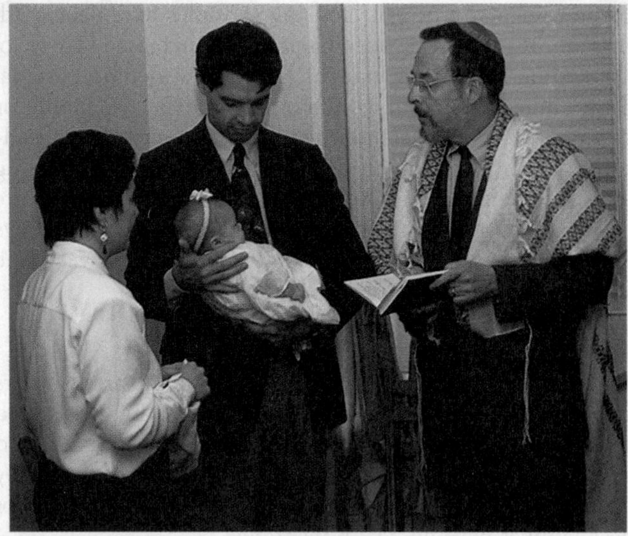

Fig. 32-3 Soon after an infant is born, many families have special religious ceremonies.

male and female role identity, and beliefs regarding their ultimate destiny (Fig. 32-3). Religion may also be a factor in determining the school the children attend, the companions with whom they associate, and often their mate selection. In a few instances, such as in the Mennonite and Amish communities, religion is the basis for a common way of life that determines where children are reared and their lifestyle (see also Religious Beliefs, p. 835).

Schools

Next to the family, schools exert the major force in providing continuity between generations by conveying a vast amount of culture from the older members to the young. In this way children are prepared to carry out the traditional social roles they are expected to assume as adults in society. School rules and regulations regarding attendance, authority relationships, and the system of sanctions and rewards based on achievement transmit to the child the behavioral expectations of the adult world of employment and relationships. School is often the only institution in which children systematically learn about the negative consequences of behaviors that deviate from social expectations. Teachers are expected to stimulate and guide the intellectual development of children and their sense of aesthetics and to foster their capacity for creative problem solving. Through education, individuals in the lower classes are offered the opportunity and the capacity to move up in the social strata.

Traditionally, the socialization process of school began when the child entered kindergarten or first grade. Today, with more than 65% of mothers of preschool children working outside the home, this socialization process begins much earlier for a significant number of children in a variety of child care settings (Annie E Casey Foundation, 2006).

Children of some cultural groups fare less well in school. They come from underrepresented groups, including African-American, Mexican-American, Puerto Rican, and Native American children (Trawick-Smith, 2006). These cultural variations can be attributed to high rates of poverty, different cognitive styles, ineffective schools, and parents' views of schools as oppressive to cultural and traditional values (Trawick-Smith, 2006).

Communities

Surveys of more than 1 million young persons in the United States in grades 6 through 12 have shown that those who experience a higher number of specific assets in their lives are more likely to make healthy choices and avoid high risk behaviors. These assets offer a framework for positive child and adolescent development. The child's or adolescent's community is made up of the family, school, neighborhood, youth organization, and other members. They all contribute to the young person's experience within any culture (Search-Institute, 2008).

Four categories of external assets that youth receive from the community include (Search-Institute, 2008):

1. **Support**—Young people need to feel support, care, and love from their families, neighbors, and others. They also need organizations and institutions that offer positive, supportive environments.
2. **Empowerment**—Young people need to feel valued by their community and be able to contribute to others. They need to feel safe and secure.
3. **Boundaries and expectations**—Young people need to know what is expected of them and what actions and behaviors are within the community boundaries and what are outside of them.
4. **Constructive use of time**—Young people need opportunities for growth through constructive, enriching opportunities and quality time at home.

Internal assets must also be nurtured in the community's young members. These internal qualities guide choices and create a sense of centeredness, purpose, and focus. The four categories of internal assets are (Search-Institute, 2008):

1. **Commitment to learning**—Young people need to develop a commitment to education and life-long learning.
2. **Positive values**—Youth need to have a strong sense of values that direct their choices.
3. **Social competencies**—Young people need competencies that help them make positive choices and build relationships.
4. **Positive identity**—Young people need a sense of their own power, purpose, worth, and promise.

Peer Cultures

Peer groups also have an impact on the socialization of children. Peer relationships become increasingly important and influential as children proceed through school. Children have what can be regarded as a culture of their own, which is most apparent in the school and in the unsupervised play group. The play group presents this culture in a much purer form than does the school, in which culture is partly produced by adults.

During their lives children are exposed to value systems such as those of the family, ethnic group, and social class. In peer-group interaction they are confronted with a variety of these sets of values. The values imposed by the peer group are especially compelling because children must accept and conform to them to be accepted as members of the group. When peer values are not too different from those of family and teachers, the mild conflict created by these small differences serves to separate children from the adults in their lives and to strengthen the feeling of belonging to the peer group. The relationships in a peer group change over time, and leadership may shift (Trawick-Smith, 2006).

The kind of socialization provided by the peer group depends on the special subculture that develops from the background, interests, and capabilities of its members. Some groups support school achievement, others focus on athletic prowess, and still others are decidedly antithetic to educative goals. Scholastic achievement is strongly related to the value system of the peer groups. Many conflicts between teachers and students and between parents and students can be attributed to fear of rejection by peers. A conflict between what is expected from parents regarding academic achievement and what is expected from the peer culture is especially pronounced in high school.

Although it has neither the traditional authority of the parents nor the legal authority of the schools for teaching information, the peer group manages to convey a substantial amount of information to its members. Peer relationships also provide an important social context for the development of body image among adolescent girls and boys. Although other subcultural forces such as the family and media influence the development of body image, adolescents' perception of what is a desirable appearance is created by norms and expectations that are modeled and reinforced within the peer group (Jones & Crawford, 2006). It is through peer relationships that children learn ways to deal with dominance and hostility and to relate with persons in positions of leadership and authority. The peer subculture relieves boredom and provides recognition that individual members do not receive from teachers and other authority figures.

The Child and Family in North America

The frontier background of the North American culture has contributed to the overall orientation to life and childrearing. There has always been a basic optimistic view of the world, a belief that things can be better and that the children can and will be better off than the parents. This hopeful outlook and a general future orientation, together with the possibility of upward social mobility, have created a pervasive attitude of optimism. Increasing development of self-confidence and autonomy in children is fostered and encouraged. Children in North America are generally permitted a greater degree of freedom than in more tradition-oriented cultures, where individuals remain in one class for life.

Family life in North America is characterized by increasing geographic and economic mobility. There is less reliance on tradition, families are fragmented, and there is limited opportunity to transmit and acquire the traditional and accepted customs of a culture. Consequently, young adults rely to a greater extent on professed experts, peers, and mass media for acquisition of acceptable patterns of behavior, including childrearing practices. Conflicting information can be a source of confusion and frustration as parents attempt to determine the comparatively stable, essential components of the culture and transmit these to their children.

Children in North America grow up with a number of adults who differ from one another but who all provide input as role models, teachers, and standards for behavior. Most children live in some form of nuclear family located in sharply differentiated neighborhoods determined by income and ethnic status within a highly technical, largely urban society. Class differences in childrearing persist, but they are becoming less divergent as a result of the increased homogeneity of the culture.

Minority-Group Membership

The United States has more racial, ethnic, and religious minority groups than any other country as a result of high immigration rates and high birth rates among these groups. Ethnic minority groups are becoming increasingly important because it is anticipated that these groups will produce children at a faster rate than will the majority Caucasian population. Consequently, the minority population is increasing, whereas the majority Caucasian population is decreasing in proportion to the whole. When people from different cultures interact, this is termed *cultural diversity* (Purnell & Paulanka, 2003).

The 2000 U.S. Census found that more than 280 million people live in the United States, with 6.8 million reporting more than two races. African-Americans alone or in combination with another race number more than 35 million, and Hispanics or Latinos of any race make up more than 35 million. The Hispanic population increased 58%, or 13 million people, from 1990 to 2000 (US Census Bureau, 2001) (see Cultural Awareness box).

CULTURAL AWARENESS

Overview of Race and Hispanic Origin in Census 2000

The federal government defines race and Hispanic origin as two separate and distinct concepts. In the 2000 U.S. Census, responders were first asked if they are of Spanish/Hispanic/Latino origin. The second question asked respondents to report the race or races they considered themselves to be. The definitions of racial groups included the following (US Census Bureau, 2001):

- **Caucasians** are people having "origins in any of the original peoples of Europe, the Middle East, or North Africa."
- **African-Americans**, sometimes referred to as **blacks**, are defined as "people having origins in any of the Black racial groups of Africa."
- An **Asian** is any person with "origins in any of the original peoples of the Far East, Southeast Asia, or the Indian subcontinent."
- **Native Hawaiians** and **Other Pacific Islanders** are "people having origins in any of the original peoples of Hawaii, Guam, Samoa, or other Pacific Islands."
- **Native Americans** (referred to as **American Indians)** and **Alaska Natives** are defined as "people having origins in any of the original peoples of North and South America (including Central America), and who maintain tribal affiliation or community attachment."

NURSING ALERT Because American cultures and subcultures can be so diverse, it is essential that nurses be aware of and knowledgeable about the predominant groups in their work community and apply the knowledge in their practice.

NURSING ALERT Generalizations made about an ethnic group may not apply to certain groups and individuals.

When minority groups immigrate to another country, a certain degree of cultural and ethnic blending occurs through the involuntary process of *acculturation*, those gradual changes produced in a culture by the influence of another culture that cause one or both cultures to be more similar to the other. This process in involuntary; the minority group member is forced to learn the new culture to survive (Spector, 2004). However, the changes occur to various degrees in different families and groups. Many groups continue to identify with their traditional heritage while adapting to the ill-defined concept of the "American way." Acculturation may be referred to as *assimilation*, which is the process of developing a new cultural identity (Spector, 2004).

Evidence indicates that changes in attitudes are slowly taking place in some groups and in some places. An attitude of cultural relativism provides for understanding behaviors in their cultural context and sees other ways of doing things as different but equally valid (Galanti, 2004). With growing awareness, interest, and understanding by increasing numbers of the majority group, which have accompanied the recent emergence of racial and ethnic pride, minority-group children are becoming more secure and confident in their racial or ethnic identity. Individuals vary in their reactions to membership in a minority group, and much of this variation can be attributed to familial factors. As with all children, the most important influences on development of a positive self-image are warm, understanding parents who take an active interest in fostering their children's growth. Parents who accept their children and react positively and constructively rather than in a negative and demeaning manner will help their children develop feelings of self-worth, self-esteem, and self-acceptance. The more adequate children feel, the more positive will be their attitudes toward both majority and minority children, the greater their ability to withstand prejudice and intolerance, and the less their need for counteraggressive behavior.

Cultural Shock and Cultural Competence

The term *cultural shock* describes the "feelings of helplessness and discomfort and a state of disorientation experienced by an outsider attempting to comprehend or effectively adapt to a different cultural group because of differences in cultural practices, values, and beliefs" (Leininger, 1978). This state occurs with both patients and health care providers who move from one cultural setting to another. It can happen to persons who immigrate to a new country (such as Asian refugees) or to those from a subcultural group who must adjust to the ways of an unfamiliar subgroup (such as children entering the school subculture or consumers entering the hospital subculture). Cultural shock is characterized by the inability to respond to or function in a new or strange situation (see Critical Thinking Exercise).

CRITICAL THINKING EXERCISE

Reducing Cultural Shock

A woman from the Middle East is visiting her child who is hospitalized for a serious illness. Her husband left for home a short time ago to wash and change clothes. She speaks little English. You need to obtain consent from her for an emergency procedure. She is hesitant and refuses to sign the consent form. What should you do?

1. Evidence—Is there sufficient information to draw any conclusions about this woman's actions?
2. Assumptions—Describe some underlying assumptions about each of the following:
   a. Arab culture
   b. Need for interpreter
   c. Approval for emergency procedures
   d. Documentation of the need for the emergency procedure
3. What priorities for nursing care should be established at this time?
4. Does the evidence support your nursing intervention(s)?
5. What alternative perspectives might you have?

Numerous factors influence reactions to a new environment. Language barriers, including dialects and jargon (such as medical language) specific to a subcultural group, inhibit effective communication. Habits and customs (such as different role behaviors or etiquette) and differences in attitudes and beliefs are puzzling to the stranger in the new environment. The outsider experiences intense feelings of isolation, loneliness, and nonrelatedness.

Nurses are challenged to overcome cultural shock and develop the dynamics of cultural sensitivity, an awareness of cultural similarities and differences. In doing so, the nurse is helped to practice culturally competent care. This requires changing the way people think about, understand, and interact within the world around them. Cultural competence is an ongoing process that is interactive and without end (Dunn, 2002). Six elements included in the process of developing cultural competence are (Dunn, 2002):

1. Working on changing one's world view by examining one's own values and behaviors and striving to reject racism and institutions that support it
2. Becoming familiar with core cultural issues by recognizing these issues and exploring them with patients
3. Becoming knowledgeable about the cultural groups we work with while learning about each individual patient's unique history
4. Becoming familiar with core cultural issues related to health and illness and communicating in a way that encourages patients to explain what an illness means to them
5. Developing a relationship of trust with patients and creating a welcoming atmosphere in the health care setting
6. Negotiating for mutually acceptable and understandable interventions of care

NURSING ALERT Cultural knowledge helps us understand the behavior of our patients and families so that we do not consider it pathologic. This knowledge does not allow us to make assumptions about their behavior clinically. A cultural assessment is a strategy to elicit the patient's and family's understanding of their illness and to individualize the patient's care plan. Cultural competence is nursing competence (Dreher & MacNaugton, 2002).

Cultural and Religious Influences on Health Care

Susceptibility to Health Problems

Some groups of people are more susceptible than others to certain illnesses. An innate susceptibility is acquired through generations of evolutionary changes that take place within constrained or segregated populations. The proximity to disease, environmental factors, and general physical status are significant factors associated with health problems.

Hereditary Factors

Advances in science have found that many diseases have a genetic basis. The access to screening for these diseases will challenge genetic testing and counseling and can present complex moral dilemmas for the individual patient and family and for society.

A number of conditions show ethnic or racial differences based on genetics. For example, Tay-Sachs disease, characterized by early neurologic deterioration and cognitive impairment, affects primarily Ashkenazi Jewish families, particularly those of Northeastern European origin, whereas Sephardic Jewish families appear to be no more at risk for the disease than are other populations. The incidence of cystic fibrosis is highest in Caucasians and almost nonexistent in Asians, and the rare affected African-Americans are usually in areas where there is likely to be mixed ancestry. A classic disorder of African-Americans is sickle cell disease; the incidence of cardiovascular disease, pneumonia, and diabetes is also high among African-Americans. Native Americans are at risk for type 2 diabetes and lactose intolerance. Racial and ethnic differences are further considered in relation to diseases and defects as they are discussed throughout the book.

Common food items and drugs may cause health problems in certain ethnic groups. For example, persons of Mediterranean, African, Near Eastern, and Asian origin frequently have glucose-6-phosphate dehydrogenase deficiency. They may develop acute hemolytic anemia after they ingest fava (horse or broad) beans or certain drugs such as aspirin preparations, sulfonamides, or primaquine. Other groups, especially Southern Europeans, Jews, Arabs, African-Americans, Asians, and Native Americans, have a deficiency of lactase, the enzyme needed to metabolize lactose. Ingestion of lactose can cause abdominal distention, flatus, and diarrhea (Purnell & Paulanka, 2003). Unknowing but well-meaning health care workers may be responsible for these symptoms in their clients when they prescribe foods or food supplements containing lactose as sources of nutrients.

Physical Characteristics

Among racial groups there are observable differences in physical appearance. The most obvious are skin and hair coloring and texture. Skin color is determined by the amount of melanin pigment present in the skin. Persons from countries located near the equator have darkly pigmented skin, which serves to protect the skin from the year-round exposure to the sun's rays. Persons from northern countries have very light skin, which provides for maximum exposure to the sun's rays (necessary for vitamin D metabolism) during the short daylight hours. There can be wide variations in skin color between these two extremes as a result of geographic origin or intermixing of persons with dark and light skin color. In patients with dark pigmentation, the detection of skin color changes (e.g., vasomotor alterations, cyanosis, jaundice) can be difficult and requires modified assessment techniques.

Variations in the newborn are often related to racial or ethnic origin. For example, newborn infants of Asian and African-American parents are smaller than infants of Caucasian parents, and bluish pigmented areas (mongolian spots) on the sacral region are a common observation in Asian, African-American, Native American, and Mexican-American infants. It is important that health care providers be familiar with these birthmarks. They should be documented at newborn examinations and subsequent visits so they are not suddenly interpreted as bruises (Garwick & Auger, 2000).

Evaluation of stature and body build reveals some racial tendencies. "Typical" growth descriptions are often based on observations of middle-class Caucasian children from the United States. Children from Asian countries are commonly smaller, falling below the 10th percentile on weight and height charts used for children in the United States, whereas African and African-American children are more advanced in physical growth (Trawick-Smith, 2006). This difference in stature can lead to misinterpretation of health status and capabilities.

Socioeconomic Factors

The most overwhelming adverse influence on health is socioeconomic status. A higher percentage of lower-class individuals are suffering from some health problem at any one time than are those in any other group. The sum of all aspects of their situation contributes to and compounds health problems; this includes crowded living conditions and poor sanitation, which facilitate transfer of disease (e.g., tuberculosis). There is a higher incidence of lead poisoning in children from families from the lower socioeconomic classes because they have greater access to lead in the environment, especially lead-based paint in old housing (Centers for Disease Control and Prevention, 2007).

In the lower classes, children are less likely to be immunized against preventable diseases than are children in the upper and middle classes. Lack of funds or inaccessibility of health services inhibits treatment for any but severe illness or injury. Sometimes health care is inadequate because of lack of information. In some areas a disorder is so commonplace that it is looked on as unavoidable; it is not recognized as something that requires (or is amenable to) treatment. The parents may not have information regarding causes, treatment, outcome of the illness, or preventive measures. The nurse can use the limited opportunities when the family does come in contact with the health care system to inquire about immunizations, screen for vision problems, provide nutritional information, and offer additional prevention and health promotion resources.

Poverty

A high correlation between poverty and the prevalence of illness has long been observed. Impoverished families suffer from poor nutrition. Without medical insurance, they have little if any preventive health care, inadequate health maintenance, and limited access to medical treatment. One of the most significant health problems related to poverty is a high infant mortality rate. Although the infant mortality rate in the United States is at an all-time low, our nation's infant survival rate remains lower than that of most industrialized nations (Annie E Casey Foundation, 2006).

Poor families are denied access to many health institutions for emergency or other hospital care. Frequently they must travel long distances to service centers that are willing to assume their care. In an emergency they must find money for taxi fare, borrow an automobile, or seek other means of transportation. They must find care for dependents, such as other infants and small children, or have them accompany them when taking the ill child for care. Families tend to delay preventive care indefinitely unless health services are relatively accessible. They are more likely to consult folk practitioners or other persons within their community. Day-to-day needs of food, clothing, and lodging take precedence over health care as long as the ailing person feels able to perform activities of daily living.

Poor nutrition accounts for many health problems in the lower classes. Lack of funds and knowledge results in a diet that may be seriously deficient in essential food substances, especially protein, vitamins, and iron. This inadequate diet often leads to nutritional deficiency disorders and growth retardation in children. In many the total intake is insufficient to support normal growth. Unstructured eating patterns and irregularly scheduled mealtimes can also contribute to erratic food intake and a proportionately larger consumption of non-nourishing snacks, which can result in excessive weight gain.

Because of deficient preventive care, dental problems are more prevalent. Lack of standard immunizations, together with reduced resistance from poor nutrition, renders the exposed children in poor segments of the population vulnerable to communicable diseases. Poor sanitation and crowded living conditions also contribute to the higher incidence and perpetuation of illness. In general, poor people become ill more frequently and remain ill for longer periods than do persons in the general population.

Homelessness

Research indicates that families are the fastest-growing subgroup of the homeless population (American Academy of Pediatrics, 2005). Homeless children experience all of the health problems associated with poverty, as well as other types of disorders. A majority of these children experience poor health. They not have a regular source of health care, and the focus of their care is not preventive. Their care is fragmented, crisis oriented, and often sought in emergency departments. Children who are homeless experience a higher incidence of trauma-related injuries, developmental delays, sinusitis, anemia, asthma, bowel dysfunction, eczema, and visual and neurologic deficits (American Academy of Pediatrics, 2005). Additionally, homeless adolescent youth are at risk for violence and victimization, substance abuse, pregnancy, and sexually transmitted infections (American Academy of Pediatrics, 2005).

Migrant Farmworker Families

Migrants generally suffer more illness, both acute and chronic, than the general population. They live in an environment of poverty, unstable and overcrowded housing, poor sanitation, unreliable transportation, and social isolation. Children of migrant farmworkers have a higher risk of respiratory tract and ear infections, gastroenteritis, intestinal parasites, skin infections, dental problems, lead and pesticide exposure, tuberculosis, short stature, undiagnosed congenital abnormalities, delayed development, and injuries (American Academy of Pediatrics, 2005).

When medical care is provided to migrant families, follow-up care is usually impossible because of their transient lifestyle. Compliance with medical therapies is primarily related to accessibility and availability. For example, medications provided by health workers are more likely to be taken than those that must be obtained at a pharmacy. In addition, medications are often discontinued after self-perceived recovery.

Immigrant Families

Children who have immigrated may have diseases such as malaria or hepatitis A that are more common in their country but rarely diagnosed in the United States. Immigrants have a higher rate of tuberculosis infections than persons in the United States. Immigrant children may not have been screened at birth for congenital diseases such as hemoglobinopathies and inborn errors of metabolism. Immunizations may not have been adequate as well (American Academy of Pediatrics, 2005).

Cultural Customs

Nurses must be aware of the need to consider cultural differences in patients when providing health care. An understanding of the various beliefs regarding the causation of illness and disease, as well as traditional health practices, is essential to successful intervention. The more nurses know about the values, beliefs, and customs of other ethnic groups, the better they are able to meet the needs of these families and to gain their cooperation and compliance.

NURSING ALERT Cultural resources that include a brief description of the culture and views on health, illness, diet, and other matters are available on the Internet; some institutions develop their own quick references. A newer approach to cultural competence focuses on educating providers to be aware of certain cross-cutting cultural and social issues and health beliefs that are present in all cultures (Betancourt et al, 2003).

Cultural Relativism

Although clinical characteristics of a disease or condition are essentially the same across cultures, how a child or family interprets or experiences it varies. Culture as an influence is one obvious explanation for variance. *Cultural relativism* is the concept that any behavior must be assessed first in the context of the culture in which it occurs (Purnell & Paulanka, 2003). Nurses must first relate to the family's perceptions and interpretations of experiences from the family's background and cultural belief system before they can effectively intervene.

Some cultures, for example, may view a chronic illness or disability as affecting only particular aspects of a child's life, and the child as a whole is viewed as normal. In contrast, Chinese families frequently describe the illness as having global effects on many aspects of the child's present and future life (Martinson, Armstrong, & Qiao, 1997). These contrasting views may result in parents having different goals and expectations for their children.

In some cultures the child's gender may influence a family's perception of the implications of an illness or disability. For example, in the Arabic and Asian cultures the male child is held in higher esteem than the female child. This also holds true for some families of Jewish, Italian, Greek, and Indian origin. The male child may receive better health care and more food because this is the child who will take care of his parents in their old age (Galanti, 2004).

Perceptions of disease or signs and symptoms of illness are also influenced by culture. Some cultures, for example, see diarrhea as a cleansing of the body that is essential for health maintenance and illness prevention or cure. Furthermore, signs or symptoms resulting from diarrhea and ensuing dehydration, such as malaise, fever, anorexia, and irritability, may be viewed as separate illness entities.

Nurses can often recognize a family's health-related cultural perceptions and interpretations through discussion and observation. Implications of these perceptions should be explored and considered when planning culturally appropriate interventions.

Relationships with Health Care Providers

Communication in the health care setting can be challenging when both parties speak the same language. It becomes even more complex when the patient and health care provider speak different languages. The same word can have different meaning in different cultures. Patients may say yes to a question they do not understand when they mean no. Communication styles can differ by style and demeanor, use of silence, eye contact, gestures, and body language (Galanti, 2004).

In relation to time, some cultures are oriented toward the clock, whereas others are more focused on activities. Conflicts can arise during an interaction involving these two orientations. For example, African-Americans tend to be flexible in their time orientation; an African-American family may be late for or miss appointments because other issues take precedence, and the family may not communicate this to the health agency. The Japanese, on the other hand, consider time to be valuable and to be used wisely.

Family roles differ by culture as well. Decision making may involve the extended family. Authority figures in a family may be a mother, father, or grandparent. Kinship structure is also determined by culture. Many cultures are unilateral in that they trace their descent from either a male or a female ancestor (Galanti, 2004).

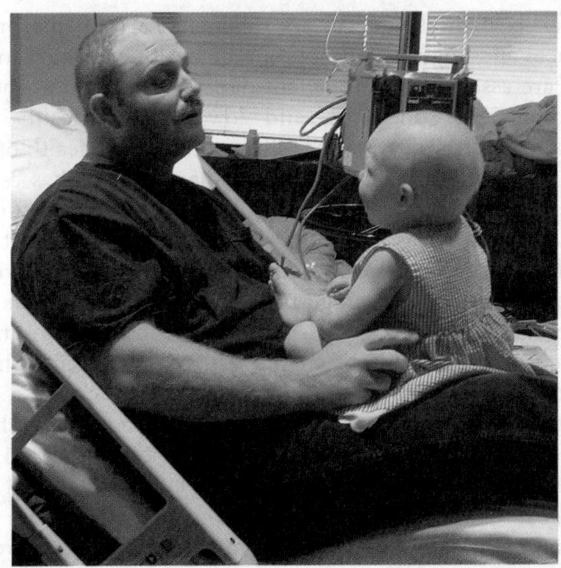

Fig. 32-4 A father with his hospitalized child. *(Courtesy E. Jacob, Texas Children's Hospital, Houston.)*

NURSING ALERT In working with families, it is essential for nurses to identify key members. Failure to include these significant individuals in teaching can seriously hinder adherence to the care plan (Fig. 32-4).

Nurses should inform themselves of any specific attitudes regarding the manner of approach to a child in a given culture. A primary social premise for Navajo Indians is that no person has the right to speak for another. They may allow a child to decide whether to take a medicine or not, whereas in other cultures this view might be viewed as irresponsible (Purnell & Paulanka, 2003). Some ethnic groups, such as the Amish, consider a child's admission to the hospital a family affair, with all members gathering to support and console the child and parents. In others, such as the Samoan family, the family is willing to relinquish the care of the child to the hospital authority without interference. Their visits with the child are short, although intense, but this behavior may be misinterpreted by the hospital staff as indifference or abandonment.

Nurses who are members of a majority culture may encounter tension and distrust in a child from a minority culture as a result of the child's learned perception or relationships with other persons in the majority group. Based on these biases, minority children may suspect that nurses have hostile feelings toward them and fear ill treatment. When such children are hospitalized, this feeling compounds the feelings of loneliness, helplessness, and retribution that accompany frightening experiences and separation from families. The reverse situation may be encountered by a nurse from a minority culture attempting to meet the needs of a child who has been conditioned to view the nurse's cultural or ethnic group as inferior.

Communication

Communication may be a source of distress and misunderstanding between persons from different ethnic groups, especially if the languages are different. Lack of interpreter services and linguistically appropriate health education materials are associated with patient dissatisfaction, poor understanding and adherence, and lower-quality health care (Betancourt et al, 2003). The Office of Minority Health of the U.S. Department of Health and Human Services has established national standards on culturally and linguistically appropriate services in health care. Health care organizations must ensure the competence of language assistance provided to persons with limited English proficiency by interpreters and bilingual staff. Family and friends should not be used for interpretation services except on request by the patient (Shaw-Taylor, 2002).

Some persons with poor or limited language comprehension may simply smile and nod in agreement if they do not understand the questions or directives. It is vital that the family fully understand all implications of a child's care and management before they sign permissions for special procedures or assume responsibility for the child's care. It is not uncommon for a Vietnamese or a Japanese family to indicate "yes" when in fact they mean "no" in order to avoid social disharmony. They tend to use indirectness rather than confrontation and may become evasive when direct questioning makes them uncomfortable.

NURSING ALERT Helpful communication tools include the following:

- Have a series of audio and audiovisual recordings in several languages designed to greet the family and familiarize them with the hospital.
- If an interpreter is not available on site, the Language Line, a national telephonic interpreter service for all languages, can be accessed by institutions as a back-up system.
- Have legal consent forms and explanations of common diagnostic tests available in several languages.
- Keep cards with common greetings, phrases, and names of body parts in the family's language with the patient's chart (e.g., miseries [pain] and locked bowels [constipation] for African-Americans; and *caida de la mollera* [fallen fontanel from dehydration]; *susto* [fright, a folk illness thought to be caused by psychologic trauma]; *dolor, duele*, or *lele* [pain]; and *la diarrhea* [diarrhea] in Hispanics).

Many Native American tribes practice nonverbal communication, and the members are highly sensitive to body language. They emphasize periods of silence to formulate thoughts in preparation for speech and often remain silent after listening to statements by others to properly assimilate what has been said. Interruption, interjection, or haste to arrive at conclusions is perceived as immature behavior.

The level of comfort with body space or distance from others varies among cultures. For example, Hispanics tend to get closer, and Asians prefer a greater distance. Eye contact is also viewed differently in cultures. Although Anglos are advised to look people straight in the eye, it is not uncommon for persons in some ethnic groups to avoid eye contact and become uncomfortable when conversing with health workers. A Vietnamese patient may not look directly into the nurse's eyes as a sign of respect. Some Native Americans will make eye contact during the initial greeting, but continued, unwavering eye contact is considered insulting and disrespectful. Asians may consider eye contact a sign of hostility or impoliteness.

Gestures also may have different meanings. For example, some Asians consider finger or foot pointing disrespectful. Native Americans consider vigorous handshaking a sign of aggression, whereas to Anglos the gesture is a sign of goodwill.

Families may be reluctant to question or otherwise initiate contact with health professionals. In the Asian cultures, for example, it is considered a sign of disrespect to question those who are viewed as persons of authority. A Japanese family may wait silently rather than ask or question. They believe that the health professionals know best and will meet their needs without being asked. It is also important to avoid criticism. Criticism can cause Asians to "lose face," to feel ashamed, which is highly undesirable.

Language and bureaucracy have been considered the biggest barriers to the use of health care services by many families (Betancourt et al, 2003). Long intake processes and wait times are also barriers for minority patients. Often families may have poor language comprehension, so it is necessary to speak slowly and carefully, not loudly, when conversing with them. Many persons are able to read and write English better than they can speak or understand it. Also, the dominant language usually takes over in anxiety-provoking situations, even among those who are able to communicate satisfactorily under ordinary circumstances.

Terms of address and use of first and last names vary among cultures and can create confusion. For example, in traditional Asian cultures the family name is given first in respect for the family and the given name follows. Therefore all siblings in a family have the same first name. Ethiopians have a complex system whereby women retain their last names after marriage and the paternal grandfather's name becomes the child's last name.

The expression of emotion also varies ethnically. In some cultures (e.g., Hispanic or Jewish) emotions are expressed openly and members are accustomed to sharing their sorrows and joys with family and friends. Conversely, Nordic and Asian groups are more restrained.

Health care providers generally ask questions and use handouts, booklets, and—particularly with children—dolls and pictures as communication aids. This is uncommon in some cultures. For example, Native American healers ask few questions and do not use forms. Nurses need to consider both verbal and nonverbal communication techniques to interact effectively with children and their families from different cultures (see Guidelines box).

Food Customs

Food customs and symbolism are an integral part of various cultural, ethnic, and religious groups. Although in a large country such as the United States most persons have adopted the eclectic food habits that have evolved over countless generations, many ethnic and geographic food traditions and preferences are retained. Special holidays, ceremonies, and life experiences such as births, birthdays, weddings, and death are often marked by special food items or feasts. In many cultures

GUIDELINES Culturally Sensitive Interactions

Nonverbal Strategies

- Invite family members to choose where they would like to sit or stand, allowing them to select a comfortable distance for personal space.
- Observe interactions with others to determine which body gestures (e.g., shaking hands) are acceptable and appropriate. Ask when in doubt.
- Avoid appearing rushed.
- Be an active listener.
- Observe for cues regarding appropriate eye contact.
- Learn appropriate use of pauses or interruptions for different cultures.
- Ask for clarification if nonverbal meaning is unclear.

Verbal Strategies

- Learn proper terms of address.
- Use a positive tone of voice to convey interest.
- Speak slowly and carefully, not loudly, when families have poor language comprehension.
- Encourage questions.
- Learn basic words and sentences of family's language, if possible.
- Avoid professional terms.
- When asking questions, tell family why the questions are being asked, the way in which the information they provide will be used, and how it might benefit their child.
- Repeat important information more than once.
- Always give the reason or purpose for a treatment or prescription.
- Use information written in family's language.
- Obtain the services of an interpreter whenever there is uncertainty regarding full comprehension in a medical encounter.
- Learn from families and representatives of their culture methods of communicating information without creating discomfort.
- Address intergenerational needs (e.g., family's need to consult with others).
- Be sincere, open, and honest and, when appropriate, share personal experiences, beliefs, and practices to establish rapport and trust.

specific food practices are followed during pregnancy in the belief that certain foods damage the developing fetus.

The distinctive food customs of ethnic groups are a product of their native environment, determined by availability. Fish is a staple food of persons living near the ocean, such as people from Japan, Polynesia, Southern Europe, and Scandinavia. Fruit and vegetable preferences are directly related to the climate in which they grow naturally or can be cultivated. The types of grain that are ethnically associated are also those that grow best in the native lands. Even in the United States there are regional favorites, such as rice, hominy grits, and okra in the Southern states. In some cultures food is highly spiced; in others, foods tend to be bland.

Children may have a number of food restrictions. Some have a physiologic origin, such as lack of dairy foods in the diets of some persons of African or Asian ancestry in whom a hereditary lactase deficiency prevents digestion of foods containing lactose. Others have religious restrictions, such as kosher foods and food preparation of the Orthodox Jewish faith, avoidance of pork by persons of Islamic faith, and the vegetarian diet of Seventh-Day Adventists.

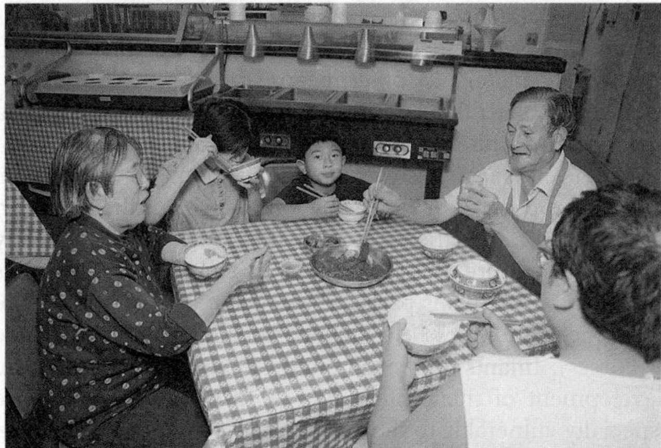

Fig. 32-5 Food customs outside the home can differ significantly from traditional cultural practices.

Children in a strange environment, such as the hospital, feel much more comfortable when they are served familiar foods (Fig. 32-5). Hospital food often tastes strange and bland. The family may be concerned that their child is not receiving foods appropriate to their culture and beliefs. When possible, it is advisable to provide children ethnic foods or allow families to bring favorite foods. Concern for differences in food habits and patterns projects an attitude of respect for the family's ethnic or religious heritage.

Health Beliefs and Practices

Health Beliefs

Beliefs related to the cause of illness and the maintenance of health are an integral part of the cultural heritage of families. Often inseparable from religious beliefs, health beliefs influence the way that families cope with health problems and the way that they respond to health care providers. Predominant among most cultures are beliefs related to natural forces, supernatural forces, and imbalance between forces.

Natural Forces

The most common natural forces held responsible for ill health if the body is not adequately protected include cold air entering the body and impurities in the air. For example, a Chinese mother may overdress her infant in an effort to keep cold wind from entering the child's body. The Chinese believe that cold weather, rain, and wind are responsible for "cold" conditions. In the African-American culture, natural phenomena such as phases of the moon, seasons of the year, and planet positions are believed to affect the body and its processes; therefore health maintenance is strongly associated with the ability to read "the signs." Most Native Americans consider health to be a state of harmony with nature and the universe.

Supernatural Forces

High on the list of causes of illness are forces beyond comprehension and logical explanation. Evil influences such as voodoo, witchcraft, or evil spirits are viewed in some cultures as causes of adverse health, especially those illnesses that cannot be explained by other means.

A health belief that is common among people from Central America, the Middle East, the Mediterranean, and some Asian and African societies is the concept of the evil eye (Galanti, 2004). The general belief is that one person inflicts evil on another and causes the victim to fall ill. The motive is usually envy. Each culture that believes in the evil eye also has ways to neutralize it. This is part of the concept of health as a state of balance, and illness as a state of imbalance (see Imbalance of Forces). Infants and small children, because of immature development of their internal strength-weakness states, are especially vulnerable to the gaze of the evil eye. Consequently, the evil eye concept serves to rationalize an inexplicable onset of illness in children who display such symptoms as restlessness, crying, diarrhea, vomiting, and fever.

Although seldom expressed to health care providers, the belief that a witch can cast a spell over others at the request of someone who wishes them ill is found in Caribbean, African, and Australian aboriginal cultures. The victim is often tortured in effigy by pins driven into a doll at the location where the intended victim is to be hurt. "Voodoo deaths" have occurred from the victim's belief in the curse and may result from dehydration as the victim gives up the will to live and refuses to drink (Chidester, 2001).

Imbalance of Forces

The concept of balance or equilibrium is widespread throughout the world. One of the most common imbalances supported by the Hispanic, Filipino, Chinese, and Arab cultures is that which exists between "hot" and "cold." This belief is reputedly derived from the Hippocratic theory of humoral pathology, which states that illness is caused by an imbalance of the four humors: phlegm, blood, black bile, and yellow bile. "Hot" and "cold" describe certain properties and conditions completely unrelated to temperature. Diseases, areas of the body, foods, and illnesses are classified as either "hot" or "cold." In Chinese health belief, the forces are termed *yin* (cold) and *yang* (hot). To maintain health, these "hot" and "cold" forces must be kept in balance.

Illness is treated by restoring normal balance through the application of appropriate "hot" or "cold" remedies. A "cold" condition such as a respiratory tract disease is believed to be caused by exposure to cold weather, rain, or cold wind entering the body; it is treated by administering "hot" foods, herbs, or drugs. Menstruation is considered to be a "hot" condition; therefore women are cautioned against ingesting "hot" foods, which might increase menstrual flow or produce cramping. Ingesting too much of either "hot" or "cold" foods can also be interpreted as a cause of illness.

Health care workers who are aware of this belief are better able to understand why some persons refuse to eat certain foods. It is possible to help families devise a diet that contains the necessary balance of basic food groups prescribed by the medical subculture while conforming to the beliefs of the ethnic subculture.

The hot-cold food classification may have adverse effects. For example, newborn infants are often started on evaporated milk formulas. Evaporated milk is considered to be a "hot" food, whereas whole milk is viewed as a "cold" food. Infants tend to develop rashes, which are believed to be caused by "hot" foods; in such cases, parents may decide to switch to whole milk. However, parents fear that it is dangerous to change too rapidly, so they often feed the child some type of neutralizing substance, which may create additional health problems. Such a problem might be averted if the family's preference is determined before discharge from the hospital, with a formula prescribed that is agreeable to both the family and the practitioner.

Health Practices

There are numerous similarities among cultures regarding prevention and treatment of illness. All cultures have some types of home remedies that they apply before seeking help from other persons. Within the ethnic community, folk healers who are endowed with the ability to "cure" maladies are sought for special situations and when home remedies are unsuccessful. There is the *curandero* (male) or *curandera* (female) of the Mexican-American community whose healing powers are believed to be a gift from God. The Asian consults an herbalist, knowledgeable in medicines, or an ethnic practitioner practiced in Asian therapies, including acupuncture (insertion of needles), acupressure (application of pressure), and moxibustion (application of heat). Native Americans consult a variety of healers with specific skills and knowledge. Specialized medicine persons diagnose illness, provide nonsacred treatments (usually by way of massage and herbs), and care for souls. Other specialists perform services or affect cures through spiritual means. Native Hawaiians consult *kahunas* and practice *ho'oponopono* to heal family imbalance or disputes.

The folk healers are powerful persons in their community. They "speak the language" of the family who seeks help and often combine their rituals and potions with prayer and entreaties to God. They also are able to create an atmosphere conducive to successful management. Furthermore, they exhibit a sincere interest in the family and their problem.

Some folk remedies are compatible with the medical regimen and can be used to reinforce the treatment plan. For example, most of the foods contraindicated for persons with peptic ulcers are "hot" foods and would be avoided because of their belief systems. Also, aspirin (a "hot" medication) is an appropriate therapy for "cold" diseases such as the common cold and arthritis. It is not uncommon to discover that a folk prescription has a scientific basis. However, no scientific basis has been found for numerous health remedies or preventive practices, such as the use of garlic or asafetida (a bad-smelling gum resin, obtained from various Asiatic plants, that looks like a dried sponge), which is worn around the neck to prevent contagious diseases. Also, wearing copper or silver bracelets to protect the wearer as he or she grows has no scientific basis.

Practices that do no harm should be respected. Overcoming the effect of the evil eye usually requires specialized rituals conducted by the appropriate practitioner. For example, the Chicano *curandera* ascertains that the condition is truly the result of the evil eye by performing an assessment ritual and then, with a confirmed diagnosis, performs a curative ritual. Sometimes the faith in the folk practitioner results in a delay in obtaining needed medical treatment, although the

BOX 32-1 Cultural Practices Possibly Considered Abusive by the Dominant Culture

Coining—An Asian practice that may produce weltlike lesions on the child's back when a coin, held on edge, is repeatedly rubbed lengthwise on the oiled skin to rid the body of a disease (Galanti, 2004).

Cupping—A practice in many parts of the world (Asia, Latin American, parts of Europe) of placing a container (e.g., tumbler, bottle, jar) containing steam against the skin surface to "draw out the poison" or other evil element. When the heated air within the container cools, a vacuum is created that produces a bruiselike blemish on the skin directly beneath the mouth of the container (Galanti, 2004).

Burning—A practice of some Southeast Asian groups whereby small areas of skin are burned to treat enuresis and temper tantrums.

Female genital mutilation (female circumcision)—Removal of or injury to any part of the female genital organ; practiced in some parts of Africa (Galanti, 2004).

Forced kneeling—A discipline measure of some Caribbean groups in which a child is forced to kneel for a long time.

Topical garlic application—A practice of Yemenite Jews in which crushed garlic cloves or garlic–petroleum jelly plaster is applied to the wrists to treat infectious disease. The practice can result in blisters or garlic burns.

Traditional remedies that contain lead—**Greta** and **azarcon** (Mexico; used for digestive problems), **paylooah** (Southeast Asia; used for rash or fever), and **surma** (India; used as a cosmetic to improve eyesight).

practitioner will usually suggest medical care if his or her ministrations are unsuccessful.

Health practices of different cultures may also present problems in assessment and interpretation. For example, certain cultural practices or remedies can be misdiagnosed as evidence of child abuse by uninformed professionals (Box 32-1). It is important to explain why these and other familiar remedies may now be considered harmful. Health care providers need to be aware of the practices so they do not misinterpret symptoms such as red welts from coining. Families need to understand how such practices can place them in jeopardy with child protective services (Galanti, 2004). Cultural health remedies that are detrimental to health include eating clay, excessive amounts of salt, or compounds that contain lead or mercury. A careful history can reveal these remedies, but it may require the collaboration of a folk healer to convince a user to stop the practice.

Faith healing and religious rituals are closely allied with many folk-healing practices. Wearing amulets, medals, and other religious relics believed by the culture to protect the individual and facilitate healing is a common practice. It is important for health workers to recognize the value of this practice and keep the items where the family has placed them or nearby. It offers comfort and support and rarely impedes medical and nursing care. If an item must be removed during a procedure, it should be replaced, if possible, when the procedure is completed. The reason for its temporary removal is explained to the family, and they are reassured that their wishes will be respected.

Nurses can be most effective by operating from a multicultural perspective. Adopting a multicultural perspective means using appropriate aspects of each culture's orientation to health to developing culturally acceptable health care interventions.

NURSING ALERT Avoid directly criticizing traditional cultural health beliefs and practices as wrong or harmful or implying that biomedical measures are uniformly correct and effective and the only way to prevent illness or treat sickness. Such criticisms usually result in rejection of both biomedical health care practitioners and their health teaching. When folk practices do not interfere with the patient's welfare, they need not be discouraged. Often a compromise can be reached that accomplishes the nurse's goal while maintaining the dignity and self-esteem of the child and family.

Religious Beliefs

Religious and spiritual dimensions are among the most important influences in many people's lives. The term *spirituality* relates to an individual's personal beliefs, transcendent experiences, and principles; *religion* refers to an organized system of beliefs or a place of worship. The pediatric nurse who learns how the patient and family view their traditions, values, and beliefs can understand how these dimensions may affect the patient's health (McEvoy, 2003). Three areas to explore for information about the family's culture, religion, or spirituality are beliefs and values, daily practices, and community involvement. An assessment tool can be easily used for integrating culture and spirituality into the nursing assessment (Box 32-2).

Religion affects the way people interpret and respond to illness (Spector, 2004). Among many groups, illness, injury, or death is believed to be sent by God as a punishment for sin. Some may believe that health workers will be unable to help a person whom God is punishing and may express a fatalistic attitude toward treatment, stating it is "the will of God." Others view it as a test of strength, like the testing of Job in the Bible, and strive to remain faithful and overcome the conflicts.

Religious affiliation has implications for many health-related functions and procedures. It is comforting for the family of an ill child to have this need recognized and respected. Nurses need to determine whether there are any special considerations, including dietary restrictions, related to spiritual practices that are important to the family. Family members are asked whether they want a clergy member present and whether they prefer hospital staff to call or prefer to do this on their own.

It is also important to determine the wishes of the family regarding baptism, rites or practices related to death, and other religious rituals (such as circumcision, communion, or use of amulets or icons). Religion, which offers families understanding and spiritual support, is a valuable asset to health care. Characteristics of selected religions with beliefs that affect health care are outlined in Table 32-1.

BOX 32-2 BELIEF Framework for Integrating Culture and Spirituality into the Nursing Assessment

Belief system—A spiritual belief system is the tenet regarding a higher power that gives structure and form to everyday lives.

Ethics or values—Ethical or personal belief systems that guide the family's everyday life. The family may not follow a formal religion but still adhere to core values.

Lifestyle—Diet, nutrition, use of caffeine and alcohol, prayer and meditation, clothing, and medicinal practices all are examples where culture, religion, and spirituality may be closely connected.

Involvement in a spiritual community—The community can provide the family the benefits of identity, socialization, and support, while keeping children and adolescents involved in safe and healthy social activities.

Education—Religious education affects the cultural, moral, and ethical development of children. The children's belief system influences their coping mechanisms, especially during chronic illness.

Future events—Knowledge of the patient and family's belief system allows the nurse to provide individualized and sensitive anticipatory guidance for future health events.

From McEvoy M: Culture and spirituality as an integrated concept in pediatric care, *MCN* 28(1):39-43, 2003.

Table 32-1 Religious Beliefs That May Affect Nursing Care

BIRTH AND DEATH	DIET AND FOOD PRACTICES	MEDICAL CARE
Buddhist		
Birth—No baptism. Infant presentation. Death—Last rite chanting is often practiced at bedside soon after death; the deceased's family or Buddhist priest should be contacted. **Organ donation/transplantation**—Organ donation is a matter of individual conscience.	Restrictions on some food combinations; extremes must be avoided. Some sects are strictly vegetarian. Discourage use of alcohol and drugs.	Illness is believed to be a trial to aid development of soul; illness results from Karmic causes. Surgery is permitted, but extremes must be avoided. Cleanliness is of great importance. Family, community, and Buddhist priest are supportive visitors.
Church of Christ, Scientist (Christian Science)		
Birth—No baptism. Death—No last rites; autopsy is not permitted except in cases of sudden death; individuals can choose burial or cremation. **Organ donation/transplantation**—Church takes no specific position on transplantation as distinct from other medical or surgical procedures. Individuals decide on organ donation.	Abstain from alcohol and some forms of tea and coffee.	Oppose human intervention with drugs or other therapies; however, accept legally required immunizations. Accept physical and moral healing. Family, friends, and members of spiritual community may visit.
Church of Jesus Christ of Latter Day Saints (Mormon)		
Birth—No baptism. Infant is blessed by church official at first opportunity after birth (in church). Baptism by immersion at 8 years. Death—Believe that it is proper to bury the dead in the ground; cremation is discouraged. **Organ donation/transplantation**—Individuals can choose whether to will organs to be used in transplants.	Prohibit tea (except herbal), coffee, and alcohol. Some individuals avoid chocolate and other products that contain caffeine. Fasting for 24 hours each month.	Devout adherents believe in divine healing. Medical therapy is not prohibited. **Spiritual items**—A "garment" (type of underwear) that is considered sacred; person may not want to remove it. Family, friends, and church members are supportive visitors.
Hindu		
Birth—No baptism. Death—Certain prescribed rites are followed after death; priest may tie thread around neck or wrist to signify blessing; family will wash the body and are particular about who touches the dead; bodies are to be cremated. **Organ donation/transplantation**—No religious laws prohibiting donation; individual decision.	Many dietary restrictions. Eating meat is forbidden.	With an amputation, loss of a limb is believed to represent sins committed in previous life. Accept most modern medical practices; some belief in faith healing. **Spiritual items**—Person may wear a thread around wrist or body; do not remove it. Family, community members, and priest are supportive visitors.

Table 32-1 Religious Beliefs That May Affect Nursing Care—cont'd

BIRTH AND DEATH	DIET AND FOOD PRACTICES	MEDICAL CARE
Islam (Muslim/Moslem)		
Birth—At birth, the first words said to the infant in his or her right ear are *Allah-o-Akbar* (Allah is great), and the remainder of the Call for Prayer is recited. An *Aqeeqa* (party) to celebrate the birth of the child is arranged by the parents. Male children are circumcised. **Death**—At the time of death, specific rituals (e.g., bathing, wrapping the body in cloth) must be done by same-sex Muslim. Before moving and handling the body, it is preferable to contact someone from the person's mosque or the local Islamic Society to perform these rituals. **Organ donation/transplantation**—Individual decides on organ donation/transplantation.	Prohibit all pork products and alcohol. Fasting is practiced during the ninth month of the Islamic year (Ramadan).	Believers are encouraged in the Qu'ran to seek treatment. It is taught that only Allah cures; however, Muslims are taught not to refuse treatment in the belief that Allah will take care of them because he also chooses at times to work through the efforts of humans. **Other practices**—Right hand is used for eating; left hand is for hygiene. Family and friends are supportive visitors.
Jehovah's Witnesses		
Birth—No baptism. **Death**—No official last rites are practiced when death occurs. **Organ donation/transplantation**—Organ donation is forbidden.	No tobacco; moderate alcohol permissible.	Blood or blood products are not allowed; volume expanders are permissible if not derived from blood.
Judaism (Orthodox and Conservative)		
Birth—No baptism. Ritual circumcision of male infants on eighth day; performed by mohel (ritual circumciser familiar with Jewish law and aseptic technique). **Death**—According to tradition, during last moments of life, relatives and close friends remain with the deceased. Amputated limbs or surgically removed tissues should be made available to family for burial. Cremation not allowed. **Organ donation/transplantation**—Organ transplantation/donation is complex issue; sometimes they are practiced.	Numerous dietary kosher laws exist; followers are allowed only meat from animals that are vegetable eaters and are ritually slaughtered; predatory fowl, shellfish, and pork are prohibited. Milk products served first can be followed by meat in a few minutes, but milk may not be consumed for several hours after eating meat. Fasting is part of Yom Kippur observance. Matzo replaces leavened bread during Passover week.	May resist surgical procedures during Sabbath, which extends from sundown Friday until sundown Saturday. Illness is grounds for violating dietary laws. **Spiritual items**—Men may wear prayer shawl, yarmulka (cap) while praying. Family, friends, and rabbi are supportive visitors.
Roman Catholic		
Birth—Infant baptism; especially urgent if poor prognosis, when it may be performed by anyone. **Death**—Sacrament of the Sick is performed if prognosis is poor while patient is alive. **Organ donation/transplantation**—Transplantation of organs is ethically and morally acceptable to Vatican; organ donation is viewed as an act of charity.	Abstaining from meat is practiced on Ash Wednesday, Good Friday, and Fridays during Lent (as a rule).	Encourage anointing of the sick. **Spiritual items**—Rosary beads, crucifix. Traditional church teaching does not approve of contraceptives or abortion.

Data from Galanti G: *Caring for patients from different cultures*, ed 3, Philadelphia, 2004, University of Pennsylvania Press; Lipson JG, Dibble SL, Minarik PA: *Culture and clinical care: a pocket guide*, San Francisco, 2005, UCSF Nursing Press; Purnell LD, Paulanka BJ: *Transcultural health care: a culturally competent approach*, Philadelphia, 2003, Davis; Spector RE: *Cultural diversity in health and illness*, ed 6, Upper Saddle River, NJ, 2004, Prentice Hall.

Importance of Culture and Religion to Nurses

A general agreement exists among nurses to raise the cultural competence of professional nursing practice. To begin to understand and deal effectively with families in a multicultural community, nurses need to recognize barriers to transcultural communication and work to remove these barriers (Muñoz & Luckmann, 2005). Nurses, too, are a product of their own cultural background. They also need to recognize that they are part of the "nursing culture." Nurses function within the framework of a professional culture with its own values and traditions and, as such, become socialized into their professional culture in their educational program and later in their work environments and professional associations.

Frequently, nurses and other health care workers are not aware of their own cultural values and how those values influence their thoughts and actions. A model for self-examination on cultural competence is the *ASKED* model (Box 32-3). Recognizing that a behavior may be characteristic of a culture rather than an "abnormal" behavior places nurses at an advantage in their relationships with families. When nurses respect a family's cultural differences, they are better able to determine whether the behavior is distinctive to the individual or a characteristic of the culture.

Cultural standards and values, family structure and function, and experience with health care influence a family's feelings and attitudes toward health, their children, and health care delivery systems. It is often difficult for nurses to be nonjudgmental and objective in working with families whose behaviors and attitudes differ from or conflict with their own. The nurse needs to understand how one's own cultural background influences the way care is delivered (American Nurses Association, 1991). Relying on one's own values and experiences for guidance can result in frustration and disappointment. It is one thing to know what is needed to deal with a health problem; it is often quite another to implement a fruitful course of action unless nurses work within the cultural and socioeconomic framework of the family.

It is beneficial to adapt ethnic practices to the family's health needs rather than to attempt to change longstanding beliefs. To aid their efforts to understand and respect the cultural beliefs of families, nurses need to develop knowledge on how cultural groups understand life processes, define health and illness, and view the causes of illness. Nurses should combine their cross-cultural knowledge with excellent communication skills to learn from the individual patient and family about issues important to their care (Betancourt et al, 2003).

Some broad characteristics of selected cultures are outlined in Table 32-2. Tables 32-1 and 32-2 are presented as beginning

evolve Skill—Providing Culturally Sensitive Care

BOX 32-3 Exploring Your Cultural Competence: ASKED Model of Cultural Competence

Awareness—Am I aware of my personal biases and prejudices toward cultural groups different from mine?

Skill—Do I have the skill to conduct a cultural assessment and perform a culturally based physical assessment in a sensitive manner?

Knowledge—Do I have knowledge of the patient's world view and the field of biocultural ecology?

Encounters—How many face-to-face encounters have I had with patients from diverse cultural backgrounds?

Desire—What is my genuine desire to "want to be" culturally competent?

Data from Campinha-Bacote J: Many faces: addressing diversity in health care, *Online J Issues Nurs* 8:1, 2003. Available at www.nursingworld.org/ojin/topic20/tpc20_2.htm (accessed May 5, 2007).

Table 32-2 Broad Cultural Characteristics Related to Health Care of Children and Families

HEALTH BELIEFS	HEALTH PRACTICES	FAMILY RELATIONSHIPS	COMMUNICATION
African			
Illness classified as: **Natural**–Affected by forces of nature without adequate protection (e.g., cold air, pollution, food and water) **Unnatural**–God's punishment for improper behavior May see illness as the "will of God"	Self-care and folk medicine prevalent Folk therapies usually religious in origin Folk therapies often not shared with the medical provider Prayer as common means for prevention and treatment	Strong kinship bonds in extended family; members come to aid of others in crisis Less likely to view illness as a burden Place strong emphasis on work and ambition Elders cared for and respected	Alert to any evidence of discrimination Place importance on nonverbal behavior Affection shown by touching and hugging Silence may indicate lack of trust Initial eye contact to show respect; maintaining eye contact can be viewed as aggressive Best to use direct but caring approach
Chinese			
A healthy body viewed as gift from parents and ancestors and must be cared for Health seen as one of the results of balance between the forces of **yin** (cold) and **yang** (hot)—energy forces that rule the world Illness caused by imbalance Blood believed to be source of life and is not regenerated **Chi** is innate energy	**Goal of therapy**–To restore balance of yin and yang Acupuncture needles applied to appropriate meridians identified in terms of yin and yang Acupressure and **tai chi** replacing acupuncture in some areas Use of **moxibustion**–application of heat to skin over specific meridians Wide use of medicinal herbs procured and applied in prescribed ways Meals may or may not be planned to balance hot and cold	Extended family pattern common Strong concept of loyalty of young to old Respect for elders taught at early age–acceptance without questioning or talking back Children's behavior a reflection on family Family and individual honor and "face" important Self-reliance and self-esteem highly valued; self-expression repressed	Open expression of emotions unacceptable Often smile when they do not comprehend Eye contact avoided as sign of respect

Table 32-2 Broad Cultural Characteristics Related to Health Care of Children and Families—cont'd

HEALTH BELIEFS	HEALTH PRACTICES	FAMILY RELATIONSHIPS	COMMUNICATION
Haitian			
Illness seen as a punishment **Natural** cause (*maladi bone die*—disease of the Lord) caused by environmental factors, movement of blood within the body, changes between hot and cold, and bone displacement **Supernatural** (*loa*—spirits' anger) Good health seen as the maintenance of equilibrium Prayer and good spiritual habits important	Health a personal responsibility Foods have properties of "hot" or "cold" and "light" or "heavy" and must be in harmony with one's life cycle and bodily states Natural illnesses treated by home and folk remedies first May use religious medallions, rosary beads, or figure of saint to pray with	Maintenance of family reputation paramount Lineal authority supreme; children in a subordinate position in family hierarchy Children valued for parental security in old age and expected to contribute to family welfare at an early age	Recent immigrants and older persons may speak only Haitian Creole Often smile and nod in agreement when do not understand Quiet and gentle communication style and lack of assertiveness lead health care providers to falsely believe they comprehend health teaching and are compliant May not ask questions if health care provider is busy or rushed
Japanese			
Shinto religious influence Human inherently good Evil caused by outside spirits Illness caused by contact with polluting agents (e.g., blood, corpses, skin diseases) Health achieved through harmony and balance between self and society Disease caused by disharmony with society and not caring for body	Energy restored by means of acupuncture, acupressure, massage, and moxibustion along affected meridians *Kampō* medicine—use of natural herbs Believe in removal of diseased parts Trend is to use both Western and Asian healing methods Care for disabled viewed as family's responsibility Take pride in child's good health Seek preventive care, medical care for illness	Close intergenerational relationships Generational categories: ***Issei***—first generation to live in United States ***Nisei***—second generation ***Sansei***—third generation ***Yonsei***—fourth generation Family tends to keep problems to self Value self-control and self-sufficiency Concept of ***haji*** (shame) imposes strong control; unacceptable behavior of children reflects on family	Make significant use of nonverbal communication with subtle gestures and facial expression Tend to suppress emotions Will often wait silently
Mexican-American			
Health controlled by environment, fate, and will of God Certain illnesses considered "hot" and "cold" states and are treated with food that complements those states Disease based on imbalance between individual and environment	Seek help from *curandero* or *curandera*, especially in rural areas *Curandero(a)* receives position by birth, apprenticeship, or a "calling" via dream or vision Treatments involve use of herbs, rituals, and religious artifacts Practice for severe illness—make promises, visit shrines, offer medals and candles, offer prayers Adhere to "hot" and "cold" food prescriptions and prohibitions for prevention and treatment of illness	Strong kinship—extended families include ***compadres*** (godparents) established by ritual kinship Children valued highly and desired, taken everywhere with family Elderly treated with respect	Spanish speaking or bilingual May have a strong preference for native language and revert to it in times of stress May shake hands or engage in introductory embrace Interpret prolonged eye contact as disrespectful Relaxed concept of time; may be late to appointments
Native American			
Believe health is state of harmony with nature and universe Respect bodies through proper management Depend on individual belief in traditional culture Traditional health beliefs holistic and wellness oriented	Distinction made between indigenous health problem requiring native healer or practice and Western disease requiring other medical care Health practices include self-sufficiency and harmonious living Participation in religious ceremonies and prayer promotes health	Cultures vary in kinship structure Extended family structure—usually includes relatives from both sides of family Elder members assume leadership roles	Use anecdotes or metaphors to discuss a situation Long pauses indicate careful consideration Nonverbal communication Respect indicated by avoiding eye contact Individuals usually speak for themselves

Continued

Table 32-2 Broad Cultural Characteristics Related to Health Care of Children and Families—cont'd

HEALTH BELIEFS	HEALTH PRACTICES	FAMILY RELATIONSHIPS	COMMUNICATION
Puerto Rican			
Subscribe to the "hot-cold" theory of causation of illness Believe some illness caused by evil forces Destiny (*Si Dios quiere*–if God wants) is in control of health	Infrequent use of health care system Seek folk healers (*espiritistas*)–use of herbs, rituals Treatment classified as "hot" or "cold" Many varieties of herbal teas used to treat illness and promote healing	Family usually large and home centered–the core of existence Father has authority in family Great respect for elders Children valued–seen as a gift from God Children taught to obey and respect parents	Spanish speaking or bilingual Strong sense of family privacy–may view questions regarding family as impudent
Vietnamese			
Good health considered to be balance between yin and yang Concept of health based on harmony and balance Rituals used to prevent illness	Family uses all means possible before using outside agencies for health care Regard health as family responsibility; outside aid sought when resources run out Use herbal medicine, spiritual practices, and acupuncture May consider head sacred and feet profane; avoid touching head after feet May use cupping, coin rubbing, or pinching skin May inhale aromatic oils, take herbal teas, or wear strings tied on body	Family is revered institution Multigenerational families Family is chief social network Children highly valued Individual needs and interests subordinate to those of a family group Father is main decision maker Women taught submission to men Parents expect respect and obedience from children	May hesitate to ask questions Questioning authority is sign of disrespect; asking questions considered impolite May avoid eye contact with health professionals as a sign of respect

From Galanti G: *Caring for patients from different cultures,* ed 3, Philadelphia, 2004, University of Pennsylvania Press; Lipson JG, Dibble SL, Minarik PA: *Culture and clinical care: a pocket guide,* San Francisco, 2005, UCSF Nursing Press; Purnell LD, Paulanka BJ: *Transcultural health care: a culturally competent approach,* Philadelphia, 2003, Davis; Spector RE: *Cultural diversity in health and illness,* ed 6, Upper Saddle River, NJ, 2004, Prentice Hall.

frameworks for practicing transcultural nursing. Nurses must assess the cultural and religious practices of families to identify how these practices are similar to and different from those of their own cultural and religious backgrounds.

NURSING ALERT These generalizations are presented to help nurses learn the unique beliefs and practices of various groups and are not meant to be used as stereotypes of any group. A stereotype is an end point, and the nurse does not attempt to learn where the individual fits the statement. A generalization provides a beginning point from which the nurse can inquire further to obtain more information and individualize the patient's care (Galanti, 2004).

Key Points

- Culture is the sum total of mores, traditions, and beliefs about how people function and encompasses other products of human works and thoughts specific to members of an intergenerational group, community, or population.
- Nurses have a responsibility to continually develop cultural competence. This includes understanding and respecting the influence of culture, race, and ethnicity on the development of social and emotional relationships, childrearing practices, and attitudes toward health.
- A child's self-concept evolves from ideas about his or her social roles.
- Important subcultural influences on children include ethnicity, socioeconomic class, poverty, homelessness, immigration, religion, schools, community, and peers.
- A trend that has significantly influenced the American family is increasing geographic and economic mobility.

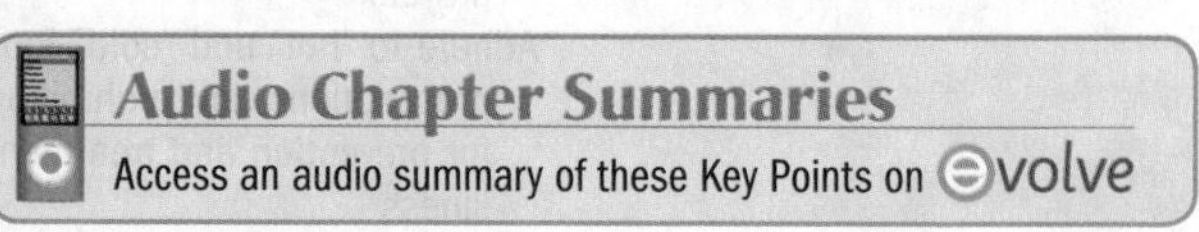
Audio Chapter Summaries
Access an audio summary of these Key Points on evolve

- Membership in a minority group presents special challenges for children, although changes in societal attitudes are slowly taking place.
- A child's physical characteristics and susceptibility to health problems can be related to ethnic and cultural variations of hereditary and socioeconomic forces.
- Groups of children suffering from greater physical and mental health problems are those living in poverty, those who are homeless, those who live in migrant farm families, and those who are recent immigrants to the United States.

- Because verbal and nonverbal communication is an important cultural consideration, nurses need to acknowledge and respect their patient's practices for productive interaction to occur.
- Cultural beliefs related to cause of illness and maintenance of health may focus on natural forces, supernatural forces, or imbalance of forces.
- In planning and implementing patient care, nurses need to strive to adapt ethnic practices to the family's health needs rather than attempt to change longstanding beliefs.
- No cultural group is homogeneous; every racial and ethnic group contains great diversity.

References

American Academy of Pediatrics, Committee on Community Health Services: Providing care for immigrant, homeless, and migrant children, *Pediatrics* 115(4):1095-1100, 2005.

American Nurses Association: *Position statement: cultural diversity in nursing practice,* 1991. Available from http://nursingworld.org/readroom/position/ethics/etcldv.htm (accessed April 15, 2007).

Annie E Casey Foundation: One out of five U.S. children is living in an immigrant family, *Data Snapshot,* no. 4, March 2007. Available from www.kidscount.org/sld/snapshot_immigrant.pdf (accessed April 15, 2007).

Annie E Casey Foundation: *2006 Kids count data book: state profiles of child well-being,* 2006. Available from www.aecf.org/upload/PublicationFiles/DA36221056.pdf (accessed April 20, 2007).

Betancourt JR: Cultural competence—marginal or mainstream movement, *N Engl J Med* 351(10):953-954, 2004.

Betancourt JR et al: Defining cultural competence: a practical framework for addressing racial/ethnic disparities in health and healthcare, *Pub Health Rep* 118:292-302, 2003.

Centers for Disease Control and Prevention: *Childhood lead poisoning prevention program,* 2007. Available from www.cdc.gov/nceh/publications/factsheets/ChildhoodLeadPoisoningPreventionProgram.pdf (accessed April 22, 2007).

Chidester D: *Patterns of transcendence: religion, death, and dying,* ed 2, Belmont, CA, 2001, Wadsworth.

Dreher M, MacNaugton N: Cultural competence in nursing: foundation or fallacy? *Nurs Outlook* 50:181-186, 2002.

Dunn AM: Culture competence and the primary care provider, *J Pediatr Health Care* 16:105-111, 2002.

Galanti G: *Caring for patients from different cultures,* ed 3, Philadelphia, 2004, University of Pennsylvania Press.

Garwick A, Auger S: What do providers need to know about American Indian culture? Recommendations from urban Indian family caregivers, *Fam Systems Health* 18:177-189, 2000.

Giger JN, Davidhizar RE: *Transcultural nursing: assessment and intervention,* ed 5, St Louis, 2008, Mosby.

Jones DC, Crawford JK: The peer appearance culture during adolescence: gender and body mass variations, *J Youth Adolesc* 2:257-269, 2006.

Leininger M: *Transcultural nursing,* New York, 1978, John Wiley & Sons.

Martinson IM, Armstrong V, Qiao J: The experience of the family of children with chronic illness at home in China, *Pediatr Nurs* 23(4):371-375, 1997.

McEvoy M: Culture and spirituality as an integrated concept in pediatric care, *MCN* 28(1):39-43, 2003.

Meléndez L: Parental beliefs and practices around early self-regulation: the impact of culture and immigration, *Infants Young Child* 18(2):136-146, 2005.

Muñoz C, Luckmann J: *Transcultural communication in nursing,* ed 2, Clifton Park, NY, 2005, Thomson Delmar Learning.

Purnell LD, Paulanka BJ: *Transcultural health care: a culturally competent approach,* ed 2, Philadelphia, 2003, Davis.

Scruggs L, Allan JP: The material consequences of welfare states: benefit generosity and absolute poverty in 16 OECD countries, *Comp Pol Studies* 39:880-904, 2006.

Search-Institute: *What kids need: developmental assets,* 2008. Available from www.search-institute.org/assets/forty.htm (accessed March 31, 2009).

Shaw-Taylor Y: Culturally and linguistically appropriate health care for racial or ethnic minorities: analysis of the US Office of Minority Health's recommended standards, *Health Policy* 62:211-221, 2002.

Spector RE: *Cultural diversity in health and illness,* ed 6, Upper Saddle River, NJ, 2004, Prentice-Hall.

Trawick-Smith J: *Early childhood development: a multicultural perspective,* ed 4, Upper Saddle River, NJ, 2006, Pearson Education.

Tropello PD: The many faces of homelessness. In Kelley ML, Fitzsimons VM (editors): *Understanding cultural diversity,* Sudbury, MA, 2000, Jones & Bartlett.

US Census Bureau: *Overview of race and Hispanic origin: census 2000 brief,* 2001. Available from www.census.gov/prod/2001pubs/c2kbr01-1.pdf (accessed May 5, 2007).

Unit 7

33 Developmental Influences on Child Health Promotion

Learning Objectives

On completion of this chapter the reader will be able to:

- Describe major trends in growth and development.
- Explain the alterations in the major body systems that take place during the process of growth and development.
- Discuss the development and relationships of personality, cognition, language, morality, spirituality, and self-concept.
- Describe the role of play in the growth and development of children.
- Demonstrate an understanding of the role of innate and environmental factors in the physical and emotional development of children.

Electronic Resources

Additional information related to the content in Chapter 33 can be found on

evolve the Companion Website at http://evolve.elsevier.com/Perry/maternal/

- NCLEX Review Questions
- Critical Thinking Exercise—Growth Trends During Infancy

Growth and Development

Foundations of Growth and Development

Growth and development, usually referred to as a unit, express the sum of the numerous changes that take place during the lifetime of an individual. The entire course is a dynamic process that encompasses several interrelated dimensions:

Growth—An increase in number and size of cells as they divide and synthesize new proteins; results in increased size and weight of the whole or any of its parts

Development—A gradual change and expansion; advancement from lower to more advanced stages of complexity; the emerging and expanding of the individual's capacities through growth, maturation, and learning

Maturation—An increase in competence and adaptability; aging; usually used to describe a qualitative change; a change in the complexity of a structure that makes it possible for that structure to begin functioning; to function at a higher level

Differentiation—Processes by which early cells and structures are systematically modified and altered to achieve specific and characteristic physical and chemical properties; sometimes used to describe the trend of mass to specific; development from simple to more complex activities and functions

All these processes are interrelated, simultaneous, and ongoing; none occurs apart from the others. The processes depend on a sequence of endocrine, genetic, constitutional, environmental, and nutritional influences (Seidel et al, 2006). The child's body becomes larger and more complex; the personality simultaneously expands in scope and complexity. Very simply, growth can be viewed as a quantitative change, and development as a qualitative change.

Stages of Development

Most authorities in the field of child development conveniently categorize child growth and behavior into approximate age stages or in terms that describe the features of an age group. The age ranges of these stages are admittedly arbitrary and, because they do not take into account individual differences, cannot be applied to all children with any degree of precision. However, categorization affords a convenient means to describe the characteristics associated with the majority of children at periods when distinctive developmental changes appear and specific developmental tasks must be accomplished. (A developmental task is a set of skills and competencies peculiar to each developmental stage that children must accomplish or master to deal effectively with their environment.) It is also significant for nurses to know that there are characteristic health problems peculiar to each major phase of development. The sequence of descriptive age periods and subperiods that are used here and elaborated on in subsequent chapters is listed in Box 33-1.

Patterns of Growth and Development

There are definite and predictable patterns in growth and development that are continuous, orderly, and progressive.

BOX 33-1 Developmental Age Periods

Prenatal Period—Conception to Birth

Germinal—Conception to approximately 2 weeks
Embryonic—2 to 8 weeks
Fetal—8 to 40 weeks (birth)

A rapid growth rate and total dependency make this one of the most crucial periods in the developmental process. The relationship between maternal health and certain manifestations in the newborn emphasizes the importance of adequate prenatal care to the infant's health and well-being.

Infancy Period—Birth to 12 Months

Neonatal—Birth to 27 or 28 days
Infancy—1 to approximately 12 months

The infancy period is one of rapid motor, cognitive, and social development. Through mutuality with the caregiver (parent), the infant establishes a basic trust in the world and the foundation for future interpersonal relationships. The critical first month of life, although part of the infancy period, is often differentiated from the remainder because of the infant's major physical adjustments to extrauterine existence and the parent's psychologic adjustment.

Early Childhood—1 to 6 Years

Toddler—1 to 3 years
Preschool—3 to 6 years

This period, which extends from the time children attain upright locomotion until they enter school, is characterized by intense activity and discovery. It is a time of marked physical and personality development. Motor development advances steadily. Children at this age acquire language and wider social relationships, learn role standards, gain self-control and mastery, develop increasing awareness of dependence and independence, and begin to develop a self-concept.

Middle Childhood—6 to 11 or 12 Years

Frequently referred to as the *school age*, this period of development is one in which the child is directed away from the family group and centered around the wider world of peer relationships. There is steady advancement in physical, mental, and social development, with emphasis on developing skill competencies. Social cooperation and early moral development take on more importance with relevance for later life stages. This is a critical period in the development of a self-concept.

Later Childhood—11 to 19 Years

Prepubertal—10 to 13 years
Adolescence—13 to approximately 18 years

The tumultuous period of rapid maturation and change known as adolescence is considered to be a transitional period that begins at the onset of puberty and extends to the point of entry into the adult world—usually high school graduation. Biologic and personality maturation are accompanied by physical and emotional turmoil, and there is redefining of the self-concept. In the late adolescent period the young person begins to internalize all previously learned values and to focus on an individual, rather than a group, identity.

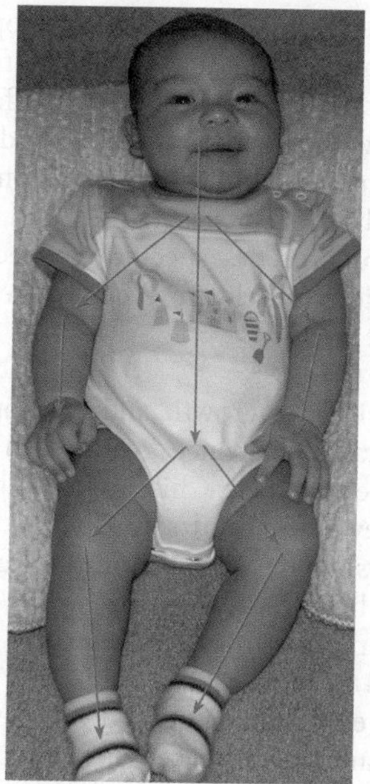

Fig. 33-1 Directional trends in growth.

These patterns, or trends, are universal and basic to all human beings, but each human being accomplishes these in a manner and time unique to that individual.

Directional Trends

Growth and development proceed in regular, related directions or gradients and reflect the physical development and maturation of neuromuscular functions (Fig. 33-1). The first pattern is the cephalocaudal, or head-to-tail, direction. The head end of the organism develops first and is large and complex, whereas the lower end is small and simple and takes shape at a later period. The physical evidence of this trend is most apparent during the period before birth, but it also applies to postnatal behavior development. Infants achieve structural control of the head before they have control of the trunk and extremities, hold their back erect before they stand, use their eyes before their hands, and gain control of their hands before they have control of their feet.

Second, the proximodistal, or near-to-far, trend applies to the midline-to-peripheral concept. A conspicuous illustration is the early embryonic development of limb buds, which is followed by rudimentary fingers and toes. In the infant, shoulder control precedes mastery of the hands, the whole hand is used as a unit before the fingers can be manipulated, and the central nervous system develops more rapidly than the peripheral nervous system.

These trends or patterns are bilateral and appear symmetric—each side develops in the same direction and at the same rate as the other. For some of the neurologic functions, this symmetry is only external because of unilateral differentiation of function at an early stage of postnatal development. For example, by the age of approximately 5 years the child has demonstrated a decided preference for the use of one hand over the other, although previously either one had been used.

The third trend, differentiation, describes development from simple operations to more complex activities and functions. From broad, global patterns of behavior, more specific,

evolve Critical Thinking Exercise—Growth Trends During Infancy

refined patterns emerge. All areas of development (physical, mental, social, and emotional) proceed in this direction. Through the process of development and differentiation, early embryonal cells with vague, undifferentiated functions progress to an immensely complex organism composed of highly specialized and diversified cells, tissues, and organs. Generalized development precedes specific or specialized development; gross, random muscle movements take place before fine muscle control.

Sequential Trends

In all dimensions of growth and development there is a definite, predictable sequence, with each child normally passing through every stage. Children crawl before they creep, creep before they stand, and stand before they walk. Later facets of the personality are built on the early foundation of trust. The child babbles, then forms words and, finally, sentences; writing emerges from scribbling.

Developmental Pace

Although development has a fixed, precise order, it does not progress at the same rate or pace. There are periods of accelerated growth and periods of decelerated growth in both total body growth and the growth of subsystems. Not all areas develop at the same pace. When a spurt occurs in one area such as gross motor, minimal advances may take place in language, fine motor, or social skills. Once the gross motor skill has been achieved, then development focus will shift to another area. The rapid growth before and after birth gradually levels off throughout early childhood. Growth is relatively slow during middle childhood, markedly increases at the beginning of adolescence, and levels off in early adulthood. Each child grows at his or her own pace. Distinct differences are observed between children as they reach developmental milestones.

Sensitive Periods

There are limited times during the process of growth when the organism will interact with a particular environment in a specific manner. Periods termed *critical, sensitive, vulnerable,* and *optimal* are those times in the life of an organism when it is more susceptible to positive or negative influences.

The quality of interactions during these sensitive periods determines whether the effects on the organism will be beneficial or harmful. For example, physiologic maturation of the central nervous system is influenced by adequacy and timing of contributions from the environment such as stimulation and nutrition. The first 3 months of prenatal life are sensitive periods for physical growth of the fetus.

Psychologic development also appears to have sensitive periods, when an environmental event has maximal influence on the developing personality. For example, primary socialization occurs during the first year when the infant makes the initial social attachments and establishes a basic trust in the world. A warm relationship with a parent figure is fundamental to a healthy personality. The same concept might be applied to readiness for learning skills such as toilet training or reading. In these instances there appears to be an opportune time when the skill is best learned.

Individual Differences

Each child grows in his or her own unique and personal way. Great individual variation exists in the age at which developmental milestones are reached. The sequence is predictable; the exact timing is not. Rates of growth vary, and measurements are defined in terms of ranges to allow for individual differences. Some children are fast growers, others are moderate, and some are slower to reach maturity. Periods of fast growth, such as the pubescent growth spurt, may begin earlier or later in some children than in others. Children may grow fast or slowly during the spurt and may finish sooner or later than other children. Gender is an influential factor because girls seem to be more advanced in physiologic growth at all ages.

Biologic Growth and Physical Development

As children grow, their external dimensions change. These changes are accompanied by corresponding alterations in structure and function of internal organs and tissues that reflect the gradual acquisition of physiologic competence. Each part has its own rate of growth, which may be directly related to alterations in the child's size (e.g., the heart rate). Skeletal muscle growth approximates whole body growth; brain, lymphoid, adrenal, and reproductive tissues follow distinct and individual patterns (Fig. 33-2). When growth deficiency has a secondary cause, such as severe illness or acute malnutrition, recovery from the illness or establishment of an adequate diet will produce a dramatic acceleration of the growth rate that usually continues until the child's individual growth pattern is resumed.

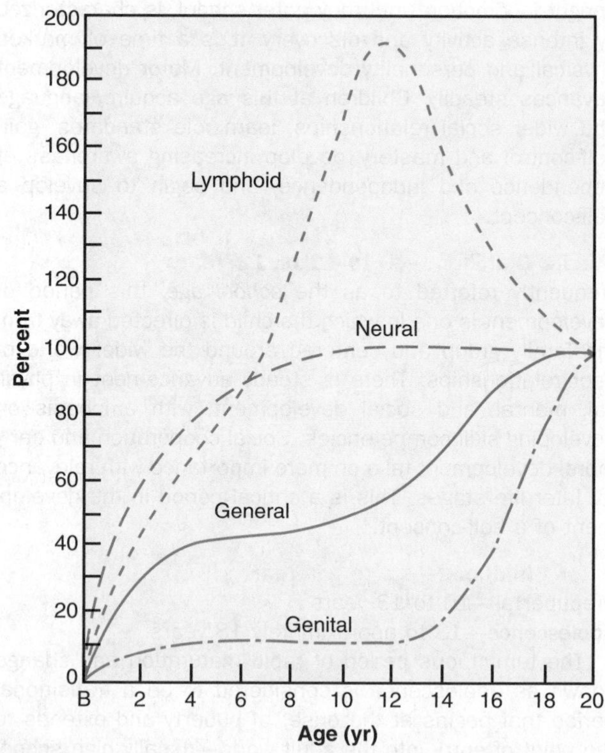

Fig. 33-2 Growth rates for the body as a whole and three types of tissues. *Lymphoid:* thymus, lymph nodes, and intestinal lymph masses. *Neural:* brain, dura, spinal cord, optic apparatus, and head dimensions. *General:* body as a whole; external dimension; and respiratory, digestive, renal, circulatory, and musculoskeletal systems. *B,* Birth. (From Jackson JA, Patterson DG, Harris RE: *The measurement of man*, Minneapolis, 1930, University of Minnesota Press.)

External Proportions

Variations in the growth rate of different tissues and organ systems produce significant changes in body proportions during childhood. The cephalocaudal trend of development is most evident in total body growth as indicated by these changes. During fetal development the head is the fastest-growing body part, and at 2 months of gestation the head constitutes 50% of total body length. During infancy growth of the trunk predominates; the legs are the most rapidly growing part during childhood; in adolescence, the trunk once again elongates. In the newborn infant the lower limbs are one third the total body length but only 15% of the total body weight; in the adult the lower limbs constitute one half of the total body height and 30% or more of the total body weight. As growth proceeds, the midpoint in head-to-toe measurements gradually descends from a level even with the umbilicus at birth to the level of the symphysis pubis at maturity.

Biologic Determinants of Growth and Development

The most prominent feature of childhood and adolescence is physical growth (Fig. 33-3). Throughout development various tissues in the body undergo changes in size, composition, and structure. In some tissues the changes are continuous (e.g., bone growth and dentition); in others, significant alterations occur at specific stages (e.g., appearance of secondary sex characteristics). When these measurements are compared with standardized norms, a child's developmental progress can be determined with a high degree of confidence (Table 33-1). Growth in children with Down syndrome differs from that in other children. They have slower growth velocity between 6 months and 3 years and then again in adolescence. Puberty occurs earlier, and they achieve shorter stature. This population of patients are frequent users of the health care system, often with multiple providers, and benefit from the use of the Down syndrome growth chart to monitor their growth (Cronk et al, 1988; Myrelid et al, 2002).

Linear growth, or height, occurs almost entirely as a result of skeletal growth and is considered a stable measurement of general growth. Growth in height is not uniform throughout life but ceases when maturation of the skeleton is complete. The maximum rate of growth in length occurs before birth, but the newborn continues to grow at a rapid, though slower, rate.

NURSING ALERT Double the child's height at the age of 2 years to estimate how tall he or she may be as an adult.

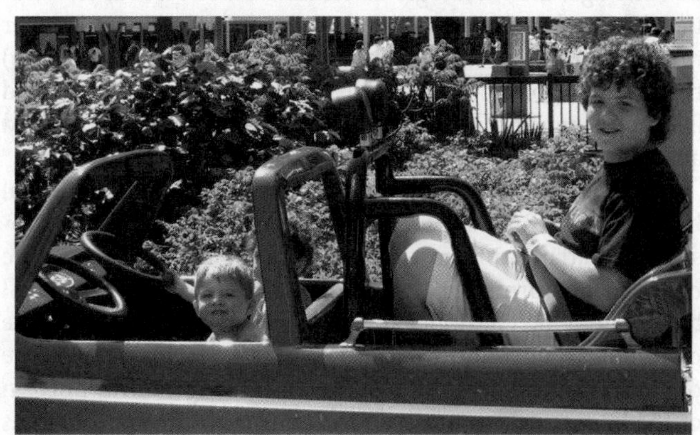

Fig. 33-3 Changes in body proportions occur dramatically during childhood.

Table 33-1 General Trends in Height and Weight Gain During Childhood

AGE GROUP	WEIGHT*	HEIGHT*
Infants		
Birth-6 mo	Weekly gain–140-200 g (5-7 oz) Birth weight doubles by end of first 4-7 mo†	Monthly gain–2.5 cm (1 inch)
6-12 mo	Weight gain–85-140 g (3-5 oz) Birth weight triples by end of first year	Monthly gain–1.25 cm (0.5 inch) Birth length increases by approximately 50% by end of first year
Toddlers	Birth weight quadruples by age 2½	Height at age 2 yr is approximately 50% of eventual adult height Gain during second year–about 12 cm (4.7 inches) Gain during third year–about 6-8 cm (2.4-3.1 inches)
Preschoolers	Yearly gain–2-3 kg (4.4-6.6 lb)	Birth length doubles by age 4 yr Yearly gain–5-7.5 cm (2-3 inches)
School-age children	Yearly gain–2-3 kg (4.4-6.6 lb)	Yearly gain after age 7 yr–5 cm (2 inches) Birth length triples by about age 13
Pubertal growth spurt		
Females–10-14 yr	Weight gain–7-25 kg (15.4-55 lb) Mean–17.5 kg (38.6 lb)	Height gain–5-25 cm (2-10 inches); approximately 95% of mature height achieved by onset of menarche or skeletal age of 13 yr Mean–20.5 cm (8 inches)
Males–11-16 yr	Weight gain–7-30 kg (15.4-66 lb) Mean–23.7 kg (52.2 lb)	Height gain–10-30 cm (4-12 inches); approximately 95% of mature height achieved by skeletal age of 15 yr Mean–27.5 cm (11 inches)

*Yearly height and weight gains for each age group represent averaged estimates from a variety of sources.
†Jung FE, Czajka-Narins DM: Birth weight doubling and tripling times: an updated look at the effects of birth weight, sex, race, and type of feeding, *Am J Clin Nutr* 42:182-189, 1985.

At birth, weight is more variable than height and is, to a greater extent, a reflection of the intrauterine environment. The average newborn weighs from 3175 to 3400 g (7 to 7.5 lb). In general, the birth weight doubles by 4 to 7 months of age and triples by the end of the first year. By the age of 2 to 2½ years the birth weight usually quadruples. After this point the "normal" rate of weight gain, just as the growth in height, assumes a steady annual increase of approximately 2 to 2.75 kg (4.4 to 6 lb) per year until the adolescent growth spurt.

Both bone age determinants and state of dentition are used as indicators of development. Because both are discussed elsewhere, neither is elaborated here (see next section for bone age; see also Chapters 36 and 38 for dentition).

Skeletal Growth and Maturation

The most accurate measure of general development is skeletal or bone age, the radiologic determination of osseous maturation. Skeletal age appears to correlate more closely with other measures of physiologic maturity (such as onset of menarche) than with chronologic age or height. Bone age is determined by comparing the mineralization of ossification centers and advancing bony form to age-related standards.

Bone formation begins during the second month of fetal life when calcium salts are deposited in the intercellular substance (matrix) to form calcified cartilage first and then true bone. Bone formation exhibits some differences. In small bones the bone continues to form in the center and cartilage continues to be laid down on the surfaces. In long bones the ossification begins in the diaphysis (the long central portion of the bone) and continues in the epiphysis (the end portions of the bone). Between the diaphysis and the epiphysis, an epiphyseal cartilage plate (or growth plate) unites with the diaphysis by columns of spongy tissue, the metaphysis. Active growth in length takes place in the epiphyseal growth plate. Interference with this growth site by trauma or infection can result in deformity.

The first centers of ossification appear in the 2-month-old embryo, and at birth the number is approximately 400, about half the number at maturity. New centers appear at regular intervals during the growth period and provide the basis for assessment of bone age. Postnatally the earliest centers to appear (at 5 to 6 months of age) are those of the capitate and hamate bones in the wrist. Therefore radiographs of the hand and wrist provide the most useful areas for screening to determine skeletal age, especially before age 6 years. These centers appear earlier in girls than in boys.

Nurses must understand that the growing bones of children possess many unique characteristics. Bone fractures occurring at the growth plate may be difficult to discover and may significantly affect subsequent growth and development (Urbanski & Hanlon, 1996). Factors that may influence skeletal muscle injury rates and types in children and adolescents include (Kaczander, 1997; Caine, DiFiori, & Maffulli, 2006):

- Less use of protective sports equipment for children
- Less emphasis on conditioning, especially flexibility
- In adolescents, fractures being more common than ligamentous ruptures because of the rapid growth rate of the physeal (segment of tubular bone that is concerned mainly with growth) zone of hypertrophy

Neurologic Maturation

In contrast to other body tissues, which grow rapidly after birth, the nervous system grows proportionately more rapidly before birth. Two periods of rapid brain cell growth occur during fetal life: a dramatic increase in the number of neurons between 15 and 20 weeks of gestation and another increase at 30 weeks, which extends to 1 year of age. The rapid growth of infancy continues during early childhood and then slows to a more gradual rate during later childhood and adolescence.

Postnatal growth consists of increasing the amount of cytoplasm around the nuclei of existing cells, increasing the number and intricacy of communications with other cells, and advancing their peripheral axons to keep pace with expanding body dimensions. This allows for increasingly complex movement and behavior. Neurophysiologic changes also provide the foundation for language, learning, and behavior development. Neurologic or electroencephalographic development is sometimes used as an indicator of maturational age in the early weeks of life.

Lymphoid Tissues

Lymphoid tissues contained in the lymph nodes, thymus, spleen, tonsils, adenoids, and blood lymphocytes follow a growth pattern unlike that of other body tissues. These tissues are small in relation to total body size, but they are well developed at birth. They increase rapidly to reach adult dimensions by 6 years of age and continue to grow. At about age 10 to 12 years they reach a maximum development that is approximately twice their adult size. This is followed by a rapid decline to stable adult dimensions by the end of adolescence.

Development of Organ Systems

All tissues and organ systems undergo changes during development. Some are striking; others are subtle. Many have implications for assessment and care. Because the major importance of these changes relates to their dysfunction, the developmental characteristics of various systems and organs are discussed throughout the book as they relate to these areas. Physical characteristics and physiologic changes that vary with age are included in age group descriptions.

Physiologic Changes

Physiologic changes that take place in all organs and systems are discussed as they relate to dysfunction. Other changes such as pulse and respiratory rates and blood pressure are an integral part of physical assessment (see Chapter 34). In addition, changes occur in basic functions, including metabolism, temperature, and patterns of sleep and rest.

Metabolism

The rate of metabolism when the body is at rest (basal metabolic rate, or BMR) demonstrates a distinctive change throughout childhood. Highest in the newborn infant, the BMR closely relates to the proportion of surface area to body mass, which changes as the body increases in size. In both sexes the proportion decreases progressively to maturity. The BMR is slightly higher in boys at all ages and further increases during pubescence over that in girls.

The rate of metabolism determines the child's caloric requirements. The basal energy requirement is about 108 kcal/kg of body weight in infancy and decreases to 40 to 45 kcal/kg at maturity. Water requirements throughout life remain at approximately 1.5 ml/calorie of energy expended. Children's energy needs vary considerably at different ages and with changing circumstances. The energy requirement to build tissue steadily decreases with age, following the general growth curve; however, energy needs vary with the individual child and may be considerably higher. For short periods (e.g., during strenuous exercise) and more prolonged periods (e.g., illness), the needs can be very high.

Temperature

Body temperature, reflecting metabolism, decreases over the course of development. Thermoregulation is one of the most important adaptation responses of the infant during the transition from intrauterine to extrauterine life. In the healthy neonate hypothermia can result in several negative metabolic consequences such as hypoglycemia, elevated bilirubin levels, and metabolic acidosis. Skin-to-skin care, also referred to as *kangaroo care,* is an effective way to prevent neonatal hypothermia in infants. Unclothed, diapered infants are placed on the parent's bare chest after birth, promoting thermoregulation and attachment (Galligan, 2006). After the unstable regulatory ability in the neonatal period, heat production steadily declines as the infant grows into childhood. Individual differences of 0.5° to 1° F are normal, and occasionally a child normally displays an unusually high or low temperature. Beginning at approximately 12 years of age, girls display a temperature that remains relatively stable, whereas the temperature in boys continues to fall for a few more years. Females maintain a temperature slightly above that of males throughout life.

Even with improved temperature regulation, infants and young children are highly susceptible to temperature fluctuations. Body temperature responds to changes in environmental temperature and is increased with active exercise, crying, and emotional stress. Infections can cause a higher and more rapid temperature increase in infants and young children than in older children. In relation to body weight, an infant produces more heat per unit than adolescents. Consequently, during active play or when heavily clothed, an infant or small child is likely to become overheated.

Sleep and Rest

Sleep, a protective function in all organisms, allows for repair and recovery of tissues after activity. As in most aspects of development, there is wide variation among individual children in the amount and distribution of sleep at various ages. As children mature, there is a change in the total time they spend in sleep and the amount of time they spend in deep sleep.

Newborn infants sleep much of the time that is not occupied with feeding and other aspects of their care. As infants grow older, the total time spent in sleep gradually decreases, they remain awake for longer periods, and they sleep longer at night. For example, the length of a sleep cycle increases from approximately 50 to 60 minutes in the newborn infant to approximately 90 minutes in adolescence (Anders, Sadeh, & Appareddy, 2005). During the latter part of the first year, most children sleep through the night and take one or two naps during the day. By the time they are 12 to 18 months old, most children have eliminated the second nap. After age 3 years the child has usually given up daytime naps, except in cultures in which an afternoon nap or siesta is customary. Sleep time declines slightly from ages 4 to 10 and then increases somewhat during the pubertal growth spurt.

The quality of sleep changes as children mature. As children develop through adolescence, their need for sleep does not decline, but their opportunity for sleep may be affected by social, activity, and academic schedules. The time spent in deep, restful sleep increases from 50% in infancy to 80% in the older child.

Temperament

Temperament is defined as "the manner of thinking, behaving, or reacting characteristic of an individual" (Chess & Thomas, 1999) and refers to the way in which a person deals with life. From the time of birth, children exhibit marked individual differences in the way they respond to their environment and the way others, particularly the parents, respond to them and their needs. A genetic basis has been suggested for some differences in temperament. Nine characteristics of temperament have been identified through interviews with parents (Box 33-2). Temperament refers to behavioral tendencies, not to discrete behavioral acts. There are no implications of good or bad. Most children can be placed into one of three common categories based on their overall pattern of temperamental attributes:

BOX 33-2 Attributes of Temperament

Activity—Level of physical motion during activity such as sleep, eating, play, dressing, and bathing

Rhythmicity—Regularity in the timing of physiologic functions such as hunger, sleep, and elimination

Approach-withdrawal—Nature of initial responses to new stimuli such as people, situations, places, foods, toys, and procedures (**Approach** responses are positive and are displayed by activity or expression; **withdrawal** responses are negative expressions or behaviors.)

Adaptability—Ease or difficulty with which the child adapts or adjusts to new or altered situations

Threshold of responsiveness (sensory threshold)—Amount of stimulation, such as sounds or light, required to evoke a response in the child

Intensity of reaction—Energy level of the child's reactions, regardless of quality or direction

Mood—Amount of pleasant, happy, friendly behavior compared with unpleasant, unhappy, crying, unfriendly behavior exhibited by the child in various situations

Distractibility—Ease with which a child's attention or direction of behavior can be diverted by external stimuli

Attention span and persistence—Length of time a child pursues a given activity (**attention**) and the continuation of an activity in spite of obstacles (**persistence**)

1. **The easy child**—Easy-going children are even tempered, are regular and predictable in their habits, and have a positive approach to new stimuli. They are open and adaptable to change and display a mild to moderately intense mood that is typically positive. Approximately 40% of children fall into this category.
2. **The difficult child**—Difficult children are highly active, irritable, and irregular in their habits. Negative withdrawal responses are typical, and they require a more structured environment. These children adapt slowly to new routines, people, or situations. Mood expressions are usually intense and primarily negative. They exhibit frequent periods of crying, and frustration often produces violent tantrums. This group represents about 10% of children.
3. **The slow-to-warm-up child**—Slow-to-warm-up children typically react negatively and with mild intensity to new stimuli and, unless pressured, adapt slowly with repeated contact. They respond with only mild but passive resistance to novelty or changes in routine. They are inactive and moody but show only moderate irregularity in functions. Fifteen percent of children demonstrate this temperament pattern.

Thirty-five percent of children either have some, but not all, of the characteristics of one of the categories or are inconsistent in their behavioral responses. Many normal children demonstrate this wide range of behavioral patterns.

Significance of Temperament

Observations indicate that children who display the difficult or slow-to-warm-up patterns of behavior are more vulnerable to the development of behavior problems in early and middle childhood. Any child can develop behavior problems if there is dissonance between the child's temperament and the environment. Demands for change and adaptation that are in conflict with the child's capacities can become excessively stressful. However, authorities emphasize that it is not the children's temperament patterns that place them at risk; it is the degree of fit between children and their environment, specifically their parents, that determines the degree of vulnerability. The potential for optimum development exists when environmental expectations and demands fit with the individual's style of behavior and the parents' ability to navigate this period (Chess & Thomas, 1999) (see Growth Failure [Failure to Thrive], Chapter 36).

Early identification of temperament provides a useful tool for caregivers in anticipating probable areas of difficulty or risk associated with development. For example, "difficult" children may be prone to colic in infancy, active children require more vigilance to prevent injury, and school entry requires different approaches for children with different temperaments.

Research indicates that irritable and inadaptable infants can raise doubts in mothers about their competence (Beck, 1996). Additional research indicates that a child's temperament can affect parent-child interactions and influence the parents' self-esteem, marital harmony, mood, and overall satisfaction as parents (Carey, 1998). Studies on the relationship between temperament and the ability to perform a task successfully (mastery motivation) have found that infants with high mastery are more cooperative and less difficult (Morrow & Camp, 1996). Principles that nurses can use in direct patient care and anticipatory guidance are listed in Box 33-3.

BOX 33-3 Activities to Promote Mastery Motivation

- Provide inconspicuous assistance during play.
- Share pleasure with infant in accomplishments.
- Do not give immediate assistance during tasks.
- Do not interrupt infant during tasks.
- Let infant initiate activities.
- Limit controlling feedback during play.
- Provide audio and visually responsive toys.
- Provide early kinesthetic stimulation (picking up, rocking).

From Morrow JD, Camp BW: Mastery motivation and temperament of 7-month-old infants, *Pediatr Nurs* 22(3):211-217, 1996.

Development of Personality and Mental Function

Personality and cognitive skills develop in much the same manner as biologic growth—new accomplishments build on previously mastered skills. Many aspects depend on physical growth and maturation. This is not a comprehensive account of the multiple facets of personality and behavior development. Many aspects are integrated with later discussion of the child's emotional and social development at various ages. Table 33-2 summarizes some of the developmental theories.

Theoretic Foundations of Personality Development

Psychosexual Development (Freud)

According to Freud, all human behavior is energized by psychodynamic forces, and this psychic energy is divided among three components of personality: the id, the ego, and the superego. The *id*, the *unconscious mind*, is the inborn component that is driven by instincts. The id obeys the pleasure principle of immediate gratification of needs, regardless of whether the object or action can actually do so. The *ego*, the *conscious mind*, serves the reality principle. It functions as the conscious or controlling self that is able to find realistic means for gratifying the instincts while blocking the irrational thinking of the id. The superego, the conscience, functions as the moral arbitrator and represents the ideal. It is the mechanism that prevents individuals from expressing undesirable instincts that might threaten the social order.

Freud considered the sexual instincts to be significant in the development of the personality. However, he used the term *psychosexual* to describe any *sensual pleasure*. During childhood certain regions of the body assume a prominent psychologic significance as the source of new pleasures and new conflicts gradually shifts from one part of the body to another at particular stages of development:

Oral stage (birth to 1 year)—During infancy the major source of pleasure seeking is centered on oral activities

Table 33-2 Summary of Personality, Cognitive, and Moral Development Theories

PSYCHOSEXUAL (FREUD)	PSYCHOSOCIAL (ERIKSON)	COGNITIVE (PIAGET)	MORAL JUDGMENT (KOHLBERG)	SPIRITUAL (FOWLER)
I. Infancy—Birth–1 Yr				
Oral-sensory	Trust vs. mistrust	Sensorimotor (birth–2 yr)		Undifferentiated
II. Toddlerhood—1-3 Yr				
Anal-urethral	Autonomy vs. shame and doubt	Preoperational thought, preconceptual phase (transductive reasoning [e.g., specific to specific]) (2-4 yr)	Preconventional (premoral) level Punishment and obedience orientation	Intuitive-projective
III. Early Childhood—3-6 Yr				
Phallic-locomotion	Initiative vs. guilt	Preoperational thought, intuitive phase (transductive reasoning) (4-7 yr)	Preconventional (premoral) level Naive instrumental orientation	Mythical-literal
IV. Middle Childhood—6-12 Yr				
Latency	Industry vs. inferiority	Concrete operations (inductive reasoning and beginning logic) (7-11 yr)	Conventional level Good-boy, nice-girl orientation Law-and-order orientation	Synthetic-convention
V. Adolescence—12-18 Yr				
Genitality	Identity vs. role confusion	Formal operations (deductive and abstract reasoning) (11-15 yr)	Postconventional or principled level Social-contract orientation Universal ethical principle orientation	Individuating-reflexive

such as sucking, biting, chewing, and vocalizing. Children may prefer one of these over the others, and the preferred method of oral gratification can provide some indication of the personality they develop.

Anal stage (1 to 3 years)—Interest during the second year of life centers in the anal region as sphincter muscles develop and children are able to withhold or expel fecal material at will. At this stage the climate surrounding toilet training can have lasting effects on children's personalities.

Phallic stage (3 to 6 years)—During the phallic stage the genitalia become an interesting and sensitive area of the body. Children recognize differences between the sexes and become curious about the dissimilarities. This is the period around which the controversial issues of the Oedipus and Electra complexes, penis envy, and castration anxiety are centered.

Latency period (6 to 12 years)—During the latency period children elaborate on previously acquired traits and skills. Physical and psychic energy are channeled into acquisition of knowledge and vigorous play.

Genital stage (age 12 and older)—The last significant stage begins at puberty with maturation of the reproductive system and production of sex hormones. The genital organs become the major source of sexual tensions and pleasures, but energies are also invested in forming friendships and preparing for marriage.

Psychosocial Development (Erikson)

The most widely accepted theory of personality development is that advanced by Erikson (1963). Although built on Freudian theory, it is known as *psychosocial* development and emphasizes a healthy personality as opposed to a pathologic approach. Erikson also uses the biologic concepts of critical periods and epigenesis, describing key conflicts or core problems that the individual strives to master during critical periods in personality development. Successful completion or mastery of each of these core conflicts is built on the satisfactory completion or mastery of the previous stage.

Each psychosocial stage has two components—the favorable and the unfavorable aspects of the core conflict—and progress to the next stage depends on resolution of this conflict. No core conflict is ever mastered completely but remains a recurrent problem throughout life. No life situation is ever secure. Each new situation presents the conflict in a new form. For example, when children who have satisfactorily achieved a sense of trust encounter a new experience (e.g., hospitalization), they must again develop a sense of trust in those responsible for their care in order to master the situation. Erikson's life-span approach to personality development consists of eight stages; however, only the first five relating to childhood are included here:

1. **Trust vs. mistrust (birth to 1 year)**—The first and most important attribute to develop for a healthy personality is basic *trust.* Establishment of basic trust dominates the first year of life and describes all of the child's satisfying experiences at this age. Corresponding to Freud's oral stage, it is a time of "getting" and "taking in" through all the senses. It exists only in relation to something or someone; therefore consistent, loving care by a mothering person is essential for development of trust. *Mistrust* develops when trust-promoting experiences are deficient or lacking or when basic needs are inconsistently or inadequately met. Although shreds of mistrust are sprinkled throughout the personality, from a basic trust in parents stems trust in the world, other people, and oneself. The result is *faith* and *optimism.*
2. **Autonomy vs. shame and doubt (1 to 3 years)**—Corresponding to Freud's anal stage, the problem of *autonomy* can be symbolized by the holding on and letting go of the sphincter muscles. The development

of autonomy during the toddler period is centered on children's increasing ability to control their bodies, themselves, and their environment. They want to do things for themselves, using their newly acquired motor skills of walking, climbing, and manipulating and their mental powers of selecting and decision making. Much of their learning is acquired by imitating the activities and behavior of others. Negative feelings of *doubt* and *shame* arise when children are made to feel small and self-conscious, when their choices are disastrous, when others shame them, or when they are forced to be dependent in areas in which they are capable of assuming control. The favorable outcomes are *self-control* and *willpower.*

3. **Initiative vs. guilt (3 to 6 years)**—The stage of *initiative* corresponds to Freud's phallic stage and is characterized by vigorous, intrusive behavior; enterprise; and a strong imagination. Children explore the physical world with all their senses and powers (Fig. 33-4). They develop a conscience. No longer guided only by outsiders, they have an inner voice that warns and threatens. Children sometimes undertake goals or activities that are in conflict with those of parents or others, and being made to feel that their activities or imaginings are bad produces a sense of *guilt.* Children must learn to retain a sense of initiative without impinging on the rights and privileges of others. The lasting outcomes are *direction* and *purpose.*
4. **Industry vs. inferiority (6 to 12 years)**—The stage of *industry* is the latency period of Freud. Having achieved the more crucial stages in personality development, children are ready to be workers and producers. They want to engage in tasks and activities that they can carry through to completion; they need and want real achievement. Children learn to compete and cooperate with others, and they learn the rules. It is a decisive period in their social relationships with others. Feelings of *inadequacy* and *inferiority* may develop if too much is expected of them or if they believe that they cannot measure up to the standards set for them by others. The ego quality developed from a sense of industry is *competence.*
5. **Identity vs. role confusion (12 to 18 years)**—Corresponding to Freud's genital period, the development of *identity* is characterized by rapid and marked physical changes. Previous trust in their bodies is shaken, and children become overly preoccupied with the way they appear in the eyes of others as compared with their own self-concept. Adolescents struggle to fit the roles they have played and those they hope to play with the current roles and fashions adopted by their peers, to integrate their concepts and values with those of society, and to come to a decision regarding an occupation. Inability to solve the core conflict results in *role confusion.* The outcome of successful mastery is *devotion* and *fidelity* to others and to values and ideologies.

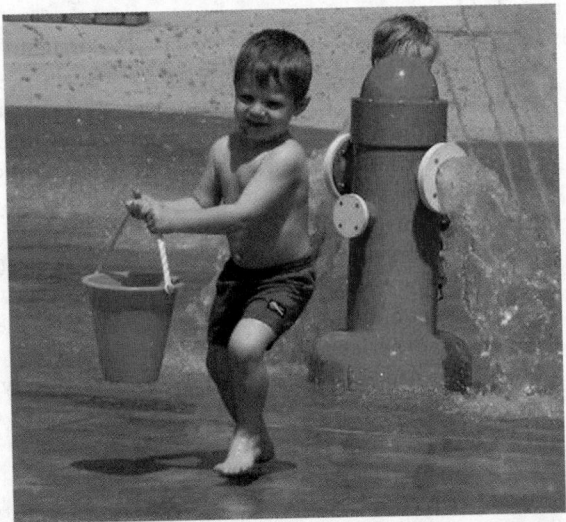

Fig. 33-4 The stage of initiative is characterized by physical activity and imagination while children explore the physical world around them.

Theoretic Foundations of Mental Development

The term *cognition* refers to the process by which developing individuals become acquainted with the world and the objects it contains. Children are born with inherited potentials for intellectual growth, but they must develop that potential through interaction with the environment. By assimilating information through the senses, processing it, and acting on it, they come to understand relationships between objects and between themselves and their world. With cognitive development, children acquire the ability to reason abstractly, to think in a logical manner, and to organize intellectual functions or performances into higher-order structures. Language, morals, and spiritual development emerge as cognitive abilities advance.

Cognitive Development (Piaget)

Cognitive development consists of age-related changes that occur in mental activities. The best-known theory regarding children's thinking, and a more comprehensive developmental theory than those already described, was developed by the Swiss psychologist Jean Piaget (1969). According to Piaget, intelligence enables individuals to make adaptations to the environment that increase the probability of survival, and through their behavior individuals establish and maintain equilibrium with the environment.

Piaget (1969) proposed three stages of reasoning: (1) intuitive, (2) concrete operational, and (3) formal operational. When they enter the stage of concrete logical thought at about age 7 years, children are able to make logical inferences, classify, and deal with quantitative relationships about concrete things. Not until adolescence are they able to reason abstractly with any degree of competence. Each stage is derived from and builds on the accomplishments of the previous stage in a continuous, orderly process. The course of intellectual development is both maturational and invariant and is divided into the following stages (ages are approximate):

Sensorimotor (birth to 2 years)—The sensorimotor stage of intellectual development consists of six substages (see pp. 958-960 and 1019-1021) that are governed by sensations in which simple learning takes place.

Children progress from reflex activity through simple repetitive behaviors to imitative behavior. They develop a sense of cause and effect as they direct behavior toward objects. Problem solving is primarily by trial and error. They display a high level of curiosity, experimentation, and enjoyment of novelty and begin to develop a sense of self as they are able to differentiate themselves from their environment. They become aware that objects have *permanence*—that an object exists even though it is no longer visible. Toward the end of the sensorimotor period, children begin to use language and representational thought.

Preoperational (2 to 7 years)—The predominant characteristic of the preoperational stage of intellectual development is egocentrism, which in this sense does not mean selfishness or self-centeredness, but the inability to put oneself in the place of another. Children interpret objects and events not in terms of general properties, but in terms of their relationships or their use to them. They are unable to see things from any perspective other than their own; they cannot see another's point of view, nor can they see any reason to do so (see Cognitive Development, Chapter 38).

Preoperational thinking is concrete and tangible. Children cannot reason beyond the observable, and they lack the ability to make deductions or generalizations. Thought is dominated by what they see, hear, or otherwise experience. However, they are increasingly able to use language and symbols to represent objects in their environment. Through imaginative play, questioning, and other interactions, they begin to elaborate concepts and to make simple associations between ideas. In the latter stage of this period their reasoning is *intuitive* (e.g., the stars have to go to bed just as children do), and they are only beginning to deal with problems of weight, length, size, and time. Reasoning is also *transductive*—because two events occur together, they cause each other, or knowledge of one characteristic is transferred to another (e.g., all women with big bellies have babies).

Concrete operations (7 to 11 years)—At this age thought becomes increasingly logical and coherent. Children are able to classify, sort, order, and otherwise organize facts about the world to use in problem solving. They develop a new concept of permanence—*conservation* (see Cognitive Development [Piaget], Chapter 39); that is, they realize that physical factors such as volume, weight, and number remain the same even though outward appearances are changed. They are able to deal with a number of different aspects of a situation simultaneously. They do not have the capacity to deal in abstraction; they solve problems in a concrete, systematic fashion based on what they can perceive. Reasoning is *inductive.* Through progressive changes in thought processes and relationships with others, thought becomes less self-centered. They can consider points of view other than their own. Thinking has become socialized.

Formal operations (11 to 15 years)—Formal operational thought is characterized by adaptability and flexibility. Adolescents can think in abstract terms, use abstract symbols, and draw logical conclusions from a set of observations. For example, they can solve the following question: If *A* is larger than *B,* and *B* is larger than *C,* which symbol is the largest? (The answer is *A*.) They can make hypotheses and test them; they can consider abstract, theoretic, and philosophic matters. Although they may confuse the ideal with the practical, most contradictions in the world can be dealt with and resolved.

Language Development

Children are born with the mechanism and capacity to develop speech and language skills. However, they do not speak spontaneously. The environment must provide a means for them to acquire these skills. Speech requires intact physiologic structure and function (including respiratory, auditory, and cerebral) plus intelligence, a need to communicate, and stimulation.

The rate of speech development varies from child to child and is directly related to neurologic competence and cognitive development. Gesture precedes speech, and in this way a small child communicates satisfactorily. As speech develops, gesture recedes but never disappears entirely. Research suggests that infants can learn sign language before vocal language and that it may enhance the development of vocal language (Thompson et al, 2007). At all stages of language development, children's comprehension vocabulary (what they understand) is greater than their expressed vocabulary (what they can say), and this development reflects a continuing process of modification that involves both the acquisition of new words and the expansion and refinement of word meanings previously learned. By the time they begin to walk, children are able to attach a name to objects and persons.

The first parts of speech used are nouns, sometimes verbs (e.g., "go"), and combination words (such as "bye-bye"). Responses are usually structurally incomplete during the toddler period, although the meaning is clear. Next they begin to use adjectives and adverbs to qualify nouns, followed by adverbs to qualify nouns and verbs. Later, pronouns and gender words are added (such as "he" and "she"). By the time children enter school, they are able to use simple, structurally complete sentences that average five to seven words.

Moral Development (Kohlberg)

Children also acquire moral reasoning in a developmental sequence. Moral development, as described by Kohlberg (1968), is based on cognitive developmental theory and consists of the following three major levels, each of which has two stages:

1. **Preconventional level**—The preconventional level of moral development parallels the preoperational level of cognitive development and intuitive thought. Culturally oriented to the labels of good/bad and right/wrong, children integrate these in terms of the physical or pleasurable consequences of their actions. At first children determine the goodness or badness of an action in terms of its consequences. They avoid

punishment and obey without question those who have the power to determine and enforce the rules and labels. They have no concept of the basic moral order that supports these consequences. Later, children determine that the right behavior consists of that which satisfies their own needs (and sometimes the needs of others). Although elements of fairness, give and take, and equal sharing are evident, they are interpreted in a practical, concrete manner without loyalty, gratitude, or justice.

2. **Conventional level**—At the conventional stage children are concerned with conformity and loyalty. They value the maintenance of family, group, or community expectations regardless of consequences. Behavior that meets with approval and pleases or helps others is considered good. One earns approval by being "nice." Obeying the rules, doing one's duty, showing respect for authority, and maintaining the social order are the correct behaviors. This level is correlated with the stage of concrete operations in cognitive development.
3. **Postconventional, autonomous, or principled level**—At the postconventional level the individual has reached the cognitive stage of formal operations. Correct behavior tends to be defined in terms of general individual rights and standards that have been examined and agreed on by the entire society. Although procedural rules for reaching consensus become important, with emphasis on the legal point of view, there is also emphasis on the possibility for changing law in terms of societal needs and rational considerations.

The most advanced level of moral development is one in which self-chosen ethical principles guide decisions of conscience. These are abstract and ethical but universal principles of justice and human rights with respect for the dignity of persons as individuals. It is believed that few persons reach this stage of moral reasoning.

Spiritual Development (Fowler)

Spiritual beliefs are closely related to the moral and ethical portion of the child's self-concept and, as such, must be considered as part of the child's basic needs assessment. Children need to have meaning, purpose, and hope in their lives. Also, the need for confession and forgiveness is present, even in very young children. Extending beyond religion (an organized set of beliefs and practices), spirituality affects the whole person: mind, body, and spirit. Fowler (1981) has identified seven stages in the development of faith, four of which are closely associated with and parallel cognitive and psychosocial development in childhood:

Stage 0: Undifferentiated—This stage of development encompasses the period of infancy during which children have no concept of right or wrong, no beliefs, and no convictions to guide their behavior. However, the beginnings of a faith are established with the development of basic trust through their relationships with the primary caregiver.

Stage 1: Intuitive-projective—Toddlerhood is primarily a time of imitating the behavior of others. Children imitate the religious gestures and behaviors of others without comprehending any meaning or significance to the activities. During the preschool years children assimilate some of their parents' values and beliefs. Parental attitudes toward moral codes and religious beliefs convey to children what they consider to be good and bad. Children still imitate behavior at this age and follow parental beliefs as part of their daily lives rather than through an understanding of their basic concepts.

Stage 2: Mythical-literal—Through the school-age years, spiritual development parallels cognitive development and is closely related to children's experiences and social interaction. Most have a strong interest in religion during the school-age years. They accept the existence of a deity, and petitions to an omnipotent being are important and expected to be answered; good behavior is rewarded, and bad behavior is punished. Their developing conscience bothers them when they disobey. They have a reverence for thoughts about spiritual matters and are able to articulate their faith. They may even question its validity.

Stage 3: Synthetic-convention—As children approach adolescence, however, they become increasingly aware of spiritual disappointments. They recognize that prayers are not always answered (at least on their own terms) and may begin to abandon or modify some religious practices. They begin to reason, to question some of the established parental religious standards, and to drop or modify some religious practices.

Stage 4: Individuating-reflexive—Adolescents become more skeptical and begin to compare their parents' religious standards with those of others. They attempt to determine which to adopt and incorporate into their own set of values. They also begin to compare religious standards with the scientific viewpoint. It is a time of searching rather than reaching conclusions. Adolescents are uncertain about many religious ideas but will not achieve profound insights until late adolescence or early adulthood.

Development of Self-Concept

Self-concept is how an individual describes himself or herself. The term *self-concept* includes all the notions, beliefs, and convictions that constitute an individual's self-knowledge and that influence that individual's relationships with others. It is not present at birth but develops gradually as a result of unique experiences within the self, with significant others, and with the realities of the world. However, an individual's self-concept may or may not reflect reality.

In infancy the self-concept is primarily an awareness of one's independent existence learned in part as a result of social contacts and experiences with others. The process becomes more active during toddlerhood as children explore the limits of their capacities and the nature of their impact on others. School-age children are more aware of differences among people, are more sensitive to social pressures, and become more preoccupied with issues of self-criticism and self-evaluation. During early adolescence children focus more on physical and emotional changes taking place and on peer acceptance. Self-concept is crystallized during later adolescence as young people organize their self-concept around a set of values, goals, and competencies acquired throughout childhood.

Body Image

A vital component of self-concept, *body image* refers to the subjective concepts and attitudes that individuals have toward their own bodies. It consists of the physiologic (the perception of one's physical characteristics), psychologic (values and attitudes toward the body, abilities, and ideals), and social nature of one's image of self (the self in relation to others). All three components interrelate with one another. Body image is a complex phenomenon that evolves and changes during the process of growth and development. Any actual or perceived deviation from the "norm" (no matter how this is interpreted) is cause for concern. The extent to which a characteristic, defect, or disease affects children's body image is influenced by the attitudes and behavior of those around them.

The significant others in their lives exert the most important and meaningful impact on children's body image. Labels that are attached to them (such as "skinny," "pretty," or "fat") or body parts (such as "ugly mole," "bug eyes," or "yucky skin") are incorporated into the body image. Because they lack the understanding of deviations from the physical standard or norm, children notice prominent differences in others and unwittingly make rude or cruel remarks about such minor deviations as large or widely spaced front teeth, large or small eyes, moles, or extreme variations in height.

Infants receive input about their bodies through self-exploration and sensory stimulation from others. As they begin to manipulate their environment, they become aware of their bodies as separate from others. Toddlers learn to identify the various parts of their bodies and are able to use symbols to represent objects. Preschoolers become aware of the wholeness of their bodies and discover the genitalia. Exploration of the genitalia and the discovery of differences between the sexes become important. They have only a vague concept of internal organs and function (Stuart & Laraia, 2000).

School-age children begin to learn about internal body structure and function and become aware of differences in body size and configuration. They are highly influenced by the cultural norms of society and current fads. Children whose bodies deviate from the norm are often criticized or ridiculed. Adolescence is the age when children become most concerned about the physical self. The unfamiliar body changes, and the new physical self must be integrated into the self-concept. Adolescents face conflicts over what they see and what they visualize as the ideal body structure. Body image formation during adolescence is a crucial element in the shaping of identity, the psychosocial crisis of adolescence.

Self-Esteem

Self-esteem is the value that an individual places on himself or herself and refers to an overall evaluation of oneself (Willoughby, King, & Polatajko, 1996). Self-esteem is described as the affective component of the self, whereas self-concept is the cognitive component; however, the two terms are almost indistinguishable and are often used interchangeably.

The term *self-esteem* refers to a personal, subjective judgment of one's worthiness derived from and influenced by the social groups in the immediate environment and individuals' perceptions of how they are valued by others. Self-esteem changes with development. Highly egocentric toddlers are unaware of any difference between competence and social approval. On the other hand, preschool and early school-age children are increasingly aware of the discrepancy between their competencies and the abilities of more advanced children. Being accepted by adults and peers outside the family group becomes more important to them. Positive feedback enhances their self-esteem; they are vulnerable to feelings of worthlessness and are anxious about failure.

As children's competencies increase and they develop meaningful relationships, their self-esteem rises. Their self-esteem is again at risk during early adolescence when they are defining an identity and sense of self in the context of their peer group. Unless children are continually made to feel incompetent and of little worth, a decrease in self-esteem during vulnerable times is only temporary. Children assess the following aspects of themselves in forming an overall evaluation of their self-esteem (Sieving & Zirbel-Donisch, 1990):

Competence—How adequate are my cognitive, physical, and social skills?

Sense of control—How well can I complete tasks needed to produce desired actions? Is someone or something specific vs. luck or chance responsible for my successes and failures?

Moral worth—How closely do my actions and behaviors meet moral standards that have been set?

Worthiness of love and acceptance—How worthy am I of love and acceptance from parents, other significant adults, siblings, and peers?

Factors that influence the formation of a child's self-esteem include (1) the child's temperament and personality, (2) abilities and opportunities available to accomplish age-appropriate developmental tasks, (3) how significant others interact with the child, and (4) social roles assumed and the expectations surrounding these roles (see also Psychosocial History, Chapter 34).

Role of Play in Development

Through the universal medium of play, children learn what no one can teach them. They learn about their world and how to deal with this environment of objects, time, space, structure, and people. They learn about themselves operating within that environment—what they can do, how to relate to things and situations, and how to adapt themselves to the demands society makes on them. Play is the *work* of the child. In play, children continually practice the complicated, stressful processes of living, communicating, and achieving satisfactory relationships with other people.

Classification of Play

From a developmental point of view, patterns of children's play can be categorized according to content and social character. In both there is an additive effect; each builds on past accomplishments, and some element of each is maintained throughout life. At each stage in development the new predominates.

Content of Play

The content of play involves primarily the physical aspects of play, although social relationships cannot be ignored. The content of play follows the directional trend of the simple to the complex:

Social-affective play—Play begins with social-affective play, wherein infants take pleasure in relationships with people. As adults talk, touch, nuzzle, and in various ways elicit a response from an infant, the infant soon learns to provoke parental emotions and responses with such behaviors as smiling, cooing, or initiating games and activities. The type and intensity of the adult behavior with children vary among cultures.

Sense-pleasure play—Sense-pleasure play is a nonsocial stimulating experience that originates from without. Objects in the environment—light and color, tastes and odors, textures and consistencies—attract children's attention, stimulate their senses, and give pleasure. Pleasurable experiences are derived from handling raw materials (water, sand, food), from body motion (swinging, bouncing, rocking), and from other uses of senses and abilities (smelling, humming) (Fig. 33-5).

Skill play—After infants have developed the ability to grasp and manipulate, they persistently demonstrate and exercise their newly acquired abilities through skill play, repeating an action over and over. The element of sense-pleasure play is often evident in practicing a new ability, but frequently the determination to conquer the elusive skill produces pain and frustration (e.g., learning to get into a play car) (Fig. 33-6).

Unoccupied behavior—In unoccupied behavior children are not playful but focusing their attention momentarily on anything that strikes their interest. Children daydream, fiddle with clothes or other objects, or walk aimlessly. This role differs from that of onlookers, who actively observe the activity of others.

Dramatic, or pretend, play—One of the vital elements in children's process of identification is dramatic play, also known as *symbolic* or *pretend play.* It begins in late infancy (11 to 13 months) and is the predominant form of play in the preschool child. After children begin to invest situations and people with meanings and to attribute affective significance to the world, they can pretend and fantasize almost anything. By acting out events of daily life, children learn and practice the roles and identities modeled by the members of their family and society. Children's toys, replicas of the tools of society, provide a medium for learning about adult roles and activities that may be puzzling and frustrating to them. Interacting with the world is one way children get to know it. The simple, imitative, dramatic play of the toddler, such as using the telephone, driving a car, or rocking a doll, evolves into more complex, sustained dramas of the preschooler, which extend beyond common domestic matters to the wider aspects of the world and the society, such as playing police officer, storekeeper, teacher, or nurse. Older children work out elaborate themes, act out stories, and compose plays.

Games—Children in all cultures engage in games alone and with others. Solitary activity involving games begins as very small children participate in repetitive activities and progress to more complicated games that challenge their independent skills such as puzzles, solitaire, and computer or video games. Very young children participate in simple, *imitative games* such as pat-a-cake and peekaboo. Preschool children learn and enjoy *formal games*, beginning with ritualistic, self-sustaining games such as ring-around-a-rosy and London Bridge. With the exception of some simple board games, preschool children do not engage in *competitive games*. Preschoolers hate to lose and will try to cheat, want to change rules, or demand exceptions and opportunities to change their moves. School-age children and adolescents enjoy competitive games, including cards, checkers, and chess, and physically active games such as baseball.

Fig. 33-5 Children derive pleasure from handling raw materials.

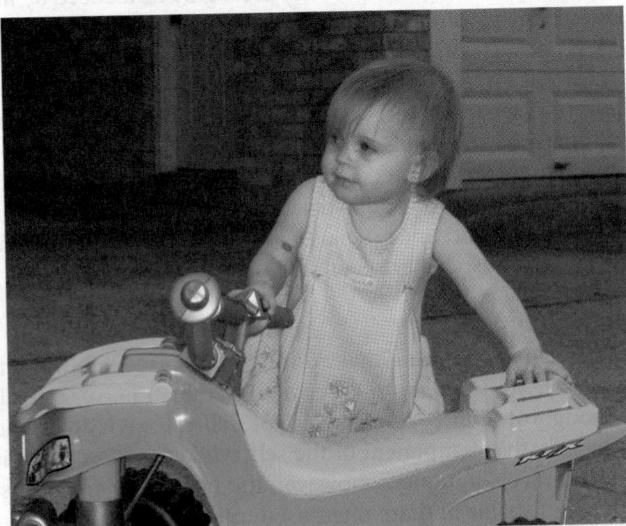

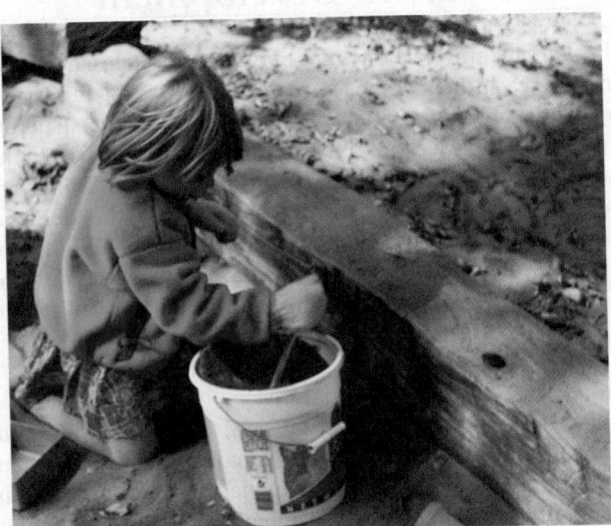

Fig. 33-6 After infants develop new skills to grasp and manipulate, they begin to conquer new abilities such as getting on a play motorcycle.

Social Character of Play

The play interactions of infancy are between the child and an adult. Children continue to enjoy the company of adults but are increasingly able to play alone. As age advances, interaction with age-mates increases in importance and becomes an essential part of the socialization process. Through interaction, highly egocentric infants, unable to tolerate delay or interference, ultimately acquire concern for others and the ability to delay gratification or even to reject gratification at the expense of another. A pair of toddlers will engage in considerable combat because their personal needs cannot tolerate delay or compromise. By the time they reach age 5 or 6 years, children are able to arrive at a compromise or make use of arbitration, usually after they have attempted but failed to gain their own way. Through continued interaction with peers and the growth of conceptual abilities and social skills, children are able to increase participation with others in the following types of play:

Onlooker play—During onlooker play, children watch what other children are doing but make no attempt to enter into the play activity. There is an active interest in observing the interaction of others but no movement toward participating. Watching an older sibling bounce a ball is a common example of the onlooker role.

Solitary play—During solitary play, children play alone with toys different from those used by other children in the same area. They enjoy the presence of other children but make no effort to get close to or speak to them. Their interest is centered on their own activity, which they pursue with no reference to the activities of the others.

Parallel play—During parallel activities children play independently but among other children. They play with toys like those the children around them are using, but as each child sees fit, neither influencing nor being influenced by the other children. Each plays beside, but not with, other children (Fig. 33-7). There is no group association. Parallel play is the characteristic play of toddlers, but it may occur in other groups of any age. Individuals who are involved in a creative craft with each person separately working on an individual project are engaged in parallel play.

Associative play—In associative play, children play together and are engaged in a similar or even identical activity, but there is no organization, division of labor, leadership assignment, or mutual goal. Children borrow and lend play materials, follow each other with wagons and tricycles, and sometimes attempt to control who may or may not play in the group. Each child acts according to his or her own wishes; there is no group goal (Fig. 33-8). For example, two children play with dolls, borrowing articles of clothing from each other and engaging in similar conversation, but neither directs the other's actions or establishes rules regarding the limits of the play session. There is a great deal of behavioral contagion: when one child initiates an activity, the entire group follows the example.

Cooperative play—Cooperative play is organized, and children play in a group *with* other children (Fig. 33-9). They discuss and plan activities for the purposes of accomplishing an end—to make something, to attain a competitive goal, to dramatize situations of adult or group life, or to play formal games. The group is loosely formed, but there is a marked sense of

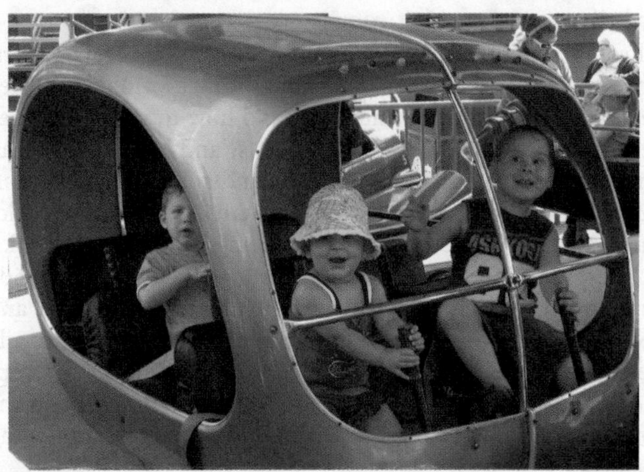

Fig. 33-8 Associative play.

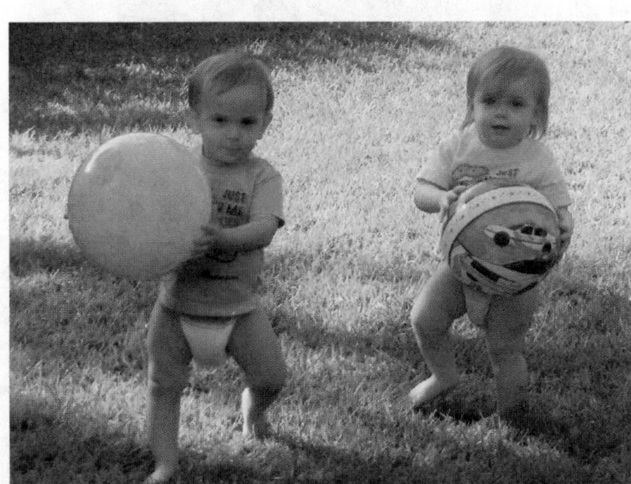

Fig. 33-7 Parallel play.

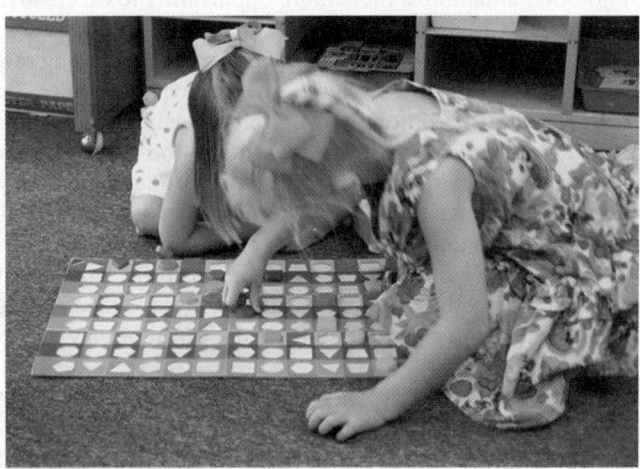

Fig. 33-9 Cooperative play.

belonging or not belonging. The goal and its attainment require organization of activities, division of labor, and role playing. The leader-follower relationship is definitely established, and the activity is controlled by one or two members who assign roles and direct the activity of the others. The activity is organized to allow one child to supplement another's function to complete the goal.

Functions of Play

Sensorimotor Development

Sensorimotor activity is a major component of play at all ages and is the predominant form of play in infancy. Active play is essential for muscle development and serves a useful purpose as a release for surplus energy. Through sensorimotor play, children explore the nature of the physical world. Infants gain impressions of themselves and their world through tactile, auditory, visual, and kinesthetic stimulation. Toddlers and preschoolers revel in body movement and exploration of objects in space. With increasing maturity, sensorimotor play becomes more differentiated and involved. Whereas very young children run for the sheer joy of body movement, older children incorporate or modify the motions into increasingly complex and coordinated activities such as racing, playing games, roller skating, and bicycle riding.

Intellectual Development

Through exploration and manipulation children learn colors, shapes, sizes, textures, and the significance of objects. They learn the significance of numbers and how to use them; they learn to associate words with objects; and they develop an understanding of abstract concepts and spatial relationships, such as *up, down, under,* and *over.* Activities such as puzzles and games help them develop problem-solving skills. Books, stories, films, and collections expand knowledge and provide enjoyment as well. Play provides a means to practice and expand language skills. Through play, children continually rehearse past experiences to assimilate them into new perceptions and relationships. Play helps children comprehend the world in which they live and distinguish between fantasy and reality.

Creativity

In no other situation is there more opportunity to be creative than in play. Children can experiment and try out their ideas in play through every medium at their disposal, including raw materials, fantasy, and exploration. Creativity is stifled by pressure toward conformity; therefore striving for peer approval may inhibit creative endeavors in the school-age or adolescent child. Creativity is primarily a product of solitary activity, yet creative thinking is often enhanced in group settings where listening to others' ideas stimulates further exploration of one's own ideas. After children feel the satisfaction of creating something new and different, they transfer this creative interest to situations outside the world of play.

Self-Awareness

Beginning with active explorations of their bodies and awareness of themselves as separate from the mother, the process of developing a self-identity is facilitated through play activities. Children learn who they are and their place in the world. They become increasingly able to regulate their own behavior, to learn what their abilities are, and to compare their abilities with those of others. Through play, children are able to test their abilities, to assume and try out various roles, and to learn the effect their behavior has on others. They learn the sex role that society expects them to fulfill, as well as approved patterns of behavior and deportment.

Therapeutic Value

Play is therapeutic at any age (Fig. 33-10). In play, children can express emotions and release unacceptable impulses in a socially acceptable fashion. Children are able to experiment and test fearful situations and can assume and vicariously master the roles and positions that they are unable to perform in the world of reality. Children reveal much about themselves in play. Through play, children are able to communicate to the alert observer the needs, fears, and desires that they are unable to express with their limited language skills. Throughout their play, children need the acceptance of adults and their presence to help them control aggression and channel their destructive tendencies.

Moral Value

Although children learn at home and at school those behaviors considered right and wrong in the culture, the interaction with peers during play contributes significantly to their moral training. Nowhere is the enforcement of moral standards as rigid as in the play situation. If they are to be members of the group, children must adhere to the accepted codes of behavior of the culture (e.g., fairness, honesty, self-control, consideration for others). Children soon learn that their peers are less

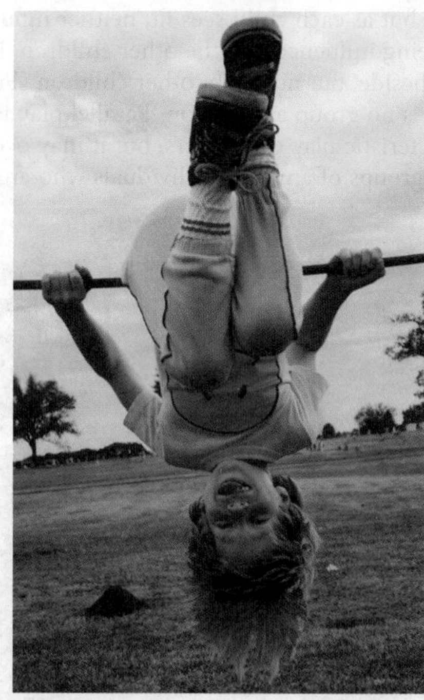

Fig. 33-10 Play is therapeutic at any age and provides a means for release of tension and stress.

tolerant of violations than are adults and that to maintain a place in the play group, they must conform to the group's standards.

Toys

The type of toys chosen by or provided for children can support and enhance the child's development in the areas just described. Although no scientific evidence shows that any toy is necessary for optimal learning, toys offer an opportunity to bring the child and parent together. Research has indicated that a positive parent-child interaction can enhance early childhood brain development (American Academy of Pediatric, Committee on Early Childhood, Adoption, and Dependent Care, 2003). Toys that are small replicas of the culture and its tools help children assimilate into their culture. Toys that require pushing, pulling, rolling, and manipulating teach them about physical properties of the items and help develop muscles and coordination. Rules and the basic elements of cooperation and organization are learned through board games.

Because they can be used in a variety of ways, raw materials with which children can exercise their own creativity and imaginations are sometimes superior to ready-made items. For example, building blocks can be used to construct a variety of structures, to count, and to learn shapes and sizes.

Toy Safety

Selection of toys and play equipment is a joint effort between parents and children, but evaluation of their safety is the adult's responsibility. Government agencies do not inspect and police all toys on the market. Therefore adults who purchase, supervise purchases, or allow children to use play equipment need to evaluate such equipment for its safety and age appropriateness. This includes toys that are gifts or those that are purchased by the children themselves (see Family-Centered Care box). A choke tube tester, about the same diameter as a child's windpipe, can be used to determine whether a toy is small enough to be a choking hazard. Parents should also be alert to notices of toys determined to be defective and recalled by the manufacturers. Parents and health workers can obtain information on a variety of recalled products and can report potentially dangerous toys and child products to the U.S. Consumer Product Safety Commission (CPSC)* or, in Canada, the Canadian Toy Testing Council.†

Selected Factors That Influence Development

Heredity

Inherited characteristics have a profound influence on development. The child's sex, determined by random selection at the time of conception, directs both the pattern of growth and the behavior of others toward the child. In all cultures, attitudes and expectations are shaped by the child's sex. Sex and other hereditary determinants strongly affect the end result of growth and the rate of progress toward it. There is a high correlation between parent and child with regard to traits such as height, weight, and rate of growth. Most physical characteristics, including shape and form of features, body build, and physical peculiarities, are inherited and can influence the way in which children grow and interact with their environment. Many dimensions of personality, such as temperament, activity level, responsiveness, and a tendency toward shyness, are believed to be inherited.

Differences in children's health and vigor may be attributed to hereditary traits. An inherited physical or mental disorder will alter or modify a child's physical or emotional growth and interactions. The extent to which disabling conditions interfere with the child's growth and well-being is considered in relation to numerous disabilities throughout the remainder of the book.

Neuroendocrine Factors

The hypothalamic-pituitary axis produces a number of releasing and inhibitory hormones that influence growth. Probably all hormones affect growth in some fashion. Three hormones—growth hormone, thyroid hormone, and androgens—when given to persons deficient in these hormones, stimulate protein anabolism and thereby produce retention of elements essential for building protoplasm and bony tissue. It appears that each of the hormones that has a significant influence on growth manifests its major effect at a different period of growth (see Chapter 52).

Nutrition

Nutrition is probably the single most important influence on growth. Dietary factors regulate growth at all stages of development, and their effects are exerted in numerous and complex ways. During the rapid prenatal growth period, poor nutrition may influence development from the time of implantation of the ovum until birth. During infancy and childhood the demand for calories is relatively great, as evidenced by the rapid increase in both height and weight. At this time protein and caloric requirements are higher than at almost any period of postnatal development. As the growth rate slows, with its concomitant decrease in metabolism, there is a corresponding reduction in caloric and protein requirements (see Table 33-2).

Growth is uneven during the periods of childhood between infancy and adolescence, when there are plateaus and small growth spurts. The child's appetite fluctuates in response to these variations until the turbulent growth spurt of adolescence, when adequate nutrition is extremely important but may be subject to numerous emotional influences. Adequate nutrition is closely related to good health throughout life, and an overall improvement in nourishment is evidenced by the gradual increase in size and early maturation of children in this century (see Community Focus box).

Interpersonal Relationships

Relationships with significant others play a critical role in development, particularly in emotional, intellectual, and per-

CPSC hotline: 800-638-2772; www.cpsc.gov (assistance is also available in Spanish).

†*1973 Baseline Road, Ottawa ON K2C 0C7, Canada; 613-228-3155; fax: 613-228-3242;* www.toy-testing.org.

FAMILY-CENTERED CARE

Toy Safety*

Selection

Select toys that suit the skills, abilities, and interests of children.

Select toys that are safe for the specific child; look for a label that indicates the intended age group. Toys that are safe for one age may not be safe for another.

For infants, toddlers, and all children who still mouth objects, avoid toys with small parts that may pose a fatal choking or aspiration hazard. Toys in this category are usually labeled, "Not recommended for children under 3 years."

For infants avoid toys with strings or cords that are 7 inches or longer because they may cause strangulation.

For all children younger than 8 years avoid electric toys with heating elements.

For children younger than 5 years avoid arrows or darts.

Check for safety labels such as "flame retardant" or "flame resistant."

Select toys durable enough to survive rough play; look for sturdy construction such as tightly secured eyes, nose, or any small parts.

Select toys light enough that they will not cause harm if one falls on a child.

Look for toys with smooth, rounded edges. Avoid toys with sharp edges that can cut or that have sharp points. Points on the inside of the toy can puncture the skin if the toy is broken.

Avoid toys with any shooting or throwing objects that can injure eyes. This includes toys with which other missiles such as sticks or pebbles might be used as substitutes for the intended projectiles.

Arrows and darts used by children should have blunt tips and be manufactured from resilient materials; make certain the tips are securely attached.

Make certain that materials in toys are nontoxic.

Avoid toys that make loud noises that might damage a child's hearing. Even some squeaking toys are too loud when held close to the ear.

If selecting caps for cap guns, look for the label required by federal law to be on boxes or packages of caps, which states: "Warning—Do not fire closer than 1 foot to the ear. Do not use indoors."

If selecting a toy gun, be certain that the barrel or the entire gun is brightly colored to avoid being mistaken for a real gun.

BB guns or pellet rifles should not be given to children under the age of 16.

Electric toys should be labeled UL, which means they have met the safety standards of the Underwriters Laboratories.

Check toy instructions for clarity. They should be clear to an adult and, when appropriate, to the child.

Supervision

Maintain a safe play environment.

Remove and discard plastic wrappings on toys immediately; they could suffocate a child.

Remove large toys, bumper pads, and boxes from playpens; an adventuresome child can use such items as a means of climbing or falling out.

Set ground rules for play.

Supervise young children closely during play.

Teach children how to use toys properly and safely.

Instruct older children to keep their toys away from younger brothers, sisters, and friends.

Keep children who are playing with riding toys away from stairs, hills, traffic, and swimming pools.

Establish and enforce rules regarding protective gear.

- Insist that children wear helmets when using bicycles, skateboards, or in-line skates.
- Insist that children wear gloves and wrist, elbow, and knee pads when using skateboards or in-line skates.

Instruct children on electrical safety.

- Teach children the proper way to unplug an electric toy—pull on the plug, not the cord.
- Teach children to beware of electrical appliances and even electrically operated playthings; often children are unfamiliar with the hazards of electricity in association with water.

Teach children the safe use of utensils or other items that under certain circumstances can cause injury—scissors, knives, needles, heating elements, loops, long string, or cord.

Maintenance

Inspect old and new toys regularly for breakage, loose parts, and other potential hazards.

Look for jagged or sharp edges or broken parts that might constitute a choking hazard.

Check movable parts to make certain they are attached securely to the toys; sometimes pieces that are safe when attached to the toy become a danger when detached.

Examine all outdoor toys regularly for rust and weak or sharp parts that could become a danger to a child.

Check electrical cords and plugs for cracked or fraying parts.

Maintain toys in good repair, without signs of possible hazards such as sharp edges, splinters, weak seams, or rust.

Make repairs immediately, or discard out of reach of children.

Sand sharp wooden toys or splintered surfaces so they are smooth.

Use only paint labeled "nontoxic" to repaint toys, toy boxes, or children's furniture.

Storage

Provide a safe place for children to store toys, and teach them how to store toys safely to prevent accidental injury from stepping, tripping, or falling on a toy.

Select a toy chest or toy box that is ventilated, is free of self-locking devices that could trap a child inside, and has a lid designed not to pinch a child's fingers or fall on a child's head.

To avoid entrapment and suffocation, containers other than toy chests used for storage purposes should be fitted with spring-loaded support devices if they have a hinged lid.

Playthings meant for older children and adults should be safely stowed away on high shelves, in locked closets, or in other areas unavailable to younger children.

*Another helpful resource is *Toy safety: guidelines for parents* from American Academy of Pediatrics, Division of Publications, 141 Northwest Point Blvd., Elk Grove Village, IL 60007-1098; *www.aap.org*.

COMMUNITY FOCUS

Healthy Food Choices

Current research indicates that new lower-fat recipes in school lunch programs are well accepted by children (Matvienko, 2007). However, less-healthy foods are still more available than more-healthy foods in our nation's schools (Delva, O'Malley, & Johnston, 2007).

sonality development. Not only do the quality and quantity of contacts with other persons exert an influence on the growing child, but the widening range of contacts is essential to learning and developing a healthy personality.

The mothering person is unquestionably the single most influential person during early infancy. This person is the one who meets the infant's basic needs of food, warmth, comfort, and love. He or she stimulates the child's senses and facilitates his or her expanding capacities. Through this person the child learns to trust the world and feel secure to venture in increasingly wider relationships.

Generally the parents are most influential in helping the child to assume sex-role identification. Parents define and reinforce acceptable sex-role behavior and provide sex-appropriate role models for the child. In the absence of a sex-role model in the family setting, the child may adopt some characteristics of the opposite-sex parent or sibling. Frequently the child identifies with a teacher or other significant person of the same sex.

Siblings are children's first peers, and the way in which they learn to relate to each other affects later interactions with peers outside the family group. The sphere of persons from whom children seek approval widens to include other members of their family, their peers, and, to a lesser extent, other authority figures (e.g., teachers). The increasing importance of the peer group in determining the behavior of school-age children and adolescents is well documented (Fig. 33-11).

When children fail to have high-quality interpersonal relationships with mothering persons, they experience *emotional deprivation*. The most prominent feature of emotional deprivation, particularly during the first year, is developmental delays. Much of the information regarding the adverse effects of interpersonal influences on development has been acquired through retrospective studies of gross deprivation and trauma. The most notable instances involved homeless infants who were placed in institutions for care. Those infants who did not receive consistent mothering care failed to gain weight even with an adequate diet; were pale, listless, and immobile; and were unresponsive to stimuli such as smiling or cooing that usually elicit a response from the normal infant. If emotional deprivation continues for a sufficient length of time, the child may not survive infancy.

Although the most remarkable examples of emotional deprivation were first recognized among infants in institutions, the term *masked deprivation* has been used to describe children reared in homes in which there is a distorted parent-child relationship or otherwise disordered home environment. Infants do not thrive if the caregiving person is hostile, fearful of handling them, or indifferent to them and their needs. Such children exhibit poor growth even though they are apparently free of physical disease. Growth delays in these children are believed to be caused by a psychologically induced endocrine imbalance that interferes with growth. These same infants and children display "catch-up" growth in a changed environment (see Growth Failure [Failure to Thrive], Chapter 36).

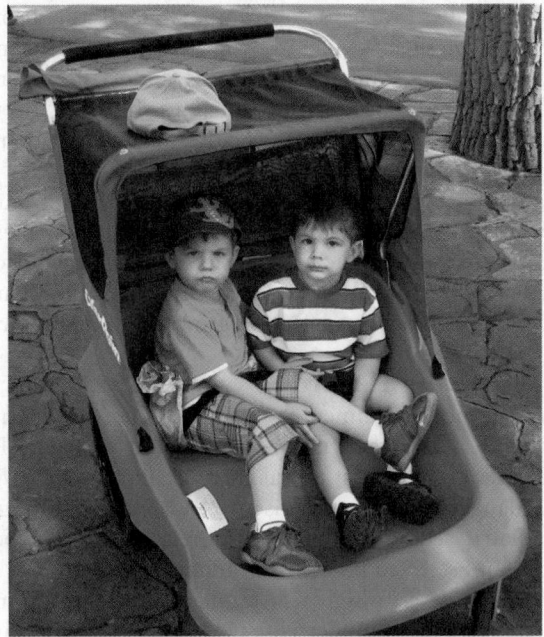

Fig. 33-11 Peers become increasingly important as children develop friendships outside the family group.

Socioeconomic Level

Evidence indicates that the families' socioeconomic level has a significant impact on children's growth and development. At all ages, children from upper- and middle-class families are taller than comparative children of families in the lower socioeconomic strata. The cause of these differences is less definite, although the poorer health and nutrition of lower socioeconomic levels are probably significant factors. Nutritious food sources (especially proteins) are scarce, and other factors (e.g., larger family size and irregularity in eating, sleeping, and exercise) may play a role.

Families from lower socioeconomic groups may lack the knowledge or resources needed to provide the safe, stimulating, and enriched environment that fosters optimum development for children. They may be unable to move from unsafe neighborhoods where drug traffic and drive-by shootings are the norm. The effects on the emotional development of children living under these conditions have been compared with those experienced by children living in war zones.

Disease

Altered growth and development are one of the clinical manifestations in a number of hereditary disorders. Growth impairment is particularly marked in skeletal disorders, such as the various forms of dwarfism and at least one of the chromosomal anomalies (Turner's syndrome). Many of the disorders of metabolism, such as vitamin D–resistant rickets, the mucopolysaccharidoses, and the numerous endocrine disorders, interfere with the normal growth pattern. In other disorders (e.g., Klinefelter's and Marfan syndromes) the tendency is toward the upper percentile of height.

Many chronic illnesses that are associated with varying degrees of growth failure are congenital cardiac anomalies and respiratory disorders such as cystic fibrosis. Any disorder characterized by the inability to digest and absorb body nutrients will have an adverse effect on growth and development.

Environmental Hazards

Hazards in the environment are a source of concern to health care providers and others interested in health and safety. Physical injuries are the most prevalent consequences of environmental dangers, and these are discussed extensively throughout the pediatric section of this book in relation to age, specific hazards, and selected physical disabilities.

Children are at a high risk for harm resulting from the chemical residues of modern life present in the environment. The hazards of these chemical residues relate to their potential carcinogenicity, enzymatic effects, and accumulation (Baum & Shannon, 1995) (see Community Focus box). The harmful agents most often associated with health risks are chemicals and radiation. Water, air, and food contamination from a variety of sources are well documented. Significant causes of exposure are substances in the immediate environment such as lead and asbestos, chemicals secreted in breast milk (especially prescribed drugs and nicotine), and contamination within well-insulated homes (especially from disinfectants or burning of substances that produce toxic fumes). Passive inhalation of tobacco smoke by infants and children is a hazard at all stages of development. The harmful effects of large doses of radiation are unquestioned, although the effects of low-dose or short-term radiation are debatable, as are the safe vs. harmful dosage levels.

COMMUNITY FOCUS

Sun Protection Basics

Skin cancer is increasing in children, accounting for about 4% of pediatric malignancies. Each Global Solar UV Index level has associated precautions, including sunglasses, sunscreens, sun protective clothing, and sun avoidance.

- Children's sunglasses must absorb at least 99% of ultraviolet radiation (UV). Choose sunglasses with the label "Blocks 99% of UV rays," "UV absorption up to 400 nm," "Special purpose," or "Meets American National Standards Institute (ANSI) requirements."
- Allow children to choose their sunglasses. A child who wears prescription glasses should also wear prescription sunglasses.
- Avoid sun exposure between 10 am and 2 pm. High altitude, sand, concrete, snow, and water increase UV exposure.
- Wear wide-brim hats and sun-protective clothing
- Apply an adequate layer of sunscreen, preferably waterproof or water resistant, and reapply at regular intervals.

From Maguire-Eisen M, Rothman K, Demierre M: The ABC's of sun protection, *Dermatol Nurs* 17(6):419-433, 2005.

Stress in Childhood

Defined from both a physiologic and an emotional point of view, essentially *stress* is "an imbalance between environmental demands and a person's coping resources that . . . disrupts the equilibrium of the person" (Masten et al, 1988).

Although all children experience stress, some youngsters appear to be more vulnerable than others. Children's age, temperament, life situation, and state of health affect their vulnerability, reactions, and ability to handle stress. Also, the responses to a stressor can be behavioral, psychologic, or physiologic. It is impossible and undesirable to protect children from stress, but providing them with interpersonal security helps them develop coping strategies for dealing with stress. The concept of an *emotional bank*, in which deposits and withdrawals can be made, can help parents and caregivers maintain a proper perspective regarding the effects of stress and coping. Children with a good, positive balance in the account can tolerate significant withdrawal experiences. For children with a low balance, even a minor withdrawal may bankrupt the account, causing it to be overdrawn.

Parents and other caregivers can try to recognize signs of stress to help children deal with stressors before they become overwhelming. Signs of stress take many forms but are typically the same ones seen in children who are abused (see Chapter 38) or depressed (see Chapter 40). If a number of stressors are imposed on children at the same time, the children are more vulnerable. When a succession of stressors produces an excessive stress load, children may experience a serious change in health or behavior.

It is important that parents and persons working with children understand the nature of childhood stress and ways it can be recognized or anticipated. Caregivers must *listen* to children so they are aware of children's fears and concerns and must let them know that they are important and that what they say matters. Physical contact is comforting and reassuring to children. Simply holding, touching, or hugging children is both relaxing and comforting and facilitates communication. Spending unhurried time with children, taking family outings or vacations, and exposing children to positive influences help build children's strength and security. Supportive interpersonal relationships are essential to children's psychologic well-being.

Coping

Coping refers to a special class of individual reactions to stressors—specifically, a reaction to a stressor that resolves, reduces, or replaces the affective state classified as stressful. *Coping strategies* are the specific ways in which children cope with stressors, as distinguished from *coping styles*, which are relatively unchanging personality characteristics or outcomes of coping (Wachs, 2006). Research indicates that, as children age, they tend toward a more internal locus of control and use more vigilant modes of coping (LaMontagne et al, 1996). Children, like adults, respond to everyday stress by trying to change the circumstances or trying to adjust to circumstances the way they are. Any strategy that provides relaxation is effective in reducing stress, and most children have their own natural methods such as withdrawing, engaging in physical activity, reading, listening to music, working on a project, or taking a nap. Some turn to parents to solve their problems, or they may develop socially unacceptable strategies, such as cheating, stealing, or lying.

Children can be taught stress-reduction techniques to use in coping. First, they must be helped to recognize signs of tension in themselves and then taught any of a variety of appropriate strategies—special exercises, relaxation and breathing, mental imagery, and numerous other simple activities. Also, parents and other caregivers can anticipate possible stress-provoking events and prepare children for coping by role playing a scenario or "talking it through" beforehand. Probably the most useful tool that children can learn is how to solve problems. When children can view any new situation as a problem to be solved and an opportunity to learn, they are not vulnerable to the control of others. It provides them with a sense of mastery over their own lives and reinforces the fact that they have within themselves the ability and information to handle whatever comes their way. Problem-solving skill gives them the confidence to know where and how to seek help when they need it.

Influence of the Mass Media

Media can have an enormous influence on the developing child. There is no doubt that the media provide children with a means for extending their knowledge about the world in which they live and have helped narrow the differences between classes. However, there is growing concern regarding the enormous influence the media can have on the developing child because of the large number of hours spent watching television. The images of risky behavior presented by the media may establish or reinforce teenagers' perceptions of their social environment. Children may identify closely with people or characters portrayed in reading materials, movies, video games, and television programs and commercials.

Reading Materials

Books, newspapers, and magazines are the oldest form of mass media. They contribute to children's competence in almost every respect and also provide enjoyment. Recognition of the impact that reading matter used in the schools has on the value system and socialization processes has prompted reevaluation of the content of textbooks in terms of the biased presentation of male and female role models, the sugar-coated view of life situations, and the biased history of minority groups.

Fairy tales, for generations the mainstay of young children's literature, for a time were condemned for being sexist; violent; and riddled with unfavorable stereotypes, such as the wicked stepmother, dwarves, and physical unattractiveness associated with evil. They are now believed to provide an excellent medium for explaining puzzling and important topics such as death, stepparents, and inner feelings and turmoil. Although they do not provide solutions, fairy tales confront children with emotional predicaments and offer suggestions for dealing with them.

Comic books and other pulp reading material have been popular in every generation, usually at the expense of literature provided by schools, libraries, and parents. Many children have nothing else to read. The easy reading, quick action, and adventure in brief episodes seem to fulfill a need for children who are striving to understand both aggression in others and their own impulses. Reading ability, intelligence, and school adjustment apparently have no relationship to the number and type of comic books read. Most comic books appear to be relatively harmless to the majority of children and may be beneficial. Comic books seem to have only a minor influence on acquisition of beliefs, values, and behaviors. The popularity of this medium has prompted some educators to encourage translations of literature into comic book form to stimulate students' interest in the classics.

Movies

Movies that are not closely bound to reality and often portray an assortment of socially approved behaviors may contribute to children's value systems and provide opportunities for desirable social learning. On the other hand, children, especially adolescents, flock to the "macho" movies and those whose heroes resort to violent resolution of problems, such as karate and wild automobile chases.

Another concern is the plethora of "slasher" and R-rated movies available to children and teenagers in theaters and through cable television and DVDs. The content of movies has changed markedly during the past few decades, with violence and mutilation being major themes. To children who are unable to distinguish between reality and fantasy, these films play on their deepest fears and result in bedtime fears, nightmares, and a fearful view of the world.

Young children can be frightened by some of the movies considered safe for family viewing. For example, *Bambi* can frighten young children, and the villainous witches in *Snow White* and *The Wizard of Oz* are terrifying figures. Also, certain classic children's movies, such as *Snow White* and *Cinderella,* depict stepmothers as evil, destructive persons; such portrayals can have a deleterious effect on children-stepmother relationships or can be confusing to children who have developed a positive relationship with a stepmother.

Movie rating categories are available on the Motion Picture Association website *(www.mpaa.org).*

Television

The medium with the most impact on children in North America today is television, which has become one of the most significant socializing agents in the lives of young children. The content of programs and commercials provides multiple sources for acquiring information, modeling behaviors, and observing value orientations. Besides producing a leveling effect on class differences in general information and vocabulary, television exposes children to a wider variety of topics and events than they encounter in day-to-day life. Television always has time to talk to children and is a form of access to the adult world.

BOX 33-4 Factors That Encourage Learning or Performing Television-Influenced Behaviors

Age—Younger children focus on behaviors rather than on motives or consequences. They view alternatives in a concrete manner, and they are unable to differentiate between central and peripheral plot information.
Identification with characters or situations—Children often imitate behaviors of persons in situations similar to those in their own lives.
Reward and punishment syndrome—Children imitate behaviors they see rewarded or not punished when it is expected. They are less likely to repeat an act they see punished; their attention is immediately attracted when they see an act committed that they know should be punished but is not.
Opportunity to reproduce behaviors—Children imitate behaviors when given the right environment or when violence seems an accepted solution. When children see a situation on television, they use this information when they encounter a similar situation that requires a solution.
Motivation to reproduce behaviors—Children imitate behavior when given the appropriate incentives: expectation of reward or lack of punishment. Some children have self-control; others do not.

Television viewing has a direct impact on child development and behavior. Several studies have found that violence on television and the mass media in general can have a negative influence on the development of unhealthy behaviors and violence in children (Earles et al, 2002; Monsen, 2002; Brown & Witherspoon, 2002). Several factors encourage the learning or performing of television-influenced behaviors (Box 33-4).

Most researchers have concluded that protracted television viewing can have detrimental effects on children. For example, in one study, television viewing was implicated as contributing to irregular sleep schedules in children under 3 years of age (Thompson & Christakis, 2005). Recognizing the negative effects of television viewing, the American Academy of Pediatrics has recommended that children older than age 2 watch less than 2 hours of high-quality television a day and that children younger than 2 years watch no television (American Academy of Pediatrics, Committee on Public Education, 2001a; Certain & Kahn, 2002). However, this warning has not been heeded, with approximately 40% of infants already watching by 3 months of age and the number increasing to 90% by 24 months. Parents reported the three primary reasons they allowed their infants to watch television was because they thought it was educational for them, they thought it was entertaining, and they needed time to get other things done. Parents did watch television with their infants more than half the time (Zimmerman, Christakis, & Meltzoff, 2007).

The passive activity associated with television viewing is frequently accompanied by eating—in many cases, high-calorie snacks. Furthermore, children may expend tremendous mental energy processing the audiovisual messages from television, which may be exhausting and make them less likely to engage in physical activity later. Andersen and colleagues (1998) found that the incidence of body fat increased in direct proportion to the number of hours of television watched by children in the United States; as viewing increased, children were less likely to participate in vigorous physical activities.

In a study to identify children at risk for heart disease, researchers found that more than half of the children with high cholesterol levels watched at least 2 hours of television each day. Using a family history of heart disease or high cholesterol as the screening indicator for cholesterol testing in children, researchers identified three out of four children with high cholesterol levels. When these families were also questioned about the time their children spent watching television, investigators were able to identify 90% of the children with high cholesterol levels by using 2 or more viewing hours as the risk factor (Goldsmith, 1990).

Television programs and commercials, like movies, contain many implicit and explicit messages that promote alcohol consumption, smoking, violence, and promiscuous or unsafe sexual activity. There is evidence documenting a relationship between television viewing and the use of alcohol or tobacco, violence and aggressive behavior, the use of guns to commit violent acts, and early sexual activity (American Academy of Pediatrics, Committee on Public Education, 2001a; Strasburger & Donnerstein, 1999).

Parents can help children evaluate television violence by pointing out the subtleties children miss, such as the aggressor's motives and intentions and the unpleasant consequences the perpetrators suffer as a result of their aggressive acts. Often the consequence is separated from the act by a commercial, and therefore children cannot make the correlation. Parents need to point out that conflicts can be resolved without resorting to violent behavior. They can also stress the program's purpose—primarily entertainment—and explain why they like or dislike something on television (e.g., "This show is trying to tell you that crime does not pay and that if one does wrong, one will go to jail"). Explanations and discussions can take place between shows (with the volume turned down), and young children can learn from both older children and adults. These discussions can be effective when begun early and carried out consistently.

It is especially important to identify at-risk children and control their viewing. House rules that specify the type and amount of television help children understand limits, and recorded selections of appropriate programs can be substituted for less desirable offerings. Parents need to carefully monitor cable and other pay-television programming because these popular options present more uncensored programming. Lockboxes, V-chips, and blocking devices are available for cable receivers to prevent children from viewing programs when unsupervised. Vessey, Yim-Chiplis, and MacKenzie (1998) suggest that parental role modeling may have a more positive influence on the child's behavior than television programming. They further recommend that parents watch television with children and help children understand the difference between their life and habits and those of persons represented on television.

Television is the medium by which most children learn of a natural disaster or act of terrorism. Research on the effects of September 11, 2001, and the Oklahoma City bombing suggests that posttraumatic stress reactions increase with increased exposure to media coverage. Reading, rather than watching the event on television, may lead to better retention of the experience (Pfefferbaum et al, 2003). After September 11, 85% of children in one study reported concerns for their safety and security (Phillips, Prince, & Schiebelhut, 2004). More than half of the children in this study coped by volunteering their time or donating materials for relief teams. In addition, parents should limit the exposure to media coverage of traumatic events, talk to their child about the event, and maintain routines as much as possible.

On the plus side, television has been shown to have a positive influence on children's abilities to deal with a variety of social issues such as divorce, the arrival of a new baby, discrimination, honesty, and helpfulness. Children who view educational programming (such as *Mister Rogers' Neighborhood* and *Sesame Street*) for a long period become more affectionate, considerate, cooperative, and helpful toward their playmates. A systematic review of preschoolers and television found that educational viewing can increase their knowledge, affect their racial attitudes, and increase their imaginative behavior (Thakkar, Garrison, & Christakis, 2006). The ways that minority and ethnic characters are portrayed on television can have an impact on the way the majority culture views minority persons and on the self-image of minority children.

Parents need to supervise the amount and type of television programs their children watch and to teach their children how to watch television (Box 33-5 and Family-Centered Care box).

NURSING ALERT During an assessment, consider that parents may not be aware of how much time their children spend watching television. Parents may also not understand the child's inability to distinguish between the "fantasy" of television and life events (Vessey, Yim-Chiplis, & MacKenzie, 1998).

Nurses and parents can be powerful forces in influencing the media. They can watch closely for an increase in violence and other undesirable programming and complain to sponsors and television stations if they believe it is not appropriate. Good programming can be both educational and entertaining.

BOX 33-5 Five Important Ideas to Teach Children and Adolescents About Television

1. You are smarter than what you see on your television.
2. Television world is not real.
3. Television teaches that some people are more important than others.
4. Television keeps showing the same things over and over again.
5. Somebody is always trying to make money with television.

Modified from Davis J: Five important ideas to teach your children about TV, *Media Values* 59/60:10-14, 1992.

FAMILY-CENTERED CARE

Television Viewing

Provide a positive role model by developing television substitutes such as reading, athletics, physical conditioning, and hobbies.

Construct a time chart of child's activities (homework, television viewing, scheduled outside activities, playing with a friend).

Discuss with child what you both believe to be a balanced set of activities.

At the beginning of each week, select appropriate programs from television schedules.

Allow child to select programs from this approved list.

Limit child's viewing to 2 hours or less per day.

Rule out television at specific times (e.g., before breakfast or on school nights).

Leave the television off at mealtimes.

Make a list of alternative activities (e.g., riding a bicycle, reading a book, or working on a hobby).

Require that child choose to do something from this list before watching television.

Watch programs with child.

Discuss program and commercial content with child:

- Distinguish between the real and the unreal.
- Correlate consequences with actions.
- Point out subtle messages.
- Explore alternatives to aggressive conflict resolution.
- Stress purpose of program (e.g., entertainment, education).
- Explain likes and dislikes.

Turn the television off after the selected program is over.

Remove televisions from children's bedrooms.

Monitor cable and pay television selections; use a lockbox if necessary.

Limit use of television as a safe distraction to potentially stressful times (e.g., keeping the children occupied while the parent gets organized after a difficult day).

Video Games

With the popularity of home gaming systems, children are spending increased hours playing video games. Unfortunately, many of the video games available are violent, portraying virtual crimes and violence against others, particularly women. Video games allow the player to be the aggressor, making an ideal environment for a child to learn violent behavior (American Academy of Pediatrics, Committee on Public Education, 2001b). Although video games come with violence and age ratings, many parents are not aware of or choose to ignore the rating appropriate for their child. The American Academy of Pediatrics (2001b) recommends that health care providers encourage parents to adhere to the game ratings and limit the amount of time spent playing games and watching television to less than 2 hours a day combined.

Video games have two ratings criteria. The front cover has the rating symbol for age appropriateness, and the back cover has a descriptor indicating the elements of the game. The ratings can be found on the Entertainment Software Rating Board website *(www.esrb.org/ratings).*

Internet

The use of computers in both the classroom and household has affected childhood learning and development. Schools offer a wide variety of computer programs that enable children of all ages to broaden their world views. Computers offer the advantage of interactive learning and improved hand-eye coordination. Parents have a wide variety of computer software choices for learning and gaming.

Although computer technology has enhanced many forms of learning and recreation, there are potential dangers to children. The Internet and e-mail have made correspondence and information available to children from around the world in minutes. Social networking sites (e.g., MySpace, FaceBook) provide opportunities for children and adolescents to express themselves through blogs, music, pictures, and videos, and the overwhelming majority of adolescents responsibly use these sites (Hinduja & Patchin, 2008; Ybarra & Mitchell, 2008). Nurses must be involved in encouraging parents to be knowledgeable of their children's Internet activities while providing appropriate learning activities unique to computers. One helpful strategy is to locate the computer in a public area of the home such as the kitchen or family room to enable parents to easily monitor its use.

Key Points

- *Growth* describes a change in quantity and occurs when cells divide and synthesize new proteins.
- *Maturation,* a qualitative change, describes the aging process or an increase in competence and adaptability.
- *Differentiation* refers to biologic processes by which early cells and structures are modified and altered to achieve specific and characteristic physical and chemical properties.
- Development involves change from a lower to a more advanced stage of complexity.
- The five major developmental periods are prenatal, infancy, early childhood, middle childhood, and later childhood (pubescence and adolescence).
- Growth and development proceed in predictable patterns of direction, sequence, and pace.
- The directional trends in growth and development are cephalocaudal, proximodistal, and mass to specific.
- Physical development includes increase in height and weight and changes in body proportion, dentition, and some body tissues.
- The three broad classifications of child temperament are the easy child, the difficult child, and the slow-to-warm-up child.
- The developmental theories most widely used in explaining child growth and development are Freud's psychosexual stages, Erikson's stages of psychosocial development, Piaget's stages of cognitive development, Kohlberg's stages of moral development, and Fowler's stages of spiritual development.
- To develop a positive self-concept, children need recognition for their achievements and the approval of others.
- Through play, children learn about their world and how to relate to objects, people, and situations.
- Play provides a means of development in the areas of sensorimotor and intellectual progress, socialization, creativity, self-awareness, and moral behavior; it serves as a means for release of tension and expression of emotions.
- Growth and development are affected by a variety of conditions and circumstances, including heredity, physiologic function, gender, disease, physical environment, nutrition, and interpersonal relationships.
- Children's vulnerability and reaction to stress depend to a large extent on their age, coping behaviors, and support systems.
- The mass media can be influential in children's learning and behavior.

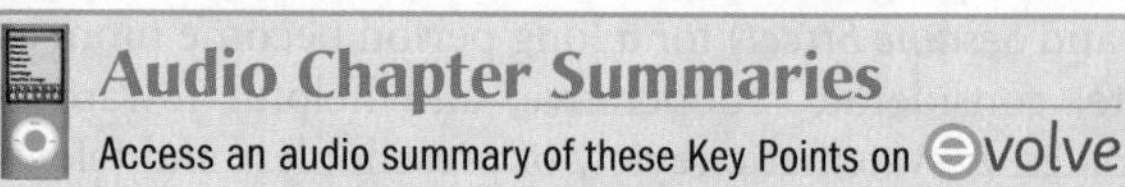
Audio Chapter Summaries
Access an audio summary of these Key Points on evolve

References

American Academy of Pediatrics, Committee on Early Childhood, Adoption, and Dependent Care: Selecting appropriate toys for young children: the pediatrician's role, *Pediatrics* 111(4):911-913, 2003.

American Academy of Pediatrics, Committee on Public Education: Children, adolescents, and television, *Pediatrics* 107(2):423-426, 2001a.

American Academy of Pediatrics, Committee on Public Education: Media violence, *Pediatrics* 108(5):1222-1226, 2001b.

Anders TF, Sadeh A, Appareddy V: Normal sleep in neonates and children. In Sheldon, S, Ferber R, Kryger M (editors): *Principles and practice of sleep medicine in the child,* Philadelphia, 2005, Saunders.

Andersen RE et al: Relationship of physical activity and television watching with body weight and level of fatness among children, *JAMA* 279(12):938-943, 1998.

Baum C, Shannon M: Environmental toxins: cutting the risks, *Contemp Pediatr* 12(7):20-43, 1995.

Beck CT: A meta-analysis of the relationship between postpartum depression and infant temperament, *Nurs Res* 45(4):225-230, 1996.

Brown JD, Witherspoon EM: The mass media and American adolescents' health, *J Adolesc Health* 31(6S):153-170, 2002.

Caine D, DiFiori J, Maffulli N: Physeal injuries in children's and youth sports: reasons for concern? *Br J Sports Med* 40(9):749-760, 2006.

Carey WB: Teaching parents about infant temperament, *Pediatrics* 102(5 Suppl E):1311-1316, 1998.

Certain LK, Kahn RS: Prevalence, correlates, and trajectory of television viewing among infants and toddlers, *Pediatrics* 109(4):634-642, 2002.

Chess S, Thomas A: *Goodness of fit: clinical applications from infancy through adult life*, London, 1999, Routledge.

Cronk C et al: Growth charts for children with Down syndrome: 1 month to 18 years of age, *Pediatrics* 81(1):102-110, 1988.

Delva J, O'Malley PM, Johnston LD: Availability of more-healthy and less-healthy food choices in American schools: a national study of grade, racial/ethnic, and socioeconomic differences, *Am J Prev Med* 33(4 Suppl):S226-S239, 2007.

Earles KA et al: Media influences on children and adolescents: violence and sex, *J Natl Med Assoc* 94(9):797-801, 2002.

Erikson EH: *Childhood and society*, ed 2, New York, 1963, Norton.

Fowler J: *Stages of faith: the psychology of human development and the quest for meaning*, New York, 1981, HarperCollins.

Galligan M: Proposed guidelines for skin to skin treatment of neonatal hypothermia, *MCN* 31(5):298-304, 2006.

Goldsmith M: Youngsters dialing up cholesterol levels? *JAMA* 264(23): 2976, 1990.

Hinduja S, Patchin JW: Personal information of adolescents on the Internet: a quantitative content analysis of MySpace, *J Adolesc* 31(1):125-146, 2008.

Kaczander BI: Pediatric sports medicine: a unique perspective, *Podiatr Manage* 16(2):53-60, 1997.

Kohlberg L: Moral development. In Sills DL (editor): *International encyclopedia of the social sciences*, New York, 1968, Macmillan.

LaMontagne LL et al: Children's preoperative coping and its effects on postoperative anxiety and return to normal activity, *Nurs Res* 45(3):141-147, 1996.

Masten AS et al: Competence and stress in school children: moderating effects of individual and family qualities, *J Child Psychol Psychiatry* 29: 747-764, 1988.

Matvienko O: Impact of a nutrition education curriculum on snack choices of children ages six and seven years, *J Nutr Educ Behav* 39(5):281-285, 2007.

Monsen RB: Children and the media, *J Pediatr Nurs* 17(4):309-310, 2002.

Morrow JD, Camp BW: Mastery motivation and temperament of 7-month-old infants, *Pediatr Nurs* 22(3):211-217, 1996.

Myrelid A et al: Growth charts for Down's syndrome from birth to 18 years of age, *Arch Dis Child* 87(2):97-103, 2002.

Pfefferbaum B et al: Media exposure in children 100 miles from a terrorist bombing, *Ann Clin Psychiatry* 15(1):1-8, 2003.

Phillips D, Prince S, Schiebelhut L: Elementary school children's responses 3 months after the September 11 terrorist attacks: a study in Washington, DC, *Am J Orthopsych* 75(4):509-528, 2004.

Piaget J: *The theory of stages in cognitive development*, New York, 1969, McGraw-Hill.

Seidel HM et al: *Mosby's guide to physical examination*, ed 6, St Louis, 2006, Mosby.

Sieving RE, Zirbel-Donisch ST: Development and enhancement of self-esteem in children, *J Pediatr Health Care* 4(6):290-296, 1990.

Strasburger VC, Donnerstein E: Children, adolescents, and the media: issues and solution, *Pediatrics* 103(1):129-139, 1999.

Stuart GW, Laraia MT: *Principles and practice of psychiatric nursing*, ed 7, St Louis, 2000, Mosby.

Thakkar R, Garrison M, Christakis D: A systematic review for the effects of television viewing by infants and preschoolers, *Pediatrics* 118(5):2025-2031, 2006.

Thompson DA, Christakis DA: The association between television viewing and irregular sleep schedules among children less than 3 years of age, *Pediatrics* 116(4):851-856, 2005.

Thompson R et al: Enhancing early communication through infant sign training, *J Appl Behav Anal* 40(1):15-23, 2007.

Urbanski LF, Hanlon DP: Pediatric orthopedics, *Top Emerg Med* 18(2): 73-90, 1996.

Vessey JA, Yim-Chiplis PK, MacKenzie NR: Effects of television viewing on children's development, *Pediatr Nurs* 23(5):483-486, 1998.

Wachs T: Contributions of temperament to buffering and sensitization processes in children's development, *Ann NY Acad Sci* 1094:28-30, 2006.

Willoughby C, King G, Polatajko H: A therapist's guide to children's self-esteem, *Am J Occup Ther* 50(2):124-132, 1996.

Ybarra ML, Mitchell KJ: How risky are social networking sites? A comparison of places online where youth sexual solicitation and harassment occurs, *Pediatrics* 121(2):e350-357, 2008.

Zimmerman F, Christakis D, Meltzoff A: Television and DVD/video viewing in children younger than 2 years, *Arch Pediatr Adolesc Med* 161: 473-479, 2007.

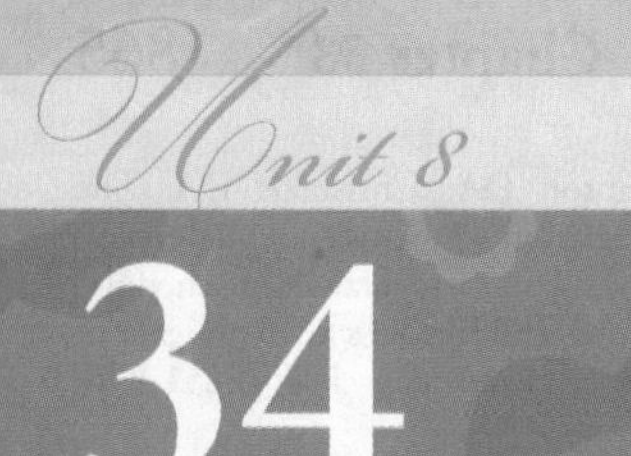

34 Communication, History, Physical, and Developmental Assessment

Learning Objectives

On completion of this chapter the reader will be able to:

- Identify communication strategies for interviewing parents.
- Formulate guidelines for using an interpreter.
- Identify communication strategies for communicating with children of different age groups.
- Describe four communication techniques that are useful with children.
- State the components of a complete health history.
- List three areas that are evaluated as part of nutritional assessment.
- Prepare a child for a physical examination based on his or her developmental needs.
- Perform a comprehensive physical examination in a sequence appropriate to the child's age.
- Recognize expected normal findings for children at various ages.
- Record the physical examination according to the head-to-toe format.

Electronic Resources

Additional information related to the content in Chapter 34 can be found on

evolve the Companion Website at

http://evolve.elsevier.com/Perry/maternal/

- NCLEX Review Questions
- Anatomy Reviews
- Animation—Abdominal Anatomy
- Animation—Cranial Nerves
- Animation—Organ Systems 3-D Tour
- Assessment Video Clips
- Case Study—Communicating with Adolescents
- Case Study—Pediatric Assessment
- Critical Thinking Exercise—Cardiovascular Assessment
- Critical Thinking Exercise—The Interview
- Skill—Communicating with Children
- Skill—Measuring Body Temperature
- Skill—Measuring Physical Growth

Guidelines for Communication and Interviewing

The most widely used method of communicating with parents on a professional basis is the interview process. Unlike social conversation, *interviewing* is a specific form of goal-directed communication. As nurses converse with children and adults, they focus on the individuals to determine the kind of persons they are, their usual mode of handling problems, whether help is needed, and the way they react to counseling. Developing interviewing skills requires time and practice, but following some guiding principles can facilitate this process. An organized approach is most effective when using interviewing skills in patient teaching.

evolve Critical Thinking Exercise—The Interview

Establishing a Setting for Communication

Appropriate Introduction

Introduce yourself to, and ask the name of, each family member who is present. Address parents or other adults by their appropriate titles, such as "Mr." and "Mrs.," unless they specify a preferred name. Record the preferred name on the medical record. Using formal address or their preferred names, rather than using first names or "mother" or "father," conveys respect and regard for the parents or other caregivers (Seidel et al, 2006).

At the beginning of the visit, include children in the interaction by asking them their name, age, and other information. Nurses often direct all questions to adults, even when children are old enough to speak for themselves. This serves to terminate one extremely valuable source of information: the patient. When the child is included, follow the general rules for communicating with children given in the Guidelines box, p. 870.

Assurance of Privacy and Confidentiality

The place where the interview is conducted is almost as important as the interview itself. The physical environment should allow for as much privacy as possible, with distractions, such as interruptions, noise, or other visible activity, kept to a minimum. At times it is necessary to turn off a television or radio. The environment should also have some play provision for young children to keep them occupied during the parent-nurse interview (Fig. 34-1). Parents who are constantly interrupted by their children are unable to concentrate fully and tend to give brief answers to finish the interview as quickly as possible.

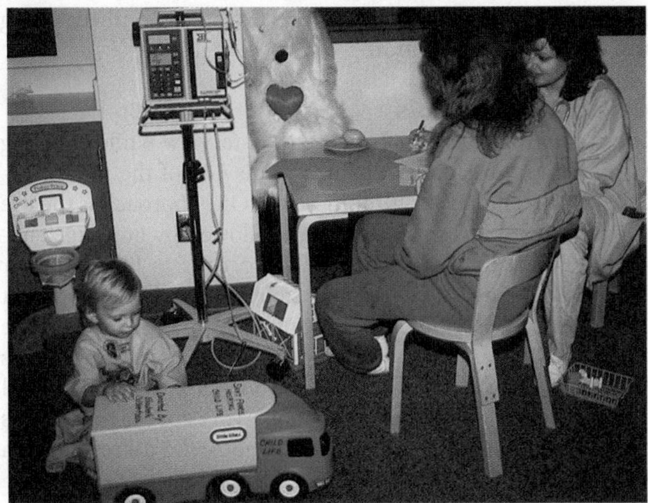

Fig. 34-1 Child plays while nurse interviews parent.

Confidentiality is another essential component of the initial phase of the interview. Since the interview is usually shared with other members of the health team care or the teacher (in the case of students), be certain to inform the family of the limits regarding confidentiality. If confidentiality is a concern in a particular situation, such as when talking to a parent suspected of child abuse or a teenager contemplating suicide, deal with this directly and inform the person that in such instances confidentiality cannot be ensured. However, the nurse judiciously protects information of a confidential nature (Sullivan, 1997).

NURSING ALERT In 2003 the Health Insurance Portability and Accountability Act (HIPAA) was implemented to ensure patient privacy and limit access to sensitive health information. Nurses and students should become familiar with their institution's policy regarding HIPAA compliance.*

Computer Privacy and Applications in Nursing

The use of computer technology to store and retrieve health information has become widespread. The privacy and security of this health information has generated a growing concern throughout the health care community. Any person accessing confidential health information is charged with managing safeguards for disclosure, since violations might incur civil damages.

In 1994 a committee of the Institute of Medicine recommended a national code of fair health information practices. It suggested that health data organizations establish data protection units to develop privacy policies and security practices for manual and automated data processing systems. Technologic safeguards, such as encryption and managerial security procedures, can be applied to computer hardware across a network to ensure protection of individual patient privacy.

Many institutions use computer and information applications in nursing (nursing informatics), such as electronic medical records, to record care and access information. Two important health care applications are record transmission, including facsimile (fax), electronic mail (e-mail), and telemedicine. The telemedicine application is capable of two-way video conferencing, transmission of radiographs, and clinical consultation between remote sites and centralized resources.†

Telephone Triage and Counseling

Nurses are increasingly responsible for assessment of children's symptoms and clinical judgment for further medical care (triage) via telephone report. Most often, health problems are assessed and prioritized according to urgency, and treatment is judiciously provided via telephone services. Successful outcomes are based on the consistency and accuracy of the information provided, and parents are empowered to participate in their child's medical care. Telephone triage care management has increased access to high-quality health care services, and patient satisfaction has significantly improved. Unnecessary emergency department and clinic visits have decreased, saving medical costs and time (with less absence from work) for families in need of health care. The most common telephone triage call is for a fever. Approximately 37% of the triage calls related to fever require emergency care, and nearly 50% benefit from home management (Deadrick & Boggess, 1996).

A well-designed telephone triage program is essential for safe, prompt, and consistent-quality health care (Rutenberg, 2000). Telephone triage is more than "just a phone call," since a child's life is a high price to pay for poorly managed or incompetent telephone assessment skills. Typically, guidelines for telephone triage include asking screening questions; determining when to immediately refer to emergency medical services (dial 911); and determining when to refer to same-day appointments, appointments in 24 to 72 hours, appointments in 4 days or more, or home care (Box 34-1).

Communicating with Families

Communicating with Parents

Although the parent and child are separate and distinct individuals, the nurse's relationship with the child is frequently mediated by the parent, particularly in the case of younger children. For the most part, information about the child is acquired by direct observation or is communicated to the nurse by the parents. Usually it can be assumed that because of the close contact with the child, the parent gives reliable information. Making an assessment of the child requires input from the child (verbal and nonverbal), information from the parent, and the nurse's own observations of the child and interpretation of the relationship between the child and the parent. Counseling and guidance must be directed to the caregiver of infants and small children; when children are old enough to be active participants in their own health maintenance, the parent becomes a collaborator in health care.

**For more information, visit* www.hhs.gov/ocr/hipaa.

†*Resources: Nicoll LH:* Nurses' guide to the Internet, *ed 3, Philadelphia, 2001, Lippincott. Also available is a bimonthly publication,* CIN: Computers, Informatics, Nursing. *To order, call 800-638-3030; fax: 301-223-2400; e-mail: CustomerService@LWW.com;* www.cinjournal.com.

BOX 34-1 Telephone Triage Guidelines

Date and time
Background
- Name, age, sex
- Chronic illness
- Allergies, current medications, treatments, or recent immunizations

Chief complaint
General symptoms
- Severity
- Duration
- Other symptoms
- Pain

Systems review
Steps taken
- Advised to call emergency medical services (911)
- Advised to see practitioner
- Advice given for home care
- Call back if symptoms worsen or fail to improve

Resources for Telephone Triage Protocols

Briggs JK: *Telephone triage protocols for nurses*, ed 3, Philadelphia, 2006, Lippincott Williams & Wilkins.

Schmitt BD: *Pediatric telephone protocols: office version*, ed 12, Elk Grove Village, IL, 2009, American Academy of Pediatrics.

Encouraging the Parent to Talk

Interviewing parents not only offers the opportunity to determine the child's health and developmental status, but also offers information about factors that influence the child's life. Whatever the parent sees as a problem should be a concern of the nurse. These problems are not always easy to identify. Nurses need to be alert for clues and signals by which a parent communicates worries and anxieties. Careful phrasing with broad, open-ended questions such as "What is Jimmy eating now?" provides more information than several single-answer questions, such as "Is Jimmy eating what the rest of the family eats?"

Sometimes the parent will take the lead without prompting. At other times it may be necessary to direct another question on the basis of an observation, such as "Connie seems unhappy today" or "How do you feel when David cries?" If the parent appears to be tired or distraught, consider asking, "What do you do to relax?" or "What help do you have with the children?" A comment such as "You handle the baby very well. What kinds of experience have you had with babies?" to new parents who appear comfortable with their first child gives positive reinforcement and provides an opening for any questions they might have regarding the infant's care. Often all that is required to keep parents talking is a nod or saying "yes" or "uh-huh."

When attempting to elicit feelings and covert problem areas, avoid closed-ended questions that begin with "Does . . .," "Did . . .," or "Is . . .," which usually require only a single response. In addition, asking questions such as "Does your son have any problems at school?" subtly implies a lack of parental skills and evokes defensiveness. Instead, say, "What . . .," "How . . .," or "Tell me about . . .," and encourage elaboration with "You were saying . . ." or "You say that . . .," or by reflecting back a key word. Open-ended questions are nonthreatening and encourage description.

Directing the Focus

The ability to direct the focus of the interview while allowing for maximum freedom of expression is one of the most difficult goals in effective communication. One approach is the use of open-ended or broad questions, followed by guiding statements. For example, if the parent proceeds to list the other children by name, say, "Tell me their ages, too." If the parent continues to describe each child in depth, which is not the purpose of the interview, redirect the focus by stating, "Let's talk about the other children later. You were beginning to tell me about Paul's activities at school." This approach conveys interest in the other children but focuses the assessment on the patient.

Listening and Cultural Awareness

Listening is the most important component of effective communication. When listening is truly aimed at understanding the client, it is an active process that requires concentration and attention to all aspects of the conversation—verbal, nonverbal, and abstract. Major blocks to listening are environmental distraction and premature judgment.

The nurse's attitudes and feelings are easily injected into an interview. Often nurses' perceptions of a parent's behavior are influenced by their own perceptions, prejudices, and assumptions, which may include racial, religious, and cultural stereotypes. What may be interpreted as a parent's passive hostility or lack of interest may be shyness or an expression of anxiety. For example, in Western cultures eye contact and directness are signs of paying attention. However, in many non-Western cultures, including that of Native Americans, directness, such as looking someone in the eye, is considered rude. Children are taught to avert their gaze and to look down when being addressed by an adult, especially one with authority (Seidel et al, 2006). Therefore judgments about listening and verbal interactions need to be made with an appreciation of cultural differences (see Guidelines box, p. 833, and Chapter 32).

Although it is necessary to make some preliminary judgments, listen with as much objectivity as possible by clarifying meanings and attempting to see the situation from the parent's point of view. Effective interviewers consciously control their reactions, responses, and the techniques they use.

Minimum verbal activity with active listening facilitates parent involvement. It is tempting to spend time explaining, describing, and interpreting health information when the opportunity presents itself. However, it is possible to provide effective health education by timing the information properly and presenting only as much as is necessary at the moment.

Careful listening facilitates the use of clues, verbal leads, or signals from the interviewee to move the interview along. Frequent references to an area of concern, repetition of certain key words, or a special emphasis on something or someone serves as cues to the interviewer for the direction of inquiry. Concerns and anxieties are often mentioned in a casual, offhand manner. Even though they are casual, they are important and deserve careful scrutiny to identify problem areas. For example, a parent who is concerned about a child's habit of bed-wetting may casually mention that the child's bed was "wet this morning."

Using Silence

Silence as a response is often one of the most difficult interviewing techniques to learn. It requires a sense of confidence and comfort on the part of the interviewer to allow the interviewee space in which to think without interruptions. Silence permits the interviewee to sort out thoughts and feelings and search for responses to questions. Silence can also be a cue for the interviewer to go more slowly, reexamine the approach, and not push too hard (Seidel et al, 2006).

Sometimes it is necessary to break the silence and reopen communication. Do this in a way that encourages the person to continue talking about what is considered important. Breaking a silence by introducing a new topic or by prolonged talking essentially terminates the interviewee's opportunity to use the silence. Suggestions for breaking the silence include statements such as "Is there anything else you wish to say?" "I see you find it difficult to continue; how may I help?" or "I don't know what this silence means. Perhaps there is something you would like to put into words but find difficult to say."

Being Empathic

Empathy is the capacity to understand what another person is experiencing from within that person's frame of reference; it is often described as the ability to put oneself in another's shoes. The essence of empathic interaction is accurate understanding of another's feelings (Price & Archbold, 1997; White, 1997; Reynolds, Scott, & Jessiman, 1999). Empathy differs from sympathy, which is *having* feelings or emotions in common with another person, rather than *understanding* those feelings. Sympathy is not therapeutic in the helping relationship because it leads to overinvolvement emotionally and potentially to professional burnout (Yegdich, 1999).

Providing Anticipatory Guidance

The ideal way to handle a situation is to deal with it *before* it becomes a problem. The best preventive measure is anticipatory guidance. Traditionally, anticipatory guidance has focused on providing families information on normal growth and development, as well as nurturing childrearing practices. For example, one of the most significant areas in pediatrics is injury prevention. Beginning prenatally, parents need specific instructions on home safety. Because of the child's maturing developmental skills, home safety changes must be implemented early to minimize risks to the child.

Many normal developmental changes can disturb unprepared parents, such as a toddler's diminished appetite, negativism, altered sleeping patterns, and anxiety toward strangers. Such topics are discussed in the chapters on health promotion to provide the nurse with information for counseling parents.

However, anticipatory guidance should extend beyond giving information to empowering families to use the information as a means of building competence in their parenting abilities. To achieve this level of anticipatory guidance (Desselle & Pearlmutter, 1997), the nurse should:

- Base interventions on needs identified by the family, not by the professional
- View the family as competent or as having the ability to be competent
- Provide opportunities for the family to achieve competence

Avoiding Blocks to Communication

A number of blocks to communication can adversely affect the quality of the helping relationship. Many of these blocks are initiated by the interviewer, such as giving unrestricted advice or forming prejudged conclusions. Another type of block occurs primarily with the interviewees and concerns information overload. When individuals are presented with too much information or information that is overwhelming, they will often demonstrate signs of increasing anxiety or decreasing attention. Such signals should alert the interviewer to give less information or to clarify what has been said. Some of the more common blocks to communication, including signs of information overload, are listed in Box 34-2.

Communicating with Families Through an Interpreter

Sometimes communication is impossible because two people speak different languages. In this case it is necessary to obtain information through a third party, the interpreter. When an interpreter is used, the same interviewing guidelines apply. Specific guidelines for using an adult interpreter are presented in the Guidelines box.

GUIDELINES Using an Interpreter

- Explain to interpreter the reason for the interview and the type of questions that will be asked.
- Clarify whether a detailed or brief answer is required and whether the translated response can be general or literal.
- Introduce interpreter to family and allow some time before the interview for them to become acquainted.
- Communicate directly with family members when asking questions to reinforce interest in them and to observe nonverbal expressions, but do not ignore interpreter.
- Pose questions to elicit only one answer at a time, such as "Do you have pain?" rather than "Do you have any pain, tiredness, or loss of appetite?"
- Refrain from interrupting family member and interpreter while they are conversing.
- Avoid commenting to interpreter about family members, since they may understand some English.
- Be aware that some medical words, such as ***allergy,*** may have no similar word in another language; avoid medical jargon whenever possible.
- Be aware that cultural differences may exist regarding views on sex, marriage, or pregnancy.
- Allow time after the interview for interpreter to share something that he or she thought could not be said earlier; ask about the interpreter's impression of nonverbal clues to communication and family members' reliability or ease in revealing information.
- Arrange for family to speak with same interpreter on subsequent visits whenever possible.

BOX 34-2 Blocks to Communication

Communication Barriers (Nurse)
Socializing
Giving unrestricted and sometimes unasked for advice
Offering premature or inappropriate reassurance
Giving overready encouragement
Defending a situation or opinion
Using stereotyped comments or clichés
Limiting expression of emotion by asking directed, closed-ended questions
Interrupting and finishing the person's sentence
Talking more than the interviewee
Forming prejudged conclusions
Deliberately changing the focus

Signs of Information Overload (Patient)
Long periods of silence
Wide eyes and fixed facial expression
Constant fidgeting or attempting to move away
Nervous habits (e.g., tapping, playing with hair)
Sudden disruptions (e.g., asking to go to the bathroom)
Looking around
Yawning, eyes drooping
Frequently looking at a watch or clock
Attempting to change topic of discussion

Communicating with families through an interpreter requires sensitivity to cultural, legal, and ethical considerations. For example, in some cultures using a child as an interpreter is considered an insult to an adult because children are expected to show respect by not questioning their elders. In some cultures class differences between the interpreter and the family may cause the family to feel intimidated and less inclined to offer information. Therefore it is important to choose the translator carefully and provide time for the interpreter and family to establish rapport.

Issues of legal and ethical concerns may also arise. For example, in obtaining informed consent through an interpreter, it is important that the family be fully informed of all aspects of the particular procedure to which they are consenting. Issues of confidentiality may arise when family members related to another patient are asked to interpret for the family, thus revealing sensitive information that may be shared with other families on the unit. With increased sensitivity toward patient rights and confidentiality, many institutions now require consent forms to be produced in the patient's primary language.

When no one else is available to translate, children within the family are often asked to assume this role. In this situation it is important to stress *literal* translation of parent responses. To ensure correct translations, it may be necessary to interrupt the parent and ask the child to translate every few sentences. When using children as interpreters, ask questions directed at specific answers and assess the interpreted translation in terms of nonverbal expressions of communication. It should be noted that some institutions prohibit or discourage the use of children as interpreter; check institutional policy for compliance.

Communicating with Children

Although the greatest amount of verbal communication is usually carried out with the parent, do not exclude the child during the interview. Pay attention to infants and younger children through play or by occasionally directing questions or remarks to them. Include older children as active participants.

In communication with children of all ages, the nonverbal components of the communication process convey the most significant messages. It is difficult to disguise feelings, attitudes, and anxiety when relating to children. They are alert to surroundings and attach meaning to every gesture and move that is made; this is particularly true of very young children.

Active attempts to make friends with children before they have had an opportunity to evaluate an unfamiliar person tend to increase their anxiety. It is helpful to continue to talk to the child and parent but go about activities that do not involve the child directly, thus allowing the child to observe from a safe position. If the child has a special toy or doll, "talk" to the doll first. Ask simple questions such as "Does your teddy bear have a name?" to ease the child into conversation. Other guidelines for communicating with children are presented in the Guidelines box.

GUIDELINES Communicating with Children

- Allow children time to feel comfortable.
- Avoid sudden or rapid advances, broad smiles, extended eye contact, or other gestures that may be seen as threatening.
- Talk to the parent if child is initially shy.
- Communicate through transition objects such as dolls, puppets, and stuffed animals before questioning a young child directly.
- Give older children the opportunity to talk without the parents present.
- Assume a position that is at eye level with child (Fig. 34-2).
- Speak in a quiet, unhurried, and confident voice.
- Speak clearly, be specific, and use simple words and short sentences.
- State directions and suggestions positively.
- Offer a choice only when one exists.
- Be honest with children.
- Allow them to express their concerns and fears.
- Use a variety of communication techniques.

Communication Related to Development of Thought Processes

The normal development of language and thought offers a frame of reference for communicating with children. Thought processes progress from sensorimotor to perceptual to concrete and finally to abstract, formal operations. The early social communicative development of children has been divided into three stages: (1) *perlocutionary stage*—unintentional communication behavior; (2) *illocutionary stage*—true intent in communication efforts; and (3) *locutionary stage*—intentional communication behaviors and use of symbols (Hoge & Parette, 1995). An understanding of the typical characteristics of these

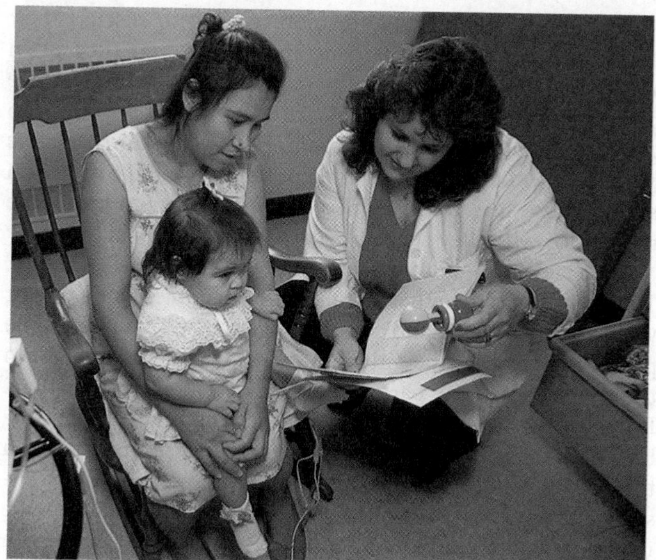

Fig. 34-2 Nurse assumes position at child's level.

BOX 34-3 Characteristics of Communicative Development in Young Children

Perlocutionary Stage (0 to 8-9 Months)
Child is reflexive to stimuli.
Child shows increasing purpose in action.

Emerging Illocutionary Stage (8-9 to 12-15 Months)
Child communicates intentionally with signals and gestures.

Conventional Illocutionary–Emerging Locutionary Stage (12-15 to 18-24 Months)
Child communicates intentionally with gestures, vocalizations, and verbalizations.

Modified from Hoge DR, Parette HP: Facilitating communicative development in young children with disabilities, *Transdisc J* 5(2):113-130, 1995.

stages provides the nurse with a framework to facilitate social communication (Box 34-3).

Infancy

Because they are unable to use words, infants primarily use and understand nonverbal communication. Infants communicate their needs and feelings through nonverbal behaviors and vocalizations that can be interpreted by someone who is around them for a sufficient time. Infants smile and coo when content and cry when distressed. Crying is provoked by unpleasant stimuli from inside or outside, such as hunger, pain, body restraint, or loneliness. Adults interpret this to mean that an infant needs something and consequently try to alleviate the discomfort and reduce tension. Crying (or the desire to cry) persists as a part of everyone's communication repertoire.

Infants respond to adults' nonverbal behaviors. They become quiet when they are cuddled, are patted, or receive other forms of gentle physical contact. They derive comfort from the sound of a voice, even though they do not understand the words that are spoken. Until infants reach the age at which they experience stranger anxiety, they readily respond to any firm, gentle handling and quiet, calm speech. Loud, harsh sounds and sudden movements are frightening.

Older infants' attention is centered on themselves and their parents; therefore any stranger is a potential threat until proved otherwise. Holding out the hands and asking the child to come is seldom successful, especially if the infant is with the parent. If infants must be handled, simply pick them up firmly without gestures. Observe the position in which the parent holds the infant. Most infants learn to prefer a particular position and manner of handling. In general, infants are more at ease upright than horizontal. Also, hold infants so they can see their parents. Until they develop the understanding that an object (in this case the parent) removed from sight can still be present, they have no way of knowing the object is still there.

Early Childhood

Children younger than 5 years of age are egocentric. They see things only in relation to themselves and from their point of view. Therefore focus communication on them. Tell them what they can do or how they will feel. Experiences of others are of no interest to them. It is futile to use another child's experience in an attempt to gain the cooperation of small children. Allow them to touch and examine articles that will come in contact with them. A stethoscope bell will feel cold; palpating a neck might tickle. Although they have not yet acquired sufficient language skills to express their feelings and wants, toddlers are able to communicate effectively with their hands to transmit ideas without words. They push an unwanted object away, pull another person to show them something, point, and cover the mouth that is saying something they do not wish to hear.

Everything is direct and concrete to small children. They are unable to work with abstractions and interpret words literally. Analogies escape them because they are unable to separate fact from fantasy. For example, they attach literal meaning to such common phrases as "two-faced," "sticky fingers," or "coughing your head off." Children who are told they will get "a little stick in the arm" may not be able to envision an injection (Fig. 34-3). Therefore avoid using a phrase that might be misinterpreted by a small child.

Young children assign human attributes to inanimate objects. Consequently they fear that objects may jump, bite, cut, or pinch all by themselves. Children do not know that these devices are unable to perform without human direction. To minimize their fear, keep unfamiliar equipment out of view until it is needed.

School-Age Years

Younger school-age children rely less on what they see and more on what they know when faced with new problems. They want explanations and reasons for everything but require no verification beyond that. They are interested in the functional aspect of all procedures, objects, and activities. They want to know why an object exists, why it is used, how it works, and the intent and purpose of its user. They need to know what is going to take place and why it is being done to them specifically. For example, to explain a procedure such as taking blood pressure (BP), show the child how squeezing the bulb pushes air into the cuff and makes the "silver" in the tube go up. Let the child operate the bulb. An explanation for the procedure

evolve Skill—Communicating with Children

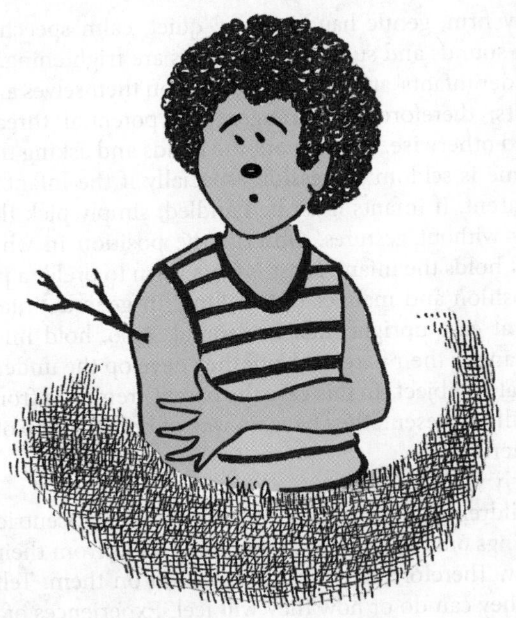

Fig. 34-3 A young child may take the expression "a little stick in the arm" literally.

might be as simple as, "I want to see how far the silver goes up when the cuff squeezes your arm." The child then becomes an enthusiastic participant.

School-age children have a heightened concern about body integrity. Because of the special importance they place on their body, they are sensitive to anything that constitutes a threat or suggestion of injury to it. This concern extends to their possessions, so that they may appear to overreact to loss or threatened loss of treasured objects. Helping children voice their concerns enables the nurse to provide reassurance and to implement activities that reduce their anxiety. For example, if a shy child dislikes being the center of attention, ignore that particular child by talking and relating to other children in the family or group. When children feel more comfortable, they will usually interject personal ideas, feelings, and interpretations of events.

Older children have an adequate and satisfactory use of language. They still require relatively simple explanations, but their ability to think concretely can facilitate communication and explanation. Commonly, they have sufficient experience with health and health care workers to understand what is transpiring and what is generally expected of them.

evolve Case Study—Communicating with Adolescents

Adolescence

As children move into adolescence, they fluctuate between child and adult thinking and behavior. They are riding a current that is moving them rapidly toward a maturity that may be beyond their coping ability. Therefore, when tensions rise, they may seek the security of the more familiar and comfortable expectations of childhood. Anticipating these shifts in identity allows the nurse to adjust the course of interaction to meet the needs of the moment. No single approach can be relied on consistently, and encountering cooperation, hostility, anger, bravado, and a variety of other behaviors and attitudes can be expected. It is as much a mistake to regard the adolescent as an adult with an adult's wisdom and control as it is to assume that the teenager has the concerns and expectations of a child.

Frequently adolescents are more willing to discuss their concerns with an adult outside the family, and they often welcome the opportunity to interact with a nurse outside the presence of their parents. They are accepting of anyone who displays a genuine interest in them. However, adolescents are quick to reject persons who attempt to impose their values on them, whose interest is feigned, or who appear to have little respect for who they are and what they think or say.

Interviewing the adolescent presents some special issues. The first may be whether to talk with the adolescent alone or with the adolescent and parents together. Of course, if the parent is not there, the only question is whether to suggest to the teenager that the parents be interviewed at another time. If the parents and teenager are together, talking with the adolescent first has the advantage of immediately identifying with the young person, thus fostering the interpersonal relationship. However, talking with the parents initially may provide insight into the family relationship. In either case, give both parties an opportunity to be included in the interview. If time constraints are important, such as during history taking, clarify this at the onset to avoid appearing to "take sides" by talking more with one person than with the other.

Confidentiality is of great importance when interviewing adolescents. Explain to parents and teenagers the limits of confidentiality, specifically that young persons' disclosures will not be shared unless they indicate a need for intervention, as in the case of suicidal behavior.

Another dilemma in interviewing adolescents is that two views of a problem frequently exist—the teenager's and the parents'. Clarification of the problem is a major task. However, providing both parties an opportunity to discuss their perceptions in an open and unbiased atmosphere can, by itself, be therapeutic. Demonstrating positive communication skills can help families communicate more effectively (see Guidelines box).

GUIDELINES Communicating with Adolescents

Build a Foundation

Spend time together.
Encourage expression of ideas and feelings.
Respect their views.
Tolerate differences.
Praise good points.
Respect their privacy.
Set a good example.

Communicate Effectively

Give undivided attention.
Listen, listen, listen.
Be courteous, calm, and open minded.
Try not to overreact. If you do, take a break.
Avoid judging or criticizing.
Avoid the "third degree" of continuous questioning.
Choose important issues when taking a stand.
After taking a stand:
- Think through all options.
- Make expectations clear.

BOX 34-4 Creative Communication Techniques with Children

Verbal Techniques

"I" Messages

Relate a feeling about a behavior in terms of "I."
Describe effect behavior had on the person.
Avoid use of "you."
"You" messages are judgmental and provoke defensiveness.

Example—"You" message: "You are being uncooperative about doing your treatments."

Example—"I" message: "I am concerned about how the treatments are going because I want to see you get better."

Third-Person Technique

Express a feeling in terms of a third person ("he," "she," "they"). This is less threatening than directly asking children how they feel because it gives them an opportunity to agree or disagree without being defensive.

Example—"Sometimes when a person is sick a lot, he feels angry and sad because he cannot do what others can." Either wait silently for a response or encourage a reply with a statement such as "Did you ever feel that way?"

Approach allows children three choices: (1) to agree and, one hopes, express how they feel; (2) to disagree; or (3) to remain silent, which means they probably have such feelings but are unable to express them at this time.

Facilitative Response

Listen carefully and reflect back to patients the feelings and content of their statements.
Responses are empathic and nonjudgmental and legitimize the person's feelings.
Formula for facilitative responses: "You feel ___________ because ___________."

Example—If child states, "I hate coming to the hospital and getting needles," a facilitative response is, "You feel unhappy because of all the things that are done to you."

Storytelling

Use the language of children to probe into areas of their thinking while bypassing conscious inhibitions or fears.
The simplest technique is asking children to relate a story about an event, such as "being in the hospital."
Other approaches:

- Show children a picture of a particular event, such as a child in a hospital with other people in the room, and ask them to describe the scene.
- Cut out comic strips, remove words, and have child add statements for scenes.

Mutual Storytelling

Reveal child's thinking and attempt to change child's perceptions or fears by retelling a somewhat different story (more therapeutic approach than storytelling).
Begin by asking child to tell a story about something, then tell another story that is similar to child's tale but with differences that help child in problem areas.

Example—Child's story is about going to the hospital and never seeing his or her parents again. Nurse's story is also about a child (using different names but similar circumstances) in a hospital whose parents visit every day, but in the evening after work, until the child is better and goes home with them.

Bibliotherapy

Use books in a therapeutic and supportive process.
Provide children with an opportunity to explore an event that is similar to their own but sufficiently different to allow them to distance themselves from it and remain in control.
General guidelines for using bibliotherapy are:

1. Assess child's emotional and cognitive development in terms of readiness to understand the book's message.
2. Be familiar with the book's content (intended message or purpose) and the age for which it is written.
3. Read the book to the child if child is unable to read.
4. Explore the meaning of the book with the child by having child:
   - Retell the story
   - Read a special section with the nurse or parent
   - Draw a picture related to the story and discuss the drawing
   - Talk about the characters
   - Summarize the moral or meaning of the story

Dreams

Dreams often reveal unconscious and repressed thoughts and feelings.
Ask child to talk about a dream or nightmare.
Explore with child what meaning the dream could have.

"What If" Questions

Encourage child to explore potential situations and to consider different problem-solving options.

Example—"What if you got sick and had to go the hospital?" Children's responses reveal what they know already and what they are curious about, providing an opportunity for them to learn coping skills, especially in potentially dangerous situations.

Three Wishes

Ask, "If you could have any three things in the world, what would they be?"
If child answers, "That all my wishes come true," ask child for specific wishes.

Rating Game

Use some type of rating scale (numbers, sad to happy faces) to have child rate an event or feeling.

Example—Instead of asking youngsters how they feel, ask how their day has been "on a scale of 1 to 10, with 10 being the best."

Word Association Game

State key words and ask children to say the first word they think of when they hear the word.

Continued

BOX 34-4 Creative Communication Techniques with Children—cont'd

Verbal Techniques—cont'd

Word Association Game—cont'd

Start with neutral words and then introduce more anxiety-producing words, such as "illness," "needles," "hospitals," and "operation."

Select key words that relate to some relevant event in the child's life.

Sentence Completion

Present a partial statement and have the child complete it. Some sample statements are:

- The thing I like best (least) about school is ________.
- The best (worst) age to be is ________.
- The most (least) fun thing I ever did was ________.
- The thing I like most (least) about my parents is ________.
- The one thing I would change about my family is ________.
- If I could be anything I wanted, I would be ________.
- The thing I like most (least) about myself is ________.

Pros and Cons

Select a topic, such as "being in the hospital," and have child list "five good things and five bad things" about it.

This is an exceptionally valuable technique when applied to relationships, such as things family members like and dislike about each other.

Nonverbal Techniques

Writing

Writing is an alternative communication approach for older children and adults.

Specific suggestions include:

- Keep a journal or diary.
- Write down feelings or thoughts that are difficult to express.
- Write "letters" that are never mailed (a variation is making up a pen pal to write to).

Keep an account of child's progress from both a physical and an emotional viewpoint.

Drawing

Drawing is one of the most valuable forms of communication—both nonverbal (from looking at the drawing) and verbal (from child's story of the picture).

Children's drawings tell a great deal about them because they are projections of their inner selves.

Spontaneous drawing involves giving child a variety of art supplies and providing the opportunity to draw.

Directed drawing involves a more specific direction, such as "draw a person" or the "three themes" approach (state three things about child and ask child to choose one and draw a picture).

Guidelines for Evaluating Drawings

Use spontaneous drawings and evaluate more than one drawing whenever possible.

Interpret drawings in light of other available information about child and family, including the child's age and stage of development.

Interpret drawings as a whole rather than focusing on specific details of the drawing.

Consider individual elements of the drawing that may be significant:

- **Sex of figure drawn first**—Usually relates to child's perception of own sex role.
- **Size of individual figures**—Expresses importance, power, or authority.
- **Order in which figures are drawn**—Expresses priority in terms of importance.
- **Child's position in relation to other family members**—Expresses feelings of status or alliance.
- **Exclusion of a member**—May denote feeling of not belonging or desire to eliminate.
- **Accentuated parts**—Usually express concern for areas of special importance (e.g., large hands may be a sign of aggression).
- **Absence of or rudimentary arms and hands**—Suggest timidity, passivity, or intellectual immaturity; tiny, unstable feet may express insecurity, and hidden hands may mean guilt feelings.
- **Placement of drawing on the page and type of stroke**—Free use of paper and firm, continuous strokes express security, whereas drawings restricted to a small area and lightly drawn in broken or wavering lines may be a sign of insecurity.
- **Erasures, shading, or cross-hatching**—Expresses ambivalence, concern, or anxiety with a particular area.

Magic

Use simple magic tricks to help establish rapport with child, encourage compliance with health interventions, and provide effective distraction during painful procedures.

Although the magician talks, no verbal response from child is required.

Play

Play is the universal language and "work" of children.

It tells a great deal about children because they project their inner selves through the activity.

Spontaneous play involves giving child a variety of play materials and providing the opportunity to play.

Directed play involves a more specific direction, such as providing medical equipment or a dollhouse for focused reasons, such as exploring child's fear of injections or exploring family relationships.

Communication Techniques

In addition to such conventional interviewing methods as reflection and open-ended questions, a number of techniques encourage family members to express their thoughts and feelings in a less directive and confrontational manner. Several approaches are *projective*—they present nonspecific material that enables individuals to externalize or project inner aspects of themselves to others.

A variety of verbal techniques can be used to encourage communication. Some of these techniques can be used to pose questions or explore concerns in a less threatening manner. Others can be presented as "word games," which are often well received by children. However, for many children and adults, talking about feelings is difficult, and verbal communication may be more stressful than supportive. In such instances several nonverbal techniques can be used to encourage communication.

Both verbal and nonverbal techniques are described in Box 34-4. Because of the importance of play in communicating with children, play is discussed more extensively below. Any of the verbal or nonverbal techniques can give rise to strong feelings that surface unexpectedly. Be prepared to handle them or to recognize when issues go beyond your ability to deal with them. At that point, consider an appropriate referral.

History Taking

Performing a Health History

The format used for history taking may be (1) *direct,* where the nurse asks for information via direct interview with the informant; or (2) *indirect,* where the informant supplies the information by completing some type of questionnaire. The direct method is superior to the indirect approach or a combination of both. However, in view of time constraints, the direct approach is not always practical. If the direct approach cannot be used, review parents' written responses and question them regarding any unusual answers. The categories listed in Box 34-5 encompass children's current and past health status and information about their psychosocial environment.

Identifying Information

Much of the identifying information may already be available from other recorded sources. However, if the parent and youngster seem anxious, use this opportunity to ask about such information to help them feel more comfortable.

Informant

One of the important elements of identifying information is the informant, the person(s) who furnish the information. Record (1) who the person is (child, parent, or other), (2) an impression of reliability and willingness to communicate, and (3) any special circumstances such as the use of an interpreter or conflicting answers by more than one person.

Chief Complaint

The chief complaint is the specific reason for the child's visit to the clinic, office, or hospital. It may be viewed as the theme, with the present illness viewed as the description of the problem. The chief complaint is elicited by asking open-ended, neutral questions such as "What seems to be the matter?" "How may I help you?" or "Why did you come here today?"

BOX 34-5 Outline of a Pediatric Health History

Identifying information
1. Name
2. Address
3. Telephone
4. Birth date and place
5. Race/ethnic group
6. Sex
7. Religion
8. Date of interview
9. Informant

Chief complaint (CC)—To establish the major specific reason for the child's and parents' seeking professional health attention

Present illness (PI)—To obtain all details related to the chief complaint

Past history (PH)—To elicit a profile of the child's previous illnesses, injuries, or operations
1. Birth history (pregnancy, labor and delivery, perinatal history)
2. Previous illnesses, injuries, or operations
3. Allergies
4. Current medications
5. Immunizations
6. Growth and development
7. Habits

Review of systems (ROS)—To elicit information concerning any potential health problem
1. General
2. Integument
3. Head
4. Eyes
5. Ears
6. Nose
7. Mouth
8. Throat
9. Neck
10. Chest
11. Respiratory
12. Cardiovascular
13. Gastrointestinal
14. Genitourinary
15. Gynecologic
16. Musculoskeletal
17. Neurologic
18. Endocrine

Family medical history—To identify genetic traits or diseases that have familial tendencies and to assess exposure to a communicable disease in a family member and family habits that may affect the child's health, such as smoking and chemical use

Psychosocial history—To elicit information about the child's self-concept

Sexual history—To elicit information concerning the child's sexual concerns or activities and any pertinent data regarding adults' sexual activity that influences the child

Family history—To develop an understanding of the child as an individual and as a member of a family and a community
1. Family composition
2. Home and community environment
3. Occupation and education of family members
4. Cultural and religious traditions
5. Family function and relationships

Nutritional assessment—To elicit information on the adequacy of the child's nutritional intake and needs
1. Dietary intake
2. Clinical examination

evolve Case Study—Pediatric Assessment

Avoid labeling-type questions such as "How are you sick?" or "What is the problem?"; it is possible that the reason for the visit is not an illness or problem.

Occasionally, it is difficult to isolate one symptom or problem as the chief complaint because the parent may identify many. In this situation be as specific as possible when asking questions. For example, asking informants to state which *one* problem or symptom prompted them to seek help now may help them focus on the most immediate concern.

Present Illness

The history of the present illness* is a narrative of the chief complaint from its earliest onset through its progression to the present. Its four major components are (1) the details of onset, (2) a complete interval history, (3) the present status, and (4) the reason for seeking help now. The focus of the present illness is on all factors relevant to the main problem, even if they have disappeared or changed during the onset, interval, and present.

Analyzing a Symptom

Because pain is often the most characteristic symptom denoting the onset of a physical problem, it is used as an example for analysis of a symptom. Assessment includes (1) type, (2) location, (3) severity, (4) duration, and (5) influencing factors (see Guidelines box; see also Pain Assessment, Chapter 35).

GUIDELINES Analyzing the Symptom: Pain

Type

Be as specific as possible. With young children, asking the parents how they know the child is in pain may help describe its type, location, and severity. For example, a parent may state, "My child must have a severe earache because she pulls at her ears, rolls her head on the floor, and screams. Nothing seems to help." Help older children describe the "hurt" by asking them if it is sharp, throbbing, dull, or stabbing. Record whatever words they use in quotes.

Location

Be specific. "Stomach pains" is too general a description. Children can better localize the pain if they are asked to "point with one finger to where it hurts" or to "point to where Mommy or Daddy would put a Band-Aid." Determine if the pain radiates by asking, "Does the pain stay there or move? Show me with your finger where the pain goes."

Severity

Severity is best determined by finding out how it affects the child's usual behavior. Pain that prevents a child from playing, interacting with others, sleeping, and eating is most often severe. Assess pain intensity using a rating scale, such as a numeric or FACES scale (see Chapter 35).

Duration

Include the duration, onset, and frequency. Describe this in terms of activity and behavior, such as "pain reported to last all night, child refused to sleep and cried intermittently."

Influencing Factors

Include anything that causes a change in the type, location, severity, or duration of the pain: (1) precipitating events (those that cause or increase the pain), (2) relieving events (those that lessen the pain, such as medications), (3) temporal events (times when the pain is relieved or increased), (4) positional events (standing, sitting, lying down), and (5) associated events (meals, stress, coughing).

History

The history contains information relating to all previous aspects of the child's health status and concentrates on several areas that are ordinarily passed over in the history of an adult, such as birth history, detailed feeding history, immunizations, and growth and development. Since a great deal of information is included in this section, use a combination of open-ended and fact-finding questions. For example, begin interviewing for each section with an open-ended statement such as "Tell me about your child's birth" to provide the informants with the opportunity to relate what they think is most important. Ask fact-finding questions related to specific details whenever necessary to focus the interview on certain topics.

Birth History

The birth history includes all data concerning (1) the mother's health during pregnancy, (2) the labor and delivery, and (3) the infant's condition immediately after birth. Since prenatal influences have significant effects on a child's physical and emotional development, a thorough investigation of the birth history is essential. Because parents may question what relevance pregnancy and birth have on the child's present condition, particularly if the child is past infancy, explain why such questions are included. An appropriate statement may be, "I will be asking you some questions about your pregnancy and ____'s [refer to child by name] birth. Your answers will give me a more complete picture of his [or her] overall health."

Because emotional factors also affect the outcome of pregnancy and the subsequent parent-child relationship, investigate (1) concurrent crises during pregnancy and (2) prenatal attitudes toward the fetus. It is best to approach the topic of parental acceptance of pregnancy through indirect questioning. Asking parents if the pregnancy was planned is a leading statement because they may respond affirmatively for fear of criticism if the pregnancy was unexpected. Rather, encourage parents to disclose their true reactions by referring to specific facts relating to the pregnancy, such as the spacing between offspring, an extended or short interval between marriage and conception, or the concurrent experience of pregnancy and adolescence. The parent can choose to explore such statements with further explanations or, for the moment, may not be able to reveal such feelings. If the parent remains silent, return to this topic later in the interview.

**The term* illness *is used in its broadest sense to denote any problem of a physical, emotional, or psychosocial nature. It is actually a history of the chief complaint.*

Dietary History

Because parental concerns are common and nursing interventions are important in ensuring optimum nutrition, the dietary history is discussed in detail later in this chapter under Nutritional Assessment.

Previous Illnesses, Injuries, and Operations

When inquiring about past illnesses, begin with a general statement such as "What other illnesses has your child had?" Since parents are most likely to recall serious health problems, ask specifically about colds; earaches; and childhood diseases such as measles, rubella (German measles), chickenpox, mumps, pertussis (whooping cough), diphtheria, tuberculosis, scarlet fever, strep throat, tonsillitis, or allergic manifestations.

In addition to illnesses, ask about injuries that required medical intervention, operations, and any other reason for hospitalization, including the dates of each incident. It is important to focus on injuries such as accidental falls, poisoning, choking, or burns, since these may be potential areas for parental guidance.

Allergies

Ask about commonly known allergic disorders such as hay fever and asthma; unusual reactions to drugs, food, or latex products; and reactions to other contact agents such as poisonous plants, animals, household products, or fabrics. If asked appropriate questions, most people can give reliable information about drug reactions (see Guidelines box).

GUIDELINES Taking an Allergy History

- Has your child ever taken any drugs or tablets that have disagreed with him or her or caused an allergy? If yes, can you remember the name(s) of these drugs?
- Can you describe the reaction?
- Was the drug taken by mouth (as a tablet or syrup), or was it an injection?
- How soon after starting the drug did the reaction happen?
- How long ago did this happen?
- Did anyone tell you it was an allergic reaction, or did you decide for yourself?
- Has your child ever taken this drug, or a similar one, again? If yes, did your child experience the same problems?
- Have you told the doctors or nurses about your child's reaction or allergy?

Modified from Cantrill JA, Cottrell WN: Accuracy of drug allergy documentation, *Am J Health Syst Pharm* 54:1627-1629, 1997.

NURSING ALERT Information about allergic reactions to drugs or other products is essential. Failure to document a serious reaction places the child at risk if the agent is given.

Current Medications

Inquire about current drug regimens, including vitamins, antipyretics (especially aspirin), antibiotics, antihistamines, decongestants, or antitussives. List all medications, including name, dose, schedule, duration, and reason for administration. Often parents are unaware of the drug's actual name. Whenever possible, ask parents to bring the containers with them to the next visit, or ask for the name of the pharmacy and call for a list of all the child's recent prescription medications. However, this list will not include over-the-counter medications, which are important to know.

Immunizations

A record of all immunizations is essential. Since many parents are unaware of the exact name and date of each immunization, the most reliable source of information is a hospital, clinic, or private practitioner's record. All immunizations and "boosters" are listed, stating (1) the name of the specific disease, (2) the number of injections, (3) the dosage (sometimes lesser amounts are given if a reaction is anticipated), (4) the ages when administered, and (5) the occurrence of any reaction following the immunization.

Growth and Development

The most important previous growth patterns to record are:

- Approximate weight at 6 months, 1 year, 2 years, and 5 years of age
- Approximate length at ages 1 and 4 years
- Dentition, including age of onset, number of teeth, and symptoms during teething

Developmental milestones include:

- Age of holding up head steadily
- Age of sitting alone without support
- Age of walking without assistance
- Age of saying first words with meaning
- Present grade in school
- Scholastic grades
- Interactions with other children, peers, and adults

Use specific and detailed questions when inquiring about each developmental milestone. For example, "sitting up" can mean many different activities, such as sitting propped up, sitting in someone's lap, sitting with support, sitting up alone but in a hyperflexed position for assisted balance, or sitting up unsupported with the back slightly rounded. A clue to misunderstanding of the requested activity may be an unusually early age of achievement (see Developmental Assessment, p. 923).

Habits

Habits are an important area to explore (Box 34-6). Parents frequently express concerns during this part of the history. Encourage their input by saying, "Please tell me any concerns you have about your child's habits, activities, or development." Investigate further any concerns that are expressed.

One of the most common concerns relates to sleep. Many children develop a normal sleep pattern, and all that is required during the assessment is a general overview of nighttime sleep and nap schedules. However, a number of children also develop sleep problems (see Sleep Problems, Chapters 36 and 38). When sleep problems occur, a more detailed sleep history is required to guide appropriate interventions.*

**A sleep history and a sleep chart for the family to record the child's daily sleep and wake activities is available in Wilson D, Hockenberry M: Wong's clinical manual of pediatric nursing, ed 7, St Louis, 2008, Mosby.*

BOX 34-6 Habits to Explore During Health Interview

- Behavior patterns such as nail biting, thumb sucking, pica (habitual ingestion of nonfood substances), rituals ("security" blanket or toy), and unusual movements (head banging, rocking, overt masturbation, walking on toes)
- Activities of daily living, such as hour of sleep and arising, duration of nighttime sleep and naps, type and duration of exercise, regularity of stools and urination, age of toilet training, and daytime or nighttime bed-wetting
- Unusual disposition; response to frustration
- Use or abuse of alcohol, drugs, coffee, or tobacco

Habits related to use of chemicals apply primarily to older children and adolescents. If a youngster admits to smoking, drinking, or drug use, ask about the quantity and frequency. Questions such as "Have you ever had a drinking or drug problem?" or "When was the last time you had a drink or took drugs?" may yield more reliable data than questions such as "How much do you drink?" or "How often do you drink or take drugs?" Clarify that "drinking" includes all types of alcohol, such as beer and wine. When quantities such as a "glass" of wine or a "can" of beer are given, ask about the size of the container.

If older children deny use of chemical substances, inquire about past experimentation. Asking, "You mean you never tried to smoke or drink?" implies that the nurse expects some such activity, and the youngster may be more inclined to answer truthfully. Be aware of the confidential nature of such questioning, the adverse effect that the parents' presence may have on the adolescent's willingness to answer, and the fact that self-reporting may not be an accurate account of chemical abuse.

Sexual History

The sexual history is an essential component of adolescents' health assessment. The history uncovers areas of concern related to sexual activity; alerts the nurse to circumstances that may indicate screening for sexually transmitted infections or testing for pregnancy; and provides information related to the need for sexual counseling, such as safe sex practices. Guidelines for anticipatory guidance topics for parents and adolescents are found in Box 34-7.

One approach to initiating a conversation about sexual concerns is to begin with a history of peer interactions. Open-ended statements such as "Tell me about your social life" or "Who are your closest friends?" generally lead into a discussion of dating and sexual issues. To probe further, include questions about the adolescent's attitudes on such topics as sex education, going steady, living together, and premarital sex. Phrase questions to reflect concern rather than judgment or criticism of sexual practices.

In any conversation regarding sexual history, be aware of the language that is used in either eliciting or conveying sexual information. For example, avoid asking whether the adolescent is "sexually active," because this term is broadly defined. "Are you having sex with anyone?" is probably the most direct and best understood question. Since same-sex experimentation may occur, refer to all sexual contacts in nongender terms, such as "anyone" or "partners," rather than "girlfriends" or "boyfriends."

A detailed account of sexual partners is needed if the patient has a history of, displays any symptoms of, or asks for treatment of a sexually transmitted infection. A difficult but necessary part of the interview is to determine the sites of possible infection. Since sexual diseases can be contracted in any of the body orifices, inform the adolescent that a sexually transmitted infection can be acquired without visible signs of disease at nongenital sites.

BOX 34-7 Anticipatory Guidance—Sexuality

Ages 12 to 14 Years

Have adolescent identify supportive adult to discuss sexuality issues and concerns with.
Discuss advantages of delaying sexual activity.
Discuss making responsible decisions regarding normal sexual feelings.
Discuss role of gender, peer pressure, and the media in sexual decision making.
Discuss contraceptive options (advantages and disadvantages).
Provide education regarding sexually transmitted infections (STIs) and human immunodeficiency virus (HIV) infection; clarify risks and discuss condoms.
Discuss abuse prevention: avoiding dangerous situations, role of drugs and alcohol, and use of self-defense.
Have adolescent clarify values, needs, and ability to be assertive.
If adolescent is sexually active, discuss limiting partners, use of condoms, and contraceptive options.
Have confidential interview with adolescent (including a sexual history).
Discuss the evolution of sexual identity and expression.
Discuss breast examination or testicular examination.

Ages 15 to 18 years

Support delaying sexual activity.
Discuss alternatives to intercourse.
Discuss "When are you ready for sex?"
Clarify values; encourage responsible decision making.
Discuss consequences of unprotected sex: early pregnancy; STIs, including HIV infection.
Discuss negotiating with partner and barriers to safer sex.
If adolescent is sexually active, discuss limiting partners, use of condoms, and contraceptive options.
Emphasize that sex should be safe and pleasurable for both partners.
Have confidential interview with adolescent.
Discuss concerns about sexual expression and identity.

Modified from Wright K: Anticipatory guidance: developing a healthy sexuality, *Pediatr Ann* 26(2 Suppl):S142-S144, C3, 1997.

Family Medical History

The family medical history is used primarily for discovering the potential existence of hereditary or familial diseases in the parents and child. In general, it is confined to first-degree relatives (parents, siblings, grandparents, and immediate aunts and uncles). Information for each family member includes age, marital status, state of health if living, cause of death if deceased, and any evidence of the following conditions: heart disease, hypertension, cancer, diabetes mellitus, obesity, congenital anomalies, allergy, asthma, seizures, tuberculosis, sickle cell disease, cognitive impairment, mental disorders such as depression or psychosis, emotional problems, syphilis, or rheumatic fever. Confirm the accuracy of the reported disorders by inquiring about the symptoms, course, treatment, and sequelae of each diagnosis.

Geographic Location

One of the important areas to explore when assessing the family health history is geographic location, including the birthplace and travel to different areas in or outside of the country, for identification of possible exposure to endemic diseases. Although the primary interest focuses on the child's temporary residence in various localities, also inquire about close family members' travel, especially during tours of military service or business trips. Children are especially susceptible to parasitic infestation in areas of poor sanitary conditions and to vector-borne diseases, such as those from mosquitoes or ticks in warm and humid or heavily wooded regions.

Family Structure

Assessment of the family, both its structure and function, is an important component of the history-taking process. Because the quality of the functional relationship between the child and family members is a major factor in emotional and physical health, family assessment is discussed separately and in greater detail apart from the more traditional health history.

Family assessment is the collection of data about the family's composition and the relationships among its members. In its broadest sense, *family* refers to all those individuals who are considered by the family member to be significant to the nuclear unit, including relatives, friends, and social groups such as the school and church. Although family assessment is not family therapy, it can and frequently is therapeutic. Involving family members in discussing family characteristics and activities can provide insight into family dynamics and relationships.

Because of the time involved in performing an in-depth family assessment as presented here, be selective in deciding when knowledge of family function may facilitate nursing care (see Guidelines box). During brief contacts with families, a full assessment is not appropriate, and screening with one or two questions from each category may reflect the health of the family system or the need for additional assessment.

Family structure refers to the family's composition—who lives in the home and those social, cultural, religious, and economic characteristics that influence the child's and family's overall psychobiologic health (see also Chapters 31 and 32). Since the information elicited in this part of the history is often the most personal and confidential, include it toward the end of the interview when rapport is well established.

The most common method of eliciting information on the family structure is to interview family members. The principal areas of concern (Box 34-8) are (1) family composition, (2) home and community environment, (3) occupation and education of family members, and (4) cultural and religious traditions.

NURSING ALERT In assessing family composition, it is sometimes difficult to ascertain the status of the adult relationships. If the parent fails to mention the other parent, ask, "Where is the child's father [or mother]?" Avoid saying "husband" or "wife" because this assumes that only marital relationships exist.

Psychosocial History

The traditional medical history includes a personal and social section that concentrates on children's personal status, such as school adjustment and any unusual habits, and the family and home environment. Since several personal aspects are covered under development and habits, only those issues related to children's ability to cope and their self-concept are presented here.

Through observation, obtain a general idea of how children handle themselves in terms of confidence in dealing with others, answering questions, and coping with new situations. Observe the parent-child relationship for the types of messages sent to children about their coping skills and self-worth. Do the parents treat the child with respect, focusing on strengths, or is the interaction one of constant reprimands, with emphasis on weaknesses and faults? Do the parents help the child learn new coping strategies or support the ones the child uses?

Messages about body image are also conveyed through the parent-child interaction. Do the parents label the child and body parts, such as "bad boy," "skinny legs," or "ugly scar"? Do the parents handle the child gently, using soothing touch to calm an anxious child, or do they treat the child roughly, using slaps or restraint to force compliance? If the child touches certain parts of the body, such as the genitalia, do the parents make negative comments?

GUIDELINES Initiating a Comprehensive Family Assessment

Perform a comprehensive assessment on:

- Children receiving comprehensive well-child care
- Children experiencing major stressful life events (e.g., chronic illness, disability, parental divorce, death of a family member)
- Children requiring extensive home care
- Children with developmental delays
- Children with repeated accidental injuries and those with suspected child abuse
- Children with behavioral or physical problems that could be caused by family dysfunction

BOX 34-8 Family Assessment Interview

General Guidelines

Schedule the interview with the family at a time that is most convenient for all parties; include as many family members as possible; clearly state the purpose of the interview.

Begin the interview by asking each person's name and their relationship to one another.

Restate the purpose of the interview and the objective.

Keep the initial conversation general to put members at ease and to learn the "big picture" of the family.

Identify major concerns and reflect these back to the family to be certain that all parties receive the same message.

Terminate the interview with a summary of what was discussed and a plan for additional sessions if needed.

Structural Assessment Areas

Family Composition

Immediate members of the household (names, ages, and relationships)

Significant extended family members

Previous marriages, separations, death of spouses, or divorces

Home and Community Environment

Type of dwelling, number of rooms, occupants

Sleeping arrangements

Number of floors, accessibility of stairs and elevators

Adequacy of utilities

Safety features (fire escape, smoke and carbon monoxide detectors, guardrails on windows, use of car restraint)

Environmental hazards (e.g., chipped paint, poor sanitation, pollution, heavy street traffic)

Availability and location of health care facilities, schools, play areas

Relationship with neighbors

Recent crises or changes in home

Child's reaction and adjustment to recent stresses

Occupation and Education of Family Members

Types of employment

Work schedules

Work satisfaction

Exposure to environmental or industrial hazards

Sources of income and adequacy

Effect of illness on financial status

Highest degree or grade level attained

Cultural and Religious Traditions

Religious beliefs and practices

Cultural and ethnic beliefs and practices

Language spoken in home

Assessment questions include:

- Does the family identify with a particular religious or ethnic group? Are both parents from that group?
- How is religious or ethnic background part of family life?
- What special religious or cultural traditions are practiced in the home (e.g., food choices and preparation)?
- Where were family members born, and how long have they lived in this country?
- What language does the family speak most often?
- Do they speak and understand English?
- What do they believe causes health or illness?
- What religious or ethnic beliefs influence the family's perception of illness and its treatment?
- What methods are used to prevent or treat illness?
- How does the family know when a health problem needs medical attention?
- Whom does the family contact when a member is ill?
- Does the family rely on cultural or religious healers or remedies? If so, ask them to describe the type of healer or remedy.
- Whom does the family go to for support (clergy, medical healer, relatives)?
- Does the family experience discrimination because of their race, beliefs, or practices? Ask them to describe.

Functional Assessment Areas

Family Interactions and Roles

Interactions refer to ways family members relate to each other.

Chief concern is the amount of intimacy and closeness among the members, especially spouses.

Roles refer to behaviors of people as they assume a different status or position.

Observations include:

- Family members' responses to each other (cordial, hostile, cool, loving, patient, short tempered)
- Obvious roles of leadership vs. submission
- Support and attention shown to various members

Assessment questions include:

- What activities does the family perform together?
- Whom do family members talk to when something is bothering them?
- What are members' household chores?
- Who usually oversees what is happening with the children, such as at school or health care?
- How easy or difficult is it for the family to change or accept new responsibilities for household tasks?

Power, Decision Making, and Problem Solving

Power refers to individual member's control over others in family; it is manifested through family decision making and problem solving.

Chief concern is clarity of boundaries of power between parents and children.

One method of assessment involves offering a hypothetical conflict or problem, such as a child failing school, and asking family how they would handle this situation.

Assessment questions include:

- Who usually makes the decisions in the family?
- If one parent makes a decision, can the child appeal to the other parent to change it?
- What input do children have in making decisions or discussing rules?

BOX 34-8 Family Assessment Interview—cont'd

Functional Assessment Areas—cont'd

Power, Decision Making, and Problem Solving—cont'd

- Who makes and enforces the rules?
- What happens when a rule is broken?

Communication

Communication is concerned with clarity and directness of communication patterns.

Further assessment includes periodically asking family members if they understood what was just said and to repeat the message.

Observations include:

- Who speaks to whom
- If one person speaks for another or interrupts
- If members appear uninterested when certain individuals speak
- If there is agreement between verbal and nonverbal messages

Assessment questions include:

- How often do family members wait until others are through talking before "having their say"?
- Do parents or older siblings tend to lecture and preach?
- Do parents tend to "talk down" to the children?

Expression of Feelings and Individuality

Expressions are concerned with personal space and freedom to grow with limits and structure needed for guidance.

Observing patterns of communication offers clues to how freely feelings are expressed.

Assessment questions include:

- Is it OK for family members to get angry or sad?
- Who gets angry most of the time? What do they do?
- If someone is upset, how do other family members try to comfort this person?
- Who comforts specific family members?
- When someone wants to do something, such as try out for a new sport or get a job, what is the family's response (offer assistance, discouragement, or no advice)?

With older children many of the communication strategies discussed earlier in the chapter are useful in eliciting more definitive information about their coping and self-concept. Children can write down five things they like and dislike about themselves. The nurse can use sentence completion statements, such as "The thing I like best (or worst) about myself is ____________," "If I could change one thing about myself, it would be ____________," or "When I am scared, I ____________."

Review of Systems

The review of systems is a specific review of each body system, following an order similar to that of the physical examination (see Guidelines box). Often the history of the present illness provides a complete review of the system involved in the chief complaint. Since asking questions about other body systems may appear unrelated and irrelevant to the parents or child, precede the questioning with an explanation of why the data are needed (similar to the explanation concerning the relevance of the birth history) and reassure the parents that the child's main problem has not been forgotten.

Begin the review of a specific system with a broad statement such as "How has your child's general health been?" or "Has your child had any problems with his eyes?" If the parent states that the child has had problems with some body function, pursue this with an encouraging statement such as "Tell me more about that." If the parent denies any problems, query for specific symptoms (e.g., "No headaches, bumping into objects, or squinting?"). If the parent reconfirms the absence of such symptoms, record positive statements in the history, such as "Mother denies headaches, bumping into objects, or squinting." In this way, anyone who reviews the health history is aware of exactly what symptoms were investigated.

Nutritional Assessment

Dietary Intake

Food consumption patterns of children have changed over the past 30 years (Nicklas et al, 2004). The prevalence of overweight and obesity among children and adolescents has significantly increased (Hedley et al, 2004). Knowledge of the child's dietary intake is an essential component of a nutritional assessment. However, it is also one of the most difficult factors to assess. Individuals' recall of food consumption, especially amounts eaten, is frequently unreliable. The food intake history of children and adolescents is prone to reporting error, mostly in the form of underreporting (Livingstone, Robson, & Wallace, 2004). People from different cultures may have difficulty adequately describing the types of food they eat. Despite these obstacles, a dietary evaluation is an important component of the child's assessment.

The dietary reference intakes (DRIs) are a set of four nutrient-based reference values that provide quantitative estimates of nutrient intake for use in assessing and planning dietary intake (American Academy of Pediatrics, 2004; Murphy & Poos, 2002). The specific DRIs include:

Estimated average requirement (EAR)—Nutrient intake estimated to meet the requirement of half the healthy individuals (50%) for a specific age and gender group. Used to examine the possibility of inadequacy.

Recommended dietary allowance (RDA)—Average daily dietary intake sufficient to meet the nutrient requirement of nearly all (97% to 98%) of healthy individuals for a specific age and gender group. Dietary intake at or above this level usually has a low probability of inadequacy.

GUIDELINES Review of Systems

General—Overall state of health, fatigue, recent or unexplained weight gain or loss (period of time for either), contributing factors (change of diet, illness, altered appetite), exercise tolerance, fevers (time of day), chills, night sweats (unrelated to climatic conditions), frequent infections, general ability to carry out activities of daily living

Integument—Pruritus, pigment or other color changes, acne, eruptions, rashes (location), tendency for bruising, petechiae, excessive dryness, general texture, disorders or deformities of nails, hair growth or loss, hair color change (for adolescent, use of hair dyes or other potentially toxic substances, such as hair straighteners)

Head—Headaches, dizziness, injury (specific details)

Eyes—Visual problems (behaviors indicative of blurred vision, such as bumping into objects, clumsiness, sitting close to television, holding a book close to face, writing with head near desk, squinting, rubbing the eyes, bending head in an awkward position), cross-eyes (strabismus), eye infections, edema of lids, excessive tearing, use of glasses or contact lenses, date of last optic examination

Ears—Earaches, discharge, evidence of hearing loss (ask about behaviors, such as need to repeat requests, loud speech, inattentive behavior), results of any previous auditory testing

Nose—Nosebleeds (epistaxis), constant or frequent runny or stuffy nose, nasal obstruction (difficulty breathing), alteration or loss of sense of smell

Mouth—Mouth breathing, gum bleeding, toothaches, toothbrushing, use of fluoride, difficulty with teething (symptoms), last visit to dentist (especially if temporary dentition is complete), response to dentist

Throat—Sore throats, difficulty swallowing, choking (especially when chewing food—may be from poor chewing habits), hoarseness or other voice irregularities

Neck—Pain, limitation of movement, stiffness, difficulty holding head straight (torticollis), thyroid enlargement, enlarged nodes or other masses

Chest—Breast enlargement, discharge, masses, enlarged axillary nodes (for adolescent girl, ask about breast self-examination)

Respiratory—Chronic cough, frequent colds (number per year), wheezing, shortness of breath at rest or on exertion, difficulty breathing, sputum production, infections (pneumonia, tuberculosis), date of last chest x-ray examination, and skin reaction from tuberculin testing

Cardiovascular—Cyanosis or fatigue on exertion, history of heart murmur or rheumatic fever, anemia, date of last blood count, blood type, recent transfusion

Gastrointestinal (questions in regard to appetite, food tolerance, and elimination habits are asked elsewhere)—Nausea, vomiting (not associated with eating, may be indicative of brain tumor or increased intracranial pressure), jaundice or yellowing skin or sclera, belching, flatulence, recent change in bowel habits (blood in stools, change of color, diarrhea, or constipation)

Genitourinary—Pain on urination, frequency, hesitancy, urgency, hematuria, nocturia, polyuria, unpleasant odor to urine, force of stream, discharge, change in size of scrotum, date of last urinalysis (for adolescent, sexually transmitted infection, type of treatment; for male adolescent, ask about testicular self-examination)

Gynecologic—Menarche, date of last menstrual period, regularity or problems with menstruation, vaginal discharge, pruritus, date and result of last Papanicolaou (Pap) smear (include obstetric history, as discussed under birth history, when applicable); if sexually active, type of contraception, sexually transmitted disease and type of treatment

Musculoskeletal—Weakness, clumsiness, lack of coordination, unusual movements, back or joint stiffness, muscle pains or cramps, abnormal gait, deformity, fractures, serious sprains, activity level

Neurologic—Seizures, tremors, dizziness, loss of memory, general affect, fears, nightmares, speech problems, any unusual habits

Endocrine—Intolerance to weather changes, excessive thirst or urination, excessive sweating, salty taste to skin, signs of early puberty

Adequate intake (AI)—Recommended intake level based on estimates of nutrient intake by healthy groups of individuals. Dietary intake at or above this level usually has a low probability of inadequacy.

Tolerable upper intake level (UL)—Highest average daily nutrient intake level likely to pose no risk of adverse health effects. As intake increases above the UL, risk of adverse effects increases. Dietary intake above this level usually places an individual at risk of adverse effects from excessive nutrient intake.

MyPyramid for Kids describes dietary intake in children *(www.mypyramid.gov)*. Specific questions used to conduct a nutritional assessment are also included in Box 34-9. Every nutritional assessment should begin with a dietary history. The exact questions used to elicit a dietary history vary with the child's age. In general, the younger the child, the more specific and detailed the history should be.

The overview elicited from the dietary history can be helpful in evaluating food frequency records. The history is also concerned with financial and cultural factors that influence food selection and preparation (see Cultural Awareness box).

The most common and probably easiest method of assessing daily intake is the 24-hour recall. The child or parent recalls every item eaten in the past 24 hours and the approximate amounts. The 24-hour recall is most beneficial when it represents a typical day's intake. Some of the difficulties with a daily recall are the family's inability to remember exactly what was eaten and inaccurate estimation of portion size. To increase accuracy of reporting portion sizes, the use of food models and additional questioning are recommended. In general, this method is most useful in providing *qualitative* information about the child's diet.

To improve the reliability of the daily recall, the family can complete a food diary by recording every food and liquid

BOX 34-9 Dietary Reference Intakes for an Individual

Dietary History

What are the family's usual mealtimes?
Do family members eat together or at separate times?
Who does the family grocery shopping and meal preparation?
How much money is spent to buy food each week?
How are most foods prepared—baked, broiled, fried, other?
How often does the family or your child eat out?
- What kinds of restaurants do you go to?
- What kinds of food does your child typically eat at restaurants?

Does your child eat breakfast regularly?
Where does your child eat lunch?
What are your child's favorite foods, beverages, and snacks?
- What are the average amounts eaten per day?
- What foods are artificially sweetened?
- What are your child's snacking habits?
- When are sweet foods usually eaten?
- What are your child's toothbrushing habits?

What special cultural practices are followed? What ethnic foods are eaten?
What foods and beverages does your child dislike?
How would you describe your child's usual appetite (hearty eater, picky eater)?
What are your child's feeding habits (breast, bottle, cup, spoon, eats by self, needs assistance, any special devices)?
Does your child take vitamins or other supplements? Do they contain iron or fluoride?
Does your child have any known or suspected food allergies? Is your child on a special diet?
Has your child lost or gained weight recently?
Are there any feeding problems (excessive fussiness, spitting up, colic, difficulty sucking or swallowing)? Are there any dental problems or appliances, such as braces, that affect eating?
What types of exercise does your child do regularly?
Is there a family history of cancer, diabetes, heart disease, high blood pressure, or obesity?

Additional Questions for Infants

What was the infant's birth weight? When did it double? Triple?
Was the infant preterm?
Are you breastfeeding or have you breastfed your infant? For how long?
If you use a formula, what is the brand?
- How long has the infant been taking it?
- How many ounces does the infant drink a day?

Are you giving the infant cow's milk (whole, low fat, skim)?
- When did you start?
- How many ounces does the infant drink a day?

Do you give your infant extra fluids (water, juice)?
If the infant takes a bottle to bed at nap or nighttime, what is in the bottle?
At what age did the child start on cereal, vegetables, meat or other protein sources, fruit or juice, finger food, table food?
Do you make your own baby food or use commercial foods, such as infant cereal?
Does the infant take a vitamin or mineral supplement? If so, what type?
Has the infant had an allergic reaction to any food(s)? If so, list the foods and describe the reaction.
Does the infant spit up frequently; have unusually loose stools; or have hard, dry stools? If so, how often?
How often do you feed your infant?
How would you describe your infant's appetite?

Modified from Murphy SP, Poos MI: Dietary reference intakes: summary of applications in dietary assessment, *Pub Health Nutr* 5(6A):843-849, 2002.

CULTURAL AWARENESS

Food Practices

Because cultural practices are prevalent in food preparation, consider carefully the kinds of questions that are asked and the judgments made during counseling. For example, some cultures, such as Hispanic, African-American, and Native American, include many vegetables, legumes, and starches in their diet that together provide sufficient essential amino acids, even though the actual amount of meat or dairy protein is low (see Food Customs, Chapter 32).

consumed for a certain number of days. A 3-day record consisting of 2 weekdays and 1 weekend day is representative for most people. Providing specific charts to record intake can improve compliance. The family should record items immediately after eating.

A food frequency questionnaire or record provides information about the number of times in a day, week, or month a child consumes items from the different food groups. In general, it provides a qualitative overview but has the advantage of avoiding recall based on a "typical" day. It can be especially useful when verifying a food history or diary.

Clinical Examination

A significant amount of information regarding nutritional deficiencies is elicited from a clinical examination, especially from assessing the skin, hair, teeth, gums, lips, tongue, and eyes. Hair, skin, and mouth are vulnerable because of the rapid turnover of epithelial and mucosal tissue. Table 34-1 summarizes clinical signs of possible nutritional deficiency or excess. Few are diagnostic for a specific nutrient, and if suspicious signs are found, they must be confirmed with dietary and biochemical data. Generally, the clinical examination does not reveal children *at risk* for a deficiency or excess.

Table 34-1 Clinical Assessment of Nutritional Status

EVIDENCE OF ADEQUATE NUTRITION	EVIDENCE OF DEFICIENT OR EXCESS NUTRITION	DEFICIENCY OR EXCESS*
General Growth		
Between 5th and 95th percentiles for height, weight, and head circumference	Below 5th or above 95th percentile for growth	Protein, calories, fats, and other essential nutrients, especially vitamin A, pyridoxine, niacin, calcium, iodine, manganese, zinc
Steady gain with expected growth spurts during infancy and adolescence	Absence of or delayed growth spurts; poor weight gain	
Sexual development appropriate for age	Delayed sexual development	Excess vitamins A, D
Skin		
Smooth, slightly dry to touch Elastic and firm Absence of lesions Color appropriate to genetic background	Hardening and scaling	Vitamin A
	Seborrheic dermatitis	Excess niacin
	Dry, rough, petechiae	Riboflavin
	Delayed wound healing	Vitamin C
	Scaly dermatitis on exposed surfaces	Riboflavin, vitamin C, zinc
	Wrinkled, flabby	Niacin
	Crusted lesions around orifices, especially nares	Protein, calories, zinc
	Pruritus	Excess vitamin A, riboflavin, niacin
	Poor turgor	Water, sodium
	Edema	Protein, thiamine Excess sodium
	Yellow tinge (jaundice)	Vitamin B_{12} Excess vitamin A, niacin
	Depigmentation	Protein, calories
	Pallor (anemia)	Pyridoxine, folic acid, vitamins B_{12}, C, E (in preterm infants), iron Excess vitamin C, zinc
	Paresthesia	Excess riboflavin
Hair		
Lustrous, silky, strong, elastic	Stringy, friable, dull, dry, thin	Protein, calories
	Alopecia	Protein, calories, zinc
	Depigmentation	Protein, calories, copper
	Raised areas around hair follicles	Vitamin C
Head		
Even molding, occipital prominence, symmetric facial features	Softening of cranial bones, prominence of frontal bones, skull flat and depressed toward middle	Vitamin D
Fused sutures after 18 mo	Delayed fusion of sutures	Vitamin D
	Hard, tender lumps in occiput	Excess vitamin A
	Headache	Excess thiamine
Neck		
Thyroid not visible, palpable in midline	Thyroid enlarged, may be grossly visible	Iodine
Eyes		
Clear, bright	Hardening and scaling of cornea and conjunctiva	Vitamin A
Good night vision	Night blindness	Vitamin A
Conjunctiva—Pink, glossy	Burning, itching, photophobia, cataracts, corneal vascularization	Riboflavin
Ears		
Tympanic membrane—Pliable	Calcified (hearing loss)	Excess vitamin D
Nose		
Smooth, intact nasal angle	Irritation and cracks at nasal angle	Riboflavin Excess vitamin A

*Nutrients listed are deficient unless specified as excess.

Table 34-1 Clinical Assessment of Nutritional Status—cont'd

EVIDENCE OF ADEQUATE NUTRITION	EVIDENCE OF DEFICIENT OR EXCESS NUTRITION	DEFICIENCY OR EXCESS*
Mouth		
Lips—Smooth, moist, darker color than skin	Fissures and inflammation at corners	Riboflavin Excess vitamin A
Gums—Firm, coral pink, stippled	Spongy, friable, swollen, bluish red or black, bleed easily	Vitamin C
Mucous membranes—Bright pink, smooth, moist	Stomatitis	Niacin
Tongue—Rough texture, no lesions, taste sensation	Glossitis	Niacin, riboflavin, folic acid
	Diminished taste sensation	Zinc
Teeth—Uniform white color, smooth, intact	Brown mottling, pits, fissures	Excess fluoride
	Defective enamel	Vitamins A, C, D, calcium, phosphorus
	Caries	Excess carbohydrates
Chest		
In infants, shape almost circular	Depressed lower portion of rib cage	Vitamin D
In children, lateral diameter increased in proportion to anteroposterior diameter	Sharp protrusion of sternum	Vitamin D
Smooth costochondral junctions	Enlarged costochondral junctions	Vitamins C, D
Breast development—Normal for age	Delayed development	See under General Growth; especially zinc
Cardiovascular System		
Pulse and blood pressure (BP) within normal limits	Palpitations	Thiamine
	Rapid pulse	Potassium Excess thiamine
	Arrhythmias	Magnesium, potassium Excess niacin, potassium
	Increased BP	Excess sodium
	Decreased BP	Thiamine Excess niacin
Abdomen		
In young children, cylindric and prominent	Distended, flabby, poor musculature	Protein, calories
	Prominent, large	Excess calories
In older children, flat	Potbelly, constipation	Vitamin D
Normal bowel habits	Diarrhea	Niacin Excess vitamin C
	Constipation	Excess calcium, potassium
Musculoskeletal System		
Muscles—Firm, well developed, equal strength bilaterally	Flabby, weak, generalized wasting	Protein, calories
	Weakness, pain, cramps	Thiamine, sodium, chloride, potassium, phosphorus, magnesium Excess thiamine
	Muscle twitching, tremors	Magnesium
	Muscular paralysis	Excess potassium
Spine—Cervical and lumbar curves (double S curve)	Kyphosis, lordosis, scoliosis	Vitamin D
Extremities—Symmetric; legs straight with minimum bowing	Bowing of extremities, knock-knees	Vitamin D, calcium, phosphorus
	Epiphyseal enlargement	Vitamins A, D
	Bleeding into joints and muscles, joint swelling, pain	Vitamin C
Joints—Flexible, full range of motion, no pain or stiffness	Thickening of cortex of long bones with pain and fragility, hard tender lumps in extremities	Excess vitamin A
	Osteoporosis of long bones	Calcium Excess vitamin D

Continued

Table 34-1 Clinical Assessment of Nutritional Status—cont'd

EVIDENCE OF ADEQUATE NUTRITION	EVIDENCE OF DEFICIENT OR EXCESS NUTRITION	DEFICIENCY OR EXCESS*
Neurologic System		
Behavior—Alert, responsive, emotionally stable	Listless, irritable, lethargic, apathetic (sometimes apprehensive, anxious, drowsy, mentally slow, confused)	Thiamine, niacin, pyridoxine, vitamin C, potassium, magnesium, iron, protein, calories Excess vitamins A, D, thiamine, folic acid, calcium
Absence of tetany, convulsions	Masklike facial expression, blurred speech, involuntary laughing	Excess manganese
	Convulsions	Thiamine, pyridoxine, vitamin D, calcium, magnesium Excess phosphorus (in relation to calcium)
Intact peripheral nervous system	Peripheral nervous system toxicity (unsteady gait, numb feet and hands, fine motor clumsiness)	Excess pyridoxine
Intact reflexes	Diminished or absent tendon reflexes	Thiamine, vitamin E

*Nutrients listed are deficient unless specified as excess.

Anthropometry, an essential parameter of nutritional status, is the measurement of height, weight, head circumference, proportions, skin fold thickness, and arm circumference in young children. Height and head circumference reflect past nutrition, whereas weight, skin fold thickness, and arm circumference reflect present nutritional status, especially of protein and fat reserves. Skin fold thickness is a measurement of the body's fat content because approximately half the body's total fat stores are directly beneath the skin. The upper arm muscle circumference is correlated with measurements of total muscle mass. Since muscle serves as the body's major protein reserve, this measurement is considered an index of the body's protein stores. Ideally, growth measurements are recorded over time, and comparisons are made regarding the *velocity* of growth based on previous and present values. Numerous biochemical tests available for assessing nutritional status include analysis of plasma; blood cells; urine; and tissues from liver, bone, hair, and fingernails. Many of these tests are complicated and are not performed routinely. Common laboratory procedures for nutritional status include measurement of hemoglobin, hematocrit, transferrin, albumin, creatinine, and nitrogen. Laboratory values for these tests and more specific nutrient measurements are given in Appendix D.

Evaluation of Nutritional Assessment

After collecting the data needed for a thorough nutritional assessment, evaluate the findings to plan appropriate counseling. From the data, assess whether the child is (1) malnourished, (2) at risk for becoming malnourished, or (3) well nourished with adequate reserves.

Analyze the daily food diary for the variety and amounts of foods suggested in MyPyramid *(www.mypyramid.gov)*. For example, if the list includes no vegetables, inquire about this rather than assuming that the child dislikes vegetables, since it could be that none were served that day. Also, evaluate the information in terms of the family's ethnic practices and financial resources. Encouraging increased protein intake with additional meat may be unfeasible for families on a limited budget or in conflict with food practices that use meat sparingly, such as in Asian meal preparation.

General Approaches Toward Examining the Child

Sequence of the Examination

Ordinarily, the sequence for examining patients follows a head-to-toe direction. The main function of such a systematic approach is to avoid omitting segments of the examination. The standard recording of data also facilitates exchange of information among different professionals. This orderly sequence is frequently altered to accommodate the child's developmental needs, although the examination is recorded following the head-to-toe model. Using developmental and chronologic age as the main criteria for assessing each body system accomplishes several goals:

- Minimizes stress and anxiety associated with assessment of various body parts
- Fosters a trusting nurse-child-parent relationship
- Allows for maximum preparation of the child
- Preserves the essential security of the parent-child relationship, especially with young children
- Maximizes the accuracy and reliability of assessment findings

Preparation of the Child

Although the physical examination consists of painless procedures, to a child the use of a tight arm cuff, probes in the ears and mouth, pressure on the abdomen, and a cold piece of metal to listen to the chest can be stressful. Therefore the same considerations discussed in Chapter 45 for preparing children for procedures are followed here. In addition to that discussion, general guidelines related to the examining process are presented in the Guidelines box.

The physical examination should be as pleasant as possible and educational. For example, the nurse can use a detailed drawing or anatomically correct doll to help preschoolers and older children learn about their bodies (Vessey, 1995). The paper-doll technique is a useful approach to teaching children about the body part that is being examined (Fig. 34-4). At the conclusion of the visit, the child can bring home the paper doll as a memento of the experience.

GUIDELINES Performing Pediatric Physical Examination

Perform examination in appropriate, nonthreatening area.
- Have room well lit and decorated with neutral colors.
- Have room temperature comfortably warm.
- Place all strange and potentially frightening equipment out of sight.
- Have some toys, dolls, stuffed animals, and games available for child.
- If possible, have rooms decorated and equipped for different-age children.
- Provide privacy, especially for school-age children and adolescents.

Provide time for play and becoming acquainted.

Observe behaviors that signal child's readiness to cooperate:
- Talking to the nurse
- Making eye contact
- Accepting the offered equipment
- Allowing physical touching
- Choosing to sit on examining table rather than parent's lap

If signs of readiness are not observed, use the following techniques:
- Talk to parent while essentially "ignoring" child; gradually focus on child or a favorite object, such as a doll.
- Make complimentary remarks about child, such as appearance, dress, or a favorite object.
- Tell a funny story or play a simple magic trick.
- Have a nonthreatening "friend" available, such as a hand puppet to "talk" to child for the nurse (see Fig. 34-25, *A*).

If child refuses to cooperate, use the following techniques:
- Assess reason for uncooperative behavior; consider that a child who is unduly afraid may have had a traumatic experience.
- Try to involve child and parent in process.
- Avoid prolonged explanations about examining procedure.
- Use a firm, direct approach regarding expected behavior.
- Perform examination as quickly as possible.
- Have attendant gently restrain child.
- Minimize any disruptions or stimulation.
- Limit number of people in room.
- Use isolated room.
- Use quiet, calm, confident voice.

Begin examination in a nonthreatening manner for young children or children who are fearful:
- Use activities that can be presented as games, such as test for cranial nerves (see Table 34-13) or parts of developmental screening tests (p. 923).
- Use approaches such as Simon Says to encourage child to make a face, squeeze a hand, stand on one foot, and so on.
- Use paper-doll technique:
  1. Lay child supine on an examining table or floor that is covered with a large sheet of paper.
  2. Trace around child's body outline.
  3. Use body outline to demonstrate what will be examined, such as drawing a heart and listening with stethoscope before performing activity on child.

If several children in the family will be examined, begin with most cooperative child to model desired behavior.

Involve child in examination process:
- Provide choices, such as sitting on table or in parent's lap.
- Allow child to handle or hold equipment.
- Encourage child to use equipment on a doll, family member, or examiner.
- Explain each step of the procedure in simple language.

Examine child in a comfortable and secure position:
- Sitting in parent's lap
- Sitting upright if in respiratory distress

Proceed to examine the body in an organized sequence (usually head to toe) with the following exceptions:
- Alter sequence to accommodate needs of different-age children (see Table 34-2).
- Examine painful areas last.
- In emergency situation, examine vital functions (airway, breathing, and circulation) and injured area first.

Reassure child throughout examination, especially about bodily concerns that arise during puberty.

Discuss findings with family at end of examination.

Praise child for cooperation during examination; give reward such as a small toy or sticker.

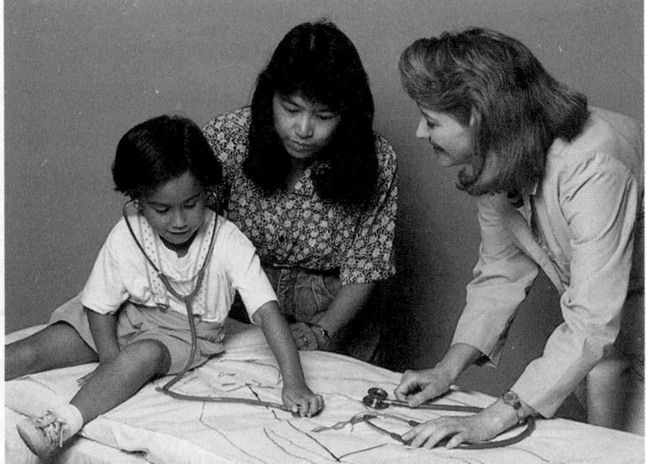

Fig. 34-4 Using paper-doll technique to prepare child for physical examination.

Table 34-2 summarizes guidelines for positioning, preparing, and examining children at various ages. Because no child fits precisely into one age category, it may be necessary to vary the approach after a preliminary assessment of the child's developmental achievements and needs. Even with the best approach, many toddlers are uncooperative and inconsolable for much of the physical examination. However, some seem intrigued by the new surroundings and unusual equipment and respond more like preschoolers than toddlers. Likewise, some early preschoolers may require more of the "security measures" employed with younger children, such as continued parent-child contact, and less of the preparatory measures used with preschoolers, such as playing with the equipment before and during the actual examination (Fig. 34-5).

Although the variations in the general approaches are numerous, some common ones are elaborated on here. For

Table 34-2 Age-Specific Approaches to Physical Examination During Childhood

POSITION	SEQUENCE	PREPARATION
Infant		
Before able to sit alone—Supine or prone, preferably in parent's lap; before 4-6 mo, can place on examining table **After able to sit alone**—Sitting in parent's lap whenever possible; if on table, place with parent in full view	If quiet, auscultate heart, lungs, abdomen. Record heart and respiratory rates. Palpate and percuss same areas. Proceed in usual head-to-toe direction. Perform traumatic procedures last (eyes, ears, mouth [while crying]). Elicit reflexes as body part is examined. Elicit Moro reflex last.	Completely undress if room temperature permits. Leave diaper on male infant. Gain cooperation with distraction, bright objects, rattles, talking. Smile at infant; use soft, gentle voice. Pacify with bottle of sugar water or feeding. Enlist parent's aid for restraining to examine ears, mouth. Avoid abrupt, jerky movements.
Toddler		
Sitting or standing on or by parent Prone or supine in parent's lap	Inspect body area through play: "count fingers," "tickle toes." Use minimum physical contact initially. Introduce equipment slowly. Auscultate, percuss, palpate whenever quiet. Perform traumatic procedures last (same as for infant).	Have parent remove outer clothing. Remove underwear as body part is examined. Allow to inspect equipment; demonstrating use of equipment is usually ineffective. If uncooperative, perform procedures quickly. Use restraint when appropriate; request parent's assistance. Talk about examination if cooperative; use short phrases. Praise for cooperative behavior.
Preschool Child		
Prefer standing or sitting Usually cooperative prone or supine Prefer parent's closeness	If cooperative, proceed in head-to-toe direction. If uncooperative, proceed as with toddler.	Request self-undressing. Allow to wear underpants if shy. Offer equipment for inspection; briefly demonstrate use. Make up story about procedure (e.g., "I'm seeing how strong your muscles are"[blood pressure]). Use paper-doll technique. Give choices when possible. Expect cooperation; use positive statements (e.g., "Open your mouth").
School-Age Child		
Prefer sitting Cooperative in most positions Younger child prefers parent's presence Older child may prefer privacy	Proceed in head-to-toe direction. May examine genitalia last in older child.	Respect need for privacy. Request self-undressing. Allow to wear underpants. Give gown to wear. Explain purpose of equipment and significance of procedure, such as otoscope to see eardrum, which is necessary for hearing. Teach about body function and care.
Adolescent		
Same as for school-age child Offer option of parent's presence	Same as older school-age child. May examine genitalia last.	Allow to undress in private. Give gown. Expose only area to be examined. Respect need for privacy. Explain findings during examination: "Your muscles are firm and strong." Matter-of-factly comment about sexual development: "Your breasts are developing as they should be." Emphasize normalcy of development. Examine genitalia as any other body part; may leave to end.

example, the suggested sequence may change considerably when the child is in pain or when obvious physical defects are present. In either situation, examine the affected area last to minimize distress early in the examination and to focus on normal, healthy, functioning body parts.

Physical Examination

Although the approach to and sequence of the physical examination differ according to the child's age, the following discussion outlines the traditional model for physical assessment.

The focus includes all pediatric age groups, but the reader is referred to Chapter 25 for a detailed discussion of a newborn assessment. Because the physical examination is a vital part of preventive pediatric care, a schedule for periodic health visits is given in Fig. 34-6.

Growth Measurements

Measurement of physical growth in children is a key element in evaluating their health status. Physical growth parameters include weight, height (length), skin fold thickness, arm circumference, and head circumference. Values for these growth parameters are plotted on percentile charts, and the child's measurements in percentiles are compared with those of the general population.

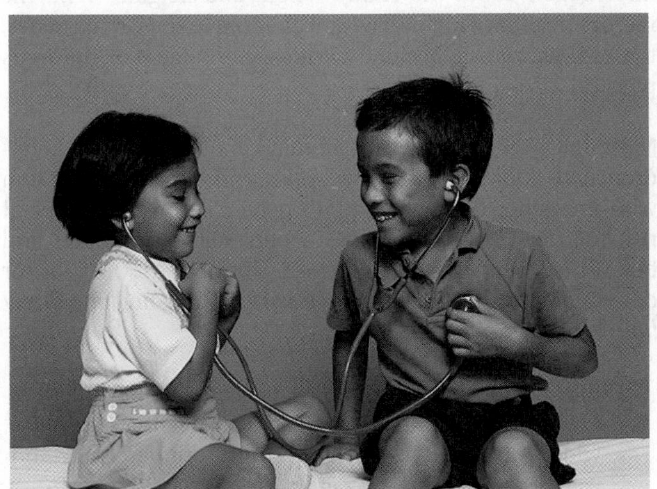

Fig. 34-5 Preparing children for physical examination.

Growth Charts

The most commonly used growth charts in the United States are from the National Center for Health Statistics (NCHS) (Kuczmarski et al, 2000). The growth charts have been revised to include the body mass index–for-age (BMI-for-age) charts, 3rd and 97th smoothed percentiles for all charts, and the 85th percentile for the weight-for-stature and BMI-for-age charts (see the EVOLVE site). The data were collected from five national surveys between 1963 and 1994. The revised charts have eliminated the disjunctions between the curves for infants and other children and have been extended for children and adolescents to 20 years.

The weight-for-age percentile distributions are now continuous between the infant and the older child charts at 24 to 36 months. The length-for-age to stature-for-age and weight-for-length to weight-for-stature curves are parallel in the overlapping ages of 24 to 36 months. The revised weight-for-stature charts provide a smoother transition from the weight-for-length charts for preschool-age children.

The most prominent change to the complement of growth charts for older children and adolescents is the addition of the

evolve Skill—Measuring Physical Growth

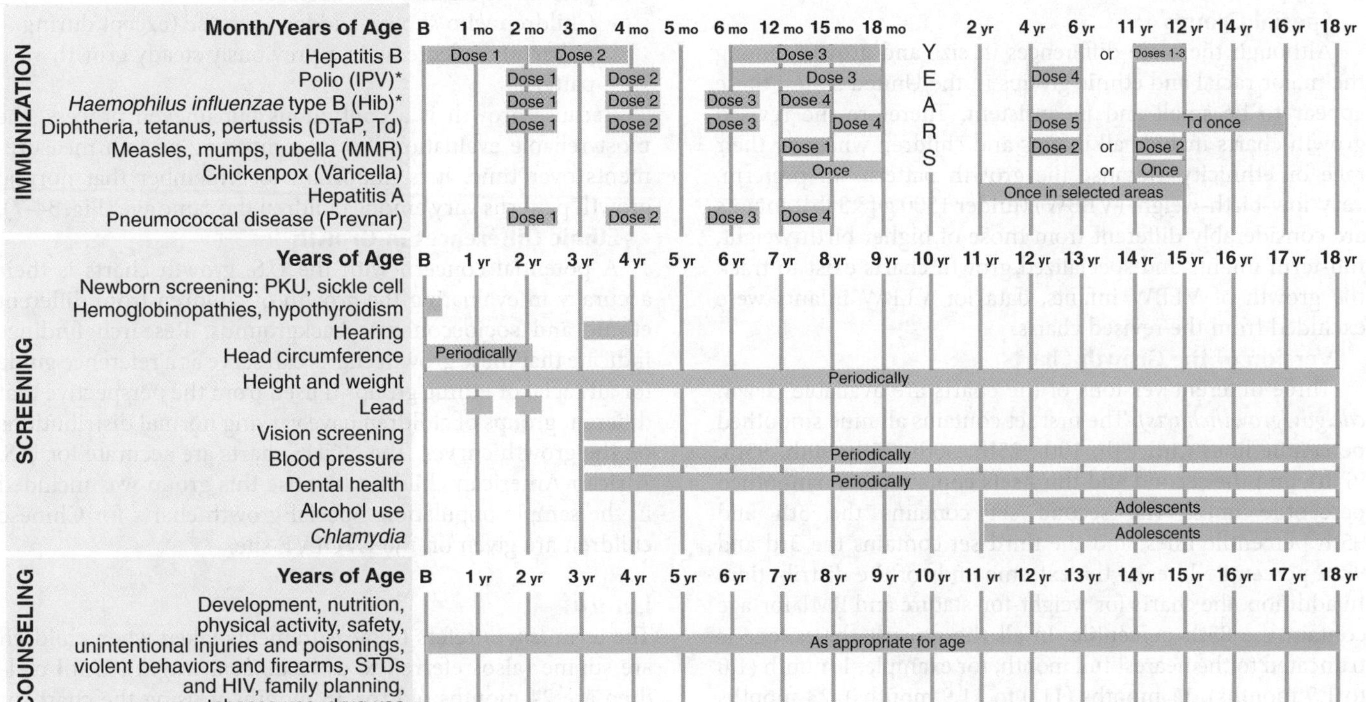

Fig. 34-6 Child preventive care time line. The information on immunizations is based on recommendations issued by Advisory Committee on Immunization Practices, American Academy of Pediatrics, and American Academy of Family Physicians. *B,* Birth; *HIV,* human immunodeficiency virus; *PKU,* phenylketonuria; *STDs,* sexually transmitted diseases. (From US Department of Health and Human Services: *Child health guide: put prevention into practice*, Washington, DC, January 2003 [rev], The Department.)

BMI-for-age growth curves. The BMI-for-age charts were developed with national survey data (1963 to 1994), excluding data from the 1988 to 1994 National Health and Nutrition Examination Surveys III (NHANES III) for children older than 6 years because an increase in body weight and BMI occurred between NHANES III and previous national surveys. Without this exclusion, the 85th and 95th percentile curves would have been higher, and fewer children and adolescents would have been classified as at risk of or overweight. Therefore the BMI-for-age growth curves do not represent the current population of children older than 6 years of age.

NURSING ALERT The sex-specific BMI-for-age charts for ages 2 to 20 years replace the 1977 NCHS weight-for-stature charts that were limited to prepubescent boys younger than 11½ years and with statures less than 145 cm (4 feet, 9 inches), and to prepubescent girls younger than 19 years and with statures less than 135 cm (4 feet, 5 inches).

Breastfed and Formula-Fed Infants

The national survey data better represent the combined size and growth patterns of the general U.S. population (1971 to 1994). Over the past 30 years in the United States, approximately half of all infants were reported to have been breastfed, and approximately one third were breastfed for 3 months or more. Therefore, compared with the 1977 NCHS growth charts, the nationally representative data on which the revised infant growth charts are based better represent the combined growth patterns of breastfed and formula-fed infants in the U.S. population.

Special Groups

Although there are differences in size and growth among the major racial and ethnic groups in the United States, these appear to be small and inconsistent. Therefore the revised growth charts include all infants and children whatever their race or ethnicity. Because the growth patterns of preterm, very-low-birth-weight (VLBW) (under 1500 g [3.3 lb]) infants are considerably different from those of higher birth-weight, full-term infants and specialized growth charts exist to track the growth of VLBW infants, data for VLBW infants were excluded from the revised charts.

Version of the Growth Charts

Three different versions of the charts are available *(www.cdc.gov/growthcharts)*. The first set contains all nine smoothed percentile lines (3rd, 5th, 10th, 25th, 50th, 75th, 90th, 95th, 97th), and the second and third sets contain seven smoothed percentile lines. The second set contains the 5th and 95th percentile lines, and the third set contains the 3rd and 97th percentile lines at the extreme ends of the distribution. In addition, the charts for weight-for-stature and BMI-for-age contain the 85th percentile. In all the growth charts, age is truncated to the nearest full month, for example, 1 month (1.0 to 1.9 months), 11 months (11.0 to 11.9 months), 23 months (23.0 to 23.9 months).

The three sets of charts are provided to meet the needs of various users. Set 1 shows all the major percentile curves but may have limitations when the curves are close together, especially at the youngest ages. Most users in the United States may wish to use the format shown in set 2 for the majority of routine clinical applications. Pediatric endocrinologists and others dealing with special populations, such as children with failure to thrive, may wish to use the format in set 3.

Nurses are often responsible for measuring growth in children, so it is essential that they understand the revised growth charts. Several important differences exist between the 1977 and the revised charts with significant implications for classifying children as underweight or overweight. Nurses need to become familiar with determining BMI, which only requires information about the child's weight and height.* With the increasing number of overweight children in the United States, the BMI charts will become a critical component of children's physical assessment.

NURSING ALERT BMI-for-age may be used to identify children and adolescents at the upper end of the distribution who are either overweight (95th percentile or greater) or at risk for being overweight (85th percentile and above and below the 95th percentile) (Roche & Guo, 2001). Formulas for determining BMI are available at *www.cdc.gov/nccdphp/dnpa/bmi*, below, and on p. 1129.

Children whose growth may be questionable include:

- Children whose height and weight percentiles are widely disparate (e.g., height in the 10th percentile and weight in the 90th percentile, especially with above-average skin fold thickness)
- Children who fail to show the expected growth rates in height and weight, especially during the rapid growth periods of infancy and adolescence
- Children who show a sudden increase (except during puberty) or decrease in a previously steady growth pattern

Because growth is a continuous but uneven process, the most reliable evaluation lies in comparing growth measurements over time. It is important to remember that normal growth patterns vary among children the same age (Fig. 34-7).

Ethnic Differences in Growth

A potential concern with the U.S. growth charts is their accuracy in evaluating the growth of children from different ethnic and socioeconomic backgrounds. Research findings indicate that these growth charts can serve as a reference guide for all racial or ethnic groups if used from the perspective that different groups of children have varying normal distributions on the growth curves. The NCHS charts are accurate for U.S. African-American children because this group was included in the sample population. Special growth charts for Chinese children are given on the EVOLVE site.

Length

The term *length* refers to measurements taken when children are supine (also referred to as *recumbent length*). Until children are 24 months old (or 36 months if using the chart for

**BMI = [Weight in pounds ÷ (Height in inches × Height in inches)] × 703. NOTE: Formula is BMI calculation for adults, used in some pediatric settings; for child and adolescent BMI table and plotting, see the EVOLVE site.*

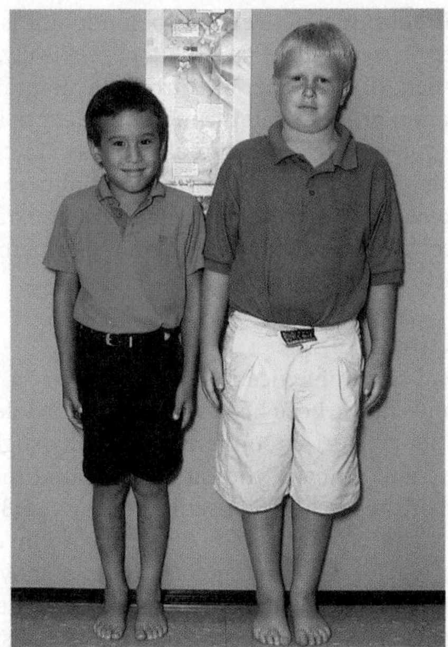

Fig. 34-7 These children of identical age (8 years) are markedly different in size. Child on left, of Asian descent, is at 5th percentile for height and weight. Child on right is above 95th percentile for height and weight. However, both children demonstrate normal growth patterns.

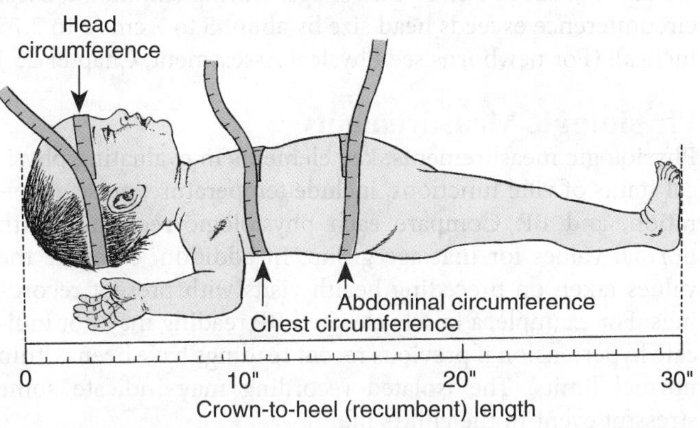

Fig. 34-8 Measurement of head, chest, and abdominal circumference and crown-to-heel (recumbent) length.

birth to 36 months), measure recumbent length. Because of the normally flexed position during infancy, fully extend the body by (1) holding the head in midline, (2) grasping the knees together gently, and (3) pushing down on the knees until the legs are fully extended and flat against the table. If using a measuring board, place the head firmly at the top of the board and the heels of the feet firmly against the footboard.

If such a measuring device is not available, measure length by placing the child on a paper-covered surface, marking the end points of the top of the head and the heels of the feet, and measuring between these two points (Fig. 34-8). For accurate measurement, hold the writing utensil at a right angle to the table when marking the cephalic point; position the feet with the toes pointing directly to the ceiling when marking the heel point. Regardless of the method used, have someone assist in holding the child's head in midline while you extend the legs and take the measurements.

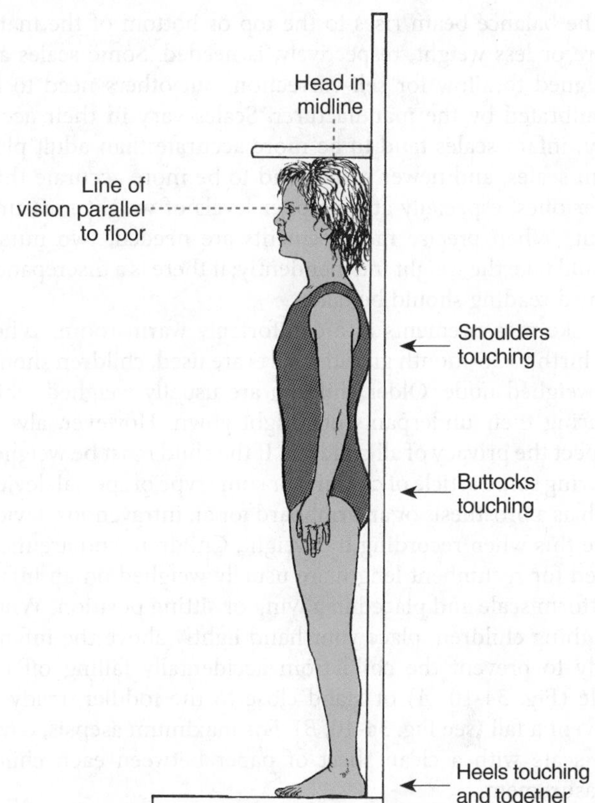

Fig. 34-9 Measurement of height. (Redrawn from *Human growth and growth disorders: an update*, San Francisco, 1989, Genentech.)

Height

The term *height* (or *stature*) refers to the measurement taken when children are standing upright. Measure height by having the child, with shoes removed, stand as tall and straight as possible, with the head in midline and the line of vision parallel to the ceiling and floor. Be certain the child's back is to the wall or other vertical flat surface, with the heels, buttocks, and back of the shoulders touching the wall and the medial malleoli touching if possible (Fig. 34-9). Check for and correct bending of the knees, slumping of the shoulders, or raising of the heels.

For the most accurate measurement, use a wall-mounted unit (stadiometer; see Fig. 34-9). The movable measuring rod of platform scales is accurate only if it maintains a parallel position to the floor and rests securely on the topmost part of the head. To improvise a flat surface for measuring length, attach a paper or metal tape or yardstick to the wall, position the child adjacent to the tape, and place a three-dimensional object, such as a thick book or box, on top of the head. Rest the side of the object firmly against the wall to form a right angle. Measure length or stature to the nearest 1 mm or ⅛ inch.

Weight

Weight is measured with an appropriately sized beam balance scale, which measures weight to the nearest 10 g (0.35 oz) for infants and 100 g (0.22 lb) for children. Before the child is weighed, balance the scale by setting it at 0 and noting if the balance registers exactly in the middle of the mark. If the end of the balance beam rises to the top or bottom of the mark, more or less weight, respectively, is needed. Some scales are designed to allow for self-correction, but others need to be recalibrated by the manufacturer. Scales vary in their accuracy; infant scales tend to be more accurate than adult platform scales, and newer scales tend to be more accurate than older ones, especially at the upper levels of weight measurement. When precise measurements are needed, two nurses should take the weight independently; if there is a discrepancy, a third reading should be taken.

Take measurements in a comfortably warm room. When the birth to 36-month growth charts are used, children should be weighed nude. Older children are usually weighed while wearing their underpants or a light gown. However, always respect the privacy of all children. If the child must be weighed wearing some article of clothing or some type of special device, such as a prosthesis or an armboard for an intravenous device, note this when recording the weight. Children who are measured for recumbent length are usually weighed on an infant platform scale and placed in a lying or sitting position. When weighing children, place your hand lightly above the infant's body to prevent the child from accidentally falling off the scale (Fig. 34-10, *A*) or stand close to the toddler, ready to prevent a fall (see Fig. 34-10, *B*). For maximum asepsis, cover the scale with a clean sheet of paper between each child's measurement.

Skin Fold Thickness and Arm Circumference

Measures of relative weight and stature cannot distinguish between adipose (fat) tissue and muscle. One convenient measure of body fat is skin fold thickness, which is increasingly recommended as a routine measurement. Skin fold thickness is measured with special calipers, such as the Lange calipers. The most common sites for measuring skin fold thickness are the triceps (most practical for routine clinical use), subscapula, suprailiac, abdomen, and upper thigh. For greatest reliability the exact procedure for measurement must be followed and the average of at least two measurements of one site recorded.

Arm circumference is an indirect measure of muscle mass. Measurement of arm circumference follows the same procedure for skin fold thickness except the midpoint is measured with a paper or steel tape. Place the tape vertically, along the posterior aspect of the upper arm from the acromial process to the olecranon process; half the measured length is the midpoint. Percentiles for triceps skin fold and arm circumference in children are listed on the EVOLVE site and may be used as reference data. However, the percentiles are not standards or norms, since values between the 5th and 95th percentiles are not ranges of normal.

Head Circumference

Measure head circumference in children up to 36 months of age and in any child whose head size is questionable. Measure the head at its greatest circumference, usually slightly above the eyebrows and pinna of the ears and around the occipital prominence at the back of the skull (see Fig. 34-8). Because head shape can affect the location of the maximum circumference, more than one measurement at points above the eyebrows may be needed to obtain the most accurate measure. Use a paper or metal tape, since a cloth tape can stretch and give a falsely small measurement. For greatest accuracy, use devices with tenths of a centimeter, since the percentile charts have only 0.5-cm increments.

Plot the head size on the appropriate growth chart under head circumference. Generally, head and chest circumferences are equal at about 1 to 2 years of age. During childhood, chest circumference exceeds head size by about 5 to 7 cm (2 to 2.75 inches). (For newborns see Physical Assessment, Chapter 25.)

Physiologic Measurements

Physiologic measurements, key elements in evaluating physical status of vital functions, include temperature, pulse, respiration, and BP. Compare each physiologic recording with normal values for that age group. In addition, compare the values taken on preceding health visits with present recordings. For example, a falsely elevated BP reading may not indicate hypertension if previous recent readings have been within normal limits. The isolated recording may indicate some stressful event in the child's life.

As in most procedures carried out with children, older children and adolescents are treated much the same as adults.

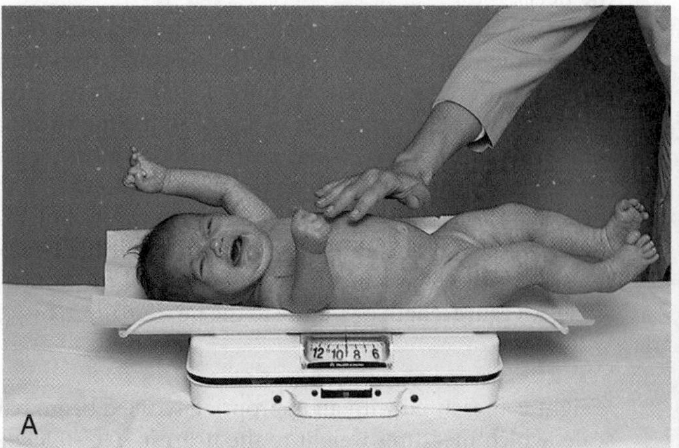

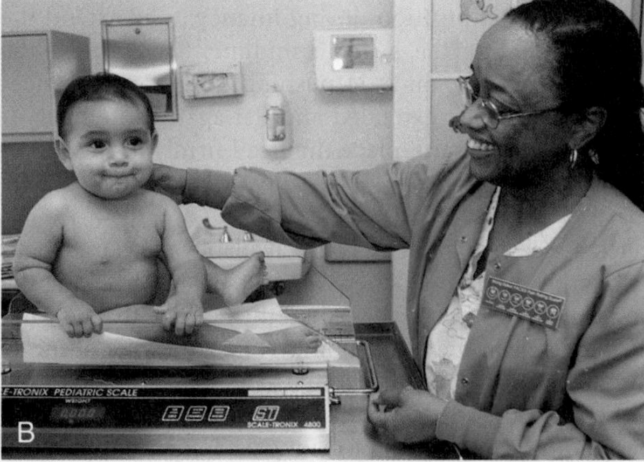

Fig. 34-10 A, Infant on scale. B, Toddler on scale. Note presence of nurse to prevent falls. *(B, Courtesy Paul Vincent Kuntz, Texas Children's Hospital, Houston.)*

However, special consideration must be given to preschool children (see Atraumatic Care box).

ATRAUMATIC CARE

Reducing Young Children's Fears

Young children, especially preschoolers, fear intrusive procedures because of their poorly defined body boundaries. Therefore avoid invasive procedures, such as measuring rectal temperature, whenever possible. Also, avoid using the word "take" when measuring vital signs, since young children interpret words literally and may think that their temperature or other function will be taken away. Instead, say, "I want to know how warm you are."

For best results in taking vital signs of infants, count respirations first (before the infant is disturbed), take the pulse next, and measure temperature last. If vital signs cannot be taken without disturbing the child, record the child's behavior (e.g., crying) along with the measurement.

Temperature

Temperature is the measure of heat content within an individual's body. The core temperature most closely reflects the temperature of the blood flow through the carotid arteries to the hypothalamus. Core temperature is relatively constant despite wide fluctuations in the external environment. When a child's temperature is altered, receptors in the skin, spinal cord, and brain respond in an attempt to achieve normothermia, a normal temperature state. In pediatrics, there is a lack of consensus regarding what temperature constitutes normothermia for every child. For rectal temperatures in children, 37° to 37.5° C (98.6° to 99.5° F) is an acceptable range, where heat loss and heat production are balanced. For neonates, a core body temperature between 36.5° and 37.6° C (97.7° and 99.7° F) is a desirable range. In the neonate, temperature measurements are obtained for monitoring adequacy of thermoregulation, not fever; therefore temperature measurements in each infant should be carefully considered in the context of the *purpose* and the environment. Temperature definitions of fever based on age are found in Box 34-10.

Temperature in healthy children can be measured at several body sites via oral, rectal, axillary, ear canal, tympanic membrane, temporal artery, or skin route (Box 34-11). For the ill child other sites for temperature measurement that have been investigated include the urinary bladder, pulmonary artery, and esophageal and nasopharyngeal sites (Martin & Kline, 2004) (Box 34-12). One of the most important influences on the accuracy of temperature is improper temperature-taking technique. Detailed discussion of temperature-taking methods and visual examples of proper techniques are shown in Table 34-3. For a critical review of the evidence on temperature taking methods, see the Evidence-Based Practice box.

NURSING ALERT Glass mercury thermometers used in many studies as the "gold standard" are no longer recommended for use (Goldman & Shannon, 2001).

BOX 34-10 Fever in Infants and Children

Temperature depends on the time of day, age and physical activity. In general fever is defined as:

In infants less than 3 months of age: below 38° C (100.4° F)

For infants older than 3 months of age: below 39° C (102.2° F)

BOX 34-11 Recommended Temperature Screening Routes in Infants and Children

Birth to 2 Years

Axillary

Rectal—if definitive temperature reading is needed for infants over 1 month of age

2 to 5 Years

Axillary

Tympanic

Oral—when child can hold thermometer under tongue

Rectal—if definitive temperature reading is needed

Over 5 Years

Oral

Axillary

Tympanic

The most frequently used temperature measurement devices in infants and children are as follows (Healthcare Product Comparison System, 2004a, 2004b):

Electronic intermittent thermometers—Measure the patient's temperature at oral, rectal, and axillary sites and are used as primary diagnostic indicators

Infrared thermometers—Measure the patient's temperature by collecting emitted thermal radiation from a particular site (e.g., ear canal)

Electronic continuous thermometers—Measure the patient's temperature during the administration of general anesthesia, treatment of hypothermia or hyperthermia, and other situations that require continuous monitoring

A detailed description of these devices is found in Box 34-13.

NURSING ALERT The belief that core temperature can be estimated by adding 1° C to the temperature taken in the axilla is incorrect. Do not add a degree to the finding obtained by taking a temperature by the axillary route (Craig et al, 2000).

Pulse

A satisfactory pulse can be taken radially in children older than 2 years of age. However, in infants and young children, the apical impulse (heard through a stethoscope held to the chest at the apex of the heart) is more reliable (see Fig. 34-32 for location of pulses). Count the pulse for 1 full minute in infants and young children because of possible irregularities

evolve Skill—Measuring Body Temperature

BOX 34-12 Alternative Temperature Measurement Sites for the Ill Child

Skin

Probe is placed on the skin to determine heat output in response to changes in the patient's skin temperature.

Skin temperature sensors are most often used for neonates and infants placed in radiant heat warmers or isolettes (using servocontrol feature of the apparatus). In turn, the heater unit warms to a set point to maintain the infant's temperature within a specified range.

ThermoSpot is an example of a device allowing continuous thermal monitoring in neonates.

Urinary Bladder

A thermistor or thermocouple is placed within the indwelling bladder catheter. The catheter tip immersed in the bladder provides a continuous temperature read-out on the bedside monitor.

This is not a true measure of core temperature but responds better than rectal and skin temperatures to core body changes.

Because of thermistor sizes, this method is unusable with neonates and small infants.

Pulmonary Artery

A catheter is placed into the heart to obtain a reading in the pulmonary artery.

It is used in critical care settings or operating rooms only in patients requiring aggressive monitoring.

Catheter is not available in sizes for neonates or small infants.

Esophageal Site

Probe is inserted into the lower third of the esophagus at the level of the heart.

This is used in critical care settings or operating rooms.

Several companies have esophageal stethoscopes with temperature probe monitors that show a continuous temperature reading for patients in the operating room.

Nasopharyngeal Site

Probe is inserted into the nasopharynx, posterior to the soft palate, and provides an estimate of hypothalamic temperature.

This is used in critical care settings or operating rooms.

Data from Kumar PR, Nisarga R, Gowda B: Temperature monitoring in newborns using ThermoSpot, *Indian J Pediatr* 71(9):795-796, 2004; Martin SA, Kline AM: Can there be a standard for temperature measurement in the pediatric intensive care unit? *AACN Clin Issues* 15(2):254-266, 2004; Maxton FJC, Justin L, Gilles D: Estimating core temperature in infants and children after cardiac surgery: a comparison of six methods, *J Adv Nurs* 45(2):214-222, 2004.

Table 34-3 Temperature Measurement Locations for Infants and Children

TEMPERATURE SITE
Oral Place tip under tongue in right or left posterior sublingual pocket, not in front of tongue. Have child keep mouth closed, without biting on thermometer. Pacifier thermometers measure intraoral or supralingual temperature and are available but lack support in the literature. Several factors affect mouth temperature: eating and mastication, hot or cold beverages, open-mouth breathing, ambient temperature. 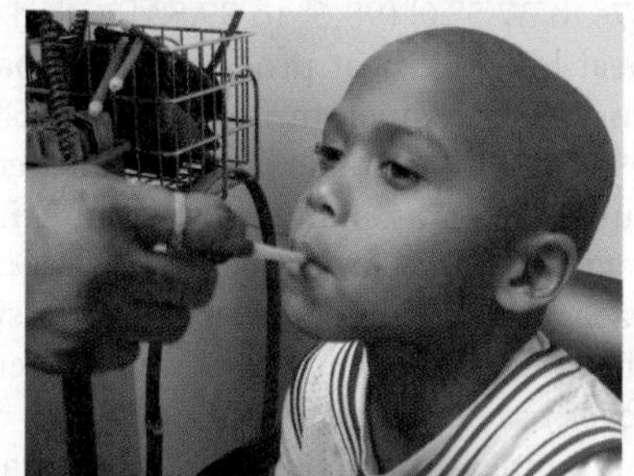
Axillary Place tip under arm in center of axilla and keep close to skin, not clothing. Hold child's arm firmly against side. Temperature may be affected by poor peripheral perfusion (results in lower value), clothing or swaddling, use of radiant warmer, or amount of brown fat in cold-stressed neonate (results in higher value). Advantage: avoids intrusive procedure and eliminates risk of rectal perforation. 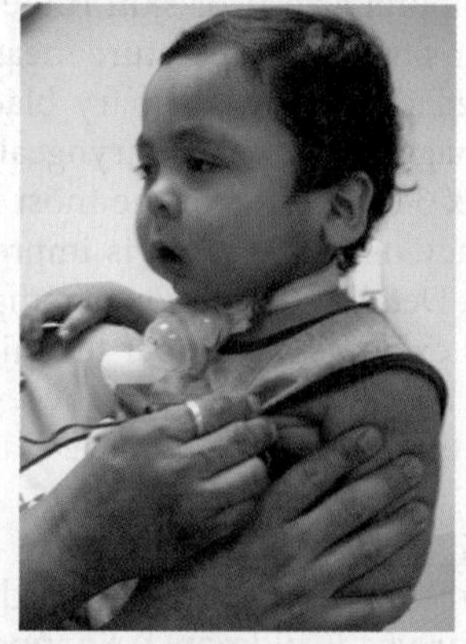

Table 34-3 Temperature Measurement Locations for Infants and Children—cont'd

TEMPERATURE SITE	
Ear Based (Aural) Insert small infrared probe deeply into canal to allow sensor to obtain measurement. Size of probe (most are 8 mm) may influence accuracy of result. In young children this may be a problem because of small diameter of canal. Proper placement of ear is controversial related to whether the pinna should be pulled in manner similar to that used during otoscopy (see p. 910).	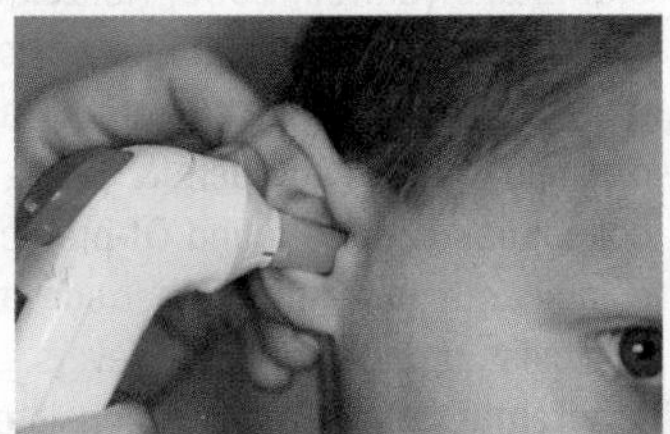
Rectal Place well-lubricated tip at maximum 2.5 cm (1 inch) into rectum for children and 1.5 cm (0.6 inch) for infants; securely hold thermometer close to anus. Child may be placed in side-lying, supine, or prone position (i.e., supine with knees flexed toward abdomen); cover penis, since procedure may stimulate urination. A small child may be placed prone across parent's lap.	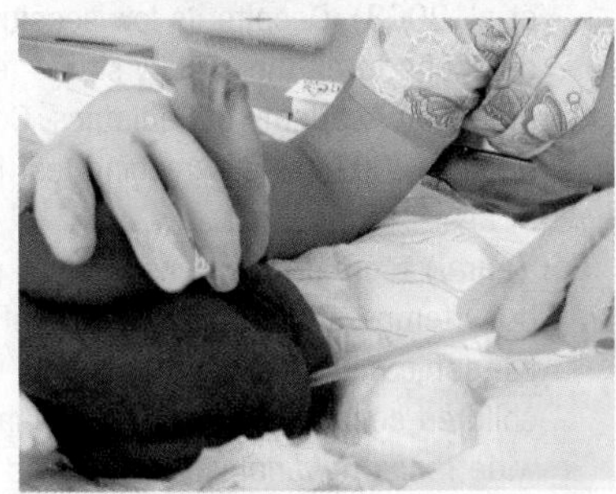
Temporal Artery An infrared sensor probe scans across forehead, capturing heat from arterial blood flow. Temporal artery is only artery close enough to skin's surface to provide access for accurate temperature measurement.	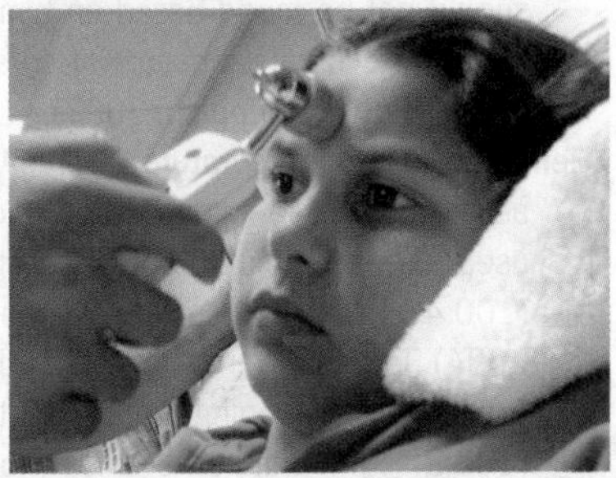

Data from Martin SA, Kline AM: Can there be a standard for temperature measurement in the pediatric intensive care unit? *AACN Clin Issues* 15(2):254-266, 2004; Falzon A et al: How reliable is axillary temperature measurement? *Acta Paediatr* 92(3):309-313, 2003. Oral, axillary, rectal, and temporal artery images courtesy Paul Vincent Kuntz, Texas Children's Hospital, Houston.

EVIDENCE-BASED PRACTICE Temperature Measurement in Pediatrics

Ask the Question

In infants and children, what is the most accurate method for measuring temperature?

Search for Evidence

Search Strategies

English publications, published within past 10 years, research-based articles (level 3 or lower), infant and child populations, comparisons to gold standard: rectal thermometry

Databases Searched

PubMed, Cochrane Collaboration, MD Consult, Joanna Briggs Institute, National Guideline Clearinghouse (AHRQ), TRIP Database Plus, PedsCCM, BestBETs

Critically Analyze the Evidence

Rectal temperature–Rectal measurement remains the clinical gold standard for the precise diagnosis of fever in infants and children (Greenes & Fleisher, 2004; Riddell & Eppich, 2003; University of Michigan, 2003). However, this procedure is more invasive and is contraindicated for infants less than 1 month old, children with recent rectal surgery, children with diarrhea or anorectal lesions, and children receiving chemotherapy (cancer treatment usually affects mucosa and causes neutropenia). Findings are affected by depth of insertion and presence of stool. Rectal temperatures are slow to change in relation to changing core temperature. Many parents are uncomfortable with this method, and children may resent it. It has capacity to spread contaminants found in stool.

Oral temperature (OTs)–OT indicates rapid changes in core body temperature, but accuracy may be an issue when compared with rectal site (Jensen et al, 2000). OTs are considered the standard for temperature measurement (Gilbert, Barton, & Counsell, 2002), but are contraindicated in children who have an altered level of consciousness, are receiving oxygen, are mouth breathing, are experiencing mucositis, had recent oral surgery or trauma, or are under 5 years of age (Carroll, 2000; Holtzclaw, 1998; El-Radhi & Barry, 2006). Limitations of OTs include the effect of ambient room temperature and recent

Continued

EVIDENCE-BASED PRACTICE Temperature Measurement in Pediatrics—cont'd

Critically Analyze the Evidence—cont'd

oral intake (Carroll, 2000; Holtzclaw, 1998; Martin & Kline, 2004). Even patients with no obvious mouth breathing were found to have OTs in the normal range despite the presence of clinical fever (Tandberg & Sklar, 1983). O'Brien and colleagues (2000) found OT-predictive thermometers to read significantly lower than other core temperature measurements and miss one out of seven fevers.

Axillary temperature—This is inconsistent and insensitive in infants and children over 1 month old (Jean-Mary et al, 2002; Falzon et al, 2003). Despite its low sensitivity and specificity in detecting fever, the axillary site is recommended by the American Academy of Pediatrics, Committee on Environmental Health (2001) as a screening test for fever in infants 1 month of age.

Ear (aural) temperature—This is not a precise measurement of body temperature. Meta-analysis of 101 studies comparing tympanic membrane temperatures with rectal temperatures in children concluded that the tympanic method demonstrated a wide range of variability, limiting its application in a pediatric setting (Craig et al, 2002). Diagnosis of fever without a focus should not be made based on tympanic thermometry, since it is not an accurate measure of core temperature (Craig et al, 2002; Riddell & Eppich, 2003).

Temporal artery temperature (TAT)—TAT was not reliable in the assessment of fever in children under 3 months but could be used as a screening tool for detecting fever less than 38° C (100.4° F) in children 3 to 24 months old (Schuh et al, 2004). Temporal temperature can be used as a rapid assessment screening tool to identify rectal fever over 39° C (102.2° F) in children 3 to 24 months old, but is unreliable as a screening tool for infants under 3 months (Siberry et al, 2002). These published studies examining the accuracy and precision of TATs in infants and children are limited by small sample sizes. Previous samples included subjects primarily under the age of 36 months, although one abstract was found of a study that examined 75 TATs in children 6 to 12 years old (Pidwell et al, 2000). Settings that have been used to study TATs in pediatric patients include the emergency department (Greenes & Fleisher, 2001; Pidwell et al, 2000; Schuh et al, 2004; Siberry et al, 2002), physician's office (Callanan, 2003), pediatric intensive care unit (Hebbar et al, 2005), and operating room (Al-Mukhaizeem et al, 2004).

Apply the Evidence: Nursing Implications

No single site used for temperature assessment provides unequivocal estimates of core body temperature. Studies show that the axillary and tympanic measures demonstrate poor agreement when these modes are compared with more accurate core temperature methods. The differences are more evident as temperature increases, regardless of age. When an accurate method for obtaining a correct reflection of core temperature is needed, the rectal temperature is recommended in younger children and the oral route in older children. For infants less than 1 month of age, the American Academy of Pediatrics, Committee on Environmental Health (2001) recommends axillary temperatures.

References

Al-Mukhaizeem F et al: Comparison of temporal artery, rectal and esophageal core temperatures in children: results of a pilot study, *Paediatr Child Health* 9(7):461-465, 2004.

American Academy of Pediatrics, Committee on Environmental Health: Technical report: mercury in the environment: implications for pediatricians, *Pediatrics* 108(1):197-205, 2001.

Callanan D: Detecting fever in young infants: reliability of perceived, pacifier, and temporal artery temperatures in infants younger than 3 months of age, *Pediatr Emerg Care* 19(4):240-243, 2003.

Carroll M: An evaluation of temperature measurement, *Nurs Stand* 14(44):39-43, 2000.

Craig JV et al: Infrared ear thermometry compared with rectal thermometry in children: a systemic review, *Lancet* 360:603-609, 2002.

El-Radhi AS, Barry W: Thermometry in paediatric practice, *Arch Dis Child* 91(4):351-356, 2006.

Falzon A et al: How reliable is axillary temperature measurement? *Acta Paediatr* 92(3):309-313, 2003.

Gilbert M, Barton AJ, Counsell CM: Comparison of oral and tympanic temperatures in adult surgical patients, *Appl Nurs Res* 15(1):42-47, 2002.

Greenes DS, Fleisher GR: When body temperature changes, does rectal temperature lag? *J Pediatr* 144(6):824-826, 2004.

Greenes DS, Fleisher GR: Accuracy of a noninvasive temporal artery thermometer for use in infants, *Arch Pediatr Adolesc Med* 155(3):376-381, 2001.

Hebbar K et al: Comparison of temporal artery thermometer to standard temperature measurement in pediatric intensive care unit patients, *Pediatr Crit Care Med* 6(5):557-561, 2005.

Holtzclaw BJ: New trends in thermometry for the patient in the ICU, *Crit Care Nurs Q* 21(3):12-25, 1998.

Jean-Mary MB et al: Limited accuracy and reliability of infrared axillary and aural thermometers in a pediatric outpatient population, *J Pediatr* 141(5):671-676, 2002.

Jensen BN et al: Accuracy of digital tympanic, oral, axillary, and rectal thermometers compared with standard rectal mercury thermometers, *Eur J Surg* 166(11):848-851, 2000.

Martin SA, Kline AM: Can there be a standard for temperature measurement in the pediatric intensive care unit? *AACN Clin Issues* 15(2):254-266, 2004.

O'Brien DL et al: The accuracy of oral predictive and infrared emission detection tympanic thermometers in an emergency department setting, *Acad Emerg Med* 7(9):1061-1064, 2000.

Pidwell WB et al: Accuracy of temporal artery thermometer (abstract), *Ann Emerg Med* 36(4):S5, 2000.

Riddell A, Eppich W: *Should tympanic temperature measurement be trusted?* BestBETs, 2003. Available at www.bestbets.org/cgi-bin/bets.pl?record=00340 (accessed April 2005).

Schuh S et al: Comparison of the temporal artery and rectal thermometry in children in the emergency department, *Pediatr Emerg Care* 20(11):736-741, 2004.

Siberry GK et al: Comparison of temple temperatures with rectal temperatures in children under 2 years of age, *Clin Pediatr* 41(6):405-414, 2002.

Tandberg D, Sklar D: Effect of tachypnea on the estimation of body temperature by an oral thermometer, *N Engl J Med* 308(16):945-946, 1983.

University of Michigan: *Rectal temperature is still the gold standard for determining the presence or absence of fever*, Evidence-Based Pediatrics website, 2003. Available at www.med.umich.edu/pediatrics/ebm/cats/fever.htm (accessed April 2005).

BOX 34-13 Types of Thermometers Used to Measure Temperature in Infants and Children

Electronic Thermometer

Temperature is sensed with an electronic component called thermistor mounted at the tip of a plastic and stainless steel probe, which is connected to an electronic recorder. A disposable plastic cover is used for infection control.

Temperature measurement appears on digital display within 60 seconds.

Probe can be placed in mouth, axilla, or rectum.

Infrared Thermometer

Thermal radiation is measured from axilla, ear canal, or tympanic membrane.

Temperature measurement appears on digital display in approximately 1 second.

Three types are available for ear-based use: tympanic, ear canal, and arterial heat balance via the ear canal (AHBE).

Often these devices are all inappropriately referred to as *tympanic thermometers*.

Temperatures measured in this way reflect arterial (bloodstream) temperature.

Ear-Based Temperature Sensor

Although this is frequently used in pediatric settings (especially ambulatory clinics), debate still continues on the reliability of ear-based thermometry in screening febrile children.

Most models use "offsets" for internal calculations that transform ear temperature into supposedly equivalent oral or rectal temperatures.

Ear Sensor (LighTouch LTX)

This measures the infrared heat energy radiating from canal opening, scans canal for highest temperature reading, and then calculates arterial temperature (correlates highly with core or internal body temperature).

It is available in two sizes; smaller size of LighTouch Pedi-Q is for infants and toddlers.

Axillary Sensor (LighTouch LTN)

This measures the infrared heat energy radiating from the axilla.

It can be used on wet skin; in incubators; or under radiant heaters, warming pads, or other heat sources.

Digital Thermometer

A probe is connected to a microprocessor chip, which translates signals into degrees and sends temperature measurement to digital display.

It is used like an oral electronic thermometer and can be used for measuring oral, rectal, and axillary temperature.

It is more accurate and easier to read, but somewhat more expensive, than plastic strip thermometer.

Liquid Crystal Skin Contact Thermometer (Chemical Dot Thermometer)

This single-use, disposable, flexible thermometer has a specific chemical mixture in each circle that changes color to measure temperature increments of $\frac{2}{10}$ of a degree.

There are two types:

1. Kept in mouth (1 minute), axilla (3 minutes), or rectum (3 minutes); color change is read 10 to 15 seconds after removing thermometer
2. Wearable, continuous-use thermometer, which is placed under axilla; may be read within 2 to 3 minutes after placement and continuously thereafter; discard and replace every 48 hours

Table 34-4 Grading of Pulses

GRADE	DESCRIPTION
0	Not palpable
+1	Difficult to palpate, thready, weak, easily obliterated with pressure
+2	Difficult to palpate, may be obliterated with pressure
+3	Easy to palpate, not easily obliterated with pressure (normal)
+4	Strong, bounding, not obliterated with pressure

in rhythm. However, when frequent apical rates are needed, use shorter counting times (e.g., 15- or 30-second intervals). For greater accuracy, measure the apical rate while the child is asleep; record the child's behavior along with the rate. Pulses may be graded according to the criteria in Table 34-4. Compare radial and femoral pulses at least once during infancy to detect the presence of circulatory impairment, such as coarctation of the aorta.

Respiration

Count the respiratory rate in children in the same manner as for the adult patient. However, in infants observe abdominal movements, since respirations are primarily diaphragmatic. Because the movements are irregular, count them for 1 full minute for accuracy (see also Appendix E).

Blood Pressure

BP measurement by noninvasive methods is part of a routine vital sign determination. BP should be measured annually in children 3 years of age through adolescence and in children with symptoms of hypertension, children in emergency departments and intensive care units, and high risk infants (National High Blood Pressure Education Program Working Group on High Blood Pressure in Children and Adolescents, 2004). Ambulatory BP monitoring in children and adolescents is a valuable method for assessing and managing suspected hypertension (Bald, 2002).

Measurement Devices

BP can also be measured using electronic devices that employ oscillometric or Doppler techniques. In oscillometry, pressure changes are transmitted through the arterial wall to

Table 34-5 Normative Dinamap Blood Pressure Values (Systolic/Diastolic; Mean Arterial Pressure in Parentheses)

AGE GROUP	MEAN	90th PERCENTILE	95th PERCENTILE
Newborn (1-3 days)	65/41 (50)	75/49 (59)	78/52 (62)
1 mo–2 yr	95/58 (72)	106/68 (83)	110/71 (86)
2-5 yr	101/57 (74)	112/66 (82)	115/68 (85)

From Park M, Menard S: Normative oscillometric blood pressure values in the first 5 years in an office setting, *Am J Dis Child* 143(7):860-864, 1989.

the pressure cuff, and the oscillations are detected by a pressure-sensitive indicator. Oscillometers have digital read-outs for systolic, diastolic, and mean arterial pressures (MAP) and for pulse. The MAP is not the same as the mean BP (arithmetic average of systolic and diastolic pressures). Rather, it is a value somewhat lower than the arithmetic mean. BP readings using oscillometry, such as Dinamap, are generally higher (10 mm Hg higher) than measurements using auscultation (Park, Menard, & Yuan, 2001) (Table 34-5). Differences between Dinamap and auscultatory readings prevent the interchange of the readings by the two methods. The oscillometric BP monitoring method is a reliable screening tool used in a variety of age groups (Mattu, Heran, & Wright, 2004a, 2004b).

Doppler ultrasound translates changes in ultrasound frequency caused by blood movement within the artery to audible sound by means of a transducer in the cuff. This technique is useful for systolic pressure measurement but is unreliable for diastolic pressure measurement. Oscillometric and Doppler instruments are useful in measuring BP in infants and have largely replaced the flush method, which reflects only the mean BP, and the auscultatory method.

Selection of Cuff

No matter what type of noninvasive technique is used, the most important factor in accurately measuring BP is the use of an appropriately sized cuff (cuff size refers only to the inner inflatable bladder, not the cloth covering). A technique to establish an appropriate cuff size is to choose a cuff having a bladder width that is approximately 40% of the arm circumference midway between the olecranon and the acromion. This will usually be a cuff bladder that covers 80% to 100% of the circumference of the arm (Fig. 34-11) (Beevers, Lip, & O'Brien, 2001; National Institutes of Health & National Heart, Lung, and Blood Institute, 1996). Researchers have found that selection of a cuff with a bladder width equal to 40% of the upper arm circumference most accurately reflects directly measured radial arterial pressure (Clark et al, 2002) (Table 34-6).

Using limb circumference for selecting cuff width more accurately reflects direct arterial BP than using limb length, since this method takes into account variations in arm thickness and the amount of pressure required to compress the artery (Gillman & Cook, 1995). For measurement sites other than the upper arms, the limb circumference guidelines can be used, although the shape of the limb (e.g., conical shape of the thigh) may prevent appropriate placement of the cuff and inaccurately reflect intraarterial BP.

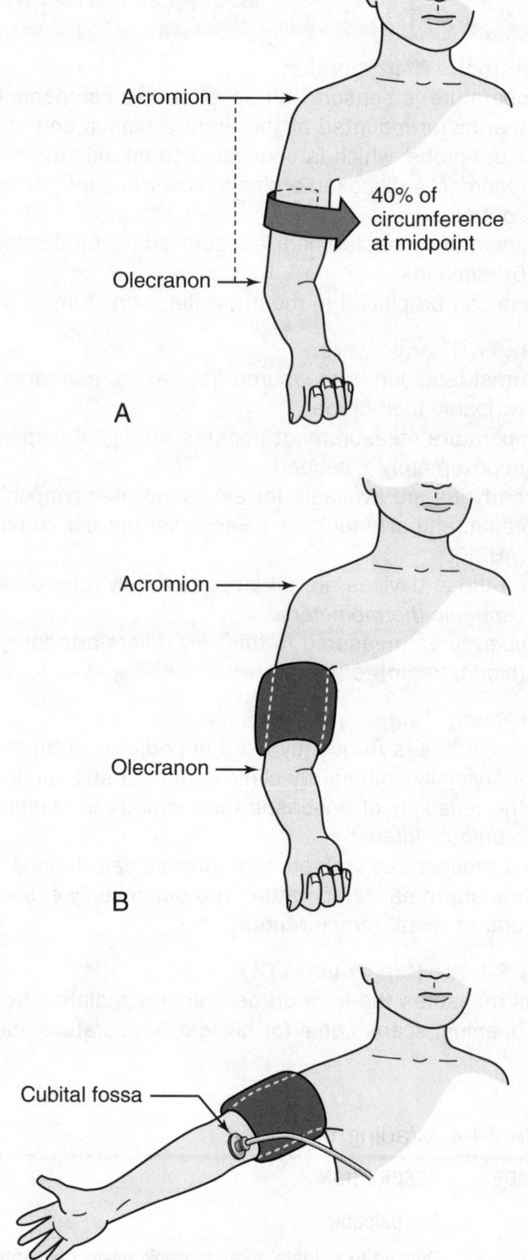

Fig. 34-11 Determination of proper cuff size. **A,** Cuff bladder width should be approximately 40% of circumference of arm measured at a point midway between olecranon and acromion. **B,** Cuff bladder length should cover 80% to 100% of circumference of arm. **C,** Blood pressure should be measured with cubital fossa at heart level. Arm should be supported. Stethoscope bell is placed over brachial artery pulse, proximal and medial to cubital fossa and below bottom edge of cuff. (From National Institutes of Health, National Heart, Lung, and Blood Institute: *Update on the Task Force Report [1987] on high blood pressure in children and adolescents: a working group report from the National High Blood Pressure Education Program*, NIH Pub No 96-3790, Bethesda, MD, September 1996, The Institutes.)

Table 34-6 Recommended Dimensions for Blood Pressure Cuff Bladders

AGE RANGE	WIDTH (cm)	LENGTH (cm)	MAXIMUM ARM CIRCUMFERENCE (cm)*
Newborn	4	8	10
Infant	6	12	15
Child	9	18	22
Small adult	10	24	26
Adult	13	30	34
Large adult	16	38	44
Thigh	20	42	52

From National High Blood Pressure Education Program Working Group on High Blood Pressure in Children and Adolescents: The fourth report on the diagnosis, evaluation, and treatment of high blood pressure in children and adolescents, *Pediatrics* 114(2 Suppl 4th Rep):555-576, 2004.
*Calculated so that largest arm would still allow bladder to encircle arm by at least 80%.

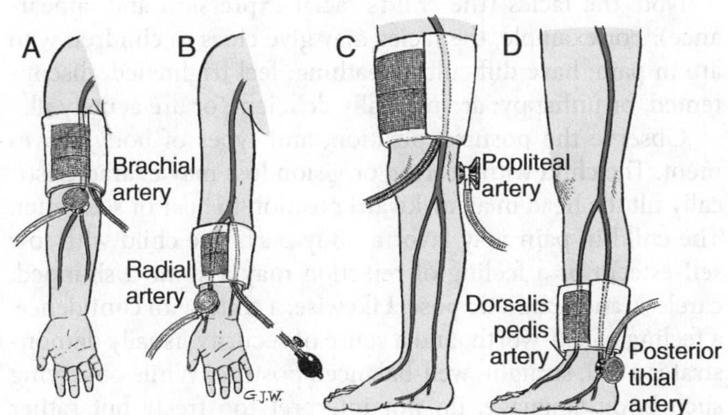

Fig. 34-12 Sites for measuring blood pressure. **A,** Upper arm. **B,** Lower arm or forearm. **C,** Thigh. **D,** Calf or ankle.

Cuffs that are either too narrow or too wide affect the accuracy of BP measurements. If the cuff size is too small, the reading on the device is falsely high. If the cuff size is too large, the reading is falsely low (Clark et al, 2002).

When another site is used, BP measurements using noninvasive techniques may differ. Generally, systolic pressure in the lower extremities (thigh or calf) is greater than pressure in the upper extremities, and systolic BP in the calf is higher than that in the thigh (Fig. 34-12). These differences are listed in Table 34-7 and apply to oscillometric measurements taken on the right extremities with the child supine and the cuff size based on the circumference method (Park, Lee, & Johnson, 1993).

NURSING ALERT When taking BP, use an appropriately sized cuff. When the correct size is not available, use an oversized cuff rather than an undersized one or use another site that more appropriately fits the cuff size. Do not choose a cuff based on the name of the cuff (e.g., an "infant" cuff may be too small for some infants).

Table 34-7 Differences in Oscillometric Systolic Blood Pressure Between Arm and Lower Extremity Sites in Normal Children

	Systolic Blood Pressure × (Mean ± SD)	
AGE GROUP (yr)	ARM-THIGH	ARM-CALF
4-8	−7.1 ± 6.8	−9.3 ± 7.4
9-16	−2.4 ± 7.7	−5.0 ± 26.9

From Park M, Lee D, Johnson GA: Oscillometric blood pressures in the arm, thigh, and calf in healthy children and those with aortic coarctation, *Pediatrics* 91(4):761-765, 1993.

NURSING ALERT Compare BP in the upper and lower extremities at least once to detect abnormalities, such as coarctation of the aorta, in which the lower extremity pressure is less than the upper extremity pressure.

Measurement and Interpretation

Measuring and interpreting BP in infants and children requires additional attention to correct procedure because (1) limb sizes vary and cuff selection must accommodate the circumference; (2) excessive pressure on the antecubital fossa affects the Korotkoff sounds; (3) children easily become anxious, which can elevate BP; and (4) BP values change with age and growth. In children and adolescents the normal range of BP is determined by body size and age. BP standards that are based on gender, age, and height provide a more precise classification of BP according to body size. This approach avoids misclassifying children who are very tall or very short. The revised BP tables now include the 50th, 90th, 95th, and 99th percentiles (with standard deviations) by gender, age, and height.

To use the tables in a clinical setting, the height percentile is determined by using the newly revised Centers for Disease Control and Prevention growth charts *(www.cdc.gov/growthcharts)*. The child's measured systolic BP and diastolic BP are compared with the numbers provided in the table (boys or girls) according to the child's age and height percentile. The child is normotensive if the BP is below the 90th percentile. If the BP is at or above the 90th percentile, the BP measurement should be repeated at that visit to verify an elevated BP. BP measurements between the 90th and 95th percentiles indicate prehypertension and warrant reassessment and consideration of other risk factors. In addition, if an adolescent's BP is more than 120/80 mm Hg, the patient should be considered prehypertensive even if this value is below the 90th percentile. This BP level typically occurs for systolic BP at 12 years old and for diastolic BP at 16 years old. If the child's BP (systolic or diastolic) is at or above the 95th percentile, the child may be hypertensive, and the measurement must be repeated on at least two occasions to confirm diagnosis (National High Blood Pressure Education Program Working Group on High Blood Pressure in Children and Adolescents, 2004) (see Guidelines box).

Orthostatic Hypotension

Orthostatic hypotension (OH), also called *postural hypotension* or *orthostatic intolerance,* is often manifested as syncope

GUIDELINES Using the Blood Pressure Tables

1. Use the standard height charts to determine the height percentile.
2. Measure and record the child's systolic blood pressure (SBP) and diastolic blood pressure (DBP).
3. Use the correct gender table for SBP and DBP.
4. Find the child's age on the left side of the table. Follow the age row horizontally across the table to the intersection of the line for the height percentile (vertical column).
5. There, find the 50th, 90th, 95th, and 99th percentiles for SBP in the left columns and for DBP in the right columns.
   - BP less than 90th percentile is normal.
   - BP between the 90th and 95th percentile is prehypertension. In adolescents, BP of 120/80 mm Hg or greater is prehypertension, even if this figure is less than the 90th percentile.
   - BP over 95th percentile may be hypertension.
6. If the BP is over the 90th percentile, the BP should be repeated twice at the same office visit, and an average SBP and DBP should be used.
7. If the BP is over the 95th percentile, BP should be staged. If stage 1 (95th to 99th percentile plus 5 mm Hg), BP measurements should be repeated on two more occasions. If hypertension is confirmed, evaluation should proceed. If BP is stage 2 (greater than 99th percentile plus 5 mm Hg), prompt referral should be made for evaluation and therapy. If the patient is symptomatic, immediate referral and treatment are indicated.

From National High Blood Pressure Education Program Working Group on High Blood Pressure in Children and Adolescents: The fourth report on the diagnosis, evaluation, and treatment of high blood pressure in children and adolescents, *Pediatrics* 114(2 Suppl 4th Rep):555-576, 2004.

(fainting), vertigo (dizziness), or lightheadedness and is caused by decreased blood flow to the brain (cerebral hypoperfusion). Normally blood flow to the brain is maintained at a constant level by a number of compensating mechanisms that regulate systemic BP. When one assumes a sitting or standing position from a supine or recumbent position, peripheral capillary vasoconstriction occurs, and blood that was pooling in the lower vasculature is returned to the heart for redistribution to the head and remainder of the body. When this mechanism fails or is slow to respond, the person may experience vertigo or syncope. One of the most common causes of OH is hypovolemia, which may be induced by medications such as diuretics, vasodilators, and prolonged immobility or bed rest. Other causes of OH include dehydration, diarrhea, emesis, fluid loss from sweating and exertion, alcohol intake, dysrhythmias, diabetes mellitus, sepsis, and hemorrhage.

BP measurements taken with the child supine then standing (at least 2 minutes in each position) may demonstrate variability and assist in the diagnosis of OH. The child with a sustained drop in systolic pressure of more than 20 mm Hg or in diastolic pressure of more than 10 mm Hg after standing for 2 minutes without an increase in heart rate of more than 15 beats/min most likely has an autonomic deficit. Nonneurogenic causes of OH have a compensatory increase in pulse of more than 15 beats/min as well as a drop in BP, as noted previously. For the child or adolescent who is seen with vertigo, lightheadedness, nausea, syncope, diaphoresis, and pallor, it is important to monitor BP and heart rate to determine the original cause. BP is an important diagnostic measurement in children and adolescents and must be a part of the routine monitoring of vital signs.

NURSING ALERT Published norms for BP, such as those located in Appendix E, are valid only if the same method of measurement (auscultation and cuff size determination) is used in clinical practice.

General Appearance

The child's general appearance is a cumulative, subjective impression of the child's physical appearance, state of nutrition, behavior, personality, interactions with parents and nurse (also siblings if present), posture, development, and speech. Although general appearance is recorded at the beginning of the physical examination, it encompasses all the observations of the child during the interview and physical assessment.

Note the facies (the child's facial expression and appearance). For example, the facies may give clues to children who are in pain; have difficulty breathing; feel frightened, discontented, or unhappy; are mentally deficient; or are acutely ill.

Observe the posture, position, and types of body movement. The child with hearing or vision loss may characteristically tilt the head in an awkward position to hear or see better. The child in pain may favor a body part. The child with low self-esteem or a feeling of rejection may assume a slumped, careless, and apathetic pose. Likewise, a child with confidence, a feeling of self-worth, and a sense of security usually demonstrates a tall, straight, well-balanced posture. While observing such body language, do not interpret too freely but rather record objectively.

Note the child's hygiene in terms of cleanliness; unusual body odor; the condition of the hair, neck, nails, teeth, and feet; and the condition of the clothing. Such observations are excellent clues to possible instances of neglect, inadequate financial resources, housing difficulties (e.g., no running water), or lack of knowledge concerning children's needs.

Behavior includes the child's personality, activity level, reaction to stress, requests, frustration, interactions with others (primarily the parent and nurse), degree of alertness, and response to stimuli. Some mental questions that serve as reminders for observing behavior include: What is the child's overall personality? Does the child have a long attention span, or is he or she easily distracted? Can the child follow two or three commands in succession without the need for repetition? What is the youngster's response to delayed gratification or frustration? Is eye contact used during conversation? What is the child's reaction to the nurse and family members? Is the child quick or slow to grasp explanations?

Development can be assessed by carefully observing the child, but verify your impressions with screening tests. Various tests for assessing development, speech, vision, and hearing are discussed later in this chapter and in Chapter 42.

Under general appearance, record an overall estimate of the child's speech development, motor skills, coordination, and recent area of achievement. For example, the following statement may apply to an 18-month-old child: "Motor development advanced for age; climbs, runs, jumps (most recent motor skill), manipulates small objects with ease; excellent coordination and balance; beginning to name many objects; uses two-word phrases; and enjoys 'talking' to self and others."

Skin

Skin is assessed for color, texture, temperature, moisture, and turgor. Examination of the skin and its accessory organs primarily involves inspection and palpation. Touch allows the nurse to assess the texture, turgor, and temperature of the skin (Turnbull, 2000). The normal color in light-skinned children varies from a milky white and rose to a deeply hued pink. Dark-skinned children, such as those of Native American, Hispanic, or African descent, have inherited various brown, red, yellow, olive green, and bluish tones in their skin. Asian persons have skin that is normally of a yellow tone. Several variations in skin color can occur, some of which warrant further investigation. The types of color change and their appearance in children with light or dark skin are summarized in Table 34-8.

Normally the skin texture of young children is smooth, slightly dry, and not oily or clammy. Evaluate skin temperature by symmetrically feeling each part of the body and comparing upper areas with lower ones. Note any difference in temperature.

Determine tissue turgor, or elasticity in the skin, by grasping the skin on the abdomen between the thumb and index finger, pulling it taut, and quickly releasing it. Elastic tissue immediately assumes its normal position without residual marks or creases. In children with poor skin turgor, the skin remains suspended or tented for a few seconds before slowly falling back on the abdomen. Skin turgor is one of the best estimates of adequate hydration and nutrition.

Accessory Structures

Inspection of the accessory structures of the skin may be performed while the skin is being examined or when the scalp and extremities are being assessed.

Inspect the hair for color, texture, quality, distribution, and elasticity. Children's scalp hair is usually lustrous, silky, strong, and elastic. Genetic factors affect the appearance of hair. For example, the hair of African-American children is usually curlier and coarser than that of Caucasian children. Hair that is stringy, dull, brittle, dry, friable, and depigmented may suggest poor nutrition. Record any bald or thinning spots. Loss of hair in infants may indicate lying in the same position and may be a clue for counseling parents concerning the child's stimulation needs.

Inspect the hair and scalp for general cleanliness. Persons in various ethnic groups condition their hair with oils or lubricants that, if not thoroughly washed from the scalp, clog the sebaceous glands, causing scalp infections. Also examine the area for lesions; scaliness; evidence of infestation, such as lice or ticks; and signs of trauma, such as ecchymosis, masses, or scars.

In children who are approaching puberty, look for growth of secondary hair as a sign of normally progressing pubertal changes. Note precocious or delayed appearance of hair growth because, although not always suggestive of hormonal dysfunction, it may be of great concern to the early- or late-maturing adolescent.

Inspect the nails for color, shape, texture, and quality. Normally the nails are pink, convex, smooth, and hard but flexible (not brittle). The edges, which are usually white, should extend

Table 34-8 Differences in Color Changes of Racial Groups

DESCRIPTION	APPEARANCE IN LIGHT SKIN	APPEARANCE IN DARK SKIN
Cyanosis–Bluish tone through skin; reflects reduced (deoxygenated) hemoglobin	Bluish tinge, especially in palpebral conjunctiva (lower eyelid), nail beds, earlobes, lips, oral membranes, soles, and palms	Ashen gray lips and tongue
Pallor–Paleness; may be sign of anemia, chronic disease, edema, or shock	Loss of rosy glow in skin, especially face	Ashen gray appearance in black skin More yellowish brown color in brown skin
Erythema–Redness; may be result of increased blood flow from climatic conditions, local inflammation, infection, skin irritation, allergy, or other dermatoses, or may be caused by increased numbers of red blood cells as compensatory response to chronic hypoxia	Redness easily seen anywhere on body	Much more difficult to assess; rely on palpation for warmth or edema
Ecchymosis–Large, diffuse areas, usually black and blue, caused by hemorrhage of blood into skin; typically result of injuries	Purplish to yellow-green areas; may be seen anywhere on skin	Very difficult to see unless in mouth or conjunctiva
Petechiae–Same as ecchymosis except for size: small, distinct, pinpoint hemorrhages $\leq$2 mm in size; can denote some type of blood disorder, such as leukemia	Purplish pinpoints most easily seen on buttocks, abdomen, and inner surfaces of arms or legs	Usually invisible except in oral mucosa, conjunctiva of eyelids, and conjunctiva covering eyeball
Jaundice–Yellow staining of skin usually caused by bile pigments	Yellow staining seen in sclerae of eyes, skin, fingernails, soles, palms, and oral mucosa	Most reliably assessed in sclerae, hard palate, palms, and soles

over the fingers. Dark-skinned individuals may have more deeply pigmented nail beds. Short, ragged nails are typical of habitual biting. Uncut, dirty nails are a sign of poor hygiene.

The palm normally shows three flexion creases (Fig. 34-13, *A*). In some situations such as Down syndrome, the two distal horizontal creases are fused to form a single horizontal crease (the single palmar crease, or transpalmar crease) (see Fig. 34-13, *B*). If grossly abnormal lines or folds are observed, sketch a picture to describe them and refer the finding to a specialist for further investigation.

Lymph Nodes

Lymph nodes are usually assessed when the part of the body in which they are located is examined. The body's lymphatic drainage system is extensive; the usual sites for palpating accessible lymph nodes are shown in Fig. 34-14.

evolve Anatomy Review–Structures of the Neck

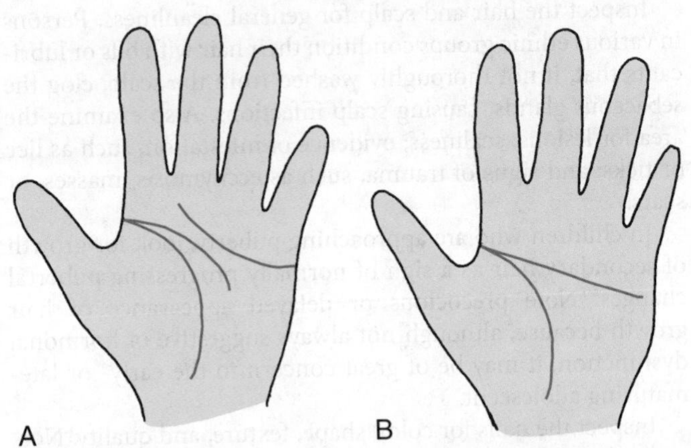

Fig. 34-13 Examples of flexion creases on palm. **A**, Normal. **B**, Transpalmar crease.

Palpate nodes using the distal portion of the fingers and gently but firmly pressing in a circular motion along the regions where nodes are normally present. During assessment of the nodes in the head and neck, tilt the child's head upward slightly but without tensing the sternocleidomastoid or trapezius muscles. This position facilitates palpation of the submental, submandibular, tonsillar, and cervical nodes. Palpate the axillary nodes with the child's arms relaxed at the sides but slightly abducted. Assess the inguinal nodes with the child in the supine position. Note size, mobility, temperature, and tenderness, as well as reports by the parents regarding any visible change of enlarged nodes. In children, small, nontender, movable nodes are usually normal. Tender, enlarged, warm lymph nodes generally indicate infection or inflammation close to their location. Report such findings for further investigation.

Head and Neck

Observe the head for general shape and symmetry. A flattening of one part of the head, such as the occiput, may indicate that the child continually lies in this position. Marked asymmetry is usually abnormal and may indicate premature closure of the sutures (craniosynostosis).

NURSING ALERT Significant head lag after 6 months of age strongly indicates cerebral injury and is referred for further evaluation.

Note head control in infants and head posture in older children. Most infants by 4 months of age should be able to hold the head erect and in midline when in a vertical position.

Evaluate range of motion by asking the older child to look in each direction (to either side, up, and down) or by manually

evolve Anatomy Review–Superficial Lymph Nodes

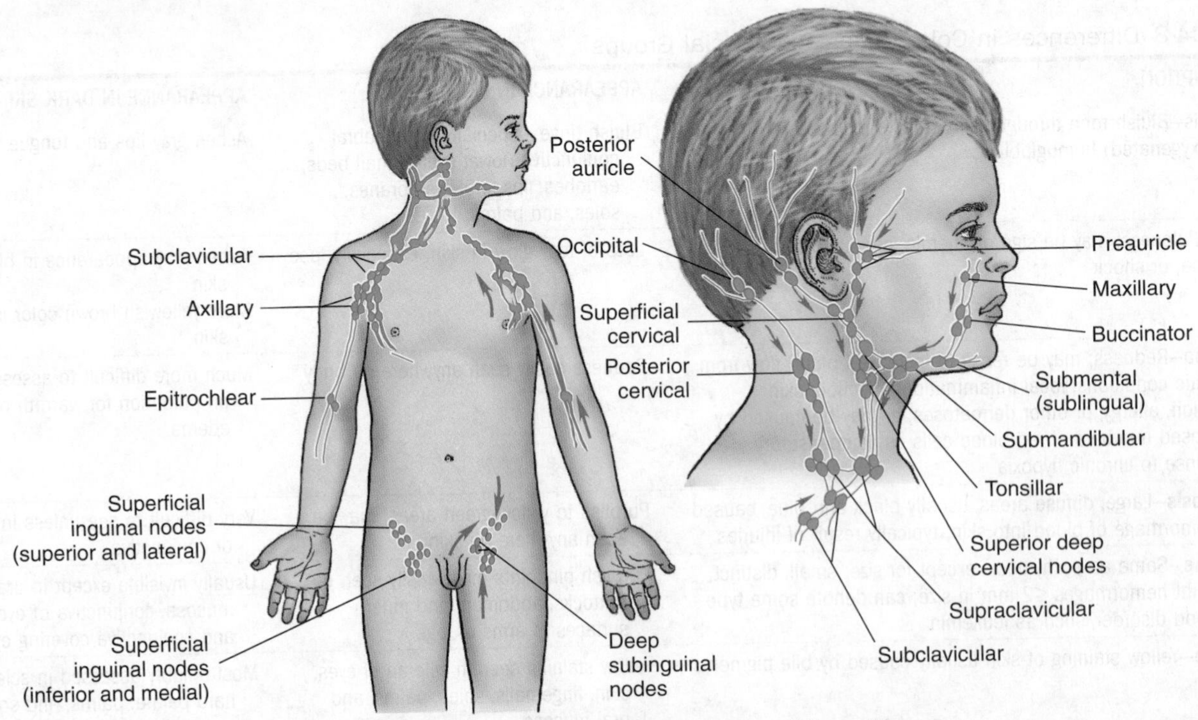

Fig. 34-14 Location of superficial lymph nodes. *Arrows* indicate directional flow of lymph.

putting the younger child through each position. Limited range of motion may indicate wryneck, or torticollis, in which the child holds the head to one side with the chin pointing toward the opposite side as a result of injury to the sternocleidomastoid muscle.

NURSING ALERT Hyperextension of the head (opisthotonos) with pain on flexion is a serious indication of meningeal irritation and is referred for immediate medical evaluation.

Palpate the skull for patent sutures, fontanels, fractures, and swellings. Normally the posterior fontanel closes by the second month of life, and the anterior fontanel fuses between 12 and 18 months of age. Early or late closure is noted, since either may be a sign of a pathologic condition.

While examining the head, observe the face for symmetry, movement, and general appearance. Ask the child to "make a face" to assess symmetric movement and disclose any degree of paralysis. Note any unusual facial proportion, such as an unusually high or low forehead; wide- or close-set eyes; or a small, receding chin.

In addition to assessment of the head and neck for movement, inspect the neck for size and palpate its associated structures. The neck is normally short, with skin folds between the head and shoulders during infancy; however, it lengthens during the next 3 to 4 years.

NURSING ALERT If any masses are detected in the neck, report them for further investigation. Large masses can block the airway.

Eyes

Inspection of External Structures

Inspect the lids for proper placement on the eye. When the eye is open, the upper lid should fall near the upper iris. When the eyes are closed, the lids should completely cover the cornea and sclera (Fig. 34-15).

Determine the general slant of the palpebral fissures or lids by drawing an imaginary line through the two points of the medial canthus and across the outer orbit of the eyes and aligning each eye on the line. Usually the palpebral fissures lie horizontally. However, in Asians the slant is normally upward.

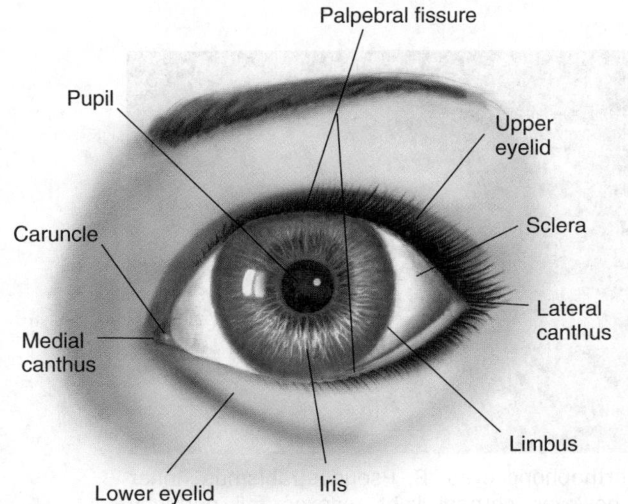

Fig. 34-15 External structures of eye.

Also inspect the inside lining of the lids, the palpebral conjunctiva. To examine the lower conjunctival sac, pull the lid down while the patient looks up. To evert the upper lid, hold the upper lashes and gently pull *down* and *forward* as the child looks down. Normally the conjunctiva appears pink and glossy. Vertical yellow striations along the edge are the meibomian, or sebaceous, glands near the hair follicle. Located in the inner or medial canthus and situated on the inner edge of the upper and lower lids is a tiny opening, the lacrimal punctum. Note any excessive tearing, discharge, or inflammation of the lacrimal apparatus.

The bulbar conjunctiva, which covers the eye up to the limbus, or junction of the cornea and sclera, should be transparent. The sclera, or white covering of the eyeball, should be clear. Tiny black marks in the sclera of heavily pigmented individuals are normal.

The cornea, or covering of the iris and pupil, should be clear and transparent. Record opacities because they can be signs of scarring or ulceration, which can interfere with vision. The best way to test for opacities is to illuminate the eyeball by shining a light at an angle (obliquely) toward the cornea.

Compare the pupils for size, shape, and movement. They should be round, clear, and equal. Test their reaction to light by quickly shining a light toward the eye and removing it. As the light approaches, the pupils should constrict; as the light fades, the pupils should dilate. Test the pupil for any response of accommodation by having the child look at a bright, shiny object at a distance and quickly moving the object toward the face. The pupils should constrict as the object is brought near the eye. Normal findings on examination of the pupils may be recorded as *PERRLA,* which stands for "*P*upils *E*qual, *R*ound, *R*eact to *L*ight, and *A*ccommodation."

Inspect the iris and pupil for color, size, shape, and clarity. Permanent eye color is usually established by 6 to 12 months of age. While inspecting the iris and pupil, look for the lens. Normally the lens is not visible through the pupil.

Inspection of Internal Structures

The ophthalmoscope permits visualization of the interior of the eyeball with a system of lenses and a high-intensity light. The lenses permit clear visualization of eye structures at different distances from the nurse's eye and correct visual acuity differences in the examiner and child. Use of the ophthalmoscope requires practice to know which lens setting produces the clearest image.

The ophthalmic and otic heads are usually interchangeable on one "body" or handle, which encloses the power source, either disposable or rechargeable batteries. The nurse should practice changing the heads, which snap on and are secured with a quarter turn, and replacing the batteries and light bulbs. Nurses who are not directly involved in physical assessment are often responsible for ensuring that the equipment functions properly.

Preparing the Child

The nurse can prepare the child for the ophthalmoscopic examination by showing the child the instrument, demonstrating the light source and how it shines in the eye, and explaining the reason for darkening the room. For infants and young children who do not respond to such explanations, it is best to use distraction to encourage them to keep their eyes open. Forcibly parting the lids results in an uncooperative, watery eyed child and a frustrated nurse. Usually, with some practice, the nurse can elicit a red reflex almost instantly while approaching the child and may also gain a momentary inspection of the blood vessels, macula, or optic disc.

Funduscopic Examination

Fig. 34-16 shows the structures of the back of the eyeball, or the fundus. The fundus is immediately apparent as the red reflex. The intensity of the color increases in darkly pigmented individuals.

NURSING ALERT A brilliant, uniform red reflex is an important sign because it rules out many serious defects of the cornea, aqueous chamber, lens, and vitreous chamber. Any dark shadows or opacities are recorded because they indicate some abnormality in any of these structures.

As the ophthalmoscope is brought closer to the eye, the most conspicuous feature of the fundus is the optic disc, the area where the blood vessels and optic nerve fibers enter and exit from the eye. The color of the disc is creamy pink; it is

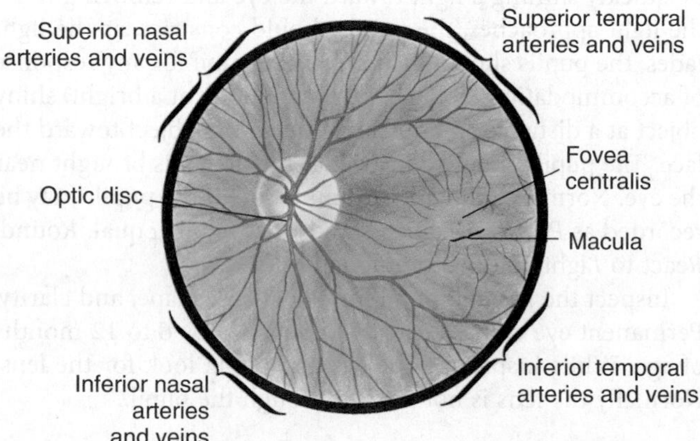

Fig. 34-16 Structures of fundus. (From Seidel HM et al: *Mosby's guide to physical examination*, ed 6, St Louis, 2006, Mosby.)

lighter in color than the surrounding fundus. Normally it is round or vertically oval.

After the optic disc is located, the area is inspected for blood vessels. The central retinal artery and vein appear in the depths of the disc and emanate outward with visible branching. The veins are darker and about one fourth larger than the arteries. Normally the branches of the arteries and veins cross one another.

Other structures that may be seen are the macula, the area of the fundus with the greatest concentration of visual receptors; and, in the center of the macula, a minute glistening spot of reflected light called the fovea centralis, which is the area of most perfect vision.

Vision Testing

Several tests are available for assessing vision. This discussion focuses on four areas: (1) ocular alignment, (2) visual acuity, (3) peripheral vision, and (4) color vision. Vision screening should be performed at the earliest possible age and at regular intervals (American Academy of Pediatrics, Committee on Practice and Ambulatory Medicine, Section on Ophthalmology, 2003; Wall et al, 2002). Behavioral and physical signs of visual impairment are discussed in Chapter 42.

Ocular Alignment

Normally, by the age of 3 to 4 months, children are able to fixate on one visual field with both eyes simultaneously (binocularity). One of the most important tests for binocularity is alignment of the eyes to detect nonbinocular vision, or strabismus (Halle, 2002). In strabismus, or cross-eye, one eye deviates from the point of fixation. If the misalignment is constant, the weak eye becomes "lazy," and the brain eventually suppresses the image produced by that eye. If strabismus is not detected and corrected by ages 4 to 6 years, blindness from disuse, known as *amblyopia,* may result.

Tests commonly used to detect misalignment are the corneal light reflex and the cover tests. To perform the corneal light reflex test, or Hirschberg test, shine a flashlight or the light of the ophthalmoscope directly into the patient's eyes from a distance of about 40.5 cm (16 inches). If the eyes are orthophoric, or normal, the light falls symmetrically within each pupil (Fig. 34-17, *A*). If the light falls off center in one

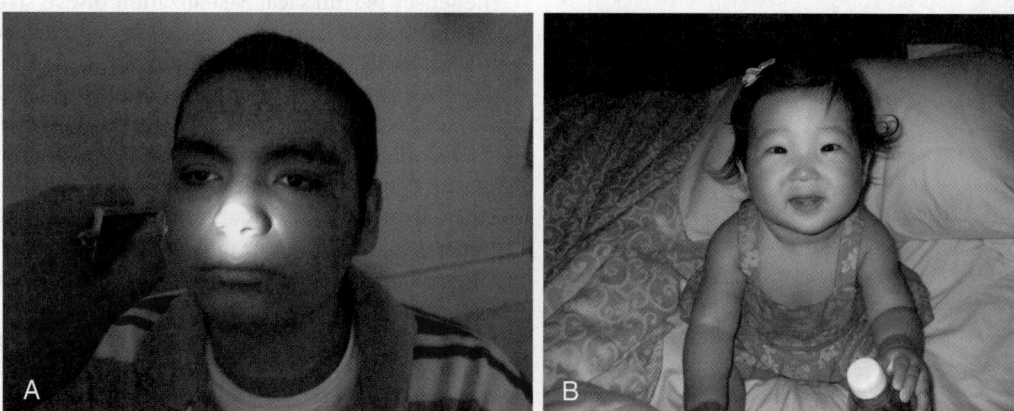

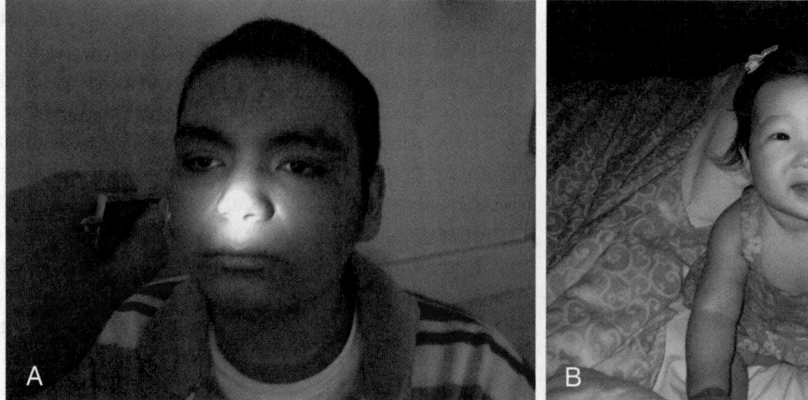

Fig. 34-17 A, Corneal light reflex test demonstrating orthophoric eyes. **B,** Pseudostrabismus. Inner epicanthal folds cause eyes to appear misaligned; however, corneal light reflexes fall perfectly symmetrically.

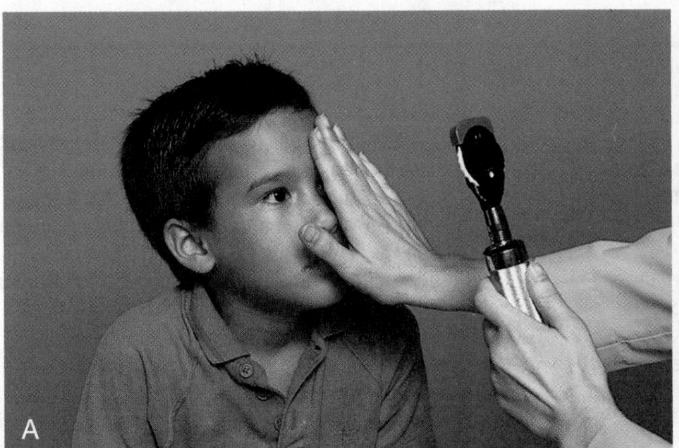

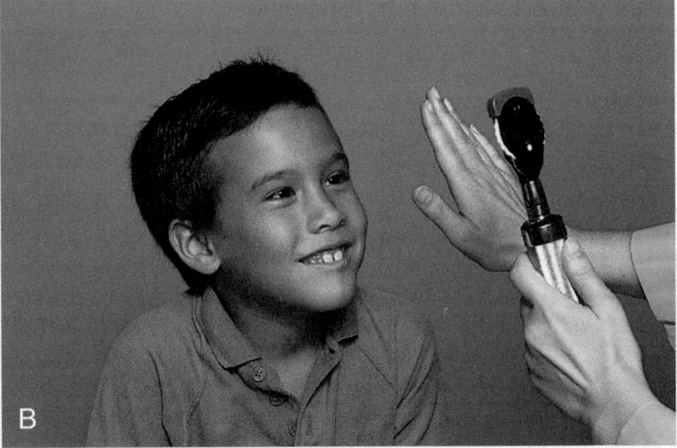

Fig. 34-18 Alternate cover test to detect amblyopia in patient with strabismus. **A,** Eye is occluded, and child is fixating on light source. **B,** If eye does not move when uncovered, eyes are aligned.

eye, the eyes are misaligned. Epicanthal folds, excess folds of skin that extend from the roof of the nose to the inner termination of the eyebrow and that partially or completely overlap the inner canthus of the eye, may give a false impression of misalignment (pseudostrabismus) (see Fig. 34-18, *B*). Epicanthal folds are often found in Asian children.

In the cover test, one eye is covered, and the movement of the *uncovered* eye is observed while the child looks at a near (33 cm [13 inches]) or distant (6 m [20 feet]) object. If the uncovered eye does not move, it is aligned. If the uncovered eye moves, a misalignment is present because, when the stronger eye is temporarily covered, the misaligned eye attempts to fixate on the object.

In the alternate cover test, occlusion shifts back and forth from one eye to the other, and movement of the eye that was *covered* is observed as soon as the occluder is removed while the child focuses on a point in front of him or her (Fig. 34-18). If normal alignment is present, shifting the cover from one eye to the other will not cause the eye to move. If misalignment is present, eye movement will occur when the cover is moved. This test takes more practice than the other cover test because the occluder must be moved back and forth quickly and accurately to see the eye move. Because deviations can occur at different ranges, it is important to perform the cover tests at both close and far distances.

NURSING ALERT The cover test is usually easier to perform if the examiner uses his or her own hand rather than a card-type occluder (see Fig. 34-18). Attractive occluders fashioned like an ice cream cone or happy-face lollipop cut from cardboard are also well received by young children.

Photoscreening is a technique used to screen for amblyopia, refractive disorders, and media opacities (American Academy of Pediatrics, Committee on Practice and Ambulatory Medicine, Section on Ophthalmology, 2003; Berry et al, 2001). Using a camera, the nurse obtains images of the pupillary reflexes (reflections) and red reflexes (Bruckner test) (American Academy of Pediatrics, Committee on Practice and Ambulatory Medicine, Section on Ophthalmology, 2003). Photoscreening offers an effective way to screen infants, preverbal children, and those with developmental delays who are difficult to screen.

Visual Acuity Testing in Children Beyond Infancy

The most common test for measuring visual acuity is the Snellen letter chart, which consists of lines of letters of decreasing size (see the EVOLVE site). During testing, the American Academy of Pediatrics, Committee on Practice and Ambulatory Medicine, Section on Ophthalmology (2003) now recommends that children stand 10 feet from the chart with their heels at the 10-foot line. When screening for visual acuity in children, the nurse tests the child's right eye first by covering the left. Children who wear glasses should be screened with them on. Tell the child to keep both eyes open during the examination. If the child fails to read the current line, move up the chart to the next larger line. Continue up the chart until a line is found that the child can pass. Then begin moving down the chart again until the child fails to read the line. To pass each line, the child must correctly identify four of six symbols on the line. Repeat the procedure, covering the right eye. Table 34-9 provides a list of visual screening tests for children and guidelines for referral recommended by the American Academy of Pediatrics, Committee on Practice and Ambulatory Medicine, Section on Ophthalmology (2003).

For children unable to read letters and numbers, the tumbling E or HOTV test is useful (Coats & Jenkins, 1997). The tumbling E test uses the capital letter E pointing in four different directions. The child is asked to point in the direction the E is facing. The HOTV test consists of a wall chart composed of the letters H, O, T, and V. The child is given a board containing a large H, O, T, and V. The examiner points to a letter on the wall chart, and the child matches the correct letter on the board held in his or her hand. The tumbling E and HOTV are excellent tests for preschool-age children.

When a child is unable to perform the tumbling E or HOTV test, the LEA symbol or Allen card test may be used. The Allen card test uses common figures to test the child's vision. It is important to assess whether the child is able to identify the pictures before actual vision testing. The examiner walks backward slowly, flipping through the cards and presenting different pictures to the child. The examiner continues to move

Table 34-9 Eye Examination Guidelines*

FUNCTION	RECOMMENDED TESTS	REFERRAL CRITERIA	COMMENTS
Ages 3-5 Yr			
Distance visual acuity	Snellen letters Snellen numbers Tumbling E HOTV Picture test Allen figures LEA symbols	1. Fewer than 4 of 6 correct on 20-foot line with either eye tested at 10 foot monocularly (i.e., <10/20 or 20/40) or 2. Two-line difference between eyes, even within passing range (i.e., 10/12.5 and 10/20 or 20/25 and 20/40)	1. Tests are listed in decreasing order of cognitive difficulty; highest test that child is capable of performing should be used; in general, tumbling E or HOTV test should be used for children 3-5 yr of age and Snellen letters or numbers for children 6 yr and older. 2. Testing distance of 10 feet is recommended for all visual acuity tests. 3. Line of figures is preferred over single figures. 4. Nontested eye should be covered by occluder held by examiner or by adhesive occluder patch applied to eye; examiner must ensure that it is not possible to peek with nontested eye.
Ocular alignment	Cross cover test at 10 feet (3 m) Random dot E stereo test at 40 cm Simultaneous red reflex test (Bruckner test)	Any eye movement Fewer than 4 of 6 correct Any asymmetry of pupil color, size, brightness	Child must be fixing on a target while cross cover test is performed. Use direct ophthalmoscope to view both red reflexes simultaneously in a darkened room from 2-3 feet away; detects asymmetric refractive errors as well.
Ocular media clarity (cataracts, tumors, etc.)	Red reflex	White pupil, dark spots, absent reflex	Use direct ophthalmoscope in a darkened room. View eyes separately at 12-18 inches; white reflex indicates possible retinoblastoma.
6 Yr and Older			
Distance visual acuity	Snellen letters Snellen numbers Tumbling E HOTV Picture test Allen figures LEA symbols	1. Fewer than 4 of 6 correct on 15-foot line with either eye tested at 10 feet monocularly (i.e., <10/15 or 20/30) or 2. Two-line difference between eyes, even within the passing range (i.e., 10/10 and 10/15 or 20/20 and 20/30)	1. Tests are listed in decreasing order of cognitive difficulty; highest test that child is capable of performing should be used; in general, tumbling E or HOTV test should be used for children 3-5 yr of age and Snellen letters or numbers for children 6 yr and older. 2. Testing distance of 10 feet is recommended for all visual acuity tests. 3. Line of figures is preferred over single figures. 4. Nontested eye should be covered by occluder held by examiner or by adhesive occluder patch applied to eye; examiner must ensure that it is not possible to peek with nontested eye.
Ocular alignment	Cross cover test at 10 feet (3 m) Random dot E stereo test at 40 cm Simultaneous red reflex test (Bruckner test)	Any eye movement Fewer than 4 of 6 correct Any asymmetry of pupil color, size, brightness	Child must be fixing on target while cross cover test is performed. Use direct ophthalmoscope to view both red reflexes simultaneously in a darkened room from 2-3 feet away; detects asymmetric refractive errors as well.
Ocular media clarity (cataracts, tumors, etc.)	Red reflex	White pupil, dark spots, absent reflex	Use direct ophthalmoscope in a darkened room. View eyes separately at 12-18 inches; white reflex indicates possible retinoblastoma.

From American Academy of Pediatrics, Committee on Practice and Ambulatory Medicine, Section on Ophthalmology: Eye examination in infants, children, and young adults by pediatricians, *Pediatrics* 111(4):902-907, 2003.

*Assessing visual acuity (vision screening) is one of the most sensitive techniques for detection of eye abnormalities in children. The American Academy of Pediatrics Section on Ophthalmology, in cooperation with American Association for Pediatric Ophthalmology and Strabismus and American Academy of Ophthalmology, has developed these guidelines to be used by physicians, nurses, educational institutions, public health departments, and other professionals who perform vision evaluation services.

backward as the child correctly calls out the figures. When the child begins to miss the figure on the cards, the examiner moves forward to confirm that the child is able to identify the figures at that point. All Allen card figures are 20/30 in size. The farthest distance at which the child is able to accurately identify the pictures becomes the numerator, and 30 becomes the denominator. For example, if the child is able to identify the pictures accurately at 15 feet, the visual acuity is recorded as 15/30. This is equivalent to 20/40 or 10/20 visual acuity.

Visual Acuity Testing in Infants and Difficult-to-Test Children

In newborns, vision is tested mainly by checking for light perception by shining a light into the eyes and noting responses such as pupillary constriction, blinking, following the light to midline, increased alertness, or refusal to open the eyes after exposure to the light. Although the simple maneuver of checking light perception and eliciting the pupillary light reflex indicates that the anterior half of the visual apparatus is intact, it does not confirm that the infant can see. In other words, this test does not assess whether the brain receives the visual message and interprets the signals.

Another test of visual acuity is the infant's ability to fix on and follow a target. Although any brightly colored or patterned object can be used, the human face is excellent. Hold the infant upright while moving your face slowly from side to side.

NURSING ALERT If visual fixation and following are not present by 3 to 4 months of age, further ophthalmologic evaluation is needed.

Other signs that may indicate visual loss or other serious eye problems include fixed pupils, strabismus, constant nystagmus, the setting-sun sign, and slow lateral movements. Unfortunately, it is difficult to test each eye separately; the presence of such signs in one eye could indicate unilateral blindness.

Special tests are available for testing infants and other difficult-to-test children to assess acuity or confirm blindness. For example, in visually evoked potentials, the eyes are stimulated with a bright light or pattern, and electrical activity to the visual cortex is recorded through scalp electrodes. Acuity is assessed by using progressively smaller patterns.

Peripheral Vision

In children who are old enough to cooperate, estimate peripheral vision, or the visual field of each eye, by having the children fixate on a specific point directly in front of them as an object, such as a finger or a pencil, is moved from beyond the field of vision into the range of peripheral vision. Check each eye separately and for each quadrant of vision. As soon as children see the object, have them say "stop." At that point measure the angle from the anteroposterior axis of the eye (straight line of vision) to the peripheral axis (point at which the object is first seen). Normally children see about 50 degrees upward, 70 degrees downward, 60 degrees nasalward, and 90 degrees temporally. Limitations in peripheral vision may indicate blindness from damage to structures within the eye or to any of the visual pathways.

Color Vision

Another important test is for color vision. It is estimated that 8% to 10% of Caucasian males and less than half that percentage of African-American males inherit the X-linked disorder known as *color vision deficit* (also known as *color blindness,* a less acceptable term). From 0.5% to 1% of Caucasian females are affected. Although the severity of impaired perception of color varies considerably, the two most common types are protanomaly, in which the child confuses gray with pink or pale blue with green, and deuteranomaly, in which the child confuses gray with pale purple or green. In most of these individuals the color vision deficit causes no major problems. However, some individuals with more severe deficits may be unable to distinguish amber or red traffic lights, fail to see a red brake light on the rear of a car, have difficulty distinguishing green traffic lights from certain types of incandescent street lamps, and have a poor sense of color coordination of clothing. For school-age children the greatest difficulty lies in performance of academic skills that use color as a visual aid. Adolescents may be ineligible for certain vocational opportunities, such as electronics, photography, printing, interior decorating, pharmaceuticals, textiles, police work, and several types of military service.

The tests available for color vision include the Ishihara test and the Hardy-Rand-Rittler test. Each consists of a series of cards (pseudoisochromatic) on which is printed a color field composed of spots of a certain "confusion" color. Against the field is a number or symbol similarly printed in dots but of a color likely to be confused with the field color by the person with a color vision deficit. As a result, the figure or letter is invisible to an affected individual but is clearly seen by a person with normal vision.

Ears

Inspection of External Structures

The entire external earlobe is called the *pinna,* or *auricle*; one is located on each side of the head. Measure the height alignment of the pinna by drawing an imaginary line from the outer orbit of the eye to the occiput, or most prominent protuberance of the skull. The top of the pinna should meet or cross this line. Low-set ears are commonly associated with renal anomalies or cognitive impairment. Measure the angle of the pinna by drawing a perpendicular line from the imaginary horizontal line and aligning the pinna next to this mark. Normally the pinna lies within a 10-degree angle of the vertical line (Fig. 34-19). If it falls outside this area, record the deviation and look for other anomalies.

Normally the pinna extends slightly outward from the skull. Except in newborn infants, ears that are flat against the head or protruding away from the scalp may indicate problems. Flattened ears in an infant may suggest a frequent side-lying position and, just as with isolated areas of hair loss, may indicate a need to investigate parents' understanding of the child's stimulation needs.

Inspect the skin surface around the ear for small openings, extra tags of skin, or sinuses. If a sinus is found, note this because it may represent a fistula that drains into some area of the neck or ear. Cutaneous tags represent no pathologic process but may cause parents concern in terms of the child's appearance.

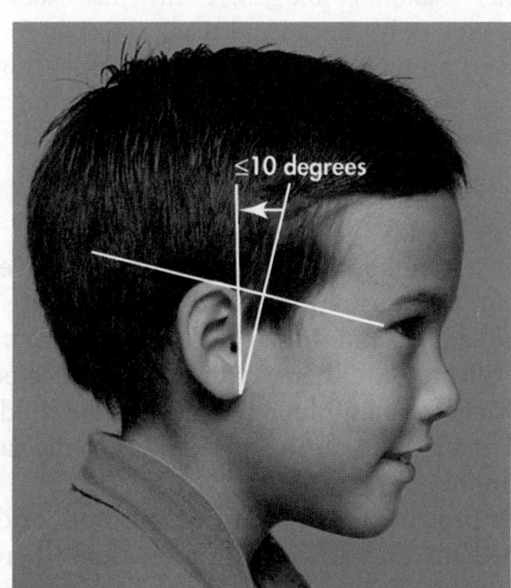

Fig. 34-19 Ear alignment.

evolve Anatomy Review—Landmarks of the Pinna

Also assess the ear for hygiene. An otoscope is not necessary for looking into the external canal to note the presence of cerumen, a waxy substance produced by the ceruminous glands in the outer portion of the canal. Cerumen is usually yellow-brown and soft. If an otoscope is used and any discharge is seen, its color and odor are noted. Avoid transmitting potentially infectious material to the other ear or to another child through hand washing and using disposable specula or sterilizing reusable specula between each examination.

Inspection of Internal Structures

The head of the otoscope permits visualization of the tympanic membrane by use of a bright light, a magnifying glass, and a speculum. Some otoscopes have an attachment for a pneumonic device to insert air into the canal to determine membrane compliance (movement). The speculum, which is inserted into the external canal, comes in a variety of sizes to accommodate different canal widths. The largest speculum that fits comfortably into the ear is used to achieve the greatest area of visualization. The lens, or magnifying glass, is movable, allowing the examiner to insert an object, such as a curette, into the ear canal through the speculum while still viewing the structures through the lens.

Positioning the Child

Before beginning the otoscopic examination, position the child properly and restrain if necessary. Older children usually cooperate and do not need restraint. However, prepare them for the procedure by allowing them to play with the instrument, demonstrating how it works, and stressing the importance of remaining still. A helpful suggestion is to let them observe you examining the parent's ear. Restraint is needed for younger children because the ear examination upsets them (see Atraumatic Care box).

> **ATRAUMATIC CARE**
>
> *Reducing Distress from Otoscopy in Young Children*
>
> Make examining the ear a game by explaining that you are looking for a "big elephant" in the ear. This kind of make-believe is an absorbing distraction and usually elicits cooperation. After examining the ear, clarify that "looking for elephants" was only pretend and thank the child for letting you look in his or her ear. Another great distraction technique is asking the child to put a finger on the opposite ear to keep the light from getting out.

As you insert the speculum into the meatus, move it around the outer rim to accustom the child to the feel of something entering the ear. If examining a painful ear, touch a nonpainful part of the affected ear, then examine the unaffected ear, and finally return to the painful ear. By this time the child is usually less fearful of anything causing discomfort to the ear and will cooperate more.

For their protection and safety, infants and toddlers must be restrained for the otoscopic examination. There are two general positions of restraint. In one the child is seated sideways in the parent's lap with one arm hugging the parent and the other arm at the side. The ear to be examined is toward the nurse. With one arm the parent holds the child's head firmly against his or her chest, and with the other arm hugs the child, thereby securing the child's free arm (Fig. 34-20, *A*). The ear is examined using the same procedure for holding the otoscope as described later.

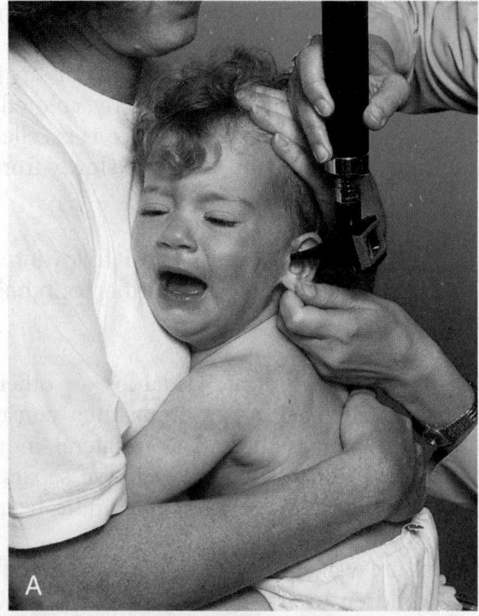

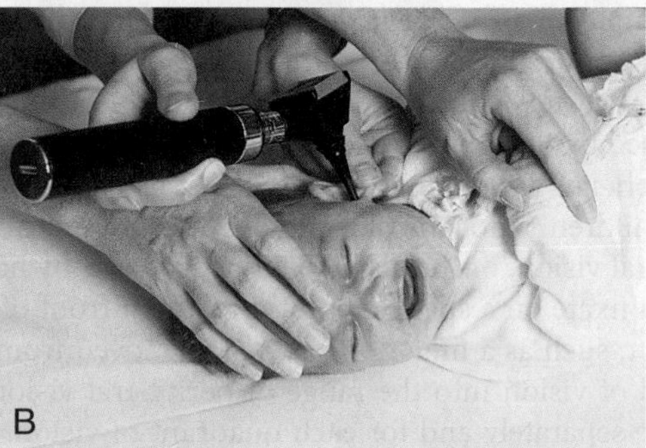

Fig. 34-20 Position for restraining child (**A**) and infant (**B**) during otoscopic examination.

The other position involves placing the child on the side, back, or abdomen with the arms at the side and the head turned so that the ear to be examined points toward the ceiling. Lean over the child, use the upper part of the body to restrain the arms and upper trunk movements, and use the examining hand to stabilize the head. This position is practical for young infants or for older children who need minimum restraint, but it may not be feasible for other children who protest vigorously. For safety enlist the parent's or an assistant's help in immobilizing the head by firmly placing one hand above the ear and the other on the child's side, abdomen, or back (see Fig. 34-20, *B*).

With cooperative children, examine the ear with the child in a side-lying, sitting, or standing position. One disadvantage to standing is that the child may "walk away" as the otoscope enters the canal. If the child is standing or sitting, tilt the head slightly toward the child's opposite shoulder to achieve a better view of the drum (Fig. 34-21).

With the thumb and forefinger of the free (usually non-dominant) hand, grasp the auricle. For the two positions of restraint, hold the otoscope upside down at the junction of its head and handle with the thumb and index finger. Place the other fingers against the skull to allow the otoscope to move with the child in case of sudden movement. In examining a cooperative child, hold the handle with the otic head upright or upside down. Use the dominant hand to examine both ears or reverse hands for each ear, whichever is more comfortable.

Before using the otoscope, visualize the external ear and the tympanic membrane as being superimposed on a clock (Fig. 34-22). The numbers become important geographic landmarks. Introduce the speculum into the meatus between the 3 and 9 o'clock positions in a *downward* and *forward* position. Because the canal is curved, the speculum does not permit a panoramic view of the tympanic membrane unless the canal is straightened. In infants the canal curves upward. Therefore pull the pinna *down* and *back* to the 6 to 9 o'clock range to straighten the canal (Fig. 34-23, *A*).

With older children, usually those older than 3 years of age, the canal curves downward and forward. Therefore pull the pinna *up* and *back* toward a 10 o'clock position (see Fig. 34-24, *B*). If you have difficulty visualizing the membrane, try repositioning the head, introducing the speculum at a different angle, and pulling the pinna in a slightly different direction. Do not insert the speculum past the cartilaginous (outermost) portion of the canal, usually a distance of 0.60 to 1.25 cm (0.23 to 0.5 inch) in older children. Insertion of the speculum into the posterior or bony portion of the canal causes pain.

In neonates and young infants the walls of the canal are pliable and floppy because of the underdeveloped cartilaginous and bony structures. Therefore the very small 2-mm speculum usually needs to be inserted deeper into the canal

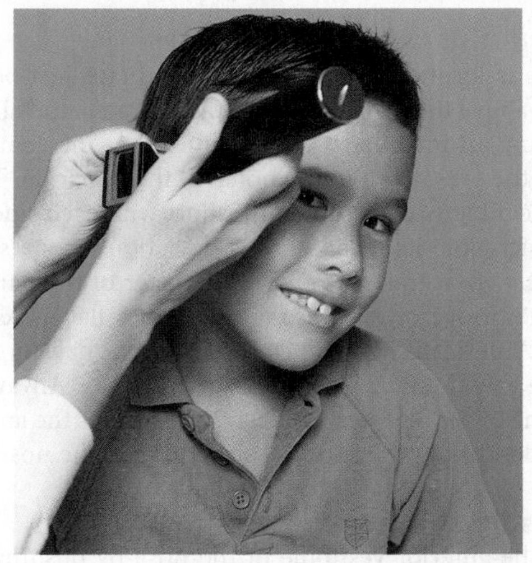

Fig. 34-21 Positioning head by tilting it toward opposite shoulder for full view of tympanic membrane.

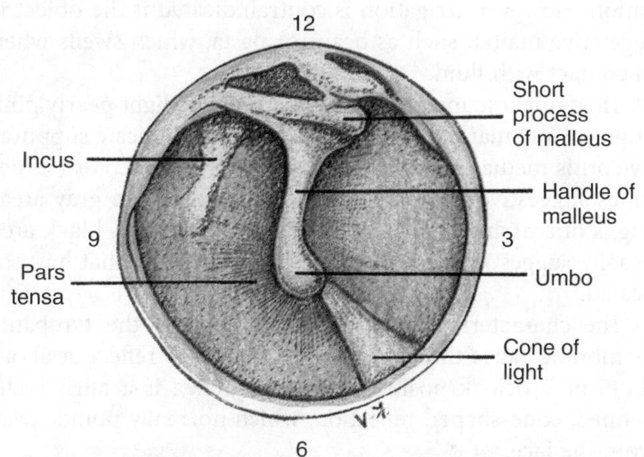

Fig. 34-22 Landmarks of tympanic membrane with "clock" superimposed. (Modified from Potter PA, Perry AG: *Basic nursing: essentials for practice*, ed 6, St Louis, 2006, Mosby.)

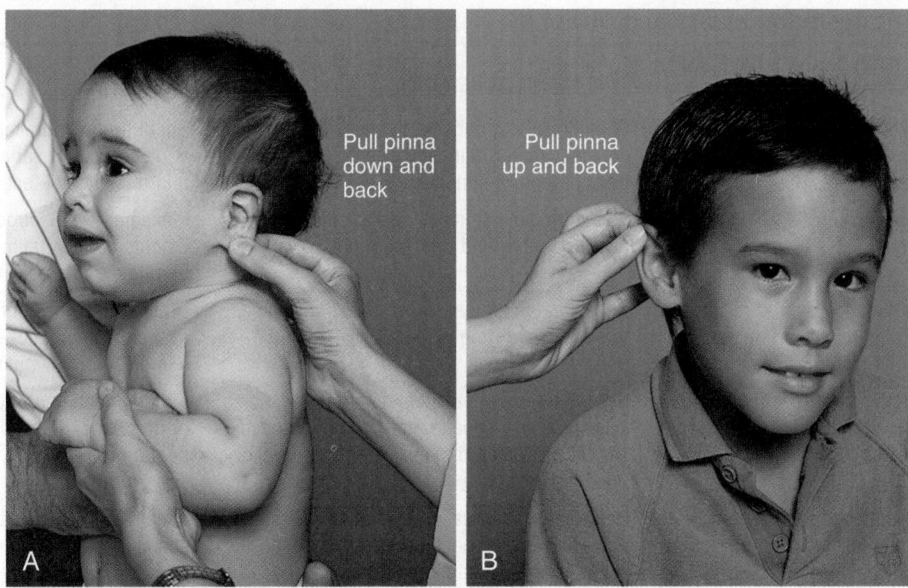

Fig. 34-23 Positioning for visualizing eardrum in infant (**A**) and in child older than 3 years of age (**B**).

evolve Anatomy Review—External, Middle, and Inner Ear

than in older children. Great care must be exercised not to damage the walls or drum. For this reason, only an experienced examiner should insert an otoscope into the ears of very young infants.

Otoscopic Examination

As you introduce the speculum into the external canal, inspect the walls of the canal, the color of the tympanic membrane, the light reflex, and the usual landmarks of the bony prominences of the middle ear. The walls of the external auditory canal are pink, although they are more pigmented in dark-skinned children. Minute hairs are evident in the outermost portion, where cerumen is produced. Note signs of irritation, foreign bodies, or infection.

Foreign bodies in the ear are not uncommon in children and range from erasers to beans. Symptoms may include pain, discharge, and affected hearing. Soft objects, such as paper or insects, can be removed with forceps. Small, hard objects, such as pebbles, can be removed with a suction tip, a hook, or irrigation. However, irrigation is contraindicated if the object is vegetative matter, such as beans or pasta, which swells when in contact with fluid.

The tympanic membrane is a translucent, light pearly pink or gray. Note marked erythema (which may indicate suppurative otitis media), a dull nontransparent grayish color (sometimes suggestive of serous otitis media), or ashen gray areas (signs of scarring from a previous perforation). A black area usually suggests a perforation of the membrane that has not healed.

The characteristic tenseness and slope of the tympanic membrane cause the light of the otoscope to reflect at about the 5 or 7 o'clock position. The light reflex is a fairly well-defined, cone-shaped reflection, which normally points away from the face.

The bony landmarks of the drum are formed by the umbo, or tip of the malleus. It appears as a small, round, opaque, concave spot near the center of the drum. The manubrium (long process or handle) of the malleus appears to be a whitish line extending from the umbo upward to the margin of the membrane. At the upper end of the long process near the 1 o'clock position (in the right ear) is a sharp, knoblike protuberance, representing the short process of the malleus. Note the absence of the light reflex or loss or abnormal prominence of any of these landmarks.

Auditory Testing

Several types of hearing tests are available and recommended for screening in infants and children (American Academy of Pediatrics, Committee on Practice and Ambulatory Medicine, Section on Otolaryngology and Bronchoesophagology, 2003) (Table 34-10). The nurse must operate under a high index of suspicion for those children who may have conditions associated with hearing loss and who may have developed behaviors that indicate auditory impairment (Cunningham & Cox, 2003).

Nose

Inspection of External Structures

The nose is located in the middle of the face just below the eyes and above the lips. Compare its placement and alignment by drawing an imaginary vertical line from the center point between the eyes down to the notch of the upper lip. The nose should be directly centered on this line, with each side exactly symmetric. Note its location, any deviation to one side, and asymmetry in overall size and in diameter of the nares (nostrils). The bridge of the nose is sometimes flat in Asian and African-American children. Observe the alae nasi for any sign of flaring, which indicates respiratory difficulty. Always report any flaring of the alae nasi. Fig. 34-24 illustrates the landmarks used in describing the external structures of the nose.

Inspection of Internal Structures

Inspect the anterior vestibule of the nose by pushing the tip upward, tilting the head backward, and illuminating the cavity

Table 34-10 Audiologic Tests for Infants and Children

AGE	AUDITORY TEST AND AVERAGE TIME	TYPE OF MEASUREMENT	PROCEDURE
All ages	Evoked otoacoustic emissions, 10-min test	Physiologic test specifically measuring cochlear (outer hair cell) response to presentation of stimulus	Small probe containing sensitive microphone is placed in ear canal for stimulus delivery and response detection.
Birth–9 mo	Auditory brainstem response, 15-min test	Electrophysiologic measurement of activity in auditory nerve and brainstem pathways	Placement of electrodes on child's head detects auditory stimuli presented though earphones one ear at a time
9 mo–2½ yr	Conditioned oriented responses or visual reinforced audiometry, 30-min test	Behavioral tests measuring child's responses to speech and frequency-specific stimuli presented through speakers	Both techniques condition child to associate speech or frequency-specific sound with reinforcement stimulus, such as lighted toy.
2½-4 yr	Play audiometry, 30-min test	Behavioral test measuring auditory thresholds in response to speech and frequency-specific stimuli presented through earphones and/or bone vibrator	Child is conditioned to put peg in peg board or drop block in a box when stimulus tone is heard.
4 yr–adolescence	Conventional audiometry, 30-min test	Behavioral test measuring auditory thresholds in response to speech and frequency-specific stimuli presented through earphone and/or bone vibrator	Patient is instructed to raise hand when stimulus is heard.

Modified with permission from Bachmann KR, Arvedson JC: Early identification and intervention for children who are hearing impaired, *Pediatr Rev* 19:155-165, 1998.

with a flashlight or otoscope without the attached ear speculum. Note the color of the mucosal lining, which is normally redder than the oral membranes, as well as any swelling, discharge, dryness, or bleeding. There should be no discharge from the nose.

On looking deeper into the nose, inspect the turbinates, or concha, plates of bone that jut into the nasal cavity and are enveloped by mucous membrane. The turbinates greatly increase the surface area of the nasal cavity as air is inhaled. The spaces or channels between the turbinates are called the *meatus* and correspond to each of the three turbinates. Normally the front end of the inferior and middle turbinate and the middle meatus are seen. They should be the same color as the lining of the vestibule.

Inspect the septum, which should divide the vestibules equally. Note any deviation, especially if it causes an occlusion of one side of the nose. A perforation may be evident within the septum. If this is suspected, shine the light of the otoscope into one naris and look for admittance of light to the other. Because olfaction is an important function of the nose, testing for smell may be done at this point or as part of cranial nerve assessment (see Table 34-13).

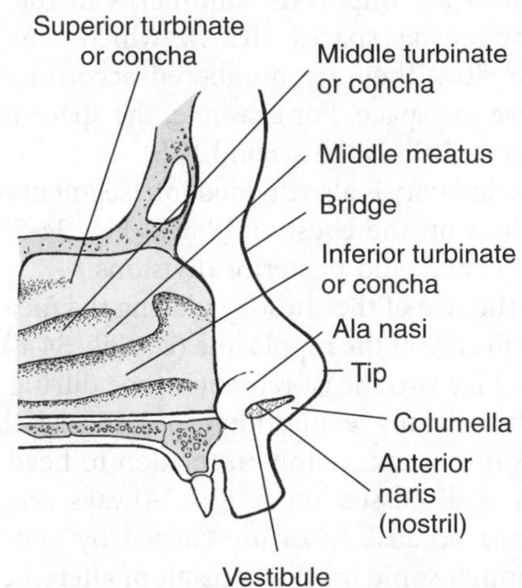

Fig. 34-24 External landmarks and internal structures of nose.

Mouth and Throat

With a cooperative child, almost the entire examination of the mouth and throat can be accomplished without the use of a tongue blade. Ask the child to open the mouth wide; to move the tongue in different directions for full visualization; and to say "ahh," which depresses the tongue for full view of the back of the mouth (tonsils, uvula, and oropharynx) (Fig. 34-25, *B*). For a closer look at the buccal mucosa, or lining of the cheeks, ask children to use their fingers to move the outer lip and cheek to one side (see Atraumatic Care box).

ATRAUMATIC CARE

Encouraging Opening the Mouth for Examination

- Perform the examination in front of a mirror.
- Let child first examine someone else's mouth, such as the parent, the nurse, or a puppet (see Fig. 34-25, *A*), and then examine child's mouth.
- Instruct child to tilt the head back slightly, breathe deeply through the mouth, and hold the breath; this action lowers the tongue to the floor of the mouth without the use of a tongue blade.
- Lightly brushing the palate with a cotton swab also may open the mouth for assessment.

Infants and toddlers usually resist attempts to keep the mouth open. Because inspecting the mouth is upsetting, leave it for the end of the physical examination (along with examination of the ears) or do it during episodes of crying. However, the use of a tongue blade (preferably flavored) to depress the tongue is necessary. Place the tongue blade along the *side* of the tongue, not in the center back area where the gag reflex is elicited. Fig. 34-25, *B*, illustrates proper positioning of the child for the oral examination.

The major structure of the exterior of the mouth is the lips. The lips should be moist, soft, smooth, and pink, or a deeper hue than the surrounding skin. The lips should be symmetric when relaxed or tensed. Assess symmetry when the child talks or cries.

evolve Anatomy Review—External and Internal Structures of the Nose
evolve Anatomy Review—Location of the Sinuses

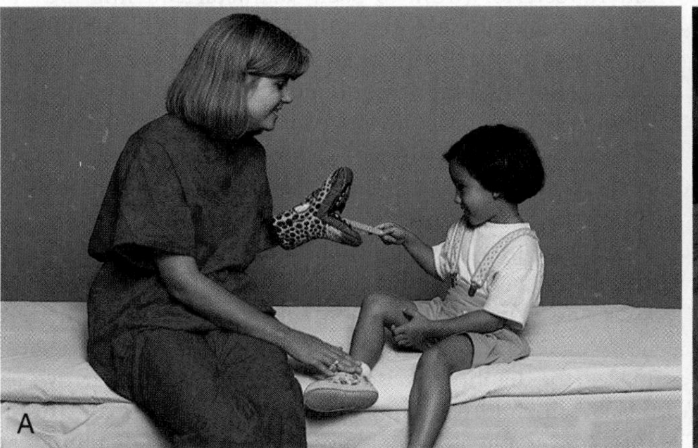

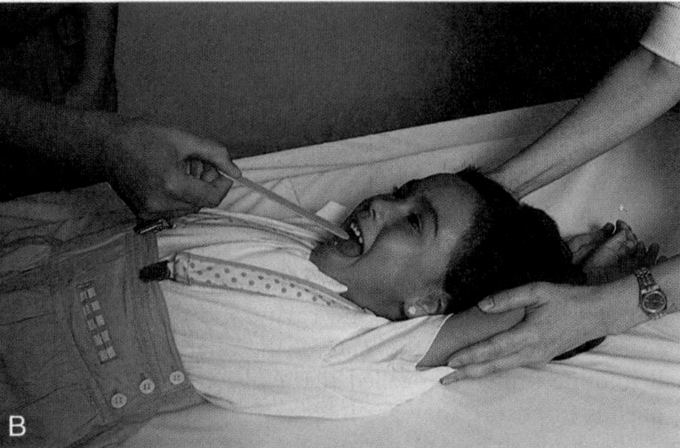

Fig. 34-25 **A**, Encouraging child to cooperate. **B**, Positioning child for examination of mouth.

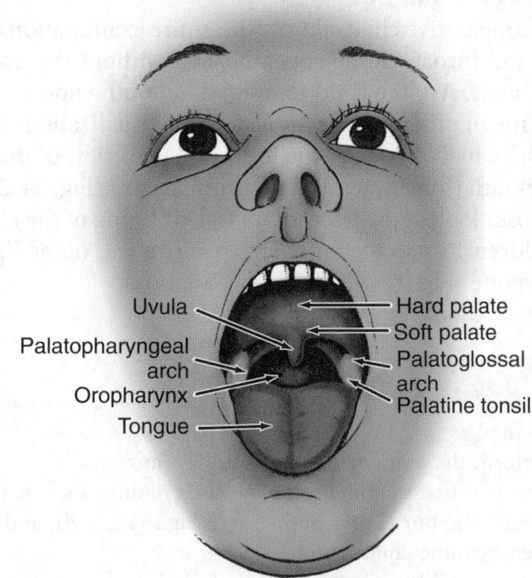

Fig. 34-26 Interior structures of mouth.

evolve Anatomy Review—Interior Structures of the Mouth

Inspection of Internal Structures

The major structures that are visible within the oral cavity and oropharynx are the mucosal lining of the lips and cheeks, gums (or gingiva), teeth, tongue, palate, uvula, tonsils, and posterior oropharynx (Fig. 34-26). Inspect all areas lined with mucous membranes (inside the lips and cheeks, gingiva, underside of the tongue, palate, and back of the pharynx) for color, any areas of white patches or ulceration, bleeding, sensitivity, and moisture. The membranes should be bright pink, smooth, glistening, uniform, and moist.

Inspect the teeth for number in each dental arch, for hygiene, and for occlusion or bite. Discoloration of tooth enamel with obvious plaque (whitish coating on the surface of the teeth) is a sign of poor dental hygiene and indicates a need for counseling. Brown spots in the crevices of the crown of the tooth or between the teeth may be caries (cavities). Chalky white to yellow or brown areas on the enamel may indicate fluorosis (excessive fluoride ingestion). Teeth that appear greenish black may be stained temporarily from ingestion of supplemental iron.

Examine the gums (gingiva) surrounding the teeth. The color is normally coral pink, and the surface texture is stippled, similar to the appearance of an orange peel. In dark-skinned children the gums are more deeply colored, and a brownish area is often observed along the gum line.

Inspect the tongue for papillae, small projections that contain several taste buds and give the tongue its characteristic rough appearance. Note the size and mobility of the tongue. Normally the tip of the tongue should extend to the lips or beyond.

The roof of the mouth consists of the hard palate, which is located near the front of the oral cavity, and the soft palate, which is located toward the back of the pharynx and has a small midline protrusion called the uvula. Carefully inspect the palates to ensure they are intact. The arch of the palate should be dome shaped. A narrow, flat roof or a high, arched palate affects the placement of the tongue and can cause feeding and speech problems. Test movement of the uvula by eliciting a gag reflex. It should move upward to close off the nasopharynx from the oropharynx.

Examine the oropharynx and note the size and color of the palatine tonsils. They are normally the same color as the surrounding mucosa; glandular, rather than smooth in appearance; and barely visible over the edge of the palatoglossal arches. The size of the tonsils varies considerably during childhood. However, report any swelling, redness, or white areas on the tonsils.

Chest

Inspect the chest for size, shape, symmetry, movement, breast development, and the bony landmarks formed by the ribs and sternum. The rib cage consists of 12 ribs on each side and the sternum, or breast bone, located in the midline of the trunk (Fig. 34-27). The sternum is composed of three main parts. The manubrium, the uppermost portion, can be felt at the base of the neck at the suprasternal notch. The largest segment of the sternum is the body, which forms the sternal angle (angle of Louis) as it articulates with the manubrium. At the end of the body is a small, movable process called the xiphoid. The angle of the costal margin as it attaches to the sternum is called the costal angle and is normally about 45 to 50 degrees. These bony structures are important landmarks in the location of ribs and intercostal spaces (ICSs), which are the spaces between the ribs. They are numbered according to the rib directly *above* the space. For example, the space immediately below the second rib is the second ICS.

The thoracic cavity is also divided into segments by drawing imaginary lines on the chest and back. Fig. 34-28 illustrates the anterior, lateral, and posterior divisions.

Measure the size of the chest by placing the measuring tape around the rib cage at the nipple line (see Fig. 34-8). For greatest accuracy, take two measurements—one during inspiration and the other during expiration—and record the average. Chest size is important mainly in relation to head circumference, which is discussed on p. 892. Always report marked disproportions because most are caused by abnormal head growth, although some may be a result of altered chest shape, such as barrel chest (chest is round) or pigeon chest (sternum protrudes outward).

During infancy the chest's shape is almost circular, with the anteroposterior (front-to-back) diameter equaling the transverse, or lateral (side-to-side), diameter. As the child grows, the chest normally increases in the transverse direction, causing the anteroposterior diameter to be less than the lateral diameter. Note the angle made by the lower costal margin and the sternum, and palpate the junction of the ribs with the costal cartilage (costochondral junction) and sternum, which should be fairly smooth.

Movement of the chest wall should be symmetric bilaterally and coordinated with breathing. During inspiration the chest rises and expands, the diaphragm descends, and the costal angle increases. During expiration the chest falls and decreases in size, the diaphragm rises, and the costal angle narrows (Fig. 34-29). In children younger than 6 or 7 years of age, respiratory movement is principally abdominal or diaphragmatic. In older children, particularly girls, respirations are chiefly

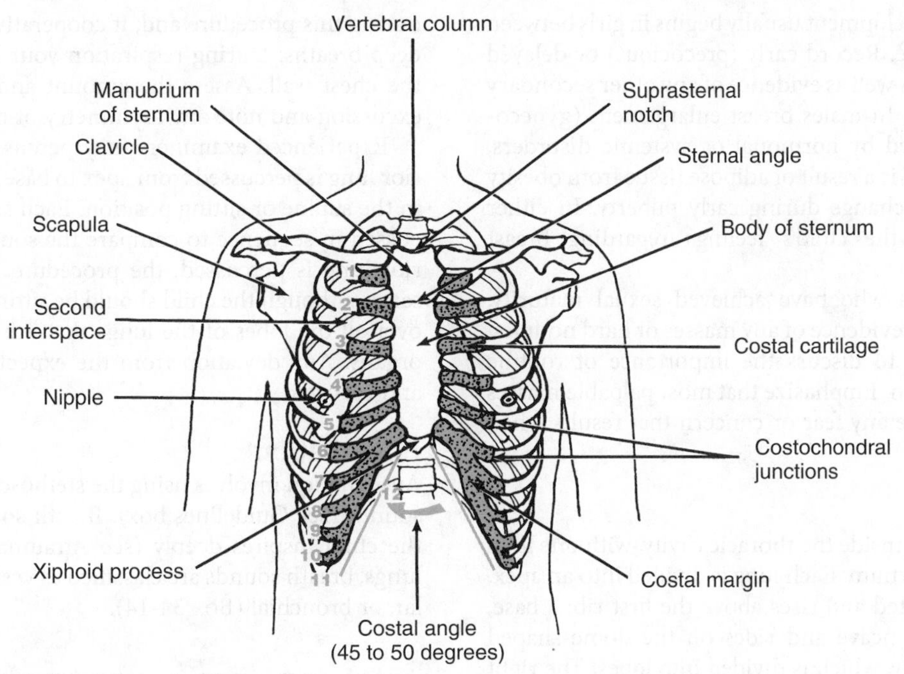

Fig. 34-27 Rib cage.

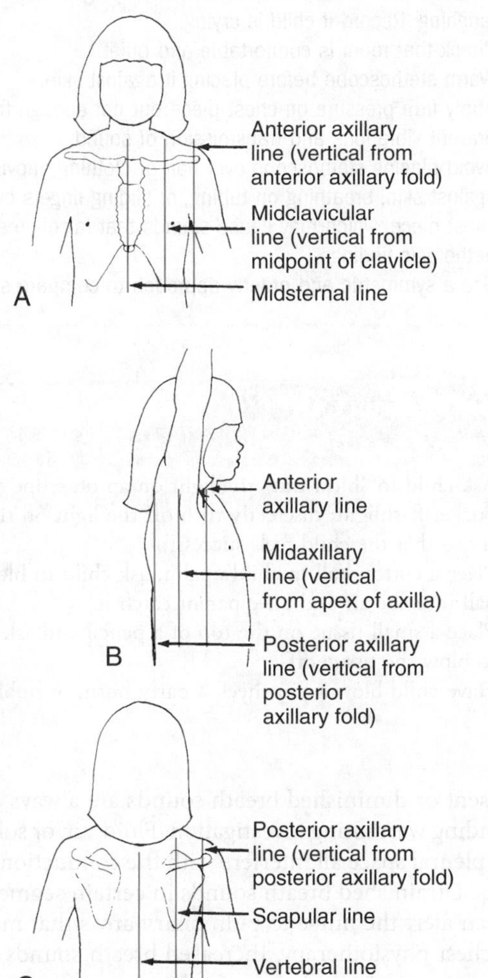

Fig. 34-28 Imaginary landmarks of chest. A, Anterior. B, Right lateral. C, Posterior.

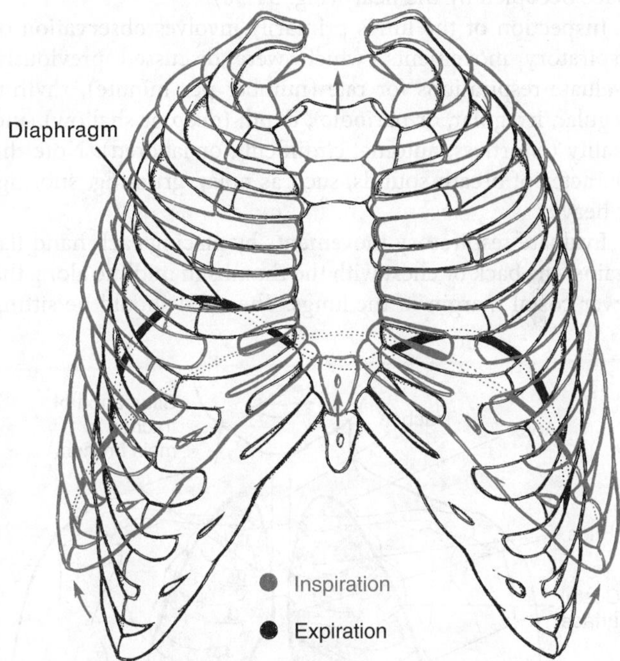

Fig. 34-29 Movement of chest during respiration.

thoracic. In either type the chest and abdomen should rise and fall together. Always report any asymmetry of movement.

While inspecting the skin surface of the chest, observe the position of the nipples and any evidence of breast development. Normally the nipples are located slightly lateral to the midclavicular line between the fourth and fifth ribs. Note symmetry of nipple placement and normal configuration of a darker pigmented areola surrounding a flat nipple in the prepubertal child.

evolve Anatomy Review—Rib Cage

evolve Anatomy Review—Imaginary Landmarks of the Chest

Pubertal breast development usually begins in girls between 10 and 14 years of age. Record early (precocious) or delayed breast development, as well as evidence of any other secondary sexual characteristics. In males breast enlargement (gynecomastia) may be caused by hormonal or systemic disorders, but more commonly it is a result of adipose tissue from obesity or a transitory body change during early puberty. In either situation investigate the child's feelings regarding breast enlargement.

In adolescent girls who have achieved sexual maturity, palpate the breasts for evidence of any masses or hard nodules. Use this opportunity to discuss the importance of routine breast self-examination. Emphasize that most palpable masses are benign to decrease any fear or concern that results when a mass is felt.

Lungs

The lungs are situated inside the thoracic cavity, with one lung on each side of the sternum. Each lung is divided into an apex, which is slightly pointed and rises above the first rib; a base, which is wide and concave and rides on the dome-shaped diaphragm; and a body, which is divided into lobes. The right lung has three lobes: the upper, middle, and lower. The left lung has only two lobes, the upper and lower, because of the space occupied by the heart (Fig. 34-30).

Inspection of the lungs primarily involves observation of respiratory movements, which were discussed previously. Evaluate respirations for rate (number per minute), rhythm (regular, irregular, or periodic), depth (deep or shallow), and quality (effortless, automatic, difficult, or labored). Note the character of breath sounds, such as noisy, grunting, snoring, or heavy.

Evaluate respiratory movements by placing each hand flat against the back or chest with the thumbs in midline along the lower costal margin of the lungs. The child should be sitting during this procedure and, if cooperative, should take several deep breaths. During respiration your hands will move with the chest wall. Assess the amount and speed of respiratory excursion and note any asymmetry of movement.

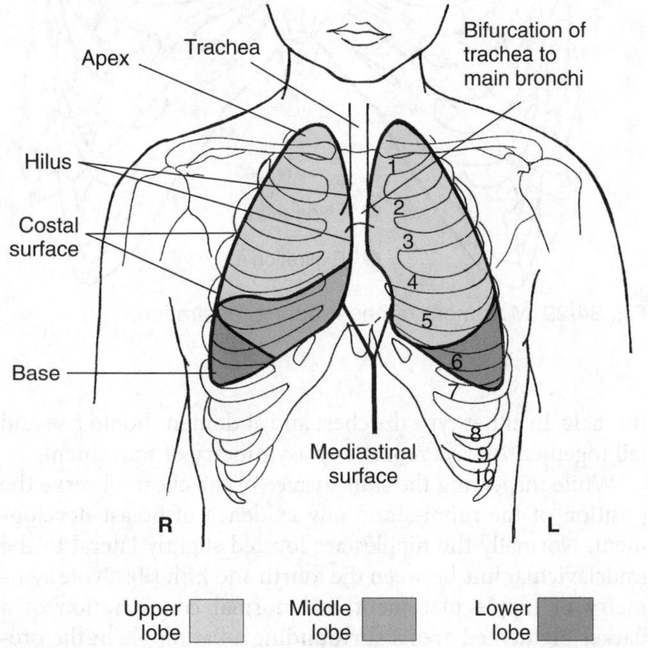

Fig. 34-30 Location of lobes of lungs within thoracic cavity.

Experienced examiners may percuss the lungs. The anterior lung is percussed from apex to base, usually with the child in the supine or sitting position. Each side of the chest is percussed in sequence to compare the sounds. When the posterior lung is percussed, the procedure and sequence are the same, although the child should be sitting. Resonance is heard over all the lobes of the lungs that are not adjacent to other organs. Any deviation from the expected sound is recorded and reported.

Auscultation

Auscultation involves using the stethoscope to evaluate breath sounds (see Guidelines box). Breath sounds are best heard if the child inspires deeply (see Atraumatic Care box). In the lungs, breath sounds are classified as vesicular, bronchovesicular, or bronchial (Box 34-14).

GUIDELINES *Effective Auscultation*

- Make certain child is relaxed and not crying, talking, or laughing. Record if child is crying.
- Check that room is comfortable and quiet.
- Warm stethoscope before placing it against skin.
- Apply firm pressure on chest piece but not enough to prevent vibrations and transmission of sound.
- Avoid placing stethoscope over hair or clothing, moving it against skin, breathing on tubing, or sliding fingers over chest piece, which may cause sounds that falsely resemble pathologic findings.
- Use a symmetric and orderly approach to compare sounds.

ATRAUMATIC CARE

Encouraging Deep Breaths

- Ask child to "blow out" the light on an otoscope or pocket flashlight; discreetly turn off the light on the last try so that the child feels successful.
- Place a cotton ball in child's palm; ask child to blow the ball into the air and have parent catch it.
- Place a small tissue on the top of a pencil and ask child to blow the tissue off.
- Have child blow a pinwheel, a party horn, or bubbles.

Absent or diminished breath sounds are always an abnormal finding warranting investigation. Fluid, air, or solid masses in the pleural space all interfere with the conduction of breath sounds. Diminished breath sounds in certain segments of the lung can alert the nurse to pulmonary areas that may benefit from chest physiotherapy. Increased breath sounds after pulmonary therapy indicate improved passage of air through the respiratory tract. Terms used to describe various respiration patterns are found in Box 34-15.

BOX 34-14 Classification of Normal Breath Sounds

Vesicular Breath Sounds

Heard over entire surface of lungs, with exception of upper intrascapular area and area beneath manubrium.

Inspiration is louder, longer, and higher pitched than expiration.

Sound is soft, swishing noise.

Bronchovesicular Breath Sounds

Heard over manubrium and in upper intrascapular regions where trachea and bronchi bifurcate.

Inspiration is louder and higher pitched than in vesicular breathing.

Bronchial Breath Sounds

Heard only over trachea near suprasternal notch.

Inspiratory phase is short, and expiratory phase is long.

BOX 34-15 Various Patterns of Respiration

Tachypnea—Increased rate

Bradypnea—Decreased rate

Dyspnea—Distress during breathing

Apnea—Cessation of breathing

Hyperpnea—Increased depth

Hypoventilation—Decreased depth (shallow) and irregular rhythm

Hyperventilation—Increased rate and depth

Kussmaul respiration—Hyperventilation, gasping and labored respiration; usually seen in diabetic coma or other states of respiratory acidosis

Cheyne-Stokes respiration—Gradually increasing rate and depth with periods of apnea

Biot respiration—Periods of hyperpnea alternating with apnea (similar to Cheyne-Stokes except that depth remains constant)

Seesaw (paradoxic) respirations—Chest falls on inspiration and rises on expiration

Agonal—Last gasping breaths before death

Various pulmonary abnormalities produce adventitious sounds that are not normally heard over the chest. These sounds occur in addition to normal or abnormal breath sounds. They are classified into two main groups: crackles, which result from the passage of air through fluid or moisture; and wheezes, which are produced as air passes through narrowed passageways, regardless of the cause, such as exudate, inflammation, spasm, or tumor. Considerable practice with an experienced tutor is necessary to differentiate the various types of lung sounds. Often it is best to describe the type of sound heard in the lungs rather than trying to label it. Always report any abnormal sounds for further medical evaluation.

Heart

The heart is situated in the thoracic cavity between the lungs in the mediastinum and above the diaphragm (Fig. 34-31). About two thirds of the heart lies within the left side of the rib

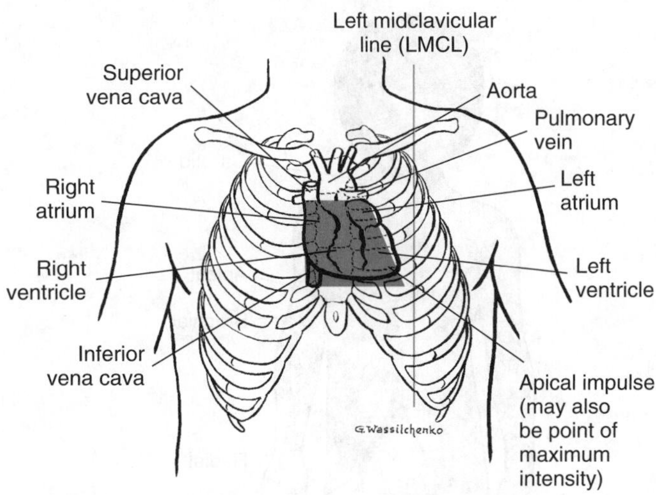

Fig. 34-31 Position of heart within thorax.

cage, with the other third on the right side as it crosses the sternum. The heart is positioned in the thorax like a trapezoid:

- *Vertically* along the right sternal border (RSB) from the second to the fifth rib
- *Horizontally* (long side) from the lower right sternum to the fifth rib at the left midclavicular line (LMCL)
- *Diagonally* from the left sternal border (LSB) at the second rib to the LMCL at the fifth rib
- *Horizontally* (short side) from the RSB and LSB at the second ICS—base of the heart

Inspection is best done with the child sitting in a semi-Fowler position. Look at the anterior chest wall from an angle, comparing both sides of the rib cage with each other. Normally they should be symmetric. In children with thin chest walls, a pulsation may be visible. Because comprehensive evaluation of cardiac function is not limited to the heart, also consider other findings such as the presence of all pulses (especially the femoral pulses) (Fig. 34-32), distended neck veins, clubbing of the fingers, peripheral cyanosis, edema, BP, and respiratory status.

Use palpation to determine the location of the apical impulse (AI), the most lateral cardiac impulse that may correspond to the apex. The AI is found:

- Just lateral to the LMCL and fourth ICS in children over 7 years of age
- At the LMCL and fifth ICS in children less than 7 years of age

Although the AI gives a general idea of the size of the heart (with enlargement, the apex is lower and more lateral), its normal location is variable, making it an unreliable indicator of heart size.

The point of maximum intensity (PMI), as the name implies, is the area of most intense pulsation. Usually the PMI is located at the same site as the AI, but it can occur elsewhere. For this reason, the two terms should not be used synonymously.

Assess capillary refill time, an important test for peripheral circulation, by pressing the skin lightly on a central site, such as the forehead, or a peripheral site, such as the top of the

evolve Critical Thinking Exercise—Cardiovascular Assessment

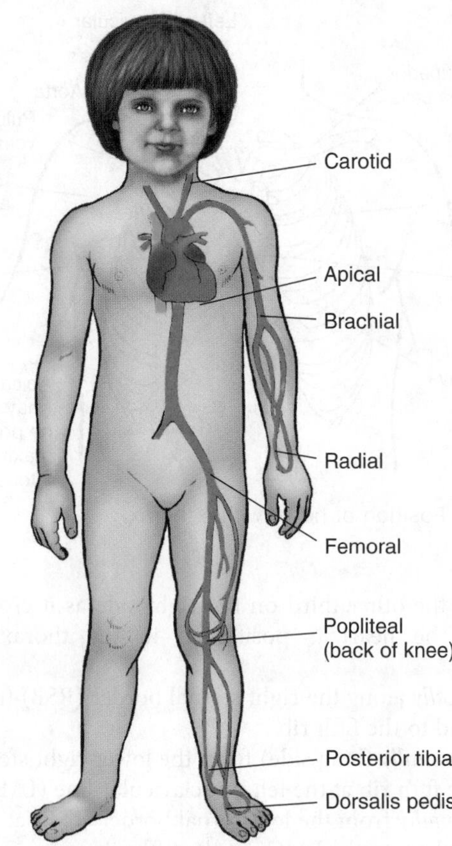

Fig. 34-32 Location of pulses.

evolve Anatomy Review—Location of Pulses

hand, to produce a slight blanching. The time it takes for the blanched area to return to its original color is the capillary refill time.

NURSING ALERT Capillary refill should be brisk–less than 2 seconds; prolonged refill may be associated with poor systemic perfusion or a cool ambient temperature.

Auscultation

Origin of Heart Sounds

The heart sounds are produced by the opening and closing of the valves and the vibration of blood against the walls of the heart and vessels. Normally two sounds—S_1 and S_2—are heard, which correspond, respectively, to the familiar "lub dub" often used to describe the sounds. S_1 is caused by closure of the tricuspid and mitral valves (sometimes called the *atrioventricular valves*). S_2 is the result of closure of the pulmonic and aortic valves (sometimes called *semilunar valves*). Normally the split of the two sounds in S_2 is distinguishable and widens during inspiration. Physiologic splitting is a significant normal finding.

evolve Anatomy Review—Direction of Heart Sounds

NURSING ALERT *Fixed splitting,* in which the split in S_2 does not change during inspiration, is an important diagnostic sign of atrial septal defect.

Two other heart sounds—S_3 and S_4—may be produced. S_3 is normally heard in some children; S_4 is rarely heard as a normal heart sound; it usually indicates the need for further cardiac evaluation.

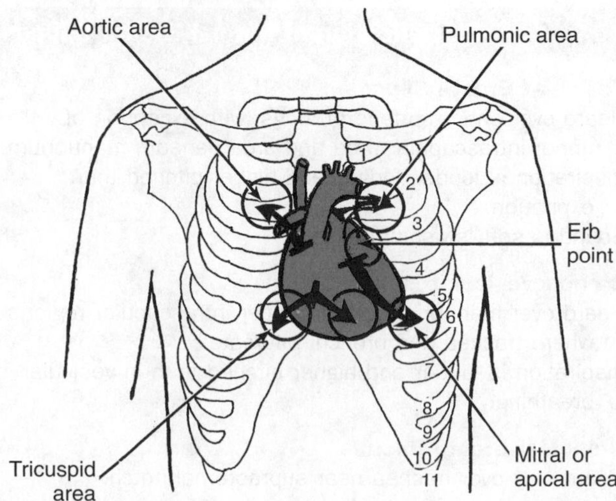

Fig. 34-33 Direction of heart sounds for anatomic valve sites and areas *(circled)* for auscultation.

Differentiating Normal Heart Sounds

Fig. 34-33 illustrates the approximate anatomic position of the valves within the heart chambers. Note that the anatomic location of valves does not correspond to the area where the sounds are heard best. The auscultatory sites are located in the direction of the blood flow through the valves. Normally S_1 is louder at the apex of the heart in the mitral and tricuspid area, and S_2 is louder near the base of the heart in the pulmonic and aortic area (Table 34-11). Listen to each sound by inching down the chest. The following areas should also be auscultated for sounds, such as murmurs, which may radiate to these sites: sternoclavicular area above the clavicles and manubrium, area along the sternal border, area along the left midaxillary line, and area below the scapulae.

NURSING ALERT To distinguish between S_1 and S_2 heart sounds, simultaneously palpate the carotid pulse with the index and middle fingers and listen to the heart sounds; S_1 is synchronous with the carotid pulse.

Auscultate the heart with the child in at least two positions: sitting and reclining. If adventitious sounds are detected, further evaluate them with the child standing, sitting and leaning forward, and lying on the left side. For example, atrial sounds such as S_4 are heard best with the person in a recumbent position and usually fade if the person sits or stands.

Evaluate heart sounds for (1) quality (they should be clear and distinct, not muffled, diffuse, or distant); (2) intensity, especially in relation to the location or auscultatory site (they should not be weak or pounding); (3) rate (they should have the same rate as the radial pulse); and (4) rhythm (they should be regular and even). A particular arrhythmia that occurs normally in many children is sinus arrhythmia, in which the heart rate increases with inspiration and decreases with expiration. Differentiate this rhythm from a truly abnormal arrhythmia by having children hold their breath. In sinus

Table 34-11 Sequence of Auscultating Heart Sounds*

AUSCULTATORY SITE	CHEST LOCATION	CHARACTERISTICS OF HEART SOUNDS
Aortic area	Second right intercostal space close to sternum	S_2 heard louder than S_1; aortic closure heard loudest
Pulmonic area	Second left intercostal space close to sternum	Splitting of S_2 heard best, normally widens on inspiration; pulmonic closure heard best
Erb's point	Second and third left intercostal spaces close to sternum	Frequent site of innocent murmurs and those of aortic or pulmonic origin
Tricuspid area	Fifth right and left intercostal spaces close to sternum	S_1 heard as louder sound preceding S_2 (S_1 synchronous with carotid pulse)
Mitral or apical area	Fifth intercostal space, left midclavicular line (third to fourth intercostal space and lateral to left midclavicular line in infants)	S_1 heard loudest; splitting of S_1 may be audible because mitral closure is louder than tricuspid closure S_1 heard best at beginning of expiration with child in recumbent or left side-lying position; occurs immediately after S_2; sounds like word S_1 S_2 S_3: "Ken-tuc-ky" S_4 heard best during expiration with child in recumbent position (left side-lying position decreases sound); occurs immediately before S_1; sounds like word S_4 S_1 S_2: "Ten-nes-see"

*Use both diaphragm and bell chest pieces when auscultating heart sounds. Bell chest piece is necessary for low-pitched sounds of murmurs, S_3, and S_4.

arrhythmia, cessation of breathing causes the heart rate to remain steady.

Heart Murmurs

Another important category of the heart sounds is murmurs, which are produced by vibrations within the heart chambers or in the major arteries from the back-and-forth flow of blood. Murmurs are classified as:

Innocent—No anatomic or physiologic abnormality exists.

Functional—No automatic cardiac defect exists, but a physiologic abnormality such as anemia is present.

Organic—A cardiac defect with or without a physiologic abnormality exists.

The description and classification of murmurs are skills that require considerable practice and training. In general, recognize murmurs as distinct swishing sounds that occur in addition to the normal heart sounds and record the (1) location, or the area of the heart in which the murmur is heard best; (2) time of the occurrence of the murmur within the S_1-S_2 cycle; (3) intensity (evaluate in relationship to the child's position); and (4) loudness. The usual subjective method of grading the loudness or intensity of a murmur is listed in Table 34-12.

Table 34-12 Grading of the Intensity of Heart Murmurs

GRADE	DESCRIPTION
I	Very faint; often not heard if child sits up
II	Usually readily heard; slightly louder than grade I; audible in all positions
III	Loud, but not accompanied by a thrill
IV	Loud, accompanied by a thrill
V	Loud enough to be heard with a stethoscope barely touching the chest; accompanied by a thrill
VI	Loud enough to be heard with the stethoscope not touching the chest; often heard with the human ear close to the chest; accompanied by a thrill

Abdomen

Examination of the abdomen involves inspection, followed by auscultation and then palpation. Perform palpation last because it may distort the normal abdominal sounds. Knowledge of the anatomic placement of the abdominal organs is essential to differentiate normal, expected findings from abnormal ones (Fig. 34-34).

For descriptive purposes, the abdominal cavity is divided into four quadrants by drawing a vertical line midway from the sternum to the symphysis pubis and a horizontal line across the abdomen through the umbilicus. The sections are named:

- Left upper quadrant
- Left lower quadrant
- Right upper quadrant
- Right lower quadrant

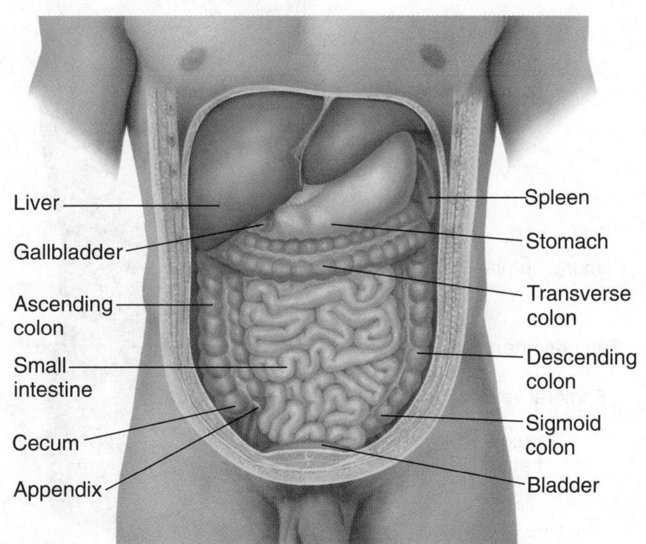

Fig. 34-34 Location of structures in abdomen. (From Seidel HM et al: *Mosby's guide to physical examination*, ed 6, St Louis, 2006, Mosby.)

evolve Anatomy Review—Abdominal Anatomy

Inspection

Inspect the contour of the abdomen with the child erect and supine. Normally the abdomen of infants and young children is cylindric and, in the erect position, fairly prominent because of the physiologic lordosis of the spine. In the supine position the abdomen appears flat. A midline protrusion from the xiphoid to the umbilicus or symphysis pubis is usually diastasis recti, or failure of the rectus abdominis muscles to join in utero. In a healthy child a midline protrusion is usually a variation of normal muscular development.

NURSING ALERT A tense, boardlike abdomen is a serious sign of paralytic ileus and intestinal obstruction.

The skin covering the abdomen should be uniformly taut, without wrinkles or creases. Sometimes silvery, whitish striae ("stretch marks") are seen, especially if the skin has been stretched as in obesity. Superficial veins are usually visible in light-skinned, thin infants, but distended veins are an abnormal finding.

Observe movement of the abdomen. Normally chest and abdominal movements are synchronous. In infants and thin children peristaltic waves may be visible through the abdominal wall; they are best observed by standing at eye level to and across from the abdomen. Always report this finding.

Examine the umbilicus for size, hygiene, and evidence of any abnormalities, such as hernias. The umbilicus should be flat or only slightly protruding. If a herniation is present, palpate the sac for abdominal contents and estimate the approximate size of the opening. Umbilical hernias are common in infants, especially in African-American children.

Hernias may exist elsewhere on the abdominal wall (Fig. 34-35). An inguinal hernia is a protrusion of peritoneum through the abdominal wall in the inguinal canal. It occurs mostly in males, is frequently bilateral, and may be visible as a mass in the scrotum. To locate a hernia, slide the little finger into the external inguinal ring at the base of the scrotum and ask the child to cough. If a hernia is present, it will hit the tip of the finger.

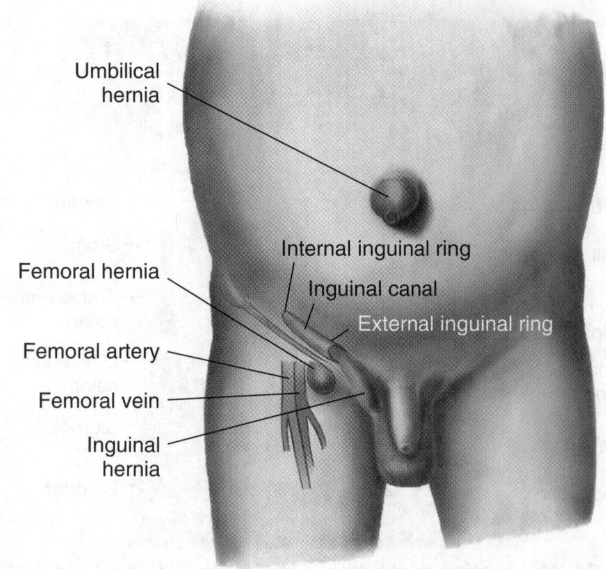

Fig. 34-35 Location of hernias.

A femoral hernia, which occurs more frequently in girls, is felt or seen as a small mass on the anterior surface of the thigh just below the inguinal ligament in the femoral canal (a potential space medial to the femoral artery). Feel for a hernia by placing the index finger of your right hand on the child's right femoral pulse (left hand for left pulse) and the middle finger flat against the skin toward the midline. The ring finger lies over the femoral canal, where the herniation occurs. Palpation of hernias in the pelvic region is often part of the genital examination.

Auscultation

The most important finding to listen for is peristalsis, or bowel sounds, which sound like short metallic clicks and gurgles. Their frequency per minute should be recorded (e.g., 5 sounds/min). Bowel sounds may be stimulated by stroking the abdominal surface with a fingernail. Report absence of bowel sounds or hyperperistalsis, since either usually denotes an abdominal disorder.

Palpation

Two types of palpation are performed: superficial and deep. For superficial palpation, lightly place your hand against the skin and feel each quadrant, noting any areas of tenderness, muscle tone, and superficial lesions such as cysts. Because superficial palpation is often perceived as tickling, several techniques can be used to minimize this sensation and relax the child (see Atraumatic Care box). Admonishing the child

ATRAUMATIC CARE

Promoting Relaxation During Abdominal Palpation

- Position child comfortably, such as in a semireclining position in the parent's lap, with knees flexed.
- Warm the hands before touching the skin.
- Use distraction, such as telling stories or talking to child.
- Teach child to use deep breathing and to concentrate on an object.
- Give infant a bottle or pacifier.
- Begin with light, superficial palpation and gradually progress to deeper palpation.
- Palpate any tender or painful areas last.
- Have child hold the parent's hand and squeeze it if palpation is uncomfortable.
- Use the nonpalpating hand to comfort child, such as placing the free hand on the child's shoulder while palpating the abdomen.
- To minimize sensation of tickling during palpation:
  - Have children "help" with palpation by placing a hand over the palpating hand.
  - Have them place a hand on the abdomen with the fingers spread wide apart, and palpate between their fingers.

to stop laughing only draws attention to the sensation and decreases cooperation.

Deep palpation is used for palpating organs and large blood vessels and for detecting masses and tenderness that were not discovered during superficial palpation. Palpation usually begins in the lower quadrants and proceeds upward to avoid missing the edge of an enlarged liver or spleen. Except for palpating the liver, successful identification of other organs, such as the spleen, kidney, and part of the colon, requires considerable practice with tutored supervision. Report any questionable mass. The lower edge of the liver is sometimes felt in infants and young children as a superficial mass 1 to 2 cm (0.4 to 0.8 inch) below the right costal margin (the distance is sometimes measured in fingerbreadths). Normally, the liver descends during inspiration as the diaphragm moves downward. Do not mistake this downward displacement as a sign of liver enlargement.

NURSING ALERT If the liver is palpable 3 cm (1.2 inch) below the right costal margin or the spleen is palpable more than 2 cm (0.8 inch) below the left costal margin, these organs are enlarged—a finding that is always reported for further medical investigation.

Palpate the femoral pulses by placing the tips of two or three fingers (index, middle, or ring) along the inguinal ligament about midway between the iliac crest and symphysis pubis. Feel both pulses simultaneously to make certain that they are equal and strong (Fig. 34-36).

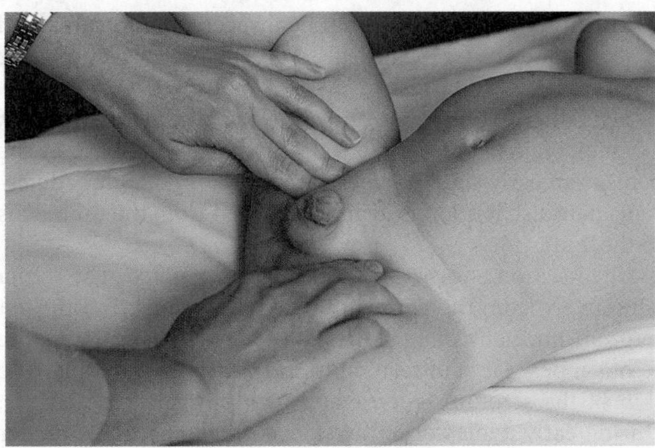

Fig. 34-36 Palpating femoral pulses.

NURSING ALERT Absence of femoral pulses is a significant sign of coarctation of the aorta and is referred for medical evaluation.

Genitalia

Examination of genitalia conveniently follows assessment of the abdomen while the child is still supine. In adolescents inspection of the genitalia may be left to the end of the examination. The best approach is to examine the genitalia matter-of-factly, placing no more emphasis on this part of the assessment than on any other segment. It helps to relieve children's and parents' anxiety by telling them the results of the findings; for example, the nurse might say, "Everything looks fine here."

If it is necessary to ask questions, such as about discharge or difficulty urinating, respect the child's privacy by covering the lower abdomen with the gown or underpants. To prevent embarrassing interruptions, keep the door or curtain closed and post a "do not disturb" sign. Have a drape ready to cover the genitalia if someone enters the room.

In examining the genitalia, wear gloves when touching body substances. It might be helpful for the adolescent to know that wearing gloves also prevents skin-to-skin contact.

The genital examination is an excellent time for eliciting questions or concern about body function or sexual activity. Also use this opportunity to increase or reinforce the child's knowledge of reproductive anatomy by naming each body part and explaining its function. This part of the health assessment is an opportune time to teach testicular self-examination to boys.*

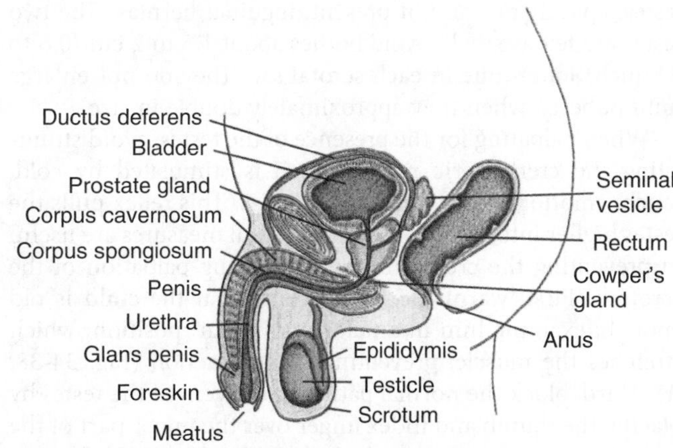

Fig. 34-37 Major structures of genitalia in uncircumcised postpubertal male. (From Potter PA, Perry AG: *Basic nursing: essentials for practice*, ed 6, St Louis, 2006, Mosby.)

Male Genitalia

Note the external appearance of the glans and shaft of the penis, the prepuce, the urethral meatus, and the scrotum (Fig. 34-37). The penis is generally small in infants and young boys until puberty, when it begins to increase in both length and width. In an obese child the penis often looks abnormally small because of the folds of skin partially covering it at the base. Be familiar with normal pubertal growth of the external male genitalia to compare the findings with the expected sequence of maturation.

Examine the glans (head of the penis) and shaft (portion between the perineum and prepuce) for signs of swelling, skin lesions, inflammation, or other irregularities. Any of these signs may indicate underlying disorders, especially sexually transmitted infections.

**For free information on testicular cancer, contact Jason A. Struble Memorial Cancer Fund, Inc., 1544 Mammoth Drive, Saint Paul, MO 63366; 636-227-3996;* www.testicularcancer.org.

The urethral meatus is carefully inspected for location and evidence of discharge. Normally it is centered at the tip of the glans.

Hair distribution is also noted. Normally, before puberty, no pubic hair is present. Soft, downy hair at the base of the penis is an early sign of pubertal maturation. In older adolescents hair distribution is diamond-shaped from the umbilicus to the anus.

The location and size of the scrotum are noted. The scrota hang freely from the perineum behind the penis, and the left scrotum normally hangs lower than the right. In infants the scrota appear large in relation to the rest of the genitalia. The skin of the scrotum is loose and highly rugated (wrinkled). During early adolescence the skin normally becomes redder and coarser. In dark-skinned children the scrota are usually more deeply pigmented.

Palpation of the scrotum includes identification of the testes, epididymis, and, if present, inguinal hernias. The two testes are felt as small, ovoid bodies about 1.5 to 2 cm (0.6 to 0.8 inch) long—one in each scrotal sac. They do not enlarge until puberty, when they approximately double in size.

When palpating for the presence of the testes, avoid stimulating the cremasteric reflex, which is stimulated by cold, touch, emotional excitement, or exercise. This reflex pulls the testes higher into the pelvic cavity. Several measures are useful in preventing the cremasteric reflex during palpation of the scrotum. First, warm the hands. Second, if the child is old enough, examine him in a tailor or "Indian" position, which stretches the muscle, preventing its contraction (Fig. 34-38, *A*). Third, block the normal pathway of ascent of the testes by placing the thumb and index finger over the upper part of the scrotal sac along the inguinal canal (see Fig. 34-38, *B*). If there is any question concerning the existence of two testes, place the index and middle fingers in a scissors fashion to separate the right and left scrota. If, after using these techniques, you have not palpated the testes, feel along the inguinal canal and perineum to locate masses that may be undescended testes. Although undescended testes may descend at any time during childhood and are checked at each visit, failure to palpate testes is reported.

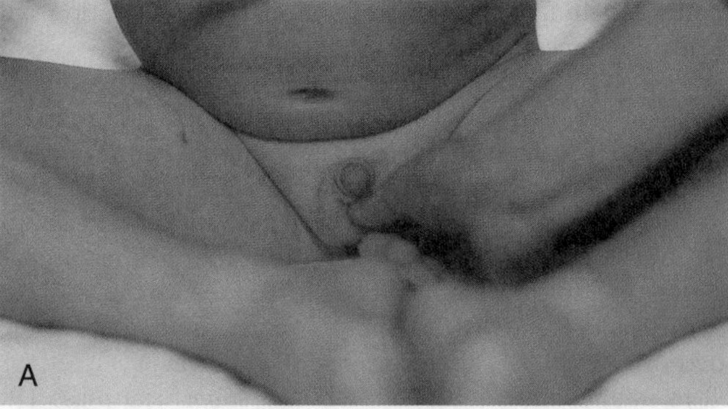

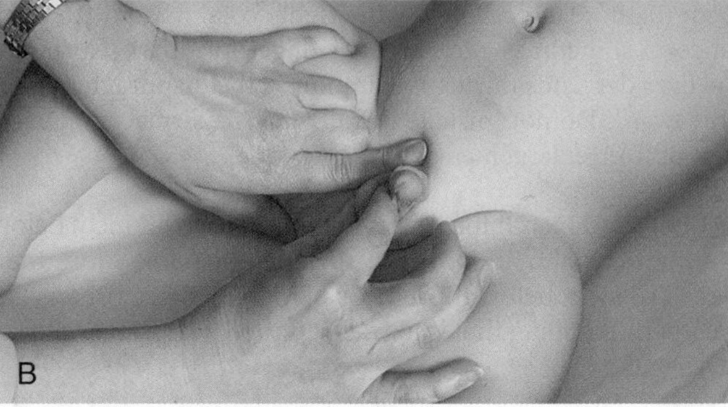

Fig. 34-38 A, Preventing cremasteric reflex by having child sit in "tailor" position. **B,** Blocking inguinal canal during palpation of scrotum for descended testes.

Female Genitalia

The examination of female genitalia is limited to inspection and palpation of external structures. If a vaginal examination is required, an appropriate referral is made unless the nurse is qualified to perform the procedure. A convenient position for examination of the genitalia involves placing the young child supine on the examining table or in a semireclining position on the parent's lap with the feet supported on your knees as you sit facing the child. Divert the child's attention from the examination by instructing her to try to keep the soles of her feet pressed against each other. Separate the labia majora with the thumb and index finger and retract outward to expose the labia minora, urethral meatus, and vaginal orifice.

Examine the female genitalia for size and location of the structures of the vulva, or pudendum (Fig. 34-39). The mons pubis is a pad of adipose tissue over the symphysis pubis. At puberty the mons is covered with hair, which extends along the labia. The usual pattern of female hair distribution is an

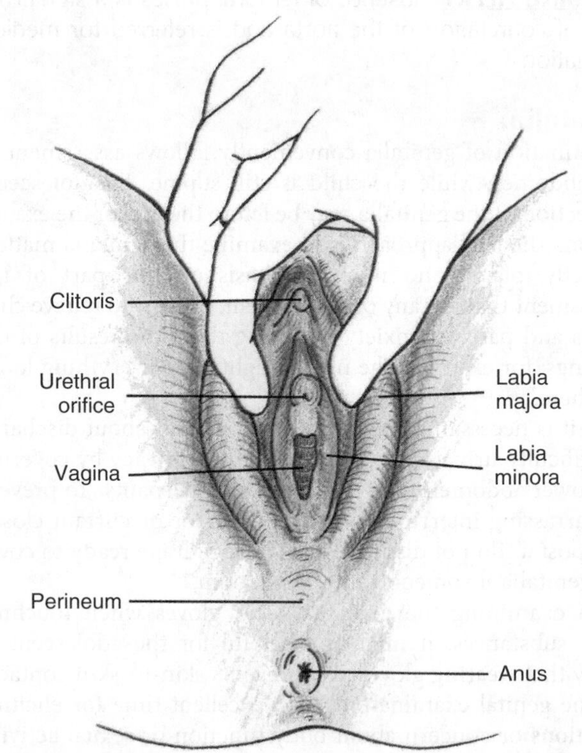

Fig. 34-39 External structures of genitalia in postpubertal female. Labia are spread to reveal deeper structures. (From Potter PA, Perry AG: *Basic nursing: essentials for practice*, ed 6, St Louis, 2006, Mosby.)

inverted triangle. The appearance of soft, downy hair along the labia majora is an early sign of sexual maturation. Note the size and location of the clitoris, a small, erectile organ located at the anterior end of the labia minora. It is covered by a small flap of skin, the prepuce.

The labia majora are two thick folds of skin running posteriorly from the mons to the posterior commissure of the vagina. Internal to the labia majora are two folds of skin called the labia minora. Although the labia minora are usually prominent in the newborn, they gradually atrophy, which makes them almost invisible until their enlargement during puberty. The inner surface of the labia should be pink and moist. Note the size of the labia and any evidence of fusion, which may suggest male scrota. Normally no masses are palpable within the labia.

The urethral meatus is located posterior to the clitoris and is surrounded by Skene's glands and ducts. Although not a prominent structure, the meatus appears as a small V-shaped slit. Note its location, especially if it opens from the clitoris or inside the vagina. Gently palpate the glands, which are common sites of cysts and sexually transmitted lesions.

The vaginal orifice is located posterior to the urethral meatus. Its appearance varies depending on individual anatomy and sexual activity. Ordinarily, examination of the vagina is limited to inspection. In virgins a thin crescent-shaped or circular membrane, called the hymen, may cover part of the vaginal opening. In some instances it completely occludes the orifice. After rupture, small rounded pieces of tissue called caruncles remain. Although an imperforate hymen denotes lack of penile intercourse, a perforate one does not necessarily indicate sexual activity.

NURSING ALERT In girls who have been circumcised, the genitalia will appear different. Do not show surprise or disgust, but note the appearance and discuss the procedure with the young woman.

Surrounding the vaginal opening are Bartholin's glands, which secrete a clear, mucoid fluid into the vagina for lubrication during intercourse. Palpate the ducts for cysts. Also note the discharge from the vagina, which is usually clear or white.

Anus

After examination of the genitalia, the anal area is easily examined, although the child should be placed on the abdomen. Note the general firmness of the buttocks and symmetry of the gluteal folds. Assess the tone of the anal sphincter by eliciting the anal reflex. Gently scratching the anal area results in an obvious quick contraction of the external anal sphincter.

Back and Extremities

Spine

The general curvature of the spine is noted. Normally the back of a newborn is rounded or C shaped from the thoracic and pelvic curves. The development of the cervical and lumbar curves approximates development of various motor skills, such as cervical curvature with head control, and gives the older child the typical double S curve.

Marked curvatures in posture are abnormal. Scoliosis, lateral curvature of the spine, is an important childhood problem, especially in girls. Although scoliosis may be identified by observing and palpating the spine and noting a sideways displacement, more objective tests include:

- With the child standing erect, clothed only in underpants (and bra if older girl), observe from behind, noting asymmetry of the shoulders and hips.
- With the child bending forward so that the back is parallel to the floor, observe from the side, noting asymmetry or prominence of the rib cage.

A slight limp, a crooked hemline, or complaints of a sore back are other signs and symptoms of scoliosis.

Inspect the back, especially along the spine, for any tufts of hair, dimples, or discoloration. Mobility of the vertebral column is easily assessed in most children because of their propensity for constant motion during the examination. However, mobility can be tested by asking the child to sit up from a prone position or to do a modified sit-up exercise.

Movement of the cervical spine is an important diagnostic sign of neurologic problems, such as meningitis. Normally movement of the head in all directions is effortless.

NURSING ALERT Hyperextension of the neck and spine, or opisthotonos, which is accompanied by pain when the head is flexed, is always referred for immediate medical evaluation.

Extremities

Inspect each extremity for symmetry of length and size; refer any deviation for orthopedic evaluation. Count the fingers and toes to be certain of the normal number. This is so often taken for granted that an extra digit (polydactyly) or fusion of digits (syndactyly) may go unnoticed.

Inspect the arms and legs for temperature and color, which should be equal in each extremity, although the feet may normally be colder than the hands.

Assess the shape of bones. Several variations of bone shape may be observed in children. Although many of them cause parents concern, most are benign and require no treatment. Bowleg, or genu varum, is lateral bowing of the tibia. It is clinically present when the child stands with the medial malleoli (rounded prominence on either side of the ankle) opposite each other and the space between the knees is greater than approximately 5 cm (2 inches) (Fig. 34-40). Toddlers are usually bowlegged after beginning to walk until all their lower back and leg muscles are well developed. Unilateral or asymmetric bowlegs that are present beyond the age of 2 to 3 years, particularly in African-American children, may represent pathologic conditions requiring further investigation.

Knock-knee, or genu valgum, appears as the opposite of bowleg, in that the knees are close together but the feet are spread apart. It is determined clinically by using the same method as for genu varum but by measuring the distance between the malleoli, which normally should be less than 7.5 cm (3 inches) (Fig. 34-41). Knock-knee is normally present in children from about 2 to 7 years of age. Knock-knee that is excessive, asymmetric, accompanied by short stature, or evident in a child nearing puberty requires further evaluation.

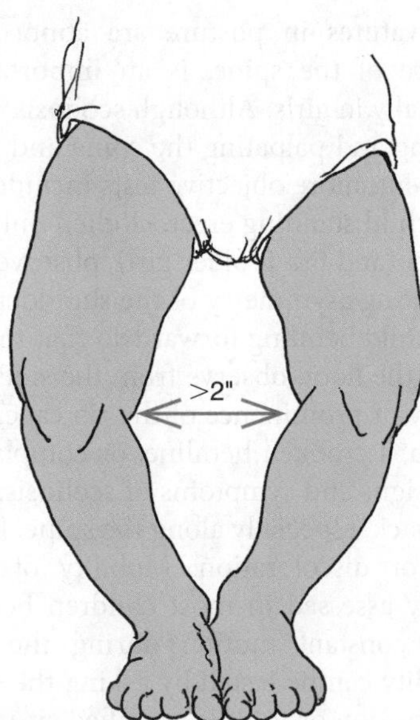

Fig. 34-40 Bowleg.

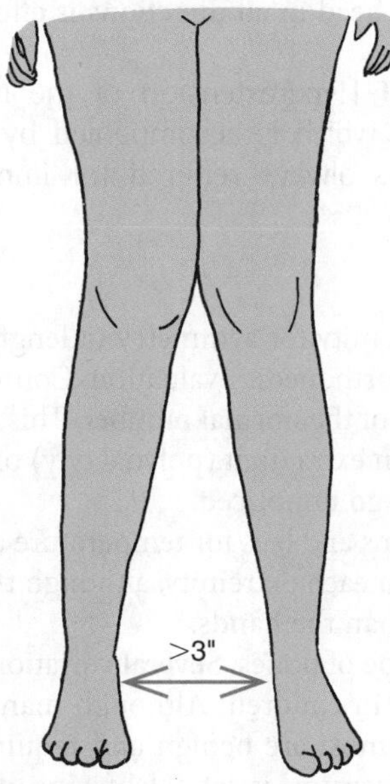

Fig. 34-41 Knock-knee.

Next inspect the feet. Infants' and toddlers' feet appear flat because the foot is normally wide and the arch is covered by a fat pad. Development of the arch occurs naturally from the action of walking. Normally, at birth the feet are held in a valgus (outward) or varus (inward) position. To determine whether a foot deformity at birth is a result of intrauterine position or development, scratch the outer, then inner, side of the sole. If the foot position is self-correctable, it will assume a right angle to the leg. As the child begins to walk, the feet turn outward less than 30 degrees and inward less than 10 degrees.

Toddlers have a "toddling" or broad-based gait, which facilitates walking by lowering the center of gravity. As the child reaches preschool age, the legs are brought closer together. By school age the walking posture is much more graceful and balanced.

The most common gait problem in young children is pigeon toe, or toeing in, which usually results from torsional deformities, such as internal tibial torsion (abnormal rotation or bowing of the tibia). Tests for tibial torsion include measuring the thigh-foot angle, which requires considerable practice for accuracy.

Elicit the plantar or grasp reflex by exerting firm but gentle pressure with the tip of the thumb against the lateral sole of the foot from the heel upward to the little toe and then across to the big toe. The normal response in children who are walking is flexion of the toes. Babinski sign, dorsiflexion of the big toe and fanning of the other toes, is normal during infancy but abnormal after about 1 year of age or when locomotion begins (see Fig. 36-6).

Joints

Evaluate the joints for range of motion. Normally this requires no specific testing if the nurse has observed the child's movements during the examination. However, the hips should be routinely investigated in infants for congenital dislocation. Report any evidence of joint immobility or hyperflexibility.

Palpate the joints for heat, tenderness, and swelling. These signs, as well as redness over the joint, warrant further investigation.

Muscles

Note symmetry and quality of muscle development, tone, and strength. Observe development by looking at the shape and contour of the body in both a relaxed and a tensed state. Estimate tone by grasping the muscle and feeling its firmness when it is relaxed and contracted. A common site for testing tone is the biceps muscle of the arm. Children are usually willing to "make a muscle" by clenching their fist.

Estimate strength by having the child use an extremity to push or pull against resistance, as in the following examples:

Arm strength—Child holds the arms outstretched in front of the body and tries to raise the arms while downward pressure is applied.

Hand strength—Child shakes hands with nurse and squeezes one or two fingers of the nurse's hand.

Leg strength—Child sits on a table or chair with the legs dangling and tries to raise the legs while downward pressure is applied.

Note symmetry of strength in the extremities, hands, and fingers, and report evidence of paresis, or weakness.

Neurologic Assessment

The assessment of the nervous system is the broadest and most diverse part of the examination process, since every human function, both physical and emotional, is controlled by neurologic impulses. Much of the neurologic examination has already been discussed, such as assessment of behavior, sensory testing, and motor function. The following focuses on a general appraisal of cerebellar function, deep tendon reflexes, and the cranial nerves.

Cerebellar Function

The cerebellum controls balance and coordination. Much of the assessment of cerebellar function is included in observing

BOX 34-16 Tests for Cerebellar Function

Finger-to-nose test—With child's arm extended, ask child to touch the nose with the index finger with eyes open and then closed.

Heel-to-shin test—Have child stand and run the heel of one foot down the shin or anterior aspect of the tibia of the other leg, both with eyes opened and then closed.

Romberg test—Have child stand with eyes closed and heels together; falling or leaning to one side is abnormal and is called *Romberg sign.*

the child's posture, body movements, gait, and development of fine and gross motor skills. Tests such as balancing on one foot and the heel-to-toe walk assess balance. Test coordination by asking the child to reach for a toy, button clothes, tie shoes, or draw a straight line on a piece of paper (provided the child is old enough to do these activities). Coordination can also be tested by any sequence of rapid, successive movements, such as quickly touching each finger with the thumb of the same hand.

Several tests for cerebellar function can be performed as games (Box 34-16). When a Romberg test is done, stay beside the child if there is a possibility that the child may fall. School-age children should be able to perform these tests, although in the finger-to-nose test preschoolers normally can only bring the finger within 5 to 7.5 cm (2 to 3 inches) of the nose. Difficulty in performing these exercises indicates poor sense of position (especially with the eyes closed) and incoordination (especially with the eyes opened).

Reflexes

Testing reflexes is an important part of the neurologic examination. Persistence of primitive reflexes, loss of reflexes, or hyperactivity of deep tendon reflexes is usually a result of a cerebral insult.

Elicit reflexes by using the rubber head of the reflex hammer, flat of the finger, or side of the hand. If the child is easily frightened by equipment, use your hand or finger. Although testing reflexes is a simple procedure, the child may inhibit the reflex by unconsciously tensing the muscle. To avoid tensing, distract younger children with toys or talk to them. Older children can concentrate on the exercise of grasping their two hands in front of them and trying to pull them apart. This diverts their attention from the testing and causes involuntary relaxation of the muscles.

Deep tendon reflexes are stretch reflexes of a muscle. The most common deep tendon reflex is the knee jerk, or patellar reflex (sometimes called the quadriceps reflex). The reflexes normally elicited are described in Figs. 34-42 to 34-45. Report any diminished or hyperreflexive response for further evaluation.

Cranial Nerves

Assessment of the cranial nerves is an important area of neurologic assessment (Table 34-13). With young children, present the tests as games to foster trust and security at the beginning of the examination. Or include the cranial nerve test when each system is examined, such as tongue movement and strength, gag reflex, swallowing, cardinal positions of gaze (Fig. 34-46), and position of the uvula during examination of the mouth.

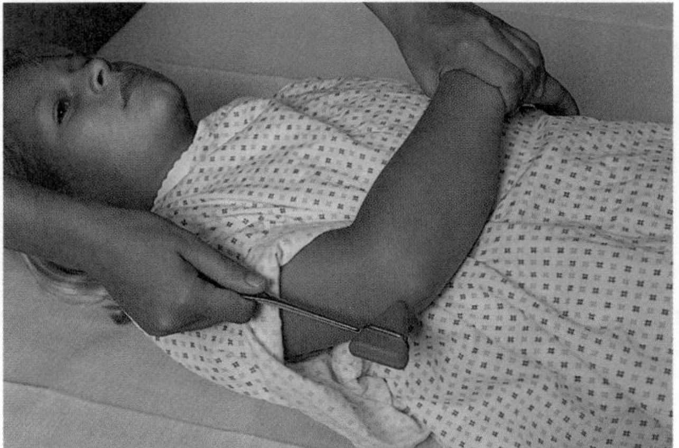

Fig. 34-42 Testing for triceps reflex. Child is placed supine, with forearm resting over chest, and triceps tendon is struck. Alternate procedure: child's arm is abducted, with upper arm supported and forearm allowed to hang freely. Triceps tendon is struck. Normal response is partial extension of forearm.

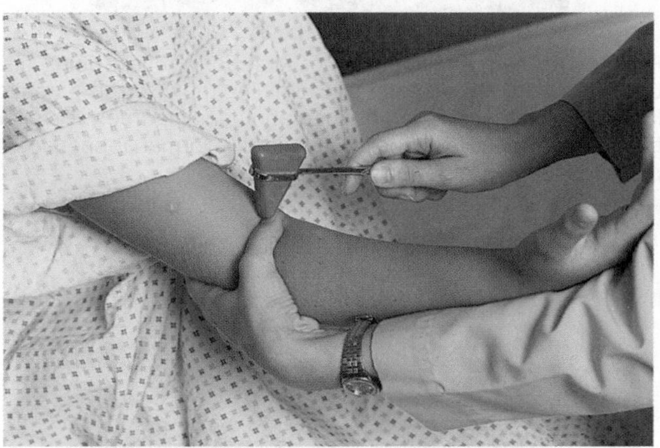

Fig. 34-43 Testing for biceps reflex. Child's arm is held by placing partially flexed elbow in examiner's hand with thumb over antecubital space. Examiner's thumbnail is struck with hammer. Normal response is partial flexion of forearm.

Developmental Assessment

One of the most essential components of a complete health appraisal is assessment of developmental function. Screening procedures are designed to identify quickly and reliably those children whose developmental level is below normal for their age and who therefore require further investigation. They also provide a means of recording objective measurements of present developmental function for future reference. Since the passage of Public Law 99-457, the Education of the Handicapped Act Amendments of 1986, much greater emphasis is placed on developmental assessment of children with disabili-

evolve Animation—Cranial Nerves

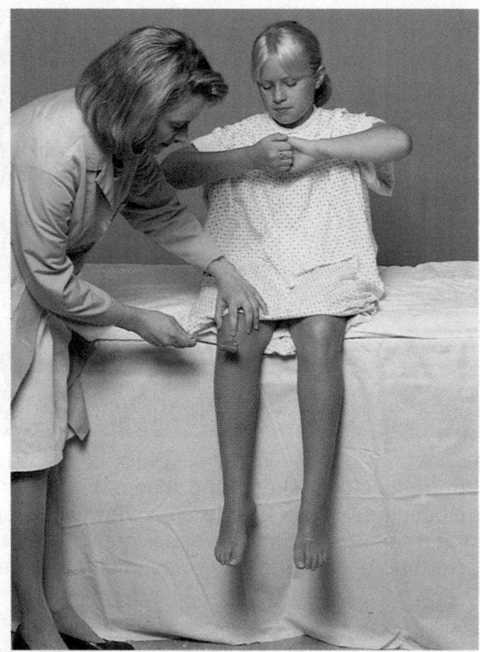

Fig. 34-44 Testing for patellar, or knee jerk, reflex, using distraction. Child sits on edge of examining table (or on parent's lap) with lower legs flexed at knee and dangling freely. Patellar tendon is tapped just below kneecap. Normal response is partial extension of lower leg.

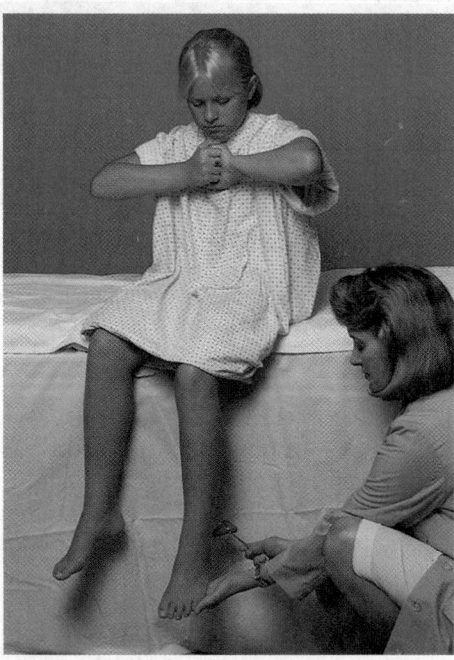

Fig. 34-45 Testing for Achilles reflex. Child should be in same position as for knee jerk reflex. Foot is supported lightly in examiner's hand, and Achilles tendon is struck. Normal response is plantar flexion of foot (foot pointing downward).

ties, and nurses can play a vital role in providing this service. All the procedures discussed in this section can be administered in a variety of settings: home, school, day care center, hospital, practitioner's office, or clinic.

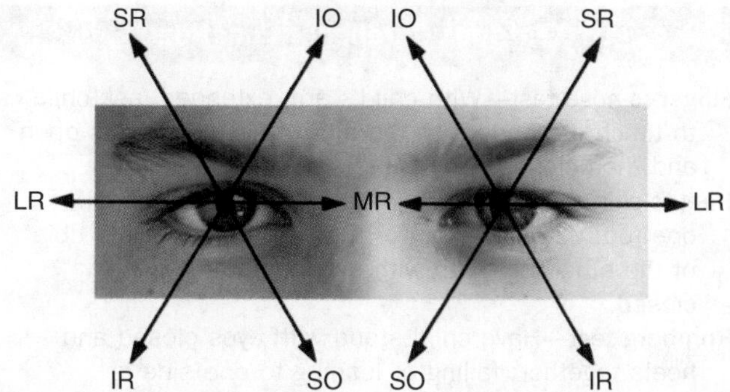

Fig. 34-46 Testing cardinal positions of gaze. Muscles responsible for movement: *SR,* Superior rectus; *IR,* inferior rectus; *MR,* medial rectus; *IO,* inferior oblique; *SO,* superior oblique; *LR,* lateral rectus.

Denver II

The most widely used developmental screening tests for young children are the series of tests developed by Dr. William Frankenburg and his colleagues in Denver. The oldest and best known, the Denver Developmental Screening Test (DDST), and its revision, the DDST-R, have been revised, restandardized, and renamed the Denver II. Before administering the Denver II, the examiner should be trained by, and receive certification from, a master instructor who has been trained by the Denver faculty.* The Denver II differs from the DDST in items, test form, interpretation, and referral (see Appendix B). The previous total of 105 items has been increased to 125, including an increase from 21 DDST to 39 Denver II language items. Previous items that were difficult to administer or interpret have been either modified or eliminated. Many items that were previously tested by parental report now require observation by the examiner.

Each item was evaluated to determine whether significant differences exist on the basis of sex, ethnic group, maternal education, and place of residence. Items for which clinically significant differences exist were replaced or, if retained, are discussed in the technical manual. When evaluating children delayed on one of these items, the examiner can look up norms for the subpopulations to consider whether the delay may be caused by sociocultural or environmental differences.

The items on the test form are arranged in the same format as the DDST-R. The norms for the distribution bars were updated with the new standardization data but retain the 25th, 50th, 75th, and 90th percentile divisions. The test form contains a place to rate the child's behavioral characteristics (compliance, interest in surroundings, fearfulness, and attention span).

To determine relative areas of advancement and delay, enough items should be administered to establish the basal and ceiling levels in each sector. By scoring appropriate items

**Forms and complete instructions are available from Denver Developmental Materials, PO Box 371075, Denver, CO 80237-5075; 303-355-4729 or 800-419-4729;* www.denverii.com. *The DDST and DDST-R are no longer available.*

Table 34-13 Assessment of Cranial Nerves

DESCRIPTION AND FUNCTION	TESTS
I—Olfactory Nerve	
Olfactory mucosa of nasal cavity Smell	With eyes closed, have child identify odors such as coffee, alcohol from a swab, or other smells; test each nostril separately.
II—Optic Nerve	
Rods and cones of retina, optic nerve Vision	Check for perception of light, visual acuity, peripheral vision, color vision, and normal optic disc.
III—Oculomotor Nerve	
Extraocular muscles of eye: Superior rectus (SR)–moves eyeball up and in Inferior rectus (IR)–moves eyeball down and in Medial rectus (MR)–moves eyeball nasally Inferior oblique (IO)–moves eyeball up and out	Have child follow an object (toy) or light in six cardinal positions of gaze (see Fig. 34-46).
Pupil constriction and accommodation	Perform *PERRLA* (*P*upils *E*qual, *R*ound, *R*eact to *L*ight, and *A*ccommodation).
Eyelid closing	Check for proper placement of lid.
IV—Trochlear Nerve	
Superior oblique muscle (SO)–moves eye down and out	Have child look down and in (see Fig. 34-46).
V—Trigeminal Nerve	
Muscles of mastication	Have child bite down hard and open jaw; test symmetry and strength.
Sensory–face, scalp, nasal and buccal mucosa	With child's eyes closed, see if child can detect light touch in mandibular and maxillary regions. Test corneal and blink reflex by touching cornea lightly (approach from side so that child does not blink before cornea is touched).
VI—Abducens Nerve	
Lateral rectus (LR) muscle–moves eye temporally	Have child look toward temporal side (see Fig. 34-46)
VII—Facial Nerve	
Muscles for facial expression	Have child smile, make funny face, or show teeth to see symmetry of expression.
Anterior two thirds of tongue (sensory)	Have child identify sweet or salty solution; place each taste on anterior section and sides of protruding tongue; if child retracts tongue, solution will dissolve toward posterior part of tongue.
VIII—Auditory, Acoustic, or Vestibulocochlear Nerve	
Internal ear Hearing and balance	Test hearing; note any loss of equilibrium or presence of vertigo.
IX—Glossopharyngeal Nerve	
Pharynx, tongue	Stimulate posterior pharynx with a tongue blade; child should gag.
Posterior third of tongue Sensory	Test sense of sour or bitter taste on posterior segment of tongue.
X—Vagus Nerve	
Muscles of larynx, pharynx, some organs of gastrointestinal system, sensory fibers of root of tongue, heart, and lung	Note hoarseness of voice, gag reflex, and ability to swallow. Check that uvula is in midline; when stimulated with tongue blade, it should deviate upward and to stimulated side.
XI—Accessory Nerve	
Sternocleidomastoid and trapezius muscles of shoulder	Have child shrug shoulders while applying mild pressure; with examiner's hands placed on shoulders, have child turn head against opposing pressure on either side; note symmetry and strength.
XII—Hypoglossal Nerve	
Muscles of tongue	Have child move tongue in all directions; have child protrude tongue as far as possible; note any midline deviation. Test strength by placing tongue blade on one side of tongue and having child move it away.

as "pass," "fail," "refusal," or "no opportunity," and relating such scores to the child's age, the examiner can interpret each item as described in Box 34-17. To identify "cautions," all items intersected by the age line are administered. To screen solely for developmental delays, only the items located totally to the *left* of the child's age line are administered. Criteria for referral are based on the availability of resources in the community.

Research on the Denver II's validity and accuracy is limited. One study found that it identified most children with even subtle developmental problems. However, almost half the

BOX 34-17 Denver II Scoring

Interpretation of Denver II Scores

Advanced—Passed an item completely to the right of the age line (passed by less than 25% of children at an age older than the child)

OK—Passed, failed, or refused an item intersected by the age line between the 25th and 75th percentiles

Caution—Failed or refused items intersected by the age line on or between the 75th and 90th percentiles

Delay—Failed an item completely to the left of the age line; refusals to the left of the age line may also be considered delays, since the reason for the refusal may be inability to perform the task

Interpretation of Test

Normal—No delays and a maximum of one caution

Suspect—One or more delays or two or more cautions

Untestable—Refusals on one or more items completely to the left of the age line or on more than one item intersected by the age line in the 75th to 90th percentile area

Recommendations for Referral for Suspect and Untestable Tests

Rescreen in 1 to 2 weeks to rule out temporary factors.

If rescreen is suspect or untestable, use clinical judgment based on the following: number of cautions and delays; which items are cautions and delays; rate of past development; clinical examination and history; availability of referral resources.

children without developmental problems received suspect scores, resulting in a high rate of overreferrals (Glascoe et al, 1992). To minimize overreferrals, a decision for referral depends not only on the results of the Denver II, but also on the practitioner's clinical judgment after considering the child's developmental history; general health status; and social, cultural, and emotional environment and the availability of local resources for diagnosis and treatment (Frankenburg, 1994a, 1994b).

Although it is not the purpose of this discussion to detail the instruction manual, some points concerning preparation, administration, and interpretation of the Denver II are important to stress. Before beginning the screening, ask whether the child was born prematurely and correctly calculate the adjusted age. Up to 24 months of age, allowances are made for infants born prematurely by subtracting the number of weeks of missed gestation from their present age and testing them at the adjusted age. For example, a 16-week-old infant who was born 4 weeks early is tested at a 12-week adjusted age level.

Explain to the parents and child, if appropriate, that the screenings are *not* intelligence tests but rather are a method of showing what the child can do at a particular age. Emphasize that the child is *not* expected to perform each item on the test. Tell the parent before the screening begins that the results of the child's performance will be explained after all the items have been concluded. It is the nurse's responsibility to properly inform parents of any testing or screening procedure before its administration so that they are fully aware of its purpose and intent.

Prepare toddlers and preschoolers for the procedure by presenting it as a game. Frequently, the Denver II is an excellent way to begin a health appraisal because it is nonthreatening, requires no painful or unfamiliar procedures, and capitalizes on the child's natural activity of play. Because children are easily distracted, perform each item quickly and present only one toy from the kit at a time. After that toy's purpose is concluded, such as building a tower of blocks or identifying its color, replace the toy in the bag and take out another one. Other temporary factors that may interfere with the child's performance include fatigue, illness, fear, hospitalization, separation from the parent, or general unwillingness to perform the activities. In addition, undiagnosed cognitive impairment, hearing loss, vision loss, neurologic impairment, or a familial pattern of slow development greatly influences the child's performance.

After completion of the Denver II, ask the parent whether the child's performance was typical of behavior at other times. If the parent replies affirmatively and the child's cooperation was satisfactory, explain the results, emphasizing all successful items first, then those items the child failed but was not expected to pass, and finally those items that represent delays. If the parent replies that the child's performance was not typical of usual behavior, it is best to defer any scoring or discussion of results, especially if the refusals yield a suspect score. In this situation reschedule testing for a time when the child is more likely to cooperate.

In explaining a normal score, focus on how well the child performed and reinforce the parents' efforts in satisfactorily stimulating their child. In addition to assessing the child's present developmental level, the Denver II can be used to guide parents toward those activities that are appropriate, although not necessarily expected, for the child's age. By testing for items to the right of the age line (ones the child is not expected to perform), the examiner can identify children with advanced development, who may be gifted.

In explaining delays, carefully note the parent's response, especially casual acceptance such as "He'll catch up" or questions such as "Does this mean my child is retarded?" Be aware of personal anxieties during these situations and refrain from giving glib reassurances such as "I'm sure he will do better next time." Rather, respond honestly to parents' questions, yet with appropriate flexibility and concern, stressing the need for further developmental testing.

Denver II Prescreening Developmental Questionnaire

The Prescreening Developmental Questionnaire (PDQ II) is a further revision of the PDQ and the R-PDQ. This version uses the norms (90th and 75th percentiles) from the Denver II. The PDQ II is a parent-answered prescreen consisting of 91 questions from the Denver II, although only a subset of questions is asked for each age group. The form may need to be read to parents and caregivers who are less educated.

Four different forms are available and are selected based on age: orange (0 to 9 months), purple (9 to 24 months), cream

(2 to 4 years), and white (4 to 6 years). The caregiver answers questions until (1) three "no's" are circled (they do not have to be consecutive) or (2) all the questions on both sides of the form have been answered. Scoring is based on the number of delays or cautions (see Box 34-17). Children who have no delays or cautions are considered to be developing normally. If a child has one delay or two cautions, the caregiver is provided with age-appropriate developmental activities to pursue with the child, and a rescreen with the PDQ II is done 1 month later. If on rescreening the child has one or more delays, the Denver II is administered as soon as possible. If a child has two or more delays or three or more cautions on the first screening with the PDQ II, the Denver II is administered as soon as possible.

Key Points

- To effectively establish a setting for communication, nurses must make an appropriate introduction and ensure privacy and confidentiality.
- When communicating with parents, nurses need to encourage parental involvement, listen carefully, use silence, and be empathic.
- Communication with children must reflect their developmental stage.
- Nonverbal communication with children may take the form of writing, drawing, and play.
- The objectives of performing a health history are to identify pertinent information, determine the chief complaint, analyze the present illness, secure the patient's health history, review biologic systems, and record a family medical history and child psychosocial and sexual history.
- Family assessment is the collection of data about family composition and relationships among its members; it also focuses on home and community environment, parents' occupation and education, and cultural and religious traditions.
- Nutritional assessment is performed by determination of dietary intake, clinical examination, and biochemical analysis.
- Growth measurements during the physical examination focus on length or height, weight, skin fold thickness, and arm and head circumference. Assessment of growth is measured against standard growth charts to determine a child's status in comparison with that of other children the same age.
- Measurements of temperature, pulse, respiration, and BP constitute the physiologic approach to assessment.
- The general appearance of a child is a cumulative, subjective impression of physical appearance, state of nutrition, behavior, personality, interactions with parents and nurse, posture, development, and speech.

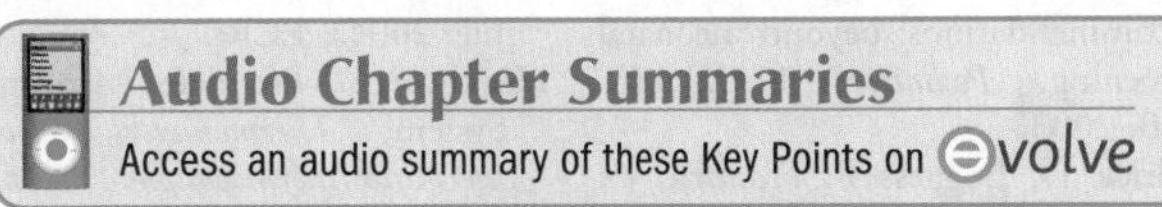
Audio Chapter Summaries
Access an audio summary of these Key Points on evolve

- Assessment of the skin, which primarily involves inspection and palpation, focuses on color, texture, temperature, moisture, and turgor. The nurse needs to be aware of both physiologic and ethnic factors that may affect these areas.
- In assessment of the lymph nodes, the nurse examines, by palpation, the part of the body in which the glands are located.
- The head is inspected for shape, symmetry, mobility, and muscle control.
- Examination of the eyes includes placement and alignment, inspection of external and internal structures, and vision testing.
- The ear examination encompasses placement and alignment, external and internal structures, and auditory testing.
- The lungs are examined by inspection, palpation, percussion, and auscultation.
- Auscultation is the most important procedure for examining the heart.
- Abdominal assessment follows an orderly sequence of inspection, auscultation, and palpation, since palpation may distort normal abdominal sounds.
- Examination of the genitalia may provoke anxiety in the child, and the nurse must avoid any transference of anxiety.
- Neurologic assessment addresses behavior; motor, sensory, and cerebellar function; reflexes; and cranial nerves.
- The Denver II, a major revision and a restandardization of the DDST, differs from the DDST in items included in the test, the test form, and the interpretation of scoring.

References

American Academy of Pediatrics: *Pediatric nutrition handbook*, ed 5, Elk Grove Village, IL, 2004, The Academy.

American Academy of Pediatrics, Committee on Practice and Ambulatory Medicine, Section on Ophthalmology: Eye examination in infants, children, and young adults by pediatricians, *Pediatrics* 111(4):902-907, 2003.

American Academy of Pediatrics, Committee on Practice and Ambulatory Medicine, Section on Otolaryngology and Bronchoesophagology: Hearing assessment in infants and children: recommendations beyond neonatal screening, *Pediatrics* 111(2): 436-440, 2003.

Bald M: Ambulatory blood pressure monitoring in children and adolescents, *Minerva Pediatr* 54(1):13-24, 2002.

Beevers G, Lip GYH, O'Brien E: ABC of hypertension blood pressure measurement, part I, Sphygmomanometry: factors common to all techniques, *BMJ* 322(7292):981-985, 2001.

Berry BE et al: Preschool vision screening using the MTI-Photoscreener, *Pediatr Nurs* 27(1):27-34, 2001.

Clark JA et al: Discrepancies between direct and indirect blood pressure measurements using various recommendations for arm cuff selection, *Pediatrics* 110(5):920-923, 2002.

Coats DK, Jenkins RH: Vision assessment of the pediatric patient: refinements, *Am Acad Ophthalmol* 1(1):1-12, 1997.

Craig JV et al: Temperature measured at the axilla compared with rectum in children and young people: systematic review, *BMJ* 320(7243):1174-1178, 2000.

Cunningham M, Cox EO: Hearing assessment in infants and children: recommendations beyond neonatal screening, *Pediatrics* 111(2):436-440, 2003.

Deadrick D, Boggess P: *Pediatrics on telephone line*, paper presented at the First Annual National Conference for Advanced Practice Nurses, New Brunswick, NJ, November 6-8, 1996, Rutgers University.

Desselle DD, Pearlmutter L: Navigating two cultures: deaf children, self-esteem, and parents' communication patterns, *Soc Work Educ* 19(1):23-30, 1997.

Frankenburg WK: Preventing developmental delays: is developmental screening sufficient? part I, Developmental screening and the Denver II, *Pediatrics* 93(4):586-589, 1994a.

Frankenburg WK: Preventing developmental delays: is developmental screening sufficient? part II, Partners in health care, *Pediatrics* 93(4):589-593, 1994b.

Gillman MW, Cook NR: Blood pressure measurement in childhood epidemiological studies, *Circulation* 92(4):1049-1057, 1995.

Glascoe FP et al: Accuracy of the Denver-II in developmental screening, *Pediatrics* 89(6 Pt 2):1221-1225, 1992.

Goldman LR, Shannon MW: Technical report: mercury in the environment: implications for pediatricians, *Pediatrics* 108(1):197-205, 2001.

Halle C: Achieve new vision screening objectives, *Nurse Pract* 27(3):15-35, 2002.

Healthcare Product Comparison System: *Thermometers, electronic, infrared*, Plymouth Meeting, PA, July 2004a, ECRI.

Healthcare Product Comparison System: *Thermometers, electronic, thermistor/thermocouple, patient*, Plymouth Meeting, PA, July 2004b, ECRI.

Hedley AA et al: Prevalence of overweight and obesity among US children, adolescents, and adults, 1999-2002, *JAMA* 291(23):2847-2850, 2004.

Hoge DR, Parette HP: Facilitating communicative development in young children with disabilities, *Transdisc J* 5(2):113-130, 1995.

Kuczmarski RJ et al: CDC growth charts: United States, *Adv Data* 314:1-27, 2000.

Livingstone MBE, Robson PJ, Wallace MW: Issues in dietary intake assessment of children and adolescents, *Br J Nutr* 92(Suppl 2):S213-S222, 2004.

Martin SA, Kline AM: Can there be a standard for temperature measurement in the pediatric intensive care unit? *AACN Clin Issues* 15(2):254-266, 2004.

Mattu GS, Heran BS, Wright JM: Comparison of the automated non-invasive oscillometric blood pressure monitor (BpTRU™) with the auscultatory mercury sphygmomanometer in a paediatric population, *Blood Pressure Monit* 9(1):39-45, 2004a.

Mattu GS, Heran BS, Wright JM: Overall accuracy of the BpTRU™—an automated electronic blood pressure device, *Blood Press Monit* 9(1):47-52, 2004b.

Murphy SP, Poos MI: Dietary reference intakes: summary of applications in dietary assessment, *Public Health Nutr* 5(6A):843-849, 2002.

National High Blood Pressure Education Program Working Group on High Blood Pressure in Children and Adolescents: The fourth report on the diagnosis, evaluation, and treatment of high blood pressure in children and adolescents, *Pediatrics* 114(2 Suppl 4th Rep):555-576, 2004.

National Institutes of Health, National Heart, Lung, and Blood Institute: *Update on the Task Force Report (1987) on high blood pressure in children and adolescents: a working group report from the National High Blood Pressure Education Program*, NIH Pub No 96-3790, Bethesda, MD, September 1996, The Institutes.

Nicklas TA et al: Children's food consumption patterns have changed over 2 decades (1973-1994): the Bogalusa heart study, *J Am Diet Assoc* 104(7):1127-1140, 2004.

Park M, Lee D, Johnson GA: Oscillometric blood pressures in the arm, thigh, and calf in healthy children and those with aortic coarctation, *Pediatrics* 91(4):761-765, 1993.

Park MK, Menard SW, Yuan C: Comparison of auscultatory and oscillometric blood pressures, *Arch Pediatr Adolesc Med* 155(1):50-53, 2001.

Price V, Archbold J: What's it all about, empathy? *Nurs Educ Today* 17(2):106-110, 1997.

Reynolds WH, Scott B, Jessiman WC: Empathy has not been measured in clients' terms or effectively taught: a review of the literature, *J Adv Nurs* 30(5):1177-1185, 1999.

Roche AF, Guo S: The new growth charts, *Pediatr Basics* 94:2-13, 2001.

Rutenberg CD: Telephone triage, *Am J Nurs* 100(3):77-78, 80-81, 2000.

Seidel HM et al: *Mosby's guide to physical examination*, ed 6, St Louis, 2006, Mosby.

Sullivan GH: Protecting patient's privacy, *RN* 60(6):55-56, 58-59, 1997.

Turnbull R: Skin assessment in children: a methodical approach, *Nurs Times* 96(41):33-34, 2000.

Vessey JA: Developmental approaches to examining young children, *Pediatr Nurs* 21(1):53-56, 1995.

Wall TC et al: Compliance with vision-screening guidelines among a national sample of pediatricians, *Ambul Pediatr* 2(6):449-455, 2002.

White SJ: Empathy: a literature review and concept analysis, *J Clin Nurs* 6(4):253-257, 1997.

Yegdich T: On the phenomenology of empathy in nursing: empathy or sympathy? *J Adv Nurs* 30(1):83-93, 1999.

Unit 8

35 Pain Assessment and Management

Learning Objectives

On completion of this chapter the reader will be able to:

- Identify measures to assess pain in children.
- List various types of pain assessment tools for use with children.
- Outline essential pain management strategies to reduce pain in children.
- Review common types of pain experienced by children.
- Discuss evidence to support specific pain management strategies.

Electronic Resources

Additional information related to the content in Chapter 35 can be found on

evolve the Companion Website at

http://evolve.elsevier.com/Perry/maternal/

- NCLEX Review Questions
- Nursing Care Plan—The Child in Pain
- Skill—Calculating Safe Dosages for Children
- Skill—Managing Pain

Pain Assessment

Although the ability to measure pain in children has improved dramatically in recent years, assessment of pain in children continues to be complex and challenging. Children's ability to describe pain changes as they grow older and as they cognitively and linguistically mature (Box 35-1). Three types of measures—behavioral, physiologic, and self-report—have been developed to measure children's pain, and their applicability depends on the child's cognitive and linguistic ability.

Behavioral Measures

Distress behaviors, such as vocalization, facial expression, and body movement, have been associated with pain (Figs. 35-1 and 35-2). These behaviors are helpful in evaluating pain in infants and children with limited communication skills. However, discriminating between pain behaviors and reactions from other sources of distress, such as hunger, anxiety, or other types of discomfort, is not always easy. These factors decrease the specificity and sensitivity of behavioral measures (Table 35-1).

Behavioral assessment is useful for measuring pain in infants and preverbal children who do not have the language skills to communicate that they are in pain, or in children with mental clouding and confusion that limit their ability to communicate meaningfully (McGrath, 1998). Behavior provides important information that cannot be obtained from self-report. Behavioral assessment may provide a more complete picture of the total pain experience when administered in conjunction with a subjective self-report measure. However, behavioral pain scales may be more time-consuming than self-reports. These measures depend on a trained observer to watch and record children's behaviors such as vocalization, facial expression, and body movements that suggest discomfort.

Behavioral measures are most reliable when measuring short, sharp procedural pain, such as during injections or lumbar punctures. They are less reliable when measuring longer-lasting pain. In older children pain scores on behavioral measures do not always correlate with the children's own reports of pain intensity.

The four most commonly used behavioral pain measures are the FLACC, CHEOPS, TPPPS, and PPPRS. The *FLACC Pain Assessment Tool* is an interval scale that includes five categories of behavior: *F*acial expression, *L*eg movement, *A*ctivity, *C*ry, and *C*onsolability (Manworren & Hynan, 2003) (Table 35-2). It measures pain by quantifying pain behaviors with scores ranging from 0 (no pain behaviors) to 10 (most possible pain behaviors). The FLACC observational pain tool has been revised and validated to include behaviors specific to those with cognitive impairment (Malviya et al, 2006).

Physiologic Measures

Physiologic measures are not able to distinguish between physical responses to pain and other forms of stress to the body (Sweet & McGrath, 1998). Profound physiologic changes often accompany the experience of pain. Physiologic parameters such as heart rate, respiratory rate, blood pressure, palmar sweating, cortisone levels, transcutaneous oxygen, vagal tone, and endorphin concentrations reflect a generalized and complex response to stress. They are not localized response to pain, but they provide useful information about general distress levels of children experiencing pain. Like

BOX 35-1 Developmental Characteristics of Children's Responses to Pain

Young Infant

Generalized body response of rigidity or thrashing, possibly with local reflex withdrawal of stimulated area
Loud crying
Facial expression of pain (brows lowered and drawn together, eyes tightly closed, mouth open and squarish)
No association demonstrated between approaching stimulus and subsequent pain

Older Infant

Localized body response with deliberate withdrawal of stimulated area
Loud crying
Facial expression of pain or anger
Physical resistance, especially pushing the stimulus away after it is applied

Young Child

Loud crying, screaming
Verbal expressions such as "Ow," "Ouch," "It hurts"
Thrashing of arms and legs
Attempts to push stimulus away before it is applied
Lack of cooperation; need for physical restraint
Requests for termination of procedure
Clinging to parent, nurse, or other significant person
Requests for emotional support, such as hugs or other forms of physical comfort
Becoming restless and irritable with continuing pain
Behaviors occurring in anticipation of actual painful procedure

School-Age Child

May see all behaviors of young child, especially during actual painful procedure, but less in anticipatory period
Stalling behavior, such as "Wait a minute" or "I'm not ready"
Muscular rigidity, such as clenched fists, white knuckles, gritted teeth, contracted limbs, body stiffness, closed eyes, wrinkled forehead

Adolescent

Less vocal protest
Less motor activity
More verbal expressions, such as "It hurts" or "You're hurting me"
Increased muscle tension and body control

Data from Craig KD et al: Developmental changes in infant pain expression during immunization injections, *Soc Sci Med* 19(12):1331-1337, 1984; and Katz ER, Kellerman J, Siegel SE: Behavioral distress in children with cancer undergoing medical procedures: developmental considerations, *J Consult Clin Psychol* 48(3):356-365, 1980.

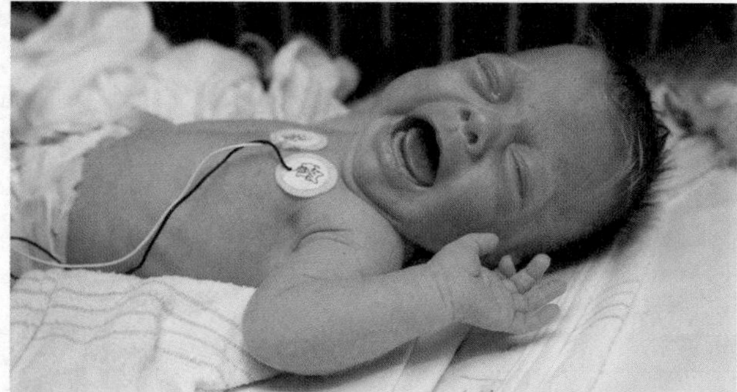

Fig. 35-1 Full, robust crying of preterm infant after heel stick. *(Courtesy Halbouty Premature Nursery, Texas Children's Hospital, Houston, TX; photo by Paul Vincent Kuntz.)*

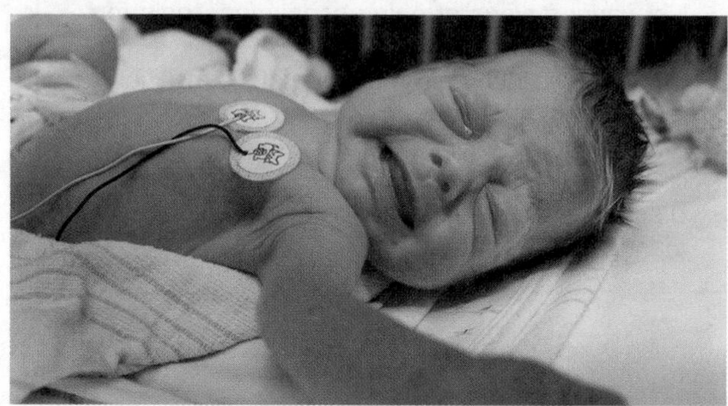

Fig. 35-2 The face of pain after heel stick. Note eye squeeze, brow bulge, nasolabial furrow, and widespread mouth. *(Courtesy Halbouty Premature Nursery, Texas Children's Hospital, Houston, TX; photo by Paul Vincent Kuntz.)*

behavioral scales, physiologic measures may be useful for infants and children who are not able to communicate verbally. The physiologic parameters provide indirect estimates of pain, and the presence and strength of pain can only be inferred from the changes in these parameters. Most of the studies on the physiologic parameters involved predominantly infants.

Self-Report Measures

Although children who are 4 or 5 years old are able to use self-report measures (Table 35-3), their ability to use them may be influenced by the cognitive characteristics of the preoperational stage (Stanford, Chambers, & Craig, 2006). The child's thinking tends to be egocentric, concrete, and perceptually dominated. Simple, concrete anchor words, such as "no hurt" to "biggest hurt," are more appropriate than "least pain sensation to worst intense pain imaginable."

The ability to discriminate degrees of pain in facial expressions appears to be reasonably established by 3 years of age (Stanford, Chambers, & Craig, 2006). *Faces pain scales* that were developed for young children may be a measure of pain intensity, pain affect, or both, particularly when the faces are anchored by a smiling face on one end and a face with tears on the other end (Chambers et al, 1999; Chambers et al, 2005). Although clinicians may think that the smiling face anchor confounds the emotion of "feeling happy" with being "pain free," there is no evidence to support this notion. Researchers looked at the effects of the smiling face (e.g., the Wong-Baker [WB] FACES Pain Scale) vs. those of the neutral anchor faces (e.g., Bieri Faces Pain Scale–Revised) on measurement of pain. Chambers and colleagues (2005) demonstrated a high correlation between the two forms of faces scales, with r = 0.91

Table 35-1 Selected Behavioral Pain Assessment Scales for Infants and Young Children

AGES OF USE	INSTRUMENT
4 mo-18 yr	Objective Pain Score (OPS) (Hannallah et al, 1987)
1-5 yr	Children's Hospital of Eastern Ontario Pain Scale (CHEOPS) (McGrath et al, 1985)
Newborn-16 yr	Nurses Assessment of Pain Inventory (NAPI) (Stevens, 1990)
3-36 mo	Behavioral Pain Score (BPS) (Robieux et al, 1991)
4-6 mo	Modified Behavioral Pain Scale (MBPS) (Taddio et al, 1995)
<36 mo and children with cerebral palsy	Riley Infant Pain Scale (RIPS) (Schade et al, 1996)
2 mo-7 yr	FLACC Postoperative Pain Tool (Merkel et al, 1997)
1-7 mo	Postoperative Pain Score (POPS) (Barrier et al, 1987)
Average gestational age 33.5 wk	Neonatal Infant Pain Scale (NIPS) (Lawrence et al, 1993)
27 wk gestational age to full term	Pain Assessment Tool (PAT) (Hodgkinson et al, 1994)
1-36 mo	Pain Rating Scale (PRS) (Joyce et al, 1994)
32-60 wk gestational age	CRIES (Krechel & Bildner, 1995)
28-40 wk gestational age	Premature Infant Pain Profile (PIPP) (Stevens et al, 1996)
0-28 days	Scale for Use in Newborns (SUN) (Blauer & Gerstmann, 1998)
Birth (23 wk gestational age) and full-term newborns up to 100 days	Neonatal Pain, Agitation, and Sedation Scale (NPASS) (Puchalski & Hummel, 2002)

Table 35-2 FLACC Scale

	0	1	2
Face	No particular expression or smile	Occasional grimace or frown, withdrawn, disinterested	Frequent to constant frown, clenched jaw, quivering chin
Legs	Normal position or relaxed	Uneasy, restless, tense	Kicking, or legs drawn up
Activity	Lying quietly, normal position, moves easily	Squirming, shifting back and forth, tense	Arched, rigid, or jerking
Cry	No cry (awake or asleep)	Moans or whimpers, occasional complaint	Crying steadily, screams or sobs, frequent complaints
Consolability	Content, relaxed	Reassured by occasional touching, hugging, or talking to; distractible	Difficult to console or comfort

From Merkel S et al: The FLACC: a behavioral scale for scoring postoperative pain in young children, *Pediatr Nurs* 23(3):293-297, 1997. Used with permission of Jannetti Publications, Inc., and the University of Michigan Health System. Can be reproduced for clinical and research use.

between the Bieri Faces (neutral anchor) and WB-FACES Pain Scale (smiling anchor). These data suggest that children are able to use either scale for communicating the amount of pain they experience.

Multidimensional Measures

Several cognitive skills, such as measurement, classification, and seriation (the ability to accurately place in ascending or descending order), become explicit between approximately 7 and 10 years of age. Older children are able to use the 0 to 10 numeric rating scale that is currently used by adolescents and adults. However, use of this scale is only an assessment of pain intensity, which may not change in some pain states (Jacob et al, 2003a). Other dimensions such as pain quality, pain location, and spatial distribution of pain may change without a change in pain intensity.

Two multidimensional assessment tools that have been well validated in children 8 years and older assess not only pain intensity, but also pain location and pain quality. Modeled after the McGill Pain Questionnaire (Melzack, 1975), the *Adolescent Pediatric Pain Tool (APPT)* is a multidimensional pain instrument for children and adolescents that is used to assess three dimensions of pain: location, intensity, and quality. The *Pediatric Pain Questionnaire (PPQ)* is a multidimensional pain instrument to assess patient and parental perceptions of the pain experience in a manner appropriate for the cognitive-developmental level of children and adolescents. The PPQ represents an attempt to assess the complexities of pediatric chronic, recurrent pain and targeted chronic musculoskeletal pain in children with juvenile rheumatoid arthritis. It consists of eight questions: (1) the pain history, (2) pain language, (3) the colors children associate with pain, (4) the emotions they experience, (5) their worst pain experiences, (6) the ways they cope with pain, (7) the positive aspects of pain, and (8) the location of their current pain.

Table 35-3 Pain Rating Scales for Children

PAIN SCALE, DESCRIPTION	RECOMMENDED AGE, COMMENTS
FACES Pain Rating Scale (Wong & Baker, 1988) Uses six cartoon faces ranging from smiling face for "no pain" to tearful face for "worst pain"	Children as young as 3 yr. Using original instructions without affect words, such as *happy* or *sad,* or brief words resulted in same range of pain rating, probably reflecting child's rating of pain intensity. For coding purposes, numbers 0, 2, 4, 6, 8, 10 can be substituted for 0-5 system to accommodate 0-10 system. Provides three scales in one: facial expressions, numbers, and words. Research supports cultural sensitivity of FACES for Caucasian, African-American, Hispanic, Thai, Chinese, and Japanese children.
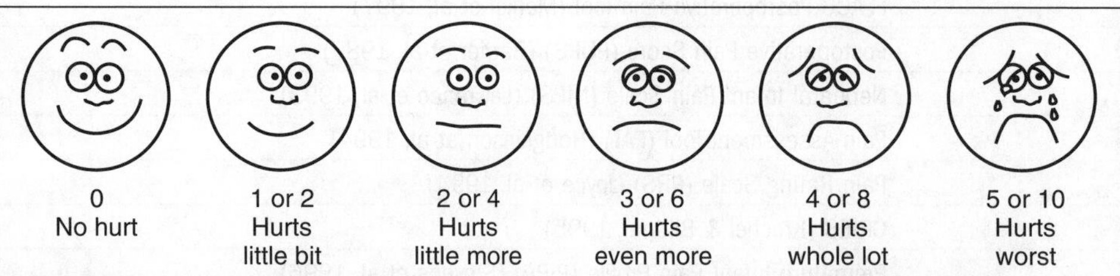 	
Oucher (Beyer, Denyes, & Villarruel, 1992) Uses six photographs of Caucasian child's face representing "no hurt" to "biggest hurt you could ever have"; also includes vertical scale with numbers from 0-100; scales for African-American and Hispanic children have been developed (Villarruel & Denyes, 1991)	Children 3-13 yr. Use numeric scale if child can count to 100 by ones and identify the larger of any two numbers, or by tens (Jordan-Marsh et al, 1994). Determine whether child has cognitive ability to use photographic scale; child should be able to rate six geometric shapes from largest to smallest. Determine which ethnic version of Oucher to use. Allow child to select version of Oucher, or use version that most closely matches child's physical characteristics. NOTE: Child may not prefer ethnically similar scale when given choice of ethnically neutral cartoon scale (Luffy & Grove, 2003).
Poker Chip Tool (Hester et al, 1998) Uses four red poker chips placed horizontally in front of child to denote varying intensities of pain	Children as young as 4 yr. Determine whether child has cognitive ability to use numbers by identifying larger of any two numbers.
Word-Graphic Rating Scale (Tesler et al, 1991) Uses descriptive words (may vary in other scales) to denote varying intensities of pain	Children 4-17 yr.
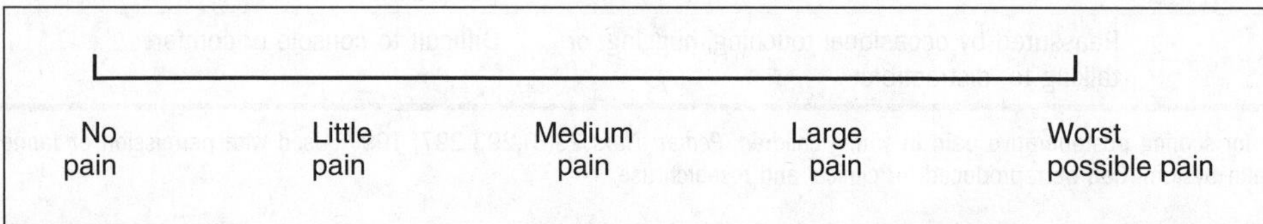 	
Numeric Scale Uses straight line with end points identified as "no pain" and "worst pain" and sometimes "medium pain" in the middle; divisions along line marked in units from 0-10 (high number may vary)	Children as young as 5 yr, as long as they can count and have some concept of numbers and their values in relation to other numbers. Scale may be used horizontally or vertically. Number coding should be same as in other scales used in facility.
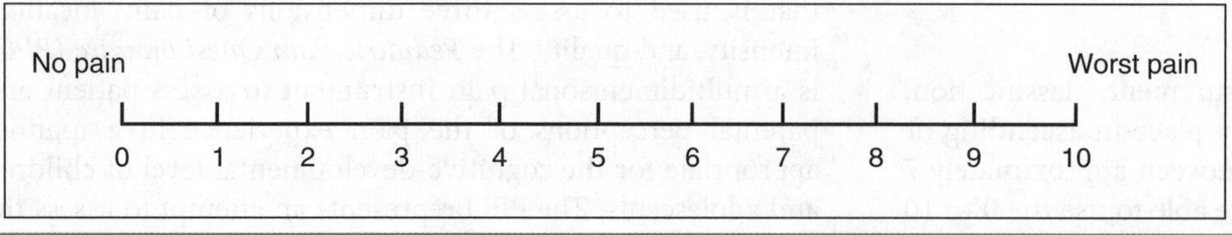 	

Table 35-3 Pain Rating Scales for Children—cont'd

PAIN SCALE, DESCRIPTION	RECOMMENDED AGE, COMMENTS
Visual Analog Scale (VAS) (Cline et al, 1992) A vertical or horizontal line drawn to a certain length, such as 10 cm (4 inches) and anchored by items that represent extremes of the subjective phenomenon, such as pain, that is measured 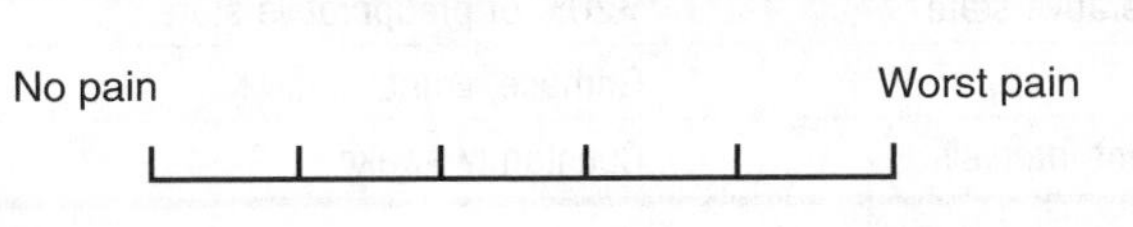	Children as young as 4½ yr, preferably 7 yr. Vertical or horizontal scale may be used. Research shows that children ages 3-18 yr prefer VAS less than other scales (Luffy & Grove, 2003; Wong & Baker, 1988).
Color Tool (Eland & Banner, 1999) Uses markers for child to construct own scale that is used with body outline; different colored markers denote different levels of pain in different body areas	Children as young as 4 yr, provided they know their colors, are not color blind, and are able to construct the scale if in pain.

BOX 35-2 Manifestations of Acute Pain in the Neonate

Physiologic Responses

Vital signs—Observe for variations.
- Increased heart rate
- Increased blood pressure
- Rapid, shallow respirations

Oxygenation
- Decreased transcutaneous oxygen saturation ($tcPo_2$)
- Decreased arterial oxygen saturation (Sao_2)

Skin—Observe color and character.
- Pallor or flushing
- Diaphoresis
- Palmar sweating

Laboratory evidence of metabolic or endocrine changes
- Hyperglycemia
- Lowered pH
- Elevated corticosteroids

Other observations
- Increased muscle tone
- Dilated pupils
- Decreased vagal nerve tone
- Increased intracranial pressure

Behavioral Responses

Vocalizations—Observe quality, timing, and duration.
- Crying
- Whimpering
- Groaning

Facial expression—Observe characteristics, timing, orientation of eyes and mouth.
- Grimaces
- Brow furrowed
- Chin quivering
- Eyes tightly closed
- Mouth open and squarish

Body movements and posture—Observe type, quality, and amount of movement or lack of movement; relationship to other factors.
- Limb withdrawal
- Thrashing
- Rigidity
- Flaccidity
- Fist clenching

Changes in state—Observe sleep, appetite, activity level.
- Changes in sleep-wake cycles
- Changes in feeding behavior
- Changes in activity level
- Fussiness, irritability
- Listlessness

Pain Assessment in Specific Populations

Pain in Neonates

Assessment of pain is difficult in the preverbal child, especially the neonate, since the most reliable indicator of pain, self-report, is not possible. Evaluation must be based on physiologic changes and behavioral observations (Box 35-2). Although behaviors such as vocalizations, facial expressions, and body movements are common to all infants, they vary with different situations. Crying associated with pain is more intense and sustained (see Fig. 35-1). Facial expression is the most consistent and specific characteristic; scales are available to systematically evaluate facial features, such as eye squeeze, brow bulge, open mouth, and taut tongue (Hadjistavropoulos et al, 1997). Most infants respond with increased body movements, but the infant may be experiencing pain even when lying quietly with eyes closed. The preterm infant's response to pain may be behaviorally blunted or absent; however, there is ample evidence that such infants are neurologically capable of feeling pain. In addition, infants in awake or alert states demonstrate a more robust reaction to painful stimuli than infants in sleep states. Also, an infant receiving a muscle-paralyzing agent such as vecuronium will be incapable of a behavioral or visible pain response.

Although regular use of pain assessment tools can assist caregivers in determining whether the infant is in pain, caregivers must consider the infant's maturity, behavioral state,

Table 35-4 CRIES Neonatal Postoperative Pain Scale

	0	1	2
Crying	No	High pitched	Inconsolable
Requires oxygen for saturation >95%	No	<30%	>30%
Increased vital signs	Heart rate and blood pressure ≤ preoperative state	Heart rate and blood pressure increase <20% of preoperative state	Heart rate and blood pressure increase >20% of preoperative state
Expression	None	Grimace	Grimace, grunt
Sleepless	No	Wakes at frequent intervals	Constantly awake

energy resources available to respond, and risk factors for pain. In infants with diminished ability to respond robustly to pain, it is imperative to presume that pain exists in all situations that are usually considered painful for adults and children, even in the absence of behavioral or physiologic signs (Sweet & McGrath, 1998).

Several pain assessment tools have been developed for the assessment of pain in the neonate. One pain assessment tool used by nurses who work with preterm and full-term infants in the neonatal intensive care setting is called *CRIES*, which is an acronym for the tool's physiologic and behavioral indicators of pain: *C*rying, *R*equires increased oxygen, *I*ncreased vital signs, *E*xpression, and *S*leeplessness (Table 35-4). Each indicator is scored from 0 to 2—similar to the Apgar score for neonates. The total possible pain score, representing the worst pain, is 10. A pain score greater than 4 should be considered significant. This tool has been tested for reliability and validity for postoperative pain in infants between the ages of 32 weeks of gestation up to 20 weeks postterm (60 weeks) (Sweet & McGrath, 1998).

The *Premature Infant Pain Profile (PIPP)* is unique because it has been developed specifically for preterm infants (Sweet & McGrath, 1998). The category "gestational age at time of observation" gives a higher pain score to infants with lower gestational age. Infants who are asleep 15 seconds before the painful procedure also receive additional points for their blunted behavioral responses to painful stimuli.

Children with Communication and Cognitive Impairment

The assessment of pain in children with communication and cognitive impairment can be challenging. Children who have significant difficulties communicating with others about their pain include those with significant neurologic impairments (e.g., cerebral palsy), cognitive impairment, metabolic disorders, autism, severe brain injury, and communication barriers (e.g., critically ill children who are on ventilators or heavily sedated or have neuromuscular disorders, loss of hearing, or loss of vision). These children are at greater risk than other children for undertreatment of pain because they have medical problems that may cause pain and they undergo painful procedures. Their behaviors include moaning, inconsistent patterns of play and sleep, changes in facial expression, and other physical problems that may mask expression of pain and be difficult to interpret (Hadden & von Baeyer, 2002). These children may experience spasticity, contractures, and orthopedic surgical treatment that may be painful.

The mother or primary caregiver is an important source of information during assessment (Breau et al, 2003). Up to 60% of parents of children with severe cognitive impairment reported that their child experienced pain or severe discomfort that was not being effectively managed (Lenton et al, 2001; Stallard et al, 2002a). The most frequently reported pain behaviors are crying; being less active; seeking comfort; moaning; not cooperating; being irritable; being stiff, spastic, tense, or rigid; sleeping less; being difficult to satisfy or pacify; flinching or moving body part away; and being agitated or fidgety (Hadden & von Baeyer, 2002). Parents also reported pain during some daily living activities such as assisted stretching and walking; independent standing; toileting; putting on splints; and doing occupational therapy, range-of-motion exercises, or physical therapy.

The *Non-communicating Children's Pain Checklist* is a pain measurement tool specifically designed for children with cognitive impairments (Breau et al, 2002). The scale discriminates between periods of pain and calm and can predict behavior during subsequent episodes of pain. The scale consists of six subscales (vocal, social, facial, activity, body and limbs, physiologic), which are scored based on the number of times the items are observed over a 10-minute period (0 = not at all; 1 = just a little; 2 = fairly often; 3 = very often).

Another tool, the *Pain Indicator for Communicatively Impaired Children (PICIC)*, distinguishes between pain and nonpain in communicatively impaired children with life-threatening illness (Stallard et al, 2002a, 2002b). The PICIC has six core pain cues: (1) crying with or without tears; (2) screaming, yelling, groaning, or moaning; (3) screwed up or distressed looking face; (4) body appearing stiff or tense; (5) difficulty in comforting or consoling; and (6) flinching or moving away if touched. The items are rated using a 4-point Likert scale (1 = not at all, 2 = a little, 3 = often, 4 = all the time).

Cultural Issues in Pain Assessment

A major challenge in the assessment and management of pain in children is the *cultural appropriateness* of pain assessment tools that have been validated only in Caucasian and English-speaking children. Observational scales and interview questionnaires for pain may not be as reliable for pain assessment as self-report scales in Hispanic children. In Chinese children who learned to read Chinese characters vertically downward and from right to left, the use of vertically oriented visual analog scales resulted in less error than horizontally oriented scales. Cultural background may therefore influence the reliability of pain assessment tools developed in a single cultural context (Bernstein & Pachter, 2003).

The *Oucher Pain Scale* (see Table 35-3), originally developed and validated as a self-report of pain intensity for Caucasian children 3 to 12 years old, now features culturally specific photographs of children who better represent the physical characteristics of African-American and Hispanic children (Beyer & Knott, 1998). The Oucher Pain Scale consists of six photographs on the right side and a 0 to 100 scale marked off in tens on the left side. The photographs show the face of one child with the pictures arranged to show increasing levels of discomfort. Each version has been tested primarily with children in the ethnic group (Caucasian, African-American, Hispanic) depicted in the photographs. Children ages 3 to 12 years old use the Oucher by selecting a photograph or number that most closely represents the level of pain intensity they are experiencing (Beyer & Knott, 1998). This tool is designed to promote cultural sensitivity during pain assessment for minority or non-Caucasian children.

Children with Chronic Illness and Complex Pain

Questionnaires and pain assessment scales do not always provide the most meaningful means of assessing pain in children, particularly for those with complex pain. Some children cannot relate to a face or a number that describes their pain and may not be able to isolate pain from other symptoms they are experiencing. Children with cancer experience multiple symptoms, making it difficult to isolate the pain symptom from other symptoms. Rating the pain does not always accurately convey to others how they really feel (Woodgate & Yanofsky, 2004).

In children with chronic illness, particularly those with complex pain, the most important aspect of assessment is to develop a trusting relationship with the child and the family, so that a deeper understanding of the pain experience may be obtained. The pain experience may be complicated by pain processes that occur in the central nervous system (such as hyperalgesia, central sensitization, windup), by other symptoms (such as fatigue, nausea, vomiting, diarrhea, constipation) that accompany medical treatments, and by complications (such as infections, unexpected development of fistulas, typhlitis) from disease or treatments (Turner, 2005). The pain experience may interfere with the child's ability to eat, sleep, and perform daily activities and routines (Miaskowski & Lee, 1999; Morin, Gibson, & Wade, 1998).

Other important components of assessment include the onset of pain; pain duration or pattern; the effectiveness of the current treatment; factors that aggravate or relieve the pain; other symptoms and complications concurrently felt; and interference with the child's mood, function, and interactions with family (Turner, 2005). In addition to asking the child or parent when the pain started and how long the pain lasts, the nurse can assess variations and rhythms by asking if the pain is better or worse at certain times during the day or night. If the child has had pain for a while, the child or parent may know which medications and doses are helpful. They may also have found some nonpharmacologic methods that have helped. The nurse may ask the child or parent if there are activities, positions, and other events that may increase the pain. Pain may be accompanied by other symptoms such as nausea and poor appetite.

Other factors warranting careful assessment that may pose barriers to effective management include family issues and relationships, fears and concerns about addiction (see Family-Centered Care box), the clinician's and family's lack of knowledge about pain, inappropriate use of pain medications, ineffective management of adverse effects from medications, and the use of different pain interventions (Turner, 2005).

Pain Management

Unrelieved pain may lead to potential long-term physiologic, psychosocial, and behavioral consequences (Goldschneider & Anand, 2003; Weisman, Bernstein, & Schechter, 1998). Management of pain should be a priority for all clinicians.

Nonpharmacologic Management

Pain is often associated with fear, anxiety, and stress (Kain et al, 2006). A number of *nonpharmacologic techniques* (see Guidelines box), such as distraction, relaxation, guided imagery, and cutaneous stimulation, provide coping strategies that may help reduce pain perception, make pain more tolerable, decrease anxiety, and enhance the effectiveness of analgesics or reduce the dosage required (Rusy & Weisman, 2000). In addition, these techniques decrease the perceived threat of pain, provide a sense of control, enhance comfort, and promote rest and sleep (Greco & Berde, 2005). Although there is a paucity of research on the effectiveness of many of these interventions, the strategies are safe, noninvasive, and inexpensive, and most are independent nursing functions. Environmental and psychologic factors may exert a powerful influence on children's pain perceptions and may be modified by using psychosocial strategies, education, parental support, and cognitive-behavioral interventions. For children undergoing repeated painful procedures, cognitive-behavioral interventions are effective for decreasing anxiety and distress (McGrath & Hillier, 2003).

If the child cannot identify a familiar coping technique, the nurse can describe several strategies and let the child select the most appealing one. Experimentation with several strategies that are suitable to the child's age, pain intensity, and abilities is often necessary to determine the most effective approach. Parents should be involved in the selection process; they may be familiar with the child's usual coping skills and can help identify potentially successful strategies. Involving parents also encourages their participation in learning the skill with the child and acting as coach. If the parent cannot assist the child, other appropriate persons may include a grandparent, older sibling, nurse, or child life specialist (McGrath & Hillier, 2003).

Children should learn to use a specific strategy before pain occurs or before it becomes severe. Children are responsive to pain-controlling strategies that involve their imaginations and

evolve Nursing Care Plan—The Child in Pain
evolve Skill—Managing Pain

FAMILY-CENTERED CARE

Fear of Opioid Addiction

One of the reasons for the unfounded but prevalent fear of addiction from opioids used to relieve pain is a misunderstanding of the differences between physical dependence, tolerance, and addiction. Health care professionals and the community often confuse addiction with the physiologic effects of opioids, when in reality physical dependence, tolerance, and addiction are unrelated. The American Society of Addiction Medicine defines these terms as follows:

Physical dependence on an opioid is a physiologic state in which abrupt cessation of the opioid, or administration of an opioid antagonist, results in withdrawal syndrome. Physical dependence on opioids is an expected occurrence in all individuals who continuously use opioids for therapeutic or nontherapeutic purposes. It does not, in and of itself, imply addiction.

Tolerance is a form of neuroadaptation to the effects of chronically administered opioids (or other medications) that is indicated by the need for increasing or more frequent doses of the medication to achieve the initial effects of the drug. A person may develop tolerance both to the analgesic effects of opioids and to some of the unwanted side effects, such as respiratory depression, sedation, or nausea. Tolerance is variable in occurrence, but it does not, in and of itself, imply addiction.

Addiction in the context of pain treatment with opioids is characterized by a persistent pattern of dysfunctional opioid use that may involve any or all of the following:

- Adverse consequences associated with the use of opioids
- Loss of control over the use of opioids
- Preoccupation with obtaining opioids, despite the presence of adequate analgesia

Unfortunately, individuals who have severe, unrelieved pain may become intensely focused on finding relief. Sometimes behaviors such as "clock watching" make patients appear to others to be preoccupied with obtaining opioids. However, this preoccupation centers on finding relief of pain, not on using opioids for reasons other than pain control. This phenomenon has been termed *pseudoaddiction* and must not be confused with real addiction.

Nurses must educate older children, parents, and health professionals about the extremely low risk of real addiction (less than 1%) from the use of opioids to treat pain. Infants, young children, and comatose or terminally ill children simply cannot become addicted because they are incapable of a consistent pattern of drug-seeking behavior, such as stealing, drug dealing, prostitution, or use of family income, to obtain opioids for nonanalgesic reasons.

Data from American Society of Addiction Medicine: *Public policy statement on definitions related to the use of opioids for pain treatment*, February 2001. Internet document available from http://www.asam.org/Pain.html (accessed May 7, 2007).

senses of play (Gerik, 2005). To reduce the child's effort, instructions for a strategy, such as distraction or relaxation, can be audiotaped and played during a period of comfort. However, even after they have learned an intervention, children often need help using it during a painful procedure. The intervention can also be used after the procedure. This gives the child a chance to recover, feel mastery, and cope more effectively (McGrath & Hillier, 2003).

Virtual reality has been identified as a potentially effective tool for pain distraction (Gold et al, 2006). The participant's attention is drawn away from the "real world" and into the "virtual world" with the incorporation of visual, auditory, and tactile stimuli.

Several studies have documented the effectiveness of nonpharmacologic analgesia, such as containment, positioning, nonnutritive sucking (Fig. 35-3), and kangaroo holding during painful procedures in neonates. *Containment* is achieved through positioning and blanket rolls (Cole & Jorgensen, 1997). It provides a "nest" that enhances the infant's feelings of security and decreases stress. Comforting measures and *swaddling* have been demonstrated to reduce crying and heart rate after procedures such as heel punctures and injections. In infants between 27 and 34 weeks of gestational age, those infants who were swaddled after a routine heel stick procedure were able to calm crying immediately, decrease heart rate, and return to a sleep state; in comparison, infants who were not swaddled took a minimum of 10 minutes to return to baseline physiologic and behavioral levels (Fearon et al, 1997). *Proper positioning* with the infant held in a midline orientation, hand to mouth activity, and proper flexion can promote self-soothing behaviors. *Facilitated tucking*, which is holding the infant's extremities flexed and contained close to the trunk, during heel lance procedures has been demonstrated to decrease heart rate, decrease crying time, and promote stability in the sleep-wake cycles after the lance.

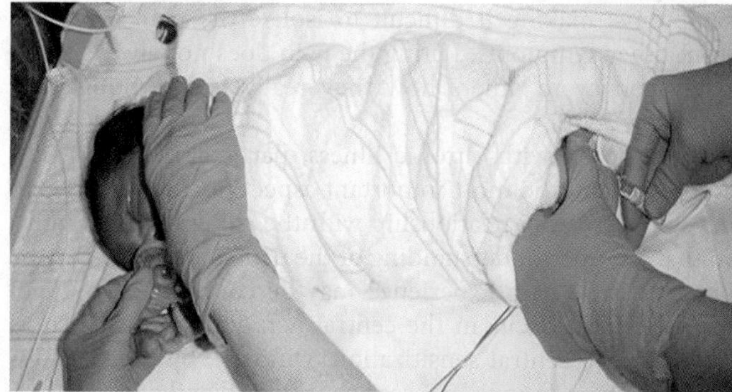

Fig. 35-3 Sucking following oral sucrose can enhance analgesia before a heel stick in a preterm infant.

Nonnutritive sucking (pacifier) attenuates behavioral, physiologic, and hormonal responses to pain from procedures, such as heel punctures, venipuncture, and immunization injections. The administration of concentrated sucrose with or without nonnutritive sucking has been demonstrated to have calming and pain-relieving effects for invasive procedures in

GUIDELINES Nonpharmacologic Strategies for Pain Management

General Strategies

Use nonpharmacologic interventions to supplement, not replace, pharmacologic interventions, and use for mild pain and pain that is reasonably well controlled with analgesics.

Form a trusting relationship with child and family.

Express concern regarding their reports of pain and intervene appropriately.

Take an active role in seeking effective pain management strategies.

Use general guidelines to prepare child for procedure.

Prepare child before potentially painful procedures, but avoid "planting" the idea of pain.

- For example, instead of saying, "This is going to (or may) hurt," say, "Sometimes this feels like pushing, sticking, or pinching, and sometimes it doesn't bother people. Tell me what it feels like to you."
- Use "nonpain" descriptors when possible (e.g., "It feels like heat" rather than "It's a burning pain"). This allows for variation in sensory perception, avoids suggesting pain, and gives the child control in describing reactions.
- Avoid evaluative statements or descriptions (e.g., "This is a terrible procedure" or "It really will hurt a lot").

Stay with child during a painful procedure.

- Allow parents to stay with child if child and parent desire; encourage parent to talk softly to child and to remain near child's head.
- Involve parents in learning specific nonpharmacologic strategies and in assisting child with their use.

Educate child about the pain, especially when explanation may lessen anxiety (e.g., that pain may occur after surgery and does not indicate something is wrong); reassure the child that he or she is not responsible for the pain.

For long-term pain control, give child a doll, which represents "the patient," and allow child to do everything to the doll that is done to the child; pain control can be emphasized through the doll by stating, "Dolly feels better after the medicine."

Teach procedures to child and family for later use.

Specific Strategies

Distraction

Involve parent and child in identifying strong distracters.

Involve child in play; use radio, tape recorder, CD player, or computer game; have child sing or use rhythmic breathing.

Have child take a deep breath and blow it out until told to stop.

Have child blow bubbles to "blow the hurt away."

Have child concentrate on yelling or saying "ouch," with instructions to "yell as loud or soft as you feel it hurt; that way I know what's happening."

Have child look through kaleidoscope (type with glitter suspended in fluid-filled tube) and encourage him or her to concentrate by asking, "Do you see the different designs?"

Use humor, such as watching cartoons, telling jokes or funny stories, or acting silly with child.

Have child read, play games, or visit with friends.

Relaxation

With an infant or young child:

- Hold in a comfortable, well-supported position, such as vertically against the chest and shoulder.
- Rock in a wide, rhythmic arc in a rocking chair or sway back and forth, rather than bouncing child.
- Repeat one or two words softly, such as "Mommy's here."

With a slightly older child:

- Ask child to take a deep breath and "go limp as a rag doll" while exhaling slowly; then ask child to yawn (demonstrate if needed).
- Help child assume a comfortable position (e.g., pillow under neck and knees).
- Begin progressive relaxation: starting with the toes, systematically instruct child to let each body part "go limp" or "feel heavy"; if child has difficulty relaxing, instruct child to tense or tighten each body part and then relax it.
- Allow child to keep eyes open, since children may respond better if eyes are open rather than closed during relaxation.

Guided Imagery

Have child identify some highly pleasurable real or imaginary experience.

Have child describe details of the event, including as many senses as possible (e.g., "feel the cool breezes," "see the beautiful colors," "hear the pleasant music").

Have child write down or tape record script.

Encourage child to concentrate only on the pleasurable event during the painful time; enhance the image by recalling specific details through reading the script or playing the tape.

Combine with relaxation and rhythmic breathing.

Positive Self-Talk

Teach child positive statements to say when in pain (e.g., "I will be feeling better soon," "When I go home, I will feel better, and we will eat ice cream").

Thought Stopping

Identify positive facts about the painful event (e.g., "It does not last long").

Identify reassuring information (e.g., "If I think about something else, it does not hurt as much").

Condense positive and reassuring facts into a set of brief statements and have child memorize them (e.g., "short procedure, good veins, little hurt, nice nurse, go home").

Have child repeat the memorized statements whenever thinking about or experiencing the painful event.

Behavioral Contracting

Informal—May be used with children as young as 4 or 5 years of age:

- Use stars, tokens, or cartoon character stickers as rewards.
- Give a child who is uncooperative or procrastinating during a procedure a limited time (measured by a visible timer) to complete the procedure.
- Proceed as needed if child is unable to comply.
- Reinforce cooperation with a reward if the procedure is accomplished within specified time.

Formal—Use written contract, which includes:

- Realistic (seems possible) goal or desired behavior
- Measurable behavior (e.g., agreeing not to hit anyone during procedures)
- Date and signature of all persons involved in any of the agreements
- Identified rewards or consequences that are reinforcing
- Goals that can be evaluated
- Commitment and compromise requirements for both parties (e.g., while timer is used, nurse will not nag or prod child to complete procedure)

neonates. The amount of time crying was decreased with the oral administration of 2 ml of a 12% to 24% sucrose solution, 2 minutes before a heel lance or venipuncture (Stevens, Yamada, & Ohlsson, 2005).

Kangaroo care is skin-to-skin holding of infants dressed only in diapers against their mother's or father's chest (Gray, Watt, & Blass, 2000; Johnston et al, 2003). Infants who spent 1 to 3 hours in kangaroo care showed increased frequency in quiet sleep, longer duration of quiet sleep, and decreased crying in the neonatal intensive care unit. They also cried less at age 6 months when compared with neonates who did not receive skin-to-skin contact. Significant differences were found in pain responses during heel lancing between infants who were kangaroo held and those who were not. In the study by Gray, Watt, and Blass (2000), heart rate increased by 8 to 10 beats/min in the kangaroo care group vs. an increase by 36 to 38 beats/min in the control group of neonates who were swaddled in bassinets. Grimacing was 64% less, and crying was 82% less frequent.

In another study, infant responses to pain during heel lance procedures were compared using kangaroo holding (Fig. 35-4), with the neonate held upright at a 60-degree angle between the mother's breasts for maximal skin-to-skin contact (Johnston et al, 2003). A blanket was placed over the neonate's back, and the mother's clothes were wrapped around the neonate for 30 minutes before the lancing procedure, during, and at least 30 minutes after the heel stick. Another group remained in the isolette in a prone position, swaddled with a blanket and the heel accessible, for 30 minutes before the heel lancing procedure. Pain scores were significantly lower in kangaroo-held infants.

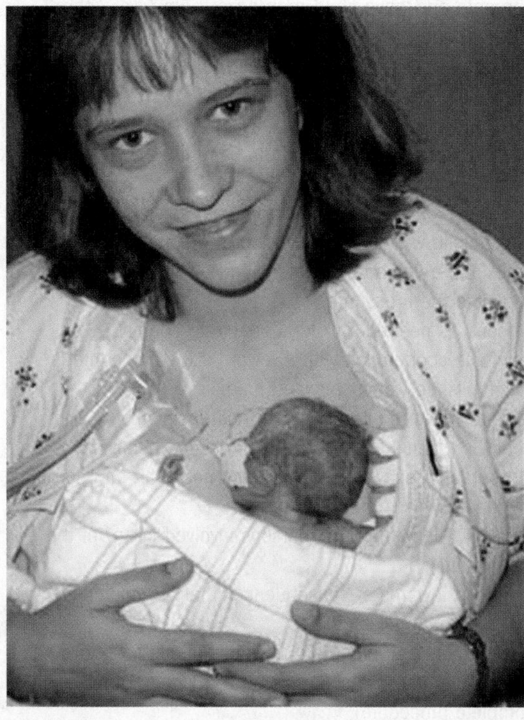

Fig. 35-4 Mother using kangaroo hold with her newborn infant. Note placement of the infant directly on the mother's skin.

Complementary Pain Medicine

Many terms are used to describe approaches to health care that are outside the realm of conventional medicine as practiced in the United States. *Complementary and alternative medicine (CAM)*, as defined by the National Center for Complementary and Alternative Medicine, is a group of diverse medical and health care systems, practices, and products that are not currently considered part of conventional medicine (Myers et al, 2005). Although some scientific evidence exists regarding the efficacy of some CAM therapies, questions are yet to be answered through well-designed scientific studies, such as whether these therapies are safe and whether they work for the diseases or medical conditions for which they are used.

CAM therapies may be grouped into five classes:

1. **Biologically based**—Foods, special diets, herbal or plant preparations, vitamins, other supplements
2. **Manipulative treatments**—Chiropractic, osteopathy, massage
3. **Energy based**—Reiki, bioelectric or magnetic treatments, pulsed fields, alternating and direct currents
4. **Mind-body techniques**—Mental healing, expressive treatments, spiritual healing, hypnosis, relaxation
5. **Alternative medical systems**—Homeopathy; naturopathy; ayurvedic; and traditional Chinese medicine, including acupuncture and moxibustion

Current estimates of pediatric CAM use range from 10% to 15%, derived from children sampled at health care facilities, with chronic conditions, and/or from countries other than the United States. For the U.S. population, pediatric CAM use was estimated to be 31% to 84% (Myers et al, 2005; Rusy & Weisman, 2000). Those who used CAM were found in each age group, and the mean age was 10.3 years. The majority used unconventional therapy for chronic, as opposed to life-threatening, medical conditions. The therapies that are increasingly used include herbal medicine, massage, megavitamins, self-help groups, folk remedies, energy healing, and homeopathy (Myers et al, 2005; Rusy & Weisman, 2000).

Pharmacologic Management

Nonopioids, including acetaminophen (Tylenol, Paracetamol) and nonsteroidal antiinflammatory drugs (NSAIDs), are suitable for mild to moderate pain (Table 35-5); *opioids* are needed for moderate to severe pain (Table 35-6). A combination of the two analgesics acts on the pain system on two levels: nonopioids primarily act at the peripheral nervous system, and opioids primarily act at the central nervous system. The combination of NSAIDs and opioids provides increased analgesia without increased side effects. Several combinations, such as acetaminophen with codeine, may have increasing doses of the opioid but a constant dose of the nonopioid Before increasing the opioid, it may be preferable to increase the nonopioid component, for example, by adding one regular-strength acetaminophen tablet (325 mg) to acetaminophen 300 mg with codeine 15 mg (Tylenol No. 2) before advancing to acetaminophen 300 mg with codeine 30 mg (Tylenol No. 3) or codeine 60 mg (Tylenol No. 4). However, if this approach is not successful, pain management will require a stronger opioid (see Table 35-6). Oxycodone is available without a nonopioid in an immediate release and con-

evolve Skill—Calculating Safe Dosages for Children

Table 35-5 Nonsteroidal Antiinflammatory Drugs (NSAIDs) Approved for Children*

DRUG	DOSAGE	COMMENTS
Acetaminophen (Tylenol)	10-15 mg/kg/dose q4-6hr not to exceed 5 doses in 24 hr or 75 mg/kg/day, PO	Available in numerous preparations Nonprescription Higher dosage range may provide increased analgesia
Choline magnesium trisalicylate (Trilisate)	Children <37 kg (81.5 pounds)–50 mg/kg/day divided into 2 doses Children >37 kg (81.5 pounds)–2250 mg/day divided into 2 doses	Available in suspension, 500 mg/5 ml Prescription
Ibuprofen (children's Motrin, children's Advil)	Children >6 mo–5-10 mg/kg/dose q6-8hr; maximum: 40 mg/kg/day	Available in numerous preparations Available in suspension (100 mg/5 ml) and drops (100 mg/2.5 ml) Nonprescription
Naproxen (Naprosyn)	Children >2 yr–10 mg/kg/day divided into 2 doses	Available in suspension (125 mg/5 ml) and several different dosages for tablets Nonprescription
Tolmetin (Tolectin)	Children >2 yr–20 g/kg/day divided into 3-4 doses	Available in 200-mg, 400-mg, and 600-mg tablets Prescription

Data from *Drug facts and comparisons*, Philadelphia, 2008, Lippincott Williams & Wilkins.
PO, Orally; *q*, every.
NOTE: Newer formulations of NSAIDs selectively inhibit one of the enzymes of cyclooxygenase (COX-2, which is responsible for pain transmission) but do not inhibit the other (COX-1). Inhibition of COX-1 decreases prostaglandin production, which is necessary for normal organ function. For example, prostaglandins help maintain gastric mucosal blood flow and barrier protection, regulate blood flow to the liver and kidneys, and facilitate platelet aggregation and clot formation. Theoretically, the COX-2 NSAIDs provide similar analgesic and antiinflammatory benefits with fewer gastric and platelet side effects than the nonselective agents. COX-2 NSAIDs are approved for use in patients >18 yr of age.
*All NSAIDs in this table (except acetaminophen) have significant antiinflammatory, antipyretic, and analgesic actions. Acetaminophen has a weak antiinflammatory action, and its classification as an NSAID is controversial. Patients respond differently to various NSAIDs; therefore changing from one drug to another may be necessary for maximum benefit.
Acetylsalicylic acid (aspirin) is also an NSAID but is not recommended for children because of its possible association with Reye's syndrome. The NSAIDs in this table have no known association with Reye's syndrome. However, caution should be exercised in prescribing any salicylate-containing drug (e.g., choline magnesium trisalicylate) for children with known or suspected viral infection.
Side effects of ibuprofen, naproxen, and tolmetin include nausea, vomiting, diarrhea, constipation, gastric ulceration, bleeding nephritis, and fluid retention.
Acetaminophen and choline magnesium trisalicylate are well tolerated in the gastrointestinal tract and do not interfere with platelet function. NSAIDs (except acetaminophen) should not be given to patients with allergic reactions to salicylates. All the NSAIDs should be used cautiously in patients with renal impairment.

trolled release preparation (OxyContin). The oxycodone dose can be safely increased without the risk of toxicity from excessive acetaminophen use.

Actions of various opioids differ. Morphine is considered the gold standard for the management of severe pain. When morphine is not a suitable opioid, drugs such as hydromorphone (Dilaudid) and fentanyl (Sublimaze) are effective substitutes. Although fentanyl is used as an anesthetic in the operating room, it is classified as an analgesic. It can be safely administered by nurses by the intravenous (IV), intramuscular (IM), transmucosal, and transdermal routes (Algren et al, 1998).

Several drugs, known as *coanalgesics* or *adjuvant analgesics*, may be used alone or with opioids to control pain symptoms and opioid side effects. Drugs frequently used to relieve anxiety, cause sedation, and provide amnesia are diazepam (Valium) and midazolam (Versed); however, these drugs are not analgesics and should be used to enhance the effects of analgesics, not as a substitute for analgesics. Other adjuvants include tricyclic antidepressants (e.g., amitriptyline, imipramine) and antiepileptics (e.g., gabapentin, carbamazepine, clonazepam) for neuropathic pain (Table 35-7), stool softeners and laxatives for constipation, antiemetics for nausea and vomiting, diphenhydramine for itching, steroids for inflammation and bone pain, and dextroamphetamine and caffeine for possible increased analgesia and decreased sedation (Greco & Berde, 2005).

The use of *placebos* to determine whether the patient is having pain is unjustified and unethical. A positive response to a placebo, such as a saline injection, is common in patients who have a documented organic basis for pain. Therefore the deceptive use of placebos does not provide useful information about the presence or severity of pain. The use of placebos can cause side effects similar to those of opioids, can destroy the patient's trust in the health care staff, and raises serious ethical and legal questions. The American Society for Pain Management Nursing has issued a position statement against the use of placebos to treat pain (McCaffery & Pasero, 1999).

NURSING ALERT The optimum dosage of an analgesic is one that controls pain without causing severe side effects. This usually requires titration, the gradual adjustment of drug dosage (usually by increasing the dose) until optimum pain relief without excessive sedation is achieved. Dosage recommendations are only safe initial dosages (see Tables 35-5 and 35-6), not optimum dosages.

Children (except infants younger than about 3 to 6 months) metabolize drugs more rapidly than adults; younger children may require higher doses of opioids to achieve the same analgesic effect. Therefore the therapeutic effect and duration of analgesia vary. Children's dosages are usually calculated according to body weight, except in children with a weight

Table 35-6 Dosage of Selected Opioids for Children

DRUG	APPROPRIATE EQUIANALGESIC	APPROXIMATE EQUIANALGESIC PARENTERAL DOSE	Recommended Starting Dosage (Children <50 kg [110 Pounds] Body Weight)* ORAL	PARENTERAL*
Morphine	30 mg q3-4hr	10 mg q3-4hr	0.2-0.4 mg/kg q3-4hr 0.3-0.6 mg/kg time released q12hr	0.1-0.2 mg/kg IM q3-4hr 0.02-0.1 mg/kg IV bolus q2hr 0.015 mg/kg q8min PCA 0.01-0.02 mg/kg/hr IV infusion (neonates) 0.01-0.06 mg/kg/hr IV infusion (child)
Fentanyl (Sublimaze) (oral mucosal form [Actiq])†	Not available	0.1 mg IV	5-15 mcg/kg; maximum dose: 400 mcg	0.5-1.5 mcg/kg IV bolus q30min 1-2 mcg/hr IV infusion
Codeine‡	200 mg q3-4hr	130 mg q3-4hr	1 mg/kg q3-4hr	Not recommended
Hydromorphone§ (Dilaudid)	7.5 mg q3-4hr	1.5 mg q3-4hr	0.04-0.1 mg/kg q3-4hr	0.02-0.1 mg/kg q3-4hr 0.005-0.2 mg/kg IV bolus q2hr
Hydrocodone and acetaminophen (Lorcet, Lortab, Vicodin)	30 mg q3-4hr	Not available	0.2 mg/kg q3-4hr	Not available
Levorphanol (Levo-Dromoran)	4 mg q6-8hr	2 mg q6-8hr	0.04 mg/kg q6-8hr	0.02 mg/kg q6-8hr
Methadone (Dolophine)	20 mg q6-8hr	10 mg q6-8hr	0.2 mg/kg q6-8hr	0.1 mg/kg q6-8hr
Oxycodone (Roxicodone, OxyContin; also in Percocet, Percodan, Tylox)	20 mg q3-4hr	Not available	2 mg/kg q3-4hr‖	Not available

Data from Acute Pain Management Guideline Panel: *Acute pain management: operative or medical procedures and trauma: clinical practice guideline,* AHCPR Pub No 92-0032, Rockville, MD, 1992, Agency for Health Care Policy and Research, Public Health Service, US Department of Health and Human Services; and Berde C et al: American Academy of Pediatrics report of the Subcommittee on Disease-Related Pain in Childhood Cancer, *Pediatrics* 86(5 Pt 2):818-825, 1990. Codeine dosages from McCaffery M, Pasero C: *Pain: a clinical manual,* ed 2, St Louis, 1999, Mosby.

IM, Intramuscular; *IV,* intravenous; *PCA,* patient-controlled analgesia; *q,* every.

NOTE: Published tables vary in suggested doses that are equianalgesic to morphine. Clinical response is criterion that must be applied for each patient; titration to clinical response is necessary. Because there is not complete cross-tolerance among these drugs, it is usually necessary to use a lower than equianalgesic dose when changing drugs and to retitrate to response.

CAUTION: Recommended dosages do not apply to patients with renal or hepatic insufficiency or other conditions affecting drug metabolism and kinetics.

*CAUTION: Dosages listed for patients with body weight <50 kg (110 pounds) cannot be used as initial starting doses in infants <6 mo of age. For nonventilated infants younger than 6 mo, the initial opioid dose should be about one fourth to one third of the dose recommended for older infants and children. For example, morphine could be used at a dose of 0.03 mg/kg instead of the traditional 0.1 mg/kg.

†Actiq is indicated only for management of breakthrough cancer pain in patients with malignancies who are already receiving and are tolerant to opioid therapy, but it can be used for preoperative or preprocedural sedation and analgesia.

‡CAUTION: Codeine doses above 65 mg often are not appropriate because of diminishing incremental analgesia with increasing doses along with continually increasing constipation and other side effects.

§For morphine, hydromorphone, and oxymorphone, rectal administration is an alternate route for patients unable to take oral medications, but equianalgesic doses may differ from oral and parenteral doses because of pharmacokinetic differences.

‖CAUTION: Doses of aspirin and acetaminophen in combination with opioid or nonsteroidal antiinflammatory drug preparations must also be adjusted to patient's body weight. Daily dose of acetaminophen should not exceed 75 mg/kg or 4000 mg.

greater than 50 kg (110 pounds), where the weight formula may exceed the average adult dosage. In this case the adult dosage is used.

A reasonable starting dose of opioid for infants under 6 months who are not mechanically ventilated is one fourth to one third of the recommended starting dose for older children. The infant is monitored closely for signs of pain relief and respiratory depression. The dose is titrated to effect. Because tolerance can develop rapidly, large doses may be needed for continued severe pain (Greco & Berde, 2005). If pain relief is inadequate, the initial dose is increased (usually by 25% to 50% if pain is moderate, or by 50% to 100% if pain is severe) to provide greater analgesic effectiveness. Decreasing the interval between doses may also provide more continuous pain relief. A major difference between opioids and nonopioids is that nonopioids have a *ceiling effect,* which means that dosages higher than the recommended dosage will not produce greater pain relief. Opioids do not have a ceiling effect other than that imposed by side effects; therefore larger dosages can be safely given for increasing severity of pain.

Parenteral and oral dosages of opioids are not the same. Because of the *first-pass effect,* an oral opioid is rapidly absorbed from the gastrointestinal tract and is partially metabolized in the liver before reaching the central circulation. Therefore oral dosages must be larger to compensate for the partial loss of analgesic potency to achieve *equianalgesia* (equal analgesic effect). Conversion factors (Table 35-8) for selected opioids must be used when a change is made from IV (preferred) or IM to oral administration. Immediate conversion from IM or IV to the suggested equianalgesic oral dose may result in a substantial error. For example, the dose may be significantly more or less than what the child requires. Small changes ensure small errors. Several routes of analgesic administration can be used (Box 35-3); the most effective and least traumatic should be selected.

Table 35-7 Coanalgesic Adjuvant Drugs

DRUG	DOSAGE	INDICATIONS	COMMENTS
Antidepressants			
Amitriptyline	0.2-0.5 mg/kg PO hs Titrate upward by 0.25 mg/kg q 5-7 days prn Available in 10- and 25-mg tablets Usual starting dose–10-25 mg	Continuous neuropathic pain with burning, aching, dysthesia with insomnia	Provides analgesia by blocking reuptake of serotonin and norepinephrine, possibly slowing transmission of pain signals Helps with pain related to insomnia and depression (use nortriptyline if patient is oversedated) Analgesic effects seen earlier than antidepressant effects Side effects include dry mouth, constipation, urinary retention
Nortriptyline	0.2-1.0 mg/kg PO AM or bid Titrate up by 0.5 mg q 5-7 days Maximum–25 mg/dose	Neuropathic pain as above without insomnia	
Anticonvulsants			
Gabapentin	5 mg/kg PO hs Increase to bid on day 2, tid on day 3 Maximum–300 mg/day	Neuropathic pain	Mechanism of action unknown Side effects include sedation, ataxia, nystagmus, dizziness
Carbamazepine	*<6 years:* 2.5-5 mg/kg PO bid initially Increase 20 mg/kg/24 hr, divide bid every week prn Maximum–100 mg bid *6-12 years:* 5 mg/kg PO bid initially Increase 10 mg/kg/24 hr, divide bid every week prn to usual maximum–100 mg bid *>12 years:* 200 mg PO bid initially Increase 200 mg/24 hr, divide bid every week prn to maximum–1.6-2.4 g/24 hr	Sharp, lancinating neuropathic pain Peripheral neuropathies Phantom limb pain	Similar analgesic effect to amitriptyline Monitor blood levels for toxicity only Side effects include decreased blood counts, ataxia, gastrointestinal irritation
Anxiolytics			
Lorazepam	0.03-0.1 mg/kg q 4-6 hr PO or IV Maximum–2 mg/dose	Muscle spasm Anxiety	May increase sedation in combination with opioids Can cause depression with prolonged use
Diazepam	0.1-0.3 mg/kg q 4-6 hr PO or IV Maximum–10 mg/dose		
Corticosteroids			
Dexamethasone	Dose dependent on clinical situation; higher bolus doses in cord compression, then lower daily dose Try to wean to NSAIDs if pain allows Cerebral edema–1-2 mg/kg load then 1-1.5 mg/kg/day divided q 6 hr Maximum–4 mg/dose Antiinflammatory–0.08-0.3 mg/kg/day divided q 6-12 hr	Pain from increased intracranial pressure Bony metastasis Spinal or nerve compression	Side effects include edema, gastrointestinal irritation, increased weight, acne Use gastroprotectants such as H_2-blockers (ranitidine) or proton pump inhibitors such as omeprazole for long-term administration of steroids or NSAIDs in end-stage cancer with bony pain
Others			
Clonidine	2-4 mcg/kg PO q 4-6 hr May also use a 100 mcg transdermal patch q 7 days for patients >40 kg (88 pounds)	Neuropathic pain Lancinating, sharp, electrical, shooting pain Phantom limb pain	α_2-Adenoreceptor agonist modulates ascending pain sensations Routes of administration: oral, transdermal, and spinal Management of withdrawal symptoms Monitor for orthostatic hypertension, decreased heart rate Sedation common
Mexiletine	2-3 mg/kg/dose PO tid, may titrate 0.5 mg/kg q 2-3 wk prn Maximum–300 mg/dose		Similar to lidocaine, longer acting Stabilizes sodium conduction in nerve cells, reduces neuronal firing Can enhance action of opioids, antidepressants, anticonvulsants Side effects include dizziness, ataxia, nausea, vomiting May measure blood levels for toxicity

bid, Twice a day; *hs,* at bedtime; *IV,* intravenous; *NSAIDs,* nonsteroidal antiinflammatory drugs; *PO,* by mouth; *prn,* as needed; *q,* every; *tid,* three times a day.

Table 35-8 Equianalgesia of Selected Analgesics

DRUG*	EQUAL TO ORAL MORPHINE (mg)	EQUAL TO IM OR IV MORPHINE (mg)
Hydromorphone (Dilaudid) 1 mg	4	1.3
Codeine 30 mg	4.5	1.5
Meperidine (Demerol) 50 mg	4.8	1.6
Codeine 30 mg, acetaminophen 300 mg (Tylenol No. 3)	7.2	2.4
Oxycodone 5 mg, acetaminophen 325 mg (Percocet)	7.2	2.4
Oxycodone 5 mg, aspirin 325 mg (Percodan)	7.2	2.4
Hydrocodone 5 mg, acetaminophen 500 mg (Vicodin, Lortab)	9	3
Oxycodone 5 mg, acetaminophen 500 mg (Tylox)	9	3
Methadone (Dolophine) 10 mg	15	7.5
Acetaminophen 325 mg (Tylenol)	2.7	0.9
Aspirin 325 mg	2.7	0.9
Acetaminophen 500 mg (Tylenol Extra Strength)	4	1.3
Codeine 60 mg, acetaminophen 300 mg (Tylenol No. 4)	11.7	3.9
Fentanyl transdermal patch (Duragesic) (based on 25 mcg/hr patch applied q3days = 50 mg oral morphine q24hr or divided into 6 doses = 8.3 mg) or use:	8.3	2.77

Recommended Initial Duragesic Dose Based on Daily Oral Morphine Dose†

ORAL 24-HR MORPHINE (mg/day)	DURAGESIC DOSE (mg/hr)
45-134	25
135-224	50
225-314	75
315-404	100
405-494	125
495-584	150
585-674	175
675-764	200
765-854	225
855-944	250
945-1034	275
1035-1124	300

Courtesy Betty R. Ferrell, PhD, FAAN, 1999. Used with permission.
IM, Intramuscular; *IV,* intravenous; *q,* every.
NOTE: When converting to oral oxycodone from oral morphine, an appropriate conservative estimate is 15-20 mg oxycodone per 30 mg morphine; however, when converting to oral morphine from oral oxycodone, an appropriate conservative estimate is 30 mg morphine per 30 mg oxycodone (McCaffery M, Pasero C: *Pain: a clinical manual,* ed 2, St Louis, 1999, Mosby).
*Oral medication with exception of fentanyl.
†Data from Duragesic package insert, Janssen Pharmaceutical Products, Titusville, NJ, 2001.

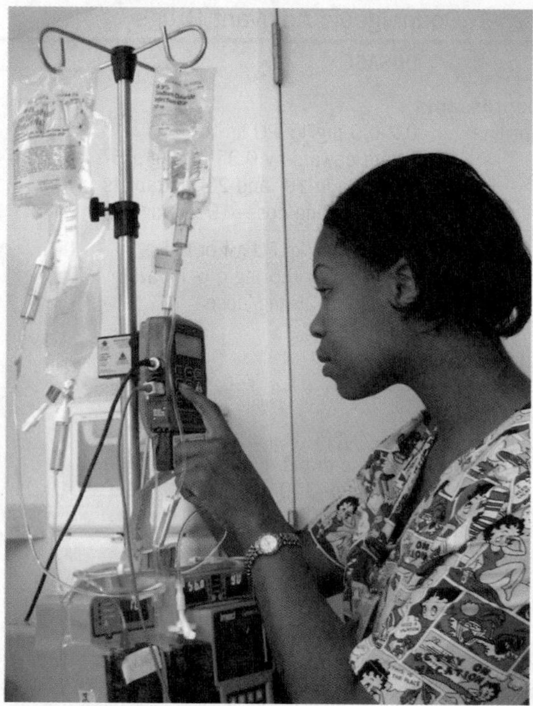

Fig. 35-5 Nurse programming a patient-controlled analges pump to administer analgesic.

Patient-Controlled Analgesia

A significant advance in the administration of IV, epidural, c subcutaneous analgesics is the use of patient-controlled ana gesia (PCA). As the name implies, the patient controls th amount and frequency of the analgesic, which is typical delivered through a special infusion device. Children who a physically able to "push a button" (i.e., 5 to 6 years of age) an who can understand the concept of pushing a button to obtai pain relief can use PCA (Maxwell & Yaster, 2000). Althoug it is controversial, parents and nurses have used the IV PC system for the child. Nurses can efficiently use the infusio device on a child of any age to administer analgesics to avoi signing for and preparing opioid injections every time one needed (Fig. 35-5). When PCA is used as "nurse- or paren controlled" analgesia, the concept of patient control is negate and the inherent safety of PCA needs to be monitore Research has reported safe and effective analgesia in childre when the PCA was controlled by patient, parent, or nurs (Algren et al, 1998; Maxwell & Yaster, 2000).

PCA infusion devices typically allow for three methoc or modes of drug administration to be used alone or i combination:

1. Patient-administered boluses that can only be infused according to the preset amount and *lockout interval* (time between doses). More frequent attempts at self-administration usually mean the patient may need the dose and time adjusted for better pain control.
2. Nurse-administered boluses that are typically used to give an initial loading dose to increase blood levels rapidly and to relieve *breakthrough pain* (pain not relieved with the usual programmed dose).

BOX 35-3 Routes and Methods of Analgesic Drug Administration

Oral

Oral route preferred because of convenience, cost, and relatively steady blood levels

Higher dosages of oral form of opioids required for equivalent parenteral analgesia

Peak drug effect after 1 to 2 hours for most analgesics

Delay in onset a disadvantage when rapid control of severe pain or of fluctuating pain is desired

Sublingual, Buccal, or Transmucosal

Tablet or liquid placed under tongue (sublingual), between cheek and gum (buccal), or through the mucous membrane in general

Highly desirable because more rapid onset than oral route

- Produced less first-pass effect through liver than oral route, which normally reduces analgesia from oral opioids (unless sublingual or buccal form is swallowed, which occurs often in children)

Few drugs commercially available in this form

Many drugs able to be compounded into sublingual troche or lozenge

Actiq—Oral transmucosal fentanyl citrate in hard confection base on a plastic holder; indicated only for management of breakthrough cancer pain in patients with malignancies who are already receiving and are tolerant to opioid therapy, but can be used for preoperative or preprocedural sedation and analgesia

Intravenous (Bolus)

Preferred for rapid control of severe pain

Provides most rapid onset of effect, usually in about 5 minutes

Advantage for acute pain, procedural pain, and breakthrough pain

Needs to be repeated hourly for continuous pain control

Preferable for drugs with short half-life (morphine, fentanyl, hydromorphone) to avoid toxic accumulation of drug

Intravenous (Continuous)

Preferred over bolus and intramuscular injection for maintaining control of pain

Provides steady blood levels

Easy to titrate dosage

Subcutaneous (Continuous)

Used when oral and intravenous (IV) routes not available

Provides equivalent blood levels to continuous IV infusion

Suggested initial bolus dose to equal 2-hour IV dose; total 24-hour dose usually requires concentrated opioid solution to minimize infused volume; use smallest gauge needle that accommodates infusion rate

Patient-Controlled Analgesia

Generally refers to self-administration of drugs, regardless of route

Typically uses programmable infusion pump (IV, epidural, subcutaneous [SC]) that permits self-administration of boluses of medication at preset dose and time interval (*lockout interval* is time between doses)

Patient-controlled analgesia (PCA) bolus administration often combined with initial bolus and continuous (basal or background) infusion of opioid

Optimum lockout interval not known but must be at least as long as time needed for onset of drug

- Should effectively control pain during movement or procedures
- Longer lockout requires larger dose

Family-Controlled Analgesia

One family member (usually a parent) or other caregiver designated as child's primary pain manager with responsibility for pressing PCA button

Guidelines for selecting a primary pain manager for family-controlled analgesia:

- Spends a significant amount of time with the patient
- Is willing to assume responsibility of being primary pain manager
- Is willing to accept and respect patient's reports of pain (if able to provide) as best indicator of how much pain the patient is experiencing; knows how to use and interpret a pain rating scale
- Understands the purpose and goals of patient's pain management plan
- Understands concept of maintaining a steady analgesic blood level
- Recognizes signs of pain and side effects and adverse reactions to opioid

Nurse-Activated Analgesia

Child's primary nurse designated as primary pain manager and is only person who presses PCA button during that nurse's shift

Guidelines for selecting primary pain manager for family-controlled analgesia also applicable to nurse-activated analgesia

May be used in addition to a basal rate to treat breakthrough pain with bolus doses; patients assessed every 30 minutes for the need for a bolus dose

May be used without a basal rate as a means of maintaining analgesia with around-the-clock bolus doses

Intramuscular

NOTE: Not recommended for pain control; not current standard of care

Painful administration (hated by children)

Tissue and nerve damage possible with some drugs

Wide fluctuation in absorption of drug from muscle

Faster absorption from deltoid than from gluteal sites

Shorter duration and more expensive than oral drugs

Time-consuming for staff and unnecessary delay for child

Intranasal

Available commercially as butorphanol (Stadol NS); approved for those older than 18 years of age

Should not be used in patient receiving morphinelike drugs because butorphanol is partial antagonist that will reduce analgesia and may cause withdrawal

Intradermal

Used primarily for skin anesthesia (e.g., before lumbar puncture, bone marrow aspiration, arterial puncture, skin biopsy)

Local anesthetics (e.g., lidocaine) cause stinging, burning sensation

Continued

BOX 35-3 Routes and Methods of Analgesic Drug Administration—cont'd

Intradermal—cont'd

Duration of stinging dependent on type of "caine" used

To avoid stinging sensation associated with lidocaine:

- Buffer the solution by adding 1 part sodium bicarbonate (1 mEq/ml) to 9 or 10 parts 1% or 2% lidocaine with or without epinephrine

Normal saline with preservative, benzyl alcohol, used to anesthetize venipuncture site

Use same dose as for buffered lidocaine

Topical or Transdermal

EMLA (eutectic mixture of local anesthetics [lidocaine and prilocaine]) cream and anesthetic disk or LMX4 (4% lidocaine cream)

- Eliminates or reduces pain from most procedures involving skin puncture
- Must be placed on intact skin over puncture site and covered by occlusive dressing or applied as anesthetic disk for 1 hour or more before procedure

LAT (lidocaine-adrenaline-tetracaine) or tetracaine-phenylephrine (tetraphen)

- Provides skin anesthesia about 15 minutes after application on nonintact skin
- Gel (preferable) or liquid placed on wounds for suturing
- Adrenaline not for use on end arterioles (fingers, toes, tip of nose, penis, earlobes) because of vasoconstriction

Numby Stuff

- Uses iontophoresis to transport lidocaine 2% and epinephrine 1:100,000 (Iontocaine) into the skin
- Current delivered by small battery-powered device that has an electrode with Iontocaine and a ground electrode
- Produces local dermal anesthesia in about 10 minutes to a depth of approximately 10 mm at maximum setting
- May be frightening to young children when they see the device and feel the current
- Observe child during iontophoresis and remove all metal, such as jewelry, from application site to prevent burns

Transdermal fentanyl (Duragesic)

- Available as patch for continuous pain control
- Safety and efficacy not established in children younger than 12 years of age
- Not appropriate for initial relief of acute pain because of long interval to peak effect (12 to 24 hours); for rapid onset of pain relief, give an immediate-release opioid
- Orders for "rescue doses" of an immediate-release opioid recommended for breakthrough pain (a flare of severe pain that breaks through the medication being administered at regular intervals for persistent pain)
- Has duration of up to 72 hours for prolonged pain relief
- If respiratory depression occurs, possible need for several doses of naloxone

Vapocoolant

- Use of prescription spray coolant, such as fluorimethane (Spray and Stretch) or ethyl chloride (Pain Ease)
- Applied to the skin for 10 to 15 seconds immediately before the needle puncture; anesthesia lasts about 15 seconds
- Cold disliked by some children; may be more comfortable to spray coolant on a cotton ball and then apply this to the skin
- Application of ice to the skin for 30 seconds found to be ineffective

Rectal

Alternative to oral or parenteral routes

Variable absorption rate

Generally disliked by children

Many drugs able to be compounded into rectal suppositories*

Regional Nerve Block

Use of long-acting local anesthetic (bupivacaine or ropivacaine) injected into nerves to block pain at site

Provides prolonged analgesia postoperatively, such as after inguinal herniorrhaphy

May be used to provide local anesthesia for surgery, such as dorsal penile nerve block for circumcision or for reduction of fractures

Inhalation

Use of anesthetics, such as nitrous oxide, to produce partial or complete analgesia for painful procedures

Side effects (e.g., headache) possible from occupational exposure to high levels of nitrous oxide

Epidural or Intrathecal

Involves catheter placed into epidural, caudal, or intrathecal space for continuous infusion or single or intermittent administration of opioid with or without a long-acting local anesthetic (e.g., bupivacaine, ropivacaine)

Analgesia primarily from drug's direct effect on opioid receptors in spinal cord

Respiratory depression rare but may have slow and delayed onset; can be prevented by checking level of sedation and respiratory rate and depth hourly for initial 24 hours and decreasing dose when excessive sedation is detected

Nausea, itching, and urinary retention common dose-related side effects from the epidural opioid

Mild hypotension, urinary retention, and temporary motor or sensory deficits common unwanted effects of epidural local anesthetic

Catheter for urinary retention inserted during surgery to decrease trauma to child; if inserted when child is awake, anesthetize urethra with lidocaine

Data primarily from American Pain Society: *Principles of analgesic use in the treatment of acute pain and chronic cancer pain*, ed 4, Skokie, IL, 1999, The Society; and McCaffery M, Pasero C: *Pain: a clinical manual*, ed 2, St Louis, 1999, Mosby.

*For further information about compounding drugs in troche or suppository form, contact Professional Compounding Centers of America (PCCA), 9901 S. Wilcrest Drive, Houston, TX 77009; 800-331-2498; *www.pccarx.com.*

Table 35-9 Suggested Intravenous Patient-Controlled Analgesia Opioid Infusion Orders

DRUG	BASAL RATE (mcg/kg/hr)	BOLUS RATE (mcg/kg/dose)	LOCKOUT PERIOD (min)	MAXIMUM DOSE/HOUR (mg/kg)
Morphine	10-30	10-30	6-10	0.1-0.15
Hydromorphone	3-5	6-10	0.015-0.02	3-5
Fentanyl	0.5-1.0	0.5-1.0	6-10	0.002-0.004

From Yaster M et al: *Pediatric pain management and sedation handbook*, St Louis, 1997, Mosby.

3. Continuous basal rate infusion that delivers a constant amount of analgesic and prevents pain from returning during those times, such as sleep, when the patient cannot control the infusion.

As with any type of analgesic management plan, continued assessment of the child's pain relief is essential for the greatest benefit from PCA. Typical uses of PCA are for controlling pain from surgery, sickle cell crisis, trauma, and cancer. Morphine is the drug of choice for PCA and is usually prepared in a concentration of 10 mcg/ml (Table 35-9). Other options are hydromorphone (2 mcg/ml) and fentanyl (0.1 mcg/ml). Hydromorphone is often used when patients are not able to tolerate side effects such as pruritus and nausea from the morphine PCA (Algren et al, 1998; Maxwell & Yaster, 2000).

Some physicians may still prescribe meperidine. However, meperidine is the least potent and shortest-acting of the synthetic opioids and the least effective in providing analgesia for severe pain. More important, it may increase the risk of seizures when administered chronically because of the excitatory effects on the nervous system of its metabolite, normeperidine.

Epidural Analgesia

Epidural analgesia may also be used to manage pain in selected cases. Although an epidural catheter may be inserted at any vertebral level, it is usually placed into the epidural space of the spinal column at the lumbar or caudal level (Fig. 35-6). The thoracic level is usually reserved for older children or adolescents who have had an upper abdominal or thoracic procedure, such as a lung transplant. An opioid (usually fentanyl, hydromorphone, or preservative-free morphine, which is often combined with a long-acting local anesthetic such as bupivacaine or ropivacaine) is instilled via single or intermittent bolus, continuous infusion, or patient-controlled epidural analgesia. Analgesia results from the drug's effect on opiate receptors in the dorsal horn of the spinal cord, rather than the brain. As a result, respiratory depression is rare, but if it occurs, it develops slowly, typically 6 to 8 hours after administration (Golianu et al, 2000). Properly securing the epidural catheter with an occlusive dressing decreases the possibility of soiling or inadvertently displacing the catheter. Careful monitoring of sedation level and respiratory status is critical to prevent opioid-induced respiratory depression. Assessment of pain and the skin condition around the catheter site is an important aspect of nursing care.

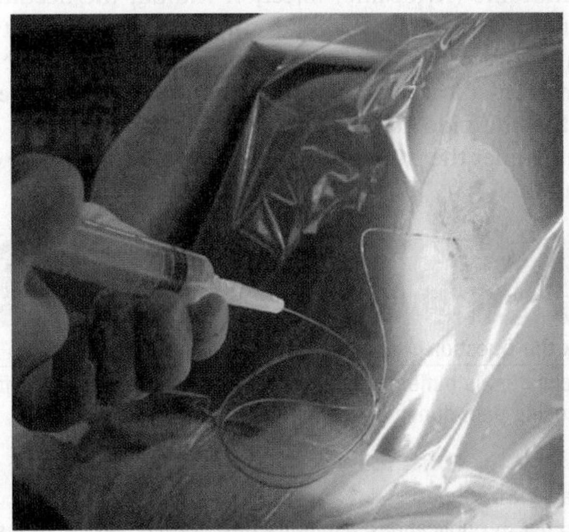

Fig. 35-6 Epidural analgesia catheter placement.

Transmucosal and Transdermal Analgesia

Fentanyl is also available as a transdermal patch (Duragesic). Although contraindicated for acute pain management, it may be used for older children and adolescents who have cancer pain or sickle cell pain or for patients who are opioid tolerant.

One of the most significant improvements in the ability to provide atraumatic care to children is the *anesthetic cream* LMX (a 4% liposomal lidocaine cream) or EMLA (an eutectic mixture of local anesthetics) (Abdelkefi et al, 2004; Choi et al, 2003; Egekvist & Bjerring, 2000; Gad et al, 2005; Rogers & Ostrow, 2004; Santiago et al, 2000; Uziel et al, 2003). The eutectic mixture (lidocaine 2.5% and prilocaine 2.5%), whose melting point is lower than that of the two anesthetics alone, permits effective concentrations of the drug to penetrate intact skin (see Evidence-Based Practice box and Fig. 35-7).

A needle free-system containing 0.5 mg of sterile lidocaine powder (Zingo) is now available and provides a rapid onset of action to reduce pain associated with peripheral IV insertions or blood draws. Two randomized, double-blind, placebo-controlled studies conducted at 15 centers across the United States found significant reduction in procedural pain compared with placebo in children 3 to 18 years of age (Migdal et al, 2006; Zempsky et al, 2008).

In some situations *refrigerant sprays* such as ethyl chloride and fluorimethane can be used (Reis & Holubkov, 1997). When sprayed on the skin, these sprays vaporize, rapidly cooling the area and providing superficial anesthesia. Hospital formularies may have other products with lidocaine, prilocaine, or amethocaine topical preparations that require less time for application.

The LidoSite Topical System is another method to help reduce needlestick pain associated with procedures such as IV cannulation, venipuncture, or laser ablation of superficial skin lesions for patients ages 5 years and older. The LidoSite system delivers numbing medication to the procedure site quickly and effectively after a 10-minute application. The system consists of a single-use, prefilled LidoSite patch, filled with lidocaine hydrochloride 10% and epinephrine 0.1%, and the LidoSite controller, an easy-to-use preprogrammed device that activates the patch. It provides pain reduction equivalent to that of a lidocaine (Xylocaine) injection without the needlestick. Through iontophoresis, a mild current from the controller activates the patch to accelerate delivery of lidocaine—the anesthetic medication—to the injection site. Epinephrine contained in the LidoSite patch helps focus the anesthetic effect directly under the patch and extends the duration of the effect for an hour.

The *intradermal route* is sometimes used to inject a local anesthetic, typically lidocaine, into the skin to reduce the pain from a lumbar puncture, bone marrow aspiration, or venous or arterial access. One problem with the use of lidocaine is the stinging and burning that initially occur. However, the use of buffered lidocaine with sodium bicarbonate (see Evidence-Based Practice box) reduces the stinging sensation (Wong & Pasero, 1997a, 1997b). Warming the lidocaine to 37° C (98.6° F) may accomplish the same effect.

Timing of Analgesia

The right timing for administering analgesics depends on the type of pain. For *continuous pain control,* such as for postoperative or cancer pain, a preventive schedule of medication *around the clock (ATC)* is effective. The ATC schedule avoids the low concentrations of medications in plasma that permit breakthrough pain. If analgesics are administered only when

EVIDENCE-BASED PRACTICE Buffered Lidocaine for Pain Reduction During Peripheral Intravenous Access in Children

—Angela C. Morgan

Ask the Question

In children, is buffered lidocaine an appropriate anesthetic for reducing pain during peripheral intravenous (PIV) access?

Search for Evidence

Search Strategies

English publications within the past 5 years, research-based articles (level 3 or lower) on children undergoing PIV access; two articles more than 5 years old included based on the limited literature in this area

Databases Searched

PubMed, Cochrane Collaboration, MD Consult, Joanna Briggs Institute, National Guideline Clearinghouse (AHQR), TRIP Database, PedsCCM, Best BETs

Critically Analyze the Evidence

A review of the literature revealed 10 studies evaluating buffered lidocaine given before PIV access from 1991 through 1999 (Murphy, 2000). Four of the studies were specific to pediatrics. Findings from the pediatric studies support buffered lidocaine as a pain reduction measure in children before PIV access.

- A randomized trial consisting of 69 subjects ranging from 4 to 17 years of age (61% female) evaluated buffered lidocaine vs. LMX (liposomal lidocaine cream) before PIV access. Results showed both interventions decreased pain and resulted in no significant differences in pain levels. The LMX group stated that the pain came with the removal of the occlusive dressing from the site (Luhmann et al, 2004).
- Fein and colleagues (1998) evaluated buffered lidocaine vs. no pain control measures in a group of 99 children requiring PIV access in the emergency department (ED). PIV access without buffered lidocaine was significantly more painful than PIV access with buffered lidocaine.
- Sacchetti and Carraccio (1996) evaluated subcutaneous lidocaine vs. no pain control measures in 110 children less than 2 years of age before PIV access in the ED. No significant differences in pain levels were found in the groups. A weakness to this trial was that it was not blinded or randomized.
- A randomized clinical trial of 59 children requiring PIV access in the ED evaluated the use and nonuse of subcutaneous lidocaine before PIV access. PIV access without lidocaine was significantly more painful than PIV access with lidocaine regardless of catheter size. Trial weaknesses included a small sample size with wide confidence levels and no randomization (Klein et al, 1995).

Apply the Evidence: Nursing Implications

Age–More than 2 years
Time of onset–Immediate
Duration–1 hour
Multiple sites–Yes
Use with abraded skin–No
Impact on PIV access difficulty–Possibility of some vasoconstriction
Timing–Do not use within 2 hours before vesicants
Dose–0.1 to 0.5 ml buffered 1% lidocaine, to a maximum of 0.45 ml/kg/dose; can repeat dose after 2 hours
Considerations–An "extra stick" and ineffective buffered lidocaine administration may result in pain during both local administration and PIV access. Expertise in administering buffered lidocaine is an important factor related to its effectiveness.

References

Fein JA et al: Saline with benzyl alcohol as intradermal anesthesia for intravenous line placement in children, *Pediatr Emerg Care* 14(2):119-122, 1998.

Klein EJ et al: Buffered lidocaine: analgesia for intravenous line placement in children, *Pediatrics* 95(5):709-712, 1995.

Luhmann J et al: A comparison of buffered lidocaine versus ELA-Max before peripheral intravenous catheter insertions in children, *Pediatrics* 113(3 Pt 1):217-220, 2004.

Murphy R: Prior injection of local anaesthetic and the pain and success of intravenous cannulation, 2000. Available at www.bestbets.org (accessed March 2005).

Sacchetti AD, Carraccio C: Subcutaneous lidocaine does not affect the success rate of intravenous access in children less than 24 months of age, *Acad Emerg Med* 3(11):1016-1019, 1996.

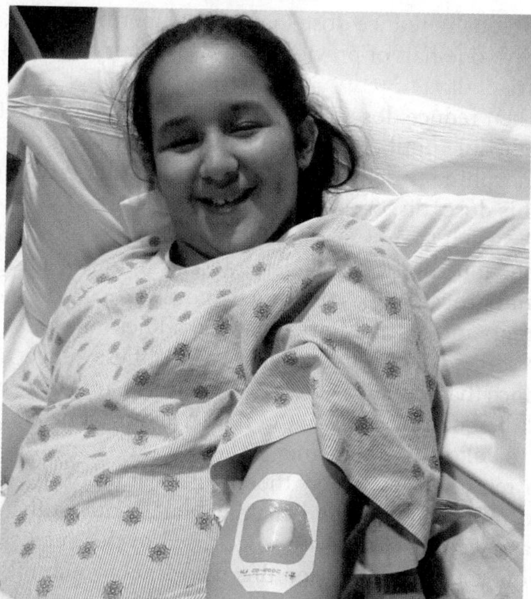

Fig. 35-7 LMX is an effective analgesic before intravenous insertion or blood draw.

pain returns (a typical use of the prn, or "as needed," order), pain relief may take several hours. This may require higher doses, leading to a cycle of undermedication of pain alternating with periods of overmedication and drug toxicity. This cycle of erratic pain control also promotes *"clock watching,"* which may be erroneously equated with addiction. Nurses can effectively use prn orders by giving the drug at regular intervals, since "as needed" should be interpreted as "as needed to prevent pain," not "as little as possible."

Preventive pain control is best provided through continuous IV infusion rather than intermittent boluses. If intermittent boluses are given, the intervals between doses should not exceed the drug's expected duration of effectiveness. For extended pain control with fewer administration times, drugs that provide longer duration of action (e.g., some NSAIDs, time-released morphine or oxycodone, methadone, levorphanol) can be used.

Continuous analgesia is not always appropriate, since not all pain is continuous. Frequently, temporary pain control or conscious sedation is needed to provide analgesia before a scheduled procedure. When pain can be predicted, the drug's *peak effect* should be timed to coincide with the painful event. For example, with opioids the peak effect is approximately a half hour for the IV route; with nonopioids the peak effect occurs about 2 hours after oral administration. For rapid onset and peak of action, opioids that quickly penetrate the blood-brain barrier (e.g., IV fentanyl) provide excellent pain control.

Monitoring Side Effects

Both NSAIDs and opioids have side effects, although the major concern is with those from opioids (Box 35-4). *Respiratory depression* is the most serious complication and is most likely to occur in sedated patients. The respiratory rate may decrease gradually, or respirations may cease abruptly. Lower limits of normal are not established for children, but any significant change from a previous rate calls for increased vigilance. A slower respiratory rate does not necessarily reflect decreased arterial oxygenation; an increased depth of ventilation may compensate for the altered rate. If respiratory depression or arrest occurs, the nurse must be prepared to intervene quickly (see Guidelines box).

Although respiratory depression is the most feared side effect, *constipation* is a common, and sometimes serious, side effect of opioids, which decrease peristalsis and increase anal sphincter tone. Prevention with stool softeners and laxatives is more effective than treatment once constipation occurs. Dietary treatment, such as increased fiber, is usually not sufficient to promote regular bowel evacuation. However, dietary measures, such as increased fluid and fruit intake, and physical activity are encouraged. *Pruritus* from epidural or IV infusion can be treated with low doses of IV naloxone, nalbuphine, or diphenhydramine. *Nausea, vomiting,* and *sedation* usually subside after 2 days of opioid administration; however, oral or rectal antiemetics may be necessary.

Both tolerance and physical dependence can occur with prolonged use of opioids (see Family-Centered Care box,

BOX 35-4 Side Effects of Opioids

General

Constipation (possibly severe)
Respiratory depression
Sedation
Nausea and vomiting
Agitation, euphoria
Mental clouding
Hallucinations
Orthostatic hypotension
Pruritus
Urticaria
Sweating
Miosis (may be sign of toxicity)
Anaphylaxis (rare)

Signs of Tolerance

Decreasing pain relief
Decreasing duration of pain relief

Signs of Withdrawal Syndrome in Patients with Physical Dependence

Initial Signs of Withdrawal

Lacrimation
Rhinorrhea
Yawning
Sweating

Later Signs of Withdrawal

Restlessness
Irritability
Tremors
Anorexia
Dilated pupils
Gooseflesh
Nausea, vomiting

GUIDELINES Managing Opioid-Induced Respiratory Depression

If Respirations Are Depressed

Assess sedation level.

Reduce infusion by 25% when possible.

Stimulate patient (shake shoulder gently, call by name, ask to breathe).

If Patient Cannot Be Aroused or Is Apneic

Administer naloxone (Narcan).

- For children weighing less than 40 kg (88 pounds), dilute 0.1 mg naloxone in 10 ml sterile saline to make 10 mcg/ml solution, and give 0.5 mcg/kg.
- For children weighing more than 40 kg, dilute 0.4-mg ampule in 10 ml sterile saline, and give 0.5 ml.

Administer bolus by slow intravenous push every 2 minutes until effect is obtained.

Closely monitor patient. Naloxone's duration of antagonist action may be shorter than that of opioid, requiring repeated doses of naloxone.

NOTE: Respiratory depression caused by benzodiazepines (e.g., diazepam [Valium] or midazolam [Versed]) can be reversed with flumazenil (Romazicon). Pediatric dosing experience suggests 0.01 mg/kg (0.1 ml/kg); if no (or inadequate) response after 1 to 2 minutes, administer same dose and repeat as needed at 60-second intervals for maximum dose of 1 mg (10 ml).

Adapted from Yaster M et al: *Pediatric pain management and sedation handbook*, St Louis, 1997, Mosby.

p. 936). *Physical dependence* is a normal, natural, physiologic state of neuroadaptation. When opioids are abruptly discontinued without weaning, *withdrawal symptoms* occur. Symptoms of withdrawal occur at 24 hours after abrupt discontinuation and reach a peak within 72 hours. Symptoms of withdrawal include signs of neurologic excitability (irritability, tremors, seizures, increased motor tone, insomnia), gastrointestinal dysfunction (nausea, vomiting, diarrhea, abdominal cramps), and autonomic dysfunction (sweating, fever, chills, tachypnea, nasal congestion, rhinitis). Withdrawal symptoms can be anticipated and prevented by weaning patients from opioids that were administered for more than 5 to 10 days. Adherence to a weaning protocol to prevent or minimize withdrawal symptoms from opioids will be required. A weaning flow sheet may be used to assess the efficacy of opioid weaning in neonates (Franck & Vilardi, 1995; Franck et al, 1998) (Fig. 35-8).

Tolerance occurs when the dose of an opioid needs to be increased to achieve the same analgesic effects that was previously achieved at a lower dose. Tolerance may develop after 10 to 21 days of morphine administration. Treatment of tolerance involves increasing the dose or decreasing the duration between doses. Treatment of physical dependence involves gradually reducing the dose over several days to prevent withdrawal symptoms. The following are guidelines for treating physical dependence from morphine:

- Gradually reduce dose (similar to tapering of steroids).
- Give one half of previous daily dose every 6 hours for first 2 days.
- Then reduce dose by 25% every 2 days. Continue this schedule until total daily dosage of 0.6 mg/kg/day of morphine (or equivalent) is reached. After 2 days on this dose, discontinue opioid.
- A switch to oral methadone may also be done, using one fourth of equianalgesic dose as initial weaning dose and proceeding as described above.

Parents and older children may fear addiction when opioids are prescribed. The nurse should address these concerns with assurance that any such risk is extremely low. It may be helpful to ask the question, "If you did not have this pain, would you want to take this medicine?" The answer is invariably no, which reinforces the solely therapeutic nature of the drug. It is also important to avoid making statements to the family such as "We don't want you to get used to this medicine," or "By now you shouldn't need this medicine," which may reinforce the fear of becoming addicted. Whereas both physical dependence and tolerance are physiologic states, *addiction* or *psychologic dependence* is a psychologic state and implies a "cause-effect" mode of thinking, such as "I need the drug because it makes me feel better." Infants and children do not have the cognitive ability to make the cause-effect association and therefore cannot become addicted. The use of opioid analgesics early in life has not been demonstrated to increase the risk for addiction later in life. Nurses need to explain to parents the differences among physical dependence, tolerance, and addiction and allow parents to express concerns about the use and duration of use of opioids. Infants and children, when treated appropriately with opioids, may be at risk for physical tolerance and physical dependence, but not psychologic dependence or addiction (Turner, 2005; Greco & Berde, 2005).

Evaluation of Effectiveness of Pain Regimen

The effectiveness of analgesics can be enhanced by a supportive attitude toward the child. By reinforcing the cause and effect of the medication and analgesia, the nurse can condition the child to expect pain relief, provided the regimen is likely to be effective. A pain relief scale or periodic ratings of pain intensity should be used for evaluation of effectiveness of pain regimens.

The response to therapy should be evaluated 15 to 30 minutes after each dose, and titration should continue to the highest achievable amount of relief. Even though The Joint Commission required documentation of pain assessments with vital signs, evidence of pain relief was not documented in 41.4% of the episodes. Titration methods in the emergency department or during the course of hospitalization, if used, were not reflected in the amount of medications received by the children (Jacob et al, 2003a, 2003b).

Several harmful effects occur with unrelieved pain, particularly when pain is prolonged. A number of *physiologic stress responses* in the body are triggered during pain, and they lead to negative consequences that involve multiple systems. Unrelieved pain may prolong the stress response and adversely

Children's Hospital Oakland Opioid Weaning Flowsheet and Guidelines for Use of the Form
Analgesia/sedation orders (drug/dose/frequency)

Date			
Drug			
Administration time			
Dose ↑ or ↓ or freq change			
	Time:		
Choose one: Crying/agitated 25%-50% of interval Crying/agitated >50% of interval	 2 3		
Choose one: Sleeps ≤25% of interval Sleeps 26%-75% of interval Sleeps >75% of interval	 3 2 1		
Choose one: Hyperactive Moro Markedly hyperactive Moro	 2 3		
Choose one: Mild tremors, disturbed Moderate/severe tremors, disturbed	 1 2		
Increased muscle tone	2		
Temperature 37.2°-38.4°C	1		
Temperature >38.4°C	2		
Respiratory rate >60 (extubated)	2		
Suction >twice/interval (intubated)	2		
Sweating	1		
Frequent yawning (>3-4/interval)	1		
Sneezing (>3-4/interval)	1		
Nasal stuffiness	1		
Emesis	2		
Projectile vomiting	3		
Loose stools	2		
Watery stools	3		
TOTAL SCORE			
ADJUSTED SCORE			
INITIALS OF PERSON SCORING			

Directions: Score every 2-4 hours per guideline
Score greater than 8-12 may indicate withdrawal

Guidelines for use of the flow sheet

Use of form

Use the flowsheet for all infants who have received continuous or around-the-clock opioid medication for 3 days or more, or more than 3 doses per day for more than 5 days. This patient population will most often include postoperative patients, agitated intubated infants, and all post-ECMO patients.

Instructions

1. Write drug, dose, and frequency of analgesics and sedatives ordered
2. Enter date, name of drug (abbreviated MS=morphine sulfate or FENT=fentanyl), and administration time of drugs given in the appropriate boxes; indicate if dose frequency given is an increase or decrease from the ordered dose
3. Scoring must be performed every 4 hours during weaning of opioids, every 2 hours if score is 8 or greater. The score for each item indicates the presence of the sign during the previous 2-4 hours (depending on the scoring interval). Every 4-hour scoring should continue until the patient is off all opioids for 48-72 hours. Place a "0" in the column after the sign if it is not seen during the scoring period.

Central nervous system

Crying behavior: Score 2 points if patient exhibits crying or cry behavior for a duration of ≤50% of the scoring interval. Score 3 points if cumulative crying behavior totals >50% of the scoring interval.
NOTE: Crying behavior is accompanied by the facial expressions associated with crying, but without audible sounds because of endotracheal intubation.
Sleeping: Score 3 points if patient sleeps for ≤25% of the scoring interval. Score 2 points if patient sleeps for 26%-75% of the scoring interval. Score 1 point if patient sleeps for >75% of the scoring interval.
Moro (startle) reflex: Score 2 points if patient has some arm and/or leg extension when touched or when disturbed by loud noises. Score 3 points if patient has marked arm and/or leg extension that is accompanied by crying behavior, hyperalert state, or continued arm and/or leg tremors after being startled.
Tremors—disturbed: Score 1 point if patient has mild tremors when disturbed. Score 2 points if patient has moderate to severe tremors when disturbed. NOTE: Tremors are alternating movements that are rhythmic, of equal rate and amplitude, and can usually be stopped by flexion of the limb.
Increased muscle tone: Score 2 points if patient exhibits fisting or tight flexion of extremities that are difficult to extend.

Metabolic

Temperature: Score 1 point if patient's temperature is 37.2°-38.4°C. Score 2 points if patient's temperature is >38.4°C.
Respiratory rate: Score 1 point if patient's spontaneous respiratory rate is >60/minute. Score 2 points if patient's spontaneous respiratory rate is >60/minute and accompanied by retractions.
Suction: Score 2 points if patient is suctioned more than twice during a 4-hour period.
Sweating: Score 1 point if patient exhibits any type of sweating, including beads of sweat, or if skin is moist to touch.
Yawning: Score 1 point if patient yawns >3-4 times in succession or yawns 1-2 times often during a 4-hour period.
Sneezing: Score 1 point if patient sneezes >3-4 times in succession or sneezes 1-2 times during a 4-hour period.
Nasal stuffiness: Score 1 point for nasal stuffiness.

Gastrointestinal

Emesis of formula/stomach contents: Score 2 points if patient has 1 or more episodes of emesis during a 4-hour period.
Projectile vomiting: Score 3 points if patient has 1 or more episodes of projectile vomiting.
Loose stools: Score 2 points if patient has loose stools characterized by a water ring around some solid stool. The stools will often be frequent. NOTE: Do not score for "breast milk" stools: frequent, small, seedy, yellow stools.
Watery stools: Score 3 points if patient has stools that consist of only liquid. The stools will often be frequent.

Total score: Add up all the scores in the column and place the total score in this box. Clinical signs that appear continuously, such as respiratory rate >60 or regular poor feeding, should be included in the total score.
Adjusted score: The adjusted score is used when a sign is detected that is expected to occur independently of withdrawal, due to a preexisting condition (high respiratory rate in infant with bronchopulmonary dysplasia). The decision to adjust the score should be made after discussion with the healthcare team during rounds, and the rationale should be recorded in a problem-oriented note. Circle the signs to be excluded and deduct the points from the total score to obtain the adjusted score.
Initials of person scoring: The person scoring should write his/her initials in this space.

Fig. 35-8 Weaning flow sheet to monitor opioid weaning in neonates.

affect an infant or child's recovery, whether it is from trauma, surgery, or disease. In a landmark study by Anand and Hickey (1992), 30 neonates received deep intraoperative anesthesia with high doses of the opioid sufentanil, followed postoperatively by an infusion of opioids for 24 hours, and 15 neonates received lighter anesthesia with halothane and morphine followed postoperatively by intermittent morphine and diazepam. The 15 neonates who received the lighter anesthesia and intermittent postoperative opioids had more severe hyperglycemia and lactic acidemia, and four postoperative deaths occurred in the group. The 30 neonates who received deep anesthesia had a lower incidence of complications (sepsis, metabolic acidosis, disseminated intravascular coagulation) and no deaths.

Poorly controlled acute pain can predispose patients to *chronic pain syndromes*. A guiding principle in pain management is that prevention of pain is always better than treatment (Benjamin, Swinson, & Nagel, 2000). Pain that is established and severe is often more difficult to control. When pain is unrelieved, sensory input from injured tissues reaches spinal cord neurons and may enhance subsequent responses. Long-lasting changes in cells within spinal cord pain pathways may occur after a brief painful stimulus and may lead to the development of chronic pain conditions. Basbaum (1999a, 1999b) reported a series of studies that emphasize a distinct neurochemistry of acute and persistent pain and concluded that persistent pain is not merely a prolonged acute pain symptom of some other disease. Underlying physiologic mechanisms lead to the persistence of pain (Marx, 2004; Woolf & Salter, 2000).

In a study of nursing practice related to pain assessment and management in different pediatric specialty units, Jacob and Puntillo (2000) noted nurses were aware of complaints of pain but seldom documented patient-specific pain scores or notations about responses to analgesics after administration. Pain scores were not available before and after analgesics, and it was therefore not possible to conclude whether analgesics were effective. Nurses need to evaluate and monitor pain in a timely fashion after administration of analgesics; titrate dosage to effect; or make recommendations for an alternate analgesic, for addition of another analgesic, or for a combination of analgesics, adjuvants, and nonpharmacologic strategies.

Key Points

- Although the ability to measure pain in children has improved dramatically in recent years, assessment of pain in children continues to be complex and challenging.
- Behavioral assessment is useful for measuring pain in infants and preverbal children who do not have the language skills to communicate that they are in pain, or when mental clouding and confusion limit a child's ability to communicate.
- Physiologic measures are not able to distinguish between physical responses to pain and other forms of stress to the body.
- The number of pain measures that are available for use in infants and young children has increased dramatically and adds a layer of complexity to the assessment of pain in children.
- Important components of assessment include the onset of pain; pain duration or pattern; effectiveness of the current treatment; factors that aggravate or relieve the pain; other symptoms and complications concurrently felt; and interference with the child's mood, function, and interactions with family.
- The administration of sucrose with or without nonnutritive sucking has been demonstrated to have calming and pain-relieving effects for invasive procedures in neonates.
- One of the most significant improvements in the ability to provide atraumatic care to children is the anesthetic creams LMX and EMLA.

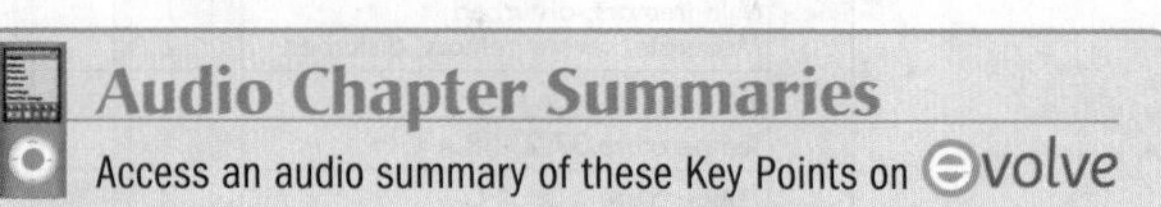
Audio Chapter Summaries
Access an audio summary of these Key Points on evolve

- Nonopioids, including acetaminophen and NSAIDs, are suitable for mild to moderate pain; opioids are needed for moderate to severe pain.
- Several drugs, known as *coanalgesics* or *adjuvant analgesics,* may be used alone or with opioids to control pain symptoms and opioid side effects.
- A significant advance in the administration of IV, epidural, or subcutaneous analgesics is the use of PCA.
- Although respiratory depression is the most feared side effect of opioids, constipation is a common, and sometimes serious, side effect, which decreases peristalsis and increases anal sphincter tone.
- Several harmful effects occur with unrelieved pain, particularly when pain is prolonged.
- Surgery and traumatic injuries generate a catabolic state as a result of increased secretion of catabolic hormones and lead to alterations in blood flow, coagulation, fibrinolysis, substrate metabolism, and water and electrolyte balance, and increase the demands on the cardiovascular and respiratory systems.

References

Abdelkefi A et al: Effectiveness of fixed 50% nitrous oxide oxygen mixture and EMLA cream for insertion of central venous catheters in children, *Pediatr Blood Cancer* 43(7):777-779, 2004.

Algren JT et al: The effect of nitrous oxide diffusion on laryngeal mask airway cuff inflation in children, *Paediatr Anaesth* 8(1):31-36, 1998.

Anand KJ, Hickey PR: Halothane-morphine compared with high-dose sufentanil for anesthesia and postoperative analgesia in neonatal cardiac surgery, *N Engl J Med* 326(1):1-9, 1992.

Barrier G et al: Measurement of post-operative pain and narcotic administration in infants using a new clinical scoring system, *Anesthesiology* 67(3A):A532, 1987.

Basbaum AI: Distinct neurochemical features of acute and persistent pain, *Proc Natl Acad Sci USA* 96(14):7739-7743, 1999a.

Basbaum AI: Spinal mechanisms of acute and persistent pain, *Reg Anesth Pain Med* 24(1):59-67, 1999b.

Benjamin L, Swinson G, Nagel R: Sickle cell anemia day hospital: an approach for the management of uncomplicated painful crises, *Blood* 95:1130-1137, 2000.

Bernstein B, Pachter L: Cultural considerations in children's pain. In Schechter N, Berde C, Yaster M (editors): *Pain in infants, children, and adolescents,* Philadelphia, 2003, Lippincott Williams & Wilkins.

Beyer JE, Denyes MJ, Villarruel AM: The creation, validation and continuing development of the Oucher: a measure of pain intensity in children, *J Pediatr Nurs* 7(5):335-346, 1992. Internet document available from http://www.oucher.org (accessed May 3, 2007).

Beyer JE, Knott CB: Construct validity estimation for the African-American and Hispanic versions of the Oucher scale, *J Pediatr Nurs* 13(1): 20-31, 1998.

Blauer T, Gerstmann D: A simultaneous comparison of three neonatal pain scales during common NICU procedures, *Clin J Pain* 14(1):39-47, 1998.

Breau LM et al: Caregivers' beliefs regarding pain in children with cognitive impairment: relation between pain sensation and reaction increases with severity of impairment, *Clin J Pain* 19(6):335-344, 2003.

Breau LM et al: Psychometric properties of the Non-communicating Children's Pain Checklist–Revised, *Pain* 99:349-357, 2002.

Chambers CT et al: Faces scales for the measurement of postoperative pain intensity in children following minor surgery, *Clin J Pain* 21(3):277-285, 2005.

Chambers CT et al: A comparison of faces scales for the measurement of pediatric pain: children's and parents' ratings, *Pain* 83:25-35, 1999.

Choi WY et al: EMLA cream versus dorsal penile nerve block for postcircumcision analgesia in children, *Anesth Analg* 96(2):396-399, 2003.

Cline ME et al: Standardization of the visual analogue scale, *Nurs Res* 41(6):378-380, 1992.

Cole J, Jorgensen K: Medical, developmental, and pharmacologic intervention: the essence of collaboration, *Neonatal Netw* 16:56-58, 1997.

Egekvist H, Bjerring P: Effect of EMLA cream on skin thickness and subcutaneous venous diameter: a randomized, placebo-controlled study in children, *Acta Dermatol Venereol* 80(5):340-343, 2000.

Eland JA, Banner W: Analgesia, sedation, and neuromuscular blockage in pediatric critical care. In Hazinski ME (editor): *Manual of pediatric critical care*, St Louis, 1999, Mosby.

Fearon I et al: Swaddling after heel lance: age-specific effects on behavioral recovery in preterm infants, *Develop Behav Pediatr* 18:222-232, 1997.

Franck L, Vilardi J: Assessment and management of opioid withdrawal in ill neonates, *Neonatal Netw* 14(2):39-48, 1995.

Franck LS et al: Opioid withdrawal in neonates after continuous infusions of morphine or fentanyl during extracorporeal membrane oxygenation, *Am J Crit Care* 7(5):364-369, 1998.

Gad LN et al: Optimized use of EMLA cream in children—secondary publication: a randomized, prospective, controlled comparison of two application regimes, *Ugeskr Laeger* 167(4):404-407, 2005.

Gerik SM: Pain management in children: developmental considerations and mind-body therapies, *South Med J* 98(3):295-302, 2005.

Gold JI et al: Effectiveness of virtual reality for pediatric pain distraction during i.v. placement, *Cyberpsychol Behav* 9(2):207-212, 2006.

Goldschneider K, Anand K: Long-term consequences of pain in neonates. In Schechter N, Berde C, Yaster M (editors): *Pain in infants, children, and adolescents*, Philadelphia, 2003, Lippincott Williams & Wilkins.

Golianu B et al: Pediatric acute pain management, *Pediatr Clin North Am* 47(3):559-587, 2000.

Gray L, Watt L, Blass E: Skin-to-skin contact is analgesic in healthy newborns, *Pediatrics* 105(1):110-111, 2000.

Greco C, Berde C: Pain management for the hospitalized pediatric patient, *Pediatr Clin North Am* 52(4):995-1027, 2005.

Hadden KL, von Baeyer CL: Pain in children with cerebral palsy: common triggers and expressive behaviors, *Pain* 99(1-2):281-288, 2002.

Hadjistavropoulos HD et al: Judging pain in infants: behavioural, contextual, and developmental determinants, *Pain* 73(3):319-324, 1997.

Hannallah RS et al: Comparison of caudal and ilioinguinal/iliohypogastric nerve blocks for control of post-orchiopexy pain in pediatric ambulatory surgery, *Anesthesiology* 66:832-834, 1987.

Hester NO et al: Putting pain measurement into clinical practice. In Finley GA, McGrath PJ (editors): *Measurement of pain in infants and children*, vol 10, Seattle, 1998, IASP Press.

Hodgkinson K et al: Measuring pain in neonates: evaluating an instrument and developing a common language, *Aust J Adv Nurs* 12(1):17-22, 1994.

Jacob E, Puntillo KA: Variability of analgesic practices for hospitalized children on different pediatric specialty units, *J Pain Symptom Manage* 20(1):59-67, 2000.

Jacob E et al: Changes in intensity, location, and quality of vaso-occlusive pain in children with sickle cell disease, *Pain* 102(1-2):187-193, 2003a.

Jacob E et al: Management of vaso-occlusive pain in hospitalized children with sickle cell disease, *J Pediatr Hematol Oncol* 25(4):307-311, 2003b.

Johnston CC et al: Kangaroo care is effective in diminishing pain response in preterm neonates, *Arch Pediatr Adolesc Med* 157(11):1084-1088, 2003.

Jordan-Marsh M et al: Alternate Oucher form testing: gender, ethnicity, and age variations, *Res Nurs Health* 17:111-118, 1994.

Joyce BA et al: Reliability and validity of preverbal pain assessment tools, *Issues Comp Pediatr Nurs* 17:121-135, 1994.

Kain ZN et al: Preoperative anxiety, postoperative pain, and behavioral recovery in young children undergoing surgery, *Pediatrics* 118(2):651-658, 2006.

Krechel SW, Bildner J: CRIES: a new neonatal postoperative pain measurement score: initial testing of validity and reliability, *Pediatr Anaesth* 5:53-61, 1995.

Lawrence J et al: The development of a tool to assess neonatal pain, *Neonatal Netw* 12(6):59-66, 1993.

Lenton S et al: Prevalence and morbidity associated with non-malignant, life-threatening conditions in childhood, *Child Care Health Devel* 27(5):389-398, 2001.

Luffy R, Grove SK: Examining the validity, reliability, and preference of three pediatric pain measurement tools in African-American children, *Pediatr Nurs* 29(1):54-60, 2003.

Malviya S et al: The revised FLACC observational pain tool: improved reliability and validity for pain assessment in children with cognitive impairment, *Pediatr Anaesth* 16(3):258-265, 2006.

Manworren R, Hynan L: Clinical validation of FLACC: Preverbal Patient Pain Scale, *Pediatr Nurs* 29(2):140-146, 2003.

Marx J: Pain research: prolonging the agony, *Science* 305(5682):326-329, 2004.

Maxwell L, Yaster M: Perioperative management issues in pediatric patients, *Anesthesiol Clin North Am* 18(3):601-632, 2000.

McCaffery M, Pasero C: *Pain clinical manual*, ed 2, St Louis, 1999, Mosby.

McGrath P: Behavioral measures of pain. In Finley G, McGrath P (editors): *Measurement of pain in infants and children*, Seattle, 1998, IASP Press.

McGrath P, Hillier L (editors): *Modifying the psychologic factors that intensify children's pain and prolong disability*, Philadelphia, 2003, Lippincott Williams & Wilkins.

McGrath PJ et al: The CHEOPS: a behavioral scale to measure postoperative pain in children. In Fields H, Dubner R, Cervero F (editors): *Advances in pain research and therapy*, New York, 1985, Raven Press.

Melzack R: The McGill pain questionnaire: major properties and scoring methods, *Pain* 1:277-299, 1975.

Merkel SI et al: The FLACC: a behavioral scale for scoring postoperative pain in young children, *Pediatr Nurs* 23(3):293-297, 1997.

Miaskowski C, Lee K: Pain, fatigue, and sleep disturbances in oncology outpatients receiving radiation therapy for bone metastasis: a pilot study, *J Pain Symptom Manage* 17(5):320-332, 1999.

Migdal M et al: Rapid, needle-free delivery of lidocaine for reducing the pain of venipuncture among pediatric subjects, *Pediatrics* 115(4):e393-e398, 2006.

Morin C, Gibson D, Wade J: Self-reported sleep and mood disturbance in chronic pain patients, *Clin J Pain* 14(4):311-314, 1998.

Myers C et al: Complementary therapies and childhood cancer, *Cancer Control* 12(3):172-180, 2005.

Puchalski M, Hummel P: The reality of neonatal pain, *Adv Neonatal Care* 2(5):233-244, 2002.

Reis E, Holubkov R: Vapocoolant spray is equally effective as EMLA cream in reducing immunization pain in school-aged children, *Pediatrics* 100(6):E5, 1997.

Robieux I et al: Assessing pain and analgesia with a lidocaine-prilocaine emulsion in infants and toddlers during venipuncture, *J Pediatr* 118(6):971-973, 1991.

Rogers TL, Ostrow CL: The use of EMLA cream to decrease venipuncture pain in children, *J Pediatr Nurs* 19(1):33-39, 2004.

Rusy L, Weisman S: Complementary therapies for acute pediatric pain management, *Pediatr Clin North Am* 47(3):589-599, 2000.

Santiago A et al: Premedication with EMLA cream for ambulatory surgery in children, *Ambul Surg* 8(3):157, 2000.

Schade JG et al: Comparison of three preverbal scales for postoperative pain assessment in a diverse pediatric sample, *J Pain Symptom Manage* 12(6):348-359, 1996.

Stallard P et al: The development and evaluation of the pain indicator for communicatively impaired children (PICIC), *Pain* 98(1-2):145-149, 2002a.

Stallard P et al: Intervening factors in caregivers' assessments of pain in non-communicating children, *Devel Med Child Neurol* 44(3):213-214, 2002b.

Stanford EA, Chambers CT, Craig KD: The role of developmental factors in predicting young children's use of a self-report scale for pain, *Pain* 120(1-2):16-23, 2006.

Stevens B: Development and testing of a pediatric pain management sheet, *Pediatr Nurs* 16(6):543-548, 1990.

Stevens B, Yamada J, Ohlsson A: *Sucrose for analgesia in newborn infants undergoing painful procedures* (review), 2005. In Cochrane Neonatal Collaboration, Internet document available from http://www.thecochranelibrary.com (accessed May 4, 2007).

Stevens B et al: Premature Infant Pain Profile: development and initial validation, *Clin J Pain* 12:13-22, 1996.

Sweet S, McGrath P: Physiological measures of pain. In Finley G, McGrath P (editors): *Measurement of pain in infants and children*, Seattle, 1998, IASP Press.

Taddio A et al: A revised measure of acute pain in infants, *J Pain Symptom Manage* 10(6):456-463, 1995.

Tesler MD et al: The word-graphic rating scale as a measure of children's and adolescents' pain intensity, *Res Nurs Health* 14:361-371, 1991.

Turner HN: Complex pain consultations in the pediatric intensive care unit, *AACN Clin Issues* 16(3):388-395, 2005.

Uziel Y et al: Evaluation of eutectic lidocaine/prilocaine cream (EMLA) for steroid joint injection in children with juvenile rheumatoid arthritis: a double blind, randomized, placebo controlled trial, *J Rheumatol* 30(3):594-596, 2003.

Villarruel AM, Denyes MJ: Pain assessment in children: theoretical and empirical validity, *Adv Nurs Sci* 14(2):32-41, 1991.

Weisman S, Bernstein B, Schechter N: Consequences of inadequate analgesia during painful procedures in children, *Arch Pediatr Adolesc Med* 152:147-149, 1998.

Wong DL, Baker CM: Pain in children: comparison of assessment scales, *Pediatr Nurs* 14(1):9-17, 1988.

Wong D, Pasero CL: Reducing the pain of lidocaine, *Am J Nurs* 97(1):17-18, 1997a.

Wong D, Pasero CL: Using local anesthetics to control procedural pain, *Am J Nurs* 97(1):17, 1997b.

Woodgate R, Yanofsky R: A different perspective to approaching cancer symptoms in children, *J Pain Symptom Manage* 26(3):800-817, 2004.

Woolf CJ, Salter MW: Neuronal plasticity: increasing the gain in pain, *Science* 288(5472):1765-1769, 2000.

Zempsky WT et al: Needle-free powder lidocaine delivery system provides rapid effective analgesic for ven puncture or cannulation pain in chi dren: randomized, double-blin comparison of venipuncture an venous cannulation pain after fast onset needle-free powder lidocain or placebo treatment trial, *Pediatri* 121(5):978-987, 2008.

36

The Infant and Family

Learning Objectives

On completion of this chapter the reader will be able to:

- Identify the major biologic, psychosocial, cognitive, and social developments during the first year of life.
- Relate parent-child attachment, separation anxiety, and stranger fear to developmental achievements during infancy.
- Provide anticipatory guidance to parents regarding common parental concerns during infancy.
- Provide anticipatory guidance to parents regarding recommendations for feeding infants.
- Outline immunization requirements during infancy, early childhood, and adolescence.
- List general contraindications, precautions, and administration routes for immunizations.
- Provide anticipatory guidance to parents regarding injury prevention based on the infant's developmental achievements.
- Provide principles of anticipatory guidance in the care of the family with an infant who is experiencing colic.
- Plan nursing care that meets the physical and emotional needs of the child and family with growth failure.
- Provide nursing care that meets the immediate and long-term needs of the family that lost a child from sudden infant death syndrome.
- Provide anticipatory guidance for the prevention of sudden infant death syndrome.
- Identify the needs of the family whose child is home monitored for apnea.

Electronic Resources

Additional information related to the content in Chapter 36 can be found on

evolve the Companion Website at

http://evolve.elsevier.com/Perry/maternal/

- NCLEX Review Questions
- Assessment Video Clips
- Case Study—Child Abuse
- Case Study—Health Problems of Infants
- Case Study—Immunizations
- Case Study—Infant Growth and Development
- Critical Thinking Exercise—Infant Safety
- Skill—Fostering Healthy Sleep Patterns in Children

Promoting Optimum Growth and Development

Biologic Development

At no other time in life are physical changes and developmental achievements as dramatic as during infancy. All major body systems undergo progressive maturation, and there is concurrent development of skills that increasingly allow infants to respond to and cope with the environment. Acquisition of these fine and gross motor skills occurs in an orderly head-to-toe and center-to-periphery (cephalocaudal and proximodistal) sequence.

Proportional Changes

Growth is very rapid during the first year, especially the initial 6 months. Infants gain 150 to 200 g (5 to 7 oz) weekly until approximately age 5 to 6 months, when the birth weight has at least doubled. An average weight for a 6-month-old child is 7.26 kg (16 lb). Weight gain slows during the second 6 months. By 1 year of age the infant's birth weight has tripled, for an average weight of 9.75 kg (21.5 lb). *Height* increases by 2.5 cm (1 inch) a month during the first 6 months and also slows during the second 6 months. Increases in length occur in sudden spurts, rather than in a slow, gradual pattern. Average height is 65 cm (25½ inches) at 6 months and 74 cm (29 inches) at 12 months. By 1 year the birth length has increased by almost 50%. This increase occurs mainly in the trunk, rather than in the legs, and contributes to the infant's characteristic physique. Standardized National Center for Health Statistics growth charts (see Appendix C) should be used to monitor the infant's growth.

Head growth is also rapid. During the first 6 months head circumference increases approximately 1.5 cm (3/5 inch) a month, but the rate of increase falls to only 0.5 cm (1/5 inch) monthly during the second 6 months. The average size is 43 cm (17 inches) at 6 months and 46 cm (18 inches) at 12 months. By 1 year, head size has increased by almost 33%. Closure of the cranial sutures occurs, with the posterior fontanel closing by 6 to 8 weeks of age and the anterior fontanel closing by 12 to 18 months of age (the average age being 14 months).

Expanding head size reflects the growth and differentiation of the *nervous system.* By the end of the first year the brain has increased in weight about 2½ times. Maturation of the brain is exhibited in the dramatic developmental achievements of infancy (see Table 36-2). Primitive reflexes are replaced by voluntary, purposeful movement, and new reflexes that influence motor development appear.

The *chest* assumes a more adult contour, with the lateral diameter becoming larger than the anteroposterior diameter. The chest circumference approximately equals the head circumference by the end of the first year. The heart grows less rapidly than the rest of the body. Its weight is usually doubled by 1 year of age; in comparison, body weight triples during the same period. The size of the heart is still large in relation to the chest cavity; its width is approximately 55% of the chest width.

Maturation of Systems

Other organ systems also change and grow during infancy. The *respiratory* rate slows somewhat (see Appendix E) and is relatively stable. Respiratory movements continue to be abdominal. Several factors predispose the infant to more severe and acute respiratory problems. The close proximity of the trachea to the bronchi and its branching structures rapidly transmits infectious agents from one anatomic location to another. The short, straight eustachian tube closely communicates with the ear, allowing infection to ascend from the pharynx to the middle ear. In addition, the inability of the immune system to produce sufficient immune globulin A (IgA) in the mucosal lining provides less protection against infection in infancy than during later childhood.

The *heart rate* slows (see Appendix E), and the rhythm is often *sinus arrhythmia* (i.e., rate increases with inspiration and decreases with expiration). Blood pressure also changes during infancy (see Appendix E). Systolic pressure rises during the first 2 months as a result of the increasing ability of the left ventricle to pump blood into the systemic circulation. Diastolic pressure decreases during the first 3 months, then gradually rises to values close to those at birth. Fluctuations in blood pressure occur during varying states of activity and emotion.

Significant *hematopoietic changes* occur during the first year (see Appendix D). Fetal hemoglobin (HgbF) is present in large quantities for the first 5 months, with adult hemoglobin steadily increasing through the first half of infancy. Fetal hemoglobin has a shorter life span than adult hemoglobin; therefore there is an increased turnover of these cells and a gradual decrease in hemoglobin. This process results in a *physiologic anemia* around 3 to 6 months of age. High levels of HgbF depress the production of erythropoietin, a hormone released by the kidney that stimulates red blood cell production. Hemoglobin levels decrease to a certain point at which tissue oxygenation needs stimulate erythropoietin, and erythropoiesis resumes, forming new red blood cells (Blackburn, 2007).

Maternal iron stores are present for the first 5 to 6 months and gradually diminish, which also accounts for lowered hemoglobin levels toward the end of the first 6 months. The occurrence of physiologic anemia is not affected by an adequate supply of iron. However, when erythropoiesis is stimulated, iron supplies are necessary for the formation of hemoglobin.

The *digestive processes* are immature at birth. Saliva is secreted in small amounts, but the majority of the digestive processes do not begin functioning until age 3 months, when drooling is common because of the poorly coordinated swallowing reflex. The enzyme *amylase* is present in small amounts but usually has little effect on the foodstuffs because of the small amount of time the food stays in the mouth. Gastric digestion in the stomach consists primarily of the action of hydrochloric acid and rennin, an enzyme that acts specifically on the casein in milk to cause the formation of curds (i.e., coagulated semisolid particles of milk). The curds cause the milk to be retained in the stomach long enough for digestion to occur.

Digestion also takes place in the duodenum, where pancreatic enzymes and bile begin to break down protein and fat. Secretion of the pancreatic enzyme *amylase,* which is needed for digestion of complex carbohydrates, is deficient until about the fourth to sixth month of life. *Lipase* is also limited, and infants do not achieve adult levels of fat absorption until 4 to 5 months of age. *Trypsin* is secreted in sufficient quantities to catabolize protein into polypeptides and some amino acids.

The immaturity of the digestive processes is evident in the appearance of stools. During infancy, solid foods (e.g., peas, carrots, corn, and raisins) are passed incompletely broken down in the feces. An excess quantity of fiber easily disposes the child to loose, bulky stools. During infancy the stomach enlarges to accommodate a greater volume of food. By the end of the first year the infant is able to tolerate three meals a day and an evening bottle and may have one or two bowel movements daily. With any type of gastric irritation, however, the infant is vulnerable to diarrhea, vomiting, and dehydration (see Chapter 47).

The *liver* is the most immature of all the gastrointestinal organs throughout infancy. The ability to conjugate bilirubin and secrete bile is achieved after the first couple of weeks of life. However, the capacities for gluconeogenesis, formation of plasma protein and ketones, storage of vitamins, and deamination of amino acids remain relatively immature for the first year of life.

Maturation of the suckling, sucking, and swallowing reflexes and the eruption of teeth (see Teething, p. 971) parallel the changes in the gastrointestinal tract and prepare the infant for the introduction of solid foods.

The *immunologic system* undergoes numerous changes during the first year. IgA is present in large amounts in colostrum; this is believed to have a protective role in the gastrointestinal tract against many bacteria such as *Escherichia coli* and viruses such as poliovirus. The function and quantity of T-lymphocytes, lymphokines, and complement are reduced in early infancy, thus preventing optimal response to certain bacteria and viruses.

The full-term newborn receives significant amounts of maternal IgG, which for approximately 3 months confers immunity against antigens to which the mother was exposed. During this time the infant begins to synthesize IgG; approximately 40% of adult levels are reached by 1 year of age. Significant amounts of IgM are produced at birth, and adult levels are reached by 9 months of age. The production of IgA, IgD, and IgE is much more gradual, and maximum levels are not attained until early childhood.

During infancy, *thermoregulation* becomes more efficient; the ability of the skin to contract and of muscles to shiver in response to cold increases. The peripheral capillaries respond to changes in ambient temperature to regulate heat loss. The capillaries constrict in response to cold, conserving core body temperature and decreasing potential evaporative heat loss from the skin surface. The capillaries dilate in response to heat, decreasing internal body temperature through evaporation, conduction, and convection. Shivering *(thermogenesis)* causes the muscles and muscle fibers to contract, generating metabolic heat that is distributed throughout the body. Increased adipose tissue during the first 6 months insulates the body against heat loss.

A shift in the *total body fluid* occurs. At birth 75% of the term infant's body weight is water, and there is an excess of extracellular fluid (ECF). As the percentage of body water decreases, so does the amount of ECF—from 40% at term to 20% in adulthood. The high proportion of ECF, which is composed of blood plasma, interstitial fluid, and lymph, predisposes the infant to a more rapid loss of total body fluid and, consequently, dehydration.

The immaturity of the *renal structures* also predisposes the infant to dehydration. Complete maturity of the kidney occurs during the latter half of the second year, when the cuboidal epithelium of the glomeruli becomes flattened. Before this time the glomeruli's filtration capacity is reduced. Urine is voided frequently and has a low specific gravity (i.e., 1.000 to 1.010).

Auditory acuity is at adult levels during infancy. Visual acuity begins to improve, and binocular fixation is established. *Binocularity,* or the fixation of two ocular images into one cerebral picture *(fusion),* begins to develop by 6 weeks of age and should be well established by age 4 months. *Depth perception (stereopsis)* begins to develop by age 7 to 9 months but may exist earlier as an innate safety mechanism against accidental falling.

Fine Motor Development

Fine motor behavior includes the use of the hands and fingers in the prehension (grasp) of an object. Grasping occurs during the first 2 to 3 months as a reflex and gradually becomes voluntary. At 1 month of age the hands are predominantly closed, and by 3 months they are mostly open. By this time infants demonstrate a desire to grasp an object, but they "grasp" it more with the eyes than with the hands. If a rattle is placed in the hand, the infant will actively hold onto it. By 4 months of age the infant regards both a small pellet and the hands and then looks from the object to the hands and back again. By 5 months the infant is able to voluntarily grasp an object.

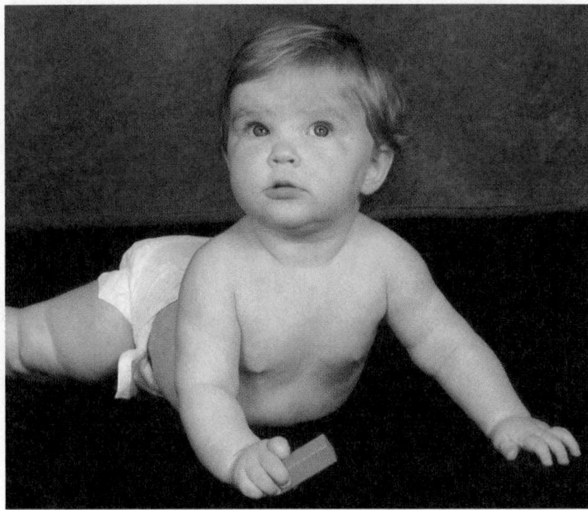

Fig. 36-1 Crude pincer grasp at 8 to 10 months. *(Photo by Paul Vincent Kuntz, Texas Children's Hospital, Houston.)*

Gradually the palmar grasp (using the whole hand) is replaced with a pincer grasp (using the thumb and index finger). The infant uses a crude pincer grasp by 8 to 9 months of age and has progressed to a neat pincer grasp by 11 months (Fig. 36-1).

By 6 months of age infants have increased manipulative skill: they hold their bottle, grasp their feet and pull them to their mouth, and feed themselves a cracker. By 7 months they transfer objects from one hand to the other, use one hand for grasping, and hold a cube in each hand simultaneously. They enjoy banging objects and will explore the movable parts of a toy.

By 10 months of age the pincer grasp is sufficiently established to enable infants to pick up a raisin and other finger foods. They can deliberately let go of an object and will offer it to someone. By 11 months they put objects into a container and like to remove them. By age 1 year, infants try to build a tower of two blocks but fail.

Gross Motor Development

Head Control

The full-term newborn can momentarily hold the head in midline and parallel when the body is suspended ventrally and can lift and turn the head from side to side when prone. This is not the case when the infant is lying prone on a pillow or soft surface; infants do not have the head control to lift their head out of the depression of the object and therefore risk possible suffocation in the prone position early in infancy (see Sudden Infant Death Syndrome, p. 1005). Marked head lag is evident when the infant is pulled from a lying to a sitting position. By 3 months of age infants can hold their head well beyond the plane of the body. By 4 months of age infants can

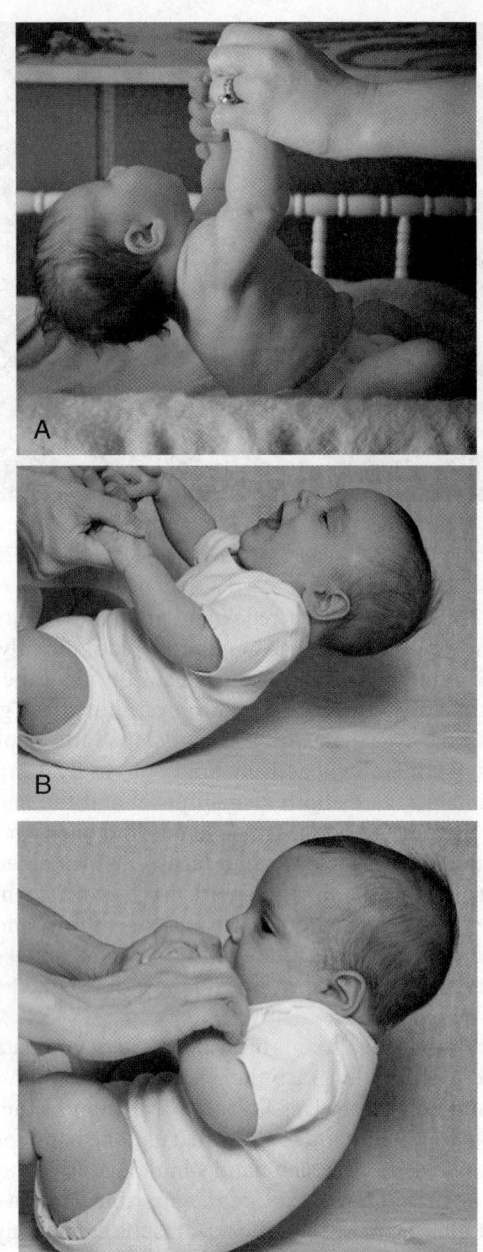

Fig. 36-2 Head control while pulled to sitting position. A, Complete head lag at 1 month. B, Partial head lag at 2 months. C, Almost no head lag at 4 months.

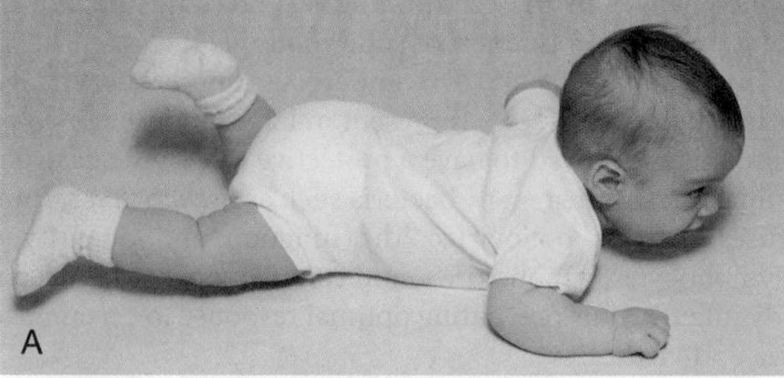

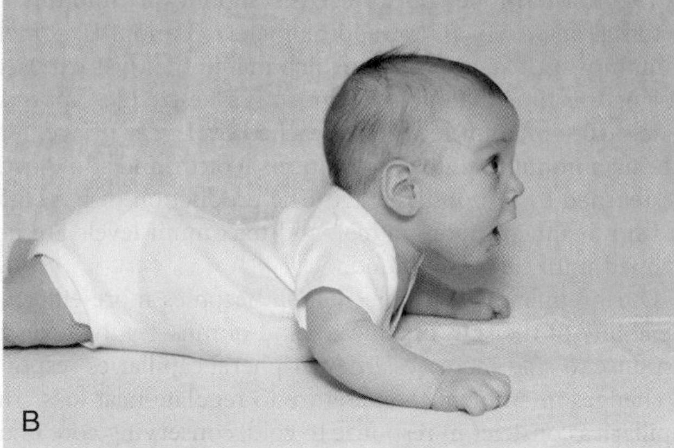

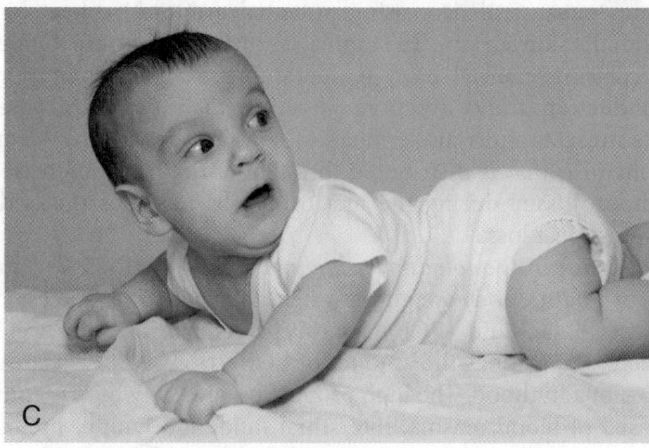

Fig. 36-3 Head control while prone. A, Infant momentarily lifts head at 1 month. B, Infant lifts head and chest 90 degrees and bears weight on forearms at 4 months. C, Infant lifts head, chest, and upper abdomen and can bear weight on hands at 6 months. Note how this position facilitates turning from abdomen to back.

lift the head and front portion of the chest approximately 90 degrees above the table, bearing their weight on the forearms. Only slight head lag is evident when the infant is pulled from a lying to a sitting position, and by 4 to 6 months head control is well established (Figs. 36-2 and 36-3).

NURSING ALERT An infant who displays head lag at 6 months of age should have a developmental and neurologic evaluation.

Rolling Over

Newborns may roll over accidentally because of their rounded back. The ability to willfully turn from the abdomen to the back occurs at 5 months, and the ability to turn from the back to the abdomen occurs at 6 months. Infants put to sleep on their sides may easily roll over to a prone (face-down) position, thus placing them at higher risk for sudden infant death syndrome (SIDS). It is therefore important to place infants in a supine position for sleep. While the infant is awake, a prone position is acceptable to enhance achievement of milestones such as head control, crawling, creeping, and turning over. It is noteworthy that the parachute reflex (Fig. 36-4), a protective response to falling, appears at 7 months.

Sitting

The ability to sit follows progressive head control and straightening of the back (Fig. 36-5). For the first 2 to 3 months

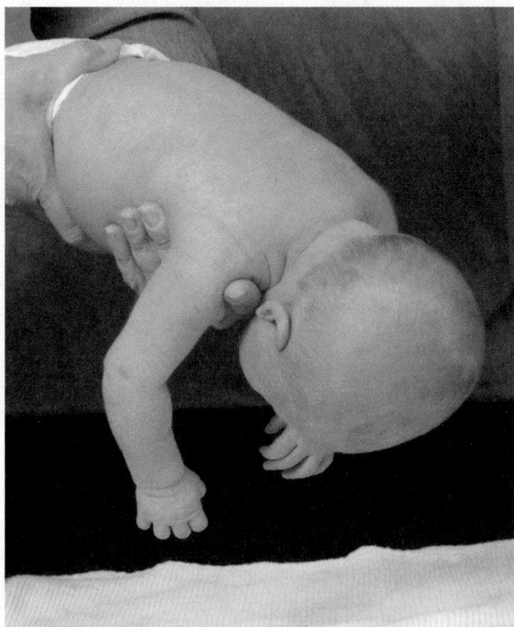

Fig. 36-4 Parachute reflex. *(Photo by Paul Vincent Kuntz, Texas Children's Hospital, Houston, TX.)*

the back is uniformly rounded. The convex cervical curve forms at approximately 3 to 4 months of age, when head control is established. The convex lumbar curve appears when the child begins to sit, at about age 4 months. As the spinal column straightens, the infant can be propped in a sitting position. By age 7 months infants can sit alone, leaning forward on their hands for support. By age 8 months they can sit well while unsupported and begin to explore their surroundings in this position rather than in a lying position. By 10 months they can maneuver from a prone to a sitting position.

Locomotion

Locomotion involves acquiring the ability to bear weight, propel forward on all four extremities, stand upright with support, and, finally, walk alone (Fig. 36-6). Following a cephalocaudal pattern, infants 4 to 6 months old have increasing coordination in their arms. Initial locomotion results in infants propelling themselves backward by pushing with the arms. By 6 to 7 months of age they are able to bear all their weight on their legs with assistance. *Crawling* (propelling forward with belly on floor) progresses to *creeping* (on hands and knees with belly off floor) by 9 months. At this time they stand while holding onto furniture and can pull themselves to the standing position, but they are unable to maneuver back down except by falling. By 11 months they walk while holding onto furniture or with both hands held, and by age 1 year they may be able to walk with one hand held. A number of infants attempt their first independent steps by their first birthday.

NURSING ALERT An infant who does not pull to a standing position by 11 to 12 months of age should be further evaluated for possible developmental dysplasia of the hip. Although there is considerable variation among infants for the achievement of these milestones, they provide guidelines for early intervention.

Psychosocial Development

Developing a Sense of Trust (Erikson)

Erikson's (1963) phase I (birth to 1 year) is concerned with *acquiring a sense of trust* while *overcoming a sense of mistrust.* The trust that develops is a trust of self, of others, and of the world. Infants "trust" that their feeding, comfort, stimulation, and caring needs will be met. The crucial element for the achievement of this task is the quality of both the parent-child (or caregiver-child) relationship and the care the infant receives. The provision of food, warmth, and shelter by itself is inadequate for the development of a strong sense of self. The infant and parent must jointly learn to satisfactorily meet their needs in order for mutual regulation of frustration to occur. When this synchrony fails to develop, mistrust is the eventual outcome.

Failure to learn *delayed gratification* leads to mistrust. Mistrust can result either from too much or too little frustration. If parents always meet their children's needs before the children signal their readiness, infants will never learn to test their ability to control the environment. If the delay is prolonged, infants experience constant frustration and eventually mistrust others in their efforts to satisfy them. Therefore consistency of care is essential.

The trust acquired in infancy provides the foundation for all succeeding phases. Trust allows infants a feeling of physical comfort and security, which assists them in experiencing unfamiliar situations with a minimum of fear. Erikson has divided the first year of life into two oral/social stages. During the first 3 to 4 months, food intake is the most important social activity in which the infant engages. The newborn can tolerate little frustration or delay of gratification. Primary *narcissism* (total concern for oneself) is at its height. However, as bodily processes such as vision, motor movements, and vocalization become better controlled, infants use more advanced behaviors to interact with others. For example, rather than cry, infants may put their arms up to signify a desire to be held.

The next social modality involves a mode of reaching out to others through *grasping.* Grasping is initially reflexive, but even as a reflex it has a powerful social meaning for the parents. The reciprocal response to the infant's grasping is the parents' holding on and touching. There is pleasurable tactile stimulation for both the child and the parents.

Tactile stimulation is extremely important in the total process of acquiring trust. The degree of mothering skill, the quantity of food, or the length of sucking does not determine the quality of the experience. Rather, it is the overall quality of the interpersonal relationship that influences the infant's formulation of trust.

During the second stage the more active and aggressive modality of *biting* occurs. Infants learn that they can hold onto what is their own and can more fully control their environment. During this stage infants may be confronted with one of their first conflicts. If they are breastfeeding, they quickly learn that biting causes the mother to become upset and withdraw the breast. Yet biting also brings internal relief from teething discomfort and a sense of power or control.

This conflict may be solved in a variety of ways. The mother may wean the infant from the breast and begin

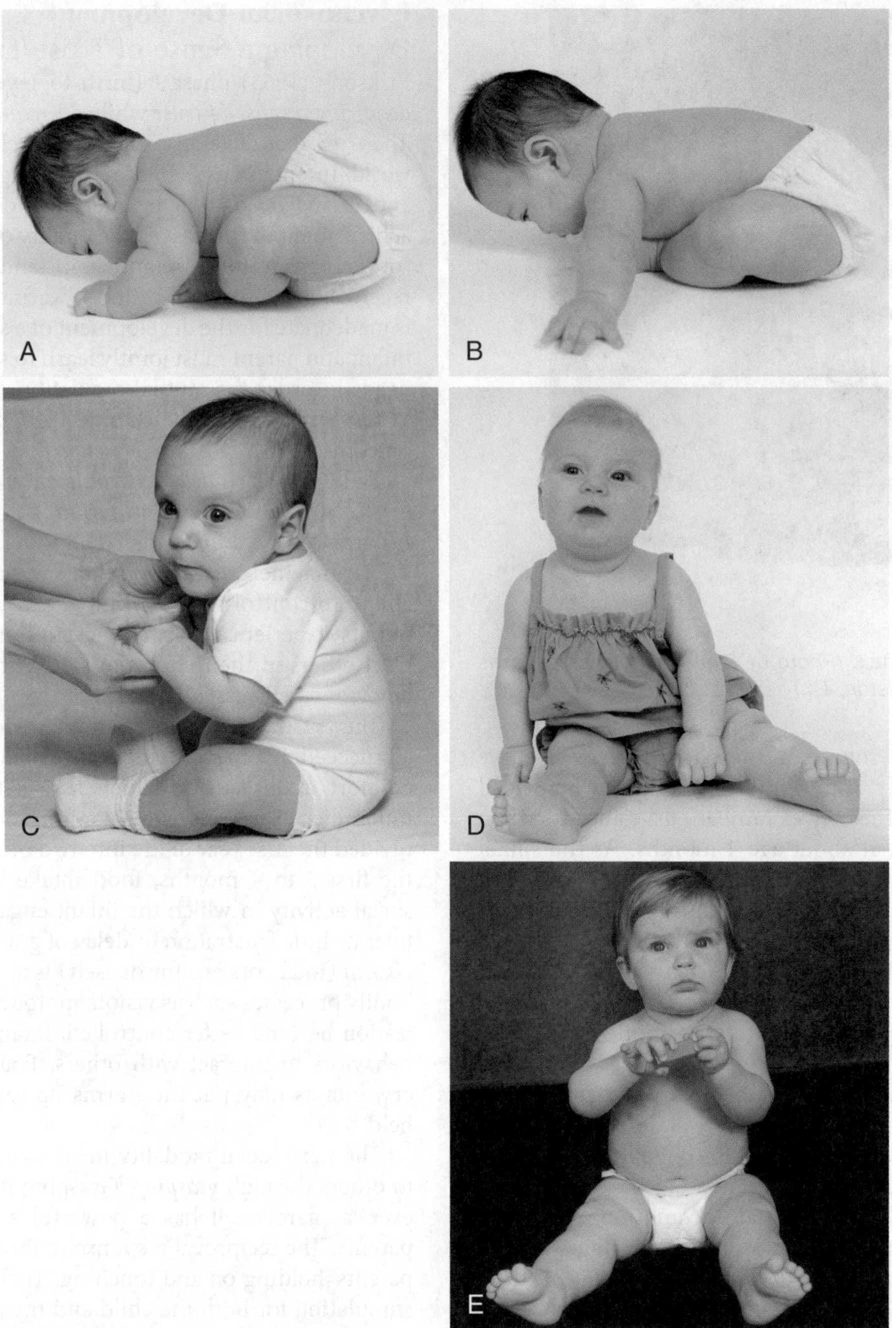

Fig. 36-5 Development of sitting. **A,** Back is completely rounded, and infant has no ability to sit upright at 1 month. **B,** At 2 months, infant exhibits more control; back is still rounded, but infant can sit up momentarily with some head control. **C,** Back is rounded only in lumbar area, and infant is able to sit erect with good head control at 4 months. **D,** Infant can sit alone, leaning on hands for support, at 7 months. **E,** Infant sits without support at 8 months. Note the transferring of objects that occurs beginning at 7 months. *(Photos by Paul Vincent Kuntz, Texas Children's Hospital, Houston, TX.)*

bottle-feeding, or the infant may learn to bite substitute "nipples," such as a pacifier, and retain pleasurable breastfeeding. The successful resolution of this conflict strengthens the mother-child relationship because it occurs at a time when infants are recognizing the mother as the most significant person in their life.

Cognitive Development

Sensorimotor Phase (Piaget)

The theory most commonly used to explain *cognition,* or the ability to know, is that of Piaget (1952). The period from birth to 24 months is termed the *sensorimotor phase* and is composed of six stages; however, because this discussion is con-

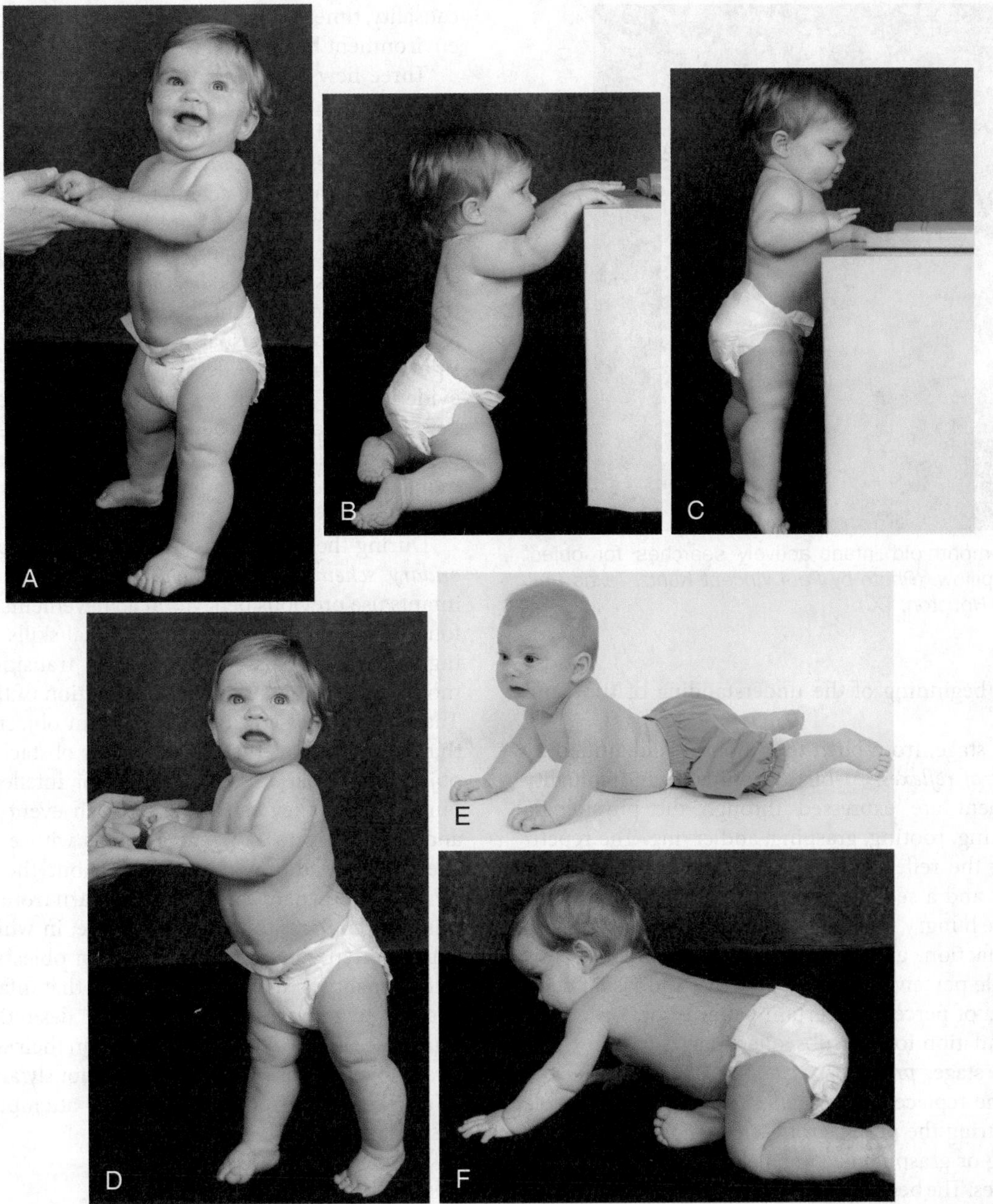

Fig. 36-6 Development of locomotion. A, Infant bears full weight on feet by 7 months. B, Infant can maneuver from sitting to kneeling position. C, Infant can stand holding onto furniture at 9 months. D, While standing, infant takes deliberate step at 10 months. E, Infant crawls with abdomen on floor and pulls self forward, and then, F, creeps on hands and knees at 9 months. *(Photos by Paul Vincent Kuntz, Texas Children's Hospital, Houston, TX.)*

cerned with ages birth to 12 months, only the first four stages are discussed. The last two stages occur during the toddler period of 12 to 24 months and are discussed in Chapter 37.

During the sensorimotor phase infants progress from reflex behaviors to simple repetitive acts to imitative activity. Three crucial events take place during this phase. The first event involves *separation,* in which infants learn to separate themselves from other objects in the environment. They realize that others besides themselves control the environment and that certain readjustments must take place for mutual satisfaction to occur. This coincides with Erikson's concept of the formation of trust.

The second major accomplishment is achieving the concept of *object permanence,* or the realization that objects that leave the visual field still exist. A typical example of the development of object permanence is when infants are able to pursue objects they observe being hidden under a pillow or behind a chair (Fig. 36-7). This skill develops at approximately 9 to 10 months of age, which corresponds to the time of increased locomotion skills.

The last major intellectual achievement of this period is the ability to use *symbols,* or *mental representation.* The use of symbols allows the infant to think of an object or situation without actually experiencing it. The recognition of

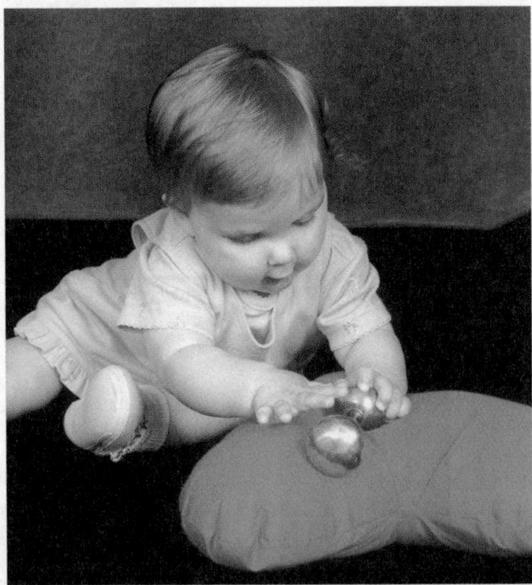

Fig. 36-7 Nine-month-old infant actively searches for object hidden behind pillow. *(Photo by Paul Vincent Kuntz, Texas Children's Hospital, Houston, TX.)*

symbols is the beginning of the understanding of time and space.

Piaget's first stage, from birth to 1 month, is identified by the infant's *use of reflexes.* At birth the infant's individuality and temperament are expressed through the physiologic reflexes of sucking, rooting, grasping, and crying. The repetitious nature of the reflexes is the beginning of associations between an act and a sequential response. When infants cry because they are hungry, a nipple is put in the mouth, and they suck, feel satisfaction, and sleep. They are assimilating this experience while perceiving auditory, tactile, and visual cues. This experience of perceiving certain patterns, or "ordering," provides a foundation for the subsequent stages.

The second stage, *primary circular reactions,* marks the beginning of the replacement of reflexive behavior with voluntary acts. During the period from 1 to 4 months, activities such as sucking or grasping become deliberate acts that elicit certain responses. The beginning of accommodation is evident. Infants incorporate and adapt their reactions to the environment and recognize the stimulus that produced a response. Previously they would cry until the nipple was brought to the mouth. Now they associate the nipple with the sound of the parent's voice. They accommodate this new piece of information and adapt by ceasing to cry when they hear the voice—before receiving the nipple. What is taking place is a realization of causality and a recognition of an orderly sequence of events. The environment is taken in with all of the senses and with whatever motor ability is present.

The *secondary circular reactions* stage is a continuation of primary circular reactions and lasts until 8 months of age. In this stage the primary circular reactions are repeated and prolonged for the response that results. Grasping and holding now become shaking, banging, and pulling. Shaking is performed to hear a noise, not solely for the pleasure of shaking. The quality and quantity of an act become evident. More or less shaking produces different responses. Understanding of causality, time, deliberate intention, and separateness from the environment begins to develop.

Three new processes of human behavior occur. *Imitation* requires the differentiation of selected acts from several events. By the second half of the first year, infants can imitate sounds and simple gestures. *Play* becomes evident as they take pleasure in performing an act after they have mastered it. Many of the infant's waking hours are absorbed in sensorimotor play. *Affect* (the outward manifestation of emotion and feeling) is seen as infants begin to develop a sense of permanency. During the first 6 months infants believe that an object exists only for as long as they can visually perceive it. In other words, out of sight, out of mind. Affect in relation to external objects is evident when the object continues to be present or remembered even though it is beyond the range of perception. Object permanence is a critical component of parent-child attachment and is seen in the development of separation anxiety at 6 to 8 months of age (see p. 962).

During the fourth sensorimotor stage, *coordination of secondary schematas and their application to new situations,* infants use previous behavioral achievements primarily as the foundation for adding new intellectual skills to their expanding repertoire. This stage is largely transitional. Increasing motor skills allow for greater exploration of the environment. They begin to discover that hiding an object does not mean that it is gone but that removing an obstacle will reveal the object. This marks the beginning of intellectual reasoning. Furthermore, they can experience an event by observing it, and they begin to associate symbols with events (e.g., "bye-bye" with "Daddy goes to work"), but the classification is purely their own. In this stage they learn from the object itself; this is in contrast to the second stage, in which infants learn from the type of interaction between objects or individuals. Intentionality is further developed in that infants now actively attempt to remove a barrier to the desired (or undesired) action (see Fig. 36-7). If something is in their way, they attempt to climb over it or push it away. Previously an obstacle would cause them to give up any further attempt to achieve the desired goal.

Development of Body Image

The development of body image parallels sensorimotor development. Infants' kinesthetic and tactile experiences are the first perceptions of their body, and the mouth is the principal area of pleasurable sensations. Other parts of the body are primarily objects of pleasure—the hands and fingers to suck and the feet to play with. As physical needs are met, they feel comfort and satisfaction with their body. Messages conveyed by the caregivers reinforce these feelings. For example, when infants smile, they receive emotional satisfaction from others who smile back.

Achieving the concept of object permanence is basic to the development of self-image. By the end of the first year infants recognize that they are distinct from their parents. At the same time, they have increasing interest in their image, especially in the mirror (Fig. 36-8). As motor skills develop, they learn that parts of the body are useful; for example, the hands bring objects to the mouth, and the legs help them move to different locations. All of these achievements transmit messages to

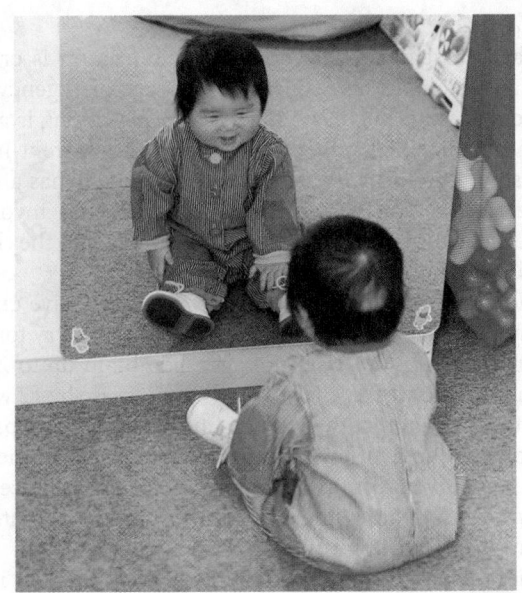

Fig. 36-8 Nine-month-old infant enjoying own image in mirror.

them about themselves. Therefore it is important to transmit positive messages to infants about their bodies.

Social Development

Infants' social development is initially influenced by their reflexive behavior, such as the grasp, and eventually depends primarily on the interaction between them and the principal caregivers. *Attachment* to the parent is increasingly evident during the second half of the first year. In addition, tremendous strides are made in communication and personal-social behavior. Whereas crying and reflexive behavior are methods to meet one's needs in the neonatal period, the social smile is an early step in social communication. This has a profound effect on family members and is a tremendous stimulus for evoking continued responses from others. By 4 months infants laugh aloud.

Play is a major socializing agent and provides stimulation needed to learn from and interact with the environment. By age 6 months infants are personable. They play games such as peekaboo when their head is hidden in a towel, they signal their desire to be picked up by extending their arms, and they show displeasure when a toy is removed or their face is washed.

Attachment

The importance to infants of human physical contact cannot be overemphasized. Parenting is not an instinctual ability but a learned, acquired process. The attachment of parent and child, which begins before birth, assumes even more importance at birth and continues during the first year. In the following discussion of attachment, the term *mother* is used in the broad context of the consistent caregiver with whom the child relates more than anyone else. However, in society's changing social climate and sex-role stereotypes, this person may very well be the father or a grandparent. Studies on paternal-infant attachment demonstrate that stages similar to those in maternal attachment occur and that fathers are often more involved in child care when mothers are employed (although mothers continue to do the majority of infant care). Additional research has shown that inexperienced, first-time fathers are as capable as experienced fathers of developing a close attachment with their infants. It has been shown that fathers develop feelings of attachment with their offspring and that their relationship with the infant is an important factor in the mother's emotional well-being. Breastfeeding mothers reported that the most important factor in establishing and maintaining breastfeeding in early infancy was the father's acceptance of breastfeeding and support for the mother (Arora et al, 2000).

Attachment progresses during infancy, with the child assuming an increasingly significant role. Two components of cognitive development are required for attachment: (1) the ability to discriminate the mother from other individuals, and (2) the achievement of object permanence. Both of these processes prepare the infant for an equally important aspect of attachment: separation from the parent. Separation-individuation should occur as a harmonious, parallel process with emotional attachment.

During the formation of attachment to the parent, the infant progresses through four distinct but overlapping stages. For the first few weeks infants respond indiscriminately to anyone. Beginning at approximately 8 to 12 weeks of age, they cry, smile, and vocalize more to the mother than to anyone else but continue to respond to others, whether familiar or not. At approximately 6 months of age, infants show a distinct preference for the mother. They follow her more, cry when she leaves, enjoy playing with her more, and feel most secure in her arms. About 1 month after showing attachment to the mother, many infants begin attaching to other members of the family, most often the father.

Infants acquire other developmental behaviors that influence the attachment process. These include (1) differential crying, smiling, and vocalization (more to the mother than to anyone else); (2) visual-motor orientation (looking more at the mother, even if she is not close); (3) crying when the mother leaves the room; (4) approaching through locomotion (crawling, creeping, or walking); (5) clinging (especially in the presence of a stranger); and (6) exploring away from the mother while using her as a secure base.

Reactive attachment disorder (RAD) is a psychologic and developmental problem that stems from maladaptive or absent attachment between the infant and parent (or primary caregiver) and may persist into childhood and even adulthood (Wilson, 2001; Zeanah & Fox, 2004). Infants at risk for RAD include those who have been victims of physical abuse, sexual abuse, or neglect; infants exposed to parental alcoholism, mental illness, and substance abuse; and infants who have experienced the absence of a consistent primary caregiver as a result of foster care, institutionalization, parental abandonment, and parental incarceration. Two different patterns of RAD have emerged: the emotionally withdrawn–inhibited pattern and an indiscriminate-disinhibited pattern (Hornor, 2008; Zeanah & Fox, 2004). Signs of RAD are usually seen before the age of 5 years in infants who had insecure attachments to the mother or other primary caretaker (American Psychiatric Association, 2000). The child may manifest behaviors such as not being cuddly with parents, failing to make eye

evolve Case Study—Child Abuse

contact with significant others, having poor impulse control, and being destructive to self and others. Without early intervention, some of these children fail to develop a conscience and suffer from an antisocial personality disorder that may lead to criminal acts. The American Psychiatric Association (2002) position statement on RAD strongly recommends against the use of coercive holding therapies or rebirthing techniques for the treatment of RAD. It is not within the scope of this text to discuss the full array of attachment disorders and associated therapies.

Separation Anxiety

Between ages 4 and 8 months the infant progresses through the first stage of separation-individuation and begins to have some awareness of self and mother as separate beings. At the same time, object permanence is developing, and the infant is aware that the parent can be absent. Therefore separation anxiety develops and is manifested through a predictable sequence of behaviors.

During the early second half of the first year, infants protest when placed in their crib, and a short time later they object when the mother leaves the room. Infants may not notice the mother's absence if they are absorbed in an activity. However, when they realize her absence, they protest. From this point on, they become very alert to her activities and whereabouts. By 11 to 12 months they are able to anticipate her imminent departure by watching her behaviors, and they begin to protest before she leaves. At this point many parents learn to postpone alerting the child to their departure until just before leaving.

Stranger Fear

As infants demonstrate attachment to one person, they correspondingly exhibit less friendliness to others. Between ages 6 and 8 months, fear of strangers and stranger anxiety become prominent and are related to infants' ability to discriminate between familiar and unfamiliar people. Behaviors such as clinging to the parent, crying, and turning away from the stranger are common (Fig. 36-9).

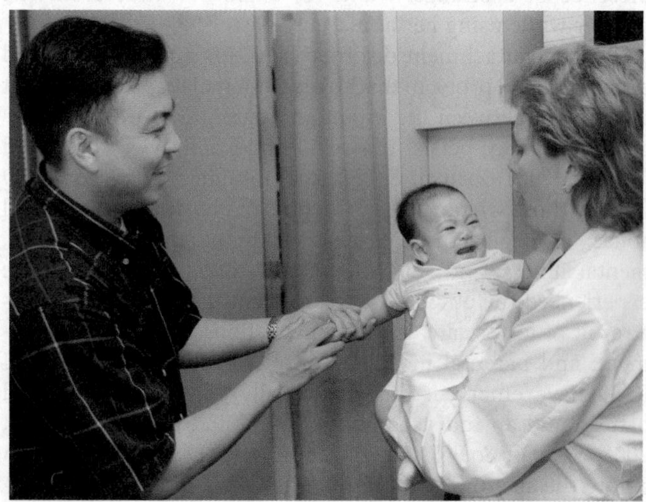

Fig. 36-9 Behaviors related to fear of strangers include clinging to the parent and turning away from the stranger. *(Photo by Paul Vincent Kuntz, Texas Children's Hospital, Houston, TX.)*

Language Development

The infant's first means of verbal communication is crying. Crying as a biologic sign conveys a message of urgency and signals displeasure, such as hunger. However, crying is also a social event that affects the development of the parent-infant relationship—either by its absence, which usually has a positive effect on parents, or its presence, which may involve a negative response or persuade parents to minister to the child's physical or emotional needs.

In the first few weeks of life, crying has a reflexive quality and is mostly related to physiologic needs. Infants cry for 1 to 1½ hours a day up to 3 weeks of age, then build up to 2 and even 4 hours by 6 weeks. Crying tends to decrease by 12 weeks of age. It is thought that the increase in crying for no apparent reason during the first few months may be related to the discharge of energy and the maturational changes in the central nervous system. During the end of the first year, infants cry for attention; from fear (especially stranger fear); and from frustration, usually in response to their developing but inadequate motor skills.

NURSING ALERT Be alert to parents' reports about maternal postpartum depression and infant crying, since these concerns may indicate a stressed mother-infant relationship.

Vocalizations heard during crying eventually become syllables and words (e.g., the "mama" heard during vigorous crying). Infants vocalize as early as 5 to 6 weeks of age by making small throaty sounds. By 2 months they make single vowel sounds such as *ah, eh,* and *uh.* By 3 to 4 months the consonants *n, k, g, p,* and *b* are added, and the infants coo, gurgle, and laugh aloud. By 8 months they imitate sounds; add the consonants *t, d,* and *w*; and combine syllables (e.g., "dada"), but they do not ascribe meaning to the word until 10 to 11 months of age (see Family-Centered Care box). By 9 to 10 months they comprehend the meaning of the word "no" and obey simple commands. By age 1 year they can say three to five words with meaning.

FAMILY-CENTERED CARE

Child's Developing Language Skills

During the acquisition of new language skills the child temporarily may stop using other recently learned sounds or words. This is often distressing for parents, who have waited in anticipation for the words "dada" or "mama," because these sounds are commonly replaced by other vocalizations and may not be repeated for several weeks. Nurses can reassure parents that the child will again say these special words, and with increased meaning.

Play

Play during infancy represents the various social modalities observed during cognitive development. Infants' activity is primarily narcissistic and revolves around their own body. As discussed under Development of Body Image (p. 960), body parts are primarily objects of play and pleasure.

During the first year, play becomes more sophisticated and interdependent. From birth to 3 months, infants' responses to the environment are global and largely undifferentiated. Play is dependent; pleasure is demonstrated by a quieting attitude (1 month), a smile (2 months), or a squeal (3 months). From 3 to 6 months, infants show more discriminate interest in stimuli and begin to play alone with a rattle or a soft stuffed toy or with someone else. There is much more interaction during play. By 4 months of age they laugh aloud, show a preference for certain toys, and become excited when food or a favorite object is brought to them. They recognize an image in a mirror, smile at it, and vocalize to it.

By 6 months to 1 year, play involves sensorimotor skills. Actual games such as peekaboo and pat-a-cake are played. Verbal repetition and imitation of simple gestures occur in response to demonstration. Play is much more selective, not only in terms of specific toys, but also in terms of "playmates." Although play is solitary or one-sided, infants choose with whom they will interact. At 6 to 8 months they usually refuse to play with strangers. Parents are definite favorites, and infants know how to attract their attention. At 6 months they extend the arms to be picked up, at 7 months cough or squeal to make their presence known, at 10 months pull the parent's clothing, and at 12 months call them by name. This represents a tremendous advance from the newborn who signaled biologic needs by crying to express displeasure.

Stimulation is as important for psychosocial growth as food is for physical growth. Knowledge of developmental milestones allows nurses to guide parents regarding proper play for infants. It is not sufficient to place a mobile over a crib and toys in a playpen for a child's optimum social, emotional, and intellectual development. Play must provide interpersonal contact and recreational and educational stimulation. Infants need to be *played with,* not merely *allowed to play.* Although the type of play infants engage in is called *solitary,* this is a figurative, not literal, term to denote one-sided play. The type of toys given to the child is much less important than the quality of personal interaction that occurs.

Table 36-1 lists play activities appropriate for the developmental level of the infant in view of motor, language, and personal-social achievements. Although the activities are grouped according to the major mode of stimulation provided, there is overlap in many instances. In addition, play activities suggested for one age group may be appropriate for older infants but inappropriate for younger infants.

Temperament

The infant's temperament or behavioral style influences the type of interaction that occurs between the child and parents, especially the mother, and other family members (see general discussion of temperament in Chapter 33). In assessments of a child's temperament, it is the parents' perception of the child and the degree of fit between their expectations and the child's actual temperament that are important. The more dissonance, or lack of harmony, between the child's temperament and the parent's ability to accept and deal with the behavior, the more risk for subsequent parent-child conflicts.

Although most behavioral researchers agree that there is a strong biologic component to temperament, researchers also suggest that temperament may be modified by the environment, particularly the family (Wilson et al, 2000). Family interaction with the infant is perceived as a circular process wherein each family member affects each other and the family as a unit. With these concepts in mind, the nurse has an important role in helping the family understand the infant's temperament as it relates to family dynamics and the eventual well-being of the child and family unit (Wilson et al, 2000).

The Revised Infant Temperament Questionnaire (RITQ) (Carey & McDevitt, 1978) can be used as a screening tool with parents. The questionnaire focuses on nine temperament variables, but the 95 questions relate specifically to activities such as sleeping, feeding, playing, diapering, and dressing. The scores from the RITQ help identify the child's temperamental style. Use of the RITQ is well accepted by parents and should be accompanied by an adequate explanation of the results. In discussing the results, the nurse should avoid descriptors such as *difficult* and describe such infants in terms such as *intense* or *less predictable.* The Early Infancy Temperament Questionnaire is a 76-item parent questionnaire that was adapted from the RITQ to specifically evaluate temperament characteristics of infants 1 to 4 months old, whereas the RITQ is best suited for infants 4 months old and older (Medoff-Cooper, Carey, & McDevitt, 1993).

With knowledge of the infant's temperament, nurses are better able to (1) provide parents with background information that will help them see their child in a better perspective, (2) offer a more organized picture of their child's behavior and possibly reveal distortions in their perceptions of the behavior, and (3) guide parents regarding appropriate childrearing techniques.

Childrearing Practices Related to Temperament

Most parents realize that their infant is born with unique characteristics, and few parents of difficult infants need to be told of the challenge of caring for them. However, few parents are aware of the significance of the temperamental characteristics and of constructive approaches to dealing with them. The following are examples of interventions that promote more positive parenting of infants with different temperament styles.*

"Difficult" children may respond better to scheduled feedings and structured caregiving routines than to demand feedings and frequent changes in daily routines. These children sleep less and may need more structured approaches to bedtime to prevent bedtime problems. "Highly distractible" children may require additional soothing measures such as swinging, rocking, or being carried in a pack worn across the parent's chest or back. Children with "high activity" levels require vigilant watching, and parents need to take extra precautions in safeguarding the home. These children benefit

**Recommended resources for parents are Turecki SK, Tonner L:* The difficult child, *New York, 2000, Bantam Books; and Chess S, 2 A:* Know your child: an authoritative guide for today's parents, *Lanham, MD, 1996, Jason Aronson.*

Table 36-1 Play During Infancy

AGE (mo)	VISUAL STIMULATION	AUDITORY STIMULATION	TACTILE STIMULATION	KINETIC STIMULATION
Suggested Activities				
Birth-1	Look at infant at close range. Hang bright, shiny object within 20-25 cm (8-10 inches) of infant's face and in midline. Hang mobiles with black-and-white designs.	Talk to infant; sing in soft voice. Play music box, tape, or CD. Have ticking clock or metronome nearby.	Hold, caress, cuddle. Keep infant warm. May like to be swaddled.	Rock infant; place in cradle. Use stroller for walks.
2-3	Provide bright objects. Make room bright with pictures or mirrors. Take infant to various rooms while doing chores. Place infant in infant seat for vertical view of environment.	Talk to infant. Include in family gatherings. Expose to various environmental noises other than those of home. Use rattles, wind chimes.	Caress infant while bathing, at diaper change. Comb hair with a soft brush. Give massage.	Use infant swing. Take in car for rides. Exercise body by moving extremities in swimming motion. Use cradle gym.
4-6	Place infant in front of unbreakable mirror. Give brightly colored toys to hold (small enough to grasp).	Talk to infant; repeat sounds infant makes. Laugh when infant laughs. Call infant by name. Crinkle different papers by infant's ear. Place rattle or ball in hand.	Give infant soft squeeze toys of various textures. Allow to splash in bath. Place nude on soft, furry rug and move extremities.	Use swing or stroller. Bounce infant in lap while holding in standing position. Support infant in sitting position; let infant lean forward to balance self. Place infant on floor to crawl, roll over, sit.
6-9	Give infant large toys with bright colors, movable parts, and noisemakers. Place unbreakable mirror where infant can see self. Play peekaboo, especially hiding face in a towel. Make funny faces to encourage imitation. Give ball of yarn or string to pull apart.	Call infant by name. Repeat simple words such as "dada," "mama," "bye-bye." Speak clearly. Name parts of body, people, and foods. Tell infant what you are doing. Use "no" only when necessary. Give simple commands. Show how to clap hands, bang a drum.	Let infant play with fabrics of various textures. Have bowl with foods of different sizes and textures to feel. Let infant "catch" running water. Encourage "swimming" in large bathtub or shallow pool. Give wad of sticky tape to manipulate.	Hold upright to bear weight and bounce. Pick up, say "up." Put down, say "down." Place toys out of reach; encourage infant to get them. Play pat-a-cake.
9-12	Show infant large pictures in books. Take infant to places where there are animals, many people, different objects (e.g., shopping center). Play ball by rolling it to child, demonstrate "throwing" it back. Demonstrate building a two-block tower.	Read infant simple nursery rhymes. Point to body parts and name each one. Imitate sounds of animals.	Give infant finger foods of different textures. Let infant mess and squash food. Let infant feel cold (ice cube) or warm objects; say what temperature each is. Let infant feel a breeze (fan blowing).	Give large push-pull toys. Place furniture in a circle to encourage cruising. Turn in different positions.
Suggested Toys				
Birth-6	Nursery mobiles Unbreakable mirrors See-through crib bumpers Contrasting colored sheets	Music boxes Musical mobiles Crib dangle bells Small-handled, clear rattle	Stuffed animals Soft clothes Soft or furry quilt Soft mobiles	Rocking crib or cradle Weighted or suction toy Infant swing
6-12	Various colored blocks Nested boxes or cups Books with rhymes and bright pictures Strings of big beads Simple take-apart toys Large ball Cup and spoon Large puzzles Jack-in-the-box	Rattles of different sizes, shapes, tones, and bright colors Squeaky animals and dolls Light, rhythmic music	Soft, different-texture animals and dolls Sponge toys, floating toys Squeeze toys Teething toys Books with textures or objects, such as fur and zipper	Activity box for crib Push-pull toys Wind-up swing

from increased opportunities for gross motor activity to constructively channel their energy.

The child who is "slow to warm up" may demonstrate more stranger fear than other children and may require gradual and frequent preparation for new situations, such as substitute child care. Even the "easy child" can present problems in that the parents may need reminders to feed the infant who sleeps for prolonged intervals and rarely cries. They may need to "retrain" the child because of the ease of developing habits such as keeping the child up late or sleeping with the youngster, which may later become troublesome.

Appropriate counseling based on awareness of the child's temperament can greatly enhance the quality of interaction between parents and infant. Even just letting parents know that "difficult" traits are innate can relieve feelings of guilt and incompetence.

Because of the complexity of the developmental process during the first 12 months, Table 36-2 is presented to help organize and clarify the data already discussed. Although all milestones are important, some represent essential integrative aspects of development that lay the foundation for achievement of more advanced skills. These essential milestones are designated by an asterisk in the table. The table represents the average monthly age at which various skills are attained. It must be remembered that although the sequence is the same, the rate will vary among children.

Coping with Concerns Related to Normal Growth and Development

Separation and Stranger Fear

A number of fears can appear during infancy. However, the fear that causes parents the most concern is fear related to strangers and separation. Although erroneously interpreted by some as a sign of undesirable, antisocial behavior, stranger fear and separation anxiety are important components of a strong, healthy, parent-child attachment. Nevertheless, this period can present difficulties for the parent and child. Parents may experience guilt at having to leave the infant because he or she violently protests having a baby-sitter. To accustom the infant to new people, parents are encouraged to have close friends or relatives visit often. This provides other persons with whom the child is comfortable and who can give parents time for themselves.

Infants also need opportunities to safely experience strangers. Usually toward the end of the first year, infants begin to venture away from the parent and demonstrate curiosity about strangers. If allowed to explore at their own rate, many infants eventually "warm up." If parents hold the child away from their face, the infant can observe while maintaining close physical contact.

The best approach for the stranger (who may be the nurse) is to talk softly; meet the child at eye level (to appear smaller); maintain a safe distance from the infant; and avoid sudden, intrusive gestures, such as holding the arms out and smiling broadly.

Parents also may wonder whether they should encourage the child's clinging, dependent behavior, especially if there is pressure from others who view this as "spoiling" (see the following discussion). Parents need to be reassured that such behavior is healthy, desirable, and necessary for the child's optimum emotional development. If parents can reassure the infant of their presence, the infant will learn to realize that they are still there even if not physically present. Talking to infants when leaving the room, allowing them to hear one's voice on the telephone, and using transitional objects (e.g., a favorite blanket or toy) reassures them of the parent's continued presence.

Alternative Child Care Arrangements

For many parents, especially working mothers, locating safe and competent child care facilities for the infant is an increasingly difficult problem—one that is compounded by the number of mothers working outside the home. Over the past 40 years there has been a marked shift in child care arrangements; whereas the majority of children are cared for in group centers or other settings, an increasing number of children are being cared for in home settings.

The basic types of care are in-home care, either in the parents' or caregivers' home (family day care), and center-based care, usually in a day care center. *In-home care* may consist of a full-time baby-sitter who lives in the home, a full-time baby-sitter who comes to the home, cooperative arrangements such as exchange baby-sitting, and family day care. A licensed *small family child day care home* typically provides care and protection for up to six children for part of a day and does not include informal arrangements such as exchange baby-sitting or caregivers in the child's own home. The six children include the family day care provider's own children younger than 5 years of age living in the home. *Large family child care homes* may provide care for eight to twelve children. Unfortunately, many family day care homes operate without a license and may care for large numbers of infants without adequate staff and facilities.

Child center-based care usually refers to a licensed day care facility that provides care for six or more children, for 6 or more hours a day. *Work-based group care* is another option that is becoming increasingly popular as employers recognize the benefit of providing high-quality and convenient child care to their employees. *Sick-child care* may also be available for times when the youngster is ill. Such programs are often located in community hospitals or in work settings.

A major nursing responsibility is guiding parents in locating suitable facilities that have a well-qualified staff. State licensing agencies can help parents identify day care centers that accept children of specific age groups and that are convenient to home and work. Their records are available to the public and provide reports from the health, safety, and fire departments; periodic evaluations from the licensing agency; complaints filed against the center; and qualifications of the center's employees. State-licensed programs are supposed to abide by established standards, which represent the minimum requirements and safeguards; however, enforcement of the standards is sometimes inadequate. Early childhood programs

Text continued on p. 970

Table 36-2 Growth and Development During Infancy

AGE (mo)	PHYSICAL	GROSS MOTOR	FINE MOTOR
1	Weight gain of 150-200 g (5-7 oz) weekly for first 6 mo Height gain of 2.5 cm (1 inch) monthly for first 6 mo Head circumference increases by 1.5 cm (6⁄10 inch) monthly for first 6 mo Primitive reflexes present and strong Doll's eye reflexes and dance reflex fading Obligatory nose breathing (most infants)	Assumes flexed position with pelvis high but knees not under abdomen when prone (at birth, knees flexed under abdomen)* Can turn head from side to side when prone; lifts head momentarily from bed (see Fig. 36-3, *A*)* Has marked head lag, especially when pulled from lying to sitting position (see Fig. 36-2, *A*) Holds head momentarily parallel and in midline when suspended in prone position Assumes asymmetric tonic neck reflex position when supine When held in standing position, body is limp at knees and hips In sitting position, back is uniformly rounded, absence of head control	Hands predominantly closed Grasp reflex strong Hand clenches on contact with rattle
2	Posterior fontanel closed Crawling reflex disappears	Assumes less flexed position when prone—hips flat, legs extended, arms flexed, head to side* Less head lag when pulled to sitting position (see Fig. 36-2, *B*) Can maintain head in same plane as rest of body when held in ventral suspension When prone, can lift head almost 45 degrees off table When moved to sitting position, head is held up but bends forward (see Fig. 36-5, *B*) Assumes asymmetric tonic neck reflex position intermittently	Hands often open Grasp reflex fading
3	Primitive reflexes fading	Able to hold head more erect when sitting, but still bobs forward Has only slight head lag when pulled to sitting position Assumes symmetric body positioning Able to raise head and shoulders from prone position to a 45- to 90-degree angle from table; bears weight on forearms When held in standing position, able to bear slight fraction of weight on legs Regards own hand	Actively holds rattle but will not reach for it* Grasp reflex absent Hands kept loosely open Clutches own hand; pulls at blankets and clothes
4	Drooling begins Moro, tonic neck, and rooting reflexes have disappeared*	Has almost no head lag when pulled to sitting position (see Fig. 36-2, *C*)* Balances head well in sitting position (see Fig. 36-5, *C*)* Back less rounded, curved only in lumbar area Able to sit erect if propped up Able to raise head and chest off surface to angle of 90 degrees (see Fig. 36-3, *B*) Assumes predominant symmetric position Rolls from back to side*	Inspects and plays with hands; pulls clothing or blanket over face in play* Tries to reach objects with hand but overshoots Grasps object with both hands Plays with rattle placed in hand, shakes it, but cannot pick it up if dropped Can carry objects to mouth
5	Beginning signs of tooth eruption Birth weight doubles	No head lag when pulled to sitting position When sitting, able to hold head erect and steady Able to sit for longer periods when back is well supported Back straight When prone, assumes symmetric positioning with arms extended Can turn over from abdomen to back* When supine, puts feet to mouth	Able to grasp objects voluntarily* Uses palmar grasp, bidextrous approach Plays with toes Takes objects directly to mouth Holds one cube while regarding a second one

*Milestones that represent essential integrative aspects of development that lay the foundation for the achievement of more advanced skills.

SENSORY	VOCALIZATION	SOCIALIZATION/COGNITION
Able to fixate on moving object in range of 45 degrees when held at a distance of 20-25 cm (8-10 inches) Visual acuity approaches 20/100† Follows light to midline Quiets when hears a voice	Cries to express displeasure Makes small, throaty sounds Makes comfort sounds during feeding	Is in sensorimotor phase—stage I, use of reflexes (birth–1 mo), and stage II, primary circular reactions (1-4 mo) Watches parent's face intently as parent talks to infant
Binocular fixation and convergence to near objects beginning When supine, follows dangling toy from side to point beyond midline Visually searches to locate sounds Turns head to side when sound is made at level of ear	Vocalizes, distinct from crying* Crying becomes differentiated Coos Vocalizes to familiar voice	Demonstrates social smile in response to various stimuli*
Follows object to periphery (180 degrees)* Locates sound by turning head to side and looking in same direction* Begins to have ability to coordinate stimuli from various sense organs	Squeals aloud to show pleasure* Coos, babbles, chuckles Vocalizes when smiling "Talks" a great deal when spoken to Less crying during periods of wakefulness	Displays considerable interest in surroundings Ceases crying when parent enters room Can recognize familiar faces and objects, such as feeding bottle Shows awareness of strange situations
Able to accommodate to near objects Binocular vision fairly well established Can focus on a 1.25 cm (½-inch) block Beginning eye-hand coordination	Makes consonant sounds *n, k, g, p, b* Laughs aloud* Vocalization changes according to mood	Is in stage III, secondary circular reactions Demands attention by fussing; becomes bored if left alone Enjoys social interaction with people Anticipates feeding when sees bottle or mother if breastfeeding Shows excitement with whole body, squeals, breathes heavily Shows interest in strange stimuli Begins to show memory
Visually pursues a dropped object Is able to sustain visual inspection of an object Can localize sounds made below ear	Squeals Makes cooing vowel sounds interspersed with consonant sounds (e.g., *ah-goo*)	Smiles at mirror image Pats bottle or breast with both hands More enthusiastically playful, but may have rapid mood swings Is able to discriminate strangers from family Vocalizes displeasure when object is taken away Discovers parts of body

†Degree of visual acuity varies according to vision measurement procedure used.

Continued

Table 36-2 Growth and Development During Infancy—cont'd

AGE (mo)	PHYSICAL	GROSS MOTOR	FINE MOTOR
6	Growth rate may begin to decline Weight gain of 90-150 g (3-5 oz) weekly for next 6 mo Height gain of 1.25 cm (½ inch) monthly for next 6 mo Teething may begin with eruption of two lower central incisors* Chewing and biting occur*	When prone, can lift chest and upper abdomen off surface, bearing weight on hands (see Fig. 36-3, *C*) When about to be pulled to a sitting position, lifts head Sits in high chair with back straight Rolls from back to abdomen When held in standing position, bears almost all of weight Hand regard absent	Resecures a dropped object Drops one cube when another is given Grasps and manipulates small objects Holds bottle Grasps feet and pulls to mouth
7	Eruption of upper central incisors	When supine, spontaneously lifts head off surface Sits, leaning forward on hands (see Fig. 36-5, *D*)* When prone, bears weight on one hand Sits erect momentarily Bears full weight on feet (see Fig. 36-6, *A*) When held in standing position, bounces actively	Transfers objects from one hand to the other (see Fig. 36-5, *E*)* Has unidextrous approach and grasp Holds two cubes more than momentarily Bangs cube on table Rakes at a small object
8	Begins to show regular patterns in bladder and bowel elimination Parachute reflex appears (see Fig. 36-4)	Sits steadily unsupported (see Fig. 36-5, *E*)* Readily bears weight on legs when supported; may stand holding onto furniture Adjusts posture to reach an object	Has beginning pincer grasp using index, fourth, and fifth fingers against lower part of thumb Releases objects at will Rings bell purposely Retains two cubes while regarding third cube Secures an object by pulling on a string Reaches persistently for toys out of reach
9	Eruption of upper lateral incisor may begin	Creeps on hands and knees Sits steadily on floor for prolonged time (10 min) Recovers balance when leaning forward but cannot do so when leaning sideways Pulls self to standing position and stands holding onto furniture (see Fig. 36-6, *B* and *C*)*	Uses thumb and index fingers in crude pincer grasp (see Fig. 36-1)* Preference for use of dominant hand now evident Grasps third cube Compares two cubes by bringing them together
10	Labyrinth-righting reflex is strongest—when infant is in prone or supine position, is able to raise head	Can change from prone to sitting position Stands while holding onto furniture, sits by falling down Recovers balance easily while sitting While standing, lifts one foot to take a step (see Fig. 36-6, *D*)	Crude release of an object beginning Grasps bell by handle
11	Eruption of lower lateral incisor may begin	When sitting, pivots to reach toward back to pick up an object Cruises or walks holding onto furniture or with both hands held*	Explores objects more thoroughly (e.g., clapper inside bell) Has neat pincer grasp Drops object deliberately for it to be picked up Puts one object after another into a container (sequential play) Able to manipulate an object to remove it from tight-fitting enclosure
12	Birth weight tripled* Birth length increased by 50%* Head and chest circumference equal (head circumference 46 cm [18 inches]) Has total of six to eight deciduous teeth Anterior fontanel almost closed Landau reflex fading Babinski reflex disappears Lumbar curve develops; lordosis evident during walking	Walks with one hand held* Cruises well May attempt to stand alone momentarily; may attempt first step alone* Can sit down from standing position without help	Releases cube in cup Attempts to build two-block tower but fails Tries to insert a pellet into a narrow-necked bottle but fails Can turn pages in a book, many at a time

SENSORY	VOCALIZATION	SOCIALIZATION/COGNITION
Adjusts posture to see an object Prefers more complex visual stimuli Can localize sounds made above ear Will turn head to the side, then look up or down	Begins to imitate sounds* Babbling resembles one-syllable utterances—*ma, mu, da, di, hi** Vocalizes to toys, mirror image Takes pleasure in hearing own sounds (self-reinforcement)	Recognizes parents; begins to fear strangers Holds arms out to be picked up Has definite likes and dislikes Begins to imitate (cough, protrusion of tongue) Excites on hearing footsteps Laughs when head is hidden in a towel Briefly searches for a dropped object (object permanence beginning)* Frequent mood swings—from crying to laughing with little or no provocation
Can fixate on very small objects* Responds to own name Localizes sound by turning head in a curving arch Beginning awareness of depth and space Has taste preferences	Produces vowel sounds and chained syllables—*baba, dada, kaka** Vocalizes four distinct vowel sounds "Talks" when others are talking	Increasing fear of strangers; shows signs of fretfulness when parent disappears* Imitates simple acts and noises Tries to attract attention by coughing or snorting Plays peekaboo Demonstrates dislike of food by keeping lips closed Exhibits oral aggressiveness in biting and mouthing Demonstrates expectation in response to repetition of stimuli
	Makes consonant sounds *t, d, w* Listens selectively to familiar words Utterances signal emphasis and emotion Combines syllables, such as *dada*, but does not ascribe meaning to them	Increasing anxiety over loss of parent, particularly mother, and fear of strangers Responds to word "no" Dislikes dressing, diaper change
Localizes sounds by turning head diagonally and directly toward sound Depth perception increasing	Responds to simple verbal commands Comprehends "no-no"	Parent (mother) is increasingly important for own sake Shows increasing interest in pleasing parent Begins to show fears of going to bed and being left alone Puts arms in front of face to avoid having it washed
	Says "dada,""mama" with meaning* Comprehends "bye-bye" May say one word (e.g., "hi,""bye," "no")	Inhibits behavior to verbal command of "no-no" or own name Imitates facial expressions; waves bye-bye Extends toy to another person but will not release it Develops object permanence* Repeats actions that attract attention and cause laughter Pulls clothes of another to attract attention Plays interactive game such as pat-a-cake Reacts to adult anger; cries when scolded Demonstrates independence in dressing, feeding, locomotive skills, and testing of parents Looks at and follows pictures in a book
	Imitates definite speech sounds	Experiences joy and satisfaction when a task is mastered Reacts to restrictions with frustration Rolls ball to another on request Anticipates body gestures when a familiar nursery rhyme or story is being told (e.g., holds toes and feet in response to "This little piggy went to market") Plays game up-down, "so big," or peekaboo Shakes head for "no"
Discriminates simple geometric forms (e.g., circle) Amblyopia may develop with lack of binocularity Can follow rapidly moving object Controls and adjusts response to sound; listens for sound to recur	Says three to five words besides "dada,""mama"* Comprehends meaning of several words (comprehension always precedes verbalization) Recognizes objects by name Imitates animal sounds Understands simple verbal commands (e.g., "Give it to me,""Show me your eyes")	Shows emotions such as jealousy, affection (may give hug or kiss on request), anger, fear Enjoys familiar surroundings and explores away from parent Is fearful in strange situation; clings to parent May develop habit of "security blanket" or favorite toy Has increasing determination to practice locomotor skills Searches for an object even if it has not been hidden, but searches only where object was last seen*

may also belong to a voluntary accreditation system, the National Association for the Education of Young Children, which serves as a model for optimum care.* References from other parents are also helpful, provided that they have investigated the center carefully and have remained involved with the agency's activities.

The same attention should be applied to locating competent baby-sitters. References from other parents are essential, and there is no substitute for observing the interaction between the individual and the child. Although very young infants need little if any preparation for the introduction of a new caregiver, older infants may benefit from a gradual placement to reduce stranger anxiety. At all times the parent should have the right to visit the child, and regular conferences should be established to review the child's progress. Some child care centers provide a service whereby the parent may log on to the Internet from work and view the child's activity at the center for reassurance that the child is well.

One of the areas that is increasingly important in selecting child care is the center's health practices; however, parents often do not check the center for health and safety features. Children in day care centers, especially under age 3 years, have more illnesses—especially diarrhea, otitis media, respiratory tract infections (especially if the caregiver smokes), hepatitis A, meningitis, and cytomegalovirus—than children cared for in their home (National Institute of Child Health and Human Development Early Child Care Research Network, 2001). The strongest predictor of risk of illness is the number of unrelated children in the room. Proactive infection control measures and education of staff have been effective in reducing the incidence of upper respiratory tract infections, diarrhea, and rotavirus (Kotch et al, 2007). It has been reported that families who have children in out-of-home child care lose an estimated 13 days of work per year as a result of infections (Brady, 2005). Parents should inquire about the center's policy regarding the attendance and care of sick children.

Limit Setting and Discipline

As infants' motor skills advance and mobility increases, parents face the need to set safe limits to protect the child and establish a positive and supportive parent-child relationship (see Nurse's Role in Injury Prevention, p. 998). Although there are numerous disciplinary techniques, some are more appropriate for this age than others. An effective approach used in disciplining a child is the use of "time-out." The basic principles are the same as those discussed in Chapter 31, except that the place for time-out needs to be commensurate with the child's abilities. For example, the playpen is better for most infants than a chair. Although parents may be concerned with instituting discipline during infancy, it is important to stress that the earlier effective disciplinary methods are employed, the easier it is to continue these approaches.

Parents must recognize the child's cognitive and behavioral limitations; adequate protection from hazards must be implemented because infants and toddlers do not understand a cause-effect relationship between dangerous objects and physical harm. Children will innately test limits and explore during the exploratory phase of growth; instead of discouraging exploration, parents should provide safe alternatives, put away dangerous household items, and provide consistent discipline and nurturing.

Thumb-Sucking and Use of a Pacifier

Sucking is the infant's chief pleasure and may not be satisfied by breastfeeding or bottle-feeding. It is such a strong need that infants who are deprived of sucking, such as those with a cleft lip repair, will suck on their tongue. Some newborns are born with sucking blisters on their hands from in utero sucking activity. The benefits of nonnutritive sucking in preterm infants, such as increased weight gain, decreased length of stay, and improved pain management, have been documented (Pickler & Frankel, 1995; Pinelli & Symington, 2000; Pinelli, Symington, & Ciliska, 2002). There is currently no evidence that pacifier use and nonnutritive sucking in *preterm* infants has any effect on the initiation and length of breastfeeding. Nonnutritive sucking should not be withheld from preterm infants, especially when performed in conjunction with the use of concentrated sucrose for pain management (see p. 936-938).

Pacifier use, particularly in the early days after birth and in the birth hospital, has gained considerable attention in the scientific literature. Some experts now state that "nontherapeutic" pacifier use should be discouraged, since there are no known benefits to its use other than for nonnutritive sucking and for managing pain. There is evidence that pacifier use in the breastfeeding pair may lead to early weaning from the breast and decreased amount of exclusive breastfeeding. The use of a pacifier has been associated with a slight increase in the incidence of otitis media, and prolonged pacifier use into preschool years has been shown to be detrimental to dental and oral health.

Biancuzzo (2003) suggests that it cannot be stated with absolute certainty that pacifier use is bad in every situation but warns of a potential harm in the use of pacifiers based on available evidence. Furthermore, she admonishes health care workers to be informed regarding potential harm in pacifier use and to inform parents of the potential. Lawrence and Lawrence (2005), as well as other experts in breastfeeding, recommend that health care workers not introduce pacifiers

---

**Information about accreditation criteria and procedures of the NAEYC Academy for Early Childhood Program Accreditation is available from the National Association for the Education of Young Children, 1313 L St. NW, Suite 500, Washington, DC 20005; 800-424-2460 or 202-232-8777;* w. *These criteria are excellent guidelines for evaluating child care facilities. Other resources are (1)* Child Care: What's Best for Your Family *and a number of other child care articles and pamphlets from American Academy of Pediatrics, 141 Northwest Point Blvd., Elk Grove Village, IL 60007; 847-434-4000;* http://aap.org; *to access online, enter the Medem Network,* www.medem.com, *then enter "Medical Library" for pamphlet titles; and (2) Child Care Aware, 800-424-2246;* www.childcareaware.org.

to breast-fed infants unless at the request of the parent. Pacifier use is not recommended as part of the Baby-Friendly Hospital Initiative (see p. 699).

A review of studies by the Joanna Briggs Institute (2005) found an association between pacifier use in infancy and a reduction in breastfeeding and exclusive breastfeeding. However, the authors concluded that pacifier use did not cause a reduction in breastfeeding; rather it was a "marker for socio-economic, demographic, psychosocial and cultural factors that determine pacifier use and breastfeeding." In addition, the researchers examined studies related to pacifier use and prevention of SIDS; infants put to sleep with a pacifier had a *reduced* risk of SIDS. Because of the limited number of studies correlating pacifier use and increased risk of infections or dental malocclusion, the authors were unable to make any recommendations for or against pacifier use in relation to these practices (Joanna Briggs Institute, 2005).

The American Academy of Pediatrics, Task Force on Sudden Infant Death Syndrome (2005), recommends limited pacifier use in infants, citing the strong evidence for pacifier use and its protective effect in SIDS reduction. The exact mechanism involved in the protection for SIDS is not known. Still, pacifier use should not replace actual feeding or suckling; prohibiting pacifier use will not absolutely ensure an increase in the length of breastfeeding; and there should be an emphasis on allowing the infant to control the pace, frequency, and termination of feeding rather than allowing the pacifier (or anything else) to become the focus of the interaction.

The use of a pacifier in infants has also been suggested as a causative factor in the increase in episodes of acute otitis media (Niemela, Uhari, & Mottonen, 1995). However, a later study showed a significant decrease in the incidence of acute otitis media when a pacifier was used only at bedtime (Niemela et al, 2000).

To decrease dependence on nonnutritive sucking in young infants, sucking pleasure can be increased by prolonging feeding time. Also, the parent's excessive use of the pacifier to calm the child should be explored. It is not unusual for parents to place a pacifier in the infant's mouth as soon as crying begins, thus reinforcing a pattern of distress-relief.

If the child uses a pacifier, safety considerations in purchasing one must be stressed. Parents should be cautioned against altering a pacifier, thus making it more dangerous (see Aspiration of Foreign Objects, p. 991). During infancy and early childhood there is no need to restrain nonnutritive sucking of the fingers. Malocclusion may occur if thumb-sucking persists past 4 to 6 years of age, or when the permanent teeth erupt. Pacifiers may be perceived by some parents as less damaging because they are discarded by 2 to 3 years of age, whereas thumb-sucking may persist well into school-age years. Both pacifier use and thumb-sucking may also have significant cultural variations. Thumb-sucking reaches its peak at age 18 to 20 months and is most prevalent when the child is hungry, tired, or feeling insecure. Persistent thumb-sucking in a listless, apathetic child always warrants investigation. It may be a sign of an emotional problem between parent and child or of boredom, isolation, and lack of stimulation.

Teething

One of the more difficult periods in the infant's (and parents') life is the eruption of the deciduous (primary) teeth, often referred to as *teething*. The age of tooth eruption shows considerable variation among children, but the order of their appearance is fairly regular and predictable (Fig. 36-10). The first primary teeth to erupt are the lower central incisors, which appear at approximately 6 to 10 months of age (average 8 months). These are followed closely by the upper central incisors. The following is a quick guide to assessment of deciduous teeth during the first 2 years:

Age of the child in months − 6 = Number of teeth

For example: 8 months of age − 6 = 2 teeth

Teething is a physiologic process; some discomfort is common as the crown of the tooth breaks through the periodontal membrane. Some children show minimum evidence of teething, such as drooling, increased finger sucking, or biting on hard objects. Others are very irritable, have difficulty sleeping, and refuse to eat. Generally, signs of illness such as fever, vomiting, or diarrhea are not symptoms of teething but of illness and may warrant further investigation. Anderson (2004) suggests that frequent waking periods are related to environmental, behavioral, or developmental changes rather than teething. The author also cautions parents (and health

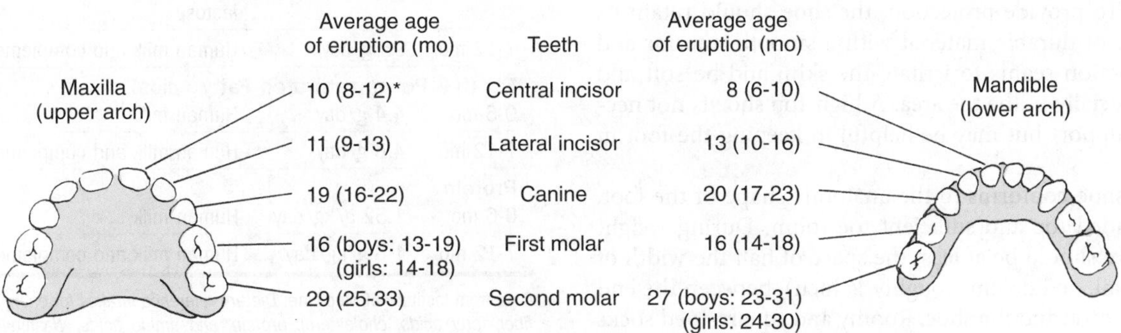

Fig. 36-10 Sequence of eruption of primary teeth. *Range represents ±1 standard deviation, or 67% of subjects studied. (Data from McDonald RE, Avery DR: *Dentistry for the child and adolescent*, ed 6, St Louis, 1994, Mosby.)

care workers) to not overdiagnose teething; the ill-appearing child or child with a temperature over 38° C (100.4° F) should be evaluated by the practitioner.

Because teething pain is a result of inflammation, cold is soothing. Giving the child a frozen teething ring helps relieve the inflammation. Several nonprescription topical anesthetic ointments are available, such as Baby Ora-Jel, although parents and health care workers should be aware of the risks of using topical anesthetic products (absorption rates vary in infants) (Anderson, 2004). The active ingredient in most of these is benzocaine. If such products are used, parents are advised to apply them correctly. In the event of persistent irritability that affects sleeping and feeding, systemic analgesics such as acetaminophen or ibuprofen (age-appropriate dose) can be given (if age appropriate) for no more than 3 days; however, parents should know that this is a temporary measure and should contact the practitioner if symptoms persist or if the child's condition changes.

NURSING ALERT The use of teething powders or procedures, such as cutting the gums or rubbing them with aspirin, is discouraged because ingestion of the powder, infection or irritation of the tissue, or aspiration of the aspirin can occur. Hard candy may cause accidental choking or aspiration and should be avoided at this age.

Infant Shoes

Many parents are unaware of the type of shoes that are appropriate for the older infant and buy expensive infant shoes because of misleading advertising claims. Inflexible shoes that have hard soles can be detrimental. They can delay walking, aggravate intoeing or outtoeing, and impede the development of supportive foot muscles. Therefore the counseling of parents regarding footwear should begin when infants are 6 months old—well before they are walking.

It is helpful to begin by explaining to parents that changes in the feet occur during infancy and early childhood as locomotion and weight bearing progress. At birth the feet are flat because the arches are protected by fat pads on the soles. As the bones in the arches develop, the pads disappear and the feet begin to assume a mature shape. A normal arch is determined by proper alignment of all the bones and development of the surrounding musculature, not by the height of the arch.

When children begin walking, the main reason for shoes is protection. To provide protection, the shoe should retain its fit; be made of durable material with a smooth interior and few construction seams to irritate the skin; and be soft and flexible, especially in the toe area. A high-top shoe is not necessary for support but may be helpful in keeping the foot in the shoe.

A good shoe conforms to the anatomic shape of the foot, with a rounded toe and sufficient toe room. During weight bearing there should be at least the space of half the width of the thumbnail, or 1.25 cm (roughly ½ inch), between the end of the longest toe and the shoe. Roomy and square-toed socks allow for proper growth and alignment. Inexpensive but well-constructed sneakers or soft-leather moccasin-type shoes are suggested as adequate footgear for walking infants.Even if the shoes are fitted properly, frequent changes are needed to accommodate the infant's rapidly growing feet. Shoe size changes at approximately 3-month intervals between 12 and 36 months; during this time the child's foot should be measured every 3 months. Curled toes when shoes are removed, and redness and irritation of the skin on the bottom of the toes, indicate the need for a larger shoe size.

Promoting Optimum Health During Infancy

Nutrition

Ideally, discussion of optimum nutrition should begin prenatally with the decision to breastfeed or bottle-feed the infant. The choice for either is highly individual and is discussed in Chapter 26. This section is primarily concerned with infant nutrition up to the age of 12 months, when growth needs and developmental milestones ready the child for the introduction of solid foods. Table 36-3 shows the Dietary Reference Intake Adequate Intakes for infants for carbohydrate, fat, and protein intake during the first year of life.

There is concern that, despite adequate availability of optimal nutrient sources, infants are not being fed appropriately. These practices may have far-reaching, long-term health consequences for infants. It has been shown that infant health practices have an impact on the child's life. Certain chronic health conditions have been linked to feeding practices in infancy. Nurses must be proactive in teaching parents about what constitutes appropriate infant nutrition and nutritional habits, which provide the opportunity to grow and develop into a healthy child and adult.

Health care professionals have become more aware of the use of complementary and alternative medical therapies in children that may not be as beneficial as touted in various media sources. One concern is children's intake of megavitamins and herbs; parents may assume that the word *natural* in

Table 36-3 Dietary Reference Intake (DRI): Adequate Intake (AI)* for Infants

AGE	AI	COMMENTS
Carbohydrate		
0-6 mo	60 g/day	Human milk; predominant source is lactose
7-12 mo	95 g/day	Human milk and complementary foods
Fat (n-6 Polyunsaturated Fatty Acids)		
0-6 mo	4.4 g/day	Human milk
7-12 mo	4.6 g/day	Human milk and complementary foods
Protein		
0-6 mo	1.52 g/kg/day	Human milk
7-12 mo	1.6 g/kg/day	Human milk and complementary foods

Data from Institute of Medicine: *Dietary reference intakes for energy, carbohydrate, fiber, fatty acids, cholesterol, protein, and amino acids,* Washington, DC, 2005, Food and Nutrition Board, Institute of Medicine, National Academies Press.

*AI–The recommended average daily intake level based on observed or experimentally determined approximations or estimates of nutrient intake by a group (or groups) of apparently healthy individuals that are assumed to be adequate; used when a recommended dietary allowance cannot be determined.

reference to ingredients means the product is safe, when this may not be the case. One report cited the home administration of star anise tea to treat colic as the cause of adverse neurologic reactions in seven infants (Ize-Ludlow et al, 2004). It is important for nurses to be aware of the effects, availability, and practice of complementary therapies and to be able to cogently discuss their use with parents.

The First 6 Months

Human milk is the most desirable complete diet for the infant during the first 6 months. The healthy term infant receiving breast milk from a well-nourished mother usually requires no specific vitamin and mineral supplements, with a few exceptions. Daily supplements of vitamin D and vitamin B_{12} may be indicated if the mother's intake of these vitamins is inadequate. The American Academy of Pediatrics (2008) issued a recommendation that all infants (including those exclusively breastfed) receive a daily supplement of 400 International Units of vitamin D beginning in the first few days of life to prevent rickets and vitamin D deficiency. Vitamin D supplementation should occur until the infant is consuming at least 1 L/day (or 1 qt/day) of vitamin-D fortified formula (American Academy of Pediatrics, 2008). Nonbreastfed infants who are taking less than 1 L/day of vitamin D–fortified formula should also receive a daily vitamin D supplement of 400 International Units. If the infant is being exclusively breastfed after 4 to 6 months (when fetal iron stores are depleted), iron supplementation, which may be accomplished with iron-fortified cereal, is recommended to offset the decrease in iron available in human milk at this time and to enhance erythropoiesis. Infants, whether breastfed or bottle-fed, do not require additional fluids, especially water or juice, during the first 4 months of life. Excessive intake of water in infants may result in water intoxication and hyponatremia.

Employed mothers can continue breastfeeding with guidance and encouragement. Mothers are encouraged to set realistic goals for employment and breastfeeding, with accurate information regarding the costs, risks, and benefits of available feeding options. The working mother is also encouraged to develop and implement a strategic plan, such as a set routine for feeding and pumping and a backup contingency for successful feeding. Barriers encountered by working breastfeeding mothers include lack of employer or co-worker support, unavailable or inadequate facilities for pumping and storing milk, and insufficient time allowed during work time to pump (Rojjanasrirat, 2004). Important themes that emerged in the study by Rojjanasrirat (2004) of working breastfeeding mothers included support (emotional, informational, and instrumental), attitude, and psychologic distress. Many mothers may find that a program of breast pumping when away from home and bottle-feeding the infant the expressed milk with or without formula supplementation is successful.

Expressed breast milk may be stored in the refrigerator (4° C [39° F]) without danger of bacterial contamination for up to 5 days (Lawrence & Lawrence, 2005). Although feeding the infant at home may occur on a demand basis, pumping milk away from home may be needed every 3 to 4 hours to maintain adequate supply. Breast milk may be expressed by hand or pump (manual or electric) and stored in an appropriate air-tight glass or plastic container. Expressed breast milk may be frozen (−18° C [0° F] or lower) for up to 12 months (depending on the type of freezer used), but care should be taken to prevent freezer burn (see Appendix P, protocol no. 8, in Lawrence & Lawrence, 2005, for further guidelines on storing and freezing human milk). Health care workers and new mothers may find the booklet *Working and Breastfeeding—Can You Do It? Yes, You Can!* by Johnson & Johnson helpful.*

In addition to efficient breast pumping, mothers also need child care by a trusted individual or agency and support and assistance from significant others. As with all breastfeeding mothers, these women must have proper nutrition and rest for adequate lactation. Maternal fatigue is considered the biggest threat to successful breastfeeding in employed mothers (Corbett-Dick & Bezek, 1997).

Warming expressed milk in a microwave decreases the availability of antiinfective properties and vitamin C and causes a separation of milk layers, which affects fat content (Lawrence & Lawrence, 2005). To prevent oral burns from uneven warming of the milk, breast milk should never be thawed or rewarmed in a microwave oven. To thaw the frozen milk, either place the container under a lukewarm water bath (less than 40.5° C [105° F]) or place it in the refrigerator overnight. Although microwaving bottles and baby food is not recommended, it remains a common practice. Guidelines have been developed for microwave heating of refrigerated formula, and these should be given to the family (see Patient Teaching box).

PATIENT TEACHING Microwave Heating of Refrigerated Infant Formula

Before heating:
- Heat only 4 oz or more.
- Heat only *refrigerated* formula.
- Always *stand* the bottle up.
- Always leave the bottle top *uncovered* to allow heat to escape.

Heating instructions (full power):
- Heat 4-oz bottles for no more than 30 seconds.
- Heat 8-oz bottles for no more than 45 seconds.

Serving instructions:
- Always replace nipple assembly; *invert* 10 times (vigorous shaking is unnecessary).
- Formula should be cool to the touch; formula warm to the touch may be too hot to serve.
- Always *test* formula; place several drops on your tongue or on the back of the hand (not the inside wrist).

Modified from Sigman-Grant M, Bush G, Anantheswaran R: Microwave heating of infant formula: a dilemma resolved, *Pediatrics* 90(3):414, 1992.

Developed by National Healthy Mothers, Healthy Babies Coalition, 2000 N. Beauregard St., 6th floor, Alexandria, VA 22311; 703-837-4792; www.hmhb.org.

An acceptable alternative to breastfeeding is commercial iron-fortified formula. Like human milk, it supplies all of the nutrients needed by the infant for the first 6 months.

Unmodified whole cow's milk, low-fat cow's milk, skim milk, other animal milks, and imitation milks are not acceptable as a major source of nutrition for infants because of their limited ability to be digested, an increased risk of contamination, and a lack of nutritional components needed for appropriate growth. Pasteurized whole cow's milk is deficient in iron, zinc, and vitamin C and has a high renal solute load, which makes it undesirable for infants less than 12 months of age (American Academy of Pediatrics, 2009).

Dietary fat should not be restricted in infancy unless under medical supervision. Substituting skim or low-fat milk is unacceptable because the essential fatty acids are inadequate and the solute concentration of protein and electrolytes, such as sodium, is too high.

The amount of formula per feeding and the number of feedings per day vary among infants. Infants on demand feeding usually determine their own feeding schedule, but some infants may need a more planned schedule based on average feeding patterns to ensure sufficient nutrients. In general, the number of feedings decreases from six at 1 month of age to four or five at 6 months. Regardless of the number of feedings, the total amount of formula ingested will usually level off at about 32 oz (960 ml/day). Parents should be cautioned concerning the use of juices and nonnutritive drinks such as fruit-flavored drinks or carbonated beverages (soda or pop) during this period. Many juices and nonnutritive drinks, although readily available to consumers, do not provide sufficient caloric intake for infants less than 12 months of age; such drinks may replace the nutrients in milk (formula) and lead to growth or health problems.

Bottled water for mixing powdered or concentrated formula is a relatively safe alternative to tap water if available tap water has a high content of contaminants such as lead. Bottled water, however, should not be assumed to be sterile unless specifically stated on the container. Fluoridated bottled water is not necessary for mixing powdered formula unless the local water source is low in fluoride, in which case fluoride supplementation is recommended after age 6 months (see Dental Health, p. 978).

The addition of solid foods before 4 to 6 months of age is not recommended. During the early months solid foods are not compatible with the ability of the gastrointestinal tract and the infant's nutritional needs. Developmentally, infants are not ready for solid food. The extrusion (protrusion) reflex is strong and causes food to be pushed out of the mouth. Early introduction of solids is a type of forced feeding that may lead to excessive weight gain and increased predisposition to allergies and iron deficiency anemia. Despite these recommendations, and lacking evidence-based information to support such practices, many parents introduce solids as early as 2 weeks of age. In such cases, rice cereal is often added to the formula to help the infant sleep better at night or to enhance weight gain; however, this practice is not substantiated by any scientific evidence (Morin, 2004). Fruit juices are not recommended during the first 6 months of life; there are no studies demonstrating benefits of giving fruit juices, yet parents may perceive this practice as beneficial.

The Second 6 Months

During the second half of the first year, human milk or formula continues to be the primary source of nutrition. Fluoride supplementation should begin, depending on the infant's intake of fluoridated tap water (see Dental Health, p. 978). If breastfeeding is discontinued, a commercial iron-fortified formula should be substituted. Follow-up or transition formulas specially marketed for older infants offer no special advantages over other infant formulas (American Academy of Pediatrics, 2009).

The major change in feeding habits is the addition of solid foods to the infant's diet. Physiologically and developmentally, the infant 4 to 6 months of age is in a transition period. By this time the gastrointestinal tract has matured sufficiently to handle more complex nutrients and is less sensitive to potentially allergenic foods. Tooth eruption is beginning and facilitates biting and chewing. The extrusion reflex has disappeared, and swallowing is more coordinated to allow the infant to accept solids easily. Head control is well developed, which permits infants to sit with support and purposely turn the head away to communicate disinterest in food. Voluntary grasping and improved eye-hand coordination gradually allow infants to pick up finger foods and feed themselves. Their increasing sense of independence is evident in their desire to hold the bottle and try to "help" during feeding.

Selection and Preparation of Solid Foods

The choice of solid foods to introduce first is variable but should meet the reasons for feeding solids, such as supplying nutrients not found in formula or breast milk. Iron-fortified infant cereal is generally introduced first because of its high iron content (7 mg/3 tbsp of prepared dry cereal). Commercially prepared ready-to-serve dry cereals for infants include rice, barley, oatmeal, and high-protein cereals; rice is usually suggested as an initial food because of its easy digestibility and low allergenic potential. Cereals such as cream of farina are not used because infant commercial cereals are a better source of iron. Some of the commercial baby cereals are combined with fruit. There is little nutritional benefit from these preparations, they are more expensive, and some may contain additional calories. New foods should be added one at a time; therefore parents should avoid cereal combinations when beginning a new grain.

Infant cereal (iron fortified) is mixed with formula until whole milk is given. If the infant is breastfed, the cereal is mixed with expressed breast milk or water. The addition of solid foods to the exclusively breastfed infant's diet does not significantly increase overall caloric intake or weight gain (Dewey, 2001). After 6 months of age, small amounts of fruit juices can be mixed with the dry cereal; the vitamin C content of the juice enhances the absorption of iron in the cereal. Because of their benefit as a source of iron, infant cereals should be continued until the child is 18 months of age.

Fruit juice can be offered from a cup for its rich source of vitamin C and as a substitute for milk for one feeding a day. Large quantities of certain juices (e.g., apple, pear, prune, sweet cherry, peach, grape) are avoided because they may cause abdominal pain, diarrhea, or bloating in some children. White grape juice is reported to be better absorbed and safe for infants this age (less than 6 oz/day) without causing gastrointestinal distress. Avoid fruit-flavored drinks, which may be marketed as juices but contain high concentrations of complex sugars. The American Academy of Pediatrics (2009) recommends that fruit juice intake not exceed 4 to 6 oz per day and that juices not be given to infants less than 6 months old; only 100% fruit juice should be given. Because vitamin C is naturally destroyed by heat, juice is not warmed. Juice containers are always kept covered and refrigerated to prevent further vitamin loss. Offer fruit juice from a cup, rather than a bottle, to prevent the development of nursing caries (see Low-Cariogenic Diet, Chapter 37).

The addition of other foods is arbitrary. A common sequence is to introduce strained fruits, followed by vegetables, and finally meats. If foods are introduced early, citrus fruits, meats, and eggs are delayed until after 6 months of age because of their potential to result in allergy. At 6 months, foods such as a cracker or zwieback can be offered as a type of finger and teething food. By 8 to 9 months, junior foods and nutritious finger foods such as a firmly cooked vegetable, raw pieces of fruit (except grapes), or cheese can be given. By 1 year, well-cooked table foods are served.

Commercially prepared baby foods are the most commonly used types of food served to infants in the United States. They are convenient and usually contain no added salt or sugar, but they are relatively expensive. An alternative is to prepare baby foods at home, which is a simple and inexpensive process. Fruits and vegetables can be steamed in a small amount of water and pureed in a blender or food processor. Many of them, such as ripe banana, can be mashed fine with a fork. Fruits such as apples or pears require little or no water in the cooking process. Vegetables such as carrots, potatoes, or string beans require additional water in the cooking and blending process.

Preferably, infant foods prepared at home should start with fresh or frozen foods, since canned foods, other than those prepared for infants, may contain excessive sodium or sugar or be a source of lead from the container. If sweetening is needed, refined sugar can be used, but honey and corn syrup are avoided because of the risk of infant botulism. There is no evidence that the addition of salt to foods such as vegetables increases the infant's acceptance of the new food. Additional guidelines for the home preparation of baby foods are provided by Morin (2005).

Parents are cautioned to avoid reliance on foods and supplements marketed as iron- or vitamin-fortified as primary sources of minerals. Instead encourage parents to offer the child a variety of fruits, vegetables, whole grains, and those known to naturally be rich in iron.

Low-calorie foods should be avoided in infants and toddlers unless a strict, medically prescribed diet is required. The infant's growth during this phase is crucial to future development, and curtailing dietary fat should be done with great caution. Many parents may be concerned that their child is getting too much dietary fat; in such cases the primary practitioner should be consulted before dietary substitutions are made. On the other hand, making an infant or toddler finish a bottle or "clean up the plate" may lead to unhealthy eating habits (see Obesity, Chapter 40).

Introduction of Solid Foods

When the spoon is first introduced, infants often push it away and appear dissatisfied. Patience and skill are required to overcome this initial response. A small-bowled, straight, long-handled spoon, similar to a demitasse spoon, allows a small portion of food to be placed toward the back of the tongue. Food that is placed on the front of the tongue and pushed out is simply scooped up and refed. As infants become accustomed to the spoon, they more eagerly accept the food and eventually will open the mouth in anticipation (or keep it closed in dislike). Because the first introduction of food is a new experience, spoon feeding should be attempted after ingestion of some breast milk or formula to associate this activity with a pleasurable and satisfying experience. Trying to introduce a food *after* the entire milk feeding is usually useless because the infant is satiated and has no inclination to try something new.

After several spoon feedings, food can be introduced at the beginning of a meal. It is best to introduce many foods during the first year, when the infant is more likely to eat them because of a hearty appetite resulting from a rapid growth rate. During the toddler years eating becomes less of an adventure, and strong food preferences become evident.

One food item is introduced at intervals of 4 to 7 days to allow for identification of food allergies. New foods are fed in small amounts, from 1 tsp to a few tablespoons. As the amount of solid food increases, the quantity of milk is decreased to less than 1 L daily to prevent overfeeding.

Because feeding is a learning process, as well as a means of nutrition, new foods are given alone to allow the child to learn new tastes and textures. Food should not be mixed in the bottle and fed through a nipple with a large hole; this deprives the child of the pleasure of learning new tastes and of developing a discriminating palate. It can also cause problems with poor chewing of food later in life because of lack of experience. Guidelines for the introduction of new foods are given in the Patient Teaching box.

The infant's first, second, and often twentieth try at self-feeding or cup feeding is a sloppy experience. Finger foods such as soft fruits or vegetables are just as good as playthings as food; they can be squeezed, smeared, squashed, and thoroughly painted on oneself, others, and the surrounding environment. However, all of this is part of learning, and mastery follows many accidents.

Parents are encouraged to interpret the infant's signals of discomfort and intervene in ways other than through feeding. Crying, fussiness, and sucking do not necessarily indicate hunger. Rocking, stroking, holding, and offering a toy or a pacifier may be more appropriate than automatically responding with food.

PATIENT TEACHING Introducing Solid Foods to Infants

- Introduce solids when infant is hungry.
- Begin spoon feeding by pushing food to back of tongue because of infant's natural tendency to thrust the tongue forward.
- Use a small spoon with a straight handle; begin with 1 or 2 tsp of food; gradually increase to a couple of tablespoons per feeding.
- Introduce one food at a time, usually at intervals of 4 to 7 days to allow for identification of food allergies.
- As the amount of solid food increases, decrease the quantity of milk to prevent overfeeding.
- Do not introduce foods by mixing them with formula in the bottle.

Weaning

Defined as the process of giving up one method of feeding for another, *weaning* usually refers to relinquishing the breast or bottle for a cup. In Western societies this is generally regarded as a major task for infants and is often seen as a potentially traumatic experience. It is psychologically significant because the infant is required to give up a major source of oral pleasure and gratification.

There is no one time for weaning that is best for every child, but most infants show signs of readiness during the second half of the first year. They have learned that good things come from a spoon. Their increasing desire for freedom of movement may lessen their desire to be held close for feedings. They are acquiring more control over their actions and can easily manipulate a cup to their lips (even if it is held upside down!). Imitation becomes a powerful motivator by age 8 or 9 months, and they enjoy using a cup or glass like others do. It is recommended that weaning be accomplished with the infant's needs as a guide (Lawrence & Lawrence, 2005).

Weaning should be gradual, replacing one bottle-feeding or breastfeeding at a time. The nighttime feeding is usually the last feeding to be discontinued. It is advisable never to begin allowing a child to take a bottle of milk to bed; this is a major cause of nursing caries in deciduous teeth. If breastfeeding is terminated before 5 or 6 months of age, weaning should be to a bottle to provide for the infant's continued sucking needs. If breastfeeding is discontinued later, weaning can be directly to a cup, especially by age 12 to 14 months. Any sweet liquid, such as fruit juice, should be given in a cup.

Sleep and Activity

Sleep patterns vary among infants, with active infants typically sleeping less than placid children. Generally, by 3 to 4 months of age most infants have developed a nocturnal pattern of sleep that lasts 9 to 11 hours. The total daily sleep is approximately 15 hours. The number of naps per day varies, but infants may take one or two naps by the end of the first year. Breastfed infants usually sleep for less prolonged periods, with more frequent waking, especially during the night, than do bottle-fed infants. Because of the trend toward breastfeeding, sleep norms such as those previously described, which were based primarily on bottle-fed infants, may not be relevant.

Most infants are naturally active and need no encouragement to be mobile. However, problems can arise when devices such as playpens, strollers, commercial swings, and walkers are used excessively. These items restrict movement and prevent infants from exploring and developing gross motor skills. Contrary to popular belief, walkers do not enhance coordination and are dangerous if tipped over or placed near stairs. The American Academy of Pediatrics, Committee on Injury and Poison Prevention (2001), recommended a ban on the sale of infant walkers because of the large number of injuries. Newer models of infant walkers have been designed without wheels to decrease infant injuries (see Falls, p. 995).

Formal infant exercise programs do not provide any long-term benefit to normal infants, and the possibility for damage to the infant's skeletal system exists. For these reasons, such programs are not recommended (American Academy of Pediatrics, Committee on Sports Medicine, 1988).

Sleep Problems

A number of sleep problems are identified in small children. One of the two major categories is dyssomnia: the child has trouble either falling or staying asleep at night, or has difficulty staying awake during the day. The second category, parasomnias, are characterized as confusional arousals, sleep-walking, sleep terrors, nightmares, and rhythmic movement disorders; these typically occur in children 3 to 8 years old (Dahl, 1998) and decline in incidence as the child matures (Davis, Parker, & Montgomery, 2004). This discussion focuses on minor sleep issues in infants such as refusal to go to sleep or frequent waking during the night (Table 36-4). Other sleep disturbances such as obstructive sleep apnea and sleep terrors are discussed elsewhere in this text.

Concerns regarding sleep are common during infancy (see Cultural Awareness box). Sometimes these concerns are as basic as parents' questioning whether the infant needs additional sleep. In this case it is best to investigate the reason for their concern, stressing each child's individual needs. Infants who are active during wakeful periods and growing normally are sleeping a sufficient amount of time.

Sleep problems in early infancy have also been positively correlated with higher maternal depression scores (Hiscock & Wake, 2001; Hawkins-Walsh, 2003) and poorer general and mental health in both mother and father (Martin et al, 2007). Therefore nurses must discuss infant sleep problems with the mother (and family) in addition to other developmental aspects of newborn care.

When a sleeping problem exists, a careful assessment is essential. Charting sleep habits both before and after interventions is also an important strategy. Questions regarding the frequency and duration of waking, the usual bedtime routine, the number of nighttime feedings, the perceived problem (e.g., how much disruption the behavior generates), and the attempted interventions are important in planning effective approaches designed for the specific sleep problem. A common suggestion given for any type of sleep problem—"Let the child cry until he or she falls asleep"—is very difficult to implement

Table 36-4 Selected Sleep Disturbances During Infancy and Early Childhood

DISORDER/DESCRIPTION	MANAGEMENT
Nighttime Feeding	
Child has a prolonged need for middle-of-night bottle-feeding or breastfeeding. Child goes to sleep at breast or with a bottle. Awakenings are frequent (may be hourly). Child returns to sleep after feeding; other comfort measures (e.g., rocking or holding) are usually ineffective.	Increase daytime feeding intervals to 4 hr or more (may need to be done gradually). Offer last feeding as late as possible at night; may need to gradually reduce amount of formula or length of breastfeeding. Offer no bottles in bed. Put to bed *awake*. When child is crying, check at progressively longer intervals each night; reassure child but do not hold, rock, take to parent's bed, or give bottle or pacifier.
Developmental Night Crying	
Child age 6-12 mo with undisturbed nighttime sleep now awakes abruptly; may be accompanied by nightmares.	Parents should be reassured that this phase is temporary. Enter room immediately to check on child but keep reassurances *brief*. Avoid feeding, rocking, taking to parent's bed, or any other routine that may initiate trained night crying.
Trained Night Crying (Inappropriate Sleep Associations)	
Child typically falls asleep in place other than own bed (e.g., rocking chair or parent's bed) and is taken to own bed while asleep; on awakening, cries until usual routine is instituted (e.g., rocking).	Put child in own bed when *awake*. If possible, arrange sleeping area separate from other family members. When child is crying, check at progressively longer intervals each night; reassure child but do not resume usual routine.
Refusal to Go to Sleep	
Child resists bedtime and comes out of room repeatedly. Nighttime sleep may be continuous, but frequent awakenings and refusal to return to sleep may occur and become a problem if parent allows child to deviate from usual sleep pattern.	Evaluate whether hour of sleep is too early (child may resist sleep if not tired). Parents should be assisted in establishing consistent before-bedtime routine and enforcing consistent limits regarding child's bedtime behavior. If child persists in leaving bedroom, close door for progressively longer periods. Use reward system with child to provide motivation.
Nighttime Fears	
Child resists going to bed or wakes during the night because of fears. Child seeks parent's physical presence and falls asleep easily with parent nearby, unless fear is overwhelming.	Evaluate whether hour of sleep is too early (child may fantasize when nothing to do but think in dark room). Calmly reassure the frightened child; keeping a night light on may help. Use reward system with child to provide motivation to deal with fears. Avoid patterns that can lead to additional problems (e.g., sleeping with child or taking child to parent's room). If child's fear is overwhelming, consider desensitization (e.g., progressively spending longer periods of time alone; consult professional help for protracted fears). Distinguish between nightmares and sleep terrors (confused partial arousals).

Modified from Ferber R: Behavioral "insomnia" in the child, *Psychiatr Clin North Am* 10(4):641-653, 1987.

and is inappropriate for certain conditions. Once the parents relent and console the child, they have only reinforced the crying.

An equally effective and more atraumatic approach to night crying, known as *graduated extinction,* is to let the child cry for progressively longer times between brief parental interventions that consist only of reassurance—not rocking, holding, or using a bottle or pacifier. For example, the parents may check on the child every 5 minutes during the first night and progressively extend this interval by 5 minutes on successive nights.

Families who cannot tolerate unexpected crying spells while everyone else is asleep can try the two-step approach. Graduated extinction is used during naps and at bedtime until the parents retire. If the child cries during the night, the parents use comforting measures. However, once the child is partially trained, step 2 is initiated—the use of graduated extinction at all times.

Children who learn to fall asleep on their own at bedtime have longer sustained sleep periods than those who fall asleep with a parent present (Davis, Parker, & Montgomery, 2004). In addition, comforting children outside their own bed at night once they awaken was associated with poor sleep consolidation. Feeding the 5-month-old after awakening at night has been associated with fewer consecutive sleep hours (Touchette et al, 2005). The authors of this study recommend parental presence at bedtime until the child is drowsy, then placing the child in his or her own bed for a night's sleep.

The best way to prevent sleep problems is to encourage parents to establish bedtime rituals that do not foster problematic patterns. One of the most constructive is placing infants *awake* in their own crib. When infants are accustomed to falling asleep somewhere else, such as in their parent's arms, and then being transferred to their crib, they awaken in unfamiliar surroundings and are unable to fall asleep until the routine is repeated. In addition, the bed should be used for sleeping only—not as a playpen. It is advisable to not hang playthings over or on the bed; in this way the child associates the bed with sleep, not with activity. Although the interventions described previously and in Table 36-4 are usually successful, it is much easier to prevent the problem with

evolve Skill—Fostering Healthy Sleep Patterns in Children

appropriate counseling during the early months of the infant's life.

Dental Health

Good dental hygiene begins with appropriate maternal dental health and counseling during early infancy regarding dietary intake for the promotion of optimal oral hygiene (Douglass, Douglass, & Silk, 2004). Parents are counseled early regarding the risk of feeding practices that increase the risk of poor dental health. Some of these have been previously mentioned and include avoiding propping the milk bottle or giving the milk bottle in the bed, and avoiding fruit juices in a bottle, especially before 6 months of age. Once the primary teeth erupt, cleaning should begin. The teeth and gums are initially cleaned by wiping with a damp cloth; toothbrushing is too harsh for the tender gingiva. The caregiver can stabilize the infant by cradling the child with one arm and using the free hand to cleanse the teeth. Oral hygiene can be made pleasant by singing or talking to the infant. There are no clear guidelines regarding when toothbrushing should begin; however, it is recommended that the infant have an oral health examination by 6 months of age from a qualified pediatric health practitioner. Infants at high risk for dental caries should be seen by a dentist between 6 months and 1 year of age (American Academy of Pediatric Dentistry, 2008b). It is generally recommended that a small, soft-bristled toothbrush be used as more teeth erupt and the infant adjusts to the routine of cleaning. Water is preferred to toothpaste, which the infant will swallow (and if the toothpaste is fluoridated, the infant will ingest excessive amounts of fluoride).

Fluoride, an essential mineral for building caries-resistant teeth, is needed beginning at 6 months of age if the infant does not receive water with an adequate fluoride content. The American Academy of Pediatric Dentistry recommends fluoride supplementation begin at 6 months. The fluoride dosage has been decreased from earlier recommendations because of an increased occurrence of dental fluorosis from excessive fluoride ingestion. The latest recommendation is to give children 6 months to 3 years of age 0.25 mg fluoride daily if water fluoride content is less than 0.3 ppm (parts per million) (American Academy of Pediatric Dentistry, 2008a). If bottled water is used to reconstitute powdered or concentrated formula, it should either be fluoride free or contain low levels of fluoride (American Dental Association, 2007).

Dietary considerations are also important because habits begun during infancy tend to continue into later years. Foods with added concentrated sugar are used sparingly (if at all) in the infant's diet. The practice of coating pacifiers with honey or using commercially available hard-candy pacifiers is discouraged. Besides being cariogenic, honey also may cause infant botulism, and parts of the candy pacifier can be aspirated (see Aspiration of Foreign Objects, p. 991). Parents need to be counseled regarding the detrimental effects of frequent and prolonged bottle-feeding or breastfeeding during sleep, when the sweet milk or other fluid, such as juice, bathes the teeth, producing nursing caries. In addition, carbonated beverages should be avoided in infancy. (See Chapter 37 for a more extensive discussion of dental care, including nursing caries.)

evolve Case Study—Immunizations

Immunizations

Perhaps one of the most dramatic advances in pediatrics has been the decline of infectious diseases during the twentieth century because of the widespread use of immunization for preventable diseases. However, childhood vaccines have been widely criticized in recent years, and fear related to vaccine components has prompted some families to avoid childhood vaccines. In addition, many of the diseases for which children are vaccinated are rarely seen on a large scale basis, leading some parents to believe that such vaccines are no longer necessary in the twenty-first century. The Internet provides a variety of information suggesting parents avoid childhood vaccines; a number of "vaccine myths" exist, which are based on erroneous information. A variety of websites that include objective and scientifically accurate information are provided in the Resources on this text's website. It is the nurse's responsibility to provide parents with accurate information regarding childhood illnesses and available vaccines; the parent must then make an informed decision regarding the child's vaccinations. Nurses should address parents' concerns about childhood vaccines and avoid judgmental attitudes regarding the parents' decision to not vaccinate children.

Although many of the immunizations can be given to individuals of any age, the recommended primary schedule begins during infancy and, with the exception of boosters, is completed during early childhood. Therefore the discussion of childhood immunizations for diphtheria, tetanus, pertussis; polio; measles, mumps, rubella; *Haemophilus influenzae* type b; hepatitis A virus (HAV), hepatitis B virus (HBV); pneumococcus; influenza; meningococcus; and chickenpox is included under health promotion during infancy. Selected vaccines generally reserved for children considered at high risk for the disease are discussed here and as appropriate throughout the text. (See also Communicable Diseases, Chapter 38, for a discussion of several of the diseases for which vaccines are available.)

Schedule for Immunizations

In the United States, two organizations—the Advisory Committee on Immunization Practices of the Centers for Disease Control and Prevention and the Committee on Infectious Diseases of the American Academy of Pediatrics—govern the recommendations for immunization policies and procedures. In Canada, recommendations are from the National Advisory Committee on Immunization under the authority of the Minister of Health and Public Health Agency of Canada. The policies of each committee are *recommendations,* not rules, and they change as a result of advances in the field of immunology. Nurses need to keep informed of the latest advances and changes in policy.

In the United States the recommended age for beginning primary immunizations of infants is within 2 weeks of birth or, in special circumstances, at birth (Figs. 36-11 and 36-12). Infants born preterm should receive the full dose of each vaccine at the appropriate chronologic age. Catch-up immunizations for children who do not receive vaccines according to the recommended schedule in Figs. 36-11 and 36-12 are

Text continued on p. 982

Recommended Immunization Schedule for Persons Aged 0 Through 6 Years—United States • 2009

For those who fall behind or start late, see the catch-up schedule

Vaccine ▼ Age ►	Birth	1 month	2 months	4 months	6 months	12 months	15 months	18 months	19–23 months	2–3 years	4–6 years
Hepatitis B[1]	HepB	HepB		*see footnote 1*			HepB				
Rotavirus[2]			RV	RV	*RV*[2]						
Diphtheria, Tetanus, Pertussis[3]			DTaP	DTaP	DTaP	*see footnote 3*	DTaP				DTaP
Haemophilus influenzae type b[4]			Hib	Hib	*Hib*[4]	Hib					
Pneumococcal[5]			PCV	PCV	PCV	PCV				PPSV	
Inactivated Poliovirus			IPV	IPV			IPV				IPV
Influenza[6]								Influenza (Yearly)			
Measles, Mumps, Rubella[7]						MMR			*see footnote 7*		MMR
Varicella[8]						Varicella			*see footnote 8*		Varicella
Hepatitis A[9]								HepA (2 doses)		HepA Series	
Meningococcal[10]										MCV	

Range of recommended ages

Certain high-risk groups

This schedule indicates the recommended ages for routine administration of currently licensed vaccines, as of December 1, 2008, for children aged 0 through 6 years. Any dose not administered at the recommended age should be administered at a subsequent visit, when indicated and feasible. Licensed combination vaccines may be used whenever any component of the combination is indicated and other components are not contraindicated and if approved by the Food and Drug Administration for that dose of the series. Providers should consult the relevant Advisory Committee on Immunization Practices statement for detailed recommendations, including high-risk conditions: http://www.cdc.gov/vaccines/pubs/acip-list.htm. Clinically significant adverse events that follow immunization should be reported to the Vaccine Adverse Event Reporting System (VAERS). Guidance about how to obtain and complete a VAERS form is available at http://www.vaers.hhs.gov or by telephone, 800-822-7967.

1. Hepatitis B vaccine (HepB). ***(Minimum age: birth)***

At birth:

- Administer monovalent HepB to all newborns before hospital discharge.
- If mother is hepatitis B surface antigen (HBsAg)-positive, administer HepB and 0.5 mL of hepatitis B immune globulin (HBIG) within 12 hours of birth.
- If mother's HBsAg status is unknown, administer HepB within 12 hours of birth. Determine mother's HBsAg status as soon as possible and, if HBsAg-positive, administer HBIG (no later than age 1 week).

After the birth dose:

- The HepB series should be completed with either monovalent HepB or a combination vaccine containing HepB. The second dose should be administered at age 1 or 2 months. The final dose should be administered no earlier than age 24 weeks.
- Infants born to HBsAg-positive mothers should be tested for HBsAg and antibody to HBsAg (anti-HBs) after completion of at least 3 doses of the HepB series, at age 9 through 18 months (generally at the next well-child visit).

4-month dose:

- Administration of 4 doses of HepB to infants is permissible when combination vaccines containing HepB are administered after the birth dose.

2. Rotavirus vaccine (RV). ***(Minimum age: 6 weeks)***

- Administer the first dose at age 6 through 14 weeks (maximum age: 14 weeks 6 days). Vaccination should not be initiated for infants aged 15 weeks or older (i.e., 15 weeks 0 days or older).
- Administer the final dose in the series by age 8 months 0 days.
- If Rotarix® is administered at ages 2 and 4 months, a dose at 6 months is not indicated.

3. Diphtheria and tetanus toxoids and acellular pertussis vaccine (DTaP). ***(Minimum age: 6 weeks)***

- The fourth dose may be administered as early as age 12 months, provided at least 6 months have elapsed since the third dose.
- Administer the final dose in the series at age 4 through 6 years.

4. *Haemophilus influenzae* type b conjugate vaccine (Hib). ***(Minimum age: 6 weeks)***

- If PRP-OMP (PedvaxHIB® or Comvax® [HepB-Hib]) is administered at ages 2 and 4 months, a dose at age 6 months is not indicated.
- TriHiBit® (DTaP/Hib) should not be used for doses at ages 2, 4, or 6 months but can be used as the final dose in children aged 12 months or older.

5. Pneumococcal vaccine. ***(Minimum age: 6 weeks for pneumococcal conjugate vaccine [PCV]; 2 years for pneumococcal polysaccharide vaccine [PPSV])***

- PCV is recommended for all children aged younger than 5 years. Administer 1 dose of PCV to all healthy children aged 24 through 59 months who are not completely vaccinated for their age.
- Administer PPSV to children aged 2 years or older with certain underlying medical conditions (see *MMWR* 2000;49[No. RR-9]), including a cochlear implant.

6. Influenza vaccine. ***(Minimum age: 6 months for trivalent inactivated influenza vaccine [TIV]; 2 years for live, attenuated influenza vaccine [LAIV])***

- Administer annually to children aged 6 months through 18 years.
- For healthy nonpregnant persons (i.e., those who do not have underlying medical conditions that predispose them to influenza complications) aged 2 through 49 years, either LAIV or TIV may be used.
- Children receiving TIV should receive 0.25 mL if aged 6 through 35 months or 0.5 mL if aged 3 years or older.
- Administer 2 doses (separated by at least 4 weeks) to children aged younger than 9 years who are receiving influenza vaccine for the first time or who were vaccinated for the first time during the previous influenza season but only received 1 dose.

7. Measles, mumps, and rubella vaccine (MMR). ***(Minimum age: 12 months)***

- Administer the second dose at age 4 through 6 years. However, the second dose may be administered before age 4, provided at least 28 days have elapsed since the first dose.

8. Varicella vaccine. ***(Minimum age: 12 months)***

- Administer the second dose at age 4 through 6 years. However, the second dose may be administered before age 4, provided at least 3 months have elapsed since the first dose.
- For children aged 12 months through 12 years the minimum interval between doses is 3 months. However, if the second dose was administered at least 28 days after the first dose, it can be accepted as valid.

9. Hepatitis A vaccine (HepA). ***(Minimum age: 12 months)***

- Administer to all children aged 1 year (i.e., aged 12 through 23 months). Administer 2 doses at least 6 months apart.
- Children not fully vaccinated by age 2 years can be vaccinated at subsequent visits.
- HepA also is recommended for children older than 1 year who live in areas where vaccination programs target older children or who are at increased risk of infection. See *MMWR* 2006;55(No. RR-7).

10. Meningococcal vaccine. ***(Minimum age: 2 years for meningococcal conjugate vaccine [MCV] and for meningococcal polysaccharide vaccine [MPSV])***

- Administer MCV to children aged 2 through 10 years with terminal complement component deficiency, anatomic or functional asplenia, and certain other high-risk groups. See *MMWR* 2005;54(No. RR-7).
- Persons who received MPSV 3 or more years previously and who remain at increased risk for meningococcal disease should be revaccinated with MCV.

The Recommended Immunization Schedules for Persons Aged 0 Through 18 Years are approved by the Advisory Committee on Immunization Practices (www.cdc.gov/vaccines/recs/acip), the American Academy of Pediatrics (http://www.aap.org), and the American Academy of Family Physicians (http://www.aafp.org).

DEPARTMENT OF HEALTH AND HUMAN SERVICES • CENTERS FOR DISEASE CONTROL AND PREVENTION

CS103164

Fig. 36-11 Recommended immunization schedule for persons ages 0 through 6 years. (From Centers for Disease Control and Prevention: Recommended immunization schedules for persons aged 0 through 18 years—United States, 2009, *Morb Mortal Wkly Rep* 57(51-52):Q-2, 2008.)

Recommended Immunization Schedule for Persons Aged 7 Through 18 Years—United States • 2009

For those who fall behind or start late, see the schedule below and the catch-up schedule

Vaccine ▼ Age ▶	7–10 years	11–12 years	13–18 years
Tetanus, Diphtheria, Pertussis[1]	see footnote 1	Tdap	Tdap
Human Papillomavirus[2]	see footnote 2	HPV (3 doses)	HPV Series
Meningococcal[3]	MCV	MCV	MCV
Influenza[4]	Influenza (Yearly)		
Pneumococcal[5]	PPSV		
Hepatitis A[6]	HepA Series		
Hepatitis B[7]	HepB Series		
Inactivated Poliovirus[8]	IPV Series		
Measles, Mumps, Rubella[9]	MMR Series		
Varicella[10]	Varicella Series		

Range of recommended ages

Catch-up immunization

Certain high-risk groups

This schedule indicates the recommended ages for routine administration of currently licensed vaccines, as of December 1, 2008, for children aged 7 through 18 years. Any dose not administered at the recommended age should be administered at a subsequent visit, when indicated and feasible. Licensed combination vaccines may be used whenever any component of the combination is indicated and other components are not contraindicated and if approved by the Food and Drug Administration for that dose of the series. Providers should consult the relevant Advisory Committee on Immunization Practices statement for detailed recommendations, including high-risk conditions: http://www.cdc.gov/vaccines/pubs/acip-list.htm. Clinically significant adverse events that follow immunization should be reported to the Vaccine Adverse Event Reporting System (VAERS). Guidance about how to obtain and complete a VAERS form is available at http://www.vaers.hhs.gov or by telephone, 800-822-7967.

1. Tetanus and diphtheria toxoids and acellular pertussis vaccine (Tdap). ***(Minimum age: 10 years for BOOSTRIX® and 11 years for ADACEL®)***
- Administer at age 11 or 12 years for those who have completed the recommended childhood DTP/DTaP vaccination series and have not received a tetanus and diphtheria toxoid (Td) booster dose.
- Persons aged 13 through 18 years who have not received Tdap should receive a dose.
- A 5-year interval from the last Td dose is encouraged when Tdap is used as a booster dose; however, a shorter interval may be used if pertussis immunity is needed.

2. Human papillomavirus vaccine (HPV). ***(Minimum age: 9 years)***
- Administer the first dose to females at age 11 or 12 years.
- Administer the second dose 2 months after the first dose and the third dose 6 months after the first dose (at least 24 weeks after the first dose).
- Administer the series to females at age 13 through 18 years if not previously vaccinated.

3. Meningococcal conjugate vaccine (MCV).
- Administer at age 11 or 12 years, or at age 13 through 18 years if not previously vaccinated.
- Administer to previously unvaccinated college freshmen living in a dormitory.
- MCV is recommended for children aged 2 through 10 years with terminal complement component deficiency, anatomic or functional asplenia, and certain other groups at high risk. See *MMWR* 2005;54(No. RR-7).
- Persons who received MPSV 5 or more years previously and remain at increased risk for meningococcal disease should be revaccinated with MCV.

4. Influenza vaccine.
- Administer annually to children aged 6 months through 18 years.
- For healthy nonpregnant persons (i.e., those who do not have underlying medical conditions that predispose them to influenza complications) aged 2 through 49 years, either LAIV or TIV may be used.
- Administer 2 doses (separated by at least 4 weeks) to children aged younger than 9 years who are receiving influenza vaccine for the first time or who were vaccinated for the first time during the previous influenza season but only received 1 dose.

5. Pneumococcal polysaccharide vaccine (PPSV).
- Administer to children with certain underlying medical conditions (see *MMWR* 1997;46[No. RR-8]), including a cochlear implant. A single revaccination should be administered to children with functional or anatomic asplenia or other immunocompromising condition after 5 years.

6. Hepatitis A vaccine (HepA).
- Administer 2 doses at least 6 months apart.
- HepA is recommended for children older than 1 year who live in areas where vaccination programs target older children or who are at increased risk of infection. See *MMWR* 2006;55(No. RR-7).

7. Hepatitis B vaccine (HepB).
- Administer the 3-dose series to those not previously vaccinated.
- A 2-dose series (separated by at least 4 months) of adult formulation Recombivax HB® is licensed for children aged 11 through 15 years.

8. Inactivated poliovirus vaccine (IPV).
- For children who received an all-IPV or all-oral poliovirus (OPV) series, a fourth dose is not necessary if the third dose was administered at age 4 years or older.
- If both OPV and IPV were administered as part of a series, a total of 4 doses should be administered, regardless of the child's current age.

9. Measles, mumps, and rubella vaccine (MMR).
- If not previously vaccinated, administer 2 doses or the second dose for those who have received only 1 dose, with at least 28 days between doses.

10. Varicella vaccine.
- For persons aged 7 through 18 years without evidence of immunity (see *MMWR* 2007;56[No. RR-4]), administer 2 doses if not previously vaccinated or the second dose if they have received only 1 dose.
- For persons aged 7 through 12 years, the minimum interval between doses is 3 months. However, if the second dose was administered at least 28 days after the first dose, it can be accepted as valid.
- For persons aged 13 years and older, the minimum interval between doses is 28 days.

The Recommended Immunization Schedules for Persons Aged 0 Through 18 Years are approved by the Advisory Committee on Immunization Practices (www.cdc.gov/vaccines/recs/acip), the American Academy of Pediatrics (http://www.aap.org), and the American Academy of Family Physicians (http://www.aafp.org).

DEPARTMENT OF HEALTH AND HUMAN SERVICES • CENTERS FOR DISEASE CONTROL AND PREVENTION

CS103164

Fig. 36-12 Recommended immunization schedule for persons ages 7 through 18 years. (From Centers for Disease Control and Prevention: Recommended immunization schedules for persons aged 0 through 18 years—United States, 2009, *Morb Mortal Wkly Rep* 57(51-52):Q-3, 2008.)

Catch-up Immunization Schedule for Persons Aged 4 Months Through 18 Years Who Start Late or Who Are More Than 1 Month Behind—United States • 2009

The table below provides catch-up schedules and minimum intervals between doses for children whose vaccinations have been delayed. A vaccine series does not need to be restarted, regardless of the time that has elapsed between doses. Use the section appropriate for the child's age.

CATCH-UP SCHEDULE FOR PERSONS AGED 4 MONTHS THROUGH 6 YEARS					
Vaccine	**Minimum Age for Dose 1**	**Minimum Interval Between Doses**			
		Dose 1 to Dose 2	**Dose 2 to Dose 3**	**Dose 3 to Dose 4**	**Dose 4 to Dose 5**
Hepatitis B[1]	**Birth**	**4 weeks**	**8 weeks** (and at least 16 weeks after first dose)		
Rotavirus[2]	**6 wks**	**4 weeks**	**4 weeks[2]**		
Diphtheria, Tetanus, Pertussis[3]	**6 wks**	**4 weeks**	**4 weeks**	**6 months**	**6 months[3]**
***Haemophilus influenzae* type b[4]**	**6 wks**	**4 weeks** if first dose administered at younger than age 12 months **8 weeks (as final dose)** if first dose administered at age 12-14 months **No further doses needed** if first dose administered at age 15 months or older	**4 weeks[4]** if current age is younger than 12 months **8 weeks (as final dose)[4]** if current age is 12 months or older and second dose administered at younger than age 15 months **No further doses needed** if previous dose administered at age 15 months or older	**8 weeks (as final dose)** This dose only necessary for children aged 12 months through 59 months who received 3 doses before age 12 months	
Pneumococcal[5]	**6 wks**	**4 weeks** if first dose administered at younger than age 12 months **8 weeks** (as final dose for healthy children) if first dose administered at age 12 months or older or current age 24 through 59 months **No further doses needed** for healthy children if first dose administered at age 24 months or older	**4 weeks** if current age is younger than 12 months **8 weeks** (as final dose for healthy children) if current age is 12 months or older **No further doses needed** for healthy children if previous dose administered at age 24 months or older	**8 weeks (as final dose)** This dose only necessary for children aged 12 months through 59 months who received 3 doses before age 12 months or for high-risk children who received 3 doses at any age	
Inactivated Poliovirus[6]	**6 wks**	**4 weeks**	**4 weeks**	**4 weeks[6]**	
Measles, Mumps, Rubella[7]	**12 mos**	**4 weeks**			
Varicella[8]	**12 mos**	**3 months**			
Hepatitis A[9]	**12 mos**	**6 months**			
CATCH-UP SCHEDULE FOR PERSONS AGED 7 THROUGH 18 YEARS					
Tetanus, Diphtheria/ Tetanus, Diphtheria, Pertussis[10]	**7 yrs[10]**	**4 weeks**	**4 weeks** if first dose administered at younger than age 12 months **6 months** if first dose administered at age 12 months or older	**6 months** if first dose administered at younger than age 12 months	
Human Papillomavirus[11]	**9 yrs**	**Routine dosing intervals are recommended[11]**			
Hepatitis A[9]	**12 mos**	**6 months**			
Hepatitis B[1]	**Birth**	**4 weeks**	**8 weeks** (and at least 16 weeks after first dose)		
Inactivated Poliovirus[6]	**6 wks**	**4 weeks**	**4 weeks**	**4 weeks[6]**	
Measles, Mumps, Rubella[7]	**12 mos**	**4 weeks**			
Varicella[8]	**12 mos**	**3 months** if the person is younger than age 13 years **4 weeks** if the person is aged 13 years or older			

1. Hepatitis B vaccine (HepB).
- Administer the 3-dose series to those not previously vaccinated.
- A 2-dose series (separated by at least 4 months) of adult formulation Recombivax HB® is licensed for children aged 11 through 15 years.

2. Rotavirus vaccine (RV).
- The maximum age for the first dose is 14 weeks 6 days. Vaccination should not be initiated for infants aged 15 weeks or older (i.e., 15 weeks 0 days or older).
- Administer the final dose in the series by age 8 months 0 days.
- If Rotarix® was administered for the first and second doses, a third dose is not indicated.

3. Diphtheria and tetanus toxoids and acellular pertussis vaccine (DTaP).
- The fifth dose is not necessary if the fourth dose was administered at age 4 years or older.

4. *Haemophilus influenzae* type b conjugate vaccine (Hib).
- Hib vaccine is not generally recommended for persons aged 5 years or older. No efficacy data are available on which to base a recommendation concerning use of Hib vaccine for older children and adults. However, studies suggest good immunogenicity in persons who have sickle cell disease, leukemia, or HIV infection, or who have had a splenectomy; administering 1 dose of Hib vaccine to these persons is not contraindicated.
- If the first 2 doses were PRP-OMP (PedvaxHIB® or Comvax®), and administered at age 11 months or younger, the third (and final) dose should be administered at age 12 through 15 months and at least 8 weeks after the second dose.
- If the first dose was administered at age 7 through 11 months, administer 2 doses separated by 4 weeks and a final dose at age 12 through 15 months.

5. Pneumococcal vaccine.
- Administer 1 dose of pneumococcal conjugate vaccine (PCV) to all healthy children aged 24 through 59 months who have not received at least 1 dose of PCV on or after age 12 months.
- For children aged 24 through 59 months with underlying medical conditions, administer 1 dose of PCV if 3 doses were received previously or administer 2 doses of PCV at least 8 weeks apart if fewer than 3 doses were received previously.
- Administer pneumococcal polysaccharide vaccine (PPSV) to children aged 2 years or older with certain underlying medical conditions (see *MMWR* 2000;49[No. RR-9]), including a cochlear implant, at least 8 weeks after the last dose of PCV.

6. Inactivated poliovirus vaccine (IPV).
- For children who received an all-IPV or all-oral poliovirus (OPV) series, a fourth dose is not necessary if the third dose was administered at age 4 years or older.
- If both OPV and IPV were administered as part of a series, a total of 4 doses should be administered, regardless of the child's current age.

7. Measles, mumps, and rubella vaccine (MMR).
- Administer the second dose at age 4 through 6 years. However, the second dose may be administered before age 4, provided at least 28 days have elapsed since the first dose.
- If not previously vaccinated, administer 2 doses with at least 28 days between doses.

8. Varicella vaccine.
- Administer the second dose at age 4 through 6 years. However, the second dose may be administered before age 4, provided at least 3 months have elapsed since the first dose.
- For persons aged 12 months through 12 years, the minimum interval between doses is 3 months. However, if the second dose was administered at least 28 days after the first dose, it can be accepted as valid.
- For persons aged 13 years and older, the minimum interval between doses is 28 days.

9. Hepatitis A vaccine (HepA).
- HepA is recommended for children older than 1 year who live in areas where vaccination programs target older children or who are at increased risk of infection. See *MMWR* 2006;55(No. RR-7).

10. Tetanus and diphtheria toxoids (Td) and tetanus and diphtheria toxoids and acellular pertussis vaccine (Tdap).
- Doses of DTaP are counted as part of the Td/Tdap series
- Tdap should be substituted for a single dose of Td in the catch-up series or as a booster for children aged 10 through 18 years; use Td for other doses.

11. Human papillomavirus vaccine (HPV).
- Administer the series to females at age 13 through 18 years if not previously vaccinated.
- Use recommended routine dosing intervals for series catch-up (i.e., the second and third doses should be administered at 2 and 6 months after the first dose). However, the minimum interval between the first and second doses is 4 weeks. The minimum interval between the second and third doses is 12 weeks, and the third dose should be given at least 24 weeks after the first dose.

Information about reporting reactions after immunization is available online at **http://www.vaers.hhs.gov** or by telephone, **800-822-7967**. Suspected cases of vaccine-preventable diseases should be reported to the state or local health department. Additional information, including precautions and contraindications for immunization, is available from the National Center for Immunization and Respiratory Diseases at **http://www.cdc.gov/vaccines** or telephone, **800-CDC-INFO (800-232-4636)**.

DEPARTMENT OF HEALTH AND HUMAN SERVICES • CENTERS FOR DISEASE CONTROL AND PREVENTION

CS113897

Fig. 36-13 Catch-up immunization schedule for persons ages 4 months through 18 years who start late or who are more than 1 month behind. (From Centers for Disease Control and Prevention: Recommended immunization schedules for persons aged 0 through 18 years—United States, 2009, *Morb Mortal Wkly Rep* 57(51-52):Q-4, 2008.)

included in Fig. 36-13. Immunization schedules for Canadian children are available from the Public Health Agency of Canada *(www.phac-aspc.gc.ca/im/is-cv/index-eng.php).*

Children who began primary immunization at the recommended age, but fail to receive all of the doses, do not need to begin the series again but instead receive only the missed doses. For situations in which there is doubt that the child will return for immunization according to the optimum schedule, any of the recommended vaccines can be administered simultaneously. Parenteral vaccines are given in separate syringes in different injection sites.

Recommendations for Routine Immunizations*

Hepatitis B Virus

HBV is a significant pediatric disease because HBV infections that occur during childhood and adolescence can lead to fatal consequences from cirrhosis or liver cancer during adulthood. Up to 90% of infants infected perinatally and 25% to 50% of children infected before age 5 years become HBV carriers. In addition, the incidence of HBV infection increases rapidly during adolescence (American Academy of Pediatrics, Committee on Infectious Diseases, 2009). It is recommended that newborns receive the hepatitis B vaccine (HepB) before hospital discharge if the mother is hepatitis B surface antigen (HBsAg) negative. Monovalent HepB should be given as the birth dose, whereas combination vaccine containing HepB may be given for subsequent doses in the series. Both full-term and preterm infants born to mothers whose HBsAg status is positive or unknown should receive HepB and hepatitis B immune globulin (HBIG), 0.5 ml, within 12 hours of birth at two different injection sites. Because the immune response to HepB is not optimum in newborns weighing less than 2000 g (4.4 lb), the first HepB dose should be given to such infants at 1 month, as long as the mother's HBsAg status is negative (American Academy of Pediatrics, Committee on Infectious Diseases, 2009). In the event that the preterm infant is given a dose at birth, the current recommendation is that the infant be given the full series (three additional doses) at 1, 2, and 6 months of age. The American Academy of Pediatrics, Committee on Infectious Diseases (2009), also encourages immunization of all children by age 11 years.

In the late 1990s HepB contained small amounts of mercury (thimerosal) as a preservative, which generated concern regarding possible mercury poisoning in infants and led to a subsequent decrease in HepB immunization rates in newborns. However, a preservative-free HepB (Recombivax HB, pediatric/adolescent formulation) is available, and the Centers for Disease Control and Prevention (2005a) strongly recommend that HepB immunization occur in newborns before discharge from the birth hospital. To date studies have not found any association between thimerosal in vaccines and neurologic developmental disorders such as autism spectrum disorder (DeStefano, 2007; Heron, Golding, & ALSPAC Study Team, 2004). The American Academy of Pediatrics, Committee on Infectious Diseases (2009), also encourages immunization of all children by age 11 years.

The vaccine is given intramuscularly in the vastus lateralis in newborns or in the deltoid for older infants and children. Regardless of age, the dorsogluteal site is avoided because it has been associated with low antibody seroconversion rates, indicating a reduced immune response (Zuckerman, Cockcroft, & Zuckerman, 1992). No data exist regarding the seroconversion when the ventrogluteal site is used. The vaccine can be safely administered simultaneously at a separate site with DTaP, MMR, and Hib vaccines.

Hepatitis A Virus

HAV has been recognized as a significant child health problem, particularly in communities where widespread childhood HepA immunization has not been historically recommended. HAV is spread by the fecal-oral route and from person-to-person contact, by ingestion of contaminated food or water, and rarely by blood transfusion. The illness has an abrupt onset, with fever, malaise, anorexia, nausea, abdominal discomfort, dark urine, and jaundice being the most common clinical signs of infection. In children under 6 years of age the disease may be asymptomatic, and jaundice is rarely evident.

HepA vaccine is now recommended for all children beginning at age 1 year (i.e., 12 months to 23 months); the second dose in the two-dose series may be administered no sooner than 6 months after the first dose. Since the implementation of widespread childhood HepA vaccination, infection rates among children ages 5 to 14 years have declined significantly (Centers for Disease Control and Prevention, 2006a). For further information see Fig. 36-11, footnote 9.

Diphtheria

Although cases of diphtheria are rarely seen in the United States, the disease can result in significant morbidity. Respiratory manifestations include respiratory nasopharyngitis or obstructive laryngotracheitis with upper airway obstruction. The cutaneous manifestations of the disease include vaginal, otic, conjunctival, or cutaneous lesions, which are primarily seen in the tropics (American Academy of Pediatrics, Committee on Infectious Diseases, 2009). Diphtheria vaccine is commonly administered (1) in combination with tetanus and pertussis vaccines (DTaP) or DTaP and Hib vaccines for children younger than 7 years of age, (2) in combination with a conjugate *H. influenzae* type B vaccine (see Fig. 36-11), (3) in a combined vaccine with tetanus (DT) for children younger than 7 years of age who have some contraindication to receiving pertussis vaccine, or (4) as a single antigen when combined antigen preparations are not indicated. Although the diphtheria vaccine does not produce absolute immunity, protective antitoxin persists for 10 years or more when given according to the recommended schedule, and boosters are given every

**Because of constant changes in the pharmaceutical industry, trade names of some single and combination vaccines in this section may differ from those currently available. The reader is encouraged to access the Vaccine page of the Center for Biologics Evaluation and Research (CBER) of the Food and Drug Administration for the latest licensed vaccine trade names:* www.fda.gov/cber/vaccines/htm.

10 years for life (see discussion below for adolescent diphtheria and acellular pertussis and tetanus toxoid recommendation). Several vaccines contain diphtheria toxoid (Hib, meningococcal, pneumococcal), but this does not confer immunity to the disease.

Tetanus

Three forms of tetanus vaccine—tetanus toxoid, tetanus immune globulin (TIG) (human), and tetanus antitoxin (equine antitoxin)—are available; however, tetanus antitoxin is no longer available in the United States. Tetanus toxoid is used for routine primary immunization, usually in one of the combinations listed for diphtheria, and provides protective antitoxin levels for approximately 10 years.

Tetanus and diphtheria toxoids as well as acellular pertussis vaccine (Tdap–adolescent formulation) are now recommended for children 11 to 12 years who have completed the recommended DTaP/DTP vaccine series yet have not received the tetanus (Td) booster dose. Adolescents who are 13 to 18 years of age and have not received the Td/Tdap booster should receive a single Tdap booster, provided the routine DTaP/DTP childhood immunization series has been previously received (see Fig. 36-12, footnote 1). Boostrix (Tdap) is currently licensed for children 10 to 18 years of age, whereas Adacel (Tdap) is licensed for individuals 11 to 64 years of age.

For wound management, passive immunity is available with TIG. In persons with a history of two previous doses of tetanus toxoid, a booster dose of the toxoid can be given. Separate syringes and different sites are used when tetanus toxoid and TIG are given concurrently. For children over 7 years who require wound prophylaxis, tetanus immunization may be accomplished by administering Td (adult-type diphtheria and tetanus toxoids).

Pertussis

Pertussis vaccine is recommended for all children 6 weeks through 6 years of age (up to the seventh birthday) who have no neurologic contraindications to its use. Concerns over outbreaks of the disease in the past decade have prompted discussion about vaccinating infants and adults; many cases of pertussis have been seen in children less than 6 months or persons over 7 years, both groups falling in the category for which there was inadequate vaccine protection from pertussis infection (Centers for Disease Control and Prevention, 2005c). The tetanus and diphtheria toxoids and acellular pertussis vaccine (Tdap) is now recommended at ages 11 to 12 years for children who have completed the DTaP/DTP childhood series; the Tdap is also recommended for adolescents 13 to 18 years old who have not received a tetanus booster (Td) or Tdap dose and have completed the childhood DTaP/DTP series. When the Tdap is used as a booster dose, it may be administered 5 years from the last Td dose or earlier if pertussis immunity is necessary (Centers for Disease Control and Prevention, 2009).

Currently, two forms of pertussis vaccine are available in the United States. The whole-cell pertussis vaccine is prepared from inactivated cells of *Bordetella pertussis* and contains multiple antigens. In contrast, the acellular pertussis vaccine contains one or more immunogens derived from the *B. pertussis* organism. The highly purified acellular vaccine is associated with fewer local and systemic reactions than those occurring with the whole-cell vaccine in children of similar age. The acellular pertussis vaccine is recommended by the American Academy of Pediatrics, Committee on Infectious Diseases (2009), for the first three immunizations and is usually given at 2, 4, and 6 months of age with diphtheria and tetanus (DTaP). Several forms of acellular pertussis vaccine are currently licensed for use in infants: Tripedia, Daptacel, Pediarix, and Infanrix (diphtheria, tetanus toxoid, and acellular pertussis conjugate). Pentacel is licensed for use in infants 4 weeks old and older; in addition to acellular pertussis, diphtheria, and tetanus, this vaccine also contains inactivated poliovirus (IPV) and Hib conjugate. TriHIBit may be used for the fourth dose after three doses of DTaP and after a primary series of any Hib vaccine. Either the acellular or whole-cell vaccine may be given for the fourth and fifth doses, but the acellular is preferred. It is also recommended that the first three DTaP vaccinations be from the same manufacturer; the fourth dose may be from a different manufacturer. The child who has received one or more whole-cell vaccines may complete the series of five with the acellular vaccine.

Health care workers who may be susceptible to pertussis as a result of waning immunity and who have potential exposure to children or adults with pertussis should take the necessary protective precautions against droplet contamination (wear procedural or surgical masks and practice hand washing). The diagnosis of pertussis may be missed or delayed in unvaccinated infants, who often are seen with respiratory distress and apnea without the typical cough (Centers for Disease Control and Prevention, 2005b). Additional guidelines for prevention and treatment of pertussis among health care workers and close contacts are found in the *2009 Red Book: Report of the Committee on Infectious Diseases* (American Academy of Pediatrics, Committee on Infectious Diseases, 2009).

Polio

An all-IPV schedule for routine childhood polio vaccination is now recommended; oral poliovirus (OPV) is no longer used in the United States. All children should receive four doses of IPV at 2 months, 4 months, 6 to 18 months, and 4 to 6 years of age (American Academy of Pediatrics, Committee on Infectious Diseases, 2009).

The change from the exclusive use of OPV to the exclusive use of IPV is related to the rare risk of vaccine-associated polio paralysis (VAPP) from OPV. The exclusive use of IPV eliminates the risk of VAPP but is associated with an increased number of injections and increased cost. Since IPV usage was instituted in the United States in 2000, no new cases of VAPP have occurred. Pediarix is a combination vaccine containing DTaP, HepB, and IPV; this may be used as the primary immunization beginning at 2 months of age (American Academy of Pediatrics, Committee on Infectious Diseases, 2009).

Measles

The measles (rubeola) vaccine is given at 12 to 15 months of age. During the course of measles outbreaks, the vaccine can be given any time after 6 months of age, followed by a second inoculation after age 12 months. The second measles immunization is recommended at 4 to 6 years of age (at school entry) but may be given earlier provided that 4 weeks have lapsed since the administration of the previous dose. Revaccination should occur by 11 to 12 years of age if the measles vaccine was not administered at school entry (4 to 6 years). Any child who is vaccinated before 12 months of age should receive two additional doses beginning at 12 to 15 months and separated by at least 4 weeks (American Academy of Pediatrics, Committee on Infectious Diseases, 2009). Revaccination should include all individuals born after 1956 who have not received two doses of measles vaccine after 12 months of age. Individuals born before this date are thought to be immune from exposure to natural measles virus. Because of the continuing occurrence of measles in older children and young adults, potentially susceptible adolescents and young adults should be identified and immunized if two doses of measles vaccine have not been administered previously or the person had a confirmed case of the illness.

Mumps

Mumps virus vaccine is recommended for children at 12 to 15 months of age and is typically given in combination with measles and rubella. It should not be administered to infants younger than 12 months because persisting maternal antibodies can interfere with the immune response.

Because of recent outbreaks of the disease, especially in children 10 to 19 years of age, mumps immunization is recommended for all individuals born after 1957 who may be susceptible to mumps (i.e., those who have no history of having had the disease or vaccine and who have no laboratory evidence of immunity).

Rubella

Rubella is a relatively mild infection in children, but in a pregnant woman the actual infection presents serious risks to the developing fetus. Therefore the aim of rubella immunization is actually protection of the unborn child rather than the recipient of the immunization.

Rubella immunization is recommended for all children at 12 to 15 months of age and is administered in a combined form with measles and mumps vaccine. Increased emphasis should also be placed on vaccinating all unimmunized prepubertal children and susceptible adolescents and adult women in the childbearing age group. Because the live attenuated virus may cross the placenta and theoretically present a risk to the developing fetus, rubella vaccine is currently not given to any pregnant woman.

Pneumococcal

A seven-valent *Streptococcus pneumoniae* conjugate vaccine (PCV7, or Prevnar) has been used for children under 2 years of age since 2000. Streptococcal pneumococci are responsible for a number of bacterial infections in children under 2 years, which may cause serious morbidity and mortality. Among these are generalized infections such as septicemia and meningitis or localized infections such as otitis media, sinusitis, and pneumonia. These illnesses are particularly problematic in children who attend day care facilities (the incidence in day care children is two to three times higher than in children not attending out-of-home day care) and in those who are immunocompromised.

The vaccine is administered at 2, 4, and 6 months, with a fourth dose at 12 to 15 months of age; children 7 to 11 months old may receive three doses as long as they are 6 to 8 weeks apart and a fourth dose at 12 to 15 months; children 12 to 23 months who have not been immunized with the pneumococcal vaccine may be given two doses, 6 to 8 weeks apart. PCV7 is also recommended for all children under 24 months and in older children (24 to 59 months) with sickle cell disease; functional or anatomic asplenia; nephrotic syndrome or chronic renal failure; conditions associated with immunosuppression, such as solid organ transplantation, drug therapy, or cytoreduction therapy (including long-term systemic corticosteroid therapy); diabetes mellitus; cochlear implants; congenital immunodeficiency; human immunodeficiency virus (HIV) infection; cerebrospinal fluid leaks; chronic cardiovascular disease (e.g., congestive heart failure or cardiomyopathy); chronic pulmonary disease (e.g., emphysema or cystic fibrosis, but not asthma); chronic liver disease (e.g., cirrhosis); or exposure to living environments or social settings in which the risk of invasive pneumococcal disease or its complications is very high (e.g., Alaskan Native, African-American, and certain Native American populations) (American Academy of Pediatrics, Committee on Infectious Diseases, 2009). Low-birth-weight infants (1500 g [3.3 lb] or less) should receive the vaccine when they reach a chronologic age of 6 to 8 weeks regardless of calculated gestational age. The PCV7 vaccine may be administered in conjunction with all other immunizations in a separate syringe and at a separate intramuscular site.

The PPV (pneumococcal polysaccharide [23-valent] vaccine) is not recommended for children younger than 24 months who do not have one of the high risk conditions described previously. One dose of PPV is recommended in children older than 23 months who have one of the high risk conditions after primary immunization with PCV7. (See American Academy of Pediatrics, Committee on Infectious Diseases, 2009, for PCV7 and PPV schedule.)

Haemophilus influenzae Type B

Hib conjugate vaccines protect against a number of serious infections caused by Hib, especially bacterial meningitis, epiglottitis, bacterial pneumonia, septic arthritis, and sepsis (Hib is not associated with the viruses that cause influenza, or "flu"). Hib vaccines that are currently available include PedvaxHIB, Pentacel, and Comvax, which are combination vaccines, and HibTITER and ActHIB. Pentacel is described in the previous section on pertussis. These conjugate vaccines connect Hib to a nontoxic form of another organism, such as meningococcal protein or diphtheria protein. There is no antibody response to these nontoxic proteins, but they significantly improve the antibody response to Hib, especially in infants. The use of combination vaccines provides equivalent immunogenicity and decreases the number of injections an infant receives; however, it is important that they be given to the appropriate-age child. The DTaP/Hib combination vaccine (TriHIBit) should not be used for the first three doses at 2, 4, or 6 months but may be used as a booster after any Hib vaccine.

The 2009 CDC immunization guidelines indicate there are limited data for administering the Hib vaccine to persons 5 years and older; however, children with sickle cell disease, leukemia, or HIV infection, or children who have had a splenectomy, may benefit from one dose of the Hib vaccine (Centers for Disease Control and Prevention, 2009).

When possible, the Hib conjugate vaccine used at the first vaccination should be used for all subsequent vaccinations in the primary series. All Hib vaccines are administered by intramuscular injection using a separate syringe and at a site separate from any concurrent vaccinations.

Varicella

Administration of the cell-free live-attenuated varicella vaccine (Varivax) is recommended for any susceptible child (one who lacks proof of varicella vaccination or has a reliable history of varicella infection). The first dose of varicella vaccine is recommended for children ages 12 to 15 months, and to ensure adequate protection a second varicella vaccine is recommended for children at 4 to 6 years of age (American Academy of Pediatrics, Committee on Infectious Diseases, 2008). The second varicella vaccine may be administered prior to age 4 as long as a period of 3 months occurs between the first and second doses.

A single dose of 0.5 ml should be given by subcutaneous injection. Children 13 years of age or older who are susceptible should receive two doses administered at least 4 weeks apart (American Academy of Pediatrics, Committee on Infectious Diseases, 2009). The vaccine should be kept frozen in the lyophilic form (stable particles that readily go into solution) and used within 30 minutes of being reconstituted to ensure viral potency. Varicella vaccine may be administered simultaneously with MMR. However, separate syringes and injection sites should be used. If they are not administered simultaneously, the interval between administration of varicella vaccine and MMR should be at least 1 month. Varicella vaccine may also be given simultaneously with DTaP, IPV, HBV, or Hib (American Academy of Pediatrics, Committee on Infectious Diseases, 2009).

The varicella vaccine is reported to be effective in preventing varicella for at least 11 years (American Academy of Pediatrics, Committee on Infectious Diseases, 2009).

Influenza

The influenza vaccine is now recommended annually for children 6 months to 18 years. Influenza vaccine (trivalent inactivated influenza vaccine [TIV]) may be given to all healthy children 6 months old and older. Children who have a reported anaphylactic hypersensitivity to eggs should not receive the vaccine. The vaccine is administered in early fall before the flu season begins and is repeated yearly for ongoing protection. The intramuscular vaccine is administered as two separate doses 4 weeks apart in first-time recipients under the age of 9 years. The dose is 0.25 ml for children ages 6 to 35 months and 0.5 ml for children 3 years and above. The vaccine may be given simultaneously with other vaccines but at a separate site. The vaccine is administered yearly because different strains of influenza are used each year in the manufacture of the vaccine.

The live attenuated influenza vaccine (LAIV) is an acceptable alternative to the intramuscular trivalent vaccine in specific age groups. The vaccine is given nasally as two doses at least 28 days apart in healthy persons ages 2 to 49 years. Although it is an alternative to the injection, there is a cost increase, and insurance may not cover the cost of the nasal vaccine. Either TIV or LAIV may be given to healthy, nonpregnant persons ages 2 to 49 years (American Academy of Pediatrics, Committee on Infectious Diseases, 2008). Yearly influenza vaccine should be administered to children ages 6 to 59 months with medical conditions that place them at risk for influenza-related complications (including asthma, cardiac disease, HIV, diabetes, and sickle cell disease) and health care workers.

Meningococcal

Invasive meningococcal disease continues to be the cause of high morbidity in children in the United States. Infants younger than 1 year of age are particularly susceptible, yet the highest fatalities occur in adolescents (approximately 20%). There is also evidence that the risk of meningococcal infections is high in college freshmen living in dormitories. Meningococcal infections are also responsible for significant morbidities, including limb or digit amputation, skin scarring, hearing loss, and neurologic disabilities (American Academy of Pediatrics, Committee on Infectious Diseases, 2009).

Neisseria meningitidis is the leading cause of bacterial meningitis in the United States. It is not recommended that children routinely receive the quadrivalent conjugate vaccine MCV4 (Menactra) at age 2 through 10 years, except those in certain high risk groups; these include children with terminal complement component deficiency, with anatomic or functional asplenia, with HIV, or who travel to or reside in countries where *N. meningitidis* is hyperendemic or epidemic (American Academy of Pediatrics, Committee on Infectious Diseases, 2009). Children and adolescents 11 to 18 years of age should receive a single immunization of MCV4; others at high risk who should receive MCV4 include military recruits and college freshmen living in dormitories (American Academy of Pediatrics, Committee on Infectious Diseases, 2009).

MCV4 is administered as an intramuscular injection (0.5 ml) and may be administered in conjunction with other vaccines in a separate syringe and at a separate site. Immunization with MCV4 is contraindicated in persons with hypersensitivity to any components of the vaccine, including diphtheria toxoid, and to rubber latex (part of vial stopper).

There have been recent concerns regarding reports of an association between MCV4 (Menactra) and cases of Guillain-Barré syndrome in vaccinated persons ages 11 to 19 years of age; onset of symptoms occurred within 2 to 23 days of vaccination. A preliminary survey by the Centers for Disease Control and Prevention (2006b) indicates there are insufficient data to change the 2005 recommendation for adolescents, college freshmen residing in dormitories, and other high risk populations.

The meningococcal vaccine Menomune (A, C, Y, W-135; MPSV4), which has been available since the early 1980s, was historically used in younger children but is no longer the recommended primary meningococcal vaccine for children.

Recommendations for Selected Immunizations

Two additional vaccines are recommended for children and adolescents at high risk for particular diseases. Two rotavirus vaccines, RotaTeq and Rotarix, have received a license from the U.S. Food and Drug Administration for distribution in the

United States. Rotavirus is one of the leading causes of severe diarrhea in infants and young children. RotaTeq is licensed for administration to infants at 6 to 12 weeks of age, with two additional doses administered at 4- to 10-week intervals but not after 32 weeks of age; the dose is 2 ml, and the product must be protected from light until administration (American Academy of Pediatrics, Committee on Infectious Diseases, 2008). Rotarix (1 ml) may be administered beginning at 6 weeks of age with a second dose at least 4 weeks after the first dose but before 24 weeks of age. Both vaccines are administered orally.

A quadrivalent human papillomavirus (HPV) vaccine, Gardasil, has been approved and is recommended for female children and adolescents to prevent HPV-related cervical cancer. The vaccine is administered intramuscularly in three separate doses; the first dose in the series may be given at 11 to 12 years of age (minimum age 9 years), the second dose is administered 2 months after the first, and the third dose is given 6 months after the first dose (Centers for Disease Control and Prevention, 2007b).

Immunizations that may be used in older children and adolescents in the future and that are being evaluated include vaccines for preventing diseases such as herpes simplex virus, human cytomegalovirus, and Epstein-Barr virus. Others, such as the rabies vaccine, are discussed elsewhere in this text.

Reactions

Vaccines used for routine immunizations are among the safest and most reliable drugs available. However, minor side effects do occur after many of the immunizations, and, rarely, a serious reaction may result from the vaccine.

With inactivated antigens, such as DTaP, side effects are most likely to occur within a few hours or days of administration and are usually limited to local tenderness, erythema, and swelling at the injection site; low-grade fever; and behavioral changes (e.g., drowsiness, fretfulness, eating less, and prolonged or unusual cry). Local reactions tend to be less severe when the deltoid (except in small infants) rather than the vastus lateralis site is used and when a needle of sufficient length to deposit the vaccine in the muscle is used (see Atraumatic Care box). Rarely, more severe reactions may occur, especially with pertussis (Table 36-5). Reactions to DTaP tend to be more severe if they occurred with a previous immunization.

Hib vaccine is one of the safest vaccines available but may be associated with low-grade fever and mild local reactions at the site of injection, which resolve rapidly. Fever (temperature higher than 38.5° C [101.3° F]) may rarely occur.

A number of inactive components are incorporated in vaccines to enhance their effectiveness and safety. Some of these components include preservatives, stabilizers, adjuvants, antibiotics, and purified culture medium proteins to enhance effectiveness. A child may react to the preservative in the vaccine rather than the vaccine component; an example of this is the HepB vaccine, which is prepared from yeast cultures. Yeast hypersensitivity would preclude one from receiving that particular vaccine (Schuval, 2003). Trace amounts of neomycin are used to decrease bacterial growth within certain vaccine preparations, and persons with documented anaphylactic reactions to neomycin should avoid those vaccines. Most vaccine preparations now contain vial stoppers with a synthetic rubber to prevent latex allergy reactions. In the event that an individual has a severe reaction to a vaccine and subsequent immunizations are required, an allergist may be consulted to determine the best course of action (Schuval, 2003).

Unlike the inactivated antigens, live attenuated virus vaccines such as MMR multiply for days or weeks, and unfavorable reactions and vaccine-associated disorders can occur for 30 to 60 days. These reactions are usually mild, although reactions to rubella tend to be more troublesome in older children and adults.

Studies in the United States and in various European countries (Denmark, Finland) have found no association between the MMR vaccine and the incidence of autism (Campion, 2002; DeStefano, 2007; Dales, Hammer, & Smith, 2001; Hviid et al, 2003; Institute of Medicine, 2004).

Contraindications and Precautions

Nurses need to be aware of the reasons for withholding immunizations—both for the child's safety in terms of avoiding reactions and for the child's maximum benefit from receiving the vaccine. Unfounded fears and lack of knowledge regarding contraindications can needlessly prevent a child from having protection from life-threatening diseases. Issues that have surfaced regarding vaccines include the misconception that administering combination vaccines may overload the child's immune system; the combined vaccines have undergone rigorous study in relation to side effects and immunogenicity rates following administration. Parents must be given appropriate information regarding vaccine safety, benefits, and risks so they can make informed decisions regarding vaccinations for their children (Koslap-Petraco & Parsons, 2003). The advantage of widespread media via television and the Internet is that information is readily available at any given moment; the disadvantage is that some of this information may be incorrect, incomplete, or misleading and may influence parents to make decisions that may have deleterious consequences on their children's health.

In one survey of parents, fear of side effects was the most commonly expressed reason (52%) for vaccination refusal; other common reasons included the belief that the disease was not harmful (26%), religious beliefs (28%), and philosophical reasons (26%) (Fredrickson et al, 2004).

For the contraindications to the usual childhood vaccines, see Table 36-5.

Administration

The principal precautions in administering immunizations include proper storage of the vaccine to protect its potency and institution of recommended procedures for injection. The nurse must be familiar with the manufacturer's directions for storage and reconstitution of the vaccine. For example, if the vaccine is to be refrigerated, it should be stored on a center shelf and not in the door, where frequent temperature increases from opening the refrigerator can alter the vaccine's potency. For protection against light, the vial can be wrapped in aluminum foil. Periodic checks are scheduled to ensure that no vaccine is used after its expiration date.

Table 36-5 Contraindications and Precautions to Vaccinations[a]

TRUE CONTRAINDICATIONS	PRECAUTIONS[b]	NOT CONTRAINDICATIONS (VACCINES MAY BE ADMINISTERED)
General for All Vaccines (DTaP, IPV, MMR, Hib, HepB, Varicella, PCV, HepA, Influenza, Meningococcal)		
Anaphylactic reaction to vaccine contraindication to further doses of that vaccine or to use of vaccines containing that substance Moderate or severe illnesses with or without fever		Mild to moderate local reaction (soreness, redness, swelling) after a dose of injectable antigen Mild acute illness with or without low-grade fever Current antimicrobial therapy Convalescent phase of illnesses Prematurity (same dosage and indications as for normal, full-term infants) Recent exposure to infectious disease History of penicillin or other nonspecific allergies or family history of such allergies
Diphtheria, Tetanus, and Pertussis or Acellular Pertussis Vaccine (DTP or DTaP)		
Encephalopathy within 7 days of administration of previous dose of DTaP	Fever of ≥40.5° C (105° F) within 48 hr after vaccination with prior dose of DTaP Collapse or shocklike state (hypotonic-hyporesponsive episode) within 48 hr of receiving prior dose of DTaP Seizures within 3 days of receiving prior dose of DTaP[c] Persistent, inconsolable crying lasting ≥3 hr within 48 hr of receiving prior dose of DTaP	Temperature of <40.5° C (105° F) after previous dose of DTaP Family history of seizures[c] Family history of sudden infant death syndrome Family history of adverse event after DTaP administration
Diphtheria, Tetanus (DT, Td)		
Severe allergic reaction after a previous dose or to a vaccine component	GBS ≤6 wk after previous dose of tetanus toxoid–containing vaccine Moderate or severe acute illness with or without fever	Same as DTaP or DTP
Inactivated Poliovirus Vaccine (IPV)		
Anaphylactic reaction to neomycin or streptomycin	Pregnancy	Breastfeeding Diarrhea
Measles, Mumps, Rubella Vaccine (MMR)		
Pregnancy Known altered immunodeficiency (hematologic and solid tumors, congenital immunodeficiency, and long-term immunosuppressive therapy)	Recent immune globulin administration Immune globulin products and MMR should not be given simultaneously; if unavoidable, give at different sites and revaccinate or test for seroconversion in 3 mo; if immune globulin is given first, MMR should not be given for at least 3-6 mo, depending on dose; if MMR is given first, immune globulin should not be given for 2 wk Thrombocytopenia or thrombocytopenic purpura	Tuberculosis or positive tuberculin skin test Simultaneous tuberculosis skin testing[d] Breastfeeding Pregnancy of mother of recipient Immunodeficient family member or household contact Infection with HIV Nonanaphylactic reactions to eggs or neomycin Consider MMR for mildly symptomatic HIV-infected children (American Academy of Pediatrics, Committee on Infectious Diseases, 2009)
***Haemophilus influenzae* Type b Vaccine (Hib)**		
None identified		History of Hib disease
Hepatitis B Virus Vaccine (HepB)		
Anaphylactic reaction to common baker's yeast	Preterm birth[e]	Pregnancy
Pneumococcal Vaccine (PCV)		
Severe allergic reaction after a previous dose or to a vaccine component	Moderate or severe acute illness with or without fever A child who has received pneumococcal polysaccharide vaccine (PPV) previously should wait at least 2 mo before receiving PCV	Minor illnesses with or without fever Mild upper respiratory tract infection Allergic rhinitis

[a]This information is based on the recommendations of Advisory Committee on Immunization Practices (ACIP) and those of Committee on Infectious Diseases (Red Book Committee) of American Academy of Pediatrics. Sometimes these recommendations vary from those contained in manufacturer's package inserts. For more detailed information, consult published recommendations of ACIP and American Academy of Pediatrics and manufacturer's package inserts.

[b]Events or conditions listed as precautions, although not contraindications, should be carefully reviewed. Benefits and risks of administering a specific vaccine to an individual under the circumstances should be considered. If risks are believed to outweigh benefits, vaccination should be withheld; if benefits are believed to outweigh risks (e.g., during an outbreak or foreign travel), vaccination should be administered. Whether and when to administer DTaP to children with proven or suspected underlying neurologic disorders should be decided on individual basis. It is prudent on theoretical grounds to avoid vaccinating pregnant women.

[c]Acetaminophen given before administering DTaP and thereafter every 4 hr for 24 hr should be considered for children with personal history of seizures or family history of seizures in siblings or parents.

[d]Measles vaccination may temporarily suppress tuberculin reactivity. If testing cannot be done the day of MMR vaccination, the test should be postponed for 4-6 wk.

[e]Birth weight <2000 g (4.4 lb) and unknown or hepatitis B surface antigen–positive mother is not a contraindication for vaccination.

Continued

Table 36-5 Contraindications and Precautions to Vaccinations[a]—cont'd

TRUE CONTRAINDICATIONS	PRECAUTIONS[b]	NOT CONTRAINDICATIONS (VACCINES MAY BE ADMINISTERED)
Varicella Vaccine		
Severe allergic reaction after a previous dose or to a vaccine component (e.g., neomycin or gelatin) Infection with HIV Known altered immunodeficiency (hematologic and solid tumors, congenital immunodeficiency, and long-term immunosuppressive therapy) Pregnancy Children receiving corticosteroids	Recent immune globulin administration (see *Measles* in American Academy of Pediatrics, Committee on Infectious Diseases, 2009) Family history of immunodeficiency	Breastfeeding
Rotavirus Vaccine		
Severe allergic reaction after a previous dose or to a vaccine component Infants born to HIV-positive mother Known or suspected weakened immune system caused by radiation; drugs; or conditions such as leukemia, blood disorders, cancer	Altered immunocompetence Moderate to severe acute gastroenteritis Moderate to severe febrile illness Chronic gastrointestinal diseases Intussusception	Pregnancy Previous history of rotavirus infection; history of intussusception; temperature ≥38° C (100.4° F); close contact with immunocompromised person(s); blood transfusion or immune globulins within previous 42 days
Influenza Vaccine (Inactivated/Live-Attenuated)[f]		
Severe allergic reaction after a previous dose or to a vaccine component, including eggs Egg hypersensitivity LAIV should not be administered to persons taking salicylates, with known or suspected immunodeficiency, with a history of GBS, or with a reactive airway disease or other chronic disorder considered high risk for severe influenza	GBS within 6 wk after previous influenza immunization	Pregnancy
Meningococcal Vaccine		
MCV4—Allergy to vaccine components, including diphtheria toxoid, and possible reaction to latex stopper; history of GBS		Pregnancy
MPSV4—Allergy to vaccine components		Pregnancy
Tetanus (Booster Toxoid), Reduced Diphtheria Toxoid, Acellular Pertussis Adsorbed (Tdap)		
Serious reaction to any vaccine component History of encephalopathy (e.g., coma, prolonged seizures) within 7 days of administration of a pertussis vaccine that is not attributable to another identifiable cause	GBS ≤6 wk after previous dose of a tetanus toxoid vaccine Progressive neurologic disorder, uncontrolled epilepsy, or progressive encephalopathy until the condition has stabilized	Temperature ≥40.5° C (105° F) within 48 hr after DTP/DTaP immunization not attributable to another cause Collapse or shocklike state within 48 hr after DTP/DTaP immunization Persistent crying lasting ≥3 hr, occurring within 48 hr after DTP/DTaP immunization Seizures with or without fever, occurring within 3 days after DTaP/DTP immunization History of entire limb swelling reaction after pediatric DTaP/DTP or Td immunization that was not an Arthus hypersensitivity reaction Stable neurologic disorder, including well-controlled seizures, history of seizure disorder, and CP Brachial neuritis Latex allergy other than anaphylactic allergies (e.g., history of contact to latex gloves) Immunosuppression, including persons with HIV Antibiotic use Intercurrent minor illness
Human Papillomavirus Vaccine		
Pregnancy Hypersensitivity to yeast or any vaccine component		Immunosuppressed female Minor acute illness Lactation

Modified from American Academy of Pediatrics, Committee on Infectious Diseases, Pickering L (editor): *Red book: 2009 report of the Committee on Infectious Diseases,* ed 28, Elk Grove Village, IL, 2009, The Academy.

CP, Cerebral palsy; *GBS,* Guillain-Barré syndrome; *HIV,* human immunodeficiency virus; *LAIV,* live-attenuated influenza vaccine; *PPD,* purified protein derivative.

[f]See James JM et al: Safe administration of influenza vaccine to patients with egg allergies, *J Pediatr* 133(5):624-628, 1998.

ATRAUMATIC CARE

Immunizations

Needle length is an important factor and must be considered for each individual child; fewer reactions to immunizations are observed when the vaccine is given deep into the muscle rather than into subcutaneous tissue. Contrary to previous belief, deep intramuscular tissue has a better blood supply and fewer pain receptors than adipose tissue, thus providing an optimum site for immunizations with fewer side effects (Zuckerman, 2000).

To minimize local reactions from vaccines:

- Recommended needle length for newborn to 2 months is ⅝ inch.
- Select a needle of adequate length (2.5 cm [1 inch] in infants) to deposit the antigen deep in the muscle mass.
- Toddlers and older children require a needle length of ⅝ to 1 inch for deltoid, or 1 to 1¼ inches for vastus lateralis (Schechter et al, 2007).
- Adolescents require a needle length of 1 to 2 inches in deltoid or vastus lateralis (Schechter et al, 2007).
- Inject into the vastus lateralis or ventrogluteal muscle; the deltoid may be used in children 18 months of age or older.
- Use an air bubble to clear the needle after injecting the vaccine (theoretically beneficial but unproved).

To minimize pain:

- Apply the topical anesthetic EMLA (lidocaine-prilocaine) to the injection site and cover with an occlusive dressing for at least 1 hour.* *OR*
- Apply the topical anesthetic LMX4 (4% lidocaine) to the injection site 30 minutes before the injection; there is no evidence that an occlusive dressing is required except to prevent ingestion or accidental application to the eyes in infants (Wong, 2003). To date, the studies for LMX4 have only discussed pain from procedures such as venipuncture, not injections. *OR*
- Apply a vapocoolant spray (e.g., ethyl chloride or FluoriMethane) directly to the skin or to a cotton ball, which is placed on the skin for 15 seconds immediately before the injection (Reis & Holubkov, 1997).
- There is evidence that a concentrated oral sucrose solution (24%) and nonnutritive sucking (pacifier) decrease the pain related to minor invasive procedures in neonates (Stevens et al, 1999; Stevens, Yamada, & Ohlsson, 2001). Most studies have focused on heel lance, venipuncture, and circumcision (neonatal period), but one institution has incorporated a neonatal oral sucrose pain protocol for painful procedures, including injections (Thompson, 2005). Hatfield (2008) found that 2- and 4-month-old infants who received a 0.6 ml/kg dose of 24% sucrose and NNS 2 minutes before immunization administration had decreased pain behavioral responses in comparison to a control group of infants who received only sterile water and NNS 2 minutes before the injection. Therefore it is recommended that a concentrated oral sucrose solution (1 to 2 ml) be administered orally 2 minutes before the injection, during the injection, and up to 3 minutes after the procedure to decrease neonatal pain with immunizations.
- In preschool children, use distraction, such as telling the child to "take a deep breath and blow and blow and blow until I tell you to stop."
- Two studies in adult patients receiving intramuscular injections documented a decrease in pain sensation at the time of the injection when manual pressure was applied to the site before the injection; pressure was applied for 10 seconds in both studies (Barnhill et al, 1996; Chung, Ng, & Wong, 2002). To date, there are no published studies involving the use of this technique in children.
- The use of a needless system to deliver lidocaine to the skin has been used in older children for venipuncture; the J-Tip delivers 1% buffered lidocaine, which numbs the skin within 1 to 3 minutes (Jimenez et al, 2006; Spanos et al, 2008; Zempsky, 2008).
- NOTE: Changing the needle on the syringe after drawing up the vaccine and before injecting it has not been shown to decrease local reactions. In children 4 to 6 years of age, the administration of sequential injections or simultaneous injections of vaccines did not alter their perceptions of distress, but parents preferred the simultaneous method (Horn & McCarthy, 1999).

*The use of the EMLA patch before administration of diphtheria-tetanus-acellular pertussis–inactivated poliovirus–*Haemophilus influenzae* type b (DTaP-IPV-Hib) and hepatitis B vaccines did not decrease antibody titers in immunized infants and was effective in reducing pain in 6-month-old children (Halperin et al, 2002). The EMLA patch is no longer commercially available in the United States.

The DTaP vaccines contain the adjuvant alum to retain the antigen at the injection site and prolong the stimulatory effect. One of the most important features of injecting vaccines is adequate penetration of the muscle for deposition of the drug intramuscularly and not subcutaneously. The use of appropriate needle length is an essential component of administering vaccines. In two studies, the use of longer needles significantly decreased the incidence of localized edema and tenderness when vaccines were administered to a group of infants (Diggle & Deeks, 2000; Diggle, Deeks, & Pollard, 2006). Because subcutaneous or intracutaneous injection of the adjuvant can cause local irritation, inflammation, or abscess formation, attention to excellent intramuscular injection technique must be used (see Atraumatic Care box above).

The total series requires several injections, and every attempt is made to rotate the sites and administer the injections as painlessly as possible (see discussion on intramuscular injections in Chapter 45). When two or more injections are given at separate sites, the order of injections is arbitrary. Some practitioners suggest injecting the less painful one first. Some believe this is DTaP, whereas others suggest the MMR or Hib vaccine. Still others advocate injecting at two sites simultaneously (which requires two operators).

One study found that children ages 4 to 6 years rated sequential injections for immunizations vs. simultaneous injections as being equally successful (Horn & McCarthy, 1999). Parents in the study preferred simultaneous immunization injections.

Because allergic reactions can occur after injection of vaccines, appropriate precautions are taken (see Anaphylaxis, Chapter 48).

Because nurses often administer vaccines, they have the responsibility for adequately informing parents of the nature, prevalence, and risks of the disease; the type of immunization product to be used; the expected benefits and the risk of side effects of the vaccine; and the need for accurate immunization records. Referring to immunizations as "baby shots" and limiting the discussion to vague statements about the vaccines are unacceptable practices.

Another important nursing responsibility is accurate documentation. Each child should have an immunization record for parents to keep, especially for families who move often. A survey of the accuracy of parental recall of children's immunizations found that parents underestimated the number of polio, DTaP, and MMR vaccines. The accuracy rate was not related to ethnic background, education level, or insurance coverage. Although immunization rates have increased significantly, health professionals should use every opportunity to encourage complete immunization of all children (see Family-Centered Care box). Blank immunization records may be downloaded from a number of websites, including the Immunization Action Coalition *(www.immunize.org)*, which has vaccine information and records in a number of languages.

The following information is documented on the medical record: day, month, and year of administration; manufacturer and lot number of vaccine; expiration date of vaccine; and the name, work address, and title of the person administering the vaccine. Additional data to record are the site and route of administration and evidence that the parent or legal guardian gave informed consent before the immunization was administered. Any adverse reactions after the administration of any vaccine are reported to the Vaccine Adverse Event Reporting System.*

An additional source of vaccine information that must be given to parents (by law, per the National Childhood Vaccine Injury Act of 1986) before the administration of certain vaccines is the *vaccine information statement* (VIS) for the particular vaccine being administered. Practitioners are required to fully inform families of the risks and benefits of the vaccines. VISs are designed to provide updated information to the adult vaccinee or parents or legal guardians of children being vaccinated regarding the risks and benefits of each vaccine. Questions regarding the information in the VISs should be answered by the practitioner. VISs are available for the following vaccines: anthrax, DTaP, Td, MMR, IPV, varicella, Hib, influenza, meningococcal, pneumococcal (PCV and PPV), and hepatitis A and B. An updated VIS should be provided to the primary caregiver, and documentation in the patient's chart should include the VIS title and the VIS publication date. VISs are available from state or local health departments and the following websites:

Immunization Coalition—*www.immunize.org/vis*

Centers for Disease Control and Prevention—*www.cdc.gov/vaccines/pubs/vis/default.htm*

In response to the concerns of manufacturers, practitioners, and parents of children with serious vaccine-associated injuries, the National Childhood Vaccine Injury Act of 1986 and the Vaccine Compensation Amendments of 1987 were

**For information call 800-822-7967;* www.fda.gov/cber/vaers/vaers.htm.

FAMILY-CENTERED CARE

Improving Immunization Rates Among Children and Adolescents

Strategies that may increase compliance include giving parents vaccine information at the time of the newborn's discharge, mailing reminder cards, making immunization services readily available, removing barriers to vaccination (such as long waiting times and appointment-only systems), and taking every opportunity to immunize children when they enter a health care facility (such as emergency departments, clinics, private offices, and hospitals).

Despite improvements in vaccination rates among infants and young children, adolescents are often incompletely immunized. An immunization update is an important part of adolescent preventive care, especially at 11 to 12 years of age. With the exception of pregnant teenagers, all adolescents should receive a second dose of the measles, mumps, and rubella (MMR) vaccine unless they have documentation of two MMR vaccinations after the first 12 months of life. Two doses of varicella vaccine are recommended for persons 13 years of age or older; these should be administered at least 4 weeks apart. All adolescents who have not previously completed the three-dose series of the hepatitis B vaccine should initiate or complete the series at age 11 to 12 years.

Adolescents ages 11 to 12 years and no later than 16 years should receive a dose of the tetanus and diphtheria toxoids and acellular pertussis (TdaP) vaccine if they have received the primary series of vaccinations and if no dose was received during the previous 5 years.

Hepatitis A vaccine should be given to all adolescents who have not yet been vaccinated for hepatitis A and to those who are traveling or living in countries where the hepatitis A virus is endemic or in communities with high rates of hepatitis A, persons with chronic liver disease, intravenous drug users, or men who have sex with other men. Adolescents who have chronic disorders or underlying medical conditions that place them at high risk for complications associated with the disease, such as influenza, should receive the appropriate vaccines (see p. 980). The meningococcal vaccine (MCV4) is now recommended for all older children (ages 11 and older) and adolescents who have not previously received the polysaccharide meningococcal vaccine (MPSV4); they should be vaccinated before or when entering college, especially if planning to live in a college dormitory.

Finally, the human papillomavirus (HPV) vaccine may be offered to girls 11 to 12 years of age to prevent cervical cancer. The vaccine is given in a series of three intramuscular injections, with the second dose 2 months after the first, and the third and final dose 6 months after the first. Adolescents 13 to 18 years of age may also complete the three-dose series if not previously immunized for HPV.

passed. These laws are designed to provide fair compensation for children who are inadvertently injured and provide greater protection from liability for vaccine manufacturers and providers.

In response to population-based studies indicating noncompliance with vaccination and confusion regarding vaccine schedules, it has been suggested that local or national computerized registries and improved record tracking systems be established to improve communication; additional recommendations include improving provider knowledge of immunization status and contraindications for administering vaccines and simplifying the immunization guidelines (Lee & Bernstein, 2005).

Injury Prevention

Injuries are a major cause of death during infancy, especially for children 6 to 12 months old. According to a Canadian survey (Pickett et al, 2003), the top leading causes of injury to infants were falls, ingestion injuries, and burns. The three leading causes of accidental death injury in infants in the United States were suffocation, motor vehicle–related accidents, and drowning (Centers for Disease Control and Prevention, 2007a). Constant vigilance, awareness, and supervision are essential as the child gains increased locomotor and manipulative skills that are coupled with an insatiable curiosity about the environment. Box 36-1 lists the major developmental achievements of each period during infancy and the appropriate injury prevention plan.

Aspiration of Foreign Objects

Asphyxiation by foreign material in the respiratory tract, combined with mechanical suffocation, is one of the leading causes of fatal injury in children younger than 1 year of age. The most common foreign bodies ingested and found in the gastrointestinal tract include both food and nonfood items. The size, shape, and consistency of foods or objects are important determinants of fatal obstruction. For example, small spheric or cylindric and pliable objects (less than 3.2 cm [1.25 inches]) are more likely to completely obstruct the airway. Unfortunately, common household items can be deadly to infants.

As soon as infants have the ability to find their mouth, they are vulnerable to aspiration of small objects, such as those left within reach or removable parts of objects that may on initial inspection appear safe. All toys must be carefully inspected for potential danger. Rattles, for example, have small beads in them to produce noise. A broken or cracked rattle can be dangerous because the beads can easily be aspirated while the infant has the toy in the mouth. Stuffed animals are another potentially dangerous toy if any of the parts, such as the eyes or nose, are removable buttons or plastic pieces. An active infant can grab a low-hanging mobile and quickly chew off a small piece. As soon as the infant crawls or plays on the floor, the floor must be kept free of any small articles that can be picked up and swallowed, such as coins, buttons, or small round batteries.

When infant *clothes* are purchased, the type of closure is important. A front button can easily be pulled off and swallowed. Safety pins for diapers are kept closed and away from the dressing table. Even though a young infant may not search for them, practicing this good habit from the beginning prevents future injuries.

Food items are a common cause of aspiration, and the most common offenders are hot dogs, candy, nuts, and grapes. When new foods are given to the child, nuts, hard candies, marshmallows, large amounts of peanut butter, and fruits with pits or seeds are avoided. When traveling or entertaining, parents must keep snack foods such as peanuts and popcorn away from young children. If given to young children, hot dogs must be cut into small, irregular pieces rather than served whole or in slices, since their size (diameter), round shape, and consistency allow for complete occlusion of the airway. Perhaps the most dangerous foods are dried beans, which, if aspirated, enlarge when they come in contact with the wet mucosa and block the airway.

Pacifiers can also be dangerous because the entire object may be aspirated if it is small, or the nipple and shield may become detached from the handle and become lodged in the pharynx. Improvised pacifiers, such as those made in hospitals from a padded nipple, also present dangers. The nipple may separate from the plastic collar and be aspirated. In addition, parents may continue to offer this pacifier to the infant at home. To eliminate the hazards of improvised pacifiers, hospitals should use only safe, commercial types. Pacifiers should not be altered from their original shape to encourage or discourage usage. Candy pacifiers pose dangers because the candy portion can dislodge from the circular base and be aspirated. To be safe, pacifiers should have:

- Sturdy, one-piece construction with material that is nontoxic, flexible, and firm but not brittle
- An easily grasped handle
- A mouthguard that cannot be separated from the nipple, that has two ventilating holes, and that is too large to be aspirated
- No detachable ribbon or string
- A label warning against tying the pacifier around the infant's neck

Using a syringe to accurately measure and dispense oral liquid medications to young children has become common practice. However, the *syringe cap* is a potential aspiration hazard. As a precaution, keep parts of medication devices out of the reach of children and be certain the cap is removed before dispensing medication. Medication administration syringes without caps are now available; syringes with caps should not be used for medication administration.

Another hazardous substance if aspirated is *baby powder,* which is usually a mixture of talc (hydrous magnesium silicate) and other silicates. Although the use of talc has been discouraged, it is a common baby care product and can cause severe and often fatal aspiration pneumonia. One of the factors involved in talc aspiration is the similar appearance of baby powder containers and nursing bottles. Talc containers often become favorite playthings and are placed in the mouth. Improperly using powder by sprinkling it directly on the skin creates a cloud of talc dust that is easily inhaled. Parents are advised of the danger of baby powder and are discouraged from using it. If they prefer to use a powder, a cornstarch preparation can be substituted (see Diaper Dermatitis, Chapter 53).

BOX 36-1 Injury Prevention During Infancy

Birth to 4 Months

Major Developmental Accomplishments

Exhibits involuntary reflexes (e.g., crawling reflex may propel infant forward or backward; startle reflex may cause the body to jerk)
May roll over
Has increasing eye-hand coordination and voluntary grasp reflex

Injury Prevention

Aspiration

Aspiration is not as great a danger to this age group as in older infants, but parents should begin practicing safeguarding early (see under Age 4 to 7 Months).
Never shake baby powder directly on infant; place powder in hand and then on infant's skin; store container closed and out of infant's reach.
Hold infant for feeding; do not prop bottle.
Know emergency procedures for choking.
Use pacifier with one-piece construction and loop handle.

Burns

Install smoke detectors in home.
Use caution when warming formula in microwave oven; always check temperature of liquid before feeding.
Check bathwater.
Do not pour hot liquids when infant is close by, such as sitting on lap.
Beware of cigarette ashes that may fall on infant.
Do not leave infant in sun for more than a few minutes; keep skin covered.
Wash flame-retardant clothes according to label directions.
Use cool-mist vaporizers.
Do not leave child in parked car.
Check surface heat of car restraint before placing child in seat.

Suffocation and Drowning

Keep all plastic bags stored out of infant's reach; discard large plastic garment bags after tying in a knot.
Do not cover mattress with plastic.
Use firm mattress and loose blankets, with no pillows.
Make certain crib design follows federal regulations and mattress fits snugly—crib slats 2⅜ inches (6 cm) apart.*
Position crib away from other furniture and away from radiators.
Do not tie pacifier on a string around infant's neck.
Remove bibs at bedtime.
Never leave infant alone in bath.
Do not leave infant under 12 months alone on adult or youth mattress or "beanbag" type seats.

Motor Vehicles

Transport infant in federally approved, rear-facing car seat, preferably in back seat.†
Do not place infant on seat (of car) or in lap.
Do not place child in a carriage or stroller behind a parked car.
Do not place infant or child in front passenger seat with an activated air bag.
Do not leave infant unattended in car, especially in environmental temperatures above 21° C (70° F).

Falls

Always raise crib rails.
Never leave infant alone on a raised, unguarded surface.
When in doubt as to where to place child, use floor.
Restrain child in infant seat, and never leave child unattended while the seat is resting on a raised surface.
Avoid using a high chair until child can sit well with support.

Poisoning

Poisoning is not as great a danger in this age group as in older infants, but parents should begin practicing safeguards early (see under Age 4 to 7 Months)

Bodily Damage

Keep sharp or jagged objects such as knives and broken glass out of child's reach.
Keep diaper pins closed and away from infant.

Age 4 to 7 Months

Major Developmental Accomplishments

Rolls over
Sits momentarily
Grasps and manipulates small objects
Resecures a dropped object
Has well-developed eye-hand coordination
Can focus on and locate very small objects
Has prominent mouthing (oral fixation)
Can push up on hands and knees
Crawls backward

Injury Prevention

Aspiration

Keep buttons, beads, syringe caps, and other small objects out of infant's reach.
Keep floor free of any small objects.
Do not feed infant hard candy, nuts, food with pits or seeds, or whole or circular pieces of hot dog.
Exercise caution when giving teething biscuits, since large chunks may be broken off and aspirated.
Do not feed infant while he or she is lying down.
Inspect toys for removable parts.
Use only cornstarch baby powder, if necessary, and keep out of reach.
Avoid storing large quantities of cleaning fluid, paints, pesticides, and other toxic substances.
Discard used containers of poisonous substances.
Do not store toxic substances in food or drink containers.
Discard used button-size batteries; store new batteries in safe area.
Know telephone number of local poison control center (800-222-1222) (usually listed in front of telephone directory).

Suffocation

Keep all latex balloons out of reach.
Remove all crib toys that are strung across crib or playpen when child begins to push up on hands or knees or is 5 months old.

BOX 36-1 Injury Prevention During Infancy—cont'd

Age 4 to 7 Months—cont'd

Injury Prevention—cont'd

Burns

Keep water faucets out of reach.

Place hot objects (cigarettes, candles, incense) on high surface out of child's reach.

Limit exposure to sun; apply sunscreen.

Falls

Restrain in a high chair.

Keep crib rails raised to full height.

Motor Vehicles

See under Birth to 4 Months.

Poisoning

Make certain that paint for furniture or toys does not contain lead.

Place toxic substances on a high shelf or in locked cabinet.

Hang plants or place on high surface rather than on floor.

Know telephone number of local poison control center (800-222-1222) (usually listed in front of telephone directory).

Bodily Damage

Give toys that are smooth and rounded, preferably made of wood or plastic.

Avoid long, pointed objects as toys.

Avoid toys that are excessively loud.

Keep sharp objects out of infant's reach.

Age 8 to 12 Months

Major Developmental Accomplishments

Crawls or creeps

Stands, holding onto furniture

Stands alone

Cruises around furniture

Walks

Climbs

Pulls on objects

Throws objects

Is able to pick up small objects; has pincer grasp

Explores by putting objects in mouth

Dislikes being restrained

Explores away from parent

Increasingly understands simple commands and phrases

Injury Prevention

Aspiration

Keep small objects off floor, off furniture, and out of reach of children.

Take care in feeding solid table food to give very small pieces.

Do not use beanbag toys or allow child to play with dried beans.

See also under Age 4 to 7 Months.

Bodily Damage

See under Age 4 to 7 Months.

Avoid placing televisions or other large objects on top of furniture, which may be overturned when infant pulls self to standing position.

Falls

Avoid walkers, especially near stairs.*

Ensure that furniture is sturdy enough for child to pull self to standing position and cruise.

Fence stairways at top and bottom if child has access to either end.*

Dress infant in safe shoes and clothing (soles that do not "catch" on floor, tied shoelaces, pant legs that do not touch floor).

Suffocation and Drowning

Keep doors of oven, dishwasher, refrigerator, cooler, and front-loading clothes washer and dryer closed at all times.

If storing an unused large appliance, such as a refrigerator, lock or remove the door.

Supervise contact with inflated balloons; immediately discard popped balloons, and keep uninflated balloons out of reach.

Fence swimming pools and other bodies of standing water such as decorative fountains; lock gate to swimming pools so only adult can access.

Always supervise when near any source of water, such as cleaning buckets, drainage areas, toilets.

Keep bathroom doors closed.

Eliminate unnecessary pools of water.

Keep one hand on child at all times when in tub.

Poisoning

Administer medications as a drug, not as a candy.

Do not administer medications unless prescribed by a practitioner.

Return medications and poisons to safe storage area immediately after use; replace caps properly if a child-protector cap is used.

Have poison control center number (800-222-1222) on telephone and refrigerator.

Burns

Place guards in front of or around any heating appliance, fireplace, or furnace.

Keep electrical wires hidden or out of reach.

Place plastic guards over electrical outlets; place furniture in front of outlets.

Keep hanging tablecloths out of reach (child may pull down hot liquids or heavy or sharp objects).

*Information on many items such as cribs or walkers is available from U.S. Consumer Product Safety Commission, 800-638-2722; *www.cpsc.gov*.

†See footnote on p. 994.

Suffocation

Mechanical suffocation includes suffocation by covering of the airway (i.e., mouth and nose); by pressure on the throat and chest; and by exclusion of air, such as by refrigerator entrapment. Nonfood items cause the majority of deaths in young children. *Latex balloons,* whether partially inflated, uninflated, or popped, are a leading cause of pediatric choking deaths from children's products. They should be kept away from infants and young children. Even the practice of inflating latex gloves to amuse children in health care settings may pose a danger, especially if the child is latex sensitive.

Encourage adults to blow up balloons for children, supervise children's balloon play, pick up and dispose of broken balloon pieces, warn older children of dangers of chewing or sucking on balloons, and substitute Mylar or paper balloons for latex balloons.

The accessibility of the plastic linings of diapers used on the infant or on dolls is especially dangerous to young children.

The *bed* or *crib* poses a number of hazards. An infant who is placed in a bed under tucked-in blankets and sheets can be caught under them and unable to wriggle free. Baby pillows filled with plastic foam beads, resembling small beanbags, are dangerous; very young infants are suffocated when the pillow contours to the face and blocks the airway. There are potential dangers when adults sleep with a small infant because of the possibility of rolling over and smothering the child (overlaying). The most common causes of infant suffocation are wedging between a bed or mattress and a wall and oronasal obstruction by a plastic bag.

Infant strangulation may occur if the infant's head becomes caught between the crib slats and mattress or other objects close to the crib. Suffocation deaths are not confined to cribs; ill-fitting mattresses in adult or youth beds, bunk beds, and waterbeds have also been reported. According to U.S. federal regulation, the distance between crib slats should not be more than 2⅜ inches (approximately 6 cm), roughly the width of three adult fingers. Mattresses and bumper pads should fit snugly against the slats. A general rule is that the mattress is too small if two adult fingers can be placed between the mattress and crib or bed side. A temporary solution is to place large, rolled towels in the space to create a snug fit. Corner post extensions on cribs are another source of strangulation. Children have died when their clothing caught on raised corner posts as they climbed out of the crib. Voluntary manufacturing standards state that corner post extensions must not exceed $\frac{1}{16}$ inch; however, the safety of any extension is questionable. Decorative extensions need to be removed from cribs. Ideally, information regarding correct crib design should be given prenatally, before parents have purchased or borrowed a crib.*

Mesh-sided playpens and cribs can result in death if the sides are left in the lowered position. Infants have suffocated when they fell off the edge of the mattress and the head or chest was compressed between the floorboard and mesh side. Parents should be advised of this danger and encouraged to always keep the sides locked securely in the up position whenever the child is in the playpen or crib.

The crib should be positioned away from large furniture, since children who crawl out of the crib may become caught between the two objects. Cribs should also be located away from windows, where drape or blind cords can become wrapped around the infant's neck.

Another cause of suffocation is *plastic bags.* Plastic bags are very lightweight and can easily and quickly be wrapped around the head of an active infant or pressed against the face. For this reason, pillows and mattresses should not be covered with plastic. Older infants may play with a plastic bag and accidentally pull it over their heads. Because plastic is nonporous, suffocation occurs in a matter of minutes.

Cords (e.g., drapery or window blinds) located near the infant are a potential cause of strangulation. Bibs are removed at bedtime, and objects such as pacifiers are never hung on a string around the infant's neck. This is a common practice in some cultures that can be remedied by tying a *short* string to a pacifier and clipping the string to the child's shirt.

Toys that have strings attached (e.g., a telephone) or toys that are tied to cribs or playpens can be hazards because the string can become wrapped around the child's neck or the child can become entrapped in the toy. As a precaution, all cords should be less than 30 cm (12 inches) long. Crib toys should be hung high enough that the infant cannot become entangled in them and should no longer be used once the child is able to reach them.

If applied too loosely or left unfastened, restraining straps can be a hazard. For example, a child may slide off a high chair beneath the tray and become strangled on the loose strap. All straps should be fastened securely.

Motor Vehicle Injuries

Automobile injuries are the leading cause of accidental death in children between the ages of 1 and 9 years (Centers for Disease Control and Prevention, 2007a). A significant number of nonfatal vehicle-related injuries in children between 1 and 4 years of age occur as a result of back-over while children are playing in a driveway (Centers for Disease Control and Prevention, 2005b). In addition, a significant number of infants are injured or die from improper restraint within the vehicle, most often from riding on the lap of another occupant or from riding unrestrained in the back seat of the vehicle. Reports indicate that child restraint use decreases with increasing age of children and increasing number of occupants. Lack of proper child restraint continues to be a major factor in fatal accidents involving children. All infants must be secured in a U.S. federally approved restraint rather than held or placed on the seat of the car. There is no safe alternative.

Infant restraints are designed either as an infant-only model or as a convertible infant-toddler model (Fig. 36-14). Either restraint is a semireclined seat that faces the rear of the car. A rear-facing car seat provides the best protection for the disproportionately heavy head and weak neck of a young child. This position minimizes the stress on the neck by spreading the forces of a frontal crash over the entire back, neck, and head; the spine is supported by the back of the car seat. If the seat were faced forward, the head would whip forward because of the force of the crash, creating enormous stress on the neck.

A recent study indicated that children 0 to 3 years of age riding properly restrained in the middle of the back seat had

---

**A number of parent education pamphlets—such as* Crib Safety Tips *and* Is Your Used Crib Safe?*—are available in English and Spanish from the U.S. Consumer Product Safety Commission, Publication Request, Washington, DC 20207; 800-638-2772;* www.cpsc.gov.

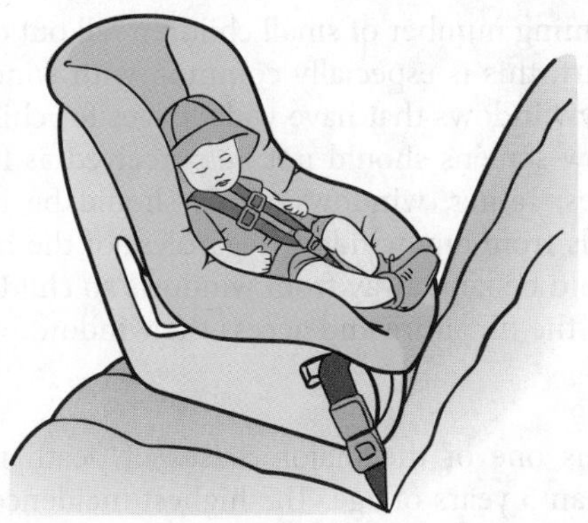

Fig. 36-14 A federally approved rear-facing infant car restraint in the back seat provides the best protection.

a 43% lower risk of injury than children riding in the outboard (window) seat during a crash (Kallan et al, 2008). Another study has shown that children 0 to 23 months riding in a rear-facing restraint were less likely to be injured than those riding in a forward-facing restraint (Henary et al, 2007).

The restraint is anchored to the vehicle with the vehicle's seat belt, and the restraint has a harness system for securing the infant. The five-point harness system provides the most effective support for infant restraint; the three-point harness system secures only the upper body. Many infant seats have a plastic base that can be left in the car; the seat latches or clicks into the base so that the base does not have to be installed each time the car seat is removed. The LATCH (lower anchor and tether for children) system provides car seat anchors between the front cushion and backrest so the seat belt does not have to be used. Some automobiles have tether anchors for rear-facing infant-only seats as well (see Chapter 37). Although many infant restraints can be recliners, they are used in the car only in the position specified by the manufacturer.

NURSING ALERT Infants should ride in rear-facing car seat from birth to 9070 g (20 lb) and as close to 1 year of age as possible. If the child weighs 20 lb but is not 1 year old, the rear-facing position is still recommended.

Severe injuries and deaths in children have occurred from air bags deploying on impact in the front passenger seat. The back seat is the safest area of the car. If the back seat is not an option, an infant restraint may be positioned in the front seat provided that the seat belt can be locked into position and there is no passenger-side air bag. If there is a passenger-side air bag and the child has special health care needs or constant observation is recommended by the practitioner and no other adult is available to ride in the back seat with the child, an on/off switch may be installed to prevent the air bag from deploying and injuring the child. Another condition that may arise is the use of vehicles without a back seat; in such cases it is best that the front passenger seat be placed as far back as possible and appropriate child safety restraint employed. With advanced technology, new, "smart" air bags include features that make them a safer alternative for children.*

For restraints to be effective, they must be used properly. Dressing the infant in an outfit with sleeves and legs allows the harness to hold the child securely in the seat. A small blanket or towel rolled tightly can be placed on either side of the head to minimize movement and keep the infant's hips against the back of the seat. Padding between the infant's legs and crotch is added to prevent slouching. Thick, soft padding is not placed under the infant or behind the back because during the impact the padding will compress, leaving the harness straps loose. Preterm infants being discharged home should be placed in an appropriate car seat restraint as it would be placed in the car and the infant's oxygen saturations monitored for a determined period to detect any potential problems with airway occlusion. (For further discussion of car seat restraints, see Chapter 37; for preterm infant car restraint test guidelines, see Community Focus box on p. 738.)

Another automobile-related hazard for infants is *overheating* (hyperthermia) and subsequent death when left in a vehicle in hot weather (over 26.4° C [80° F]). Infants dissipate heat poorly, and an increase in body temperature may cause death in a few hours. Parents are cautioned against leaving infants in a vehicle alone for *any reason.* A small sign or placard has been designed to hang in the rear-view mirror to remind the parent that there is a child in the back seat. Busy parents may forget the child in the back when preoccupied with errands, children's school and extracurricular activities, and busy work schedules.

evolve Critical Thinking Exercise—Infant Safety

Falls

Residential injuries, especially falls, accounted for the highest incidence of unintentional injuries to children seen in emergency departments in the United States (Phelan et al, 2005). Falls are most common after 4 months of age when the infant has learned to roll over, but they can occur at any age.

The best advice for prevention of falls is to never place a child of any age unattended on a raised surface that is not designed to protect the child from accidentally falling. When in doubt, the safest place is the floor. Even though young infants cannot climb over a partially raised crib rail, it is best to form a habit of raising the rail all the way, since someday that infant will be able to climb out. Crib sides should have a latching device that cannot be easily released. The welds attaching the crib corner locks to the corner posts should not be cracked or broken. If the welds are damaged, the bedspring could fall to the floor. Ideally, cribs should be placed on carpeted, not hard, floors.

Another danger area for falling is the *changing table,* which is usually high and narrow. Although these tables have a restraining belt, children are never left unattended, even

**An air bag safety fact sheet is available from the American Academy of Pediatrics, 141 Northwest Point Blvd., Elk Grove Village, IL 60009;* www.aap.org. *For car seat information, contact* www.aap.org/family/carseatguide.htm; *and the Insurance Institute for Highway Safety, 1005 N. Glebe Road, Suite 800, Arlington, VA 22201; 703-247-1500; fax: 703-247-1588;* www.highwaysafety.org. *The National Highway Traffic Safety Administration,* www.nhtsa.gov, *also provides child passenger safety and air bag safety information for parents.*

when restrained. The best way to avoid needing to leave is to arrange the area with all necessary articles within easy reach so that the child is always in full sight of the caregiver. It takes only a fraction of a second for an infant to fall off. During the latter half of the first year, infants usually resist dressing and diapering and may be difficult to manage. If there is danger that the child is strong enough to resist restraining, the infant should be changed on a safer surface, such as a clean floor.

Infant seats, high chairs, walkers, and swings present additional opportunities for falls. If the *infant seat* is placed on a table, the child should never be left unrestrained or unattended. The same rule is essential for other baby equipment, particularly when the child has learned to crawl and to stand up. *High chairs* are designed for older infants who can sit well and who are tall enough to have the tray at the level of their chest or abdomen. Small infants can slip through a high chair if a protective harness is not used. *Infant walkers* are responsible for a number of different types of injuries that occur because the walker tipped over or fell down stairs. Parents need to be warned of these dangers and encouraged to keep a constant vigil on their child's activities. The American Academy of Pediatrics, Committee on Injury and Poison Prevention (2001), does not recommend the use of mobile infant walkers. In response to the large number of accidents and deaths associated with mobile infant walkers, several manufacturers modified these products to prevent falls down stairs. The new models should have a label or sign indicating "meets new safety standard," must be wider than 36 inches, or must have a braking mechanism to stop the walker. Mobile infant walkers may still pose a risk for climbing up to reach dangerous objects and should be carefully supervised. One alternative is to use a stationary play station with a seat similar to that in a walker. There is no evidence that use of infant walkers helps infants walk sooner.

Once infants are mobile, they should not be allowed to crawl unsupervised on any raised surface, near stairs, or near any water reservoir. Gates should be used at the *bottom* and *top of stairs,* since both present dangers to the crawling and climbing infant. However, certain types of gates can present hazards. Freestanding enclosures constructed of crisscrossed wood slats that expand and contract can trap the head or neck when children attempt to climb over them. If these types of gates are used, they must be securely fastened to prevent mobility of the slats.

As children begin to pull themselves to a standing position, *heavy objects,* such as unsturdy furniture or any freestanding item (e.g., wrought iron fish tank stands or televisions), can be extremely dangerous if pulled down on top of the child. To prevent such injury, televisions should be placed on lower furniture and as far back as possible, and angle braces or anchors can secure furniture to walls.

Even when the environment is made safe, infants may sometimes literally trip over their own feet from *clothing.* Slippery socks; hard, slick soles on shoes or rubber soles that can catch, especially on a carpet; and long pants or pajama bottoms can easily upset a child's balance. Such dangers need to be pointed out to parents, especially when infants are taking their first steps.

An alarming number of small children fall out of windows and are hurt; this is especially common with window ledges such as bay windows that have wide ledges for children to sit on. Window screens should not be perceived as fall-prevention devices; rather, window guards should be installed to prevent falls from any window, regardless of the height. Furniture should be kept away from windows so children cannot climb onto the furniture and access the window.

Poisoning

Poisoning is one of the major causes of death in children younger than 5 years of age. The highest incidence occurs in the 2-year-old group, with the second highest incidence occurring in 1-year-old children. Infants who do not crawl are relatively free from danger of poisonous agents by virtue of immobility. However, once locomotion begins, danger from poisoning is present almost everywhere. The average home contains more than 500 toxic substances, and approximately one third of all poisonings occur in the kitchen.

The major reason for ingestion of poisons is *improper storage.* To protect the infant, toxic agents should not be placed on a low shelf, a low table, or the floor. Drugs that are kept in a purse pose additional dangers; if the handbag is given to infants to play with, they may open it and ingest the drug. Another unrecognized hazard occurs during diaper changes, when infants are near many toxic substances such as ointments, creams, oils, and talc. Common household over-the-counter medications such as acetaminophen and cold and cough preparations, cosmetics and personal care products, and cleaning products are also sources of childhood poisoning (Wilkerson, Northington, & Fisher, 2005).

Parents may even hand infants a potentially poisonous object to quiet them. Such dangers need to be stressed to parents, and toys need to be kept at diapering areas to minimize risks.

Plants are another source of poisoning for infants. Plants are commonly placed on the floor, and the leaves or flowers are attractive and easy to pull off. More than 700 species of plants are known to have caused illness or death.

Another danger is ingestion of the *button-sized batteries* used in devices such as hearing aids, calculators, watches, and cameras. Because they are bright and shiny, they are attractive to children. However, they can cause severe morbidity, even death, if lodged in the esophagus. The strong alkali in a battery can leak and cause a severe caustic burn. As a precaution, small batteries must be safely stored and discarded where young children cannot easily retrieve them.

Not all poisonings result from ingestion—*inhalation* is another possible route, such as inhaling chlorine vapors from household cleaning or pool supplies. Passive cocaine toxicity has occurred in young children exposed to freebase cocaine ("crack") smoking by adults. Children should be protected from environments in which airborne toxins exist. (For a discussion of passive secondhand tobacco smoke, see Chapter 46.)

The production of methamphetamines, a common central nervous system stimulant also known as ice, speed, or crystal, involves the use of a number of chemicals that may be toxic alone (contact or ingestion) or during the production (cooking) of the drug itself. Methamphetamine laboratories are commonly in household areas where children may be exposed to harmful inhalants as well as open fires where meth is "cooked." Methamphetamine laboratories are also often mobile, and children may be similarly exposed to dangerous chemicals. Methamphetamine use and exposure have been shown to cause developmental problems and short- and long-term brain damage, particularly in children. Reports of the number of children exposed daily to methamphetamine laboratories in the United States and Canada are alarming; such children are also at high risk for abuse and neglect because their caretakers are preoccupied with production, sale, and use of the drug (Bellemare, 2008; Matteucci et al, 2007; Mecham & Melini, 2002). Children should be protected from environments in which inhaled toxins exist (see Chapter 28 for discussion of effects of chemical substances on the fetus and neonate).

The only sure way to prevent poisoning is to remove toxic agents; this means placing containers out of the infant's reach or contact. Because crawling infants soon become climbing toddlers, it is best to keep all toxic agents, especially drugs, in a locked cabinet. Special plastic hooks can be attached to the inside of cabinet doors to keep them securely closed (Fig. 36-15). Firm thumb pressure is required to unlatch the hook, and small children are usually unable to manipulate them. Locks are best, but for frequently used cleaning agents, such as those often kept under a kitchen sink, hooks are a practical alternative.

With several hundred toxic substances in each house, locking up all potentially toxic substances can present a problem; however, careful planning can help. A large surplus of cleaning agents, furniture polishes, laundry additives, paints, insecticides, and solvents should be avoided. Used poison containers should be promptly discarded and not used to store another poison without adequately marking the package. Potentially hazardous substances should not be stored in any type of food container. A popular container used to store toxic liquids is a soda, or pop, bottle. A child unaware of the dangerous contents is vulnerable to poisoning.

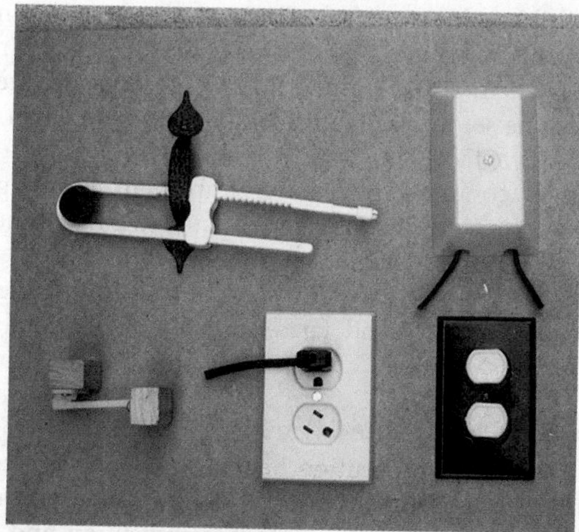

Fig. 36-15 Safety demonstration board. *Clockwise from lower left:* Two types of cabinet latches, a shock guard for an electrical outlet in use, and two types of outlet covers (the one with the white cover has passive devices that automatically cover the outlet when a plug is removed).

NURSING ALERT Parents should know the telephone number of the local poison control center–800-222-1222– and call this number in the event of a suspected poisoning. Ipecac, used to induce vomiting, is no longer a standard recommendation. If the child is not breathing, the parent should call 911 immediately.

Emergency measures for poisoning are discussed in Chapter 47.

Burns

Scalding from water that is too hot; excessive sunburn; and burns from house fires, electrical wires, sockets, and heating elements such as radiators, registers, and floor furnaces cause a significant number of deaths and many more injuries in infants. The infant's skin is particularly sensitive to irritation, and the mechanisms for temperature perception are not completely developed. As a general precaution, all homes should have smoke alarms installed near the bedroom areas and on each level of the building.

Scald burns from *hot tap water* can be prevented by lowering the water heater to a safe temperature of 49° C (120° F). In addition, the bathwater should be checked before the infant is immersed. The most common type of scald injury is from the infant pulling a hot pan of water off a stove or an elevated surface onto herself or himself (Drago, 2005). Scalds can also occur from bathing infants in the kitchen sink when the garbage disposal, occluded with debris, causes the draining dishwasher effluent to back up into the sink. The temperature of the effluent from a dishwasher is typically that of the maximum water temperature of the household water heater, but many dishwashers are equipped with heating elements that heat water to an even higher temperature. As a precaution, instruct caregivers to avoid bathing small children in the kitchen sink while the dishwasher is running.

If formula or food is warmed in a *microwave oven*, it must be checked before feeding because the container may remain cool while the contents are hot. Another danger is explosion of the container from the buildup of steam. Because of these dangers, microwaving infant formula or food should be avoided or done using the guidelines in the Patient Teaching box on p. 973. The handles of cooking utensils should be turned toward the back of the stove. When the infant is underfoot, pouring hot liquids and cooking with hot oil are avoided. Hanging tablecloths are also placed out of the infant's reach to prevent pulling hot items off the table.

Sunburn can be a source of a first- or second-degree burn. Exposure to direct sunlight should be avoided for the first 6 months. When infants are in the sun, the body, especially the face and head, should be covered. Sunscreen can be used on older infants, but should be used on small areas of the body and only sparingly in infants under 6 months (see Sunburn, Chapter 53). Although infants burn less readily, their thin skin can become sunburned and needs protection.

Electrical outlets should be covered with protective plastic caps that prevent the child from putting objects such as hairpins into the outlet (see Fig. 36-15). Extension cords are placed out of reach so that curious infants cannot chew on them and break the rubber coating (Fig. 36-16). Infants should not be

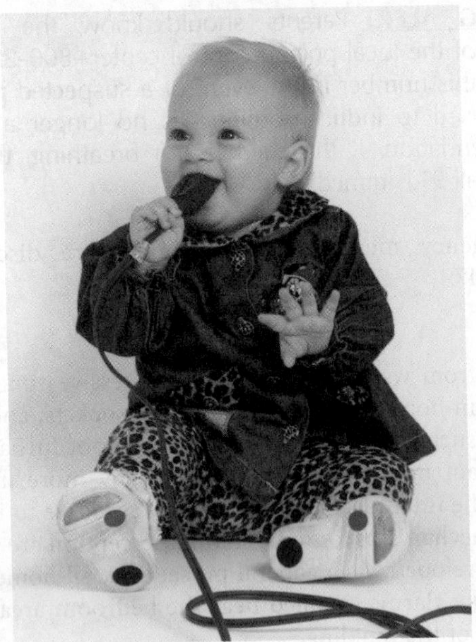

Fig. 36-16 Infants can find hazardous electrical wires. *(Photo by Paul Vincent Kuntz, Texas Children's Hospital, Houston, TX.)*

allowed to play near television sets, stereo units, or other appliances.

Any *heat-producing element* should have a guard placed in front of it. Fireplaces should be well screened because they are appealing and within easy access. Small, portable heaters should be placed on a high surface. Floor furnaces should have barrier gates to prevent children from crawling or walking over them. Burning cigarettes, candles, and incense should be kept out of reach, and infants should not be held by a smoking adult because falling ashes are a hazard, especially to the eyes. Heated-mist vaporizers are a source of burns and should not be used. If humidity is needed, only cool-mist vaporizers are safe. Handheld curling irons are also a common source of hand burns in small children.

By law, all infant sleepwear must be flame retardant. Unfortunately, this does not apply to all *infant clothing*. Flame-retardant fabric must never be viewed as the ultimate protection against burns. Repeated washing reduces the flame-retardant properties, and the use of soap or bleach destroys the protection. If sleepwear is home sewn, parents are advised to look for specially treated, flame-retardant fabric.

Children can also be burned by overheated metal hardware and vinyl seats in cars parked in the sun. As a precaution, the surface heat of car restraints should be determined before placing children in them. Covering the restraints and hardware (such as metal latches on seat belts) may be necessary to prevent skin burns. An additional safeguard is buying a light-colored restraint, which absorbs less heat.

Drowning

Drowning in this age group can occur in just an inch or two of water. Consequently, infants should always be supervised in a bathtub and near a source of water such as a swimming pool, hot tub, lake, toilet, or bucket. Most unintentional infant drownings occur in the home setting; most infants younger than age 1 year drowned in a toilet, bathtub, or bucket (Brenner & American Academy of Pediatrics, Committee on Injury, Violence, and Poison Prevention, 2003; Lassman, 2002); 5-gallon buckets are particularly dangerous because the child may inadvertently fall in head first and, because of the weight of the upper body at this age, cannot withdraw from the bucket. Inadequate supervision is often associated with childhood drowning. Organized swimming instruction is not recommended for children younger than 4 years of age because it may lead to a false sense of security (American Academy of Pediatrics, Committee on Sports Medicine and Committee on Injury and Poison Prevention, 2000). No infant can be expected to learn the elements of water safety or to react appropriately in an emergency. Therefore all young children need to be considered at risk when near water. Infants and toddlers are also at increased risk of infection and seizures from swallowing large amounts of water.

Bodily Damage

Injuries in children may occur in numerous ways. Sharp, jagged-edged objects can cause wounds in the skin. Long, pointed articles, such as the common toothpick or fork, can be poked into the eye or ear, causing serious damage. Such articles should be safely stored away from the infant's reach; forks are best avoided for self-feeding until the child has mastered the spoon, usually by age 18 months.

In addition to hazards such as aspiration, small articles can be placed in the ear or nose, and excessive noise from toys can result in sensorineural hearing loss. Although toys with the highest noise levels are model airplanes, air guns, and toy cap guns, even common squeaking toys used by young children may be harmful if placed close to the ear.

An alarming trend is the increasing number of infant deaths attributed to homicide. In one study 6.4% of 10,370 infant injury deaths occurred as a result of homicide (Brenner et al, 1999). A high rate of battering injury has been reported in infants 0 to 5 months (Agran et al, 2003). The Centers for Disease Control and Prevention (2008) recently reported that 19% of child maltreatment fatalities occurred among infants; in addition, homicide statistics suggest the fatality risk is greatest in the first week of the infant's life. Specific interventions must be set in place to protect infants from harm, especially in preventable situations.

Another common and often unrecognized danger to infants is animal attacks. As newcomers to the home, helpless infants can provoke jealousy in animals, especially dogs and cats. Parents must be constantly vigilant to protect the child from household pets and farm animals (see Animal Bites, Chapter 53).

Nurse's Role in Injury Prevention

The task of injury prevention begins to be appreciated only when the potential environmental dangers to which infants are vulnerable are considered. Injury prevention and parent education should be handled on a growth and developmental basis. It is simply impossible to completely protect infants and small children from all potential dangers without placing them in a sterile, impractical environment. However, a large percentage of childhood deaths continue to occur as a result of preventable injuries. Nurses must be aware of the possible causes of injury in each age group in order for anticipatory preventive teaching to occur. For example, the guidelines for injury prevention during infancy presented in Box 36-1 should be discussed before the child reaches the susceptible age group. Preventive teaching ideally occurs during pregnancy. Two thirds of all injuries to children occur in the home, and therefore the importance of safety cannot be overemphasized. The Patient Teaching box contains a home safety checklist that can be presented to parents to increase their awareness of danger areas in the home and assist them in implementing safety devices and practices before their absence can inflict injury on infants. In addition, displays such as a safety demonstration board can be helpful in familiarizing parents with inexpensive commercial devices that can be used in the home to prevent injuries. To help parents appreciate the dangers present in their home to young children, suggest that they get eye level with the floor to survey the environment from a child's viewpoint.

Injury prevention requires protection of the child and education of the caregiver. Nurses in ambulatory care settings, health maintenance centers, or visiting nurse agencies are in a favorable position for injury education. This does not exclude nurses in inpatient facilities, who could use visiting times as an excellent opportunity for discussing this topic.

One approach to teaching injury prevention is to relate why children in various age groups are prone to specific types of injuries. Stressing prevention is just as important as emphasizing the "why" of the injury. However, injury prevention must also be practical. Asking parents for their ideas leads to realistic suggestions that can be followed.

If an injury has occurred, the nurse should not be too quick to admonish the parent; injuries do not always indicate neglect. It is a difficult task to watch children carefully without overprotecting or unnecessarily confining them. Allowing children to explore while maintaining consistent, age-appropriate limits is sound advice.

Parents need to remember that infants and young children cannot anticipate danger or understand when it is or is not present. A dead electrical wire may present no actual harm; but if the child is allowed to play with it, a poor behavior is enforced and will be practiced when the child encounters a live wire. Although it is always wise to explain why something is dangerous, it must be remembered that small children need to be physically removed from the situation.

It is not easy to teach safety, supervise closely, and refrain from saying "no" a hundred times a day. Parents become acutely aware of this dilemma as soon as the infant learns to crawl. Preventing injuries to children is usually the first reason for limit setting and discipline, but limits are also set to prevent danger to valuable household objects. When small children are in the home, dangerous objects must be removed or guarded and valuable articles placed out of reach.

When children are taught the meaning of "no," they should also be taught what "yes" means. Children should be praised for playing with suitable toys, their efforts at behaving or listening should be reinforced, and innovative and creative recreational toys should be provided for them. Infants love to tear paper and avidly pursue books, magazines, or newspapers left on the floor. Instead of always scolding them for destroying a valued book, child-safe books (such as those constructed of fabric) can be kept available for them to play with. If they enjoy pots and pans, a cabinet can be arranged with safe utensils for them to explore.

One additional factor must be stressed concerning injury prevention and education. Children are imitators; they copy what they see and hear. *Practicing safety teaches safety.* This applies to parents and their children and to nurses and their patients. Saying one thing but doing another confuses children and can lead to difficulties as the child grows older.

Anticipatory Guidance–Care of Families

Childrearing is no easy task; it presents challenges to both new and "seasoned" parents. Society's changing roles and mores, combined with a highly mobile population, leave little stability for traditional role models and time-honored methods of raising children. As a result, parents look to professionals for guidance. Nurses are in an advantageous position to render assistance and offer suggestions. Every phase of a child's life has its particular traumas—toilet training for toddlers, unexplained fears for preschoolers, and identity crises for adolescents. For parents of an infant, some challenges center around dependency, discipline, increased mobility, and safety. Major areas for parental guidance during the first year are listed in the Patient Teaching box.

SPECIAL HEALTH PROBLEMS

Feeding Difficulties

Regurgitation and "Spitting Up"

The return of small amounts of food after a feeding is a common occurrence during infancy. It should not be confused with actual vomiting, which can be associated with a number of disturbances that may be insignificant or serious. It is usually benign, although persistent regurgitation necessitates medical evaluation to rule out gastroesophageal reflux. For clarification, the following terms are defined:

Regurgitation—Return of undigested food from the stomach, usually accompanied by burping

Spitting up—Dribbling of unswallowed formula from the infant's mouth immediately after a feeding

The normal occurrence of regurgitation or spitting up should be explained to parents, especially to those who are unduly concerned about it. Regurgitation can be reduced by some simple measures such as frequent burping during and after feeding, minimum handling during and after feeding, and positioning the child on the right side with the head slightly elevated after feeding. The inconvenience of spitting up can be managed with the use of absorbent bibs on the infant and protective cloths on the parent.

Sometimes frequent dribbling of formula causes excoriation of the corners of the mouth, the chin, and the neck.

PATIENT TEACHING Child Safety Home Checklist

Safety: Fire, Electrical, Burns

- ☐ Guards in front of or around any heating appliance, fireplace, or furnace (including floor furnace)*
- ☐ Electrical wires hidden or out of reach*
- ☐ No frayed or broken wires; no overloaded sockets
- ☐ Plastic guards or caps over electrical outlets, furniture in front of outlets*
- ☐ Hanging tablecloths out of reach, away from open fires*
- ☐ Smoke detectors tested and operating properly
- ☐ Kitchen matches stored out of child's reach*
- ☐ Large, deep ashtrays throughout house (if used)
- ☐ Small stoves, heaters, and other hot objects (cigarettes, candles, coffee pots, slow cookers) placed where they cannot be tipped over or reached by children
- ☐ Hot water heater set at 49° C (120° F) or lower
- ☐ Pot handles turned toward back of stove, center of table
- ☐ No loose clothing worn near stove
- ☐ No cooking or eating hot foods or liquids with child standing nearby or sitting in lap
- ☐ All small appliances, such as iron, turned off, disconnected, and placed out of reach when not in use
- ☐ Cool, not hot, mist vaporizer used
- ☐ Fire extinguisher available on each floor and checked periodically
- ☐ Electrical fuse box and gas shutoff accessible
- ☐ Family escape plan in case of a fire practiced periodically; fire escape ladder available on upper-level floors
- ☐ Telephone number of fire or rescue squad and address of home with nearest cross street posted near phone

Safety: Suffocation and Aspiration

- ☐ Small objects stored out of reach*
- ☐ Toys inspected for small removable parts or long strings*
- ☐ Hanging crib toys and mobiles placed out of reach
- ☐ Plastic bags stored away from young child's reach, large plastic garment bags discarded after tying in knots*
- ☐ Mattress or pillow not covered with plastic or in manner accessible to child*
- ☐ Crib design according to federal regulations (crib slats less than 2⅜ inches [6 cm] apart) with snug-fitting mattress*†
- ☐ Crib positioned away from other furniture or windows*
- ☐ Portable playpen gates up at all times while in use*
- ☐ Accordion-style gates not used*
- ☐ Bathroom doors kept closed and toilet seats down*
- ☐ Faucets turned off firmly*
- ☐ Pool fenced with locked gate
- ☐ Proper safety equipment at poolside
- ☐ Electric garage door openers stored safely and garage door adjusted to rise when door strikes object
- ☐ Doors of oven, trunks, dishwasher, refrigerator, and front-loading clothes washer and dryer kept closed*
- ☐ Unused appliance, such as a refrigerator, securely closed with lock or doors removed*
- ☐ Food served in small, noncylindric pieces*
- ☐ Toy chests without lids or with lids that securely lock in open position*
- ☐ Buckets and wading pools kept empty when not in use*
- ☐ Clothesline above head level
- ☐ At least one member of household trained in basic life support (cardiopulmonary resuscitation), including first aid for choking

Safety: Poisoning

- ☐ Toxic substances, including batteries, placed on a high shelf, preferably in locked cabinet
- ☐ Toxic plants hung or placed out of reach*
- ☐ Excess quantities of cleaning fluids, paints, pesticides, drugs, and other toxic substances not stored in home
- ☐ Used containers of poisonous substances discarded where child cannot obtain access
- ☐ Telephone number of local poison control center and address of home with nearest cross street posted near phones
- ☐ Medicines clearly labeled in childproof containers and stored out of reach
- ☐ Household cleaners, disinfectants, and insecticides kept in their original containers, separate from food, and out of reach
- ☐ Smoking in areas away from children, avoiding smoking in child's room or bed

Safety: Falls

- ☐ Nonskid mats, strips, or surfaces in tubs and showers
- ☐ Exits, halls, and passageways in rooms kept clear of toys, furniture, boxes, or other items that could be obstructive
- ☐ Stairs and halls well lighted, with switches at both top and bottom
- ☐ Sturdy handrails for all steps and stairways
- ☐ Nothing stored on stairways
- ☐ Treads, risers, and carpeting in good repair
- ☐ Glass doors and walls marked with decals
- ☐ Safety glass used in doors, windows, and walls
- ☐ Gates on top and bottom of staircases and elevated areas, such as porch, fire escape*
- ☐ Guardrails on upstairs windows with locks that limit height of window opening and access to areas such as fire escape*
- ☐ Crib side rails raised to full height; mattress lowered as child grows*
- ☐ Restraints used in high chairs or other baby furniture; preferably walkers with wheels not used*
- ☐ Scatter rugs secured in place or used with nonskid backing
- ☐ Walks, patios, and driveways in good repair

Safety: Bodily Injury

- ☐ Knives, power tools, and unloaded firearms stored safely or placed in locked cabinet
- ☐ Garden tools returned to storage racks after use
- ☐ Pets properly restrained and immunized for rabies
- ☐ Swings, slides, and other outdoor play equipment kept in safe condition
- ☐ Yard free of broken glass, nail-studded boards, other litter
- ☐ Cement birdbaths placed where young child cannot tip them over*

*Safety measures are specific for homes with young children. All safety measures should be implemented in homes where children reside and visit frequently, such as those of grandparents or baby-sitters.

†Federal regulations are available from U.S. Consumer Product Safety Commission, 800-638-2772; *www.cpsc.gov.*

PATIENT TEACHING Guidance During Infant's First Year

First 6 Months

Teach car safety with use of federally approved restraint, facing rearward, in the middle of the back seat—not in a front seat with an air bag.
Understand each parent's adjustment to the newborn, especially mother's postpartum emotional needs.
Teach care of infant and help parents understand his or her individual needs and temperament and that the infant expresses wants through crying.
Reassure parents that infant cannot be spoiled by too much attention during the first 4 to 6 months.
Encourage parents to establish a schedule that meets needs of child and themselves.
Help parents understand infant's need for stimulation in environment.
Support parents' pleasure in seeing child's growing friendliness and social response, especially smiling.
Plan anticipatory guidance for safety.
Stress need for immunizations.
Prepare for introduction of solid foods.

Second 6 Months

Prepare parents for child's "stranger anxiety."
Encourage parents to allow child to cling to them and avoid long separation from either.
Guide parents concerning discipline because of infant's increasing mobility.
Encourage use of negative voice and eye contact rather than physical punishment as a means of discipline.
Encourage showing most attention when infant is behaving well, rather than when infant is crying.
Teach injury prevention because of child's advancing motor skills and curiosity.
Encourage parents to leave child with suitable caregiver to allow some free time.
Discuss readiness for weaning (as desired).
Explore parents' feelings regarding infant's sleep patterns.

Keeping the area dry promotes healing but can be difficult to maintain. Helpful suggestions include applying a thin film of a moisture barrier cream such as A&D emollient ointment to the affected areas after cleansing and using absorbent, non-plastic-lined terry cloth bibs.

Colic (Paroxysmal Abdominal Pain)

Colic is reported to occur in 5% to 30% of all infants (Neu & Robinson, 2003), yet has no particular affinity with regard to the gender, race, or socioeconomic status of the infant and family (Ellett, 2003). The condition is generally described as paroxysmal abdominal pain or cramping that is manifested by loud crying and drawing the legs up to the abdomen. Other definitions include variables such as duration of cry greater than 3 hours a day, occurring more than 3 days per week, and parental dissatisfaction with the child's behavior. Some studies report an increase in symptoms (fussiness and crying) in the late afternoon or evening; however, in some infants the onset of symptoms occurs at another time. Colic is more common in infants under 3 months of age than in older infants, and infants with so-called difficult temperaments are more likely to be colicky. Despite the obvious behavioral indications of pain, the child tolerates breast milk or some type of infant formula well, gains weight, and usually thrives. There is no evidence of a residual effect of colic on older children, except perhaps a strained parent-child relationship in some cases; in other words, infants who are colicky grow up to be normal children and adults.

Among the theories that have been investigated as potential causes are too rapid feeding, overeating, swallowing excessive air, improper feeding technique (especially in positioning and burping), and emotional stress or tension between parent and child. Although all of these may occur, there is no evidence that one factor is consistently present. In some infants colic may be a sign of cow's milk allergy (CMA) or intolerance, and eliminating cow's milk products from the diets of infants and lactating mothers can reduce the symptoms; in some infants soy milk may cause the same discomfort as cow's milk. Parental smoking, strained parent-infant interaction, lactase deficiency, difficult infant temperament, difficulty regulating emotions, central nervous system immaturity, and neurochemical dysregulation in the brain have also been proposed as potential causes of colic (Ellett, 2003; Neu & Robinson, 2003). A positive association between consumption of fruit juices (carbohydrate malabsorption) and colic has been demonstrated in some cases (Duro et al, 2002). The consensus of most experts who study colic is that it is multifactorial in nature and that no single treatment for every colicky infant will be effective in alleviating the symptoms.

Therapeutic Management

Management of colic should begin with an investigation of possible organic causes, such as CMA, intussusception, or other gastrointestinal problem. If a sensitivity to cow's milk is strongly suspected, a trial substitution of another formula such as an extensively hydrolyzed (Nutramigen, Alimentum, Pregestimil), whey hydrolysate, or amino acid (Neocate, EleCare) formula is warranted. Soy formulas are usually avoided because of the possibility of sensitivity to soy protein as well. Oral administration of *Lactobacillus reuteri* to colicky breastfed infants decreased symptoms within 1 week of initiation in one small study (Savino et al, 2007).

The use of drugs, including sedatives, antispasmodics, antihistamines, and antiflatulents, is sometimes recommended. The most commonly used sedatives are phenobarbital, hydroxyzine hydrochloride (Atarax), and chloral hydrate. Simethicone (Mylicon) may also help allay the symptoms of colic. However, in most controlled studies none of these drugs completely reduced the symptoms of colic. Herbal (chamomile) tea offered at the onset of crying and up to three times daily has proved effective in relieving the symptoms of colic in some infants (Weizman et al, 1993); however, parents are to be cautioned regarding the unknown safety of this treatment (Crotteau, Wright, & Eglash, 2006). Behavioral interventions have not proved effective at reducing symptoms of colic but have helped parents deal with the crying infant in a more positive manner. The addition of lactase to infant formula has produced mixed results as far as abatement of overall symptoms.

One study found that a combination of interventions—massage, herbal tea, sucrose solution, and hydrolyzed formula—decreased crying in reported colicky infants; the administration of the hydrolyzed formula achieved best results, whereas massage was least effective at reducing crying (Arikan et al, 2008).

An extensive review of a wide variety of interventions for colic indicates there are no specific safe remedies to alleviate symptoms of colic in every infant; dietary changes such as eliminating cow's milk protein from the lactating mother's diet and behavioral interventions were shown to be effective in helping parents reduce stimulation and respond to the infant's crying, yet these interventions are perceived only as moderately effective (Joanna Briggs Institute, 2004).

Nursing Care Management

The initial step in managing colic is to take a thorough, detailed history of the usual daily events. Areas that should be stressed include (1) the infant's diet; (2) the diet of the breastfeeding mother; (3) the time of day when crying occurs; (4) the relationship of the crying to feeding time; (5) the presence of specific family members during the crying and habits of family members, such as smoking; (6) activity of the mother or usual caregiver before, during, and after the crying; (7) characteristics of the cry (e.g., duration, intensity); (8) measures used to relieve the crying and their effectiveness; and (9) the infant's stooling, voiding, and sleeping patterns. Of special emphasis is a careful assessment of the feeding process via demonstration by the parent.

If cow's milk sensitivity is suspected, breastfeeding mothers should follow a milk-free diet for a minimum of 3 to 5 days in an attempt to reduce the infant's symptoms. Mothers need to be cautioned that some nondairy creamers may contain calcium caseinate, a cow's milk protein. If a milk-free diet is helpful, lactating mothers may need calcium supplements to meet the body's requirement. Bottle-fed infants may improve with the same dietary modifications as for the child with CMA.

Perhaps the most important nursing intervention (once the diagnosis of colic is established) is reassurance of both parents that they are not doing anything wrong and that the infant is not experiencing any physical or emotional harm. Parents, especially mothers, become easily frustrated with the infant's crying and perceive this as a sign that there is something horribly wrong. An empathetic, gentle, and reassuring attitude, in addition to suggestions about remedies for treatment, will help allay parents' anxieties, which are usually exacerbated by loss of sleep and preoccupation over the infant's welfare. Other support persons and extended family members may be enlisted to help support the parents during this difficult time.

When no cause can be identified, helping parents understand the infant's crying behavior and modifying parent interventions to promptly attend to the infant's needs can decrease the length of fussiness and crying. Other approaches for managing colic are listed in the Patient Teaching box. Parents are encouraged to try as many of these approaches as possible, since not all are effective for every infant.

One author suggests that a problem-solving discussion with the parents, in addition to acknowledgment that the infant has colic, is an optimal strategy for helping parents manage the infant with colic until a cure is found (Ellett, 2003). Nurses must also be aware that once colic symptoms are resolved, family function may be negatively impacted by residual feelings and emotions experienced during the acute phase of the colic (Ellett, Schuff, & Davis, 2005). Practical parental support interventions include the provision of a colic hotline (mother-to-nurse practitioner or nurse) and nurse-managed colic support groups (Ellett, Schuff, & Davis, 2005).

PATIENT TEACHING Managing the Colicky Infant

- Place awake infant prone over a covered hot-water bottle, heated towel, or covered heating pad.
- Massage infant's abdomen.
- Respond immediately to the crying.
- Change infant's position frequently; walk with child's face down and with body across parent's arm, with parent's hand under infant's abdomen, applying gentle pressure (Fig. 36-17).
- Use a front carrier for transporting infant.
- Swaddle infant tightly with a soft, stretchy blanket.
- Place infant in a wind-up swing.
- Take infant for car rides or outside for a change in environment.
- Use bottles that minimize air swallowing (curved bottle or inner collapsible bag).
- Use a commercial device* in the crib that simulates the vibration and sound of a car ride or plays soothing "noise," in utero sounds, or music.†
- Provide smaller, frequent feedings; burp infant during and after feedings using the shoulder position or sitting upright, and place infant in an upright seat after feedings.
- Introduce a pacifier for added sucking.
- For breastfed infants, mother should avoid all milk products for a trial period.
- If household members smoke, avoid smoking near infant; preferably confine smoking activity to outside of home.
- Give appropriate dose of acetaminophen elixir or suppository if suggested by health professional; not recommended for daily use.
- If nothing reduces the crying, place infant in crib and allow to cry; periodically hold and comfort child and put down again.

*Sweet Dreems, Inc., Sleep Tight Order Department, 4710 E. Walnut St., Westerville, OH 43081; 800-NO COLIC, 800-662-6542; *www.sleeptightinfantsoother.com.*

†Suggested infant relaxation music: *Heartbeat Lullabies,* by Terry Woodford. Available from Baby-Go-To-Sleep Center, Audio Therapy Innovations, Inc., PO Box 550, Colorado Springs, CO 80901; 800-537-7748; *www.babygotosleep.com.*

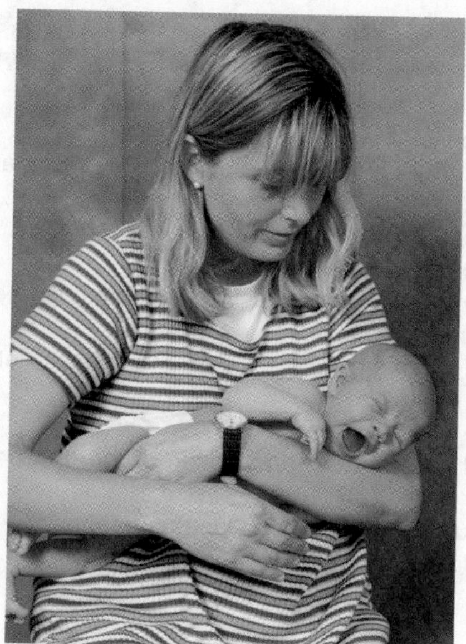

Fig. 36-17 The "colic carry" may be comforting to an infant with colic. *(Photo by Paul Vincent Kuntz, Texas Children's Hospital, Houston, TX.)*

Growth Failure (Failure to Thrive)

Growth failure, or FTT, is a sign of inadequate growth resulting from inability to obtain or use calories required for growth. FTT has no universal definition, although one of the more common parameters is a weight (and sometimes height) that falls below the 5th percentile for the child's age. Another definition of FTT includes a weight for age (height) *z* value of less than −2.0 (a *z* value is a standard deviation value that represents anthropometric data normalizing for sex and age with greater precision than growth percentile curves [Markowitz & Duggan, 2003]). A third way to define FTT is a weight curve that crosses more than two percentile lines on the National Center for Health Statistics growth charts after previous achievement of a stable growth pattern. Growth measurements alone are not used to diagnose children with FTT. Rather, the finding of a pattern of persistent deviation from established growth parameters is cause for concern. In addition to lack of consensus on the precise definition of FTT, there are those who advocate for a change in terminology; thus terms such as *growth failure* and *pediatric undernutrition* are used in the literature for FTT (Locklin, 2005).

Some experts, however, suggest that the previously used classifications of organic FTT and nonorganic FTT are too simplistic because most cases of growth failure have mixed causes; they suggest that FTT be classified according to pathophysiology in the following categories: (1) inadequate caloric intake—incorrect formula preparation, neglect, food fads, excessive juice consumption, poverty, behavioral problems affecting eating, or central nervous system problems affecting intake; (2) inadequate absorption—cystic fibrosis, celiac disease, vitamin or mineral deficiencies, biliary atresia, or hepatic disease; (3) increased metabolism—hyperthyroidism, congenital heart defects, or chronic immunodeficiency; and (4) defective utilization—genetic anomaly such as trisomy 21 or 18, congenital infection, or metabolic storage diseases (Krugman & Dubowitz, 2003). The cause of growth failure is often multifactorial and involves a combination of infant organic disease, dysfunctional parenting behaviors, subtle neurologic or behavioral problems, and disturbed parent-child interactions (Block, Krebs, & American Academy of Pediatrics, Committee on Child Abuse and Neglect and Committee on Nutrition, 2005).

Other factors that can lead to inadequate caloric intake in infancy include poverty, health or childrearing beliefs such as fad diets, inadequate nutritional knowledge, family stress, feeding resistance, and insufficient breast milk.

Diagnostic Evaluation

Diagnosis is initially made from evidence of growth failure. If FTT is recent, the weight, but not the height, is below accepted standards (usually the 5th percentile); if FTT is longstanding, both weight and height are low, indicating chronic malnutrition. Perhaps as important as anthropometric measurements are a complete health and dietary history (including perinatal history), physical examination for evidence of organic causes, developmental assessment, and family assessment. A dietary intake history, either a 24-hour food intake or a history of food consumed over a 3- to 5-day period, is also essential. In addition, the child's activity level, parental height, perceived food allergies, and dietary restrictions should be explored. An assessment of household organization and mealtime behaviors and rituals is important in the collection of pertinent data. Other tests (lead toxicity, anemia, stool-reducing substances, occult blood, ova and parasites, alkaline phosphatase, and zinc levels) are selected only as indicated to rule out organic problems. To prevent the overuse of diagnostic procedures, FTT should be considered early in the differential diagnosis. To avoid the social stigma of FTT during the early investigative phase, many health care workers use the term *growth delay* (or *failure*) until the actual cause is established.

Therapeutic Management

The primary management of FTT is aimed at reversing the cause of the growth failure. If malnutrition is severe, the initial treatment is directed at reversing the malnutrition. The goal is to provide sufficient calories to support "catch-up" growth—a rate of growth greater than the expected rate for age. Any coexisting medical problems are treated.

In most cases of FTT an interdisciplinary team of physician, nurse, dietitian, child life specialist, occupational therapist, pediatric feeding specialist, and social worker or mental health professional is needed to deal with the multiple problems. Efforts are made to relieve any additional stresses on the family by offering referrals to welfare agencies or supplemental food programs. In some cases family therapy may be required; temporary placement in a foster home may relieve the family's stress, protect the child, and allow the child some stability if insurmountable obstacles are preventing appropriate family function. Behavior modification aimed at mealtime rituals (or lack thereof) and family social time may be required. Hospitalization admission is indicated for (1) evidence (anthropometric) of severe acute malnutrition, (2) child abuse or neglect, (3) significant dehydration, (4) caretaker substance abuse or psychosis, (5) serious intercurrent infection, and (6) outpatient management that does not result in weight gain (American Academy of Pediatrics, 2009; Block, Krebs, & American Academy of Pediatrics, Committee on Child Abuse and Neglect and Committee on Nutrition, 2005).

Prognosis

The prognosis for FTT is related to the cause. There are few long-term studies that provide sufficient data for children with FTT; however, some studies indicate that children who had FTT as infants had shorter heights, lower weights, and lower scores on measures of psychomotor development than peers (Rudolf & Logan, 2005). The authors of the analysis caution widespread generalization of these findings. Factors related to poor prognosis are severe feeding resistance, lack of awareness in and cooperation from the parent(s), low family income, low maternal educational level, adolescent mother, and early age of onset of FTT. Because later cognitive and motor function is affected by malnourishment in infancy, many of these children may be below normal in intellectual development, have poorer language development and less developed reading skills, attain lower social maturity, and have a higher incidence of behavioral disturbances. Such findings indicate that a long-term plan and follow-up care are needed for the optimum development of these children.

Nursing Care Management

Caring for the child with FTT presents many nursing challenges, whether treatment takes place in the hospital, clinic, or home. Providing a positive feeding environment, teaching the parents successful feeding strategies, and supporting the child and family are essential components of care.

Nurses play a critical role in the diagnosis of FTT through their assessment of the child, parents, and family interactions. Knowledge of the characteristics of children with FTT and their families is essential in helping identify these children and hastening the confirmation of a diagnosis (Box 36-2). Accurate assessment of initial weight and height and daily weight, as well as recording of all food intake, is essential. The nurse documents the child's feeding behavior and the parent-child interaction during feeding, other caregiving activities, and play. An excellent feeding observation instrument is the Nursing Child Assessment Satellite Training Feeding Scale, which is designed to assess the feeding interaction of infants up to 12 months of age (Barnard et al, 1993).*

A feature of many children with FTT is their irregularity (low rhythmicity) in activities of daily living. Some children with FTT may typify the difficult temperament pattern. However, another type is the passive, sleepy, lethargic infant who does not wake up for feedings. Parents who have been advised to adhere to on-demand feeding schedules may be unsure of whether to wake the child or let the child sleep. Because of their inexperience and lack of guidance, parents may develop a pattern of infrequent feeding that is inadequate to meet the infant's nutritional needs. Such a pattern is particularly detrimental with the breastfeeding infant, for whom frequent nursing is essential to an adequate milk supply.

Some parents are at increased risk for attachment problems because of (1) isolation and social crisis; (2) inadequate support systems, such as for teenage and single mothers; and (3) poor parenting role models as a child. Other factors that should be considered are lack of education; physical and mental health problems such as physical and sexual abuse, depression, or drug dependence; immaturity, especially in adolescent parents; and lack of commitment to parenting, such as giving priority to entertainment or employment. Often these parents and their families are under stress and in multiple chronic emotional, social, and financial crises.

Because part of the difficulty between parent and child is dissatisfaction and frustration, the child should have a primary core of nurses (Fig. 36-18). The nurses caring for the child can learn to perceive the child's cues and reverse the cycle of dissatisfaction, especially in the area of feeding. Depending on the cause of FTT, children may be treated on an outpatient basis.

Because many of these children are responding to stimuli that have led to the negative feeding patterns, the first goal is to structure the feeding environment to encourage eating. Initially staff members and a feeding specialist may need to feed these children to assess thoroughly the difficulties encountered during the feeding process and to devise strategies that eliminate or minimize such problems. General guidelines for the feeding process are outlined in the Guidelines box.

Four primary goals in the nutritional management of FTT are to (1) correct nutritional deficiencies and achieve ideal weight for height, (2) allow for catch-up growth, (3) restore optimum body composition, and (4) educate the parents or primary caregivers regarding the child's nutritional require-

BOX 36-2 Clinical Manifestations of Growth Failure

- Growth failure (see p. 1003 for definitions)
- Malnutrition
- Developmental delays—social, motor, adaptive, language
- Apathy
- Poor hygiene in some cases
- Withdrawn behavior
- Feeding or eating disorders, such as vomiting, feeding resistance, anorexia
- No fear of strangers (at age when stranger anxiety is normal)
- Avoidance of eye contact
- Wide-eyed gaze and continual scan of the environment ("radar gaze")
- Stiff and unyielding or flaccid and unresponsive
- Minimal smiling

**Training is required to use the feeding scale. For information, contact Jean F. Kelly, PhD, Executive Director, NCAST-AVENUW, University of Washington, PO Box 357920, Seattle, WA 98195; 206-543-8528; e-mail: ncast@u.washington.edu; www.ncast.org.*

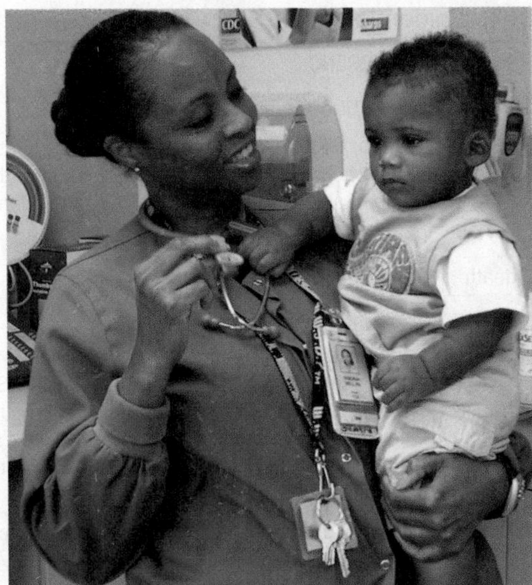

Fig. 36-18 Consistent nursing contact is important in developing trust in infants with failure to thrive.

ments and appropriate feeding methods (Corrales & Utter, 2005; Maggioni & Lifshitz, 1995). To increase caloric intake in formula-fed infants, supplements such as Polycose or medium-chain triglycerides may be added slowly. For infants, 24 kcal/oz formulas may be provided to increase caloric intake; older children (1 to 6 years) may benefit from a 30 kcal/oz formula (American Academy of Pediatrics, 2009). Other carbohydrate additives include fortified rice cereal and vegetable oil. Because vitamin and mineral deficiencies may occur, multivitamin supplementation, including zinc and iron, is recommended. Usually only in extreme cases of malnourishment are tube feedings or intravenous therapy required.

Besides attending to the physical needs of the child, the interdisciplinary team must plan care for appropriate developmental stimulation. After an approximate developmental age is established, a planned program of play is begun. Ideally a child life specialist is involved to implement and supervise the stimulation program. Every effort is made to teach the parent how to play and interact with the child.

Nursing care of these children involves a family systems approach. In other words, for the entire family to become healthy, each member must be helped to change. Care of the parents is aimed at helping them increase their feelings of self-esteem through positive, successful parenting skills. Initially this necessitates providing an environment in which they feel welcomed and accepted. Because these parents are often distrustful of authority figures, it may take some time before they trust the nurse. One approach is to empathize with the parent about the difficulties of childrearing. For example, the nurse may state that many parents find adjusting to parenthood a trying time or that the demands of caring for an infant can become overwhelming.

The nurse teaches infant care techniques to the parents through example and demonstration rather than by lecturing. As the nurse perceives the infant's cues, he or she emphasizes these to the parents. For example, during a feeding the nurse might comment that the infant is still hungry because the child sucks vigorously and looks at the nurse. When the infant is satisfied, the nurse points out that the infant is signaling this by releasing the strong suck, closing the eyes, and breathing deeply and more slowly.

Plans are made to implement these interventions at home. A home health referral is made, and if a foster grandparent was included, this person should also visit the family. Social agencies that can provide financial or housing assistance to lessen the stress of everyday life are also contacted.

GUIDELINES Feeding Children with Growth Failure

Provide a primary core of staff to feed the child. The same nurses are able to learn the child's cues and respond consistently.

Provide a quiet, unstimulating atmosphere. A number of these children are very distractible, and their attention is diverted with minimal stimuli. Older children do well at a feeding table; younger children should always be held.

Maintain a calm, even temperament throughout the meal. The child may have a habit of negative outbursts. Limits on eating behavior definitely need to be provided, but they should be stated in a firm, calm tone. If the nurse is hurried or anxious, the feeding process will not be optimized.

Talk to the child by giving directions about eating. "Take a bite, Lisa" is appropriate and directive. The more distractible the child, the more directive the nurse should be to refocus attention on feeding. Positive comments about feeding are actively given.

Be persistent. This is perhaps one of the most important guidelines. Parents often give up when the child begins negative feeding behavior. Calm perseverance through 10 to 15 minutes of food refusal will eventually diminish negative behavior. Although forced feeding is avoided, "strictly encouraged" feeding is essential.

Maintain a face-to-face posture with the child when possible. Encourage eye contact and remain with the child throughout the meal.

Introduce new foods slowly. Often these children have been exclusively bottle-fed. If acceptance of solids is a problem, begin with pureed food and, once accepted, advance to junior and regular solid foods.

Follow the child's rhythm of feeding. The child will set a rhythm when the previous conditions are met.

Develop a structured routine. Disruptions in their other activities of daily living have great impact on feeding responses, so bathing, sleeping, dressing, and playing, as well as feeding, are structured. The nurse should feed the child in the same way and place as often as possible. The length of the feeding should also be established (usually 30 minutes).

Disorders of Unknown Etiology

Sudden Infant Death Syndrome

SIDS is defined as the sudden death of an infant younger than 1 year of age that remains unexplained after a complete postmortem examination, including an investigation of the death scene and a review of the case history. Since 1992, the incidence of SIDS in the United States has decreased by 53% to an all-time low of 0.57 per 1000 live births in 2002 (American Academy of Pediatrics, Task Force on Sudden Infant Death Syndrome, 2005). The dramatic decrease is attributed to the Back to Sleep campaign.* SIDS is the third leading cause of infant deaths (birth to 12 months) and the first leading cause of postneonatal deaths (between 1 and 12 months). SIDS claimed the lives of 2162 infants in 2003 (Heron & Smith, 2007). Table 36-6 summarizes the major epidemiologic characteristics of SIDS.

Table 36-6 Epidemiology of SIDS

FACTORS	OCCURRENCE
Incidence	0.57:1000 live births (2002)
Peak age	2-3 mo; 95% occur by 6 mo; infants born preterm died from SIDS at mean age of 6 wk later than mean age of death from SIDS for term infants
Sex	Higher percentage of males affected
Time of death	During sleep
Time of year	Increased incidence in winter
Racial	Greater incidence in African-Americans, Native Americans, and Hispanics. In 2001 rate of SIDS in African-Americans was 2.5 times higher than in Caucasians; prone positioning rates were also higher in African-Americans in 2001 (21% in African-Americans vs. 11% in Caucasians)
Socioeconomic	Increased occurrence in lower socioeconomic class
Birth	Higher incidence in: Preterm infants, especially infants of extremely and very low birth weight Multiple births* Neonates with low Apgar scores Infants with central nervous system disturbances and respiratory disorders such as bronchopulmonary dysplasia Increasing birth order (subsequent siblings as opposed to firstborn child) Infants with a recent history of illness
Sleep habits	Highest risk associated with prone position; use of soft bedding; overheating (thermal stress); cosleeping with adult, especially on sofa, or noninfant bed
	Infants cosleeping with adult at higher risk if <11 wk old
Feeding habits	Lower incidence in breastfed infants
Pacifier	Lower incidence in infants put to sleep with pacifier
Siblings	May have greater incidence in siblings of SIDS victims
Maternal	Young age; cigarette smoking, especially during pregnancy; poor prenatal care; substance abuse (heroin, methadone, cocaine); a few studies have shown an increased risk in infants exposed to second-hand environmental tobacco smoke

Data from American Academy of Pediatrics, Task Force on Sudden Infant Death Syndrome: The changing concept of sudden infant death syndrome: diagnostic coding shifts, controversies regarding the sleeping environment, and new variables to consider in reducing risk, *Pediatrics* 116(5):1245-1255, 2005; American Academy of Pediatrics, Task Force on Infant Sleep Position and Sudden Infant Death Syndrome: Changing concepts of sudden infant death syndrome: implications for infant sleeping environment and sleep position, *Pediatrics* 105(3):650-656, 2000.
*Although a rare event, simultaneous death of twins from SIDS can occur.

Etiology

Numerous theories have been proposed regarding the etiology of SIDS; however, the cause remains unknown. One compelling hypothesis is that SIDS is related to a brainstem abnormality in the neurologic regulation of cardiorespiratory control. Abnormalities include prolonged sleep apnea, increased frequency of brief inspiratory pauses, excessive periodic breathing, and impaired arousal responsiveness to increased carbon dioxide or decreased oxygen. However, sleep apnea is not the cause of SIDS. The vast majority of infants with apnea do not die, and only a minority of SIDS victims have documented *apparent life-threatening events (ALTEs)* (see Apnea and Apparent Life-Threatening Events, p. 1010). Numerous studies indicate that there is no association between SIDS and any childhood vaccine.

A genetic predisposition to SIDS has been postulated as a cause. In one study a genetic mutation on chromosome 6q 22.1-22.31 was positively linked to a syndrome of SIDS and dysgenesis of the testis (Puffenberger et al, 2004).

Maternal smoking during pregnancy has emerged in numerous epidemiologic studies as a major factor in SIDS, and tobacco smoke in the infant's environment after birth has also been shown to have a possible relationship with the incidence of SIDS (American Academy of Pediatrics, Task Force on Sudden Infant Death Syndrome, 2005). Data show that exposure to tobacco smoke increased an infant's risk for SIDS 1.9 times over infants not exposed; 59% of SIDS deaths in smoke-exposed infants were attributed to maternal smoking (Anderson, Johnson, & Batal, 2005). It has been postulated that 12% of all SIDS deaths could be prevented with prenatal maternal smoking cessation (Pollack, 2001). One mechanism that has been proposed as a link between maternal smoking and SIDS is a decrease in the infant's ability to arouse to auditory stimuli in mothers who smoked prenatally (Franco et al, 1999). Increased nicotine concentrations in lung tissue were found in children who died from SIDS compared with a group of control children (McMartin et al, 2002).

Cosleeping, or an infant sharing a bed with an adult or older child on a noninfant bed, has been reported to have a positive association with SIDS. One survey found a high association between infant deaths, nonstandard beds (sofa, day bed), and bed sharing; a large percentage of infants were found dead on their backs when bed sharing, suggesting suffocation (Unger et al, 2003). A study from Scotland indicates that the risk for SIDS when bed sharing is significantly increased for infants less than 11 weeks of age (Tappin, Ecob, & Brooke,

Back to Sleep materials may be ordered by contacting NICHD Information Resource Center, Back to Sleep, PO Box 3006, Rockville, MD 20847; 800-370-2943; fax: 866-760-5947; www.nichd.nih.gov/sids.

2005). Other studies have correlated higher incidences of SIDS and infant cosleeping with maternal smoking, cosleeping with multiple family members, maternal overweight, soft bedding, and unintentional asphyxiation resulting from adult intoxication (overlaying) (American Academy of Pediatrics, Task Force on Infant Sleep Position and Sudden Infant Death Syndrome, 2000; American Academy of Pediatrics, Task Force on Sudden Infant Death Syndrome, 2005; Hauck et al, 2003; Carroll-Pankhurst & Mortimer, 2001; Person, Lavezzi, & Wolf, 2002; McGarvey et al, 2003).

A study by Hauck and colleagues (2003) found that bed sharing and SIDS correlated positively only in cases where the infant was sleeping with someone other than the parent; a high number of SIDS cases involved sleeping on a sofa.

Cosleeping with infants in the age range when most SIDS deaths occur has not been shown to be preventive. The latest recommendation for cosleeping from the American Academy of Pediatrics is that the infant's crib or bassinette be placed in close proximity to the mother's bed and that the infant be placed in the adult bed only for breastfeeding, then placed to sleep in his or her own crib once the feeding session is completed (American Academy of Pediatrics, Task Force on Sudden Infant Death Syndrome, 2005).

Mesich (2005) notes that the current scientific literature fails to provide definitive guidance regarding mother-infant sleeping together in relation to safety or nonsafety (see Cultural Awareness box); certain sleep environments (prone sleeping, tobacco smoke exposure, soft bedding, noninfant bed surface, use of certain drugs by cosleeper, and thermal stress), however, are known to increase the risk for SIDS.

Studies from countries other than the United States link sleep habits with an increased risk of SIDS. Prone sleeping may cause oropharyngeal obstruction or affect thermal balance or arousal state. One study found that healthy full-term infants had significantly impaired arousal from active and quiet sleep states when sleeping prone (Horne et al, 2001). Rebreathing of carbon dioxide by infants in the prone position is also a possible cause for SIDS. Infants sleeping prone and on soft bedding may not be able to move their heads to the side, thus increasing the risk of suffocation and lethal rebreathing. Evidence from other countries and the United States shows an increased incidence of SIDS in infants placed in a side-lying position; thus the side-lying position is no longer recommended for infants sleeping at home, day care, or hospitals (unless medically indicated).

Soft bedding such as waterbeds, sheepskins, beanbags, pillows, or quilts should be avoided for infant sleeping surfaces. Bedding items such as stuffed animals or toys should be removed from the crib while the infant is asleep. Most preterm infants being discharged from the hospital should be placed in a supine sleeping position unless special factors predispose them to airway obstruction. One postulated cause of SIDS has been a prolonged Q-T interval; however, at the time of this writing no strong evidence supports this as a cause of SIDS or universal testing of newborns for prolonged Q-T interval (American Academy of Pediatrics, Task Force on Sudden Infant Death Syndrome, 2005). Head covering by a blanket has also been found to be a risk factor for SIDS, thus supporting the recommendation to avoid extra bed linens or other items (Mitchell et al, 2008).

One study indicated that breastfeeding during the first 16 weeks of life decreased the likelihood of SIDS (Alm et al, 2002). Some studies have found pacifier use in infants to be a protective factor against the occurrence of SIDS; the data for pacifier use in this population of infants (first year of life) is said to be more compelling than data linking pacifier use to the development of dental complications and the inhibition of breastfeeding (American Academy of Pediatrics, Task Force on Sudden Infant Death Syndrome, 2005). Therefore the American Academy of Pediatrics recommendations are to use a pacifier at naptime and bedtime, use pacifier only if infant is breastfeeding successfully, use no sweetened coating on the pacifier, and avoid forcing the infant to use the pacifier.

The American Academy of Pediatrics, Task Force on Sudden Infant Death Syndrome (2005), recommends that healthy infants be placed to sleep in the supine (on the back) position. There is an increased risk of SIDS in infants placed in the side-lying position, primarily because of their ability to turn to a prone position; therefore the side-lying sleep position is no longer recommended.

Although the etiology is unknown, autopsies reveal consistent pathologic findings such as pulmonary edema and intrathoracic hemorrhages that confirm the diagnosis of SIDS. Consequently, autopsies should be performed on all infants suspected of dying of SIDS, and the findings should be shared with the parents as soon as possible after the death.

Whether subsequent siblings of one SIDS infant are at increased risk for SIDS is unclear. Even if the increased risk is correct, families have a 99% chance that their subsequent child will *not* die of SIDS. A review of recurrent sibling deaths attributed to SIDS in England failed to ascertain a precise risk of recurrence; previous studies suggested a recurrence risk range of 1.7 to 10.1, yet the researchers concluded the studies had too many methodologic flaws to draw any firm conclusions (Bacon et al, 2008). Others report that recurrence risks for a SIDS death in a family with a previous infant SIDS death range from 2% to 6% (American Academy

CULTURAL AWARENESS

The Family Bed

Cosleeping, or sharing the "family bed," in which parents allow the children to sleep with them, is a relatively common and accepted practice, especially among African-American, Hispanic, and Asian families such as the Japanese (Schachter et al, 1989). One survey indicates the practice is growing in some parts of the United States, especially among young (less than 18 years of age) African-American and Asian women in the Southern states; infants in the survey who coslept with an adult were less than 8 weeks old (Willinger et al, 2003). Other groups that practice cosleeping include (1) single parents, whose need for company may encourage this practice; (2) working parents, who desire the closeness at night that was lost during the day; and (3) parents who have had an issue about sleep or separation in their own past (Brazelton, 1990).

of Pediatrics, Task Force on Sudden Infant Death Syndrome, 2005). Home monitoring is not recommended for this group of children, but it is often used by practitioners and may even be requested by parents. Monitoring is best initiated on an individual basis.

Nursing Care Management

Nurses have a vital role in preventing SIDS by educating families about the risk of prone sleeping position in infants from birth to 6 months of age, the use of appropriate bedding surfaces, the association with maternal smoking, and the dangers of cosleeping on noninfant surfaces with adults or other children. Additionally nurses have an important role in modeling behaviors for parents to foster the implementation of practices that decrease the risk of SIDS: placing infants in a supine sleeping position in the hospital and limiting pacifier use to naps and bedtime only. Data indicate that a small percentage of nurses still place healthy infants in a side-lying position in the hospital (Bullock et al, 2004; Thompson, 2005). Statistics for infants being placed in a prone sleeping position in the United States decreased from 70% in 1992 to 13% in 2004 (American Academy of Pediatrics, Task Force on Sudden Infant Death Syndrome, 2005). Nurses must be proactive in further decreasing the incidence of SIDS; postpartum discharge planning, newborn discharges, follow-up home visits, well-baby clinic visits, and immunization visits provide excellent opportunities to educate parents in these matters.

A concern of many health care workers is that infants placed on the back to sleep will aspirate emesis or mucus; yet studies fail to show an increase in infant deaths, spitting up during sleep, aspiration, asphyxia, or respiratory failure as a result of supine sleep positioning (Malloy, 2002; Tablizo et al, 2007).

Loss of a child from SIDS presents several crises with which the parents must cope. In addition to grief and mourning the death of their child, the parents must face a tragedy that was sudden, unexpected, and unexplained. The psychologic intervention for the family must deal with these additional variables. This discussion focuses primarily on the objectives of care for families experiencing SIDS, rather than on the process of grief and mourning, which is explored in Chapter 41.

Research findings have important implications for practices that may reduce the risk of SIDS, such as avoiding smoking during pregnancy and near the infant; encouraging the supine sleeping position; avoiding soft, moldable mattresses, blankets, and pillows; discouraging bed sharing; encouraging breastfeeding; and avoiding overheating during sleep. The infant's head position should be varied to prevent flattening of the skull (positional plagiocephaly).

Finding the Infant

Usually it is the mother who finds the child dead in the crib. Typically the child is in a disheveled bed, with blankets over the head, and huddled in a corner. Frothy, blood-tinged fluid fills the mouth and nostrils, and the infant may be lying face down in the secretions, suggesting that he or she bled to death. The diaper is wet and full of stool, which is consistent with a cataclysmic type of death. The hands may be clutching the sheets, as if the child were in distress before death. The child's initial appearance, combined with the shock of such an unexpected event, adds to the horror that the parents must face.

Often the mother is alone and must deal with her initial shock, panic, grief, questions of the other siblings, and the decision of where to find help. The first persons to arrive may be the police and ambulance attendants. Ideally, they will handle the situation by asking few questions; giving no indication of wrongdoing, abuse, or neglect; making sensitive judgments concerning any resuscitation efforts for the child; and comforting the members of the family as much as possible. These individuals should be properly informed about SIDS in order to recognize its characteristic signs and tell parents that their child probably died of a disease called *sudden infant death syndrome*. A compassionate, sensitive approach to the family during the first few minutes can help spare them some of the overwhelming guilt and anguish that commonly follow this type of death.

Arriving at the Emergency Department

The first contact that nurses typically have with these families is in the emergency department, when the infant is seen by a physician to be pronounced dead. Usually there is no attempt at resuscitation. During the time in the emergency department several aspects warrant special consideration. Parents are asked only factual questions, such as when they found the infant, how he or she looked, and whom they called for help. Any remarks that may suggest responsibility, such as why they did not check on the child earlier, why they did not hear the infant cry out, whether the head was buried in a blanket, or whether other siblings were jealous of this child, are avoided.

The discussion of an autopsy should be presented at this time, emphasizing that a diagnosis cannot be confirmed until the postmortem examination is completed. If the mother was breastfeeding, she needs information about abrupt discontinuation of lactation.

A review of 60 studies shows that parents experiencing perinatal death perceive health care workers' responses as having a significant impact on the parents' grieving process; many health care workers' behaviors were perceived as thoughtless or insensitive. The findings suggest that nurses and physicians would benefit from more bereavement training (Gold, 2007).

Another important aspect of compassionate care for these parents is allowing them to say good-bye to their child. A debriefing session may help health care workers who dealt with the family and deceased infant to cope with feelings that are often engendered when a SIDS victim is brought into the acute care facility.

Comprehensive guidelines have been published for health professionals involved in SIDS investigations to assist the family and at the same time to determine that the infant's death was not the result of other factors such as child maltreatment (American Academy of Pediatrics, Committee on Child Abuse and Neglect, 2001).

Returning Home

When the parents return home, they should be visited by a competent, qualified professional as soon after the death as possible. Printed material that contains excellent information about SIDS (available from national organizations*) should be provided.

Ideally, the number of visits and plans for subsequent intervention need to be flexible. For example, the siblings may initially appear accepting of the explanation and well adjusted, but may later refuse to go to sleep or ask questions about graves or funerals, indicating their need for further help in dealing with the death. Parents facing the question of a subsequent child will need support. Both the birth of a subsequent child and the survival of that child, especially past the age of death of the previous child, are important transitional stages for parents.

Because the mourning process continues *for at least a year,* and because most health plans do not cover periodic visits to the family to evaluate their progress, referrals to other parents who have lost a child to SIDS should be considered.

Positional Plagiocephaly

Since the Back to Sleep campaign began in 1992 advocating nonprone sleeping for infants to prevent SIDS, an increase in the incidence of positional plagiocephaly has been observed (American Academy of Pediatrics, Task Force on Sudden Infant Death Syndrome, 2005; Littlefield, Saba, & Kelly, 2004). The term *plagiocephaly* connotes an oblique or asymmetric head; *positional plagiocephaly, deformational plagiocephaly*, or *nonsynostotic plagiocephaly* implies an acquired condition that occurs as a result of cranial molding during infancy (American Academy of Pediatrics, 2003; Hummel & Fortado, 2005). Because the infant's sutures are not closed, the skull is pliable and, when the infant is placed on the back to sleep, the posterior occiput flattens over time (Fig. 36-19, *A*); a typical bald spot will develop, which is usually transient. As a result of prolonged pressure on one side of the skull, that side becomes misshapen; mild facial asymmetry may develop. The sternocleidomastoid muscle may tighten on the preferential side, and torticollis may also develop. Congenital or acquired torticollis may cause plagiocephaly; this discussion centers only on plagiocephaly caused by supine sleeping position.

Diagnostic Evaluation

The diagnosis of positional plagiocephaly may be made on physical examination of the infant's head; the infant's head is viewed frontally and from above. The typical infant's head

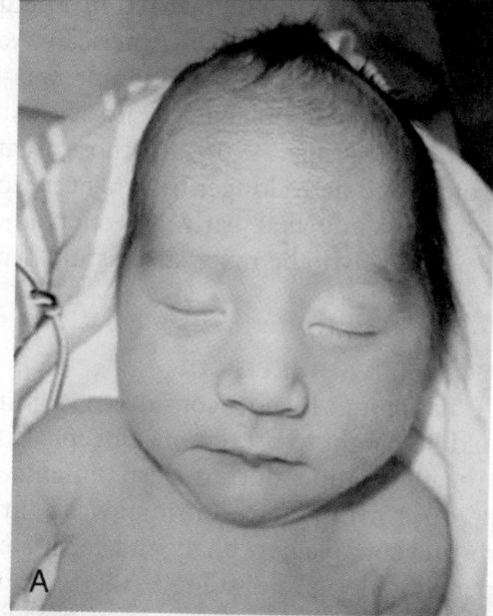

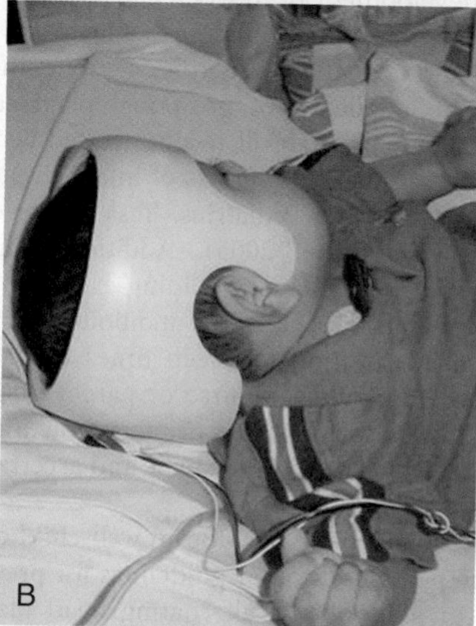

Fig. 36-19 **A**, Plagiocephaly. **B**, Helmet used to correct plagiocephaly. *(Courtesy Dr. Gerardo Cabrera-Meza, Department of Neonatology, Baylor College of Medicine, Houston, TX.)*

shape will resemble a parallelogram, with unilateral flattening of the occiput, frontal and parietal bossing, a prominent cheekbone, and an anterior ear displacement (American Academy of Pediatrics, 2003). An evaluation of neck movement and range of motion is also made to determine the presence of torticollis. In most cases skull films and further radiologic studies (computed tomographic scan) are used only to rule out craniosynostosis or other cranial deformity that may affect brain growth.

Therapeutic Management

Treatment of torticollis and plagiocephaly initially involves exercises to loosen the tight muscle and switching head position sides during feeding, carrying, and sleep. If the plagiocephaly is not resolved within 4 to 8 weeks of physical therapy, a customized helmet may be worn to decrease the pressure on the affected side of the skull (Biggs, 2003). If no improvement occurs with physical therapy or a molded helmet over

American SIDS Institute, 509 Augusta Dr., Marietta, GA 30067; 800-232-SIDS, 770-426-8746; www.sids.org; First Candle, 1314 Bedford Ave., Suite 210, Baltimore, MD 21208; 800-221-7437; www.sidsalliance.org; National Sudden and Unexpected Infant/Child Death and Pregnancy Loss Resource Center, Georgetown University, Box 571272, Washington, DC 20057-1272; 866-866-7437, 202-687-7466; www.sidscenter.org.

a given period, the infant may be referred to a pediatric neurosurgeon or craniofacial surgeon (American Academy of Pediatrics, 2003). In one study repositioning was not found to be as helpful in reducing plagiocephaly as was the use of an orthotic helmet (see Fig. 36-19, *B*); those treated with a helmet were older and had a longer treatment period, leading the authors to conclude that early detection and orthotic intervention were likely to be more successful (Graham et al, 2005).

✱ Nursing Care Management

Minor skull flattening is not considered significant, but parents should be taught to prevent plagiocephaly by altering the infant's head position during sleep. Infants should be placed prone on a firm surface during awake time (tummy time), which prevents plagiocephaly and facilitates development of upper shoulder girdle strength; the latter helps in the progressive development of movements such as rolling over and starting to rise up on all fours, which are precursors to crawling and eventually walking. Despite the reported increase in the incidence of positional plagiocephaly, the supine sleeping position is still recommended because it has led to a significant decrease in loss of infant lives from SIDS (American Academy of Pediatrics, Task Force on Sudden Infant Death Syndrome, 2005). Additional measures to prevent plagiocephaly include avoiding excessive time spent in car restraint seats or infant seats and bouncers. Alternating the infant's head position for sleep times can also prevent unilateral molding. When a nurse or parent notices plagiocephaly, a consultation with the primary practitioner is recommended to evaluate the head shape and ascertain the need for early intervention.

Nurses are in a unique position in well-child care settings to encourage parents to follow guidelines for preventing plagiocephaly, to demonstrate alternating head placement for sleeping, to demonstrate sternocleidomastoid muscle exercises (as appropriate to the condition), and to encourage tummy time for infants during awake periods. Most important, nurses should continue to encourage parents to place the infant in a supine sleep position despite the development of plagiocephaly. Parents should not become so alarmed by plagiocephaly that they abandon supine sleeping position for the infant but should consult with the practitioner for further advice.

Apnea and Apparent Life-Threatening Events

Apnea is defined as a cessation of breathing for 20 seconds. *Apnea of infancy* is defined as an unexplained respiratory pause of 20 seconds or more, or pauses of less than 20 seconds that are accompanied by pallor, cyanosis, bradycardia, or hypotension in the term infant. The latter is a distinct entity from apnea of prematurity. Apnea of prematurity is the cessation of breathing longer than 20 seconds, or any period if accompanied by bradycardia and cyanosis; it is not associated with any predisposing conditions (Dudell & Stoll, 2007). An *apparent life-threatening event (ALTE)*, formerly referred to as *aborted SIDS death* or *near-miss SIDS*, generally refers to an event that is sudden and frightening to the observer, in which the infant exhibits a combination of apnea, change in color (pallor, cyanosis, redness), change in muscle tone (usually hypotonia), choking, gagging, or coughing, and which usually involves a significant intervention and even cardiopulmonary resuscitation (CPR) by the caregiver who witnesses the event (National Institutes of Health, 1987). The definition of ALTE may include apnea, but ALTE may occur without apnea (Silvestri & Weese-Mayer, 2003).

Apnea during infancy can be a symptom of any one of many disorders—including sepsis, seizures or other neurologic disorder, upper or lower airway infection or abnormality, gastroesophageal reflux, hypoglycemia or other metabolic problems, and impaired regulation of breathing during sleep or feeding—or a result of intentional harm by an adult caregiver. Delayed ventilatory responses to hypercapnia and hypoxia were observed in one study of 69 infants with apnea of infancy (Katz-Salamon, 2004). Abusive head injury has been reported in a small percentage (2.5%) of children with ALTE (Altman et al, 2003). Intentional suffocation and Munchausen syndrome by proxy cases have also been reported with ALTE (Hall & Zalman, 2005). However, in about half the cases no cause is identified.

Infants with a history of ALTEs may be at increased risk for SIDS, but these children constitute only approximately 7% to 12% of all SIDS victims. Most infants with ALTE are less than 6 months of age, and although there has been a significant decrease in SIDS since 1992, the incidence of ALTE has not changed (Hall & Zalman, 2005). A diagnosis of apnea of infancy or idiopathic ALTE is often made when no cause is found.

Results from the Collaborative Home Infant Monitoring Evaluation study found that apnea and bradycardia occurred at conventional and extreme alarm thresholds in all groups of infants studied: siblings of SIDS infants, infants with ALTEs, symptomatic (of apnea and bradycardia) and asymptomatic preterm infants weighing less than 1750 g (3.8 lb) at birth, and healthy term infants. The researchers concluded that many infants experience apnea and bradycardia in each of these groups yet do not die (Jobe, 2001; Ramanathan et al, 2001). Furthermore, it was reported that apnea does not appear to be an immediate precursor to SIDS and that cardiorespiratory monitoring is not an effective tool for identifying infants at greater risk for SIDS (American Academy of Pediatrics, Committee on Fetus and Newborn, 2003). CHIME data indicate that infants with ALTE did not have some of the typical characteristics associated with SIDS infants; these include fewer infants with low birth weight and who are small for gestational age at birth, fewer teenage pregnancies, and a younger infant age at the time of ALTE. The researchers concluded that despite some similar characteristics between ALTE and SIDS, the differences warrant a separate focus on ALTE events (Esani et al, 2008).

Diagnostic Evaluation

An essential component of the diagnostic process includes a detailed description of the event—who witnessed the event, where the infant was during the event, and what, if any, activities were involved (such as during or after a feeding, riding in a car seat restraint, presence of siblings or any minor children, what clothing the infant was wearing). In addition, a prenatal and postnatal history must be obtained. A short period of observation in the emergency department may be appropriate to observe the infant's respiratory pattern and response to feeding. A careful evaluation of the preterm infant in a car restraint is essential; upper airway occlusion and subsequent apnea and cyanosis may occur if the infant is not positioned properly. Reported diagnoses in infants with ALTE include a neurologic event such as a seizure (30% of cases seen); gastrointestinal problem, including gastroesophageal reflux (50%); respiratory conditions (20%); and metabolic, cardiac, or child abuse (each less than 5%). In some cases, multiple diagnoses may be made (Hall & Zalman, 2005).

In the event that an underlying diagnosis such as those mentioned previously is not established, home monitoring may be recommended. The most commonly used monitoring is continuous recording of cardiorespiratory patterns (cardiopneumogram, or pneumocardiogram). Four-channel pneumocardiograms (or multichannel pneumogram) monitor heart rate, respirations (chest impedance), nasal airflow, and oxygen saturation. A more sophisticated test, polysomnography (sleep study), also records brain waves, eye and body movements, esophageal manometry, and end-tidal carbon dioxide measurements. However, none of these tests can predict risk. Some children with normal results may still have subsequent apneic episodes.

Therapeutic Management

The treatment of the infant with an ALTE depends on the underlying condition (see above). Treatment of recurrent apnea (without an underlying organic problem) usually involves continuous home monitoring of cardiorespiratory rhythms and in some cases the use of methylxanthines (respiratory stimulant drugs, such as theophylline or caffeine). The decision to discontinue the monitoring is based on the infant's clinical condition. A general guideline for discontinuation is when infants with ALTEs have gone 2 or 3 months without significant numbers of episodes requiring intervention.

Newer home apnea monitors allow download of information that assists the practitioner in deciding when to discontinue home monitoring. It is imperative to remember, however, that the home apnea monitor will not predict or prevent SIDS deaths. Furthermore, impedance-based monitors detect chest wall movement and will not detect obstructive apnea unless the episode involves significant bradycardia (see Patient Teaching box).

Nursing Care Management

The diagnosis of an ALTE engenders great anxiety and concern in parents, and the institution of home monitoring presents additional physical and emotional burdens. Parents of infants on home apnea monitors report experiencing emotional distress, especially depression and hostility, during the first few weeks after hospital discharge (Abendroth et al, 1999). For parents of a SIDS victim who have a new infant on home apnea monitoring, the anxiety is compounded by the uncertainty of the future of the living child and grief for the lost child. Home apnea monitoring may offer some predictability and control over the current child's survival through the period of uncertainty.

PATIENT TEACHING Using Apnea Monitors

Use the monitor as instructed by the practitioner.

Do not adjust the monitor to eliminate false alarms. Adjustments could compromise the monitor's effectiveness.

Place the monitor on a firm surface away from the crib and drapes; plug power cord directly into a wall socket with a three-pronged outlet.

Do not sleep in the same bed as a monitored infant.

Keep pets and children away from the monitor and infant.

Keep the monitor away from possible electrical interferences such as appliances (e.g., electric blankets, televisions, air conditioners, remote telephones [including cellular phones]).

Check the monitor several times a day to be sure the alarm is working and that it can be heard from room to room. Be certain the caregiver can reach the monitor quickly (in less than 30 seconds).

Periodically check the monitor's breath detection indicator and battery or charger connections.

Be aware that strong signals from nearby radio and television stations, airports, ham radios, cellular phones, or police stations could interfere with the monitor. Check for interference if the monitor is to be operated in these areas.

Read the monitor's user manual carefully; report problems promptly.

Inform community utility and rescue squads of home monitoring as appropriate.

Keep emergency rescue numbers near phones in the home.

Practice safety precautions:
- Remove leads when infant is not attached to the monitor.
- Unplug the power cord from the electrical outlet when the cord is not plugged into the monitor.
- Use safety covers on electrical outlets to prevent children from inserting objects into a socket.

Data primarily from *FDA safety alert: important tips for apnea monitor users,* Rockville, MD, 1990, US Department of Health and Human Services.

If monitoring is required, the nurse can be a major source of support to the family in terms of education about the equipment; observation of the infant's status; and immediate intervention during apneic episodes, including CPR. Several reports indicate that the first week to month after discharge is the most stressful for parents, particularly when the rate of false alarms is high (Bennett, 2002). To help the family cope with the numerous procedures they must learn, adequate preparation before discharge and written instructions are essential. In the first few weeks after discharge, parents may benefit by having a practitioner readily available to answer questions regarding false alarms and for other technical assistance (Abendroth et al, 1999).

Several types of home monitors are available and are set up by either a home monitor equipment company or home health staff. Nurses, especially those involved in the care at home, must become familiar with the equipment, including its advantages and disadvantages. Safety is a major concern because monitors can cause electrical burns and electrocution. The following precautions are recommended:

- Remove leads from infant when not attached to monitor.
- Unplug power cord from electrical outlet when cord is not plugged into monitor.
- Use safety covers on electrical outlets to discourage children from inserting objects into a socket.

Siblings should also be supervised when near the infant and taught that the monitor is not a toy. Other safety practices include informing local utility and rescue squads of the home monitoring in case of an emergency. Telephone numbers for these services should be posted near all telephones in the home.

NURSING ALERT If the infant is apneic, gently stimulate the trunk by patting or rubbing it. If the infant is prone, turn to the back and flick the feet. If there is still no response, begin CPR and activate the emergency medical service–"Call 911!" Never vigorously shake the child. No more than 10 to 15 seconds are spent on stimulation before implementing CPR.

Caregivers need detailed information regarding proper attachment of the electrodes to the infant's chest with impedance monitors that detect chest movement. The electrodes are placed in the midaxillary line, at a space one or two fingerbreadths below the nipple. For home use, electrodes attached to a belt that is placed around the child's trunk are preferred (Fig. 36-20). The belt is positioned so that the electrodes contact the skin in the same area. Monitors may have memory chips that allow for event recording, which can be an effective tool in evaluating the use of the monitor, events immediately before and after the event, and reported frequency of alarms.

Monitors are effective only if they are used. They do not prevent death but alert the caregiver to the ALTE in time to intervene. The need to use the monitor and to respond appropriately to alarms must be stressed. Noncompliance can result in the infant's death.

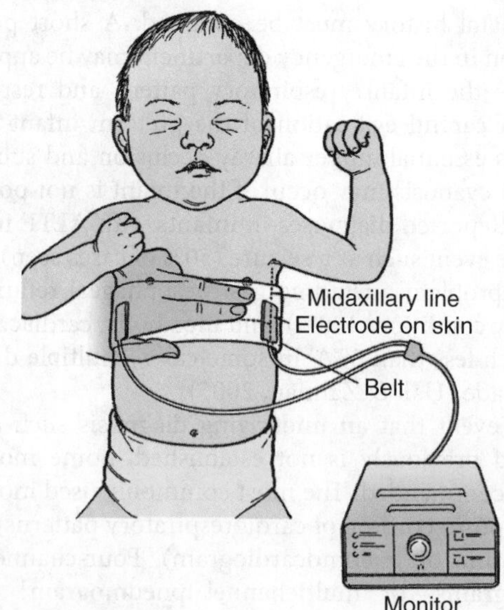
Midaxillary line
Electrode on skin
Belt
Monitor

Fig. 36-20 Electrode placement for apnea monitoring. In small infants one fingerbreadth may be used.

Family Support

Many of the stresses observed during the monitoring period are characteristic of those of families with chronically ill children. The child with an apnea or cardiorespiratory monitor may have additional health care needs such as a gastrostomy, tracheostomy, ostomy, and myriad medications or treatments that exacerbate the parents' stress. Parents report increased stress, including concern for the child's survival, fear of incompetence in assuming home responsibility, inadequate respite care, lack of time for other children and spouse, social isolation from friends and extended family, constant work, and fatigue. The monitored child is at risk for vulnerable child syndrome, which may lead to lack of parental separation and preferential treatment, causing further family disruption (Bennett, 2002). To deal with these potential effects, nurses need to employ the same interventions as those discussed for children with chronic illness and be aware of the need for referral when difficulties are suspected.

To lessen the continuous responsibility of monitoring, other family members, such as grandparents, should be taught how to manipulate the equipment, read and interpret the signals, and administer CPR. They are encouraged to stay with the infant for regular periods to allow parents respite. Support groups of other families who have successfully completed monitoring can also be of benefit. Because baby-sitters are difficult to locate, support group members or nursing students may be potential sources of qualified caregivers.

Key Points

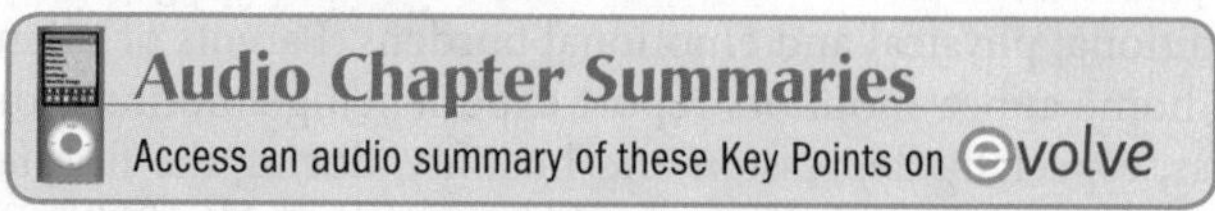
Audio Chapter Summaries
Access an audio summary of these Key Points on evolve

- Biologic development of the child encompasses proportional changes; sensory changes, including binocularity, depth perception, and visual preference; maturation of biologic systems; fine motor development; and gross motor development.
- Erikson's theory of psychosocial development (birth to 1 year) is concerned with acquiring a sense of trust while overcoming a sense of mistrust.
- Piaget's theory of cognitive development, as it applies to the infant, focuses on the sensorimotor phase, which includes the use of reflexes, primary circular reactions, secondary circular reactions, and coordination of secondary schemata and their application to new situations.

- Development of body image begins in infancy; by 1 year of age infants recognize that they are distinct from their parents.
- Social development of the infant is guided by attachment, language development, personal-social behavior, and participation in play.
- Temperament influences the type of interaction that occurs between the child and parents and siblings.
- Parents are faced with many concerns, including selecting an appropriate day care, limit setting and discipline, thumb-sucking and pacifier use, teething, and choice of infant shoes.
- Breast milk provides optimal nutrition for the infant during the first 6 months, followed by gradual introduction of solid food during the second 6 months. Commercial iron-fortified infant formula is a safe alternative to human milk. Whole milk is not recommended until after 12 months.
- Common sleep problems that develop during infancy—and that are easily prevented—are associated with night crying and feeding. Nurses should instruct the parents, after careful assessment, in strategies to deal with the specific problem.
- Cleaning the teeth regularly in early childhood and appropriate dietary intake promote good dental health.
- Recommended routine immunizations include those for HBV, HAV, diphtheria, influenza, tetanus, pertussis, polio, measles, mumps, rubella, pneumococcus, meningococcus, chickenpox, and Hib.
- Recommended immunizations for selected groups of children are rotavirus and HPV vaccines.
- Because injuries are a major cause of death during infancy, parents should be alerted to aspiration of foreign objects, suffocation, falls, poisoning, burns, motor vehicle injuries, and bodily damage, as well as preventive actions needed to make the environment safe for infants.
- Treatment of colic may involve change in feeding practices, correction of a stressful environment, behavior modification, and support of the parent.
- Growth failure, or FTT, may occur in children who have a chronic illness, or it may occur in a family environment wherein healthy infant feeding practices are poorly managed or understood. FTT is not always associated with a pattern of disturbed maternal-infant relationship.
- SIDS is the third leading cause of infant death in the United States.
- Factors that place the infant at high risk for SIDS include prone sleeping position, soft bedding, sleeping in a noninfant bed with an adult or older child, and maternal prenatal smoking.
- Positional plagiocephaly can be easily prevented by allowing the awake infant to have periods of tummy time and by alternating the infant's head position during sleep.
- The primary nursing responsibility in care associated with sudden infant death is educating the family of newborns about the risks for SIDS, modeling appropriate behaviors in the hospital such as placing the infant in a supine sleep position, and providing emotional support of the family that has experienced a SIDS loss.
- Infants with ALTEs are carefully evaluated for clues to the underlying cause.
- Home apnea or cardiorespiratory monitors do not prevent SIDS.

References

Abendroth D et al: Do apnea monitors decrease emotional distress in parents of infants at high risk for cardiopulmonary arrest? *J Pediatr Health Care* 13(2):50-57, 1999.

Agran PF et al: Rates of pediatric injuries by 3-month intervals for children 0 to 3 years of age, *Pediatrics* 111(6): e683-e692, 2003.

Alm B et al: Breast-feeding and the sudden infant death syndrome in Scandinavia, 1992-1995, *Arch Dis Child* 86(6):400-402, 2002.

Altman RL et al: Abusive head injury as a cause of apparent life-threatening events in infancy, *Arch Pediatr Adolesc Med* 157(10):1011-1015, 2003.

American Academy of Pediatric Dentistry: Clinical guidelines: fluoride therapy, *AAPD Reference Manual 2007-2008*, 2008a. Available at www.aapd.org/media/policies_Guidelines/G_Fluoridetherapy.pdf (accessed July 1, 2008).

American Academy of Pediatric Dentistry: Clinical guidelines: guideline on infant oral health care, *AAPD Reference Manual 2007-2008*, 29(7):81-83, 2008b. Available at www.aapd.org/media/Policies_Guidelines/G_InfantOralHealth.pdf (accessed July 1, 2008).

American Academy of Pediatrics: *Pediatric nutrition handbook*, ed 6, Elk Grove Village, IL, 2009, The Academy.

American Academy of Pediatrics: Prevention of rickets and vitamin D deficiency in infants, children, and adolescents, *Pediatrics* 122(5):1142-1148, 2008.

American Academy of Pediatrics: Prevention and management of positional skull deformities in infants (clinical report), *Pediatrics* 112(1): 199-202, 2003.

American Academy of Pediatrics, Committee on Child Abuse and Neglect: Distinguishing sudden infant death syndrome from child abuse fatalities, *Pediatrics* 107(2):437-441, 2001.

American Academy of Pediatrics, Committee on Fetus and Newborn: Apnea, sudden infant death syndrome, and home monitoring, *Pediatrics* 111(4):914-917, 2003.

American Academy of Pediatrics, Committee on Infectious Diseases, Pickering L (editor): *2009 red book: report of the Committee on Infectious Diseases*, ed 28, Elk Grove Village, IL, 2009, The Academy.

American Academy of Pediatrics, Committee on Infectious Diseases: Recommended immunization schedules for children and adolescents—United States, 2008, *Pediatrics* 121(1):219-220, 2008.

American Academy of Pediatrics, Committee on Injury and Poison Prevention: Injuries associated with infant walkers, *Pediatrics* 108(3):790-792, 2001.

American Academy of Pediatrics, Committee on Sports Medicine: Infant exercise programs, *Pediatrics* 82(5): 800, 1988.

American Academy of Pediatrics, Committee on Sports Medicine and Committee on Injury and Poison Prevention: Swimming programs for infants and toddlers, *Pediatrics* 105(4, Pt 1 of 2):868-869, 2000.

American Academy of Pediatrics, Task Force on Infant Sleep Position and Sudden Infant Death Syndrome: Changing concepts of sudden infant death syndrome: implications for infant sleeping environment and sleep position, *Pediatrics* 105(3):650-656, 2000.

American Academy of Pediatrics, Task Force on Sudden Infant Death Syndrome: The changing concept of sudden infant death syndrome: diagnostic coding shifts, controversies regarding the sleeping environment, and new variables to consider in reducing risk, *Pediatrics* 116(5): 1245-1255, 2005.

American Dental Association: For the dental patient ... infants, formula and fluoride, *JADA* 138(1):132, 2007.

American Psychiatric Association: *Position statement: reactive attachment disorder*, 2002. Available at www.psych.org/public_info/libr_publ/position.cfm (accessed June 2005).

American Psychiatric Association: *Diagnostic and statistical manual of mental disorders*, ed 4, Washington, DC, 2000, The Association.

Anderson JE: "Nothing but the tooth": dispelling myths about teething, *Contemp Pediatr* 21(7):75-83, 2004.

Anderson ME, Johnson DC, Batal HA: Sudden infant death syndrome and prenatal maternal smoking: rising attributed risk in the Back to Sleep era, *BMC Med* 3(1):4, 2005.

Arikan D et al: Effectiveness of massage, sucrose solution, herbal tea or hydrolyzed formula in the treatment of infantile colic, *J Clin Nurs* 17(13):1754-1761, 2008.

Arora S et al: Major factors influencing breastfeeding rates: mother's perception of father's attitude and milk supply, *Pediatrics* 106(5):e67, 2000.

Bacon CJ et al: How common is repeat sudden infant death syndrome? *Arch Dis Child* 93(4):323-326, 2008.

Barnard K et al: Measurement and meaning of parent-child interaction. In Morrison F, Lord C, Keating D (editors): *Applied developmental psychology*, vol 3, New York, 1993, Academic Press.

Barnhill BJ et al: Using pressure to decrease the pain of intramuscular injections, *J Pain Symptom Manage* 12(1):52-58, 1996.

Bellemare S: Dangers for children in the care of drug users, *CMAJ* 179(2):164, 2008.

Bennett AD: Home apnea monitoring for infants: a discussion of primary care issues, *Adv Nurs Pract* 10(3):48-53, 2002.

Biancuzzo M: *Breastfeeding the newborn: clinical strategies for nurses*, ed 2, St Louis, 2003, Mosby.

Biggs WS: Diagnosis and management of positional head deformity, *Am Fam Physician* 67(9):1953-1956, 2003.

Blackburn ST: *Maternal, fetal, and neonatal physiology: a clinical perspective*, ed 3, St Louis, 2007, Saunders.

Block RW, Krebs NF, American Academy of Pediatrics, Committee on Child Abuse and Neglect and Committee on Nutrition: Failure to thrive as a manifestation of child neglect, *Pediatrics* 116(5):1234-1237, 2005.

Brady MT: Infectious disease in pediatric out-of-home child care, *Am J Infect Control* 33(5):276-285, 2005.

Brazelton T: Parent-infant cosleeping revisited, *Brazelton Center Newsletter*, vol 2, Boston, 1990.

Brenner RA, American Academy of Pediatrics, Committee on Injury, Violence, and Poison Prevention: Prevention of drowning in infants, children, and adolescents, *Pediatrics* 112(2):440-445, 2003.

Brenner RA et al: Deaths attributable to injuries in infants, United States, 1983-1991, *Pediatrics* 103(5 Pt 1):968-974, 1999.

Bullock LFC et al: Are nurses acting as role models for the prevention of SIDS? *MCN* 29(3):172-177, 2004.

Campion EW: Suspicions about the safety of vaccines, *N Engl J Med* 347(19):1474-1475, 2002.

Carey WB, McDevitt SC: Revision of the infant temperament questionnaire, *Pediatrics* 61(5):735-739, 1978.

Carroll-Pankhurst C, Mortimer EA: Sudden infant death syndrome, bedsharing, parental weight, and age of death, *Pediatrics* 107(3):530-536, 2001.

Centers for Disease Control and Prevention: Recommended immunization schedules for persons aged 0 through 18 years—United States, 2009, *Morb Mortal Wkly Rep* 57(51):Q-1-Q-4, 2009.

Centers for Disease Control and Prevention: Nonfatal maltreatment of infants—United States, October 2005–September 2006, *Morb Mortal Wkly Rep* 57(13):336-339, 2008.

Centers for Disease Control and Prevention: Fatal injuries among children by race and ethnicity—United States, 1999-2002, *Morb Mortal Wkly Rep* 56(SS05):1-16, 2007a.

Centers for Disease Control and Prevention: Quadrivalent human papillomavirus vaccine, *Morb Mortal Wkly Rep* 56(RR-2):1-24, 2007b.

Centers for Disease Control and Prevention: Prevention of hepatitis A through active or passive immunization, *Morb Mortal Wkly Rep* 55(RR07):1-23, 2006a.

Centers for Disease Control and Prevention: Update: Guillain-Barré syndrome among recipients of Menactra meningococcal conjugate vaccine—United States, June 2005-September 2006, *Morb Mortal Wkly Rep* 55(41):1120-1124, 2006b.

Centers for Disease Control and Prevention: A comprehensive immunization strategy to eliminate transmission of hepatitis B virus infection in the United States, *Morb Mortal Wkly Rep* 54(RR16):1-23, 2005a.

Centers for Disease Control and Prevention: Nonfatal motor-vehicle-related backover injuries among children—United States, 2001-2003, *Morb Mortal Wkly Rep* 54(06):144-146, 2005b.

Centers for Disease Control and Prevention: Outbreaks of pertussis associated with hospitals—Kentucky, Pennsylvania, and Oregon, 2003, *Morb Mortal Wkly Rep* 54(3):67-71, 2005c.

Chung JWY, Ng WMY, Wong TKS: An experimental study on the use of manual pressure to reduce pain in intramuscular injections, *J Clin Nurs* 11:457-461, 2002.

Corbett-Dick P, Bezek SK: Breastfeeding promotion for the employed mother, *J Pediatr Health Care* 11(1):12-19, 1997.

Corrales KM, Utter SL: Growth failure. In Samour PQ, King K (editors): *Handbook of pediatric nutrition*, ed 3, Sudbury, MA, 2005, Jones & Bartlett.

Crotteau CA, Wright ST, Eglash A: What is the best treatment for infants with colic? *J Fam Pract* 55(7):634-636, 2006.

Dahl RE: The development and disorders of sleep, *Adv Pediatr* 45:73-90, 1998.

Dales L, Hammer SJ, Smith NJ: Time trends in autism and in MMR immunization coverage in California, *JAMA* 285(9):1183-1185, 2001.

Davis KF, Parker K, Montgomery GL: Sleep in infants and young children, part 2, Common sleep problems, *J Pediatr Health Care* 18(3):130-137, 2004.

DeStefano F: Vaccines and autism: evidence does not support a causal association, *Clin Pharmacol Ther* 82(6):756-759, 2007.

Dewey KG: Nutrition, growth, and complementary feeding of the breastfed infant, *Pediatr Clin North Am* 48(1):87-104, 2001.

Diggle L, Deeks J: Effect of needle length on incidence of local reactions to routine immunizations in infants aged 4 months: randomized controlled trial, *BMJ* 321(7266):931-993, 2000.

Diggle L, Deeks JJ, Pollard AJ: Effect of needle size and immunogenecity and reactogenecity of vaccines in infants: a randomized controlled trial, *BMJ* 333(7568):571, 2006.

Douglass JM, Douglass AB, Silk HJ: A practical guide to infant oral health, *Am Fam Physician* 70(11):2113-2120, 2004.

Drago DA: Kitchen scalds and thermal burns in children five years and younger, *Pediatrics* 115(1):10-16, 2005.

Dudell GG, Stoll BJ: Respiratory tract disorders. In Kliegman RM et al (editors): *Nelson textbook of pediatrics*, ed 18, Philadelphia, 2007, Saunders.

Duro D et al: Association between infantile colic and carbohydrate malabsorption from fruit juices in infancy, *Pediatrics* 109(5):797-805, 2002.

Ellett MLC: What is known about colic? *Gastroenterol Nurs* 26(2):60-65, 2003.

Ellett M, Schuff E, Davis JB: Parental perceptions of the lasting effects of infant colic, *MCN* 30(2):127-132, 2005.

Erikson EH: *Childhood and society*, ed 2, New York, 1963, Norton.

Esani N et al: Apparent life-threatening events and sudden infant death syndrome: comparison of risk factors, *J Pediatr* 152(3):A2, 2008.

Franco P et al: Prenatal exposure to cigarette smoking is associated with a decrease in arousal in infants, *J Pediatr* 135(1):34-38, 1999.

Fredrickson DD et al: Childhood immunization refusal: provider and parent perceptions, *Fam Med* 36(6):431-438, 2004.

Gold KJ: Navigating care after a baby dies: a systematic review of parent experiences with health providers, *J Perinatol* 27(4):230-237, 2007.

Graham JM et al: Management of deformational plagiocephaly: repositioning versus orthotic therapy, *J Pediatr* 146(2):258-262, 2005.

Hall KL, Zalman B: Evaluation and management of apparent life threatening events in children, *Am Fam Physician* 71(12):2301-2308, 2005.

Halperin BA et al: Use of lidocaine-prilocaine patch to decrease intramuscular injection pain does not adversely affect the antibody response to diphtheria–tetanus–acellular pertussis–inactivated poliovirus–*Haemophilus influenzae* type b conjugate and hepatitis B vaccines in infants from birth to 6 months of age, *Pediatr Infect Dis* 21(5):399-405, 2002.

Hatfield LA: Sucrose decreases infant neurobehavioral pain response to immunizations: a randomized controlled trial, *J Nurs Scholarship* 40(3):219-225, 2008.

Hauck FR et al: Sleep environment and the risk of sudden infant death syndrome in an urban population: the Chicago Infant Mortality Study, *Pediatrics* 111(5 Pt 2):1207-1214, 2003.

Hawkins-Walsh E: A behavioural infant sleep intervention resolved sleep problems, *Evidence-Based Nurs* 6(1):10-12, 2003.

Henary B et al: Car safety seats for children: rear facing for best protection, *Inj Prev* 13(6):398-402, 2007.

Heron J, Golding J, ALSPAC Study Team: Thimerosal exposure in infants and developmental disorders: a prospective cohort study in the United Kingdom does not support a causal association, *Pediatrics* 114(3):577-583, 2004.

Heron MP, Smith BL: Deaths: leading causes for 2003, *Natl Vital Stat Rep* 55(10):1-92, 2007.

Hiscock H, Wake M: Infant sleep problems and postnatal depression: a community-based study, *Pediatrics* 107(6):1317-1322, 2001.

Horn MI, McCarthy AM: Children's responses to sequential versus simultaneous immunization injections, *J Pediatr Health Care* 13(1):18-23, 1999.

Horne RS et al: The prone sleeping position impairs arousability in term infants, *J Pediatr* 138(6):793-795, 2001.

Hornor G: Reactive attachment disorder, *J Pediatr Health Care* 22(4):234-239, 2008.

Hummel P, Fortado D: Impacting infant head shapes, *Adv Neon Care* 5(6):329-342, 2005.

Hviid A et al: Association between thimerosal-containing vaccine and autism, *JAMA* 290(13):1763-1766, 2003.

Institute of Medicine: *Immunization safety review: vaccines and autism*, Washington, DC, 2004, National Academies Press.

Ize-Ludlow D et al: Neurotoxicities in infants seen with the consumption of star anise tea, *Pediatrics* 114(5):e653, 2004.

Jimenez N et al: A comparison of a needle-free injection system for local anesthesia versus EMLA for intravenous catheter insertion in the pediatric patient, *Anesth Analag* 102(2): 411-414, 2006.

Joanna Briggs Institute: Early childhood pacifier use in relation to breastfeeding, SIDS, infection, and dental occlusion, *Best Practice* 9(3):1-6, 2005.

Joanna Briggs Institute: Best practice information sheet: the effectiveness of interventions for infant colic, *Best Practice* 8(2):1-6, 2004.

Jobe AH: What do home monitors contribute to the SIDS problem? (editorial), *JAMA* 285(17):2244-2245, 2001.

Kallan MJ et al: Seating patterns and corresponding risk of injury among 0- to 3-year-old children in child safety seats, *Pediatrics* 121(5):e1342-e1347, 2008.

Katz-Salamon M: Delayed chemoreceptor responses in infants with apnoea, *Arch Dis Child* 89(3):261-266, 2004.

Koslap-Petraco MB, Parsons T: Communicating the benefits of combination vaccines to parents and health care providers, *J Pediatr Health Care* 17(2):53-57, 2003.

Kotch JB et al: Hand-washing and diapering equipment reduces disease among children in out-of-home child care centers, *Pediatrics* 120(1):e29-36, 2007.

Krugman SD, Dubowitz H: Failure to thrive, *Am Fam Physician* 68(5):879-886, 2003.

Lassman J: Water safety, *J Emerg Nurs* 28(3):241-243, 2002.

Lawrence RA, Lawrence RM: *Breastfeeding: a guide for the medical profession*, ed 6, St Louis, 2005, Mosby.

Lee MS, Bernstein HH: Immunizations, neonatal jaundice and animal-induced injuries, *Curr Opin Pediatr* 17(3):418-429, 2005.

Littlefield TR, Saba NM, Kelly KM: On the current incidence of deformational plagiocephaly: an estimation based on prospective registration at a single center, *Semin Pediatr Neurol* 11(4):301-304, 2004.

Locklin M: The redefinition of failure to thrive from a case study perspective, *Pediatr Nurs* 31(6):474-479, 495, 2005.

Maggioni A, Lifshitz F: Nutritional management of failure to thrive, *Pediatr Clin North Am* 42(4):791-810, 1995.

Malloy MH: Trends in postneonatal aspiration deaths and reclassification of sudden infant death syndrome: impact of the "Back to Sleep" program, *Pediatrics* 109(4):661-665, 2002.

Markowitz R, Duggan C: Failure to thrive: malnutrition in the pediatric setting. In Walker WA, Watkins JB, Duggan C, editors: *Nutrition in pediatrics*, ed 3, Hamilton, Ontario, Canada, 2003, Decker.

Martin J et al: Adverse associations of infant and child sleep problems and parent health: an Australian population study, *Pediatrics* 119(5):947-955, 2007.

Matteucci MJ et al: Methamphetamine exposures in young children, *Pediatr Emerg Care* 23(9):638-640, 2007.

McGarvey C et al: Factors relating to the infant's last sleep environment in sudden infant death syndrome in the Republic of Ireland, *Arch Dis Child* 88(12):1058-1064, 2003.

McMartin KI et al: Lung tissue concentrations of nicotine in sudden infant death syndrome, *J Pediatr* 140(2): 205-209, 2002.

Mecham N, Melini J: Unintentional victims: development of a protocol for the care of children exposed to chemicals at methamphetamine laboratories, *Pediatr Emerg Care* 18(4):327-332, 2002.

Medoff-Cooper B, Carey WB, McDevitt SC: The early infancy temperament questionnaire, *J Dev Behav Pediatr* 14(4):230-235, 1993.

Mesich HM: Mother-infant cosleeping: understanding the debate and maximizing infant safety, *MCN* 30(1):30-37, 2005.

Mitchell EA et al: Head covering and the risk for SIDS: findings from the New Zealand and German SIDS case-control studies, *Pediatrics* 121(6):e1478-e1483, 2008.

Morin K: Infant nutrition: preparing baby food at home safely, *MCN* 30(1):67, 2005.

Morin K: Infant nutrition: solids—when and why, *MCN* 29(4):259, 2004.

National Institute of Child Health and Human Development Early Child Care Research Network: Child care and common communicable illnesses: results from the National Institute of Child Health and Human Development Study of Early Child Care, *Arch Pediatr Adolesc Med* 155(4):481-488, 2001.

National Institutes of Health: Consensus Development Conference on Infantile Apnea and Home Monitoring, Sept 29 to Oct 1, 1986, *Pediatrics* 79(2):292-299, 1987.

Neu M, Robinson JA: Infants with colic: their childhood characteristics, *J Pediatr Nurs* 18(1):12-20, 2003.

Niemela M, Uhari M, Mottonen M: A pacifier increases the risk of recurrent acute otitis media in children in day care centers, *Pediatrics* 96(5 Pt 1): 884-888, 1995.

Niemela M et al: Pacifier as a risk factor for acute otitis media: a randomized, controlled trial of parental counseling, *Pediatrics* 106(3):483-488, 2000.

Person TL, Lavezzi WA, Wolf BC: Cosleeping and sudden unexpected death in infancy, *Arch Pathol Lab Med* 126(3):343-345, 2002.

Phelan KJ et al: Residential injuries in U.S. children and adolescents, *Pub Health Rep* 120(1):63-70, 2005.

Piaget J: *The origins of intelligence in children*. New York, 1952, International Universities Press.

Pickett W et al: Injuries experienced by infant children: a population-based epidemiological analysis, *Pediatrics* 111(4 Pt 1):e365-e370, 2003.

Pickler R, Frankel H: The effect of non-nutritive sucking on preterm infants' behavioral organization and feeding performance, *Neonatal Netw* 14(2):83, 1995.

Pinelli J, Symington A: Non-nutritive sucking for promoting physiologic stability and nutrition in preterm infants, *Cochrane Database Syst Rev* (2):CD001071, 2000.

Pinelli J, Symington A, Ciliska D: Nonnutritive sucking in high-risk infants: benign intervention or legitimate therapy? *J Obstet Gynecol Neonatal Nurs* 31(5):582-591, 2002.

Pollack HA: Sudden infant death syndrome, maternal smoking during pregnancy and effectiveness of smoking cessation intervention, *Am J Public Health* 91(3):432-436, 2001.

Puffenberger EG et al: Mapping of sudden infant death with dysgenesis of the testis syndrome (SIDDT) by a SNP genome scan and identification of TSPYL loss of function, *Proc Natl Acad Sci USA* 101(32):11,689-11,694, 2004.

Ramanathan R et al: Cardiorespiratory events recorded on home monitors: comparison of healthy infants with those at increased risk for SIDS, *JAMA* 285(17):2199-2243, 2001.

Reis EC, Holubkov R: Vapocoolant spray is equally effective as EMLA cream in reducing immunization pain in school-aged children, *Pediatrics* 100(6):1025, 1997.

Rojjanasrirat W: Working women's breastfeeding experiences, *MCN* 29(4):222-227, 2004.

Rudolf MCJ, Logan S: What is the long term outcome for children who fail to thrive? A systematic review, *Arch Dis Child* 90(9):925-931, 2005.

Savino F et al: *Lactobacillus reuteri* (American type culture collection strain 55730) versus simethicone in the treatment of infantile colic: a prospective randomized study, *Pediatrics* 119(1):e124-e130, 2007.

Schachter F et al: Cosleeping and sleep problems in Hispanic-American urban young children, *Pediatrics* 84(3):522-530, 1989.

Schechter NL et al: Pain reduction during pediatric immunizations: evidence-based review and recommendations, *Pediatrics* 119(5):e1184-e1198, 2007.

Schuval S: Avoiding allergic reactions to childhood vaccines (and what to do when they occur), *Contemp Pediatr* 22(4):29-49, 53, 2003.

Silvestri JM, Weese-Mayer D: Disorders of respiratory control: apnea and SIDS. In Rudolph CD, Rudolph AM, Hostetter MK (editors): *Rudolph's pediatrics*, ed 21, New York, 2003, McGraw-Hill.

Spanos S et al: Jet injection of 1% buffered lidocaine versus topical ELA-Max for anesthesia before peripheral intravenous catheterization in children: a randomized controlled trial, *Pediatr Emerg Care* 24(8):511-515, 2008.

Stevens B, Yamada J, Ohlsson A: Sucrose for analgesia in newborn infants undergoing painful procedures, *Cochrane Database Syst Rev* (4):CD001069, 2001.

Stevens B et al: The efficacy of developmentally sensitive interventions and sucrose for relieving procedural pain in very low birth weight neonates, *Nurs Res* 48(1):35-43, 1999.

Tablizo MA et al: Supine sleeping position does not cause clinical aspiration in neonates in hospital newborn nurseries, *Arch Pediatr Adolesc Med* 161(5):507-510, 2007.

Tappin D, Ecob R, Brooke H: Bedsharing, roomsharing, and sudden infant death syndrome in Scotland: a case-control study, *J Pediatr* 147(1):32-37, 2005.

Thompson DG: Safe sleep practices for hospitalized infants, *Pediatr Nurs* 31(5):400-403, 409, 2005.

Touchette E et al: Factors associated with fragmented sleep at night across early childhood, *Arch Pediatr Adolesc Med* 159(3):242-249, 2005.

Unger B et al: Racial disparity and modifiable risk factors among infants dying suddenly and unexpectedly, *Pediatrics* 111(2):E127-E131, 2003.

Weizman Z et al: Efficacy of herbal tea preparation in infantile colic, *J Pediatr* 122(4):650-652, 1993.

Wilkerson R, Northington LD, Fisher W: Ingestion of toxic substances by infants and children: what we don't know can hurt, *Crit Care Nurs* 25(4):35-44, 2005.

Willinger M et al: Trends in infant bed sharing in the United States, 1993-

2000: the National Infant Sleep Position Study, *Arch Pediatr Adolesc Med* 157(1):43-49, 2003.

Wilson ME et al: Family dynamics, parental-fetal attachment and infant temperament, *J Adv Nurs* 31(1):204-210, 2000.

Wilson S: Attachment disorders: review and current status, *J Psychol* 135(1): 37-51, 2001.

Wong DL: Topical local anesthetics: two products for pain relief during minor procedures, *Am J Nurs* 103(6): 42-45, 2003.

Zeanah CH, Fox NA: Temperament and attachment disorders, *J Clin Child Adolesc Psychol* 33(1):82-87, 2004.

Zempsky WT: Pharmacologic approaches for reducing venous access pain in children, *Pediatrics* 122(Suppl 3):S140-S153, 2008.

Zuckerman J: The importance of injecting vaccines into muscle, *BMJ* 321(7271):1237-1238, 2000.

Zuckerman JN, Cockcroft A, Zuckerman AJ: Site of injection for vaccination, *BMJ* 305(6862):1158, 1992.

Unit 9

37 The Toddler and Family

Learning Objectives

On completion of this chapter the reader will be able to:

- Identify the major biologic, psychosocial, cognitive, and social developments during the toddler years.
- Relate separation anxiety and negativism to developmental tasks.
- Recognize readiness for toilet training and offer parents guidelines.
- Prepare parents of toddlers for the birth of a sibling.
- Provide parents with guidelines for handling temper tantrums.
- Provide parents with feeding recommendations for the toddler.
- Outline a preventive dental hygiene plan for toddlers.
- Provide anticipatory guidance to parents regarding injury prevention based on the toddler's developmental achievements.

Electronic Resources

Additional information related to the content in Chapter 37 can be found on

evolve the Companion Website at http://evolve.elsevier.com/Perry/maternal/

- NCLEX Review Questions
- Assessment Video Clips
- Case Study—Heavy Metal Poisoning
- Case Study—Ingestion of an Injurious Agent
- Case Study—Salicylate Ingestion
- Case Study—Toilet Training/Toddler Development
- Skill—Car Seat Safety

Promoting Optimum Growth and Development

The term *terrible twos* has often been used to describe the toddler years, the period from 12 to 36 months of age. Although the term may be often used to describe the toddler's *behavior*, it is not meant to typify or label the child. It is a time of intense exploration of the environment as children attempt to find out how things work and how to control others through temper tantrums, negativism, and obstinacy. Although this can be a challenging time for parents and child as each learns to know the other better, it is an extremely important period for developmental achievement and intellectual growth. Toddlers are in fact very lovable at times, but because of their search for autonomy, they may test parents' and caregivers' patience.

Biologic Development

Proportional Changes

Growth slows considerably during toddlerhood. The average *weight* gain is 1.8 to 2.7 kg (4 to 6 lb). The birth weight is quadrupled by 2½ years of age. The rate of increase in height also slows. The usual increment is an addition of 7.5 cm (3 inches) per year and occurs mainly in elongation of the legs rather than the trunk. The average *height* of a 2-year-old is 86.6 cm (34 inches). In general, adult height is about twice the 2-year-old child's height. Accurate measurement of height and weight during the toddler years should reveal a steady growth curve that is *steplike* in nature rather than linear (straight), which is characteristic of the growth spurts during the early childhood years.

The rate of increase in *head circumference* slows somewhat by the end of infancy, and head circumference is usually equal to chest circumference by 1 to 2 years of age. The usual total increase in head circumference during the second year is 2.5 cm (1 inch). Then the rate of increase slows until, at age 5 years, the increase is less than 1.25 cm (½ inch) per year. The anterior fontanel closes between 12 and 18 months of age.

Chest circumference continues to increase in size and exceeds head circumference during the toddler years. Its shape also changes as the transverse, or lateral, diameter exceeds the anteroposterior diameter. After the second year the chest circumference exceeds the abdominal measurement; this, in addition to the growth of the lower extremities, gives the child a taller, leaner appearance. However, the toddler still appears relatively squat and "pot-bellied" because of the less well-developed abdominal musculature and short legs. The legs remain slightly bowed or curved during the second year from the weight of the relatively large trunk.

Sensory Changes

Visual acuity of 20/40 is considered acceptable during the toddler years. Full binocular vision is well developed, and any evidence of persistent strabismus requires professional attention as early as possible to prevent amblyopia. Depth perception continues to develop but, because of the child's lack of motor coordination, falls from heights are a persistent danger.

The senses of *hearing, smell, taste,* and *touch* become increasingly well developed, coordinated with each other, and associated with other experiences. All of the senses are used to explore the environment. Toddlers will visually inspect an object by turning it over; they may taste it, smell, it, and touch it several times before they are satisfied with their investigation. They will shake it to see if it makes noise and vigorously test its durability.

Another example of the integrated function of the senses is the toddler's development of specific *taste preferences.* The toddler is much less likely than an infant to try a new food because of its appearance, texture, or smell, not just its taste.

Maturation of Systems

Most of the physiologic systems are relatively mature by the end of toddlerhood. Volume of the *respiratory tract* and growth of associated structures continue to increase during early childhood, lessening some of the factors that predisposed the child to frequent and serious infections during infancy. The internal structures of the ear and throat continue to be short and straight, and the lymphoid tissue of the tonsils and adenoids continues to be large. As a result, otitis media, tonsillitis, and upper respiratory tract infections are common. The respiratory and heart rates slow, and the blood pressure increases (see Appendix E). Respirations continue to be abdominal.

Under conditions of moderate variation in temperature, the toddler rarely has the difficulties of the young infant in maintaining *body temperature.* The mature functioning of the renal system serves to conserve fluid under times of stress, decreasing the risk of dehydration.

The *digestive processes* are fairly complete by the beginning of toddlerhood. The acidity of the gastric contents continues to increase and has a protective function, since it is capable of destroying many types of bacteria. Stomach capacity increases to allow for the usual schedule of three meals a day.

One of the more prominent changes of the gastrointestinal system is the voluntary control of elimination. With complete myelination of the spinal cord, control of the anal and urethral sphincters is gradually achieved. The *physiologic* ability to control the sphincters probably occurs somewhere between ages 18 and 24 months. Bladder capacity also increases considerably, and by 14 to 18 months of age the child is able to retain urine for up to 2 hours or longer.

The *defense mechanisms* of the skin and blood, particularly phagocytosis, are much more efficient in toddlers than in infants. The production of antibodies is well established. However, many young children demonstrate a sudden increase in colds and minor infections when they enter preschool or other group situations, such as day care, because of their exposure to pathogens and the lack of understanding of general hygiene measures such as handwashing.

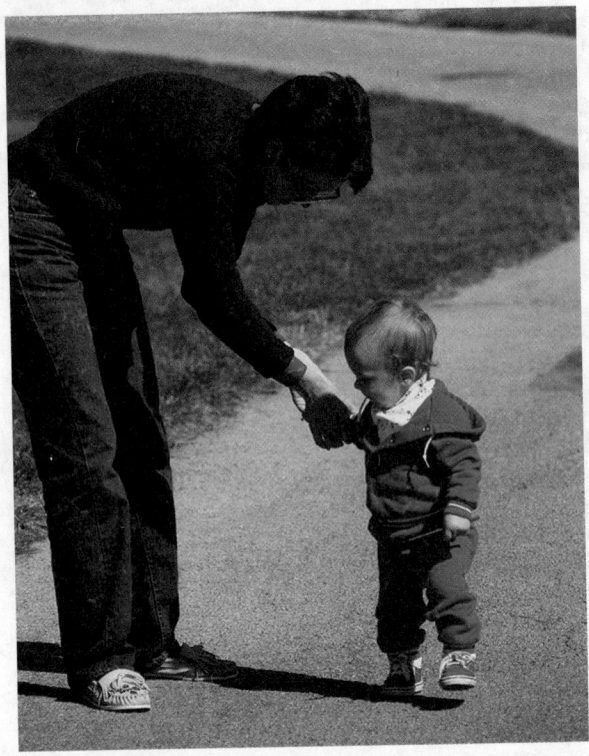

Fig. 37-1 Typical toddling gait.

Gross and Fine Motor Development

The major *gross motor skill* during the toddler years is the development of locomotion. By 12 to 13 months of age toddlers walk alone using a wide stance for extra balance, and by 18 months they try to run but fall easily (Fig. 37-1). Between 2 and 3 years of age, refinement of the upright, biped position is evident in improved coordination and equilibrium. At age 2 years, toddlers can walk up and down stairs; by age 2½ years they can jump using both feet, stand on one foot for a second or two, and manage a few steps on tiptoe. By the end of the second year they can stand on one foot, walk on tiptoe, and climb stairs with alternate footing.

Fine motor development is demonstrated in increasingly skillful manual dexterity. For example, by age 12 months toddlers are able to grasp a very small object but are unable to release it at will. At 15 months they can drop a pellet into a narrow-necked bottle. Casting or throwing objects and retrieving them become almost obsessive activities at about 15 months. By 18 months of age toddlers can throw a ball overhand without losing their balance.

Mastery of gross and fine motor skills is evident in all phases of the child's activity, such as play, dressing, language comprehension, response to discipline, social interaction, and propensity for injuries. Activities occur less in isolation and more in conjunction with other physical and mental abilities to produce a purposeful result. For example, the toddler walks to reach a new location, releases a toy to pick it up or to choose a new one, and scribbles to look at the image produced. The possibilities of the exploration, investigation, and manipulation of the environment—and its hazards—are endless.

Psychosocial Development

Toddlers are faced with the mastery of several important tasks. If the need for basic trust has been satisfied, they are ready to give up dependence for control, independence, and autonomy. Some of the specific tasks to be dealt with include:

- Differentiation of self from others, particularly the mother
- Toleration of separation from parent
- Ability to delay gratification
- Control over bodily functions
- Acquisition of socially acceptable behavior
- Verbal means of communication
- Ability to interact with others in a less egocentric manner

Mastery of these goals is only begun during late infancy and the toddler years, and tasks such as developing interpersonal relationships with others may not be completed until adolescence. However, crucial foundations for successful completion of such developmental tasks are established during these early formative years.

Developing a Sense of Autonomy (Erikson)

According to Erikson, the developmental task of toddlerhood is acquiring a sense of *autonomy* while overcoming a sense of *doubt and shame.* As infants gain trust in the predictability and reliability of their parents, environment, and interaction with others, they begin to discover that their behavior is their own and that it has a predictable, reliable effect on others. However, although they realize their will and control over others, they are confronted with the conflict of exerting autonomy and relinquishing the much-enjoyed dependence on others. Exerting their will has definite negative consequences, whereas retaining dependent, submissive behavior is generally rewarded with affection and approval. At the same time, continued dependency creates a sense of doubt regarding their potential capacity to control their actions. This doubt is compounded by a sense of shame for feeling this urge to revolt against others' will and a fear that they will exceed their own capacity for manipulating the environment.

Just as the infant has the social modalities of grasping and biting, the toddler has the newly gained modality of holding on and letting go. To hold on and let go is evident with the use of the hands, mouth, eyes, and eventually the sphincters, when toilet training is begun. These social modalities are expressed constantly in the child's play activities, such as casting or throwing objects; taking objects out of boxes, drawers, or cabinets; holding on tighter when someone says, "No, don't touch"; and spitting out food as taste preferences become strong.

Several characteristics, especially negativism and ritualism, are typical of toddlers in their quest for autonomy. As toddlers attempt to express their will, they often act with *negativism,* the persistent negative response to requests. The words "no" or "me do" can be the sole vocabulary. Emotions are strongly expressed, usually in rapid mood swings. One minute, toddlers can be engrossed in an activity, and the next minute they might be extremely frustrated because they are unable to manipulate a toy or open a door. If scolded for doing something wrong, they can have a temper tantrum and almost instantaneously pull at the parent's legs to be picked up and comforted. Understanding and coping with these swift changes in behavior is often difficult for parents. Many parents find the negativism exasperating and, instead of dealing constructively with it, give in to it, which further threatens children in their search for learning acceptable methods of interacting with others (see Temper Tantrums and Negativism, p. 1028).

In contrast to negativism, which often disrupts the environment, *ritualism,* the need to maintain sameness and reliability, provides a sense of comfort. Toddlers can venture out with security when they know that familiar people, places, and routines still exist. One can easily understand why change such as hospitalization represents such a threat to these children. Without the comfortable rituals, there is little opportunity to exert autonomy. Consequently, dependency and regression occur (see Regression, p. 1029).

Erikson focuses on the development of the *ego,* which may be thought of as reason or common sense, during this phase of psychosocial development. There is a struggle as the child deals with the impulses of the *id* and attempts to tolerate frustration and learn socially acceptable ways of interacting with the environment. The *ego* is evident as the child is able to tolerate delayed gratification.

There is also a rudimentary beginning of the *superego,* or conscience, which is the incorporation of the morals of society and the process of acculturation. With the development of the ego, children further differentiate themselves from others and expand their sense of trust within themselves. But as they begin to develop awareness of their own will and capacity to achieve, they also become aware of their ability to fail. This ever-present awareness of potential failure creates doubt and shame. Successful mastery of the task of autonomy necessitates opportunities for self-mastery while withstanding the frustration of necessary limit setting and delayed gratification. Opportunities for self-mastery are present in appropriate play activities, toilet training, the crisis of sibling rivalry, and successful interactions with significant others.

Cognitive Development

Sensorimotor and Preoperational Phase (Piaget)

The period from 12 to 24 months of age is a continuation of the final two stages of the sensorimotor phase. During this time the cognitive processes develop rapidly and at times seem similar to those of mature thinking. However, reasoning skills are still primitive and need to be understood to effectively deal with the typical behaviors of a child of this age.

Tertiary Circular Reactions

In the fifth stage of the sensorimotor phase (13 to 18 months of age), the child uses active experimentation to achieve previously unattainable goals. Newly acquired physical skills are increasingly important for the function they serve rather than for the acts themselves. The child incorporates the old learning of secondary circular reactions with new skills and applies the combined knowledge to new situations, with emphasis on the results of the experimentation. In this way there is the beginning of rational judgment and intellectual reasoning. During this stage there is further differentiation of one's self from objects. This is evident in the child's increasing ability to venture away from the parent and to tolerate longer periods of separation.

Awareness of a causal relationship between two events is apparent. After flipping a light switch, toddlers are aware that a reciprocal response occurs. However, they are not able to transfer that knowledge to new situations. Therefore, every time they see what appears to be a light switch, they must reinvestigate its function. Such behavior demonstrates the beginning of categorizing data into distinct classes and subclasses. Examples of this type of behavior are innumerable as toddlers continuously explore the same object each time it appears in a new place.

Because classification of objects is still rudimentary, the appearance of an object denotes its function. For example, if the child's toys are stored in a paper bag or large container, that toy receptacle is no different from the garbage pail or laundry basket. If allowed to turn over the toy receptacle, the child will just as quickly do the same to other similar containers because, in the child's mind, there is no difference. Expecting the child to judge which receptacles are permissible to explore and which are not is inappropriate for this age group. Instead, the forbidden object, such as the garbage pail, should be placed out of reach. This has significance in relation to protecting the toddler from injury; the toddler is not able to differentiate between what is a safe object to play with in any given situation and what is unsafe in another. For example, if the child is allowed to throw a toy ball, he or she does not necessarily understand why a different toy that may harm someone cannot be thrown as well.

The discovery of objects as objects leads to the awareness of their spatial relationships. Children are able to recognize different shapes and their relationship to each other. For example, they can fit slightly smaller boxes into each other (nesting) and can place a round object into a hole, even if the board is turned around, upside down, or reversed. Children are also aware of space and the relationship of their body to dimensions such as height. They will stretch, stand on a low stair or stool, and pull a string to reach an object.

Object permanence has also advanced. Although they still cannot find an object that has been invisibly displaced or moved from under one pillow to another without their seeing the change, toddlers are increasingly aware of the existence of objects behind closed doors, in drawers, on countertops, and under tables. Parents are usually acutely aware of this developmental achievement and find high places and locked cabinets the only places inaccessible to toddlers.

Invention of New Means Through Mental Combinations

From ages 19 to 24 months the child is in the final sensorimotor stage. During this stage the child completes the more primitive, autistic-like thought processes of infancy and is prepared for the more complex mental operations that occur during the phase of preoperational thought. One of the most dramatic achievements of this stage is in the area of object permanence. Children will now actively search for an object in several potential hiding places. In addition, they can infer a cause when only experiencing the effect. They can infer that an object was hidden in any number of places even if they only saw the original hiding place.

Imitation displays deeper meaning and understanding. There is greater symbolization to imitation. The child is acutely aware of others' actions and attempts to copy them in gestures and in words. *Domestic mimicry* (imitating household activities) and gender-role behavior become increasingly common during this stage, especially during the second year. Identification with the parent of the same gender becomes apparent by the second year and represents the child's intellectual ability to identify different models of behavior and to imitate them appropriately (Fig. 37-2).

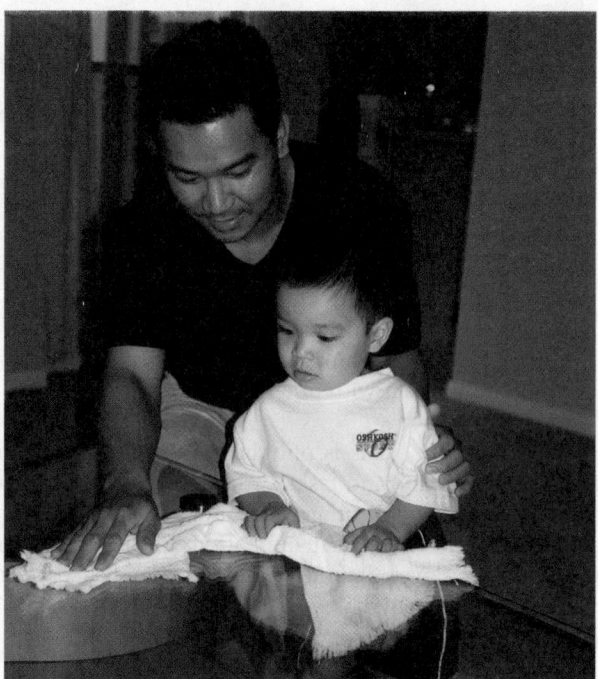

Fig. 37-2 Domestic mimicry and sex-role behavior are common during toddlerhood.

The concept of time is still embryonic, but children have some sense of timing in terms of anticipation, memory, and a limited ability to wait. They may listen to the command, "Just a minute," and behave appropriately. However, their sense of time is exaggerated—1 minute can seem like an hour. Toddlers' limited attention spans also indicate their sense of immediacy and concern for the present.

Preoperational Phase

At approximately 2 years of age the child enters the preconceptual phase of cognitive development, which lasts until about age 4 years. The preconceptual phase is a subdivision of the preoperational phase, which spans ages 2 to 7 years. The preconceptual phase is primarily one of transition that bridges the purely self-satisfying behavior of infancy and the rudimentary socialized behavior of latency. *Preoperational thought* implies that children cannot think in terms of *operations*—the ability to manipulate objects in relation to each other in a logical fashion. Rather, toddlers think primarily on the basis of their perception of an event. Problem solving is based on what they see or hear directly rather than on what they recall about objects and events. Several characteristics are unique to preoperational thought (Box 37-1).

Within the second year the child increasingly uses language symbolically and is concerned with the "why" and "how" of things. For example, a pencil is "something to write with," and food is "something to eat." However, such mental sym-

BOX 37-1 Characteristics of Preoperational Thought

Egocentrism—Inability to envision situations from perspectives other than one's own
- *Example*—If a person is positioned between the toddler and another child, the toddler, who is facing the person, will explain that both children can see the middle person's face. The young child is unable to realize that the other person views the middle person from a different perspective, the back.
- *Implication*—Avoid moralizing about "why" something is wrong if it requires an understanding of someone else's feelings or opinion. Telling a child to stop hitting because hitting hurts the other person is often ineffective because, to the aggressor, it feels good to hit someone else. Instead, emphasize that hitting is not allowed.

Transductive reasoning—Reasoning from the particular to the particular
- *Example*—Child refuses to eat a food because something previously eaten did not taste good.
- *Implication*—Accept child's reasoning; offer refused food at different time.

Global organization—Reasoning that changing any one part of the whole changes the entire whole
- *Example*—Child refuses to sleep in room because location of bed is changed.
- *Implication*—Accept child's reasoning; use same bed position or introduce change slowly.

Centration—Focusing on one aspect rather than considering all possible alternatives.
- *Example*—Child refuses to eat a food because of its color, even though its taste and smell are acceptable.
- *Implication*—Accept child's reasoning.

Animism—Attributing lifelike qualities to inanimate objects
- *Example*—Child scolds stairs for making child fall down.
- *Implication*—Join child in the "scolding." Keep frightening objects out of view.

Irreversibility—Inability to undo or reverse the actions initiated physically
- *Example*—When told to stop doing something, such as talking, child is unable to think of positive activity.
- *Implication*—State requests or instructions *positively* (e.g., "Be quiet.")

Magical thinking—Believing that thoughts are all-powerful and can cause events
- *Examples*—Child wishes someone died; then if the person dies, child feels at fault because of the "bad" thought that made the death happen.
  - Calling children "bad" because they did something wrong makes children feel as if they are bad.
- *Implications*—Clarify that thoughts do not make things happen and that child is not responsible.
  - Use "I" messages rather than "you" messages to communicate thoughts, feelings, expectations, or beliefs without imposing blame or criticism. Emphasize that the act is bad, not the child.

Inability to conserve—Inability to understand the idea that a mass can be changed in size, shape, volume, or length without losing or adding to the original mass (instead, children judge what they see by the immediate perceptual clues given to them)
- *Example*—If two lines of equal length are presented in such a way that one appears longer than the other, child will state that one line is longer even if child measures both lines with a ruler or yardstick and finds that each has the same length.
- *Implications*—Change the most obvious perceptual clue to reorient child's view of what is seen. For example, give medicine in a small medicine cup, rather than a large cup, since child will imagine that the large vessel contains more liquid. If child refuses the medicine in the small cup, pour it into a large cup, because the liquid will appear to be less in a tall, wide container.
  - Give a large, flat cookie rather than a thick, small one, or do the reverse with meat or cheese; child will usually eat larger size of favorite food and smaller size of less favorite food.

bolization is closely associated with prelogical reasoning. For instance, a needle is "something that hurts." Such painful experiences take on new significance because memory is associated with the specific event, and fears are likely to develop, such as resistance to people who wear a uniform or rooms that look like the practitioner's office. Because of the vulnerability of these early years, it is essential to prepare children for any new experience, whether it is a new baby-sitter or a visit to the practitioner or dentist.

Spiritual Development

Spiritual development in children is often discussed in terms of the child's developmental level because the evolution of spirituality often parallels cognitive development (Elkins & Cavendish, 2004). The child's family and environment strongly influence the child's perception of the world around him or her, and this often includes spirituality. Furthermore, family values, beliefs, customs, and expressions of these will influence the child's perception of his or her spiritual self (Elkins & Cavendish, 2004). The relationship between spirituality, illness in childhood, and nursing has been studied in the context of suffering, terminal illness such as cancer, and end-of-life care. In the past two decades there has been an increased interest in and focus on spiritual care in adults and children as further understanding of the influence of one's spirituality on health, illness, and well-being has progressed.

Toddlers learn about God through the words and the actions of those closest to them. They have only a vague idea of God and religious teachings because of their immature cognitive processes; however, if God is spoken about with reverence, young children associate God with something special. During this period the designation of powerful religious symbols and images is strongly influenced by the manner in which they are presented; therein lies the potential for the development of guilt and fear or, conversely, love and companionship with religious symbols (Roehlkepartain et al, 2006).

Toddlers begin to assimilate behaviors associated with the divine (folding hands in prayer). Routines such as saying prayers before meals or at bedtime can be important and comforting. Near the end of toddlerhood, when children use preoperational thought, there is some advancement of their understanding of God. Religious teachings, such as reward or fear of punishment (heaven or hell) and moral development (see Chapter 32), may influence their behavior (Fosarelli, 2003).

Development of Body Image

As in infancy, the development of body image closely parallels cognitive development. Developing psychologic understanding provides greater self-awareness, and young children learn to answer the question "Who am I?" During the second year, children recognize themselves in a mirror and make verbal references to themselves ("Me big"). With increasing motor ability, toddlers recognize the usefulness of body parts and gradually learn their names. They also learn that certain parts of the body have various meanings; for example, during toilet training the genitalia become significant and cleanliness is emphasized. By 2 years of age there is recognition of gender differences and reference to self by name and then by pronoun. Gender identity is developed by age 3 years. Also by this time the child begins to remember events with reference to their personal significance, forming an autobiographic memory that helps establish a continuous identity throughout life's events (Thompson, 2001).

Once they begin preoperational thought, toddlers can use symbols to represent objects, but their thinking may lead to inaccuracies. For example, if someone who is pregnant is called "fat," they will describe all "fat" women as having babies. There is a beginning recognition of words used to describe physical appearance, such as "pretty," "handsome," or "big boy." Such expressions eventually influence how children view their own bodies.

Although little research has been done on body-image development in young children, it is evident that body integrity is poorly understood and that intrusive experiences are threatening (Dahlquist et al, 2002). For example, toddlers forcefully resist procedures such as examining the ear or mouth and taking an axillary temperature. The procedure itself (e.g., taking vital signs) is not hurting the child, but it represents an intrusion into the child's personal space, which will elicit a strong protest. Toddlers also have unclear body boundaries and may associate nonviable parts, such as feces, with essential body parts. This can be seen in a toddler who is upset by flushing the toilet and watching the stool disappear.

Nurses can assist parents in fostering a positive body image in their child by encouraging them to avoid negative labels, such as "skinny arms" or "chubby legs," self-perceptions that can last a lifetime. Body parts, especially those related to elimination and reproduction, should be called by their correct names. Respect for the body should be practiced.

Development of Gender Identity

Just as toddlers explore their environment, they also explore their bodies and find that touching certain body parts is pleasurable. Masturbation can occur and involves manual stimulation of genitalia and posturing movements against objects. If performed in public, the behavior should be ignored. The child should be taught that it is more acceptable to perform the behavior in private (Meyer, 2002). Other demonstrations of pleasurable activities include rocking, sucking on fingers, swinging, and hugging people and toys. During the activity the child may perspire, and the activity may be difficult to interrupt.

Children in this age group are learning vocabulary associated with anatomy, elimination, and reproduction. Certain associations between words and functions become significant and can influence future sexual attitudes. For example, if parents refer to the genitalia as dirty, especially in the context of elimination, this association between "genitalia" and "dirty" may be transferred to sexual functions. Sex-role differences become obvious to children and are evident in much of their imitative play. A sense of maleness or femaleness, *gender identity,* is formed by age 3 years. Early attitudes are formed about affectionate behaviors between adults from observing parental and other adult intimate behaviors such as kissing and hugging (see also Sex Education, Chapter 38). The quality of relationships with parents is important to the child's capacity for sexual and emotional relationships later in life (DeLamater & Friedrich, 2002).

Social Development

A major task of the toddler period is differentiation of self from significant others, usually the mother. The differentiation process consists of two phases: *separation,* the child's emergence from a symbiotic fusion with the mother; and *individuation,* those achievements that mark the child's expressions of his or her individual characteristics in the environment. Although the process begins during the latter half of infancy, the major achievements occur during the toddler years.

Toddlers have an increased understanding and awareness of object permanence and some ability to withstand delayed gratification and tolerate moderate frustration. As a result, toddlers react differently to strangers than do infants. The appearance of unfamiliar persons does not represent such a significant threat to their attachment to mother. They have learned from experience that parents still exist when physically absent. Repetition of events such as going to bed without the parents but waking to find them there again (in the household) reinforces the reliability of such brief separations. Consequently toddlers are able to venture away from their parents for brief periods.

According to Harpaz-Rotem and Bergman (2006), the separation-individuation phase encompasses the phenomenon of *rapprochement;* as the toddler separates from the mother and begins to make sense of experiences in the environment, he or she is drawn back to the mother for assistance in verbally articulating the meaning of the experiences. Developmentally the term *rapprochement* means the child moves away and returns for reassurance. If the mother's response to the toddler is inappropriate, the toddler may experience insecurity and confusion.

Transitional objects, such as a favorite blanket or toy, provide security for children, especially when they are sepa-

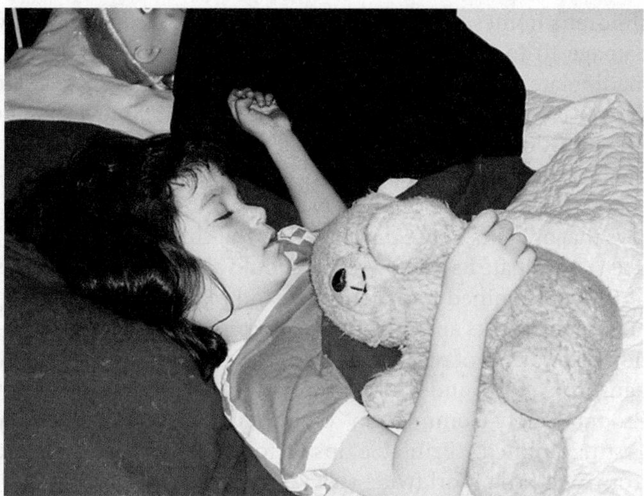

Fig. 37-3 Transitional objects, such as a fuzzy stuffed animal, are sources of security to a toddler.

rated from parents, dealing with a new stress, or just fatigued (Fig. 37-3). Security objects often become so important to toddlers that they refuse to have them taken away. Such behavior is normal; there is no need to discourage this tendency. During separations such as day care, hospitalization, or even overnight stays with relatives, transitional objects should be provided to minimize any feelings of fear or loneliness.

Learning to tolerate and master brief periods of separation is an important developmental task of children in this age group. In addition, it is a necessary component of parenting, since brief periods of separation allow parents to regain their energy and patience and to minimize any tendency to direct their irritations and frustrations at the children.

Language

The most striking characteristic of language development during early childhood is the increasing level of comprehension. Although the number of words acquired—from about 4 at 1 year of age to approximately 300 at age 2 years—is notable, *the ability to comprehend and understand speech is much greater than the number of words the child can say.* Bilingual children also achieve their early linguistic milestones in each of the languages at the same time and produce a substantial number of semantically corresponding words in each of their two languages from the very first words or signs (Petitto et al, 2001).

At age 1 year the child uses one-word sentences or holophrases. The word "up" can mean "pick me up" or "look up there." For the child, the one word conveys the meaning of a sentence, but to others it may mean many things or nothing. At this age about 25% of the vocalizations are intelligible. By the age of 2 years the child uses multiword sentences by stringing together two or three words, such as the phrases, "mama go bye-bye" or "all gone," and approximately 65% of the speech is understandable. By 3 years the child puts words together into simple sentences, begins to master grammatical rules, and acquires five or six new words daily.

Gestures precede or accompany each of the language milestones up to 30 months of age (putting phone to ear, pointing). Once language is sufficiently mastered, gestures phase out and the pace of word learning increases (Bates & Dick, 2002).

Personal-Social Behavior

One of the most dramatic aspects of development in the toddler is personal-social interaction. Parents often wonder why their manageable, docile, lovable infant has turned into a determined, strong-willed, volatile little tyrant. In addition, the tyrant of the terrible twos can swiftly and unpredictably revert back to the adorable, cuddly child. All of this is part of growing up and is evident in such areas as dressing, feeding, playing, and establishing self-control.

Toddlers are developing skills of independence, and these are evident in all areas of behavior. By 15 months children feed themselves, drink well from a covered cup, and manage a spoon with considerable spilling. By 24 months they use a spoon well and by 36 months may be using a fork. Between ages 2 and 3 years they eat with the family and like to help with chores such as setting the table or removing dishes from the dishwasher. However, they lack table manners and may find it difficult to sit through the family's entire meal.

In dressing, toddlers also demonstrate strides in independence. The 15-month-old child helps by putting the arm or foot out for dressing and pulls shoes and socks off. The 18-month-old child removes gloves, helps with pullover shirts, and may be able to unzip. By age 2 years the toddler removes most articles of clothing and puts on socks, shoes, and pants without regard to right or left and back or front. Help is still needed to fasten clothes.

Toddlers also begin to develop concern for the feelings of others and develop an understanding of how adult expectations for behavior apply to specific situations (e.g., causing a sibling to cry while playing rough) (Thompson, 2001). As parents foster their understanding, they are able to develop control. Age-appropriate discipline contributes to healthy social and emotional development. Positive reinforcement, redirecting, and time-out are appropriate for most toddlers. Social and emotional problems can develop in the youngest children. Early screening and intervention promote more positive developmental outcomes as the young child grows and develops.

Play

Play magnifies the toddler's physical and psychosocial development. Interaction with people becomes increasingly important. The solitary play of infancy progresses to *parallel play*—the toddler plays alongside, not with, other children. Although sensorimotor play is still prominent, there is much less emphasis on the exclusive use of one sensory modality. The toddler inspects the toy, talks to the toy, tests its strength and durability, and invents several uses for it. Imitation is one of the most distinguishing characteristics of play and enriches the child's opportunity to engage in fantasy. With less emphasis on gender-stereotyped toys, play objects such as dolls, carriages, dollhouses, dishes, balls, clay, cooking utensils, child-size furniture, trucks, and dress-up clothes (Fig. 37-4) are suitable for both genders; however, boys may be more interested than girls in activities related to trucks, trailers, cars, miniature plastic soldiers or super

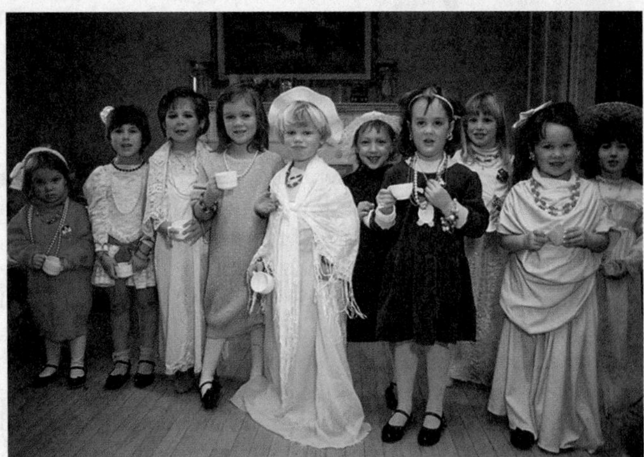

Fig. 37-4 Young children enjoy dressing up.

heroes, and building blocks, whereas girls may prefer doll-related activities.

Increased locomotive skills make push-pull toys, straddle trucks or cycles, a small gym and slide, balls of various sizes, and rocking horses appropriate for the energetic toddler. Finger paints; thick crayons; chalk; a blackboard; paper; and puzzles with large, simple pieces use the child's developing fine motor skills. Interlocking blocks in various sizes and shapes provide hours of fun and, during later years, are useful objects for creative and imaginative play. The most educational toy is the one that fosters the interaction of an adult with a child in supportive, unconditional play. Toys are never substitutes for the attention of devoted caregivers, but toys can enhance these interactions (Glassy, Romano, & Committee on Early Childhood, Adoption, and Dependent Care, 2003).

Certain aspects of play are related to emerging linguistic abilities. Talking is a form of play for toddlers who enjoy musical toys such as age-appropriate cassette tape players, "talking" dolls and animals, and toy telephones. Appropriate children's television programs are excellent for children in this age group, who learn to associate words with visual images. However, total media time should be limited to 1 to 2 hours of quality programming per day (American Academy of Pediatrics, Committee on Public Health, 2001). Toddlers also enjoy "reading" stories from a picture book and imitating the sounds of animals.

Tactile play is also important for the exploring toddler. Water toys, a sandbox with pail and shovel, finger paints, soap bubbles, and clay provide excellent opportunities for creative and manipulative recreation. Adults sometimes forget the fascination of feeling slippery cream, mud, or pudding; catching airy bubbles; squeezing and reshaping clay; or smearing paints. These types of unstructured activities are as important as educational play to allow children freedom of expression.

Selection of appropriate toys must involve safety factors, especially in relation to size and sturdiness. Toddlers' oral activity puts them at risk for aspirating small objects or for ingesting toxic substances. Parents need to be especially vigilant of toys of older siblings or those played with in other children's homes. Toys are a potential source of serious bodily damage to toddlers, who may have the physical strength to manipulate them but not the knowledge to appreciate their danger (see Family-Centered Care box, p. 858). Government agencies do not inspect and police all toys on the market. Therefore adults who purchase play equipment, supervise purchases, or allow children to use play equipment (including toys that are gifts or are purchased by the children themselves) need to evaluate its safety. Adults should also be alert to notices of toys determined to be defective and recalled by the manufacturers. Parents and health care workers can obtain information on a variety of recalled products and can report potentially dangerous toys and child products to the U.S. Consumer Product Safety Commission* or, in Canada, the Canadian Toy Testing Council.† Printable tips on toy safety are also available from Safe Kids Worldwide *(www.safekids.org)*.

The major features of growth and development for the age groups of 15, 18, 24, and 30 months are summarized in Table 37-1.

Coping with Concerns Related to Normal Growth and Development

Toilet Training

One of the major tasks of toddlerhood is toilet training. Voluntary control of the anal and urethral sphincters is achieved sometime after the child is walking, probably between ages 18 and 24 months. However, complex psychophysiologic factors are required for readiness. The child must be able to recognize the urge to let go and hold on and be able to communicate this sensation to the parent. In addition, there may be some necessary motivation in the desire to please the parent by holding on, rather than pleasing oneself by letting go.

Schmitt (2004) notes that comparative studies over the past five decades indicate that children in the 1990s in the United States were toilet trained at a later age (18 months in the 1960s vs. 36 months in the 1990s). One possible contributing factor is the availability and convenience of disposable diapers.

Five markers signal a child's readiness to toilet train: bladder readiness, bowel readiness, cognitive readiness, motor readiness, and psychologic readiness (Schmitt, 2004). According to some experts, physiologic and psychologic readiness is not complete until ages 22 to 30 months (Schum et al, 2002). However, Schmitt (2004) emphasizes that parents should begin preparing the child for toilet training earlier than 30 months. By this time the child has mastered the majority of essential gross motor skills, can communicate intelligibly, is in less conflict with parents in terms of self-assertion and negativism, and is aware of the ability to control the body and please the parent. There is no universal right age to begin toilet training or an absolute deadline to complete training. One of the nurse's most important responsibilities is to help

evolve Case Study–Toilet Training/Toddler Development

*800-638-2772; www.cpsc.gov *(assistance is also available in Spanish)*.
†*1973 Baseline Road, Ottawa ON K2C 0C7 Canada; 613-228-3155; fax: 613-228-3242;* www.toy-testing.org.

Table 37-1 Growth and Development During Toddler Years

AGE (mo)	PHYSICAL	GROSS MOTOR	FINE MOTOR	SENSORY	LANGUAGE	SOCIALIZATION
15	Steady growth in height and weight Head circumference 48 cm (19 inches) Weight 11 kg (24 lb) Height 78.7 cm (31 inches)	Walks without help (usually since age 13 mo) Creeps up stairs Kneels without support Cannot walk around corners or stop suddenly without losing balance Cannot throw ball without falling Runs clumsily; falls often	Constantly casting objects to floor Builds tower of two cubes Holds two cubes in one hand Releases a pellet into a narrow-necked bottle Scribbles spontaneously Uses cup well but rotates spoon before it reaches mouth	Able to identify geometric forms; places round object into appropriate hole Binocular vision well developed Displays an intense and prolonged interest in pictures	Uses expressive jargon Says four to six words, including names "Asks" for objects by pointing Understands simple commands May use head-shaking gesture to denote "no" Uses "no" even while agreeing to the request Uses common repetitive gestures such as putting cup to mouth when empty	Tolerates some separation from parent Less likely to fear strangers Beginning to imitate parents, such as cleaning house (sweeping, dusting), folding clothes May discard bottle Kisses and hugs parents; may kiss pictures in a book
18	Picky eater from decreased growth needs Anterior fontanel closed Physiologically able to control sphincters	Assumes standing position without support Walks up stairs with one hand held Pulls and pushes toys Jumps in place with both feet Seats self on chair Throws ball overhand without falling	Builds tower of three or four cubes Release, prehension, and reach well developed Turns pages in a book two or three at a time In drawing, makes stroke imitatively Manages spoon without rotation		Says 10 or more words Points to a common object, such as a shoe or ball, and to two or three body parts Forms word combinations Forms gesture-word combinations Forms gesture-gesture combinations	Expresses emotions; has temper tantrums Great imitator (domestic mimicry) Takes off gloves, socks, and shoes and unzips Temper tantrums may be more evident Beginning awareness of ownership ("my toy") May develop dependence on transitional objects, such as "security blanket"
24	Head circumference 49-50 cm (19.3-20 inches) Chest circumference exceeds head circumference Lateral diameter of chest exceeds anteroposterior diameter Usual weight gain of 1.8-2.7 kg (4-6 lb) Usual gain in height of 10-12.5 cm (4-5 inches) Adult height approximately double height at 2 years of age May have achieved readiness for beginning daytime control of bowel and bladder Primary dentition of 16 teeth	Goes up and down stairs alone with two feet on each step Runs fairly well, with wide stance Picks up object without falling Kicks ball forward without overbalancing	Builds tower of six or seven cubes Aligns two or more cubes like a train Turns pages of book one at a time In drawing, imitates vertical and circular strokes Turns doorknob; unscrews lid	Accommodation well developed In geometric discrimination, able to insert square block into oblong space	Has vocabulary of approximately 300 words Uses two- or three-word phrases Uses pronouns "I," "me," "you" Understands directional commands Gives first name; refers to self by name Verbalizes need for toileting, food, or drink Talks incessantly	Stage of parallel play Has sustained attention span Temper tantrums decreasing Pulls people to show them something Increased independence from parent Dresses self in simple clothing Develops visual recognition and verbal self-reference ("Me big")

Continued

Table 37-1 Growth and Development During Toddler Years—cont'd

AGE (mo)	PHYSICAL	GROSS MOTOR	FINE MOTOR	SENSORY	LANGUAGE	SOCIALIZATION
30	Birth weight quadrupled Primary dentition (20 teeth) completed May have daytime bowel and bladder control	Jumps with both feet Jumps from chair or step Stands on one foot momentarily Takes a few steps on tiptoe	Builds tower of eight cubes Adds chimney to train of cubes Good hand-finger coordination; holds crayon with fingers rather than fist Moves fingers independently In drawing, imitates vertical and horizontal strokes; makes two or more strokes for cross		Gives first and last name Refers to self by appropriate pronoun Uses plurals Names one color	Separates more easily from parent In play, helps put things away; can carry breakable objects; pushes with good steering Begins to notice sex differences; knows own sex May attend to toilet needs without help except for wiping Emotions expand to include pride, shame, guilt, embarrassment

parents identify the readiness signs in their child (see Guidelines box).* On average, girls are developmentally ready to begin toilet training 2 to 2½ months before boys (Schum et al, 2002).

GUIDELINES Assessing Toilet Training Readiness

Physical Readiness

Voluntary control of anal and urethral sphincters, usually by 18 to 24 months of age

Ability to stay dry for 2 hours; decreased number of wet diapers; waking dry from nap

Regular bowel movements

Gross motor skills of sitting, walking, and squatting

Fine motor skills to remove clothing

Mental Readiness

Recognizing urge to defecate or urinate

Verbal or nonverbal communicative skills to indicate when wet or has urge to defecate or urinate

Cognitive skills to imitate appropriate behavior and follow directions

Psychologic Readiness

Expressing willingness to please parent

Ability to sit on toilet for 5 to 10 minutes without fussing or getting off

Curiosity about adults' or older sibling's toilet habits

Impatience with soiled or wet diapers; desire to be changed immediately

Parental Readiness

Recognizing child's level of readiness

Willingness to invest the time required for toilet training

Absence of family stress or change, such as a divorce, moving, new sibling, or imminent vacation

**A helpful book is* Guide to Toilet Training, *available from the American Academy of Pediatrics, 847-434-4000;* www.aap.org/bookstore. *Additional resources are listed in the Schmitt (2004) reference.*

Nighttime bladder control normally takes several months to years after daytime training. This is because the sleep cycle needs to mature so the child can awake in time to urinate. Few children will have night wetting episodes after daytime dryness is achieved; however, those children who do not have nighttime dryness by the age of 6 years are likely to require intervention (Mercer, 2003).

Bowel training is usually accomplished before bladder training because of its greater regularity and predictability. There is a stronger sensation for defecation than for urination, and the sensation of defecation can be brought to the child's attention. A well-balanced diet that includes dietary fiber helps keep stool soft and supports the development and maintenance of regular bowel movements.

A number of techniques can be helpful when initiating training, and cultural differences should be considered. Parents should begin the readiness phase of toilet training by teaching the child how the body functions in relation to voiding and having a stool. Schmitt (2004) suggests that parents talk about how adults and animals perform such functions on a routine basis. Another suggestion is to make toilet training as easy and simple as possible. The selection of the child's clothing is an important consideration, as is the potty chair or use of the toilet. A freestanding potty chair allows children a feeling of security. Planting the feet firmly on the floor also facilitates defecation. Another option is a portable seat attached to the regular toilet, which may ease the transition from potty chair to regular toilet (Fig. 37-5). Placing a small bench under the feet helps stabilize the child's position. It is probably best to keep the potty in the bathroom and to let the child observe the excreta being flushed down the toilet to associate these activities with usual practices. If a potty chair is not available, having the child sit facing the toilet tank provides added support.

Practice sessions should be limited to 5 to 8 minutes, and a parent should stay with the child, practicing sanitary habits after every session. Children should be praised for cooperative behavior and successful evacuation. Dressing children in easily removed clothing; using training pants, "pull-on"

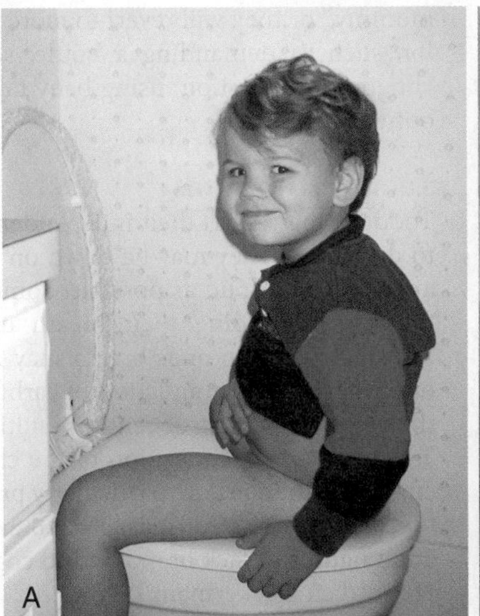

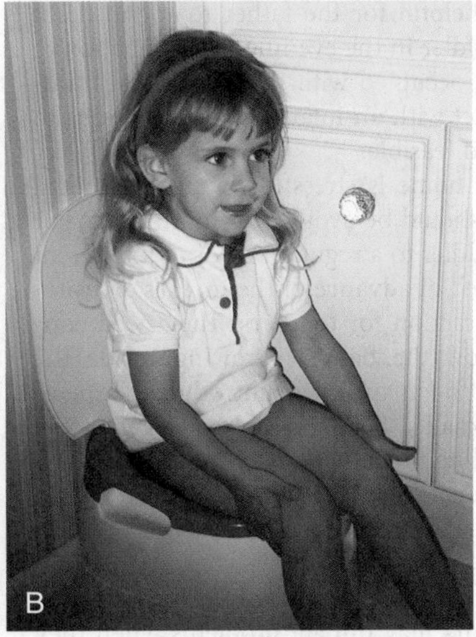

Fig. 37-5 **A,** Sitting in reverse fashion on a regular toilet provides additional security to a young child. **B,** Children may begin toilet training sitting on a small potty chair.

diapers, or underwear; and encouraging imitation by watching others are other helpful suggestions.

When the child begins to experience regular daytime dryness, parents may experiment with underwear during the day. Daytime accidents are common, particularly during periods of intense activity. Young children become so engrossed in play that, if they are not reminded, they will wait until it is too late to reach the bathroom. Therefore frequent reminders and trips to the toilet are necessary. Parents often forget to plan ahead when the toddler is being toilet trained; before trips outside the house it is important to remind the child to at least try to urinate to decrease the chance of needing to use the toilet while the car is stuck in traffic.

As the child develops each step of toileting (discussion, undressing, going, wiping, dressing, flushing, and handwashing), he or she gains a sense of accomplishment that parents should reinforce. If the parent-child relationship becomes strained, both may need a break from toilet training to focus on enjoyable activities together. Regression may coincide with a stressful family situation or may occur if the child is being pushed too hard and too fast. Regression is a normal part of toilet training and does not mean failure but should be viewed as a temporary setback to a more comfortable place for the child.

Day care providers also play a role in the support and education of parents regarding toilet training practices. It is important for parents to inform all caregivers of their individual family values and the child's specific needs when planning for training away from home. Ensuring consistency in care of the toddler and healthy practices in a sanitary environment allows for safe and effective toilet practices in all settings.

Once the child has been successfully toilet trained for bladder control, sudden wetting accidents and frequent urinating urges may require further investigation for a possible urinary tract infection (UTI), especially in girls. Younger children often have a UTI without accompanying fever or painful urination.

Sibling Rivalry

The natural jealousy and resentment of children to a new child in the family is referred to as *sibling rivalry.* The arrival of a new infant represents a crisis for even the best-prepared toddlers. It is not the infant that toddlers resent but the changes that this additional sibling produces, especially the separation from mother during the birth. The parents now share their love and attention with someone else, the usual routine is disrupted, and toddlers may lose their crib or room, all at a time when they thought they were in control of their world. Sibling rivalry tends to be most pronounced in the firstborn, who experiences *dethronement* (i.e., loss of sole parental attention). It also seems to be most difficult for young children, particularly in terms of mother-child interaction.

Preparation of children for the birth of a sibling is individual, but age dictates some important considerations. Time for toddlers is a vague concept. Tomorrow could be yesterday or next week, and a month from now could be never. Preparing children too soon for the birth may lessen their interest by the time the event occurs. A good time to start talking about the new baby is when the toddler becomes aware of the pregnancy and the changes taking place in the home in anticipation of the new member.

Toddlers need to have a realistic idea of what the newborn will be like. Telling them that a new playmate will come home soon sets up unrealistic expectations. Rather, parents should stress the activities that will take place when the baby arrives home, such as diapering, bottle-feeding or breastfeeding, bathing, and dressing. At the same time, parents should emphasize which routines will stay the same, such as reading stories or going to the park. The disruption of the toddler's routine is significant but can be restored with some effort by the parents. It may be helpful for the father to spend more quality time with the toddler in the evening in anticipation of the mother's time being occupied with the new baby. If toddlers have had no contact with an infant, it is a good idea to introduce them to one, if feasible.

A new sibling in the home is stressful, so any additional stresses for the toddler should be avoided or minimized. For example, moving the toddler to a regular bed or to a different room should be done well in advance of the infant's arrival.

Pregnancy is an abstraction for toddlers. They need concrete illustrations of how the baby is growing inside the mother. It is an excellent opportunity for introducing aspects of reproduction and sexuality. Seeing simple pictures of the uterus and fetus and feeling the fetus move help the child feel involved in the experience (see Fig. 11-3). Children also benefit from classes for siblings that may be part of prenatal sessions (see Fig. 11-4).

When the newborn arrives, toddlers keenly feel the changed focus of attention. Visitors may initiate problems when they inadvertently shower the infant with attention and presents while neglecting the older child. Parents can minimize this by alerting visitors to the toddler's needs and by including the child in the visits as much as possible. The toddler can also help with the care of the newborn by getting diapers and doing other small tasks (Fig. 37-6).

How children exhibit jealousy is complex. Some will overtly hit the infant, push the child off the mother's lap, or pull the bottle or breast from the infant's mouth. For this reason, infants must be protected by parental supervision of the interaction between the siblings. More often the expressions of hostility and resentment are more subtle and covert. Toddlers may verbally express a wish that the infant "go back inside mommy," or they will revert to more infantile forms of behavior, such as demanding a bottle, soiling their underpants, clinging for attention, using baby talk, or aggressively acting out toward others.

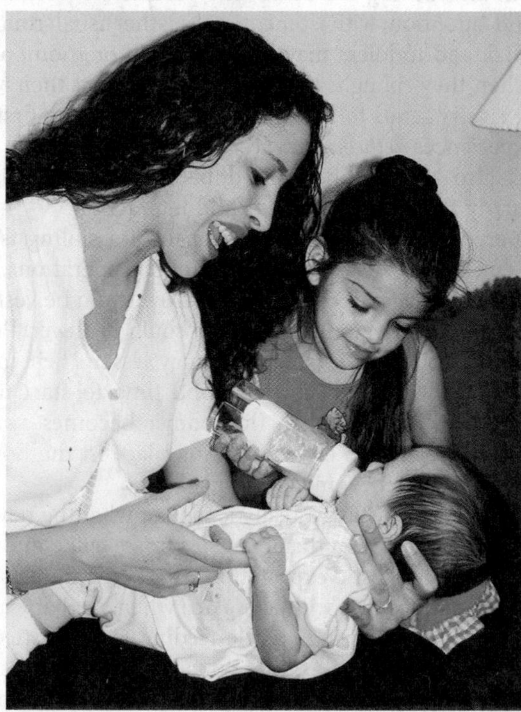

Fig. 37-6 To minimize sibling rivalry, parents should include the toddler during caregiving activities.

Temper Tantrums

Toddlers may assert their independence by violently objecting to discipline. They may lie down on the floor, kick their feet, and scream as loud as possible. Some have learned the effectiveness of holding their breath until the parent relents. Although holding one's breath may cause fainting from lack of oxygen, the accumulation of carbon dioxide will stimulate the respiratory control center, resulting in no physical harm. Tantrums are an indication of the child's inability to control emotions; toddlers are particularly prone to tantrums because their strong drive for mastery and autonomy is frustrated by adult figures or lack of motor and cognitive skills (Needlman, Howard, & Zuckerman, 1995).

The best approach toward tapering temper tantrums requires consistency and developmentally appropriate expectations and rewards. Ensuring consistency among all caregivers in expectations, prioritizing what rules are important, and developing consequences that are reasonable for the child's level of development help manage the behavior. For example, a popular time for a tantrum is before bed. Active toddlers often have trouble slowing down and, when placed in bed, resist staying there. Parents can reinforce consistency and expectations by stating, "After this story it is bedtime." Starting at 18 months, time-outs work well for managing temper tantrums.

During tantrums ignore the behavior, provided the behavior is not injurious to the child, such as violently banging the head on the floor. Continue to be present to provide a feeling of control and security to the child once the tantrum has subsided. At this time a toy or a favorite activity can be substituted for the request. (See also Limit Setting and Discipline, Chapter 31.) During periods of no tantrums, practice developmentally appropriate positive reinforcement.

Other suggestions for handling tantrums include (Needlman, Howard, & Zuckerman, 1995):

- Offering the child options instead of an "all or none" position
- Picking one's battles carefully and ignoring small skirmishes over unimportant issues
- Giving comfort once the child is able to control emotions but not giving in to the original request
- Praising the child for positive behavior when he or she is not having a tantrum

Temper tantrums are common during the toddler years and essentially represent normal developmental behaviors. However, temper tantrums can be signs of serious problems. Nurses should be alert to situations that require further evaluation.

Negativism

One of the more difficult aspects of rearing children in this age group is their persistent "no" response to every request. The negativism is not an expression of being stubborn or insolent, but a necessary assertion of self-control. One method of dealing with the negativism is to reduce the opportunities for a "no" answer. Asking the child, "Do you want to go to sleep now?" is an almost certain example of a question that will be answered with an emphatic "no." Instead, tell the child that it is time to go to sleep and proceed accordingly.

In their attempt to exert control, children like to make choices. When confronted with appropriate choices, such as "You may have a peanut-butter-and-jelly sandwich or chicken-noodle soup for lunch," they are more likely to choose one rather than automatically say no. However, if their response is negative, parents should make the choice for the child.

Regression

The retreat from one's present pattern of functioning to past levels of behavior is referred to as *regression.* It usually occurs in instances of discomfort or stress when one attempts to conserve psychic energy by reverting to patterns of behavior that were successful in earlier stages of development. Regression is common in toddlers because almost any additional stress hinders their ability to master present developmental tasks. Any threat to their autonomy, such as illness, hospitalization, separation from parents, or adjustment to a new sibling, represents a need to revert to earlier forms of behavior, such as increased dependency; refusal to use the potty chair; temper tantrums; demand for the bottle, stroller, or crib; and loss of newly learned motor, language, social, and cognitive skills.

At first, such regression appears acceptable and comfortable for children, but the loss of newly acquired achievements is actually frightening and threatening because children are aware of their helplessness. Parents become concerned about regressive behavior and often, in their efforts to deal with it, force the child to cope with an additional source of stress—the pressure to live up to expected standards. Brazelton (1999) suggests that these predictable times of regression, or *touchpoints,* are an opportunity to prepare parents for the next step in their child's development.

When regression does occur, the best approach is to ignore it while praising existing patterns of appropriate behavior. Regression is a child's way of saying, "I can't cope with this present stress and perfect this skill as well, but I will if given patience and understanding." For this reason, it is advisable not to attempt new areas of learning when an additional crisis is present or expected, such as beginning toilet training shortly before a sibling is born or attempting new areas of learning during a brief period of hospitalization.

Promoting Optimum Health During Toddlerhood

Nutrition

During the period from 12 to 18 months of age, the growth rate slows, decreasing the child's need for calories, protein, and fluid. However, the protein (13 g/day) and energy requirements are still relatively high to meet the demands for muscle tissue growth and high activity level. Estimated energy requirements (EER) for toddlers vary by age, gender, and feeding method; for example, an 18-month-old boy weighing 11.7 kg (25.8 lb) would have an EER of 961 kcal/day, whereas an 18-month-old girl with a weight of 10.9 kg (24.2 lb) would have an EER of 899 kcal/day (Institute of Medicine, 2005). The need for minerals such as iron, calcium, and phosphorus may be difficult to meet, considering the characteristic food habits of children in this age group.

At approximately 18 months of age, most toddlers manifest this decreased nutritional need with a decrease in appetite, a phenomenon known as *physiologic anorexia.* They become picky, fussy eaters with strong taste preferences. Toddlers are increasingly aware of the nonnutritive function of food: the pleasure of eating, the social aspect of mealtime, and the control of refusing food. They are influenced by factors other than taste when choosing food. If a family member refuses to eat something, toddlers are likely to imitate that response. If the plate is overfilled, they are likely to push it away, overwhelmed by its size. In essence, mealtime is more closely associated with psychologic components than with nutritional ones.

The ritualism of this age also dictates certain principles in feeding practices. Toddlers like to have the same dish, cup, or spoon every time they eat. They may reject a favorite food simply because it is served in a different dish. If one food touches another, they often refuse to eat it. Mixed foods, such as stews or casseroles, are rarely favorites. For some children a regular mealtime schedule also contributes to their desire and need for predictability and ritualism.

Many authorities consider this period of picky eating to be a developmental phase and stress that most toddlers will consume the necessary amount of food required for growth (Cathey & Gaylord, 2004).

Developmentally, by 12 months of age most children are eating the same food prepared for the rest of the family. Some may have mastered using a cup with occasional spilling, although most cannot adeptly use a spoon until 18 months of age or later and generally prefer using their fingers. Because toddlers have unpredictable table manners, it is best to use plastic dishes and cups, for both economic and safety reasons.

Nutritional Counseling

The emphasis on preventing childhood obesity and subsequent cardiovascular disease in the United States has prompted a number of changes in dietary recommendations for children and adults alike. It is now recognized that lifetime eating habits may be established in early childhood, and health care workers are increasingly emphasizing the role of food selection choices, exercise, stress reduction, and other lifestyle choices (such as tobacco and alcohol use) on the quality of adult life and survival. Conditions such as obesity and cardiovascular disease can be prevented by encouraging healthy eating habits in toddlers and their families.

If food is used as a reward or sign of approval, a child may overeat for nonnutritive reasons. If food is forced and mealtime is consistently unpleasant, the usual pleasure associated with eating may not develop. Mealtimes should be enjoyable rather than times for discipline or family arguments. The social aspect of mealtime may be distracting for young children; therefore an earlier feeding hour may be appropriate. Young children are unable to sit through a long meal and become restless and disruptive. This is particularly common when children are brought to the table just after active play. Calling them in from play 15 minutes before mealtime allows them ample opportunity to get ready for eating while settling down their active minds and bodies.

The method of serving food also takes on more importance during this period. Toddlers need to have a sense of control and achievement in their abilities. Giving them large, adult-size portions can be overwhelming. In general, what is eaten is much more significant than how much is consumed. Small amounts of meat and vegetables supply greater food value than a large consumption of bread or potato. Serving sizes need to be appropriate for age (Box 37-2). Substitutions can be provided for foods that they do not enjoy, although this practice should not cater to all of their desires. Frequent nutritious *planned* snacks may provide adequate caloric intake at this age. *Grazing*—nibbling and snacking—is a good way to ensure proper nutrition, provided that appropriate foods are offered; giving the child something to eat merely to pacify is not recommended.

BOX 37-2 Sample Menu for Toddlers Based on MyPyramid for Kids*

Breakfast

½ cup dry, unsweetened cereal
½ cup orange juice
2 oz low-fat milk†

Snack

½-1 whole banana (cut in small slices)

Lunch

1 slice cheese
2 tsp all-fruit preserves
1 slice whole-wheat bread
2 tbsp peas
2 oz low-fat milk†

Snack

2 graham crackers
2 oz low-fat milk†

Dinner

1 chicken leg, roasted without skin
¼-½ cup macaroni and cheese
2 tbsp green beans, cooked
2 tbsp carrots, cooked
2-3 oz low-fat milk†

Snack

½ cup frozen yogurt

Total (Per Day)

Bread, cereal, rice, pasta: 6 oz
Vegetable: 2½ cups
Fruit (vitamin A and C sources): 1½ cups
Milk, yogurt, cheese, pudding: 2 cups
Meat, poultry, fish, dried beans, eggs, nuts: 5 oz

*Use fats, oils, and sweets sparingly; obtain oils from fish or liquid oils such as corn oil, soybean oil, canola oil. Increase fluids with servings of water. Serving sizes are minimums for nutritional adequacy. Many children eat more. Menu is based on 1800-calorie diet.

†Substitute whole milk (vitamin D fortified) if child is younger than 24 months.

To determine serving size for young children, use the following guidelines:

- A general guide to the serving size of food is 1 tbsp of solid food per year of age, or one fourth to one third of the adult portion size.
- Use the tablespoon guide for easily measured foods such as vegetables or rice.
- Use the fraction guide for bread or milk.

Most children by 12 months of age are eating the same food prepared for the rest of the family. However, mastication skills continue to mature, putting children at risk for choking. Large round foods (hot dogs, grapes, peas, carrots, popcorn, fruit gel snacks) should be avoided. Active play while eating should be discouraged to prevent choking. Appetite and food preferences are sporadic. Often the interest in food parallels a growth spurt, so that periods of good eating are interspersed with phases of poor eating. If exposed to the same food every day, a young toddler does not learn how to manage the complex sensory information needed to eat new, more difficult foods (vegetables with a different texture vs. pureed, slippery fruits). To help prevent "food jags," it is recommended that parents present food in various physical forms. The child may need to progress to eating new foods in a stepwise fashion: visually tolerating the food, interacting with the food, smelling the food, touching the food, tasting, and then eating the food.

This period can be trying for parents and child alike. Because eating habits are established in early life and affect not only the child's future eating habits but also the child's health as an adolescent and adult, it is recommended that toddlers not be forced to eat foods they are reluctant to eat. Evidence indicates that toddlers are able to regulate their hunger and satiety needs internally and that forcing foods during this period may exacerbate or lead to future eating problems (Cathey & Gaylord, 2004). It has also been suggested that parents plan a nutritionally balanced week instead of day because of the way toddlers will restrict food intake in their effort to exert control over their environment (Morin, 2007).

Dietary Guidelines

Dietary guidelines are necessary to promote adequate energy and nutrient intake to support physical, emotional, psychologic, and cognitive development. A number of new dietary guidelines have been developed to address the issue of childhood obesity, sedentary lifestyles, and increase in cardiovascular disease mortality in the United States. Guidelines such as the 2005 American Heart Association Dietary Guidelines provide suggestions for children ages 2 years and up and are discussed in Chapter 47. See also Chapter 47 (pp. 1366-1367) regarding the MyPyramid for Kids food guide, which applies to children as young as 2 years of age.

Nutrition during toddlerhood involves a transition as a young toddler is weaned off milk- or formula-based diets. Milk intake, the chief source of calcium and phosphorus, should average two or three servings (24 to 30 oz) a day. More than a quart of milk consumption daily considerably limits the intake of solid foods, resulting in a deficiency of dietary iron and other nutrients. After 2 years of age children can be given low-fat milk to reduce daily total fat to less than 30% of calories, saturated fatty acids to less than 10% of calories, and cholesterol to less than 300 mg. Fat restriction, other than *trans* fatty acids and saturated fats, is not appropriate for toddlers (Allen & Myers, 2006). Other measures to reduce dietary fat include using lean meats, fat-modified products (such as low-fat cheese), and low-fat cooking. Because less fat in children's diet can also mean fewer calories and nutrients, caregivers must know what kinds of food to choose.

Iron-fortified cereals and iron-rich foods are recommended for all children beyond 6 months of age. Parents are encouraged to provide an iron-rich diet that includes heme and nonheme iron sources (red meats, poultry, fish, green leafy vegetables, dried fruit, beans) and limit whole-milk consumption. Iron supplementation may be necessary in some cases.

Calcium and vitamin D are essential for healthy bone development. Adequate intake of calcium for the child 1 to 3 years of age is 500 mg. Whole milk, cheese, yogurt, legumes (beans), and vegetables (broccoli, collard greens, kale) are good sources for calcium. Popular calcium-fortified foods include waffles, cereals and cereal bars, orange juice, and some white breads. Adequate vitamin D intake is essential to prevent rickets; it is now recommended that children and adolescents have an intake of at least 400 International Units of vitamin D daily (American Academy of Pediatrics, 2009b). Multivitamin preparations containing 400 International Units of vitamin D are adequate if food intake is poor or exposure to sunlight is minimal; vitamin D–only preparations containing 400 International Units are also available commercially (Wagner, Greer, & American Academy of Pediatrics, Section on Breastfeeding and Committee on Nutrition, 2008). Sources of vitamin D include fish, fish oils, and egg yolks; additionally, the consumption of 1 qt of vitamin D–fortified milk will provide 400 International Units of vitamin D. Fortified cereals, dairy products, and meat are also good sources of zinc and vitamin E.

The American Heart Association (2005) recommends that toddlers have 1 cup of fruit each day. Vitamin C enhances iron absorption. Toddlers should consume approximately 4 to 6 oz of juice per day. It tastes good to toddlers and is readily available. A 6-oz glass of fruit juice equals one fruit serving; however, juices lack the fiber of whole fruit and should not be used as a substitute. High intake of juice can contribute to diarrhea, overnutrition or undernutrition, and the development of caries; thus only 4 to 6 oz of 100% fruit juice per day are recommended (American Academy of Pediatrics, 2009b). Fruit-flavored drinks advertised as juices may not actually contain 100% juice and should be avoided.

Sleep and Activity

Total sleep decreases only slightly during the second year and averages about 12 hours a day. Most children take one nap a day, and by the end of the second or third year many relinquish this habit. Children reach an adult pattern of sleep by 3 years of age (Howard & Wong, 2001).

The activity level is high, and too little physical exercise is rarely a problem provided inappropriate restrictions are not instituted. With increasing numbers of young children being cared for outside the home, attention to the kinds of activity provided is important. For example, children with high activity levels may benefit from an environment in which outdoor play is encouraged.

Sleep problems are common, especially going to bed and falling asleep, and are probably related to fears of separation. Bedtime rituals (e.g., same hour of sleep, snack, and quiet activity) are helpful; and transitional objects, such as a favorite stuffed animal or blanket, can help ease the child's insecurity at bedtime (see Fig. 37-3).

Dental Health

Regular Dental Examinations

The American Academy of Pediatric Dentistry (2009a), now recommends that every child have an oral health examination by a practitioner by the age of 12 months. Initial visits to the dentist should be nontraumatizing. Because toddlers react negatively to new and potentially frightening experiences, the initial visit can center around meeting the dentist, seeing the equipment, and sitting in the chair. If the child is cooperative, the dentist may just look at the teeth but reserve a more thorough examination for another visit. Modeling, in which the child observes procedures performed on the parent or a cooperative sibling, can also be effective.

Removal of Plaque

Oral hygiene measures should be implemented as noted above to remove plaque, soft bacterial deposits that adhere to the teeth and cause *dental caries* (decay or cavities) and *periodontal* (gum) *disease*. Poor oral hygiene and poor dietary habits are associated with the development of caries in children. The most effective methods for plaque removal are brushing and flossing. Several brushing techniques exist, although there is no universal agreement regarding the best method. One that is suitable for cleaning the primary teeth is the scrub method. The tips of the bristles are placed firmly at a 45-degree angle against the teeth and gums and moved back and forth in a vibratory motion. The ends of the bristles should be wiggling but not moving forcefully back and forth, which can damage the gums and enamel. All the surfaces of the teeth are cleaned in this manner except the lingual (inner) surfaces of the anterior teeth. To clean these surfaces, the toothbrush is placed vertical to the teeth and moved up and down. Only a few teeth are brushed at one time, using six to eight strokes for each section. A systematic approach is used so that all surfaces are thoroughly cleaned (Fig. 37-7).

For young children, the most effective cleaning is done by parents (Fig. 37-8). Several positions can be used that facilitate access to the mouth and help stabilize the head for comfort:

- Stand with child's back toward adult. (When done in front of a bathroom mirror, both child and adult can see what is being done in the mirror.)
- Sit on a couch or bed with child's head resting in adult's lap.
- Sit on the floor or a stool with child's head resting between adult's thighs.

With all positions, use one hand to cup the chin and the other to brush the teeth. For easier access to back teeth, hold the mouth partially open.

For effective cleaning, a small toothbrush with soft, rounded, multitufted nylon bristles that are short and uniform

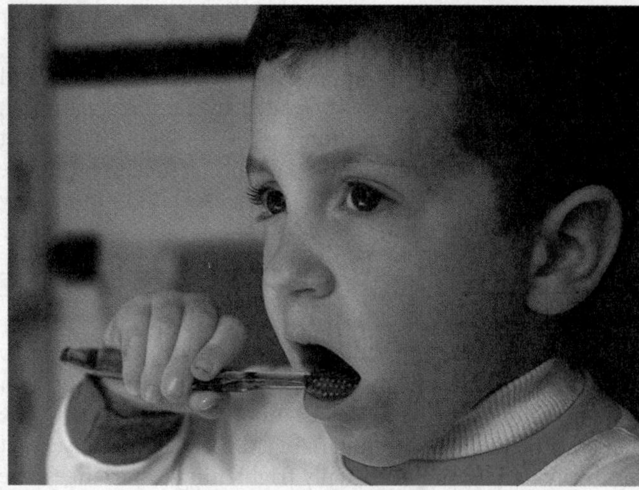
Fig. 37-7 Young children can participate in toothbrushing, but parents need to brush all the child's teeth thoroughly.

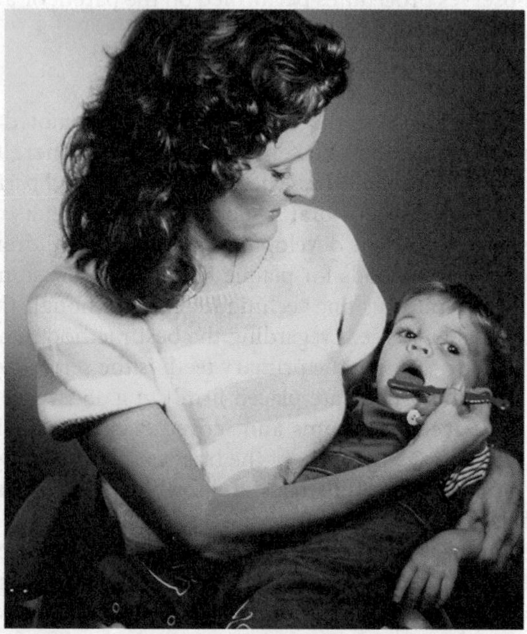
Fig. 37-8 The most effective cleaning of the teeth is done by parents.

in length is recommended. Nylon bristles dry more rapidly after use and retain their shape better than natural bristles. Toothbrushes are replaced as soon as the bristles are frayed or bent. With young children, brushing may be more easily accomplished using only water, since many children dislike the foam from toothpaste and the foam interferes with visibility. There is also the danger of swallowing fluoridated toothpaste (see following discussion under Fluoride). When using toothpaste, children should select the flavor they like to encourage the brushing habit.

After the teeth have been cleaned, flossing with dental floss is done to remove plaque and debris from between the teeth and below the gum margin, where brushing is ineffective.

Table 37-2 Fluoride Supplementation*

	Water Fluoride Content (ppm)†		
AGE	<0.3	0.3-0.6	>0.6
Birth-6 mo	0	0	0
6 mo-3 yr	0.25	0	0
3-6 yr	0.50	0.25	0
6-16 yr	1.00	0.50	0

From American Academy of Pediatric Dentistry: Guideline on fluoride therapy. In *AAPD reference manual 2008-2009,* Chicago, The Academy, 2009.
*Fluoride daily doses are given in milligrams.
†Parts per million (ppm).

Since young children do not have the dexterity to manipulate the floss, parents are taught the procedure.

A disclosing agent is helpful in identifying those areas of the teeth where plaque accumulates. It also helps motivate children to clean their teeth because plaque is difficult to see. After cleaning, the mouth is inspected to ensure that all traces of plaque have been removed. Where plaque remains, the teeth are rebrushed.

Ideally, the teeth should be cleaned after each meal and especially before bedtime, and the child should be given nothing to eat or drink after the night brushing except water. When brushing is impractical, the "swish-and-swallow" method of cleaning the mouth is taught: with a mouthful of water the child rinses the mouth and swallows, repeating the procedure three or four times.*

Fluoride

Fluoride supplementation should be considered for any child over the age of 6 months whose drinking water is deficient in fluoride. Supplementation based on a fluoride concentration of water supply at less than 0.3 parts per million is 0.25 mg for a child age 6 months to 3 years of age (American Academy of Pediatric Dentistry, 2009b).

Fluoride, a mineral, is found in water, foods, or drinks in which fluoridated water was used as part of the processing system. Because the water fluoridation process and manufacturing of fluoride toothpaste are almost impossible to standardize in the United States, the dosage of fluoride supplements has been lowered to reduce the incidence of fluorosis (Table 37-2). Increased fluoride ingestion leads to enamel protein retention, hypomineralization of the enamel and dentin, and disturbance of crystal formation. The effects caused by this change range from barely discernible white fiberlike lines or spots to gray-brown stains or pitted areas. Parents should be cautioned against regular use of fluoridated water or beverages such as bottled water containing fluoride if the community water supply already has an adequate amount of fluoride.

Supplements should remain in the mouth for 30 seconds before swallowing and be taken on an empty stomach. Afterward the child should not drink or eat for 30 minutes. All

**More detailed information can be obtained from the American Academy of Pediatric Dentistry, www.aapd.org.*

fluoride products (toothpaste, supplements, and rinse) need to be stored away from young children to prevent poisoning by accidental ingestion. If the water supply is adequately fluoridated, parents are encouraged to use tap water to prepare drinks and foods.

Low-Cariogenic Diet

Diet is critical to developing good teeth because carious development depends primarily on fermentable sugars, especially sucrose. Refined table sugar, honey, molasses, corn syrup, and dried fruits such as raisins are highly cariogenic.

Ideally, highly cariogenic foods, especially those containing complex sugars, should be eliminated. However, since this is impractical, some suggestions can be helpful. First, *the frequency with which sugar is consumed is more important than the total amount eaten.* Therefore, when sweets are eaten, they are less damaging if consumed immediately after a meal rather than as a snack between meals. When sweets are served as the dessert, the teeth can be cleaned afterward, decreasing the amount of time the sugar is in the mouth.

Second, the form of sugar (sucrose) is important. The more cariogenic foods are those that are sticky or hard, since they remain in the mouth longer. Consequently, sucking on lollipops is more cariogenic than eating a chocolate bar. Sometimes the source of the sugar is "hidden," as in numerous prescription and nonprescription drugs and in many popular cereals, including the "all-natural" variety. Sugarless gum chewed after eating may actually protect against cavities by stimulating saliva that neutralizes acid. The artificial sweeteners saccharin, aspartame, and Splenda are noncariogenic; sorbitol has low cariogenic potential. Reading food labels is essential in identifying and eliminating sources of sucrose.

A special form of tooth decay in infants and toddlers is *nursing caries* (also called *nursing bottle caries* or *bottle-mouth caries*); this occurs when the child is routinely given a bottle of milk or juice at naptime or bedtime or uses the bottle as a pacifier while awake. Frequent nocturnal breastfeeding for prolonged periods also leads to extensive destruction of the teeth. The practice of coating pacifiers in honey can also contribute to caries and may be a potential source of botulism poisoning in infants. As the sweet liquid pools in the mouth, the teeth are bathed for several hours in this cariogenic environment. The maxillary (upper) incisors and molars are affected most, since the mandibular (lower) incisors are protected by the lower lip, tongue, and saliva (Fig. 37-9). Severely decayed teeth may require the application of stainless steel bands to preserve the spacing until the permanent teeth erupt.

Prevention involves eliminating the bedtime bottle completely, feeding the last bottle before bedtime, substituting a bottle of water for milk or juice, not using the bottle as a pacifier, and never coating pacifiers in sweet substances. Juice in bottles, especially commercially available ready-to-use bottles, is discouraged; these beverages are especially damaging because the sugar is more readily converted to acid. Juice should always be offered in a cup to avoid prolonging the bottle-feeding habit. Toddlers should be encouraged to drink from a cup at the first birthday and weaned from a bottle by 14 months of age. Nurses are in an excellent position to counsel parents regarding the dangers of poor dietary habits and other aspects of dental care.*

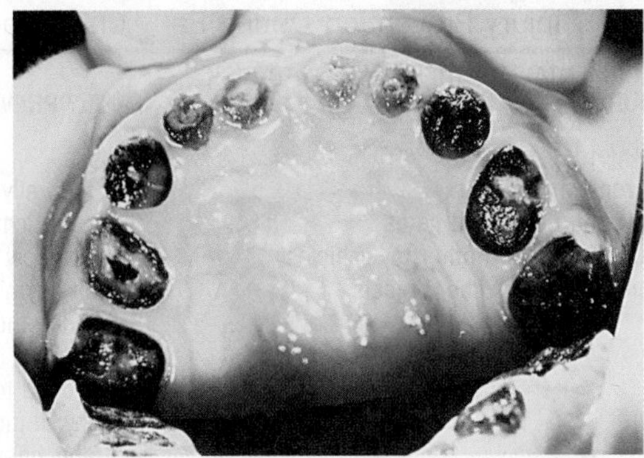

Fig. 37-9 Nursing caries. Note extensive carious involvement of maxillary primary incisors. *(Courtesy Bruce Carter, DDS, Texas Children's Hospital, Houston, TX.)*

Injury Prevention

Injuries cause more deaths in children between the ages of 1 and 4 years than in any other childhood age group except adolescence. Agran and colleagues (2003) found that the highest rate of childhood injury was in children ages 15 to 17 months; the next highest rate was in children 15 years and older. The injury death rate has remained relatively unchanged during the past decade; however, the corresponding rates from all other causes of death combined have declined significantly. Traumatic injury is the leading cause of childhood hospitalization, and infants and younger children are at higher risk because of their small size and inability to protect themselves (Dowd, Keenan, & Bratton, 2002). Child protection (adapting environment, society regulations and laws) and parent and child education are key determinants in injury prevention.

A major factor in the critical increase of injuries during early childhood is the unrestricted freedom achieved through locomotion combined with an unawareness of danger within the environment. Specific categories of injuries and appropriate prevention are best understood by associating them with the major developmental achievements of young children (Table 37-3). The discussions of injuries in Chapters 29 and 36 are also relevant to safety concerns at this age.

Motor Vehicle Injuries

Motor vehicle injuries cause more accidental deaths in all pediatric age groups after age 1 year than any other type of injury or disease and are responsible for almost half of all accidental deaths among children ages 1 to 4 years. Many of the deaths are caused by injuries within the car when restraints

**Sources of information about nursing caries and other aspects of child dental health include the National Institute of Dental and Craniofacial Research, National Institutes of Health, Bethesda, MD 20892-2190; 301-402-7364;* www.nidcr.nih.gov; *American Academy of Pediatric Dentistry, 211 E. Chicago Ave., Suite 1700, Chicago, IL 60611; 312-337-2169;* www.aapd.org; *American Dental Association, 211 E. Chicago Ave., Chicago, IL 60611; 312-440-2500;* www.ada.org, *and Canadian Dental Association, 1815 Alta Vista Drive, Ottawa, Ontario K1G 3Y6; 613-523-1770;* www.cda-adc.ca.

Table 37-3 Injury Prevention During Early Childhood

DEVELOPMENTAL ABILITIES RELATED TO RISK OF INJURY	INJURY PREVENTION
Motor Vehicles	
Walks, runs, and climbs Able to open doors and gates Can ride tricycle and other toy vehicles Can throw ball and other objects	Use federally approved car restraint. Supervise child while playing outside. Do not allow child to play on curb or behind a parked car. Do not permit child to play in pile of leaves, snow, or large cardboard container in trafficked area. Supervise tricycle riding. Lock fences and doors if not directly supervising children. Teach child to obey pedestrian safety rules: • Obey traffic regulations; cross only at crosswalks and only when traffic signal indicates it is safe. • Stand back a step from the curb until it is time to cross. • Look left, right, and left again and check for turning cars before crossing street. • Use sidewalks; when there is no sidewalk, walk on the left, facing traffic. • Wear light colors at night and attach fluorescent material to clothing.
Drowning	
Able to explore if left unsupervised Has great curiosity Helpless in water; unaware of its danger—may consider "play" in any body of water same as in bath; depth of water has no significance	Supervise closely when near any source of water regardless of depth, including buckets. Keep bathroom doors closed and lid down on toilet (or install latch). Have fence around swimming pool and lock gate. Teach swimming and water safety (this is, however, not a substitute for safety).
Burns	
Able to reach heights by climbing, stretching, and standing on toes Pulls objects Explores any holes or opening Can open drawers and closets Unaware of potential sources of heat or fire Plays with mechanical objects	Turn pot handles toward back of stove. Place electrical appliances, such as coffee maker and popcorn machine, toward back of counter. Place guardrails in front of radiators, fireplaces, or other heating elements. Store matches and cigarette lighters in locked or inaccessible area; discard carefully. Place burning candles, incense, hot foods, and cigarettes out of reach. Do not let tablecloth hang within child's reach. Do not let electric cord from iron, curling iron or other appliance hang within child's reach. Cover electrical outlets with protective plastic caps. Keep electrical wires hidden or out of reach. Do not allow child to play with electrical appliance, wires, or lighters. Stress danger of open flames; teach what "hot" means. Always check bathwater temperature; adjust water heater temperature to 49° C (120° F) or lower; do not allow children to play with faucets. Apply a sunscreen when child is exposed to sunlight.
Poisoning	
Explores by putting objects in mouth Can open drawers, closets, boxes, and most containers Climbs Cannot read labels Does not know safe dose or amount	Place all potentially toxic agents out of reach or in a locked cabinet. Caution against eating nonedible items, such as plants. Replace medications or poisons immediately in proper storage and out of child's reach; replace child-guard caps properly. Administer medications as a drug, not as a candy. Do not store surplus toxic agents. Promptly discard empty poison containers; never reuse to store a food item or other poison. Teach child not to play in trash containers. Never remove labels from containers of toxic substances. Do not store toxic liquids in containers not specifically intended for their storage (e.g., empty soda bottle that child may drink from, unaware of difference in contents). Know number of nearest poison control center **(800-222-1222)**.
Falls	
Able to open doors and some windows Goes up and down stairs Depth perception unrefined Climbs on higher surfaces	Use window guardrail; fasten securely. Place gates at top and bottom of stairs. Keep doors locked or use child-proof doorknob covers at entry to stairs, high porch, or other elevated area, including laundry chute. Remove unsecured or scatter rugs. Apply nonskid decals in bathtub or shower. Keep crib rails fully raised and mattress at lowest level. Place carpeting under crib and in bathroom. Keep large toys and bumper pads out of crib or playpen (child can use these as "stairs" to climb out), then move child to youth bed when he or she is able to climb out of crib. Avoid using wheeled walkers, especially near stairs and floor furnace. Dress in safe clothing (soles that do not "catch" on floor, tied shoelaces, pant legs that do not touch floor). Keep child restrained in vehicles; never leave unattended in shopping cart. Supervise at playgrounds; select play areas with soft ground cover and safe equipment.

Table 37-3 Injury Prevention During Early Childhood—cont'd

DEVELOPMENTAL ABILITIES RELATED TO RISK OF INJURY	INJURY PREVENTION
Choking and Suffocation	
Puts things in mouth May swallow hard or nonedible pieces of food	Avoid large, round chunks of meat, such as whole hot dogs (slice lengthwise into short pieces). Avoid fruit with pits, fish with bones, dried beans, hard candy, chewing gum, nuts, popcorn, grapes, marshmallows. Choose large, sturdy toys without sharp edges or small removable parts. Discard old refrigerators, ovens, and so on after removing door. Select safe toy boxes or chests without heavy, hinged lids. Keep Venetian blind (or shade) cords out of child's reach. Use split cords. Remove drawstrings from clothing.
Bodily Damage	
Still clumsy in many skills Easily distracted from tasks Unaware of potential danger from strangers or other people	Avoid giving sharp or pointed objects, such as knives, scissors, or toothpicks, especially when walking or running. Do not allow lollipops or similar objects in mouth when walking or running. Teach safety precautions (e.g., to carry knife or scissors with pointed end away from face). Store all dangerous tools, garden equipment, and firearms in locked cabinet. Be alert to danger of supervised animals and household pets. Use safety glass and decals on large glassed areas, such as sliding glass doors. Teach child name, address, and phone number and to ask for help from appropriate people (cashier, security guard, policeman) if lost; have identification on child (sewn in clothes, inside shoe). Teach stranger safety: • Avoid personalized clothing in public places. • Never go with a stranger. • Tell parents if anyone makes child feel uncomfortable in any way. Always listen to child's concerns regarding others' behavior. Teach child to say "no" when confronted with uncomfortable situations.

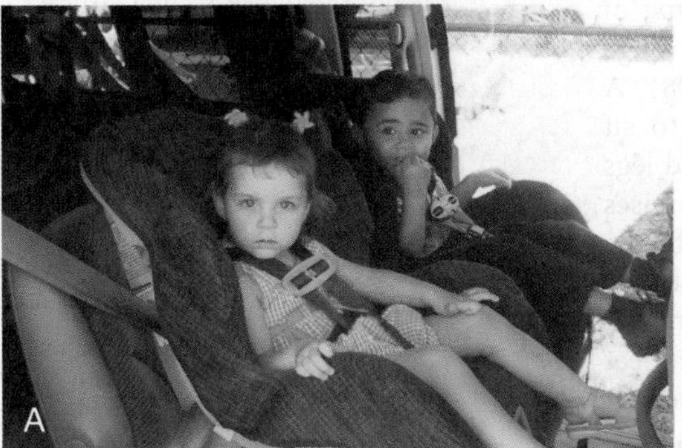

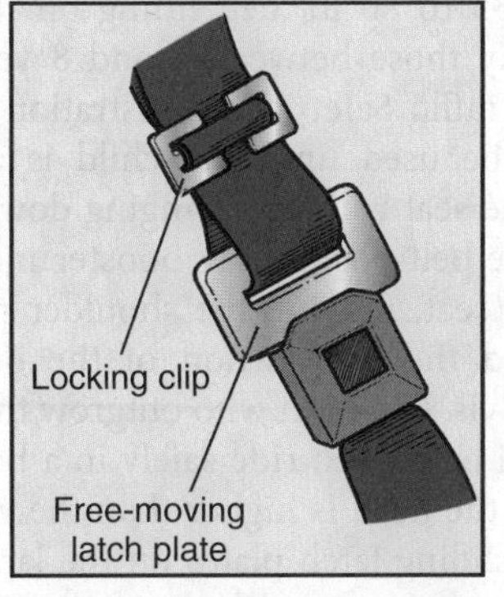

Fig. 37-10 A, Convertible car safety seat in forward-facing position. **B,** Use of locking clip.

have not been used or have been used improperly. Unrestrained children riding in the vehicle's front seat are at highest risk for injury (Durbin et al, 2005). Approved restraints properly installed and applied can prevent many fatalities and injuries (Schnitzer, 2006; American Academy of Pediatrics, 2009a).

Nurses have a responsibility for educating parents regarding the importance of car restraints and their proper use. Five types of restraints are available: (1) infant-only devices, (2) convertible models for both infants and toddlers, (3) boosters, (4) safety belts, and (5) devices for children with special needs (see Chapter 41). Infant-type restraints are discussed in Chapter 36; convertible restraints and boosters are included here. The *convertible restraint* is suitable for infants in the rear-facing position and for toddlers in the forward-facing position. The transition point for switching to the forward-facing position is defined by the manufacturer but is generally at a body weight of at least 9 kg (20 lb) and 1 year of age. Infants who weigh 9 kg before 1 year of age should continue to ride in a rear-facing seat (American Academy of Pediatrics, 2009a). One recent study has shown that children from birth to 23 months experienced fewer injuries when riding in rear-facing car restraints (Henary et al, 2007). Another study indicated that children 0 to 3 years of age riding properly restrained in the middle of the back seat had a 43% lower risk of injury than children riding in the outboard (window) seat during a crash (Kallan et al, 2008).

A convertible safety seat is positioned semireclined and facing the rear of the car for a child younger than 1 year weighing less than 9 kg. The seat is positioned upright and facing forward for an older and heavier child (up to 18 kg [40 lb]) (Fig. 37-10, *A*). Convertible safety seats should be used until the child weighs at least 13.6 kg (30 lb) or more regardless of age and as long as the child fits properly into the seat (American Academy of Pediatrics, 2009a). Convertible restraints use different types of harness systems: a five-point harness that consists of a strap over each shoulder, one on each side of the pelvis, and one between the legs (all five come together at a common buckle); and a padded shield that uses shoulder straps attached to a shield that is held in place by a crotch strap. With both the infant and toddler restraints, it is important not to add extra blankets, head cushions, or padding between the child and the restraint straps that did not come as original equipment because these "add-ons" create spaces of air between the child and the restraint and decrease support for the back, head, and neck.

Booster seats are not restraint systems like the convertible devices because they depend on the vehicle belts to hold the child and booster seat in place. Three booster models have been approved by the National Highway Traffic Safety Administration (2008): the high-back belt-positioning seat, which provides head and neck support for the child riding in a vehicle seat without a head rest; the no-back belt-positioning seat, which should be used only if the vehicle seat has a head rest; and a combination seat, which converts from a forward-facing toddler seat to a booster seat. This last model is equipped with a harness for use by toddlers; the harness may be removed and a shoulder-lap belt used when the child outgrows the harness. Booster seats are used for children who are less than 145 cm (4 feet, 9 inches) tall and who weigh 15.9 kg to 36.3 kg (35 to 80 lb, depending on the type of booster seat), typically those between 4 and 8 years of age (National Highway Traffic Safety Administration, 2008). A booster seat should be used until the child is able to sit against the back of the seat with feet hanging down and legs bent at the knees. The belt-positioning booster model raises a child higher in the seat, moving the shoulder part of the belt off the neck and the lap portion of the belt off the abdomen onto the pelvis. Children who outgrow the convertible restraint may still be able to ride safely in a booster seat until the midpoint of the head is higher than the vehicle seat back. Cars with free-sliding latch plates on the lap or shoulder belt require the use of a metal locking clip to keep the belt in a tight-holding position. The locking clip is threaded onto the belt above the latch plate (see Fig. 37-10, *B*). If parents have newer cars with automatic lap and shoulder belts, they need to have additional lap belts installed to properly secure the restraint.

Children should use specially designed car restraints until they are 145 cm (4 feet, 9 inches) in height or are 8 to 12 years old (American Academy of Pediatrics, 2009a). *Shoulder-lap safety belts* should be worn low on the hips, snug, and not on the abdominal area. Children should be taught to sit up straight to allow for proper fit. The shoulder belt is used only if it does not cross the child's neck or face.

Shoulder-only automatic belts are designed to protect adults. Children should use the manual shoulder belts in the rear seat. Air bags do not take the place of child safety seats or seat belts and can be lethal to young children. The safest area of the car for children is the back seat. Children who must ride in the passenger side of the front seat with an activated air bag should be positioned as far back as possible.

Built-in seats are available in some cars and vans. They may be used for children who are at least 1 year of age and weigh at least 9 kg (20 lb). Built-in seats eliminate installation problems. However, weight and height limits vary. Reinforce that owners must verify with vehicle manufacturers details about built-in seats.

For any restraint to be effective, it must be used consistently and properly. Examples of misuse include misrouting the vehicle seat belt through the restraint; failing to use the vehicle seat belt to secure the restraint; failing to use a tether strap; failing to use the restraint's harness system; and incorrectly positioning the child, especially by facing infants forward instead of rearward. To address these issues, nurses must stress correct use of car restraints and rules that ensure compliance (see Family-Centered Care box). Children riding in car safety seats are generally much better behaved than children left unrestrained, which can be a major benefit to parents and should be emphasized as an additional advantage of restraints. Additional information about child safety restraints is available from various sources.*

FAMILY-CENTERED CARE

Using Car Safety Seats

- Read manufacturer's directions and follow them exactly.
- Anchor safety seat securely to car's seat and apply harness snugly to child.
- Do not start the car until everyone is properly restrained.
- *Always* use the restraint, even for short trips.
- If child begins to climb out or undo the harness, firmly say, "No." It may be necessary to stop the car to reinforce the expected behavior. Use rewards, such as stars or stickers, to encourage cooperative behavior.
- Encourage child to help attach buckles, straps, and shields, but always double-check fastenings.
- Decrease boredom on long trips. Keep soft toys in the car for quiet play; talk to child; point out objects and teach child about them. Stop periodically. If child wishes to sleep, make certain child stays in the restraint.
- Insist that others who transport children also follow these safety rules.

The LATCH (lower anchors and tethers for children) universal child safety seat system was implemented as a requirement starting in 2002 for all new automobiles and child safety seats. This system provides uniform anchorage consisting of

**American Academy of Pediatrics, 141 Northwest Point Blvd., Elk Grove Village, IL 60007; 847-434-4000;* www.aap.org; *and local division of traffic safety or National Highway Traffic Safety Administration, 1200 New Jersey Ave. SE, West Building, Washington, DC 20590; 888-327-4236;* www.nhtsa.gov.

Upper anchorage
Lower anchorage
Flexible attachment on child seat
Bars installed in vehicle seat
Lower anchorage
A

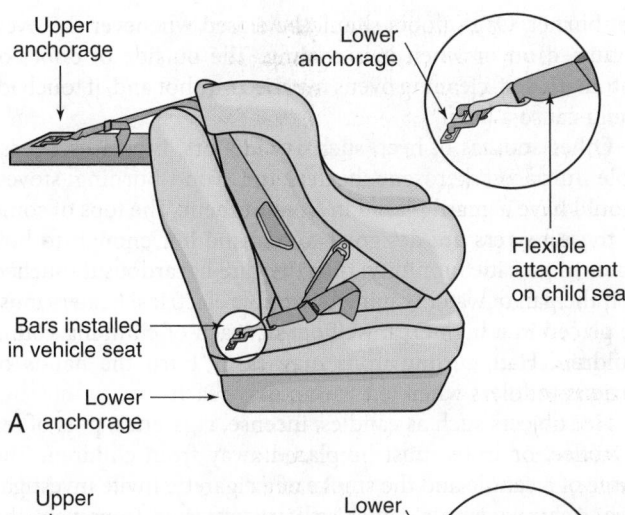

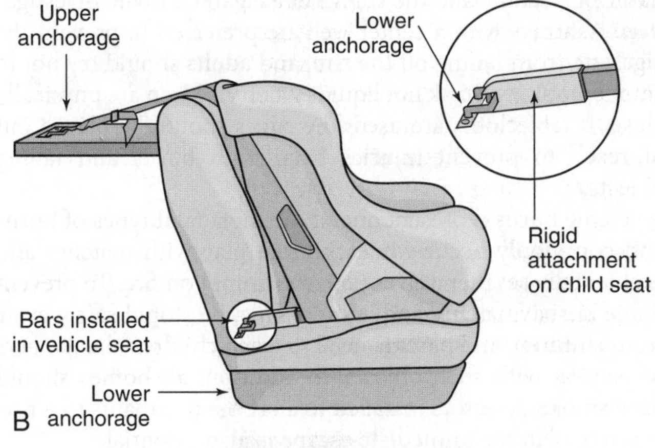

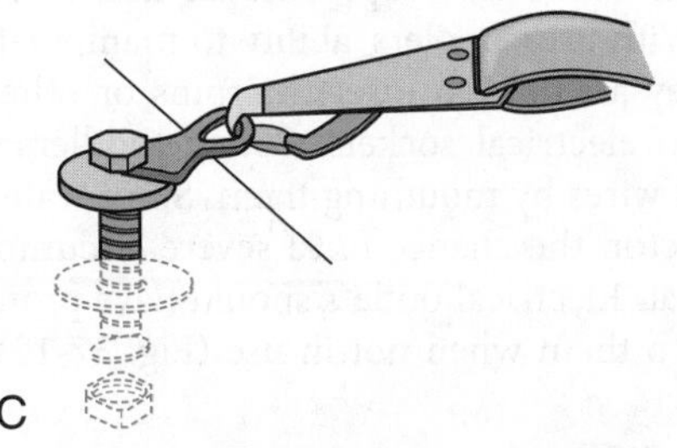

Fig. 37-11 Lower anchors and tethers for children (LATCH). **A,** Flexible 2-point attachment with top tether. **B,** Rigid 2-point attachment with top tether. **C,** Top tether. *(Courtesy US Department of Transportation, National Highway Traffic Safety Administration.)*

two lower anchorages and one upper anchorage in the rear seat of the vehicle (Fig. 37-11). When used appropriately, the top anchor (tether) strap prevents the child from pitching forward in a crash. If the tether strap is not used, up to 90% of the restraint's protection is lost. Instructions for proper installation of the tether strap and permanent bracket are included with the car restraint. New child safety seats will have a hook, buckle, strap, or other connector that attaches to the anchorage. Seat belts will no longer be used to anchor child safety seats to newer vehicles. The first phase required all new cars to have an upper anchorage. After fall 2002, all new cars were required to have the entire LATCH system.

Children with special needs may require a restraint system that secures them appropriately in the event of a crash. Examples of such devices include car bed restraints for infants who cannot tolerate a semireclining position and specially adapted molded-plastic chairs for children who have spica casts.* The E-Z-On vest is a special safety harness for larger children with poor trunk control. Additional safety restraints and a listing of distributors are available at the SafetyBeltSafe U.S.A. website *(www.carseat.org)*. See also Chapter 27 for discussion of preterm infants being discharged home and car seat evaluation.

Injuries may also occur during sudden stops when objects are left unrestrained. On sudden impact, a loose toy or package becomes a projectile missile. Therefore all items should be secured or stored in the trunk.

Children over 3 years of age are often involved in pedestrian traffic injuries. Motor vehicle back-over injuries and deaths, along with deaths or serious injury resulting from heat stroke when left in a car, account for a large number of motor vehicle–related injuries in children (Centers for Disease Control and Prevention, 2005; McLaren, Null, & Quinn, 2005). Because of their gross motor skills of walking, running, and climbing, and their fine motor skills of opening doors and fence gates, children are likely to be in hazardous areas when unsupervised. Unaware of danger and unable to approximate the speed of a car, they are often hit by moving vehicles. Running after a ball, riding a tricycle, and playing behind a parked car are common activities that may result in a vehicular tragedy. Toddlers playing in driveways or farmyards are at risk of back-over injury from vehicles in reverse gear. From 2001 to 2003, 7475 children 1 to 14 years of age were involved in motor vehicle back-over (nonfatal) injuries; the highest incidence of injuries occurred in driveways or parking lots, and most children injured were pedestrians (as opposed to riding a bicycle or tricycle) (Centers for Disease Control and Prevention, 2005). A precaution when children are playing in driveways is attaching to the tricycle a pole with a bright flag that is high enough to be visible through an automobile's back window. Another safeguard is the use of a device that beeps loudly when the vehicle is driven in reverse to alert children to the oncoming car, van, tractor, or truck. Some models now come equipped with rearview motion cameras so the driver can see the driveway clearly while backing out.

One type of injury that has become more commonplace occurs when children crawl into an open trunk and pull it closed. Asphyxia may occur in such cases; therefore car trunks should not be left open when children are not being supervised. Some cars are equipped with a safety switch that can be activated from inside the trunk to open a closed trunk door.

Preventing vehicular injuries involves protecting and educating children and adults about the danger of moved or parked vehicles. Children should never ride in the open back of a truck; the danger of falls can be compounded by another vehicle striking the child or by the truck rolling over. In addition, leaving children unsupervised in a parked vehicle, especially in a private driveway, provides an opportunity for the

*Britax Hippo by Snug Seat.

child to release the brake or put the car in gear. Children in bicycle-towed trailers or bicycle-mounted child seats can also be injured by collisions or falls.

Another automobile-related hazard for toddlers is overheating (hyperthermia) and subsequent death when left in a vehicle in hot weather (more than 27° C [80° F]). Small children dissipate heat poorly, and an increase in body temperature can cause death in a few hours. In 2003 a total of 42 children died as a result of overheating when left alone in a parked car; in 2004 the total number of child deaths was 35 (McLaren, Null, & Quinn, 2005). It is estimated that with the ambient temperature at 22° to 35.5° C (72° to 96° F), the vehicle interior temperature rises by 10.5° to 11° C (19° to 20° F) for each 10 minutes, even with a window cracked (Null, 2007). In a recent study of 171 child fatalities from overheating in a car, 50% of adults who left a child in a car either forgot or were unaware that the child was still in the car. A significant number of those children (32) were left by family members who intended to take the child to day care but forgot the child in the car at the workplace; 22 children were left in the car by a day care worker or driver (Guard & Gallagher, 2005). Parents are cautioned against leaving infants in a vehicle alone for *any reason.*

Preventing vehicular injuries involves protecting and educating children about the danger of moving or parked vehicles. Although preschool children are too young to be trusted to always obey, the parent should emphasize looking for moving vehicles before crossing the street, recognizing the stop and go colors of traffic lights, and following traffic officers' signals. Physical barriers limiting children from playing near vehicles help prevent these injuries. Most important, what is preached must be practiced. Children learn through imitation, and consistency reinforces learning.

Drowning

Drowning, not including drowning from water transportation (boats), ranks second among boys and third among girls ages 1 to 4 years as a cause of accidental death. With well-developed skills of locomotion, toddlers are able to reach potentially dangerous areas, such as bathtubs, toilets, buckets, swimming pools, hot tubs, and lakes. Their intense drive for exploration and investigation, combined with an unawareness of the danger of water and their helplessness in water, makes drowning always a viable threat. It is also one category of injuries that results in death within minutes, diminishing the chance for rescue and survival. Adult supervision of children when near any source of water is essential; teaching swimming and water safety can be helpful but cannot be regarded as sufficient protection.

Burns

Burns rank second among girls and third among boys in this age group as a cause of accidental death. Toddlers' ability to climb, stretch, and reach objects above their heads makes any hot surface a potential source of danger. Scalds from children pulling pots on top of themselves are a major source of burns. As a precaution, pot handles should be turned toward the back of the stove. Ideally, the knobs for controlling the range burners should be out of reach, not on the front panel where nimble fingers can turn them on and accidentally touch the hot burner. Oven doors should be closed whenever the oven is turned on or when it is cooling. The outside of doors of automatic self-cleaning ovens may become hot and, if touched, could cause a burn.

Other sources of heat, such as radiators, fireplaces, accessible furnaces, kerosene heaters, or wood-burning stoves, should have a guard placed in front of them. The tops of some of these heaters are designed to become hot enough to boil water to provide humidity; thus they are hazardous if touched or if the pan of water is spilled. Portable electrical heaters must be placed in a high area, well out of reach of climbing young children. Hair curling irons may easily burn the hands of curious toddlers when left within easy reach.

Hot objects such as candles, incense, cigarettes, pots of tea or coffee, or irons must be placed away from children. The flame of a candle and the smoke of a cigarette invite investigation. Ashtrays with a center well are preferred to prevent the cigarette from falling off the rim, and adults should try not to smoke, cook, or drink hot liquids when children are physically close. If tablecloths are used, the edges should be placed out of reach to prevent injuries from both burns and falling objects.

Flame burns represent one of the most fatal types of burns and commonly occur when children play with matches and accidentally set themselves (and the home) on fire. To prevent flame burns, matches and lighters must be stored safely away from children, and parents need to teach children the dangers of playing with such objects. In addition, all homes should have smoke detectors installed to alert the occupants to a fire. A safety plan for immediate escape is also essential.

Electrical burns also represent an immediate danger to children. With preschoolers' ability to manipulate small, thin objects, they are able to insert hairpins or other conductive articles into electrical sockets. Young toddlers may explore outlets and wires by mouthing them. Since water is an excellent conductor, the chance for a severe circumoral electrical burn is great. Electrical outlets should have protective guards plugged into them when not in use (Fig. 37-12) or be made

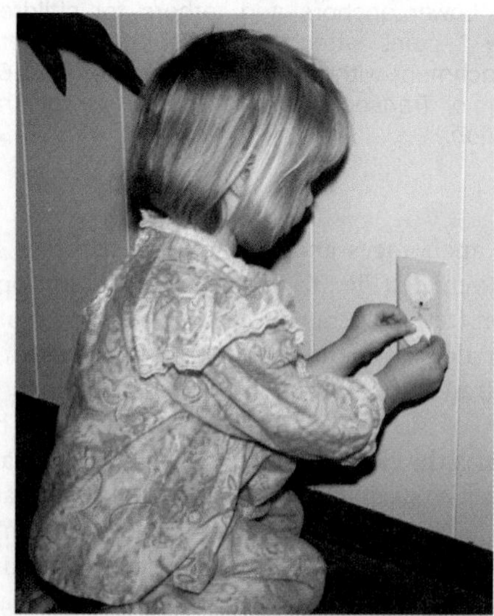

Fig. 37-12 Special plastic caps in electrical sockets prevent young fingers from exploring dangerous areas.

inaccessible by having furniture placed in front of them when feasible. Children should not be allowed to play with electrical cords or appliances, which should be kept out of reach as much as possible.

Scald burns are the most common type of thermal injury in small children. A scalding burn is often caused by high-temperature tap water, which children come in contact with as a result of turning on the hot-water faucet, falling into a bathtub of hot water, or deliberate abuse. Always supervising youngsters when they are near tap water and checking bathwater temperatures are methods of prevention. Limiting household water temperatures to less than 49° C (120° F) is also recommended. At this temperature it takes 10 minutes of exposure to the water to cause a full-thickness burn. Conversely, water temperatures of 54° C (130° F), the usual setting of most water heaters, expose household members to the risk of full-thickness burns within 30 seconds. Nurses can help prevent such burns by advising parents of this common household danger and recommending that they readjust the water heater to a safe temperature. An easy-to-read hot-water gauge that changes color to show water temperatures between 49° C and 54° C (120° and 130° F) is also available; it shows a "hot," "cool," or "OK" water temperature. A special device can also be added to the faucet that reduces the water flow once the set temperature is reached. Scalding also often occurs when a curious child tries to sip a parent's coffee or tea and spills the boiling liquid down the chin and chest.

Poisoning

Toddlers are at the highest risk for poisoning. Mouthing activity continues to be prevalent after 1 year of age, and exploring objects by tasting them is part of children's curious investigation. Many household products, medications, and plants can be poisonous if swallowed, if in contact with the skin or eyes, or if inhaled. Although in many instances poisoning does not result in death, it may cause significant morbidity, such as esophageal stricture from lye ingestion. Toddlers are able to climb most heights, open most drawers or closets, and unscrew most lids. By trial and error, younger children also manage to undo tops of bottles, plastic containers, aerosol cans, and jars, including those with child-resistant lids. In addition, drugs are often transferred to regular containers for the elderly, who may have difficulty with child-resistant lids. Newer forms of drugs, such as transdermal patches and cough-suppressant lozenges, have created additional dangers, since they are not packaged with safety caps and the lozenges look like candy.

The major reason for poisoning is improper storage (Fig. 37-13). The guidelines suggested in Chapter 36 apply to children in this age group as well. However, unlike the infant, who was confined to certain heights and unable to unlatch inventive locks, young children manage to find access to many high-level, tight-security places. For this age group, only a locked cabinet is safe.

Emergency and preventive measures for accidental poisoning are discussed in Chapter 36.

NURSING ALERT Parents should have ready access to the telephone number for the poison control center, 800-222-1222, and be prepared to act on the center's advice.

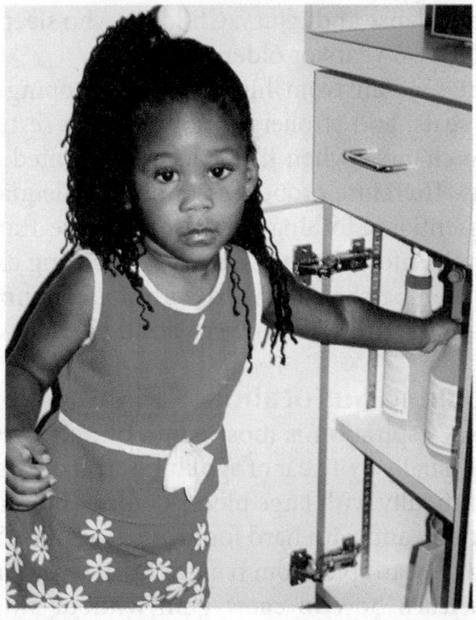

Fig. 37-13 Children are most likely to ingest substances that are on their level, such as cleaning agents stored under sinks, rat poison, plants, or diaper pail deodorants.

Falls

Falls are still a hazard to children in this age group, although by the later part of early childhood, gross and fine motor skills are well developed, decreasing the incidence of falls down stairs or from chairs. However, playground injuries are common. Children need to be taught safety at play areas, such as no horseplay on high slides or jungle gyms, *sitting* on swings, and staying away from moving swings. Passive prevention includes placement of grass, sand, or wood chips under play equipment. Swing seats should be made of plastic, canvas, or rubber and have smooth or rounded edges. Slides should not exceed an incline of 30 degrees and should have evenly spaced rungs for climbing and protective "tunnels."

The climbing and running of the typical toddler are complicated by the child's total neglect for and lack of appreciation of danger. Gates must be placed at both ends of stairs. Accessible windows that are left open during warm weather must be guarded with a rail. Falling from open windows is a major cause of accidental death in children from urban, lower socioeconomic groups; parents are advised that a screened window is not a safety device to prevent falls. Doors leading to stairwells or porches must be locked because preschoolers can easily open them. A convenient type of lock is a sliding bar or hook that can be attached to the door and frame at a level higher than the child can reach; such locks also have safety clasps or devices that prevent children from opening them.

Cribs and vehicles are other sources of falls. To avoid injury, crib rails should be fully raised, the mattress should be kept at the lowest position, and toys or bumper pads that may be used as steps to climb out should be removed. Once children reach a height of 89 cm (35 inches), they should sleep in a bed rather than a crib. If a bunk bed is selected, parents should be aware of possible dangers such as falls and head entrapment between the mattress and guardrail or between the supporting mattress slats. If the beds are constructed of tubular metal, parents should check for breaks or cracks in the metal and welds that

evolve Case Study—Salicylate Ingestion

evolve Case Study—Heavy Metal Poisoning

may lead to collapse and injury. Children who sleep on the top bunk should be 6 years or older.

Children can fall from high chairs, shopping carts, carriages, car seats, and strollers if not properly restrained or if the balance changes when the object is weighted down with heavy items. Therefore proper restraint and adequate supervision are essential. Clothing can also increase the chance of falling. Simple safety measures, such as checking clothing and shoes and keeping shoelaces tied with double knots or using self-adhering closures, can prevent accidents.

Aspiration and Suffocation

evolve Case Study—Ingestion of an Injurious Agent

Foreign body aspiration is most common during the second year of life. Usually by 1 year of age children chew well, but they may have difficulty with large pieces of food, such as meat and whole hot dogs, and with hard foods, such as nuts. Young children cannot discard pits from fruit or bones from fish. It takes practice to learn how to chew gum without swallowing it. Therefore the same precautions as discussed for infants regarding food selection must be implemented (see Chapter 36).

Play objects for toddlers must still be chosen with an awareness of danger from small parts. Large, sturdy toys without sharp edges or removable parts are safest. Coins, paper clips, pins, bells, button (round) batteries, pull-tabs on cans, thumbtacks, nails, screws, jewelry (especially pierced earrings), and all types of pins are common household objects that can cause significant harm if swallowed or aspirated. Small items such as colored beads, green peas, pellets, or beans are often placed into the nose by toddlers and may present a danger if aspirated into the airway. Because of the danger of aspiration, parents should be taught emergency procedures for choking (see Airway Obstruction, Chapter 46).

Suffocation from causes seen during infancy is less frequent, but old refrigerators, ovens, and other large appliances are a threat. Toddlers can climb inside these appliances and, if they close the door behind them, can be trapped inside. Removing all doors before discarding or storing old appliances prevents such tragic deaths. Toddlers may also suffocate when unsafe toy box lids accidentally close on their head or neck. Parents should be advised of this danger and be encouraged to buy storage chests with lightweight, removable covers.

Hollow, semirigid hemispherical or ellipsoidal objects can form suction and cupping around a small child's face, causing complete airway obstruction. Several different types of objects have been involved with choking incidents, including toys, components of toys, and containers (Nakamura, Pollack-Nelson, & Chidekel, 2003).

Bodily Damage

Toddlers are still clumsy in many of their skills and can seriously harm themselves by walking while holding a sharp or pointed object or by having food or objects such as spoons in their mouths. Preventing such occurrences is the best approach with toddlers. The child should be taught that, when walking with a pointed object such as a knife or scissors, to hold the pointed end away from the face. Dangerous garden or workshop equipment and all firearms should be stored in a locked cabinet. Power lawnmowers are especially dangerous, and young children should not be allowed in an area where a mower is being used, nor should they be taken for a ride on a mower or allowed to operate that device. Toddlers have the dexterity, curiosity, patience, and ability to find hidden items. Safety education for older toddlers should include respect for firearms and their proper and appropriate use, including nonpowder guns, such as air guns and rifles, which cause serious penetrating injuries. In addition, the child should be warned of and protected against potential danger from animals (see Animal Bites, Chapter 53).

Toys can be a source of danger, and safety must be a prime consideration when selecting toys (see Family-Centered Care box, p. 858). Most toys have age ranges written on them to designate their safety, but this information must be used with knowledge of the specific child's readiness.

Household safety should be practiced and includes the usual precautions recommended for any age group (see Family-Centered Care box, p. 1000). An additional safeguard for young children is the use of safety glass in doors, windows, and tabletops; and the application of decals on glassed areas to reduce the likelihood of running through glass. Also, children should not be allowed to run, jump, wrestle, or play ball near glass structures.

Anticipatory Guidance—Care of Families

Understanding toddlers is fundamental to successful childrearing. Nurses, particularly those in ambulatory or child health centers, are in a favorable position to assist parents in facilitating the tasks and meeting the needs of children in this age group. Prevention yields better results than treatment. Anticipatory guidance is paramount if one wishes to prevent future problems (see Family-Centered Care box). Advice is sometimes not the sole answer. Actual assistance, such as being available for telephone consulting, should be part of the nurse's flexible repertoire of interventions. Whether parents are experiencing the childrearing dilemmas of a first or a subsequent child, they benefit from sharing their feelings, frustrations, and satisfactions. They need adult companionship, occasional freedom from childrearing responsibilities, and periodic separations from their children. Part of a nurse's responsibility is to provide opportunities for parents to express their feelings and to meet their physical, mental, and spiritual needs.

FAMILY-CENTERED CARE

Guidance During Toddler Years

Ages 12 to 18 Months

Prepare parents for expected behavioral changes of toddler, especially negativism and ritualism.

Assess present feeding habits and encourage gradual weaning from bottle and increased intake of solid foods.

Stress expected feeding changes of picky eating habits, food fads and strong taste preferences, need for scheduled routine at mealtimes, inability to sit through an entire meal, and lack of table manners.

Prepare parents for potential dangers of the home, particularly motor vehicle injuries, poisoning, and falling injuries; give appropriate suggestions for safety proofing the home.

Discuss need for firm but gentle discipline and ways to deal with negativism and temper tantrums; stress positive benefits of appropriate discipline.

Emphasize importance for both child and parents of brief, periodic separations.

Discuss new toys that use developing gross and fine motor, language, cognitive, and social skills.

Emphasize need for dental supervision, types of basic dental hygiene at home, and food habits that predispose to caries; stress importance of supplemental fluoride (according to age [greater than 6 months] and fluoride content of local water supply).

Ages 18 to 24 Months

Stress importance of peer companionship in play.

Explore need for preparation for additional sibling (as appropriate); stress importance of preparing child for new experiences.

Assess sleep patterns at night, particularly the habit of a bedtime bottle, which is a major cause of dental caries, and behaviors that delay hour of sleep.

Discuss present discipline methods, their effectiveness, and parents' feelings about child's negativism; stress that negativism is important aspect of developing self-assertion and independence and is not a sign of spoiling.

Discuss signs of readiness for toilet training; emphasize importance of waiting for physical and psychologic readiness.

Discuss development of fears, such as fear of darkness or loud noises, and of habits, such as security blanket or thumb-sucking; stress normalcy of these transient behaviors.

Prepare parents for signs of regression in time of stress.

Assess child's ability to separate easily from parents for brief periods under familiar circumstances.

Allow parents opportunity to express their feelings of weariness, frustration, and exasperation; be aware that it is often difficult to love toddlers when they are not asleep!

Point out some of the expected changes of the next year, such as longer attention span, somewhat less negativism, and increased concern for pleasing others.

Ages 24 to 36 Months

Discuss importance of imitation and domestic mimicry and need to include child in activities.

Discuss approaches toward toilet training, particularly realistic expectations and attitude toward accidents.

Stress uniqueness of toddlers' thought processes, especially through their use of language, poor understanding of time, view of causal relationships in terms of proximity of events, and inability to see events from another's perspective.

Stress that discipline still must be structured and concrete and that relying solely on verbal reasoning and explanation leads to injuries, confusion, and misunderstanding.

Discuss investigation of preschool or day care center toward completion of second year.

Key Points

- The toddler stage, extending from 12 to 36 months, is a period of intense exploration of the environment.
- Biologic development during the toddler years is characterized by the acquisition of fine and gross motor skills that allow children to master a wide range of activities.
- Although most of the physiologic systems are mature by the end of toddlerhood, development of certain areas of the brain is still occurring, allowing for greater intellectual capacity.
- Locomotion is the major gross motor skill acquired during toddlerhood, followed by increased eye-hand coordination.
- Specific tasks in the psychosocial development of a toddler include differentiating self from others, tolerating separation from parent, coping with delayed gratification, controlling bodily functions, acquiring socially acceptable behavior, communicating verbally, and interacting with others in a less egocentric manner.

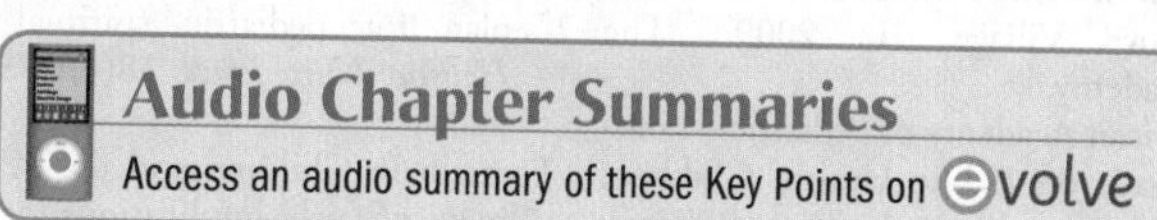
Audio Chapter Summaries
Access an audio summary of these Key Points on evolve

- According to Erikson, the major developmental task of toddlerhood is acquiring a sense of autonomy while overcoming a sense of doubt and shame.
- In Piaget's sensorimotor and preconceptual phases of development, the toddler experiments by incorporating the old learning of secondary circular reactions with new skills and applies this knowledge to new situations. There is the beginning of rational judgment, an understanding of causal relationships, and discovery of objects as objects.
- Preconceptual thought is characterized by egocentrism, centration, global organization of thought processes, animism, and irreversibility.
- Language is the major cognitive achievement in toddlerhood.

- The most striking characteristic of language development during early childhood is the increasing level of comprehension.
- Development of body image occurs with increasing motor ability, at which point toddlers recognize the importance and capacity of body parts.
- The two phases of differentiation of self from significant others are separation and individuation.
- Parental concerns during the toddler years include toilet training; coping with sibling rivalry; limit setting and discipline; and dealing with temper tantrums, negativism, and regression.
- Effective discipline techniques for toddlers include reward, ignoring or extinction, and time-out.
- Nutrition is important during the toddler stage because eating habits established in this period have lasting effects in subsequent years.
- Regular dental examinations, fluoride supplementation, removal of plaque, and provision of a low-cariogenic diet promote optimum dental health.
- Because of increased locomotion, toddlers are at high risk for sustaining injuries. Fatal injuries are primarily a result of motor vehicle accidents, drownings, and burns.

References

Agran PF et al: Rates of pediatric injuries by 3-month intervals for children 0 to 3 years of age, *Pediatrics* 111(6 Pt 1):e683-e692, 2003.

Allen RE, Myers AL: Nutrition in toddlers, *Am Fam Physician* 74(9):1527-1532, 1533-1534, 2006.

American Academy of Pediatric Dentistry: Policy on the dental home. In *AAPD Reference Manual 2008-2009*, 2009a, Chicago, The Academy. Available at www.aapd.org/media/Policies_Guidelines/P_Dentalhome.pdf (accessed April 6, 2009).

American Academy of Pediatric Dentistry: Policy on use of fluoride. In *AAPD Reference Manual 2008-2009*, 2009b, Chicago, The Academy. Available at www.aapd.org/media/Policies_Guidelines/G_Fluoride-Therapy.pdf (accessed April 6, 2009).

American Academy of Pediatrics: *Car safety seats: a guide for families 2009*, 2009a. Available at www.aap.org/family/carseatguide.htm (accessed April 6, 2009).

American Academy of Pediatrics: *Pediatric nutrition handbook*, ed 6, Elk Grove Village, IL, 2009b, The Academy.

American Academy of Pediatrics, Committee on Public Health: Children, adolescents, and television, *Pediatrics* 107(2):423-426, 2001.

American Heart Association: *Dietary recommendations for children and adolescents*, 2005. Available at www.americanheart.org/presenter.jhtml?identifier=3033999 (accessed January 3, 2008).

Bates E, Dick F: Language, gesture, and the developing brain, *Dev Psychobiol* 40(3):293-310, 2002.

Brazelton TB: How to help parents of young children: the touchpoints model, *J Perinatol* 19(6 Pt 2):S6-S7, 1999.

Cathey M, Gaylord N: Picky eating: a toddler's approach to mealtime, *Pediatr Nurs* 30(2):101-107, 2004.

Centers for Disease Control and Prevention: Nonfatal motor-vehicle-related backover injuries among children—United States, 2001-2003, *Morb Mortal Wkly Rep* 54(06):144-146, 2005.

Dahlquist LM et al: Distraction for children of different ages who undergo repeated needle sticks, *J Pediatr Oncol Nurs* 19(1):22-34, 2002.

DeLamater J, Friedrich WN: Human sexual development, *J Sex Res* 39(1):10-14, 2002.

Dowd DM, Keenan HT, Bratton SL: Epidemiology and prevention of childhood injuries, *Crit Care Med* 30(11):S385-S392, 2002.

Durbin DR et al: Effects of seating position and appropriate restraint use on the risk of injury to children in motor vehicle crashes, *Pediatrics* 115(3):e305-e309, 2005.

Elkins M, Cavendish R: Developing a plan for pediatric spiritual care, *Holistic Nurs Pract* 18(4):179-184, 2004.

Fosarelli P: Children and the development of faith: implications for pediatric practice, *Contemp Pediatr* 20(1):85-98, 2003.

Glassy D, Romano J, Committee on Early Childhood, Adoption, and Dependent Care: Selecting appropriate toys for young children: the pediatrician's role, *Pediatrics* 111(4):911-913, 2003.

Guard A, Gallagher SS: Heat related deaths in young children in parked cars: an analysis of 171 fatalities in the United States, 1995-2002, *Inj Prev* 11(1):33-37, 2005.

Harpaz-Rotem I, Bergman A: On an evolving theory of attachment: rapprochement-theory of a developing mind, *Psychoanal Study Child* 61:170-189, 2006.

Henary B et al: Car safety for children: rear facing for best protection, *Inj Prev* 13(6):398-402, 2007.

Howard BJ, Wong J: Sleep disorders, *Pediatr Rev* 22(10):327-342, 2001.

Institute of Medicine: *Dietary reference intakes for energy, carbohydrate, fiber, fat, fatty acids, cholesterol, protein, and amino acids*, Washington, DC, 2005, The Institute, National Academies Press.

Kallan MJ et al: Seating patterns and corresponding risk of injury among 0- to 3-year-old children in child safety seats, *Pediatrics* 121(5):e1342-e1347, 2008.

McLaren C, Null J, Quinn J: Heat stress from enclosed vehicles: moderate ambient temperatures cause significant temperature rise in enclosed vehicles, *Pediatrics* 116(1):e109-e112, 2005.

Mercer R: Treating nocturnal enuresis, *Adv Nurs Pract* 11(2):26-31, 2003.

Meyer TL: Unveiling the secrecy behind masturbation, *Pediatr Rev* 23(4):148-149, 2002.

Morin K: Infant nutrition: toddlers: start off on the right foot, *MCN* 32(2):122, 2007.

Nakamura SW, Pollack-Nelson C, Chidekel AS: Suction-type suffocation incidents in infants and toddlers, *Pediatrics* 111(1):e12-e16, 2003.

National Highway Traffic Safety Administration: *A parent's guide to booster seats (pamphlet)*, Washington, DC, 2008, The Administration. Available at www.nhtsa.gov.org (accessed July 15, 2008).

Needlman R, Howard B, Zuckerman B: Helping parents get beyond the terrible 2's, *Patient Care* 29(1):52-61, 1995.

Null J: *Hyperthermia deaths of children in vehicles*, San Francisco, 2007, San Francisco State University. Available at www.ggweather.com/heat (accessed July 2007).

Petitto LA et al: Bilingual signed and spoken language acquisition from birth: implications for the mechanisms underlying early bilingual language acquisition, *J Child Lang* 28(2):453-496, 2001.

Roehlkepartain EC et al (editors): *The handbook of spiritual development in childhood and adolescence*, Thousand Oaks, CA, 2006, Sage.

Schmitt BD: Toilet training: getting it right the first time, *Contemp Pediatr* 21(3):105-108, 111-112, 115-116, 2004.

Schnitzer PG: Prevention of unintentional childhood injuries, *Am Fam Physician* 74(11):1864-1869, 2006.

Schum TR et al: Sequential acquisition of toilet-training skills: a descriptive study of gender and age differences in normal children, *Pediatrics* 109(3):e48, 2002.

Thompson RA: Caring for infants and toddlers, *Future Child* 11(1):21-33, 2001.

Wagner CL, Greer FR, American Academy of Pediatrics, Section on Breastfeeding and Committee on Nutrition: Prevention of rickets and vitamin D deficiency in infants, children, and adolescents, *Pediatrics* 122(5):1142-1148, 2008.

Unit 9

38 The Preschooler and Family

Learning Objectives

On completion of this chapter the reader will be able to:

- Identify the major biologic, psychosocial, cognitive, moral, spiritual, and social developments that occur during the preschool years.
- List the benefits of imaginary playmates.
- Prepare preschoolers for preschool or day care experience.
- Provide parents with guidelines for sex education.
- Provide parents with guidelines for dealing with a child's fears, stresses, aggression, and sleep problems.
- Recognize the causes of stuttering during the preschool years.
- Offer parents suggestions for preventing speech problems.
- Recognize feeding patterns of preschoolers.
- Provide anticipatory guidance to parents regarding injury prevention based on the preschooler's developmental achievements.

Electronic Resources

Additional information related to the content in Chapter 38 can be found on

evolve the Companion Website at

http://evolve.elsevier.com/Perry/maternal/

- NCLEX Review Questions
- Assessment Video Clips
- Case Study—Bacterial Conjunctivitis
- Case Study—Chickenpox (Varicella)
- Case Study—Sleep Problems
- Case Study—Varicella in Spite of Vaccine
- Critical Thinking Exercise—Conjunctivitis
- Critical Thinking Exercise—Imitative Play
- Nursing Care Plan—The Child Who Is Maltreated
- Nursing Care Plan—The Child with a Communicable Disease

Promoting Optimal Growth and Development

The combined biologic, psychosocial, cognitive, spiritual, and social achievements during the *preschool period* (3 to 5 years of age) prepare preschoolers for their most significant change in lifestyle: entrance into school. Their control of bodily functions, experience of brief and prolonged periods of separation, ability to interact cooperatively with other children and adults, use of language for mental symbolization, and increased attention span and memory prepare them for the next major period: the school years. Successful achievement of previous levels of growth and development is essential for preschoolers to refine many of the tasks that were mastered during the toddler years.

Biologic Development

The rate of physical growth slows and stabilizes during the preschool years. The average *weight* is 14.5 kg (32 lb) at 3 years, 16.7 kg (36⅗ lb) at 4 years, and 18.8 kg (41½ lb) at 5 years. The average weight gain per year remains approximately 2 to 3 kg (4½ to 6½ lb). Growth in *height* also remains steady, with a yearly increase of 6.5 to 9 cm (2½ to 3½ inches), and generally occurs by elongation of the legs rather than of the trunk. The average height is 95 cm (37½ inches) at 3 years, 103 cm (40½ inches) at 4 years, and 110 cm (43½ inches) at 5 years.

Physical proportions no longer resemble those of the squat, pot-bellied toddler. The preschooler is slender but sturdy, graceful, agile, and posturally erect. There is little difference in physical characteristics according to gender, except as dictated by such factors as dress and hairstyle.

Most organ systems can adjust to moderate stress and change. During this period, most children are toilet trained. For the most part, motor development consists of increases in strength and refinement of previously learned skills, such as walking, running, and jumping. However, muscle development and bone growth are still far from mature. Excessive activity and overexertion can injure delicate tissues. Good posture, appropriate exercise, and adequate nutrition and rest are essential for optimal development of the musculoskeletal system.

Gross and Fine Motor Skills

Walking, running, climbing, and jumping are well established by age 36 months. Refinement in eye-hand and muscle coordination is evident in several areas. At age 3, the preschooler

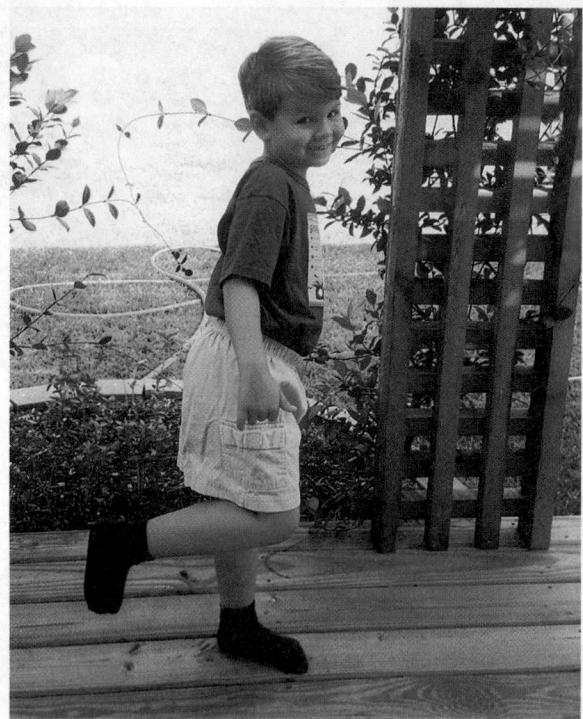

Fig. 38-1 A 4-year-old child has sufficient balance to stand or hop on one foot.

rides a tricycle, walks on tiptoe, balances on one foot for a few seconds, and broad jumps. By age 4, the child skips and hops proficiently on one foot (Fig. 38-1) and catches a ball reliably. By age 5, the child skips on alternate feet, jumps rope, and begins to skate and swim.

Fine motor development is evident in the child's increasingly skillful manipulation, such as in drawing and dressing. These skills provide readiness for learning and independence for entry into school.

Psychosocial Development

Developing a Sense of Initiative (Erikson)

After preschoolers have mastered the tasks of the toddler period, they are ready to face the developmental endeavors of the preschool period. Erikson maintained that the chief psychosocial task of this period is acquiring a sense of *initiative*. Children are in a stage of energetic learning. They play, work, and live to the fullest and feel a real sense of accomplishment and satisfaction in their activities. Conflict arises when children overstep the limits of their ability and inquiry and experience a sense of *guilt* for not having behaved appropriately. Feelings of guilt, anxiety, and fear may also result from thoughts that differ from expected behavior.

A particularly stressful thought is wishing one's parent dead. As a sense of rivalry or competition develops between the child and same-sex parent, the child may think of ways to get rid of the interfering parent. In most situations, this rivalry is resolved when the child strongly identifies with the same-sex parent and peers during the school years. However, if that parent dies before the identification process is completed, the preschooler may be overwhelmed with guilt for having wished and therefore "caused" the death. Clarifying for children that wishes cannot and do not make events occur is essential in helping them overcome their guilt and anxiety.

Development of the *superego*, or *conscience*, begins toward the end of the toddler years and is a major task for preschoolers (see Cultural Awareness box). Learning right from wrong and good from bad is the beginning of morality (see section on Moral Development).

> **CULTURAL AWARENESS**
>
> *Learning Sociocultural Mores*
>
> Developing a conscience implies learning the sociocultural mores of the family's heritage. Depending on the type of attitudes conveyed, children will learn not only appropriate behaviors, but also tolerant, biased, or prejudicial values concerning their ethnic, religious, and social background and those of other groups. Much of this influence may remain dormant until they associate with children or adults of a different heritage. Then, depending on the particular group, they may be accepted or ostracized for their attitudes.

Cognitive Development

One of the tasks related to the preschool period is readiness for school and scholastic learning. Many of the thought processes of this period are crucial for achieving such readiness, and it is intentional that the child begins school between ages 5 and 6 rather than at an earlier age.

Preoperational Phase (Piaget)

Piaget's cognitive theory does not include a period specifically for children who are 3 to 5 years old. The *preoperational phase* covers the age span from 2 to 7 years and is divided into two stages: the *preconceptual phase*, ages 2 to 4, and the phase of *intuitive thought*, ages 4 to 7. One of the main transitions during these two phases is the shift from totally egocentric thought to social awareness and the ability to consider other viewpoints. However, egocentricity is still evident.

Language continues to develop during the preschool period. Speech remains primarily a vehicle of egocentric communication. Preschoolers assume that everyone thinks as they do and that a brief explanation of their thinking makes the entire thought understood by others. Because of this self-referenced, egocentric verbal communication, it is often necessary to explore and understand the young child's thinking through other, nonverbal approaches. For children in this age group, the most enlightening and effective method is *play*, which becomes the child's way of understanding, adjusting to, and working out life's experiences.

Preschoolers increasingly use language without comprehending the meaning of words, particularly concepts of right and left, causality, and time. Children may use the concepts correctly but only in the circumstances in which they have learned them. For example, they may know how to put on shoes by remembering that the buckle is always on the outside of the foot. However, if different shoes have no buckles, they cannot reason which shoe fits which foot. In other words, they do not understand the concept of *right and left*.

Superficially, *causality* resembles logical thought. Preschoolers explain a concept as they heard it described by others, but their understanding is limited. An example is the concept of time. Because *time* is still incompletely understood, the child interprets it according to his or her own frame of reference, such as "A long time means until Christmas." Consequently, time is best explained in relationship to an event, such as "Your mother will visit you after you finish your lunch." Avoiding words such as *yesterday, tomorrow, next week,* or *Tuesday* to express when an event is expected to occur and instead associating time with expected daily events help children learn about temporal relationships while increasing their trust in others' predictions.

Preschoolers' thinking is often described as *magical thinking*. Because of their egocentrism and transductive reasoning, they believe that thoughts are all-powerful. Such thinking places them in the vulnerable position of feeling guilty and responsible for bad thoughts, which may coincide with the occurrence of a wished event. Their inability to logically reason the cause and effect of an illness or injury makes it especially difficult for them to understand such events.

NURSING ALERT Counseling children whose parents are going through a divorce or separation should involve a discussion with the child about her or his role. Because of magical thinking, the child may believe he or she wished the other parent away. The child should be reassured that this is not the case.

Preschoolers believe in the power of words and accept their meaning literally. An example of this type of thinking is calling children "bad" because they did something wrong. In the preschooler's mind, calling them bad means they are a bad person; thus it is better to say that their actions were bad by saying, for example, "That was a bad thing to do."

Moral Development

Preconventional or Premoral Level (Kohlberg)

Young children's development of moral judgment is at the most basic level. They have little, if any, concern about why something is wrong. They behave because of the freedom or restriction that is placed on actions. In the *punishment and obedience orientation*, children (from about 2 to 4 years) judge whether an action is good or bad depending on whether it results in reward or punishment. If children are punished for it, the action is bad. If they are not punished, the action is good, regardless of the meaning of the act. For example, if parents allow hitting, the child will perceive that hitting is good because it is not associated with punishment.

From approximately 4 to 7 years of age, children are in the stage of *naive instrumental orientation*, in which actions are directed toward satisfying their needs and, less frequently, the needs of others. They have a concrete sense of justice and fairness during this period of development.

Spiritual Development

Children's knowledge of faith and religion is learned from significant others in their environment, usually from parents and their religious beliefs and practices (Fosarelli, 2003). However, young children's understanding of spirituality is influenced by their cognitive level. Preschoolers have a concrete concept of a God with physical characteristics, often like an imaginary friend. They understand simple Bible stories and memorize short prayers, but their understanding of the meaning of these rituals is limited. Preschoolers benefit from concrete representations of religious practices, such as picture Bible books and small statues, such as those of the Nativity scene. They will imitate the religious practices of their parents without fully understanding the significance of these acts.

Development of the conscience is strongly linked to spiritual development. At this age, children are learning right from wrong and behaving correctly to avoid punishment. Wrongdoing provokes feelings of guilt, and preschoolers often misinterpret illness as a punishment for real or imagined transgressions. It is important that children view God as one who bestows unconditional love, rather than as a judge of good or bad behavior. Observing religious traditions and participating in a religious community can help children cope during stressful periods, such as illness, hospitalization, and other traumatic events (Barnes et al, 2000). In many religious faiths, cultural practices and religion are closely intertwined (McEvoy, 2003) and are an important part of the child and family's life.

Development of Body Image

The preschool years play a significant role in the development of body image. With increasing comprehension of language, preschoolers recognize that individuals have undesirable and desirable appearances. They recognize differences in skin color and racial identity and are vulnerable to learning prejudices and biases. They are aware of the meaning of words such as *pretty* or *ugly,* and they reflect the opinions of others regarding their own appearance. By 5 years of age, children compare their size with that of their peers and can become conscious of being large or short, especially if others refer to them as "so big" or "so little" for their age. In one study, negative associations between weight status and self-concept were identified in girls as young as 5 years of age (Davison & Birch, 2001).

Despite the advances in body image development, preschoolers have poorly defined body boundaries and little knowledge of their internal anatomy. Intrusive experiences are frightening, especially those that disrupt the integrity of the skin, such as injections and surgery. They fear that if their skin is "broken," all of their blood and "insides" can leak out. Therefore bandages are critical to "keep everything from coming out."

Development of Sexuality

Sexual development during these years is an important phase in the formation of a person's overall sexual identity and beliefs. Preschoolers are forming strong attachments to the opposite-sex parent while identifying with the same-sex parent. *Sex-typing*, or the process by which an individual develops the behavior, personality, attitudes, and beliefs appropriate for his or her culture and sex, occurs through several mechanisms during this period. Probably the most powerful mechanisms are childrearing practices and imitation. Gender identification is a result of complex prenatal and postnatal psychologic factors, as well as biologic or genetic factors. Most children are aware of their gender and the expected sets of related behaviors by 1½ to 2½ years of age.

As sexual identity develops beyond gender recognition, modesty may become a concern. Sex-role imitation and "dressing up" like Mommy or Daddy are important activities. Attitudes and responses of others to role-playing can condition the child to accept the views of others. For example, comments such as "Boys shouldn't play with dolls" can influence a boy's self-concept of masculinity.

Sexual exploration may be more pronounced now than ever before, particularly in terms of exploring and manipulating the genitalia. Questions about sexual reproduction may come to the forefront in the preschooler's search for understanding (see Chapters 39 and 40).

Social Development

During the preschool period, the *separation-individuation process* is completed. Preschoolers have overcome much of the anxiety associated with strangers and the fear of separation of earlier years. They relate to unfamiliar people easily and tolerate brief separations from parents with little or no protest. However, they still need parental security, reassurance, guidance, and approval, especially when entering preschool or elementary school. Prolonged separation, such as that imposed by illness and hospitalization, is difficult, but preschoolers respond to anticipatory preparation and concrete explanation. They can cope with changes in daily routine much better than toddlers, although they may develop more imaginary fears. Preschoolers gain security and comfort from familiar objects, such as toys, dolls, or photographs of family members. They are able to work through many of their unresolved fears, fantasies, and anxieties through play, especially if guided with appropriate play objects (e.g., dolls, puppets) that represent family members, health care professionals, and other children.

Language

During the preschool years, language becomes more sophisticated and complex. Both cognitive ability and environment—particularly, consistent role models—influence vocabulary, speech, and comprehension. Language becomes a major mode of communication and social interaction, and its development during the preschool period sets the stage for later success in school (Needlman, 2004) (Fig. 38-2). Vocabulary increases dramatically, from 300 words at age 2 to more than 2100 words at the end of age 5. Sentence structure, grammatical usage, and intelligibility also advance to a more adult level. Through language, preschool children learn to express feelings of frustration or anger without acting them out.

Children between the ages of 3 and 4 years form sentences of about three or four words and include only the most essential words to convey a meaning. Such speech is often termed *telegraphic* for its brevity. Three-year-old children ask many questions and use plurals, correct pronouns, and the past tense of verbs. They name familiar objects, such as animals, parts of the body, relatives, and friends. They can give and follow simple commands. They talk incessantly, regardless of whether anyone is listening or answering them. They enjoy musical or talking toys or dolls and imitate new words proficiently.

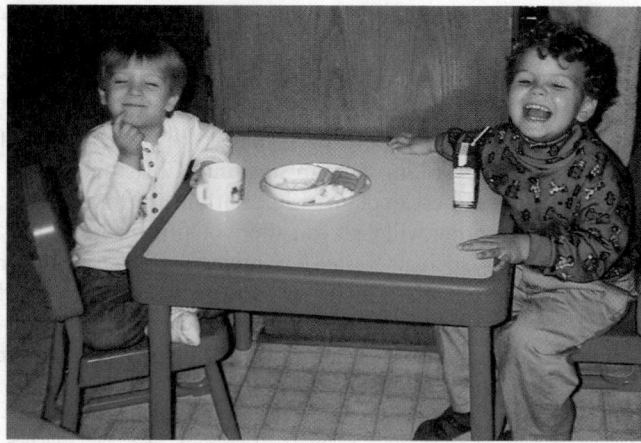

Fig. 38-2 Preschool children enjoy friends and often use nonverbal messages to communicate.

From ages 4 to 5 years, preschoolers use longer sentences of four or five words and use more words to convey a message, such as prepositions, adjectives, and a variety of verbs. They follow simple directional commands, such as "Put the ball on the chair," but can carry out only one request at a time. They answer questions such as "What do you do when you are hungry?" by describing the appropriate action. The pattern of asking questions is at its peak, and children will usually repeat a question until they receive an answer.

By age 6, children can use all parts of speech correctly, except for deviations from the rule. They can define simple things by describing their use, shape, or general category of classification, rather than simply describing their outward appearance. For example, they define a ball as "round," "something you bounce," or "a toy," rather than only describing its color. They can give some opposites, such as "If Mommy is a woman, Daddy is a man." They can also describe an object according to its composition, such as "A spoon is made of metal."

Personal-Social Behavior

The pervasive ritualism and negativism of toddlerhood gradually diminish during the preschool years. Although self-assertion is still a major theme, preschoolers demonstrate their sense of autonomy differently. They are able to verbalize their request for independence and perform independently because of their much-refined physical and cognitive development. By 4 or 5 years of age, they need little if any assistance with dressing, eating, or toileting (Fig. 38-3). They can also be trusted to obey warnings of danger, although 3- or 4-year-old children may exceed their boundaries at times.

They are much more sociable and willing to please. They have internalized many of the standards and values of the family and culture. However, by the end of early childhood they begin to question parental values and compare them with those of their peer group and other authority figures. As a result, they may be less willing to abide by the family's code of conduct. Preschoolers become increasingly aware of their position and role within the family. Although this is a more secure age for experiencing the addition of another sibling, relinquishing the position of only or youngest is still difficult

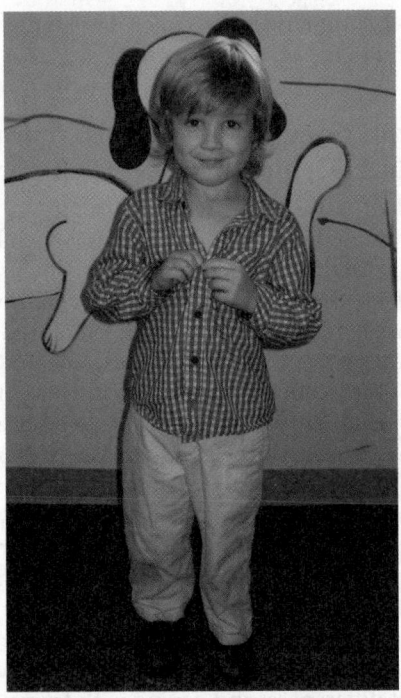

Fig. 38-3 Most preschoolers are able to dress themselves but need help with more difficult items of clothing.

and requires special parental attention to prevent feelings of desertion and resentment (Brazelton & Sparrow, 2001) (see Sibling Rivalry, Chapter 37).

Play

Various types of play are typical of this period, but preschoolers especially enjoy *associative play*—group play in similar or identical activities but without rigid organization or rules. Play should provide for physical, social, and mental development.

Play activities for physical growth and refinement of motor skills include jumping, running, and climbing. Tricycles, wagons, gym and sports equipment, sandboxes, wading pools, and activities at water parks can help develop muscles and coordination (Fig. 38-4). Activities such as swimming and skating teach safety as well as muscle development and coordination. Children involved in the work of play do not require expensive toys and gadgets to keep them entertained but often enjoy playing with common household items such as a broom handle or even items adults consider junk (boxes, sticks, rocks, and dirt). The preschooler's imaginative mind enjoys playing for its own sake.

Manipulative, constructive, creative, and educational toys provide for quiet activities, fine motor development, and self-expression. Easy construction sets, large blocks of various sizes and shapes, a counting frame, alphabet or number flash cards, paints, crayons, simple carpentry tools, musical toys, illustrated books, simple sewing or handicraft sets, large puzzles, and clay are suitable toys. Electronic games and computer programs are especially valuable in helping children learn basic skills, such as letters and simple words.

Probably the most characteristic and pervasive preschool activity is *imitative, imaginative,* and *dramatic play*. Dress-up clothes, dolls, housekeeping toys, dollhouses, play store toys,

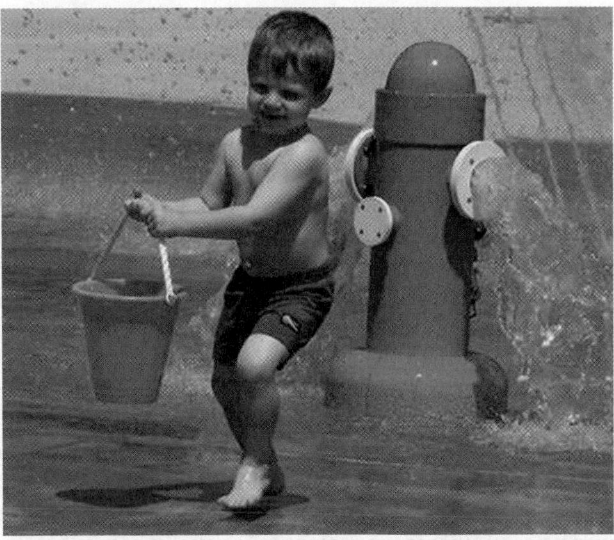

Fig. 38-4 Preschoolers enjoy play activities that promote motor skills such as jumping and running. Water play is an exciting activity for preschooler.

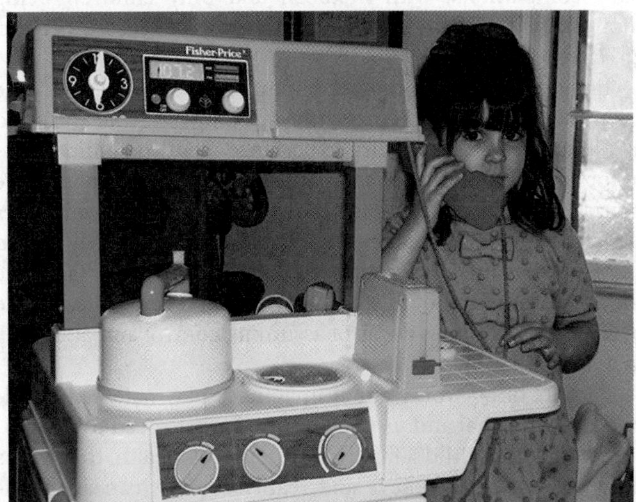

Fig. 38-5 Imaginative and imitative play is typical of preschoolers.

telephones, farm animals and equipment, village sets, trains, trucks, cars, planes, hand puppets, and medical kits provide hours of self-expression (Fig. 38-5). Probably at no other time is the reproduction of adult behavior so faithful and absorbing as in 4- and 5-year-old children. Toward the end of the preschool period, children are less satisfied with make-believe or pretend objects and enjoy doing the actual activity, such as cooking and carpentry.

Television and videos also have their place in children's play, although each should be only one part of children's total repertoire of social and recreational activities. Parents and other caregivers should supervise the selection of programs, watch and discuss programs with their children, schedule limited time for television viewing, and set a good example of television viewing (Yalçin et al, 2002; American Academy of Pediatrics, Committee on Public Education, 2001). Children also enjoy and learn from educational programs; however,

evolve Critical Thinking Exercise—Imitative Play

television viewing may limit time spent in other meaningful activities such as reading, physical activity, and socialization (American Academy of Pediatrics, Committee on Public Education, 2001).

Television can become an interactive activity when adults view programs with children and discuss program content. In one study, viewing educational programs as preschoolers was associated with higher grades, more book reading, greater emphasis on achievement, increased creativity, and less aggression in adolescent years (Anderson et al, 2001). The researchers emphasize that the content of television viewing appeared more important than the amount viewed.

Play is so much a part of the young child's life that reality and fantasy become blurred. Make-believe is reality during play and only becomes fantasy when the toys are put away or the dress-up clothes are removed. It is no wonder that *imaginary playmates* are so much a part of this age period. The appearance of imaginary companions usually occurs between ages 2½ and 3 years, and, for the most part, such playmates are relinquished when the child enters school. The birth order and number of siblings may influence the creation of imaginary companions, with firstborn and only children being more likely to create imaginary playmates (Gleason, Sebanc, & Hartup, 2000).

Imaginary companions serve many purposes: they become friends in times of loneliness, they accomplish what the child is still attempting, and they experience what the child wants to forget or remember. It is not unusual for the "friend" to have myriad vices and to be blamed for wrongdoing. Sometimes the child hopes to escape punishment by saying, "My friend George broke the glass." At other times, the child may fantasize that the companion misbehaved and play the role of the parent. This becomes a way of assuming control and authority in a safe situation.

Parents often worry about imaginary playmates, not realizing how normal and useful they are. Parents need to be reassured that the child's fantasy is a sign of health that helps differentiate make-believe and reality. Parents can acknowledge the imaginary companion's presence by calling him or her by name and even agreeing to simple requests such as setting an extra place at the table, but they should not allow the child to use the playmate to avoid punishment or responsibility. For example, if the child blames the companion for messing up a room, parents need to state clearly that the child is the only one they see; therefore the child is responsible for cleaning up.

Children also benefit from play that occurs between them and a parent. *Mutual play* fosters development from birth through the school years and provides enriched opportunities for learning. Through mutual play, parents can provide tactile and kinesthetic experiences, can maximize verbal and language abilities, and can offer praise and encouragement for exploration of the world. In addition, mutual play encourages positive interactions between the parent and child, strengthening their relationship.*

**Recommended books for suggestions on mutual play include* Quick and Fun Learning Activities *books, by Teacher Created Resources, 6421 Industry Way, Westminster, CA 92683; 800-662-4321 or 714-891-7895;* www.teachercreated.com.

Table 38-1 summarizes the major developmental achievements for children 3, 4, and 5 years of age.

Coping with Concerns Related to Normal Growth and Development

Preschool and Kindergarten Experience

Some children are home schooled, but many children attend some type of early childhood program, usually preschool or a day care center. Group care has become commonplace with the large number of parents currently employed outside the home (see Alternative Child Care Arrangements, Chapter 36). The effects of early education and stimulation on children have increasingly gained recognition. (For a discussion of the effects of day care on young children, see Working Mothers, Chapter 31.) Because social development widens to include age-mates and other significant adults, preschool provides an excellent vehicle for expanding children's experiences with others. It is also excellent preparation for entrance into elementary school.

In preschool or day care centers, children are exposed to opportunities for learning group cooperation; adjusting to sociocultural differences; and coping with frustration, dissatisfaction, and anger. If activities are tailored to provide mastery and achievement, children increasingly have feelings of success, self-confidence, and personal competence. Whether structured learning is imposed is less important than the social climate, type of guidance, and attitude toward the children that is fostered by the teacher or leader. With a teacher who is aware of preschoolers' developmental abilities and needs, children will learn from the activity that is provided. Most programs incorporate a daily schedule of quiet play, active outdoor activity, group activities such as games and projects, creative or free play, and snack and rest periods. Preschool is particularly beneficial for children who lack a peer-group experience, such as an only child, and for children from impoverished homes.

One of the issues that parents face is the child's readiness for preschool or kindergarten. There are no absolute indicators for school readiness, but the child's social maturity, especially attention span, is as important as his or her academic readiness. Using a developmental screening tool that addresses cognitive (especially language), social, and physical milestones can identify children who may benefit from diagnostic testing and early intervention programs before starting school. Parents play an integral role in their children's school readiness. They should promote a positive attitude toward learning, read to their children, encourage their children to participate in a variety of activities to explore their talents, and choose appropriate child care or preschool programs (Jellinek, Patel, & Froehle, 2002).

Nurses and other health care workers can guide parents in selecting enriched social and educational early intervention programs, schools, and child care centers. Careful selection of early childhood education is intrinsic to future learning and development. Licensed and regulated programs are mandated to abide by established standards, which represent minimum requirements and safeguards. Regulation is important to protect children from harm and to promote the conditions essential for a child's healthy development and learning. The National Association for the Education of Young Children serves as the model for optimal care of small children.*

Areas for parents to evaluate include the facility's daily program, teacher qualifications, staff-to-student ratio, discipline policy, environmental safety precautions, provision of meals, sanitary conditions, adequate indoor and outdoor space per child, and fee schedule. References from other parents help in evaluating a facility, but personal observation of the facility is recommended. Encourage parents to meet the director and some of the employees at a few facilities to make an informed choice.

Evaluation of the facility's health practices is extremely important. Children in day care centers have more illnesses than children not in day care centers, especially gastrointestinal tract infections; respiratory tract infections; and hepatitis A, varicella-zoster virus, and cytomegalovirus infections (Rafanello, 2001). Nurses play an important role in infection control. Not only can they advise parents regarding the evaluation of a facility's sanitary practices, but they can also take an active part in educating staff in measures to minimize transmission of infection (Fig. 38-6).

Children need preparation for the preschool or kindergarten experience. For young children it represents a change from their usual home environment and prolonged separation from parents. Before children begin school, parents should present the idea as exciting and pleasurable. Talking to children about

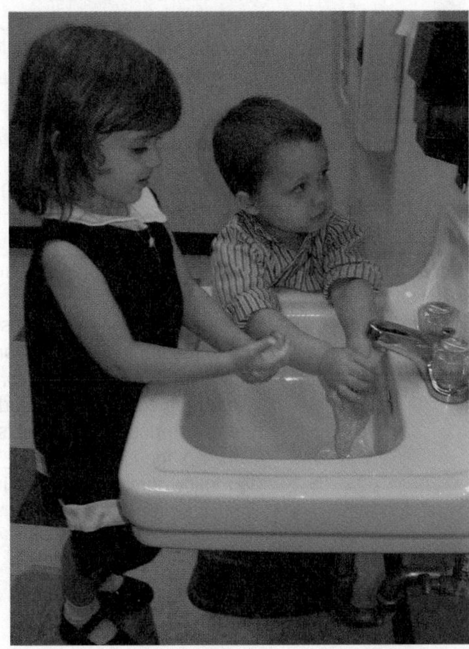

Fig. 38-6 Thorough handwashing is the single most effective method of preventing infection.

**Information about accreditation criteria and procedures of the NAEYC Academy for Early Childhood Program Accreditation is available from the National Association for the Education of Young Children, 1313 L St. NW, Suite 500, Washington, DC 20005; 800-424-2460 or 202-232-8777; www.naeyc.org. These criteria are excellent guidelines for evaluating preschools or day care centers.*

activities such as painting, building with blocks, or enjoying swings and other outdoor equipment allows children to fantasize about the forthcoming event in a positive manner. When the first day of school arrives, parents should behave confidently. Such behavior requires parents to have resolved their own feelings regarding the experience.

Parents should introduce their child to the teacher and the facility. In some instances, it is helpful for parents to remain with the child for at least part of the first day until the child is comfortable and at ease. Other specific actions that can help reduce separation anxiety include providing the school with detailed information about the child's home environment, such as familiar routines, favorite activities, food preferences, names of siblings or pets, and personal habits. Such information helps the child feel familiar in the strange surroundings. When schools automatically request this information, the parent has a valuable clue to the quality of the program because the request represents the staff's awareness of each child's needs. Transitional objects, such as a favorite toy, may also help the child bridge the gap from home to school.

Sex Education

Preschoolers have assimilated a tremendous amount of information during their short lifetimes. Although their thinking may not be mature, they search constantly for explanations and reasons that are logical and reasonable to them. The word "why" seems to supplant the word "no," which was common in toddlerhood. It is only natural that as they learn about "me," they will also want to know "why me" and "how me." Questions such as "Where do babies come from?" are as casual as "What makes it rain?" or "Who is that?" It is the *way* in which questions about procreation are answered that conditions children, even the youngest, to separate these questions from others about their world.

Two rules govern answering sensitive questions about topics such as sex. The first is to *find out what children know and think.* By investigating the theories children have produced as a reasonable explanation, parents can give correct information and help children understand why their explanation is inaccurate. Another reason for ascertaining what the child thinks before offering any information is that the "unasked for" answer may be given. For example, 4-year-old Sally asked her father, "Where did I come from?" Both parents quickly took this inquiry as a clue for offering sex education. After the explanation, Sally exclaimed, "I don't know about all that! All I know is Mary came from New York, and I want to know where I was born."

The second rule for giving information is to *be honest.* It is true that the preschooler will forget or misunderstand much of the correct information, but the correct information can be restated until the child absorbs and comprehends the facts. Even though the correct anatomic words may be hard to pronounce or even more difficult to remember, they become foundational content for explaining other concepts later on.

Honesty does not imply imparting to children every fact of life or allowing excessive permissiveness in sexual curiosity. When children ask one question, they are looking for one answer. When they are ready, they will ask about the other "unfinished" parts of the story. Sooner or later they will wonder

Table 38-1 Growth and Development During Preschool Years

PHYSICAL	GROSS MOTOR	FINE MOTOR	LANGUAGE
Age 3 Yr			
Usual weight gain of 1.8-2.7 kg (4-6 lb) Average weight of 14.5 kg (32 lb) Usual gain in height of 7.5 cm (3 inches) per year Average height of 95 cm (37½ inches) May have achieved nighttime control of bowel and bladder	Rides tricycle Jumps off bottom step Stands on one foot for a few seconds Goes up stairs using alternate feet; may still come down using both feet on step Broad jumps May try to dance, but balance may not be adequate	Builds tower of 9-10 cubes Builds bridge with three cubes Adeptly places small pellets in narrow-necked bottle In drawing, copies a circle, imitates a cross, names what has been drawn; cannot draw stick figure but may make circle with facial features	Has vocabulary of about 900 words Uses primarily telegraphic speech Uses complete sentences of three or four words Talks incessantly regardless of whether anyone is paying attention Repeats sentence of six syllables Asks many questions
Age 4 Yr			
Pulse and respiration rates decrease slightly Growth rate is similar to that of previous year Average weight of 16.7 kg (36⅘ lb) Average height of 103 cm (40½ inches) Length at birth is doubled Maximum potential for development of amblyopia	Skips and hops on one foot Catches ball reliably Throws ball overhead Walks down stairs using alternate footing	Uses scissors successfully to cut out picture following outline Can lace shoes but may not be able to tie bow In drawing, copies a square, traces a cross and diamond, adds three parts to stick figure	Has vocabulary of 1500 words or more Uses sentences of four or five words Questioning is at peak Tells exaggerated stories Knows simple songs May be mildly profane if associates with older children Obeys four prepositional phrases, such as under, on top of, beside, in back of, or in front of Names one or more colors Comprehends analogies, such as, "If ice is cold, fire is ______"
Age 5 Yr			
Pulse and respiration rates decrease slightly Average weight of 18.7 kg (41.2 lb) Average height of 110 cm (43½ inches) Eruption of permanent dentition may begin Handedness is established (about 90% are right-handed)	Skips and hops on alternate feet Throws and catches ball well Jumps rope Skates with good balance Walks backward with heel to toe Jumps from height of 12 inches and lands on toes Balances on alternate feet with eyes closed	Ties shoelaces Uses scissors, simple tools, or pencil very well In drawing, copies a diamond and triangle; adds seven to nine parts to stick figure; prints a few letters, numbers, or words, such as first name	Has vocabulary of about 2100 words Uses sentences of six to eight words, with all parts of speech Names coins (e.g., nickel, dime) Names four or more colors Describes drawing or pictures with much comment and elaboration Knows days of week, months, and other time-associated words Knows composition of objects, such as "A shoe is made of ______." Can follow three commands in succession

how the "sperm meets the egg" and "how the baby gets out," but during this period, it is best to wait until they ask.

Regardless of whether children are given sex education, they will engage in games of sexual curiosity and exploration. At about 3 years of age, children are aware of the anatomic differences between the sexes and are concerned with how the other "works." This is not really "sexual" curiosity because many children are still unaware of the reproductive function of the genitalia. Their curiosity is for the eliminative function of the anatomy. Little boys wonder how girls can urinate without a penis, so they watch girls go to the bathroom. Because they cannot see anything but the stream of urine

SOCIALIZATION	COGNITION	FAMILY RELATIONSHIPS
Dresses self almost completely if helped with back buttons and told which shoe is right or left Pulls on shoes Has increased attention span Feeds self completely Can prepare simple meals, such as cold cereal and milk Can help to set table; can dry dishes without breaking any May have fears, especially of dark and going to bed Knows own gender and gender of others Play is parallel and associative; begins to learn simple games, but often follows own rules; begins to share	Is in preconceptual phase Is egocentric in thought and behavior Has beginning understanding of time; uses many time-oriented expressions, talks about past and future as much as about present, pretends to tell time Has improved concept of space, as demonstrated by understanding of prepositions and ability to follow directional command Has beginning ability to view concepts from another perspective	Attempts to please parents and conform to their expectations Is less jealous of younger sibling; may be opportune time for birth of additional sibling Is aware of family relationships and sex-role functions Boys tend to identify more with father or other male figure Has increased ability to separate easily and comfortably from parents for short periods
Very independent Tends to be selfish and impatient Aggressive physically and verbally Takes pride in accomplishments Has mood swings Shows off dramatically, enjoys entertaining others Tells family tales to others with no restraint Still has many fears Play is associative Imaginary playmates are common Uses dramatic, imaginative, and imitative devices Sexual exploration and curiosity demonstrated through play, such as being "doctor" or "nurse"	Is in phase of intuitive thought Causality is still related to proximity of events Understands time better, especially in terms of sequence of daily events Unable to conserve matter Judges everything according to one dimension, such as height, width, or order Immediate perceptual clues dominate judgment Is beginning to develop less egocentrism and more social awareness May count correctly but has poor mathematic concept of numbers Obeys because parents have set limits, not because of understanding of right or wrong	Rebels if parents expect too much, such as impeccable table manners Takes aggression and frustration out on parents or siblings Do's and don'ts become important May have rivalry with older or younger siblings; may resent older sibling's privileges and younger sibling's invasion of privacy and possessions May "run away" from home Identifies strongly with parent of opposite sex Is able to run simple errands outside the home
Less rebellious and quarrelsome than at age 4 yr More settled and eager to get down to business Not as open and accessible in thoughts and behavior as in earlier years Independent but trustworthy, not foolhardy; more responsible Has fewer fears; relies on outer authority to control world Eager to do things right and to please; tries to "live by the rules" Has better manners Cares for self totally, occasionally needing supervision in dress or hygiene Not ready for concentrated close work or small print because of slight farsightedness and still unrefined eye-hand coordination Play is associative; tries to follow rules but may cheat to avoid losing	Begins to question what parents think by comparing them with age-mates and other adults May notice prejudice and bias in outside world Is more able to view other's perspective, but tolerates differences rather than understanding them May begin to show understanding of conservation of numbers through counting objects regardless of arrangement Uses time-oriented words with increased understanding Cautious about accepting or believing information	Gets along well with parents May seek out parent more often than at age 4 yr for reassurance and security, especially when entering school Begins to question parents' thinking and principles Strongly identifies with parent of same sex, especially boys with their fathers Enjoys activities such as sports, cooking, and shopping with parent of same sex

coming out, they want to observe further. "Doctor play" is often a game invented for just such investigation. Little girls are no less curious about boys' anatomy. It is intriguing to closely inspect this "thing" that girls do not have.

One question that parents often have is how to handle such sexual curiosity. A positive approach is to neither condone nor condemn it but to express that if children have questions, they should ask the parents; the parents should then encourage them to engage in some other activity. In this way, children can be helped to understand that there are ways to satisfy their sexual curiosity other than through investigative games. This in no way condemns the act but stresses alternate methods to seek solutions and answers. Allowing children unrestricted permissiveness only intensifies their anxiety and concern, since exploring and searching usually yield little evidence to satisfy their curiosity.

Many excellent books on sex education are available for preschool children at public libraries. The Sexuality Information and Education Council of the United States,* local chapters of the Planned Parenthood Federation of America,† and the American Academy of Pediatrics‡ have bibliographies of suggested reading material. Parents should read the book themselves *before* giving or reading it to a child.

Another concern for some parents is *masturbation*, or self-stimulation of the genitalia. This occurs at any age for a variety of reasons and, if not excessive, is normal and healthy. It is most common at 4 years of age and during adolescence. For preschoolers, it is a part of sexual curiosity and exploration. If parents are concerned about their children masturbating, it is essential for nurses to investigate the circumstances associated with the activity because it may be an expression of anxiety, boredom, or unresolved conflicts. Children who openly and publicly masturbate are inviting a reaction, such as discipline, punishment, or criticism. They may be overwhelmed by their sexual feelings and are asking others to help channel them into more constructive outlets. Masturbation, like other forms of sex play, is a private act, and parents should emphasize this to children when teaching them socially acceptable behavior.

Fears

A great number and variety of real and imagined fears are present during the preschool years, including fear of the dark, being left alone (especially at bedtime), animals (particularly large dogs), ghosts, sexual matters (castration), and objects or persons associated with pain. The exact cause of children's fears is often unknown. Parents often become perplexed about handling the fears because no amount of logical persuasion, coercion, or ridicule will send away the ghosts, boogeymen, monsters, and devils. Inappropriate television viewing by preschoolers may increase fears and anxieties because of the inability to separate reality-based experiences from fantasy portrayed on television.

The concept of *animism*, ascribing lifelike qualities to inanimate objects, helps explain why children fear objects. For example, a child may refuse to use the toilet after watching a television commercial in which the toilet bowel is portrayed as turning into a monster.

Preschoolers also experience fear of annihilation. Because of poorly defined body boundaries and improved cognitive abilities, young children develop concerns related to loss of body parts. They fear losing body parts with certain medical procedures such as an intravenous insertion or cast application on a limb and may see these procedures as real threats to their existence.

The best way to help children overcome their fears is by actively involving them in finding practical methods to deal with the frightening experience. This may be as simple as keeping a night-light on in the child's bedroom for assurance that no monsters lurk in the dark. Exposing children to the feared object in a safe situation also provides a type of conditioning, or *desensitization*. For instance, children who are afraid of dogs should never be forced to approach or touch one, but they may be gradually introduced to the experience by watching other children play with the animal. This type of modeling, with others demonstrating fearlessness, can be effective if the child is allowed to progress at his or her own rate.

Usually by 5 or 6 years of age, children relinquish many of their fears. Explaining the developmental sequence of fears and their gradual disappearance may help parents feel more secure in handling preschoolers' fears. Sometimes fears do not subside with simple measures or developmental maturation. When children experience severe fears that disrupt family life, professional help is required.

Stress

Although for parents the preschool years generally are less troublesome than toddlerhood, this period of life presents children with many unique stresses. Some, such as fears, are innate and stem from preschoolers' unique understanding of the world. Others, such as beginning school, are imposed. Although minimal amounts of stress are beneficial during the early years to help children develop effective coping skills, excessive stress is harmful. Young children are especially vulnerable because of their limited capacity to cope. Expression of frustration, fear, or anxiety is hampered by inadequate expressive language.

To help parents deal with stress in their child's life, they must be aware of signs of stress (see Stress in Childhood, Chapter 33) and be helped to identify the source. Any number of stressors may be present, such as the birth of a sibling, marital discord, divorce and separation, relocation, or illness.

The best approach to dealing with stress is prevention—monitoring the amount of stress in children's lives so that levels do not exceed their coping ability. In many instances, structuring children's schedules to allow rest and preparing them for change, such as entering school, are sufficient measures.

Aggression

The term *aggression* refers to behavior that attempts to hurt a person or destroy property. Aggression differs from anger, which is a temporary emotional state, but anger may be expressed through aggression. Hyperaggressive behavior in preschoolers is characterized by unprovoked physical attacks on other children and adults, destruction of others' property, frequent intense temper tantrums, extreme impulsivity, disrespect, and noncompliance. Aggression is influenced by a complex set of biologic, sociocultural, and familial variables. Factors that tend to increase aggressive behavior are gender, frustration, modeling, and reinforcement.

Evidence indicates that gender differences exist and that boys are more aggressive than girls (Bendersky, Bennett, &

**90 John St., Suite 104, New York, NY 10038; 212-819-9770; fax: 212-819-9776;* www.siecus.org.

†*434 W. 33rd St., New York, NY 10001; 212-541-7800 or 800-230-7526; fax: 212-245-1845;* www.plannedparenthood.org.

‡*141 Northwest Point Blvd., Elk Grove Village, IL 60007; 847-434-4000; fax: 847-434-8000;* www.aap.org.

Lewis, 2006). *Frustration*, or the continual thwarting of self-satisfaction by disapproval, humiliation, punishment, or insults, can lead children to act out against others as a means of release. Especially if they fear their parents, these children will displace their anger on others, particularly peers and other authority figures. This type of aggression often applies to the child who is well behaved at home but a discipline problem at school or a bully among playmates.

Modeling, or imitating the behavior of significant others, is a powerful influencing force in preschoolers. Children who see their parents as physically abusive are observing behavior that they come to know as acceptable and therefore may exhibit this behavior with others (Gershoff, 2002). Another aspect of modeling is the "double standard" for acceptable conduct. For example, in some families, aggression is synonymous with masculinity, and boys are encouraged to defend themselves. Television is also a significant source for modeling at this age. Numerous studies have found a positive correlation between viewing violent programs and developing aggression; therefore parents need encouragement to supervise programs viewed by their preschool children, especially those with aggressive tendencies (Brown & Hamilton-Giachritsis, 2005). The American Academy of Pediatrics, Committee on Public Education (2001), offers a list of recommendations for healthy television viewing.

Reinforcement can also shape aggressive behavior. Sometimes the reward for aggression is negative (e.g., punishment), yet reinforcing because it brings attention; for example, children who are ignored by a parent until they hit a sibling or the parent learn that this act garners attention.

When children exhibit extreme behaviors, such as aggression, parents may be concerned about the need for professional help. Generally, the difference between "normal" and "problematic" behavior is not the behavior itself but its *quantity* (number of occurrences), *severity* (interference with social or cognitive functioning), *distribution* (different manifestations), *onset* (when behavior started), and *duration* (at least 4 weeks).*

Speech Problems

The most critical period for speech development occurs between 2 and 4 years of age. During this period, children are using their rapidly growing vocabulary faster than they can produce the words. Failure to master sensorimotor integrations results in *stuttering* or *stammering* as children try to say the word they are already thinking about. This dysfluency in speech pattern is a *normal* characteristic of language development in children ages 2 to 5 years, affects boys more frequently than girls, and usually resolves during childhood (National Institute on Deafness and Other Communication Disorders, 2002). When parents or other significant persons place undue emphasis on a child's dysfluency, an abnormal speech pattern may develop. The National Institute on Deafness and Other Communication Disorders (2002) encourages parents and caregivers of children who stutter to speak slowly and clearly, refrain from correcting or criticizing the child's speech, resist the temptation to complete the child's sentences, and take time to listen attentively.

The best therapy for speech problems is prevention and early detection. Common causes of speech problems are hearing loss, developmental delay, autism, and lack of verbal or psychosocial stimulation (Feldman, 2005). Referral for further evaluation and treatment may be necessary to prevent a problem from interfering with learning. Anticipatory preparation of parents for expected developmental norms may allay caregiver concerns.

Children pressured into producing sounds ahead of their developmental level may develop *dyslalia* (articulation problems) or revert to using infantile speech. Prevention involves educating parents regarding the usual achievement of speech production during childhood. The *Denver Articulation Screening Exam* is an excellent tool for assessing articulation skills in the child and for explaining to parents the expected progression of sounds (see the EVOLVE site).

**Information on child development and behavior can be obtained through Developmental Behavioral Pediatrics Online,* www.dbpeds.org.

Promoting Optimal Health During the Preschool Years

Nutrition

Nutritional requirements for preschoolers are fairly similar to those for toddlers (Story, Holt, & Sofka, 2002). The requirement for calories per unit of body weight continues to decrease slightly to 90 kcal/kg, for an average daily intake of 1800 calories. Fluid requirements may also decrease slightly to approximately 100 ml/kg/day but depend on the activity level, climatic conditions, and state of health. Protein requirements increase with age, and the recommended intake for preschoolers is 13 to 19 g/day (0.45 to 0.67 oz/day) (Food and Nutrition Board, 2003).

The American Academy of Pediatrics recommends the following fat intake levels for children over the age of 2 years: saturated fatty acid consumption should be less than 10% of total caloric intake, and total fat over several days should be between 20% and 30% of total caloric intake (Kleinman, 2004). Evidence is increasing that the incidence of coronary heart disease, obesity, and chronic health problems such as diabetes mellitus can be influenced by early eating patterns (Barlow & Expert Committee, 2007). Research supports the efficacy of limiting fat intake, and negative health effects have not been reported (Johnson, 2000). Preschoolers may have decreased fat intake with substitutes such as soy-enriched foods without affecting overall food taste, energy, and nutrient value (Endres et al, 2003). Parents and others who provide soy substitutes should ensure that the products are vitamin enriched and low in fat content (Endres et al, 2003).

It is important that all diets contain adequate nutrients such as calcium. The recommendation for daily calcium intake for children 1 to 3 years of age is 500 mg, and the recommendation for children 4 to 8 years of age is 800 mg (Food and Nutrition Board, 2003). Milk and dairy products are excellent sources of calcium and vitamin D (fortified). Low-fat milk may be substituted so the quantity of milk may remain the same while limiting fat intake overall.

Excessive consumption of fruit juices has been associated with adverse health effects such as dental caries and gastrointestinal symptoms; therefore the American Academy of Pediatrics, Committee on Nutrition (2001), recommends limiting the intake of fruit juice to 4 to 6 oz/day for children ages 1 to 6 years. Parents should be educated regarding nonnutritious fruit drinks, which usually contain less than 10% fruit juice, yet are often advertised as healthy and nutritious; sugar content is dramatically increased and often precludes an adequate intake of milk by the child. While counseling parents regarding moderation in fruit juice consumption, providers should offer suggestions for more appropriate sources of nutrients such as ascorbic acid, folate, and potassium. Intake of high sugar content or acidic carbonated beverages in young children is also known to contribute to dental caries and large amounts of nonnutritive calories that may displace or preclude intake of nutrients necessary for growth.

MyPyramid for Kids is appropriate for preschoolers. This new system is comprehensive and applicable to children as young as 2 years of age. The foods depicted are those commonly eaten by children in this age group, and the illustrations emphasize the importance of physical activity. Parents and caregivers can provide opportunities for children to learn to like a variety of nutritious foods by exposing them to these foods. The importance of role-modeling by parents cannot be overemphasized in regard to food intake and dietary habits; if the parent will not eat a particular food or if their dietary habits are poor, children are likely to develop the same habits.

NURSING ALERT Obesity has increased over the past several decades in young children. Efforts to provide a healthy diet and to encourage physical activity should begin early to help children achieve optimal health (Spear et al, 2007; Johnson, 2000).

Some preschoolers still have food habits that are typical of toddlers, such as food fads and strong taste preferences. When children reach 4 years of age, they seem to enter another period of finicky eating, which is generally characteristic of the more rebellious behavior of children in this age group. As with the toddler, small portions should be offered of each item being served. The practice of having the child remain at the table until the "plate is clean" should be avoided because this may contribute to overeating and the development of poor eating habits that contribute to poor health later in life. By age 5 years, children are more agreeable to trying new foods, especially if they are encouraged by an adult who allows them to help with food preparation or experiment with a new taste or different dish (Fig. 38-7). Mealtimes can become battlegrounds if parents expect perfect table manners.* Usually the 5-year-old child is ready for the "social" side of eating, but the 3- or 4-year-old child still has difficulty sitting quietly through a long family meal.

The amount and variety of foods consumed by young children vary greatly from day to day. Consequently, parents sometimes worry about the quantity and quality of food preschoolers consume. In general, the quality is much more important than the quantity, a fact that should be stressed during nutritional counseling.

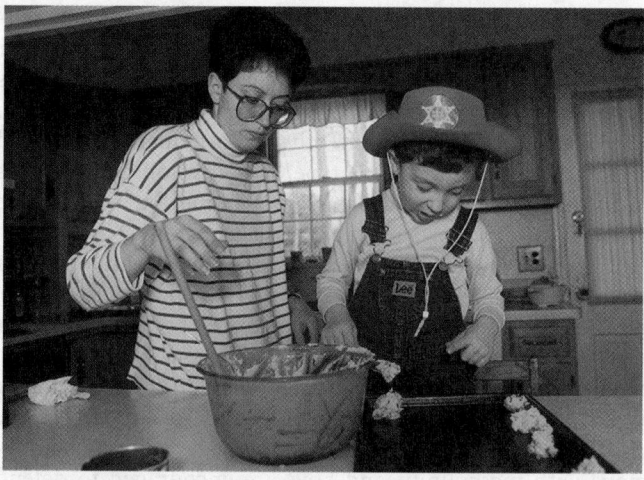

Fig. 38-7 Preschool-age children enjoy helping adults and are more likely to try new foods if they can assist in the preparation.

One way to lessen parental concern is advising parents to keep a weekly record of everything the child eats. In particular, the parents can measure the amount of food, such as setting aside a half cup of vegetables and serving the child from this premeasured amount, to provide a more accurate estimate of food intake at each meal. When parents look at the food chart at the end of the week, they are usually amazed by how much the child has consumed. In general, preschoolers consume only slightly more than toddlers, or about half an adult's portion.

Sleep and Activity

Sleep patterns vary widely, but the average preschooler sleeps about 12 hours a night and infrequently takes daytime naps. Waking during the night is common throughout early childhood and may be related to social rather than developmental factors (Thiedke, 2001). Motor activity levels continue to be high and allow preschoolers to explore their environment, begin learning physical games and sports, and interact with others. Sedentary activities, such as television and video or computer games, are increasingly appealing and can become an unhealthy substitute for active play.

Preschoolers' increased gross motor abilities and coordination allow them to engage in many physical activities, if only at a novice level. Whether young children should begin formalized training in an activity at this early age is controversial. Training programs must consider the child's physical and psychologic immaturity, and readiness to participate in organized sports should be determined individually. The decision to participate should be based on the child's, not the parent's, motivation and enjoyment. The American Academy of Pediatrics, Committee on Sports Medicine and Fitness and Committee on School Health (2001), encourages free play and a variety of physical activities; however, the academy also supports organized play when it is developmentally

**An excellent resource for parents related to mealtimes with toddlers and preschoolers is Satter E:* How to get your kid to eat … but not too much, *Palo Alto, CA, 1987, Bull Publishing.*

appropriate and occurs in a nonthreatening, fun, and safe environment.

Sleep Problems

The preschool years are a prime time for sleep disturbances. As toddlers and preschoolers cope with autonomy, separation, and object permanence, they begin to have more sleep problems (Thiedke, 2001). Some have trouble going to sleep, especially after so much activity and stimulation during the day. Others may develop bedtime fears, wake during the night, or have nightmares or sleep terrors. Still others may prolong the inevitable through elaborate rituals.

Recommendations for handling a sleep disturbance are offered only *after* a thorough assessment of the problem. Cultural traditions may dictate sleep practices that are contrary to certain well-accepted professional recommendations; therefore parents may not perceive a particular sleep practice as a problem (see Cultural Awareness box in Chapter 36, p. 1007).

Interventions differ greatly; for example, *nightmares* (frightening dreams that are followed by full arousal) and *sleep terrors* (partial arousal from deep, nondreaming sleep) require different approaches.

For children who delay going to bed, a recommended approach involves counseling parents about the importance of a consistent bedtime ritual and emphasizing the normalcy of this type of behavior in young children. Parents should ignore attention-seeking behavior and not take the child into the parents' bed or allow the child to stay up past a reasonable hour. Other measures that may be helpful include keeping a light on in the room, providing transitional objects such as a favorite toy, or leaving a drink of water by the bed.

Helping children slow down *before* bedtime also reduces the resistance to going to bed. One strategy is to establish limited rituals that signal readiness for bed, such as a bath or story. Parents can reinforce the pattern by stating, "After this story, it is bedtime," and consistently carrying out the routine. If anticipated extra stimulation, such as having visitors arrive at bedtime, disrupts this routine, it is advisable to settle children in bed beforehand. Television viewing before bedtime may cause bedtime resistance and delay sleep.

Dental Health

By the beginning of the preschool period, the eruption of the deciduous (primary) teeth is complete. Dental care is essential to preserve these temporary teeth and to teach good dental habits (see Chapter 37). Although preschoolers' fine motor control is improved, they still require assistance and supervision with brushing, and parents should floss the teeth. Professional care and prophylaxis, especially fluoride supplements (if needed), should be continued. Routine dental care should be well established during preschool years and is recommended at 6- to 12-month intervals depending on the family history, the child's dental development, and the presence or absence of dental caries (Martof, 2001). For children cared for away from home, parents should be encouraged to monitor the dental care provided by others, including minimizing cariogenic foods in the diet. Trauma to teeth during this period is not uncommon, and prompt evaluation by a dentist is warranted if oral trauma occurs. Preservation of the space previously occupied by an avulsed tooth is necessary for proper eruption of the secondary tooth.

Injury Prevention

Because of improved gross and fine motor skills, coordination, and balance, preschoolers are less prone to falls than are toddlers. They tend to be less reckless; listen more to parental rules; and are aware of potential dangers, such as hot objects, sharp instruments, and dangerous heights. Putting objects in the mouth as part of exploration has all but ceased, although accidental poisoning is still a danger. Pedestrian motor vehicle injuries increase because of activities such as playing in the parking lot, driveway, or street; riding tricycles, bicycles, and other play vehicles; running after balls; or forgetting safety regulations when crossing streets.

In general, the guidelines suggested for injury prevention in Table 37-3 apply to children in this age group as well. However, emphasis is now on *education* concerning safety and potential hazards, in addition to appropriate protection. This is an excellent time to start enforcing the use of safety items such as bicycle helmets to prevent head trauma; children are less likely to warm to the idea later in life because of peer pressure. Because preschoolers are great imitators, it is essential that parents set a good example by "practicing what they preach." Children quickly observe discrepancies in what they are told to do and what they see others do. Establishing habits at this time, such as wearing protective equipment, can create long-term safety behaviors.

Anticipatory Guidance—Care of Families

The preschool years present fewer childrearing difficulties than do earlier years, and this stage of development is facilitated by appropriate anticipatory guidance in the areas already discussed (see Family-Centered Care box). There is a shift in childrearing practices from protection to education. Whereas injury prevention previously focused on safeguarding the immediate environment, with less emphasis on reasoning, now the protective guardrails or electrical outlet caps may replaced by verbal explanations of why danger exists and how to avoid it.

During this period, an emotional transition between parent and child occurs. Although children are still attached to their parents and accept all their values and beliefs, they are nearing the period of life when they will question previous teachings and prefer the companionship of peers. Entry into school marks a separation for parents and for children. Parents may need help in adjusting to this change, particularly if one parent has focused his or her daily activities primarily on home responsibilities. All family members must adjust to changes, which is part of the process of growth and development.

Infectious Disorders

Communicable Diseases

The incidence of childhood communicable diseases has declined significantly since the advent of immunizations. Serious complications resulting from such infections have been further reduced with the use of antibiotics and antitox-

FAMILY-CENTERED CARE

Guidance During Preschool Years

Age 3 Years

Prepare parents for child's increasing interest in widening relationships.

Encourage enrollment in preschool.

Emphasize importance of setting limits.

Prepare parents to expect exaggerated tension-reduction behaviors, such as need for a "security blanket."

Encourage parents to offer child choices.

Prepare parents to expect marked changes at 3½ years, when child becomes insecure and exhibits emotional extremes.

Prepare parents for normal dysfluency in speech and advise them to avoid focusing on the pattern.

Prepare parents to expect extra demands on their attention as a reflection of child's emotional insecurity and fear of loss of love.

Warn parents that the equilibrium of a 3-year-old will change to the aggressive, out-of-bounds behavior of a 4-year-old.

Inform parents to anticipate a more stable appetite with more food selections.

Stress need for protection and education of child to prevent injury (see Injury Prevention, Chapter 37).

Age 4 Years

Prepare parents for more aggressive behavior, including motor activity and offensive language.

Prepare parents to expect resistance to parental authority.

Explore parental feelings regarding child's behavior.

Suggest some type of respite for primary caregivers, such as placing child in preschool for part of the day.

Prepare parents for child's increasing sexual curiosity.

Emphasize the importance of realistic limit setting on behavior and appropriate disciplinary techniques.

Prepare parents for the highly imaginative 4-year-old who indulges in "tall tales" (to be differentiated from lies) and develops imaginary playmates.

Prepare parents to expect nightmares or an increase in them.

Provide reassurance that a period of calmness begins at 5 years of age.

Age 5 Years

Inform parents to expect a tranquil period at 5 years of age.

Help parents prepare children for entrance into school environment.

Make certain that immunizations are up to date before child enters school.

Suggest that unemployed parental caregivers consider own activities when children begin school.

Suggest swimming lessons for the child.

ins. However, infectious diseases do occur, and nurses must be familiar with the infectious agent to recognize the disease and to institute appropriate preventive and supportive interventions (Table 38-2).

Nursing Care Management

The more common communicable diseases of childhood, their therapeutic management, and specific nursing care are described in Table 38-2. The following is a general discussion of nursing care management for communicable diseases. Identification of the infectious agent is of primary importance to prevent exposure to susceptible individuals. Nurses in ambulatory care settings, child care centers, and schools are often the first persons to see signs of a communicable disease, such as a rash or sore throat. The nurse must operate under a high index of suspicion for common childhood diseases to identify potentially infectious cases and to recognize diseases that require medical intervention. An example is the common complaint of sore throat. Although most often a symptom of a minor viral infection, it can signal diphtheria or a streptococcal infection, such as scarlet fever. Each of these bacterial conditions requires appropriate medical treatment to prevent serious sequelae.

When a communicable disease is suspected, it is important to assess (1) recent exposure to a known case; (2) *prodromal symptoms* (symptoms that occur between early manifestations of the disease and its overt clinical syndrome) or evidence of constitutional symptoms, such as a fever or rash (see Table 38-2); (3) immunization history; and (4) history of having the disease. Immunizations are available for many diseases, and infection usually confers lifelong immunity; therefore the possibility of many infectious agents can be eliminated based on these two criteria.

Prevent Spread

Prevention consists of two components: prevention of the disease and control of its spread to others. Primary prevention rests almost exclusively on immunization. (The nurse's role in immunization of children is discussed in Chapter 36.)

Control measures to prevent spread of disease should include techniques to reduce risk of cross-transmission of infectious organisms between patients and to protect health care workers from organisms harbored by patients. If the child is hospitalized, the facility's policies for infection control are followed (see Chapter 45). The most important procedure is handwashing. Persons directly caring for the child or handling contaminated articles must wash their hands and practice effective Standard Precautions between care of their patients.

The child is instructed to practice good handwashing technique after toileting and before eating. For those diseases spread by droplets, the nurse instructs parents in measures to reduce airborne transmission. The child who is old enough covers the face with a tissue during coughing or sneezing; otherwise, the parent should cover the child's mouth with a tissue and then discard it. The usual hygiene measures of not sharing eating and drinking utensils are stressed to the family.

NURSING ALERT If a child is admitted to the hospital with an undiagnosed exanthema, strict Transmission-based Precautions (Contact, Airborne, and Droplet) and Standard Precautions are instituted until a diagnosis is confirmed. Childhood communicable diseases requiring these precautions include diphtheria, chickenpox, measles, tuberculosis, adenovirus, *Haemophilus influenzae* type b, influenza, mumps, *Mycoplasma pneumoniae,* pertussis, plague, streptococcal pharyngitis, pneumonia, and scarlet fever (American Academy of Pediatrics, Committee on Infectious Diseases, 2006).

Prevent Complications

Although most children recover without difficulty, certain groups are at risk for serious, even fatal, complications from communicable diseases, especially the viral diseases chickenpox and erythema infectiosum (EI, fifth disease) caused by human parvovirus (HPV) B19. Whereas most healthy children are less likely to become infected from either of these viruses, children with immunodeficiency—those receiving steroid or other immunosuppressive therapy, those with a generalized malignancy such as leukemia or lymphoma, or those with an immunologic disorder—are at risk for viremia from replication of the *varicella-zoster virus (VZV)** in the blood. VZV is so named because it causes two distinct diseases: *varicella (chickenpox)* and *zoster (herpes zoster,* or *shingles).* Varicella occurs primarily in children younger than 15 years of age. However, it leaves the threat of herpes zoster, an intensely painful varicella that is localized to a single dermatome (body area innervated by a particular segment of the spinal cord). In children the dermatomes most likely affected by herpes zoster are the cervical and sacral dermatomes (Leung, Robson, & Leong, 2006). Immunocompromised patients and healthy infants younger than 1 year of age (who also have reduced immunity) are at a higher risk for reactivation of VZV causing herpes zoster, probably as a result of a deficiency in cellular immunity (Chen et al, 2002). Complications of VZV in children include secondary bacterial infection, depigmentation, and scarring; postherpetic neuralgia in children is uncommon (Leung, Robson, & Leong, 2006).

Children with hemolytic disease, such as sickle cell disease, are at risk for aplastic anemia from EI. HPV B19 infects and lyses red blood cell precursors, thus interrupting the production of red blood cells. Therefore the virus may precipitate a severe aplastic crisis in patients who need increased red blood cell production to maintain normal red blood cell volumes; thrombocytopenia and neutropenia may also occur as a result of parvovirus B19 infection. The fetus has a relatively high rate of red blood cell production and an immature immune system; it may develop severe anemia and hydrops as a result of maternal HPV infection. Fetal death rates as a result of HPV B19 have been estimated to be between 2% and 6% (American Academy of Pediatrics, Committee on Infectious Diseases, 2006).

NURSING ALERT Children at risk for contracting these communicable diseases are referred to the practitioner immediately in case of known exposure or outbreaks.

The past decade has seen an increase in the incidence of pertussis, particularly in infants less than 6 months old and children 10 to 14 years of age. Early clinical manifestations of pertussis in infants may include gagging, coughing, emesis, and apnea; the typical whoop associated with the disease is absent (American Academy of Pediatrics, Committee on Infectious Diseases, 2006). In older children the disease may manifest as a common cold (see Table 38-2). It is now recommended that children ages 11 to 18 receive a booster pertussis vaccine (Tdap) to prevent the disease (see Chapter 36, Immunizations). Because pertussis is very contagious, especially among close household members, pertussis should be identified early and treatment initiated for the child and those who have been exposed. Azithromycin (for infants under 1 month) and erythromycin are administered to infants and children with pertussis (American Academy of Pediatrics, Committee on Infectious Diseases, 2006).

Prevention of complications from diseases such as diphtheria, pertussis, and scarlet fever requires compliance with antibiotic therapy. With oral preparations the need to complete the entire course of therapy is stressed (see Compliance, Chapter 45). The use of varicella-zoster immune globulin (VariZIG) or immune globulin intravenous (IGIV) is recommended for children who are immunocompromised, who have no previous history of varicella, and who are likely to contract the disease and have complications as a result (American Academy of Pediatrics, Committee on Infectious Diseases, 2006). The antiviral agent acyclovir (Zovirax) may be used to treat varicella infections in susceptible immunocompromised persons; it is effective in decreasing the number of lesions; shortening the duration of fever; and decreasing itching, lethargy, and anorexia. Oral acyclovir should be considered for susceptible pregnant women, immunocompromised children without a history of varicella disease, newborns whose mother had varicella within 5 days before delivery or within 48 hours after delivery, and hospitalized preterm infants with significant varicella exposure (American Academy of Pediatrics, Committee on Infectious Diseases, 2006).

There is evidence that vitamin A supplementation reduces both morbidity and mortality in measles and that all children with severe measles should be given vitamin A supplements. A single oral dose of 200,000 International Units for children at least 1 year old (or half that dose for children 6 to 12 months of age) is recommended. The higher dose may be associated with vomiting and headache for a few hours. The dose should be repeated the next day and at 4 weeks for children with ophthalmologic evidence of vitamin A deficiency (American Academy of Pediatrics, Committee on Infectious Diseases, 2006).

NURSING ALERT Although the risk of vitamin A toxicity from these doses (they are 100 to 200 times the recommended dietary allowance) is relatively low, nurses should instruct parents on safe storage of the drug. Ideally, vitamin A should be dispensed in the age-appropriate unit dose to prevent excessive administration and possible toxicity.

Provide Comfort

Many communicable diseases cause skin manifestations that are bothersome to the child. The chief discomfort from most rashes is itching, and measures such as cool baths (usually without soap) and lotions (e.g., calamine) are helpful.

Text continued on p. 1066

Educational materials may be obtained from the National Shingles Foundation, 590 Madison Ave., 21st Floor, New York, NY 10022, www.vzvfoundation.org.

evolve Critical Thinking Exercise—Conjunctivitis

evolve Case Study—Bacterial Conjunctivitis

evolve Case Study–Chickenpox (Varicella)

evolve Case Study–Varicella in Spite of Vaccine

Table 38-2 Communicable Diseases of Childhood

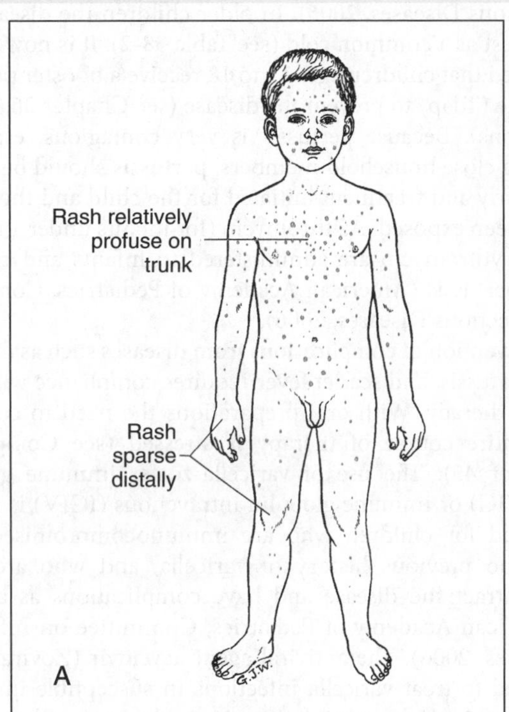

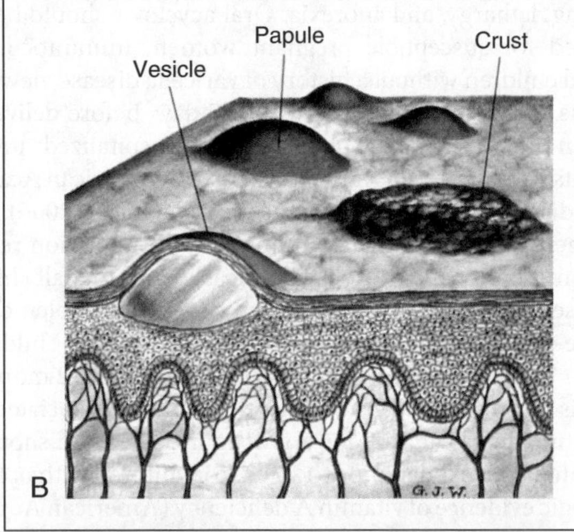

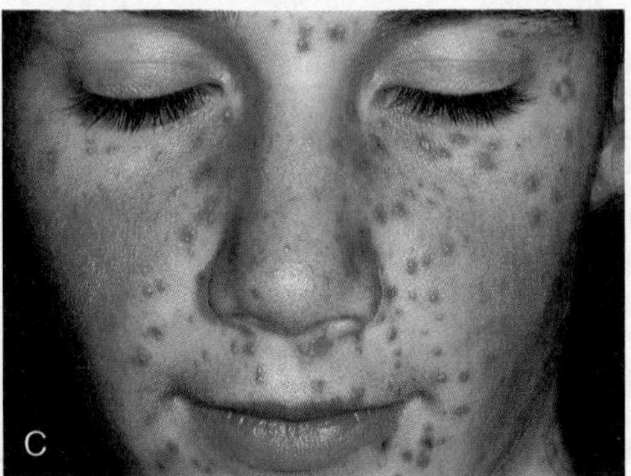

Fig. 38-8 Chickenpox (varicella). **A,** Progression of disease. **B,** Simultaneous stages of lesions. **C,** Clinical view. (**C,** From Habif TP: *Clinical dermatology: a color guide to diagnosis and therapy*, ed 4, St Louis, 2004, Mosby.)

DISEASE

Chickenpox (Varicella) (Fig. 38-8)

Agents—Varicella-zoster virus (VZV)

Source—Primary secretions of respiratory tract of infected persons; to a lesser degree, skin lesions (scabs not infectious)

Transmission—Direct contact, droplet (airborne) spread, and contaminated objects

Incubation period—2-3 wk, usually 14-16 days

Period of communicability—Probably 1 day before eruption of lesions (prodromal period) to 6 days after first crop of vesicles when crusts have formed

Diphtheria

Agent—*Corynebacterium diphtheriae*

Source—Discharges from mucous membranes of nose and nasopharynx, skin, and other lesions of infected person

Transmission—Direct contact with infected person, a carrier, or contaminated articles

Incubation period—Usually 2-5 days, possibly longer

Period of communicability—Variable; until virulent bacilli are no longer present (identified by three negative cultures); usually 2 wk but as long as 4 wk

Erythema Infectiosum (Fifth Disease) (Fig. 38-9)

Agent—Human parvovirus (HPV) B19

Source—Infected persons, mainly school-age children

Transmission—Respiratory secretions, blood, blood products

Incubation period—4-14 days; may be as long as 21 days

Period of communicability—Uncertain but before onset of symptoms in children with aplastic crisis

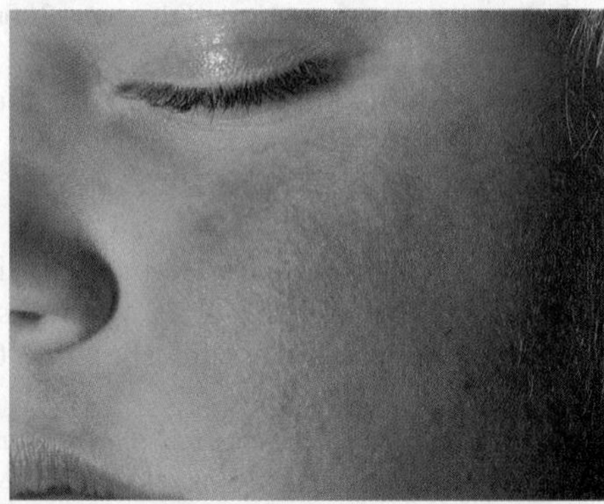

Fig. 38-9 Erythema infectiosum. (From Habif TP: *Clinical dermatology: a color guide to diagnosis and therapy*, ed 4, St Louis, 2004, Mosby.)

CLINICAL MANIFESTATIONS	THERAPEUTIC MANAGEMENT AND COMPLICATIONS	NURSING CARE MANAGEMENT
Prodromal stage—Slight fever, malaise, and anorexia for first 24 hr; rash highly pruritic; begins as macule, rapidly progresses to papule and then vesicle (surrounded by erythematous base, becomes umbilicated and cloudy, breaks easily and forms crusts); all three stages (papule, vesicle, crust) present in varying degrees at one time **Distribution**—Centripetal, spreading to face and proximal extremities but sparse on distal limbs and less on areas not exposed to heat (i.e., from clothing or sun) **Constitutional signs and symptoms**—Elevated temperature from lymphadenopathy, irritability from pruritus	**Specific**—Antiviral agent acyclovir (Zovirax); varicella-zoster immune globulin (VariZIG) or immune globulin intravenous (IGIV) after exposure in high risk children **Supportive**—Diphenhydramine hydrochloride or antihistamines to relieve itching; skin care to prevent secondary bacterial infection **Complications**—Secondary bacterial infections (abscesses, cellulitis, necrotizing fasciitis, pneumonia, sepsis) Encephalitis Varicella pneumonia (rare in normal children) Hemorrhagic varicella (tiny hemorrhages in vesicles and numerous petechiae in skin) Chronic or transient thrombocytopenia	Maintain Standard, Airborne, and Contact Precautions if hospitalized until all lesions are crusted; for immunized child with mild breakthrough varicella, isolate until no new lesions are seen. Keep child in home away from susceptible individuals until vesicles have dried (usually 1 wk after onset of disease), and isolate high risk children from infected children. Administer skin care; give bath and change clothes and linens daily; administer topical calamine lotion; keep child's fingernails short and clean; apply mittens if child scratches. Keep child cool (may decrease number of lesions). Lessen pruritus; keep child occupied. Remove loose crusts that rub and irritate skin. Teach child to apply pressure to pruritic area rather than scratching it. Avoid use of aspirin (possible association with Reye syndrome).
Vary according to anatomic location of pseudomembrane **Nasal**—Resembles common cold, serosanguineous mucopurulent nasal discharge without constitutional symptoms; may be frank epistaxis **Tonsillar/pharyngeal**—Malaise; anorexia; sore throat; low-grade fever; pulse increased above expected for temperature within 24 hr; smooth, adherent, white or gray membrane; lymphadenitis possibly pronounced ("bull's neck"); in severe cases, toxemia, septic shock, and death within 6-10 days **Laryngeal**—Fever, hoarseness, cough, with or without previous signs listed; potential airway obstruction, apprehensive, dyspneic retractions, cyanosis	Equine antitoxin (usually intravenously); preceded by skin or conjunctival test to rule out sensitivity to horse serum Antibiotics (penicillin G procaine or erythromycin) in addition to equine antitoxin Complete bed rest (prevention of myocarditis) Tracheostomy for airway obstruction Treatment of infected contacts and carriers **Complications**—Toxic cardiomyopathy (second to third week) Toxic neuropathy	Follow Standard and Droplet Precautions until two cultures are negative for *C. diphtheriae*; Contact Precautions with cutaneous manifestations. Administer antibiotics in timely manner. Participate in sensitivity testing; have epinephrine available. Administer complete care to maintain bed rest. Use suctioning as needed. Observe respiration for signs of obstruction Administer humidified oxygen as prescribed.
Rash appearing in three stages: I—Erythema on face, chiefly on cheeks, "slapped face" appearance; disappears by 1-4 days II—About 1 day after rash appears on face, maculopapular red spots appear, symmetrically distributed on upper and lower extremities; rash progresses from proximal to distal surfaces and may last a week or more III—Rash subsiding but reappearing if skin is irritated or traumatized (sun, heat, cold, friction) In children with aplastic crisis, rash is usually absent and prodromal illness includes fever, myalgia, lethargy, nausea, vomiting, and abdominal pain Child with sickle cell disease may have concurrent vasoocclusive crisis	**Symptomatic and supportive**—Antipyretics, analgesics, antiinflammatory drugs Possible blood transfusion for transient aplastic anemia **Complications**—Self-limited arthritis and arthralgia (arthritis may become chronic); more common in adult women May result in serious complications (anemia, hydrops) or fetal death if mother infected during pregnancy (primarily second trimester) Aplastic crisis in children with hemolytic disease or immunodeficiency Myocarditis (rare)	Isolation of child is not necessary, except hospitalized child (immunosuppressed or with aplastic crises) suspected of HPV infection is placed on respiratory isolation and Standard Precautions. Pregnant women need not be excluded from workplace where HPV infection is present; they should not care for patients with aplastic crises; explain low risk of fetal death to those in contact with affected children; assist with routine fetal ultrasound for detection of fetal hydrops.

Continued

Table 38-2 Communicable Diseases of Childhood—cont'd

DISEASE

Exanthem Subitum (Roseola) (Fig. 38-10)

Agent–Human herpesvirus type 6 (HHV-6; rarely HHV-7)

Source–Possibly acquired from saliva of healthy adult; entry via nasal, buccal or conjunctival mucosa

Transmission–Year round; no reported contact with infected individual in most cases (virtually limited to children under 3 yr but peak age is between 6 and 15 mo of life)

Incubation period–Usually 5-15 days

Period of communicability–Unknown

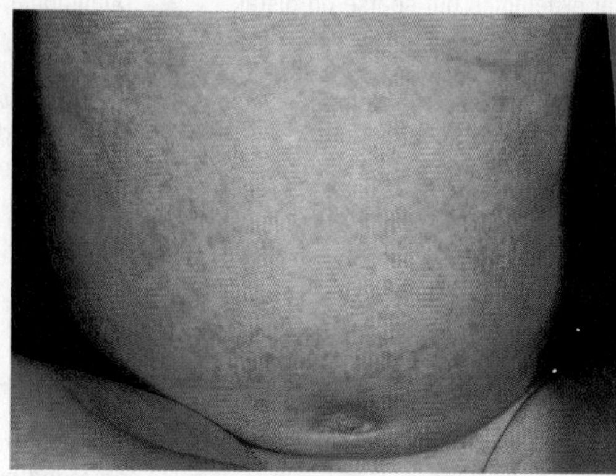

Fig. 38-10 Roseola infantum. (From Habif TP: *Clinical dermatology: a color guide to diagnosis and therapy*, ed 4, St Louis, 2004, Mosby.)

Measles (Rubeola) (Fig. 38-11)

Agent–Virus

Source–Respiratory tract secretions, blood, and urine of infected person

Transmission–Usually by direct contact with droplets of infected person; primarily in the winter

Incubation period–10-20 days

Period of communicability–From 4 days before to 5 days after rash appears but mainly during prodromal (catarrhal) stage

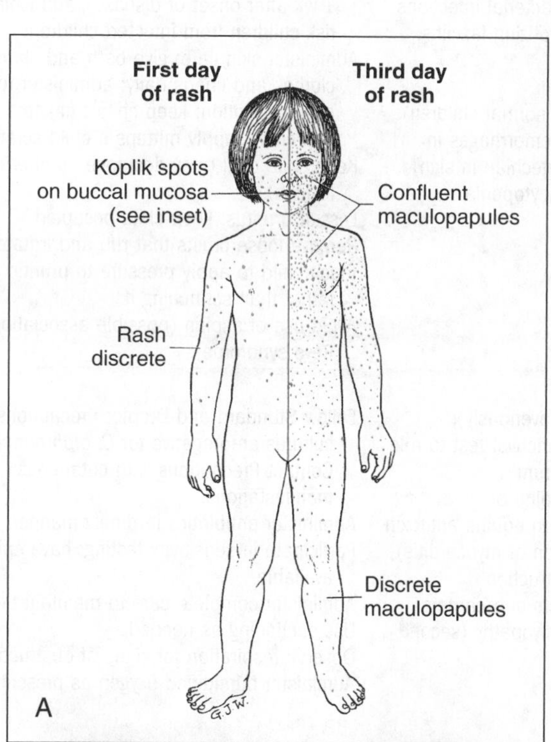

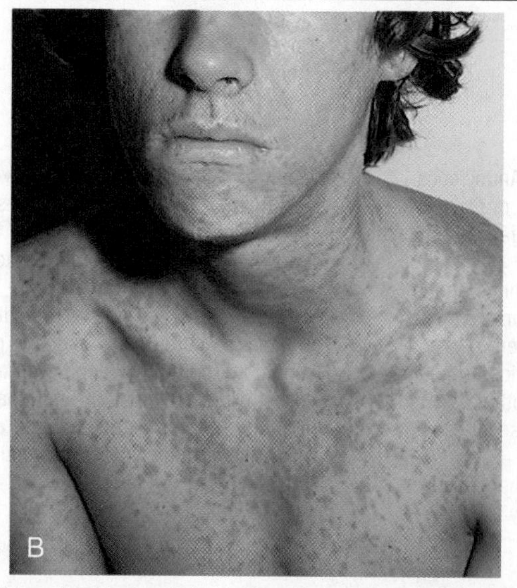

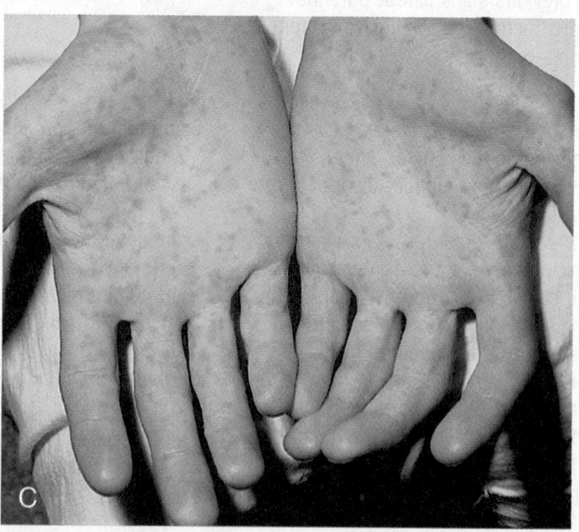

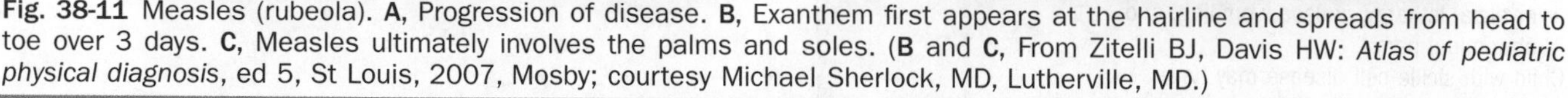

Fig. 38-11 Measles (rubeola). **A**, Progression of disease. **B**, Exanthem first appears at the hairline and spreads from head to toe over 3 days. **C**, Measles ultimately involves the palms and soles. (**B** and **C**, From Zitelli BJ, Davis HW: *Atlas of pediatric physical diagnosis*, ed 5, St Louis, 2007, Mosby; courtesy Michael Sherlock, MD, Lutherville, MD.)

CLINICAL MANIFESTATIONS	THERAPEUTIC MANAGEMENT AND COMPLICATIONS	NURSING CARE MANAGEMENT
Persistent high fever for 3-4 days in child who appears well Precipitous drop in fever to normal with appearance of rash **Rash**—Discrete rose-pink macules or maculopapules appearing first on trunk, then spreading to neck, face, and extremities; nonpruritic, fades on pressure, lasts 1-2 days **Associated signs and symptoms**—Cervical/postauricular lymphadenopathy, inflamed pharynx, cough, coryza	Nonspecific Antipyretics to control fever **Complications**—Recurrent febrile seizures (possibly from latent infection of central nervous system that is reactivated by fever) Encephalitis (rare)	Teach parents measures for lowering temperature (antipyretic drugs); ensure adequate parental understanding of specific antipyretic dosage to prevent accidental overdose. If child is prone to seizures, discuss appropriate precautions and possibility of recurrent febrile seizures.
Prodromal (catarrhal) stage—Fever and malaise, followed in 24 hr by coryza, cough, conjunctivitis, Koplik's spots (small, irregular red spots with a minute, bluish white center first seen on buccal mucosa opposite molars 2 days before rash); symptoms gradually increasing in severity until second day after rash appears, when they begin to subside **Rash**—Appears 3-4 days after onset of prodromal stage; begins as erythematous maculopapular eruption on face and gradually spreads downward; more severe in earlier sites (appears confluent) and less intense in later sites (appears discrete); after 3-4 days assumes brownish appearance, and fine desquamation occurs over area of extensive involvement **Constitutional signs and symptoms**—Anorexia, abdominal pain, malaise, generalized lymphadenopathy	Vitamin A supplementation (see p. 1057) **Supportive**—Bed rest during febrile period; antipyretics Antibiotics to prevent secondary bacterial infection in high risk children **Complications**—Otitis media Pneumonia (bacterial) Obstructive laryngitis and laryngotracheitis Encephalitis (rare but has high mortality)	Isolate until fifth day of rash; if hospitalized, institute Droplet Precautions. Encourage rest during prodromal stage; provide quiet activity. **Fever**—Instruct parents to administer antipyretics; avoid chilling; if child is prone to seizures, institute appropriate precautions. **Eye care**—Dim lights if photophobia present; clean eyelids with warm saline solution to remove secretions or crusts; keep child from rubbing eyes. **Coryza, cough**—Use cool-mist vaporizer; protect skin around nares with layer of petrolatum; encourage fluids and soft, bland foods. **Skin care**—Keep skin clean; use tepid baths as necessary.

Continued

Table 38-2 Communicable Diseases of Childhood—cont'd

DISEASE
Mumps **Agent**–Paramyxovirus **Source**–Saliva of infected persons **Transmission**–Direct contact with or droplet spread from an infected person **Incubation period**–14-21 days **Period of communicability**–Most communicable immediately before and after swelling begins
Pertussis (Whooping Cough) **Agent**–*Bordetella pertussis* **Source**–Discharge from respiratory tract of infected person **Transmission**–Direct contact or droplet spread from infected person; indirect contact with freshly contaminated articles **Incubation period**–6-20 days, usually 7-10 days **Period of communicability**–Greatest during catarrhal stage before onset of paroxysms
Poliomyelitis **Agent**–Enteroviruses, three types: type 1, most frequent cause of paralysis, both epidemic and endemic; type 2, least frequently associated with paralysis; type 3, second most frequently associated with paralysis **Source**–Feces and oropharyngeal secretions of infected persons, especially young children **Transmission**–Direct contact with persons with apparent or inapparent active infection; spread is via fecal-oral and pharyngeal-oropharyngeal routes Vaccine-acquired paralytic polio may occur as a result of the live oral polio vaccination (no longer available in the United States) **Incubation period**–Usually 7-38 days, with range of 5-35 days **Period of communicability**–Not exactly known; virus present in throat and feces shortly after infection and persists for about 1 wk in throat and 4-6 wk in feces

CLINICAL MANIFESTATIONS	THERAPEUTIC MANAGEMENT AND COMPLICATIONS	NURSING CARE MANAGEMENT
Prodromal stage—Fever, headache, malaise, and anorexia for 24 hr, followed by "earache" that is aggravated by chewing **Parotitis**—Parotid gland(s) (either unilateral or bilateral) enlarges and reaches maximum size in 1-3 days; accompanied by pain and tenderness; other exocrine glands (submandibular) may also be swollen	**Symptomatic and supportive**—Analgesics for pain and antipyretics for fever Intravenous fluid may be necessary for child refusing to drink or vomiting because of meningoencephalitis **Complications**—Sensorineural deafness Postinfectious encephalitis Myocarditis Arthritis Hepatitis Epididymoorchitis Oophoritis Pancreatitis Sterility (extremely rare in adult males) Meningitis	Isolate during period of communicability; institute Droplet and Contact Precautions during hospitalization. Encourage rest and decreased activity during prodromal phase until swelling subsides. Give analgesics for pain; if child is unwilling to swallow pills or tablets medication, use elixir form. Encourage fluids and soft, bland foods; avoid foods requiring chewing. Apply hot or cold compresses to neck, whichever is more comforting. To relieve orchitis, provide warmth and local support with tight-fitting underpants.
Catarrhal stage—Begins with symptoms of upper respiratory tract infection, such as coryza, sneezing, lacrimation, cough, and low-grade fever; symptoms continue for 1-2 wk, when dry, hacking cough becomes more severe **Paroxysmal stage**—Cough most often occurs at night and consists of short, rapid coughs followed by sudden inspiration associated with a high-pitched crowing sound or "whoop"; during paroxysms, cheeks become flushed or cyanotic, eyes bulge, and tongue protrudes; paroxysm may continue until thick mucous plug is dislodged; vomiting frequently follows attack; stage generally lasts 4-6 wk, followed by convalescent stage Infants under 6 mo of age may not have characteristic whoop cough, but have difficulty maintaining adequate oxygenation with amount of secretions, frequent vomiting of mucus and formula or breast milk (see also Immunization, Chapter 36 for discussion of pertussis in adolescents)	Antimicrobial therapy (e.g., erythromycin, clarithromycin, azithromycin) **Supportive treatment**—Hospitalization sometimes required for infants, children who are dehydrated, or those who have complications Increased oxygen intake and humidity Adequate fluids Intensive care and mechanical ventilation may be necessary for infant <6 mo **Complications**—Pneumonia (usual cause of death) Atelectasis Otitis media Seizures Hemorrhage (scleral, conjunctival, epistaxis; pulmonary hemorrhage in neonate) Weight loss and dehydration Hernias (umbilical and inguinal) Prolapsed rectum	Isolate during catarrhal stage; if hospitalized, institute Droplet Precautions. Obtain nasopharyngeal culture for diagnosis. Encourage oral fluids; offer small amount of fluids frequently. Ensure adequate oxygenation during paroxysms; position infant on side to decrease chance of aspiration with vomiting. Provide high humidity (humidifier or croup tent); suction as needed to prevent choking on secretions. Observe for signs of airway obstruction (increased restlessness, apprehension, retractions, cyanosis). Encourage compliance with antibiotic therapy for household contacts. Encourage adolescents to obtain pertussis booster (Tdap) (see also Chapter 36, Immunizations). Use Standard Precautions and mask in health care workers exposed to children with persistent cough and high suspicion of pertussis.
May be manifested in three different forms: **Abortive or inapparent**—Fever, uneasiness, sore throat, headache, anorexia, vomiting, abdominal pain; lasts a few hours to a few days **Nonparalytic**—Same manifestations as abortive but more severe, with pain and stiffness in neck, back, and legs **Paralytic**—Initial course similar to nonparalytic type, followed by recovery and then signs of central nervous system paralysis	Treatment is supportive Complete bed rest during acute phase Mechanical or assisted ventilation in case of respiratory paralysis Physical therapy for muscles following acute stage **Complications**—Permanent paralysis Respiratory arrest Hypertension Kidney stones from demineralization of bone during prolonged immobility	Administer mild sedatives as necessary to relieve anxiety and promote rest. Participate in physical therapy procedures (use of moist hot packs and range-of-motion exercises). Position child to maintain body alignment and prevent contractures or skin breakdown; use footboard or appropriate orthoses to prevent footdrop; use pressure mattress for prolonged immobility. Encourage child to perform activities of daily living to capability; early ambulation with adjuncts; administer analgesics for maximum comfort during physical activity. Provide high-protein diet and bowel management for prolonged immobility. Observe for respiratory paralysis (difficulty in talking, ineffective cough, inability to hold breath, shallow and rapid respirations); report such signs and symptoms to practitioner.

Continued

DISEASE

Rubella (German Measles) (Fig. 38-12)

Agent—Rubella virus

Source—Primarily nasopharyngeal secretions of person with apparent or inapparent infection; virus also present in blood, stool, and urine

Incubation period—14-21 days

Period of communicability—7 days before to about 5 days after appearance of rash

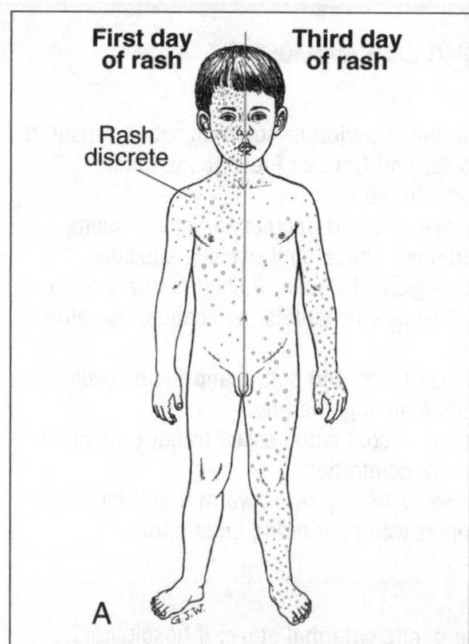

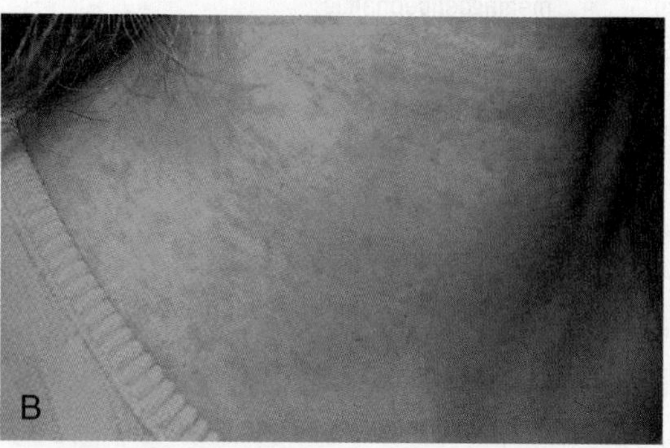

Fig. 38-12 Rubella (German measles). **A**, Progression of rash. **B**, Clinical view. (**B**, From Zitelli BJ, Davis HW: *Atlas of pediatric physical diagnosis*, ed 5, St Louis, 2007, Mosby; courtesy Michael Sherlock, MD, Lutherville, MD.)

Scarlet Fever (Fig. 38-13)

Agent—Group A β-hemolytic streptococci

Source—Usually from nasopharyngeal secretions of infected persons and carriers

Transmission—Direct contact with infected person or droplet spread; indirectly by contact with contaminated articles or ingestion of contaminated milk or other food

Incubation period—2-5 days, with range of 1-7 days

Period of communicability—During incubation period and clinical illness, approximately 10 days; during first 2 wk of carrier phase, although may persist for months

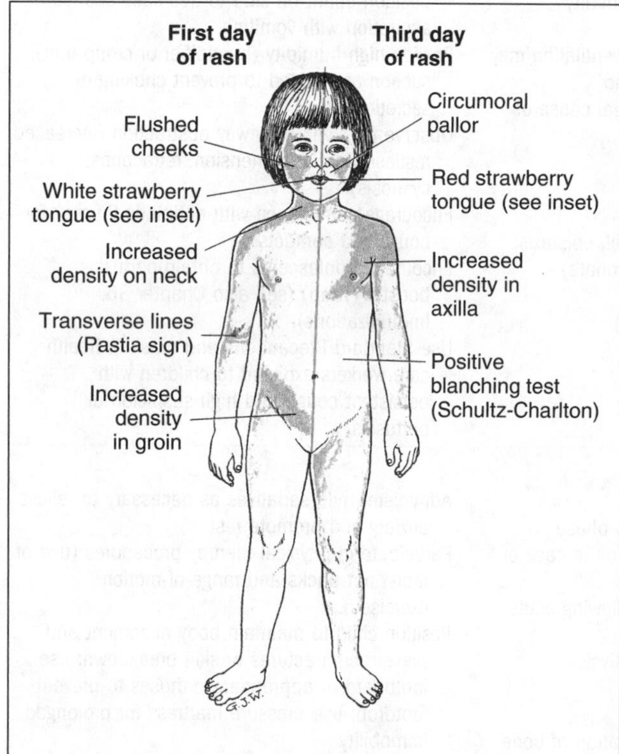

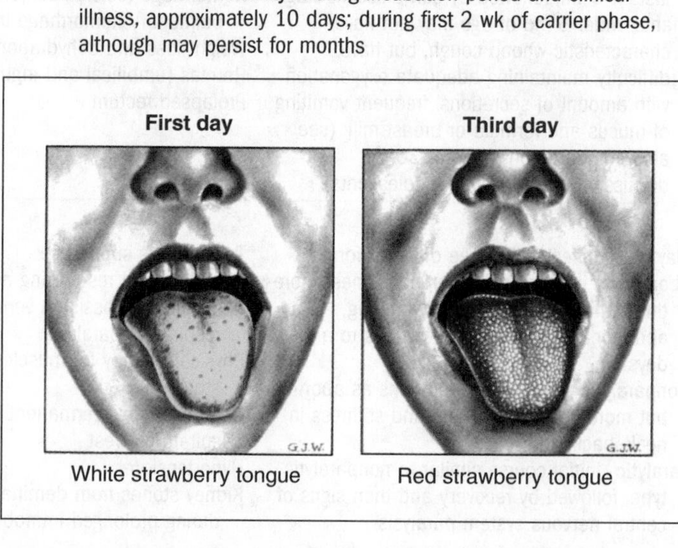

Fig. 38-13 Scarlet fever.

CLINICAL MANIFESTATIONS	THERAPEUTIC MANAGEMENT AND COMPLICATIONS	NURSING CARE MANAGEMENT
Constitutional signs and symptoms—Occasionally low-grade fever, headache, malaise, and lymphadenopathy **Prodromal stage**—Absent in children, present in adults and adolescents; consists of low-grade fever, headache, malaise, anorexia, mild conjunctivitis, coryza, sore throat, cough, and lymphadenopathy; lasts 1-5 days, subsides 1 day after appearance of rash **Rash**—First appears on face and rapidly spreads downward to neck, arms, trunk, and legs; by end of first day, body is covered with discrete, pinkish red maculopapular exanthema; disappears in same order as it began and is usually gone by third day	No treatment necessary other than antipyretics for low-grade fever and analgesics for discomfort **Complications**—Rare (arthritis, encephalitis, or purpura); most benign of all childhood communicable diseases; greatest danger is teratogenic effect on fetus	Reassure parents of benign nature of illness in affected child. Use comfort measures as necessary. Avoid contact with pregnant woman. Monitor rubella titer in pregnant adolescent.
Prodromal stage—Abrupt high fever, pulse increased out of proportion to fever, vomiting, headache, chills, malaise, abdominal pain, halitosis **Enanthema**—Tonsils enlarged, edematous, reddened, and covered with patches of exudates; in severe cases appearance resembles membrane seen in diphtheria; pharynx edematous and beefy red; during first 1-2 days tongue coated and papillae become red and swollen (white strawberry tongue); by fourth or fifth day white coat sloughs off, leaving prominent papillae (red strawberry tongue); palate covered with erythematous punctate lesions **Exanthema**—Rash appears within 12 hr after prodromal signs; red pinhead-sized punctate lesions rapidly become generalized but are absent on face, which becomes flushed with striking circumoral pallor; rash more intense in folds of joints; by end of first week desquamation begins (fine, sandpaper-like on torso; sheetlike sloughing on palms and soles), which may be complete by 3 wk or longer	**Treatment of choice**—Full course of penicillin (or erythromycin in penicillin-sensitive children), or oral cephalosporin Antibiotic therapy for newly diagnosed carriers (nose or throat cultures positive for streptococci) **Supportive measures**—Rest during febrile phase, analgesics for sore throat; antipruritics for rash if bothersome **Complications**—Peritonsillar and retropharyngeal abscess Sinusitis Otitis media Acute glomerulonephritis Acute rheumatic fever Polyarthritis (uncommon)	Institute Standard and Droplet Precautions until 24 hr after initiation of treatment. Ensure compliance with oral antibiotic therapy; intramuscular benzathine penicillin G [Bicillin] may be given if parents' reliability in giving oral drugs is questionable. Encourage rest during febrile phase; provide quiet activity during convalescent period. Relieve discomfort of sore throat with analgesics, gargles, lozenges, antiseptic throat sprays, and inhalation of cool mist. Encourage fluids during febrile phase; avoid irritating liquids (certain citrus juices) or rough foods (chips); when child is able to eat, begin with soft diet. Advise parents to consult practitioner if fever persists after beginning therapy. Discuss procedures for preventing spread of infection—discard toothbrush; avoid sharing drinking and eating utensils.

NURSING ALERT When lotions with active ingredients such as diphenhydramine in Caladryl are used, they are applied sparingly, especially over open lesions, where excessive absorption can lead to drug toxicity. These lotions should be used with caution in children who are simultaneously receiving an oral antihistamine. Cooling the lotion in the refrigerator beforehand often makes it more soothing on the skin than at room temperature.

To avoid overheating, which increases itching, children should wear lightweight, loose, nonirritating clothing and keep out of the sun. If the child persists in scratching, the nails are kept short and smooth; mittens and clothes with long sleeves or legs may be needed. For severe itching, antipruritic medication, such as diphenhydramine (Benadryl) or hydroxyzine (Atarax), may be required, especially when the child has trouble sleeping because of itching. Loratadine, cetirizine, and fexofenadine do not cause drowsiness and may be preferred for urticaria during the day.

An elevated temperature is common, and both antipyretic medicine (acetaminophen or ibuprofen) and environmental manipulation are implemented (see Controlling Elevated Temperatures, Chapter 45). The acetaminophen is effective in lowering the fever but does not significantly reduce the symptoms of itching, anorexia, abdominal pain, fussiness, or vomiting.

A sore throat, another frequent symptom, is managed with lozenges, saline rinses (if the child is old enough to cooperate), and analgesics. Because most children are anorectic during an illness, bland foods and increased liquids are usually preferred. During the early stages of the disease, children voluntarily curtail their activity, and although bed rest is beneficial, it should not be imposed unless specifically indicated. During periods of irritability, quiet activity (e.g., reading, music, television, video games, puzzles, coloring) helps distract children from the discomfort.

Support Child and Family

Most communicable diseases are benign, but may produce considerable concern and anxiety for parents. Often the occurrence of a disease such as chickenpox is the first time the child is acutely uncomfortable. Parents need assistance to cope with manifestations of the illness, such as intense itching.

The family and child need reassurance that recovery is generally rapid. However, visible signs of the dermatosis may be present for some time after the child is well enough to resume usual activities.

NURSING ALERT The occurrence of a communicable disease provides the opportunity to ask parents about the child's immunization status and reinforce the benefits of vaccines for children.

Child Maltreatment

The broad term *child maltreatment* includes intentional physical abuse or neglect, emotional abuse or neglect, and sexual abuse of children, usually by adults. It is one of the most significant social problems affecting children. In 2005 Child Protective Service (CPS) agencies in the United States confirmed that an estimated 900,000 children were victims of child maltreatment. Of the confirmed cases, 17% suffered physical abuse, 9% sexual abuse, 63% neglect, and 7% emotional abuse. In 2006 estimates indicated that 1530 children died as a result of child abuse and neglect (US Department of Health and Human Services, Administration on Children, Youth, and Families, 2006). Reported statistics only partially represent the actual incidence of child maltreatment, since many cases are believed to go unreported.*

Child Neglect

Child neglect is the most common form of maltreatment. More than half of all reported cases are associated with deprivation of necessities, and 40% of deaths from maltreatment are in this group (US Department of Health and Human Services, Administration on Children, Youth, and Families, 2006). Neglect is generally defined as the failure of a parent or other person legally responsible for the child's welfare to provide for the child's basic needs and an adequate level of care.

Important factors contributing to child neglect are lack of knowledge of child's needs, lack of resources, and caretaker substance abuse. For example, neglectful parents often demonstrate poor parenting skills. They may be unaware that an infant needs to be fed every 3 to 4 hours, may not know what to feed the child, and may have insufficient funds to buy food. Another serious lack of knowledge is failure to recognize emotional nurturing as an essential need of children. (See also Growth Failure [Failure to Thrive], Chapter 36.)

Types of Neglect

Neglect takes many forms and can be classified broadly as physical or emotional maltreatment. *Physical neglect* involves the deprivation of necessities, such as food, clothing, shelter, supervision, medical care, and education. *Emotional neglect* generally refers to failure to meet the child's needs for affection, attention, and emotional nurturance.

Neglect may also include lack of intervention for or fostering of maladaptive behavior, such as delinquency or substance abuse. *Emotional abuse,* an even more difficult aspect of maltreatment to define, refers to the deliberate attempt to destroy or significantly impair a child's self-esteem or competence. Emotional abuse may take the following forms: rejecting, isolating, terrorizing, ignoring, corrupting, verbally assaulting, or overpressuring the child.

Physical Abuse

The deliberate infliction of physical injury on a child, usually by the child's caregiver, is termed *physical abuse.* State and federal statutes provide legal definitions of physical abuse. The federal definition of abuse is "any recent act or failure to act that results in imminent risk of serious harm, death, serious physical or emotional harm of a child (less than 18 years of age) by a parent or caretaker who is responsible for the child's welfare" (Child Abuse Prevention and Treatment Act, 1996, Public Law 104-235, 10/1996). Each state defines abuse according to its reporting laws. Minor physical injury is responsible for more reported cases of maltreatment than

**Additional information is available from the Child Welfare Information Gateway at* www.childwelfare.gov/.

major physical injury, but major physical abuse causes more deaths. Despite the importance of the problem, a universally accepted definition of what constitutes minor and major physical abuse does not exist. Rather, each state in the United States defines abuse according to its individual reporting laws.

Shaken Baby Syndrome

Shaken baby syndrome (SBS) is a serious form of child abuse caused by violent shaking of infants and young children. This violent shaking would be easily recognized by others as dangerous (American Academy of Pediatrics, Committee on Child Abuse and Neglect, 2001), and is most often a result of the caregiver's frustration with crying. Every year in America an estimated 1200 to 1400 children are shaken, and of these victims, 25% to 30% die as a result of their injuries. The rest will have life-long complications.*

It is important to understand what happens in SBS. Infants have a large head-to-body ratio, weak neck muscles, and a large amount of water in the brain. Violent shaking causes the brain to rotate within the skull, resulting in shearing forces tearing blood vessels and neurons. The characteristic injuries that occur are intracranial bleeding (subdural and subarachnoid hematomas) and retinal hemorrhages, but may also include fractures of the ribs and long bones. Most often there are no signs of external injury. SBS is often not an isolated event, and in one study 45% of the children with inflicted traumatic brain injury caused by shaking showed some evidence of prior injury (Ewing-Cobb et al, 1998).

Victims of SBS can manifest a variety of symptoms, from generalized flulike symptoms to unresponsiveness with impending death (Miehl, 2005). Many of the presenting symptoms, such as vomiting, irritability, poor feeding, and listlessness, are often mistaken for common infant and childhood ailments. In more severe forms, presenting symptoms may include seizures, posturing, alterations in level of consciousness, apnea, bradycardia, or death. The long-term outcomes of SBS include seizure disorder; visual impairments, including blindness; developmental delays; hearing loss; cerebral palsy; and mild to profound mental, cognitive, and motor impairments (Walls, 2006). Nurses can take an active role in prevention of SBS by teaching all caregivers about crying and techniques to cope with inconsolable crying (Carbaugh, 2004).

NURSING ALERT Nurses should emphasize to parents the danger of shaking infants (shaking can cause SBS). Education must include coping mechanisms on caring for children with inconsolable crying.

Munchausen Syndrome by Proxy

Munchausen syndrome by proxy (MSBP), also known as factitious disorder by proxy or medical child abuse, is a rare but serious form of child abuse in which caretakers deliberately exaggerate or fabricate histories and symptoms or induce symptoms. It is a form of child maltreatment that may include physical, emotional, and psychologic abuse for the gratification of the caretaker. In most cases the perpetrator is the biologic mother, with some degree of health care knowledge and training. Health care providers can become easily misled and unknowingly enable the perpetrator (Leider et al, 2005). As a result of the history of symptoms provided by the caretaker, the child endures painful and unnecessary medical testing and procedures. Common symptoms are seizures, nausea and vomiting, diarrhea, and altered mental status; these symptoms are usually witnessed only by the perpetrator. Considerations when determining whether a child is a victim of MSBP include:

- Is the child's condition consistent with the reported history?
- Does diagnostic evidence support reported history?
- Has anyone other than the caretaker witnessed the symptoms?
- Is treatment being provided primarily because of the caretaker's demands?

The resolution of symptoms after separation from the perpetrator confirms the diagnosis.

National Center on Shaken Baby Syndrome: www.dontshake.com.

Factors Predisposing to Physical Abuse

The causes of child abuse are multifaceted. Child maltreatment occurs across all socioeconomic, religious, cultural, racial, and ethnic groups (Goldman et al, 2003). Three risk factors are commonly identified in child abuse: parental characteristics, characteristics of the child, and environmental characteristics. However, no single factor or group of factors is predictive of abuse. Rather, the interaction of these factors is thought to increase the risk of abuse occurring in a particular family.

Parental Characteristics

Certain identified characteristics occur more frequently in parents who abuse their children and are therefore considered risk factors. Younger parents more often are abusers of their children. One-parent families are at higher risk for abuse, and in single-parent families that include an unrelated partner, the partner is frequently the abuser.

Abusive families are often more socially isolated and have fewer supportive relationships. These parents are often from low-income circumstances, with concurrent undereducation and substance abuse problems. With little or no available support system and concurrent stressors imposed by the child or environment, these parents are vulnerable to additional crises of any nature and may strike out at the child as a method of releasing their increasing frustration and anxiety.

Other factors identified in abusive parents include low self-esteem and little knowledge of appropriate parenting skills. Parenting skills are learned behaviors, and parents who grew up with poor parental role models may have difficulty parenting their own children. Approximately one third of parents who were maltreated as children will subject their children to similar maltreatment (Gara et al, 2000).

Characteristics of the Child

The onus for child abuse is always on the abuser; however, children who are abused have some common characteristics. Children from birth to 3 years of age are at highest risk for being abused (US Department of Health and Human Services, Administration on Children, Youth, and Families, 2006). Infants and small children require constant attention and must have all their needs met by others. This can result in parental or caretaker fatigue with resultant striking out at the child with physical force, shaking the child, or ignoring the child's needs.

The physical and emotional demands placed on the parents or caretaker of an unwanted, brain-damaged, hyperactive, or physically disabled child may overwhelm them, resulting in abuse. Disabled children may not understand that abusive behaviors are not appropriate, so do not tell others or defend themselves. Preterm infants may be at risk for maltreatment because of failure of parent-child bonding during early infancy, increased physical needs, or irritability.

One child in the family may be singled out in an abusive family. Removing that child from the home often places the other siblings at risk for abuse. Therefore no child is safe if left in the abusive environment unless the parents can be helped to learn new parenting skills and to meet their needs and release their frustration through alternatives other than attacking their children.

Environmental Characteristics

The environment is a significant part of the potential abusive situation. A typical environment is one of chronic stress, including problems of divorce, poverty, unemployment, poor housing, frequent relocation, alcoholism, and drug addiction. Increased exposure between children and parents, such as that which occurs in crowded living conditions, also increases the likelihood of abuse.

Although most reporting of abuse has been from lower socioeconomic populations, as stated before, child abuse is not a problem of any one societal group. Stresses imposed by poverty predispose lower socioeconomic families to abusive situations, and abuse in these groups is more apt to be reported. However, concealed crises may also be present in upper-class families. Families who have substitute caregivers such as day care providers and baby-sitters may also be at risk for child abuse, especially if the family has not fully evaluated the caregiver. Nurses need to be aware of all these factors to identify the less obvious examples of child abuse and neglect.

Sexual Abuse

Sexual abuse is one of the most devastating types of child maltreatment, and estimates indicate that it has increased significantly during the past decade (US Department of Health and Human Services, Administration on Children, Youth, and Families, 2006). Child sexual abuse constitutes approximately 10% of officially substantiated child maltreatment cases. Some of the apparent increase can be attributed to increased awareness (Putnam, 2003).

As with all forms of child maltreatment, no universal definition for sexual abuse exists. Definitions of sexual abuse cover a range of acts, including involvement of children in sexual acts that they do not understand, that they cannot give consent to, or that violate social taboo (Finkel & DeJong, 2001). The Child Abuse Prevention and Treatment Act (Public Law 104-235) defines *sexual abuse* as "the use, persuasion, or coercion of any child to engage in sexually explicit conduct (or any simulation of such conduct) or producing any visual depiction of such conduct, or rape, molestation, prostitution, or incest with children."

Sexual abuse includes the following types of sexual maltreatment:

Incest—Any physical sexual activity between family members; blood relationship not required (abusers can include stepparents, unrelated siblings, grandparents, uncles, and aunts); does not include sexual relations between legally sanctioned partners, such as spouses

Molestation—A vague term that includes "indecent liberties," such as touching, fondling, kissing, single or mutual masturbation, or oral-genital contact

Exhibitionism—Indecent exposure, usually exposure of the genitalia by an adult man to children or women

Child pornography—Arranging and photographing, in any media, sexual acts involving children, alone or with adults or animals, regardless of consent by the child's legal guardian; also may denote distribution of such material in any form with or without profit

Child prostitution—Involving children in sex acts for profit and usually with changing partners

Pedophilia—Literally means "love of child" and does not denote a type of sexual activity but the preference of an adult for prepubertal children as the means of achieving sexual excitement

Characteristics of Abusers and Victims

Anyone, including siblings and mothers, can be sexual abusers, but a typical abuser is a male whom the victim knows. Offenders come from all levels of society. Adults make up 80% of offenders of sexual abuse, with the remaining 20% being adolescents and preadolescents (Johnson, 2003). Many offenders hold full-time jobs and are active in community affairs, and they may not have prior criminal records (Finkel & DeJong, 2001). Offenders often are employed in or volunteer for positions that will bring them into contact with young girls and boys, such as teaching or coaching. Child sexual abuse may be generational unless discovered and stopped (Johnson, 2003). Offenders may commit many assaults before being caught.

Incestuous relationships between father or stepfather and daughter are generally prolonged, and the victims are usually reluctant to report the situation because of fear of retaliation and fear that they will not be believed. Typically, incestuous relationships begin later than other forms of child abuse. The eldest daughter is usually abused, but in her absence another sister may be substituted. Sibling incest may also occur. Sexual abuse by relatives with a strong emotional bond with the victim is the most devastating to the child.

Boys are also victims of both intrafamilial and extrafamilial abuse. Male victims are much less likely to report abuse, and they may suffer much greater emotional harm from incestuous relationships, especially between mother and son, than female victims. Boys are likely to be subjected to anal penetration and oral-genital contact; to have subtle physical findings; and to be abused by a father, stepfather, or mother's boyfriend.

Initiation and Perpetuation of Sexual Abuse

Considerable evidence exists to show that at least 20% of American women and 5% to 10% of American men experienced some form of sexual abuse as children. Race and socioeconomic status do not seem to be major risk factors. Significant risk factors for child sexual abuse include parental unavailability, lack of emotional closeness, social isolation, emotional deprivation, and communication difficulties. Most sexual abuse is committed by men and by persons known to the child, with family members constituting up to two thirds of the perpetrators (Christian et al, 2000). Approximately 20% to 25% of child sexual abuse cases involve penetration or oral-genital contact. The mean age of vulnerability is 9 years, with a range from infancy to 17 years of age (Berlinger & Elliott, 2002). The cycle of sexual abuse often starts insidiously unless it involves an isolated attack, such as rape. Often offenders spend time with the victims to gain their trust before initiating any sexual contact. Most victims are then pressured into being an accessory to the sexual activity through various means (Box 38-1) and may be unaware that sexual activity is part of the offer. Children may not reveal the truth for fear that their parents would not believe them if they told, especially if the offender is a trusted member of the family. Some fear that they will be blamed for the situation, and many young children with limited vocabulary have difficulty describing the activity when they do have the courage or opportunity to reveal the abuse.

Incest most frequently occurs between fathers and daughters, but may be between grandfather and granddaughter or brother and sister. Brother-sister incest has been found to be just as damaging as father-daughter abuse (Cyr et al, 2002). Victims may take years to disclose this abuse. However, not all incestuous relationships follow this pattern of silence. Reports of father-daughter incest during child custody conflicts have become more common and have raised serious concerns regarding the possibility of false accusation. Rather than tolerating or denying the child's sexual abuse, the other parent (usually the mother) is typically the chief accuser.

Nursing Care of the Maltreated Child

A critical responsibility of health professionals is identifying abusive situations as early as possible. The characteristics that may predispose members of some families to commit abuse can serve as a framework for assessing vulnerability but are never predictive of actual abuse. A careful, detailed history and interview combined with a thorough physical examination are the diagnostic tools needed to identify abuse. Nurses have a special role because they may be the first person to see the child and parent and are the consistent caregivers if the child is hospitalized (see Guidelines box).

BOX 38-1 Methods Used to Pressure Children into Sexual Activity

- The child is offered gifts or privileges.
- The adult misrepresents moral standards by telling the child that it is "okay to do."
- Isolated and emotionally and socially impoverished children are enticed by adults who meet their needs for warmth and human contact.
- The successful sex offender pressures the victim into secrecy regarding the activity by describing it as a "secret between us" that other people may take away if they find out.
- The offender plays on the child's fears, including fear of punishment by the offender, fear of repercussions if the child tells, and fear of abandonment or rejection by the family.

GUIDELINES Talking with Children Who Reveal Abuse

- Provide a private time and place to talk.
- Do not promise not to tell; tell them that you are required by law to report the abuse.
- Do not express shock or criticize their family.
- Use their vocabulary to discuss body parts.
- Avoid using any leading statements that can distort their report.
- Reassure them that they have done the right thing by telling.
- Tell them that the abuse is not their fault, that they are not bad or to blame.
- Determine their immediate need for safety.
- Let the child know what will happen when you report.

During the interview with the child and family, the nurse must be careful to avoid biasing the child's retelling of the events. Some experts suggest that health professionals limit the interview to the child's physical and mental health concerns and leave topics of the family's social, legal, or other problems to the police or CPS (McClain et al, 2000). If this is not possible, an effort should be made to coordinate the interview process so that all pertinent health care professionals can be present.

NURSING ALERT Nurses must be aware of their biases regarding child abuse. Nurses are often less likely to report abuse when the child is a girl and from a middle-income, as opposed to lower-income, family; are significantly less comfortable dealing with sexual abuse, abuse of infants, and fathers as the abusers; and experience greater discomfort when dealing with abusers of children with disabilities than with abusers of children without disabilities.

Recognition of abuse or neglect necessitates a familiarity with both physical and behavioral signs that suggest maltreatment (Box 38-2). No one indicator can be used to diagnose maltreatment. It is a pattern or combination of indicators that should arouse suspicion and further investigation. It is important to note that some situations may be misinterpreted as abuse, such as bleeding disorders, osteogenesis imperfecta, sudden infant death syndrome, and cultural practices such as cupping or coin rubbing that may mimic physical abuse (see Health Practices, Chapter 32). Unintentional injuries, such as burns from metal buckles on car seats, bruising from seat belts, or spiral fractures from a twist and fall injury, may also be wrongly diagnosed as abuse. Normal variants, such as Mongolian spots and congenital anomalies of genitalia, can be mistaken for abuse.

BOX 38-2 Warning Signs of Abuse

- Physical evidence of abuse or neglect, including previous injuries
- Conflicting stories about the "accident" or injury from the parents or others
- Cause of injury blamed on sibling or other party
- An injury inconsistent with the history, such as a concussion and broken arm from falling off a bed
- History inconsistent with child's developmental level, such as a 6-month-old turning on the hot water
- A complaint other than the one associated with signs of abuse (e.g., a chief complaint of a cold when there is evidence of first- and second-degree burns)
- Inappropriate response of caregiver, such as an exaggerated or absent emotional response, refusal to sign for additional tests or agree to necessary treatment, excessive delay in seeking treatment, or absence of the parents for questioning
- Inappropriate response of child, such as little or no response to pain, fear of being touched, excessive or lack of separation anxiety, indiscriminate friendliness to strangers
- Child's report of physical or sexual abuse
- Previous reports of abuse in the family
- Repeated visits to emergency facilities with injuries

Caregiver-Child Interaction

The nurse can use the initial contact with the family to assess the interaction between the caregiver and the child. Certain behavioral responses of the parents to their child and to the interviewer should alert the nurse to the possibility of maltreatment. Abusive parents may have difficulty showing concern toward their child. They may be unable or unwilling to comfort the child. Abusers may blame the child for the injuries or belittle them for being clumsy or stupid. When interacting with the health care workers, the parent may become hostile or uncooperative. During the child's hospitalization they may not participate in the child's care and may show little concern for his or her progress, eventual discharge, or need for follow-up care. Although caregivers and children may vary in responses to a stressful event, an unusual caregiver-child relationship should be noted and factored into the overall evaluation of the child.

Abused children's responses to their parents or the injury may also support the suspicion of abuse. Although no one pattern is typical, extremes of behavior may be observed. Children may be unresponsive to the parent or excessively clinging and intolerant of separation. They may be overly attached to the abusive parent, possibly in the hope of preventing any upset that may precipitate anger and another attack. During care of the injury, children may be passive and accepting of the discomfort or uncooperative and fearful of any physical contact. They may avoid eye contact. Some children maintain a wary watchfulness of all strangers; some shy away from strangers as if frightened; others are unusually affectionate and outgoing.

History and Interview

Child Physical Abuse

It is often difficult to distinguish child maltreatment from accidental injuries. Caregivers whose history of events may be deceptive or incomplete and/or children who are nonverbal may make the assessment more complex. A purposeful, skilled history and appropriate interview questions will help the nurse to ensure the right course of action. Knowledge of mechanism of injury and child development is essential. Cases of abuse are often detected by inconsistencies in child or caregiver history of events compared with physical findings. Children who are verbal can often give a history of the injury. Separating the child from the caregiver may provide a more reliable history. It is important to ask nonleading, open-ended questions. The history should include a narrative of the injury from both caregiver and child (if verbal). Date, time, and location where injury took place along with who was present at time of the injury are essential questions. Family history for bleeding or bone disorders is important. Areas of history that are concerns for abuse are outlined in Box 38-3.

Neglect and Emotional Abuse

Each child may manifest different responses to neglect depending on the situation and the child's developmental age. The goal of the interview is to determine whether the child is in a safe environment and whether the caregiver has the skills and resources to care for the child. It is often difficult to determine whether the circumstances constitute poor parenting skills or true neglect. Warning signals for behaviors to look for are found in Box 38-2.

Sexual Abuse

An essential component to identifying sexual abuse is the interview. Several dynamics may impede the child's revelation of sexual abuse. Child sexual abuse is often perpetrated by someone known to the child, including family members. In some cases the children may have been sworn to secrecy. They may have been told that no one will believe them or their family would be harmed if they tell someone about the abuse. Small children may imitate behaviors they have had perpetrated on themselves or have seen others do. The nurse must be able to recognize normal, age-related sexual curiosity and self-stimulating behaviors. Typically, children do not act out specific details of the sexual act or perform intrusive acts on others unless they have sexual knowledge beyond their normal age-related development (Johnson, 2003).

Children's reports of sexual abuse may vary from contradictory stories to unwavering versions of the experience. Stories that sound contradictory may reflect the child's experiences in several instances of abuse. Also, children who repeatedly tell identical facts may have been prompted to do so. Increasing evidence suggests that the types of interrogation children are exposed to after reports of sexual abuse shape their thinking. To avoid biasing the interaction, nurses must be very skillful interviewers when questioning children who may be victims of abuse. Medical records should include verbatim statements made by the child and interviewer that reflect appropriate nonleading questions and statements (Hornor, 2001; McClain et al, 2000).

The child may not be emotionally ready to discuss the abuse. Establishing rapport with the child is essential to

BOX 38-3 Clinical Manifestations of Potential Child Maltreatment

Physical Neglect

Suggestive Physical Findings

Growth failure
Signs of malnutrition, such as thin extremities, abdominal distention, lack of subcutaneous fat
Poor personal hygiene
Unclean or inappropriate dress
Evidence of poor health care, such as delayed immunization, untreated infections, frequent colds
Frequent injuries from lack of supervision

Suggestive Behaviors

Dull and inactive affect; excessively passive or sleepy
Self-stimulatory behaviors, such as finger sucking or rocking
Begging or stealing food
Absenteeism from school
Substance abuse
Vandalism or shoplifting

Emotional Abuse and Neglect

Suggestive Physical Findings

Growth failure
Eating or feeding disorder
Enuresis
Sleep disorder

Suggestive Behaviors

Self-stimulatory behaviors, such as biting, rocking, sucking
During infancy, lack of social smile and stranger anxiety
Withdrawal from environment and people
Unusual fearfulness
Antisocial behavior, such as destructiveness, stealing, cruelty to animals or people
Extremes of behavior, such as overcompliant and passive, or aggressive and demanding
Lags in emotional and intellectual development, especially language
Suicide attempts

Physical Abuse

Suggestive Physical Findings

Bruises and welts
- On face, lips, mouth, back, buttocks, thighs, or areas of torso
- Regular patterns descriptive of object used, such as belt buckle, hand, wire hanger, chain, wooden spoon, squeeze or pinch marks
- May be present in various stages of healing

Burns
- On soles of feet, palms of hands, back, or buttocks
- Patterns descriptive of object used, such as round cigar or cigarette burns; sharply demarcated areas from immersion in scalding water; rope burns on wrists or ankles from being bound; burns in the shape of an iron, radiator, or electric stove burner
- Absence of "splash" marks and presence of symmetric burns
- Stun gun injury: lesions circular, fairly uniform (up to 0.5 cm), and paired about 5 cm apart

Fractures and dislocations
- Skull, nose, or facial structures
- Injury denoting type of abuse, such as spiral fracture or dislocation from twisting of an extremity or whiplash from shaking the child
- Multiple new or old fractures in various stages of healing

Lacerations and abrasions
- On backs of arms, legs, torso, face, or external genitalia
- Unusual symptoms, such as abdominal swelling, pain, and vomiting from punching
- Descriptive marks such as from human bites or pulling out of hair

Chemical
- Unexplained repeated poisoning, especially drug overdose
- Unexplained sudden illness, such as hypoglycemia from insulin administration

Suggestive Behaviors

Wary of physical contact with adults
Apparent fear of parents or going home
Lying very still while surveying environment
Inappropriate reaction to injury, such as failure to cry from pain
Lack of reaction to frightening events
Apprehension when hearing other children cry
Indiscriminate friendliness and displays of affection
Superficial relationships
Acting-out behavior, such as aggression, to seek attention
Withdrawal behavior

Sexual Abuse

Suggestive Physical Findings

Bruises, bleeding, lacerations, or irritation of external genitalia, anus, mouth, or throat
Torn, stained, or bloody underclothing
Pain on urination or pain, swelling, and itching of genital area
Penile discharge
Sexually transmitted infection, nonspecific vaginitis, or venereal warts
Difficulty in walking or sitting
Unusual odor in the genital area
Recurrent urinary tract infections
Presence of sperm
Pregnancy in young adolescent

Suggestive Behaviors

Sudden emergence of sexually related problems, including excessive or public masturbation, age-inappropriate sexual play, promiscuity, or overtly seductive behavior
Withdrawn behavior, excessive daydreaming
Preoccupation with fantasies, especially in play
Poor relationships with peers
Sudden changes, such as anxiety, loss or gain of weight, clinging behavior

Continued

BOX 38-3 Clinical Manifestations of Potential Child Maltreatment—cont'd

Sexual Abuse—cont'd

Suggestive Behaviors—cont'd

In incestuous relationships, excessive anger at mother for not protecting daughter
Regressive behavior, such as bed-wetting or thumb-sucking
Sudden onset of phobias or fears, particularly fears of the dark, men, strangers, or particular settings or situations (e.g., undue fear of leaving the house or staying at the day care center or the baby-sitter's house)
Running away from home
Substance abuse, particularly of alcohol or mood-elevating drugs
Profound and rapid personality changes, especially extreme depression, hostility, and aggression (often accompanied by social withdrawal)
Rapidly declining school performance
Suicidal attempts or ideation

gaining his or her trust. Interviews should not be rushed. Engaging the child in play activities while encouraging conversation may help the child discuss the abuse. It may take several interviews or psychologic counseling for the child to be forthcoming about the abuse.

Information regarding the last sexual contact is important because it determines the need for a forensic evaluation. Children who have had sexual abuse that has occurred within the past 72 to 96 hours should be considered for forensic testing.

Unfortunately, there is no typical profile of the victim, and there must be a high index of suspicion to identify these children. Physical signs vary and may include any of those listed for sexual abuse. The victim may exhibit various behavioral manifestations, none of which is diagnostic. When abused children exhibit these behaviors, the signs may be incorrectly attributed to the normal stresses of childhood, especially in older school-age children or adolescents. Even signs considered most predictive of sexual abuse, such as certain genital findings, sexually inappropriate behavior for age, enactment of adult sexual activity, and intense focus on sexual activity (e.g., masturbation), do not always indicate that sexual abuse has occurred. Conversely, abused children may not demonstrate more knowledge of sexual activity than nonabused children. However, one difference in the abused children's explanation of sexual activity may be unusual affective responses. For example, abused children may have an increased incidence of sleep disorders, temper tantrums, and depression (Calam et al, 1998).

NURSING ALERT When children report potentially sexually abusive experiences, their reports need to be taken seriously, but also cautiously, to avoid alarming the child or falsely accusing someone.

Physical Assessment

Child Physical Abuse

The goal of the physical assessment for child physical abuse is identification of all injuries. A systems approach ensures the whole body is evaluated. In instances of severe abuse and injuries, the assessment should begin with a rapid assessment of airway, breathing, circulation, and neurologic systems. A systematic head-to-toe examination follows. Attention to areas often overlooked, such as the scalp, behind the ears, and the lingual frenulum, is essential. The child's exterior genitalia and posterior surface should be completely examined.

Record the location and a detailed description of all injuries. Note color, size, and location of all bruising. Burn documentation should include location, pattern, demarcation lines, and presence of eschar or blisters. Diagrams of the injuries using a body diagram form are helpful. If available, photographs of the injuries using a measurement tool should be obtained.

Not all forms of physical abuse have obvious signs. Intraabdominal organ injury from blunt trauma to the abdomen can occur without signs of external abdominal bruising. Nurses should consider intraabdominal injury in infants and children who have any other signs of abuse.

NURSING ALERT Incompatibility between the history and the injury is probably the most important criterion on which to base the decision to report suspected abuse.

Neglect and Emotional Abuse

Neglect from deprivation of necessities is easier to identify than emotional neglect or abuse because physical signs are usually evident. Assessment of the child's height, weight, nutritional status, hygiene, and age-appropriate interactions is important for the overall picture of potential neglect. Emotional maltreatment may be readily suspected, but it is difficult to substantiate. Physical signs are often nonspecific, and nurses must rely on behavioral indicators, which range from depression to acting-out behavior, to help identify a possibly abusive situation. Any persistent and unexplained change in the child's behavior is an important clue to possible emotional abuse.

Sexual Abuse

Identifying instances of sexual abuse is particularly difficult because, often, few if any obvious physical indications of the activity exist. Physical signs vary and may include any of those listed in Box 38-3 for sexual abuse. The goal of the physical examination is to document genital findings. In most cases the genital examination is normal, which does not mean that sexual abuse did not occur. Fondling or genital-to-genital contact without penetration may leave no physical findings. Forensic evidence collection should be considered for any child with known or suspected sexual contact within 72 hours. Forensic evidence obtained directly from a prepubertal victim's body diminishes greatly after 24 hours, with the best chance for evidence collection coming from bed linens or the child's underwear (Christian et al, 2000). The female genital

evolve Nursing Care Plan–The Child Who Is Maltreated

examination should include a description of the vulva, hymen, and surrounding tissue. Abnormal findings of concern are injuries to the posterior vulva or the lower half of the hymenal ring, or abrasions, bruising, or bleeding of the genital or anal tissue. It is often helpful to use a magnifying instrument (colposcope) to detect subtle injuries. There are many variants of normal findings for female genital anatomy, so it is recommended that the examination be done by a practitioner experienced with these types of cases. Contrary to popular myth, the size of the hymenal opening is not predictive of the likelihood of sexual abuse (Christian & Rubin, 2002). For male victims, presence of swelling, abrasions, or bruising of the genital tissue is of concern for abuse. The anal area should be examined for symmetry, tone, fissures, or scars. Genital tissue heals quickly and most often without scars. Therefore, unless seen within a few days of injury, the genital tissue may appear normal. In addition, the vaginal and anal mucosa is elastic; therefore penetration without disruption of tissue is possible. This defies another myth that there is always evidence of female virginity.

Nursing Care Management

Protect Child from Further Abuse

Initially, identification of instances of suspected abuse or neglect is essential. The nurse may come in contact with abused children in an emergency department, practitioner's office, home, day care center, or school.

NURSING ALERT The priority is to remove the child from the abusive situation to prevent further injury.

All states and provinces in North America have laws for mandatory reporting of child maltreatment. Suspected child abuse is reported to the local authorities.* Referrals usually come to the state child welfare department and are assigned to a caseworker in an agency such as CPS. After a referral has been made, a caseworker is assigned to investigate the report. Based on the findings, the child is left in the home or temporarily removed.

A court proceeding may be necessary before the child can be placed outside the home or when parental rights are to be terminated. When the courts are involved, they usually require firsthand testimony by the referring parties. Nurses may be subpoenaed to appear in court, or their notes may be introduced as evidence in court hearings. Accurate and factual documentation is essential. Behaviors are described, not interpreted, and are recorded daily to establish a progress record (see Guidelines box). Conversations among the nurse, child, and parent are recorded verbatim as much as possible.

Support Child

Children suspected of being abused are often hospitalized for medical management of their injuries and to allow further assessment of their safety needs. The needs of these children are the same as those of any hospitalized child. The child should be treated as a child with the usual physical needs, developmental tasks, and play interests—not as a victim of abuse. The goal of the nurse-child relationship is to provide a role model for the parents in helping them relate positively and constructively to their child and to foster a therapeutic environment for the child in his or her reprieve from the abusing situation.

Support Family

The nurse also encourages the child's relationship with the nonoffending parent. The nurse does not become a substitute parent, but rather acts as a role model for parents in helping them to relate positively and constructively to their child. When parental ignorance of childrearing practices has played a part in the abuse, the nurse can educate the parent regarding children's physical and emotional needs. Because of the parents' own childrearing, they may not be aware of nonviolent methods of discipline, such as time-out. They may also need help in dealing with their frustration so that they do not vent anger on the child. Because these parents may be sensitive to criticism or perceptions of domination, teaching is implemented through demonstration and example rather than through lecturing. Any competent parenting abilities they demonstrate are praised to promote their sense of parental adequacy.

Family members are advised to encourage the child to resume normal activities and observe the child for signs of distress. Children express their feelings primarily through behavior. Parents should be alert for changes in behavior that indicate distress resulting from the incident, such as remaining in the house, refusing to go to school, changing sleeping

GUIDELINES Recording Assessment Data in Suspected Abuse

History of Injury

Date, time, and place of occurrence
Sequence of events with recorded times
Presence of witnesses, especially person caring for child at time of incident
Time lapse between occurrence of injury and initiation of treatment
Interview with child when appropriate, including verbal quotations and information from drawing or other play activities
Interview with parent, witnesses, or other significant persons, including verbal quotations
Description of parent-child interactions (verbal interactions, eye contact, touching, parental concern)
Name, age, and condition of other children in home (if possible)

Physical Examination

Location, size, shape, and color of bruises; approximate location, size, and shape on drawing of body outline
Distinguishing characteristics, such as a bruise in the shape of a hand; round burn (possibly caused by cigarette)
Symmetry or asymmetry of injury; presence of other injuries
Degree of pain; any bone tenderness
Evidence of past injuries; general state of health and hygiene
Developmental level of child; perform screening test (see Developmental Assessment, Chapter 34)

**Telephone numbers are usually listed under "Child Abuse" in the business white pages of the local directory, or call the emergency child abuse hotline: 800-422-4453 (800-4-A-CHILD).*

patterns, and having more frequent dreams and nightmares. Children are encouraged to talk about these feelings and nightmares, because the more they talk about the experience, the more they are able to gain control over it.

Referral to appropriate social service agencies is also essential. Many abusive parents live in poverty, and the daily stresses imposed by their circumstances are overwhelming. Resources for financial aid, improved housing, and child care should be sought. Self-help groups also provide important services. Groups such as *Parents Anonymous** (a group for parents who have abused or fear that they may abuse their child, but only in terms of physical abuse, not sexual abuse) and *Parents United International, Inc.*† (a group devoted to helping sexually abused families) are accepting and nonjudgmental.

Plan for Discharge

Discharge planning should begin as soon as the legal disposition for placement has been decided, which may be temporary foster home placement, return to the parents, or permanent termination of parental rights. The latter is the most drastic solution, but it is necessary in situations of life-threatening abuse. Whenever children are sent to a foster home or juvenile institution, they must be allowed an opportunity to express their feelings. No matter how severe the abuse, they usually mourn the loss of their parents. They need help to understand why they must not return home and that this new home is in no way a punishment. Whenever possible, foster parents are encouraged to visit in the hospital, and the nurse should take an active role in helping these new parents understand the child.

It is unfortunate that some abused children live in torment as they are sent from one foster home to another, sometimes enduring worse circumstances than those that existed in their original home. Only through constant evaluation of the placement residence and the child's adjustment to a new environment can the vicious circle of abuse, abandonment, and neglect be stopped.

Prevent Abuse

Prevention of child maltreatment has been an extremely difficult goal. Programs aimed at identifying potential abusers and instituting supportive intervention before the occurrence of an abusive act have met with variable success. However, nurses have played an important role in such programs. For example, home visits by nurses to primiparas who were either teenagers, unmarried, or of low socioeconomic status was noted to be an effective preventive measure (Eckenrode et al, 2000; McMillian, 2000). The nurses provided information on normal child growth and development and routine health care needs, served as informal support persons, and referred families to appropriate services when a need for assistance was identified.

Such programs provide models that can be used to reduce factors that increase the risk of abuse. Nurses in a variety of settings can implement similar activities. For example, nurses in prenatal clinics can prepare expectant families for adjustment to parenthood. Nursery and postpartum nurses can foster the attachment process by encouraging parents to hold and look at their infant, as well as teaching coping mechanisms for prolonged crying. Nurses in neonatal intensive care units can minimize the effects of separation by encouraging parents to visit and can help parents become comfortable caring for their child. Nurses in ambulatory settings can teach parents appropriate methods of bathing, feeding, toileting, disciplining, and preventing injuries, while stressing the normal needs and developmental characteristics of children. Nurses must be sensitive to parental needs for attention, reassurance, and reinforcement, and refer parents to community services and self-help groups.

Unlike preventive efforts for neglect and physical abuse, which have been aimed at the potential offender, *prevention of child sexual abuse* has centered on education of children to protect themselves. Materials are available for parents that describe sexual abuse and its prevention.‡ Supporting parental qualities of respect, affection, empathy, and ability to set boundaries, and providing high-quality child care and education, represent the true preventive approach to sexual abuse. Helpful games such as "What if the baby-sitter wants to wrestle and hug but tells you to keep it a secret?" can be used to explore dangerous situations in advance and help children learn the importance of saying "no." They need reassurance that no matter what the other person says or does, the parents want to know about it and will not punish them. Even if children participate in the activity before telling the parents, they must be reassured that it was not their fault.

It is equally important to teach children safety in terms of potential risk situations. Several suggestions for parents regarding protecting and educating children against possible molestation are presented in the Family-Centered Care box. The nurse is frequently in a position to discuss the topic of abuse with parents and to provide guidelines. In addition, parents need to be made aware that "nice" people, including friends and relatives, can be offenders; parents should carefully observe how others act toward the child. A sudden change in the child's behavior and a response such as "I don't like Uncle anymore" are clues to investigate the relationship. In the event of any doubt, further solitary encounters with this person and the child should be prevented. It is sometimes to the child's great misfortune that parents do not take certain comments seriously, such as "He hugs me too tight" or "I don't want to go with him." Casual parental statements such as "He just loves you" or "You do whatever adults tell you to do" can place children in jeopardy. Health professionals must alert parents to such dangers and guide them toward an appreciation of the problem, providing concrete guidelines toward child education and protection.

**675 West Foothill Blvd., Suite 220, Claremont, CA 91711; 909-621-6184;* www.parentsanonymous.org.

†*615 15th St., Modesto CA 95354; 209-572-3446;* www.parentsunited.info.

‡*Sources of information are Prevent Child Abuse America, Publishing Department, 500 N. Michigan Ave., Suite 200, Chicago, IL 60611-3703; 312-663-3520 or 800-Children;* www.preventchildabuse.org; *The Kempe Center and Foundation, The Gary Pavilion at The Children's Hospital, Anschutz Medical Campus, 13123 E. 16th Ave. B390, Aurora, CO 80045; 303-864-5300;* www.kempe.org; *American Humane, Children's Division, 63 Inverness Drive East, Englewood, CO 80112; 800-227-4645 (outside Colorado) or 303-792-9900;* www.americanhumane.org.

FAMILY-CENTERED CARE

Preventing or Dealing with Sexual Abuse of Children

Sexual assault of children is much more common than most people realize. It may be preventable if children have good preparation. *To provide protection and preparation:*

- Pay careful attention to who is around children. (Unwanted touch may come from someone liked and trusted.)
- Back up a child's right to say "no."
- Encourage communication by taking seriously what children *say.*
- Take a second look at signals of potential danger.
- Refuse to leave children in the company of those not trusted.
- Include information about sexual assault when teaching about safety.
- Provide specific definitions and examples of sexual assault.
- Remind children that even "nice" people sometimes do mean things.
- Urge children to tell about *anybody* who causes them to be uncomfortable.
- Prepare children to deal with bribes, threats, and possible physical force.
- Virtually eliminate secrets between children and parents.
- Teach children how to say "no," ask for help, and control who touches them and how.
- Model self-protective and limit-setting behavior for children.

Should it ever become necessary to help a child recover from a sexual assault:

- Listen carefully to understand children.
- Support the child for telling through praise, belief, sympathy, and lack of blame.
- Know local resources and choose help carefully.
- Provide opportunities to talk about the assault.
- Provide opportunities for the entire family to go through a recovery process.

Sexual assault affects everyone. To help deal with this social problem:

- Provide care and support to those who have been victimized.
- Recognize that offenders do not change without intervention.
- Organize neighborhood programs to support each other's efforts to protect children.
- Encourage schools to provide information about sexual assault as a problem of health and safety.
- Organize community groups to support educational treatment and law enforcement programs.

Modified from Adams C, Fay J: *No more secrets: protecting your child from sexual assault,* San Luis Obispo, CA, 1981, Impact.

Key Points

- The preschool years consist of the period from 3 to 5 years of age, a time that is considered critical for emotional and psychologic development.
- Biologic development in the preschool period is characterized by mature body systems and refinement in gross and fine motor behavior, as evidenced by activities such as running, riding a tricycle, and drawing.
- According to Erikson, acquiring a sense of initiative is the chief psychosocial task of the preschooler. Development of the superego occurs during this period, as conscience begins to emerge.
- According to Piaget, the preschool age is characterized by intuitive (or prelogical) thinking and a move toward logical thought processes through advanced, complex learning; language; and understanding of causality.
- The seeds of moral development are planted during the preschool period. According to Kohlberg, these children are in the stage of naive instrumental orientation, in which they are concerned with satisfying their own needs and, less frequently, the needs of others.
- Social development includes further separation-individuation; more sophisticated language; greater independence; and more complex, imaginative forms of play.

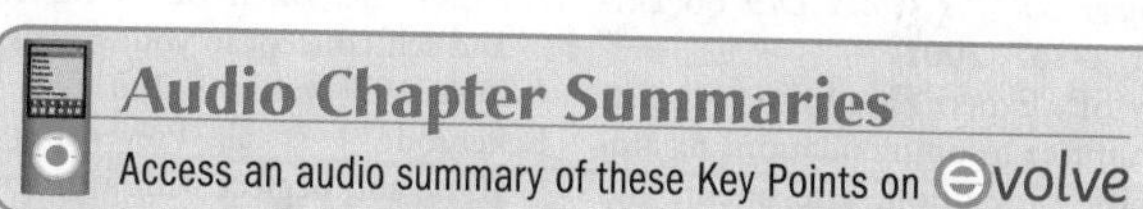
Audio Chapter Summaries
Access an audio summary of these Key Points on evolve

- Areas of special concern to parents during the preschool period are the preschool and kindergarten experience, sex education, fears, stress, and speech problems.
- In selecting an early learning program, parents should inquire about daily activities, teacher qualifications, accreditation, student-staff ratio, safety, meals, fees, and health practices.
- Two rules that govern how parents answer questions about sex and other sensitive issues are to find out what the child knows and to be honest.
- Fears constitute a great part of the preschool period; fear of objects or potential annihilation and parent-induced fears are common.
- Preschool aggression may result from frustration, modeling behavior, and reinforcement.
- Hesitancy or dysfluency in speech patterns is a normal characteristic of language development. Speech problems can occur when parents express excessive concern over this pattern.

- Health promotion continues to be directed toward proper nutrition, adequate sleep, proper dental care, and injury prevention.
- Child maltreatment may take the form of physical abuse or neglect, emotional abuse or neglect, or sexual abuse.
- Parental, child, and environmental characteristics are criteria that may predispose children to maltreatment.
- Identification of abuse entails securing evidence of maltreatment, taking a history pertaining to the incident, and assessing parental and child behaviors.
- The reported incidence of sexual abuse has increased in the past decade; common forms are incest, molestation, rape, exhibitionism, child pornography, child prostitution, and pedophilia.

References

American Academy of Pediatrics, Committee on Child Abuse and Neglect: Shaken baby syndrome: rotational cranial injuries—technical report, *Pediatrics* 108(1):206-210, 2001.

American Academy of Pediatrics, Committee on Infectious Diseases, Pickering L (editor): *2006 red book: report of the Committee on Infectious Diseases*, ed 27, Elk Grove Village, IL, 2006, The Academy.

American Academy of Pediatrics, Committee on Nutrition: The use and misuse of fruit juices in pediatrics, *Pediatrics* 107(5):1210-1213, 2001.

American Academy of Pediatrics, Committee on Public Education: Children, adolescents, and television, *Pediatrics* 107(2):423-426, 2001.

American Academy of Pediatrics, Committee on Sports Medicine and Fitness and Committee on School Health: Organized sports for children and preadolescents, *Pediatrics* 107(6):1459-1462, 2001.

Anderson DR et al: Early childhood television viewing and adolescent behavior: the recontact study, *Monogr Soc Res Child Dev* 66(1):I-VIII, 1-147, 2001.

Barlow SE, Expert Committee: Expert committee recommendations regarding the prevention, assessment, and treatment of child and adolescent overweight and obesity: summary report, *Pediatrics* 120(Suppl 4):S164-S192, 2007.

Barnes LL et al: Spirituality, religion, and pediatrics: intersecting worlds of healing, *Pediatrics* 104(6):899-908, 2000.

Bendersky M, Bennett D, Lewis M: Aggression at age 5 as a function of prenatal exposure to cocaine, gender, and environmental risk, *J Pediatr Psychol Adv Access* 31(1):71-84, 2006.

Berlinger L, Elliott D: Sexual abuse of children. In Myers JEB et al (editors): APSAC handbook on child maltreatment, ed 2, Thousand Oaks, CA, 2002, Sage.

Brazelton TB, Sparrow JD: *Touchpoints 3 to 6: your child's emotional and behavioral development*, Cambridge, MA, 2001, Da Capo Press.

Brown KD, Hamilton-Giachritsis C: The influence of violent media on children and adolescents: a public-health approach, *Lancet* 365(9460):702-710, 2005.

Calam R et al: Psychological disturbances and child sexual abuse: a follow-up study, *Child Abuse Negl* 22(9):901-913, 1998.

Carbaugh SF: The long road home: understanding shaken baby syndrome, *Adv Neonat Care* 4:105-117, 2004.

Chen TM et al: Clinical manifestations of varicella-zoster virus infection, *Dermatol Clin* 20(2):267-282, 2002.

Christian C et al: Forensic evidence findings in prepubertal victims of sexual assault, *Pediatrics* 106:100-104, 2000.

Christian CW, Rubin DM: Sexual abuse. In Giardino AP, Giardino ER (editors): *Recognition of child abuse for the mandated reporter*, St Louis, 2002, GW Medical.

Cyr M et al: Intrafamilial sexual abuse: brother-sister incest does not differ from father-daughter incest and stepfather-stepdaughter incest, *Child Abuse Neglect* 26(9):957-973, 2002.

Davison KK, Birch LL: Weight status and self-concept in young girls, *Pediatrics* 107(1):46-53, 2001.

Eckenrode J et al: Preventing child abuse and neglect with a program of nurse home visitation: the limiting effects of domestic violence, *JAMA* 284(11):1385-1391, 2000.

Endres J et al: Soy-enhanced lunch acceptance by preschoolers, *J Am Diet Assoc* 103(3):346-351, 2003.

Ewing-Cobb L et al: Neuroimaging, physical, and developmental findings after inflicted and noninflicted traumatic brain injury in young children, *Pediatrics* 102:300-307, 1998.

Feldman HM: Evaluation and management of language and speech disorders in preschool children, *Pediatr Rev* 26(4):131-142, 2005.

Finkel MA, DeJong AR: Medical findings in child sexual abuse. In Reece RM, Ludwig S (editors): *Child abuse medical diagnosis and management*, Philadelphia, 2001, Lippincott Williams & Wilkins.

Food and Nutrition Board: *Dietary reference intakes: guiding principles for nutrition labeling and fortification*, Washington, DC, 2003, National Academies Press.

Fosarelli P: Children and the development of faith: implications for pediatric practice, *Contemp Pediatr* 20(1):85-98, 2003.

Gara MA et al: The abused child as parent: the structure and content of physically abused mothers' perceptions of their babies, *Child Abuse Negl* 24(5):627-639, 2000.

Gershoff ET: Corporal punishment by parents and associated child behaviors and experiences: a meta-analytic and theoretical review, *Psychol Bull* 128(4):539-579, 2002.

Gleason TR, Sebanc AM, Hartup WW: Imaginary companions of preschool children, *Dev Psychol* 36(4):419-428, 2000.

Goldman J et al: What factors contribute to child abuse and neglect? In Goldman J et al: *A coordinated response to child abuse and neglect: the foundation for practice*, Washington, DC, 2003, Child Welfare Information 2003. Available at www.childwelfare.gov/pubs/usermanuals/foundation/foundatione.cfm (accessed June 4, 2007).

Hornor G: Repeated sexual abuse allegations: a problem for primary care providers, *J Pediatr Health Care* 15(2):71-76, 2001.

Jellinek M, Patel BP, Froehle MC (editors): *Bright futures in practice: mental health*, vol 1, Arlington, VA, 2002, National Center for Education in Maternal and Child Health.

Johnson M: Child sexual abuse. In Thomas DO, Bernardo LM, Herman B (editors): *Core curriculum for pediatric emergency nursing*, Sudbury, MA, 2003, Jones & Bartlett.

Johnson RK: Changing eating and physical activity patterns of U.S. children, *Proc Nutr Soc* 59(2):295-301, 2000.

Kleinman RE (editor): *Pediatric nutrition handbook*, ed 5, Elk Grove Village, IL, 2004, American Academy of Pediatrics.

Leider HS et al: Munchausen syndrome by proxy: a case report, *AACN Clin Issues* 16(2):178-184, 2005.

Leung AK, Robson WL, Leong AG: Herpes zoster in childhood, *J Pediatr Health Care* 20(5):1783-1785, 2006.

Martof A: Consultation with the specialist: dental care, *Pediatr Rev* 22(1):13-15, 2001.

McClain N et al: Evaluation of sexual abuse in the pediatric patient, *J Pediatr Health Care* 14(3):93-102, 2000.

McEvoy M: Culture and spirituality as an integrated concept in pediatric care, *MCN* 28(1):39-43, 2003.

McMillian H: Child maltreatment: what we know in the year 2000, *Can J Psychiatry* 45(8):702-709, 2000.

Miehl NJ: Shaken baby syndrome, *J Forensic Nurs* 1(3):111-117, 2005.

National Institute on Deafness and Other Communication Disorders: *Stuttering*, 2002, National Institutes of Health. Available at www.nidcd.nih.gov/health/voice/stutter (accessed March 2007).

Needlman R: Growth and development: preschool years. In Behrman RE, Kliegman RM, Jenson HB (editors): *Nelson textbook of pediatrics*, ed 17, Philadelphia, 2004, Saunders.

Putnam FW: Ten year update review: child sexual abuse, *J Am Acad Child Adolesc Psychiatry* 42(3):269-278, 2003.

Rafanello D: Controlling the spread of infectious disease in child care programs, *Healthy Child Care Am* Winter:1-11, 2001.

Spear BA et al: Recommendations for treatment of child and adolescent overweight and obesity, *Pediatrics* 120(Suppl 4):S254-S288, 2007.

Story M, Holt K, Sofka D (editors): *Bright futures in practice: nutrition*, ed 2, Arlington, VA, 2002, National Center for Education in Maternal and Child Health.

Thiedke CC: Sleep disorders and sleep problems in childhood, *Am Fam Physician* 63(2):277-284, 2001.

US Department of Health and Human Services, Administration on Children, Youth, and Families: Child maltreatment, Washington, DC, 2006, Government Printing Office. Available at www.acf.hhs.gov (accessed April 20, 2009).

Walls C: Shaken baby syndrome education: a role for nurse practitioners working with families of small children, *J Pediatr Health Care* 20(5):304-310, 2006.

Yalçin SS et al: Factors that affect television viewing time in preschool and primary schoolchildren, *Pediatr Int* 44(6):622-627, 2002.

Unit 9

39 The School-Age Child and Family

Learning Objectives

On completion of this chapter the reader will be able to:

- Describe the physical, cognitive, and moral changes that take place during the middle childhood years.
- Describe ways to help a child develop a sense of accomplishment.
- Demonstrate an understanding of the changing interpersonal relationships of school-age children.
- Discuss the role of the peer group in the socialization of the school-age child.
- Discuss the role of schools in the development and socialization of the school-age child.
- Demonstrate an understanding of the types, causes, and prevention of sports injuries in middle childhood.
- Describe the most common causes of growth and maturation failure in later childhood.
- Discuss the manifestations and nursing management of selected emotional and behavioral problems.
- Outline an appropriate health teaching plan for the school-age child.
- Plan a sex education session for a group of school-age children.
- Identify the causes and discuss the preventive aspects of injury in middle childhood.

Electronic Resources

Additional information related to the content in Chapter 39 can be found on

evolve the Companion Website at http://evolve.elsevier.com/Perry/maternal/

- NCLEX Review Questions
- Assessment Video Clips
- Case Study—Attention-Deficit/Hyperactivity Disorder
- Case Study—Injury Prevention
- Critical Thinking Exercise—Turner Syndrome

Promoting Optimal Growth and Development

The segment of the life span that extends from age 6 years to approximately 12 years has a variety of labels, each of which describes an important characteristic of the period. These middle years are most often referred to as *school age* or the *school years.* This period begins with entrance into the school environment, which has a significant impact on development and relationships.

Physiologically the middle years begin with the shedding of the first deciduous tooth and end at puberty with the acquisition of the final permanent teeth (with the exception of the wisdom teeth). Before 5 or 6 years of age, children have progressed from helpless infants to sturdy, complicated individuals with an ability to communicate, conceptualize in a limited way, and become involved in complex social and motor behaviors. Physical growth is also rapid during the preschool-age years. In contrast, the period of middle childhood, between the rapid growth of early childhood and the prepubescent growth spurt, is a time of gradual growth and development with more even progress in both physical and emotional aspects.

Biologic Development

During middle childhood, growth in height and weight assumes a slower but steady pace as compared with the earlier years. Between ages 6 and 12, children will grow an average of 5 cm (2 inches) per year to gain 30 to 60 cm (1 to 2 feet) in height and will almost double their weight, increasing 2 to 3 kg (4½ to 6½ lb) per year. The average 6-year-old child is about 116 cm (45⁷⁄₁₀ inches) tall and weighs about 21 kg (46 lb); the average 12-year-old child is about 150 cm (59 inches) tall and weighs approximately 40 kg (88 lb). During this period, girls and boys differ little in size, although boys tend to be slightly taller and heavier than girls. Toward the end of the school-age years, both boys and girls begin to increase in size, although most girls begin to surpass boys in both height and weight, to the acute discomfort of both girls and boys.

Proportional Changes

School-age children are more graceful than they were as preschoolers, and they are steadier on their feet. Their body proportions take on a slimmer look, with longer legs, varying body proportion, and a lower center of gravity. Posture improves over that of the preschool period to facilitate locomotion and efficiency in using the arms and trunk. These proportions make climbing, bicycle riding, and other activities easier. Fat gradually diminishes, and its distribution patterns change, contributing to the thinner appearance of the child during the middle years.

Accompanying the skeletal lengthening and fat diminution is an increase in the percentage of body weight represented by muscle tissue. By the end of this age period, both boys and girls double their strength and physical capabilities, and their steady and relatively consistent development of coordination increases their poise and skill. However, this increased strength can be misleading. Although strength increases, muscles are still functionally immature when compared with those of the adolescent, and they are more readily damaged by muscular injury caused by overuse.

The most pronounced changes that indicate increasing maturity in children are a decrease in head circumference in relation to standing height, a decrease in waist circumference in relation to height, and an increase in leg length in relation to height. These observations often provide a clue to a child's degree of physical maturity and have proved useful in predicting readiness for meeting the demands of school. There appears to be a correlation between physical indications of maturity and success in school.

Specific physiologic and anatomic characteristics are typical of children in middle childhood. Facial proportions change as the face grows faster in relation to the remainder of the cranium. The skull and brain grow very slowly during this period and increase little in size. Because all of the primary (deciduous) teeth are lost during this age span, middle childhood is sometimes known as the *age of the loose tooth* (Fig. 39-1). The early years of middle childhood, when the new secondary (permanent) teeth appear too large for the face, are known as the *ugly duckling stage.*

Maturation of Systems

Maturity of the gastrointestinal system is reflected in fewer stomach upsets; better maintenance of blood glucose levels; and an increased stomach capacity, which permits retention of food for longer periods. The school-age child does not need to be fed as carefully, as promptly, or as frequently as the preschool-age child. Caloric needs are less than they were in the preschool years.

Physical maturation is evident in other body tissues and organs. *Bladder capacity*, although differing widely among individual children, is generally greater in girls than in boys.

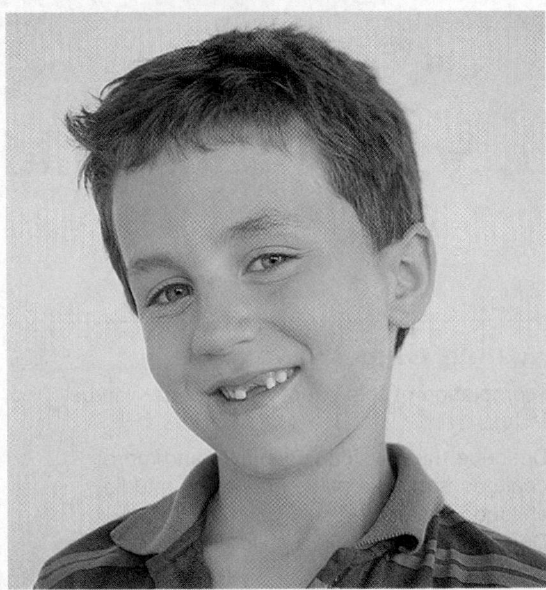

Fig. 39-1 Middle childhood is the stage of development when deciduous teeth are shed.

The *heart* grows more slowly during the middle years and is smaller in relation to the rest of the body than at any other period of life. Heart and respiratory rates steadily decrease and blood pressure increases from ages 6 to 12 (see Appendix E).

The *immune system* becomes more competent in its ability to localize infections and to produce an antibody-antigen response. However, children have several infections in the first 1 to 2 years of school because of increased exposure to other children.

Bones continue to ossify throughout childhood but yield to pressure and muscle pulls more readily than with mature bones. Children need ample opportunity to move around, but they should observe caution in carrying heavy loads. For example, they should shift books or tote bags from one arm to the other. Backpacks distribute weight more evenly than tote bags.

Wider differences between children are observed at the end of middle childhood than at the beginning. These differences become increasingly apparent and, if they are extreme or unique, may create emotional problems. The associated characteristics of height and weight relationships, rapid or slow growth, and other important features of development should be explained to children and their families. Physical maturity is not necessarily correlated with emotional and social maturity. Seven-year-old children who look like 10-year-old children will, in fact, think and act like 7-year-old children. To expect behaviors appropriate for the older age is unrealistic and can be detrimental to their development of competence and self-esteem. Conversely, to treat 10-year-old children who look young physically as though they were younger is an equal disservice to them.

Prepubescence

Preadolescence is the period of approximately 2 years that begins at the end of middle childhood and ends with the thirteenth birthday. Because puberty signals the beginning of the development of secondary sex characteristics, *prepubescence* typically occurs during preadolescence.

Toward the end of middle childhood the discrepancies in growth and maturation between boys and girls become apparent. On the average, there is a difference of approximately 2 years between girls and boys in the age of onset of pubescence. This is a period of rapid growth in height and weight, especially for girls.

There is no universal age at which children assume the characteristics of prepubescence. The first physiologic signs appear at about 9 years of age (particularly in girls) and are usually clearly evident in 11- to 12-year-old children. Although preadolescent children do not want to be different, variability in physical growth and physiologic changes between children of the same sex and between the two sexes is often striking at this time. This variability, especially in relation to the onset of secondary sexual characteristics, is of great concern to the preadolescent. Either early or late appearance of these characteristics is a source of embarrassment and uneasiness to both sexes.

Preadolescence is a period of considerable overlapping of developmental characteristics of both middle childhood and early adolescence. However, several unique characteristics set this period apart from others. Generally, puberty begins at 10 years in girls and 12 years in boys, but can be normal for either sex after the age of 8 years. Boys experience little visible sexual maturation during preadolescence.

Psychosocial Development

Freud described middle childhood as the *latency period*, a time of tranquility between the Oedipal phase of early childhood and the eroticism of adolescence. During this time children experience relationships with same-sex peers following the indifference of earlier years and preceding the heterosexual fascination that occurs for most boys and girls in puberty.

Developing a Sense of Industry (Erikson)

Successful mastery of Erikson's first three stages of psychosocial development is important in terms of development of a healthy personality. Successful completion of these stages requires a loving environment within a stable family unit. These experiences prepare the child to engage in experiences and relationships beyond the intimate family group.

A *sense of industry*, or a *stage of accomplishment*, is achieved somewhere between age 6 and adolescence. School-age children are eager to develop skills and participate in meaningful and socially useful work. They acquire a sense of personal and interpersonal competence; receive the systematic instruction prescribed by their individual cultures; and develop the skills needed to become useful, contributing members of their social communities.

Interests expand in the middle years, and with a growing sense of independence, children want to engage in tasks that can be carried through to completion (Fig. 39-2). They gain satisfaction from independent behavior in exploring and manipulating their environment and from interaction with peers. Often the acquisition of skills provides a way to achieve success in social activities. Reinforcement in the form of grades, material rewards, additional privileges, and recognition provides encouragement and stimulation.

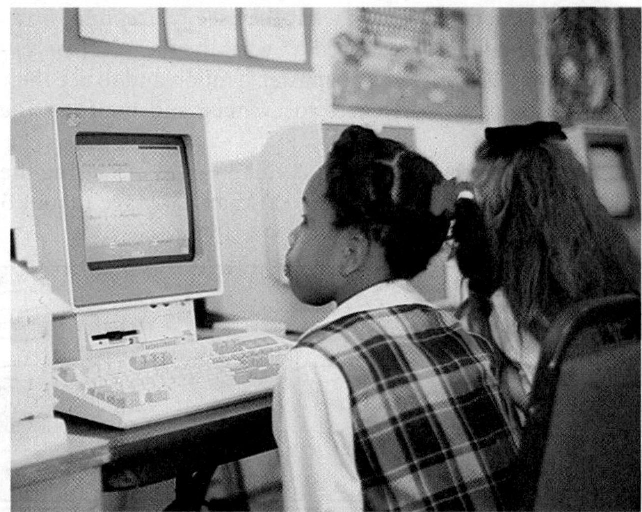

Fig. 39-2 School-age children are motivated to complete tasks working alone.

A sense of accomplishment also involves the ability to cooperate, to compete with others, and to cope effectively with people. Middle childhood is the time when children learn the value of doing things with others and the benefits derived from division of labor in the accomplishment of goals. Peer approval is a strong motivating power.

The danger inherent in this period of development is the occurrence of situations that might result in a sense of *inferiority*. Children with physical and mental limitations may be at a disadvantage in the acquisition of certain skills. When the reward structure is based on evidence of mastery, children who are incapable of developing these skills risk feeling inadequate and inferior. Even children without chronic disabilities may experience feelings of inadequacy in some areas. No child is able to do everything well, and children must learn that they will not be able to master every skill they attempt. All children, even children who usually have positive attitudes toward work and their own abilities, will feel some degree of inferiority when they encounter specific skills that they cannot master.

Children need and want real achievement. Children achieve a sense of industry when they have access to tasks that need to be done and they are able to complete the tasks well despite individual differences in their innate capacities and emotional development.

Cognitive Development (Piaget)

When children enter the school years, they begin to acquire the ability to relate a series of events to mental representations that can be expressed both verbally and symbolically. This is the stage Piaget describes as *concrete operations*, when children are able to use thought processes to experience events and actions. The rigid, egocentric view of the preschool years is replaced by mental processes that allow children to see things from another's point of view.

During this stage, children develop an understanding of relationships between things and ideas. They progress from making judgments based on what they see *(perceptual thinking)* to making judgments based on what they reason *(conceptual thinking)*. They are able to master symbols and to use their memories of past experiences to evaluate and interpret the present.

One cognitive task of school-age children is mastering the concept of conservation (Fig. 39-3). At an early age (about 5 to 7 years), children grasp the concept of reversibility of numbers as a basis for simple mathematics problems (e.g., 2 + 4 = 6 and 6 − 4 = 2). They learn that simply altering their arrangement in space does not change certain properties of the environment, and they are able to resist perceptual cues that suggest alterations in the physical state of an object. For example, they recognize that changing the shape of a sub-

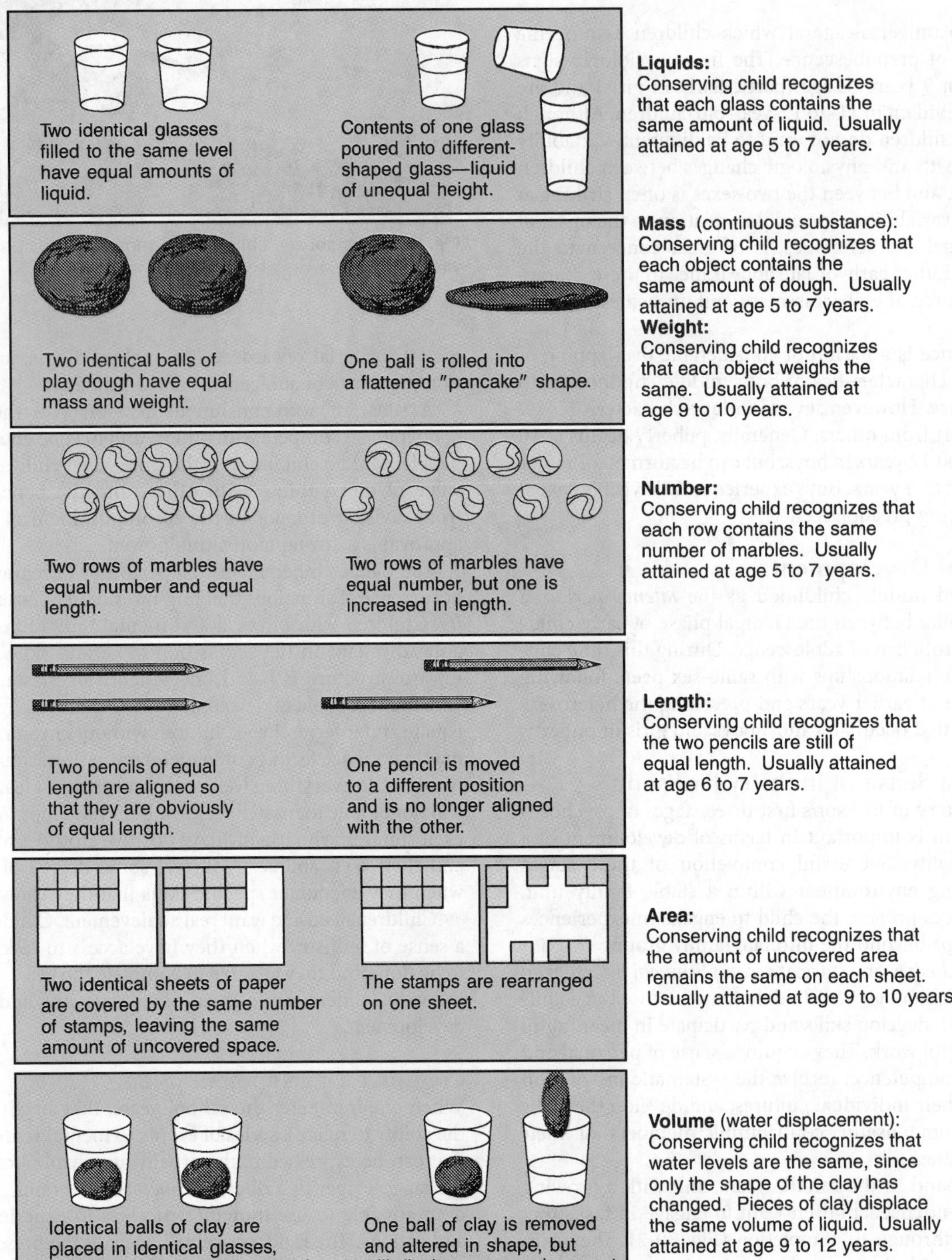

Two identical glasses filled to the same level have equal amounts of liquid.
Contents of one glass poured into different-shaped glass—liquid of unequal height.
Liquids:
Conserving child recognizes that each glass contains the same amount of liquid. Usually attained at age 5 to 7 years.
Two identical balls of play dough have equal mass and weight.
One ball is rolled into a flattened "pancake" shape.
Mass (continuous substance):
Conserving child recognizes that each object contains the same amount of dough. Usually attained at age 5 to 7 years.
Weight:
Conserving child recognizes that each object weighs the same. Usually attained at age 9 to 10 years.
Two rows of marbles have equal number and equal length.
Two rows of marbles have equal number, but one is increased in length.
Number:
Conserving child recognizes that each row contains the same number of marbles. Usually attained at age 5 to 7 years.
Two pencils of equal length are aligned so that they are obviously of equal length.
One pencil is moved to a different position and is no longer aligned with the other.
Length:
Conserving child recognizes that the two pencils are still of equal length. Usually attained at age 6 to 7 years.
Two identical sheets of paper are covered by the same number of stamps, leaving the same amount of uncovered space.
The stamps are rearranged on one sheet.
Area:
Conserving child recognizes that the amount of uncovered area remains the same on each sheet. Usually attained at age 9 to 10 years.
Identical balls of clay are placed in identical glasses, displacing the same amount of liquid.
One ball of clay is removed and altered in shape, but will displace an equal amount when replaced in the liquid.
Volume (water displacement):
Conserving child recognizes that water levels are the same, since only the shape of the clay has changed. Pieces of clay displace the same volume of liquid. Usually attained at age 9 to 12 years.

Fig. 39-3 Common examples that demonstrate the child's ability to conserve (ages are only approximate).

stance such as a lump of clay does not alter its total mass. They no longer perceive a tall, thin glass of water as containing a greater volume than a short, wide glass; they can distinguish between the weight of items regardless of their size. They recognize that size is not necessarily related to weight or volume. There is a developmental sequence in children's capacity to conserve matter. Conservation of mass usually is accomplished first, weight some time later, and volume last.

School-age children also develop *classification* skills. They can group and sort objects according to the attributes they share, place things in a sensible and logical order, and hold a concept in mind while making decisions based on that concept. Another characteristic of middle childhood is that children derive enjoyment from classifying and ordering their environment. They become occupied with collections of objects, such as stickers, shells, dolls, cars, cards, and stuffed animals. They may even begin to order friends and relationships (e.g., best friend, second best friend).

They develop the ability to understand relational terms and concepts, such as bigger and smaller; darker and paler; heavier and lighter; to the right of and to the left of; first, last, and intermediate relationships; and more than and less than. They view family relationships in terms of reciprocal roles (e.g., to be a brother, one must have a sibling).

School-age children learn the alphabet and the world of symbols called *words,* which can be arranged in terms of structure and their relationship to the alphabet. They learn to tell time, to see the relationship of events in time (history) and places in space (geography), and to combine time and space relationships (geology and astronomy).

The *ability to read* is acquired during the school years and becomes the most significant and valuable tool for independent inquiry. Children's capacity to explore, imagine, and expand their knowledge is enhanced by reading.

Moral Development (Kohlberg)

As children move from egocentrism to more logical patterns of thought, they also move through stages in the development of conscience and moral standards. Young children do not believe that standards of behavior come from within themselves but that rules are established and set down by others. During the preschool years children adopt and internalize the moral values of their parents. They learn standards for acceptable behavior, act according to these standards, and feel guilty when they violate them. Although children 6 or 7 years of age know the rules and behaviors expected of them, they do not understand the reasons behind them. Rewards and punishments guide their judgment; a "bad act" is one that breaks a rule or causes harm. Young children believe that what other people tell them to do is right and that what they themselves think is wrong. Consequently, children 6 or 7 years old may interpret accidents or misfortunes as punishment for "bad" acts.

Older school-age children are able to judge an act by the intentions that prompted it rather than just its consequences. Rules and judgments become less absolute and authoritarian, and begin to be founded on the needs and desires of others. For older children, a rule violation is likely to be viewed in relation to the total context in which it appears. The situation, as well as the morality of the rule itself, influences reactions. Although younger children judge an act only according to whether it is right or wrong, older children take into account a different point of view. They are able to understand and accept the concept of treating others as they would like to be treated.

Spiritual Development

Children at this age think in concrete terms, but are avid learners and have a great desire to learn about their God. They picture God as human and use adjectives such as "loving" and "helping" to describe their deity. They are fascinated by the concepts of hell and heaven, with a developing conscience and concern about rules. They may fear going to hell for misbehavior. School-age children want and expect to be punished for misbehavior and, when given the option, tend to choose a punishment that "fits the crime." However, they may view illness or injury as a punishment for a real or imagined misdeed. The beliefs and ideals of family and religious persons are more influential than those of their peers in matters of faith.

School-age children begin to learn the difference between the natural and the supernatural but have difficulty understanding symbols. Consequently, religious concepts must be presented to them in concrete terms. Prayer or other religious rituals comfort them, and if these activities are a part of their daily lives, they can help them cope with threatening situations. Their petitions to their God in prayers tend to be for tangible rewards. Although younger children expect their prayers to be answered, as they get older, they begin to recognize that this does not always occur and become less concerned when prayers are not answered. They are able to discuss their feelings about their faith and how it relates to their lives (see Cultural Awareness box).

CULTURAL AWARENESS

Religious Orientation

Many schools and communities have a Judeo-Christian orientation toward prayer, holidays, and values. This may result in conflict and discomfort for children of other religious or ethnic groups. Sensitivity must be exercised so as not to offend and confuse children from other religious backgrounds, such as the Buddhist, Hindu, and Muslim faiths, or no religious backgrounds.

Social Development

One of the most important socializing agents in the school-age years is the peer group. In addition to parents and the schools, the peer group conveys a substantial amount of information to its members. Peer groups have a culture of their own, with secrets, traditions, and codes of ethics that promote feelings of solidarity and detachment from adults. Through peer relationships, children learn how to deal with dominance and hostility, how to relate to persons in positions of leadership and authority, and how to explore ideas and the physical environment.

Peer group identification is an important factor in gaining independence from parents. The aid and support of the group provide the child with enough security to risk the moderate parental rejection brought about by small victories in the development of independence.

A child's concept of the appropriate sex role is also influenced by relationships with peers. During the early school years few gender differences exist in the play experiences of children. Both girls and boys share games and other activities. However, in the later school years the differences in the play of boys and girls becomes more marked.

Social Relationships and Cooperation

Daily relationships with peers provide important social interactions for school-age children. For the first time, children join group activities with unrestrained enthusiasm and steady participation. Previous interactions were limited to short periods under considerable adult supervision. With increased skills and wider opportunities, children become involved with one or more peer groups in which they can gain status as respected members.

Valuable lessons are learned from daily interaction with age-mates. First, children learn to appreciate the numerous and varied points of view that are represented in the peer group. As children interact with peers who see the world in ways that are somewhat different from their own, they become aware of the limits of their own point of view. Because age-mates are peers and are not forced to accept each other's ideas as they are expected to accept those of adults, other children have a significant influence on decreasing the egocentric outlook of the child. Consequently, children learn to argue, persuade, bargain, cooperate, and compromise to maintain friendships.

Second, children become increasingly sensitive to the social norms and pressures of the peer group. The peer group establishes standards for acceptance and rejection, and children are often willing to modify their behavior to be accepted by the group. The need for peer approval becomes a powerful influence toward conformity. Children learn to dress, talk, and behave in a manner acceptable to the group. A variety of roles, such as class joker or class hero, may be assumed by individual children to gain approval from the group.

Third, the interaction among peers leads to the formation of intimate friendships between same-sex peers. The school-age period is the time when children have "best friends" with whom they share secrets, private jokes, and adventures; they come to one another's aid in times of trouble. In the course of these friendships children also fight, threaten each other, break up, and reunite. These relationships, in which the child experiences love and closeness for a peer, may be important as a foundation for relationships in adulthood (Fig. 39-4).

Clubs and Peer Groups

One of the outstanding characteristics of middle childhood is the formation of formalized groups, or clubs. A prominent feature of these groups is the rigid rules imposed on the members. There is exclusiveness in the selection of persons who have the privilege of joining. Acceptance in the group is often determined on a pass-fail basis according to social or behavioral criteria. Conformity is the core of the group structure. There are often secret codes, shared interests, and special modes of dress, and each child must abide by a standard of behavior established by the members. Conforming to the rules provides children with feelings of security and relieves them of the responsibility of making decisions. By merging their identities with those of their peers, children are able to move from the family group to an outside group as a step toward seeking further independence. Peer groups and clubs allow children to substitute conformity to a peer group for conformity to a family at a time when children are still too insecure to function independently.

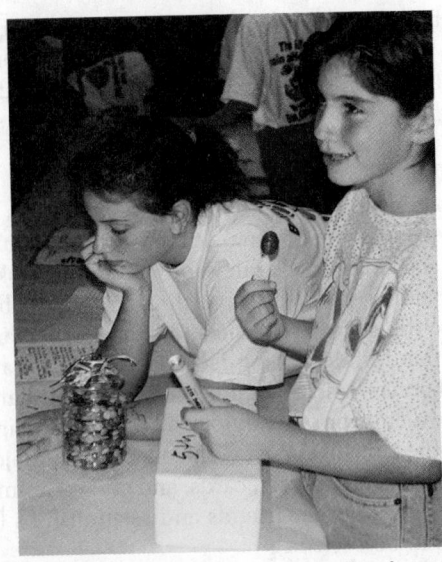

Fig. 39-4 School-age children enjoy engaging in activities with a "best friend."

During the early school years, groups are usually small and loosely organized, with changing membership and no formal structure. The clubs and groups usually do not display elements of cooperation and order that are seen in groups of older children. In general, girls' groups are less formalized than boys' are, and although there may be a mixture of both sexes in the early school years, the groups of later school years are composed predominantly of children of the same sex. Common interests are the basis around which the group is structured.

Peer-group identification and association are essential to a child's socialization. Poor relationships with peers and a lack of group identification can contribute to bullying. *Bullying* is any recurring activity that is intended to harm or bother someone where there is a perceived imbalance of power between the aggressor and the victim (Glew et al, 2005). Bullying occurs most frequently at school during unstructured times, with recess being the most common opportunity for bullying, followed by gym classes, lunchrooms, hallways, and buses (Glew et al, 2005). Bullies may be from any ethnic, racial, or socioeconomic group. They are generally defiant toward adults, antisocial, and likely to break school rules. They have little anxiety, strong self-esteem, and dominant personalities; may come from homes where parental involvement and nurturing are lacking; and may experience or witness violence or abuse at home (Lyznicki, McCaffree, & Robinowitz, 2004). Boys who bully tend to use physical force, whereas girls who bully employ psychologic methods such as ostracism or rumors. Bullying by boys is more common than by girls. Children who are targeted for bullying often have characteristics different from the group norm (e.g., children who are short or obese; have facial deformities; or have attention-deficit/hyperactivity disorder, cognitive impairment, or other developmental disabilities) (Vessey, Carlson, & David, 2003).

The long-term consequences of bullying are significant. Chronic bullies seem to continue their behaviors into adulthood, negatively influencing their ability to develop and maintain relationships. Victims of bullying often feel socially rejected and can fear school, which can develop into school phobia or long-term problems of depression and low self-esteem (Vreeman & Carroll, 2007). School personnel play an important role in implementing antibullying interventions in the elementary schools before bullying becomes a part of the school culture (Glew et al, 2005).

There are also dangers in peer-group attachments that are too strong. Peer pressures force some children to take risks or engage in behaviors that are against their better judgment. A child's membership in a gang is associated with marked increases in serious delinquent behavior (Dishion, Nelson, & Yasui, 2005). Peer-group activities that result in unlawful or criminal *gang violence* are increasing in the United States. An integration of family-centered and school-based programs is needed to reduce the influences for children to become affiliated with gangs (Dishion, Nelson, & Yasui, 2005).

Relationships with Families

Although the peer group is influential and necessary to normal child development, parents are the primary influence in shaping the child's personality, setting standards for behavior, and establishing value systems. Family values usually take precedence over peer value systems. Although children may appear to reject parental values while testing the new values of the peer group, ultimately they retain and incorporate into their own value systems the parental values they have found to be of worth.

In the middle school years, children want to spend more time in the company of peers and they often prefer peer-group activities to family activities. This can be disturbing to parents. Children become intolerant and critical of their parents, especially when their parents' ways deviate from those of the group. They discover that parents can be wrong, and they begin to question the knowledge and authority of their parents, who were previously considered to be all-knowing and all-powerful.

Although increased independence is the goal of middle childhood, children are not prepared to abandon all parental control. They need and want restrictions placed on their behavior, and they are not prepared to cope with all the problems of their expanding environment. They feel more secure knowing there is an authority figure to implement controls and restrictions. Children may complain loudly about restrictions and try to break down parental barriers, but they are uneasy if they succeed in doing so. They respect adults who prevent them from acting on every urge. Children view this behavior as an expression of love and concern for their welfare.

Children also need their parents as adults, not as friends. Sometimes parents, hurt by their children's rejection, attempt to maintain their love and gratitude by assuming the role of "pals." Children need the stable, secure strength provided by mature adults to whom they can turn during troubled relationships with peers or stressful changes in their world. With a secure base in a loving family, children are able to develop the self-confidence and maturity needed to break loose from the group and stand independently.

Play

Play takes on new dimensions that reflect a new stage of development in the school years. Play involves increased physical skill, intellectual ability, and fantasy. In addition, children develop a sense of belonging to a team or club by forming groups and cliques.

Rules and Rituals

The need for conformity in middle childhood is strongly manifested in the activities and games of school-age children. In the preschool years, children's games were either invented for them or played in the company of a friend or an adult. Now children begin to see the need for rules, and their games have fixed and unvarying rules that may be bizarre and extraordinarily rigid. Part of the enjoyment of the game is knowing the rules because knowing means belonging. Conformity and ritual permeate their play and are also evident in their behavior and language. Childhood is full of chants and taunts, such as "Eeeny, meeny, miney, mo," "Last one is a rotten egg," and "Step on a crack, break your mother's back." Children derive a sense of pleasure and power from such sayings, which have been handed down with few changes through generations.

Team Play

A more complex form of play that evolves from the need for peer interaction is team games and sports. A referee, umpire, or person of authority may be required so that the rules can be followed more accurately. Team play teaches children to modify or exchange personal goals for goals of the group; it also teaches them that division of labor is an effective strategy for attaining a goal. Children learn about competition and the importance of winning—an attribute highly valued in the United States.

Team play can also contribute to children's social, intellectual, and skill growth. Children work hard to develop the skills needed to become team members, to improve their contribution to the group, and to anticipate the consequences of their behavior for the group. Team play helps stimulate cognitive growth because children are called on to learn many complex rules, make judgments about those rules, plan strategies, and assess the strengths and weaknesses of members of their own team and members of the opposing team.

Quiet Games and Activities

Although play at this age is highly active, school-age children also enjoy quiet and solitary activities. The middle years are the time for collections, which constitute another ritual. Young school-age children's collections are an odd assortment of unrelated objects in messy, disorganized piles. Collections of later school years are more orderly; selective; and organized in scrapbooks, on shelves, or in boxes.

School-age children become fascinated with complex board, card, or computer games that they can play alone, with a best friend, or with a group. As in all games, adherence to

FAMILY-CENTERED CARE

Guidance During School Years

Age 6 Years

Prepare parents to expect strong food preferences and frequent refusal of specific food items.

Prepare parents to expect increasingly ravenous appetite.

Prepare parents for emotionality as child experiences erratic mood changes.

Help parents anticipate continued susceptibility to illness.

Teach injury prevention and safety, especially bicycle safety.

Encourage parents to respect child's need for privacy and to provide a separate bedroom for child, if possible.

Prepare parents for child's increasing interests outside the home.

Help parents understand the need to encourage child's interactions with peers

Ages 7 to 10 Years

Prepare parents to expect improvement in health with fewer illnesses, but warn them that allergies may increase or become apparent.

Prepare parents to expect an increase in minor injuries.

Emphasize caution in selecting and maintaining sports equipment, and reemphasize safety.

Prepare parents to expect increased involvement with peers and interest in activities outside the home.

Emphasize the need to encourage independence while maintaining limit setting and discipline.

Prepare mothers to expect more demands at 8 years.

Prepare fathers to expect increasing admiration at 10 years; encourage father-child activities.

Prepare parents for prepubescent changes in girls.

Ages 11 to 12 Years

Help parents prepare child for body changes of pubescence.

Prepare parents to expect a growth spurt in girls.

Make certain child's sex education is adequate with accurate information.

Prepare parents to expect energetic but stormy behavior at 11 years, becoming more even-tempered at 12 years.

Encourage parents to support child's desire to "grow up" but to allow regressive behavior when needed.

Prepare parents to expect an increase in child's masturbation.

Instruct parents that the amount of rest the child needs may increase.

Help parents educate child regarding experimentation with potentially harmful activities.

Health Guidance

Help parents understand the importance of regular health and dental care for the child.

Encourage parents to teach and model sound health practices, including diet, rest, activity, and exercise.

Stress the need to encourage children to engage in appropriate physical activities.

Emphasize providing a safe physical and emotional environment.

Encourage parents to teach and model safety practices.

the rules is fanatic. Disagreements over rules can cause much discussion and argument, but are easily resolved by reading the rules of the game.

The newly acquired skill of reading becomes increasingly satisfying as school-age children expand their knowledge of the world through books (Fig. 39-5). School-age children never tire of stories and, as with preschool children, love to have stories read aloud. Sewing, cooking, carpentry, gardening, and creative activities such as painting are other activities enjoyed. Many creative skills such as music and art, as well as athletic skills such as swimming, karate, dancing, and skating, are learned during these years and continue to be enjoyed into adolescence and adulthood (Fig. 39-6).

Ego Mastery

Play affords children the means to acquire mastery over themselves, their environment, and others. Through play, children can feel as big, as powerful, and as skillful as their imaginations will allow. They can also feel in control and attain vicarious mastery and power over whomever and whatever they choose. School-age children still need the opportunity to use large muscles in exuberant outdoor play and the freedom to exert their newfound autonomy and initiative. They need space in which to exercise large muscles and to deal with tensions, frustrations, and hostility. Physical skills practiced and mastered in play help them develop a feeling of personal competence, which contributes to a sense of accomplishment and provides status in their peer group.

Developing a Self-Concept

The term *self-concept* refers to a conscious awareness of self-perceptions, such as one's physical characteristics, abilities, values, self-ideals and expectations, and idea of self in relation to others. It also includes one's body image, sexuality, and self-esteem. Although primary caregivers continue to exert influence on children's self-evaluation, the opinions of peers and teachers provide valuable input during middle childhood. With the emphasis on skill building and broadened social relationships, children are continually engaged in the process of self-evaluation.

Significant adults can often manage to unobtrusively manipulate the environment so that children experience success. Each small success increases a child's self-image. The more positive children feel about themselves, the more confident they will be in trying for success in the future. All children profit from feeling that they are in some way special to a significant adult. A positive self-concept makes children feel likable, worthwhile, and capable of significant contributions. These feelings lead to self-respect, self-confidence, and happiness. Negative feelings lead to self-doubt.

Developing a Body Image

School-age children have a relatively accurate and positive perception of their physical selves, but in general they like their physical selves less as they grow older. The head appears to be the most important part of the school-age child's per-

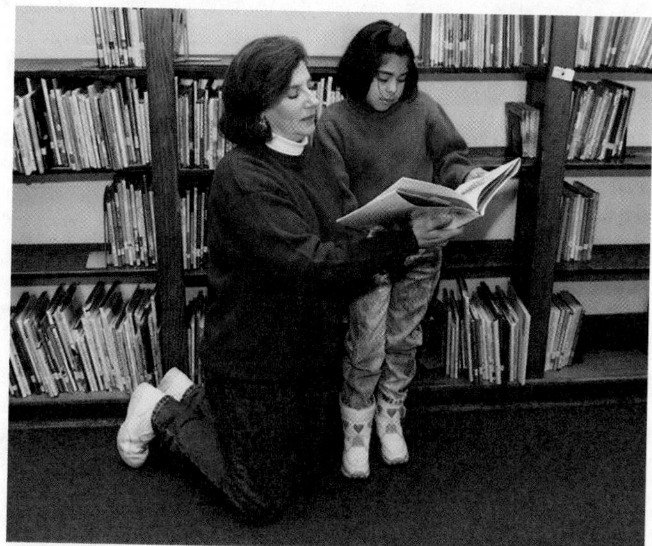

Fig. 39-5 Selecting a book with the assistance of an adult.

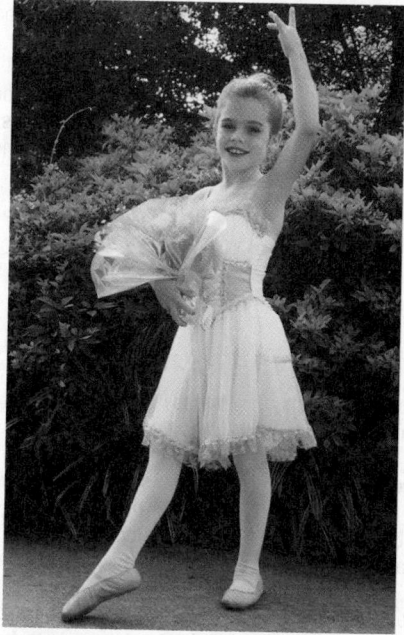

Fig. 39-6 School-age children take pride in learning new skills.

ceived image of self, with hair and eye color the characteristics used most frequently to describe the physical self.

Body image is influenced, but not solely determined, by significant others. The number of significant others influencing one's perception of the physical self increases with age. Children are acutely aware of their own body, the bodies of their peers, and those of adults. They are also aware of deviations from the norm. It is important that children learn about bodily functions and that adults provide correct information.

Physical impairments, such as hearing or visual defects, ears that "stick out," or birthmarks, assume great importance. Increasing awareness of these differences, especially when accompanied by unkind comments and taunts from others, may cause a child to feel inferior and less desirable. This is especially true if the defect interferes with the child's ability to participate in games and activities.

Table 39-1 summarizes the major developmental achievements of the school-age years.

Coping with Concerns Related to Normal Growth and Development

School Experience

School serves as the agent for transmitting the values of society to each succeeding generation of children. School is also the setting for relationships with peers. After the family, schools are the second most important socializing agent in the lives of children.

Entrance into school causes a sharp break in the structure of the child's world. For many children it is their first experience in conforming to a group pattern imposed by an adult who is not a parent and who has responsibility for too many children to be constantly aware of each child as an individual. Children want to go to school and usually adapt to the new conditions with little difficulty. Successful adjustment is related to the child's physical and emotional maturity and the parent's readiness to accept the separation associated with school entrance. Unfortunately, some parents express their unconscious attempts to delay the child's maturity by clinging behavior, particularly with their youngest child.

By the time they enter school, most children have a fairly realistic concept of what school involves. They receive information regarding the role of a student from parents, siblings, playmates, and the media. In addition, most children have had some experience with day care, preschool, or kindergarten. Middle-class children have fewer adjustments to make and less to learn about expected behavior, since schools tend to reflect dominant middle-class customs and values. If the child has attended a preschool program, the focus of the preschool program also affects the child's adjustment. Some preschool programs provide custodial care only, whereas others emphasize emotional, social, and intellectual development.

Classmates have a significant impact on the socialization of children. School is the first time that some children become members of a large group of individuals their own age. Peer relationships become increasingly important and influential as children proceed through school. The specific influence exerted by the peer group depends on the individual child's background, interests, and abilities.

Teachers

Children respond best to teachers who possess the characteristics of a warm, loving parent. Teachers in the early grades perform many of the activities formerly assumed by the parent, such as recognizing the child's personal needs (e.g., the need to go to the bathroom, need for help with clothing) and helping to develop their social behavior (e.g., manners).

Teachers, like parents, are concerned about the child's psychologic and emotional welfare. Although the functions of teachers and parents differ, both place constraints on behavior and both are in a position to enforce standards of conduct. However, the teacher's primary responsibility involves stimulating and guiding children's intellectual development, as

Table 39-1 Growth and Development During School-Age Years

PHYSICAL AND MOTOR	MENTAL	ADAPTIVE	PERSONAL-SOCIAL
Age 6 Yr			
Height and weight gain continues slowly Weight 16-26.3 kg (35½-58 lb) Height 106.7-122 cm (42-48 inches) Central mandibular incisors erupt Loses first tooth Gradual increase in dexterity Active age; constant activity Often returns to finger feeding More aware of hand as a tool Likes to draw, print, color Vision reaches maturity	Develops concept of numbers Can count 13 pennies Knows whether it is morning or afternoon Defines common objects such as fork and chair in terms of their use Obeys three commands in succession Knows right and left hands Says which is pretty and which is ugly of a series of drawings of faces Describes the objects in a picture rather than simply enumerating them Attends first grade	At table, uses knife to spread butter or jam on bread At play, cuts, folds, pastes paper; sews crudely if needle is threaded Takes bath without supervision; performs bedtime activities alone Reads from memory; enjoys oral spelling game Likes table games, checkers, simple card games Giggles a lot Sometimes steals money or attractive items Has difficulty owning up to misdeeds Tries out own abilities	Can share and cooperate better Has great need for children of own age Will cheat to win Often engages in rough play Often jealous of younger brother or sister Does what adults are seen doing May have occasional temper tantrums Is a boaster Is more independent, probably influenced by school Has own way of doing things Increases socialization
Age 7 Yr			
Begins to grow at least 5 cm (2 inches) in height per year Weight 17.7-30 kg (39-66 lb) Height 112-130 cm (44-51 inches) Maxillary central incisors and lateral mandibular incisors erupt More cautious in approaches to new activities Repeats performances to master them Jaw begins to expand to accommodate permanent teeth	Notices that certain items are missing from pictures Can copy a diamond Repeats three numbers backward Develops concept of time; reads ordinary clock or watch correctly to nearest quarter hour; uses clock for practical purposes Attends second grade More mechanical in reading; often does not stop at the end of a sentence; skips words such as "it," "the," and "he"	Uses table knife for cutting meat; may need help with tough or difficult pieces Brushes and combs hair acceptably without help Likes to help and have a choice Is less resistant and stubborn	Is becoming a real member of the family group Takes part in group play Boys prefer playing with boys; girls prefer playing with girls Spends a lot of time alone; does not require a lot of companionship
Ages 8-9 Yr			
Continues to gain 5 cm (2 inches) in height per year Weight 19.5-39.5 kg (43-87 lb) Height 117-142 cm (46-56 inches) Lateral incisors (maxillary) and mandibular cuspids erupt Movement fluid; often graceful and poised Always on the go; jumps, chases, skips Increased smoothness and speed in fine motor control; uses cursive writing Dresses self completely Likely to overdo; hard to quiet down after recess More limber; bones grow faster than ligaments	Gives similarities and differences between two things from memory Counts backward from 20 to 1; understands concept of reversibility Repeats days of the week and months in order; knows the date Describes common objects in detail, not merely their use Makes change out of a quarter Attends third and fourth grades Reads more; may plan to wake up early just to read Reads classic books, but also enjoys comics More aware of time; can be relied on to get to school on time Can grasp concepts of parts and whole (fractions) Understands concepts of space, cause and effect, nesting (puzzles), conservation (permanence of mass and volume) Classifies objects by more than one quality; has collections Produces simple paintings or drawings	Makes use of common tools such as hammer, saw, screwdriver Uses household and sewing utensils Helps with routine household tasks such as dusting, sweeping Assumes responsibility for share of household chores Looks after all of own needs at table Buys useful articles; exercises some choice in making purchases Runs useful errands Likes pictorial magazines Likes school; wants to answer all the questions Is afraid of failing a grade; is ashamed of bad grades Is more critical of self Takes music and sport lessons	Is easy to get along with at home Likes the reward system Dramatizes Is more sociable Is better behaved Is interested in boy-girl relationships but will not admit it Goes about home and community freely, alone or with friends Likes to compete and play games Shows preference in friends and groups Plays mostly with groups of own sex but is beginning to mix Develops modesty Compares self with others Enjoys organizations, clubs, and group sports

Table 39-1 Growth and Development During School-Age Years—cont'd

PHYSICAL AND MOTOR	MENTAL	ADAPTIVE	PERSONAL-SOCIAL
Ages 10-12 Yr			
Weight 24.5-58 kg (54-128 lb) Height 127-162.5 cm (50-64 inches) Posture is more similar to an adult's; will overcome lordosis Remainder of teeth will erupt and tend toward full development (except wisdom teeth) Girls—Pubescent changes may begin to appear; body lines soften and round out Boys—Slow growth in height and rapid weight gain; may become obese in this period	Writes brief stories Attends fifth to seventh grades Writes occasional short letters to friends or relatives on own initiative Uses telephone for practical purposes Responds to magazine, radio, or other advertising Reads for practical information or own enjoyment—stories or library books of adventure or romance, animal stories	Makes useful tools or does easy repair work Cooks or sews in small way Raises pets Washes and dries own hair; is responsible for a thorough job of cleaning hair, but may need reminding to do so Is sometimes left alone at home for an hour or so Is successful in looking after own needs or those of other children left in his or her care	Loves friends; talks about them constantly Chooses friends more selectively; may have a "best friend" Enjoys conversation Develops beginning interest in opposite sex Is more diplomatic Likes family; family really has meaning Likes mother and wants to please her in many ways Demonstrates affection Likes father, who is admired and may be idolized Respects parents

opposed to providing for their physical welfare beyond the school setting.

Teachers serve as models that children try to emulate. Children seek their teachers' approval and avoid their disapproval. The teacher is a significant person in the life of the early schoolchild, and hero worship of a teacher may extend into late childhood and preadolescence. Teachers who make supportive statements that reassure or commend children, use accepting and clarifying statements that help children refine ideas and feelings, and provide assistance that aids children with their own problem solving contribute to the development of a positive self-concept in the school-age child.

Parents

Parents share responsibility for helping children achieve their maximum potential. Parents can supplement the school program in numerous ways (see Patient Teaching box). Cultivating responsibility is the goal of parental assistance. Being responsible for schoolwork helps children learn to keep promises, meet deadlines, and succeed at their jobs as adults. Responsible children may occasionally ask for help (e.g., with a spelling list), but usually they prefer to think through their work by themselves. Excessive pressure or lack of encouragement from parents may inhibit the development of these desirable traits.

Latchkey Children

The term *latchkey children* is used to describe children in elementary school who are left to care for themselves before or after school without the supervision of an adult. The increasing numbers of single-parent families and working mothers, together with the lack of available child care, have created a stress-provoking situation for many school-age children. Some of these children may have a chronic illness as well.

Inadequate adult supervision after school leaves children at greater risk for injury and delinquent behavior. In some instances outside activities are curtailed and relationships with peers may be significantly diminished. Latchkey children may feel more lonely, isolated, and fearful than children who have someone to care for them. To cope with their fears and anxieties while alone, these children may devise strategies such as hiding, playing the television at loud volume, or using pets for comfort.

Many communities and persons concerned about the welfare of latchkey children are trying to help these children and their parents deal with this potentially serious problem. Some communities and employers have implemented after-school programs or telephone "hotlines" that provide check-in and reassurance for children. Nurses should be aware of these community services and encourage parents to teach self-help skills to these children.

Limit Setting and Discipline

Many factors influence the amount and manner of discipline and limit setting imposed on school-age children. Some of these factors are the parents' psychosocial maturity, the parents' childhood and childrearing experiences, the children's temperament, the context of the children's misconduct, and the children's response to rewards and punishments. When children develop an ability to see a situation from another's point of view, they are also able to understand the effects of their reactions on others and themselves.

Discipline should take place in a positive, supportive environment with the use of strategies to instruct and guide desired behaviors and eliminate undesired behaviors (Ateah, 2003). Reasoning is an effective technique for older school-age children. With advancing cognitive skills, they are able to benefit from more complex disciplinary strategies. For example, withholding privileges, requiring compensation, imposing penalties, and contracting can be used with great success. Problem solving is the best approach to limit setting, and children themselves can be included in the process of determining appropriate disciplinary measures.

Dishonest Behavior

During middle childhood, children may engage in what is considered to be antisocial behavior. Previously well-behaved children may engage in lying, stealing, and cheating. Such behaviors are disturbing and challenging to parents.

PATIENT TEACHING Helping Children in School

General Guidelines

Be supportive—provide companionship; share ideas and thoughts.
Be positive—every child should experience some success each day.
Share an interest in reading—use the library; discuss books they are reading.
Support and encourage activity rather than passivity.
Encourage originality—help children make their own projects from discarded articles or other available materials.
Foster the development of hobbies and collections.
Encourage children to wonder and reflect during free time.
Encourage family experiences and trips to places of interest.
Encourage questions—help children discover sources for information or places to explore and investigate.
Stimulate creative thinking and problem solving—help children try out new solutions to problems without fear of making mistakes.
Use rewards rather than punishment.

Specific Guidelines

Meet the teacher at the beginning of school and plan to visit the school to see what is taught and expected.
Send the child to school every day. Teachers are concerned when parents make other plans for their children; it conveys the impression that school is unimportant.
Demonstrate an interest in what the child is learning.
Demonstrate an interest in content and growth more than in grades.
Make it clear to the child that schoolwork is between the child and the teacher; teacher and child should set goals for better school performance to allow the child to feel responsible for school successes and failures.
Take advantage of situations that support and reinforce school learning.
Share information with teachers that will help them understand the child better.
Communicate with the teacher if there appears to be a problem; avoid waiting for a scheduled conference.
Provide a quiet, well-lit area for study that is safe from interruption; do not allow television or radio.
Avoid dictating a study time, but do enforce rules, such as no television until homework is done; accept the child's word that work is complete.
Help with homework should focus on explaining the question, not giving the answer.
Teach the child to break large tasks (e.g., a report) into smaller, manageable tasks spread over the allotted time rather than attempting the entire project the night before it is to be completed.
Limit home tutoring to special circumstances, such as when the teacher requests parental assistance after a child's prolonged absence.
Request special help for children with learning problems.
Support the school staff by showing respect for both the school system and the teacher, at least in the child's presence.

Lying can occur for a number of reasons. By the time children enter school, they still "tell stories," often exaggerating a story or situation as a means of impressing their family or friends. However, during middle childhood, children become able to distinguish between fact and fantasy. If children do not develop this characteristic, parents need to teach them what is real and what is make-believe.

Young children may lie to escape punishment or to get out of some difficulty even when their misbehavior is evident. Older children may lie to meet expectations set by others to which they have been unable to measure up. However, most children know that lying and cheating are wrong, and they are concerned when it is observed in their friends. They are quick to tell on others when they detect cheating.

Parents need to be reassured that all children lie occasionally and that sometimes children may have difficulty separating fantasy from reality. Parents should be helped to understand the importance of being truthful in their relationships with children.

Cheating is most common in young children 5 to 6 years of age. They find it difficult to lose at a game or contest, so they may cheat to win. They have not yet realized that this behavior is wrong, and they do it almost automatically. This behavior usually disappears as they mature. However, because children model observed behaviors, parents need to be aware of their own behavior. When parents set examples of honesty, children are more likely to conform to these standards.

As with other ethically related behavior, *stealing* is not unexpected in the younger child. Between 5 and 8 years of age, children's sense of property rights is limited, and they tend to take something simply because they are attracted to it or to take money for what it will buy. They are equally likely to give away something valuable that belongs to them. When young children are caught and punished, they are penitent—they "didn't mean to" and "promise to never do it again"—but they are likely to repeat the performance the following day. Often they not only steal but also lie about their behavior or attempt to justify it with excuses. It is seldom helpful to trap children into admission by asking directly if they committed the offense. Children do not take responsibility for these behaviors until the end of middle childhood.

Children steal for several reasons. Young children may lack a sense of property rights, attempt to acquire a specific object to bribe favors from other children, have a strong desire to own a coveted item, or have a desire for revenge to "get back at someone" (usually a parent for unfair treatment). Older children may steal to supplement an inadequate allowance. Stealing can be an indication that something is seriously wrong or lacking in the child's life. For example, children may steal to make up for love or another satisfaction that they feel is lacking. In most situations it is wise not to attempt to attach a hidden or deep meaning to the stealing. An admonition, together with an appropriate and reasonable punishment, such as having the older child pay back the money or return the stolen items, takes care of most cases. Most children can be taught to respect the property rights of others with little difficulty despite numerous temptations and opportunities. If children's personal rights are respected, they are likely to respect the rights of others. Some children simply need more time to learn the rules regarding private property.

Stress and Fear

Children today experience significant amounts of stress, which can cause long-term adjustment and health problems. Stress in childhood comes from a variety of sources such as conflict within the family, interpersonal relationships, poverty, and chronic illness. The school environment and participation in multiple organized activities can be additional sources of stress. The demands from coaches and parents, in addition to school requirements and pressure from teachers to do well on proficiency testing, can cause unrealistic expectations on the school-age child (Ryan-Wenger, Sharrer, & Campbell, 2005). In addition, with the increased exposure to sexuality and provocative clothing and behaviors, children of this age group may feel pressured to have a girlfriend or boyfriend, which their maturity level cannot handle and which causes additional stress (Ryan-Wenger, Sharrer, & Campbell, 2005).

The increasing violence in society has also spilled over into the school setting. In the present information age, in which tragedy is broadcast daily in the media, children come to school knowing more about the latest world events than any previous generation of children. In addition, today's children are often personally aware of violence in their families or communities. Many children know other children who have been killed or children who have brought weapons to school. School-age children can be victims of teasing, bullying, and physical abuse in the school environment (Nansel et al, 2003).

To help children cope with stress, parents, teachers, and health care providers need to frequently reassure children that they are safe, have honest and open communication, encourage children to express their feelings, and promote a daily routine (Nansel et al, 2003). Adults must recognize signs that indicate a child is undergoing stress, identify the source of the stress promptly, and refer those children who need specialized treatment.

NURSING ALERT The nurse who observes the following signs of stress in a child should explore the situation further:

- Stomach pains or headache
- Changes in sleep patterns or nightmares
- Bed-wetting
- Changes in eating habits
- Aggressive or stubborn behavior
- Withdrawal or reluctance to participate
- Regression to earlier behaviors (e.g., thumb-sucking)
- Trouble concentrating or changes in academic performance

Children 7 to 12 years of age are capable of identifying their own physiologic responses to stress with terms that have meaning to them. Some words or phrases used by children to describe their body's reaction to stress include *tight muscles*, *hot* or *red in the face*, *tingling*, *chills or goose bumps*, *shakiness*, *heart beating fast*, *headache*, and *stomachache* (Sharrer & Ryan-Wenger, 2002). Children should be taught to recognize these signs as indicators of stress and to use techniques to manage their stress. Children can learn relaxation techniques such as deep-breathing exercises, progressive relaxation of muscle groups, and positive imagery to immediately reduce stress (Mortweet & Christophersen, 2004). Encouraging them to "blow off steam" through physical activity reduces tension and anxiety. Children can be encouraged to observe effective coping strategies in others and adopt them for their own use (Mortweet & Christophersen, 2004). When an effective strategy has been developed for one situation, parents can show the child how to transfer the coping strategy or technique to other situations.

In addition to stress, school-age children experience a wide variety of fears, including fear of the dark, excessive worry about past behavior, self-consciousness, social withdrawal, and an excessive need for reassurance. These fears are considered normal for children this age. During the middle range of the school-age years, children become less fearful of body safety than they were as preschoolers, but they still fear being hurt, being kidnapped, or having to undergo surgery. They also fear death and are fascinated by all the aspects of death and dying. The fears of noises, darkness, storms, and dogs lessen, but new fears related predominantly to school and family bother children during this time.

Promoting Optimal Health During the School Years

Nutrition

Although caloric needs are diminished in relation to body size during middle childhood, resources are being laid down at this time for the increased growth needs of adolescence. Parents and children need to be aware of the value of a balanced diet to promote growth because children usually eat what their family members eat. The quality of the child's diet depends on the family's pattern of eating.

Likes and dislikes established at an early age continue in middle childhood, although preferences for single foods subside and children develop a taste for a variety of foods. However, the easy availability of fast-food restaurants, the influence of the mass media, and the temptation of "junk food" make it easy for children to fill up on empty calories. Foods that do not promote growth, such as sugars, starches, and excess fats, are common in the school-age child's diet. The easy availability of high-calorie foods, combined with the tendency toward more sedentary activities, has contributed to an epidemic of childhood obesity. This problem is discussed further in Chapter 40.

Parents are unable to monitor what their children eat when they are away from home. A parent may pack a lunch for school but be unaware of how much is eaten, traded, sold, or thrown away. Nutrition education can and should be integrated in the curriculum throughout the school years. Important aspects of nutrition education include the U.S. Food and Drug Administration's MyPyramid; elements of a wholesome diet; and how food products are grown, processed, and prepared. However, the school cafeteria may not always provide healthy, nutritious meals. The school nurse can take an active role in nutrition education by working with teachers to plan and implement units on nutrition instruction and by working with parents and children to give nutritional guidance.

Sleep and Rest

The amount of sleep and rest required during middle childhood is highly individualized. The amount of sleep depends on the child's age, activity level, and state of health. The growth rate slows in the school-age years, and less energy is expended in growth than during preceding years.

School-age children usually do not require a nap, and they sleep during the night approximately 11 hours at age 5 years and 9¼ hours at age 12 years (Carno et al, 2003). Although fewer bedtime problems occur during these years, occasional difficulties are still associated with the bedtime ritual. Usually children 6 or 7 years old exhibit few bedtime problems, and encouraging quiet activity before bedtime, such as coloring or reading, facilitates the task of going to bed. However, most children in middle childhood must be reminded frequently to go to bed; 8- to 9-year-old children and 11-year-old children are particularly resistant. Often these children are unaware that they are tired; if they are allowed to remain up later than usual, they are fatigued the following day. Sometimes, bedtime resistance can be resolved by allowing a later bedtime as the child gets older. Twelve-year-old children usually offer no resistance at bedtime; some even retire early to read a book or listen to music.

Exercise and Activity

The improved capabilities and adaptability of the school-age child permit greater speed and effort in motor activities. Larger, stronger muscles permit longer and increasingly strenuous play without exhaustion. School-age children acquire the coordination, timing, and concentration that are required to participate in adult-type activities, but they may lack the strength, stamina, and control of the adolescent and adult. They can engage in a greater amount of physical activity during the school years. However, parents, teachers, and coaches must remember that, although children this age are large and appear strong, they may not be ready for strenuous competitive athletics.

All growing children need regular exercise and opportunities for satisfying experiences consistent with individual likes and dislikes. Appropriate activities during the school-age years include running, jumping rope, swimming, roller skating, ice skating, dancing, and bicycle riding. Positive reinforcement achieved by experiencing increasingly smooth, rhythmic, and efficient use of the body conditions the child toward regular physical activity. Exercise is essential for muscle development and tone, refinement of balance and coordination, increased strength and endurance, and stimulation of body functions and metabolic processes. Children need ample space to run, jump, skip, and climb, in addition to safe indoor and outdoor facilities and equipment. Most children have abundant energy and need little encouragement to engage in physical activity. Children with disabling conditions or those who hesitate to become involved in active play (such as obese children) require special assessment and help so that activities appeal to them and are compatible with their limitations while also meeting their developmental needs.

Sports

Considerable controversy surrounds the trend toward early participation in competitive athletics and the amount and type of competitive sports that are appropriate for children in the elementary grades. The current view is that virtually every child is suited for some sport, and authorities do not discourage participation if children are matched to the type of sport appropriate to their abilities and to their physical and emotional constitution. School-age children enjoy competition (Fig. 39-7). However, teachers and coaches must understand the physical limitations of children this age and teach them the proper techniques and safety measures needed to avoid injuries. A safe and appropriate sport can be identified for even the most unskilled and uncompetitive child, including children with chronic illnesses and cognitive impairments. Common activities for school-age children include baseball, soccer, gymnastics, and swimming. Equipment must be maintained in safe condition, and protective apparatus should be worn to prevent serious injury (see Traumatic Injury, Chapter 54).

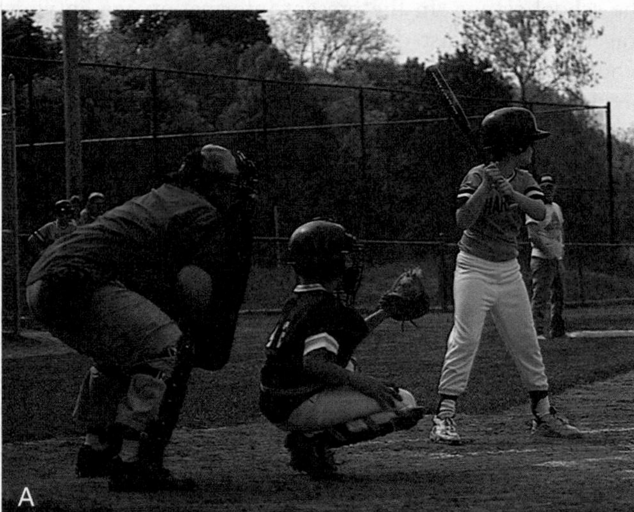

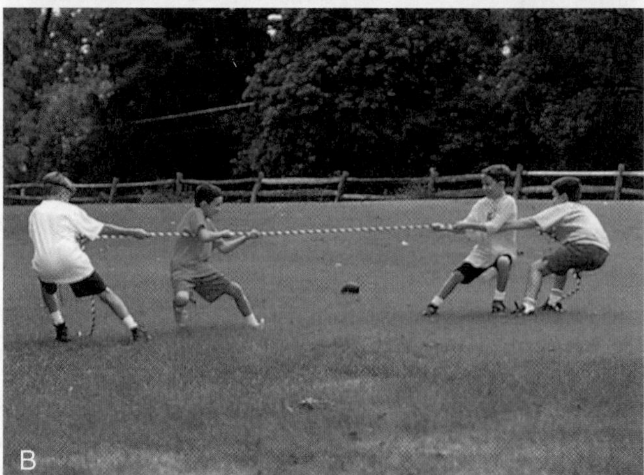

Fig. 39-7 The activities engaged in by school-age children vary according to interest and opportunity. **A,** Little League competitors. **B,** Playing tug-of-war.

During the school-age years girls have the same basic body structure as boys and have a similar response to systematic exercise training. However, at puberty, boys become larger and have more muscle mass, and at this stage, it is usually recommended that girls compete only against other girls. Before puberty there is no essential difference in strength and size between girls and boys, making these precautions unnecessary.

Preadolescence is a time to teach fundamental motor skills; develop fitness in a practical, safe, and gradual manner; and promote healthy attitudes and values. Activities should include both practice sessions and unstructured play; the actual game or event should be managed in a manner that stresses mastery of the sport and enhancement of self-image rather than winning or pleasing others. All children should have an opportunity to participate, and special ceremonies should recognize all participants, not just individuals who excel in sports or athletics.

Acquisition of Skills

School-age children demonstrate increasing fine motor abilities and complex artistic skills. Handedness is well established by the beginning of the school years, and children make great strides in writing and drawing during this period. It is a time of energetic and vibrant creative productivity. With the tools of language and reading, children create poems, stories, and plays. With more advanced fine motor skills, they are able to master an unlimited variety of handicrafts, such as ceramics, needlework, wood carving, and beadwork. They avidly pursue these skills in solitude; with a friend; or through organized groups such as boys' or girls' clubs or special interest groups that use crafts or other activities as a means to occupy, entertain, and educate children.

School-age children are capable of assuming responsibility for their own needs, although their distaste for soap and water and "dress" clothes is legendary. School-age children can and want to assume their share of household tasks, which usually are related to the male and female roles that have been defined by their culture. Many children also assume responsibility for tasks outside the home, such as baby-sitting, mowing lawns, or paper routes.

Dental Health

The first permanent (secondary) teeth erupt at about 6 years of age, beginning with the 6-year molar, which erupts posterior to the deciduous molars. Other permanent teeth appear in approximately the same order as eruption of the primary teeth and follow shedding of the deciduous teeth (Fig. 39-8). With the appearance of the second permanent (12-year) molar, most permanent teeth are present. Permanent dentition is more advanced in girls than in boys.

Because the permanent teeth erupt during the school-age years, dental hygiene and regular attention to dental caries are important parts of health supervision during this period. Correct brushing techniques should be taught or reinforced, and the role that fermentable carbohydrates play in production of dental caries should be emphasized. It is important to be alert to possible malocclusion problems that may result from irregular eruption of permanent teeth and that may

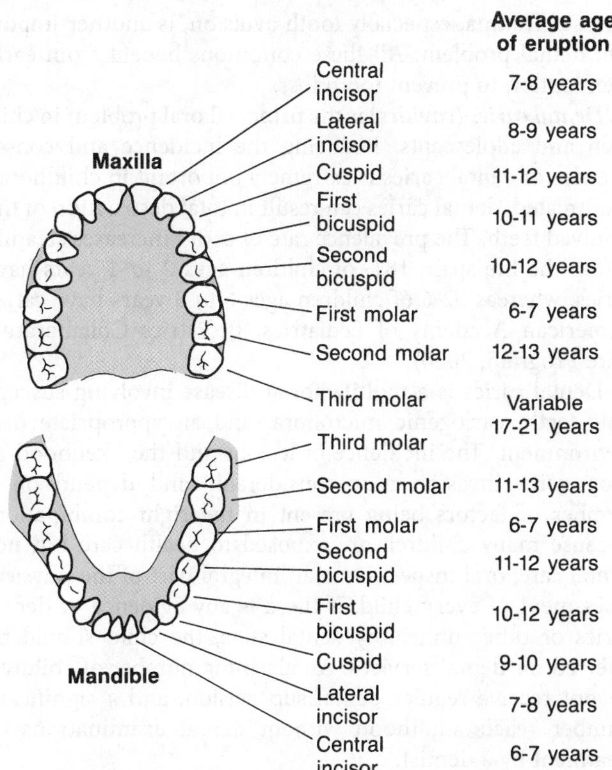

Fig. 39-8 Sequence of eruption of secondary teeth. (Data from McDonald RE, Avery DR: *Dentistry for the child and adolescent*, ed 6, St Louis, 1994, Mosby.)

impair function. Regular dental supervision and continued fluoride supplementation are integral parts of the health maintenance program.

The most effective means of preventing dental caries is proper oral hygiene. Children should be taught to perform their own dental care with the supervision and guidance of the parents. Parents should learn the correct brushing technique with their children, and they should monitor their child's efforts until the child can assume full responsibility.

Teeth should be brushed after meals, after snacks, and at bedtime. Children who brush their teeth frequently and become accustomed to the feel of a clean mouth at an early age usually maintain the habit throughout life. For the school-age child with mixed and permanent dentition, the best toothbrush is one with soft nylon bristles and should be comfortable for your child to hold and reach all teeth. Several methods of brushing have been described and recommended for children, but there is no conclusive evidence that one method is superior to another. Thorough cleaning is more important than the specific technique used. The dentist should assess factors such as the child's manipulative skills and special needs, and suggest the most appropriate brushing technique and regimen. Flossing follows brushing. Parents should perform the flossing until children acquire the manual dexterity required (usually at about 8 or 9 years of age).

Dental Problems

Limited or inadequate dental care results in the most common dental problems: dental caries, malocclusion, and periodontal disease. Trauma, especially tooth avulsion, is another important dental problem. All these conditions benefit from early intervention to prevent tooth loss.

Dental caries (cavities) is the principal oral problem in children and adolescents. Reducing the incidence and consequences of dental caries is extremely important in childhood. If untreated, dental caries can result in total destruction of the involved teeth. The prevalence rate of caries increases steadily across the life span; 18% of children ages 2 to 4 years have caries, whereas 52% of children ages 6 to 8 years have caries (American Academy of Pediatrics, Pediatrics Collaborative Care Program, 2000).

Dental caries is a multifactorial disease involving susceptible teeth, cariogenic microflora, and an appropriate oral environment. The incidence of lesions and the likelihood of progressive invasion vary considerably and depend on a number of factors being present in the right combination. Because many children are exposed to health care but not dental care, oral inspection is an integral part of the physical assessment of every child. If there is any evidence of dental caries or other unhealthy dental state, the child should be referred for dental services. An alarming number of children do not receive regular dental supervision, and a significant number reach adulthood without dental examinations or treatment by a dentist.

Periodontal disease, an inflammatory and degenerative condition involving the gums and tissues supporting the teeth, often begins in childhood and accounts for a significant amount of tooth loss in adulthood. The more common periodontal problems are *gingivitis* (simple inflammation of the gums) and *periodontitis* (inflammation of the gums and loss of connective tissue and bone in the supporting structures of the teeth).

Gingivitis, the most prevalent periodontal disease, is a reversible inflammatory disease that can begin in early childhood and is most often associated with the buildup of plaque on the teeth. Changes take place in the plaque bacteria, in both the type and number of organisms, causing them to release destructive exotoxins, enzymes, and other noxious agents. These substances produce an inflammatory reaction in the gingival tissues, causing the gums to become red, edematous, tender, and subject to bleeding at the slightest irritation. Management is directed toward prevention by conscientious brushing and flossing, including the use of fluoride. The child should see the dentist at any signs of inflammation or irritation.

Malocclusion occurs when teeth of the upper and lower dental arches do not approximate in the proper relationships. As a result, the physiologic function of chewing is less effective and the cosmetic effect is displeasing. Teeth that are uneven, crowded, or overlapping are unable to meet their counterparts in the opposite jaw in the appropriate relationships and may be predisposed to disease in later years.

Orthodontic treatment is most successful when it is started in the late school-age or early teenage years, after the last primary teeth have been shed and before growth ceases. However, referral should be made as soon as malocclusion is evident, since some deformities can be corrected at an earlier age or require treatment in stages over the years.

Dental injury may occur in childhood and includes fractures of varying degrees of severity, chipping, dislocation, or avulsion. All tooth injuries require prompt treatment by a competent dentist to prevent permanent displacement or loss. Delayed examination and diagnosis of tooth damage can result in infection or pulp involvement. Because it can affect the remaining teeth, replacement of the lost tooth is needed to maintain normal alignment and position of the other teeth.

A tooth that is *avulsed* (exarticulated, or "knocked out") should be replanted by the child, parent, or nurse and stabilized as soon as possible so that the blood supply to the tooth can be reestablished and the tooth kept alive (see Emergency box). A tooth that is replanted within 15 minutes has a 98% survival rate (Krause-Parello, 2005). Avulsed primary teeth are usually not reimplanted.

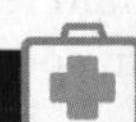

EMERGENCY

Avulsed Permanent Tooth

Recover tooth.

Hold tooth by crown; avoid touching root area.

If tooth is dirty, rinse it gently under running water or saline; be certain to insert stopper in sink or basin (to avoid tooth loss).

To Reimplant Tooth

Insert tooth into socket; be certain that the lip-side (or convex surface) is facing front.

Have child maintain tooth in place by slowly biting down on a piece of gauze.

Transport child to dentist immediately.

Avoid sudden stops or sharp turns to prevent dislodging tooth.

If Reluctant to Reimplant Tooth

Place avulsed tooth in suitable medium for transport:

- Cold milk
- Saliva—under child's or parent's tongue

If child is holding tooth in the mouth, avoid sudden stops to prevent swallowing tooth.

DON'T FORGET TO TAKE THE TOOTH.

As with all injuries to the mouth, an avulsed tooth causes a large amount of bleeding, which is frightening to children and their families; therefore the nurse or anyone faced with dental trauma should be prepared to provide support and reassurance during the dental trauma.

Sex Education

Many children experience some form of sex play during or before preadolescence as a response to normal curiosity, not as a result of love or sexual urges. Children are experimentalists by nature, and sex play is incidental and transitory. Any adverse emotional consequences or guilt feelings depend on how the behavior is managed by the parents; whether it is discovered; or whether children view their actions as wrong in the eyes of significant persons, particularly the parents.

The child's attitude toward sex is acquired indirectly at an early age. Initial curiosity about differences in body structure between boys and girls and between children and adults arises in the preschool years. Middle childhood is an ideal time for formal sex education, and many authorities believe that the topic is best presented from a life span approach. Information about sexual maturation and the process of reproduction minimizes the child's uncertainty, embarrassment, and feelings of isolation that often accompany puberty.

An important component of ongoing sex education is effective communication with parents. If parents either repress the child's sexual curiosity or avoid dealing with it, the sexual information that the child receives may be acquired almost entirely from peers. When peers are the primary source of sexual information, it is transmitted and exchanged in secret conversation and contains a large amount of misinformation.

Nurse's Role in Sex Education

No matter where nurses practice, they can provide information on human sexuality to both parents and children. To discuss the topic adequately, nurses must have an understanding of the physiologic aspects of sexuality; knowledge of the cultural and societal values; and an awareness of their own attitudes, feelings, and biases about sexuality.

When presenting sexual information to school-age children, nurses should treat sex as a normal part of growth and development. They should answer questions honestly, matter-of-factly, and to the same extent as questions about other topics. Answers should be at the child's level of understanding. There may be times when boys and girls should be taught content separately.

Children need help to differentiate sex and sexuality. Exercises on clarifying values, identifying role models, engaging in problem-solving skills, and practicing responsibility are important to prepare children for early adolescence and puberty. In addition, children need explanations of sexual information that is provided via the media or jokes. Information concerning pregnancy; contraceptives; and sexually transmitted infections, including human immunodeficiency virus and human papillomavirus, should be presented in simple, accurate terms.

Preadolescents need precise and concrete information that will allow them to answer questions such as "What if I start my period in the middle of class?" or "How can I keep people from telling I have an erection?" It is important to tell children what they want to know and what they can expect to happen as they become mature sexually.

During encounters with parents, nurses can be open and available for questions and discussion. They can set an example by the language they use in discussing body parts and their function and by the way in which they deal with problems that have emotional overtones, such as exploratory sex play and masturbation. Parents need help to understand normal behaviors and to view sexual curiosity in their children as a part of the developmental process. Assessing the parents' level of knowledge and understanding of sexuality provides cues to their need for supplemental information that will prepare them for the increasingly complex explanations they will need to provide as their children grow older.

School Health

Child health maintenance is ultimately the responsibility of the parents; however, the public schools and health departments in the United States have contributed to the improvement of child health by providing a healthful school environment, health services, and health education that emphasize sound health practices. Most of these functions constitute major components of community health services and involve large amounts of public funds and large numbers of health professionals, including nurses.

A school health program is involved in ongoing health maintenance through assessment, screening, and referral activities. Routine health services provided by most schools include health appraisal, emergency care, safety education, communicable disease control, counseling, and follow-up care. Health education of school-age children is directed toward providing knowledge of health and influencing habits, attitudes, and conduct in relation to health and injury prevention.

Traditionally, school nurses were viewed as the individuals who detected diseases in the school, applied bandages, and cared for students who were ill or injured. Although these functions remain important parts of the school nurse's job, the role has expanded considerably in recent years. Today, school nurses manage and coordinate all the care required by regular students and students with special health care needs. In many settings, school health services have enlarged into family health centers that meet the needs of not only school-age children, but also their families and the community. In these settings, school nurse practitioners provide health care that includes assessment of physical, psychomedical, psychoeducational, behavioral, and learning problems, as well as comprehensive well-child care (Hackbarth & Gall, 2005).

The passage of the Education for All Handicapped Children Act and its amendments (Public Laws 94-142 and 99-457) mandated the integration of children with chronic illness or disability into the least restrictive environments, including regular classrooms whenever possible. School nurses are responsible for the medical and nursing needs of these children while they are in the school setting. School nurses develop, implement, and evaluate individualized health care plans for these children. Unfortunately, not all schools have a school nurse, and the use of unlicensed assistive personnel (UAP) is increasing. In many schools, nurses are faced with the task of delegating to and supervising UAP (Potter & Grant, 2004). Delegation and supervision of UAP requires skillful nursing assessment, effective communication, and professional judgment.

Injury Prevention

evolve Case Study—Injury Prevention

Because school-age children have developed more refined muscular coordination and control and can apply their cognitive capacities to their behavior, the number of injuries in middle childhood is diminished compared with the number in early childhood. The most common cause of severe injury and death in school-age children is motor vehicle accidents—either as a pedestrian or passenger (Schnitzer, 2006). It is important that nurses continue to emphasize three automobile safety measures that have been found to reduce the severity of injuries: effective car restraint systems, door-lock mechanisms, and appropriate passenger-seating locations in the motor vehicle. The American Academy of Pediatrics advises health professionals and parents that the rear vehicle seat is the safest place for children under the age of 13 years (Durbin et al, 2005).

The school-age child's desire for riding bicycles increases the risk of injury on streets. Other serious injuries include accidents on skateboards, roller skates, in-line skates, scooters, and other sports equipment. All-terrain vehicles (ATVs), popular with children younger than 16 years of age, are unstable, difficult to handle, and responsible for an increasing number of childhood injuries. The Consumer Product Safety Commission has outlined ATV recommendations that include free driver training, no passengers, use of helmets, no roadway traveling, and adult supervision for children under the age of 16 years (Humphries et al, 2006).

Most injuries occur in or near the home or school. The most effective means of prevention is education of the child and family regarding the hazards of risk taking and the improper use of equipment. Safety helmets, protective eye and mouth shields, and protective padding are strongly recommended for children engaging in active sports, even though they may not be required equipment. Falls from bicycles, ATVs, and skating devices are the cause of a significant number of head injuries in school-age children. Because head injury is the major cause of bicycle-related fatalities, the most important aspect of bicycle safety is to encourage the rider to wear a protective helmet (Fig. 39-9) (Khambalia, MacArthur, & Parkin, 2005).

Physically active school-age children are also highly susceptible to cuts and abrasions, and the incidence of childhood fractures, strains, and sprains is high. Trampoline injuries are highest in children 5 through 14 years and account for numerous fractures, sprains, and head injuries. Trampolines in the home environment, routine physical education classes, or outdoor playgrounds are not recommended for children of any age (Nysted & Drogset, 2006). Serious injuries are discussed elsewhere in the book: burns (Chapter 53), eye trauma (Chapter 42), near-drowning (Chapter 51), and head injuries (Chapter 51). The prevalence of injuries depends on the dangers in the environment, the protection offered by adults, and the children's behavior patterns. Table 39-2 lists characteristics of the school-age child that make them prone to injury and suggestions for injury prevention. Family-Centered Care boxes provide guidelines for bicycle, skateboard, and in-line skate safety and guidance during the school years.

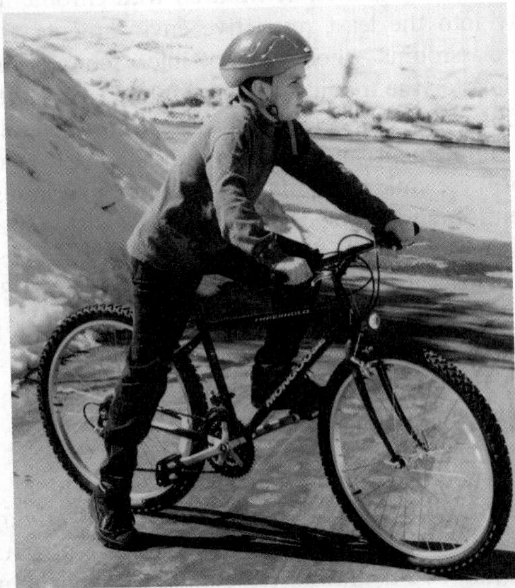

Fig. 39-9 The right size bike is important; the child should be able to sit on the bike and place the balls of both feet on the ground. The foot should comfortably reach and manipulate the pedal in the down position. Wearing a protective helmet is mandatory. The helmet should be positioned so it sits low on the forehead and parallel to the ground when the head is held upright. It should not rock back and forth or shift from side to side. The strap should fasten securely under the chin.

FAMILY-CENTERED CARE

Bicycle Safety

- Always wear a properly fitted bicycle helmet that is approved by the U.S. Consumer Product Safety Commission (CPSC); encourage parents to look for the CPSC approval sticker on the inside liner of the helmet.
- Replace a helmet every 5 years or sooner if manufacturer recommends it. **Never use a damaged or outgrown helmet.**
- Ride bicycles with traffic and away from parked cars.
- Ride single file.
- Walk bicycles through busy intersections only at crosswalks.
- Give hand signals well in advance of turning or stopping.
- Keep as close to the curb as practical.
- Watch for drain grates, potholes, soft shoulders, loose dirt, or gravel.
- Keep both hands on handlebars, except with signaling.
- Never ride double on a bicycle.
- Do not carry packages that interfere with vision or control; do not drag objects behind bike.
- Watch for and yield to pedestrians.
- Watch for cars backing up or pulling out of driveways; be especially careful at intersections.
- Look left, right, then left before turning into traffic or roadway.
- Never hitch a ride on a truck or other vehicle.
- Learn rules of the road and respect for traffic officers.
- Obey all local ordinances.
- Wear shoes that fit securely while riding.
- Wear light colors at night and attach fluorescent material to clothing and bicycle.
- Equip bicycle with proper lights and reflectors.
- Be certain the bicycle is the correct size for rider (see Fig. 39-9).
- Have bicycle inspected to ensure good mechanical condition.
- Children riding as passengers must wear appropriate-size helmets and sit in specially designed protective seats.

Modified from American Academy of Pediatrics, Committee on Injury and Poison Prevention: Bicycle helmets, *Pediatrics* 108(4):1030-1032, 2001.

Table 39-2 Injury Prevention During School-Age Years

DEVELOPMENTAL ABILITIES RELATED TO RISK OF INJURY	INJURY PREVENTION
Motor Vehicle Accidents	
Is increasingly involved in activities away from home Is excited by speed and motion Is easily distracted by environment Can be reasoned with	Educate child regarding proper use of seat belts while a passenger in a vehicle. Maintain discipline while a passenger in a vehicle (e.g., keep arms inside, do not lean against doors, do not interfere with driver). Remind parents and children that no one should ride in the bed of a pickup truck. Emphasize safe pedestrian behavior. Insist on child wearing safety apparel (e.g., helmet) when applicable, such as riding bicycle, motorcycle, moped, or all-terrain vehicle (see Family-Centered Care box, p. 1094).
Drowning	
Is apt to overdo May work hard to perfect a skill Has cautious, but not fearful, gross motor actions Likes swimming	Teach child to swim. Teach basic rules of water safety. Select safe and supervised places to swim. Check sufficient water depth for diving. Swim with a companion. Use an approved flotation device. Advocate for legislation requiring fencing around pools. Learn cardiopulmonary resuscitation.
Burns	
Has increasing independence Is adventurous Enjoys trying new things	Make certain home has smoke detectors. Set water heaters to 48.9° C (120° F) to avoid scald burns. Instruct child in behavior in areas involving contact with potential burn hazards (e.g., gasoline, matches, bonfires or barbecues, lighter fluid, firecrackers, cigarette lighters, cooking utensils, chemistry sets). Instruct child to avoid climbing or flying kite around high-tension wires. Instruct child in proper behavior in the event of fire (e.g., fire drills at home and school). Teach child safe cooking (use low heat; avoid any frying; be careful of steam burns, scalds, or exploding foods, especially from microwaving).
Poisoning	
Adheres to group rules May be easily influenced by peers Has strong allegiance to friends	Educate child regarding hazards of taking nonprescription drugs and chemicals, including aspirin and alcohol. Teach child to say "no" if offered illegal or dangerous drugs or alcohol. Keep potentially dangerous products in properly labeled receptacles, preferably out of reach.
Bodily Damage	
Has increased physical skills Needs strenuous physical activity Is interested in acquiring new skills and perfecting attained skills Is daring and adventurous, especially with peers Frequently plays in hazardous places Confidence often exceeds physical capacity Desires group loyalty and has strong need for friends' approval Attempts hazardous feats Accompanies friends to potentially hazardous facilities Is likely to overdo Growth in height exceeds muscular growth and coordination	Help provide facilities for supervised activities. Encourage playing in safe places. Keep firearms safely locked up except under adult supervision. Teach proper care of, use of, and respect for devices with potential danger (e.g., power tools, firecrackers). Teach children not to tease or surprise dogs, invade their territory, take dogs' toys, or interfere with dogs' feeding. Stress eye, ear, or mouth protection when using potentially hazardous objects or devices or when engaging in potentially hazardous sports. Do not permit use of trampolines except as part of supervised training. Teach safety regarding use of corrective devices (glasses); if child wears contact lenses, monitor duration of wear to prevent corneal damage. Stress careful selection, use, and maintenance of sports and recreation equipment, such as skateboards and in-line skates (see Family-Centered Care box, p. 1096). Emphasize proper conditioning, safe practices, and use of safety equipment for sports or recreational activities. Caution against engaging in hazardous sports, such as those involving trampolines. Use safety glass and decals on large glassed areas, such as sliding glass doors. Use window guards to prevent falls. Teach name, address, and phone number and emphasize that child should ask for help from appropriate people (e.g., cashier, security guard, police) if lost; have identification on child (e.g., sewn in clothes, inside shoe). Teach stranger safety: Avoid personalized clothing in public places. Caution child to never go with a stranger. Have child tell parents if anyone makes child feel uncomfortable in any way. Always listen to child's concerns regarding others' behavior. Teach child to say "no" when confronted by uncomfortable situations.

FAMILY-CENTERED CARE

Skateboard and In-Line Skate Safety

- Children younger than 5 years of age should not use skateboards or in-line skates because they are not developmentally prepared to protect themselves from injury. Children ages 6 to 10 years should use these only with close adult supervision.
- Children who ride skateboards or in-line skates should wear helmets and other protective equipment, especially on knees, wrists, and elbows, to prevent injury.
- Skateboards and in-line skates should never be used near traffic. Their use should be prohibited on streets and highways. Activities that bring skateboards together (e.g., "catching a ride") are especially dangerous.
- Some types of use, such as riding homemade ramps on hard surfaces, may be particularly hazardous.

Data from American Academy of Pediatrics, Committee on Injury and Poison Prevention: Skateboard injuries, *Pediatrics* 109(3):542-543, 2002; and American Academy of Pediatrics, Committee on Injury and Poison Prevention: In-line skating injuries in children and adolescents, *Pediatrics* 117(5):1846-1847, 2006.

SPECIAL HEALTH PROBLEMS

Health Problems Related to Sports Participation

Every sport has the potential for injury to the participant—whether the youngster engages in serious competition or participates for enjoyment. Serious injury occurs most often during rough contact sports or to persons who are not physically prepared for the activity. Injuries also occur to children or adolescents when their body is not suited to the sport, when their muscles and body systems (respiratory and cardiovascular) are not conditioned to endure physical stress, or when they lack the insight and judgment to recognize that an activity exceeds their physical abilities. More injuries occur during recreational sports participation than during organized athletic competition.

The environment and the sports or recreational equipment can also present risks. Children who participate in physical activity or sports do so in many different environments: indoors and outdoors, on floors, on the ground and snow, on or beneath water surfaces, and sometimes in free air space. Most of these activities also involve equipment.

Acute overload injuries are those that occur suddenly during an activity and produce immediate symptoms. A blow or overstretching, twisting, or sudden stress to tissues can cause these injuries. For descriptions and management of traumatic injuries, see Chapter 54.

Overuse Syndromes

To excel in sports, the young athlete is forced to train longer, harder, and earlier in life than previously. The rewards are an increased level of fitness, better performances, faster times, and the satisfaction of attaining a personal goal. However, the risk of overuse injury is always present and is related to several factors: training errors, muscle-tendon imbalance, anatomic malalignment, incorrect footwear or playing surface, an associated disease state, and growth.

A common feature in overuse injuries is the *repetitive microtrauma* that occurs to a particular anatomic structure when the same movements are performed over a long period. The result is inflammation of the involved structure with complaints of chronic pain, tenderness, swelling, and disability. Examples of overuse syndromes include "Little League elbow" (tendinitis and osteochondritis from repetitive throwing), "tennis elbow" (lateral epicondylitis from repetitive elbow strain), and Osgood-Schlatter disease (traction apophysitis of the tibial tubercle).

Stress Fractures

Stress fractures occur as a result of repeated muscle contraction and are seen most often in repetitive weight-bearing sports such as running, gymnastics, and basketball. They occur less often in swimmers. The most common symptoms are a sharp, persistent, progressive pain or a deep, persistent, dull ache located over the bone. Sometimes there is pain on impact (heel strike), but the most important clinical sign is pain over the involved bony surface. Diagnosis is established on the basis of clinical observation, but occasionally a bone scan is performed.

Therapeutic Management

Inflammation is common in all overuse syndromes, and management is directed toward rest or alteration of activities, physical therapy, and medication. Rest is the primary therapy and is usually interpreted as reduced activity and the use of alternative exercise—*not* bed rest or immobilization with casting. The primary purpose is to alleviate the repetitive stress that initiated the symptoms. It is important to keep the youngster mobile, and training can be continued. Alternative exercise that maintains conditioning without aggravating the injury is selected. For example, pool running (treading water in the deep end of a pool) is an excellent alternative to running. Pool running uses the same movements as running without weight bearing. Other therapies include cryotherapy; cold whirlpools; and sometimes taping, bracing, splinting, or other orthoses. Treatment is specific to the injury. Nonsteroidal anti-inflammatory medications are prescribed to reduce pain and inflammation. Topical medications are of questionable value.

Nurse's Role in Sports for Children and Adolescents

Nurses are often involved in sports activities in the areas of preparation and evaluation for activities, prevention of injury, treatment of injuries, and rehabilitation after injury. Selecting an appropriate sport for both recreation and competition is a joint effort of the youngster, parents, and health professionals. The best approach to counseling children and parents regarding sports participation is to encourage activities that are most likely to provide pleasure and physical benefits throughout childhood and into adulthood. Exposure to a variety of activities is better for young children than limiting them to one sport. Parents should be cautioned against overcommitting children to sports activities so that they have time for other activities.

When children sustain athletic injuries, nurses are often responsible for instructions regarding care. Instructions (e.g., schedule for appointments, application of ice, and any restrictions in activity) should be clear and accompanied by written directions. The importance of taking medications as prescribed is emphasized, especially if medications are needed for an extended period and if adherence is an issue. Medications given an hour before practice or competition may be advantageous to children who are continuing their activities.

Prevention of sports injuries is the most important aspect of athletic programs. Children should be suited to the activity; the environment and the equipment must be safe. Children should be prepared for the sport, especially if it requires strenuous or continuous physical exertion. Nurses, coaches, and athletic trainers must collaborate to ensure that safety measures are implemented. Stretching exercises, warm-up and cool-down activities, and appropriate training are requirements for safe participation. Protective measures such as pads, taping, and wrapping are also important to prevent injury. Finally, nurses must be aware of environmental safety risks.

Altered Growth and Maturation

The absence of physical or sexual maturation at a time when other children are experiencing positive evidence of sexual development and its associated spurt in growth and physical strength is an important concern to both the parents and their affected child. Fortunately, in most instances the delay in development is a simple physiologic or *constitutional delay* that represents one end of the normal genetically influenced variation of pubertal growth. These children will go through a delayed but normal puberty and finally catch up, in their late teens, with their more rapidly developing age-mates. Less benign causes of delayed development may be the result of endocrine disorders or chromosomal abnormalities. Delayed development can also be a result of chronic diseases (such as malabsorption or chronic asthma) that are serious enough to retard development or a result of environmental factors (such as stress or poor nutrition).

The rate of maturation is important during the school years, but at puberty it assumes gigantic proportions to both teens and their parents. Girls or boys who lag behind their peers in physical maturation are painfully aware of their difference in growth. Adolescent girls with delayed maturation feel out of place among companions whose hips and breasts are developing, feel cheated if they have not yet menstruated, and feel left out when their friends giggle and talk about boys. Adolescent boys with delayed maturation feel weak and small compared to their more muscular companions, with whom they can no longer compete. Slow-maturing youngsters need support and reassurance that they are not abnormal and that they will develop the physical characteristics they desire.

Serial measurements of growth are plotted periodically on standard growth charts to determine the pattern of growth and to compare the individual child with the norms for his or her age group. When children are in the extremes of height ranges, it is important to compare their height with that of their parents and siblings.

Tall or Short Stature

Tall Stature

Despite the fact that the average height of both boys and girls is steadily increasing, there is a small group of children who, because of some organic disorder or a familial tendency, are excessively tall compared with their peers. To boys, this may be a source of pride; to girls, it may cause intense anxiety and be a severe social handicap.

When the rate of height change before puberty suggests the probability of excessive adult height, treatment with hormones may be considered, although there is considerable controversy regarding the use of hormones for this purpose. The use of estrogens is effective in controlling height when therapy is initiated before menarche and before the end of the adolescent growth spurt that normally precedes menarche. The selection of children for hormonal therapy is made on the basis of a careful evaluation of physical, psychologic, and social factors.

Short Stature

Short stature is a nonspecific finding that may be the first manifestation of a serious disorder, or it may be of no consequence medically. On a worldwide scale, the most common cause of short stature or delayed development is inadequate nutrition. The major physical disorders that produce delayed development are chronic diseases, endocrine dysfunction, and syndromes of primary gonadal failure.

Chronic diseases can interfere with growth, but unless the illness is unduly prolonged, catch-up growth occurs. Diseases and disorders that cause some degree of growth delay include asthma, cystic fibrosis, gastrointestinal diseases (such as parasitic infections), malabsorption syndromes, cardiac anomalies, and chronic renal disturbances. The duration of the illness is more significant than the intensity in terms of the effect on growth, although the precise length of time necessary to affect growth permanently has not been determined.

Skeletal disorders that affect growth in stature are those described as dwarfism. Most disorders are caused by congenital defects and disorders, such as achondroplasia, and by inborn errors of metabolism, such as Hurler's syndrome or Hunter's syndrome.

Psychosocial, or *deprivation, dwarfism* is a stress-induced growth failure. It is defined as growth retardation in children over 2 years of age that is caused by environmental (emotional) stress and is associated with a marked delay in physical growth, delayed developmental skills, and immature behavior. When these children are removed from the deprived environment, their growth proceeds at a normal or increased rate. (See also Growth Failure [Failure to Thrive], Chapter 36, and Child Maltreatment, Chapter 38.)

Management involves continued medical observation, attention to general health and nutrition, and psychologic support. When growth delay is accompanied by poor self-esteem, many authorities recommend hormonal therapy. Testosterone in carefully regulated doses is effective in some cases. Growth hormone is capable of increasing height and is used to treat growth hormone deficiency (see Hypopituitarism, Chapter 52). Its use with children who have constitutional delay is highly controversial.

Nursing Care Management

Deviation from the normal course of puberty is a significant concern for affected adolescents. For some teens, this concern assumes monumental proportions. Most cases of delayed development are caused by simple constitutional delay of puberty, and the child can be assured that normal development will eventually take place.

One difficulty related to size being incongruent with chronologic and mental age is the manner in which others relate to the child. People often respond to children with short stature as though they are younger than their age. Consequently, these children may react with babyish or juvenile behavior, thus establishing a circular pattern of behavior and response. Conversely, children who are tall or physically advanced for their age are frequently treated as though they are more advanced than their years. They are often considered to be cognitively impaired or immature when they perform according to the normal behavioral expectations for their age.

Listening to distressed adolescents and conveying interest and concern are important interventions. Counseling and therapy are individualized for each youth. Encouraging these children to focus on the positive aspects of their bodies and personalities and to adopt sound health practices and practice good grooming fosters a more positive self-image.

Sex Chromosome Abnormalities

Most sex chromosome abnormalities are caused by an alteration in sex chromosome number (Table 39-3). The majority of these conditions are due to nondisjunction. An alteration in the number of sex chromosomes usually does not produce the profound defects that are associated with the autosomal trisomies. Intelligence may be normal or low normal or the child may have some learning disabilities. Moderate or severe cognitive impairment is less common.

Turner's Syndrome

Turner's syndrome is caused by absence of one of the X chromosomes. Most girls who have this disorder have one X chromosome missing from all cells (45,X). This disorder is often recognized at birth if the newborn has a webbed neck, low posterior hairline, widely spaced nipples, and edema of the hands and feet. It can also be diagnosed at puberty because of three features: short stature, sexual infantilism, and amenorrhea. Girls with Turner's syndrome are generally infertile. They may also have difficulty with peer relationships and understanding social cues. They frequently exhibit behavioral problems, especially in relation to their immature, socially isolated behavior. Diagnosis is confirmed on the basis of a negative sex chromatin test.

Therapy is individualized for these girls and consists primarily of hormone treatment and psychologic counseling for both the child and parents. Linear growth can be increased by the administration of growth hormone if therapy is begun early. Estrogen therapy is initiated during the usual time for puberty to promote the development of secondary sex characteristics. Responses to estrogen therapy vary from girl to girl, but gradual feminization is accomplished to some degree in most individuals.

Klinefelter's Syndrome

Klinefelter's syndrome, the most common of all sex chromosome abnormalities, is caused by the presence of one or more additional X chromosomes. Most males with this syndrome have a chromosome complement of 47,XXY. The disorder is seldom recognized before puberty, at which time varying degrees of failure of adolescent virilization occur. Some males are not diagnosed until they appear for evaluation for infertility. All have absence of sperm in the semen (azoospermia), small testes, and defective development of secondary sex characteristics. In 80% of these boys there is a chromatin-positive buccal smear, and the extra chromosome is apparent on chromosome analysis.

Cognitive impairment is a frequent clinical finding and appears to be related to the number of X chromosomes. Boys may also have gross motor skill difficulties, a developmental language delay, poor verbal skills, reduced auditory memory, shyness, passivity, behavioral problems, and school difficulties. Therapy is directed toward enhancing the masculine characteristics through administration of testosterone.

Nursing Care Management

The nursing care of children with Turner's syndrome or Klinefelter's syndrome is primarily supportive. Nurses assist in diagnosis, explain tests and therapies, and provide support and

evolve Critical Thinking Exercise–Turner Syndrome

Table 39-3 Common Sex Chromosome Abnormalities

SYNDROME	CHROMOSOMAL NOMENCLATURE	PHENOTYPE	INCIDENCE (LIVE BIRTHS)	CLINICAL MANIFESTATIONS
Turner's	45,X or 45XO	Female	1:2500 female births*	Short stature; webbed neck; low posterior hairline; shield-shaped chest with widely spaced nipples; sterile; no development of secondary sex characteristics
Triple X, or superfemale	47,XXX (can also be 48,XXXX or 49,XXXXX)	Female	1:850-1250 female births	Normal female characteristics; usually tall; variable mental capacity and behavior; at risk for impaired language, learning difficulties; fertile
XYY male	47,XYY (can also be 48,XYYY or mosaic)	Male	1:900 male births*	Usually normal sexual development; tendency to be tall with long head; poor coordination; may demonstrate aberrant behavior
Klinefelter's	47,XXY (48,XXYY, 48,XXXY, 49,XXXXY, and so on, mosaics)	Male	1:850 male births*	Tall with long legs; hypogenitalism; sterile; male secondary sex characteristics may be deficient; may demonstrate aberrant behavior; learning disabled; possible gynecomastia

*Data from Nora JJ, Fraser FC: *Medical genetics: principles and practice*, ed 3, Philadelphia, 1989, Lea & Febiger.

encouragement to the child and the family. Because both disorders render the individual unable to reproduce, psychologic counseling is an important aspect of care. Marriage and sexual relationships are possible, but alternative reproductive options, such as artificial insemination and adoption, should be discussed.

Disorders with Behavioral Components

Attention-Deficit/Hyperactivity Disorder and Learning Disability

Attention-deficit/hyperactivity disorder (ADHD) refers to developmentally inappropriate degrees of inattention, impulsiveness, and hyperactivity. To be diagnosed as ADHD, the symptoms must have been present before age 7 years and must be present in at least two settings. In addition, the persistence of developmentally inappropriate and marked inattention must not be a symptom of another disorder (American Psychiatric Association, 2000). A *learning disability (LD)* refers to a heterogeneous group of disorders manifested by significant difficulties in the acquisition and use of listening, speaking, reading, writing, reasoning, or mathematic skills.

ADHD and LDs affect every aspect of the child's life but are most obvious in the classroom. Early identification of affected children is important because the characteristics of these disorders significantly interfere with the normal course of emotional and psychologic development. Many children develop maladaptive behavior patterns that impede psychosocial adjustment while they try to cope with cognitive dysfunction. Their behavior evokes negative responses from others, and repeated exposure to negative feedback adversely affects their self-concept. The characteristics of ADHD affect the child's written and adaptive skills, social status, and self-esteem (Myers, Eisenhauer, & Ryan, 2003).

Diagnostic Evaluation

The behaviors exhibited by the child with ADHD are not unusual aspects of behavior. The difference lies in the quality of motor activity and developmentally inappropriate inattention, impulsivity, and hyperactivity that the child displays. The manifestations may be numerous or few, mild or severe, and will vary with the child's developmental level. Any given child will not have every symptom of the condition. A comprehensive battery of tests is needed to confirm a learning disability. These include intelligence tests (many children have normal or above average intelligence quotients [IQs]); hand-eye coordination tests; and measurements of auditory and visual perception, comprehension, and memory. Often there is a wide gap between verbal and performance scores on IQ tests.

Therapeutic Management

Management of the child with ADHD usually involves multiple approaches that include family education and counseling, medication, proper classroom placement, environmental manipulation, and sometimes behavioral therapy or psychotherapy for the child. Interventions for children with LDs are primarily educational.

Medication

Stimulant medications and behavioral therapy are appropriate for the school-age child with ADHD (American Academy of Pediatrics, Subcommittee on Attention-Deficit/Hyperactivity Disorder and Committee on Quality Improvement, 2001). The most frequently prescribed medications are the psychostimulants methylphenidate hydrochloride (Ritalin) and dextroamphetamine sulfate (Dexedrine). These medications increase dopamine and norepinephrine levels, which leads to stimulation of the inhibitory system of the central nervous system. Tricyclic antidepressants, bupropion, and the α_2-adrenergic agonists (clonidine and guanfacine) are second-line medications. In addition, atomoxetine, a presynaptic norepinephrine transport inhibitor, is available for use in children (Aschenbrenner, 2003; Michelson et al, 2001).

Regularly scheduled evaluations of the child are essential with all of these medications. Children taking stimulant medication may have side effects that include nervousness, insomnia, increased blood pressure, and decreased appetite with subsequent weight loss. Long-term use of dextroamphetamine may result in suppression of growth.

Environmental Manipulation

In ADHD the child's environment is simplified by decreasing external stimuli and distractions, reducing alternatives, increasing consistency in routines, and encouraging desired patterns of behavior. Parents need to develop firm but reasonable limits and to provide a stable and predictable environment with regular routines of sleeping, eating, working, and playing.

Classroom Education

Special activities are designed to address learning deficits that involve visual perception, auditory perception, and other areas involving integration and coordination. The purpose of programs for children with LDs is to assist them to move toward more successful achievement and personal adjustment in the regular classroom. According to the Education for All Handicapped Children Act, children with ADHD or LDs must receive free public education in the least restrictive environment.

Prognosis

ADHD is relatively stable through early adolescence for most children. Some children experience decreased symptoms during late adolescence and adulthood, but a significant number of these children carry their symptoms into adulthood. The goal for children with LDs is to help them identify their areas of weakness and learn to compensate for them.

Nursing Care Management

Nurses are active participants in all aspects of management of the child with ADHD or LD. Nurses in the community work with families and school personnel on a long-term basis to help plan and implement therapeutic regimens and to evaluate the effectiveness of therapy. They should teach parents and children to take stimulant medication in the morning to maximize its effectiveness in the classroom and to decrease its insomnia-producing potential. If decreased appetite is a concern, giving the psychostimulant with or after meals rather than before is helpful. Parents also benefit from practical, specific strategies that help children with ADHD, such as the

evolve Case Study—Attention-Deficit/Hyperactivity Disorder

provision of structure and consistency in dressing, meals, sleep, and discipline.

Nurses must understand which type of LD a child has to provide direction for the child, parents, and teachers. Children with an auditory perceptual deficit are often unable to follow directions or to comprehend large amounts of verbal teaching. These children need diagrams, pictures, demonstration, and written lists. Children with visual perceptual deficits may have difficulty reading, lining up numbers for mathematic operations, or judging distance. These children may have dyslexia (letter reversals) and do better with demonstration and a verbal approach. Children with an integrative deficit may have difficulty sequencing data or storing and retrieving sensory data. Multisensory techniques should be used, and comprehension should be checked frequently throughout instruction. Children with dysgraphia often benefit from computers in the classroom, because their handwriting will *not* improve. They need to find an alternative to physical competition that requires coordination of movement (Selekman & Snyder, 2000).

Enuresis

Enuresis (bed-wetting) is a common and troublesome disorder that is defined as intentional or involuntary passage of urine into bed (usually at night) or into clothes during the day in children who are beyond the age when voluntary bladder control should normally have been acquired. The inappropriate voiding of urine must occur are least twice a week for at least 3 months, and the chronologic or developmental age of the child must be at least 5 years. The predominant symptom is urgency that is immediate and accompanied by acute discomfort, restlessness, and urinary frequency. Enuresis is more common in boys; nocturnal bed-wetting usually ceases between 6 and 8 years of age.

Organic causes that may be related to enuresis should be ruled out before psychogenic factors are considered. Organic causes include structural disorders of the urinary tract; urinary tract infection; neurologic deficits; disorders that increase the normal output of urine, such as diabetes; and disorders that impair the concentrating ability of the kidneys, such as chronic renal failure or sickle cell disease. A bladder volume of 300 to 350 ml is sufficient to hold a night's urine. (To determine a child's bladder capacity, have the child void in a measuring cup after holding urine for as long as possible. Normal bladder capacity [in ounces] is the child's age plus 2 [e.g., a 6-year-old's normal capacity is 8 oz].) In other cases the enuresis is influenced by emotional factors, although it is doubtful that they are causative factors. Parents report that these children sleep more soundly than other children; however, the depth of sleep has not been identified as the cause of nocturnal enuresis. Enuresis has a strong familial tendency.

Therapeutic techniques used to manage enuresis include medications, bladder training, restriction or elimination of fluids after the evening meal, interruption of sleep to void, and various devices designed to establish a conditioned reflex response to waken the child at the initiation of voiding.

Three types of drugs are used to treat enuresis: tricyclic antidepressants, antidiuretics, and antispasmodics. The drug used most frequently to inhibit urination is the tricyclic antidepressant imipramine (Tofranil). Another anticholinergic drug, oxybutynin, reduces uninhibited bladder contractions and may be helpful for children with daytime urinary frequency. Desmopressin (DDAVP) nasal spray, an analog of vasopressin, reduces nighttime urine output to a volume less than functional bladder capacity.

✱Nursing Care Management

No matter what techniques are used, the nurse can help both children and parents to understand the problem of enuresis, the treatment plan, and the difficulties they may encounter in the process. The nurse can also provide consistent support and encouragement to help sustain both the child and the parents through the inconsistent and unpredictable treatment process. Parents need to understand that punishment is contraindicated because of its negative emotional impact and limited success in reducing the behavior. Children need to believe that they are helping themselves, and they need to sustain feelings of confidence and hope.

Encopresis

Encopresis is the repeated voluntary or involuntary passage of feces of normal or near-normal consistency into places not appropriate for that purpose according to the individual's own sociocultural setting. The event must occur at least once a month for at least 3 months, and the child's chronologic or developmental age must be at least 4 years. The fecal incontinence must not be caused by any physiologic effect, such as a laxative, or a general medical condition.

Primary encopresis is identified by age 4 when the child has not achieved fecal continence. *Secondary encopresis* is fecal incontinence occurring in a child over 4 years of age after a period of established fecal continence. The disorder is more common in boys than in girls.

One of the most common causes of encopresis is constipation, which may be precipitated by environmental change. Chronic, severe constipation has a tendency to impair the usual movement and contractions of the colon, which can lead to fecal obstruction. Abnormalities in the digestive tract can also lead to encopresis.

Children with encopresis often feel ashamed and may wish to avoid situations that might lead to embarrassment. School performance and attendance are affected as the child's offensive odor becomes a target for scorn and ridicule from classmates. Therapeutic management consists of determining the cause of the soiling and using appropriate interventions to correct the problem. Interventions may involve dietary changes, relief of a fecal impaction, or behavioral therapy. Psychotherapeutic intervention with the child and the family is often necessary.

✱Nursing Care Management

The nursing care of the child with encopresis involves education and support of the family, as well as treatment of existing constipation. Education regarding the physiology of normal defecation, toilet training as a developmental process, and the treatment outlined for the particular family is essential to a successful outcome. Family counseling is directed toward reassurance that most problems resolve successfully, although relapses during periods of stress are possible.

Posttraumatic Stress Disorder

Posttraumatic stress disorder (PTSD) refers to the development of characteristic symptoms after exposure to an extremely traumatic experience or catastrophic event. The traumatic experience is typically life threatening to self or a significant other and may involve grotesque mutilation or death, serious injury, or physical coercion (e.g., an assault, a natural disaster, sexual abuse, or witnessing violence). It is important to note that PSTD is not limited to children who have lived in "war-torn" countries. Events such as automobile, school, or recreational accidents and bullying have been identified as causes of PTSD (Sundelin-Wahlsten, Ahmad, & von Knorring, 2001). The characteristic symptoms are persistent reexperiencing of the traumatic event, avoidance of stimuli associated with the event or trauma, numbing of general responsiveness, and increased arousal.

The response to the event takes place in three stages. The *initial response* involves intense arousal, which usually lasts for a few minutes to 1 or 2 hours. The stress hormones are at the maximum as the individual prepares for "fight" or "flight." A prolonged arousal phase may indicate psychosis.

The *second phase,* which lasts approximately 2 weeks, is one in which defense mechanisms are mobilized. It is a period of quiescence in which the event appears to have produced no impression. The child feels numb, and stress hormone secretion is absent. Defense mechanisms are less adaptive to specific situations and may not be what the situation demands. Denial that anything is wrong is a frequently observed defense mechanism.

The *third phase* is one of coping and consciously directed inquiry, which normally extends over 2 to 3 months. The victims want to know what happened and appear to be getting worse, when actually they are getting better. Numerous psychologic symptoms, such as depression, phobia, anxiety, and conversion reactions, may be present. Children frequently display repetitive actions. They play out the situation over and over again in an attempt to come to terms with their fear. Flashbacks are common. This phase can be self-perpetuating, and a prolonged reaction can develop into an obsession with the traumatic event. Some traumatic effects remain indefinitely.

❋Nursing Care Management

Children need to deal with any traumatic event. Their reactions depend heavily on their social environment and the way in which their caretaking adults react to the event. In the second phase of PTSD, the appropriateness of the defense mechanism must be assessed, and children must be assisted in application of their defense. If children do not engage in some catharsis, or if their defense phase is prolonged, they need referral for special psychologic help.

Coping is a learned response, and children in the third phase can be helped to deal with their fear. Children usually are willing to accept reasoning. Those who are assisted in their catharsis and allowed expression will survive without serious lasting effects. They should be encouraged to play out the stress and to discuss their feelings about the event. If they are unable to do this, they may become obsessed with the traumatic event and require professional help. Conversion reactions are common obsessive behaviors in children suffering from PTSD.

Children need professional help if any of the phases of PTSD are prolonged. Boys tend to have a prolonged defense phase more often than girls. Occasionally the event will be unrecognized, and the affected child will engage in what is considered to be unusual behavior. Children exhibiting any sudden change in behavior need to be assessed for a traumatic event. When the change in behavior is traced to a traumatic event, treatment can be implemented.

School Phobia

Children, other than beginning students, who resist going to school or who demonstrate extreme reluctance to attend school for a sustained period as a result of severe anxiety or fear of school-related experiences are said to have *school phobia.* The terms *school refusal* and *school avoidance* are also used to describe this behavior. School-avoidance behaviors occur in both boys and girls and in children from all socioeconomic levels.

Physical symptoms are prominent and may affect any part of the body (e.g., anorexia, nausea, vomiting, diarrhea, dizziness, headache, leg pains, abdominal pains, or even a low-grade fever). A striking feature of school phobia is the prompt subsidence of symptoms when it is evident that the child can remain at home. Another significant observation is absence of symptoms on weekends and holidays unless they are related to other places such as Sunday school or parties. Occasional mild reluctance is not uncommon among schoolchildren, but if the fear continues for longer than a few days, it must be considered a serious problem.

❋Nursing Care Management

Treatment for school phobia depends on the cause. The primary goal is to *return the child to school.* The longer a child is permitted to stay out of school, the more difficult it is for the child to reenter. Parents must be convinced gently but firmly that *immediate* return is essential and that it is their responsibility to insist on school attendance.

A school reentry protocol may be necessary for the child with severe symptoms. In reentry programs, the child role-plays routines involved in getting ready for school and that occur at school. Relaxation techniques are also used. The child usually goes to school initially for a half day and then progresses to a full day. Often the school nurse is asked to provide support to the parents and the teacher during the reentry process. If the problem persists, professional help is recommended.

Recurrent Abdominal Pain

Recurrent abdominal pain (RAP) is a complaint that is often attributed to a psychogenic etiology, although it can be a symptom of either psychosomatic or organic disease. RAP is defined as three or more separate episodes of abdominal pain during a 3-month period, similar to the "spastic" or "irritable" colon syndrome of adulthood. Children with RAP have real pain that is usually located in the periumbilical or epigastric area (or both). On palpation the pain is likely to be experienced in the epigastric area or in the lower right or left quadrant and is accompanied by vague tenderness without muscle guarding. The pain is irregular in time, duration, and intensity and associated with either loose or pellet-formed stools. Other symptoms that may accompany the pain are headache, pallor, dizziness, dysuria, flushing, vomiting, diarrhea, and fatigue.

Children at risk for RAP tend to be high achievers who have extensive personal goals or whose parents have unusually high expectations. They are described as sensitive and overly concerned about what others think of them. They are uncomfortable with expressions of anger or argument, especially in those persons who are significant in their life. School attendance is adversely affected, and these children may exhibit poor learning performance. It is not uncommon for symptoms to be aggravated during school days.

Treatment involves providing reassurance and reducing or eliminating the symptoms. Hospitalization may be necessary, and the child frequently shows improvement in the hospital. Initial efforts are directed toward ruling out organic causes of the pain, relieving discomfort, and attempting to determine the situations that precipitate attacks. A high-fiber diet, psyllium bulk agents, lubricants such as mineral oil, and bowel training are emphasized. Other therapies include cognitive-behavioral therapy, biofeedback, and medications such as famotidine and propantheline bromide (an antispasmodic).

Nursing Care Management

Once the diagnosis has been established, the parents and the child need an explanation of the pain, which can be compared to a skeletal muscle cramp or "charley horse." Reassurance that the symptoms are not unique to their child and that the pain can be expected to subside is helpful in relieving parental fears and anxieties.

The simple measure of having the child rest in a peaceful, quiet environment and providing comfort will often relieve the symptoms in a short time. A heating pad may also help ease the discomfort (see Nonpharmacologic Management, Chapter 35). When pain is not relieved by these simple measures, the parents are taught how to administer antispasmodics, if prescribed. For example, if pain is precipitated by meals, having the child take the medication 20 to 30 minutes before mealtime may prevent an episode.

The most valuable assistance that the nurse can provide is support and reassurance to the family. When open communication is established and families appreciate the relationship between stress-provoking situations and the child's symptoms, the chance for remedial action is enhanced. Follow-up care and continued support are essential, since the symptoms tend to remit and exacerbate. The availability of a supportive health professional is a source of comfort to the child and family.

Conversion Reaction

Conversion reaction, also known as *hysteria, hysterical conversion reaction,* and *childhood hysteria,* is a psychophysiologic disorder with a sudden onset that can usually be traced to a precipitating environmental event. In childhood the disorder is observed with equal frequency in both sexes, but girls outnumber boys during adolescence.

The manifestations involve primarily the voluntary musculature and special senses. Symptoms include abdominal pain, fainting, pseudoseizures, paralysis, headaches, and visual field restriction. The most common symptom is seizure activity, which can be differentiated from symptoms of neurogenic origin by formal tests. A normal electroencephalogram indicates that the origin is not neurogenic. Many children with a conversion reaction have experienced a major family crisis (such as the loss of a parent or other significant person through death, divorce, or moving) before the onset of symptoms.

Nursing Care Management

Nursing care is similar to that for the child with RAP. If significant personality problems are evident, psychiatric consultation is indicated.

Childhood Depression

Depression in childhood is often difficult to detect because children may be unable to express their feelings and tend to act out their problems and concerns. Some states of depression are temporary (e.g., acute depression precipitated by a traumatic event). This might be related to a period of hospitalization; loss of a parent through death or separation; or loss of a significant relationship with something (a pet), someone (a friend or family member), or a place (move from a familiar home, neighborhood, or city). Children with depression may demonstrate a variety of behaviors (Box 39-1). Most responses in children are not sustained and can be modified with social and family support.

More serious and less common are the depressive responses to chronic stress and loss; these are frequently observed in children with chronic illness or disability when other family members are in denial and often depressed. There is no apparent

BOX 39-1 Characteristics of Children with Depression

Behavior

- Predominantly sad facial expression with absence or diminished range of affective response
- Solitary play or work; tendency to be alone; lack of interest in play
- Withdrawal from previously enjoyed activities and relationships
- Lowered grades in school; lack of interest in doing homework or achieving in school
- Diminished motor activity; tiredness
- Tearfulness or crying
- Dependent and clinging or aggressive and disruptive

Internal States

- Utterance of statements reflecting lowered self-esteem, sense of hopelessness, or guilt
- Suicidal ideations

Physiology

- Constipation
- Nonspecific complaints of not feeling well
- Change in appetite resulting in weight loss or gain
- Alterations in sleeping pattern; sleeplessness or hypersomnia

precipitating event, but there is often a history of frequent disruptions in important relationships. Often, there is also a history of depressive illness in one or both parents. Manifestations in the child are similar to those observed in acute depression, but they occur more frequently and extend over a longer time.

Nursing Care Management

Depressed children are managed by a health team especially prepared in the care of children with mental disorders. Treatment is highly individualized and undertaken in the least restrictive environment. Suicidal children are admitted to the hospital for protection if the family is unable to provide constant monitoring. Pharmacotherapy may involve tricyclic antidepressants or serotonin reuptake inhibitors such as fluoxetine (Prozac), trazodone (Desyrel), sertraline (Zoloft), paroxetine (Paxil), bupropion (Wellbutrin), and venlafaxine (Effexor). Nurses should be aware that depression can easily be overlooked in the child and can interrupt normal growth and development. Recognizing depression and suicidal tendencies in depressed adolescents and making appropriate referrals is an important nursing function. Identification of the depressed child requires a careful history (health, growth and development, social, and family health); interviews with the child; and observations by the nurse, parents, and teachers. (See also Suicide, Chapter 40.)

Childhood Schizophrenia

Childhood schizophrenia is a term that refers to severe deviations in ego functioning and is generally reserved for psychotic disorders that appear in children younger than 15 years of age. Childhood schizophrenia is a rare illness among children in the general population, and among children with mental illness, only about 2 in every 1000 have childhood schizophrenia.

Childhood schizophrenia is characterized by symptoms that last for at least 6 months and that seriously interfere with the child's functioning in school, at home, or in social situations. The basic disturbance is a lack of contact with reality and the subsequent development of a world of the child's own. Other areas of development that may be impaired include cognition, perception, emotion, language, and physical motor control. The most common manifestations involve language disturbances, impaired interpersonal relationships, and inappropriate affect (outward expression of emotion). Treatment involves management of the symptoms, prevention of relapse, and social and occupational rehabilitation of the young person. Antipsychotic drugs that are used to treat schizophrenia include haloperidol, chlorpromazine, and risperidone.

Nursing Care Management

Nursing care of psychotic children is a highly specialized area. However, nurses should be alert to the possibility that schizophrenia can occur in children, and refer children who consistently demonstrate abnormal behavior to a psychiatrist for evaluation. In addition, nurses will need to teach family members of children taking antipsychotic drugs to observe for possible side effects.

Key Points

- Middle childhood, also known as the school years, is the period of life that extends from 6 to 12 years of age.
- Although growth is slower than in previous years, there is a steady gain in height and weight, with maturation of body systems; primary teeth are lost and replaced by permanent teeth.
- A major task during the middle school years is developing a sense of industry or accomplishment (Erikson).
- Piaget's period of concrete operations refers to the school-age period, when children are able to use their thought processes to experience events and actions and make judgments based on reasoning.
- The child develops a conscience and is able to understand and adhere to rules and standards set by others.
- Entertaining different points of view, becoming sensitive to social norms, and forming peer friendships are important features of social development during the school years.
- Cooperative play, team activities, and the acquisition of skills are prime elements of play during the school years; rules and rituals assume greater importance.
- Parental concerns during middle childhood include lying, cheating, stealing, and school achievement.
- The availability of junk foods, irregular family meals, and schedules of working parents often interfere with optimal nutrition.

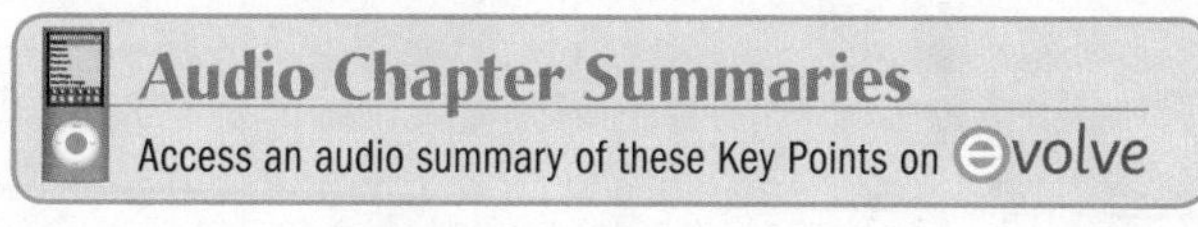
Audio Chapter Summaries
Access an audio summary of these Key Points on evolve

- Dental care is important during this time; potential dental problems include caries, periodontal disease, malocclusion, and dental injury.
- Increased socialization and media exposure make the school years an ideal time for sex education.
- School health programs ideally include health appraisal, emergency care, safety education, communicable disease control, counseling, guidance, and health education with adjustment to individual student needs.
- Injury prevention is directed toward safety education, provision of safe play areas and equipment, and well-supervised sports activities.
- Alterations in growth and maturation may be manifested as short or tall stature, or delayed sexual development.
- Behavior problems in middle childhood can result from ADHA, enuresis, encopresis, school phobia, RAP, childhood depression, conversion reaction, and childhood schizophrenia.

References

American Academy of Pediatrics, Pediatrics Collaborative Care Program: *Oral health risk assessment training for pediatricians and other child health professionals,* Rockville, MD, 2000, National Institutes of Health.

American Academy of Pediatrics, Subcommittee on Attention-Deficit/Hyperactivity Disorder and Committee on Quality Improvement: Clinical Practice Guideline: treatment of the school-aged child with attention-deficit/hyperactivity disorder, *Pediatrics* 108(4):1033-1044, 2001.

American Psychiatric Association: *Diagnostic and statistical manual of mental disorders,* ed 4 (text rev) (DSM-IV TR), Washington, DC, 2000, The Association.

Aschenbrenner DS: New drug for ADHD, *Am J Nurs* 103(4):63, 2003.

Ateah CA: Disciplinary practices with children: parental sources of information, attitudes, and educational needs, *Issues Compr Pediatr Nurs* 26:89-101, 2003.

Carno MA et al: Developmental stages of sleep from birth to adolescence, common childhood sleep disorders: overview and nursing implications, *J Pediatr Nurs* 18(4):274-283, 2003.

Dishion TJ, Nelson SE, Yasui M: Predicting early adolescent gang involvement from middle school adaptation, *J Clin Child Adolesc Psychol* 34(1):62-73, 2005.

Durbin DR et al: Effects of seating position and appropriate restraint use on the risk of injury to children in motor vehicle crashes, *Pediatrics* 115(3):305-309, 2005.

Glew GM et al: Bullying, psychosocial adjustment, and academic performance in elementary school, *Arch Pediatr Adolesc Med* 159:1026-1031, 2005.

Hackbarth D, Gall GB: Evaluation of school-based health center programs and services: the whys and hows of demonstrating program effectiveness, *Nurs Clin North Am* 40(4):711-724, 2005.

Humphries RL et al: An assessment of pediatric all-terrain vehicle injuries, *Pediatr Emerg Care* 22(7):491-494, 2006.

Khambalia A, MacArthur C, Parkin PC: Peer and adult companion helmet use is associated with bicycle helmet use by children, *Pediatrics* 116(4):939-942, 2005.

Krause-Parello CA: Tooth avulsion in the school setting, *J School Nurs* 21(5):279-282, 2005.

Lyznicki JM, McCaffree MA, Robinowitz CB: Childhood bullying: implications for physicians, *Am Fam Physician* 70(9):1723-1728, 2004.

Michelson D et al: Atomoxetine in the treatment of children and adolescents with attention-deficit/hyperactivity disorder: a randomized, placebo-controlled, dose-response study, *Pediatrics* 108:E83, 2001.

Mortweet SL, Christophersen E: Coping skills for the angry/impatient/clamorous child: a home/office practicum, *Contemp Pediatr* 21(6):43-45, 2004.

Myers SM, Eisenhauer NJ, Ryan ME: ADHD: it is real, and it can be treated, *Clin Advisor* 6(3):15-25, 2003.

Nansel TR et al: Relationships between bullying and violence among US youth, *Arch Pediatr Adolesc Med* 157(4):348-353, 2003.

Nysted M, Drogset JO: Trampoline injuries, *Br J Sports Med* 40:984-987, 2006.

Potter P, Grant E: Understanding RN and unlicensed assistive personnel working relationships in designing care delivery strategies, *J Nurs Admin* 34(1):19-24, 2004.

Ryan-Wenger NA, Sharrer VW, Campbell KK: Changes in children's stressors over the past 30 years, *Pediatr Nurs* 31(4):282-288, 2005.

Schnitzer PG: Prevention of unintentional childhood injuries, *Am Fam Physician* 74(11):1864-1869, 2006.

Selekman J, Snyder M: Learning disabilities and/or attention deficit disorder. In Jackson P, Vessey JA, editors: *Primary care of children with chronic conditions,* ed 3, St Louis, 2000, Mosby.

Sharrer VW, Ryan-Wenger NA: School-age children's self-reported stress symptoms, *Pediatr Nurs* 28(1):21-27, 2002.

Sundelin-Wahlsten V, Ahmad A, von Knorring A-L: Traumatic experiences and post-traumatic stress reactions in children from Kurdistan and Sweden, *Acta Paediatr* 90:563-568, 2001.

Vessey JA, Carlson K, David J: Helping children who are being teased and bullied, *Nurs Spectrum* 13:16-18, 2003.

Vreeman RC, Carroll AE: A systematic review of school-based interventions to prevent bullying, *Arch Pediatr Adolesc Med* 161(1):78-88, 2007.

Unit 9

40

The Adolescent and Family

Learning Objectives

On completion of this chapter the reader will be able to:

- Describe the physical changes that occur at puberty.
- Discuss the reactions of the adolescent to physical changes that take place at puberty.
- Demonstrate an understanding of the processes by which the adolescent develops a sense of identity.
- Discuss the significance of the changing interpersonal relationships and the role of the peer group during adolescence.
- Outline a health teaching plan for adolescents.
- Identify the causes and discuss the preventive aspects of injuries during adolescence.
- Demonstrate an understanding of common disorders of the male and female reproductive systems.
- Demonstrate an understanding of health problems related to adolescent sexuality.
- Outline a care plan for the child or adolescent with an eating disorder.
- Discuss the manifestations and nursing management of selected emotional and/or behavioral problems.

Electronic Resources

Additional information related to the content in Chapter 40 can be found on

evolve the Companion Website at http://evolve.elsevier.com/Perry/maternal/

- NCLEX Review Questions
- Assessment Video Clips
- Case Study—Behaviors Indicative of Future Child Abuse
- Case Study—Interviewing Adolescents
- Case Study—Teen Smoking
- Critical Thinking Exercise—Depression
- Critical Thinking Exercise—Obesity
- Nursing Care Plan—The Adolescent with an Eating Disorder

Promoting Optimum Growth and Development

Adolescence is a period of transition between childhood and adulthood—a time of rapid physical, cognitive, social, and emotional maturing as the boy prepares for manhood and the girl prepares for womanhood. The precise boundaries of adolescence are difficult to define, but this period is customarily viewed as beginning with the gradual appearance of secondary sex characteristics at about 11 or 12 years of age and ending with cessation of body growth at 18 to 20 years.

Several terms are used to refer to this stage of growth and development. *Puberty* refers to the maturational, hormonal, and growth process that occurs when the reproductive organs begin to function and the secondary sex characteristics develop. This process is sometimes divided into three stages: *prepubescence,* the period of about 2 years immediately before puberty when the child is developing preliminary physical changes that herald sexual maturity; *puberty,* the point at which sexual maturity is achieved, marked by the first menstrual flow in girls but by less obvious indications in boys; and *postpubescence,* a 1- to 2-year period following puberty during which skeletal growth is completed and reproductive functions become fairly well established. *Adolescence,* which literally means "to grow into maturity," is generally regarded as the psychologic, social, and maturational process initiated by the pubertal changes. It involves three distinct subphases: *early adolescence* (ages 11 to 14), *middle adolescence* (ages 15 to 17), and *late adolescence* (ages 18 to 20). The term *teenage years* is used synonymously with *adolescence* to describe ages 13 through 19.

Biologic Development

The physical changes of puberty are primarily the result of hormonal activity under the influence of the central nervous system, although all aspects of physiologic functioning are mutually interacting. The obvious physical changes are noted in increased physical growth and in the appearance and development of secondary sex characteristics; less obvious are physiologic alterations and neurogonadal maturity, accompanied by the ability to procreate. Physical distinction between the sexes is made on the basis of distinguishing characteristics. *Primary sex characteristics* are the external and internal organs that carry out the reproductive functions (e.g., ovaries, uterus, breasts, penis). *Secondary sex characteristics* are the changes that occur throughout the body as a result of hormonal changes (e.g., voice alterations, development of facial and pubertal hair, fat deposits) but that play no direct part in reproduction.

Hormonal Changes of Puberty

The events of puberty are caused by hormonal influences and controlled by the anterior pituitary (adenohypophysis) in response to a stimulus from the hypothalamus. Stimulation of the gonads has a dual function: (1) production and release of gametes—production of sperm in the male and maturation and release of ova in the female; and (2) secretion of sex-appropriate hormones—estrogen and progesterone from the ovaries (female) and testosterone from the testes (male).

The ovaries, testes, and adrenals secrete sex hormones. These hormones are produced in varying amounts by both sexes throughout the life span. The adrenal cortex is responsible for the small amounts secreted before the pubescent years, but the sex hormone production that accompanies maturation of the gonads is responsible for the biologic changes observed during puberty.

Estrogen, the feminizing hormone, is found in low quantities during childhood. This hormone is secreted in slowly increasing amounts until about age 11 years. In males this gradual increase continues through maturation. In females the onset of estrogen production in the ovary causes a pronounced increase that continues until about 3 years after the onset of menstruation, at which time it reaches a maximum level that continues throughout the reproductive life of the female.

Androgens, the masculinizing hormones, are also secreted in small and gradually increasing amounts up to about 7 or 9 years of age, at which time there is a more rapid increase in both sexes, especially boys, until about age 15 years. These hormones appear to be responsible for most of the rapid growth changes of early adolescence. With the onset of testicular function, the level of androgens (principally *testosterone*) in males increases over that in females and continues to increase until a maximum level is attained at maturity.

Sexual Maturation

The visible evidence of sexual maturation is achieved in an orderly sequence, and the state of maturity can be estimated on the basis of the appearance of these external manifestations. The age at which these changes are observed and the time required to progress from one stage to another may vary among children. The time from the appearance of breast buds to full maturity may be 1½ to 6 years for adolescent girls. It may take 2 to 5 years for male genitalia to reach adult size. The stages of development of secondary sex characteristics and genital development have been defined as a guide for estimating sexual maturity and are referred to as the *Tanner stages.* The usual sequence of appearance of maturational changes is presented in Box 40-1.

BOX 40-1 Usual Sequence of Maturational Changes

Girls

Breast changes
Rapid increase in height and weight
Growth of pubic hair
Appearance of axillary hair
Menstruation (usually begins 2 years after first signs)
Abrupt deceleration of linear growth

Boys

Enlargement of testicles
Growth of pubic hair, axillary hair, hair on upper lip, hair on face and elsewhere on body (facial hair usually appears about 2 years after appearance of pubic hair)
Rapid increase in height
Changes in the larynx and consequently the voice (usually take place along with growth of penis)
Nocturnal emissions
Abrupt deceleration of linear growth

Sexual Maturation in Girls

In most girls the initial indication of puberty is the appearance of breast buds, an event known as *thelarche,* which occurs between 9 and 13½ years of age (Fig. 40-1). This is followed in approximately 2 to 6 months by growth of pubic hair on the mons pubis, known as *adrenarche* (Fig. 40-2). In a minority of normally developing girls, however, pubic hair may precede breast development.

The initial appearance of menstruation, or *menarche,* occurs about 2 years after the appearance of the first pubescent changes, approximately 9 months after attainment of peak height velocity and 3 months after attainment of peak weight velocity. Menarche has been related to a critical gain in body fat content (more fat content, earlier menarche), although this is controversial. The normal age range of menarche is usually 10½ to 15 years, with the average age being 12 years, 9½ months for North American girls. Ovulation and regular menstrual periods usually occur 6 to 14 months after menarche. Girls may be considered to have *pubertal delay* if breast development has not occurred by age 13 or if menarche has not occurred within 4 years of the onset of breast development.

Sexual Maturation in Boys

The first pubescent changes in boys are testicular enlargement accompanied by thinning, reddening, and increased looseness of the scrotum (Fig. 40-3). These events usually occur between 9½ and 14 years of age. Early puberty is also characterized by the initial appearance of pubic hair. Penile enlargement begins, and testicular enlargement and pubic hair growth continue throughout midpuberty. During this period there is also increasing muscularity, early voice changes, and development of early facial hair. Temporary breast enlargement and tenderness, *gynecomastia,* are common during midpuberty, occurring in up to one third of boys. The spurts in height and weight occur concurrently toward the end of midpuberty. For most boys, breast enlargement disappears within 2 years. By late puberty there is a definite increase in the length and width of the penis, testicular enlargement continues, and

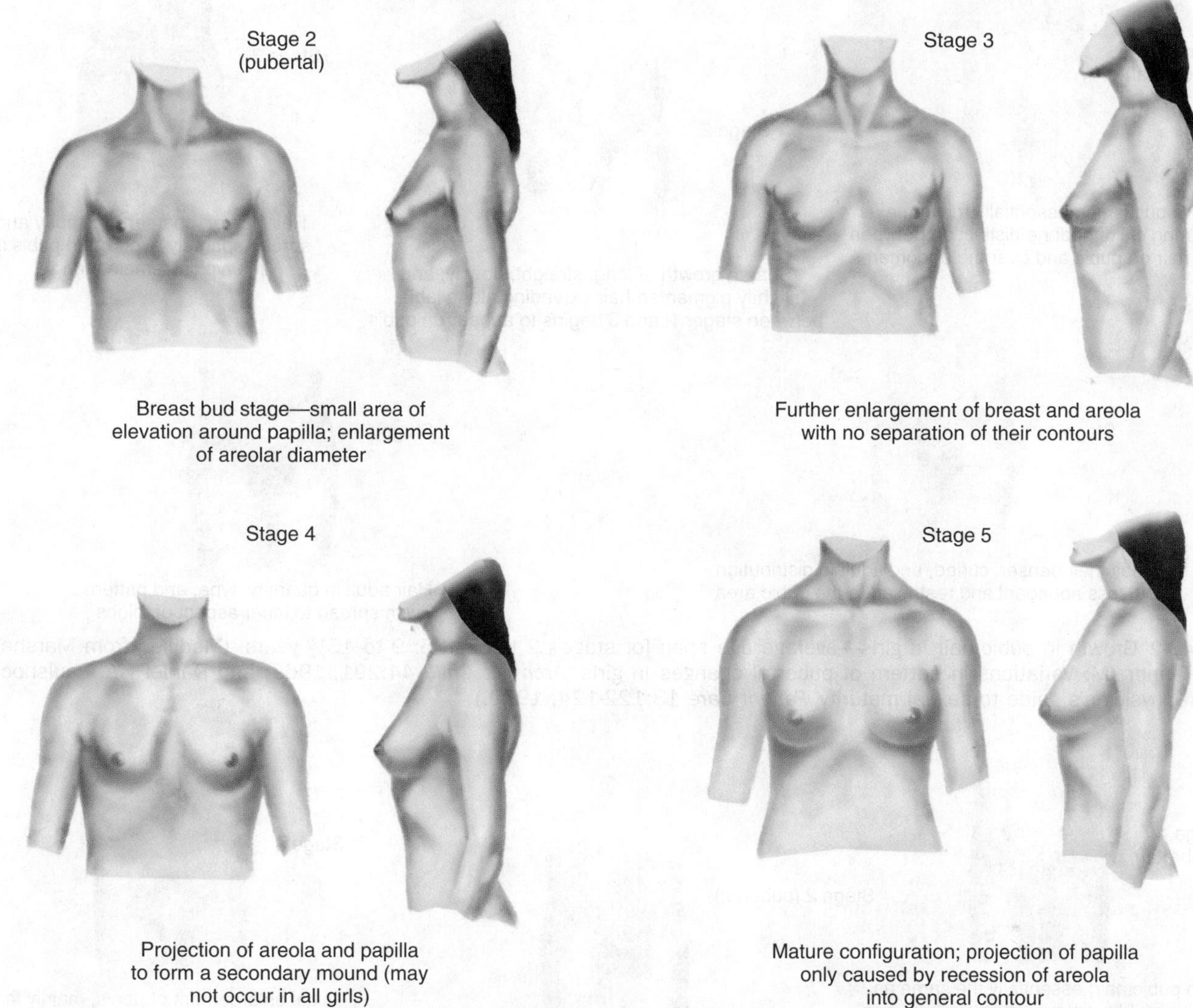

Stage 2
(pubertal)
Breast bud stage—small area of elevation around papilla; enlargement of areolar diameter
Stage 3
Further enlargement of breast and areola with no separation of their contours
Stage 4
Projection of areola and papilla to form a secondary mound (may not occur in all girls)
Stage 5
Mature configuration; projection of papilla only caused by recession of areola into general contour

Fig. 40-1 Development of the breast in girls—average age span: 9 to 13½ years. Stage 1 (prepubertal, elevation of papilla only) is not shown. (Modified from Marshall WA, Tanner JM: Variations in pattern of pubertal changes in girls, *Arch Dis Child* 44:291, 1969; and Daniel WA, Paulshock BZ: A physician's guide to sexual maturity, *Patient Care* 13:122-124, 1979.)

first ejaculation occurs. Axillary hair develops, and facial hair extends to cover the anterior neck. Final voice changes occur secondary to the growth of the larynx. Concerns about *pubertal delay* should be considered for boys who exhibit no enlargement of the testes or scrotal changes by 13½ to 14 years of age, or if genital growth is not complete 4 years after the testicles begin to enlarge.

Physical Growth

A constant phenomenon associated with sexual maturation is a dramatic increase in growth. The final 20% to 25% of height is achieved during puberty, and most of this growth occurs during a 24- to 36-month period—the adolescent *growth spurt*. This accelerated growth occurs in all children but, as in other areas of development, is highly variable in age of onset, duration, and extent. The growth spurt begins earlier in girls, usually between ages 9½ and 14½ years; on the average it begins between ages 10½ and 16 years in boys. During this period, the average boy gains 10 to 30 cm (4 to 12 inches) in height and 7 to 30 kg (15½ to 66 lb) in weight. The average girl, in whom the growth spurt is slower and less extensive, gains 5 to 20 cm (2 to 8 inches) in height and 7 to 25 kg (15½ to 55 lb) in weight. Growth in height typically ceases 2 to 2½ years after menarche in girls and at age 18 to 20 years in boys.

This increase in size is acquired in a characteristic sequence. Growth in length of the extremities and neck precedes growth in other areas, and since these parts are the first to reach adult length, the hands and feet appear larger than normal during adolescence. Increases in hip and chest breadth take place in a few months, followed several months later by an increase in shoulder width. These changes are followed by increases in length of the trunk and depth of the chest. This sequence of changes is responsible for the characteristic long-legged, gawky appearance of the early adolescent child.

Sex Differences in General Growth Patterns

Sex differences in general growth and distribution patterns are apparent in skeletal growth, muscle mass, adipose tissue, and skin. Skeletal growth differences between boys and girls

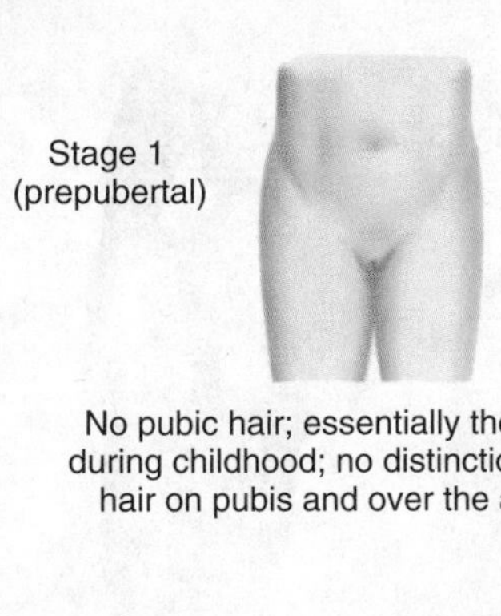

Stage 1 (prepubertal)

No pubic hair; essentially the same as during childhood; no distinction between hair on pubis and over the abdomen

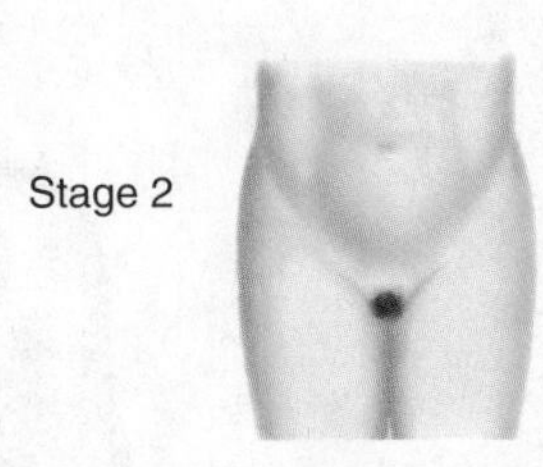

Stage 2

Sparse growth of long, straight, downy, and slightly pigmented hair extending along labia; between stages 2 and 3 begins to appear on pubis

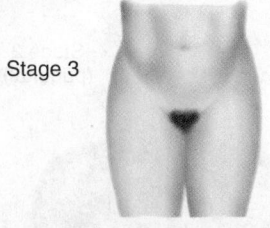

Stage 3

Hair darker, coarser, and curly and spread sparsely over entire pubis in the typical female triangle

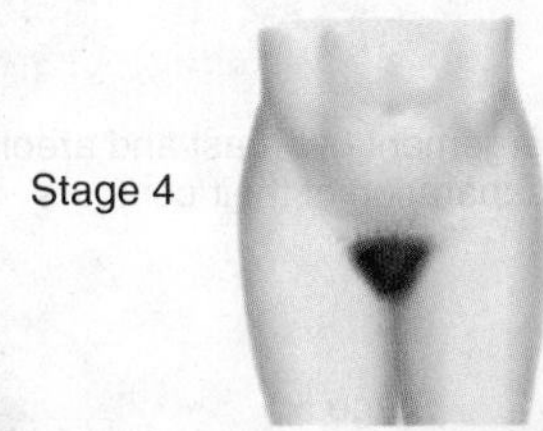

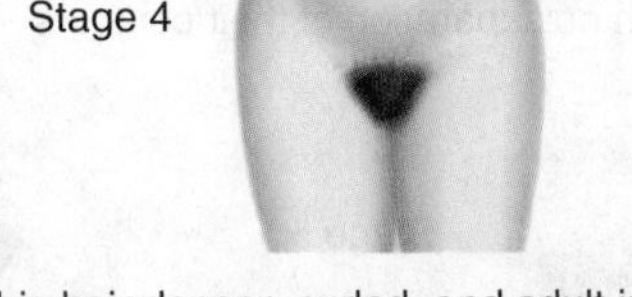

Stage 4

Pubic hair denser, curled, and adult in distribution but less abundant and restricted to the pubic area

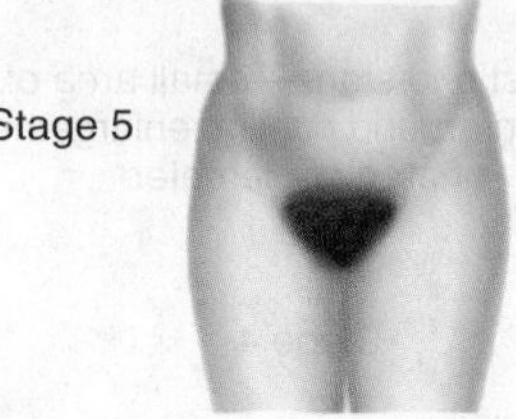

Stage 5

Hair adult in quantity, type, and pattern with spread to inner aspect of thighs

Fig. 40-2 Growth in pubic hair in girls—average age span for stages 2 through 5: 9 to 13½ years. (Modified from Marshall WA, Tanner JM: Variations in pattern of pubertal changes in girls, *Arch Dis Child* 44:291, 1969; and Daniel WA, Paulshock BZ: A physician's guide to sexual maturity, *Patient Care* 13:122-124, 1979.)

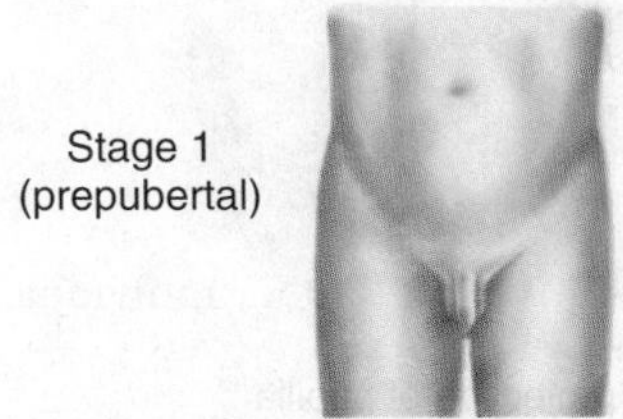

Stage 1 (prepubertal)

No pubic hair; essentially the same as during childhood; no distinction between hair on pubis and over the abdomen

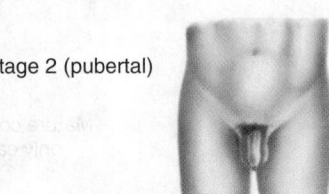

Stage 2 (pubertal)

Initial enlargement of scrotum and testes; reddening and textural changes of scrotal skin; sparse growth of long, straight, downy, and slightly pigmented hair at base of penis

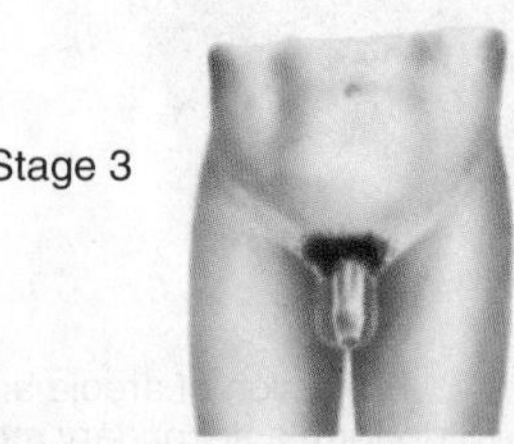

Stage 3

Initial enlargement of penis, mainly in length; testes and scrotum further enlarged; hair darker, coarser, and curly and spread sparsely over entire pubis

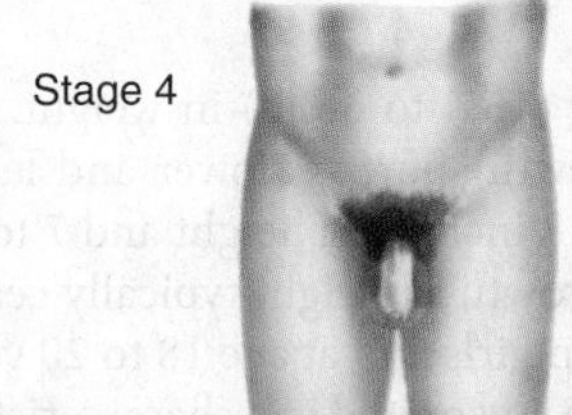

Stage 4

Increased size of penis with growth in diameter and development of glans; glans larger and broader; scrotum darker; pubic hair more abundant with curling but restricted to pubic area

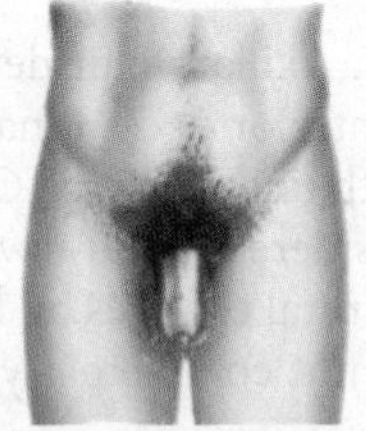

Stage 5

Testes, scrotum, and penis adult in size and shape; hair adult in quantity and type with spread to inner surface of thighs

Fig. 40-3 Developmental stages of secondary sex characteristics and genital development in boys—average age span, 9½ to 14 years. (Modified from Marshall WA, Tanner JM: *Arch Dis Child* 44:291, 1969; and Daniel WA, Paulshock BZ: *Patient Care*, pp 122-124, May 13, 1979.)

are apparently a function of hormonal effects at puberty and are evident primarily in limb length. The earlier cessation of growth in girls is caused by epiphyseal unity under the potent effect of estrogen secretion, and the hormonal effect on female bone growth is much stronger than the similar effect of testosterone in boys. In boys the prolonged growth period before puberty and the less rapid epiphyseal closure are reflected in their greater overall height and longer arms and legs. Other skeletal differences are increased shoulder width in boys and broader hip development in girls.

Hypertrophy of the laryngeal mucosa and enlargement of the larynx and vocal cords occur in both boys and girls to produce voice changes. Girls' voices become slightly deeper and considerably fuller, but the effect in boys is striking. The change in the voice of adolescent boys occurs between Tanner stages 3 and 4, with the voice often shifting uncontrollably from deep to high tones in the middle of a sentence.

Growth of lean body mass, principally muscle, which tends to occur after the bone growth spurt, takes place steadily during adolescence. Lean body mass is both quantitatively and qualitatively greater in boys than in girls at comparable stages of pubertal development. Muscle development, under the influence of androgenic hormones, increases steadily. Muscles become remarkably well developed in boys, whereas in girls, muscle mass increase is proportionate to general tissue growth.

Nonlean body mass, primarily fat, is also increased but follows a less orderly pattern. There may be a transient increase in subcutaneous fat just before the skeletal growth spurt, especially in boys. This is followed 1 to 2 years later by a modest-to-marked decrease, which is again more notable in boys. Later, variable amounts of fat are deposited to fill out and contour the mature physique in patterns characteristic of the adolescent's sex, particularly in the regions over the thighs, hips, and buttocks and around the breast tissue. It should be noted, however, that pediatric obesity has increased in the United States, and obesity can change the timing of puberty. Girls with thelarche as the first sign of puberty have earlier menarche and greater body fat and body mass index (BMI) at menarche than girls with adrenarche as the first pubertal sign. This may have long-term effects for increased risk of adult adiposity and obesity (Biro et al, 2003); however, the relationship between early pubescence and obesity has yet to be fully understood (Kaplowitz, 2008).

Hormonal influences during puberty cause acceleration in growth and maturation of the skin and its structural appendages. Sebaceous glands become extremely active at this time, especially those on the genitalia and in the "flush areas" of the body (i.e., face, neck, shoulders, upper back, and chest). This increased activity and the structural nature of the glands are extremely important in the pathogenesis of a common problem of puberty: acne (see Chapter 53). The eccrine sweat glands, present almost everywhere on the human skin, become fully functional and respond to emotional and thermal stimulation. Heavy sweating appears to be more pronounced in boys than in girls. The apocrine sweat glands, nonfunctional in childhood, reach secretory capacity during puberty. Unlike the eccrine sweat glands, the apocrine glands are limited in distribution and grow in conjunction with hair follicles in the axillae, around the areola of the breast, around the umbilicus, on the external auditory canal, and in the genital and anal regions. Apocrine glands secrete a thick substance as a result of emotional stimulation that, when acted on by surface bacteria, becomes highly odoriferous.

Body hair assumes very characteristic distribution patterns and changes texture during puberty. Under the influence of gonadal and adrenal androgens, hair coarsens, darkens, and lengthens at sites related to secondary sex characteristics. Pubic and axillary hair appears in both sexes, although pubic hair is more extensive in males than in females. Beard, mustache, and body hair on the chest, upward along the linea alba, and sometimes on other areas (e.g., back and shoulders) appears in males and is androgen dependent. Extremity hair appears in varying amounts in both males and females but is also more prolific in the male.

Physiologic Changes

A number of physiologic functions are altered in response to some of the pubertal changes. The size and strength of the heart, blood volume, and systolic blood pressure increase, whereas the pulse rate and basal heat production decrease (see Appendix E). Blood volume, which has increased steadily during childhood, reaches a higher value in boys than in girls, a fact that may be related to the increased muscle mass in pubertal boys. Adult values are reached for all formed elements of the blood. Respiratory rate and basal metabolic rate, decreasing steadily throughout childhood, reach the adult rate in adolescence. Respiratory volume and vital capacity are increased and to a far greater extent in males than in females. During this period, physiologic responses to exercise change drastically: performance improves, especially in boys, and the body is able to make the physiologic adjustments needed for normal functioning after exercise is completed. These capabilities are a result of the increased size and strength of muscles and the increased level of cardiac, respiratory, and metabolic functioning.

Psychosocial Development

Developing a Sense of Identity (Erikson)

Traditional psychosocial theory holds that the developmental crisis of adolescence leads to the formation of a sense of identity (Erikson, 1963). Throughout childhood, individuals have been going through the process of identification as they concentrate on various parts of the body at specific times. During infancy children identify themselves as being separate from the mother; during early childhood they establish a gender-role identification with the appropriate-sex parent; and in later childhood they establish who they are in relation to others. In adolescence they come to see themselves as distinct individuals, somehow unique and separate from every other individual.

Adolescence begins with the onset of puberty and extends to relative physical and emotional stability at or near graduation from high school. During this time the adolescent is faced with the crisis of *group identity vs. alienation.* In the period that follows, the individual strives to attain autonomy from the family and develop a sense of *personal identity* as opposed to *role diffusion.* A sense of group identity appears to be essential to the development of a sense of personal identity. Young adolescents must resolve questions concerning relationships with a peer group before they are able to resolve questions about who they are in relation to family and society.

Group Identity

During the early stage of adolescence, pressure to belong to a group is intensified. Teenagers find it essential to have a group to which they feel they can belong and that provides them with status. Belonging to a crowd helps adolescents establish the differences between themselves and their parents. They dress as the group dresses and wear makeup and hairstyles according to group criteria, all of which are different from those of the parental generation. Language, music, and dancing reflect a culture that is exclusive to the adolescent. When adults begin to emulate these fashions and interests, the style changes immediately. The evidence of adolescent conformity to the peer group and nonconformity to the adult group provides teenagers with a frame of reference in which they can display their own self-assertion while they reject the identity of their parents' generation. To be different is to be unaccepted and alienated from the group.

Individual Identity

The quest for personal identity is part of the ongoing identification process. As adolescents establish identity within a group, they also attempt to incorporate multiple body changes into a concept of the self. Body awareness is part of self-awareness. In their search for identity, adolescents consider the relationships that have developed between themselves and others in the past, as well as the directions they hope to take in the future.

Significant others hold expectations for the adolescent's behavior. Often these expectations or demands are persistent enough to result in certain decisions that might be made differently or not at all if the individual could be solely responsible for identity formation. It is all too easy to slip into the roles that are expected by these external influences without incorporating personal goals or questioning these decisions. Thus individuals may become what parents or others wish them to be, based on these premature decisions. Young persons might form a negative identity when society or their culture provides them with a self-image that is contrary to the values of the community. Labels such as "loser," "juvenile delinquent," "hoodlum," or "failure" are applied to certain adolescents, who then accept and live up to these labels with behaviors that validate and strengthen them.

The process of evolving a personal identity is time-consuming and fraught with periods of confusion, depression, and discouragement. Determining an identity and a place in the world is a critical and perilous feature of adolescence (see Critical Thinking Exercise). However, as the pieces gradually shift and settle into place, a positive identity eventually emerges. Role diffusion results when the individual is unable to formulate a satisfactory identity from the multiplicity of aspirations, roles, and identifications.

Sex-Role Identity

Adolescence is the time for consolidation of a sex-role identity. During early adolescence the peer group begins to communicate expectations regarding heterosexual relationships, and as development progresses, adolescents encounter expectations for mature sex-role behavior from both peers and adults. Expectations vary from culture to culture, among geographic areas, and among socioeconomic groups.

Emotionality

Adolescents vacillate in their emotional states between considerable maturity and childlike behavior. One minute they are exuberant and enthusiastic; the next minute they are depressed and withdrawn. Unpredictable, but essentially normal, mood swings are common during this time. As the tension is relieved, emotion is brought under control and individuals retreat to review what has happened, to attempt to master their anger, and to increase their ability to control their emotions and gain from the new experience. Because of these mood swings, adolescents are frequently labeled as unstable, inconsistent, and unpredictable. Little things can cause an emotional upheaval and, depending on the teenager's interpretation, can mean a great deal.

Teenagers are better able to control their emotions in later adolescence. They can approach problems more calmly and rationally, and although they are still subject to periods of sadness, their feelings are less vulnerable and they begin to demonstrate more mature emotions. Whereas early adolescents react immediately and emotionally, older adolescents can control their emotions until socially acceptable times and places for expression present themselves. They are still subject to heightened emotion, and when it is expressed, their behavior reflects feelings of insecurity, tension, and indecision.

CRITICAL THINKING EXERCISE

Discussing the Future

Jeremy, age 17, will be graduating from high school in the spring. His mother, a single parent, tells you that she is concerned because graduation is quickly approaching and Jeremy has made no plans for what he will do with his life after graduation. Whenever Jeremy mentions the topic, his mother tells him, "This is what you must do," and begins to outline the steps he must take. Jeremy just walks away. She asks, "What should I do?" What advice should you give Jeremy's mother?

1. Evidence—Is there sufficient evidence to draw any conclusions about what advice the nurse should give Jeremy's mother?
2. Assumptions—Describe an underlying assumption about each of the following issues:
   a. Adolescents and the search for personal identity
   b. The influence of others on the adolescent's search for personal identity
   c. Ways to communicate with adolescents
3. What implications and priorities for nursing care can be drawn at this time?
4. Does the evidence objectively support your argument (conclusion)?
5. Are there alternative perspectives to your arguments? What are they?

Cognitive Development (Piaget)

Cognitive thinking culminates with the capacity for *abstract thinking.* This stage, the period of *formal operations,* is Piaget's fourth and last stage. Adolescents are no longer restricted to the real and actual, which was typical of the period of concrete thought; they are also concerned with the possible. They now think beyond the present. Without having to center attention on the immediate situation, they can imagine a sequence of events that might occur, such as college and occupational possibilities; how things might change in the future, such as relationships with parents; and the consequences of their actions, such as dropping out of school. At this time their thoughts can be influenced by logical principles rather than

evolve Case Study—Behaviors Indicative of Future Child Abuse

just their own perceptions and experiences. They become increasingly capable of scientific reasoning and formal logic.

Adolescents are capable of mentally manipulating more than two categories of variables at the same time. For example, they can consider the relationship between speed, distance, and time in planning a trip. They can detect logical consistency or inconsistency in a set of statements and evaluate a system or set of values in a more analytic manner. For instance, they question the parent who insists on honesty in the teenager but at the same time cheats on an income tax report or expense account.

In adolescence, young people begin to think about both their own thinking and the thinking of others. They wonder what opinion others have of them, and they are able to imagine the thoughts of others. With this capacity comes the ability to differentiate between others' thoughts and their own and to interpret the thoughts of others more accurately. They are able to understand that few concepts are absolute or independent of other influencing factors. As they become aware that other cultures and communities have different norms and standards from their own, it becomes easier for them to accept members of these other cultures, and the decision to behave in their own culture in an accepted manner becomes a more conscious commitment.

Moral Development (Kohlberg)

Although younger children merely accept the decisions or point of view of adults, adolescents, to gain autonomy from adults, must substitute their own set of morals and values. When old principles are challenged but new independent values have not yet emerged to take their place, young people search for a moral code that preserves their personal integrity and guides their behavior, especially in the face of strong pressure to violate the old beliefs. Their decisions involving moral dilemmas must be based on an *internalized set of moral principles* that provides them with the resources to evaluate the demands of the situation and to plan actions that are consistent with their ideals.

Late adolescence is characterized by serious questioning of existing moral values and their relevance to society and the individual. Adolescents can easily take the role of another. They understand duty and obligation based on reciprocal rights of others, as well as the concept of justice that is founded on making amends for misdeeds and repairing or replacing what has been spoiled by wrongdoing. However, they seriously question established moral codes, often as a result of observing that adults verbally ascribe to a code but do not adhere to it.

Spiritual Development

As adolescents move toward independence from parents and other authorities, some begin to question their families' values and ideals. Others cling to these values as a stable element in their lives as they struggle with the conflicts of this turbulent period. Adolescents need to work out these conflicts for themselves, but they also need support from authority figures and/or peers for their resolution.

Adolescents are capable of understanding abstract concepts and of interpreting analogies and symbols. They are able to empathize, philosophize, and think logically. Most teens search for ideals and speculate about illogical statements and conflicting ideologies. Their tendency toward introspection and emotional intensity often makes it difficult for others to know what they are thinking. They tend to keep their thoughts private, fearing that no one will understand these feelings that they perceive to be unique and special. However, they may reveal deep spiritual concerns. They need support and encouragement in their struggle for understanding and the freedom to question without censure.

Greater levels of religiosity and spirituality are associated with fewer high risk behaviors and more health-promoting behaviors. Nurses play an important role for teens by providing an opportunity to discuss issues regarding spirituality.

Social Development

To achieve full maturity, adolescents must free themselves from family domination and define an identity independent of parental authority. However, this process is fraught with ambivalence on the part of both teenagers and their parents. Adolescents want to grow up and be free of parental restraints, but they are fearful as they try to comprehend the responsibilities that are linked with independence. Feelings of immortality and exemption from the consequences of risk-taking behavior, although viewed as negative, can serve an important developmental function at this time. These feelings give adolescents the courage to separate from their parents and become independent. Part of this emancipation involves developing social relationships outside the family that help teenagers identify their role in society. Adolescence is a time of intense sociability and often a time of equally intense loneliness. Acceptance by peers, a few close friends, and the secure love of a supportive family are requisites for interpersonal maturation.

Relationships with Parents

During adolescence the parent-child relationship changes from one of protection-dependency to one of *mutual affection and equality*. The process of achieving independence often involves turmoil and ambiguity as both parent and adolescent learn to play new roles and work toward this end while, at the same time, resolving the often painful series of rifts essential to establishing the ultimate relationship.

Most behavior observed in the adolescent is related to the struggle for independence and the external restrictions and checks that are placed on this spontaneous maturation process. On the one hand, adolescents are accepted as maturing preadults. They are allowed privileges heretofore denied, and they are provided with increasing responsibilities. On the other hand, because of their unpredictability and insecurity in evaluating situations and making sound judgments, they must conform to regulations and restrictions set by adults. This state of affairs is particularly exemplified by the struggle between parents and adolescents concerning the nightly curfew.

As teenagers assert their rights for grown-up privileges, they frequently create tensions within the home. They resist parental control, and conflicts can arise from almost any situation or any subject. Favorite topics of dispute include use of the home telephone, Internet use, a personal cellular telephone, manners, dress, chores and duties, homework, disrespectful behavior, friendships, dating and relationships, money, automobiles, alcohol and other substance abuse, and time schedules. Present in these areas of conflict is the overriding argument that "everyone else has one" or is allowed the desired item or privilege and the ever-present assertions that "you don't understand me or trust me" and "you always treat me like a baby." Spoken or unspoken, parents' reactions consist of "Is this all the thanks I get for what I have done for you?"

Teenagers' earliest attempts to achieve emancipation from parental controls are manifested in a period of rejection of the parents. They absent themselves from home and family activities and spend increasing time with the peer group. They confide less in their parents, but parents continue to play an important role in their personal and health-related decision making.

With advancing adolescence, teenagers become more competent, and with this competence comes a need for more autonomy. Although they may be psychologically prepared for independence, they are often thwarted in their efforts by lack of money or other parental barriers. Conflict arises in relation to the teenager's outside activities and the elements of privacy and trust. Parental supervision remains important throughout adolescence and may have a direct influence on adolescent sexual and substance use behavior. Parents should be guided toward an authoritative style of parenting in which authority is used to guide the adolescent while allowing developmentally appropriate levels of freedom and providing clear, consistent messages regarding expectations. Authoritative style of parenting has been shown to have both immediate and long-term protective effects toward adolescent risk reduction (DeVore & Ginsburg, 2005). However, to gain the trust of adolescents, parents must respect their adolescent's privacy and show an honest and sincere interest in what the adolescent believes and feels (see Family-Centered Care box).

Relationships with Peers

Although parents remain the primary influence in their lives, for the majority of teenagers, peers assume a more significant role in adolescence than they did during childhood. The peer group serves as a strong support to teenagers, individually and collectively, providing them with a sense of belonging and a feeling of strength and power. The peer group forms the transitional world between dependence and autonomy.

Peer Group

Adolescents are usually social, gregarious, and group minded. Thus the peer group has an intense influence on adolescents' self-evaluation and behavior. To gain acceptance by a group, younger teenagers tend to conform completely in such things as mode of dress, hairstyle, taste in music, and vocabulary. Teenagers use the peer group as a yardstick of what is normal.

The school is psychologically important to adolescents as a focus of social life. Teenagers usually distribute themselves into a relatively predictable social hierarchy. They know to which groups they and others belong. A sense of school connectedness has been found to predict decreased risk-taking behaviors in adolescents (Bond et al, 2007). School connectedness is correlated with caring teachers and the absence of prejudice or discrimination from peers. A sense of school connectedness is less dependent on class size, attendance, academic preparation, and parental involvement (Maes & Lievens, 2003).

Within the larger groups are smaller, distinct, and rather exclusive crowds or cliques of selected close friends who are emotionally attached to each other. The selection is based on common tastes, interests, and background. Although cliques may become formalized, most remain informal and small. However, each has an identifying feature that proclaims its difference from others and its solidarity within itself, in much the same manner as the adolescent generation as a whole sets itself apart from the adult generation. Cliques are usually made up of one gender, and girls tend to be more cliquish than boys and to have a greater need for close friendships (Fig. 40-4). Within the intimacy of the group, adolescents gain support in learning about themselves, consideration for the feelings of others, and increased ego development and self-reliance.

To belong is of utmost importance; thus adolescents behave in a way that will ensure their establishment in a group. Adolescents are highly susceptible to social approval, acceptance, and demands. To be ignored or criticized by peers creates feelings of inferiority, inadequacy, and incompetence.

Best Friends

Personal friendships of the one-on-one variety usually develop between same-sex adolescents. This relationship is closer and more stable than it is in middle childhood, and it is important in the quest for identity. A best friend is the best audience on whom to try out possible roles and identities that an adolescent wants to test. Best friends may try a role together, each supporting the other. Each cares about what the other

FAMILY-CENTERED CARE

Communication with Teens: The Art of Listening

Conflicts between parents and their adolescents are often a result of a natural characteristic of parenthood: the desire to protect one's offspring from harm or from simply doing something "stupid" or embarrassing or something they may later regret. Teenagers sometimes "bounce" their thoughts and ideas off adults. At times they really want some feedback; at other times they simply want to elicit a reaction.

I found it easy to listen openly, thoughtfully, and without interrupting when my teenagers' friends discussed troublesome topics. However, one day, when one of my own teenagers had a similar conversation with me, the parent part kicked in. I felt responsible and spoke my piece on the spot. This brought communication to a halt and resulted in defensiveness. It was a long time before my child tried to talk to me about anything controversial again. The next time one of my teenagers started a similar conversation, I decided to try to trick myself.

Throughout the entire conversation, I told myself over and over again to act as if this were not my teenager, but rather someone else's child. I found this actually worked quite well, and I was able to listen without interrupting. I continued to use the system, sometimes with more success than at other times.

—Mother of Four

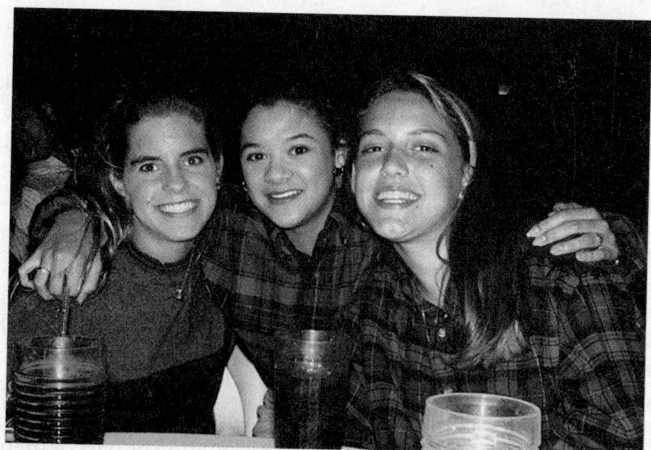

Fig. 40-4 Teenagers like to gather in small groups.

thinks and feels. Since a sense of intimacy grows within a permanent relationship, the stability of this same-gender friendship is an important link in the progress toward an intimate relationship in young adulthood.

Interests and Activities

Adolescents spend a large amount of time engaging in leisure-time activities. As teenagers progress through the developmental stages of adolescence, these leisure-time activities move from being family centered to being peer centered. In addition to providing teenagers with fun and enjoyment, leisure-time activities assist in the development of social, physical, and cognitive skills. Leisure-time activities also allow teenagers the opportunity to learn to set priorities and structure their time (Fig. 40-5).

Today, many adolescents must learn to juggle their time between school, activities, and the responsibilities of a job. Adolescent work experiences provide many benefits, including time management, teamwork skills, and increased income. However, many jobs available to teenagers do not provide opportunities to apply the skills they learn in school, and jobs often have high demands for quick work with low rewards. Few apprentice opportunities are available for teenagers. It is generally recommended that adolescents limit their work to no more than 20 hours per week during the school year.

Adolescent Sexuality

Sexual activity rates have been decreasing for teens since the 1990s, including a decline in the rate among early adolescents (Santelli et al, 2007). Among teenagers who have initiated sexual intercourse at an age younger than 14 years, the incidence of sexual abuse is high. In 2002 about half of all teenagers had had sexual intercourse at least once (Abma et al, 2004). Teens engage in a wide range of sexual activity, including kissing and petting (fondling), oral sex, and vaginal and rectal sex. Data indicate that more adolescents are engaging in sexual activity such as oral sex and delaying vaginal intercourse (Mosher, Chandra, & Jones, 2005); whether this is intended to preserve female virginity or to presumably avoid sexually transmitted infection is not known.

Adolescence represents a critical time in the development of sexuality. Hormonal, physical, cognitive, and social changes

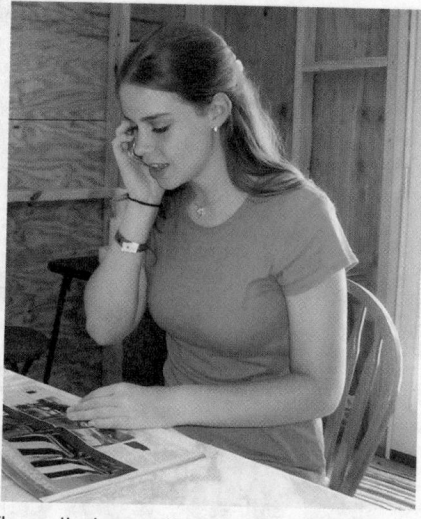

Fig. 40-5 The cell phone allows adolescents to talk for hours with peers.

that occur during adolescence all have an impact on sexual development. Of all the developmental changes that affect adolescent sexuality, none is more obvious than the impact of puberty. Adolescents must come to terms with hormonal influences, physiologic manifestations such as menstruation and ejaculation, and physical changes such as breast and genital development. All these changes have a profound impact on the way teenagers perceive their bodies (i.e., body image). In addition to transitions in body image, increasing levels of pubertal hormones contribute to increased levels of sexual motivation among both boys and girls.

Changes in sexual motivations and feelings, happening at the same time as shifts in cognitive skills, contribute to painful conjectures ("Is what I'm feeling normal?"), self-conscious concern ("Am I good looking enough?"), and hypothetical thinking ("What if she wants to have sex?"). The emergence of formal operational thinking also increases adolescents' decision-making capabilities concerning sexual issues. As they mature, teenagers become better able to think through potential risks and benefits of sexual behaviors before they engage in any behavior. Older adolescents may also be able to conceptualize more long-term consequences of present behaviors. One of the important tasks of adolescence is to incorporate sexuality successfully into close, intimate relationships. This task is made possible by the advanced cognitive abilities that emerge over the course of adolescence.

Part of adolescent identity formation involves the development of sexual identity. As they begin to integrate changes involved with puberty, young adolescents also develop emotional and social identities separate from their families. For young adolescents, the process of sexual identity development usually involves forming close friendships with same-sex peers, with whom they may experiment sexually, often to satisfy curiosity. Sexual activity among young teenagers varies by gender. Masturbation provides an opportunity for sexual self-exploration; participation in this behavior is influenced by learned cultural attitudes and sex-role expectations.

Many teenagers begin to make a shift from relationships with same-sex peers to intimate relationships with members

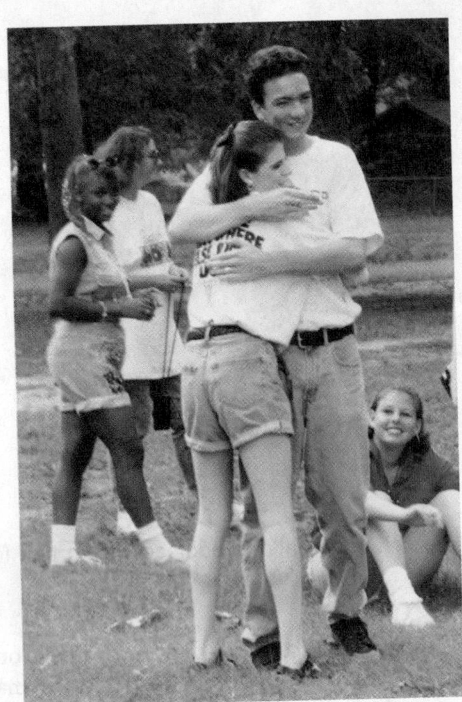

Fig. 40-6 Relationships with peers of the opposite gender are an important part of adolescence.

of the opposite sex during middle adolescence (Fig. 40-6). Opposite-sex relationships typically begin with peer activities involving both boys and girls. Pairing off as couples becomes more common as middle adolescence progresses. The type and degree of seriousness of partner relationships vary. Initial relationships are usually noncommittal, extremely mobile, and seldom characterized by any deep romantic attachments. Sexual activity becomes more common during middle adolescence. The relationship between love and sexual expression is brought into focus during middle adolescence. Most young people oppose exploitation, pressure, or force in sex, as well as sex solely for the sake of physical enjoyment without a personal relationship. Adolescents find it hard to believe that sex can exist without love; therefore they view each relationship as real love.

An integrated sexual identity often emerges during late adolescence as individuals incorporate sexual experiences, feelings, and knowledge. For most, this identity is consistent with their own physical and mental capacities and with societal limits and expectations. Most older adolescents identify themselves as being predominantly heterosexual or bisexual, with a smaller number self-identifying as homosexual and an even smaller group still unsure of their sexual orientation, although this varies somewhat by ethnicity (Saewyc et al, 1998; Russell, Seif, & Truong, 2001). Whatever their sexual orientation, many older teenagers possess the capacity to have intimate relationships that satisfy the emotional and sexual needs of both partners.

Sexual orientation is an important aspect of sexual identity. Sexual orientation is defined as a pattern of sexual arousal or romantic attraction toward persons of the opposite gender (heterosexual), of the same gender (homosexual, often called *gay* or *lesbian*), or of both genders (bisexual). Sexual orientation encompasses several dimensions, including attraction, fantasy, actual sexual behavior, and self-labeling or group affiliation. In individuals the direction and intensity of each dimension are not necessarily consistent with any of the others. For example, individuals may be attracted most strongly to their same gender, fantasize about both genders, have sexual activity only with the opposite gender, and identify as gay or lesbian. Other individuals may engage in same-gender sexual behavior, fantasize about both genders, but identify as heterosexual. As with all aspects of sexual identity, the dimensions of sexual orientation are influenced by cultural meaning and expectation, by gender, by peer groups, and by other environmental contexts.

Adolescence is the period during which individuals commonly begin to identify their sexual orientation as part of their developing sexual identity. However, this identification process can be profoundly influenced by cultural beliefs and values, by societal and family pressures, or by a lack of similar peers. The majority of adolescents eventually report an orientation toward exclusively heterosexual relationships. For adolescents whose orientation encompasses any same-gender dimensions, the identity process during adolescence can be complicated, especially when community norms disapprove of orientations other than heterosexual. Adolescents who have witnessed harassment or violence directed at gay, lesbian, and bisexual people, for example, may be reluctant to self-identify, even when their attractions and behaviors are exclusively same-gender or bisexual.

The development of sexual orientation as part of sexual identity includes several developmental milestones during late childhood and throughout adolescence. These milestones do not necessarily occur in the same order for everyone, nor are they completed in the same amount of time. They include (1) the realization of romantic or erotic attraction to people of one (or both) genders; (2) erotic daydreaming about one or both genders; (3) romantic partners or dates without sexual activity; (4) sexual activity with people of the preferred gender or genders (also, for some teens, sexual activity with a nonpreferred gender, out of curiosity or through social pressure); (5) self-identification of the orientation that best fits one's current circumstances and understanding; (6) publicly self-identifying that orientation, usually to intimate friends and family first, then the wider social group; and (7) an intimate, committed, sexual relationship with a person of the gender appropriate to one's orientation.

There is no evidence that gay, lesbian, or bisexual adults are more or less likely to create long-term, stable relationships than are heterosexual couples. It should be noted that bisexual adolescents and adults do not generally engage in sexual relationships with both genders concurrently; self-identification as bisexual usually refers to the ability to be attracted to either gender but does not imply that such a person requires partners of both genders, or that one must be equally attracted to and have sexual experience with both genders.

Although the order of these milestones varies greatly among adolescents, adolescents who identify as gay, lesbian, or bisexual tend to publicly self-identify later than heterosexual peers. Without positive gay, lesbian, or bisexual role models or a supportive peer group, sexual minority teens can feel isolated, and they may not share their orientation with anyone for fear of rejection or violence (see Critical Thinking Exercise). When adolescents who would otherwise identify as bisexual can only find a peer group of gay and lesbian teens, they may focus on their same-gender dimensions of orientation and adopt the label of lesbian or gay; later, they may self-label as bisexual. Likewise, some gay and lesbian adolescents may first identify as heterosexual, then bisexual, before identifying as gay or lesbian.

CRITICAL THINKING EXERCISE

Discussing Sexual Orientation with Adolescents

John, a 17-year-old adolescent, comes into the school-based clinic and tells the nurse practitioner that he thinks he is homosexual. What is the most appropriate response for the nurse practitioner?

1. Evidence—Is there sufficient evidence to draw any conclusions about John's sexual orientation at this time?
2. Assumptions—Describe an underlying assumption about each of the following issues:
   a. Sexual orientation in adolescents
   b. Society's reaction to homosexuality
   c. Health care professionals and sexuality
3. What implications and priorities for nursing care can be drawn at this time?
4. Does the evidence support your argument (conclusion)?
5. Are there alternative perspectives to your arguments? What are they?

Development of Self-Concept and Body Image

The sudden growth that takes place in early adolescence creates feelings of confusion for adolescents. They have lost the security of a familiar body and feel uncomfortable with their altered body. Consequently, they may try to either hide their body or advertise it, or they may alternate between the two extremes. Teenagers are acutely aware of their appearance as they begin to acquire images of themselves as adults, but they see discrepancies between their ideal and actual skills and abilities.

Adolescents are continually comparing themselves with their peers and making judgments about their own normality based on these observations. Pubertal children feel most comfortable when they are just like their friends and age-mates. Perceived defects or deviations from the group average are threatening to their idealized image. Any blemish is likely to be magnified out of proportion, and any delay of the visible evidence of maturity is cause for worry. Unfortunately, this is also the time when the hormonal effect of the sebaceous glands produces acne, which creates problems for many adolescents. To the adolescent, even the most insignificant pimple may be viewed as a gross disfigurement. The diagnosis of chronic disease or a permanent physical disability has special significance during adolescence and creates additional stresses for both adolescents with the condition and health care providers.

Experts have determined that the body image established during adolescence is the one that individuals retain throughout life. Much of adolescents' search for identity takes place before a mirror as they try to read from the reflected features just who they are and what they look like to other people. Adolescents practice facial expressions and postures, try out hair arrangements, worry about a pimple, and in other ways attempt to assess the best means to achieve a maximum effect—to reveal the "true self."

The self-concept becomes more differentiated as adolescents acquire a more complex picture of themselves, one that takes situational factors into account. The self-concept gradually becomes more individualized and more distinct from the concepts of others. Although younger teenagers describe themselves in terms of similarities with peers, as adolescence advances, young people describe themselves in terms of their special characteristics.

Responses to Puberty

The response to the physical changes of pubertal growth and development is manifested differently depending on the stage of development. During early adolescence, young adolescents become preoccupied with the rapid changes in their body and are interested in the anatomy, physiology, and function of their sexual organs. Boys must also confront the sexual feelings and tensions that accompany puberty, and the appearance of nocturnal emissions may be puzzling, troublesome, or embarrassing. Unless the boy has been prepared in advance, he may find it difficult to discuss his feelings with his parents and may turn to his friends for information and guidance. Many girls also find the rapid changes in their body to be sources of concern. Some girls perceive the increase in weight and associated fat deposition as evidence of obesity and may indulge in fad diets. Although many girls look forward to menstruation and take this event in stride, others may find the first menstrual period a distressing and frightening event. All teenagers, regardless of gender, are concerned with the question, "Am I normal?" To answer this question, they compare their body with those of their peers and with images in the media. This leads to a great deal of uncertainty about their appearance and attractiveness.

If an adolescent does not enter puberty at the same time as his or her peers, considerable inner conflict may occur. Early-maturing girls and boys have higher rates of sexual risk-taking behaviors, delinquency, and substance abuse than their on-time peers (Costello et al, 2007; Lynne et al, 2007). Nurses who work with adolescents must provide teaching and health care interventions that are appropriate for the adolescent's chronologic and cognitive development rather than the stage of physical maturation.

As growth and development proceed through middle adolescence, the rapid body changes diminish, and the adolescent has time to try to make the body more attractive. Adolescents strive to achieve the perfect body within their own cultural norms. The "right" clothes and hairstyle become very important. By late adolescence the heightened concern with body image has ended and is replaced by a general comfort with the body.

The changes that occur during the early, middle, and late phases of adolescence are summarized in Table 40-1.

Table 40-1 Growth and Development During Adolescence

EARLY ADOLESCENCE (11-14 yr)	MIDDLE ADOLESCENCE (15-17 yr)	LATE ADOLESCENCE (18-20 yr)
Growth		
Rapidly accelerating growth Reaches peak velocity Secondary sex characteristics appear	Growth decelerating in girls Stature reaches 95% of adult height Secondary sex characteristics well advanced	Physically mature Structure and reproductive growth almost complete
Cognition		
Explores newfound ability for limited abstract thought Clumsy groping for new values and energies Comparison of "normality" with peers of same sex	Developing capacity for abstract thinking Enjoys intellectual powers, often in idealistic terms Concern with philosophic, political, and social problems	Established abstract thought Can perceive and act on long-range options Able to view problems comprehensively Intellectual and functional identity established
Identity		
Preoccupied with rapid body changes Trying out of various roles Measurement of attractiveness by acceptance or rejection of peers Conformity to group norms	Modifies body image Very self-centered; increased narcissism Tendency toward inner experience and self-discovery Has a rich fantasy life Idealistic Able to perceive future implications of current behavior and decisions; variable application	Body image and gender-role definition nearly secured Mature sexual identity Phase of consolidation of identity Stability of self-esteem Comfortable with physical growth Social roles defined and articulated
Relationships with Parents		
Defining independence-dependence boundaries Strong desire to remain dependent on parents while trying to detach No major conflicts over parental control	Major conflicts over independence and control Low point in parent-child relationship Greatest push for emancipation; disengagement Final and irreversible emotional detachment from parents; mourning	Emotional and physical separation from parents completed Independence from family with less conflict Emancipation nearly secured
Relationships with Peers		
Seeks peer affiliations to counter instability generated by rapid change Upsurge of close, idealized friendships with members of the same sex Struggle for mastery takes place within peer group	Strong need for identity to affirm self-image Behavioral standards set by peer group Acceptance by peers extremely important—fear of rejection Exploration of ability to attract opposite sex	Peer group recedes in importance in favor of individual friendship Testing of romantic relationships against possibility of permanent alliance Relationships characterized by giving and sharing
Sexuality		
Self-exploration and evaluation Limited dating, usually group Limited intimacy	Multiple plural relationships Internal identification of heterosexuality, homosexual, or bisexual attractions Exploration of "self appeal" Feeling of "being in love" Tentative establishment of relationships	Forms stable relationships and attachment to another Growing capacity for mutuality and reciprocity Dating as a romantic pair May publicly identify as gay, lesbian, or bisexual Intimacy involves commitment rather than exploration and romanticism
Psychologic Health		
Wide mood swings Intense daydreaming Anger outwardly expressed with moodiness, temper outbursts, and verbal insults and name-calling	Tendency toward inner experiences; more introspective Tendency to withdraw when upset or feelings are hurt Vacillation of emotions in time and range Feelings of inadequacy common; difficulty in asking for help	More constancy of emotion Anger more apt to be concealed

Promoting Optimum Health During Adolescence

The major causes of morbidity and mortality in adolescence are not diseases, but health-damaging behaviors. New sources of morbidity in adolescence include injury, depression, violence, sexually transmitted infections, and pregnancy; obesity may begin in childhood or adolescence, but the health consequences are more evident in early and middle adulthood. Health promotion for this age group consists mainly of teaching and guidance to avoid risk-taking activities and health-damaging behaviors. Adolescence provides an opportunity for teenagers to incorporate healthy lifestyle behaviors that will benefit them not only during the teenage years, but also throughout the life span.

Effective health education for adolescents should incorporate a developmentally appropriate, multifaceted approach. Motivational interviewing has been shown to improve adherence to health care advice by using a collaborative approach (Gance-Cleveland, 2007). In this process the adolescent is encouraged to introspectively explore ambivalence and develop solutions for effecting change. Education alone is not enough to change behavior. Effective programs for adolescents must include opportunities to improve communication skills and enhance their social network to make more positive connections (Tuttle, Campbell-Heider, & David, 2006).

As adolescents progress through adolescence, they are able to assume additional responsibility for their own health, including maintaining health practices, taking prescribed medications, keeping appointments, and performing procedures when necessary. Health professionals who work with adolescents should consider the adolescent's increasing independence and responsibility while maintaining privacy and ensuring confidentiality (see Guidelines box and Critical Thinking Exercise). Parents should also respect their teenager's independence and move toward the role of consultant about health issues while also maintaining some level of parental involvement throughout adolescence.

GUIDELINES Interviewing Adolescents

- Ensure confidentiality and privacy; interview adolescent without parents.
- Show concern for adolescent's perspective: "First, I'd like to talk about your main concerns" and "I'd like to know what you think is happening."
- Offer a nonthreatening explanation for the questions you ask: "I'm going to ask a number of questions to help me better understand your health."
- Maintain objectivity; avoid assumptions, judgments, and lectures.
- Ask open-ended questions when possible; move to more directive questions if necessary.
- Begin with less sensitive issues and proceed to more sensitive ones.
- Use language that both the adolescent and you understand. Clarify terms, such as "having sex."
- Restate: reflect back to adolescents what they have said, along with feelings that may be associated with their descriptions.

In response to changes in adolescent morbidity and mortality, the American Medical Association (1997) developed the Guidelines for Adolescent Preventive Services (GAPS), which provide a framework for health care providers to use in their clinical practice. The following discussion provides information on specific GAPS topics and recommendations related to screening, guidance, and immunizations.

Immunizations

Immunization updates are a significant part of adolescent preventive care. Adolescents 11 to 18 years of age should receive a single tetanus-diphtheria–acellular pertussis (Tdap) vaccine if they have received the recommended childhood series of DTaP immunizations. This vaccine is now required because of the increased incidence of pertussis seen in adolescents and adults who were previously immunized with the DTaP series yet developed the condition as adolescents. The adolescent who has received Td but not Tdap vaccine should also receive a single dose of the Tdap vaccine, provided 5 years have elapsed between the Td and Tdap vaccination (American Academy of Pediatrics, Committee on Infectious Diseases, 2006). Meningococcal vaccine (MCV4) should be given to adolescents 11 to 12 years of age or at 15 years of age if previous immunization with MPSV4 occurred in childhood and at least 3 to 5 years have passed since primary immunization. The MCV4 vaccine is now preferred over the MPSV4 vaccine (American Academy of Pediatrics, Committee on Infectious Diseases, 2008). College students living in dormitories are at increased risk for meningococcal disease and should therefore be immunized with MCV4 (American Academy of Pediatrics, Committee on Infectious Diseases, 2005).

The human papillomavirus vaccine series is recommended only for girls based on research results at this time. Additional recommendations may be made for boys if it is determined to be safe and effective. The series may be started as early as 9 years of age, with the second and third doses at 2 months and 6 months, respectively.

With the exception of pregnant teenagers, all adolescents should receive a second measles-mumps-rubella (MMR) vaccine unless they have documentation of two MMR vaccinations during childhood.

All adolescents who have not previously received three doses of hepatitis B vaccine should be vaccinated against hepatitis B virus. The hepatitis A vaccine should be given to all adolescents as part of the routine immunization schedule; the two-dose series may be completed in childhood, and a catch-up schedule for those who have not been previously immunized is recommended. Annual influenza vaccination with either the live attenuated influenza vaccine or trivalent influ-

CRITICAL THINKING EXERCISE

Respecting Privacy

Jamie, a 17-year-old girl, arrives at the adolescent clinic with her mother, Mrs. S, for a routine history and physical examination with the nurse practitioner. As the nurse practitioner walks with Jamie to an examination room, Mrs. S whispers to the nurse practitioner, "I need to speak with you in private." How should the nurse practitioner respond to Mrs. S's request?

1. Evidence—Is there sufficient evidence to formulate a response to Jamie's mother?
2. Assumptions—Describe an underlying assumption about each of the following topics:
   a. The role of the adolescent in health care
   b. The role of the parents in the health of their adolescent
   c. Adolescents and confidentiality
3. What implications for nursing care should be established at this time?
4. Does the evidence support your conclusion?
5. Are there alternative perspectives that you should consider?

evolve Case Study—Interviewing Adolescents

enza vaccine is now encouraged for all children and adolescents. All adolescents should also be assessed for previous history of varicella infection or vaccination. Vaccination with the varicella vaccine is recommended for those with no previous history; for those with no previous infection or history, the varicella vaccine may be given in two doses 4 or more weeks apart to adolescents 13 years or older (American Academy of Pediatrics, Committee on Infectious Diseases, 2008). Any adolescent who has not completed the immunization series for hepatitis A, hepatitis B, poliovirus, and influenza should receive these immunizations according to the latest catch-up schedule (see also Immunizations, Chapter 36).

Nutrition

The rapid and extensive increase in height, weight, muscle mass, and sexual maturity of adolescence is accompanied by increased nutritional requirements. Because nutritional needs are closely related to the increase in body mass, the peak requirements occur in the years of maximum growth, during which the body mass almost doubles. The caloric and protein requirements during this time are higher than at almost any other time of life. As a result of this increased anabolic need, the adolescent is highly sensitive to caloric restrictions.

Current guidelines for caloric intake are provided by a number of sources. The Dietary Reference Intakes provide age-specific guidelines for nutrients (see Chapter 47). Another guideline has been developed by the American Heart Association (2005) aimed at promoting balanced nutrient intake in children and adolescents with an overall decrease in fat intake and discretionary calories or snacks that increase the propensity for obesity and cardiovascular disease. Caloric intake can be tailored to meet the adolescent's increased growth needs and activity level such as involvement in sports. The guidelines also encourage limiting sweetened beverage consumption and moderating caloric intake to activity levels. Another resource for optimal nutrition guidelines is the U.S. Department of Agriculture MyPyramid *(www.mypyramid.gov)*.

Adolescents may normally have sufficient intake of protein to meet their needs, except for people who limit their food intake because of economic problems or in an attempt to lose weight. The need for the minerals calcium, iron, and zinc substantially increases during periods of rapid growth: calcium for skeletal growth, iron for expansion of muscle mass and blood volume, and zinc for the generation of both skeletal and bone tissue. Girls with heavy or frequent menses may be especially susceptible to iron deficiency due to blood loss. Calcium intake from food sources is essential during adolescence to assist in the prevention of osteoporosis. Eventual bone mass is a balance between the amount of bone laid down during adolescence and the amount later lost with aging. Maximum bone mass is also acquired during adolescence; therefore the calcium deposited during these years determines the risk of osteoporosis. Overall, osteoporosis is a result of polygenic and multiple environmental factors such as nutrition, economics, and exercise (Ongphiphadhanakul, 2007). Dietary intervention should promote the regular consumption of breakfast and a balanced intake of a variety of foods.

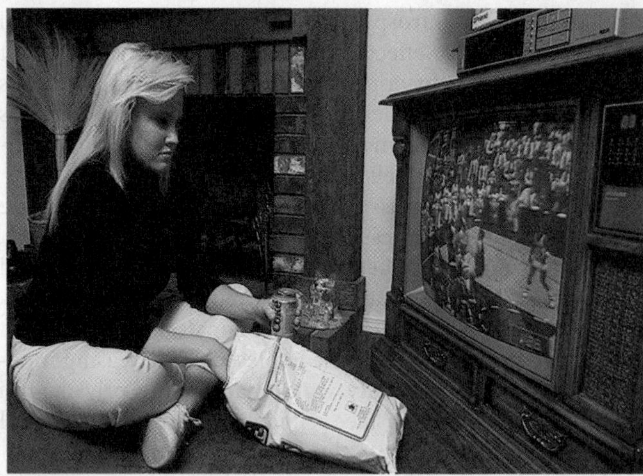

Fig. 40-7 Snacking on empty calories is common among adolescents, especially during inactivity.

Eating Habits and Behavior

Eating and attitudes toward food are primarily family centered during early and middle childhood, and food habits are largely related to cultural and individual family preferences and patterns. With adolescence and the move toward independence, family influences on the individual may change. Adolescent's interests, attitudes, and routines are altered as an increasing number of meals are eaten away from home. These changes are largely a result of the high value that teenagers place on peer acceptability and sociability and an increased amount of time spent away from home. Peers may easily influence the adolescent's eating habits.

Pressure for time and commitments to activities adversely affect the teenager's eating habits. Omitting breakfast or eating a breakfast that is nutritionally poor is frequently a problem. Snacks, usually selected on the basis of accessibility rather than nutritional merit, become more and more a part of the habitual eating pattern during adolescence (Fig. 40-7). Excess intake of calories, sugar, fat, cholesterol, and sodium is common among adolescents and is found in all income and racial or ethnic groups and both genders. Inadequate intake of certain vitamins (folic acid, vitamin B_6, vitamin A) and minerals (iron, calcium, zinc) is also evident, particularly among girls and teenagers of low socioeconomic status. In combination with other factors, these dietary patterns could result in increased risk for obesity and chronic diseases such as heart disease, osteoporosis, and some types of cancer later in life.

Overeating or undereating during adolescence presents special problems. When they experience the normal increase in weight and fat deposition of the growth spurt, teenage girls often resort to dieting. The desire for a slim figure and a fear of becoming "fat" prompt teenage girls to embark on nutritionally inadequate reducing regimens that drain their energy and deprive their growing bodies of essential nutrients. They resort to diets on their own or with peers in an effort to conform. Many adopt current fad diets and are victims of food misinformation. Boys may be less inclined to undereat. They are more concerned about gaining size and strength. However, they tend to eat foods high in calories but low in other essential nutrients.

Obesity has increased significantly among both children and adolescents in the United States. The obesity currently seen is not a result of metabolic disturbances, but of poor dietary habits and sedentary lifestyles. Childhood obesity often results in obesity in adulthood. Adolescent obesity poses both immediate and long-term problems for adolescents. Obesity is directly linked to the development of cardiovascular disease and other chronic illnesses such as type 2 diabetes. Anorexia nervosa (AN) and bulimia nervosa (BN) also commonly occur during the adolescent and young adult years. If left untreated, these disorders, like obesity, can lead to considerable morbidity and mortality. Over the past two decades the overall portion size for foods has increased. The largest portions for most foods are found at fast-food restaurants. However, portion sizes for desserts and hamburgers are reportedly the largest at home (Nielsen & Popkin, 2003). Lifestyle changes necessary for adolescents to lose weight require the involvement of family members who provide support and encourage active participation.

Nursing Care Management

Adolescents should receive at a minimum an annual assessment of weight, height, and BMI for age, plotted on a standard growth chart (see Appendix C). Healthy dietary habits should be discussed with all adolescents. The frequency of eating at fast-food and other restaurants, consumption of sweetened beverages, and consumption of excessive portion sizes should be identified. A growing concern among children and adolescents is the availability of high-fat, high-carbohydrate snack foods and drinks within the school environment, which may further contribute to obesity; such foods compete with school meals yet are favorites of adolescents (Story, Nanney, & Schwartz, 2009). In addition to food intake, the nurse should assess the level of physical activity and sedentary behaviors. Readiness to change; environmental supports and barriers; and family history of diabetes, heart disease, and early stroke must be considered when planning nutritional education and guidance. Nurses in the school setting can assist in advocating for comprehensive nutritional services for preschool through grade 12 students. Comprehensive nutrition education with access to nutritious meals and snacks and physical activity at school will begin to reverse the trend of childhood obesity (Briggs, Safaii, & Beall, 2003).

To help teenagers select a nutritious diet, it is best to begin with their present diet and actively involve them in the process. Adolescents do not respond well to judgmental attitudes and dislike lectures, but they do respond when their independence is respected and they are given the opportunity to make their own decisions regarding food choices.

In general, adolescents are body conscious and concerned about their appearance. Concrete messages about the relationship between an attractive appearance and the benefits of a healthy lifestyle are most effective. However, helping adolescents arrive at a decision for change is more difficult than providing information. They respond best when the counselor provides straightforward information, uses instructional methods that actively involve them, talks *with* them and not *at* them, and listens to what they have to say.

Sleep and Rest

Adolescents vary in their need for sleep and rest. Rapid physical growth, the tendency toward overexertion, and the overall increased activity of this age contribute to fatigue in adolescents. During growth spurts the need for sleep is increased. Their propensity for staying up late makes it difficult to arise in the morning, and they may sleep late at every opportunity. Adequate sleep and rest at this time are important to a total health regimen.

Exercise and Activity

Although today's youth are said to be less fit than children 20 years ago, adolescents probably spend more time and energy practicing and participating in sports activities than members of any other age group. Many adolescents participate in sports within school settings (Fig. 40-8). School-based, health-oriented physical education may provide both immediate effects of the activity and sustained effects through encouragement of lifelong activity patterns. High schools continue to cut physical education classes, with only half of high school students attending at least one day of physical education classes in 2007. Less than half of students attended these classes daily, and the majority of classes included only 20 minutes of exercise (Centers for Disease Control and Prevention, 2008). To improve health outcomes, school-age children and adolescents should engage in 60 minutes or more of moderate to vigorous physical activity daily (Strong et al, 2005).

The practice of sports, games, and even dancing contributes significantly to growth and development, the education process, and better health. These activities provide exercise for growing muscles, interactions with peers, and a socially acceptable means of enjoying stimulation and conflict. In addition, competitive activities help the teenager in the process of self-appraisal and the development of self-respect and concern for others. Because physical fitness appears to be a major influence on one's lifelong health status, children and adolescents should be encouraged to participate in activities

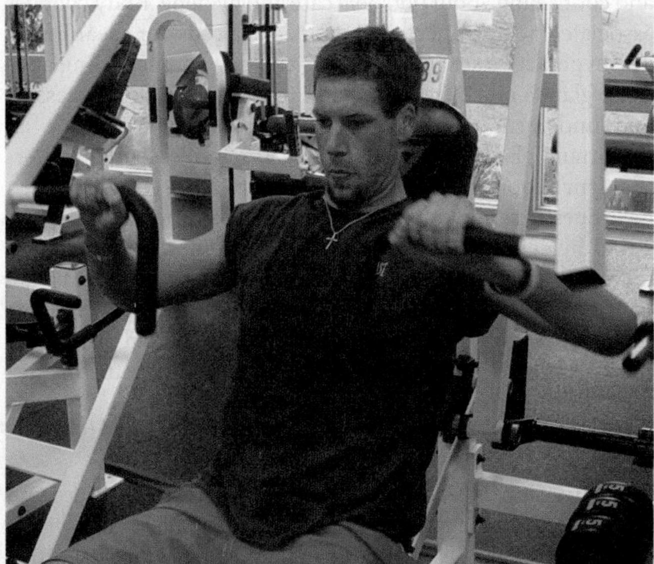

Fig. 40-8 Adolescents should be encouraged to participate in activities that contribute to lifelong physical fitness.

that contribute to lifelong physical fitness. Nurses can encourage participation as a way to promote health and build self-esteem. However, adolescents should not be encouraged to engage in physical activities that are beyond their physical or emotional capacity (see Health Problems Related to Sports Participation, Chapter 39).

Dental Health

Dental health should not be neglected during adolescence; the rate of caries formation may be significant due to poor nutritional habits (e.g., increased intake of cariogenic substances) and lack of compliance with routine oral hygiene. Flossing and regular tooth brushing in adolescence serve to remove plaque and prevent periodontal disease. Additional oral health considerations for adolescents include the initiation of tobacco use, pregnancy, eating disorders, increased risk for traumatic dental injury and periodontal disease, and increased awareness of appearance (American Academy of Pediatric Dentistry, 2009). Dental care is an aspect of preventive care that substantial proportions of children in the United States do not receive.

Early adolescence is usually when corrective orthodontic appliances are worn, and these may be a source of embarrassment and concern; however, in some cases these may be considered trendy, depending on the peers' attitudes toward their cosmetic effects. Reassurance regarding the temporary nature of the annoyance and anticipation of an improved appearance help make the inconvenience tolerable. It is also important to reinforce the orthodontist's directions regarding use and care of the appliances and to emphasize careful attention to toothbrushing during this time (see also Chapters 37 and 39).

Fluoride continues to be important, but after the age of 16 years this need may be met through fluoridated water and prescribed compounds (instead of via systemic supplementation).

Personal Care

The body-conscious teenager is highly amenable to discussion and counseling about personal care and hygiene. Body changes associated with puberty bring special needs for cleanliness. The hyperactive sebaceous glands and newly functioning apocrine glands make frequent bathing or showering a necessity, and underarm deodorants and antiperspirants assume an important place in personal care. The adolescent discovers that hair requires more frequent shampooing, and girls often have questions about hair removal, use of cosmetics, and menstrual hygiene. Peer group discussions center on the advantages of particular products or methods. Adolescents are continually bombarded with messages from the media regarding the best way to enhance their popularity and attractiveness. Nurses are in a position to help them evaluate the relative merits of commercial products.

Vision

Regular vision testing is an important part of health care and supervision during adolescence. During this time, visual refractive difficulties reach a high level that is not exceeded until the fifth decade of life. The increased demands of schoolwork make adequate vision essential for academic success. Consequently, teenagers are more likely to be referred for visual evaluation. The need for corrective lenses can create psychologic problems for teenagers if they believe that glasses spoil their appearance or do not fit their body image. Contact lenses may be a preferred solution; a wide variety of lenses are now available at fairly reasonable prices. For some, the impact of a visual defect, no matter how slight, may be stressful.

Hearing

Considerable concern has focused on current teenage practices that cause hearing damage. Cochlear damage from relatively continuous exposure to the loud sound levels of music has been documented. The popularity of compact personal music players and compact disc (CD) players with lightweight earphones are of particular concern to health care professionals. When these units are used for extended periods, permanent hearing loss can occur. Although appeals for more judicious use are not always successful, teenagers should be informed of the risk. Efforts directed toward legislating legal limits to the noise exposure that can be achieved through the sets may be another possible solution. (See Chapter 42 for a discussion of noise-related hearing loss.)

Posture

Many adolescents demonstrate altered posture. Rapid skeletal growth is often associated with slower muscular growth, and as a result, some teenagers may appear awkward or slump and fail to stand or sit upright. However, some postural defects of adolescence require early medical intervention. Scoliosis is a defect of the spine that occurs frequently in adolescence and is more common in girls than in boys (see Idiopathic Scoliosis, Chapter 54). The majority of the cases are idiopathic, and the defect manifests as a painless curvature of the spine. Fortunately, most of these spinal curvatures will not require treatment. However, because there is no way to predict which curvatures will progress, all curvatures of the spine should be referred for further evaluation.

Body Art

Body art (piercing and tattooing) is used to assist with adolescent identity formation. The skin has become the latest source of parent-adolescent conflict. The adolescent often seeks body art as an expression of his or her personal identity and style. Tattoos are often obtained to mark significant life events such as new relationships, births, and deaths. Piercing the ear, nose, nipple, navel, penis, or tongue may sometimes create a health problem. It is a nursing responsibility to caution girls and boys against having piercings performed by friends, mothers, or themselves. Although most cases of piercing are accompanied by few if any serious side effects, there is always a danger of complications such as infection, abscess formation, cyst or keloid formation, bleeding, dermatitis, or metal allergy. Using the same unsterilized needle to pierce body parts of multiple teenagers presents the same risk of human immunodeficiency virus (HIV), hepatitis C, and hepatitis B virus transmission as occurs with other needle-sharing activities.

A qualified operator using proper sterile technique should perform the procedure. This is especially important if the adolescent has a history of diabetes, allergies, or skin disorders.

Adolescents should be informed about the approximate time for healing after body piercing and the care of the pierced area during and after healing. Some body sites require extra precautions. For example, cartilage (ear, nose) has a poor blood supply and heals slowly and scars easily; nipple piercing puts the adolescent at risk for breast abscess. Penile piercing often penetrates the urethra, requiring the male to sit to void thereafter. Finally, migration of the piercing is common with naval and other flat skin surface piercing. Piercing guns should not be used for piercing anything other than the earlobe because guns place the piercing too deeply.

It is estimated that 3% to 5% of people in Western society have a tattoo and that 13% of the population in the United States has at least one tattoo. Studies of distinct populations of young adults and adolescents report body art rates as high as 23% (Braverman, 2006). Professionals as well as amateur artists administer tattoos. The risk to the adolescent receiving a tattoo is low. The greatest risk is for the tattoo artist who comes in contact with the client's blood. Adolescents who are amateur tattoo artists benefit from discussions about Standard Precautions and the hepatitis B vaccination. Many states either have no regulations or do not enforce existing regulations of piercing and tattooing facilities. The local health department is a source of information about local regulatory requirements. The Centers for Disease Control and Prevention has an excellent website that outlines safety concerns for persons performing and receiving body art *(www.cdc.gov/Features/BodyArt)*.

Tanning

The quest for an attractive appearance leads many teenagers to excessive sunbathing and artificial means for tanning. However, this practice has serious long-term risks, and the adolescent should be educated regarding the detrimental effects of sunlight on the skin (see Sunburn, Chapter 53). Long-term effects include premature aging of the skin; increased risk of skin cancer; and, in susceptible individuals, phototoxic reactions.

The increasing popularity of artificial tanning has prompted concern among health professionals regarding the use of sunlamps and tanning machines. The long-term effects of tanning machines are similar to those of the sun; dermatologists do not recommend tanning by these means. Those who insist on using tanning equipment should be warned that goggles must be worn in tanning booths to prevent serious corneal burning. Education on the use of sunscreens, including hypoallergenic products, with a sun protective factor (SPF) of at least 15 and a nonalcohol base without lanolin, parobens, or fragrance is important. Broad-spectrum sunscreens that protect against both ultraviolet A and B are the most effective. Self-tanning creams safely simulate the appearance of a tan; however, teens using these products should be cautioned that sun protection is still required. Targeting health education messages to adolescents and incorporating educational components relating to sun protection behaviors in school health curricula and in health care visits will increase adolescent knowledge and awareness.

A large cross-sectional study of 12- to 18-year-olds in the United States found that teens are not following these recommendations; 34% used sunscreen routinely in the past summer and 14% used a tanning bed at least once (Geller et al, 2002). Cutaneous melanoma, the most common fatal form of skin cancer, is associated with ultraviolet light exposure and continues to affect a significant amount of individuals yearly (Geller & Annas, 2003; Leiter & Garbe, 2008; Rigel, 2008).

Stress Reduction

The multiple changes occurring in adolescence can result in great stress (Fig. 40-9 and Box 40-2). Adolescents are faced with pressures from peers that often involve flouting adult authority and taking serious health risks. Health risks include pressures for sexual experimentation and use of drugs, alcohol, and tobacco, as well as potentially dangerous physical activities.

Early-maturing girls and late-maturing children are especially sensitive to the stresses of being different from their peers. Many feel intense anxiety over their identity. Both early- and late-maturing children feel out of place among their classmates, but slow-maturing children appear to suffer the most pronounced inner turmoil and may be hesitant to voice their concerns.

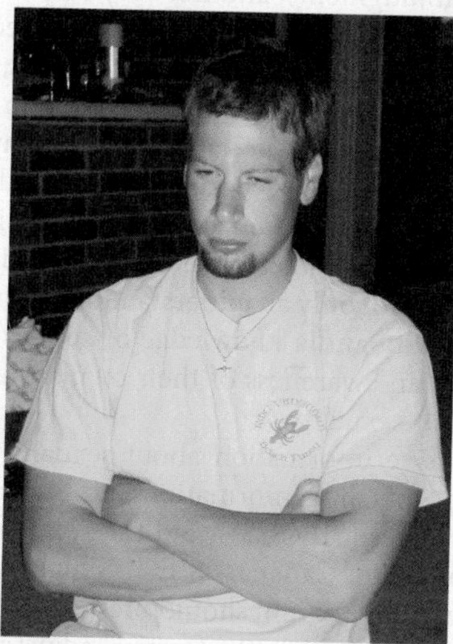

Fig. 40-9 Adolescents use being alone as a method of coping with stress. Health care professionals need to assess whether this indicates clinical depression.

BOX 40-2 Areas of Stress in Adolescence

- Body image
- Sexuality conflicts
- Scholastic pressures
- Competitive pressures
- Relationships with parents
- Relationships with siblings
- Relationships with peers
- Dating
- Finances
- Decisions about present and future roles
- Career planning
- Ideologic conflicts

Sexuality Education and Guidance

Contemporary adolescents are constantly exposed to sexual symbolism and erotic stimulation from the mass media. At the same time, the development of primary and secondary sex characteristics and the increased sensitivity of the genitalia produce thoughts and fantasies about sexual relationships. Sexual aspects of interpersonal relationships become particularly important. Societal expectations push adolescents toward dating, and their own inner sex drive urges them toward exploration. This is often exacerbated by peer pressure to be involved in sexual relationships and the adolescents' need to fit in.

North American society continues to do a poor job of educating adolescents about pubertal growth and development. Omar, McElderry, and Zakharia (2003) found that 36% of males and 2% of females never were spoken to about pubertal development or sexuality issues. Girls received sex education at a mean age of 13 years and boys at a mean age of 15 years. A large portion of their knowledge relating to sex is acquired from their peers, television, Internet, movies, and magazines. In addition, information obtained from their parents may be inaccurate. As a result, the information they accumulate may be incomplete, inaccurate, riddled with cultural and moral judgments, and not very helpful.

The responsibility for providing sexuality education has been assumed by parents; schools; churches; community agencies such as Planned Parenthood Federation of America*; and health professionals, especially nurses. Many adolescents perceive nurses, especially school nurses, as individuals who possess important information and who are willing to discuss sex with them. To be able to discuss the topic adequately, nurses must have not only an understanding of the physiologic aspects of sexuality and a knowledge of cultural and societal values, but also an awareness of their own attitudes, feelings, and biases about sexuality.

Comprehensive information about sexuality education is offered by the Sexuality Information and Education Council of the United States (SIECUS)† and the Sex Information and Education Council of Canada.‡ SIECUS maintains that every sexuality education program should present the topic from six aspects: biologic, social, health, personal adjustments and attitudes, interpersonal associations, and the establishment of values.

Whether nurses counsel young people on an individual basis, in mixed groups, or in groups segregated by gender makes little difference. Ideally, boys and girls should be able to discuss sexuality objectively with one another and in groups, but this is not always possible. The differences in the rate of maturation between boys and girls and between different members of the same sex often make it desirable to discuss certain aspects of sexuality in segregated groups. As a rule, the need for separate discussion groups diminishes as young people mature.

*434 W. 33rd St., New York, NY 10001; 212-541-7800; www.plannedparenthood.org.

†90 John St., Suite 704, New York, NY 10038; 212-819-9770; www.siecus.org.

‡850 Coxwell Ave., Toronto, Ontario M4C 5R1; 416-466-5304; www.sieccan.org.

Sexuality education should consist of instruction concerning normal body functions and should be presented in a straightforward manner using correct terminology. When discussing sex and sexual activities, nurses should use simple but correct language, not street language, highly scientific terminology, or euphemisms. Once the meanings of biologic terms such as *uterus, testicles,* and *vagina* are understood, most teenagers prefer to use them in their discussions.

Many girls arrive at menarche with ambivalent attitudes, myths, and illogical beliefs. Even girls adequately prepared for menstruation do not always understand its relationship to the total process of reproduction. Many are under the incorrect impression that the "safe" time for sexual intercourse is midway between menstrual periods.

Teenagers' curiosity and desire for information extend beyond the need for anatomic and physiologic knowledge. They need to know more than the mechanics of conception, pregnancy, and birth. Adolescents, girls in particular, want answers to questions such as "What is it like?" "Does it hurt?" "What happens when ...?" and "Is it all right if you ...?" Boys are often concerned about the fallacy that a relationship exists between penis size and sexual function. They need reassurance that masturbation is a normal and common practice, that some degree of homosexuality is not unusual in early adolescence, and that oral-genital relations can be normal substitutes for intercourse.

Teenagers need to discuss intercourse, alternative methods of sexual satisfaction, and how to resist peer pressure. With the increased incidence of sexually transmitted infections, especially HIV infection, the topic of "safe sex," especially abstinence or the use of condoms and abstinence, is essential. Role-playing can help teenagers learn effective approaches to dealing with difficult situations. Sex and sexuality cannot be taught without discussions of mature decision making, sexual responsibility, and values clarification. Adolescents may receive inaccurate and ambiguous messages regarding sexual behavior; for example, an adolescent may be told that abstinence from vaginal intercourse will prevent transmission of a sexually transmitted infection. Accurate and unbiased information regarding sexual practices should be provided in a setting where the adolescent feels comfortable asking questions without being degraded or made to feel uncomfortable.

Adolescents need role models and life experiences with delayed gratification. Most important, they need problem-solving experience and decision-making skills so that they can anticipate the positive and negative outcomes of a decision. With these types of assistance, teenagers can become sexually responsible young adults.

Injury Prevention

Physical injuries are the greatest single cause of death in the adolescent age group and claim more lives than all other causes combined. The most vulnerable ages are the years 15 to 24, when accidental injuries account for about 60% of deaths in boys and 40% of deaths in girls. These figures remain fairly constant from year to year and are significant because almost all fatal injuries are preventable.

During adolescence, peak physical, sensory, and psychomotor function gives teenagers a feeling of strength and confidence that they have never experienced before, and the physiologic changes of puberty give impetus to many basic instinctual forces. One manifestation of this is an increase in energy that simply must be discharged through action, often at the expense of logical thinking and other control mechanisms. Their propensity for risk-taking behavior plus feelings of indestructibility makes adolescents especially prone to injuries. Some of the developmental characteristics of teenagers and the common injuries associated with this age group are outlined in Box 40-3.

Vehicle-Related Injuries

The adolescent's newly acquired ability to drive and the normal developmental need for independence and freedom make the automobile an attractive part of an adolescent's life. Thirty-six percent of all teen deaths in the United States are the result of motor vehicle crashes (Centers for Disease Control and Prevention, 2006). Many factors contribute to the higher rate of crashes among teen drivers, including lacking driving experience and maturity, following too closely, driving too fast, having other teen passengers in the car, and using alcohol (Williams & Ferguson, 2002). Approximately 40 states have enacted graduated driver license laws with restrictions on younger adolescent driving. In Missouri, for example, the adolescent between 15 and 18 years of age must obtain an instruction permit and then an intermediate license before obtaining a full driver license. The goal is to increase the adolescent driver's driving experience before giving her or him a free rein to drive without more driver training in order to decrease the number of traffic fatalities among teenagers. According to data from the 2007 Youth Risk Behavior Survey, 11% of adolescent respondents reported not wearing a seat belt in a car, 29%

BOX 40-3 Injury Prevention During Adolescence

Developmental Abilities Related to Risk of Injury

Need for independence and freedom
Testing independence
Age permitted to drive a motor vehicle (varies)
Inclination for risk taking
Feeling of indestructibility
Need for discharging energy, often at expense of logical thinking and other control mechanisms
Strong need for peer approval
Desire to attempt hazardous feats
Peak incidence for practice and participation in sports
Access to more complex tools, objects, and locations
Can assume responsibility for own actions

Injury Prevention

Motor or Nonmotor Vehicles

Pedestrian—Emphasize and encourage safe pedestrian behavior.

- At night, walk with a friend.
- If someone is following you, go to nearest place with people.
- Do not walk in secluded areas; take well-traveled walkways.

Passenger—Promote appropriate behavior while riding in a motor vehicle.

Driver—Provide competent driver education; encourage judicious use of vehicle; discourage drag racing, "playing chicken"; discourage text messaging; maintain vehicle in proper condition (brakes, tires, etc.).

Teach and promote safety and maintenance of two-wheeled vehicles

Encourage wearing of safety apparel such as helmet, long trousers.

Reinforce the dangers of drugs, including alcohol, when operating a motor vehicle.

Falls

Teach and encourage general safety measures in all activities.

Drowning

Teach nonswimmer to swim.

Teach basic rules of water safety:

- Judicious selection of place to swim
- Sufficient water depth for diving
- Swimming with companion
- Wear life vest with water sports (e.g., boating, skiing)
- Avoid swimming, boating, or other water sports after alcohol consumption

Burns

Reinforce proper behavior in areas involving contact with burn hazards (gasoline, electric wires, fires).

Advise regarding excessive exposure to natural or artificial sunlight (ultraviolet burn).

Discourage smoking.

Encourage use of sunscreen.

Poisoning

Educate in hazards of drug use, including alcohol.

Bodily Damage

Promote acquisition of proper instruction in sports and use of sports equipment.

Instruct in safe use of and respect for firearms and other devices with potential danger (e.g., power tools, fireworks).

Provide and encourage use of protective equipment when using potentially hazardous devices (e.g., motorcycles, power tools).

Promote access to and/or provision of safe sports and recreational facilities.

Be alert for signs of depression (potential suicide).

Discourage use and availability of hazardous sports equipment (e.g., trampoline, surfboards).

Instruct regarding proper use of corrective devices (e.g., glasses, contact lenses, hearing aids).

Encourage and foster judicious application of safety principles and prevention.

reported riding in a vehicle with someone who had been drinking alcohol, and 10.5% reported driving a car while drinking alcohol (Centers for Disease Control and Prevention, 2008).

Because of the significant increase in the number of accidents when adolescents drive at night, many states have effectively enacted driving curfews, decreasing fatal crashes by 38% and crashes involving injury by 40% for adolescents (Baker, Chen, & Li, 2007).

Nurses should educate teenagers and their parents about the risk of driving while drinking alcohol or when intoxicated, or of riding in an automobile with a drunk driver. Many families have developed a plan to arrange a no-questions-asked ride home to prevent an adolescent from riding with a drunk driver. Families should also require adolescents to log several hours of supervised practice driving before taking the car out alone. The major risk for death in a motor vehicle accident is failure to use a safety restraint. Teenage seat belt use, especially among boys, is lower than adult seat belt usage. Belt use as a passenger is low for teens even when the driver is an adult. Continued efforts to ensure teenage seat belt use should be focused at the individual educational level and through tough enforcement laws (Williams, McCartt, & Geary, 2003).

Nonautomotive Vehicle Injuries

The increasing use of motorized bicycles, all-terrain vehicles, jet skis, and snowmobiles has caused an increase in injuries among teenagers below the legal age for driving automobiles. Many adolescents ride bicycles without helmets and without lights at night, and the overwhelming majority of deaths from bicycle injuries (primarily head injuries) involve teenagers.

Firearms

Firearms are the major cause of intentional fatal injuries in the United States. Adolescence is the peak age for being either a victim or an offender in an injury involving a firearm. Gun carrying among adolescents is on the rise and is not limited to the stereotypic inner-city youth. Family members and acquaintances are a common source of guns for young people. Gun availability in the home is strongly linked to unintentional death and injury to children (Glatt, 2005). In addition, the presence of a gun in the home increases the risk of adolescent suicide and homicide. All families should be assessed for the presence of a gun in the home and informed of the increased risk for suicide and homicide. When guns are present in the home, families must take preventive action to be certain that the guns are never loaded, that they are locked up in a safe place, and that ammunition is stored and locked up separately in a location where only appropriate adults have access to it.

Nonpowder Firearms

Guns that do not use powder (e.g., air rifles, BB guns), although viewed as toys by many, account for almost as many injuries as powder guns. The regulations regarding nonpowder guns are relaxed; they can be purchased legally by adolescents and are labeled as suitable for children as young as 8 years of age. Few states regulate their use. Nurses should act as child advocates and urge passage of laws to regulate the sale of these potentially dangerous "toys."

Sports Injuries

Because the degree of physical maturity, size, coordination, and endurance varies greatly among adolescents of the same age, sports competition among young people who differ greatly in strength and agility is unfair and hazardous. Matching candidates for sports should be done relative to physical maturity, height, weight, and physical fitness and skills, particularly in a sport involving rigorous body contact. Age is a less important consideration.

Every sport has some potential for injury, whether one participates in serious competition or for pure enjoyment. Overuse injuries are common in adolescents and result in more time missed from the activity than fractures. A large number of severe or fatal injuries occur to youths who are not physically prepared for the activity. The increase in strength and vigor in adolescence may tempt adolescents to overextend themselves, especially boys who are urged on by teammates or stimulated by the admiration of female observers. The range of injuries sustained in sports or recreational activities can involve any part of the body and extend from relatively minor cuts, bruises, and abrasions to totally incapacitating central nervous system injuries or death. The leading cause of serious sports injuries among boys is participation in football, whereas most girls are injured while participating in gymnastics and cheerleading. With the increase in girl's competitive sports in high schools in the United States, there has been an increase in sports-related injuries among this population.

Nursing Care Management

Injury prevention is an ongoing part of nursing responsibility throughout the childhood years. Anticipatory guidance to parents and children regarding the expected problems and hazards related to growth and development does not end as children approach maturity. They need education in basic safety precautions and instruction in skills required in the performance of activities such as sports, instruction in handling motor vehicles, proper protective equipment, and instruction in proper maintenance of equipment. During adolescence, however, health and safety education and guidance are more effective when the young people are involved directly. Parents and health professionals can emphasize the importance of safety during performance of activities and the proper conditioning and preparation for sports.

Prevention can occur on a variety of levels. Safety advocacy, changes in public policy, and legislation can curtail injuries. Examples of such approaches are laws that mandate wearing seat belts, requiring helmets be worn while driving moving vehicles other than automobiles, keeping the legal drinking age at 21 years, and instituting curfews for teen drivers. In addition to improving the environment, health education for teenagers and significant adults is essential. Helping adolescents understand their need for engaging in risky behavior, exploring possible negative outcomes, and weighing possible alternatives are critical components of injury prevention.

Anticipatory Guidance—Care of Families

Both adolescents and their parents are often confused and perplexed about the changes and behavior of this stage of development. Parents need support and guidance to help them through this trying time. They need to understand the changes taking place and to accept the expected behaviors that accompany the process of detachment. Parents may need help to "let go" and to promote the changed relationship from one of dependence to one of mutuality (see Patient Teaching box).

PATIENT TEACHING Guidance During Adolescence

Encourage Parents to:

- Accept adolescent as a unique individual
- Respect adolescent's ideas, likes and dislikes, and wishes
- Be involved with school functions and attend adolescent's performances, whether it be a sporting event or a school play
- Listen and try to be open to teenager's views, even when they disagree with parental views
- Avoid criticism about no-win topics
- Provide opportunity for choosing options and accept natural consequences of these choices
- Allow young person to learn by doing, even when choices and methods differ from those of adults
- Provide adolescent with clear, reasonable limits
- Clarify house rules and consequences for breaking them
- Let society's rules and consequences teach responsibility outside the home
- Allow increasing independence within limitations of safety and well-being
- Be available but avoid pressing teenager too far
- Respect adolescent's privacy
- Try to share adolescent's feelings of joy or sorrow
- Respond to feelings, as well as words
- Be available to answer questions, give information, and provide companionship
- Try to make communication clear
- Avoid comparisons with siblings
- Assist adolescent in selecting appropriate career goals and preparing for adult role
- Welcome adolescent's friends into the home and treat them with respect
- Provide unconditional love
- Be willing to apologize when mistaken

Be Aware That Adolescents:

- Are subject to turbulent, unpredictable behavior
- Are struggling for independence
- Are extremely sensitive to feelings and behavior that affect them
- May receive a different message from what was sent
- Consider friends extremely important
- Have a strong need to belong

SPECIAL HEALTH PROBLEMS

Disorders Related to the Reproductive System

Amenorrhea

Menarche, or the first menstrual period, occurs relatively late in female pubertal development. Although girls vary in the onset and rate of progression of pubertal development, the sequence and tempo should be the same. When an adolescent is seen with a complaint of absence of menses, a careful history of the timing of her pubertal development will help determine if there is a need for further evaluation or if reassurance is all that is necessary.

Primary amenorrhea is an absence of secondary sex characteristics and no uterine bleeding by 14 to 15 years of age, or absence of uterine bleeding with secondary sex characteristics by 16 years of age (Master-Hunter & Heiman, 2006). No uterine bleeding after attaining sexual maturity rating 5 (Tanner; see Figs. 40-1 and 40-2) for 1 year, or after breast development for 4 years, is also considered primary amenorrhea (American Academy of Pediatrics & American College of Obstetricians and Gynecologists, 2006). The cause of primary amenorrhea may be anatomic, hormonal, genetic, or idiopathic. A thorough patient and family history and physical examination will provide clues to the etiology.

Secondary amenorrhea is defined as the absence of menses for 6 months or at least three cycles after menstruation was previously established. Irregular menstrual cycles are common within the first year or two after menarche. These early cycles may be anovulatory, resulting in regular, irregular, or absent bleeding; however, cycle lengths outside the range of 21 to 45 days should be investigated (American Academy of Pediatrics & American College of Obstetricians and Gynecologists, 2006). Girls with a later onset of menarche will take longer to establish regular ovulatory cycles.

Pregnancy is the most common cause of secondary amenorrhea and should be ruled out in both types of amenorrhea, even if the adolescent denies sexual activity. Other factors that disturb the hypothalamic-pituitary-gonadal axis and cause secondary amenorrhea include physical or emotional stress; sudden environmental change; hyperthyroidism or hypothyroidism; polycystic ovary disease; chronic illness; extreme weight loss or gain; intensive exercise; AN or BN; ovarian disturbance; and extrinsic pharmacologic agents, especially phenothiazines, contraceptive steroids, and heroin.

Dysmenorrhea

A certain amount of discomfort during the first day or two of the menstrual flow is extremely common. Most girls experience cramping, abdominal pain, backache, and leg ache, but in a few cases the pain is intolerable and incapacitating. *Primary dysmenorrhea* is painful menses not related to any pelvic disease. *Secondary dysmenorrhea* is defined as painful menses with a pathologic condition such as endometriosis, salpingitis, or congenital anomalies of the müllerian system.

Primary dysmenorrhea usually begins at the time of menarche or within 6 to 12 months. The pain begins with menstrual flow or hours before the onset of bleeding each month, usually continuing for 48 to 72 hours. The exact etiology is widely debated. The pain is clearly related to ovulatory cycles. The overproduction of uterine prostaglandins has been implicated, and women with dysmenorrhea have higher levels of prostaglandins. Overproduction of vasopressin (a hormone that stimulates the contraction of muscular tissue) may also contribute to dysmenorrhea.

A careful history should include the onset of symptoms, the duration, type of pain and relationship to menstrual flow, age at menarche, family history of dysmenorrhea, and sexual history. The nurse should also ask about previous treatment that has been tried, including dosages of medications. Associated symptoms such as nausea, vomiting, diarrhea, and leg and back pain are helpful for diagnosis and treatment. Depending on the results of the history, the physical examination may include a gynecologic examination.

Therapeutic Management

First-line treatment for adolescents with dysmenorrhea is the administration of nonsteroidal antiinflammatory drugs that block the formation of prostaglandins for 2 or 3 days of the menstrual cycle. The girl should be instructed to begin the medication at the first sign of cramping or bleeding. Girls with vomiting at the time of menstruation benefit from beginning the medication 1 or 2 days before the onset of their menses. The medication should be taken with food.

Cyclic estrogen therapy and oral contraceptives are also effective. Simple exercises such as pelvic rocking, assuming the knee-chest position, and breathing exercises may be beneficial. Adequate personal hygiene, participation in regular activities, and methods to decrease stress should be discussed with the adolescent. Dietary changes, supplements, and herbal medications are often used to treat dysmenorrhea. Randomized controlled clinical trials have demonstrated that vitamins B_1 and E are effective in the treatment of dysmenorrhea (Dennehy, 2006).

Nursing Care Management

All adolescent girls need reassurance that menstruation is a normal function. When nurses are asked for advice regarding menstrual problems, they have a valuable opportunity to engage in health teaching concerning menstrual physiology and hygiene, as well as the importance of a well-balanced diet, exercise, and general health maintenance. Health teaching can dispel myths about menstruation and femininity. When assessment indicates a potential problem and the need for evaluation, referral to an appropriate practitioner, health service, or clinic may be necessary.

One of the most difficult experiences facing the adolescent girl is the gynecologic examination. Whether it is her first experience or not, she is often filled with apprehension. Almost all adolescents are extremely self-conscious about their bodies and the changes taking place. They need continuing support in the form of anticipatory guidance regarding what to expect and suggestions of what to do to relax during the procedure. Most girls favor a semisitting position, which has the additional advantage of allowing eye contact during the procedure. Sometimes a pillow helps the patient feel more comfortable and less vulnerable. The provision of a mirror for the girl to see what is taking place if she so desires helps the examiner explain various aspects of anatomy. When possible, it is important to respect the adolescent's request for a female provider.

Vaginitis

Vaginitis can be caused by physical, chemical, or infectious agents. Physical causes may include a forgotten tampon; chemical irritants include bubble bath, douching, deodorant pads, and tampons. Removing the offending material or discontinuing use of the irritating substance is usually all that is necessary to treat physical or chemical vaginitis. Infectious vaginitis can be caused by *Candida* fungi (yeast), *Trichomonas* protozoa parasites, or bacteria. Diagnosis is confirmed with microscopic evaluation of vaginal secretions. Treatment varies depending on the infectious agent.

Health teaching is important in the prevention and management of vaginitis. Adolescent girls need reassurance that increased vaginal mucus can occur at the time of ovulation, before menstruation, or with sexual excitement. Many teenage girls mistake these variations as signs of infection. Girls should be taught to wipe from front to back after toileting and to realize that vaginitis can result from irritation, foreign objects, and sexual activity. Nurses should stress the importance of a medical evaluation to determine the exact cause.

Disorders of the Male Reproductive System

Most obvious anomalies, such as hypospadias, hydrocele, phimosis, and cryptorchidism, have been identified and corrective measures instituted during early childhood. The most frequent problems related to the reproductive organs in later childhood are (1) infections, such as urethritis (see Urinary Tract Infection, Chapter 50); (2) hematuria; (3) penile problems, such as nonretractable foreskin in uncircumcised males, carcinoma, and trauma; (4) scrotal conditions, such as varicocele (elongation, dilation, and tortuosity of the veins superior to the testicle); and (5) testicular torsion (a condition in which the testicle hangs free from its vascular structures, which can result in partial or complete venous occlusion with rotation).

Tumors of the testes are not common, and not all testicular tumors are cancerous, but when one is manifested in adolescence, immediate evaluation is required. Testicular cancer is the most common solid tumor in men 20 to 34 years of age with a higher incidence in Caucasians than in African-Americans (Gray & Moore, 2009). The usual presenting symptom for testicular cancer is a heavy, hard, painless mass (either smooth or nodular) the size of a pea that is palpated on the front or the side of the testis. Additional symptoms may include testicular enlargement, groin pain, or sudden accumulation of fluid or blood in the scrotum. Treatment depends on the tumor stage and type and may involve surgical removal of the affected testicle (orchiectomy), often followed by radiation and chemotherapy (Gray & Moore, 2009).

Nursing Care Management

The adolescent boy is extremely self-conscious about his changing body and needs preparation for a genital examination. The most successful approach is to assume a matter-of-fact attitude toward the examination, explain precisely what will take place, and maintain a continuous commentary about what is being done and the findings at each phase of the examination.

The routine health assessment of every adolescent boy should include teaching about testicular cancer and how to perform a testicular self-examination (TSE) every month. This rare malignancy is curable if detected early. Nurses are in an ideal position to teach TSE in a manner that is respectful of the adolescent boy's anxieties and promotes early treatment (see Critical Thinking Exercise).

CRITICAL THINKING EXERCISE

Testicular Self-Examination

At a recent faculty meeting, Paul, the pediatric nurse practitioner who runs the school-based health clinic, presented his plan for a class on testicular self-examination (TSE) to be delivered to the sophomore boys. Several teachers questioned the value of providing such a class when time to deliver content relating to "routine academic subjects" is limited. What important issues regarding testicular cancer and TSE should Paul use to justify providing this class to the sophomore boys?

1. Evidence—Is there sufficient evidence to justify teaching sophomore boys about TSE?
2. Assumptions—Describe the underlying assumption about each of the following:
   a. Detection of testicular cancers in adolescence
   b. Usual presenting symptom of testicular cancer
   c. Knowledge of genital anatomy among adolescent boys
   d. Ways to teach adolescent boys about their anatomy
3. What priorities for nursing care can be drawn at this time?
4. Does the evidence support your nursing intervention?
5. What alternative perspectives might you have?

The normal testicle is a firm organ with a smooth, egg-shaped contour; the epididymis is palpated as a raised swelling on the superior aspect of the testicle and should not be confused with an abnormality.

Gynecomastia

The male breast, although not strictly part of the male reproductive system, responds to hormonal changes. Some degree of bilateral or unilateral breast enlargement occurs frequently in boys during puberty. It is estimated that approximately half of adolescent boys have transient gynecomastia, usually subsiding spontaneously within 1 to 2 years of onset. A careful assessment of the pubertal stage at the onset of gynecomastia; medication history, including anabolic steroids; and the exclusion of renal, liver, thyroid, and endocrine disorders or dysfunction allow the examiner to reassure the adolescent that the changes are pubertal gynecomastia and no further assessment is indicated.

If the condition persists or is extensive enough to cause embarrassment or to produce doubts about gender identity in the young boy, plastic surgery may be indicated for cosmetic and psychologic considerations. Administration of testosterone has no effect on breast development or regression and may aggravate the condition.

Nursing Care Management

Treatment usually consists of assuring the adolescent and his parents that this is a benign and temporary situation. Adolescents who are distressed about physical integrity and masculinity may benefit from the knowledge that this condition occurs in more than 50% to 65% of all adolescent boys.

Eating Disorders

Obesity

Few problems in childhood and adolescence are so obvious to others, are so difficult to treat, and have such long-term effects on health as obesity. Several different definitions have been proposed for obesity and overweight. *Obesity* has been defined as an increase in body weight resulting from an excessive accumulation of body fat relative to lean body mass. *Overweight* refers to the state of weighing more than average for height and body build. Currently, the *BMI* measurement is recommended as the most accurate method for screening children and adolescents for obesity. The BMI measurement is strongly associated with subcutaneous and total body fat and also with skin fold thickness measurements. It is also highly specific for children with the greatest amount of body fat. Pediatric growth charts that include BMI for age and gender are available from Centers for Disease Control and Prevention (*www.cdc.gov/growthcharts*). Children with a BMI between the 85th and 95th percentiles are considered overweight, and obesity is defined by a BMI greater than the 95th percentile (Skelton & Rudolph, 2007).

The number of overweight children in the United States has increased dramatically and has reportedly reached epidemic status (Spear, 2005). According to 2003-2004 National Health and Nutrition Examination Survey (NHANES), 17% of children and adolescents 2 to 19 years of age were overweight, and 32% of adults were obese (Ogden et al, 2006). This represents a significant increase in childhood and adolescent overweight data from previous NHANES studies. A study of 9464 Native-American schoolchildren ages 5 to 18 years found that 39% were overweight, and a further review of tribes across the United States found that 30% to 46% of Native Americans were at risk for overweight (85th percentile or higher) (Hardy, Harrell, & Bell, 2004).

Research indicates that overweight children and adolescents are at risk of continuing to be obese as adults, thereby experiencing the health and social consequences of obesity much earlier than children and adolescents of normal weight. Parental obesity increases the risk of overweight by twofold to threefold (Baker et al, 2005). The probability that overweight school-age children will become obese adults is estimated at 50%, whereas the likelihood that overweight adolescents will become obese adults is estimated at 70% to 80% (National Institute for Health Care Management Foundation, 2003). Children who were overweight in toddler and preschool years (BMI greater than 85th percentile) were five times as likely to be overweight at age 12 years than those who had a BMI below the 85th percentile during the preschool years (Nader et al, 2006).

Obesity in childhood and adolescence has been related to elevated blood cholesterol, high blood pressure, respiratory disorders, orthopedic conditions (Taylor et al, 2006; Falkner et al, 2006), cholelithiasis, some types of adult-onset cancer (MacKenzie, 2000), nonalcoholic fatty liver disease (Baker et al, 2005; Angulo, 2002), and type 2 diabetes mellitus (Ehtisham, Barrett, & Shaw, 2000). The incidence of metabolic syndrome was 50% in a study group of overweight and obese adolescents (Weiss et al, 2004). Common emotional conse-

evolve Critical Thinking Exercise—Obesity

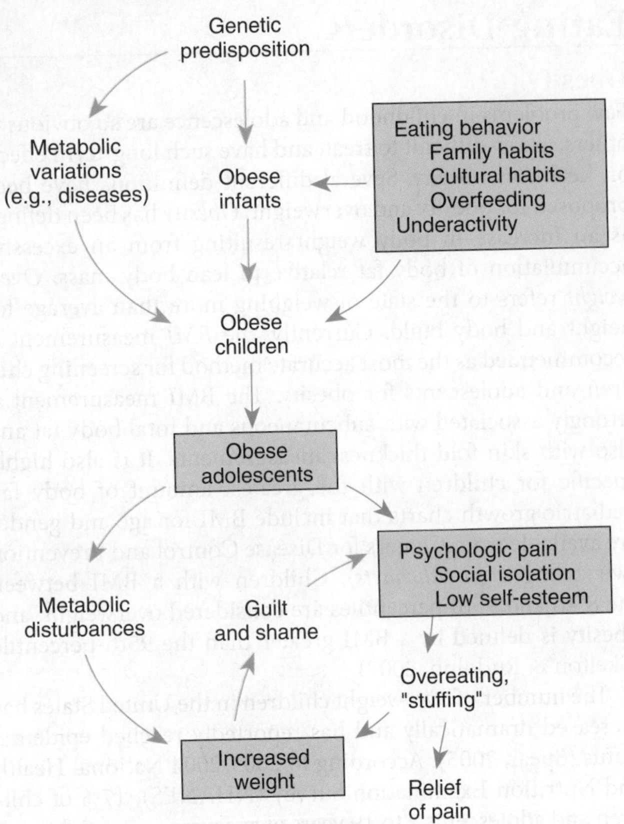

Fig. 40-10 Complex relationships in obesity.

quences of obesity include poor body image, low self-esteem, social isolation, and feelings of depression and rejection (Sjöberg, Nilsson, & Leppert, 2005).

Etiology and Pathophysiology

Obesity results from a caloric intake that consistently exceeds caloric requirements and expenditure and may involve a variety of interrelated influences, including metabolic, hypothalamic, hereditary, social, cultural, and psychologic factors (Fig. 40-10). Because the etiology of obesity is multifactorial, the treatment requires multilevel interventions.

Birth weight is not considered a contributing factor in detection and prediction of childhood obesity; obese children do not have higher birth weights than nonobese children. There is, however, a high correlation between childhood adiposity and parental adiposity. The strongest predictor of childhood overweight and future adult obesity is parental overweight (Skelton & Rudolph, 2007).

A balance between *energy intake* and *energy expenditure* is a critical factor in regulating body weight. Factors that raise energy intake or decrease energy expenditure by even small amounts can have a long-term impact on the development of overweight and obesity. For example, a positive balance of one serving of a sweetened juice or soft drink (about 120 kcal) per day would produce a 50 kg (110 lb) increase in body mass over a 10-year period (Hill et al, 2003).

Familial influence is an epidemiologic consideration in regard to a child weight. Twin studies suggest that approximately 50% to 70% of the tendency toward obesity is inherited (Kiess et al, 2001). Twin studies have also suggested that this tendency is based on a combination of genetic and environmental factors. If both parents are lean, the likelihood of the child becoming overweight is just 9%. When both parents are obese, there is a 60% to 80% increase in the likelihood of the child becoming obese (Koeppen-Schomerus, Wardle, & Plomin, 2001). The specific influences of genes and environment within the developing child is not well defined. The increasing rates of obesity within genetically stable populations suggest that environmental and some perinatal factors (e.g., bottle feeding) are contributors to the current increases in childhood obesity (National Institute for Health Care Management Foundation, 2003).

Fewer than 5% of the cases of childhood obesity can be attributed to an underlying *disease.* Such diseases include hypothyroidism; adrenal hypercorticoidism; hyperinsulinism; and dysfunction or damage to the central nervous system as a result of tumor, injury, infection, or vascular accident. Obesity is a frequent complication of muscular dystrophy, paraplegia, Down syndrome, spina bifida, and other chronic illnesses that limit mobility.

A major focus of obesity research has been on *appetite regulation.* The expression of appetite is chemically coded in the hypothalamus by distinctive circuitry. Orexigenic substances produce signals that promote eating behaviors, and anorexigenic substances promote the cessation of eating behaviors. Feedback loops between signals have been identified where one signal peptide is able to alter the secretion of another signal peptide. No one signal has been identified as the gatekeeper of appetite. It is apparent that an entire network of signals, including their frequency and amplitude, is responsible for triggering eating behaviors.

There is little evidence to support a relationship between obesity and "low metabolism." Small differences may exist in regulation of dietary intake or metabolic rate between obese and nonobese children that could lead to an energy imbalance and inappropriate weight gain, but these small differences are difficult to accurately quantify. No differences in basal metabolic rate, sleeping metabolic rate, respiratory quotient, heart rate, or total energy expenditure have been found in normal weight children with or without a familial predisposition to overweight (Baker et al, 2005). In childhood, overeating is the dominant feature in obesity, whereas in adult life, reduced physical activity with normal intake is more likely.

The tendency toward obesity is manifested whenever *environmental conditions* are favorable to excessive caloric intake, such as an abundance of food, limited access to low-fat foods, reduced or minimum physical activity, and snacking combined with excessive television viewing. Family and cultural eating patterns, as well as psychologic factors, play an important role; many families and cultures consider fat to be an indication of good health. It is not uncommon for obese children to have families that emphasize large meals or admonish children for leaving food on their plates. Parents may have an exaggerated concept of the amount of food children require and expect them to eat more than they need. The prevalence of obesity shows a marked difference between upper- and lower-class children, with differences often becoming apparent before 6 years of age. Lower socioeconomic groups have a greater prevalence of obesity, especially in girls. Physical activity may also be influenced by sociocultural factors.

Some *community factors* that influence activity patterns include unsafe neighborhoods that keep children from playing outside. Many communities lack affordable and accessible areas for low-income youth to be active, thus limiting opportunities for young people to participate in physical activities. Social policies also contribute to obesity. The increased availability of high-fat foods, pricing strategies that promote unhealthy food choices, and overzealous food advertising that targets children and adolescents with high-fat and high-sugar foods are some examples.

Institutional factors also influence patterns of obesity and decreased physical activity. Many secondary school policies allow students to leave school for lunch. Vending machines in school often are filled with high-fat and high-calorie foods and soft drinks. Although well-balanced, nutritious school lunches may be available to students, they will often opt for less nutritious choices such as high-fat snacks.

Physical inactivity has also been identified as an important contributing factor in the development and maintenance of childhood overweight. There is little doubt that physical activity has decreased in elementary and secondary schools in the United States. Consequently, most of a child's physical activity must occur within the family or outside of school. Decreased physical activity within the family is a powerful influence on children, since children imitate their parents and other adults. Parental obesity and low levels of physical activity are correlated with decreased physical activity in children. Research has shown that children who are more active after school and who spend less time watching TV are much less likely to be overweight by age 12 than sedentary children (O'Brien et al, 2007). A recent study found that children at age 9 years engaged in approximately 3 hours of daily moderate to vigorous physical activity; by age 15 years children were only engaging in 49 minutes of moderate to vigorous physical activity. Boys were more active than girls, and the cut-off period for a marked decrease in activity was 13.1 years for girls and 14.7 years for boys (Nader et al, 2008).

Psychologic factors also affect eating patterns. In infancy, children experience relief from discomfort through feeding and learn to associate eating with a sense of well-being, security, and the comforting presence of a nurturing person. Eating is soon associated with the feeling of being loved. In addition, the pleasurable oral sensation of sucking provides a connection between emotions and early eating behavior. Many parents use food as a positive reinforcer for desired behaviors. This practice may become a habit, and the child may continue to use food as a reward, a comfort, and a means of dealing with depression or hostility. Many individuals eat when they are not hungry or in response to boredom, loneliness, sadness, depression, or tiredness. Difficulty determining feelings of satiety can lead to weight problems and may compound the factor of eating in response to emotional rather than physical hunger cues.

Eating behaviors are closely related to memory. Memory and appetite are chemically encoded, with each individual having his or her own circuitry relating to eating behaviors. Like memory, the circuitry can be modified over time (Feldman, Friedman, & Sleisenger, 2002).

Diagnostic Evaluation

A careful history is obtained regarding the development of obesity, and a physical examination is performed to differentiate simple obesity from increased fat that results from organic causes. A family history of obesity, diabetes, coronary heart disease, and dyslipidemia should be obtained for all children who are overweight or at risk for overweight. For some, psychologic assessment, by interviews and standardized personality tests, may provide insight into the personality and emotional problems that contribute to obesity and that might interfere with therapy.

The history is an important guide to determine the workup. The physical examination should focus on identifying comorbid conditions and identifiable causes of obesity. Some areas to focus on include (1) skin for stretch markings and discolorations (e.g., acanthosis nigricans), (2) joints for swelling and evidence of pain, and (3) airway for evidence of obstruction and enlarged tonsils. Basic laboratory studies include a fasting lipid panel; fasting insulin level; fasting glucose hepatic enzymes, including γ-glutamyltransferase; and, in some institutions, hemoglobin A_{1c}. Other studies, such as a sleep study, metabolic studies, and radiographic evaluations, may be added based on the history and physical examination.

It is useful to estimate the degree of obesity to determine the component of body weight that can be modified. All the following methods have been used to assess obesity: BMI, body weight, weight-height ratios, weight-age ratios, hydrostatic (underwater) weight, skin fold measurements, bioelectrical analysis, computed tomography, magnetic resonance imaging, and neutron activation. Each of these methods has advantages and disadvantages. Hydrostatic, or underwater, weighing provides the most accurate measurement of lean body weight.

BMI is currently considered the best method to assess weight in children and adolescents. The calculation is based on the individual's height and weight. In adults, BMI definitions are fixed measures without regard for sex and age. The BMI in children and adolescents varies to accommodate age- and gender-specific changes in growth. The formula for BMI calculation is:

$$[(\text{Weight in pounds} \div \text{Height in inches}) \div \text{Height in inches}] \times 703$$

or

$$\text{Weight in kilograms} \div [\text{Height in meters}]^2$$

BMI measures in children and adolescents are plotted on growth charts that enable heath care professionals to determine the patient's BMI-for-age (see the EVOLVE site).

Therapeutic Management

The best approach to the management of obesity is a preventive one. Early recognition and control measures are essential before the child or adolescent reaches an obese state. Health care providers must educate families about the medical complications of obesity, and families are encouraged to be involved in the treatment plan.

The treatment of obesity is difficult. Many approaches do not achieve long-term success. The average individual only loses about 5% to 10% of his or her weight with available therapies. Losing weight can have a significant positive effect on many comorbidities, but unfortunately the lost weight is frequently regained in a year or two (Yanovski & Yanovski, 2002).

Diet modification is an essential part of weight-reduction programs. Dietary counseling is directed toward improving the nutritional quality of the diet rather than dietary restriction. Children should avoid fad diets. Most dietitians and nutrition experts recommend a diet with low-saturated fat, moderate total fat (30% or less), and five servings of fruits and vegetables, consistent with the MyPyramid food guide for children. Also, promoting high-fiber foods and avoiding highly refined starches and sugars will decrease caloric intake. The 2005 Dietary Guidelines for Americans *(www.health.gov/DietaryGuidelines/dga2005/document/default.htm)* may be used as a guide for caloric intake for adolescents concerned about weight control; the guidelines also emphasize daily exercise in weight management for children and adolescents. Many programs recommend using a food diary as a helpful tool to increase awareness of food choices and eating behaviors. The goal is to encourage the individual to make healthier choices in foods selection and discourage eating food by habit or to appease boredom.

In patients with severe obesity, strict diets have been used, such as the protein-sparing modified fast, a hypocaloric, ketogenic diet that is designed provide enough protein to minimize loss of lean body mass during weight loss. Such diets need to be closely monitored and should be used only with multidisciplinary teams that include a physician, nutritionist, and behavioral therapist. Generally, the diet consists of 1.5 to 2.5 g of protein per kilogram. The intake of carbohydrates is low enough to induce ketosis. The benefits of the diet are relatively rapid weight loss and anorexia induced by ketosis. Potential complications include protein losses, hypokalemia, hypoglycemia, inadequate calcium intake, and orthostatic hypotension. It is difficult to sustain such diets over the long term, and the long-term outcomes of using these diets have not been established.

Some drugs have been used to promote weight loss in children with certain conditions; examples include metformin in obese adolescents with insulin resistance and hyperinsulinism, octreotide for hypothalamic obesity caused by intracranial tumors, growth hormone in children with Prader-Willi syndrome, and leptin for congenital leptin deficiency. The drug sibutramine, in addition to behavioral therapy, significantly reduced BMI and body weight more than placebo; however, the drug was associated with side effects (tachycardia and hypertension) (Berkowitz et al, 2006).

Bariatric surgery may be the only practical alternative for increasing numbers of severely overweight adolescents who have failed organized attempts to lose or maintain weight loss through conventional nonoperative approaches and who have serious life-threatening conditions. Some preliminary studies suggest that adolescents with severe obesity have successful weight loss up to 14 years after bariatric surgery; most adolescents were reported to have a significant change in lifestyle as a result of the weight loss after surgery (Sugerman et al, 2003). Other researchers suggest that bariatric surgery in adolescents is safe and they have fewer postoperative complications than adults, but the procedure is relatively uncommon in comparison to the number of adults having surgery for obesity (Tsai, Inge, & Burd, 2007). In general, bariatric surgery should be reserved for severely obese adolescents with comorbidities after careful consideration. Candidates for surgery should be referred to centers that offer a multidisciplinary team experienced in the management of childhood and adolescent obesity, and the surgery should be performed by surgeons who have participated in subspecialty training in bariatric medical and surgical care as detailed by the American College of Surgeons and the American Society for Metabolic and Bariatric Surgery.

Nursing Care Management

Nurses play a key role in the adherence and maintenance phases of many weight-reduction programs. Nurses assess, manage, and evaluate the progress of many overweight adolescents. They also play an important role in recognizing potential weight problems and assisting parents and adolescents in preventing obesity. The nursing process in the care of the adolescent who is overweight is outlined in the Nursing Process box.

The presence of obesity may not be obvious from appearance alone. Regular assessment of height and weight and computation of the BMI facilitate early recognition. Children with a BMI greater than or equal to the 95th percentile for age and sex should receive in-depth medical assessment. Children with a BMI in the 85th to 95th percentile range should be evaluated for secondary complications, such as hypertension and hyperlipidemia, and family history (Greaser & Whyte, 2004). Evaluation includes a height and weight history of the adolescent and family members, eating habits, appetite and hunger patterns, and physical activities. A psychosocial history is also helpful in understanding the impact of obesity on the child's life.

Before initiating a treatment plan, it is important to be certain that the family is ready for change. Lack of readiness may result in failure, frustration, and reluctance to address the problem in the future. The nurse should explore with adolescents the reasons behind the desire to lose weight, since motivation to lose weight is the key to success. Adolescents need to take a personal responsibility for dietary habits and physical activity. Teens who are forced by their parents to seek help are seldom motivated, become rebellious, and are unwilling to control their dietary intake.

Nutritional Counseling

Preventing an increase in body fat during growth is a realistic approach. This is often accomplished by adjusting three aspects of eating:

1. Reducing the quantity eaten by purchasing, preparing, and serving smaller portions
2. Altering the quality consumed by substituting low-calorie, low-fat foods for high-calorie foods (especially for snacks)
3. Altering situations by severing associations between eating and other stimuli, such as eating while watching television

NURSING PROCESS: THE CHILD OR ADOLESCENT WHO IS OVERWEIGHT

Assessment

The nurse assists in determining the child or adolescent's body mass index, gathers appropriate anthropometric data, uses standardized growth charts to plot growth, and obtains a comprehensive health history. Further information that is appropriate to obtain in the assessment includes a 24-hour food intake history, family health history, and lifestyle practices that affect the child or adolescent's well-being. The health interview and nutritional assessment often provide clues and guidelines for further investigation.

Nursing Diagnoses (Problem Identification)

Several nursing diagnoses are identified after a thorough assessment:

- Situational low self-esteem
- Imbalanced nutrition: more than body requirements
- Risk for injury
- Risk-prone health behavior
- Disturbed personal identity

Planning

Expected patient outcomes for the adolescent with an eating disorder include:

- Child or adolescent will develop a positive self-image.
- Adolescent will willingly engage in behaviors to reverse effects of cardiovascular disease.
- Healthy personal identity will be achieved.
- Healthy eating patterns will be adopted.
- Adolescent will assume control for changes in lifestyle designed to lose weight.
- Child or adolescent will remain injury free.

Implementation

Numerous intervention strategies are discussed on pp. 1130-1132.

Evaluation

The effectiveness of nursing interventions is determined by continual reassessment and evaluation of nursing care based on the following observational guidelines:

- Perform nutritional assessment; measure weight; review diet and nutritional intake (e.g., log); interview adolescent regarding food and eating behaviors; observe eating behaviors.
- Interview adolescent regarding self-perceptions; observe behavior; confer with psychologist and other members of the interdisciplinary team regarding evidence of progress.
- Observe adolescent's behavior, and interview him or her regarding attitudes, concerns, and behaviors.

The most successful diets are those that use ordinary foods in controlled portions rather than diets that require the avoidance of specific foods. Low-carbohydrate diets such as the Atkins diet have been promoted for weight loss in adults and adolescents (Sondike, Copperman, & Jacobson, 2003). However, low-carbohydrate diets can result in ketosis, insulin resistance, and glucose intolerance. More research is needed to evaluate the long-term safety and efficacy of these diets for children and adolescents.

The nurse teaches adolescents and parents how to incorporate favorite foods into their diet and to select satisfying substitutes. The dieting teen should eat what the rest of the family eats, but less of it. When parents buy and prepare smaller amounts, they eliminate tempting second helpings and leftovers. To maintain a healthy diet, it is necessary to encourage the consumption of high-nutrient foods such as fruits, vegetables, whole grains, and low-fat dairy protein products. Calories and fat should be kept to a healthy level without being significantly restricted. To be successful, a dietary program should be nutritionally sound with sufficient satiety value, produce the desired weight loss, and be accompanied by nutrition education and continued support. Children and adolescents should not initiate a reduction diet without health assessment and counseling (Schwimmer, 2004).

Behavioral Therapy

Altering eating behavior and eliminating inappropriate eating habits are essential to weight reduction, especially in maintaining long-term weight control. Most behavioral modification programs include the following concepts:

- A description of the behavior to be controlled, such as eating habits
- Attempts to modify and control the stimuli that govern eating
- Development of eating techniques designed to control speed of eating
- Positive reinforcement for these modifications through a suitable reward system

Specific strategies to modify eating habits are included in Box 40-4.

Group Involvement

Commercial groups (e.g., Weight Watchers) or diet workshops composed primarily of adults may be helpful to some teenagers; however, a group of other adolescents is often more effective. Teenage groups include summer camps designed for obese young people and conducted by health professionals, school groups organized and led by a school nurse, and groups associated with special clinics.

These groups are concerned not only with weight loss but also with the development of a positive self-image and the encouragement of physical activity. Nutrition education, diet planning, and the improvement of social skills are essential components of these groups. Improvement is determined by positive changes in all aspects of behavior.

Family Involvement

There is a definite connection between family environment, interaction, and obesity. The nurse needs to educate parents in the purposes of the therapeutic measures and their role in management. The family needs nutrition education and counseling regarding the reinforcement plan, alterations in the food environment, and ways to maintain proper attitudes. They can support their child in efforts to change eating behaviors, food intake, and physical activity.

BOX 40-4 Helpful Suggestions to Promote Healthy Eating Habits

Identify current eating patterns and behaviors by keeping a food diary to look for areas to change. Record everything eaten, including where, when, and associated activities.

Change eating patterns.

- Choose sugar-free beverages or low-fat milk only.
- Limit fast-food consumption to no more than once a week.
- Do not skip meals.
- Eat three meals and one or two snacks per day.
- Try the plate method: one half plate of vegetables, one fourth plate of lean meat, and one fourth plate of starch or starchy vegetables (potatoes, peas).
- Take second helpings of fruits and vegetables (not potatoes) only.
- Avoid low-fat food (these are usually high in sugars).
- Use whole-grain breads, cereals, and pastas.
- Pack your lunch for school.
- Buy healthy foods for snacking.

Change the act of eating.

- Eat meals at the family dinner table.
- Avoid distractions (e.g., television).
- Slow down; meals may last at least 20 to 30 minutes.

Substitute other activities for managing stress, such as hobbies, walking, listening to music, talking to friends on the phone, reading, playing a game.

Provide alternative rewards for reinforcement or accomplishments (e.g., CDs, movie, concert, new clothes, new games).

Think positively.

Enlist family involvement and support.

evolve Nursing Care Plan—The Adolescent with an Eating Disorder

Physical Activity

Regular physical activity is incorporated into all weight-reduction programs. Any form of increased physical activity is beneficial, provided that the activities are age appropriate and enjoyable. Recommendations for physical activity need to consider the current health status and developmental level of the child or adolescent. The best choice for exercise is any form that is enjoyable and likely to be sustainable. Aerobic and endurance exercises help oxidize body fats. Light exercises like walking may provide an opportunity for the family to increase time together and increase caloric expenditure. Walking for 30 minutes each day and decreasing caloric intake by 500 calories per day may significantly reduce the risk of chronic disease. Weight training can increase basal metabolic rate and replace fat mass with muscle mass. However, weight training is not generally recommended for prepubertal children until they have reached physical and skeletal maturity. In prepubertal children increasing outdoor playtime is likely to be beneficial. Many children find exercise videos and treadmills boring and may not continue these activities. There are a great variety of physical activities to choose from that are likely to appeal to different people. Team sports and individual sports such as dance, bike riding, swimming, and karate are some. Limiting sedentary activities such as television viewing (while eating snacks!) is the most effective way to encourage physical activity.

Prevention

Weight loss programs do not enjoy the success of therapeutic interventions for other disorders. Gradual accumulation of adipose tissue during childhood establishes a pattern of eating that is difficult to reverse in adolescence. Prevention of obesity should begin in early childhood with the development of healthy eating habits, regular exercise patterns, and a positive relationship between parents and children. Prevention of adolescent obesity is best accomplished by early identification of obesity in the preschool, school-age, and preadolescent periods. Health care professionals should encourage frequent health care visits for children who are overweight or obese and incorporate a dietary history and counseling into each well-infant, well-child, and well-adolescent visit.

Anorexia Nervosa and Bulimia Nervosa

AN is an eating disorder characterized by a refusal to maintain a minimally normal body weight and by severe weight loss in the absence of obvious physical causes. Approximately 5% of adolescent females in the United States have AN, and 5% to 10% of all cases occur in males (American Academy of Pediatrics, Committee on Adolescence, 2003). The average age of onset is 13 years, but the disorder can occur as early as 10 years of age and as late as 25 years of age. Individuals with AN are described as perfectionists, academically high achievers, conforming, and conscientious. Typically, they have high energy levels, even with marked emaciation. Patients with AN may eventually develop bulimia (Mehler, 2001).

Bulimia (from the Greek meaning "ox hunger") refers to an eating disorder similar to AN. BN is observed more commonly in older adolescent girls and young women; males with bulimia are less common. BN patients may be of average or slightly above average weight. BN is characterized by repeated episodes of binge eating followed by inappropriate compensatory behaviors, such as self-induced vomiting; misuse of laxatives, diuretics, or other medications; fasting; or excessive exercise (American Psychiatric Association, 2000). The binge behavior consists of secretive, frenzied consumption of large amounts of high-calorie (or "forbidden") foods during a brief time (usually less than 2 hours). The binge is counteracted by a variety of weight control methods *(purging)*. These binge-purge cycles are followed by self-deprecating thoughts, a depressed mood, and an awareness that the eating pattern is abnormal.

Although persons with BN have many issues in common with those who have other eating disorders, impulse control and satiety regulation are important problems in BN. Many individuals with BN begin with only occasional binges and purges "just for fun," enjoying the control over their weight while eating amounts of food that would normally produce obesity. As the condition progresses, the frequency of binges increases, the amount of food consumed increases, and they gradually lose control over the binge-purge cycle. The frequency of binging can be anywhere from once per week to seven or eight times per day. Because persons with BN usually binge on high-calorie foods, especially sweets, ice cream, and pastries, insulin production is stimulated to cope with the added carbohydrates. When the food is vomited, the unused insulin stimulates hunger and the desire to eat.

A third eating disorder, identified as *EDNOS (eating disorder not otherwise specified),* has components of both AN and BN with varying degrees of symptomatology that are not always characteristic of the established diagnostic criteria for AN and BN (American Dietetic Association, 2006). *Binge eating disorder (BED)* is a type of EDNOS. Persons with BED may diet in an attempt to control their weight but without the extreme weight-control compensatory practices of vomiting, laxative use, diuretics, and excessive exercise (American Dietetic Association, 2006; Forman, 2007).

Etiology and Pathophysiology

The cause of these disorders remains unclear. There is a distinct psychologic component, and the diagnosis is based primarily on psychologic and behavioral criteria. Dieting appears to be common to the initiation of both AN and BN. The disorders appear to be caused by a combination of genetic, neurochemical, psychodevelopmental, and sociocultural factors. The dominant aspects of AN are a relentless pursuit of thinness and a fear of fatness, usually preceded by a period of mood disturbances and behavior changes.

Weight loss may be triggered by a typical adolescent crisis such as the onset of menstruation or a traumatic interpersonal incident that precipitates serious, out-of-control dieting. Situations of severe family stress (such as parental separation or divorce) or circumstances in which the adolescent perceives a lack of personal control (such as teasing at school, changing schools, or going to college) may precipitate a desire for control and the decision not to eat. Frequently, there is an exaggerated misinterpretation of the normal fat deposition characteristic of early adolescence or anxiety because of comments that the adolescent is putting on weight.

Many experts have associated the development of an eating disorder with family characteristics such as an adolescent perception of high parental expectations for achievement and appearance, difficulty managing conflict and poor communication styles, enmeshment and occasionally estrangement between family members, devaluation of the mother or the maternal role, and marital tension. Families struggling with an eating disorder have been characterized as often having difficulties responding positively to the adolescent's changing physical and emotional needs. Family stress of any kind may become a significant factor in the development of an eating disorder (Forman, 2007).

Society's emphasis and the media's focus on tall, thin individuals may also play a role. Studies evaluating the possible association of eating disorders and sexual abuse have been conflicting. Childhood sexual abuse may be a factor in some cases of AN.

Patients with eating disorders commonly have psychiatric problems, including affective disorder, anxiety disorder, obsessive-compulsive disorder, and personality disorder. Adult women with eating disorders were found to have higher than average rates of obsessive-compulsive behavior traits in their childhood. Patients with eating disorders have also been found to have higher than average reported rates of substance abuse, with alcohol problems being more common in those with BN than AN (Forman, 2007). It is important to note that many of the clinical findings are directly related to the state of starvation and improve with weight gain.

Many sports and artistic endeavors that emphasize leanness (e.g., ballet and running) and sports in which the scoring is partly subjective (e.g., skating and gymnastics) have been associated with a higher incidence of eating disorders such as AN. The term *female athlete triad,* characterized by disordered eating behavior, amenorrhea, and osteoporosis, has been applied to young women with restrictive eating disorders and amenorrhea (Rome et al, 2003).

A genetic role has been postulated for eating disorders; a significant number of young females with a first-degree relative having an eating disorder had a significantly higher rate of eating disorders (Forman, 2007).

Diagnostic Evaluation

Diagnosis of AN is made on the basis of clinical manifestations (Box 40-5) and conformity to the criteria established by the American Psychiatric Association (2000) (Box 40-6). Diagnosis of BN is confirmed, according to the American Psychiatric Association's *Diagnostic and Statistical Manual of Mental Disorders* (2000) (Box 40-7), by at least two binge-eating episodes per week for the preceding 3 months.

A complete history and physical examination are important to rule out other causes for weight loss. The medical assessment of an eating disorder focuses on the complications of altered nutritional status and purging. A careful history assesses weight changes, dietary patterns, and the frequency and severity of purging and excessive exercise. The patient's weight and height should be measured and evaluated for appropriateness according to standard weight for height, age, and sex charts, determined according to the percentile of his or her expected body weight or BMI.

Additional diagnostic measures may include a complete blood count to evaluate for anemia and other hematologic abnormalities; erythrocyte sedimentation rate or C-reactive protein to detect evidence of inflammation; electrolytes, calcium, magnesium, phosphorus, blood urea nitrogen, and creatinine; urinalysis, including specific gravity; and bone density studies for osteopenia, which is commonly observed in patients with AN. In patients with prolonged amenorrhea, human chorionic gonadotropin is assessed to check for pregnancy. Other tests for patients with amenorrhea include

BOX 40-5 Clinical Manifestations of Anorexia Nervosa

Severe and profound weight loss
Signs of altered metabolic activity:

- Secondary amenorrhea (if menarche attained)
- Primary amenorrhea (if menarche not attained)
- Bradycardia
- Lowered body temperature
- Decreased blood pressure
- Cold intolerance
- Dry skin and brittle nails
- Appearance of lanugo hair

BOX 40-6 Diagnostic Criteria for Anorexia Nervosa

1. Refusal to maintain body weight over a minimal normal weight for age and height (e.g., weight loss leading to maintenance of body weight less than 85% of that expected; or failure to make expected weight gain during period of growth, leading to body weight less than 85% of that expected)
2. Intense fear of gaining weight or becoming fat, even though underweight
3. Disturbance of body image, undue influence of shape or weight on evaluation, or denial of the seriousness of the current low body weight
4. In postmenarcheal females, amenorrhea (i.e., the absence of at least three consecutive menstrual cycles); a woman is considered to have amenorrhea if her periods occur only following hormone (i.e., estrogen) administration

Specify Type:

Restricting type—No regular binging or purging behavior (i.e., self-induced vomiting or the misuse of laxatives, diuretics, or enemas)

Binge eating/purging type—During the current episode of AN, the person has regularly engaged in binge eating or purging behavior (i.e., self-induced vomiting or the misuse of laxatives, diuretics, or enemas)

From American Psychiatric Association: *Diagnostic and statistical manual of mental disorders,* ed 4 (DSM-IV TR), Washington, DC, 2000, The Association.

BOX 40-7 Diagnostic Criteria for Bulimia

1. Recurrent episodes of binge eating. An episode of binge eating is characterized by both of the following:
   a. Eating, in a discrete period of time (e.g., within any 2-hour period), an amount of food that is definitely larger than most people would eat during a similar period of time and under similar circumstances
   b. A sense of lack of control over eating during the episode (e.g., a feeling that one cannot stop eating or control what or how much one is eating)
2. Recurrent inappropriate compensatory behavior in order to prevent weight gain, such as self-induced vomiting; misuse of laxatives, diuretics, enemas, or other medications; fasting; or excessive exercise
3. The binge eating and inappropriate compensatory behaviors both occur, on average, at least twice a week for 3 months
4. Self-evaluation is unduly influenced by body shape and weight
5. The disturbance does not occur exclusively during episodes of AN

Specify Type:

Purging type—During the current episode of bulimia nervosa, the person has regularly engaged in self-induced vomiting or the misuse of laxatives, diuretics, or enemas

Nonpurging type—During the current episode of bulimia nervosa, the person has used other inappropriate compensatory behaviors, such as fasting or excessive exercise, but has not regularly engaged in self-induced vomiting or the misuse of laxatives, diuretics, or enemas

From American Psychiatric Association: *Diagnostic and statistical manual of mental disorders,* ed 4 (DSM-IV TR), Washington, DC, 2000, The Association.

thyroid function tests and measurement of serum prolactin and follicle-stimulating hormone to help rule out prolactinoma (hormone-secreting pituitary tumor), hyperthyroidism, hypothyroidism, or ovarian failure. In addition, a comprehensive cardiac evaluation is often recommended in those with AN. Further diagnostic tests may be required based on the history and findings from above diagnostic tests.

Therapeutic Management

The treatment of AN involves four major goals:

1. Restoration of a healthy weight
2. Establishment of healthy eating patterns
3. Resolution of disturbed patterns of family interaction
4. Individual psychotherapy to correct deficits and distortions in psychologic functioning

Most adolescents are treated on an outpatient basis, but those with problems requiring immediate medical attention, such as severe malnutrition or electrolyte or psychiatric disturbances (severe depression or suicidal ideation), require hospitalization. A multidisciplinary team of dietitians, physicians, nurses, and counselors provide the interventions.

Persons with BN may benefit from cognitive behavioral therapy, other psychotherapy, antidepressant medications, or a combination of antidepressant medication and psychotherapy (Forman, 2007). Nutrition education and meal planning may help the BN patient maintain an adequate weight and accept foods that are often considered bad or forbidden (Spear, 2005).

Nutrition Therapy

The most important goal is to treat any life-threatening malnutrition and to restore dietary stability and weight gain. This may require the administration of tube feedings or intravenous fluids if the malnutrition is severe. In most cases, it is best to reintroduce food and snacks slowly in a stepwise manner. A reasonable goal is to reach an eventual intake of 2000 to 3000 kcal/day and a weight gain of 0.22 to 0.45 kg (½ to 1 lb) per week (American Dietetic Association, 2006). When restoring nutrition, health professionals must avoid the *refeeding syndrome,* which consists of cardiovascular, neurologic, and hematologic complications that occur when nutritional replacement is given too rapidly. This syndrome can be avoided with slow refeeding and the addition of phosphorus when total body phosphorus is depleted. Treatment goal weights are individualized and based on age, height, stage of puberty, premorbid weight, and previous growth charts. In girls who have reached menarche, resumption of menses is an objective measure of return to biologic health.

Dietary interventions are combined with psychotherapy to improve the underlying psychologic misconceptions about weight loss. Another aspect of treatment is to relieve the anxiety related to eating and the depression that accompanies the disorder. The administration of antianxiety or antidepressant medications is beneficial. However, when these drugs are used, patients should be carefully monitored for cardiovascular side effects.

Psychotherapy

Behavioral interventions are often necessary to encourage patients to accomplish the desired caloric intake and weight gain. Weight restoration as an outpatient is accomplished with behavioral contracts negotiated between the therapists and patient. The goal is to increase the patient's feelings of control and responsibility for achieving recovery. The contract can stipulate at what weight tube feedings will be implemented. Individual psychotherapy is aimed at helping the young person resolve the adolescent identity crisis, particularly as it relates to a distorted body image. If the disorder is related to a dysfunctional family situation, therapy is most successful when it is started soon after the onset of illness and directed toward disengagement and redirection of malfunctioning processes in the family.

Pharmacologic Therapy

Pharmacotherapy in the treatment of AN has been disappointing so far. The few studies that have been done have primarily evaluated medications' efficacy in the treatment of comorbid disorders such as obsessive-compulsive disorders and depression. Anxiolytic medications may be helpful before meals to relieve some patients' anxiety.

Tricyclic antidepressants and fluoxetine belong to a group of medications known as selective serotonin reuptake inhibitors, which have been more successful when used with BN. There is also some evidence that tricyclic antidepressants such as desipramine, imipramine, and amitriptyline; monoamine oxidase inhibitors; and buspirone are more effective compared with a placebo in decreasing binging and vomiting in patients with BN. Topiramate, an antiepileptic agent, and the selective serotonin antagonist ondansetron may have some benefit in treating BN.

Nursing Care Management

Nurses must maintain a kind and supportive yet firm manner in managing the care of the adolescent with eating disorders without creating a passive-dependent attitude. The individual requires sustained support and reassurance to cope with ambivalent feelings related to body concept and the desire to be seen as cooperative, reliable, and worthy of receiving kindness. Encouraging the adolescent with education and activities that strengthen self-esteem facilitates the resocialization process and promotes social acceptance among peers.

It is important for nurses to be aware of the physical side effects of AN. Patients frequently limit their fluid intake. Urinary tract problems are common, and ketones and protein may be detected in the urine as a result of breakdown of fat and protein. Vital sign instability can be severe and can include orthostatic hypotension; the pulse becomes irregular, and the rate decreases markedly. Bradycardia and hypothermia can result in cardiac arrest (see Critical Thinking Exercise).

The health care team responsible for the management of young people with AN arranges a carefully structured environment. First, there must be consistency. The team decides on an approach and adheres to it. The plan is structured with reality testing regarding caloric intake and body-image perception as an essential component. The team members provide a unified front to avoid any possibility of manipulation or inconsistency. Second, all team members are involved; responsibility for the program cannot be left to one person. The role and boundaries of each member are clearly spelled out. Third, continuity of team members is important; it is helpful to have the same team members all the time.

Fourth, communication among team members is essential. Communication with the patient regarding what is expected is also important. Sometimes the limit setting may seem unreasonable; if the adolescent does not understand the rationale for the limits, he or she may sabotage the entire program. It is also important to communicate with the family. Fifth, the plan must provide for support of the adolescent, the family, and team members. The adolescent's efforts should be supported, and positive feedback should be provided for accomplishments made in normalizing eating habits. Meetings are held to discuss the feelings and concerns of the patient, immediate caregivers, and team members.

A *behavioral contract*, an agreement that the adolescent makes with others to change a maladaptive behavior, has proved to be effective in some cases. The written contract is

CRITICAL THINKING EXERCISE

Anorexia Nervosa

Jane is a 13-year-old whose grades have been excellent and whom the teachers describe as a "model student." Recently, Jane's teacher told the nurse practitioner that Jane's parents were in the middle of a "messy divorce." In addition, several of Jane's friends told the nurse practitioner that they are concerned about Jane because she runs every day at lunchtime and seldom eats lunch with them. Jane told her friends that she gained weight over the winter months and that she is running because she wants to qualify for the track team this spring. At the time of her routine health interview and sports physical, the nurse practitioner notes that Jane's oral temperature is 36° C (96.8° F) and she weighs 34 kg (75 lb). Jane has lost 9 kg (20 lb) since her last sports physical. When discussing her menstrual periods with the nurse practitioner, Jane states that she has not had her period for 3 months.

1. Evidence—Is there sufficient evidence to draw any conclusions about Jane's behavior?
2. Assumptions—Describe some underlying assumptions about the following:
   a. Personality characteristics of individuals with anorexia nervosa (AN)
   b. Factors influencing the development of AN
   c. Clinical manifestations of AN
   d. Treatment of AN
3. What implications for nursing care should be established for Jane at this time?
4. Does the evidence support your conclusion?
5. Are there alternative perspectives that you should consider?

constructed by the therapeutic team and approved and signed by the adolescent. Unless the adolescent agrees to its terms, the contract can become the source of a power struggle. However, it can be an effective tool that places the responsibility for weight gain or other behavioral change on the adolescent.

Nursing care of the adolescent with BN is similar to care of the patient with AN. Acute care involves careful monitoring of fluid and electrolyte alterations and observation for signs of cardiac complications. Nutritional consultation and follow-up care are essential. The nurse should encourage the adolescent and family members to structure the environment to reduce the binging behavior. Getting rid of binge foods; restricting eating to one room of the house; not engaging in other activities while eating; and substituting exercise, crafts, visualization, and relaxation techniques for binging are helpful interventions.

Health professionals, patients, and families can find assistance and information from several organizations. The National Association of Anorexia Nervosa and Associated Disorders* and the National Eating Disorders Association† provide counseling, referrals, and self-help programs.

Serious Health Problems with a Behavioral Component

Tobacco

evolve Case Study–Teen Smoking

Cigarette smoking has continued to decline since the late 1990s, in part due to increased costs, changes in community attitudes about smoking among adults, decreased advertising of cigarettes to children, and increased antismoking advertising as a result of the government lawsuits against tobacco companies (Johnston et al, 2005). In 2007 50% of adolescents attending grades 9 to 12 reported ever trying to smoke a cigarette; 20% of all adolescents surveyed reported smoking on at least 1 day of the previous 30, and of the 20%, 10% reported smoking more than 10 cigarettes per day (Centers for Disease Control and Prevention, 2008).

Although the number of adult and adolescent smokers has declined in recent years, cigarette smoking is still considered the chief avoidable cause of death. The hazards of smoking at any age are undisputed; however, a preventive approach to teenage smoking is especially important. Because of its addictive nature, smoking begun in childhood and adolescence can result in a lifetime habit, with increased morbidity and early mortality. Smoking in adolescence has also been related to other risk behaviors: approximately three times as many adolescents who smoke report carrying weapons and drinking alcohol compared with adolescents who do not smoke; other associated risks in Caucasians include using smokeless tobacco, using marijuana, having multiple sexual partners, not using bicycle helmets, and binge drinking. Research also indicates an association between current use of tobacco and the development of depression (Goodman & Capitman, 2000) and sleep problems (Patten et al, 2000) in adolescence. Cigarettes are considered to be a gateway drug, and teenagers who smoke are 11.4 times more likely to use illicit drugs (Gordon, 2000).

The effects of second-hand smoke exposure are also well known and include increased incidence of low birth weight and subsequent illness, increased incidence of sudden infant death syndrome (if mother smoked during pregnancy), increased incidence of acute lower respiratory tract infections, and exacerbation of asthma symptoms (wheezing, cough, phlegm, breathlessness) in asthmatic children (US Department of Health and Human Services, 2006).

Etiology

Teenagers begin smoking for a variety of reasons, including imitation of adult behavior; peer pressure; a desire to imitate behaviors and lifestyles portrayed in movies and advertisements; and a desire to control weight, especially among females. Teenagers who do not smoke usually have family members and friends who do not smoke or who oppose smoking. Most teens who refrain from smoking have a desire to succeed in academics or athletics (particularly high-performance sports, such as basketball, swimming, and track) and plans to go to college (see Community Focus box). Although smoking among college students has increased in recent years, rates of smoking are highest among adolescents who do not complete high school.

Smokeless Tobacco

The term *smokeless tobacco* refers to tobacco products that are placed in the mouth but not ignited (e.g., chewing tobacco). This substitute for cigarettes continues to pose a hazard to adolescents, although use has declined by about 50% since the peak prevalence in 1995; in 2004 only 16.7% of teens tried smokeless tobacco by the twelfth grade (Johnston et al, 2005). Many children and adolescents believe that smokeless tobacco is a safe alternative to cigarette smoking and is not addictive, and they believe they can stop using it at any time. However, the number of adolescents who identify it as a health risk has increased since the mid-1990s, with nearly half now agreeing it has health risks (Johnston et al, 2005). These products have also been proved to be carcinogenic, and regular use can cause dental problems, foul-smelling breath, and tooth erosion or loss.

Nursing Care Management

Prevention of regular smoking in teenagers is the most effective way to reduce the overall incidence of smoking. A variety of methods have been employed. Posters, charts, displays, statistics, and the use of examples of actual damaged lungs to communicate the hazards of smoking all have their supporters and doubters. Some schools also use films and demonstrations in science classes.

For the most part, smoking-prevention programs that focus on the negative, long-term effects of smoking on health have been ineffective. Youth-to-youth programs and those emphasizing the immediate consequences are more effective

**PO Box 7, Highland Park, IL 60035; 847-831-3438; e-mail: anadhelp@anad.org;* www.anad.org.

†603 Stewart St., Suite 803, Seattle, WA 98101; 800-931-2237; www.nationaleatingdisorders.org.

COMMUNITY FOCUS

Early Sexual Maturation, Alcohol, and Cigarettes

Smoking cigarettes and drinking alcohol among adolescents are complex behaviors that are not explained by any one factor. Some theorists and investigators believe there is a relationship between biologic maturation and risk-taking behaviors. For example, young girls who are sexually mature at an earlier age than their peers are often attracted to older girls and boys who may engage in risk-taking behaviors. If older teens smoke, drink, and drive while under the influence of alcohol with no adverse consequences (e.g., no motor vehicle accidents), young girls may believe that they, too, will be safe while smoking, drinking, or riding in an automobile with friends who are drinking.

Although parents and nurses cannot influence the time of biologic maturation, they can identify young girls who are at risk for the initiation of risk-taking behaviors because of early puberty. Parents need to understand that an early-maturing daughter might be uncomfortable with her body, and they should take advantage of opportunities to build her self-esteem. Parental sensitivity to the importance of peer-group acceptance and parental support of a teenage daughter who feels left out or different are crucial. School nurses can provide anticipatory guidance to these girls and help them role-play coping strategies for situations that involve offers to smoke and drink. In addition, school nurses can provide information about physical development during puberty and emphasize that not all teenagers mature at the same time or rate.

Teachers, coaches, and community and church leaders can provide opportunities for these girls to "fit in" with their same-age peers through activities that stress mutual goals. For example, an early-maturing girl is typically taller than her age-mates and can be an asset in sports such as basketball and track-and-field events.

but primarily in improving teenagers' attitudes toward not smoking. Because smoking and smoking-related behaviors are social symbols, antismoking campaigns must address the norms of potential smokers. Anything that ridicules or threatens the social norms of the peer group can be unproductive or counterproductive. Investigators have found that teaching resistance to peer pressure to smoke is effective in early adolescence. Although the effects of these programs may decrease with time, the effects can be enhanced in older adolescents by presenting information in class instead of simply handing out written material to the students (Adelman et al, 2001).

Two areas of focus for antismoking programs are peer-led programs and use of media in smoking prevention (e.g., CDs, videotapes, and films). Peer-led programs emphasizing the social consequences of smoking have proved most successful. If a significant number of influential peers can "sell" their classmates on the idea that the habit is not popular, the followers will imitate their behavior. Such programs emphasize short-term rather than long-term consequences (e.g., the effects of smoking on personal appearance, such as unattractive stains on teeth and hands and unpleasant odor of breath and clothing).

The impact of school-based antismoking programs can be strengthened by expanding these programs to include parents, mass media, youth groups, and community organizations. For example, mass media efforts that involve antismoking radio campaigns have been identified as the most cost-effective mass media intervention.

Smoking bans in schools accomplish several goals: (1) they discourage students from starting to smoke, (2) they reinforce knowledge of the health hazards of cigarette smoking and exposure to environmental tobacco smoke, and (3) they promote a smoke-free environment as the norm (see Community Focus box).

Substance Abuse

Although experimentation with drugs during childhood and adolescence is widespread, most children and teens do not become high risk users. National and statewide surveys indicate that despite a steady increase in the incidence of adolescents using tobacco, alcohol, and marijuana between the ages of 12 and 18, experimentation is limited to one adolescent in eight for stimulants and inhalants and to less than one adolescent in 10 for "hard" drugs such as hallucinogens, sedatives, and crack cocaine. It has been reported that as many as 51% of American youth have tried an illegal drug by the time of high school graduation (American Academy of Pediatrics, 2005). Although surveys demonstrate a modest decrease in the use of certain substances among youth (marijuana, amphetamines, barbiturates, and tranquilizers), abuse of other drugs (cocaine, steroids, heroine, flunitrazepam [Rohypnol]) has remained steady (American Academy of Pediatrics, 2005; Centers for Disease Control and Prevention, 2008).

Drug abuse, misuse, and *addiction* are culturally defined and are voluntary behaviors. *Drug tolerance* and *physical dependence* are involuntary physiologic responses to the pharmacologic characteristics of the drugs, such as opioids and alcohol. Consequently, an individual can be addicted to a narcotic with or without being physically dependent. A person can also be physically dependent on a narcotic without being addicted (e.g., patients who use opioids to control pain).

Motivation

Most drug use begins with experimentation. The drug may be used only once, may be used occasionally, or may become part of a drug-centered lifestyle. Children and adolescents initiate drug use out of curiosity. Adolescents who use drugs may fall into one of two broad categories—experimenters and compulsive users—or they may fall into a third category somewhere on the continuum between these extremes as recreational users, principally of drugs such as marijuana, cocaine, alcohol, and prescription drugs. For many the goal is peer acceptance; these users fit more closely with the experimenting, intermittent users. For others the goal is intoxication or the sustained intense effects from using a particular drug; these users resemble the compulsive users. These users may engage in periodic heavy use, or binges. The groups of greatest concern to health care workers are those whose patterns of use involve high doses or mixed drugs with the danger of overdose, and those compulsive users with the threat of dependence, withdrawal syndromes, and altered lifestyle.

COMMUNITY FOCUS

Nonsmoking Strategies

Nurses who work in schools, hospitals, and community agencies can take advantage of all opportunities to provide education about the dangers of smoking, to discourage smoking initiation by children and adolescents, to encourage smoking cessation, and to promote smoke-free environments. In particular, school nurses must be alert to the vulnerability of young preteens when they enter junior high or middle school. These nurses are in an ideal position to assess stress, personal conflict, weight concerns, peer pressures, and other factors that place preteens at risk for smoking initiation. Nurses should serve as counselors to student, teacher, and parent groups and as advocates for antismoking legislative efforts. The following additional strategies are recommended*:

- Provide only brief information about long-term health consequences (e.g., cardiovascular and cancer risks).
- Discuss immediate physiologic consequences (e.g., changes in heart rate, blood pressure, respiratory symptoms, and blood carbon monoxide concentrations).
- Mention alternatives to smoking that also establish a self-image that appears independent, mature, or sophisticated (e.g., weight lifting; jogging; dancing; joining a boys' or girls' club; engaging in volunteer work for a hospital, political, religious, or community group).
- Mention the negative effects in detail (e.g., earlier wrinkling of skin; yellow stains on teeth and fingers; tobacco odor on breath, hair, and clothing).
- Mention the increasing ostracism of smokers by nonsmokers, both legal and informal, in the workplace and in public places.
- Mention the increasing evidence that secondhand smoke is injurious to the health of nonsmokers who are regularly exposed, especially small children.
- Acknowledge that many adults, who were enticed to start smoking as teenagers because of its social benefits, now wish they could stop smoking.
- Give cooperative adolescents effective arguments to deal with peer pressure (e.g., by not smoking, a teenager demonstrates independence and nonconformity, traits normally prized by youth).
- Request posters or pamphlets from local agencies (e.g., American Cancer Society, American Heart Association, and American Lung Association) to display in prominent places at school.

*The Centers for Disease Control and Prevention has information on the effects of tobacco, smoking cessation, and tobacco control programs; 1600 Clifton Road, Atlanta, GA 30333; 800-232-4636; e-mail: tobaccoinfo@cdc.gov; *www.cdc.gov/tobacco*.

Types of Drugs Abused

Any drug can be abused, and most are potentially harmful to adolescents still going through formative life experiences. Although rarely considered drugs by society, the chemically active substances frequently abused are the xanthines and theobromines contained in chocolate, tea, coffee, and colas. Ethyl alcohol and nicotine are other drugs that are legal and socially sanctioned. Any of these substances can produce mild to moderate euphoric or stimulant effects and can lead to physical and psychologic dependence.

Drugs with mind-altering abilities that are available on the "street" and are of medical and legal concern are the hallucinogenic, narcotic, hypnotic, and stimulant drugs. In addition, there has been a notable increase in the use of alcohol and volatile substances that are inhaled to achieve altered sensation (such as gasoline, antifreeze, plastic model airplane cement, typewriter correction fluid, and organic solvents). Abuse of prescription and synthetic drugs such as oxycodone, alprazolam (Xanax), and amphetamine-dextroamphetamine (Adderall) has become a concern for professionals who work with children and adolescents. Many of the prescription drugs are available at a decreased cost in comparison to the more exotic drugs of abuse and are often found in the medicine cabinet at home. Internet websites also promote the "safe use" of some psychoactive drugs and supply information on new "designer" drugs that are not detectable on a standard urine drug screening test.

Alcohol

Acute or chronic abuse of alcohol (ethanol) is responsible for many acts of violence, suicide, accidental injury, and death. Alcohol drinking is likely to begin in the middle school years and increases with age. By 18 years of age, 80% to 90% of adolescents have tried alcohol. Ethanol is a depressant that reduces inhibitions against aggressive and sexual acting out. Severe physical and psychologic symptoms accompany abrupt withdrawal, and long-term use leads to slow tissue destruction, especially of the brain and liver cells. The most noticeable effects of alcohol occur within the central nervous system and include changes in cognitive and autonomic functions such as judgment, memory, learning ability, and other intellectual capacities. Young alcoholics often drink alone and cannot control their use of alcohol. They often rely on the substance as a defense against depression, anxiety, fear, or anger. Not all of these characteristics are observed in the adolescent who is abusing alcohol, but if several signs are evident, the child or adolescent should be considered at risk. Referral to a health care professional and detoxification therapy may be necessary. Information about alcohol and answers to questions are available through the Alcohol Hotline (800-ALCOHOL). Other groups that provide support and counseling for families are Al-Anon, Ala-Teen, Ala-Tot, and Alcoholics Anonymous (an organization that has listings in all local telephone directories).

Cocaine

Although cocaine is not pharmacologically considered a narcotic, it is legally categorized as such. Cocaine is available in two forms: water-soluble cocaine hydrochloride, which is administered by "snorting" or intravenous injection, and non-soluble alkaloid (freebase) cocaine, which is used primarily for smoking. Crack, or "rock," is a purer, more menacing form of the drug. It can be produced cheaply and smoked in either water pipes or mentholated cigarettes. The use of cocaine has increased in recent years because of its availability and affordability, its association with persons in glamorous occupations, peer pressure, and its reputation as a sexually enhancing drug.

Cocaine creates a sense of euphoria, or an indefinable high. Withdrawal does not produce the dramatic symptoms observed in withdrawal from other substances. The effects are those commonly seen in depression, including lack of energy and motivation, irritability, appetite changes, psychomotor retardation, and irregular sleep patterns. More serious symptoms include cardiovascular manifestations and seizures. Physical withdrawal should not be confused with the so-called crash after a cocaine high, which consists of a long period of sleep. Answers to questions about the risks of using cocaine are available at the National Cocaine Hotline (800-COCAINE), which also provides referrals to support groups and treatment centers.

Narcotics

Narcotic drugs include opiates such as heroin and morphine, and opioids (opiate-like drugs), such as hydromorphone (Dilaudid), hydrocodone, fentanyl, meperidine (Demerol), and codeine. These drugs produce a state of euphoria by removing painful feelings and creating a pleasurable experience and a sense of success accompanied by clouding of the consciousness and a dreamlike state. Physical signs of narcotic abuse include constricted pupils, respiratory depression, and, often, cyanosis. Needle marks may be visible on the arms or legs in chronic users. Physical withdrawal from opiates is extremely unpleasant unless controlled with supervised tapering doses of the opioid or substitution of methadone.

As important as the physical effects are the indirect consequences related to the illegal status of narcotic use and the problems associated with securing the drug (e.g., the time-consuming searches to obtain the drug and the often illegal methods used to meet the high cost of purchasing it). Health problems also result from self-neglect of physical needs (nutrition, cleanliness, dental care); overdose; contamination; and infection, including HIV and hepatitis B and C infection.

Central Nervous System Depressants

Central nervous system depressants include a variety of hypnotic drugs that produce physical dependence and withdrawal symptoms on abrupt discontinuation. They create a feeling of relaxation and sleepiness but impair general functioning. Drugs in this category include barbiturates, nonbarbiturates, and alcohol. Barbiturates combined with alcohol produce a profound depressant effect. Flunitrazepam, known as the "date rape drug," is a recent hypnotic drug abused by adolescents. Many women report being raped after unknowingly being given flunitrazepam in a drink. Flunitrazepam is 10 times more powerful than diazepam (Valium). It produces prolonged sedation, a feeling of well-being, and short-term memory loss.

Central Nervous System Stimulants

Amphetamines and cocaine do not produce strong physical dependence and can be withdrawn without much danger. However, psychologic dependence is strong, and acute intoxication can lead to violent aggressive behavior or psychotic episodes characterized by paranoia, uncontrollable agitation, and restlessness. When combined with barbiturates, the euphoric effects are particularly addictive.

Methamphetamine can be snorted, injected, swallowed, or smoked and produces a burst of energy in its users, along with intense, alternating attacks of boldness and paranoia. It provokes excitement far more intense than that caused by cocaine. The drug, with the street names *speed, crank, meth, ice*, and *crystal*, is inexpensive and has a longer period of action than cocaine. Instead of a short (few minutes) high, as achieved with cocaine, a user can remain "up" for hours on a similar dose of crank.

Health care professionals are concerned about the use of various volatile substances, or *inhalants* such as gasoline, model airplane cement, and organic solvents; these substances are inhaled by the user to achieve an altered sensation, and recent surveillance has indicated a modest increase in use, after nearly a decade of decline. Adolescents breathe or place these substances into paper or plastic bags or soda cans from which they rebreathe the fumes to produce a feeling of euphoria and altered consciousness. These substances contain chemical solvents and are extremely hazardous. Dusters contain Freon, a substance that can cause fatal cardiac arrhythmias. The use of inhalants is increasing, and inhalants are becoming a gateway drug for young children and preteens, who often progress to other harder drugs such as marijuana, heroin, and cocaine. Many young children are unaware of the dangers of "sniffing" or "huffing." In addition to rapid loss of consciousness and respiratory arrest, these substances may cause visual scanning problems, language deficiencies, motor instability, memory deficits, and attention and concentration problems.

Mind-Altering Drugs

Hallucinogens (psychedelics, psychotomimetics, psychotropics, or illusionogenics) are drugs that produce vivid hallucinations and euphoria. These drugs do not produce physical dependence, and they can be abruptly withdrawn without ill effect. However, the acute and long-term effects are variable, and in some individuals the dissociative behavior may be prolonged. Cannabis (marijuana, hashish) and lysergic acid diethylamide (LSD) are also included in this category of drugs. Marijuana was the highest (19.7%) reported drug used within the last 30 days by high school students (Centers for Disease Control and Prevention, 2008).

Nursing Care Management Related to Therapeutic Management

Nurses who have contact with children and adolescents are in an excellent position to provide information about substance abuse and to serve as patient advocates. The nurse most often encounters young drug abusers when they are (1) experiencing overdose or withdrawal symptoms, (2) manifesting bizarre behavior or confusion secondary to drug ingestion, (3) worried that they are or will become addicted, or (4) worried about a friend or family member who is addicted.

In particular, nurses who care for hospitalized adolescents need to know if these youths use drugs compulsively. Drug withdrawal can seriously complicate other illnesses. Nurses should be alert for any physical or behavioral clues that indicate the onset of withdrawal or the effects of drugs. Nurses who work in schools or the community play an essential role in identifying children, adolescents, and families with substance abuse problems. The school nurse may be the first to identify a child or adolescent who has ingested a particular drug by the child's erratic behavior in class or on the school grounds. Early identification of those at risk for substance abuse problems is an essential aspect of prevention. Pediatric health care professionals also prevent substance abuse by creating trusting relationships so that children and adolescents feel comfortable asking questions about drugs and health professionals can alert them to websites and other aspects of society that encourage experimentation with drugs.

Acute Care

Adolescents experiencing toxic drug effects or withdrawal symptoms are usually seen initially in the emergency department. Experienced emergency department personnel are familiar with the management of acute drug toxicity and the signs, symptoms, and behavioral characteristics associated with a variety of substances. When the drug is questionable or unknown, knowledge of these factors facilitates management and treatment. Often, observation or description of the child or adolescent's behavior is more valuable than reports by patients or their friends.

The treatment for drug toxicity or withdrawal varies according to the drug and the method used. Every effort is made to determine the type, the time of ingestion, the amount of drug taken, the mode of administration, and factors related to the onset of presenting symptoms. It is helpful to know the individual's pattern of use. For example, if two types of drugs are involved, they may require different treatments. Gastric lavage may be employed when the drug has been ingested recently and the cough reflex is intact, but it is of little value when the drug has been administered by the intravenous ("mainlined") or intranasal ("sniffed") route. Because the actual content of most street drugs is highly questionable, other pharmaceutical agents are administered with caution, except perhaps the narcotic antagonists in cases of suspected opiate overdoses. It is also necessary to assess for possible trauma sustained while the patient was under the influence of the drug.

Long-Term Management

A major factor in the treatment and rehabilitation of young drug users is careful assessment in the nonacute stage to determine the function that the drug plays in the adolescent's life. The motivation phase is directed toward exploring the factors that influence drug use. It also involves establishing a feeling of self-worth and a commitment to self-help in the teen.

Rehabilitation begins when adolescents decide that they can and are willing to change. *Rehabilitation* involves fostering healthy interdependent relationships with caring and supportive adults and exploring alternate mechanisms for problem solving while simultaneously reducing or eliminating drug use. Persons working with troubled youth must be prepared for *recidivism*, or the tendency to relapse, and maintain a plan for reentry into the treatment process.

Family Support

Most treatment programs for substance abusers are based on adult 12-step models such as Alcoholics Anonymous. Research is needed to determine whether these adult models are effective for adolescents. Tough Love *(www.toughlove.com)* is one program that is based on the conviction that parents have the right and responsibility to be the policymakers in the family, to set limits on their children's behavior, and to take control of the household from out-of-control adolescents. The premise is that allowing teenagers to experience the negative consequences of their behavior will bring them closer to accepting help or changing their behavior. Another group that provides support and counseling for families experiencing substance abuse and seeking strategies to cope with their children is Parents Anonymous.* Another source of information is the Substance Abuse and Mental Health Services Administration's National Clearinghouse for Alcohol and Drug Information.†

Prevention

Nurses play an important role in education efforts, as well as in individual observation, assessment, and therapy related to substance abuse. In recent years a variety of educational programs have been applied with promising results. The most effective prevention strategies are those that are part of a broader, more general effort to promote overall health and success. Health-compromising behaviors are often interconnected and have common antecedents. Prevention efforts that focus on changing only one behavior (e.g., alcohol, other drug use) are less likely to be successful. Successful programs are those that have promoted parenting skills, social skills among distractible children, academic achievement, and skills to resist peer pressure.

Peer pressure is a powerful tool and can be used effectively in substance abuse prevention. A group that has had some success in reducing injury from drunk driving is Students Against Destructive Decisions (SADD).‡ Techniques used by this group include peer counseling, parental guidelines for teenage parties, and community awareness. Nurses should encourage the formation of SADD chapters in the high schools in their communities.

Suicide

Suicide is defined as the deliberate act of self-injury with the intent that the injury results in death. Most experts distinguish between suicidal ideation, suicide attempt (or parasuicide), and suicide. *Suicidal ideation* involves a preoccupation with thoughts about committing suicide and may be a precursor to suicide. Although it is not uncommon for adolescents to experience occasional suicidal thoughts, expressions of preoccupation with suicide should be taken seriously, and an assessment should be conducted for appropriate referral. A *suicide attempt* is intended to cause injury or death. The term *parasuicide* refers to behaviors ranging from gestures to serious attempts to kill oneself. *Parasuicide* is a preferred term because it makes no reference to intent and because a person's motive may be too difficult or complex to determine. However, all parasuicidal activity should be taken seriously.

NURSING ALERT A history of a previous suicide attempt is a serious indicator for possible suicide completion in the future. Studies of adolescent suicides have found that as many as half of the adolescents had made previous attempts.

*675 W. Foothill Blvd., Suite 220, Claremont, CA 91711; 909-621-6184; www.parentsanonymous.org.

†PO Box 2345, Rockville, MD 20847; 800-729-6686; e-mail: info@health.org; http://ncadi.samhsa.gov.

‡255 Main St., Marlborough, MA 01752; 877-SADD-INC; www.sadd.org.

Results from the 2007 Youth Risk Behavior Surveillance, indicated that 6.9% of students nationwide had attempted suicide at least once during the 12 months preceding the survey; the range of suicide attempts by adolescents across the states varied from 4.8% to 14.3% (Centers for Disease Control and Prevention, 2008). The overall incidence of youth suicide has decreased since 1992, yet the Centers for Disease Control and Prevention notes the incidence is still too high. Approximately 11% of the students in this survey reported that they had made a specific plan to attempt suicide in the 12 months preceding the survey. Suicide is currently the third leading cause of death in adolescents aged 15 to 19 years, surpassed only by death from motor vehicle crash and homicide (see Chapter 29).

Etiology

Individual, family, and social or environmental factors have all been implicated in suicide. The single most important individual factor is the presence of an active psychiatric disorder (depression, bipolar disorder, psychosis, substance abuse, or conduct disorder). Comorbidity of an affective disorder and substance abuse also increases the risk for suicide. Approximately 90% of adolescents who completed suicide met criteria for a psychiatric disorder before the suicide (Shain & AAP Committee on Adolescence, 2007). Depression is considered the highest single risk factor for adolescent suicide (American Academy of Child and Adolescent Psychiatry & American Psychiatric Association, 2004). Mental health problems that may predispose to suicide include depression; bipolar disorder; substance abuse or dependence; panic attacks; posttraumatic stress disorder; and a history of aggression, severe anger, or impulsivity (Shain & AAP Committee on Adolescence, 2007). Gay and lesbian adolescents are at particularly high risk for suicide completion, especially if raised in an environment in which they are denied support systems (see Community Focus box). Family factors influencing suicide include parental loss; family disruption; a family history of suicide, depression, substance abuse, or emotional disturbance; child abuse or neglect; unavailable parents; poor communication and isolation within the family; family conflict; and unrealistically high parental expectations or parental indifference with low expectations. Social or environmental factors include incarceration, isolation, acute loss of a boyfriend or girlfriend, lack of future options, and availability of firearms in the home.

Methods

Firearms are by far the most commonly used instruments (54%) in completed suicides among males (Shain & AAP Committee on Adolescence, 2007). For adolescent males, the second and third most common means of suicide are hanging and overdose, respectively; for females the most common means are overdose and strangulation, respectively.

The most common method of suicide attempt is overdose or ingestion of a potentially toxic substance, such as drugs. The second most common method of suicide attempt is self-inflicted laceration.

NURSING ALERT Given what is known about youth suicide, nurses should ask parents, especially those with at-risk teenagers, if firearms are available in the house and, if so, recommend their removal. Parents must ensure that their children—especially those who are depressed, have poor problem-solving skills, or use drugs or alcohol—do not have access to firearms. Parents must also be educated on the warning signs of suicide (Box 40-8).

COMMUNITY FOCUS

Suicide, Sexual Identity, and Sexual Orientation

A significant number of teenage suicides occur among homosexual youths. Gay or lesbian adolescents who live in families or communities that do not accept homosexuality are likely to suffer low self-esteem, self-loathing, depression, and hopelessness as a result. Such internalization, without treatment and support, can lead to substance abuse and, eventually, suicide. Youths most at risk are those who struggle with gender identity issues such as gay identity formation at a young age, intrapersonal conflict regarding sexuality, and nondisclosure of orientation to others.

Supportive parents, friends, or relationships serve as protective factors against suicide. However, many gay, lesbian, and bisexual adolescents do not feel supported, understood, or accepted by their friends, parents, and families. Nurses who interact with adolescents must be aware of the association between suicide and adolescent homosexuality and gender nonconformity. School nurses may be the first individuals to discuss issues of sexual identity and orientation with adolescents or their families. In their professional capacity, nurses can serve as support persons for these adolescents. Nurses can also provide guidance and resources to families so that they understand how best to nurture and support their child.

Nurses must also capitalize on opportunities or experiences that promote the healthy development of self-esteem in youths who choose nontraditional sexual orientation. Educational programs to raise the level of consciousness about the risk factors for and warning signs of suicide are one example. Another possibility could be programs conducted in or outside of school that are designed to foster peer relationships and competency in social skills among high-risk adolescents and young adults, such as support groups and social organizations for these young people.

Motivation

Suicidal ideation is not uncommon in adolescents. It represents numerous fantasies, such as relief from suffering, a means of gaining comfort and sympathy, or a means of revenge against those who have hurt them. Adolescents have the erroneous perception that the act of suicide will evoke remorse and pity and that they will be able to return and witness the grief. Angry children who are unable to directly punish those who have injured or insulted them may take revenge on those who love them through self-destruction ("They'll be sorry when they find me dead"; "They'll be sorry they were mean to me").

For adolescents who are severely depressed, suicide seems to be the only release from their despair. These adolescents rarely provide evidence of their intent and frequently conceal their suicidal thoughts. Many adolescents, however, tell their

BOX 40-8 Warning Signs of Suicide

- Preoccupation with themes of death—focuses on morbid thoughts
- Wants to give away cherished possessions
- Talks of own death, desire to die
- Loss of energy, loss of interest, listlessness
- Exhaustion without obvious cause
- Changes in sleep patterns—too much or too little
- Increased irritability, argumentativeness, or stubbornness
- Physical complaints—recurrent stomachaches, headaches
- Repeated visits to physician, nurse practitioner, or emergency department for treatment of injuries
- Reckless behavior
- Antisocial behavior—engages in drinking, uses drugs, fights, commits acts of vandalism, runs away from home, becomes sexually promiscuous
- Sudden change in school performance—lowered grades, cutting classes, dropping out of activities
- Resists or refuses to go to school
- Remains distant, sad, remote—flat affect, frozen facial expression
- Describes self as worthless
- Sudden cheerfulness following deep depression
- Social withdrawal from friends, activities, interests that were previously enjoyed
- Impaired concentration
- Dramatic change in appetite

BOX 40-9 Characteristics of Children or Adolescents with Depression

Behavior

Predominantly sad facial expression with absence or diminished range of affective response (most of the day)
Solitary play or work; tendency to be alone; lack of interest in play with friends
Withdrawal from previously enjoyed activities and relationships
Lowered grades in school; lack of interest in doing homework or achieving in school; refuses to wake up for school
Diminished motor activity; tiredness
Tearfulness or crying
Inability to concentrate
Dependent and clinging or aggressive and disruptive
Recurrent suicidal thoughts or talk

Internal States

Utterance of statements reflecting lowered self-esteem, sense of hopelessness, or guilt
Suicidal ideations

Physiology

Constipation
Loss of energy; fatigue
Nonspecific complaints of not feeling well
Change in appetite resulting in weight loss or gain
Alterations in sleeping pattern, sleeplessness, or hypersomnia

evolve Critical Thinking Exercise—Depression

peers of their suicidal thoughts or plans but avoid telling adults. Social isolation is a significant factor in distinguishing adolescents who will kill themselves from those who will not. It is also more characteristic of those who complete suicide than of those who make attempts or threats.

The frequency of *contagion*, or *copycat suicides* (i.e., an increase in youth suicide that occurs after the suicide of one teenager is publicized) is disturbing and may indicate that teenagers perceive suicide as glamorous. In addition, young people may not realize the finality of suicide because they have become desensitized from constantly viewing violence and death on television, in video games, or in movies.

Diagnostic Evaluation

Depression is common among adolescents who attempt suicide. It is estimated that approximately 5% of children and adolescents experience some form of depression (American Academy of Child and Adolescent Psychiatry & American Psychiatric Association, 2004). Depression is characterized by both subjective symptoms and objective signs that reflect the adolescent's sadness and despair. Adolescents describe feelings of sadness, despair, helplessness, hopelessness, boredom, loss of interest, and isolation. They may also feel self-reproach, self-deprecation, and guilt. Subjective symptoms of depression or specific changes in behavior place an adolescent at risk for suicide (Box 40-9).

Therapeutic Management

Threats of suicide should always be taken seriously. There has been a tendency to dismiss a suicide attempt as an impulsive act resulting from a temporary crisis or depression. If a suicide attempt fails to draw attention to their problems or makes them worse, the child or adolescent may conclude that suicide is the only answer. Children and adolescents need to know that someone cares and must be provided with swift and efficient crisis intervention. Although ordinary practitioners can manage an acute depressive reaction without difficulty, the adolescent who has made a serious attempt or has a specific plan for suicide should receive immediate attention and competent psychiatric care.

The American Academy of Child and Adolescent Psychiatry (2001) has published a practice parameter for the assessment and treatment of child and adolescent suicide.

NURSING ALERT Adolescents who express suicidal feelings and have a specific plan should be monitored at all times. They should not have access to firearms, prescription or over-the-counter drugs, belts, scarves, shoestrings, sharp objects, matches, or lighters. If they are intoxicated, they must be restrained or placed in a protective environment until a psychiatrist or psychologist can assess them.

Nursing Care Management

Nurses play a pivotal role in reducing adolescent suicide. Nurses have the opportunity to provide anticipatory guidance to parents and adolescents. They can teach parents to be supportive and to develop positive communication patterns that help teens feel connected with and loved by their families. To foster healthy development, parents can be encouraged to provide teens with creative outlets and to assist young people in accepting strong emotions—pain, anger, and frustration—as a normal part of the human experience.

Nurses may question parents about signs of depression for young children. At one hospital adolescents are screened for depression by asking eight yes-no questions; if the adolescent reports five or more signs of depression, the nurse implements a screening for suicidal ideation (Weeks et al, 2004). The depression screening questions consider whether the adolescent reports:

- Feeling sad or crying often
- Perceiving that nothing is fun anymore
- Frequently losing his or her temper
- Preferring to be alone than with friends
- Sleeping a lot or too little
- Feeling restless or tired much of the time
- Eating infrequently or too often
- Having difficulty making a decision

If the adolescent is considered a suicide risk as a result of the screening, close observation is implemented by the staff and the primary practitioner is notified of the screening results (Weeks et al, 2004).

Care of the suicidal adolescent includes early recognition, management, and prevention. The most important aspect of management is the recognition of warning signs that indicate an adolescent is troubled and might attempt suicide. Health professionals must be alert to the signs of depression, and anyone who exhibits such behavior should be referred for thorough psychologic assessment. Depression is manifested differently in children and adolescents than in adults. In teens it may be masked by impulsive aggressive behaviors. Defiance, disobedience, behavior problems, and psychosomatic disturbances can indicate underlying depression, suicidal ideation, and impending suicide attempts.

No threat of suicide should be ignored or challenged. Threats are a symptom that must be taken seriously. Too often, suicidal threats or minor attempts are confused with bids for attention. It is also a mistake to be lulled into a false sense of security when the adolescent's depression is apparently relieved. The improvement in attitude may mean that the adolescent has made the decision and found the means to carry out the threat.

Peers or other confidants are valuable observers and excellent sources of information about potential suicide attempts. They may not be able to diagnose depression, but they are able to sense when a friend has undergone a marked personality change. It is important to emphasize that the peer who detects any changes in a friend is a potential rescuer and should not remain silent about the observations. Friendship does not imply collusion. A peer who believes that a friend may be suicidal should alert someone who can help (e.g., a parent, teacher, guidance counselor, school nurse).

Routine health assessments of adolescents should include questions that assess the presence of suicidal ideation or intent. The following questions can be asked (Greydanus & Pratt, 1995):

- Do you consider yourself more a happy person, an unhappy person, or somewhere in the middle?
- Have you ever been so unhappy or upset that you felt like being dead?
- Have you ever thought about hurting yourself?
- Have you ever developed a plan to hurt yourself or kill yourself?
- Have you ever attempted to kill yourself?

If children or adolescents express suicidal intent, nurses make a contract, asking them to sign an agreement that they will not attempt suicide during an agreed-on period and that they will call the 24-hour crisis line immediately if they feel that they cannot keep their contract. The amount of time an adolescent feels comfortable contracting is usually an indication of his or her risk and stability.

Because a suicide attempt is frequently an outgrowth of family distress, it is essential to intervene with the family. It is important to assess family interactions and to recognize disturbed relationships. The most effective approach is recognition of susceptible adolescents during the early stages of family distress so that family counseling can be started. Prevention must be directed toward improving childrearing practices through support and education of parents and changing societal conditions that generate defeat, despair, and maladaptive behavior.

Although confidentiality is an essential part of adolescent counseling, in the case of self-destructive behaviors confidentiality cannot be honored. Suicidal behavior is reported to the family and other professionals, and adolescents are informed that this will be done. Such action conveys an important message to the youth: that the professionals understand and care.

Many schools have instituted suicide prevention programs. These programs include services such as drop-in counseling and a peer-counseling telephone line. Information can also be obtained from the American Association of Suicidology.*

5221 Wisconsin Ave. NW, Washington, DC 20015; 202-237-2280; www.suicidology.org.

Key Points

- The pubescent growth spurt that begins around age 10 in girls and age 12 in boys signals the beginning of adolescence.
- Biologic development during puberty is characterized by increased activity of the pituitary gland, which results in sexual maturity and the appearance of secondary sex characteristics.
- According to Erikson, the major developmental crisis of adolescence is establishing a sense of identity.
- Spiritual development is characterized by the questioning of family values and ideals, a move to more philosophic thinking, and emphasis on personal religion.
- Adolescent relationships with parents may be strained; the influence of the peer group increases and intimate relationships assume importance.
- Teenagers demonstrate a wide variety of interests, and their increased physical and cognitive skills allow them to engage in increasingly difficult and complex activities.
- Adolescents' emotions fluctuate.
- Nutritional needs may not be met by teenagers' eating habits, such as snacking and irregular mealtimes.
- Motor vehicle injuries are the primary cause of death from injury in the adolescent years.
- The rapid changes, growth, and stress accompanying the transition to adulthood may predispose adolescents to faulty problem solving.
- Cognitive development in adolescence includes abstract thought, thinking beyond the present, logical reasoning, and a sense of idealism.

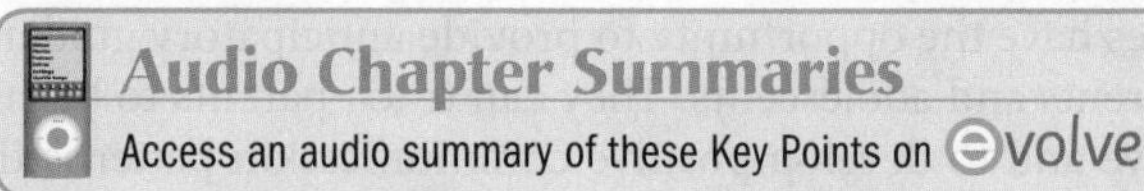
Audio Chapter Summaries
Access an audio summary of these Key Points on evolve

- Development of body image is closely tied to body changes and social interactions.
- According to Kohlberg's theory of moral development, adolescents begin to question existing moral values and learn to make choices.
- The most common health problems related to the female reproductive system involve menstrual dysfunction.
- Eating disorders observed in middle and late childhood are obesity, AN, and BN.
- Tobacco smoking is a widespread problem among teenagers. Reasons for smoking include social pressure, mass media influence, and a need to develop a self-concept.
- The substances abused by children and adolescents are alcohol, marijuana, narcotics, central nervous system depressants, central nervous system stimulants, hydrocarbons and fluorocarbons, and mind-altering drugs.
- Suicide, the deliberate act of self-injury with the intent to kill, may occur because of difficulties coping with stress, disturbed family environment, substance abuse or dependency, or mental health disorder.
- No threat of suicide by an adolescent should be ignored or challenged.

References

Abma JC et al: Teenagers in the United States: sexual activity, contraceptive use, and childbearing, 2002, *Vital Health Stats* 23(24):1-48, 2004.

Adelman WP et al: Effectiveness of a high school smoking cessation program, *Pediatrics* 107(4):e50, 2001.

American Academy of Child and Adolescent Psychiatry: Practice parameter for the assessment and treatment of children and adolescents with suicidal behavior, *J Am Acad Child Adolesc Psychiatry* 40(7 Suppl):24S-51S, 2001.

American Academy of Child and Adolescent Psychiatry, American Psychiatric Association: *Joint statement from the American Academy of Child and Adolescent Psychiatry and American Psychiatric Association for the Senate Substance Abuse and Mental Health Services Committee of the Health, Education, Labor and Pensions Hearing Committee Hearing on Suicide Prevention and Youth: Saving lives*, March 3, 2004. Available at www.aacap.org/galleries/legislaticeaction/suicideH.pdf (retrieved July 15, 2008).

American Academy of Pediatric Dentistry: Adolescent oral health care. *AAPD Reference Manual 2008-2009* 30(7):94-101, 2009. Available at www.aapd.org/media/Policies_Guidelines/G_Adolescenthealth.pdf (accessed April 12, 2009).

American Academy of Pediatrics: Tobacco, alcohol, and other drugs: the role of the pediatrician in prevention, maintenance, and identification of substance abuse, *Pediatrics* 115(3):816-821, 2005.

American Academy of Pediatrics, Committee on Adolescence: Identifying and treating eating disorders, *Pediatrics* 111(1):204-211, 2003.

American Academy of Pediatrics, Committee on Infectious Diseases: Recommended immunization schedules for children and adolescents—United States, 2008, *Pediatrics* 121(1):219-220, 2008.

American Academy of Pediatrics, Committee on Infectious Diseases, Pickering L (editor): *Red book: 2006 report of the Committee on Infectious Diseases*, ed 27, Elk Grove Village, IL, 2006, The Academy.

American Academy of Pediatrics, Committee on Infectious Diseases: Prevention and control of meningococcal disease: recommendations for use of meningococcal vaccines in pediatric patients, *Pediatrics* 116(2):496-505, 2005.

American Academy of Pediatrics, American College of Obstetricians and Gynecologists: Menstruation in girls and adolescents: using the menstrual cycle as a vital sign, *Pediatrics* 118(5):2245-2250, 2006.

American Dietetic Association: Position of the American Dietetic Association: nutrition intervention in the treatment of anorexia nervosa, bulimia nervosa, and other eating disorders, *J Am Diet Assoc* 106(12):2073-2082, 2006.

American Heart Association: Dietary recommendations for children and adolescents, 2005. Available at www.americanheart.org/presenter.jhtml?identifier=3033999 (accessed January 24, 2008).

American Medical Association: *Guidelines for adolescent preventive services (GAPS)*, Chicago, 1997, The Association.

American Psychiatric Association: *Diagnostic and statistical manual of mental disorders*, ed 4 (DSM-IV TR), Washington, DC, 2000, The Association.

Angulo P: Nonalcoholic fatty liver disease, *N Engl J Med* 346(16):1221-1231, 2002.

Baker SP, Chen L, Li G: *Nationwide review of graduated driver licensing*, Washington, DC, 2007, AAA Foundation for Traffic Safety.

Baker S et al: Overweight children and adolescents: a clinical report of the North American Society for Pediatric Gastroenterology, Hepatology and Nutrition, *J Pediatr Gastroenterol Nutr* 40:533-543, 2005.

Berkowitz RI et al: Effects of sibutramine treatment in obese adolescents, *Ann Intern Med* 145(2):81-90, 2006.

Biro FM et al: Pubertal maturation in girls and the relationship to anthropometric changes: pathways through puberty, *J Pediatr* 142(6):643-646, 2003.

Bond L et al: Social and school connectedness in early secondary school as predictors of late teenage substance use, mental health, and academic outcomes, *J Adolesc Health* 40(4):357.e9-357.e18, 2007.

Braverman PK: Body art: piercing, tattooing, and scarification, *Adolesc Med* 17:505-519, 2006.

Briggs M, Safaii S, Beall DL: Nutrition services an essential component of comprehensive school health programs, *J Am Diet Assoc* 103(4):505-514, 2003.

Centers for Disease Control and Prevention: Youth Risk Behavior Surveillance—United States, 2007, *Morbid Mortal Wkly Rep* 57(SS04):1-131, 2008.

Centers for Disease Control and Prevention: *Welcome to WISQARS*, 2006. Available at www.cdc.gov/ncipc/wisqars (accessed January 24, 2008).

Costello EJ et al: Pubertal maturation and the development of alcohol use and abuse, *Drug Alcohol Depend* 88(4 Suppl 1):S50-S59, 2007.

Dennehy CE: The use of herbs and dietary supplements in gynecology: an evidence-based review, *J Midwifery Womens Health* 51(6):402-409, 2006.

DeVore ER, Ginsburg KR: The protective effects of good parenting on adolescents, *Curr Opin Pediatr* 17(4):460-465, 2005.

Ehtisham S, Barrett TG, Shaw NJ: Type 2 diabetes mellitus in UK children—an emerging problem, *Diabetes Med* 17(12):867-871, 2000.

Erikson EH: *Childhood and society*, ed 2, New York, 1963, WW Norton.

Falkner B et al: The relationship of body mass index and blood pressure in primary care pediatric patients, *J Pediatr* 148(2):195-200, 2006.

Feldman M, Friedman LS, Sleisenger MH: Obesity: a historical perspective and disease prevalence estimates. In Feldman M, Friedman LS, Sleisenger MH (editors): *Sleisenger and Fordtran's gastrointestinal and liver disease*, ed 7, Philadelphia, 2002, Saunders.

Forman SF: Eating disorders: epidemiology, pathogenesis, and clinical features, *UpToDate*, 2007. Available at www.uptodate.com (accessed July 31, 2007).

Gance-Cleveland B: Motivational interviewing: improving patient education, *J Pediatr Health* 21(2):81-88, 2007.

Geller AC, Annas GD: Epidemiology of melanoma and nonmelanoma skin cancer, *Semin Oncol Nurs* 19(1):2-11, 2003.

Geller AC et al: Use of sunscreen, sunburning rates and tanning bed use among more than 10,000 U.S. children and adolescents, *Pediatrics* 109(6):1009-1014, 2002.

Glatt K: Child-to-child unintentional injury and death from firearms in the United States: what can be done? *J Pediatr Nurs* 10(6):448-452, 2005.

Goodman E, Capitman J: Depressive symptoms and cigarette smoking among teens, *Pediatrics* 106(4):748-755, 2000.

Gordon SM: *Adolescent drug use: trends in abuse, treatment and prevention*, Wernersville, PA, 2000, Caron Foundation.

Gray M, Moore KN: *Urologic disorders: adult and pediatric care*, St Louis, 2009, Mosby.

Greaser J, Whyte JJ: Childhood obesity: is there effective treatment? *Consult Pediatr* 4(10):474-478, 2004.

Greydanus DE, Pratt HD: Emotional and behavioral disorders of adolescence, part 2, *Adolesc Health Update* 8(1):1-8, 1995.

Hardy LR, Harrell JS, Bell RA: Overweight in children: definitions, measurements, confounding factors, and health consequences, *J Pediatr Nurs* 19(6):376-383, 2004.

Hill JO et al: Obesity and the environment: where do we go from here? *Science* 299(5608):853-855, 2003.

Johnston LD et al: *Monitoring the future national results on adolescent drug use: overview of key findings, 2004*, NIH Pub No 05-5726, Bethesda, MD, 2005, National Institute on Drug Abuse.

Kaplowitz PB: Link between body fat and the timing of puberty, *Pediatrics* 121(Suppl 3): S208-S217, 2008.

Kiess W et al: Clinical aspects of obesity in childhood and adolescence, *Obesity Rev* 1:29-36, 2001.

Koeppen-Schomerus G, Wardle J, Plomin R: A genetic analysis of weight and overweight in 4-year-old twin pairs, *Int J Obes Relat Metab Dis* 25(6):838-844, 2001.

Leiter U, Garbe C: Epidemiology of melanoma and nonmelanoma skin cancer—the role of sunlight, *Adv Exp Med Biol* 624(1):89-103, 2008.

Lynne SD et al: Links between pubertal timing, peer influences and externalizing behaviors among urban students followed through middle school, *J Adolesc Health* 40(2):181.e7-e13, 2007.

MacKenzie NR: Childhood obesity: strategies for prevention, *Pediatr Nurs* 26(5):527-530, 2000.

Maes L, Lievens J: Can the school make a difference? A multilevel analysis of adolescent risk and health behaviour, *Soc Sci Med* 56(3):517-529, 2003.

Master-Hunter T, Heiman DL: Amenorrhea: evaluation and treatment, *Am Fam Physician* 73(8):1374-1382, 2006.

Mehler PS: Diagnosis and care of patients with anorexia nervosa in primary care settings, *Ann Intern Med* 134:1048-1059, 2001.

Mosher WD, Chandra A, Jones J: Sexual behavior and selected health measures: men and women 15-44 years of age, United States, 2002, *Adv Data*, September 15(362):1-55, 2005.

Nader PR et al: Moderate-to-vigorous activity from ages 9 to 15 years, *JAMA* 300(3):295-305, 2008.

Nader PR et al: Identifying risk for obesity in early childhood, *Pediatrics* 118(3):e594-e601, 2006.

National Institute for Health Care Management Foundation: *Childhood obesity: advancing effective prevention and treatment: an overview for health professionals*, prepared for National Institute for Health Care Management Foundation Forum, April 9, 2003, Washington, DC.

Nielsen SJ, Popkin BM: Patterns and trends in food portion sizes, 1977-1998, *JAMA* 289(4):450-453, 2003.

O'Brien M et al: The ecology of childhood overweight: a 12-year longitudinal analysis, *Int J Obesity* (Lond) 31(9):1469-1478, 2007.

Ogden CL et al: Prevalence of overweight and obesity in the United States, 1999-2004, *JAMA* 295(13):1549-1555, 2006.

Omar H, McElderry D, Zakharia R: Educating adolescents about puberty: what are we missing? *Int J Adolesc Med Health* 15(1):79-83, 2003.

Ongphiphadhanakul B: Osteoporosis: the role of genetics and the environment, *Forum Nutr* 60:158-167, 2007.

Patten LH et al: Depressive symptoms and cigarette smoking predict development and persistence of sleep problems in US adolescents, *Pediatrics* 106(2):E23, 2000.

Rigel DS: Cutaneous ultraviolet exposure and its relationship to the development of skin cancer, *J Am Acad Dermatol* 58(5 Suppl 2):S129-S132, 2008.

Rome ES et al: Children and adolescents with eating disorders: the state of the art, *Pediatrics* 111(1):e98-e108, 2003.

Russell ST, Seif H, Truong NL: School outcomes of sexual minority youth in the United States: evidence from a national study, *J Adolesc* 24(1):111-127, 2001.

Saewyc EM et al: Gender differences in health and risk behaviors among bisexual and homosexual adolescents, *J Adolesc Health* 23(3):181-188, 1998.

Santelli JS et al: Explaining recent declines in adolescent pregnancy in the United States: the contribution of abstinence and improved contraceptive use, *Am J Pub Health* 97(1):150-156, 2007.

Schwimmer JB: Managing overweight in older children and adolescents, *Pediatr Ann* 33(1):39-44, 2004.

Shain B, AAP Committee on Adolescence: Suicide and suicide attempts in adolescents, *Pediatrics* 120(3):669-676, 2007.

Sjöberg RL, Nilsson KW, Leppert J: Obesity, shame, and depression in school-aged children: a population-based study, *Pediatrics* 116(3):e389-e393, 2005.

Skelton JA, Rudolph C: Overweight and obesity. In Kliegman RM et al (editors): *Nelson textbook of pediatrics*, ed 18, Philadelphia, 2007, Saunders.

Sondike S, Copperman N, Jacobson MS: Effects of a low-carbohydrate diet on weight loss and cardiovascular risk factors in overweight adolescents, *J Pediatr* 142(3):253-258, 2003.

Spear B: Weight management: obesity to eating disorders. In Samour PQ, King K (editors): *Handbook of pediatric nutrition*, ed 3, Sudbury, MA, 2005, Jones & Bartlett.

Story M, Nanney MS, Schwartz MB: Schools and obesity prevention: creating school environments and policies to promote healthy eating and physical activity, *Milbank Q* 87(1):71-100, 2009.

Strong WB et al: Evidence based physical activity for school-aged youth, *J Pediatr* 146:732-737, 2005.

Sugerman HJ et al: Bariatric surgery for severely obese adolescents, *J Gastrointest Surg* 7(1):102-107, 2003.

Taylor ED et al: Orthopedic complications of overweight in children and adolescents, *Pediatrics* 117(6):2167-2173, 2006.

Tsai WS, Inge TH, Burd RS: Bariatric surgery in adolescents: recent national trends in use and in-hospital outcomes, *Arch Pediatr Adolesc Med* 161(3):217-221, 2007.

Tuttle J, Campbell-Heider N, David TM: Positive adolescent life skills training for high-risk teens: results of a group intervention study, *J Pediatr Health* 20(3):184-191, 2006.

US Department of Health and Human Services: *The health consequences of involuntary exposure to tobacco smoke: a report of the surgeon general*, Washington, DC, 2006, The Department.

Weeks SK et al: Getting inside depression and suicide ideation, *Nurs Manage* 35(10):42-46, 2004.

Weiss R et al: Obesity and the metabolic syndrome in children and adolescents, *N Engl J Med* 350(23):2362-2374, 2004.

Williams AF, Ferguson SA: Rationale for graduated licensing and the risks it should address, *Injury Prev* 8(Suppl 2):ii9-ii16, 2002.

Williams AF, McCartt AF, Geary L: Seatbelt use by high school students, *Injury Prev* 9(1):25-28, 2003.

Yanovski SZ, Yanovski JA: Obesity, *N Engl J Med* 346(8):591-602, 2002.

Unit 10

41 Chronic Illness, Disability, and End-of-Life Care

Learning Objectives

On completion of this chapter the reader will be able to:

- Identify the scope of and changing trends in care of children with special needs.
- Identify the major reactions of and effects on the family of a child with a special need.
- Define the stages of adjustment to the diagnosis of a chronic condition.
- Recognize the impact of the illness or disability on the developmental stages of childhood.
- Outline nursing interventions that promote the family's optimal adjustment to the child's chronic disorder.
- Outline nursing interventions that support the family at the time of death.
- Define the usual symptoms of normal grief.

Electronic Resources

Additional information related to the content in Chapter 41 can be found on

evolve the Companion Website at

http://evolve.elsevier.com/Perry/maternal/

- NCLEX Review Questions
- Case Study—The Dying Child
- Critical Thinking Exercise—Neonatal Loss
- Nursing Care Plan—The Child Who Is Terminally Ill or Dying

Perspectives on the Care of Children with Special Needs

Scope of the Problem

A number of terms and defining characteristics have been used to describe chronic illness and disability in children (Box 41-1). In recent years there have been continuing efforts to develop a definition that better identifies the number of children living with chronic conditions and the impact on health and social services (Jackson, 2000; van Dyck et al, 2004a). Currently children with special health care needs are defined as children who have or are at increased risk for a chronic physical, developmental, behavioral, or emotional condition and who also require health and related services of a type or amount beyond that generally required by children (Msall et al, 2003; Newacheck et al, 1998).

Ongoing progress in medical and technologic disease management has contributed to the growing number of children with special health care needs (Palfrey et al, 2005). The estimated number of newly diagnosed U.S. children under the age of 13 with acquired immunodeficiency syndrome (AIDS) declined by 62% between 2003 and 2007 and increased slightly for children ages 15 to 19 (Centers for Disease Control and Prevention, 2009). Technologic advances have substantially increased the survival of extremely-low- and very-low-birth-weight infants (Jackson, 2000). Children with disabilities are more likely to be in poor health than children without disabilities (Newacheck & Halfon, 1998). The result of such progress is that an estimated 15% to 18% of the children in the United States live with a chronic illness or disability and require specialized health care of a type or amount beyond that generally required by children (Perrin, 2004).

The most commonly occurring conditions causing disability are diseases of the respiratory tract and impairments of speech, special senses, and intelligence. Mental and nervous system disorders account for about one sixth of all childhood disability (Newacheck & Halfon, 1998).

The impact of chronic illness and disability in children is wide ranging. Chronic conditions in children present most families with additional tasks, responsibilities, and concerns (Ray, 2002). A child's activity level and developmental opportunities can be affected. Days can be lost from school. Children with chronic illness or disability may be at increased risk for behavior or emotional problems. Parents may lose days from work, experience financial strain, and be challenged both emotionally and physically as they cope with care of the child.

Siblings are also affected by having a "different" brother or sister and may simultaneously feel guilt and anger or jealousy toward their ill sibling. Additionally, they suffer secondary losses such as the ability to participate in extracurricular activities or social events because of routines imposed by the affected child's chronic condition.

BOX 41-1 Common Terms Regarding Children with Special Needs

Chronic illness—A condition that interferes with daily functioning for more than 3 months in a year, causes hospitalization of more than 1 month in a year, or (at time of diagnosis) is likely to do either of these

Congenital disability—A disability that has existed since birth but is not necessarily hereditary

Developmental delay—A maturational lag; an abnormal, slower rate of development in which a child demonstrates a functioning level below that observed in normal children of the same age

Developmental disability—Any mental or physical disability that is manifested before age 22 years and is likely to continue indefinitely

Disability—A functional limitation that interferes with a person's ability, for example, to walk, lift, hear, or learn

Handicap—A condition or barrier imposed by society, the environment, or one's own self; not a synonym for disability

Impairment—A loss or abnormality of structure or function

Life-limiting illness—Any illness or condition developed in childhood whereby the child is likely to die before adulthood or with a limited expectation of life thereafter

Technology-dependent child—A child from birth to 21 years with a chronic disability that requires the routine use of a medical device to compensate for the loss of a life-sustaining body function; requires daily ongoing care or monitoring by trained personnel

Data from Westbrook LE, Silver EJ, Stein RE: Implications for estimates of disability in children: a comparison of definitional components, *Pediatrics* 101(6):1025-1030, 1998; Newacheck PW, Halfon N: Prevalence and impact of disabling chronic conditions in childhood, *Am J Public Health* 88(4):610-617, 1998; Danvers L et al: Providing seamless service for children with life-limiting illness: experiences and recommendations of professional staff at the Diana Princess of Wales Children's Community Service, *J Clin Nurs* 12(3):351-359, 2003.

Trends in Care

Developmental Focus

Focusing on the child's *developmental level* rather than chronologic age or diagnosis emphasizes the child's abilities and strengths rather than disabilities. Attention is directed to normalizing experiences, adapting the environment, and promoting coping skills. Nurses often are in vital positions to redirect attention from the pathologic model with its focus on weaknesses and problems to the developmental model to meet the unique needs of the child and family.

A developmental focus also considers family development. The life cycle of the family unit reflects changing ages and needs of family members, as well as changing external demands. A family member's serious illness or disability can cause significant stress or crisis at any stage of the family life cycle. Just as with individual development, family development may be interrupted or even regress to an earlier level of functioning. Nurses can use the concept of family development to plan meaningful interventions and evaluate care.

Family-Centered Care

Children's physical and emotional health, as well as cognitive and social functioning, is strongly influenced by how well their families function (Schor, 2003). The importance of family-centered care—a philosophy that considers the family as the constant in the child's life—is especially evident in the care of children with special needs. As parents learn about the youngster's health care needs, they often become experts in delivering care. Health care providers, including nurses, are adjuncts to the child's care and need to form partnerships with parents. Effective communication and negotiation between parents and nurses are essential to forming trusting and effective partnerships and finding the best ways to meet the needs of the child and family (Corlett & Twycross, 2006). Collaborative relationships are characterized by communication, dialogue, active listening, awareness, and acceptance of differences (Schor, 2003).

Family–Health Care Provider Communication

The disclosure of a child's serious acute or chronic illness is one of the most stressful aspects of communication between families and health care professionals. Often, parents have suspected for some time that something is wrong with their child and believe that their concerns were minimized or ignored by health care professionals (Whitehead & Gosling, 2003; Thomlinson, 2002; Cohen, 1995). After a diagnosis is made, numerous studies have shown that parents are not always satisfied with the way in which information is given. Factors that influence parent dissatisfaction with communication include unsympathetic and brief diagnostic interviews, lack of privacy during diagnostic discussions, and lack of opportunity to ask questions. Conversely, parents report satisfaction when they perceive the health care providers giving information in an open and honest manner with respect for the parents' need for privacy and time to express emotions and ask questions (Davies, Davis, & Sibert, 2003). Similar factors are important in communication of changes in the child's condition throughout the course of the illness.

Providing information to families with a chronically ill child should be a process of repeated discussions to allow the family to process the information and their reactions to that information, and allow them to ask for clarification and further information. Nurses play an important role in ensuring that families' needs are met during discussions related to the child's diagnosis, condition, and treatment. This requires assessment regarding how much information the family is comfortable with, what they understand of the information already given to them, and how they are coping with the information both cognitively and emotionally. Nurses should ensure that the appropriate health care professionals address any concerns or further questions that families may have.

Establishing Therapeutic Relationships

Another important aspect of family-centered care of chronically ill children is establishing a therapeutic relationship with the child and family, which has been shown to predict improved health-related outcomes (Denboba et al, 2006). Families, most often the mother, take on enormous responsibility in providing technical care and symptom management of their child's condition outside the health care institution (O'Brien & Wegner, 2002; Raina et al, 2005; Swallow & Jacoby, 2001). To build successful therapeutic relationships with families, it is necessary for nurses to recognize parents' expertise with regard to their child's condition and needs. Care conferences, especially multidisciplinary meetings that include the family and key health professionals, provide an opportunity for sharing ideas and expressing feelings or concerns.

The Role of Culture in Family-Centered Care

Issues of culture, ethnicity, and race affect access to services, utilization, and follow-through with referrals and recommendations (van Dyck et al, 2004b; Wise et al, 2002; Wood et al, 2002; Zuvekas & Taliaferro, 2003). For some ethnic and minority populations, cultural understandings of illness and disability, the structure of family life, social roles for individuals who are disabled, and other factors related to the perception of children may differ from those of mainstream American culture. These factors may affect family needs and family choices regarding the care of their child with special needs.

Although culture cannot completely explain how an individual will think and act, understanding cultural perspectives can help the nurse anticipate and understand why families may make certain decisions. Cultural attributes such as values and beliefs regarding illness or disability and its causation, social roles for the ill or disabled, family structure, the role of children, childrearing practices, self vs. group orientation, spirituality, and time orientation also affect a family's response to illness or disability in a child (Carnevale et al, 2006; Carter, 2002; Marshall et al, 2003; Rehm, 1999; Sterling & Peterson, 2003).

When parents are informed of their child's chronic illness, interpreters familiar with both culture and language should be used. Children, family members, and friends of the family should not be used as translators because their presence may prevent parents from openly discussing the issues. When working with people of cultural backgrounds different from their own, nurses must listen carefully with an initial goal of understanding and articulating the family's perspective. The ability to interpret the mainstream medical culture to the family is also important. Furthermore, every effort is made to incorporate a family's traditional cultural beliefs into treatment plans. Developing a care plan in conjunction with the family, considering their preferences and priorities, is an important first step in formulating a plan that best meets the family's needs, no matter what their cultural background (Ahmann, 1994; Ochieng, 2003).

Shared Decision Making

Shared decision making among the child, family, and health care team can result from open, honest, culturally sensitive communication and the establishment of a therapeutic relationship between the family and health care providers. In a shared decision-making model the health care professionals provide honest, clear information regarding diagnosis, prognosis, treatment options, and risk-benefit assessment. The patient and/or family then shares information with the health care team regarding important family values, acceptable levels of discomfort or inconvenience, and the ability to comply with treatments being recommended (Charles, Gafni, & Whelan, 1997). This process allows them to discuss all options in terms of the risks and benefits to the child and family, the prognosis or expected course of the illness, and the impact on the family's resources (Box 41-2).

BOX 41-2 Facilitating Shared Decision Making

- Continually assess the impact of the child's illness and treatment on the family.
- Provide honest, accurate information regarding the trajectory of the disease, anticipated complications, and prognostic information.
- Discuss what the family desires for the child's quality of life.
- Avoid personal opinion or judgment of the family's questions and decisions.

Normalization

Normalization refers to behaviors and intentions of the disabled to integrate into society by living life as persons without a disability would (Morse, Wilson, & Penrod, 2000). For the chronically ill or disabled child, such behaviors could include attending school, pursuing hobbies and recreational interests, and achieving employment and a level of independence. For their families, it may entail adapting the family routine to accommodate the ill or disabled child's health and physical needs (McDougal, 2002).

Children with chronic illness and disability and their families face numerous challenges in achieving normalization. Families move between the "normal" of living with the experience of chronic childhood illness and the "normal" of the healthy outside world; they often redefine "normal" based on their particular experiences, needs, and circumstances (Nelson, 2002; Deatrick, Knafl, & Murphy-Moore, 1999).

Nurses can assist families in normalizing their lives by assessing the family's everyday life, social support systems, coping strategies, family cohesiveness, and family and community resources. Interventions could include encouraging families to reduce stress through delegation of care and family tasks, identifying ways to incorporate care into current routines, structuring the home environment to foster the child's engagement in age-appropriate activities, and ensuring families have access to appropriate community support services (Jokinen, 2004; Shepard & Mahon, 2000). Being supportive of the child's illness and treatment and actively including the family in all aspects of care will improve their self-esteem and promote further development (Shepard & Mahon, 2000).

Home care represents the return to a system and set of priorities in which family values are as important in the care of a child with a chronic health problem as they are in the care of other children. Home care seeks to achieve goals that are consistent with the developmental model (Stein, 1985).

Goals for Home Care

- Normalize the life of a child with special needs, including those with technologically complex care, in a family and community context and setting.

- Minimize the disruptive impact of the child's condition on the family.
- Foster the child's maximum growth and development.

Paralleling normalization and home care is the process of *mainstreaming*, or integrating children with special needs into regular classrooms. Just as the home is the natural environment for children, so school must also be included as an essential component of the children's overall physical, intellectual, and social development. Children who attend school have the advantages of learning and socializing with a wide group of peers. There is an increased focus on individualization as plans are made to meet the academic needs of these children along with those of the rest of the students.

A variety of supplemental programs have been designed in the school system to accommodate special needs, both at school age and younger, through *early intervention*, which consists of any sustained and systematic effort to assist children from birth to age 3 years who are disabled and developmentally vulnerable. This change and increasing opportunities for normalization for children with special needs in large part have resulted from the passage of (1) the Education for All Handicapped Children Act of 1975 (Public Law 94-142) and its 1990 amendments (Public Law 101-476), which changed the name of the act to the Individuals with Disabilities Education Act (IDEA); (2) the Education of the Handicapped Act Amendments of 1986 (Public Law 99-457), which directs states to develop and implement statewide comprehensive, coordinated, multidisciplinary interagency programs of early intervention services for infants and toddlers with disabilities, as well as support services for their families; and (4) the Americans with Disabilities Act of 1990. Nurses can provide parents with information about these laws and in some cases may participate in the development of individualized educational programs or individualized family service plans for children with special needs.

Managed Care

Managed care programs have become the major form of health care provision in the United States (Jackson, 2000). The transition to this model of care presents both opportunities and challenges with respect to the care of children with special health care needs. Managed care may promote continuity and coordination of care. Children rely on adults for access to health care and follow-up with treatment regimens, making it necessary to manage the child's care in the context of the family (McPherson et al, 2004; van Dyck et al, 2004b).

The Family of the Child with Special Needs

A major goal in working with the family of a child with special needs is to support the family's coping and promote their optimal functioning throughout the child's life. Long-term, comprehensive, family-centered approaches extend beyond supporting the child and family during the critical periods of diagnosis and hospitalization. Rather, comprehensive care involves forming parent-professional partnerships that can support a family's adaptation to the many changes that may be necessary in day-to-day life, determine expectations of and for the child, and provide a long-term perspective (Box 41-3).

BOX 41-3 Adaptive Tasks for Parents of Children with Chronic Conditions

- Accept the child's condition.
- Manage the child's condition on a day-to-day basis.
- Meet the child's normal developmental needs.
- Meet the developmental needs of other family members.
- Cope with ongoing stress and periodic crises.
- Assist family members in managing their feelings.
- Educate others about the child's condition.
- Establish a support system.

From Canam C: Common adaptive tasks facing parents of children with chronic conditions, *J Adv Nurs* 18:46-53, 1993.

The impact of a child's medical or developmental condition is often experienced over time, initially as a crisis at the time of diagnosis, which may occur at birth, after a long period of physical or psychologic testing, or immediately after a tragic injury. The impact may also be felt before the diagnosis is made, when parents are aware that something is wrong with their child but before medical confirmation (Whitehead & Gosling, 2003; Thomlinson, 2002; Cohen, 1995).

The diagnosis and initial discharge home are critical times for parents (Coffey, 2006). Several factors can make it particularly difficult, including a long duration of uncertainty in the diagnostic process, negative perceptions of chronic illness or disability, insufficient information, and lack of mutual trust between parents and their child's health care team (Cohen, 1995; Garwick et al, 1995; Nuutila & Salanterä, 2006). Parental feelings of shock, helplessness, isolation, fear, and depression are common (Coffey, 2006; Nuutila & Salanterä, 2006). Throughout the first year, parents struggle to accept the child's diagnosis, care, and uncertainty of the future (Coffey, 2006). Providing explicit and uncomplicated information to parents in an empathic way (Nuutila & Salanterä, 2006); assessing the family's daily routine, living conditions, background knowledge, skills and abilities, and coping behaviors; and evaluating the family's understanding of the information can encourage optimal support at the time of diagnosis and initial discharge home. It is also necessary to reassess parental needs for information and support on a routine basis (Nuutila & Salanterä, 2006).

Impact of the Child's Chronic Illness or Disability

Each member of a family who has a child with special needs is affected by the experience (Sullivan-Bolyai et al, 2003). The effects on the parents and their responses are so critical that they directly influence the other members' reactions and the child's own coping.

Parents

In addition to the stress of grieving for the loss of a perfect child, parents are affected by whether or not they receive positive feedback from transactions with their child. Many parents

BOX 41-4 Anticipated Parental Stress Points

Diagnosis of the condition—Parents require considerable education while dealing with an emotional response.
Developmental milestones—Times that children normally achieve walking, talking, and self-care are delayed or impossible for the child.
Start of schooling—Particularly stressful are situations in which appropriate schooling will not be in a regular class placement.
Reaching the ultimate attainment—Parents must handle situations such as realizing that ambulation will be impossible or that the child will not learn to read.
Adolescence—Issues such as sexuality and independence become prominent.
Future placement—Decisions about placement must be made when the child becomes an adult or when the parents can no longer care for the child.
Death of the child

feel satisfaction and fulfillment from the parenting role. For others, parenting may be a series of unrewarding experiences that contribute to feelings of inadequacy and failure (Box 41-4). These responses may be most evident in parents who are responsible for the child's care. For example, parents may become preoccupied with their ability to carry out certain procedures, overlooking the child's personal comfort and satisfaction or failing to offer praise for anything less than perfect cooperation or performance. They may pursue a frustrating activity until they achieve "success"—long after the child has become irritable and uncooperative. As a result, parents can become caught in a pattern of interaction that is mutually unrewarding and minimally productive. For these parents, several strategies may be helpful: education regarding what can reasonably be expected of their child, assistance in identifying the child's strengths, praise for a parental job well done, and respite care so that parents can renew their energies.

Parental Roles

Parenting a child with a chronic illness or disability requires much more than raising a typical child. In addition to attending to the routine aspects of parenting, parents of chronically ill children take on the added responsibility of performing complex technical care and symptom management, advocating for their child, and seeking and coordinating health and social services for their ill or disabled child. These added responsibilities must then be balanced with the needs of other family members, extended family and friends, and personal health and obligations to minimize consequences to the overall functioning of the family (Coffey, 2006; Ray, 2002).

Enormous demands may be placed on parental time, energy, and financial resources. The nurse can assist parents in avoiding role conflicts by providing anticipatory guidance early on. Teaching should address stressors often identified as having an impact on the marriage: (1) the burden of care at home assumed by primarily one parent, (2) the financial burden, (3) the fear of the child dying, (4) pressure from relatives, (5) the hereditary nature of the disease (if applicable), and (6) fear of pregnancy. Other causes of tension may center on the inconveniences associated with care, such as long waits for an appointment, lack of parking near care facilities, or lack of overnight accommodations. Certainly, these last stressors are within health professionals' domain to minimize, if not eliminate.

Mother-Father Differences

Mothers and fathers in the same family often adjust and cope differently as parents of a child with special needs. Some mothers experience a peaks-and-valleys periodic crisis pattern, whereas most fathers tend to experience a steady, gradual recovery. Some research suggests that mothers of children with certain conditions may be more susceptible to psychologic distress and fatigue than fathers (Tong et al, 2002). Mothers are most often the primary caregiver and are more likely than fathers to give up their job to care for their child, often resulting in social isolation (Coffey, 2006). Mothers often have greater needs for social support and positive appraisal of the situation, whereas fathers are more likely to use self-controlling behaviors to cope (Goldbeck, 2001; Mastroyannopoulou et al, 1997).

The father of a child with special needs struggles with issues that may be distinct from those of the mother. He may think that his role of protector is challenged because he does not know how to help and cannot protect the family from the seemingly overwhelming recurring problems. With today's increased emphasis on fathers' involvement in the lives of their children, this loss is felt more profoundly than in the past. The extensive stresses in the family can leave the father feeling depressed, weak, guilty, powerless, isolated, embarrassed, and angry. Fearful that he will lose control or be viewed as weak or ineffectual, however, the father often hides his feelings and displays an outward confidence that may lead others to believe that everything is fine. Fathers worry about what the future holds for their children, their ability to manage the increasing financial burden, and the daily disruptions of the entire family (Davies et al, 2004). Some fathers escape in their work as a means of dulling the pain. Common coping strategies are problem oriented and include praying, getting information, looking at options, and weighing choices, in addition to withdrawal (Mastroyannopoulou et al, 1997).

Single-Parent Families

Single-parent families are of special concern. The absence of a parent may result from divorce or death, or the parents may never have married. As the only parent of a child who may require extensive, sophisticated, and lifelong care, the single parent may feel an enormous burden. Available financial and emotional resources may already be stretched to the limit. A special effort should be made to assist the single parent in finding financial and support services that can ease the burden of care. Nurses can also assist the single parent in identifying helping roles that may be acceptable to relatives and friends.

Siblings

Results of studies on how siblings (almost exclusively European Americans) are affected by having a brother or sister with special needs are unclear (Barlow & Ellard, 2006). Generally, the evidence reveals a negative effect on siblings of children with a chronic illness when compared with siblings of healthy children. This effect appears, however, to be decreasing in

BOX 41-5 Supporting Siblings of Children with Special Needs

Promote Healthy Sibling Relationships

Value each child individually and avoid comparisons. Remind each child of his or her positive qualities and contribution to other family members.

Help siblings see the differences and similarities between themselves and a child with special needs. Create a climate in which children can achieve successes without feeling guilty.

Teach siblings ways to interact with the child.

Seek to be fair in terms of discipline, attention, and resources; require the affected child to do as much for himself or herself as possible.

Let siblings settle their own differences; intervene only to prevent siblings from hurting one another.

Legitimize reasonable anger. Even children with special needs behave badly sometimes.

Respect a sibling's reluctance to be with or to include the child with special needs in activities.

Help Siblings Cope

Listen to siblings to let them know that their thoughts and suggestions are valued.

Praise siblings when they have been patient, have sacrificed, or have been particularly helpful. Do not expect siblings to always act in this manner.

Acknowledge the personal strengths siblings have and their ability to cope with stress successfully.

Provide age-appropriate information about the child's condition, and update when appropriate.

Let teachers know what is happening so they can be understanding and helpful.

Recognize special stress times for siblings and plan to minimize negative effects.

Schedule special time with siblings; have a friend or family member substitute when parent is unavailable.

Encourage siblings to join or help establish a sibling support group.

Use the services of professionals when needed. If a parent thinks that such a service is necessary, it should be provided in as vigorous a manner as a service for the child with special needs.

Involve Siblings

Seek out ways to realistically include siblings in the care and treatment of the child with special needs.

Limit caregiving responsibilities and give recognition when siblings perform them.

Develop a library of children's books on special needs.

Invite siblings to attend meetings to develop plans for the child with special needs (e.g., individualized educational program, individualized family service plan).

Discuss future plans with them.

Solicit their ideas on treatment and service needs.

Have them visit professionals who work with the child.

Help them develop competencies to teach the child new skills.

Provide opportunities for siblings to advocate for the child.

Allow siblings to set their own pace for learning and involvement.

Data from Powell T, Ogle P: *Brothers and sisters—a special part of exceptional families,* Baltimore, 1985, Paul H Brooks; Spokane Washington Deaconess Medical Center, Pediatric Oncology Unit: Tips for dealing with siblings, *Candlelighters Childhood Cancer Found Q Newslett* 11(3,4):7, 1987; and Carlson J, Leviton A, Mueller M: Services to siblings: an important component of family-centered practice, *ACCH Advocate* 1(1):53-56, 1993.

significance in recent years—most likely because of changes in public attitudes toward the ill and disabled (Sharpe & Rossiter, 2002). Siblings of children with chronic illness or disability report depression and anxiety more often than their peers (Rossiter & Sharpe, 2001). However, most investigators do agree that brothers and sisters of children with special needs are no more at risk for *severe* psychiatric problems than are siblings of children without chronic or disabling conditions. A number of factors increase the risk of negative effects for siblings of ill children. Responsibility for caregiving, differential treatment by parents, and limitations in family resources and recreational time are often the experience of siblings of ill or disabled children (Lobato & Kao, 2002) (Box 41-5).

An important factor in sibling adjustment and coping is information and knowledge regarding their brother or sister's illness or disability. What siblings piece together or overhear is often much worse than the truth. Often they imagine gruesome things regarding the experiences related to the illness, treatment, and hospitalization (Shepard & Mahon, 2000). Latino siblings have reported less accurate information about their sibling's condition than non-Latino siblings (Lobato, Kao, & Plante, 2005). Parents are usually in the best position to impart information, although they are often overwhelmed with the medical crisis at hand (Fleitas, 2000). Nurses can encourage parents to talk with the siblings about how they perceive their sick brother or sister and to be accepting of the siblings' feelings. Nurses can be ideal educators and counselors of siblings during the course of their brother's or sister's illness (Shepard & Mahon, 2000).

FAMILY-CENTERED CARE

Reflection of an Older Brother

My youngest sister, Kerry, was on an apnea monitor 3 years ago, when I was 15. I was never embarrassed about Kerry being on the monitor, except for the time it went off in church and everyone turned around to look at us.

–Joey Bellino, Oldest Sibling of an Infant on an Apnea Monitor Washington, DC

Coping with Ongoing Stress and Periodic Crises

Professionals can help families cope with stress by providing anticipatory guidance, providing emotional support, assisting the family in assessing and identifying specific stressors, aiding the family in developing coping mechanisms and problem-solving strategies, and working collaboratively with parents so that they become empowered in the process.

Concurrent Stresses Within the Family

The ability to deal with the overwhelming stress of a lifelong disability or illness is challenged further when additional stresses are present. Stressors may be situational or developmental. They may be related to marital difficulties, sibling needs, homelessness, or social isolation. Some families may simultaneously be struggling with a family member's alcohol or other drug problem. Even relatively minor stressors, such as arranging care for siblings, managing the home, and traveling to distant treatment centers, can challenge a family's ability to cope successfully.

Most families, regardless of their income or insurance coverage, have financial concerns. The costs of caring for a child with special needs can be overwhelming. Nurses and social workers can help a family review various options for financial assistance, including insurance, managed care, or health maintenance organization policies; Medicaid; Supplemental Security Income; Women, Infants, and Children program (WIC); the state Program for Children with Special Health Needs; disease-related associations; and local philanthropic organizations.

Coping Mechanisms

Coping mechanisms are behaviors aimed at reducing the tension caused by a crisis. *Approach behaviors* are coping mechanisms that result in movement toward adjustment and resolution of the crisis. *Avoidance behaviors* result in movement away from adjustment and represent maladaptation to the crisis. Several approach and avoidance behaviors used in coping with a chronic illness or disability are listed in the Guidelines box. None of the indices can be used singly to assess the possible success or failure in resolving the crisis. Each behavior must be viewed in the context of all of the variables affecting the family. For example, the observation of several avoidance behaviors in an emotionally healthy family may denote significantly less risk to the successful resolution of the crisis than an equal number of avoidance behaviors in an individual who has few available supports.

Parental Empowerment

Empowerment can be seen as a process of recognizing, promoting, and enhancing competence. For parents of children with chronic conditions, empowerment may occur gradually as strength and capabilities are drawn on to master the child's care, manage family life, and plan for the future. Advocating for the child and developing parent-professional partnerships are part of taking charge (Ray, 2002).

Assisting Family Members in Managing Their Feelings

Although some previous research has postulated stages of adaptation to a chronic illness or disability, there is a great deal of individual variation in responses to the diagnosis, adjustments made, and time frames for coming to terms with a diagnosis. It is important that professionals recognize and respect a wide range of reactions and coping mechanisms. In fact, members of the family of a child with a chronic illness or disability may experience a number of difficult emotions, including fear, guilt, anger, resentment, and anxiety. Learning to manage these emotions promotes adaptive coping (see Guidelines box above). Support from professionals, other family members, and friends can assist family members in managing their feelings. The following discussion examines some common phases of adjustment and emotional reactions.

GUIDELINES Assessing Coping Behaviors

Approach Behaviors

- Asks for information regarding diagnosis and child's present condition
- Seeks help and support from others
- Anticipates future problems; actively seeks guidance and answers
- Endows the illness or disability with meaning
- Shares burden of disorder with others
- Plans realistically for the future
- Acknowledges and accepts child's awareness of diagnosis and prognosis
- Expresses feelings such as sorrow, depression, and anger and realizes reason for the emotional reaction
- Realistically perceives child's condition; adjusts to changes
- Recognizes own growth through passage of time, such as earlier denial and nonacceptance of diagnosis
- Verbalizes possible loss of child

Avoidance Behaviors

- Fails to recognize seriousness of child's condition despite physical evidence
- Refuses to agree to treatment
- Intellectualizes about the illness, but in areas unrelated to child's condition
- Is angry and hostile to members of the staff, regardless of their attitude or behavior
- Avoids staff, family members, or child
- Entertains unrealistic future plans for child, with little emphasis on the present
- Is unable to adjust to or accept a change in progression of disease
- Continually looks for new cures with no perspective toward possible benefit
- Refuses to acknowledge child's understanding of disease and prognosis
- Uses magical thinking and fantasy; may seek "occult" help
- Places complete faith in religion to point of relinquishing own responsibility
- Withdraws from outside world; refuses help
- Punishes self because of guilt and blame
- Makes no change in lifestyle to meet needs of other family members
- Resorts to excessive use of alcohol or drugs to avoid problems
- Verbalizes suicidal intents
- Is unable to discuss possible loss of child or previous experiences with death

Shock and Denial

The initial diagnosis of a chronic illness or disability is often met with intense emotion and is characterized by shock, disbelief, and sometimes denial, especially if the disorder is not obvious, as in chronic illness. Denial as a defense mechanism is a necessary cushion to prevent disintegration and is a normal response to grieving for any type of loss. Probably all family members experience various degrees of adaptive denial as they learn of the impact that the diagnosis has on their lives.

In children, the importance of denial has repeatedly been demonstrated as a factor in their positive coping with the diagnosis. Denial allows the child to maintain hope in the face of overwhelming odds and to function adaptively and productively. Like hope, denial may be an adaptive mechanism for dealing with loss that persists until a family or patient is ready or needs other responses.

Denial is probably the least understood and most poorly dealt-with reaction. Health professionals typically label denial as maladaptive and act inappropriately by attempting to strip it away by repeated and sometimes blunt explanations of the prognosis. However, denial becomes maladaptive only when it prevents recognition of treatment or rehabilitative goals necessary for the child's optimal survival or development.

Adjustment

For most families, adjustment gradually follows shock and is usually characterized by an open admission that the condition exists. This stage may be accompanied by several responses, which are normal parts of the adaptation process. Probably the most universal of these feelings are *guilt and self-accusation*. Guilt is often greatest when the cause of the disorder is directly traceable to the parent, as in genetic diseases or accidental injury. However, it can occur even without any scientific or realistic basis for parental responsibility. Frequently the guilt stems from a false assumption that the disability is a result of personal failure or wrongdoing, such as not doing something correctly during pregnancy or the birth. Guilt may also be associated with cultural or religious beliefs. Some parents are convinced that they are being punished for some previous misdeed. Others may see the disorder as a trial sent by God to test their religious strength and faith. With correct information, support, and time, most parents master guilt and self-accusation. The ability to master resentful and self-accusatory feelings of having "caused" the child's disorder is a crucial factor in determining the parents' acceptance of their child.

Other common and normal reactions to a diagnosis are *bitterness* and *anger.* Anger directed inward may be evident as self-reproaching or punitive behavior, such as neglecting one's health and verbally degrading oneself. Anger directed outward may be manifested in either open arguments or withdrawal from communication and may be evident in the person's relationship with any number of individuals, such as the spouse, the child, and siblings. Passive anger toward the ill child may be evident in decreased visiting, refusal to believe how sick the child is, or inability to provide comfort. Among the most common targets for parental anger are members of the staff. Parents may complain about the nursing care, the insufficient time physicians spend with them, or the lack of skill of those who draw blood or start intravenous infusions.

Children are likely to respond with anger as well, and this includes the affected child and the well siblings. Children are aware of the loss engendered by their illness or disability and may react angrily to the restrictions imposed or the feelings of being different. Siblings may also feel anger and resentment toward the ill child and parents for the loss of routine and parental attention. It is difficult for older children and almost impossible for younger children to comprehend the plight of the affected child. Their perception is of a brother or sister who has the undivided attention of their parents, is showered with cards and gifts, and is the focus of everyone's concern.

During the period of adjustment, four types of parental reactions to the child influence the child's eventual response to the disorder:

1. Overprotection, in which the parents fear letting the child achieve any new skill, avoid all discipline, and cater to every desire to prevent frustration (Box 41-6)
2. Rejection, in which the parents detach themselves emotionally from the child but usually provide adequate physical care or constantly nag and scold the child
3. Denial, in which parents act is if the disorder does not exist or attempt to have the child overcompensate for it
4. Gradual acceptance, in which parents place necessary and realistic restrictions on the child, encourage self-care activities, and promote reasonable physical and social abilities

Reintegration and Acknowledgment

For many families the adjustment process culminates in the development of realistic expectations for the child and

BOX 41-6 Characteristics of Parental Overprotection

- Sacrifices self and rest of family for the child
- Continually helps the child, even when the child is capable
- Is inconsistent with regard to discipline or employs no discipline; frequently applies different rules to the siblings
- Is dictatorial and arbitrary, making decisions without considering the child's wishes, such as keeping the child from attending school
- Hovers and offers suggestions; calls attention to every activity, overdoes praise
- Protects the child from every possible discomfort
- Restricts play, often because of fear that the child will be injured
- Denies the child opportunities for growing up and assuming responsibility, such as learning to give own medications or perform treatments
- Does not understand the child's capabilities and sets goals too high or too low
- Monopolizes the child's time, such as sleeping with the child, permitting few friends, or refusing participation in social or educational activities

reintegration of family life with the illness or disability in a manageable perspective. Because a large portion of this phase is one of grief for a loss, total resolution is not possible until the child dies or leaves home as an independent adult. Therefore one can regard adjustment as "increased comfort" with everyday living rather than a complete resolution.

This adjustment phase also involves social reintegration in which the family broadens its activities to include relationships outside of the home, with the child as an accepted and participating member of the group. This last criterion often differentiates the reaction of gradual acceptance during the adjustment period from total acceptance, or perhaps is more descriptive of the acknowledgment process.

Many parents of children with chronic illnesses experience chronic sorrow, feelings of sorrow and loss that recur in waves over time. As the child's condition progresses, parents experience repeated losses that represent further declines and new caregiving demands. Consequently, families must be assessed on an ongoing basis and offered appropriate support and resources as their needs change over time (Gravelle, 1997).

BOX 41-7 Concept of Functional Burden

Impact of the Child with Special Needs

The child's need for medical and nursing care
The child's fixed deficits
The child's age-appropriate dependency in activities of daily living
The disruptions in the family routine caused by the care
The psychologic burden of the prognosis on the family

Family Resources and Ability to Cope

The family's physical resources
The family's emotional resources
The family's educational resources
The family's social supports and available help
The competing demands for family members' time and energy

Data from Stein REK: Home care: a challenging opportunity, *Child Health Care* 14(2):90-95, 1985.

Establishing a Support System

The diagnosis of a child with a serious health problem or disability is a major situational crisis that affects the entire family system. However, families can experience positive outcomes as they successfully deal with the many challenges that accompany a child with chronic illness or disability.

One nursing goal is to assess which families are at greater or lesser risk for succumbing to the effects of the crisis. Several variables—available support system, perception of the event, coping mechanisms, reactions to the child, available resources, and concurrent stresses within the family—influence the resolution of a crisis. Although most families cope well, the needs of families at risk are great. If they receive emotional support and guidance early, there is an increased likelihood that they will also cope successfully.

Although it is easy to assume that families of children with the most severe illnesses or disabilities would have the poorest adjustment, the severity of the condition reflects only one part of the overall picture. The level of adjustment is significantly influenced by the *functional burden* on the individual family (Stein, 1985). This concept considers the issues related to caring for and living with the child in relation to the family's resources and ability to cope (Box 41-7). The family of a child with multiple disabilities demanding complex care, yet having many resources and coping skills, may adjust more successfully to the child's situation than the family of a child with a less serious condition and few resources to counterbalance.

Intrafamilial resources, social support from friends and relatives, parent-to-parent support, parent-professional partnerships, and community resources interweave to provide a flexible web of support for the family of a child with a chronic condition.

The Child with Special Needs

The child's reaction to chronic illness or disability depends to a great extent on his or her developmental level, temperament, and available coping mechanisms; on the reactions of family members or significant others; and, to a lesser extent, on the condition itself. A child's conceptual understanding of his or her own illness is based not only on age and developmental level, but also on the duration and type of experience accumulated with the disease. Knowledge of these variables is essential in providing the kind of information and support these children need to cope with a sometimes overwhelming situation.

Developmental Aspects

The impact of a chronic illness or disability is influenced by the age at onset. Chronic illness affects children of all ages, but the developmental aspects of each age group dictate particular stresses and risks for the child. The nurse must also recognize that children need to redefine their condition and its implications as they develop and grow. For example, appearance, skills, and abilities are highly valued by peers (Fig. 41-1); a teenager who is limited in any of these qualities is subject to rejection. This is especially marked when a physical disability interferes with sexual attractiveness. Developmental effects of chronic illness or disability on children are described in Table 41-2.

Coping Mechanisms

Children with chronic conditions tend to use five distinct patterns of coping (Box 41-8). Children with more positive and accepting attitudes about their chronic illness use a more adaptive coping style characterized by optimism, competence, and compliance. They show fewer behavior problems at home and at school. The two maladaptive coping patterns—"Feels different and withdraws" and "Is irritable, is moody, and acts out"—are associated with poorer adaptation; children using these strategies have poorer self-concepts, more negative attitudes about their conditions, and more behavior problems at home and at school.

Well-adapted children gradually learn to accept their physical limitations and find achievement in a variety of compensatory motor and intellectual pursuits. They function well at home, at school, and with peers. They have an understanding

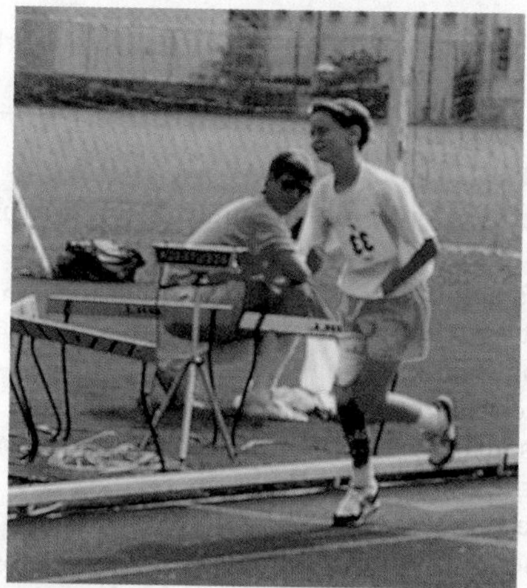

Fig. 41-1 Children with any type of impairment should have the opportunity to develop their skills. *(Courtesy Poyo/Hinton Photography.)*

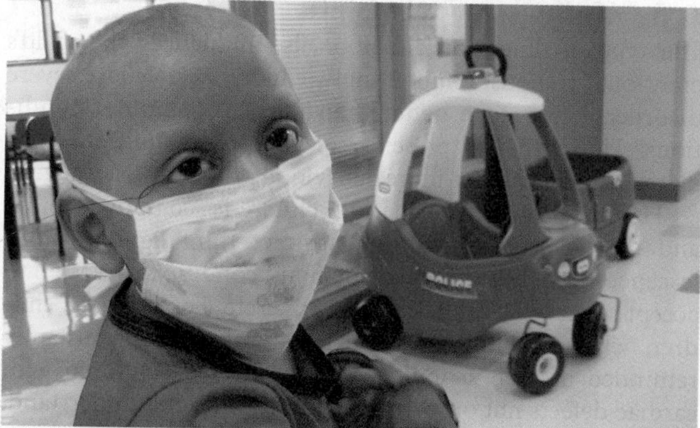

Fig. 41-2 Periods of sadness and anger are appropriate in the child's adjustment to a chronic illness or disability, especially during exacerbations of the disorder.

BOX 41-8 Coping Patterns Used by Children with Special Needs

Develops competence and optimism—Accentuates the positive aspects of the situation and concentrates more on what he or she has or can do than on what is missing or on what he or she cannot do; is as independent as possible

Feels different and withdraws—Sees self as being different from other children because of the chronic health condition; views being different as negative; sees self as less worthy than others; focuses on things he or she cannot do and sometimes overrestricts activities needlessly

Is irritable, is moody, and acts out—Uses proactive and self-initiated coping behaviors, although usually counterproductive in that the behaviors are not ego enhancing or socially responsible and do not result in desired outcomes; acts out irritability, which may or may not be associated with condition's symptoms

Complies with treatment—Takes necessary medications, treatments; adheres to activity restrictions; also uses behaviors that indicate developing independence (e.g., assumes responsibility for taking medication)

Seeks support—Talks with adults, children, physicians, and nurses; develops plans to handle problems as they occur; uses downward comparison (i.e., realizes that others have it worse)

Modified from Austin J, Patterson J, Huberty T: Development of the Coping Health Inventory for children, *J Pediatr Nurs* 6(3):166-174, 1991.

of their disorder that allows them to accept their limitations, assume responsibility for care, and assist in treatment and rehabilitation regimens. They express appropriate emotions, such as sadness, anxiety, and anger, at times of exacerbations but confidence and guarded optimism during periods of clinical stability (Fig. 41-2). They are able to identify with other similarly affected individuals, promoting positive self-images and displaying pride and self-confidence in their ability to lead a productive, successful life despite the disability.

Hopefulness

Children, particularly adolescents, function well or poorly depending on the presence or absence of hope. Hopefulness is an internal quality that mobilizes humans into goal-directed action that may be satisfying and life sustaining. A sense of hopefulness can produce increased participation in health-seeking behaviors and an improved sense of well-being (Ritchie, 2001).

Health Education and Self-Care

Health education is an intervention that promotes coping. Children need information about their condition, the therapeutic plan, and how the disease or the therapy might affect their particular situation. Children nearing puberty also need to understand the maturation process and how their disability may alter this event. For example, a youngster with Crohn's disease should understand that this disorder is associated with growth failure and delayed puberty; a child with diabetes needs to know that hormonal changes and increased growth needs will alter food and insulin requirements at this time; and a sexually active girl with sickle cell anemia or systemic lupus erythematosus needs to be aware of the risks of pregnancy. The information should not be given all at once but should be timed appropriately to meet the changing needs of the youngsters, and it should be described and repeated as often as the situation demands.

Responses to Parental Behavior

Parental behavior toward the child is one of the most important factors influencing the child's adjustment. Children's perceptions of their mothers' support and maternal perceptions of the psychosocial impact of the child's chronic illness on the family were shown to be two of the greatest predictors of children's psychologic adjustment (Immelt, 2006). In addition, family organization and illness-related support and involvement of parents influence children's adjustment to chronic illness (Schor, 2003). They often display pride and confidence in their ability to cope successfully with the challenges imposed by their disorder. Anticipatory guidance by the nurse and encouragement of normalizing practices may assist parents in facilitating their child's adjustment.

Type of Illness or Disability

The type of illness or disability also influences the child's emotional response. Interestingly, children with *more* severe disorders often cope better than those with milder conditions. However, the presence of multiple conditions may place a child at risk for more behavioral problems (Newacheck & Halfon, 1998). Considering children's cognitive ability and their delay in achieving abstract thinking until adolescence, it is likely that an obvious condition is easier to accept because its limitations are concrete. For example, children who are blind or physically disabled are constantly reminded of their inability to run. However, children with cardiac defects not only live by rules they do not understand, but also only vaguely and occasionally sense their illness, such as when they try to run and experience dyspnea and fatigue. Therefore some chronic illnesses pose special threats to children.

The onset of a disabling condition may generate a state of confusion for children, who may have trouble differentiating between actual bodily functions and their image of their bodies. They may also experience problems in identifying themselves and those extensions of self (e.g., wheelchairs, braces, crutches, other mechanical or prosthetic devices) and may have difficulty in accepting functional aids.

Nursing Care of the Family and Child with Special Needs

Assessment

Because the nurse may meet a family during any phase of the adjustment process, several assessment areas are important. The family's ability to cope with previous stresses influences the current situation, and answers to questions about their usual coping skills are enlightening. Knowledge of concurrent stresses, such as financial, marital, and career or unemployment, helps identify families who may have fewer resources to cope with the child's needs.

Finally, awareness of family members' reactions to the child and the illness or disability is important. Sample questions that the nurse and family can use to evaluate the support system, perception of the illness, coping mechanisms, resources, and concurrent stresses are listed in Table 41-1. Because factors affecting the family's response may change at any point during the illness, assessment must be a continual process.

Special challenges exist in assessing the child's feelings about having a disability. Chapter 34 presents several approaches to encourage a child to discuss feelings about the condition. The nurse should use a variety of communication

Table 41-1 Assessment of Factors Affecting Family Adjustment

FACTORS AFFECTING ADJUSTMENT	ASSESSMENT QUESTIONS
Available Support System	
Status of marital relationship	To whom do you talk when you have something on your mind? (If answer is not the spouse, ask for the reason.)
Alternate support systems	When something is worrying you, what do you do? What helps you most when you are upset?
Ability to communicate	Does talking seem to help when you feel upset?
Perception of the Illness or Disability	
Previous knowledge of disorder	Have you ever heard the word (name of diagnosis) before? Tell me about it (if answer is yes).
Imagined cause of disorder	What are your thoughts about the causes of the disorder?
Effects of illness or disability on family	How has your child's illness or disability affected you and your family? How has your lifestyle changed?
Coping Mechanisms	
Reactions to previous crises	Tell me one time you've had another crisis (problem, bad time) in your family. How did you solve that problem?
Reactions to the child	Do you find yourself being a little more cautious with this child than with your other children?
Childrearing practices	Do you feel as comfortable disciplining this child as your other children?
Influence of religion	Has your religion or faith been of help to you? Tell me how (if answer is yes).
Attitudes	How is this child different from the siblings or other children of similar age? Describe your child's personality. Is it easy, difficult, or in between? When you think of your child's future, what thoughts come to mind?
Available Resources	
	What parts of your child's care are causing the most difficulty for you or your family? What services are available to help? What services do you need that currently are not available?
Concurrent Stresses	
	What other problems are you facing now? (Be specific; ask about financial, marital, sibling, and extended family or friends concerns.)

techniques, such as drawing and play, as assessment tools rather than relying solely on parental reports. Often, children are neglected partners in their care, and their unique needs are not identified (Young et al, 2003; Dixon-Woods, Young, & Henry, 1999).

The needs of working parents and siblings also should be assessed, a goal that requires flexibility in scheduling appointments to include these important family members. When working parents know that their input is valuable, they will often change their work schedule to meet with a health professional. Because siblings can be of any age, the use of appropriate communication strategies for assessment must be considered. Nonverbal techniques such as those discussed in Chapter 34 should be considered for these children.

The main objective in working with the family is to help them cope effectively with those stresses imposed by the child's special needs. To achieve this goal, the entire family should be considered in every aspect of the implementation process (see Family-Centered Care box).

FAMILY-CENTERED CARE

Identifying Family Needs

To ensure an effective care plan, attention to family-identified needs and priorities is essential. For example, a family may have difficulty focusing on treatment issues if their current priority is obtaining enough food to feed their children.

Provide Support at the Time of Diagnosis

The diagnosis is a critical time for parents and can influence how they perceive their health care providers throughout care. Although they may not hear or remember all that is said to them, they frequently sense a certain attitude of acceptance, rejection, hope, or despair that may influence their ability to absorb the shock and begin adapting to the family's altered future.

Parents may be encouraged to be together when they are informed of their child's condition, thus avoiding the problem of one parent having to interpret complex findings and deal with the initial emotional reaction of the other. The informing session should take place in a private, comfortable setting free of distractions and interruptions, in an atmosphere in which the parents feel free to express their emotions (Fig. 41-3). Their emotional needs are acknowledged by showing acceptance of such expressions as crying, sadness, anger, and disappointment. Emotional support is offered by having tissues available if a family member cries and demonstrating through facial and body language that indeed this is a difficult and painful period. Although touching is a powerful expression of empathy, it must be used wisely. For example, it can prematurely terminate free expression of feelings, especially when combined with statements such as "Everything will be all right." Nurses should also be aware of cultural issues regarding touching.

Parents should receive the kind of information they desire. This can be assessed by asking questions such as, "Do you prefer to hear detailed information?" Parents or other family members may have different preferences regarding the amount of information they wish to hear. Most parents want a clear, simple explanation of the diagnosis; a prediction of possible futures for the child; advice on what to do next; an opportunity to ask questions; a warm, sympathetic listener; and, most important, time. Understanding of explanations is elicited with such questions as "Do you see what I mean?" or "Is this clear to you?" Technical terms are used with simple definitions. If the parents are unaware of the term, they are given written literature or at least a written summary of the diagnosis.

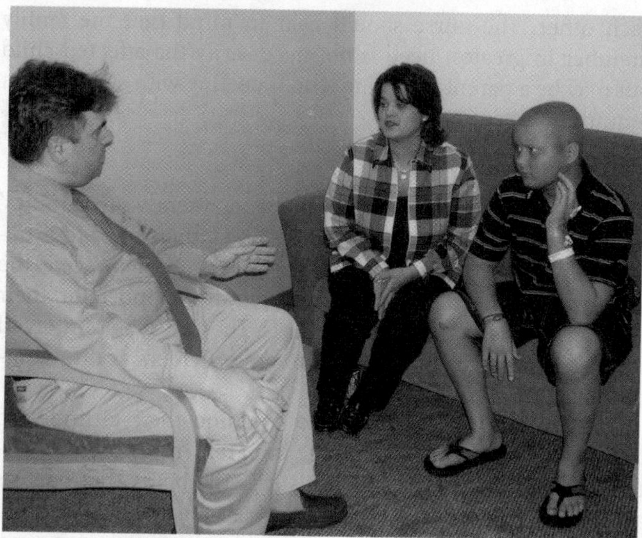

Fig. 41-3 Informing session should take place in a private, comfortable setting free of distractions and interruptions.

NURSING ALERT Develop a glossary of commonly used terms, acronyms, and abbreviations to distribute to parents. The list can stand alone or become a part of patient or parent handbooks.

Finally, the informing conference does not end with the presentation of devastating news. Instead, the child's strengths, appealing behaviors, and potential for development are stressed, as are available rehabilitation efforts or treatment. Parents can be encouraged to view their experiences as a series of challenges that they are capable of handling, particularly with available professional feedback. The parents are assured that the nurse will be available to answer questions and to provide further assistance as needed.

The preceding discussion relates primarily to the initial informing interview. However, because of the need for long-term follow-up, it is only one in a series of continuing discussions. In all interactions the family's input is solicited and incorporated into the care plan. Some situations require consideration of special problems.

Support Family's Coping Methods

For the family to meet the stresses of optimally adjusting to the child's condition, each member must be individually supported so that the family system is strong. Although the family can indefinitely support a member who is in need of assistance, its greatest strength lies in every member supporting each other. The nurse should bear in mind that the family member in greatest need is not necessarily the affected child but may be a parent or sibling who is dealing with stresses that require intervention.

Parents

The nurse can provide support by being attentive to families' responses to their children. Mothers and fathers need to experience success, joy, and pride in their children to give the support they need. Children, too, require support for their interactions, adjustments, and efforts. They must be reinforced for attempts to get to know their care providers and to communicate their needs to them.

It is important for nurses to examine their attitudes to determine their ability to engage in parent-professional partnerships. An essential characteristic is the belief that parents are equal to professionals and are experts regarding their child (see Patient Teaching box).

PATIENT TEACHING Developing Successful Parent-Professional Partnerships

- Promote primary nursing; in nonhospital settings designate a case manager.
- Acknowledge parents' overall competence and their unique expertise with their child.
- Respect parents' time as having value equal to that of other members of child's health care team.
- Explain or define any medical, technical, or discipline-specific terms.
- Tell families, "I am not sure" or "I don't know," when appropriate.
- Facilitate family's effectiveness in team meetings (e.g., provide parents with same information as other participants).

Communication among all family members is encouraged. Parent group sessions can help parents verbalize thoughts and feelings to each other but often do not take into account siblings' or the child's viewpoint. Therefore the nurse may need to set up a family session, such as during a home or clinic visit. Although the ideal situation is to have all the members present at one time, often this is not possible. Inviting members to participate at various visits is an appropriate alternative.

Parents can be encouraged to discuss their feelings toward the child, the impact of this event on their marriage, and associated stresses such as financial burdens. For most families, regardless of their income or insurance coverage, financial concerns exist. The costs of caring for a child with special needs can be overwhelming. In addition, the family wage earner may have to sacrifice job opportunities to remain close to a medical facility or to avoid losing insurance benefits.*

**Information regarding financial issues is available from the Federation for Children with Special Needs, 1135 Tremont St., Suite 420, Boston, MA 02120; 617-236-7210;* www.fcsn.org.

The nurse regards fathers as able, effective parents, competent and capable of coping with the challenges they face. Every effort is made to include the father in visits, such as to the nursery, clinic, special school, and stimulation programs. The father is included in the assessment process, with specific emphasis on having him describe the child's strengths and difficulties. It is not unusual to find two parents who have differing views of the child's abilities, especially in the area of developmental disabilities.

Numerous volunteer and community resources are available that provide assistance, rehabilitation, equipment, and funding for a variety of health problems.* National and local disease-oriented organizations may provide needed assistance and support to families that qualify. Many of these are discussed elsewhere in the text under the specific diagnosis. State and federal departments of health, mental health, social services, and labor may be able to help locate appropriate regional resources. For example, state programs for Children with Special Health Needs (formerly Crippled Children's Services) provide financial assistance for children with many disabling conditions. Local and national sources of respite care and medical day care may be useful to families. Nurses should become acquainted with those in their communities and with vocational programs for special groups.

Parent-to-Parent Support

Just being with another parent who has shared similar experiences is helpful. It may not need to be a parent of a child with the same diagnosis, since parents in the process of adjusting to a child with special needs—or finding respite services, educational or rehabilitative services, special equipment vendors, and financial counseling—tread a common path. The parent self-help group is another way to promote parent-to-parent support. Group members feel less alone and have the opportunity to observe both coping and mastery role modeling from other members. Parents' groups are rich resources for information. Even if parents are unable to attend meetings, they can still benefit from group newsletters and other literature that often accompany membership. The nurse can foster parent participation in self-help groups by serving as a referral agent, a group advisory board member, a resource person, a group member, or an assistant in founding a group. Sometimes all that is required in starting a group is identifying one or two parents as leaders; sharing with them the names, telephone numbers, and addresses of other families who have expressed both an interest and a willingness to release this information; and guiding them in how to initiate a first meeting.

**General sources of information are the Clearinghouse on Disability Information, 550 12th St. SW, Room 5133, Washington, DC 20202-2550; 202-245-7307;* www.ed.gov; *National Dissemination Center for Children with Disabilities, PO Box 1492, Washington, DC 20013; 800-695-0285;* www.nichcy.org. *A comprehensive list of books and pamphlets for parents and teachers is available from the Easter Seals, 233 S. Wacker Drive, Suite 2400, Chicago, IL 60606; 800-221-6827;* www.easterseals.com. *In Canada: Council of Canadians with Disabilities, 926-294 Portage Ave., Winnipeg, Manitoba R3C 0B9; 204-947-0303;* www.ccdonline.ca.

Advocate for Empowerment

Nurses can advocate for methods that foster opportunities for parent empowerment. For example, nurses can suggest reimbursement for travel and child care, plus stipends to enable parents' voices to be heard at meetings and conferences. They can encourage parent membership on staff, committees, and boards. They can keep parents informed of pending legislation on child health issues or take action when parents inform them.

The Child

Through ongoing contacts with the child, the nurse (1) observes the child's responses to the disorder, ability to function, and adaptive behaviors within the environment and with significant others; (2) explores the child's own understanding of his or her illness or condition; and (3) provides support while the child learns to cope with his or her feelings. Children are encouraged to express their concerns rather than allowing others to express them for them, since open discussions may reduce anxiety.

One of the most important interventions is alleviating the child's feeling of being different and normalizing his or her life as much as possible (see Patient Teaching box). Whenever possible, the nurse assists the family in assessing the child's daily routine for indications of a need for normalizing practices. For example, the child who remains in a bedroom all day requires a restructured daily routine to provide activities in different parts of the house, such as eating in the kitchen or dining room with the family. Such children may also be deprived of social, recreational, and academic activities that can be better accommodated by applying normalization practices. For example, home and out-of-home health-related treatments should be planned at times that least interfere with normal daily activities.

Children who are concerned that their condition detracts from their physical attractiveness need attention focused on the normal aspects of appearance and capabilities. Health professionals help strengthen and consolidate the self-image by emphasizing the normal, while allowing children to express anger, isolation, fear of rejection, feelings of sadness, and loneliness. The children need positive reinforcement for compliance and any evidence of improvement. Anything that might improve attractiveness and contribute to a positive self-image is employed, such as makeup for a teenager with a scar, clothing that disguises a prosthesis, or a hairstyle or wig to cover a deformity or lost hair.

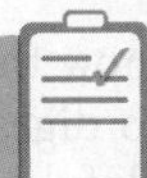

PATIENT TEACHING Promoting Normalization

Preparation—Prepare child in advance for changes that may occur from the illness or disability.

Example—Tell the child in advance the possible side effects of drug therapy.

Participation—Include child in as many decisions as possible, especially those relating to his or her care regimen.

Example—The child is responsible for taking medications or scheduling home treatments.

Sharing—Allow both family members and child's peers to be a part of the care regimen whenever possible.

Examples—Give the child his or her medication when the other siblings receive their vitamins.

The parent cooks the same menu for the whole family.

If the child is invited to another's home, the parent advises the family of the child's dietary restrictions.

Control—Identify areas where child can be in control to decrease feelings of uncertainty, passivity, and helplessness.

Example—The child identifies activities that are appropriate to his or her energy level and chooses to rest when fatigued.

Expectation—Apply the same family rules to the child with a chronic illness or disability as to the well siblings or peers.

Example—The child is disciplined, is expected to fulfill household responsibilities, and attends school in accordance with abilities.

Siblings

The presence of a child with special needs in a family may result in parents paying less attention to the other children. Siblings may respond by developing negative attitudes toward the child or by expressing anger in different forms. The nurse can help by using anticipatory guidance, questioning the parents about what they believe is the best way to have siblings respond to the child and guiding them through ways to meet their other children's needs for attention. This questioning should take place before serious negative effects occur.

Siblings may also experience embarrassment associated with having a brother or sister with an illness or disability. Parents are then faced with the difficulty of responding to this embarrassment in an understanding and appropriate manner without punishing the siblings for how they feel. Parents are encouraged to talk with the siblings about how they view their affected sibling. For example, siblings of a child who is cognitively impaired may express fears about their ability to bear normal children. Adolescents in particular may not be able to discuss these vital issues with their parents and may prefer to consult with the nurse. Many siblings benefit from sharing their concerns with other young people who are in a similar situation. Support groups for siblings can help decrease isolation, promote expression of feelings, and provide examples of effective coping skills.

The nurse is sensitive to the reactions of siblings and whenever possible intervenes to promote more positive adjustment. For example, siblings often mention that they are expected to take on additional responsibilities to help the parents care for the child. It is not unusual for them to express a positive reaction to assuming the extra duties but a negative response to feeling unappreciated for doing so. Such feelings can often be minimized by encouraging siblings to discuss this with the parents and by suggesting to parents ways of showing gratitude, such as an increase in allowance, special privileges, and, most significantly, verbal praise.

Educate About the Disorder and General Health Care

Educating the family about the disorder is actually an extension of revealing the diagnosis. Education involves not only supplying technical information, but also discussing how the condition will affect the child. Parents may be able to digest only so much information at a time. It may be helpful to provide essential information and then follow by asking, "What else would you like to know about your child's condition?" Responding to parents' questions and concerns ensures that their information needs are met.

Activities of Daily Living

Parents also need guidance in how the condition may interfere with or alter activities of daily living, such as eating, dressing, sleeping, and toileting. One area frequently affected is nutrition. Common problems are undernutrition resulting from food being inappropriately restricted or loss of appetite, vomiting, or motor deficits that interfere with feeding; overnutrition may also occur, usually because of a caloric intake in excess of energy expenditure or boredom and lack of stimulation in other areas. Although the child requires the same basic nutrients as other children, the daily requirements may differ. Special nutritional considerations are discussed as appropriate throughout the text.

Safe Transportation

Modifications may also be needed regarding car safety. Children with conditions such as low birth weight or orthopedic, neuromuscular, or respiratory problems often cannot safely use conventional car restraints. For example, children with hip spica casts cannot sit properly in child safety seats (see Developmental Dysplasia of the Hip, Chapter 54). Modifications can be made to some commercial models, and for older children a special vest is available that secures the child to the back seat in a lying-down position.*

If a child requires a wheelchair, the family should consult the wheelchair manufacturer for specific instructions regarding safe car transportation. Considerations for wheelchairs used with vehicle transportation include securing both the wheelchair and the occupant in the wheelchair. Wheelchairs should be secured facing forward with tie downs at four points. The tie-down system should be dynamically crash tested, as should the occupant securement system that secures the child in the wheelchair. For example, use of trays would not be recommended for transportation. With children who must travel with additional medical equipment (e.g., oxygen, monitors, or ventilators), this equipment should be anchored to the floor or underneath the vehicle seat or wheelchair. Soft padding should be added around the equipment to reduce movement. A second adult should be present to monitor the condition of a medically fragile child while traveling.

Primary Health Care

Children with special needs require all the usual health care recommended for any child. Attention to injury prevention, immunizations, dental health, and regular physical examinations is essential. Nurses can play an important role in reminding parents of these aspects of care that are so often neglected when the concern is focused on the child's illness or disability. Specific discussions of nutrition, sleep and activity, dental health, and injury prevention are presented in the chapters on health promotion for specific age groups. Immunizations are discussed in Chapter 36.

Parents also need to be aware of the importance of communicating the child's condition in the event of a medical emergency. Young children are unable to give information about their disorder, and although older children may be reliable sources, after an accident they may be physically unable to speak. Therefore all children with any type of chronic condition that may affect medical care should wear some type of identification, such as a MedicAlert bracelet,* or carry a card in their wallet that lists the medical condition and a phone number for emergency medical records and other personal information.

Promote Normal Development

Aside from knowledge of the condition and its effect on the child's abilities, the family must be guided toward fostering appropriate development in their child. Although each stage may take longer to achieve, parents are guided toward helping the child fully realize his or her potential in preparation for the next developmental stage. Table 41-2 outlines developmental aspects of chronic illness or disability and supportive interventions. With appropriate planning and knowledge of strategies to improve the child's functional abilities, most children can live fulfilling and productive lives.

One important aspect of promoting normal development is to encourage the child's self-care abilities in both activities of daily living and the medical regimen. An assessment of the child's age and physical, emotional, and mental capacities, as well as the support and structure provided by the family, should be considered in determining the appropriate level of self-care in the medical regimen. Even toddlers can be involved in their own care by holding supplies for the parent during a procedure. Over time, children should be encouraged toward greater autonomy in the self-care arena.

Early Childhood

During infancy the child is achieving basic *trust* through a satisfying, intimate, consistent relationship with his or her parents. However, the affected child's early existence may be stressful, chaotic, and unsatisfying. Consequently, he or she may need more parental support and expressions of affection to achieve trust. Likewise, the parents require assistance in finding ways to meet the infant's needs, such as how to hold a rigid or flaccid infant, how to feed a child with tongue thrust or episodes of dyspnea, and how to stimulate a child who seems incapable of achieving any skills.

During early childhood the goal is to achieve *separation* from parents, *autonomy,* and *initiative.* However, the natural parental response to having a sick child is overprotection. Parents need help in realizing the importance of allowing brief separations of the child from them and from others involved

---

Footnotes

***Information on car safety restraints for children with special needs is available from the Automotive Safety Program, 575 West Drive, Room 004, Indianapolis, IN 46202; 800-543-6227 or 317-274-2997; www.preventinjury.org.*

***MedicAlert Foundation International, 2323 Colorado Ave., Turlock, CA 95382; 888-633-4298; www.medicalert.org.*

Table 41-2 Developmental Effects of Chronic Illness or Disability on Children

DEVELOPMENTAL TASKS	POTENTIAL EFFECTS OF CHRONIC ILLNESS OR DISABILITY	SUPPORTIVE INTERVENTIONS
Infancy		
Develop a sense of trust	Multiple caregivers and frequent separations, especially if hospitalized Deprived of consistent nurturing	Encourage consistent caregivers in hospital or other care settings. Encourage parental presence, "rooming in" during hospitalization, and participation in care.
Bond, or attach, to parent	Delayed because of separation; parental grief for loss of "dream" child; parental inability to accept the condition, especially a visible defect	Emphasize healthy, perfect qualities of infant. Help parents learn special care needs of infant for them to feel competent.
Learn through sensorimotor experiences	More exposure to painful experiences than pleasurable ones Limited contact with environment from restricted movement or confinement	Expose infant to pleasurable experiences through all senses (touch, hearing, sight, taste, movement). Encourage age-appropriate developmental skills (e.g., holding bottle, finger feeding, crawling).
Begin to develop a sense of separateness from parent	Increased dependency on parent for care Overinvolvement of parent in care	Encourage all family members to participate in care to prevent overinvolvement of one member. Encourage periodic respite from demands of care responsibilities.
Toddlerhood		
Develop autonomy	Increased dependency on parent	Encourage independence in as many areas as possible (e.g., toileting, dressing, feeding).
Master locomotor and language skills	Limited opportunity to test own abilities and limits	Provide gross motor skill activity and modification of toys or equipment, such as modified swing or rocking horse.
Learn through sensorimotor experience; beginning preoperational thought	Increased exposure to painful experiences	Give choices to allow simple feeling of control (e.g., choice of what book to look at, what kind of sandwich to eat). Institute age-appropriate discipline and limit setting. Recognize that negative and ritualistic behaviors are normal. Provide sensory experiences (e.g., water play, sandbox play, finger painting).
Preschool		
Develop initiative and purpose Master self-care skills	Limited opportunities for success in accomplishing simple tasks or mastering self-care skills	Encourage mastery of self-help skills. Provide devices that make task easier (e.g., self-dressing).
Begin to develop peer relationships	Limited opportunities for socialization with peers; may appear "like a baby" to age-mates Protection within tolerant and secure family causing child to fear criticism and withdraw	Encourage socialization (e.g., inviting friends to play, day care experience, trips to park). Provide age-appropriate play, especially associative play opportunities. Emphasize child's abilities; dress appropriately to enhance desirable appearance.
Develop sense of body image and sexual identification	Awareness of body centering on pain, anxiety, and failure Sex-role identification focused primarily on mothering skills	Encourage relationships with same-sex and opposite-sex peers and adults.
Learn through preoperational thought (magical thinking)	Guilt (thinking he or she caused the illness or disability or is being punished for wrongdoing)	Help child deal with criticisms; realize that too much protection prevents child from learning to cope with realities of world. Clarify that child's illness or disability is not his or her fault or a punishment.
School Age		
Develop a sense of accomplishment	Limited opportunities to achieve and compete (e.g., many school absences, inability to join regular athletic activities)	Encourage school attendance; schedule medical visits at times other than school; encourage child to make up missed work.
Form peer relationships	Limited opportunities for socialization	Educate teachers and classmates about child's condition, abilities, and special needs. Encourage sports activities (e.g., Special Olympics). Encourage socialization (e.g., Girl Scouts, Campfire, Boy Scouts, 4-H Club; having a best friend or club membership).
Learn through concrete operations	Incomplete comprehension of the imposed physical limitations or treatment of the disorder	Provide child with information about his or her condition. Encourage creative activities (e.g., VSA Arts).

Continued

Table 41-2 Developmental Effects of Chronic Illness or Disability on Children—cont'd

DEVELOPMENTAL TASKS	POTENTIAL EFFECTS OF CHRONIC ILLNESS OR DISABILITY	SUPPORTIVE INTERVENTIONS
Adolescence		
Develop personal and sexual identity	Increased sense of feeling different from peers and reduced ability to compete with peers in appearance, abilities, special skills	Help child realize that many of the difficulties the teenager is experiencing are part of normal adolescence (rebelliousness, risk taking, lack of cooperation, hostility toward authority).
Achieve independence from family	Increased dependency on family; limited job or career opportunities	Provide instruction on interpersonal and coping skills. Encourage increased responsibility for care and management of the disease or condition (e.g., assuming responsibility for making and keeping appointment [ideally alone], sharing assessment and planning stages of health care delivery, contacting resources). Discuss planning for future and how condition can affect choices.
Form heterosexual relationships	Limited opportunities for heterosexual friendships; less opportunity to discuss sexual concerns with peers Increased concern with issues such as why did he or she get the disorder, can he or she marry and have a family	Encourage socialization with peers, including peers with special needs and those without special needs. Encourage activities appropriate for age (e.g., attending mixed-sex parties, sports activities, driving a car). Be alert to cues that signal readiness for information regarding implications of condition on sexuality and reproduction. Emphasize good appearance and wearing stylish clothes, use of makeup. Understand that adolescent has same sexual needs and concerns as any other teenager.
Learn through abstract thinking	Decreased opportunity for earlier stages of cognition impeding achievement of level of abstract thinking	Provide instruction on decision making, assertiveness, and other skills necessary to manage personal plans.

in the child's care and of providing social experiences outside the home whenever possible. Respite care, which provides temporary relief for family members, can be essential in allowing caregivers time away from the daily burdens.

Young children also need the opportunity to develop *independence*. Frequently the child is able to learn self-help skills, such as holding the bottle, finger feeding, and removing simple articles of clothing, but the parent continues to perform the act. The nurse can guide parents to the usual milestones expected from the child. When a child is unable to perform a skill independently, functional aids should be used. With innovation, many adaptations can be implemented in children's environments to increase their mobility and independence and allow them to play like other children their age. For example, with slight modifications, a child with physical limitations may be able to ride a tricycle (Fig. 41-4).

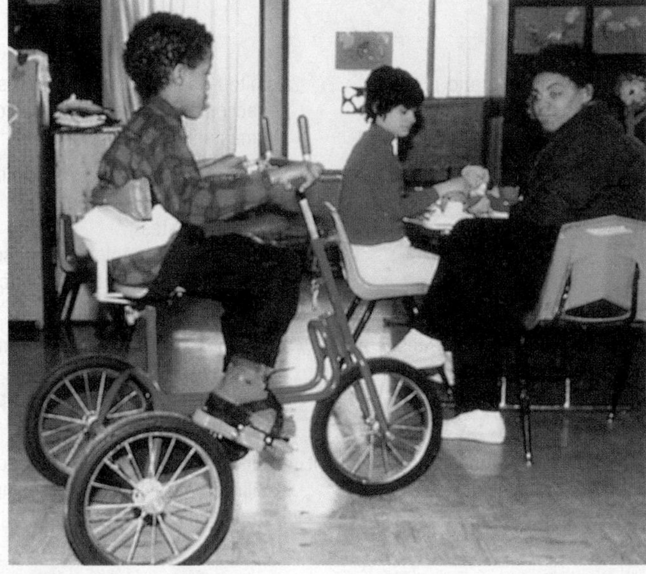

Fig. 41-4 A modified tricycle with block pedals, self-adhesive straps for support, and modified seat and handle bars can help a child with disabilities gain mobility.

Another critical component for normal child development is *discipline*. Discipline and guidance serve several purposes, such as providing children with boundaries on which to test out their behavior and teaching them socially acceptable behavior. Resentment and hostility can arise among siblings if different standards are applied to each child. The nurse's responsibility is to help parents learn successful methods of managing a child's behaviors before they become problems.

School Age

For school-age children the major tasks are entry into school and achieving a sense of *industry*. Although the importance of school in the life of all children is well known, school absences are significantly higher among children with chronic illness than among their healthy peers. The more school absences the child experiences, the more difficult it is to resume attendance, and school phobia may result. The child should return to school as soon as possible after diagnosis or treatments.

Preparation for entry into or resumption of school is best accomplished through a team approach with the parents, child, teacher, school nurse, and primary nurse in the hospital. Ideally, this planning should begin before hospital discharge,

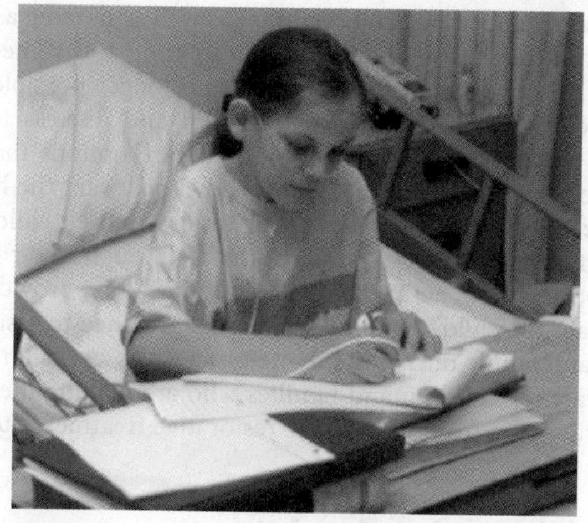

Fig. 41-5 Children with special needs should continue their schooling as soon as their condition permits.

provided that the child is well enough to resume usual activities. A structured plan should be developed, with attention to those aspects of care that must be continued during school hours, such as administration of medication or other treatments.

Children also need preparation before entering or resuming school. Having a tutor in the hospital or home as soon as children are physically able helps them realize that school will continue and gives them time to consider this prospect (Fig. 41-5). They need to investigate possible answers to the many questions others will ask. One method of anticipatory preparation is to role-play, with the child as the "returned pupil" and the nurse or parent as "other schoolmates." If the child returns to school with some obvious physical change, such as hair loss, amputation, or visible scar, the nurse might also ask questions about these alterations to prompt preparatory responses from the child.

Classroom peers also need preparation, and a joint plan of the teacher, nurse, and child is best. At a minimum, classmates should be given a description of the child's condition, prepared for any visible changes in the child, and allowed an opportunity to ask questions. The child should have the option of attending this session. As the child's condition changes, particularly if the illness is potentially fatal, school personnel, including the students, need periodic apprisal of the child's status and preparation for what to expect.

Children with special needs are encouraged to maintain or reestablish relationships with peers and to participate according to their capabilities in any age-appropriate activities. Alternative activities may be substituted for those that are impossible or that place a strain on the child's condition. Programs such as the Special Olympics* offer children an opportunity to compete with their peers and to achieve athletic skill. Summer camps* allow children to associate with peers and develop a wide variety of skills. Children with special needs can derive enormous benefits from expressive activities, such as art, music, poetry, dance, and drama. With adaptive equipment and imagination, children can participate in a variety of activities. Organizations such as VSA Arts allow children to celebrate and share their accomplishments.† Children need the opportunity to interact with healthy peers and to engage in activities with groups or clubs composed of similarly affected age-mates. Such organizations as ostomy clubs, diabetes clubs, and cerebral palsy groups share information and provide support related to the special problems the members face.

Adolescence

Adolescence can be a particularly difficult period for the teenager and family. All of the needs discussed previously apply to this age group as well. Developing *independence* or *autonomy*, however, is a major task for the adolescent as planning for the future becomes a prominent concern. Although the emphasis in the past has been on achieving independence from physical assistance, recent developments in the fields of special education, adolescent development, and family systems suggest redefining autonomy in terms of individuals' capacities to take responsibility for their own behavior, to make decisions regarding their own lives, and to maintain supportive social relationships. Given this understanding, even individuals with severe impairment can be viewed as autonomous if they perceive their own needs and take responsibility for meeting them, either directly or by engaging the assistance of others. As adolescents become more autonomous, the nurse can help them articulate needs, participate in developing their own care plan, and discover and express how others can be of greatest assistance.

Physical symptoms are high on the teenager's list of health-related concerns. Because adolescence is a time of enormous physical and emotional changes, it is important for the nurse to distinguish between body changes that are related to disability and those that are a result of normal body development. It can be a great comfort for teenagers with disabling conditions to know that many of the changes they experience are normal developmental outcomes.

A sense of feeling different from peers can lead to loneliness, isolation, and depression. Participation in groups of teenagers with chronic conditions or disabilities can alleviate feelings of isolation and smooth the transition to a meaningful relationship with one person in adulthood.

Establish Realistic Future Goals

One of the most difficult adjustments is setting realistic future goals for the child and for those involved in his or her contin-

1133 19th St. NW, Washington, DC 20036; 202-628-3630; www.specialolympics.org. Several pamphlets on sports and recreation for children with disabilities are available from Easter Seals (see footnote, p. 1158) and American Alliance for Health, Physical Education, Recreation and Dance, 1900 Association Drive, Reston, VA 20191; 703-476-3400 or 800-213-7193; www.aahperd.org.

**A directory of private, paying camps for children with a variety of chronic illnesses or general physical disabilities is available from the American Camp Association, 5000 State Road 67 North, Martinsville, IN 46151-7902; 765-342-8456; www.acacamps.org.*

†VSA Arts has affiliate chapters in all 50 states and in selected sites internationally; yearly festivals are held throughout the world. Information is available from VSA Arts, 818 Connecticut Ave. NW, Suite 600, Washington, DC 20006; 202-628-2800 or 800-933-8721; www.vsarts.org.

ued care. Sometimes the impact of this decision does not surface until the child finishes school or the parents approach retirement, when a crisis can arise because of disruption of all of the family roles and relationships that maintained stability.

Planning for the future should be a gradual process. All along, the parents should cultivate realistic vocations for the child. For example, if children have physical disabilities, they are directed to intellectual, artistic, or musical pursuits. Children with developmental disabilities are taught manual skills. In this way, the child's development proceeds in the direction of self-support through gainful employment.

With prolonged survival, young people with chronic illnesses must deal with new decisions and problems, such as marriage, employment, and insurance coverage. With appropriate guidance, individuals with disabilities can attain gainful employment, marriage, and a family. For those whose conditions are genetic, counseling is needed regarding future offspring. Prospective spouses often benefit from an opportunity to discuss their feelings regarding marriage to an individual with continued health needs and possibly a limited life span. Health insurance coverage is a critical issue because some private carriers may no longer insure a young person who leaves home or may be unwilling to reinsure the person who is independent. Life insurance is another dilemma, especially when children have serious defects, such as congenital heart anomalies.

Perspectives on the Care of Children at the End of Life

evolve Nursing Care Plan—The Child Who Is Terminally Ill or Dying

Although most childhood illnesses and many injuries and other trauma respond favorably to treatment, some do not. When a child and family face a prolonged and possibly terminal illness, health professionals must confront the challenge of providing the best possible care to meet the physical, psychologic, spiritual, and emotional needs of the child and family during the uncertain course of the illness and at the time of death. When death is sudden and unexpected, nurses are challenged to respond to grief and shock in families and provide comfort and support in the absence of a prior relationship.

Many factors affect the causes of death that nurses are likely to encounter in children: developmental factors, medical advances and technology, and changing social patterns. In infants the leading causes of death are congenital anomalies, respiratory distress syndrome, disorders related to short gestation and low birth weight, and sudden infant death syndrome (Arias et al, 2003). The leading causes of death in children 5 to 9 years of age include injuries (accidents), malignant neoplasms, congenital anomalies, assault (homicide), and heart disease. In children 10 to 14 years of age, suicide is the third leading cause of death, after injuries (accidents) and malignant neoplasms. In youths 15 to 19 years of age, assault (homicide), suicide, malignant neoplasms, and heart disease follow accidents as the most prevalent causes of death (Anderson & Smith, 2005).

A child who is diagnosed with a life-threatening illness or who is suffering serious, life-threatening trauma needs medical diagnosis and intervention, as well as nursing assessment and care—sometimes for a short time and sometimes over a lengthy period. When cure is no longer possible and life-prolonging measures result in pain and distress to the child, parents need information about care options that are available to assist them in deciding how they want the health care team to manage the remaining time with their child. It is important to reassure families that, although their child cannot be cured, active care will continue to be provided to maintain the child's comfort. Support is provided to assist the child and family during the dying process. As a result, nurses may care for children and families who are making the difficult transition from curative or restorative treatments to palliative care.

Principles of Palliative Care

Palliative care involves a multidisciplinary approach to the management of a terminal illness or the dying process that focuses on symptom control and support rather than on cure or life prolongation in the absence of the possibility of a cure (Field & Behrman, 2004). The World Health Organization (1996) defines *palliative care* as the "active total care of patients whose disease is not responsive to curative treatment. Control of pain, of other symptoms, and of psychological, social and spiritual problems is paramount. The goal of palliative care is the achievement of the best possible quality of life for patients and their families."

Palliative care interventions do not serve to hasten death; rather, they provide pain and symptom management, attention to issues faced by the child and family with regard to death and dying, and promotion of optimal functioning and quality of life during the time the child has remaining. The implementation of neonatal and pediatric palliative care consulting services within hospitals has led to enhanced quality of life and end-of-life care for children and their families and support for their care providers (Jennings, 2005; Pierucci, Kirby, & Leuthner, 2001). Several principles are hallmarks of palliative care.

The child and family are considered the unit of care. The death of a child is an extremely stressful event for a family because it is out of the natural order of things. Children represent health and hope, and their death calls into question the understanding of life. A multidisciplinary team of health care professionals consisting of social workers, chaplains, nurses, personal care aides, and physicians skilled in caring for dying patients assist the family by focusing care on the complex interactions between physical, emotional, social, and spiritual issues.

Palliative care seeks to create a therapeutic environment, as homelike as possible, if not in the child's own home. Through education and support of family members, an atmosphere of open communication is provided regarding the child's dying process and its impact on all members of the family (see Evidence-Based Practice box).

Decision Making at the End of Life

Discussions concerning the possibility that a child's illness or condition is not curable and that death is an inevitable outcome cause everyone involved a great deal of stress. Physicians,

EVIDENCE-BASED PRACTICE Pediatric Pain and Symptom Management at the End of Life

Ask the Question

In children, what is the pain and symptom experience at the end of life?

Search for Evidence

Search Strategies

Published studies from 2000 to 2005 using the subject terms *child, palliative care, pain,* and *symptoms;* findings dominated by retrospective descriptive studies describing infants and children's end-of-life experiences through the use of medical record reviews and provider and parental surveys

Databases Searched

PubMed, CINAHL

Critically Analyze the Evidence

Children experienced an average of 11 symptoms during their last week of life (Drake, Frost, & Collins, 2003). Pain, dyspnea, and fatigue were the most frequently documented symptoms, experienced by most children at the end of life (Bradshaw et al, 2005; Carter et al, 2004; Drake, Frost, & Collins, 2003; Hongo et al, 2003). Children and their parents reported high distress with pain and symptoms at the end of life. Parents reported pain and suffering as one of the most important factors in deciding to withhold or withdraw life support from their child in the pediatric intensive care unit (Meert, Thurston, & Sarnaik, 2000).

Documentation was scarce related to symptom management. Morphine was the most commonly prescribed pain medication (Drake, Frost, & Collins, 2003; Hongo et al, 2003). Parents reported their children as experiencing high levels of pain near the end of life (Contro et al, 2002). Physicians were more likely than nurses or parents to report that a child's pain and symptoms were well managed at the end of life, whereas the majority of both provider groups believed the child's physical management was difficult (Andresen, Seecharan, & Toce, 2004; Wolfe et al, 2000).

Barriers to the adequate provision of pediatric palliative care include developmental issues specific to infants and children; symptoms, their causes, how they are related, and effective treatment strategies; lack of education; and reimbursement issues (Harris, 2004). Physicians reported reliance on trial and error as they learned to care for children at the end of life and the need for specialty consults with palliative care service providers (Hilden et al, 2001).

Apply the Evidence: Nursing Implications

Although the philosophy of palliative care encompasses pain and symptom management for infants and children who may not outlive their disease, the provision of that care to ease suffering and provide comfort to those who will die continues to lag. Studies show that children experience significant pain and other distressing symptoms at the end of life that are not well managed. Discrepancies in perceptions of infant and child pain and suffering continue to exist between providers and parents. Barriers to the provision of pediatric palliative care exist. Improvements are needed in the management of pain and symptoms at the end of life for infants and children.

References

Andresen EM, Seecharan GA, Toce SS: Provider perceptions of child deaths, *Arch Pediatr Adolesc Med* 158:430-435, 2004.

Bradshaw G et al: Cancer-related deaths in children and adolescents, *J Palliat Med* 8(1):86-95, 2005.

Carter BS et al: Circumstances surrounding the deaths of hospitalized children: opportunities for pediatric palliative care, *Pediatrics* 114(3):361-366, 2004.

Contro N et al: Family perspectives on the quality of pediatric palliative care, *Arch Pediatr Adolesc Med* 156:1-29, 2002.

Drake R, Frost J, Collins JJ: The symptoms of dying children, *J Pain Symptom Manage* 26(1):594-603, 2003.

Harris B: Palliative care in children with cancer: which child and when? *J Natl Cancer Institute Mono* 32:144-149, 2004.

Hilden JM et al: Attitudes and practices among pediatric oncologists regarding end-of-life care: results of the 1998 American Society of Clinical Oncology Survey, *J Clin Oncol* 19(1):205-212, 2001.

Hongo T et al: Analysis of the circumstances at the end of life in children with cancer: symptoms, suffering and acceptance, *Pediatr Int* 45:60-64, 2003.

Meert KL, Thurston CS, Sarnaik AP: End-of-life decision-making and satisfaction with care: parental perspectives, *Pediatr Crit Care Med* 1(2):179-185, 2000.

Wolfe J et al: Symptoms and suffering at the end of life in children with cancer, *N Engl J Med* 342(5):326-333, 2000.

other members of the health care team, and families must consider all information regarding the child's situation and make decisions that all parties agree to and that will have a profound impact on the child and family.

Ethical Considerations in End-of-Life Decision Making

A number of ethical concerns arise when parents and health care professionals are deciding on the best course of care for the dying child. Many parents and health care providers are concerned that not offering treatment that would cause potential pain and suffering, but might extend life, would be considered euthanasia or assisted suicide. To eliminate such concerns, it is necessary to understand the various terms. *Euthanasia* involves an action carried out by a person other than the patient to end the life of the patient suffering from a terminal condition. This action is based on the belief that the act is "putting the patient out of his [or her] misery"; this action has also been called *mercy killing. Assisted suicide* occurs when someone provides the patient with the means to end his or her life and the patient uses that means to do so. The important distinction between these two actions involves who is actually acting to end the person's life.

The American Nurses Association *Code of Ethics for Nurses* (2001) does not support the active intent on the part of a nurse to end a person's life. However, it does permit the nurse to provide interventions to relieve symptoms in the dying patient even when the interventions involve substantial risks of hastening death. When the prognosis for a patient is poor and death is the expected outcome, it is ethically acceptable to withhold or withdraw treatments that may cause pain and suffering and provide interventions that promote comfort and quality of life. Therefore providing palliative care for patients is the ethically correct choice in such a circumstance.

Physician–Health Care Team Decision Making

Decisions by physicians regarding care are often made on the basis of the progression of the disease or amount of trauma, the availability of treatment options that would provide cure from disease or restoration of health, the impact of such treatments on the child, and the child's overall prognosis (Davis & Eng, 1998). Often the main determinants prompting physicians to discuss end-of-life issues and options for children with critical illnesses include the child's age, premorbid cognitive condition and functional status, pain or discomfort, probability of survival, and quality of life (Masri et al, 2000). When the physician discusses this information openly with families, a shared decision-making process can occur regarding *do-not-resuscitate (DNR) orders* and care that is focused on the comfort of the child and family during the dying process.

Unfortunately, many families are not given the option of terminating treatment and pursuing care that is focused on comfort and quality of life when cure is unlikely, and staff may be reluctant to raise the question of DNR orders. This occurs for a number of reasons, including the belief that not being able to "save" a child is a "failure." Also, the physician and other members of the health care team may lack knowledge of and experience with the principles of palliative care (Field & Behrman, 2004; Sumner, 2003; Sahler et al, 2000).

Parental Decision Making

Rarely are families prepared to cope with the numerous decisions that must be made when a child is dying. When the death is unexpected, as in the case of an accident or trauma, the confusion of emergency services and possibly an intensive care setting presents challenges to parents as they are asked to make difficult choices. If the child has either experienced a life-threatening illness such as cancer or lived with a chronic illness that has now reached its terminal phase, parents are often unprepared for the reality of their child's impending death (see Family-Centered Care box). Numerous studies have found that families facing the impending death of a child depend on information provided to them by the health care team, particularly an honest appraisal of the child's prognosis, to make difficult decisions regarding care options for their child (Wolfe, Friebert, & Hilden, 2002; Hinds et al, 2001; James & Johnson, 1997).

As the group of health professionals who are most involved with families, nurses are in an excellent position to ensure that families are presented with the options available to them. The nurse's first responsibility is to explore the family's wishes. This is best done in concert with the physician, but at times may need to be initiated by the nurse. Statements such as "Tell me about your thoughts for the type of care you want your child to receive when he is dying" or "Have you considered the types of interventions you would like us to use when your child is near death?" can begin discussion of this sensitive but critical aspect of terminal care.

FAMILY-CENTERED CARE

Family of the Dying Child

No matter whether you have a PhD or many children, when your child dies, it is a new experience and nothing can prepare you for it. Like so many things in life, experience is the best teacher.

Three of our children have died, and by the time the third was dying, we handled many things differently. We learned a lot about dignity and the rights of the child and family. For example, at first, we didn't know that we had a right to have our child die at home. We also didn't understand pain medications and that if children are taking these medicines and are still in agony, they have not overdosed on the medication.

We learned a lot about case management. With our first two children, lots of different people were making decisions and disagreeing about what was best and what should be done. No one had primary authority. With our third child, one doctor took a primary role. Any questions and problems were handled by one person. I could call him 24 hours a day. It made a lot of difference, and I felt our concerns and needs were better heard and respected.

The nurses caring for our third child at home enabled me to step back and just be his mommy. When I could do this, I realized that we were fighting so hard for his life that we weren't really letting him die. His nurses had worked with him for a long time and really loved him. It was hard for them when we decided to let him die. In his last several days we wanted a lot of family time with our son, and I think the nurses felt left out. Something about their reaction to our increased time with him in the last few days made us feel guilty. If we had all been able to communicate a little more openly, I would have understood that they needed more time with him at the end, too. Everyone's needs could have been met.

–Jeni Stepanek, Mother
Upper Marlboro, MD

The Dying Child

Children need honest and accurate information about their illness, treatments, and prognosis; this information needs to be given in clear, simple language. In most situations this best occurs as a gradual process over time, characterized by increasingly open dialogue between parents, professionals, and the child (Young et al, 2003). Providing an atmosphere of open communication early in the course of an illness facilitates answering difficult questions as the child's condition worsens. Providing appropriate literature about the disease and the experience of illness and possible death is also helpful. Exactly how and when to involve children in decisions regarding care during their dying process and death is an individual matter. The child's age or developmental level is an important consideration in the process (Table 41-3). In general, parents should be asked how they would like their child to be told of the prognosis, and they should be included in his or her care. Some parents may request that their child not be told that he or she is dying, even if the child asks. This often places health care providers in a difficult situation. Children, even at a young age, are perceptive. Even if they are not told outright that they are dying, they realize that something is seriously wrong and that it involves them. Often, helping parents

evolve Case Study–The Dying Child

Table 41-3 Children's Understanding of and Reactions to Death

CONCEPTS OF DEATH	REACTIONS TO DEATH	NURSING CARE MANAGEMENT
Infants and Toddlers		
Death has least significance to children <6 mo of age. After parent-child attachment and trust are established, the loss, even if temporary, of the significant person is profound. Prolonged separation during the first several years is thought to be more significant in terms of future physical, social, and emotional growth than at any subsequent age. Toddlers are egocentric and can only think about events in terms of their own frame of reference—living. Their egocentricity and vague separation of fact and fantasy make it impossible for them to comprehend absence of life. Instead of understanding death, this age group is affected more by any change in lifestyle.	With the death of someone else, they may continue to act as though the person is alive. As children grow older, they will be increasingly able and willing to let go of the dead person. Ritualism is important; a change in lifestyle could be anxiety producing. This age group reacts more to the pain and discomfort of a serious illness than to the probable fatal prognosis. This age group also reacts to parental anxiety and sadness.	Help parents deal with their feelings, allowing them greater emotional reserves to meet the needs of their children. Encourage parents to remain as near to child as possible, yet be sensitive to parents' needs. Maintain as normal an environment as possible to retain ritualism. If a parent has died, promote arrangements for consistent caregiver for child. Promote primary nursing.
Preschool Children		
Preschoolers believe their thoughts are sufficient to cause death; the consequence is the burden of guilt, shame, and punishment. Their egocentricity implies a tremendous sense of self-power and omnipotence. They usually have some understanding of the meaning of death. Death is seen as a departure, a kind of sleep. They may recognize the fact of physical death but do not separate it from living abilities. Death is seen as temporary and gradual; life and death can change places with one another. They have no understanding of the universality and inevitability of death.	If they become seriously ill, they conceive of the illness as a punishment for their thoughts or actions. They may feel guilty and responsible for the death of a sibling. Greatest fear concerning death is separation from parents. They may engage in activities that seem strange or abnormal to adults. Because they have fewer defense mechanisms to deal with loss, young children may react to a less significant loss with more outward grief than to the loss of a very significant person. The loss is so deep, painful, and threatening that the child must deny it for a time to survive its overwhelming impact. Behavior reactions such as giggling, joking, attracting attention, or regressing to earlier developmental skills indicate children's need to distance themselves from tremendous loss.	Help parents deal with their feelings, allowing them greater emotional reserves to meet the needs of their children. Help parents understand their children's behavioral reactions. Encourage parents to remain near the child as much as possible, to minimize the child's great fear of separation from parents. If a parent has died, promote arrangements for a consistent caregiver for child. Promote primary nursing.
School-Age Children		
The children still associate misdeeds or bad thoughts with causing death and feel intense guilt and responsibility for the event. Because of their higher cognitive abilities, they respond well to logical explanations and comprehend the figurative meaning of words. They have a deeper understanding of death in a concrete sense. They particularly fear the mutilation and punishment they associate with death. They personify death as the devil, a monster, or the bogeyman. They may have naturalistic or physiologic explanations of death. By age 9-10, children have an adult concept of death, realizing that it is inevitable, universal, and irreversible.	Because of their increased ability to comprehend, they may have more fears, for example: The reason for the illness Communicability of the disease to themselves or others Consequences of the disease The process of dying and death itself Their fear of the unknown is greater than their fear of the known. The realization of impending death is a tremendous threat to their sense of security and ego strength. They are likely to exhibit fear through verbal uncooperativeness rather than physical aggression. They are interested in postdeath services. They may be inquisitive about what happens to the body.	Help parents deal with their feelings, allowing them greater emotional reserves to meet their children's needs. Encourage parents to remain near child as much as possible, yet be sensitive to parents' needs. Because of children's fear of the unknown, anticipatory preparation is important. Because the developmental task of this age is industry, interventions of helping children maintain control over their bodies and increasing their understanding allow them to achieve independence, self-worth, and self-esteem and avoid a sense of inferiority. Encourage children to talk about their feelings and provide aggressive outlets. Encourage parents to honestly answer questions about dying rather than avoiding the subject or fabricating euphemisms. Encourage parents to share their moments of sorrow with their children. Provide preparation for postdeath services.

Continued

Table 41-3 Children's Understanding of and Reactions to Death—cont'd

CONCEPTS OF DEATH	REACTIONS TO DEATH	NURSING CARE MANAGEMENT
Adolescents		
Adolescents have a mature understanding of death. They are still influenced by remnants of magical thinking and are subject to guilt and shame. They are likely to see deviations from accepted behavior as reasons for their illness.	Adolescents straddle transition from childhood to adulthood. They have the most difficulty in coping with death. They are least likely to accept cessation of life, particularly if it is their own. Concern is for the present much more than for the past or the future. They may consider themselves alienated from their peers and unable to communicate with their parents for emotional support, feeling alone in their struggle. Adolescents' orientation to the present compels them to worry about physical changes even more than the prognosis. Because of their idealistic view of the world, they may criticize funeral rites as barbaric, money making, and unnecessary.	Help parents deal with their feelings, allowing them greater emotional reserves to meet their children's needs. Avoid alliances with either parent or child. Structure hospital admission to allow for maximum self-control and independence. Answer adolescents' questions honestly, treating them as mature individuals and respecting their needs for privacy, solitude, and personal expressions of emotions. Help parents understand their child's reactions to death and dying, especially that concern for present crises, such as loss of hair, may be much greater than for future ones, including possible death.

understand that honesty and shared decision making between them and their child are important to the child and family's emotional health will encourage parents to allow discussion of dying with their child. Parents may require professional support and guidance in this process from a nurse, social worker, or child life specialist who has a good relationship with the child and family.

If given the opportunity, children will tell others how much they want to know. Asking questions such as "If the disease came back, would you want to know?" "Do you want others to tell you everything, even if the news isn't good?" or "If someone were not getting better [or more directly, "were dying"], do you think he would want to know?" helps children set the limits of how much truth they can accept and cope with. Children need time to process many feelings and much information so that they can assimilate and ideally accept the inevitable fact of mortality.

Care of the dying adolescent requires the nurse to become knowledgeable about any possible delays or alterations in normal growth and development. Legal and ethical issues also come to the forefront with respect to the age at which an adolescent should have autonomy in decision making about care and treatment. Effective communication between the patient, family, and health care team is an important part of optimal care for the dying adolescent (Freyer, 2004).

Treatment Options for Terminally Ill Children

Based on the child and family's decision regarding their wishes for terminal care, they have several options from which to choose.

Hospital Care

Families may choose to remain in the hospital to receive care if the child's illness or condition is unstable and home care is not an option or the family is uncomfortable with providing care at home. If a family chooses to remain at the hospital for terminal care, the setting should be made as homelike as possible. Families are encouraged to bring familiar items from the child's room at home. In addition, there should be a consistent and coordinated care plan for the child and family's comfort.

Home Care

Some families prefer to take their child home and receive services from a home care agency. Generally, these services entail periodic nursing visits to administer a treatment or provide medications, equipment, or supplies. The child's care continues to be directed by the primary physician. Home care is often the option chosen by physicians and families because of the traditional view that a child must be considered to have a life expectancy of less than 6 months to be referred to hospice care. Fortunately, a number of hospice organizations are expanding their services to children based on the presence of a life-limiting disease process for which cure is not possible, rather than on the sole criterion of a limited time projected prognosis.

Hospice Care

Parents should be offered the option of caring for their child at home during the final phases of an illness with the assistance of a hospice organization. *Hospice* is a community health care organization that specializes in the care of dying patients by combining the hospice philosophy with the principles of palliative care. *Hospice philosophy* regards dying as a natural process and care of dying patients as including management of the physical, psychologic, social, and spiritual needs of the patient and family. Care is provided by a multidisciplinary group of professionals in the patient's home or an inpatient facility that employs the hospice philosophy. Hospice care for children was introduced in the 1970s, and a number of community hospice organizations now accept children into their care (Davies, Davis, & Sibert, 2003; Forrester, 2003; Winkler & Mardegian, 2001; Faulkner & Armstrong-Dailey, 1997). Collaboration between the child's primary treatment team and the hospice care team is essential to the success of hospice care. Families may continue to see their primary care physicians as they choose.*

Hospice care is based on a number of important concepts that significantly set it apart from hospital care:

- Family members are usually the principal caregivers and are supported by a team of professional and volunteer staff.
- The priority of care is comfort. The child's physical, psychologic, social, and spiritual needs are considered. Pain and symptom control are primary concerns, and no extraordinary efforts are used to attempt a cure or prolong life.
- The family's needs are considered to be as important as those of the patient.
- Hospice is concerned with the family's postdeath adjustment, and care may continue for a year or more.

The goal of hospice care is for children to live life to the fullest without pain, with choices and dignity, in the familiar environment of their home, and with the support of their family. Hospice care is covered under state Medicaid programs and by most insurance plans. The service provides home visits from nurses, social workers, chaplains, and, in some cases, physicians. Medications, medical equipment, and any necessary medical supplies are all provided by the hospice organization providing care.

With children, the home has been the more common environment for implementing the hospice concept; it benefits the family in a variety of ways. Children who are dying are allowed to remain with those they love and with whom they feel secure. Many children who were thought to be in imminent danger of death have gone home and lived longer than expected. Siblings can feel more involved in the care and often have more positive perceptions of the death. Parental adaptation is often more favorable, demonstrated by their perceptions of how the experience at home affected their marriage, social reorientation, religious beliefs, and views on the meaning of life and death.

If the home is chosen for hospice care, the child may or may not die in the home. Reasons for final admission to a hospital vary but may be related to the parents' or siblings' wish to have the child die outside the home; exhaustion on the part of the caregivers; and physical problems such as sudden, acute pain or respiratory distress.

Nursing Care of the Child and Family at the End of Life

Regardless of where the child is cared for during the terminal stage of illness, both the child and the family usually experience fear of (1) pain and suffering, (2) dying alone (child) or not being present when the child dies (parent), and (3) actual death. Nurses can help reduce families' fears through attention to the care needs of the child and family.

Fear of Pain and Suffering

The presence of unrelieved pain in a terminally ill child can have detrimental effects on the quality of life experienced by the child and family. Parents believe that having their child in pain is unendurable and results in feelings of helplessness and a sense that they must be present and vigilant to get the necessary pain medications. Persistent pain also has an impact on the family as a whole. Nurses can alleviate the fear of pain and suffering by providing interventions aimed at treating the pain and symptoms associated with the terminal process in children.

Pain and Symptom Management

Pain control for children in the terminal stages of illness or injury must be given the highest priority. Despite ongoing efforts to educate physicians and nurses on pain management strategies in children, studies have reported that children continue to be undermedicated for their pain (Wolfe et al, 2000). Nearly all children experience some amount of pain in the terminal phase of their illness. The current standard for treating children's pain follows the World Health Organization's analgesic stepladder (1996), which promotes tailoring the pain interventions to the child's level of reported pain. Children's pain should be assessed frequently, and medications adjusted as necessary. Pain medications should be given on a regular schedule, and extra doses for breakthrough pain should be available to maintain comfort. Opioid drugs such as morphine should be given for severe pain, and the dose should be increased as necessary to maintain optimal pain relief. Techniques such as distraction, relaxation techniques, and guided imagery (Lambert, 1999) should be combined with drug therapy to provide the child and family strategies to control pain (see Chapter 35 for further discussion of pain management strategies).

In addition to pain, children experience a variety of symptoms during their terminal course as a result of their disease process or as a side effect of medicines used to manage pain or other symptoms. These symptoms include fatigue, nausea and vomiting, constipation, anorexia, dyspnea, congestion, seizures, anxiety, depression, restlessness, agitation, and confusion (Wolfe, Friebert, & Hilden, 2002; Hellsten et al, 2000). Each of these symptoms should be aggressively managed with appropriate medications or treatments and with interventions such as repositioning, relaxation, massage, and other measures to maintain the child's comfort and quality of life.

Occasionally, children require very high doses of opioids to control pain. This may occur for several reasons. The child on long-term opioid pain management can become *tolerant* of the drug, meaning that it is necessary to give more drugs to maintain the same level of pain relief. This should not be confused with *addiction*, which is a psychologic dependence on the side effects of opioids. Addiction is not a factor in managing terminal pain in children. Other obvious reasons for requiring increased doses of opioids include progression of disease and other physiologic experiences of pain. It is important to understand that there is no maximum dose that can be given to control pain. However, nurses often express

**For more information, contact National Hospice and Palliative Care Organization, 1731 King St., Suite 100, Alexandria, VA 22314; 703-837-1500; fax: 703-837-1233;* www.nhpco.org; *and Children's Hospice International, 1101 King St., Suite 360, Alexandria, VA 22314; 703-684-0330 or 800-24-CHILD;* www.chionline.org.

BOX 41-9 Ethical Principle of Double Effect

An action that has one good (intended) effect and one bad (unintended but foreseeable) effect is permissible if the following conditions are met:

- The action itself must be good or indifferent. Only the good consequences of the action must be sincerely intended.
- The good effect must not be produced by the bad effect.
- There must be a compelling or proportionate reason for permitting the foreseeable bad effect to occur.

concern that administering doses of opioids that exceed what they are familiar with will hasten the child's death. The *principle of double effect* (Box 41-9) addresses such concerns. It provides an ethical standard that supports the use of interventions intended to relieve pain and suffering even though there is a foreseeable possibility that death may be hastened (Rousseau, 2001). In cases in which the child is terminally ill and in severe pain, using large doses of opioids and sedatives to manage pain is justified when no other treatment options are available that would relieve the pain but make the risk of death less likely (Hawryluck & Harvey, 2000).

Parents' and Siblings' Need for Education and Support

Parents are the primary caregivers when the child is at home, and nurses providing care to the child and family need to teach the family about the medications being given to the child, how to administer medications, and the use of nonpharmacologic techniques to control pain. Parents are kept informed of all medications and treatments given to a child in the hospital, and they encouraged to participate in the child's care to the extent that they desire. This empowers parents and provides a sense of control over the child's comfort and well-being, reducing their fear that their child will be in pain or suffering as he or she is dying. Additionally, better bereavement outcomes (e.g., adaptive coping; family cohesion; less anxiety, stress, and depression) have been reported by parents who were actively involved in their child's care (Goodenough et al, 2004; Lauer et al, 1989). The grief work of fathers in particular seems to be facilitated when their child dies in the home setting. This finding may be related to the increased opportunity of working fathers to provide care to and spend time with their child at home vs. the hospital setting.

Siblings may feel isolated and displaced while their brother or sister is dying. Parents devote the majority of their time to the dying child's care and comfort, causing siblings to feel left out of the parent–sick child relationship. Siblings may become resentful of their sick sibling and begin to feel guilty or ashamed about such feelings (Murray, 1999). Nurses can assist the family by helping the parents identify ways to involve siblings in the caring process, perhaps by bringing some supplies or favorite toy, game, or food item. Parents should also be encouraged to schedule time to spend with the other children where their focus is on them. Helping parents identify a trusted friend or family member who can sit with the ill child for a short period will allow them to attend to their own needs or those of their other children.

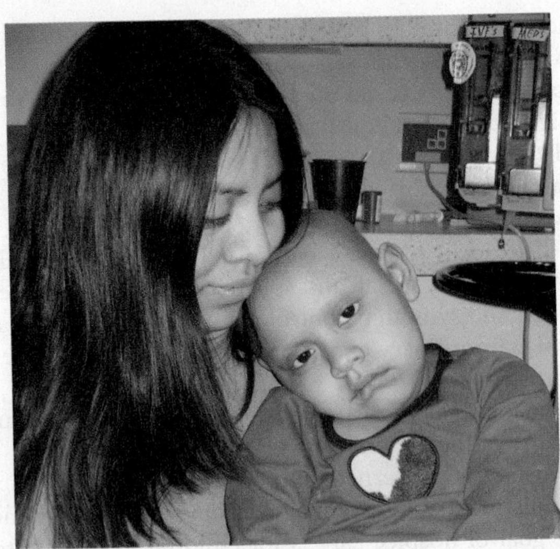

Fig. 41-6 For the dying child there is no greater comfort than the security and closeness of a parent.

Fear of Dying Alone or of Not Being Present When the Child Dies

When a child is being cared for at home, the burden of care on parents and family members can be great. Often, as the child's condition declines, family members begin the "death vigil." Rarely is a child left alone for any length of time. This can be exhausting for family members, and nurses can assist the family by helping them arrange shifts so that friends or family members can be present with the child and allow others to rest. If the family has limited resources, community organizations such as hospice or churches often have volunteers who are willing to visit and sit with children. It is important that whoever is sitting with the child be aware of when the parent(s) would like to be notified to return to the child's bedside (Fig. 41-6).

When a child is dying in the hospital, parents should be given full access to the child at all times. If parents need to leave, they should be provided with a pager or other means of immediate communication and alerted if staff members note any change in the child that may indicate imminent death. Nurses advocate for parents' presence in intensive care and emergency departments and attend to the parents' needs for food, drinks, comfortable chairs, blankets, and pillows.

Fear of Actual Death

Home Deaths

The majority of children receiving hospice care die at home, often in their own room with family, pets, and other loved possessions around them. The physical process of dying can be distressing to parents because often the child slowly become less alert in the days before the actual death. The nurse can assist the family by providing them with information about what changes will occur as the child progresses through the dying process (Box 41-10). During this time, nursing visits often become more frequent and longer in duration to provide the family with additional support as the death nears. The most distressing change for parents to observe is the change

BOX 41-10 Physical Signs of Approaching Death

Loss of sensation and movement in the lower extremities, progressing toward the upper body
Sensation of heat, although body feels cool
Loss of senses:
- Tactile sensation decreasing
- Sensitivity to light
- Hearing the last sense to fail

Confusion, loss of consciousness, slurred speech
Muscle weakness
Loss of bowel and bladder control
Decreased appetite and thirst
Difficulty swallowing
Change in respiratory pattern:
- Cheyne-Stokes respirations (waxing and waning of depth of breathing with regular periods of apnea)
- "Death rattle" (noisy chest sounds from accumulation of pulmonary and pharyngeal secretions)

Weak, slow pulse; decreased blood pressure

in the respiratory pattern. In the final hours of life, the dying patient's respirations may become labored, with deep breaths and long periods of apnea, referred to as Cheyne-Stokes respirations. Families are reassured that this is not distressing to the child and that it is a normal part of the dying process. However, the use of opioids can slow the respirations to make the child breathe more easily, and scopolamine, usually applied as a topical patch, can help reduce noisy respirations, known as the "death rattle." Noisy respirations are more likely to occur if the child is overhydrated.

All families have the option of admitting their child to the hospital if they feel unable to deal with the death. The child who dies at home must be pronounced dead; hospice programs typically have provisions so that this proceeds smoothly. In some circumstances the police may be notified, with an explanation of the circumstances to prevent unnecessary concern regarding abuse. Providing the police with the number of the responsible practitioner is usually all that is necessary to confirm the cause of death.

Hospital Deaths

Children dying in the hospital of terminal illnesses who are receiving supportive care interventions will experience a similar process. Again, increased nursing presence and attendance to the child and family's needs provide comfort and support for many families.

Death resulting from accident, trauma, or acute illness in settings such as the emergency department or intensive care unit often requires the active withdrawal of some form of life-supporting intervention, such as a ventilator or bypass machine. These situations often raise difficult ethical issues (Sine et al, 2001), and parents are often less prepared for the actual moment of death. Nurses can assist these parents by providing detailed information about what will happen as supportive equipment is withdrawn, ensuring that appropriate pain medications are administered to prevent pain during the dying process, and allowing the parents time before the start of the withdrawal to be with and speak to their child. It is important that the nurse attempt to control the environment around the family at this time by providing privacy, asking if they would like to play music, softening lights and monitor noises, and arranging for any religious or cultural rituals that the family may want performed.

After the child's death, the family should be allowed to remain with the body and hold or rock the child if they desire. After the nurse has removed all tubes and equipment from the body, parents should be given the option of assisting with the preparation of the body, such as bathing and dressing. It is important for the nurse to determine whether the family has any specific needs, since many cultures have adopted specific methods for coping with and mourning death and impeding these practices may interfere with the grieving process (Clements et al, 2003).

At some point the nurse discusses whether the family has made preparations for the burial service and whether the staff can help in any way. Parents often have concerns about the funeral, such as siblings' involvement in the death rituals. Although no absolute answers exist regarding the question of siblings attending the funeral or burial services, the consensus is that the surviving children benefit from being involved in these events. However, children need preparation for post-death services. They should be told what to expect, particularly how the deceased person will look if the coffin is open; allowed their private time to say good-bye; and permitted to stay as long as they wish. Ideally, the parents should prepare the siblings. If the parents' grief prevents this communication, a significant family member or friend should substitute (see Family-Centered Care box).

FAMILY-CENTERED CARE

Children Need to Say Good-bye

As a nurse and grief counselor, I conduct grief workshops with children who have experienced the death of someone special. Children often communicate their feelings of being excluded through drawings. They may draw a picture of the dying person in a hospital bed that is raised too high for them to see the person's face clearly. Sometimes children reveal that they did not get to say good-bye because a family member told them, for example, "You don't want to see your grandma this way. She is too sick for you to visit." If the special person died at home, the children had to stay in their room when the funeral home staff took away the body.

I have learned to never underestimate the importance of allowing children to be involved with the dying person and the significance of a child's loss. Once, when I asked a 6-year-old girl to draw a picture with the theme "This is what I was doing when my __________ died," she drew a picture and completed the sentence with "when my home died." Her grandmother had been like her mother; to the child, her home was gone. We need to give children the choice of being included in the family's activities of saying good-bye.

–Barbara Bilderback, MS, MA, RN, Bereavement Supervisor, Saint Francis Hospice Tulsa, OK

Organ or Tissue Donation and Autopsy

For some families organ or tissue donation may be a meaningful act—one that benefits another human being despite the loss of their child. Unfortunately, initiating a discussion about tissue donation is often stressful for staff, and there may be confusion regarding whose responsibility this is. In centers in which transplants are performed, a full-time transplant coordinator is usually available to inform the family about organ donation and to take care of details. If such services are not available, the staff needs to determine which members should discuss this topic with the family. Ideally, the person who knows the family best, knows when the death is expected, or has the opportunity to spend time with the family when the death is unexpected takes the role. Often nurses are in an optimal position to suggest tissue donation after consultation with the attending physician. When possible, the topic should be raised before death occurs. The request should be made in a private and quiet area of the hospital and should be simple and direct, with questions such as "Are you a donor family?" or "Have you ever considered organ donation?"

Many states have legislated a mandatory request for organ or tissue donation when a child dies, especially if the patient is brain dead. Written consent from the family is required before donation can proceed. When requests for organ donation are made, health care practitioners must address common misunderstandings families have about brain death and organ donation (Franz et al, 1997). Training health care professionals on sensitive approaches to requests for organ donation has been shown to increase families' willingness to consent to organ donation (American Academy of Pediatrics, Committee on Hospital Care and Section on Surgery, 2002; Evanisko et al, 1998). The option to donate organs should always be separate from the communication of impending or actual death.

Nurses need to be aware of common questions about organ donation to help families make an informed decision. Healthy children who die unexpectedly are excellent candidates for organ donation. Children with cancer, chronic disease, or infection or those who have suffered prolonged cardiac arrest may not be suitable candidates, although this is individually determined. The nurse should ask whether organ donation was discussed with the child or whether the child ever expressed such a wish. Any number of body tissues or organs can be donated (skin, corneas, bone, kidney, heart, liver, pancreas), and their removal does not mutilate or desecrate the body or cause any suffering. The family may have an open casket, and there is no delay in the funeral. There is no cost to the donor family, but organ donation does not eliminate funeral or cremation responsibilities. Most religions permit organ donation as long as the recipient benefits from the transplant, although Orthodox Judaism forbids it (see Table 32-1).

In cases of unexplained death, violent death, or suspected suicide, autopsy is required by law. In other instances it may be optional, and parents should be informed of this choice. The procedure, as well as forms that require signing, should be explained. The family should know that the child can be in an open casket after an autopsy.

Grief and Mourning

Grief is a process, not an event, of experiencing physiologic, psychologic, behavioral, social, and spiritual reactions to the loss of a child. Grief is highly individualized, encompassing a broad range of manifestations from person to person. It is a natural and expected reaction to loss. It is neither orderly nor predictable. Grieving in any form is necessary for healing to occur. When death is the expected or a possible outcome of a disorder, the child and family members may experience *anticipatory grief*. Anticipatory grief may be manifested in varying behaviors and intensities and may include denial, anger, depression, and other psychologic and physical symptoms.

Anticipatory guidance may assist grieving family members. Health care professionals should emphasize that grief reactions such as hearing the dead person's voice, feeling distant from others, or seeking reassurance that they did everything possible for the lost person are normal, necessary, and expected. They in no way signify poor coping, insanity, or an approaching mental breakdown. On the contrary, such behaviors signify that the survivor is working through the acute grief. Anticipatory guidance regarding the mourning process may help families recognize the normalcy of their experiences.

It is important to recognize that some family members may experience complicated grief. *Complicated grief reactions* (more than a year after the loss) include such symptoms as intense intrusive thoughts, pangs of severe emotion, distressing yearnings, feelings of excessive loneliness and emptiness, unusual sleep disturbance, and maladaptive levels of loss of interest in personal activities (Horowitz et al, 1997). Bereaved persons experiencing such prolonged and complicated grief should be referred to an expert in grief and bereavement counseling.

Another important aspect of grief is the individual nature of the grief experience. Each member of the family will experience the grief of the child's death in his or her own way based on the particular relationship with that child. This can create potential conflict for families, since each family member has expectations that the other family members should feel and grieve as they do. Nurses caring for families experiencing grief should be aware of the different grieving styles and help the family learn to recognize and support the uniqueness of each other's grief.

Parental Grief

Parental grief after the death of a child can be the most intense, complex, long-lasting, and fluctuating grief experience when compared with that of other bereaved individuals. Although parents experience the primary loss of their child, many secondary losses are felt such as the loss of part of one's self, hopes and dreams for the child's future, the family unit, prior social and emotional community supports, and often spousal support. It is common for parents of the same child to experience different grief reactions.

Studies with bereaved parents have shown that grieving does not end with the severing of the bond with the deceased child, but rather involves a continuing bond between the parent and the deceased child (Klass, 2001). Parental resolution of grief is a process of integrating the dead child into daily life where the pain of losing a child is never completely gone, but lessens. There are occasions of brief relapse, but not to the degree experienced when the loss initially occurred. Thus parental grief work is never completed and is a timeless process of accommodating the new reality of being without a child, as it changes over time (Davies, 2004). A child's death can also challenge the marital relationship in several ways. Maternal and paternal reactions often differ (Birenbaum, Stewart, & Phillips, 1996; Moriarty, Carroll, & Cotroneo, 1996; Vance et al, 1995). Different grieving styles between the couple may hinder communication and support for each other. Differing needs and expectations can place a strain on the marriage.

Sibling Grief

Each child grieves in his or her own way and on his or her own timeline. Children, even adolescents, grieve differently than adults. Adults and children differ more widely in their reactions to death than in their reactions to any other phenomenon. Children of all ages grieve the loss of a loved one, and their understanding and reactions to death depend on their age and developmental level. Children grieve for a longer duration, revisiting their grief as they grow and develop new understandings of death. However, they do not grieve 100% of the time. They grieve in spurts and can be emotional and sad in one instance and then, just as quickly, off and playing. Children express their grief though play and behavior. Children can be exquisitely attuned to their parents' grief and will try to protect them by not asking questions or by trying not to upset them. This can set the stage for the sibling to try to become the "perfect child." Children exhibit many of the grief reactions of adults, including physical sensations and illnesses, anger, guilt, sadness, loneliness, withdrawal, acting out, sleep disturbances, isolation, and search for meaning. Again, nurses should be attentive for signs that siblings are struggling with their grief and provide guidance to parents when possible.

At times family members may need assistance in their grieving (see Guidelines box). Communication with the bereaved family is essential, but often nurse do not know what to say and feel helpless in offering words of comfort. The most supportive approach is to avoid judging the family's reactions or offering advice or rationalizations and to focus on feelings. Perhaps the most valuable supportive measure the nurse can perform for families is to listen. Families understand that no words will relieve their pain; all they want is acceptance, understanding, and respect for their grief.

It is important for families to understand that mourning takes a long time. Whereas acute grief may last only weeks or months, resolving the loss is measured in years. Holidays and anniversaries can be particularly difficult, and people who previously had been supportive may now expect the family to have "adjusted." Consequently, prolonged mourning is often silent and lonely.

Many families never receive the support and guidance that could help them resolve the loss. A plan for regular follow-up with bereaved families can be beneficial. At minimum, one follow-up phone call or meeting with the family should be arranged. Families can also be referred to self-help groups. When such groups are not available, nurses can be instrumental in bringing families together or facilitating parent and sibling groups. Formal bereavement programs or bereavement counseling can be helpful as well.

For more information on end-of-life care, visit these websites:

GUIDELINES Supporting Grieving Families*

General

- Stay with the family; sit quietly if they prefer not to talk; cry with them if desired.
- Accept the family's grief reactions; avoid judgmental statements (e.g., "You should be feeling better by now").
- Avoid offering rationalizations for the child's death (e.g., "Your child isn't suffering anymore").
- Avoid artificial consolation (e.g., "I know how you feel," or "You are still young enough to have another baby").
- Deal openly with feelings such as guilt, anger, and loss of self-esteem.
- Focus on feelings by using a feeling word in the statement (e.g., "You're still feeling all the pain of losing a child").
- Refer the family to an appropriate self-help group or for professional help if needed.

At the Time of Death

- Reassure the family that everything possible is being done for the child, if they want lifesaving interventions.
- Do everything possible to ensure the child's comfort, especially relieving pain.
- Provide the child and family with the opportunity to review special experiences or memories in their lives.
- Express personal feelings of loss or frustrations (e.g., "We will miss him so much," "We tried everything; we feel so sorry that we couldn't save her").
- Provide information that the family requests and be honest.
- Respect the emotional needs of family members, such as siblings, who may need brief respites from the dying child.
- Make every effort to arrange for family members, especially parents, to be with the child at the moment of death, if they want to be present.
- Allow the family to stay with the dead child for as long as they wish and to rock, hold, or bathe the child.
- Provide practical help when possible, such as collecting the child's belongings.
- Arrange for spiritual support, based on the family's religious beliefs; pray with the family if no one else can stay with them.

After Death

- Attend the funeral or visitation if there was a special closeness with the family.
- Initiate and maintain contact (e.g., sending cards, telephoning, inviting them back to the unit, making a home visit).
- Refer to the dead child by name; discuss shared memories with the family.
- Discourage the use of drugs or alcohol as a method of escaping grief.
- Encourage all family members to communicate their feelings rather than remaining silent to avoid upsetting another member.
- Emphasize that grieving is a painful process that often takes years to resolve.

*"Family" refers to all significant persons involved in the child's life, such as the parents, siblings, grandparents, or other close relatives or friends.

Americans for Better Care of the Dying—*www.abcd-caring.org*
End of Life/Palliative Education Resource Center—*www.eperc.mcw.edu*
Growth House—*www.growthhouse.org*
Robert Wood Johnson Foundation—*www.rwjf.org*

Nurses' Reactions to Caring for Dying Children

The death of a patient is one of the most stressful aspects of critical care or oncology nursing (see Family-Centered Care box).* Nurses experience reactions to a fatal illness that are very similar to the responses of family members, including denial, anger, depression, guilt, and ambivalent feelings.

Strategies that can assist the nurse in remaining able to work effectively in these settings include maintaining good general health, developing well-rounded interests, using distancing techniques such as taking time off when needed, developing and using professional and personal support systems, cultivating the capacity for empathy, focusing on the positive aspects of the caregiver role, and basing nursing interventions on sound theory and empiric observations. Attending shared-remembrance rituals assists some nurses in resolving grief (Davis & Eng, 1998). Similarly, attending the funeral services can be a supportive act for both the family and the nurse and in no way detracts from the professionalism of care.

FAMILY-CENTERED CARE

A Dying Child: A Nurse's Perspective

Claire was unresponsive with slow, gasping breathing. Her mother asked me what I thought was happening. I replied honestly, "Your baby is dying because of her brain tumor." The mother put her arms around me and cried. We arranged for Claire to be baptized.

Honesty. As painful as the loss of a child is, my job is to assist the family through this experience. Although I usually wait until a private moment, such as driving home, I found tears streaming down my face as family and friends gathered for Claire's baptism. I went into the kitchen to compose myself, only to find several of my colleagues crying as well. Saying good-bye to a dying child will always be a difficult but shared experience.

–Jeanne O'Connor Egan, RN, MSN, Pediatric Clinical Specialist, Children's Hospital Washington, DC

Key Points

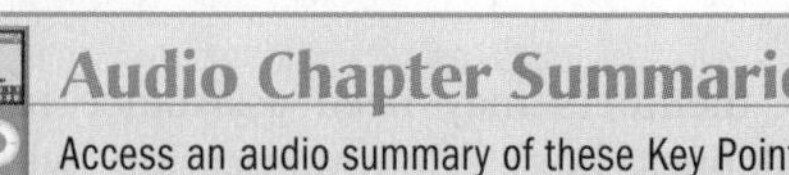
Audio Chapter Summaries
Access an audio summary of these Key Points on evolve

- Trends in the treatment of children with chronic illness or disability have focused on developmental age, the child's strengths and uniqueness, family-centered care, normalization, early discharge, home care, mainstreaming, and early intervention.
- In response to the child with chronic illness or disability, parents may be affected by feelings of inadequacy and failure; excessive demands on time, energy, and financial resources; and strain on the marital relationship.
- Families' reactions to disability or chronic illness are manifested in the following stages: shock and denial, adjustment, reintegration, and acknowledgment.
- The child's reaction to illness or disability depends on the child's developmental level, coping mechanisms, others' reactions, and the illness itself.
- Assessment of the family's adjustment to a child's chronic illness, disability, or death includes the availability of a support system, their perception of the event, their coping mechanisms, concurrent stressors, and their response to the child.
- To help parents cope with their child's chronic illness or disability, nurses must offer attentiveness, humanistic support, solicitation of suggestions for care, facilitation of communication, an opportunity to verbalize feelings, and referral to volunteer and community agencies.
- Supporting the child involves encouraging self-expression, alleviating feelings of being different, and strengthening the child's self-image.
- Children's concept of death is determined by their cognitive ability and their experience with life-threatening illness.
- Young children see death as temporary and reversible and mainly fear separation.
- School-age children view death as irreversible but not necessarily inevitable and may fear mutilation.
- Children beyond 9 to 10 years of age realize that death is irreversible, universal, and inevitable but may resist the thought of their own death.
- Siblings have special needs, including the need for information, reassurance about their own health status, assurance that they are not responsible for the illness or death, and support for their own grieving process.

**Other sources of publications on life-threatening illness and death are the Compassionate Friends, PO Box 3696, Oak Brook, IL 60522-3696; 630-990-0010 or 877-969-0010;* www.compassionatefriends.org; *Centering Corporation, 7230 Maple St., Omaha, NE 68134; 866-218-0101;* www.centering.org; *Children's Hospice International (see footnote, p. 1169); and National Cancer Institute Public Inquiries Office, 6116 Executive Blvd., Room 3036A, Bethesda, MD 20892-8322; 800-422-6237;* www.cancer.gov.

- Special needs of the family facing the unexpected death of a child include support while awaiting news of the child's status; a sensitive pronouncement of death; acknowledgment of feelings of denial, guilt, and anger; an opportunity to view the body; and referrals for support.
- Special decisions at the time of dying and death may involve hospital or hospice care, visualization of the body, tissue donation and autopsy, and siblings' attendance at the funeral.
- Acute grief is a syndrome with intense and distressing psychologic and somatic symptoms that appear at the time of death.
- In dealing with stress related to the dying patient, the nurse can cope successfully through self-awareness, consciousness raising, knowledge and practice, an available support system, and maintenance of general good health, and by focusing on the positive rewards of involvement with dying children and their families.

References

Ahmann E: "Chunky stew": appreciating cultural diversity while providing health care for children, *Pediatr Nurs* 20(3):320-324, 1994.

American Academy of Pediatrics, Committee on Hospital Care and Section on Surgery: Pediatric organ donation and transplantation, *Pediatrics* 109(5):982-984, 2002.

American Nurses Association: *Code of ethics for nurses with interpretive statements*, Washington, DC, 2001, ANA Publishing.

Anderson RN, Smith BL: Deaths: leading causes, *Natl Vital Stat Rep* 53(17):1-89, 2005.

Arias E et al: Annual summary of vital statistics—2002, *Pediatrics* 112(6): 1215-1230, 2003.

Barlow JH, Ellard DR: The psychosocial well-being of children with chronic disease, their parents and siblings: an overview of the research evidence base, *Child Care Health Dev* 32(1):19-31, 2006.

Birenbaum LK, Stewart BJ, Phillips DS: Health status of bereaved parents, *Nurs Res* 45(2):105-109, 1996.

Carnevale FA et al: Daily living with distress and enrichment: the moral experience of families with ventilator-assisted children at home, *Pediatrics* 117(1):e48-e60, 2006.

Carter B: Chronic pain in childhood and the medical encounter: professional ventriloquism and hidden voices, *Qual Health Res* 12:28-41, 2002.

Centers for Disease Control and Prevention: *HIV/AIDS surveillance report, 2007*, Vol 19, Atlanta, 2009, U.S. Department of Health and Human Services and The Centers.

Charles C, Gafni A, Whelan T: Shared decision making in the medical encounter: what does it mean? *Soc Sci Med* 44:681-692, 1997.

Clements PT et al: Cultural perspectives of death, grief, and bereavement, *J Psychosoc Nurs Ment Health Serv* 41(7):18-26, 2003.

Coffey JS: Parenting a child with chronic illness: a metasynthesis, *Pediatr Nurs* 32(1):51-59, 2006.

Cohen MH: The stages of the prediagnostic period in chronic life-threatening childhood illness: a process analysis, *Res Nurs Health* 18(1):39-48, 1995.

Corlett J, Twycross A: Negotiation of parental roles within family-centered care: a review of the research, *J Clin Nurs* 15(10):1308-1316, 2006.

Davies B et al: "Living in the dragon's shadow": fathers' experiences of a child's life-limiting illness, *Death Studies* 28(2):111-135, 2004.

Davies R: New understandings of parental grief: literature review, *J Adv Nurs* 46(5):506-513, 2004.

Davies R, Davis B, Sibert J: Parents' stories of sensitive and insensitive care by paediatricians in the time leading up to and including diagnostic disclosure of a life-limiting condition in their child, *Child Care Health Dev* 29(1):77-82, 2003.

Davis B, Eng B: Special issues in bereavement and staff support. In Doyle D, Hanks GWC, MacDonald N (editors): *Oxford textbook of palliative medicine*, ed 2, New York, 1998, Oxford University Press.

Deatrick JA, Knafl KA, Murphy-Moore C: Clarifying the concept of normalization, *Image J Nurs Sch* 31:209-214, 1999.

Denboba D et al: Achieving family and provider partnerships for children with special health care needs, *Pediatrics* 118(4):1607-1615, 2006.

Dixon-Woods M, Young B, Henry D: Partnerships with children, *Br J Med* 319:778-780, 1999.

Evanisko MJ et al: Readiness of critical care physicians and nurses to handle requests for organ donation, *Am J Crit Care* 7(1):4-12, 1998.

Faulkner KW, Armstrong-Dailey A: Care of the dying child. In Pizzo PA, Poplack DG (editors): *Principles and practice of pediatric oncology*, Philadelphia, 1997, Lippincott-Raven.

Field MJ, Behrman RE (editors): *When children die: improving palliative and end-of-life care for children and their families*, Washington, DC, 2004, National Academies Press.

Fleitas J: When Jack fell down ... Jill came tumbling after: siblings in the web of illness and disability, *MCN* 25:267-273, 2000.

Forrester L: One to one care in children's hospice, *Nurs Times* 99(16): 44-45, 2003.

Franz HG et al: Explaining brain death: a critical feature of the donation process, *J Transplant Coord* 7(1):14-21, 1997.

Freyer DR: Care of the dying adolescent: special considerations, *Pediatrics* 113(2):381-388, 2004.

Garwick AW et al: Breaking the news: how families first learn about their child's chronic condition, *Arch Pediatr Adolesc Med* 149(9):991-997, 1995.

Goldbeck L: Parental coping with the diagnosis of childhood cancer: gender effects, dissimilarity within couples, and quality of life, *Psychooncology* 10:325-335, 2001.

Goodenough B et al: Bereavement outcomes for parents who lose a child to cancer: are place of death and sex of parent associated with differences in psychological functioning? *Psychooncology* 13(11):779-791, 2004.

Gravelle AM: Caring for a child with a progressive illness during the complex chronic phase: parents' experience of facing adversity, *J Adv Nurs* 25:738-745, 1997.

Hawryluck LA, Harvey WR: Analgesia, virtue, and the principle of double effect, *J Palliative Care* 16(Suppl):S24-S30, 2000.

Hellsten MB et al: *End-of-life care for children*, Austin, TX, 2000, Texas Cancer Council.

Hinds PS et al: End-of-life decision making by adolescents, parents, and healthcare providers in pediatric oncology: research to evidence-based practice guidelines, *Cancer Nurs* 24:122-134, 2001.

Horowitz MJ et al: Diagnostic criteria for complicated grief disorder, *Am J Psychiatry* 154(7):904-910, 1997.

Immelt S: Psychological adjustment in young children with chronic medical conditions, *J Pediatr Nurs* 21(5):362-377, 2006.

Jackson PL: The primary care provider and children with chronic conditions. In Jackson PL, Vessey PA (editors): *Primary care of the child with a chronic condition*, ed 3, St Louis, 2000, Mosby.

James L, Johnson B: The needs of parents of pediatric oncology patients during the palliative care phase, *J Pediatr Oncol Nurs* 14(2):83-95, 1997.

Jennings PD: Providing pediatric palliative care through a pediatric supportive care team, *Pediatr Nurs* 31(3): 195-200, 2005.

Jokinen P: The family life-path theory: a tool for nurses working in partnership with families, *J Child Health Care* 8(2):124-133, 2004.

Klass D: The inner representation of the dead child in the psychic and social narratives of bereaved parents. In RA Neimeyer (editor): *Meaning reconstruction and the experience of loss*, Washington, DC, 2001, American Psychological Association.

Lambert S: Distraction, imagery, and hypnosis techniques for management of children's pain, *J Child Fam Nurs* 2(1):5-15, 1999.

Lauer ME et al: Long-term follow-up of parental adjustment following a child's death at home or hospital, *Cancer* 63(5):988-994, 1989.

Lobato DJ, Kao BT: Integrated sibling-parent group intervention to improve sibling knowledge and adjustment to chronic illness and disability, *J Pediatr Psychol* 27:711-716, 2002.

Lobato DJ, Kao BT, Plante W: Latino sibling knowledge and adjustment to chronic illness, *J Fam Psychol* 19(4): 625-632, 2005.

Marshall ES et al: "This is a spiritual experience": perspectives of Latter-Day Saint families living with a child with disabilities, *Qual Health Res* 13:57-76, 2003.

Masri C et al: Decision making and end-of-life care in critically ill children, *J Palliative Care* 16(Suppl):S45-S52, 2000.

Mastroyannopoulou K et al: The impact of childhood non-malignant life threatening illness on parents: gender differences and predictors of parental adjustment, *J Child Psychol Psychiatry* 38(7):823-829, 1997.

McDougal J: Promoting normalization in families with preschool children with type 1 diabetes, *J Specialty Pediatr Nurs* 7(3):113-120, 2002.

McPherson M et al: Implementing community-based systems of services for child and youths with special health care needs: how well are we doing? *Pediatrics* 113(5):1538-1544, 2004.

Moriarty H, Carroll R, Cotroneo M: Differences in bereavement reactions within couples following the death of a child, *Res Nurs Health* 19:461-469, 1996.

Morse JM, Wilson S, Penrod J: Mothers and their disabled children: refining the concept of normalization, *Health Care Woman Int* 21(8):659-676, 2000.

Msall ME et al: Functional disability and school activity limitations in 41,300 school-age children: relationship to medical impairments, *Pediatrics* 111:548-553, 2003.

Murray JS: Siblings of children with cancer: a review of the literature, *J Pediatr Oncol Nurs* 16(1):25-34, 1999.

Nelson AM: A metasynthesis: mothering other-than-normal children, *Qual Health Res* 12:515-530, 2002.

Newacheck PW, Halfon N: Prevalence and impact of disabling chronic conditions in childhood, *Am J Public Health* 88(4):610-617, 1998.

Newacheck PW et al: An epidemiologic profile of children with special health care needs, *Pediatrics* 102(1):117-123, 1998.

Nuutila L, Salanterä S: Children with a long-term illness: parents' experiences of care, *J Pediatr Nurs* 21(2):153-160, 2006.

O'Brien ME, Wegner CB: Rearing the child who is technology dependent: perceptions of parents and home care nurses, *J Spec Pediatr Nurs* 7:7-15, 2002.

Ochieng BM: Minority ethnic families and family-centered care, *J Child Health Care* 7(2):123-132, 2003.

Palfrey JS et al: Introduction: addressing the millennial morbidity—the context of community pediatrics, *Pediatrics* 115(4 Suppl):1121-1123, 2005.

Perrin JM: Chronic illness in childhood. In Behrman RE, Kleigman RM, Jensen HB (editors): *Nelson textbook of pediatrics*, ed 17, Philadelphia, 2004, Saunders.

Pierucci RL, Kirby RS, Leuthner SR: End-of-life for neonates and infants: the experience and effects of a palliative care consultation service, *Pediatrics* 108(3):653-660, 2001.

Raina P et al: The health and well-being of caregivers of children with cerebral palsy, *Pediatrics* 115(6):e626-e636, 2005.

Ray LD: Parenting and childhood chronicity: making visible the invisible work, *J Pediatr Nurs* 17(6):424-438, 2002.

Rehm RS: Religious faith in Mexican-American families dealing with chronic childhood illness, *Image J Nurs Sch* 31:33-38, 1999.

Ritchie MA: Self-esteem and hopefulness in adolescents with cancer, *J Pediatr Nurs* 16:35-42, 2001.

Rossiter L, Sharpe D: The siblings of individuals with mental retardation: a quantitative integration of the literature, *J Child Fam Studies* 10(1):65-84, 2001.

Rousseau P: Ethical and legal issues in palliative care, *Prim Care* 28:391-400, 2001.

Sahler O et al: Medical education about end-of-life care in the pediatric setting: principles, challenges, and opportunities, *Pediatrics* 105:575-584, 2000.

Schor EL: Family pediatrics: report of the Task Force on the Family, *Pediatrics* 111:1541-1571, 2003.

Sharpe D, Rossiter L: Siblings of children with a chronic illness: a meta-analysis, *J Pediatr Psychol* 27:699-710, 2002.

Shepard MP, Mahon MM: Chronic conditions and the family. In Jackson PL, Vessey JA (editors): *Primary care of the child with a chronic condition*, ed 3, St Louis, 2000, Mosby.

Sine D et al: Pediatric extubation: "pulling the tube," *J Palliative Med* 4:519-524, 2001.

Stein REK: Home care: a challenging opportunity, *Child Health Care* 14(2):90-95, 1985.

Sterling YM, Peterson JW: Characteristics of African American women caregivers of children with asthma, *MCN* 28:32-38, 2003.

Sullivan-Bolyai S et al: Great expectations: a position description for parents as caregivers, part I, *Pediatr Nurs* 29(6):52-56, 2003.

Sumner LH: Lighting the way: improving the way children die in America, *Caring* 22:14-18, 2003.

Swallow VM, Jacoby A: Mothers' evolving relationships with doctors and nurses during the chronic childhood illness trajectory, *J Adv Nurs* 36:755-764, 2001.

Thomlinson EH: The lived experience of families of children who are failing to thrive, *J Adv Nurs* 39:537-545, 2002.

Tong H et al: Physical functioning in female caregivers of children with physical disabilities compared with female caregivers of children with a chronic medical condition, *Arch Pediatr Adolesc Med* 156:1138-1142, 2002.

Vance JC et al: Psychological changes in parents eight months after the loss of an infant from stillbirth, neonatal death, or sudden infant death syndrome—a longitudinal study, *Pediatrics* 96(5):933-938, 1995.

van Dyck P et al: The national survey of children's health: a new data resource, *Matern Child Health J* 8(3):183-188, 2004a.

van Dyck PC et al: Prevalence and characteristics of children with special health care needs, *Arch Pediatr Adolesc Med* 158(9):884-890, 2004b.

Whitehead LC, Gosling V: Parent's perceptions of interactions with health professionals in the pathway to gaining a diagnosis of tuberous sclerosis (TS) and beyond, *Res Dev Disabil* 24:109-119, 2003.

Winkler WD, Mardegian CA: Completing the continuum of care: the growth of a pediatric hospice program, *Caring* 20:22-25, 2001.

Wise PH et al: Chronic illness among poor children enrolled in the temporary assistance for needy families program, *Am J Public Health* 92:1458-1461, 2002.

Wolfe J, Friebert S, Hilden J: Caring for children with advanced cancer integrating palliative care, *Pediatr Clin North Am* 49(5):1043-1062, 2002.

Wolfe J et al: Symptoms and suffering at the end of life in children with cancer, *N Engl J Med* 342(5):326-333, 2000.

Wood PR et al: Relationships between welfare status, health insurance status, and health and medical care among children with asthma, *Am J Public Health* 92:1446-1452, 2002.

World Health Organization: *Cancer pain relief and palliative care*, Geneva, 1996, The Organization.

Young B et al: Managing communication with young people who have a potentially life threatening chronic illness: qualitative study of patients and parents, *BMJ* 326:1-5, 2003.

Zuvekas SH, Taliaferro GS: Pathways to access: health, insurance, the health care delivery system and racial/ethnic disparities, 1996-1999, *Health Affairs* 22(2):139-153, 2003.

Unit 10

42 Cognitive and Sensory Impairment

Learning Objectives

On completion of this chapter the reader will be able to:

- Define the classifications of cognitive impairment.
- Outline nursing interventions for the child with cognitive impairment that promote optimum development, including during hospitalization.
- Identify the major biologic and cognitive characteristics of the child with Down syndrome.
- Outline nursing interventions for the child with Down syndrome.
- Identify the major characteristics associated with fragile X syndrome.
- List the general classifications of hearing impairment and the effect on speech.
- Outline nursing interventions for the child with hearing impairment, including during hospitalization.
- List the common types of visual disorders in children.
- Outline nursing interventions for the child with visual impairment, including during hospitalization.
- Outline nursing interventions for the child with retinoblastoma.
- Outline nursing interventions for the child with autism spectrum disorder.

Electronic Resources

Additional information related to the content in Chapter 42 can be found on

evolve the Companion Website at

http://evolve.elsevier.com/Perry/maternal/

- NCLEX Review Questions
- Case Study—Down Syndrome
- Critical Thinking Exercise—Down Syndrome
- Critical Thinking Exercise—Fragile X Syndrome
- Nursing Care Plan—The Child with Hearing Impairment
- Nursing Care Plan—The Child with Cognitive Impairment

Cognitive Impairment

General Concepts

Cognitive impairment (CI) is a general term that encompasses any type of mental difficulty or deficiency. Although the family's needs and concerns are a primary focus throughout the chapter, the reader is encouraged to review Chapter 41, which details the family's adjustment to disabilities in general.

The definition of intellectual disability in children consists of three components: intellectual functioning, functional strengths and weaknesses, and age younger than 18 years at time of diagnosis. A disability in intellectual functioning is measured by the intelligence quotient (IQ) of 70 to 75 or below. The child with an intellectual disability must demonstrate functional impairment in at least two of 10 different adaptive skill areas: communication, self-care, home living, social skills, leisure, health and safety, self-direction, functional academics, community use, and work (American Psychiatric Association, 2000). The classification system by the American Association on Intellectual and Developmental Disabilities allows for identification of the individual's specific needs in four established dimensions of care (Box 42-1). Careful evaluation to identify the needs of individuals with CI is focused on promoting habilitation for each person. It is anticipated that the functional capabilities of children with CI will improve over time when support is provided.

Diagnosis and Classification

The diagnosis of CI is usually made after a period of suspicion, by professionals or the family, that the child's developmental progress is delayed. In some cases it is confirmed at birth because of recognition of distinct syndromes, such as Down syndrome and fetal alcohol syndrome. At the other extreme, the diagnosis is made when problems such as speech delays arouse concern. In all cases a high index of suspicion for developmental delay and behavioral signs (Box 42-2) is necessary for early diagnosis; routine developmental screening can assist in early identification (see Chapter 33). Delays are

BOX 42-1 Dimensions of Care for the Intellectually Disabled

Dimension I—Intellectual functioning and adaptive skills
Dimension II—Psychologic and emotional considerations
Dimension III—Physical, health, and etiology considerations
Dimension IV—Environmental considerations

BOX 42-2 Early Behavioral Signs Suggestive of Cognitive Impairment

- Dysmorphic features (e.g., Down syndrome, fragile X syndrome)
- Irritability or unresponsiveness to contact
- Abnormal eye contact during feeding
- Gross motor delay
- Decreased alertness to voice or movement
- Language difficulties or delay
- Feeding difficulties

From Crocker A, Nelson R: Mental retardation. In Levine M, Carey WB, Crocker AC (editors): *Developmental-behavioral pediatrics*, ed 3, Philadelphia, 1999, Saunders; and Shapiro B, Batshaw M: Mental retardation. In Behrman RE, Kliegman RM, Jenson HB (editors): *Nelson textbook of pediatrics*, ed 17, Philadelphia, 2004, Saunders.

typically seen in gross and fine motor and speech development, although the latter is most predictive. *Developmental delay* can be described as any significant lag in a child's physical, cognitive, behavioral, emotional, or social development, when compared against developmental norms. CI is a permanent impairment encompassing cognitive ability and adaptive behavior that are functioning significantly below average (see Box 42-2). In the absence of clear-cut evidence of CI, it is more appropriate to use a diagnosis of developmental delay (Biasini et al, 1999).

Results of standardized tests are used in making the diagnosis of intellectual disability based on cognitive deficits. Tests for assessing adaptive behaviors include the Vineland Social Maturity Scale and the AAMR Adaptive Behavior Scale. Informal appraisal of adaptive behavior may be made by those fully acquainted with the child (e.g., teachers, parents, other care providers). Frequently these observations lead parents to seek evaluation of the child's development.

A more useful approach for clinical application is classification based on educational potential or symptom severity. For educational purposes the term *educable CI* corresponds to the mildly impaired group, which constitutes about 85% of all people with CI. *Trainable CI* generally applies to children with moderate levels of CI and accounts for about 10% of the intellectually disabled population (American Psychiatric Association, 2000; Walker & Johnson, 2006) (Table 42-1). Although nurses may be familiar with the approximate range of IQ for classifying severity, they should refrain from using numbers as the criterion for assessing or evaluating the child's abilities, since numbers are of little value in counseling parents or training these children.

evolve Nursing Care Plan—The Child with Cognitive Impairment

Etiology

The causes of severe CI are primarily genetic, biochemical, and infectious. Although the etiology is unknown in the majority of cases, familial, social, environmental, and organic causes may predominate. Among individuals with CI, a sizable proportion of the cases are linked to Down syndrome, fragile X syndrome, or fetal alcohol syndrome. General categories of events that may lead to cognitive impairment include (Walker & Johnson, 2006; Kabra & Gulati, 2003):

- Infection and intoxication, such as congenital rubella, syphilis, maternal drug consumption (e.g., fetal alcohol syndrome), chronic lead ingestion, or kernicterus
- Trauma or physical agent (i.e., injury to the brain suffered during the prenatal, perinatal, or postnatal period)
- Inadequate nutrition and metabolic disorders, such as phenylketonuria or congenital hypothyroidism
- Gross postnatal brain disease, such as neurofibromatosis and tuberous sclerosis
- Unknown prenatal influence, including cerebral and cranial malformations, such as microcephaly and hydrocephalus
- Chromosomal abnormalities resulting from radiation; viruses; chemicals; parental age; and genetic mutations, such as Down syndrome and fragile X syndrome
- Gestational disorders, including prematurity, low birth weight, and postmaturity
- Psychiatric disorders that have their onset during the child's developmental period up to age 18 years, such as autism spectrum disorders
- Environmental influences, including evidence of a deprived environment associated with a history of intellectual disability among parents and siblings

Nursing Care of Children with Impaired Cognitive Function

Nurses play a major role in identifying children with CI. In the newborn and early infancy periods, few signs are present, with the exception of Down syndrome (p. 1183). After this age, however, delayed developmental milestones are the major clues to CI. In addition, nurses must have a high index of suspicion for early behavior patterns that may suggest CI (see Box 42-2). Parental concerns, such as delayed development compared with siblings, need to be taken seriously. All children should receive regular developmental assessment, and the nurse is often the person responsible for performing such assessments (see Chapter 33). When delays are found, the nurse must use sensitivity and discretion in revealing this finding to parents.

Nursing Care Management

Educate Child and Family

To teach children with CI, it is necessary to investigate their learning abilities and deficits. This is important for the nurse who may be involved in a home care program or who may be caring for the child in a health care setting. The nurse who understands how these children learn can effectively teach them basic skills or prepare them for various health-related procedures.

Children with CI have a marked deficit in their ability to discriminate between two or more stimuli because of difficulty in recognizing the relevance of specific cues. However, these

Table 42-1 Classification of Cognitive Impairment

LEVEL (IQ)*	PRESCHOOL (BIRTH-5 YR)—MATURATION AND DEVELOPMENT	SCHOOL AGE (6-21 YR)—TRAINING AND EDUCATION	ADULT (≥21 YR)—SOCIAL AND VOCATIONAL ADEQUACY
Mild—50-55 to approximately 70-75	Often not noticed as delayed by casual observer but is slower to walk, feed self, and talk than most children; follows same sequence in development as normal children	Can acquire practical skills and useful reading and arithmetic to a third- to sixth-grade level with special education; can be guided toward social conformity; achieves mental age of 8-12 yr	Can usually achieve social and vocational skills adequate for self-maintenance; may need occasional guidance and support when under unusual social or economic stress; can adjust to marriage but not childrearing
Moderate—35-40 to 50-55	Noticeable delays in motor development, especially in speech; responds to training in various self-help activities	Can learn simple communication, elementary health and safety habits, and simple manual skills; does not progress in functional reading or arithmetic; achieves mental age of 3-7 yr	Can perform simple tasks under sheltered conditions; participates in simple recreation; travels alone in familiar places; usually incapable of self-maintenance
Severe—20-25 to 35-40	Marked delay in motor development; little or no communication skills; may respond to training in elementary self-care (e.g., self-feeding)	Usually walks, barring specific disability; has some understanding of speech and some response; can profit from systematic habit training; achieves mental age of toddler	Can conform to daily routines and repetitive activities; needs continuing direction and supervision in protective environment
Profound—below 20-25	Gross delay; minimum capacity for functioning in sensorimotor areas; needs total care	Obvious delays in all areas of development; shows basic emotional responses; may respond to skillful training in use of legs, hands, and jaws; needs close supervision; achieves mental age of young infant	May walk; needs complete custodial care; has primitive speech; usually benefits from regular physical activity

*Data from American Psychiatric Association: *Diagnostic and statistical manual of mental disorders*, ed 4 (text rev) (DSM-IV TR), Washington, DC, 2000, The Association; and Rittey CD: Learning difficulties: what the neurologist needs to know, *J Neurol Neurosurg Psychiatry* 74(Suppl 1):30-36, 2005.
IQ, Intelligence quotient.

children can learn to discriminate if the cues are presented in an exaggerated, concrete form and if all extraneous stimuli are eliminated. For example, the use of colors to emphasize visual cues or the use of singing or rhymes to stress auditory cues can help them learn. Their deficit in discrimination also implies that concrete ideas are learned much more effectively than abstract ideas. Therefore demonstration is preferable to verbal explanation, and learning should be directed toward mastering a skill rather than understanding the scientific principles underlying a procedure.

Another cognitive deficit is in short-term memory. Whereas children of average intelligence can remember several words, numbers, or directions at one time, children with CI are less able to do so. Therefore they need simple, one-step directions. Learning through a step-by-step process requires a *task analysis*, in which each task is separated into its necessary components and each step is taught completely before proceeding to the next activity.

One critical area of learning that has had a tremendous impact on education for cognitively impaired individuals is *motivation*. Programs based on the motivational principles of behavior modification, employing positive reinforcement for specific tasks or behaviors, have demonstrated marked improvement in children's ability to learn. Advances in technology have greatly aided in providing reinforcement, especially in children who are severely disabled and who may have physical disabilities that limit their range of capabilities. For example, with the use of specially designed switches, children are given control of some event in the environment, such as turning on the television (Fig. 42-1). The television picture becomes reinforcement for activating the switch. Repetitive use of these switches provides an early, simplistic association with a technical device that may progress to increasingly complex aids.

Early intervention program is a systematic program of therapy, exercises, and activities designed to address developmental delays in disabled children to help achieve their full potentials (American Academy of Pediatrics, Committee on Genetics, 2001; National Down Syndrome Society, 2006). There is considerable evidence that these programs are valuable for cognitively impaired children. Nurses working with these families need to be aware of the types of programs in their community. Under the Individuals with Disabilities Education Act (IDEA) of 1990 (Public Law 101-476), states are encouraged to provide full early intervention services and are required to provide educational opportunities for all children with disabilities from birth to 21 years of age. Services may be provided under state Programs for Children with Special Health Needs or Head Start, or by private organizations such as National Down Syndrome Society,* Easter Seals,† or The Arc of the United States.‡ Parents should inquire about these programs by contacting the appropriate agencies. The child's education should begin as soon as possible. As children grow

**Information on early intervention programs in each state is available from the National Down Syndrome Society, 666 Broadway, 8th Floor, New York, NY 10012-2317; 800-221-4602;* www.ndss.org.

†233 S. Wacker Drive, Suite 2400, Chicago, IL 60606; 800-221-6827; TTY: 312-726-4258; fax: 312-726-1494; www.easterseals.com.

‡1010 Wayne Ave., Suite 650, Silver Spring, MD 20910; 301-565-3842 or 800-433-5255; fax: 301-565-5342; www.thearc.org.

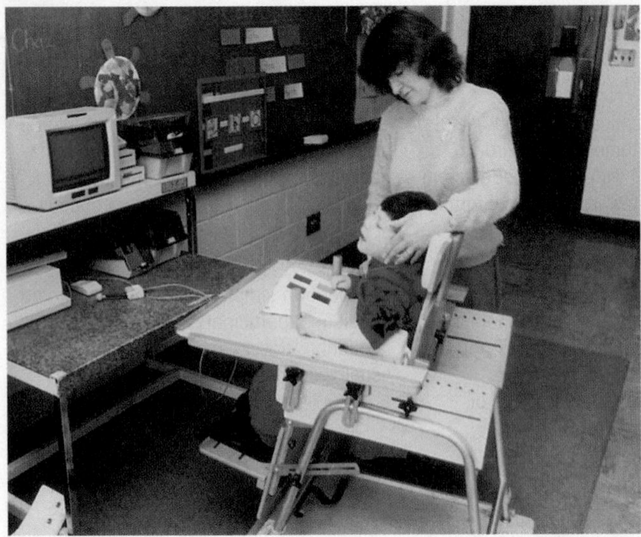

Fig. 42-1 A push panel allows a child with cognitive impairment to turn a computer on and off.

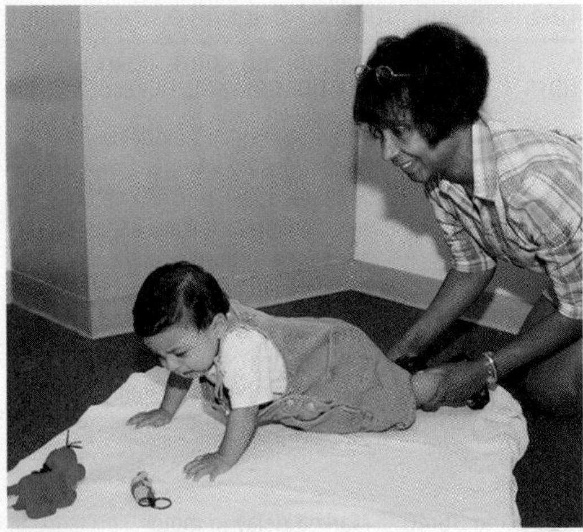

Fig. 42-2 Placing an attractive object outside the child's reach encourages crawling movements. *(Courtesy James DeLeon, Texas Children's Hospital, Houston, TX.)*

older, their education should be directed toward vocational training that prepares them for as independent a lifestyle as possible within their scope of abilities.

Teach Child Self-Care Skills

When a child with CI is born, parents need assistance in promoting normal developmental skills that are almost automatically learned by other children. These include self-care skills such as feeding, toileting, dressing, and grooming. Teaching these skills requires a basic knowledge of the developmental sequence in learning the skills demonstrated by children of average intelligence. For example, children with subaverage intelligence would not be expected to dress themselves as early as unaffected youngsters.

Teaching self-care skills also necessitates a working knowledge of the individual steps needed to master a skill. For example, before beginning a self-feeding program, the nurse performs a task analysis. After a task analysis, the child is observed in a particular situation, such as eating, to determine what skills are possessed and the child's developmental readiness to learn the task. Family members are included in this process because their "readiness" is as important as the child's. Numerous self-help aids, such as a plate with suction cups to prevent accidental spills, are available to facilitate independence and can help eliminate some of the difficulties of learning.*

Promote Child's Optimal Development

Optimal development involves more than achieving independence. It requires appropriate guidance for establishing acceptable social behavior and personal feelings of self-esteem, worth, and security. These attributes are not simply learned through a stimulation program. Rather, they must arise from the genuine love and caring that exist among family members. However, families need guidance in providing an environment that fosters optimal development. Often it is the nurse who can provide assistance in these areas of childrearing.

Another important area for promoting optimal development and self-esteem is ensuring the child's physical well-being. Any congenital defects, such as cardiac, gastrointestinal, or orthopedic anomalies, should be repaired. Plastic surgery may be considered when the child's appearance can be substantially improved. Dental health is significant, and orthodontic and restorative procedures can improve facial appearance immensely.

Encourage Play and Exercise

Children who are cognitively impaired have the same needs for recreation and exercise as other children. However, because of the children's slower development, parents may be less aware of the need to provide such activities. Therefore the nurse guides parents toward selection of suitable play and exercise activities. Because play has been discussed for children in each age group in earlier chapters, only the exceptions are presented here (Fig. 42-2).

The type of play is based on the child's developmental age, although the need for sensorimotor play may be prolonged for several years. Parents should use every opportunity to expose the child to as many different sounds, sights, and sensations as possible. Appropriate play includes musical mobiles, stuffed toys, water play, floating toys, a rocking chair or horse, a swing, bells, and rattles. The child should be taken on outings, such as trips to the grocery store or shopping center; other people should be encouraged to visit in the home; and the child should be related to directly, such as by cuddling, holding, rocking, talking to the child in the *en face* (face-to-face) position, and giving "rides" on the parents' shoulders.

Toys are selected for their recreational and educational value. For example, a large inflatable beach ball is a good water toy; it encourages interactive play and can be used to learn motor skills, such as balance, rocking, kicking, and throwing. A doll with removable clothes and different types of closures can help the child learn dressing skills. Musical toys that mimic animal sounds or respond with social phrases are

**A resource for a variety of self-help equipment is Sammons Preston, 1000 Remington Blvd., Suite 210, Bolingbrook, IL 60440-5117; 800-323-5547; fax: 800-547-4333;* www.sammonspreston.com. *In Canada: 800-665-9200.*

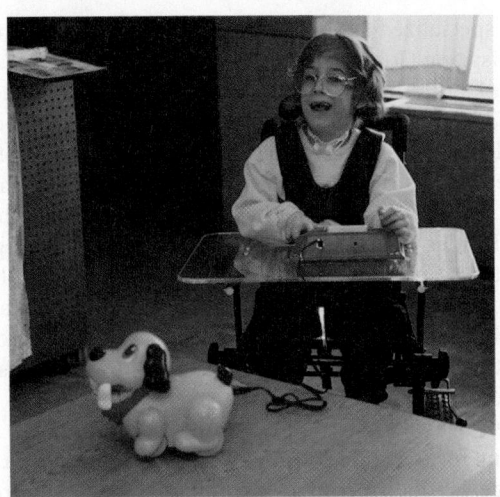

Fig. 42-3 A manual switch allows a child with cognitive impairment to play with a battery-operated toy.

excellent ways of encouraging speech. Toys should be simple in design so that the child can learn to manipulate them without help. For children with severe cognitive and physical impairment, electronic switches can be used to allow them to operate toys (Fig. 42-3).

Suitable activities for physical activity are based on the child's size, coordination, physical fitness and maturity, motivation, and health (Fig. 42-4). Some children may have physical problems that prevent participation in certain sports, such as atlantoaxial instability in children with Down syndrome (p. 1183). These children often have greater success in individual and dual sports than in team sports and enjoy themselves most with children of the same developmental level. The Special Olympics* provides these children with a unique competitive opportunity.

Safety is a major consideration in selecting recreational and exercise activities. For example, toys that may be appropriate developmentally may present dangers to a child who is strong enough to break them or use them incorrectly.

Provide Means of Communication

Verbal skills are typically delayed more than other physical skills. Speech requires hearing and interpretation *(receptive skills)* and facial muscle coordination *(expressive skills)*. Because both types of skills may be impaired, these children need frequent audiometric testing and should be fitted with hearing aids if indicated. In addition, they may need help in learning to control their facial muscles. For example, some children may need tongue exercises to correct the tongue thrust or gentle reminders to keep the lips closed.

Nonverbal communication may be appropriate for some of these children, and various devices are available. For the child without associated physical disabilities, a talking picture board is helpful. For children with physical limitations, several

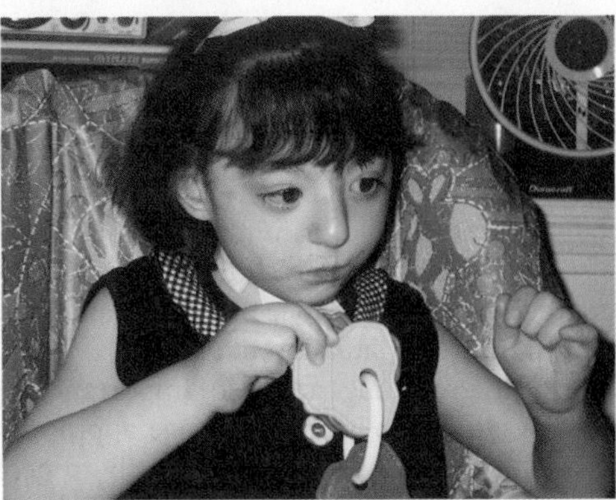

Fig. 42-4 A favorite toy provides stimulation for a young child.

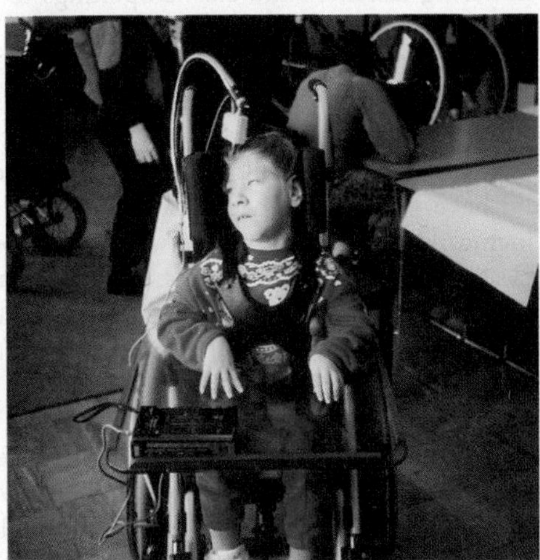

Fig. 42-5 A child with cognitive and physical impairments can activate electronic/communication equipment by moving a device near her head.

adaptations or types of communication devices are available to facilitate selection of the appropriate picture or word (Fig. 42-5). Some children may be taught sign language or *Blissymbols*—a highly stylized system of graphic symbols that represent words, ideas, and concepts. Although the symbols require education to learn their meaning, no reading skill is needed. The symbols are usually arranged on a board, and the person points or uses some type of selector to convey a message.

Establish Discipline

Discipline must begin early. Limit-setting measures need to be simple, consistently applied, and appropriate for the child's mental age. Control measures are based primarily on teaching a specific behavior rather than on understanding the reasons behind it. Stressing moral lessons is of little value to a child who lacks the cognitive skills to learn from self-criticism or from a lesson based on previous wrong-doing. Behavior modification, especially reinforcement of desired actions, and time-out are appropriate forms of behavior control.

Encourage Socialization

Acquiring social skills is a complex task, as is learning self-care procedures. Active rehearsal with role-playing and practice sessions and positive reinforcement for desired behavior

**1133 19th St. NW, Washington, DC 20036; 800-700-8585 or 202-628-3630; fax: 202-824-0200;* www.specialolympics.org. *(Website includes listing of state offices.) In Canada: Special Olympics Canada, 60 St. Clair Ave. E, Suite 700, Toronto, Ontario M4T 1N5; 416-927-9050; fax: 416-927-8475;* www.specialolympics.ca.

have been the most successful approaches. Parents should be encouraged early to teach their child socially acceptable behavior: waving goodbye, saying "hello" and "thank you," responding to his or her name, greeting visitors, and sitting modestly. The teaching of socially acceptable sexual behavior is especially important to minimize sexual exploitation. Parents also need to expose the child to strangers so that he or she can practice manners, since there is no automatic transfer of learning from one situation to another.

Dressing and grooming are also important aspects of socialization. A child who is dressed in age-appropriate clothing and is well groomed is much more likely to be accepted and to develop good self-esteem. Clothes should be clean, up-to-date, and well fitted. Many attractive outfits can be adapted with self-adhering fasteners and elastic openings to facilitate self-dressing.

As soon as possible, parents should enroll the child in appropriate preschool programs. Not only do these programs provide education and training, but they also offer an opportunity for social experiences among the children. As children grow older, they should have peer experiences similar to those of other children, including group outings, sports, and organized activities such as scouts and Special Olympics. Nurses can assess the child's abilities and encourage others (e.g., parents, teachers) to promote developmentally appropriate peer interaction (Johnson & Walker, 2006; Rehm & Bradley, 2006).

Provide Information on Sexuality

Adolescence may be a particularly difficult time for the family, especially in terms of the child's sexual behavior, possibility of pregnancy, future plans to marry, and ability to be independent. Frequently, little anticipatory guidance has been offered parents to prepare the child for physical and sexual maturation. The nurse can help in this area by providing parents with information about sexuality education that is geared to the child's developmental level. For example, the adolescent girl needs a *simple* explanation of menstruation and instructions on personal hygiene during the menstrual cycle.

These adolescents also need practical sexual information regarding anatomy, physical development, and conception. Because of their easy persuasion and lack of judgment, they need a well-defined, concrete code of conduct. The subtleties of social sexual behavior are less beneficial than specific instructions for handling certain situations. For example, an adolescent should be firmly told never to go alone anywhere with any person she does not know well. To protect him or her from abusive sexual activities, parents must closely observe their teenager's activities and associates. The question of contraceptive protection for these adolescents is often a parental concern.

Parents of these adolescents are often concerned about the advisability of marriage between two individuals with an intellectual disability. There is no conclusive answer; each situation must be judged individually. In some instances marriage is possible, but parenthood may not desirable because of the complexity of childrearing and the potential problem of perpetuating mental deficiency. The nurse should discuss this topic with parents and with the prospective couple, stressing suitable living accommodations and contraceptive methods to prevent pregnancy. If children are conceived, these parents require specialized assistance in learning to meet the needs of their offspring (Johnson & Walker, 2006).

Help Family Adjust to Future Care

Not all families are able to cope with home care of their affected child, especially one who is severely or profoundly impaired or has multiple disabilities. Older parents may not be able to assume care responsibilities after they reach retirement or older age. For these parents, the decision regarding residential placement is a difficult one, and the availability of such facilities varies widely. The nurse working with a family should help them investigate and evaluate various programs, in addition to assisting them in adjusting to the decision for placement.

Care for Child During Hospitalization

Caring for the child during hospitalization can be a special challenge. Frequently, nurses are unfamiliar with children who are cognitively impaired, and they may cope with their feelings of insecurity and fear by ignoring or isolating the child. Not only is this approach nonsupportive, but it may also be destructive for the child's sense of self-esteem and optimal development, and it may hamper the parents' ability to cope with the stress of the experience. One method that successfully avoids this nontherapeutic approach is the use of the mutual participation model in planning the child's care. Parents are encouraged to stay with their child but should not be made to feel as if the responsibility is totally theirs.

When the child is admitted, a detailed history is taken (see Chapter 34), especially in terms of all self-care activity. During the interview the child's developmental age is assessed. It is best to avoid asking directly about IQ levels, since this may make the parents uncomfortable and often tells little about the child's actual abilities. Questions are approached positively. For example, rather than asking, "Is your child toilet trained yet?" the nurse may state, "Tell me about your child's toileting habits." The assessment should also focus on any special devices the child uses, effective measures of limit setting, unusual or favorite routines, and any behaviors that may require intervention. If the parent states that the child engages in self-injurious activities (such as head banging or self-biting), the nurse should inquire about events that precipitate them and techniques that the parents use to manage them (Bosch & Ringdahl, 2001; Walker & Johnson, 2006).

The nurse also assesses the child's functional level of eating and playing; ability to express needs verbally; progress in toilet training; and relationship with objects, toys, and other children. The child is encouraged to be as independent as possible in the hospital.

Realizing that the child may be lonely in the hospital, the nurse makes certain that toys and other activities are provided. The child is placed in a room with other children of approximately the same developmental age, preferably a room with only two beds to avoid overstimulation. The nurse discusses with the other parents the child's abilities and introduces the parents and children to each other. By the nurse's example of treating the child with dignity and respect, others who may be fearful of what they do not understand are encouraged to accept the child.

Procedures are explained to the child through methods of communication that are at the appropriate cognitive level.

Generally, explanations should be simple, short, and concrete, emphasizing what the child will experience *physically.* Demonstration either through actual practice or with visual aids is always preferable to verbal explanation. The nurse repeats instructions often and evaluates the child's understanding by asking questions such as "What will it feel like?" "Show me how you must lie," or "Where will the dressing be?" Parents are included in preprocedural teaching for their own learning and to help the nurse learn effective methods of communicating with the child.

During hospitalization the nurse should also focus on growth-promoting experiences for the child. For example, hospitalization may be an excellent opportunity to emphasize to parents abilities that the child does have but has not had the opportunity to practice, such as self-dressing. It may also be an opportunity for social experiences with peers, group play, or new educational and recreational activities. For example, one child who had the habit of screaming and kicking demonstrated a definite decrease in those behaviors after he learned to pound pegs and use a punching bag. Through social services the parents may become aware of specialized programs for the child. Hospitalization may also offer parents a respite from everyday care responsibilities and an opportunity to discuss their feelings with a concerned professional.

Assist in Measures to Prevent Cognitive Impairment

Besides having a responsibility to families with a child with CI, nurses also need to be involved in programs aimed at preventing CI. Many of the familial, social, and environmental factors known to cause mild impairment are preventable. Counseling and education can reduce or eliminate such factors (e.g., poor nutrition, cigarette smoking, chemical abuse), which increase the risk of prematurity and intrauterine growth restriction. Interventions are directed toward improving maternal health by educating women regarding the dangers of chemicals, including prenatal alcohol exposure, which affects organogenesis, craniofacial development, and cognitive ability (Wilton & Plane, 2006). Other preventive strategies that play an important role include adequate prenatal care; optimal medical care of high risk newborns; rubella immunization; genetic counseling and prenatal screening, especially in terms of Down or fragile X syndrome; use of folic acid supplements to prevent neural tube defects during pregnancy and during the childbearing years; newborn screening for treatable inborn errors of metabolism, such as congenital hypothyroidism, phenylketonuria, and galactosemia; and early appropriate therapies and rehabilitation services for children with developmental disabilities.

Down Syndrome

Down syndrome is the most common chromosomal abnormality of a generalized syndrome, occurring in one in every 800 to 1000 live births (National Down Syndrome Society, 2006; Skotko, 2005). It occurs slightly more often in Caucasians than in African-Americans, although the incidence is unchanged in various socioeconomic classes.

Etiology

The cause of Down syndrome is not known, but evidence from cytogenetic and epidemiologic studies supports the concept of multiple causality. Approximately 95% of all cases of Down syndrome are attributable to an extra chromosome 21 (group G), thus the name *nonfamilial trisomy 21* (National Down Syndrome Society, 2006; Walker & Johnson, 2006). Although children with trisomy 21 are born to parents of all ages, there is a statistically greater risk in older women, particularly those older than 35 years of age. For example, in women 35 years of age the chance of conceiving a child with Down syndrome is about 1 in 400 live births, but in women age 40 it is about 1 in 110. However, the majority (about 80%) of infants with Down syndrome are born to women younger than age 35. About 3% to 4% of the cases may be caused by *translocation* of chromosomes 15 and 21 or 22. This type of genetic aberration is usually hereditary and is not associated with advanced parental age. From 1% to 2% of affected persons demonstrate ***mosaicism,*** which refers to mixture of normal and abnormal cell types. The degree of cognitive and physical impairment is related to the percentage of cells with the abnormal chromosome makeup.

Diagnostic Evaluation

Down syndrome can usually be diagnosed by the clinical manifestations alone (Box 42-3 and Fig. 42-6), but a chromosome analysis should be done to confirm the genetic abnormality.

Several physical problems are associated with Down syndrome. Many of these children have congenital heart malformations, the most common being septal defects. Respiratory tract infections are prevalent and, when combined with cardiac anomalies, are the chief causes of death, particularly during the first year of life. Hypotonicity of chest and abdominal muscles and dysfunction of the immune system probably predispose the child to the development of respiratory tract infection. Other physical problems include thyroid dysfunction, especially congenital hypothyroidism, and an increased incidence of leukemia.

evolve Case Study—Down Syndrome

Therapeutic Management

Although no cure exists for Down syndrome, a number of therapies are advocated, such as surgery to correct serious congenital anomalies (e.g., heart defects, strabismus). These children also benefit from an evaluative echocardiogram soon

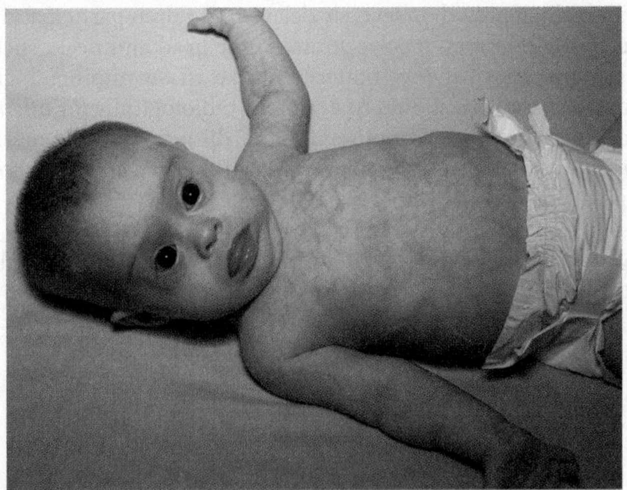

Fig. 42-6 Down syndrome in an infant. Note small, square head with upward slant to eyes, flat nasal bridge, protruding tongue, mottled skin, and hypotonia.

BOX 42-3 Clinical Manifestations of Down Syndrome

Head and Eyes
*Separated sagittal suture
Brachycephaly
Rounded and small skull
Flat occiput
Enlarged anterior fontanel
*Oblique palpebral fissures (upward, outward slant)
Inner epicanthal folds
Speckling of iris (Brushfield's spots)

Nose and Ears
*Small nose
*Depressed nasal bridge (saddle nose)
Small ears and narrow canals
Short pinna (vertical ear length)
Overlapping upper helices
Conductive hearing loss

Mouth and Neck
*High, arched, narrow palate
Protruding tongue
Hypoplastic mandible
Delayed tooth eruption and microdontia
Alignment teeth abnormalities common
Periodontal disease
*Neck skin excess and laxity
Short and broad neck

Chest and Heart
Shortened rib cage
Twelfth rib anomalies
Pectus excavatum or carinatum
Congenital heart defects common (e.g., atrial septal defect, ventricular septal defect)

Abdomen and Genitalia
Protruding, lax, and flabby abdominal muscles
Diastasis recti abdominis
Umbilical hernia
Small penis
Cryptorchidism
Bulbous vulva

Hands and Feet
Broad, short hands and stubby fingers
Incurved little finger (clinodactyly)
Transverse palmar crease
*Wide space between big and second toes
*Plantar crease between big and second toes
Broad, short feet and stubby toes

Musculoskeleton and Skin
Short stature
*Hyperflexibility and muscle weakness
Hypotonia
Atlantoaxial instability
Dry, cracked, and frequent fissuring
Cutis marmorata (mottling)

Other
Reduced birth weight
Learning difficulty (average intelligence quotient of 50)
Hypothyroidism common
Impaired immune function
Increased risk of leukemia
Early-onset dementia (in one third)

*Most common findings in modified chart (Pueschel, 1999).

after birth and regular medical care. Evaluation of sight and hearing is essential, and treatment of otitis media is required to prevent auditory loss, which can influence cognitive function. Periodic testing of thyroid function is recommended, especially if growth is severely delayed. Children participating in sports that may involve stress on the head and neck, such as gymnastics, diving, butterfly stroke in swimming, high jump, and soccer, should be evaluated radiologically for *atlantoaxial instability*. Symptoms of the disorder include neck pain, weakness, and torticollis. Affected children are at risk for spinal cord compression.

NURSING ALERT Report immediately any child with the following signs of spinal cord compression:
- Persistent neck pain
- Loss of established motor skills and bladder or bowel control
- Changes in sensation

Prognosis

Life expectancy for those with Down syndrome has improved in recent years but remains lower than for the general population. More than 80% survive to age 55 years and beyond. As the prognosis continues to improve for these individuals, it will be important to provide for their long-term health care, social, and leisure needs (National Down Syndrome Society, 2006; Van Riper, 2003).

Nursing Care Management

Support Family at Time of Diagnosis

Because of the unique physical characteristics, the infant with Down syndrome is usually diagnosed at birth if a prenatal diagnosis had not been established. Parents should be informed of the diagnosis at this time. Parents usually prefer that both of them be present during the informing interview so that they can support one another emotionally. They appreciate receiving reading material about the syndrome* and being referred

*Sources of information include The Arc of the United States (see footnote, p. 1179); American Association on Intellectual and Developmental Disabilities, 501 3rd St. NW, Suite 200, Washington, DC 20001; 800-424-3688; fax: 202-387-2193; www.aamr.org; National Down Syndrome Society (see footnote, p. 1179); and National Down Syndrome Congress, 1370 Center Drive, Suite 102, Atlanta, GA 30338; 800-232-6372 or 770-604-9500; www.ndsccenter.org.

to others for help or advice, such as parent groups or professional counseling.

After parents are aware of the diagnosis, they are confronted with the crisis of losing their perfect or dream child and grieving for and accepting their reality child. Consequently, the parents' responses to the child may greatly influence decisions regarding future care. Whereas some families willingly take the child home, others consider immediate residential placement. The nurse must carefully answer questions regarding developmental potential. Institutionalization is no longer an option. For families unable or unready to choose taking the newborn home, specialized foster care or adoption are other options (see Critical Thinking Exercise).

CRITICAL THINKING EXERCISE

Diagnosis of Down Syndrome

The parents of Melissa, a newborn diagnosed as having Down syndrome, ask the nurse, "What are we supposed to do with her?" They further state that they already have three other children at home.

1. Evidence—Is there sufficient evidence to draw conclusions about the parents' concerns regarding their newborn daughter?
2. Assumptions—Describe an underlying assumption about each of the following:
   a. Newborn diagnosed with Down syndrome
   b. Parental care of a newborn with Down syndrome
   c. Newborn with Down syndrome and older siblings
3. What priorities for the nursing response should be established?
4. Does the evidence support your nursing intervention?
5. What alternative perspectives might you have?

Assist Family in Preventing Physical Problems

Many of the physical characteristics of Down syndrome present nursing problems. The hypotonicity of muscles and hyperextensibility of joints complicate positioning. The limp, flaccid extremities resemble the posture of a rag doll; as a result, holding the infant is difficult and cumbersome. Sometimes parents perceive this lack of molding to their bodies as evidence of inadequate parenting. The extended body position promotes heat loss because more surface area is exposed to the environment. Parents are encouraged to swaddle or wrap the infant tightly in a blanket before picking up the child to provide security and warmth. The nurse also discusses with parents their feelings concerning attachment to the child, emphasizing that the child's lack of clinging or molding is a physical characteristic, not a sign of detachment or rejection.

Decreased muscle tone compromises respiratory expansion. In addition, the underdeveloped nasal bone causes a chronic problem of inadequate drainage of mucus. The constant stuffy nose forces the child to breathe by mouth, which dries the oropharyngeal membranes, increasing the susceptibility to upper respiratory tract infections. Measures to lessen these problems include clearing the nose with a bulb-type syringe, rinsing the mouth with water after feedings, increasing fluid intake, and using a cool-mist vaporizer to keep the mucous membranes moist and the secretions liquefied. Other helpful measures include changing the child's position frequently, performing postural drainage with percussion if necessary, practicing good handwashing, and properly disposing of soiled articles such as tissues. If antibiotics are ordered, the nurse stresses the importance of completing the full course of therapy for successful eradication of the infection and prevention of growth of resistant organisms.

Inadequate drainage resulting in pooling of mucus in the nose also interferes with feeding. Because the child breathes by mouth, sucking for any length of time is difficult. When eating solids, the child may gag on the food because of mucus in the oropharynx. Parents are advised to clear the nose before each feeding; give small, frequent feedings; and allow opportunities for rest during mealtime.

The protruding tongue also interferes with feeding, especially of solid foods. Parents need to know that the tongue thrust is not an indication of refusal to feed, but a physiologic response. Parents are advised to use a small but long, straight-handled spoon to push the food toward the back and side of the mouth. If food is thrust out, it should be refed.

Dietary intake needs supervision. Decreased muscle tone affects gastric motility, predisposing the child to constipation. Dietary measures such as increased fiber and fluid promote evacuation. The child's eating habits may need careful scrutiny to prevent obesity. Height and weight measurements should be obtained on a serial basis, especially during infancy. Because these children grow more slowly than the general pediatric population's trends, special growth charts developed for these children should be used (American Academy of Pediatrics, Committee on Genetics, 2001).

During infancy the child's skin is pliable and soft. However, it gradually becomes rough and dry and is prone to cracking and infection. Skin care involves the use of minimum soap and application of lubricants. Lip balm is applied to the lips, especially when the child is outdoors, to prevent excessive chapping.

Assist in Prenatal Diagnosis and Genetic Counseling

Prenatal diagnosis of Down syndrome is possible through chorionic villus sampling and amniocentesis, since chromosome analysis of fetal cells can detect the presence of trisomy or translocation. However, analysis will not identify sporadic cases in young women when there is no indication for prenatal testing. Testing for low maternal serum alpha-fetoprotein, high chorionic gonadotropin, low unconjugated estriol levels, and maternal serum fetal cell markers may identify an affected fetus, and the woman can then undergo amniocentesis (National Down Syndrome Society, 2006; Peterson, 2006; Hall, 2004).

Prenatal testing and genetic counseling should be offered to women of advanced maternal age or those who have a family history of the disorder. If prenatal testing indicates the fetus is affected, the nurse must allow the parents to express their feelings concerning elective abortion and support their decision to terminate or proceed with the pregnancy.

Fragile X Syndrome

Fragile X syndrome is the most common inherited cause of CI and the second most common genetic cause of CI after Down syndrome. It has been described in all ethnic groups and races; the incidence of affected males is 1 in 3600; the incidence of affected females is 1 in 4000 to 6000; and the incidence of carrier females is 1 in 100 to 260 and the incidence of carrier males is 1 in 250 to 800 worldwide (National Fragile X Foundation, 2006; Phalen, 2005; Crawford, 2001).

The syndrome is caused by an abnormal gene on the lower end of the long arm of the X chromosome. Chromosome analysis may demonstrate a *fragile site* (a region that fails to condense during mitosis and is characterized by a nonstaining gap or narrowing) in the cells of affected males and females and in carrier females. This fragile site has been determined to be caused by a gene mutation that results in excessive repeats of nucleotide in a specific deoxyribonucleic acid (DNA) segment of the X chromosome. The number of repeats in a normal individual is between 6 and 50. An individual with 50 to 200 base-pair repeats is said to have a *permutation* and is therefore a carrier. When passed from a parent to a child, these base-pair repeats can expand from 200 or more, which is termed a *full mutation*. This expansion occurs only when a carrier mother passes the mutation to her offspring; it does not occur when a carrier father passes the mutation to his daughters. Prenatal diagnosis of the fragile X gene mutation is now possible with direct DNA testing in a family with an established history, using amniocentesis or chorionic villus sampling (Centers for Disease Control and Prevention, 2002; Crawford, 2001). Both affected sexes are fertile and therefore capable of transmitting the fragile X disorder.

evolve Critical Thinking Exercise—Fragile X Syndrome

Clinical Manifestations

The classic trend of physical findings in adult men with fragile X syndrome consists of a long face with a prominent jaw (prognathism); large, protruding ears; and large testes (macroorchidism). In prepubertal children, however, these features may be less obvious, and behavioral manifestations may initially suggest the diagnosis (Box 42-4). In carrier females the clinical manifestations are extremely varied.

Therapeutic Management

No cure exists for fragile X syndrome. Medical treatment may include the use of serotonin agents such as carbamazepine (Tegretol) or fluoxetine (Prozac) to control violent temper outbursts and the use of central nervous system stimulants or clonidine (Catapres) to improve attention span and decrease hyperactivity. Protein replacement and gene therapy are treatment options that are being investigated (Phalen, 2005).

All affected children require referral to early intervention program (speech and language therapy, occupational therapy, and special education assistance) and multidisciplinary assessment, including cardiology (i.e., mitral valve prolapse), neurology (i.e., seizures), and orthopedic anomalies (Alanay et al, 2007).

Prognosis

Individuals with fragile X syndrome are expected to live a normal life span. Their CI may be improved by behavioral and educational interventions.

Nursing Care Management

Because CI is a fairly consistent finding in individuals with fragile X syndrome, the care given to these families is the same as for any child with CI. Because the disorder is hereditary, genetic counseling is necessary to inform parents and siblings of the risks of transmission. In addition, any male or female with unexplained or nonspecific mental impairment should be referred for genetic testing and, if needed, counseling. Families with a member affected by the disorder should be referred to the National Fragile X Foundation.*

BOX 42-4 Clinical Manifestations of Fragile X Syndrome

Physical Features
- Increased head circumference
- Long, wide, and/or protruding ears
- Long, narrow face with prominent jaw
- Strabismus
- Mitral valve prolapse, aortic root dilation
- Hypotonia
- Enlarged testicles (especially postpubertally)

Behavioral Features
- Mild to severe cognitive impairment
- Speech delay; may have rapid speech with stuttering, word repetition
- Short attention span, hyperactivity
- Hypersensitivity to taste, sounds, touch
- Intolerance to change in routine
- Autistic-like behaviors

Sensory Impairment

Hearing Impairment

Hearing impairment is one of the most common disabilities in the United States. An estimated 3 in 1000 well infants have hearing loss of varying degrees (Gregg, Wiorek, & Arvedson, 2004). For infants admitted to the neonatal intensive care unit, the incidence rises sharply to approximately 2 to 4 per 100 neonates (Cunningham, Cox, & Committee on Practice and Ambulatory Medicine and the Section on Otolaryngology and Bronchoesophagology, 2003; American Academy of Pediatrics, Task Force on Newborn and Infant Hearing, 1999). In the United States there are about 1 million children with hearing impairment ranging in age from birth to 21 years, and almost a third of these children have other disabilities, such as visual or cognitive deficits.

Definition and Classification

Hearing impairment is a general term indicating disability that may range in severity from mild to profound and includes the subsets of deaf and hard-of-hearing. *Deaf* refers to a person whose hearing disability precludes successful processing of linguistic information through audition, with or without a hearing aid. *Hard-of-hearing* refers to a person who, generally with the use of a hearing aid, has residual

*PO Box 37, Walnut Creek, CA 94597; 800-688-8765 or 925-938-9300; fax: 925-938-9315; www.fragilex.org.

hearing sufficient to enable successful processing of linguistic information through audition. Other terms, such as *deaf and dumb, mute,* or *deaf-mute,* are unacceptable. Hearing-impaired persons are not dumb and, if mute, have no physical speech defect other than that caused by the inability to hear.

Hearing defects may be classified according to etiology, pathology, or symptom severity. Each is important in terms of treatment, possible prevention, and rehabilitation.

Etiology

Hearing loss may be caused by a number of prenatal and postnatal conditions. These include a family history of childhood hearing impairment, anatomic malformations of the head or neck, low birth weight, severe perinatal asphyxia, perinatal infection (cytomegalovirus, rubella, herpes, syphilis, toxoplasmosis, bacterial meningitis), chronic ear infection, cerebral palsy, Down syndrome, or administration of ototoxic drugs (Smith, Bale, & White, 2005; Gregg, Wiorek, & Arvedson, 2004).

In addition, high risk neonates who survive formerly fatal prenatal or perinatal conditions may be susceptible to hearing loss from the disorder or its treatment. For example, sensorineural hearing loss may be a result of continuous humming noises or high noise levels associated with incubators, oxygen hoods, or intensive care units, especially when combined with the use of potentially ototoxic antibiotics.

Environmental noise is a special concern. Sounds loud enough to damage sensitive hair cells of the inner ear can produce irreversible hearing loss. Very loud, brief noise, such as gunfire, can cause immediate, severe, and permanent loss of hearing. Longer exposure to less intense but still hazardous sounds, such as loud persistent music via headphones, sound systems, concerts, or industrial noises, can also produce hearing loss (Daniel, 2007; Kenna, 2004; Segal et al, 2003). Loud noises combined with the toxic substances of smoking produces a synergistic effect on hearing that causes hearing loss (Mizoue, Miyamoto, & Shimizu, 2003).

Pathology

Disorders of hearing are divided according to the location of the defect. *Conductive* or *middle-ear hearing loss* results from interference of transmission of sound to the middle ear. It is the most common of all types of hearing loss and most frequently a result of recurrent serous otitis media. Conductive hearing impairment involves mainly interference with loudness of sound.

Sensorineural hearing loss, also called *perceptive* or *nerve deafness,* involves damage to the inner ear structures or the auditory nerve. The most common causes are congenital defects of inner ear structures or consequences of acquired conditions, such as kernicterus, infection, administration of ototoxic drugs, or exposure to excessive noise. Sensorineural hearing loss results in distortion of sound and problems in discrimination. Although the child hears some of everything going on around him or her, the sounds are distorted, severely affecting discrimination and comprehension.

Mixed conductive-sensorineural hearing loss results from interference with transmission of sound in the middle ear and along neural pathways. It frequently results from recurrent otitis media and its complications.

Table 42-2 Intensity of Sounds Expressed in Decibels

DECIBELS	REPRESENTATIVE SOUND
0	Softest sound normal ear can hear
10	Heartbeat, rustling of leaves
20	Whisper at 1.5 m (5 feet)
30-45	Normal conversation
60	Noise in average restaurant
70-80	Street noises
80	Loud radio in home
90-100	Train
120	Thunder, loud music (e.g., rock concerts)
140	Jet plane during departure
>140	Pain threshold

Central auditory imperception includes all hearing losses that are not linked to defects in the conductive or sensorineural structures. They are usually divided into organic or functional losses. In the *organic* type of central auditory imperception, the defect involves the reception of auditory stimuli along the central pathways and the expression of the message into meaningful communication. Examples are *aphasia,* the inability to express ideas in any form, either written or verbal; *agnosia,* the inability to interpret sound correctly; and *dysacusis,* difficulty in processing details or discriminating among sounds. In the *functional* type of hearing loss, no organic lesion exists to explain a central auditory loss. Examples of functional hearing loss are conversion hysteria (an unconscious withdrawal from hearing to block remembrance of a traumatic event), infantile autism, and childhood schizophrenia.

Symptom Severity

Hearing impairment is expressed in terms of a *decibel (db),* a unit of loudness (Table 42-2); hearing is measured at various frequencies, such as 500, 1000, and 2000 cycles/sec, the critical listening speech range. Hearing impairment can be classified according to *hearing threshold level* (the measurement of an individual's hearing threshold by means of an audiometer) and the degree of symptom severity as it affects speech (Table 42-3). These classifications offer only general guidelines regarding the effect of the impairment on any individual child, since children differ greatly in their ability to use residual hearing.

Therapeutic Management

Conductive Hearing Loss

Treatment of hearing loss depends on the cause and type of hearing impairment. Many conductive hearing defects respond to medical or surgical treatment, such as antibiotic therapy for acute otitis media or insertion of tympanostomy tubes for chronic otitis media. When the conductive loss is permanent, hearing can be improved with the use of a hearing aid to amplify sound.

The nurse should be familiar with the types, basic care, and handling of hearing aids, especially when the child is

evolve Nursing Care Plan—The Child with Hearing Impairment

Table 42-3 Classification of Hearing Loss Based on Symptom Severity

HEARING LEVEL (db)	EFFECT
Slight—16-25	Has difficulty hearing faint or distant speech Usually is unaware of hearing difficulty Likely to achieve in school but may have problems No speech defects
Mild to moderate—26-55	May have speech difficulties Understands face-to-face conversational speech at 0.9-1.5 m (3-5 feet)
Moderately severe—56-70 (hard of hearing)	Unable to understand conversational speech unless loud Considerable difficulty with group or classroom discussion Requires special speech training
Severe—71-90 (deaf)	May hear a loud voice if nearby May be able to identify loud environmental noises Can distinguish vowels but not most consonants Requires speech training
Profound—91 (deaf)	May hear only loud sounds Requires extensive speech training

hospitalized.* Types of aids include those worn in or behind the ear, models incorporated into an eyeglass frame, or types worn on the body with a wire connection to the ear (Fig. 42-7). One of the most common problems with a hearing aid is *acoustic feedback,* an annoying whistling sound usually caused by improper fit of the ear mold. Sometimes the whistling may be at a frequency that the child cannot hear but that is annoying to others. In this case, if children are old enough, they are told of the noise and asked to readjust the aid.

NURSING ALERT To reduce or eliminate whistling from a hearing aid, try reinserting the aid, making certain that no hair is caught between the ear mold and the canal, cleaning the ear mold or ear, or lowering the volume of the aid.

As children grow older, they may be self-conscious about the device. Every effort is made to make the aid inconspicuous, such as an appropriate hairstyle to cover behind-the-ear or in-the-ear models; attractive frames for glasses; and placement of the on-the-body type where it is not seen, such as under a blouse or sweater. Children are given responsibility for the care of the device as soon as they are able, since fostering independence is a primary goal of rehabilitation.

NURSING ALERT When parents express concern about their child's hearing and speech development, refer the child for a hearing evaluation. Absence of well-formed syllables *(da, na, yaya)* by 11 months of age should result in immediate referral.

Information about hearing aids is available from the International Hearing Society, 16880 Middlebelt Road, Suite 4, Livonia, MI 48154; 734-522-7200; fax: 734-522-0200; http://ihsinfo.org.

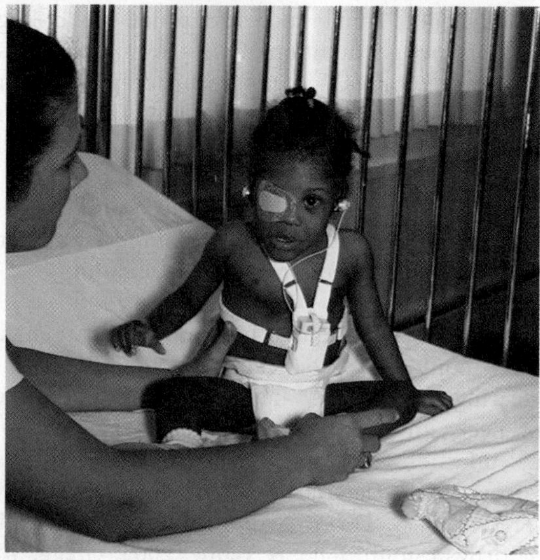

Fig. 42-7 On-the-body hearing aids are convenient for young children, such as this child with severe bilateral hearing loss. Note eye patching for strabismus.

Sensorineural Hearing Loss

Treatment for sensorineural hearing loss is much less satisfactory. Because the defect is not one of intensity of sound, hearing aids are of less value in this type of defect. The use of *cochlear implants** (a surgically implanted prosthetic device) provides a sensation of hearing for individuals who have severe or profound hearing loss (Zeng & Liu, 2006; Downs & Buchman, 2005). Children with sensorineural hearing loss have lost or damaged some or all of their hair cells or auditory nerve fibers. Often these children cannot benefit from conventional hearing aids because they only amplify sound that cannot be processed by a damaged inner ear. A cochlear implant bypasses the hair cells to directly stimulate surviving auditory nerve fibers so that they can send signals to the brain. These signals can be interpreted by the brain to produce sound and sensations (Zeng & Liu, 2006; Gregg, Wiorek, & Arvedson, 2004).

Multichanneled implants are now available. This more sophisticated device stimulates the auditory nerve at a number of locations with differently processed signals. This type of stimulation allows a person to use the pitch information present in speech signals, leading to better understanding of speech. The trend is toward early use of cochlear implants, usually by 18 months of age, to give the child maximum opportunity to develop listening, language, and speaking skills.

Nursing Care Management

Assessment of children for hearing impairment is a critical nursing responsibility. Early detection of hearing loss, preferably within the first 3 to 6 months of life, is essential to improve the language and educational outcomes of those with hearing

Hearing Enrichment Language Program of the Hough Ear Institute, 3434 N.W. 56th St., Oklahoma City, OK 73112; 405-945-7186; fax: 405-945-7188; www.integris-health.com/INTEGRIS/en-US/Specialties/EarInstitute/HELP.

impairments (Gregg, Wiorek, & Arvedson, 2004; Kenna, 2004). To accomplish this goal, the current recommendation is universal newborn hearing screening before discharge from the newborn nursery (Gregg, Wiorek, & Arvedson, 2004; Cunningham, Cox, & Committee on Practice and Ambulatory Medicine and Section on Otolaryngology and Bronchoesophagology, 2003; American Academy of Pediatrics, Task Force on Newborn and Infant Hearing, 1999). This discussion focuses on developmental and behavioral indices associated with hearing impairment. Auditory testing is presented in Chapter 34.

Infancy

At birth the nurse can observe the neonate's response to auditory stimuli, as evidenced by the startle reflex, head turning, eye blinking, and cessation of body movement. The infant may vary in the intensity of the response, depending on the state of alertness. However, a consistent absence of a reaction should lead to suspicion of hearing loss. Box 42-5 summarizes other clinical manifestations of hearing impairment in the infant.

Childhood

The child who is profoundly deaf is much more likely to be diagnosed during infancy than the less severely affected one. If the defect is not detected during early childhood, it likely will become evident during entry into school, when the child has difficulty learning. Unfortunately, some of these children are mistakenly placed in special classes for students with learning disabilities or CI. Therefore it is essential that the nurse suspect a hearing impairment in any child who demonstrates the behaviors listed in Box 42-5.

Of primary importance is the effect of hearing impairment on speech development.* A child with a mild conductive hearing loss may speak fairly clearly but in a loud, monotone voice. A child with a sensorineural defect usually has difficulty in articulation. For example, inability to hear higher frequencies may result in the word *spoon* being pronounced "poon." Children with articulation problems need to have their hearing tested.

NURSING ALERT Stress to parents the importance of storing batteries for hearing aids in a safe location and teaching children not to remove the battery from the hearing aid (or supervising young children to prevent the removal). Ingestion of batteries is most often of those from hearing aids, including the child's own aid.

Lipreading

Even though the child may become an expert at lipreading, only about 40% of the spoken word is understood, and less if the speaker has an accent, mustache, or beard. Exaggerating pronunciation or speaking in an altered rhythm further reduces comprehension. Parents can help the child understand the spoken word by using the suggestions in the Guidelines box. The child learns to supplement the spoken word with sensitivity to visual cues, primarily body language and facial expression (e.g., tightening the lips, muscle tension, eye contact).

Other sources of information on several aspects of hearing loss are the Alexander Graham Bell Association for the Deaf and Hard of Hearing, 3417 Volta Place NW, Washington, DC 20007; voice: 202-337-5220; TTY: 202-337-5221; fax: 202-337-8314; www.agbell.org; and Canadian Hearing Society, voice: 877-347-3427; TTY: 877-347-3429; www.chs.ca.

BOX 42-5 Clinical Manifestations of Hearing Impairment

Infants

- Lack of startle or blink reflex to a loud sound
- Failure to be awakened by loud environmental noises
- Failure to localize a source of sound by 6 months of age
- Absence of babble or voice inflections by age 7 months
- Lack of response to the spoken word; failure to follow verbal directions
- Response to loud noises as opposed to the voice

Children

- Use of gestures rather than verbalization to express desires
- Failure to develop intelligible speech by age 24 months
- Monotone and unintelligible speech; lessened laughter
- Vocal play, head banging, or foot stamping for vibratory sensation
- Yelling or screeching to express pleasure, needs, or annoyance (tantrum)
- Asking to have statements repeated or answering them incorrectly
- Greater response to facial expression and gestures than to verbal explanation
- Avoidance of social interaction; preference for playing alone
- Inquiring, sometimes confused facial expression
- Suspicious alertness alternating with cooperation
- Frequently stubbornness because of lack of comprehension
- Irritability at not making themselves understood
- Shy, timid, and withdrawn behavior
- Often appearing "dreamy," "in a world of their own," or exhibiting inattentiveness

GUIDELINES Facilitating Lipreading

- Attract child's attention before speaking; use light touch to signal speaker's presence.
- Stand close to child.
- Face child directly or move to a 45-degree angle.
- Stand still; do not walk back and forth or turn away to point or look elsewhere.
- Establish eye contact and show interest.
- Speak at eye level and with good lighting on speaker's face.
- Be certain nothing interferes with speech patterns, such as chewing food or gum.
- Speak clearly and at a slow and even rate.
- Use facial expression to assist in conveying messages.
- Keep sentences short.
- Rephrase message if child does not understand the words.

Cued Speech

This method of communication is an adjunct to straight lipreading. It uses hand signals to help the child with a hearing impairment distinguish between words that look alike when formed by the lips (e.g., mat, bat). It is most often used by children with hearing impairments who are using speech rather than those who are nonverbal.

Sign Language

Sign language, such as *American Sign Language (ASL)* or *British Sign Language (BSL),* is a visual gestural language that uses hand signals that roughly correspond to specific words and concepts in the English language. Family members are encouraged to learn signing because using or watching hands requires much less concentration than lipreading or talking. Also, a symbol method enables some children to learn more and to learn faster. Learning a language promotes cognitive development.

Speech Language Therapy

The most formidable task in the education of a child who is profoundly hearing impaired is learning to speak. Speech is learned through a multisensory approach, using visual, tactile, kinesthetic, and auditory stimulation. Parents are encouraged to participate fully in the learning process.

Additional Aids

Everyday activities present problems for older children with hearing impairment. For example, they may not be able to hear the telephone, doorbell, or alarm clock. Several commercial devices are available to help them adjust to these dilemmas. Flashing lights can be attached to a telephone or doorbell to signal its ringing. Trained hearing ear dogs can provide great assistance because they alert the person to sounds, such as someone approaching, a moving car, a signal to wake up, or a child's cry. Special *teletypewriters* or *telecommunications devices for the deaf (TDD* or *TTY)* help people with impaired hearing communicate with each other over the telephone; the typed message is conveyed via the telephone lines and displayed on a small screen.*

Any audiovisual medium presents dilemmas for these children, who can see the picture but cannot hear the message. However, with *closed captioning* a special decoding device is attached to the television, and the audio portion of a program is translated into subtitles that appear on the screen.†

Socialization

Because socialization is extremely important to the child's development, the nurse discusses with the family methods of fostering social contact. If children attend a special school for the deaf, they are able to socialize with peers in that setting. Classmates become a potential source of close friendships because they communicate more easily among themselves. Parents are encouraged to promote these relationships whenever possible.

Children with a hearing impairment may need special help with school or social activities. For children wearing hearing aids, background noise should be kept to a minimum. Because many of these children are able to attend regular classes, the teacher may need assistance in adapting methods of teaching for the child's benefit. The school nurse is often in an optimal position to emphasize methods of facilitated communication, such as lipreading (see Guidelines box, p. 1189). Because group projects and audiovisual teaching aids may hinder the child's learning, these educational methods should be carefully evaluated.

Support Child and Family

After the diagnosis of hearing impairment is made, parents need extensive support to adjust to the shock of learning about their child's disability and an opportunity to realize the extent of the hearing loss. If the hearing loss occurs during childhood, the child also requires sensitive, supportive care during the long and often difficult adjustment to this sensory loss. Early rehabilitation is one of the best strategies for fostering adjustment. However, progress in learning communication may not always coincide with emotional adjustment. Depression or anger is common, and such feelings are a normal part of the grieving process.

Care for Child During Hospitalization

The needs of the hospitalized child with impaired hearing are the same as those of any other child, but the disability presents special challenges to the nurse. For example, verbal explanations must be supplemented by tactile and visual aids, such as books or actual demonstration and practice. Children's understanding of the explanation needs to be constantly reassessed. If their verbal skills are poorly developed, they can answer questions through drawing, writing, or gesturing. For example, if the nurse is attempting to clarify where a spinal tap is done, the child is asked to point to where the procedure will be done on the body. Because these children often need more time to grasp the full meaning of an explanation, the nurse needs to be patient, allowing ample time for understanding.

When communicating with the child, the nurse should use the same principles as those outlined for facilitating lipreading. Ideally, nurses without foreign accents should be assigned to the child. The child's hearing aid is checked to ensure that it is working properly. If it is necessary to awaken the child at night, the nurse gently shakes the child or turns on the hearing aid before arousing the child. The nurse always makes certain that the child can see him or her before any procedures, even routine ones such as changing a diaper or regulating an infusion. It is important to remember that the child may not be aware of one's presence until alerted through visual or tactile cues.

Ideally, parents are encouraged to room with the child. However, it must be conveyed to them that this is not to serve as a convenience to the nurse but as a benefit to the child. Although the parents' aid can be enlisted in familiarizing the child with the hospital and explaining procedures, the nurse also talks directly to the youngster, encouraging expression of

---

**Directory listings stating "TDD or TTY only" before a phone number indicate that regular telephone use is not possible; "TDD or TTY and voice" indicates that both TDD/TYY users and speaking, hearing people can use the telephone number.*

†Additional information is available from the National Captioning Institute, 1900 Gallows Road, Suite 3000, Vienna, VA 22182; 703-917-7600; fax: 703-917-9853; www.ncicap.org.

feelings about the experience. If the child's speech is difficult to understand, the nurse makes an effort to become familiar with his or her pronunciation of words. Parents often can be helpful by explaining the child's usual speech habits. Nonverbal communication devices that employ pictures or words that the child can point to are also available. Such boards can also be made by drawing pictures or writing the words of common needs on cardboard, such as *parent, food, water,* or *toilet.*

The nurse has a special role as child advocate and is in a strategic position to alert other health team members and other patients to the child's special needs regarding communication. For example, the nurse should accompany other practitioners on visits to the child's room to ensure that they speak to the child and that the child understands what is said. Caregivers sometimes forget that the child has the abilities to perceive and learn despite a hearing loss, and consequently they communicate only with the parents. As a result, the child's needs and feelings remain unrecognized and unmet.

Because children with impaired hearing may have difficulty forming social relationships with other children, the child is introduced to roommates and encouraged to engage in play activities. The hospital setting can provide growth-promoting opportunities for social relationships. With the assistance of a child life specialist, the child can learn new recreational activities, experiment with group games, and engage in therapeutic play. The use of puppets, dollhouses, role-playing with dress-up clothes, building with a hammer and nails, finger painting, and water play can help the child express feelings that previously were suppressed.

Assist in Measures to Prevent Hearing Impairment

A primary nursing role is prevention of hearing loss. Because the most common cause of impaired hearing is chronic otitis media, it is essential that appropriate measures be instituted to treat existing infections and prevent recurrences. Children with a history of ear or respiratory tract infections or any other condition known to increase the risk of hearing impairment should receive periodic auditory testing.

To prevent the causes of hearing loss that begin prenatally and perinatally, pregnant women need counseling regarding the necessity of early prenatal care, including genetic counseling for known familial disorders; avoidance of all ototoxic drugs, especially during the first trimester; tests to rule out syphilis, rubella, or blood incompatibility; medical management of maternal diabetes; strict control of alcohol intake; adequate dietary intake; and avoidance of smoke exposure. The necessity of routine immunization during childhood to eliminate the possibility of acquired sensorineural hearing loss from rubella, mumps, or measles (encephalitis) is stressed.

Excessive noise pollution with or without smoke exposure causes sensorineural hearing loss (Daniel, 2007). The nurse should routinely assess the possibility of environmental pollution (e.g. loud noise and smoking) and advise children and parents of the potential danger of hearing loss. When individuals engage in activities associated with high-intensity noise, such as flying model airplanes, target shooting, or snowmobiling, they should wear ear protection such as earmuffs or earplugs. Even common household equipment, such as lawn mowers, vacuum cleaners, and cordless telephones, may cause noise-induced hearing loss.

NURSING ALERT Suspect hazardous noise if the listener experiences (1) difficulty in communication while hearing the sound, (2) ringing in the ears (tinnitus) after exposure to the sound, or (3) muffled hearing after leaving the sound.

Visual Impairment

Visual impairment is a common problem during childhood. In the United States the prevalence of blindness and serious visual impairment in the pediatric population is estimated at 30 to 64 children per 100,000 population. Vision problems occur in 5% to 10% of all preschoolers and include refractive error, strabismus, and amblyopia (Tingley, 2007). The nurse's role is clearly one of early assessment and detection, prevention, referral, and, in some instances, rehabilitation.

Definition and Classification

Visual impairment is a general term that refers to visual loss that cannot be corrected with regular prescription lenses. However, more useful definitions for classifying visual impairments exist. *School vision* (also known as *partially sighted*) refers to visual acuity between 20/70 and 20/200. The child should be able to obtain an education in the usual public school system with the use of normal-sized print. Near vision is almost always better than distance vision. *Legal blindness,* visual acuity of 20/200 or less and/or a visual field of 20 degrees or less in the better eye, is useful only as a legal definition, not as a medical diagnosis. It allows special considerations with regard to taxes, entrance into special schools, eligibility for aid, and other benefits.

Etiology

Visual impairment can be caused by a number of genetic and prenatal or postnatal conditions. These include perinatal infections (herpes, chlamydia, gonococci, rubella, syphilis, toxoplasmosis); retinopathy of prematurity; trauma; postnatal infections (meningitis); and disorders such as sickle cell disease, juvenile rheumatoid arthritis, Tay-Sachs disease, albinism, and retinoblastoma. In many instances, such as with refractive errors, the cause of the defect is unknown.

Refractive errors are the most common types of visual disorders in children. The term *refraction* means bending and refers to the bending of light rays as they pass through the lens of the eye. Normally, light rays enter the lens and fall directly on the retina. However, in refractive disorders the light rays either fall in front of the retina *(myopia)* or beyond it *(hyperopia).* Other eye problems, such as strabismu[illegible] may or may not include refractive errors, but they are i[illegible]portant because, if untreated, they result in blindness fr[illegible] amblyopia. These, along with other less frequent visu[illegible] disorders, are summarized in Box 42-6. In addition t[illegible]ese disorders, other visual problems can be a result of i[illegible]ction or trauma.

Trauma

Trauma is a co[illegible]n cause of blindness in children. Injuries to the ey[illegible] and adnexa (supporting or accessory structures, suc[illegible] eyelids, conjunctiva, or lacrimal glands) can

BOX 42-6 Types of Visual Impairment

Refractive Errors

Myopia

Nearsightedness—Ability to see objects clearly at close range but not at a distance

Pathophysiology

Results from eyeball that is too long, causing image to fall in front of retina

Clinical Manifestations

Excessive eye rubbing
Head tilt or forward head thrusts
Difficulty in reading or doing other close work
Headaches
Dizziness
Clumsiness; walking into objects
Blinking more than usual or irritability when doing close work
Inability to see objects clearly
Poor school performance, especially in subjects that require demonstration, such as arithmetic

Treatment

Corrected with biconcave lenses that focus rays on retina
May be corrected with laser surgery

Hyperopia

Farsightedness—Ability to see objects at a distance

Pathophysiology

Results from eyeball that is too short, causing image to focus beyond retina

Clinical Manifestations

Because of accommodative ability, usually an ability to see objects at all ranges
Most children normally hyperopic until about 7 years of age

Treatment

When required, corrected with convex lenses that focus rays on retina
May be corrected with laser surgery

Astigmatism

Unequal curvatures in refractive apparatus

Pathophysiology

Results from unequal curvatures in cornea or lens that cause light rays to bend in different directions

Clinical Manifestations

Depend on severity of refractive error in each eye
Possible clinical manifestations of myopia

Treatment

Corrected with special lenses that compensate for refractive errors
May be corrected with laser surgery

Anisometropia

Different refractive [illegible]trength in each eye

Pathophysiology

May develop amblyopia a[illegible]weaker eye is used less

Clinical Manifestations

Depend on severity of refractive [illegible]or in each eye
Possible clinical manifestations of [illegible]pia

Treatment

Treated with corrective lenses, preferably [illegible]act lenses, to improve vision in each eye so they work [illegible]unit
May be corrected with laser surgery

Amblyopia

Lazy eye—Reduced visual acuity in one eye

Pathophysiology

Results when one eye does not receive sufficient stimulation
Each retina receives different images, resulting in diplopia (double vision)
Brain accommodates by suppressing less intense image
Visual cortex eventually does not respond to visual stimulation, with resultant loss of vision in that eye

Clinical Manifestations

Poor vision in affected eye

Treatment

Preventable if treatment of primary visual defect, such as anisometropia or strabismus, begins before 6 years of age

Strabismus

"Squint" or cross-eye—Malalignment of eyes
Estropia—Inward deviation of eye
Exotropia—Outward deviation of eye

Pathophysiology

May result from muscle imbalance or paralysis, poor vision, or congenital defect
Because visual axes are not parallel, brain receives two images, and amblyopia can result

Clinical Manifestations

Squints eyelids together or frowns
Has difficulty focusing from one distance to another
Inaccurate judgment in picking up objects
Unable to see print or moving objects clearly
Closes one eye to see
Tilts head to one side
If combined with refractive errors, may see any of the manifestations listed for refractive errors
Diplopia
Photophobia
Dizziness
Headaches
Crossed eyes

Treatment

Depends on cause of strabismus
May involve occlusion therapy (patching stronger eye) or surgery to increase visual stimulation to weaker eye
Early diagnosis essential to prevent vision loss

Cataracts

Opacity of crystalline lens

Pathophysiology

Prevents light rays from entering eye and refracting on retina

Clinical Manifestations

Gradual decrease in ability to see objects clearly
Possible loss of peripheral vision
Nystagmus (with complete blindness)
Gray opacities of lens
Strabismus
Absence of red reflex

BOX 42-6 Types of Visual Impairment—cont'd

Cataracts—cont'd

Treatment

Requires surgery to remove cloudy lens and replace lens (with intraocular lens implant, removable contact lens, prescription glasses)

Must be treated early to prevent blindness from amblyopia

Glaucoma

Increased intraocular pressure

Pathophysiology

Congenital type results from defective development of some component related to flow of aqueous humor

Increased pressure on optic nerve causes eventual atrophy and blindness

Clinical Manifestations

Loss of peripheral vision—mostly seen in acquired types

Possible bumping into objects

Perception of halos around objects

Possible complaint of pain or discomfort (pain, nausea, or vomiting if sudden rise in pressure)

Eye redness

Excessive tearing (epiphora)

Photophobia

Spasmodic winking (blepharospasm)

Corneal haziness

Enlargement of eyeball (buphthalmos)

Treatment

Requires surgical treatment (goniotomy) to open outflow tracts

May require more than one procedure

be classified as penetrating or nonpenetrating. *Penetrating wounds* are most often a result of sharp instruments, such as sticks, knives, or scissors; propulsive objects, such as firecrackers, bullets from guns, arrows, or rocks from slingshots; or a powerful contusion by a blunt object, which may occur during a fight or from a serious car accident. *Nonpenetrating injuries* may be a result of foreign objects in the eyes, lacerations, a blow from a blunt object such as a ball (from baseball, softball, basketball, or racquet sports) or fist, or thermal or chemical burns.

Treatment is aimed at preventing further ocular damage and is primarily the responsibility of the ophthalmologist. It involves adequate examination of the injured eye (with the child sedated or anesthetized in severe injuries); appropriate immediate intervention, such as removal of the foreign body or suturing of the laceration; and prevention of complications, such as administration of antibiotics or steroids and complete bed rest to allow the eye to heal and blood to reabsorb (see Emergency box). The prognosis varies according to the type

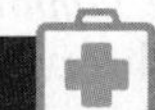

EMERGENCY

Eye Injuries

Foreign Object

Examine eye for presence of a foreign body (evert upper lid to examine upper eye).

Remove a freely movable object with pointed corner of gauze pad lightly moistened with water.

Do not irrigate eye or attempt to remove a penetrating object (see following section).

Caution child against rubbing eye.

Chemical Burns

Irrigate eye copiously with tap water for 20 minutes.

Evert upper lid to flush thoroughly.

Hold child's head with eye under tap of running lukewarm water.

Take to emergency department.

Have child rest with eyes closed.

Keep room darkened.

Ultraviolet Burns

If skin is burned, patch both eyes (make certain lids are completely closed); secure dressing with Kling bandages wrapped around head rather than tape.

Have child rest with eyes closed.

Refer to an ophthalmologist.

Hematoma ("Black Eye")

Use a flashlight to check for gross *hyphema* (hemorrhage into anterior chamber; visible fluid meniscus across iris; more easily seen in light-colored than in brown eyes).

Apply ice for first 24 hours to reduce swelling if no hyphema is present.

Refer to an ophthalmologist immediately if hyphema is present.

Have child rest with eyes closed.

Penetrating Injuries

Take child to emergency department.

Never remove an object that has penetrated eye.

Follow strict aseptic technique in examining eye.

Observe for:

- Aqueous or vitreous leaks (fluid leaking from point of penetration)
- Hyphema
- Shape and equality of pupils, reaction to light, prolapsed iris (not perfectly circular)

Apply a Fox shield if available (not a regular eye patch) and apply patch over unaffected eye to prevent bilateral movement.

Maintain bed rest with child in 30-degree Fowler's position.

Caution child against rubbing eye.

Refer to ophthalmologist.

of injury. It is usually guarded in all cases of penetrating wounds because of the high risk of serious complications.

Infections

Infections of the adnexa and structures of the eyeball or globe may occur in children. The most common eye infection is *conjunctivitis*. Treatment is usually with ophthalmic antibiotics. Severe infections may require systemic antibiotic therapy. Steroids are used cautiously because they exacerbate viral infections such as herpes simplex, increasing the risk of damage to the involved structures.

Nursing Care Management

Assessment of children for visual impairment is a critical nursing responsibility. Discovery of a visual impairment as early as possible is essential to prevent social, physical, and psychologic damage to the child. Assessment involves (1) identifying those children who by virtue of their history are at risk, (2) observing for behaviors that indicate a vision loss, and (3) screening all children for visual acuity and signs of other ocular disorders such as strabismus. This discussion focuses on clinical manifestations of various types of visual problems (see Box 42-6). Vision testing is discussed in Chapter 34.

Infancy

At birth the nurse should observe the neonate's response to visual stimuli, such as following a light or object and cessation of body movement. The infant may vary in the intensity of the response, depending on the state of alertness.

Of special importance in detecting visual impairment during infancy are the parents' concerns regarding visual responsiveness in their child. Their concerns, such as lack of eye contact from the infant, must be taken seriously. During infancy the child should be tested for strabismus. Lack of binocularity after 4 months of age is considered abnormal and must be treated to prevent amblyopia.

NURSING ALERT Suspect blindness if the infant does not react to light or if parents of a child at any age express concern.

Childhood

Because the most common visual impairment during childhood is refractive errors, testing for visual acuity is essential. The school nurse usually assumes major responsibility for vision testing in schoolchildren. In addition to refractive errors, the nurse should be aware of signs and symptoms that indicate other ocular problems.

Promote Parent-Child Attachment

A crucial time in the life of blind infants is when they and their parents are getting acquainted with each other. Pleasurable patterns of interaction between the infant and parents may be lacking if there is not enough reciprocity. For example, if the parent gazes fondly at the infant's face and seeks eye contact but the infant fails to respond because he or she cannot see the parent, a troubled cycle of responses may occur. The nurse can help parents learn to look for other cues that indicate the infant is responding to them, such as whether the eyelids blink; whether the activity level accelerates or slows; whether respiratory patterns change, such as faster or slower breathing, when the parents come near; and whether the infant makes throaty sounds when they speak to the infant. In time parents learn that the infant has unique ways of relating to them. They are encouraged to show affection using nonvisual methods, such as talking or reading, cuddling, and walking the child.

Promote Child's Optimum Development

Promoting the child's optimum development requires rehabilitation in a number of important areas. These include learning self-help skills and appropriate communication techniques to become independent. Although nurses may not be directly involved in such programs, they can provide direction and guidance to families regarding the availability of programs and the need to promote these activities in their child.

Development and Independence

Motor development depends on sight almost as much as verbal communication depends on hearing. From earliest infancy, parents are encouraged to expose the infant to as many visual-motor experiences as possible, such as sitting supported in an infant seat or swing and being given opportunities for holding up the head, sitting unsupported, reaching for objects, and crawling.

Despite visual impairment, the child can become independent in all aspects of self-care. The same principles used for promoting independence in sighted children apply, with additional emphasis on nonvisual cues. For example, the child may need help in dressing, such as special arrangement of clothing for style coordination and braille tags to distinguish colors and prints.

The blind child also must learn to become independent in navigational skills. The two main techniques are the *tapping method* (use of a cane to survey the environment for direction and to avoid obstacles) and *guides,* such as a sighted human guide or a dog guide, such as a Seeing Eye dog. Children who are partially sighted may benefit from ocular aids, such as a monocular telescope.

Play and Socialization

Blind children do not learn to play automatically. Because they cannot imitate others or actively explore the environment as sighted children do, they depend much more on others to stimulate and teach them how to play. Parents need help in selecting appropriate play material, especially those that encourage fine and gross motor development and stimulate the senses of hearing, touch, and smell. Toys with educational value are especially useful, such as dolls with various clothing closures.

Blind children have the same needs for socialization as sighted children. Because they have little difficulty in learning verbal skills, they are able to communicate with age-mates and participate in suitable activities. The nurse discusses with parents opportunities for socialization outside the home, especially regular preschools. The trend is to include these children with sighted children to help them adjust to the outside world for eventual independence.

To compensate for inadequate stimulation, these children may develop *blindisms* (self-stimulatory activities, such as body rocking, finger flicking, or arm twirling). Such habits restrict the child's social acceptance and are discouraged. Behavior modification is often successful in reducing or eliminating blindisms.

Education

The main obstacle to learning is the child's total dependence on nonvisual cues. Although the child can learn via verbal lecturing, he or she is unable to read the written word or to write without special education. Therefore the child must rely on *braille*, a system that uses raised dots to represent letters and numbers. The child can then read the braille with the fingers and can write a message using a braille writer. However, unless others read braille, this system is not useful for communicating with others. A more portable system for written communication is the use of a braille slate and stylus or a microcassette tape recorder. A recorder is especially helpful for leaving messages for others and taking notes during classroom lectures. For mathematic calculations, portable calculators with voice synthesizers are available.*

Records and tapes are significant sources of reading material other than braille books, which are large and cumbersome. The Library of Congress† has talking books, braille books, and a special records program, which are available at many local and state libraries and directly from the Library of Congress. The talking book machine and tape player are provided at no cost to families, and there is no postage fee for returning the materials. Recording for the Blind and Dyslexic‡ also provides texts and tapes of books, which are helpful for secondary and college students who are blind.

Learning to use a regular typewriter is another form of writing but has the disadvantage of the blind person's being unable to check what he or she has written. Computers eliminate this drawback; a home computer with a voice synthesizer can be adapted to speak each letter or word that has been typed.

The child with partial sight benefits from specialized visual aids that produce a magnified retinal image. The basic devices are accommodation (e.g., bringing the object closer), special plus lenses, handheld and stand magnifiers, telescopes, video projection systems, and large print. Special equipment is available to enlarge print. Information about services for the partially sighted is available from the National Association for Visually Handicapped and American Foundation for the Blind. Children with diminished vision often prefer to do close work without their glasses and compensate by bringing the object very near to their eyes. This should be allowed. The exception is the child with vision in only one eye, who should always wear glasses for protection.

Care for the Child During Hospitalization

Because nurses are more likely to care for children who are hospitalized for procedures that involve temporary loss of vision than for children who are blind, the following discussion concentrates primarily on the needs of such children. The nursing care objectives in either situation are to (1) reassure the child and family throughout every phase of treatment, (2) orient the child to the surroundings, (3) provide a safe environment, and (4) encourage independence. Whenever possible, the same nurse should care for the child to ensure consistency in the approach.

When sighted children temporarily lose their vision, almost every aspect of the environment becomes bewildering and frightening. They are forced to rely on nonvisual senses for help in adjusting to the blindness without the benefit of any special training. Nurses have a major role in minimizing the effects of temporary loss of vision. They need to talk to the child about everything that is occurring, emphasizing aspects of procedures that are felt or heard. They should approach the child by always identifying themselves as soon as they enter the room. Because unfamiliar sounds are especially frightening, these are explained. Parents are encouraged to room with their child and participate in the care. Familiar objects, such as a teddy bear or doll, should be brought from home to help lessen the strangeness of the hospital. As soon as the child is able to be out of bed, he or she is oriented to the immediate surroundings. If the child is able to see on admission, this opportunity is taken to point out significant aspects of the room. The child is encouraged to practice ambulation with the eyes closed to become accustomed to this experience.

The room is arranged with safety in mind. For example, a stool or chair is placed next to the bed to help the child climb in and out of bed. The furniture is always placed in the same position to prevent collisions. Cleaning personnel are reminded of the need to keep the room in order. If the child has difficulty navigating by feeling the walls, a rope can be attached from the bed to the point of destination, such as the bathroom. Attention to details such as well-fitting slippers or robes that do not drag on the floor is important in preventing tripping. Unlike the child who is blind, these children are not familiar with navigating with a cane.

The child is encouraged to be independent in self-care activities, especially if the visual loss may be prolonged or potentially permanent. For example, during bathing the nurse sets up all the equipment and encourages the child to participate. At mealtime the nurse explains where each food item is on the tray, opens any special containers, prepares cereal or toast, and encourages the child in self-feeding. Favorite finger foods, such as sandwiches, hamburgers, hot dogs, or pizza, may be good selections. The child is praised for efforts at being cooperative and independent. Any improvements made in self-care, no matter how small, are stressed.

Appropriate recreational activities are provided, and if a child life specialist is available, such planning is done jointly. Because children with temporary blindness have a wide variety of play experiences to draw on, they are encouraged to select activities. For example, if they like to read, they may enjoy being read to. If they prefer manual activity, they may appreciate playing with clay or building blocks or feeling different textures and naming them. If they need an outlet for aggression, activities such as pounding or banging on a drum can be helpful. Simple board and card games can be played with a

---

**A catalog of numerous products for people with vision problems is available from American Foundation for the Blind from Lighthouse International, 111 E. 59th St., New York, NY 10022-1202; 212-821-9200 or 800-829-0500;* www.lighthouse.org.

†National Library Service for the Blind and Physically Handicapped, 888-657-7323; TTD: 202-707-0744; fax: 202-707-0712; www.loc.gov/nls. *(A state-by-state listing of libraries for blind and physically handicapped readers, as well as other reference circulars, is available from this office.)*

‡20 Roszel Road, Princeton, NJ 08540; 800-221-4792 or 866-RFBD-585; www.rfbd.org.

"seeing partner" or an opponent who helps with the game. They should have familiar toys from home to play with, since familiar items are more easily manipulated than new ones. If parents want to bring presents, they should be objects that stimulate hearing and touch, such as a radio, music box, or stuffed animal.

Occasionally, children who are blind come to the hospital for procedures to restore their vision. Although this is an extremely happy time, it also requires intervention to help them adjust to sight. They need an opportunity to take in all that they see. They should not be bombarded with visual stimuli. They may need to concentrate on people's faces or their own to become accustomed to this experience. They often need to talk about what they see and to compare the visual images with their mental ones. The children may also go through a period of depression, which must be respected and supported. The nurse or parents should refrain from statements such as "How can you be so sad when you can see again?" Instead the children should be encouraged to discuss how it feels to see, especially in terms of seeing themselves.

Newly sighted children also need time to adjust to the ability to engage in activities that were impossible before. For example, they may prefer to use braille to read, rather than learning a new "visual approach," because of familiarity with the touch system. Eventually, as they learn to recognize letters and numbers, they will integrate these new skills into reading and writing. However, parents and teachers must be careful not to push them before they are ready. This applies to social relationships and physical activities as well as learning situations.

Assist in Measures to Prevent Visual Impairment

An essential nursing goal is to prevent visual impairment. This involves many of the same interventions discussed under hearing impairments:

- Prenatal screening for pregnant women at risk, such as those with rubella or syphilis infection and family histories of genetic disorders associated with visual loss
- Adequate prenatal and perinatal care to prevent prematurity
- Periodic screening of all children, especially newborns through preschoolers, for congenital blindness and visual impairments caused by refractive errors, strabismus, and other disorders
- Rubella immunization of all children
- Safety counseling regarding the common causes of ocular trauma and safe practices when working with, playing with, or carrying objects such as scissors, knives, and balls

NURSING ALERT A helmet with a face mask should be required for children playing football, hockey, or baseball.

After detection of eye problems, the nurse has a responsibility to prevent further ocular damage by ensuring that corrective treatment is used. For the child with strabismus, this often necessitates occlusion patching of the stronger eye. Compliance with the procedure is greatest during the early preschool years. It is more difficult to encourage school-age children to wear the occlusive patch because the poor visual acuity of the uncovered weaker eye interferes with school work and the patch sets them apart from their peers. In school they benefit from being positioned favorably (closer to the chalkboard or other visual media) and allowed extra time to read or complete an assignment. If treatment of the eye disorder requires instillation of ophthalmic medication, the family is taught the correct procedure (see Chapter 45).

For the child with refractive errors, the nurse helps the child adjust to wearing *glasses*. Young children who often pull glasses off benefit from temporal pieces that wrap around the ears or an elastic strap attached to the frames and around the back of the head to hold the glasses on securely. After children appreciate the value of clear vision, they are more likely to wear the corrective lenses.

Glasses should not interfere with any activity. Special protective guards are available during contact sports to prevent accidental injury, and all corrective lenses should be made from safety glass, which is shatterproof. Often, corrective lenses improve visual acuity so dramatically that children are able to compete more effectively in sports. This in itself is a tremendous inducement to continue wearing glasses.

Contact lenses are a popular alternative, especially for adolescents. Several types are available, such as hard lenses, including gas-permeable ones, and soft lenses, which may be designed for daily or extended wear. Contact lenses offer several advantages over glasses, such as greater visual acuity, total corrected field of vision, convenience (especially with the extended-wear type), and optimal cosmetic benefit. Unfortunately, they are usually more expensive and require much more care than glasses, including considerable practice to learn techniques for insertion and removal. If they are prescribed, the nurse can be helpful in teaching parents or older children how to care for the lenses.

Because trauma is the leading cause of blindness, the nurse has the major responsibility of preventing further eye injury until specific treatment is instituted. The major principles to follow when caring for an eye injury are outlined in the Emergency box on p. 1193. Because patients with a serious eye injury fear blindness, the nurse should stay with the child and family to provide support and reassurance.

Deaf-Blind Children

The most traumatic sensory impairment is loss of sight and hearing. Obviously, auditory and visual disabilities have profound effects on the child's development. They interfere with the normal sequence of physical, intellectual, and psychosocial growth. Although such children often achieve the usual motor milestones, their rate of development is slower. These children learn communication only with specialized training. *Finger spelling* is one desirable method often taught to these children. Some deaf-blind children, especially those with residual hearing or sight, can learn to speak. Whenever possible, speech is encouraged because it allows communication with other individuals.

The future prospects for deaf-blind children are, at best, unpredictable. Congenital blindness or deafness may be accompanied by other physical or neurologic problems, which further diminish the child's learning potential. The most favorable prognosis is for children who have acquired deafness and blindness and have few, if any, associated disabilities. Their learning capacity is greatly potentiated by their developmental progress before the sensory impairments. Although total independence, including gainful vocational training, is the goal, some deaf-blind children are unable to develop to this level. They may require lifelong parental or residential care. The nurse working with such families helps them deal with future goals for the child, including possible alternatives to home care during the parents' advancing years.

Retinoblastoma

Retinoblastoma, which arises from the retina, is the most common congenital malignant intraocular tumor of childhood. Approximately 11 cases per million occur annually, primarily in children younger than 5 years of age. Retinoblastoma is caused by a mutation in a gene and may occur sporadically or be inherited (Hurwitz et al, 2006). Retinoblastoma develops when the mutated gene is unable to produce the natural signals to stop the growth of retinal cells. The majority of cases are nonhereditary and unilateral, with the remainder divided between hereditary and unilateral, and hereditary and bilateral. Hereditary retinoblastomas are transmitted as an autosomal dominant trait with 90% penetrance (Hurwitz et al, 2006).

Diagnostic Evaluation

Retinoblastoma has few grossly obvious signs (Box 42-7). Typically the most common sign is observed by the parent as a whitish "glow" in the pupil, known as the white reflex or *leukokoria*. Leukokoria represents visualization of the tumor as the light momentarily falls on the mass. The second most common sign of retinoblastoma is acquired strabismus (Hurwitz et al, 2006).

The first step in diagnosis is carefully listening to and recognizing the significance of reports from family members regarding suspected abnormalities within the eye. Eye abnormalities, including white reflex, strabismus, decreased vision, and persistent painful erythematous eyes, are referred to an ophthalmologist. Definitive diagnosis is usually based on ophthalmoscopic examination with the patient under general anesthesia. Imaging studies, including ultrasonography and computed tomography of the orbit, are done to determine the extent of the disease.

Therapeutic Management

The aim of therapy is to preserve useful vision and eradicate the tumor. Treatment of retinoblastoma depends chiefly on the stage of the tumor at the time of diagnosis. Some of the common focal therapies are (1) plaque brachytherapy (surgical radioactive implant on the sclera until maximum dose has been delivered to the tumor), (2) laser photocoagulation (laser beam to coagulate blood supply to the tumor), (3) cryotherapy (freezing the tumor by destroying the microcirculation to the tumor through microcrystal formation), and (4) thermotherapy (using microwaves or infrared radiation to deliver heat to the tumor) (Melamud, Palekar, & Singh, 2006; De Potter, 2002; Schouten–van Meeteren et al, 2002). Chemoreduction and chemoprevention minimize the use of external beam radiation treatment and therefore reduce the risk of radiation-induced malignancies and facial disfigurement.

With advanced tumor growth into the optic nerve, choroid, orbit, and anterior chamber or no hope for useful vision, *enucleation* (removal) of the affected eye is the treatment of choice. After enucleation, an orbital implant is placed to provide a more natural cosmetic appearance, minimize sinking of the prosthesis, and enable motility of the prosthesis. With bilateral disease, every attempt is made to preserve useful vision in both eyes. Chemotherapy, external beam, radiotherapy, and other treatments (i.e., cryotherapy, laser, plaque brachytherapy, thermotherapy) to both eyes may prevent the need for enucleation.

Prognosis

The overall prognosis for retinoblastoma is favorable, with a survival rate of nearly 90% for both unilateral and bilateral tumors. Retinoblastoma is one of the tumors that may spontaneously regress. Of major concern in long-term survivors is the development of decreased visual acuity; facial disfiguration; and secondary tumors, especially osteogenic sarcoma, other sarcomas, and melanoma. Children with bilateral disease (hereditary form) are more likely to develop secondary cancers than are children with unilateral disease. It is thought that these individuals are predisposed to developing cancer and that radiation increases their risk.

BOX 42-7 Clinical Manifestations of Retinoblastoma

- White eye reflex (most common sign)
- Strabismus (second most common sign)
- Red, painful eye, often with glaucoma
- Blindness (late sign)

Nursing Care Management

One of the most important nursing goals is to have a high index of suspicion for this rare malignancy. If parents report noticing a strange light in the eye or expression, these concerns must be taken seriously. Families with a history of retinoblastoma require follow-up, and the nurse can be instrumental in reminding parents of appointments.

Because the tumor is usually diagnosed in infants or very young children, most of the preparation for diagnostic tests and treatment involves parents. After indirect ophthalmoscopy, the child may not see clearly, or the eyes may be sensitive to light because of pupillary dilation. Parents are made aware of these normal reactions before the procedure. Screening tests, such as bone surveys and bone marrow aspiration, are rarely performed unless metastatic disease is suspected.

The treatment plan may include focal intraocular therapy with or without chemotherapy, external beam radiation, and, if necessary, enucleation. Enucleation is the treatment of choice if there is extensive disease threatening metastasis or no chance for useful vision. The enucleation procedure and the positive benefits of a prosthesis are explained to the parents. Showing them pictures of another child with an artificial eye may help them adjust to the thought of disfigurement.

After surgery the parents are prepared for the child's facial appearance. An eye patch is in place, and the child's face may be edematous or ecchymotic. Parents often fear seeing the surgical site because they imagine a cavity in the skull. A surgically implanted sphere maintains the shape of the eyeball, and the implant is covered with conjunctiva. When the lids are open, the exposed area resembles the mucosal lining of the mouth. After the child is fitted for a prosthesis, usually within 3 weeks, the facial appearance returns to normal. Initial instructions for care of the prosthesis are given by the ocularist who fits and manufactures the device.

Care of the socket is minimal and easily accomplished. The wound itself is clean and has little or no drainage. If an antibiotic ointment is prescribed, it is applied in a thin line on the surface of the tissues of the socket. To cleanse the site, an irrigating solution may be ordered and is instilled daily or more frequently, *before* application of the antibiotic ointment. The dressing, consisting of an eye pad taped over the surgical site, is changed daily. After the socket has healed completely, a dressing is no longer necessary, although it is a preventive measure against infection.

Autism Spectrum Disorders

Autism spectrum disorders (ASDs) are complex neurodevelopmental disorders of brain function accompanied by intellectual and social behavioral deficits. ASDs include autistic disorder, Asperger's syndrome, and pervasive developmental disorder not otherwise specified, which are impairments ranging from mild to severe (Croen et al, 2006). ASD is typically noticed during early childhood, primarily from 24 to 48 months of age. It occurs in 1 in 166 children; is about four times more common in males than in females (although females are more severely affected); and is not related to socioeconomic level, race, or parenting style (Courtney-Manning, 2007; Schaefer & Lutz, 2006; Fombonne, 2003).

Etiology

ASD is now recognized as a genetic disorder of prenatal and postnatal brain development (Bloom-DiCicco et al, 2006). Immune and environmental factors (e.g., viral infections) may interact with the genetic susceptibility to increase the incidence of ASD (Bloom-DiCicco et al, 2006). Individuals with ASD may have abnormal electroencephalograms, epileptic seizures, delayed development of hand dominance, persistence of primitive reflexes, metabolic abnormalities (elevated blood serotonin), cerebellar vermal hypoplasia (part of the brain involved in regulating motion and some aspects of memory), and infantile abnormal head enlargement (Dawson, 2007; Bloom-DiCicco et al, 2006).

The strong evidence for a genetic basis in twins is consistent with an autosomal recessive pattern of inheritance. Twin studies demonstrate a high concordance (60% to 96%) for monozygotic (identical) twins and less than 5% concordance for dizygotic (nonidentical) twins. In addition, between 5% and 16% of males with ASD are positive for the fragile X chromosome.

There is a relatively high risk of recurrence of ASD in families with one affected child (Schaefer & Lutz, 2006; Muhle, Trentacoste, & Rapin, 2004). Although several genes have been suggested as possible causative factors in ASD, no specific gene for the disorder has been identified (Dawson, 2007; Kolevzon, Gross, & Reichenberg, 2007; Schanen, 2006).

Contrary to previous reports, autism does not appear to be caused by the measles-mumps-rubella (MMR) and thimerosal-containing vaccines (D'Souza, Fombonne, & Ward, 2006; DeStefano et al, 2004; Muhle, Trentacoste, & Rapin, 2004) (see Evidence-Based Practice box). ASD has been reported in association with a number of conditions such as fragile X syndrome, tuberous sclerosis, metabolic disorders, fetal rubella syndrome, *Haemophilus influenzae* meningitis, and structural brain anomalies (Dawson, 2007; Muhle, Trentacoste, & Rapin, 2004). Recent reports have retrospectively tied ASD to prenatal and perinatal events such as maternal and paternal ages over 40 years (for fathers, 1 in 116 births; for mothers, 1 in 123 births), uterine bleeding during pregnancy, low Apgar score, fetal distress, and neonatal hyperbilirubinemia (Croen et al, 2007; Kolevzon, Gross, & Reichenberg, 2007; Muhle, Trentacoste, & Rapin, 2004). These same researchers, however, urge caution in interpreting these findings.

Clinical Manifestations and Diagnostic Evaluation

Children with ASD demonstrate several peculiar and often seemingly bizarre characteristics, primarily in social interactions, communication, and behavior. One hallmark characteristic is the inability to maintain eye contact with another person. Parents of autistic children have noted their infants had difficulties with eye contact, avoidance of body contact, and language delay at a very early age (Belschner, 2007; Dawson, 2007). Children with ASD also display limited functional play and may interact with toys in an unusual or odd manner (Belschner, 2007). ASD children may have significant gastrointestinal symptoms. Constipation is a common symptom and can be associated with acquired megarectum in children with ASD (Afzal et al, 2003). Other clinical manifestations typically seen in children with autism are described in Box 42-8.

Children with autism do not always have the same manifestations; cases vary from mild forms requiring minimal supervision, to severe forms in which self-abusive behavior is common. The majority (50% to 70%) of children with autism have some degree of CI, with scores typically in the moderate to severe range. More females than males tend to have very low intelligence scores. Despite their relatively moderate to severe disability, some children with autism (known as *savants*) excel in particular areas, such as art, music, memory, mathematics, or perceptual skills such as puzzle building.

Speech and language delays are also common in ASD children. Any child who does not display such language skills as babbling or gesturing by 12 months, single words by 16 months, and two-word phrases by 24 months is recommended for immediate hearing and language evaluation (Grizzle & Simms, 2005). A sudden deterioration in extant expressive speech is also a red-flag event for further evaluation.

Early recognition, referral, diagnosis, and intensive early intervention tend to improve outcomes for children with ASD (Belschner, 2007; Courtney-Manning, 2007). Unfortunately, diagnosis is often not made until 2 to 3 years after symptoms

EVIDENCE-BASED PRACTICE Thimerosal-Containing Vaccines and Autism Spectrum Disorders

Ask the Question

Is the incidence of autism spectrum disorders (ASDs) or other neurodevelopmental disorders increased in children receiving vaccines containing thimerosal?

Search for Evidence

Search Strategies

English language publications within the past 15 years, research-based articles (level 3 or lower), and child populations

Databases Searched

PubMed, Cochrane Collaboration, MD Consult, Vaccine Adverse Events Reporting System (VAERS) database, American Academy of Pediatrics, Autism Research Institute

Critically Analyze the Evidence

A two-phased retrospective study used computerized health maintenance organization (HMO) databases to assess the possible toxicity of thimerosal-containing vaccines among infants. Phase I screened for associations between neurodevelopmental disorders and thimerosal exposure in 124,170 infants born from 1992 to 1999. Phase II screened for the most common disorders found during phase I in 16,717 children born from 1991 to 1997 in another HMO database. In the analyses of the data, no significant associations were found between receipt of thimerosal-containing vaccines and neurodevelopmental outcomes (Verstraeten et al, 2003).

A cohort study of 467,450 children in Denmark compared the incidence of ASDs in children vaccinated with thimerosal-containing vaccines with that in children vaccinated with a thimerosal-free formulation of the same vaccine. Results found no relationship between childhood vaccination with thimerosal-containing vaccines and the development of ASDs (Hviid et al, 2003).

A retrospective cohort study involving 109,863 children in the United Kingdom from 1988 to 1997 was designed to investigate the relationship between the amount of thimerosal in a diphtheria- tetanus-pertussis (DTP) or diphtheria-tetanus (DT) vaccination administered at a young age and the subsequent occurrence of neurodevelopmental disorders. The study found no evidence that thimerosal exposure from DTP or DT vaccines causes neurodevelopmental disorders, except for tics (Andrews et al, 2004).

In a longitudinal study evaluating more than 14,000 children in the United Kingdom, the mercury exposure from thimerosal-containing vaccines was recorded and calculated at age 3, 4, and 6 months and compared to cognitive and behavioral-developmental assessments performed from 6 to 91 months of age. Researchers found no evidence that early exposure to thimerosal had any deleterious effect on neurologic or psychologic outcome (Heron, Golding, & ALSPAC Study Team, 2004).

Between 1985 and 1989 and again during the late 1990s, Stehr-Green and colleagues (2003) compared the incidence and prevalence of autism-like disorders in California, Sweden, and Denmark. Findings indicated that the incidence and prevalence of autism-like disorders began to rise from 1985 to 1989 and increased in incidence until the early 1990s. In the United States the thimerosal level in vaccines increased throughout the 1990s, whereas in Sweden and Denmark the already low thimerosal level in the vaccines steadily decreased in the 1980s and was virtually eliminated from all vaccines in the early 1990s. This study concludes that an increased exposure to thimerosal-containing vaccines does not correlate with the increased rates of autism in young children observed in Sweden and Denmark.

Madsen and colleagues (2003) studied 956 children diagnosed with autism from 1971 to 2000 and showed that the incidence was stable until 1990 with increased rates thereafter, in spite of the decreased amount of thimerosal used from 1970 to 1992. The rise in the incidence of autism continued even in children born after discontinuation of thimerosal-containing vaccines in Denmark in 1992.

In 2004 the Institute of Medicine completed an update to the review of the evidence and concluded that the epidemiologic evidence supports the rejection of a causal relationship between thimerosal exposure from childhood vaccines and the onset of autism. The Institute of Medicine supported the effort to remove thimerosal from vaccines to reduce any mercury exposure to infants and children.

Apply the Evidence: Nursing Implications

Decisions about the total elimination of thimerosal (even traces) from vaccines must balance the potential benefit of no exposure to mercury against the risks of decreased vaccine coverage because of higher cost of the thimerosal-free vaccine, the risks of sepsis due to the potential bacterial contamination of the preservative-free formulations, and the risk of exposure to alternative preservatives that might replace the thimerosal preservative.

Thimerosal as a preservative has been removed or reduced to trace amounts in all vaccines routinely administered to children except influenza vaccine. The maximum total exposure during the first 6 months of life is less than 3 mcg of mercury. Based on guidelines established by the U.S. Food and Drug Administration (2007) and other government monitoring agencies, no children will be exposed to excessive mercury from childhood vaccines.

References

Andrews N et al: Thimerosal exposure in infants and developmental disorders: a retrospective cohort study in the United Kingdom does not support a causal association, *Pediatrics* 114(3):584-591, 2004.

Heron J, Golding J, ALSPAC Study Team: Thimerosal exposure in infants and developmental disorders: a prospective cohort study in the United Kingdom does not support a causal association, *Pediatrics* 114(3):577-583, 2004.

Hviid A et al: Association between thimerosal-containing vaccine and autism, *JAMA* 290(13):1763-1766, 2003.

Institute of Medicine: *Immunization safety review: vaccines and autism*, Washington, DC, 2004, National Academy Press.

Madsen KM et al: Thimerosal and the occurrence of autism: negative ecological evidence from Danish population-based data, *Pediatrics* 112(3):604-606, 2003.

Stehr-Green P et al: Autism and thimerosal-containing vaccines: lack of consistent evidence for an association, *Am J Prev Med* 25(2):101-106, 2003.

US Food and Drug Administration: *Thimerosal in vaccines*, 2007. Available from www.fda.gov/cber/vaccine/thimerosal.htm (accessed March 7, 2008).

Verstraeten T et al: Safety of thimerosal-containing vaccines: a two-phased study of computerized health maintenance organization databases, *Pediatrics* 112(5):1039-1048, 2003.

BOX 42-8 Diagnostic Criteria for Autistic Disorder

A. A total of six (or more) items from (1), (2), and (3), with at least two from (1), and one each from (2) and (3):
   (1) Qualitative impairment in social interaction, as manifested by at least two of the following:
      (a) Marked impairment in the use of multiple nonverbal behaviors such as eye-to-eye gaze, facial expression, body postures, and gestures to regulate social interaction
      (b) Failure to develop peer relationships appropriate to developmental level
      (c) A lack of spontaneous seeking to share enjoyment, interests, or achievements with other people (e.g., by a lack of showing, bringing, pointing out objects of interest)
      (d) Lack of social or emotional reciprocity
   (2) Qualitative impairments in communication as manifested by at least one of the following:
      (a) Delay in, or total lack of, the development of spoken language (not accompanied by an attempt to compensate through alternative modes of communication such as gestures or mime)
      (b) In individuals with adequate speech, marked impairment in the ability to initiate or sustain a conversation with others
      (c) Stereotyped and repetitive use of language or idiosyncratic language
      (d) Lack of varied, spontaneous make-believe play or social imitative play appropriate to developmental level
   (3) Restricted repetitive and stereotyped patterns of behavior, interests, and activities, as manifested by at least one of the following:
      (a) Encompassing preoccupation with one or more stereotyped and restricted patterns of interest that is abnormal either in intensity or focus
      (b) Apparently inflexible adherence to specific, nonfunctional routines or rituals
      (c) Stereotyped and repetitive motor mannerisms (e.g., hand or finger flapping or twisting, complex whole-body movements)

B. Delays or abnormal functioning in at least one of the following areas, with onset before age 3 years: (1) social interaction, (2) language as used in social communication, or (3) symbolic or imaginative play

C. The disturbance is not better accounted for by Rett's disorder or childhood disintegrative disorder

From American Psychiatric Association: *Diagnostic and statistical manual of mental disorders*, ed 4, rev trans (DSM-IV TR), Washington, DC, 2000, The Association.

are first recognized. The American Academy of Neurology report has a comprehensive set of suggested diagnostic criteria to be used to either rule out or establish the diagnosis of childhood ASD (Belschner, 2007; Filipek et al, 2000) (see Box 42-8).

Prognosis

ASD is usually a severely disabling condition. However, some children improve with acquisition of language skills and communication with others (Bloom-DiCicco et al, 2006). Some ultimately achieve independence, but most require lifelong adult supervision. Aggravation of psychiatric symptoms occurs in about half of the children during adolescence, with girls having a tendency for continued deterioration.

Early recognition of behaviors associated with ASD is critical to implement appropriate interventions and family involvement. The prognosis is most favorable for children with communicative speech development by age 6 years and an IQ above 50 at the time of diagnosis.

Nursing Care Management

Therapeutic intervention for the child with ASD is a specialized area involving professionals with advanced training. Although there is no cure for ASD, numerous therapies have been used. The most promising results have been through highly structured and intensive behavior modification programs. In general, the objective in treatment is to promote positive reinforcement, increase social awareness of others, teach verbal communication skills, and decrease unacceptable behavior. Providing a structured routine for the child to follow is a key in the management of ASD.

When these children are hospitalized, the parents are essential to planning care and ideally should stay with the child as much as possible. Nurses should recognize that not all children with ASD are the same, and they will require individual assessment and treatment. Decreasing stimulation by using a private room, avoiding extraneous auditory and visual distractions, and encouraging the parents to bring in possessions the child is attached to may lessen the disruptiveness of hospitalization. Because physical contact often upsets these children, minimum holding and eye contact may be necessary to avoid behavioral outbursts. Care must be taken when performing procedures on, administering medicine to, or feeding these children, since they may be either fussy eaters who willfully starve themselves or gag to prevent eating or indiscriminate hoarders, swallowing any available edible or inedible items, such as a thermometer. Eating habits of ASD children may be particularly problematic for families and may involve food refusal, mouthing objects, eating nonedibles, and smelling and throwing food (Belschner, 2007; Caronna, Augustyn, & Zuckerman, 2007).

Children with ASD need to be introduced slowly to new situations, with visits with staff caregivers kept short whenever possible. Because these children have difficulty organizing their behavior and redirecting their energy, they need to be told directly what to do. Communication should be at the child's developmental level, brief, and concrete.

Family Support

ASD, as with so may other chronic conditions, involves the entire family and often becomes "a family disease." Nurses can help alleviate the guilt and shame often associated with this disorder by stressing what is known from a biologic standpoint and by providing family support. It is imperative to help parents understand that they are not the cause of the child's condition.

Parents need expert counseling early in the course of the disorder and should be referred to the Autism Society of America.* The society provides information about education, treatment programs and techniques, and facilities such as camps and group homes. Other helpful resources for parents of children with ASD are the local and state departments of mental health and developmental disabilities; these organizations provide important programs for ASD children and in-school programs throughout the United States.

As much as possible, the family is encouraged to care for the child in the home. With the help of family support programs in many states, families are often able to provide home care and assist with the educational services the child needs. As the child approaches adulthood and parents become older, the family may require assistance in locating a long-term placement facility.

**7910 Woodmont Ave., Suite 300, Bethesda, MD 20814-3067; 301-657-0881 or 800-328-8476; www.autism-society.org.*

Key Points

- The American Association on Intellectual and Developmental Disabilities defines intellectual disability as significantly subaverage general intellectual functioning existing concurrently with deficits in adaptive behavior and manifested during the developmental period.
- Causes of severe CI are primarily genetic, biochemical, and infectious. Mild CI is associated primarily with familial, social, and environmental causes, whereas severe CI is more likely to be associated with specific syndromes.
- Education of children with CI emphasizes sensory and verbal discrimination, improvement of short-term memory, motivation, and technologic support.
- Optimal development may be promoted through family guidance regarding play, communication, discipline, socialization, and sexuality.
- Prevention of CI focuses on support for the preterm neonate and other high risk newborns, rubella immunization, genetic counseling, and maternal education regarding the risks of chemical use (e.g., alcohol ingestion) and the importance of adequate nutrition.
- Down syndrome, a chromosomal abnormality, is characterized by mild to moderate range of CI (most often), physical characteristics, slowed language development, congenital anomalies, sensory problems, and diminished growth and sexual development.
- Fragile X syndrome is characterized by CI and phenotypic findings in affected males. It is considered the most common hereditary cause and the second leading chromosomal cause of CI after Down syndrome.
- Hearing disorders may be classified according to the location of the defect: conductive, sensorineural, mixed conductive-sensorineural, and central auditory imperception.

Audio Chapter Summaries

Access an audio summary of these Key Points on evolve

- Rehabilitation for hearing loss involves parent education and support, hearing aids, lipreading, sign language, speech therapy, and promotion of socialization.
- Prevention of hearing loss includes treatment of infection, universal newborn screening and child auditory testing, immunization, pregnancy and genetic counseling, and reduction of noise pollution.
- Common visual impairments in childhood include refractive errors, amblyopia, strabismus, cataracts, glaucoma, trauma, and infections.
- Prevention of visual impairment focuses on prenatal screening, prenatal and perinatal care, periodic vision screening, immunization, and safety counseling.
- Nursing goals in visual rehabilitation include helping the family and child adjust to the child's visual impairment, promoting parent-child attachment, fostering optimal development and independence, providing for play and socialization, and being aware of educational facilities.
- For the child undergoing ocular surgery, nursing care is aimed at reassuring the child and family throughout treatment, orienting the child to the surroundings, providing a safe environment, and encouraging independence.
- Retinoblastoma is a rare congenital malignant tumor; its most common clinical manifestations are white pupil reflex and strabismus.
- ASDs are a complex neurodevelopmental disorder of brain function accompanied by a broad range and severity of intellectual and behavioral deficits.

References

Afzal N et al: Constipation with acquired megarectum in children with autism, *Pediatrics* 112(4):939-942, 2003.

Alanay Y et al: Multidisciplinary approach to the management of individuals with fragile X syndrome, *J Intellect Disabil Res* 51:151-161, 2007.

American Academy of Pediatrics, Committee on Genetics: Health supervision for children with Down syndrome, *Pediatrics* 107(2):442-449, 2001.

American Academy of Pediatrics, Task Force on Newborn and Infant Hearing: Newborn and infant hearing loss: detection and intervention, *Pediatrics* 103(2):527-530, 1999.

American Psychiatric Association: *Diagnostic and statistical manual of mental disorders,* ed 4 (text rev) (DSM-IV TR), Washington, DC, 2000, The Association.

Belschner RA: Stop, assess and motivate: the SAM approach to autism spectrum disorder, *Am J Nurse Pract* 11(4):43-50, 2007.

Biasini FJ et al: Mental retardation: a symptom and a syndrome. In Netherton SD, Holmes D, Walker E (editors): *Child and adolescent psychological disorders: a comprehensive textbook*, vol 4, New York, 1999, Oxford University Press.

Bloom-DiCicco E et al: The development neurobiology of autism spectrum disorder, *J Neurosci* 26(26): 6897-6906, 2006.

Bosch JJ, Ringdahl J: Functional analysis of problem behavior in children with mental retardation: what is it, and why should pediatric nurses care? *MCN* 26(6):307-311, 2001.

Caronna EB, Augustyn M, Zuckerman B: Revisiting parental concerns in the age of autism spectrum disorders, *Arch Pediatr Adolesc Med* 161:406-407, 2007.

Centers for Disease Control and Prevention: Delayed diagnosis of fragile X syndrome—United States, 1990-1999, *Morbid Mortal Wkly Rep* 51(33):740-742, 2002.

Courtney-Manning P: Addressing the crisis in access to autism treatment using health care improvement science, *Arch Pediatr Adolesc Med* 161:414-415, 2007.

Crawford DC: FMR1 and the fragile X syndrome, *CDC fact sheet*, 2001. Available at www.cdc.gov/genomics/hugenet/factsheets/FS_FragileX.htm (accessed February 28, 2008).

Croen LA et al: Maternal and paternal age and the risk of autism spectrum disorders, *Arch Pediatr Adolesc Med* 161:334-340, 2007.

Croen LA et al: A comparison of health care utilization and costs of children with and without autism spectrum disorders in a large group-model health plan, *Pediatrics* 118(4):1203-1211, 2006.

Cunningham M, Cox EO, Committee on Practice and Ambulatory Medicine and the Section on Otolaryngology and Bronchoesophagology: Hearing assessment in infants and children: recommendations beyond neonatal screening, *Pediatrics* 111(2): 436-440, 2003.

Daniel E: Noise and hearing loss: a review, *J School Health* 77(5):225-231, 2007.

Dawson G: Despite major challenges, autism research continues to offer hope, *Arch Pediatr Adolesc Med* 161:411-412, 2007.

De Potter P: Current treatment of retinoblastoma, *Curr Opin Ophthalmol* 13(5):331-336, 2002.

DeStefano F et al: Age at first measles-mumps-rubella vaccination in children with autism and school-matched control subjects: a population-based study in metropolitan Atlanta, *Pediatrics* 113(2):259-266, 2004.

Downs BW, Buchman CA: External auditory canal translocation for cochlear implantation, *Laryngoscope* 115:555-556, 2005.

D'Souza Y, Fombonne E, Ward BJ: No evidence of persisting measles virus in blood mononuclear cells from children with autism spectrum disorder, *Pediatrics* 118:1664-1675, 2006.

Filipek P et al: Practice parameter: screening and diagnosis of autism: report of the Quality Standards Subcommittee of the American Academy of Neurology and the Child Neurology Society, *Neurology* 55(2 of 2):468-479, 2000.

Fombonne E: The prevalence of autism, *JAMA* 289:87-89, 2003.

Gregg RB, Wiorek MA, Arvedson JC: Pediatric audiology: a review, *Pediatr Rev* 25(7):224-234, 2004.

Grizzle KL, Simms MD: Early language development and language learning disabilities, *Pediatr Rev* 26(8):274-283, 2005.

Hall JG: Chromosomal clinical abnormalities. In Behrman RE, Kliegman RM, Jenson HB (editors): *Nelson textbook of pediatrics*, ed 17, Philadelphia, 2004, Saunders.

Hurwitz RL et al: Retinoblastoma. In Pizzo PA, Poplack DG (editors): *Principle and practice of pediatric oncology*, ed 5, Philadelphia, 2006, Lippincott.

Johnson CP, Walker WO: Mental retardation: management and prognosis, *Pediatr Rev* 27(7):249-256, 2006.

Kabra M, Gulati S: Mental retardation, *Indian J Pediatr* 70(2):153-158, 2003.

Kenna MA: Medical management of childhood hearing loss, *Pediatr Ann* 33(12):822-832, 2004.

Kolevzon A, Gross R, Reichenberg A: Prenatal and perinatal risk factors for autism: a review and integration of findings, *Arch Pediatr Adolesc Med* 161:326-333, 2007.

Melamud A, Palekar R, Singh A: Retinoblastoma, *Am Fam Physician* 73(6):1041-1044, 2006.

Mizoue T, Miyamoto R, Shimizu T: Combined effect of smoking and occupational exposure to noise on hearing loss in steel factory workers, *J Occup Environ Med* 60(10):56-59, 2003.

Muhle E, Trentacoste SV, Rapin I: The genetics of autism, *Pediatrics* 113(5): e472-e486, 2004.

National Down Syndrome Society: About Down syndrome, 2006. Available at www.ndss.org (accessed March 7, 2008).

National Fragile X Foundation: *Prevalence of fragile X syndrome*, 2006. Available at www.fragilex.org/html/prevalence.htm (accessed January 21, 2007).

Peterson CC: A review of biochemical and ultrasound markers in detection of Down syndrome, *J Perinatal Educ* 15(1):19-25, 2006.

Phalen JA: Fragile X syndrome, *Pediatr Rev* 26(5):181-182, 2005.

Pueschel SM: The child with Down syndrome. In Levine MD, Carey WB, Crocker AC (editors): *Developmental-behavioral pediatrics*, ed 3, Philadelphia, 1999, Saunders.

Rehm RS, Bradley JF: Social interactions at school of children who are medically fragile and developmentally delayed, *J Pediatr Nurs* 21(4): 299-307, 2006.

Schaefer GB, Lutz RE: Diagnostic yield in the clinical genetic evaluation of autism spectrum disorders, *Genet Med* 8(9):549-556, 2006.

Schanen NC: Epigenetics of autism spectrum disorders, *Hum Molec Genet* 15(R1-2):R138-R150, 2006.

Schouten–van Meeteren AYN et al: Overview chemotherapy for retinoblastoma: an expanding area of clinical research, *Med Pediatr Oncol* 38:428-438, 2002.

Segal S et al: Inner ear damage in children due to noise exposure from toy cap pistols and firecrackers: a retrospective review of 53 cases, *Noise Health* 5(18):13-18, 2003.

Skotko B: Mothers of children with Down syndrome reflect on their postnatal support, *Pediatrics* 115(1):64-77, 2005.

Smith RJH, Bale JF, White KR: Sensorineural hearing loss in children, *Lancet* 365:879-890, 2005.

Tingley DH: Vision screening essentials: screening today for eye disorders in the pediatric patient, *Pediatr Rev* 28(2):54-61, 2007.

Van Riper M: A change of plans: the birth of a child with Down syndrome doesn't have to be a negative experience, *Am J Nurs* 103(6):71-74, 2003.

Walker WO, Johnson CP: Mental retardation: overview and diagnosis, *Pediatr Rev* 27(6):204-212, 2006.

Wilton G, Plane MB: The family empowerment network: a service model to address the needs of children and families affected by fetal alcohol spectrum disorders, *Pediatr Nurs* 32(4):299-305, 2006.

Zeng FG, Liu S: Speech perception in individuals with auditory neuropathy, *J Speech Lang Hearing Res* 49:367-380, 2006.

Unit 10

43 Family-Centered Home Care

Learning Objectives

On completion of this chapter the reader will be able to:

- Differentiate home care from hospice care.
- List at least three factors contributing to the increasing emphasis on home care services.
- Describe case management/care coordination and its importance in home care.
- List general principles of a family-centered assessment and planning process.
- Identify five key characteristics of collaborative relationships.
- Describe approaches to promoting optimum development, self-care, and education in home care.
- Outline six areas in need of attention for promoting safety in home care.

Electronic Resources

Additional information related to the content in Chapter 43 can be found on

evolve the Companion Website at
http://evolve.elsevier.com/Perry/maternal/

- NCLEX Review Questions
- Case Study—Home Care

General Concepts of Home Care

Definition

Home care nursing has become a routine option for the pediatric patient in today's health care environment. Advances in medical technology have produced a large population of children with a variety of health care needs. The growing demand for home care services came in part as the result of increasing costs of institutionalized care. More important, home-based health care recognizes the family's valuable contribution to the child's overall health in his or her natural environment. Although there is limited evidence on the ability of home care to reduce hospital admissions and emergency department visits, home care programs lead to greater parent satisfaction, improved quality of life, and a reduction in length of hospital stay (Cooper et al, 2006).

Home care is not a new concept in pediatrics. Over time the term has referred to parents caring for mildly ill children at home; to nursing home visits after children are discharged from the hospital; to hospice care; and, more recently, to care at home for children with more serious chronic illness and dependence on medical technology. As discussed in this chapter, *home care* refers to care provided for children with simple or complex health care needs and their families in their places of residence for the purpose of promoting, maintaining, or restoring health or for maximizing the level of independence while minimizing the effects of disability and illness, including terminal illness.

Home care differs from *hospice care,* which is a program of palliative and supportive care services providing physical, psychologic, social, and spiritual care for dying persons, their families, and other loved ones. Hospice services are available in both the home and inpatient settings. *End-of-life care* and planning should be considered for any child with a terminal diagnosis. Some patients may be admitted for end-of-life home care services before being ready for admission to hospice services. Many hospice programs have admission criteria that do not permit therapies such as intravenous antibiotics, total parenteral nutrition, or enteral feedings that the family may wish to continue. It is therefore important to discuss the type of care the family wishes for the child early in discharge planning to clarify expectations for home care.

Home Care Trends

The shift toward home-based health care is propelled by numerous factors. Providing quality home health care for children generally requires parental desire and ability, professional assistance, and community preparedness. A natural family environment optimizes growth and development when stress is minimal and support is optimal.

Advances in medical technology have resulted in increased survival for children with congenital and acquired illnesses. Preterm infants or children who are ventilator dependent were once cared for indefinitely in an intensive care unit or long-term care facility. These children are now able to live with their families in their own home (Feudtner et al, 2005).

Children with cancer, kidney disorders, cystic fibrosis, spina bifida, cardiac and respiratory disorders, gastrointestinal disorders, neurodegenerative diseases, and human immunodeficiency virus infection may have ongoing health care needs as a result of the disease, its treatment, or side effects of treatment (Magrabi et al, 2005; Davis, 2006; Nazer et al, 2006; Stevens et al, 2006). Parents frequently have ongoing stressors after a child's hospitalization for diagnosis and treatment. Subsequent needs may include reinforcing teachings about the disease process, addressing the child's physical care needs, providing emotional support during this change in parental role, and teaching in a low-stress environment. Home-based nutrition programs are useful, safe, and well tolerated in children. There is sufficient evidence that these programs provide a better quality of life, decrease cost of therapy, and improve survival (Howard, 2006; Daveluy et al, 2006).

Improving the quality of life for both the child and the family is one of the driving forces in the efforts to move technology-dependent children from the hospital to the home setting. The concept of *normalization* describes the process whereby families of children with chronic illness over time begin to perceive the child and their family life as normal (Knafl & Deatrick, 2002). This has important implications for pediatric home care nurses in relation to the assessment of family function and in helping home care nurses gain a better understanding of family dynamics. The normalized family tends to be more flexible with treatments and incorporates the child with a disability or illness into the usual routines of daily living (Knafl & Deatrick, 2002).

The *cost of care* is another important factor in the health care delivery system today. Shorter inpatient stays are due in part to the overwhelming cost of lengthy hospitalizations. Children are either not admitted to the hospital at all or are returned home as soon as possible after their illness. Home-based nursing care has decreased the length of hospital stay (Cooper et al, 2006). Length of stay has been evaluated using bed days, inpatient stay, and use of hospital-based services. The length of hospital stay was significantly reduced when children received home-based care (Bagust et al, 2002; Dougherty, Soderstrom, & Schiffrin, 1998; Strawczynski et al, 1973). Likewise, a portion of the financial burden is shifted to the family. The family may be forced to absorb the costs of certain medications, supplies, transportation, shelter, utilities, food, laundry, housekeeping, and a portion of the nursing care. Over time chronically ill children can cause a financial burden to the family.

Home health care of children is not restricted to children with chronic health care needs. Several short-term, intermittent therapies such as phototherapy, chemotherapy, apnea monitoring, and intravenous antibiotic administration may be successfully treated in a home setting, where the child may remain with the family, rather than in an acute care setting. One study found that home health nurses providing asthma education to families of children hospitalized for an asthma exacerbation increased the family's and caregiver's knowledge about asthma symptoms, triggers, and management (Navaie-Waliser et al, 2004). A number of strategies can be implemented in the home setting to reduce the triggers that cause acute asthma exacerbations and often result in hospitalization (see Asthma, Chapter 46).

With the increased demand for nurses in home health and continued, pervasive short supply, there has been an increased focus on the role of the *family caregiver* in providing home care. A survey by the National Alliance for Caregiving (2005) revealed that 21% of U.S. households have a person being cared for by another family member; this represents care above and beyond the daily routine care of the family household.

Sullivan-Bolyai and colleagues (2003) explored the literature on adult and pediatric family caregivers' responsibilities in the care of a family member who has a chronic illness. Their review of the literature revealed four family-related caregiving responsibilities adapted from the adult literature that may be applied to children's caregivers as well:

Managing the illness—Providing daily hands-on care, monitoring the child's medical condition, and educating others to care for the child

Identifying, accessing, and coordinating resources—Locating appropriate resources in the community to meet the needs of the child and of the family as the child's caregiver

Maintaining the family unit—Continuing to nurture the family unit: siblings' needs, husband-wife relationships, and household maintenance

Maintaining self—Grieving the loss of the healthy child; balancing caregiver responsibilities with own physical, emotional, mental, and personal needs; recognizing stressors and potential caregiver burnout

The researchers developed a multifaceted list of parent caregiving management responsibilities and associated activities that the home health nurse may use to facilitate discussions with parents and families regarding caregiving in the home and its unique requirements (Sullivan-Bolyai et al, 2004). Nurses can use the results of this research to better understand the magnitude of responsibilities facing the caregiving family and assist in finding resources to provide the family some respite from caring for the child to care for each other and maintain self and family integrity.

The American Academy of Pediatrics supports the philosophy of *permanency planning*, wherein children with special health care needs obtain permanent family placement and ongoing relationship with caring adults (Johnson, Kastner, & American Academy of Pediatrics, Committee on Children with Disabilities, 2005). Within this framework, the home environment with the child's family is perceived as the best place for the child to be reared. Should the family be unable to support the child as a result of poor resources or family structure, options include extended family members, birth family plus an unrelated family sharing parental responsibilities, or two unrelated families sharing parental responsibilities. In addition, adoptive families may participate in care of the child with special health care needs. The American Academy of Pediatrics further stresses the importance of providing the child's family with adequate resources and support to promote family well-being (Johnson, Kastner, & American Academy of Pediatrics, Committee on Children with Disabilities, 2005). In addition, primary care physicians play a vital role in the process of care coordination in collaboration with the family and nursing home care team (American Academy of Pediatrics, 2005).

Respite care for caregivers of children with special care needs has been slow in its development and availability, although respite care centers are now common for adults. Such care for ventilator-dependent children and those with skilled technologic care requirements is lacking throughout the United States. Respite care provides temporary relief to parents and allows for a break from the responsibilities of caring for the child on a daily basis. Nurses can play an important role in advocating for the provision of high-quality respite care so families and caregivers can maintain appropriate family function, care for themselves, and continue to provide for the care of the child as necessary (Parra, 2003).

Effective Home Care

Providing home-based care for children gives the nurse an opportunity to assess and interact with the family in their environment. This assessment can provide the health care team with valuable information about safety, support systems, nutrition, parenting ability, and actual health care practices. This valuable information will determine future decisions for individualized care and realistic outcomes (Thompson, 2000).

The pediatric home care nurse has two distinct arrangements for implementation of care. Nurses who perform *intermittent skilled nursing visits* may see different types and numbers of patients each day. These nurses typically have an assigned patient caseload and accept responsibility for implementing the care plan. This mode of nursing care is the one most often used today as a result of shortage of personnel and decreased reimbursements. Most home visits now focus on helping the patient and caregiver achieve independence with care in the home, including home care by therapists, home infusion teaching by nurses, and care management, rather than direct provision of physical care. Nurses who perform *private-duty nursing,* or block nursing, are usually assigned individual patients, and they remain in the home for a predetermined time (e.g., 8- or 12-hour block of time) providing patient care. The care plan is implemented over the course of the time in the home. Required nursing skills are determined by patient need, parental ability, complexity of family, and the home environment. In both types of home care, the pediatric nurse is responsible for patient and family assessment, evaluating the appropriateness of the care plan (Petit de Mange, 1998) (Box 43-1).

A major issue in providing home care in this era is the *nursing shortage.* Agencies and families are facing much more difficulty in staffing required home care services; thus more and more of the home care must be carried out by family members or other caregivers. According to Page (2001), the lack of pediatric training in some nursing programs, increased acuity of home care patients, and increased pay for nurses working in acute care settings have contributed to a greater than ever nursing shortage in pediatric home health care. An increasing trend resulting from the nursing shortage and limitations in reimbursement is to have patients receive short-term treatment in nonhospital ambulatory settings (such as ambulatory infusion centers).

BOX 43-1 Intermittent Skilled Nursing

Health Care Need

- Child at risk—Parental substance abuse, failure to thrive, social or family situation potentially detrimental to child's well-being
- Chronically ill, but medically stable child with multiple care needs
- Education and competency validation of caregiver skills
- Skilled procedures—regularly scheduled injections or infusions, dressing changes, phototherapy
- Reinforcement of home care teaching; evaluation of caregiver's skills
- Technology-dependent child (e.g., ventilator or tracheostomy, home total parenteral nutrition, or enteral feedings by pump)
- Chronically ill child with multiple skilled nursing needs

Intervention

- Regularly scheduled visits to assess patient status, evaluate home environment, teach care provider skills, determine status of growth and development, set goals with family for positive health outcomes
- As-needed home visits during illness exacerbation to assess physical status and determine appropriate intervention
- Assistance with transportation of child to ambulatory center or practitioner's office for evaluation and diagnostic services
- Regular visits of limited duration to perform skilled nursing intervention, assess parental ability and desire to perform procedure, teach procedure technique, supervise parental performance of procedure
- Assessment of patient status; evaluation of safety of home environment; teaching, evaluation, and reinforcement of caregivers' skills; determination of status of growth and development; goal setting with family for positive health outcomes

Consideration of the caregiver's willingness, ability, and limitations are of utmost importance when assessing the appropriateness of the care plan (Box 43-2). It is vital to ensure that patients and families have adequate back-up support and access to resources such as social services. An increasing concern in pediatric home health care is obtaining a managing practitioner. Declining reimbursement and short hospital stays have increased patients' rapid movement through the continuum of care; a patient may be seen in the emergency department or neonatal intensive care unit, then discharged to home health without ever seeing a primary care physician. It is therefore imperative that the provision of care for home patients involve multidisciplinary cooperation and communication among health care workers.

Discharge Planning and Selection of a Home Care Agency

Identifying appropriate local community resources is critical to a successful transfer to home care (Box 43-3). The ultimate goal of discharge planning is for the family to become familiar

BOX 43-2 Services That Support Effective Home Care

- Adequate family training and preparation
- Primary care physician willing to oversee medical aspects of home care
- Professional caregivers trained in relevant nursing and communication skills
- Developmental intervention (e.g., physical, occupational, and speech therapy; early intervention)
- Appropriately designed and well-maintained equipment
- Supportive therapies (e.g., respiratory therapy, pharmacy, rehabilitation services, parenteral therapy, physical therapy, durable medical/infusion supplies, nutritional support)
- Adequate social and psychologic support services
- High-quality respite care
- Appropriate home renovation
- Telephone service in the home
- Appropriate transportation
- Appropriate locally available emergency facilities
- Competent case management services
- Safe environment (electricity, refrigeration, cleanliness)

Modified from Office of Technology Assessment (OTA), Congress of the United States: *Technology dependent children: hospital v. home care—a technical memorandum* (OTA-TM-H-38), Washington, DC, 1987, US Government Printing Office; and Bakewell-Sachs S, Porth S: Discharge planning and home care of the technology-dependent infant, *J Obstet Gynecol Neonatal Nurs* 24(1):77-83, 1995.

BOX 43-3 Characteristics of a High-Quality Pediatric Home Care Agency

- Fully trained pediatric staff to provide for all aspects of care (nursing, rehabilitation therapies, pharmacy, nutrition, social work, home medical equipment)
- Prompt, responsive staff with 24-hour availability
- Family-centered care
- Comprehensive continuing education programs
- Certification of local, state, and federal regulatory agencies
- Accreditation by The Joint Commission or Community Health Accreditation Program

Data from Dittbrenner H: Pediatric home care as a viable new service, *Caring* 18(2):12-15, 1999; and Lovejoy D: *Making the transition to home health nursing: a practical guide*, New York, 1997, Springer.

with the child's needs and to be competent in providing that care. A discharge plan should include emergency management and provision of social and emotional support. The American Academy of Pediatrics (Johnson, Kastner, & American Academy of Pediatrics, Committee on Children with Disabilities, 2005) emphasizes that the goal for a home health care program for infants, children, or adolescents with chronic conditions or disabilities is the provision of community-based, culturally effective, comprehensive, and cost-effective health care within a nurturing home environment that maximizes the capabilities of the individual and minimizes the effects of the disabilities.

NURSING ALERT If home care equipment is different from hospital equipment, have the portable equipment delivered to the hospital to allow family use before discharge.

Much of the success of home care, particularly for the child who is dependent on medical technology or who has complex medical problems, depends on careful planning and preparation. Discharge planning must begin early; should be based on criteria of child and family readiness; must be a multidisciplinary process, including representatives from acute care, home care, and community settings; and must involve the family. Predischarge assessment (Box 43-4) and planning should include:

- The child's medical, nursing, educational, and other therapeutic needs
- Family members' (including siblings') education and training, coping skills, and adjustment needs
- Community readiness in areas such as availability of equipment, appropriate nursing and other personnel, educational and developmental services, respite care, and emergency plans
- Financial arrangements

Creative financial planning, including negotiating arrangements with the insurance company, health maintenance or managed care organization, and public programs, may be required.

Early involvement of the home care agency in the discharge planning process promotes continuity of care and a smooth transition from hospital to home (Box 43-5). Before discharge, a general plan, sometimes called an *individualized home care plan*, should be developed with multidisciplinary input. This care plan should address the range of needs identified as part of the comprehensive predischarge assessment.

NURSING ALERT An excellent method of providing home care instructions is with video recordings. Once the family masters the procedures, consider video recording their performance. Visual learning is most helpful for people who cannot read or who are not fluent in English.

The plans for transition from hospital to home should include at least two family members learning and demonstrating all aspects of the child's care in the hospital. An in-hospital trial period during which parents provide total care for the child (such as rooming-in) is generally beneficial as well. After a successful trial, the family may benefit from taking the child home on a brief pass before making final discharge plans. (This arrangement may need to be negotiated with the insurance company before implementation.) The home care nurse plays an important role in assessing this experience with the family. A predischarge home visit allows the home care nurse to meet the family, help them assess their preparedness and the preparedness of the home environment, discuss plans for arranging the child's equipment at home (Fig. 43-1), reinforce prior discharge teaching, and implement any additional teaching that may be necessary (Bakewell-Sachs et al, 2000). Additional factors that should be considered in discharge planning include working parents, extended family, and child care arrangements.

BOX 43-4 Example of Predischarge Assessment for Technology-Dependent Infant

The Child's Family
Identification and training of primary caretakers
Identification and training of caretakers for respite and emergency care
Parent employment status while caring for child at home
Family financial picture, especially if one parent must stop working
Sibling preparation
Availability of psychosocial support services

Technical Equipment and Supplies for the Home
Home care company's availability and experience
Home care company's coordination of services with local health care provider and others
24-Hour availability and coverage for unexpected situations

Community Nursing and Support Services
Availability, training, and experience
Adequacy of number of personnel to meet needs
Additional training of staff, if needed
24-Hour availability of ambulance services and emergency medical services

Physical Environment of the Home
Adequacy of space for equipment and supplies
Heavy equipment (e.g., ventilator, oxygen tanks, compressor) accessibility
Layout of home (e.g., number of floors, stairways, room accessibility, room sizes)
Location and layout of bedrooms
Adequacy of apartment building elevator and fire escape
Telephone access
Type of transportation family uses
Possibility of modifying living space to minimize invasiveness of technology without isolating child
Adequacy of heating and cooling systems
Adequacy of electrical system to accommodate equipment

Emergency Plan
Identification and training of those involved
Written implementation plan: who, what, where, when, how (include telephone numbers)
Notification of utility companies for priority repairs and maintenance
Notification of emergency medical unit (911)
Emergency drill

Primary Care Provider
Identification of local primary provider or pediatrician who is able to assume direct care responsibility and coordinate other care providers
Inclusion of local provider in discharge planning
Information needs of local provider before child's discharge

From Bakewell-Sachs S, Porth S: Discharge planning and home care of the technology-dependent infant, *J Obstet Gynecol Neonatal Nurs* 24(1):77-83, 1995.

BOX 43-5 Critical Home Care Referral Information

- Scheduled medications
- Durable medical equipment
- Medical supplies
- Transportation needs
- Adaptive equipment
- Rehabilitation therapies (occupational, physical, and speech therapy)
- Psychologic counseling
- Social work referral
- Nursing care
- Respite plans
- Key family members
- Demographic information
- Reimbursement information

Modified from Townsend JL: Assessment of the child and family. In Votroubek WL, Townsend JL (editors): *Pediatric home care*, ed 2, Gaithersburg, MD, 1997, Aspen.

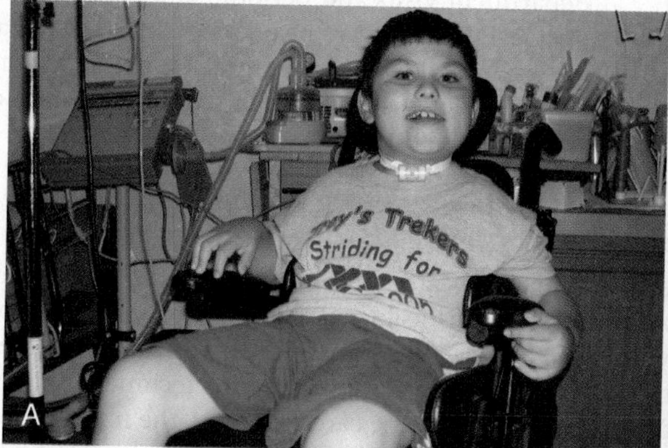

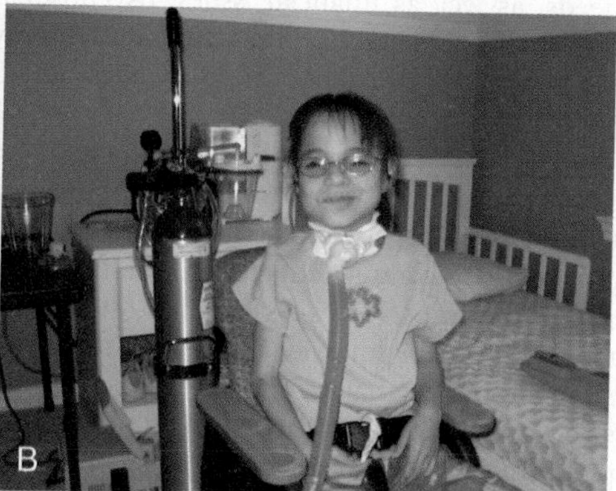

Fig. 43-1 A, An essential aspect of preparation for home care is the arrangement of equipment and supplies. **B,** The nurse in the home care setting requires expertise to care for a child who is technology dependent.

Care Coordination (Case Management)

Traditional definitions of *case management* generally focus on cost control, attainment of desired clinical outcomes, and monitoring and evaluation of care provided. However, for optimal home care of the child who is technology dependent, case management—or *care coordination*—should be viewed more broadly.

Changes in health care over the past three decades not only have improved survival and decreased morbidity among children with special health care needs, but also have heralded higher costs for health care and services provided. As a result, insurance companies have focused on reducing services to contain costs. The advent of managed care and fee-for-service reimbursement has changed the outlook for families desiring to have the child in the home. Often services are provided by multiple organizations and multiple vendors with different missions and a consistent lack of single systems linking home health care. In addition, eligibility criteria for funding and services are complex and vary from one state to another. As a result, coordination of home care can be challenging, frustrating, and complicated for the family (American Academy of Pediatrics, 2005).

The concept of *care coordination* is to link children with special home health care needs (and their families) to services and resources in a coordinated effort to provide the child with optimum care (American Academy of Pediatrics, 2005). Care coordination has several purposes. Its primary goal is ensuring continuity for the child and family across hospital, home, educational, therapeutic, and other settings. Other goals involve facilitating timely access to services and enhancing child and family well-being (Lindeke et al, 2002). Care should be coordinated among multiple providers to reduce the complexity of care for the child, reduce fragmentation of care, prevent duplication of services, and decrease the burden of care for the family. Case managers from a number of agencies may be involved in the patient's care, which may add to the parents' confusion; the home care nurse should try to coordinate meetings between all case managers and the family and a nurse care coordinator to minimize confusion and prevent duplication. Lindeke and colleagues (2002) proposed that the ideal situation is when the family serves as lead care coordinator within the context of family-centered care. Care coordination should ensure that the child's medical, nursing, and health maintenance needs, as well as financial issues, psychosocial concerns, and educational needs of the child and family, are addressed (American Academy of Pediatrics, 2005; Dittbrenner, 1999).

Care coordination is most effective if a single person works with the family to accomplish the many tasks and responsibilities involved (Box 43-6). The nurse case coordinator should have a minimum of a baccalaureate degree in nursing and 3 years' experience (American Nurses Association, 1998). The nurse case manager should be knowledgeable about community resources, including primary, secondary, and tertiary health care services; speech, language, hearing, and vision resources; respite care services; financial assistance programs; parent groups; advocacy groups; local, state, and federal public officials; transportation services; and private-sector individuals with an interest in children with disabilities (Thompson, 2000). With a greater focus on outcomes of care in home health care, the nurse case manager is challenged to be resourceful and skilled in communication at a number of levels (Rice, 2006).

BOX 43-6 Care Coordination for Children with Special Health Care Needs

- Facilitate timely access to services and resources.
- Promote continuity of care.
- Ensure high-quality care is performed in the home.
- Provide family support and enhance family well-being.
- Improve health, developmental, educational, vocational, psychosocial, and functional outcomes.
- Maximize efficient, effective use of resources.

Modified from Presler B: Care coordination for children with special health care needs, *Orthop Nurs* 17(25 Suppl):45-51, 1998.

A valuable tool for nurse case managers is the *care path*, which is a multidisciplinary care plan aimed at measuring the quality of patient care outcomes derived from standardized patient outcomes; the care path evaluates the quality of patient care with respect to cost-effectiveness and timeliness. (For samples of home care clinical care paths, see Rice, 2006.) Care paths may also be used to help nurses and other health care workers learn home care and should be shared with the family members involved in patient care to provide direction and help the family see the eventual goals of care (Rice, 2006).

Although professionals must always see part of their role as ensuring that integrated, coordinated care is provided, care coordination should promote the family's role as primary decision maker and enhance the family's capability to meet the special needs of the child and the family unit. Families may choose to be involved to varying degrees in coordinating their child's care. Many parents take on increasing responsibility for care coordination over time; they should be encouraged and supported in this role. Home care nurses and case managers should be aware that the termination of private-duty or home care nursing can be a difficult transition for which families may need preparation. A gradual reduction in services allows patients and families to adjust favorably to the changes. Care coordination by office-based nurses for children and youth with special health care needs decreases emergency department visits and periodic office visits, thus significantly decreasing the cost of health care. Increased health care costs are associated with more physician-dependent care coordination activities among such children (Antonelli, Stille, & Antonelli, 2008).

Role of the Nurse, Training, and Standards of Care

The home care nurse must share a level of technical expertise with the critical care nurse while being able to adapt equipment, procedures, and the nursing process to the home setting. (See Chapter 45 for specific technical skills that may be required in home care practice.) The need for technical expertise must be matched by a knowledge of child development and the ability to work creatively with the child challenged by chronic illness and technology dependence. When caring for

BOX 43-7 Qualities of a Pediatric Home Care Nurse

- Shows competence in skills and case management
- Recognizes that the nurse is a guest in the home
- Respects family culture and adapts appropriately
- Works as a multidisciplinary team member
- Demonstrates expertise in pediatric care (assessment and technical skills)
- Possesses and uses effective communication skills

patients in the home setting, the nurse must be comfortable making independent nursing judgments and solving problems with no immediate assistance. At the same time, the nurse must have excellent interpersonal skills; an ability to work with other professionals and the family; and, most important, an ability to respect family autonomy. Patient outcomes are more readily achievable with a balance of nursing skills that demonstrate clinical excellence; adaptability; accountability; and the development of positive relationships with physicians, patients, and families (Box 43-7).

When working with a home care agency, nurses should expect to receive patient placements appropriate to their expertise. They should also expect to receive orientation to the skills and knowledge base of the home health care nursing specialty and subsequent continuing education to develop as expert practitioners. The minimum initial orientation should include the individual patient's care plan and equipment needs; the agency's policies and procedures, including procedures for addressing any problems that may occur when care is provided in the home; legal liability issues; and documentation procedures. Stronger emphasis should be placed on issues specific to home care.

Supervision of practice, including occasional site visits by a nursing supervisor, should be provided. Mentoring or precepting is ideal. Because of the unique practice environment of home health nurses, it is important for an agency to facilitate sharing among peers to decrease work-related stress, increase job satisfaction, and support high-quality patient care.

Nurses in pediatric home health face increasing demands for providing high-quality care with fewer resources to achieve positive patient outcomes. In doing so, nurses often must rely on *delegation* skills to ensure the patient and family receive the necessary care. Delegation often involves assigning nursing tasks to other health care professionals (Timm, 2003).

Public or private home care agencies that participate in the Medicare or Medicaid programs must be certified by a federally designated state certification body and abide by federal and state regulations. Additionally, the American Nurses Association has developed standards of nursing practice for both (community) public health and home health nurses (American Nurses Association, 1999b, 1999c). Generalist and clinical specialist certification in both home health and community health is offered by the American Nurses Credentialing Center,* a subsidiary of American Nurses Association. The Hospice and Palliative Nurses Association offers certification in hospice nursing. Despite important differences between pediatric and adult care in the home, as of this writing no national standards specific to pediatric home care practice have been developed. Nursing practice in pediatric home care should be guided by published guidelines, textbooks, peer-reviewed articles, and written standards of care for pediatric patients. Professional nursing organizations such as Infusion Nurses Society, National Association of Neonatal Nurses, Society of Pediatric Nurses, Association of Pediatric Hematology/Oncology Nurses, National Association of Pediatric Nurse Practitioners, and others have published standards of care that apply to pediatric home health nursing practice (see Resources on this text's website).

A *quality improvement program* is an important component of an effective home care agency. *Evidence-based practice* is rapidly becoming an important aspect of home health care, as is *benchmarking*, in which the product or practice (in this case, patient outcome) is compared with other agencies' outcomes and practices to determine best practice; this allows agencies to see how they measure in comparison to other similar agencies (Wilson, 2003; Yoder-Wise, 2007). The *OASIS (Outcome and Assessment Information Set)*, as part of Medicare, has been established for adults in home health care; however, as of this writing no such data exist for children younger than age 18 years. As a part of OASIS, home health care quality measures have been established to measure patient care outcomes for Medicare reimbursement purposes. Other certification and licensing organizations that may oversee and regulate practice in home health include The Joint Commission, Centers for Medicare and Medicaid Services (formerly the Health Care Financing Administration), Occupational Safety and Health Administration, and Community Health Accreditation Program. The Health Insurance Portability and Accountability Act of 1996 guidelines affect the manner in which patient records are handled in home health care to ensure patient confidentiality (Wilson, 2004).

Family-Centered Home Care

Technology dependence, chronic illness, and complex care requirements cross social, cultural, spiritual, and economic boundaries. Regardless of a family's background, family values must be respected in the provision of home care services. *The home is the family's domain,* and the child is at home because the family's central role is to nurture and raise their child. The ultimate responsibility for managing the child's health, developmental, and emotional needs lies with the family. Roush and Cox (2000) developed a framework for helping the home health care nurse understand the significance of the home to the family. The three central concepts of the model are:

Home as familiar—The environment where one is comfortable and at ease because of the familiarity with living arrangements and routines of home

Home as center—The location of everyday experiences related to time, space, and one's social life

Home as protector—The environment that preserves privacy, safety, and identity

8515 Georgia Ave., Suite 400, Silver Spring, MD 20910-3492; 800-284-2378; www.nursecredentialing.org.

evolve Case Study—Home Care

The nurse must respect and encourage the family's central role in the care of the child and must collaborate with the family in efforts to care for the child. Family-centered nursing practice is essential in the home setting. Family-centered care has become acknowledged as the standard of care for children with special health care needs (Johnson, 2000).

The philosophic basis for family-centered practice is the recognition that the family is the constant in the child's life, whereas the service systems and personnel within those systems fluctuate. Professionals working with the families of children with complex chronic problems must respect the family's central, caring role; their knowledge; and their particular and unique expertise. Families have the most intimate knowledge of the child's strengths and abilities, the challenges of providing care, and the abilities and needs of other family members. Believing that no one knows the child better than the family is critical to the success of any health care plan.

Respect for Diversity

Respect for varied family structures and for racial, ethnic, cultural, spiritual, and socioeconomic diversity among families is essential in home care (see also Chapters 31 and 32). Home care nurses work in close relationship with family members and in the family's own domain. The nurse shares in these relationships, participating in care throughout the course of illness (see Family-Centered Care box). The family's background and their lifestyle choices are respected. Particular attention is given to communication. The meaning of words used and the way they are said may affect various cultural groups in different ways. Volume of speech and language style must be taken into consideration as part of a family cultural assessment. The home health care nurse must pay particular attention to nonverbal communication. Body language, eye contact, and degree of physical contact have different meanings within particular cultures.

NURSING ALERT One should not assume that everyone who speaks English can read the language. Color-coded medication bottles, written schedules, and pillboxes or oral syringes may aid compliance with prescription administration. Pictures or special symbols may be helpful when providing instructions for procedures and medication administration.

Families may also differ in their cultural views of children; health care; childrearing practices; and illness, its causes, and its meaning. The family's health care practices and beliefs may influence the level of investment a family will make in the child's care. The family's *religion* or spirituality is another factor that can have a major influence on a family's response to the child's special health care needs. Some families will look for spiritual meaning and purpose for the illness. Other families may choose to reject past religious ties. In some cultures, religion and beliefs about health care and illness are closely intertwined (McEvoy, 2003); thus it is important that home care nurses assess the relationships among culture, religion, and the family's beliefs about the child's illness (see Community Focus box).

A variety of cultural assessment tools are available (Giger & Davidhizar, 2002; Spruhan, 1996). The home care nurse, aware that *personal values* drive behavior, must learn about the family's culture, ask questions without implying judgment, interpret the mainstream medical culture, and help families design interventions that meet their preferences. When possible, culture-specific teaching materials should be used. Increased emphasis in health care in the United States has been placed on health care workers—including home care nurses—becoming culturally competent to better understand the patient populations they serve and effectively deliver holistic care to their patients (National Center for Cultural Competence, 2002).

Respect for family diversity and awareness of both family developmental stages (see Chapter 31) and the stages of a fam-

FAMILY-CENTERED CARE

Developing Relationships with Culturally Diverse Families

I work in the inner city, and my home care patients come from a variety of racial and ethnic backgrounds. I am Caucasian, from Australia. Often, when I first visit a family, there is an initial coolness or apprehension toward me. This is understandable because I am a stranger, and perhaps families think I'll judge them in one way or another. By the end of the first visit, however, there is usually a smile as I leave; by the second visit they often greet me with a smile at the door; and by the third visit we usually have a friendship, a trust, and an ease of communication.

If I'm working on a case for an extended time, I use a holistic nursing approach. This involves being aware of how the child's illness affects the entire family. As I listen over many weeks to their fears and questions, and often as I share faith perspectives, a bond begins to form. I find it a privilege to share in their joys and their pain, and I feel rewarded by the trust that they invest in me.

—Julie Edgerton, RN, Home Care Nurse
Children's National Medical Center
Washington, DC

Modified from Ahmann E: Thinking critically about family-centered home care nursing, *Pediatr Nurs* 20(6):588-590, 1994.

COMMUNITY FOCUS

Spiritual Assessment

The mnemonic BELIEF was developed by McEvoy (2003) for pediatric nurses to initiate discussions with parents and children about their faith or religious values and beliefs. The components of the assessment tool are:

Belief system
Ethics or values
Lifestyle
Involvement in a spiritual community (church, synagogue, mosque)
Education
Future events

The tool may be used to develop a culturally sensitive dialogue regarding spiritual matters and practices that affect the child and family.

ily's adjustment to illness in a child (see Chapter 41) will assist the home care nurse in recognizing and promoting family strengths and in respecting varied coping mechanisms. Labels such as "dysfunctional," "difficult," and "noncompliant" can reinforce negative expectations and shape behaviors of both parents and professionals. On the other hand, emphasizing, identifying, and building on family strengths and coping mechanisms are strategies that promote a central goal in nursing care of the child and family: *family empowerment* (see Chapter 29).

Parent-Professional Collaboration

Family-centered nursing practice is built on a foundation of parent-professional collaboration, which represents a shift from the traditional unidirectional relationships between health care providers and families. The *Collaborative Family Health Care Coalition** has developed core competencies for professionals collaborating with families.

Collaborative caring allows the nurse and family to work together and share outcomes in a deep and meaningful way. This approach, essential in the home care setting, is characterized by (Kellett & Mannion, 1999):

- Encouraging activities to develop self-confidence and self-esteem
- Displaying increased awareness of and respect for family caregivers
- Recognizing that families vary in defining their role
- Demonstrating an ability to understand the family's approach to caregiving
- Sharing perspectives, not just tasks and functions
- Supporting family members in their primary, irreplaceable role as caregivers
- Exchanging expertise in providing care to the child
- Assisting families in recognizing their contributions as worthwhile
- Identifying strengths and resources of child and family
- Negotiating options, priorities, and preferences
- Assisting with coping by allowing families to find meaning in caring for patient at home

Communication with the family should not be intrusive. There is no need to collect information from the family that can be obtained from the child's records. The nurse should explain to families the reason for questions, particularly those they may perceive as intrusive, and should tell families who will have access to the information (see Critical Thinking Exercise). The nurse must also assure families that they have a right to expect confidentiality in regard to the data collected. When working in the home, the nurse must respect the privacy of family communications that may be overheard.

Communication with family members should include sharing with the family, in a supportive manner, complete and unbiased information about all aspects of the child's condition and care. Parents often feel overwhelming frustration related to obtaining accurate information about their child's illness and its management. Parents want information given slowly and repeated as necessary over time; they want explanations in terms they can understand; and they want the opportunity to ask questions, which should be answered in a straightforward manner. Stating "I don't know" or "I'll find out" is better than pretending to know or giving excuses. Unfortunately, the home health care nurse may become a source of added stress on the caregiver or family when the nurse displays unprofessional attitudes or fails to show proper respect for the family's knowledge of the child's needs and care (Harrigan et al, 2002).

A plan can be made with the parents to gather relevant information when necessary (Hanson & Randall, 1999; Newton, 2000). Information should be shared with families in a way that has meaning in their cultural context (Davidhizar, Havnes, & Bechtel, 1999). Many parents report a preference for interactions with professionals who communicate empathy and concern (Harrigan et al, 2002). Families vary in the amount and delivery of information they can tolerate regarding their child's status.

*Collaborative Family Healthcare Coalition, Collaborative Family Healthcare Association, PO Box 23980, Rochester, NY 14692-3980; 585-482-8210; fax: 585-482-2901; www.cfha.net.

CRITICAL THINKING EXERCISE

Family-Centered Home Care and Conflicts

A family wants to begin oral feeding with a tracheostomy of their 3-year-old daughter, Sarah, who is ventilator dependent and is being tube fed through a skin-level gastrostomy feeding tube (MIC-KEY). The mother, who has assumed the role of Sarah's primary caretaker, is adamant about starting oral feedings so Sarah can be more like other children her age. One day the mother asks you, the nurse case manager overseeing the child's home care, to feed Sarah baby food by mouth to see how she tolerates the feeding. The child is alert and sociable yet cannot communicate her wishes except through crying and whining. She has a seizure disorder and has had several episodes of aspiration pneumonia since birth. Sarah appears to have a considerable amount of tongue thrusting and copious amounts of oral mucus that must be suctioned frequently to prevent aspiration; her cough reflex is compromised and usually elicited only with tracheal suctioning.

1. Evidence—Is there sufficient evidence to draw any conclusions about the issue of feeding Sarah at this time?
2. Assumptions—Describe some underlying assumptions about the following:
   a. Sarah's readiness for oral feedings
   b. Sarah's ability to tolerate oral feedings
   c. The mother's request for Sarah to start oral feedings
3. What implications and priorities for nursing care may be drawn at this time?
4. Does the evidence objectively support your argument (conclusion)?
5. Are there alternative perspectives to your arguments? What are they?

NURSING ALERT Home care nurses should restrict their communications with other professionals to clinically relevant information about the family.

On occasion, disagreements may arise between parents and nurses over proper procedures for the child's care. Nurses should respect parental preferences in any situation that does not pose danger or risk for the child (see Family-Centered Care box). If parents wish to alter a treatment plan that is part of medical orders, the nurse should ask that they negotiate the change with the practitioner because the nurse must follow the written medical orders. If disagreements cannot be resolved, a home care supervisor or case manager (care coordinator) should be contacted to assist with problem solving. Increasingly, home care agencies are developing ethics committees and policies for managing difficult situations such as treatment refusal (see Critical Thinking Exercise, p. 1211).

FAMILY-CENTERED CARE

Knowledgeable Parents

It is not unusual for parents, particularly those whose children have chronic illnesses or complex care regimens, to be more knowledgeable about their child's condition than a nurse who is assigned to the child's care. This can be disconcerting for both the parents and the nurse. It is important to remember and reinforce that, regardless of the condition, parents will always know more about their child than the professional caring for the child. The nurse and parents can set goals for care in an atmosphere of mutual respect. If the parents' goal is respite from prolonged caregiving, they are less likely to want to give long explanations about their child's care, and assistance from an experienced peer may be more appropriate for the nurse to seek. If the parents wish to maintain maximum participation in care delivery, the nurse and the parents can negotiate the collaboration.

When teaching parents to perform complex chronic care regimens at home, include teaching them to expect to know more about their child's care than professionals who may come to assist them, whether that be home health, hospital, or outpatient personnel. At the same time, assure them that what various professionals who work with them will have from working with a multitude of families is a scientific knowledge base and a wealth of options for addressing and solving care problems.

–Teresa L. Hall, MS, RN
Hathaway Children's Services
Sylmar, CA

A tool that might be helpful to the pediatric home care nurse is the Caregiver Strain Index, a 13-item assessment designed to ascertain caregiver stress and subsequently develop appropriate strategies for individual and family coping (Sullivan, 2003).

The Nursing Process

In the home the family is a partner in each step of the nursing process. Assessment should address family strengths and resources* (Box 43-8). The principles of communication discussed previously guide data collection.

Self-report instruments to help families identify concerns, priorities, resources, and sources of support include Family Needs Survey, which is available from FPG Child Development Institute, University of North Carolina at Chapel Hill, CB 8180, Chapel Hill, NC 27599; 919-966-2622; or can be downloaded from www.fpg.unc.edu.

BOX 43-8 Sample Family Assessment Questions

- What are the child and family's experiences and expectations of the disease or illness?
- How does that affect the current situation?
- Is the current coping status a reflection of a new condition, the same chronic condition, or a new phase in a chronic condition?
- How can the nurse address family needs and promote health among all family members?
- What specific nursing interventions will facilitate a healthy response to child and family limitations caused by the illness?

Modified from Gedaly-Duff V, Heims ML: Family child health nursing. In Hanson SMH, Boyd ST (editors): *Family health care nursing*, Philadelphia, 1996, Davis.

All the information gathered as part of the assessment process is shared with the family. The nurse should recognize that the family's perception of their most important need will generally guide their behavior and consume their attention and energy. Family priorities should guide the planning process.

Both short- and long-term goals should be outlined and agreed on by the child, family, and professionals involved. The care plan should integrate various disciplines that may be involved with the child to eliminate duplication and coordinate and consolidate care requirements. Cross-training of professionals and a transdisciplinary mode of treatment can also be useful when a child has multiple and complex care requirements. For example, certain physical or occupational therapy routines may be incorporated into the child's morning nursing procedures, or speech therapy interventions may be conducted by the parent or nurse around eating times so that the entire day is not occupied by procedures. A written schedule of daily routines should be developed and followed by all caregivers.

NURSING ALERT At each home visit, physically handle and look at all medications. Check them against the medical orders and read the labels. There may be discrepancies, duplications, or changes between hospitalizations. Clarify medication purpose, effect, and dosages for the family.

Goals of care and achievement of established outcomes are supported by intervention strategies that reflect normalization (see Chapter 41) and the interests and abilities of the child and family. Nurses can help the family explore a range of alternative strategies, services, and resources so that the family can choose the best match for their situation.

Families can participate in evaluating a home care plan on several levels. Families and care providers should regularly review the goals of care and update the care plan as required. The nurse can ask the family open-ended questions at regular intervals to assess their opinions on the effectiveness of care. As part of the evaluation process, families should be acknowledged for their successes and accomplishments. Finally, families should be given an opportunity to evaluate individual home care nurses, the home care agency, and other service providers periodically. The evaluation should address the nurse's knowledge, skills, and respect for the family's choices. The agency should use the evaluations to improve quality of care (see Family-Centered Care box).

In addition to maintaining a sense of control over their child's care, families need to control their home and personal lives. For this reason, nurses should discuss "house rules" with the family and address issues such as the physical environment, private areas in the home, responsibility for maintaining the child's environment, and interactions with siblings (see Guidelines box). Home care nursing encourages a close and rewarding relationship with the family. One of the most important aspects of this relationship is maintaining professional boundaries and a therapeutic role that is supportive but not intrusive (McKlindon & Barsteiner, 1999) (see Critical Thinking Exercise).

Technologic trends that influence the nursing process in home care include the use of *laptop computers* (notebooks) to document the home visit; *personal data assistants*, or small hand-held computers that store large amounts of data, includ-

FAMILY-CENTERED CARE

What I Learned About Home Care

I learned many things as a result of having home care for four children over a period of 8 years. Two of the major areas I learned about were communication and families' rights. It took a long time to learn some of these things.

Initially I tried very hard to be sensitive to the professionals and often put my own feelings and needs aside. It took a while to learn that I could stand up for myself and my family and that my child could continue to receive good care. One area that was important to me was to have nurses withhold judgment on our parenting style, even if they might have parented differently.

Communication needs to be open and two way. Families and nurses ought to tell each other what is going well. For example, "Thanks for keeping the room so neat while you're here" can help a nurse see a family's appreciation. There was so little I could do as just "Mommy" that it really meant a lot to me when nurses would say, "That's such a cute outfit you picked out for him today." Communicating about little things, even inconsequential topics such as favorite TV shows, makes it easier to communicate about more important things and about problems. Communication has to be open about problems, too.

—Jeni Stepanek, Mother
Upper Marlboro, MD

GUIDELINES Negotiating "House Rules" for Home Care

House Rules

Parking—Identify where to park and community regulations.

Access—State where to enter the home. Is knocking preferred or ringing the bell?

Personal belongings—Where does the nurse store own coat, boots, etc.? Does the family prefer slippers to shoes in the home?

Meals—Where may the nurse store own food? NOTE: This is very important given cultural diversity of clients.

Radio and television—Identify preferences regarding usage. Remember, this may help nurses to remain awake at night.

Patient room—The nurse is responsible for the child's immediate environment. Maintaining a clean working area and cleaning up the room at the end of the shift is the nurse's responsibility.

Telephone—Agency policy may dictate that all personal calls be limited to brief periods and charged to the nurse making them. NOTE: Many nurses do need to check in with home at some interval during the evening.

Visitors—Identify who may enter the home when the parents are away (e.g., child's friends or grandparents). A list of names should be available.

Privacy—Describe what parts of the home are off-limits to the nurse and at what times.

Child

Routine—Specify times for playtime, bathtime, and bedtime. What does the parent want to participate in regarding these routines?

Mealtime—Specify where the family wants the child fed; if tube fed, specify a preference as to how and where it is done.

Clothing—Identify who picks out the child's clothes. Identify where the laundry is and who is responsible for washing the sick child's clothing.

Discipline—Discuss specific guidelines for discipline.

Homework—Discuss when it should be done and who is responsible for it being completed.

Siblings

Discipline—Establish guidelines regarding how parents should be informed of siblings' conflicts and how discipline should be handled. NOTE: Parents or another caregiver must be in the home when siblings are home.

Patient care—Be specific regarding how children have helped with the child's care. Discuss any concerns regarding behavior that may compromise the child's or siblings' safety.

Nursing

Parental notification—Specify what information the family wishes to be aware of immediately and what can wait until they are home.

Limits of responsibility—Specify duties the nurse may not perform, such as transportation of the child to care facilities or baby-sitting the siblings.

Environment—Discuss the need to have adequate lighting and a comfortable working area.

Modified from Klug R: Clarifying roles and expectations in home care, *Pediatr Nurs* 19(4):375, 1993.

CRITICAL THINKING EXERCISE

Maintaining Therapeutic Boundaries

As the home care nurse who has been working with a 4-year-old ventilator-dependent child, Derek, weekly for about 5 months, you are aware that the parents have become increasingly argumentative with each other. Most of the arguments are about whether Mr. J helps enough with the child's care and the house cleaning. Mr. J works full time at one job, then supplements the family income by working at a part-time job every weekend. Ms. J approaches you to complain about her husband's lack of involvement with the child and his care. Derek requires constant care, and the family has many expenses related to his physical care; the child is severely developmentally impaired and is not expected to improve significantly despite numerous medical interventions. He is the only child, although Ms. J stated at one time they wanted to have many children.

1. Evidence—Is there sufficient evidence to draw any conclusions about the family situation at this time?
2. Assumptions—Describe some underlying assumptions about the following:
   a. Home care of the child with a chronic, terminal condition (see p. 1203)
   b. Impact of the chronic condition, child's prognosis, and required care on the parents
   c. Status of the marriage relationship between Mr. and Ms. J
3. What implications and priorities for nursing care may be drawn at this time?
4. Does the evidence objectively support your argument (conclusion)?
5. Are there alternative perspectives to your arguments? What are they?

ing addresses, appointments, patient tracking systems, textbooks, and pharmacologic databases (Lewis & Sommers, 2003); *Internet* and *e-mail* services, which increase patient-practitioner accessibility and communication; and *telemedicine* or *telehealth*, which has various features, including electronic systems that can transmit physiologic data directly to the practitioner via the telephone. The American Nurses Association (1999a) has established a list of competencies for nurses involved in telehealth technology. *Telephone triage* has become standard in many health care institutions, and standards for triage have been published elsewhere. Concerns with the increasing use of technology in health care are cost, governmental regulations and patient care standards, liability and malpractice issues, ethics, and confidentiality matters (Rice, 2006). In addition, concerns regarding the nurse-patient relationship (high tech–low touch) and the nurse's role are raised with the use of any technology.

Promotion of Optimal Development, Self-Care, and Education

There is little question that living at home offers most children with complex medical problems great social and emotional advantages over living in the hospital or other institutional setting. However, in infancy and throughout the developmental stages, a child's medical condition and dependence on medical technology can place constraints on and pose challenges to *normal development*. For example, the child may have lengthy and repeated hospitalizations; developmental regression can occur in response to stress; fatigue may result from an underlying pathologic condition, the exacerbation of an illness, or medication side effects; and equipment requirements may impede mobility, exploration, and independence. The challenge of providing support for normal development in a child who is chronically ill and technology dependent requires optimizing opportunities for developmentally appropriate experiences within these constraints.

Home care plans are designed to promote optimum child development through assessment, planning, and referrals and through interventions that address normalization issues and self-care (Box 43-9). General principles for a family-centered assessment and planning process are addressed earlier in this chapter and are also applied in developmental assessment and planning.

BOX 43-9 Incorporating Developmental Support into the Home Care Plan

Example

A 6-month-old infant with a history of 24-week prematurity and bronchopulmonary dysplasia: currently using cardiorespiratory monitor, oxygen via nasal cannula, and skin-level (MIC-KEY) gastrostomy feedings

Outcome Criteria

Age-appropriate growth—developmental activities promoted with normal parameters achieved

Absence of growth and development deficits for age within limits imposed by illness

Intervention

Assess growth and development with the Denver II Developmental Assessment.

Reassess growth and development every 4 weeks.

Provide consistent caregiver.

Instruct parents in normal growth and development for child's age, reasons for delay, and anticipated outcomes.

Inform parents of age-related play and other activities that enhance growth and development and provide stimulation.

Consult with physical, occupational, and speech therapists to incorporate recommendations in daily routines.

Provide visual, auditory, and tactile stimulation, including mobiles with or without color, music, toys, books, television.

Hold, rock, pat, and talk to child.

Data from Klijanowicz AS: Care of high-risk infant. In Votroubek WL, Townsend JL (editors): *Pediatric home care*, ed 2, Gaithersburg, MD, 1997, Aspen; Jaffe M: *Pediatric nursing care plans*, ed 2 Englewood, CO, 1998, Skidmore-Roth; and Luxner K, Jaffe M: *Delmar's pediatric nursing care plans*, ed 3, Clifton Park, NY, 2004, Thomson Delmar Learning.

Some parents may not pursue early developmental intervention because they do not believe their child needs the services. In this case professionals need to explain the child's developmental needs to parents in ways that are meaningful from the parents' own cultural and socioeconomic perspectives. Only then can parents make truly informed decisions. Once parents have been fully informed of the child's condition, likely developmental sequelae, and the expected benefits of intervention, developmental goals outlined by the child and family should guide planning and intervention.

The impact of chronic illness on development is discussed in Chapter 41. Behaviors that may be observed in children receiving home care that need to be addressed by the nurse include:

Infants—Crying, withdrawal, detachment, inability to achieve developmental milestones

Toddlers—Inactivity; sadness; screaming; regressive behavior; delays in motor, speech, social skills

Preschoolers—Temper tantrums, refusal to comply with routines, refusal to eat or participate in self-care

School-age children—Expression of loneliness, boredom, isolation, depression, and worry about school absences; altered physical growth

Adolescents—Dependency, uncooperativeness, withdrawal, fear of loss of peer status or acceptance at school, altered image

Promoting coping and capability can buffer stress and contribute to mental health and self-esteem in a child with a chronic illness. The extent to which a child is involved in his or her own care depends on many factors, including parental comfort and support and the child's developmental age, level of interest, and physical ability. Self-care, both in activities of daily living and in regard to the medical condition, is important. The goal for self-care in activities of daily living should be attainment of age-appropriate competence. Some modifications in the environment, the medical equipment, or the techniques for daily activities are often required to promote and support self-care (Fig. 43-2). Effective teaching for self-care is focused at the child's own level of conceptual understanding and may be augmented by the use of dolls, other models and diagrams, simple explanations, and repetition.

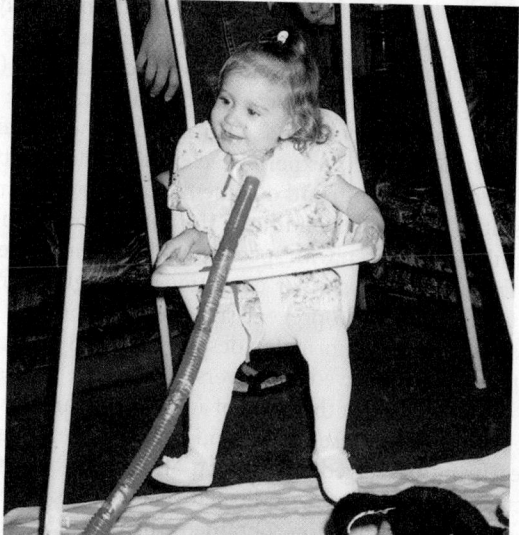

Fig. 43-2 Use of lengthy tubing facilitates a child's freedom of movement.

Educational planning is important for the child who has a chronic medical condition. Federal laws ensure that all children receive a public education. Before age 3 years, children with developmental delays are eligible for an early intervention program. The child can receive rehabilitation therapies as appropriate (physical, occupational, or speech therapy). After age 3 years, the local school system is responsible for providing this education. Some children may be eligible for special education preschools. The home care nurse should refer the family to local educational programs.

Each family is entitled to an individual family service plan (IFSP), or individualized care plan, to help ensure early intervention. All states in the United States provide agencies that develop IFSPs; each state's plan can easily be accessed via the Internet by entering the term *individual family service plan* in an Internet search engine such as Yahoo or Google. The IFSP provides the child with a disability, from birth to age 3 years, with a plan for integrating early intervention and rehabilitation, based on the child's and family's needs.

When a child requiring special medical care is to be placed in an educational setting, the parents, child, school health coordinator, educational evaluation team, and education and administrative staff should meet to determine safe and appropriate placement and the necessary services and personnel to enable the child to attend school in the least restrictive environment. Training of education staff and caregivers is essential to ensuring the child's safety in the educational setting.* Special assistance can also be beneficial in reintegrating previously schooled children, such as those with cancer, into the school setting. The home care nurse may need to assist parents in developing the skills to advocate effectively for their child in the educational system.

Safety Issues in the Home

Safety is an important consideration in pediatric home care and should be addressed in the home care plan.

NURSING ALERT Arrangements should be made to ensure that in an emergency the family has adequate methods of communicating with properly trained emergency medical personnel (e.g., a telephone). A cellular phone may be used in place of a landline, but it is advisable to check with the local emergency facilities regarding policies for cell phone use and emergency 911 calls.

The telephone and electric companies (if the use of medical equipment requires electricity) must be notified that the family needs to be placed on a priority service list. In this way the family will learn of any anticipated interruptions in service and will receive priority in reinstatement of interrupted services. Prior contact with rescue squad and local emergency

A thorough discussion of training issues, content, and guidelines for care in the school is provided in Porter S et al (editors): Children and youth assisted by medical technology in educational settings: guidelines for care, *ed 2, Baltimore, 1997, Paul H. Brookes.*

facility personnel can help ensure prompt and appropriate interventions if required. This is especially important if the family lives in a rural location that may not be familiar to local emergency responders. It is recommended that local authorities be given a map marked with key landmarks and intersections for rapid access to the home.

Before hospital discharge, emergency protocols are developed and reviewed with the parents and professional caregivers. Cardiopulmonary resuscitation guidelines, if appropriate, should be posted near the child's bedside or in another accessible location. A list of emergency telephone numbers can be placed near each home phone and should include those of the rescue squad, emergency department, managing physician(s), nursing agency, and equipment vendor(s) or providers. Additional issues to consider are advance directives and out-of-hospital do-not-resuscitate (OHDNR) orders (may vary by state), as indicated. If the patient and family desire enforcement of an *advance directive*, they must follow specific guidelines, which could prevent undesired lifesaving measures for children with terminal illnesses.

Another aspect of safety relates to the provision of care by appropriately trained individuals. Family members should receive thorough training in the child's care requirements and have the opportunity to demonstrate knowledge and confidence before hospital discharge. Children with complex medical care needs are often admitted to an acute care center for nonmedical reasons, including lack of parent training and parents' inability to care for a child with complex medical needs (Schanwald, 2005). One study found that although technology-dependent children cared for in the home received adequate care, the time demands of such care had negative effects on the caregiver's school, employment, and social life. Furthermore, a shortage of skilled caregivers often leads to disrupted sleep patterns and increased stress (Heaton et al, 2005). Professional staff caring for the child should have the appropriate background and training for the child's particular care needs. Because of the child's body size, special skill and caution are required in the performance of procedures (e.g., gastrostomy feedings, suctioning) and in monitoring the use of equipment (e.g., ventilator settings, intravenous flow rates, and total fluid volumes).

The activity level and curiosity of young children raise additional safety considerations in the provision of home care. All medications, needles, syringes, and contaminated materials must be securely stored well out of the reach of curious hands. Arrangements for the disposal of sharp items or contaminated materials can be made with the home health agency. Special attention is given to childproofing the control panels on ventilators, pumps, monitors, and other equipment. The use of clear plastic tape, covers, or panels to cover control knobs or buttons reduces the risk of accidental changes in settings. Much of the medical equipment now in use has special lock-out capabilities that may be used to prevent accidentally altering settings. Electrical cords are kept short and out of reach, and safety covers are used on any open outlets. Equipment is unplugged when not in use, and any wires (e.g., lead wires for an apnea monitor) are stored out of reach.

Care at night poses other safety concerns. Parents or other caregivers need to be able to clearly hear monitor, ventilator, or pump alarms at night; an inexpensive intercom system or baby monitor can be used. Steps must be taken to prevent accidental strangulation by apnea, oximeter, or cardiac monitor wires or lengthy intravenous tubing during sleep.

NURSING ALERT Coiling extra tubing and taping it at the exit site, as well as running wires or tubes out the bottoms of pajamas or one-piece infant suits, are precautions against strangulation.

Safe transportation is a vital concern. Wheelchairs and other medical equipment must be properly secured to the vehicle, including vans and buses. Appropriate child restraints must be used. If necessary, an extra adult should be present to monitor the child while in transit. Information on car seat safety and transportation for children with special needs is available from the American Academy of Pediatrics (1999) reference, which provides guidelines for wheelchairs in cars, supine car seats, and equipment transportation. (See also Chapter 37, Motor Vehicle Injuries, for discussion of transportation of children with special needs.)

Family-to-Family Support

Family-to-family support networks can be an important source of emotional and instrumental support and empowerment for families of children with chronic health problems. Family-to-family support does not replace professional sources of support but rather is a unique resource that promotes family strengths through shared experience.

Families will most likely experience increased emotional stress as the result of living with and caring for a child with special needs. Other issues that are likely to arise as a result of the child's illness and the constant attention required include labeling the child as being vulnerable, or *vulnerable child syndrome,* wherein parents may spend too much time preoccupied with the child's welfare while ignoring other family members' needs (Bennett, 2002). As the child with special health care needs develops and grows, parents should impose the same disciplinary rules on the child receiving home care as on siblings to avoid further conflict within the family.

Identifying meaningful sources of support can make a difference in coping abilities. Montagnino and Mauricio (2004) surveyed a group of mothers caring for children in the home who had a tracheostomy and gastrostomy. The researchers found that the mothers experienced significant anxiety, and social interaction within and outside the family was disrupted as a result of the child's condition. The authors recommended that families of children with special health care needs network with other parents in similar conditions through online and local support groups to prevent social disruption and maintain a sense of family normalcy despite the child's condition.

Baum (2004) surveyed caregivers of children with special health care needs about the value of an Internet parent support group; the researcher used stress and coping theory as a guide for measuring perceived satisfaction and a number of other characteristics. The survey indicated that parents were satisfied with the information obtained through the Internet support group, and improved caregiver-child relationship was the strongest outcome factor. The author suggests that undesirable results may also be obtained via such Internet groups and that parents should carefully evaluate the quality of such support groups.

The nurse can assist the family in increasing their involvement in community social networks. For example, a referral to a parent support group may meet an individual family's needs. The nurse should inform the parents of the group's goals so that they can determine whether they might benefit from this connection. In addition, informal support networks can be extremely beneficial. A link to a family in the same or a similar situation allows the sharing of common experiences. This in itself may decrease the sense of isolation and provide a connection with someone who can really identify with family struggles. Positive outcomes can include understanding, empathizing, problem solving, or just talking to someone who will listen.

The nurse should remember that each family member's needs differ. The care plan should acknowledge the needs of each family member (mother, father, siblings, grandparents). Peer support for school-age children and adolescents with complex care needs may be beneficial. These connections can be expanded to include letter writing, e-mails, telephone calls, or specialty camping programs (Johnson, Ravert, & Everton, 2001). Most school-age children and adolescents just want to be accepted by their peers and fit in as a part of the group. Same-age peers may at first be standoffish to children with disabilities, but this is likely out of fear and lack of understanding; helping others see that they have the same dreams, desires, goals, and interests promotes group cohesiveness and understanding.

Key Points

- Effective home care depends on many factors, including the child's medical stability; the family's willingness, training, and ability to accommodate the child's care requirements; and professional, financial, and community support.
- Comprehensive, multidisciplinary discharge planning should begin early and should include the family and a home care coordinator in addition to hospital personnel.
- Thorough education and training of the family or primary caregiver can ease the transition to home.
- Care coordination ensures continuity of care, prevents duplication of services, and reduces fragmentation of services. The family may assume responsibility for varying degrees of care coordination over time.
- The home care nurse must possess a high level of technical expertise while being able to adapt equipment, procedures, and the nursing process to the home setting.
- Federal standards apply to agencies that participate in Medicare or Medicaid; standards of practice by the American Nurses Association and other professional nursing organizations can guide nurses in the home setting.
- Family-centered nursing practice is applied in the home setting; diversity in family structures, cultural backgrounds, strengths, and coping mechanisms is respected.

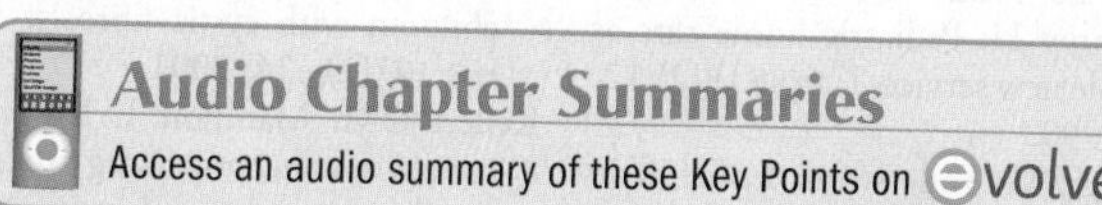
Audio Chapter Summaries
Access an audio summary of these Key Points on evolve

- Collaborative relationships between parents and home care providers are characterized by communication, dialog, active listening, awareness and acceptance of differences, and negotiation.
- The nursing process is adapted to involve the family in each step and to preserve the family's central role in decision making.
- House rules agreed on by the nurse, child, and family allow the family to maintain a feeling of control over their own environment when professionals are present.
- Individualized home care plans are designed to promote optimum development of the child and to focus on normalization—the impact of the child's medical condition and technologic requirements on development, self-care, and educational needs.
- Safety in the provision of home care services involves emergency preparations and protocols, appropriate training of family and home care personnel, and the safe use and childproofing of medical equipment.
- Family-to-family support networks can provide emotional and instrumental support and foster family empowerment.

References

American Academy of Pediatrics: Care coordination in the medical home: integrating health and related systems of care for children with special health care needs, *Pediatrics* 116(5): 1238-1244, 2005.

American Academy of Pediatrics: Transporting children with special health care needs, *Pediatrics* 104(4): 988-992, 1999.

American Nurses Association: *Competencies for telehealth technologies in nursing*, Washington, DC, 1999a, The Association.

American Nurses Association: *Standards of home health nursing practice*, Washington, DC, 1999b, The Association.

American Nurses Association: *Standards of public health nursing practice*, Washington, DC, 1999c, The Association.

American Nurses Association: *Nursing case management*, Washington, DC, 1998, The Association.

Antonelli RC, Stille CJ, Antonelli DM: Care coordination for children and youth with special health care needs: a descriptive, multisite study of activities, personnel, costs, and outcomes, *Pediatrics* 122(1):e209-e216, 2008.

Bagust A et al: Economic evaluation of an acute paediatric hospital at home clinical trial, *Arch Dis Child* 87:489-492, 2002.

Bakewell-Sachs S et al: Home care considerations for chronic and vulnerable populations, *Nurse Pract Forum* 11(1):65-72, 2000.

Baum LS: Internet parent support groups for primary caregivers of a child with special health care needs, *Pediatr Nurs* 30(5):381-388, 401, 2004.

Bennett AD: Home apnea monitoring for infants: a discussion of primary care issues, *Adv Nurs Pract* 10(3):48-53, 2002.

Cooper C et al: Specialist home-based nursing services for children with acute and chronic illnesses, *Cochrane Database Syst Rev* 18(4):CD004383, 2006.

Daveluy W et al: Dramatic changes in home-based enteral nutrition practices in children during an 11-year period, *J Pediatr Gastroenterol Nurs* 43(2):240-244, 2006.

Davidhizar R, Havnes R, Bechtel G: Assessing culturally diverse pediatric clients, *Pediatr Nurs* 25(4):371-376, 1999.

Davis C: Safe on the home watch, *Nurs Stand* 20(34):20-22, 2006.

Dittbrenner H: Pediatric home care as a viable new service, *Caring* 18(2):12-15, 1999.

Dougherty G, Soderstrom L, Schiffrin A: An economic evaluation of home care for children with newly diagnosed diabetes: results from a randomized controlled trial, *Med Care* 36(4):586-598, 1998.

Feudtner C et al: Technology-dependence among patients discharged from a children's hospital: a retrospective cohort study, *BMC Pediatrics* 5(8):1-8, 2005.

Giger JN, Davidhizar R: The Giger and Davidhizar Transcultural Assessment Model, *J Transcult Nurs* 13(3):185-188, 2002.

Hanson JL, Randall VF: Evaluating and improving the practice of family-centered care, *Pediatr Nurs* 25(4):445-449, 1999.

Harrigan RC et al: Medically fragile children: an integrative review of the literature and recommendations for future research, *Issues Compr Pediatr Nurs* 25(1):1-20, 2002.

Heaton J et al: Families' experiences of caring for technology-dependent children: a temporal perspective, *Health Soc Care Community* 13(5):441-450, 2005.

Howard L: Home parenteral nutrition: survival, cost, and quality of life, *Gastroenterology* 130(2 Suppl 1):S52-S59, 2006.

Johnson BH: Family-centered care: facing the new millennium: interview by Elizabeth Ahmann, *Pediatr Nurs* 26(1):87-90, 2000.

Johnson CP, Kastner TA, American Academy of Pediatrics, Committee on Children with Disabilities: Helping families raise children with special health care needs at home, *Pediatrics* 115(2):507-511, 2005.

Johnson KB, Ravert RD, Everton A: Hopkins Teen Central: assessment of an Internet-based support system for children with cystic fibrosis, *Pediatrics* 107(2):e24, 2001.

Kellett UM, Mannion J: Meaning in caring: reconceptualizing the nurse–family carer relationship in community practice, *J Adv Nurs* 29(3):697-703, 1999.

Knafl KA, Deatrick JA: The challenges of normalization for families of children with chronic conditions, *Pediatr Nurs* 28(1):49-53, 56, 2002.

Lewis JA, Sommers CO: Personal data assistants: using new technology to enhance nursing practice, *MCN* 28(2):66-71, 2003.

Lindeke LL et al: Family-centered care coordination for children with special needs across multiple settings, *J Pediatr Health Care* 16(6):290-297, 2002.

Magrabi F et al: Designing home telecare: a case study in monitoring cystic fibrosis, *Telemed J e-health* 11(6):707-719, 2005.

McEvoy M: Culture and spirituality as an integrated concept in pediatric care, *MCN* 28(1):39-43, 2003.

McKlindon D, Barsteiner JH: Therapeutic relationships, *MCN* 24(5):237-243, 1999.

Montagnino BA, Mauricio RV: The child with a tracheostomy and gastrostomy: parental stress and coping in the home—a pilot study, *Pediatr Nurs* 30(5):373-380, 401, 2004.

National Alliance for Caregiving: *Family caregiving in the U.S.: findings from a national survey*, 2005, The Alliance. Available at www.caregiving.org/data/04execsumm.pdf (accessed April 22, 2009).

National Center for Cultural Competence: Developing cultural competence in health care settings, *Pediatr Nurs* 28(2):133-137, 2002.

Navaie-Waliser M et al: Evaluating the needs of children with asthma in home care: the vital role of nurses as caregivers and educators, *Pub Health Nurs* 21(4):306-315, 2004.

Nazer D et al: Home versus hospital intravenous antibiotic therapy for acute pulmonary exacerbations in children with cystic fibrosis, *Pediatr Pulmonol* 41(8):744-749, 2006.

Newton MS: Family-centered care: current realities in parent participation, *Pediatr Nurs* 26(2):164-168, 2000.

Page DR: Pediatric home care: nursing the shortage, *Caring* 20(6):46-47, 2001.

Parra MM: Nursing and respite care services for ventilator-assisted children, *Caring* 22(5):6-9, 2003.

Petit de Mange EA: Pediatric considerations in home care, *Crit Care Nurs Clin North Am* 10(3):339-346, 1998.

Rice R: Case management and leadership strategies for home care nurses. In Rice R (editor): *Home care nursing practice: concepts and application*, ed 4, St Louis, 2006, Mosby.

Roush CV, Cox JE: The meaning of home: how it shapes the practice of home and hospice care, *Home Healthc Nurse* 18(6):388-394, 2000.

Schanwald PR: Gaps in pediatric care, *Caring* 25(9):20-25, 2005.

Spruhan JB: Beyond traditional nursing care: cultural awareness and successful home healthcare nursing, *Home Healthc Nurse* 14(6):445-449, 1996.

Stevens B et al: Children receiving chemotherapy at home: perceptions of children and parents, *J Pediatr Oncol Nurs* 23(5):276-285, 2006.

Strawczynski H et al: Delivery of care to hemophilic children: home care versus hospitalization, *Pediatrics* 51(6):986-991, 1973.

Sullivan T: Caregiver Strain Index, *Home Healthc Nurse* 21(3):197-198, 2003.

Sullivan-Bolyai S et al: Great expectations: a position description for parents as caregivers, part II, *Pediatr Nurs* 30(1):52-56, 2004.

Sullivan-Bolyai S et al: Great expectations: a position description for parents as caregivers, part I, *Pediatr Nurs* 29(6):457-460, 2003.

Thompson J: Pediatric assessment in the home, *Home Healthc Nurse* 18(10):639-646, 2000.

Timm S: Effectively delegating nursing activities in home care, *Home Healthc Nurse* 21(4):260-265, 2003.

Wilson A: Understanding benchmarks, *Home Healthc Nurse* 21(2):102-107, 2003.

Wilson H: HIPAA: the big picture for home care and hospice, *Home Health Care Manage Pract* 16(2):127-137, 2004.

Yoder-Wise P: *Leading and managing in nursing*, ed 4, St Louis, 2007, Mosby.

Unit 10

44 Reaction to Illness and Hospitalization

Learning Objectives

On completion of this chapter the reader will be able to:

- Identify the stressors of illness and hospitalization for children during each developmental stage.
- List essential priorities of nursing care for a child on admission to the hospital.
- Outline nursing interventions that prevent or minimize the stress of separation during hospitalization.
- Outline nursing interventions that minimize the stress of loss of control during hospitalization.
- Outline nursing interventions that minimize the fear of bodily injury during hospitalization.
- Outline nursing interventions that support parents, siblings, and family during a child's illness and hospitalization.
- Describe nursing interventions needed when children are admitted to special units such as the emergency department.

Electronic Resources

Additional information related to the content in Chapter 44 can be found on

evolve the Companion Website at

http://evolve.elsevier.com/Perry/maternal/

- NCLEX Review Questions
- Critical Thinking Exercise—Discharge Planning
- Nursing Care Plan—The Child in the Hospital
- Nursing Care Plan—The Child Undergoing Surgery
- Nursing Care Plan—The Family of the Ill or Hospitalized Child
- Skill—Admitting a Child to the Health Care System
- Skill—Preparing the Child for Surgery
- Skill—Therapeutic Play

Stressors of Hospitalization and Children's Reactions

Often, illness and hospitalization are the first crises children must face. Especially during the early years, children are particularly vulnerable to the crises of illness and hospitalization because (1) stress represents a change from the usual state of health and environmental routine and (2) children have a limited number of coping mechanisms to resolve *stressors* (those events that produce stress). Major stressors of hospitalization include separation, loss of control, bodily injury, and pain. Children's reactions to these crises are influenced by their developmental age; their previous experience with illness, separation, or hospitalization; their innate and acquired coping skills; the seriousness of the diagnosis; and the support system available.

Separation Anxiety

The major stress from middle infancy throughout the preschool years, especially for children ages 6 to 30 months, is separation anxiety, also called *anaclitic depression.* The principal behavioral responses to this stressor during early childhood are summarized in Box 44-1. During the phase of *protest,* children react aggressively to the separation from the parent. They cry and scream for their parents, refuse the attention of anyone else, and are inconsolable in their grief (Fig. 44-1). During the phase of *despair,* the crying stops and depression is evident. The child is much less active, is uninterested in play or food, and withdraws from others (Fig. 44-2).

The third stage is *detachment,* also called *denial.* Superficially it appears that the child has finally adjusted to the loss. The child becomes more interested in the surroundings, plays with others, and seems to form new relationships. However, this behavior is the result of resignation and is not a sign of contentment. The child detaches from the parent in an effort to escape the emotional pain of desiring the parent's presence and copes by forming shallow relationships with others, becoming increasingly self-centered, and attaching primary importance to material objects. This is the most serious stage in that reversal of the potential adverse effects is less likely to occur after detachment is established. However, in most situations, the temporary separations imposed by hospitalization do not cause such prolonged parental absences that the child enters into detachment. In addition, considerable evidence suggests that even with stressors such as separation, children are remarkably adaptable and permanent ill effects are rare.

Although progression to the stage of detachment is uncommon, the initial stages are frequently observed even with brief separations from either parent. Unless health team members

BOX 44-1 Manifestations of Separation Anxiety in Young Children

Phase of Protest

Behaviors observed during later infancy include:

- Crying
- Screaming
- Searching for parent with eyes
- Clinging to parent
- Avoiding and rejecting contact with strangers

Additional behaviors observed during toddlerhood include:

- Verbally attacking strangers (e.g., "Go away")
- Physically attacking strangers (e.g., kicking, biting, hitting, pinching)
- Attempting to escape to find parent
- Attempting to physically force parent to stay

Behaviors may last from hours to days.

Protest, such as crying, may be continuous, ceasing only with physical exhaustion.

Approach of stranger may precipitate increased protest.

Phase of Despair

Observed behaviors include:

- Being inactive
- Withdrawing from others
- Being depressed, sad
- Lacking interest in environment
- Being uncommunicative
- Regressing to earlier behavior (e.g., thumb sucking, bed-wetting, use of pacifier, use of bottle)

Behaviors may last for variable length of time.

Child's physical condition may deteriorate from refusal to eat, drink, or move.

Phase of Detachment

Observed behaviors include:

- Showing increased interest in surroundings
- Interacting with strangers or familiar caregivers
- Forming new but superficial relationships
- Appearing happy

Detachment usually occurs after prolonged separation from parent; it is rarely seen in hospitalized children.

Behaviors represent a superficial adjustment to loss.

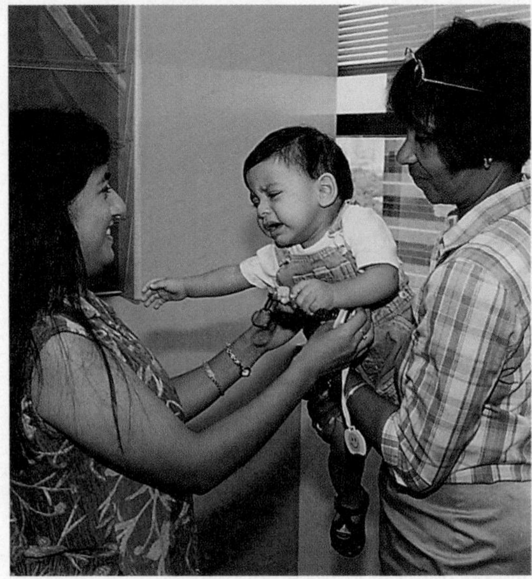

Fig. 44-1 In the protest phase of separation anxiety, children cry loudly and are inconsolable in their grief for the parent. *(Courtesy James DeLeon, Texas Children's Hospital, Houston, TX.)*

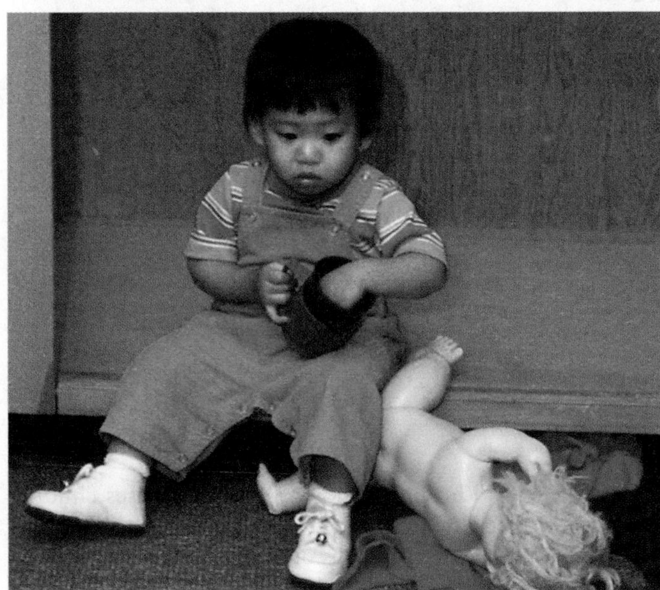

Fig. 44-2 During the despair phase of separation anxiety, children are sad, lonely, and uninterested in food and play.

understand the meaning of each stage of behavior, they may erroneously label the behaviors as positive or negative. For example, they may see the loud crying of the protest phase as "bad" behavior. Because the protests increase when a stranger approaches the child, they may interpret that reaction as meaning they should stay away. During the quiet, withdrawn phase of despair, health team members may think that the child is finally "settling in" to the new surroundings, and they may see the detachment behaviors as proof of a "good adjustment." The faster this stage is reached, the more likely it is that the child will be regarded as the "ideal patient."

Because children seem to react "negatively" to visits by their parents, uninformed observers feel justified in restricting parental visiting privileges. For example, during the protest stage, children outwardly do not appear happy to see their parents (Fig. 44-3). In fact, they may even cry louder. If they are depressed, they may reject their parents or begin to protest again. Often they cling to their parents in an effort to ensure their continued presence. Consequently, such reactions may be regarded as "disturbing" the child's adjustment to the new surroundings. If the separation has progressed to the phase of detachment, children will respond no differently to their parents than they would to any other person.

Such reactions are distressing to parents, who are unaware of their meaning. If parents are regarded as intruders, they will see their absence as "beneficial" to the child's adjustment and recovery. They may respond to the child's behavior by staying for only short periods, visiting less frequently, or deceiving the child when it is time to leave. The result is a destructive cycle of misunderstanding and unmet needs.

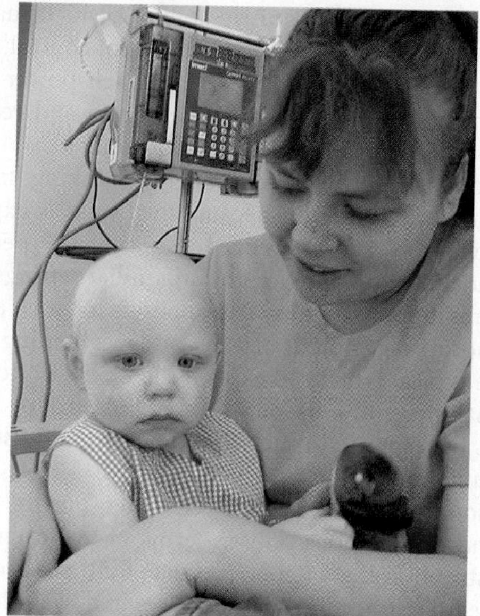

Fig. 44-3 Young children may appear withdrawn and sad even in the presence of a parent. *(Courtesy E. Jacob, Texas Children's Hospital, Houston, TX.)*

Early Childhood

Separation anxiety is the greatest stress imposed by hospitalization during early childhood. If separation is avoided, young children have a tremendous capacity to withstand any other stress. During this period, the typical reactions just described are seen. However, children in the toddler stage demonstrate more goal-directed behaviors. For example, they may plead with the parents to stay and physically try to keep the parents with them or try to find parents who have left. They may demonstrate displeasure on the parents' return or departure by having temper tantrums; refusing to comply with the usual routines of mealtime, bedtime, or toileting; or regressing to more primitive levels of development. However, temper tantrums, bed-wetting, or other behaviors may also be expressions of anger, a physiologic response to stress, or symptoms of illness.

Because preschoolers are more secure interpersonally than toddlers, they can tolerate brief periods of separation from their parents and are more inclined to develop substitute trust in other significant adults. However, the stress of illness usually renders preschoolers less able to cope with separation; as a result, they manifest many of the stage behaviors of separation anxiety, although in general the protest behaviors are more subtle and passive than those seen in younger children. Preschoolers may demonstrate separation anxiety by refusing to eat, experiencing difficulty in sleeping, crying quietly for their parents, continually asking when the parents will visit, or withdrawing from others. They may express anger indirectly by breaking their toys, hitting other children, or refusing to cooperate during usual self-care activities. Nurses need to be sensitive to these less obvious signs of separation anxiety in order to intervene appropriately.

Later Childhood and Adolescence

Previous research, usually based on adult recollections, indicated that the family does not play as important a role for school-age children as it does during the toddler and preschool years. However, in a recent study that asked children about their fears when hospitalized, children listed their greatest fears regarding hospitalization as being separated from family and friends, being in an unfamiliar environment, receiving investigations or treatments, and losing self-determination or choices (Coyne, 2006).

Although school-age children are better able to cope with separation in general, the stress and often accompanying regression imposed by illness or hospitalization may increase their need for parental security and guidance. This is particularly true for young school-age children who have only recently left the safety of the home and are struggling with the crisis of school adjustment. Middle and late school-age children may react more to the separation from their usual activities and peers than to the absence of their parents. These children have a high level of physical and mental activity that frequently finds no suitable outlets in the hospital environment, and even when they dislike school, they admit to missing its routine and worry that they will not be able to compete or "fit in" with their classmates when they return. Feelings of loneliness, boredom, isolation, and depression are common. Such reactions may occur more as a result of separation than of concern over the illness, treatment, or hospital setting.

School-age children may need and desire parental guidance or support from other adult figures but may be unable or unwilling to ask for it. Because the goal of attaining independence is so important to them, they are reluctant to seek help directly, fearing that they will appear weak, childish, or dependent. Cultural expectations to "act like a man" or to "be brave and strong" weigh heavily on these children, especially boys, who tend to react to stress with stoicism, withdrawal, or passive acceptance. Often the need to express hostile, angry, or other negative feelings finds outlets in alternate ways, such as irritability and aggression toward parents, withdrawal from hospital personnel, inability to relate to peers, rejection of siblings, or subsequent behavioral problems in school.

For adolescents, separation from home and parents may produce varied emotions, ranging from difficulty coping to welcoming the event. However, loss of peer-group contact may pose a severe emotional threat because of loss of group status, inability to exert group control or leadership, and loss of group acceptance. Deviations within peer groups are poorly tolerated, and although group members may express concern for the adolescent's illness or need for hospitalization, they continue their group activities, quickly filling the gap of the absent member. During the temporary separation from their usual group, ill adolescents may benefit from group associations with other hospitalized teens.

Loss of Control

One of the factors influencing the amount of stress imposed by hospitalization is the amount of control that persons perceive themselves as having. Lack of control increases the perception of threat and can affect children's coping skills. Many hospital situations decrease the amount of control a child feels. Although the usual sensory stimulations are lacking, the additional hospital stimuli of sight, sound, and smell may be overwhelming. Without an insight into the type of environment conducive to children's optimal growth, the hospital experience can at best temporarily slow development and at worst permanently restrict it. Because children's needs vary greatly depending on their age, the major areas of loss of control in terms of physical restriction, altered routine or rituals, and dependency are discussed for each age group.

Infants

Infants are developing the most important attribute of a healthy personality—trust. Trust is established through consistent, loving care by a nurturing person. Infants attempt to control their environment through emotional expressions, such as crying or smiling. In the hospital setting, cues may be missed or misinterpreted, and routines may be established to meet the hospital staff's needs instead of the infant's needs. Inconsistent care and deviations from the infant's daily routine may lead to mistrust and a decreased sense of control.

Toddlers

Toddlers are striving for autonomy, and this goal is evident in most of their behaviors: motor skills, play, interpersonal relationships, activities of daily living, and communication. When their egocentric pleasures meet with obstacles, toddlers react with negativism, especially temper tantrums. Any restriction or limitation of movement, such as the simple act of making toddlers lie down, can cause forceful resistance and noncompliance.

Loss of control also results from altered routines and rituals. Toddlers rely on the consistency and familiarity of daily rituals to provide a measure of stability and control in their complex world of growing and developing. The experience of hospitalization or illness severely limits their sense of expectation and predictability, since practically every detail of the hospital environment differs from that of the home.

Toddlers' main areas for rituals include eating, sleeping, bathing, toileting, and play. When the routines are disrupted, difficulties can occur in any or all of these areas. The principal reaction to such change is regression. For example, when mealtime and food choices differ from those at home, toddlers often refuse to eat, demand a bottle, or ask others to feed them. Although regression to earlier forms of behavior may seem to increase toddlers' security and comfort, in reality it is threatening for them to relinquish their most recently acquired achievements.

Enforced dependency is a chief characteristic of the sick role and accounts for the numerous instances of toddler negativism. For example, rigid schedules, different clothes, altered caregiving activities, unfamiliar surroundings, separation from parents, and medical procedures usurp toddlers' control over their world. Although most toddlers initially react negatively and aggressively to such dependency, prolonged loss of autonomy may result in passive withdrawal from interpersonal relationships and regression in all areas of development. Therefore the effects of the sick role are most severe in instances of chronic, long-term illnesses or in those families who foster the sick role despite the child's improved health.

Preschoolers

Preschoolers also suffer from loss of control caused by physical restriction, altered routines, and enforced dependency. However, their specific cognitive abilities, which make them feel all-powerful, also make them feel out of control. This loss of control in the context of their sense of self-power is a critical influencing factor in their perception of and reaction to separation, pain, illness, and hospitalization.

Preschoolers' egocentric and magical thinking limits their ability to understand events because they view all experiences from their own self-referenced (egocentric) perspective. Without adequate preparation for unfamiliar settings or experiences, preschoolers' fantasy explanations for such events are usually more exaggerated, bizarre, and frightening than the facts. One typical fantasy to explain the illness or hospitalization is that it represents punishment for real or imagined misdeeds. In response to such thinking the child usually feels shame, guilt, and fear.

Preschoolers' preoperational thinking means that they understand explanations only in terms of real events. Purely verbal instructions are often inadequate for them because they are unable to abstract and synthesize beyond what their senses tell them. When combined with their egocentric and magical thinking, this characteristic may lead them to interpret messages according to their particular past experiences. Even with the best preparation for a procedure, they may misconstrue the details.

School-Age Children

Because of their striving for independence and productivity, school-age children are particularly vulnerable to events that may lessen their feeling of control and power. In particular, altered family roles; physical disability; fears of death, abandonment, or permanent injury; loss of peer acceptance; lack of productivity; and inability to cope with stress according to perceived cultural expectation may result in loss of control.

Because of the nature of the patient role, many routine hospital activities usurp individual power and identity. For school-age children, dependent activities such as enforced bed rest, use of a bedpan, inability to choose a menu, lack of privacy, help with a bed bath, or transport by a wheelchair or stretcher can be a direct threat to their security. Although all these procedures seem routine and inconsequential, they allow no freedom of choice to children who want to "act grown-up." However, when children are allowed to exert a measure of control, regardless of how limited it may be, they generally respond well to any procedure. For example, some of the most cooperative, satisfied, and contented patients are school-age children who help make their beds, choose their schedule of activities, and assist in their own care. An increased sense of control usually results from a feeling of usefulness and productivity.

In addition to the hospital environment, illness may also cause a feeling of loss of control. One of the most significant problems of children in this age group is boredom. When physical or enforced limitations curtail their usual ability to care for themselves or to engage in favorite activities, school-age children generally respond with depression, hostility, or frustration. Keeping a normally active child on bed rest is difficult. However, emphasizing areas of control and capitalizing on quiet activities, particularly hobbies such as building models or playing age-appropriate video or board games, promotes their adjustment to physical restriction.

Adolescents

Adolescents' struggle for independence, self-assertion, and liberation centers on the quest for personal identity. Anything that interferes with this poses a threat to their sense of identity and results in a loss of control. Illness, which limits one's physical abilities, and hospitalization, which separates one from one's usual support systems, constitute major situational crises.

The patient role fosters dependency and depersonalization. Adolescents may react to dependency with rejection, uncooperativeness, or withdrawal. They may respond to depersonalization with self-assertion, anger, or frustration. Regardless of the response elicited, hospital personnel often regard them as difficult, unmanageable patients. Parents may not be a source of help because these behaviors serve to isolate them further from understanding the adolescent. Although peers may visit, they may not be able to offer the kind of support and guidance needed. Sick adolescents often voluntarily isolate themselves from age-mates until they feel they can compete on an equal basis and meet group expectations. As a result, ill adolescents may be left with virtually no support system.

Loss of control also occurs for many of the reasons discussed for school-age children. However, adolescents are more sensitive to potential instances of loss of control and dependency than are younger children. For example, both groups seek information about their physical status and rely heavily on anticipatory preparation to decrease fear and anxiety. However, adolescents react not only to the kinds of information supplied them, but also to the means by which it is conveyed. They may feel threatened by others who relay facts in a condescending manner. Adolescents want to know that others can relate to them on their own level. This necessitates a careful assessment of their intellectual abilities, previous knowledge, and present needs. It may also require the nurse to learn the adolescent's language.

Effects of Hospitalization on the Child

Children may react to the stresses of hospitalization before admission, during hospitalization, and after discharge. A child's concept of illness is even more important than age and intellectual maturity in predicting the level of anxiety before hospitalization (Clatworthy, Simon, & Tiedeman, 1999). This may or may not be affected by the duration of the condition or prior hospitalizations; therefore nurses should avoid overestimating the illness concepts of children with prior medical experience (Box 44-2).

BOX 44-2 Posthospital Behaviors in Children

Young Children

They show initial aloofness toward parents; this may last from a few minutes (most common) to a few days.

This is frequently followed by dependency behaviors:

- Tendency to cling to parents
- Demands for parents' attention
- Vigorous opposition to any separation (e.g., staying at preschool or with a baby-sitter)

Other negative behaviors include:

- New fears (e.g., nightmares)
- Resistance to going to bed, night waking
- Withdrawal and shyness
- Hyperactivity
- Temper tantrums
- Food finickiness
- Attachment to blanket or toy
- Regression in newly learned skills (e.g., self-toileting)

Older Children

Negative behaviors include:

- Emotional coldness, followed by intense, demanding dependence on parents
- Anger toward parents
- Jealousy toward others (e.g., siblings)

Individual Risk Factors

A number of risk factors make certain children more vulnerable than others to the stresses of hospitalization (Box 44-3). Rural children may exhibit significantly greater degrees of psychologic upset than urban children, possibly because urban children have opportunities to become familiar with a local hospital. Because separation is such an important issue surrounding hospitalization for young children, children who are active and strong willed tend to fare better when hospitalized than youngsters who are passive. Consequently, nurses should be alert to children who passively accept all changes and requests; these children may need more support than the "oppositional" child.

BOX 44-3 Risk Factors That Increase Children's Vulnerability to the Stresses of Hospitalization

- "Difficult" temperament
- Lack of fit between child and parent
- Age (especially between 6 months and 5 years)
- Male gender
- Below-average intelligence
- Multiple and continuing stresses (e.g., frequent hospitalizations)

The stressors of hospitalization may cause young children to experience short- and long-term negative outcomes. Adverse outcomes may be related to the length and number of admissions, multiple invasive procedures, and the parents' anxiety. Common responses include regression, separation anxiety, apathy, fears, and sleep disturbances, especially for children younger than 7 years of age (Melnyk, 2000). Supportive practices, such as family-centered care and frequent family visiting, may lessen the detrimental effects of such admissions. Research also indicates that a child's pain experience determines how the overall hospitalization is experienced (Woodgate & Kristjanson, 1996). Consequently nurses should attempt to identify children at risk for poor coping strategies (Small, 2002).

Changes in the Pediatric Population

With a growing trend toward shortened hospital stays and outpatient surgery, a greater percentage of the children hospitalized today have more serious and complex problems than those hospitalized in the past. Many of these children are fragile newborns and children with severe injuries or disabilities who have survived because of major technologic advances, yet have been left with chronic or disabling conditions that require frequent and lengthy hospital stays. The nature of their conditions increases the likelihood that they will experience more invasive and traumatic procedures while they are hospitalized. These factors make them more vulnerable to the emotional consequences of hospitalization and result in their needs being significantly different from those of the short-term patients of the past (see Chapter 41 for further discussion on children with special needs). The majority of these children are infants and toddlers, the age group most vulnerable to the effects of hospitalization.

Concern in recent years has focused on the increasing length of hospitalization because of complex medical and nursing care, elusive diagnoses, and complicated psychosocial issues. Without special attention devoted to meeting the child's psychosocial and developmental needs in the hospital environment, the detrimental consequences of prolonged hospitalization may be severe.

Beneficial Effects of Hospitalization

Although hospitalization usually is stressful for children, it can also be beneficial. The most obvious benefit is the recovery from illness, but hospitalization also can present an opportunity for children to master stress and feel competent in their coping abilities. The hospital environment can provide children with new socialization experiences that can broaden their interpersonal relationships. The psychologic benefits need to be considered and maximized during hospitalization.

Stressors and Reactions of the Family of the Hospitalized Child

Parental Reactions

The crisis of childhood illness and hospitalization affects every member of the family. Parents' reactions to illness in their child depend on a variety of factors. Although one cannot predict which factors are most likely to influence their response, a number of variables have been identified (Box 44-4).

BOX 44-4 Factors Affecting Parents' Reactions to Their Child's Illness

- Seriousness of the threat to the child
- Previous experience with illness or hospitalization
- Medical procedures involved in diagnosis and treatment
- Available support systems
- Personal ego strengths
- Previous coping abilities
- Additional stresses on the family system
- Cultural and religious beliefs
- Communication patterns among family members

Recent research has identified common themes among parents whose children were hospitalized, including feeling an overall sense of helplessness, questioning the skills of staff, accepting the reality of hospitalization, needing to have information explained in simple language, dealing with fear, coping with uncertainty, and seeking reassurance from caregivers. This reassurance involves staff being compassionate, expressing concern for the child, and attending to detail in the child's care (Stranton, 2004).

Sibling Reactions

Siblings' reactions to a sister's or brother's illness or hospitalization are discussed in Chapter 41 and differ little when a child becomes temporarily ill. Siblings experience loneliness, fear, and worry, as well as anger, resentment, jealousy, and guilt. Various factors have been identified that influence the effects of the child's hospitalization on siblings. Although these factors are similar to those seen when a child has a chronic illness, Craft (1993) reported that siblings can feel greater effects from the hospital experience based on the following factors:

- Being younger and experiencing many changes
- Being cared for outside the home by care providers who are not relatives
- Receiving little information about their ill brother or sister
- Perceiving that their parents treat them differently compared with before their sibling's hospitalization

Parents are often unaware of the number of effects that siblings experience during the sick child's hospitalization and the benefit of simple interventions to minimize such effects, such as explicit explanations about the illness and provisions for the siblings to remain at home. Sibling visitation is usually beneficial to the patient, sibling, and parent but should be evaluated on an individual basis. Siblings should be prepared for the visit with developmentally appropriate information and be given the opportunity to ask questions.

Altered Family Roles

In addition to the effects of separation on family roles, loss of parenting, sibling, and offspring roles may affect each family member differently. One of the most common reactions of parents is specialized and intensified attention toward the sick child. The other siblings may regard this as unfair and interpret the parents' attitude toward them as rejection. Although such responses are usually unconscious and unintended, they place unique burdens on ill children. For example, the ill child may feel obligated to play the sick role to meet parents' expectations, especially those children who have had limited physical ability and regain normal health status, such as after corrective heart surgery. Parents may be unable to perceive the child's recovery and therefore continue the pattern of overprotection and indulgent attention.

Ill children may also feel jealousy and resentment from other siblings. Because of their singular position in the family, they may be denied the companionship of their brothers and sisters. Rivalry between siblings tends to be greatest for the sibling who is nearest in age to the ill child. Without an understanding of the interpersonal dynamics between siblings, parents are likely to blame the well children for antisocial behavior. Illness may also result in children's loss of status within either their family or social group. For example, illness in the oldest child may temporarily terminate special privileges as "big" brother or sister.

Nursing Care of the Hospitalized Child

Preparation for Hospitalization

Children and families require individualized care to minimize the potential negative effects of hospitalization. One method that can decrease negative feelings and fear in children is preparation for hospitalization. The rationale for preparing children for the hospital experience and related procedures is based on the principle that fear of the unknown (fantasy) exceeds fear of the known. When children do not have paralyzing fear to cope with, they are able to direct their energies toward dealing with the other, unavoidable stresses of hospitalization.

Although preparation for hospitalization is a common practice, there is no universal standard or program for all settings. The preparation process may be elaborate with tours, puppet shows, and playtime with miniature hospital equipment; it may involve the use of books, videos, or films; or it may be limited to a brief description of the major aspects of any hospital stay (Stewart, Algren, & Arnold, 1994). No consensus exists on the timing of preparation. Some authorities recommend preparing children 4 to 7 years of age about 1 week in advance so that they can assimilate the information and ask questions. For older children the time may be longer. However, for young children, who may begin to fantasize about what they observed, 1 or 2 days before admission is sufficient time for anticipatory preparation. The length of the session should be tailored to the children's attention span—the younger the child, the shorter the program. The optimal approach is one that is individualized for each child and family.

Regardless of the specific type of program, all children, even those who have been hospitalized before, benefit from an introduction to the environment and routine of the unit. Sometimes it is not possible to prepare children and families for hospitalization, as in the event of sudden, acute illness. However, care should be taken to orient the child and family to hospital routines, establish expectations, and allow for questions.

NURSING ALERT In many hospitals, child life specialists—health care professionals with extensive knowledge of child growth and development and of the special psychosocial needs of children who are hospitalized and their families—help prepare children for hospitalization, surgery, and procedures. A collaborative effort between the nurse, child life specialist, and other members of the child's health care team helps ensure the best possible hospital experience for the child and family.

Admission Assessment

The nursing admission history refers to a systematic collection of data about the child and family that allows the nurse to plan individualized care. The nursing admission history presented in Box 44-5 is organized according to the Functional Health Patterns outlined by Gordon (1994, 2002). This assessment framework is a guideline for formulating nursing diagnoses. One of the main purposes of the history is to assess the child's usual health habits at home to promote a more normal environment in the hospital. Therefore questions related to activities of daily living in the nutrition-metabolic, elimination, sleep-rest, and activity-exercise patterns are a major part of the assessment. The questions found under the health perception–health management pattern are directed toward evaluation of the child's preparation for hospitalization and are key factors in determining whether additional preparation is needed. The questions included in the self-perception–self-concept and role-relationship patterns offer insight into the child's potential reaction to hospitalization, especially in terms of separation.

The nurse should also inquire about the use of any medications at home, including complementary medicine practices (Box 44-6). In a study of children with cancer, 42% had used alternative or complementary therapies simultaneously with or after conventional treatments (Fernandez, Pyesmany, & Stutzer, 1999). It is important that the use of any herbal or complementary therapy be noted in a preoperative assessment because of possible anesthesia or surgical complications related to herbal products (Flanagan, 2001).

After collecting the admission data, the nurse must apply the information to the nursing process and communicate it to other staff. Information gathered in the nursing admission assessment can offer insight into family dynamics, assist in normalization of the hospital environment, and aid staff members in meeting the child and family's needs. Asking questions and seeking information directly from the child in an age-appropriate manner can yield a wealth of information regarding understanding of their illness and hospitalization.

Besides completing the nursing admission history, nurses should also perform a physical assessment (see Chapter 34) before planning care. At the very least, the nurse's physical assessment of the child should include observation of the body for any bruises, rashes, signs of neglect, deformities, or physical limitations. The nurse should also listen to the heart and lungs to assess overall physical status. For example, it is impossible to evaluate improvement in respiratory function in a child admitted with pulmonary disease unless there are baseline data with which to compare subsequent findings.

Preparing Child for Admission

The preparation that children require on the day of admission depends on the kind of prehospital counseling they have received. If they have been prepared in a formalized program, they will usually know what to expect in terms of initial medical procedures, inpatient facilities, and nursing staff. However, prehospital counseling does not preclude the need for support during procedures such as obtaining blood specimens, x-ray tests, or physical examination. For example, undressing young children before they feel comfortable in their new surroundings can be upsetting. Causing needless anxiety and fear during admission may adversely affect the nurse's establishment of trust with these children. Therefore nursing assistance during the admission procedure is vital, regardless of how well prepared any child is for the experience

evolve Skill—Admitting a Child to the Health Care System

BOX 44-5 Nursing Admission History According to Functional Health Patterns*

Health Perception–Health Management Pattern

Why has your child been admitted?

How has your child's general health been?

What does your child know about this hospitalization?

- Ask the child why he or she came to the hospital.
- If the answer is "For an operation or for tests," ask the child to tell you about what will happen before, during, and after the operation or tests.

Has your child ever been in the hospital before?

- How was that hospital experience?
- What things were important to you and your child during that hospitalization? How can we be most helpful now?

What medications does your child take at home?

- Why are they given?
- When are they given?
- How are they given (if a liquid, with a spoon; if a tablet, swallowed with water; or other)?
- Does your child have any trouble taking medication? If so, what helps?
- Is your child allergic to any medications?

What, if any, forms of complementary medicine practices are being used?

Nutrition-Metabolic Pattern

What are the family's usual mealtimes?

Do family members eat together or at separate times?

What are your child's favorite foods, beverages, and snacks?

- Average amounts consumed or usual size of portions
- Special cultural practices, such as family eating only ethnic food

What foods and beverages does your child dislike?

What are your child's feeding habits (bottle, cup, spoon, eating by self, needing assistance, any special devices)?

How does your child like the food served (warmed, cold, one item at a time)?

How would you describe your child's usual appetite (hearty eater, picky eater)?

- Has being sick affected your child's appetite? In what ways?

Are there any known or suspected food allergies?

Is your child on a special diet?

Are there any feeding problems (excessive fussiness, spitting up, colic); any dental or gum problems that affect feeding?

- What do you do for these problems?

Elimination Pattern

What are your child's toilet habits (diaper, toilet trained—day only or day and night, use of word to communicate urination or defecation, potty chair, regular toilet, other routines)?

What is your child's usual pattern of elimination (bowel movements)?

Do you have any concerns about elimination (bed-wetting, constipation, diarrhea)?

- What do you do for these problems?

Have you ever noticed that your child sweats a lot?

Sleep-Rest Pattern

What is your child's usual hour of sleep and awakening?

What is your child's schedule for naps; length of naps?

Is there a special routine before sleeping (bottle, drink of water, bedtime story, night-light, favorite blanket or toy, prayers)?

Is there a special routine during sleep time, such as waking to go to the bathroom?

What type of bed does your child sleep in?

Does your child have a separate room or share a room; if shares, with whom?

Does you child sleep with someone or alone (sibling, parent, other person)?

What is your child's favorite sleeping position?

Are there any sleeping problems (falling asleep, waking during night, nightmares, sleep walking)?

Are there any problems in awakening and getting ready in the morning?

- What do you do for these problems?

Activity-Exercise Pattern

What is your child's schedule during the day (preschool, day care center, regular school, extracurricular activities)?

What are your child's favorite activities or toys (both active and quiet interests)?

What is your child's usual television-viewing schedule at home?

What are your child's favorite programs?

Are there any television restrictions?

Does your child have any illness or disabilities that limit activity? If so, how?

What are your child's usual habits and schedule for bathing (bath in tub or shower, sponge bath, shampoo)?

What are your child's dental habits (brushing, flossing, fluoride supplements or rinses, favorite toothpaste); schedule of daily dental care?

Does your child need help with dressing or grooming, such as hair combing?

Are there any problems with these patterns (dislike of or refusal to bathe, shampoo hair, or brush teeth)?

- What do you do for these problems?

Are there special devices that your child requires help in managing (eyeglasses, contact lenses, hearing aid, orthodontic appliances, artificial elimination appliances, orthopedic devices)?

NOTE: Use the following code to assess functional self-care level for feeding, bathing-hygiene, dressing-grooming, toileting:

0—Full self-care

I—Requires use of equipment or device

II—Requires assistance or supervision from another person

III—Requires assistance or supervision from another person and equipment or device

IV—Is totally dependent and does not participate

BOX 44-5 Nursing Admission History According to Functional Health Patterns—cont'd

Cognitive-Perceptual Pattern

Does your child have any hearing difficulty?
- Does the child use a hearing aid?
- Have "tubes" been placed in your child's ears?

Does your child have any vision problems?
- Does the child wear glasses or contact lenses?

Does your child have any learning difficulties?
What is the child's grade in school?

Self-Perception–Self-Concept Pattern

How would you describe your child (e.g., takes time to adjust, settles in easily, shy, friendly, quiet, talkative, serious, playful, stubborn, easygoing)?
What makes your child angry, annoyed, anxious, or sad? What helps?
How does your child act when annoyed or upset?
What have been your child's experiences with and reactions to temporary separation from you (parent)?
Does your child have any fears (places, objects, animals, people, situations)?
- How do you handle them?

Do you think your child's illness has changed the way he or she thinks about self (e.g., more shy, embarrassed about appearance, less competitive with friends, stays at home more)?

Role-Relationship Pattern

Does your child have a favorite nickname?
What are the names of other family members or others who live in the home (relatives, friends, pets)?
Who usually takes care of your child during the day and night (especially if other than parent, such as babysitter, relative)?
What are the parents' occupations and work schedules?
Are there any special family considerations (adoption, foster child, stepparent, divorce, single parent)?
Have any major changes in the family occurred lately (death, divorce, separation, birth of a sibling, loss of a job, financial strain, mother beginning a career, other)? Describe child's reaction.
Who are your child's play companions or social groups (peers, younger or older children, adults, prefers to be alone)?
Do things generally go well for your child in school or with friends?
Does your child have "security" objects at home (pacifier, bottle, blanket, stuffed animal or doll)? Did you bring any of these to the hospital?
How do you handle discipline problems at home? Are these methods always effective?
Does your child have any condition that interferes with communication? If so, what are your suggestions for communicating with your child?
Will your child's hospitalization affect the family's financial support or care of other family members?
What concerns do you have about your child's illness and hospitalization?
Who will be staying with your child while hospitalized?
How can we contact you or another close family member outside of the hospital?

Sexuality-Reproductive Pattern

(Answer questions that apply to your child's age group.)
Has your child begun puberty (developing physical sexual characteristics, menstruation)? Have you or your child had any concerns?
Does your daughter know how to do breast self-examination?
Does your son know how to do testicular self-examination?
How have you approached topics of sexuality with your child?
Do you think you might need some help with some topics?
Has your child's illness affected the way he or she feels about being a boy or a girl? If so, how?
Do you have any concerns with behaviors in your child, such as masturbation, asking many questions or talking about sex, not respecting others' privacy, or wanting too much privacy?
Initiate a conversation about an adolescent's sexual concerns with open-ended to more direct questions and using the terms "friends" or "partners" rather than "girlfriend" or "boyfriend":
- Tell me about your social life.
- Who are your closest friends? (If one friend is identified, could ask more about that relationship, such as how much time they spend together, how serious they are about each other, if the relationship is going the way the teenager hoped.)
- Might ask about dating and sexual issues, such as the teenager's views on sexuality education, "going steady," "living together," or premarital sex.
- Which friends would you like to have visit in the hospital?

Coping-Stress Tolerance Pattern

(Answer questions that apply to your child's age group.)
What does your child do when tired or upset?
- If upset, does your child want a special person or object?
- If so, explain.

If your child has temper tantrums, what causes them and how do you handle them?
Whom does your child talk to when worried about something?
How does your child usually handle problems or disappointments?
Have there been any big changes or problems in your family recently? If so, how have you handled them?
Has your child ever had a problem with drugs or alcohol or tried to commit suicide?
Do you think your child is "accident prone"? If so, explain.

Value-Belief Pattern

What is your religion?
How is religion or faith important in your child's life?
What religious practices would you like continued in the hospital (e.g., prayers before meals or bedtime; visit by minister, priest, or rabbi; prayer group)?

*The focus of the admission history is the child's psychosocial environment. Most of the questions are worded in terms of parental responses. Depending on the child's age, they should be addressed directly to the child when appropriate.

BOX 44-6 Complementary Medicine Practices and Examples

Nutrition, diet, and lifestyle or behavioral health changes—Macrobiotics, megavitamins, diets, lifestyle modification, health risk reduction and health education, wellness

Mind-body control therapies—Biofeedback, relaxation, prayer therapy, guided imagery, hypnotherapy, music or sound therapy, massage, aromatherapy, education therapy

Traditional and ethnomedicine therapies—Acupuncture, ayurvedic medicine, herbal medicine, homeopathic medicine, Native American medicine, natural products, traditional Asian medicine

Structural manipulation and energetic therapies—Acupressure, chiropractic medicine, massage, reflexology, rolfing, therapeutic touch, Qi Gong

Pharmacologic and biologic therapies—Antioxidants, cell treatment, chelation therapy, metabolic therapy, oxidizing agents

Bioelectromagnetic therapies—Diagnostic and therapeutic application of electromagnetic fields (e.g., transcranial electrostimulation, neuromagnetic stimulation, electroacupuncture)

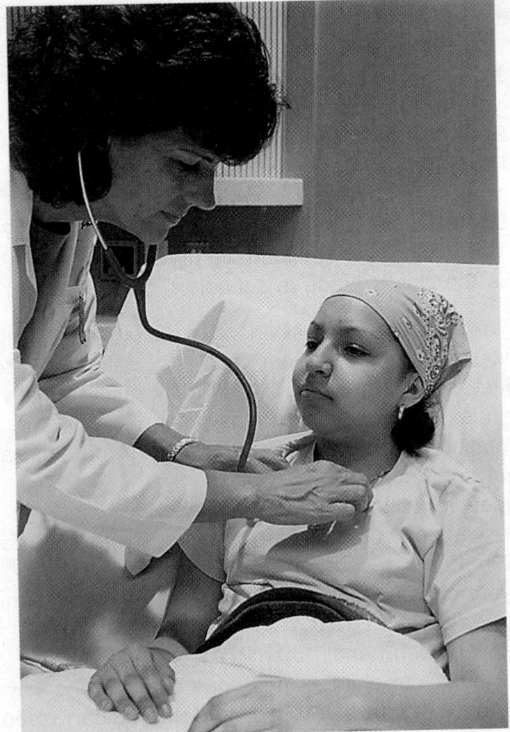

Fig. 44-4 The initial admission procedures give the nurse an opportunity to get to know the child and to assess the child's understanding of the hospital experience.

of hospitalization. In addition, spending this time with the child gives the nurse an opportunity to evaluate the child's understanding of subsequent procedures (Fig. 44-4). Ideally, a primary nurse is assigned whenever possible to allow for individualized care and to provide a substitute support person for the child.

When a child is admitted, nurses follow several fairly universal admission procedures (Box 44-7). One particularly important decision is room assignment. The minimum considerations for room assignment are age, sex, and nature of the illness. No absolute rules govern room selection, but, in general, placing children of the same age group and with similar types of illness in the same room is both psychologically and medically advantageous. However, there are many exceptions. For example, a child in traction may be therapeutic for another child confined to bed because of a serious illness. A child who is independent despite physical disabilities may help another child with similar or different limitations, and the parents of the child with disabilities may achieve deeper insight and acceptance of their child's disorder.

Age-grouping is especially important for adolescents. Many hospitals make an effort to place teenagers on their own unit or in a separate, designated section of the pediatric or general unit whenever possible.

Nursing Interventions

Preventing or Minimizing Separation

A primary nursing goal is to prevent separation, particularly in children younger than 5 years of age. Changes in hospitals' policies over recent years reflect a changed attitude toward parents; many hospitals no longer consider parents "visitors" and welcome their presence at all times throughout the child's hospitalization. Many hospitals have developed a system of *family-centered care*. This philosophy of care recognizes the integral role of the family in a child's life and acknowledges the family as an essential part of the child's care and illness experience. The family is considered to be partners in the child's care (Smith & Conant Rees, 2000) (see Chapter 29). Family-centered care also supports the family by establishing priorities based on the needs and values of the family unit (Lewandowski & Tesler, 2003).

At the very least, most hospitals welcome parents at any time. Many provide facilities such as a chair or bed for at least one person per child, unit kitchen privileges, and other amenities that create a welcoming atmosphere for parents. However, not all hospitals provide such amenities, and parents' own schedules may prevent rooming-in. In such instances, strategies to minimize the effects of separation must be implemented.

Nurses must have an appreciation of the child's separation behaviors. As discussed earlier, the phases of protest and despair are normal. The child is allowed to cry. Even if the child rejects strangers, the nurse provides support through physical presence. *Presence* is defined as spending time being physically close to the child while using a quiet tone of voice, appropriate choice of words, eye contact, and touch in ways that establish rapport and communicate empathy. If behaviors of detachment are evident, the nurse maintains the child's contact with the parents by frequently talking about them; encouraging the child to remember them; and stressing the significance of their visits, telephone calls, or letters. The use of cellular phones can increase the contact between the hospitalized child and parents or other significant family members

BOX 44-7 Guidelines for Admission

Preadmission

Assign a room based on developmental age, seriousness of diagnosis, communicability of illness, and projected length of stay.

Prepare roommate(s) for the arrival of a new patient; when children are too young to benefit from this consideration, prepare parents.

Prepare room for child and family, with admission forms and equipment nearby to eliminate need to leave child.

Admission

Introduce primary nurse to child and family.

Orient child and family to inpatient facilities, especially to assigned room and unit; emphasize positive areas of pediatric unit.

- **Room**—Explain call light, bed controls, television, bathroom, telephone, etc.
- **Unit**—Direct to playroom, desk, dining area, or other areas.

Introduce family to roommate and his or her parents.

Apply identification band to child's wrist, ankle, or both (if not already done).

Explain hospital regulations and schedules (e.g., visiting hours, mealtimes, bedtime, limitations [give written information if available]).

Perform nursing admission history (see Box 44-5).

Take vital signs, blood pressure, height, and weight.

Obtain specimens as needed and order needed laboratory work.

Support child and assist practitioner with physical examination (for purposes of nursing assessment).

and friends. However, many cell phone signals are not compatible with medical equipment, and use may be restricted in certain areas within the hospital.

Separation may be equally difficult for parents, especially when they do not understand the behaviors of separation anxiety. To avoid the immediate protest, parents may sneak out or lie to the child about leaving. As a result, instead of learning that absence is associated with a guaranteed return, the child learns that absence means loss of parents. Helping parents recognize that separation behaviors are normal and expected can decrease the parents' anxiety and may ease their fears about leaving their child. Explaining to parents how the child reacts after they leave may also be helpful. Many parents imagine that the child cries for hours after they leave, whereas in reality the child may cry for a few minutes but settle down when comforted by someone else.

Toddlers and preschoolers have a limited concept of time. Time is measured in associations, such as eating dinner "when Daddy comes home." Therefore, when helping parents with children's fears of separation, nurses need to suggest ways of explaining leaving and returning. For example, if parents must leave to go to work or to make meals for other family members, they should tell the child the reason for leaving. They also need to convey the expected time of return in terms of anticipated events. For example, if the parents will return in the morning,

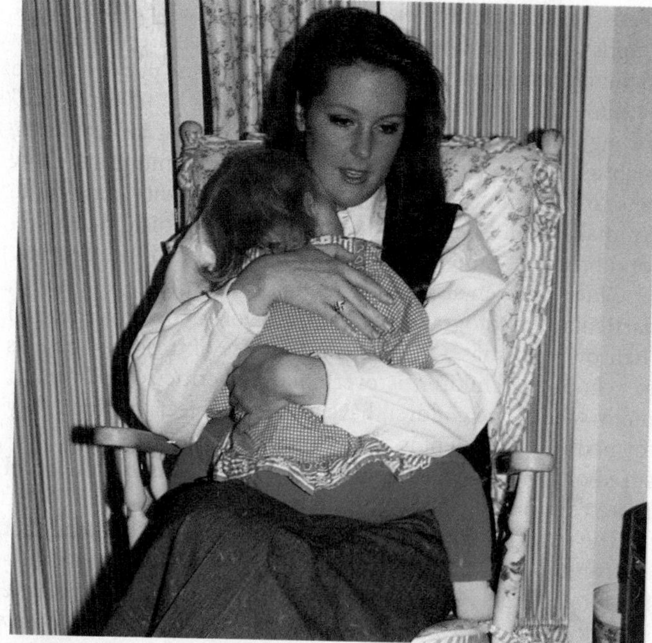

Fig. 44-5 When parents cannot visit, other significant persons can provide comfort to the hospitalized child.

they can say to the child, "We'll see you after the sun comes up" or "We'll come back when [a favorite program] is on television."

The young child's ability to tolerate parental absence is limited. Therefore parental visits should be frequent (e.g., visiting three times a day for short periods rather than once a day for an extended time). This may necessitate that each parent visit at different times to lessen the length of separation. When parents cannot visit, the presence of other significant people can be most comforting for the child (Fig. 44-5).

If parents leave after the child is asleep, they still need to communicate their absence. The parents of a 5-year-old boy solved this problem by devising a sign; on one side they drew a picture of a telephone, and on the other they drew a hamburger. Before they left, they turned the sign to the appropriate side to tell the child when he awoke that they were out using the telephone or eating.

Older children who know how to tell time may find it helpful to have a clock or watch. However, these children have the same need for honesty from their parents regarding visiting schedules. Because their peer groups are important, adolescents often appreciate planning visiting hours with their parents to ensure that the patient has some private time for friends.

Familiar surroundings also increase the child's adjustment to separation. If parents cannot stay with the child, they should leave favorite articles from home with the child, such as a blanket, toy, bottle, feeding utensil, or article of clothing. Because young children associate such inanimate objects with significant people, they gain comfort and reassurance from these possessions. They make the association that if the parents left this, the parents will surely return. Placing an identification band on the toy lessens the chances of its being misplaced and provides a symbol that the toy is experiencing the same needs as the child. Other mementos of home include photographs and audiotape or videocassette recordings of family members reading a story, singing a song, saying prayers before bedtime, relating events at home, or taking a "talking walk" through the home. The tapes can be played at lonely times, such as on awakening or before sleeping. Some units allow pets to visit, which can have therapeutic benefits for a child. Animals should be carefully screened for medical or behavioral problems, and patients should be screened for allergies.

Older children also appreciate familiar articles from home, particularly photographs, a radio, a favorite toy or game, and their own pajamas. Often the importance of treasured objects to school-age children is overlooked or criticized. However, many school-age children have a special object to which they formed an attachment in early childhood. Therefore such treasured or transitional objects can help even older children feel more comfortable in a strange environment.

The strange sights, smells, and sounds in the hospital that are commonplace for the nurse can be frightening and confusing for children. It is important for the nurse to try to evaluate stimuli in the environment from the child's point of view (considering also what the child may see or hear happening to other patients) and to make every effort to protect the child from frightening and unfamiliar sights, sounds, and equipment. The nurse should offer explanations or prepare the child for those experiences that are unavoidable. Combining familiar or comforting sights with the unfamiliar can relieve much of the harshness of medical equipment.

Helping children maintain their usual contacts also minimizes the effects of separation imposed by hospitalization. This includes continuing school lessons during the illness and confinement, visiting with friends either directly or through letter writing or telephone calls, and participating in stimulating projects whenever possible (Fig. 44-6). For extended hospitalizations, youngsters enjoy personalizing the hospital room to make it "home" by decorating the walls with posters and cards, rearranging the furniture (when possible), and displaying a collection or hobby.

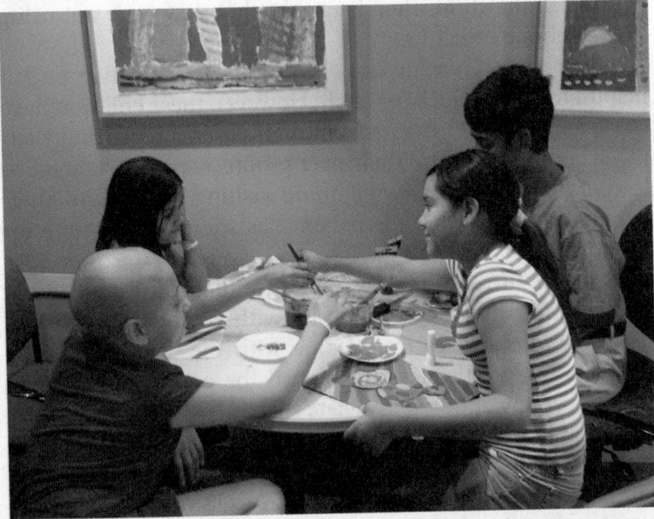

Fig. 44-6 For extended hospitalizations children enjoy having projects with other patients to occupy time.

Minimizing Loss of Control

Feelings of loss of control result from separation, physical restriction, changed routines, enforced dependency, and magical thinking. Although some of these cannot be prevented, most can be minimized through individualized planning of nursing care.

Promoting Freedom of Movement

Younger children react most strenuously to any type of physical restriction or immobilization. Although temporary immobilization may be necessary for some interventions such as maintaining an intravenous line, most physical restriction can be prevented if the nurse gains the child's cooperation.

For young children, particularly infants and toddlers, preserving parent-child contact is the best means of decreasing the need for or stress of restraint. For example, almost the entire physical examination can be done with the child in a parent's lap, with the parent hugging the child for procedures such as otoscopy. For painful procedures, the nurse should assess the parents' preferences for assisting, observing, or waiting outside the room.

Environmental factors may also restrict movement. Keeping children in cribs or playpens may not represent immobilization in a concrete sense, but it certainly limits sensory stimulation. Increasing mobility by transporting children in carriages, wheelchairs, carts, or wagons provides them with a sense of freedom.

In some cases, physical restraint or isolation is necessary due to the child's medical diagnosis. In these cases, the environment can be altered to increase sensory freedom (e.g., moving the bed toward the window; opening window shades; providing musical, visual, or tactile activities).

Maintaining Child's Routine

Altered daily schedules and loss of rituals are particularly stressful for toddlers and early preschoolers and may increase the stress of separation. The nursing admission history provides a baseline for planning care around the child's usual home activities. A frequently neglected aspect of altered routines is the change in the child's daily activities. A nonhospitalized child's day, especially during the school years, is structured with specific times for eating, dressing, going to school, playing, and sleeping. However, this time structure vanishes when the child is hospitalized. Although nurses have a set schedule, the child is frequently unaware of it, and the new schedules that are imposed may be rigid. For example, some units have uniform nap times and bedtimes for all children, whereas others allow children to stay up late at night. Many children obtain significantly less sleep in the hospital than at home; the primary causes are delay in sleep onset and early termination of sleep because of hospital routines. Not only are hours of sleep disrupted, but waking hours are spent in passive activities. For example, few institutions impose any limits on the amount of time the child spends watching television. This may lead to the child being less "tired" at bedtime and delay the onset of sleep.

One technique that can minimize the disruption in the child's routine is establishing a daily schedule. This approach is most suitable for the non–critically ill school-age or adolescent child who has mastered the concept of time. It involves scheduling the child's day to include all those activities that

Eric's Daily Schedule

7:30 AM	– Breakfast, morning bath	3:00 PM	– Tutor (M, W, F) – Study time (T, Th)
9:00	– Medications, dressing change	4:00	– Physical therapy
		5:30	– Dinner
11:00	– Physical therapy	9:00	– Medications, dressing change
12:00 PM	– Lunch	9:15	– Bedtime

Fig. 44-7 Time structuring is an effective strategy for normalizing the hospital environment and increasing the child's sense of control.

are important to the child and nurse, such as treatment procedures, schoolwork, exercise, television, playroom, and hobbies. Together, the nurse, parent, and child then plan a daily schedule with times and activities written down (Fig. 44-7). This is left in the child's room, and a clock or watch is available for the child's use. Whenever possible, a calendar is also constructed with special events marked, such as favorite television programs, visits by friends or relatives, events in the playroom, and holidays or birthdays. If specific changes in treatment are expected (e.g., "beginning physical therapy in 2 days"), these are added.

NURSING ALERT Ask the young child to select or draw pictures or symbols to represent daily or weekly fun activities (e.g., favorite television programs, family visits, playroom times). Draw a clock face with the hands of the clock depicting the time each event will occur next to the child's representation. Have the child compare the clock on the schedule with a clock or watch in the room. When the two match, the child knows it is time for a favorite activity.

Encouraging Independence

The dependent role of the hospitalized patient imposes tremendous feelings of loss on older children. Principal interventions should focus on respect for individuality and the opportunity for decision making. Although these sound simple, their efficacy lies with nurses who are flexible and tolerant. It is also important for the nurse to empower the patient while not feeling threatened by a sense of lessened control.

Enabling children's control involves helping them maintain independence and promoting the concept of self-care. *Self-care* refers to the practice of activities that individuals personally initiate and perform on their own behalf in maintaining life, health, and well-being (Orem, 2001). Although self-care is limited by the child's age and physical condition, most children beyond infancy can perform some activities with little or no help. Whenever possible, these activities are encouraged in the hospital. Other approaches include jointly planning care, time structuring, wearing street clothes, making choices in food selections and bedtime, continuing school activities, and rooming with an appropriate age-mate.

Promoting Understanding

Loss of control can occur from feelings of having too little influence on one's destiny or from sensing overwhelming control or power over fate. Although preschoolers' cognitive abilities predispose them most to magical thinking and delusions of power, all children are vulnerable to misinterpreting causes for stresses such as illness and hospitalization.

Most children feel more in control when they know what to expect, since the element of fear is reduced. Anticipatory preparation and provision of information help to lessen stress and increase understanding (see Preparation for Diagnostic and Therapeutic Procedures, Chapter 45).

Informing children of their rights while hospitalized fosters greater understanding and may relieve some of the feelings of powerlessness they typically experience. Hospitals providing services to children should have a hospital-wide policy on the rights and responsibilities of these patients and of their parents or guardians (Joint Commission on Accreditation of Healthcare Organizations, 2004). An increasing number of hospitals and organizations have developed a patient "bill of rights" that is prominently displayed throughout the hospital or is presented to children and their families on admission (Box 44-8).

BOX 44-8 Bill of Rights for Children and Teens

In this hospital you and your family have the right to:
- Respect and personal dignity
- Care that supports you and your family
- Information you can understand
- Quality health care
- Emotional support
- Care that respects your need to grow, play, and learn
- Make choices and decisions

From Association for the Care of Children's Health: *A pediatric bill of rights*, Bethesda, MD, 1991, The Association.

Preventing or Minimizing Fear of Bodily Injury

Beyond early infancy, all children fear bodily injury from mutilation, bodily intrusion, body-image change, disability, or death. In general, preparation of children for painful procedures decreases their fears and increases cooperation. Manipulating procedural techniques for children in each age group also minimizes fear of bodily injury. For example, because toddlers and young preschoolers are traumatized by insertion of a rectal thermometer, axillary temperatures or temperatures taken with electronic or tympanic membrane devices can effectively be substituted. Whenever procedures are performed on young children, the most supportive intervention is to do the procedure as quickly as possible while maintaining parent-child contact.

Because of toddler and preschool children's poorly defined body boundaries, the use of bandages may be particularly helpful. For example, telling children that the bleeding will stop after the needle is removed does little to relieve their fears, whereas applying a small Band-Aid usually reassures them. The size of bandages is also significant to children in this age group; the larger the bandage, the more importance is attached to the wound. Watching their surgical dressings become successively smaller is one way young children can measure healing and improvement. Prematurely removing a dressing may cause these children considerable concern for their well-being. Specific pain management strategies are discussed in Chapter 35.

For children who fear mutilation of body parts, it is essential that the nurse repeatedly stress the reason for a procedure and evaluate their understanding. For example, explaining cast removal to preschoolers may seem simple enough, but children's comprehension of the details may vary considerably. Asking them to draw a picture of what they think will happen presents substantial evidence of how they perceive events.

Children may fear bodily injury from a great variety of sources. Imaging machines, strange equipment used for examination, unfamiliar rooms, or awkward positions can be perceived as potentially hazardous. In addition, thoughts and actions can be imagined sources of bodily damage. Therefore it is important to investigate imagined reasons, particularly of a sexual nature, for illness. Because children may fear revealing such thoughts, using techniques such as drawing or doll play may elicit previously undisclosed misconceptions.

Older children fear bodily injury of both internal and external origins. For example, school-age children are aware of the significance of the heart and may fear the actual operation as much as the pain, the stitches, and the possible scar. Adolescents may express concern about the actual procedure but be much more anxious over the resulting scar.

Children can grasp information only if it is presented on or close to their level of cognitive development. This necessitates an awareness of the words used to describe events or processes. For example, young children told that they are going to have a CAT (i.e., CT, computed tomography) scan may wonder, "Will there be cats? Or something that scratches?" It is clearer to describe the procedure in simple terms and explain what the letters of the common name stand for. Therefore, to prevent or alleviate fears, nurses must be keenly aware of the medical terminology and vocabulary that they use every day.

When children are upset about their illness, their perception can be changed by (1) providing a somewhat different and less negative account of the disease or (2) offering an explanation that is characteristic of the next stage of cognitive development. An example of the first strategy is reassuring a preschooler who fears that, after a tonsillectomy, another sore throat means a second operation. Explaining that after tonsils are "fixed" they do not need fixing again can help relieve the fear. An example of the latter strategy is to explain that germs made the tonsils sick and even though germs can cause another sore throat, they cannot cause the tonsils to ever be sick again. This higher-level explanation is based on the school-age child's concept of germs as a cause of disease.

Providing Developmentally Appropriate Activities

A primary goal of nursing care for the child who is hospitalized is to minimize threats to the child's development. Many strategies (e.g., minimizing separation) have been discussed and may be all that the short-term patient requires. However, children who experience prolonged or repeated hospitalization are at greater risk for developmental delays or regression. The nurse who provides opportunities for the child to participate in developmentally appropriate activities further normalizes the child's environment and helps reduce interference with the child's development.

Interference with normal development may have long-term implications for the infant and toddler. The nurse plays a primary role in identifying children at risk and helping to plan, implement, and evaluate developmental interventions.

School is an integral part of the school-age child's and adolescent's development. Accreditation standards for hospitals serving children consider access to appropriate educational services a key factor in the accreditation decision process when a child's treatment requires a significant absence from school (Joint Commission on Accreditation of Healthcare Organizations, 2004). The nurse can encourage children to resume schoolwork as quickly as their condition permits, help them schedule and protect a selected time for studies, and help the family coordinate hospital educational services with their children's schools. Children should have the opportunity to continue art and music classes, as well as their academic subjects.

To meet the unique developmental needs of adolescents, special units may be designated that provide privacy, increased socialization, and appropriate activities for these young people. Typically these units can be set apart from the general pediatric facility so that the teenagers do not share space with younger children, who are often perceived as a threat to their maturity.

In caring for the adolescent patient, it is essential to provide flexible routines and activities, such as more group activity, wearing of street clothes, and access to the items so critical to adolescents—telephones, compact disc players, DVD players, videocassette recorders, computers, e-mail, video games, and televisions. Because adolescents' food habits are rarely limited to the three traditional meals a day, a ready supply of snacks should be available. However, the most important benefit of these units is increased socialization with peers. In addition, staff members usually enjoy working with this age group and are able to establish the trust so essential for communication.

NURSING ALERT When adolescents must share a common activity room with younger patients, referring to the area as the "activity room" rather than the "playroom" may entice them to visit the room and participate in activities.

Although regression is expected and normal for all age groups, nurses have the responsibility for fostering the child's growth and development. Hospitalization can become a significant opportunity for learning and advancing. Extended hospitalizations for long-term chronic illness or situations of failure to thrive, abuse, or neglect represent instances in which regression must be seen as an adjustment period, to be followed by plans for promoting appropriate developmental skills.

Providing Opportunities for Play and Expressive Activities

Play is one of the most important aspects of a child's life and one of the most effective tools for managing stress. Because illness and hospitalization constitute crises in a child's life and often involve overwhelming stresses, children need to act out

BOX 44-9 Functions of Play in the Hospital

- Provides diversion and brings about relaxation
- Helps the child feel more secure in a strange environment
- Lessens the stress of separation and the feeling of homesickness
- Provides a means for release of tension and expression of feelings
- Encourages interaction and development of positive attitudes toward others
- Provides an expressive outlet for creative ideas and interests
- Provides a means for accomplishing therapeutic goals (see Use of Play in Procedures, Chapter 45)
- Places child in active role and provides opportunity to make choices and be in control

their fears and anxieties as a means of coping with these stresses. Play is essential to children's mental, emotional, and social well-being. As with their other developmental needs, play does not stop when children are ill or in the hospital. On the contrary, play in the hospital serves many functions (Box 44-9). Of all hospital facilities, no room probably alleviates the stressors of hospitalization more than the playroom (or activity room). In the playroom, children temporarily distance themselves from their illness, hospitalization, and the associated stressors. This room should be a safe haven for children, free from medical or nursing procedures (including medication administration), strange faces, and probing questions. The playroom then becomes a sanctuary in an otherwise frightening environment.

Engaging in play activities gives children a sense of control. In the hospital environment, most decisions are made for the child; play and other expressive activities offer the child much-needed opportunities to make choices for themselves. Even if a child chooses not to participate in a particular activity, the nurse has offered the child a choice, perhaps one of only a few real choices the child has had that day.

The hospitalized child typically has lower energy levels than healthy children of the same age. Therefore children may not appear engaged and enthusiastic about an activity, even though they are enjoying the experience. Activities may need to be adjusted or limited based on the child's age, endurance, and special needs.

Diversional Activities

Almost any form of play can be used for diversion and recreation, but the activity should be selected on the basis of the child's age, interests, and limitations (Fig. 44-8). Children do not necessarily need special direction for using play materials. All they require is the raw materials with which to work and adult approval and supervision to help keep their natural enthusiasm or expression of feelings from getting out of control. Small children enjoy a variety of small, colorful toys that they can play with in bed or in their room, or more elaborate play equipment, such as playhouses, sandboxes, rhythm instruments, or large boxes and blocks, that may be a part of the hospital playroom.

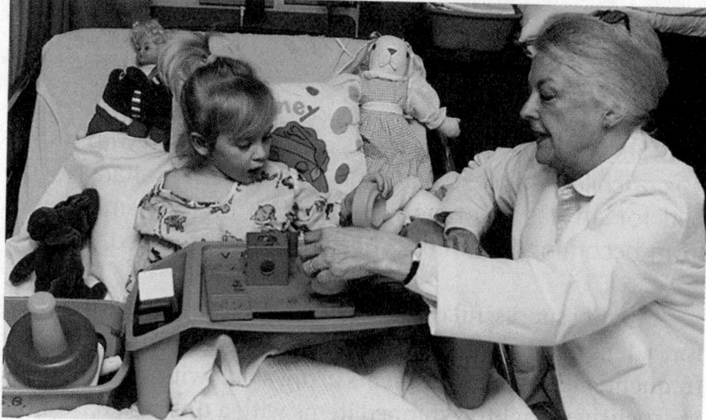

Fig. 44-8 Play materials for children in the hospital need to be appropriate for their age, interests, and limitations.

Games that can be played alone or with another child or an adult are popular with older children, as are puzzles; reading material; quiet, individual activities, such as sewing, stringing beads, and weaving; and Lego blocks and other building materials. Assembling models is an excellent pastime, but one should make certain that all pieces and necessary materials are included in the package so that the child is not disappointed and frustrated.

Well-selected books are of infinite value to the child. Children never tire of stories; having someone read aloud gives them endless hours of pleasure and is of special value to the child who has limited energy to expend in play. A radio, DVD player, electronic games, and television, included among most hospital room equipment, are useful tools for entertaining a child. Computers with access to the Internet can provide diversion, educational opportunities, and online support groups.

When supervising play for ill or convalescent children, it is best to select activities that are simpler than would normally be chosen for the child's specific developmental level. These children usually do not have the energy to cope with more challenging activities. Other limitations also influence the type of activities. Special consideration must be given to the child who is confined in terms of movement, has a restricted extremity, or is isolated. Toys for isolated children must be disposable or need to be disinfected after every use. Therefore toys that are not able to be disinfected (e.g., stuffed animals) cannot be used as community toys.

Toys

Parents of hospitalized children often ask nurses about the types of toys that would be best to bring for their child. Although parents often want to buy new toys for the hospitalized child to offer cheer and comfort, it is often better to wait to bring new things, especially in the case of younger children. Small children need the comfort and reassurance of familiar things, such as the stuffed animal the child hugs and takes to bed at night. These familiar items are a link with home and the world outside the hospital. All toys brought into the hospital should be assessed for safety.

Large numbers of toys often confuse and frustrate a small child. A few small, well-chosen toys are usually preferred to one large, expensive one. Children who are hospitalized for an

evolve Skill—Therapeutic Play

extended time benefit from changes. Rather than a confusing accumulation of toys, older toys should be replaced periodically as interest wanes.

NURSING ALERT Have parents provide the child with a shoe box, a child's small suitcase, or a backpack to attach to the bed for an easy storage receptacle to prevent small items from becoming lost in the sheets or under the bed.

A highly successful diversion for a child who is hospitalized for a length of time and whose parents are unable to visit frequently is having the parents bring a box with several small, inexpensive, brightly wrapped items with a different day of the week printed on the outside of each package. The child will eagerly anticipate the time for opening each one. If the parents know when their next visit will be, they can provide the number of packages that corresponds to the time between visits. In this way the child knows that the diminishing packages also represent the anticipated visit from the parent.

Expressive Activities

Play and other expressive activities provide one of the best opportunities for encouraging emotional expression, including the safe release of anger and hostility. Nondirective play that allows children freedom for expression can be tremendously therapeutic. Therapeutic play, however, should not be confused with *play therapy,* a psychologic technique reserved for use by trained and qualified therapists as an interpretative method with emotionally disturbed children. *Therapeutic play,* on the other hand, is an effective, nondirective modality for helping children deal with their concerns and fears, and at the same time it often helps the nurse gain insights into children's needs and feelings.

Tension release can be facilitated through almost any activity; with younger ambulatory children, large-muscle activity such as use of tricycles and wagons is especially beneficial. Much aggression can be safely directed into pounding and throwing games or activities. Beanbags are often thrown at a target or open receptacle with surprising vigor and hostility. A pounding board is employed with enthusiasm by young children; clay and Play-Doh are beneficial for use at any age.

Creative Expression

Although all children derive physical, social, emotional, and cognitive benefits from engaging in art or other creative activities, children's need for such activities is intensified when they are hospitalized. Drawing and painting are excellent media for expression. Children are more at ease expressing their thoughts and feelings through art, since humans think first in images and later learn to translate these images into words. The child needs only to be supplied with the raw materials, such as crayons and paper; large brushes and an ample supply of newsprint supported on easels; or materials for finger painting (Fig. 44-9). Children can work individually or work together on a group project, such as a mural painted on a long piece of paper.

Although interpretation of children's drawing requires special training, observing changes in a series of the child's drawings over time can be helpful in assessing psychosocial adjustment and coping. The nurse can use children's drawings, stories, poetry, and other products of creative expression as a springboard for discussion of thoughts, fears, and understanding of concepts or events (see Communication Techniques, Chapter 34). A child's drawing before surgery, for example, may reveal unvoiced concerns about mutilation, body changes, and loss of self-control.

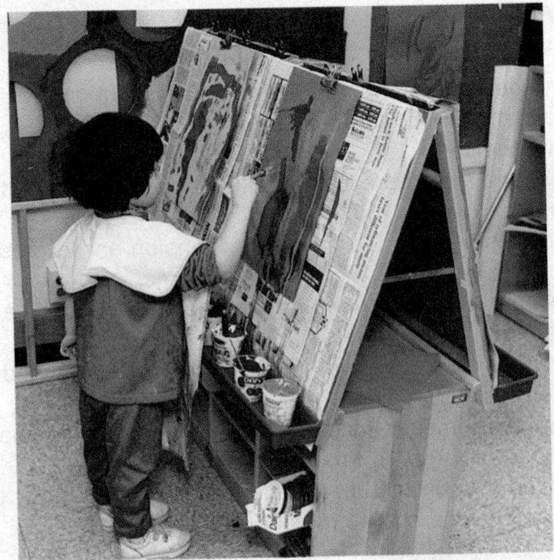

Fig. 44-9 Drawing and painting are excellent media for expression.

Nurses can incorporate opportunities for musical expression into routine nursing care. For example, simple musical instruments, such as bracelets with bells, can be placed on infants' legs for them to shake to accompany mealtime music or dressing changes. Dance and movement suggestions may encourage a child to ambulate.

Holidays provide stimulus and direction for unlimited creative projects. Children can participate in decorating the pediatric unit; making pictures and decorations for their rooms gives them a sense of pride and accomplishment. This is especially beneficial for children who are immobilized and isolated. Making gifts for someone at home helps to maintain interpersonal ties.

Dramatic Play

Dramatic play is a well-recognized technique for emotional release, allowing children to reenact frightening or puzzling hospital experiences. Through use of puppets, replicas of hospital equipment, or some actual hospital equipment, children can act out the situations that are a part of their hospital experience. Dramatic play enables children to learn about procedures and events that concern them and to assume the roles of the adults in the hospital environment.

Puppets are universally effective for communicating with children. Most children see them as peers and readily communicate with them. Children will tell the puppet feelings that they hesitate to express to adults. Puppets can share children's own experiences and help them find solutions to their problems. Puppets dressed to represent figures in the child's environment—for example, a physician, nurse, child patient, therapist, and members of the child's own family—are especially useful. Small, appropriately attired dolls are equally effective in encouraging the child to play out situations, although puppets are usually best for direct conversation.

NURSING ALERT Make a simple puppet using a large handkerchief. Place some cotton balls in the center of the cloth and wrap a rubber band over the handkerchief and cotton balls to form a "head." Place the head over the index finger with the rubber band securing it to the finger. Let the cloth drape over the front and back of the hand. The cloth forms four parts of the puppet: the index finger is the head, the thumb and other fingers are the arms, and the draped cloth is the body. Decorate the head by drawing features on it.

Play must consider medical needs, but at times a procedure can be postponed briefly to allow the child to complete a special activity (see Critical Thinking Exercise). Play must consider any limitations imposed by the child's condition. For example, small children may eat paste and other creative media; therefore a child who is allergic to wheat should not be given finger paint made from wallpaper paste or modeling dough made with flour. A child on restricted salt intake should not play with modeling dough because salt is one of its major constituents. At home the play program can be planned around the therapy regimen. However, play can be satisfactorily incorporated into the child's care if the nurse and others involved allow some flexibility and use creativity in planning for play.

CRITICAL THINKING EXERCISE

Playroom and Hospital Procedures

Hannah, a 7-year-old with cystic fibrosis, has been hospitalized numerous times with complications from the condition. She is playing Candyland with her brother, sister, and several other children in the playroom on the pediatric unit. A pediatric phlebotomist enters the playroom and says, "Hannah, I need to take some blood. I can see that you are playing a game, so I'll just do it while you play. It will just take a minute." Hannah nods her head indicating that she agrees to let the phlebotomist draw the blood at this time. The playroom is usually off-limits for invasive procedures. As Hannah's nurse, you are aware that Dr. Lung wants the results of the laboratory studies as soon as possible to make a decision about her course of therapy.

1. Evidence—Is there sufficient evidence to draw any conclusions about this situation at this time?
2. Assumptions—What are some underlying assumptions about the following?
   a. Children and painful procedures such as venipunctures
   b. The function of play for a hospitalized child
   c. The priority in performing the procedure
   d. Implications of performing the procedure in the playroom
3. What implications and priorities for nursing care can be drawn at this time (i.e., what will you do)?
4. Does the evidence objectively support your argument (conclusion)?
5. Are there alternative perspectives to your conclusions? If so, what are they?

Maximizing Potential Benefits of Hospitalization

Although hospitalization generally represents a stressful time for children and families, it also represents an opportunity for facilitating positive change within the child and among family members. For some families the stress of a child's illness, hospitalization, or both can lead to strengthening of family coping behaviors and the emergence of new coping strategies.

Fostering Parent-Child Relationships

The crisis of illness or hospitalization can mobilize parents into more acute awareness of their child's needs. For example, hospitalization provides opportunities for parents to learn more about their children's growth and development. When parents are helped to understand children's usual reactions to stress, such as regression or aggression, they are not only better able to support the child through the hospital experience, but also may extend their insights into childrearing practices after discharge.

Difficulties in parent-child relationships that existed before hospitalization that are characterized by feeding problems, negative behavior, and sleep disturbances may decrease during hospitalization. The temporary cessation of such problems sometimes alerts parents to the role they may be playing in propagating the negative behavior. With assistance from health professionals, parents can restructure ways of relating to their children to foster more positive behavior.

Hospitalization may also represent a temporary reprieve or refuge from a disturbed home. Typically, abused or neglected children's dramatic physical and social improvement during hospitalization is proof of the benefits and potential growth that can occur during such times. These children temporarily are able to seek support, reassurance, and security from new relationships, particularly with nurses and hospitalized peers.

Providing Educational Opportunities

Illness and hospitalization represent excellent opportunities for children and other family members to learn more about their bodies, each other, and the health professions. For example, during a hospital admission for a diabetic crisis, the child may learn about the disease; the parents may learn about the child's needs for independence, normalcy, and appropriate limits; and each of them may find a new support system in the hospital staff.

Illness or hospitalization can also help older children in choosing a career. Frequently, children have impressions of physicians or nurses that are disproportionately positive or negative. Actual experience with different health professionals can influence their attitude about health professionals and even a decision regarding a career in health care.

Promoting Self-Mastery

The experience of facing a crisis such as illness or hospitalization, coping successfully with it, and maturing as a result of it constitutes an opportunity for self-mastery. Younger children have the chance to test fantasy vs. reality of their fears. They realize that they were not abandoned, mutilated, or punished. In fact, they were loved, cared for, and treated with respect for their individual concerns. It is not unusual for children who have undergone hospitalization or surgery to tell others that "it was nothing" or to display proudly their scars or bandages. For older children, hospitalization may represent an opportunity for decision making, independence, and self-

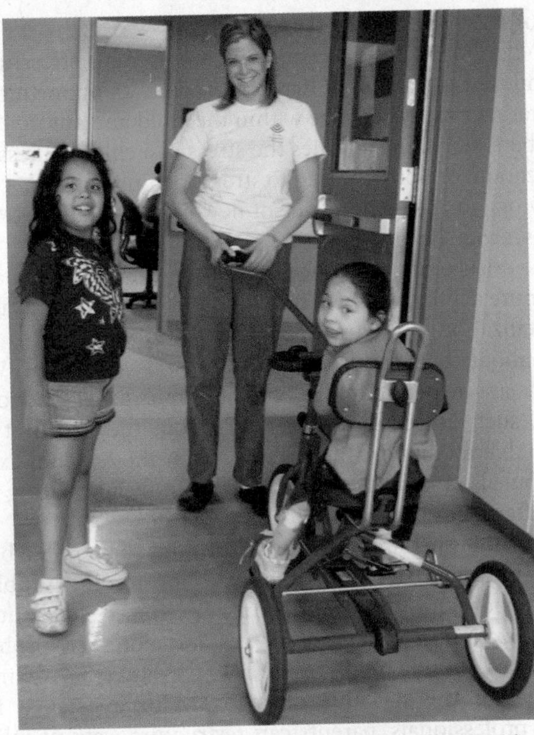

Fig. 44-10 Placing children of the same age group with similar illnesses near each other on the unit is both psychologically and medically supportive. *(Courtesy E. Jacob, Texas Children's Hospital, Houston, TX.)*

reliance. They are proud of having survived the experience and may feel a genuine self-respect for their achievements. Nurses can facilitate such feelings of self-mastery by emphasizing aspects of personal competence in the child and not focusing on uncooperative or negative behavior.

Providing Socialization

Hospitalization may offer children a special opportunity for social acceptance. Lonely, asocial, and even delinquent children find a sympathetic environment in the hospital. Children who have a physical handicap or are in some other way "different" from their age-mates may find an accepting social peer group (Fig. 44-10). Although this does not always spontaneously occur, nurses can structure the environment to foster a supportive child group. For example, selection of a compatible roommate can help children gain a new friend and learn more about themselves. Forming relationships with significant members of the health care team, such as the physician, nurse, child life specialist, or social worker, can greatly enhance children's adjustment in many areas of life.

Parents may also encounter a new social group in other parents who have similar problems. The waiting room or hallway "self-help" groups are inherent to every institution. Parents meet while in the hospital or clinic and discuss their children's illnesses and treatments. Nurses can capitalize on this informal gathering by encouraging parents to discuss collectively their concerns and feelings. Nurses can also refer parents to organized parent groups or can use the help and support of parents of recovered hospitalized patients. It is important that nurses emphasize to families that each child responds differently to disease, treatments, and care. Any questions raised during group discussions should be clarified with a nurse or physician.

Nursing Care of the Family

Although it is not possible to predict exactly which factors are most likely to have an effect on the family's reactions, important variables are (1) the seriousness of the child's illness, (2) the family's previous experience with hospitalization, and (3) the medical procedures involved in the diagnosis and treatment. Important information is also obtained in the nursing admission history (see Box 44-5).

Supporting Family Members

Support involves the willingness to stay and listen to parents' verbal and nonverbal messages. Sometimes the nurse does not give this support directly. For example, the nurse may offer to stay with the child to allow the parents time alone or may discuss with other family members the parents' need for extra relief. Often relatives and friends want to help but do not know how. Suggesting ways, such as baby-sitting, preparing meals, doing laundry, or transporting the siblings to school, can prompt others to help reduce the responsibilities that burden parents.

Support may also be provided through the clergy. Parents with deep religious beliefs may appreciate the counsel of a clergy member, but because of their stress they may not have sufficient energy to initiate the contact. Nurses can be supportive by arranging for clergy to visit, upholding parents' religious beliefs, and respecting the individual meaning and significance of those beliefs (Feudtner, Haney, & Dimmers, 2003).

Support involves accepting cultural, socioeconomic, and ethnic values. For example, health and illness are defined differently by various ethnic groups. For some, a disorder that has few outward manifestations of illness, such as diabetes, hypertension, or cardiac problems, is not a sickness. Consequently, following a prescribed treatment may be seen as unnecessary. Nurses who appreciate the influences of culture are more likely to intervene therapeutically. (See also Cultural and Religious Influences on Health Care, Chapter 32.)

Parents need help in accepting their own feelings toward the ill child. If given the opportunity, parents often disclose their feelings of loss of control, anger, and guilt. They often resist admitting to such feelings because they expect others to disapprove of behavior that is less than perfect. Unfortunately, health personnel, including nurses, sometimes do exercise little tolerance for deviation from the norm. This only increases the psychologic impact of a child's illness on family members. Helping parents identify the specific reason for such feelings and emphasizing that each is a normal, expected, and healthy response to stress may reduce the parents' emotional burden.

Family-centered care also addresses the needs of siblings. Support may involve preparing siblings for hospital visits, assessing their adjustment, and providing appropriate interventions or referrals when needed. The Family-Centered Care box suggests ways that parents can support siblings during hospitalization.

evolve Nursing Care Plan–The Family of the Ill or Hospitalized Child

FAMILY-CENTERED CARE

Supporting Siblings During Hospitalization

Trade off staying at the hospital with spouse or have a surrogate who knows the siblings well stay in the home.

Offer information about the child's condition to young siblings as well as older siblings; respect the sibling who avoids information as a means of coping with the situation.

Arrange for children to visit their brother or sister in the hospital if possible.

Encourage phone visits and mail between brothers and sisters; provide children with phone numbers, writing supplies, and stamps.

Help each sibling identify an extended family member or friend to be their support person and provide extra attention during parental absence.

Make or buy inexpensive toys or trinkets for siblings, one gift for each day the child will be hospitalized.

- Wrap each gift separately and place in a basket, box, or other container at each child's bedside.
- Instruct siblings to open one gift each night at bedtime and to remember that he or she is in the parent's thoughts.

If the child's condition is stable and distance is not prohibitive, plan a special time at home with the siblings or have spouse or another relative or friend bring the children to meet parent(s) at a restaurant or other location near the hospital.

- Have extended family members or friends schedule a visit to the child in the hospital during parental absence.
- Arrange a pass for the child to leave the hospital to join the family if the child's condition permits.

Data from Craft M, Craft J: Perceived changes in siblings of hospitalized children: a comparison of sibling and parent reports, *Child Health Care* 18(1):42-48, 1989; and Rollins J: *Brothers and sisters: a discussion guide for families,* Landover, MD, 1992, Epilepsy Foundation of America.

Providing Information

One of the most important nursing interventions is providing information about (1) the disease, its treatment, the prognosis, and home care; (2) the child's emotional and physical reactions to illness and hospitalization; and (3) the probable emotional reactions of family members to the crisis.

For many families the child's illness is the first contact they have with the hospital experience. Often parents are not prepared for the child's behavioral reactions to hospitalization, such as separation behaviors, regression, aggression, and hostility. Providing the parents with information about these normal and expected behavioral responses can lessen the parents' anxiety during the hospitalization. The family is equally unfamiliar with hospital rules, which often compounds their confusion and anxiety. Therefore the family needs clear explanations about what to expect and what is expected of them.

Parents also need to be aware of the effects of illness on the family and strategies that prevent negative changes. Specifically, parents should keep the family well informed and communicate with everyone as much as possible. They should treat all the children equally and as normally as before the illness occurred. Discipline, which initially may be lessened for the ill child, should be continued to provide a measure of security and predictability. When ill children know that their parents expect certain standards of conduct from them, they feel certain that they will recover. Conversely, when all limits are removed, they fear that something catastrophic will happen.

Helping parents understand the meaning of posthospitalization behaviors in the sick child is necessary for them to tolerate and support such behaviors. In addition, parents should be forewarned of the common reactions following discharge (see Box 44-2). Parents who do not expect such reactions may misinterpret them as evidence of the child's "being spoiled" and demand perfect behavior at a time when the child is still reacting to the stress of illness and hospitalization. If the behaviors, especially the demand for attention, are dealt with in a supportive manner, most children are able to relinquish them and assume precrisis levels of functioning.

Nurses should also prepare parents for the reactions of siblings—particularly anger, jealousy, and resentment. Older siblings may deny such reactions because they provoke feelings of guilt. However, everyone needs outlets for emotions, and the repressed feelings may surface as problems in school or with age-mates, as psychosomatic illnesses, or in delinquent behavior.

Probably one of the most neglected areas of communication involves giving information to siblings. Frequently, age becomes the only factor that leads to an awareness of this problem, since older children may begin to ask questions or request explanations. Even in this situation, however, the information may be seriously inadequate. Children in every age group deserve some explanation of the sibling's illness or hospitalization. Although the exact wording may differ, the explanation should focus on the following concerns: (1) "Will I get sick and have to go to the hospital?" (2) "Did I cause the illness?" (for actual or imagined reasons), and (3) "Will my parents abandon me if my brother or sister doesn't recover?" If parents or nurses address these three questions, the siblings' own fears of illness, guilt, and abandonment are minimized (Melnyk & Alpert-Gillis, 1998).

Encouraging Parent Participation

Preventing or minimizing separation is a key nursing goal with the child who is hospitalized, but maintaining parent-child contact is also beneficial for the family. One of the best approaches is encouraging parents to stay with their child and to participate in the care whenever possible. Although some health facilities provide special accommodations for parents, the concept of rooming-in can be instituted anywhere. The first requirement is the staff's positive attitude toward parents. A negative attitude toward parent participation can create barriers to collaborative working relationships.

When hospital staff genuinely appreciates the importance of continued parent-child attachment, they foster an environment that encourages parents to stay. When parents are included in the care planning and understand that they are contributing to the child's recovery, they are more inclined to remain with their child and have more emotional reserves to support themselves and the child through the crisis. An empowerment model of helping allows the nurse to focus on parents' strengths and seek ways to promote growth and family functioning so that the parents become empowered in caring for their child.

Because the mother tends to be the family caregiver, she usually spends more time in the hospital than the father. However, not all mothers (or fathers) feel equally comfortable assuming responsibility for their child's care. Some may be under such great emotional stress that they need a temporary reprieve from total participation in caregiving activities. Others may feel insecure in participating in specialized areas of care, such as bathing the child after surgery. On the other hand, some mothers may feel a great need to control their child's care. This seems particularly true of young mothers, who have recently established their role as a parent; mothers of children too young to verbalize their needs; and ethnic minority mothers when the hospital setting is predominantly staffed by nonminority personnel. Individual assessment of each parent's preferred involvement is necessary to prevent the effects of separation while supporting parents in their needs as well.

With lifestyles and gender roles changing, fathers may assume all or some of the usual "mothering" roles in the household. In this case it may be the father-child relationship that requires preservation. Fathers need to be included in the care plan and respected for their parental role. For some fathers the child's hospitalization may represent an opportunity to alter their usual caregiving role and increase their involvement. In single-parent families the caregiver may not be a parent but an extended family member, such as a grandparent or aunt.

One of the potential problems with continuous parent involvement is neglect of the parent's need for sleep, nutrition, and relaxation. Often the sleeping accommodations are limited to a chair, and sleep is disrupted by nursing procedures. Encouraging the parents to leave for brief periods, arranging for sleeping quarters on the unit but outside the child's room, and planning a schedule of alternating visits with another family member can minimize the stresses for the parent.

All too often, nurses respond to parent participation by abandoning their patient responsibilities. Nurses need to restructure their roles to complement and augment the parents' caregiving functions. Even in units structured to provide care by parents, parents frequently feel anxiety in their caregiving responsibilities; those more involved in direct care may feel more anxiety than those less involved in direct care. Therefore 24-hour responsibility may be too much for some parents. Assistance and relief by nursing personnel should always be available to these families, and nurses may need to work diligently to establish the strong bond of trust some parents need to take advantage of these opportunities.

evolve Critical Thinking Exercise—Discharge Planning

Preparing for Discharge and Home Care

Most hospitalizations necessitate some type of discharge preparation. Often this involves education of the family for continued care and follow-up in the home. Depending on the diagnosis, this may be relatively simple or highly complex. Preparing the family for home care demands a high degree of competence in planning and implementing discharge instructions. This usually is best accomplished using an *interdisciplinary team approach*, which requires a shift from the *multidisciplinary team approach* used during an acute phase of a child's illness (Hornick, 1996).

Nurses are often key individuals in initiating and carrying out the discharge process. They collaborate with others in the planning and implementation phases to ensure appropriate care after hospitalization. Throughout the hospitalization the nurse should be aware of the need for discharge planning and those assessment factors that affect the family's ability to provide home care. A thorough assessment of the family and home environment should be performed to ensure that the family's emotional and physical resources are sufficient to manage the tasks of home care. In addition to adequate family resources, an investigation of community services, including respite care, is needed to ensure that appropriate support agencies are available, such as emergency facilities, home health agencies, and equipment vendors. Financial resources are also a consideration. To coordinate the immense task of assessment and to plan implementation, a care coordinator or manager should be appointed early in the discharge process.

The preparation for hospital discharge and home care begins during the admission assessment. Short- and long-term goals are established to meet the child's physical and psychosocial needs. For children with complex care needs, discharge planning focuses on obtaining appropriate equipment and health care personnel for the home. Discharge planning is also concerned with those treatments that parents or children are expected to continue at home. In planning appropriate teaching, nurses need to assess (1) the actual and perceived complexity of the skill, (2) the parents' or child's ability to learn the skill, and (3) the parents' or child's previous or present experience with such procedures.

The teaching plan incorporates levels of learning, such as observing, participating with assistance, and, finally, acting without help or guidance. The skill is divided into discrete steps, and each step is taught to the family member until it is learned. Return demonstration of the skill is requested before new skills are introduced. A record of teaching and performance provides an efficient checklist for evaluation. All families need to receive detailed *written* instructions about home care, with telephone numbers for assistance, before they leave the hospital. Communication between the nurse performing discharge planning and home health care is essential for ensuring a smooth transition for the child and family.

After the family is competent in performing the skill, they are given responsibility for the care. When possible, the family should have a transition or trial period to assume care with minimal health care supervision. This may be arranged on the unit; during a home pass; or in a facility, such as a motel, near the hospital. Such transitions provide a safe practice period for the family, with assistance readily available when needed, and are especially valuable when the family lives far from the hospital.

In many instances parents need only simple instructions and understanding of follow-up care. However, the often overwhelming care assumed by some families, coupled with other stressors they may be experiencing, necessitates continued professional support after discharge. A follow-up home visit or telephone call gives the nurse an opportunity to individualize care and provide information in perhaps a less stressful learning environment than the hospital. Appropriate referrals and resources may include visiting nurse or home health agencies, private nurse services, the school system, a physical therapist, a mental health counselor, a social worker, and any number of community agencies. Sharing the important issues surrounding the child's and family's needs is essential. Referral summaries should be concise, specific, and factual. When numerous support services are required, periodic collaboration among the professionals involved and the family is an excellent strategy to ensure efficient usage and comprehensive delivery of services.

Care of the Child and Family in Special Hospital Situations

In addition to a general pediatric unit, children may be admitted to special facilities such as an ambulatory or outpatient setting, an isolation room, or intensive care.

Ambulatory or Outpatient Setting

The ambulatory or outpatient setting provides needed medical services for the child while eliminating the necessity of overnight admission. Among the benefits of ambulatory care are (1) minimization of the stressors of hospitalization, especially separation from the family; (2) reduced chance of infection; and (3) cost savings. Admission to the ambulatory or outpatient hospital setting usually is for surgical or diagnostic procedures, such as insertion of tympanostomy tubes, hernia repair, adenoidectomy, tonsillectomy, cystoscopy, or bronchoscopy.

In the ambulatory or outpatient setting, adequate preparation is particularly challenging. Ideally, the child and parents should receive preadmission preparation, including a tour of the facility and a review of the day's events (Brewer & Lambert, 1997). Parents need information in advance to help prepare the child and themselves for surgery and enable them to care for the child at home after the procedure. Parents also appreciate suggestions for items to bring to the hospital, such as blankets or stuffed animals. When preadmission preparation is not possible, time should be allowed on the day of the procedure for children to become acquainted with their surroundings and for nurses to assess, plan, and implement appropriate teaching.

Waiting is usually inevitable in ambulatory settings. Families frequently report waiting to be the most stressful part of the experience. Providing a pager is one way to allow the family (and at times the child) to leave the area and then be paged to return when needed (Ashenberg et al, 1996).

Explicit discharge instructions are important after outpatient surgery (see Family-Centered Care box and Preparing for Discharge and Home Care, p. 1238). Parents need guidelines on when to call their practitioner regarding a change in the child's condition. A follow-up telephone call system allows for nurses to check on the child's progress within 48 to 72 hours after discharge. It also provides an opportunity for the nurse to review discharge information and answer questions.

Isolation

Admission to an isolation room increases all of the stressors typically associated with hospitalization. There is further separation from familiar persons; additional loss of control; and added environmental changes, such as sensory deprivation and the strange appearance of visitors. Orientation to time and place is affected. These stressors are compounded by children's limited understanding of isolation. Preschool children have difficulty understanding the rationale for isolation because they cannot comprehend the cause-and-effect relationship between germs and illness. They are likely to view isolation as punishment. Older children understand the causality better but still require information to decrease fantasizing or misinterpretation.

When a child is placed in isolation, preparation is essential for the child to feel in control. With young children the best approach is a simple explanation, such as "You need to be in this room to help you get better. This is a special place to make all the germs go away. The germs made you sick, and you could not help that."

All children, but especially younger ones, need preparation in terms of what they will see, hear, or feel in isolation. Therefore they are shown the mask, gloves, and gown and are encouraged to "dress up" in them. Playing with the strange apparel lessens the fear of seeing "ghostlike" people walk into the room. Before entering the room, nurses and other health personnel should introduce themselves and let the child see their face before donning a mask. In this way the child associates them with significant experiences and gains a sense of familiarity in an otherwise strange and lonely environment.

When the child's condition improves, appropriate play activities are provided to minimize boredom, stimulate the senses, provide a real or perceived sense of movement, orient the child to time and place, provide social interaction, and reduce depersonalization. For example, the environment can be manipulated to increase sensory freedom by moving the bed toward the door or window. Opening window shades; providing musical, visual, or tactile toys; and increasing interpersonal contact can substitute mental mobility for the limitations of physical movement. Rather than dwelling on the negative aspects of isolation, the child can be encouraged to view this experience as challenging and positive. For example, the nurse can help the child look at isolation as a method of keeping others out and letting only special people in. Children often think of intriguing signs for their doors, such as "Enter at your own risk." These signs also encourage people "on the outside" to talk with the child about the ominous greeting.

NURSING ALERT Have the child select a place he or she would like to visit. Help the child decorate the bed and equipment to suit the theme (e.g., truck, circus tent, spaceship, sky). At a set time each day pretend to go with the child to the special place. Consider including props such as a suitcase or picnic basket.

Emergency Admission

One of the most traumatic hospital experiences for the child and parents is an emergency admission. The sudden onset of

FAMILY-CENTERED CARE

Discharge from Ambulatory Settings

Before beginning, explain that all instructions will also be presented in writing for the family to refer to later.

Provide an overview of the typical trajectory (expected pattern) of recovery.

Discuss expected progression of the child's activity level during the postdischarge period (e.g., "Mary will probably sleep for the rest of the day, feel kind of tired most of tomorrow, but be back to her usual activities the next day").

Explain which activities the child is allowed and what is not permitted (e.g., bed rest, bathing).

Discuss dietary restrictions, being very specific and giving examples of "clear fluids" or what is meant by a "full liquid diet."

Discuss nausea and vomiting, if applicable, explaining how much is "normal" and what to do if more occurs (e.g., "Juan may be sick to his stomach and vomit. This is normal. However, if he vomits more than three times, please call us at this number right away.").

Discuss fever and appropriate comfort measures, explaining how much fever is considered "normal," and specifically what to do if the child goes beyond the range.

Explain the amount, location, and kind of pain or discomfort the child may experience.

Give any prescribed medication before leaving the facility.

Send a pain scale home with the family.

Explain how much pain and discomfort is "normal" and what to do if the child surpasses that level or if pain management interventions are unsuccessful.

Discuss pain management, including dosage for pain medications and details on how to administer them.

Describe appropriate nonpharmacologic comfort measures, such as holding, rocking, or swaddling.

Provide information about each medication that the child will be taking at home.

- Review the details, including dose and route.
- Demonstrate how to administer medications, if necessary (e.g., how to take wrapping off suppositories, how to insert).

Discuss guidelines for requesting other medications.

Request that all prescriptions be filled and given to the family before discharge.

Make certain the family has all of the equipment and supplies (e.g., gauze and tape for dressing changes) they will need at home.

Discuss complications that may occur and the steps to take if they do.

Ensure that appropriate measures are in place for safe transport home.

- Remind family to use a seat belt or car seat for the child.
- Determine whether there will be one person whose sole responsibility is helping ensure the child's safety and comfort during transport.
- Discuss measures the driver may need to take if this is impossible (e.g., be certain a basin is within the child's reach should vomiting occur; take a route that permits slower traffic and has places along the roadside to stop if necessary).
- Determine the availability of a blanket, pillow, and cup with a lid and straw for the child's use in the car.
- Provide a basin or plastic bag in case of vomiting.

Provide emergency phone numbers for the family to call with any concerns.

Explain that the family will be contacted (give an approximate time) to follow up on the child but that they should not hesitate to call if concerns arise before then.

Ask the family and child, if appropriate, if they have any questions, and problem solve with family members to meet their unique needs.

an illness or the occurrence of an injury leaves little time for preparation and explanation. Sometimes the emergency admission is compounded by admission to an intensive care unit (ICU) or the need for immediate surgery. However, even in those instances requiring only outpatient treatment, the child is exposed to a strange, frightening environment and to experiences that may elicit fear or cause pain.

There is a wide discrepancy between what constitutes a medically defined emergency and a client-defined emergency. A growing concern is the use of major emergency departments for routine primary care health visits. To offset overcrowding in emergency departments, many facilities have minor emergency units or pediatric minor emergency units for after-hours health care. Telephone triage for minor illnesses for patients is also emerging as a health care delivery mode to differentiate illnesses such as a common cold from true life-threatening conditions that require immediate practitioner attention and intervention. Other factors contributing to the overuse of emergency departments (as opposed to the primary practitioner's office) include the increasing number of uninsured persons and households where both parents work full time and cannot afford to take off during the daytime to take the sick child to a practitioner.

In pediatric populations most visits to an emergency department are for respiratory tract infections; skin conditions, gastrointestinal disorders, and trauma such as poisoning account for most of the remainder of cases. The most common reason parents give for bringing the child to the emergency department is concern about the illness worsening. However, practitioners may not think that the progressive symptoms necessitate immediate or emergency care. One of the nurse's primary goals is to assess the parents' perception of the event and their reasons for considering it serious or life threatening.

Lengthy preparatory admission procedures are often inappropriate for emergency situations. In such instances, nurses must focus their nursing interventions on the essential components of admission counseling (Box 44-10) and complete the process as soon as the child's condition has stabilized.

Unless an emergency is life threatening, children need to participate in their care to maintain a sense of control. Because emergency departments are frequently hectic, there is a ten-

BOX 44-10 Guidelines for Special Hospital Admission*

Emergency Admission

Lengthy preparatory admission procedures are often impossible and inappropriate for emergency situations.

Focus assessment on airway, breathing, and circulation; weigh child whenever possible for calculation of drug dosages.

Unless an emergency is life threatening, children need to participate in their care to maintain a sense of control.

Focus on essential components of admission counseling, including:

- Appropriate introduction to the family
- Use of child's name, not terms such as "honey" or "dear"
- Determination of child's age and some judgment about developmental age (If the child is of school age, asking about the grade level will offer some evidence of intellectual ability.)
- Information about child's general state of health, any problems that may interfere with medical treatment (e.g., allergies), and previous experience with hospital facilities
- Information about the chief complaint from both the parents and the child

Admission to Intensive Care Unit

Prepare child and parents for elective intensive care unit (ICU) admission, such as for postoperative care after cardiac surgery.

Prepare child and parents for unanticipated ICU admission by focusing primarily on the sensory aspects of the experience and on usual family concerns (e.g., persons in charge of child's care, schedule for visiting, area where family can stay).

Prepare parents regarding child's appearance and behavior when they first visit child in ICU.

Accompany family to bedside to provide emotional support and answer questions.

Prepare siblings for their visit; plan length of time for sibling visitation; monitor siblings' reactions during visit to prevent them from becoming overwhelmed.

Encourage parents to stay with their child:

- If visiting hours are limited, allow flexibility in schedule to accommodate parental needs.
- Give family members a written schedule of visiting times.
- If visiting hours are liberal, be aware of family members' needs and suggest periodic respites.
- Assure family they can call the unit at any time.

Prepare parents for expected role changes and identify ways for parents to participate in child's care without overwhelming them with responsibilities:

- Help with bath or feeding.
- Touch and talk to child.
- Help with procedures.

Provide information about child's condition in understandable language:

- Repeat information often.
- Seek clarification of understanding.
- During bedside conferences, interpret information for family members and child or, if appropriate, conduct report outside room.

Prepare child for procedures, even if this involves explanation while procedure is performed.

Assess and manage pain; recognize that a child who cannot talk, such as an infant or child in a coma or on mechanical ventilation, can be in pain.

Establish a routine that maintains some similarity to daily events in child's life whenever possible:

- Organize care during normal waking hours.
- Keep regular bedtime schedules, including quiet times when television or radio is lowered or turned off.
- Provide uninterrupted sleep cycles (60 minutes for infant, 90 minutes for older child).
- Close and open drapes and dim lights to allow for day-night.
- Place curtain around bed for privacy.
- Orient child to day and time; have clocks or calendars in easy view for older children.

Schedule a time when child is left undisturbed (e.g., during naps, visit with family, playtime, or favorite program).

Provide opportunities for play.

Reduce stimulation in environment:

- Refrain from loud talking or laughing.
- Keep equipment noise to a minimum:
  — Turn alarms as low as safely possible.
  — Perform treatments requiring equipment at one time.
  — Turn off bedside equipment that is not in use, such as suction and oxygen.
- Avoid loud, abrupt noises.

*See also Box 44-7.

dency to rush through procedures to save time. However, the extra few minutes needed to allow children to participate may save many more minutes of useless resistance and uncooperativeness during subsequent procedures. Other supportive measures include ensuring privacy, accepting various emotional responses to fear or pain, preserving parent-child contact, explaining all events before or as they occur, and personally remaining calm. Pain management strategies are discussed in Chapter 35.

At times, because of the child's physical condition, little or no preparatory counseling for emergency hospitalization can be done. In such situations the implementation of *postvention,* or counseling subsequent to the event, has therapeutic value. The process of postvention involves evaluating children's thoughts regarding admission and related procedures. It is similar to precounseling techniques; however, instead of supplying information, the nurse listens to the explanations offered by the child. Projective techniques such as drawing,

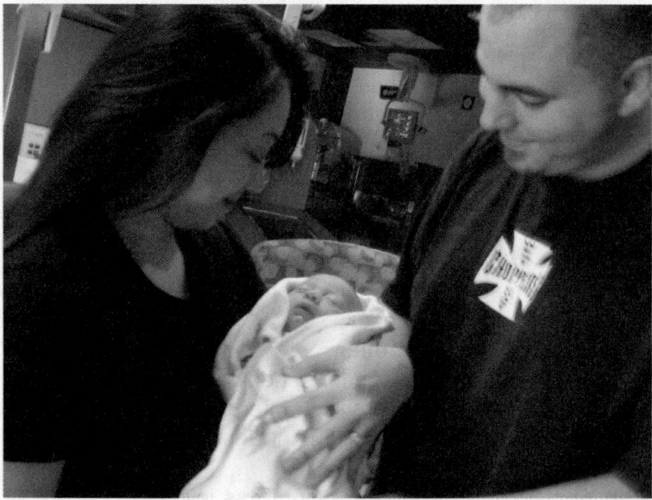

Fig. 44-11 Parental presence during hospitalization provides emotional support for the child and increases the parent's sense of empowerment in the caregiver role. *(Courtesy E. Jacob, Texas Children's Hospital, Houston, TX.)*

doll play, or storytelling are especially effective. The nurse then bases additional information on what has already been understood.

Intensive Care Unit

Admission to an ICU can be traumatic for both the child and parents (Fig. 44-11). The nature and severity of the illness and the circumstances surrounding the admission are major factors, especially for parents. Parents experience significantly more stress when the admission is unexpected rather than expected. One study found that parental anxiety reached near panic levels initially (Huckabay & Tilem-Kessler, 1999). Stressors for the child and parent are described in Box 44-11. Although several studies have described what parents perceive as most stressful, the most effective strategy may be to simply ask parents what is stressful and implement interventions that will enhance their ability to cope (Board & Ryan-Wenger, 2003; Melnyk & Alpert-Gillis, 1998). Assessment should be repeated periodically to account for changes in perceptions over time.

The family's emotional needs are paramount when a child is admitted to an ICU. Although the same interventions discussed earlier for the stressors of separation and loss of control apply here, additional interventions may also benefit the family and child (see Box 44-11 and Family-Centered Care box). In a qualitative study of 19 parents of 10 children in an ICU, parents reported that they simply wanted nurses to nurture the child in the same way the family would (Harbaugh, Tomlinson, & Kirschbaum, 2004). Nurse behaviors that exemplified caring and affection were perceived as helpful in decreasing stress. Behaviors perceived as not helpful included separating the child from the parents and communicating poorly with parents. Therefore even critical care must be centered on the family. It is important that visiting hours be liberal and flexible enough to accommodate parental needs and involvement (Hazinski, 1999).

BOX 44-11 Neonatal or Pediatric Intensive Care Unit Stressors for the Child and Family

Physical Stressors

Pain and discomfort (e.g., injections, intubation, suctioning, dressing changes, other invasive procedures)
Immobility (e.g., use of restraints, bed rest)
Sleep deprivation
Inability to eat or drink
Changes in elimination habits

Environmental Stressors

Unfamiliar surroundings (e.g., crowding)
Unfamiliar sounds
- Equipment noise (e.g., monitors, telephone, suctioning, computer printout)
- Human sounds (e.g., talking, laughing, crying, coughing, moaning, retching, walking)

Unfamiliar people (e.g., health care professionals, patients, visitors)
Unfamiliar and unpleasant smells (e.g., alcohol, adhesive remover, body odors)
Constant lights (disturb day-night rhythms)
Activity related to other patients
Sense of urgency among staff
Unkind or thoughtless comments from staff

Psychologic Stressors

Lack of privacy
Inability to communicate (if intubated)
Inadequate knowledge and understanding of situation
Severity of illness
Parental behavior (expression of concern)

Social Stressors

Disrupted relationships (especially with family and friends)
Concern with missing school or work
Play deprivation

Data primarily from Tichy AM et al: Stressors in pediatric intensive care units, *Pediatr Nurs* 14(1):40-42, 1988.

Critically ill children become the focus of the parents' lives, and parents' most pressing need is for information (Scott, 1998). They want to know if their child will live and, if so, whether the child will be the same as before. They need to know why various interventions are being done for the child, that the child is being treated for pain or is comfortable, and that the child may be able to hear them even though not awake. When parents first visit the child in the ICU, they need preparation regarding the child's appearance. Ideally, the nurse should accompany the parents to the bedside to provide emotional support and answer any questions.

Despite the stresses normally associated with ICU admission, a special security develops from being carefully monitored and receiving individualized care. Therefore planning for transition to the regular unit is essential and should include:

FAMILY-CENTERED CARE

Artists as Partners in Care

A teenage boy with a rare genetic disorder, having made steady progress after awakening from a coma, relapsed and seemed very depressed. When told that a musician was visiting the pediatric intensive care unit, he immediately perked up and asked to have his room lights turned on. He whispered endless song requests to the musician. Family members and staff were treated to some of his first smiles in days; his biggest came when the musician held his hand and guided it across the guitar strings while they sang "Born to Be Wild" together at the boy's request. His dad was misty eyed as he thanked the musician for the visit.

A few weeks later the boy's condition worsened and he again lapsed into a coma. There was nothing more to be done. His parents began the necessary preparations to take their son home to die.

We continued to visit our friend and his family, offering a song, a story, or a simple hello. I hold a vivid picture of our final visit. We stood around the boy's bed with his parents singing together songs they remembered from their youth, from more carefree times. Song and laughter filled the boy's room.

Perhaps the boy heard his parents' laughter and knew then that they would be okay. He died a few days later on the morning he was to have been discharged.

–Judy Rollins, MS, RN
Washington, DC

Modified from Rollins J: *Placed in our keeping*, 1995, Unpublished.

- Assignment of a primary nurse on the regular unit
- Continued visits by the ICU staff to assess the child's and parents' adjustment and to act as a temporary liaison with the nursing staff
- Explanation of the differences between the two units and the rationale for the change to less intense monitoring of the child's physical condition
- Selection of an appropriate room, such as one that is close to the nursing station, and a compatible roommate

Key Points

- Children are particularly vulnerable to the stressors of illness and hospitalization because stress represents a change from the usual state of health and routine and because they possess limited coping mechanisms.
- The three phases of separation anxiety are protest, despair, and detachment.
- Feelings of loss of control are caused by unfamiliar environmental stimuli, physical restriction, altered routine, and dependency.
- Fear of bodily pain may be manifested in the following ways: infants—facial expressions, body movements; toddlers—intense emotional upset, physical resistance; preschoolers—aggression, verbal expression, dependency; school-age children—precise verbalization of pain, passive requests for support or help, procrastination technique; adolescents—self-control, limited movement.
- Because of their separation from significant people, children who are hospitalized may lack the opportunity to form new attachments in the strange environment of the hospital and exhibit negative behaviors after discharge.
- Nursing care of the child in the hospital is aimed at preventing or minimizing separation, decreasing loss of control, minimizing fear of bodily injury, using play or expressive activities to lessen stress, and maximizing the potential benefits of hospitalization.
- The nurse can maximize potential benefits of hospitalization by fostering parent-child relations, providing educational opportunities, promoting self-mastery, and encouraging socialization.

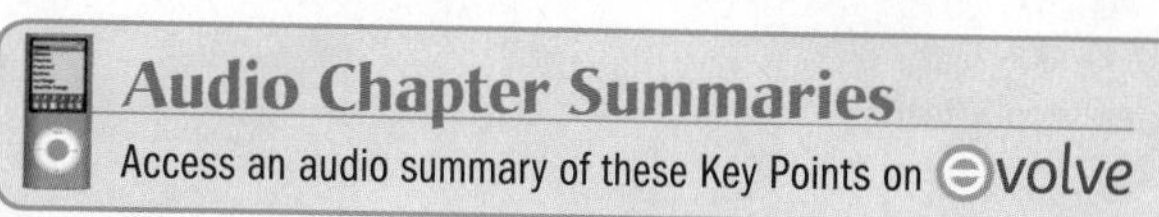
Audio Chapter Summaries
Access an audio summary of these Key Points on evolve

- Family reactions are influenced by the seriousness of the illness, experience with illness or hospitalization and diagnostic or therapeutic procedures, available support systems, personal ego strengths, coping abilities, presence of additional stressors, cultural and religious beliefs, and family communication patterns.
- Fear of contracting illness, their younger age, a close relationship with the ill sibling, substitute child care, minimal explanation of the illness, and perceived changes in parenting all increase the deleterious effects of a brother's or sister's illness and hospitalization on siblings.
- Nursing care of the family involves listening to parents' verbal and nonverbal messages; providing clergy support; accepting cultural, socioeconomic, and ethnic values; giving information to families and siblings; and preparing for discharge and home care.
- Admission to an outpatient setting, emergency department, isolation room, or ICU requires additional intervention strategies to meet the child's and family's needs.

References

Ashenberg MD et al: Easing the wait: development of a pager program for families, *Pediatr Nurs* 22(2):103-107, 1996.

Board R, Ryan-Wenger N: Stressors and symptoms of mothers with children in the PICU, *J Pediatr Nurs* 18(3):195-201, 2003.

Brewer S, Lambert C: Preparing children for same day surgery: innovative approaches, *J Pediatr Nurs* 12(4):257-259, 1997.

Clatworthy S, Simon K, Tiedeman ME: Child drawing: hospital—an instrument designed to measure the emotional status of hospitalized school-aged children, *J Pediatr Nurs* 14(1):2-9, 1999.

Coyne I: Children's experiences of hospitalization, *J Child Health Care* 10(4):326-336, 2006.

Craft MJ: Siblings of hospitalized children: assessment and intervention, *J Pediatr Nurs* 8(5):289-297, 1993.

Fernandez C, Pyesmany A, Stutzer C: Alternative therapies in childhood cancer, *N Engl J Med* 340(7):569-570, 1999.

Feudtner HJ, Haney J, Dimmers MA: Spiritual care needs of hospitalized children and their families: a national survey of pastoral care providers' perceptions, *Pediatrics* 111(1):e67-e72, 2003.

Flanagan K: Preoperative assessment: safety considerations for patients taking herbal products, *J Perianesth Nurs* 16(1):19-26, 2001.

Gordon M: *Manual of nursing diagnosis*, ed 10, St Louis, 2002, Mosby.

Gordon M: *Nursing diagnosis: process and application*, ed 3, St Louis, 1994, Mosby.

Harbaugh BL, Tomlinson PS, Kirschbaum M: Parents' perceptions of nurses' caregiving behaviors in the pediatric intensive care unit, *Issues Compr Pediatr Nurs* 27(3):163-178, 2004.

Hazinski MF: *Manual of pediatric critical care*, St Louis, 1999, Mosby.

Hornick R: Discharge teams. In Gunter K, Manago R (editors): *Beyond discharge: interdisciplinary perspectives for transitioning children with complex medical needs from hospital to home*, Bethesda, MD, 1996, Association for the Care of Children's Health.

Huckabay LMD, Tilem-Kessler D: Patterns of parental stress in PICU emergency admission, *Dimens Crit Care Nurs* 18(2):36-42, 1999.

Joint Commission on Accreditation of Healthcare Organizations: *AMH92 accreditation manual for hospitals*, Chicago, 2004, The Commission.

Lewandowski LA, Tesler MD: *Family centered care: putting it into action*, Washington, DC, 2003, American Nurses Association.

Melnyk BM: Intervention studies involving parents of hospitalized young children: an analysis of the past and future recommendations, *J Pediatr Nurs* 15(1):4-13, 2000.

Melnyk B, Alpert-Gillis L: The COPE Program: a strategy to improve outcomes of critically ill young children and their parents, *Pediatr Nurs* 24(6):521-527, 1998.

Orem D: *Nursing: concepts of practice*, ed 5, New York, 2001, Mosby.

Scott LD: Perceived needs of parents of critically ill children, *J Soc Pediatr Nurs* 3(1):4-12, 1998.

Small L: Early predictors of poor coping outcomes in children following intensive care hospitalization and stressful medical encounters, *Pediatr Nurs* 28(4):393-401, 2002.

Smith T, Conant Rees HL: Making family-centered care a reality, *Semin Nurs Manage* 8(3):136-142, 2000.

Stewart E, Algren C, Arnold S: Preparing children for a surgical experience, *Today's OR Nurse* 16(2):9-14, 1994.

Stranton KM: Parents' experiences of their child's care during hospitalization, *J Cult Divers* 11(1):4-11, 2004.

Woodgate R, Kristjanson L: "Getting better from my hurts": toward a model of the young child's pain experience, *J Pediatr Nurs* 11(4):233-242, 1996.

45

Pediatric Variations of Nursing Interventions

Learning Objectives

On completion of this chapter the reader will be able to:

- Identify those instances in which informed consent is required and in which minors may be considered emancipated.
- Formulate general guidelines for preparing children for procedures, including surgery.
- Implement play in therapeutic procedures.
- List general strategies for enhancing compliance in children and families.
- Outline general hygiene and care procedures for hospitalized children.
- Implement feeding techniques that encourage food and fluid intake.
- Describe methods of reducing temperature of child with fever or hyperthermia.
- Describe systems that can be used for infection control.
- Describe safe methods of administering oral, parenteral, rectal, optic, otic, and nasal medications to children.
- Identify nursing responsibilities in maintaining fluid balance.
- Demonstrate correct procedures for postural drainage and tracheostomy care.
- Describe the procedures involved in providing nutrition via gavage, gastrostomy, and parenteral routes.
- Describe the procedures involved in administering an enema and ostomy care to children.

Electronic Resources

Additional information related to the content in Chapter 45 can be found on

evolve the Companion Website at http://evolve.elsevier.com/Perry/maternal/

- NCLEX Review Questions
- Animation—Central Venous Access
- Animation—Foley Catheter Insertion
- Animation—IV Line Placement
- Animation—Lumbar Puncture, Infant
- Animation—PICC Line Placement
- Case Study—Pediatric Procedures
- Critical Thinking Exercise—Central Venous Access Device
- Nursing Care Plan—The Child Undergoing Surgery
- Nursing Care Plan—The Child with Elevated Body Temperature
- Skill—Administering Oral Medications
- Skill—Measuring Oxygen Saturation
- Skill—Preparing the Child for Procedures
- Skill—Urine Specimen Collection

General Concepts Related to Pediatric Procedures

Informed Consent

Before undergoing any invasive procedure, the patient or the patient's legal surrogate must receive sufficient information on which to make an informed health care decision. *Informed consent* should include the expected care or treatment, potential risks, benefits, alternatives, and what might happen if the patient chooses not to consent. To obtain valid informed consent, the following three conditions must be met:

1. The person must be capable of giving consent; he or she must be over the age of majority (usually age 18) and must be considered competent (i.e., possessing the mental capacity to make choices and understand their consequences).
2. The person must receive the information needed to make an intelligent decision.
3. The person must act voluntarily when exercising freedom of choice without force, fraud, deceit, duress, or other forms of constraint or coercion.

The patient has the right to accept or refuse any health care. If the patient is treated without consent, the hospital or health care provider may be charged with assault and held liable for damages.

Requirements for Obtaining Informed Consent

Written informed consent of the parent or legal guardian is usually required for medical or surgical treatment, including many diagnostic procedures. One universal consent is not sufficient. Separate informed permissions must be obtained for each surgical or diagnostic procedure, including major or minor surgery, diagnostic tests with an element of risk (e.g., bronchoscopy), and medical treatments with an element of risk (e.g., blood transfusion, radiotherapy).

Other situations that require parental consent include:

- Photographs for medical, educational, or public use
- Removal of the child from the health care institution against medical advice
- Postmortem examinations, except in unexplained deaths, such as sudden infant death, violent death, or suicide
- Release of medical information

Decision making involving the care of older children and adolescents should include, to the extent feasible, the patient's *assent* as well as that of the parents. Assent means the child or adolescent has been informed about what will happen during the treatment or procedure and is willing to permit a health care provider to perform it. Assent should include the following elements:

- Helping the patient achieve a developmentally appropriate awareness of the nature of his or her condition
- Telling the patient what he or she can expect
- Making a clinical assessment of the patient's understanding
- Soliciting an expression of the patient's willingness to accept the proposed procedure of care

Multiple methods should be used to provide information, including age-appropriate methods (e.g., videotapes, peer discussion, diagrams, and written materials). An assent form should be provided to each child to sign, and the child should keep a copy (Broome, 1999). By including children in the decision-making process and gaining their acceptance, staff members demonstrate respect for the child. Assent is not a legal requirement but an ethical one to protect the rights of children.

Eligibility for Giving Informed Consent

Informed Consent of Parents or Legal Guardians

Parents have full responsibility for the care and rearing of their minor children, including legal control over them. As long as children are minors, their parents or legal guardians are required to give informed consent before medical treatment is rendered or any procedure is performed. If parents are married to each other, consent from only one parent is required for nonurgent pediatric care. If the parents are divorced, consent usually rests with the parent who has legal custody (Berger & AAP Committee on Medical Liability, 2003). Parents also have a right to withdraw consent at any time.

Evidence of Consent

Obtaining informed consent varies from state to state, and policies differ at each health care facility. It is the physician's responsibility to explain the procedure, risks, benefits, and alternatives. The nurse witnesses the patient's, parent's, or legal guardian's signature on the consent form and may reinforce what the patient has been told. A signed consent form is the legal document that signifies that the process of informed consent has occurred. If parents are unavailable to sign consent forms, verbal consent may be obtained via the telephone in the presence of two witnesses. Both witnesses record that informed consent was given and by whom. Their signatures indicate that they witnessed the verbal consent.

Informed Consent of Mature and Emancipated Minors

State laws differ with regard to the so-called *age of majority*, the age at which a person is considered to have all the legal rights and responsibilities of an adult. In most states, 18 is the age of majority. Competent adults can give informed consent on their own behalf. An *emancipated minor* is one who is legally under the age of majority but is recognized as having the legal capacity of an adult under circumstances prescribed by state law, such as pregnancy, marriage, high school graduation, independent living, or military service.

Treatment Without Parental Consent

Exceptions to requiring parental consent before treating minor children occur when children need urgent medical or surgical treatment and a parent is not readily available or refuses to give consent. For example, a child may be brought to an emergency department accompanied by a grandparent, child care provider, teacher, or others. In the absence of parents or legal guardians, persons in charge of the child may be given permission by the parents to give informed consent by proxy. In emergencies, including danger to life or the possibility of permanent injury, appropriate care should not be withheld or delayed because of problems obtaining consent (Berger & AAP Committee on Medical Liability, 2003; American Academy of Pediatrics, 2003). Efforts made to obtain consent should be documented.

Refusal to give consent can occur when the treatment, such as blood transfusions, conflicts with the parents' religious beliefs. All states recognize such exceptions and have statutory procedures to permit treatment if the life or health of such a minor is in jeopardy or if delayed treatment would create a risk to the minor's health. Evaluation for child abuse or neglect can occur without parental consent and without prior notification to the state in most states.

Adolescents, Consent, and Confidentiality

The Health Insurance Portability and Accountability Act of 1996 (HIPAA) was passed to help protect and safeguard the security and confidentiality of a person's health information. Because adolescents are not yet adults, parents have the right to make most decisions on their behalf and receive information. Adolescents, however, are more likely to seek care in a setting in which they believe their privacy will be maintained. All 50 states have enacted legislation that entitles adolescents to consent to treatment without their parents' knowledge for one or more "medically emancipated" conditions, such as sexually transmitted infections, alcohol and drug abuse, and need for contraceptive advice (Anderson, Schaechter, & Brosco, 2005; Tillett, 2005). Consent to abortion is controversial, and statutes vary widely by state. State law preempts HIPAA regardless of whether that law prohibits, mandates, or allows discretion about a disclosure.

Informed Consent and Parental Right to the Child's Medical Chart

Some state statutes give parents the unrestricted right to a copy of children's medical records. In states without statutes the best practice is to allow parents to review or have a copy of minors' charts under reasonable circumstances. Practitioners should avoid restrictive requirements such as review permitted only in the presence of a clinician. Rather, an appropriate practitioner should be available to answer any questions that parents may have during reviews.

Preparation for Diagnostic and Therapeutic Procedures

Technologic advances and changes in health care have resulted in more pediatric procedures being performed in a variety of settings. Many procedures are both stressful and painful experiences. For most procedures the focus of care is psychologic preparation of the child and family. However, some procedures require the administration of sedatives or analgesics.

Psychologic Preparation

Preparing children for procedures decreases their anxiety, promotes their cooperation, supports their coping skills and may teach them new ones, and facilitates a feeling of mastery in experiencing a potentially stressful event. Many institutions have developed preadmission teaching programs designed to educate the pediatric patient and family by offering hands-on experience with hospital equipment, information about the procedure to be performed, and an overview of departments they may visit (Algren, Ireland, & Stewart, 1998). Preparatory methods may be formal, such as group preparation for hospitalization. Most preparation strategies used by nurses are informal, focus on providing information about the experience, and are directed at stressful or painful procedures. The most effective preparation includes providing sensory-procedural information and helping the child develop coping skills, such as imagery, distraction, or relaxation (Broome, Rehwaldt, & Fogg, 1998).

General guidelines for preparing children for procedures are described in Box 45-1, and age-specific guidelines that consider children's developmental needs and cognitive abilities are presented in Box 45-2. In addition to these suggestions, nurses should consider the child's temperament, existing coping strategies, and previous experiences. Children who are distractible and highly active, as well as those who are "slow to warm up," may need individualized sessions that are shorter for the active child but more slowly paced for the shy child. Youngsters who tend to cope well may need more emphasis on using their present skills, whereas those who appear to cope less adequately can benefit from more time devoted to simple coping strategies, such as relaxing, breathing, counting, squeezing a hand, or singing.

The exact timing of the preparation for a procedure varies with the child's age and type of procedure. No exact guidelines govern timing, but in general the younger the child, the closer the explanation should be to the actual procedure to prevent undue fantasizing and worrying. With complex procedures, more time may be needed for assimilation of information, especially with older children. For example, the explanation for an injection can immediately precede the procedure for all ages, whereas preparation for surgery may begin the day before for young children and a few days before for older children (although older children's preferences should be elicited).

BOX 45-1 General Guidelines for Preparing Children for Procedures

- Determine details of exact procedure to be performed.
- Review parents' and child's present understanding.
- Base teaching on developmental age and existing knowledge.
- Incorporate parents in the teaching if they desire, especially if they plan to participate in care.
- Inform parents of their supportive role during procedure, such as standing near child's head or in child's line of vision and talking softly to child.
- Allow for ample discussion to prevent information overload and ensure adequate feedback.
- Use concrete, not abstract, terms and visual aids to describe procedure. For example, use a simple line drawing of a boy or girl and mark the body part that will be involved in the procedure. Use nonthreatening but realistic models.*
- Emphasize that no other body part will be involved.
- If the body part is associated with a specific function, stress the change in or noninvolvement of that ability (e.g., after tonsillectomy, child can still speak).
- Use words appropriate to child's level of understanding
- Avoid words and phrases with dual meanings unless child understands such words.
- Clarify all unfamiliar words (e.g., "Anesthesia is a *special* sleep").
- Emphasize sensory aspects of procedure—what child will feel, see, hear, smell, and touch and what child can do during procedure (e.g., lie still, count out loud, squeeze a hand, hug a doll).
- Allow child to practice procedures that require cooperation (e.g., turning, deep breathing, incentive spirometry).
- Introduce anxiety-laden information last (e.g., starting an intravenous line).
- Be honest with child about unpleasant aspects of a procedure but avoid creating undue concern. When discussing that a procedure may be uncomfortable, state that it feels differently to different people.
- Emphasize end of procedure and any pleasurable events afterward (e.g., going home, seeing parents).
- Stress positive benefits of procedure (e.g., "After your tonsils are fixed, you won't have as many sore throats").

*Soft-sculptured dolls and customized adapters and overlays for preparing children and families about procedures and as teaching models for technical care are available from Legacy Products, Inc., 508 S. Green St., PO Box 267, Cambridge City, IN 47327; 800-238-7951; e-mail: info@legacyproductsinc.com; *www.legacyproductsinc.com.*

Establish Trust and Provide Support

The nurse who has spent time with and established a positive relationship with a child will usually find it easier to gain cooperation. If the relationship is based on trust, the child will associate the nurse with caregiving activities that give comfort and pleasure most of the time rather than discomfort and stress. If the nurse does not know the child, it is best to be introduced by another staff person whom the child trusts. The first visit with the child should not include any painful

evolve Case Study—Pediatric Procedures

BOX 45-2 Age-Specific Preparation of Children for Procedures Based on Developmental Characteristics

Infant: Developing a Sense of Trust and Sensorimotor Thought

Attachment to Parent
Involve parent in procedure if desired.*
Keep parent in infant's line of vision.
If parent is unable to be with infant, place familiar object with infant (e.g., stuffed toy).

Stranger Anxiety
Have usual caregivers perform or assist with procedure.*
Make advances slowly and in nonthreatening manner.
Limit number of strangers entering room during procedure.*

Sensorimotor Phase of Learning
During procedure use sensory soothing measures (e.g., stroking skin, talking softly, giving pacifier).
Use analgesics (e.g., topical anesthetic, intravenous opioid) to control discomfort.*
Cuddle and hug infant after stressful procedure; encourage parent to comfort infant.

Increased Muscle Control
Expect older infant to resist.
Restrain adequately.
Keep harmful objects out of reach.

Memory for Past Experiences
Realize that older infants may associate objects, places, or persons with prior painful experiences and will cry and resist at the sight of them.
Keep frightening objects out of view.*
Perform painful procedures in a separate room, not in crib (or bed).*
Use nonintrusive procedures whenever possible (e.g., axillary temperatures, oral medications).*

Imitation of Gestures
Model desired behavior (e.g., opening mouth).

Toddler: Developing a Sense of Autonomy and Sensorimotor to Preoperational Thought

Use same approaches as for infant plus the following.

Egocentric Thought
Explain procedure in relation to what child will see, hear, taste, smell, and feel.
Emphasize those aspects of procedure that require cooperation (e.g., lying still).
Tell child it is okay to cry, yell, or use other means to express discomfort verbally.

Negative Behavior
Expect treatments to be resisted; child may try to run away.
Use firm, direct approach.
Ignore temper tantrums.
Use distraction techniques (e.g., singing a song *with* a child).
Restrain adequately.

Animism
Keep frightening objects out of view (young children believe objects have lifelike qualities and can harm them).

Limited Language Skills
Communicate using behaviors.
Use a few, simple terms familiar to child.
Give one direction at a time (e.g., "Lie down," then "Hold my hand").
Use small replicas of equipment; allow child to handle equipment.
Use play; demonstrate on doll but avoid child's favorite doll, since child may think doll is really "feeling" procedure.
Prepare parents separately to avoid child's misinterpreting words.

Limited Concept of Time
Prepare child shortly or immediately before procedure.
Keep teaching sessions short (about 5 to 10 minutes).
Have preparations completed before involving child in procedure.
Have extra equipment nearby (e.g., alcohol swabs, new needle, adhesive bandages) to avoid delays.
Tell child when procedure is completed.

Striving for Independence
Allow choices whenever possible; child may still be resistant and negative.
Allow child to participate in care and to help whenever possible (e.g., drink medicine from a cup, hold a dressing).

Preschooler: Developing Initiative and Preoperational Thought

Egocentric
Explain procedure in simple terms and in relation to how it affects child (as with toddler, stress sensory aspects).
Demonstrate use of equipment.
Allow child to play with miniature or actual equipment.
Encourage "playing out" experience on a doll both before and after procedure to clarify misconceptions.
Use neutral words to describe the procedure.

Increased Language Skills
Use verbal explanation; avoid overestimating comprehension.
Encourage child to verbalize ideas and feelings.

Limited Concept of Time and Frustration Tolerance
Implement same approaches as for toddler but may plan longer teaching session (10 to 15 minutes); may divide information into more than one session.

Illness and Hospitalization Viewed as Punishment
Clarify why each procedure is performed; a child will find it difficult to understand how medicine can make him or her feel better and can taste bad at the same time.
Ask child thoughts regarding why a procedure is performed.
State directly that procedures are never a form of punishment.

Animism
Keep equipment out of sight, except when shown to or used on child.

Skill—Preparing the Child for Procedures

BOX 45-2 Age-Specific Preparation of Children for Procedures Based on Developmental Characteristics—cont'd

Preschooler: Developing Initiative and Preoperational Thought—cont'd

Fears of Bodily Harm, Intrusion, and Castration

Point out on drawing, doll, or child where procedure is performed.
Emphasize that no other body part will be involved.
Use nonintrusive procedures whenever possible (e.g., axillary temperature, oral medication).
Apply an adhesive bandage over puncture site.
Encourage parental presence.
Realize that procedures involving genitalia provoke anxiety.
Allow child to wear underpants with gown.
Explain unfamiliar situations, especially noises or lights.

Striving for Initiative

Involve child in care whenever possible (e.g., hold equipment, remove dressing).
Give choices whenever possible but avoid excessive delays.
Praise child for helping and attempting to cooperate; never shame child for lack of cooperation.

School-Age Child: Developing Industry and Concrete Thought

Increased Language Skills; Interest in Acquiring Knowledge

Explain procedures using correct scientific or medical terminology.
Explain reason for procedure using simple diagrams.
Explain function and operation of equipment in concrete terms.
Allow child to manipulate equipment; use doll or another person as model to practice using equipment whenever possible (doll play may be considered childish by older school-age child).
Allow time before and after procedure for questions and discussion.

Improved Concept of Time

Plan for longer teaching sessions (about 20 minutes).
Prepare before procedure.

Increased Self-Control

Gain child's cooperation.
Tell child what is expected.
Suggest ways of maintaining control (e.g., deep breathing, relaxation, counting).

Striving for Industry

Allow responsibility for simple tasks (e.g., collecting specimens).
Include child in decision making (e.g., time of day to perform procedure, preferred site).
Encourage active participation (e.g., removing dressings, handling equipment, opening packages).

Developing Relationships with Peers

Prepare two or more children for same procedure or encourage one peer to help prepare another.
Provide privacy from peers during procedure to maintain self-esteem.

Adolescent: Developing Identity and Abstract Thought

Increasing Abstract Thought and Reasoning

Supplement explanations with reasons why procedure is necessary or beneficial.
Explain long-term consequences of procedures.
Realize adolescent may fear death, disability, or other risks.
Encourage questioning regarding fears, options, and alternatives.

Consciousness of Appearance

Provide privacy.
Discuss how procedure may affect appearance (e.g., scar) and what can be done to minimize it.
Emphasize any physical benefits of procedure.

Concern More with Present Than with Future

Realize that immediate effects of procedure are more significant than future benefits.

Striving for Independence

Involve in decision making and planning (e.g., time, place, individuals present during procedure, clothing).
Impose as few restrictions as possible.
Suggest methods of maintaining control.
Accept regression to more childish methods of coping.
Realize that adolescent may have difficulty accepting new authority figures and may resist complying with procedures.

Developing Peer Relationships and Group Identity

Same as for school-age child but assumes greater significance.
Allow adolescents to talk with other adolescents who have had same procedure.

*Applies to any age.

procedure and ideally should focus on the child first, then on the explanation of the procedure.

Parental Presence and Support

Children need support during procedures, and for young children the greatest source of support is the parents. They represent security, safety, and comfort. Controversy exists regarding the role parents should assume during the procedure, especially if discomfort is involved. Parental presence is preferable, however, since it can reduce patient and parent anxiety and decrease the need for sedation (Nelson, 1999). The nurse should assess the parents' preferences for assisting, observing, or waiting outside the room, as well as the child's preference for parental presence. The child's and parents' choice should be respected. Parents who wish to stay should be given appropriate explanation about the procedure and coached about what to do, where to sit or stand, and what to say to help the child through the procedure. Simple instructions such as clarifying where parents can stand or sit in the room and positioning them where they have eye contact with the child provide support and lessen anxiety. Parents who do not want to be present or participate are supported in their decision and encouraged to remain close by so that they can be available to console the child immediately after the procedure. Parents should also know that someone will be with their child to provide support. Ideally, this person should inform the parents after the procedure about how the child did.

Provide an Explanation

Age-appropriate explanations are one of the most widely used interventions for reducing anxiety in children undergoing procedures. Before performing a procedure, explain what is to be done and what is expected of the child. The explanation should be short, simple, and geared to the child's level of comprehension. Long explanations may increase anxiety in a young child. When explaining the procedure to parents with the child present, the nurse uses language appropriate to the child because unfamiliar words can be misunderstood. If the parents need additional preparation, this is done in an area away from the child. Teaching sessions are planned at times most conducive to the child's learning (e.g., after a rest period) and for the usual span of attention. Allowing children to handle actual items that will be used in their care, such as a stethoscope, sphygmomanometer, or oxygen mask, helps them develop familiarity with these items and reduces the threat often associated with their use. Written and illustrated materials are also valuable aids to preparation.

Physical Preparation

One area of special concern is the administration of sedation and analgesia before stressful procedures. Refer to Chapter 35 for information on sedating children.

Performance of the Procedure

Supportive care continues during the procedure and can be a major factor in a child's ability to cooperate. Ideally, the same nurse who explains the procedure should perform or assist with the procedure. Before beginning, all equipment is assembled and the room is readied to prevent unnecessary delays and interruptions that increase the child's anxiety.

NURSING ALERT To avoid a delay during a procedure, have extra supplies handy. For example, have tape, bandages, alcohol swabs, and an extra needle when performing an injection or venipuncture.

If possible, procedures should be performed in a special treatment room rather than the child's hospital room. Traumatic procedures should never be performed in "safe" areas, such as the playroom. If the procedure is lengthy, avoid conversation that could be misinterpreted by the child. As the procedure is nearing completion, inform the child that it is almost over in language the child understands.

Expect Success

Nurses who approach children with confidence and who convey the impression that they expect to be successful are less likely to encounter difficulty. It is best to approach a child as though cooperation is expected. Children sense anxiety and uncertainty in an adult and respond by striking out or actively resisting. Although it is not possible to eliminate such behavior in every child, a firm approach with a positive attitude tends to convey a feeling of security to most children.

Involve the Child

Involving children helps to gain their cooperation. Permitting choices gives them some measure of control. However, a choice is given only in situations in which one is available. Asking children, "Do you want to take your medicine now?" leads them to believe they have an option and provides them with the opportunity to legitimately refuse or delay the medication. This places the nurse in an awkward, if not impossible, position. It is much better to state firmly, "It's time to drink your medicine now." Children usually like to make choices, but the choice must be one that they do indeed have (e.g., "It's time for your medicine. Do you want to drink it plain or with a little water?"). Many children respond to tactics that appeal to their maturity or courage. This also gives them a sense of participation and achievement. For example, preschool children will be proud that they can hold the dressing during the procedure or remove the tape. The same is true for the school-age child, who often cooperates with minimal resistance.

Provide Distraction

Distraction is a powerful coping strategy during painful procedures (Algren & Algren, 1997). It is accomplished by focusing the child's attention on something other than the procedure. Singing favorite songs, listening to music, counting aloud, or blowing bubbles to "blow the hurt away" are effective techniques. For other nonpharmacologic interventions that may lessen discomfort, see Pain Management, Chapter 35.

Allow Expression of Feelings

The child should be allowed to express feelings of anger, anxiety, fear, frustration, or any other emotion. It is natural for children to strike out in frustration or to try to avoid stress-provoking situations. The child needs to know that it is all right to cry. Behavior is children's primary means of communication and coping and should be permitted unless it inflicts harm on them or those caring for them.

Postprocedural Support

After the procedure, the child continues to need reassurance that he or she performed well and is accepted and loved. If the parents did not participate, the child is united with them as soon as possible so that they can provide comfort.

Encourage Expression of Feelings

Planned activity after the procedure is helpful in encouraging constructive expression of feelings. For verbal children, reviewing the details of the procedure can clarify misconceptions and garner feedback for improving the nurse's preparatory strategies. Play is an excellent activity for all children. Infants and young children are given the opportunity for gross motor movement. Older children are able to vent their anger and frustration in acceptable pounding or throwing activities. Play-Doh is a remarkably versatile medium for pounding and shaping. Dramatic play provides an outlet for anger and places the child in a position of control, in contrast to the position of helplessness in the real situation. Puppets can also allow the child to communicate feelings in a nonthreatening way. One

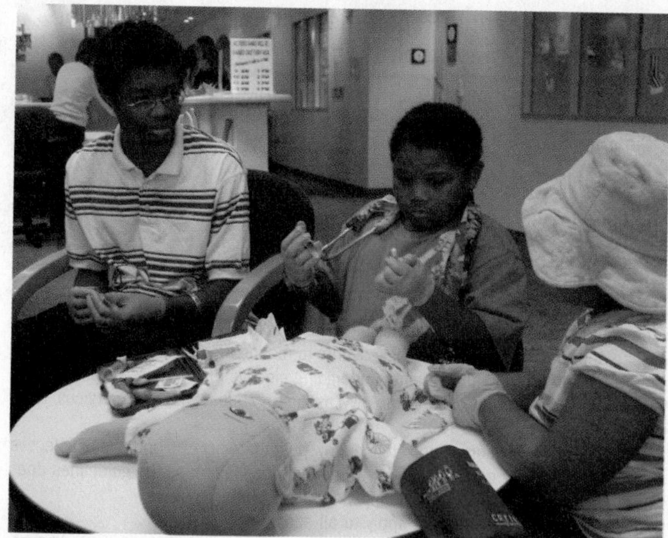

Fig. 45-1 Playing with hospital equipment provides children the opportunity to play out fears and concerns.

of the most effective interventions is *therapeutic play*, which includes well-supervised activities such as permitting the child to give an injection to a doll or stuffed toy to reduce the stress of injections (Fig. 45-1).

Provide Positive Reinforcement

Children need to hear from adults that they know the youngsters did the best they could in the situation, no matter how they behaved. It is important for children to know that their worth is not being judged on the basis of their behavior in a stressful situation. Reward systems, such as earning stars, stickers, or a badge of courage, are appealing to children.

Returning to the child a short while after the procedure helps the nurse strengthen a supportive relationship. Relating with the child in a relaxed and nonstressful period allows the child to see the nurse not only as someone associated with stressful situations but as someone with whom to share pleasurable experiences.

Use of Play in Procedures

The use of play is an integral part of relationships with children. As such, its value in specific situations is discussed throughout this book, such as in Chapter 44, in relation to hospitalization. Many institutions have elaborate and well-organized play areas and programs under the direction of child life specialists; other institutions have limited facilities. No matter what the institution provides for children, nurses can include play activities as part of nursing care. Play can be used to teach, express feelings, or achieve a therapeutic goal. Consequently, it should be included in preparing children for and encouraging their cooperation during procedures. Play sessions after procedures can be structured, such as directed toward needle play, or general, with a wide variety of equipment available for children to play with. Routine procedures such as measuring blood pressure and administering oral medication may be of concern to children. Box 45-3 offers suggestions for incorporating play into nursing procedures and activities for the hospitalized child that facilitate learning and adjustment to a new situation.

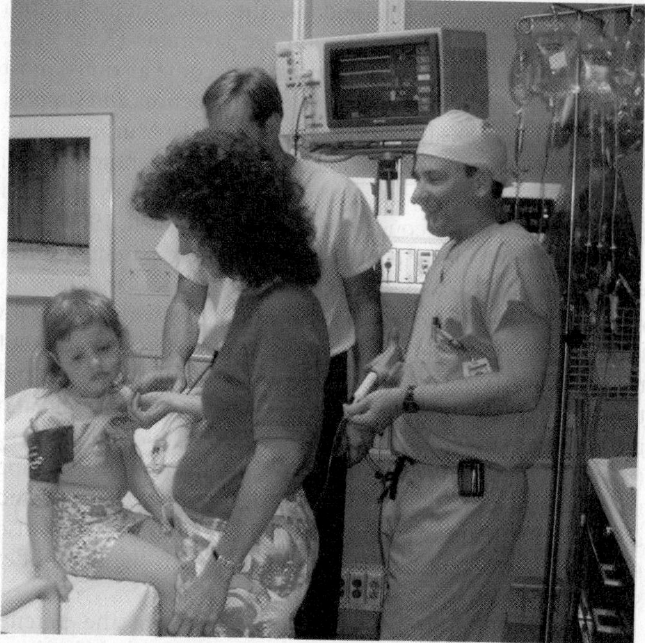

Fig. 45-2 Parental presence during induction of anesthesia can minimize child's and parents' anxiety during the preoperative period.

Surgical Procedures

Preoperative Care

Children experiencing surgical procedures require both psychologic and physical preparation. In general, psychologic preparation is similar to that previously discussed for any procedure and employs many of the same techniques used in preparing a child for hospitalization, such as films, books, brochures, play, and tours. However, some important differences exist. Even though children are asleep for the actual surgical intervention, they are subjected to numerous preoperative and postoperative procedures. Stress points before and after surgery include the admission process, blood tests, injection of preoperative medication (if prescribed), transport to the operating room, and the stay in the postanesthesia care unit (PACU).

Surprisingly little research has been conducted on children's perception of the surgical experience and their fears of the event. Although fear of anesthesia is thought to be a major concern among children, little evidence exists. School-age children report few remembered events and even fewer fears. Those events recalled most often were riding to and arriving in the operating room, receiving the preoperative or induction injection, waking up in pain, and not being allowed to eat or drink. The most feared events were the preoperative injection and the mask on the face.

Parental presence during induction of anesthesia is allowed in some institutions (Fig. 45-2). Potential benefits include minimizing the need for premedication and reducing the struggle that often occurs during separation (Kain, Caldwell-Andrews, & Wang, 2002). Other benefits are controversial but may include decreasing the child's anxiety during induction (e.g., breath holding and laryngospasm) and decreasing long-term behavioral effects of surgery (Romino et al, 2005).

evolve Nursing Care Plan—The Child Undergoing Surgery

Although few institutions endorse the policy, reports from parents who attend the induction are favorable (Kain et al, 2004). Even though some parents may become anxious, most control their anxiety, do not disrupt the induction, and support the child (Hall et al, 1995; LaRosa-Nash & Murphy, 1997; Munro & D'Errico, 2000). Clinical observations show parental presence decreases anxiety in the child and reduces the need for heavy doses of preoperative sedation (Fennell, 1999).

Appropriate education is essential to help parents understand the stages of anesthesia, what to expect, and how to support their child (Fennell, 1999), combined with a program that prepares them for what to expect and what is expected of them. When parents choose not to or are not allowed to attend this induction, leaving a favorite possession with the child and uniting the child and parents as soon as possible after surgery (preferably in the PACU) are important interventions. During surgery the family should have a designated place to wait and should be kept informed of the child's progress. They also should know where and when they can visit the child after surgery.

Aside from possibly being separated from the parents before and after surgery, children may be cared for by a number of unfamiliar practitioners, which promotes fear and uncertainty. Although the same supportive nurse should remain with the child through as many of the procedures as possible, the child may have other nurses, especially if the patient returns to a special care unit postoperatively. Many hospitals have surgical tours for children and parents to familiarize them with the strange environment and to introduce them to other individuals who will be involved in their care.

An important concern is restriction of food and fluids before surgery to avoid aspiration during anesthesia. Infants require special attention to fluid needs. They should not be without oral fluids for an extended period preoperatively to avoid glycogen depletion and dehydration. Current preoperative fasting guidelines are found in Table 45-1.

Table 45-1 Fasting Recommendations to Reduce the Risk of Pulmonary Aspiration*

INGESTED MATERIAL	MINIMUM FASTING PERIOD (hr)†
Clear liquids‡	2
Breast milk	4
Infant formula	6
Nonhuman milk§	6
Light meal¶	6

From American Society of Anesthesiologists: Practice guidelines for preoperative fasting and the use of pharmacologic agents to reduce the risk of pulmonary aspiration: application to healthy patients undergoing elective procedures, *Anesthesiology* 90(3):896-905, 1999. Available at www.asahq.org/publicationsAndServices/NPO.pdf (accessed June 15, 2009).

*These recommendations apply to healthy patients who are undergoing elective procedures. They are not intended for women in labor. Following the guidelines does not guarantee a complete gastric emptying has occurred.

†Fasting periods noted in chart apply to all ages.

‡Examples of clear liquids include water, fruit juices without pulp, carbonated beverages, clear tea, and black coffee.

§Because nonhuman milk is similar to solids in gastric emptying time, the amount ingested must be considered when determining appropriate fasting period.

¶A light meal typically consists of toast and clear liquids. Meals that include fried or fatty foods or meat may prolong gastric emptying time. Both the amount and type of foods ingested must be considered when determining appropriate fasting period.

Preoperative Sedation

Historically the most upsetting event for children has been the preoperative injection. Significant increases have recently occurred in the number of anesthesiologists who use preoperative sedatives, usually midazolam (Versed), and parental presence for children undergoing surgery (Kain et al, 2004). When drugs are administered, they should be delivered atraumatically via oral or intravenous (IV) routes. Numerous preanesthetic drug regimens are used with children, and no consensus exists on the optimal method. The goals for using preoperative medications include (1) anxiety reduction, (2) amnesia, (3) sedation, (4) antiemetic effect, and (5) reduction of secretions (Landsman & Cook, 1998; Manworren & Fledderman, 2000). Midazolam provides excellent preoperative anxiety reduction, amnesia, and sedation. It is popular because of its short duration, predictable onset, and rare occurrence of respiratory depression. Oral transmucosal fentanyl (OTFC, or Oralet) is available as a sweetened lozenge on a plastic stick. When first approved, this appeared to be an excellent, atraumatic route of administration. However, associated nausea and vomiting, respiratory depression, and the need for more intensive monitoring and observation than with other oral sedatives have limited its popularity (Klein et al, 2002). If children have no preoperative pain, are well prepared psychologically for surgery, and have their parents nearby, preoperative medication may be unnecessary.

Anesthesia induction of the pediatric patient is commonly accomplished by administering inhalation agents in combination with nitrous oxide and oxygen by mask. Children may fear induction of anesthesia by mask. Practices that can minimize anxiety related to inhalation anesthesia are (1) disguising the unpleasant odor of anesthetic gases by applying a pleasant-smelling substance on the mask; (2) using a transparent plastic mask rather than an opaque black mask and gradually bringing it toward the face; (3) directing a stream of gas toward the child's face from the bare tube until the child becomes drowsy, then using the mask; (4) allowing the child to sit up rather than lie down for anesthesia induction; and (5) allowing preoperative play with a mask and a doll or manikin.

Postoperative Care

Various psychologic and physical interventions and observations are required to prevent or minimize possible untoward effects from anesthesia and the surgical procedure (see Guidelines box). Although the incidence of serious postoperative complications in healthy children undergoing surgery is less than 1% (Maxwell & Yaster, 2000), continuous monitoring of cardiopulmonary status is essential during the immediate postoperative period. Postanesthesia complications such as airway obstruction, postextubation croup, laryngospasm, and bronchospasm make maintaining a patent airway and maximum ventilation critical.

Monitoring oxygen saturation and providing supplemental oxygen as needed, maintaining body temperature, and promoting fluid and electrolyte balance are important aspects of immediate postoperative care. Vital signs are continuously monitored, and each vital sign is evaluated in terms of side effects from anesthesia, shock, or respiratory compromise (Table 45-2).

GUIDELINES Postoperative Care

Ensure that preparations are made to receive child:
- Bed or crib is ready.
- Intravenous pumps and poles, suction apparatus, and oxygen flow meter are at bedside.

Obtain baseline information:
- Take vital signs, including blood pressure; keep blood pressure cuff in place and deflated to lessen amount of disturbance to child.
- Take and record vital signs more frequently if any value fluctuates.
- Inspect operative area.
- Check dressing if present: (1) outline any bleeding area on dressing or cast with pen; (2) reinforce, but do not remove, loose dressing; (3) observe areas below surgical site for blood that may have drained toward bed; and (4) assess for bleeding and other symptoms in areas not covered with a dressing, such as throat after tonsillectomy.
- Assess skin color and characteristics.
- Assess level of consciousness and activity.

Notify physician of any irregularities in child's condition.

Assess for evidence of pain (see Pain Assessment, Chapter 35).

Review surgeon's orders after completing initial assessment, and check that any preoperative orders, such as seizure or cardiac medications, have been reordered and can be given by available routes (oral preparations may be contraindicated).

Monitor vital signs as ordered and more often if indicated.

Check dressings for bleeding or other abnormalities.

Check bowel sounds.

Observe for signs of shock, abdominal distention, and bleeding.

Assess for bladder distention.

Observe for signs of dehydration.

Detect presence of infection:
- Take vital signs every 2 to 4 hours, as ordered.
- Collect or request needed specimens.
- Inspect wound for signs of infection—redness, swelling, heat, pain, and purulent drainage.

A change in vital signs that demands immediate attention in the perioperative period is caused by *malignant hyperthermia* (MH), a potentially fatal genetic myopathy. In susceptible children, anesthetics such as succinylcholine and halothane trigger the disorder, producing hypermetabolism, muscle rigidity, and an elevated temperature. Early symptoms of MH include tachycardia and tachyarrhythmias, tachypnea, hypercarbia, and metabolic and respiratory acidosis. An elevated temperature is considered by many to be a late sign of the disorder (Redmond, 2001). A family or previous history of sudden high fever associated with a surgical procedure and certain neuromuscular disorders increase risk for MH; children who have successfully undergone prior surgery without adverse effects may still be considered susceptible. Treatment includes immediate discontinuation of the triggering agent and surgical procedure, hyperventilation with 100% oxygen, and IV dantrolene sodium. Infusions of cool saline, cooling blankets, gastric or peritoneal lavage, packed ice bags in the axillae and groin, and, possibly, cardiopulmonary bypass reduce core temperature (Redmond, 2001). The patient should be transferred to an intensive care unit and closely monitored for stabilization of vital signs, metabolic state, and possible recurrence of symptoms.

Managing pain is a major nursing responsibility after surgery (see Chapter 35). The nurse should assess pain frequently and administer analgesics to provide comfort and facilitate cooperation with postoperative care such as ambulation and deep breathing. Opioids are the most commonly used analgesics. Routinely scheduled IV analgesics, patient-controlled analgesia, and epidural infusions, rather than as needed (PRN) orders, provide excellent analgesia in postoperative pediatric patients.

Because respiratory infections are a potential complication, every effort is taken to aerate the lungs and remove secretions. The lungs are auscultated regularly to identify abnormal sounds or any areas of diminished or absent breath sounds. To prevent hypostatic pneumonia, respiratory movement can be encouraged with incentive spirometers or other motivating activities (see Box 45-3). If these measures are presented as games, the child is more likely to comply. The child's position is changed every 2 hours, and deep breathing is encouraged.

Compliance

Compliance, also termed *adherence*, refers to the extent to which the patient's behavior coincides with the prescribed regimen in terms of taking medication, following diets, or executing other lifestyle changes. In developing strategies to promote compliance, the nurse must first assess level of compliance. Because many children are too young to assume partial or total responsibility for their care, parents are usually primarily responsible for home management.

Factors relating to the care setting are important in ensuring compliance and should be considered in planning strategies to improve compliance. Basically, any aspect of the health care environment that increases the family's satisfaction with the physical setting and the relationship with the practitioner positively influences adherence to the treatment regimen. However, the more complex, expensive, inconvenient, and disruptive the treatment protocol, the less likely the family is to comply. Long-term conditions that involve multiple treatments and considerable rearrangement of lifestyle severely affect compliance.

Although it is helpful to know those factors that influence compliance, assessment must include more direct measurement techniques. A number of methods exist, each with advantages and disadvantages. The most successful approach includes a combination of at least two of the following methods:

Clinical judgment—This is subject to bias and inaccuracy unless the nurse carefully evaluates the criteria used in assessment.

Self-reporting—Most people overestimate compliance by about 20% even when they admit to lapses.

Direct observation—This is difficult to employ outside the health care setting, and awareness of being observed frequently affects performance.

Table 45-2 Potential Causes of Postoperative Vital Sign Alterations in Children

ALTERATION	POTENTIAL CAUSE	COMMENTS
Heart Rate		
Increase	Decreased perfusion (shock) Elevated temperature Pain Respiratory distress (early) Medications (atropine, morphine, epinephrine)	Heart rate may increase to maintain cardiac output.
Decrease	Hypoxia Vagal stimulation Increased intracranial pressure Respiratory distress (late) Medications	In the young child, bradycardia is of more concern than tachycardia.
Respiratory Rate		
Increase	Respiratory distress Fluid volume excess Hypothermia Elevated temperature Pain	Body responds to respiratory distress primarily by increasing rate.
Decrease	Anesthetics, opioids Pain	Decreased respiratory rate from opioids may be compensated for by increase depth of respiration.
Blood Pressure		
Increase	Excess intravascular volume Increased intracranial pressure Carbon dioxide retention Pain Medication (ketamine, epinephrine)	This is serious in preterm infants because it increases risk of intraventricular hemorrhage.
Decrease	Vasodilating anesthetic agents (halothane, isoflurane, enflurane) Opioids (morphine)	Decreased blood pressure is late sign of shock because of elasticity and constriction of vessels to maintain cardiac output.
Temperature		
Increase	Shock (late sign) Infection Environmental causes (warm room, excess coverings) Malignant hyperthermia	Fever associated with infection usually occurs later than fever of noninfectious origin. Absence of fever does not rule out infection, especially in infants.
Decrease	Vasodilating anesthetic agents (halothane, isoflurane, enflurane) Muscle relaxants Environmental causes (cool room) Infusion of cool fluids or blood	Malignant hyperthermia requires immediate treatment. Neonates are especially susceptible to hypothermia, with serious or fatal consequences.

From Smith DP: *Comprehensive child and family nursing skills*, St Louis, 1991, Mosby.

Monitoring appointments—Keeping appointments indirectly indicates compliance with the prescribed care.

Monitoring therapeutic response—Few treatments yield directly measurable results (e.g., decreased blood pressure, weight loss); record on a graph or chart.

Pill counts—The nurse counts the number of pills remaining in the original container and compares the number missing with the number of times the medication should have been taken. Families may forget to bring the container or deliberately alter the number of pills to avoid detection. This method is also poorly suited to liquid medication. Another technique is the use of pill container caps that record every opening as a presumptive dose.

Chemical assay—For certain drugs, such as digoxin and phenytoin, measurement of plasma drug levels provides information on the amount of drug recently ingested. However, this method is expensive, indicates only short-term compliance, and requires precise timing of the assay for accurate results.

Compliance Strategies

Strategies to improve compliance are composed of interventions that encourage families to follow the prescribed treatment regimen. Some evidence suggests that higher levels of self-esteem and increased autonomy favorably affect adolescent compliance (KyngAs, Kroll, & Duffy, 2000). However, family factors are also important, and characteristics associated with good compliance include family support, family reminders, good communication, and expectations for successful completion of the therapeutic regimen (KyngAs, Kroll, & Duffy, 2000). No one approach is always successful, and the best results occur when at least two strategies are used.

BOX 45-3 Play Activities for Specific Procedures*

Fluid Intake

Make ice pops using child's favorite juice.
Cut gelatin into fun shapes.
Make a game out of taking a sip when turning page of a book or in games such as Simon Says.
Use small medicine cups; decorate the cups.
Color water with food coloring or powdered drink mix.
Have a tea party; pour at a small table.
Let child fill a syringe and squirt into mouth or use to fill small cups.
Cut straws in half and place in a small container (much easier for child to suck liquid).
Use a "crazy" straw.
Make a "progress poster"; give rewards for drinking a predetermined quantity.

Deep Breathing

Blow bubbles with a bubble blower.
Blow bubbles with a straw (no soap).
Blow on a pinwheel, feather, whistle, harmonica, balloon, horn, party blower.
Practice band instruments.
Have blowing contest using balloons,* boats, cotton balls, feathers, marbles, Ping-Pong balls, pieces of paper; blow objects on a table top over a goal line, over water, through an obstacle course, into the air, against an opponent, or up and down a string.
Suck paper or cloth from one container to another using a straw.
Use blow bottles with colored water to transfer water from one side to the other.
Dramatize stories such as "I'll huff and puff and blow your house down" from the Three Little Pigs.
Do straw-blowing painting.
Take a deep breath and "blow out the candles" on a birthday cake.
Use a little paint brush to "paint" nails with water and blow nails dry.

Range of Motion and Use of Extremities

Throw beanbags at a fixed or movable target or throw wadded-up paper into a wastebasket.
Touch or kick Mylar balloons held or hung in different positions (if child is in traction, hang balloon from a trapeze).
Play "tickle toes"; have child wiggle them on request.
Play Twister game or Simon Says.
Play pretend and guessing games (e.g., imitate a bird, butterfly, horse).
Have tricycle or wheelchair races in safe area.
Play kickball or catch with a soft foam ball in a safe area.
Position bed so that child must turn to view television or doorway.
Climb wall like a "spider."
Pretend to teach "aerobic" dancing or exercises; encourage parents to participate.
Encourage swimming if feasible.
Play video games or pinball (fine motor movement).
Play "hide and seek": hide toy somewhere in bed (or room if ambulatory) and have child find it using specified hand or foot.
Provide clay to mold with fingers.
Paint or draw on large sheets of paper placed on floor or wall.
Encourage combing own hair; play "beauty shop" with "customer" in different positions.

Soaks

Play with small toys or objects (cups, syringes, soap dishes) in water.
Wash dolls or toys.
Pick up marbles or pennies* from bottom of bath container.
Make designs with coins on bottom of container.
Pretend a boat is a submarine by keeping it immersed.
During soaks, read to child; sing with child; or play game, such as cards, checkers, or other board game (if both of the child's hands are immersed, move board pieces for child).
During a sitz bath, give child something to listen to (music, stories) or look at (View-Master, book).
Punch holes in bottom of plastic cup, fill with water, and let it "rain" on child.

Injections

Let child handle syringe, vial, and alcohol swab, and give an injection to doll or stuffed animal.
Use syringes to decorate cookies with frosting, squirt paint, or target shoot into a container.
Draw a "magic circle" on area before injection; draw smiling face in circle after injection, but avoid drawing on puncture site.
Allow child to have a "collection" of syringes (without needles); make "wild" creative objects with syringes.
If child has multiple injections or venipunctures, make a "progress poster"; give rewards for predetermined number of injections.
Have child count to 10 or 15 during injection.

Ambulation

Give child something to push.
- **Toddler**—Push-pull toy
- **School-age child**—Wagon or a doll in a stroller or wheelchair
- **Adolescent**—Decorated intravenous stand

Have a parade; make hats, drums, etc.

Extending Environment (e.g., for Patients in Traction)

Make bed into a pirate ship or airplane with decorations.
Put up mirrors so patient can see around room.
Move bed frequently to playroom, hallway, or outside.

*Small objects such as marbles or coins, as well as Latex gloves or balloons, are unsafe for young children because of possible aspiration. Latex products also carry the risk of an allergic reaction.

BOX 45-4 Factors That Positively Influence Compliance

Individual and Family Factors
High self-esteem
Positive body image
High degree of autonomy (increased locus of control)
Supportive and well-adjusted family
Effective family communication
Family expectation for successful completion of therapy

Care Setting Factors
Perceived satisfaction with care
Positive interactions with practitioners
Continuity of care
Individualized care
Minimum waiting time for appointments
Convenient care setting

Treatment Factors
Simple regimen
Minimum disruption in usual lifestyle
Short duration
Inexpensive
Visible benefits
Tolerable side effects

Organizational strategies involve the care setting and the therapeutic plan. They include manipulating the factors listed in Box 45-4 that positively affect compliance. *Educational strategies* instruct the family about the treatment plan. Although education is an important factor in enhancing compliance and patients who are more knowledgeable about their condition are more likely to comply, education alone does not ensure compliant behavior. The nurse should incorporate teaching principles known to enhance understanding and retention of material. Written materials are essential, especially in any regimen requiring multiple or complex treatments, and they need to be understandable to the average individual, who reads at about the fourth-grade level. *Treatment strategies* relate to the child's refusal or inability to take the prescribed medication. The family may also have difficulty following a prescribed treatment regimen. They may remember and understand the instructions but may not be able to give the medicine as prescribed. Assess the reason for refusal. For example, the child may not be able to swallow pills. In this case, perhaps pills can be crushed or a liquid medication substituted (always review medication to ensure that crushing is acceptable before giving this instruction).

Assess the treatment and medication schedule to determine if it is reasonable for a home situation. Although an every-6-hour or every-8-hour schedule is reasonable for hospitals, a parent would have difficulty getting up once or twice nightly; instead a medication could be given during the day at times that would be easy to remember.

Behavioral strategies are designed to modify behavior directly. Several strategies encouraging the desired behavior are effective with children. Ideally, positive reinforcement should be employed to strengthen the behavior and may consist of earning stars or tokens, which gains the child a special privilege or gift. At times, however, disciplinary techniques such as time-out for young children or withholding privileges for older children may be needed to improve compliance (see Limit Setting and Discipline, Chapter 31). *Contracting,* a formal process in which exact elements of desired behavior are explicitly outlined along with rewards or negative consequences, is an effective method with older children.

General Hygiene and Care

Maintaining Healthy Skin

Maintaining an IV line, removing a dressing, positioning a child in bed, changing a diaper, using electrodes, and using restraints have the potential to contribute to skin injury. Skin care must go beyond the daily bath and become a part of each nursing intervention (see Guidelines box). Specific guidelines for skin care of neonates are provided in Sponge Bathing, Cord Care, and Skin Care, Chapter 25.

Assessment of the skin is most easily accomplished during the bath. Examine for early signs of injury. Risk factors include impaired mobility, protein malnutrition, edema, incontinence, sensory loss, anemia, infection, failure to turn the patient, and intubation. Critically ill children often are at high risk of pressure ulcers and skin breakdown, since they often have several risk factors combined. Identification of risk factors helps to determine those children who need a more thorough skin assessment. Assessment should occur within 24 hours of admission so that pressure ulcers and wounds that occurred before admission can be identified (Ratliff & Rodheaver, 1999; Quigley & Curley, 1996).

When capillary blood flow is interrupted by pressure, the blood flows back into the tissue when the pressure is relieved. As the body attempts to reoxygenate the area, a bright red flush appears. This *reactive hyperemia,* or flush, is the earliest sign of tissue compromise and pressure-related ischemia. If pressure is prolonged, reactive hyperemia will not be sufficient to revitalize ischemic tissue (Calianno, 1999).

Staging of pressure ulcers is used to classify the amount of tissue damage.* Necrotic tissue must be removed so that the tissue depth can accurately be assessed. Accurate documentation of redness or obvious skin breakdown is essential. Color, size (diameter and depth), location, presence of sinus tracts, odor, exudate, and response to treatment are observed and recorded at least daily.

Pressure ulcers can develop when the pressure on the skin and underlying tissues is greater than the capillary closing pressure, causing capillary occlusion. If the pressure remains unrelieved, vessels can collapse, resulting in tissue anoxia and cellular death. Pressure ulcers most often occur over bony prominences and are usually very deep, extending into subcutaneous tissue or even deeper into muscle, tendon, or bone. A *pressure-reduction device* reduces pressure but does not prevent pressure from causing capillary closure; therefore turning and repositioning are always included when using these devices. Most of these items are overlays that are placed on top of the

**Staging of pressure ulcers and guidelines for prevention and management of pressure ulcers can be found at* wocn.org.

GUIDELINES Skin Care

- Cleanse skin with mild nonalkaline soap or soap-free cleaning agents for routine bathing.
- Provide daily cleansing of eyes, oral and diaper or perineal areas, and any areas of skin breakdown.
- Apply moisturizing agents during or immediately after bathing; cleanse skin of old cream before adding a new layer.
- Use minimum tape and adhesives. On very sensitive skin, use a protective, pectin-based or hydrocolloid skin barrier between skin and tape or adhesives.
- Use water or adhesive remover (if skin is not fragile) when removing tape or adhesives.
- Place pectin-based or hydrocolloid skin barriers directly over excoriated skin. Leave barrier undisturbed until it begins to peel off, or for 5 to 7 days. With wet, oozing excoriations, place a small amount of stoma powder on site, remove excess powder, and apply skin barrier. Hold barrier in place for several minutes to allow barrier to soften and mold to skin surface.
- Alternate electrode placement and thoroughly assess skin underneath electrodes at least every 24 hours. Alcohol-free skin sealant under leads protects skin from epidermal stripping.
- Be certain fingers or toes are visible whenever extremity is used for intravenous (IV) or arterial line.
- Keep skin dry (may apply absorbent powder [e.g., cornstarch]) and use soft, smooth bed linen and clothes.
- Use a draw sheet to move a child in bed or onto a gurney; do not drag the child from under the arms.
- Identify children at risk for skin breakdown before it occurs. Employ measures such as pressure-reducing or pressure-relieving devices (e.g., mattress overlay, low-air-loss bed, gel pillows).
- Do not massage reddened bony prominences, since this can cause deep tissue damage; provide pressure relief to those areas instead.
- Keep skin free of excess moisture (e.g., urine or fecal incontinence, wound drainage, excessive perspiration).
- Routinely assess the child's nutritional status. A child who is NPO (nothing by mouth) for several days and is receiving only IV fluid is nutritionally at risk, which can also affect the skin's ability to maintain its integrity. Consider parenteral nutrition.

regular mattress. A *pressure-relief device* maintains pressure below that which would cause capillary closure. These devices are usually high-technology beds that are used for patients who have multiple problems and cannot be turned effectively.

Friction and shear contribute to pressure ulcers. *Friction* occurs when the skin's surface rubs against another surface, such as the bed sheets. Skin damage most often occurs over the elbows, heels, or occiput; is usually limited to the epidermal and upper layers; and may have the appearance of an abrasion. Prevention of friction injury includes the use of protective sheepskin over the elbows or heels; gel pillows under the head of infants and toddlers; moisturizing agents; transparent dressings over susceptible areas; and soft, smooth bed linen and clothing. *Shear* is the result of the force of gravity pushing down on the body and friction of the body against a surface, such as the bed or chair. For example, when a patient is in the semi-Fowler position and begins to slide to the foot of the bed, the skin over the sacral area remains in the same place because of the resistance of the bed surface. The blood vessels in the area are stretched and may cause small-vessel thrombosis and tissue death (Bryant & Doughty, 2000). Prevention of shear injury includes using *lift sheets* when repositioning a patient, elevating the bed no more than 30 degrees for short periods, and using the knee gatch to interrupt the pull of gravity on the body toward the foot of the bed.

Epidermal stripping results when the epidermis is unintentionally removed with tape removal. These lesions are usually shallow and irregularly shaped and may blister or weep. Babies are at increased risk for epidermal injury. Prevention includes using no tape when possible, securing dressings with laced binders (Montgomery straps) or stretchy netting (Spandage or stockinette). Using porous or low-tack tapes (e.g., Medipore, paper, hydrogel), using alcohol-free skin sealants (No Sting Barrier Film), or picture framing wounds with hydrocolloid or wafer barriers (e.g., DuoDERM, Coloplast, Stomahesive) and then taping on top of the barrier will also reduce epidermal stripping.

Tape is placed so that there is no tension, traction, or wrinkles on the skin. To remove tape, slowly peel the tape away while stabilizing the underlying skin. Adhesive remover may be used to break the adhesive bond but may be drying to the skin; adhesive removers should be avoided in preterm neonates, since absorption rates vary and toxicity may occur. The adhesive is removed with water to prevent absorption and irritation. Wetting the tape with water or alcohol-based foam hand cleansers may facilitate removal.

Chemical factors can also lead to skin damage. Fecal incontinence, especially when mixed with urine; wound drainage; or gastric drainage around gastrostomy tubes can erode epidermis. The skin can quickly progress from redness to denudement if exposure continues. Moisture barriers, gentle cleansing as soon after exposure as possible, and skin barriers can be used to prevent damage caused by chemical factors (see also Diaper Dermatitis, Chapter 53). In addition, foam dressings that wick moisture away from the skin are helpful around gastrostomy tubes and tracheostomy sites.

Bathing

Most infants and children can be bathed in a basin at the bedside, on the bed, or in a standard bathtub or shower. For infants and young children confined to bed, the towel method can be used. Two towels are immersed in a diluted soap solution and wrung damp. With the child lying supine on a dry towel, one damp towel is placed on top of the child and used to gently clean the body. This towel is discarded, and the child is dried and turned prone. The procedure is repeated using the second damp towel. Commercially available bath cloths may also be used.

Infants and small children are *never* left unattended in a bathtub, and infants who are unable to sit alone are securely held with one hand during the bath. The nurse should securely support the infant's head with one hand, or grasp the farther arm firmly while the head rests comfortably on the nurse's arm. Children who are able to sit without assistance need only close supervision and a pad placed in the bottom of the tub to prevent slipping and loss of balance.

School-age children and adolescents may shower or bathe. Nurses need to use judgment regarding the amount of supervision the child requires. Some can assume this responsibility unaided, whereas others will need someone in constant attendance. Children with cognitive impairments, physical limitations, or suicidal or psychotic problems (who may commit bodily harm) require close supervision.

Children who are ill or debilitated need more extensive assistance with bathing, but should be encouraged to perform as much as they can without overtaxing their energies. Expect increasing involvement with improved strength and endurance.

Oral Hygiene

Mouth care is an integral part of daily hygiene and should be continued in the hospital. Infants and debilitated children require the nurse or a family member to perform mouth care. Although young children can manage a toothbrush and are encouraged to use it, most need assistance to perform satisfactorily. Older children, although capable of brushing and flossing without assistance, sometimes need to be reminded. (See Dental Health, Chapters 36 and 37, for specific oral hygiene techniques; mouth care of children with mucosal ulcers is discussed under nursing care of the child with leukemia in Chapter 49.)

Hair Care

Children should have their hair brushed and combed at least once daily. The hair is styled for comfort and in a manner pleasing to the child and parents. The hair should not be cut without parental permission, although clipping hair to provide access to a scalp vein for IV insertion may be necessary.

If children are hospitalized for more than a few days, the hair may need shampooing. With infants the hair may be washed during the daily bath or less frequently. For most children, washing the hair and scalp once or twice weekly is sufficient unless there is an indication for more frequent washing, such as following a high fever and profuse sweating. Adolescents normally have increased oily sebaceous secretions that require frequent hair care and more frequent shampoos.

Most children can be transported to an accessible sink for shampooing. Those who are unable to be transported can receive a shampoo in their beds with adequate protection, specially adapted equipment or positioning, or dry shampoo caps. When necessary, a shampoo basin may be used or the child may be positioned near the edge of the bed, towels placed under the shoulders, a large plastic garbage bag draped at the edge of the bed with one open end under the shoulders, and the hair placed inside the opening. The other end is opened and placed in a collection container. Water can be transported in a basin.

Feeding the Sick Child

Loss of appetite is a symptom common to most childhood illnesses. Because an acute illness is usually short, the nutritional state is seldom compromised. Urging foods on the sick child may precipitate nausea and vomiting, and in most cases children can be permitted to determine their own need for food.

Refusing to eat may also be one way children can exert power and control in an otherwise helpless situation. For young children, loss of appetite may be related to the depression caused by separation from their parents. Parents' concern with eating can intensify the problem. Forcing a child to eat meets with rebellion and reinforces the behavior as a control mechanism. Parents are encouraged to relax any pressure during an acute illness. Although it is best to encourage high-quality nutritious foods, the child may desire foods and liquids that contain mostly empty or nonnutritional calories. Some well-tolerated foods include gelatin, diluted clear soups, carbonated drinks, flavored ice pops, dry toast, and crackers. Even though these substances are not nutritious, they can provide necessary fluid and calories.

Dehydration is always a hazard when children are febrile or anorexic, especially when accompanied by vomiting or diarrhea. Offer small amounts of favored fluids at frequent intervals and provide salty foods (which increase thirst) if allowed. If diarrhea is present, avoid high-carbohydrate liquids (e.g., carbonated beverages, gelatin, flavored ice pops) because they may aggravate the diarrhea by an osmotic effect. Replacing abnormal losses with plain water or undiluted broth may worsen the electrolyte imbalance. Fluids should not be forced, and the child is not awakened to take fluids. Forcing fluids may create the same difficulties as urging unwanted food. Gentle persuasion with preferred beverages will usually meet with success. Using play techniques can also be effective (see Guidelines box).

Once the child is feeling better, appetite usually begins to improve. It is best to take advantage of any hungry period by serving high-quality foods and snacks. If the child still refuses to eat, nutritious fluids, such as prepared breakfast drinks, should be encouraged. Parents can help by bringing in food items from home, especially if the family's cultural eating habits differ from the hospital food. A clinical dietitian may also be consulted for alternative food choices.

When children are placed on special diets, such as clear liquids after surgery or during episodes of diarrhea, assessment of their intake and readiness to advance to more complex foods is essential. Regardless of the type of diet, charting of the amount consumed is an important nursing responsibility. Descriptions need to be detailed and accurate, such as "4 oz of orange juice, one pancake, and 8 oz of milk." Comments such as "ate well" or "ate poorly" are inadequate. Charting the percentage of the meal eaten is also inadequate unless food is measured before serving.

If parents are involved in the child's care, they are encouraged to keep a list of everything eaten. Using a premeasured cup for fluids ensures a more accurate estimate of intake. A comparison of the intake at each meal can isolate food deficiencies, such as insufficient intake of meat or vegetables. Behaviors associated with mealtime also may point to possible factors influencing appetite. For example, the observation that "child eats well when with other children but plays with food if left alone in room" helps the nurse plan mealtime activities that stimulate the appetite.

GUIDELINES Feeding the Sick Child

Take a dietary history (see Chapter 34) and use information to make eating time as much like home as possible.
Encourage parents or other family members to feed child or to be present at mealtimes.
Make mealtimes pleasant; avoid any procedures immediately before or after eating; make certain child is rested and pain free.
Serve small, frequent meals rather than three large meals, or serve three meals and nutritious between-meal snacks.
Provide finger foods for young children.
Involve children in food selection and preparation whenever possible.
Serve small portions, and serve each course separately, such as soup first; followed by meat, potatoes, and vegetables; and ending with dessert.
- With young children, camouflage size of food by cutting meat thicker so that less appears on plate or by folding a cheese slice in half.
- Offer second helpings.

Ensure a variety of foods, textures, and colors.
Provide food selections that are favorites of most children, such as peanut butter and jelly sandwiches, hot dogs, hamburgers, macaroni and cheese, pizza, spaghetti, tacos, fried chicken, corn, and fruit yogurt.
Avoid foods that are highly seasoned, have strong odors, or are all mixed together, unless typical of cultural practices.
Provide fluid selections that are favorites of most children, such as fruit punch, cola, ginger ale, sweetened tea, flavored ice pops, sherbet, ice cream, milk, milkshakes, eggnog, pudding, gelatin, clear broth, or creamed soups.
Offer nutritious snacks, such as frozen yogurt or pudding, ice cream, oatmeal or peanut butter cookies, hot cocoa, cheese slices, pieces of raw vegetable or fruit, and dried fruit or cereal.
Make food attractive and different; for example:
- Serve a "picnic lunch" in a paper bag.
- Pack food in a Chinese take-out container; decorate container.
- Put a "face" or a "flower" on a hamburger or sandwich with pieces of vegetable.
- Use a cookie cutter to shape a sandwich.
- Serve pudding, yogurt, or juice frozen as an ice pop.
- Make Slurpies or snow cones by pouring flavored syrup on crushed ice.
- Add food coloring to water or milk.
- Serve fluids through brightly colored or unusually shaped straws.
- Make "bowtie" sandwiches by cutting them in triangles and placing two points together.
- Slice sandwiches into "fingers."
- Grate mounds of cheese.
- Cut apples horizontally to make circles.
- Put a banana on a hot dog bun and spread with peanut butter.
- Break uncooked spaghetti into toothpick lengths and skewer cheese, cold meat, vegetables, or fruit chunks.

Praise children for what they do eat.
Do not punish children for not eating by removing their dessert or putting them to bed.

Controlling Elevated Temperatures

An elevated temperature, most frequently from fever but occasionally caused by hyperthermia, is one of the most common symptoms of illness in children. This manifestation is of great concern to parents. To facilitate an understanding of fever, the following terms are defined:

Set point—The temperature around which body temperature is regulated by a thermostat-like mechanism in the hypothalamus

Fever (hyperpyrexia)—An elevation in set point such that body temperature is regulated at a higher level; may be arbitrarily defined as temperature above 38° C (100.4° F)

Hyperthermia—Body temperature exceeding the set point, which usually results from the body or external conditions creating more heat than the body can eliminate, as in heatstroke, aspirin toxicity, seizures, or hyperthyroidism

Body temperature is regulated by a thermostat-like mechanism in the hypothalamus. This mechanism receives input from centrally and peripherally located receptors. When temperature changes occur, these receptors relay the information to the thermostat, which either increases or decreases heat production to maintain a constant set point temperature. However, during an infection, pyrogenic substances cause an increase in the body's normal set point, a process that is mediated by prostaglandins. Consequently, the hypothalamus increases heat production until the core temperature reaches the new set point.

Most fevers in children are of brief duration with limited consequences and are viral in origin. When fever is caused by bacteria, endotoxins are produced that activate the inflammatory process and produce fever (Rote, Huether, & McCance, 2000). Contrary to popular belief, neither the rise in temperature nor its response to antipyretics indicates the severity or cause of infection, which casts doubt on the value of using fever as a diagnostic or prognostic indicator.

Therapeutic management of elevated temperature depends on whether it is due to a fever or hyperthermia. Because the set point is normal in hyperthermia but increased in fever, different approaches must be used to lower body temperature successfully.

Fever

The principal reason for treating fever is the relief of discomfort. Relief measures include pharmacologic or environmental intervention. The most effective intervention is the use of antipyretics to lower the set point.

Antipyretic drugs include acetaminophen, aspirin, and nonsteroidal antiinflammatory drugs (NSAIDs). Acetaminophen is the preferred drug; aspirin should *not* be given to children because of the association between aspirin use in

evolve Nursing Care Plan—The Child with Elevated Body Temperature

children and influenza virus or chickenpox and Reye's syndrome. One nonprescription NSAID, ibuprofen, is approved for fever reduction in children as young as 6 months of age. Dosage is based on the initial temperature level: 5 mg/kg of body weight for temperatures less than 39.2° C (102.6° F) or 10 mg/kg for temperatures greater than 39.2° C. The recommended dosage for pain is 10 mg/kg every 6 to 8 hours, and the recommended maximum daily dose for pain and fever is 40 mg/kg. The duration of fever reduction is generally 6 to 8 hours and is longer with the higher dose. It may be given every 4 hours but no more than five times in 24 hours. Because body temperature normally decreases at night, three or four doses in 24 hours will control most fevers. The nurse should retake the temperature 30 minutes after the antipyretic is given to assess its effect, but temperature should not be repeatedly measured; the child's level of discomfort is the best indication for continued treatment.

Environmental measures to reduce fever may be used if tolerated by the child and if they do not induce shivering. Shivering is the body's way of maintaining the elevated set point by producing heat. Compensatory shivering greatly increases metabolic requirements above those already caused by the fever.

Traditional cooling measures, such as wearing minimum clothing, exposing the skin to the air, reducing room temperature, increasing air circulation, and applying cool, moist compresses to the skin (e.g., the forehead), are effective if employed approximately 1 hour *after* an antipyretic is given so that the set point is lowered. Cooling procedures such as sponging or tepid baths are ineffective in treating febrile children (these measures are effective for hyperthermia) when used either alone or in combination with antipyretics, and they cause considerable discomfort (Sharber, 1997).

Seizures associated with a fever occur in 3% to 4% of all children, usually those 3 months to 5 years of age. Although most children never have febrile seizures after the first occurrence, a younger age at onset and a family history of febrile seizures are associated with recurring episodes (Berg et al, 1999; Shinnar et al, 2001). There is little evidence to support the use of antipyretic drugs to prevent febrile seizures; nursing interventions should focus on ways to provide care and comfort during a febrile illness (Purssell, 2000).

Hyperthermia

Unlike fever, antipyretics are of no value in hyperthermia because the set point is already normal. Consequently, cooling measures are used. Cool applications to the skin help reduce the core temperature. Cooled blood from the skin surface is conducted to inner organs and tissues, and warm blood is circulated to the surface, where it is cooled and recirculated. The surface blood vessels dilate as the body attempts to dissipate heat to the environment and facilitate the cooling process.

Commercial cooling devices, such as cooling blankets or mattresses, are available to reduce body temperature. Place on the bed and cover with a sheet or lightweight blanket. Frequent temperature monitoring is essential to prevent excessive cooling of the body.

Traditionally, cool compresses have been used to decrease high temperature. For tepid tub baths it is usually best to start with warm water and gradually add cool water until the desired water temperature of 37° C (98.6° F) is reached to accustom the child to the lower water temperature. Generally, the temperature of the water only has to be 1° C or 2° F less than the child's temperature to be effective. The child is placed directly in the tub of tepid water for 15 to 20 minutes while water is gently squeezed from a washcloth over the back and chest or gently sprayed over the body from a sprayer. In the bed or crib, cool washcloths or towels are used, exposing only one area of the body at a time. The sponging is continued for approximately 20 minutes. After the tub or sponge bath, the child is dried and dressed in lightweight pajamas, a nightgown, or a diaper and placed in a dry bed. The child is dried by gently rubbing the skin surface with a towel to stimulate circulation. The temperature is retaken 30 minutes after the tub bath or sponge bath. The tub or sponge bath should not be continued or restarted until the skin surface is warm or if the child feels chilled. Chilling causes vasoconstriction, which defeats the purpose of the cool applications. In this condition, little blood is carried to the skin surface; the blood remains primarily in the viscera to become heated.

Whether a temperature elevation in the critically ill child is caused by fever or hyperthermia, it should be treated aggressively. The metabolic rate increases 10% for every 1° C increase in temperature and three to five times during shivering, thus increasing oxygen, fluid, and caloric requirements. If the child's cardiovascular or neurologic system is already compromised, these increased needs are especially hazardous. In all children with elevated temperature, attention to adequate hydration is essential. Most children's needs can be met through additional oral fluids.

Family Teaching and Home Care

Although most children have learned self-care and hygiene in the home or at school, many have not. For some young children, this is their first introduction to the use of a toothbrush. Much health teaching can be accomplished even when the child is hospitalized for only a short time. The daily bath, handwashing before meals and after bowel and bladder evacuation, and conscientious dental hygiene are taught during routine care. Positive reinforcement of good hygiene practices helps create a positive body image, enhances self-esteem, and prevents health problems (e.g., teaching girls to wipe the genital area from front to back after toileting).

Although sick children's appetites may be poor and not characteristic of their home eating habits, the hospital stay provides numerous opportunities for nurses to assess the family's knowledge of good nutrition and to implement teaching as needed to improve nutritional intake.

Fever is one of the most common problems for which parents seek health care. Parental anxiety increases with temperature elevation and its management (Liebman & Barnsteiner, 2001). Parents need to know that sponging is indicated for elevated temperatures from hyperthermia rather than fever and that ice water and alcohol are inappropriate, potentially dangerous solutions (Axelrod, 2000). Parents should know how to take the child's temperature and read the thermometer accurately and should have guidelines for seeking professional care (see Patient Teaching box). Some of the newer temperature-measuring devices, such as plastic strips or digital thermometers, may be better suited for home use than hospital use (see Temperature, Chapter 34). If acetaminophen or ibuprofen is indicated, the parents need instruction in administering the drug. Emphasize accuracy in both the amount of drug given and the time intervals at which the drug is administered.

PATIENT TEACHING The Child with Fever

Call the Office Immediately If:

Your child is younger than 2 months old.

The fever is over 40.6° C (105° F).

Your child looks or acts very sick: stiff neck, persistent vomiting, purplish spots on skin, confusion, trouble breathing after you have cleaned his or her nose, or inability to be comforted.

Call Within 24 Hours If:

The fever is between 40° and 40.6° C (104° and 105° F), especially if your child is younger than 2 years old.

Your child has:

- Had a fever for more than 24 hours without an obvious cause or location of infection
- Had a fever for more than 3 days
- Burning or pain with urination
- A history of febrile seizures

The fever went away for more than 24 hours and then returned.

You have other concerns or questions.

Modified from Schmitt BD: *Instructions for pediatric patients*, ed 2, Philadelphia, 1999, Saunders.

Safety

Safety is an essential component of any patient's care, but children have special characteristics that require an even greater concern for safety. Because small children in the hospital are separated from their usual environment and do not possess the capacity for abstract thinking and reasoning, it is the responsibility of everyone who comes in contact with them to maintain protective measures throughout their hospital stay. Nurses need to understand the age level at which each child is operating and plan for safety accordingly.

Identification bands are particularly important for children. Infants and unconscious patients are unable to tell or respond to their names. Toddlers may answer to any name or to a nickname only. Older children may exchange places, give an erroneous name, or choose not to respond to their own names as a form of joke, unaware of the hazards of such practices.

Environmental Factors

All of the environmental safety measures for the protection of adults apply to children, including good illumination, floors clear of fluid or objects that might contribute to falls, and nonskid surfaces in showers and tubs. All staff members should be familiar with the area-specific fire plan. Staff members should practice proper care and disposal of small objects such as syringe caps, needle covers, and temperature probe covers (Fig. 45-3).

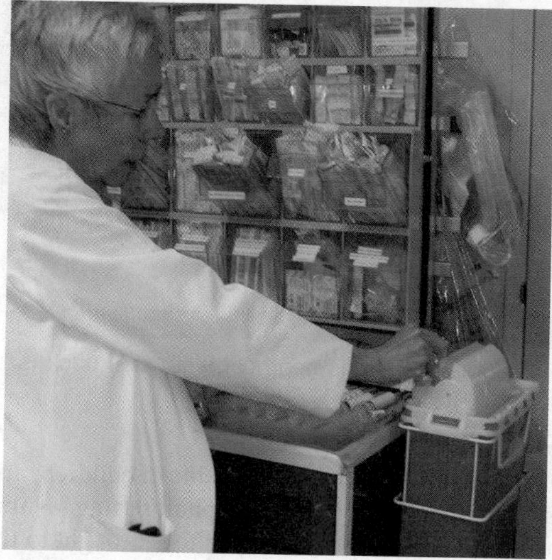

Fig. 45-3 To prevent needlestick injuries, used needles (and other sharp instruments) are not capped or broken and are disposed of in a rigid, puncture-resistant container located near the site of use. Note placement of the container to prevent children's access to the contents.

Bathwater is carefully checked before placing the child in it, and children must never be left alone in a bathtub. Infants are helpless in water, and small children (and some older ones) may turn on the hot water faucet and be severely burned.

Furniture is safest when it is scaled to the child's proportions, is sturdy, and is well balanced to prevent its being easily tipped over. A special hazard for children is the danger of entrapment under an electronically controlled bed when it is activated to descend. Infants and small children must be securely strapped into infant seats, feeding chairs, and strollers. Baby walkers should not be used because they provide access to hazards and can cause injuries by tipping over. Infants; young children; and those who are weak, paralyzed, agitated, confused, sedated, or cognitively impaired are never left unattended on treatment tables, on scales, or in treatment areas. Even preterm infants are capable of surprising mobility; therefore portholes in incubators must be securely fastened when not in use. Beds of ambulatory patients should remain locked in place and at a height that allows easy access to the floor.

Crib sides are kept up and fastened securely unless an adult is at the bedside. It is safer to leave crib sides up, regardless of the child's ability to get out and even when the crib is unoccupied, to remove the child's temptation to climb in. Anyone attending an infant or small child in a crib with the sides down should never turn away without maintaining hand contact with the child; that is, one hand should be kept on the child's back or abdomen to prevent the child from rolling, crawling, or jumping from the open crib (Fig. 45-4). A child who is likely to or has demonstrated the inclination to climb over the sides of the crib is safest when placed in a specially constructed crib with a cover.

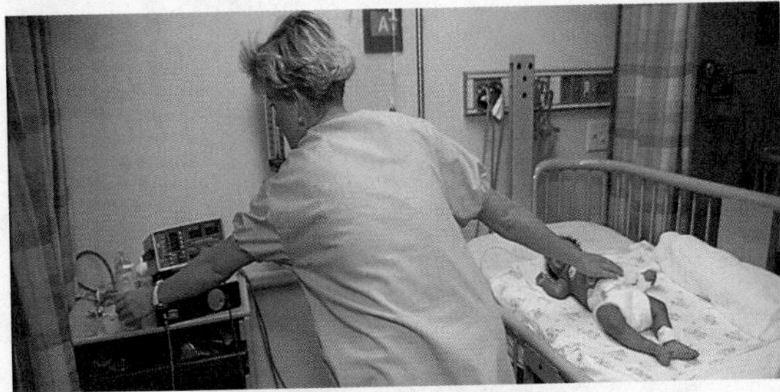

Fig. 45-4 Nurse maintains hand contact when back is turned.

Toy Safety

Toys play a vital role in the everyday life of children, and they are no less important in the hospital setting. Nurses are responsible for assessing the safety of toys brought to the hospital by well-meaning parents and friends. Toys should be appropriate to the child's age, condition, and treatment. For example, if the child is receiving oxygen, electrical or friction toys are not safe, since sparks can cause oxygen to ignite. Inspect toys to ensure they are nonallergenic, washable, and unbreakable and have no small, removable parts that can be aspirated or swallowed or in other ways injure a child. All objects within reach of children younger than 3 years should pass the choke tube test. A toilet paper roll is a handy guide. If a toy or object fits into the cylinder (items less than 1¼ inches across or balls smaller than 1¾ inches), it is a potential choking danger to the child. Latex balloons pose a serious threat to children of all ages. If the balloon breaks, a child may put a piece of the latex in his or her mouth. If it is aspirated or swallowed, the latex piece is difficult to remove, resulting in choking. Latex balloons should *never* be permitted in the hospital setting.

Preventing Falls

Multiple interventions are needed to minimize pediatric patients' risk of falling. Once individual children are identified as at risk for falling, visual identification and communication of the risk among all health care providers is essential. Reduce the risk of falling through patient, family, and staff education.

1. Identify children at risk of falling. Perform a fall risk assessment on patients on admission and throughout hospitalization to identify patients at high risk for falls. Risk factors for hospitalized children include:
   - Medication effects—postanesthesia or sedation; analgesics or narcotics, especially in those who have never had narcotics in the past and in whom effects are unknown
   - Altered mental status—secondary to seizures, brain tumors, or medications
   - Altered or limited mobility—reduced skill at ambulation secondary to developmental age, disease process, tubes, drains, casts, splints, or other appliances; new to ambulation with assistive devices such as walkers or crutches
   - Postoperative children—risk of hypotension or syncope secondary to large blood loss, a heart condition, or extended bed rest
   - History of falls
   - Infants or toddlers in cribs with side rails down or on the daybed with family members
2. Visually identify patients at risk with one or more of the following:
   - Post signs on the door and at the bedside.
   - Apply a special colored armband labeled "Fall Precautions."
   - Label the chart with a sticker.
   - Document information on the chart.
3. Alter the environment:
   - Keep bed in lowest position, breaks locked, and side rails up.
   - Place call bell within reach.
   - Ensure that all necessary and desired items are within reach (e.g., water, glasses, tissues, snacks).
   - Offer toileting on a regular basis, especially if patient is taking diuretics or laxatives.
   - Keep lights on at all times, including dim lights while sleeping.
   - Lock wheelchairs before transferring patients.
   - Ensure that patient has appropriate size gown and nonskid footwear. Do not allow gowns or ties to drag on the floor when ambulating.
   - Keep floor clean and free of clutter. Post "wet floor" sign if floor is wet.
   - Ensure that patient has glasses on if he or she normally wears them.
4. Educate patients (as age appropriate):
   - Assist with ambulation even though the child may have ambulated well before hospitalization.
   - Patients who have been lying in bed will need to get up slowly, sitting on the side of the bed before standing.
5. Educate family members:
   - Call the nursing staff for assistance, and do not allow patients to get up independently.
   - Keep the side rails of the crib or bed up whenever patient is in the crib or bed.
   - Do not leave infants on the daybed; put them in the crib with the side rails up.
   - When all family members need to leave the bedside, notify staff and ensure the patient is in the bed or crib with side rails up and call bell within reach (if appropriate).

Infection Control

According to the Centers for Disease Control and Prevention, approximately 2 million patients each year develop nosocomial (hospital-acquired) infections. These infections occur when there is interaction among patients, health care personnel, equipment, and bacteria (Quality, equipment hold keys to infection control, 2006). Nosocomial infections are preventable if caregivers practice meticulous cleaning and disposal techniques. *Standard Precautions* synthesize the major features of universal (blood and body fluid) precautions (designed to reduce the risk of transmission of blood-borne pathogens) and body substance isolation (designed to reduce the risk of transmission of pathogens from moist body substances). Standard Precautions involve the use of *barrier protection*, such as gloves, goggles, gown, or mask, to prevent contamination from (1) blood; (2) all body fluids, secretions, and excretions *except sweat,* regardless of whether they contain visible blood; (3) nonintact skin; and (4) mucous membranes. Standard Precautions are designed for the care of all patients to reduce the risk of transmission of microorganisms from both recognized and unrecognized sources of infection.

Transmission-based precautions are designed for patients with documented or suspected infection or colonization (presence of microorganism in or on patient but without clinical signs and symptoms of infection) with highly transmissible or epidemiologically important pathogens for which additional precautions beyond Standard Precautions are needed to interrupt transmission in hospitals. There are three types of transmission-based precautions: Airborne Precautions, Droplet Precautions, and Contact Precautions. They may be combined for diseases that have multiple routes of transmission (Box 45-5). They are to be used in addition to Standard Precautions.

Airborne Precautions reduce the risk of airborne transmission of infectious agents. Airborne transmission occurs by dissemination of either airborne droplet nuclei (small-particle residue [5 µm or smaller in size] of evaporated droplets that may remain suspended in the air for long periods) or dust particles containing the infectious agent. Microorganisms carried in this manner can be dispersed widely by air currents and may become inhaled by or deposited on a susceptible host within the same room or over a longer distance from the source patient, depending on environmental factors. Special air handling and ventilation are required to prevent airborne transmission. Airborne Precautions apply to patients with known or suspected infection with pathogens transmitted by the airborne route such as measles, varicella, and tuberculosis.

Droplet Precautions reduce the risk of droplet transmission of infectious agents. Droplet transmission involves contact of the conjunctivae or the mucous membranes of the nose or mouth of a susceptible person with large-particle droplets (larger than 5 µm in size) containing microorganisms generated from a person who has a clinical disease or who is a carrier of the microorganism. Droplets are generated from the source person primarily during coughing, sneezing, or talking and during procedures such as suctioning and bronchoscopy. Transmission requires close contact between source and recipient persons, since droplets do not remain suspended in the air and generally travel only short distances, usually 3 feet or less, through the air. Because droplets do not remain suspended in the air, special air handling and ventilation are not required to prevent droplet transmission. Droplet Precautions apply to any patient with known or suspected infection with

BOX 45-5 Types of Precautions and Patients Requiring Them

Standard Precautions

Use Standard Precautions for the care of all patients.

Airborne Precautions

In addition to Standard Precautions, use Airborne Precautions for patients known or suspected to have serious illnesses transmitted by airborne droplet nuclei. Examples of such illnesses include measles, varicella (including disseminated zoster), and tuberculosis.

Droplet Precautions

In addition to Standard Precautions, use Droplet Precautions for patients known or suspected to have serious illnesses transmitted by large-particle droplets. Examples of such illnesses include:

- Invasive *Haemophilus influenzae* type b, including meningitis, pneumonia, epiglottitis, and sepsis
- Invasive *Neisseria meningitidis*, including meningitis, pneumonia, and sepsis
- Other serious bacterial respiratory tract infections spread by droplet transmission, including diphtheria (pharyngeal), mycoplasmal pneumonia, pertussis, pneumonic plague, streptococcal pharyngitis, pneumonia, or scarlet fever in infants and young children
- Serious viral infections spread by droplet transmission, including adenovirus, influenza, mumps, parvovirus B19, rubella

Contact Precautions

In addition to Standard Precautions, use Contact Precautions for patients known or suspected to have serious illnesses easily transmitted by direct patient contact or by contact with items in the patient's environment. Examples of such illnesses include:

- Gastrointestinal, respiratory tract, skin, or wound infections or colonization with multidrug-resistant bacteria judged by the infection control program, based on current state, regional, or national recommendations, to be of special clinical and epidemiologic significance
- Enteric infections with a low infectious dose or prolonged environmental survival, including *Clostridium difficile;* for diapered or incontinent patients: enterohemorrhagic *Escherichia coli* O157:H7, *Shigella* sp., hepatitis A, or rotavirus
- Respiratory syncytial virus, parainfluenza virus, or enteroviral infections in infants and young children
- Skin infections that are highly contagious or that may occur on dry skin, including diphtheria (cutaneous), herpes simplex virus (neonatal or mucocutaneous), impetigo, major (noncontained) abscesses, cellulitis or decubiti, pediculosis, scabies, staphylococcal furunculosis in infants and young children, zoster (disseminated or in the immunocompromised host)
- Viral or hemorrhagic conjunctivitis
- Viral hemorrhagic infections (Ebola, Lassa, or Marburg)

From Garner JS: Guidelines for isolation precautions in hospitals, *Infect Control Hosp Epidemiol* 17(1):66, 1996.

pathogens that can be transmitted by infectious droplets (see Box 45-5).

Contact Precautions reduce the risk of transmission of microorganisms by direct or indirect contact. Direct-contact transmission involves a skin-to-skin contact and physical transfer of microorganisms to a susceptible host from an infected or colonized person, such as occurs when turning or bathing patients. Direct-contact transmission also can occur between two patients (e.g., by hand contact). Indirect-contact transmission involves contact of a susceptible host with a contaminated intermediate object, usually inanimate, in the patient's environment. Contact Precautions apply to specified patients known or suspected to be infected or colonized with microorganisms that can be transmitted by direct or indirect contact.

NURSING ALERT The most common piece of medical equipment, the stethoscope, can be a potent source of harmful microorganisms and nosocomial infections. One study found that 80% of 200 stethoscopes were contaminated with at least one microbe (Eckler, 1997).

Nurses caring for young children are frequently in contact with body substances, especially urine, feces, and vomitus. They should exercise judgment concerning those situations when gloves, gowns, or masks are necessary. For example, gloves and possibly gowns should be worn for changing diapers when there are loose or explosive stools. Otherwise, the plastic lining of disposable diapers provides a sufficient barrier between the hands and body substances. The type of diaper may be an important aspect of infection control. Super absorbent disposable diapers with elastic legs contain urine and feces better than cloth diapers.

Antimicrobial-resistant organisms are causing increasing numbers of nosocomial infections. Nearly 70% of nosocomial infections can be attributed to seven pathogens: the gram-positive organisms *Staphylococcus aureus,* coagulase-negative staphylococci, and enterococci; and the gram-negative organisms *Escherichia coli, Pseudomonas aeruginosa, Enterobacter* organisms, and *Klebsiella pneumoniae.* In hospitals, patients are the most significant sources of methicillin-resistant *S. aureus*, and the main mode of transmission is patient to patient via the hands of a health care provider (Eaton, 2005; Quality, equipment hold keys to infection control, 2006).

NURSING ALERT Handwashing is the most critical infection-control practice.

During feedings, gowns should be worn if the child is likely to vomit or spit up, which often occurs during burping. When gloves are worn, wash hands thoroughly after removing the gloves, since gloves fail to provide complete protection. The absence of visible leakage does not indicate gloves are intact.

Another essential practice of infection control is that all needles (uncapped and unbroken) are disposed of in a rigid, puncture-resistant container located near the site of use. Consequently, these containers are installed in patients' rooms. Since children are naturally curious, extra attention is needed in selecting a suitable type of container and a location that prevents access to disposed needles (see Fig. 45-3). The use of needleless systems allows secure syringe or IV tubing attachment to vascular access devices without the risk of needlestick injury to the child or nurse.

Transporting Infants and Children

Infants and children usually need to be transported within the unit and to areas outside the pediatric unit. Infants and small children can be carried for short distances within the unit, but for more extended trips the child should be securely transported in a suitable conveyance.

Small infants can be held or carried in the horizontal position with the back supported and the thigh grasped firmly by the carrying arm (Fig. 45-5, *A*). In the football hold, the infant is carried on the nurse's arm with the head supported by the hand and the body held securely between the nurse's body and elbow (see Fig. 45-5, *B*). Both of these holds leave the nurse's other arm free for activity. The infant also can be held in the upright position with the buttocks on the nurse's forearm and the front of the body resting against the nurse's chest. The

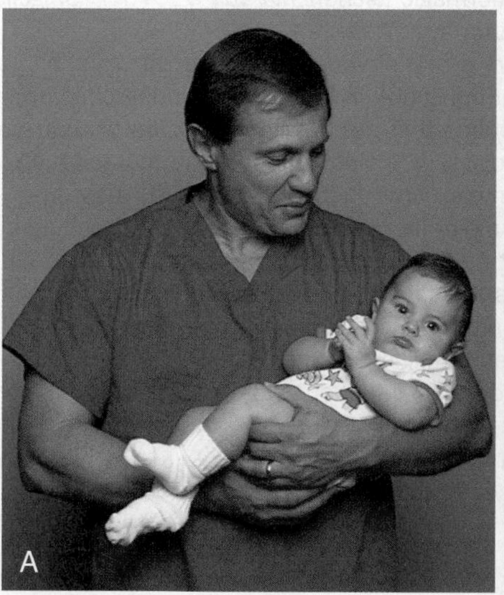

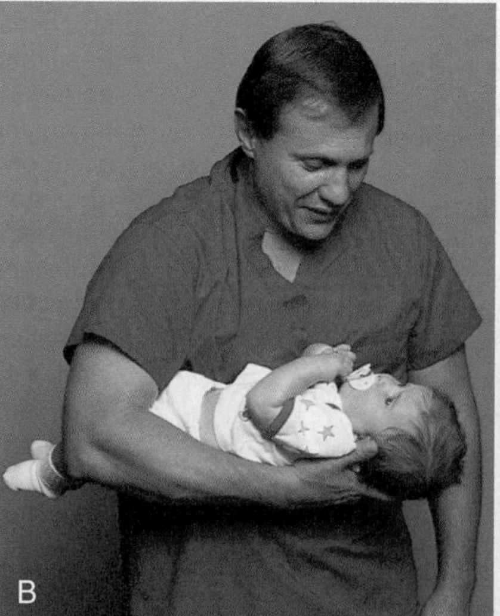

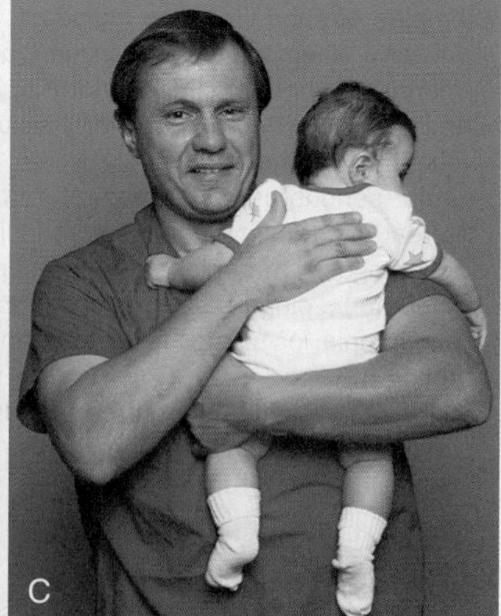

Fig. 45-5 Transporting infants. **A,** Infant's thigh firmly grasped in nurse's hand. **B,** Football hold. **C,** Back supported.

infant's head and shoulders are supported by the nurse's other arm in case the infant moves suddenly (see Fig. 45-5, *C*). Older infants are able to hold their heads erect but are still subject to sudden movements.

Infants can be transported to other areas, such as the radiology department, in their bassinet or crib. Strollers and wheeled feeding chairs or tables are also convenient transporters in some situations, such as trips to the playroom or nurse's station.

The method of transporting children is determined by their age, condition, and destination. Older children are safe in wheelchairs or on stretchers. Younger children can be transported in a crib, on a stretcher, in a wagon with raised sides, or in a wheelchair with a safety belt. Stretchers should be equipped with high sides and a safety belt, both of which are secured during transport.

Restraining Methods and Therapeutic Holding

A restraint is any method, physical or mechanical, that restricts a person's movement, physical activity, or normal access to his or her body. Before initiating restraints, the nurse completes a comprehensive assessment of the patient to determine whether the need for a restraint outweighs the risk of not using one. Restraints can result in loss of dignity, violation of patient rights, psychologic harm, physical harm, and even death. Alternative methods should first be considered and documented in the patient's record. The nurse is responsible for selecting the least restrictive type of restraint. Using less restrictive restraints is often possible by gaining the cooperation of the child and parents.

The two types of restraints used with children are classified as nonbehavioral and behavioral restraints (Joint Commission on Accreditation of Healthcare Organizations, 2009). When a standard or protocol states that immobilization is required 100% of the time as a part of the procedure or postprocedural care process, the restraint device is considered a part of routine care. For example, the postoperative use of elbow restraints after a cleft lip repair, if written in the protocol or standard of care and used for 100% of patients, would not fall under The Joint Commission or Centers for Medicare and Medicaid Services mandates for restraints.

Nonbehavioral (medical-surgical) restraints are used for children with an artificial airway or airway adjunct for delivery of oxygen, indwelling catheters, tubes, drains, lines, pacemaker wires, or suture sites. The nonbehavioral restraint is used to ensure that safe care is given to the patient. The potential risks of the restraint are offset by the potential benefit of providing safer care. Nonbehavioral restraints may be instituted for any of the following reasons:

- Risk for interruption of therapy used to maintain oxygenation or airway patency
- Risk of harm if indwelling catheter, tube, drain, line, pacemaker wire, or sutures are removed, dislodged, or ruptured
- Patient confusion, agitation, unconsciousness, or developmental inability to understand direct requests or instructions

Nonbehavioral restraints can be initiated by an individual order or by protocol; the use of the protocol must be authorized by an individual order. Continued use of restraints must be renewed each day. Patients are monitored at least every 2 hours.

Behavioral restraints are limited to situations with a significant risk of patients physically harming themselves or others because of behavioral reasons and when nonphysical interventions are not effective. Before initiating a behavioral restraint, the nurse should assess the patient's mental, behavioral, and physical status to determine the cause for the child's behavior that may be harmful to the patient or others. If behavioral restraints are indicated, a collaborative approach involving the patient (if appropriate), the family, and the health care team should be used. An order must be obtained as soon as possible, but no longer than 1 hour after the initiation of behavioral restraints. Behavioral restraints for children must be reordered every 1 to 2 hours, based on age. A licensed independent practitioner must conduct an in-person evaluation within 1 hour and again every 4 hours until restraints are discontinued. Children in behavioral restraints must be *continuously* observed and assessed every 15 minutes. Assessment components include signs of injury associated with applying restraint, nutrition and hydration, circulation and range-of-motion of extremities, vital signs, hygiene and elimination, physical and psychologic status and comfort, and readiness for discontinuation of restraint. The nurse must use clinical judgment in setting a schedule for when each of these parameters needs to be evaluated because every parameter must be assessed during each 15-minute physical assessment.

Restraints with ties must be secured to the bed or crib frame, not the side rails. Suggestions for increasing safety and comfort while the child is in a restraint include leaving one finger breadth between skin and the device; tying knots that allow for quick release; ensuring the restraint does not tighten as the child moves; decreasing wrinkles or bulges in the restraint; placing jacket restraints over an article of clothing; placing limb restraints below waist level, below knee level, or distal to the IV; and tucking in dangling straps (Selekman & Snyder, 1997).

An alternative approach for temporary restraint is therapeutic holding. *Therapeutic holding* is the use of a secure, comfortable, temporary holding position that provides close physical contact with the parent or caregiver for 30 minutes or less (Fig. 45-6).

The use of restraints can often be avoided with adequate preparation of the child; parental or staff supervision of the child; or adequate protection of a vulnerable site, such as an infusion device. The nurse needs to assess the child's development, mental status, potential to hurt others or self, and safety. The nurse should carefully consider alternatives to using restraints. Some examples of alternative measures include bringing a child to the nurses' station for continuous observation, providing diversional activities such as music, or encouraging the participation of the parents.

Jacket Restraint

A jacket restraint is sometimes used to keep the child safe in various chairs. The jacket is put on the child with the ties in back so that the child is unable to manipulate them. The long tapes, secured to the understructure of the crib, keep the child

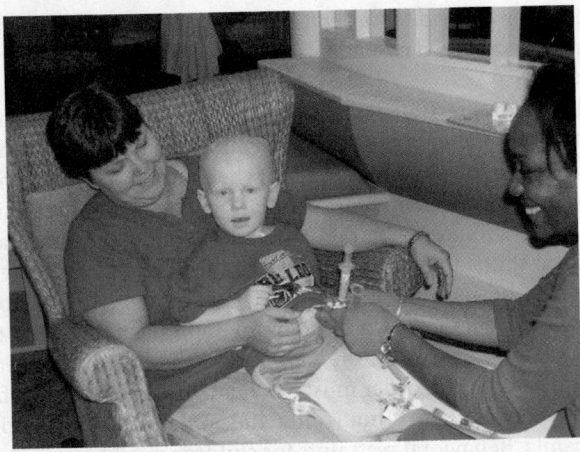

Fig. 45-6 Therapeutic holding of child for extremity venipuncture with parental assistance.

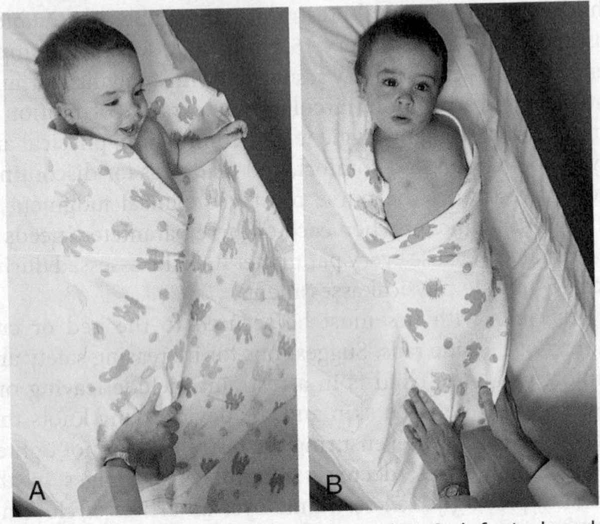

Fig. 45-7 Application of mummy restraint. **A,** Infant placed on folded corner of blanket and one corner of blanket brought across body and secured beneath body. **B,** Second corner brought across body and secured, and lower corner folded and tucked or pinned in place; modified mummy restraint with chest uncovered.

inside the crib. The jacket restraint is also useful as a means of maintaining the child in a desired horizontal position.

Mummy Restraint or Swaddle

When an infant or small child requires short-term restraint for examination or treatment that involves the head and neck, such as venipuncture, throat examination, and gavage feeding, a papoose board with straps or a mummy wrap effectively controls the child's movements. A blanket or sheet is opened on the bed or crib with one corner folded to the center. The infant is placed on the blanket with shoulders at the fold and feet toward the opposite corner. With the infant's right arm straight down against the body, the right side of the blanket is pulled firmly across the infant's right shoulder and chest and secured beneath the left side of the body (Fig. 45-7, *A*). The left arm is placed straight against the infant's side, and the left side of the blanket is brought across the shoulder and chest and locked beneath the body on the right side. The lower corner is folded and brought over the body and tucked or fastened securely with safety pins. Safety pins can be used to fasten the blanket in place at any step in the process.

To modify the mummy restraint for chest examination, the folded edge of the blanket is brought over each arm and under the back, after which the loose edge is folded over and secured at a point below the chest to allow visualization of and access to the chest (see Fig. 45-7, *B*).

Arm and Leg Restraints

Occasionally, one or more extremities must be restrained or limited in motion. Several commercial restraining devices are available, including disposable wrist and ankle restraints. The restraints must be appropriate to the child's size and padded to prevent undue pressure, constriction, or tissue injury; and the extremity must be observed frequently for signs of irritation or impairment of circulation. The ends of the restraints are never tied to the side rails, since lowering the rail will disturb the extremity, frequently with a jerk that may hurt or injure the child.

Elbow Restraint

Sometimes it is important to prevent the child from reaching the head or face (e.g., after lip surgery, when a scalp vein infusion is in place, or to prevent scratching in skin disorders). Elbow restraints fashioned from a variety of materials function well. Commercial elbow restraints are available. An improvised form of elbow restraint consists of a piece of muslin long enough to reach comfortably from just below the axilla to the wrist with a number of vertical pockets into which tongue depressors are inserted. The restraint is wrapped around the arm and secured with tape or pins. It may be necessary to pin the top of the restraint to the undershirt sleeve to prevent the restraint from slipping.

Positioning for Procedures

Infants and small children are unable to cooperate for many procedures; therefore the nurse is responsible for minimizing their movement and discomfort with proper positioning. Older children usually need only minimal, if any, restraint. Careful explanation and preparation beforehand and support and simple guidance during the procedure are usually sufficient. For painful procedures the child should receive adequate analgesia and sedation to minimize pain and the need for excessive restraint. For local anesthesia, use buffered lidocaine to reduce the stinging sensation or a topical anesthetic (see Pain Management, Chapter 35).

Femoral Venipuncture

The nurse places the child supine with the legs in a frog position to provide extensive exposure of the groin area. The infant's legs can be effectively controlled by the nurse's forearms and hands (Fig. 45-8). Only the side used for the venipuncture is uncovered, so the practitioner is protected should the infant urinate during the procedure. Apply pressure to the site to prevent oozing from the site.

Extremity Venipuncture

The most common sites of venipuncture are the veins of the extremities, especially the arm and hand. A convenient position

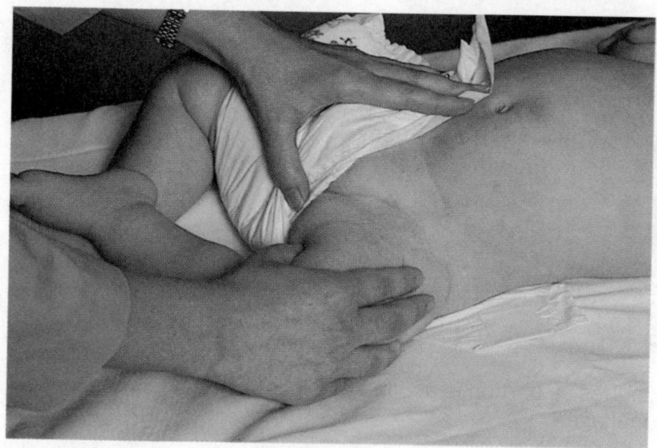

Fig. 45-8 Restraining infant for femoral venipuncture.

is to place the child in the parent's (or assistant's) lap, with the child facing the parent and in the straddle position. Next, place the child's arm for venipuncture on a firm surface, such as a treatment table. The child's outstretched arm is partially stabilized by the technician drawing the blood. Then have the parent hug the child's upper body, preventing movement, and use an arm to immobilize the venipuncture site. This type of restraint also comforts the child because of the close body contact and allows each person to maintain eye contact (see Fig. 45-6).

Lumbar Puncture

Pediatric lumbar puncture (LP) sets contain smaller spinal needles, but sometimes the practitioner will specify a different size or type of needle. The technique for LP in infants and children is similar to that in the adult, although modifications are suggested in neonates, who have less distress in a side-lying position with modified neck extension than in flexion or a sitting position.

Children are usually controlled best in the side-lying position, with the head flexed and the knees drawn up toward the chest. Even cooperative children need to be held gently to prevent possible trauma from unexpected, involuntary movement. They can be reassured that, although they are trusted, the holding will serve as a reminder to maintain the desired position. It also provides a measure of support and reassurance to them.

The child is placed on the side with the back close to the edge of the examining table on the side from which the practitioner is working. Maintain the child's spine in a flexed position by holding the child with one arm behind the neck and the other behind the thighs (Fig. 45-9). The flexed position enlarges the spaces between the lumbar vertebrae, which facilitates access to the spinal fluid space. It is helpful to wrap the legs before positioning to decrease leg movement.

An alternate position used with small infants and some older children is the sitting position. The child is placed with the buttocks at the edge of the table and with the neck flexed so that the chin rests on the child's chest or the nurse's arm. The infant's arms and legs are immobilized by the nurse's hands.

Specimens and spinal fluid pressure are obtained, measured, and sent for analysis in the same manner as for the adult patient. Vital signs are taken as ordered, and the child is observed for any changes in level of consciousness, motor activity, or other neurologic signs. Post-LP headache may occur and is related to postural changes; this is less severe when the child lies flat. Headache is seen much less frequently in young children than in adolescents.

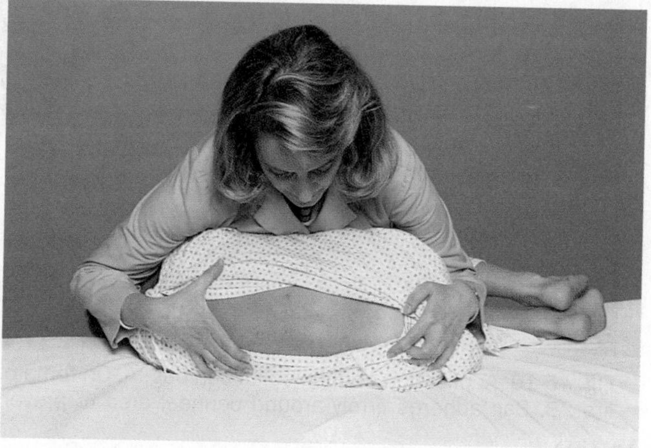

Fig. 45-9 Child in side-lying position for lumbar puncture.

Bone Marrow Aspiration or Biopsy

The position for a bone marrow aspiration or biopsy depends on the chosen site. In children the posterior or anterior iliac crest is most frequently used, although in infants the tibia may be selected because of easy access to the site and holding of the child. The sternum, which is the most frequent site in adults, is generally avoided in children because the bone is more fragile and adjacent to vital organs.

If the posterior iliac crest is used, the child is positioned prone. Sometimes a small pillow or folded blanket is placed under the hips to facilitate obtaining the bone marrow specimen. Children should receive adequate analgesia or anesthesia to relieve pain. If the child may awaken, holding may be needed and is best done with two people—one person to immobilize the upper body and a second person to immobilize the lower extremities (see Atraumatic Care box).

ATRAUMATIC CARE

Lumbar Puncture and Bone Marrow Test

Apply EMLA (an eutectic mixture of lidocaine and prilocaine) to the puncture site at least 60 minutes or LMX cream (lidocaine) at least 30 minutes before the procedure. To identify the lumbar puncture site, draw an imaginary line from the posterior iliac crest across the spine to the opposite iliac crest. The puncture site is intersected by the line at approximately L4. For additional anesthesia, buffered lidocaine with a 30-gauge needle can be used. *Sedation* with agents such as propofol (Diprivan) or ketamine is recommended for bone marrow biopsy and aspiration.

Collection of Specimens

Urine Specimens

Older children and adolescents can use a bedpan or urinal or can be trusted to follow directions for collection in the bathroom. However, they may have special needs. School-age

Animation—Lumbar Puncture, Infant

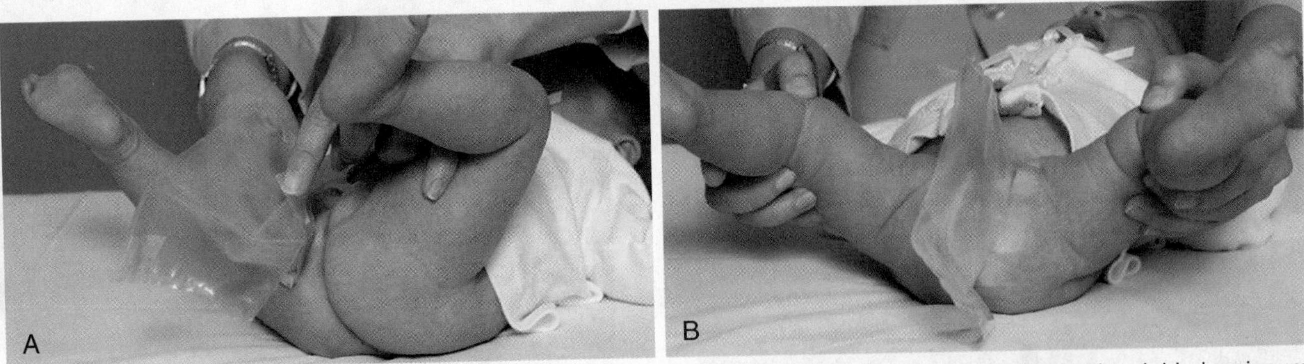

Fig. 45-10 Application of urine collection bag. **A,** On female infants, adhesive portion is applied to exposed and dried perineum first. **B,** Bag adheres firmly around perineal area to prevent urine leakage.

children are cooperative but curious. They are concerned about the reasons behind things and are likely to ask questions regarding the disposition of their specimen and what one expects to discover from it. Self-conscious adolescents may be reluctant to carry a specimen through a hallway or waiting room and appreciate a paper bag or other means for disguising the container. The presence of menses may be an embarrassment or a concern to teenage girls; therefore it is a good idea to ask if they are menstruating and to make adjustments as necessary. The specimen can be delayed or a notation made on the laboratory slip to explain the presence of red blood cells.

Preschoolers and toddlers are usually unable to void on request. It is often best to offer them water or other liquids that they enjoy and wait about 30 minutes until they are ready to void voluntarily.

Children will better understand what is expected if the nurse uses familiar terms, such as "pee-pee," "wee-wee," "tee-tee," or "tinkle." Some will have difficulty voiding in an unfamiliar receptacle. Potty chairs or a potty hat placed on the toilet is usually satisfactory. Toddlers who have recently acquired bladder control may be especially reluctant, since they undoubtedly have been admonished for "going" in places other than those approved by parents. A useful approach is to enlist the help of parents; they are likely to be successful.

For infants and toddlers who are not toilet trained, special urine collection bags with self-adhering material round the opening at the point of attachment are used. To prepare the infant, the genitalia, perineum, and surrounding skin are washed and dried thoroughly because the adhesive will not stick to a moist, powdered, or oily skin surface. The collection bag is easiest to apply if attached first to the perineum, progressing to the symphysis pubis (Fig. 45-10). With girls, the perineum is stretched taut during application to that area to ensure a leak-proof fit. With boys the penis and sometimes the scrotum are placed inside the bag. The adhesive portion of the bag must be firmly applied to the skin all around the genital area to avoid leakage. For low-birth-weight infants, small bags with adhesive that is gentle to the skin are available.* Anatomically correct urine collection bags are also available.† The diaper is carefully replaced. The bag is checked frequently and removed as soon as the specimen is available, since the moist bag may become loosened on an active child. When urine is collected for culture, the bag is removed immediately. For some types of urine testing, such as specific gravity, ketones, glucose, and protein, urine can be aspirated directly from the diaper. If the urine is not tested within 30 minutes, the specimen is refrigerated or placed in a sterile container with a preservative.

Available from Hollister, Inc., 2000 Hollister Drive, Libertyville, IL 60048; 888-740-8999; www.hollister.com.

†*Available from ConvaTec, 100 Headquarters Park Drive, Skillman, NJ 08558; 800-422-8811;* www.convatec.com.

Urine obtained from disposable diapers can be tested accurately for glucose, ketones, protein, blood, and urea. In one study, urine obtained from a disposable diaper provided a valid sample for diagnosing urinary tract infections (Cohen et al, 1997). Superabsorbent disposable diapers may produce a false crystalluria. Specific gravity measurements are accurate for up to 4 hours provided that the disposable diapers are kept folded. Urine samples collected by the cotton ball method were accurate for pH and specific gravity and were atraumatic to the skin of newborns (Burke, 1995).

NURSING ALERT

- When using a urine collection bag, cut a small slit in the diaper and pull the bag through to allow room for urine to collect and to facilitate checking on the contents.
- To obtain small amounts of urine, use a syringe without a needle to aspirate urine directly from the diaper; if diapers with absorbent gelling material that trap urine are used, place a small gauze dressing, some cotton balls, or a urine collection device* inside the diaper to collect urine and aspirate the urine with a syringe.

*The Bard Sure Catch is available from Bard Urological Division, C.R. Bard, Inc., 13183 Harland Drive, Covington, GA 30014; 888-367-2273; *www.crbard.com*.

At times parents may be asked to bring a urine sample to a health care facility for examination, especially when infants are unable to void during an outpatient visit. In this instance parents need instruction on applying the collection device and storing the specimen. Ideally, the specimen should be brought to the designated place as soon as possible; if there is a delay, the sample is refrigerated and the lapsed time reported to the examiner.

evolve Skill—Urine Specimen Collection

Clean-Catch Specimens

Clean-catch specimens traditionally refer to a urine sample obtained for culture after the urethral meatus is cleaned and the first few milliliters of urine are voided before the urine is collected *(midstream specimen)*. In girls, the perineum is wiped with an antiseptic-soaked cotton ball or pad from front to back at least three times, using a new cotton ball or pad each time. In boys, the tip of the penis is cleansed. The area may be wiped with sterile water to prevent accidental contamination of the urine with a solution that may destroy pathogens.

Twenty-Four–Hour Collection

Collection bags are required to collect specimens from infants and small children. Older children require special instruction about notifying someone when they need to void or have a bowel movement so that urine can be collected separately and not discarded. Some older school-age children and adolescents can take responsibility for collection of their own 24-hour specimens and can keep output records and transfer each voiding to the 24-hour collection container.

The collection period always starts and ends with an empty bladder. At the time the collection begins, the child is instructed to void and the specimen is discarded. All urine voided in the subsequent 24 hours is saved in a container with a preservative or is placed on ice. Twenty-four hours from the time the precollection specimen was discarded, the child is again instructed to void, the specimen is added to the container, and the entire collection is taken to the laboratory.

Infants and small children who are bagged for a 24-hour urine collection require a special collection bag. Frequent removal and replacement of adhesive collection devices can produce skin irritation. A thin coating of sealant, such as Skin-Prep, applied to the skin helps to protect it and aids adhesion, unless its use is contraindicated, such as in a preterm infant or a child with irritated skin. Plastic collection bags with collection tubes attached are ideal when the container must be left in place for a time. These can be connected to a collecting device or emptied periodically by aspiration with a syringe. When such devices are not available, a regular bag with a feeding tube inserted through a puncture hole at the top of the bag serves as a satisfactory substitute. However, care is taken to empty the bag as soon as the infant urinates to prevent leakage and loss of contents. An indwelling catheter may also be placed for the collection period.

Bladder Catheterization and Other Techniques

Bladder catheterization or suprapubic aspiration is employed when a specimen is urgently needed or when the child is unable to void or otherwise provide an adequate specimen. Catheterization is used to obtain a sterile urine specimen and when urethral obstruction or anuria caused by renal failure is believed to be the cause of the child's failure to void. The American Academy of Pediatrics recommends that urine collected by the bag can be used to determine whether it is necessary to obtain a catheterized urine specimen for culture (Wald, 2005). Suprapubic aspiration is useful in clarifying the diagnosis of suspected urinary tract infection in acutely ill infants.

Preparation for catheterization includes instruction on pelvic muscle relaxation. The toddler, preschooler, or younger child is taught to blow a pinwheel and to press the hips against the bed or procedure table during catheterization to relax the pelvic and periurethral muscles. The location and function of the pelvic muscles are described briefly to the older child or adolescent. The patient is then taught to contract and relax the pelvic muscles, and the relaxation procedure is repeated during catheter insertion. If the patient vigorously contracts the pelvic muscles when the catheter reaches the striated sphincter (proximal urethra in boys and midurethra in girls), catheter insertion is temporarily stopped. The catheter is neither removed nor advanced; instead, the child is helped to press the hips against the bed or examining table and relax the pelvic muscles. The catheter is then gently advanced into the bladder (Gray, 1996).

Children and adolescents experience some discomfort and anxiety during this procedure. Assistance and gentle holding may be necessary, especially for the younger child. Most children prefer to have the parents remain with them during the procedure. Encourage the parent to talk softly and hold the child's hand as the catheter is inserted. Using distractions such as reading a book, singing a song, or playing with small toys may decrease the child's anxiety. Older children and adolescents may wish to listen to music with headphones. Adolescents should be asked if they would like a parent to remain with them during the procedure. The decision should be made before the perineum is exposed and the sterile field is prepared.

Catheterization is a sterile procedure, and Standard Precautions for body substance protection should be followed. When placing a catheter to obtain a sterile urine specimen or to check for residual urine, the nurse may use a sterile feeding tube if a catheter is unavailable. If the catheter is to remain in place, a Foley catheter is used. Table 45-3 gives guidelines for choosing the appropriately sized catheter and length of insertion. The supplies needed for this procedure include sterile gloves, sterile lubricant anesthetic, an appropriately sized catheter, povidone-iodine (Betadine) swabs or an alternative cleansing agent and 4 × 4 inch gauze squares, a sterile drape, and a syringe with sterile water if a Foley catheter is used. Test the balloon of the Foley catheter by injecting sterile water before catheter insertion.

evolve Animation—Foley Catheter Insertion

NURSING ALERT Identify patients who have allergies to povidone-iodine or latex before using these items in catheterization.

Table 45-3 Straight Catheter or Foley Catheter*

	SIZE (LENGTH OF INSERTION [cm]) FOR GIRLS	SIZE (LENGTH OF INSERTION [cm]) FOR BOYS
Term neonate	5-6 (5)	5-6 (6)
Infant-3 yr	5-8 (5)	5-8 (6)
4-8 yr	8 (5-6)	8 (6-9)
8 yr-prepubertal	10-12 (6-8)	8-10 (10-15)
Pubertal	12-14 (6-8)	12-14 (13-18)

*Foley catheters are approximately 1 French size larger because of the circumference of the balloon. Example: 10 French Foley = approximately 12 French calibration.

Adolescent boys and children with a history of urethral surgery may be catheterized using a coudé-tipped catheter. The child with myelodysplasia or one who has been identified as being sensitive or allergic to latex is catheterized with a catheter manufactured from an alternative material. When an indwelling catheter is indicated for urinary drainage, a lubricious-coated or silicone catheter is selected because these materials produce less irritation of the urethral mucosa when compared with a Silastic or latex catheter when the catheter is left in place for more than 72 hours.

A 2% lidocaine lubricant with applicator is assembled according to the manufacturer's instructions,* and several drops of the lubricant are placed at the meatus. Advise the child that the lubricant is used to reduce discomfort associated with inserting the catheter and that introduction of the lubricant and catheter into the urethra will produce a sensation of pressure and a desire to urinate (Gray, 1996).

In male patients, grasp the penis with the nondominant hand and retract the foreskin. In uncircumcised newborns and infants the foreskin may be adhered to the shaft; use care when retracting. If the penis is pendulous, place a sterile drape under the penis. Using the sterile hand, swab the glans and meatus three times with povidone-iodine. Gently introduce the tip of the lidocaine jelly applicator into the urethra 1 to 2 cm (0.4 to 0.8 inch) so that the lubricant flows only into the urethra; insert 5 to 10 ml 2% lidocaine lubricant into the urethra and hold in place for 2 to 3 minutes by gently squeezing the distal penis. Lubricate the catheter and insert into the urethra while gently stretching the penis and lifting it to a 90-degree angle to the body. Resistance may occur when the catheter meets the urethral sphincter. Ask the patient to inhale deeply and advance the catheter. Do not force a catheter that does not easily enter the meatus, particularly if the child has had corrective surgery. For indwelling catheters, once urine is obtained, advance the catheter to the hub, inflate the balloon with sterile water, pull it back gently to test inflation, and connect it to the closed drainage system. Cleanse the glans and meatus and replace retracted foreskin. If blood is seen at any time during the procedure, discontinue the procedure and notify the practitioner.

In female patients, place a sterile drape under the buttocks. Use the nondominant hand to gently separate and pull up the labia minora to visualize the meatus. Swab the meatus from front to back three times, using a different povidone-iodine swab each time. Place 1 to 2 ml 2% lidocaine lubricant on the periurethral mucosa, and insert 1 to 2 ml into the urethral meatus. Delay catheterization for 2 to 3 minutes to maximize absorption of the anesthetic into the periurethral and intraurethral mucosa. Add lubricant to the catheter, and gently insert into the urethra until urine returns then advance the catheter an additional 2.5 to 5 cm (1 to 2 inches). When using a Foley catheter, inflate the balloon with sterile water and gently pull back, then connect to a closed drainage system. Cleanse the meatus and labia (see Cultural Awareness box). Because the use of lidocaine jelly can increase the volume of intraurethral lubricant, urine return may not be as rapid as when minimal lubrication is used.

Lidocaine hydrochloride 2% jelly is available from International Medication Systems, Ltd., 1886 Santa Anita Ave., South El Monte, CA 91733; 800-423-4136; www.ims-limited.com; and from AstraZeneca, 1800 Concord Pike, Wilmington, DE 19801; 800-236-9933; www.astrazeneca-us.com.

CULTURAL AWARENESS

Bladder Catheterization

Parents may be upset when their child is catheterized. Aside from the trauma the child experiences, some parents may fear that the procedure affects the daughter's virginity. To correct this misconception, the family may benefit from a detailed explanation of the genitourinary anatomy, preferably with a model that shows the separate vaginal and urethral openings. The nurse can also indicate that catheterization has no effect on virginity.

Suprapubic aspiration is mainly used when the bladder cannot be accessed through the urethra (such as with some congenital urologic birth defects) or to reduce the risk of contamination that may be present when passing a catheter. With the advent of small catheters (5 and 6 French), the need for suprapubic aspiration has decreased. Access to the bladder via the urethra has a much higher success rate than suprapubic aspiration, where success depends on the practitioner's skill at assessing the location of the bladder and the amount of urine in the bladder. Suprapubic aspiration involves aspirating bladder contents by inserting a 20- or 21-gauge needle in the midline approximately 1 cm (0.4 inch) above the symphysis pubis and directed vertically downward. The skin is prepared as for any needle insertion, and the bladder should contain an adequate volume of urine. This can be assumed if the infant has not voided for at least 1 hour or the bladder can be palpated above the symphysis pubis. This technique is useful for obtaining sterile specimens from young infants, since the bladder is an abdominal organ and is easily accessed. Suprapubic aspiration is painful, and therefore pain management during the procedure is important.

Stool Specimens

Stool specimens are frequently collected in children to identify parasites and other organisms that cause diarrhea, to assess gastrointestinal function, and to check for occult (hidden) blood. Ideally, stool should be collected without contamination with urine, but in children wearing diapers this is difficult unless a urine bag is applied. Children who are toilet trained should urinate first, flush the toilet, then defecate in the toilet, a bedpan (preferably one that is placed on the toilet to avoid embarrassment), or a commercial potty hat.

NURSING ALERT To obtain a stool specimen, place plastic wrap over the toilet bowl to collect the stool. Use a tongue depressor or disposable spoon or knife to collect the stool.

Stool specimens should be large enough to obtain an ample sampling, not merely a fecal fragment. Specimens are placed in an appropriate container, which is covered and labeled. If several specimens are needed, the containers are marked with the date and time and kept in a specimen refrigerator. Care is exercised in handling the specimen because of the risk of contamination.

Blood Specimens

Whether the specimen is collected by the nurse or others, the nurse is responsible for making certain that specimens, such as serial examinations and fasting specimens, are collected on time and that the proper equipment is available. Collecting, transporting, and storing specimens can have a major impact on laboratory results.

Venous blood samples can be obtained by venipuncture or by aspiration from a peripheral or central access device. Withdrawing blood specimens through peripheral lock devices in small peripheral veins has met with varying degrees of success. Although it avoids an additional venipuncture for the child, attempting to aspirate blood from the peripheral lock may shorten the life of the device. When using an IV infusion site for specimen collection, consider the type of fluid being infused. For example, a specimen collected for glucose level would be inaccurate if removed from a catheter through which glucose-containing solution was being administered.

NURSING ALERT

- To obtain a blood specimen from a peripheral lock when the infusion solution may interfere with tests results, first aspirate a quantity of blood equal to the volume of fluid in the catheter and discard; then aspirate the blood sample.
- For a blood culture, use the first sample of blood, since organisms are most likely to collect within the catheter itself.

NURSING ALERT On small or anemic children, keep track of the amount drawn and discarded over time. Frequent taking of blood specimens can rapidly decrease a child's blood volume. Coordinate blood samples and ask the laboratory to save as much blood as possible to reduce the frequency.

Arterial blood samples are sometimes needed for blood gas measurement, although noninvasive techniques, such as transcutaneous oxygen monitoring and pulse oximetry, are used frequently. Arterial samples may be obtained by arterial puncture using the radial, brachial, or femoral arteries; by deep heel puncture; or from indwelling arterial catheters. Adequate circulation should be assessed before arterial puncture by observing capillary refill or performing the *Allen test*, a procedure that assesses the circulation of the radial, ulnar, or brachial arteries. Because unclotted blood is required, only heparinized collection tubes are used. In addition, no air bubbles should enter the tube, since they can alter blood gas concentration. Crying, fear, and agitation also affect blood gas values; therefore every effort is made to comfort the child. The nurse should pack the sample in ice to reduce blood cell metabolism and take it to the laboratory for immediate analysis.

Capillary blood samples are taken from children by a finger stick. A common method for taking peripheral blood samples from infants younger than 6 months of age is by a heel stick. Before the blood sample is taken, the heel is warmed for 3 minutes. The area is cleansed with alcohol, the infant's foot firmly restrained with the free hand, and the heel punctured with an automatic lancet device. An automatic device delivers a more precise puncture depth and is less painful than using a lance (Vertanen et al, 2001). A surgical blade of any kind is contraindicated. An example of a safe device is the BD Quickheel Safety Lancet. The Tenderfoot Preemie device was compared with the Monolet lancet and was found to be safer than the lancet and required fewer heel punctures, less collection time, and lower recollection rates (Kellam et al, 2001). Shepherd and colleagues (2006) reported the Tenderfoot device was more effective and safer than a lancet for newborn screening tests. Although obtaining capillary blood gases is a common practice, these measures may not accurately reflect arterial values.

The most serious complications of infant heel puncture are necrotizing osteochondritis from lancet penetration of the underlying calcaneus bone, infection, or abscess (Meehan, 1998). To avoid osteochondritis, the puncture should be no deeper than 2 mm and should be made at the outer aspect of the heel. The boundaries of the calcaneus can be marked by an imaginary line extending posteriorly from a point between the fourth and fifth toes and running parallel to the lateral aspect of the heel and another line extending posteriorly from the middle of the great toe and running parallel to the medial aspect of the heel (Fig. 45-11). Repeated trauma to the walking surface of the heel can cause fibrosis and scarring that may interfere with locomotion.

The specimens are quickly collected, and pressure is applied to the puncture site with dry gauze until bleeding stops. The arm is kept extended, not flexed, while pressure is applied for a few minutes after venipuncture in the antecubital fossa to reduce bruising. The site is covered with an adhesive bandage. In young children, adhesive bandages pose an aspiration hazard; they should be avoided or removed as soon as the bleeding stops. Applying warm compresses to ecchymotic areas increases circulation, helps remove extravasated blood, and decreases pain.

No matter how or by whom the specimen is collected, children, even some older ones, fear the loss of their blood. This is particularly true for children whose condition requires frequent blood specimens. They mistakenly believe that blood

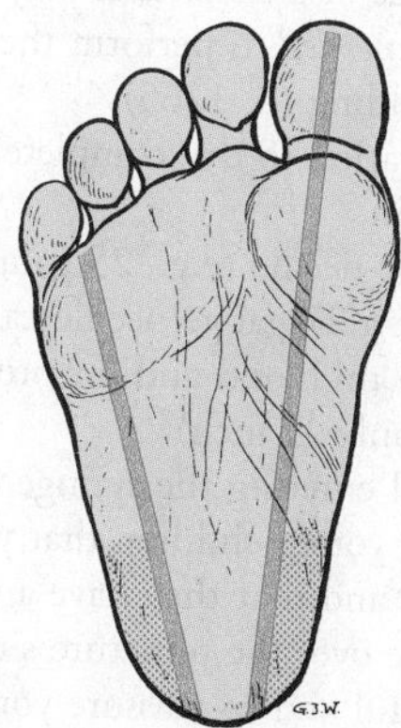

Fig. 45-11 Puncture site *(colored stippled area)* on sole of infant's foot.

removed from their bodies is a threat to their lives. Explaining to them that their body is continuously producing blood provides them with a measure of reassurance. When the blood is drawn, a comment such as "Just look how red it is. You're really making a lot of nice red blood," confirms this information and affords them an opportunity to express their concern. An adhesive bandage gives them added reassurance that the vital fluids will not leak out.

Children also dislike the discomfort associated with venous, arterial, or capillary punctures. Children have identified these procedures as the ones most frequently causing pain during hospitalization and arterial punctures as being one of the most painful of all procedures experienced (Van Cleve, Johnson, & Pothier, 1996). The ones most distressed by venipunctures are toddlers, followed by school-age children and then adolescents. Consequently nurses need to institute pain reduction techniques to lessen the discomfort of these procedures (see Atraumatic Care box).

Respiratory Secretion Specimens

Collection of sputum or nasal discharge is sometimes required for diagnosis of respiratory infections, especially tuberculosis and respiratory syncytial virus (RSV). Older children and adolescents are able to cough and supply sputum specimens when given proper directions. It must be made clear to them that a coughed specimen, not mucus that is cleared from the throat, is needed. It is helpful to demonstrate a deep cough. Infants and small children are unable to follow directions to cough and will swallow any sputum produced; therefore gastric washings (lavage) may be used to collect a sputum specimen. Sometimes a satisfactory specimen can be obtained using a suction device such as a mucus trap if the catheter is inserted into the trachea and the cough reflex is elicited. A catheter inserted into the back of the throat is not sufficient. For children with a tracheostomy, a specimen is easily aspirated from the trachea or major bronchi by attaching a collecting device to the suction apparatus.

ATRAUMATIC CARE

Guidelines for Skin and Vessel Punctures

For Reduction of Pain Associated with Heel, Finger, Venous, or Arterial Punctures

Apply EMLA (an eutectic mixture of lidocaine and prilocaine) topically over the site if time permits (at least 60 minutes). LMX (lidocaine) cream also may be used and requires a shorter application time (30 minutes).

To remove the Tegaderm dressing atraumatically, grasp opposite sides of the film and pull the sides away from each other to stretch and loosen the film. After the film begins to loosen, grasp the other two sides of the film and pull.

Use iontophoresis (Numby Stuff) over the site if time permits (8 to 20 minutes, depending on the amount of current), a vapocoolant spray, or buffered lidocaine (injected intradermally near the vein with a 30-gauge needle) to numb the skin.

Use nonpharmacologic methods of pain and anxiety control (e.g., ask child to take a deep breath when the needle is inserted and again when the needle is withdrawn; exhale a large breath or blow bubbles to "blow hurt away"; count slowly and then faster and louder if pain is felt).

Keep all equipment out of sight until used.

Enlist parents' presence or assistance if they wish.

Restrain child *only as needed* to perform the procedure safely; use therapeutic holding (p. 1265).

Allow the skin preparation to dry completely before penetrating the skin.

Use the smallest-gauge needle (e.g., 25 gauge) that permits free flow of blood; a 27-gauge needle can be used for obtaining 1 to 1.5 ml blood and for prominent veins (needle length is only ½ inch).

Emphasize that blood entering the syringe or tube does not hurt, and reassure young children that you did not "take their blood" away and that they have a lot more inside.

Place a small bandage over the puncture site to make removal easy and less painful and to reassure young children that their blood will not "leak out."

Have a "two-try" only policy to reduce excessive insertion attempts—two operators each have two insertion attempts; if insertion is not successful after four punctures, consider alternative venous access, such as a peripherally inserted central catheter (PICC); have a policy for identifying children with difficult access and appropriate interventions (e.g., most experienced operator for the first attempt).*

For Multiple Blood Samples

Use an intermittent infusion device (saline lock) to collect additional samples; consider PICC lines early, not as a last resort.

Coordinate care to allow several tests to be performed on one blood sample using micromethods of testing.

Anticipate tests (e.g., drug levels, chemistry, immunoglobulin levels) and ask the laboratory to save blood for additional testing.

For Heel Lancing in Newborns

Heel lancing has been shown to be more painful than venipuncture (Larsson et al, 1998); consider venipuncture when the amount of blood from the heel would require much squeezing (e.g., genetic screening tests).

The effectiveness of EMLA is controversial, although application of 0.5 g for 30 minutes four times a day in preterm infants was found to be safe (Essink-Tebbes et al, 1999).

Place diapered newborn against mother's bare chest in skin-to-skin contact 10 to 15 minutes before and during heel lance (Gray, Watt, & Blass, 2000).

During the procedure, allow newborn to suck a pacifier coated with a slurry of sucrose. When commercially manufactured 24% sucrose solution is unavailable, add 1 tsp of table sugar to 4 tsp of sterile water. Use this solution to coat the pacifier, or administer 2 ml to the tongue 2 minutes before the procedure (Blass & Watt, 1999).

*For an example of one hospital's guidelines for reducing excessive IV insertion attempts, see Catudal (1999).

Nasal washings are usually obtained to diagnose an infection of RSV. The child is placed supine, and 1 to 3 ml sterile normal saline is instilled with a sterile syringe (without needle) into one nostril. The contents are aspirated using a small, sterile bulb syringe and are placed in a sterile container. Another method uses a syringe with 5 cm (2 inches) of 18- to 20-gauge tubing. The saline is quickly instilled and then aspirated to recover the nasal specimen. To prevent additional discomfort, all of the equipment should be ready before beginning the procedure.

Other respiratory secretion collection methods include nasopharyngeal swabs to diagnose *Bordetella pertussis* and throat cultures. The nurse swabs both the tonsils and the posterior pharynx when obtaining a throat culture. The swab stick is inserted into the culture tube. Some culture kits require squeezing an ampule to release the culture medium.

Administration of Medication

Determination of Drug Dosage

Nurses must have an understanding of the safe dosage of medications they administer to children, as well as the expected action, possible side effects, and signs of toxicity (Kennedy, 1996). Unlike with adult medications, there are few standardized pediatric dosage ranges, and with a few exceptions, drugs are prepared and packaged in average adult-dosage strengths.

Factors related to growth and maturation significantly alter an individual's capacity to metabolize and excrete drugs. Immaturity or defects in any of the important processes of absorption, distribution, biotransformation, or excretion can significantly alter the effects of a drug. Newborn and preterm infants with immature enzyme systems in the liver (where most drugs are broken down and detoxified), lower plasma concentrations of protein for binding with drugs, and immaturely functioning kidneys (where most drugs are excreted) are particularly vulnerable to the harmful effects of drugs. Beyond the newborn period, many drugs are metabolized more rapidly by the liver, necessitating larger doses or more frequent administration. This is particularly important in pain control, since the dosage of analgesics may need to be increased or the interval between doses decreased.

Various formulas involving age, weight, and body surface area (BSA) have been devised to determine children's drug dosage. Because the administration of medication is a nursing responsibility, nurses need knowledge of not only drug action and patient responses, but also some resources for estimating safe dosages for children. The method most often used to determine children's dosage is based on a specific dose per kilogram of body weight, such as 0.1 mg/kg.

The most reliable method for determining children's dosage is to calculate the proportional amount of *BSA* to body weight. The ratio of BSA to weight varies inversely with length; therefore the infant who is shorter and weighs less than an older child or adult has relatively more surface area than would be expected from the weight. The usual determination of BSA requires the use of the *West nomogram* or an electronic calculator (widely available on the Internet). The BSA is estimated from the child's height and weight.

Checking Dosage

Administering the correct dosage of a drug is a shared responsibility between the practitioner who orders the drug and the nurse who carries out that order. Children react with unexpected severity to some drugs, and ill children are especially sensitive to drugs. When a dose is ordered that is outside the usual range or when there is some question regarding the preparation or the route of administration, the nurse should always check with the prescribing practitioner before proceeding with the administration, since the nurse is legally liable for any drug administered.

Even when it has been determined that the dosage is correct for a particular child, many drugs are potentially hazardous or lethal. Most facilities have regulations requiring specified drugs to be double-checked by another nurse before they are given to the child. Among drugs that require such safeguards are antiarrhythmics, anticoagulants, chemotherapeutic agents, electrolytes, and insulin. Others frequently included are epinephrine, opioids, and sedatives. Even if this precaution is not mandatory, nurses are wise to observe it. Errors in decimal point placement may occur and result in a tenfold or greater dosage error.

Identification

Before the administration of any medication, the child must be correctly identified. Two identifiers (e.g., name and medical record number or birth date) are required before medication administration.

Oral Administration

The oral route is preferred for administering medications to children because of the ease of administration. Most are dissolved or suspended in liquid preparations. Although some children are able to swallow or chew solid medications at an early age, solid preparations are not recommended for young children because of the danger of aspiration.

Most pediatric medications come in palatable and colorful preparations for ease of administration. Some have a slightly unpleasant aftertaste, but most children will swallow these liquids with little if any resistance. The nurse can taste a minute amount of an oral preparation to ascertain whether it is palatable or bitter. Complaints of dislike from the child can be accepted and the taste camouflaged whenever possible. Most pediatric units have preparations available for this purpose (see Atraumatic Care box).

Preparation

The devices available to measure medicines are not always sufficiently accurate for measuring the small amounts needed in pediatric nursing practice. Although molded plastic calibrated cups offer reasonable accuracy in measuring moderate doses of liquids, paper cups are likely to have irregular shapes or crumpled bottoms. Considerable amounts of thick medication may remain in the cup. Measures of less than a teaspoon are impossible to determine accurately with a cup.

The teaspoon is an inaccurate measuring device and is subject to error. Teaspoons vary greatly in capacity, and different persons using the same spoon will pour different amounts. Therefore a drug ordered in teaspoons should be

evolve Skill—Administering Oral Medications

ATRAUMATIC CARE

Encouraging a Child's Acceptance of Oral Medication

- Give child a flavored ice pop or small ice cube to suck to numb the tongue before giving the drug.
- Mix the drug with a small amount (about 1 tsp) of sweet-tasting substance, such as honey (except in infants because of the risk of botulism), flavored syrups, jam, fruit purees, sherbet, or ice cream; avoid essential food items, since the child may later refuse to eat them.
- Give a "chaser" of water, juice, soft drink, ice pop, or frozen juice bar after the drug.
- If nausea is a problem, give a carbonated beverage poured over finely crushed ice before or immediately after the medication.
- When medication has an unpleasant taste, have child pinch the nose and drink the medicine through a straw. Much of what we taste is associated with smell.
- Flavorings such as apple, banana, and bubble gum can be added at many pharmacies (e.g., FLAVORx) at nominal additional cost. An alternative is to have the pharmacist prepare the drug in a flavored, chewable troche or lozenge.*
- Infants will suck medicine from a needleless syringe or dropper in small increments (0.25 to 0.5 ml) at a time. Use a nipple or special pacifier with a reservoir for the drug.

*For information about compounding drugs, contact Technical Staff, Professional Compounding Centers of America (PCCA), 9901 S. Wilcrest Drive, Houston, TX 77099; 800-331-2498; *www.pccarx.com*.

measured in milliliters; the established standard is 5 ml per teaspoon. A convenient hollow-handled medicine spoon is available to accurately measure and administer the drug. Household *measuring* spoons can also be used when other devices are not available. A device called the Medibottle has been shown to be more effective in delivering oral medication to infants than the oral syringe (Kraus et al, 2001).

Another unreliable device for measuring liquids is the dropper, which varies to a greater extent than the teaspoon or measuring cup. Droppers are available in numerous sizes, but even with the standard USP dropper, the volume of a drop will vary according to the viscosity (thickness) of the liquid measured; viscous fluids produce much larger drops than thin liquids. Many medications are supplied with caps or droppers designed for measuring each specific preparation. These are accurate when used to measure that specific medication but are not reliable for measuring other liquids. Emptying dropper contents into a medicine cup invites additional error. Because some of the liquid clings to the sides of the cup, a significant amount of the drug can be lost.

The most accurate means for measuring small amounts of medication is the plastic disposable syringe, especially the tuberculin syringe for volumes less than 1 ml. Not only does the syringe provide a reliable measure, but it also serves as a convenient means for transporting and administering the medication. The medication can be placed directly into the child's mouth from the syringe.

Young children and some older children have difficulty swallowing tablets or pills. Because a number of drugs are not available in pediatric preparations, the tablet needs to be crushed before it can be given to these children. Commercial devices* are available, or simple methods can be employed for crushing tablets. Not all drugs can be crushed (e.g., medication with an enteric or protective coating or formulated for slow release).

Children who must take oral medication for an extended period can be taught to swallow tablets or capsules. Training sessions include verbal instruction, demonstration, reinforcement for swallowing progressively larger candy or capsules, no attention for inappropriate behavior, and gradual withdrawal of guidance once children can swallow their medication.

Because pediatric doses often require dividing adult preparations of medication, the nurse may be faced with the dilemma of accurate dosage. With tablets, only those that are scored can be halved or quartered accurately. If the medication is soluble, the tablet or contents of a capsule can be mixed in a small, premeasured amount of liquid and the appropriate portion given. For example, if half a dose is required, the tablet is dissolved in 5 ml water or flavored liquid and 2.5 ml is given.

Administration

Although administering liquids to infants is relatively easy, the nurse must be careful to prevent aspiration. With the infant held in a semireclining position, the medication is placed in the mouth from a spoon, plastic cup, dropper, or syringe (without needle). The dropper or syringe is best placed along the side of the infant's tongue, and the liquid is administered slowly in small amounts, allowing the child to swallow between deposits.

NURSING ALERT In infants up to 11 months of age and children with neurologic impairments, blowing a small puff of air in the face frequently elicits a swallow reflex.

Medicine cups can be used effectively for older infants who are able to drink from a cup. Because of the natural outward tongue thrust in infancy, medications may need to be retrieved from the lips or chin and refed. Allowing the infant to suck medication that has been placed in an empty nipple or inserting the syringe or dropper into the side of the mouth, parallel to the nipple, while the infant nurses are other convenient methods for giving liquid medications to infants. Medication is not added to the infant's formula feeding because the child may subsequently refuse the formula. Dispose of any plastic covers that may be on the ends of syringes. These covers are small enough to be aspirated by young children.

The young child who refuses to cooperate or resists consistently despite explanation and encouragement may require mild physical coercion. If so, it is carried out quickly and carefully. Every effort is made to determine why the child resists, and the reasons for the coercion are explained to the

**Trademark Medical manufactures a pill crusher and has compiled a list of more than 190 medications that should not be crushed or chewed. Both are available from Trademark Medical, 449 Sovereign Court, St. Louis, MO 63011; 800-325-9044; www.trademarkmedical.com.*

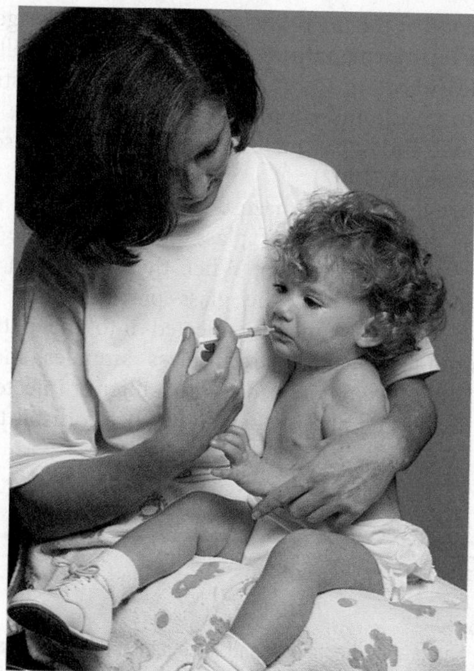

Fig. 45-12 Nurse partially restrains child for easy and comfortable administration of oral medication.

child in such a way that the child will know that it is being carried out for his or her well-being and is not a form of punishment. There is always a risk in using even mild forceful techniques. A crying child can aspirate a medication, particularly when lying on the back. If the nurse holds the child in the lap with the child's right arm behind the nurse, the left hand firmly grasped by the nurse's left hand, and the head securely restrained between the nurse's arm and body, the medication can be slowly poured into the mouth (Fig. 45-12).

Intramuscular Administration

Selecting the Syringe and Needle

The volume of medication prescribed for small children and the small amount of tissue available for injection require that a syringe be selected that can measure small amounts of solution. For volumes of less than 1 ml, the tuberculin syringe, calibrated in 1/100-ml increments, is appropriate. Minute doses may require the use of a 0.5-ml, low-dose syringe. These syringes, along with specially constructed needles, minimize the possibility of inadvertently administering incorrect amounts of a drug because of *dead space*, which allows fluid to remain in the syringe and needle after the plunger is pushed completely forward. A minimum of 0.2 ml of the solution remains in a standard needle hub; therefore, when very small amounts of two drugs are combined in the syringe, such as mixtures of insulin, the ratio of the two drugs can be altered significantly. Measures that minimize the effect of dead space are:

- When two drugs are combined in the syringe, always draw them up in the same order to maintain a consistent ratio between the drugs.
- Use the same brand of syringe (dead space may vary between brands).
- Use one-piece syringe units (needle permanently attached to the syringe).

Dead space is also an important factor to consider when injecting medication, since flushing the syringe with an air bubble adds an additional amount of medication to the prescribed dose. This can be hazardous when very small amounts of a drug are given. Consequently, flushing is not advisable, especially when less than 1 ml of medication is given. Syringes are calibrated to deliver a prescribed drug dose, and the amount of medication left in the hub and needle is not part of the syringe barrel calibrations. Certain drugs such as iron dextran and diphtheria and tetanus toxoid may cause irritation when tracked into the subcutaneous tissue. The Z-track method is recommended for use in infants and children rather than an air bubble. Changing the needle after withdrawing the fluid from the vial is another technique to minimize tracking.

The *needle length* must be sufficient to penetrate the subcutaneous tissue and deposit the medication into the body of the muscle. The needle gauge should be as small as possible to deliver fluid safely. Smaller-diameter (25- to 30-gauge) needles cause the least discomfort, but larger diameters are needed for viscous medication and prevention of accidental bending of longer needles (Table 45-4).

Determining the Site

Older children and adolescents usually pose few problems in selecting a suitable site for intramuscular (IM) injections, but infants, with their small and underdeveloped muscles, have fewer available sites. It is sometimes difficult to assess the amount of fluid that can be safely injected into a single site. Usually 1 ml is the maximum volume that should be administered in a single site to small children and older infants. The muscles of small infants may not tolerate more than 0.5 ml. As the child approaches adult size, volumes approaching those given to adults may be used. However, the larger the amount of solution, the larger the muscle must be into which it is injected.

Major nerves and blood vessels must be avoided. The preferred site for infants is the vastus lateralis (the rectus femoris is not an acceptable site). The ventrogluteal site is relatively free of major nerves and blood vessels, is a relatively large muscle with less subcutaneous tissue than the dorsal site, has well-defined landmarks for safe site location, is less painful than the vastus lateralis, and is easily accessible in several positions. Cook and Murtagh's (2006) research into IM injection sites in children indicates that the ventrogluteal site has not been associated with complications and is the preferred site in children of all ages (see Table 45-4). In clinical practice, this site has been safely used in children as young as newborns. The deltoid muscle, a small muscle near the axillary and radial nerves, can be used for small volumes of fluid in children as young as 18 months of age. Its advantages are less pain and fewer side effects from the injectate (as observed with immunizations), compared with the vastus lateralis (Ipp et al, 1989). Table 45-4 summarizes the three major injection sites and illustrates the location of the preferred IM injection sites for children.

Administration

Although injections that are executed with care seldom cause trauma to the child, there have been reports of serious disability related to IM injections in children. Repeated use of a single site has been associated with fibrosis of the muscle with subsequent muscle contracture. Injections close to large nerves, such as the sciatic nerve, have been responsible for permanent disability, especially when potentially neurotoxic drugs are administered. There are several reports of tissue damage from penicillin. One of the difficulties in administering the opaque preparations, such as penicillin G (Bicillin), is that aspirated blood cannot be detected at the bottom of the syringe, thus increasing the risk of injecting into a blood vessel. When such drugs are injected, great care must be used in locating the correct site. When aspirating, the nurse should look for blood at the *top* of the syringe near the plunger, since blood may be drawn up through the column of penicillin. One study of IM injection techniques revealed that the straighter the path of needle insertion (e.g., 90-degree angle), the less displacement and shear to tissue, thus reducing discomfort (Katsma & Smith, 1997).

A reported potential hazard with medication in glass ampules is the presence of glass particles in the ampule after the container is broken. When the medication is withdrawn into the syringe, the glass particles may also be withdrawn and subsequently injected into the patient. As a precaution, medication from glass ampules should be drawn up only through a needle with a filter or injected intravenously through a site in the tubing that is distal to an IV filter.

Table 45-4 Intramuscular Injection Sites in Children

SITE	DISCUSSION
Vastus Lateralis GREATER TROCHANTER* Sciatic nerve Femoral artery **Site of injection** (vastus lateralis) Rectus femoris KNEE JOINT*	*Location** Palpate to find greater trochanter and knee joints; divide vertical distance between these two landmarks into thirds; inject into middle third. *Needle Insertion and Size* Insert needle perpendicular to knee in infants and young children or perpendicular to thigh or slightly angled toward anterior thigh. 22-25 gauge, ⅝-1 inch† *Advantages* Large, well-developed muscle that can tolerate larger quantities of fluid (0.5 ml [infant] to 2.0 ml [child]) Easily accessible if child is supine, side lying, or sitting *Disadvantages* Thrombosis of femoral artery from injection in midthigh area Sciatic nerve damage from long needle injected posteriorly and medially into small extremity More painful than deltoid or gluteal sites
Ventrogluteal 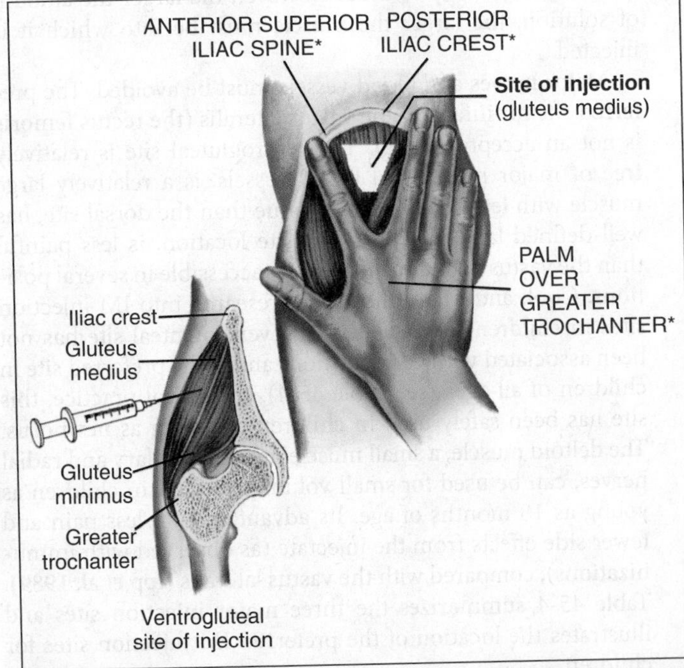 Ventrogluteal site of injection	*Location** Palpate to locate greater trochanter, anterior superior iliac tubercle (found by flexing thigh at hip and measuring up to 1-2 cm above crease formed in groin), and posterior iliac crest; place palm of hand over greater trochanter, index finger over anterior superior iliac tubercle, and middle finger along crest of ileum posteriorly as far as possible; inject into center of V formed by fingers. *Needle Insertion and Size* Insert needle perpendicular to site but angled slightly toward iliac crest. 22-25 gauge, ½-1 inch† *Advantages* Free of important nerves and vascular structures Easily identified by prominent bony landmarks Thinner layer of subcutaneous tissue than in dorsogluteal site, thus reducing chance of depositing drug subcutaneously rather than intramuscularly Can accommodate larger quantities of fluid (0.5 ml [infant] to 2.0 ml [child]) Easily accessible if child is supine, prone, or side lying Less painful than vastus lateralis *Disadvantages* Health professionals' unfamiliarity with site

Table 45-4 Intramuscular Injection Sites in Children—cont'd

SITE	DISCUSSION
Deltoid Clavicle ACROMION PROCESS* Site of injection (deltoid) Axilla Brachial artery Humerus Radial nerve	***Location**** Locate acromion process; inject only into upper third of muscle that begins about 2 fingerbreadths below acromion. ***Needle Insertion and Size*** Insert needle perpendicular to site but angled slightly toward shoulder. 22-25 gauge, ½-1 inch ***Advantages*** Faster absorption rates than gluteal sites Easily accessible with minimal removal of clothing Less pain and fewer local side effects from vaccines as compared with vastus lateralis ***Disadvantages*** Small muscle mass; can accommodate only limited amounts of drug (0.5-1.0 ml) Small margins of safety with possible damage to radial nerve and axillary nerve (not shown; lies under deltoid at head of humerus)

*Locations are indicated by asterisks on illustrations.
†Research has shown that a 1-inch needle is needed for adequate muscle penetration in infants 4 mo old and possibly in infants as young as 2 mo (Cook & Murtagh, 2002).

Most children are unpredictable and few are totally cooperative when receiving an injection. Even children who appear to be relaxed and constrained can lose control under the stress of the procedure. It is advisable to have someone available to help hold the child if needed. Because children often jerk or pull away unexpectedly, the nurse should carry an extra needle to exchange for a contaminated one so that the delay is minimal. The child, even a small one, is told that he or she is receiving an injection (preferably using a phrase such as "putting medicine under the skin"), and then the procedure is carried out as quickly and skillfully as possible to avoid prolonging the stressful experience. Invasive procedures such as injections are especially anxiety provoking in young children, who may associate any assault to the "behind" area with punishment. Because injections are painful, the nurse should employ excellent injection technique and effective pain reduction measures to reduce discomfort (see Guidelines box).

Small infants offer little resistance to injections. Although they squirm and may be difficult to hold in position, they can usually be restrained without assistance. The body of a larger infant can be securely held between the nurse's arm and body (Fig. 45-13). To inject into the body of the muscle, the nurse firmly grasps the muscle mass between the thumb and fingers to isolate and stabilize the site. In obese children, however, it is preferable to first spread the skin with the thumb and index finger to displace subcutaneous tissue and then grasp the muscle deeply on each side.

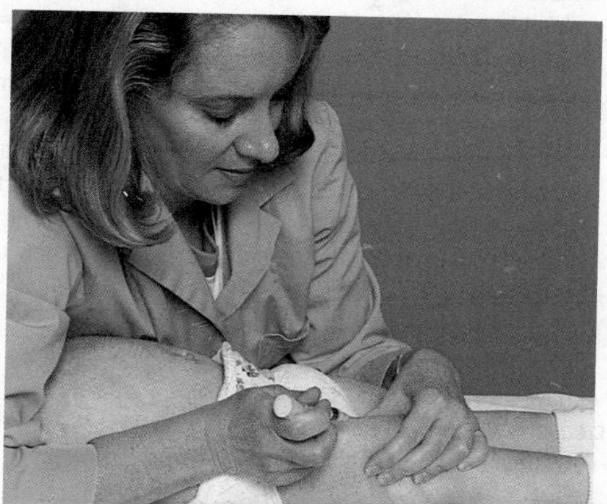

Fig. 45-13 Holding small child for intramuscular injection. Note how nurse isolates and stabilizes muscle.

If the medication is given around the clock, the nurse must wake the child. Although it may seem to be easier to surprise the sleeping child and do it quickly, this can cause the child to fear going back to sleep. When awakened first, children know that nothing will be done unless they are forewarned. See Guidelines box for techniques that maximize safety and minimize discomfort.

A needless injection system delivers IM or subcutaneous injections without the use of a needle and eliminates the risk

GUIDELINES Intramuscular Administration of Medication

Use safety precautions in administering medication (e.g., check child's identification).

Apply EMLA (an eutectic mix of lidocaine and prilocaine) topically over site if time permits (at least 60 minutes, preferably 2 to 2½ hours for (intramuscular [IM] injection). LMX (lidocaine) cream may be applied for a shorter interval (see Pain Management, Chapter 35).

Prepare medication:

- Select needle and syringe appropriate to the following: (1) amount of fluid to be administered (syringe size), (2) viscosity of fluid to be administered (needle gauge), and (3) amount of tissue to be penetrated (needle length).
- Maximum volume to be administered in a single site is 1 ml for older infants and small children.

Determine site of injection (see Table 45-4), making certain that muscle is large enough to accommodate volume and type of medication.

- Acceptable sites for infants and small or debilitated children are the vastus lateralis muscle and the ventrogluteal muscle.
- The dorsogluteal muscle is insufficiently developed to be a safe site for infants and small children.

Administer medication.

- Obtain sufficient help in restraining child; children are often uncooperative, and their behavior is usually unpredictable.
- Explain briefly what is to be done and, if appropriate, what child can do to help.
- Expose injection area for unobstructed view of landmarks.
- Select a site where skin is free of irritation and danger of infection; palpate for and avoid sensitive or hardened areas. With multiple injections, rotate sites.
- Place child in a lying or sitting position; child is not allowed to stand because (1) landmarks are more difficult to assess, (2) restraint is more difficult, and (3) child may faint and fall.
- Use a new, sharp needle with smallest diameter that permits free flow of the medication.
- Grasp muscle firmly between thumb and fingers to isolate and stabilize muscle for deposition of drug in its deepest part; in obese children, spread skin with thumb and index finger to displace subcutaneous tissue and grasp muscle deeply on each side.
- Allow skin preparation to dry completely before skin is penetrated.
- Have medication at room temperature.

Decrease perception of pain.

- Distract child with conversation.
- Give child something on which to concentrate (e.g., squeezing a hand or side rail, pinching own nose, humming, counting, yelling "Ouch!").
- Spray vapocoolant (e.g., ethyl chloride or fluorimethane) on site 11 to 15 seconds before injection or place a cold compress or wrapped ice cube on site about a minute before injection, or apply cold to contralateral site.
- Say to child, "If you feel this, tell me to take it out, please."
- Have child hold a small adhesive bandage and place it on puncture site after IM injection is given.

Insert needle quickly, using a dartlike motion at a 90-degree angle unless contraindicated.

- Use new needle, not one that has pierced rubber stopper on vial.

Avoid tracking any medication through superficial tissues:

- Replace needle after withdrawing medication, or wipe medication from needle with sterile gauze.
- If withdrawing medication from an ampule, use a needle equipped with a filter that removes glass particles; then use a new, nonfilter needle for injection.
- Use the Z-track or air-bubble technique as indicated.
- Avoid depressing the plunger during insertion of the needle.

Aspirate for blood.

- If blood is found, remove syringe from site, change needle, and reinsert into new location.
- If no blood is found, inject into a relaxed muscle:

  Ventrogluteal—Place child on side with upper leg flexed and placed in front of lower leg.

  Vastus lateralis—Child can be supine, lying on the side, or sitting.

Inject medication slowly.

Remove needle quickly; hold gauze sponge firmly against skin near needle when removing it to avoid pulling on tissue.

Apply firm pressure to site after injection; massage site to hasten absorption unless contraindicated, as with irritating drugs.

Place a small adhesive bandage on puncture site; with young children decorate it by drawing a smiling face or other symbol of acceptance.

Hold and cuddle young child and encourage parents to comfort child; praise older child.

Allow expression of feelings.

Discard syringe and uncapped, uncut needle in puncture-resistant container located near site of use.

Record time of injection, drug, dose, and injection site.

of accidental needle puncture. This needle-free injection system involves a carbon dioxide cartridge that provides the power to deliver the medication through the skin. Although it is not painless, it may reduce pain and also the anxiety of seeing the needle (Polillio & Killy, 1997).

Subcutaneous and Intradermal Administration

Subcutaneous and intradermal injections are frequently administered to children, but the technique differs little from the method used with adults. Examples of *subcutaneous injections* include insulin, hormone replacement, allergy desensitization, and some vaccines. Tuberculin testing, local anesthesia, and allergy testing are examples of frequently administered *intradermal injections.*

Techniques to minimize the pain associated with these injections include changing the needle if it pierced a rubber stopper on a vial, using 26- to 30-gauge needles (only to inject the solution), and injecting small volumes (up to 0.5 ml). The angle of the needle for the subcutaneous injection is typically 90 degrees. In children with little subcutaneous tissue, some practitioners insert the needle at a 45-degree angle. However, the benefit of using the 45-degree angle rather than the 90-degree angle remains controversial.

Although subcutaneous injections can be given anywhere there is subcutaneous tissue, common sites include the center third of the lateral aspect of the upper arm, the abdomen, and the center third of the anterior thigh. Some practitioners believe it is not necessary to aspirate before injecting subcutaneously; for example, this is an accepted practice in the administration of insulin. Automatic injector devices do not aspirate before injecting.

When giving an intradermal injection into the volar surface of the forearm, the nurse should avoid the medial side of the arm, where the skin is more sensitive.

NURSING ALERT Families often need to learn subcutaneous injection techniques to administer medications, such as insulin, at home. Begin teaching as early as possible to allow the family the maximum amount of practice time possible.

Intravenous Administration

The IV route for administering medications is frequently used in pediatric therapy. For some drugs it is the only effective route. This method is used for giving drugs to children who have poor absorption as a result of diarrhea, dehydration, or peripheral vascular collapse; who need a high serum concentration of a drug; who have resistant infections that require parenteral medication over an extended time; who need continuous pain relief; and who require emergency treatment.

Insertion sites and observation of the IV infusion are discussed on p. 1286. Several factors need to be considered in relation to IV medication. When a drug is administered intravenously, the effect is almost instantaneous and further control is limited. Most drugs for IV administration require a specified minimum dilution and/or rate of flow, and many are highly irritating or toxic to tissues outside the vascular system. In addition to the precautions and nursing observations related to IV therapy, factors to consider when preparing and administering drugs to infants and children by the IV route include:

- Amount of drug to be administered
- Minimum dilution of drug and whether child is fluid restricted
- Type of solution in which drug can be diluted
- Length of time over which drug can be safely administered
- Rate of infusion that child and vessels can tolerate safely
- IV tubing volume capacity
- Time that this or another drug is to be administered
- Compatibility of all drugs that child is receiving intravenously
- Compatibility with infusion fluids

Before any IV infusion, the site of insertion is checked for patency. Medications are never administered with blood products. Only one antibiotic should be administered at a time.

IV infusion is suitable for children who can tolerate the necessary infusion rate and the extra fluid needed to administer the medication. For the very small infant or fluid-restricted child who is not able to tolerate the increased rate of fluids, special delivery systems, such as syringe pumps, are used. Regardless of the technique, the nurse must know the minimum dilutions for safe administration of IV medications to infants and children.

Peripheral Intermittent Infusion Device

The *peripheral lock,* also known as an *intermittent infusion device* or *saline* or *heparin lock,* is an alternative to a keep-open infusion when extended access to a vein is required without the need for continuous fluid. It is most frequently employed for intermittent infusion of medication into a peripheral venous route. A short, flexible catheter is used as the lock device, and a site is selected where there will be minimal movement, such as the forearm. The catheter is inserted and secured in the same manner as for any IV infusion device, but the hub is occluded with a stopper or injection cap.

The type of device used may vary, and the care and use of the peripheral lock are carried out according to the protocol of the institution or unit. However, the general concept is the same. The catheter remains in place and is flushed with saline after infusion of the medication. See the Evidence-Based Practice box on flushing with normal saline or heparin.

Children may be discharged with a peripheral lock in place to continue receiving medications without hospitalization. This is usually reserved for children who require medications on a short-term basis. They are referred to a home-based infusion company. Those with chronic illnesses who require repeated blood sampling or medications, long-term chemotherapy, or frequent hyperalimentation or antibiotic therapy are best managed with a central venous catheter.

Central Venous Access Device

Central venous access devices (VADs) have several different characteristics. Factors that can influence the type of VAD include the reason for placement of the catheter (diagnosis), length of therapy, risk to the patient in placement of the catheter, and availability of resources to assist the family in maintaining the catheter.

Short-term or *nontunneled catheters* are used in acute care, emergency, and intensive care units. These catheters are made of polyurethane and are placed in large veins such as the subclavian, femoral, or jugular. Insertion is by surgical incision or large percutaneous threading. A chest x-ray film should be taken to verify placement of the catheter tip before administration of fluids or medications.

Peripherally inserted central catheters (PICCs) can be used for short-term to moderate-length therapy. These catheters consist of silicone or polymer material and are placed by specially trained nurses, physicians, or interventional radiologists (Gamulka, Mendoza, & Connolly, 2005). The most common insertion site is above the antecubital area using the median, cephalic, or basilic vein. The catheter is threaded either with or without a guidewire into the superior vena cava. PICCs can be trimmed before insertion, and the decision can be made to insert the catheter midline, which is considered between the insertion site and the axilla. The midline has a dwell time of 2 to 4 weeks. If the catheter is threaded midline, total parenteral

evolve Animation—Central Venous Access

evolve Critical Thinking Exercise—Central Venous Access Device

EVIDENCE-BASED PRACTICE Normal Saline or Heparinized Saline Flush Solution in Pediatric Intravenous Lines

—David Wilson

Ask the Question

Is there a significant difference in the longevity of intravenous (IV) intermittent infusion locks in children when normal saline (NS) is used instead a heparinized saline (HS) solution as a flush?

Search for Evidence

Search Strategies

English-language publications with the following terms: saline vs. heparin intermittent flush, children's heparin lock flush, heparin lock patency, and peripheral venous catheter in children

Databases Searched

CINAHL, PubMed

Critically Analyze the Evidence

A Cochrane systematic review by Shah and Sinha (2002) revealed eight studies that were randomized or quasirandomized trials of HS administration vs. NS, placebo, or no treatment in neonates. The authors of the review concluded that, because of the studies' heterogeneity and variability in methodologic quality, clinical details, and reporting outcomes, they provided no strong evidence regarding the effectiveness and safety of heparin to prolong catheter life in neonates.

No significant statistical difference was found between HS and NS flushes for maintaining catheter patency in children (Hanrahan, Kleiber, & Fagan, 1994; Kotter, 1996; Schultz, Drew, & Hewitt, 2002; Hanrahan, Kleiber, & Berends, 2000; Heilskov et al, 1998).

Several studies reported increased incidence of pain or erythema with HS flushing of infusion devices (Hanrahan, Kleiber, & Fagan, 1994; Robertson, 1994; Nelson & Graves, 1998; McMullen et al, 1993).

Several studies found increased patency and/or longer dwell times with HS solutions vs. NS in 24-gauge catheters (Mudge, Forcier, & Slattery, 1998; Danek & Noris, 1992; Beecroft et al, 1997; Gyr et al, 1995; Hanrahan, Kleiber, & Berends, 2000).

Younger age in children and lower gestational age in preterm neonates were associated with shorter patency of IV catheters (Paisley et al, 1997; Robertson, 1994; McMullen et al, 1993).

Infusion devices flushed with NS lasted longer than those flushed with HS (Nelson & Graves, 1998; Le Duc, 1997; Goldberg et al, 1999).

When measured and reported, length of time between flushing peripheral devices affected dwell time (Crews et al, 1997; Gyr et al, 1995).

None of the studies cited anticoagulation-associated complications with HS, which is a concern in preterm neonates who are at higher risk for development of clotting problems as a result of heparin (Klenner et al, 2003).

Apply the Evidence: Nursing Implications

Further research is needed with larger samples of children, especially preterm neonates, using small-gauge catheters (24 gauge) and other gauge catheters, flushed with NS and HS as intermittent infusion devices only (no continuous infusions).

NS is a safe alternative to HS flush in infants and children with intermittent IV locks larger than 24 gauge; smaller neonates may benefit from HS flush (longer dwell time), but the evidence is inconclusive for all weight ranges and gestational ages.

References

Beecroft PC et al: Intravenous lock patency in children: dilute heparin versus saline, *J Pediatr Pharmacol Practice* 2(4):211-223, 1997.

Crews BE et al: Effects of varying intervals between heparin flushes on pediatric catheter longevity, *Pediatr Nurs* 23(1):87-91, 1997.

Danek GD, Noris EM: Pediatric IV catheters: efficacy of saline flush, *Pediatr Nurs* 18(2):111-113, 1992.

Goldberg M et al: Maintaining patency of peripheral intermittent infusion devices with heparinized saline and saline: a randomized double blind controlled trial in neonatal intensive care and a review of literature, *Neonatal Intensive Care* 12(1):18-22, 1999.

Gyr P et al: Double blind comparison of heparin and saline flush solutions in maintenance of peripheral infusion devices, *Pediatr Nurs* 21(4):383-389, 1995.

Hanrahan KS, Kleiber C, Berends S: Saline for peripheral intravenous locks in neonates: evaluating a change in practice, *Neonatal Netw* 19(2):19-24, 2000.

Hanrahan KS, Kleiber C, Fagan C: Evaluation of saline for IV locks in children, *Pediatr Nurs* 20(6):549-552, 1994.

Heilskov J et al: A randomized trial of heparin and saline for maintaining intravenous locks in neonates, *J Soc Pediatr Nurs* 3(3):111-116, 1998.

Klenner AF et al: Benefit and risk of heparin for maintaining peripheral venous catheters in neonates: a placebo-controlled trial, *J Pediatr* 143(6):741-745, 2003.

Kotter RW: Heparin vs. saline for intermittent intravenous device maintenance in neonates, *Neonatal Netw* 15(6):43-47, 1996.

Le Duc K: Efficacy of normal saline solution versus heparin solution for maintaining patency of peripheral intravenous catheters in children, *J Emerg Nurs* 23(4):306-309, 1997.

McMullen A et al: Heparinized saline or normal saline as a flush solution in intermittent intravenous lines in infants and children, *MCN* 18(2):78-85, 1993.

Mudge B, Forcier D, Slattery MJ: Patency of 24-gauge peripheral intermittent infusion devices: a comparison of heparin and saline flush solutions, *Pediatr Nurs* 24(2):142-149, 1998.

Nelson TJ, Graves SM: 0.9% Sodium chloride injection with and without heparin for maintaining peripheral indwelling intermittent infusion devices in infants, *Am J Health Syst Pharm* 55:570-573, 1998.

Paisley MK et al: The use of heparin and normal saline flushes in neonatal intravenous catheters, *J Pediatr Nurs* 23(5):521-527, 1997.

Robertson J: Intermittent intravenous therapy: a comparison of two flushing solutions, *Contemp Nurs* 3(4):174-179, 1994.

Schultz AA, Drew D, Hewitt H: Comparison of normal saline and heparinized saline for patency of IV locks in neonates, *Appl Nurs Res* 15(1):28-34, 2002.

Shah PS, Sinha AK: Heparin for prolonging peripheral intravenous catheter use in neonates, *Cochrane Database Syst Rev* (2):1-26, 2002.

evolve Animation—IV Line Placement

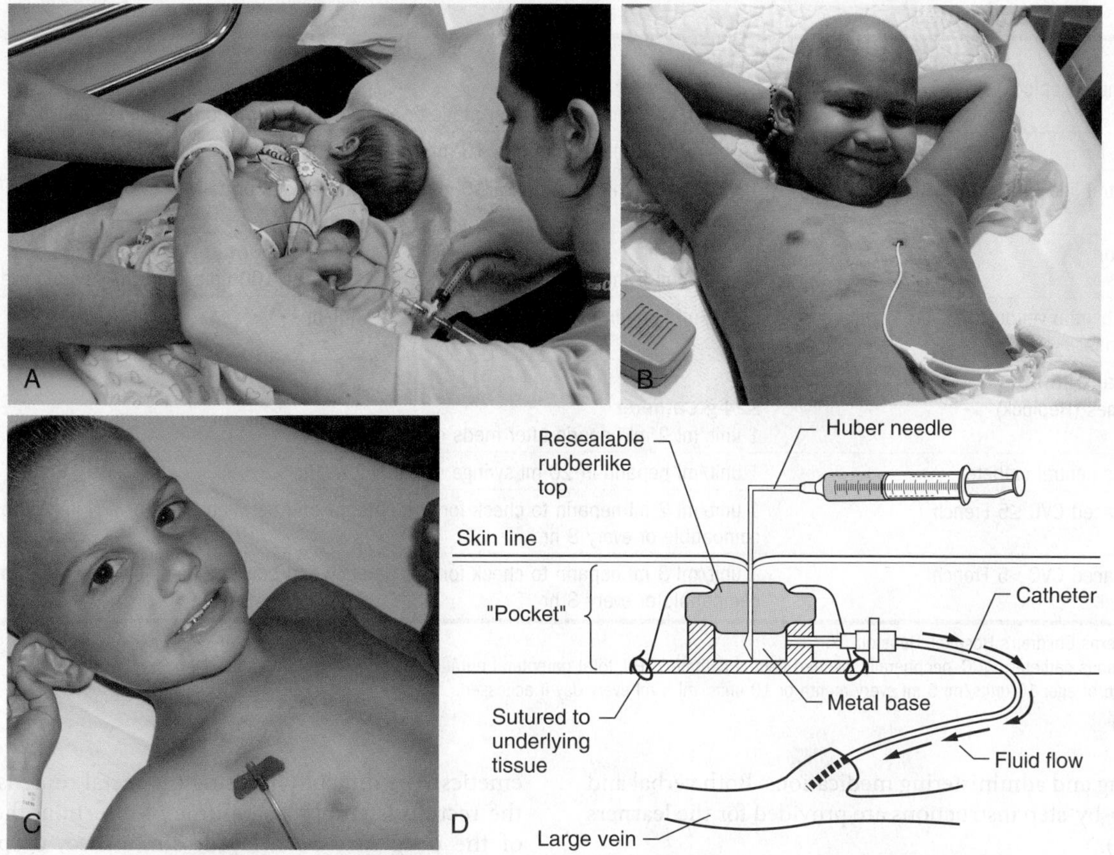

Fig. 45-14 Venous access devices. **A,** Blood being drawn from a central venous catheter. **B,** Child with external central venous catheter. **C,** Child with implanted port with Huber needle in place. **D,** Side view of implanted port.

evolve Animation—PICC Line Placement

nutrition (TPN) or any drug known to irritate a peripheral vein (e.g., chemotherapy drugs) should not be administered. The high concentration of glucose in TPN makes it irritating to the vessel; it should be infused through a central catheter.

NURSING ALERT Most PICC lines are not sutured into place, so care is needed when changing the dressing.

Long-term central VADs include tunneled catheters and implanted infusion ports (Fig. 45-14). They may have single, double, or triple lumens. Several lumens (multilumen) catheters allow more than one therapy to be administered at the same time. Reasons to use multilumen catheters include repeated blood sampling, TPN, administration of blood products or infusion of large quantities and/or concentrations of fluids, administration of incompatible drugs or fluids at the same time (through different lumens), and central venous pressure monitoring.

With any of the central venous catheters, medication is easily instilled through the injection cap. Maintenance of the catheter includes dressing changes, flushing to maintain patency, and prevention of occlusion or dislodgment.

NURSING ALERT When working with tunneled catheters, PICCs, and peripheral intravenous lines (PIVs), avoid using scissors around the tubing or dressing. Removal is best accomplished using fingers and much patience. In the event that a tunneled catheter is cut, use a padded clamp to clamp the catheter proximal to the exit site to avoid blood loss. Repair kits are available, which may save the catheter and avoid surgery to replace a cut catheter.

With the implanted device the port must be palpated for placement and stabilized, the overlying skin cleansed, and only special noncoring Huber needles used to pierce the port's diaphragm on the top or side, depending on the style. To avoid repeated skin punctures, a special infusion set with a Huber needle and extension tubing with a Luer connection can be used (see Fig. 45-14). With this attached, the injection procedure is the same as for an intermittent infusion device or a central venous catheter. To prevent infection, meticulous aseptic technique must be used any time the devices are entered, including instillation of heparin or saline to prevent clotting (Harris & Maguire, 1999). There should be a protocol stating that the Huber needle needs to be changed at established intervals, usually 5 to 7 days.

The children and parents are taught the procedure for care of the VAD before discharge from the hospital, including preparation and injection of the prescribed medication, the flush, and dressing changes. A protective device may be recommended for some active children to prevent accidental dislodgment of the needle. Many children take responsibility

Table 45-5 Flush Guidelines

Children		
Peripheral lines (Heplock)	*≤24-g Catheter* 10 units/ml 2 ml heparin after meds or every 8 hr	*>24-g Catheter* 5 ml normal saline after meds or every 8 hr
Midline	10 units/ml 3 ml heparin in a 10-ml syringe after meds or every 8 hr	
External central line (nonimplanted, tunneled, or PICC)	10 units/ml 3 ml heparin in a 10-ml syringe after meds or daily	
Implanted port	*Intermittent* 10 units/ml 5 ml heparin after meds	*Dormant* 100 units/ml 5 ml heparin every month*
Arterial and central venous pressure continuous monitored lines	1 unit/ml heparin in 55-ml syringes run at 1 ml/hr	
Neonates and Infants		
Peripheral lines (Heplock)	*≤24-g Catheter* 1 unit/ml 2 ml heparin after meds or every 8 hr	
Percutaneous central catheter	1 unit/ml heparin in 20-ml syringe run at 0.2 ml/hr	
Surgically placed CVC ≤5 French	1 unit/ml 2 ml heparin to check for line patency and between meds or TPN known to be compatible or every 8 hr	
Surgically placed CVC >5 French	1 unit/ml 3 ml heparin to check for line patency and between meds or TPN known to be compatible or every 8 hr	

Modified from Texas Children's Hospital, Houston, TX.
CVC, Central venous catheter; *PICC*, peripherally inserted central catheter; *TPN*, total parenteral nutrition.
*Patients <6 mo of age: 10 units/ml 5 ml every month or 10 units/ml 5 ml every day if accessed.

for preparing and administering medications. Both verbal and written step-by-step instructions are provided for the learners (Table 45-5).

Infection and catheter occlusion are two of the most common complications of central venous catheters. They require treatment with antibiotics for infection and a fibrinolytic agent, such as alteplase, for clots (Fisher et al, 2004; Shen et al, 2003). Uncapping can be prevented by taping the cap securely to the catheter and the clamped line to the dressing. Leaks can be prevented by using a smooth-edged clamp only. Parents are cautioned to keep scissors away from the child to prevent accidental cutting of the catheter. If the catheter leaks, they are instructed to tape it above the leak and then clamp the catheter at the taped site. The child should be taken to the practitioner as soon as possible to prevent infection or clotting after a catheter leak.

Nasogastric, Orogastric, or Gastrostomy Administration

When a child has an indwelling feeding tube or a gastrostomy, oral medications are usually given via that route. An advantage of this method is the ability to administer oral medications around the clock without disturbing the child. A disadvantage is the risk of occluding or clogging the tube, especially when giving viscous solutions through small-bore feeding tubes. The most important preventive measure is adequate flushing after the medication is instilled (see Guidelines box).

Rectal Administration

The rectal route for administration is less reliable but is sometimes used when the oral route is difficult or contraindicated. It is also used when oral preparations are unsuitable to control vomiting. Some of the drugs available in suppository form are acetaminophen, sedatives, analgesics (morphine), and antiemetics. The difficulty in using the rectal route is that, unless the rectum is empty at the time of insertion, the absorption of the drug may be delayed, diminished, or prevented by the presence of feces. Sometimes the drug is later evacuated, securely surrounded by stool.

The wrapping on the suppository is removed and the suppository lubricated with water-soluble jelly or warm water. Rectal suppositories are traditionally inserted with the apex (pointed end) foremost. Reverse contractions or the pressure gradient of the anal canal may help the suppository slip higher into the canal. Using a glove or finger cot, quickly but gently insert the suppository into the rectum, beyond both of the rectal sphincters. The buttocks are then held together firmly to relieve pressure on the anal sphincter until the urge to expel the suppository has passed—5 to 10 minutes. Sometimes the amount of drug ordered is less than the dosage available. The irregular shape of most suppositories makes the process of dividing them into a desired dose difficult if not dangerous. If the suppository must be halved, it should be cut lengthwise. However, there is no guarantee that the drug is evenly dispersed throughout the petrolatum base.

Optic, Otic, and Nasal Administration

There are few differences between administering eye, ear, and nose medication to children and to adults. The major difficulty is in gaining children's cooperation. Older children need only explanation and direction. Although the administration of optic, otic, and nasal medication is not painful, these drugs can cause unpleasant sensations that can be eliminated with various techniques.

NURSING ALERT The following steps help reduce unpleasant sensations when administering medications:

Eye–Apply finger pressure to the lacrimal punctum at the inner aspect of the lid for 1 minute to prevent drainage

GUIDELINES Nasogastric, Orogastric, or Gastrostomy Medication Administration in Children

Use elixir or suspension (rather than tablet) preparations of medication whenever possible.
Dilute viscous medication or syrup with a small amount of water if possible.
If administering tablets, crush tablet to a fine powder and dissolve drug in a small amount of warm water.
Never crush enteric-coated or sustained-release tablets or capsules.
Avoid oily medications because they tend to cling to side of tube.
Do not mix medication with enteral formula unless fluid is restricted. If adding a drug:
- Check with pharmacist for compatibility.
- Shake formula well and observe for any physical reaction (e.g., separation, precipitation).
- Label formula container with name of medication, dosage, date, and time infusion started.

Have medication at room temperature.
Measure medication in a calibrated cup or syringe.
Check for correct placement of nasogastric or orogastric tube (see Guidelines box, p. 1296).
Attach syringe (with adaptable tip but without plunger) to tube.
Pour medication into syringe.
Unclamp tube and allow medication to flow by gravity.
Adjust height of container to achieve desired flow rate (e.g., increase height for faster flow).
As soon as syringe is empty, pour in water to flush tubing.
Amount of water depends on length and gauge of tubing. Determine amount before administering any medication by using a syringe to fill completely an unused nasogastric or orogastric tube with water. Amount of flush solution is usually 1.5 times this volume.
With certain drug preparations (e.g., suspensions) more fluid may be needed.
If administering more than one drug at the same time, flush tube between each medication with clear water.
Clamp tube after flushing, unless tube is left open.

of medication to the nasopharynx and the unpleasant "tasting" of the drug.

Ear—Allow medications stored in the refrigerator to warm to room temperature before instillation.

Nose—Position the child with the head hyperextended to prevent strangling sensations caused by medication trickling into the throat rather than up into the nasal passages.

To instill eye medication, the child is placed supine or sitting with the head extended, and the child is asked to look up. One hand is used to pull the lower lid downward; the hand that holds the dropper rests on the head so that it may move synchronously with the child's head, thus reducing the possibility of trauma to a struggling child or of dropping medication on the face (Fig. 45-15). As the lower lid is pulled down, a small conjunctival sac is formed; the solution or ointment is

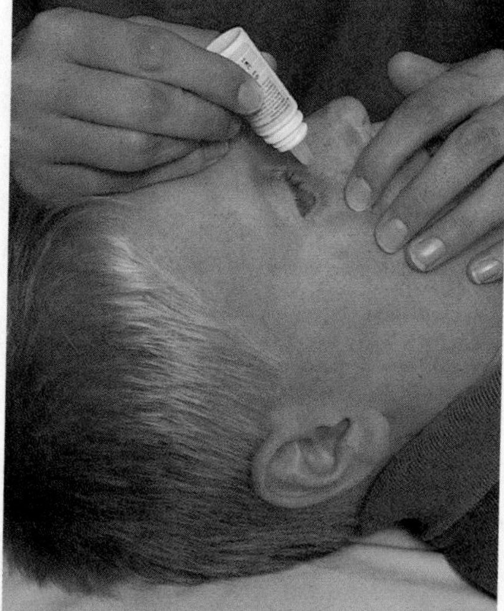

Fig. 45-15 Administering eye drops.

applied to this area, never directly on the eyeball. Another effective technique is to pull the lower lid down and out to form a cup effect, into which the medication is dropped. The lids are gently closed to prevent expression of the medication, and the child is asked to look in all directions to enhance even distribution of the preparation. Excess medication is wiped from the inner canthus outward to prevent contamination to the contralateral eye.

Instilling eye drops in infants can be difficult, since they often clench the lids tightly closed. One approach is to place the drops in the nasal corner where the lids meet. The medication pools in this area, and when the infant opens the lids, the medication flows onto the conjunctiva. For young children, playing a game can be helpful, such as instructing the child to keep the eyes closed until the count of three and then open them, at which time the drops are quickly instilled. Ointment can be applied by gently pulling down the lower lid and placing the ointment in the lower conjunctival sac.

NURSING ALERT If both eye ointment and drops are ordered, give drops first, wait 3 minutes, and then apply the ointment to allow each drug to work. When possible, administer eye ointments before bedtime or naptime, since the child's vision will be blurred temporarily.

Ear drops are instilled with the child in the prone or supine position and the head turned to the appropriate side. For children younger than 3 years of age, the external auditory canal is straightened by gently pulling the pinna downward and straight back. The pinna is pulled upward and back in children older than 3 years of age. To place the drops deep in the ear canal without contaminating the tip of the dropper, place a disposable ear speculum in the canal and administer the drops through the speculum. After instillation, the child should remain lying on the unaffected side for a few minutes. Gentle massage of the area immediately anterior to the ear facilitates the entry of drops into the ear canal. The use of cotton pledgets prevents medication from flowing out of the external canal. However, the pledgets should be loose enough to allow any discharge to exit from the ear. Premoistening the

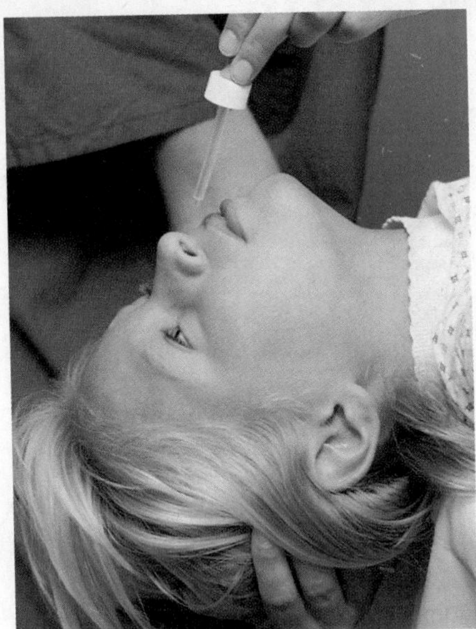

Fig. 45-16 Proper position for instilling nose drops.

cotton with a few drops of medication prevents the wicking action from absorbing the medication instilled in the ear.

Nose drops are instilled in the same manner as in the adult patient. Unpleasant sensations associated with medicated nose drops are minimized when care is taken to position the child with the head extended well over the edge of the bed or a pillow (Fig. 45-16). Depending on size, the infant can be positioned in the football hold (see Fig. 45-5, *B*); in the nurse's arm with the head extended and stabilized between the nurse's body and elbow, and the arms and hands immobilized with the nurse's hands; or as shown in Fig. 45-16. After instillation of the drops, the child should remain in position for 1 minute to allow the drops to come in contact with the nasal surfaces.

Nasal spray dispensers are inserted into the naris vertically and then angled nasally to avoid trauma to the septum and to direct medication toward the inferior turbinate.

Family Teaching and Home Care

The nurse usually assumes the responsibility for preparing families to administer medications at home. The family should understand why the child is receiving the medication and the effects that might be expected, as well as the amount, frequency, and length of time the drug is to be administered. Instruction should be carried out in an unhurried, relaxed manner, preferably in an area away from a busy ward or office.

The caregiver is carefully instructed regarding the correct dosage. Some persons have difficulty understanding medical terminology from the pharmacy; just because they nod or otherwise indicate an understanding, it cannot be assumed that the message is clear. It is important to ascertain their interpretation of a teaspoon, for example, and to be certain they have acceptable devices for measuring the drug. If the drug is packaged with a dropper, syringe, or plastic cup, the nurse should show or mark the point on the device that indicates the prescribed dose and demonstrate how the dose is drawn up into a dropper or syringe, measured, and the bubbles eliminated. If the nurse has any doubts about the parent's ability to administer the correct dose, the parent should be asked to give a return demonstration. This is essential when the drug has potentially serious consequences from incorrect dosage, such as insulin or digoxin, or when more complex administration is required, such as parenteral injections. When teaching a parent to give an injection, the nurse must allot adequate time for instruction and practice.

Home modifications are often necessary because the availability of equipment or assistance can differ from the hospital setting. For example, the parent may need guidance in devising methods that allow for one person to hold the child and safely give the drug.

PATIENT TEACHING Administering Oral, Nasal, or Optic Medication

To administer oral, nasal, or optic medication when only one person is available to hold the child, use the following procedure:

- Place child supine on flat surface (bed, couch, floor).
- Sit facing child so that child's head is between operator's thighs and child's arms are under operator's legs.
- Place lower legs over child's legs to restrain lower body, if necessary.
- To administer oral medication, place small pillow under child's head to reduce risk of aspiration.
- To administer nasal medication, place small pillow under child's shoulders to aid flow of liquid through nasal passages.

The time that the drug is to be administered is clarified with the parent. For instance, when a drug is prescribed in association with meals, the number of meals that the family is accustomed to eating influences the amount of drug the child receives. Does the child have meals twice a day or five times a day? When a drug is to be given several times during the day, together the nurse and parents can work out a schedule that accommodates the family's routine. This is particularly significant if the drug must be given at equal intervals throughout a 24-hour period. For example, telling parents that the child needs 1 teaspoon of medicine four times a day is subject to misinterpretation, since parents may routinely schedule the doses at incorrect times. Instead, a preplanned schedule based on 6-hour intervals should be set up with the number of days required for therapeutic dosage listed. Written instruction should accompany all drug prescriptions.

PATIENT TEACHING Color-Coded Instructions

If parents have difficulty reading or understanding English, use colors to convey instructions. For example, mark each drug with a color and place the appropriate color on a calendar chart or on a drawing of a clock to identify when the drug needs to be given. If a liquid medication and syringe are used, also mark the syringe with color-coded tape at the place the plunger needs to be.

Maintaining Fluid Balance

Measurement of Intake and Output

Accurate measurements of fluid intake and output (I&O) are essential to the assessment of fluid balance. Measurements from all sources—including gastrointestinal and parenteral I&O from urine, stools, vomitus, fistulas, nasogastric suction, sweat, and drainage from wounds—must be taken and considered. Although the practitioner usually indicates when I&O measurements are to be recorded, it is a nursing responsibility to keep an accurate I&O record on certain children, including those:

- Receiving IV therapy
- Who underwent major surgery
- Receiving diuretic or corticosteroid therapy
- With severe thermal burns or injuries
- With renal disease or damage
- With congestive heart failure
- With dehydration
- With diabetes mellitus
- With oliguria
- In respiratory distress
- With chronic lung disease

Infants or small children who are unable to use a bedpan or those who have bowel movements with every voiding require the application of a collecting device (p. 1268). If collecting bags are not used, wet diapers or pads are carefully weighed to ascertain the amount of fluid lost. This includes liquid stool, vomitus, and other losses. The volume of fluid in milliliters is equivalent to the weight of the fluid measured in grams. The specific gravity as a measure of osmolality is determined with a refractometer or urine dipsticks and assists in assessing the degree of hydration.

NURSING ALERT

1 g of wet diaper weight = 1 ml urine

In infants with diapers, weigh all dry diapers to be used and note in an indelible marker the dry weight of the diaper; when there is fluid (urine or liquid stool) in the diaper, the amount of output can be approximated by subtracting the weight of the dry diaper from the weight of the wet diaper.

Disadvantages of the weighed-diaper method of fluid measurement include (1) inability to differentiate one type of loss from another because of admixture, (2) loss of urine or liquid stool from leakage or evaporation (especially if the infant is under a radiant warmer), and (3) additional fluid in the diaper (superabsorbent disposable type) from absorption of atmospheric moisture (in high-humidity incubators).

Special Needs When the Child Is NPO

Infants or children who are unable or not permitted to take fluids by mouth (NPO) have special needs. To ensure that they do not receive fluids, a sign can be placed in some obvious place, such as over their beds or on their shirts, to alert others to the NPO status. To prevent the temptation to drink, fluids should not be left at the bedside.

Oral hygiene, a part of routine hygienic care, is especially important when fluids are restricted or withheld. For the young child who cannot brush the teeth or rinse the mouth without swallowing fluid, the mouth and teeth can be cleaned and kept moist by swabbing with saline-moistened gauze.

NURSING ALERT To keep the mouth feeling moist when the child is NPO, give ice chips (if this is permitted by the practitioner) or spray the mouth from an atomizer. To meet the need to suck, the infant is provided with a safe commercial pacifier.

The child who is fluid restricted presents an equal challenge. Limiting fluids is often more difficult for the child than being NPO, especially when IV fluids are also eliminated. To make certain the child does not drink the entire amount allowed early in the day, the daily allotment is calculated to provide fluids at periodic intervals throughout the child's waking hours. Serving the fluids in small containers gives the illusion of larger servings. No extra liquid is left at the bedside.

Parenteral Fluid Therapy

Site and Equipment

The site selected for PIV infusion depends on accessibility and convenience. Although it is possible to use any accessible vein in older children, the child's developmental, cognitive, and mobility needs must be considered when selecting a site. Ideally, in older children, the superficial veins of the forearm should be used, leaving the hands free. An older child can help select the site and thereby maintain some measure of control. For veins in the extremities it is best to start with the most distal site and avoid the child's favored hand to reduce the disability related to the procedure. Restrict the child's movements as little as possible—avoid a site over a joint in an extremity, such as the antecubital space. In small infants a superficial vein of the hand, wrist, forearm, foot, or ankle is usually most convenient and most easily stabilized (Fig. 45-17). Foot veins should be avoided in children learning to walk or already walking. Superficial veins of the scalp have no valves, insertion is easy, and they can be used in infants up to about 9 months of age, but they should be used only when other site attempts have failed. A transilluminator can aid in finding and evaluating veins for access (Fig. 45-18).

Selection of a scalp vein may require clipping the area around the site to better visualize the vein and provide a smoother surface on which to tape the catheter hub and tubing. Clipping a portion of the infant's hair is upsetting to parents; therefore they should be told what to expect and reassured that the hair will grow in again rapidly (save the hair because parents often wish to keep it). Remove as little as possible, directly over the insertion site and taping surface. A rubber band slipped onto the head from brow to occiput will usually suffice as a tourniquet, although if the vessel is visible, a tourniquet may not be necessary.

NURSING ALERT A tab of tape should be placed on the rubber band to help grasp it when removing it from the infant's head. The rubber band should be cut to avoid accidentally dislodging the catheter when moving the rubber

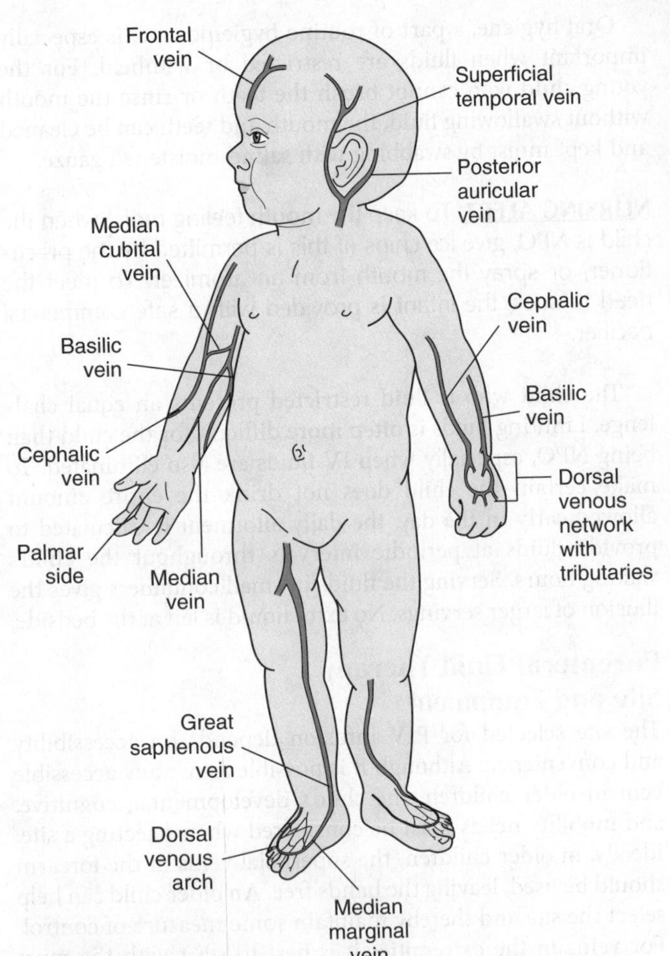

Fig. 45-17 Preferred sites for venous access in infants.

band over the IV insertion site. The tape tab will lift the rubber band and allow it to be cut. Hold the rubber band in two places and cut between these areas to prevent the rubber band from snapping on the head.

Situations may occur in which rapid establishment of systemic access is vital, and venous access may be hampered by peripheral circulatory collapse, hypovolemic shock (secondary to vomiting or diarrhea, burns, or trauma), cardiopulmonary arrest, or other conditions (Dubick & Holcomb, 2000). *Intraosseous infusion* provides a rapid, safe, and lifesaving alternate route for administration of fluids and medications until intravascular access can be obtained, especially in children who are 6 years of age and younger.

A large-bore needle, such as a bone marrow aspiration needle (e.g., Jamshidi) or an intraosseous needle (e.g., Cook), is inserted into the medullary cavity of a long bone, most often the proximal tibia. This procedure is usually reserved for children who are unconscious or for those who are receiving analgesia, since the procedure is painful. Local anesthesia should be used for a semiconscious patient. Observe the dependent tissue closely for swelling, since extravasation may be hidden under the leg and compartment syndrome may result.

For most IV infusions in children, a 22- to 24-gauge catheter may be used if therapy is expected to last less than 5 days.

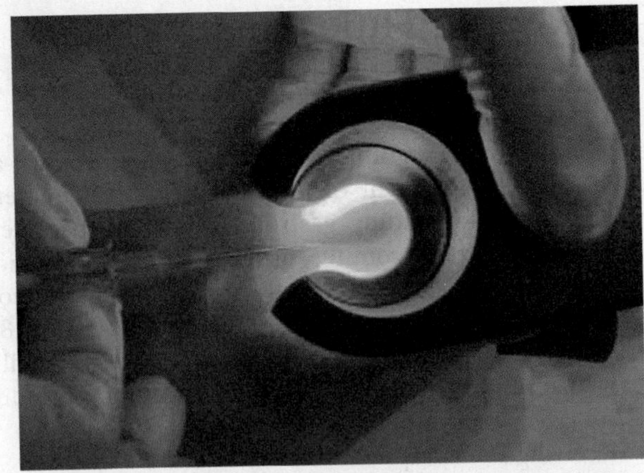

Fig. 45-18 Transilluminator: low-heat light-emitting diode (LED) light placed on the skin to illuminate veins; an opening allows cannulation of vein.

The smallest-gauge and shortest-length catheter that will accommodate the prescribed therapy should be chosen. The length of the catheter may be directly related to infection and/or embolus formation—the shorter the catheter, the fewer the complications (Maki, 1994). The gauge of the catheter should maintain adequate flow of the infusate into the cannulated vein while allowing adequate blood flow around the catheter walls to promote proper hemodilution of the infusate.

Determining the best catheter for the patient early in the therapy provides the best chance of avoiding catheter-related complications (Moureau, 1999). As the length of therapy increases, decisions regarding the type of infusion device (short peripheral, midline, PICC, or central venous catheter) should be explored. Guidelines such as flow charts or algorithms are available to help in these decisions (Catudal, 1999).

Safety Catheters and Needleless Systems

Over-the-needle IV catheters with hollow-bore needles carry a high risk for transmission of blood-borne pathogens from needlestick injuries. Safety catheters prevent accidental needlesticks with the use of over-the-needle IV catheters.

Needleless IV systems are designed to prevent needlestick injuries during administration of IV push medications and IV piggyback medications. Some needleless devices can be used with any tubing, whereas others require use of the entire IV delivery system for compatibility. Needleless IV systems rely on prepierced septa that are accessed by blunted plastic cannulas or systems that use valves that open and close a fluid path when activated by insertion of a syringe.

Blunt plastic cannulas and preslit injection port sites (Fig. 45-19) eliminate the need for steel needles and conventional injection port sites but remain accessible via hypodermic needles, a drawback except in emergent situations. Systems that do not permit needled access enhance safety by preventing health care workers from attempting to use needles. A syringe with a blue spike is available to access a single-dose vial (see Fig. 45-19, *A*). The preslit injection port sites are identified by a white ring surrounding the port; this ring alerts users that the system is needleless (see Fig. 45-19, *B*). Syringes are available with the blunt plastic cannula for accessing these sites (see Fig. 45-19, *C*). A lever lock (see Fig. 45-19, *D*) or

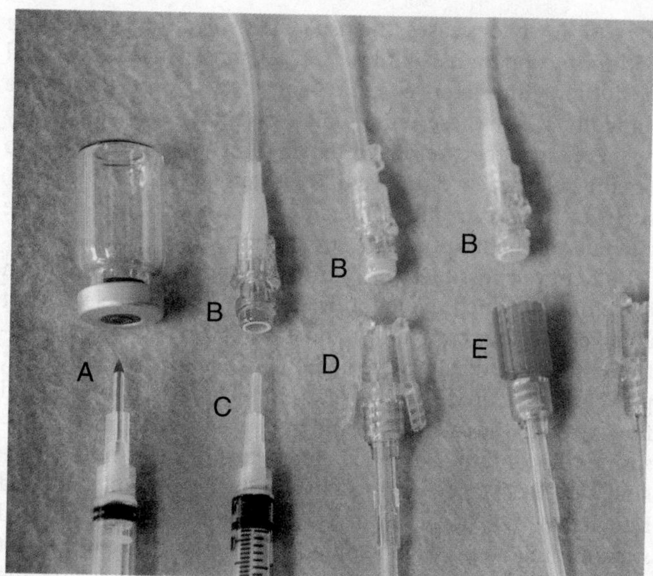

Fig. 45-19 Interlink intravenous access systems. A, Blue spike syringe. B, Preslit injection port (needleless). C, Blunt plastic cannula syringe. D, Lever lock cannula. E, Threaded lock cannula.

threaded lock cannula (see Fig. 45-19, *E*) attaches to an IV line, IV Y site, or peripheral intermittent infusion device. A preslit universal vial adapter (not pictured) provides access to standard multiple-dose vials, and syringe cannulas are then used to access the adapter. Valve technology allows syringes and IV tubing to connect directly in-line without the use of an adapter.

NURSING ALERT Misconnections of tubing have occurred, resulting in patient deaths. Many needleless IV systems allow other types of tubing such as blood pressure and oxygen tubing to connect and instill air directly into the IV line. Before tubing is connected or reconnected to a patient, trace it completely from the patient to the point of origin for verification (Institute for Safe Medication Practices, 2004).

Infusion Pumps

A variety of infusion pumps are available and used in nearly all pediatric infusions to accurately administer medication and minimize the possibility of overloading the circulation. It is important to calculate the amount to be infused in a given length of time, set the infusion rate, and monitor the apparatus frequently (at least every 1 to 2 hours) to make certain that the desired rate is maintained, the integrity of the system remains intact, the site remains intact (free of redness, edema, infiltration, or irritation), and the infusion does not stop. Continuous infusion pumps, although convenient and efficient, are not without risks. Overreliance on the accuracy of the machine can cause either too much or too little fluid to be infused; therefore its use does not eliminate the need for careful periodic assessment by the nurse. Excess pressure can build up if the machine is set at a rate faster than the vein is able to accommodate (or continues to pump when the needle is out of the lumen).

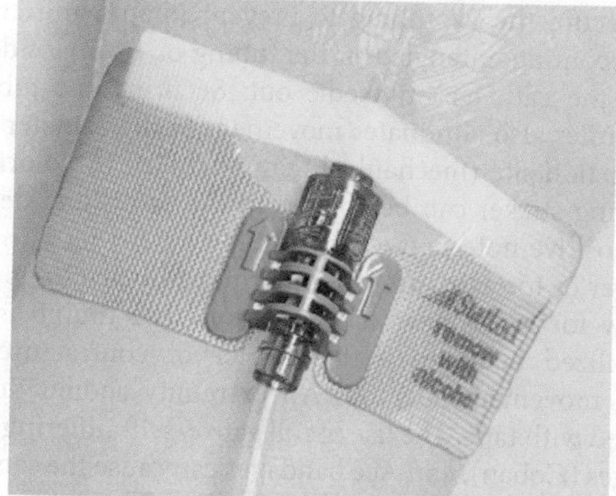

Fig. 45-20 StatLock securement devices enhance peripheral intravenous line dwell time and decrease phlebitis.

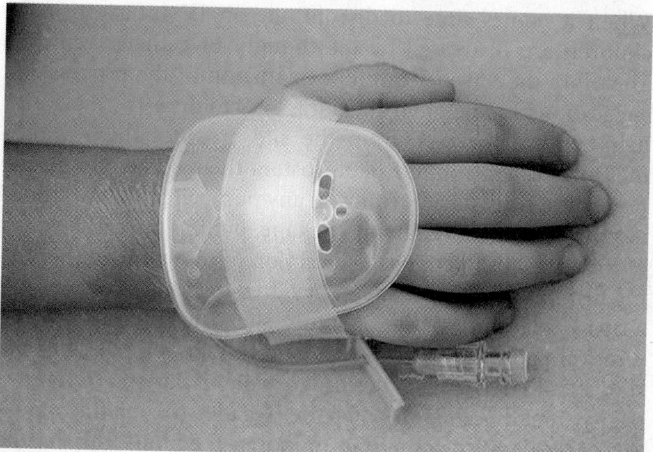
Fig. 45-21 I.V. House used to protect intravenous site.

Securement of a Peripheral Intravenous Line

To maintain the integrity of the IV line, adequate protection of the site is required. The catheter hub is firmly secured at the puncture site with a transparent dressing and commercial securement device (e.g., StatLock) (Fig. 45-20) or clear, nonallergenic tape. Transparent dressings are ideal because the insertion site is easily observed. Minimal tape should be used at the puncture site and on about 1 to 2 inches of skin beyond the site to avoid obscuring the insertion site for early detection of infiltration.

A protective cover is applied directly over the catheter insertion site to protect the infusion site. Easy access to the IV site for frequent (1- to 2-hour) assessments must be considered. Improvised plastic cups that are cut in half with the ridged edges covered with tape should not be used, since they have injured patients. A commercial site protector, I.V. House, is available in different sizes (Fig. 45-21). Its ventilation holes prevent moisture from accumulating under the dome (Lee & Vallino, 1996). This device is designed to protect the IV site; allow for visibility of the site; minimize use of padded boards, splints, or other restraints and tape; and maintain skin integrity. The connector tubing or extension tubing can be looped to make it small enough to fit under the protective cover to prevent accidental snagging of the catheter. It is important to safely secure the IV tubing to prevent infants and children from becoming entangled in the tubing or from accidentally pulling the catheter or needle out. Securing the tubing in this manner also eliminates movement of the catheter hub at the insertion site (mechanical manipulation). A colorful and interesting sticker can be applied to the protecting device to add a positive note to the procedure.

Finger or toe areas are left unoccluded by dressings or tape to allow for assessment of circulation. The thumb is never immobilized because of the danger of contractures with limited movement later on. An extremity should never be encircled with tape. The use of roll gauze, self-adhering stretch bandages (Coban), and Ace bandages can cause the same constriction and hide signs of infiltration (Infusion Nurses Society, 2000a).

Removal of a Peripheral Intravenous Line

When it comes time to discontinue an IV infusion, many children are distressed by the thought of catheter removal. Therefore they need a careful explanation of the process and suggestions for helping. Encouraging children to remove or help remove the tape from the site provides them with a measure of control and often fosters their cooperation. The procedure consists of turning off any pump apparatus, occluding the IV tubing, removing the tape, pulling the catheter out of the vessel in the opposite direction of insertion, and exerting firm pressure at the site. A dry dressing (adhesive bandage strip) is placed over the puncture site. The use of adhesive-removal pads can decrease the pain of tape removal, but the skin should be washed after use to avoid irritation. To remove transparent dressings (e.g., OpSite, Tegaderm), pull the opposing edges parallel to the skin to loosen the bond. Inspect the catheter tip to ensure the catheter is intact and that no portion remains in the vein.

NURSING ALERT Consider the child's age, development, neurologic status, and predictability (how the child responds to painful treatments) when determining the need for assistance to maintain safety. Manual removal of tape is the preferred method. Only if absolutely necessary should a small cut be made in the tape, using bandage scissors, to facilitate its removal. Before cutting the tape:

- Ensure that all digits are visible.
- Remove any barrier that hinders visibility, such as a protective covering.
- Protect the child's skin and digits by sliding own finger(s) between the tape and the child's skin so that the scissors do not touch the patient.
- Place a cut on the tape located on the medial aspect (thumb side) of the extremity.

Complications

The same precautions regarding maintenance of asepsis, prevention of infection, and observation for infiltration are carried out with patients of any age. However, infiltration is more difficult to detect in infants and small children than in adults. The increased amount of subcutaneous fat and the amount of tape used to secure the catheter often obscure the early signs of infiltration. When the fluid appears to be infusing too slowly or ceases, the usual assessment for obstruction within the apparatus—kinks, screw clamps, shutoff valve, and positioning interference (e.g., a bent elbow)—often locates the difficulty. When these actions fail to detect the problem, it may be necessary to carefully remove some of the dressing to obtain a clear view of the venipuncture site. Dependent areas, such as the palm and undersides of the extremity or the occiput and behind the ears, are examined.

Whenever possible, the IV infusion should be placed in an extremity to which the identification band (or bracelet) is not attached. Serious circulatory impairment can result from infiltrated solution distal to the band, which acts as a tourniquet, preventing adequate venous return. To check for return blood flow through the catheter, the tubing is removed from the infusion pump, and the bag is lowered below the level of the infusion site. Resistance during flushing or aspiration for blood return also indicates that the IV infusion may have infiltrated surrounding tissue. A good blood return, or lack thereof, is not always an indicator of infiltration in small infants. Flushing the catheter and observing for edema, redness, or streaking along the vein are appropriate for assessment of the IV.

IV therapy in pediatrics tends to be difficult to maintain because of mechanical factors such as vascular trauma resulting from the catheter, the insertion site, vessel size, vessel fragility, pump pressure, the patient's activity level, operator skill and insertion technique, forceful administration of boluses of fluid, and infusion of irritants or vesicants through a small vessel (Pettit & Hughes, 1999). These factors cause infiltration and extravasation injuries. *Infiltration* is defined as inadvertent administration of a nonvesicant solution or medication into surrounding tissue. *Extravasation* is defined as inadvertent administration of vesicant solution or medication into surrounding tissue (Infusion Nurses Society, 2000a, 2000b). A *vesicant* or *sclerosing agent* causes varying degrees of cellular damage when even minute amounts escape into surrounding tissue. Guidelines are available for determining the severity of tissue injury by staging characteristics, such as the amount of redness, blanching, the amount of swelling, pain, the quality of pulses below infiltration, capillary refill, and warmth or coolness of the area (Infusion Nurses Society, 2000a, 2000b; Montgomery et al, 1999).*

Treatment of infiltration or extravasation varies according to the type of vesicant. Guidelines are available outlining the sequence of interventions and specific treatment of infiltration or extravasation with antidotes (Oncology Nursing Society, 1998; Montgomery et al, 1999).†

NURSING ALERT When infiltration or extravasation is observed (signs include erythema, pain, edema, blanching, streaking on the skin along the vein, and darkened area at the insertion site), immediately stop the infusion, elevate the

**Guidelines for determining tissue injury severity are available from the Infusion Nurses Society, 315 Norwood Park South, Norwood, MA 02062; 781-440-9408; fax: 781-440-9409;* www.ins1.org.

†Guidelines on interventions for infiltration and extravasation are available from the Oncology Nursing Society, 125 Enterprise Drive, Pittsburgh, PA 15275; 866-257-4ONS or 412-859-6100; fax: 412-859-6162; www.ons.org.

extremity, notify the practitioner, and initiate the ordered treatment as soon as possible. Remove the IV line when it is no longer needed (e.g., after infusing an antidote).

Procedures for Maintaining Respiratory Function

Inhalation Therapy

Oxygen Therapy

Oxygen is administered for hypoxemia and may be delivered by mask, nasal cannula, tent, hood, face mask, or ventilator. Oxygen therapy is frequently administered in the hospital, although increasing numbers of children are receiving oxygen in the home. Oxygen delivered to infants is well tolerated by using a *plastic hood* (Fig. 45-22). The humidified oxygen should not be blown directly into the infant's face. Older, cooperative infants and children can use a *nasal cannula* or *prongs*, which can supply a concentration of oxygen of about 50%. A *mask* is not well tolerated by children.

For children beyond early infancy, the *oxygen tent* is a satisfactory means for administration of oxygen (Fig. 45-23). A tent does not require any device to come into direct contact with the face, but the concentration of oxygen within the tent is difficult to control and to maintain above 30% to 50%. A major difficulty with the use of the tent is keeping the tent closed so that the oxygen concentration is maintained.

To reduce oxygen loss, nursing care is planned carefully so that the tent is opened as little as possible. Because oxygen is heavier than air, loss will be greater at the bottom of the tent; therefore the tent is tucked in snugly without open edges. The bottom of the tent should be examined more often when the child is restless and fussy and liable to pull the covers loose. Some tents are even open at the top. Because of the rapidly diffusing qualities of carbon dioxide, the levels of the gas do not build up within these enclosures.

After the tent has been opened for an extended period, it is flushed with oxygen by increasing the flow meter for a few minutes to quickly raise the oxygen and mist concentration. The flow meter is then reset to the prescribed number of liters per minute.

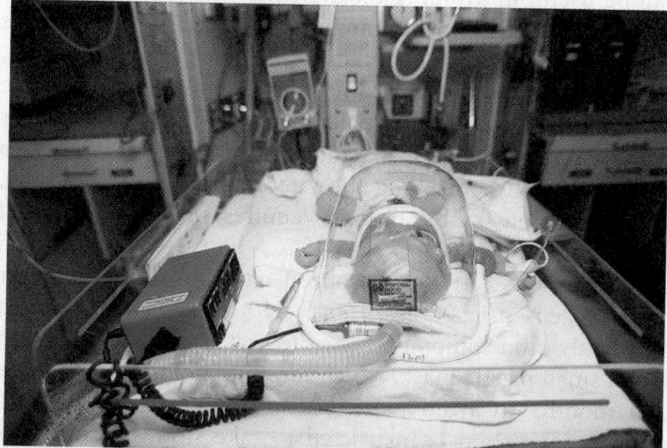

Fig. 45-22 Oxygen administered to infant by means of a plastic hood. Note oxygen analyzer (*blue machine*).

The enclosed tent becomes warm; therefore some type of cooling mechanism is provided. The temperature inside the tent must be checked periodically to be certain that it is maintained at the desired level. Although the cool environment can reduce fever and airway inflammation, it can also produce hypothermia and cold stress. It is important to make certain that the child is kept warm and dry. Because oxygen is drying to the tissues, the gas is humidified, which causes moisture to condense on the tent walls.

NURSING ALERT Keep the child warm and dry by checking the temperature inside the tent and the child's bedding and clothing frequently. Adjust the temperature and change clothing as often as needed.

In some instances the child can be removed from the oxygen tent for activities such as feeding and bathing, whereas in other cases the child is placed in the tent only during periods of rest. Still other children may require oxygen continuously and can be removed from the tent or incubator only if an oxygen source is held close to the child's face. Any change in color, increased respiratory effort, or restlessness is an indication to return the child to the oxygen tent.

Oxygen Toxicity

Prolonged exposure to high oxygen tensions can damage some body tissues and functions. The organs most vulnerable to the adverse effects of excessive oxygenation are the retina of the extremely preterm infant and the lungs of persons at any age.

Oxygen-induced carbon dioxide narcosis is a physiologic hazard of oxygen therapy that may occur in persons with chronic pulmonary disease, such as cystic fibrosis. In these patients the respiratory center has adapted to the continuously higher arterial carbon dioxide tension ($Paco_2$) levels, and therefore hypoxia becomes the more powerful stimulus for respiration. When the arterial oxygen tension (Pao_2) level is elevated during oxygen administration, the hypoxic drive is removed, causing progressive hypoventilation and increased

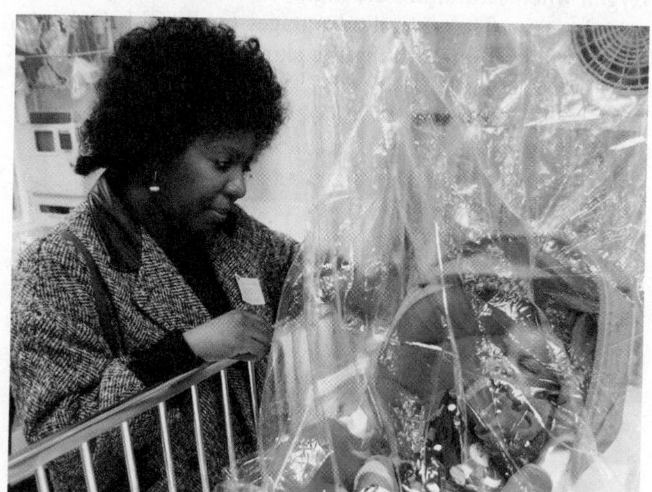

Fig. 45-23 The tent provides a comfortable method for oxygen administration. (From Wilson SF, Thompson JM: *Respiratory disorders*, St Louis, 1990, Mosby.)

$Paco_2$ levels, and the child rapidly becomes unconscious. Carbon dioxide narcosis can also be induced by the administration of sedation in these patients.

Monitoring Oxygen Therapy

Pulse oximetry is a continuous, noninvasive method of determining oxygen saturation (Sao_2) to guide oxygen therapy. A sensor composed of a light-emitting diode (LED) and a photodetector is placed in opposition around a foot, hand, finger, toe, or earlobe, with the LED placed on top of the nail when digits are used (Fig. 45-24). The diode emits red and infrared lights that pass through the skin to the photodetector. The photodetector measures the amount of each type of light absorbed by functional hemoglobins. Hemoglobin saturated with oxygen (oxyhemoglobin) absorbs more infrared light than does hemoglobin not saturated with oxygen (deoxyhemoglobin). Pulsatile blood flow is the primary physiologic factor that influences accuracy of the pulse oximeter. In infants, reposition the probe at least every 3 to 4 hours to prevent pressure necrosis; poor perfusion and very sensitive skin may necessitate more frequent repositioning.

Another noninvasive method is *transcutaneous monitoring (TCM),* which provides continuous monitoring of transcutaneous partial pressure of oxygen in arterial blood ($tcPao_2$) and, with some devices, of carbon dioxide in arterial blood ($tcPaco_2$). An electrode is attached to the warmed skin to facilitate arterialization of cutaneous capillaries. The site of the electrode must be changed every 3 to 4 hours to avoid burning the skin, and the machine must be calibrated with every site change. TCM is used frequently in neonatal intensive care units, but it may not reflect Pao_2 in infants with impaired local circulation or in older infants whose skin is thicker.

evolve Skill—Measuring Oxygen Saturation

Oximetry is insensitive to hyperoxia because hemoglobin approaches 100% saturation for all Pao_2 readings greater than approximately 100 mm Hg, which is a dangerous situation for the preterm infant at risk for developing retinopathy of prematurity (see Chapter 27). Therefore the preterm infant being monitored with oximetry should have upper limits identified, such as 90% to 95%, and a protocol established for decreasing oxygen when saturations are high.

Oximetry offers several advantages over TCM. Oximetry (1) does not require heating the skin, thus reducing the risk of burns; (2) eliminates a delay period for transducer equilibration; and (3) maintains an accurate measurement regardless of the patient's age or skin characteristics or the presence of lung disease.

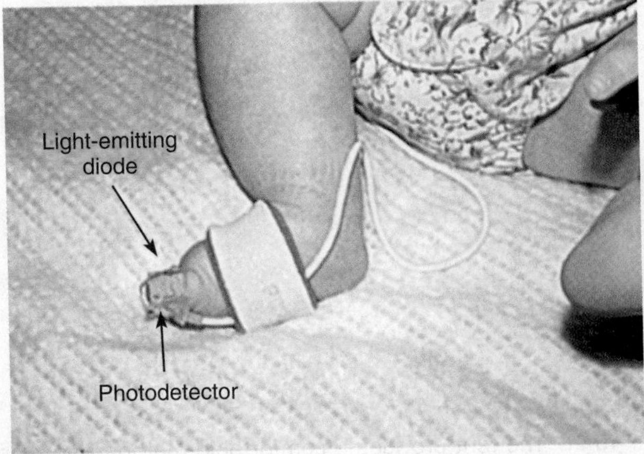

Fig. 45-24 Pulse oximeter sensor. Note the sensor is positioned with light-emitting diode (LED) opposite photodetector.

NURSING ALERT It is important to make certain that sensor connectors and oximeters are compatible. Wiring that is incompatible can generate considerable heat at the tip of the sensor, causing second- and third-degree burns under the sensors. Pressure necrosis can also occur from sensors attached too tightly. Therefore inspect the skin under the sensor frequently.

Applying the sensor correctly is essential for accurate Sao_2 measurements. Because the sensor must identify every pulse beat to calculate the Sao_2, movement can interfere with sensing. Some devices synchronize the Sao_2 reading with the heartbeat, thereby reducing the interference caused by motion. Sensors are not placed on extremities used for blood pressure monitoring or with indwelling arterial catheters, since pulsatile blood flow may be affected.

Infant—Secure the sensor to the great toe and tape the wire to the sole of the foot (or use a commercial holder that fastens with a self-adhering closure). Place a snugly fitting sock over the foot, but check the site frequently for color, temperature, and pulse.

Child—Secure the sensor securely to the index finger and tape the wire to the back of the hand.

Ambient light from ceiling lights and phototherapy, as well as high-intensity heat and light from radiant warmers, can interfere with readings. Therefore the sensor should be covered to block these light sources. IV dyes; green, purple, or black nail polish; nonopaque synthetic nails; and possibly ink used for footprinting can also cause inaccurate Sao_2 measurements. The dyes should be removed or, in the case of porcelain nails, a different area used for the sensor. Skin color, thickness, and edema do not affect the readings.

Aerosol Therapy

Aerosol therapy can be effective in depositing medication directly into the airway. The value of aerosolized water, or "mist therapy," is controversial. This route of administration can be useful in avoiding the systemic side effects of certain drugs and in reducing the amount of drug necessary to achieve the desired effect. Bronchodilators, steroids, and antibiotics, suspended in particulate form, can be inhaled so that the medication reaches the small airways. Aerosol therapy is particularly challenging in children who are too young to cooperate with controlling the rate and depth of breathing. Administration of this therapy requires skill, patience, and creativity.

Medications can be aerosolized or nebulized with air or with oxygen-enriched gas. *Handheld nebulizers* are the most frequently used equipment. The medicated mist is discharged into a small plastic mask, which the child holds over the nose and mouth. To avoid particle deposition in the nose and pharynx, the child is instructed to take slow, deep breaths through an open mouth during the treatment. For home use an air compressor is necessary to force air through the liquid medication to form the aerosol. Compact, portable units can be obtained from health equipment companies. The *metered-dose inhaler (MDI)* is a self-contained, handheld device that allows for intermittent delivery of a specified amount of medication. Many bronchodilators are available in this form and are successfully used by children with asthma. For children under the age of 5 or 6 years, a *spacer device* attached to the MDI can help with coordination of breathing and aerosol delivery. It allows the aerosolized particles to remain in suspension longer. (See also Asthma, Chapter 46.)

Assessment of breath sounds and work of breathing should be done before and after treatments. Young children who become upset by having a mask held close to the face may become fatigued with fighting the procedure and may actually appear worse during and immediately after the therapy. It may be necessary to spend a few minutes calming the child after the procedure and allowing the vital signs to return to baseline to accurately assess changes in breath sounds and work of breathing.

Bronchial (Postural) Drainage

Bronchial drainage is indicated whenever excessive fluid or mucus in the bronchi is not being removed by normal ciliary activity and cough. Positioning the child to take maximum advantage of gravity facilitates removal of secretions. Postural drainage can be effective in children with chronic lung disease characterized by thick mucus, such as cystic fibrosis.

Postural drainage is carried out three or four times daily and is more effective when it follows other respiratory therapy, such as bronchodilator or nebulization medication. Bronchial drainage is generally performed before meals (or 1 to 1½ hours after meals) to minimize the chance of vomiting and is repeated at bedtime. The duration of treatment depends on the child's condition and tolerance; it usually lasts 20 to 30 minutes. Several positions facilitate drainage from all major lung segments; all positions are not employed at each session. Children will usually cooperate for four to six positions. Older children can tolerate longer periods.

In the hospital an older child can be positioned over an elevated knee rest. Small children and infants can be positioned with pillows or on the therapist's lap and legs. Infants should not be placed in the Trendelenburg position because they do not have an autonomic regulation of blood flow to the head. Special modifications of the techniques are required in children whose conditions, such as head injuries, some types of surgical incisions or burns, and casts, contraindicate the standard positioning.

Chest physical therapy (CPT) usually refers to the use of postural drainage in combination with adjunctive techniques that are thought to enhance the clearance of mucus from the airway. These techniques include manual percussion, vibration, and squeezing of the chest; cough; forceful expiration; and breathing exercises. Special mechanical devices (e.g., ThAIRapy Vest) are also currently used to perform CPT. Postural drainage in combination with forced expiration has been shown to be beneficial. Noninvasive inspiratory nasal pressure–support ventilation during CPT has demonstrated a significant improvement in respiratory muscle performance and a reduction in oxygen desaturation (Fauroux et al, 1999).

The most common technique used in association with postural drainage is manual percussion of the chest wall. The patient is dressed in a lightweight shirt and placed in a postural drainage position. CPT is contraindicated when patients have pulmonary hemorrhage, pulmonary embolism, end-stage renal disease, increased intracranial pressure, osteogenesis imperfecta, or minimal cardiac reserves.

Artificial Ventilation

Artificial Airways

An artificial airway is usually used in association with mechanical ventilation and in children with upper airway obstruction. Endotracheal intubation can be accomplished by the nasal (nasotracheal), oral (orotracheal), or direct tracheal (tracheostomy) routes. Although it is more difficult to place, nasotracheal intubation is preferred to orotracheal intubation because it facilitates oral hygiene and provides more stable fixation, which reduces the complication of tracheal erosion and the danger of accidental extubation. Only uncuffed endotracheal tubes should be used in children younger than 8 years of age (Curley & Moloney-Harmon, 2001). Air or gas delivered directly to the trachea must be humidified.

Tracheostomy

A tracheostomy is a surgical opening in the trachea; the procedure may be done on an emergency basis or may be an elective one, and it may be combined with mechanical ventilation. Pediatric tracheostomy tubes are usually made of plastic or Silastic (Fig. 45-25). The most common types are the Hollinger, Jackson, Aberdeen, and Shiley tubes. These tubes are constructed with a more acute angle than adult tubes, and they soften at body temperature, conforming to the contours of the trachea. Because these materials resist the formation of crusted respiratory secretions, they are made without an inner cannula.

Children who have undergone a tracheostomy must be closely monitored for complications such as hemorrhage, edema, aspiration, accidental decannulation, tube obstruction, and the entrance of free air into the pleural cavity. Nursing care focuses on maintaining a patent airway, facilitating the removal of pulmonary secretions, providing humidified air or oxygen, cleansing the stoma, monitoring the child's

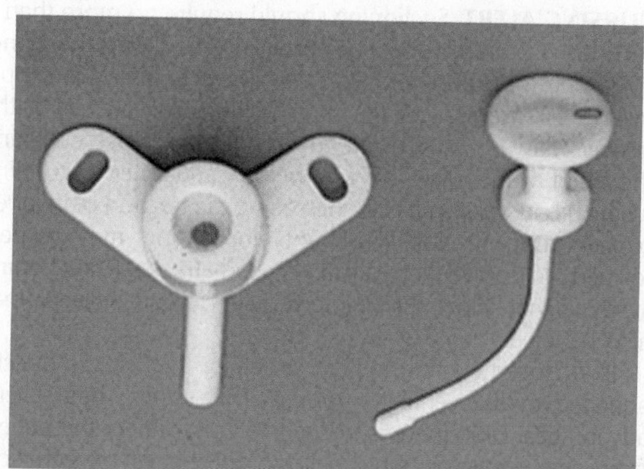

Fig. 45-25 Silastic pediatric tracheostomy tube and obturator.

ability to swallow, and teaching while simultaneously preventing complications.

Because the child may be unable to signal for help, direct observation and use of respiratory and cardiac monitors are essential. Respiratory assessments include breath sounds and work of breathing, vital signs, tightness of the tracheostomy ties, and the type and amount of secretions. Large amounts of bloody secretions are uncommon and should be considered a sign of hemorrhage. The practitioner should be notified immediately if this occurs.

The child is positioned with the head of the bed raised or in the position most comfortable to the child, with the call light easily available. Suction catheters, suction source, gloves, sterile saline, sterile gauze for wiping away secretions, scissors, an extra tracheostomy tube of the same size with ties already attached, another tracheostomy tube one size smaller, and the obturator are kept at the bedside. A source of humidification is provided because the normal humidification and filtering functions of the airway have been bypassed. IV fluids ensure adequate hydration until the child is able to swallow sufficient amounts of fluids.

Suctioning

The airway must remain patent and requires frequent suctioning during the first few hours after a tracheostomy to remove mucous plugs and excessive secretions. Proper vacuum pressure and suction catheter size are important to prevent atelectasis and decrease hypoxia from the suctioning procedure. Vacuum pressure should range from 60 to 100 mm Hg for infants and children and from 40 to 60 mm Hg for preterm infants. Unless secretions are thick and tenacious, the lower range of negative pressure is recommended. Tracheal suction catheters are available in a variety of sizes. The catheter selected should have a diameter one-half the diameter of the tracheostomy tube. If the catheter is too large, it can block the airway. The catheter is constructed with a side port so that the catheter is introduced without suction and removed while simultaneous intermittent suction is applied by covering the port with the thumb (Fig. 45-26). The catheter is inserted to 0.5 cm beyond or just to the end of the tracheostomy tube. The practice of instilling sterile saline in the tracheostomy tube before suctioning is not supported by research and is no longer recommended (see Evidence-Based Practice box).

NURSING ALERT Suctioning should require no more than 5 seconds. Counting one one-thousand, two one-thousand, three one-thousand, and so on while suctioning is a simple means for monitoring the time. Without a safeguard, the airway may be obstructed for too long. Hyperventilating the child with 100% oxygen before and after suctioning (using a bag-valve-mask or increasing the fraction of inspired oxygen concentration [FiO_2] ventilator setting) may be performed to prevent hypoxia. Closed tracheal suctioning systems that allow for uninterrupted oxygen delivery may also be used.

In a closed suction system, a suction catheter is directly attached to the ventilator tubing. This system has several advantages. First, there is no need to disconnect the patient from the ventilator, which allows for better oxygenation. Second, the suction catheter is enclosed in a plastic sheath, which reduces the risk of the nurse being exposed to the patient's secretions (Carroll, 1998).

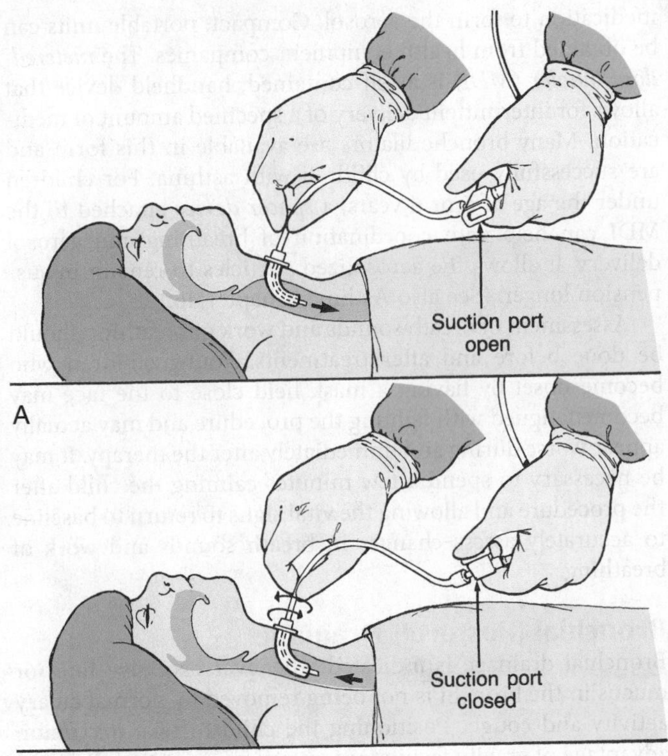

Fig. 45-26 Tracheostomy suctioning. **A**, Insertion, port open. **B**, Withdrawal, port occluded. Note that catheter is inserted just slightly beyond end of tracheostomy tube.

The child is allowed to rest for 30 to 60 seconds after each aspiration to allow oxygen saturation to return to normal; then the process is repeated until the trachea is clear. Suctioning should be limited to about three aspirations in one period. Oximetry is used to monitor suctioning and prevent hypoxia.

NURSING ALERT Suctioning is carried out only as often as needed to keep the tube patent. Signs of mucus partially occluding the airway include an increased heart rate, a rise in respiratory effort, a drop in SaO_2, cyanosis, and an increase in the positive inspiratory pressure on the ventilator.

In the acute care setting, aseptic technique is used during care of the tracheostomy. Secondary infection is a major concern, since the air entering the lower airway bypasses the natural defenses of the upper airway. Gloves are worn during the aspiration procedure, although a sterile glove is needed only on the hand touching the catheter. A new tube, gloves, and sterile saline solution are used each time.

Routine Care

The tracheostomy stoma requires daily care. Assessments of the stoma area include observations for signs of infection and breakdown of the skin. The skin is kept clean and dry, and crusted secretions around the stoma may be gently removed with half-strength hydrogen peroxide. Hydrogen peroxide should not be used with sterling silver tracheostomy tubes

EVIDENCE-BASED PRACTICE Normal Saline Instillation Before Suctioning—Helpful or Harmful?

—Marilyn J. Hockenberry

Ask the Question

In intubated children and those with tracheostomy, is normal saline instillation before suctioning helpful or harmful?

Search for Evidence

Search Strategies

English-language publications and research-based articles on suctioning intubated children and those with a tracheostomy

Databases Searched

PubMed, Cochrane Collaboration, MD Consult, BestBETs, PedsCCM

Critically Analyze the Evidence

Instillation of normal saline before endotracheal (ET) tube suctioning has been used for years as a method to loosen and dilute secretions, lubricate the suction catheter, and promote cough. In recent years the possible adverse effects of this procedure have been explored. Adult studies have found decreased oxygen saturation, increased frequency of nosocomial pneumonia, and increased intracranial pressure after instillation of normal saline before suctioning (O'Neal et al, 2001; Kinlock, 1999; Hagler & Traver, 1994; Reynolds et al, 1990; Ackerman, 1993; Ackerman & Gugerty, 1990; Bostick & Wendelgass, 1987).

Two of the first research studies evaluating the effect of normal saline instillation before suctioning in neonates found no deleterious effects. Shorten, Byrne, and Jones (1991) found no significant differences in oxygenation, heart rate, or blood pressure before or after suctioning in a group of 27 intubated neonates. In a second study of nine neonates acting as their own controls, no adverse effects on lung mechanics were found after normal saline instillation and suctioning (Beeram & Dhanireddy, 1992).

A study evaluating the effects of normal saline instillation before suctioning in children found results similar to those in the previously published adult studies. Ridling, Martin, and Bratton (2003) evaluated the effects of normal saline instillation before suctioning in a group of 24 critically ill children, ages 10 weeks to 14 years (level 1 evidence). A total of 104 suctioning episodes were analyzed. Children experienced significantly greater oxygen desaturation after suctioning if normal saline was instilled.

The American Thoracic Society's (2005) official position statement on the care of children with tracheostomies now states that normal saline should not be instilled before suctioning.

Apply the Evidence: Nursing Implications

Studies support that the adverse effects of normal saline instillation before suctioning in children are similar to those found for adults. This technique causes a significant reduction in oxygen saturation that can last up to 2 minutes after suctioning. The evidence does not support the use of normal saline instillation before ET suctioning in children.

References

Ackerman MH: The effect of saline lavage prior to suctioning, *Am J Crit Care* 2(4):326-330, 1993.

Ackerman MH, Gugerty B: The effect of normal saline bolus instillation in artificial airways, *Journal: Society of Otorhinolaryngology Head-Neck Nurses* 8(2):14-17, 1990.

American Thoracic Society: *Care of the child with a chronic tracheostomy*, 2005. Available at www.thoracic.org/sections/publications/statements/pages/respiratory-disease-pediatric/childtrach1-12.html (accessed April 17, 2006).

Beeram MR, Dhanireddy R: Effects of saline instillation during tracheal suction on lung mechanics in newborn infants, *J Perinatol* 12(2):120-123, 1992.

Bostick J, Wendelgass ST: Normal saline instillation as part of the suctioning procedure: effects of Pao2 and amount of secretions, *Heart Lung* 16(5):532-537, 1987.

Hagler DA, Traver GA: Endotracheal saline and suction catheters: sources of lower airway contamination, *Am J Crit Care* 3(6):444-447, 1994.

Kinlock D: Instillation of normal saline during endotracheal suctioning: effects on mixed venous oxygen saturation, *Am J Crit Care* 8(4):231-240, 1999.

O'Neal PV et al: Level of dyspnoea experienced in mechanically ventilated adults with and without saline instillation prior to endotracheal suctioning, *Intensive Crit Care Nurs* 17(6):356-363, 2001.

Reynolds P et al: Effects of normal saline instillation on secretion volume, dynamic compliance, and oxygen saturation (abstract), *Am Rev Respir Dis* 141:A574, 1990.

Ridling DA, Martin LD, Bratton SL: Endotracheal suctioning with or without instillation of isotonic sodium chloride in critically ill children, *Am J Crit Care* 12(3):212-219, 2003.

Shorten DR, Byrne PJ, Jones RL: Infant responses to saline instillations and endotracheal suctioning, *J Obstet Gynecol Neonatal Nurs* 20(6):464-469, 1991.

because it tends to pit and stain the silver surface. The nurse should be aware of wet tracheostomy dressings, which can predispose the peristomal area to skin breakdown. Several products are available to prevent or treat excoriation. The Allevyn tracheostomy dressing is a hydrophilic sponge with a polyurethane back that is highly absorptive. Other possible barriers to help maintain skin integrity include the use of hydrocolloid wafers (e.g., DuoDERM CGF, Hollister Restore) under the tracheostomy flanges, as well as extra-thin hydrocolloid wafers under the chin.

The tracheostomy tube is held in place with tracheostomy ties made of a durable, nonfraying material. The ties are changed daily and when soiled. New ties are looped through the flanges and tied snugly in a triple knot at the side of the neck *before* the soiled ties are cut and removed. Some nurses have found that threading the ties through a piece of ¼-inch surgical tubing cushions the ties; others have found the tubing irritating to the skin. The ties should be tight enough to allow just a fingertip to be inserted between the ties and the neck (Fig. 45-27). It is easier to ensure a snug fit if the child's head is flexed rather than extended while the ties are being secured. Ties fastened with self-adhering closures are also available. These devices, such as the Dale tracheostomy tube holder, are made of a soft, cushioning, and slightly stretchy material that is very comfortable. They are becoming increasingly popular because of their ease of use and ability to maintain better skin

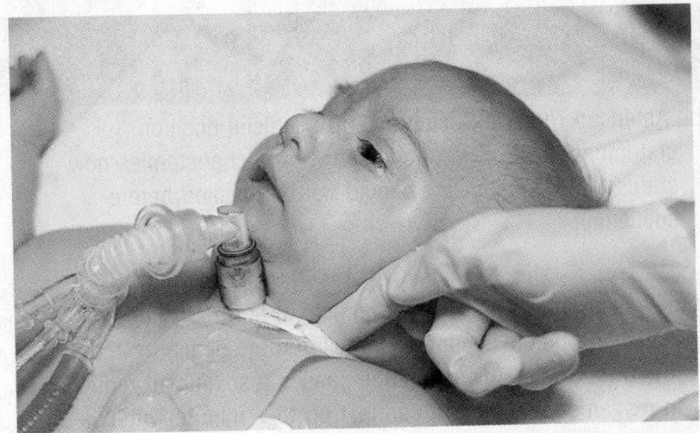

Fig. 45-27 Tracheostomy ties are snug but allow one finger to be inserted.

integrity. However, nurses and family members must consider the safety factor and use them only on a child who will not pull and undo the fastener.

Routine tracheostomy tube changes are usually carried out weekly after a tract has been formed to minimize the formation of granulation tissue. The first change is usually performed by the surgeon; subsequent changes are performed by the nurse and, if the child is discharged home with the tracheostomy, by either a parent or a visiting nurse. Ideally, two caregivers participate in the procedure to assist with positioning the child.

Changing the tracheostomy tube is accomplished using sterile technique. Tube changes should occur before meals or 2 hours after the last meal. Continuous feedings should be turned off at least an hour before a tube change. The new, sterile tube is prepared by inserting the obturator and attaching new ties. The child is suctioned before the procedure to minimize secretions, then restrained and positioned with the neck slightly extended. One caregiver cuts the old ties and removes the tube from the stoma. The new tube is inserted gently into the stoma (using a downward and forward motion that follows the curve of the trachea), the obturator is removed, and the ties are secured. The adequacy of ventilation must be assessed after a tube change because the tube can be inserted into the soft tissue surrounding the trachea; therefore breath sounds and respiratory effort are carefully monitored.

Supplemental oxygen is always delivered with a humidification system to prevent drying of the respiratory mucosa. Humidification of room air for an established tracheostomy can be intermittent if secretions remain thin enough to be coughed or suctioned from the tracheostomy. Direct humidification via a tracheostomy mask can be provided during naps and at night so that the child is able to be up and around unencumbered during much of the day. Room humidifiers are also used successfully.

The inner cannula, if used, should be removed with each suctioning, cleaned with sterile saline and pipe cleaners to remove crusted material, dried thoroughly, and reinserted.

Emergency Care: Tube Occlusion and Accidental Decannulation

Occlusion of the tracheostomy tube is life threatening, and infants and children are at greater risk than adults because of the smaller diameter of the tube. Patency of the tube is maintained with suctioning and routine tube changes to prevent the formation of crusts that can occlude the tube.

NURSING ALERT Life-threatening occlusion is apparent when the child displays signs of respiratory distress and a suction catheter cannot be passed to the end of the tube despite several attempts and instillation of saline. This situation requires an immediate tube change.

Accidental decannulation also requires immediate tube replacement. Some children have a fairly rigid trachea, so the airway remains partially open when the tube is removed. However, others have malformed or flexible tracheal cartilage, which causes the airway to collapse when the tube is removed or dislodged. Because many infants and children with upper airway problems have little airway reserve, if replacement of the dislodged tube is impossible, a smaller-sized tube should be inserted. If the stoma cannot be cannulated with another tracheostomy tube, oral intubation should be performed.

Procedures Related to Alternative Feeding Techniques

Some children are unable to take nourishment by mouth because of anomalies of the throat, esophagus, or bowel; impaired swallowing capacity; severe debilitation; respiratory distress; or unconsciousness. These children are frequently fed by way of a tube inserted orally or nasally into the stomach *(orogastric* or *nasogastric gavage)* or duodenum-jejunum *(enteral gavage)*, or by a tube inserted directly into the stomach *(gastrostomy)* or jejunum *(jejunostomy)*. Such feedings may be intermittent or by continuous drip.

Feeding resistance is a problem that may result from any long-term feeding method that bypasses the mouth. During gavage or gastrostomy feedings, infants are given a pacifier. Nonnutritive sucking has several advantages, such as increased weight gain and decreased crying. However, to prevent the possibility of aspiration, only pacifiers with a safe design may be used. Using improvised pacifiers made from bottle nipples is not a safe practice.

NURSING ALERT When a child is concurrently receiving continuous-drip gastric or enteral feedings and parenteral (IV) therapy, the potential exists for inadvertent administration of the enteral formula through the circulatory system, especially when the parenteral solution is a fat emulsion, which looks milky. Safeguards to prevent this potentially serious error include:

- Use a separate, specifically designed enteral feeding pump mounted on a separate pole for continuous-feeding solutions.
- Label all tubing for continuous enteral feeding with brightly colored tape or labels.
- Use specifically designed continuous-feeding bags to contain the solutions instead of parenteral equipment, such as a burette.

Gavage Feeding

Infants and children can be fed simply and safely by a tube passed into the stomach through either the nares or the mouth. The tube can be left in place or inserted and removed with each feeding. In older children it is usually less traumatic to tape the tube securely in place between feedings. When this alternative is used, the tube should be removed and replaced with a new tube according to hospital policy, specific orders, and the type of tube used. Meticulous handwashing is practiced during the procedure to prevent bacterial contamination of the feeding, especially during continuous-drip feedings (see Atraumatic Care box).

ATRAUMATIC CARE

Reducing the Distress of Nasogastric Tube Insertion

Numerous strategies can be used to decrease discomfort during nasogastric (NG) tube insertion. Most important, the nurse performing the procedure should be competent in NG tube placement. The nurse should discuss the procedure with the child in a developmentally appropriate way and give family members the details of what to expect during the procedure. Administration of sedation and analgesia should be considered before NG insertion. The use of topical lidocaine and phenylephrine for the nose and tetracaine and benzocaine spray for the throat before NG insertion has been found to reduce pain and discomfort in a group of adult patients (Singer & Konia, 1999). A smaller-caliber, soft, flexible tube should be used. To prevent the trauma of reinsertion, make certain the NG tube is well secured after placement.

Data from Maglinte C: Strategies for reducing the pain and discomfort of nasogastric intubation, *Acad Emerg Med* 6(3):166-168, 1999.

Not all feeding tubes are the same. Polyethylene and polyvinylchloride types lose their flexibility and need to be replaced frequently, usually every 3 or 4 days. The polyurethane and silicone tubes are indwelling and remain flexible, so they can remain in place longer and afford more patient comfort. Use of these small-bore tubes for continuous feeding has reduced the incidence of complications such as pharyngitis, otitis media, and incompetence of the lower esophageal sphincter. Although the increased softness and flexibility of the tubes are advantages, they also have disadvantages such as difficult insertion (may require a stylet or metal guidewire), collapse of the tube during aspiration of gastric contents to test for correct placement, dislodgment during forceful coughing, and unsuitability for thick feedings. Traditional methods for verifying placement are less reliable with the small-bore tubes.

Infants will be easier to control if they are first wrapped in a mummy restraint (see Fig. 45-7). Even tiny infants with random movements can grasp and dislodge the tube. Preterm infants do not ordinarily require restraint, but if they do, a small blanket folded across the chest and secured beneath the shoulders is usually sufficient. Care must be taken so that breathing is not compromised.

Whenever possible, the infant should be held and provided a means of nonnutritive sucking during the procedure to associate the comfort of physical contact with the feeding. When this is not possible, gavage feeding is carried out with the infant or child on the back or toward the right side with the head and chest elevated. Feeding the child in a sitting position helps maintain the placement of the tube in the lowest position, thus increasing the likelihood of correct placement in the stomach (see Guidelines box).

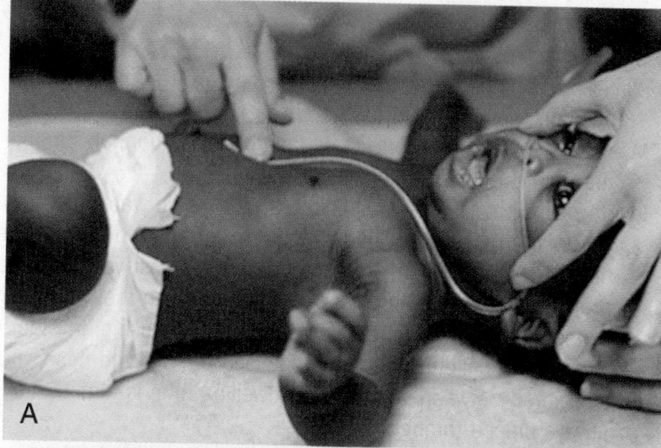

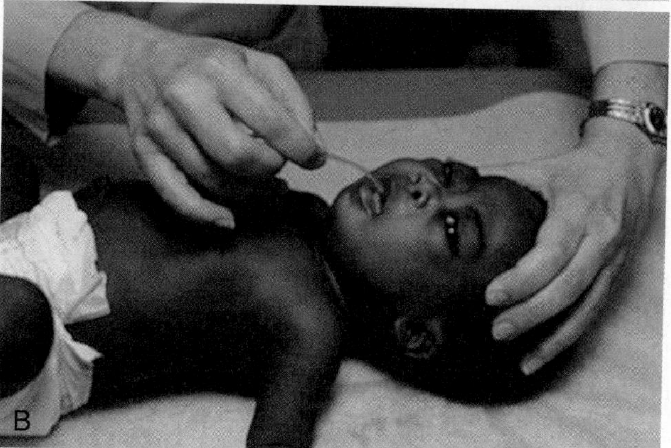

Fig. 45-28 Gavage feeding. **A,** Measuring tube for orogastric feeding from tip of nose to earlobe and to midpoint between end of xiphoid process and umbilicus. **B,** Inserting tube.

Table 45-6 Recommended Minimum Insertion Lengths for Orogastric Tubes in Very-Low-Birth-Weight Infants

	Daily Weight (g)			
	<750	750-999	1000-1249	1250-1499
Insertion length (cm)	13	15	16	17

From Gallaher KJ et al: Orogastric tube insertion length in very-low-birth-weight infants (<1500 g), *J Perinatol* 13(2):128-131, 1993.

Two standard methods of measuring tube length for insertion are (1) measuring from the nose to the bottom of the earlobe and then to the end of the xiphoid process or (2) measuring from the nose to the earlobe and then to a point midway between the xiphoid process and the umbilicus (Fig. 45-28, *A*). For very-low-birth-weight infants, weight can be used to predict insertion length (Table 45-6). See Evidence-Based Practice box for placement verification techniques.

GUIDELINES Nasogastric Tube Feedings in Children

Place child supine with head slightly hyperflexed or in a sniffing position (nose pointed toward ceiling).

Measure the tube for approximate length of insertion, and mark the point with a small piece of tape.

Insert a tube that has been lubricated with sterile water or water-soluble lubricant through either the mouth or one of the nares to the predetermined mark. Because most young infants are obligatory nose breathers, insertion through the mouth causes less distress and helps to stimulate sucking. In older infants and children the tube is passed through the nose and alternated between nostrils. An indwelling tube is almost always placed through the nose.

- When using the nose, slip the tube along the base of the nose and direct it straight back toward the occiput.
- When entering through the mouth, direct the tube toward the back of the throat (see Fig. 45-28, *B*).
- If the child is able to swallow on command, synchronize passing the tube with swallowing.
- Confirm placement by x-ray examination, if available. Document pH and color of aspirate (see Evidence-Based Practice box, p. 1297).

Stabilize the tube by holding or taping it to the cheek, not to the forehead, because of possible damage to the nostril. To maintain correct placement, measure and record the amount of tubing extending from the nose or mouth to the distal port when the tube is first positioned. Recheck this measurement before each feeding.

Warm the formula to room temperature. Do not microwave! Document pH and color of aspirate before each feeding to confirm tube placement. Pour formula into the barrel of the syringe attached to the feeding tube. To start the flow, give a gentle push with the plunger, but then remove the plunger and allow the fluid to flow into the stomach by gravity. The rate of flow should not exceed 5 ml every 5 to 10 minutes in preterm and very small infants and 10 ml/min in older infants and children to prevent nausea and regurgitation. The rate is determined by the diameter of the tubing and the height of the reservoir containing the feeding and is regulated by adjusting the height of the syringe. A usual feeding may take 15 to 30 minutes to complete.

Flush the tube with sterile water (1 or 2 ml for small tubes to 5 to 15 ml or more for large ones), or see discussion of flushing for administering medication through nasogastric tubes in the Guidelines box (p. 1283), to clear it of formula.

Cap or clamp indwelling tubes to prevent loss of feeding. If the tube is to be removed, first pinch it firmly to prevent escape of fluid as the tube is withdrawn. Withdraw the tube quickly.

Position the child with the head elevated about 30 degrees and on the right side or abdomen for at least 1 hour in the same manner as after any infant feeding to minimize the possibility of regurgitation and aspiration. If the child's condition permits, bubble the youngster after the feeding.

Record the feeding, including the type and amount of residual, the type and amount of formula, and how it was tolerated.

For most infant feedings, any amount of residual fluid aspirated from the stomach is refed to prevent electrolyte imbalance, and the amount is subtracted from the prescribed amount of feeding. For example, if the infant is to receive 30 ml and 10 ml is aspirated from the stomach before the feeding, the 10 ml of aspirated stomach contents is refed along with 20 ml of feeding. Another method can be used in children. If residual fluid is more than one fourth of the last feeding, return the aspirate and recheck in 30 to 60 minutes. When residual fluid is less than one fourth of the last feeding, give the scheduled feeding. If large amounts of aspirated fluid persist and the child is due for another feeding, notify the practitioner.

Gastrostomy Feeding

Feeding by way of a gastrostomy tube is a variation of tube feeding that is often used for children in whom passage of a tube through the mouth, pharynx, esophagus, and cardiac sphincter of the stomach is contraindicated or impossible. It is also used to avoid the constant irritation of a gastric tube in children who require tube feeding over an extended period. Placement of a gastrostomy tube may be performed with the patient under general anesthesia or percutaneously using an endoscope with the patient sedated and under local anesthesia (percutaneous endoscopic gastrostomy [PEG]). The tube is inserted through the abdominal wall into the stomach about midway along the greater curvature and, when surgically placed, is secured by a purse-string suture. The stomach is anchored to the peritoneum at the operative site. The tube used can be a Foley, wing-tip, or mushroom catheter. Immediately after surgery the catheter is left open and attached to gravity drainage for 24 hours or more.

Postoperative care of the wound site is directed toward prevention of infection and irritation. The area is cleansed at least daily or as often as needed to keep the area free of drainage. After healing takes place, meticulous care is needed to keep the area surrounding the tube clean and dry to prevent excoriation and infection. Daily applications of antibiotic ointment or other preparations may be prescribed to aid in healing and prevent irritation. Care is exercised to prevent excessive pull on the catheter that might cause widening of the opening and subsequent leakage of highly irritating gastric juices. The tube is securely taped to the abdomen, leaving a small loop of tubing at the exit site to prevent tension on the site.

Granulation tissue may grow around a gastrostomy site (Fig. 45-29). This moist, beefy red tissue is not a sign of infection. However, if it continues to grow, the excess moisture can irritate the surrounding skin.

For children receiving long-term gastrostomy feeding, a *skin-level device* (e.g., MIC-KEY, Bard Button) offers several advantages. The small, flexible silicone device protrudes slightly from the abdomen, is cosmetically pleasing in appearance, affords increased comfort and mobility to the child, is easy to care for, and is fully immersible in water. The one-way valve at the proximal end minimizes reflux and eliminates the need for clamping. However, the button requires a well-established gastrostomy site and is more expensive than the conventional tube. In addition, the valve may become clogged.

EVIDENCE-BASED PRACTICE Assessing Correct Placement of Nasogastric or Orogastric Tubes in Children

—Marilyn J. Hockenberry

Ask the Question

In children, how do we assess for correct placement of nasogastric or orogastric tubes?

Search for Evidence

Search Strategies

English-language publications, research-based articles (level 3 or lower), children or adult populations, comparisons to gold standard (x-ray examination)

Databases Searched

PubMed, Cochrane Collaboration, MD Consult, Joanna Briggs Institute, National Guideline Clearinghouse (AHQR), TRIP Database Plus, PedsCCM, BestBETs

Critically Analyze the Evidence

Studies compared various methods used to evaluate placement of the tube with the gold standard, x-ray examination. Nine articles were found, with five adult and four child sample populations:

- pH-assisted feeding tubes, child (Krafte-Jacobs et al, 1996)
- Bilirubin, adult and child (Westhus, 2004; Metheny et al, 1999; Metheny, Smith, & Stewart, 2000)
- Enzyme tests, child and adult (Westhus, 2004; Metheny et al, 1997)
- Bedside sonography for tube placement, adult (Hernandez-Socorro et al, 1996)
- Aspiration of insufflated air for tube placement, adult (Neumann et al, 1995; Harrison et al, 1997)

Most reliable tests for determining tube placement in the nine published studies (other than the gold standard of x-ray examination) were the combination of:

- pH testing (Huffman et al, 2004; Metheny et al, 1999; Westhus, 2004; Gharpure et al, 2000)
- Visual inspection of aspirate
- Bilirubin and enzyme tests

Bilirubin and enzyme measures are not currently available at the bedside.

Sensitivity and specificity of the bedside tests for children need further evaluation.

Auscultation is an unreliable method to confirm tube placement because of the similarity of sounds produced by air in the bronchus, esophagus, or pleural space.

Apply the Evidence: Nursing Implications

Use x-ray to confirm initial placement. Document pH and color of aspirate with initial placement.

A pH of 5 or less supports the conclusion that the tip of the tube is in a gastric location.

A pH greater than 5 does not reliably predict the correct distal tip location. It may indicate respiratory or esophageal placement, or presence of medications to suppress acid secretion.

If pH is greater than 5, use other measures to evaluate tube placement. If bilirubin and enzyme testing is not available, check color of aspirate. Gastric contents are clear, off-white, or tan; they may be brown tinged if blood is present. Respiratory secretions may look the same. Intestinal contents are often bile stained, light to dark yellow, or greenish brown. It may also be necessary to obtain an x-ray.

A change in pH may indicate tube dislodgment. Check external markings and tube length to ensure tube has not moved. If uncertain about placement, obtain an x-ray.

pH and color of aspirate can be checked before medication or feeding. For continuous feedings, it is recommended that tube placement be checked every 4 hours.

A *Visual Bilirubin Scale*, effective in determining bilirubin content in feeding tube aspirates, has been published (Metheny, Smith, & Stewart, 2000). Evaluation of the accuracy of the scale is needed with children.

Risk factors for improper tube placement are comatose or semicomatose state, swallowing problems, and recurrent retching or vomiting.

Experience of the individual inserting the tube is always important.

References

Gharpure V et al: Indicators of postpyloric feeding tube placement in children, *Crit Care Med* 28(8):2962-2966, 2000.

Harrison AM et al: Nonradiographic assessment of enteral feeding tube position, *Crit Care Med* 25(12):2055-2059, 1997.

Hernandez-Socorro CR et al: Bedside sonographic-guided versus blind nasoenteric feeding tube placement in critically ill patients, *Crit Care Med* 24(10):1690-1694, 1996.

Huffman S et al: Methods to confirm feeding tube placement: application of research in practice, *Pediatr Nurs* 30(1):10-13, 2004.

Krafte-Jacobs B et al: Rapid placement of transpyloric feeding tubes: a comparison of pH-assisted and standard insertion techniques in children, *Pediatrics* 98(2 Pt 1):242-248, 1996.

Metheny NA, Smith L, Stewart BJ: Development of a reliable and valid bedside test for bilirubin and its utility for improving prediction of feeding tube location, *Nurs Res* 49(6):302-309, 2000.

Metheny NA et al: pH and concentration of bilirubin in feeding tube aspirates as predictors of tube placement, *Nurs Res* 48(4):189-197, 1999.

Metheny NA et al: pH and concentrations of pepsin and trypsin in feeding tube aspirates as predictors of tube placement, *JPEN* 21:279-285, 1997.

Neumann MJ et al: Hold that x-ray: aspirate pH and auscultation prove tube placement, *J Clin Gastroenterol* 20(4):293-295, 1995.

Westhus N: Methods to test feeding tube placement in children, *MCN Am J Maternal/Child Nurs* 29(5):282-291, 2004.

When functioning, the valve prevents air from escaping; therefore the child may require frequent bubbling. With some devices, during feedings the child must remain fairly still because the tubing easily disconnects from the opening if the child moves. With other devices, extension tubing can be securely attached to the opening (Fig. 45-30). The feeding is instilled at the other end of the tubing in a manner similar to that for a regular gastrostomy. The extension tubing may also have a separate medication port. Both the feeding and the medication ports have plugs attached. Some skin-level devices require a special tube to decompress the stomach (to check residual or release air).

Feeding of water, formula, or pureed foods is carried out in the same manner and rate as in gavage feeding. A mechanical pump may be used to regulate the volume and rate of feeding. After feedings, the infant or child is positioned on the

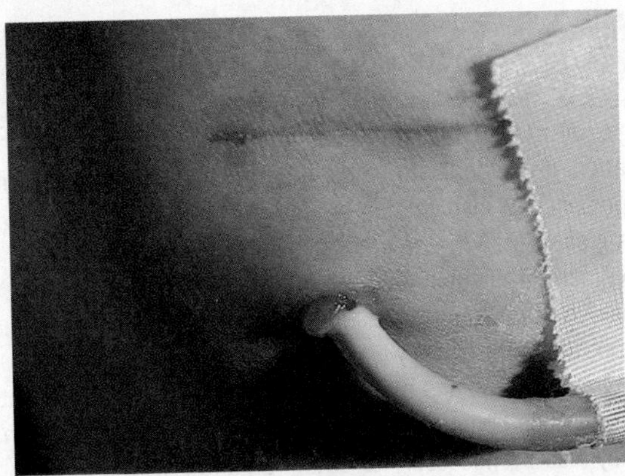

Fig. 45-29 Appearance of healthy granulation tissue around stoma.

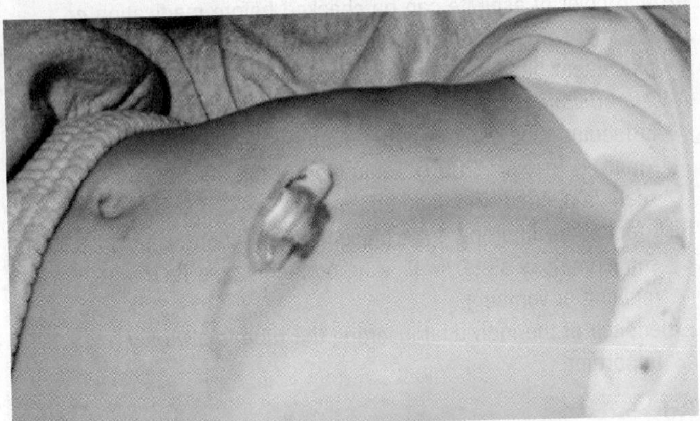

Fig. 45-30 Child with skin-level gastrostomy device (MIC-KEY), which provides for secure attachment of extension tubing to gastrostomy opening.

right side or in Fowler's position, and the tube may be clamped or left open and suspended between feedings, depending on the child's condition. A clamped tube allows more mobility but is appropriate only if the child can tolerate intermittent feedings without vomiting or prolonged backup of feeding into the tube. Sometimes a Y tube is used to allow for simultaneous decompression during feeding. If a Foley catheter is used as the gastrostomy tube, very slight tension is applied. The tube is securely taped to maintain the balloon at the gastrostomy opening to prevent leakage of gastric contents and to prevent the tube's progression toward the pyloric sphincter, where it may occlude the stomach outlet. As a precaution, the length of the tube should be measured postoperatively and then remeasured each shift to be certain it has not slipped. A mark can be made above the skin level to further ensure its placement. When the gastrostomy tube is no longer needed, it is removed; the skin opening usually closes spontaneously by contracture.

Nasoduodenal and Nasojejunal Tubes

Children at high risk for regurgitation or aspiration such as those with gastroparesis, mechanical ventilation, or brain injuries may require placement of a postpyloric feeding tube. Insertion of a nasoduodenal or nasojejunal tube is done by a trained practitioner because of the risk of misplacement and potential for perforation in tubes requiring a stylet. Accurate placement is verified by radiography. Small-bore tubes may easily clog. Flush tube when feeding is interrupted, before and after medication administration, and routinely every 4 hours or as directed by institutional policy. Tube replacement should be considered monthly to ensure optimal tube patency. Continuous feedings are delivered by mechanical pump to regulate volume and rate. Bolus feeds are contraindicated. Tube displacement is suspected in the child showing signs of feeding intolerance such as vomiting. Stop feedings and notify the practitioner.

Total Parenteral Nutrition

TPN provides for the total nutritional needs of infants or children when feeding by the gastrointestinal tract is impossible, inadequate, or hazardous. Some common conditions include chronic intestinal obstruction, inadequate intestinal length, and prophylactically after surgery or during critical illness.

TPN therapy involves IV infusion of highly concentrated solutions of carbohydrates, lipids, amino acids, vitamins, minerals, water, trace elements, and other additives in a single container (Teitelbaum et al, 2005). The highly concentrated solutions require infusion into a vessel with sufficient volume and turbulence to allow for rapid dilution. The wide-diameter vessels selected are the superior vena cava and innominate or intrathoracic subclavian veins approached by way of the external or internal jugular veins. The highly irritating nature of concentrated glucose precludes the use of the small peripheral veins in most instances. However, dilute glucose-protein hydrolysates that are appropriate for infusing into peripheral veins are being used with increasing frequency.

The major nursing responsibilities are the same as for any IV therapy: control of sepsis, monitoring of the infusion rate, and assessment of the patient's tolerance of the solution. The TPN solution must be prepared under sterile conditions. The infusion is maintained at a constant rate by an infusion pump. The TPN infusion rate should not be increased or decreased without the practitioner being informed, since alterations can cause hyperglycemia or hypoglycemia.

General assessments, such as vital signs, I&O measurements, and laboratory tests, facilitate early detection of infection or fluid and electrolyte imbalance. Hyperglycemia may occur during the first day or two as the child adapts to the high-glucose load of the hyperalimentation solution. Although hyperglycemia occurs infrequently, insulin may be required to assist the body's adjustment. To prevent hypoglycemia at the time the hyperalimentation is disconnected, the rate of the infusion and the amount of insulin are decreased gradually.

Family Teaching and Home Care

When alternative feedings are needed for an extended period, the family may need to learn how to feed the child with a nasogastric, gastrostomy, or TPN feeding regimen. Because of the numerous skills the family must learn for home TPN, ample time must be allowed for the family to learn and perform the procedures under supervision before assuming full responsibility for the child's care.

Procedures Related to Elimination

Enema

The procedure for giving an enema to an infant or child does not differ essentially from that for an adult, except for the type and amount of fluid administered and the distance for inserting the tube into the rectum. Depending on the volume, a syringe with rubber tubing, an enema bottle, or an enema bag should be used (see Guidelines box).

GUIDELINES Administration of Enemas to Children

Age	Amount (ml)	Insertion Distance
Infant	120-240	2.5 cm (1 inch)
2-4 yr	240-360	5 cm (2 inches)
4-10 yr	360-480	7.5 cm (3 inches)
11 yr	480-720	10 cm (4 inches)

An isotonic solution is used in children. Plain water is not used because, being hypotonic, it can cause rapid fluid shift and fluid overload. The Fleet enema (pediatric or adult sized) is not advised for children because of the harsh action of its ingredients (sodium biphosphate and sodium phosphate). Commercial enemas can be dangerous to patients with megacolon and to dehydrated or azotemic children. The osmotic effect of the Fleet enema may produce diarrhea, which can lead to metabolic acidosis. Other potential complications are extreme hyperphosphatemia, hypernatremia, and hypocalcemia, which may lead to neuromuscular irritability and coma (Walton et al, 2000).

Because infants and young children are unable to retain the solution after it is administered, the buttocks must be held together for a short time to retain the fluid. The enema is administered and expelled while the child is lying with the buttocks over the bedpan and with the head and back supported by pillows. Older children are usually able to hold the solution if they understand what to do and if they are not expected to hold it for too long. The nurse should have the bedpan handy or, for the ambulatory child, ensure that the bathroom is available before beginning the procedure. An enema is an intrusive procedure and thus threatening to the preschool child; therefore a careful explanation is especially important to ease possible fear.

A preoperative bowel preparation solution given orally or through a nasogastric tube is increasingly being used instead of an enema. The polyethylene glycol–electrolyte lavage solution (GoLYTELY) mechanically flushes the bowel without significant absorption, thereby avoiding potential fluid and electrolyte imbalance. Another effective oral cathartic is magnesium citrate solution.

Ostomies

Children may require stomas for various health problems. The most frequent causes in the infant are necrotizing enterocolitis and imperforate anus (less often, Hirschsprung's disease). In the older child the most frequent causes are inflammatory bowel disease, especially Crohn's disease (regional enteritis), and ureterostomies for distal ureter or bladder defects.

Care and management of ostomies in the older child differ little from the care of ostomies in the adult patient. The major emphases in pediatric care are preparing the child for the procedure and teaching care of the ostomy to the child and family. The basic principles of preparation are the same as for any procedure (see p. 1247). Simple, straightforward language is most effective, together with the use of illustrations and a replica model (e.g., drawing a picture of a child with a stoma on the abdomen and explaining it as "another opening where bowel movements [or any other term the child uses] will come out"). At another time the nurse can draw a pouch over the opening to demonstrate how the contents are collected. Using a doll to demonstrate the process is an excellent teaching strategy, and special books are available.

Children with ileostomies are fitted immediately after surgery with an appliance to protect the skin from the proteolytic enzymes in the liquid stool. Infants may not be fitted with a pouch in the immediate postoperative period. When stomal drainage is minimal, a gauze dressing will suffice. Parents are usually given a choice of caring for the colostomy with or without an appliance. Pediatric appliances are available in a variety of sizes to ensure an adequate fit.

Ostomy equipment consists of a one- or two-piece system with a hypoallergenic skin barrier to maintain peristomal skin integrity. The pouch should be large enough to contain a moderate amount of stool and flatus but not so large as to overwhelm the infant or child. A backing helps minimize the risk of skin breakdown from moisture trapped between the skin and pouch. Small clips or rubber bands should be avoided to prevent choking in the young child. Granulation tissue may grow around an ostomy site (see Fig. 45-29). This moist, beefy red tissue is not a sign of infection. However, if it continues to grow, the excess moisture can irritate the surrounding skin.

Protection of the peristomal skin is a major aspect of stoma care. Well-fitting appliances are important to prevent leakage of contents. Before the appliance is applied, the skin is prepared with a skin sealant that is allowed to dry. Then stoma paste is applied around the base of the stoma or the back of the wafer. The sealant and paste work together to prevent peristomal breakdown.

In infants with a colostomy left unpouched, skin care is similar to that of any diapered infant. However, the peristomal skin is protected with a wafer barrier, such as a hydrocolloid dressing (e.g., DuoDERM) or a barrier substance (e.g., zinc oxide ointment [Desitin], or a mixture of the zinc oxide ointment and stoma [Stomahesive] powder). A gauze dressing may be applied over the stoma and wafer to absorb stomal drainage. If the skin becomes inflamed, denuded, or infected, the care is similar to the interventions used for diaper dermatitis (see Chapter 53). A product that helps protect healthy skin, heal excoriated skin, and minimize pain associated with skin breakdown is Proshield Plus. The skin protectant adheres to denuded, weeping skin. Proshield Plus can be applied over topical antifungal and antibacterial agents if infection is present. No Sting Barrier Film is a skin sealant that has no alcohol base and can be used on open skin without stinging.

With young children, protecting the pouch from being pulled off is also an important consideration. One-piece outfits keep exploring hands from reaching the pouch, and the loose waist prevents any pressure on the appliance. Keeping the child occupied with toys during the pouch change is also helpful. As children mature, their participation in ostomy care is encouraged. Even preschoolers can assist by holding supplies, pulling paper backings from the appliance, and helping clean the stoma area. Toilet training for bladder control needs to begin at the appropriate time as for any other child.

Older children and adolescents should eventually have total responsibility for ostomy care just as they would for usual bowel function. During adolescence, concerns for body image and the ostomy's impact on intimacy and sexuality emerge. The nurse should stress to teenagers that the presence of a stoma need not interfere with their activities. These youngsters can choose which ostomy equipment is best suited to their needs. Attractively designed and decorated pouch covers are well liked by teenagers.

An enterostomal therapy nurse specialist is an important member of the health care team and will have additional suggestions and skin care information and ostomy pouching options. Further information may be obtained by contacting the Wound, Ostomy and Continence Nurses Society.*

Family Teaching and Home Care

Because these children are almost always discharged with a functioning colostomy, preparation of the family should begin as early as possible in the hospital. The family is instructed in the application of the device (if used), care of the skin, and appropriate action in case skin problems develop. Early evidence of skin breakdown or stomal complications, such as ribbonlike stools, excessive diarrhea, bleeding, prolapse, or failure to pass flatus or stool, is brought to the attention of the physician, the nurse, or the stoma specialist. The same principles are applied as discussed earlier in this chapter for compliance, especially in terms of education (p. 1254), and in Chapter 44 for discharge planning and home care.

*888-224-9626; www.wocn.org.

Key Points

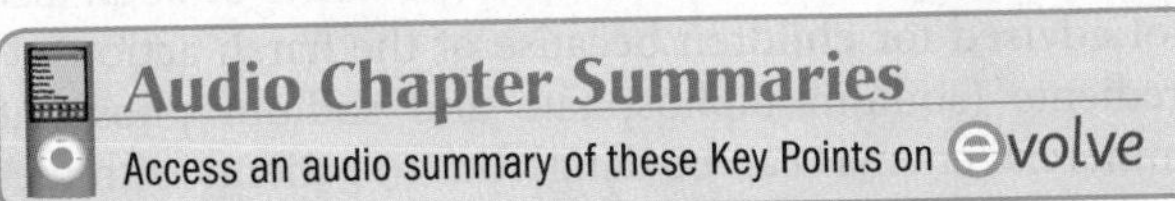
Audio Chapter Summaries
Access an audio summary of these Key Points on evolve

- Informed consent is valid when the person is capable of giving consent (is over the age of majority and is competent), is supplied with information needed to make an intelligent decision, and acts voluntarily when exercising freedom of choice.
- Informed consent is needed for major surgery, minor surgery, and diagnostic tests and medical treatments with an element of risk.
- The major principles in psychologic preparation of the child for procedures are to establish trust, provide support, and give an explanation in easy-to-understand terms.
- Preparation for procedures should be based on developmental characteristics of the child and family, emphasizing the importance of the parents' role.
- Most parents and children want to be together during stressful procedures and should be offered this opportunity, with guidance on how the parent can comfort the child.
- In performing a procedure, the nurse should expect success, involve the child when possible in the procedure, provide distraction, and allow for expression of feelings.
- Proper positioning of infants and small children for procedures is essential to minimize movement and discomfort.
- In giving postprocedural support, the nurse should encourage children to express feelings and should give praise for completion of the procedure.
- Stressful times before and after surgery that produce anxiety in children are admission, blood tests, injection of preoperative medication (if used), transportation to the operating room, and return from the PACU.
- Assessment of compliance entails measuring factors that affect compliance through clinical judgment, self-reporting, direct observation, monitoring of appointments and therapeutic response, pill counts, and chemical assays.
- Compliance strategies may be classified as organizational, educational, and behavioral.
- Knowledge of the ill child's eating habits and favorite foods can help in maintaining adequate nutrition.
- Skin care is essential to prevent skin breakdown.
- Control of fever may be accomplished by administration of antipyretics; hyperthermia is controlled by environmental means (minimum clothing, increased air circulation, hypothermia mattress, or cool compresses).
- Infection control is based on two systems. Standard Precautions provide protection when the infected person is undiagnosed. Transmission-based precautions add extra interventions for patients diagnosed with or suspected of having an infection.
- Ensuring safety in the hospital setting is a major concern and can be achieved through environmental measures, limit setting, infection control, and safe transportation.
- Restraints are used cautiously and require a medical order. Therapeutic hugging can avoid the use of restraints.
- Factors that affect drug dosage determination are growth and maturation, difficulty in evaluating drug response, and BSA.
- Family teaching regarding medication administration includes telling parents why the child is receiving the drug; its possible effects; and the amount, frequency, and length of time the drug is to be administered.

- The preferred sites for intramuscular injection in children are the vastus lateralis and ventrogluteal areas.
- Intermittent venous access is accomplished by a peripheral intermittent infusion device, a peripherally inserted central catheter, a central venous catheter, or an implanted port.
- Several safety catheters and needleless device systems are available to reduce the risk of needlestick injuries in patients and caregivers.
- Nursing assessment of fluid and electrolyte disturbances entails observation of general appearance, vital signs, and measurement of I&O.
- Oxygen can be administered by hood, mask, nasal cannula, incubator, or oxygen tent.
- Tracheostomy suctioning involves premeasured insertion of the catheter, application of suction for 5 seconds when withdrawing the catheter, and supplemental oxygen before and after suctioning.
- Alternative forms of feeding include gavage feeding, gastrostomy feeding, and TPN.
- In the care of children with ostomies, nurses play an important role in family support and instruction in care of the stoma site.

References

Algren C, Algren J: Pediatric sedation essentials for the preoperative nurse, *Nurs Clin North Am* 32(1):17-30, 1997.

Algren C, Ireland D, Stewart E: Perioperative and perianesthesia care of the child. In Albers AC, Schwartz P (editors): *Comprehensive care of the pediatric patient: prehospital through rehabilitation*, Park Ridge, IL, 1998, Emergency Nurses Association.

American Academy of Pediatrics: Consent for emergency medical services for children and adolescents, *Pediatrics* 111(3):703-705, 2003.

Anderson SL, Schaechter J, Brosco JP: Adolescent patients and their confidentiality: staying within legal bounds, *Contemp Pediatr* 22(7):54, 2005.

Axelrod P: External cooling in the management of fever, *Clin Infect Dis* 31(Suppl 5):S224-S229, 2000.

Berg AT et al: Childhood-onset epilepsy with and without preceding febrile seizures, *Neurology* 53(8): 1742-1748, 1999.

Berger JE, AAP Committee on Medical Liability: Consent by proxy for nonurgent pediatric care, *Pediatrics* 112(5):1186-1195, 2003.

Blass EM, Watt L: Suckling- and sucrose-induced analgesia in human newborns, *Pain* 83(3):611-623, 1999.

Broome M: Consent (assent) for research with pediatric patients, *Semin Oncol Nurs* 15(2):96-103, 1999.

Broome M, Rehwaldt M, Fogg L: Relationship between cognitive behavioral techniques, temperament, observed distress, and pain reports in children and adolescents during lumbar puncture, *J Pediatr Nurs* 13(1):48-54, 1998.

Bryant RA, Doughty D, editors: *Acute and chronic wounds: nursing management*, ed 2, St Louis, 2000, Mosby.

Burke N: Alternative methods for newborn urine sample collection, *Pediatr Nurs* 21(6):546-549, 1995.

Calianno C: Patient hygiene, part II, Skin care: keeping the outside healthy, *Nursing* 29(12 Suppl):1-11, 1999.

Carroll P: Closing in on safer suctioning, *RN* 61(5):22-27, 1998.

Catudal R: Pediatric IV therapy: actual practice, *J Vasc Access Devices* 4(2):27-29, 1999.

Cohen HA et al: Urine samples from disposable diapers: an accurate method for urine cultures, *J Fam Pract* 44(3):290-292, 1997.

Cook IF, Murtagh J: Ventroluteal area: a suitable site for intramuscular vaccination of infants and toddlers, *Vaccine* 24(13):2403-2408, 2006.

Cook IF, Murtagh J: Needle length required for intramuscular vaccination of infants and toddlers: an ultrasonographic study, *Aust Fam Physician* 31(3):295-297, 2002.

Curley MAQ, Moloney-Harmon PA: *Critical care nursing of infants and children*, ed 2, Philadelphia, 2001, Saunders.

Dubick MA, Holcomb JB: A review of intraosseous vascular access: current status and military application, *Mil Med* 165(7):552-559, 2000.

Eaton L: Hand washing is more important than cleaner wards in controlling MRSA, *BMJ* 330(7497):922, 2005.

Eckler J: Combating infection, *Nursing* 27(10):20, 1997.

Essink-Tebbes CM et al: Safety of lidocaine-prilocaine cream application four times a day in premature neonates: a pilot study, *Eur J Pediatr* 158(5):421-423, 1999.

Fauroux B et al: Chest physiotherapy in cystic fibrosis: improved tolerance with nasal pressure support ventilation, *Pediatrics* 103(3):E32, 1999.

Fennell ME: Parents in the OR? You bet! *RN* 62(12):38-40, 1999.

Fisher AA et al: The use of alteplase for restoring patency to occluded central venous access devices in infants and children, *J Infus Nurs* 27(3):171-174, 2004.

Gamulka B, Mendoza C, Connolly B: Evaluation of a unique, nurse-inserted, peripherally inserted central catheter program, *Pediatrics* 115(6): 1602-1606, 2005.

Gray L, Watt L, Blass EM: Skin-to-skin contact is analgesic in healthy newborns, *Pediatrics* 105(1):110-111, 2000. Available at www.pediatrics.org/cgi/content/full/105/1/E14 (accessed July 7, 2007).

Gray M: Atraumatic urethral catheterization of children, *Pediatr Nurs* 22(4):306-310, 1996.

Hall PA et al: Parents in the recovery room: survey of parental and staff attitudes, *BMJ* 310(6973):163-164, 1995.

Harris J, Maguire D: Developing a protocol to prevent and treat pediatric central venous catheter occlusions, *J Intraven Nurs* 22(4):194-198, 1999.

Infusion Nurses Society: *Policies and procedures for infusion nursing*, Norwood, MA, 2000a, The Society.

Infusion Nurses Society: Revised infusion nursing standards of practice, *J Intraven Nurs* 23(6 Suppl):S17, S39, S41, S45, S49-S50, S60, 2000b.

Institute for Safe Medication Practices: Problems persist with life-threatening tubing misconnections, *ISMP Medication Safety Alert* June 17, 2004. Available at www.ismp.org/newsletters/acutecare/articles/20040617.asp (accessed June 15, 2009).

Ipp MM et al: Adverse reactions to diphtheria, tetanus, pertussis–polio vaccination at 18 months of age: effect of injection site and needle length, *Pediatrics* 83(5):679-682, 1989.

Joint Commission on Accreditation of Healthcare Organizations: *2009 Hospital accreditation standards*, Oakbrook Terrace, IL, 2009, Joint Commission Resources.

Kain Z, Caldwell-Andrews A, Wang S: Psychological preparation of the parent and pediatric surgical patient, *Anesthesia Clin North Am* 20(1):29-44, 2002.

Kain ZN et al: Trends in the practice of parental presence during induction of anesthesia and the use of preoperative sedative premedication in the United States, 1995-2002: results of a follow-up national survey, *Anesth Analg* 98(5):1252-1259, 2004.

Katsma D, Smith G: Analysis of needle path during intramuscular injection, *Nurs Res* 46(5):288-292, 1997.

Kellam B et al: Tenderfoot Preemie vs a manual lancet: a clinical evaluation, *Neonatal Netw* 20(7):31-36, 2001.

Kennedy D: Medication "safety checks" in pediatric acute care, *J Intraven Nurs* 19(6):295-302, 1996.

Klein EJ et al: A randomized, clinical trial of oral midazolam plus placebo versus oral midazolam plus oral transmucosal fentanyl for sedation during laceration repair, *Pediatrics* 109(5):894-897, 2002.

Kraus D et al: Effectiveness and infant acceptance of the Rx Medibottle versus the oral syringe, *Pharmacotherapy* 21(4):416-423, 2001.

KyngAs H, Kroll T, Duffy M: Compliance in adolescents with chronic diseases: a review, *J Adolesc Health* 26:379-388, 2000.

Landsman IS, Cook DR: Pediatric anesthesia. In O'Neill J et al (editors): *Pediatric surgery*, St Louis, 1998, Mosby.

LaRosa-Nash PA, Murphy JM: An approach to pediatric perioperative care: parent-present induction, *Nurs Clin North Am* 32(1):183-199, 1997.

Larsson BA et al: Alleviation of the pain of venipuncture in neonates, *Acta Paediatr* 87(7):774-779, 1998.

Lee WE, Vallino LM: Intravenous insertion site protection: moisture accumulation in intravenous site protectors, *J Intraven Nurs* 29(4):194-197, 1996.

Liebman M, Barnsteiner J: Fever education: does it reduce parent fever anxiety? *Pediatr Emerg Care* 17(1):47-51, 2001.

Maki DG: Infections caused by intravascular devices used for infusion therapy: pathogenesis, prevention, and management. In Bisno AL, Waldvogel FA (editors): *Infections associated with indwelling medical devices*, ed 2, Washington, DC, 1994, American Society for Microbiology.

Manworren R, Fledderman M: Preparation of the child and family for surgery. In Wise BV et al (editors):

Nursing care of the general pediatric surgical patient, Gaithersburg, MD, 2000, Aspen.

Maxwell LG, Yaster M: Perioperative management issues in pediatric patients, *Anesthesiol Clin North Am* 18(3):601-632, 2000.

Meehan RM: Heelsticks in neonates for capillary blood sampling, *Neonatal Netw* 17(1):17-24, 1998.

Montgomery LA et al: Guidelines for IV infiltrations in pediatric patients, *Pediatr Nurs* 25(2):167-180, 1999.

Moureau N: Practical access, a back-to-basics review of intravenous therapy, *J Vasc Access Devices* 4(2 Suppl):1-4, 1999.

Munro H, D'Errico FC: Parental involvement in perioperative anesthetic management, *J Perianesth Nurs* 15(6):397-400, 2000.

Nelson D: Procedural sedation in the emergency department. In Krauss B, Brustowicz RM (editors): *Pediatric procedural sedation and analgesia*, Philadelphia, 1999, Lippincott Williams & Wilkins.

Oncology Nursing Society: *Cancer chemotherapy guidelines and recommendations for practice*, ed 2, Pittsburgh, 1998, Oncology Nursing Press.

Pettit J, Hughes K: Neonatal intravenous therapy practices, *J Vasc Access Devices* 4:7-16, 1999.

Polillio AM, Killy J: Does a needleless injection system reduce anxiety in children receiving intramuscular injections? *Pediatr Nurs* 23(1):46-49, 1997.

Purssell E: The use of antipyretic medications in the prevention of febrile convulsions in children, *J Pediatr Nurs* 9(4):473-480, 2000.

Quality, equipment hold keys to infection control, *ED Manage* 18(2):19-21, 2006.

Quigley SM, Curley MAQ: Skin integrity in the pediatric population: preventing and managing pressure ulcers, *J Soc Pediatr Nurses* 1(1):7, 1996.

Ratliff CR, Rodheaver GT: Pressure ulcer assessment and management, *Lippincott's Primary Care Pract* 3:242-258, 1999.

Redmond MC: Malignant hyperthermia: perianesthesia recognition, treatment, and care, *J Perianesth Nurs* 16(4):259-270, 2001.

Romino SL et al: Parental presence during anesthesia induction in children, *AORN J* 81(4):780-792, 2005.

Rote N, Huether S, McCance K: Hypersensitivities, infection, and immunodeficiencies. In Huether S, McCance K (editors): *Understanding pathophysiology*, ed 2, St Louis, 2000, Mosby.

Selekman J, Snyder B: Institutional policies on the use of physical restraints on children, *Pediatr Nurs* 23(5):531-537, 1997.

Sharber J: The efficacy of tepid sponge bathing to reduce fever in young children, *Am J Emerg Med* 15(2):188-192, 1997.

Shen V et al: Recombinant tissue plasminogen activator (alteplase) for restoration of function to occluded central venous catheters in pediatric patients, *J Pediatr Hematol Oncol* 25(1):38-45, 2003.

Shepherd AJ et al: A Scottish study of heel-prick blood sampling in newborn babies, *Midwifery* 22(2):158-168, 2006.

Shinnar S et al: Short-term outcomes of children with febrile status epilepticus, *Epilepsia* 42(1):47-53, 2001.

Singer AJ, Konia N: Comparison of topical anesthetics and vasoconstrictors vs lubricants prior to nasogastric intubation: a randomized, controlled trial, *Acad Emerg Med* 6(3):184-190, 1999.

Teitelbaum D et al: Definition of terms, style, and conventions used in A.S.P.E.N. guidelines and standards, *Nutr Clin Pract* 20(2):281-285, 2005.

Tillett J: Adolescents and informed consent: ethical and legal issues, *J Perinatal Neonatal Nurs* 19(2):112-121, 2005.

Van Cleve L, Johnson L, Pothier P: Pain responses of hospitalized infants and children to venipuncture and intravenous cannulation, *J Pediatr Nurs* 11:169-174, 1996.

Vertanen H et al: An automatic incision device for obtaining blood samples from the heels of the preterm infants causes less damage than a conventional manual lancet, *Arch Dis Child Fetal Neonatal Ed* 84:F53-F55, 2001.

Wald ER: To bag or not to bag, *J Pediatr* 174(4):418-419, 2005.

Walton DM et al: Morbid hypocalcemia associated with phosphate enema in a six-week-old infant, *Pediatrics* 106(3):e37, 2000.

Unit 11

46

Respiratory Dysfunction

Learning Objectives

On completion of this chapter the reader will be able to:

- Identify the factors leading to respiratory tract infection in the infant or young child.
- Contrast the effects of various respiratory infections observed in infants and children.
- Describe the postoperative nursing care of the child with an adenotonsillectomy.
- Outline a nursing care plan for a child with croup.
- Outline a nursing care plan for a child with acute otitis media.
- Demonstrate an understanding of the ways in which inhalation of noninfectious irritants produce pulmonary dysfunction.
- Describe the ways in which the various therapeutic measures relieve the symptoms of asthma.
- Outline a plan for teaching home care for the child with asthma.
- Describe the physiologic effects of cystic fibrosis on the gastrointestinal and pulmonary systems.
- Outline a plan of care for the child with cystic fibrosis.
- List the major signs of respiratory distress in infants and children.
- Describe the nursing care for a child with respiratory failure.

Electronic Resources

Additional information related to the content in Chapter 46 can be found on

evolve the Companion Website at http://evolve.elsevier.com/Perry/maternal/

- NCLEX Review Questions
- Anatomy Review—Location of Retractions
- Anatomy Review—Location of Tonsillar Masses
- Animation—Asthma
- Animation—Bag Ventilation
- Animation—Bronchi and Bronchioles
- Animation—Intubation
- Animation—Lung Sounds
- Animation—Respiratory Failure, Infant
- Case Study—Acute Epiglottitis
- Case Study—Bronchiolitis
- Case Study—Cystic Fibrosis
- Case Study—Mononucleosis
- Case Study—Tonsillitis
- Critical Thinking Exercise—Cystic Fibrosis Inheritance Risks
- Critical Thinking Exercise—Ingestion of a Foreign Body
- Nursing Care Plan—The Child with Acute Respiratory Infection
- Nursing Care Plan—The Child with Asthma
- Nursing Care Plan—The Child with Respiratory Failure

Respiratory Infection

General Aspects of Respiratory Infections

Infections of the respiratory tract are described according to the anatomic area of involvement. The *upper respiratory tract,* or *upper airway,* consists of the oronasopharynx, pharynx, larynx, and upper part of the trachea. The *lower respiratory tract* consists of the lower trachea, mainstem bronchi, segmental bronchi, subsegmental bronchioles, terminal bronchioles, and alveoli. In this discussion the trachea is considered with lower tract disorders, and infections of the epiglottis and larynx are categorized as croup syndromes. However, respiratory infections seldom fall into discrete anatomic areas. Infections often spread from one structure to another because of the contiguous nature of the mucous membrane lining the entire tract. Consequently, respiratory tract infections involve several areas rather than a single structure, although the effect on one area may predominate in any given illness.

Etiology and Characteristics

Respiratory infections account for the majority of acute illnesses in children. The etiology and course of these infections are influenced by the age of the child, the season, living conditions, and preexisting medical problems.

Infectious Agents

The respiratory tract is subject to a wide variety of infective organisms. Most infections are caused by viruses, particularly respiratory syncytial virus (RSV), nonpolio enteroviruses (coxsackieviruses A and B), adenoviruses, parainfluenza viruses, and human meta-pneumoviruses. Other agents involved in primary or secondary invasion include group A β-hemolytic streptococci (GABHS), staphylococci, *Haemophilus influenzae, Chlamydia trachomatis, Mycoplasma* organisms, and pneumococci.

Age

Infants younger than age 3 months of age have a lower infection rate than older children, presumably because of the protective function of maternal antibodies. The infection rate increases from 3 to 6 months of age, the time between the disappearance of maternal antibodies and the infant's own antibody production. The viral infection rate remains high during the toddler and preschool years. By 5 years of age, viral respiratory infections are less frequent, but the incidence of *Mycoplasma pneumoniae* and GABHS infections increases.

Some viral agents produce a mild illness in older children but severe lower respiratory tract illness or croup in infants. For example, RSV often causes nothing more than upper respiratory symptoms in older children but can cause severe respiratory compromise in infants.

Size

Anatomic differences influence the response to respiratory tract infections. The diameter of the airways is smaller in young children and subject to considerable narrowing from edematous mucous membranes and increased production of secretions. The distance between structures within the respiratory tract is also shorter in the young child, and organisms may move rapidly down the respiratory tract, causing more extensive involvement. The relatively short and open eustachian tube in infants and young children allows pathogens easy access to the middle ear.

Resistance

The ability to resist invading organisms depends on several factors. Deficiencies of the immune system place the child at risk for infection. Other conditions that decrease resistance are malnutrition, anemia, fatigue, and chilling of the body. Conditions that weaken defenses of the respiratory tract and predispose children to infection also include allergies (e.g., allergic rhinitis), preterm birth, bronchopulmonary dysplasia (BPD), asthma, history of RSV infection, cardiac anomalies that cause pulmonary congestion, and cystic fibrosis (CF). Day care attendance, especially if the caregivers smoke, increases the likelihood of infection.

Seasonal Variations

The most common respiratory pathogens appear in epidemics during the winter and spring months. Mycoplasmal infections occur more often in autumn and early winter. Infection-related asthma (e.g., asthmatic bronchitis) occurs more frequently during cold weather, whereas winter and spring are typically the "RSV seasons."

Clinical Manifestations

Infants and young children, especially those between 6 months and 3 years of age, react more severely to acute respiratory tract infection than older children. Young children display a number of generalized signs and symptoms and local manifestations (Box 46-1).

Nursing Care Management

Assessment of the respiratory system follows the guidelines described in Chapter 34 (for assessment of the nose, mouth and throat, chest, and lungs). Special attention should also be given to the components and observations listed in Box 46-2. The nursing process for the care of the child with acute respiratory tract infection is outlined in the Nursing Process box.

Ease Respiratory Efforts

Many acute respiratory infections are mild and cause few symptoms. Although children may feel uncomfortable and have a "stuffy" nose (congestion) and some mucosal swelling, respiratory distress occurs infrequently. Interventions delivered at home are usually sufficient to relieve minor discomfort and ease respiratory efforts. However, children with croup or epiglottitis can develop sufficient swelling to obstruct the airway and may require hospitalization and more complex therapy.

Warm or cool mist is a common therapeutic measure for symptomatic relief of respiratory discomfort. The moisture soothes inflamed membranes and is beneficial when there is hoarseness or laryngeal involvement. However, the use of steam vaporizers in the home is often discouraged because of the hazards related to their use and limited evidence to support their efficacy. Shallow pans with wide surface areas for evaporation increase humidity but should be placed where they do not pose a safety hazard.

A time-honored method (albeit not evidence based!) of producing warm mist is the shower. Running a shower of hot water into the empty bathtub or open shower stall with the bathroom door closed produces a quick source of steam. Keeping a child in this environment for 10 to 15 minutes provides the same advantages as the mist tent without the fear and restraint associated with the confines of a tent. A small child can be held on the parent's lap. Older children can sit in the bathroom under the supervision of an adult.

Promote Rest

Children who have an acute febrile illness should be placed on bed rest. This is usually not difficult while the temperature is elevated but may become a problem when children begin to feel better. Often children will comply with bed rest if they are allowed to lie quietly on a couch where they can watch television, play a video game, or participate in a quiet activity. If children protest, allowing them to play quietly serves the purpose of rest better than allowing them to cry excessively in bed.

Promote Comfort

Older children are usually able to manage nasal secretions with little difficulty. Parents are instructed in the correct administration of nose drops and throat irrigations, if ordered. For very young infants, who normally breathe through their noses, an infant nasal aspirator or a rubber ear syringe is helpful in removing nasal secretions before feeding. This practice, followed by instillation of saline nose drops, may clear nasal passages and promote feeding. For older infants and children who can tolerate decongestants, vasoconstrictive nose drops may be administered 15 to 20 minutes before feeding and at bedtime. Two drops are instilled; because this shrinks only the anterior mucous membranes, two more drops are instilled 5 to 10 minutes later. Older cooperative children often prefer nasal sprays. They are taught to compress the plastic container at the moment of inspiration. Bottles of nose drops should be used for only one child and one illness because

BOX 46-1 Signs and Symptoms Associated with Respiratory Infections in Infants and Small Children

Fever

May be absent in newborn infants
Greatest at ages 6 months to 3 years
Temperature may reach 39.5° to 40.5° C (103° to 105° F) even with mild infections
Often appears as first sign of infection
May be listless and irritable or somewhat euphoric and more active than normal temporarily; some children talk with unaccustomed rapidity
Tendency to develop high temperatures with infection in certain families
May precipitate febrile seizures (see Chapter 51)
Febrile seizures uncommon after 3 or 4 years of age

Meningismus

Meningeal signs without infection of the meninges
Occurs with abrupt onset of fever
Accompanied by the following:

- Headache
- Pain and stiffness in the back and neck
- Presence of Kernig and Brudzinski signs

Subsides as the temperature decreases

Anorexia

Common with most childhood illnesses
Frequently the initial evidence of illness
Persists to a greater or lesser degree throughout febrile stage of illness; often extends into convalescence

Vomiting

Small children vomit readily with illness
Clue to onset of infection
May precede other signs by several hours
Usually short-lived but may persist during the illness
Frequent cause of dehydration if fluid intake is impaired

Diarrhea

Usually mild, transient diarrhea but may become severe
Often accompanies viral respiratory infections
Frequent cause of dehydration

Abdominal Pain

Common complaint
Sometimes indistinguishable from pain of appendicitis
Mesenteric lymphadenitis may be cause
Muscle spasms from vomiting may be a factor, especially in nervous, tense child

Nasal Blockage

Small nasal passages of infants easily blocked by mucosal swelling and exudation
Can interfere with respiration and feeding in infants
May contribute to the development of otitis media and sinusitis

Nasal Discharge

Frequent occurrence
May be thin and watery (rhinorrhea) or thick and purulent
Depends on the type or stage of infection
Associated with itching
May irritate upper lip and skin surrounding the nose

Cough

Common feature
May be evident only during acute phase
May persist several months after a disease

Respiratory Sounds

Sounds associated with respiratory disease:

- Cough
- Hoarseness
- Grunting
- Stridor
- Wheezing

Auscultation:

- Wheezing
- Crackles
- Absence of breath sounds

Sore Throat

Frequent complaint of older children
Young children (unable to describe symptoms) may not complain even when highly inflamed
Child will often refuse to take oral fluids or solids

evolve Animation—Lung Sounds

they are easily contaminated with bacteria. To avoid rebound congestion, nose drops or sprays should not be administered for more than 3 days.

Hot or cold applications sometimes provide relief for children with painful cervical adenitis. An ice bag or heating pad applied to the neck may decrease the discomfort, but safety precautions must be observed to prevent burns. The ice bag or heating device must be covered, and the heating pad should not be set at high ranges.

Prevent Spread of Infection

Children and families are taught to use a tissue or their hand to cover their nose and mouth when they cough or sneeze, dispose of tissues properly, and wash their hands. Remembering to cover the nose or mouth is often difficult for toddlers; therefore frequent handwashing is encouraged to prevent the spread of infection. Used tissues should be thrown into the wastebasket immediately, and tissues should not be allowed to accumulate in a pile. Children with respiratory infections should not share drinking cups, washcloths, or towels. To avoid contamination with respiratory viruses, nurses should wash hands and should not touch their eyes or nose.

Efforts should be made to separate affected children from contact with other children. Parents should keep affected children out of school and day care settings to prevent the spread of infection. Ideally, ill children should be isolated in a separate bedroom at the first sign of illness. However, this is a problem when living arrangements are crowded and there are

NURSING PROCESS: THE CHILD WITH ACUTE RESPIRATORY TRACT INFECTION

Assessment

Assessment of the respiratory system follows the guidelines described in Chapter 34 (for nose, ears, mouth and throat, chest, and lungs). In addition, special attention is given to the observations outlined in Box 46-1 and the components in Box 46-2.

- Assess respiratory effort (respiratory rate, accessory muscle use, retractions, nasal flaring).
- Assess oxygenation (pulse oximetry, color).
- Assess body temperature.
- Assess child's activity level.
- Assess child's level of comfort.

Nursing Diagnoses

After a thorough assessment, several nursing diagnoses are evident. Other nursing diagnoses may be apparent in individual cases.

Ineffective breathing pattern related to
- inflammatory process

Ineffective airway clearance related to
- mechanical obstruction
- inflammation
- increased secretions

Risk for infection related to
- presence of infectious organisms
- presence of optimum medium (mucus, sputum) for growth of infectious agents

Activity intolerance related to
- inflammatory process
- imbalance between oxygen supply and demand

Interrupted family processes related to
- child's illness

Planning

Expected patient outcomes include:

- Child will have adequate oxygenation.
- Child will demonstrate effective clearance of secretions.
- Optimum patient comfort will be achieved.
- Child will have effective respirations.
- Child will have adequate fluid and nutrient intake.
- Child will remain euthermic.

Implementation

Numerous intervention strategies are discussed on pp. 1304-1307.

Evaluation

The effectiveness of nursing interventions is determined by continual reassessment and evaluation of care based on the following observational guidelines:

- Observe child's respiratory effort and chest movements.
- Observe child's behavior and activity.
- Observe other family members and contacts for evidence of infection.
- Take temperature, respiratory rate, pulse oximetry reading, blood pressure, and heart rate.
- Observe for signs of adequate hydration.
- Assess complications such as dehydration, weight loss, or spread of infection to other areas of the body.
- Observe family's behavior and interview members regarding their feelings and concerns.

several children in the family. Well children should be told to stay away from ill children.

Reduce Temperature

If the child has a significantly elevated temperature, controlling the fever is important. Parents should know how to take a child's temperature and read the thermometer accurately. Nurses should not assume that all parents can read a thermometer. Parents who cannot perform this skill should receive instruction.

If the practitioner prescribes acetaminophen or ibuprofen, parents may need help giving the drug. Most parents can read the label and calculate the desired dose, but some may require careful instruction. It is important to emphasize accuracy in determining both the amount of drug to be given and the time intervals for administration. Cool liquids are given to reduce the temperature and minimize the chances of dehydration. (See Controlling Elevated Temperatures, Chapter 45.)

NURSING ALERT Parents are cautioned regarding over-the-counter combination "cold" remedies, since these often include acetaminophen. Careful calculation of both the acetaminophen given separately and the acetaminophen in combination medications is necessary to avoid an overdose.

Promote Hydration

Dehydration is a potential complication when children have respiratory tract infections and are febrile or anorexic, especially when vomiting or diarrhea is present. Infants are especially prone to fluid and electrolyte deficits when they have a respiratory illness because a rapid respiratory rate that accompanies such illnesses precludes adequate fluid intake. In addition, the presence of fever increases the total body fluid turnover in infants. If the infant has nasal secretions, this further prevents adequate respiratory effort by blocking the narrow nasal passages when the infant reclines to bottle-feed or breastfeed and ceases the compensatory mouth breathing effort, thus causing the child to limit intake of fluids. Adequate fluid intake is encouraged by offering small amounts of favorite fluids (clear liquids if vomiting) at frequent intervals. High-calorie liquids—such as colas, fruit juice drinks, water flavored and sweetened with corn syrup, or similar drinks—help prevent catabolism and dehydration but should be avoided, especially if diarrhea is present. Oral rehydration solutions such as Infalyte or Pedialyte should be considered for infants; sports drinks such as Gatorade should be considered for older children. Fluids with caffeine (tea, coffee) are avoided because these may act as a diuretic and promote fluid loss. Breastfeeding infants should continue to be breastfed because human

BOX 46-2 Components for Assessing Respiratory Function

Respirations

The pattern of respirations is observed for rate, depth, ease, and rhythm of breathing:

- **Rate**—Rapid *(tachypnea),* normal, or slow for the particular child
- **Depth**—Normal depth, too shallow *(hypopnea),* too deep *(hyperpnea);* usually estimated from the amplitude of thoracic and abdominal excursion
- **Ease**—Effortless; labored *(dyspnea); orthopnea* (difficult breathing except in upright position); associated with intercostal or substernal retractions (inspiratory "sinking in" of soft tissues in relation to the cartilaginous and bony thorax); flaring nares; head bobbing (head of sleeping child with suboccipital area supported on caregiver's forearm bobs forward in synchrony with each inspiration); grunting; or wheezing
- **Labored breathing**—Continuous, intermittent, becoming steadily worse, sudden onset, at rest or on exertion, associated with wheezing or grunting, associated with pain
- **Rhythm**—Variation in rate and depth of respirations

Other Observations

In addition to respirations, particular attention is addressed to the following:

- **Evidence of infection**—Check for elevated temperature; enlarged cervical lymph nodes; inflamed mucous membranes; and purulent discharges from the nose, ears, or lungs (sputum).
- **Cough**—Observe characteristics of cough (if present); under what circumstances cough is heard (e.g., night only, on arising), nature of cough (paroxysmal with or without wheeze, "croupy" or "brassy"), frequency of cough, associated with swallowing or other activity, character of cough (moist and dry), productivity.
- **Wheeze**—Note if expiratory or inspiratory, high-pitched or musical, prolonged, slowly progressive or sudden, associated with labored breathing.
- **Cyanosis**—Note distribution (peripheral, perioral, facial, trunk, and face), degree, duration, associated with activity.
- **Abdominal pain**—May be a complaint in preschooler and school-age children; probably represents referred pain from chest; may be a complaint in children with pneumonia.
- **Chest pain**—May be a complaint of older children; note location and circumstances: localized or generalized, referred to base of neck or abdomen, dull or sharp, deep or superficial, associated with rapid, shallow respirations or grunting.
- **Sputum**—Older children may provide sputum sample by coughing, whereas young children may need use of bulb suction to provide a sample; note volume, color, viscosity, and odor.
- **Bad breath**—May be associated with some lung infections.

milk confers some degree of protection from infection (see Chapter 26). Fluids should not be forced, and children should not be awakened to take fluids. Forcing fluids creates the same problem as urging unwanted food. Gentle persuasion with preferred beverages or sugar-free popsicles is usually more successful.

To assess their child's level of hydration (see also Chapter 47), parents are advised to observe the frequency of voiding and to notify the nurse or practitioner if there is insufficient voiding. Counting the number of wet diapers in a 24-hour period is a satisfactory method to assess output in infants and toddlers.

Provide Nutrition

Loss of appetite is characteristic of children with acute infections. In most cases children can be permitted to determine their own need for food. Many children show no decrease in appetite, and others respond well to foods such as gelatin, soup, and puddings (see Feeding the Sick Child, Chapter 45). Urging foods on anorexic children may precipitate nausea and vomiting and cause an aversion to feeding that may extend into the convalescent period and beyond.

Encourage Family Support and Home Care

Young children with respiratory tract infections are irritable and difficult to comfort; therefore the family needs support, encouragement, and practical suggestions concerning comfort measures and administration of medication. In addition to antipyretics and nose drops, the child may require antibiotic therapy. Parents of children receiving oral antibiotics must understand the importance of regular administration and continuing the drug for the prescribed length of time, regardless of whether the child appears ill. Parents are cautioned against giving their child any medications that are not approved by the health practitioner and to avoid giving antibiotics left over from a previous illness or prescribed for another child. Administering unprescribed antibiotics can produce serious side effects and adverse reactions (see Chapter 45 for administration of medications and teaching parents). See also the Nursing Care Plan.

Upper Respiratory Tract Infections

Nasopharyngitis

Acute nasopharyngitis (the equivalent of the "common cold") is caused by rhinovirus, RSV, adenovirus, influenza virus, and parainfluenza virus. Symptoms are more severe in infants and children than in adults. Fever is common in young children, and older children have low-grade fevers, which appear early in the course of the illness. Other clinical manifestations are listed in Box 46-3.

Therapeutic Management

Children with nasopharyngitis are managed at home. There is no specific treatment, and effective vaccines are not available. Antipyretics are prescribed for mild fever and discomfort (see Chapter 45 for management of fever). Rest is recommended

evolve Anatomy Review—Location of Retractions

until the child is free of fever for at least 1 day. Decongestants may be prescribed for children older than 5 years of age to shrink swollen nasal passages. The decongestants that exert their effect by vasoconstriction are usually less effective when taken orally than when applied topically as nose drops. Because these drugs affect all vascular beds, they should be given with caution to children with diabetes.

Cough suppressants may be prescribed for a dry, hacking cough in older children. However, cough preparations can cause adverse effects such as confusion, hyperexcitability, and sedation; therefore parents should monitor the child carefully for potential adverse effects.

Antihistamines are largely ineffective in treatment of nasopharyngitis. These drugs have a weak atropine-like effect that dries secretions, but they can cause drowsiness or, paradoxically, have a stimulatory effect on children. There is no support for the usefulness of expectorants, and antibiotics are usually not indicated because most infections are viral.

Recent concerns regarding serious side effects of cough and cold preparations in young children, particularly infants, and

NURSING CARE PLAN ✤ The Child with Acute Respiratory Tract Infection

Nursing Diagnosis	Expected Patient Outcomes	Nursing Interventions	Rationale
Ineffective breathing pattern related to inflammatory process **Child's/Family's Defining Characteristics** *(Subjective and Objective Data)* Use of accessory muscles to breathe Dyspnea Shortness of breath Nasal flaring Altered chest excursion Assumption of three-point position (tripod) Respiratory rate outside normal parameter for child's age (increased or decreased rate)	Child's respirations will be nonlabored. **The Following NOC Concepts Apply to These Outcomes** Respiratory Status: Airway Patency, Ventilation	Position child for maximal ventilatory efficiency and airway patency.	To allow increased chest expansion
		Position child to facilitate drainage of secretions.	To maintain patent airway and prevent airway obstruction
		Provide humidified oxygen as necessary.	To improve oxygenation
		Monitor oxygenation status, including vital signs, for changes in condition.	To determine need for additional interventions
		Suction airway (nose, trachea) as necessary.	To remove secretions and maintain airway patency
		Provide gentle chest percussion and chest physical therapy (CPT) as necessary.	To facilitate secretion removal
		Administer bronchodilator medications.	To promote bronchodilation and improve ventilation
		Administer antiinflammatory medications.	To decrease airway inflammation
		Administer antibiotics (if bacterial).	To decrease inflammatory response
		The Following NIC Concepts Apply to These Interventions Aspiration Precautions Positioning Respiratory Monitoring Surveillance Oxygen Therapy Airway Suctioning Vital Signs Monitoring Cough Enhancement	
Ineffective airway clearance related to inflammation, mechanical obstruction, increased secretions **Child's/Family's Defining Characteristics** *(Subjective and Objective Data)* Dyspnea Difficulty vocalizing Orthopnea Adventitious breath sounds (crackles, wheezing, rhonchi) Cough ineffective or absent Restlessness Changes in respiratory rate and rhythm	Child's airways will remain patent. **The Following NOC Concepts Apply to These Outcomes** Aspiration Control Airway Patency	Position child to facilitate drainage of secretions.	To prevent airway obstruction
		Perform CPT.	To loosen and remove secretions
		Suction airway as necessary.	To remove secretions
		Provide humidified oxygen.	To moisten secretions and prevent airway drying
		Assist with coughing (as developmentally or age appropriate).	To remove secretions
		Avoid throat examination if epiglottitis is suspected.	To prevent airway compromise
		Assure child (as appropriate) that all measures will be taken to ensure adequate airway is maintained.	To allay anxiety
		Implement comfort measures such as allowing parental presence, parental holding, favorite blanket or stuffed animal at side; explain all procedures beforehand.	To reduce anxiety and decrease effects of medical therapy, including hospitalization if required
		The Following NIC Concepts Apply to These Interventions Cough Enhancement Positioning Chest Physiotherapy Vital Signs Monitoring Anxiety Reduction	

NURSING CARE PLAN ✤ The Child with Acute Respiratory Tract Infection—cont'd

Nursing Diagnosis	Expected Patient Outcomes	Nursing Interventions	Rationale
Risk for injury related to presence (only as indicated) of infective organisms **Child's/Family's Defining Characteristics** ***(Subjective and Objective Data)*** Tissue hypoxia Abnormal blood profile People or provider (nosocomial agents) Mode of transport Developmental age	Child will remain free from complications of infection. **The Following NOC Concept Applies to These Outcomes** Risk Control	Maintain aseptic environment using sterile suction equipment and technique.	To prevent spread of infectious organisms in child and family
		Implement and practice standard precautions.	
		Implement contact and airborne precautions as necessary.	
		Obtain (secretion, tissue, or blood) specimen as indicated.	To identify infective organism
		Encourage child and family contacts to practice frequent handwashing and avoid hand-to-eye and hand-to-mouth contact.	To prevent spread of infection
		Teach child (as age appropriate) and family how to decrease spread of organisms through coughing and other secretions (e.g., by covering mouth when coughing; disposing of secretions to avoid cross-contamination).	To prevent spread of infection
		Administer antibiotic or antiviral medications.	To treat infection source
		Administer fever reduction medication(s) as appropriate.	To promote comfort if fever is present
		Monitor and assess for signs and symptoms of secondary complications: hypoxia, skin breakdown, poor nutrient and fluid intake, increased work of breathing, deteriorating cardiorespiratory status. **The Following NIC Concepts Apply to These Interventions** Risk Identification Environmental Management Infection Control Parent Education	To implement therapy for prevention of secondary complications
Interrupted family processes related to child's illness, hospitalization, and medical or therapeutic regimen **Child's/Family's Defining Characteristics** ***(Subjective and Objective Data)*** Communication patterns Participation in decision making Availability for emotional support Expressions of conflict within family Patterns and rituals	Family will demonstrate ability to cope with child's illness. **The Following NOC Concepts Apply to These Outcomes** Family Functioning Family Normalization Parenting	Allow family to remain with child.	To decrease effects of separation
		Promote family-centered care.	To promote family integrity
		Explain procedures and therapeutic regimen to family.	To provide accurate information regarding therapy and child's condition
		Keep family informed of child's status.	To promote family sense of control and involvement in care
		Encourage family involvement in child's care.	
		Provide support and referral for continued support as necessary. **The Following NIC Concepts Apply to These Interventions** Caregiver Support Family Support Coping Enhancement Emotional Support Financial Resource Assistance	

lack of convincing evidence that such medications are effective in reducing symptoms have prompted recommendations by health experts to carefully evaluate the benefits and risks of using such preparations in children under 6 years of age (Ryan, Brewer, & Small, 2008).

Prevention

Nasopharyngitis is so widespread in the general population that it is impossible to prevent. Children are more susceptible because they have not yet developed resistance to many viruses. Very young infants are subject to serious complications such as pneumonia, and attempts should be made to protect them from exposure.

✤ Nursing Care Management

A cold is often the parents' first introduction to an illness in their infant. Most discomfort of nasopharyngitis is related to

BOX 46-3 Clinical Manifestations of Nasopharyngitis and Pharyngitis

Nasopharyngitis

Younger Child
Fever
Irritability, restlessness
Sneezing
Vomiting or diarrhea

Older Child
Dryness and irritation of nose and throat
Sneezing, chilling sensation
Muscular aches
Cough, sometimes

Physical Signs
Edema and vasodilation of mucosa

Pharyngitis

Younger Child
Fever
General malaise
Anorexia
Moderate sore throat
Headache

Older Child
Fever (may reach 40° C [104° F])
Headache
Anorexia
Dysphagia
Abdominal pain
Vomiting

Physical Signs
Younger Child
Mild to moderate hyperemia
Older Child
Mild to fiery red, edematous pharynx
Hyperemia of tonsils and pharynx; may extend to soft palate and uvula
Often abundant follicular exudate that spreads and coalesces to form pseudomembrane on tonsils
Cervical glands enlarged and tender

BOX 46-4 Early Evidence of Respiratory Complications

Parents are instructed to notify the health professional if any of the following are noted:

- Evidence of earache (see p. 1314)
- Respirations faster than 50 to 60 breaths/min
- Fever over 38.3° C (101° F)
- Listlessness
- Increasing irritability with or without fever
- Persistent cough for 2 days or more
- Wheezing
- Crying
- Refusal to eat
- Restlessness and poor sleep patterns

Modified from National Association of Pediatric Nurse Associates and Practitioners (NAPNAP): *Baby's first cold*, New York, 1989, Winthrop Consumer Products. Copies available from NAPNAP, 1101 Kings Hwy. N., No. 206, Cherry Hill, NJ 08034; phone: 609-667-1773; website: *www.napnap.org*.

the nasal obstruction, especially in small infants. Elevating the head of the bed or crib mattress assists with drainage of secretions. Nasopharyngeal suctioning and vaporization may also provide relief. Saline nose drops and gentle suctioning with a bulb syringe before feeding are useful.

Maintaining adequate fluid intake is essential. Although a child's appetite for solid foods is usually diminished for several days, it is important to offer favorite fluids to prevent dehydration. Fluids can be cool or warm, depending on individual preference.

Because nasopharyngitis is spread from secretions, the best means for prevention is avoiding contact with affected persons. This goal is difficult to accomplish in family settings, classrooms, and day care centers. Family members with a cold should try to "keep it to themselves" by carefully disposing of tissues; not sharing towels, glasses, or eating utensils; covering the mouth and nose with tissues when coughing or sneezing; and washing the hands thoroughly after nose blowing or sneezing. The most frequent carriers of infection are the human hands, which deposit viruses on doorknobs, faucets, toys, and other everyday objects. Children should be taught to wash their hands thoroughly before putting them near their eyes, nose, or mouth.

Family Support

Support and reassurance are important elements of care for families of young children with recurrent upper respiratory infections (URIs). Because URIs are common in children less than 3 years of age, families may feel as if they are on an endless roller coaster of illness. They need reassurance that frequent colds are a normal part of childhood and that by 5 years of age their children will have developed immunity to many viruses. Parents who work outside the home should expect to take time off to care for ill children during the fall and winter months. When children spend time routinely in day care centers, their infection rate is higher than if they are cared for in the home. Parents should know the signs of respiratory complications and should notify a health professional if complications occur or if the child does not improve within 2 or 3 days (Box 46-4).

Pharyngitis

Children who experience GABHS infection of the upper airway *(strep throat)* are at risk for *rheumatic fever (RF)*, an inflammatory disease of the heart, joints, and central nervous system (see Chapter 48), and *acute glomerulonephritis (AGN)*, an acute kidney infection (see Chapter 50). Permanent damage can result from these sequelae, especially RF.

Clinical Manifestations

GABHS is generally a relatively brief illness that varies in severity from subclinical (no symptoms) to severe toxicity. The onset is often abrupt and characterized by pharyngitis, headache, fever, and abdominal pain (especially in small children).

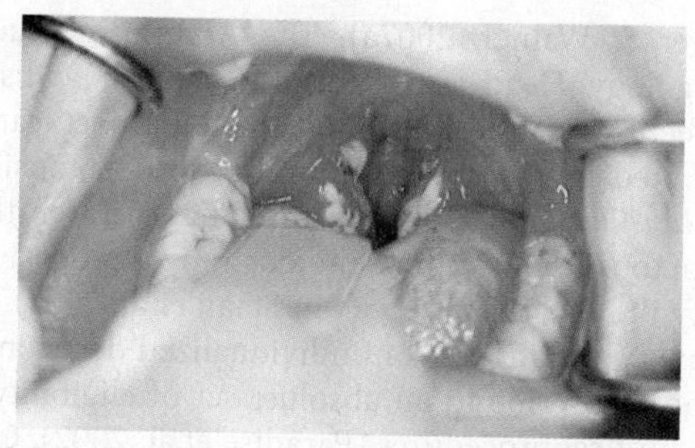

Fig. 46-1 Tonsillitis and pharyngitis. *(Courtesy Dr. Edward L. Applebaum, Head, Department of Otolaryngology, University of Illinois Medical Center, Chicago.)*

The tonsils and pharynx may be inflamed and covered with exudate (Fig. 46-1), which usually appears by the second day of illness. However, streptococcal infections should be suspected in children older than 2 years of age who have pharyngitis without exudate. Anterior cervical lymphadenopathy (in about 30% to 50% of cases) usually occurs early, and the nodes are often tender. Pain can be relatively mild to severe enough to make swallowing difficult. Clinical manifestations usually subside in 3 to 5 days unless complicated by sinusitis or parapharyngeal, peritonsillar, or retropharyngeal abscess. Nonsuppurative complications may appear after the onset of GABHS (i.e., AGN in about 10 days and RF in an average of 18 days).

Diagnostic Evaluation

Although 80% to 90% of all cases of acute pharyngitis are viral, a throat culture should be performed to rule out GABHS. Most streptococcal infections are short-term illnesses, and antibody responses appear later than symptoms and are useful only for retrospective diagnosis.

Rapid identification of GABHS with diagnostic test kits (rapid antigen detection test) is possible in the office or clinic setting. Because of the high specificity of these rapid tests, a positive test result generally does not require throat culture confirmation. However, the sensitivities of these kits vary considerably, and a confirmatory throat culture is recommended in patients who have a negative test result (American Academy of Pediatrics, Committee on Infectious Diseases, 2009).

Therapeutic Management

If streptococcal sore throat infection is present, oral penicillin is prescribed in a dose sufficient to control the acute local manifestations and maintain an adequate level for at least 10 days to eliminate any organisms that might remain to initiate RF symptoms. Penicillin does not prevent the development of AGN in susceptible children; however, it may prevent the spread of a nephrogenic strain of GABHS to others in the family. Penicillin usually produces a prompt response within 24 hours. Patients who have a history of RF or who remain symptomatic after a full course of antibiotics may require a follow-up throat swab.

Intramuscular (IM) benzathine penicillin G is an appropriate therapy, but it is painful and is not the first choice for children. Oral erythromycin is indicated for children allergic to penicillin. Other antibiotics used to treat GABHS are azithromycin, clarithromycin, oral cephalosporins, amoxicillin, and amoxicillin with clavulanic acid (American Academy of Pediatrics, Committee on Infectious Diseases, 2009; Gerber, 2005).

Nursing Care Management

The nurse often obtains a throat swab for culture and instructs the parents about administering penicillin and analgesics as prescribed. Cold or warm compresses to the neck may provide relief. In children who can cooperate, warm saline gargles offer relief of throat discomfort. Pain may interfere with oral intake, and children should not be forced to eat. Cool liquids or ice chips are usually more acceptable than solids.

Special emphasis is placed on correct administration of oral medication and completing the course of antibiotic therapy (see Administration of Medication, Chapter 45). If injections are required, they must be administered deep into a large muscle mass (e.g., vastus lateralis or ventrogluteal muscle). To prevent pain, application of a topical analgesic such as EMLA or LMX 4 over the injection site before the injection is helpful (see Administration of Medication: Intramuscular Administration, Chapter 45). Parents also need to be aware of residual tenderness at the injection site, which may cause the child to limp for a day or two. Local applications of heat are helpful in relieving this discomfort.

Nurses play a key role in preventing the spread of disease. Children are considered noninfectious to others 24 hours after initiation of antibiotic therapy, but they should not return to school or day care until they have been taking antibiotics for a full 24-hour period. Nurses should remind the children to discard their toothbrush and replace it with a new one after they have been taking antibiotics for 24 hours. Parents are cautioned to prevent other household members, especially if immunocompromised, from having close contact with the sick child and avoid sharing drinking or eating items.

Tonsillitis

The tonsils are masses of lymphoid tissue located in the pharyngeal cavity. They filter and protect the respiratory and alimentary tracts from invasion by pathogenic organisms and play a role in antibody formation. Although their size varies, children generally have much larger tonsils than adolescents or adults. This difference is thought to be a protective mechanism because young children are especially susceptible to URIs.

evolve Case Study—Tonsillitis

Pathophysiology

Several pairs of tonsils are part of a mass of lymphoid tissue encircling the nasal and oral pharynx, known as the *Waldeyer tonsillar ring* (Fig. 46-2). The *palatine* or *faucial tonsils* are located on either side of the oropharynx, behind and below the pillars of the fauces (opening from the mouth). A surface of the palatine tonsils is usually visible during oral examination. The palatine tonsils are those removed during tonsillectomy. The *pharyngeal tonsils,* also known as the *adenoids,* are located above the palatine tonsils on the posterior wall of the nasopharynx. Their proximity to the nares and eustachian tubes causes difficulties in instances of inflammation. The *lingual tonsils* are located at the base of the tongue. The *tubal*

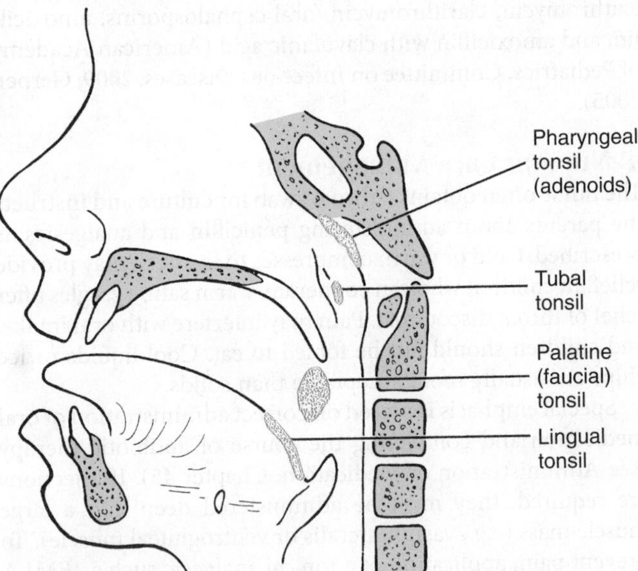

Fig. 46-2 Location of various tonsillar masses.

evolve Anatomy Review–Location of Tonsillar Masses

tonsils, found near the posterior nasopharyngeal opening of the eustachian tubes, are not part of the Waldeyer tonsillar ring.

Etiology

Tonsillitis often occurs with pharyngitis. The causative agent may be viral or bacterial. Because of the abundant lymphoid tissue and the frequency of URIs, tonsillitis is a common cause of morbidity in young children.

Clinical Manifestations

The manifestations of tonsillitis are caused by inflammation. As the palatine tonsils enlarge from edema, they may meet in the midline (kissing tonsils), obstructing the passage of air or food. The child has difficulty swallowing and breathing. When the adenoids enlarge, the space behind the posterior nares becomes blocked, making it difficult or impossible for air to pass from the nose to the throat. As a result, the child breathes through the mouth.

Therapeutic Management

Because tonsillitis is self-limiting, treatment of viral pharyngitis is symptomatic. Throat cultures positive for GABHS infection warrant antibiotic treatment. It is important to differentiate between viral and streptococcal infection in febrile exudative tonsillitis. Because most infections are of viral origin, early rapid tests can eliminate unnecessary antibiotic administration.

Tonsillectomy is the surgical removal of the palatine tonsils. Absolute indications for a tonsillectomy are malignancy, recurrent peritonsillar abscess, and airway obstruction. *Adenoidectomy* (the surgical removal of the adenoids) is recommended for children who have hypertrophied adenoids that obstruct nasal breathing; additional indications for adenoidectomy include recurrent adenoiditis and sinusitis, otitis media (OM) with effusion, airway obstruction and subsequent sleep-disordered breathing, and recurrent rhinorrhea (Benninger & Walner, 2007a). The American Academy of Otolaryngology–Head and Neck Surgery (2000) lists "3 or more infections of the tonsils or adenoids per year despite adequate medical therapy" as an indication for tonsillectomy or *adenotonsillectomy.* However, for some children the effectiveness of tonsillectomy or adenoidectomy is modest and may not justify the risk of surgery (van Staaij et al, 2004). In practice, many physicians rely on individualized decision making and do not subscribe to an absolute set of eligibility criteria for these surgical procedures (Paradise et al, 2002). Contraindications to either tonsillectomy or adenoidectomy are (1) cleft palate because tonsils help minimize escape of air during speech, (2) acute infections at the time of surgery because locally inflamed tissues increase the risk of bleeding, and (3) uncontrolled systemic diseases or blood dyscrasias.

Nursing Care Management

Nursing care involves providing comfort and minimizing activities or interventions that precipitate bleeding. A soft to liquid diet is preferred. A cool-mist vaporizer keeps the mucous membranes moist during periods of mouth breathing. Warm salt-water gargles, throat lozenges, and analgesic-antipyretic drugs such as acetaminophen are used to promote comfort. Often opioids are needed to reduce pain for the child to drink. Combination nonopioid and opioid elixirs or tablets such as acetaminophen with codeine or with hydrocodone (Lortab) relieve pain and should be given routinely every 4 hours.

If surgery is required, the child requires the same psychologic preparation and physical care as for any other surgical procedure (see Chapters 44 and 45). Most tonsillectomy and adenoidectomy (T&A) surgeries now take place in outpatient settings; however, the priorities of preoperative and postoperative care remain the same. The following discussion focuses on postoperative nursing care for T&A, although both procedures may not be performed.

Until they are fully awake, children are placed on their abdomen or side to facilitate drainage of secretions. Routine suctioning is avoided, and, when performed, it is done carefully to avoid trauma to the oropharynx. When alert, children may prefer sitting up. They are discouraged from coughing frequently, clearing their throat, blowing their nose, or any other activity that may aggravate the operative site.

Some secretions are common, particularly dried blood from surgery. All secretions and vomitus are inspected for evidence of fresh bleeding (some blood-tinged mucus is expected). Dark brown (old) blood is usually present in the emesis, in the nose, and between the teeth. If parents do not expect this, they often become frightened at a time when they need to be calm and reassuring.

The throat is sore after surgery. An ice collar provides relief, but many children find it bothersome and refuse to use it. Most children experience moderate pain after a T&A and need pain medication for at least the first 24 hours. Analgesics may be given rectally or intravenously to avoid the oral route. Because pain is continuous, analgesics should be administered at regular intervals. An antiemetic such as ondansetron (Zofran) may be administered postoperatively (see Pain Management, Chapter 35).

Food and fluids are restricted until children are fully alert and there are no signs of hemorrhage. Cool water, crushed ice, flavored ice pops, or diluted fruit juice may be given, but fluids with a red or brown color are avoided to distinguish fresh or old blood in emesis from the ingested liquid. Citrus juice may cause discomfort and is usually poorly tolerated. Soft foods, particularly gelatin, cooked fruits, sherbet, soup, and mashed potatoes, are started on the first or second postoperative day or as the child tolerates feeding. The pain from surgery often inhibits fluid intake, reinforcing the need for adequate pain control. Milk, ice cream, and pudding are usually not offered, since milk products coat the mouth and throat and may cause the child to clear the throat, which can initiate bleeding.

Postoperative hemorrhage is uncommon but can occur. The nurse observes the throat directly for evidence of bleeding, using a good source of light and, if necessary, carefully inserting a tongue depressor. Other signs of hemorrhage are tachycardia, pallor, frequent clearing of the throat or swallowing by a younger child, and vomiting of bright red blood. Restlessness, an indication of hemorrhage, may be difficult to differentiate from general discomfort after surgery. Decreasing blood pressure is a late sign of shock.

Surgery may be required to cauterize or ligate a bleeding vessel. Airway obstruction may also occur as a result of edema or accumulated secretions and is indicated by signs of respiratory distress, such as stridor, drooling, restlessness, agitation, increasing respiratory rate, and progressive cyanosis. Suction equipment and oxygen should be available after tonsillectomy.

NURSING ALERT The most obvious early sign of bleeding is the child's continuous swallowing of the trickling blood. While the child is sleeping, note the frequency of swallowing. If continuous bleeding is suspected, notify the surgeon immediately.

Family Support and Home Care

Discharge instructions include (1) avoiding irritating or highly seasoned foods; (2) avoiding gargles or vigorous toothbrushing; (3) avoiding coughing, clearing the throat, or putting objects in the mouth; (4) using analgesics or an ice collar for pain; and (5) limiting activity to decrease the potential for bleeding. Objectionable mouth odor and slight ear pain with a low-grade fever are common for a few days postoperatively. However, persistent severe earache, fever, or cough requires medical evaluation. Most children are ready to resume normal activity within 1 to 2 weeks after the operation.

Hemorrhage may occur up to 10 days after surgery as a result of tissue sloughing from the healing process. Any sign of bleeding warrants immediate medical attention.

Influenza

Influenza, or flu, is caused by three orthomyxoviruses, which are antigenically distinct: types A and B, which cause epidemic disease, and type C, which is unimportant from an epidemiologic standpoint. Influenza is spread from one individual to another by direct contact (large-droplet infection) or by articles recently contaminated by nasopharyngeal secretions. There is no predilection for a specific age group, but attack rates are highest in young children who have had no previous contact with a strain. Influenza is frequently most severe in infants. During epidemics, infection among school-age children is believed to be a major source of transmission in a community. The disease is more common during the winter months and has a 1- to 3-day incubation period. Affected persons are most infectious for 24 hours before and after the onset of symptoms. The virus has a peculiar affinity for epithelial cells of the respiratory tract mucosa, where it destroys ciliated epithelium with metaplastic hyperplasia of the tracheal and bronchial epithelium with associated edema. The alveoli may also become distended with a hyaline-like material. The viruses can be isolated from nasopharyngeal secretions early after the onset of infection, and serologic tests identify the type by complement fixation or the subgroups by hemagglutination inhibition.

Avian Influenza Virus

Several types of influenza were identified in Asian countries that caused mild to severe disease in adults and children. The avian influenza that has resulted in several deaths in Hong Kong, Vietnam, and Thailand has been identified as subtypes H5 and H7 and has as its host chickens and wild ducks, in which the mortality rates range from 90% to 100% (Lee & Krilov, 2005). The virus has also been reported to spread among other animals such as pigs and tigers. In humans the viral manifestations of avian influenza often consist of fever and respiratory symptoms—sore throat, rhinorrhea, and cough—occurring within 3 to 5 days of illness (Chokephaibulkit, 2004). Laboratory findings include leukopenia and thrombocytopenia, and moderately elevated liver transaminases are often identified. Patients may rapidly progress to acute respiratory distress syndrome (ARDS) with acute lung injury. In some children the virus is manifest only as an eye infection (conjunctivitis).

Treatment is aimed at prompt diagnosis and intervention to reduce the onset of ARDS. The virus may respond to influenza drugs such as amantadine, rimantadine, oseltamivir, and zanamivir; but cases of avian flu in Southeast Asia were resistant to amantadine and rimantadine (Lee & Krilov, 2005). Rimantadine is not indicated for children. At present laboratory testing in the United States is indicated only in the case of a hospitalized patient with a severe respiratory illness without a diagnosis who has traveled to a country with documented avian influenza (Lee & Krilov, 2005). To obtain updated information on the emergence of and progress in treatment of these and other respiratory viruses, the reader is encouraged to visit the Centers for Disease Control and Prevention website *(www.cdc.gov).*

Clinical Manifestations

The manifestations of influenza may be subclinical, mild, moderate, or severe. Most patients have a dry throat and nasal mucosa, a dry cough, and a tendency toward hoarseness. A flushed face, photophobia, myalgia, hyperesthesia, and sometimes exhaustion and lack of energy accompany a sudden onset of fever and chills. Subglottal croup is common, especially in infants. The symptoms of influenza last for 4 or 5 days.

Complications include severe viral pneumonia (often hemorrhagic); encephalitis; and secondary bacterial infections such as OM, sinusitis, or pneumonia.

Therapeutic Management

Uncomplicated influenza in children usually requires only symptomatic treatment: acetaminophen or ibuprofen for fever and sufficient fluids to maintain hydration. Amantadine hydrochloride (Symmetrel) has been effective in reducing symptoms associated with type A disease if administered within 24 to 48 hours after their onset; the symptoms associated with influenza are reportedly shortened by 24 hours, but the drug does not cure the disease. It is ineffective against type B or C influenza or other viral diseases. It should not be given to children under 1 year of age but is recommended for unvaccinated high risk children.

Zanamivir and rimantadine have been approved for the treatment of flu symptoms in children under 18 years of age. Both medications must also be started within 48 hours of symptom onset. Zanamivir is an inhaled medication effective for type A and B influenza. The drug is taken twice daily for 5 days and is administered by a specially designed oral inhaler (Diskhaler). Zanamivir cannot be used for children younger than 7 years of age. A fourth drug, oseltamivir (Tamiflu), is a neuroaminidase inhibitor that may be administered orally for 5 days to children over 1 year (and adults) to decrease the flu symptoms; as with other antiviral drugs, it must be taken within 2 days of the onset of symptoms. It is reported to be effective for types A and B influenza (American Academy of Pediatrics, Committee on Infectious Diseases, 2009). Bronchospasm and a decline in lung function can occur when zanamivir is used in patients with underlying airway disease such as asthma or chronic obstructive pulmonary disease. Rimantadine is effective only for type A virus; this drug is taken orally by tablet or syrup twice daily for 7 days; it cannot be used for children younger than 1 year of age. Children with influenza (or other similar viruses) should not receive aspirin because of its possible link with Reye syndrome.

Prevention

Two vaccines may be administered to prevent influenza. Inactivated trivalent influenza viral (TIV) vaccines are safe and effective provided the antigens in the vaccine correlate with the circulating influenza viruses (see Immunizations, Chapter 36). The live-attenuated influenza vaccine (LAIV) is a nasal spray flu vaccine approved by the U.S. Food and Drug Administration that is licensed for administration in children 2 years of age and older. However, this preparation contains a live virus and should not be used in individuals who are immunocompromised, have anaphylactic reactions to egg protein, have reactive airway disease, are receiving immunosuppressive therapy, have a chronic respiratory condition, or have a history of Guillain-Barré syndrome.

Nursing Care Management

Nursing care is the same as that for any child with a URI, including implementing measures to relieve symptoms. The greatest danger to affected children is development of a secondary infection. Prolonged fever or appearance of fever during early convalescence is a sign of secondary bacterial infection and should be reported to the practitioner for antibiotic therapy.

Otitis Media

OM is one of the most prevalent diseases of early childhood. Its incidence is highest in the winter months. Many cases of bacterial OM are preceded by a viral respiratory infection. The two viruses most likely to precipitate OM are RSV and influenza. Most episodes of acute otitis media (AOM) occur in the first 24 months of life, but the incidence decreases with age, except for a small increase at age 5 or 6 years when children enter school. OM occurs infrequently in children older than 7 years of age. Preschool-age boys are affected more frequently than preschool-age girls. Children who have siblings or parents with a history of chronic OM have a higher incidence of OM. Children living in households with many members (especially smokers) are more likely to have OM than those living with fewer persons. Passive smoking increases the risk of persistent middle ear effusion by enhancing attachment of the pathogens that cause otitis to the respiratory epithelium in the middle ear space, prolonging the inflammatory response, and impeding drainage through the eustachian tube (American Academy of Pediatrics, 2004a). Family socioeconomic status and extent of exposure to other children are the two most important identifiable risk factors for the occurrence of OM (American Academy of Pediatrics 2004a; Kershner, 2007).

OM has been defined in a variety of ways. The standard terminology used to define it is outlined in Box 46-5, and AOM treatment guidelines have been published (American Academy of Pediatrics, 2004a, 2004b).

Etiology

Streptococcus pneumoniae, H. influenzae, and *Moraxella catarrhalis* are the three most common bacteria causing AOM. The etiology of noninfectious OM is unknown, although OM may occur because of blocked eustachian tubes from the edema of URIs, allergic rhinitis, or hypertrophic adenoids. Chronic OM is frequently an extension of an acute episode.

A relationship has been observed between the incidence of OM and infant feeding methods. Infants fed breast milk have a lower incidence of OM compared with formula-fed infants. Breastfeeding may protect infants against respiratory viruses and allergy because it contains secretory immune globulin A, which limits the exposure of the eustachian tube and middle ear mucosa to microbial pathogens and foreign proteins. Reflux of milk up the eustachian tubes is less likely in breast-fed infants because of the semivertical positioning

BOX 46-5 Standard Terminology for Otitis Media

Otitis media (OM)—An inflammation of the middle ear without reference to etiology or pathogenesis

Acute otitis media (AOM)—An inflammation of the middle ear space with a rapid onset of the signs and symptoms of acute infection (i.e., fever and otalgia [ear pain])

Otitis media with effusion (OME)—Fluid in the middle ear space without symptoms of acute infection

during breastfeeding compared with positioning during bottle-feeding.

Pathophysiology

OM is primarily a result of malfunctioning eustachian tubes. The eustachian tube is part of a contiguous system composed of the nares, nasopharynx, eustachian tube, middle ear, and mastoid antrum and air cells. Eustachian tubes have three functions relative to the middle ear: (1) protection of the middle ear from nasopharyngeal secretions, (2) drainage of secretions produced in the middle ear into the nasopharynx, and (3) ventilation of the middle ear to equalize air pressure within the middle ear and atmospheric pressure in the external ear canal and to replenish oxygen that has been absorbed.

Mechanical or functional obstruction of the eustachian tube causes accumulation of secretions in the middle ear. Intrinsic obstruction can be caused by infection or allergy; extrinsic obstruction is usually a result of enlarged adenoids or nasopharyngeal tumors. Persistent collapse of the tube during swallowing can cause functional obstruction associated with decreased stiffness or an inefficient opening mechanism. Eustachian tube obstruction results in negative middle ear pressure and, if persistent, produces a transudative middle ear effusion. Drainage is inhibited by sustained negative pressure and impaired ciliary transport within the tube. When the passage is not totally obstructed, contamination of the middle ear can take place by reflux, aspiration, or insufflation during crying, sneezing, nose blowing, and swallowing when the nose is obstructed.

Diagnostic Evaluation

Careful assessment of tympanic membrane mobility with a pneumatic otoscope is essential to differentiate AOM from OM with effusion (OME) (American Academy of Pediatrics, 2004b). A diagnosis of AOM is made if visual inspection of the tympanic membrane reveals a purulent discolored effusion and a bulging or full, opacified, or reddened immobile membrane. Some practitioners also consider the presence of acute onset of less than 48 hours of ear pain with the preceding criteria to be a diagnostic factor in AOM (Powers, 2007). An immobile tympanic membrane or an orange discolored membrane indicates OME. Clinical symptoms of otitis are also helpful in making the diagnosis (Box 46-6). In AOM, symptoms such as acute onset of ear pain, fever, and a bulging yellow or red tympanic membrane are usually present. In OME, these symptoms may be absent, and other nonspecific symptoms such as rhinitis, cough, or diarrhea are often present (American Academy of Pediatrics, 2004a, 2004b).

BOX 46-6 Clinical Manifestations of Otitis Media

Acute Otitis Media

Follows an upper respiratory infection
Otalgia (earache)
Fever
Purulent discharge (otorrhea) may or may not be present

Infant or Very Young Child

Crying
Fussy, restless, irritable
Tendency to rub, hold, or pull affected ear
Rolls head from side to side
Difficulty comforting child
Loss of appetite

Older Child

Crying or verbalizing feelings of discomfort
Irritability
Lethargy
Loss of appetite

Chronic Otitis Media

Hearing loss
Difficulty communicating
Possible feeling of fullness, tinnitus, or vertigo

Therapeutic Management

Treatment for AOM is one of the most common reasons for antibiotic use in the ambulatory setting. However, recently concerns about drug-resistant *S. pneumoniae* and other drug resistances have led infectious disease authorities to recommend careful and judicious use of antibiotics for treatment of this illness. Current literature indicates that waiting up to 72 hours for spontaneous resolution is safe and appropriate management of AOM in healthy infants over 6 months and children (American Academy of Pediatrics, 2004a; Bhetwal & McConaghy, 2007). Furthermore some reviews of the treatment of AOM reveal no clear evidence that antibiotics improve outcomes in children younger than 2 years of age with uncomplicated AOM. However, the watchful waiting approach is not recommended for children younger than 2 years who have persistent acute symptoms of fever and severe ear pain (Kershner, 2007). In addition, all cases of AOM in infants younger than 6 months of age should be treated with antibiotics because of the infant's immature immune system and the potential for infection with bacteria other than the three most common organisms found in older infants and children with AOM.

When antibiotics are warranted, oral amoxicillin in high doses (80 to 90 mg/kg/day, divided twice daily) is the treatment of choice for initial episodes of AOM in children who have not received antibiotics within the past month (American Academy of Pediatrics, 2004a; Bhetwal & McConaghy, 2007; Pichichero & Casey, 2005). The recommendation for the duration of antibiotic therapy is 5 to 7 days in children 6 years and older with uncomplicated AOM (American Academy of Pediatrics, Committee on Infectious Diseases, 2009).

Second-line antibiotics used to treat OM include amoxicillin-clavulanate; azithromycin; and cephalosporins such as cefdinir, cefuroxime, and cefpodoxime. IM ceftriaxone is used if the causative organism is a highly resistant pneumococcus or if the parents are noncompliant with the therapy. An important consideration with the use of single-dose IM injections is the pain involved in this therapy. One strategy to minimize pain at the injection site is to reconstitute the cephalosporin with 1% lidocaine. The use of steroids, decongestants, and antihistamines to treat AOM is not recommended.

Supportive care or symptomatic treatment of AOM includes treating the fever and pain. For fever or discomfort associated with OM, analgesic-antipyretic drugs such as acetaminophen or ibuprofen may be given. Topical pain relief is recommended by external application of heat or cold, or the practitioner may prescribe topical pain relief drops such as benzocaine drops. Antihistamines and decongestants are not recommended. Antibiotic ear drops have no value in treating AOM.

Myringotomy, a surgical incision of the eardrum, may be necessary to alleviate the severe pain of AOM. A myringotomy is also performed to provide drainage of infected middle ear fluid in the presence of complications (mastoiditis, labyrinthitis, or facial paralysis) or to allow purulent middle ear fluid to drain into the ear canal for culture. A minimally invasive laser-assisted myringotomy procedure may be performed in outpatient settings.

Tympanostomy tube placement and adenoidectomy are surgical procedures that may be done to treat recurrent OM. Tympanostomy tubes or pressure-equalizer (PE) tubes are grommets that facilitate continued drainage of fluid and allow ventilation of the middle ear. Adenoidectomy is not recommended for treatment of AOM and is performed only in children with recurrent AOM or chronic OME with postnasal obstruction, adenoiditis, or chronic sinusitis.

In some children residual middle ear effusions remain after episodes of AOM. Some children have fluid that persists in the middle ear for weeks or months. Antibiotics are not required for initial treatment of OME but may be indicated for children with persistent effusion for more than 3 months (American Academy of Pediatrics, 2004a). Placement of tympanostomy tubes is recommended after a total of 4 to 6 months of bilateral effusion with a bilateral hearing deficit (American Academy of Pediatrics, 2004b). This therapy allows for mechanical drainage of the fluid, which promotes healing of the membrane and prevents scar formation and loss of elasticity. Myringotomy with or without insertion of PE tubes should not be performed for initial management of OME but may be recommended for children who have recurrent episodes of OME with a long cumulative duration (American Academy of Pediatrics, 2004b). Tonsillectomy either alone or with adenoidectomy is not considered an effective treatment for OME (American Academy of Pediatrics, 2004b).

OME is frequently associated with mild to moderate impairment of hearing; therefore a hearing test should also be performed 3 months after the acute episode of AOM, if OME persists for 3 months or more, or if there is evidence of language or learning delays. Follow-up examinations of children with chronic OME should be maintained on a 3- to 6-month basis until the OME is resolved, a significant hearing loss is identified, or structural defect of the tympanic membrane or middle ear is identified (American Academy of Pediatrics, 2004a). Children with hearing loss should be referred to an otolaryngologist and should receive a speech and language evaluation as necessary.

Prevention

The pneumococcal conjugate vaccine (PCV) has significantly decreased the incidence of invasive pneumococcal infections in children under 5 years of age since the year 2000 (American Academy of Pediatrics, Committee on Infectious Diseases, 2009).

Parents are encouraged to reduce risk factors for AOM by breastfeeding infants for at least the first 6 months of life, avoiding propping the bottle, decreasing or discontinuing pacifier use after 6 months, and preventing exposure to tobacco smoke (American Academy of Pediatrics, 2004a).

Nursing Care Management

Nursing objectives for the child with AOM include (1) relieving pain, (2) facilitating drainage when possible, (3) preventing complications or recurrence, (4) educating the family in care of the child, and (5) providing emotional support to the child and family.

Analgesic drugs such as acetaminophen and ibuprofen are used to treat mild pain. For more severe pain the American Academy of Pediatrics (2004a) guidelines recommend a stronger analgesic such as codeine.

If the ear is draining, the external canal may be cleaned with sterile cotton swabs or pledgets coupled with topical antibiotic treatment. If ear wicks or lightly rolled sterile gauze packs are placed in the ear after surgical treatment, they should be loose enough to allow accumulated drainage to flow out of the ear; otherwise, infection may be transferred to the mastoid process. The wicks need to stay dry during shampoos or baths. Occasionally, drainage is so profuse that the auricle and the skin surrounding the ear become excoriated from the exudate. This is usually prevented by frequent cleansing and application of various moisture barriers (e.g., Proshield Plus) or petrolatum jelly (e.g., Vaseline).

Tympanostomy tubes may allow water to enter the middle ear, but recommendations for earplugs are inconsistent. Research indicates that swimming without earplugs poses a slightly increased risk of infection (Goldstein et al, 2005). However, lake and river water is potentially contaminated, and wearing earplugs while swimming in a lake prevents total flooding of the external canal. Bathwater and shampoo water should be kept out of the ear, if possible, because soap reduces the surface tension of water and facilitates entry through the tube. Parents should be aware of the appearance of a grommet (usually a tiny, white, plastic spool-shaped tube) so that they can recognize it if it falls out. They are reassured that this is normal and requires no immediate intervention, although they should notify the practitioner.

Prevention of recurrence requires adequate education regarding antibiotic therapy. The symptoms of pain and fever usually subside within 24 to 48 hours, but nurses must emphasize that all of the prescribed medication should be taken. Parents should be aware that potential complications of OM, such as hearing loss, can be prevented with adequate treatment and follow-up care.

Parents also need anticipatory guidance regarding methods to reduce the risks of OM, especially in children under 2 years of age. Reducing the chances of OM is possible with simple measures, such as sitting or holding an infant upright for feedings, maintaining routine childhood immunizations, and exclusively breastfeeding until at least 6 months of age. Propping bottles is discouraged to avoid pooling of milk while the child is in the supine position and to encourage human contact during feeding. Eliminating tobacco smoke and known allergens is also recommended. Early detection of middle ear effusion is essential to prevent complications. Infants and preschool children should be screened for effusion, and all schoolchildren, especially those with learning disabilities, should be tested for middle ear effusion. Frequent audiologic evaluations, medical consultation, and education of parents and children are advised when middle ear effusion is detected.

Infectious Mononucleosis

Infectious mononucleosis is an acute, self-limiting infectious disease that is common among adolescents. The illness is characterized by an increase in the mononuclear elements of the blood and by general symptoms of an infectious process. The course is usually mild but occasionally can be severe or, rarely, accompanied by serious complications.

Etiology and Pathophysiology

The herpes-like Epstein-Barr virus (EBV) is the principal cause of infectious mononucleosis. It appears in both sporadic and epidemic forms, but the sporadic cases are more common. The mechanism of spread has not been proved, but it is believed to be transmitted in saliva by direct intimate contact. It is mildly contagious, but the period of communicability is unknown. There is evidence that the virus is spread through sexual contact, especially when multiple partners are involved (Rimsza & Kirk, 2005). The incubation period following exposure is approximately 30 to 50 days (American Academy of Pediatrics, Committee on Infectious Diseases, 2009).

Diagnostic Tests

The onset of symptoms may be acute or insidious and may appear anywhere from 10 days to 6 weeks after exposure. The presenting symptoms vary greatly in type, severity, and duration (Box 46-7). The clinical manifestations of infectious mononucleosis are usually less severe (often subclinical or unapparent), and the convalescent phase is shorter in younger children than in older children and young adults. The leukocyte count may be normal or low. Usually lymphocytic leukocytosis develops, and there is an increase in atypical leukocytes in the peripheral blood smear. The heterophil antibody test determines the extent to which the patient's serum will agglutinate sheep red blood cells; the response in this test is primarily to immune globulin M, which is present in the first 2 weeks of the illness in adolescents.

The *spot test (Monospot)* is a slide test of venous blood that has high specificity. It is rapid, sensitive, inexpensive, and easy to perform and has an advantage over the heterophil antibody test (i.e., it can detect significant agglutinins at lower levels, thus allowing earlier diagnosis). Blood is usually obtained for the test by finger puncture or venous sampling and is placed on special paper. If the blood agglutinates, forming fragments or clumps, the test is positive for the infection.

Therapeutic Management

No specific treatment exists for infectious mononucleosis. Simple remedies ordinarily relieve the symptoms. A mild analgesic is often sufficient to relieve the headache, fever, and malaise. Rest is encouraged for fatigue but is not imposed for any specific period. Affected persons are instructed to regulate activities according to their own tolerance unless complicating factors are present. Contact sports are discouraged in the presence of splenomegaly.

BOX 46-7 Clinical Manifestations of Infectious Mononucleosis

Early Signs
Headache
Malaise
Fatigue
Chills
Low-grade fever
Loss of appetite
Puffy eyes

Acute Disease

Cardinal Features
Fever
Sore throat
Cervical adenopathy

Common Features
Splenomegaly (may persist for several months)
Palatine petechiae
Macular eruption (especially on trunk)
Exudative pharyngitis or tonsillitis

Antibiotics are contraindicated unless GABHS are present. If sore throat is severe, effective therapies include gargles; hot drinks; anesthetic troches; or analgesics, including opioids. Corticosteroids have been used to treat respiratory distress from significant tonsillar inflammation, hemolytic anemia, thrombocytopenia, and neurologic complications; however, routine use of steroids is not recommended (American Academy of Pediatrics, Committee on Infectious Diseases, 2009).

Prognosis

The course of this disease is usually self-limiting and uncomplicated. Acute symptoms often disappear within 7 to 10 days, and persistent fatigue subsides within 2 to 4 weeks. Some adolescents may need to restrict vigorous activities for 2 to 3 months, but the disease rarely extends for longer periods. Complications are uncommon but can be serious and require appropriate management.

Nursing Care Management

Nursing responsibilities are directed toward providing comfort measures to relieve symptoms and helping affected adolescents and their families determine appropriate activities for the stage of the disease. The child is advised to limit exposure to persons outside the family, especially during the acute phase of illness. Children and adolescents may need diet counseling to select foods that contain sufficient calories to meet growth and energy needs but are easy to swallow. It may be more comfortable to limit intake to liquids during the acute phase; milk shakes are a good alternative to solid foods on a temporary basis. Throat pain may be severe enough to require a mild analgesic such as codeine. Careful nursing assessment of swallowing ability is essential because the edema may cause serious airway compromise in some children.

evolve Case Study—Mononucleosis

NURSING ALERT Advise the family to seek medical evaluation of the child or adolescent if:

- Breathing becomes difficult.
- Severe abdominal pain develops.
- Sore throat pain is so severe that the child is unable drink liquids.
- Respiratory stridor is observed.

Croup Syndromes

Croup is a general term applied to a symptom complex characterized by hoarseness, a resonant cough described as "barking" or "brassy" (croupy), varying degrees of inspiratory stridor, and varying degrees of respiratory distress resulting from swelling or obstruction in the region of the larynx. Acute infections of the larynx are important in infants and small children because of their increased incidence in these age groups and because the small diameter of the airway in infants and children places them at risk for significant narrowing with inflammation.

Croup syndromes can affect the larynx, trachea, and bronchi. However, laryngeal involvement often dominates the clinical picture because of the severe effects on the voice and breathing. Croup syndromes are described according to the primary anatomic area affected (i.e., epiglottitis [or supraglottitis], laryngitis, laryngotracheobronchitis [LTB], and tracheitis). In general, LTB occurs in very young children, and epiglottitis is more common in older children. A comparison of croup syndromes is provided in Table 46-1.

With widespread immunization programs aimed at preventing *H. influenzae* type b, the cause of most cases of croup in the United States is attributed to viruses (i.e., parainfluenza virus, human meta-pneumovirus, influenza types A and B, adenovirus, and measles).

Acute Epiglottitis

Acute epiglottitis, or *acute supraglottitis*, is a serious obstructive inflammatory process that occurs predominantly in children 2 to 8 years of age (Rotta & Wiryawan, 2003) but can occur from infancy to adulthood. The disorder requires immediate attention. The obstruction is supraglottic as opposed to the subglottic obstruction of laryngitis. The responsible organism is usually *H. influenzae.* LTB and epiglottitis do not occur together.

Clinical Manifestations

The onset of epiglottitis is abrupt and can rapidly progress to severe respiratory distress. The child usually goes to bed asymptomatic to awaken later, complaining of sore throat and pain on swallowing. The child has a fever; appears sicker than clinical findings suggest; and insists on sitting upright and leaning forward with the chin thrust out, mouth open, and tongue protruding *(tripod position).* Drooling of saliva is common because of the difficulty or pain on swallowing and excessive secretions (see Critical Thinking Exercise).

NURSING ALERT Three clinical observations that have been found to be predictive of epiglottitis are absence of spontaneous cough, presence of drooling, and agitation.

The child is irritable and extremely restless and has an anxious, apprehensive, and frightened expression. The voice is thick and muffled, with a froglike croaking sound on inspiration, but the child is not hoarse. Suprasternal and substernal retractions may be visible. The child seldom struggles to breathe, and slow, quiet breathing provides better air exchange. The throat is red and inflamed, and a distinctive large, cherry-red, edematous epiglottis is visible on careful throat inspection.

Table 46-1 Comparison of Croup Syndromes

	ACUTE EPIGLOTTITIS	ACUTE LTB	ACUTE SPASMODIC LARYNGITIS	ACUTE TRACHEITIS
Age group affected	2-8 yr	Infant or child under 5 yr	1-3 yr	1 mo–6 yr
Etiologic agent	Bacterial	Viral	Viral with allergic component	Viral with allergic component
Onset	Rapidly progressive	Slowly progressive	Sudden; at night	Moderately progressive
Major symptoms	Dysphagia Stridor aggravated when supine Drooling High fever Toxic appearance Rapid pulse and respirations	URI Stridor Brassy cough Hoarseness Dyspnea Restlessness Irritability Low-grade fever Nontoxic appearance	URI Croupy cough Stridor Hoarseness Dyspnea Restlessness Symptoms awakening child Symptoms disappearing during day Tendency to recur	URI Croupy cough Purulent secretions High fever No response to LTB therapy
Treatment	Airway protection Racemic epinephrine Corticosteroids Fluids Reassurance	Racemic epinephrine Corticosteroids Fluids Reassurance	Cool mist	Antibiotics Fluids

LTB, Laryngotracheobronchitis; *URI,* upper respiratory infection.

evolve Case Study—Acute Epiglottitis

CRITICAL THINKING EXERCISE

Croup Syndrome

Kim, a 4-year-old, is admitted to the emergency department with a sore throat, pain on swallowing, drooling, and a fever of 39° C (102.2° F). She looks ill, is agitated, and prefers to sit up leaning on her arms. What nursing interventions should the nurse implement in this situation?

1. Evidence—Is there sufficient evidence to draw any conclusions about Kim's condition at this time?
2. Assumptions—Describe some underlying assumptions about each of the following:
   a. Epiglottitis in children
   b. Symptoms of epiglottitis
   c. Precautions to be taken when a child has suspected epiglottitis
   d. Immediate nursing interventions when caring for a child with epiglottitis
3. What priorities for nursing care can be drawn at this time?
4. Does the evidence objectively support your argument (conclusion)?
5. Are there alternative perspectives to your arguments? What are they?

NURSING ALERT Throat inspection should be attempted only when immediate endotracheal intubation can be performed if needed.

Therapeutic Management

The course of epiglottitis may be fulminant, with respiratory obstruction appearing suddenly. Progressive obstruction leads to hypoxia, hypercapnia, and acidosis followed by decreased muscle tone; reduced level of consciousness; and, when obstruction becomes more or less complete, a rather sudden death. A presumptive diagnosis of epiglottitis constitutes an emergency.

The child who is suspected of having epiglottitis should be examined in a setting where emergency airway equipment is readily available. Examination of the throat with a tongue depressor is contraindicated until experienced personnel and equipment are available to proceed with immediate intubation or tracheostomy in the event that the examination precipitates further or complete obstruction.

If a lateral neck film is indicated, experienced personnel should accompany the child to the radiology department. It is preferable that a young child, who is likely to become more agitated by the procedure, not be transported but remain on the parent's lap in the examination area during portable radiology. Other procedures, such as insertion of an intravenous (IV) line, that are likely to further agitate the child may need to be delayed until adequate airway is maintained.

Nasotracheal intubation or tracheostomy is usually considered for the child with epiglottitis with severe respiratory distress. It is recommended that the intubation or tracheostomy and any invasive procedure, such as starting an IV infusion, be performed in an area where emergency airway maintenance can be easily and quickly accomplished. Humidified oxygen is administered as necessary either via mask in older children or flowby in younger children to avoid further agitation. Whether or not there is an artificial airway, the child requires intensive observation by experienced personnel. The epiglottal swelling usually decreases after 24 hours of antibiotic therapy, and the epiglottis is near normal by the third day. Intubated children are generally extubated at this time. Additional treatment for children with moderate or severe disease includes administration of nebulized epinephrine (racemic epinephrine) or a mixture of helium and oxygen (heliox) to decrease edema. The use of corticosteroids for reducing edema has become a mainstay in the treatment of epiglottitis. Oral corticosteroid is preferred, but other routes of administration include IM, IV, and nebulized (Wright et al, 2005).

Children with suspected bacterial epiglottitis are given antibiotics intravenously, followed by oral administration, to complete a 7- to 10-day course.

Nursing Care Management

Epiglottitis is a serious and frightening disease for the child and family. It is important to act quickly but calmly and to provide support without increasing anxiety. The child is allowed to remain in the position that provides the most comfort and security, and parents are reassured that everything possible is being done to obtain relief for their child.

NURSING ALERT When epiglottitis is suspected, the nurse should not attempt to visualize the epiglottis directly with a tongue depressor or take a throat culture but should refer the child for medical evaluation immediately.

Acute care of the child is the same as that described later for the child with LTB. Continuous monitoring of respiratory status, including pulse oximetry (and blood gases if the patient is intubated), is an important part of nursing observations, and the IV infusion is maintained as described in Chapter 45.

Acute Laryngitis

Acute infectious laryngitis is a common illness in older children and adolescents. Infants and smaller children experience more generalized involvement (see the following section on LTB). Viruses are the usual causative agents; and the principal complaint is hoarseness, which may be accompanied by other upper respiratory symptoms (e.g., rhinitis, sore throat, nasal congestion) and systemic manifestations (e.g., fever, headache, myalgia, malaise). Associated complaints vary with the infecting virus. Adenoviruses, human meta-pneumoviruses, and influenza viruses are responsible for more systemic involvement; parainfluenza viruses, rhinoviruses, and RSV cause milder illness.

Therapeutic Management and Nursing Care Management

The disease is usually self-limited without long-term sequelae. Treatment is symptomatic with fluids and humidified air (see Nursing Care Plan, pp. 1308-1309).

Acute Laryngotracheobronchitis

LTB is the most common croup syndrome. It primarily affects children younger than 5 years of age, and the causative organisms are the parainfluenza virus types 2 and 3, human metapneumovirus, RSV, influenza A and B, and *M. pneumoniae.* The disease is usually preceded by a URI, which gradually descends to adjacent structures. It is characterized by gradual onset of low-grade fever, and the parents often report that the child went to bed and later awoke with a barky, brassy cough. Inflammation of the mucosa lining the larynx and trachea causes a narrowing of the airway. When the airway is significantly narrowed, the child struggles to inhale air past the obstruction and into the lungs, producing the characteristic inspiratory stridor and suprasternal retractions; other classic manifestations include cough and hoarseness. Respiratory distress in infants and toddlers may be manifested by nasal flaring, intercostal retractions, tachypnea, and continuous stridor. The typical child with LTB is a toddler who develops the classic barking or seal-like cough and acute stridor after several days of rhinitis. When the child is unable to inhale a sufficient volume of air, symptoms of hypoxia become evident. Obstruction that is severe enough to prevent adequate ventilation and exhalation of carbon dioxide can cause respiratory acidosis and eventually respiratory failure. The progression of symptoms is outlined in Box 46-8.

BOX 46-8 Progression of Symptoms in Laryngotracheobronchitis

Stage I
Fear
Hoarseness
Croupy cough
Inspiratory stridor when disturbed

Stage II
Continuous respiratory stridor
Lower rib retraction
Retraction of soft tissue of neck
Use of accessory muscles of respiration
Labored respiration

Stage III
Signs of anoxia and carbon dioxide retention
Restlessness
Anxiety
Pallor
Sweating
Rapid respirations

Stage IV
Intermittent cyanosis
Permanent cyanosis
Cessation of breathing

From Walter EB, Shurin PA: Acute respiratory infections. In Krugman S et al: *Infectious diseases of children,* ed 9, St Louis, 1992, Mosby.

Therapeutic Management

The major objective in medical management is maintaining the airway and providing adequate respiratory exchange. Children with mild croup (no stridor at rest) can be managed at home. Parents are taught the signs of respiratory distress and instructed to summon professional help early if needed. Children who progress to stage II respiratory symptoms should receive medical attention (see Box 46-8).

High humidity with cool mist provides relief for most children. A cool-air vaporizer can be used at home. In the hospital a nebulized mist for older infants and toddlers may be used to provide increased humidity and supplemental oxygen. However, controversy surrounds the use of mist therapy to treat croup. Studies have failed to demonstrate any improvement in subglottic edema with mist therapy (Moore & Little, 2006).

Nebulized epinephrine (racemic epinephrine) is often used in children with severe disease, stridor at rest, retractions, or difficulty breathing. The α-adrenergic effects cause mucosal vasoconstriction and subsequently decrease subglottic edema. The onset of action is rapid, and the peak effect is observed in 2 hours. Children may be discharged home following racemic epinephrine after a 2- to 3-hour period of observation for return of acute symptoms.

Oral steroids have proved effective in the treatment of croup; IM dexamethasone may be given to children who are unable to tolerate oral dosing. Nebulized budesonide may be administered in conjunction with IM dexamethasone. A single dose of oral corticosteroid has been shown to decrease hospitalizations and the need for multiple racemic epinephrine treatments in children with mild croup.

In severe cases of LTB the administration of heliox may serve to reduce the work of breathing and relieve airway obstruction. Because helium has a lower density than room air, it forms a respirable gas (with oxygen) that reduces airway turbulence.

evolve Animation—Intubation

Nursing Care Management

The most important nursing function in the care of children with LTB is continuous, vigilant observation and accurate assessment of respiratory status. Pulse oximetry is commonly used for monitoring oxygenation status. Changes in therapy are frequently based on the nurses' observations and assessments, the child's response to therapy, and tolerance of procedures. The trend away from early intubation of children with LTB emphasizes the importance of nursing observations and the ability to recognize impending respiratory failure so that intubation can be implemented without delay. Intubation equipment must be readily accessible and taken with the child during transport to other areas (e.g., radiology, operating room).

NURSING ALERT Early signs of impending airway obstruction include increased pulse and respiratory rate; substernal, suprasternal, and intercostal retractions; flaring nares; and increased restlessness.

Infants or small children find that being enclosed in a tent, coughing, having laryngeal spasms, and needing IV therapy are additional sources of distress. In many acute care facilities the mist tent has been abandoned, and the parent is allowed to hold the infant; if cool mist is used in the treatment, it can be administered through a tube held in front of the patient while the child is held on the parent's lap.

Children with mild croup are allowed to drink beverages they like as long as respiratory status is stable, and parents are encouraged to try whatever comforting measures work best (e.g., holding their child, rocking, singing). If the child is unable to take oral fluids, IV fluids may be required in addition to IV medications (dexamethasone).

The rapid progression of croup, the alarming sound of the cough and stridor, and the child's apprehensive behavior and ill appearance combine to create a frightening experience for the parents. Parents need reassurance regarding their child's progress and an explanation of treatments. The family should be allowed to remain with their child as much as possible.

The nurse should provide the parents with an opportunity to express their feelings and should provide them with referrals as necessary. Parents need frequent reassurance provided in a calm, quiet manner and education regarding what they can do to make their child more comfortable. Home care includes continued humidity, adequate hydration, and nourishment.

Acute Spasmodic Laryngitis

Acute spasmodic laryngitis (*spasmodic croup*, "midnight croup," or "twilight croup") is distinct from laryngitis and LTB and is characterized by paroxysmal attacks of laryngeal obstruction that occur chiefly at night. Signs of inflammation are absent or mild, and there is often a history of previous attacks lasting 2 to 5 days, followed by uneventful recovery. This condition usually affects children ages 1 to 3 years. Some children appear to be predisposed to the condition; allergies may be implicated in some cases.

The child goes to bed feeling well or with mild respiratory symptoms but awakens suddenly with characteristic barking, metallic cough; hoarseness; noisy inspirations; and restlessness. The child appears anxious and frightened. Dyspnea is aggravated by excitement, but there is no fever, the attack subsides in a few hours, and the child appears well the next day.

✱ Therapeutic Management and Nursing Care Management

Spasmodic croup is usually self-limiting, and most children are managed at home. A cool mist humidifier may be recommended for home treatment. Sometimes the spasm is relieved by sudden exposure to cold air (as when the child is taken out into the night air to see the practitioner). Parents are usually advised to have the child sleep in humidified air until the cough has subsided to prevent subsequent episodes. Children with moderately severe symptoms may be hospitalized for observation and therapy with cool mist and racemic epinephrine, as for LTB. Some patients respond to corticosteroid therapy.

Bacterial Tracheitis

Bacterial tracheitis, an infection of the mucosa of the upper trachea, is a distinct entity with features of both croup and epiglottitis. The disease occurs more commonly in children under 3 years of age and may be a serious cause of airway obstruction that is severe enough to cause respiratory arrest. It is believed to be a complication of LTB, and although *Staphylococcus aureus* is the most frequent organism responsible, *M. catarrhalis, S. pneumonia*, and *H. influenzae* have also been implicated.

Many of the manifestations of bacterial tracheitis are similar to those of LTB but are unresponsive to LTB therapy. There is a history of previous URI with croupy cough, stridor unaffected by position, toxicity, absence of drooling, and high fever. A prominent manifestation is the production of thick, purulent tracheal secretions. Respiratory difficulties are secondary to these copious secretions. Children with this condition may develop a life-threatening upper airway obstruction, respiratory failure, ARDS, and multiple organ dysfunction (Hopkins et al, 2006).

✱ Therapeutic Management and Nursing Care Management

Bacterial tracheitis requires vigorous management with antipyretics and antibiotics. Many children require endotracheal intubation and mechanical ventilation; patients are closely monitored for impending respiratory failure if not intubated. Early recognition to prevent life-threatening airway obstruction is essential.

Lower Respiratory Tract Infections

The *reactive portion* of the lower respiratory tract includes the bronchi and bronchioles in children. Cartilaginous support of the large airways is not fully developed until adolescence. Consequently, the smooth muscle in these structures represents a major factor in the constriction of the airway, particularly in the *bronchioles*, the portion that extends from the bronchi to the alveoli. Table 46-2 compares some of the major features of bronchial and bronchiolar infections.

Bronchitis

Bronchitis (sometimes referred to as *tracheobronchitis*) is inflammation of the large airways (trachea and bronchi), which is frequently associated with a URI. Viral agents are the primary cause of the disease, although *M. pneumoniae* is a common cause in children older than 6 years of age. A dry, hacking, nonproductive cough that worsens at night and becomes productive in 2 or 3 days characterizes this condition.

Bronchitis is a mild, self-limiting disease that requires only symptomatic treatment, including analgesics, antipyretics, and humidity. Cough suppressants may be useful to allow rest but can interfere with clearance of secretions. Most patients recover uneventfully in 5 to 10 days.

Respiratory Syncytial Virus and Bronchiolitis

Bronchiolitis is an acute viral infection with maximum effect at the bronchiolar level. Although most cases of bronchiolitis are caused by RSV, adenoviruses and parainfluenza viruses are also implicated; recently, human meta-pneumovirus has also been associated with bronchiolitis in children. The infection occurs primarily in winter and spring. By age 3 years most children have been infected at least once. RSV infection is the most frequent cause of hospitalization in children less than 1 year old. In addition, severe RSV infections in the first year of

evolve Case Study–Bronchiolitis

Table 46-2 Comparison of Conditions Affecting the Bronchi

	ASTHMA*	BRONCHITIS	BRONCHIOLITIS
Description	Exaggerated response of bronchi to a trigger such as URI, dander, cold air, exercise Bronchospasm, exudation, and edema of bronchi	Usually occurs in association with URI Seldom an isolated entity	Most common infectious disease of lower airways Maximum obstructive impact at bronchiolar level
Age group affected	Infancy to adolescence	First 4 yr of life	Usually children 2-12 mo of age; rare after age 2 yr Peak incidence approximately age 6 mo
Etiologic agents	Most often viruses such as RSV in infants but may be any of a variety of URI pathogens	Usually viral Other agents (e.g., bacteria, fungi, allergic disorders, airborne irritants) can trigger symptoms	Viruses, predominantly RSVs; also adenoviruses, parainfluenza viruses, human meta-pneumovirus, and *Mycoplasma pneumoniae*
Predominant characteristics	Wheezing, cough	Persistent dry, hacking cough (worse at night) becoming productive in 2-3 days	Labored respirations, poor feeding, cough, tachypnea, retractions and flaring nares, emphysema, increased nasal mucus, wheezing, may have fever
Treatment	Inhaled corticosteroids, bronchodilators, leukotriene modifiers, allergen, and control of triggers	Cough suppressants if needed	Provide supplemental oxygen if saturations ≤90%; bronchodilators (optional) Suction nasopharynx Ensure adequate fluid intake Maintain adequate oxygenation

*See Asthma, p. 1334.
RSV, Respiratory syncytial virus; *URI*, upper respiratory infection.

life represent a significant risk factor for the development of asthma up to age 13 (Chávez-Bueno et al, 2005). RSV infection may also occur in children older than 1 year who have a chronic or serious disabling illness.

Pathophysiology

RSV affects the epithelial cells of the respiratory tract. The ciliated cells swell, protrude into the lumen, and lose their cilia. RSV produces a fusion of the infected cell membrane with cell membranes of adjacent epithelial cells, thus forming a giant cell with multiple nuclei. At the cellular level this fusion results in multinucleated masses of protoplasm, or *syncytia*.

The bronchiolar mucosa swells, and lumina are subsequently filled with mucus and exudate. The walls of the bronchi and bronchioles are infiltrated with inflammatory cells, and peribronchiolar interstitial pneumonitis is usually present. Because luminal epithelial cells are shed into the bronchioles when they die, the lumina are frequently obstructed, particularly on expiration. The varying degrees of obstruction produced in small air passages lead to hyperinflation, obstructive emphysema resulting from partial obstruction, and patchy areas of atelectasis. Dilation of bronchial passages on inspiration allows sufficient space for intake of air, but narrowing of the passages on expiration prevents air from leaving the lungs. Thus air is trapped distal to the obstruction and causes progressive overinflation (emphysema).

Clinical Manifestations

The illness usually begins with a URI after an incubation of about 5 to 8 days. Symptoms such as rhinorrhea and low-grade fever often appear first. OM and conjunctivitis may also be present. In time a cough may develop. If the disease progresses, it becomes a lower respiratory tract infection and manifests typical symptoms (Box 46-9). Infants may have several days of URI symptoms or no symptoms except slight lethargy, poor feeding, or irritability.

BOX 46-9 Signs and Symptoms of Respiratory Syncytial Virus

Initial
- Rhinorrhea
- Pharyngitis
- Coughing/sneezing
- Wheezing
- Possible ear or eye drainage
- Intermittent fever

With Progression of Illness
- Increased coughing and wheezing
- Tachypnea and retractions
- Cyanosis

Severe Illness
- Tachypnea greater than 70 breaths/min
- Listlessness
- Apneic spells
- Poor air exchange; poor breath sounds

Once the lower airway is involved, classic manifestations include signs of altered air exchange, such as wheezing, retractions, crackles, dyspnea, tachypnea, and diminished breath sounds. Apnea may be the first recognized indicator of RSV infection in very young infants.

Diagnostic Evaluation

Identification has been simplified by the development of tests done on nasal or nasopharyngeal secretions, using either rapid immunofluorescent antibody–direct fluorescent antibody staining (DFA), or enzyme-linked immunosorbent assay (ELISA) techniques for RSV antigen detection (see Respiratory Secretion Specimens, Chapter 45).

Therapeutic Management

Bronchiolitis is treated symptomatically with cool humidified oxygen, adequate fluid intake, airway maintenance, and medications. Most children with bronchiolitis can be managed at home. Hospitalization is usually recommended for children with respiratory distress or those who cannot maintain adequate hydration. Other reasons for hospitalization include complicating conditions, such as underlying lung or heart disease or associated debilitated states, or a home environment where adequate management is questionable. The infant who is tachypneic or apneic, has marked retractions, seems listless, or has a history of poor fluid intake should be admitted.

Humidified oxygen is administered in concentrations sufficient to maintain adequate oxygenation (Spo_2) at or above 90% as measured by pulse oximetry. The administration of humidified mist is controversial. Routine chest physical therapy (CPT) is not recommended; infants with abundant nasal secretions benefit from periodic suctioning. Fluids by mouth may be contraindicated because of tachypnea, weakness, and fatigue; therefore IV fluids are preferred until the acute stage of the disease has passed.

Clinical assessments and noninvasive oxygen monitoring guide therapy. Medical therapy for bronchiolitis is primarily supportive and aimed at decreasing airway hyperresonance and inflammation and promoting adequate fluid intake. Bronchodilators may provide short-term benefits, yet overall significant improvement in the child's condition is not always appreciable. Racemic epinephrine has been shown to produce modest improvement in ventilation status. Corticosteroids and antihistamines have not been shown to be effective in controlled studies and are not recommended for routine use. Antibiotics are not part of the treatment of RSV unless there is a coexisting bacterial infection such as OM (American Academy of Pediatrics, 2006). Additional treatment recommendations in the American Academy of Pediatrics practice guideline (2006) are to encourage breastfeeding; avoid passive tobacco smoke exposure; and promote preventive measures, including handwashing and the administration of palivizumab (Synagis) to high risk infants.

Ribavirin, an antiviral agent (synthetic nucleoside analog), is the only specific therapy approved for hospitalized children; however, use of this drug in infants with RSV is controversial because of concerns about the high cost, aerosol route of administration, potential toxic effects among exposed health care personnel, and conflicting results of efficacy trials (American Academy of Pediatrics, 2006; Chávez-Bueno et al, 2005; Ventre & Randolph, 2007). This drug is aerosolized and delivered via a small-particle aerosol generator. It may be administered by hood, tent, or mask or through ventilator tubing for 12 to 20 hours daily; average duration of therapy is 3 days.

Prevention of Respiratory Syncytial Virus Infection

The only product available in the United States for prevention of RSV is palivizumab, a monoclonal antibody, which is given monthly in an IM injection. According to the American Academy of Pediatrics practice guideline (2006), candidates for palivizumab include infants born before 32 weeks of gestation who required medical therapy such as supplemental oxygen or mechanical ventilation. Infants and children younger than 2 years of age with BPD who have received medical therapy (supplemental oxygen, bronchodilator, diuretic, or corticosteroid therapy) for BPD within 6 months before the anticipated RSV season may benefit from palivizumab prophylaxis. Children with more severe BPD may benefit from palivizumab prophylaxis for two RSV seasons. Children with severe immunodeficiencies (e.g., severe combined immunodeficiency or acquired immunodeficiency syndrome [AIDS]) may also benefit from prophylaxis. Infants and children younger than 2 years of age with hemodynamically significant congenital heart disease benefit from 5 monthly IM injections of palivizumab. Prophylaxis for RSV should be initiated at the onset of the RSV season and terminated at the end of the season (November to March). Additional age and condition recommendations are outlined in the American Academy of Pediatrics practice guideline (2006). The lyophilized powder form of palivizumab should be administered within 6 hours of being reconstituted with sterile water because it is preservative free.

A second-generation monoclonal antibody, motavizumab (Numax), is currently undergoing phase III clinical trials; this drug is reported to be more effective in the prevention of RSV than palivizumab (DeVincenzo, 2008).

❀ Nursing Care Management

Children admitted to the hospital with suspected RSV infection may be assigned separate rooms or grouped with other RSV-infected children. Contact and standard precautions are used, including handwashing, not touching the nasal mucosa or conjunctiva, and using gloves and gowns when entering the patient's room. Other isolation procedures of potential benefit are those aimed at diminishing the number of hospital personnel, visitors, and uninfected children in contact with the child. Another measure is to make patient assignments so that nurses assigned to children with RSV are not caring for other patients who are considered high risk.

Infants with RSV often have copious nasal secretions, making breathing and nursing or bottle-feeding difficult. This engenders concerns that the child will lose weight or stop breastfeeding altogether. Encourage breastfeeding mothers to continue feeding the infant, or if feedings are contraindicated because of the acuity of the illness, mothers should pump their milk and store appropriately for later use (see Chapter 26). Parents are taught how to instill normal saline drops into the nares and suction the mucus with a bulb syringe before feedings and before bedtime so the child may eat and rest better; unfortunately no medications appropriate for infants can help with these symptoms. To address the issue of decreased fluid intake, parents may offer small amounts of clear fluids, 5 to 10 ml at a time, with a medication syringe every 10 minutes or so to maintain adequate hydration. Infants may cough or vomit as the secretions settle in the stomach and make them prone to emesis of such secretions.

Additional nursing care is aimed at monitoring oxygenation with pulse oximetry, ensuring that bronchodilator therapy is optimized by using a small mask for delivery, and providing information for the parent regarding the infant's status. The unpredictability of the infant's individual response to the disease compounds parental anxiety when they hear about children who had serious morbidity or died from RSV. However, for the most part infants recover quickly from the disease and resume normal daily activities, including fluid intake. Such infants are at risk for further episodes of wheezing that may or may not involve an RSV infection; however, parents may be concerned that the infant has another serious case of RSV.

Pneumonias

Pneumonia, inflammation of the pulmonary parenchyma, is common in childhood but occurs more frequently in infancy and early childhood. Clinically, pneumonia may occur either as a primary disease or as a complication of another illness. The various types of pneumonia include:

Lobar pneumonia—All or a large segment of one or more pulmonary lobes is involved.

Bronchopneumonia—This begins in the terminal bronchioles, which become clogged with mucopurulent exudate to form consolidated patches in nearby lobules; also called *lobular pneumonia.*

Interstitial pneumonia—The inflammatory process is more or less confined within the alveolar walls (interstitium) and the peribronchial and interlobular tissues.

Although the morphologic classification is typically used, the most useful classification of pneumonia is based on the etiologic agent (i.e., viral, bacterial, mycoplasmal, or aspiration of foreign substances) (see Aspiration Pneumonia, p. 1330). Histomycosis, coccidioidomycosis, and other fungi also cause pneumonia. The causative agent is identified from the clinical history, the child's age, the general health history, the physical examination, radiography, and the laboratory examination. Other terms that describe pneumonias are hemorrhagic, fibrinous, and necrotizing. *Pneumonitis* is a localized acute inflammation of the lung without the toxemia associated with lobar pneumonia.

The clinical manifestations of pneumonia vary depending on the etiologic agent, the child's age, the child's systemic reaction to the infection, the extent of the lesions, and the degree of bronchial and bronchiolar obstruction. The causative agent is identified from the clinical history, the child's age, the general health history, the physical examination, radiography, and the laboratory examination.

Viral Pneumonia

Viral pneumonias, which occur more frequently than bacterial pneumonias, are seen in children of all ages and are often associated with viral URIs. Viruses that cause pneumonia include RSV in infants and parainfluenza, influenza, human meta-pneumovirus, and adenovirus in older children. Few clinical symptoms are unique to a specific virus, and differentiation among viruses is usually made by clinical features such as child's age, past medical history, season of the year, and radiographic and laboratory examination (Box 46-10).

The prognosis is generally good, although viral infections of the respiratory tract render the affected child more susceptible to secondary bacterial invasion, especially when there is denuded bronchial mucosa. Treatment is symptomatic and includes measures to promote oxygenation and comfort, such as oxygen administration with cool mist, CPT and postural drainage, antipyretics for fever management, fluid intake, and family support. Some authorities recommend antimicrobial therapy in the hopes of reducing or preventing secondary bacterial infection, but this therapy should be reserved for children in whom a bacterial infection is demonstrated by appropriate cultures.

BOX 46-10 General Signs of Pneumonia

Fever—Usually quite high

Respiratory
- Cough—Nonproductive to productive with whitish sputum
- Tachypnea
- Breath sounds—Rhonchi or fine crackles
- Dullness with percussion
- Chest pain; abdominal pain with lower lobe involvement
- Retractions
- Nasal flaring
- Pallor to cyanosis (depends on severity)

Chest x-ray film—Diffuse or patchy infiltration with peribronchial distribution

Behavior—Irritable, restless, lethargic

Gastrointestinal—Anorexia, vomiting, diarrhea, abdominal pain

Primary Atypical Pneumonia

Atypical pneumonia refers to pneumonia that is caused by pathogens other than the traditionally most common and readily cultured bacteria (e.g., *S. pneumoniae*). In the category of atypical pneumonias, *M. pneumoniae* and *Chlamydia pneumoniae* are the most common causes of community-acquired pneumonia in children 5 years old or older (Rafei & Lichenstein, 2006). It occurs in the fall and winter months and is more prevalent in crowded living conditions. Most affected persons recover from acute illness in 7 to 10 days with symptomatic treatment followed by a week of convalescence. Hospitalization is rarely necessary.

Bacterial Pneumonia

S. pneumoniae is the most common bacterial pathogen responsible for community-acquired pneumonia in both children and adults (Rafei & Lichenstein, 2006). Other bacteria that cause pneumonia in children are group A streptococcus, *S. aureus, M. catarrhalis, M. pneumoniae,* and *C. pneumoniae.*

Beyond the neonatal period, bacterial pneumonias display distinct clinical patterns that facilitate their differentiation from other forms of pneumonia. The onset of illness is abrupt and generally follows a viral infection that disturbs the natural defense mechanisms of the upper respiratory tract.

The child with bacterial pneumonia usually appears ill. Symptoms include fever, malaise, rapid and shallow respirations, cough, and chest pain. The pain of pneumonia may be referred to the abdomen and confused with appendicitis. Chills and meningeal symptoms *(meningism)* are common.

Most older children with pneumonia can be treated at home if the condition is recognized and treatment is initiated early. Antibiotic therapy, bed rest, liberal oral intake of fluid, and administration of an antipyretic for fever are the principal therapeutic measures. Follow-up examination is recommended for small infants and toddlers. Hospitalization is indicated when pleural effusion or empyema accompanies the disease, when compliance with therapy is estimated to be poor, in infants less than 1 month old, and when there are chronic illnesses such as congenital heart disease or BPD (Rafei & Lichenstein, 2006). IV fluids may be necessary to ensure adequate hydration, and oxygen is required if the child is in respiratory distress; some children may require initial therapy with parenteral antibiotics due to the severity of illness.

Complications

At present the classic features and clinical course of pneumonia are seen infrequently because of early and vigorous antibiotic and supportive therapy. However, some children, especially infants, with staphylococcal pneumonia develop empyema, pyopneumothorax, or tension pneumothorax. AOM and pleural effusion are common in children with pneumococcal pneumonia.

Continuous closed-chest drainage may be instituted when purulent fluid is aspirated. If a large amount of purulent drainage is obtained, an appropriate antibiotic is instilled into the pleural space, and active chest drainage is discontinued for approximately 1 hour after the instillation. Closed drainage is continued until drainage fluid is free of pathogens, which rarely requires more than 5 to 7 days. Sometimes, repeated pleural taps are sufficient to remove fluid; however, if the purulent drainage accumulates rapidly and is highly viscous, continuous chest drainage is preferred. Thoracotomy with open debridement of the infected lung tissue may be required; if empyema and pneumothorax tend to recur, a partial thoracoscopic lobectomy may be performed.

Prognosis

The prognosis for pneumonia is generally good, with rapid recovery when symptoms are recognized and treated early. Streptococcal infections vary in duration but usually resolve spontaneously. The course of staphylococcal pneumonia is generally prolonged. The prognosis varies with the length of illness before treatment is begun, although early recognition and treatment are usually effective.

Prevention

The use of the heptavalent pneumococcal conjugate vaccine (PCV; Prevnar) is recommended for infants and children younger than 23 months of age to be administered at 2, 4, 6, 12, and 15 months of age; studies have demonstrated a decrease in pneumococcal pneumonia in children younger than 24 months. The polyvalent pneumococcal polysaccharide vaccine (PPSV) provides protection from pneumococcal serotypes in children 24 months old and older (American Academy of Pediatrics, Committee on Infectious Diseases, 2009) (see Immunizations, Chapter 36).

✱ Nursing Care Management

For the child being cared for at home the nurse educates the parent regarding antibiotic and antipyretic administration, assessment of respiratory status, and oral fluid intake. If the child is ill, solid foods may be rejected; fluid intake is encouraged until the he or she feels well enough to eat solids. Parents are reassured that the child's appetite will return once the acute phase of the illness has passed. If the cough is disturbing, judicious use of antitussives, especially at bedtime, is often helpful. Most sick children are adept at self-regulation of activity and rest; parents are encouraged to allow the child appropriate rest and discourage vigorous activities until the he or she has been afebrile for 24 hours or more. Return to school or day care is usually permitted according to the type of pneumonia, severity of illness, and practitioner recommendation. It should be emphasized that the infection may be transmitted to other children with close contact.

Nursing care of the hospitalized child with pneumonia is primarily supportive and symptomatic but necessitates thorough respiratory assessment, antibiotics, and evaluation of hydration status; supplemental oxygen may be required if oxygenation status is compromised. The child's respiratory rate and oxygenation status, as well as vital signs, pain level, and general disposition and level of activity, are frequently assessed. Isolation procedures are implemented according to hospital policy, but standard and contact precautions are recommended initially for all children with a URI until the exact cause is known. To prevent dehydration, fluids are frequently administered intravenously during the acute phase.

Nursing care of the child with a chest tube requires close attention to respiratory status as noted previously; the chest tube and drainage device used are monitored for proper function (i.e., drainage is not impeded, vacuum setting is correct, tubing is free of kinks, dressing covering chest tube insertion site is intact, water seal is maintained [if used], and chest tube remains in place). Movement in bed and ambulation with a chest tube are encouraged according to the child's respiratory status, but children often require a mild analgesic such as acetaminophen.

If needed, supplemental oxygen may be administered by nasal cannula or face mask (or face tent [bucket]); small infants may be given humidified oxygen via a plastic head hood or rarely via a mist tent. Children are usually more comfortable in a semierect position (Fig. 46-3) but should be allowed to determine the position of comfort. Lying on the affected side (if pneumonia is unilateral) splints the chest on that side and reduces the pleural rubbing that often causes discomfort. Fever is controlled by the cool environment and administration of antipyretic drugs.

Children, especially infants, with ineffectual cough or difficulty handling secretions require suctioning to maintain a patent airway. A simple bulb suction syringe is usually sufficient for clearing the nares and nasopharynx of infants, but mechanical suction should be readily available if needed. A noninvasive suction device may be used to suction the infant's nares without the danger of causing nasal trauma; the device may be connected to mechanical suction for best results. Older children can usually handle secretions without assistance. Postural drainage, CPT, and nebulized bronchodilator

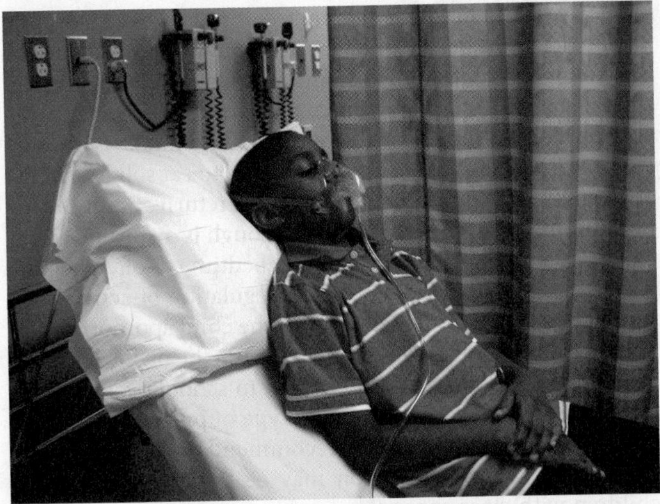

Fig. 46-3 Child placed in semierect position is often more comfortable, and this position enhances diaphragmatic expansion.

treatments may be prescribed, depending on the child's condition.

The hospitalized child may be apprehensive, and the treatments and tests are frightening and stress producing. Reducing anxiety and apprehension reduces psychologic distress, and when the child is more relaxed, the respiratory efforts are lessened. Easing respiratory efforts makes the child less apprehensive, and encouraging the presence of a caregiver provides the child with a source of comfort and support. It is important to involve the entire family in the care as appropriate and to encourage questions and facilitate effective communication. Allowing the child to be involved in regular activities such as quiet play may help reduce the anxiety of hospitalization and separation from friends and family.

Other Respiratory Tract Infections

Pertussis (Whooping Cough)

Pertussis, or whooping cough, is an acute respiratory tract infection caused by *Bordetella pertussis* that in the past primarily occurred in children younger than 4 years of age who were not immunized. It is highly contagious and is particularly threatening in young infants, who have a higher morbidity and mortality rate. Infants less than 6 months of age may not come in to the practitioner with the typical cough; in this age group, apnea is a common presenting manifestation (American Academy of Pediatrics, Committee on Infectious Diseases, 2009). Likewise, older children are known to manifest the disease with a persistent cough and the absence of the characteristic whoop (see Table 38-2 for clinical manifestations of pertussis and Chapter 36 for immunization). The incidence is highest in the spring and summer months, and a single attack confers lifetime immunity. The resurgence of pertussis in the United States, particularly among children 10 years old and older, has prompted concerns of the long-term effects of the pertussis vaccine. Consequently two acellular pertussis booster vaccines have been approved for older children: Boostrix (for children ages 10 to 18 years) and Adacel (for persons ages 11 to 64 years).

Tuberculosis

Tuberculosis (TB) is the second leading cause of death from an infectious disease. Ten million to 15 million persons in the United States are infected with TB. Case rates of TB for all ages are higher in urban, low-income areas and among non-Caucasian racial and ethnic groups. In recent years, foreign-born children have accounted for more than one fourth of newly diagnosed cases of TB in children 14 years of age or younger in the United States (American Academy of Pediatrics, Committee on Infectious Diseases, 2009).

TB is caused by *Mycobacterium tuberculosis*, an acid-fast bacillus not readily decolorized by acids after staining. Children are susceptible to the human *(M. tuberculosis)* and the bovine *(Mycobacterium bovis)* organisms. In parts of the world where TB in cattle is not controlled or milk is not pasteurized, the bovine type is a common source of infection.

Although the causative agent for TB is the tubercle bacillus, other factors influence the degree to which the organism produces an altered state in the host. These factors include heredity (resistance to the infection may be genetically transmitted), gender (higher rates in adolescent girls), age (lower resistance in infants, higher incidence during adolescence), stress (emotional or physical), nutritional state, and intercurrent infection (especially human immunodeficiency virus [HIV], measles, and pertussis). Children with HIV infection have an increased incidence of TB disease, and all children with TB should be tested for HIV.

The source of TB infection in children is usually an infected member of the household or a frequent visitor to the home such as a baby-sitter or domestic worker. The lung is the usual portal of entry for the organism. In the lungs a proliferation of epithelial cells surrounds and encapsulates the multiplying bacilli in an attempt to wall it off, thus forming the typical tubercle. Extension of the primary lesion at the original site causes progressive tissue destruction as it spreads within the lung, discharges material from foci to other areas of the lungs (e.g., bronchi, pleura), or produces pneumonia. Erosion of blood vessels by the primary lesion can cause widespread dissemination of the tubercle bacillus to near and distant sites (miliary TB). Extrapulmonary TB may be manifested as superior lymphadenitis, meningitis, and osteoarthritis and may appear in the middle ear and mastoid and on the skin (American Academy of Pediatrics, Committee on Infectious Diseases, 2009). With the exception of meningitis, treatment for extrapulmonary TB may be the same drug regimen as for pulmonary TB.

Diagnostic Evaluation

Diagnosis is based on information derived from physical examination, history, tuberculin skin testing, radiographic examinations, and cultures of the organism. The clinical manifestations of the disease are extremely variable (Box 46-11).

The *tuberculin skin test (TST)* is the most important indicator of whether a child has been infected with the tubercle bacillus. The standard dose of purified protein derivative (PPD) is 5 tuberculin units, which is administered using a

BOX 46-11 Clinical Manifestations of Tuberculosis

May be asymptomatic or produce a broad range of symptoms:
- Fever
- Malaise
- Anorexia
- Weight loss
- Cough (may or may not be present; progresses slowly over weeks to months)
- Aching pain and tightness in the chest
- Hemoptysis (rare)

With progression:
- Increased respiratory rate
- Poor expansion of lung on the affected side
- Diminished breath sounds and crackles
- Dullness on percussion
- Persistent fever
- Generalized symptoms
- Pallor, anemia, weakness, and weight loss

27-gauge needle and a 1-ml syringe intradermally into the volar aspect of the forearm. Creation of a visible wheal is crucial to accurate testing. A change in TB screening procedures has been recommended by the American Academy of Pediatrics, Committee on Infectious Diseases (2009); universal testing of all children for TB is no longer recommended. Subsequently a targeted testing method is used wherein only children and adolescents at high risk for contracting the disease, in addition to patients at risk for progression to TB disease, are screened. A risk factor questionnaire (available from the Pediatric Tuberculosis Collaborative Group [2004]), has been developed to facilitate screening pediatric populations at high risk; factors on the questionnaire include a close association with persons having latent or active disease, foreign birth, or foreign travel. Recommendations for TST of children are listed in Box 46-12.

A *positive reaction* indicates that the individual has been infected and has developed sensitivity to the tubercle bacillus. However, it does not confirm the presence of active disease. Once an individual reacts positively, he or she will always react positively. A previously negative reaction that becomes positive indicates that the person has been infected since the last test. Guidelines for interpreting the TST are listed in Box 46-13. Prompt radiographic evaluation of all children with a positive TST reaction is recommended. The American Academy of Pediatrics, Committee on Infectious Diseases (2009) recommends that administration of the TST and interpretation of the results be performed and read only by trained health care professionals.

The term *latent tuberculosis infection* (LTBI) is used to indicate infection in a person who has a positive TST, no physical findings of disease, and normal chest radiograph findings. The term *tuberculosis disease* is used when a child has clinical symptoms or radiographic manifestations caused by the *M. tuberculosis* organism. A diagnosis of LTBI or TB disease in a child is a sentinel event usually representing recent transmission of the *M. tuberculosis* organism.

Therapeutic Management

Medical management of TB disease in children consists of adequate nutrition, pharmacotherapy, general supportive measures, prevention of unnecessary exposure to other infections that further compromise the body's defenses, prevention of reinfection, and sometimes surgical procedures.

The recommended drug regimen for LTBI in children and adolescents includes a daily dose of isoniazid (INH) for 9 months or alternatively two or three times per week with direct observation of therapy (DOT). DOT means that a health care worker or other responsible, mutually agreed-on individual is present when medications are administered to the patient. Rifampin (daily for 6 months; alternatively DOT twice weekly for 6 months) may be used to treat the child or adolescent who is INH resistant (American Academy of Pediatrics, Committee on Infectious Diseases, 2009).

For the child with clinically active TB, the goal is to achieve sterilization of the tuberculous lesion. Recommended drug therapy for treating TB disease includes combinations of INH, rifampin, and pyrazinamide (PZA). The American Academy of Pediatrics, Committee on Infectious Diseases (2009) recommends a 6-month regimen consisting of INH, rifampin, and PZA given daily for the first 2 months, followed by INH and rifampin given two or three times a week by DOT for the remaining 4 months. DOT decreases the rates of relapse, treatment failures, and drug resistance and is recommended for treatment of children and adolescents with TB in the United States.

If the child is suspected of having multidrug-resistant TB, a fourth medication such as streptomycin (IM injection only) or ethambutol is added. Optimal therapy for TB in children with HIV infection has not been established, and consultation with a specialist is advised. Therapy should always include at least three drugs initially and be continued for at least 9 months. INH, rifampin, and PZA usually with ethambutol or an aminoglycoside should be given for at least the first 2 months. The three-drug regimen can be used after drug-resistant disease is excluded.

Surgical procedures may be required to remove the source of infection in tissues that are inaccessible to pharmacotherapy or that are destroyed by the disease. Orthopedic procedures may be performed for correction of bone deformities, and bronchoscopy may be done for removal of a tuberculous granulomatous polyp.

Prognosis

Most children recover from primary TB infection and are often unaware of its presence. However, very young children have a higher incidence of disseminated disease. TB is a serious disease during the first 2 years of life, during adolescence, and in children who are HIV positive. Except in cases of tuberculous meningitis, death seldom occurs in treated children. Antibiotic therapy has decreased the death rate and the hematogenous spread from primary lesions.

Prevention

The only definite means to prevent TB is to avoid contact with the tubercle bacillus. Maintaining an optimal state of health with adequate nutrition and avoiding fatigue and debilitating infections promote natural resistance but do not prevent infection. Pasteurization and routine testing of milk

BOX 46-12 Tuberculin Skin Test (TST) Recommendations for Infants, Children, and Adolescents*

Children for Whom Immediate TST Is Indicated

- Contact with persons with confirmed or suspected contagious tuberculosis (contact investigation)
- Children with radiographic or clinical findings suggesting tuberculosis disease
- Children immigrating from endemic countries (e.g., Asia, Middle East, Africa, Latin America)
- Children with travel histories to endemic countries or significant contact with indigenous persons from such countries†

Children Who Should Have Annual TST‡

- Children infected with HIV
- Incarcerated adolescents

Children Who Some Experts Recommend Should Be Tested Every 2 to 3 Years

- Children with ongoing exposure to the following people: HIV-infected people, homeless people, residents of nursing homes, institutionalized adolescents or adults, users of illicit drugs, incarcerated adolescents or adults and migrant farm workers; foster children with exposure to adults in the preceding high-risk groups

Children Who Some Experts Recommend Should Be Considered for Tuberculin Skin Test at 4 to 6 and 11 to 16 Years

- Children whose parents immigrated (with unknown TST status) from regions of the world with high prevalence of tuberculosis; continued potential exposure by travel to the endemic areas or household contact with persons from the endemic areas (with unknown TST status) should be an indication for repeat TST

Children at Increased Risk for Progression of Infection to Disease

- Children with other medical risk factors, including diabetes mellitus, chronic renal failure, malnutrition, and congenital or acquired immunodeficiencies, deserve special consideration. Without recent exposure these people are not at increased risk of acquiring tuberculosis infection. Underlying immune deficiencies associated with these conditions theoretically would enhance the possibility for progression to severe disease. Initial histories of potential exposure to tuberculosis should be included for all of these patients. If these histories or local epidemiologic factors suggest a possibility of exposure, immediate and periodic TST should be considered. **An initial TST should be performed before initiation of immunosuppressive therapy, including prolonged steroid administration, for any child with an underlying condition that necessitates immunosuppressive therapy.**

From American Academy of Pediatrics, Committee on Infectious Diseases, Pickering L, editor: *Red book: 2006 report of the Committee on Infectious Diseases*, ed 27, Elk Grove Village, Ill, 2006, The Academy.

*Bacille Calmette-Guérin (BCG) immunization is not a contraindication to TST.

†If child is well, TST should be delayed for up to 10 weeks after return.

‡Initial tuberculin skin testing is done at the time of diagnosis or circumstance, beginning as early as 3 months of age.

and elimination of diseased cattle have reduced the incidence of bovine TB.

Limited immunity can be produced by administration of bacille Calmette-Guérin (BCG), a live vaccine containing bovine bacilli with reduced virulence (attenuated). In most instances positive tuberculin reactions develop after inoculation with BCG. The distribution of BCG is controlled by local or state health departments, and the vaccine is not used extensively, even in areas with a high prevalence of disease. BCG vaccination is not generally recommended for use in the United States. However, it may be recommended for long-term protection of infants and children with a negative TST who are not infected with HIV and who (1) are at high risk for continuing exposure to persons with infectious pulmonary TB, or (2) are continuously exposed to persons with TB who have bacilli resistant to both INH and rifampin when the child cannot be removed from the environment or given anti-TB drug therapy (American Academy of Pediatrics, Committee on Infectious Diseases, 2009).

Nursing Care Management

Children with TB receive their nursing care in ambulatory settings, outpatient departments, schools, and public health settings. Most children are not contagious and require only standard precautions. Children with no cough and negative sputum smears can be hospitalized in a regular patient room. However, airborne precautions and a negative-pressure room are required for children who are contagious and hospitalized with active TB disease. Infection control for hospital personnel in contagious cases should include the use of a personally fitted air-purifying N95 or N100 respirator for all patient contacts.

Asymptomatic children with TB can attend school or day care facilities if they are receiving pharmacotherapy. They can return to regular activities as soon as effective therapy has been instituted, adherence to therapy has been documented, and clinical symptoms have diminished. Children receiving pharmacotherapy for TB can receive measles and other age-appropriate live virus vaccines unless they are receiving high-dose corticosteroids, are severely ill, or have specific contraindications to immunization. Children with TB should also receive optimal nutrition and adequate rest.

Nurses assume several roles in management of the disease, including helping the family understand the rationale for diagnostic procedures, assisting with radiographic examinations, performing and interpreting skin tests, and obtaining specimens for laboratory examination. Skin tests must be carried out correctly to obtain accurate results. The tuberculin is injected intradermally with the bevel of the needle pointing upward. A wheal 6 to 10 mm in diameter should form between the layers of the skin when the solution is injected properly. If the wheal is not formed, the procedure is repeated. The volar

BOX 46-13 Definition of Positive Tuberculin Skin Test (TST) Results in Infants, Children, and Adolescents*

Induration 5 mm or Greater

Children in close contact with known or suspected contagious cases of tuberculosis (TB) disease

Children suspected of having TB disease:

- Findings on chest x-ray film consistent with active or previously active TB
- Clinical evidence of TB disease†

Children receiving immune suppressive therapy‡ or who have immunosuppressive conditions, including human immunodeficiency virus (HIV) infection

Induration 10 mm or Greater

Children at increased risk of disseminated disease:

- Those younger than 4 years of age
- Those with other medical risk conditions, including Hodgkin's disease, lymphoma, diabetes mellitus, chronic renal failure, or malnutrition

Children at increased risk of exposure to TB disease:

- Those born, or whose parents were born, in high-prevalence (TB) regions of the world
- Those frequently exposed to adults who are HIV infected, homeless, users of illicit drugs, residents of nursing homes, incarcerated or institutionalized, or migrant farm workers
- Those who travel to high-prevalence (TB) regions of the world

Induration 15 mm or Greater

Children 4 years of age or older without any risk factors

From American Academy of Pediatrics, Committee on Infectious Diseases, Pickering L, editor: *Red book: 2006 report of the Committee on Infectious Diseases*, ed 27, Elk Grove Village, Ill, 2006, The Academy.

*These definitions apply regardless of previous Bacille Calmette-Guérin (BCG) immunization; erythema at TST site does not indicate a positive test result. TSTs should be read at 48 to 72 hours after placement.

†Evidence by physical examination or laboratory assessment that would include tuberculosis in the working differential diagnosis (e.g., meningitis).

‡Including immunosuppressive doses of corticosteroids.

or dorsal surface of the forearm is the usual injection site. The reaction to the skin test is determined in 48 to 72 hours; however, reactions occurring after 72 hours should be measured and considered the result (American Academy of Pediatrics, Committee on Infectious Diseases, 2009). The size of the transverse diameter of induration, not the erythema, is measured. The diameter transverse to the long axis of the forearm is the only one standardized for measurement purposes (American Academy of Pediatrics, Committee on Infectious Diseases, 2009).

Sputum specimens are difficult or impossible to obtain from an infant or young child because they swallow any mucus coughed from the lower respiratory tract. The best means for obtaining material for smears or culture is by gastric washing (i.e., aspiration of lavaged contents from the fasting stomach). The procedure is carried out, and the specimen obtained early in the morning before the customary breakfast time. In some cases an induced sputum specimen may be obtained by administering aerosolized normal saline for 10 to 15 minutes, followed by CPT and suctioning of the nasopharynx for sputum collection.

Because the success of therapy depends on compliance with the drug regimen, parents are instructed about the importance and rationale for DOT. Case finding in the community and follow-up of known contacts—individuals from whom the affected child may have acquired the disease and persons who may have been exposed to the child with the disease—are essential control measures.

Severe Acute Respiratory Syndrome

A severe form of atypical pneumonia identified as severe acute respiratory syndrome (SARS) was first reported in Asia in 2003. SARS is caused by a previously unrecognized coronavirus called SARS-associated coronavirus (SARS Co-V). Additional human coronavirus types have since been identified in Canada, Hong Kong, and the Netherlands. Clinical manifestations of this disorder include a fever greater than 38° C (100.4° F); headache; cough; shortness of breath; difficulty breathing; and after 2 to 7 days, a dry, nonproductive cough and dyspnea. In some patients the symptoms are severe enough to require intubation and mechanical ventilation. The disease is spread by close contact with a person with SARS. Most cases have involved people who have cared for or lived with someone with SARS or people who have traveled to areas with reported cases of SARS.

In children, two distinct forms of the illness have been observed. Adolescents have malaise, myalgia, chills, and rigor, whereas young children have mainly cough and runny nose. In younger children the clinical course seems to be milder, and the disease resolves more quickly than in adolescents or adults (Denison, 2005; Stockman et al, 2007).

Laboratory findings include lymphopenia; leukopenia; thrombocytopenia; and elevated lactate dehydrogenase, aspartate aminotransferase, and creatinine kinase levels. The most reliable laboratory diagnostic test is positive antibodies for the SARS Co-V. Chest radiographs in a substantial number of patients reveal focal interstitial infiltrates that progress to more generalized, patchy interstitial infiltrates.

Treatment of SARS involves predominantly supportive care measures. Other therapies such as antibiotics, antiviral drugs such as ribavirin, and steroids have been used with mixed results (O'Connor, 2003).

Nursing Care Management

The Centers for Disease Control and Prevention (2004b) recommends that patients with SARS receive the same treatment as any patient with serious community-acquired atypical pneumonia. This includes the use of strict handwashing, contact precautions, and airborne precautions (e.g., an isolation room with negative pressure relative to the surrounding area and the use of an N95 filtering disposable respirator for persons entering the room). Recommendations for stopping the spread of SARS have also been developed. When triaging patients, nurses should place a surgical mask on any patient who has had close contact with someone who has SARS or who has a history of international travel to an area with cases of SARS. Health care workers who have had high risk, unpro-

evolve Critical Thinking Exercise–Ingestion of a Foreign Body

tected exposure to SARS should be excluded from duty and remain home from work to monitor their health for 10 days.

Pulmonary Dysfunction Caused by Noninfectious Irritants

Foreign Body Aspiration

Small children characteristically explore matter with their mouths and are prone to aspirate a foreign body (FB). They also place objects such as beads, paper clips, small magnets, or food items in the nose, which can easily be aspirated into the trachea. FB aspiration can occur at any age but is most common in children 1 to 3 years of age. Severity is determined by the location, type of object aspirated, and extent of obstruction. For example, dry vegetable matter, such as a seed, nut, or piece of carrot or popcorn, that does not dissolve and that may swell when wet creates a particularly difficult problem. The high fat content of potato chips and peanuts may cause the added risk of lipoid pneumonia. "Fun foods" are the worst offenders in terms of potential for aspiration. Offending foods in the order of frequency of aspiration are hot dog, round candy, peanut or other nut, grape, cookie or biscuit, other meat, carrot, peas, apple, and peanut butter. Other items include plastic or glass beads, button or disc batteries, and coins. Objects such as small lithium or cadmium batteries may cause esophageal or tracheal corrosion.

Diagnostic Evaluation

The diagnosis of FB aspiration is suspected on the basis of the history and physical signs. Initially, an FB in the air passages produces choking, gagging, wheezing, or coughing. Laryngotracheal obstruction most commonly causes dyspnea, cough, stridor, and hoarseness because of decreased air entry. Up to half of all children with FB ingestion may be asymptomatic (Uyemura, 2005). Cyanosis may occur if the obstruction becomes worse. Bronchial obstruction usually produces cough (frequently paroxysmal), wheezing, asymmetric breath sounds, decreased airway entry, and dyspnea. When an object is lodged in the larynx, the child is unable to speak or breathe. If the obstruction progresses, the child's face may become livid; if the obstruction is total, the child can become unconscious and die of asphyxiation. If obstruction is partial, hours, days, or even weeks may pass without symptoms after the initial period. Secondary symptoms are related to the anatomic area in which the object is lodged and are usually caused by a persistent respiratory tract infection distal to the obstruction. FB aspiration should also be suspected in the presence of acute or chronic pulmonary lesions. Often, by the time secondary symptoms appear, the parents have forgotten the initial episode of coughing and gagging.

Radiographic examination reveals opaque FBs but is of limited use in localizing nonradiographic matter. Bronchoscopy is required for a definitive diagnosis of objects in the larynx and trachea. Fluoroscopic examination is valuable in detecting FBs in the bronchi. The mainstay of diagnosis and management of FBs is endoscopy. If there is doubt about the presence of an FB, endoscopy can be diagnostic and therapeutic.

Therapeutic Management

FB aspiration may result in life-threatening airway obstruction, especially in infants (because of the small diameter of their airways). Current recommendations for the emergency treatment of the choking child include the use of abdominal thrusts for children older than 1 year of age and back blows and chest thrusts for those younger than 1 year of age (see Airway Obstruction, p. 1358).

An FB is rarely coughed up spontaneously. Most frequently, it must be removed instrumentally by endoscopy. Endoscopy and bronchoscopy require sedation with an agent such as IV propofol or midazolam. The procedure is carried out as quickly as possible because the progressive local inflammatory process triggered by the foreign material hampers removal. A chemical pneumonia soon develops, and vegetable matter begins to macerate within a few days, making it even more difficult to remove. After removal of the FB, the child is usually observed for any complications such as laryngeal edema and discharged home within a matter of hours if vital signs are stable and recovery is satisfactory.

Nursing Care Management

A major role of nurses caring for a child who has aspirated an FB is to recognize the signs of FB aspiration and implement immediate measures to relieve the obstruction. All persons working with children must be prepared to deal effectively with aspiration of an FB. Choking on food or other material should not be fatal. Back blows and chest thrusts in infants and abdominal thrusts in children are simple procedures that can be used by both health professionals and laypersons to save lives (see Figs. 46-16 and 46-17). It is the responsibility of nurses to learn these techniques and to teach them to parents and other groups. To aid a child who is choking, nurses must recognize the signs of distress. Not every child who gags or coughs while eating is truly choking.

NURSING ALERT The child in severe distress (1) cannot speak, (2) becomes cyanotic, and (3) collapses. These three signs indicate that the child is truly choking and requires immediate action. The child can die within 4 minutes.

Prevention

Nurses are in a position to teach prevention in a variety of settings. They can educate parents singly or in groups about hazards of aspiration in relation to the developmental level of their children and encourage them to teach their children safety. Parents should be cautioned about behaviors that their children might imitate (e.g., holding foreign objects, such as pins, nails, and toothpicks, in their lips or mouth). (Prevention based on the child's age is discussed in Chapters 36, 37, and 38.)

Aspiration Pneumonia

Aspiration pneumonia occurs when food, secretions, inert materials, volatile compounds, or liquids enter the lung and cause inflammation and a chemical pneumonitis. Aspiration of fluid or foods is a particular hazard in the child who has difficulty swallowing; is unable to swallow because of paralysis, weakness, debility, congenital anomalies, or absent cough reflex; or is force-fed, especially while crying or breathing rapidly. Clinical signs of the aspiration of oral secretions may not be distinguishable from those of other forms of acute bacterial pneumonia. For example, if vegetable matter has been aspirated, manifestations may not appear for several weeks after the event. Classic symptoms include an increasing cough or fever with foul-smelling sputum, deteriorating chest radiographs, and other signs of lower airway involvement. However, these deviations may persist for weeks while the child starts to feel better. Rarely, aspiration causes immediate death from asphyxia; more often the irritated mucous membrane becomes a site for secondary bacterial infection. In addition to fluids, food, vomitus, and nasopharyngeal secretions, other substances that may cause pneumonia are hydrocarbons, lipids, powder, and barium.

Nursing Care Management

Care of the child with aspiration pneumonia is the same as that described for the child with pneumonia from other causes. However, the major focus of nursing care is on prevention of aspiration. Proper feeding techniques should be carried out for weak, debilitated, and uncooperative children, and preventive measures should be used to prevent aspiration of any material that might enter the nasopharynx. Nasogastric tubes used for feedings are checked before the initiation of bolus feedings; continuous nasogastric tube feedings are also evaluated periodically for proper tube placement. Children who are at risk for swallowing difficulties as a result of illness, physical debilitation, anesthesia, or sedation are kept NPO (nothing by mouth) until they can properly swallow fluids effectively. The child who is at risk for vomiting and incapable of protecting the airway should be positioned in a side-lying recovery position (see Fig. 46-18).

Acute Respiratory Distress Syndrome/ Acute Lung Injury

ARDS is recognized in children and adults and has been associated with clinical conditions and injuries such as sepsis, trauma, viral pneumonia, fat emboli, drug overdose, reperfusion injury after lung transplantation, smoke inhalation, and near-drowning. It is characterized by respiratory distress and hypoxemia that occur within 72 hours of a serious injury or surgery in a person with previously normal lungs. Acute lung injury (ALI) is said to involve a spectrum of inflammatory disease responses to a precipitating event (Frye, 2005). ARDS and ALI cause acute respiratory failure and account for significant morbidity and mortality in critically ill patients (Matthay et al, 2003). Acute pulmonary inflammation with alveolar capillary membrane destruction results in significant hypoxemia, and mechanical ventilation is often required. ARDS is the most severe in the spectrum of illnesses in relation to the degree of hypoxemia. Hypoxemia is expressed as the ratio of partial pressure of oxygen (Pao_2) to fraction of inspired oxygen (Fio_2), or P/F ratio, with the P/F ratio for ALI being 300 or less and the P/F ratio for ARDS being 200 or less. Both ALI and ARDS demonstrate radiographic evidence of bilateral alveolar infiltrates without evidence of left-sided heart failure (Rice & Bernard, 2006).

The hallmark of ARDS is increased permeability of the alveolar-capillary membrane that results in pulmonary edema. During the acute phase of ARDS, the alveolocapillary membrane is damaged, with an increasing pulmonary capillary permeability and resulting interstitial edema. Later stages are characterized by pneumocyte and fibrin infiltration of the alveoli, with the start of either the healing process or fibrosis. When fibrosis occurs, the child may demonstrate respiratory distress and the need for mechanical ventilation. In ARDS the lungs become stiff as a result of surfactant inactivation, gas diffusion is impaired, and eventually bronchiolar mucosal swelling and congestive atelectasis occur. The net effect is decreased functional residual capacity, pulmonary hypertension, and increased intrapulmonary right-to-left shunting of pulmonary blood flow. Surfactant secretion is reduced, and the atelectasis and fluid-filled alveoli provide an excellent medium for bacterial growth.

The criteria for diagnosis of ARDS in children are an acute antecedent illness or injury, acute respiratory distress or failure, no evidence of prior cardiopulmonary disease, and diffuse bilateral infiltrates evidenced on chest radiography. The child with ARDS may first demonstrate only symptoms caused by an injury or infection, but as the condition deteriorates, hyperventilation, tachypnea, increasing respiratory effort, cyanosis, and decreasing oxygen saturation occur. At times the developing hypoxemia is not responsive to oxygen administration.

Therapeutic Management

Treatment involves supportive measures such as maintenance of adequate oxygenation and pulmonary perfusion, treatment of infection (or the precipitating cause), maintenance of adequate cardiac output and vascular volume, hydration, adequate nutritional support, comfort measures, prevention of complications such as gastrointestinal ulceration and aspiration, and psychologic support. Prone positioning may be used to improve oxygenation; this requires close communication and coordination among the health care team (Frye, 2005). Definitive therapy is directed toward improvement of oxygenation. The use of endotracheal intubation, positive end-expiratory pressure, and low tidal volume may be required to ensure maximum oxygen delivery by increasing functional residual capacity, reducing intrapulmonary shunting, and reducing pulmonary fluid. Ventilation with low tidal volume (6 ml/kg of ideal body weight) has been associated with lower mortality rates in children with ALI (Hanson & Flori, 2006). Additional supportive strategies in the treatment of ARDS in children include the use of permissive hypercapnia, inhaled nitric oxide, exogenous surfactant administration, high-frequency ventilation, partial liquid ventilation, and extracorporeal life support (extracorporeal membrane oxygenation, or ECMO). Exogenous surfactant therapy has increased oxygenation status in infants and children with ARDS/ALI and decreased disease severity (Willson, Chess, & Notter, 2008). Once the underlying cause is identified, specific treatment (e.g., antibiotics for infection) is initiated.

Prognosis

In spite of advances in understanding and treating ARDS/ALI, mortality in children ranges from 22% (after severe trauma) to 88% (after bone marrow transplant) (Flori et al, 2005; Frankel & DiCarlo, 2004). The precipitating disorder influences the outcome; the worst prognosis is associated with uncontrolled sepsis, bone marrow transplantation, cancer, and multisystem involvement with hepatic failure. Children who recover may have persistent cough and exertional dyspnea.

Nursing Care Management

The child with ARDS is cared for in intensive care during the acute stages of illness. Nursing care involves close monitoring of cardiac output, perfusion, fluid and electrolyte balance, and renal function (urinary output), as well as assessment of oxygenation and respiratory status. Blood gas analysis and pulse oximetry are important evaluation tools. Parenteral and enteral nutritional support is often required because of the length of the acute phase of the illness. Diuretics may be administered to reduce pulmonary fluid, and vasodilators may be administered to decrease pulmonary vascular pressure. Nursing management also includes managing pain, monitoring the effects of the numerous parenteral fluids and drugs used to stabilize the child, and monitoring for changes in the child's hemodynamic status. Most children with ARDS require invasive monitoring via a central venous line and possibly a pulmonary artery catheter to monitor oxygenation and administer medications. The nursing care of the child with ARDS also involves close observance of skin condition and prevention of breakdown, passive range of motion for prevention of muscle atrophy and contractures, and nutritional support. Respiratory distress is a frightening situation for both the child and the parents, and attention to their psychologic needs is a major element in the care of these children. The child is often sedated during the acute phase of the illness, and weaning from sedation requires close monitoring for anxiety reduction and comfort.

Smoke Inhalation Injury

A number of noxious substances that may be inhaled are toxic to humans. They are primarily products of incomplete combustion and cause more deaths from fires than flame injuries. The severity of the injury depends on the nature of the substances generated by the material burned, whether the victim is confined in a closed space, and the duration of contact with the smoke. Smoke inhalation results in three types of injury: heat, chemical, and systemic. Three distinct stages occur in the child suffering from inhalation injury:

1. Pulmonary insufficiency, usually during the initial 12 hours
2. Pulmonary edema, usually after 6 to 72 hours, with an increase in the lung fluid and interstitial edema
3. Bronchopneumonia, usually after 72 hours, with a resulting airway obstruction or atelectasis

Heat injury involves thermal injury to the upper airway. Air has low specific heat; therefore the injury goes no farther than the upper airway. Reflex closure of the glottis prevents injury to the lower airway.

Chemical injury involves gases that may be generated during the combustion of materials such as clothing, furniture, and floor coverings. Acids, alkalis, and their precursors in smoke can produce chemical burns. These substances can be carried deep into the respiratory tract, including the lower respiratory tract, in the form of insoluble gases. Soluble gases tend to dissolve in the upper respiratory tract.

Synthetic materials are especially toxic, producing gases such as oxides of sulfur and nitrogen, acetaldehyde, formaldehyde, hydrocyanic acid, and chlorine. Heated plastics are the source of extremely toxic vapors, including chlorine and hydrochloric acid from polyvinylchloride and hydrocarbons, aldehydes, ketones, and acids from polyethylene. Irritant gases such as nitrous oxide or carbon dioxide combine with water in the lungs to form corrosive acids; aldehydes cause denaturation of proteins, cellular damage, and edema of pulmonary tissues. Chemical burns to the airways are similar to burns on the skin except that they are painless because the tracheobronchial tree is relatively insensitive to pain.

Inhalation of small amounts of noxious irritants produces alveolar and bronchiolar damage that can lead to obstructive bronchiolitis. Severe exposure causes further injury, including alveolocapillary damage with hemorrhage, necrotizing bronchiolitis, inhibited secretion of surfactant, and formation of hyaline membranes—manifestations of ARDS.

Systemic injury occurs from gases that are nontoxic to the airways (e.g., carbon monoxide [CO], hydrogen cyanide). However, these gases cause injury and death by interfering with or inhibiting cellular respiration. CO is responsible for more than half of all fatal inhalation poisonings in the United States. It is a colorless, odorless gas with an affinity for hemoglobin 230 times greater than that of oxygen. When it enters the bloodstream, CO combines readily with hemoglobin to form carboxyhemoglobin (COHb). Because it is released less readily, tissue hypoxia reaches dangerous levels before oxygen is available to meet tissue needs.

NURSING ALERT The oxygen saturation (Sao_2) obtained by pulse oximetry will be normal because the device measures only oxygenated and deoxygenated hemoglobin; it does not measure dysfunctional hemoglobin such as COHb.

Accidental CO poisoning is most often a result of exposure to fumes of heaters or smoke from structural fires, although poorly ventilated recreational vehicles with improperly operated or maintained gas lamps or stoves and cooking in underventilated areas with charcoal grills are also frequent causes. CO is produced by incomplete combustion of carbon or carbonaceous material such as wood or charcoal.

The signs and symptoms of CO poisoning are secondary to tissue hypoxia and vary with the level of COHb. Mild manifestations include headache, visual disturbances, irritability, and nausea, whereas more severe intoxication causes confusion, hallucinations, ataxia, and coma. The bright, cherry-red lips and skin often described are less often observed; pallor and cyanosis are seen more frequently.

Therapeutic Management

Treatment of children with smoke inhalation injury is largely symptomatic. The most widely accepted treatment is placing the child on humidified 100% oxygen as quickly as possible and monitoring for signs of respiratory distress and impending failure. Baseline arterial blood gases (ABGs) and COHb levels are obtained. Pao_2 may be within normal limits unless there is marked respiratory depression. If CO poisoning is confirmed, 100% oxygen is continued until COHb levels fall to the nontoxic range of about 10%. If CO poisoning is severe, the patient may benefit from hyperbaric oxygen therapy; however, the benefits and risks of treatment are debatable (Kao & Nañagas, 2004); at this time there are no published clinical practice guidelines for the therapy, especially in children. Hyperbaric oxygen therapy may be useful in the treatment of neurologic complications related to CO poisoning.

Respiratory distress may occur early in the course of smoke inhalation as a result of hypoxia, or patients who are breathing well on admission may suddenly develop respiratory distress. Therefore intubation equipment should be readily available. Transient edema of the airways can occur at any level in the tracheobronchial tree. Assessment and localization of the obstruction should be accomplished before severe swelling of the head, neck, or oropharynx occurs. Intubation is often necessary when (1) severe burns in the area of the nose, mouth, and face increase the likelihood of developing oropharyngeal edema and obstruction; (2) vocal cord edema causes obstruction; (3) the patient has difficulty handling secretions; and (4) progressive respiratory distress requires artificial ventilation. Controversy surrounds tracheostomy, but many prefer this procedure when the obstruction is proximal to the larynx and reserve nasotracheal intubation for lower tract involvement.

Nursing Care Management

Nursing care of the child with inhalation injury is the same as that for any child with respiratory distress. Vital signs and other respiratory assessments are performed frequently, and the pulmonary status is carefully observed and maintained. Pulmonary physiotherapy is often part of the therapy, as well as mechanical ventilation if needed. Fluid requirements for children experiencing inhalation injury are greater than for those with surface burns alone; however, one concern is the development of pulmonary edema. Therefore accurate monitoring of intake and output is essential.

In addition to observation and management of the physical aspects of inhalation injury, the nurse also deals with the psychologic needs of a frightened child and distraught parents. As with any accidental injury, the parents feel overwhelming guilt, even when the injury occurred through no fault of their own. Parents need support, reassurance, and information regarding the child's condition, treatment, and progress.

Environmental Tobacco Smoke Exposure

Numerous investigations indicate that parental smoking is an important cause of morbidity in children. Children exposed to passive or environmental tobacco smoke have an increased number of respiratory illnesses, increased respiratory symptoms (e.g., cough, sputum, and wheezing), and reduced performance on pulmonary function tests. AOM and OME are also increased in children who have smoking parents. Indoor exposure to environmental tobacco smoke has been linked to asthma in children. Among children with asthma, there is an association between parental cigarette smoking and asthma exacerbations, trips to the emergency department, medication use, and impaired recovery after hospitalization for acute asthma. Maternal cigarette smoking is associated with increased respiratory symptoms and illnesses in children; decreased fetal growth; increased deliveries of low-birth-weight, preterm, and stillborn infants; and a greater incidence of sudden infant death syndrome (SIDS). Antenatal maternal smoking has emerged as a significant risk factor for SIDS (American Academy of Pediatrics, Task Force on Sudden Infant Death Syndrome, 2005). The risk for diagnosis of early-onset asthma in the first 3 years of life is associated with in utero exposure to maternal smoking; grandmaternal smoking was also associated with an increased risk of early-onset asthma in the grandchild even if the mother did not smoke during pregnancy (Li et al, 2005). Exposure to tobacco smoke during childhood may also contribute to the development of chronic lung disease in the adult.

Nursing Care Management

Nurses must provide information about the hazards of environmental smoke exposure in all their interactions with children and their family members. This information is especially important for children with respiratory and allergic illnesses. In families in which smokers refuse to quit, appropriate guidance is provided for reducing smoke in the child's environment (see Family-Centered Care box). Nurses should set an example for children and families and become advocates for "no smoking" ordinances in public places, prohibition of advertising tobacco products in the media, and inclusion of health warnings of sidestream smoke on tobacco products.* Nurses also have an important role in providing parents with affordable smoking cessation education resources, including the appropriate use of smoking cessation pharmacologic aids (Sheahan & Free, 2005).

FAMILY-CENTERED CARE

Decreasing Childhood Exposure to Environmental Tobacco Smoke

- Maintain a smoke-free home.
- Avoid exposing an infant to environmental smoke.
- Use an air-purifying filter in the home where smoking is unavoidable.
- Encourage exclusive breastfeeding for the first 6 months.
- If smoking cessation is in progress by breastfeeding mother, suggest she change upper clothing after smoking and before breastfeeding infant.
- Do not smoke around children.
- Change clothing after smoking and before holding an infant in close proximity.
- Restrict smoking to an isolated area of the house where the children do not play or sleep.
- Do not smoke in motor vehicles with children.
- Do not smoke in rooms children use.
- Do not allow visitors to smoke in the home.

*For further information on the effects of second-hand smoke on child health go to www.cdc.gov/tobacco/secondhand_smoke/index.htm.

Animation—Asthma

Long-Term Respiratory Dysfunction

Asthma

Asthma is a chronic inflammatory disorder of the airways in which many cells (mast cells, eosinophils, and T lymphocytes) play a role. In susceptible children, inflammation causes recurrent episodes of wheezing, breathlessness, chest tightness, and cough, especially at night or in the early morning. These asthma episodes are associated with airflow limitation or obstruction that is reversible either spontaneously or with treatment. The inflammation also causes an increase in bronchial hyperresponsiveness to a variety of stimuli (National Asthma Education and Prevention Program, 2007). Recognition of the importance of inflammation has made the use of antiinflammatory agents, especially inhaled steroids, a key component in the treatment of asthma.

Asthma is classified into four categories based on the symptom indicators of disease severity. These categories are intermittent, mild persistent, moderate persistent, and severe persistent. The intermittent category has the least number of symptoms; symptoms increase in frequency or intensity until the last category of severe persistent asthma (Box 46-14). These categories provide a stepwise approach to the pharmacologic management, environmental control, and educational interventions needed for each category (National Asthma Education and Prevention Program, 2007). A new component of the asthma severity classification system includes the domains of impairment and risk for each category; these categories emphasize the multifaceted aspect of the disease for consideration of the effects of symptoms on present quality of life and functional capacity and the future risk of adverse events (National Asthma Education and Prevention Program, 2007).

Asthma prevalence, morbidity, and mortality are increasing in the United States, especially among African-Americans (Linzer, 2007). These increases may result from worsening air pollution, poor access to medical care, or underdiagnosis and undertreatment. Asthma is the most common chronic disease of childhood, the primary cause of school absences, and the third leading cause of hospitalizations in children under the age of 15. Although the onset of asthma may occur at any age, 80% to 90% of children have their first symptoms before 4 or 5 years of age. Boys are affected more frequently than girls until adolescence, when the trend reverses.

BOX 46-14 Asthma Severity Classification in Children: Ages 0 to 11*

Step 5 or 6—Severe Persistent Asthma

Continual symptoms throughout the day
Frequent nighttime symptoms
Peak expiratory flow (PEF)—Less than 60%
Forced expiratory volume in 1 second (FEV_1)—Less than 75% of predicted value
Interference with normal activity—Extremely limited
Use of short-acting β-agonist for symptom control—Several times a day

Step 3 or 4—Moderate Persistent Asthma

Daily symptoms
Nighttime symptoms—Three to four times a month (ages 0 to 4); more than one per week but not nightly (ages 5 to 11)
PEF—60% to 80% of predicted value
FEV_1—75% to 80%
PEF variability—More than 30%
Interference with normal activity—Some limitation
Use of short-acting β-agonist for symptom control—Daily

Step 2—Mild Persistent Asthma

Symptoms more than two times a week but less than one time a day
Nighttime symptoms—One to two times a month (ages 0 to 4); three to four times a month (ages 5 to 11)
PEF or FEV_1—80% or more of predicted value
PEF variability—20% to 30%
Interference with normal activity—Minor limitation
Use of short-acting β-agonist for symptom control—More than 2 days a week but not daily

Step 1—Intermittent Asthma

Symptoms fewer than 2 days/week
Nighttime symptoms (awakenings)—None (ages 0 to 4); fewer than two times a month (ages 5 to 11)
PEF or FEV_1—80% or more of predicted value
PEF variability—Less than 20%
Interference with normal activity—None
Use of short-acting β-agonist for symptom control—Fewer than 2 days/week

From National Asthma Education and Prevention Program: *Guidelines for the diagnosis and management of asthma: summary report 2007.* Available at www.nhlbi.nih.gov/guidelines/asthma/index.htm (accessed March 8, 2008).
*The presence of one clinical feature of severity is sufficient to place a patient in that category. An individual should be assigned to the most severe grade in which any feature occurs. The characteristics in this table are general and may overlap because asthma is highly variable. An individual's classification may change over time. Risk factors for each category are not presented in this table. See the original table (referenced above) for additional classification data. Asthma treatment should not be based on this table.

Etiology

Studies of children with asthma indicate that allergy influences both the persistence and the severity of the disease. In fact, atopy, or the genetic predisposition for the development of an immune globulin E (IgE)–mediated response to common aeroallergens, is the strongest identifiable predisposing factor for developing asthma (National Asthma Education and Prevention Program, 2007). Although allergens play an important role in asthma, 20% to 40% of children with asthma have no evidence of allergic disease. In addition to allergens, other substances and conditions can serve as triggers that may exacerbate asthma (Box 46-15). It is a complex disorder involving biochemical, genetic, immunologic, environmental, infectious, endocrine, and psychologic factors. Evidence shows that viral respiratory infections may have a significant role in the development and expression of asthma (National Asthma Education and Prevention Program, 2007).

BOX 46-15 Triggers Tending to Precipitate or Aggravate Asthmatic Exacerbations

Allergens
- **Outdoor**—Trees, shrubs, weeds, grasses, molds, pollens, air pollution, spores
- **Indoor**—Dust or dust mites, mold, cockroach antigen

Irritants—Tobacco smoke, wood smoke, odors, sprays
Exposure to occupational chemicals
Exercise
Cold air
Changes in weather or temperature
Environmental change—Moving to new home, starting new school, etc.
Colds and infections
Animals—Cats, dogs, rodents, horses
Medications—Aspirin, nonsteroidal antiinflammatory drugs (NSAIDs), antibiotics, β-blockers
Strong emotions—Fear, anger, laughing, crying
Conditions—Gastroesophageal reflux, tracheoesophageal fistula
Food additives—Sulfite preservatives
Foods—Nuts, milk/dairy products
Endocrine factors—Menses, pregnancy, thyroid disease

Pathophysiology

There is general agreement that inflammation contributes to heightened airway reactivity in asthma. The mechanisms contributing to airway inflammation are multiple and involve a number of different pathways. It is unlikely that asthma is caused by either a single cell or a single inflammatory mediator; rather, it appears that asthma results from complex interactions among inflammatory cells, mediators, and the cells and tissues present in the airways (National Asthma Education and Prevention Program, 2007). However, recognition of the importance of inflammation has made the use of antiinflammatory agents a key component of asthma therapy.

Another important component of asthma is bronchospasm and obstruction. The mechanisms responsible for the obstructive symptoms in asthma (Fig. 46-4) include (1) inflammatory response to stimuli; (2) airway edema and accumulation and secretion of mucus; and (3) spasm of the smooth muscle of the bronchi and bronchioles, which decreases the caliber of the bronchioles.

Bronchial constriction is a normal reaction to foreign stimuli, but in the child with asthma it is abnormally severe, producing impaired respiratory function. The smooth muscle arranged in spiral bundles around the airway causes narrowing and shortening of the airway, which significantly increases airway resistance to airflow. Airflow is determined by the size of the airway lumen, degree of bronchial wall edema, mucus production, smooth muscle contraction, and muscle hypertrophy.

Because the bronchi normally dilate and elongate during inspiration and contract and shorten on expiration, the respiratory difficulty is more pronounced during the expiratory phase of respiration.

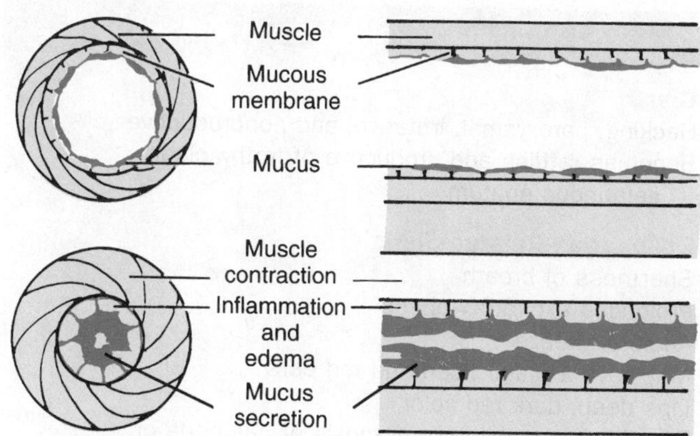

Fig. 46-4 Mechanisms of obstruction in asthma.

Increased resistance in the airway causes forced expiration through the narrowed lumen. The volume of air trapped in the lungs increases as airways are functionally closed at a point between the alveoli and the lobar bronchi. This trapping of gas forces the individual to breathe at higher and higher lung volumes. Consequently, the person with asthma fights to inspire sufficient air. This expenditure of effort for breathing causes fatigue, decreased respiratory effectiveness, and increased oxygen consumption. The inspiration occurring at higher lung volumes hyperinflates the alveoli and reduces the effectiveness of the cough. As the severity of obstruction increases, there is reduced alveolar ventilation with carbon dioxide retention, hypoxemia, respiratory acidosis, and eventually respiratory failure.

Chronic inflammation may also cause permanent damage (airway remodeling) to airway structures; this remodeling cannot be prevented by and is not responsive to current treatments (National Asthma Education and Prevention Program, 2007).

evolve Animation—Bronchi and Bronchioles

Diagnostic Evaluation

The classic manifestations of asthma are dyspnea, wheezing, and coughing. However, children may experience symptoms that range from acute episodes of shortness of breath, wheezing, and cough, followed by a quiet period, to a relatively continuous pattern of chronic symptoms that fluctuate in severity (Box 46-16). An attack may develop gradually or appear abruptly and may be preceded by a URI. The age of the child is often a significant factor, since the first attack frequently occurs before the age of 5 years, with some children manifesting clinical signs and symptoms in infancy. In infancy an attack usually follows a respiratory infection. Some children may experience a prodromal itching at the front of the neck or over the upper part of the back just before an attack.

NURSING ALERT Shortness of breath with air movement in the chest restricted to the point of absent breath sounds accompanied by a sudden rise in respiratory rate is an ominous sign indicating ventilatory failure and imminent respiratory arrest.

The diagnosis is determined primarily on the basis of clinical manifestations, history, physical examination, and to a

BOX 46-16 Clinical Manifestations of Asthma

Cough

Hacking, paroxysmal, irritative, and nonproductive
Becomes rattling and productive of frothy, clear, gelatinous sputum

Respiratory-Related Signs

Shortness of breath
Prolonged expiratory phase
Audible wheeze
May have a malar flush and red ears
Lips deep, dark red color
Possible progression to cyanosis of nail beds or circumoral cyanosis
Restlessness
Apprehension
Sweating may be prominent as the attack progresses
Posture—Older children may sit upright with shoulders in a hunched-over position, hands on the bed or chair, and arms braced (tripod position)
Speech—May speak in short, panting, broken phrases

Chest

Hyperresonance on percussion
Coarse, loud breath sounds
Wheezes throughout the lung fields
Prolonged expiration
Crackles
Generalized inspiratory and expiratory wheezing; increasingly high pitched

With Repeated Episodes

Barrel chest
Elevated shoulders
Use of accessory muscles of respiration
Facial appearance: flattened malar bones, circles beneath the eyes, narrow nose, prominent upper teeth

lesser extent laboratory tests. Generally, chronic cough in the absence of infection or diffuse wheezing during the expiratory phase of respiration is sufficient to establish a diagnosis.

Pulmonary function tests (PFTs) provide an objective method of evaluating the presence and degree of lung disease and the response to therapy. Spirometry can generally be performed reliably on children by the age of 5 or 6 years and includes either the traditional and simple mechanical spirometer often used in clinics, offices, and the home or new computerized versions. The National Asthma Education and Prevention Program (2007) recommends that spirometry testing be done at the time of initial assessment of asthma, after treatment is initiated and symptoms have stabilized, and at least every 1 to 2 years to assess the maintenance of airway function.

Another key measurement is the *peak expiratory flow rate (PEFR)*, which measures the maximum flow of air that can be forcefully exhaled in 1 second. PEFR is measured in liters per minute using a *peak expiratory flow meter (PEFM)*. Three zones of measurement are typically used to interpret PEFR. The zone system is patterned after a traffic light to make the categories easy to understand and remember (see Guidelines box). Each child needs to establish his or her personal best value. A personal best value should be established during a 2- to 3-week period when the child's asthma is stable. During this period the child records the PEFR at least twice a day. After the personal best value has been established, the child's current PEFR on any occasion can be compared with the personal best value.

GUIDELINES Interpreting Peak Expiratory Flow Rates*

- **Green (80% to 100% of personal best)** signals all clear. Asthma is under reasonably good control. No symptoms are present, and the routine treatment plan for maintaining control can be followed.
- **Yellow (50% to 79% of personal best)** signals caution. Asthma is not well controlled. An acute exacerbation may be present. Maintenance therapy may need to be increased. Call the practitioner if the child stays in this zone.
- **Red (below 50% of personal best)** signals a medical alert. Severe airway narrowing may be occurring. A short-acting bronchodilator should be administered. Notify the practitioner if the peak expiratory flow rate does not return immediately and stay in yellow or green zones.

*These zones are guidelines only. Specific zones and management should be individualized for each child.

Bronchoprovocation testing (i.e., direct exposure of the mucous membranes to a suspected antigen in increasing concentrations) helps to identify inhaled allergens. Exposure to methacholine, histamine, or cold or dry air may be performed to assess airway responsiveness or reactivity. Exercise challenges may be used to identify children with exercise-induced bronchospasm (Liu et al, 2007). Although these tests are highly specific and sensitive, they place the child at risk for an asthmatic episode and should be done under close observation in a qualified laboratory or clinic.

Skin testing is useful in identifying specific allergens, and those obtained by the puncture technique correlate better than intracutaneous tests with symptoms and measurements of specific IgE antibody. The radioallergosorbent test (RAST) helps identify antigens against various foods and is often useful in determining appropriate therapy. It is recommended that all patients with year-round asthma symptoms be tested with skin tests or laboratory blood analysis to determine sensitization to perennial allergens (e.g., house dust mites, cats, dogs, cockroaches, molds, and fungus) (National Asthma Education and Prevention Program, 2007) (see Atraumatic Care box).

In addition to these tests, other important tests include laboratory tests (complete blood count with differential) and chest radiographs. The complete blood count may show a slight elevation in the white blood cell count during acute asthma, but elevations to more than 12,000/mm^3 or an increased percentage of band cells may indicate respiratory tract infection. On the other hand, the presence of eosino-

ATRAUMATIC CARE

Skin Testing

To help allay children's fears of skin tests, give them a careful and thorough explanation of what is to be done and how many "pricks" are involved (usually a series of eight on each site, for a total of 30 tests). Very young, anxious patients may benefit from one prick on the arm to demonstrate how it feels. The skin is pierced with a stylet rather than a regular needle and syringe; then a drop of allergen is placed on the site. Another helpful strategy is to have the child count off the number of pricks with the nurse as a distraction. For intradermal skin injection, EMLA or LMX4, both topical anesthetics, reduce or eliminate pain without altering test results.

philia greater than 500/mm^3 tends to suggest an allergic or inflammatory disorder.

Frontal and lateral radiographs show infiltrates and hyperexpansion of the airways, with the anteroposterior diameter on physical examination indicating an increased diameter (suggestive of barrel chest). Additional diagnostic tests for conditions such as gastroesophageal reflux may be carried out to determine whether they may contribute to asthma symptoms. Radiography may assist in ruling out a respiratory tract infection.

Therapeutic Management

The overall goals of asthma management are to maintain normal activity levels, maintain normal pulmonary function, prevent chronic symptoms and recurrent exacerbations, provide optimal drug therapy with minimal or no adverse effects, and assist the child in living as normal and happy a life as possible. This includes facilitating the child's social adjustments in the family, school, and community and normal participation in recreational activities and sports. To accomplish these goals, several treatment principles need to be followed (National Asthma Education and Prevention Program, 2007):

- A continuous care approach with regular visits (at least every 1 to 6 months) to the health care provider is necessary to control symptoms and prevent exacerbations.
- Prevention of exacerbations includes avoiding triggers, avoiding allergens, and using medications as needed.
- Therapy includes efforts to reduce underlying inflammation and relieve or prevent symptomatic airway narrowing.
- Therapy includes patient education, environmental control, pharmacologic management, and the use of objective measures to monitor the severity of disease and guide the course of therapy.

Allergen Control

Nonpharmacologic therapy is aimed at the prevention and reduction of exposure to airborne allergens and irritants. *House dust mites* and other components of house dust are frequent agents identified in children allergic to inhalants. The *cockroach*, another common household inhabitant, is an important allergen in many locations. Exterminating live cockroaches, carefully cleaning kitchen floors and cabinets, putting food away after eating, and taking trash out in the evening are essential measures to control cockroaches. The mouse allergen is the most recent allergen to be identified in the homes of inner-city children with asthma. The role of cat and dog dander in allergen-induced asthma has also been studied. Sensitized persons should carefully evaluate having such pets in the household; there are inconclusive data on cat dander, but there is some evidence that dog dander either has no effect or may be protective (Sharma et al, 2007). Additional sources of pollutants include ozone, particulate matter produced by tobacco smoke, wood-burning stoves, pesticides, lead, mold spores, nitrogen dioxide, and sulfur dioxide; these are believed to contribute to asthma morbidity in children and should be avoided or minimized. Exposure to tobacco smoke is a significant contributing factor in the development of asthma in infants and small children (Sharma et al, 2007). Recommendations for controlling allergens are found in the Patient Teaching box.

Skin testing identifies specific allergens so steps can be taken to eliminate or avoid them. Often, simply removing the offending environmental allergens or irritants (e.g., removing carpeting from the home of a child sensitive to mold and dust particles) decreases the frequency of asthma episodes. Dehumidifiers or air conditioners control nonspecific factors, such as extremes of temperature, that trigger an episode.

Despite the proven association between the incidence of asthma and exposure to these residential hazards, little evidence-based research demonstrates an overall reduction in symptoms, even with significant interventions aimed at environmental (housing) modifications such as removal of carpeting, cleaning, and extermination (Sandel et al, 2004; Sharma et al, 2007).

Drug Therapy

Pharmacologic therapy is used to prevent and control asthma symptoms, reduce the frequency and severity of asthma exacerbations, and reverse airflow obstruction. A stepwise approach is recommended based on the severity of the child's asthma. Because inflammation is considered an early and persistent feature of asthma, therapy is directed toward long-term suppression of inflammation.

Asthma medications are categorized into two general classes: *long-term control medications (preventive medications)* to achieve and maintain control of inflammation and *quick-relief medications (rescue medications)* to treat symptoms and exacerbations (National Asthma Education and Prevention Program, 2007).

Quick-relief and long-term medications are often used in combination. Inhaled corticosteroids, cromolyn sodium and nedocromil, long-acting β_2-agonists, methylxanthines, and leukotriene modifiers are used as long-term control medications. Short-acting β_2-agonists, anticholinergics, and systemic corticosteroids are used as quick-relief or rescue medications. Bronchodilators that relax bronchial smooth muscle and dilate the airways include β_2-agonists, methylxanthines, and anticholinergics that can be used as both quick-relief and long-term medications.

Many asthma medications are given by inhalation with a nebulizer or *a metered-dose inhaler (MDI)*. The MDI should always be attached to a spacer when an inhaled corticosteroid

PATIENT TEACHING "Allergy-Proofing" the Home and Community

- Keep humidity between 30% and 50%; use dehumidifier or air conditioner if available; keep air conditioners clean and free of mold; do not use vaporizers or humidifiers.
- Encase pillows in zippered allergen-impermeable covers or wash pillows in hot water (at least 54.4° C [130° F]) every week.
- Encase mattress and box springs in zippered allergen-impermeable cover.
- Use foam rubber mattress and pillows or Dacron pillows and synthetic blankets.
- Wash bed linens every 7 to 10 days in hot water (at least 54.4° C).
- Encase polyester comforters in allergen-impermeable covers or wash in hot water (at least 54.4° C) every week; if possible, do not use comforters and use cotton blankets.
- Do not use a canopy above the bed; children should not sleep on the bottom bunk of a bunk bed.
- Store nothing under the bed; keep clothing in a closet with the door shut.
- Use washable window shades; avoid heavy curtains; if curtains are used, launder them frequently.
- Remove all carpeting if possible; if not possible, vacuum carpet once or twice a week while the child wears a mask; have child remain out of the room while vacuuming occurs and for 30 minutes after vacuuming.
- If possible, use a central vacuum cleaner with a collecting bag outside of the home or use cleaner filters (e.g., high-efficiency particulate air [HEPA] filters).
- Have air and heating ducts cleaned annually; change or clean filters monthly; cover heating vents with filter material (e.g., cheesecloth) to prevent circulation of dust, especially when heat is turned on after summer.
- Remove unnecessary furniture, rugs, stuffed or real animals, toys, books, upholstered furniture, plants, aquariums, and wall hangings from child's room.
- Use wipeable furniture (wood, plastic, vinyl, or leather) in place of upholstered furniture; avoid rattan or wicker furniture.
- Cover walls with washable paint or wallpaper.
- Limit child's exposure to animals (rabbits, gerbils, hamsters) at school; teach child to stay away from zoos, petting farms, and neighbor's pets.
- Change child's clothes after playing outdoors; wash child's hair nightly if child is outside and pollen count is high.
- Keep child indoors while lawn is being mowed, bushes/trees are being trimmed, or pollen count is high.
- Keep windows and doors closed during pollen season; use air conditioner if possible or go to places that are air conditioned, such as libraries and shopping malls, when the weather is hot.
- Wet-mop bare floors weekly; wet-dust and clean child's room weekly; child should not be present during cleaning activities.
- Wash showers and shower curtains with bleach or Lysol at least once a month.
- Limit or avoid child's exposure to tobacco and wood smoke; do not allow cigarette smoking in the house or car; select day care centers, play areas, and shopping malls that are smoke free.
- Avoid odors or sprays (e.g., perfumes, talcum powder, room deodorizers, chalk dust at school, fresh paint, cleaning solutions).
- Avoid cellar (basement) as a play area if it is damp and use a dehumidifier in damp basement.
- Cover all food, including pet food, and put food away in cabinets.
- Store garbage in closed containers.
- Use pesticide sprays, roach bait traps, and boric acid powder to kill cockroaches; if living in an apartment or adjacent housing, encourage neighbors to work together to get rid of cockroaches and mice.
- Repair leaking or dripping faucets; seal cracks and crevices in cabinets and pantry areas.

is administered to prevent yeast infections in the mouth. Spacers are also important for children who have difficulty coordinating or learning proper inhalation technique (Pongracic, 2003). The spacer and holder can be equipped with a mask or a mouthpiece. Pharmaceutical companies are currently mandated to produce inhalers that do not contain chlorofluorocarbons (CFCs) as the propellant because CFCs have been linked to damage and depletion of the earth's ozone level. An alternative propellant to the CFCs is hydrofluoroalkanes; the purported advantages include delivery of more fine particles and less oral deposition (Pongracic, 2003). The U.S. Food and Drug Administration mandated December 2008 as the targeted cessation date for MDIs containing CFCs to be produced and sold (US Food and Drug Administration, Center for Drug Evaluation and Research, 2005). Several currently available CFC-free MDI devices use dry powder (and also called *dry powder inhalers* [DPIs]); these include the Diskus inhaler and the Turbuhaler. These devices are breath activated, and the child needs to inhale as quickly and deeply as possible to use them effectively. The Diskhaler and Aerosolizer are similar, but with the Aerosolizer the medication must be loaded into the inhaler before use. Infants and very young children who have difficulty using MDIs or other inhalers can receive their asthma medications via a *nebulizer.* When this device is used, the medication is mixed with saline (also available in premixed form) and nebulized with compressed air. Children are instructed to breathe normally with the mouth open to provide a direct route to the trachea.

Corticosteroids are antiinflammatory drugs used to treat reversible airflow obstruction and control symptoms and reduce bronchial hyperresponsiveness in chronic asthma. A major change in the last two revisions of the National Asthma Education and Prevention Program guidelines is the recommendation that inhaled corticosteroids be used as first-line therapy in children over 5 years of age. Clinical studies of corticosteroids have indicated significant improvement of all asthma parameters, including decreases in symptoms, emergency visits, and medication requirements (National Asthma Education and Prevention Program, 2007).

Corticosteroids may be administered parenterally, orally, or by inhalation. Oral medications are metabolized slowly, with an onset of action up to 3 hours after administration and peak effectiveness occurring within 6 to 12 hours. Oral systemic steroids may be given for short periods of time (e.g., 3- or 10-day "bursts") to gain prompt control of inadequately controlled persistent asthma or to manage severe persistent asthma. These drugs should be given in the lowest effective dose. They have few side effects (cough, dysphonia, and oral thrush), and there is strong evidence that they improve the long-term outcomes for children of all ages with mild or moderate persistent asthma. Evidence from clinical trials that monitored children for 6 years indicates that the use of inhaled corticosteroids at recommended doses does not have long-term significant effects on growth, bone mineral density, ocular toxicity, or suppression of the adrenal-pituitary axis (National Asthma Education and Prevention Program, 2007). However, primary care providers should frequently monitor (at least every 3 to 6 months) the growth of children and adolescents taking corticosteroids to assess the systemic effects of these drugs and make appropriate reductions in dosages or changes to other types of asthma therapy when necessary. The inhaled corticosteroids include budesonide and fluticasone.

Cromolyn sodium is a nonsteroidal antiinflammatory drug (NSAID) for asthma. It stabilizes mast cell membranes; inhibits activation and release of mediators from eosinophil and epithelial cells; and inhibits the acute airway narrowing after exposure to exercise, cold dry air, and sulfur dioxide. There is no way to reliably predict whether a child will respond to the drug. Cromolyn sodium has minimal side effects (occasional coughing on inhalation of the powder formulation) and may be given via nebulizer or MDI. *Nedocromil sodium* inhibits the bronchoconstrictor response to inhaled antigens and inhibits the activity of and release of histamine, leukotrienes, and prostaglandins from inflammatory cells associated with asthma. The drug has few side effects and is used for maintenance therapy in asthma; it is not effective for reversal of acute exacerbations and is not used in children under 5 years of age.

β-Adrenergic agonists (short acting) (primarily albuterol, levalbuterol [Xopenex], and terbutaline) are used for treatment of acute exacerbations and for the prevention of exercise-induced bronchospasm. These drugs bind with the β-receptors on the smooth muscle of airways, where they activate adenylate cyclase and convert adenosine monophosphate (AMP) to cyclic AMP (cAMP). It is believed that the increased cAMP enhances binding of intracellular calcium to the cell membrane, reducing the availability of calcium and thus allowing smooth muscle to relax. Other effects of the drug help stabilize mast cells to prevent release of mediators. Most β-adrenergics used in asthma therapy affect predominantly the β_2-receptors, which help eliminate bronchospasm. β_1-Effects such as increased heart rate and gastrointestinal disturbances have been minimized. These drugs can be given via inhalation or as oral or parenteral preparations. The inhaled drug has a more rapid onset of action than the oral form. Inhalation also reduces troublesome systemic side effects: irritability, tremor, nervousness, and insomnia. Levalbuterol reportedly causes fewer side effects; however, its overall effectiveness in childhood asthma is controversial (Linzer, 2007). The 2007 National Asthma Education and Prevention Program guidelines recommend the addition of a long-acting β_2-agonist to a low- or medium-dose inhaled corticosteroid to improve lung function and asthma symptoms and decrease the need for a short-acting β_2-agonist. There is some evidence that this combination may actually allow the practitioner to lower the corticosteroid dose and manage asthma symptoms just as effectively (Mintz, 2004). Inhaled β-adrenergic agents should not be taken more than three or four times daily for acute symptoms.

Salmeterol (Serevent) is a long-acting β_2-agonist (bronchodilator) that is used twice a day (no more frequently than every 12 hours). This drug is added to antiinflammatory therapy and used for long-term prevention of symptoms, especially nighttime symptoms, and exercise-induced bronchospasm. Salmeterol is not used in children younger than 12 years of age, and it is not used to treat acute symptoms or exacerbations.

Theophylline was used for decades to relieve symptoms and prevent asthma attacks; however, it is now used primarily in the emergency department when the child is not responding to maximal therapy (Linzer, 2007). Therapeutic levels should be obtained with this drug because it has a narrow therapeutic window.

Leukotrienes are mediators of inflammation that cause increases in airway hyperresponsiveness. Leukotriene modifiers (such as zafirlukast [Accolate] and montelukast sodium [Singulair]) block inflammatory and bronchospasm effects. These drugs are not used to treat acute episodes but are given orally in combination with β-agonists and steroids to provide long-term control and prevent symptoms in mild persistent asthma. Montelukast is approved for children 12 months old and older, whereas zafirlukast is approved for children 7 years and older.

Anticholinergics (atropine and ipratropium [Atrovent]) may also be used for relief of acute bronchospasm. However, these drugs have adverse side effects that include drying of respiratory secretions, blurred vision, and cardiac and central nervous system stimulation. The primary anticholinergic drug used is ipratropium, which does not cross the blood-brain barrier and therefore elicits no central nervous system effects. Ipratropium, when used in combination with albuterol, has been shown to be effective during acute severe asthma in significantly improving lung function and reducing hospitalizations in children coming to the emergency department (Liu et al, 2007).

A fairly new asthma drug, omalizumab (Xolair), is a monoclonal antibody that blocks the binding of IgE to mast cells. Blocking this interaction eventually inhibits the inflammation that is associated with asthma. Because many patients with asthma are atopic and possess specific IgE antibodies to allergens responsible for airway inflammation, this drug is a promising adjunct to the treatment of asthma. It has been approved for use in children 12 years and older. The drug is administered once or twice a month by subcutaneous injection. Efficacy of omalizumab is not immediate, and clinical trials report that response to the drug was not evident before 12 weeks (Strunk & Bloomberg, 2006). Clinical trials of the drug indicate that it can be an effective therapy for patients with symptomatic moderate to severe allergic asthma that is poorly controlled with inhaled corticosteroids. However, it is expensive (Courtney, McCarter, & Pollart, 2005), and there have been reported cases of severe anaphylactic reactions. In early 2007 the Food and

Drug Administration added a "black box warning" to the drug, which highlights the risk of anaphylaxis.

The use of complementary and alternative medicine (CAM) in children with asthma is reported by several sources; most common are the use of herbal products, breathing techniques, homeopathy, and acupuncture (Slader et al, 2006). The use of CAM should be evaluated carefully in conjunction with other therapies in the overall management of asthma.

Exercise

Exercise-induced bronchospasm (EIB) is an acute, reversible, usually self-terminating airway obstruction that develops during or after vigorous activity, reaches its peak 5 to 10 minutes after stopping the activity, and usually stops in another 20 to 30 minutes. Patients with EIB have cough, shortness of breath, chest pain or tightness, wheezing, and endurance problems during exercise, but an exercise challenge test in a laboratory is necessary to make the diagnosis.

The problem is rare in activities that require short bursts of energy (e.g., baseball, sprints, gymnastics, skiing) and more common in those that involve endurance exercise (e.g., soccer, basketball, distance running). Swimming is well tolerated by children with EIB because they are breathing air fully saturated with moisture and because of the type of breathing required in swimming.

Children with asthma are often excluded from exercise by parents, teachers, and practitioners, as well as by the children themselves, because they are reluctant to provoke an attack. However, this practice can seriously hamper peer interaction and physical health. Exercise is advantageous for children with asthma, and most children can participate in activities at school and in sports with minimal difficulty, provided their asthma is under control. Participation should be evaluated on an individual basis. Appropriate prophylactic treatment with β-adrenergic agents or cromolyn sodium before exercise usually permits full participation in strenuous exertion.

Chest Physiotherapy

CPT includes breathing exercises and physical training. These therapies help produce physical and mental relaxation, improve posture, strengthen respiratory musculature, and develop more efficient patterns of breathing. For the motivated child, breathing exercises and controlled breathing are of value in preventing overinflation and improving efficiency of the cough. However, CPT is not recommended during acute, uncomplicated exacerbations of asthma.

Hyposensitization

The role of hyposensitization in childhood asthma has become controversial. In the past, immunotherapy was used for seasonal allergies and when single substances were identified as the offending allergen. It is not recommended for allergens that can be eliminated, such as foods, drugs, and animal dander.

The National Asthma Education and Prevention Program guidelines (2007) recommend immunotherapy for asthma patients in the following situations:

- When there is evidence of a relationship between asthma symptoms and unavoidable exposure to an allergen to which the patient is sensitive
- When symptoms occur all year or at least during a major portion of the year
- When symptom control is difficult with drug therapy because multiple medications are required, the patient is not responsive to available drugs, or the patient refuses to take the medications

Injection therapy is usually limited to clinically significant allergens. The initial dose of the offending allergen(s), based on the size of the skin reaction, is injected subcutaneously. The amount is increased at weekly intervals until a maximum tolerance is reached, after which a maintenance dose is given at 4-week intervals. This may be extended to 5- or 6-week intervals during the off-season for seasonal allergens. Successful treatment is continued for a minimum of 3 years and then stopped. If no symptoms appear, acquired immunity is assumed; if symptoms recur, treatment is reinstituted. Hyposensitization injections should be administered only with emergency equipment and medications readily available in the event of an anaphylactic reaction.

Prognosis

The outlook for children with asthma varies widely. Some children's asthma symptoms may improve at puberty, but up to two thirds of children with asthma continue to have symptoms through puberty and into adulthood. The prognosis for control or disappearance of symptoms varies in children from those who have rare and infrequent attacks to those who are constantly wheezing or are subject to status asthmaticus. In general, when symptoms are severe and numerous, when symptoms have been present for a long time, and when there is a family history of allergy, there is a greater likelihood of a poor prognosis. Risk factors that may predict persistence of symptoms into childhood (from infancy) include atopy, male gender, exposure to environmental tobacco, and maternal history of asthma (Ross, Mjaanes, & Lemanske, 2003). Many children who outgrow their exacerbations continue to have airway hyperresponsiveness and cough as adults. Furthermore, airway hyperresponsiveness in adults appears to be associated with decreased lung function.

Although deaths from asthma have been relatively uncommon (especially in the young age groups) since the 1980s, the rate of death from asthma has increased steadily in the United States and other countries. Data indicate a significant increase in asthma symptoms, emergency department visits, and hospitalization among children from birth to 4 years of age in 2003 to 2004. Most asthma deaths for the same period were in children ages 11 to 17 years, with significant increases seen in non-Hispanic African-Americans (Linzer, 2007). Mortality and morbidity for asthma are especially high among African-American children, whose hospitalization and death rates are three times higher than those of Caucasian and Hispanic children (Liu et al, 2007).

The adolescent age group appears to be the most vulnerable, with the greatest increase occurring in children 10 to 14 years of age. No reliable data exist to explain this increase. Factors that have been postulated include exposure of atopic persons to more allergens (particularly in large urban centers), change in severity of the disease, abuse of drug therapy (toxicity), failure of families and practitioners to recognize the severity of asthma, and psychologic factors such as denial and refusal to accept the disease.

Risk factors for asthma deaths include early onset, frequent attacks, difficult-to-manage disease, adolescence, history of respiratory failure, psychologic problems (refusal to take medications), dependency on or misuse of asthma drugs (high use), presence of physical stigmata (barrel chest, intercostal retractions), and abnormal PFTs.

Status Asthmaticus

Status asthmaticus is a medical emergency that can result in respiratory failure and death if unrecognized and untreated. Children who continue to display respiratory distress despite vigorous therapeutic measures, especially the use of sympathomimetics (e.g., albuterol, epinephrine), are considered to be in status asthmaticus. The condition may develop gradually or rapidly, often coincident with complicating conditions, such as pneumonia or a respiratory virus, that can influence the duration and treatment of the exacerbation.

Therapy for status asthmaticus is aimed at improving ventilation, decreasing airway resistance and relieving bronchospasm, correcting dehydration and acidosis, allaying child and parent anxiety related to the severity of the event, and treating any concurrent infection. Humidified oxygen is recommended and should be given to maintain an oxygen saturation greater than 90%. Inhaled aerosolized short-acting β_2-agonists are recommended for all patients. Three treatments of β_2-agonists spaced 20 to 30 minutes apart are usually given as initial therapy, and continuous administration of β_2-agonists may be initiated. A systemic corticosteroid (oral, IV, or IM) may also be given to decrease the effects of inflammation. An anticholinergic such as ipratropium bromide may be added to the aerosolized solution of the β_2-agonist. Anticholinergics have been shown to result in additional bronchodilation in patients with severe airflow obstruction. An IV infusion is often initiated to provide a means for hydration and to administer medications. Correction of dehydration, acidosis, hypoxia, and electrolyte disturbance is guided by frequent determination of arterial pH, blood gases, and serum electrolytes.

Additional therapies in acute asthma attacks include the use of IV magnesium sulfate, a potent muscle relaxant that acts to decrease inflammation and improves pulmonary function and peak flow rate among pediatric patients treated in the emergency department with moderate to severe asthma. Heliox may be administered to decrease airway resistance and thereby decrease the work of breathing; it can be delivered via a nonrebreathing face mask from premixed tanks, which may be blended in a stand-alone unit or within a ventilator. It may be used in acute exacerbations as an adjunct to β_2-agonist and IV corticosteroid therapy to improve pulmonary function until the two latter medications have time to take full effect in decreasing bronchospasm; the effects of heliox are usually seen within 20 minutes of administration, whereas other drugs may take longer to exert the desired effect. Ketamine, a dissociative anesthetic, is believed to cause smooth muscle relaxation and decrease airway resistance caused by severe bronchospasm in acute asthma (Linzer, 2007); it may be administered as an adjunct to other therapies mentioned previously. Inhaled magnesium sulfate used in addition to a β_2-agonist for acute asthma attacks has also been effective in treating acute asthma exacerbation (Blitz et al, 2005).

Antibiotics should not be used to treat acute asthma attacks except when a bacterial infection resulting from another condition such as pneumonia or sinusitis is present (National Asthma Education and Prevention Program, 2007).

A child suspected of having status asthmaticus is usually seen in the emergency department and is often admitted to a pediatric intensive care unit for close observation and continuous cardiorespiratory monitoring. A key component in the prevention of morbidity is helping the child, parents, teachers, coaches, and other adults recognize features of deteriorating respiratory status, use the correct rescue drugs effectively, and immediately place the child with deteriorating respiratory status into the care of trained health care professionals instead of waiting to see if the asthma gets better on its own. The child going into early status asthmaticus is no different from the adult who is having a myocardial infarction in terms of needing trained medical assistance before the condition deteriorates to irreversible respiratory failure and possible death. Community education regarding asthma recognition and management is an important component of nursing care.

❋ Nursing Care Management

The nursing care of the child with asthma begins with a review of the child's health history; the home, school, and play environment; parent and child attitudes about the child's condition; and a comprehensive physical assessment with focus on the respiratory system. Nursing care of children with asthma involves both acute and long-term care. Nurses who are involved with children in the home, hospital, school, outpatient clinic, or practitioner's office play an important role in helping children and their families learn to live with the condition. The disease can be managed so that it does not require hospitalization or interfere with family life, physical activity, or school attendance. The nursing process in the care of the child with asthma is outlined in the Nursing Care Plan.

Physical assessment of asthma involves the same observations and techniques described in Chapter 34. In addition, the nurse notes and evaluates physical characteristics of chronic respiratory involvement, including chest configuration (e.g., barrel chest), posturing (tripod), and type of breathing. A history of the current and previous episodes and precipitating factors or events provides important information.

Nurses may perform a variety of functions in asthma care, including asthma education in the primary care setting and in schools and other community settings, care of the child with asthma in the acute care setting, ambulatory care, and intensive care. Nurses also obtain information on how asthma affects the child's everyday activities and self-concept, the child's and family's adherence to the prescribed therapy, and their personal treatment goals. Every effort is made to build a partnership between the child and family and the health care team. Communication is an essential part of this partnership, and health care providers should routinely assess the effectiveness of patient-provider communication. In particular, the child and family's satisfaction with asthma control and with the quality of care should be assessed. The nurse should also assess their perception of the severity of the disease and their level of social support.

NURSING CARE PLAN ✤ The Child with Asthma

Nursing Diagnosis	Expected Patient Outcomes	Nursing Interventions	Rationale
Risk for suffocation related to interaction between individual and triggering factors (allergens, respiratory tract infection, exercise, irritants, emotions, temperature changes) **Child's/Family's Defining Characteristics** ***(Subjective and Objective Data)*** Wheezing Dry cough Labored respirations Dyspnea Intercostal retractions Complaints of tightness in chest, shortness of breath Bronchial inflammation and airway constriction	Child will have adequate airway exchange. Family and child will assume responsibility for asthma symptom management. **The Following NOC Concepts Apply to These Outcomes** Asthma Control Anxiety Control Child Development	Assist child and family in recognizing factors such as allergens, irritants, temperature changes, and upper respiratory infections that trigger asthma symptoms. Assist child (according to developmental age) and family in recognizing early signs of an asthmatic episode (use peak expiratory flow meter [PEFM]). Educate child and family in the use of inhaled corticosteroids and bronchodilator. Educate child and family regarding proper use of rescue medications in case of disease exacerbation. Educate child and family regarding the proper use of metered-dose inhaler with spacer, aerosolized nebulizer, and PEFM (know child's personal best). **The Following NIC Concepts Apply to These Interventions** Respiratory Monitoring Administering Inhaled Medications Risk Identification Family Integrity Promotion Energy Management Coping Enhancement Environmental Management	To avoid asthma exacerbations To control symptoms with medication To control symptoms and minimize shortness of breath To prevent illness exacerbations and hospitalization; to prevent side effects from improper use of certain asthma drugs To help child and family effectively manage asthma symptoms independently
Interrupted family processes related to child with a chronic illness **Child's/Family's Defining Characteristics** ***(Subjective and Objective Data)*** Anxiety Disruptive family interactions with child and members Family conflicts Inadequate child support Child's health status ignored Family ignoring other members' needs for those of the child with asthma	Family will cope with effects of the disease. Family will provide child an appropriate protective environment. **The Following NOC Concepts Apply to These Outcomes** Family support Family normalization	Provide family and child (as age appropriate) with explanations about the disease and management. Cooperate with family to develop a written action plan for asthma management. Discuss facilitators and barriers to effective asthma management. Encourage family and child (as age appropriate) to discuss the impact of the illness on the family's lifestyle. Evaluate family resources for asthma management in relation to the following: ✤ Access to health care ✤ Medication availability in home and school (or day care as appropriate) ✤ Allergen exposure control and eradication **The Following NIC Concepts Apply to These Interventions** Emotional Support Anticipatory Guidance Family Involvement Promotion Financial Resource Assistance Decision-Making Support Mutual Goal Setting	To provide adequate information To provide realistic expectations To provide family and child sense of control To assist family members in understanding their role as being vital in the management of asthma To provide opportunity to verbalize frustrations and challenges of having a child with a chronic illness To enhance family's ability to cope with child's chronic illness

One of the major emphases of nursing care is outpatient management by the family. Parents are taught how to avoid allergens, recognize and respond to symptoms of bronchospasm, maintain health and prevent complications, and promote normal activities. The nurse should determine any cultural or ethnic beliefs or practices that influence self-management and that may necessitate modifications in educational approaches to meet the family's needs.

Avoid Allergens

One goal of asthma management is avoidance of an exacerbation. Parents need to know how to avoid allergens that precipitate asthma episodes. The nurse assists the parent in modifying the environment to reduce contact with the offending allergen(s) (see Patient Teaching box, p. 1338). Parents are cautioned to avoid exposing a sensitive child to excessive cold, wind, or other extremes of weather; smoke; sprays; or other irritants. Foods known to provoke symptoms should be eliminated from the diet.

Approximately 2% to 6% of children with asthma are sensitive to aspirin; therefore nurses should caution parents to use other analgesic-antipyretic drugs for discomfort or fever and to read package labeling. Although aspirin is rarely given to children in the United States, salicylate compounds are in other common medicines such as Pepto-Bismol. Children with aspirin-induced asthma may also be sensitive to NSAIDs and tartrazine (yellow dye number 5, a common food coloring).

NURSING ALERT Parents are encouraged to avoid administering aspirin to *any* child unless specifically recommended by and under the supervision of a health practitioner. Acetaminophen is safe for children and is the analgesic of choice.

Relieve Bronchospasm

Parents and older children are taught to recognize early signs and symptoms of an impending attack so that it can be controlled before symptoms become distressing. Most children can recognize prodromal symptoms well before an attack (about 6 hours) and implement preventive therapy. Objective signs that parents may observe include rhinorrhea, cough, low-grade fever, irritability, itching (especially in front of the neck and chest), apathy, anxiety, sleep disturbance, abdominal discomfort, and loss of appetite. A variety of easy-to-use, inexpensive PEFMs are available for use in the home and at school to assess changes in pulmonary function (see Patient Teaching box). In general, children 5 years of age and older are able to use a PEFM successfully. However, young children need to be supervised while they are learning to use their PEFM, and their technique should be checked frequently to ensure that it is correct. Children should use the same PEFM over time, and they should bring it for use at every follow-up visit. Using the same brand of meter is recommended because different brands can give significantly different values. The use of a PEFM provides objective monitoring regarding the severity of asthma and can decrease asthma episodes, health care visits, and missed school days (Burkhart et al, 2007).

Children who use a nebulizer, MDI, Diskus, or Turbuhaler to deliver drugs need to learn how to use the device correctly. A study of school-age children with asthma indicated that only 7% of these children had effective MDI skills (Winkelstein et al, 2000). The MDI device (Fig. 46-5) delivers medication directly to the airways; therefore the child needs to learn to breathe slowly and deeply for better distribution to narrowed airways (see Patient Teaching box).

Young children and those who are unable to manipulate the MDI or coordinate breathing should use spacers. These devices allow the parent or child to deliver the medication from the MDI into the spacer, from which the child then inhales the medication. Spacers also prevent yeast infections in the mouth when corticosteroids are inhaled via an MDI.

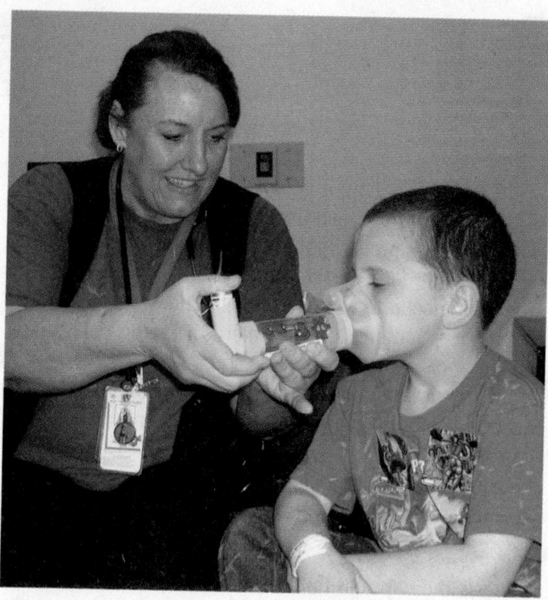

Fig. 46-5 Child using metered-dose inhaler with spacer and face mask.

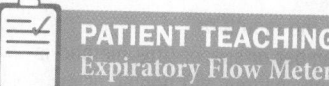

PATIENT TEACHING Use of a Peak Expiratory Flow Meter

1. Before each use, make sure the sliding marker or arrow on the peak expiratory flow meter points to zero or is at the bottom of the numbered scale.
2. Stand up straight.
3. Remove gum or any food from the mouth.
4. Close your lips tightly around the mouthpiece. Be sure to keep your tongue away from the mouthpiece.
5. Blow out as hard and as quickly as you can, a "fast hard puff."
6. Note the number by the marker on the numbered scale.
7. Repeat entire routine three times; wait 30 seconds between each routine.
8. Record the highest of the three readings, not the average.
9. Measure the peak expiratory flow rate (PEFR) close to the same time and same way each day (e.g., morning and evening; before or 15 minutes after taking medication).
10. Keep a chart of your PEFRs.

The child and parents also need to be cautioned about the adverse effects of prescribed drugs and the dangers of overuse of β_2-agonists. They should know that it is important to use these drugs when needed but not indiscriminately or as a substitute for avoiding the symptom-provoking allergen. Parents are cautioned against purchasing over-the-counter preparations because these medications can place the children at risk for increased dosage of a drug and toxicity.

NURSING ALERT Caution parents of children with asthma and adolescents that long-acting β-adrenergic inhalers (salmeterol) should be used only as directed (usually every 12 hours) and not more frequently. They are not intended to relieve acute asthmatic symptoms.

PATIENT TEACHING Use of a Metered-Dose Inhaler*

Steps for Checking How Much Medicine Is in the Canister

1. If the canister is new, it is full.
2. If the canister has been used repeatedly, it might be empty. (Check product label to see how many inhalations should be in each canister.)
3. The most accurate way to determine how many doses remain in a metered-dose inhaler (MDI) is to count and record each actuation as it is used.
4. Many dry-powder inhalers have a dose-counting device or dose indicator on the canister to let you know when the canister is empty.
5. Placing dry-powder inhalers or MDIs with hydrofluoroalkanes in water will destroy these inhalers.

Steps for Using the Inhaler

1. Remove the cap and hold the inhaler upright.
2. Shake the inhaler.
3. Tilt the head back slightly and breathe out slowly.
4. With the inhaler in an upright position, position the mouthpiece as follows:
   a. About 3 to 4 cm from the mouth *or*
   b. Insert into an AeroChamber *or* spacer (this method is recommended for young children and people using corticosteroids)
5. At the end of a normal expiration, depress the top of the inhaler canister firmly to release the medication (into either the AeroChamber or the mouth) and breathe in slowly (about 3 to 5 seconds). Relax the pressure on the top of the canister.
6. Hold the breath for at least 5 to 10 seconds to allow the aerosol medication to reach deeply into the lungs.
7. Remove the inhaler and breathe out slowly through the nose.
8. Wait 1 minute between puffs (if an additional one is needed).

Adapted from National Asthma Education and Prevention Program: *Expert panel report II: guidelines for the diagnosis and management of asthma,* Pub No 97-4051, Bethesda, Md, 1997, National Heart, Lung, and Blood Institute.

*NOTE: Some dry-powder inhalers require a different inhalation technique. To use these dry-powder inhalers, it is important to close the mouth tightly around the mouthpiece of the inhaler and inhale rapidly and deeply.

The family should obtain a PEFM and learn to use this device to monitor the child's asthma. A written asthma action plan that includes the three peak flow meter zones and the child's asthma medications may be obtained from the child's primary care provider. Medications used for asthma exacerbations are also included in the asthma plan. This action plan should be used to make decisions about asthma management at home and at school. The nurse may assist the child and family in preparing this plan, emphasizing that they, and not the health professionals, determine the success of the plan.

Foods known to provoke symptoms should be eliminated from the diet, and parents are advised to read labels on prepared foods and snacks to determine the presence of allergens.

The child should be protected from a respiratory tract infection that can trigger an attack or aggravate the asthmatic state, especially in young children whose airways are mechanically smaller and more reactive. Annual influenza vaccinations are recommended for children with persistent asthma (American Academy of Pediatrics, Committee on Infectious Diseases, 2008). Equipment used for the child, such as nebulizers, must be kept absolutely clean to decrease the chances of contamination with bacteria and fungi.

Breathing exercises and controlled breathing are taught and encouraged for motivated children, and the nurse should provide information concerning activities that promote diaphragmatic breathing, side expansion, and improved mobility of the chest wall. Play techniques that can be used for younger children to extend their expiratory time and increase expiratory pressure include blowing cotton balls or a Ping-Pong ball on a table, blowing a pinwheel, blowing bubbles, or preventing a tissue from falling by blowing it against the wall. Self-care and asthma self-management programs are important in helping the child and family cope with asthma. Most asthma self-management programs for children convey several principles. First, asthma is a common disease that can be controlled with appropriate drug therapy, environmental control, education, and management skills. Second, it is much easier to prevent than to treat an asthma episode; adherence to a therapeutic program is necessary to prevent exacerbations. Third, children with asthma can live full and active lives.

Asthma camps provide an opportunity for children with asthma to engage in physical activity while learning about their disease in a controlled environment with their peers and health professionals. Children who attend asthma camps often demonstrate improved asthma self-management skills.

Self-contained programs and brochures for patient education are available from the Asthma and Allergy Foundation of America* and the American Lung Association.† The National Heart, Lung, and Blood Institute‡ provides educational materials for asthma education in the school setting and also copies of the *Guidelines for the Diagnosis and Management of Asthma* for the practitioner (National Asthma Education and Prevention Program, 2007). Another publication designed for health care practitioners, *Pediatric Asthma: Promoting Best Practice,* can be obtained from the American Academy of Allergy Asthma and Immunology.§

Provide Acute Asthma Care

Children who are admitted to the hospital with acute asthma are ill, anxious, and uncomfortable. The progression or resolution of status asthmaticus is variable. The importance of continual observation and assessment cannot be overemphasized.

**1233 20th St., NW, Suite 402, Washington, DC 20036; 800-7-Asthma; www.aafa.org.*

†61 Broadway, 6th Floor, New York, NY 10006; 800-548-8252; national headquarters: 212-315-8700; www.lungusa.org.

‡NHLBI Health Information Center, PO Box 30105, Bethesda, MD 20824-0105; 301-592-8573; fax: 240-629-3246; www.nhlbi.nih.gov.

§555 E. Wells St., Suite 1100, Milwaukee, WI 53202; 414-272-6071; http://aaaai.org.

When β_2-agonists and corticosteroids are given, the child is monitored closely and continuously for relief of respiratory distress and signs of side effects or toxicity. Oral fluid intake may be limited during the acute phase; IV fluid replacement may be required to provide adequate tissue hydration.

Older children may be more comfortable standing (Fig. 46-6), sitting upright, or leaning slightly forward (Fig. 46-7). When possible, the nurse communicates in such a way that a child can reply in a few words to avoid fatigue. Shortness of breath makes talking difficult.

Children with acute asthma are apprehensive and anxious. The calm, efficient presence of a nurse helps reassure them that they are safe and will be cared for during this stressful period. It is important to assure children that they will not be left alone and that their parents are allowed to remain with them.

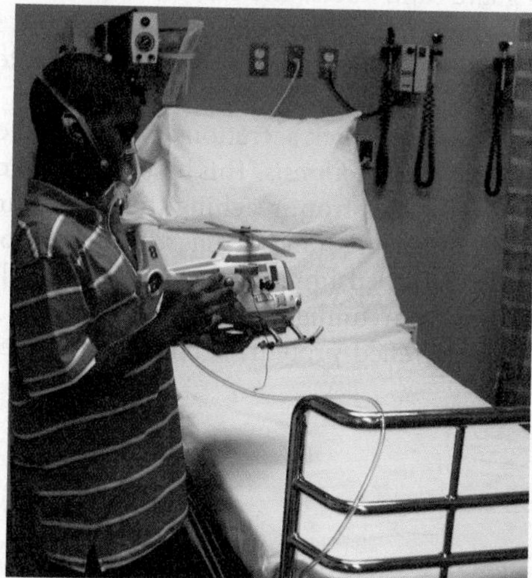

Fig. 46-6 Child with asthma is allowed play activity as tolerated.

Parents need reassurance and want to be informed of their child's condition and therapies. They may believe that they have in some way contributed to the child's condition or could have prevented the episode. Reassurance regarding their efforts expended on the child's behalf and their parenting capabilities can help alleviate their stress. Efforts to reduce parental apprehension also reduce the child's distress. Anxiety is easily communicated to the child from parents and members of the staff.

Support Child or Adolescent and Family

The nurse working with children with asthma can provide support in a number of ways. Many children voice frustration because their exacerbations interfere with their daily activities and social lives. They need education about what to do to prevent an asthma episode. These children also need reassurance from the health team that they can learn to control and cope with their asthma and live a normal life. Be aware of children, especially adolescents, who demonstrate signs of depression and may not comply with therapy as a means of passive suicide.

Children in disruptive family situations (divorce, separation, violence, custodial battles) may disregard daily asthma medication regimen or may be at higher risk as a result of neglect by adults who are in charge of their care. Adolescents struggling with a sense of identity and body image often regard asthma as a condition that will "go away," especially if there is a time lapse between symptoms, and may abandon the therapeutic regimen. In some cases adolescents find themselves in charge of other siblings in blended family situations and may ignore their own health needs. Referral for counseling and guidance is appropriate when the child or adolescent's life is potentially in harm's way and the therapeutic regimen for asthma is abandoned due to other crises.

The short- and long-term adaptation of children with asthma often depends on the family's acceptance of the disor-

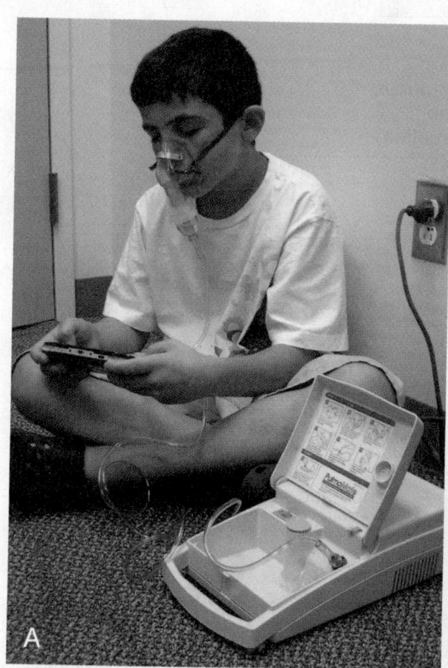

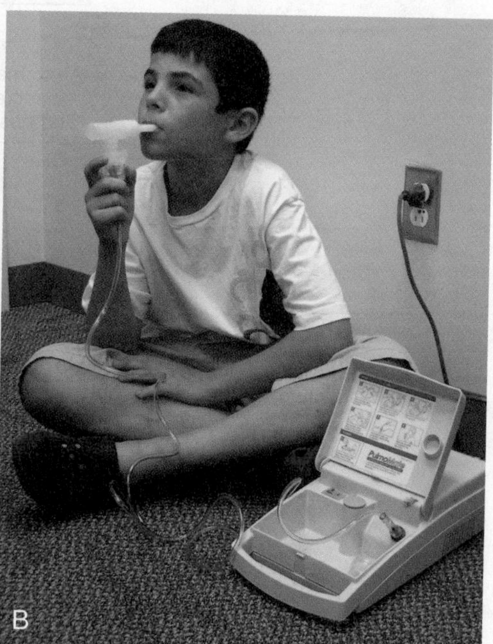

Fig. 46-7 Children with asthma may take a nebulized aerosol treatment with a mask (**A**) or mouthpiece (**B**). *(Courtesy Texas Children's Hospital, Houston, TX.)*

der. The task of living day-to-day with affected children involves the entire family. There are periodic crises and the ever-present threat of a crisis, requiring parental vigilance; sleepless nights; frequent trips to the physician, emergency department, or hospital; and often overwhelming medical expenses. Throughout these stresses, parents are encouraged to promote as normal a life as possible for their children.

Cystic Fibrosis

CF is inherited as an autosomal recessive trait; the affected child inherits the defective gene from both parents, with an overall incidence of 1:4. The mutated gene responsible for CF is located on the long arm of chromosome 7. This gene codes a protein of 1480 amino acids called the *cystic fibrosis transmembrane regulator (CFTR)*. The CFTR protein is related to a family of membrane-bound glycoproteins. The glycoproteins constitute a cAMP-activated chloride channel and also regulate other chloride and sodium channels at the surfaces of the epithelial cells.

Pathophysiology

CF is characterized by several clinical features: increased viscosity of mucous gland secretions, a striking elevation of sweat electrolytes, an increase in several organic and enzymatic constituents of saliva, and abnormalities in autonomic nervous system function. Although both sodium and chloride are affected, the defect appears to be primarily a result of abnormal chloride movement; the CFTR appears to function as a chloride channel. Children with CF demonstrate decreased pancreatic secretion of bicarbonate and chloride and an increase in sodium and chloride in both saliva and sweat. This characteristic is the basis for the sweat chloride diagnostic test. The sweat electrolyte abnormality is present from birth, continues throughout life, and is unrelated to the severity of the disease or the extent to which other organs are involved.

The primary factor, and the one that is responsible for many of the clinical manifestations of the disease, is mechanical obstruction caused by the increased viscosity of mucous gland secretions (Fig. 46-8). Instead of forming a thin, freely flowing secretion, the mucous glands produce a thick mucoprotein that accumulates and dilates them. Small passages in organs such as the pancreas and bronchioles become obstructed as secretions precipitate or coagulate to form concretions in glands and ducts. The earliest postnatal manifestation of CF is often *meconium ileus* in the newborn, in which the small intestine is blocked with thick, puttylike, tenacious, mucilaginous meconium.

In the pancreas the thick secretions block the ducts, eventually causing *pancreatic fibrosis*. This blockage prevents essential pancreatic enzymes from reaching the duodenum, which causes marked impairment in the digestion and absorption of nutrients. The disturbed function is reflected in bulky stools that are frothy from undigested fat *(steatorrhea)* and foul smelling from putrefied protein *(azotorrhea)*. The endocrine

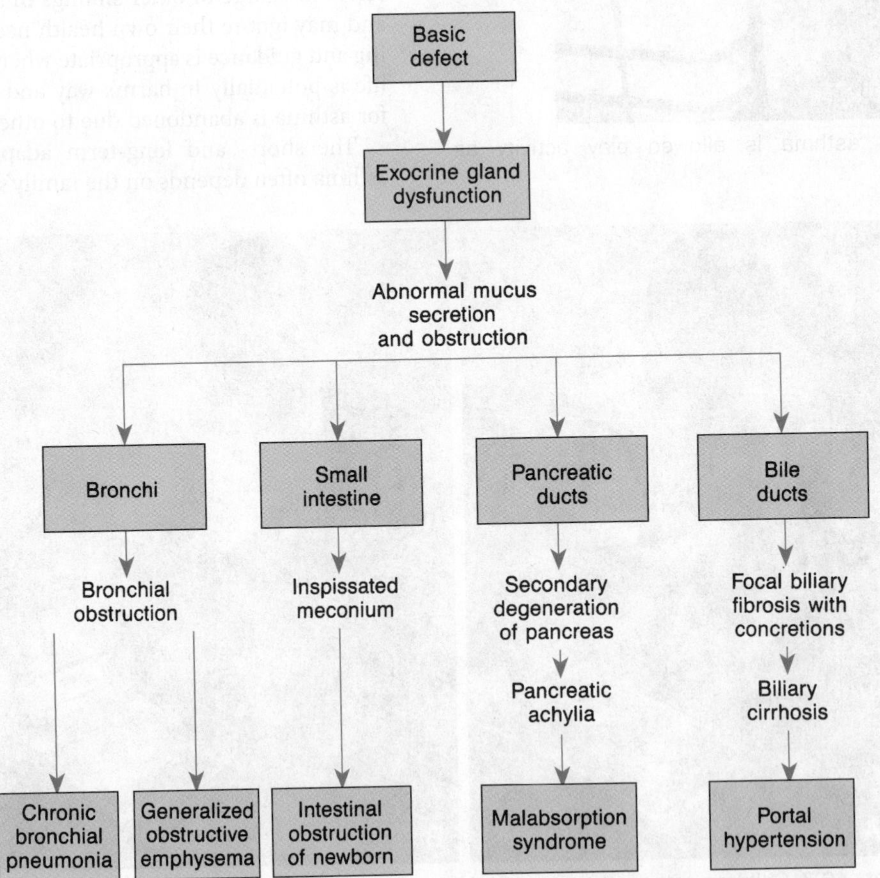

Fig. 46-8 Various effects of exocrine gland dysfunction in cystic fibrosis.

function of the pancreas often remains unchanged because the islets of Langerhans are normal but may decrease in number as pancreatic fibrosis progresses. The incidence of diabetes mellitus (cystic fibrosis–related diabetes [CFRD]) is greater in CF children than in the general population (Balinsky & Zhu, 2004), which may be caused by changes in pancreatic architecture and diminished blood supply over time. Consequently, with increased survival and primarily in adolescents and adults, type 1 diabetes is becoming a more frequent finding. There is no relationship between the progression of pulmonary disease and the development of diabetes mellitus in CF. In the liver, localized biliary obstruction and fibrosis are common and become more extensive with time.

A common gastrointestinal complication associated with CF is *prolapse of the rectum*, which occurs in infancy and childhood and is related to large, bulky stools; malnutrition; and increased intraabdominal pressure secondary to paroxysmal cough. Affected children of all ages are subject to intestinal obstruction from inspissated or impacted feces. Gumlike masses can obstruct the bowel and produce a partial or complete obstruction, a condition that is referred to as *distal intestinal obstruction syndrome.*

Pulmonary complications are present in almost all children with CF, but the onset and extent of involvement are variable. Symptoms are produced by stagnation of mucus in the airways, with eventual bacterial colonization leading to destruction of lung tissue. The abnormally viscous and tenacious secretions are difficult to expectorate and gradually obstruct the bronchi and bronchioles, causing scattered areas of bronchiectasis, atelectasis, and hyperinflation. The stagnant mucus offers a favorable environment for bacterial growth.

The reproductive systems of both males and females with CF are affected. Females with CF have normal fallopian tubes and ovaries, but fertility can be inhibited by highly viscous cervical secretions, which act as a plug, blocking sperm entry. Women with CF who become pregnant have an increased incidence of premature labor and delivery and low birth weight in the infant. Favorable nutritional status and pulmonary function are positively correlated with favorable pregnancy outcomes. Most adult men (95%) with CF are sterile, which may be caused by blockage of the vas deferens with abnormal secretions or by failure of normal development of the wolffian duct structures (vas deferens, epididymis, and seminal vesicles), resulting in decreased or absent sperm production.

Growth and development are often affected in children with moderate to severe forms of CF. Physical growth may be restricted as a result of decreased absorption of nutrients, including vitamins and fat; increased oxygen demands for pulmonary function; and delayed bone growth. The usual pattern is one of growth failure (failure to thrive), with increased weight loss despite an increased appetite and gradual deterioration of the respiratory system. Clinical manifestations of CF are listed in Box 46-17.

Diagnostic Evaluation

Traditionally the diagnosis of CF was based on a positive sweat chloride test, absence of pancreatic enzymes, radiography, chronic obstructive pulmonary disease, and family history.

BOX 46-17 Clinical Manifestations of Cystic Fibrosis

Meconium Ileus*
Abdominal distention
Vomiting
Failure to pass stools
Rapid development of dehydration

Gastrointestinal Manifestations
Large, bulky, loose, frothy, extremely foul-smelling stools
Voracious appetite (early in disease)
Loss of appetite (later in disease)
Weight loss
Marked tissue wasting
Failure to grow
Distended abdomen
Thin extremities
Sallow skin
Evidence of deficiency of fat-soluble vitamins A, D, E, and K
Anemia

Pulmonary Manifestations
Initial signs:
- Wheezing respirations
- Dry, nonproductive cough

Eventually:
- Increased dyspnea
- Paroxysmal cough
- Evidence of obstructive emphysema and patchy areas of atelectasis

Progressive involvement:
- Overinflated, barrel-shaped chest
- Cyanosis
- Clubbing of fingers and toes
- Repeated episodes of bronchitis and bronchopneumonia

*In about 10% of cases.

Newer diagnostic methods make it possible to diagnose CF early in infancy so therapies can be implemented to increase the child's overall survival and quality of life. In addition to the sweat chloride test and factors listed previously, diagnosis may be confirmed by any one of the following: newborn screening, deoxyribonucleic acid (DNA) identification of mutant genes, and abnormal nasal potential difference measurement.

Universal newborn screening for CF has been proposed yet remains controversial, since many states lack the resources for such screening programs. In 2009 all but two states offered some type of CF newborn screening (National Newborn Screening and Genetics Resource Center, 2009). The Centers for Disease Control and Prevention (2004a) emphatically recommends newborn screening for CF. The newborn screening test consists of an immunoreactive trypsinogen (IRT) analysis performed on a dried spot of blood, which may be followed by direct analysis of DNA for the presence of the ΔF508 mutation or other mutations on the same dried blood spot. Benefits

evolve Critical Thinking Exercise–Cystic Fibrosis Inheritance Risks

of early screening and detection include earlier nutritional intervention for identified infants (Farrell et al, 2007; Southern et al, 2009); disadvantages include the parental anxiety false-positive results may generate. Children who were identified and treated early in infancy with aggressive nutritional support had improved height and weight well into adolescence. Although the technology is available to conduct carrier screening for the general population, this issue remains controversial, and widespread implementation of carrier screening programs is not recommended. An in utero diagnosis of CF is also possible based on detection of two CF mutations in the fetus.

The consistent finding of abnormally high sodium and chloride concentrations in the sweat is a unique characteristic of CF. Parents may report that their infant tastes "salty" when they kiss him or her. The quantitative sweat chloride test (pilocarpine iontophoresis) involves stimulating the production of sweat with a special device (involves stimulation with 3-mA electric current), collecting the sweat on filter paper, and measuring the sweat electrolytes. The quantitative analysis requires a sufficient volume of sweat (more than 75 mg). Two separate samples are collected to ensure the reliability of the test for any individual. Normally sweat chloride content is less than 40 mEq/L, with a mean of 18 mEq/L. A chloride concentration greater than 60 mEq/L is diagnostic of CF; in infants younger than 3 months a sweat chloride concentration greater than 40 mEq/L is highly suggestive of CF. In some situations DNA testing may be substituted for the sweat test. The presence of a mutation known to cause CF on each CFTR gene predicts with a high degree of certainty that the individual has CF; however, multiple CFTR mutations may also be present and detected with DNA assay.

Chest radiography reveals characteristic patchy atelectasis and obstructive emphysema. PFTs are sensitive indexes of lung function, providing evidence of abnormal small airway function in CF. Other diagnostic tools that may aid in diagnosis include stool fat or enzyme analysis. Stool analysis requires a 72-hour sample with accurate recording of food intake during that time. Radiographs, including barium enema, are used for diagnosis of meconium ileus.

Therapeutic Management

Improved survival among patients with CF during the past two decades can be attributed largely to antibiotic therapy and improved nutritional management. Goals of CF therapeutic management are to (1) prevent or minimize pulmonary complications, (2) ensure adequate nutrition for growth, (3) encourage appropriate physical activity, and (4) promote a reasonable quality of life for the child and the family. A multidisciplinary approach to treatment is needed to accomplish these goals.

Management of Pulmonary Problems

Management of pulmonary problems is directed toward prevention and treatment of pulmonary infection by improving ventilation, removing mucopurulent secretions, and administering antimicrobial agents. Many children develop respiratory symptoms by 3 years of age. The large amounts and viscosity of respiratory secretions in children with CF contribute to the likelihood of respiratory tract infections. Recurrent pulmonary infections in the child with CF result in greater damage to the airways; small airways are destroyed, causing bronchiectasis.

The most common pathogens responsible for pulmonary infections are *P. aeruginosa, B. cepacia, S. aureus, H. influenzae, E. coli,* and *K. pneumoniae. P. aeruginosa* and *B. cepacia* are particularly pathogenic for children with CF, and infections with these organisms are difficult to clear. In addition, children with CF who are chronically colonized with these organisms have poorer survival rates than children who are not colonized. Colonization and infection with methicillin-resistant *S. aureus* (MRSA) has recently emerged as a critical factor in lung infection and pulmonary function in patients with CF. Patients with MRSA required longer hospitalization and multiple antibiotic regimens (Ren et al, 2007). Fungal colonization with *Candida* or *Aspergillus* organisms in the respiratory tract is also common in CF patients.

Prevention of infection involves a daily routine of CPT to maintain pulmonary hygiene. CPT is usually performed on average twice daily (on rising and in the evening) and more frequently if needed, especially during pulmonary infection. The *Flutter mucus clearance device* is a small, handheld plastic pipe with a stainless-steel ball on the inside that facilitates removal of mucus (Fig. 46-9). It has the advantage of increasing sputum expectoration and being used without an assistant. Handheld percussors may be used to loosen secretions. Another method to clear mucus is high-frequency chest compression, in which the child temporarily wears a mechanical vest device that provides high-frequency chest wall oscillation. Some children and adolescents with an implantable port may experience localized pain with the vest.

Patients with CF have been found to regress when conventional CPT is discontinued. Therefore, although it is time consuming for the child and family, CPT remains the cornerstone of pulmonary therapy. Forced expiration, or "huffing," with the glottis partially closed helps move secretions from the small airways so that subsequent coughing can move secretions forcefully from the large airways. Several studies indicate that this maneuver enhances the pulmonary function of patients with CF. Autogenic drainage involves a variety of breathing techniques, which the older child can use to force

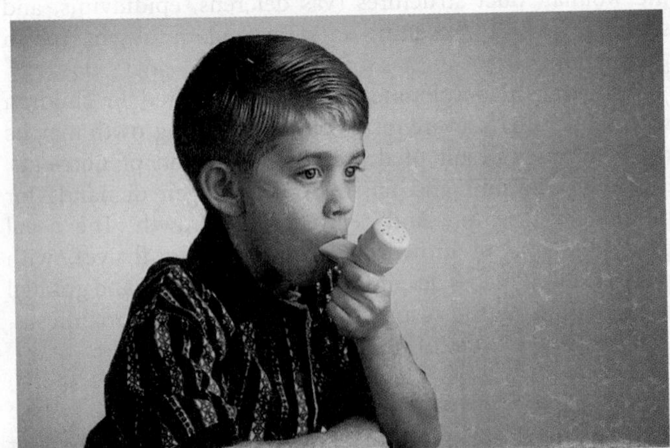

Fig. 46-9 Child using Flutter mucus clearance device. *(Courtesy Scandipharm, Inc.)*

mucus in lower lobes up into the airways so it can be successfully expelled. Another mucus-clearing technique involves use of a positive expiratory pressure mask; this technique involves breathing into a mask attached to a one-way valve, which creates resistance—as the patient exhales, the airway is kept open by the pressure, and mucus is forced into the upper airway for expulsion.

Bronchodilator medication delivered in an aerosol opens bronchi for easier expectoration and is administered before CPT when the patient exhibits evidence of reactive airway disease or wheezing. Another aerosolized medication is recombinant human deoxyribonuclease (DNase, known generically as dornase alfa [Pulmozyme]), which decreases the viscosity of mucus. It is well tolerated and has no major adverse effects; minor reactions are voice alterations and laryngitis. This medication, given daily via nebulization, has resulted in improvements in spirometry, PFTs, dyspnea scores, and perceptions of well-being and has reduced the viscosity of sputum.

Physical exercise is an important adjunct to daily CPT. Exercise stimulates mucus excretion and provides a sense of well-being and increased self-esteem. Any aerobic exercise that the patient enjoys should be encouraged. The ultimate aim of exercise is to increase lung vital capacity, remove secretions, increase pulmonary blood flow, and maintain healthy lung tissue for effective ventilation.

Pulmonary infections are treated as soon as they are recognized. In CF patients characteristic signs of pulmonary infection—fever, tachypnea, and chest pain—may be absent; therefore a careful history and physical examination are essential. The presence of anorexia, weight loss, and decreased activity alert the practitioner to pulmonary infection and the need for an antibiotic regimen (Boat & Acton, 2007). Aerosolized antibiotics such as tobramycin, ticarcillin, and gentamicin are beneficial for patients with frequent pulmonary exacerbations. It is not uncommon for the hospitalized child with CF to be placed on as many as two or three antibiotics and one antifungal medication to treat coexisting pulmonary infections.

IV antibiotics may be administered at home as an alternative to hospitalization. The use of peripherally inserted central catheters (PICCs) for the administration of antibiotics in children with CF is a viable option with limited complications and fewer needle punctures to obtain blood specimens and to maintain often lengthy treatment with parenteral antibiotics (Tolomeo & Mackey, 2003). Alternatively, an implanted port offers the advantage of access for blood draws and antibiotic infusion. Patients may receive antibiotic therapy at home and continue daily activities with minimum disruptions. However, when pulmonary function does not improve with outpatient management, hospitalization may be recommended for continued antibiotic therapy and vigorous CPT and postural drainage. Oxygen administration is used for children with acute episodes but must be used cautiously because many children with CF have chronic carbon dioxide retention and the unsupervised use of oxygen can be harmful (see Oxygen Therapy, Chapter 45). With repeated infection and inflammation, bronchial cysts and emphysema may develop. These cysts may rupture, resulting in a pneumothorax.

NURSING ALERT Signs of a pneumothorax are usually nonspecific and include tachypnea, tachycardia, dyspnea, pallor, and cyanosis. A subtle drop in oxygen saturation (measured by pulse oximetry) may be an early sign of pneumothorax.

Blood streaking of the sputum is usually associated with increased pulmonary infection and often requires no specific treatment. Hemoptysis greater than 250 ml/24 hr for the older child (less for a younger child) indicates a potentially life-threatening event and needs to be treated immediately. Sometimes bleeding can be controlled with bed rest, IV antibiotics, replacement of acute blood loss, IV conjugated estrogens (Premarin) or vasopressin (Pitressin), and correction of any coagulation defects with vitamin K or fresh frozen plasma. If hemoptysis persists, the site of bleeding should be localized via bronchoscopy and cauterized or embolized.

Treatment of nasal polyps includes intranasal corticosteroids, oral antihistamines, and decongestants. If these measures are ineffective, surgical interventions may be necessary.

Because pulmonary damage in patients with CF is believed to be caused by the inflammatory process that occurs with frequent infections, the use of corticosteroids has been studied; however, treatment with corticosteroids for prolonged periods has been associated with linear growth restriction, glucose tolerance abnormalities, and cataract formation. Antiinflammatory medications such as ibuprofen are becoming more important in the treatment of CF, but careful monitoring for adverse effects (gastrointestinal bleeding) is essential.

Management of Gastrointestinal Problems

The principal treatment for pancreatic insufficiency is replacement of pancreatic enzymes, which are administered with meals and snacks to ensure that digestive enzymes are mixed with food in the duodenum. Enteric-coated products prevent the neutralization of enzymes by gastric acids, thus allowing activation to occur in the alkaline environment of the small bowel. The amount of enzymes depends on the severity of the insufficiency, the child's response to enzyme replacement, and the practitioner's philosophy. Usually one to five capsules are administered with a meal, and fewer are taken with snacks. Capsules can be swallowed whole or taken apart, and the contents sprinkled on a small amount of food to be taken at the beginning of the meal. The amount of enzyme is adjusted to achieve normal growth and a decrease in the number of stools to one or two per day. Pancreatic enzymes should be taken within 30 minutes of eating. The enteric-coated beads should not be chewed or crushed, since destroying the enteric coating can lead to inactivation of the enzymes and excoriation of oral mucosa. The powder form should be used cautiously because inhalation of the powder may precipitate acute bronchospasm. Enzymes are mixed into cereal or fruit such as applesauce. Because the uptake of fat-soluble vitamins is decreased, water-miscible forms of these vitamins (A, D, E, and K) are given, along with multivitamins and the pancreatic enzymes. When high-fat foods are eaten, the child is encouraged to add extra enzymes.

Children with CF require a well-balanced, high-protein, high-caloric diet (because of the impaired intestinal absorption). In the patient with minimal pulmonary disease, energy requirements up to 5% to 10% above the recommended daily allowances are necessary; for those with severe lung disease, energy requirements may be as high as 20% to 50% or more of the recommended daily allowance (American Academy of Pediatrics, 2009). Breastfeeding with enzyme supplementation should be continued whenever possible and, when necessary, supplemented with a higher-calorie-per-ounce (e.g., 24 kcal/oz) formula. For formula-fed infants, commercial cow's milk–based formulas may be adequate to achieve desired growth, but if growth is inadequate, additional caloric intake may be required. In older children with CF, three daily meals and three snacks are recommended to meet energy and growth requirements (American Academy of Pediatrics, 2009). Growth failure despite adequate nutritional support may indicate deterioration of pulmonary status. Patients with CF may experience frequent anorexia as a result of the copious amounts of mucus produced and expectorated, persistent cough, effect of medications, fatigue, and sleep disruption. They may be placed on nighttime supplemental gastrostomy feedings or parenteral alimentation in an effort to build up nutritional reserves if there has been a history of inability to maintain weight. Enzyme supplementation is encouraged with gastrostomy feedings; these may be given at the initiation of the infusion, at bedtime, and at the conclusion of the feeding infusion (American Academy of Pediatrics, 2009).

Meconium ileus and meconium ileus equivalent, or total or partial intestinal obstruction, can occur at any age. Constipation is often the result of a combination of malabsorption (either from inadequate pancreatic enzyme dosage or a failure to take the enzymes), decreased intestinal motility, and abnormally viscous intestinal secretions. These problems usually do not require surgical interventions and may be treated with GoLYTELY or Colyte (osmotic solutions given orally or by nasogastric tubes), other laxatives, stool softeners, or rectal administration of meglumine diatrizoate (Gastrografin).

Rectal prolapse occurs in about 20% to 25% of children with CF (McMullen & Bryson, 2004). The first episode of rectal prolapse is frightening to both parents and child. Its reduction usually requires immediate guidance and intervention, which is managed by simply guiding the rectum back into place with a gloved, lubricated finger. Further management usually involves attempting to decrease the bulk of daily stools through enzyme replacement.

Children with CF often experience transient or chronic gastroesophageal reflux, which should be treated with the appropriate histamine-receptor antagonist and gastrointestinal motility drug, dietary modifications, and an upright position after feedings or meals (McMullen & Bryson, 2004).

Management of Endocrine Problems

The management of CFRD is critical in the therapeutic treatment of the child with CF. CFRD presents a combination of insulin resistance and insulin deficiency, with unstable glucose homeostasis in the presence of acute lung infection and treatment. Children with CFRD require close monitoring of blood glucose, administration of oral glucose-lowering agents or insulin injections, and diet and exercise management; children with CF may be at increased risk for glucose management problems as a result of decreased nutrient absorption, anorexia, and severity of pulmonary illness. The prevalence of CFRD increases with age, and there is increased morbidity and mortality among children with CFRD compared to those without (Strausbaugh & Davis, 2007). Microvascular complications such as retinopathy and nephropathy may occur in children and adolescents with CFRD (Schwarzenberg et al, 2007). However, ketoacidosis is reported to be rare in individuals with CFRD (Boat & Acton, 2007).

Bone health is of concern in children and adults with CF. The pancreatic insufficiency of CF and chronic steroid use present potential risks for less than optimum bone growth in such children. Assessment of bone health by history and bone mass density evaluation should be considered in assessing the child's (8 years old and older) health status to detect and prevent osteoporosis or osteopenia (Borowitz, Baker, & Stallings, 2002).

The administration of growth hormone (somatropin [Nutropin]) is being investigated as a nutritional adjunct in children with CF to achieve optimum growth; one small study sample suggests an improvement in CF clinical status (Hardin et al, 2005). One randomized study indicates that the drug is well tolerated but does not result in short-term improvement of forced expiratory volume (FEV) in CF patients (Schnabel et al, 2007).

Prognosis

The median predicted survival age for the CF patient in 2008 was 37.4 years, and approximately 45% of all patients with CF are 18 years or older (Cystic Fibrosis Foundation, 2007). Lung, heart, pancreas, and liver transplantation have increased survival rates among some CF patients. Heart-lung and double-lung procedures have been successfully performed in children with advanced pulmonary vascular disease and hypoxia. The obstacles surrounding this technique are availability of donated organs; complications from surgery; pulmonary infections; and recurrence of obstructive bronchiolitis, which decreases transplanted lung function.

Despite considerable progress and a recent surge in new treatment modalities, CF remains a progressive and incurable disease. The pulmonary involvement ultimately determines the patient's outcome because pancreatic enzyme deficiency is less of a problem if adequate nutrition is ensured. With advances in technology, parents and adolescents are challenged to set future goals that may include college, careers, social relationships, and marriage. Concurrently they are faced with increasing morbidity and higher rates of CF complications as they grow older.

Nursing Care Management

Assessment of the child with CF involves both pulmonary and gastrointestinal observations. Pulmonary assessment is the same as that described for asthma, with special attention to lung sounds, observation of cough, and evidence of decreased activity or fatigue. Gastrointestinal assessment primarily involves observing the frequency and nature of the stools and abdominal distention. The observer is also alert to evidence of growth failure (e.g., weight loss, muscle wasting, pallor, anorexia, decreased activity [from baseline norm]). Family members are interviewed to determine the child's eating and eliminating habits and confirm a history of frequent respiratory tract infections or bowel obstruction in infancy.

The nurse assesses the newborn for feeding and stooling patterns, which may indicate a potential problem such as meconium ileus. The nurse also participates in diagnostic testing such as the initial newborn screening, IRT, DNA analysis, or sweat chloride test.

Parents are often anxious and puzzled about the diagnostic tests and the possible implications of the test results. They need careful explanations of the disease, how it might affect their family, and what they can do to provide the best possible care for their child. It is crucial to involve the parents in the follow-up for early diagnostic testing; the neonate may require several follow-up visits in the first few weeks of life if initial test results are not conclusive.

The uncertainty, fear, and initial shock associated with the diagnosis are overwhelming to parents. They must face the impact of the chronic, life-threatening nature of the disease and the prospect of intensive treatment, for which they must assume a major part of the responsibility and for which they are ill prepared. They often fear that they will be unable to provide the care the child needs. One of the most difficult aspects of the diagnosis is the implication inherent in its etiology (i.e., the recognition that each parent contributed the gene responsible for the defect).

Hospital Care

Most patients with CF require hospitalization only for treatment of pulmonary infection, uncontrolled diabetes, or a coexisting medical problem that cannot be treated on an outpatient basis. Therefore, when patients with CF are hospitalized, standard precautions with meticulous handwashing should be implemented to decrease the nosocomial spread of organisms to the CF patient and between hospitalized CF patients (especially when MRSA is prevalent). Contact precautions may be required for specific infections.

When the child with CF is hospitalized for diagnosis or treatment of pulmonary complications, aerosol therapy, chest percussion therapy, and postural drainage are instituted or continued. Respiratory therapists often initiate, supervise, and provide these treatments; however, it is the nurse's responsibility to monitor the patient's tolerance to the procedure and evaluate its effectiveness in relation to treatment goals. The nurse may at times administer aerosol therapy, perform CPT, assist with mucus removal interventions such as the mechanical vest, and teach breathing exercises. CPT should not be performed before or immediately after meals. Planning CPT so that it does not coincide with meals is difficult in the hospital situation but is essential to the effectiveness of this treatment.

Supplemental oxygen therapy is administered to the child with mild or moderate respiratory distress, and the child requires frequent assessment of the tolerance to the procedure. Noninvasive pulse oximetry provides valuable data about the patient's oxygenation status, but nursing assessments, including observation of respiratory pattern, work of breathing, and lung auscultation, are vital.

One of the nursing challenges in the care of the child with CF is encouraging compliance with the therapeutic medication regimen, which often involves a significant number of medications; pancreatic enzymes; vitamins A, D, E, and K; oral antifungals for *Candida* infection; antihistamines; antiinflammatory agents; and oral antibiotics. This may be overwhelming to the child. Factor in multiple inhaled bronchodilators, CPT and aerosol treatments, blood glucose monitoring and insulin administration, various other medications, and increased mucus production during the acute phase, and it is not uncommon for the child with CF to rebel and be noncompliant with this regimen. Gentle coaxing, positive reinforcement, and frank negotiation may be required to enlist cooperation for effective medication compliance.

The child's sleep is disrupted frequently by hospital routines; therefore nursing care should be flexible enough to allow him or her some quiet time without affecting vital care. In some cases a daily schedule of events, including medication administration, CPT, aerosolized therapy, and dressing changes, may need to be mutually developed with the child, nurses, and physician so that the child feels he or she has some control of the care.

The diet for the child with CF represents another challenge; careful planning with a pediatric dietitian and the child's input may help decrease the loss of appetite and weight loss that are often part of the condition. Patients with CF, especially adolescents, enjoy foods brought from home or an occasional fast food of choice (provided these meet therapeutic requirements). Children in the early stages of CF often have a good appetite. With infection and increased lung involvement, their appetite diminishes, and eventually it becomes a challenge to tempt failing appetites. When dietary intake fails to meet the child's needs for growth, enteral feedings or supplements may be considered (Borowitz, Baker, & Stallings, 2002). These feedings may be administered via gastrostomy tube during the night to minimize the disruption of daily activities, including school. A skin-level feeding gastrostomy affords the child few activity restrictions and minimum disruption of body image in comparison to a nasogastric tube or conventional gastrostomy tube. The child and parents are encouraged to perceive this therapy not as a last-ditch effort but as an adjunct therapy to maintain optimum growth and prevent excessive weight loss (Borowitz, Baker, & Stallings, 2002).

The child needs support during the many treatments and tests that are a part of the hospitalization. IV fluids, IV antibiotics and antifungals, and blood tests are almost always a part of the acute care treatment, and the child soon associates hospitalization with these stress-provoking procedures.

Depression, anxiety, and disturbed self-image may occur in children and adolescents with CF; young adults with severe symptoms may be especially prone to depression as a result of the realization of the poor prognosis and the reality of unmet life expectations and goals.

Providing support to both the child and the family is essential. The progressive nature of the disease makes each illness requiring hospitalization a potentially life-threatening event. Skilled nursing care and sympathetic attention to the emotional needs of the child and family help them cope with the stresses associated with repeated respiratory tract infections and hospitalizations.

The child or adolescent who is immobilized as a result of CF requires the same care and attention as the child with immobility from any other chronic or acute illness, including skin care, bowel management, passive range of motion, and positioning.

Home Care

Most children and adolescents with CF can be managed at home. The goals of care include normalization and daily activities, including school and peer involvement. The care plan should be flexible so that family activities are disrupted as little as possible. Parents may initially require assistance finding and contacting durable medical equipment companies that provide home care equipment. They also need opportunities to learn how to use the equipment and to solve problems they may encounter while delivering therapy at home. The many aspects of home care for the child with CF are similar to those of home care for other children and are discussed in Chapter 43.

Patients and family members need education about the preferred diet of nutritious meals with tolerated fat, increased protein and carbohydrate, and the administration of pancreatic enzymes. For infants and young children, the enzymes can be mixed with pureed fruit such as applesauce and fed with a spoon. Capsules are usually suitable for older children. It is important to stress to parents that the enzymes, in the amount regulated to the child's needs, should be administered at the beginning of all meals and snacks.

One of the most important aspects of educating parents for home care is teaching techniques for the removal of mucus (CPT, vest, forced expiration) and breathing exercises. The success of a therapy program depends on conscientious performance of these treatments regularly as prescribed. The number of times these therapies are performed each day is determined on an individual basis, and often parents readily learn to adjust the number and intensity of the treatments to the child's needs. For pulmonary infection home IV antibiotics may be prescribed. Home IV care may be preferred for willing and competent families, since it reduces tension and usually brings a sense of belonging to the family members; however, this option depends on a number of factors, including availability of an agency with adequate staff to perform multiple daily home antibiotic infusions. With use of the venous access devices such as PICC lines and implanted ports, the parents and child can be taught the technique of direct administration into the IV line. Around-the-clock administration may be difficult for families and requires certain adjustments such as waking at least once during the night to give the drug.

Families also need information about medications and possible side effects. If a child is receiving ibuprofen, serum drug levels need to be monitored closely to establish therapeutic dosages, and observations for side effects such as gastrointestinal irritation are essential.

Children and adolescents with CF should receive routine primary care with special attention to diet, growth and development, and immunizations. Primary care providers should be alert to any weight loss or flattening in the growth curve associated with loss of appetite, which could indicate a pulmonary exacerbation in children with CF (McMullen & Bryson, 2004). In addition to all the recommended routine immunizations, CF patients should be immunized against influenza starting at age 6 months and followed by an annual booster (American Academy of Pediatrics, Committee on Infectious Diseases, 2009). Anticipatory guidance concerning issues of discipline, how to incorporate aspects of the treatment regimen into the school environment, and delayed pubertal development are also important considerations for the primary care provider.

Home palliative care for the child or adolescent with CF who is in the terminal stages may be carried out with the assistance of hospice (see Chapter 41).

The nurse can assist the family in contacting resources that provide help to families with affected children. Various special child health services, many local clinics, private agencies, service clubs, and other community groups often offer equipment and medications either free or at reduced rates. The Cystic Fibrosis Foundation* has chapters throughout the United States to provide education and services to families and professionals.

Family Support

The most challenging aspect of providing care for the family of a child or adolescent with CF is meeting the emotional needs of the child and family. The diagnosis, treatment, and prognosis for CF are often associated with many problems and frustrations. The diagnosis can evoke feelings of guilt and self-recrimination in parents.

The long-range problems for an infant, child, or adolescent with CF are those encountered in any chronic illness (see Chapter 41). Both the child and the family must make many adjustments, the success of which depends on their ability to cope and also on the quality and quantity of support they receive from outside sources. Combined efforts of a variety of health professionals are needed to provide the most comprehensive services to families. It is often the nurse who assesses the home situation, organizes and coordinates these services, and collects the data needed to evaluate the effectiveness of the services.

The persistent need for treatment several times a day places tremendous strain on the family. When the child is young, a family member must perform postural drainage and CPT. Children often balk at these treatments, and the parents are placed in the position of insisting on adherence. The stress and anxiety related to this routine may produce feelings of resentment in both the child and the family members. When possible, occasional trusted respite care should be available to allow parents to leave the situation for short periods without undue anxiety about the child's welfare.

The affected child or adolescent may become resentful about the disease, its relentless routine of therapy, and the necessary curtailment it places on activities and relationships. The child's activities are interrupted or built around treat-

---

**6931 Arlington Road, Bethesda, MD 20814-3205; 301-951-4422 or 800-FIGHT CF;* www.cff.org. *In Canada: Canadian Cystic Fibrosis Foundation, 2221 Yonge St., Suite 601, Toronto, Ontario M4S 2B4;* www.cysticfibrosis.ca. *Two excellent publications available from the Cystic Fibrosis Foundation are* What Everyone Should Know About Cystic Fibrosis, *and* Cystic Fibrosis: A Summary of Symptoms, Diagnosis, and Treatment. *For information about specialized medications, especially dornase alfa, and equipment for CF and other pulmonary diseases, contact Cystic Fibrosis Pharmacy, HHCS Health Group, 3901 E. Colonial Drive, Orlando, FL 32803; 800-741-4427;* www.cfpharmacy.com.

ments, medications, and diet. This imposes hardships and influences his or her quality of life. The child should be encouraged to attend school and join age-appropriate peer groups to foster a life that is as normal and productive as possible. Sports are often an important part of the child and adolescent's life; interaction with peers is a valuable life experience, especially to adolescents. The child or adolescent with CF should be encouraged to participate in sports activities as much as physical and pulmonary health allows. Exercise is encouraged to increase pulmonary vital capacity, promote muscle development, and enhance cardiovascular function.

As the disease progresses, however, family stress should be expected, and the patient may become angry and noncompliant. It is important for the nurse to recognize the family's changing needs and the grief they may experience as the CF worsens. Families should be made aware of sources for counseling. Patients need to be guided into activities that enable them to express anger, sorrow, and fear without guilt.

Transition to Adulthood

As life expectancy continues to rise for children and adolescents with CF, issues related to marriage, sexuality, childbearing, and career choice become more pressing. Males must be informed at some point that they will often be unable to produce offspring. It is important that the distinction be made between sterility and impotence. Normal sexual relationships can be expected. Female patients may be able to bear children but should be informed of the possible deleterious effects on the respiratory system created by the burden of pregnancy. They also need to know that their children will be carriers of the CF gene. Adolescent females may need counseling concerning the use of oral contraceptives and other contraceptive options (McMullen & Bryson, 2004).

Adolescents with CF are encouraged to take personal ownership and management of the illness to maximize their life's potential. Many adolescents and young persons with the illness enroll in college or vocational and technical training school and complete degrees by either distance learning or attending a local school. Young people are encouraged to set life goals and live normal lives to the extent their illness allows.

Life as an independent adult should be encouraged for children with CF. From the time that children can take partial responsibility for their own care (e.g., CPT and taking enzymes), independence and accountability should be fostered. Although the prognosis for these children has improved, many will need continued support as they cope with the demands of surviving with CF.

Anticipatory grieving and other aspects related to care of a child with a terminal illness are also part of nursing care. For example, it is important to prepare the child and family members for end-of-life decisions and care.

Obstructive Sleep-Disordered Breathing

Pediatric obstructive sleep-disordered breathing reportedly affects between 10% and 12% of children ages 2 to 8 years; obstructive sleep apnea may occur in as many as 2% of all children (Benninger & Walner, 2007b). Obstructive sleep-disordered breathing is said to form a continuum of sleep-disordered breathing ranging from partial obstruction of the upper airway to continuous episodes of complete upper airway obstruction, with the most severe form being *obstructive sleep apnea syndrome (OSAS)* (Benninger & Walner, 2007b). OSAS is defined by the American Thoracic Society (1996) as a disorder of breathing during sleep with prolonged partial upper airway obstruction and/or complete obstruction that disrupts normal respiration during sleep and normal sleep patterns. Common symptoms include nightly snoring, interrupted or disturbed sleep patterns, enuresis, and daytime neurobehavioral problems (American Academy of Pediatrics, 2002; Chan, Edman, & Koltai, 2004). OSAS is to be distinguished from primary snoring, which is snoring without obstructive apnea, frequent sleep arousals, or abnormalities in gas exchange (American Academy of Pediatrics, 2002). Interestingly, children with OSAS do not exhibit daytime sleepiness as do adults; the exception may be obese children (Chan, Edman, & Koltai, 2004). If left untreated, obstructive sleep-disordered breathing may result in complications such as growth failure, cor pulmonale, pulmonary hypertension, poor learning, behavioral problems, attention-deficit/hyperactivity disorder, and death.

The diagnosis of obstructive sleep-disordered breathing is made by a sleep study (polysomnography), which provides evidence of sleep disturbance, respiratory pauses, and changes in oxygenation. The six-channel polysomnography can be performed in children of all ages with videotaping or audiotaping, and abbreviated (vs. full-night sleep study) polysomnography may be useful; however, this latter method does not predict the severity of OSAS (American Academy of Pediatrics, 2002).

A common treatment for sleep-disordered breathing in children is adenotonsillectomy, provided there is evidence of adenotonsillar hypertrophy (Benninger & Walner, 2007b). Complications of these surgical interventions are discussed previously in this chapter. Continuous positive airway pressure (CPAP) and bilevel (cycles between high and low pressure) positive airway pressure (BiPAP) may be helpful in older children with sleep-disordered breathing whose condition persists after surgical intervention. CPAP is a long-term therapy with frequent assessments to evaluate the required amount of pressure and the overall effectiveness of the intervention.

Surgical interventions such as tracheotomy may be required for children with craniofacial syndromes such as Goldenhar, Pierre Robin, Apert, and Crouzon, in which there is partial or complete upper airway obstruction (Chan, Edman, & Koltai, 2004).

Nursing care of the child with sleep-disordered breathing involves early detection by observation of the infant's or child's sleep patterns and active participation in the diagnostic polysomnography. Important nursing roles are inserting the pH probe into the esophagus, ensuring accurate placement by radiography, and monitoring the sleep study and the patient's response to diagnostic therapy. Counseling families of children with sleep-disordered breathing may involve dietary counseling for exercise programs and weight management, use of the CPAP or BiPAP equipment, and direct postoperative care after the surgical intervention of tonsillectomy or adenoidectomy. The nurse can be instrumental in helping the child and family cope with the chronic illness diagnosis should intervention such as CPAP or BiPAP be required.

Respiratory Emergency

Respiratory Failure

In general, the term *respiratory insufficiency* is applied to two situations: (1) when there is increased work of breathing but gas exchange function is near normal, and (2) when normal blood gas tensions cannot be maintained and hypoxemia and acidosis develop secondary to carbon dioxide retention.

Respiratory failure is defined as the inability of the respiratory apparatus to maintain adequate oxygenation of the blood, with or without carbon dioxide retention. This process involves pulmonary dysfunction that generally results in impaired alveolar gas exchange, which can lead to hypoxemia or hypercapnia. Respiratory failure is the most common cause of cardiopulmonary arrest in children (Rotta & Wiryawan, 2003). *Respiratory arrest* is the cessation of respiration. *Apnea* is the cessation of breathing for more than 20 seconds or for a shorter period when associated with hypoxemia or bradycardia (Curley & Moloney-Harmon, 2001). Apnea can be (1) central, in which respiratory efforts are absent; (2) obstructive, in which respiratory efforts are present; and (3) mixed, in which both central and obstructive components are present.

Effective pulmonary gas exchange requires clear airways, normal lungs and chest wall, and adequate pulmonary circulation. Anything that affects these functions or their relationships can compromise respiration.

evolve Animation—Respiratory Failure, Infant

Diagnostic Evaluation

Respiratory dysfunction may have an abrupt or an insidious onset. Respiratory failure can occur as an emergency situation or may be preceded by gradual and progressive deterioration of respiratory function. Most clinical manifestations are nonspecific and are affected by variations among individual patients and differences in the severity and duration of inadequate gas exchange.

The diagnosis of respiratory failure is determined by the combined application of three sources of information:

1. Presence or history of a condition that might predispose the patient to respiratory failure
2. Observation of respiratory failure
3. Measurement of arterial blood gases (ABGs) and pH

Nursing observation and judgment are vital to the recognition and early management of respiratory failure. Nurses must be able to assess a situation and initiate appropriate action within moments. Signs of respiratory failure are listed in Box 46-18.

Therapeutic Management

The interventions used in the management of respiratory failure are often dramatic, requiring special skills and emergency procedures. If respiratory arrest occurs, the primary objectives are to recognize the situation and immediately initiate resuscitative measures such as airway positioning, administration of oxygen, cardiopulmonary resuscitation (CPR), suctioning, or intubation. When the situation is not an arrest, the suspicion of respiratory failure is confirmed by assessment; the severity may be defined by ABG analysis. Interventions such as administering supplemental oxygen, positioning, stimulation, suctioning, providing positive pressure ventilation by bag and mask, and early intubation may avert an arrest. When severity is established, an attempt is made to determine the underlying cause by thorough evaluation.

BOX 46-18 Clinical Manifestations of Respiratory Failure

Cardinal Signs

Restlessness
Tachypnea
Tachycardia
Diaphoresis

Early but Less Obvious Signs

Mood changes such as euphoria or depression
Headache
Altered depth and pattern of respirations
Hypertension
Exertional dyspnea
Anorexia
Increased cardiac output and renal output
Central nervous system symptoms (decreased efficiency, impaired judgment, anxiety, confusion, restlessness, irritability, depressed level of consciousness)
Flaring nares
Chest wall retractions
Expiratory grunt
Wheezing or prolonged expiration

Signs of More Severe Hypoxia

Hypotension or hypertension
Dimness of vision
Somnolence
Stupor
Coma
Dyspnea
Depressed respirations
Bradycardia
Cyanosis, peripheral or central

Treatment of respiratory dysfunction involves both specific and nonspecific therapy. Specific therapies are directed toward reversal of the causative factors. However, nonspecific measures are needed to maintain adequate oxygenation and enhance carbon dioxide removal until specific methods take effect. The major reasons for implementing nonspecific treatments are (1) unknown etiology, (2) lack of specific treatment for a known cause, (3) lack of time for a specific treatment to take effect, and (4) need for specialized personnel or equipment for specific treatment.

The principles of management are to (1) maintain ventilation and maximize oxygen delivery, (2) correct hypoxemia and hypercapnia, (3) treat the underlying cause, (4) minimize extrapulmonary organ failure, (5) apply specific and nonspecific therapy to control oxygen demands, and (6) anticipate complications. Monitoring the patient's condition is critical.

Nursing Care Management

For families whose child has a respiratory arrest, support is aimed at keeping the family informed of the child's status and helping them cope with a near-death experience or an actual death (see Chapter 41). Knowing that their child requires CPR is a frightening and often overwhelming experience for parents. Uncertainty regarding the outcome—both mortality and morbidity—is a primary concern. Traditionally family members are not allowed to be present during resuscitation efforts in the emergency department. However, studies indicate that family presence during emergencies alleviates the family's anger about being separated from the patient during a crisis, reduces their anxiety, eliminates doubts about what was done to help the patient, and facilitates the grieving process when the patient dies (Mangurten et al, 2006).

Regardless of whether an institution permits parental presence during CPR, nurses must consider the needs, fears, and concerns of family members during an arrest situation. If family presence is not permitted, nurses should arrange for someone to remain with the family during the code. After the child's recovery or death, the family will continue to need support and thorough medical information regarding lifesaving measures, the prognosis if the child survives, and the cause of death if the child dies.

Cardiopulmonary Resuscitation

Cardiac arrest in children is less often of cardiac origin than from prolonged hypoxemia secondary to inadequate oxygenation, ventilation, and circulation (shock). Some causes of cardiac arrest include injuries, suffocation (e.g., FB aspiration), smoke inhalation, or infection. In small infants the small size of the airway may easily be compromised by improper positioning with the chin resting on the chest; this can easily be remedied by positioning the infant with the chin elevated (but not hyperextended) so the airway is open. This is common in infants who are not positioned properly in an infant seat or car restraint seat. Respiratory arrest is associated with a better survival rate than cardiac arrest. After cardiac arrest occurs, the outcome of resuscitative efforts is poor.

Complete apnea signals the need for rapid, vigorous action to prevent cardiac arrest. In such situations nurses must initiate action immediately. In the hospital emergency equipment must be available and easily accessible in all patient care areas. The status of emergency equipment must be checked at least once daily. Regardless of the cause of the arrest, basic procedures are carried out and modified somewhat according to the child's size.

Optimally, mouth-to-mouth resuscitation should be performed with a barrier device or mask with a one-way valve to prevent infection transmission in both the victim and rescuer. When CPR is anticipated in the workplace or other out-of-hospital settings, rescuers should have access to these devices.

Outside of the hospital the first action in an emergency is to quickly assess the extent of any injury and determine whether the child is unconscious. A child who is struggling to breathe but conscious should be transported immediately to an *advanced life support (ALS)* facility, with the child maintaining whatever position affords the most comfort. Attempting to transport a child by automobile wastes valuable time in obtaining help. Transportation by an *emergency medical service (EMS)* is recommended. Services in most large communities can institute ALS immediately or en route to a medical facility.

An unconscious child is managed with care to prevent additional trauma if a head or spinal cord injury has been sustained (see Spinal Cord Injuries, Chapter 55). The circumstances in which the child is found offer clues to a possible injury. For example, a child who has been thrown from a bicycle or fallen from a tree is more likely to sustain trauma than a child who is discovered in bed.

Resuscitation Procedure

The American Heart Association (2005) implemented several changes in CPR guidelines that incorporate the use of the automatic external defibrillator (AED) as part of the treatment of cardiorespiratory arrest in children 1 year of age and older. The 2005 guidelines state that AEDs can be safely and effectively used in children ages 1 to 8 years; however, there are insufficient data to support or refute the use of AEDs in children younger than 1 year old. Appropriate-sized pediatric pads must be used for small children. Health care providers are advised to give children 1 year and older a defibrillatory shock after providing approximately five cycles of CPR (approximately 2 minutes) of cycles of 30 compressions and two ventilations by the lone rescuer), provided the AED is sensitive to pediatric rhythms, the device is capable of delivering a pediatric dosage of 2 joules/kg, and a shockable rhythm (usually ventricular fibrillation) is present. In a hospital situation, where weight-based defibrillation dosing is possible, manual defibrillation is the mode of choice instead of AED (Samson et al, 2003). When using an AED, health care providers are advised to give adults and children older than 8 years a defibrillatory shock within 5 minutes of collapse outside the hospital and within 3 minutes in the hospital.

Changes in resuscitation procedure for the lay rescuer are discussed in the text. The sequence of CPR steps for the health care provider is discussed in both the text and Fig. 46-10.

If two rescuers are present, one rescuer should begin CPR while the second rescuer activates the EMS system by calling 911 and obtaining an AED. Pediatric rescuers provide five cycles of basic life support (approximately 2 minutes) before activating EMS; each cycle consists of 30 chest compressions and two ventilations. Because pediatric arrests are most commonly caused by respiratory arrest, maintaining ventilation is primary.

Open the Airway

For effective CPR the victim is placed on the back on a firm, flat surface, using appropriate precautions. With loss of consciousness the tongue, which is attached to the lower jaw, relaxes and falls back, obstructing the airway. To open the airway, the head is positioned with a head tilt–chin lift maneuver by the lay rescuer. Health professionals should open the airway using either a head tilt–chin lift or jaw thrust maneuver. A head tilt is accomplished by placing one hand on the victim's forehead and applying firm, backward pressure with the palm to tilt the head back. The fingers of the free hand are placed under the bony portion of the lower jaw near the chin to lift and bring the chin forward (chin lift). This supports the jaw and helps tilt the head back (Fig. 46-11).

evolve Nursing Care Plan—The Child with Respiratory Failure

Maneuver	**Adult** **Lay rescuer:** ≥8 yr **HCP:** Adolescent and older	**Child** **Lay rescuer:** 1–8 yr **HCP:** 1 yr to adolescence	**Infant** <1 yr of age
Activate Emergency response Number (1 rescuer)	Activate when victim found unresponsive. **HCP:** If asphyxial arrest likely, call after 5 cycles (2 min) of CPR.	Activate after performing 5 cycles of CPR. For sudden, witnessed collapse, activate after verifying that victim unresponsive.	
Airway	Head tilt–chin lift (**HCP: suspected trauma, use jaw thrust**)		
Breaths Initial	2 breaths at 1 sec/breath	2 effective breaths at 1 sec/breath	
HCP: Rescue breathing without chest compressions	10-12 breaths/min (approximately 1 breath every 5-6 sec)	12-20 breaths/min (approximately 1 breath every 3-5 sec)	
HCP: Rescue breaths for CPR with advanced airway	8-10 breaths/min (approximately 1 breath every 6-8 sec)		
Foreign-body airway obstruction	Abdominal thrusts		Back blows and chest thrusts
Circulation **HCP:** Pulse check (≤10 sec)	Carotid (**HCP** can use femoral in child)		Brachial or femoral
Compression landmarks	Center of chest, between nipples		Just below nipple line
Compression method Push hard and fast Allow complete recoil	**2 Hands:** Heel of 1 hand, other hand on top	**2 Hands:** Heel of 1 hand with second on top *or* **1 Hand:** Heel of 1 hand only	**1 Rescuer:** 2 fingers **HCP, 2 rescuers:** 2 thumb-encircling hands
Compression depth	1½-2 inches	Approximately 1/3-1/2 the depth of the chest	
Compression rate	Approximately 100/min		
Compression-ventilation ratio	30:2 (1 or 2 rescuers)	30:2 (1 rescuer) **HCP:** 15:2 (2 rescuers)	
Defibrillation (AED)	Use adult pads. Do not use child pads/child system. **HCP:** For out-of-hospital response, may provide 5 cycles/2 min of CPR before shock if response >4-5 min and arrest not witnessed.	**HCP:** Use AED as soon as available for sudden collapse and in-hospital. **All:** Use after 5 cycles of CPR (out-of-hospital). If available, use child pads/child system for child 1-8 yr. If pads/system not available, use adult AED pads.	No recommendation for infants <1 yr of age.

Fig. 46-10 Summary of basic life support maneuvers for infants, children, and adults (newborn-neonatal information not included). *CPR,* Cardiopulmonary resuscitation; *HCP,* maneuvers used only by health care provider; *AED,* automated external defibrillator. (From American Heart Association: 2005 American Heart Association guidelines for cardiopulmonary resuscitation and emergency cardiovascular care, *Circulation* 112(24 Suppl 1):IV-166, 2005.)

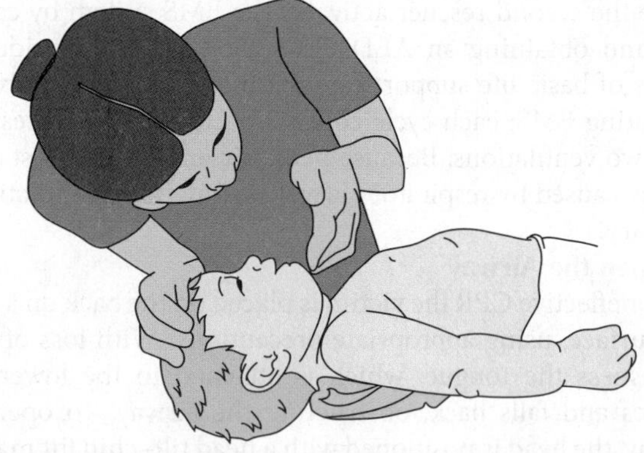

Fig. 46-11 Open airway using the head tilt–chin lift maneuver, and check breathing.

evolve Animation—Bag Ventilation

The jaw thrust is accomplished by grasping the angles of the victim's lower jaw and lifting with both hands, one on each side, displacing the mandible upward and outward. *The jaw thrust is recommended for use only by health care workers.* In suspected neck injuries the jaw thrust method should be used while the cervical spine is completely immobilized. After a patent airway has been restored by removal of foreign material and secretions (if indicated) and if the child is not breathing, maintenance of the airway is continued, and rescue breathing is initiated.

Give Breaths

To ventilate the lungs in the infant (from birth to 1 year of age), the bag-valve mask or operator's mouth is placed in such a way that both the mouth and the nostrils are covered (Fig. 46-12). Children (over 1 year of age) are ventilated through the mouth while the nostrils are firmly pinched for airtight contact.

The volume of air in an infant's lungs is small, and the air passages are considerably smaller, with resistance to flow potentially higher than in adults. The rescuer should deliver small puffs of air and assess the rise of the chest to ensure that overinflation does not occur. A gentle rise of the chest is a sufficient indicator of adequate inflation.

The correct volume for each breath is the volume that causes the chest to rise. If air enters freely and the chest rises, the airway is assumed to be clear. Breaths should be given slowly with sufficient volume to make the chest rise.

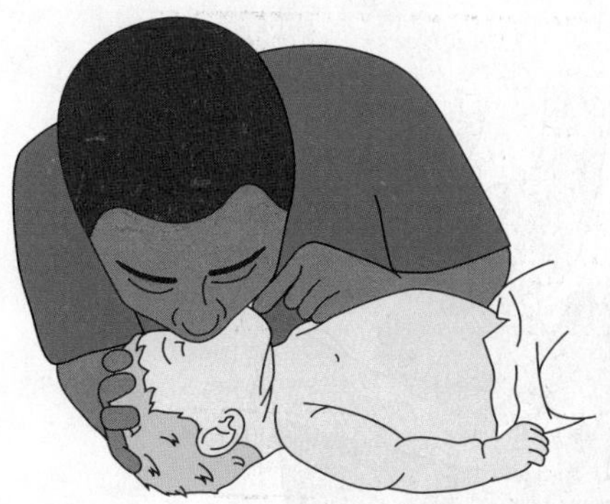

Fig. 46-12 Mouth-to-mouth and nose breathing for infant.

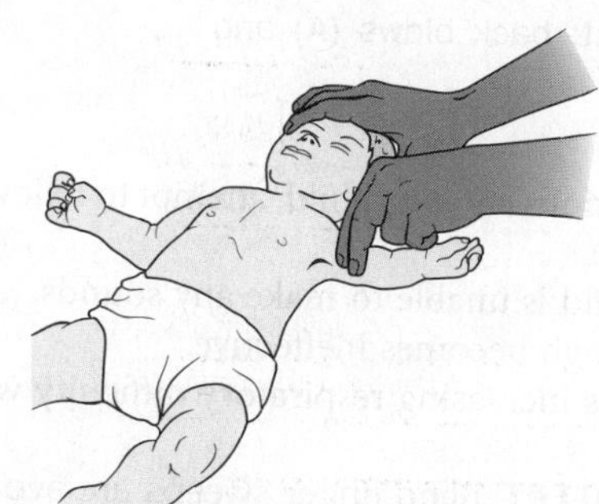

Fig. 46-13 Locating brachial pulse in infant.

Check Pulse

After an initial two breaths, the health care provider palpates the pulse to ascertain the presence of a heartbeat. The carotid is the most central and accessible artery in children over 1 year of age. However, the infant's short and often fat neck makes the carotid pulse difficult to palpate. Therefore in the infant it is preferable to use the brachial pulse, located on the inner side of the upper arm midway between the elbow and the shoulder (Fig. 46-13). Absence of a carotid or brachial pulse is considered sufficient indication to begin external cardiac massage. *Lay rescuers are not taught to check the pulse but are taught to look for signs of circulation (e.g., normal breathing, coughing, or air movement) in response to rescue breaths.*

Perform Chest Compression

External chest compression consists of serial, rhythmic compressions of the chest to maintain circulation to vital organs until the child achieves spontaneous vital signs or ALS can be provided. *Chest compressions are always interspersed with ventilation of the lungs.* For optimal compressions it is essential that the child's spine be supported on a firm surface during compressions of the sternum and that sternal pressure is forceful but not traumatic. For a small infant the hard surface can be the rescuer's hand or forearm, with the palm supporting the infant's back. The child's head is positioned for optimal airway opening using the head tilt–chin lift maneuver. It is essential to prevent overextension of the head of small infants because this tends to close the flexible trachea.

The placement of the fingers for compression in infants is at a point on the lower sternum just below the intersection of the sternum and an imaginary line drawn between the nipples (Fig. 46-14). Compressions on the child 1 to 8 years of age are

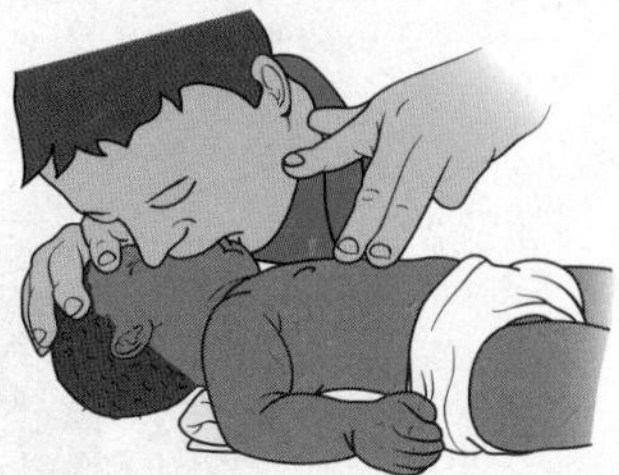

Fig. 46-14 Combining chest compressions with breathing in infant.

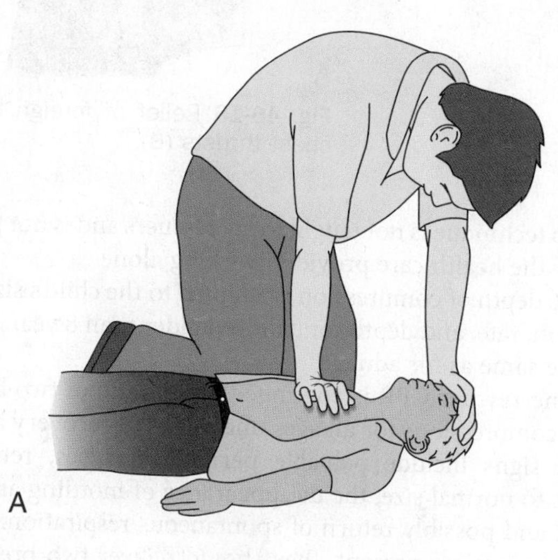

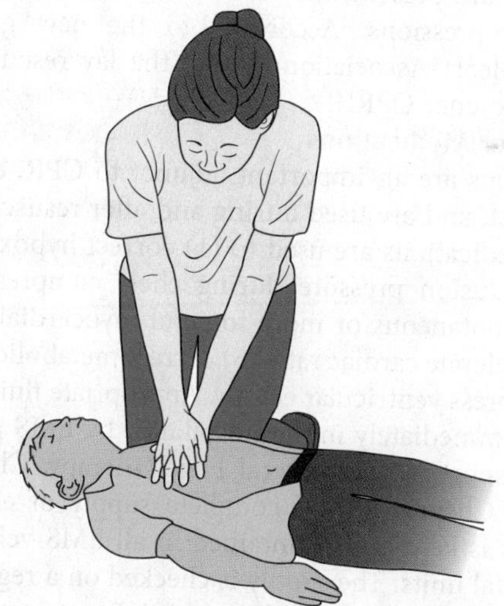

Fig. 46-15 Chest compressions in child: one hand for smaller child (A) and two hands for larger child (B).

applied to the lower half of the sternum (Fig. 46-15). Sternal compression to infants is applied with two fingers on the sternum, exerting a firm downward thrust; chest compression for children is applied with the heel of one hand or two hands, depending on the child's size. Current American Heart Association (2005) guidelines include the addition of the two-thumb technique for chest compressions for infants when two health care providers are present. In the two-thumb technique, one of the two rescuers places both thumbs side by side over the lower half of the infant's sternum; the remaining fingers encircle the infant's chest and support the back. The two-

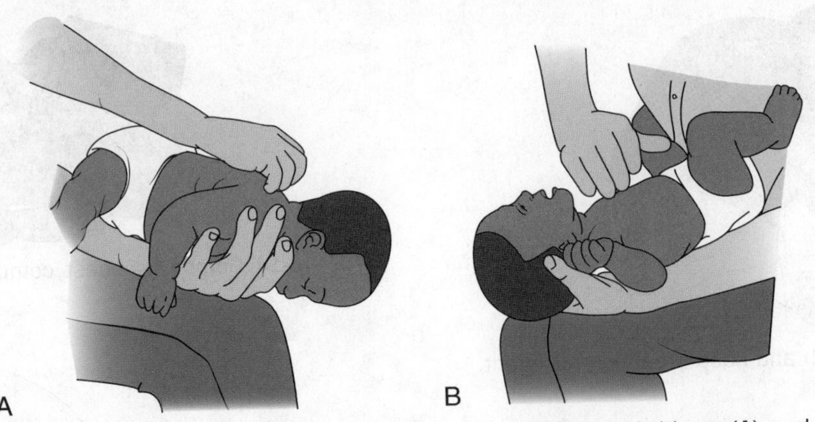

Fig. 46-16 Relief of foreign body obstruction in infant: back blows **(A)** and chest thrusts **(B)**.

thumb technique is not taught to lay rescuers and is not practical for the health care provider working alone.

The depth of compression is adapted to the child's size. The location, rate, and depth for children older than 8 years of age are the same as for adults.

Lone-rescuer CPR is continued at the ratio of two breaths to 30 compressions for all ages until signs of recovery appear. These signs include palpable peripheral pulses, return of pupils to normal size, the disappearance of mottling and cyanosis, and possibly return of spontaneous respiration. When two rescuers are present, they should deliver two breaths to each 15 compressions. According to the new guidelines (American Heart Association, 2005), the lay rescuer is not taught two-rescuer CPR.

Administer Medications

Medications are an important adjunct to CPR, especially cardiac arrest, and are used during and after resuscitation in children. Medications are used to (1) correct hypoxemia, (2) increase perfusion pressure during chest compression, (3) stimulate spontaneous or more forceful myocardial contraction, (4) accelerate cardiac rate, (5) correct metabolic acidosis, and (6) suppress ventricular ectopy. Appropriate fluid therapy is initiated immediately in the hospital or by EMS personnel during transport (see Parenteral Fluid Therapy, Chapter 45, and Shock, Chapter 48). A complete supply of emergency medications is kept and maintained in all EMS vehicles and on all hospital units. The supply is checked on a regular basis (usually once on each 8- or 12-hour shift). Resuscitation medications are listed in Table 46-3.

When administering drugs during CPR (or a "code"), use a saline flush between medications to prevent drug interactions. Document all drugs, dosages, and the time and route of administration.

Airway Obstruction

Attempts at clearing the airway should be considered for (1) children in whom aspiration of an FB is witnessed or strongly suspected and (2) unconscious, nonbreathing children whose airways remain obstructed despite the usual maneuvers to open them. When aspiration is strongly suspected, the child is encouraged to continue coughing as long as the cough remains forceful.

In a conscious choking child, attempt to relieve the obstruction only if:

- The child is unable to make any sounds.
- The cough becomes ineffective.
- There is increasing respiratory difficulty with stridor.

NURSING ALERT Blind finger sweeps are avoided in infants and children under 8 years old.

Infants

A combination of *back blows* (over the spine between the shoulder blades) and *chest thrusts* (on the sternum, same location as for chest compressions) is recommended to relieve the FB obstruction in infants (Fig. 46-16). A choking infant is placed face down over the rescuer's arm with the head supported and lower than the trunk. For additional support the rescuer should support the arm firmly against the thigh. Up to five quick, sharp, back blows are delivered between the infant's shoulder blades with the heel of the rescuer's hand. Less force is required than would be applied to an adult. After delivery of the back blows, the rescuer's free hand is placed flat on the infant's back so that the infant is "sandwiched" between the two hands, making certain the neck and chin are well supported. While the rescuer maintains support with the infant's head lower than the trunk, the infant is turned and placed supine on the rescuer's thigh, where up to five quick downward chest thrusts are applied in rapid succession in the same location as external chest compressions described for CPR. Back blows and chest thrusts are continued until the object is removed or the infant becomes unconscious.

Children

A series of *subdiaphragmatic abdominal thrusts (Heimlich maneuver)* is recommended for children older than 1 year of age. The maneuver creates an artificial cough that forces air, and with it the FB, out of the airway. The procedure is carried out with the child in a standing, sitting, or lying position (Fig. 46-17). In the conscious choking child, upward thrusts are delivered to the upper abdomen with the fisted hand at a point just below the rib cage. To prevent damage to the internal organs, the rescuer's hands should not touch the xiphoid process of the sternum or the lower margins of the ribs. Up to

Table 46-3 Drugs for Pediatric Cardiopulmonary Resuscitation

DRUG AND DOSAGE	ACTION	IMPLICATION
Epinephrine HCl* IV/IO–0.01 mg/kg/dose (1:10,000) ET–0.1 mg/kg/dose (1:1000) Repeat doses–0.1 ml/kg (1:1000)	Adrenergic Acts on both α- and β-receptor sites, especially heart and vascular and other smooth muscle	Most useful drug in cardiac arrest Disappears rapidly from bloodstream after injection; instill 5 ml saline after ET administration May produce renal vessel constriction and decreased urine formation
Sodium bicarbonate IV/IO–1 mEq/kg/dose Newborn–0.5 mEq/ml (4.2%)	Alkalinizer Buffers pH	Infuse slowly and only when ventilation is adequate; flush with saline before and after administration Do not mix with catecholamines or calcium
Atropine sulfate* 0.02 mg/kg/dose Minimum dose–0.1 mg Maximum single dose–infants and children, 0.5 mg; adolescents, 1 mg	Anticholinergic-parasympatholytic Increases cardiac output, heart rate by blocking vagal stimulation in heart	Used to treat bradycardia after ventilatory assessment Always provide adequate ventilation and monitor oxygen saturation Produces pupillary dilation, which constricts with light
Calcium chloride 10% 20 mg/kg IV 0.2 mg/kg/dose q10min	Electrolyte replacement Needed for maintenance of normal cardiac contractility	Used only for hypocalcemia, calcium blocker overdose, hyperkalemia, or hypermagnesemia Administer slowly; very sclerosing; administer in central vein Incompatible with phosphate solutions
Lidocaine HCl* 1 mg/kg/dose	Antidysrhythmic agent Inhibits nerve impulses from sensory nerves	Used for ventricular arrhythmias only
Amiodarone IV–5 mg/kg over 30 min followed by continuous infusion Starting at 5 mcg/kg/min May increase to maximum 10 mcg/kg/min	Antidysrhythmic agent Inhibits adrenergic stimulation; prolongs action potential and refractory period in myocardial tissues; decreases AV conduction and sinus node function	Recommended as first choice for shock-refractory ventricular tachycardia Contraindicated in severe sinus node dysfunction, marked sinus bradycardia, second- and third-degree AV block Monitor electrocardiogram and blood pressure
Adenosine 0.1-0.2 mg/kg as a rapid IV bolus Maximum single initial dose–6-12 mg (given over 1-2 sec) May repeat administration–double initial dose (maximum dose = 12 mg) Follow with ≥5 ml normal saline flush	Antidysrhythmic, for supraventricular tachycardia Causes temporary block through AV node and interrupts reentry circuits	Administer by rapid IV push followed by saline flush May cause transient bradycardia
Naloxone (Narcan)* 0.1 mg/kg/dose† May repeat q2-3min	Reverses respiratory arrest caused by excessive opiate administration	Evaluate level of pain after administration because analgesic effects of opioids are reversed with large doses of naloxone
Magnesium 25-50 mg/kg/dose Maximum–2 g	Inhibits calcium channels and causes smooth muscle relaxation	Given by rapid IV infusion for suspected hypomagnesemia Have calcium gluconate (IV) available as antidote
Infusions		
Epinephrine HCl infusion 0.05 mcg/kg/min	Adrenergic See above	Titrated to desired hemodynamic effect
Dopamine HCl infusion 2 mcg/kg/min	Agonist Acts on α-receptors, causing vasoconstriction Increases cardiac output	Titrated to desired hemodynamic response
Dobutamine HCl infusion 2 mcg/kg/min	Adrenergic direct-acting β_2-agonist Increases contractility and heart rate	Titrated to desired hemodynamic response Little vasoconstriction, even at high rates
Lidocaine HCl infusion 20-50 mcg/kg/min	Antidysrhythmic Increases electrical stimulation threshold of ventricle	See above Lower infusion dose used in shock

AV, Atrioventricular; *ET*, endotracheal tube; *HCl*, hydrochloride; *IO*, intraosseous; *IV*, intravenous.
*These drugs may be administered via ET tube if IV is not available.
†Dose of naloxone to reverse respiratory depression without reversing analgesia from opioids is 0.5 mcg/kg in children <40 kg (88 lb) (American Pain Society, 1999).

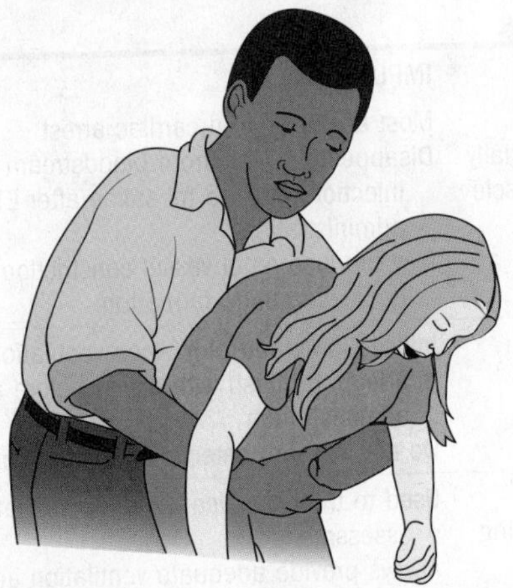

Fig. 46-17 Abdominal thrusts in standing child for relief of foreign body obstruction.

five thrusts are repeated in rapid succession until the FB is expelled.

It is neither necessary nor desirable to squeeze or compress the arms during the procedure. It is not a punch or a bear hug. The child may vomit after relief of the obstruction and should be positioned to prevent aspiration. After breathing is restored, the child should receive medical attention and be assessed for complications.

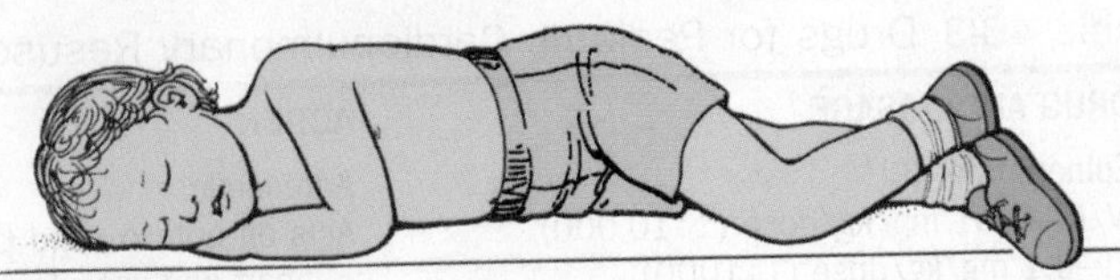

Fig. 46-18 Recovery position for child after respiratory emergency.

The success of the technique is primarily a result of the obstruction occurring at the end of a maximum respiration. The victim is most likely to choke on food during inspiration; therefore the tidal volume plus expiratory reserve volume is present in the lungs. When pressure is exerted on the diaphragm by the maneuver, the food bolus is ejected with considerable force by this trapped air.

If the victim is breathing or resumes effective breathing after emergency interventions, place in the recovery position: move the head, shoulders, and torso simultaneously and turn onto the side. The leg not in contact with the ground may be bent and the knee moved forward to stabilize the victim (Fig. 46-18). The victim should not be moved in any way if trauma is suspected and should not be placed in the recovery position if rescue breathing or CPR is required.

Key Points

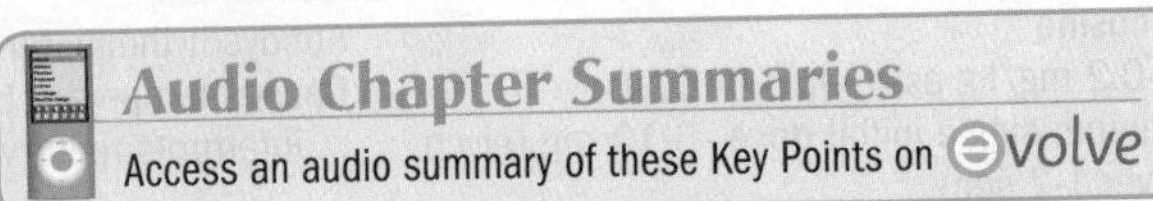
Audio Chapter Summaries
Access an audio summary of these Key Points on evolve

- Acute infection of the respiratory tract is the most common cause of illness in infancy and childhood.
- The incidence and severity of respiratory tract infections are influenced by the infectious agents involved, the child's age, and the child's natural defenses.
- Common respiratory tract infections of childhood include nasopharyngitis, pharyngitis (including tonsillitis), influenza, infectious mononucleosis, and OM.
- Croup syndromes involve acute inflammation and variable degrees of obstruction of the epiglottis, larynx, or trachea.
- The primary goals in the care of children with croup are observation for signs of respiratory distress and relief of laryngeal inflammation.
- Common infections of the lower airways are bacterial tracheitis, bronchitis, and RSV-bronchiolitis.
- Pneumonias are classified according to site (lobar, bronchial, or interstitial) or by etiologic agent (viral, bacterial, mycoplasmal), or are associated with aspiration of foreign material.
- In TB, susceptibility to the bacillus can be influenced by heredity, age, stress, poor nutrition, and intercurrent infection.
- Second-hand smoke exposure is a major environmental pollutant contributing to respiratory illness in children.
- Asthma is the leading cause of chronic illness in children.
- General therapeutic management of asthma includes assessment of asthma severity, allergen control, drug therapy, symptom management, and sometimes hyposensitization.
- Support for the family of the child with asthma includes education about the disease and its therapy and facilitation of self-management.
- CF is the most common inherited disease in children.
- The diagnosis of CF is based on newborn screening finding of elevated IRT, DNA analysis showing a CFTR mutation, and a positive sweat chloride test (increased sweat electrolyte content).
- Choking and respiratory failure are respiratory emergencies that require immediate intervention.
- Abdominal thrusts are used in children in whom FB obstruction is witnessed or strongly suspected. A combination of back blows and chest thrusts is used for infants with FB obstruction.
- In a conscious choking child, attempts to relieve the obstruction are used only if the child is unable to make any sounds, the cough becomes ineffective, or the child has increasing respiratory difficulty with stridor.

References

American Academy of Otolaryngology–Head and Neck Surgery: 2000 Clinical indicators compendium, *Bulletin* 19:6, 2000.

American Academy of Pediatrics: *Pediatric nutrition handbook*, ed 6, Elk grove Village, Ill, 2009, The Academy.

American Academy of Pediatrics: Clinical practice guideline: diagnosis and management of bronchiolitis, *Pediatrics* 118(4):1774-1793, 2006.

American Academy of Pediatrics: Clinical practice guidelines: diagnosis and management of acute otitis media, *Pediatrics* 113(5):1451-1465, 2004a.

American Academy of Pediatrics: Clinical practice guidelines: otitis media with effusion, *Pediatrics* 113(5):1412-1429, 2004b.

American Academy of Pediatrics: Clinical practice guideline: diagnosis and management of childhood obstructive sleep apnea syndrome, *Pediatrics* 109(4):704-712, 2002.

American Academy of Pediatrics, Committee on Infectious Diseases: Recommended immunization schedules for children and adolescents—United States, 2008, *Pediatrics* 121(1):219-220, 2008.

American Academy of Pediatrics, Committee on Infectious Diseases, Pickering L, editor: *Red book: 2009 report of the Committee on Infectious Diseases*, ed 28, Elk Grove Village, Ill, 2009, The Academy.

American Academy of Pediatrics, Task Force on Sudden Infant Death Syndrome: The changing concept of sudden infant death syndrome: diagnostic coding shifts, controversies regarding the sleeping environment, and new variables to consider in reducing risk, *Pediatrics* 116(5):1245-1255, 2005.

American Heart Association: 2005 American Heart Association guidelines for cardiopulmonary resuscitation and emergency cardiovascular care, *Circulation* 112(24 Suppl 1):IV-166, 2005.

American Pain Society: *Principles of analgesic use in the treatment of acute pain and chronic cancer pain*, ed 3, Glenview, Ill, 1999, The Society.

American Thoracic Society: Standards and indications for cardiopulmonary sleep studies in children, *Am J Respir Crit Care Med* 153(2):866-878, 1996.

Balinsky W, Zhu CW: Pediatric cystic fibrosis: evaluating costs and genetic testing, *J Pediatr Health Care* 18:30-34, 2004.

Benninger M, Walner D: Coblation: improving outcomes for children following adenotonsillectomy, *Clin Cornerstone* 9(Suppl 1):S13-S23, 2007a.

Benninger M, Walner D: Obstructive sleep-disordered breathing in children, *Clin Cornerstone* 9(Suppl 1):S006-SS12, 2007b.

Bhetwal N, McConaghy JR: The evaluation and treatment of children with acute otitis media, *Prim Care* 34(1):59-70, 2007.

Blitz M et al: Inhaled magnesium sulfate in the treatment of acute asthma, *Cochrane Database Syst Rev* 20(3):CD003898, 2005.

Boat TF, Acton JD: Cystic fibrosis. In Kliegman RM et al (editors): *Nelson textbook of pediatrics*, ed 18, Philadelphia, 2007, Saunders.

Borowitz D, Baker RD, Stallings V: Consensus report on nutrition for pediatric patients with cystic fibrosis, *J Pediatr Gastroenterol Nutr* 35(3): 246-259, 2002.

Burkhart PV et al: Improved health outcomes with peak flow monitoring for children with asthma, *J Asthma* 44(2):137-142, 2007.

Centers for Disease Control and Prevention: Newborn screening for cystic fibrosis, *MMWR Recomm Rep* 53(RR13):1-36, 2004a.

Centers for Disease Control and Prevention: Severe acute respiratory syndrome. Supplement I: Infection control in healthcare, home, and community setting, January 8, 2004b. Available at www.cdc.gov/ncidod/sars/guidance/I/index.htm (accessed August 2, 2008).

Chan J, Edman JC, Koltai PJ: Obstructive sleep apnea in children, *Am Fam Physician* 69(5):1147-1154, 1159-1160, 2004.

Chávez-Bueno S et al: Respiratory syncytial virus: old challenges and new approaches, *Pediatr Ann* 34(1):62-68, 2005.

Chokephaibulkit K: Q&A: avian influenza virus infection of children in Vietnam and Thailand, *Pediatr Infect Dis J* 23(8):793-794, 2004.

Courtney AU, McCarter DF, Pollart SM: Childhood asthma: treatment update, *Am Fam Physician* 71(10): 1959-1968, 2005.

Curley MA, Moloney-Harmon PA: *Critical care nursing of infants and children*, Philadelphia, 2001, Saunders.

Cystic Fibrosis Foundation: *CFF Patient Registry: annual data report 2007*, Bethesda, Md, 2007, The Foundation.

Denison MR: Severe acute respiratory syndrome coronavirus pathogenesis, disease and vaccines: an update, *Pediatr Infect Dis J* 23(Suppl 11): S207-S214, 2005.

DeVincenzo J: Passive antibody prophylaxis for RSV, *Pediatr Infect Dis J* 27(1):69-70, 2008.

Farrell PM et al: Evidence on improved outcomes with early diagnosis of cystic fibrosis through neonatal screening: enough is enough! *J Pediatr* 147(Suppl 3):S30-S36, 2007.

Flori HR et al: Pediatric acute lung injury, *Am J Respir Crit Care Med* 171(9):995-1001, 2005.

Frankel LR, DiCarlo JV: Acute (adult) respiratory distress syndrome (ARDS). In Behrman RE, Kliegman RM, Jenson HB, editors: *Nelson textbook of pediatrics*, ed 17, Philadelphia, 2004, Saunders.

Frye AD: Acute lung injury and acute respiratory distress syndrome in the pediatric patient, *Crit Care Nurs Clin North Am* 17(4):311-318, 2005.

Gerber MA: Diagnosis and treatment of pharyngitis in children, *Pediatr Clin North Am* 52(3):729-747, 2005.

Goldstein NA et al: Water precautions and tympanostomy tubes: a randomized, controlled trial, *Laryngoscope* 115(2):324-330, 2005.

Hanson JH, Flori H: Application of the acute respiratory distress syndrome network low-tidal volume strategy to pediatric acute lung injury, *Respir Care Clin N Am* 12(3):349-357, 2006.

Hardin DS et al: Growth hormone treatment enhances nutrition and growth in children with cystic fibrosis receiving enteral nutrition, *J Pediatr* 146(3):324-328, 2005.

Hopkins A et al: Changing epidemiology of life-threatening upper airway infections: the reemergence of bacterial tracheitis, *Pediatrics* 118(4):1418-1421, 2006.

Kao LW, Nañagas KA: Carbon monoxide poisoning, *Emerg Med Clin North Am* 22(4):985-1018, 2004.

Kershner JE: Otitis media. In Kliegman RM et al (editors): *Nelson textbook of pediatrics*, ed 18, Philadelphia, 2007, Saunders.

Lee PJ, Krilov LR: When animal viruses attack: SARS and avian influenza, *Pediatr Ann* 34(1):43-52, 2005.

Li YF et al: Maternal and grand maternal smoking patterns are associated with early childhood asthma, *Chest* 127(4):1232-1241, 2005.

Linzer JF: Review of asthma: pathophysiology and current treatment options, *Clin Pediatr Emerg Med* 8(2):87-95, 2007.

Liu AH et al: Childhood asthma. In Kliegman RM et al (editors): *Nelson textbook of pediatrics*, ed 18, Philadelphia, 2007, Saunders.

Mangurten J et al: Effects of family presence during resuscitation and invasive procedures in a pediatric emergency department, *J Emerg Nurs* 32(3):225-233, 2006.

Matthay MA et al: Future research directions in acute lung injury NHLBI summary, *Am J Respir Crit Care Med* 167(7):1027-1035, 2003.

McMullen AH, Bryson EA: Cystic fibrosis. In Jackson PL, Vessey JA (editors): *Primary care of the child with a chronic condition*, ed 4, St Louis, 2004, Mosby.

Mintz M: Asthma update, part II, Medical management, *Am Fam Physician* 70(6):1061-1066, 2004.

Moore M, Little P: Humidified air inhalation for treating croup, *Cochrane Database Syst Rev* 19(3): CD002870, 2006.

National Asthma Education and Prevention Program: Guidelines for the diagnosis and management of asthma, August 2007. Available at www.nhlbi.nih.gov/guidelines/asthma/index.htm (accessed March 7, 2008).

National Newborn Screening and Genetics Resource Center: *National newborn screening status report*, Austin, TX, 2009, The Center. Available online at http://genes-r-us.uthscsa.edu/nbsdisorders.pdf (accessed April 26, 2009).

O'Connor BB: SARS—the latest menacing microbe, *Nurs Spectrum* 13(12DC):12-13, April 7, 2003.

Paradise JL et al: Tonsillectomy and adenotonsillectomy for recurrent throat infection in moderately affected children, *Pediatrics* 110:7-15, 2002.

Pediatric Tuberculosis Collaborative Group: Targeted tuberculin skin testing and treatment of latent tuberculosis infection in children and adolescents, *Pediatrics* 114(Suppl 4): 1175-1201, 2004.

Pichichero ME, Casey JR: Acute otitis media: making sense of recent guidelines on antimicrobial treatment, *J Fam Pract* 54(4):313-322, 2005.

Pongracic JA: Asthma delivery devices: age-appropriate use, *Pediatr Ann* 32(1):50-54, 2003.

Powers JH: Diagnosis and treatment of acute otitis media: evaluating the evidence, *Infect Dis Clin North Am* 21(2):409-426, 2007.

Rafei K, Lichenstein R: Airway infectious disease emergencies, *Pediatr Clin North Am* 53(2):215-242, 2006.

Ren CL et al: Presence of methicillin-resistant *Staphylococcus aureus* in respiratory cultures from cystic fibrosis patients is associated with lower lung function, *Pediatr Pulmonol* 42(6):513-518, 2007.

Rice TW, Bernard GR: Acute lung injury and the acute respiratory distress syndrome: challenges in clinical trial testing, *Clin Chest Med* 27(4): 733-754, 2006.

Rimsza ME, Kirk GM: Common medical problems of the college student, *Pediatr Clin North Am* 52(1):vii, 9-24, 2005.

Ross MH, Mjaanes CM, Lemanske R: Asthma. In Rudolph CD, Rudolph AM, Hostetter MK (editors): *Rudolph's pediatrics*, ed 21, New York, 2003, McGraw-Hill.

Rotta AT, Wiryawan B: Respiratory emergencies in children, *Respir Care* 48(3):248-260, 2003.

Ryan T, Brewer M, Small L: Over-the-counter cough and cold medication use in young children, *Pediatr Nurs* 34(2):174-180, 184, 2008.

Samson RA et al: Use of automated external defibrillators for children: an update: advisory statement from the pediatric advanced life support task force, International Liaison Committee on Resuscitation, *Circulation* 107(25):3250-3255, 2003.

Sandel M et al: The effects of housing interventions on child health, *Pediatr Ann* 33(7):475-481, 2004.

Schnabel D et al: A multicenter, randomized, double-blind, placebo-controlled trial to evaluate the metabolic and respiratory effects of growth hormone in children with cystic fibrosis, *Pediatrics* 119(6):e1230-e1238, 2007.

Schwarzenberg SJ et al: Microvascular complications in cystic fibrosis–related diabetes, *Diabetes Care* 30(5):1056-1061, 2007.

Sharma HP et al: Indoor environmental influences on children's asthma, *Pediatr Clin North Am* 54(1):103-120, 2007.

Sheahan SL, Free TA: Counseling parents to quit smoking, *Pediatr Nurs* 31(2):98-108, 2005.

Slader CA et al: Complementary and alternative medicine use in asthma: who is using what? *Respirology* 11(4):373-387, 2006.

Southern KW et al: Newborn screening for cystic fibrosis, *Cochrane Database Syst Rev* (1):CD001402, 2009.

Stockman LJ et al: Severe acute respiratory syndrome in children, *Pediatr Infect Dis J* 26(1):68-74, 2007.

Strausbaugh SD, Davis PB: Cystic fibrosis: a review of epidemiology and pathobiology, *Clin Chest Med* 28(2):279-288, 2007.

Strunk RC, Bloomberg GR: Omalizumab for asthma, *N Engl J Med* 354(25):2689-2695, 2006.

Tolomeo C, Mackey W: Peripherally inserted central catheters (PICCs) in the CF population: one center's experience, *Pediatr Nurs* 29(5):355-359, 2003.

US Food and Drug Administration, Center for Drug Evaluation and Research: *Questions and answers on final rule on albuterol MDIs*, March 2005. Available at www.fda.gov/cder/mdi/mdifaqs.htm (accessed June 2007).

Uyemura MC: Foreign body ingestion in children, *Am Fam Physician* 72(2):287-291, 2005.

van Staaij BK et al: Effectiveness of adenotonsillectomy in children with mild symptoms of throat infections of adenotonsillar hypertrophy: open, randomized controlled trial, *BMJ* 329(7467):651, 2004.

Ventre K, Randolph AG: Ribavirin for respiratory syncytial virus infection of the lower respiratory tract in infants and young children, *Cochrane Database Syst Rev* 24(1):CD000181, 2007.

Willson DF, Chess PR, Notter RH: Surfactant for pediatric acute lung injury, *Pediatr Clin North Am* 55(3):545-575, 2008.

Winkelstein ML et al: Factors associated with medication self-administration in children with asthma, *Clin Pediatr* 39(6):337-345, 2000.

Wright RB et al: Current pharmacologic options in the treatment of croup, *Expert Opin Pharmacother* 6(2):255-261, 2005.

Unit 11

47

Gastrointestinal Dysfunction

Learning Objectives

On completion of this chapter the reader will be able to:

- Identify children at increased risk of developing nutritional disorders.
- Outline a nutritional counseling plan for vitamin or mineral deficiency or excess.
- Describe the characteristics of infants that affect their ability to adapt to fluid loss or gain.
- Formulate a plan of care for the infant with acute diarrhea.
- Compare and contrast the inflammatory bowel diseases.
- Identify the routes of transmission for hepatitis A, B, and C.
- Describe the nursing care of the child with hepatitis.
- Formulate a plan for teaching parents preoperative and postoperative care of the child with a cleft lip or palate.
- Formulate a plan of care for the child with an obstructive gastrointestinal disorder.
- Identify nutritional therapies for the child with a malabsorption syndrome.
- Outline a teaching plan designed to prevent transmission of intestinal parasites.
- Identify the principles in the emergency treatment of poisoning.
- Name four sources of lead in the environment.
- Describe the nursing care of the child with lead poisoning.

Electronic Resources

Additional information related to the content in Chapter 47 can be found on

evolve the Companion Website at http://evolve.elsevier.com/Perry/maternal/

- NCLEX Review Questions
- Animation—Appendicitis
- Animation—Digestive Tract, Passage of Food
- Animation—Volvulus, Pediatric
- Case Study—Acute Diarrhea (Gastroenteritis)
- Case Study—Appendicitis
- Case Study—Cleft Lip and Palate
- Case Study—Dehydration and Diarrhea
- Critical Thinking Exercise—Constipation
- Critical Thinking Exercise—Hematemesis
- Critical Thinking Exercise—Home Care for the Adolescent
- Nursing Care Plan—The Child with Appendicitis
- Nursing Care Plan—The Child with Acute Diarrhea (Gastroenteritis)

Nutritional Disturbances

Vitamin Imbalances

Although true vitamin deficiencies are rare in the United States, subclinical deficiencies are commonly seen in population subgroups in which either maternal or child dietary intake of foods containing adequate amounts of vitamins is imbalanced. *Vitamin D–deficiency rickets*, once rarely seen because of the widespread commercial availability of vitamin D–fortified milk, increased before the turn of the century. Populations at risk include:

- Children exclusively breastfed by mothers with an inadequate intake of vitamin D or who are exclusively breastfed longer than 6 months without adequate maternal vitamin D intake or supplementation
- Children with dark skin pigmentation who are exposed to minimal sunlight because of socioeconomic, religious, or cultural beliefs or housing in urban areas with high levels of pollution
- Children with diets that are low in sources of vitamin D and calcium
- Individuals who use milk products not supplemented with vitamin D (e.g., yogurt, raw cow's milk) as the primary source of milk

The American Academy of Pediatrics (2008) now recommends that infants who are exclusively breastfed should receive 400 International Units of vitamin D beginning shortly after birth to prevent rickets and vitamin D deficiency. Vitamin D supplementation should occur until the infant is consuming at least 1 L/day (or 1 qt/day) of vitamin D–fortified formula (American Academy of Pediatrics, 2008). Nonbreastfed infants who are taking less than 1 L/day of vitamin D–fortified formula should also receive a daily vitamin D supplement of 400 International Units. Inadequate maternal ingestion of cobalamin (vitamin B_{12}) may contribute to infant neurologic impairment when exclusive breastfeeding (past 6 months) is the only source of the infant's nutrition (Centers for Disease Control and Prevention, 2003a).

Children may also be at risk secondary to disorders or their treatment. For example, vitamin deficiencies of the fat-soluble vitamins A and D may occur in malabsorptive disorders. Preterm infants may develop rickets in the second month of life as a result of inadequate intake of vitamin D, calcium, and phosphorus. Children receiving high doses of salicylates may have impaired vitamin C storage. Environmental tobacco smoke exposure has been implicated in decreased concentrations of ascorbate in children; therefore increased intake of sources of vitamin C should be encouraged even in children minimally exposed to environmental tobacco smoke (Preston, Rodriguez, & Rivera, 2006; Preston et al, 2003). Children with chronic illnesses resulting in anorexia, decreased food intake, or possible nutrient malabsorption as a result of multiple medications should be carefully evaluated for adequate vitamin and mineral intake in some form (parenteral or enteral).

Children with sickle cell disease are reported to have suboptimal intakes (according to Dietary Reference Intake [DRI] recommendations) of vitamins E and D, folate, calcium, and fiber, which decrease significantly with increasing age. Poor dietary intake was a significant factor in the study's findings (Kawchak et al, 2007).

Vitamin A deficiency has been reported with increased morbidity and mortality in children with measles. However, a Cochrane review of studies wherein a single dose of vitamin A was administered to children with measles found no decrease in mortality. Children with measles under the age of 2 years who received two doses of vitamin A (200,000 International Units) on consecutive days did have decreased mortality rates and a reduced rate of pneumonia-specific mortality (Huiming, Chaomin, & Meng, 2005). Complications from diarrhea and infections are often increased in infants and children with vitamin A deficiency. The American Academy of Pediatrics, Committee on Infectious Diseases (2009b) recommends that vitamin A supplementation be considered in children hospitalized with measles and associated complications (diarrhea, croup, pneumonia), especially children between the ages of 6 months and 2 years. Although scurvy (caused by a deficiency of vitamin C) is rare in developed countries, cases have been reported in children who were fed an organic diet deficient in vegetables and fruits (Burk & Molodow, 2007).

An excessive dose of a vitamin is generally defined as 10 or more times the Recommended Dietary Allowance (RDA), although the fat-soluble vitamins, especially A and D, tend to cause toxic reactions at lower doses. With the addition of vitamins to commercially prepared foods, the potential for hypervitaminosis has increased, especially when combined with the excessive use of vitamin supplements. Hypervitaminosis of A and D presents the greatest problems, since these fat-soluble vitamins are stored in the body. High intakes of vitamin A have been linked to physeal growth arrest, which can lead to osteoporosis, fracture, and metaphyseal irregularity (Saltzman & King, 2007). Vitamin D is the most likely of all vitamins to cause toxic reactions in relatively small overdoses. The water-soluble vitamins, primarily niacin, B_6, and C, can also cause toxicity. Poor outcomes in infants (e.g., a fatal hypermagnesemia) have been associated with megavitamin therapy with high doses of magnesium oxide (McGuire, Kulkarni, & Baden, 2000), and severe anemia and thrombocytopenia have resulted from megadoses of vitamin A (Perrotta et al, 2002).

One vitamin supplement that is recommended for all women of childbearing age is a daily dose of 0.4 mg of folic acid, the usual RDA. Folic acid taken before conception and during early pregnancy can reduce the risk of neural tube defects such as spina bifida by as much as 70%. Drugs such as oral contraceptives and antidepressants may decrease folic acid absorption; thus adolescent females taking such medications should consider supplementation.

Deficiencies and excesses of vitamins A, B complex, C, D, E, and K are summarized in Table 47-1. General nursing care management is discussed later in the chapter, and specific interventions are presented in Table 47-1.

Complementary and Alternative Medicine

The misuse or overuse of vitamins as a part of *complementary and alternative medicine (CAM)* places some children at risk for health problems. One survey found that a relatively small group of parents routinely gave their children megavitamin therapy; however, the researcher recommends further research to ascertain a more realistic number of children using multivitamin preparations (Loman, 2003). Sawni and colleagues (2007) noted that of persons reportedly using CAM, the most common CAM remedies used in children seen in the emergency department were home or folk remedies (59%), herbs (41%), prayer for healing (14%), and massage therapy (10%). A survey in a Women, Infants, and Children (WIC) clinic found that child herbal use was common, especially among Hispanic children attending the clinic. Some of the herbs used by the children in the survey (St. John's wort, dong quai, and kava) have questionable safety (Lohse, Stotts, & Priebe, 2006).

There is concern among health care workers that terms often used to market supplements such as megavitamins may mislead parents regarding the actual benefits (or harm) of such therapies. The intention herein is not to discredit the use of CAM such as vitamin supplements; rather, it is to ensure safety and efficacy in children who may experience inadvertent harm. The use of various herbal therapies, or intake of herbs, is also becoming more popular; many of these supplements have been a part of medicine since early days and are beneficial in some cases.

There are reports of an increase in the use of herbs by lactating mothers to increase breast milk supply. The *galactogogues* fenugreek, blessed thistle, fennel, and chaste tree have been purported to increase maternal milk supply; however, few studies support the efficacy or safety of these herbs in breastfeeding infants. Fenugreek has been the most widely studied, yet it may have adverse effects such as colic and diarrhea in breastfeeding infants (Conover & Buehler, 2004; Lawrence & Lawrence, 2005). For a discussion of galactogogues, including those mentioned previously, see Appendix P in Lawrence and Lawrence (2005).

Herbs known to have adverse effects in children include ephedra, comfrey, and pennyroyal; some herbs may not be harmful taken alone but may counteract or potentiate prescription medications when taken concurrently (Loman, 2003). Parents should be fully informed of the use of herbs to ensure that there is more benefit than potential harm in the ingredient being used. Health care workers also need to be knowledgeable about the benefits or potential harm in herbs so that they can appropriately counsel parents and address their concerns. Little research has been performed in children on many over-the-counter herbal medicines, yet some herbs are known to cause harm in children (Kemper & Gardiner, 2007; Lanski et al, 2003; Loman, 2003). Parents should be cautioned not to exceed the upper limits of vitamin intake according to the new DRI (see p. 1366 and the Dietary Reference Intakes appendix on the Evolve site).*

Mineral Imbalances

A number of minerals are essential nutrients. The *macrominerals* refer to those with daily requirements greater than 100 mg and include calcium, phosphorus, magnesium, sodium, potassium, chloride, and sulfur. *Microminerals,* or *trace elements,* have daily requirements of less than 100 mg and include several essential minerals and those whose exact role in nutrition is still unclear. The greatest concern with minerals is deficiency, especially of iron, calcium, phosphorus, magnesium, and zinc. Low levels of zinc can cause nutritional growth failure (failure to thrive).

The regulation of mineral balance in the body is complex. Dietary extremes of mineral intake can cause a number of mineral-mineral interactions that could result in unexpected deficiencies or excesses. For example, excessive amounts of one mineral such as zinc can result in a deficiency of another mineral such as copper, even if sufficient amounts of copper are ingested. Thus megadose intake of one mineral may cause deficiency of another essential mineral by blocking its absorption in the blood or intestinal wall or by competing with binding sites on protein carriers needed for metabolism.

Deficiencies can also occur when various substances in the diet interact with minerals. For example, iron, zinc, and calcium can form insoluble complexes with *phytates* or *oxalates* (substances found in plant proteins), which impair the bioavailability of the mineral. This type of interaction is important in vegetarian diets because plant foods such as soy are high in phytates. Contrary to popular opinion, spinach is not an ideal source of iron or calcium because of its high oxalate content.

Children with certain illnesses are at greater risk for growth failure, especially in relation to bone mineral deficiency as a result of the treatment of the disease, decreased nutrient intake, or decreased absorption of necessary minerals. Those at risk for such deficiencies include children who are receiving or have received radiation and chemotherapy for cancer; children with human immunodeficiency virus (HIV), sickle cell disease, cystic fibrosis, gastrointestinal (GI) malabsorption, or nephrosis; and very low–birth-weight preterm infants.

**Helpful websites for health care and consumer information concerning herbs are National Center for Complementary and Alternative Medicine,* www.nccam.nih.gov; *American Botanical Council,* www.herbalgram.org; *and Herb Research Foundation,* www.herbs.org.

Deficiencies and excesses of the essential macrominerals and microminerals are summarized in Table 47-2. General nursing care management is discussed on p. 1366, and specific nursing interventions are discussed in the table.

Vegetarian Diets

Vegetarian diets have become increasingly popular in the United States because people are concerned about hypertension; cholesterol; obesity; cardiovascular disease; the influence of the animal rights movement, and cancer of the stomach, intestine, and colon. In one survey, adolescent vegetarians were more likely than nonvegetarians to meet the *Healthy People 2010* objectives for overall nutrient consumption (Perry et al, 2002). The American Dietetic Association and Dietitians of Canada (2003) issued a statement endorsing vegetarian diets for adults and children; the statement further notes that well-planned vegetarian diets are adequate for all stages of the life cycle and promote normal growth. Children and adolescents on vegetarian diets have the potential for lifelong healthy diets and have been shown to have lower intakes of cholesterol, saturated fat, and total fat and higher intakes of fruits, fiber, and vegetables than nonvegetarians (American Dietetic Association and Dietitians of Canada, 2003).

The major types of vegetarianism are:

Lacto-ovo vegetarians, who exclude meat from their diet but consume dairy products and rarely fish

Lactovegetarians, who exclude meat and eggs but drink milk

Pure vegetarians (vegans), who eliminate any food of animal origin, including milk and eggs

Macrobiotics, who are even more restrictive than pure vegetarians, allowing only a few types of fruits, vegetables, and legumes

Semivegetarians, who consume a lacto-ovo vegetarian diet with some fish and poultry (this is an increasingly popular form of vegetarianism and poses little or no nutritional risk to infants unless dietary fat and cholesterol intake is severely restricted)

Many individuals who are concerned about healthy diets subscribe to vegetarian diets that may not be typified by these categories. Therefore during nutritional assessment it is necessary to clearly list exactly what the diet includes and excludes.*

The major deficiencies that may occur in the stricter vegan diets are inadequate protein for growth; inadequate calories for energy and growth; poor digestibility of many of the bulky natural, unprocessed foods, especially for infants; and deficiencies of vitamin B_6, niacin, riboflavin, vitamin D, iron, calcium, and zinc. Strict vegan diets also require supplements of vitamin B_{12} and vitamin D. Vitamin D is essential if exposure to sunlight is inadequate (less than 5 to 15 min/day on the hands, arms, and face of light-skinned persons; slightly more in darker pigmented individuals) or in persons who are dark-skinned or who live in northern latitudes or cloudy or smoky areas. Many of these deficiencies can be avoided in children who are not consuming 100% of the RDA of vitamins and minerals with a multivitamin-mineral supplement (Dunham & Kollar, 2006).

**Further information regarding vegetarian diets may be found at the Vegetarian Resource Group, PO Box 1463, Baltimore, MD 21203; 410-366-8343;* www.vrg.org.

BOX 47-1 Factors That Affect Iron Absorption

Increase

Acidity (low pH)—Administer iron between meals (gastric hydrochloric acid)

Ascorbic acid (vitamin C)—Administer iron with juice, fruit, or multivitamin preparation

Vitamin A

Calcium

Tissue need

Meat, fish, poultry

Cooking in cast iron pots

Decrease

Alkalinity (high pH)—Avoid any antacid preparation

Phosphates—Milk is unfavorable vehicle for iron administration

Phytates—Found in cereals

Oxalates—Found in many fruits and vegetables (plums, currants, green beans, spinach, sweet potatoes, tomatoes)

Tannins—Found in tea, coffee

Tissue saturation

Malabsorptive disorders

Disturbances that cause diarrhea or steatorrhea

Infection

Children on strict vegetarian and macrobiotic diets should be evaluated for iron deficiency anemia and rickets; this may occur as a result of consuming plant foods such as unrefined cereals, which impair the absorption of iron, calcium, and zinc. Other factors that affect iron absorption are listed in Box 47-1.

Nursing Care Management

Identification of adequacy of nutrient intake is the initial nursing goal and requires assessment based on a dietary history and physical examination for signs of deficiency or excess. Once assessment data are collected, this information is evaluated against standard intakes to identify areas of concern.

The Dietary Reference Intakes

The Dietary Reference Intakes (DRIs*) are quantitative estimates of nutrient requirements for planning and evaluating diets for healthy infants and are comprised of four categories. These include Estimated Average Requirements (EARs) for age and gender categories, tolerable upper-limit (UL) nutrient intakes that are associated with a low risk of adverse effects, adequate intakes (AIs) of nutrients, and new standard RDAs. The guidelines present information about lifestyle factors that may affect nutrient function, such as caffeine intake and exercise, and about how the nutrient may be related to chronic disease. The first DRIs published included calcium, magnesium, phosphorus, vitamin D, and fluoride. Additional groups of nutrients include folate and other B vitamins, dietary antioxidants, micronutrients, macronutrients, trace elements, electrolytes, and food components such as dietary fiber. The comprehensive set of guidelines covers nutrient needs across the life span, including infancy. An important factor in the development of the DRIs that affects children, particularly infants 0 to 6 months, is that the AIs are based on the nutrient intake of term, healthy, breastfed infants (by well-nourished mothers), which now represents the gold standard for infant nutrition in this age group. This represents a major change in infant nutrition recommendations; specific needs to meet the nutrient requirements for formula-fed infants were not included in DRI reports (Devaney & Barr, 2002; Institute of Medicine, Food and Nutrition Board, 2000).

The American Heart Association (AHA) (2005) (see also Gidding et al, 2005) Dietary Guidelines, patterned after the 2005 Dietary Guidelines for Americans, may also be used to encourage healthy dietary intakes designed to decrease obesity and cardiovascular risk factors and subsequent cardiovascular disease, which is now known to occur in both young children and adults. The AHA Guidelines have been endorsed by the American Academy of Pediatrics (2006), but it is important to note that these guidelines are for children ages 2 years and older. The guidelines encourage a variety of fruits, vegetables, whole grains, and low-fat dairy and nonfat dairy products, in addition to fish, beans, and lean meat.

MyPyramid, developed by the U.S. Department of Agriculture, replaces the Food Guide Pyramid as a guide for adult and childhood nutrition. This interactive dietary guide aims to simplify food choices designed to decrease fat and empty calorie intake and increase consumption of grains and vegetables. The MyPyramid for Kids incorporates examples of exercise for children and suggested serving sizes. The Internet version of MyPyramid for Kids *(www.mypyramid.gov)* offers an interactive game for children (Blast Off). Suggested serving sizes for the five food groups are listed in Fig. 47-1.

A vegetarian food pyramid (rainbow for Canadian vegetarians) developed by the American Dietetic Association and Dietitians of Canada includes guidelines for meeting the minimum recommendations for nutrients, including protein, iron, zinc, calcium, vitamin D, riboflavin, and iodine. The new food guide can be adapted to different types of vegetarian diets according to specific needs (American Dietetic Association and Dietitians of Canada, 2003; Messina, Melina, & Mangels, 2003).

Achieving a nutritionally adequate vegetarian diet is not difficult (except with the strictest diets), but it requires careful planning and knowledge of nutrient sources. For children the lacto-ovo vegetarian diet is nutritionally adequate; however, the vegan diet requires supplementation with vitamins D and B_{12} for children ages 2 to 12 years. Infants should be breastfed for the first 6 months and preferably for 1 year, be introduced to some solid foods after about 4 to 6 months, and receive iron-fortified cereal for at least 18 months. Vitamin B_{12} supplementation is recommended if the breastfeeding mother's intake of the vitamin is inadequate or if she is not on vitamin supplements (Dunham & Kollar, 2006). The introduction of solids for vegetarian infants may occur using the same guidelines as for other children (see p. 975). The American Dietetic Association and Dietitians of Canada (2003) recommend iron

**For information on the DRIs go to the Institute of Medicine website,* www.iom.edu, *and click on the link for Food and Nutrition; or call 202-334-2352.*

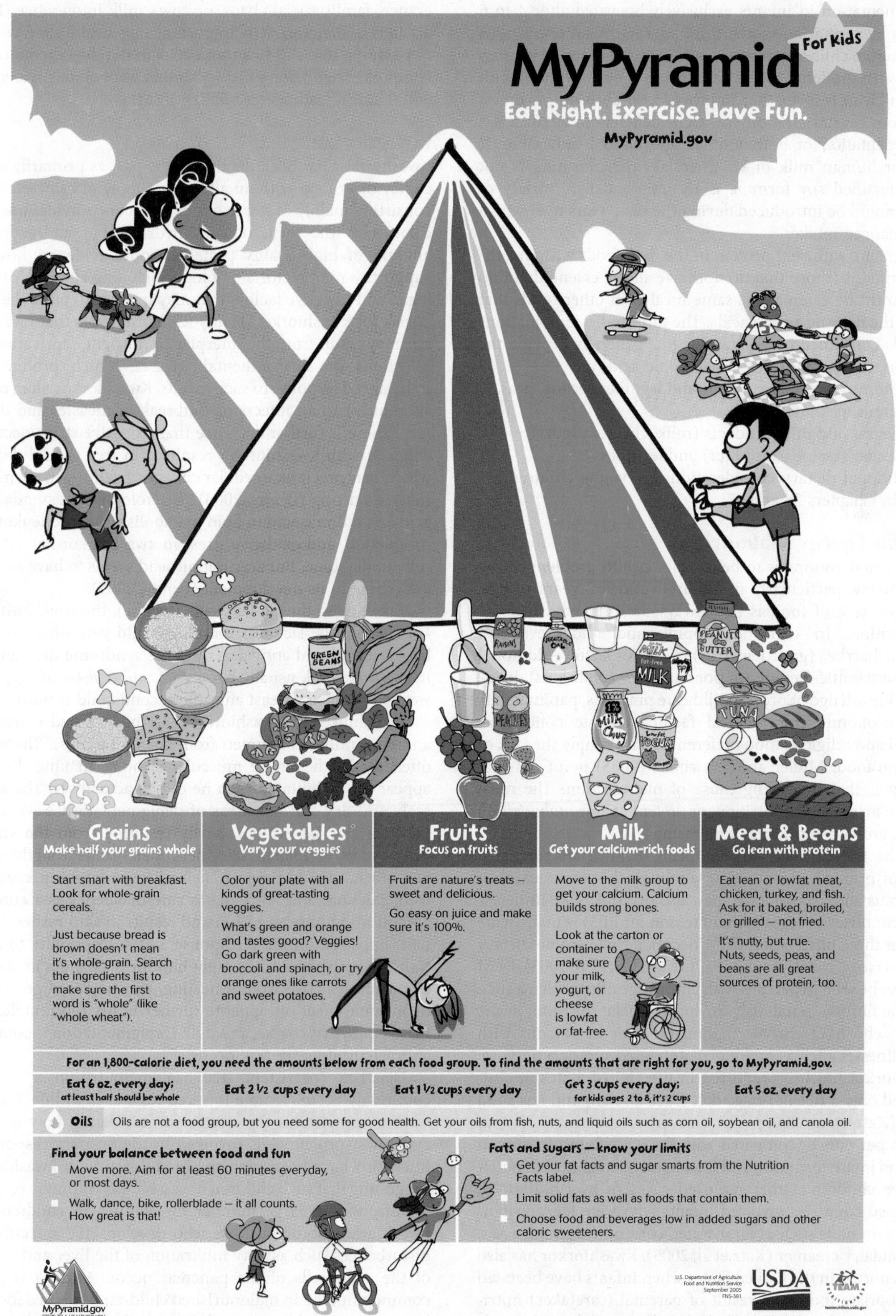

Fig. 47-1 MyPyramid for Kids. (From Food and Nutrition Service, U.S. Department of Agriculture: *MyPyramid for kids* [FNS-381], Washington, DC, April 19, 2005, The Service. Available at www.mypyramid.gov.)

supplementation in infants exclusively breastfed after 4 to 6 months by vegetarian mothers and no dietary fat restrictions in vegetarian children younger than 2 years. The use of vitamin C juices (in moderate amounts, not as a milk substitute) with foods high in iron further improves iron absorption. Breast milk from vegetarian mothers can be deficient in vitamin B_{12}; supplementation of both mother and child is advisable. If cow's or human milk or commercial infant formula is not given, fortified soy formula is recommended. A variety of foods should be introduced during the early years to ensure a well-balanced intake.

To ensure sufficient protein in the diet, foods with incomplete proteins (those that do not have all the essential amino acids) must be eaten at the same meal with other foods that supply the missing amino acids. The three basic combinations of foods consumed by vegetarians that generally provide the appropriate amounts of essential amino acids are:

1. Grains (cereal, rice, pasta) and legumes (beans, peas, lentils, peanuts)
2. Grains and milk products (milk, cheese, yogurt)
3. Seeds (sesame, sunflower) and legumes

Additional dietary considerations for young children are found in Chapters 36 and 37.

Protein-Energy Malnutrition

Malnutrition continues to be a major health problem in the world today, particularly in children under 5 years of age. However, lack of food is not always the primary cause for malnutrition. In many developing and underdeveloped nations, diarrhea (gastroenteritis) is a major factor. Additional factors are bottle-feeding (in poor sanitary conditions), inadequate knowledge of proper child care practices, parental illiteracy, economic and political factors, climate conditions, cultural and religious food preferences, and simply the lack of adequate food. Müller and Krawinkel (2005) point out that poverty is the underlying cause of malnutrition. The most extreme forms of malnutrition, or *protein-energy malnutrition (PEM),* are kwashiorkor and marasmus.

In the United States milder forms of PEM are seen as a result of primary malnutrition, although the classic cases of marasmus and kwashiorkor may also occur. Unlike in developing countries, where the main reason for PEM is inadequate food, in the United States PEM occurs despite ample dietary supplies (see Growth Failure [Failure to Thrive], p. 1003). PEM may also be seen in persons with chronic health problems such as cystic fibrosis, renal dialysis, and GI malabsorption; in the elderly who have chronic malnutrition; or in persons with acute illnesses such as prolonged, untreated anorexia nervosa. Kwashiorkor has been reported in the United States in children fed only a rice beverage diet (Rice Dream) and few solid foods (Katz et al, 2005). The rice drink contains 0.13 g of protein per ounce (compared with the 0.5 g found in human milk and infant formulas) and is an inadequate source of nutrition for children. Other reported cases of kwashiorkor in developed countries involved infants who were fed nonstandard infant diets such as flour water, corn porridge, molasses, and nondairy creamer (Katz et al, 2005). Kwashiorkor has also been reported in the United States when infants have been fed inappropriate food as a result of parental (caretaker) nutritional ignorance, a perceived cow's milk–based formula intolerance, family social chaos, or cow's milk intolerance (Liu et al, 2001). Therefore it is important that health care workers not assume that PEM cannot occur in developed countries; a comprehensive dietary history should be obtained in any child with clinical features resembling PEM.

Kwashiorkor

Kwashiorkor has been defined in the past as primarily a deficiency of protein with an adequate supply of calories. A diet consisting mainly of starch grains or tubers provides adequate calories in the form of carbohydrates but an inadequate amount of high-quality proteins. Some evidence, however, supports a multifactorial etiology, including cultural, psychologic, and infective factors that may interact to place the child at risk for kwashiorkor. Penny (2003) suggests that kwashiorkor may result from the interplay of nutrient deprivation and infectious or environmental stresses, which produces an imbalanced response to such insults. Kwashiorkor often occurs subsequent to an infectious outbreak of measles and dysentery. There is further evidence that oxidative stress occurs in children with kwashiorkor, resulting in free radical damage, which may precipitate cellular changes, resulting in edema and muscle wasting (Penny, 2003). The role of the essential fatty acid arachidonic acid in lipid metabolism, altered leukotriene production, and oxidative stress in kwashiorkor has yet to be fully understood, but arachidonic acid seems to have an interactive role in its development (Penny, 2003).

Taken from the Ga language (Ghana), the word *kwashiorkor* means "the sickness the older child gets when the next baby is born" and aptly describes the syndrome that develops in the first child, usually between 1 and 4 years of age, when weaned from the breast after the second child is born.

The child with kwashiorkor has thin, wasted extremities and a prominent abdomen from edema (ascites). The edema often masks the severe muscular atrophy, making the child appear less debilitated than he or she actually is. The skin is scaly and dry and has areas of depigmentation. Several dermatoses may be evident, partly resulting from the vitamin deficiencies. Permanent blindness often results from the severe lack of vitamin A. Mineral deficiencies are common, especially iron, calcium, and zinc. Acute zinc deficiency is a common complication of severe PEM and results in skin rashes, loss of hair, impaired immune response and susceptibility to infections, digestive problems, night blindness, changes in affective behavior, defective wound healing, and impaired growth. Its depressant effect on appetite further limits food intake. The hair is thin, dry, coarse, and dull. Depigmentation is common, and patchy alopecia may occur.

Diarrhea (persistent diarrhea malnutrition syndrome) commonly occurs from a lowered resistance to infection and further complicates the electrolyte imbalance. Low levels of cytokines (protein cells involved in the primary response to infection) have been reported in children with kwashiorkor, suggesting that such children have a blunted immune response to infection. A large number of fatalities in children with kwashiorkor occur in those who develop HIV infection. GI disturbances such as fatty infiltration of the liver and atrophy of the acini cells of the pancreas occur. Anemia is also a common finding in malnourished children. Protein deficiency increases the child's susceptibility to infection, which eventually results in death. Fatal deterioration may be caused by diarrhea and infection or by circulatory failure.

Marasmus

Marasmus results from general malnutrition of both calories and protein. It is a common occurrence in underdeveloped countries during times of drought, especially in cultures where adults eat first; the remaining food is often insufficient in quality and quantity for the children.

Marasmus is usually a syndrome of physical and emotional deprivation and is not confined to geographic areas where food supplies are inadequate. It may be seen in children with growth failure in whom the cause is not solely nutritional but primarily emotional. Marasmus may be seen in infants as young as 3 months of age if breastfeeding is not successful and there are no suitable alternatives. *Marasmic kwashiorkor* is a form of PEM in which clinical findings of both kwashiorkor and marasmus are evident; the child has edema, severe wasting, and stunted growth. In marasmic kwashiorkor the child suffers from inadequate nutrient intake and superimposed infection. Fluid and electrolyte disturbances, hypothermia, and hypoglycemia are associated with a poor prognosis.

Marasmus is characterized by gradual wasting and atrophy of body tissues, especially of subcutaneous fat. The child appears to be very old, with loose and wrinkled skin, unlike the child with kwashiorkor, who appears more rounded from the edema. Fat metabolism is less impaired than in kwashiorkor; thus deficiency of fat-soluble vitamins is usually minimal or absent. In general, the clinical manifestations of marasmus are similar to those seen in kwashiorkor with the following exceptions: with marasmus there is no edema from hypoalbuminemia or sodium retention, which contributes to a severely emaciated appearance; no dermatoses caused by vitamin deficiencies; little or no depigmentation of hair or skin; moderately normal fat metabolism and lipid absorption; and smaller head size and slower recovery after treatment.

The child is fretful, apathetic, withdrawn, and so lethargic that prostration frequently occurs. Intercurrent infection with debilitating diseases such as tuberculosis, parasitosis, HIV, and dysentery is common.

Therapeutic Management

The treatment of PEM includes providing a diet with high-quality proteins, carbohydrates, vitamins, and minerals. When PEM occurs as a result of persistent diarrhea, three management goals are identified:

1. Rehydration with an oral rehydration solution that also replaces electrolytes
2. Administration of medications such as antibiotics and antidiarrheals
3. Provision of adequate nutrition by either breastfeeding or a proper weaning diet

Local protocols are used in developing countries to deal with PEM. Penny (2003) proposes a three-phase treatment protocol: (1) acute or initial phase in the first 2 to 10 days, involving initiation of treatment for oral rehydration, diarrhea, and intestinal parasites; prevention of hypoglycemia and hypothermia; and subsequent dietary management; (2) recovery or rehabilitation (2 to 6 weeks), focusing on increasing dietary intake and weight gain; and (3) follow-up phase, focusing on care after discharge in an outpatient setting to prevent relapse and promote weight gain, provide developmental stimulation, and evaluate cognitive and motor deficits. In the acute phase care is taken to prevent fluid overload; the child is observed closely for signs of food or fluid intolerance. The refeeding syndrome may occur if intake progresses too rapidly; cardiac failure may cause sudden death in the child who has been malnourished and refed too rapidly.

Vitamin and mineral supplementation are required in most cases of PEM; vitamin A, zinc, and copper are recommended; iron supplementation is not recommended until the child is able to tolerate a steady food source. In addition, the child is observed for signs of skin breakdown, which should be treated to prevent infection. Breastfeeding is encouraged if the mother and child are able to do so effectively; in some cases partial supplementation with a modified cow's milk–based formula may be necessary (Penny, 2003). In severely malnourished children a modest energy food source is given initially, followed by a high-protein and energy food source; severely malnourished children will not tolerate a high-energy and high-protein source initially. A number of food sources may be provided to treat PEM. They include oral rehydration solutions (ReSoMal), amino acid–based elemental food, and ready-to-feed foods that do not require the addition of water (to minimize contaminated water consumption); parenteral and oral antibiotics are often part of the standard treatment for PEM (Ciliberto et al, 2005; Amadi et al, 2005).

✽ Nursing Care Management

Because PEM appears early in childhood, primarily in children 6 months to 2 years of age, and is associated with early weaning, low-protein diet, delayed introduction of complementary foods, and frequent infections (Müller & Krawinkel, 2005), it is essential that nursing care focus on prevention of PEM through parent education about feeding practices during this crucial period. Breastfeeding is the optimal method of feeding for the first 6 months. The immune properties naturally found in breast milk not only nourish the infant but aid in the prevention of opportunistic infections, which may contribute to PEM. Providing essential physiologic needs, such as appropriate nutrient intake, protection from infection, adequate hydration, skin care, and restoration of physiologic integrity, is paramount. Additional nursing care focuses on education about and administration of childhood vaccinations to prevent illness, promotion of maternal nutrition and well-being for the lactating mother, encouragement and participation in well-child visits for infants and toddlers, and education regarding sanitation practices to prevent childhood GI diseases.

Poor skin integrity further increases the chance of infections, hypothermia, water loss, and skin breakdown. Tube feedings may be required in infants too weak to breastfeed or bottle-feed. Oral rehydration with an approved oral rehydration solution is commonly used in cases of PEM in which diarrhea and infection are not immediately life threatening.

It is imperative that nurses be at the forefront in educating and reinforcing healthy nutrition habits in parents of small children to prevent malnutrition. Because children with marasmus may suffer from emotional starvation as well, care should be consistent with care of the child with growth failure (p. 1004).

Food Sensitivity

Food sensitivity is a general term that includes any type of adverse reaction to food or food additives. Food sensitivities can be divided into two broad categories:

1. **Food allergy or hypersensitivity,** which refers to reactions involving immunologic mechanisms, usually immune globulin E (IgE); the reactions may be immediate or delayed and mild or severe such as an anaphylactic reaction.
2. **Food intolerance,** which refers to reactions involving known or unknown nonimmunologic mechanisms; lactose intolerance is an example of a reaction that looks like allergy but is caused by deficiency of the enzyme lactase.

However, this classification is not universally accepted; therefore the terms *food sensitivity, hypersensitivity, allergy,* and *intolerance* are often used interchangeably. The American Academy of Allergy, Asthma, and Immunology further suggests defining food-induced reactions according to the following: adverse food reactions, food hypersensitivity (allergy), food anaphylaxis, food intolerance, food idiosyncrasy, food toxicity or poisoning, anaphylactoid reaction to food, pharmacologic food reaction, and metabolic food reaction (American Academy of Pediatrics, 2009).

The clinical manifestations of food hypersensitivity may be divided as follows (American Academy of Pediatrics, 2009):

Systemic—Anaphylactic, growth failure
Gastrointestinal—Abdominal pain, vomiting, cramping, diarrhea
Respiratory—Cough, wheezing, rhinitis, infiltrates
Cutaneous—Urticaria, rash, atopic dermatitis

Food hypersensitivities usually occur either as an IgE-mediated or non–IgE-mediated immune response; some toxic reactions may occur as a result of a toxin found within the food (Sampson, 2004). Food allergy is caused by exposure to *allergens,* usually proteins (but not the smaller amino acids) that are capable of inducing IgE antibody formation (sensitization) when ingested. *Sensitization* refers to the initial exposure of an individual to an allergen, resulting in an immune response; subsequent exposure induces a much stronger response that is clinically apparent. Consequently, food hypersensitivity typically occurs after the food has been ingested one or more times. The most common food allergens are listed in Box 47-2.

Allergies in general demonstrate a genetic component: children who have one parent with allergy have a 50% or greater risk of developing allergy; children who have two parents with allergy have up to a 100% risk of developing allergy. Allergy with a hereditary tendency is referred to as *atopy.* Some infants with atopy can be identified at birth from elevated levels of IgE in cord blood.

Deaths have been reported in children who suffered an anaphylactic reaction to food. Onset of the reactions occurred shortly after ingestion (5 to 30 minutes). In most of the children the reactions did not begin with skin signs, such as hives, red rash, and flushing, but rather mimicked an acute asthma attack (wheezing, decreased air movement in airways, dyspnea). Children with food anaphylaxis should be watched closely because a biphasic response has been recorded in a number of cases in which there is an immediate response, apparent recovery, and then acute recurrence of symptoms (Sampson, 2003). Parents, teachers, and child day care workers should be educated regarding signs and symptoms of food hypersensitivity reactions. People with food sensitivity should avoid unfamiliar foods and restaurants that do not disclose food ingredients. New labeling guidelines require that food additives such as spices and flavoring be clearly labeled on commercially sold, store-bought foods. Hidden ingredients in prepared foods have been implicated as a potential source of food hypersensitivity.

Other symptoms of anaphylaxis to food allergens include wheezing, cough, dyspnea, urticaria, abdominal cramps, vomiting, diarrhea, a drop in systemic blood pressure or shock, and in small preverbal children restlessness, urticaria, irritability, listlessness, and unresponsiveness. *Oral allergy syndrome* occurs when a food allergen is ingested (commonly fruits and vegetables) and there is subsequent edema and pruritus involving the lips, tongue, palate, and throat; recovery from symptoms is usually rapid. *Immediate GI hypersensitivity*

BOX 47-2 Hyperallergenic Foods/Sources

Milk*—Ice cream, butter, margarine (if it contains dairy products), yogurt, cheese, pudding, baked goods, wieners, bologna, canned creamed soups, instant breakfast drinks, powdered milk drinks, milk chocolate
Eggs*—Mayonnaise, creamy salad dressing, baked goods, egg noodles, some cake icing, meringue, custard, pancakes, French toast, root beer
Wheat*—Almost all baked goods, wieners, bologna, pressed or chopped cold cuts, gravy, pasta, some canned soups
Legumes—Peanuts,* peanut butter or oil, beans, peas, lentils
Nuts*—Some chocolates, candy, baked goods, cherry soda (may be flavored with a nut extract), walnut oil
Fish or shellfish*—Cod liver oil, pizza with anchovies, Caesar salad dressing, any food fried in same oil as fish
Soy*—Soy sauce, teriyaki or Worcestershire sauce, tofu, baked goods using soy flour or oil, soy nuts, soy infant formulas or milk, soybean paste, tuna packed in vegetable oil, many margarines
Chocolate—Cola beverages, cocoa, chocolate-flavored drinks
Buckwheat—Some cereals, pancakes
Pork, chicken—Bacon, wieners, sausage, pork fat, chicken broth
Strawberries, melon, pineapple—Gelatin, syrups
Corn—Popcorn, cereal, muffins, cornstarch, corn meal, corn bread, corn tortilla
Citrus fruits—Orange, lemon, lime, grapefruit; any of these in drinks, gelatin, juice, or medicines
Tomatoes—Juice, some vegetable soups, spaghetti, pizza sauce, catsup
Spices—Chili, pepper, vinegar, cinnamon

*Most common allergens.

is an IgE-mediated reaction to a food allergen; reactions include nausea, abdominal pain, cramping, diarrhea, vomiting, anaphylaxis, or all of these. Additional food hypersensitivities seen in young children include allergic eosinophilic gastritis, allergic eosinophilic gastroenterocolitis, dietary protein enterocolitis (or milk protein intolerance), and dietary protein proctitis.

Although the reason is unknown, many children "outgrow" their food allergies; children may outgrow milk and egg allergies, but peanut allergies may persist. Children who are allergic to more than one food may develop tolerance to each food at different times. Because of the tendency to lose the hypersensitivity, allergic foods should be reintroduced into the diet after a period of abstinence (usually a year or more) to evaluate whether the food can be safely added to the diet. However, foods that are associated with severe anaphylactic reactions will continue to present a lifelong risk and must be avoided. Because children with food allergies (usually two or more) are at risk for inadequate nutrient intake and growth failure, it is recommended that they have an annual nutritional assessment to prevent such problems (Christie et al, 2002).

Breastfeeding is now considered to be a primary strategy for avoiding atopy in families with known food sensitivities; however, there is some evidence that cow's milk protein is transferred via breast milk. The breastfeeding mother is encouraged to avoid foods such as peanuts, tree nuts, fish, and shellfish during the first 6 months of breastfeeding. In addition, supplementation, if required, is best with hydrolysated or amino acid formulas, *not soy* formulas. Additional recommendations to decrease the incidence of food allergies in children at higher risk for allergies is to avoid introduction of selected complementary and solid foods: dairy products should not be introduced until 12 months of age; hen's eggs at 24 months; and peanut, tree nuts, fish, and seafood at 36 months (Fiocchi et al, 2006). However, recently some authorities have now suggested that there is a lack of evidence to support maternal dietary restrictions in pregnancy or during breastfeeding to prevent atopy in the child (Greer et al, 2008). Exclusive breastfeeding is recommended for 4 months for infants at high risk of developing atopy, and exclusive breastfeeding for at least 3 months may be protective against wheezing. The researchers indicate that delaying the introduction of highly allergenic foods past 4 to 6 months may not be as protective for atopy as previously believed (Greer et al, 2008). Parents are advised to discuss infant feeding practices with the primary practitioner and obtain adequate information to make an informed decision if there is a family history of atopy. The strategies listed in the Guidelines box are those recommended by most authorities for infants with a family history of atopy.*

**Further information for parents of infants with food allergies is available from the American Academy of Allergy, Asthma, and Immunology, 555 E. Wells St., Suite 1100, Milwaukee, WI 53202; 414-272-6071;* www.aaaai.org. *Additional helpful websites for information on food allergy include MedlinePlus (sponsored by U.S. National Library of Medicine and National Institutes of Health),* http://medlineplus.gov; *Food Allergy and Anaphylaxis Network, 800-929-4040,* www.foodallergy.org; *and National Institute of Allergy and Infectious Diseases,* www3.niaid.nih.gov *and* www.allergicchild.com.

GUIDELINES Preventing Atopy in Children

Identify Children at Risk

Family history of allergy

Increased immune globulin E in cord blood and postnatal serum

Dry, flaky skin

Prenatal Precautions (Last Trimester)

Avoid any known food allergens

Avoid milk and other dairy products, peanuts, and eggs

Minimize ingestion of other hyperallergenic foods (see Box 47-2)

Postnatal Precautions

Breast milk (preferred), extensively hydrolyzed formula (Nutramigen, Pregestimil, or Alimentum), or amino acid formula (Neocate or EleCare) exclusively for at least 6 months

No solid food for first 6 months

No whole cow's milk, substitution milks, or soy formula for 12 months

Avoid hen's eggs until 24 months; peanut, tree nuts, fish, and seafood for 36 months; and chocolate for first 12 to 18 months

One new food added at 5-day intervals to identify possible reaction

Read commercial food product label carefully for ingredients, preservatives

Environmental Control

Limited exposure to dust mites, molds, furry animals, latex products, and second-hand cigarette smoke

Data from Johnstone D: Strategy for intervention of food allergy in infants, *Int Pediatr* 4(4):319-325, 1989; Zeiger RS et al: Effectiveness of dietary manipulation in the prevention of food allergy in infants, *J Allergy Clin Immunol* 78(1 Pt 2):224-238, 1986; Wood RA: Prospects for the prevention of allergy in children, *Curr Opin Pediatr* 8(6):601-605, 1995; Fiocchi A et al: Food allergy and the introduction of solid foods to infants: a consensus document, *Ann Allergy Asthma Immunol* 97(1):10-20, 2006.

NURSING ALERT Sampson (2003) suggests that indications for the administration of intramuscular epinephrine in a child with a life-threatening anaphylactic reaction or one who is experiencing severe symptoms include any one of the following: itching sensation or tightness in throat; hoarseness; "barky" cough; difficulty swallowing; dyspnea; wheezing; cyanosis; respiratory arrest; mild dysrhythmia or mild hypotension; severe bradycardia, hypotension, or cardiac arrest; or loss of consciousness.

Children with extremely sensitive food allergies should wear medical identification such as a bracelet and have an injectable epinephrine cartridge (EpiPen) readily available and know how to use it. It is also helpful for the child to have a copy of the individualized written treatment plan on hand for prompt diagnosis and treatment (such plans can be downloaded from *www.foodallergy.org* and completed by the practitioner).

Cow's Milk Allergy

Cow's milk allergy (CMA) (also referred to as cow's milk protein allergy [CMPA] or cow milk protein intolerance [CMPI]) is a multifaceted disorder representing adverse systemic and local GI reactions to cow's milk protein. (This discussion is centered on cow's milk protein found in commercial infant formulas; whole milk is not recommended for infants younger than the age of 12 months.) The hypersensitivity may be manifested within the first 4 months of life through a variety of signs and symptoms that may appear within 45 minutes of milk ingestion or after a period of several days (Box 47-3). In infants who are highly sensitive to the protein, even a small amount of cow's milk protein may induce anaphylactic reaction. Cases of contamination of non-cow's milk–based infant formula during the manufacturing process resulting in severe reactions have been documented (Levin, Motala, & Lopata, 2005). The diagnosis may initially be made from the history, although the history alone is not diagnostic; the timing and diversity of clinical manifestations vary greatly. For example, CMA may be manifested as colic (see p. 1001), diarrhea, vomiting, GI bleeding, gastroesophageal reflux (GER), chronic constipation, or sleeplessness in an otherwise healthy infant.

The incidence of CMA is reported to range from 2% to 7.5% in developed countries, although the percentage may appear to be higher because of parental report of symptoms rather than actual confirmation of CMA (Host, 2002; Salvatore & Vandenplas, 2002).

Diagnostic Evaluation

A number of diagnostic tests may be performed, including stool analysis for blood (both frank and occult bleeding can occur from the colitis), serum IgE levels, skin-prick or scratch testing, and radioallergosorbent test (measures IgE antibodies to specific allergens in serum by radioimmunoassay). Both skin and radioallergosorbent testing help identify the offending food, but the results are not always conclusive.

BOX 47-3 Common Clinical Manifestations of Cow's Milk Sensitivity

Gastrointestinal
- Diarrhea
- Vomiting
- Colic
- Abdominal pain

Respiratory
- Rhinitis
- Bronchitis
- Asthma
- Wheezing
- Sneezing
- Coughing
- Chronic nasal discharge

Other Signs and Symptoms
- Eczema
- Excessive crying
- Pallor (from anemia secondary to chronic blood loss in gastrointestinal tract)

The most definitive diagnostic strategy is elimination of milk in the diet, followed by challenge testing after improvement of symptoms. A clinical diagnosis is made when symptoms improve after removal of milk from the diet and two or more challenge tests produce symptoms (Ewing & Allen, 2005). Challenge testing involves reintroducing small quantities of milk in the diet to detect resurgence of symptoms; at times it involves the use of a placebo so that the parent is unaware of (or "blind" to) the timing of allergen ingestion. A double-blind placebo-controlled food challenge is the gold standard for diagnosing food allergies such as CMA, yet it may not be used very often for diagnosing CMA because of the expense, time involved, and risk for further exposure and anaphylactic reaction (Ewing & Allen, 2005).

Therapeutic Management

Treatment of CMA is elimination of cow's milk–based formula and all other dairy products. For infants fed cow's milk formula, this primarily involves changing the formula to a casein hydrolysate milk formula or extensively hydrolyzed formula (Pregestimil, Nutramigen, or Alimentum), in which the protein has been broken down into its amino acids through enzymatic hydrolysis. Although the American Academy of Pediatrics (2009) recommends the use of hydrolyzed formulas for CMA, many practitioners may start a soy formula instead. Approximately 10% of infants who are sensitive to cow's milk protein will also demonstrate sensitivity to soy (Assa'ad, 2006), but soy is less expensive than protein hydrolysate formula. Intolerance to soy is reported to be higher in infants under age 6 months with a family history of atopy and severe GI symptoms (Ewing & Allen, 2005). Other choices for children who are intolerant to cow's milk–based formula are the amino acid–based formulas Neocate or EleCare, but their cost is a major consideration. Goat's milk is not an acceptable substitute because it cross-reacts with cow's milk protein, is deficient in folic acid, and is unsuitable as the only source of calories. Anaphylactic reaction to goat's milk has been noted in an infant who was also allergic to cow's milk (Pessler & Nejat, 2004). Infants are maintained on the milk-free diet until after 1 year of age, after which time small quantities of milk are reintroduced; eggs and fish may be introduced at 3 years of age.

Nursing Care Management

The principal nursing objectives are to prevent and reduce exposure of infants to cow's milk protein by encouraging exclusive breastfeeding in the first 4 to 6 months of life. In addition, nurses have an important role in identifying potential CMA, appropriate counseling of parents regarding signs and symptoms of CMA, and the use of substitute formulas that are appropriate for infants with diagnosed CMA. Parents need much reassurance regarding the needs of nonverbal infants with such an array of symptoms. Endless nights of lost sleep and a crying infant may promote feelings of parenting inadequacy and role conflict, thus aggravating the situation. Nurses can reassure parents that many of these symptoms are common and the reasons are often never found, yet the child does achieve appropriate growth and development; acute symptoms are reported to the practitioner for further evaluation. The protein hydrolysate (partially hydrolyzed and extensively hydrolyzed) formulas tend to be less palatable and more expensive than milk-based formulas. Consequently, the child's reluctance to accept the new formula may be a problem. This can be overcome by adding nonnutritive, hypoallergenic flavor packets or by introducing the formula gradually over a few days, using 1 oz of new formula to 7 oz of old formula, then 2 to 6 oz, 3 to 5 oz, and as needed. Parents also need to be reassured that the infant will receive complete nutrition from the new formula and will suffer no ill effects from the absence of cow's milk.

Once solid foods are started, parents need guidance in avoiding milk products (see Box 47-2), although many children reportedly outgrow cow's milk protein sensitivity by 3 to 4 years of age (Fiocchi & Martelli, 2006).

Lactose Intolerance

Lactose intolerance refers to at least four different entities that involve a deficiency of the enzyme *lactase,* which is needed for the hydrolysis or digestion of lactose in the small intestine; lactose is hydrolyzed into glucose and galactose. *Congenital lactase deficiency* occurs soon after birth after the newborn has consumed lactose-containing milk (human milk or commercial formula). This inborn error of metabolism involves the complete absence or severely reduced presence of lactase, is rare, and requires lifelong lactose-free or extremely reduced lactose diet.

Primary lactase deficiency, sometimes referred to as *late-onset lactase deficiency,* is the most common type of lactose intolerance and is manifested usually after 4 or 5 years of age, although the time of onset varies. Ethnic groups with a high incidence of lactase deficiency include Asians, southern Europeans, Arabs, Israelis, and African Americans, whereas Scandinavians tend to have the lowest. Lactose malabsorption manifests as lactose intolerance and is characterized by an imbalance between the ability for lactase to hydrolyze the ingested lactose and the amount of lactose ingested (Heyman & American Academy of Pediatrics Committee on Nutrition, 2006).

Secondary lactase deficiency may occur secondary to damage of the intestinal lumen, which decreases or destroys the enzyme lactase. Cystic fibrosis; sprue; celiac disease; kwashiorkor; or infections such as giardiasis, HIV, or rotavirus may cause temporary or permanent lactose intolerance.

Developmental lactase deficiency refers to the relative lactase deficiency observed in preterm infants of less than 34 weeks of gestation (Heyman & American Academy of Pediatrics Committee on Nutrition, 2006).

The primary symptoms of lactose intolerance include abdominal pain, bloating, flatulence, and diarrhea after the ingestion of lactose. The onset of symptoms occurs within 30 minutes to several hours of lactose consumption. Lactose intolerance is often perceived as an allergy; and in several studies with reports of acute GI symptoms ascribed to lactose intolerance, measurement of lactase activity is normal (Goldberg, Folta, & Must, 2002).

Lactose intolerance may be diagnosed on the basis of the history and improvement with a lactose-reduced diet. The breath hydrogen test is used to positively diagnose the condition. Breath samples in lactose-deficient individuals yield a higher percentage of hydrogen (20 ppm [parts per million] or more above baseline). In infants lactose malabsorption may be diagnosed by evaluating fecal pH and reducing substances; fecal pH in infants is usually lower than in older children, but an acidic pH may indicate malabsorption (Heyman & American Academy of Pediatrics Committee on Nutrition, 2006).

Treatment of lactose intolerance is elimination of offending dairy products; however, some advocate decreasing amounts of dairy products rather than total elimination, especially in small children (Heyman & American Academy of Pediatrics Committee on Nutrition, 2006; Goldberg, Folta, & Must, 2002). In infants lactose-free or low-lactose formula offers no special advantages over lactose-containing formula, except in the severely malnourished (Heyman & American Academy of Pediatrics Committee on Nutrition, 2006).

One concern is that dairy avoidance in children and adolescents with lactose intolerance contributes to reduced bone mineral density and osteoporosis (Sibley, 2004). There is evidence that dietary lactose enhances calcium absorption and that lactose-free diets may negatively affect bone mineralization (Heyman & American Academy of Pediatrics Committee on Nutrition, 2006). It has been suggested that individuals with lactose maldigestion who do not experience lactose intolerance symptoms continue to consume small amounts of dairy products with meals to prevent reduced bone mass density and subsequent osteoporosis (Sibley, 2004). There is evidence that *probiotics* (food preparations containing microorganisms such as *Lactobacillus,* which alter the GI microflora and thus are beneficial to the host) improve lactose intolerance when live cultures are fermented in dairy products (Zeisel & Erickson, 2003). The positive attributes of probiotics for those with lactose maldigestion include delayed GI transit (slower than milk), positive effects on intestinal and colonic microflora, and a reduction of maldigestion symptoms (de Vrese et al, 2001).

Most people are able to tolerate small amounts of lactose even in the presence of deficient lactase activity (Heyman & American Academy of Pediatrics Committee on Nutrition, 2006; Goldberg, Folta, & Must, 2002) and should be encouraged to continue their intake of dairy products in small amounts to obtain much-needed nutrients. Milk taken at meals may be better tolerated than when taken alone (see Family-Centered Care box). Pretreated milk (with microbial-derived lactase) is reported to be effective in improving lactose absorption.

FAMILY-CENTERED CARE

Controlling Symptoms of Lactose Intolerance

- In infants substitute soy-based formula for cow's milk formula or human milk.
- Limit milk consumption to one glass at a time.
- Drink milk with other foods rather than alone.
- Eat hard cheese, cottage cheese, or yogurt instead of drinking milk.
- Use enzyme tablets (Lactaid, Lactrase, Dairy Ease) to metabolize the lactose in milk or supplement the body's own lactose (add tablets to milk or sprinkle on dairy products such as ice cream).
- Eat small amounts of dairy foods daily to help colonic bacteria adapt to ingested lactose.

Because dairy products are a major source of calcium and vitamin D, supplementation of these nutrients is needed to prevent deficiency. Yogurt contains inactive lactase enzyme, which is activated by the temperature and pH of the duodenum; this lactase activity substitutes for the lack of endogenous lactase. Fresh, plain yogurt may be tolerated better than frozen or flavored yogurt; hard cheeses, lactase-treated dairy products, and lactase tablets taken with dairy products are also viable options. An important distinction between lactose intolerance and food hypersensitivity is that lactose intolerance does not manifest as an anaphylactic-type reaction.

Nursing Care Management

Nursing care is similar to the interventions discussed for CMA: explaining the dietary restrictions to the family; identifying alternate sources of calcium such as yogurt and calcium supplementation; explaining the importance of supplementation; and discussing sources of lactose, especially hidden sources such as its use as a bulk agent in certain medications, and ways of controlling the symptoms (see Family-Centered Care box). Parents are advised to check with the pharmacist regarding this possibility when obtaining medication.

Text continued on p. 1380

Table 47-1 Vitamins and Their Nutritional Significance

PHYSIOLOGIC FUNCTIONS AND SOURCES	RESULTS OF DEFICIENCY OR EXCESS	NURSING CARE MANAGEMENT
Vitamin A (Retinol)*		
Functions Necessary component in formation of pigment rhodopsin (visual purple) Formation and maintenance of epithelial tissue Normal bone growth and tooth development Needed for growth and spermatogenesis Involved in thyroxine formation Antioxidant *Sources* **Natural form**—Liver, kidney, fish oils, milk and nonskim milk products, egg yolk **Provitamin A (carotene)**—Carrots, sweet potatoes, squash, apricots, spinach, collards, broccoli, cabbage, artichokes	*Deficiency* Night blindness Keratinization (hardening and scaling) of epithelium Xerophthalmia (hardening and scaling of cornea and conjunctiva) Phrynoderma (toad skin) Drying of respiratory, gastrointestinal, and genitourinary tracts Defective tooth enamel Delayed growth Impaired bone formation Decreased thyroxine formation Decreased resistance to infections *Excess* **Early signs**—Irritability, anorexia, pruritus, fissures at corners of nose and lips, dry skin **Later signs**—Hepatomegaly, jaundice, retarded growth, poor weight gain, thickening of the cortex of long bones with pain and fragility, hard tender lumps in extremities and occiput of the skull Can cause birth defects if excessive maternal intake NOTE: Overdose results from ingestion of large quantities of the vitamin only, not the provitamin; large amounts of carotene (carotenemia) cause yellow or orange discoloration of the skin (not the sclera, urine, or feces as in jaundice) but none of the above symptoms.	*Deficiency* Encourage foods rich in vitamin A, such as whole cow's milk (after 12 mo). As milk consumption decreases, encourage foods rich in vitamin A. Ensure adequate intake in preterm infants. Advise parents of safe use of supplements in child with measles. It may play a role in prevention of severity of bronchopulmonary dysplasia in preterm infants (affects growth of respiratory tract epithelial cells). *Excess* Emphasize correct use of vitamin supplements and potential hazards of excess. Evaluate child's dietary habits to calculate approximate intake; if excessive, remove supplemental source (e.g., daily feeding of liver). Advise parents of the benign nature of carotenemia; treatment is avoidance of excess pigmented fruits or vegetables, especially carrots; skin color returns to normal in 2 to 6 wk.
Vitamin B_1 (Thiamine)†		
Functions Coenzyme (with phosphorus) in carbohydrate metabolism Needed for healthy nervous system Digestion and normal appetite *Sources* Pork, beef, liver, legumes, nuts, whole or enriched grains and cereals, green vegetables, fruits, milk, brown rice	*Deficiency* **Gastrointestinal**—Anorexia, constipation, indigestion **Neurologic**—Apathy, fatigue, emotional instability, polyneuritis, tenderness of calf muscles, partial anesthesia, muscle weakness, paresthesia, hyperesthesia, decreased or absent tendon reflexes, convulsions, coma (in infants) **Cardiovascular**—Palpitations, cardiac failure, peripheral vasodilation, edema *Excess* Headache Irritability Insomnia Weakness	*Deficiency: Vitamin B Complex* Encourage foods rich in B vitamins. Stress proper cooking and storage techniques to preserve potency, such as minimum cooking of vegetables in small amount of liquid and storage of milk in opaque container. Encourage fortified breakfast cereals and soy milk (which have B_{12}) for persons on strict vegetarian diet; dairy products and eggs contain B_{12} if these are allowed; otherwise supplementation may be required. Evaluate need for vitamin supplements when dieting, when using unfortified goat's milk exclusively for infant feeding (deficient in folic acid), or when the breastfeeding mother is a strict vegetarian (vitamin B_{12}). *Excess* Emphasize correct use of vitamin supplements and potential hazards of excess. Individuals with malabsorption syndrome or being treated with hemodialysis or peritoneal dialysis may have increased need for thiamine.

Table 47-1 Vitamins and Their Nutritional Significance—cont'd

PHYSIOLOGIC FUNCTIONS AND SOURCES	RESULTS OF DEFICIENCY OR EXCESS	NURSING CARE MANAGEMENT
Vitamin B_2 (Riboflavin)† *Functions* Coenzyme (with phosphorus) in carbohydrate, protein, and fat metabolism Maintains healthy skin, especially around mouth, nose, and eyes *Sources* Milk and its products, eggs, organs (liver, kidney, heart), enriched cereals, some green leafy vegetables,‡ legumes	*Deficiency* Ariboflavinosis **Lips**–Cheilosis (fissures at corners of lips), perlèche (inflammation at corners of lips) **Tongue**–Glossitis **Nose**–Irritation and cracks at nasal angle **Eyes**–Burning, itching, tearing, photophobia, blurred vision, corneal vascularization, cataracts **Skin**–Seborrheic dermatitis, delayed wound healing and tissue repair *Excess* Paresthesia, pruritus	Same as vitamin B complex
Niacin (Nicotinic Acid, Nicotinamide)† *Functions* Coenzyme (with riboflavin) in protein and fat metabolism Needed for healthy nervous system and skin and for normal digestion May lower cholesterol *Sources* Meat, poultry, fish, peanuts, beans, peas, whole or enriched grains (except corn and rice) Milk and its products are sources of tryptophan (60 mg tryptophan = 1 mg niacin).	*Deficiency* Pellagra (rash, diarrhea, mental status changes, stomatitis) **Oral**–Stomatitis, glossitis **Cutaneous**–Scaly dermatitis on exposed areas **Gastrointestinal**–Anorexia, weight loss, diarrhea, fatigue **Neurologic**–Apathy, anxiety, confusion, depression, dementia *Excess* Release of histamine, a vasodilator (flushing, decreased blood pressure, increased cerebral blood flow; aggravates asthma) Dermatologic problems (pruritus, rash, hyperkeratosis, acanthosis nigricans) Increased gastric acidity (aggravates peptic ulcer disease) Hepatotoxicity Increased serum uric acid levels Elevated plasma glucose levels Certain cardiac arrhythmias	Same as vitamin B complex *Excess* If used as hypolipidemic agent, stress safe storage to prevent child's accidental ingestion.
Vitamin B_6 (Pyridoxine)† *Functions* Coenzyme in protein and fat metabolism Needed for formation of antibodies and hemoglobin Needed for utilization of copper and iron Aids in conversion of tryptophan to niacin *Sources* Meats, especially liver and kidney, cereal grains (wheat, corn), yeast, soybeans, peanuts, tuna, chicken, salmon	*Deficiency* Scaly dermatitis Weight loss Anemia Retarded growth Irritability Seizures Peripheral neuritis *Excess* Peripheral nervous system toxicity (unsteady gait, numb feet and hands, clumsiness of hands, sometimes perioral numbness) May cause peptic ulcer disease or seizures	Same as vitamin B complex *Deficiency* Stress proper cooking and storing techniques to preserve potency. Cook food covered in small amount of water. Do not soak food in water. Store in light-resistant container.
Folic Acid (Folacin; Reduced Form Called Folinic Acid or Citrovorum Factor)† *Functions* Coenzyme for single-carbon transfer (purines, thymine, hemoglobin) Necessary for formation of red blood cells May prevent neural tube defects (i.e., myelomeningocele) and facial clefts (cleft lip and palate) *Sources* Green leafy vegetables, beets, cabbage, asparagus, liver, kidneys, nuts, eggs, whole grain cereals, legumes, bananas	*Deficiency* Macrocytic anemia Bone marrow depression Glossitis Intestinal malabsorption Growth failure *Excess* Rare because megadoses not available over the counter May cause insomnia and irritability	Same as vitamin B complex *Deficiency* Stress proper cooking and storing techniques to preserve potency: Cook food covered in small amount of water. Do not soak food in water. Store in light-resistant container. Women of childbearing age should supplement to prevent neural tube defects and orofacial clefts.

*Fat soluble.
†Water soluble.
‡Green leafy vegetables include spinach, broccoli, kale, turnip greens, mustard greens, collards, dandelion greens, and beet greens.

Continued

Table 47-1 Vitamins and Their Nutritional Significance—cont'd

PHYSIOLOGIC FUNCTIONS AND SOURCES	RESULTS OF DEFICIENCY OR EXCESS	NURSING CARE MANAGEMENT
Vitamin B_{12} (Cobalamin)† *Functions* Coenzyme in protein synthesis; indirect effect on formation of red blood cells (particularly on formation of nucleic acids and folic acid metabolism) Needed for normal functioning of nervous tissue *Sources* Meat, liver, kidney, fish, shellfish, poultry, milk, eggs, cheese, nutritional yeast, sea vegetables	*Deficiency* Pernicious anemia (one form of deficiency from absence of intrinsic factor in gastric secretions) General signs of severe anemia Lemon-yellow tinge to skin Spinal cord degeneration Delayed brain growth *Excess* Rare	Same as vitamin B complex *Deficiency* Consider fortified foods or supplements in persons over 50 yr of age to meet RDA because malabsorption of food-bound vitamin B_{12} is common.
Vitamin C (Ascorbic Acid)† *Functions* Essential for collagen formation Increases absorption of iron for hemoglobin formation Enhances conversion of folic acid to folinic acid Affects cholesterol synthesis and conversion of proline to hydroxyproline Probably a coenzyme in metabolism of tyrosine and phenylalanine May play role in hydroxylation of adrenal steroids May have stimulating effect on phagocytic activity of leukocytes and formation of antibodies Antioxidant agent (spares other vitamins from oxidation) *Sources* Citrus fruits, strawberries, tomatoes, potatoes, cabbage, broccoli, cauliflower, spinach, papaya, mango, cantaloupe, watermelon, enriched fruit juice	*Deficiency* Scurvy **Skin**—Dry, rough, petechiae; perifollicular hyperkeratotic papules (raised areas around hair follicles) **Musculoskeletal**—Bleeding muscles and joints, pseudoparalysis from pain, swelling of joints, costochondral beading (scorbutic rosary) **Gums**—Spongy, friable, swollen, bleed easily, bluish red or black, teeth loosen and fall out **General disposition**—Irritable, anorexic, apprehensive, in pain, refuses to move, assumes semi-froglike position when supine (scorbutic pose) Signs of anemia Decreased wound healing Increased susceptibility to infection *Excess* Diarrhea Increased excretion of uric acid and acidification of urine (may cause urate precipitation and formation of oxalate stones) Hemolysis Impaired leukocytosis activity Damage to β-cells of pancreas and decreased insulin production Reproductive failure "Rebound scurvy" from withdrawal of large amounts	*Deficiency* Encourage foods rich in vitamin C. Evaluate child's diet for sources of vitamin, especially when cow's milk is principal source of nutrition. Tobacco smokers require an additional 35 mg/day; nonsmokers exposed to second-hand smoke should make sure they meet RDA. Stress proper cooking and storage techniques to preserve potency: Wash vegetables quickly; do not soak in water. Cook vegetables in covered pot with minimum water and for short time; avoid copper or cast iron cookware. Do not add baking soda to cooking water. Use fresh fruits and vegetables as soon as possible; store in refrigerator. Store juice in airtight, opaque container. Wrap cut fruit or eat soon after exposing to air. *Excess* Emphasize correct use of vitamin supplement and potential hazards of excess. Identify groups at risk for excessive vitamin C supplements (e.g., those with thalassemia or those receiving anticoagulant or aminoglycoside antibiotic therapy).
Vitamin D_2 (Ergocalciferol) and D_3 (Cholecalciferol)* *Functions* Absorption of calcium and phosphorus and decreased renal excretion of phosphorus *Sources* Direct sunlight Cod liver oil, herring, mackerel, salmon, tuna, sardines **Enriched food sources**—Milk, milk products, enriched cereals, margarine, breads, many breakfast drinks	*Deficiency* Rickets **Head**—Craniotabes (softening of cranial bones, prominence of frontal bones[bossing]), deformed shape (skull flat and depressed toward middle), delayed closure of fontanels **Chest**—Rachitic rosary (enlargement of costochondral junction of ribs), Harrison groove (horizontal depression in lower portion of rib cage), pigeon chest (sharp protrusion of sternum) **Spine**—Kyphosis, scoliosis, lordosis **Abdomen**—Pot belly, constipation **Extremities**—Bowing of arms and legs, knock knee, saber shins, instability of hip joints, pelvic deformity, enlargement of epiphyses at ends of long bones **Teeth**—Delayed calcification, especially of permanent teeth Rachitic tetany—Seizures *Excess* **Acute**—Vomiting, dehydration, fever, abdominal cramps, bone pain, seizures, coma **Chronic**—Lassitude, mental slowness, anorexia, failure to thrive, thirst, urinary urgency, polyuria, vomiting, diarrhea, abdominal cramps, bone pain, pathologic fractures **Calcification of soft tissue**—Kidneys, lungs, adrenal glands, vessels (hypertension), heart, gastric lining, tympanic membrane (deafness) Osteoporosis of long bones Elevated serum levels of calcium and phosphorus	*Deficiency* Encourage foods rich in vitamin D, especially fortified whole cow's milk (>12 mo of age). Encourage use of vitamin D supplement in all exclusively breastfed infants starting within first 2 wk of life (see text). Observe for possibility of overdose from supplements. If prescribed, supervise proper use of orthoses (splints and braces). *Excess* Same as vitamin A; may include low-calcium diet during initial therapy

Table 47-1 Vitamins and Their Nutritional Significance—cont'd

PHYSIOLOGIC FUNCTIONS AND SOURCES	RESULTS OF DEFICIENCY OR EXCESS	NURSING CARE MANAGEMENT
Vitamin E (Tocopherol)* *Functions* Production of red blood cells and protection from hemolysis Muscle and liver integrity Coenzyme factor in tissue respiration Minimizes oxidation of polyunsaturated fatty acids and vitamins A and C in intestinal tract and tissues *Sources* Vegetable oils, wheat germ oil, milk, egg yolk, fish, whole grains, nuts, legumes, spinach, broccoli	*Deficiency* Hemolytic anemia from hemolysis caused by shortened life of red blood cells, especially in preterm infants; focal necrosis of tissues *Excess* Little is known; less toxic than other fat-soluble vitamins	*Deficiency* Initiate early feeding in preterm infants; may need supplementation. Potential role as antioxidant in immune function, preventing or limiting the severity of retinopathy and prevention of hemolytic anemia, bronchopulmonary dysplasia, and intracranial hemorrhage
Vitamin K* *Functions* Catalyst for production of prothrombin and blood-clotting factors II, VII, IX, and X by the liver *Sources* Pork, liver, green leafy vegetables, cabbage, tomatoes, egg yolk, cheese	*Deficiency* Hemorrhage *Excess* Hemolytic anemia in individuals who are deficient in glucose 6-phosphate dehydrogenase	*Deficiency* Administer prophylactically to all newborns. Other indications include intestinal disease, lack of bile, prolonged antibiotic therapy; may be used in management of blood-clotting time when anticoagulants such as warfarin (Coumadin) and dicumarol (bishydroxycoumarin), which are vitamin K antagonists, are used.

Table is not intended to be all inclusive.
RDA, Recommended dietary allowance.
*Fat soluble.
†Water soluble.

Table 47-2 Minerals and Their Nutritional Significance

PHYSIOLOGIC FUNCTIONS AND SOURCES	RESULTS OF DEFICIENCY OR EXCESS	NURSING CARE MANAGEMENT
Calcium* *Functions* Bone and tooth development and maintenance (in combination with phosphorus) Muscle contractions, especially the heart Blood clotting Absorption of vitamin B_{12} Enzyme activation Nerve conduction Integrity of intracellular cement substances and various membranes *Sources* Dairy products, egg yolk, sardines, canned salmon with bones, green leafy vegetables† (except spinach), soybeans, dried beans, peas	*Deficiency* Rickets Tetany Impaired growth, especially of bones and teeth Osteoporosis *Excess* Drowsiness, extreme lethargy Impaired absorption of other minerals (iron, zinc, manganese) Calcium deposits in tissues (renal failure)	*Deficiency* Encourage foods rich in calcium, especially dairy products. Give vitamin D supplements in infants beginning by age 2 mo (see text). Caution that oxalates in leafy vegetables (spinach), oxalates in chocolates, and a high phosphorus intake (especially from carbonated beverages) can decrease calcium absorption. Discourage use of whole cow's milk or other animal milks in newborns and infants under 12 mo because the phosphorus/calcium ratio favors excretion of calcium. Advise against diets that restrict dairy products unless adequate supplementation is followed. *Excess* Emphasize correct use of calcium supplements, especially the possible interaction between megadoses of calcium and resulting deficiency states of other minerals.
Chloride* *Functions* Acid-base and fluid balance Enzyme activation in saliva Component of hydrochloric acid in stomach *Sources* Salt, meat, eggs, dairy products, many prepared and preserved foods	*Deficiency* Acid-base disturbances (hypochloremic alkalosis, dehydration); occurs mostly in combination with sodium loss *Excess* Acid-base disturbance	Deficiency and excess are unusual; most diets supply adequate chloride (usually in combination with sodium). Disease states such as excessive vomiting can necessitate chloride replacement.

*Macrominerals—required intake >100 mg/day.
†Green leafy vegetables include spinach, broccoli, kale, turnip greens, mustard greens, collards, dandelion greens, and beet greens.
‡Microminerals or trace elements—required intake <100 mg/day.

Continued

Table 47-2 Minerals and Their Nutritional Significance—cont'd

PHYSIOLOGIC FUNCTIONS AND SOURCES	RESULTS OF DEFICIENCY OR EXCESS	NURSING CARE MANAGEMENT
Copper† ***Functions*** Production of hemoglobin Essential component of several enzyme systems ***Sources*** Organ meats, oysters, nuts, seeds, legumes, corn oil margarine	***Deficiency*** Anemia, leukopenia, neutropenia ***Excess*** Severe vomiting and diarrhea Hemolytic anemia	***Deficiency*** Emphasize the correct use of any vitamin supplement with mineral because deficiency from inadequate food sources is less likely than from excess intake of other minerals, especially zinc and possibly iron. ***Excess*** Cooking acid foods in unlined copper pots can lead to chronic and toxic accumulation of copper.
Fluoride† ***Functions*** Formation of caries-resistant teeth Strong bone development ***Sources*** Fluoridated water and foods or beverages prepared with fluoridated water, fish, tea	***Deficiency*** Increased susceptibility to tooth decay ***Excess*** Fluorosis (mottling or pitting of enamel) Severe bone deformities	Fluoride has the narrowest range of safe and adequate intake; therefore stress the importance of storing supplements in a safe area. ***Deficiency*** In areas with optimally fluoridated water, encourage sufficient intake to supply recommended amount of fluoride. In areas of unfluoridated water or when ready-to-use formula, powder formula, bottled water, or breast milk is used, stress the importance of fluoride supplements (age appropriate). ***Excess*** In areas with excess fluoride in the water, consider the use of bottled water (without fluoride) in drinking and cooking to reduce the fluoride intake to safe levels.
Iodine† ***Functions*** Production of thyroid hormone Normal reproduction ***Sources*** Seafood, kelp, iodized salt, sea salt, enriched bread, milk (from dairy processing); medications, including amiodarone, povidone-iodine, and prenatal vitamins	***Deficiency*** Goiter (enlarged thyroid from decreased thyroxine formation) ***Excess*** Thyrotoxicosis; goiter; hypothyroidism	***Deficiency*** Encourage use of iodized salt for individuals living far from the sea. ***Excess*** If iodine preparations are in the home, stress the importance of safe storage.
Iron ***Functions*** Formation of hemoglobin and myoglobin Essential part of several enzymes and proteins ***Sources*** Liver, especially pork, followed by calf, beef, and chicken; kidney, red meat, poultry, shellfish, whole grains, iron-enriched infant formula and cereal, enriched cereals and bread, legumes, nuts, seeds, green leafy vegetables† (except spinach), dried fruits, potatoes, molasses, tofu, prune juice	***Deficiency*** Anemia (see Chapter 49) ***Excess*** Hemosiderosis (excess iron storage in various tissues of the body, especially the spleen, liver, lymph glands, heart, and pancreas) Hemochromatosis (excess iron storage with cellular damage)	***Deficiency*** Discourage excessive iron-fortified milk consumption, especially more than 1 L/day (cow's milk is a poor source of iron). If iron supplements are prescribed, teach parents factors that affect absorption. ***Excess*** Stress the importance of storing iron supplements in a safe area.
Magnesium* ***Functions*** Bone and tooth formation Production of proteins Nerve conduction to muscles Activation of enzymes needed for carbohydrate and protein metabolism ***Sources*** Whole grains, nuts, soybeans, meat, green leafy vegetables (uncooked), tea, cocoa, raisins	***Deficiency*** Tremors, spasm Irregular heartbeat Muscular weakness Lower extremity cramps Convulsions, delirium ***Excess*** Nervous system disturbances caused by imbalance in calcium/magnesium ratio	Deficiency and excess are unusual, except in disease states such as prolonged vomiting or diarrhea or kidney dysfunction, where replacement may be needed.

Table 47-2 Minerals and Their Nutritional Significance—cont'd

PHYSIOLOGIC FUNCTIONS AND SOURCES	RESULTS OF DEFICIENCY OR EXCESS	NURSING CARE MANAGEMENT
Phosphorus* *Functions* Bone and tooth development (in combination with calcium) Involved in numerous chemical reactions, including protein, carbohydrate, and fat metabolism Acid-base balance *Sources* Dairy products, eggs, meat, poultry, legumes, carbonated beverages	*Deficiency* Weakness, anorexia, malaise, bone pain *Excess* Produces secondary calcium deficiency from imbalanced calcium/phosphorus ratio	*Deficiency* Dietary deficiency is uncommon, although prolonged use of antacids can produce deficiency, in which case supplementation is recommended. To preserve calcium/phosphorus ratio in newborns and infants, discourage use of cow's milk.
Potassium* *Functions* Acid-base and fluid balance (major extracellular fluid areas) Nerve conduction Muscular contraction, especially the heart Release of energy *Sources* Bananas, citrus fruit, dried fruits, meat, fish, bran, legumes, peanut butter, potatoes, coffee, tea, cocoa	*Deficiency* Cardiac arrhythmias Muscular weakness Lethargy Kidney and respiratory failure Heart failure *Excess* Cardiac arrhythmias Respiratory failure Mental confusion Numbness of extremities	Dietary deficiency and excess are unlikely, although disease states such as prolonged nausea and vomiting or the use of certain diuretics can result in hypokalemia; in such instances encourage replacement with supplements of rich food sources such as bananas.
Selenium‡ *Functions* Antioxidant, especially protective of vitamin E Protects against toxicity of heavy metals Associated with fat metabolism *Sources* Seafood, organs, egg yolk, whole grains, chicken, meat, tomatoes, cabbage, garlic, mushrooms, milk	*Deficiency* Keshan disease (cardiomyopathy in children; found in China) *Excess* Eye, nose, and throat irritation Increased dental caries Liver and kidney degeneration	Deficiency and excess are uncommon in North America, although selenium deficiency can occur in patients receiving prolonged total parenteral alimentation; in these instances supplementation is required.
Sodium* *Functions* Acid-base and fluid balance (major extracellular fluid cation) Cell permeability; absorption of glucose Muscle contraction *Sources* Table salt, seafood, meat, poultry, numerous prepared foods	*Deficiency* Dehydration Hypotension Convulsions Muscle cramps *Excess* Edema Hypertension Intracranial hemorrhage	*Deficiency* Deficient intake is rare, although losses secondary to nausea, vomiting, excessive sweating, and use of diuretics can occur and require replacement. *Excess* Encourage parents to limit excessive use of salt in preparing foods and to limit commercial foods with high sodium content such as smoked meats.
Zinc† *Functions* Component of about 100 enzymes Synthesis of nucleic acids and protein in immune system and coagulation Release of vitamin A from liver Improved wound healing with vitamin C Normal taste sensitivity *Sources* Seafood (especially oysters), meat, poultry, eggs, wheat, legumes	*Deficiency* Loss of appetite Diminished taste sensation Delayed healing **Skin lesions**—Erythematous, crusted lesions around body orifices (mouth, nares, anus) Alopecia Diarrhea Growth failure Delayed sexual maturity *Excess* Vomiting and diarrhea Malaise, dizziness Anemia, gastric bleeding Impaired absorption of calcium and copper	Emphasize correct use of zinc supplements and the possible interaction with other minerals. *Deficiency* Encourage food sources rich in zinc, especially protein. Caution that fiber, phytates, oxalates, tannins (in tea or coffee), iron, and calcium adversely affect zinc absorption. Recognize groups at risk for zinc deficiency, such as vegetarians and Hispanics, whose diets may have restricted or low meat content and high fiber and phytate content; and patients with malabsorption syndromes.

Table is not intended to be all inclusive.
*Macrominerals—required intake >100 mg/day.
†Green leafy vegetables include spinach, broccoli, kale, turnip greens, mustard greens, collards, dandelion greens, and beet greens.
‡Microminerals or trace elements—required intake <100 mg/day.

Gastrointestinal Dysfunction

The extensive surface area of the GI tract and its digestive function represent the major means of exchange between the human organism and the environment. Inflammatory and malabsorptive disorders impair the functional integrity of the GI tract. In addition, the infant's intestine is extremely vulnerable to infection. Acute infectious diarrhea causes significant alterations in fluid and electrolyte balance in both infants and children.

Numerous clinical observations provide clues to specific GI problems (Box 47-4). In any disorder that involves GI losses of large amounts of fluid, dehydration poses a serious threat to life and demands immediate attention.

Dehydration

Dehydration is a common body fluid disturbance in infants and children and occurs whenever the total output of fluid exceeds the total intake, regardless of the cause. Dehydration may result from a number of diseases that cause insensible losses through the skin and respiratory tract, through increased renal excretion, and through the GI tract. Although dehydration can result from lack of oral intake (especially in elevated environmental temperatures), more often it is a result of abnormal losses, such as those that occur in vomiting or diarrhea, when oral intake only partially compensates for the abnormal losses. Other significant causes of dehydration are diabetic ketoacidosis and extensive burns.

Water Balance in Infants

Compared with older children and adults, infants and young children have a greater need for water and are more vulnerable to alterations in fluid and electrolyte balance. Infants have a greater fluid intake and output relative to size. Water and electrolyte disturbances occur more frequently and more rapidly, and infants and children adjust less promptly to these alterations.

The fluid compartments in the infant vary significantly from those in the adult, primarily because of an expanded extracellular compartment. The *extracellular fluid (ECF)* compartment constitutes more than half the total body water at birth and has a greater relative content of extracellular sodium and chloride. The infant loses a large amount of fluid at birth and maintains a larger amount of ECF than the adult until about 2 years of age. This contributes to greater and more rapid water loss during this age period.

Fluid losses create compartment deficits that are reflected throughout the duration of dehydration. In general approximately 60% of fluid lost is from the ECF, and the remaining

BOX 47-4 Clinical Manifestations of Gastrointestinal Dysfunction in Children

Growth failure—Weight consistently below the 3rd percentile, body mass index below the 5th percentile, or a decrease from established growth pattern

Spitting up or regurgitation—Passive transfer of gastric contents into the esophagus or mouth

Vomiting—Forceful ejection of gastric contents; involves a complex process under central nervous system control that causes salivation, pallor, sweating, and tachycardia; usually accompanied by nausea

Projectile vomiting—Vomiting accompanied by vigorous peristaltic waves and typically associated with pyloric stenosis or pylorospasm

Nausea—Unpleasant sensation vaguely referred to the throat or abdomen with an inclination to vomit

Constipation—Delay or difficulty with the passage of stools that is present for 2 weeks or longer; associated with symptoms that may include blood-streaked stools and abdominal discomfort

Encopresis—Involuntary overflow of incontinent stool causing soiling or incontinence secondary to fecal retention or impaction

Diarrhea—Increase in the number of stools with increased water content as a result of alterations of water and electrolyte transport by the gastrointestinal (GI) tract; may be acute or chronic

Hypoactive, hyperactive, or absent bowel sounds—Evidence of intestinal motility problems that may be caused by inflammation or obstruction

Abdominal distention—Protuberant contour of the abdomen that may be caused by delayed gastric emptying, accumulation of gas or stool, inflammation, or obstruction

Abdominal pain—Pain associated with the abdomen that may be localized or diffuse, acute or chronic; often caused by inflammation, obstruction, or hemorrhage

Gastrointestinal bleeding—May be from an upper or lower GI source and may be acute or chronic

Hematemesis—Vomiting of bright red or denatured blood that results from bleeding in the upper GI tract or from swallowed blood from the nose or oropharynx

Hematochezia—Passage of bright red blood per rectum, usually indicating lower GI tract bleeding

Melena—Passage of dark-colored, "tarry" stools resulting from denatured blood, suggesting upper GI tract bleeding or bleeding from the right colon

Jaundice—Yellow coloration of the skin and sclerae associated with liver dysfunction in infants and children over 2 months of age

Dysphagia—Difficulty swallowing caused by abnormalities in the neuromuscular function of the pharynx or upper esophageal sphincter or by disorders of the esophagus

Dysfunctional swallowing—Impaired swallowing caused by central nervous system defects or structural defects of the oral cavity, pharynx, or esophagus; can cause feeding problems or aspiration

Fever—Common manifestation of illness in children with GI disorders; usually associated with dehydration, infection, or inflammation

evolve Critical Thinking Exercise—Hematemesis

40% comes from the *intracellular fluid (ICF)*. The amount of fluid lost from the ECF increases with acute illness and decreases with chronic loss.

Fluid losses vary with age and are divided into insensible, urinary, and fecal losses. Approximately two thirds of *insensible losses* occur through the skin; the remaining one third is lost through the respiratory tract. Heat and humidity, body temperature, and respiratory rate influence insensible fluid loss. Infants and children have a greater tendency to become highly febrile than do adults. Fever increases insensible water loss approximately 7 ml/kg/24 hr for each degree rise in temperature above 37.2° C (99° F). Fever and increased surface area relative to volume are factors that contribute to greater insensible fluid losses in young patients.

Body Surface Area

The infant's relatively greater body surface area (BSA) allows larger quantities of fluid to be lost in insensible losses through the immature skin. It is estimated that the BSA of the preterm neonate is five times greater, and that of the newborn is two to three times greater, than that of the older child or adult. The proportionately longer GI tract in infancy is another source of fluid loss, especially from diarrhea.

Basal Metabolic Rate

The rate of metabolism in infancy is significantly higher than in adulthood because of the larger BSA in relation to the mass of active tissue. Consequently, a greater production of metabolic wastes must be excreted by the kidneys. Any condition that increases metabolism causes greater heat production, insensible fluid loss, and an increased need for water for excretion. The basal metabolic rate in infants and children is higher to support growth and organ function.

Kidney Function

The kidneys of the infant are functionally immature at birth and inefficient in excreting waste products of metabolism. Of particular importance for fluid balance is the inability of the infant's kidneys to efficiently concentrate or dilute urine, conserve or excrete sodium, and acidify urine. The infant is less able to handle large quantities of solute-free water than is the older child, and infants are more likely to become dehydrated when given excessively concentrated commercial formulas or overhydrated when given excessive water or dilute formula.

Fluid Requirements

Infants ingest and excrete a greater amount of fluid per kilogram of body weight than do older children. Because electrolytes are excreted with water and the infant has limited ability for conservation, maintenance requirements include both water and electrolytes. The daily exchange of ECF in the infant is greatly increased over that of older children, which leaves the infant little fluid volume reserve in dehydrated states. Fluid requirements depend on hydration status, size, environmental factors, and underlying disease. Box 47-5 lists daily maintenance fluid requirements for children.

BOX 47-5 Daily Maintenance Fluid Requirements

1. Calculate weight of child in kilograms:
   Weight of child (in pounds) ÷ 2.2 lb/kg = Weight in kilograms.
2. Allow 100 ml/kg for first 10 kg.
3. Allow 50 ml/kg for second 10 kg.
4. Allow 20 ml/kg for remainder of weight in kilograms.
5. Divide total amount by 24 hours to obtain rate in milliliters per hour.

Types of Dehydration

The pathophysiology of dehydration is understood by recognizing that the distribution of water between the ECF and ICF spaces depends on active transport of potassium into and sodium out of cells by energy-requiring processes. Sodium is the chief solute in ECF and the primary determinant of ECF volume. Potassium is primarily intracellular. When ECF volume is reduced in acute dehydration, the total body sodium content is almost always reduced as well, regardless of serum sodium measurements. Replacement of fluid volume should therefore be accompanied by sodium replacement as well. Sodium depletion in diarrhea occurs in two ways: out of the body in stool and into the ICF compartment to replace potassium to maintain electrical equilibrium.

Dehydration is classified into three categories on the basis of osmolality and depends primarily on the serum sodium concentration: (1) isotonic, (2) hypotonic, and (3) hypertonic.

Isotonic (isosmotic or *isonatremic) dehydration*, the primary form of dehydration in children, occurs in conditions in which electrolyte and water deficits are present in approximately balanced proportions. Water and salt are lost in approximately equal amounts. The observable fluid losses are not necessarily isotonic, since losses from other avenues make adjustments so that the sum of all losses, or the net loss, is isotonic. There is no osmotic force between the ICF and the ECF; thus the major loss is sustained from the ECF compartment. This significantly reduces the plasma volume and the circulating blood volume, which affects the skin, muscles, and kidneys. Shock is the greatest threat to life, and the child with isotonic dehydration displays symptoms characteristic of hypovolemic shock. Plasma sodium remains within normal limits, between 130 and 150 mEq/L.

Hypotonic (hyposmotic or *hyponatremic) dehydration* occurs when the electrolyte deficit exceeds the water deficit, leaving the serum hypotonic. Because ICF is more concentrated than ECF in hypotonic dehydration, water moves from the ECF to the ICF to establish osmotic equilibrium. This movement further increases the ECF volume loss, and shock is a frequent finding. Because there is a greater proportional loss of ECF in hypotonic dehydration, the physical signs tend to be more severe with smaller fluid losses than with isotonic or hypertonic dehydration. Serum sodium concentration is less than 130 mEq/L.

Hypertonic (hyperosmotic or *hypernatremic) dehydration* results from water loss in excess of electrolyte loss and is usually caused by a proportionately larger loss of water or a larger intake of electrolytes. This type of dehydration is the most dangerous and requires more specific fluid therapy. Hypertonic diarrhea may occur in infants who are given fluids by mouth that contain large amounts of solute or in children who receive high-protein nasogastric (NG) tube feedings that place an excessive solute load on the kidneys. In hypertonic

Table 47-3 Evaluating Extent of Dehydration

	Level of Dehydration		
CLINICAL SIGNS	MILD	MODERATE	SEVERE
Weight loss—infants	3%-5%	6%-9%	≥10%
Weight loss—children	3%-4%	6%-8%	10%
Pulse	Normal	Slightly increased	Very increased
Respiratory rate	Normal	Slight tachypnea (rapid)	Hyperpnea (deep and rapid)
Blood pressure	Normal	Normal to orthostatic (>10 mm Hg change)	Orthostatic to shock
Behavior	Normal	Irritable, more thirsty	Hyperirritable to lethargic
Thirst	Slight	Moderate	Intense
Mucous membranes*	Normal	Dry	Parched
Tears	Present	Decreased	Absent, sunken eyes
Anterior fontanel	Normal	Normal to sunken	Sunken
External jugular vein	Visible when supine	Not visible except with supraclavicular pressure	Not visible even with supraclavicular pressure
Skin*	Capillary refill >2 sec	Slowed capillary refill (2-4 sec [decreased turgor])	Very delayed capillary refill (>4 sec) and tenting; skin cool, acrocyanotic or mottled
Urine specific gravity	>1.020	>1.020; oliguria	Oliguria or anuria

Data from Jospe N, Forbes G: Fluids and electrolytes—clinical aspects, *Pediatr Rev* 17(11):395-403, 1996; and Steiner MJ, DeWalt DA, Byerley JS: Is this child dehydrated? *JAMA* 291(22):2746-2754, 2004.

*These signs are less prominent in patients who have hypernatremia.

dehydration, fluid shifts from the lesser concentration of the ICF to the ECF. Plasma sodium concentration is greater than 150 mEq/L.

Because the ECF volume is proportionately larger, hypertonic dehydration consists of a greater degree of water loss for the same intensity of physical signs. Shock is less apparent. However, neurologic disturbances, including alterations in consciousness, poor ability to focus attention, lethargy, increased muscle tone with hyperreflexia, and hyperirritability to stimuli, are more likely to occur. Cerebral changes are serious and may result in permanent damage.

Diagnostic Evaluation

Diagnosis of the type and degree of dehydration is necessary to develop an effective plan of therapy. The degree of dehydration has been described as a percentage of body weight dehydrated: mild—less than 3% in older children or less than 5% in infants; moderate—5% to 10% in infants and 3% to 6% in older children; and severe—more than 10% in infants and more than 6% in older children (Greenbaum, 2007). Water constitutes only 60% to 70% of the infant's weight. However, adipose tissue contains little water and is highly variable in individual infants and children. A more accurate means of describing dehydration is to reflect acute loss (over a period of 48 hours or less) in milliliters per kilogram of body weight. For example, a loss of 50 ml/kg is considered to be a mild fluid loss, whereas a loss of 100 ml/kg produces severe dehydration. Weight is the most important determinant of the percent of total body fluid loss in infants and younger children. However, often the preillness weight is unknown. Other predictors of fluid loss include a changing level of consciousness (irritability to lethargy), response to stimuli, decreased skin elasticity and turgor, prolonged capillary refill (longer than 2 seconds), increased heart rate, and sunken eyes and fontanels. Clinical signs provide clues to the extent of dehydration (Table 47-3). Using multiple predictors increases the sensitivity of assessing the fluid deficit, and early studies have shown a reasonably high degree of agreement between experienced observers in assessment of the level of dehydration. Objective signs of dehydration are present at a fluid deficit of less than 5%. Any two of the following signs—capillary refill greater than 2 seconds, abnormal skin turgor, and abnormal respiratory pattern—are predictors of a deficit of at least 5%. Generally, three or more clinical findings are present at a deficit of 5% to 9%, and four or more findings are found with a deficit of 10% or more (Steiner et al, 2004). Shock, tachycardia, and very low blood pressure are common features of severe depletion of ECF volume (see Shock, Chapter 48).

Therapeutic Management

See discussion on therapeutic management of diarrhea, p. 1387.

Nursing Care Management

Nursing observation and intervention are essential for detection and therapeutic management of dehydration. A variety of circumstances cause fluid losses in infants, and changes can take place quickly. An important nursing responsibility is observation for signs of dehydration. Nursing assessment should begin with observation of general appearance and proceed to more specific observations. Conditions in which dehydration may develop quickly include diarrhea; vomiting; sweating; fever; disorders such as diabetes, renal disease, and cardiac anomalies; administration of certain drugs (such as diuretics and steroids); and trauma (major surgery, burns, and other extensive injury). In addition, any condition that causes a decrease in oral intake such as herpangina, hand-foot-and-mouth disease, or thrush has the potential to cause dehydration in infants and small children.

Intake and Output

Accurate measurements of fluid intake and output are vital to the assessment of dehydration. This includes oral and parenteral intake and losses from urine, stools, vomiting, fistulas, NG suction, sweat, and wound drainage:

Urine—Frequency, color, consistency, and volume (when weighing diapers, approximately 1 g wet diaper weight equals 1 ml urine)
Stools—Frequency, volume, and consistency
Vomitus—Volume, frequency, and type
Sweating—Can be only estimated from frequency of clothing and linen changes

In addition to fluid intake and output, the following observations assist in assessment of dehydration:

Vital signs—Temperature (normal, elevated, or lowered depending on degree of dehydration), pulse (tachycardia), respirations (hyperpnea), and blood pressure (hypotension)
Skin—Color, temperature, turgor, presence or absence of edema, and capillary refill
Mucous membranes—Moisture, color, and presence and consistency of secretions
Body weight—Decreased in relation to degree of dehydration
Fontanel (infants)—Sunken, soft, or normal
Sensory alterations—Presence of thirst

For nursing interventions, see discussion under specific disorders.

Disorders of Motility

Diarrhea

Diarrhea is a symptom that results from disorders involving digestive, absorptive, and secretory functions. It is caused by abnormal intestinal water and electrolyte transport. Worldwide there are an estimated 1.3 billion episodes of diarrhea per year. Approximately 24% of all deaths in children living in developing countries are related to diarrhea and dehydration. Most children living in developing countries who develop diarrhea have mild forms. However, in the United States approximately 200,000 children younger than age 5 are hospitalized, and approximately 200 children younger than 5 years die of diarrhea and dehydration each year (Malek et al, 2006; Staat, 2006).

Diarrheal disturbances involve the stomach and intestines (gastroenteritis), the small intestine (enteritis), the colon (colitis), or the colon and intestines (enterocolitis). Diarrhea is classified as acute or chronic.

Acute diarrhea, a leading cause of illness in children younger than 5 years of age, is defined as a sudden increase in frequency and a change in consistency of stools, often caused by an infectious agent in the GI tract. It may be associated with upper respiratory or urinary tract infections, antibiotic therapy, or laxative use. Acute diarrhea is usually self-limited (less than 14 days' duration) and subsides without specific treatment if dehydration does not occur. *Acute infectious diarrhea (infectious gastroenteritis)* is caused by a variety of viral, bacterial, and parasitic pathogens (Table 47-4).

Chronic diarrhea is defined as an increase in stool frequency and increased water content with a duration of more than 14 days. It is often caused by chronic conditions such as malabsorption syndromes, inflammatory bowel disease (IBD), immunodeficiency, food allergy, lactose intolerance, or chronic nonspecific diarrhea, or it can be the result of inadequate management of acute diarrhea.

Intractable diarrhea of infancy is a syndrome that occurs in the first few months of life, persists for longer than 2 weeks with no recognized pathogens, and is refractory to treatment. The most common cause is acute infectious diarrhea that was not managed adequately.

Chronic nonspecific diarrhea (CNSD), also known as irritable colon or childhood and toddlers' diarrhea, is a common cause of chronic diarrhea in children 6 to 54 months of age. These children have loose stools, often with undigested food particles, and diarrhea greater than 2 weeks' duration. Children with CNSD grow normally and have no evidence of malnutrition, no blood in their stool, and no enteric infection. Dietary indiscretions and food sensitivities have been linked to chronic diarrhea. The excessive intake of juices and artificial sweeteners such as sorbitol, a substance found in many commercially prepared beverages and foods, may be a factor.

evolve Case Study—Acute Diarrhea (Gastroenteritis)

Etiology

Most pathogens that cause diarrhea are spread by the fecal-oral route through contaminated food or water or are spread from person to person where there is close contact (e.g., day care centers). Lack of clean water, crowding, poor hygiene, nutritional deficiency, and poor sanitation are major risk factors, especially for bacterial or parasitic pathogens. The increased frequency and severity of diarrheal disease in infants is also related to age-specific alterations in susceptibility to pathogens. For example, the immune system of infants has not been exposed to many pathogens and has not acquired protective antibodies; newborns do not have a well-developed GI mucosal barrier to many pathogens, thus increasing the predisposition to gastroenteritis. Worldwide, the most common causes of acute gastroenteritis are infectious agents, viruses, bacteria, and parasites. In developed nations viruses, primarily rotavirus, cause 70% to 80% of infectious diarrhea.

Rotavirus is the most important cause of serious gastroenteritis among children and a significant nosocomial (hospital-acquired) pathogen, accounting for 55,000 to 70,000 hospitalizations annually (Staat, 2006). Rotavirus disease is most severe in children 3 to 24 months of age. Children younger than 3 months of age have some protection from the disease because of maternally acquired antibodies. Milder disease occurs in breastfeeding infants.

evolve Case Study—Dehydration and Diarrhea

Salmonella, Shigella, and *Campylobacter* organisms are the most frequently isolated bacterial pathogens. *Salmonella* has the highest occurrence in infants; *Giardia* and *Shigella* have the highest incidence among toddlers. *Shigella* infection is uncommon in the United States, accounting for less than 5% of diarrheal illnesses in infants and toddlers. *Campylobacter* infection has a bimodal presentation (highest in children younger than 12 months of age with a second rise in incidence at age 15 to 19 years). *Giardia* and *Cryptosporidium* organisms are parasites. *Giardia* infection represents 15% of nondysen-

Table 47-4 Infectious Causes of Acute Diarrhea

ORGANISM	PATHOLOGY	CHARACTERISTICS	COMMENTS
Viral Agents			
Rotavirus Incubation: 48 hr Diagnosis: enzyme immunoassay (EIA) and latex agglutination assay	Fecal-oral transmission Seven groups (A-G): Most group A virus replicates in mature villus epithelial cells of small intestine; leads to (1) imbalance in ratio of intestinal fluid absorption to secretion and (2) malabsorption of complex carbohydrates	Mild to moderate fever Vomiting followed by the onset of watery stools Fever and vomiting generally abate in approximately 2 days, but diarrhea persists 5-7 days Adult contacts in household may develop symptomatic infection	Most common cause of diarrhea in children <5 yr of age Infants 6-12 mo are most vulnerable Peak occurrences in winter months; important cause of nosocomial infections Affects all ages; usually milder in children >3 yr of age; immune-compromised children at greater risk for complications Virus can live on toys and hard surfaces (sinks, countertops) Vaccine available for infants
Noroviruses (formerly Norwalk-like) Caliciviruses Incubation: 12-48 hr Diagnosis: EIA, reverse-transcriptase polymerase chain reaction (RT-PCR)	Fecal-oral; contaminated food or water Pathology similar to rotavirus Affects villus epithelial cells of small intestine Leads to (1) imbalance in ratio of intestinal fluid absorption to secretion and (2) malabsorption of complex carbohydrates	Abdominal cramps; nausea, vomiting, malaise, low-grade fever, watery diarrhea without blood; duration brief, 2-3 days; tends to resemble so-called food poisoning symptoms with nausea predominating	Affects all ages Multiple strains often named for the location of outbreak (e.g., Norwalk, Sapporo, Snow Mountain, Montgomery) Common in closed populations such as daycare and cruise ships
Bacterial Agents			
Escherichia coli Incubation: 3-4 days Variable depending on strain Diagnosis: sorbitol MacConkey agar (SMAC agar) + for blood but fecal leukocytes are absent or rare	Five *E. coli* strains produce diarrhea as a result of enterotoxin production, adherence, or invasion; these strains include enterotoxigenic-producing [ETEC], enteroaggregative [EAEC], Shiga toxin–producing [STEC], enteropathogenic [EPEC], and enteroinvasive [EIEC] *E. coli*	Watery diarrhea 1-2 days; then severe abdominal cramping and bloody diarrhea STEC can progress to hemolytic uremic syndrome (HUS) and postdiarrheal thrombotic thrombocytopenia (TTP); 50% require dialysis and 3%-5% die	Food-borne pathogen Traveler's diarrhea Highest incidence in summer Cause of nursery epidemics Symptomatic treatment Antibiotics may worsen course, but meta-analysis shows no harm or benefit from antibiotic therapy (American Academy of Pediatrics, Committee on Infectious Diseases, 2009b) Antimotility agents and opioids should be avoided
Salmonella groups (nontyphoidal; gram-negative rods, nonencapsulated, nonsporulating) Incubation 6-72 hr Diagnosis: gram-stained stool culture	Invasion of mucosa in the small and large intestine; edema of the lamina propria; focal acute inflammation with disruption of the mucosa and microabscesses	Nausea, vomiting, colicky abdominal pain, bloody diarrhea, fever; symptoms variable: mild to severe May have headache, cerebral manifestations (e.g., drowsiness, confusion, meningismus, seizures) Infants may be afebrile and nontoxic May result in life-threatening septicemia and meningitis Nausea/vomiting typically short duration; diarrhea may persist as long as 2-3 wk Typically shed virus for average of 5 wk; cases reported up to 1 yr	Incidence highest in warm months: July to November Food-borne outbreaks common Usually transmitted person to person but may transmit via undercooked meats, poultry Poultry and poultry products cause about half the cases In children: pets (e.g., dogs, cats, hamsters, turtles) Communicable as long as organisms are excreted Antibiotics not recommended in uncomplicated cases Antimotility agents also not recommended—prolong transit time and carrier state Incidence decreasing over past 10 yr

Table 47-4 Infectious Causes of Acute Diarrhea—cont'd

ORGANISM	PATHOLOGY	CHARACTERISTICS	COMMENTS
Salmonella typhi Produces enteric fever–systemic syndrome Incubation usually 7-14 days but could be 3-30 days, depending on size of inoculum Diagnosis: positive blood cultures; also sometimes positive stool and urine Late stage: positive bone marrow culture	Bloodstream invasion; after ingestion, organism attaches to microvilli of ileal brush borders, and bacteria invade the intestinal epithelium via Peyer's patches; is then transported to intestinal lymph nodes and enters bloodstream via thoracic ducts, and circulating organisms reach reticuloendothelial cells causing bacteremia	Manifestations depend on age Abdominal pain; diarrhea; nausea, vomiting, high fever, lethargy Must be treated with antibiotics	Incidence is much lower in developed countries; United States has about 400 cases/yr 65% of U.S. cases acquired via international cases Ingestion of foods/water contaminated with human feces is most common mode of transmission Congenital and intrapartum transmission can occur Three vaccines are available
Shigella species Gram-negative organisms Nonmotile Anaerobic bacilli Incubation: 1-7 days Diagnosis: stool culture Loaded with polymorphonuclear leukocytes	Enterotoxins: invade the epithelium with superficial mucosal ulcerations	Patients appear sick Symptoms begin with fever, fatigue, anorexia Crampy abdominal pain precedes watery or bloody diarrhea Symptoms usually subside in 5-10 days	Most cases in children younger than 9 yr with about one third of cases in children ages 1-4 wk Antibiotics shorten illness and lower mortality risk All patients are at risk for dehydration Acute symptoms may persist for 1 wk or more Antidiarrheal medications not recommended; may predispose to toxic megacolon
Yersinia enterocolitica Incubation period: dose dependent, 1-3 wk Diagnosis: stool culture serology; enzyme-linked immunosorbent assay (ELISA) Patients have leukocytosis; elevated sedimentation rate	Pathology is poorly understood; believe production of enterotoxin	Mucoid diarrhea, sometimes bloody; abdominal pain suggestive of appendicitis; fever, vomiting	Seen more frequently in winter months Transmitted by pets and food Antibiotics usually do not alter the clinical course in uncomplicated cases; they should be used in complicated infections and compromised hosts
Campylobacter jejuni and *Campylobacter coli* Microaerophilic, motile, gram-negative bacilli Incubation period: 1-7 days Ability to cause illness appears dose related Diagnosis by stool culture, sometimes in the blood Commonly found in gastrointestinal (GI) tract of wild or domestic animals	Not fully understood; possibly (1) adherence to intestinal mucosa by toxin; (2) invasion of the mucosa in the terminal ileum and colon; (3) translocation, in which the organisms penetrate the mucosa and replicate in the lamina propria	Fever, abdominal pain, diarrhea, can be bloody; vomiting Watery, profuse, foul-smelling diarrhea Clinically similar to *Salmonella* or *Shigella* Fecal-oral transmission	Most infections in humans relate to consumption of contaminated foods or water; undercooked meats, particularly chicken; unpasteurized milk Also acquired from contaminated household pets (e.g., dogs, cats, hamsters) Bimodal peaks in infants <1 yr and again at ages 15-29 mo Antibiotics do not prolong the carriage of bacteria and may eliminate organism more quickly Erythromycin and azithromycin are drugs of choice (5-7 days) Antimotility agents not recommended and tend to prolong symptoms
Vibrio cholerae Gram-negative, motile, curved bacillus living in bodies of salt water Incubation period: 1-3 days Diagnosis by stool culture	Enters via oral route in contaminated food or water; if survives acid stomach environment, travels to the small intestine, adheres to mucosa, and produces toxin	Onset abrupt; vomiting, watery diarrhea without cramping or tenesmus Dehydration can occur quickly	More prevalent in developing countries Rehydration most important treatment Antibiotics can shorten diarrhea Despite continued efforts, still no vaccine

Continued

Table 47-4 Infectious Causes of Acute Diarrhea—cont'd

ORGANISM	PATHOLOGY	CHARACTERISTICS	COMMENTS
Clostridium difficile Gram-positive anaerobic bacillus Diagnosis by detecting *C. difficile* toxin in stool culture	Produces two important toxins (A and B) Toxin binds to enterocyte surface receptor, resulting in alteration of permeability, protein synthesis, and direct cytotoxicity	Most cases: mild, watery diarrhea lasting few days Some cases: prolonged diarrhea and illness May cause pseudomembranous colitis Some individuals are extremely ill with high fever, leukocytosis, hypoalbuminemia	Associated with alteration of normal intestinal flora by antibiotics More common in hospitalized persons Adults tend to have more severe symptoms than children Treatment with antibiotics in symptomatic patients–metronidazole Resistant strains have developed Relapse common
Clostridium perfringens Incubation period: 8-24 hr; anaerobic, gram-positive, spore-producing bacilli	Toxins produced in the intestine after ingestion of organism	Acute onset: watery diarrhea, crampy abdominal pain Fever, nausea, and vomiting rare Duration of illness usually 24 hr	Transmitted by contaminated food products, most often meats and poultry Usually self-limiting and medical intervention not needed Oral rehydration usually sufficient Antibiotics serve no purpose and should not be used
Clostridium botulinum Incubation period: 12-26 hr (range, 6 hr to 8 days) Gram-positive, anaerobic, spore-producing bacilli Blood and stool culture should be obtained and transmitted to special laboratory (usually state health department) to detect toxin	Botulism caused by binding of toxin to the neuromuscular junction	Clinical presentation related to age and the strain of the botulism Abdominal pain, cramping, and diarrhea Other strains: respiratory compromise, central nervous system symptoms	Transmitted in contaminated food products Can be acquired via wound infection Treatment involves supportive care and neutralization of the toxin
Staphylococcus (food poisoning) Incubation period: generally short, 1-8 hr Gram-positive, nonmotile, aerobic, or facultative anaerobic bacteria Diagnosis by identifying organism in food, blood, pus, aspirate	Direct tissue invasion and production of toxin	Clinical presentation depends on site of entry In food poisoning: profuse diarrhea, nausea, and vomiting Low-grade fever and hypothermia may occur	GI illness transmitted in inadequately cooked or refrigerated foods Self-limiting in GI illness Symptomatic treatment Antibiotics not recommended

teric illness in the United States; *Cryptosporidium* infection is often associated with outbreaks in young children in day care centers. *Plesiomonas* and *Yersinia* are also parasites that are frequently responsible for causing diarrhea that lasts more than 10 days in a previously healthy adolescent.

Antibiotic administration is frequently associated with diarrhea because antibiotics alter the normal intestinal flora, resulting in an overgrowth of other bacteria such as *Clostridium difficile*. National rates of *C. difficile* have more than doubled since 2000 (Richards, 2006). Antibiotic-associated diarrhea can also be caused by *Salmonella* organisms, *Clostridium porringers* type A, and *Staphylococcus aureus* pathogens (Jabbar & Wright, 2003).

Pathophysiology

Invasion of the GI tract by pathogens results in increased intestinal secretion as a result of enterotoxins, cytotoxic mediators, or decreased intestinal absorption secondary to intestinal damage or inflammation. Enteric pathogens attach to the mucosal cells and form a cuplike pedestal on which the bacteria rest. The pathogenesis of the diarrhea depends on whether the organism remains attached to the cell surface, resulting in a secretory toxin (noninvasive, toxin-producing, noninflammatory type diarrhea), or penetrates the mucosa (systemic diarrhea). Noninflammatory diarrhea is the most common diarrheal illness, resulting from the action of enterotoxin that is released after attachment to the mucosa (Ramaswamy & Jacobson, 2001). The most serious and immediate physiologic disturbances associated with severe diarrheal disease are (1) dehydration, (2) acid-base imbalance with acidosis, and (3) shock that occurs when dehydration progresses to the point that circulatory status is seriously impaired.

Diagnostic Evaluation

Evaluation of the child with acute gastroenteritis begins with a careful history that seeks to discover the possible cause of diarrhea, assess the severity of symptoms and the risk of complications, and elicit information about current symptoms indicating other treatable illnesses that could be causing the diarrhea. The history should include questions about recent travel, exposure to untreated drinking or washing water sources, contact with animals or birds, day care center attendance, recent treatment with antibiotics, or recent diet changes. History questions should also explore the presence or absence of other symptoms such as fever and vomiting, frequency and character of stools (e.g., watery, bloody), urinary output, dietary habits, and recent food intake.

Extensive laboratory evaluation is not indicated in children who have uncomplicated diarrhea and no evidence of dehydration because most diarrheal illnesses are self-limiting. Laboratory tests are indicated for children who are severely dehydrated and receiving intravenous (IV) therapy. Watery, explosive stools suggest glucose intolerance; foul-smelling, greasy, bulky stools suggest fat malabsorption. Diarrhea that develops after the introduction of cow's milk, fruits, or cereal may be related to enzyme deficiency or protein intolerance. Neutrophils or red blood cells in the stool indicate bacterial gastroenteritis or IBD. The presence of eosinophils suggests protein intolerance or parasitic infection. Stool cultures should be performed only when blood, mucus, or polymorphonuclear leukocytes are present in the stool; symptoms are severe; there is a history of travel to a developing country; and a specific pathogen is suspected. Gross blood or occult blood may indicate pathogens such as *Shigella, Campylobacter,* or hemorrhagic *Escherichia coli* strains. An enzyme-linked immunosorbent assay (ELISA) may be used to confirm the presence of rotavirus or *Giardia* organisms. If there is a history of recent antibiotic use, the stool should be tested for *C. difficile* toxin. When bacterial and viral cultures are negative and diarrhea persists for more than a few days, stools should be examined for ova and parasites. A stool specimen with a pH of less than 6 and the presence of reducing substances may indicate carbohydrate malabsorption or secondary lactase deficiency. Stool electrolyte measurements may help identify children with secretory diarrhea.

Urine specific gravity should be determined if dehydration is suspected. A complete blood count (CBC), serum electrolytes, creatinine, and blood urea nitrogen (BUN) should be obtained in the child who requires hospitalization. The hemoglobin, hematocrit, creatinine, and BUN levels are usually elevated in acute diarrhea and should normalize with rehydration.

Therapeutic Management

The major goals in the management of acute diarrhea include (1) assessment of fluid and electrolyte imbalance, (2) rehydration, (3) maintenance fluid therapy, and (4) reintroduction of an adequate diet. Infants and children with acute diarrhea and dehydration should be treated first with *oral rehydration therapy (ORT).* ORT is one of the major worldwide health care advances of the past few decades. It is more effective, safer, less painful, and less costly than IV rehydration. The American Academy of Pediatrics, World Health Organization, and Centers for Disease Control and Prevention all recommend ORT as the treatment of choice for most cases of dehydration caused by diarrhea (American Academy of Pediatrics, 2009; Centers for Disease Control and Prevention, 2003b). Oral rehydration solutions (ORSs) enhance and promote the reabsorption of sodium and water, and studies indicate that these solutions greatly reduce vomiting, volume loss from diarrhea, and the duration of the illness. ORSs, including reduced osmolarity ORS, are available in the United States as commercially prepared solutions and are successful in treating the majority of infants with dehydration. Guidelines for rehydration recommended by the American Academy of Pediatrics and the Centers for Disease Control and Prevention are included in Box 47-6.

BOX 47-6 Model for Rehydration

- Rehydration solution should consist of 75 mEq of sodium (Na+) per liter.
- Give 50 to 100 ml/kg of oral rehydration solution over 3 to 4 hours for mild to moderate dehydration.
- Administer in small volumes (e.g., 5 ml [1 tsp] every 5 to 10 minutes by spoon or syringe)
- Replacement and maintenance solution should consist of 40 to 60 mEq of Na+ per liter.
- Reevaluate the need for further hydration; initiate maintenance therapy using maintenance formulations, with daily volumes not to exceed 150 ml/kg/day.
- After initial hydration continue breastfeeding (if doing so previously) or full-strength formula (resume age-appropriate diet)
- Replace fluid losses from vomiting and diarrhea on ongoing basis.

Modified from American Academy of Pediatrics, Provisional Committee on Quality Improvement, Subcommittee on Acute Gastroenteritis: Practice parameter: the management of acute gastroenteritis in young children, *Pediatrics* 97(3):424-435, 1996; Centers for Disease Control and Prevention: Managing acute gastroenteritis among children: oral rehydration, maintenance, and nutritional therapy, *MMWR* 52(RR-16):1-16, 2003.

After rehydration, ORS may be used during maintenance fluid therapy by alternating the solution with a low-sodium fluid such as water, breast milk, lactose-free formula, or half-strength lactose-containing formula. In older children ORS can be given and a regular diet continued. Ongoing stool losses should be replaced on a 1 : 1 basis with ORS. If the stool volume is not known, approximately 10 ml/kg (4 to 8 oz) of ORS should be given for each diarrheal stool.

Solutions for oral hydration are useful in most cases of dehydration, and vomiting is not a contraindication. A child who is vomiting should be given an ORS at frequent intervals and in small amounts. For young children the caregiver may give the fluid with a spoon or small syringe in 5- to 10-ml increments every 1 to 5 minutes. An ORS may also be given via NG or gastrostomy tube infusion. Infants without clinical signs of dehydration do not need ORT. However, they should receive the same fluids recommended for infants with signs of dehydration in the maintenance phase and for ongoing stool losses. The use of probiotics reduces the risk of antibiotic-associated diarrhea in children by 56% (Szajewska, Ruszczynski, & Radzikowski, 2006). *Lactobacillus* GG, *Saccharomyces boulardii,* and *L. reuteri* have been shown to decrease the duration of watery diarrhea by 1 day, particularly diarrhea as a result of rotavirus (Guandalini, 2008).

Prevention

A human-bovine pentavalent rotavirus vaccine (RotaTeq) became available in 2006, and live-attenuated human rotavirus vaccine (Rotarix) was made available in 2008 for the prevention of rotavirus. Infants should receive three doses of RotaTeq oral vaccine at 2, 4, and 6 months of age. Two doses of Rotarix, given at 2 and 4 months of age, will induce protective immunity (see Immunizations, Chapter 36).

NURSING ALERT

- Diarrhea is not managed by encouraging intake of clear fluids by mouth, such as fruit juices, carbonated soft drinks, and gelatin. These fluids usually have high carbohydrate content, very low electrolyte content, and high osmolality.
- Caffeinated soda is avoided because caffeine is a mild diuretic and may lead to increased loss of water and sodium.
- Chicken or beef broth is not given because it contains excessive sodium and inadequate carbohydrate.
- The BRATT diet (bananas, rice, applesauce, toast, and tea) is contraindicated for the child and especially for the infant with acute diarrhea because this diet has little nutritional value (low in energy and protein), is high in carbohydrates, and is low in calories (American Academy of Pediatrics, 2009).

evolve Nursing Care Plan—The Child with Acute Diarrhea (Gastroenteritis)

Early reintroduction of nutrients is desirable and is gaining more widespread acceptance. Continued feeding or early reintroduction of a normal diet has no adverse effects and actually lessens the severity and duration of the illness and improves weight gain when compared with the gradual reintroduction of foods (Zangwill, 2006). Infants who are breastfeeding should continue to do so, and ORS should be used to replace ongoing losses in these infants. Formula-fed infants should resume their formula; formula should not be diluted or mixed with additional water. In older children a regular diet, including milk, can generally be offered after rehydration has been achieved. In toddlers there is no contraindication to continuing soft or pureed foods. A diet of easily digestible foods such as cereals, cooked vegetables, and meats is adequate for the older child.

In cases of severe dehydration and shock, IV fluids are initiated whenever the child is unable to ingest sufficient amounts of fluid and electrolytes to (1) meet ongoing daily physiologic losses, (2) replace previous deficits, and (3) replace ongoing abnormal losses. Patients who usually require IV fluids are those with severe dehydration, those with uncontrollable vomiting, those who are unable to drink for any reason (e.g., extreme fatigue, coma), and those with severe gastric distention.

The IV solution is selected on the basis of what is known regarding the probable type and cause of the dehydration—usually a normal saline solution or lactated Ringer's is used to replace volume, after which a saline solution containing 5% dextrose in ¼ normal saline with potassium chloride (20 mEq/L) may be administered as maintenance therapy. Sodium bicarbonate may be added, since acidosis is usually associated with severe dehydration. Although the initial phase of fluid replacement is rapid in both isotonic and hypotonic dehydration, rapid replacement is contraindicated in hypertonic dehydration because of the risk of water intoxication, especially in the brain cells.

After the severe effects of dehydration are under control, specific diagnostic and therapeutic measures are begun to detect and treat the cause of the diarrhea. Because of the self-limiting nature of vomiting and its tendency to improve when dehydration is corrected, antiemetic agents are often not administered. Ondansetron may be administered to decrease vomiting and increase the effectiveness of oral hydration, thus potentially avoiding IV therapy and hospitalization admissions in children with mild to moderate dehydration (Roslund, Hepps, & McQuillen, 2008). Antidiarrheal medications are not recommended for children. The use of antibiotic therapy in children with acute gastroenteritis is controversial. Antibiotics may shorten the course of some diarrheal illnesses (e.g., those caused by *Shigella* organisms). However, most bacterial diarrheas are self-limiting, and the diarrhea often resolves before the causative organism can be determined. Antibiotics may prolong the carrier period for bacteria such as *Salmonella*. However, antibiotics may be considered in patients with immunosuppression, severe symptoms, or persistent disease or in patients who have had transplantation (Jabbar & Wright, 2003).

Nursing Care Management

The management of most cases of acute diarrhea takes place in the home with education of the caregiver. Caregivers are taught to monitor for signs of dehydration (especially the number of wet diapers or voidings) and the amount of fluids taken by mouth and to assess the frequency and amount of stool losses. Education relating to ORT, including the administration of maintenance fluids and replacement of ongoing losses, is important (see Critical Thinking Exercise). ORS should be administered in small quantities at frequent intervals. Vomiting is not a contraindication to ORT unless it is severe. Information concerning the introduction of a regular diet is essential. Parents need to know that a slightly higher stool output initially occurs with continuation of a normal diet and with ongoing replacement of stool losses. The benefits of a better nutritional outcome with fewer complications and a shorter duration of illness outweigh the potential increase in stool frequency. Parents' concerns should be addressed to ensure adherence to the treatment plan.

If the child with acute diarrhea and dehydration is hospitalized, an accurate weight must be obtained, and intake and output must be carefully monitored. The child may be placed on parenteral fluid therapy with reinstitution of oral fluids and soft foods; keeping the child with gastroenteritis NPO for a long period is usually avoided to prevent changes in intestinal permeability as a result of infection (Centers for Disease Control and Prevention, 2003b). Monitoring the IV infusion is an important nursing function. The nurse must ensure that the correct fluid and electrolyte concentration is infused, the flow rate is adjusted to deliver the desired volume in a given time, and the IV site is maintained.

Accurate measurement of output is essential to determine whether renal blood flow is sufficient to permit the addition of potassium to the IV fluids. The nurse is responsible for examination of stools and collection of specimens for laboratory examination (see Collection of Specimens, Chapter 45). Care should be taken when obtaining and transporting stools to prevent possible spread of infection. A clean tongue depressor can be used to obtain specimens for laboratory examination or as an applicator for transfer to a culture medium. Stool

CRITICAL THINKING EXERCISE

Diarrhea

A mother brings her 8-month-old infant, Mary, to the primary care clinic. The mother reports that Mary has had a "cold" for about 2 days and this morning she began to vomit and has had diarrhea for the past 8 hours. The mother states that Mary is still breastfeeding but that she is not taking as much fluid as usual and she is having three times as many stools as usual (the stools are watery in consistency). When the nurse practitioner examines Mary, she notes that her temperature is 100.4° F (38.0° C), her pulse and blood pressure are in the normal range, her mucous membranes are moist, and she has tears when she cries. The nurse practitioner also notes that Mary's weight has not changed from when she was seen in the clinic 2 weeks ago for her well-child visit. What interventions should the nurse practitioner include in her initial management of Mary?

1. Evidence—Is there sufficient evidence for the nurse practitioner to draw any conclusions for the initial plan of management?
2. Assumptions—Describe some underlying assumptions about the following:
   a. Clinical manifestations of various levels of dehydration
   b. Management of acute diarrhea
   c. Breastfeeding and the management of acute diarrhea
   d. Use of antidiarrheal medications for acute diarrhea in children
3. What nursing interventions should the nurse practitioner implement at this time?
4. Does the evidence support the nurse practitioner's conclusion?
5. Are there any alternative perspectives that the nurse practitioner should consider?

specimens should be transported to the laboratory in appropriate containers and media according to hospital policy.

Diarrheal stools are highly irritating to the skin, and extra care is needed to protect the skin of the perianal and perineal region from excoriation (see Diaper Dermatitis, Chapter 53). Rectal temperatures are avoided because they stimulate the bowel, increasing passage of stool.

Support for the child and family involves the same care and consideration given all hospitalized children (see Chapter 44). Parents are kept informed of the child's progress and instructed in the use of frequent and proper handwashing and the disposal of soiled diapers, clothes, and bed linen. Everyone caring for the child must be aware of "clean" areas and "dirty" areas, especially in the hospital, where the sink in the child's room is used for many purposes. Soiled diapers and linen should be discarded in receptacles close to the bedside. To remind caregivers to keep diapers and other soiled articles away from clean areas, place signs identifying "clean" (e.g., bed table) and "dirty" (e.g., sink, bathroom) areas. List the articles that may be stored in each area on these signs.

Prevention

The best intervention for diarrhea is prevention. The fecal-oral route spreads most infections, and parents need information about preventive measures such as personal hygiene, protection of the water supply from contamination, and careful food preparation.

To reduce the risk of bacteria transmitted via food, encourage parents to:

- Quickly freeze or refrigerate all ground meat and other perishable foods.
- Never thaw food on the counter or let it sit out of the refrigerator for more than 2 hours.
- Wash hands, utensils, and work areas with hot, soapy water after contact with raw meat to keep bacteria from spreading.
- Check ground meat with a fork to make certain no pink is showing before taking a bite.
- Cook all dishes made with ground meat until brown or gray inside or to an internal temperature of 71° C (160° F).

Meticulous attention to perianal hygiene, disposal of soiled diapers, proper handwashing, and isolation of infected persons also minimizes the transmission of infection (see Infection Control, Chapter 45).

Parents need information about preventing diarrhea while traveling. They are cautioned against giving their children adult medications that are used to prevent traveler's diarrhea. Until vaccines or other prophylactic measures are proven to be safe for children, the best measure during travel to areas where water may be contaminated is to allow children to drink only bottled water and carbonated beverages (from the container through a straw supplied from home). Tap water, ice, unpasteurized dairy products, raw vegetables, unpeeled fruits, meats, and seafood should also be avoided. Handwashing is an important measure in the prevention of diarrheal disease, particularly in small children with increased hand-to-mouth activity.

The *expected outcomes* for the child with diarrhea are described in the Nursing Process Box.

Constipation

Constipation is an alteration in the frequency, consistency, or ease of passing stool. Parents often define constipation as passing less than three stools per week. It may also be defined as painful bowel movements, which are often blood streaked or include the retention of stool, with or without soiling, even with a stool frequency of more than three stools per week (Loening-Baucke & Pashankar, 2006). However, the frequency of bowel movements is not considered a diagnostic criterion because it varies widely among children. Having extremely long intervals between defecation is termed *obstipation*. Constipation with fecal soiling is referred to as *encopresis*.

Constipation may arise secondary to a variety of organic disorders or in association with a wide range of systemic disorders. Structural disorders of the intestine, such as strictures, ectopic anus, and Hirschsprung disease (HD), may be associated with constipation. Systemic disorders associated with constipation include hypothyroidism, hypercalcemia resulting from hyperparathyroidism or vitamin D excess, and chronic lead poisoning. Constipation may be associated with drugs such as antacids, diuretics, antiepileptics, antihistamines, opioids, and iron supplementation. Spinal cord lesions may be associated with loss of rectal tone and sensation. Affected

evolve Critical Thinking Exercise—Constipation

NURSING PROCESS: THE CHILD WITH DIARRHEA

Assessment

Observe the infant or child's general appearance and behavior. Assess for dehydration, such as decreased urinary output; decreased weight; dry mucous membranes; poor skin turgor; sunken fontanel; and pale, cool, dry skin. With severe dehydration, increased pulse and respiration, decreased blood pressure, and a prolonged capillary refill time (longer than 2 seconds) may indicate impending shock (see Table 47-3).

A history provides information about probable etiologic agents, such as introduction of a new food, exposure to infectious agents, travel to an area of high susceptibility, contact with foods that might have been contaminated, and contact with pets known to be sources of enteric infections. An allergic, drug, and dietary history may indicate food allergies, use of laxatives or antibiotics, or sources of excess sorbitol and fructose (e.g., apple juice).

Nursing Diagnoses (Problem Identification)

After a thorough assessment, several nursing diagnoses are evident:

Deficient fluid volume related to
- diarrhea (gastrointestinal) losses
- inadequate intake

Risk for infection related to
- microorganisms invading gastrointestinal tract

Impaired skin integrity related to
- irritation caused by frequent loose stools

Planning

Expected patient outcomes include:

- Infant or child will maintain adequate hydration.
- Infant or child will maintain appropriate nutrition for age.
- Infant or child will not spread infection (if etiologic agent) to others.
- Family will receive appropriate support and education, especially regarding home care.

Implementation

Numerous intervention strategies are discussed on pp. 1388-1389.

Evaluation

The effectiveness of nursing interventions for the family and the child with diarrhea is determined by continual assessment and evaluation of care based on the following guidelines:

- Monitor fluid losses with careful intake and output measurements and daily weights.
- Monitor food intake, especially calories.
- Observe for evidence of complications from underlying disease (specify) or therapy.
- Observe and interview family to determine extent and effectiveness of care.

children are prone to chronic fecal retention and overflow incontinence.

The majority of children have *idiopathic* or *functional constipation* since no underlying cause can be identified. Chronic constipation may occur as a result of environmental or psychosocial factors or a combination of the two. Transient illness, withholding and avoidance secondary to painful or negative experiences with stooling, and dietary intake with decreased fluid and fiber all play a role in the etiology of constipation.

Newborn Period

Normally the newborn infant passes a first meconium stool within 24 to 36 hours of birth. Any infant who does not do so should be assessed for evidence of intestinal atresia or stenosis, HD, hypothyroidism, meconium plugs, or meconium ileus. *Meconium plugs* are caused by meconium that has reduced water content and are usually evacuated after digital examination but may require irrigation with a hypertonic solution or contrast medium.

Meconium ileus, the initial manifestation of cystic fibrosis, is the luminal obstruction of the distal small intestine by abnormal meconium. Treatment is the same as for a meconium plug; early surgical intervention may be needed to evacuate the small intestine.

Infancy

The onset of constipation frequently occurs during infancy and may result from organic causes such as HD, hypothyroidism, and strictures. It is important to differentiate these conditions from functional constipation. Constipation in infancy is often related to dietary practices. It is less common in breastfed infants, who have softer stools than bottle-fed infants. Breastfed infants may also have decreased stools because of more complete use of breast milk with little residue. When constipation occurs with a change from human milk or modified cow's milk to whole cow's milk, simple measures, such as adding or increasing the amount of cereal, vegetables, and fruit in the infant's diet, usually correct the problem. When a bottle-fed infant passes a hard stool that results in an anal fissure, stool-withholding behaviors may develop in response to pain on defecation (see Critical Thinking Exercise).

Childhood

Most constipation in early childhood is the result of environmental changes or normal development when a child begins to attain control over bodily functions. A child who has experienced discomfort during bowel movements may deliberately try to withhold stool. Over time, the rectum accommodates to the accumulation of stool, and the urge to defecate passes. When the bowel contents are ultimately evacuated, the accumulated feces are passed with pain, thus reinforcing the desire to withhold stool.

Constipation in school-age children may represent an ongoing problem or a first-time event. The onset of constipation at this age is often the result of environmental changes, stresses, and changes in toileting patterns. A common cause of new-onset constipation at school entry is fear of using the school bathrooms, which are noted for their lack of privacy.

CRITICAL THINKING EXERCISE

Constipation

Harry, an 8-month-old infant, is seen by the pediatric nurse practitioner for his well-child visit. Harry's mother states that he usually has one hard stool every 4 to 5 days, which causes discomfort when the stool is passed. He has also had one episode of diarrhea and two episodes of ribbonlike stools. Abdominal distention and vomiting have not accompanied the constipation, and Harry's growth has been appropriate. Currently his diet consists of cow's milk formula only. Harry's mother reports that the infrequent passage of hard stools began approximately 6 weeks ago when she stopped breastfeeding. Which interventions should the nurse practitioner include in the initial management of Harry's problem?

1. Evidence—Is there sufficient evidence for the nurse practitioner to draw any conclusions about the management of Harry's problem?
2. Assumptions—Describe some underlying assumptions about the following:
   a. Causes of constipation in infants
   b. Factors associated with functional constipation in infants
   c. Management of functional constipation in infants
3. What interventions should the nurse practitioner implement at this time?
4. Does the evidence support these interventions?
5. Are there alternative perspectives that the nurse practitioner should consider? What are they?

Early and hurried departure for school immediately after breakfast may also impede bathroom use.

The management of simple constipation consists of a plan to promote regular bowel movements. Often this is as simple as changing the diet to provide more fiber and fluids, eliminating foods known to be constipating, and establishing a bowel routine that allows for regular passage of stool. Stool-softening agents such as docusate or lactulose may also be helpful. Polyethylene glycol (PEG) 3350 without electrolytes (Miralax) is a chemically inert polymer that has been introduced as a new laxative in recent years. It is tolerated well by children because it can be mixed in a beverage of choice (Loening-Baucke & Pashankar, 2006). If other symptoms such as vomiting, abdominal distention, or pain and evidence of growth failure are associated with the constipation, the condition should be investigated further.

Nursing Care Management

Constipation tends to be self-perpetuating. A child who has difficulty or discomfort when attempting to evacuate the bowels has a tendency to retain the bowel contents, and this may initiate a vicious cycle. Nursing assessment begins with an accurate history of bowel habits; diet; events associated with the onset of constipation; drugs or other substances that the child may be taking; and the consistency, color, frequency, and other characteristics of the stool. If there is no evidence of a pathologic condition, the major tasks are to educate the parents regarding normal stool patterns and to participate in the education and treatment of the child.

BOX 47-7 High-Fiber Foods

Bread, Grains
Whole-grain bread or rolls
Whole-grain cereals
Bran
Pancakes, waffles, and muffins with fruit or bran
Unrefined (brown) rice

Vegetables
Raw vegetables, especially broccoli, cabbage, carrots, cauliflower, celery, lettuce, and spinach
Cooked vegetables, such as those listed previously and asparagus, beans, Brussels sprouts, corn, potatoes, rhubarb, squash, string beans, and turnips

Fruits
Raw fruits, especially those with skins or seeds, other than ripe banana or avocado
Raisins, prunes, or other dried fruits

Miscellaneous
Nuts, seeds, legumes, popcorn
High-fiber snack bars

Dietary modifications are essential in preventing constipation. During infancy, simply increasing the carbohydrate (dark corn syrup) in the infant's formula often relieves the problem. During childhood the diet should contain increased amounts of fiber and fluid. Parents benefit from guidance in selecting foods that facilitate bowel movements (Box 47-7). They need reassurance concerning the benign nature of the condition. It is also important to discuss their attitudes and expectations regarding toilet habits.

When constipation persists despite dietary intervention, more aggressive management may be necessary. It is important to differentiate an acute episode of constipation from chronic functional constipation, which can result from chronic stool-withholding behavior. As the rectal vault becomes distended over time, further complications such as fecal impaction and encopresis may develop (see Chapter 39).

Hirschsprung Disease

HD *(congenital aganglionic megacolon)* is a mechanical obstruction caused by inadequate motility of part of the intestine. It accounts for about one fourth of all cases of neonatal obstruction, although it may not be diagnosed until later in infancy or childhood. The incidence is 1 in 5000 live births (Wyllie, 2007a). It is four times more common in males than in females and may follow a familial pattern in about 10% of cases. HD is usually an isolated birth defect, but it has been associated with other syndromes, including Down syndrome. Mutations in the RET proto-oncogene have been found in 17% to 38% of children with short-segment HD and in 70% to 80% of those with long-segment involvement (Dasgupta & Langer, 2004). Depending on its presentation, it may be an acute, life-threatening, or chronic condition.

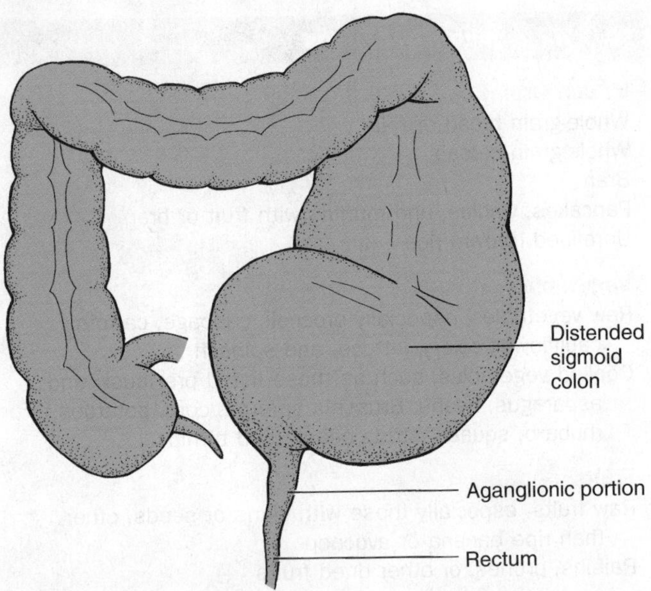

Fig. 47-2 Hirschsprung disease.

Pathophysiology

HD is a developmental disorder of the enteric nervous system that is characterized by the absence of ganglion cells, originating from the neural crest in both the Auerbach myenteric and Meissner submucosal plexuses of the distal intestine. The length of the aganglionic distal bowel depends on the timing of the arrest in craniocaudal migration of ganglion cells. The aganglionic bowel is chronically contracted. This results in absent peristalsis in the affected bowel and the development of a functional intestinal obstruction (Fig. 47-2) (Dasgupta & Langer, 2004). Intestinal distention and ischemia may also occur as a result of distention of the bowel wall, which contributes to the development of *enterocolitis* (inflammation of the small bowel and colon). Enterocolitis is characterized by fever, abdominal distention, and diarrhea that may be severe and lead to life-threatening dehydration or sepsis (Dasgupta & Langer, 2004).

Diagnostic Evaluation

Most children with HD are diagnosed in the first few months of life. Clinical manifestations vary according to the age when symptoms are recognized and the presence of complications such as enterocolitis (Box 47-8). A neonate usually is seen with distended abdomen, feeding intolerance with bilious vomiting, and delay in the passage of meconium. Typically, 95% of normal-term infants pass meconium in the first 24 hours of life, whereas fewer than 10% of infants with HD do so. In older children a careful history is helpful. Radiographs, an unprepped barium enema, and anorectal manometric examinations assist in the differential diagnosis, which is confirmed by a full-thickness rectal biopsy demonstrating the absence of ganglion cells in the myenteric and submucosal plexuses.

Therapeutic Management

Treatment is primarily surgery to remove the aganglionic portion of the bowel to relieve obstruction and restore normal bowel motility and function of the internal anal sphincter. If the bowel is not significantly distended, this is accomplished in one surgery. However, in most cases two stages are required. First, a temporary ostomy is created proximal to the aganglionic segment to relieve obstruction and allow the normally enervated and dilated bowel to return to its normal size. Complete corrective surgery is performed later. The various surgical procedures that can be performed are the Swenson, Duhamel, Boley, and Soave procedures. The Soave endorectal pull-through procedure, one of the most frequently used procedures, consists of pulling the end of the normal bowel through the muscular sleeve of the rectum, from which the aganglionic mucosa has been removed. The ostomy is usually closed at the time of the pull-through procedure.

Prognosis

Most children with HD require surgery rather than medical therapy. Once the child is stabilized with fluid and electrolyte replacement, if needed, the temporary colostomy is performed and has a high rate of success. After the later pull-through procedure, anal stricture and incontinence are potential complications, requiring further therapy, including dilation or bowel-retraining therapy.

BOX 47-8 Clinical Manifestations of Hirschsprung Disease

Newborn Period
Failure to pass meconium within 24 to 48 hours after birth
Refusal to feed
Bilious vomiting
Abdominal distention

Infancy
Growth failure
Constipation
Abdominal distention
Episodes of diarrhea and vomiting
Signs of enterocolitis
Explosive, watery diarrhea
Fever
Appears significantly ill

Childhood (Symptoms Appear More Chronic)
Constipation
Ribbonlike, foul-smelling stools
Abdominal distention
Visible peristalsis
Easily palpable fecal mass
Undernourished, anemic appearance

Nursing Care Management

The nursing concerns depend on the child's age and the type of treatment. If the disorder is diagnosed during the neonatal period, the main objectives are to (1) help the parents adjust to a congenital defect in their child, (2) foster infant-parent bonding, (3) prepare them for the medical-surgical intervention, and (4) assist them in colostomy care after discharge.

Preoperative Care

The child's preoperative care depends on the age and clinical condition. A child who is malnourished may not be able to withstand surgery until his or her physical status improves.

Often this involves symptomatic treatment with enemas; a low-fiber, high-calorie, and high-protein diet; and in severe situations the use of total parenteral nutrition (TPN).

Physical preoperative preparation includes the same measures that are common to any surgery (see Surgical Procedures, Chapter 45). In the newborn, whose bowel is sterile, no additional preparation is necessary. However, in other children, preparation for the pull-through procedure involves emptying the bowel with repeated saline enemas and decreasing bacterial flora with oral or systemic antibiotics and colonic irrigations using antibiotic solution. Enterocolitis is the most serious complication of HD. Emergency preoperative care includes frequent monitoring of vital signs and blood pressure for signs of shock; monitoring fluid and electrolyte replacements and plasma or other blood derivatives; and observing for symptoms of bowel perforation, such as fever, increasing abdominal distention, vomiting, increased tenderness, irritability, dyspnea, and cyanosis.

Because progressive distention of the abdomen is a serious sign, the nurse measures abdominal circumference with a paper tape measure, usually at the level of the umbilicus or at the widest part of the abdomen. The point of measurement is marked with a pen to ensure reliability of subsequent measurements. Abdominal measurement can be obtained with the vital sign measurements and is recorded in serial order so that any change is obvious. To reduce stress to the acutely ill child when frequent measurements of abdominal circumference are needed, the tape measure can be left in place beneath the child rather than removed each time.

The child's age dictates the type and extent of psychologic preparation. Because a colostomy is usually performed, the child who is of preschool age is told about the procedure in concrete terms with the use of visual aids (see Chapter 44). It is important to time explanations appropriately to prevent the anxiety and confusion that could result from too much information. It is also important to stress to parents and older children that the colostomy for HD is temporary, unless so much bowel is involved that a permanent ileostomy must be performed. In most instances the extent of bowel resection is known before surgery, although the nurse should be aware of cases when doubt exists concerning repair. The nurse should remember that, although a temporary colostomy is favorable in terms of future health and adjustment, it requires additional surgery, which may be stressful to parents and children.

Postoperative Care

Postoperative care is the same as that for any child or infant with abdominal surgery (see Surgical Procedures, Chapter 45). When a colostomy is part of the corrective procedure, stomal care is a major nursing task (see Ostomies, Chapter 45). To prevent contamination of an infant's abdominal wound with urine, the diaper should be pinned below the dressing. Sometimes a Foley catheter is used in the immediate postoperative period to divert the flow of urine away from the abdomen.

Discharge Care

After surgery, parents need instruction concerning colostomy care. Even a preschooler can be included in the care by handing articles to the parent, rolling up the colostomy pouch after it is emptied, or applying barrier preparations to the surrounding skin. Although the diagnosis of HD is less frequent in school-age children or adolescents, children this age can often be involved in colostomy care to the point of total responsibility.

Some institutions and communities have enterostomal therapists who provide expert assistance in planning home care. If families require financial assistance and psychologic support, referral to a social worker, home health care agency, or community health nurse provides continuity of care.

Vomiting

Vomiting is the forceful ejection of gastric contents through the mouth. It is a well-defined, complex, coordinated process that is under central nervous system control and is often accompanied by nausea and retching. Vomiting may be divided into two categories: nonbilious and bilious. Some small intestinal reflux is common in all vomiting. In nonbilious vomiting, the majority of bile drains into the more distal portions of the intestine. If an obstruction is present, nonbilious vomiting suggests a more proximal obstruction. Bilious vomiting implies a disorder of motility or distal physical blockage. Causes of nonbilious vomiting include infectious, inflammatory, metabolic or endocrinologic, neurologic, and psychologic causes and obstructive lesions. Causes of bilious vomiting include intestinal atresia and stenosis, malrotation with or without volvulus, ileus, intussusceptions, intestinal duplication, mass lesions, incarcerated inguinal hernia, and appendicitis. Vomiting may also be associated with other processes, including acute infectious diseases, increased intracranial pressure, toxic ingestions, food intolerances and allergies, mechanical obstruction of the GI tract, metabolic disorders, and psychogenic problems. It is common in childhood, is usually self-limiting, and requires no specific treatment. However, complications may occur, including dehydration and electrolyte disturbances, malnutrition, aspiration, and Mallory-Weiss syndrome (small tears in the distal esophageal mucosa).

Therapeutic Management

Management is directed toward detection and treatment of the cause of the vomiting and prevention of complications from the loss of fluid. Fluids are administered in the same manner and in a similar electrolyte composition to those administered for diarrhea. Although most children respond to these measures, antiemetic drugs may be needed. Antiemetics such as ondansetron (Zofran) and trimethobenzamide (Tigan) block receptors in the chemoreceptor trigger zone; others such as metoclopramide (Reglan) enhance gastroduodenal peristalsis; still others such as promethazine (Phenergan) compete for H_1-receptor sites. For children who are prone to motion sickness, it is helpful to administer an appropriate dose of dimenhydrinate (Dramamine) before a trip.

Nursing Care Management

The major focus of nursing care is observing and reporting vomiting behavior and associated symptoms and implementing measures to reduce the vomiting. Accurate assessment of the type of vomiting, the appearance of the vomitus, and the child's behavior in association with the vomiting helps to establish a diagnosis.

Nursing interventions are determined by the cause of the vomiting. When the vomiting is a manifestation of improper feeding methods, establishing proper techniques through teaching and example usually corrects the situation. If vomiting is believed to be an indication of obstruction, food is usually withheld, or special feeding techniques are implemented. In situations in which vomiting is related to concurrent infection, dietary indiscretion, or emotional factors, efforts are directed toward maintaining hydration or preventing dehydration.

The thirst mechanism is the most sensitive guide to fluid needs, and ad libitum administration of a glucose-electrolyte solution to an alert child restores water and electrolytes satisfactorily. It is important to include carbohydrate to spare body protein and avoid ketosis resulting from exhaustion of glycogen stores. Small, frequent feedings of fluids or foods are preferred. After vomiting has stopped, more liberal amounts of fluids are offered, followed by gradual resumption of the regular diet.

The vomiting infant or child is positioned on the side or semireclining to prevent aspiration and observed for evidence of dehydration. It is important to emphasize the need for the child to brush the teeth or rinse the mouth after vomiting to dilute hydrochloric acid that comes in contact with the teeth. A flavored mouthwash or tooth brushing freshens the mouth. Careful monitoring of fluid and electrolyte status is necessary to prevent an electrolyte disturbance.

Gastroesophageal Reflux

Gastroesophageal reflux (GER) is defined as the transfer of gastric contents into the esophagus. This phenomenon is physiologic, occurring throughout the day, most frequently after meals and at night; therefore it is important to differentiate GER from *gastroesophageal reflux disease (GERD)*. GERD represents symptoms or tissue damage that results from GER. Approximately 50% of infants younger than 2 months old are reported to have GER (Suwandhi, Ton, & Schwarz, 2006). This "physiologic" GER usually resolves spontaneously by 1 year of age. GER becomes a disease when complications such as growth failure, bleeding, or dysphagia develop. GERD is associated with respiratory symptoms, including apnea, bronchospasm, laryngospasm, and pneumonia. Heartburn is also a frequent symptom in children who are able to describe it (Box 47-9). Certain conditions predispose children to a high prevalence of GERD, including neurologic impairment, hiatal hernia, repaired esophageal atresia, and morbid obesity (Suwandhi, Ton, & Schwarz, 2006).

Sandifer syndrome is an uncommon condition, usually occurring in young children, characterized by repetitive stretching and arching of the head and neck that can be mistaken for a seizure. This maneuver likely represents a physiologic neuromuscular response attempting to prevent acid refluxate from reaching the upper portion of the esophagus (Cavataio & Guandalini, 2005).

Pathophysiology

Although the pathogenesis of GER is multifactorial, its primary causative mechanism likely involves inappropriate transient relaxation of the lower esophageal sphincter (LES) (Suwandhi, Ton, & Schwarz, 2006). Factors that increase abdominal pressure such as coughing and sneezing, scoliosis, and overeating may contribute to GERD. Esophageal symptoms are caused by inflammation from the acid in the gastric refluxate, whereas reactive airway disease may result from stimulation of airway reflexes by the acid refluxate.

BOX 47-9 Clinical Manifestations and Complications of Gastroesophageal Reflux

Symptoms in Infants

Spitting up, regurgitation, vomiting (may be forceful)
Excessive crying, irritability, arching of the back, stiffening
Weight loss, growth failure
Respiratory problems (cough, wheeze, stridor, gagging, choking with feedings)
Hematemesis
Apnea or apparent life-threatening event (ALTE)

Symptoms in Children

Heartburn
Abdominal pain
Noncardiac chest pain
Chronic cough
Dysphagia
Nocturnal asthma
Recurrent pneumonia

Complications

Esophagitis
Esophageal stricture
Laryngitis
Recurrent pneumonia
Anemia
Barrett's esophagus

Adapted from Rudolph CD et al: Guidelines for evaluation and treatment of gastroesophageal reflux in infants and children: recommendations of the North American Society for Pediatric Gastroenterology and Nutrition, *J Pediatr Gastroenterol Nutr* 32(Suppl 2):S1-S31, 2001.

Diagnostic Evaluation

The history and physical examination are usually sufficiently reliable to establish the diagnosis of GER. However, the upper GI series is helpful in evaluating the presence of anatomic abnormalities (e.g., pyloric stenosis, malrotation, annular pancreas, hiatal hernia, esophageal stricture). The 24-hour intraesophageal pH monitoring study is the gold standard in the diagnosis of GER (Suwandhi, Ton, & Schwarz, 2006). Endoscopy with biopsy may be helpful to assess the presence and severity of esophagitis, strictures, and Barrett esophagus and to exclude other disorders such as Crohn's disease. *Scintigraphy* detects radioactive substances in the esophagus after a feeding of the compound and assesses gastric emptying. It can differentiate between aspiration of gastric contents from reflux vs. aspiration from poor oropharyngeal muscle coordination.

Therapeutic Management

Therapeutic management of GER depends on its severity. No therapy is needed for the infant who is thriving and has no respiratory complications. Avoidance of certain foods that exacerbate acid reflux (e.g., caffeine, citrus, tomatoes, alcohol, peppermint, spicy or fried foods), lifestyle modifications in children (e.g., weight control if indicated; small, more frequent meals; smoking cessation [in symptomatic children]), and feeding maneuvers in infants (e.g., thickened feedings, upright positioning) can improve mild GER symptoms. Thickened feedings do not improve pH scores on 24-hour intraesophageal monitoring but may decrease the number of vomiting episodes. Feedings thickened with 1 tsp to 1 tbsp of rice cereal per ounce of formula may be recommended. This may benefit infants who are underweight as a result of GERD. Constant NG feedings may be necessary for the infant with severe reflux and growth failure until surgery can be performed. Elevating the head of the bed 30 degrees or placing the infant in an infant seat elevated 30 degrees for 1 hour after feedings may decrease GER. Prone positioning of infants also decreases episodes of GER but is recommended only with extreme caution when the risk of GERD complications exceeds the risk of sudden infant death syndrome (Cavataio & Guandalini, 2005). The American Academy of Pediatrics recommends supine positioning for sleep (see Chapter 36). If the prone position is used, parents need to be cautioned to avoid soft bedding.

Pharmacologic therapy may be used to treat infants and children with GERD. Both H_2-receptor antagonists (cimetidine [Tagamet], ranitidine [Zantac], or famotidine [Pepcid]) and proton pump inhibitors (PPIs; esomeprazole [Nexium], lansoprazole [Prevacid], omeprazole [Prilosec], pantoprazole [Protonix], and rabeprazole [Aciphex]) reduce gastric hydrochloric acid secretion and may stimulate some increase in LES tone. Use of available prokinetic drugs (e.g., bethanechol [Urecholine] and metoclopramide) remains controversial. Careful analyses of published data have failed to demonstrate clinical efficacy in modifying the natural history or therapeutic outcomes of GER in childhood (Suwandhi, Ton, & Schwarz, 2006).

Surgical management of GER is reserved for children with severe complications such as recurrent aspiration pneumonia, apnea, severe esophagitis, or growth failure and for children who have failed to respond to medical therapy. The *Nissen fundoplication* (Fig. 47-3) is the most common surgical procedure (Christian & Buyske, 2005). This surgery involves passage of the gastric fundus behind the esophagus to encircle the distal esophagus. The most recent surgical advance for GER is the introduction of the laparoscopic Nissen fundoplication (Durkin & Shaaban, 2008). Complications following fundoplication include breakdown of the wrap, small bowel obstruction, gas-bloat syndrome, infection, retching, and dumping syndrome (Rudolph et al, 2001).

Nursing Care Management

Nursing care is directed at (1) identifying children with symptoms; (2) educating parents regarding home care, including feeding, positioning, and medications; and (3) if appropriate, providing care for the child undergoing surgical repair (see Surgical Procedures, Chapter 45). Early in the treatment program, parents should be reassured that most infants and children outgrow GER and often conservative lifestyle changes are sufficient. Parents need support and reassurance to implement lifestyle changes. Although it is not known if lifestyle changes bring additional benefit to patients receiving pharmacologic interventions, some changes may be helpful. To help parents cope with the inconvenience of dealing with a child who spits up frequently, simple measures such as using bibs and protective cloths during and after feedings are beneficial. Older children and adolescents need to know that caffeine, chocolate, and spicy foods may weaken the LES and aggravate symptoms. Exposure to tobacco and alcohol are also associated with GER. Obesity increases abdominal pressure, and weight management may reduce GER symptoms. When medical management is necessary, parents need information about the medications and their potential side effects. Prokinetic medications must be given before feedings. Medications for acid control must be timed to provide coverage and given regularly and as ordered.

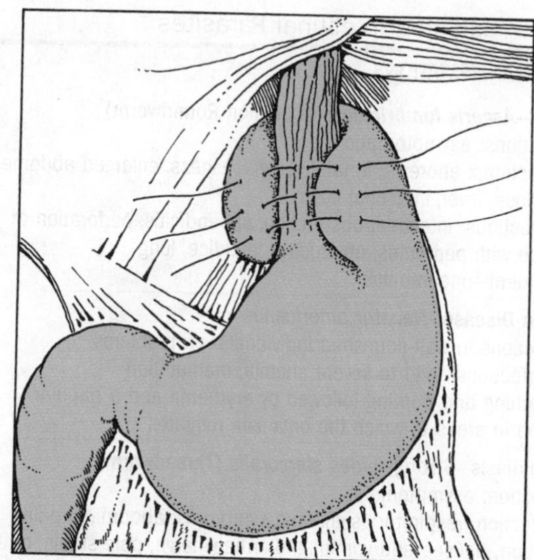

Fig. 47-3 Nissen fundoplication sutures passing through esophageal musculature. (Redrawn from Campbell A, Ferrara B: *AORN J* 57:671-679, 1993.)

Intestinal Parasitic Diseases

Intestinal parasitic diseases, including helminths (worms) and protozoa, constitute the most frequent infections in the world. In the United States the incidence of intestinal parasitic disease, especially giardiasis, has increased among young children who attend day care centers. Young children are especially at risk because of typical hand-mouth activity and uncontrolled fecal activity.

Intestinal parasitic diseases in humans are caused by various infecting organisms. This discussion is limited to the two most common parasitic infections among children in the United States: giardiasis and pinworms. Table 47-5 describes the outstanding features of selected helminths that belong to the family of nematodes.

General Nursing Care Management

Nursing responsibilities related to intestinal parasitic infections involve assistance with identification of the parasite, treatment of the infection, and prevention of initial infection or reinfection. Identification of the organism is accomplished by laboratory examination of substances containing the worm, its larvae, or ova. Most are identified by examining fecal smears from the stools of persons suspected of harboring the

Table 47-5 Selected Intestinal Parasites

CLINICAL MANIFESTATIONS	COMMENTS
Ascariasis—*Ascaris lumbricoides* (Common Roundworm) Light infections: asymptomatic Heavy infections: anorexia, irritability, nervousness, enlarged abdomen, weight loss, fever, intestinal colic Severe infections: intestinal obstruction, appendicitis, perforation of intestine with peritonitis, obstructive jaundice, lung involvement—pneumonitis	Transferred to mouth by way of contaminated food, fingers, or toys Largest of the intestinal helminths Affects principally young children 1-4 yr of age Prevalent in warm climates
Hookworm Disease—*Necator americanus* Light infections in well-nourished individuals: no problems Heavier infections: mild to severe anemia, malnutrition May be itching and burning followed by erythema and a papular eruption in areas to which the organism migrates	Transmitted by discharging eggs on the soil, which are picked up, causing infection from direct skin contact with contaminated soil Wearing shoes is recommended, although children playing in contaminated soil expose many skin surfaces
Strongyloidiasis—*Strongyloides stercoralis* (Threadworm) Light infection: asymptomatic Heavy infection: respiratory signs and symptoms; abdominal pain, distention; nausea and vomiting; diarrhea—large, pale stools, often with mucus Threat to life in children with weakened immunologic defenses Elevated eosinophils may be the only manifestation	Transmission is same as for hookworm (direct contact with human skin), except autoinfection (organism can complete its lifecycle in humans) is common Older children and adults affected more often than young children Severe infections may lead to severe nutritional deficiency Prevalent in warm climates
Visceral Larva Migrans—*Toxocara canis* (Dogs); Intestinal Toxocariasis—*Toxocara cati* (Cats) Depends on reactivity of infected individual May be asymptomatic except for eosinophilia Specific diagnosis difficult	Transmitted by ingestion of or contact with soil containing eggs from feces of infected dog or cat Dogs and cats should be kept away from areas where children play; sandboxes are especially comment transmission areas More prevalent in hot, humid environments where eggs remain in soil Periodic deworming of diagnosed dogs and cats Control of dog and cat population Continued education and laws to prevent indiscriminate canine and feline defecation
Trichuriasis—*Trichuris trichiura* (Whipworm) Light infections: asymptomatic Heavy infections: abdominal pain and distention, diarrhea	Transmitted from contaminated soil or from vegetables grown in soil where eggs are present Most frequent in warm, moist climates Occurs most often in undernourished children living in unsanitary conditions

parasite. Fresh specimens are best for revealing parasites or larvae; therefore collected specimens should be taken directly to the laboratory for examination. If this is not feasible, the specimen is placed in a container with a preservative. Parents need clear instructions on obtaining an adequate sample and the number of samples required (see Stool Specimens, Chapter 45). In most parasitic infections, examination of other family members, especially children, may be carried out to identify those who are similarly affected.

After the diagnosis is confirmed and appropriate treatment is planned, parents need further explanation and reinforcement. Compliance in terms of drug therapy and other measures, such as thorough handwashing, is essential for eradication of the parasite. The family needs to understand the nature of transmission and that in some cases the medication must be repeated in 2 weeks to 1 month to kill organisms hatched since initial treatment.

The nurse's most important function is preventive education of children and families regarding hygiene and health habits. Thorough handwashing before eating or handling food and after using the toilet is the most important precautionary method.

Giardiasis

Giardiasis is caused by the protozoan *Giardia lamblia* (also called *Giardia intestinalis, Giardia duodenalis,* and *Lamblia intestinalis*). It is the most common intestinal parasitic pathogen in the United States. Child care centers and institutions providing care for persons with developmental disabilities are common sites for urban giardiasis, and the children may pass cysts for months. Giardiasis should also be considered in those with a history of recent travel to an endemic area.

The potential for transmission is great, because the *cysts*—the nonmotile stage of the protozoa—can survive in the environment for months. Chief modes of transmission are person to person; contaminated water, especially in mountain lakes and streams and swimming or wading pools frequented by diapered infants (who have the condition); food; and animals, especially puppies. In children, person-to-person transmission is the most likely cause. Although individuals infected with giardiasis may be asymptomatic, common symptoms include abdominal cramps and diarrhea (Box 47-10).

Diagnosis of giardiasis may be made by microscopic examination of stool specimens or duodenal fluid or by identification of *G. lamblia* antigens in these specimens by techniques

BOX 47-10 Clinical Manifestations of Giardiasis

Infants and young children:
- Diarrhea
- Vomiting
- Anorexia
- Growth failure

Children older than 5 years of age:
- Abdominal cramps
- Intermittent loose stools
- Constipation
- Stools may be malodorous, watery, pale, and greasy

Most infections resolve spontaneously in 4 to 6 weeks

Rarely, chronic form occurs:
- Intermittent loose, foul-smelling stools
- Possibility of abdominal bloating, flatulence, sulfur-tasting belches, epigastric pain, vomiting, headache, and weight loss

such as enzyme immunoassay (EIA). Because the *Giardia* organisms live in the upper intestine and are excreted in a highly variable pattern, repeated microscopic examination of stool specimens may be required to identify *trophozoites* (active parasites) or cysts. Duodenal specimens are obtained by direct aspiration, biopsy, or the *string* test. In the string test, the child swallows a gelatin capsule with a nylon string attached. Several hours later, the string is withdrawn, and the contents are sent for laboratory analysis. With the availability of EIA techniques to identify *Giardia* antigens in stool specimens, other tests are being used less often.

Therapeutic Management

The drugs of choice for treatment of giardiasis are metronidazole (Flagyl), tinidazole (Tindamax), and nitazoxanide (Alinia). Tinidazole is said to have an 80% to 100% cure rate after a single dose (American Academy of Pediatrics, Committee on Infectious Diseases, 2009b). Metronidazole and tinidazole have a metallic taste and GI side effects, including nausea and vomiting; nitazoxanide has no bitter taste and should be taken with food to avoid GI symptoms. Albendazole is also used to treat the disease and reportedly has fewer side effects than metronidazole (American Academy of Pediatrics, Committee on Infectious Diseases, 2009b).

Nursing Care Management

The most important nursing consideration is prevention of giardiasis and education of parents, child care center staff, and those who are entrusted with the daily care of small children. Attention to meticulous sanitary practices, especially during diaper changes, is essential (Fig. 47-4). Nurses can play an important role in educating parents of small children and day care staff regarding appropriate sanitation practices. In addition, young children who are infected or who have diarrhea should be discouraged from swimming in community or private pools until they are infection free. Lakes and streams may contain high numbers of *Giardia* spore cysts, which can be swallowed in the water. When there is a high chance of swallowing water, children are discouraged from swimming

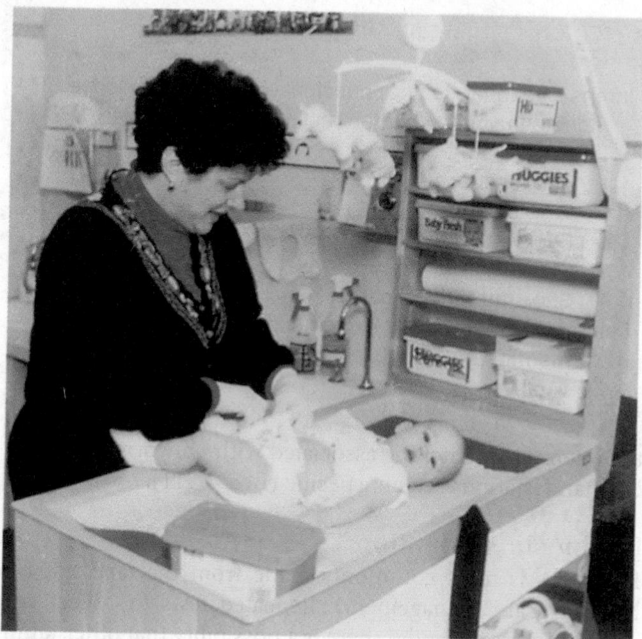

Fig. 47-4 Prevention of giardiasis, especially in day care centers, requires sanitary practices during diaper changes such as discarding paper diapers in a covered receptacle, changing paper covers on the diaper-changing surface, and having facilities for handwashing nearby. NOTE: Soiled cloth diapers and clothing should be stored in a plastic bag for transport home.

in stagnant bodies of water and in water where children who are known to be infected are swimming. *Giardia* organisms are said to be resistant to chlorine (Hlavsa, Watson, & Beach, 2005). Parents are encouraged to take small children to the restroom frequently when swimming, to avoid letting children in diapers in swimming areas, and to change diapers away from the water source (see also Centers for Disease Control information on recreational water illnesses *[www.cdc.gov/healthyswimming]*). After children are infected, family education regarding drug administration is essential.

Enterobiasis (Pinworms)

Enterobiasis, or pinworms, caused by the nematode *Enterobius vermicularis,* is the most common helminthic infection in the United States. It is universally present in temperate climatic zones and may infect more than 30% of all children at any one time. Crowded conditions such as in classrooms and day care centers favor transmission.

Infection begins when the eggs are ingested or inhaled (they float in the air). The eggs hatch in the upper intestine and then mature and migrate through the intestine. After mating, adult females migrate out the anus and lay eggs (American Academy of Pediatrics, Committee on Infectious Diseases, 2009b). The movement of the worms on skin and mucous membrane surfaces causes intense itching. As the child scratches, eggs are deposited on the hands and underneath the fingernails. The typical hand-to-mouth activity of youngsters makes them especially prone to reinfection. Pinworm eggs persist in the indoor environment for 2 to 3 weeks, contaminating anything they contact, such as toilet seats, doorknobs, bed linen, underwear, and food. Except for

BOX 47-11 Clinical Manifestations of Pinworms

Intense perianal itching (principal symptom); evidence of itching in young children includes the following:
- General irritability
- Restlessness
- Poor sleep
- Bed-wetting
- Distractibility
- Short attention span

Perianal dermatitis and excoriation secondary to itching
If worms migrate, possible vaginal and urethral infection

the intense rectal itching associated with pinworms, the clinical manifestations are nonspecific (Box 47-11).

Diagnostic Evaluation

Diagnosis is most commonly made from the tape test (see Nursing Care Management). Repeated tests to collect eggs may be necessary, and if there is a possibility that other family members may be infected, a tape test should be performed on them.

Therapeutic Management

The drugs available for treatment of pinworms include mebendazole (Vermox), pyrantel pamoate (Pin-Rid, Antiminth), and albendazole. The drug of choice is mebendazole, which is safe, effective, and convenient, with few side effects; however, it is not recommended for children younger than 2 years of age. If pyrvinium pamoate is prescribed, parents are advised that the drug stains stool and vomitus bright red, as well as clothing or skin that comes in contact with it; it is available without prescription and should not be used in children under 2 years without consulting the primary practitioner. Because pinworms are easily transmitted, all household members are treated. The dose of antiparasitic medication should be repeated in 2 weeks to completely eradicate the parasite and prevent reinfection.

evolve Animation—Appendicitis

Nursing Care Management

Nursing care is directed at identifying the parasite, eradicating the organism, and preventing reinfection. Parents need clear, detailed instructions for the *tape test.* A loop of transparent (not "frosted" or "magic") tape, sticky side out, is placed around the end of a tongue depressor, which is then firmly pressed against the child's perianal area. A convenient, commercially prepared tape is also available for this purpose. Pinworm specimens are collected in the morning as soon as the child awakens and *before* he or she has a bowel movement or bathes. The procedure may need to be performed on 3 or more consecutive days before eggs are collected. Parents are instructed to place the tongue blade in a glass jar or loosely in a plastic bag so that it can be brought in for microscopic examination. For specimens collected in the hospital, practitioner's office, or clinic, the tape is placed smoothly on a glass slide, sticky side down, for examination.

evolve Case Study—Appendicitis

Adherence to the drug regimen is usually excellent because the duration of treatment is typically only one dose. However, the family is reminded of the need to take a second dose in 2 weeks to ensure eradication of the eggs.

To prevent reinfection, washing all clothes and bed linens in hot water and vacuuming the house may be recommended. However, there is little documentation on the effectiveness of these measures because pinworms survive on many surfaces. Helpful suggestions include handwashing after toileting and before eating, keeping the child's fingernails short to minimize the chance of ova collecting under the nails, dressing children in one-piece sleeping outfits, and daily showering rather than tub bathing. Families should be informed that recurrence is common. Repeated infections should be treated in the same manner as the first one.

Inflammatory Disorders

Acute Appendicitis

Appendicitis, inflammation of the *vermiform appendix* (blind sac at the end of the cecum), is the most common cause of emergency abdominal surgery in childhood. In the United States 60,000 to 80,000 cases are diagnosed each year. The average age of children with appendicitis is 10 years, with boys and girls equally affected before puberty. Classically, the first symptom of appendicitis is periumbilical pain, followed by nausea, right lower quadrant pain, and later vomiting with fever (Kwok, Kim, & Gorelick, 2004). Perforation of the appendix can occur within approximately 48 hours of the initial complaint of pain. At the time of initial presentation, about one third of all cases involve an already perforated appendix. Complications from appendiceal perforation include major abscess, phlegmon, enterocutaneous fistula, peritonitis, and partial bowel obstruction (Kwok, Kim, & Gorelick, 2004). A *phlegmon* is an acute suppurative inflammation of subcutaneous connective tissue that spreads.

Etiology

The cause of appendicitis is obstruction of the lumen of the appendix, usually by hardened fecal material (fecalith). Swollen lymphoid tissue, frequently occurring after a viral infection, can also obstruct the appendix. Another rare cause of obstruction is a parasite such as *Enterobius vermicularis,* or pinworms, which can obstruct the appendiceal lumen.

Pathophysiology

With acute obstruction, the outflow of mucus secretions is blocked, and pressure builds within the lumen, resulting in compression of blood vessels. The resulting ischemia is followed by ulceration of the epithelial lining and bacterial invasion. Subsequent necrosis causes perforation or rupture with fecal and bacterial contamination of the peritoneal cavity. The resulting inflammation spreads rapidly throughout the abdomen *(peritonitis),* especially in young children, who are unable to localize infection. Progressive peritoneal inflammation results in functional intestinal obstruction of the small bowel *(ileus)* because intense GI reflexes severely inhibit bowel motility. Because the peritoneum represents a major portion of total body surface, the loss of ECF to the peritoneal cavity leads to electrolyte imbalance and hypovolemic shock.

Diagnostic Evaluation

Diagnosis is not always straightforward. Fever, vomiting, abdominal pain, and an elevated white blood cell (WBC) count are associated with appendicitis but are also seen in IBD, pelvic inflammatory disease, gastroenteritis, urinary tract infection, right lower lobe pneumonia, mesenteric adenitis, Meckel's diverticulum, and intussusception. Prolonged symptoms and delayed diagnosis often occur in younger children, in whom the risk of perforation is greatest because of their inability to verbalize their complaints. In addition to fever, signs of peritonitis include sudden relief from pain after perforation, subsequent increase in pain (usually diffuse and accompanied by rigid guarding of the abdomen), progressive abdominal distention, tachycardia, rapid shallow breathing, pallor, chills, and irritability.

The diagnosis is based primarily on the history and physical examination (Box 47-12). Pain, the cardinal feature, is initially generalized (usually periumbilical); however, it usually descends to the lower right quadrant. The most intense site of pain may be at *McBurney point,* located at a point midway between the anterior superior iliac crest and the umbilicus. Rebound tenderness is not a reliable sign and is extremely painful to the child. Referred pain, elicited by light percussion around the perimeter of the abdomen, indicates peritoneal irritation. Movement such as riding over bumps in an automobile or on a stretcher, aggravates the pain. In addition to pain, significant clinical manifestations include fever, a change in behavior, anorexia, and vomiting.

Laboratory studies usually include a CBC, urinalysis (to rule out a urinary tract infection), and in adolescent females serum human chorionic gonadotropin (to rule out an ectopic pregnancy). A WBC count greater than 10,000/mm^3 and a C-reactive protein (CRP) are common but are not necessarily specific for appendicitis. An elevated percentage of bands (often referred to as "a shift to the left") may indicate an inflammatory process. CRP is an acute-phase reactant that rises within 12 hours of the onset of infection.

Computed tomography (CT) scan has become the imaging technique of choice, although ultrasound may also be helpful in diagnosing appendicitis. A CT scan is considered positive in the presence of enlarged appendiceal diameter; appendiceal wall thickening; and periappendiceal inflammatory changes, including fat streaks, phlegmon, fluid collection, and extraluminal gas (Aiken & Oldham, 2007).

BOX 47-12 Clinical Manifestations of Appendicitis

- Right lower quadrant abdominal pain
- Fever
- Rigid abdomen
- Decreased or absent bowel sounds
- Vomiting (typically follows onset of pain)
- Constipation or diarrhea may be present
- Anorexia
- Tachycardia; rapid, shallow breathing
- Pallor
- Lethargy
- Irritability
- Stooped posture (guarding)

Therapeutic Management

Treatment of appendicitis before perforation includes rehydration, antibiotics, and surgical removal of the appendix *(appendectomy).* Laparoscopic surgery is now commonly used to treat nonperforated acute appendicitis. Recovery is rapid, and, if no complications occur, the hospital stay is short.

Ruptured Appendix

Management of the child diagnosed with peritonitis caused by a ruptured appendix often begins preoperatively with IV administration of fluid and electrolytes, systemic antibiotics, and NG suction. Postoperative management includes IV fluids, continued administration of antibiotics, and NG suction for abdominal decompression until intestinal activity returns. Sometimes surgeons close the wound after irrigation of the peritoneal cavity. Other times, they leave the wound open (delayed closure) to prevent wound infection. A Penrose drain may be used to permit transperitoneal drainage.

Prognosis

Complications are uncommon after a simple appendectomy. The mortality rate for perforating appendicitis has improved from nearly certain death a century ago to less than 1% (0.3%) (Aiken & Oldham, 2007). Early recognition of the illness is essential to prevent complications.

Nursing Care Management

Because abdominal pain is the most common childhood complaint with appendicitis, it is important to assess the severity of pain (see Pain Assessment, Chapter 35). One of the most reliable estimates is the degree of change in behavior. The younger, nonverbal child will assume a rigid, motionless, side-lying posture with the knees flexed on the abdomen, and there is decreased range of motion of the right hip. Older children may exhibit all of these behaviors while complaining of abdominal pain. They can always indicate a point at which the pain is worse than at any other location.

NURSING ALERT In any instance when appendicitis is suspected, be aware of the danger of administering laxatives or enemas or applying heat to the area. Such measures stimulate bowel motility and increase the risk of perforation.

evolve Nursing Care Plan—The Child with Appendicitis

Postoperative Care

Postoperative care for the nonperforated appendix is the same as for most abdominal procedures. Care of the child with a ruptured appendix and peritonitis is more complex, and the course of recovery is considerably longer (usually 3 to 5 days of hospitalization). The child is maintained on IV fluids, NPO, and the NG tube is kept on low continuous gastric decompression until there is evidence of intestinal activity. Listening for bowel sounds and observing for other signs of bowel activity (e.g., passage of stool) are part of the routine assessment. Management of IV therapy is the same as for any child receiving fluids and parenteral antibiotics. A drain is often placed in the wound during surgery, and frequent dressing changes with meticulous skin care are essential to prevent excoriation of the area surrounding the surgical site. Wound care includes irrigation with antibacterial solution. If the wound is left open, a Montgomery strap may be used to facilitate dressing changes and minimize tape removal and epidermal stripping. Early ambulation with adequate pain management assists in preventing many of the complications associated with prolonged bed rest and immobility (e.g., venous stasis, bowel hypomotility, abdominal pain from intestinal gas).

Management of pain from the incision and repeated dressing changes and irrigations are an essential part of the child's care. Psychologic care of the child and parents is similar to that used in other emergency situations (see Emergency Admission, Chapter 44). Parents and older children need to express their feelings and concerns regarding the events surrounding the illness and hospitalization. The nurse can provide education and psychosocial support to promote adequate coping and alleviate anxiety for both the child and the family.

Meckel's Diverticulum

Meckel's diverticulum is a remnant of the fetal omphalomesenteric duct that connects the yolk sac with the primitive midgut during fetal life. Normally this structure is obliterated by the fifth to seventh week of gestation, when the placenta replaces the yolk sac as the source of nutrition for the fetus (Sagar, Kumar, & Shah, 2006). Failure of obliteration may result in an *omphalomesenteric fistula*, a fibrous band connecting the small intestine to the umbilicus, known as Meckel's diverticulum.

Meckel's diverticulum is a true diverticulum because it arises from the antimesenteric border of the small intestine and contains all layers of the intestinal wall with a separate blood supply from the vitelline artery. The diverticulum is usually found within 100 cm (40 inches) of the ileocecal valve and averages 1 to 10 cm (0.4 to 4 inches) in length.

Meckel's diverticulum is the most common congenital malformation of the GI tract and is present in 2% to 4% of the population (Sagar, Kumar, & Shah, 2006). Its occurrence in males and females is equal, but the incidence of complications is three to four times greater in males. Most symptomatic cases are seen in childhood. Patients requiring surgery are generally younger than 10 years of age, and about 50% are younger than 2 years of age (Sagar, Kumar, & Shah, 2006).

Pathophysiology

The symptomatic complications of Meckel's diverticulum are ulceration, bleeding, intussusception, intestinal obstruction, diverticulitis, and perforation; bleeding is the most common problem in children. Gastric mucosa is the most common ectopic tissue found in Meckel's diverticulum. Bleeding is caused by peptic ulceration or perforation because of the unbuffered acidic gastric secretion. Several mechanisms can cause obstruction. Intussusception may be led by the diverticulum. Obstruction may also be caused by entanglement of the small intestine around a fibrous cord, trapping of a loop of intestine under the band, incarceration within a hernia sac, or volvulus of the intestinal segment containing the diverticulum. Diverticulitis occurs when peptic ulceration or obstruction leads to inflammation.

BOX 47-13 Clinical Manifestations of Meckel's Diverticulum

Abdominal Pain
Similar to appendicitis
May be vague and recurrent

Bloody Stools*
Painless
Bright or dark red with mucus ("currant jelly" stool)
In infants, bleeding may be accompanied by pain

Sometimes
Severe anemia
Shock

*Often an initial sign.

Diagnostic Evaluation

Diagnosis is usually based on the history, physical examination, and a specialized radiographic study. The most common clinical presentation in children includes painless rectal bleeding, abdominal pain, or signs of intestinal obstruction (Box 47-13). Bleeding, which may be mild or profuse, often appears as dark red or "currant jelly" stools; it may be significant enough to cause hypotension. The Meckel scan, a technetium-99m pertechnetate scan, detects the presence of gastric mucosa with an overall diagnostic accuracy of 90%. Blood studies are performed to screen for bleeding disorders and anemia.

Therapeutic Management

The standard treatment is surgical removal of the diverticulum. When severe hemorrhage increases the surgical risk, interventions to correct hypovolemic shock, such as blood replacement, IV fluids, and oxygen, may be necessary. Antibiotics may be used preoperatively to control infection. If intestinal obstruction has occurred, appropriate preoperative measures are used to reverse electrolyte imbalances and minimize abdominal distention.

Prognosis

If this condition is diagnosed and treated early, full recovery is likely. The mortality rate of untreated Meckel's diverticulum ranges from 2.5% to 15%. Complications of untreated Meckel's diverticulum include GI hemorrhage and bowel obstruction.

Nursing Care Management

Nursing objectives are similar to those for any child undergoing surgery (see Chapter 44). Because the onset of this condition is often rapid, parents require psychologic support. The massive intestinal bleeding that can accompany a Meckel's diverticulum is traumatic to both the child and the parents and may significantly affect their emotional reaction to hospitalization and surgery.

Specific preoperative considerations with intestinal bleeding include (1) frequent monitoring of vital signs and blood pressure for shock, (2) keeping the child on bed rest, and (3) recording the approximate amount of blood lost in stools. In the absence of frank hemorrhage, the nurse tests the stools for occult blood. Postoperatively, the child requires IV fluids

Table 47-6 Clinical Manifestations of Inflammatory Bowel Diseases

CHARACTERISTICS	ULCERATIVE COLITIS	CROHN'S DISEASE
Rectal bleeding	Common	Uncommon
Diarrhea	Often severe	Moderate to severe
Pain	Less frequent	Common
Anorexia	Mild or moderate	May be severe
Weight loss	Moderate	May be severe
Growth delay	Usually mild	May be severe
Anal and perianal lesions	Rare	Common
Fistulas and strictures	Rare	Common
Rashes	Mild	Mild
Joint pain	Mild to moderate	Mild to moderate

and an NG tube for the decompression and evacuation of gastric contents.

Inflammatory Bowel Disease

Inflammatory bowel disease (IBD) is a term that is used for two forms of chronic intestinal inflammation: *ulcerative colitis (UC)* and *Crohn's disease (CD)*. Although UC and CD have similar epidemiologic, immunologic, and clinical features, there are important differences (Table 47-6).

GI symptoms, extraintestinal and systemic inflammatory responses, and exacerbations and remissions without complete resolution characterize these diseases. Growth failure, particularly common in CD, is an important problem unique to the pediatric population. CD is more disabling, has more serious complications, and has less effective medical and surgical treatment than UC. Because UC is confined to the colon, theoretically it may be cured with a colectomy. Over the past 30 years, the incidence of CD has risen, whereas the incidence of UC in children has remained stable (Silbermintz & Markowitz, 2006). The incidence of UC has been estimated as 2 to 7 cases per 100,000 per year, affecting as many as 250,000 to 500,000 persons in the United States (Langan et al, 2007).

Etiology

Despite decades of research, the etiology of IBD is not completely understood, and there is no known cure. There is evidence to indicate a multifactorial etiology. Research is focused on theories of defective immunoregulation of the inflammatory response to bacteria or viruses in the GI tract in individuals with a genetic predisposition (Silbermintz & Markowitz, 2006). In CD the chronic immune process is characterized by a T helper 1 cytokine profile, whereas in UC the response is more humoral and mediated by T helper 2 cells (Silbermintz & Markowitz, 2006). An epidemiologic study by Kugathasan and colleagues (2003) found an equal distribution of IBD among all racial and ethnic groups, contrasting with earlier studies that suggested IBD typically affects Caucasians (especially Ashkenazi Jews) more than persons of Asian or African decent. The Kugathasan study also did not demonstrate a higher risk for developing IBD in urban populations, as had been reported in earlier studies.

There is an influence of genetics in the development of CD. Several CD susceptibility genes have been identified, including *NOD2/CARD15* on chromosome 16 associated with ileal disease, *IBD5* on chromosome 5, and *IBD6* on chromosome 6 (Kugathasan et al, 2004; Ahmad et al, 2002). The influence of genetics in UC appears to be smaller than in CD; however, the *MDRI* gene has been associated with UC (Schwab et al, 2003). Environmental factors appear to play a role in the development of IBD. Breastfeeding decreases the risk of developing CD, whereas infantile diarrhea seems to increase the risk. Cigarette smoking also appears to be a risk factor for CD but appears to be protective against UC.

Pathophysiology of Ulcerative Colitis

The inflammation is limited to the colon and rectum, with the distal colon and rectum the most severely affected. It affects the mucosa and submucosa and involves continuous segments along the length of the bowel with varying degrees of ulceration, bleeding, and edema. The presentation may be mild, moderate, or severe, depending on the extent of mucosal inflammation and systemic symptoms. Children with UC usually are seen with diarrhea, rectal bleeding, and abdominal pain, often associated with tenesmus and urgency (Silbermintz & Markowitz, 2006). Thickening of the bowel wall and fibrosis are unusual, but long-standing disease can result in shortening of the colon and strictures. Extraintestinal manifestations are less common in UC than in CD. Toxic megacolon is the most dangerous form of severe colitis.

Pathophysiology of Crohn's Disease

The chronic inflammatory process of CD involves any part of the GI tract from the mouth to the anus but most often affects the terminal ileum. The disease involves all layers of the bowel wall (transmural) in a discontinuous fashion, meaning that between areas of intact mucosa there are areas of affected mucosa (skip lesions). The most common symptoms are abdominal pain, diarrhea, and decrease in appetite resulting in weight loss. Perianal disease, including skin tags, fistulas, and abscesses, occur in CD. Fever, growth delay, and delayed sexual development are seen commonly (Silbermintz & Markowitz, 2006). Mild GI symptoms, poor growth, and extraintestinal manifestations may be present for several years before overt GI symptoms occur. The inflammation may result in ulcerations; fibrosis; adhesions; stiffening of the bowel wall; stricture formation; and fistulas to other loops of bowel, bladder, vagina, or skin. Extraintestinal manifestations include erythema nodosum, pyoderma gangrenosum, arthralgia and arthritis, uveitis and episcleritis, sclerosing cholangitis, autoimmune hepatitis, nephrolithiasis, and pneumonitis (Silbermintz & Markowitz, 2006).

Diagnostic Evaluation

The diagnosis of UC and CD is derived from the history, physical examination, laboratory evaluation, and other diagnostic procedures. Laboratory tests include a CBC to evaluate anemia and an erythrocyte sedimentation rate or CRP to assess the systemic reaction to the inflammatory process. Levels of total protein, albumin, iron, zinc, magnesium, vitamin B_{12}, and fat-soluble vitamins may be low in children with CD. Stools are examined for blood, leukocytes, and infectious organisms. A serologic panel is often used in combination with clinical findings to diagnose IBD and to differentiate between CD and UC. In IBD, autoantibodies called antineutrophil cytoplasmic antibodies (ANCAs) may be detected in the blood. The perinuclear antineutrophil cytoplasmic antibody (pANCA) is associated with UC. Approximately 60% of children with UC and 10% of those with CD are pANCA-positive. Anti–*Saccharomyces cerevisiae* antibodies (ASCA) and anti–outer membrane porin of *E. coli* (anti-OmpC) have been found in up to 60% of children with CD (Ruemmele et al, 1998).

In patients with CD, an upper GI series with small bowel follow-through assists in assessing the existence, location, and extent of disease. Upper endoscopy and colonoscopy with biopsies are an integral part of diagnosing IBD. Endoscopy allows direct visualization of the surface of the GI tract so that the extent of inflammation and narrowing can be evaluated. CT and ultrasound also may be used to identify bowel wall inflammation, intraabdominal abscesses, and fistulas. CD lesions may pierce the walls of the small intestine and colon, creating tracts called *fistulas* between the intestine and adjacent structures such as the bladder, anus, vagina, or skin.

Therapeutic Management

The goals of therapy are to (1) control the inflammatory process to reduce or eliminate the symptoms, (2) obtain long-term remission, (3) promote normal growth and development, and (4) allow as normal a lifestyle as possible. Treatment is individualized and managed according to the type and severity of the disease, its location, and the response to therapy.

Medical Treatment

The goal of any treatment regimen is first to induce remission of acute symptoms and then to maintain remission over time. *5-Aminosalicylates* (5-ASAs) are effective in the induction and maintenance of remission in mild to moderate UC. Mesalamine, olsalazine, and balsalazide are now preferred over sulfasalazine because of reduced side effects (headache, nausea, vomiting, neutropenia, and oligospermia). Suppository and enema preparations of mesalamine are used to treat left-sided colitis. These drugs decrease inflammation by inhibiting prostaglandin synthesis. 5-ASAs can be used to induce remission in mild CD. Corticosteroids, such as prednisone and prednisolone, are indicated in induction therapy in children with moderate to severe UC and CD. These drugs inhibit the production of adhesion molecules, cytokines, and leukotrienes. Although these drugs reduce the acute symptoms of IBD, they have side effects that relate to long-term use, including growth suppression (adrenal suppression), weight gain, and decreased bone density (Baron, 2002). High doses of IV corticosteroids may be administered in acute episodes and tapered according to clinical response. Budesonide, a synthetic corticosteroid, is designed for controlled release in the ileum and is indicated for ileal and right-sided colitis; budesonide has fewer side effects than prednisone and prednisolone (Silbermintz & Markowitz, 2006). Rectal steroid therapy (enemas and foam-based preparations) are available for both induction and maintenance therapy in left-sided colitis.

Immunomodulators, such as azathioprine and its metabolite 6-mercaptopurine (6-MP), are used to induce and maintain remission in children with IBD who are steroid resistant or steroid dependent and in treating chronic draining fistulas. They block the synthesis of purine, thus inhibiting the ability of deoxyribonucleic acid (DNA) and ribonucleic acid (RNA) to hinder lymphocyte function, especially that of T cells. Side effects include infection, pancreatitis, hepatitis, bone marrow toxicity, arthralgia, and malignancy. Methotrexate has also been shown to be useful in inducing and maintaining remission in CD patients unresponsive to standard therapies. Cyclosporine and tacrolimus have both been shown to be effective in inducing remission in severe steroid-dependent UC. 6-MP or azathioprine is then used to maintain remission. Patients on immunomodulating medications require regular monitoring of their CBC and differential to assess for changes that reflect suppression of the immune system, since many of the side effects can be prevented or managed by dose reduction or discontinuation of medication.

Antibiotics, such as metronidazole and ciprofloxacin, may be used as an adjunctive therapy to treat complications such as perianal disease or small bowel bacterial overgrowth in CD. Side effects of these drugs are peripheral neuropathy, nausea, and a metallic taste.

Biologic therapies act to regulate inflammatory and anti-inflammatory cytokines. Tumor necrosis factor-α (TNF-α) is believed to influence active inflammation. Infliximab (Remicade) is a chimeric human-murine monoclonal antibody to TNF-α that is administered intravenously. The U.S. Food and Drug Administration (FDA) has approved it for inducing and maintaining remission in adult CD patients with moderate to severe disease who have not responded sufficiently to conventional therapy. Children appear to respond to infliximab similarly to adults. Infliximab is approved for the treatment of fistulas in CD and for systemic manifestations of IBD such as ankylosing spondylitis, pyoderma gangrenosum, and chronic uveitis. Recently infliximab was approved by the FDA for the treatment of UC unresponsive to steroids. Many patients relapse if treatment is stopped; therefore long-term maintenance therapy with infliximab every 8 weeks may be required. Patients generally require concurrent maintenance with 6-MP or methotrexate to avoid the development of antibodies to infliximab, which are associated with infusion reactions and loss of efficacy. Approximately 5% of patients have acute allergic reactions to infliximab and require premedication with prednisone and diphenhydramine before infusion to prevent reactions. Long intervals between infusions may predispose patients to serum sickness (an immune response causing fever, muscle pain, arthritis, and hives) (Baron, 2002). Severe complications of this drug include lupuslike syndrome or lymphoma. Adalimumab (Humira) was introduced in 2007 for adults with IBD who have lost response or are intolerant to infliximab. To date studies demonstrate that Humira is effective in decreasing symptoms in approximately 64% of pediatric patients and is well tolerated in pediatric patients with CD (Wyneski et al, 2008). Tuberculosis and other opportunistic infections have been observed in patients receiving adalimumab (Abbott Laboratories, 2007).

Nutritional Support

Nutritional support is important in the treatment of IBD. Growth failure is a common serious complication, especially in CD. It is characterized by weight loss, alteration in body composition, retarded height, and delayed sexual maturation. Malnutrition causes the growth failure, and its etiology is multifactorial. Malnutrition occurs as a result of inadequate dietary intake, excessive GI losses, malabsorption, drug-nutrient interaction, and increased nutritional requirements. Inadequate dietary intake occurs with anorexia and episodes of increased disease activity. Excessive loss of nutrients (protein, blood, electrolytes, and minerals) occurs secondary to intestinal inflammation and diarrhea. Carbohydrate, lactose, fat, vitamin, and mineral malabsorption, as well as vitamin B_{12} and folic acid deficiencies, occur with disease episodes and with drug administration and when the terminal ileum is resected. Finally, nutritional requirements are increased with inflammation, fever, fistulas, and periods of rapid growth (e.g., adolescence).

The goals of nutritional support include (1) correction of nutrient deficits and replacement of ongoing losses, (2) provision of adequate energy and protein for healing, and (3) provision of adequate nutrients to promote normal growth. Nutritional support includes both enteral and parenteral nutrition. A well-balanced, high-protein, high-calorie diet is recommended for children whose symptoms do not prohibit an adequate oral intake. There is little evidence that avoiding specific foods influences the severity of the disease. Supplementation with multivitamins, iron, and folic acid is recommended.

Special enteral formulas, given either by mouth or continuous enteral (NG or gastrostomy) infusion (often at night), may be required. Elemental formulas are completely absorbed in the small intestine with almost no residue. Several studies have demonstrated that a diet consisting only of elemental formula not only improved nutritional status but also induced disease remission, either without steroids or with a diminished dosage of steroids required. An elemental diet is a safe and potentially effective primary therapy for patients with CD. Unfortunately, remission is not sustained when enteral feedings are discontinued unless maintenance medications are added to the treatment regimen.

TPN has also improved nutritional status in patients with IBD. Short-term remissions have been achieved after TPN, although complete bowel rest has not reduced inflammation or added to the benefits of improved nutrition by TPN. Nutritional support is less likely to induce a remission in UC than in CD. However, improvement of nutritional status is important in preventing deterioration of the patient's health status and in preparing the patient for surgery.

Surgical Treatment

Surgery is indicated for UC when medical and nutritional therapies fail to prevent complications. Surgical options include a *subtotal colectomy* and *ileostomy* that leaves a rectal stump as a blind pouch. A reservoir pouch is created in the configuration of a J or S to help improve continence postoperatively. An ileoanal pull-through preserves the normal pathway for defecation. Pouchitis, an inflammation of the surgically created pouch, is the most common late complication of this procedure and had been reported to occur in up to 50% of cases. Metronidazole and ciprofloxacin are effective in treating pouchitis (Alexander et al, 2003). In many cases UC can be cured with a total colectomy.

Surgery may be required in children with CD when complications cannot be controlled by medical and nutritional therapy. Segmental intestinal resections are performed for small bowel obstructions, strictures, or fistulas. Partial colonic resection is not curative, and the disease often recurs.

Prognosis

IBD is a chronic disease. Relatively long periods of quiescent disease may follow exacerbations. The outcome of the disease is influenced by the regions and severity of involvement, as well as by appropriate therapeutic management. Malnutrition, growth failure, and bleeding are serious complications. The overall prognosis for UC is good.

The development of colorectal cancer (CRC) is a long-term complication of IBD. In UC the cumulative incidence of CRC is 2.5% after 20 years, increasing to 10.8% after 30 years (Rutter et al, 2006). Surveillance colonoscopy with multiple biopsies should begin approximately 10 years after diagnosis of UC or CD and continue every 1 to 2 years (Rubin & Kavitt, 2006). Removal of the diseased colon prevents development of CRC. However, in CD surgical removal of the affected colon does not prevent cancer from developing elsewhere in the GI tract.

Nursing Care Management

The nursing considerations in the management of IBD extend beyond the immediate period of hospitalization. These interventions involve continued guidance of families in terms of (1) managing diet; (2) coping with factors that increase stress and emotional lability; (3) adjusting to a disease of remissions and exacerbations; and (4) when indicated, preparing the child and parents for the possibility of diversionary bowel surgery.

Because nutritional support is an essential part of therapy, encouraging the anorectic child to consume sufficient quantities of food is often a challenge. Successful interventions include involving the child in meal planning; encouraging small, frequent meals or snacks rather than three large meals a day; serving meals around medication schedules when diarrhea, mouth pain, and intestinal spasm are controlled; and preparing high-protein, high-calorie foods such as eggnog, milkshakes, cream soups, puddings, or custard (if lactose is tolerated) (see Feeding the Sick Child, Chapter 45). Foods that are known to aggravate the condition are avoided. Using bran or a high-fiber diet for active IBD is questionable. Bran, even in small amounts, has been shown to worsen the patient's condition. Occasionally the occurrence of aphthous stomatitis (mouth ulcers) further complicates adherence to dietary management. Mouth care before eating and the selection of bland foods help relieve the discomfort of mouth sores.

When NG feedings or TPN is indicated, nurses play an important role in explaining the purpose and expected outcomes of this therapy. The nurse should acknowledge the anxieties of the child and family members and give them adequate time to demonstrate the skills necessary to continue the therapy at home if needed (see Critical Thinking Exercise).

evolve Critical Thinking Exercise—Home Care for the Adolescent

CRITICAL THINKING EXERCISE

Inflammatory Bowel Disease

Susan, a 13-year-old girl, was admitted to the hospital because of bloody diarrhea, abdominal pain, and weight loss. After a thorough evaluation, including laboratory tests, radiographic studies, and gastrointestinal endoscopy procedures, the diagnosis of Crohn's disease (CD) was made. Medical treatment, including corticosteroid drugs and nutritional support, was implemented during this hospitalization.

Susan has improved considerably and is to be discharged home this week. Enteral formula administered by continuous nighttime gastrostomy infusion will be continued at home, and both Susan and her family are eager to learn how to perform these feedings. You are the nurse who is responsible for Susan's discharge planning. Which interventions relating to these feedings should you include in Susan's preparations for discharge?

1. Evidence—Are there sufficient data to formulate any specific interventions for discharge?
2. Assumptions—Describe some underlying assumptions about the following:
   a. The goals of nutritional support for children with CD
   b. Teaching required by an adolescent or family member who is administering gastrostomy tube feedings at home
   c. Psychosocial issues related to CD
3. What are the priorities for discharge planning at this time?
4. Does the evidence support your conclusion?
5. Are there alternative perspectives to your conclusion? What are they?

The importance of continued drug therapy despite remission of symptoms must be stressed to the child and family members. Failure to adhere to the pharmacologic regimen can result in exacerbation of the disease (see Compliance, Chapter 45). Unfortunately, exacerbation of IBD can occur even if the child and family are compliant with the treatment regimen; this is difficult for the child and family to accept.

Family Support

The nurse should attend to the emotional components of the disease and assess any sources of stress. Frequently, the nurse can help children adjust to problems of growth restriction, delayed sexual maturation, dietary restrictions, feelings of being "different" or "sickly," inability to compete with peers, and necessary absence from school during exacerbations of the illness.

If a permanent colectomy-ileostomy is required, the nurse can teach the child and family how to care for the ileostomy. The nurse can also emphasize the positive aspects of the surgery, particularly accelerated growth and sexual development, permanent recovery, eliminated risk of colon cancer in UC, and normality of life despite bowel diversion. Introducing the child and parents to other ostomy patients, especially those who are the same age, can be effective in fostering eventual acceptance. Whenever possible, continent ostomies should be offered as options to the child, although they are not performed in all centers in the United States.

Because of the chronic and often lifelong nature of the disease, families benefit from the educational services provided by organizations such as the Crohn's and Colitis Foundation of America (CCFA).* If diversionary bowel surgery is indicated, United Ostomy Associations of America† and the Wound, Ostomy and Continence Nurses Society‡ are available to assist with ileostomy care and provide important psychologic support through their self-help groups. Adolescents often benefit by participating in peer-support groups, which are sponsored by the CCFA.

Peptic Ulcer Disease

Peptic ulcers may be classified as acute or chronic, and peptic ulcer disease (PUD) is a chronic condition that affects the stomach or duodenum. Ulcers are described as gastric or duodenal and as primary or secondary. A *gastric ulcer* involves the mucosa of the stomach; a *duodenal ulcer* involves the pylorus or duodenum. Most *primary ulcers* occur in the absence of a predisposing factor and tend to be chronic, occurring more frequently in the duodenum. *Stress ulcers* result from the stress of a severe underlying disease or injury (e.g., severe burns, sepsis, increased intracranial pressure, severe trauma, multisystem organ failure) and are more frequently acute and gastric. About 25% of hospitalized critically ill children have evidence of gastric bleeding (Blanchard & Czinn, 2007).

About 1.7% of children in general pediatric practices have PUD, and the disease represents about 3.4% per 10,000 of pediatric hospital admissions. Primary ulcers are more common in children older than 6 years, and stress ulcers are more common in infants younger than 6 months. Except for very young children, the incidence is two to three times greater in boys than in girls.

Etiology

The exact cause is unknown, although infectious, genetic, and environmental factors are important. There is an increased familial incidence, and the disease is increased in persons with blood group O.

There is a significant relationship between the bacterium *Helicobacter pylori (H. pylori)* and ulcers. *H. pylori* is a microaerophilic, gram-negative, slow-growing, spiral-shaped, and flagellated bacterium known to colonize the gastric mucosa in about half of the population of the world (Blanchard & Czinn, 2007; Czinn, 2005). It has been identified in 90% to 100% of adult patients with PUD. *H. pylori* synthesizes the enzyme urease, which hydrolyses urea to form ammonia and carbon dioxide. Ammonia then absorbs acid to form ammonium,

**386 Park Ave. South, 17th Floor, New York, NY 10016; 800-932-2423;* www.ccfa.org. *In Canada: Crohn's and Colitis Foundation of Canada,* www.ccfc.ca.

†UOAA, PO Box 66, Fairview, TN 37062-0066; 800-826-0826; www.uoaa.org. *In Canada: United Ostomy Association of Canada, PO Box 825-50, Charles St. East, Toronto, Ontario M4Y 2N7; 416-595-5452; fax: 416-595-9924;* www.ostomycanada.ca.

‡1500 Commerce Pkwy., Suite C, Mt. Laurel, NJ; 888-224-9626; www.wocn.org.

thus raising the gastric pH. Also, its flagella allow the bacterium to swim across the viscous gastric mucus and reach the more neutral gastric pH below the mucus (Sgouros & Bergele, 2006). *H. pylori* may cause ulcers by weakening the gastric mucosal barrier and allowing acid to damage the mucosa. It is believed that it is acquired via the fecal-oral route, and this hypothesis is supported by finding viable *H. pylori* in feces.

In addition to ulcerogenic drugs, both alcohol and smoking contribute to ulcer formation. There is no conclusive evidence to implicate particular foods such as caffeine-containing beverages or spicy foods, but polyunsaturated fats and fiber may play a role in ulcer formation. Psychologic factors may play a role in the development of PUD, and stressful life events, dependency, passiveness, and hostility have all been implicated as contributing factors.

Pathophysiology

Most likely, the pathology is due to an imbalance between the destructive (cytotoxic) factors and defensive (cytoprotective) factors in the GI tract. The toxic mechanisms include acid, pepsin, medications such as aspirin and nonsteroidal antiinflammatory drugs (NSAIDs), bile acids, and infection with *H. pylori*. The defensive factors include the mucus layer, local bicarbonate secretion, epithelial cell renewal, and mucosal blood flow. Prostaglandins play a role in mucosal defense because they stimulate both mucus and alkali secretion. The primary mechanism that prevents the development of peptic ulcer is the secretion of mucus by the epithelial and mucus glands throughout the stomach. The thick mucus layer acts to diffuse acid from the lumen to the gastric mucosal surface, thus protecting the gastric epithelium. The stomach and duodenum produce bicarbonate, decreasing acidity on the epithelial cells and thereby minimizing the effects of the low pH (Chelimsky & Czinn, 2001). When abnormalities in the protective barrier exist, the mucosa is vulnerable to damage by acid and pepsin. Exogenous factors, such as aspirin and NSAIDs, cause gastric ulcers by inhibition of prostaglandin synthesis.

Zollinger-Ellison syndrome may occur in children who have multiple, large, or recurrent ulcers. This syndrome is characterized by hypersecretion of gastric acid, intractable ulcer disease, and intestinal malabsorption caused by a gastrin-secreting tumor of the pancreas.

Diagnostic Evaluation

Diagnosis is based on the history of symptoms, physical examination, and diagnostic testing. The focus is on symptoms such as epigastric abdominal pain, nocturnal pain, oral regurgitation, heartburn, weight loss, hematemesis, and melena (Box 47-14). History should include questions relating to the use of potentially causative substances such as NSAIDs, corticosteroids, alcohol, and tobacco. Laboratory studies may include a CBC to detect anemia, stool analysis for occult blood, liver function tests (LFTs), sedimentation rate, or CRP to evaluate IBD; amylase and lipase to evaluate pancreatitis; and gastric acid measurements to identify hypersecretion. A lactose breath test may be performed to detect lactose intolerance.

Radiographic studies such as an upper GI series may be performed to evaluate obstruction or malrotation. An upper endoscopy is the most reliable procedure to diagnose PUD. A biopsy is taken to determine the presence of *H. pylori*. *H. pylori* can also be diagnosed by a blood test that identifies the presence of the antigen to this organism. The C-urea breath test measures bacterial colonization in the gastric mucosa. This test is used to screen for *H. pylori* in adults and children. Polyclonal and monoclonal stool antigen tests are an accurate noninvasive method for both the initial diagnosis of *H. pylori* and the confirmation of its eradication after treatment (Gisbert, de la Morena, & Abraira, 2006).

BOX 47-14 Characteristics of Peptic Ulcer

Neonates

- Usually gastric and secondary to stress or critical illness
- Commonly has a history of preterm birth, respiratory distress, sepsis, hypoglycemia, or an intraventricular hemorrhage
- Perforation may be first sign that massive bleeding may occur

Infants to 3-Year-Old Children

- Most likely to have a secondary ulcer located equally in the stomach or duodenum
- Primary ulcers less common and usually located in stomach
- Likely to occur in relation to illness, surgery, or trauma
- Hematemesis, melena, or perforation

2- to 6-Year-Old Children

- Primary or secondary ulcers
- Located equally in stomach and duodenum
- Perforation more likely in secondary ulcers
- Periumbilical pain, poor eating, vomiting, irritability, nighttime waking, hematemesis, melena

Children 6 Years and Older

- Usually primary and most often duodenal
- More typical of adult type
- Chance of recurrence greater
- Often associated with *Helicobacter pylori*
- Epigastric or vague abdominal pain
- Possibly nighttime waking, hematemesis, melena, and anemia

Therapeutic Management

The major goals of therapy for children with PUD are to relieve discomfort, promote healing, prevent complications, and prevent recurrence. Management is primarily medical and consists of administration of medications to treat the infection and reduce or neutralize gastric acid secretion.

Antacids are beneficial medications to neutralize gastric acid.

Histamine (H_2) receptor antagonists (antisecretory drugs) act to suppress gastric acid production. Cimetidine (Tagamet), ranitidine (Zantac), and famotidine (Pepcid) are examples of these medications. They have few side effects.

PPIs, such as omeprazole and lansoprazole, act to inhibit the hydrogen ion pump in the parietal cells, thus blocking the production of acid. Controlled studies of these drugs have been done in adults, and these drugs are now commonly used to treat ulcers in children. They appear to be well tolerated and have infrequent side effects (e.g., headache, diarrhea, nausea and vomiting).

Mucosal protective agents, such as sucralfate and bismuth-containing preparations, may be prescribed for PUD. Sucralfate is an aluminum-containing agent that forms a protective barrier over ulcerated mucosa to protect against acid and pepsin. Sucralfate is available in both pill and liquid forms. Because sucralfate blocks the absorption of other medications, it should be given separately from them.

Bismuth compounds are sometimes prescribed for the relief of ulcers, but they are used less frequently than PPIs. Although these compounds inhibit the growth of microorganisms, the mechanism of their activity is poorly understood. In combination with antibiotics, bismuth is effective against *H. pylori.* Although concern has been expressed about the use of bismuth salts in children because of potential side effects, none of these side effects has been reported when these compounds have been used in the treatment of *H. pylori* infection.

Triple drug therapy is the recommended treatment regimen for *H. pylori* (Blanchard & Czinn, 2007; Ford et al, 2004). Combination therapy has demonstrated 90% effectiveness in eradication of *H. pylori* when compared with antibiotic monotherapy. Examples of drug combinations used in triple therapy are (1) bismuth, clarithromycin, and metronidazole; (2) lansoprazole, amoxicillin, and clarithromycin; and (3) metronidazole, clarithromycin, and omeprazole. Common side effects of medications include diarrhea, nausea, and vomiting. The annual relapse rate of 80% for duodenal ulcer and 60% for gastric ulcer can be reduced to less than 5% after successful *H. pylori* eradication (Ford et al, 2004).

In addition to medications, the child with PUD should be given a nutritious diet and advised to avoid caffeine. Adolescents are warned about gastric irritation associated with alcohol use and smoking.

Children with an acute ulcer who have developed complications, such as massive hemorrhage, require emergency care. The administration of IV fluids, blood, or plasma depends on the amount of blood loss. Replacement with whole blood or packed cells may be necessary for significant loss.

Surgical intervention may be required for complications such as hemorrhage, perforation, or gastric outlet obstruction. Ligation of the source of bleeding or closure of a perforation is performed. A vagotomy and pyloroplasty may be indicated in children with recurring ulcers despite aggressive medical treatment.

Prognosis

The long-term prognosis for PUD is variable. Many ulcers are treated successfully with medical therapy; however, primary duodenal peptic ulcers often recur. Complications such as GI bleeding can occur and extend into adult life. The effect of maintenance drug therapy on long-term morbidity remains to be established with further studies.

Nursing Care Management

The primary nursing goal is to promote healing of the ulcer through compliance with the medication regimen. If an analgesic-antipyretic is needed, acetaminophen, not aspirin or an NSAID, is used. Critically ill neonates, infants, and children in intensive care units should receive H_2 blockers to prevent stress ulcers. Critically ill children receiving IV H_2 blockers should have their gastric pH values checked at frequent intervals.

The role of stress in ulcer formation should be considered for nonhospitalized children with chronic illnesses. In children, many ulcers occur secondary to other conditions, and the nurse should be aware of family and environmental conditions that may aggravate or precipitate ulcers. Children may benefit from psychologic counseling and learning how to cope constructively with stress.

Hepatic Disorders

Acute Hepatitis

Etiology

Hepatitis is an acute or chronic inflammation of the liver that can result from several different causes (e.g., virus, chemical or drug reaction, or other diseases). Nonviral causes of hepatitis include autoimmune hepatitis, Wilson's disease, α_1-antitrypsin deficiency, and steatohepatitis. The following six viruses cause 90% of cases of viral hepatitis (Table 47-7):

1. Hepatitis A virus (HAV)
2. Hepatitis B virus (HBV)
3. Hepatitis C virus (HCV)
4. Hepatitis D virus (HDV)
5. Hepatitis E virus (HEV)
6. Hepatitis G virus (HGV)

Hepatitis A

HAV is the most common form of acute viral hepatitis in most parts of the world. It is a member of the picornavirus family. The virus produces a contagious disease transmitted primarily in contaminated stool spread via the fecal-oral route from person to person. HAV has been associated with miniepidemics in areas of poor hygiene and high population density. There is no chronic or carrier state. HAV infection affects individuals of all ages, but the highest incidence occurs among preschool- or school-age children younger than 15 years. Children may serve as the source of HAV infection in adults, such as in child care center exposures. Usually HAV disease in children is mild. It is frequently anicteric and often subclinical. Infected children who show no symptoms may still spread the virus to others. HAV can be severe in children with immunodeficiency disorders. The incubation period is approximately 3 weeks. Although some cases may be prolonged, the prognosis is excellent. A highly effective vaccine for HAV is currently recommended for all children and adolescents in the United States (see Chapter 36).

Hepatitis B

HBV infection can occur as an acute or chronic infection and may range from being asymptomatic and limited to causing fatal fulminant (rapid and severe) hepatitis. HBV varies greatly throughout the world. High-prevalence areas have been identified in Africa and Asia; the United States is considered a low-prevalence area. Transmission is usually via the parenteral route through the exchange of blood or any bodily secretion or fluid. Infections from blood transfusion have been reduced as a result of blood product–screening

Table 47-7 Comparison of Types A, B, and C Hepatitis

CHARACTERISTICS	TYPE A	TYPE B	TYPE C
Incubation period	15-50 days, average 25-30 days	30-180 days, average 50 days	2 wk-6 mo, average 6-7 wk
Period of communicability	Believed to be later half of incubation period to first week after onset of clinical illness	Variable Virus in blood or other body fluids during late incubation period and acute stage of disease; may persist in carrier state for years to lifetime	Begins before onset of symptoms May persist in carrier state for years
Mode of transmission	Principal route–Fecal-oral Rarely–Parenteral	Principal route–parenteral Less frequent route–oral, sexual, any body fluid Perinatal transfer–transplacental blood (last trimester), at delivery, or during breastfeeding, especially if mother has cracked nipples	Principal route–parenteral Nonparenteral spread possible
Clinical features			
Onset	Usually rapid, acute	More insidious	Usually insidious
Fever	Common and early	Less frequent	Less frequent
Anorexia	Common	Mild to moderate	Mild to moderate
Nausea and vomiting	Common	Sometimes present	Mild to moderate
Rash	Rare	Common	Sometimes present
Arthralgia	Rare	Common	Rare
Pruritus	Rare	Sometimes present	Sometimes present
Jaundice	Present (many cases anicteric)	Present	Present
Immunity	Present after one attack; no crossover to type B or C	Present after one attack; no crossover to type A or C	Present after one attack; no crossover to type A or B
Carrier state	No	Yes	Yes
Chronic infection	No	Yes	Yes
Prophylaxis			
Immune globulin (Ig)	Passive immunity Successful, especially in early incubation period and preexposure prophylaxis	May provide passive immunity Inconsistent benefits; probably of no use	Not currently recommended by Centers for Disease Control and Prevention
HAV vaccine	Two inactivated vaccines are approved for children ages 2-18 yr: Havrix and Vaqta; given in a two-dose schedule (6-12 mo between doses)		
HBV Ig (HBIg)	No benefit	Provides passive immunity Postexposure protection possible (for 3-6 months) if given immediately after definite exposure	No benefit
HBV vaccine	No benefit	Provides active immunity Universal vaccination recommended for all newborns	No benefit
Mortality rate	0.1%-0.2%	0.5%-2.0% in uncomplicated cases; may be higher in complicated cases	1%-2.0% in uncomplicated cases; may be higher in complicated case

HAV, Hepatitis A virus; *HBV*, hepatitis B virus.

procedures. Transplantation of organs, intimate physical contact, transmission from mother to infant, and the splashing of contaminated fluids into the mouth or eyes are other sources of infection. Adults whose occupations are associated with exposure to blood or blood products (such as health care workers) are at increased risk for infection and should receive HBV vaccination.

Most HBV infection in children is acquired perinatally. Newborns are at risk for hepatitis if the mother is infected with HBV or was a carrier of HBV during pregnancy. Possible routes of maternal-fetal or maternal-infant transmission include (1) leakage of virus across the placenta late in pregnancy (less than 2% of cases) or during labor, and (2) ingestion of amniotic fluid or maternal blood. Infants who have HBV infection are more than 90% likely to become chronic carriers (Broderick & Jonas, 2003). The incubation period of HBV infection varies from 45 to 160 days.

HBV infection occurs in children and adolescents in the following high risk groups:

- Individuals with hemophilia and others who have received multiple transfusions
- Children and adolescents involved in IV drug abuse
- Institutionalized children and adolescents
- Preschool-age children in endemic areas

- Individuals engaged in heterosexual or homosexual activity with infected partners

Hepatitis C

The prevalence of HCV-positive individuals in the United States during the period of 1999 to 2002 was 1.6 % or an estimated 4.1 million persons infected; the highest risk factor was history of injection drug use (Armstrong et al, 2006). About 0.2% to 0.4% of children younger than 12 years of age are infected with HCV. It is estimated that 4 million people in the United States are anti–HCV-positive. Approximately 5% to 6% of HCV-infected mothers transmit HCV to their newborns; transmission occurs only if the mother is HCV RNA positive at the time of delivery (American Academy of Pediatrics, Committee on Infectious Diseases, 2009b). Another common route of infection is by percutaneous exposure, which occurs through transfusion of blood or blood products, transplantation of organs or tissues, or sharing of used needles. Transfusion-associated HCV infection is low, but a common cause of infection is injection drug use. The American Academy of Pediatrics, Committee on Infectious Diseases (2009b) suggests screening the following groups:

- All infants born to HCV-infected women
- Individuals who received blood products or solid organ transplants before 1992
- Individuals involved in injection drug use
- Individuals who receive long-term hemodialysis
- Persons who received clotting factor concentrations before 1987
- Persons with persistently abnormal alanine aminotransferase (ALT) concentrations
- Persons in settings where HCV prevalence is high and risk factor ascertainment is poor (sexually transmitted disease clinic, correctional facilities)

The clinical course of HCV infection varies. Incubation averages 6 to 7 weeks, with a range of 2 weeks to 6 months. Both acute and chronic HCV infection often produce only mild nonspecific symptoms or no symptoms at all (American Academy of Pediatrics, Committee on Infectious Diseases, 2009b).

The length of time that maternal antibody is present in infants born to HCV-infected women must be considered, and screening should be done after the infant is 18 months old. However, a routine screening program, such as that for HBV, is not recommended. Current recommendations are to evaluate HCV-infected children at regular intervals to monitor for chronic hepatitis. Most children will be asymptomatic with evidence of chronic hepatitis on liver biopsy. Liver enzyme levels may fluctuate between periods of normal and elevated values.

Hepatitis D

HDV is an important cause of acute and chronic liver disease. HDV is a defective RNA virus that requires the presence of HBV. HDV infection occurs primarily in hemophiliac patients and IV drug abusers. The incubation period is 2 to 8 weeks. Both acute and chronic forms are more severe than HBV infection and can lead to cirrhosis. Testing for HDV infection is recommended in children with chronic HBV infection or severe liver disease and in children with acute exacerbation of a previously stable liver disease.

Hepatitis E

HEV infection is enterally transmitted. Transmission may occur through the fecal-oral route or from contaminated water. The incubation period is 2 to 9 weeks. This illness is uncommon in children, does not cause chronic liver disease, is not a chronic condition, and has no carrier state. The mortality rate resulting from submassive hepatic necrosis is low except in pregnant women in their third trimester, in whom mortality reaches 20%.

Hepatitis G

HGV is a blood-borne virus that may also be transmitted by organ transplantation. High-risk groups include transfusion recipients, IV drug users, and individuals infected with HCV. Individuals with the virus are often asymptomatic, and most infections are chronic. The incubation period is unknown.

Diagnostic Evaluation

Diagnosis is based on the history (especially regarding possible exposure to a hepatitis virus); physical examination; and serologic markers (antibodies or antigens) indicating the presence of active infection with hepatitis A, B, or C or previous infection. Because the liver has a large functional reserve, abnormal laboratory tests may be the only indication of hepatitis. However, LFTs are not specific for the diagnosis of viral hepatitis. Although serum aspartate aminotransferase (AST) and ALT levels are markedly elevated in viral hepatitis, other diseases or conditions may cause their elevation. Serum bilirubin levels peak 5 to 10 days after clinical jaundice appears. When hepatitis is severe, albumin levels are depressed, and prothrombin times are increased.

Diagnosis of viral hepatitis is based on the presence of specific viral markers. Diagnosis of acute HAV infection is based on the presence of anti-HAV immune globulin (immune globulin M [IgM]) antibody in the serum. HBV diagnosis depends on the presence of hepatitis B surface antigen (HBsAg) or anti-HBV core (anti-HBc) IgM antibody. Chronic HBV infection is associated with the persistence of HBsAg and HBV DNA markers. The diagnosis of HCV is based on the detection of anti-HCV antibodies and confirmation by polymerase chain reaction for hepatitis C RNA.

An abdominal ultrasound provides measurement of liver size, detection of cystic lesions and stones, and imaging of the gallbladder. Cholescintigraphy radionuclide imaging detects abnormalities in liver uptake, concentration, and excretory function. Finally, a liver biopsy aids in assessing the severity of the disease.

Pathophysiology

Pathologic changes occur primarily in the parenchymal cells of the liver and result in varying degrees of swelling, infiltration of liver cells by mononuclear cells, subsequent degeneration, necrosis, and fibrosis.

Hepatitis can be self-limited, and complete regeneration of liver cells without scarring may occur. However, some forms of hepatitis do not result in complete return of liver function. These include *fulminant hepatitis*, which is characterized by a severe, acute course and massive destruction of the liver, resulting in liver failure and death in 1 to 2 weeks. *Subacute* or *chronic active hepatitis* is characterized by progressive liver destruction, uncertain regeneration, scarring, and potential cirrhosis.

The initial *anicteric* (absence of jaundice) *phase* usually lasts 5 to 7 days and is often mistaken for influenza. Symptoms include nausea, vomiting, extreme anorexia, malaise, easy fatigability, arthralgia, skin rashes, slight to moderate fever, and epigastric or upper right quadrant abdominal pain. Dark urine is a symptom of the *icteric* (jaundice) *phase.* Pruritus may accompany jaundice and can be bothersome, but many children with acute viral hepatitis do not develop jaundice.

Therapeutic Management

Treatment options for viral hepatitis are limited. The goals of management include early detection, recognition of chronic liver disease, support and monitoring, and prevention of spread of the disease.

HAV infection is an acute disease that resolves with support and management of symptoms. Treatment of HBV and HCV is directed at managing the viral load to prevent further destruction of the liver. Currently, HBV and HCV are treated with interferons, naturally occurring proteins that exert antiviral, antiproliferative, and immunomodulatory effects. An interferon formulation, pegylated interferon, can be administered once a week and has been found to sustain plasma levels and enhance viral suppression (Karnam & Reddy, 2003). Lamivudine and adefovir are two other interferon analogs that suppress the replication of HBV (Yuen & Lai, 2001). A combination of α-interferon and ribavirin has resulted in a sustained response in only 50% of patients with HBV and HCV (Waters & Nelson, 2006).

Another important aspect of the therapeutic management of hepatitis involves hospitalization. Hospitalization is necessary if coagulopathy or fulminant hepatitis is present.

Prevention

Proper handwashing and standard isolation precautions can prevent the spread of hepatitis. Prophylactic use of standard immune globulin is effective in preventing HAV infection in situations of preexposure (e.g., anticipated travel to areas where HAV is prevalent) or in situations of postexposure during the early part of the incubation period. Hepatitis B immune globulin (HBIg) is effective in preventing HBV infection after exposure. Immune globulin and HBIg must be administered less than 2 weeks after exposure.

Vaccines have been developed to prevent HAV and HBV infection. HBV vaccination is recommended for all newborns and for high risk groups. HAV vaccination is also recommended for all children beginning at age 12 months and for certain high risk groups (see Immunizations, Chapter 36). Active immunizations are not available against HCV. It is possible to prevent HDV infection by preventing HBV infection.

Prognosis

The prognosis for children with hepatitis varies and depends on the type of virus. HAV usually causes a mild and brief illness with no carrier state. HBV causes a wide spectrum of acute and chronic illness. Approximately 5% of individuals develop chronic hepatitis B each year, and about half of these develop fulminant liver failure, leading to death in the absence of liver transplantation (Kim et al, 2005). Hepatocellular carcinoma is a potentially fatal complication of HBV infection. HCV causes acute hepatitis that progresses to chronic disease in more than 85% of affected individuals, with approximately 15% to 20% developing cirrhosis or hepatocellular carcinoma (Richmond, Dunning, & Desmond, 2004). HCV infection is the leading reason for liver transplantation in adults in the United States (American Academy of Pediatrics, Committee on Infectious Diseases, 2009b).

❋Nursing Care Management

Nursing objectives depend on the severity of the hepatitis, the medical management, and factors influencing the control and transmission of the disease. Children with benign viral hepatitis are frequently cared for at home, and the clinic or office nurse must explain the medical therapy and control measures. If further assistance is needed for parents to comply with therapy, a home health nursing referral may be necessary.

A well-balanced diet and a realistic schedule of rest and activity adjusted to the child's condition are encouraged. HAV is not infectious within a week after the onset of jaundice, and children may feel well enough to resume school. Parents are cautioned about administering any medication to the child, since normal dosages of many drugs may become dangerous because of the liver's inability to detoxify and excrete them. Handwashing is the single most critical measure in reducing risk of transmission. The nurse should explain to parents and children the ways in which HAV (oral-fecal route) and HBV (parenteral route) are spread.

Nurses caring for young people with HBV infection and a known or suspected history of illicit IV drug use should help these teens realize the dangers of substance abuse. Nurses should stress the parenteral mode of transmission of hepatitis and encourage them to seek counseling through a substance abuse program. HBV and HCV are chronic diseases that require frequent monitoring and management. Many communities have multidisciplinary clinics dedicated to the management of these diseases.

Cirrhosis

Cirrhosis occurs at the end stage of many chronic liver diseases, including biliary atresia (BA) and chronic hepatitis. Cirrhosis can also result from infectious, autoimmune, or toxic factors and from chronic diseases such as hemophilia and cystic fibrosis. A cirrhotic liver is irreversibly damaged.

Clinical manifestations in children are similar to those seen with all chronic liver disorders. Children exhibit jaundice, poor growth, anorexia, muscle weakness, and lethargy. Ascites, edema, GI bleeding, anemia, and abdominal pain may be present with impaired intrahepatic blood flow. Pulmonary function may be impaired because of pressure against the diaphragm from hepatosplenomegaly and ascites. Dyspnea and cyanosis may occur, especially on exertion. Intrapulmonary arteriovenous shunts may develop and cause hypoxemia. Spider angiomas and prominent blood vessels are often present on the upper torso.

Therapeutic Management

Therapy is directed toward (1) frequent assessment of liver status with physical examination and LFTs, and (2) management of specific complications. The only successful treatment for end-stage liver disease and liver failure may be *liver transplantation,* which has improved the prognosis substantially for many children with cirrhosis. Currently, the 1- and 5-year survival rate for liver transplantation in children is 87% and 77%, respectively; children under 1 year have a poorer 1-year survival (85%) rate than older children (90%) (Hurwitz & Cox, 2007). Increasing numbers of recipients are reaching their second decade after transplant. The increasing life span after transplantation is related to advances in surgical techniques and improved preoperative, intraoperative, and postoperative care.

Prognosis

Liver transplantation has revolutionized the approach to liver cirrhosis. Liver failure and cirrhosis are indications for transplantation. Liver transplantation reflects the failure of other medical and surgical measures to prevent or treat cirrhosis. Careful monitoring of the child's condition and quality of life is necessary to evaluate the need for and timing of transplantation (see Family-Centered Care box).

FAMILY-CENTERED CARE

End-Stage Liver Disease

In many cases the child and family must cope with an uncertain progression of the disease. The only hope for long-term survival may be liver transplantation. Transplantation can be very successful, but the waiting period may be long, and there are many more children in need of organs than there are donors. The procedure is very expensive and is performed only at designated medical centers that are often far from the family's home. The nurse should recognize the unique stresses of coping with end-stage liver disease and waiting for transplantation and assist the family in coping with these stressors. The assistance of social workers and support from other parents can be very beneficial.

Nursing Care Management

Nursing care of the child with cirrhosis is determined by the cause of the cirrhosis, the severity of complications, and the prognosis. The prognosis for life is poor unless successful liver transplantation occurs. Nursing care of this child is similar to that for any child with a life-threatening illness (see Chapter 41). Hospitalization is usually required when complications occur.

Biliary Atresia

BA is a destructive, idiopathic, inflammatory process that leads to fibrosis and obliteration of the biliary tree (Emerick & Whitington, 2006). BA has been detected in 3.7 in 10,000 live births (Chen et al, 2006). The disorder is more common in girls and preterm infants. In the United States the incidence is twice as high in African-Americans as in Caucasian infants and more common in Chinese than in either Japanese or Caucasian populations.

Etiology and Pathophysiology

The exact cause of BA is unknown. Because it has two distinct forms, postnatal and fetal-embryonic, different pathogenic mechanisms are suggested. Postnatal BA represents 65% to 90% of cases and is probably the result of infection or an immune-mediated mechanism. Jaundice, manifesting with yellow discoloration of the skin or sclerae, is the most common early symptom of BA. Jaundice, indicating cholestasis (the accumulation of compounds that cannot be excreted because of occlusion or obstruction of the biliary tree), can be visible at a total serum bilirubin concentration as low as 5.0 mg/dl. An abnormal direct bilirubin has been designated as greater than 1.0 mg/dl if the total bilirubin is less than 5 mg/dl or a value of direct bilirubin that represents more than 20% of the total bilirubin if it is greater than 5 mg/dl (Emerick & Whitington, 2006). Direct hyperbilirubinemia first appears after the resolution of physiologic (neonatal) jaundice. Jaundice is often associated with pale stool and dark urine. Histologic study demonstrates bile duct remnants and a progressive inflammatory process. In the fetal embryonic form of BA, which represents 10% to 35% of cases, there is a congenital absence of biliary ductal patency and an absence of bile duct remnants. Many infants have associated congenital anomalies. Varying degrees of cholestasis occur, resulting in retention of irritants and toxins. Injury to the liver occurs as the result of the inflammation caused by the cholestasis.

Diagnostic Evaluation

Early diagnosis is the key to survival of the child with BA. Infants who undergo surgery in the first 60 days of life have an 80% chance of establishing bile flow. Between 60 to 90 days of life, the chance of reestablishing flow drops to 50%, and after 90 days to 10% (Chen et al, 2006). The typical infant is thriving, appears well, and has only very mild jaundice during the first 6 to 8 weeks (Emerick & Whitington, 2006) but will soon begin failing to grow and thrive. Several clinical signs may indicate the presence of BA (Box 47-15). Blood tests should include a CBC, electrolytes, bilirubin, and liver enzymes. Additional laboratory analyses, including α_1-antitrypsin level, TORCH titers (see discussion of maternal infections in Chapter 28, p. 748), hepatitis serology, α-fetoprotein, urine cytomegalovirus, and a sweat test, are indicated to rule out

BOX 47-15 Clinical Manifestations of Extrahepatic Biliary Atresia

Jaundice
- Earliest manifestation and most striking feature of disorder
- First observed in sclera
- May be present at birth, but usually not apparent until age 2 to 3 weeks

Urine dark and stains diaper
Stools lighter than expected or white or tan
Hepatomegaly and abdominal distention common
Splenomegaly occurs later
Poor fat metabolism results in:
- Poor weight gain
- General growth failure

Pruritus
Irritability; difficulty comforting infant

other conditions that cause persistent cholestasis and jaundice. Abdominal ultrasonography allows inspection of the liver and biliary system. Hepatobiliary scintigraphy demonstrates biliary patency but does not provide diagnostic certainty. Endoscopic retrograde cholangiopancreatography (ERCP) is performed in very young infants. This procedure, which is done using general anesthesia, has an 80% reported diagnostic accuracy. Percutaneous liver biopsy is highly reliable when the biopsy contains specimens from a number of portal areas. Definitive diagnosis of BA is obtained during surgical laparotomy and an intraoperative cholangiogram.

Therapeutic Management

The primary treatment of BA is *hepatic portoenterostomy (Kasai procedure)*, in which a segment of intestine is anastomosed to the resected porta hepatis to attempt bile drainage. Bile drainage is achieved in approximately 80% to 90% of infants who undergo surgery when younger than 10 weeks of age (Ohi, 2001). However, progressive cirrhosis still occurs in many children, necessitating liver transplantation. Prophylactic antibiotics are given after the Kasai procedure to minimize the risk of ascending cholangitis.

Medical management is primarily supportive. It includes nutritional support with infant formulas that contain medium-chain triglycerides and essential fatty acids. Supplementation is usually required with fat-soluble vitamins; a multivitamin; and minerals, including iron, zinc, and selenium. Aggressive nutritional support with continuous tube feedings or TPN is indicated for moderate to severe growth failure (failure to thrive). The enteral solution should be low in sodium. Ursodeoxycholic acid is used to treat pruritus and hypercholesterolemia.

Prognosis

Untreated BA results in progressive cirrhosis and death in most children by 2 years of age. The Kasai procedure improves the prognosis but is not a cure. Biliary drainage can often be achieved if the surgery is done before the intrahepatic bile ducts are destroyed. Long-term survival has been reported in children who receive the Kasai procedure; however, even with successful bile drainage, many children ultimately develop liver failure.

Advances in surgical techniques and the use of immunosuppressive and antifungal drugs have improved the success of transplantation. The major obstacle continues to be a shortage of donor livers. Reduced-size, split-liver transplantation, retransplantation, and increased public awareness may improve donor organ availability in the future.

Nursing Care Management

Nursing interventions for the child with BA include support of the family before, during, and after surgical procedures and education regarding the treatment plan. In the postoperative period of a portoenterostomy, nursing care is similar to that after major abdominal surgery. Family members need education relating to the proper administration of medications and nutritional therapy, including special formulas, vitamin and mineral supplements, tube feedings, or parenteral nutrition. Pruritus can often be relieved by drug therapy or comfort measures such as baths; trimming fingernails may help decrease the chance of secondary infection as a result of skin breakdown.

Children and their families also need psychosocial support. The uncertain prognosis, discomfort, and waiting for transplantation produce stress, and hospitalizations, pharmacologic therapy, and nutritional therapy impose financial burdens on the family. Families can receive help from the Children's Liver Disease Foundation,* an organization that provides educational materials, programs, and support systems.

Structural Defects

Cleft Lip or Cleft Palate

Clefts of the lip (CL) and palate (CP) are facial malformations that occur during embryonic development and are the most common congenital deformities of the head and neck. They may appear separately or, more often, together. CL results from failure of the maxillary and median nasal processes to fuse; CP is a midline fissure of the palate that results from failure of the two sides to fuse.

CL may vary from a small notch to a complete cleft extending into the base of the nose (see Fig. 28-13). Clefts can be unilateral or bilateral. Deformed dental structures are associated with CL. CP alone occurs in the midline and may involve the soft and hard palates. When associated with CL, the defect may involve the midline and extend into the soft palate on one or both sides.

Cleft lip and palate (CL/P) is more common than CP alone and varies by ethnicity. The occurrence is 1 in 1000 births in Caucasians; 1 in 500 births in Native Americans and Asians, and 1 in 2000 births in African-Americans. CP occurs alone in only 1 in 2500 cases and does not display variation by ethnicity (Merritt, 2005a; Wilkins-Haug, 2008). Approximately 60% to 80% of children born with CL/P are male. Females have a higher frequency of isolated clefts of the secondary palate. Unilateral clefts are nine times more common than bilateral clefts and occur twice as frequently on the left side. Isolated bilateral CLs are uncommon; approximately 86% of those with bilateral CL also have palatal clefts. Approximately 68% of those with unilateral CLs have an associated palatal cleft (Kirschner & LaRossa, 2000). Although the majority of clefts are nonsyndromic (have no associated identifiable syndrome), associated syndromes occur in varying frequencies according to the specific defect; it is estimated that 10% to 50% of children with CL/P have an associated syndrome (Curtin & Boekelheide, 2004; Merritt, 2005a).

Etiology

Cleft deformities may be an isolated anomaly, or they may occur with a recognized syndrome. CL with or without CP is distinct from isolated CP. Clefts of the secondary palate alone are more likely to be associated with syndromes than is isolated CL or CL/P.

CL/P may be caused by exposure to teratogens such as alcohol, anticonvulsants, steroids, and retinoids. Use of phe-

*36 Great Charles St., Birmingham, B3 3JY, United Kingdom; 0121-212-3839; fax: 0121-212-4300; www.childliverdisease.org.

evolve Case Study—Cleft Lip and Palate

nytoin during pregnancy is associated with a tenfold increase in the incidence of CL. The incidence of CL among mothers who smoke during pregnancy is twice as great as the incidence in mothers who do not (Eppley et al, 2005). Alcohol consumption (especially binge drinking) in the first trimester is associated with a higher incidence of oral clefts (DeRoo et al, 2008).

Pathophysiology

Cleft deformities represent a genetic defect in cell migration that results in a failure of the maxillary and premaxillary processes to come together between the third and twelfth week of embryonic development. Although often appearing together, CL and CP are distinct malformations embryologically, occurring at different times during the developmental process. Merging of the upper lip at the midline is completed between the seventh and eleventh weeks of gestation. Fusion of the secondary palate (hard and soft palate) takes place later, between the seventh and twelfth weeks of gestation. In the process of migrating to a horizontal position, the palates are separated by the tongue for a short time. If there is delay in this movement or if the tongue fails to descend soon enough, the remainder of development proceeds, but the palate never fuses.

Diagnostic Evaluation

CL with or without CP is apparent at birth. The defect elicits significant emotional reactions in parents. CP is less obvious than CL and may not be detected without a thorough assessment of the mouth. CP is identified when the examiner places a gloved finger directly on the palate. Clefts of the hard palate form a continuous opening between the mouth and the nasal cavity. The severity of the CP has an impact on feeding; the infant is unable to generate negative pressure and create suction in the oral cavity. This impairs feeding, even though in most cases the infant's ability to swallow is normal.

Prenatal diagnosis with fetal ultrasound is not reliable until the soft tissues of the fetal face can be visualized at 13 to 14 weeks. The sensitivity of fetal ultrasound for facial clefting is almost 100% when CL/P is associated with other structural anomalies. In isolated CP, sensitivity may be 50%; an intact lip is the most difficult to diagnose prenatally (Wilkins-Haug, 2008).

Therapeutic Management

Treatment of the child with isolated CL is surgical and involves no long-term interventions other than possible scar revision. The management of CP involves the cooperative efforts of a multidisciplinary health care team, including pediatrics, plastic surgery, orthodontics, otolaryngology, speech/language pathology, audiology, nursing, and social work. Management is directed toward closure of the cleft(s), prevention of complications, and facilitation of normal growth and development in the child. Until recently, repair of cleft deformities in the neonate was not considered safe. Surgery is now possible in younger neonates because of advances in pediatric anesthesiology and neonatology. However, the infant must be free of any oral, respiratory, or systemic infections.

Surgical Correction of Cleft Lip

The two most common procedures for repair of CL are the Tennison-Randall triangular flap (Z-plasty) and the Millard rotational advancement technique; Z-plasty is used less frequently. The difference between these two is that the Tennison-Randall procedure crosses the philtral line and the Millard procedure advances a triangle of tissue in the upper third of the lip and does not cross the midline. Surgeons often use a combination of these two techniques to address individual differences. Improved surgical techniques have minimized scar retraction, and in the absence of infection or trauma, healing occurs with little scar formation. However, optimal cosmetic results are difficult to obtain in severe defects. Additional revisions of the lip may be necessary at a later age.

Surgical Correction of Cleft Palate

CP repair was previously postponed until a later age than the repair of the CL to take advantage of palatal changes that take place with normal growth. With advanced surgical and anesthesia techniques, some surgeons are currently performing palatal repairs in the neonatal period (Merritt, 2005b; Sandberg, Magee, & Denk, 2002); however, the timing of repair remains controversial and may occur at 9 to 15 months to maximize speech production and growth of the midface. Most surgeons prefer to close the cleft before the child develops faulty speech habits. Persistent velopharyngeal insufficiency, manifested by nasal regurgitation and hypernasal speech, may require a posterior pharyngeal flap procedure. Palatal bone grafting may be performed at a later time to build up bone in the alveolus.

Prognosis

Even with good anatomic closure, most children with CL/P have some degree of compensatory speech pattern that requires speech therapy. Physical problems result from inefficient functioning of the muscles of the soft palate and nasopharynx, improper tooth alignment, and varying degrees of hearing loss. Improper drainage of the middle ear as a result of inefficient function of the eustachian tube contributes to recurrent otitis media and otitis media with effusion, which can cause scarring of the tympanic membrane, leading to hearing impairment in many children with CP. Upper respiratory tract infections require immediate and meticulous attention, and extensive orthodontics and prosthodontics may be needed to correct malposition of teeth and maxillary arches.

Long-term problems are related to the child's social adjustment. The better the physical care, the better is the chance for emotional and social adjustment, although the type of the defect and the degree of residual disability are not always directly related to a satisfactory adjustment. Physical defects are a threat to the self-image, and abnormal speech quality is an impediment to social expression.

Nursing Care Management

The immediate nursing problems in the care of an infant with CL and CP deformities are related to feeding the infant and dealing with the parental reaction to the defect. Facial deformities are especially disturbing to parents; CL is a particularly disfiguring, visible defect that may generate a strong negative response in parents. During the initial phase after birth of an infant with CL or CP, it is important for the nurse to address not only the infant's physical needs but also the parents' emotional needs. The concept that infants with CL or CP are at increased risk for failure of maternal attachment has been challenged. In a few studies, maternal-infant attachment was not negatively affected when measured at 1 year (Speltz et al, 1997) and 24 months of age (Coy, Speltz, & Jones, 2002; Maris et al, 2000).

The nurse should encourage expression of parental grief and fears; such expression may promote attachment in the preoperative period. It is especially important to emphasize the positive aspects of the infant's physical appearance and to express optimism regarding surgical correction while acknowledging the parents' concern. The manner of handling the infant should convey to the parents that the infant is indeed a precious human being.

Feeding

Feeding the newborn with CL/P can be difficult, and teaching the parent to successfully feed the child is perhaps one of the most significant and challenging nursing roles. Growth failure in infants with CL and/or CP has been attributed to preoperative feeding difficulties. After surgical repair most infants with isolated CL or CP and no associated syndrome gain weight successfully or achieve adequate weight and height for age.

Clefts of the lip or palate reduce the infant's ability to suck, which interferes with compression of the areola and renders breastfeeding and bottle-feeding difficult. Liquid taken into the mouth tends to escape via the CP through the nose. Feeding is best accomplished with the infant's head in an upright position, either held in the caregiver's hand or cradled in the arm. Standard bottle nipples may be unsuitable for these infants, who are unable to generate the suction required; therefore special nipples or other feeding devices are needed.

Breastfeeding the infant with CL/P is a viable option and in some cases more successful than bottle-feeding (Merritt, 2005b). The nipple is positioned and stabilized well back in the oral cavity so that tongue action facilitates milk expression. However, the suction required to stimulate milk let-down may be absent initially; therefore a breast pump may be useful before nursing to stimulate the let-down reflex. The advantages to breastfeeding include those described in Chapter 26; in addition, there is evidence that breastfeeding infants with CL/P is protective for otitis media (Lawrence & Lawrence, 2005).

A number of special feeding devices are available for feeding the infant with CL/P, and some are more successful than others, depending on a number of factors (Fig. 47-5). One device is the Cleft Lip/Cleft Palate Nurser,* which consists of a squeezable plastic bottle and a cross-cut nipple. The Haberman Special Needs Feeder† may also be used successfully in infants with a poor or disorganized suck. The Haberman Feeder has a specially designed valve and nipple to adjust the flow of milk to the infant and prevent choking or gagging. A Gravity Flow nipple‡ attached to a squeezable plastic bottle allows formula to be deposited into the mouth of the infant with CL/P. The Pigeon bottle§ has a nipple with a Y-cut, and the nipple is slightly larger and more bulbous to fit naturally into the oral cavity. A one-way backflow valve prevents milk from flowing retrograde into the bottle to minimize the amount of air the infant swallows. The Pigeon bottle is not a squeezable feeding system.

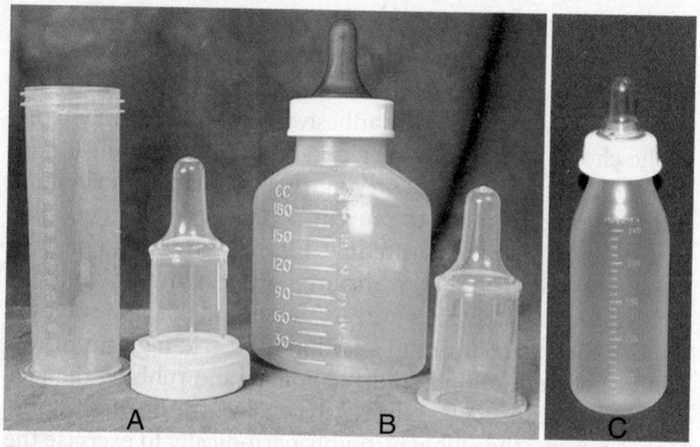

Fig. 47-5 **A,** Haberman feeder. **B,** Mead-Johnson bottle used to feed infant with cleft lip and palate. **C,** Pigeon bottle. *(A and B, Courtesy Texas Children's Hospital, Houston. C, Courtesy Paul Vincent Kuntz, Texas Children's Hospital, Houston, TX.)*

Using these various types of nipples for feeding also has the advantage of helping to meet the infant's sucking needs. Muscle development is especially important for later development of speech. The nipple is positioned in such a way that it is compressed by the infant's tongue and existing palate. If a single-slit nipple is used, the slit is placed vertically so that the infant will be able to produce and stop the flow of milk by alternately opening and closing the opening. Regardless of which type of nipple is used, gentle, steady pressure on the base of the bottle reduces the chance of choking or coughing, and the person doing the feeding should resist the temptation to remove the nipple because of the noise the infant makes or for fear that the infant will choke. An indication that the infant needs to stop feeding momentarily is the facial signal, which involves elevated eyebrows and a wrinkled forehead; the nipple may be gently removed to allow the infant to swallow formula in the mouth without getting upset. These infants need frequent burping because they have a tendency to swallow excessive amounts of air.

Regardless of the feeding method used, the mother should begin to feed the infant as soon as possible. In this way she is able to help determine the method best suited to her and the infant and to become adept in the technique before discharge.

Preoperative Care

In preparation for surgical repair, parents are frequently taught to accustom the infant to the needs of the early postoperative period, especially if surgery is delayed for several months. The infant must be positioned on the back or side postoperatively. Most infants tolerate these positions well because they are accustomed to being supine for sleeping. It is also helpful to place the infant or child in elbow restraints periodically before admission and to feed the infant with a rubber-tipped Asepto syringe or other device (e.g., soft Sipee cup) that will be used postoperatively.

**Mead Johnson, Evansville, IN.*

†Medela Inc., McHenry, IL.

‡Ross Laboratories, Columbus, OH.

§Children's Medical Ventures, South Weymouth, MA.

Postoperative Care for Cleft Lip

The major efforts in the postoperative period are directed toward protecting the operative site. After CL repair *(cheiloplasty)* a metal appliance or adhesive strips are securely taped to the cheeks to relax the surgical site and prevent tension on the suture line caused by crying or other facial movement. Efforts should be made to prevent crying as much as possible to avoid stress on the suture line. Elbow restraints to prevent the infant from rubbing or disturbing the suture line may be applied immediately after surgery. Older infants who roll over require a jacket restraint in addition to restricting arm movement to prevent rolling on the abdomen and rubbing the face on the sheet, especially if the repair involves the lip. It is important to remove the elbow restraints periodically to exercise the arms, provide relief from restrictions, observe the skin for signs of irritation, and provide an opportunity for cuddling and body contact. Sitting the infant in an infant seat provides a change of position and a different view of the environment. Adequate analgesia is required to relieve postoperative pain and to prevent restlessness.

Clear liquids are offered when the infant has fully recovered from the anesthesia, and feeding is resumed when tolerated. The suture site is carefully cleansed of formula or serosanguineous drainage as needed. A thin layer of antibiotic ointment may be prescribed for application to the suture line after cleansing. Meticulous care of the suture line is essential because inflammation or infection will interfere with optimal healing and the ultimate cosmetic effect of the surgical repair. Gentle aspiration of mouth and nasopharyngeal secretions may be necessary to prevent aspiration and respiratory complications. An upright or infant seat position is helpful in the immediate postoperative period (especially for the infant who has difficulty handling secretions).

Postoperative Care of Cleft Palate

The child with CP repair *(palatoplasty)* is allowed to lie on the abdomen immediately after surgery. The child may resume feeding by breast or cup once the child is fully awake; some surgeons prefer soft Sipee cup or asepto syringe feeding in the postoperative period.

NURSING ALERT Avoid the use of suction or other objects in the mouth, such as tongue depressors, thermometers, pacifiers, spoons, or straws following a palatoplasty to maintain the integrity of the surgically repaired palate.

Oral packing may be secured to the palate after palatoplasty; this packing is usually removed after 2 to 3 days. Sometimes the infant will have difficulty breathing after surgery because it is often necessary to alter an established pattern of breathing and adjust to breathing through the nose. This is frustrating but seldom requires more than positioning and support. The elbows may be restrained to keep the child's hands away from the mouth. Parents are instructed to maintain elbow restraints at home until the palate is healed, usually in 4 to 6 weeks. They are instructed to remove the restraints (one at a time) frequently to allow the child to exercise the arms.

The nurse must assess the infant or child's level of postoperative pain. Opioids may be prescribed initially, and acetaminophen may be given as needed thereafter. It is important to manage pain to decrease crying in infants with CL repair.

The older infant or child may be discharged on a blenderized or soft diet, and parents are instructed to continue the diet until the surgeon directs them otherwise. Parents are cautioned against allowing the child to eat hard items (such as toast, hard cookies, and potato chips) that can damage the repaired palate. The expected outcomes are described in the Nursing Process box.

Long-Term Care

Children with CL/P often require a variety of services during recovery. Family members need support and encouragement from health professionals and guidance in activities that facilitate a normal outcome for their child. Parents frequently cite financial stress as a difficult issue. With the combined efforts of the family and the health team, most children achieve a satisfactory outcome. Many children with CL/P have surgical correction that creates a near normal–appearing lip and permits good function. Parents need to understand the function of therapy, the purpose and care of all appliances, and the importance of establishing good mouth care and proper brushing habits.

Throughout the child's development, an important goal is the development of a healthy personality and self-esteem. Many communities have CP parents' groups that offer help and support to families. Agencies that provide services and information for children with CL/P and their families include the American Cleft Palate–Craniofacial Association, the Cleft Palate Foundation,* the Birth Defect Research for Children, Inc.,† and the March of Dimes.‡

Esophageal Atresia with Tracheoesophageal Fistula

Congenital atresia of the esophagus and tracheoesophageal fistula (TEF) are rare malformations that result from failed separation of the esophagus and trachea by the fourth week of gestation. These defects may occur as separate entities or in combination, and without early diagnosis and treatment they pose a serious threat to the infant's well-being (see Fig. 28-15).

Etiology

Esophageal atresia (EA) with or without an associated TEF is the most common esophageal malformation, occurring in approximately 1 in 3500 live births (Shaw-Smith, 2006). There appears to be an equal sex incidence, but the birth weight of most affected infants is significantly lower than average, and incidence of preterm birth is unusually high. A history of maternal polyhydramnios is present in approximately 50% of infants with the defects. EA/TEF is often present with the

---

**1504 E. Franklin St., Suite 102, Chapel Hill, NC 27514-2820; 919-933-9044; e-mail: info@cleftline.org;* www.cleftline.org.

†930 Woodcock Road, Suite 225, Orlando, FL 32803; 407-895-0802, 800-313-2232; e-mail: staff@birthdefects.org; www.birthdefects.org.

‡1275 Mamaroneck Ave., White Plains, NY 10605; 914 428-7100, 888-MODIMES; www.marchofdimes.com. *In Canada,* www.dimes.on.ca.

NURSING PROCESS: THE CHILD WITH A CLEFT LIP OR PALATE

Assessment

The lip defect is visible at birth, and assessment involves describing the location and extent of the defect; the cleft palate (CP) is estimated by visualization during crying. CP without cleft lip (CL) is detected by palpating the palate with the gloved finger during the newborn assessment. The emotional impact of the birth of a child with a cosmetic and functional disability is especially traumatic to the family. Consequently, nursing assessment is also concerned with the family's emotional reaction.

Diagnosis (Problem Identification)

After a thorough assessment, several nursing diagnoses are evident:

Imbalanced nutrition: less than body requirements related to
- oral physical defect
- difficulty eating following surgical procedure

Risk for impaired parenting related to
- infant with a highly visible physical defect

Risk for trauma of the surgical site related to
- infant's developmental need to suck
- increased hand-to-mouth activity

Pain related to
- surgical procedure

Interrupted family processes related to
- child with a physical defect, hospitalization

Planning

The goals of care are related to preoperative care, short-term postoperative care, and long-term management. Goals for the infant and family include:

Preoperative Care

Family will cope with the impact of an infant with a defect.
Infant will receive optimal nutrition.
Infant and family will be prepared for surgery.

Postoperative Care

Infant will experience no trauma and minimal or no pain.
Infant will receive optimal nutrition.
Infant will experience no complications.
Infant and family will receive adequate support.
Family will be prepared for care at home and long-term needs of a child with CP.

Implementation

Numerous intervention strategies are discussed on pp. 1412-1414.

Evaluation

The effectiveness of nursing interventions for the family and the child who has CP is determined by continual assessment and evaluation of care based on the following guidelines:

Preoperative Care

Observe and interview family members about their understanding, feelings, and concerns regarding the defect; any anticipated surgery; and their interactions with the infant.
Observe infant during feeding.
Complete preoperative checklist.

Postoperative Care

Inspect operative site, including the protective device.
Observe operative site for evidence of infection, bleeding, sloughing, or irritation.
Observe for behavioral and physiologic indicators of pain and response to analgesics.
Observe infant during feeding, measure intake and output, and weigh infant daily.
Observe and interview family regarding their understanding and concerns about the infant, including long-term needs.

VATER or VACTERL syndromes, acronyms for syndromes involving a combination of *V*ertebral, *A*norectal, *C*ardiovascular, *T*racheo*E*sophageal, *R*enal, and *L*imb abnormalities. The cardiac and renal anomalies occur most frequently with EA/TEF.

Pathophysiology

The cause of EA/TEF is unknown. In the most frequently encountered form of EA and TEF (80% to 95% of cases), the proximal esophageal segment terminates in a blind pouch, and the distal segment is connected to the trachea or primary bronchus by a short fistula at or near the bifurcation (see Fig. 28-15, *C*). The second most common variety (5% to 8%) consists of a blind pouch at each end, widely separated and with no communication to the trachea (see Fig. 28-15, *A*). Less frequently, an otherwise normal trachea and esophagus are connected by a common fistula (see Fig. 28-15, *E*). Extremely rare anomalies involve a fistula from the trachea to the upper esophageal segment (see Fig. 28-15, *B*) or to both the upper and lower segments (see Fig. 28-15, *D*).

BOX 47-16 Clinical Manifestations of Tracheoesophageal Fistula

Excessive salivation and drooling
Three C's of tracheoesophageal fistula:
- Coughing
- Choking
- Cyanosis

Apnea
Increased respiratory distress during and after feeding
Abdominal distention

Diagnostic Evaluation

The disorder is suspected on the basis of clinical manifestations (Box 47-16). EA should also be suspected in cases of maternal polyhydramnios. Although the diagnosis is established on the basis of clinical signs and symptoms, the exact type of anomaly is determined by radiographic studies. A radiopaque catheter is inserted into the hypopharynx and advanced until it encounters an obstruction. Chest films are taken to ascertain esophageal patency or the presence and level of a blind pouch. Sometimes fistulas are not patent, which makes them more difficult to diagnose. The presence of gas in the stomach or small bowel is indicative of a coexisting TEF.

Therapeutic Management

EA is a surgical emergency. The treatment includes maintenance of a patent airway, prevention of pneumonia, gastric or blind pouch decompression, and surgical repair of the anomaly. When EA/TEF is suspected, the infant is immediately taken off oral intake, started on IV fluids, and placed in the position least likely to cause aspiration of either mouth or stomach secretions (usually elevation of the head 30 to 45 degrees, as the infant's condition allows). Removal of secretions from the mouth and upper pouch requires frequent or continuous suction. Because aspiration pneumonia is almost inevitable and appears early, broad-spectrum antibiotic therapy is often instituted.

Primary surgical correction consists of a thoracotomy with division and ligation of the TEF and an end-to-side anastomosis of the esophagus. This may consist of one operation or be staged with two or more procedures. For infants who are preterm, have multiple anomalies, or are in poor condition, a staged procedure is preferred that involves palliative measures, including gastrostomy, ligation of the TEF, and provision of constant drainage of the esophageal pouch. A delayed esophageal anastomosis is usually attempted after several weeks to months when the upper pouch elongates. Further surgical techniques may be performed later to facilitate esophageal lengthening. If an esophageal anastomosis still cannot be accomplished, a *cervical esophagostomy* (to allow drainage of saliva) and gastrostomy are performed. In some centers, thoracoscopic repair of EA/TEF has been successful, negating the need for a thoracotomy and thus minimizing associated operative complications and morbidities (Holcomb et al, 2005).

A primary anastomosis may be impossible because of insufficient length of the two segments of the esophagus. In these cases, an esophageal replacement procedure using a part of the colon, or gastric tube interposition may be necessary to bridge the missing esophageal segment. Many infants with EA (10% to 20%) also have *tracheomalacia,* a weakness in the tracheal wall that occurs when a dilated proximal pouch compresses the trachea in early fetal life or when the trachea does not develop normally because of a loss of intratracheal pressure.

Complications of a primary repair include an anastomotic leak, strictures resulting from tension or ischemia, esophageal motility disorders causing dysphagia, and GER.

Prognosis

The prognosis is related to the birth weight, associated congenital anomalies, and time of diagnosis. The survival rate is nearly 100% in full-term infants without severe respiratory distress or other anomalies. In preterm low-birth-weight infants with associated anomalies, the incidence of complications is high.

Nursing Care Management

Nursing responsibility for detection of this malformation begins *immediately* after birth. Ideally, the diagnosis should be made before the initial feeding, but often it is not. If fed, the infant swallows normally but suddenly coughs and struggles, and the fluid is aspirated or returns through the nose and mouth. For this reason, it is customary for the nurse to give the infant the first feeding of plain water or to be present when a parent feeds the child to observe the infant's response. Early breastfeeding should not be prevented unless there is a strong suspicion of EA.

NURSING ALERT Any infant who has an excessive amount of frothy saliva in the mouth or difficulty with secretions and unexplained episodes of cyanosis should be suspected of having an EA/TEF and referred immediately for medical evaluation.

Cyanosis is usually the result of laryngospasm caused by overflow of saliva into the larynx from the proximal esophageal pouch. It normally clears after removal of the secretions from the oropharynx by suctioning. Any suspicion of TEF is reported immediately. The infant is placed in an incubator or a radiant warmer, and oxygen is administered to help relieve respiratory distress. Intubation and assisted mechanical ventilation may be necessary if the infant is in respiratory distress. When a newborn is suspected of having a TEF, the most desirable position is supine with the head elevated at least 30 degrees. This position minimizes the reflux of gastric secretions up the distal esophagus into the trachea and bronchi.

It is imperative that the source of aspiration be removed at once. Oral fluids are withheld, and the infant's fluid needs are met parenterally. Until surgery the blind pouch is kept empty by intermittent or continuous suction through an indwelling nasal catheter that extends to the end of the pouch. The catheter needs attention because it has a tendency to become clogged with mucus. It is usually replaced daily. In the event that a staged repair is performed, a gastrostomy tube is inserted and left open so that air entering the stomach through the fistula can escape, thus minimizing the danger that gastric contents will be regurgitated into the trachea. The tube empties by gravity drainage. Feedings through the gastrostomy tube and irrigations with fluid are contraindicated before surgery in the infant with a distal TEF. Nursing interventions include respiratory assessment, airway management, thermoregulation, fluid and electrolyte management, and often nutritional support.

Postoperative Care

Postoperative care is essentially the same as for any high risk newborn. The infant is returned to the radiant warmer, and the gastrostomy tube is connected to gravity drainage until the infant can tolerate feedings. At this time the tube is elevated and secured at a point above the level of the stomach. This allows gastric secretions to pass to the duodenum, and swallowed air can escape through the open tube. Tracheal suction should be done only using a premeasured catheter and with extreme caution to avoid injury to the suture line. If tolerated, gastrostomy feedings may be started and continued until the esophageal anastomosis is healed. Before oral feedings are initiated and the chest tube is removed, a contrast study or esophagram is performed to verify the integrity of the esophageal anastomosis.

The initial attempt at oral feeding must be carefully observed to make certain that the infant can swallow without choking. Oral feedings are begun with sterile water, followed by frequent small feedings of formula. Until the infant can take a sufficient amount by mouth, gastrostomy feedings or parenteral nutrition may supplement oral intake. Infants are usually not discharged until they are taking oral fluids well and the gastrostomy tube is removed. However, the infant who has palliative surgery is discharged with the gastrostomy tube in place. The nurse is responsible for making certain that the caregiver is educated and has practiced the care of the gastrostomy.

Special Problems

Upper respiratory tract complications are a threat to life in both the preoperative and postoperative periods. In addition to pneumonia, there is a constant danger of respiratory distress resulting from atelectasis, pneumothorax, and laryngeal edema. Any persistent respiratory difficulty after removal of secretions is reported to the surgeon immediately. The infant is monitored for anastomotic leaks, as evidenced by purulent chest tube drainage, increased WBC count, and temperature instability.

Periodic esophageal dilations are often necessary in infants and children to manage strictures; the infant may show signs of choking or inability to swallow, thus indicating necessity for dilation. A significant number of infants develop GER after surgery and are placed on antireflux medications. Additional complications following EA repair include tracheomalacia and recurring TEFs (Naik-Mathuria & Olutoye, 2006).

In the infant awaiting esophageal replacement surgery, the catheter is removed, and the upper esophageal segment is drained through a cervical esophagostomy. An esophagostomy is difficult to care for because the skin becomes irritated by moisture from the continuous discharge of saliva. Frequent removal of drainage and application of a layer of protective ointment may remedy the problem. A dressing or ostomy appliance may be applied to collect the drainage, and an enterostomal therapist can provide additional guidance to prevent or treat skin breakdown.

For the infant who requires esophageal replacement, nonnutritive sucking is provided by a pacifier. Sometimes small amounts of water or formula are given orally; although the liquid drains from the esophagostomy, this process allows the infant to develop mature sucking patterns. Other appropriate oral stimulation prevents feeding aversions. Infants who remain NPO for an extended period or who have not received oral stimulation have difficulty eating by mouth after corrective surgery and may develop oral hypersensitivity and food aversion. They require patient, firm guidance to learn how to take food into the mouth and swallow after repair. A referral to a multidisciplinary feeding behavior program is often necessary.

As with any congenital anomaly, parents need support in adjusting to the child's condition. One difficulty is the immediate transfer of the sick newborn to the intensive care unit and the length of hospitalization. Encouraging parents to visit the infant, participate in care when appropriate, and express their feelings regarding the infant's condition facilitates the attachment process. The nurse in the intensive care unit should assume responsibility for ensuring that the parents are kept fully informed of the infant's progress.

Preparing parents for discharge involves teaching them skills they will need at home. They are taught to observe for behaviors that indicate the need for suctioning and for signs of respiratory distress and constriction of the esophagus (e.g., poor feeding, dysphagia, drooling, regurgitation of undigested food). Discharge planning also includes obtaining the necessary equipment and home nursing services to provide home care.

Hernias

A *hernia* is a protrusion of a portion of an organ or organs through an abnormal opening. The danger from herniation arises when the organ protruding through the opening is constricted to the extent that circulation is impaired or when the protruding organs encroach on and impair the function of other structures. A hernia that cannot be reduced easily is called an *incarcerated hernia*. A *strangulated hernia* is one in which the blood supply to the herniated organ is impaired. The herniations of concern are those that protrude through the diaphragm, the abdominal wall, or the inguinal canal. The other hernias of significance to the pediatric age groups are outlined in Table 47-8.

Obstructive Disorders

Obstruction in the GI tract occurs when the passage of nutrients and secretions is impeded by a constricted or occluded lumen or when there is impaired motility *(paralytic ileus)*. Obstructions may be congenital or acquired. Many congenital obstructions such as atresia, imperforate anus, meconium plug, and meconium ileus usually appear in the neonatal period. Other obstructions of congenital etiology such as malrotation, HD, volvulus, incarcerated hernia, and Meckel's diverticulum appear after the first few weeks of life. Intestinal obstruction from acquired causes such as intussusception, pyloric stenosis, and tumors may occur in infancy or childhood. Intestinal obstructions from any cause are characterized by similar signs and symptoms (Box 47-17).

evolve Animation—Digestive Tract, Passage of Food

Hypertrophic Pyloric Stenosis

Hypertrophic pyloric stenosis (HPS) occurs when the circumferential muscle of the pyloric sphincter becomes thickened, resulting in elongation and narrowing of the pyloric channel. This produces an outlet obstruction and compensatory dilation, hypertrophy, and hyperperistalsis of the stomach. This condition usually develops in the first 2 to 5 weeks of life, causing projectile nonbilious vomiting, dehydration, metabolic alkalosis, and eventually, growth failure. The precise etiology is unknown. The reported incidence is 1 to 3 per 1000 live births in the United States (Wyllie, 2007b) with a male/female ratio of 6:1. There is a genetic predisposition, and siblings and offspring of affected persons are at increased risk of developing HPS. It is more common in full-term than in preterm infants and is seen less frequently in African-American and Asian infants than in Caucasian infants.

Table 47-8 Summary Outline of Hernias

TYPE	MANIFESTATIONS/DIAGNOSTIC EVALUATION	MANAGEMENT
Diaphragmatic (Congenital) Protrusion of abdominal organs through opening in diaphragm	**Symptoms:** Mild to severe respiratory distress within a few hours after birth; tachypnea, cyanosis, dyspnea, absent breath sounds in affected area; impaired cardiac output; possible symptoms of shock, severe acidosis **Diagnosis:** Suspected on basis of symptoms—confirmed by radiographic study; often diagnosed prenatally as early as 25th week of gestation	**Therapeutic:** Supportive treatment of respiratory distress and correction of acidosis; possible use of endotracheal intubation, GI decompression, ECMO, high-frequency ventilation and inhaled nitric oxide Surgical reduction of hernia and repair of defect after period of cardiorespiratory stabilization **Nursing** *Preoperative:* Prompt recognition; resuscitation and stabilization Maintain oxygenation and IV fluids Maintain acid-base balance Administer medications Reduce stimulation—environmental/care activities *Postoperative:* Carry out routine postoperative care and observation Relieve pain and provide comfort Support family because this is a critical illness
Hiatal **Sliding:** Protrusion of an abdominal structure (usually stomach) through esophageal hiatus	**Symptoms:** Dysphagia, growth failure, vomiting, neck contortions, frequent unexplained respiratory problems, bleeding; usually associated with GER; may cause gastric volvulus and obstruction **Diagnosis:** Made by fluoroscopy	**Therapeutic:** Management of GER symptoms; positioning; pharmacologic treatment; and dietary management Surgical treatment when complications are related to GER despite medical management **Nursing:** Be alert to significant signs and carry out routine postoperative care
Abdominal **Umbilical:** Weakness in abdominal wall around umbilicus; incomplete closure of abdominal wall, allowing intestinal contents to protrude through opening	**Symptoms:** Noted by inspection and palpation of the abdomen High incidence in preterm and African-American infants Usually closes spontaneously by 1-2 yr of age	**Therapeutic:** No treatment of small defects Operative repair if persists to age 4-6 yr or if defect is >1.5-2.0 cm by age 2 yr Strangulation requires immediate attention **Nursing:** Discourage use of home remedies (e.g., belly bands, coins) Reassure parents
Omphalocele: Protrusion of intraabdominal viscera into base of umbilical cord; sac is covered with peritoneum without skin **Gastroschisis:** Protrusion of intraabdominal contents through defect in abdominal wall lateral to umbilical ring; there is never a peritoneal sac covering the intestinal contents	**Symptoms:** Obvious on inspection Observe for other malformations such as bladder exstrophy and hypospadias	**Therapeutic:** Surgical repair of defect *Preoperative:* Large lesions—gradual reduction of defect Prophylactic antibiotic administration **Nursing (preoperative):** Keep sac or viscera moist with saline-soaked pads Use overhead warming unit Routine care of IV fluid administration Nasogastric suction NPO Nonnutritive sucking

ECMO, Extracorporeal membrane oxygenation; *GER,* gastroesophageal reflux; *GI,* gastrointestinal; *IV,* intravenous; *NPO,* nothing by mouth.

Pathophysiology

The circular muscle of the pylorus thickens as a result of hypertrophy (increased size) and hyperplasia (increased mass). This produces severe narrowing of the pyloric canal between the stomach and the duodenum, causing partial obstruction of the lumen (Fig. 47-6, *A*). Over time, inflammation and edema further reduce the size of the opening, resulting in complete obstruction. The hypertrophied pylorus may be palpable as an olivelike mass in the upper abdomen. Pyloric stenosis is not a congenital disorder. There is now substantial evidence to support decreased expression of neuronal nitric oxide synthase in the nerve fibers of the pyloric circular muscle in infants with HPS (Huang et al, 2006). In most cases HPS is an isolated lesion; however, it may be associated with intestinal malrotation, esophageal and duodenal atresia, and anorectal anomalies.

Diagnostic Evaluation

The diagnosis of HPS is often made after the history and physical examination. The olivelike mass is easily palpated when the stomach is empty, the infant is quiet, and the abdominal muscles are relaxed. Vomiting usually occurs 30 to 60 minutes after feeding and becomes projectile as the obstruction pro-

BOX 47-17 Clinical Manifestations of Mechanical/Paralytic Intestinal Obstruction

Colicky abdominal pain—From peristalsis attempting to overcome the obstruction
Abdominal distention—As a result of accumulation of gas and fluid above the level of the obstruction
Vomiting—Often the earliest sign of a high obstruction; a later sign of lower obstruction (may be bilious or feculent)
Constipation and obstipation—Early signs of low obstructions; later signs of higher obstructions
Dehydration—From losses of large quantities of fluid and electrolytes into the intestine
Rigid and boardlike abdomen—From increased distention
Bowel sounds—Gradually diminish and cease
Respiratory distress—Occurs as the diaphragm is pushed up into the pleural cavity
Shock—Plasma volume diminishes as fluids and electrolytes are lost from the bloodstream into the intestinal lumen (third spacing)
Sepsis—Caused by bacterial proliferation with invasion into the circulation

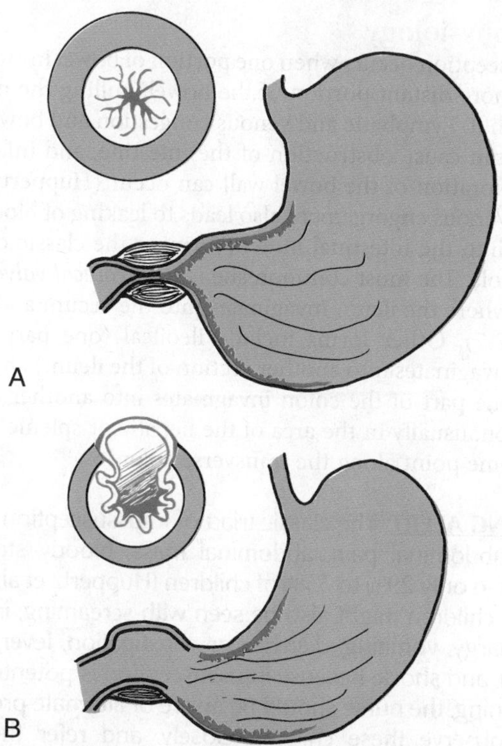

Fig. 47-6 Hypertrophic pyloric stenosis. **A**, Enlarged muscular area nearly obliterates pyloric channel. **B**, Longitudinal surgical division of muscle down to submucosa establishes adequate passageway.

gresses. Emesis is nonbilious, usually consisting of stale milk. Often these infants become dehydrated and lethargic and eventually may appear significantly malnourished.

If the diagnosis is inconclusive from the history and physical signs (Box 47-18), ultrasonography will demonstrate an elongated, sausage-shaped mass with an elongated pyloric channel. The widespread availability of diagnostic ultrasound has made the diagnosis and treatment more expedient. If ultrasound fails to demonstrate a hypertrophied pylorus, upper GI radiography should be done to rule out other causes of vomiting. Laboratory findings reflect the metabolic alterations created by severe depletion of both fluid and electrolytes in the event that vomiting is prolonged and the condition remains undiagnosed. There are decreased serum levels of both sodium and potassium, although these may be masked by the hemoconcentration from ECF depletion. Of greater diagnostic value is a decrease in serum chloride levels and increases in pH and bicarbonate (carbon dioxide content) characteristic of metabolic alkalosis. The BUN level is elevated as evidence of dehydration.

BOX 47-18 Clinical Manifestations of Hypertrophic Pyloric Stenosis

Projectile vomiting
- May be ejected 3 to 4 feet from the child when in a side-lying position, 1 foot or more when in a back-lying position
- Occurs shortly after a feeding (may not occur for several hours)
- May follow each feeding or appear intermittently
- Nonbilious vomitus; may be blood tinged

Infant hungry, avid nurser; eagerly accepts a second feeding after vomiting episode
No evidence of pain or discomfort except that of chronic hunger
Weight loss
Signs of dehydration
Distended upper abdomen
Readily palpable olive-shaped tumor in the epigastrium just to the right of the umbilicus
Visible gastric peristaltic waves that move from left to right across the epigastrium

Therapeutic Management

Surgical relief of the pyloric obstruction by *pyloromyotomy* is the standard treatment for this disorder. The procedure is performed through a right upper quadrant incision (laparotomy) and consists of a longitudinal incision through the circular muscle fibers of the pylorus down to, but not including, the submucosa (see Fig. 47-6, *B*). The procedure has a high success rate when infants receive careful preoperative preparation to correct fluid and electrolyte imbalances.

Feedings are usually begun 4 to 6 hours postoperatively, beginning with small, frequent feedings of clear liquids followed by formula or breast milk as tolerated. Another procedure, *laparoscopy,* may be performed for infants with HPS. The use of a small incision for the laparoscope results in shorter surgical time, more rapid postoperative feeding, and quicker discharge.

Prognosis

Most infants recover completely and rapidly after pyloromyotomy. Postoperative complications include persistent pyloric obstruction and wound dehiscence. Some infants also have GER.

Nursing Care Management

The diagnosis of HPS is considered in the infant less than 6 to 8 weeks of age who appears alert but often fails to gain weight and has a history of vomiting after milk consumption. Assessment is based on observation of eating behaviors and evidence of other characteristic clinical manifestations.

Preoperative Care

Preoperatively the emphasis is placed on restoring hydration and electrolyte balance, however often the condition is brought to the practitioner's attention and readily diagnosed before fluid and electrolyte problems occur. Infants are usually given no oral feedings and receive IV fluids with glucose and electrolyte replacement based on laboratory serum electrolyte values. Careful monitoring of the IV infusion and diligent attention to intake, output, and urine specific gravity measurements are important. Vomiting and the number and character of stools are observed and recorded accurately.

Observations also include assessment of vital signs, particularly those that might indicate fluid or electrolyte imbalances. These infants may have metabolic alkalosis from loss of hydrogen ions and from potassium, sodium, and chloride depletion if vomiting is prolonged. The skin, mucous membranes, and daily weight are assessed for alterations in hydration status and water gain or loss.

If stomach decompression and gastric lavage are used preoperatively, the nurse is responsible for ensuring that the tube is patent and functioning properly and for measuring and recording the type and amount of drainage. Infants who are receiving IV fluids or have an NG tube for continuous drainage must be observed to prevent the infusion device or tube from becoming dislodged.

General hygienic care, with attention to the skin and mouth in dehydrated infants, is essential. Protection from infection is also important because infants with impaired nutritional status are more susceptible than normal newborns. Parental involvement is encouraged and promoted.

Postoperative Care

Postoperative vomiting may occur, and most infants, even with successful surgery, exhibit some vomiting during the first 24 to 48 hours because of edema resulting from the surgery. IV fluids are administered until the infant can retain adequate amounts by mouth. Observation of physical signs, monitoring of IV fluids, and careful recording of intake and output are maintained. The infant is also observed for evidence of pain, and appropriate analgesics are given.

Feedings are usually instituted soon after surgery, beginning with clear liquids and advancing to formula or breast milk as tolerated. They are offered slowly, in small amounts, and at frequent intervals as ordered by the practitioner. Observation and recording of feedings and the infant's responses to them are a vital part of postoperative care. Care of the operative site consists of observation for any drainage or signs of inflammation and care of the incision as directed by the surgeon.

Parents are encouraged to remain with their child and become involved in the child's care. Vomiting of a projectile nature is frightening to parents, and they often believe that they may have done something wrong or that surgery was not successful. Most parents need support and reassurance that the condition is caused by a structural problem and is in no way a reflection on their parenting skills and capacities.

Intussusception

Intussusception is the most common cause of acute intestinal obstruction in children younger than 5 years of age. The peak age is 3 to 9 months (Huppertz et al, 2006). It is more common in boys than in girls and in children with cystic fibrosis. Although specific intestinal lesions can be found in about 3% of these children, the cause is usually not known. More than 90% of intussusceptions do not have a pathologic lead point, such as a polyp, lymphoma, or Meckel's diverticulum. The idiopathic cases are most likely a result of hypertrophy of intestinal lymphoid tissue secondary to viral infection. Some cases were associated with administration of the first licensed rotavirus vaccine, the reassortant rhesus-human tetravalent rotavirus vaccine (RRV-IV; RotaShield), which led to its voluntary withdrawal in the late 1990s. No such association has been reported to date from large phase III safety trials with the two new rotavirus vaccines currently being administered in the United States (American Academy of Pediatrics, Committee on Infectious Diseases, 2009a).

Pathophysiology

Intussusception occurs when one portion of bowel invaginates into a more distant portion of the bowel, pulling the mesentery with it. Lymphatic and venous congestion and bowel wall edema can cause obstruction of the intestine, and infarction and perforation of the bowel wall can occur (Huppertz et al, 2006). Venous engorgement also leads to leaking of blood and mucus into the intestinal lumen, forming the classic currant jelly stools. The most common site is the *ileocecal valve* (ileocolic), where the ileum invaginates into the cecum and colon (Fig. 47-7). Other forms include ileoileal (one part of the ileum invaginates into another section of the ileum) and colocolic (one part of the colon invaginates into another area of the colon, usually in the area of the hepatic or splenic flexure or at some point along the transverse colon).

NURSING ALERT The classic triad of intussusception symptoms (abdominal pain, abdominal mass, bloody stools) is present in only 29% to 33% of children (Huppertz et al, 2006). Initially children might also be seen with screaming, irritability, lethargy, vomiting, diarrhea or constipation, fever, dehydration, and shock. Because intussusception is potentially life threatening, the nurse should be aware of alternate presentations, observe these children closely, and refer them for further evaluation.

Diagnostic Evaluation

Frequently subjective findings lead to the diagnosis (Box 47-19), which can be confirmed by ultrasound. Spontaneous reduction occurs in up to 10% of patients.

Therapeutic Management

Conservative treatment consists of radiologist-guided pneumoenema (air enema) with or without water-soluble contrast

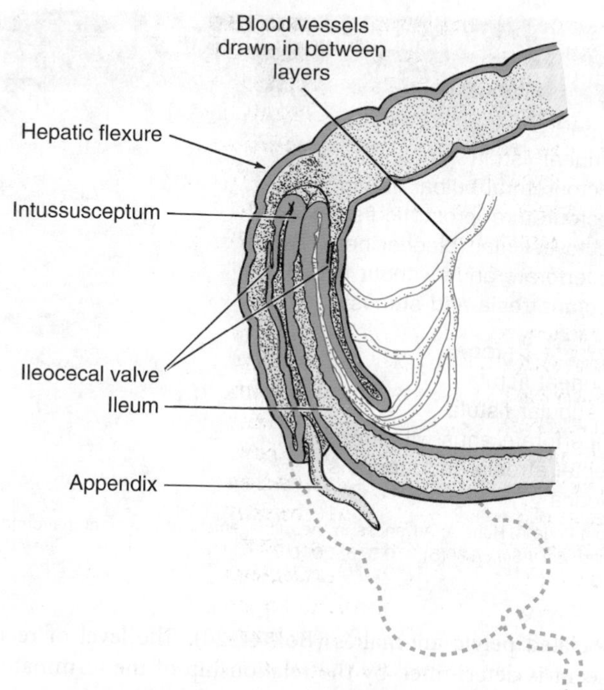

Fig. 47-7 Ileocecal (ileocolic) intussusception.

BOX 47-19 Clinical Manifestations of Intussusception

- Sudden acute abdominal pain
- Child screaming and drawing the knees toward the chest
- Child appearing normal and comfortable during intervals between episodes of pain
- Vomiting
- Lethargy
- Passage of red, currant jelly–like stools (stool mixed with blood and mucus)
- Tender, distended abdomen
- Palpable sausage-shaped mass in upper right quadrant
- Empty lower right quadrant (Dance sign)
- Eventual fever, prostration, and other signs of peritonitis

or ultrasound-guided hydrostatic (saline) enema to reduce the defect, the advantage of the latter being that no ionizing radiation is needed (Huppertz et al, 2006). Recurrence of intussusception after conservative treatment occurs in about 1 in 10 patients; no predictable risk factors for recurrence have been identified.

IV fluids, NG decompression, and antibiotic therapy may be used before hydrostatic reduction is attempted. If these procedures are not successful, the child may require surgical intervention. Surgery involves manually reducing the invagination and, when indicated, resecting any nonviable intestine.

Prognosis

Nonoperative reduction is successful in approximately 80% of cases (Huppertz et al, 2006). Surgery is required for patients in whom the contrast enema is unsuccessful. With early diagnosis and treatment, serious complications and death are uncommon.

Nursing Care Management

The nurse can help establish a diagnosis by listening to the parent's description of the child's physical and behavioral symptoms. It is not unusual for parents to state that they thought something was seriously wrong before others shared their concerns. The description of the child's severe colicky abdominal pain combined with vomiting is a significant sign of intussusception.

As soon as a possible diagnosis of intussusception is made, the nurse prepares the parents for the immediate need for hospitalization, the nonsurgical technique of hydrostatic reduction, and the possibility of surgery. It is important to explain the basic defect of intussusception. A model of the defect is easily demonstrated by pushing the end of a finger on a rubber glove back into itself or using the example of a telescoping rod. The principle of reduction by hydrostatic pressure can be simulated by filling the glove with water, which pushes the "finger" into a fully extended position.

Physical care of the child does not differ from that for any child undergoing abdominal surgery. Even though nonsurgical intervention may be successful, the usual preoperative procedures, such as maintenance of NPO status, routine laboratory testing (CBC and urinalysis), signed parental consent, and preanesthetic sedation, are performed. For the child with signs of electrolyte imbalance, hemorrhage, or peritonitis, additional preparation, such as replacement fluids, whole blood or plasma, and NG suctioning, may be needed. Before surgery the nurse monitors all stools.

NURSING ALERT Passage of a normal brown stool usually indicates that the intussusception has reduced itself. This is immediately reported to the practitioner, who may choose to alter the diagnostic and therapeutic care plan.

Postprocedural care includes observations of vital signs, blood pressure, intact sutures and dressing, and the return of bowel sounds. After spontaneous or hydrostatic reduction, the nurse observes for passage of water-soluble contrast material (if used) and the stool patterns, since the intussusception may recur. Children may be admitted to the hospital or monitored on an outpatient basis. A recurrence is treated with the conservative reduction techniques described previously, but a laparotomy is considered for multiple recurrences.

Because hospitalization may be the child's first separation from the parents, it is important to preserve the parent-child relationship by encouraging rooming-in or extended visiting. It may be the parents' first experience with hospitalization, necessitating their preparation for procedures such as IV therapy, frequent vital sign and blood pressure monitoring, dressings, and NPO. Because of the rapidity of the onset, diagnosis, and treatment, parents may feel stunned or numb. They may ask few questions, or they may constantly make inquiries, sometimes the same ones several times. If the nurse realizes the circumstances surrounding this condition, the parents' reactions are more likely to be understood and accepted.

evolve Animation—Volvulus, Pediatric

Malrotation and Volvulus

Malrotation of the intestine is caused by the abnormal rotation of the intestine around the superior mesenteric artery during embryologic development. Malrotation may manifest in utero or may be asymptomatic throughout life. Infants with malrotation may have intermittent bilious vomiting, recurrent abdominal pain, distention, or lower GI bleeding. Malrotation is the most serious type of intestinal obstruction because, if the intestine undergoes complete volvulus (the intestine twisting around itself), compromise of the blood supply will result in intestinal necrosis, peritonitis, perforation, and death.

Diagnostic Evaluation

It is imperative that malrotation and volvulus be diagnosed promptly and surgical treatment instituted quickly. An upper GI series is the definitive procedure to diagnose this condition.

Therapeutic Management

Surgery is indicated to remove the affected area. Because of the extensive nature of some lesions, short-gut syndrome is a postoperative complication.

Nursing Care Management

Preoperatively the nursing care is the same as that provided to an infant or child with intestinal obstruction. Postoperatively the nursing care is similar to that provided to the infant or child who has undergone abdominal surgery.

Anorectal Malformations

Anorectal malformations include a number of anomalies of the genitourinary and pelvic organs. These malformations are among the more common congenital malformations caused by abnormal development, with an incidence of 1 in 4000 live births (Klein & Thomas, 2007). The anus and rectum originate from an embryologic structure called the *cloaca.* Lateral growth of the cloaca forms the urorectal septum that separates the rectum dorsally from the urinary tract ventrally. The rectum and urinary tract separate completely by the seventh week of gestation. Anomalies that occur reflect the stage of development of these processes.

Imperforate anus includes several forms of malformation without an obvious anal opening. Many have a fistula from the distal rectum to the perineum or genitourinary system. Anorectal malformations may occur in isolation or as part of the VACTERL or VATER syndromes.

A *persistent cloaca* is a complex anorectal malformation in which the rectum, vagina, and urethra drain into a common channel that opens onto the perineum via the usual urethral site (Chien et al, 2005). *Cloacal exstrophy* is a rare, severe defect in which there is externalization of the bladder and bowel through the abdominal wall. Often the genitalia are indefinite, and chromosome studies are necessary to determine the child's gender, which is almost always female. The exstrophic bladder is separated into two halves by the cecum; other features may include an omphalocele, imperforate anus, and at times a neural tube defect.

Anorectal anomalies are classified according to gender and abnormal anatomic features, including genitourinary and associated pelvic anomalies (Box 47-20). The level of rectal descent is determined by the relationship of the termination of the bowel to the puborectalis sling of the levator ani musculature. Anorectal malformations may also be classified according to the level of the malformation (high, intermediate, and low), although this classification is slowly being abandoned in favor of anatomic features. About 50% of children with anorectal anomalies have a urologic problem.

BOX 47-20 Classification of Anorectal Malformations

Male Defects
Perineal fistula
Rectourethral bulbar fistula
Rectourethral prostatic fistula
Rectovesicular (bladder neck) fistula
Imperforate anus without fistula
Rectal atresia and stenosis

Female Defects
Perineal fistula
Vestibular fistula
Imperforate anus without fistula
Rectal atresia and stenosis
Cloaca

From Peña A, Hong A: Advances in the management of anorectal malformations, *Am J Surg* 180(5):370-376, 2000.

Diagnostic Evaluation

Checking for patency of the anus and rectum is a routine part of the newborn assessment and should include observations regarding the passage of meconium. Inspection of the perineal area reveals absence of the normal anal opening; however, the appearance of the perineum alone does not accurately predict the level of the lesion. Genitourinary and pelvic anomalies associated with anorectal malformations should be considered.

In the newborn the presence of meconium on the perineum does not always indicate anal patency (particularly in girls) because a fistula may be present and allow evacuation of meconium through the vagina. Fistulas may not be apparent at birth but may become obvious as peristalsis gradually forces the meconium through the fistula. Rectourinary fistulas should be suspected if there is meconium in the urine. Anal stenosis may not be identified until the child is older and comes to the physician with a history of difficult defecation, abdominal distention, and ribbonlike stools.

Abdominal ultrasound is performed to determine the existence of other malformations. An IV pyelogram and voiding cystourethrogram are recommended for an infant with a high malformation to identify anomalies of the urinary tract. Further examination is also indicated when there is evidence of urinary tract infection or other symptoms. If a syndrome is suspected, cardiac evaluation and spinal films should be obtained.

Therapeutic Management

Successful treatment for anal stenosis is generally accomplished by manual dilations. The procedure is initiated by a physician and repeated on a regular basis by the nurses in the hospital. Parents are taught to continue the dilations at home. Perineal fistulas are treated by anoplasty during the newborn period. The opening is moved to the center of the external sphincter, and dilations are begun. More extensive defects are usually managed with a colostomy, and corrective surgical repair is performed later in the first year.

The type of defect, the sacral anatomy, and the quality of muscles influence the long-term prognosis. In general, if the newborn has a deep midline groove, two well-formed buttocks, and an anal dimple, the prognosis for bowel control is better than if the infant has a flat or "rocker" bottom and no midline groove because of associated neurologic problems. A functioning interior anal sphincter is important to achieve continence. In its absence, the child may need a bowel program to achieve socially acceptable bowel continence. Other potential complications after surgical treatment include strictures, recurrent rectourinary fistula, mucosal prolapse, and constipation.

Nursing Care Management

The first nursing responsibility is identification of undetected anorectal malformations. A poorly developed anal dimple, a genitourinary fistula, or vertebral abnormalities suggest a high lesion. A newborn who does not pass a stool within 24 to 48 hours of birth requires further assessment. In addition, meconium that appears at an inappropriate orifice is reported. Preoperative care includes diagnostic evaluation, GI decompression, and IV fluids.

Nursing care after an anorectoplasty is directed toward healing the surgical site without infection or complications. Care involves keeping the anal area as clean as possible with scrupulous perineal care. A temporary dressing and drain may be placed initially to manage the continuous passage of stool. Protective ointments such as zinc oxide and occlusive dressings such as hydrocolloids decrease skin irritation from frequent loose stools. The preferred position is a side-lying prone position with the hips elevated or a supine position with the legs suspended at a 90-degree angle to the trunk to prevent pressure on perineal sutures.

There may be an NG tube for abdominal decompression and IV feedings. The infant is given formula when normal peristalsis is noted. Care of the infant with a colostomy involves frequent dressing changes, meticulous skin care, and correct application of a collection device (see Chapter 45).

Family Support, Discharge Planning, and Home Care

Long-term follow-up is important for children with high malformations. After the definitive pull-through procedure, toilet training is delayed, and complete continence is seldom achieved at the usual age of 2 to 3 years. Prevention of constipation is important, and breastfeeding is encouraged postoperatively. If a cow's milk–based formula is used, a laxative may be prescribed. Bowel habit training, diet modification, and administration of stool softeners or fiber are important aspects of bowel management. Optimum bowel function may not be achieved until late childhood or adolescence. Support and reassurance are important during the slow progression to normal function.

Parents are instructed in perineal and wound care or care of the colostomy. Anal dilations may be necessary for some infants. Parents are advised to observe stooling patterns and notify the physician if there are any signs of anal stricture or complications.

Malabsorption Syndromes

Chronic diarrhea and malabsorption of nutrients characterize malabsorption syndromes. An important complication of malabsorption syndromes in children is growth failure (failure to thrive). Most cases are classified according to the location of the supposed anatomic or biochemical defect. The term *celiac disease* is often used to describe a symptom complex with four characteristics: (1) steatorrhea (fatty, foul, frothy, bulky stools), (2) general malnutrition, (3) abdominal distention, and (4) secondary vitamin deficiencies.

Digestive defects are conditions in which the enzymes necessary for digestion are diminished or absent, such as (1) cystic fibrosis, in which pancreatic enzymes are absent; (2) biliary or liver disease, in which bile flow is affected; or (3) lactase deficiency, in which there is congenital or secondary lactose intolerance.

Absorptive defects are conditions in which the intestinal mucosal transport system is impaired. This may occur because of a primary defect (e.g., celiac disease) or secondary to IBD that results in impaired absorption because bowel motility is accelerated (e.g., ulcerative colitis). Obstructive disorders (e.g., HD) also cause secondary malabsorption from enterocolitis.

Anatomic defects, such as extensive resection of the bowel or short-bowel syndrome (SBS), affect digestion by decreasing the transit time of substances and affect absorption by severely compromising the absorptive surface.

Celiac Disease

Celiac disease, also known as *gluten-induced enteropathy, gluten-sensitive enteropathy,* and *celiac sprue,* is an immune-mediated enteropathy of the proximal small intestine triggered by inappropriate immune response to ingested gluten and gluten-related proteins found in wheat, rye, and barley. Celiac disease is one of the most common lifelong disorders affecting approximately 1% of the general population. As many as 2 million to 3 million Americans may be affected by celiac disease, but only 70,000 to 80,000 carry the diagnosis. It is second only to cystic fibrosis as a cause of malabsorption in children. The age that this condition first appears and its prevalence have changed over the past 30 to 40 years. Celiac sprue used to be considered a disease of childhood, but adult presentation is becoming more common. It is seen more frequently in Europe than in the United States and is rarely reported in Asians or African-Americans. Recent studies suggest the prevalence of celiac disease as being 1 in 322 in children and 1 in 105 adults (Rostom, Murray, & Kagnoff, 2006). The exact cause of celiac disease is unknown, but there appears to be an inherited predisposition with an influence by environmental factors.

Pathophysiology

Genetic predisposition is an essential factor in the development of celiac disease. Membrane receptors involved in preferential antigen presentation to CD4+ T cells play a crucial role in the immune response characteristic of celiac disease. Genes located on the HLA region of chromosome 6 (i.e., HLA-DQ2 or HLA-DQ8) are found in almost 100% of those affected with celiac disease (Murdock & Johnston, 2005). Once the inflammatory reaction is activated by gluten, CD4+ T cells produce cytokines, which are likely to contribute to the intestinal damage. The damage consists of infiltration of the lamina propria, crypt hyperplasia, and villous atrophy and flattening. With sufficient villous atrophy, malabsorption occurs.

Diagnostic Evaluation

Classic symptoms of celiac disease are GI manifestations usually noted several months after the introduction of gluten-containing grains into the diet, typically between the ages of 6 months and 2 years (Box 47-21). Typically, children are seen with impaired growth, chronic diarrhea, abdominal distention, muscle wasting with hypotonia, poor appetite, and lack of energy. The clinical manifestations are usually insidious and chronic. The first evidence may be growth failure and diarrhea. Less typical presentation has been observed in children ages 5 to 7 years who have abdominal pain; nausea; vomiting; bloating; constipation; or extraintestinal manifestations, including short stature, pubertal delay, iron deficiency, dental enamel defects, and abnormal LFTs. Older children have been found to have osteoporosis. Untreated celiac disease can evolve into celiac crisis, characterized by abdominal distention, explosive watery diarrhea, and dehydration with electrolyte imbalance, leading to hypotensive shock and lethargy.

BOX 47-21 Clinical Manifestations of Celiac Disease

Impaired Fat Absorption

Steatorrhea (excessively large, pale, oily, frothy stools)
Exceedingly foul-smelling stools

Impaired Absorption of Nutrients

Malnutrition
Muscle wasting (especially prominent in legs and buttocks)
Anemia
Anorexia
Abdominal distention

Behavioral Changes

Irritability
Fretfulness
Uncooperativeness
Apathy

Celiac Crisis*

Acute, severe episodes of profuse watery diarrhea and vomiting
May be precipitated by:

- Infections (especially gastrointestinal)
- Prolonged fluid and electrolyte depletion
- Emotional disturbance

*In very young children.

The diagnosis of celiac disease is based on a biopsy of the small intestine demonstrating the characteristic changes of mucosal inflammation, crypt hyperplasia, and villous atrophy (Sood, 2007). Within a day or two of instituting the gluten-free diet, most children with celiac disease demonstrate a favorable response, including weight gain and improved appetite. Within a few weeks diarrhea and steatorrhea resolve.

Commercially available serologic tests for celiac disease include antigliadin antibodies of both the immune globulin A and G classes (IgA and IgG); antiendomysium IgA; and anti-tissue transglutaminase IgA and IgG antibodies for screening first-degree relatives of known celiac disease patients and those with known celiac disease–associated disorders such as type 1 diabetes, thyroiditis, arthritis, primary biliary cirrhosis, Down syndrome, Turner's syndrome, Williams syndrome, and osteopenia or osteoporosis. False-positive results are likely when only one serologic test is used because patients with these disorders can also test positive for these antibodies. Use of more than one test increases diagnostic accuracy (Gelfond & Fasano, 2006). Ruling out total IgA deficiency is necessary to minimize false-negative results.

Therapeutic Management

Treatment of chronic celiac disease is primarily dietary. Although the diet is called *gluten free,* it is actually *low* in gluten, since it is impossible to remove every source of this protein. Because gluten is found primarily in wheat and rye, but also in smaller quantities in barley and oats, these four foods are eliminated. Corn and rice become substitute grain foods.

Children with untreated celiac disease may have associated lactose intolerance related to intestinal mucosal lesions, which usually improves with gluten withdrawal and intestinal healing. Specific nutritional deficiencies are treated with appropriate supplements, including vitamins, iron, and calories.

Prognosis

Celiac disease is regarded as a chronic disease. The most severe symptoms usually occur in early childhood and again in adult life. Strict dietary avoidance of gluten prevents symptoms and may minimize the risk of developing lymphoma, the most serious complication of the disease.

Nursing Care Management

The main nursing consideration is helping the child adhere to dietary management. Considerable time is involved in explaining to the child and parents the disease process, the specific role of gluten in aggravating the condition, and the foods that must be restricted. Also, a lactose-free diet, which necessitates eliminating all milk products, may be needed initially. It is especially difficult to maintain a diet indefinitely when the child has no symptoms and temporary transgressions result in no difficulties. However, evidence indicates that most individuals who relax their diet experience a relapse of their disease and possibly exhibit growth delay, anemia, or osteomalacia. There is also the risk of developing malignant lymphoma of the small intestine or other GI malignancies.

Although the chief source of gluten is cereal and baked goods, grains are frequently added to processed foods as thickeners or fillers. Gluten is also added to many foods as "hydrolyzed vegetable protein." The nurse must advise parents to read carefully all ingredients on labels to avoid hidden sources of gluten. Many gluten-containing products are easily eliminated from the infant's or young child's diet, but monitoring the diet of a school-age child or adolescent is more difficult. Many "favorite" foods, such as hot dogs, pizza, and spaghetti, are chief offenders. Luncheon preparation away from home is particularly difficult because bread, luncheon meats, and instant soups are not tolerated.

Generally, management includes a diet high in calories and proteins with simple carbohydrates, such as fruits and vegetables, but low in fats. Initially the bowel may be inflamed as a result of the pathologic process, so high-fiber foods, such as nuts, raisins, raw vegetables, and raw fruits with skin, are avoided until inflammation has subsided. In a survey of 253 patients with celiac disease in New York State, Lee and Newman (2003) found that 86% experienced difficulties eating out and 82% experienced difficulties traveling because of the constraints of a gluten-free diet.

Several organizations and resources are available to help families cope with this condition. The Celiac Sprue Association/United States of America* provides support, guidance, and educational materials to families concerning a gluten-free diet, food sources, recipes, and travel information. Several published cookbooks contain gluten-free recipes.†

Short-Bowel Syndrome

SBS is a malabsorptive disorder that occurs when there is decreased mucosal surface area, usually as a result of extensive resection of the small intestine. The most common causes of SBS in children include congenital anomalies (jejunal and ileal atresia, gastroschisis), ischemia (necrotizing enterocolitis), and trauma or vascular injury (volvulus [twisting of bowel on itself]). Other causes include volvulus that results in massive resection, long-segment HD, and omphalocele.

The prognosis for infants and children with SBS has dramatically improved in the past 25 years as a result of advances in parenteral nutrition and enteral feeding. Both the amount and location of bowel lost are important in determining the severity of the condition. The preservation of the terminal ileum and ileocecal valve influences fluid and nutrient absorption and may avoid problems of bacterial overgrowth by preventing the entrance of bacteria from the colon into the small intestine.

The small intestine has significant capacity for adaptation after resection. During the *adaptation process*, the villus height increases (villous hyperplasia), and the cell number and absorptive surface area also increase. As villus length and the number of enterocytes available for absorption per centimeter of bowel increase, nutrient absorption increases. Intraluminal enteral feedings stimulate the adaptation process and maintain the structural and functional integrity of the small intestine.

Therapeutic Management

The goals of treatment are to (1) preserve as much length of bowel as possible during surgery; (2) maintain the child's nutritional status, growth, and development while intestinal adaptation occurs; (3) stimulate intestinal adaptation with enteral feeding; and (4) minimize complications related to the disease process and therapy.

Nutritional support is the long-term focus of care. The *initial phase* of therapy includes TPN as the primary source of nutrition. The *second phase* is the introduction of enteral feeding, which usually begins as soon as possible after surgery. Elemental formulas containing glucose, sucrose and glucose polymers, hydrolyzed proteins, and medium-chain triglycerides facilitate absorption. Usually these formulas are given by continuous infusion through an NG or gastrostomy tube. As the enteral feedings are advanced, the TPN solution is decreased in terms of calories, amount of fluid, and total hours of infusion per day. The *final phase* of nutritional support occurs when growth and development are sustained exclusively by enteral feedings. When TPN is discontinued, there is a risk of nutritional deficiency secondary to malabsorption of fat-soluble vitamins (A, D, E, K) and trace minerals (iron, selenium, zinc). Serum vitamin and mineral levels should be obtained, and enteral supplementation of vitamins and minerals may be required. Pharmacologic agents have been used to reduce secretory losses. H_2 blockers, PPIs, and octreotide inhibit gastric or pancreatic secretion. Cholestyramine is often prescribed to improve diarrhea that is associated with bile salt malabsorption. Growth factors have also been used to hasten adaptation and enhance mucosal growth, but these uses are still experimental.

Numerous complications are associated with SBS and long-term TPN (see Chapter 45). Infectious, metabolic, and technical complications can occur. Catheter sepsis can occur after improper care of the catheter. The GI tract can also be a source of microbial seeding of the catheter. Bowel atrophy may foster increased intestinal permeability of bacteria. A lack of adequate sites for central lines may become a significant problem for the child in need of long-term TPN. Hepatic dysfunction, hepatomegaly with abnormal LFTs, and cholestasis may also occur.

Bacterial overgrowth is likely to occur when the ileocecal valve is absent or when stasis exists as a result of a partial obstruction or a dilated segment of bowel with poor motility. Alternating cycles of broad-spectrum antibiotics are used to reduce bacterial overgrowth. This treatment may also decrease the risk of bacterial translocation and subsequent central venous catheter infections. Other complications of bacterial overgrowth and malabsorption include metabolic acidosis and gastric hypersecretion.

Many surgical interventions, including intestinal valves, tapering enteroplasty or stricturoplasty, intestinal lengthening, and interposed segments, have been used to slow intestinal transit, reduce bacterial overgrowth, or increase mucosal surface area. *Intestinal transplantation* has been performed

---

**PO Box 31700, Omaha, NE 68131-0700; 877-CSA-4CSA or 402-558-0600;* www.csaceliacs.org. *In Canada: Canadian Celiac Association, 5170 Dixie Road, Suite 204, Mississauga, Ontario, L4W 1E3; 905-507-6208;* www.celiac.ca.

†A booklet, Pointers for Parents: Coping with Celiac Sprue, *provides information on shopping, cooking, and living with an affected child and is available from the Clinical Dietetics Department, Children's Memorial Hospital, 2300 Children's Plaza, Chicago, IL 60614; 773-880-4793.*

successfully in children. Only children with a permanent dependence on TPN or severe complications of long-term parenteral nutrition are candidates for transplantation.

Prognosis

The prognosis for infants with SBS has improved with advances in TPN and with the understanding of the importance of intraluminal nutrition. Improved surgical techniques for the management of therapy-related problems and the development of more specific immunosuppressive medications for transplantation have all contributed to improved management. The prognosis depends in part on the length of the residual small intestine. An intact ileocecal valve also improves the prognosis. Mortality in infants and children with SBS is usually associated with TPN-related problems, such as fulminant sepsis or severe TPN cholestasis.

Nursing Care Management

The most important components of nursing care are administration and monitoring of nutritional therapy. During TPN therapy, care must be taken to minimize the risk of complications related to the central venous access device (i.e., catheter infections, occlusions, dislodgment, or accidental removal). Care of the enteral feeding tubes and monitoring of enteral feeding tolerance are also important nursing responsibilities.

When long-term parenteral nutrition is required, preparing the family for home care is a major nursing responsibility that should be initiated early to prevent a lengthy hospitalization with subsequent problems such as family dysfunction and developmental delays. Many infants and children can be successfully cared for at home with enteral and parenteral nutrition when the family is prepared and provided with adequate support services. Follow-up by a multidisciplinary nutritional support service is essential. The nurse plays an active and important role in the success of a home nutrition program. Home infusion companies provide portable equipment, which enables the child and family to maintain a more normal lifestyle.

When hospitalization is prolonged, the child's developmental and emotional needs must be met. This often requires special planning to promote normal family adjustment and adaptation of the hospital routines. Care of the hospitalized child is discussed in Chapter 44.

Ingestion of Injurious Agents

Since the passage of the Poison Prevention Packaging Act of 1970, which requires that certain potentially hazardous drugs and household products be sold in child-resistant containers, the incidence of poisonings in children has decreased dramatically. However, despite these advances, poisoning remains a significant health concern, with most cases (51% in 2007; Bronstein et al, 2008) occurring in children younger than 6 years of age. Although pharmaceuticals such as analgesics, cough and cold preparations, topical preparations, antibiotics, vitamins, GI preparations, hormones, and antihistamines are frequently the agents of poisonings, children may be poisoned by a variety of substances. The most frequently ingested poisons include (Watson et al, 2005; Litovitz et al, 2000; Powers, 2000):

- Cosmetics and personal care products (perfume, cologne, aftershave)*
- Cleaning products (hypochlorite ["household"] bleach, pine oil disinfectants)
- Plants (nontoxic GI irritants, oxalates) (Box 47-22)
- Foreign bodies, toys, and miscellaneous substances (desiccants, thermometers, bubble-blowing solutions)

Many poisonings reflect the ready accessibility of the product in the home, where more than 90% of poisonings occur, although a significant number take place elsewhere, such as in a grandparent's or friend's home, a school, or a health care facility.

The following five commonly used and easily available drugs (first four are over-the-counter products) can cause serious or fatal consequences if as little as ¼ tsp or ½ tablet is ingested: methyl salicylate, camphor, topical imidazolines (sympathomimetics such as those contained in Visine, Afrin, and Clear Eyes), benzocaine, and diphenoxylate-atropine (e.g., Lomotil). Stress to parents the importance of keeping such drugs away from children. If these agents are ingested, advise parents to seek medical treatment immediately. Emesis should not be induced at home.The developmental characteristics of young children predispose them to poisoning by ingestion. Infants and toddlers explore their environment through oral experimentation. Because the sense of taste is not discriminating at this age, many unpalatable substances are ingested. In addition, toddlers and preschoolers are developing autonomy and initiative, which increase their curiosity and noncompliant behavior. Imitation is also a powerful motivator, especially when combined with lack of awareness of danger.

This section is primarily concerned with the immediate emergency treatment of ingestion of injurious agents. Specific management of corrosive, hydrocarbon, acetaminophen, salicylate, iron, and plant poisoning is summarized in Box 47-23. Because of the importance of lead poisoning among young children, ingestion of lead is discussed separately. Appropriate suggestions for poison prevention are discussed on p. 1431.

Principles of Emergency Treatment

A poisoning may or may not require emergency intervention, but in every instance medical evaluation is necessary to initiate appropriate action. Parents are advised to call the *poison control center (PCC) before* initiating any intervention. The local PCC telephone number (usually listed in the front of the telephone directory) should be posted near each phone in the house (see Critical Thinking Exercise and Emergency box).

NURSING ALERT The national number for the PCC is 800-222-1222; or online at American Association of Poison Control Centers, *www.aapcc.org*.

Based on the initial telephone assessment, the PCC counsels the parents to begin treatment at home or to take the child to an emergency facility. When a call is taken, the name and

**The most common substances in each category are in parentheses. Substances ingested are not necessarily most toxic but often are readily available.*

BOX 47-22 Poisonous and Nonpoisonous Plants

Poisonous Plants: Toxic Parts
Apple—Leaves, seeds
Apricot—Leaves, stem, seed pits
Azalea—All parts
Buttercup—All parts
Cherry (wild or cultivated)—Twigs, seeds, foliage
Daffodil—Bulbs
Dumb cane, Dieffenbachia—All parts
Elephant ear—All parts
English ivy—All parts
Foxglove—Leaves, seeds, flowers
Holly—Berries and leaves
Hyacinth—Bulbs
Ivy—Leaves
Mistletoe*—Berries, leaves
Oak tree—Acorn, foliage
Philodendron—All parts
Plum—Pit
Poinsettia†—Leaves, stems, sap
Poison ivy, poison oak—Leaves, fruit, stems, smoke from burning plants
Pothos—All parts
Rhubarb—Leaves
Tulip—Bulbs
Water hemlock—All parts
Wisteria—Seeds, pods
Yew—All parts

Nonpoisonous Plants
African violet
Aluminum plant
Asparagus fern
Begonia
Boston fern
Christmas cactus
Coleus
Gardenia
Grape ivy
Jade plant
Piggyback begonia
Piggyback plant
Prayer plant
Rubber tree
Snake plant
Spider plant
Swedish ivy
Wax plant
Weeping fig
Zebra plant

*Eating one or two berries or leaves is probably nontoxic.
†Mildly toxic if ingested in massive quantities.

CRITICAL THINKING EXERCISE

Poisoning

Mrs. B, a neighbor, calls you. She is very upset because her 2-year-old son has eaten several chewable multivitamins with iron. She asks you if she should give her son syrup of ipecac. What should you advise her to do?

1. Evidence–Is there sufficient evidence to formulate an answer for Mrs. B?
2. Assumptions–Answer the following questions and describe some underlying assumptions on which your answers are based:
   a. What is the best initial response when a child ingests a potentially poisonous substance?
   b. What is syrup of ipecac?
   c. What are the dangers involved in the use of syrup of ipecac?
3. What is the priority for nursing care at this time?
4. Does the evidence support your conclusion?
5. What alternative perspectives might you have?

telephone number of the caller are recorded to reestablish contact if the connection is interrupted. Because most poisonings are managed in the home, expert advice is essential in minimizing adverse effects. When the exact quantity or type of ingested toxin is not known, admission to a health care facility with pediatric emergency treatment services for laboratory evaluation and surveillance is critical after ingestion.

Assessment

The first and most important principle in dealing with a poisoning is to *treat the child first, not the poison.* This requires an immediate concern for life support. Vital signs are taken, and respiratory or circulatory support is instituted as needed. The child's condition is routinely reevaluated. Because shock is a complication of several types of household poisons, particularly corrosives, measures to reduce the effects of shock, beginning with the ABCs (airway, breathing, circulation) of resuscitation are important. Establishing and maintaining vascular access for rapid intravascular volume expansion is vital in the treatment of pediatric shock.

The emergency department nurse's responsibility is to be prepared for immediate intervention with all of the necessary equipment. Because time and speed are critical factors in recovery from serious poisonings, anticipation of potential problems and complications may mean the difference between life and death.

Gastric Decontamination

In general, the immediate treatment is to remove the ingested poison by adsorbing the toxin with activated charcoal, performing gastric lavage, or increasing bowel motility (catharsis). Because of continuing controversy regarding the use of these methods, each toxic ingestion should be treated individually (Abruzzi & Stork, 2002). Specific antidotes may be administered for certain poisonings. *Syrup of ipecac*, an emetic that exerts its action through irritation of the gastric mucosa and by stimulation of the vomiting center, is no longer recommended for immediate treatment of poison ingestion (Ameri-

BOX 47-23 Selected Poisonings in Children

Corrosives (Strong Acids or Alkali)

Drain, toilet, or oven cleaners
Electric dishwasher detergent (liquid, because of higher pH, is more hazardous than granular)
Mildew remover
Batteries
Clinitest tablets
Denture cleaners
Bleach

Clinical Manifestations

Severe burning pain in mouth, throat, and stomach
White, swollen mucous membranes; edema of lips, tongue, and pharynx (respiratory obstruction)
Violent vomiting (hemoptysis)
Drooling and inability to clear secretions
Signs of shock
Anxiety and agitation

Comments

Household bleach is a frequently ingested corrosive but rarely causes serious damage.
Liquid corrosives cause more damage than granular preparations.

Treatment

Assess child's breathing and level of consciousness.
Contact poison control center (800-222-1222) for advice.
Inducing emesis is contraindicated (vomiting redamages the mucosa).
Dilute corrosive with water or milk (usually no more than 120 ml [4 oz]).
Do not neutralize. Neutralization can cause an exothermic reaction (which produces heat and causes increased symptoms or produces a thermal burn in addition to a chemical burn).
Maintain patent airway if needed.
Administer analgesics.
Do not allow oral intake.
Esophageal stricture may require repeated dilations or surgery.

Hydrocarbons

Gasoline
Kerosene
Lamp oil
Mineral seal oil (found in furniture polish)
Lighter fluid
Turpentine
Paint thinner and remover (some types)

Clinical Manifestations

Gagging, choking, and coughing
Nausea
Vomiting
Alterations in sensorium, such as lethargy
Weakness
Respiratory symptoms of pulmonary involvement
- Tachypnea
- Cyanosis
- Retractions
- Grunting

Comments

Immediate danger is aspiration (even small amounts can cause bronchitis and chemical pneumonia).
Gasoline, kerosene, lighter fluid, mineral seal oil, and turpentine cause severe pneumonia.

Treatment

Contact poison control center (800-222-1222).
Inducing emesis is generally contraindicated.
Gastric decontamination and emptying are questionable, even when the hydrocarbon contains a heavy metal or pesticide; if gastric lavage must be performed, a cuffed endotracheal tube should be in place before lavage because of a high risk of aspiration.
Symptomatic treatment of chemical pneumonia includes high humidity, oxygen, hydration, and antibiotics for secondary infection.

Acetaminophen

Clinical Manifestations

Occurs in four stages:

1. Initial period (2 to 4 hours after ingestion)
   - Nausea
   - Vomiting
   - Sweating
   - Pallor
2. Latent period (24 to 36 hours)
   - Patient improves
3. Hepatic involvement (may last up to 7 days and be permanent)
   - Pain in right upper quadrant
   - Jaundice
   - Confusion
   - Stupor
   - Coagulation abnormalities
4. Patients who do not die in hepatic stage gradually recover

Comments

It is the most common drug poisoning in children.
It occurs from acute ingestion.
Toxic dose is 150 mg/kg or greater in children.
Because of multiple formulations and concentrations, chronic acetaminophen toxicity is a significant problem.
Parents should be counseled to read product packaging carefully and to consult a health care professional to avoid inappropriate dosing (Abruzzi & Stork, 2002).

Treatment

Antidote *N*-acetylcysteine (Mucomyst) can usually be given orally but is first diluted in fruit juice or soda because of the antidote's offensive odor.
It is given as 1 loading dose and usually 17 maintenance doses in different dosages.
It may be given intravenously, but use is investigational.

Aspirin (Acetylsalicylic Acid [ASA])

Clinical Manifestations

Acute poisoning
- Nausea
- Disorientation
- Vomiting

BOX 47-23 Selected Poisonings in Children—cont'd

Aspirin (Acetylsalicylic Acid [ASA])—cont'd

Clinical Manifestations—cont'd

- Dehydration
- Diaphoresis
- Hyperpnea
- Hyperpyrexia
- Oliguria
- Tinnitus
- Coma
- Convulsions

Chronic poisoning

- Same as for acute poisoning but subtle onset (often mistaken for viral illness)
- Dehydration, coma, and seizures may be more severe
- Bleeding tendencies

Comments

It may be caused by acute ingestion (severe toxicity occurs with 300 to 500 mg/kg).

It may be caused by chronic ingestion (i.e., more than 100 mg/kg/day for 2 or more days) and can be more serious than acute ingestion.

Time to peak serum salicylate level can vary with enteric aspirin or the presence of concretions (bezoars).

Treatment

Hospitalization is required for severe toxicity.

Emesis, lavage, activated charcoal, or cathartic measures may be used.

Lavage will not remove concretions of ASA.

Activated charcoal is important early in ASA toxicity.

Sodium bicarbonate (intravenous) to correct metabolic acidosis and urinary alkalinization may be effective in enhancing elimination; urinary alkalinization is very difficult to achieve.

Be aware of the risk for fluid overload and pulmonary edema.

Prescribe:

- External cooling for hyperpyrexia.
- Anticonvulsants.
- Oxygen and ventilation for respiratory depression.
- Vitamin K for bleeding.

In severe cases, hemodialysis (not peritoneal dialysis) may be used

Iron

Mineral supplement or vitamin containing iron

Clinical Manifestations

Occurs in five stages:

1. Initial period (0.5 to 6 hours after ingestion) (if child does not develop gastrointestinal symptoms in 6 hours, toxicity is unlikely)
   - Vomiting
   - Hematemesis
   - Diarrhea
   - Hematochezia (bloody stools)
   - Gastric pain
2. Latency (2 to 12 hours)
   - Patient improves
3. Systemic toxicity (4 to 24 hours after ingestion)
   - Metabolic acidosis
   - Fever
   - Hyperglycemia
   - Bleeding
   - Shock
   - Death (may occur)
4. Hepatic injury (48 to 96 hours)
   - Seizures
   - Coma
5. Rarely, pyloric stenosis develops at 2 to 5 weeks

Comments

Factors related to frequency of iron poisoning:

- Widespread availability
- Packaging of large quantities in individual containers
- Lack of parental awareness of iron toxicity
- Resemblance of iron tablets to candy (e.g., M&M's)

Toxic dose is based on the amount of elemental iron in various salts (sulfate, gluconate, fumarate), which ranges from 20% to 33%; ingestions of 60 mg/kg are considered dangerous.

Treatment

Emesis or lavage may be used.

For toxic doses lavage may be necessary for all chewable tablets or liquids if spontaneous vomiting has not occurred.

Chelation therapy with deferoxamine is used in severe intoxication (may turn urine a red to orange color).

If intravenous deferoxamine is given too rapidly, hypotension, facial flushing, rash, urticaria, tachycardia, and shock may occur; stop the infusion, maintain the intravenous line with normal saline, and notify the practitioner immediately.

Plants

See Box 47-22.

Clinical Manifestations

Depends on type of plant ingested

May cause local irritation of oropharynx and entire gastrointestinal tract

May cause respiratory, renal, and central nervous system symptoms

Topical contact with plants can cause dermatitis

Comments

Plants are some of the most frequently ingested substances.

Plant ingestions rarely cause serious problems, although some can be fatal.

Plants can also cause choking and allergic reactions.

Treatment

Induce emesis.

Wash from skin or eyes.

Supportive care as needed.

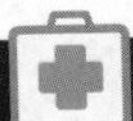

EMERGENCY

Poisoning

1. Assess the victim:
   - Take vital signs; reevaluate routinely.
   - Initiate cardiorespiratory support if needed.
   - Treat other symptoms, such as seizures.
2. Terminate exposure:
   - Empty mouth of pills, plant parts, or other material.
   - Flush eyes continuously with normal saline (or room-temperature tap water at home) for 15 to 20 minutes.
   - Flush skin and wash with soap and a soft cloth; remove contaminated clothes, especially if a pesticide, acid, alkali, or hydrocarbon is involved.
   - Bring victim of an inhalation poisoning into fresh air.
   - Give one sip of water to dilute ingested poison.
3. Identify the poison:
   - Question the victim and witnesses.
   - Look for environmental cues (empty container, nearby spill, odor on breath) and save all evidence of poison (container, vomitus, urine).
   - Be alert to signs and symptoms of potential poisoning in absence of other evidence, including symptoms of ocular or dermal exposure.
   - Call poison control center (800-222-1222) or other competent emergency facility for immediate advice regarding treatment.
4. Remove poison and prevent absorption:
   - Place child in side-lying, sitting, or kneeling position with head below chest to prevent aspiration.
   - Administer activated charcoal if ordered (unless used repeatedly, usual dose is 1 g/kg unless amount of toxin is known).

can Academy of Clinical Toxicology & European Association of Poisons Centres and Clinical Toxicologists, 2004b; American Academy of Pediatrics, Committee on Injury, Violence, and Poison Prevention, 2003). The American Academy of Pediatrics, Committee on Injury, Violence, and Poison Prevention (2003) recommends that existing ipecac in the home be disposed of safely and that the first action for a caregiver of a child who may have ingested a toxic substance is to consult the local PCC. If the PCC cannot be reached, the child should be taken to the nearest emergency department.

Ipecac is contraindicated because it may cause prolonged vomiting (up to 12 hours), which makes it relatively contraindicated in ingestions that may cause sedation, coma, or seizures (Powers, 2000). Medications such as calcium channel blockers and benzodiazepines either produce a rapid onset of adverse symptoms (e.g., sedation, seizures, coma) or exaggerate the vagal response induced by gagging, which can lead to significant bradycardia. Under either circumstance, uncontrolled vomiting becomes an undesirable and unsafe event.

No emetic or other substance should be given at home without consultation with a PCC or physician.

If the child is admitted to an emergency facility, *gastric lavage* may be performed to empty the stomach of the toxic agent; however, this procedure is associated with serious complications (GI perforation, hypoxia, aspiration), and it is no longer recommended in all cases of ingestion. There is no conclusive evidence that gastric lavage decreases morbidity (Criddle, 2007; Heard, 2005). In addition, gastric lavage may be of little use if used beyond 1 hour of ingestion (Heard, 2005). Conditions that may be appropriate for the use of gastric lavage include presentation within 1 hour of ingestion of a toxin, ingestion in patient who has decreased GI motility, the ingestion of a toxic amount of sustained-release medication, and a massive or life-threatening amount of poison (Criddle, 2007). When gastric lavage is used, the patient requires a protected airway, possible sedation, and the largest-diameter tube that can be inserted to facilitate passage of gastric contents.

A more commonly used method of GI decontamination is the use of *activated charcoal*, an odorless, tasteless, fine black powder that adsorbs many compounds, creating a stable complex. Activated charcoal may replace ipecac as the home remedy of choice (Bond, 2002), but the American Academy of Pediatrics, Committee on Injury, Violence, and Poison Prevention (2003) suggests that it is premature to recommend the administration of activated charcoal in the home. Activated charcoal is mixed with water or a saline cathartic to form a slurry. Slurries are neither gritty nor distasteful but resemble black mud. To increase the child's acceptance of activated charcoal, the nurse should mix it with diet soda and serve it through a straw in an opaque container with a cover (such as a disposable coffee cup and lid) or an ordinary cup covered with aluminum foil or placed inside a small paper bag. In one small study, healthy adolescents preferred the taste of activated charcoal mixed with Coca-Cola or chocolate milk mixture instead of water (Cheng & Ratnapalan, 2007). For small children an NG tube may be required to administer activated charcoal. Because the charcoal solution is thick, a 12-French (or larger) NG tube should be used.

Potential complications from the use of activated charcoal include aspiration (usually in patients with impaired gag reflexes), constipation, and intestinal obstruction (in multiple doses). Superactivated charcoal products for gastric decontamination are reported to be more palatable and just as effective (Criddle, 2007; Heard, 2005). Cathartics, such as sorbitol, sodium, or magnesium, may be administered to stimulate evacuation of the bowel, thus decreasing systemic absorption of the poison and aiding in the removal of the charcoal. Many commercial preparations of activated charcoal contain cathartics. However, the use of cathartics is controversial, and the American Academy of Clinical Toxicology and European Association of Poisons Centres and Clinical Toxicologists (2004a) do not recommend their use in children. The Evidence-Based Practice box reviews recent literature on the use of gastric lavage in comparison to activated charcoal when a child has ingested poison.

Specific *antidotes* are available to counteract a minority of poisonings. They are highly effective and should be available in all emergency facilities. The supply of antidotes should be checked routinely and replaced as used or according to expiration dates. Antidotes available to treat toxin ingestion include *N*-acetylcysteine for acetaminophen poisoning, oxygen for

EVIDENCE-BASED PRACTICE Gastric Lavage in Children

—*Curt Roberts and Danna Salinas*

Ask the Question

What is the effect of gastric lavage in reducing systemic absorption of toxic substances compared with the administration of activated charcoal or forced emesis?

Search for Evidence

Search Strategies

Keywords included gastric lavage, gastric decontamination, activated charcoal, and toxic ingestion. Searches were limited to English articles with human subjects.

Databases Used

PubMed, STAT!Ref, UpToDateOnline, CINAHL, EMBASE, D.A.R.E, Cochrane Library, National Guideline Clearinghouse (AHRQ)

Critically Analyze the Evidence

Eddleston, Juszczak, and Buckley (2003) completed a review of the literature to determine whether gastric lavage pushes poisons beyond the pylorus to assist with faster elimination of toxins from the body. The review examined two studies designed to measure movement of substances through the stomach and into the small intestine after gastric lavage. One study randomized 40 patients to gastric emptying by forced emesis or gastric lavage and maintained a control group of 20 patients in whom gastric emptying was not necessary. Either radiopaque pellets or radiolabeled water was used as a marker. There were no significant differences in the number of pellets in the small bowel between the emesis group and the control group or between the gastric lavage group and the control group. The second study consisted of five volunteers who were subjected to gastric lavage on three occasions. Less poison was found in the small bowel after gastric lavage than after no intervention. The researchers concluded there was no evidence that gastric lavage drives toxins into the small intestine.

Other studies have demonstrated that gastric lavage is equivalent to forced emesis as a method of gastric emptying (American Academy of Clinical Toxicology & European Association of Poisons Centres and Clinical Toxicologists, 1999, 2005; Smilkstein, 2002). A randomized crossover study with 12 volunteers who ingested paracetamol 50 mg/kg 1 hour after a standard meal demonstrated that activated charcoal administered within 1 hour of ingestion was more effective than gastric lavage followed by charcoal because there was a delay in administration of the activated charcoal (Christophersen et al, 2002). Forced emesis was superior to gastric lavage when the goal was to remove large particles and fragments. However, the literature supports that gastric emptying has limited benefit in gastrointestinal decontamination because administration of activated charcoal appears to be more effective (American Academy of Clinical Toxicology & European Association of Poisons Centres and Clinical Toxicologists, 1999, 2005; Smilkstein, 2002).

Numerous complications are reported with both gastrointestinal lavage and activated charcoal. Complications of orogastric or nasogastric intubation include esophageal tears or perforation, nasal injury, oropharyngeal injury, gastric perforation, and inadvertent tracheal intubation (American Academy of Clinical Toxicology & European Association of Poisons Centres and Clinical Toxicologists, 1999, 2005; Smilkstein, 2002; Caravati et al, 2001). Neither the American Academy of Clinical Toxicology nor the European Association of Poisons Centres and Clinical Toxicologists (2005) has recommended the routine use of gastric lavage in the management of toxic ingestions since 1997. Contraindications to the administration of charcoal also exist, including in patients who have ingested corrosive materials and in those at risk for hemorrhage or perforation due to structural abnormalities or recent surgery.

Apply the Evidence: Nursing Implications

Gastric lavage has little or no effect in reducing absorption, especially when used as an intervention more than 1 hour after ingestion. Single-dose or multidose activated charcoal is most effective when administered within 1 hour of ingestion but may have an effect up to 4 hours after ingestion, depending on the substance. Administration of activated charcoal should not be delayed by the use of forced emesis or gastric lavage.

References

American Academy of Clinical Toxicology, European Association of Poisons Centres and Clinical Toxicologists: Position paper: single-dose activated charcoal, *J Toxicol Clin Toxicol* 43:61-87, 2005.

American Academy of Clinical Toxicology, European Association of Poisons Centres and Clinical Toxicologists: Position statement and practice guidelines on the use of multi-dose activated charcoal in the treatment of acute poisoning, *J Toxicol Clin Toxicol* 37(6):731-751, 1999.

Caravati EM et al: Esophageal laceration and charcoal mediastinum complicating gastric lavage, *J Emerg Med* 20(3):273-276, 2001.

Christophersen AB et al: Activated charcoal alone or after gastric lavage: a simulated large paracetamol intoxication, *Br J Clin Pharmacol* 53(3):312-317, 2002.

Eddleston M, Juszczak E, Buckley N: Does gastric lavage really push poisons beyond the pylorus? A systematic review of the evidence, *Ann Emerg Med* 42(3):359-364, 2003.

Smilkstein MJ: Techniques used to prevent gastrointestinal absorption of toxic compounds. In Goldfrank LR et al, editors: *Goldfrank's toxicologic emergencies*, ed 7, New York, 2002, McGraw-Hill.

carbon monoxide inhalation, naloxone for opioid overdose, flumazenil (Romazicon) for benzodiazepines (diazepam [Valium], midazolam [Versed]) overdose, digoxin immune Fab (Digibind) for digoxin toxicity, amyl nitrate for cyanide, and antivenin for certain poisonous bites.

Prevention of Recurrence

The ultimate objective is to prevent poisonings from occurring or recurring. One effective counseling method is first to discuss the difficulties of constantly watching and safeguarding young children (see Family-Centered Care box). In this way the challenging task of raising children can lead to a discussion of injury prevention as part of the parental role. This approach also incorporates contributory causes for the incident, such as inadequate support systems; marital discord; discipline techniques (especially use of physical punishment); parental distress; or any disruption in the family or family activities, such as vacations, moves, visitors, illnesses, or births. A visit to the home, especially after repeat poisonings, is recommended as part of the follow-up care to assess hazards, including family factors, and to evaluate appropriate injury-proofing measures. One method of identifying risk areas is to ask specific questions or to have the parent complete a questionnaire designed to isolate factors that predispose children to poisoning. Another approach is to encourage parents to bend down to the child's eye level and survey the home environment for potential hazards. Have the parents try to open cabinets and reach shelves to access poisons.

FAMILY-CENTERED CARE

Poisoning

A poisoning is more than a physical emergency for the child—it usually represents an emotional crisis for the parents, particularly in terms of guilt, self-reproach, and insecurity in the parenting role. The emergency department is no place to admonish the family for negligence, lack of appropriate supervision, or failure to injury-proof the home. Rather, it is a time to calm and support the child and parents while unaccusingly exploring the circumstances of the injury. If the nurse prematurely attempts to discuss ways of preventing such an incident from recurring, the parents' anxiety will block out any suggestions or offered guidance. Therefore it is preferable for the nurse to delay the discussion until the child's condition is stabilized or, if the child is discharged immediately after emergency treatment, to make a public health referral or send a packet of information.

Passive measures (those that do not require active participation) have been the most successful in preventing poisoning and include using child-resistant closures and limiting the number of tablets in one container. However, these measures alone are not sufficient to prevent poisoning because most toxic agents in the home do not have safety closures. Therefore *active measures* (those that require participation) are essential. Guidelines for preventing the occurrence or recurrence of a poisoning are listed in the Guidelines box.

Heavy Metal Poisoning

Heavy metal poisoning can occur from the ingestion of a variety of substances, the most common being lead. Other sources that are important in terms of children are iron and mercury. *Mercury toxicity*, a rare form of heavy metal poisoning, has occurred in children from a variety of sources, such as broken thermometers or thermostats, broken fluorescent light bulbs, disk batteries, topical medications, gas regulators, cathartics, and interior latex house paint (Clifton, 2007; Etzel, 2001). Elemental mercury (also called *metallic mercury* or *quicksilver*) is nontoxic if ingested and if the GI tract is healthy (e.g., has no fistulas). However, mercury is volatile at room temperature and enters the bloodstream after it is inhaled, causing toxicity (tremors, memory loss, insomnia, gingivitis, diarrhea, anorexia, weight loss). The classic form of mercury poisoning is called *acrodynia* (or "painful extremities").

NURSING ALERT Mercury thermometers are no longer recommended because the inhaled vapors can cause toxicity if they are broken. To prevent inhalation, spilled mercury must be cleaned up quickly, using disposable towels and rubber gloves and washing the hands well after removing the spill.

GUIDELINES Poison Prevention

- Assess possible contributing factors in occurrence of injury, such as discipline, parent-child relationship, developmental ability, environmental factors, and behavior problems.
- Institute anticipatory guidance for possible future injuries based on child's age and maturational level.
- Refer to visiting nurse agency to evaluate home environment and need for injury-proofing measures.
- Provide assistance with environmental manipulation, such as lead removal, when necessary.
- Educate parents regarding safe storage of toxic substances.
- Advise parents to take drugs out of sight of children.
- Teach children the hazards of ingesting nonfood items.
- Advise parents against using plants for teas or medicine.
- Discuss problems of discipline and children's noncompliance and offer strategies for effective discipline.
- Instruct parents regarding correct administration of drugs for therapeutic purposes and discontinuation of drug if there is evidence of mild toxicity.
- Advise parents to contact the poison control center or practitioner immediately when a poisoning occurs.
- Post number of regional poison control center (800-222-1222) with emergency phone list by telephone.
- Include by the telephone the home address with nearest cross street in case an ambulance is needed. (In an emergency, family members may not remember the house address, and baby-sitters may not be aware of the information.)

Heavy metals have an affinity for certain essential tissue chemicals, which must remain free for adequate cell functioning. When metals are bound to these substances, cellular enzyme systems are inactivated. Treatment involves *chelation*, use of a chemical compound that combines with the metal for rapid and safe excretion.

Lead Poisoning

In the United States lead poisoning emerged as a problem in the early 1900s, when white lead was added to paints and tetraethyl lead was added to gasoline as an antiknock compound. Lead content in paint was decreased in 1950, and in 1978 the use of lead in household paint was banned. The use of lead in paint and leaded gasoline has been banned in the United States. After this change in policy, the average blood lead level (BLL) in the United States for people ages 1 to 74 years dropped from 12.8 mcg/dl in 1980 to 1.9 mcg/dl in 1999 (American Academy of Pediatrics, Committee on Environmental Health, 2005). Yet because it does not decompose or break down into smaller particles, lead deposited in the past is still present in soil near heavily trafficked areas. Coupled with deteriorating lead-based paint falling from the exterior of nearby houses, soil becomes a significant pathway by which lead poisoning can occur. Bare soil used as a play area contributes to the lead exposure of young children, since lead-contaminated dust is tracked into the home.

A child does not need to eat loose paint chips to be exposed to the toxin; normal hand-to-mouth behavior, coupled with the presence of lead dust in the environment, is the usual method of poisoning (American Academy of Pediatrics, Committee on Environmental Health, 2005; Erickson & Thompson, 2005). Cultural practices may also lead to pediatric ingestion of substances containing lead, especially when these are brought in from other countries. Children of Hispanic origin are believed to be at higher risk for lead poisoning as a result of exposure to culturally related items that contain lead (Erickson & Thompson, 2005). Other risk factors for having an elevated BLL include poverty, age younger than 6 years, dwelling in urban areas, and living in older rental homes where lead decontamination may not be a priority. Children of immigrants and internationally adopted children may have been exposed to sources of lead before arrival in the United States and should also be carefully evaluated for lead exposure (Woolf, Goldman, & Bellinger, 2007). However, any child is at risk for lead poisoning if hazardous conditions for lead are present in the environment.

Causes of Lead Poisoning

Although there are numerous sources of lead (Box 47-24), in most instances of acute childhood lead poisoning, the source is nonintact lead-based paint in an older home or lead-contaminated bare soil in the yard. Microparticles of lead gain entrance into a child's body through ingestion or inhalation and, in the case of an exposed pregnant woman, by placental transfer. When measured, a mother's lead level is nearly the same as that of her unborn child. A level of lead not harmful to an adult woman can be harmful to the fetus.

Inhalation exposure usually occurs during renovation and remodeling activities in the home, whereas ingestion happens during normal day-to-day play and mouthing activities. Sometimes a child will actually swallow loose chips of lead-based paint because it has a sweet taste. Water and food may also be contaminated with lead.

Because of family, cultural, or ethnic traditions, a source of lead may be a routine part of life for a child. Nurses must educate themselves about the practices of their patients and identify when such products may be a source of lead. The use of pottery or dishes containing lead may be an issue, as may the use of folk remedies for stomachaches or the use of some cosmetics (see Cultural Awareness box). Some hobbies and occupations of adult family members may contribute to lead hazards carried into the household on clothes, shoes, or skin (American Academy of Pediatrics, Committee on Environmental Health, 2005). Nurses are often in a position to observe or elicit information about these practices and educate families about their potential harm.

BOX 47-24 Sources of Lead*

Lead-based paint in deteriorating condition
Lead solder
Lead crystal
Battery casings
Lead fishing sinkers
Lead curtain weights
Lead bullets
The following may contain lead:

- Ceramic ware
- Water
- Pottery
- Pewter
- Dyes
- Industrial factories
- Vinyl miniblinds
- Playground equipment
- Collectible toys
- Artists' paints
- Pool cue chalk
- Some imported toys or children's metal jewelry

Occupations and hobbies involving lead:

- Battery and aircraft manufacturing
- Lead smelting
- Brass foundry work
- Radiator repair
- Construction work
- Bridge repair work
- Painting contracting
- Mining
- Ceramics work
- Stained-glass making
- Jewelry making

*The U.S. Consumer Product Safety Commission issues alerts and recalls for products that contain lead and that may unexpectedly pose a hazard to young children.

Pathophysiology and Clinical Manifestations

Lead can affect any part of the body, including the renal, hematologic, and neurologic systems (Fig. 47-8). Of most concern for young children is the developing brain and nervous system, which are more vulnerable than those of an older child or adult. Lead in the body moves via an equilibration process among the blood, the soft tissues and organs, and the bones and teeth. Lead ultimately settles in the bones and teeth, where it remains inert and in storage. This makes up the largest portion of the body burden, approximately 75% to 90%. At the cellular level it competes with molecules of calcium, interfering with the regulating action of calcium.

The neurologic system is of most concern when young children are exposed to lead. The developing brain is especially vulnerable. Lead disrupts the biochemical processes and may directly affect the release of neurotransmitters, may cause alterations in the blood-brain barrier, and may interfere with the regulation of synaptic activity (Lidsky & Schneider, 2006).

There is a relationship between anemia and lead poisoning. Children who are iron deficient absorb lead more readily than those with sufficient iron stores. Lead can interfere with the binding of iron onto the heme molecule. This sometimes creates a picture of anemia, even though the child is not iron deficient. Lead toxicity to the erythrocytes leads to the release of the enzyme erythrocyte protoporphyrin (EP). Because EP is not sensitive to BLLs of less than about 16 to 25 mcg/dl, it is no longer used as a screening test. Therefore the BLL test is currently used for screening and diagnosis. However, elevation of the EP level (above 35 mcg/dl of whole blood) is a good indicator of toxicity from lead and reflects the length of exposure and body burden of lead in the individual child.

CULTURAL AWARENESS

Sources of Lead

In some cultures the use of traditional ethnic remedies that contain lead may increase children's risk of lead poisoning. These remedies include:

Azarcon (Mexico)—For digestive problems; a bright orange powder; usual dose 0.25 to 1 tsp, often mixed with oil, milk, or sugar or sometimes given as a tea; sometimes a pinch is added to a baby bottle or tortilla dough for preventive purposes

Greta (Mexico)—A yellow-orange powder, used in the same way as azarcon

Paylooah (Southeast Asia)—Used for rash or fever; an orange-red powder given as 0.5 tsp straight or in a tea

Surma (India)—Black powder applied to the inner lower eyelid that is used as a cosmetic to improve eyesight

Unknown ayurvedic (Tibet)—Small, gray-brown balls used to improve slow development; two balls given orally three times a day

Tamarindo jellied, fruit candy (Mexico)—Fruit candy packaged in paper wrappers that contain high lead levels

Lozeena (Iraq)—A bright orange powder used to color meat and rice

Modified from Centers for Disease Control and Prevention: Lead poisoning associated with use of traditional ethnic remedies—California, 1991-1992, *MMWR* 42(27):521-524, 1993; Centers for Disease Control and Prevention: Lead poisoning associated with imported candy and powdered food coloring—California and Michigan, *MMWR* 47(48):1041-1043, 1998; Centers for Disease Control and Prevention: Childhood lead poisoning associated with tamarind candy and folk remedies—California, 1992-2000, *MMWR* 51(31):684-686, 2002.

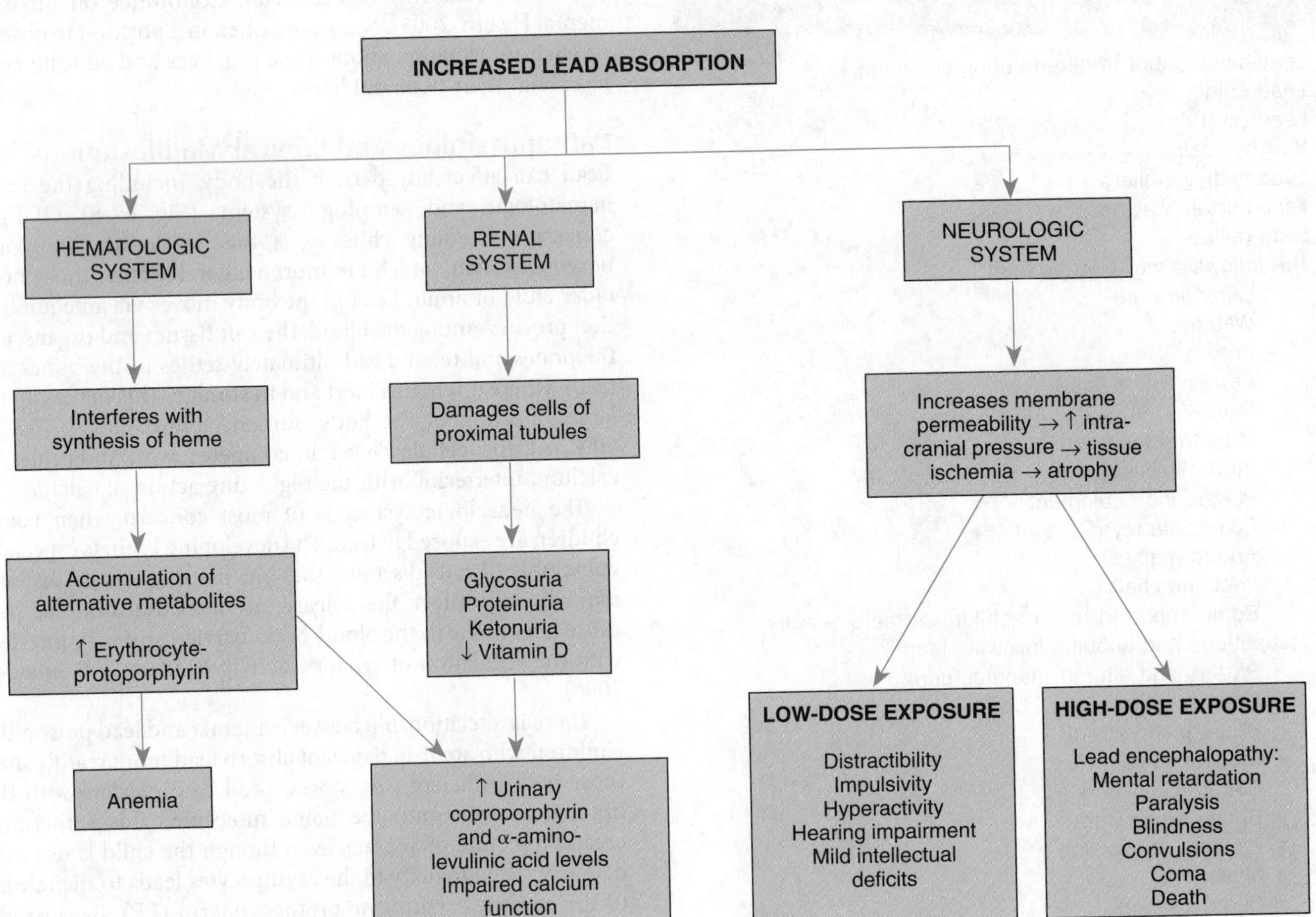

Fig. 47-8 Main effects of lead on body systems.

Although adults have been shown to suffer adverse renal effects from occupational lead exposure, few studies document renal effects in children at other than extremely high lead levels. One can hypothesize that lead can affect the renal integrity of both children and adults. Therefore the renal system of a child is still considered a potential target for its harmful effects.

The lead levels identified in children have declined since the initiation of screening for children at risk for lead poisoning. With earlier intervention the most prevalent effects have changed. Since the late 1960s, children have rarely died of lead poisoning, and seizures and cognitive impairment have become less likely. However, even mild and moderate lead poisoning can cause a number of cognitive and behavioral problems in young children, including aggression, hyperactivity, impulsivity, delinquency, disinterest, and withdrawal. Long-term neurocognitive signs of lead poisoning include developmental delays, lowered intelligence quotient (IQ), reading skill deficits, visual-spatial problems, visual-motor problems, learning disabilities, and lower academic success. Physical growth and reproductive efficiency may also be adversely affected by chronic lead toxicity (Woolf, Goldman, & Bellinger, 2007).

NURSING ALERT Acute signs of lead poisoning include nausea, vomiting, constipation, anorexia, and abdominal pain. Additional clinical manifestations are hypophosphatemia, glycosuria, and aminoaciduria (Erickson & Thompson, 2005).

Diagnostic Evaluation

Children with lead poisoning rarely have symptoms, even at levels requiring chelation therapy. A diagnosis of lead poisoning is based only on the lead testing of a venous blood specimen from a venipuncture. The collection process is important. Blood must be collected carefully to avoid contamination by lead on the skin. The level of concern for an elevated BLL has dropped from 80 mcg/dl in 1950 to 10 mcg/dl today (American Academy of Pediatrics, Committee on Environmental Health, 2005).

Anticipatory Guidance

Anticipatory guidance lends support to primary prevention efforts. The Centers for Disease Control and Prevention (2005) recommends that the following information be made available to families beginning during prenatal care, at 3 to 6 months, and at 1 year of age:

- Hazards of lead-based paint in older housing
- Ways to control lead hazards safely
- Hazards accompanying repainting and renovation of homes built before 1978
- Other exposure sources, such as traditional remedies, that might be relevant for a family

There has been recent concern regarding toys and other imported play items that have been found to contain lead. Parents should carefully evaluate the source of the toy (manufacturer) or plaything and not assume it is safe because it is sold in a U.S. market. The U.S. Consumer Product Safety Commission *(www.cpsc.gov)* is an excellent resource for parents and caretakers concerned about the safety of a given toy or product.

Screening for Lead Poisoning

When primary prevention fails, the secondary prevention effort of screening for elevated BLLs can identify children much earlier than in the past. Guidelines from the Centers for Disease Control and Prevention (2005) recommend universal or targeted screening on the basis of each state's determination of need. This need is established using blood lead surveillance and other risk factor data collected over time to establish the status and risk of children throughout the state. In areas without available data, universal screening is recommended.

Universal screening should be done at ages 1 and 2 years. Any child between the ages of 3 and 6 years who has not been previously screened should also be tested. Any child with risk factors should be screened more often.

Targeted screening is acceptable when an area has been determined by existing data to have less risk. Children should be screened when they live in a high risk geographic area or are members of a group determined to be at risk (e.g., Medicaid recipients) or if their family cannot answer "no" to the following personal risk questions:

- Does your child live in or regularly visit a house that was built before 1950?
- Does your child live in or regularly visit a house built before 1978 with recent or ongoing renovations or remodeling within the past 6 months?
- Does your child have a sibling or playmate who has or did have lead poisoning?

Therapeutic Management

The degree of concern, urgency, and need for medical intervention changes as the lead level increases. Education is one of the most important elements of the treatment process. The Centers for Disease Control and Prevention (2005) has identified several areas that should be discussed with the family of every child who has an elevated BLL (10 mcg/dl or higher):

- The child's BLL and what it means
- Potential adverse health effects of an elevated BLL
- Sources of lead exposure and suggestions on how to reduce exposure, such as importance of wet cleaning to remove lead dust on floors, window sills, and other surfaces
- Importance of good nutrition in reducing the absorption and effects of lead; for persons with poor nutritional patterns, adequate intake of calcium and iron and importance of regular meals
- Need for follow-up testing to monitor the child's BLL
- Results of an environmental investigation if applicable
- Hazards of improper removal of lead paint (dry sanding, scraping, or open-flame burning)

Treatment actions vary depending on the child's BLL. Based on a diagnosis from a venous BLL test, the Centers for Disease Control and Prevention (2002) recommends the following actions:

BLL (mcg/dl)	Action
<10	Reassess or rescreen in 1 year. If exposure status changes, do this sooner.
10-14	Provide family with lead poisoning education, follow-up testing, and social service referral if necessary.
15-19	Provide family with lead poisoning education (dietary and environmental), follow-up testing, and social service referral as needed; if BLL persists, initiate actions for BLL of 20 to 44 mcg/dl.
20-44	Provide coordination of care, clinical management, environmental investigation, and lead hazard control.
45-69	Within 48 hours provide coordination of care and clinical management, including treatment, environmental investigation, and lead hazard control. The child must not remain in a lead-hazardous environment if resolution is to occur.
≥70	*Immediately* provide medical treatment and begin coordination of care, clinical management, environmental investigation, and lead hazard control.

Chelation Therapy

Chelation is the term used for removing lead from circulating blood and, theoretically, some lead from organs and tissues. It is unclear whether chelation affects lead stores in bones. Although not an antidote in the truest sense, it does serve a similar purpose in that the toxic substance or poison is removed from the body. However, chelation does not counteract any effects of the lead. Because lead in circulating blood (the compartment most readily accessed by the chelator) is such a small part of the total body burden, the equilibration process causes blood lead to rise again after treatment.

Historically two chelating agents have been used consistently: calcium disodium edetate ($CaNa_2EDTA$ or calcium EDTA) and succimer (Chemet, *meso*-2,3 dimercaptosuccinic acid [DMSA]). British anti-Lewisite (BAL, dimercaprol, dimercaptopropanol) is used in conjunction with EDTA. All the agents have potential toxic side effects and contraindications. Renal, hepatic, and hematologic parameters must be monitored.

Because of the equilibration process among blood, soft tissues, and other sites in the body, there is often a rebound of the BLL after chelation. After the body burden of lead is reduced enough to stabilize the BLL, rebound ceases. Multiple chelation treatments may be necessary. Adequate hydration is essential during therapy because the chelates are excreted via the kidneys.

BAL must not be used in the presence of a glucose 6-phosphate dehydrogenase (G6PD) deficiency or peanut allergy, nor should it be given in conjunction with iron. It is never used as a single-agent therapy, only in conjunction with EDTA. It must be given only at a deep intramuscular site. EDTA should be given intravenously over several hours or, when necessary to restrict fluids, intramuscularly.

Succimer is given orally over a 19-day course of treatment. The capsule is opened and sprinkled on a small amount of food or may be swallowed whole. Adverse effects include nausea, vomiting, diarrhea, loss of appetite, rash, elevated LFTs, and neutropenia. Because the chelates are excreted via the kidneys, adequate hydration is essential.

An oral chelating agent, D-penicillamine, is sometimes used to treat lead poisoning, but low doses should be used in children, and monitoring of renal function and blood counts during administration is essential (Woolf, Goldman, & Bellinger, 2007).

Prognosis

Although most of the pathophysiologic effects of lead are reversible, the most serious consequences of both high and low lead exposure are the effects on the central nervous system. In children with lead encephalopathy, permanent brain damage can result in cognitive impairment, behavior changes, possible paralysis, and seizures. However, moderate- to low-dose exposure may also cause permanent neurologic deficits. Increased distractibility, short attention span, impulsivity, reading disabilities, and school failure have been associated with lead exposure (Markowitz, 2000). There is some evidence that treatment of moderate levels of lead poisoning can result in cognitive improvement (American Academy of Pediatrics, Committee on Environmental Health, 2005).

Nursing Care Management

The primary nursing goal in lead poisoning is to prevent the child's initial or further exposure to lead. For children with low-level exposure, this requires identifying the sources of lead in the environment. Careful history taking is the most useful and valuable tool and should concentrate on the personal risk questions (see p. 1435). Suggestions for reducing lead in the child's environment are listed in the Community Focus box.

Children who must undergo chelation therapy are prepared for the injections, and all efforts are made to reduce injection pain. Chelating agents are administered deeply into a large muscle mass (see Atraumatic Care box). To lessen the pain from EDTA, the local anesthetic procaine is injected with the drug. Rotation of sites is essential to prevent the formation of painful areas of fibrotic tissue. Because EDTA and lead are toxic to the kidneys, records are kept of intake and output, and the results of urinalysis are assessed to monitor renal functioning.

ATRAUMATIC CARE

Lead Chelation Therapy

To lessen the pain from intramuscular injection of CaNa2EDTA, the local anesthetic procaine is injected with the drug. Apply eutectic mixture of local anesthetic (i.e., EMLA, LMX4) cream over the puncture site 2.5 hours before the injection of EDTA and BAL. Administer intravenous EDTA whenever possible.

Use extreme caution with chelating agents. Incidences of child death from hypocalcemia have been recorded when Na_2EDTA was substituted for $CaNa_2EDTA$ and used as a che-

COMMUNITY FOCUS

Reducing Blood Lead Levels

- Make sure child does not have access to peeling paint or chewable surfaces painted with lead-based paint, especially window sills and wells.
- If a house was built before 1960 (possibly before 1980) and has hard-surface floors, wet mop them at least once per week. Wipe other hard surfaces (e.g., window sills, baseboards). If there are loose paint chips in an area, such as a window well, use a wet disposable cloth to pick up and discard them. Do not vacuum hard-surfaced floors or window sills or wells, because this spreads dust. Use vacuum cleaners with agitators to remove dust from rugs rather than vacuum cleaners with suction only. If a rug is known to contain lead dust and cannot be washed, it should be discarded.
- Wash and dry child's hands and face frequently, especially before eating.
- Wash toys and pacifiers frequently.
- If soil around home is or is likely to be contaminated with lead (e.g., if home was built before 1960 or is near a major highway), plant grass or other ground cover; plant bushes around outside of house so that child cannot play there.
- During remodeling of older homes, be sure to follow correct procedures. Be certain children and pregnant women are not in the home, day or night, until process is completed. After deleading, thoroughly clean house using cleaning solution to damp mop and dust before inhabitants return.
- In areas where lead content of water exceeds the drinking water standard and a particular faucet has not been used for 6 hours or more, "flush" the cold-water pipes by running the water until it becomes as cold as it will get (30 seconds to more than 2 minutes). The more time water has been sitting in pipes, the more lead it may contain.*
- *Use only cold water* for consumption (drinking, cooking, and especially for making infant formula).
- Hot water dissolves lead more quickly than cold water and thus contains higher levels of lead. First-flush water may be used for nonconsumption uses.
- Have water tested by a competent laboratory. This action is especially important for apartment dwellers; flushing may not be effective in high-rise buildings or in other buildings with lead-soldered central piping.
- Do not store food in open cans, particularly if cans are imported.
- Do not use pottery or ceramic ware that was inadequately fired or is meant for decorative use for food storage or service. Do not store drinks or food in lead crystal.
- Avoid folk remedies or cosmetics that contain lead.
- Make sure that home exposure is not occurring from parental occupations or hobbies. Household members employed in occupations such as lead smelting should shower and change into clean clothing before leaving work. Construction and lead abatement workers may also bring home lead contaminants.
- Make sure child eats regular meals, because more lead is absorbed on an empty stomach.
- Make sure child's diet contains sufficient iron and calcium and not excessive fat.

Modified from Centers for Disease Control and Prevention: *Preventing lead poisoning in young children,* Atlanta, 1991, The Centers.

*For more information, contact the county or state department of health or environment for information on local water quality. For general information on lead, call the EPA Safe Drinking Water Hotline, 800-426-4791, *www.epa.gov;* National Lead Information Center, 422 S. Clinton Ave., Rochester, NY 14620; 800-424-LEAD (5323); *www.epa.gov/lead/pubs/nlic.htm;* Water Quality Association, 630-505-0160; *www.wqa.org;* or NSF International, 877-867-3435; *www.nsf.org.*

lating agent (Centers for Diseases Control and Prevention, 2006).

NURSING ALERT Calcium EDTA is only administered when there is adequate urinary output. Children receiving the drug intramuscularly must be able to maintain adequate oral intake of fluids.

Discharge planning for children with lead poisoning must include thorough education of families regarding safety from lead hazards, clear instructions regarding medication administration and follow-up, and confirmation that the child will be discharged to a home without lead hazards. Although caution must be used to avoid alarming parents unnecessarily, it is important that they know the risk implications for their child's behavior and cognitive functions. Nurses should observe the development and behavior of children who are hospitalized. Any concerns that are identified should be thoroughly evaluated. Referral to a child development or speech and language specialist may be indicated.

As in any situational crisis, parents need support and understanding if their child is treated for lead poisoning. Many families at the highest risk for lead poisoning have the fewest resources to comply with measures such as relocation or removing lead from the environment where the child experiences exposure.

Key Points

- Common nutritional disorders of infancy and early childhood may result from vitamin and mineral deficiency or excess, some types of vegetarian diets, protein-energy malnutrition, and food intolerance.
- Food consumption varies among vegetarians; therefore a detailed dietary intake is essential for planning adequate intakes, particularly in children and pregnant and lactating women.
- Protein-energy malnutrition may occur as a complication of underlying disease, lack of parental education about infant nutrition, inappropriate management of food allergy, or incorrect preparation of formula.
- Food intolerance encompasses food allergies and food sensitivities, which can have a number of systemic and local clinical manifestations. CMA and lactose intolerance may occur in some children.
- Infants are subject to fluid depletion because of their greater surface area relative to body mass, high rate of metabolism, and immature kidney function.
- Dehydration can be classified as isotonic, hypotonic, and hypertonic.
- Vomiting and diarrhea account for significant fluid depletion, especially in infants and small children.
- The amount, frequency, and characteristics of stool and vomitus are important nursing observations.
- Diarrhea can be caused by an inflammatory process of infectious origin, a toxic reaction to ingestion of poisonous substances, dietary indiscretions, or infections outside the alimentary tract. The primary treatment of diarrhea is the use of an oral rehydrating solution.
- Structural disorders of the GI tract include CL, CP, EA with TEF, anorectal malformations, and BA.
- CL/P, the most common facial malformation, may involve nutritional, dental, and speech problems.
- Hernias related to the GI tract can be minor (umbilical) or life-threatening (diaphragmatic, gastroschisis, omphalocele).
- HD requires surgical removal of aganglionic segments of bowel.
- Postoperative care of the child with abdominal surgery involves assessing the abdomen and providing hydration and nutrition, intravenous fluids, proper positioning, wound care, and psychologic support.
- Nursing care of GER is aimed at identifying children with suggestive symptoms, helping parents with home care feeding and positioning, and caring for the child undergoing surgical intervention.
- Although the cause of appendicitis is poorly understood, it is typically a result of obstruction of the lumen, usually by a fecalith. Common signs and symptoms are right lower quadrant abdominal pain, tenderness, and fever.
- Meckel's diverticulum is a congenital malformation of the GI tract characterized by bloody stools.
- IBD refers to UC and CD.

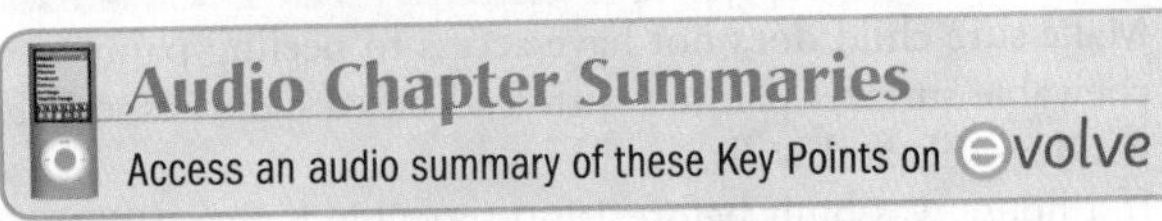
Audio Chapter Summaries
Access an audio summary of these Key Points on evolve

- Peptic ulcers are poorly understood, but contributing factors include interference with the normal protective mechanisms of the mucosal lining and the presence of *Helicobacter pylori.*
- Viral hepatitis is caused by six types of virus: HAV, HBV, HCV, HDV, HEV, and HGV.
- HAV is spread by the fecal-oral route, whereas HBV and HCV are transmitted primarily by the parenteral route. The most effective measure in prevention and control of hepatitis in any setting is handwashing.
- BA is a serious disorder, often causing progressive liver failure, which is an indication for liver transplantation.
- General signs of obstruction include colicky abdominal pain, nausea and vomiting, abdominal distention, and decreased stool output.
- HPS is recognized by characteristic projectile vomiting, malnutrition, dehydration, and a palpable mass in the epigastrium and is relieved by pyloromyotomy.
- Intussusception is one of the most common causes of intestinal obstruction during infancy and is characterized by abdominal pain and blood in stools. Treatment is either nonsurgical hydrostatic reduction or surgical reduction.
- Malabsorption syndromes are disorders associated with some degree of impaired digestion or absorption. They include digestive, absorptive, and anatomic defects.
- Celiac disease is characterized by intolerance to gluten. It is thought to be either an inborn error of metabolism or an immunologic response.
- SBS is characterized by a loss of intestine resulting in a diminished ability to absorb a regular diet normally. Specialized enteral and parenteral nutrition is a major element of care for these children.
- Intestinal parasitic diseases constitute the most common infections in the world; giardiasis and enterobiasis are the most widespread parasitic infections among children in the United States.
- Although the incidence of poisoning has decreased in the past 30 years as a result of more stringent packaging regulations, childhood poisoning remains a serious health concern.
- The major principles of treatment for poisoning include assessment and the ABCs of resuscitation (airway, breathing and cardiovascular supportive measures), minimization of poison absorption, prevention of complications, family support, and prevention of recurrence.
- Communication with the area Poison Control Center is essential in the treatment of any poisoning.

- Acetaminophen poisoning is the most common accidental drug poisoning among children and occurs primarily from acute overdose.
- The most important factor contributing to lead poisoning is its availability in the child's environment. Lead-based paint is the most toxic source of lead.
- Because of increasing awareness of the detrimental effects of low levels of lead on the developing nervous system, acceptable BLLs have been decreasing and now are at less than 10 mcg/dl.

References

Abbott Laboratories: *HUMIRA (adalimumab) for the management of moderate-to-severe Crohn's disease,* Abbott Park, Ill, 2007, The Laboratories.

Abruzzi G, Stork CM: Pediatric toxicological concerns, *Emerg Med Clin North Am* 20(1):223-247, 2002.

Ahmad T et al: The molecular classification of the clinical manifestations of Crohn's disease, *Gastroenterology* 122(4):854-866, 2002.

Aiken JJ, Oldham KT: Acute appendicitis. In Kliegman RM et al (editors): *Nelson textbook of pediatrics,* ed 18, Philadelphia, 2007, Saunders.

Alexander F et al: Fate of the pouch in 151 pediatric patients after ileal pouch anal anastomosis, *J Pediatr Surg* 38(1):328-332, 2003.

Amadi B et al: Improved nutritional recovery on an elemental diet in Zambian children with persistent diarrhoea and malnutrition, *J Trop Pediatr* 51(1):5-10, 2005.

American Academy of Clinical Toxicology, European Association of Poisons Centres and Clinical Toxicologists: position paper: cathartics, *J Toxicol* 42(3):243-253, 2004a.

American Academy of Clinical Toxicology, European Association of Poisons Centres and Clinical Toxicologists: position paper: ipecac syrup, *J Toxicol* 42(2):133-143, 2004b.

American Academy of Pediatrics: *Pediatric nutrition handbook,* ed 6, Elk Grove Village, Ill, 2009, The Academy.

American Academy of Pediatrics: Prevention of rickets and vitamin D deficiency in infants, children, and adolescents, *Pediatrics* 122(5):1142-1148, 2008.

American Academy of Pediatrics: Dietary recommendations for children and adolescents: a guide for practitioners, *Pediatrics* 117(2):544-559, 2006.

American Academy of Pediatrics, Committee on Environmental Health: Lead exposure in children: prevention, detection, and management, *Pediatrics* 116(4):1036-1046, 2005.

American Academy of Pediatrics, Committee on Infectious Diseases: Prevention of rotavirus disease: updated guidelines for use of rotavirus vaccine, *Pediatrics* 123(5):1412-1420, 2009a.

American Academy of Pediatrics, Committee on Infectious Diseases, Pickering L (editor): *Red book: 2009 report of the Committee on Infectious Diseases,* ed 28, Elk Grove Village, Ill, 2009b, The Academy.

American Academy of Pediatrics, Committee on Injury, Violence, and Poison Prevention: Poison treatment in the home, *Pediatrics* 112(5):1182-1185, 2003.

American Dietetic Association and Dietitians of Canada: Position of the American Dietetic Association and Dietitians of Canada: vegetarian diets, *J Am Diet Assoc* 103(6):748-765, 2003.

American Heart Association: *Dietary recommendations for children,* 2005. Available at www.americanheart.org/presenter.jhtml?identifier=3033999 (accessed January 3, 2008).

Armstrong GL et al: The prevalence of hepatitis C virus infection in the United States, 1999 through 2002, *Ann Intern Med* 144(10):705-714, 2006.

Assa'ad AH: Gastrointestinal food allergy and intolerance, *Pediatr Ann* 35(10):718-726, 2006.

Baron ML: Crohn's disease in children: this chronic illness can be painful and isolating, but new treatments may help, *Am J Nurs* 102(10):26-34, 2002.

Blanchard SS, Czinn SJ: Peptic ulcer disease in children. In Kliegman RM et al (editors): *Nelson textbook of pediatrics,* ed 18, Philadelphia, 2007, Saunders.

Bond GR: Activated charcoal in the home: helpful and important or simply a distraction? *Pediatrics* 109(1):145-146, 2002.

Broderick AL, Jonas MM: Hepatitis B in children, *Semin Liver Dis* 23(1):59-68, 2003.

Bronstein AC et al: 2007 Annual report of the American Association of Poison Control Center's National Poison Data System (NPDS): 25th annual report, *Clin Toxicol* 46(10):927-1057, 2008.

Burk CJ, Molodow R: Infantile scurvy: an old diagnosis revisited with a modern dietary twist, *Am J Clin Dermatol* 8(2):103-106, 2007.

Cavataio F, Guandalini S: Gastroesophageal reflux. In Guandalini S, editor: *Essential pediatric gastroenterology and nutrition,* New York, 2005, McGraw-Hill.

Centers for Disease Control and Prevention: Deaths associated with hypocalcemia from chelation therapy—Texas, Pennsylvania, and Oregon, 2003-2005, *MMWR* 55(08):204-207, 2006.

Centers for Disease Control and Prevention: *Statewide plan for childhood blood lead screening,* Atlanta, 2005, The Centers.

Centers for Disease Control and Prevention: Neurologic impairment in children associated with maternal dietary deficiency of cobalamin—Georgia, 2001, *MMWR* 52(4):61-64, 2003a.

Centers for Disease Control and Prevention: Managing acute gastroenteritis among children: oral rehydration, maintenance, and nutritional therapy, *MMWR* 52(RR-16)1-16, 2003b.

Centers for Disease Control and Prevention: *Managing elevated blood lead levels among young children: recommendations from the Advisory Committee on Childhood Lead Poisoning Prevention,* Atlanta, 2002, The Centers.

Chelimsky G, Czinn S: Peptic ulcer disease in children, *Pediatr Rev* 22(10):349-355, 2001.

Chen SM et al: Screening for biliary atresia by infant stool color card in Taiwan, *Pediatrics* 117(4):1147-1154, 2006.

Cheng A, Ratnapalan S: Improving the palatability of activated charcoal in pediatric patients, *Pediatr Emerg Care* 23(6):384-386, 2007.

Chien JC et al: Is urorectal septum malformation sequence a variant of the vertebral defects, anal atresia, tracheo-oesophageal fistula, renal defects and radial dysplasia association? Report of a case and a review of the literature, *Eur J Pediatr* 164(6):350-354, 2005.

Christian DJ, Buyske J: Current status of antireflux surgery, *Surg Clin North Am* 85(5):931-947, 2005.

Christie L et al: Food allergies in children affect nutrient intake and growth, *J Am Diet Assoc* 102(11):1648-1651, 2002.

Ciliberto MA et al: Comparison of a home-based therapy with ready-to-use therapeutic food with standard therapy in the treatment of malnourished Malawin children: a controlled, clinical effectiveness trial, *Am J Clin Nutr* 81(4):864-870, 2005.

Clifton JC: Mercury exposure and public health, *Pediatr Clin North Am* 54(2):237-269, 2007.

Conover E, Buehler BA: Use of herbal agents by breastfeeding women may affect infants, *Pediatr Ann* 33(4):235-240, 2004.

Coy K, Speltz ML, Jones K: Facial appearance and attachment in infants with orofacial clefts: a replication, *Cleft Palate Craniofac J* 39(1):66-72, 2002.

Criddle LM: An overview of pediatric poisonings, *AACN Adv Crit Care* 18(2):109-118, 2007.

Curtin G, Boekelheide A: Cleft lip and palate. In Allen PJ, Vessey JA (editors): *Primary care of the child with a chronic condition,* St Louis, 2004, Mosby.

Czinn SJ: *Helicobacter pylori* infection: detection, investigation, and management, *J Pediatr* 146(3 Suppl):S21-S26, 2005.

Dasgupta R, Langer JC: Hirschsprung disease, *Curr Probl Surg* 41(12):949-988, 2004.

DeRoo LA et al: First-trimester alcohol consumption and the risk of infant oral clefts in Norway: a population-based case-control study, *Am J Epidemiol* 168(6):638-646, 2008.

Devaney BL, Barr SI: DRI, EAR, RDA, AI, UL: Making sense of this alphabet soup, *Pediatr Basics* 97(Winter):2-9, 2002.

de Vrese M et al: Probiotics: compensation for lactase insufficiency, *Am J Clin Nutr* 73(2 Suppl):421S-429S, 2001.

Dunham L, Kollar L: Vegetarian eating for children and adolescents, *J Pediatr Health Care* 20(1):27-34, 2006.

Durkin ET, Shaaban AF: Recent advances and controversies in pediatric laparoscopic surgery, *Surg Clin North Am* 88(5):1101-1119, 2008.

Emerick KM, Whitington PF: Neonatal liver disease, *Pediatr Ann* 35(4):281-286, 2006.

Eppley BL et al: The spectrum of orofacial clefting, *Plast Reconstr Surg* 115(7):101e-114e, 2005.

Erickson L, Thompson T: A review of a preventable poison: pediatric lead poisoning, *J Soc Pediatr Nurs* 10(4):171-182, 2005.

Etzel RA: Indoor air pollutants in homes and schools, *Pediatr Clin North Am* 48(5):1153-1165, 2001.

Ewing WM, Allen PJ: The diagnosis and management of cow's milk protein intolerance in the primary care setting, *Pediatr Nurs* 31(6):486-492, 2005.

Fiocchi A, Martelli A: Dietary management of food allergy, *Pediatr Ann* 35(10):755-763, 2006.

Fiocchi A et al: Food allergy and the introduction of solid foods to infants: a consensus document, *Ann Allergy Asthma Immunol* 97(1):10-20, 2006.

Ford AC et al: Eradication therapy in *Helicobacter pylori* positive peptic ulcer disease: systematic review and economic analysis, *Am J Gastroenterol* 99(9):1833-1855, 2004.

Gelfond D, Fasano A: Celiac disease in the pediatric population, *Pediatr Ann* 35(4):275-279, 2006.

Gidding SS et al: Dietary recommendations for children and adolescents: a guide for practitioners: consensus statement from the American Heart Association, *Circulation* 112(13): 2061-2075, 2005.

Gisbert JP, de la Morena F, Abraira V: Accuracy of monoclonal stool antigen test for the diagnosis of *H. pylori* infection: a systematic review and meta-analysis, *Am J Gastroenterol* 101(8):1921-1930, 2006.

Goldberg JP, Folta SC, Must A: Milk: Can a "good" food be so bad? *Pediatrics* 110(4):826-831, 2002.

Greenbaum L: Deficit therapy. In Kliegman RM et al (editors): *Nelson textbook of pediatrics*, ed 18, Philadelphia, 2007, Saunders.

Greer FR et al: Effects of early nutritional interventions on the development of atopic disease in infants and children: the role of maternal dietary restriction, breastfeeding, timing of introduction of complementary foods, and hydrolyzed formulas, *Pediatrics* 121(1):183-191, 2008.

Guandalini S: Probiotics for children with diarrhea: an update, *J Clin Gastroenterol* 42(Suppl 2):S53-S57, 2008.

Heard K: Gastrointestinal decontamination, *Med Clin North Am* 89(6):1067-1078, 2005.

Heyman MB, American Academy of Pediatrics Committee on Nutrition: Lactose intolerance in infants, children, and adolescents, *Pediatrics* 118(3):1279-1286, 2006.

Hlavsa MC, Watson JC, Beach MJ: Giardiasis surveillance—United States, 1998-2002, *MMWR* 54(SS1): 9-16, 2005.

Holcomb GW III et al: Thoracoscopic repair of esophageal atresia and tracheoesophageal fistula: a multi-institutional analysis, *Ann Surg* 242(3): 422-428, 2005.

Host A: Frequency of cow's milk allergy in childhood, *Ann Allergy Asthma Immunol* 89(6 Suppl 1):33-37, 2002.

Huang L-T et al: Low plasma nitrite in infantile hypertrophic pyloric stenosis patients, *Dig Dis Sci* 51(5):869-872, 2006.

Huiming Y, Chaomin W, Meng M: Vitamin A for treating measles in children, Cochrane Database Syst Rev (4):CD001479, 2005.

Huppertz HI et al: Intussusception among young children in Europe, *Pediatr Infect Dis J* 25(1):S22-S29, 2006.

Hurwitz M, Cox, KL: Liver transplantation. In Kliegman RM et al (editors), *Nelson textbook of pediatrics*, ed 18, Philadelphia, 2007, Saunders.

Institute of Medicine, Food and Nutrition Board: *Dietary Reference Intakes: applications in dietary assessment*, Washington DC, 2000, National Academies Press.

Jabbar A, Wright RA: Gastroenteritis and antibiotic-associated diarrhea, *Primary Care* 30(1):63-80, 2003.

Karnam US, Reddy KR: Pegylated interferons, *Clin Liver Dis* 7(1):139-148, 2003.

Katz KA et al: Rice nightmare: kwashiorkor in two Philadelphia-area infants fed Rice Dream beverage, *J Am Acad Dermatol* 52(5 Suppl 1):S69-S72, 2005.

Kawchak DA et al: Adequacy of dietary intake declines with age in children with sickle cell disease, *J Am Diet Assoc* 107(5):843-848, 2007.

Kemper KJ, Gardiner P: Herbal medicines. In Kliegman RM et al (editors): *Nelson textbook of pediatrics*, ed 18, Philadelphia, 2007, Saunders.

Kim WR et al: Mortality and hospitalization for hepatocellular carcinoma in the United States, *Gastroenterology* 129(2):486-493, 2005.

Kirschner RE, LaRossa D: Cleft lip and palate, *Otolaryngol Clin North Am* 33(6):1191-1215, 2000.

Klein MD, Thomas RP: Surgical conditions of the anus, rectum, and colon. In Kliegman RM et al (editors), *Nelson textbook of pediatrics*, ed 18, Philadelphia, 2007, Saunders.

Kugathasan S et al: CARD15 gene mutations and risk for early surgery in pediatric-onset Crohn's disease, *Clin Gastroenterol Hepatol* 2(11): 1003-1009, 2004.

Kugathasan S et al: Epidemiologic and clinical characteristics of children with newly diagnosed inflammatory bowel disease in Wisconsin: a statewide population-based study, *J Pediatr* 143(4):525-531, 2003.

Kwok MY, Kim MK, Gorelick MH: Evidence-based approach to the diagnosis of appendicitis in children, *Pediatr Emerg Care* 20(10):690-698, 2004.

Langan RC et al: Ulcerative colitis: diagnosis and treatment, *Am Fam Physician* 76(9):1323-1330, 2007.

Lanski SL et al: Herbal therapy in a pediatric emergency department population: expect the unexpected, *Pediatrics* 111(5 pt 1):981-985, 2003.

Lawrence RA, Lawrence RM: *Breastfeeding: a guide for the medical professional*, ed 6, St Louis, 2005, Mosby.

Lee A, Newman JM: Celiac diet: its impact on quality of life, *J Am Diet Assoc* 103(11):1533-1535, 2003.

Levin ME, Motala C, Lopata AL: Anaphylaxis in a milk-allergic child after ingestion of soy formula cross-contaminated with cow's milk protein, *Pediatrics* 116(5):1223-1225, 2005.

Lidsky TI, Schneider JS: Adverse effects of childhood lead poisoning: the clinical neuropsychological perspective, *Environ Res* 100(1):284-293, 2006.

Litovitz T et al: 1999 Annual report of the American Association of Poison Control Centers Toxic Exposure Surveillance System, *Am J Emerg Med* 18(5):517-574, 2000.

Liu T et al: Kwashiorkor in the United States: fad diets, perceived and true milk allergy, and nutritional ignorance, *Arch Dermatol* 137(5):630-636, 2001.

Loening-Baucke V, Pashankar DS: A randomized, prospective, comparison study of polyethylene glycol 3350 without electrolytes and milk of magnesia for children with constipation and fecal incontinence, *Pediatrics* 118(2):528-535, 2006.

Lohse B, Stotts JL, Priebe JR: Survey of herbal use by Kansas and Wisconsin WIC participants reveals moderate, appropriate use and identifies herbal education needs, *J Am Diet Assoc* 106(2):227-237, 2006.

Loman DG: The use of complementary and alternative health care practices among children, *J Pediatr Health Care* 17(2):58-63, 2003.

Malek MA et al: Diarrhea- and rotavirus-associated hospitalizations among children less than 5 years of age: United States, 1997 and 2000, *Pediatrics* 117(6):1887-1892, 2006.

Maris CL et al: Are infants with orofacial clefts at risk for insecure mother-child attachments? *Cleft Palate Craniofac J* 37(3):257-265, 2000.

Markowitz M: Lead poisoning, *Pediatr Rev* 21(10):327-335, 2000.

McGuire JK, Kulkarni MS, Baden HP: Fatal hypermagnesemia in a child treated with megavitamin/megamineral therapy, *Pediatrics* 105(2):414, 2000.

Merritt L: Understanding the embryology and genetics of cleft lip and palate, part I, *Adv Neonat Care* 5(2):64-71, 2005a.

Merritt L: Physical assessment of the infant with cleft lip and/or palate, part II, *Adv Neonat Care* 5(3):125-134, 2005b.

Messina V, Melina V, Mangels AR: A new food guide for North American vegetarians, *J Am Diet Assoc* 103(6): 771-775, 2003.

Müller O, Krawinkel M: Malnutrition and health in developing countries, *CMAJ* 173(3):279-286, 2005.

Murdock AM, Johnston SD: Diagnostic criteria for coeliac disease: time for change? *Eur J Gastroenterol Hepatol* 17(1):41-43, 2005.

Naik-Mathuria B, Olutoye OO: Foregut abnormalities, *Surg Clin North Am* 86(2):261-284, 2006.

Ohi R: Surgery for biliary atresia, *Liver* 21(3):175-182, 2001.

Penny ME: Protein-energy malnutrition: pathophysiology, clinical consequences, and treatment. In Walker WA, Watkins JB, Duggan C (editors): *Nutrition in pediatrics*, ed 3, Hamilton, Ontario, 2003, Decker.

Perrotta S et al: Infant hypervitaminosis A causes severe anemia and thrombocytopenia: evidence of a retinol-dependent bone marrow cell growth inhibition, *Blood* 99(6):2017-2022, 2002.

Perry CL et al: Adolescent vegetarians: how well do their dietary patterns meet the Healthy People 2010 objectives? *Arch Pediatr Adolesc Med* 156(5):426-427, 2002.

Pessler F, Nejat M: Anaphylactic reaction to goat's milk in a cow's milk-allergic infant, *Pediatr Allergy Immunol* 15(2):183-185, 2004.

Powers K: Diagnosis and management of common toxic ingestions and inhalations, *Pediatr Ann* 29(6):330-342, 2000.

Preston AM, Rodriguez C, Rivera CE: Plasma ascorbate in a population of children: influence of age, gender, vitamin C intake, and smoke exposure, *P R Health Sci J* 25(2):137-142, 2006.

Preston AM et al: Influence of environmental tobacco smoke on vitamin C status in children, *Am J Clin Nutr* 77(1):167-172, 2003.

Ramaswamy K, Jacobson K: Infectious diarrhea in children, *Gastroenterol Clin* 30(3):611-624, 2001.

Richards CA: *C. difficile* epidemic continuing to spread, *Infect Dis Children* 39-41, September 2006.

Richmond J, Dunning P, Desmond P: Hepatitis C: a medical and social diagnosis, *Aust Nurs J* 12(1):23-25, 2004.

Roslund G, Hepps TS, McQuillen KK: The role of oral ondansetron in children with vomiting as a result of acute gastritis/gastroenteritis who have failed oral rehydration therapy: a randomized controlled trial, *Ann Emerg Med* 52(1): 22-29, 2008.

Rostom A, Murray JA, Kagnoff MF: American Gastroenterological Association (AGA) Institute technical review on the diagnosis and management of celiac disease, *Gastroenterology* 131(6):1981-2002, 2006.

Rubin DT, Kavitt RT: Surveillance for cancer and dysplasia in inflammatory bowel disease, *Gastroenterol Clin North Am* 35(3):581-604, 2006.

Rudolph CD et al: Guidelines for evaluation and treatment of gastroesophageal reflux in infants and children: recommendations of the North American Society for Pediatric Gastroenterology and Nutrition, *J Pediatr Gastroenterol Nutr* 32(Suppl 2):S1-S31, 2001.

Ruemmele FM et al: Diagnostic accuracy of serological assays in pediatric inflammatory bowel disease, *Gastroenterology* 115(4):822-829, 1998.

Rutter MD et al: Thirty-year analysis of colonoscopic surveillance program for neoplasia in ulcerative colitis, *Gastroenterology* 130(4):1030-1038, 2006.

Sagar J, Kumar V, Shah DK: Meckel's diverticulum: a systematic review, *J R Soc Med* 99(10):501-505, 2006.

Saltzman MD, King EC: Central physeal arrests as a manifestation of hypervitaminosis A, *J Pediatr Orthop* 27(3):351-353, 2007.

Salvatore S, Vandenplas Y: Gastroesophageal reflux and cow milk allergy: is there a link? *Pediatrics* 110(5):972-984, 2002.

Sampson HA: Update on food allergy, *J Allergy Clin Immunol* 113(5):805-819, 2004.

Sampson HA: Anaphylaxis and emergency treatment, *Pediatrics* 111(6 Pt 3):1601-1608, 2003.

Sandberg SJ, Magee WP, Denk MJ: Neonatal cleft lip and cleft palate repair, *AORN Online* 75(3):488, 490-499, 501, 503-504, 506-508, 2002.

Sawni A et al: The use of complementary/alternative therapies among children attending an urban pediatric emergency department, *Clin Pediatr* 46(1):36-41, 2007.

Schwab M et al: Association between the C3435T MDRI gene polymorphism and susceptibility for ulcerative colitis, *Gastroenterology* 124(1):26-33, 2003.

Sgouros SN, Bergele C: Clinical outcome of patients with *Helicobacter pylori* infection: the bug, the host, or the environment? *Postgrad Med J* 82(967):338-342, 2006.

Shaw-Smith C: Oesophageal atresia, tracheo-oesophageal fistula, and the VACTERL association: review of genetics and epidemiology, *J Med Genet* 43(7):545-554, 2006.

Sibley E: Carbohydrate intolerance, *Curr Opin Gastroenterol* 20(2):162-167, 2004.

Silbermintz A, Markowitz J: Inflammatory bowel diseases, *Pediatr Ann* 35(4):268-274, 2006.

Sood MR: Disorders of malabsorption. In Kliegman RM, et al (editors): *Nelson textbook of pediatrics*, ed 18, Philadelphia, 2007, Saunders.

Speltz ML et al: Early predictors of attachment in infants with cleft lip and/or palate, *Child Dev* 68(1):12-25, 1997.

Staat MA: What is the disease burden associated with rotavirus? In *The management and prevention of rotavirus*, Thorofare, NJ, 2006, Vindico Medical Education.

Steiner MJ et al: Is this child dehydrated? *JAMA* 291(22):2746-2754, 2004.

Suwandhi E, Ton MN, Schwarz SM: Gastroesophageal reflux in infancy and childhood, *Pediatr Ann* 35(4):259-266, 2006.

Szajewska H, Ruszcynski M, Radzikowski A: Probiotics in the prevention of antibiotic-associated diarrhea in children: a meta-analysis of randomized controlled trials, *J Pediatr* 149(3):367-372, 2006.

Waters L, Nelson M: New therapeutic options for hepatitis C, *Curr Opin Infect Dis* 19(6):615-622, 2006.

Watson WA et al: 2004 Annual report of the American Association of Poison Control Centers Toxic Exposure Surveillance System, *Am J Emerg Med* 23(5):589-666, 2005.

Wilkins-Haug L: Prenatal diagnosis of orofacial clefts, *Up to date*, July 2008. Available at www.uptodate.com (accessed July 31, 2008).

Woolf AD, Goldman R, Bellinger DC: Update on clinical management of childhood lead poisoning, *Pediatr Clin North Am* 54(2):271-294, 2007.

Wyllie R: Motility disorders and Hirschsprung disease. In Kliegman RM et al (editors): *Nelson textbook of pediatrics*, ed 18, Philadelphia, 2007a, Saunders.

Wyllie R: Pyloric stenosis and congenital anomalies of the stomach. In Kliegman RM et al (editors): *Nelson textbook of pediatrics*, ed 18, Philadelphia, 2007b, Saunders.

Wyneski MJ et al: Safety and efficacy of adalimumab in pediatric patients with Crohn disease, *J Pediatr Gastroenterol* 47(1):19-25, 2008.

Yuen MF, Lai CL: Treatment of chronic hepatitis B, *Lancet Infect Dis* 1(4):383-393, 2001.

Zangwill KM: Protecting against rotavirus disease and its complications. In *The management and prevention of rotavirus*, Thorofare, NJ, 2006, Vindico Medical Education.

Zeisel SH, Erickson KE: Dietary supplements (nutraceuticals). In Walker WA, Watkins JB, Duggan C (editors): *Nutrition in pediatrics*, ed 3, Hamilton, Ontario, 2003, Decker.

Unit 11

48 Cardiovascular Dysfunction

Learning Objectives

On completion of this chapter the reader will be able to:

- Design a plan for assisting a child during a cardiac diagnostic procedure.
- Demonstrate an understanding of the hemodynamics, distinctive manifestations, and therapeutic management of congenital heart disease.
- Outline a care plan for an infant or child with congestive heart failure.
- Describe the care for a child who has hypoxia.
- Describe the care for an infant or a child with a congenital heart defect and its surgical repair.
- Discuss the nurse's role in helping the child and family cope with congenital heart disease.
- Differentiate between rheumatic fever and rheumatic heart disease.
- List the criteria for selected cholesterol screening of children.
- Discuss the assessment and management of hypertension in children and adolescents.
- Outline a care plan for a child with Kawasaki disease.

Electronic Resources

Additional information related to the content in Chapter 48 can be found on

evolve the Companion Website at

http://evolve.elsevier.com/Perry/maternal/

- NCLEX Review Questions
- Anatomy Review—Changes in Circulation at Birth
- Anatomy Review—Conduction System of the Heart
- Animation—Cardiac Tamponade, Infant
- Animation—Catheter Placement, Umbilical Vein
- Animation—Heart Sounds
- Animation—Structure of the Heart
- Animation—Subaortic Stenosis
- Case Study—Patent Ductus Arteriosus
- Critical Thinking Exercise—Cardiac Catheterization
- Critical Thinking Exercise—Digoxin Administration
- Critical Thinking Exercise—Patent Ductus Arteriosus
- Nursing Care Plan—The Child with Congestive Heart Failure

Cardiovascular Dysfunction

Cardiovascular disorders in children are divided into two major groups: congenital heart disease and acquired heart disorders. *Congenital heart disease (CHD)* includes primarily anatomic abnormalities present at birth that result in abnormal cardiac function. The clinical consequences of congenital heart defects fall into two broad categories: congestive heart failure (CHF) and hypoxemia. *Acquired cardiac disorders* are disease processes or abnormalities that occur after birth and can be seen in the normal heart or in the presence of congenital heart defects. They result from various factors, including infection, autoimmune responses, environmental factors, and familial tendencies.

History and Physical Examination

Taking an accurate health history is an important first step in assessing an infant or child for possible heart disease. Parents may have specific concerns, such as an infant with poor feeding or fast breathing, or a 7-year-old who can no longer keep up with friends on the soccer field. Others may not realize that their child has a medical problem; their baby has always been pale and fussy.

Asking details about the mother's health history, pregnancy, and birth history are important in assessing infants. Mothers with chronic health conditions, such as diabetes or lupus, are more likely to have infants with heart disease. Some medications, such as phenytoin (Dilantin), are teratogenic to the fetus. Maternal alcohol use or illicit drug use increases the risk of congenital heart defects. Exposures to infections, such as rubella, early in pregnancy may result in congenital anomalies. Infants with low birth weight resulting from intrauterine growth restriction are more likely to have congenital anomalies. High-birth-weight infants have an increased incidence of heart disease.

A detailed family history is also important. There is an increased incidence of congenital cardiac defects if either parent or a sibling has a heart defect. Some diseases, such as Marfan syndrome, and some cardiomyopathies are hereditary. A family history of frequent fetal loss, sudden infant death, and sudden death in adults may indicate heart disease.

Congenital heart defects are seen in many syndromes such as Down and Turner's syndromes.

The physical assessment of suspected cardiac disease begins with observation of general appearance and proceeds with more specific observations. The following are supplementary to the general assessment techniques described for physical examination of the chest and heart in Chapter 34.

Inspection

Nutritional state—Failure to thrive or poor weight gain is associated with heart disease.

Color—Cyanosis is a common feature of CHD, and pallor is associated with poor perfusion.

Chest deformities—An enlarged heart sometimes distorts the chest configuration.

Unusual pulsations—Visible pulsations of the neck veins are seen in some patients.

Respiratory excursion—This refers to the ease or difficulty of respiration (e.g., tachypnea, dyspnea, expiratory grunt).

Clubbing of fingers—This is associated with cyanosis.

Palpation and Percussion

Chest—These maneuvers help discern heart size and other characteristics (e.g., thrills) associated with heart disease.

Abdomen—Hepatomegaly or splenomegaly may be evident.

Peripheral pulses—Rate, regularity, and amplitude (strength) may reveal discrepancies.

Auscultation

Heart rate and rhythm—Listen for fast heart rates (tachycardia), slow heart rates (bradycardia), or irregular rhythms.

Character of heart sounds—Listen for distinct or muffled sounds, murmurs, and additional heart sounds.

Diagnostic Evaluation

A variety of invasive and noninvasive tests may be used in the diagnosis of heart disease (Table 48-1). Some of the more common diagnostic tools that require nursing assessment and intervention are described here.

Electrocardiogram

Bedside cardiac monitoring with the electrocardiogram (ECG) is commonly used in pediatrics, especially in the care of children with heart disease. The bedside monitor provides valuable information about heart rate and rhythm through a graphic display of the ECG tracing and a digital display. An alarm can be set with parameters for individual patient requirements and will sound if the heart rate is above or below the set parameters. Gelfoam electrodes are commonly used and placed on the right side of the chest (above the level of the heart) and the left side of the chest, and a ground electrode is placed on the abdomen. Electrodes should be changed every 1 or 2 days because they irritate the skin. Bedside monitors are an adjunct to patient care and should never be substituted for direct assessment and auscultation of heart sounds. The nurse should assess the patient, not the monitor.

NURSING ALERT Electrodes for cardiac monitoring are often color coded: white for right, green (or red) for ground, and black for left. Always check to ensure that these colors are placed correctly.

Table 48-1 Procedures for Cardiac Diagnosis

PROCEDURE	DESCRIPTION
Chest radiograph (x-ray)	Provides information on heart size and pulmonary blood flow patterns
Electrocardiography	Graphic measure of electrical activity of heart
Holter monitor	24-hr continuous electrocardiogram (ECG) recording used to assess dysrhythmias
Echocardiography	Use of high-frequency sound waves obtained by a transducer to produce an image of cardiac structures
Transthoracic	Done with transducer on chest
M-mode	One-dimensional graphic view used to estimate ventricular size and function
Two-dimensional	Real-time, cross-sectional views of heart used to identify cardiac structures and cardiac anatomy
Doppler	Identifies blood flow patterns and pressure gradients across structures
Fetal	Imaging fetal heart in utero
Transesophageal (TEE)	Transducer placed in esophagus behind heart to obtain images of posterior heart structures or in patients with poor images from chest approach
Cardiac catheterization	Imaging study using radiopaque catheters placed in a peripheral blood vessel and advanced into heart to measure pressures and oxygen levels in heart chambers and visualize heart structures and blood flow patterns
Hemodynamics	Measures pressures and oxygen saturations in heart chambers
Angiography	Use of contrast material to illuminate heart structures and blood flow patterns
Biopsy	Use of special catheter to remove tiny samples of heart muscle for microscopic evaluation; used in assessing infection, inflammation, or muscle dysfunction disorders and to evaluate for rejection after heart transplant
Electrophysiology (EPS)	Special catheters with electrodes used to record electrical activity from within heart; used to diagnose rhythm disturbances
Exercise stress test	Monitoring of heart rate, blood pressure, ECG, and oxygen consumption at rest and during progressive exercise on a treadmill or bicycle
Cardiac magnetic resonance imaging (MRI)	Noninvasive imaging technique; used in evaluation of vascular anatomy outside of heart (e.g., coarctation of the aorta, vascular rings), estimates of ventricular mass and volume; uses for MRI are expanding

evolve Animation—Heart Sounds

evolve Animation—Structure of the Heart

Echocardiography

Echocardiography is one of the most frequently used tests for detecting cardiac dysfunction in children. Recent improvements in echocardiographic techniques have made it increasingly possible to confirm the diagnosis without resorting to cardiac catheterization. In more and more cases a prenatal diagnosis of CHD can be made by fetal echocardiography.

Echocardiography involves the use of ultrahigh-frequency sound waves to produce an image of the heart's structure. A transducer placed directly on the chest wall delivers repetitive pulses of ultrasound and processes the returned signals (echoes).

Although the test is noninvasive, painless, and associated with no known side effects, it can be stressful for children. The child must lie quietly in the standard echocardiographic positions; crying, nursing, or sitting up often leads to diagnostic errors or omissions. Therefore infants and young children may need a mild sedative; older children benefit from psychologic preparation for the test. The distraction of a video or movie is often helpful.

Cardiac Catheterization

Cardiac catheterization is an invasive diagnostic procedure in which a radiopaque catheter is inserted through a peripheral blood vessel into the heart. The catheter is usually introduced through percutaneous technique, in which the catheter is threaded through a large-bore needle that is inserted into the vein. The catheter is guided through the heart with the aid of fluoroscopy. After the tip of the catheter is within a heart chamber, contrast material is injected, and films are taken of the dilution and circulation of the material *(angiography)*. Types of cardiac catheterizations include:

Diagnostic catheterizations—These studies are used to diagnose congenital cardiac defects, particularly in symptomatic infants and before surgical repair. They are divided into right-sided catheterizations, in which the catheter is introduced through a vein (usually the femoral vein) and threaded to the right atrium (most common), and left-sided catheterizations, in which the catheter is threaded through an artery into the aorta and then into the heart.

Interventional catheterizations (therapeutic catheterizations)—A balloon catheter or other device is used to alter the cardiac anatomy. Examples include dilating stenotic valves or vessels or closing abnormal connections (Table 48-2).

Electrophysiology studies—Catheters with tiny electrodes that record the impulses of the heart directly from the conduction system are used to evaluate dysrhythmias and sometimes destroy accessory pathways that cause some tachydysrhythmias.

Nursing Care Management

Cardiac catheterization has become a routine diagnostic procedure and may be done on an outpatient basis. However, it is not without risks, especially in neonates and seriously ill infants and children. Possible complications include acute hemorrhage from the entry site (more likely with interventional procedures because larger catheters are used), low-grade fever, nausea, vomiting, loss of pulse in the catheterized extremity (usually transient, resulting from a clot, hematoma, or intimal tear), and transient dysrhythmias (generally catheter induced) (Uzark, 2001). Rare risks include stroke, seizures, tamponade, and death.

Table 48-2 Current Interventional Cardiac Catheterization Procedures in Children

INTERVENTION	DIAGNOSIS
Balloon atrioseptostomy—Use well established in newborns; may also be done under echocardiographic guidance	Transposition of great arteries Some complex single-ventricle defects
Balloon dilation—Treatment of choice	Valvular pulmonic stenosis Branch pulmonary artery stenosis Congenital valvular aortic stenosis Rheumatic mitral stenosis Recurrent coarctation of aorta Further follow-up required in: Native coarctation of aorta in patients over 7 mo old Congenital mitral stenosis
Coil occlusion—Accepted alternative to surgery	Patent ductus arteriosus (<4 mm)
Transcatheter device closure—Several devices used in clinical trials	Atrial septal defect (ASD)
Amplatzer septal occluder—Approved for ASD closure	ASD
Ventricular septal defect devices—Used in clinical trials	Ventricular septal defects
Stent placement	Pulmonary artery stenosis Coarctation of the aorta in adolescents Use to treat other lesions investigational
Radiofrequency ablation	Some tachydysrhythmias

Data from Allen HD et al: Pediatric therapeutic cardiac catheterization: AHA scientific statement, *Circulation* 97:609-625, 1998; updated data from Rome J, Kreutzer J: Pediatric interventional catheterization: reasonable expectations and outcomes, *Pediatr Clin North Am* 51:1589-1610, 2004.

Preprocedural Care

A complete nursing assessment is necessary to ensure a safe procedure with minimum complications. This assessment should include accurate height (essential for correct catheter selection) and weight. Obtaining a history of allergic reactions is important because some of the contrast agents are iodine based. Specific attention to signs and symptoms of infection is crucial. Severe diaper rash may be a reason to cancel the procedure if femoral access is required. Because assessment of pedal pulses is important after catheterization, the nurse should assess and mark pulses (dorsalis pedis, posterior tibial) before the child goes to the catheterization room. The presence and quality of pulses in both feet are clearly documented. Baseline oxygen saturation using pulse oximetry in children with cyanosis is also recorded.

Preparing the child and family for the procedure is the joint responsibility of the patient care team. School-age children and adolescents benefit from a description of the catheterization laboratory and a chronologic explanation of the procedure, emphasizing what they will see, feel, and hear. Older children and adolescents may bring earphones and favorite music so they can listen during the catheterization procedure. Preparation materials such as picture books, videotapes, or tours of the catheterization laboratory may be helpful. Preparation should be geared to the child's developmental level. The child's caregivers often benefit from the same explanations. Additional information, such as the expected length of the catheterization, description of the child's appearance after catheterization, and usual postprocedure care, should be outlined. (See also Prepare Child and Family for Invasive Procedures, p. 1469.)

Methods of sedation vary among institutions and may include oral or intravenous (IV) medications (see Chapter 45). The child's age, heart defect, clinical status, and type of catheterization procedure planned are considered when sedation is determined. General anesthesia may be needed for some interventional procedures. Children are allowed nothing by mouth (NPO) for 4 to 6 hours or more before the procedure according to institutional guidelines. Infants and patients with polycythemia may need IV fluids to prevent dehydration and hypoglycemia.

Postprocedural Care

Patients may recover from the procedure in a recovery unit, their hospital room, or occasionally intensive care. They are placed on a cardiac monitor and a pulse oximeter for the first few hours of recovery. The most important nursing responsibility is observation of the following for signs of complications:

- Pulses, especially below the catheterization site, for equality and symmetry (Pulse distal to the site may be weaker for the first few hours after catheterization but should gradually increase in strength.)
- Temperature and color of the affected extremity since coolness or blanching may indicate arterial obstruction
- Vital signs, which are taken as frequently as every 15 minutes, with special emphasis on heart rate, which is counted for 1 full minute for evidence of dysrhythmias or bradycardia
- Blood pressure (BP), especially for hypotension, which may indicate hemorrhage from cardiac perforation or bleeding at the site of initial catheterization
- Dressing, for evidence of bleeding or hematoma formation in the femoral or antecubital area
- Fluid intake, both IV and oral, to ensure adequate hydration (Blood loss in the catheterization laboratory, the child's NPO status, and diuretic actions of dyes used during the procedure put children at risk for hypovolemia and dehydration.)
- Blood glucose levels for hypoglycemia, especially in infants, who should receive dextrose-containing IV fluids

NURSING ALERT If bleeding occurs, direct continuous pressure is applied 2.5 cm (1 inch) above the percutaneous skin site to localize pressure over the vessel puncture.

Depending on hospital policy, the child may be kept in bed with the affected extremity maintained straight for 4 to 6 hours after venous catheterization and 6 to 8 hours after arterial catheterization to facilitate healing of the cannulated vessel. If younger children have difficulty complying, they can be held in the parent's lap with the leg maintained in the correct position. The child's usual diet can be resumed as soon as tolerated, beginning with sips of clear liquids and advancing as the condition allows. The child is encouraged to void to clear the contrast material from the blood. Generally, there is only slight discomfort at the percutaneous site. To prevent infection, the catheterization area is protected from possible contamination. If the child wears diapers, the dressing can be kept dry by covering it with a piece of plastic film and sealing the edges of the film to the skin with tape. However, the nurse must be careful to continue observing the site for any evidence of bleeding (see Family-Centered Care box).

FAMILY-CENTERED CARE

Care After Cardiac Catheterization

- Remove pressure dressing the day after catheterization. Cover site with an adhesive bandage strip for several days.
- Keep site clean and dry. Avoid tub baths for several days; patient may shower.
- Observe site for redness, swelling, drainage, and bleeding. Monitor for fever. Notify practitioner if these occur.
- Avoid strenuous exercise for several days; patient may attend school.
- Resume regular diet without restrictions.
- Use acetaminophen or ibuprofen for pain.
- Keep follow-up appointments per practitioner's instruction.

Modified from Children's Hospital (Boston) Cardiovascular Program, 1996.

evolve Critical Thinking Exercise—Cardiac Catheterization

Congenital Heart Disease

The incidence of CHD in children is approximately 5 to 8 per 1000 live births (Park, 2003). About 2 or 3 in 1000 infants will be symptomatic during the first year of life with significant heart disease that will require treatment (Hoffman & Kaplan, 2002). CHD is the major cause of death (other than prematurity) in the first year of life. Although there are more than 35 well-recognized cardiac defects, the most common heart anomaly is ventricular septal defect (VSD).

The exact etiology of most congenital cardiac defects is unknown. Most are thought to be a result of multifactorial inheritance: a complex interaction of genetic and environmental factors. The tremendous amount of information being discovered in molecular biology and the Human Genome Project will likely increase our understanding of the genetic causes of congenital heart defects.

Some risk factors are known to increase the incidence of congenital heart defects. Maternal factors include chronic illnesses such as diabetes or poorly controlled phenylketonuria, alcohol consumption, and exposure to environmental toxins and infections. Family history of a cardiac defect in a parent or sibling increases the likelihood of a cardiac anomaly. The risk of CHD increases if a first-degree relative (parent or sibling) is affected. The familial risk is higher with left-sided obstructive lesions.

Congenital heart anomalies are often associated with chromosome abnormalities, syndromes, or congenital defects in other body systems. Down syndrome (trisomy 21) and trisomy 13 and 18 are highly correlated with congenital heart defects.

Circulatory Changes at Birth

During fetal life, blood carrying oxygen and nutritive materials from the placenta enters the fetal system through the umbilicus via the large umbilical vein. Oxygenated blood enters the heart by way of the inferior vena cava. Because of the higher pressure of blood entering the right atrium, it is directed posteriorly in a straight pathway across the right atrium and through the *foramen ovale* to the left atrium. In this way the better-oxygenated blood enters the left atrium and ventricle to be pumped through the aorta to the head and upper extremities. Blood from the head and upper extremities entering the right atrium from the superior vena cava is directed downward through the tricuspid valve into the right ventricle. From here it is pumped through the pulmonary artery, where the major portion is shunted to the descending aorta via the *ductus arteriosus*. Only a small amount flows to and from the nonfunctioning fetal lungs (Fig. 48-1, *A*).

Before birth the high pulmonary vascular resistance created by the collapsed fetal lung causes greater pressures in the right side of the heart and the pulmonary arteries. At the same time, the free-flowing placental circulation and the ductus arteriosus produce a low vascular resistance in the remainder of the fetal vascular system. With the cessation of placental blood flow from clamping of the umbilical cord and the expansion of the lungs at birth, the hemodynamics of the fetal vascular system undergo pronounced and abrupt changes (see Fig. 48-1, *B*).

With the first breath, the lungs are expanded, and increased oxygen causes pulmonary vasodilation. With the removal of the placenta, pulmonary pressures start to fall as systemic pressures start to rise. Normally the foramen ovale closes as the pressure in the left atrium exceeds the pressure in the right atrium. The ductus arteriosus starts to close in the presence of increased oxygen concentration in the blood and other factors.

Altered Hemodynamics

To appreciate the physiology of heart defects, it is necessary to understand the role of pressure gradients, flow, and resistance within the circulation. As with any fluid, blood flows from an area of high pressure to one of lower pressure and toward the path of least resistance in response to the pumping action of the heart. In general, the higher the pressure gradient, the greater the rate of flow; the higher the resistance, the lesser the rate of flow.

Normally the pressure on the right side of the heart is lower than that on the left side, and the resistance in the pulmonary circulation is less than that in the systemic circulation. Vessels entering or exiting these chambers have corresponding pressures. Therefore, if an abnormal connection exists between the heart chambers (such as a septal defect), blood will necessarily flow from an area of higher pressure (left side) to one of lower pressure (right side). Such a flow of blood is termed a *left-to-right shunt.* Anomalies resulting in cyanosis may result from a change in pressure so that the blood is shunted from the right to the left side of the heart *(right-to-left shunt)* because of either increased pulmonary vascular resistance or obstruction to blood flow through the pulmonic valve and artery. Cyanosis may also result from a defect that allows mixing of

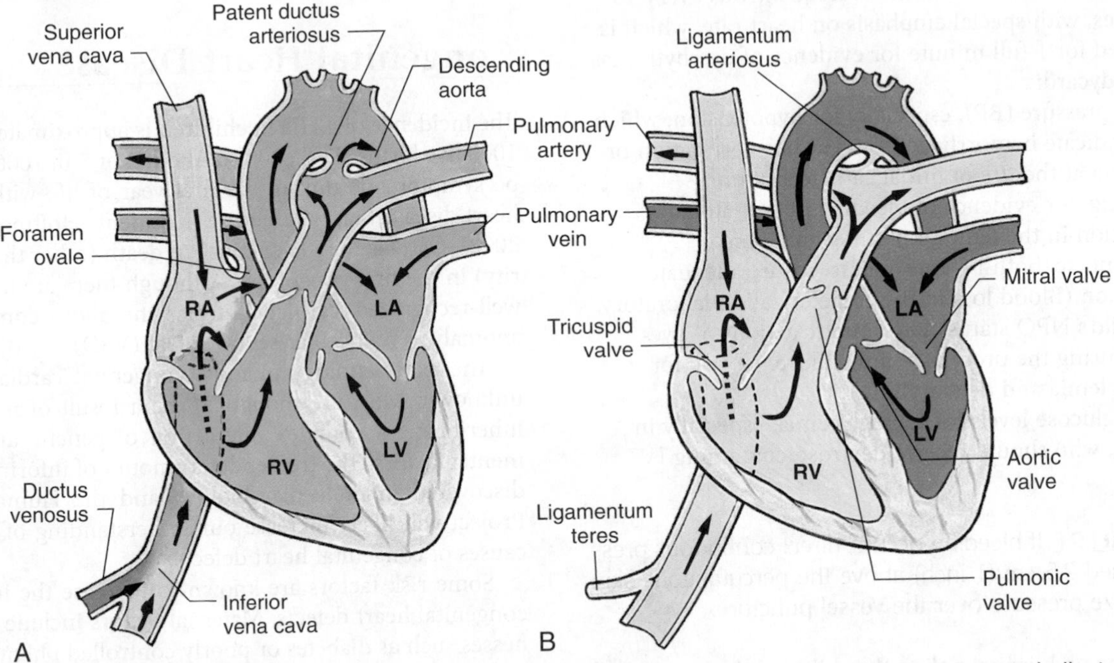

Fig. 48-1 Changes in circulation at birth. **A,** Prenatal circulation. **B,** Postnatal circulation. *Arrows* indicate direction of blood flow. Although four pulmonary veins enter the LA, for simplicity this diagram shows only two. *LA,* Left atrium; *LV,* left ventricle; *RA,* right atrium; *RV,* right ventricle.

oxygenated and deoxygenated blood within the heart chambers or great arteries, such as occurs in truncus arteriosus.

Classification of Defects

Congenital heart defects have been divided into two categories. Traditionally, cyanosis, a physical characteristic, has been used as the distinguishing feature, dividing the anomalies into *acyanotic defects* and *cyanotic defects*. In clinical practice this system is problematic because children with acyanotic defects may develop cyanosis. More often those with cyanotic defects may appear pink and have more clinical signs of CHF.

A more useful classification system is based on hemodynamic characteristics (blood flow patterns within the heart). These blood flow patterns are (1) *increased pulmonary blood flow;* (2) *decreased pulmonary blood flow;* (3) *obstruction to blood flow* out of the heart; and (4) *mixed blood flow*, in which saturated and desaturated blood mix within the heart or great arteries. As a comparison, both classification systems are outlined in Fig. 48-2.

With the hemodynamic classification system, the clinical manifestations of each group are more uniform and predictable. Defects that allow blood flow from the higher-pressure left side of the heart to the lower-pressure right side (left-to-right shunt) result in increased pulmonary blood flow and cause CHF. Obstructive defects impede blood flow out of the ventricles; obstruction on the left side of the heart results in CHF, whereas severe obstruction on the right side causes cyanosis. Defects that cause decreased pulmonary blood flow result in cyanosis. Mixed lesions present a variable clinical picture based on the degree of mixing and amount of pulmonary blood flow; hypoxemia (with or without cyanosis) and CHF usually occur together. Using this classification system, the clinical presentation and management of the most common defects are outlined in the following sections and Box 48-1.

The outcomes of surgical treatment for patients with moderate to severe disease vary. Patient risk factors for increased morbidity and mortality include prematurity or low birth weight, a genetic syndrome, multiple cardiac defects, a noncardiac congenital anomaly, and age at time of surgery (neonates are a higher risk group). For example, aortic stenosis or coarctation manifesting in the first week of life is more severe and carries a higher mortality than if it becomes apparent at 1 year of age. Outcomes for surgical repair of similar congenital heart defects also vary among treatment centers. Most mortality rates are obtained from a large multicenter database maintained by the Society of Thoracic Surgeons (Jacobs et al, 2004) to reflect the more likely outcome of present-day treatments. Individual center results may be better or worse than the Society of Thoracic Surgeons database. In general, the outcomes of surgical procedures have steadily improved in the past decade, with mortality rates for many severe defects below 10%, and the incidence of complications and length of hospital stay have declined.

Defects with Increased Pulmonary Blood Flow

In this group of cardiac defects, intracardiac communications along the septum or an abnormal connection between the great arteries allows blood to flow from the higher-pressure left side of the heart to the lower-pressure right side of the heart (Fig. 48-3). Increased blood volume on the right side of the heart increases pulmonary blood flow at the expense of systemic blood flow. Clinically, patients demonstrate signs and symptoms of CHF. Atrial septal defect (ASD), VSD, and patent ductus arteriosus are typical anomalies in this group (Box 48-1).

Obstructive Defects

Obstructive defects are those in which blood exiting the heart meets an area of anatomic narrowing *(stenosis)*, causing obstruction to blood flow. The pressure in the ventricle and great artery before the obstruction is increased, and the

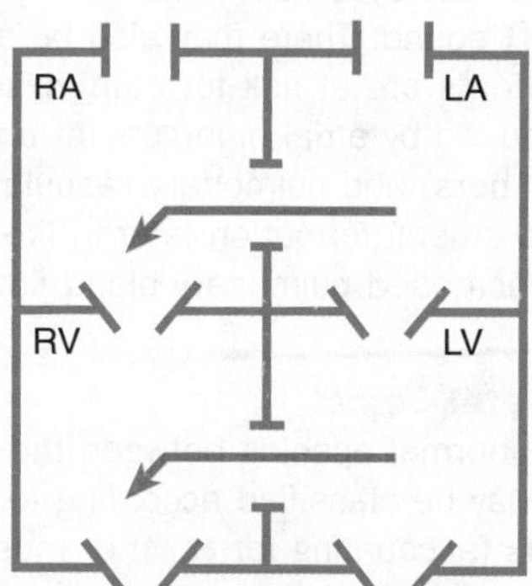

Fig. 48-3 Hemodynamics in defects with increased pulmonary blood flow. See Fig. 48-1 for abbreviations.

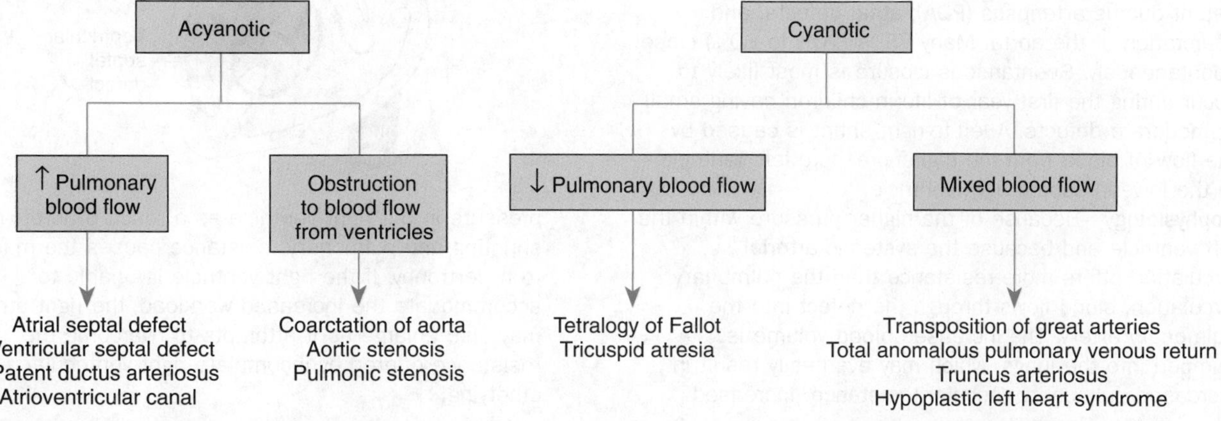

Fig. 48-2 Comparison of acyanotic-cyanotic and hemodynamic classification systems of congenital heart disease.

BOX 48-1 Defects with Increased Pulmonary Blood Flow

Atrial Septal Defect

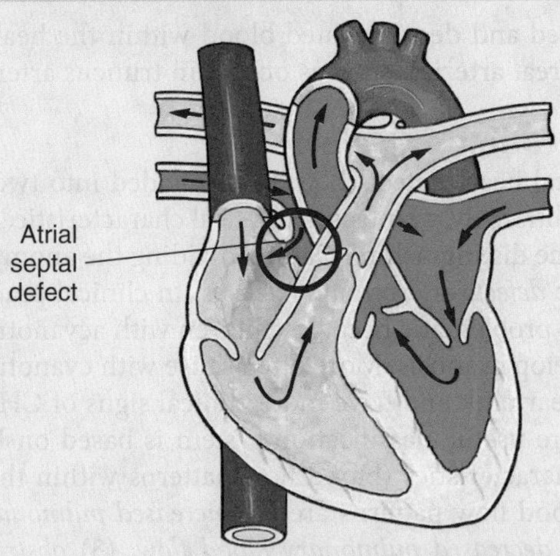

Description—Abnormal opening between the atria, allowing blood from the higher-pressure left atrium to flow into the lower-pressure right atrium. There are three types of atrial septal defects (ASDs):

Ostium primum (ASD 1)—Opening at lower end of septum; may be associated with mitral valve abnormalities

Ostium secundum (ASD 2)—Opening near center of septum

Sinus venosus defect—Opening near junction of superior vena cava and right atrium; may be associated with partial anomalous pulmonary venous connection

Pathophysiology—Because left atrial pressure slightly exceeds right atrial pressure, blood flows from the left to the right atrium, causing an increased flow of oxygenated blood into the right side of the heart. Despite the low pressure difference, a high rate of flow can still occur because of low pulmonary vascular resistance and the greater distensibility of the right atrium, which further reduces flow resistance. This volume is well tolerated by the right ventricle because it is delivered under much lower pressure than with a ventricular septal defect (VSD). Although there is right atrial and ventricular enlargement, cardiac failure is unusual in an uncomplicated ASD. Pulmonary vascular changes usually occur only after several decades if the defect is left unrepaired.

Clinical manifestations—Patients may be asymptomatic. They may develop congestive heart failure (CHF). There is a characteristic systolic murmur with a fixed split second heart sound. There may also be a diastolic murmur. Patients are at risk for atrial dysrhythmias (probably caused by atrial enlargement and stretching of conduction fibers) and pulmonary vascular obstructive disease and emboli formation later in life from chronically increased pulmonary blood flow.

Surgical treatment—Surgical patch closure (pericardial patch or Dacron patch) is done for moderate to large defects. Open repair with cardiopulmonary bypass is usually performed before school age. In addition, the sinus venosus defect requires patch placement, so the anomalous right pulmonary venous return is directed to the left atrium with a baffle. The ASD 1 type may require mitral valve repair or, rarely, replacement of the mitral valve.

Nonsurgical treatment—ASD 2 closure with a device during cardiac catheterization is becoming commonplace and can be done as an outpatient procedure. The Amplatzer Septal Occluder is most commonly used. Smaller defects that have a rim around them for attachment of the device can be closed with a device; large, irregular defects without a rim require surgical closure. Successful closure in appropriately selected patients yields results similar to those from surgery but involves shorter hospital stays and fewer complications. Patients receive low-dose aspirin for 6 months (Rome & Kreutzer, 2004).

Prognosis—Operative mortality is very low (less than 1%).

Ventricular Septal Defect

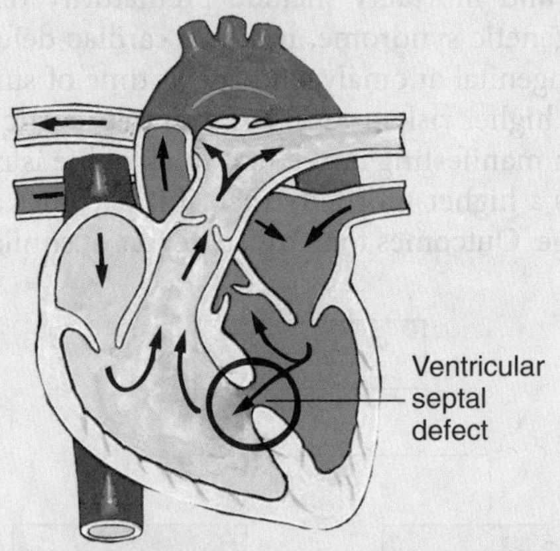

Description—Abnormal opening between the right and left ventricles. May be classified according to location: membranous (accounting for 80%) or muscular. May vary in size from a small pinhole to absence of the septum, which results in a common ventricle. VSDs are frequently associated with other defects, such as pulmonary stenosis, transposition of the great vessels, patent ductus arteriosus (PDA), atrial defects, and coarctation of the aorta. Many VSDs (20% to 60%) close spontaneously. Spontaneous closure is most likely to occur during the first year of life in children having small or moderate defects. A left-to-right shunt is caused by the flow of blood from the higher-pressure left ventricle to the lower-pressure right ventricle.

Pathophysiology—Because of the higher pressure within the left ventricle and because the systemic arterial circulation offers more resistance than the pulmonary circulation, blood flows through the defect into the pulmonary artery. The increased blood volume is pumped into the lungs, which may eventually result in increased pulmonary vascular resistance. Increased pressure in the right ventricle as a result of left-to-right shunting and pulmonary resistance causes the muscle to hypertrophy. If the right ventricle is unable to accommodate the increased workload, the right atrium may also enlarge as it attempts to overcome the resistance offered by incomplete right ventricular emptying.

Ventricular Septal Defect—cont'd

Clinical manifestations—CHF is common. A characteristic loud holosystolic murmur is heard best at the left sternal border. Patients are at risk for bacterial endocarditis and pulmonary vascular obstructive disease.

Surgical Treatment

Palliative—Pulmonary artery banding (placement of a band around the main pulmonary artery to decrease pulmonary blood flow) may be done in infants with multiple muscular VSDs or complex anatomy. Improvements in surgical techniques and postoperative care make complete repair in infancy the preferred approach.

Complete repair (procedure of choice)—Small defects are repaired with sutures. Large defects usually require that a knitted Dacron patch be sewn over the opening. Cardiopulmonary bypass is used for both procedures. The approach for the repair is generally through the right atrium and the tricuspid valve. Postoperative complications include residual VSD and conduction disturbances.

Nonsurgical treatment—Device closure during cardiac catheterization is being performed in some centers under investigational protocols. One device has been approved for closure of muscular defects. Early results are encouraging, with successful defect closure and few complications (Rome & Kreutzer, 2004).

Prognosis—Risks depend on the location of the defect, the number of defects, and the presence of other associated cardiac defects. Single membranous defects are associated with low mortality (less than 2%); multiple muscular defects can carry a higher risk (Jacobs et al, 2004).

Atrioventricular Canal Defect

Description—Incomplete fusion of the endocardial cushions. Consists of a low ASD that is continuous with a high VSD and clefts of the mitral and tricuspid valves, which create a large central atrioventricular (AV) valve that allows blood to flow between all four chambers of the heart. The directions and pathways of flow are determined by pulmonary and systemic resistance, left and right ventricular pressures, and the compliance of each chamber, although flow is generally from left to right. It is the most common cardiac defect in children with Down syndrome.

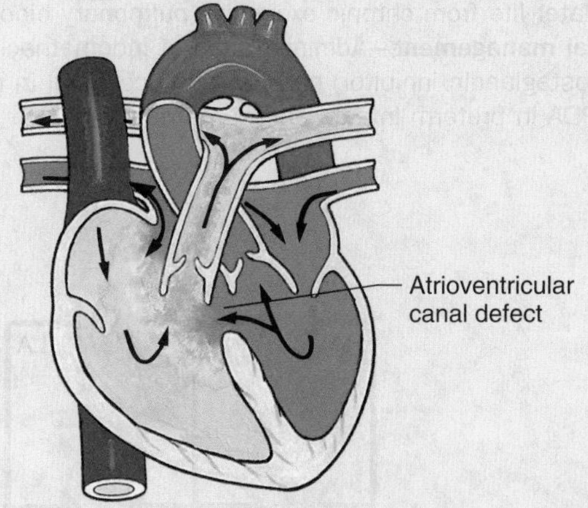

Pathophysiology—The alterations in hemodynamics depend on the severity of the defect and the child's pulmonary vascular resistance. Immediately after birth, while the newborn's pulmonary vascular resistance is high, there is minimum shunting of blood through the defect. Once this resistance falls, left-to-right shunting occurs, and pulmonary blood flow increases. The resultant pulmonary vascular engorgement predisposes the child to development of CHF.

Clinical manifestations—Patients usually have moderate to severe CHF. There is a loud systolic murmur. There may be mild cyanosis that increases with crying. Patients are at high risk for developing pulmonary vascular obstructive disease.

Surgical treatment

Palliative—Pulmonary artery banding is occasionally done in small infants with severe symptoms. Complete repair in infancy is most common.

Complete repair—Surgical repair consists of patch closure of the septal defects and reconstruction of the AV valve tissue (either repair of the mitral valve cleft or fashioning of two AV valves). Postoperative complications include heart block, CHF, mitral regurgitation, dysrhythmias, and pulmonary hypertension.

Prognosis—Operative mortality is less than 5% (Jacobs et al, 2004). A potential later problem is mitral regurgitation, which may require valve replacement.

Patent Ductus Arteriosus

Description—Failure of the fetal ductus arteriosus (artery connecting the aorta and pulmonary artery) to close within the first weeks of life. The continued patency of this vessel allows blood to flow from the higher-pressure aorta to the lower-pressure pulmonary artery, which causes a left-to-right shunt.

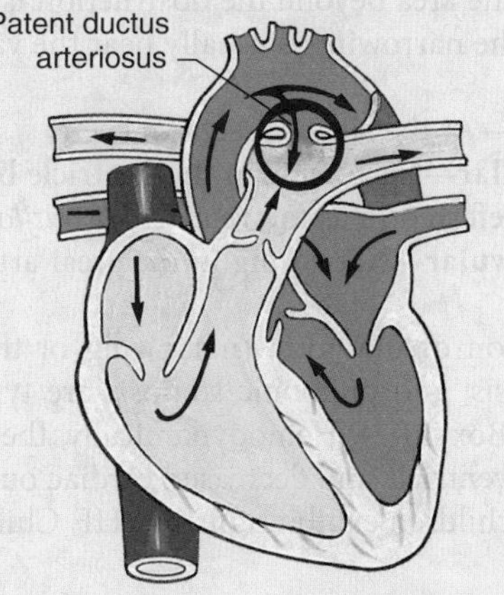

Pathophysiology—The hemodynamic consequences of PDA depend on the size of the ductus and the pulmonary vascular resistance. At birth the resistance in the pulmonary and systemic circulations is almost identical so that the resistance in the aorta and pulmonary artery is equalized. As the systemic pressure comes to exceed the pulmonary pressure,

evolve Case Study—Patent Ductus Arteriosus

Continued

BOX 48-1 Defects with Increased Pulmonary Blood Flow—cont'd

Patent Ductus Arteriosus—cont'd

blood begins to shunt from the aorta across the duct to the pulmonary artery (left-to-right shunt). The additional blood is recirculated through the lungs and returned to the left atrium and left ventricle. The effect of this altered circulation is increased workload on the left side of the heart, increased pulmonary vascular congestion and possibly resistance, and potentially increased right ventricular pressure and hypertrophy.

Clinical manifestations—Patients may be asymptomatic or show signs of CHF. There is a characteristic machinery-like murmur. A widened pulse pressure and bounding pulses result from runoff of blood from the aorta to the pulmonary artery. Patients are at risk for bacterial endocarditis and pulmonary vascular obstructive disease in later life from chronic excessive pulmonary blood flow.

Medical management—Administration of indomethacin (prostaglandin inhibitor) has proved successful in closing a PDA in preterm infants and some newborns.

Surgical treatment—Surgical division or ligation of the patent vessel is performed via a left thoracotomy. In a newer technique, video-assisted thoracoscopic surgery, a thoracoscope and instruments are inserted through three small incisions on the left side of the chest to place a clip on the ductus. The technique is used in some centers and eliminates the need for a thoracotomy, thereby speeding postoperative recovery.

Nonsurgical treatment—Coils to occlude the PDA are placed in the catheterization laboratory in many centers. Preterm or small infants (with small-diameter femoral arteries) and patients with large or unusual PDAs may require surgery.

Prognosis—Both surgical and nonsurgical procedures can be done at low risk with less than 1% mortality. PDA closure in very preterm infants has a higher mortality rate because of the additional significant medical problems.

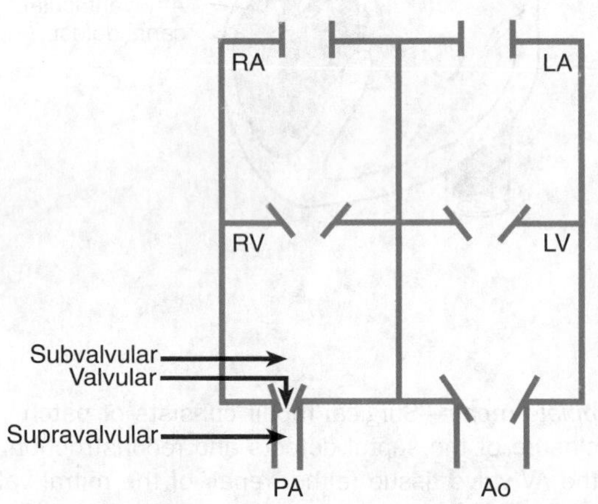

Fig. 48-4 Obstruction to ventricular ejection can occur at the valvular level (shown), below the valve (subvalvular), or above the valve (supravalvular). Pulmonary stenosis is shown here. *Ao*, Aorta; *PA*, pulmonary artery. See Fig. 48-1 for additional abbreviations.

pressure in the area beyond the obstruction is decreased. The location of the narrowing is usually near the valve (Fig. 48-4), as follows:

Valvular—At the site of the valve itself

Subvalvular—Narrowing in the ventricle below the valve (also referred to as the *ventricular outflow tract*)

Supravalvular—Narrowing in the great artery above the valve

Coarctation of the aorta (narrowing of the aortic arch), aortic stenosis, and pulmonic stenosis are typical defects in this group (Box 48-2). Hemodynamically, there is a pressure load on the ventricle and decreased cardiac output. Clinically, infants and children exhibit signs of CHF. Children with mild obstruction may be asymptomatic. Rarely, as in severe pulmonic stenosis, hypoxemia may be seen.

Defects with Decreased Pulmonary Blood Flow

In this group of defects, there is obstruction of pulmonary blood flow and an anatomic defect (ASD or VSD) between the right and left sides of the heart (Fig. 48-5). Because blood has difficulty exiting the right side of the heart via the pulmonary artery, pressure on the right side increases, exceeding left-sided pressure. This allows desaturated blood to shunt right to left, causing desaturation in the left side of the heart and in the systemic circulation. Clinically, these patients are hypoxemic and usually appear cyanotic. Tetralogy of Fallot and tricuspid atresia are the most common defects in this group (Box 48-3).

Mixed Defects

Many complex cardiac anomalies are classified together in the mixed category (Box 48-4) because survival in the postnatal period depends on mixing of blood from the pulmonary and systemic circulations within the heart chambers. Hemodynamically, fully saturated systemic blood flow mixes with the desaturated pulmonary blood flow, causing a relative desaturation of the systemic blood flow. Pulmonary congestion occurs because the differences in pulmonary artery pressure and aortic pressure favor pulmonary blood flow. Cardiac output decreases because of a volume load on the ventricle. Clinically, these patients have a variable picture that combines some degree of desaturation (although cyanosis is not always visible) and signs of CHF. Some defects, such as transposition of the great arteries, cause severe cyanosis in the first days of life and later cause CHF. Others, such as truncus arteriosus, cause severe CHF in the first weeks of life and mild desaturation.

BOX 48-2 Obstructive Defects

Coarctation of the Aorta

Description—Localized narrowing near the insertion of the ductus arteriosus, which results in increased pressure proximal to the defect (head and upper extremities) and decreased pressure distal to the obstruction (body and lower extremities).

Pathophysiology—The effect of a narrowing within the aorta is increased pressure proximal to the defect (upper extremities) and decreased pressure distal to it (lower extremities).

Clinical manifestations—The patient may have high blood pressure and bounding pulses in the arms, weak or absent femoral pulses, and cool lower extremities with lower blood pressure. There are signs of congestive heart failure (CHF) in infants. In infants with critical coarctation, the hemodynamic condition may deteriorate rapidly with severe acidosis and hypotension. Mechanical ventilation and inotropic support are often necessary before surgery. Older children may experience dizziness, headaches, fainting, and epistaxis resulting from hypertension. Patients are at risk for hypertension, ruptured aorta, aortic aneurysm, and stroke.

Surgical treatment—Surgical repair is the treatment of choice for infants younger than 6 months of age and for patients with long-segment stenosis or complex anatomy; it may be performed for all patients with coarctation. Repair is by resection of the coarctated portion with an end-to-end anastomosis of the aorta or enlargement of the constricted section using a graft of prosthetic material or a portion of the left subclavian artery. Because this defect is outside the heart and pericardium, cardiopulmonary bypass is not required, and a thoracotomy incision is used. Postoperative hypertension is treated with intravenous sodium nitroprusside, esmolol, or milrinone followed by oral medications, such as angiotensin-converting enzyme inhibitors or β-blockers. Residual permanent

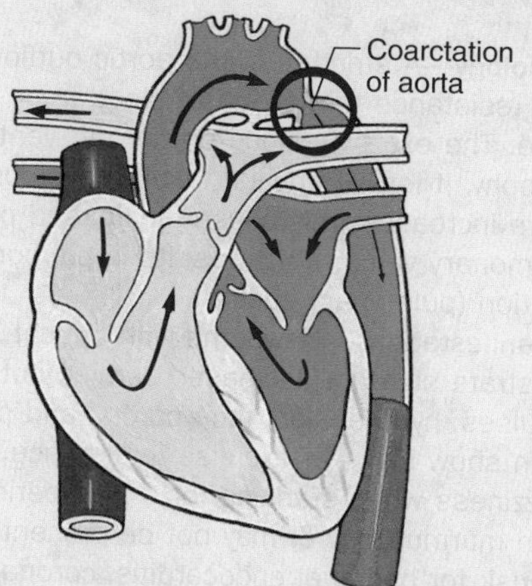

hypertension after repair of coarctation of the aorta (COA) seems to be related to age and time of repair. To prevent both hypertension at rest and exercise-provoked systemic hypertension after repair, elective surgery for COA is advised within the first 2 years of life. There is a 15% to 30% risk of recurrence in patients who underwent surgical repair as infants (Beekman, 2001). Percutaneous balloon angioplasty techniques have proved to be effective in relieving residual postoperative coarctation gradients.

Nonsurgical treatment—Balloon angioplasty is being performed as a primary intervention for COA in older infants and children. In adolescents, stents may be placed in the aorta to maintain patency. Recent studies have demonstrated that balloon angioplasty is effective in children and aneurysm formation is rare. The high restenosis rate in young infants limits its application in this group (Rome & Kreutzer, 2004).

Prognosis—Mortality is less than 5% in patients with isolated coarctation; risk is increased in infants with other complex cardiac defects (Jacobs et al, 2004).

Aortic Stenosis

Description—Narrowing or stricture of the aortic valve, causing resistance to blood flow in the left ventricle, decreased cardiac output, left ventricular hypertrophy, and pulmonary vascular congestion. The prominent anatomic consequence of aortic stenosis (AS) is the hypertrophy of the left ventricular wall, which eventually leads to increased end-diastolic pressure resulting in pulmonary venous and pulmonary arterial hypertension. Left ventricular hypertrophy also interferes with coronary artery perfusion and may result in myocardial infarction or scarring of the papillary muscles of the left ventricle, which causes mitral insufficiency. Valvular stenosis, the most common type, is usually caused by malformed cusps that result in a bicuspid rather than tricuspid valve or fusion of the cusps. Subvalvular stenosis is a stricture caused by a fibrous ring below a normal valve; supravalvular stenosis occurs infrequently. Valvular AS is a serious defect for the following reasons: (1) the obstruction tends to be progressive; (2) sudden

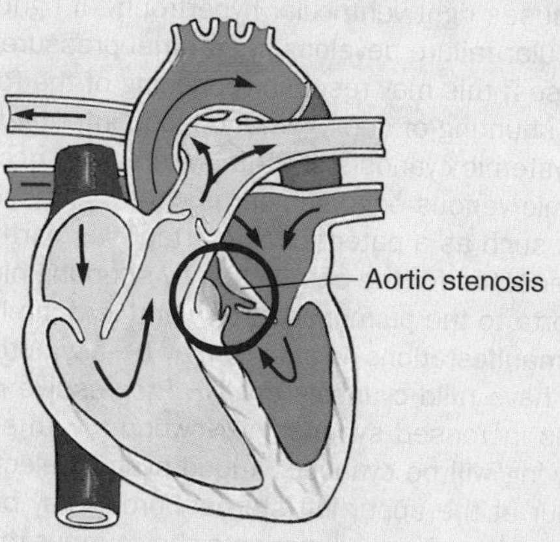

episodes of myocardial ischemia, or low cardiac output, can result in sudden death; and (3) surgical repair rarely results in a normal valve. This is one of the rare instances in which strenuous physical activity may be curtailed because of the cardiac condition.

Continued

BOX 48-2 Obstructive Defects—cont'd

Aortic Stenosis—cont'd

Pathophysiology—A stricture in the aortic outflow tract causes resistance to ejection of blood from the left ventricle. The extra workload on the left ventricle causes hypertrophy. If left ventricular failure develops, left atrial pressure increases; this causes increased pressure in the pulmonary veins, which results in pulmonary vascular congestion (pulmonary edema).

Clinical manifestations—Newborns with critical AS demonstrate signs of decreased cardiac output with faint pulses, hypotension, tachycardia, and poor feeding. Children show signs of exercise intolerance, chest pain, and dizziness when standing for a long period. A systolic ejection murmur may or may not be present. Patients are at risk for bacterial endocarditis, coronary insufficiency, and ventricular dysfunction.

Valvular Aortic Stenosis

Surgical treatment—Aortic valvotomy is performed under inflow occlusion. It is rarely used because balloon dilation in the catheterization laboratory is the first-line procedure. Newborns with critical AS and small left-sided structures may undergo a stage 1 Norwood procedure (see Hypoplastic Left Heart Syndrome, Box 48-4).

Prognosis—Aortic valve replacement offers a good treatment option and may lead to normalization of left ventricular size and function (Arnold et al, 2008). Results of aortic valvotomy in older children are very good, with mortality and morbidity close to 0% (Shanmugam, MacArthur, & Pollock, 2005). However, aortic valvotomy remains a palliative procedure, and approximately 25% of patients require additional surgery within 10 years for recurrent stenosis. A valve replacement may be required at the second procedure. An aortic homograft with a valve may also be used (extended aortic root replacement), or the pulmonary valve may be moved to the aortic position and replaced with a homograft valve (Ross procedure).

Nonsurgical treatment—The narrowed valve is dilated using balloon angioplasty in the catheterization laboratory. This procedure is usually the first intervention.

Prognosis—Complications include aortic insufficiency or valvular regurgitation, tearing of the valve leaflets, and loss of pulse in the catheterized limb.

Subvalvular Aortic Stenosis

Surgical treatment—Procedure may involve incising a membrane if one exists or cutting the fibromuscular ring. If the obstruction results from narrowing of the left ventricular outflow tract and a small aortic valve annulus, a patch may be required to enlarge the entire left ventricular outflow tract and annulus and replace the aortic valve; this is known as the Konno procedure.

Prognosis—Mortality from surgical repairs of subvalvular AS is less than 5% in major centers; however, about 20% of these patients develop recurrent subaortic stenosis and require additional surgery (Freed, 2001).

Pulmonic Stenosis

Description—Narrowing at the entrance to the pulmonary artery. Resistance to blood flow causes right ventricular hypertrophy and decreased pulmonary blood flow. Pulmonary atresia is the extreme form of pulmonic stenosis (PS) in that there is total fusion of the commissures and no blood flows to the lungs. The right ventricle may be hypoplastic.

Pathophysiology—When PS is present, resistance to blood flow causes right ventricular hypertrophy. If right ventricular failure develops, right atrial pressure increases; this may result in reopening of the foramen ovale, shunting of unoxygenated blood into the left atrium, and systemic cyanosis. If PS is severe, CHF occurs, and systemic venous engorgement is noted. An associated defect such as a patent ductus arteriosus partially compensates for the obstruction by shunting blood from the aorta to the pulmonary artery and into the lungs.

Clinical manifestations—Patients may be asymptomatic; some have mild cyanosis or CHF. Progressive narrowing causes increased symptoms. Newborns with severe narrowing will be cyanotic. A loud systolic ejection murmur at the upper left sternal border may be present. However, in severely ill patients the murmur may be much softer due to decreased cardiac output and shunting of blood. Cardiomegaly is evident on chest radiographic films. Patients are at risk for bacterial endocarditis.

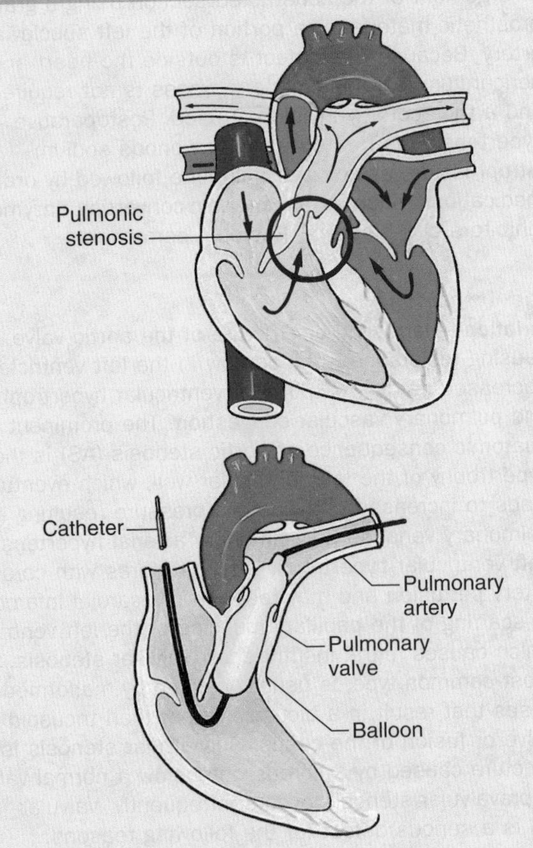

BOX 48-2 Obstructive Defects—cont'd

Pulmonic Stenosis—cont'd

Surgical treatment—In infants, transventricular (closed) valvotomy (Brock procedure). In children, pulmonary valvotomy with cardiopulmonary bypass. Need for surgical treatment is rare with widespread use of balloon angioplasty techniques.

Nonsurgical treatment—Balloon angioplasty in the cardiac catheterization laboratory to dilate the valve. A catheter is inserted across the stenotic pulmonic valve into the pulmonary artery, and a balloon at the end of the catheter is inflated and rapidly passed through the narrowed opening (see figure on p. 1452). The procedure is associated with few complications and has proved to be highly effective. It is the treatment of choice for discrete PS in most centers and can be done safely in neonates.

Prognosis—Risk is low for both surgical and nonsurgical procedures; mortality is lower than 1%, slightly higher in neonates (Latson, 2001). Both balloon dilation and surgical valvotomy leave the pulmonic valve incompetent because they involve opening the fused valve leaflets; however, these patients are clinically asymptomatic. Long-term problems with restenosis or valve incompetence may occur.

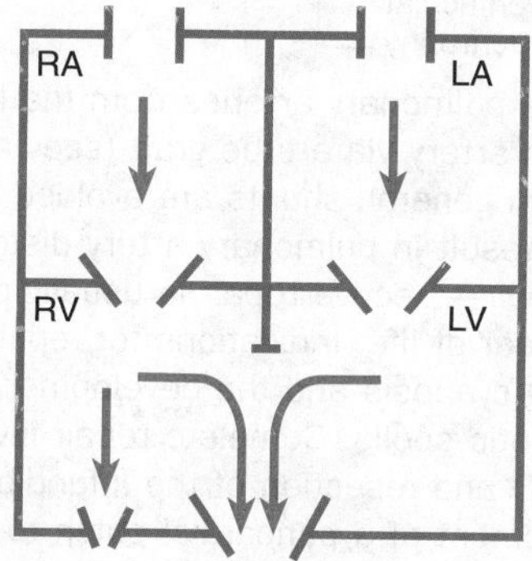

Fig. 48-5 Hemodynamic defects with decreased pulmonary blood flow. See Fig. 48-1 for abbreviations.

Clinical Consequences of Congenital Heart Disease

Congestive Heart Failure

CHF is the inability of the heart to pump an adequate amount of blood to the systemic circulation at normal filling pressures to meet the body's metabolic demands. In children, CHF most frequently occurs secondary to structural abnormalities (e.g., septal defects) that result in increased blood volume and pressure within the heart. It can also result from myocardial failure in which the contractility of the ventricle is impaired. This can occur with cardiomyopathy, dysrhythmias, or severe electrolyte disturbances. CHF can also occur because of excessive demands on a normal heart muscle, such as sepsis or severe anemia.

Pathophysiology

Heart failure is often separated into two categories: right-sided and left-sided failure. In *right-sided failure* the right ventricle is unable to pump blood effectively into the pulmonary artery, resulting in increased pressure in the right atrium and systemic venous circulation. Systemic venous hypertension causes hepatosplenomegaly and occasionally edema. In *left-sided failure* the left ventricle is unable to pump blood into the systemic circulation, resulting in increased pressure in the left atrium and pulmonary veins. The lungs become congested with blood, causing elevated pulmonary pressures and pulmonary edema.

Although each type of heart failure produces different signs and symptoms, clinically it is unusual to observe solely right- or left-sided failure in children. Because each side of the heart depends on adequate function of the other side, failure of one chamber causes a reciprocal change in the opposite chamber.

If the abnormalities precipitating CHF are not corrected, the heart muscle becomes damaged. Despite compensatory mechanisms, the heart is unable to maintain an adequate cardiac output. Decreased blood flow to the kidneys continues to stimulate sodium and water reabsorption, leading to fluid overload, increased workload on the heart, and congestion in the pulmonary and systemic circulations (Fig. 48-6).

The signs and symptoms of CHF can be divided into three groups: (1) impaired myocardial function, (2) pulmonary congestion, and (3) systemic venous congestion (Box 48-5). Because these hemodynamic changes occur from different causes and at differing times, the clinical presentation may vary among children.

Diagnostic Evaluation

Diagnosis is made on the basis of clinical symptoms such as tachypnea and tachycardia at rest, dyspnea, retractions, activity intolerance (especially during feeding in infants), weight gain caused by fluid retention, and hepatomegaly. A chest x-ray film demonstrates cardiomegaly and increased pulmonary blood flow. Ventricular hypertrophy appears on the ECG. An echocardiogram is done to determine the cause of CHF such as a congenital heart defect or poor ventricular function.

Therapeutic Management

The goals of treatment are to (1) improve cardiac function (increase contractility and decrease afterload), (2) remove accumulated fluid and sodium (decrease preload), (3) decrease cardiac demands, and (4) improve tissue oxygenation and decrease oxygen consumption. For most infants diagnosed with CHF, the cause is CHD. Infants are stabilized on medical therapy and then referred for surgical repair. For children newly diagnosed with CHF, the cause may be worsening ventricular function after a previous cardiac repair, cardiomyopathy, dysrhythmia, or other causes. In addition to

Text continued on p. 1459

BOX 48-3 Defects with Decreased Pulmonary Blood Flow

Tetralogy of Fallot

Description—The classic form includes four defects: (1) ventricular septal defect (VSD), (2) pulmonic stenosis (PS), (3) overriding aorta, and (4) right ventricular hypertrophy.

Pathophysiology—The alteration in hemodynamics varies widely, depending primarily on the degree of PS and also on the size of the VSD and the pulmonary and systemic resistance to flow. Because the VSD is usually large, pressures may be equal in the right and left ventricles. Therefore the shunt direction depends on the difference between pulmonary and systemic vascular resistance. If pulmonary vascular resistance is higher than systemic resistance, the shunt is from right to left. If systemic resistance is higher than pulmonary resistance, the shunt is from left to right. PS decreases blood flow to the lungs and consequently the amount of oxygenated blood that returns to the left side of the heart. Depending on the position of the aorta, blood from both ventricles may be distributed systemically.

Clinical manifestations—Some infants may be acutely cyanotic at birth; others have mild cyanosis that progresses over the first year of life as the PS worsens. There is a characteristic systolic murmur that is often moderate in intensity. There may be acute episodes of cyanosis and hypoxia, called *blue spells* or *tet spells* (see p. 1464). Anoxic spells occur when the infant's oxygen requirements exceed the blood supply, usually during crying or after feeding. Patients are at risk for emboli, seizures, and loss of consciousness or sudden death following an anoxic spell.

Surgical treatment

Palliative shunt—In infants who cannot undergo primary repair, a palliative procedure to increase pulmonary blood flow and increase oxygen saturation may be performed. The preferred procedure is a modified Blalock-Taussig shunt operation, which provides blood flow to the pulmonary arteries from the left or right subclavian artery via a tube graft (see Table 48-4). However, in general, shunts are avoided because they may result in pulmonary artery distortion.

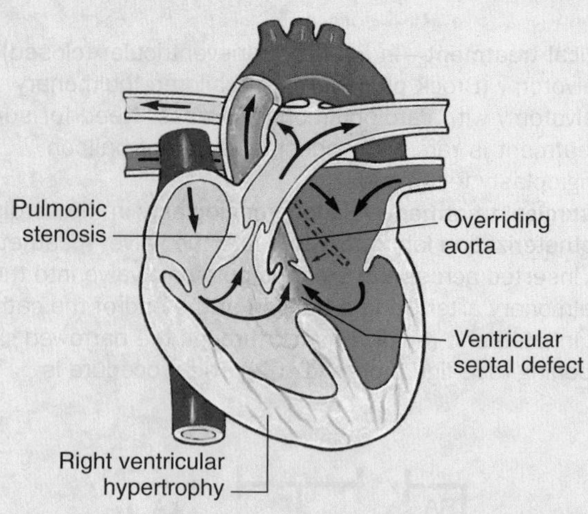

Complete repair—Elective repair is usually performed in the first year of life. Indications for repair include increasing cyanosis and the development of hypercyanotic spells. Complete repair involves closure of the VSD and resection of the infundibular stenosis, with placement of a pericardial patch to enlarge the right ventricular outflow tract. In some repairs the patch may extend across the pulmonary valve annulus (transannular patch), making the pulmonary valve incompetent. The procedure requires a median sternotomy and the use of cardiopulmonary bypass.

Prognosis—The operative mortality for total correction of tetralogy of Fallot is less than 3% (Jacobs et al, 2004). With improved surgical techniques there is a lower incidence of dysrhythmias and sudden death; surgical heart block is rare. Congestive heart failure may occur postoperatively.

Tricuspid Atresia

Description—The tricuspid valve fails to develop; consequently there is no communication from the right atrium to the right ventricle. Blood flows through an atrial septal defect (ASD) or a patent foramen ovale to the left side of the heart and through a VSD to the right ventricle and out to the lungs. The condition is often associated with PS and transposition of the great arteries. There is complete mixing of unoxygenated and oxygenated blood in the left side of the heart, which results in systemic desaturation, and varying amounts of pulmonary obstruction, which causes decreased pulmonary blood flow.

Pathophysiology—At birth the presence of a patent foramen ovale (or other atrial septal opening) is required to permit blood flow across the septum into the left atrium; the patent ductus arteriosus allows blood flow to the pulmonary artery into the lungs for oxygenation. A VSD allows a modest amount of blood to enter the right ventricle and pulmonary artery for oxygenation. Pulmonary blood flow usually is diminished.

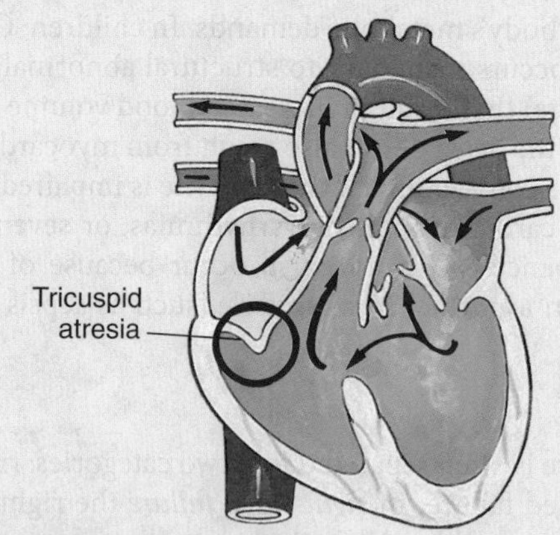

Clinical manifestations—Cyanosis is usually seen in the newborn period. There may be tachycardia and dyspnea. Older children have signs of chronic hypoxemia with clubbing.

Therapeutic management—For the neonate whose pulmonary blood flow depends on the patency of the

BOX 48-3 Defects with Decreased Pulmonary Blood Flow—cont'd

Tricuspid Atresia—cont'd

ductus arteriosus, a continuous infusion of prostaglandin E_1 is started at 0.1 mg/kg/min until surgical intervention can be arranged.

Surgical treatment—Palliative treatment is the placement of a shunt (pulmonary–to–systemic artery anastomosis) to increase blood flow to the lungs. If the ASD is small, an atrial septostomy is performed during cardiac catheterization. Some children have increased pulmonary blood flow and require pulmonary artery banding to lessen the volume of blood to the lungs. A bidirectional Glenn shunt (cavopulmonary anastomosis) may be performed at 4 to 9 months as a second stage.

Modified Fontan procedure—Systemic venous return is directed to the lungs without a ventricular pump through surgical connections between the right atrium and the pulmonary artery. A fenestration (opening) is sometimes made in the right atrial baffle to relieve pressure. The patient must have normal ventricular function and a low pulmonary vascular resistance for the procedure to be successful. The modified Fontan procedure separates oxygenated and unoxygenated blood inside the heart and eliminates the excess volume load on the ventricle but does not restore normal anatomy or hemodynamics. This operation is also the final stage in the correction of many complex defects with a functional single ventricle, including hypoplastic left heart syndrome.

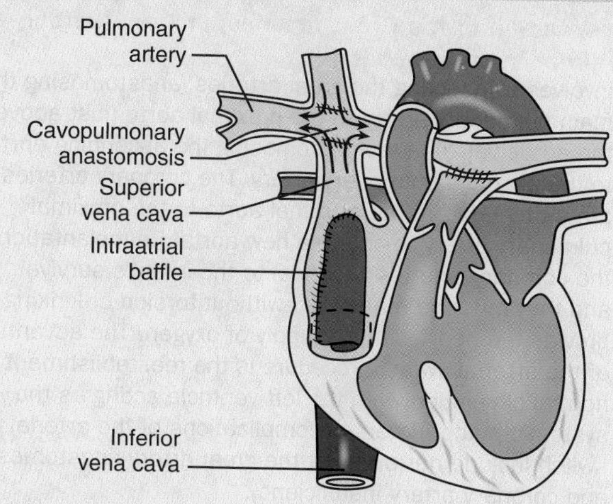

Prognosis—Surgical mortality is less than 5% (Jacobs et al, 2004); the rate increases when the anatomy is more complex and other risk factors are present. Postoperative complications include dysrhythmias, systemic venous hypertension, pleural and pericardial effusions, and ventricular dysfunction. Long-term concerns are the development of protein-losing enteropathy, atrial dysrhythmias, late ventricular dysfunction, and developmental delays.

BOX 48-4 Mixed Defects

Transposition of the Great Arteries, or Transposition of the Great Vessels

Description—The pulmonary artery leaves the left ventricle, and the aorta exits from the right ventricle, with no communication between the systemic and pulmonary circulations.

Pathophysiology—Associated defects such as septal defects or patent ductus arteriosus must be present to permit blood to enter the systemic circulation or the pulmonary circulation for mixing of saturated and desaturated blood. The most common defect associated with transposition of the great arteries (TGA) is a patent foramen ovale. At birth there is also a patent ductus arteriosus, although in most instances this closes after the neonatal period. Another associated defect may be a ventricular septal defect (VSD). The presence of a VSD increases the risk of congestive heart failure (CHF) because it permits blood to flow from the right to the left ventricle, into the pulmonary artery, and finally to the lungs. However, it also produces high pulmonary blood flow under high pressure, which can result in high pulmonary vascular resistance.

Clinical manifestations—Depend on the type and size of the associated defects. Newborns with minimum communication are severely cyanotic and have depressed function at birth. Those with large septal defects or a patent ductus arteriosus may be less cyanotic but have symptoms of CHF. Heart sounds vary according to the type of defect present. Cardiomegaly is usually evident a few weeks after birth.

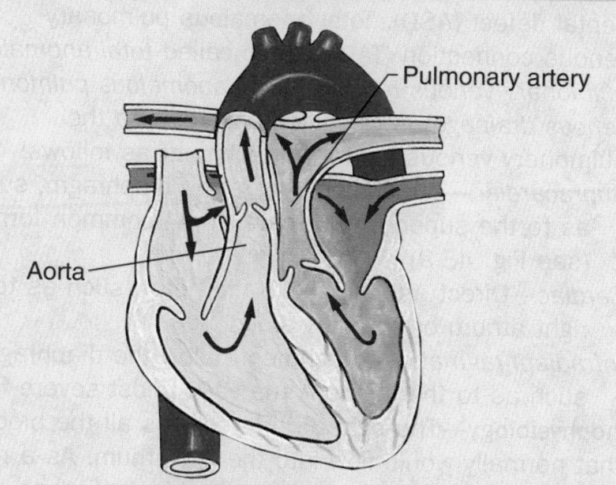

Therapeutic management (to provide intracardiac mixing)—The administration of intravenous prostaglandin E_1 may be initiated to keep the ductus arteriosus open to temporarily increase blood mixing and provide an oxygen saturation of 75% or to maintain cardiac output. During cardiac catheterization or under echocardiographic guidance, a balloon atrial septostomy (Rashkind procedure) may also be performed to increase mixing by opening the atrial septum.

Surgical treatment: An arterial switch procedure is the procedure of choice performed in the first weeks of life. It

Continued

Transposition of the Great Arteries, or Transposition of the Great Vessels—cont'd

involves transecting the great arteries, anastomosing the main pulmonary artery to the proximal aorta (just above the aortic valve), and anastomosing the ascending aorta to the proximal pulmonary artery. The coronary arteries are switched from the proximal aorta to the proximal pulmonary artery to create a new aorta. Reimplantation of the coronary arteries is critical to the infant's survival, and they must be reattached without torsion or kinking to provide the heart with its supply of oxygen. The advantage of the arterial switch procedure is the reestablishment of normal circulation, with the left ventricle acting as the systemic pump. Potential complications of the arterial switch include narrowing at the great artery anastomoses and coronary artery insufficiency.

Intraatrial baffle repairs—Intraatrial baffle repairs are rarely performed, although many adolescents and adults survive today with repairs that were done more than 15 years ago. An intraatrial baffle is created to divert venous blood to the mitral valve and pulmonary venous blood to the tricuspid valve using the patient's atrial septum (Senning procedure) or a prosthetic material (Mustard procedure). A disadvantage is the continuing role of the right ventricle as the systemic pump and the late development of right ventricular failure and rhythm disturbances. Other potential postoperative complications include loss of normal sinus rhythm, baffle leaks, and ventricular dysfunction.

Rastelli procedure—This procedure is the operative choice in infants with TGA, VSD, and severe pulmonic stenosis (PS). It involves closure of the VSD with a baffle, so left ventricular blood is directed through the VSD into the aorta. The pulmonic valve is then closed, and a conduit is placed from the right ventricle to the pulmonary artery to create a physiologically normal circulation. Unfortunately, this procedure requires multiple conduit replacements as the child grows.

Prognosis—Operative mortality is less than 2% (Jacobs et al, 2004). Potential long-term problems include suprapulmonic stenosis and neoaorta dilation and regurgitation.

Total Anomalous Pulmonary Venous Connection

Description—Rare defect characterized by failure of the pulmonary veins to join the left atrium. Instead, the pulmonary veins are abnormally connected to the systemic venous circuit via the right atrium or various veins draining toward the right atrium, such as the superior vena cava. The abnormal attachment results in mixed blood being returned to the right atrium and shunted from the right to the left through an atrial septal defect (ASD). Total anomalous pulmonary venous connection (TAPVC; also called *total anomalous pulmonary venous return* or *total anomalous pulmonary venous drainage*) is classified according to the pulmonary venous point of attachment as follows:

Supracardiac—Attachment above the diaphragm, such as to the superior vena cava (most common form) (see Fig. 48-9)

Cardiac—Direct attachment to the heart, such as to the right atrium or coronary sinus

Infradiaphragmatic—Attachment below the diaphragm, such as to the inferior vena cava (most severe form)

Pathophysiology—The right atrium receives all the blood that normally would flow into the left atrium. As a result, the right side of the heart hypertrophies, whereas the left side, especially the left atrium, may remain small. An associated ASD or patent foramen ovale allows systemic venous blood to shunt from the higher-pressure right atrium to the left atrium and into the left side of the heart. As a result, the oxygen saturation of the blood in both sides of the heart (and ultimately in the systemic arterial circulation) is the same. If the pulmonary blood flow is large, pulmonary venous return is also large, and the amount of saturated blood is relatively high. However, if there is obstruction to pulmonary venous drainage, pulmonary venous return is impeded, pulmonary venous pressure rises, and pulmonary interstitial edema develops and eventually contributes to CHF. Infradiaphragmatic TAPVC is often

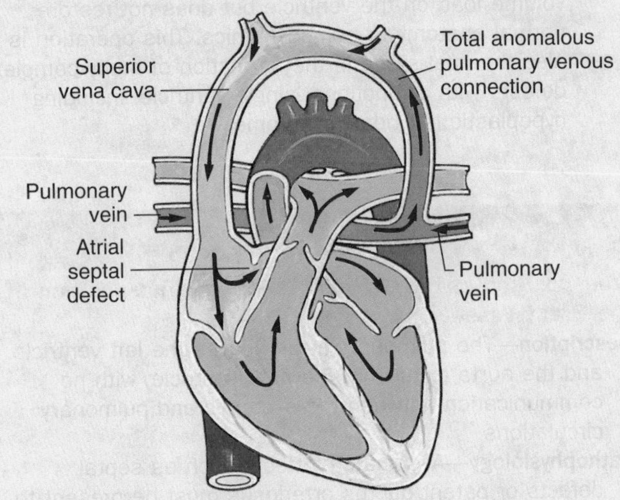

associated with obstruction to pulmonary venous drainage and is a surgical emergency.

Clinical manifestations—Most infants develop cyanosis early in life. The degree of cyanosis is inversely related to the amount of pulmonary blood flow—the more pulmonary blood, the less cyanosis. Children with unobstructed TAPVC may be asymptomatic until pulmonary vascular resistance decreases during infancy, increasing pulmonary blood flow, with resulting signs of CHF. Cyanosis becomes worse with pulmonary vein obstruction; once obstruction occurs, the infant's condition usually deteriorates rapidly. Without intervention, cardiac failure will progress to death.

Surgical treatment—Corrective repair is performed in early infancy. The surgical approach varies with the anatomic defect. However, in general, the common pulmonary vein is anastomosed to the back of the left atrium, the ASD is closed, and the anomalous pulmonary venous connection is ligated. The cardiac type is most easily repaired; the infradiaphragmatic type carries the highest

Total Anomalous Pulmonary Venous Connection—cont'd

morbidity and mortality because of the higher incidence of pulmonary vein obstruction. Potential postoperative complications include reobstruction; bleeding; dysrhythmias, particularly heart block; pulmonary artery hypertension; and persistent heart failure.

Prognosis—Mortality for all types is less than 10% (Jacobs et al, 2004) and is lowest for the cardiac type; morbidity increases with the presence of pulmonary vein obstruction.

Truncus Arteriosus

Description—Failure of normal septation and division of the embryonic bulbar trunk into the pulmonary artery and the aorta, which results in development of a single vessel that overrides both ventricles. Blood from both ventricles mixes in the common great artery, which leads to desaturation and hypoxemia. Blood ejected from the heart flows preferentially to the lower-pressure pulmonary arteries, so pulmonary blood flow is increased and systemic blood flow is reduced. There are three types:

Type I—A single pulmonary trunk arises near the base of the truncus and divides into the left and right pulmonary arteries.

Type II—The left and right pulmonary arteries arise separately but in close proximity and at the same level from the back of the truncus.

Type III—The pulmonary arteries arise independently from the sides of the truncus.

Pathophysiology—Blood ejected from the left and right ventricles enters the common trunk so that pulmonary and systemic circulations are mixed. Blood flow is distributed to the pulmonary and systemic circulations according to the relative resistances of each system. The amount of pulmonary blood flow depends on the size of the pulmonary arteries and the pulmonary vascular resistance. Generally, resistance to pulmonary blood flow is less than systemic vascular resistance, which results in preferential blood flow to the lungs. Pulmonary vascular disease develops at an early age in patients with truncus arteriosus.

Clinical manifestations—Most infants are symptomatic with moderate to severe CHF and variable cyanosis, poor growth, and activity intolerance. There is a holosystolic murmur at the left sternal murmur with a diastolic murmur present if truncal regurgitation is present. Thirty-five percent of patients have 22q11 deletions (Goldmuntz et al, 1998).

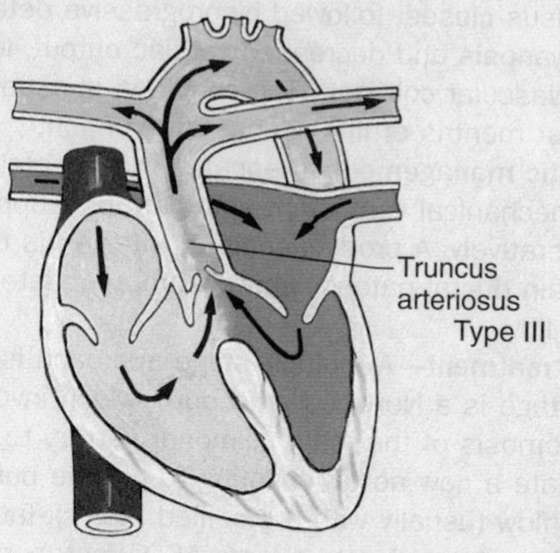

Surgical treatment—Early repair is performed in the first month of life. It involves closing the VSD so that the truncus arteriosus receives the outflow from the left ventricle, excising the pulmonary arteries from the aorta and attaching them to the right ventricle by means of a homograft. Currently homografts (segments of cadaver aorta and pulmonary artery that are treated with antibiotics and cryopreserved) are preferred over synthetic conduits to establish continuity between the right ventricle and pulmonary artery. Homografts are more flexible and easier to use during the procedure and appear less prone to obstruction. Postoperative complications include persistent heart failure, bleeding, pulmonary artery hypertension, dysrhythmias, and residual VSD. Because conduits are not living tissue, they will not grow along with the child and may also become narrowed with calcifications. One or more conduit replacements will be needed in childhood.

Prognosis—Mortality is greater than 10%; future operations are required to replace the conduits.

Hypoplastic Left Heart Syndrome

Description—Underdevelopment of the left side of the heart, resulting in a hypoplastic left ventricle and aortic atresia. Most blood from the left atrium flows across the patent foramen ovale to the right atrium, to the right ventricle, and out the pulmonary artery. The descending aorta receives blood from the patent ductus arteriosus supplying systemic blood flow.

Pathophysiology—An ASD or patent foramen ovale allows saturated blood from the left atrium to mix with desaturated blood from the right atrium and to flow through the right ventricle and out into the pulmonary artery. From the pulmonary artery, the blood flows both to the lungs and through the ductus arteriosus into the aorta and out to the body. The amount of blood flow to the pulmonary and systemic circulations depends on the

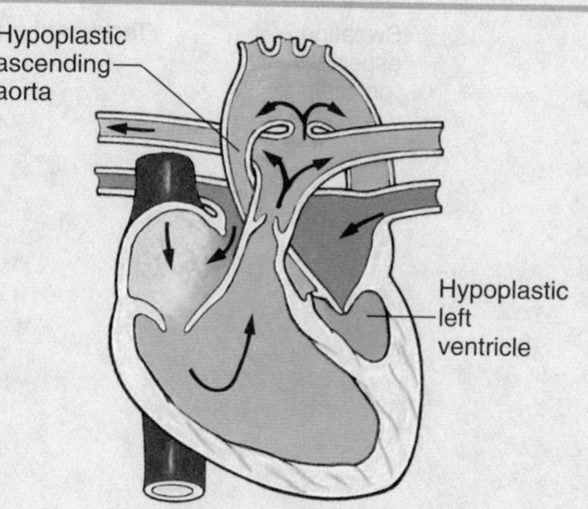

Continued

Hypoplastic Left Heart Syndrome—cont'd relationship between the pulmonary and systemic vascular resistances. The coronary and cerebral vessels receive blood by retrograde flow through the hypoplastic ascending aorta.

Clinical manifestations—The patient has mild cyanosis and signs of congestive failure until the patent ductus arteriosus closes, followed by progressive deterioration with cyanosis and decreased cardiac output, leading to cardiovascular collapse. The condition is usually fatal in the first months of life without intervention.

Therapeutic management—Neonates require stabilization with mechanical ventilation and inotropic support preoperatively. A prostaglandin E_1 infusion is needed to maintain ductal patency and ensure adequate systemic blood flow.

Surgical treatment—A multiple-stage approach is used. The first stage is a Norwood procedure, which involves an anastomosis of the main pulmonary artery to the aorta to create a new aorta, shunting to provide pulmonary blood flow (usually with a modified Blalock-Taussig shunt), and creation of a large ASD. Postoperative complications include imbalance of systemic and pulmonary blood flow, bleeding, low cardiac output, and persistent heart failure. A new modification of the first-stage repair is the use of a right ventricle–to–pulmonary artery homograft conduit instead of a shunt to supply pulmonary blood flow (Sano procedure). The second stage is often a bidirectional Glenn shunt procedure (see Fig. 48-9) or a hemi-Fontan operation. Both involve anastomosing the superior vena cava to the right pulmonary artery so superior vena cava flow bypasses the right atrium and flows directly to the lungs. The procedure is usually done at 3 to 6 months of age to relieve cyanosis and reduce the volume load on the right ventricle. The final repair is a modified Fontan procedure (see Tricuspid Atresia, Box 48-3).

Transplantation—Heart transplantation in the newborn period is another option for these infants. Problems include the shortage of newborn organ donors, risk of rejection, long-term problems with chronic immunosuppression, and infection (see Heart Transplantation, p. 1478).

Prognosis—For the first-stage repair, survival rates vary widely in different centers. Much progress has been made, and some experienced centers are reporting mortality rates of about 10% (Tweddell et al, 2002), but a large multicenter series reports a mortality of about 30% (Jacobs et al, 2004). Long-term problems with repair include worsening ventricular function, tricuspid regurgitation, recurrent aortic arch narrowing, dysrhythmias, and developmental delays. There is a risk of mortality between surgical procedures. The mortality for the later two operations is less than 5%.

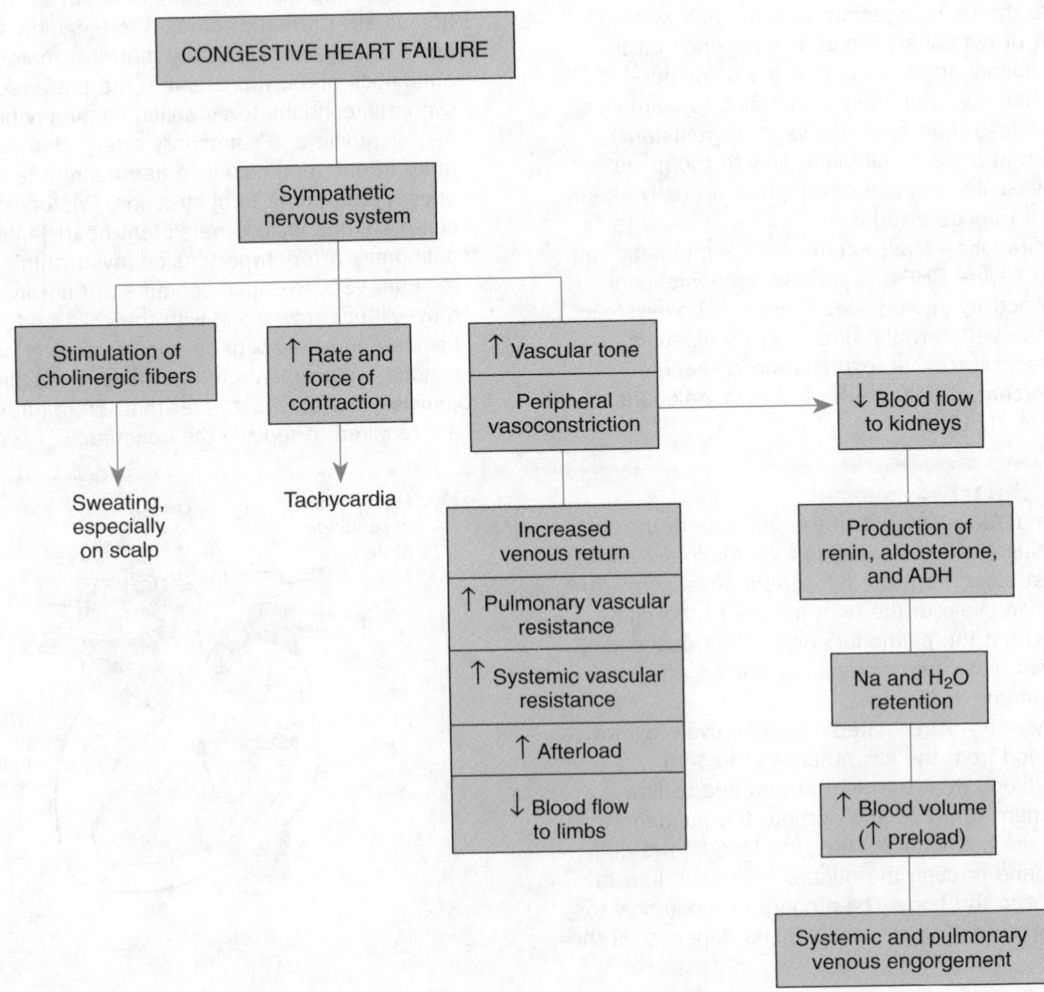

Fig. 48-6 Pathophysiology of congestive heart failure. *ADH,* Antidiuretic hormone.

BOX 48-5 Clinical Manifestations of Congestive Heart Failure

Impaired Myocardial Function
Tachycardia
Sweating (inappropriate)
Decreased urinary output
Fatigue
Weakness
Restlessness
Anorexia
Pale, cool extremities
Weak peripheral pulses
Decreased blood pressure
Gallop rhythm
Cardiomegaly

Pulmonary Congestion
Tachypnea
Dyspnea
Retractions (infants)
Flaring nares
Exercise intolerance
Orthopnea
Cough, hoarseness
Cyanosis
Wheezing
Grunting

Systemic Venous Congestion
Weight gain
Hepatomegaly
Peripheral edema, especially periorbital
Ascites
Neck vein distention (children)

management of CHF, the underlying cause is treated if possible.

Improve Cardiac Function

Myocardial efficiency is improved through administration of digitalis glycosides. The beneficial effects are increased cardiac output, decreased heart size, decreased venous pressure, and relief of edema. In pediatrics, *digoxin (Lanoxin)* is used almost exclusively because of its more rapid onset. It is available as an elixir (0.05 mg/ml) for oral administration. For infants the dose is calculated in micrograms (1000 mcg = 1 mg).

Treatment consists of a digitalizing dosage, given orally or intravenously in divided doses over 24 hours to produce optimal cardiac effects, and a maintenance dosage, given orally twice a day to maintain blood levels. During digitalization the child is monitored by means of an ECG to observe for the desired effects (prolonged PR interval and reduced ventricular rate) and detect side effects, especially dysrhythmias.

A group of drugs used in the treatment of CHF are the *angiotensin-converting enzyme (ACE) inhibitors.* As their name implies, these drugs inhibit the normal function of the renin-angiotensin system in the kidney. The ACE inhibitors block the conversion of angiotensin I to angiotensin II so that, instead of vasoconstriction, vasodilation occurs. Vasodilation results in decreased pulmonary and systemic vascular resistance, decreased BP, and a reduction in afterload. Common medications used in pediatrics are *captopril (Capoten), enalapril (Vasotec),* and lisinopril. The principal side effects of ACE inhibitors are hypotension, cough, and renal dysfunction.

Carvedilol, a β-blocker, blocks the α- and β-adrenergic receptors, causing decreased heart rate, decreased BP, and vasodilation. It has been shown to decrease morbidity and mortality in some adults with heart failure and is being used selectively in children. Side effects include dizziness, headache, and hypotension

A new and promising therapy for some patients with severe ventricular dysfunction may be biventricular pacing, also called resynchronization therapy. Both ventricles are paced to closely mimic normal ventricular conduction and thereby improve the mechanical function of the heart muscle (Rosenthal et al, 2004).

NURSING ALERT Because ACE inhibitors also block the action of aldosterone, the addition of potassium supplements or spironolactone (Aldactone) to the drug regimen of patients taking diuretics is usually not needed and may cause hyperkalemia.

Remove Accumulated Fluid and Sodium

Treatment consists of diuretics, possible fluid restriction, and possible sodium restriction. Diuretics are the mainstay of therapy to eliminate excess water and salt to prevent reaccumulation. The most frequently used agents are listed in Table 48-3. Because furosemide and the thiazides are potassium-losing diuretics, potassium supplements may be prescribed, and rich sources of the electrolyte are encouraged in the diet.

NURSING ALERT A fall in the serum potassium level enhances the effects of digitalis, increasing the risk of digoxin toxicity. Therefore serum potassium levels must be monitored carefully.

Fluid restriction may be required in the acute stages of CHF and must be calculated carefully to avoid dehydrating the child, especially if cyanotic CHD and significant polycythemia are present. Infants rarely need fluid restrictions because CHF makes feeding so difficult that they struggle to take maintenance fluids.

Sodium-restricted diets are used less often in children than in adults to control CHF because of their potential negative effects on appetite. If salt intake is restricted, additional table salt and highly salted foods are avoided.

Decrease Cardiac Demands

The workload on the heart is reduced when metabolic needs are kept to a minimum. This is accomplished by limiting physical activity (bed rest), maintaining body temperature, treating any infections, reducing the effort of breathing (semi-Fowler position), and using medication to sedate an irritable child.

Improve Tissue Oxygenation

All of the preceding measures serve to increase tissue oxygenation, by either improving myocardial function or lessen-

evolve Critical Thinking Exercise—Digoxin Administration

Table 48-3 Diuretics Used in Congestive Heart Failure

ACTIONS	COMMENTS	NURSING CARE MANAGEMENT
Furosemide (Lasix)—Blocks reabsorption of sodium and water in proximal renal tubule and interferes with reabsorption of sodium	Drug of choice in severe congestive heart failure Causes excretion of chloride and potassium (hypokalemia may precipitate digitalis toxicity)	Begin to record output as soon as drug is given. Observe for dehydration caused by profound diuresis. Observe for side effects (nausea and vomiting, diarrhea, ototoxicity, hypokalemia, dermatitis, postural hypotension). Encourage foods high in potassium and/or give potassium supplements. Monitor chloride and acid-base balance with long-term therapy. Observe for signs of digoxin toxicity.
Chlorothiazide (Diuril)—Acts directly on distal tubules to decrease sodium, water, potassium, chloride, and bicarbonate absorption	Less frequently used drug Causes hypokalemia, acidosis from large doses	Observe for side effects (nausea, weakness, dizziness, paresthesia, muscle cramps, skin eruptions, hypokalemia, acidosis). Encourage foods high in potassium and/or give potassium supplements.
Spironolactone (Aldactone)—Blocks action of aldosterone, which promotes retention of sodium and excretion of potassium	Weak diuretic Has potassium-sparing effect; frequently used with thiazides, furosemide Poorly absorbed from gastrointestinal tract Takes several days to achieve maximum actions	Observe for side effects (skin rash, drowsiness, ataxia, hyperkalemia). Do not administer potassium supplements.

ing tissue oxygen demands. In addition, supplemental cool, humidified oxygen may be administered to increase the amount of available oxygen during inspiration. Oxygen administration is especially helpful in patients with pulmonary edema, intercurrent respiratory tract infections, and increased pulmonary vascular resistance (oxygen is a vasodilator that decreases pulmonary vascular resistance).

NURSING ALERT Oxygen is a drug and is administered only with an appropriate order. In some uncommon circumstances in patients with complex hemodynamics, oxygen can be detrimental.

An oxygen hood, nasal cannula, or face tent is used to deliver oxygen. Nasal cannulas are ideal for long-term oxygen administration because the child can be ambulatory and can easily eat and drink. Cool humidification is necessary to counteract the drying effect of oxygen. The amount of cool humidity is carefully regulated to prevent chilling.

Nursing Care Management

The infant or child with CHF may be acutely ill, and some may require intensive care until the symptoms improve. Expert nursing care is essential to reduce the cardiac demands that strain the failing heart muscle. During this time the child and family require emotional support. Although the objectives of nursing care are the same, interventions differ, depending on the child's age (see Nursing Care Plan).

Assist in Measures to Improve Cardiac Function

The nurse's responsibility in administering digoxin includes calculating and administering the correct dosage, observing for signs of toxicity, and instituting parental teaching regarding drug administration at home. The child's apical pulse is always checked before administering digoxin. As a general rule, the drug is not given if the pulse is below 90 to 110 beats/min in infants and young children or below 70 beats/min in older children (the cutoff point for adults is 60 beats/min). However, because the pulse rate varies in children in different age groups, the written drug order should specify at what heart rate the drug is withheld. The nurse should also use judgment in evaluating the pulse rate. If it is significantly lower than the previous recording, the dose should be withheld until the practitioner is notified.

The apical rate is taken because a pulse deficit (radial pulse rate lower than apical) may be present with decreased cardiac output. It is auscultated for a full minute to evaluate alterations in rhythm. If the child is monitored by means of an ECG, a rhythm strip is obtained and attached to the chart for rate and rhythm analysis, such as abnormal lengthening of the PR interval (more than 50% increase over predigitalization interval) and dysrhythmias.

Digoxin is a potentially dangerous drug because of its narrow margin of safety of therapeutic, toxic, and lethal doses. Many toxic responses are extensions of its therapeutic effects. Therefore the nurse must maintain a high index of suspicion for signs of toxicity when administering digoxin (Box 48-6).

Because digoxin toxicity can occur from accidental overdose, great care must be taken in properly calculating and measuring the dosage. When converting milligrams to

BOX 48-6 Common Signs of Digoxin Toxicity in Children

Gastrointestinal
Nausea
Vomiting
Anorexia

Cardiac
Bradycardia
Dysrhythmias

micrograms to milliliters, the nurse carefully checks the placement of the decimal point, since an error causes a significant change in dosage. For example, 0.1 mg is 10 times the dosage of 0.01 mg.

NURSING ALERT Infants rarely receive more than 1 ml (50 mcg, or 0.05 mg) in one dose; a higher dose is an immediate warning of a dosage error. To ensure safety, compare the calculation with another staff member's calculation before giving the drug.

These same principles are taught to parents in preparation for discharge, although the correct dose in milliliters is usually specified on the container, thus reducing potential errors in calculation. The nurse watches the parent measure the elixir in the dropper and stresses the level mark as the meniscus of the fluid that is observed at eye level. Other instructions for administering digoxin are listed in the Family-Centered Care box and the Critical Thinking Exercise.

Parents are also advised of the signs of toxicity. According to the practitioner's preference, they may be taught to take the pulse before giving the drug. A return demonstration of the procedure from the parents or another principal caregiver is included as part of the teaching plan. Their level of anxiety in counting the pulse is assessed, since overconcern about the heart rate may result in excessive withholding of the drug.

NURSING CARE PLAN ✤ The Child with Congestive Heart Failure (CHF)

Nursing Diagnosis	Expected Patient Outcomes	Nursing Interventions	Rationale
Decreased cardiac output related to structural defect, myocardial dysfunction, altered hemodynamics **Child's/Family's Defining Characteristics** *(Subjective and Objective Data)* Tachycardia Tachypnea Ineffective peripheral circulation, cool extremities Hypotension Rapid, weak peripheral pulses Prolonged capillary refill, longer than 2 to 3 seconds Narrow pulse pressure Distended neck veins in older children Cardiomegaly revealed on chest x-ray film Gallop rhythm Edema Rapid weight gain Feeding difficulty Irritability	Child will have adequate cardiac output as evidenced by: ✤ Heart rate within acceptable range (state specific range) ✤ Respiratory rate (RR) within acceptable range (state specific range) ✤ Skin warm to touch ✤ Strong and equal peripheral pulses ✤ Blood pressure normal for age ✤ Brisk capillary refill within 2 to 3 seconds ✤ Lack of distended neck veins ✤ Normal sinus rhythm ✤ Lack of edema ✤ Adequate urinary output (state specific; 1 to 2 ml/kg/hr) Child will have age-appropriate weight gain on standardized growth curve. Infant will demonstrate successful feeding. Child and/or family will be able to state at least four characteristics of CHF such as: ✤ Rapid heart rate ✤ Fast breathing ✤ Cool extremities ✤ Puffiness (edema) ✤ Fussiness ✤ Decreased appetite Child and/or family will be able to state knowledge of care regarding: ✤ Medication administration ✤ Elevated head positioning ✤ Sufficient rest periods ✤ Monitoring intake and output ✤ When to contact health care provider **The Following NOC Concepts Apply to These Outcomes** Cardiac Pump Effectiveness Knowledge: Illness Care Tissue Perfusion: Cardiac	Assess and record heart rate, RR, blood pressure, and any signs and symptoms of decreased cardiac output (listed under defining characteristics) every 2 to 4 hours and as needed (PRN).	To assess for changes in vital signs and child's physical status that reflect altered cardiac output
		Administer cardiac drugs on schedule. Assess for and record any side effects or any signs or symptoms of toxicity. Follow hospital protocol for administration.	To improve heart function by giving drugs on time and to avoid dangers by giving as prescribed and with careful assessment before administration
		Keep accurate record of intake and output.	To assess for CHF, which causes decreased urinary output
		Weigh child or infant on same scale at same time of day. Document results and compare with previous weight.	To observe for weight increase that may indicate excess fluid accumulation
		Administer diuretics on schedule. Assess and record effectiveness and any side effects noted.	To prevent fluid retention, which commonly occurs with CHF; to eliminate excess water and salt
		Elevate head of bed at a 30- to 45-degree angle.	To promote maximum chest expansion
		Offer small, frequent feedings to infant's or child's tolerance.	To prevent fatigue during feeding and to ensure adequate nutrition since metabolic rate is greater because of poor cardiac function
		Organize nursing care to allow child or infant uninterrupted rest.	To account for decreased energy level and lower tolerance to activity
		Educate child and family about characteristics of CHF. Assess and record teaching session.	To provide parent education that can promote measures to improve cardiac function and decrease demands
		Educate child and family about care such as medication administration. Assess and record results and family's participation in care.	To educate on proper medication administration, promote safety, and minimize medication side effects
		The Following NIC Concepts Apply to These Interventions Cardiac Care Fluid Management Medication Administration Positioning Vital Signs Monitoring Respiratory Monitoring	

Continued

evolve Nursing Care Plan—The Child with Congestive Heart Failure

NURSING CARE PLAN ✤ The Child with Congestive Heart Failure (CHF)—cont'd

Nursing Diagnosis	Expected Patient Outcomes	Nursing Interventions	Rationale
Ineffective breathing pattern related to pulmonary congestion, decreased cardiac output **Child's/Family's Defining Characteristics** ***(Subjective and Objective Data)*** Tachypnea Dyspnea Retractions Crackles Shortness of breath Cyanosis Pallor Mottling Nasal flaring Grunting Head bobbing Cough Use of accessory muscles Activity intolerance	Child will have effective breathing pattern as evidenced by: ✤ RR within acceptable range (state specific range) ✤ Clear and equal breath sounds bilaterally anterior and posterior ✤ Pink or tan color ✤ Absence of nasal flaring, retractions, cough, and head bobbing ✤ Unlabored breath sounds ✤ Tolerance of activities appropriate for age Child and/or family will be able to state four characteristics of ineffective breathing pattern such as: ✤ Color change from pink or tan to pale, dusky, or blue color ✤ Fast breathing ✤ Change in amount and/or characteristics of secretions ✤ Retractions, head bobbing ✤ Ineffective cough ✤ Decreased or altered activity level Child and/or family will be able to state knowledge of care regarding: ✤ Positioning to facilitate respiratory effort ✤ Oxygen administration ✤ When to contact health care provider **The Following NOC Concepts Apply to These Outcomes** Activity Tolerance Knowledge: Illness Care Respiratory Status: Gas Exchange Tissue Perfusion: Pulmonary	Assess and record RR, breath sounds, and any signs and symptoms of ineffective pattern (listed under characteristics) every 2 to 4 hours and PRN. Administer humidified oxygen in correct amount, using correct route of delivery. Record percent of oxygen and route of delivery. Assess and record child's response to therapy. Keep head of bed elevated at a 30- to 45-degree angle. Suction if child has ineffective cough or is unable to manage secretions. Assess and record amount and characteristics of secretions. Assess and record oxygen saturation every 2 to 4 hours and PRN. Educate child and family about characteristics of ineffective breathing pattern. Assess and record results. Educate child and family about care. Assess and record results and family participation in care. **The Following NIC Concepts Apply to These Interventions** Airway Management Airway Suctioning Chest Physiotherapy Family Involvement Promotion Health Education	To assess for respiratory changes that can be indicators of worsening CHF To provide oxygen, which can reduce respiratory distress by easing respiratory effort To promote maximum chest expansion To maintain patent airway to promote respiratory expansion To evaluate pulmonary effectiveness To provide parent education that can promote measures to improve breathing effort To promote family support

FAMILY-CENTERED CARE

Administering Digoxin

- Give digoxin at regular intervals, usually every 12 hours, such as at 8 AM and 8 PM.
- Administer the drug carefully by slowly directing it to the side and back of the mouth.
- Do not mix the drug with foods or other fluids, since refusal to consume these results in inaccurate intake of the drug.
- If the child has teeth, give water after administering the drug; whenever possible, brush the teeth to prevent tooth decay from the sweetened liquid.
- If a dose is missed, do not give an extra dose or increase the dose. Stay on the same medication schedule.
- If the child vomits, do not give a second dose.
- If more than two consecutive doses have been missed, notify the physician or other designated practitioner.
- Frequent vomiting, poor feeding, or slow heart rate can be signs of toxicity; if they occur, contact the physician.
- If the child becomes ill, notify the physician or other designated practitioner immediately.
- Keep digoxin in a safe place, preferably in a locked cabinet.
- In case of accidental overdose of digoxin, call the nearest poison control center immediately.

CRITICAL THINKING EXERCISE

Digoxin Toxicity

You are visiting a 3-month-old infant at home who began receiving digoxin and furosemide (Lasix) 5 days ago for management of congestive heart failure (CHF). A brief assessment indicates that the infant appears well but is not very active, has a weak suck reflex, and does not exhibit much spontaneous movement during interaction with the mother. The mother mentions that the infant is a good baby and does not cry much except when he is very hungry. She also mentions that he vomited several times yesterday and twice this morning; this was not perceived as unusual because her 3-year-old did the same thing and was diagnosed with gastroesophageal reflux. Further assessment of the infant reveals an irregular heartbeat of 86 to 104 beats/min at rest; the heart rhythm is also noted to be irregular. No murmur or other significant sounds are auscultated.

1. Evidence—Is there sufficient evidence to draw conclusions about this infant?
2. Assumptions—Describe an underlying assumption about each of the following:
   a. Side effects of furosemide
   b. Side effects of digoxin
   c. Infants with CHF
3. What priorities for nursing care should be established for this infant?
4. Does the evidence support your nursing interventions?
5. What alternative perspectives might you have?

Monitor Afterload Reduction

For patients receiving ACE inhibitors for afterload reduction, the nurse should carefully monitor BP before and after dose administration, observe for symptoms of hypotension, and notify the practitioner if BP is low. Numerous medications affecting the kidney can potentiate renal dysfunction; thus children taking multiple diuretics and an ACE inhibitor require careful assessment of serum electrolytes and renal function.

Decrease Cardiac Demands

The infant requires rest and conservation of energy for feeding. Every effort is made to organize nursing activities to allow for uninterrupted periods of sleep. Whenever possible, parents are encouraged to stay with their infant to provide the holding, rocking, and cuddling that help children sleep more soundly. To minimize disturbing the infant, changing bed linen and complete bathing are done only when necessary. Feeding is planned to accommodate the infant's sleep and wake patterns. The child is fed at the first sign of hunger, such as when sucking on fists, rather than waiting until he or she cries for a bottle, because the stress of crying exhausts the limited energy supply. Because infants with CHF tire easily and may sleep through feedings, smaller feedings every 3 hours may be helpful. Gavage feedings may be instituted to provide adequate nutrition and allow the infant to rest.

Every effort is made to minimize unnecessary stress. Older children need an explanation of what is happening to them to decrease anxiety about their illness and necessary treatments such as cardiac monitoring, oxygen administration, and medications. Outlining a plan for the day, preparing the child for tests and procedures, providing quiet activities, and providing adequate rest periods are all helpful interventions with older children. Some infants and children require sedation during the acute phase of illness to allow them to rest.

Temperature is monitored carefully because hyperthermia or hypothermia increases the need for oxygen. Febrile states are reported to the physician, since infection must be treated promptly. Maintaining body temperature is of special importance in children who are receiving cool, humidified oxygen and in infants, who tend to be diaphoretic and lose heat by way of evaporation.

Skin breakdown from edema is prevented with a change of position every 2 hours (from side to side while in semi-Fowler position) and use of a pressure-relieving mattress or bed. The skin, especially over the sacrum, is checked for evidence of redness from pressure.

Reduce Respiratory Distress

Careful assessment, positioning, and oxygen administration can reduce respiratory distress. Respirations are counted for 1 full minute during a resting state. Any evidence of increased respiratory distress is reported, since this may indicate worsening CHF.

Infants are positioned to encourage maximum chest expansion, with the head of the bed elevated; they should sit up in an infant seat or be held at a 45-degree angle. Children prefer to sleep on several pillows and remain in a semi-Fowler or high-Fowler position during waking hours. Safety restraints, such as those used with infant seats, are applied low on the abdomen and loosely enough to provide both safety and maximum expansion.

The infant or child is often given humidified supplemental oxygen via oxygen hood or tent, nasal cannula, or mask. The child's response to oxygen therapy is carefully evaluated by noting respiratory rate, ease of respiration, color, and especially oxygen saturation as measured by oximetry.

Respiratory tract infections can exacerbate CHF and should be treated appropriately and prevented if possible. The child should be protected from persons with respiratory tract infections and have a noninfectious roommate. For an older child, it is advantageous to choose a roommate who is also confined to bed and relatively quiet to promote a restful environment. Good handwashing is practiced before and after caring for any hospitalized child. Antibiotics may be given to combat respiratory tract infection. The nurse ensures that the drug is given at equally divided times over a 24-hour schedule to maintain high blood levels of the antibiotic.

Maintain Nutritional Status

Meeting the nutritional needs of infants with CHF or serious cardiac defects is a nursing challenge. The metabolic rate of these infants is greater because of poor cardiac function and increased heart and respiratory rates. Their caloric needs are greater than those of the average infant because of their increased metabolic rate, yet their ability to take in adequate calories is hampered by their fatigue. Feeding for a fragile infant with serious CHD is similar to exercising for an adult, and these infants often do not have the energy or cardiac reserve to do extra work. The nurse seeks measures to enable the infant to feed easily without excess fatigue and to increase the caloric density of the formula.

The infant should be well rested before feeding and fed soon after awakening so as not to expend energy on crying. A 3-hour feeding schedule works well for many infants. (Feeding every 2 hours does not provide enough rest between feedings, and a 4-hour schedule requires an increased volume of feeding, which many infants are unable to take.) The feeding schedule should be individualized to the infant's needs. A feeding goal of 150 ml/kg/day and at least 120 kcal/kg/day is common for newborns with significant heart disease (Stetzler, Rudd, & Pick, 2005). A soft preemie nipple or a slit in a regular nipple to enlarge the opening decreases the infant's energy expenditure while sucking. Infants should be well supported and fed in a semiupright position. The infant may need to rest frequently and may need to have the jaw and cheeks stroked to encourage sucking. Generally, giving an infant about a half hour to complete a feeding is reasonable. Prolonging the feeding time can exhaust the infant and decrease the rest period between feedings.

Infants with feeding difficulties are often gavage fed using a nasogastric tube to supplement their oral intake and ensure adequate calories. If they are very stressed and fatigued, in respiratory distress, or tachypneic to 80 to 100 breaths/min, oral feedings may be withheld and all nutrition given by gavage feedings. Gavage feedings are usually a temporary measure until the infant's medical status improves and nutritional needs can be met through oral feedings. Some infants with severe CHF, neurologic deficits, or significant gastroesophageal reflux may need placement of a gastrostomy tube to allow adequate nutrition.

Caloric density of formulas is frequently increased by concentration and then adding Polycose, medium-chain triglyceride oil, or corn oil. Infant formulas provide 20 cal/oz, and the use of additives can increase the calories to 30 cal/oz or more. This allows the infant to obtain more calories despite a smaller volume intake of formula. The caloric density of the formula needs to be increased slowly (by 2 cal/oz/day) to prevent diarrhea or formula intolerance. Breastfeeding mothers are encouraged to provide the infant with alternating feedings of breast milk and high-calorie formulas. Some lactating mothers prefer to feed the child expressed breast milk that has been fortified with Similac or Enfamil powder, Polycose, or corn oil to increase caloric intake. A supplemental nurser may also be helpful. A diet plan specific to the individual infant's needs is calculated and prescribed by the nutritionist in collaboration with the other health personnel. The nurse needs to reinforce this information with the parents as necessary.

Assist in Measures to Promote Fluid Loss

When diuretics are given, the nurse records fluid intake and output and monitors body weight at the same time each day to evaluate benefit from the drug. Because profound diuresis may cause dehydration and electrolyte imbalance (loss of sodium, potassium, chloride, bicarbonate), the nurse observes for signs indicating either complication, as well as signs and symptoms suggesting reactions to the drugs. Diuretics should be given early in the day to children who are toilet trained to avoid the need to urinate at night. If potassium-losing diuretics are given, the nurse encourages foods high in potassium, such as bananas, oranges, whole grains, legumes, and leafy vegetables, and administers prescribed supplements. Serum potassium levels are checked frequently.

Fluid restriction is rarely necessary in infants because of their difficulty in feeding. However, if fluids are restricted, the nurse plans fluid intake schedules for a 24-hour period, allowing for most fluids during waking hours. Toddlers and preschoolers should be given small amounts of liquid in small cups so that the containers appear full. Older children's cooperation is gained by placing them in charge of recording fluid intake.

If salt is limited, the nurse discusses food sources of sodium with the family and discourages their bringing salt-containing treats to the child. At mealtime the child's tray is checked to make sure the appropriate diet is given.

Support Child and Family

CHF is a serious complication of heart disease. Parents and older children are usually acutely aware of the critical nature of the condition. Because stress places additional demands on cardiac function, the nurse should focus on reducing anxiety through anticipatory preparation, frequent communication with the parent regarding the child's progress, and constant reassurance that everything possible is being done.

Home care involves many of the same interventions discussed under Plan for Discharge and Home Care (p. 1471). The nurse teaches the family about the medications that need to be administered and alerts them to the signs of worsening CHF that require medical attention, such as increased sweating, decreased urinary output (noted in fewer wet diapers or infrequent use of the toilet), or poor feeding. Every effort is made to improve the family's adherence to the medication schedule by adapting the schedule to their usual home routines, avoiding medications during the night, making it as simple as possible, and using charts or visual aids to remember when to give medications (see Chapter 45). Written instructions regarding correct administration of digoxin are essential (see Family-Centered Care box, p. 1462), including an explanation regarding signs of toxicity.

If CHF is the end stage of a severe heart defect, the nurse cares for this child as for any child who is terminally ill, using the principles discussed in Chapter 41.

Hypoxemia

Hypoxemia refers to an arterial oxygen tension (or pressure, $Pa{O_2}$) that is less than normal and can be identified by a decreased arterial saturation or a decreased $Pa{O_2}$. *Hypoxia* is a reduction in tissue oxygenation that is caused by low oxygen saturations and $Pa{O_2}$ and results in impaired cellular processes. *Cyanosis* is a blue discoloration in the mucous membranes, skin, and nail beds of the child with reduced oxygen saturation. It results from the presence of deoxygenated hemoglobin (hemoglobin not bound to oxygen) in a concentration of 5 g/dl of blood. Cyanosis is usually apparent when arterial oxygen saturations are 80% to 85%. Determination of cyanosis is subjective. It can vary depending on skin pigment, quality of light, color of the room, or clothing worn by the child. The presence of cyanosis may not accurately reflect arterial hypoxemia because both oxygen saturation and the amount of circulating hemoglobin are involved. Children with severe anemia may not be cyanotic despite severe hypoxemia because the hemoglobin level may be too low to produce the characteristic blue color. Conversely, patients with polycythemia may appear cyanotic despite a near-normal Pao_2. Heart defects that cause hypoxemia and cyanosis result from desaturated venous blood (blue blood) entering the systemic circulation without passing through the lungs.

Clinical Manifestations

Over time, two physiologic changes occur in the body in response to chronic hypoxemia: polycythemia and clubbing. *Polycythemia,* an increased number of red blood cells, increases the oxygen-carrying capacity of the blood. However, anemia may result if iron is not readily available for the formation of hemoglobin. Polycythemia increases the viscosity of the blood and crowds out clotting factors. *Clubbing,* a thickening and flattening of the tips of the fingers and toes, is thought to occur because of chronic tissue hypoxemia and polycythemia (Fig. 48-7). Infants with mild hypoxemia may be asymptomatic except for cyanosis and exhibit near-normal growth and development. Those with more severe hypoxemia may exhibit fatigue with feeding, poor weight gain, tachypnea, and dyspnea. Severe hypoxemia resulting in tissue hypoxia is manifested by clinical deterioration and signs of poor perfusion.

Hypercyanotic spells, also referred to as *blue spells* or *tet spells* because they are often seen in infants with tetralogy of Fallot, may occur in any child whose heart defect includes obstruction to pulmonary blood flow and communication between the ventricles. The infant becomes acutely cyanotic and hyperpneic because sudden infundibular spasm decreases pulmonary blood flow and increases right-to-left shunting (the proposed mechanism in tetralogy of Fallot). Spells, rarely seen before 2 months of age, occur most frequently in the first year of life. They occur more often in the morning and may be preceded by feeding, crying, defecation, or stressful procedures (see Critical Thinking Exercise). Because profound hypoxemia causes cerebral hypoxia, hypercyanotic spells require prompt assessment and treatment to prevent brain damage or possibly death.

Persistent cyanosis as a result of cyanotic heart defects places the child at risk for significant *neurologic complications.* Cerebrovascular accident (CVA, stroke), brain abscess, and developmental delays (especially in motor and cognitive development) may result from chronic hypoxia.

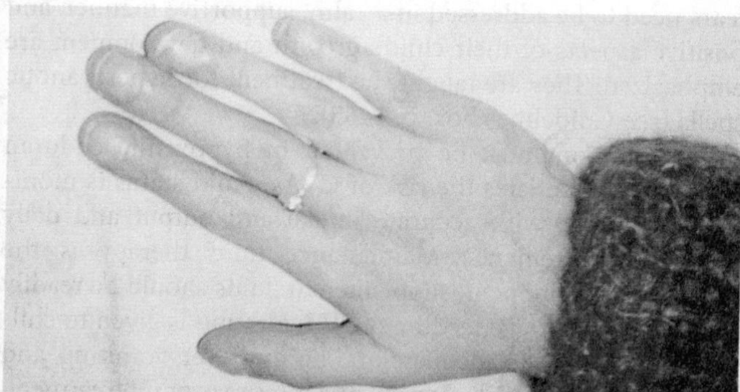

Fig. 48-7 Clubbing of the fingers.

CRITICAL THINKING EXERCISE

Hypercyanotic Spell

A 4-month-old infant known to have tetralogy of Fallot is seen in the emergency department because of a 2-day history of diarrhea, low-grade fever, and poor oral intake. When blood tests are obtained, he becomes acutely cyanotic with rapid shallow respirations.

1. Evidence—Is there sufficient evidence to draw conclusions about this infant's condition?
2. Assumptions—Describe an underlying assumption about each of the following:
   a. Symptoms associated with tetralogy of Fallot
   b. Diarrhea, low-grade fever, and poor oral intake in a 4-month-old infant
   c. Acute cyanotic episodes in a 4-month-old infant
3. What priorities for nursing care should be established for this infant?
4. Does the evidence support your nursing interventions?
5. What alternative perspectives might you have?

Therapeutic Management

Newborns generally exhibit cyanosis within the first few days of life as the ductus arteriosus, which provided pulmonary blood flow, begins to close. Prostaglandin E_1, which causes vasodilation and smooth muscle relaxation, thus increasing dilation and patency of the ductus arteriosus, is administered intravenously to reestablish pulmonary blood flow. The use of prostaglandins has been lifesaving for infants with ductus-dependent cardiac defects. The increase in oxygenation allows the infant to be stabilized and have a complete diagnostic evaluation performed before further treatment is needed.

Hypercyanotic spells occur suddenly, and prompt recognition and treatment are essential. In the hospital setting, spells are often seen during blood drawing or IV insertion, when the child is highly agitated, or after cardiac catheterization. Treatment of a hypercyanotic spell is outlined in the Guidelines box. Morphine, administered subcutaneously or through an existing IV line, helps reduce infundibular spasm. A spell indicates the need for prompt surgical treatment if possible. In infants with defects not amenable to surgical repair, a shunt may be created surgically to increase blood flow to the lungs. Several commonly used shunt procedures are described in Table 48-4 and Fig. 48-9.

The cyanotic infant and child are well hydrated to keep the hematocrit and blood viscosity within acceptable limits to

GUIDELINES Treating Hypercyanotic Spells

- Place infant in knee-chest position (Fig. 48-8).
- Use calm, comforting approach.
- Administer 100% oxygen by blow by.
- Give morphine subcutaneously or through existing intravenous (IV) line.
- Begin IV fluid replacement and volume expansion if needed.
- Repeat morphine administration.

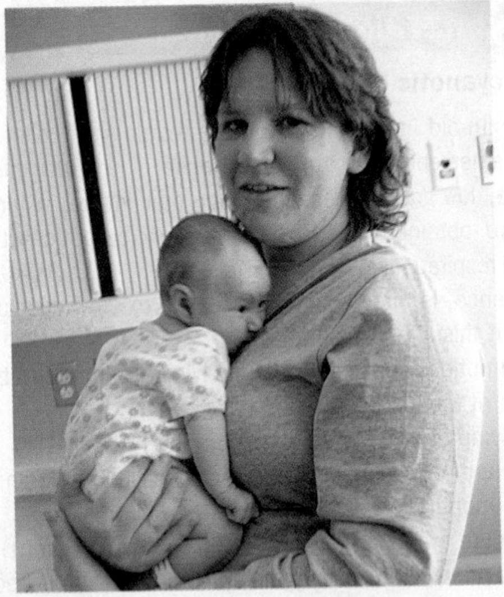

Fig. 48-8 Infant held in knee-chest position.

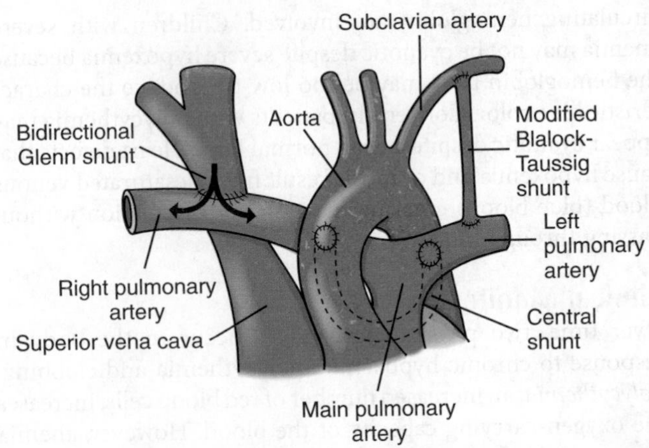

Fig. 48-9 Schematic diagram of cardiac shunts.

Table 48-4 Selected Shunt Procedures for Children with Cardiac Defects

SHUNT TYPE	COMMENTS
Modified Blalock-Taussig shunt—Subclavian artery to pulmonary artery using Gore-Tex or Impra tube graft	Shunt flow sometimes excessive, requiring use of diuretics Possibility of thrombosis; aspirin usually prescribed postoperatively Easy to ligate at time of definitive correction Shunt size fixed and may become too small as child grows
Central shunt—Ascending aorta to main pulmonary artery using Gore-Tex graft	Length of shunt acts to restrict blood flow; possibility of symptoms of congestive heart failure; diuretic therapy sometimes required Uncommon; used when modified Blalock-Taussig shunt cannot be used Easy to insert and remove at time of repair Possibility of thrombosis; aspirin usually prescribed postoperatively
Bidirectional Glenn shunt (cavopulmonary anastomosis)—Superior vena cava to side of right pulmonary artery; blood flow to both lungs	Done as a second shunt; often used as a staging step to a Fontan procedure Can be incorporated into eventual modified Fontan procedure Relieves severe cyanosis and decreases volume overload on ventricle Carries risk of embolic events (mixing defect); aspirin often prescribed Pulmonary arteriovenous fistulas may occur months or years later, causing desaturation (uncommon finding)

reduce the risk of CVAs. Fevers are carefully evaluated because bacteremia can result in bacterial endocarditis. The infant is monitored closely for anemia because of the risk of CVAs and the reduced arterial oxygen-carrying capacity that occurs. Iron supplementation and possibly blood transfusion are used as needed.

Respiratory tract infections or reduced pulmonary function from any cause can worsen hypoxemia in the cyanotic child. Aggressive pulmonary hygiene, chest physical therapy, administration of antibiotics, and use of oxygen to improve arterial saturations are important interventions.

Nursing Care Management

The general appearance of infants and children with significant cyanosis poses unique concerns. Blue lips and fingernails are obvious signs of their hidden cardiac defect. Clubbing and small, thin stature in older children further indicate severe heart disease. Adolescents are especially concerned about their body image; children with cyanosis are often teased about their appearance and singled out as different. When asked what surgery will do, many children reply, "Make me pink." Their joy and excitement after surgery are evident when they see their pink fingers. Parents are often fearful of their child's bluish color because cyanosis is usually associated with lack of oxygen and severe illness. They also must deal with comments from relatives, friends, and strangers about their child's abnormal color. They need a simple explanation of hypoxemia and cyanosis and reassurance that cyanosis does not imply a lack of oxygen to the brain. Their questions and fears need to be addressed in a calm, supportive manner, and positive aspects of their child's growth and development are emphasized. They are taught the treatment for hypercyanotic spells (see Guidelines box, p. 1465).

Dehydration must be prevented in hypoxemic children because it potentiates the risk of CVAs. Fluid status is monitored carefully, with accurate intake and output and daily weight measurements. Maintenance fluid therapy is the minimum requirement, supplemental fluids should be readily available, and gavage feeding or IV hydration is given to children unable to take adequate oral fluids. Fever, vomiting, and diarrhea can cause dehydration and require prompt treatment. Parents are instructed in the importance of adequate fluid intake and measures to prevent dehydration. An oral electrolyte solution should be available at home in the event that the infant is unable to tolerate the usual formula. The practitioner should be notified of fever, vomiting, diarrhea, or other problems.

Preventive measures and accurate assessment of respiratory infection are important nursing considerations. Any compromise in pulmonary function will increase the infant's hypoxemia. Good handwashing and protection from individuals with an obvious respiratory tract infection are important. Aggressive pulmonary hygiene, treatment with antibiotics or antiviral agents as indicated, and supplemental oxygen to decrease hypoxemia are necessary measures. Infants may need to be gavage fed or given parenteral hydration if respiratory distress prevents oral feeding.

NURSING ALERT Intracardiac shunting of blood from the right side (desaturated) to the left side of the heart allows air in the venous system to go directly to the brain, resulting in an air embolism. Therefore all IV lines should have filters in place to prevent air from entering the system, the entire tubing should be checked for air, all connections should be taped securely, and any air should be removed.

Nursing Care of the Family and Child with Congenital Heart Disease

When a child is born with a severe cardiac anomaly, the parents are faced with the immense psychologic and physical tasks of adjusting to the birth of a child with special needs. Family issues and nursing interventions to support the family are similar to those discussed in Chapter 41. The following discussion is primarily directed (1) toward the family of an infant who has a serious heart defect and requires home care before definitive repair and (2) toward preparation and care of the child and family when invasive procedures (catheterization and surgery) are performed. For nursing care related to the child with hypoxemia and CHF, see earlier discussions of these topics.

Nursing care of the child with a congenital heart defect begins as soon as the diagnosis is suspected. Prenatal diagnosis of congenital heart defects is becoming increasingly frequent. New demands are being placed on nurses to counsel and support families as they prepare for the birth of these infants.

Help Family Adjust to the Disorder

Once parents learn of the heart defect, they are initially in a period of shock, followed by high anxiety and fear that the child will die. The family needs time to grieve before they can assimilate the meaning of the defect. Unfortunately, the demands for medical treatment may not allow this, instead necessitating that the parents immediately give informed consent for diagnostic-therapeutic procedures. The nurse can be instrumental in supporting parents in their loss, assessing their level of understanding, supplying information as needed, and helping other members of the health care team understand the parents' reactions (see Family-Centered Care box).

> **FAMILY-CENTERED CARE**
>
> *Diagnosis of Heart Disease*
>
> Remember that we don't have your experience. We don't see children every day who have heart disease. We would have been upset finding out our child had to have his tonsils out. How could we ever be prepared for this? Please remember, we only know people who have trivial heart murmurs. How could we ever expect this to happen? And to us, this is the worst problem we've ever heard of.
>
> We still fear most what we don't know and understand. Be honest with us. If you don't know either, tell us. But at least don't leave us wondering about what you know and we don't. Not knowing anything really can be worse than knowing something bad. Be honest, but don't strip us of hope....
>
> Please, remember we are trying to learn complex information in a moment of time. And trying to learn it in a context of great pain and emotional investment. This is our lives you're talking about. Please be thorough, but keep it simple. Tell us again, maybe even again and again, when we can hear better.
>
> From Schrey C, Schrey M: A parent's perspective: our needs and our message, *Crit Care Nurs Clin North Am* 6(1):113-119, 1994.

Severely ill newborns usually remain in the hospital. Parent-infant attachment is supported by encouraging parents to hold, touch, and look at their child and providing time and privacy for the parents to spend with their newborn.

The effect of a child with a serious heart defect on the family is complex. No member, regardless of the degree of positive adjustment, is unaffected. Mothers frequently feel inadequate in their mothering ability because of the more complex care infants with congenital heart defects require. They often feel exhausted from the pressures of caring for these children and the other family members. Fathers and siblings may feel neglected and resentful, a reaction similar to the feelings toward family members with other chronic conditions (see Chapter 41). Often, parents do not feel confident leaving the child in another's care. This often sets up a trap for parents, especially mothers, who become locked into the child's care with no relief. Although the fears are justified, they can be minimized by gradually teaching someone (a reliable relative or neighbor) how to care for the child.

The need to maintain discipline and set consistent limits can be difficult for parents. Using behavior modification techniques in the form of either concrete awards (e.g., a favorite activity) or social reinforcement (e.g., approval) can be effective. However, these techniques are most beneficial if used *before* the child learns to control the family. It is necessary to begin discussions with parents while the child is in infancy regarding the need for discipline to prevent later problems as the child gets older.

Another issue that may develop within family relationships is the child's overdependency. This is often the result of parental fear that the child may die. The nurse can help parents recognize the eventual hazards of continuing dependency and protectiveness as the child grows older and learn ways to foster optimum development. Unless parents are shown what activities the child can do, they may focus on physical limitations and encourage dependency.

The child also needs opportunities for normal social interaction with peers. These children do not need to be prevented from playing with other children because of concern regarding overexertion. Children usually limit their activities if allowed to set their own pace.

A child with CHD may constitute a long-term family crisis. Frequently the continuing unremitting stresses of care—physical exhaustion, financial costs, emotional upset, fear of death, and concern for the child's future—are not fully appreciated by those caring for the family. Even when the child's condition is stabilized or corrected, the family may need to make adjustments in their lifestyle. Introducing them to other families with similarly affected children can help them adjust to the daily stresses.

Educate Family About the Disorder

When parents are ready to hear about the heart condition, they require a clear explanation based on their level of understanding. A review of the basic structure and function of the heart is helpful before describing the defect. A simple diagram, pictures, or a model of the heart can help parents visualize the heart and the congenital defect.* Parents appreciate receiving written information about the specific condition, and a glossary of frequently used terms is helpful. Parents also require information about prognosis and treatment options.

Increasingly, families are using the Internet as a source of information about heart disease in children.† They are also finding support through contacts with other parents and parent groups. It is important for parents to realize that not all websites offer medically accurate information and that information from other parents might not be applicable to their own situation. Some children with rare, complex heart defects require individualized treatment plans, and general information on the Internet or in books may not apply to their child. Parents should discuss with their health care team, in particular their cardiologist, information they have received from other sources.

Information given to the child must be tailored to his or her developmental age. As the child matures, the level of information is revised to meet his or her new cognitive level. Preschoolers need basic information about what they will experience more than what is actually occurring physiologically. School-age children benefit from a concrete explanation of the defect. Preadolescents and adolescents often appreciate a more detailed description of how the defect affects their heart. Children of all ages need to express their feelings concerning the diagnosis.

Help Family Manage the Illness at Home

Parents are the child's principal caregivers and need to develop a positive, supportive working relationship with the health care team. Parents should be aware of the symptoms of their child's cardiac condition and signs of worsening clinical status. Parents of children who may develop CHF should be familiar with the symptoms (see Box 48-5) and know when to contact the practitioner. Parents of children with cyanosis should be informed about fluid management and hypercyanotic spells. They should have an information sheet with their child's diagnosis, significant treatments such as surgical procedures, allergies, other health care problems, current medications, and health care providers' contact numbers available in case of emergencies and to share with other caregivers such as teachers, baby-sitters, or day care providers.

The family also needs to be knowledgeable regarding the therapeutic management of the disorder and the role that surgery, other procedures, medications, and healthy lifestyle play in maintaining good health. Medications play a critical role in managing some cardiac conditions such as dysrhythmias, severe CHF, anticoagulation for artificial valves, and antirejection medications after heart transplantation. Some patients must take multiple medications daily for their lifetime. Many medications can be dangerous if taken incorrectly and require close monitoring. Parents are taught the correct procedure for giving medications and cautioned to keep them in a safe area to prevent accidental ingestion (see Family-Centered Care box, p. 1462).

Another area of parental concern is the child's level of physical activity. Most children do not need to restrict activity, and the best approach is to treat the child normally and allow self-limited activity. Exceptions to self-determined activity primarily involve strenuous recreational and competitive sports in children with specific cardiac problems. Activities and exercise restrictions should be discussed with the child's cardiologist. Deliberately attempting to prevent crying should be avoided because it can establish a maladaptive parental pattern of relating to the infant.

Infants and children with CHD require good nutrition. Breastfeeding should be possible for many infants with CHD. Providing adequate nutrition to infants with CHF or complex congenital defects is especially difficult because of their high caloric requirements and inability to suck effectively because of fatigue and tachypnea. Instructing parents in feeding methods that decrease the infant's work and giving high-calorie formula are important interventions (see p. 1463 for a discussion on feeding the infant with CHF). Children with severe cardiac defects are often anorexic. Encouraging them to eat can be a tremendous challenge. Consultation with a dietitian is often helpful. The child should be given a choice of available high-nutrient foods.

Infants with heart disease should be immunized according to the current guidelines. Immunization schedules may need to be modified around times of acute illness or surgical procedures (Smith, 2001). Infants and children less than 2 years

The booklet If Your Child Has a Congenital Heart Defect: A Guide for Parents, *as well as other information, is available from the American Heart Association, 7272 Greenville Ave., Dallas, TX 75231; 214-373-6300 or 800-AHA-USA1;* www.americanheart.org.

†*The Congenital Heart Information Network (TCHIN), First Floor, 600 N. 3rd St., Philadelphia, PA 19123-2902; 215-627-4034; fax: 215-627-4036;* http://tchin.org.

of age with unrepaired heart defects, cyanotic lesions, pulmonary hypertension, or history of prematurity should receive the vaccine for respiratory syncytial virus (RSV) monthly during RSV season (November to April in North America) (American Academy of Pediatrics, Committee on Infectious Diseases, 2006).

Infants and children who have serious heart disease are at risk for developmental delays. Multiple factors can influence neurodevelopmental outcomes, including genetics (chromosome abnormalities and microdeletions), family background (parental intelligence quotient [IQ] and socioeconomic status), preoperative factors (including prematurity, cyanosis, shock), intraoperative factors (use of cardiopulmonary bypass, deep hypothermic circulatory arrest), and postoperative factors (hemodynamic instability, hypoxia, acidosis, cardiac arrest, stroke, ischemic events). Recent efforts to limit the time of deep hypothermic circulatory arrest and provide better neuroprotection during infant surgery may improve outcomes in the future. Although most children with serious heart disease are within the normal range for IQ, there is a higher incidence of neurodevelopmental deficits in children after heart surgery than in the normal population, specifically in speech and language, fine motor skills, and cognitive processes (Majnemer & Limperopoulos, 1999). Severe neurologic problems such as cerebral palsy, epilepsy, and cognitive impairment are uncommon.

Prepare Child and Family for Invasive Procedures

Chapter 45 provides an extensive discussion of the principles for preparing children for invasive procedures. The American Heart Association published a scientific statement, "Recommendations for Preparing Children and Adolescents for Invasive Cardiac Procedures" (LeRoy et al, 2003), which addresses issues specific to the child with heart disease. The following discussion highlights some important aspects of preparation for cardiac catheterization and cardiac surgery.

The expected outcomes for preprocedure preparation include reducing anxiety, improving patient cooperation with procedures, enhancing recovery, developing trust with caregivers, and improving long-term emotional and behavioral adjustments after procedures (LeRoy et al, 2003). Important factors to consider in planning preparation strategies are the child's cognitive development, previous hospital experiences, child's temperament and coping style, timing of preparation, and involvement of the parents. The most beneficial preparation strategies usually combine information giving and coping skills training such as conscious breathing exercises, distraction techniques, guided imagery, or other behavioral interventions.

Outpatient preoperative and precatheterization workups are common for most elective procedures. Children are then admitted on the morning of the procedure. Preprocedure teaching is often done in the clinic setting or at home and may include a tour of the intensive care unit (ICU) and inpatient facilities. Children of different ages and developmental levels require different amounts of information and different approaches. Young children should be prepared close in time to the event, whereas older children and adolescents may benefit from teaching several weeks in advance. Parents should be included in the preparation session to support their child and learn about upcoming events.

A discussion of ways the child can cope with the experience should be included. Bringing a familiar stuffed animal or comfort object will help a young child relieve anxiety, whereas advising an older child to bring headphones and favorite music to the catheterization laboratory will help distract him or her during the procedure. Recovery topics after catheterization include lying still to prevent bleeding at the catheter site, advancing diet, controlling pain, and monitoring. After surgery, the nurse reviews the importance of ambulation, coughing, deep breathing, drinking, and eating and describes pain management and monitoring routines. Simple coping strategies for use during painful procedures should be reviewed; these include distraction techniques such as counting, blowing, singing, or telling stories.

Children and their families should have a choice about an ICU tour. Exposure to the ICU environment can actually increase anxiety in some children, particularly young children, those with previous hospital experiences, and those who are highly anxious (LeRoy et al, 2003). The day before the procedure is usually ample time to allow the child to ask questions and to prevent undue fantasizing about the experience. The child should be protected from the frightening sights in the unit; equipment not in view after surgery, such as equipment located behind or below the bed, needs less attention. The child and parents are encouraged to ask questions or to explore further any equipment in the room, but they should not be pushed to assimilate more information than they are able.

Provide Postoperative Care

Immediate postoperative care is usually provided by specially trained nurses in ICUs. Many of the procedures, such as arterial pressure and central venous pressure (CVP) monitoring, and the observations related to vital functions require advanced educational training (the reader should refer to critical care texts for further information). However, nurses caring for the child before surgery and during the convalescent period need to be familiar with the major principles of care. Selected complications that may occur postoperatively are described in Box 48-7.

Observe Vital Signs

Vital signs and BP are recorded frequently until stable. Heart rate and respirations are counted for 1 full minute, compared with the ECG monitor, and recorded with activity. The heart rate is normally increased after surgery. The nurse observes cardiac rhythm and notifies the practitioner of any changes in regularity. Dysrhythmias may occur postoperatively secondary to anesthetics, acid-base and electrolyte imbalance, hypoxia, surgical intervention, or trauma to conduction pathways (p. 1476).

At least hourly, the lungs are auscultated for breath sounds. Diminished or absent sounds may indicate an area of atelectasis or a pleural effusion or pneumothorax, which necessitates further medical assessment. Temperature changes are typical during the early postoperative period. Hypothermia is expected

BOX 48-7 Selected Complications After Cardiac Surgery and Treatment Approaches

Cardiac

Congestive heart failure—Digoxin, diuretics (p. 1453)
Low cardiac output—Intravenous inotropes (Shock, p. 1482)
Dysrhythmias—Identification, drug treatment, possible pacing, cardioversion (p. 1476)
Tamponade (blood or fluid in the pericardial space constricting the heart)—Prompt removal of fluid by pericardiocentesis

Respiratory

Atelectasis—Chest physical therapy, coughing, deep breathing, ambulation
Pulmonary edema—Diuretics
Pleural effusions—Diuretics, possible chest tube drainage
Pneumothorax—Possible chest tube drainage

Neurologic

Seizures—Assessment, antiepileptic drugs
Cerebrovascular accident (stroke), cerebral edema, neurologic deficits—Assessment and treatment

Infectious Disease

Infections (especially wound, pneumonia, otitis media, and sepsis)—Antibiotics

Hematologic

Anemia—Iron supplementation, possible transfusion
Postoperative bleeding—Initially, clotting factors, blood products; may need repeat surgery to locate and ligate source of bleeding

Other

Postpericardiotomy syndrome (syndrome of fever, leukocytosis, friction rub, pericardial and pleural effusions, and lethargy seen about 7 to 21 days after cardiac surgery; possible viral or autoimmune etiologies)—Antipyretics, diuretics, antiinflammatory medications

evolve Animation—Cardiac Tamponade, Infant

immediately after surgery from hypothermia procedures, effects of anesthesia, and loss of body heat to the cool environment. During this period the child is kept warm to prevent additional heat loss. Infants may be placed under radiant heat warmers. During the next 24 to 48 hours the body temperature may rise to 37.7° C (100° F) or slightly higher as part of the inflammatory response to tissue trauma. After this period an elevated temperature is most likely a sign of infection and warrants immediate investigation for probable cause.

Intraarterial monitoring of BP is commonly done after open-heart surgery. A catheter is passed into the radial artery or other artery, and the other end is attached to an electronic monitoring system, which provides a continuous recording of the BP. The intraarterial line is maintained with a low-rate, constant infusion of heparinized saline to prevent clotting.

Several IV lines are inserted preoperatively: a peripheral IV to give fluids and medications; and a CVP, which is usually inserted in a large vessel in the neck. In addition, intracardiac monitoring lines are sometimes placed intraoperatively in the right atrium, left atrium, or pulmonary artery. Intracardiac lines allow assessment of pressures inside the cardiac chambers, providing vital information about volume status, cardiac output, and ventricular function. All lines must be cared for using strict aseptic technique, and patients must be carefully assessed for bleeding at the time of line removal.

Maintain Respiratory Status

Infants usually require mechanical ventilation in the immediate postoperative period. Early extubation in the operating room or early postoperative period is becoming more common. Children, especially those who did not require cardiopulmonary bypass, may be extubated in the operating room or in the first few postoperative hours. Suctioning is performed only as needed and is performed carefully to avoid vagal stimulation (which can trigger cardiac dysrhythmias) and laryngospasm, especially in infants. Suctioning is intermittent and maintained for no more than 5 seconds at a time to avoid depleting the oxygen supply. Supplemental oxygen is administered with a manual resuscitation bag before and after the procedure to prevent hypoxia. The heart rate is monitored after suctioning to detect changes in rhythm or rate, especially bradycardia. The child should always be positioned facing the nurse to permit assessment of the child's color and tolerance of the procedure.

<u>NURSING ALERT</u> During suctioning, observe for signs and symptoms of respiratory distress, such as tachypnea, use of accessory muscles for breathing, and restlessness.

When weaning and extubation are completed, humidified oxygen is delivered by mask, hood, or nasal cannula to prevent drying of mucosa. The child is encouraged to turn and deep breathe at least hourly. Measures such as splinting the operative site and providing analgesics are used to enhance ventilation and decrease pain. Chest tubes are inserted into the pleural or mediastinal space during surgery or in the immediate postoperative period to remove secretions and air to allow reexpansion of the lung. Drainage is checked hourly for color and quantity. Immediately after surgery the drainage may be bright red, but afterward it should be serous. The largest volume of drainage occurs in the first 12 to 24 hours and is greater in extensive heart surgery.

<u>NURSING ALERT</u> Chest tube drainage greater than 3 ml/kg/hr for more than 3 consecutive hours or 5 to 10 ml/kg in any 1 hour is excessive and may indicate postoperative hemorrhage. The surgeon is notified immediately because cardiac tamponade can develop rapidly and is life threatening.

Chest tubes are usually removed on the first to third postoperative day. Removal of chest tubes is a painful, frightening experience. Analgesics such as morphine sulfate, often combined with midazolam (Versed), should be given before the procedure. Older children are forewarned that they will feel a sharp, momentary pain. After the suture is cut, the tubes are quickly pulled out at the end of full inspiration to prevent intake of air into the pleural cavity. A purse-string suture (placed when the tubes were inserted) is pulled tight to close the opening. A petrolatum-covered gauze dressing is immediately applied over the wound and securely taped on all four sides to the skin so that an airtight seal is formed. It is left on for 1 or 2 days. Breath sounds are checked to assess for a pneumothorax.

Monitor Fluids

Intake and output of all fluids must be accurately calculated. Intake is primarily IV fluids; however, a record of fluid used to flush the arterial and CVP lines or to dilute medications is also kept. Output includes hourly recordings of urine (usually a Foley catheter is inserted and attached to a closed collecting device), drainage from chest and nasogastric tubes, and blood drawn for analysis. Urine is analyzed for specific gravity to assess the concentrating ability of the kidneys and the body's approximate degree of hydration. Renal failure is a potential risk from a transient period of low cardiac output.

NURSING ALERT The signs of renal failure are decreased urinary output (less than 1 ml/kg/hr) and elevated levels of blood urea nitrogen and serum creatinine.

Fluids are restricted during the immediate postoperative period to prevent hypervolemia, which places additional demands on the myocardium, predisposing the patient to cardiac failure. To monitor fluid retention, the child is weighed daily, and the same scale is used at approximately the same time each day to avoid errors in measurement. The child is usually given nothing by mouth for the first 24 hours. If an endotracheal (ET) tube is inserted, oral fluids are usually withheld until the child is extubated. Fluid restriction may be imposed even when oral fluids are given. The nurse calculates the distribution over a 24-hour period based on the child's preoperative weight and drinking habits. The distribution should allow for most fluid to be given during the child's most wakeful and active periods.

Provide Rest and Progressive Activity

After heart surgery, rest should be provided to decrease the workload of the heart and promote healing. The simplest way to ensure individualized, efficient, high-quality care is to plan at the beginning of the shift the nursing procedures to be done, with periods of rest identified. The schedule should be shared with parents to allow them to visit at the most advantageous times, such as after a rest period when no special treatments are anticipated.

A progressive schedule of ambulation and activity is planned, based on the child's preoperative activity patterns and postoperative cardiovascular and pulmonary function. Ambulation is initiated early, usually by the second postoperative day, when chest tubes, arterial lines, and assisted ventilatory equipment may be removed. Activity progresses from sitting on the edge of the bed and dangling the legs to standing up and sitting in a chair. Heart rate and respirations are carefully monitored to assess the degree of cardiac demand imposed by each activity. Tachycardia, dyspnea, cyanosis, desaturation, progressive fatigue, or dysrhythmias indicate the need to limit further energy expenditure.

Provide Comfort and Emotional Support

Heart surgery is both painful and frightening for children, and comfort is a primary nursing concern. Several incisions may be used for heart surgery. A median sternotomy is most common, following the sternum down the center of the chest. A ministernotomy opens the lower sternum. A thoracotomy incision is most uncomfortable because it goes through muscle tissue. It allows access to the side of the chest through an incision from under the arm around the back to the scapula.

Most patients need IV analgesics for pain control during the immediate postoperative period. Patient-controlled analgesia may be used with children old enough to understand the concept. Nonsteroidal antiinflammatory drugs (NSAIDs) such as ketorolac (Toradol) may be used intravenously. Paralyzing agents may also be used with the analgesics for children who are agitated or hemodynamically unstable.

After extubation and removal of lines and tubes, pain can be controlled satisfactorily with oral medications such as ibuprofen, codeine with acetaminophen (Tylenol No. 3), or oxycodone and acetaminophen (Tylox). Acetaminophen alone provides adequate pain relief for most children at discharge. Sternotomy incisions are usually well tolerated, with some discomfort when walking and coughing. Thoracotomy incisions are usually more painful because the incision is through muscle; a more aggressive pain management plan with around-the-clock medications for several days is often necessary to allow for adequate rest, ambulation, and pulmonary hygiene.

In addition to pharmacologic pain control, every effort is made to minimize the discomfort of procedures, such as using a firm pillow or favorite stuffed animal placed against the chest incision during movement and when performing treatments *after* pain medication is given, preferably at a time that coincides with the drug's peak effect. Nonpharmacologic measures are used to lessen the perception of pain, and parents are encouraged to comfort their child as much as possible. (See also Pain Assessment; Pain Management, Chapter 35.)

Children may become depressed after surgery. This is thought to be caused by preoperative anxiety, postoperative psychologic and physiologic stress, and sensory overstimulation. Typically the child's disposition improves on leaving the ICU. Children may also be angry and uncooperative after surgery as a response to the physical pain and the loss of control imposed by the surgery and treatments. They need an opportunity to express feelings, either verbally or through activity.

Plan for Discharge and Home Care

Ideally, discharge planning begins on admission for cardiac surgery and includes an assessment of the parents' adjustment to the child's altered state of health. Neonates need additional screening tests (such as newborn metabolic screen and hearing tests) and may need immunizations before discharge (Dodds & Merle, 2005). The family needs both verbal and written instructions on medication, nutrition, activity restrictions, subacute bacterial endocarditis, return to school, wound care, and signs and symptoms of infection or complications (see Patient Teaching box). Referrals to community agencies may be warranted to assist parents in the transition from hospital to home and to reinforce the teaching.

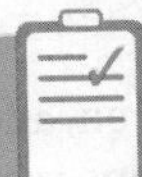

PATIENT TEACHING Topics to Include in Discharge Teaching After Cardiac Surgery

- Medication teaching (for digoxin, see Family-Centered Care box, p. 1462)
- Activity restrictions
- Diet and nutrition
- Wound care (including dressings, if any; suture removal; bathing)
- Bacterial endocarditis prophylaxis (see Box 48-9)
- Follow-up appointments (cardiologist, primary care provider)
- Community agencies as needed (visiting nurse service, early developmental intervention)
- When to call practitioner; signs and symptoms of postoperative problems
- Review of cardiac defect and surgical repair

The parents also need clear instructions on when to seek medical care for complications and how to contact the health care provider. Follow-up with the cardiologist and primary care provider is arranged before discharge. Parents should have a summary, including their child's medical condition, medications, and health care providers available for emergencies. Appropriate identification, such as a MedicAlert device, is indicated for children with a pacemaker or heart transplant and for those receiving anticoagulation therapy or antidysrhythmic medication.

Although surgical correction of heart defects has improved dramatically, it is still not possible to completely repair many of the complex anomalies. For many children, repeat procedures are required to replace conduits or grafts or to manage complications such as restenosis. Consequently, the long-term prognosis is uncertain, and full recovery is not always possible. For these families, medical follow-up and continued emotional support are essential. The nurse can often serve as an important primary health professional and as a resource for referrals when needed.

Acquired Cardiovascular Disorders

Bacterial (Infective) Endocarditis

Bacterial endocarditis (BE), or infective endocarditis (IE), also referred to as *subacute bacterial endocarditis (SBE)*, is an infection of the valves and inner lining of the heart. Although it can occur without underlying heart disease, it is most often a sequela of bacteremia in the child with acquired or congenital anomalies of the heart or great vessels. It especially affects children with valvular abnormalities, prosthetic valves, shunts, recent cardiac surgery with invasive lines, and rheumatic heart disease with valve involvement. The most common causative agent is *Streptococcus viridans;* other causative agents are *Staphylococcus aureus,* gram-negative bacteria, and fungi such as *Candida albicans.*

Pathophysiology

Organisms may enter the bloodstream from any site of localized infection. In the past, endocarditis was believed to be highly associated with invasive procedures; however, it most likely occurs from routine exposure to bacteremia associated with usual daily activities, although it can also occur after procedures such as dental work *(S. viridans);* after invasive procedures involving the gastrointestinal-genitourinary tract; after cardiac surgery, especially if synthetic material is used (valves, patches, conduits); or from long-term indwelling catheters. The microorganisms grow on the endocardium, forming vegetations (verrucae), deposits of fibrin, and platelet thrombi. The lesion may invade adjacent tissues, such as aortic and mitral valves, and may break off and embolize elsewhere, especially in the spleen, kidney, and central nervous system.

BOX 48-8 Clinical Manifestations of Infective Endocarditis

Onset usually insidious
Unexplained fever (low grade and intermittent)
Anorexia
Malaise
Weight loss
Characteristic findings caused by extracardiac emboli formation:
- Splinter hemorrhages (thin black lines) under the nails
- Osler nodes (red, painful intradermal nodes found on pads of phalanges)
- Janeway lesions (painless hemorrhagic areas on palms and soles)
- Petechiae on oral mucous membranes

May be present:
- Congestive heart failure
- Cardiac dysrhythmias
- New murmur or change in previously existing one

Diagnostic Evaluation

The diagnosis of IE is suspected on the basis of clinical manifestations (Box 48-8). Several laboratory findings may suggest IE (e.g., ECG changes [prolonged PR interval], radiographic evidence of cardiomegaly, anemia, elevated erythrocyte sedimentation rate, leukocytosis, microscopic hematuria). Vegetations on the valve and abnormal valve function can often be visualized by echocardiography. Definitive diagnosis rests on growth and identification of the causative agent in the blood.

Therapeutic Management

Treatment should be instituted immediately and consists of administration of high doses of appropriate antibiotics intravenously for 2 to 8 weeks. Blood cultures are taken periodically to evaluate response to antibiotic therapy.

Prevention involves administration of prophylactic antibiotic therapy 1 hour before procedures known to increase the risk of entry of organisms in very high risk patients. New guidelines only require prophylaxis in patients with the highest risk of poor outcome if they develop endocarditis (Box 48-9). Drugs of choice for prophylaxis include amoxicillin, ampicillin, clindamycin, cephalexin, cefadroxil, azithromycin, and clarithromycin.

BOX 48-9 Cardiac Conditions Associated with the Highest Risk of Adverse Outcome from Endocarditis

Prophylaxis with dental procedures recommended for*:
- Previous episode of infective endocarditis
- Prosthetic cardiac valve

Congenital heart disease (CHD), including only:
- Unrepaired cyanotic CHD, including palliative shunts and conduits
- Completely repaired congenital heart defect with prosthetic material or device, whether placed by surgery or catheter intervention, during the first 6 months after the procedure

Repaired CHD with residual defects at the site of or adjacent to the site of a prosthetic patch or prosthetic device (which inhibit endothelialization)

Cardiac transplantation recipients who develop cardiac valvulopathy

Adapted from Wilson W et al: Prevention of infective endocarditis: guidelines from the American Heart Association, *Circulation* 116(15):1736-1754, 2007.

*Except for the conditions listed, antibiotic prophylaxis is no longer recommended for any other form of CHD.

Nursing Care Management

Ideally, the objective of nursing care is to counsel parents of high risk children concerning the signs and symptoms of endocarditis and in certain cases the need for prophylactic antibiotic therapy before procedures such as dental work. The family's regular dentist should be advised of the child's cardiac diagnosis as an added precaution to ensure preventive treatment. SBE prophylaxis is now reserved for very high risk patients. Many patients who met criteria established in the past may not require prophylaxis under the new guidelines (Wilson et al, 2007) (see Box 48-9). It is important that all children with congenital or acquired heart disease maintain the highest level of oral health to reduce the chance of bacteremia from oral infections.

Parents should also have a high index of suspicion regarding potential infections. Without unduly alarming them, the nurse stresses that any unexplained fever, weight loss, or change in behavior (lethargy, malaise, anorexia) must be brought to the practitioner's attention. Such symptoms should not be self-diagnosed as a cold or flu. Early diagnosis and treatment are important in preventing further cardiac damage, embolic complications, and growth of resistant organisms.

Treatment of endocarditis requires long-term parenteral drug therapy. In many cases, IV antibiotics may be administered at home with nursing supervision for part of the treatment course. Nursing goals during this period are (1) preparation of the child for IV infusion, usually with an intermittent-infusion device, and several venipunctures for blood cultures; (2) observation for side effects of antibiotics, especially inflammation along venipuncture sites; (3) observation for complications, including embolism and CHF; and (4) education regarding the importance of follow-up visits for cardiac evaluation, echocardiographic monitoring, and blood cultures.

Rheumatic Fever

Rheumatic fever (RF) is a poorly understood inflammatory disease that occurs after infection with group A β-hemolytic streptococcal (GABHS) pharyngitis. It occurs most often in late school-age children or adolescents and is rare in adults. It is a self-limited illness that involves the joints, skin, brain, serous surfaces, and heart. Cardiac valve damage (referred to as *rheumatic heart disease*) is the most significant complication of RF. The mitral valve is most often affected. In developed countries RF and rheumatic heart disease have become uncommon. However, RF remains a devastating problem in developing (Third World) countries and has reappeared in some parts of the United States (Gentles et al, 2001).

Etiology

Strong evidence supports a relationship between upper respiratory tract infection with GABHS and subsequent development of RF (usually within 2 to 6 weeks). Acute RF is the result of an exaggerated immune response to bacteria in a susceptible host (Carapetis, McDonald, & Wilson, 2005). In almost all cases of RF a previous infection with GABHS can be documented by laboratory evidence of rising antibody titers. Prevention or treatment of GABHS infection prevents RF.

Diagnostic Evaluation

Diagnosis is based on a set of guidelines recommended by the American Heart Association (Newburger et al, 2004). These guidelines, known as *modifications of the Jones criteria*, suggest that the presence of two major manifestations or one major and two minor manifestations, such as fever and arthralgia, with supportive evidence of recent streptococcal infection, indicates a high probability of RF (see Guidelines box).

Children suspected of having RF are tested for streptococcal antibodies. The most reliable and best standardized test is an elevated or rising *antistreptolysin O (ASO or ASLO) titer*, which occurs in 80% of children with RF.

Therapeutic Management

The goals of medical management are (1) eradication of hemolytic streptococci, (2) prevention of permanent cardiac damage, (3) palliation of the other symptoms, and (4) prevention of recurrences of RF. Penicillin is the drug of choice, with erythromycin as a substitute in penicillin-sensitive children. Salicylates are used to control the inflammatory process, especially in the joints, and reduce the fever and discomfort. Bed rest is recommended during the acute febrile phase but need not be strict.

Prophylactic treatment against recurrence of RF is started after the acute therapy and involves monthly intramuscular injections of benzathine penicillin G (1.2 million units), two daily oral doses of penicillin (200,000 units), or one daily dose of sulfadiazine (1 g). The duration of long-term prophylaxis is uncertain, but 5 years since the last episode or age 18, longer with cardiac involvement, is suggested by the World Health Organization (Carapetis, McDonald, and Wilson, 2005).

Children who have had acute RF are susceptible to recurrent RF for the rest of their lives and should be followed

GUIDELINES Diagnosis of Initial Attack of Rheumatic Fever (Jones Criteria, 1992 Update)*

Major Manifestations

Carditis

Tachycardia out of proportion to degree of fever
Cardiomegaly
New murmurs or change in preexisting murmurs
Muffled heart sounds
Pericardial friction rub
Chest pain
Changes in electrocardiogram (especially prolonged PR interval)

Polyarthritis

Swollen, hot, red, painful joint(s)
After 1 to 2 days, different joint(s) affected
Favors large joints—knees, elbows, hips, shoulders, wrists

Erythema Marginatum

Erythematous macules with clear center and wavy, well-demarcated border
Transitory
Nonpruritic
Primarily affects trunk and extremities (inner surfaces)

Chorea (St. Vitus Dance, Sydenham Chorea)

Sudden aimless, irregular movements of extremities
Involuntary facial grimaces
Speech disturbances
Emotional lability
Muscle weakness (can be profound)
Muscle movements exaggerated by anxiety and attempts at fine motor activity; relieved by rest

Subcutaneous Nodes

Nontender swelling
Located over bony prominences
May persist for some time and then gradually resolve

Minor Manifestations

Clinical Findings

Arthralgia
Fever

Laboratory Findings

Elevated acute-phase reactants
- Erythrocyte sedimentation rate
- C-reactive protein

Supporting Evidence of Antecedent Group A Streptococcal Infection

Positive throat culture or rapid streptococcal antigen test
Elevated or rising streptococcal antibody titer

From Special Writing Group of the Committee on Rheumatic Fever, Endocarditis, and Kawasaki Disease of the Council on Cardiovascular Disease in the Young of the American Heart Association: Guidelines for the diagnosis of rheumatic fever: Jones criteria, 1992 (update), *JAMA* 268:2069-2073, 1992.

*If supported by evidence of preceding group A streptococcal infection, the presence of two major manifestations or of one major and two minor manifestations indicates a high probability of acute rheumatic fever.

medically for at least 5 years. Repeated infections are likely to result in rheumatic heart disease. Children and families must be aware of the need for continuing antibiotic prophylaxis for dental work, infection, and invasive procedures.

Nursing Care Management

The objectives of nursing care for the child with RF are to (1) encourage compliance with drug regimens, (2) facilitate recovery from the illness, (3) provide emotional support, and (4) prevent the disease. Because compliance is a major concern in long-term drug therapy, every effort is made to encourage adherence to the therapeutic plan (see Compliance, Chapter 45). When compliance is poor, monthly injections may be substituted for daily oral administration of antibiotics, and children need preparation for this often-dreaded procedure.

Interventions during home care are primarily concerned with providing rest and adequate nutrition. Usually, after the febrile stage is over, children can resume moderate activity, and their appetite improves. If carditis is present, the family must be aware of any activity restrictions and may need help in choosing less strenuous activities for the child.

One of the most disturbing and frustrating manifestations of the disease is *chorea*. The onset is gradual and may occur weeks to months after the illness; it sometimes even occurs in children who have not been diagnosed with RF. It may be mistaken for nervousness, clumsiness, behavioral changes, inattentiveness, and learning disability. It is usually a source of great frustration to the child because the movements, incoordination, and weakness severely limit physical ability. Of utmost importance is stressing to parents and schoolteachers the involuntary, sudden nature of the movements; that the chorea is transitory; and that all manifestations eventually disappear.

Nurses also have a role in prevention, primarily in screening school-age children for sore throats caused by GABHS. This may involve actively participating in throat culture screening programs or referring children with a possible streptococcal infection for testing.

Hyperlipidemia (Hypercholesterolemia)

Hyperlipidemia is a general term for excessive lipids (fat and fatlike substances); *hypercholesterolemia* refers to excessive cholesterol in the blood. High lipid or cholesterol levels play an important role in producing atherosclerosis (fatty plaque on the arteries), which eventually can lead to coronary artery disease, a primary cause of morbidity and mortality in the adult population. A presymptomatic phase of atherosclerosis can begin in childhood. Preventive cardiology is focusing on the screening and management of lipid levels in childhood. The goal is to identify children at high risk and intervene early.

Cholesterol is part of the lipoprotein complex in plasma that is essential for cellular metabolism. Triglycerides, natural fats synthesized from carbohydrates, are used for energy. Both are major lipids transported on *lipoproteins*, a combination of lipids and proteins, which include:

Low-density lipoproteins (LDLs)—These contain low concentrations of triglycerides, high levels of cholesterol, and moderate levels of protein. LDL is the major carrier of cholesterol to the cells. Cells use cholesterol for synthesis of membranes and steroid production. Elevated circulating LDL is a strong risk factor in cardiovascular disease.

High-density lipoproteins (HDLs)—These contain very low concentrations of triglycerides, relatively little cholesterol, and high levels of protein. They transport free cholesterol to the liver for excretion in the bile. High levels of HDL are thought to protect against cardiovascular disease.

Diagnostic Evaluation

Hyperlipidemia is diagnosed on the basis of analysis of blood for a full lipid profile, drawn after a 12-hour fast. A screening thyroid-stimulating hormone (TSH) is useful to rule out hypothyroidism as a cause of secondary hypercholesterolemia. In overweight children, a fasting glucose may be obtained to assess for the potential of *metabolic syndrome,* which is a combination of multiple symptoms that are associated with increased cardiovascular risk in adults. Blood samples should be collected after having the child sit for 5 minutes, and the tourniquet should be applied immediately before the needle puncture, since posture and vascular stasis may affect results. Diagnostic values for acceptable, borderline, and high total cholesterol and LDL cholesterol levels are listed in Table 48-5.

Screening children for hypercholesterolemia is a controversial issue; some authorities advocate universal screening, and others propose selective screening. Guidelines from the American Academy of Pediatrics' Committee on Nutrition (American Academy of Pediatrics, 1998) recommend a strategy that combines two complementary approaches: (1) a *population approach* that aims to lower the average levels of blood cholesterol among all American children through population-wide changes in nutrient intake and eating patterns, and (2) an *individualized approach* based on selective screening.

Therapeutic Management

The first step in the treatment of high cholesterol is oriented to lifestyle modification. The American Academy of Pediatrics (1998) guidelines advocate a heart-healthy diet for all children. Children with known elevated cholesterol should have individual nutritional counseling by a nutritionist with expertise in pediatric lipids.

Research continues to support the benefit of diets low in saturated fats (Van Horn et al, 2005). Current thinking favors a "Mediterranean"-type diet. Whole grains, fruits, and vegetables form the foundation of this diet. In addition, this diet allows the use of monounsaturated fats, such as olive oil and canola oil, which have beneficial effects on HDL cholesterol values. The use of these fats also makes the diet more realistic. Daily aerobic exercise of at least 60 minutes a day is also recommended for children with high cholesterol. In addition, patients and parents should be counseled regarding the negative effects of smoking (both first hand and second hand).

Table 48-5 Classification of Cholesterol Levels in Children from Families with a History of Heart Disease

CATEGORY	TOTAL CHOLESTEROL (mg/dl)	LDL CHOLESTEROL (mg/dl)
Acceptable	<170	<110
Borderline	170-199	110-129
High	≥200	≥130

From National Cholesterol Education Program: Report of the Expert Panel on Blood Cholesterol Levels in Children and Adolescents, *Pediatrics* 89(3 Pt 2):527, 1992.
LDL, Low-density lipoprotein.

For children with severe hypercholesterolemia who fail to respond to dietary modifications (after a 6- to 12-month trial), drug therapy may be necessary. Pharmacologic therapy is recommended for children with LDL cholesterol over 190 mg/dl without other risk factors or over 160 mg/dl in patients with two or more other risk factors. In most situations medication is reserved for boys over 10 years old and for girls once they begin their menses.

In the past bile acid–binding resins were the only class of drugs recommended for treatment of children. This class of drug acts by binding bile acids in the intestinal lumen. Because they are not absorbed by the intestine, they do not produce systemic toxicity and are safe for children. Cholestyramine (Questran) and colestipol (Colestid) are both powders that are mixed with water or juice just before ingestion. Unfortunately, bile acid–binding resins do not adequately reduce LDL cholesterol in the vast majority of patients. Many cannot tolerate the medication because of the taste; gritty texture; and side effects, the most significant being constipation, abdominal pain, gastrointestinal bloating, flatulence, and nausea. The most recent findings on lipid abnormalities in children recommend treatment with statins if pharmacologic therapy is indicated, using the previously outlined guidelines for treatment (McCrindle et al, 2007). Statins are much more effective at lowering LDL cholesterol and triglycerides and raising HDL cholesterol. They work by inhibiting the enzyme necessary for cholesterol synthesis, are most effective when taken in the evening, and are started at the lowest possible dose in young people. Blood work should be followed closely and should include a fasting lipid profile, liver function tests, and creatinine kinase repeated at 4- and 8-week intervals initially and with dosage changes.

Patients beginning therapy with a statin should be counseled regarding rare but potentially serious side effects such as rhabdomyolysis, elevated transaminases, and elevated creatinine kinase. They should discontinue their medication and contact their practitioner if they develop dark urine or new muscle aches. Finally, statin medications are not safe during pregnancy; therefore sexually active adolescents need to take adequate birth control measures. Very long–term studies are unlikely to be available over decades; however, in the shorter-term studies that have been completed, statins seem to have a similar safety profile for children as they do for adults (McCrindle et al, 2007).

✱ Nursing Care Management

Nurses play an important role in the screening, education, and support of children with hyperlipidemia and their families. When a child is referred to a lipid clinic, it is essential that the family be adequately prepared for the first visit. Generally, the parents are asked to keep a dietary history of the child before this visit. Sometimes they need to complete a questionnaire regarding the child's normal dietary habits during the preceding year. Families should be instructed to keep their child fasting for at least 12 hours before screening. It is important to schedule the blood test early in the morning and arrange for nourishment immediately thereafter. At the visit a full family history should be taken, including the health of both parents and all first-degree relatives. Specific questions should be asked regarding early heart disease, hypertension, strokes (CVAs), sudden death, hyperlipidemia, diabetes, and endocrine abnormalities.

Stringent dietary guidelines may become an issue of control and a source of great stress for many families. Children should not be viewed as having a disease. Rather, the positive aspects of healthy eating, exercising regularly, and avoiding smoking should be emphasized. Basic dietary changes should be encouraged for the whole family so that the affected child is not singled out. Cultural differences must be considered, and recommendations individualized. Substitution rather than elimination needs to be emphasized. Visual aids (e.g., test tubes depicting the amount of fat in a hot dog) are often helpful, especially for children. Diets should be flexible and individually tailored by a nutritionist experienced in combining recommendations that meet both the nutritional demands of the growing child and the lipid modifications. Parents are encouraged to participate in dietary and educational sessions, ask questions, and share ideas and experiences.

Parents of children who require pharmacologic therapy need to understand the purpose, dosage, and possible side effects of the various drugs. Medication schedules should remain flexible and should not interfere with the child's daily activities. Follow-up phone calls by the nurse between visits allow parents to discuss their concerns and ask any questions that have arisen.

Cardiac Dysrhythmias

Dysrhythmias, or abnormal heart rhythms, can occur in children with structurally normal hearts, as features of some congenital heart defects, and in patients after surgical repair of congenital heart defects. They are also seen in patients with cardiomyopathy and cardiac tumors and can occur secondary to metabolic and electrolyte imbalances. They can be classified in several ways, including by heart rate characteristics (bradycardia and tachycardia) and by the origin of the dysrhythmia in the atria or ventricles. Some dysrhythmias are well tolerated and self-limiting. Others may cause decreased cardiac output with associated symptoms, and some can cause sudden death. Treatment depends on the cause of the dysrhythmia and its severity.

Many advances have been made in the diagnosis and treatment of pediatric dysrhythmias in the past decade. Improvements in technology have allowed better diagnosis, the development of ablation techniques, and the expansion of pacemaker capabilities. New antidysrhythmic medications have proved safe and effective in children. Radiofrequency ablation has offered a cure for some dysrhythmias. Pediatric electrophysiology has become a highly specialized field, and the student should consult more detailed sources for an in-depth discussion. The following sections address diagnostic studies and provide a general discussion of the most common tachycardia (supraventricular tachycardia [SVT]) and the most common bradycardia (complete heart block) that require treatment in the pediatric population.

Diagnostic Evaluation

Nurses must be familiar with the standards of normal heart rate for the particular age group. An initial nursing responsibility is recognition of a heartbeat that is abnormal in either rate or rhythm. When a dysrhythmia is suspected, the apical rate is counted for a full minute and compared with the radial rate, which may be lower because not all of the apical beats are felt. Consistently high or low heart rates should be regarded as suspicious. The patient should be placed on a cardiac monitor with recording capabilities. A 12-lead ECG yields more information than the monitor recording and should be done as soon as possible.

The basic diagnostic procedure is the ECG, including 24-hour Holter monitoring. *Electrophysiologic cardiac catheterization* allows for identification of the conduction disturbance and immediate investigation of drugs that may control the dysrhythmia. Another procedure that may be used is *transesophageal recording.* An electrode catheter is passed to the lower esophagus and, when in position at a point proximal to the heart, is used to stimulate and record dysrhythmias.

Dysrhythmias can be classified according to various criteria, such as effect on heart rate and rhythm, as follows:

Bradydysrhythmias—Abnormally slow rate
Tachydysrhythmias—Abnormally rapid rate
Conduction disturbances—Irregular heart rate

Bradydysrhythmias

Sinus bradycardia (slower than normal rate) in children can be caused by the influence of the autonomic nervous system, as with hypervagal tone, or in response to hypoxia and hypotension. Sinus bradycardias are also known to develop after some complex cardiac surgical repairs involving extensive atrial suture lines such as atrial baffle repairs (Mustard and Senning repairs) and the Fontan procedure.

Complete atrioventricular block (AV block) is also referred to as *complete heart block.* This can be either congenital (occurring in children with structurally normal hearts) or acquired after surgery to repair cardiac defects. AV blocks are most often related to edema around the conduction system and resolve without treatment. Temporary epicardial wires are placed in most patients at surgery; if a rhythm disturbance occurs, temporary pacing can be used. Several days after surgery, the health practitioner removes the wires by pulling slowly and deliberately down on them from the site of insertion.

Some children may need a permanent pacemaker. The pacemaker takes over or assists in the heart's conduction function. The implantation of a pacemaker, in the operating room or possibly the catheterization laboratory, is usually a low risk procedure. The pacemaker is made up of two basic parts: the pulse generator and the lead. The pulse generator is composed of the battery and the electronic circuitry. The lead is an insulated, flexible wire that conducts the electrical impulse from the pulse generator to the heart. Two types of leads are available: transvenous and epicardial. After the lead has been attached to the heart, a small incision is made, and a pocket is formed under the muscle to house and protect the generator. Continuous ECG monitoring is necessary during the recovery phase to assess pacemaker function. The nurse should be aware of the programmed rate and expected individual generator variations. The pacemaker insertion site is monitored for signs of infection. Analgesics are given for pain.

Pacemaker functions have become more sophisticated, and some models can adjust heart rate to activity demands or be programmed for overdrive pacing or cardioversion (see Patient Teaching box).

PATIENT TEACHING Discharge Teaching for the Child with a Pacemaker

Discharge teaching includes information about the signs and symptoms of infection, general wound care, and activity restrictions. Parents and patients, if they are old enough, should be taught to take a pulse and know the settings of the pacemaker. If the patient's low rate is set at 80 beats/min and the heart rate is only 68 beats/min, there is a possible problem with the pacemaker that needs to be investigated. Instructions for telephone transmission of electrogram (ECG) readings are also given. Telephone transmission can be used to transmit ECG strips and also to monitor battery life and pacemaker function. The pacemaker generator will have to be replaced periodically because of battery depletion. Children with pacemakers should wear a medical alert device, and their parents should have a paper identification card with specific pacer data in case of an emergency. Cardiopulmonary resuscitation instruction is suggested for parents.

Tachydysrhythmias

Sinus tachycardia (abnormally fast heart rate) secondary to fever, anxiety, pain, anemia, dehydration, or any other etiologic factor requiring increased cardiac output should be ruled out before diagnosing an increased heart rate as pathologic. SVT is the most common tachydysrhythmia found in children and refers to a rapid regular heart rate of 200 to 300 beats/min. The onset of SVT is often sudden, the duration is variable, and the rhythm may end abruptly and convert back to a normal sinus rhythm. Clinical signs in infants and young children are poor feeding, extreme irritability, and pallor. Children may experience palpitations, dizziness, chest pain, and diaphoresis. If SVT is sustained, signs of CHF may be seen.

The treatment of SVT depends on the degree of compromise imposed by the dysrhythmia. In some cases vagal maneuvers, such as applying ice to the face, massaging the carotid artery (on one side of the neck only), or having an older child perform a Valsalva maneuver (e.g., exhaling against a closed glottis, blowing on a thumb as if it were a trumpet for 30 to 60 seconds), have terminated SVT. If vagal maneuvers fail or the child is hemodynamically unstable, adenosine (a drug that impairs AV conduction) may be used. Adenosine is given by rapid IV push with a saline bolus immediately after the drug because of its very short half-life. If this is unsuccessful or cardiac output is compromised, esophageal overdrive pacing or synchronized cardioversion (delivering an electrical shock to the heart) can be used in the intensive care setting. Sedation is needed for both procedures. Cardioversion should never be done in a conscious patient. More long-term pharmacologic treatment includes digoxin or possibly propranolol (Inderal) or amiodarone for severe or recurrent SVT.

A primary focus of nursing care is education of the family regarding the symptoms of SVT and its treatment. SVT may occur again despite therapy. Parents should be taught to take a radial pulse for a full minute. If medication is prescribed, instructions regarding accurate dosage and the importance of administering the correct dose at specified intervals are stressed.

Radiofrequency ablation has become first-line therapy for some types of SVT. The procedure is done in the cardiac catheterization laboratory and begins with mapping of the conduction system to identify the dysrhythmia focus. A catheter delivering radiofrequency current is directed at the site, and the area is heated to destroy the tissue in the area. These are lengthy procedures, often 6 to 8 hours, and sedation or general anesthesia is required. Preparation is similar to that for cardiac catheterization.

Pulmonary Artery Hypertension

Pulmonary artery hypertension (PAH) describes a group of rare disorders that result in an elevation of pulmonary artery pressure above 25 mm Hg at rest after the neonatal period (Barst, 1999). These disorders are poorly understood, and until recently there was no treatment beyond supportive care. PAH is a progressive, eventually fatal disease for which there is no known cure. It can be difficult to diagnose in the early stages. Often when patients become symptomatic and a diagnosis is made, their disease is rapidly progressing, treatment is unsuccessful, and death occurs within several years. Significant new information about the disease process, genetic links, diagnosis, and treatment has recently been learned that may improve treatments and outcomes for these patients.

PAH affects the small pulmonary arteries and is characterized by vascular narrowing leading to an increase in pulmonary vascular resistance. Why some children develop the disease and others do not is unclear. There are many possible causes of PAH. Cardiac causes occur primarily in patients with a large left-to-right shunt producing increased pulmonary blood flow. If these defects are not repaired early, the high pulmonary flow will cause changes in the pulmonary artery vessels, and the vessels will lose their elasticity. Other causes of PAH include hypoxic lung diseases, thromboembolic diseases causing pulmonary vascular obstruction, collagen vascular diseases, and exposure to toxic substances. Many of the patients have no identifiable cause for PAH and have primary or idiopathic PAH.

Clinical Manifestations

The clinical manifestations include dyspnea with exercise, chest pain, and syncope. Dyspnea is the most common symptom and is caused by impaired oxygen delivery. Chest pain is the result of coronary ischemia in the right ventricle from severe hypertrophy. Syncope reflects a limited cardiac output leading to decreased cerebral blood flow. Right-sided heart dysfunction is steadily progressive; when symptoms of venous congestion and edema are present, prognosis is poor.

Therapeutic Management

Although no cure is known, several therapies have shown promise in slowing the progression of the disease and improving quality of life. In general, situations that may exacerbate the disease and cause hypoxia, such as exercise and high altitudes, are avoided. Supplemental oxygen, especially at night while sleeping, is commonly used to relieve hypoxia. Patients are at risk for thromboembolic events leading to pulmonary emboli; thus anticoagulation with warfarin (Coumadin) is often prescribed.

Vasodilator therapy (which relaxes vascular smooth muscle and reduces pulmonary artery pressure) has prolonged the survival of patients with PAH. Oral calcium channel blockers have been successful in some children. Continuous IV prostacyclin has been used with some success in children who did not respond to oral therapy. Although promising, both these therapies have been used in only small numbers of patients and are expensive. Lung transplantation may be another treatment option.

Cardiomyopathy

Cardiomyopathy refers to abnormalities of the myocardium in which the cardiac muscles' ability to contract is impaired. Cardiomyopathies are relatively rare in children. Possible etiologic factors include familial or genetic causes, infection, deficiency states, metabolic abnormalities, and collagen vascular diseases. Most cardiomyopathies in children are considered primary or idiopathic, in which the cause is unknown and the cardiac dysfunction is not associated with systemic disease. Some of the known causes of *secondary* cardiomyopathy are anthracycline toxicity (the antineoplastic agents doxorubicin [Adriamycin] and daunomycin), hemochromatosis (from excessive iron storage), Duchenne muscular dystrophy, Kawasaki disease (KD), collagen diseases, and thyroid dysfunction.

Cardiomyopathies can be divided into three broad clinical categories according to the type of abnormal structure and dysfunction present: dilated cardiomyopathy, hypertrophic cardiomyopathy, and restrictive cardiomyopathy.

Dilated cardiomyopathy is characterized by ventricular dilation and greatly decreased contractility resulting in symptoms of CHF. This is the most common type of cardiomyopathy in children. Its cause is often unknown. The clinical findings are of CHF with tachycardia, dyspnea, hepatosplenomegaly, fatigue, and poor growth. Dysrhythmias may be present and may be more difficult to control with worsening heart failure.

Hypertrophic cardiomyopathy is characterized by an increase in heart muscle mass without an increase in cavity size, usually occurring in the left ventricle and associated with abnormal diastolic filling. It is a familial autosomal dominant genetic abnormality in most cases and is probably the most common genetically transmitted cardiovascular disease (Maron, 2001). The expression of clinical disease varies greatly among patients. Clinical symptoms usually appear in the school-age period or adolescence and may include anginal chest pain, dysrhythmias, and syncope. Sudden death is possible. Presentation in infancy includes signs of CHF and has a poor prognosis. The ECG demonstrates left ventricular hypertrophy, often with ST-T changes. The echocardiogram is most helpful and demonstrates asymmetric septal hypertrophy and an increase in left ventricular wall thickness with a small left ventricle cavity.

Restrictive cardiomyopathy, rare in children, describes a restriction to ventricular filling caused by endocardial or myocardial disease or both. It is characterized by diastolic dysfunction and absence of ventricular dilation or hypertrophy. Symptoms are similar to those of CHF (see Box 48-5).

Therapeutic Management

Treatment is directed toward correcting the underlying cause whenever feasible. However, in most affected children this is not possible, and treatment is aimed at managing CHF and dysrhythmias. Digoxin, diuretics, and aggressive use of afterload reduction agents have been found to be helpful in managing symptoms in those with dilated cardiomyopathy. Practice guidelines for the management of heart failure in children have been outlined and provide an in-depth review of available therapies (Rosenthal et al, 2004). Digoxin and inotropic agents are usually not helpful in the other forms of cardiomyopathy because increasing the force of contraction may exacerbate the muscular obstruction and actually impair ventricular ejection. β-Blockers such as propranolol or calcium channel blockers such as verapamil (Calan) have been used to reduce left ventricular outflow obstruction and improve diastolic filling in those with hypertrophic cardiomyopathy.

Careful monitoring and treatment of dysrhythmias are essential. The placement of an implantable defibrillator (AICD) should be considered for patients at high risk of sudden death from ventricular dysrhythmias. Anticoagulants may be given to reduce the risk of thromboemboli, a complication of the sluggish circulation through the heart. For worsening heart failure and signs of poor perfusion, IV inotropic or vasodilating drugs may be needed. Severely ill children may require mechanical ventilation, oxygen administration, and IV medications. Heart transplantation may be a treatment option for patients who have worsening symptoms despite maximum medical therapy.

✱ Nursing Care Management

Because of the poor prognosis in many children with cardiomyopathy, nursing care is consistent with that for any child with a life-threatening disorder (see Chapter 41). One of the most difficult adjustments for the child (especially the normally active youngster with hypertrophic cardiomyopathy) may be the realization of failing health and the need for restricted activity. The child should be included in decisions regarding activity and allowed to discuss feelings, particularly if the disease follows a progressively fatal course. After symptoms of CHF or dysrhythmias develop, the same nursing interventions are implemented. If heart transplantation is considered, the needs of the child and family are great in terms of psychologic preparation and postoperative care. The nurse plays an important role in assessing the family's understanding of the procedure and long-term consequences. Children of school age and older should be fully informed to give their assent to the procedure (see Informed Consent, Chapter 45).

Heart Transplantation

Heart transplantation has become a treatment option for infants and children with worsening heart failure and a limited life expectancy despite maximum medical and surgical management. Indications for heart transplantation in children are cardiomyopathy and end-stage CHD. It is also an option for patients with some forms of complex congenital cardiac defects, such as hypoplastic left heart syndrome, for whom conventional surgical approaches have a high mortality rate.

Before transplantation, potential recipients undergo a careful cardiac evaluation to determine whether any other medical or surgical options are available to improve the patient's cardiac status. Other organ systems are assessed to identify problems that might increase the risk of or preclude transplantation. A psychosocial evaluation of the patient and family is done to assess family function, support systems, and ability to comply with the complex medical regimen after the transplant. Support services to help the family successfully care for their child are provided when possible.

The number of heart transplants in pediatric patients has been constant for the past decade at about 400 transplants per year internationally (Boucek et al, 2007). This likely reflects a limit in the number of available donors. Infants are the largest group of pediatric transplant recipients and account for about a fourth of all procedures. The International Society for Heart and Lung Transplantation registry data for all pediatric heart transplant recipients from 1982 to 2005 demonstrated a 1-year actuarial survival rate of 85%. Early rejection within the first year posttransplant is associated with increased late mortality. There is an ongoing risk of death with time from transplant. The infant group is associated with higher early mortality and adolescents with higher late mortality. Overall survival was approximately 40% for patients up to 20 years after transplantation (Boucek et al, 2007). Surviving pediatric patients have excellent functional recovery, with less than 10% reporting activity limitations (Boucek et al, 2007).

The posttransplant course is complex. Although heart function is greatly improved or normal after transplantation, the risk of rejection is serious. The leading cause of death in the first 3 years after heart transplantation is rejection, with the greatest risk in the first 6 months (Blume, 2003). Rejection of the heart is diagnosed primarily by endomyocardial biopsy in older children. Serial echocardiograms are often used in infants and young children to reduce the need for invasive biopsies. Immunosuppressants must be taken for life and have many systemic side effects. Triple drug therapy for immunosuppression with a calcineurin inhibitor (cyclosporine or tacrolimus), steroids, and azathioprine is most commonly used in pediatric patients, although mycophenolate mofetil is being used more frequently and replacing azathioprine. Steroids are weaned in the first year and may be discontinued in some patients.

Infection is always a risk. Potential long-term problems that may limit survival include chronic rejection, causing coronary artery disease; renal dysfunction and hypertension resulting from cyclosporine administration; lymphoma; and infection. Coronary artery disease is the leading cause of death among late survivors of heart transplantation (Boucek et al, 2007).

✻ Nursing Care Management

Successfully caring for a child after a heart transplant requires the expertise and dedication of many members of the health care team. Nurses play vital roles in assessment, coordination of care, psychosocial support, and patient and family education. The heart transplant recipient must be carefully monitored for signs of rejection, infection, and the side effects of the immunosuppressant medications. The patient's and family's psychosocial well-being also needs to be assessed to identify issues such as increased family stress, depression, substance abuse, and school problems. Noncompliance with an intense medication regimen, especially during adolescence, can lead to serious medical problems and can be fatal. Care of the immunosuppressed child is reviewed in Chapter 49. Psychosocial concerns and appropriate interventions for the child with a life-threatening disorder are presented in Chapter 44.

The first 6 months to 1 year after the transplant are most intense because the risk of complications is greatest and the patient and family are adjusting to a new lifestyle. Patients are monitored closely by the health care team, with frequent visits and laboratory tests. Care is usually shared between local health care providers and the transplant center. Many patients are able to return to school and other age-appropriate activities within 2 to 3 months after the transplant.

Vascular Dysfunction

Systemic Hypertension

Hypertension is defined as the consistent elevation of BP beyond values considered to be the upper limits of normal. The two major categories are *essential hypertension* (no identifiable cause) and *secondary hypertension* (subsequent to an identifiable cause). In recent years interest in this disorder in adolescents and children has been increasing. Hypertension in children and adolescents is defined as having a systolic or diastolic BP that consistently falls at or over the 95th percentile. This group is further delineated as follows:

- Stage 1 hypertension includes patients with BP readings between the 95th and 99th percentiles.
- Stage 2 hypertension describes patients with BP readings over the 99th percentile plus 5 mm Hg.

An additional group includes children and adolescents who have prehypertension (or high-normal BP). This prehypertensive group includes those with BP readings that fall consistently between the 90th and 95th percentiles. *The Fourth Report on the Diagnosis, Evaluation, and Treatment of High Blood Pressure in Children and Adolescents* outlines in detail the identification, testing, and treatment recommendations for young people with high BP (National High Blood Pressure Education Program Working Group on High Blood Pressure in Children and Adolescents, 2004).

Etiology

Most instances of hypertension observed in young children occur secondary to a structural abnormality or an underlying pathologic process, although this is being challenged by screening programs of relatively healthy children. The most common cause of secondary hypertension is renal disease, followed by cardiovascular, endocrine, and some neurologic disorders. As a rule, the younger the child and the more severe the hypertension, the more likely it is to be secondary.

The causes of essential hypertension are undetermined, but evidence indicates that both genetic and environmental factors play a role. The incidence of hypertension has been shown to be higher in children whose parents are hypertensive. African-Americans have a higher incidence of hypertension than Caucasians, and in these persons it develops earlier, is frequently more severe, and results in death at an earlier age. Environmental factors that contribute to the risk of developing hypertension include obesity, salt ingestion, smoking, and stress.

Diagnostic Evaluation

From the increasing numbers of hypertensive or potentially hypertensive children and adolescents being identified, a BP determination should be a routine part of annual assessment in healthy children over 3 years old. BP readings should be done in children less than 3 years old who have high risk family histories or those with individual risk factors, including CHD, kidney disease, malignancy, transplant, certain neurologic problems, or systemic illnesses known to cause hypertension. Although clinical manifestations associated with hypertension depend largely on the underlying cause, some observations can provide clues to the examiner that an elevated BP may be a factor (Box 48-10). In infants and very young children who cannot communicate symptoms, observation of behavior provides clues, although gross behavioral changes may not be apparent until complications are present.

No definitive cutoff values are used in the diagnosis of hypertension in the pediatric patient. The *Fourth Report on the Diagnosis, Evaluation, and Treatment of High Blood Pressure in Children and Adolescents* (National High Blood Pressure Education Program Working Group on High Blood Pressure in Children and Adolescents, 2004) provides normative data for children (see Appendix E). BP tables now include the 50th, 90th, 95th, and 99th percentiles for BP readings based on age, gender, and height percentiles. These guidelines are based on auscultatory readings; therefore this is currently the preferred method of assessment. These charts take into account differences in body height. Therefore it is important to note that a child who is large for his or her age may normally have a higher BP than a child of average size. Before a diagnosis is made, BP should be measured on at least three separate occasions.

A careful medical and family history should be obtained to screen for other relatives with hypertension or other cardiovascular risk factors. In children with suspected hypertension, initial laboratory data include a urinalysis, renal function studies such as creatinine and blood urea nitrogen, a lipid profile, complete blood count, and electrolytes. Depending on the severity of hypertension, additional testing may be indicated. Testing may include a renal ultrasound to measure kidney size and Doppler flow to detect the possibility of a renal cause, a cardiac echocardiogram to evaluate the presence of end-organ involvement such as left ventricular hypertrophy, and a retinal examination.

BOX 48-10 Clinical Manifestations of Hypertension

Adolescents and Older Children

- Frequent headaches
- Dizziness
- Changes in vision

Infants or Young Children

- Irritability
- Head banging or head rubbing
- Waking up screaming in the night

Therapeutic Management

Therapy for secondary hypertension involves diagnosis and treatment of the underlying cause. In cases amenable to surgical repair, the nature of the condition, the type of surgery, and the child's age are all important considerations. Children or adolescents with consistently elevated BP readings from no known cause or those with secondary hypertension not amenable to surgical correction may be treated with a combination of nonpharmacologic and pharmacologic interventions. Dietary practices and lifestyle changes are important in the control of hypertension both for children and for adults. Nonpharmacologic measures, such as weight control in overweight patients, increased exercise, limited salt intake, and avoidance of stress and smoking, carry no risk and should be instituted first, except in severe cases. Because the long-term effects of antihypertensive agents on children are not known, drug treatment of asymptomatic children with mild or borderline hypertension is not recommended.

Drug therapy is instituted with caution in children with significant elevations of BP resistant to nonpharmacologic intervention. The treatment should begin with one drug; other drugs should be added only if control is not obtained. The oral antihypertensive drugs used in children include β-blockers, ACE inhibitors, calcium channel blockers, angiotensin-receptor blockers, and diuretics. The goal is to achieve a normotensive state throughout the day without accompanying drug side effects.

Nursing Care Management

BP measurement should always be a part of the routine assessment of children over 3 years old and patients under 3 years old who are considered to be at high risk for hypertension. To obtain an accurate reading, care is taken to quiet the child or relax the adolescent while the measurement is recorded to avoid false readings caused by excitement. The chief cause of falsely elevated BP readings is the use of improperly fitting, narrow cuffs. Therefore attention to correct measurement technique is essential (see Blood Pressure, Chapter 34).

Nursing counseling and guidance of affected children are challenges. Education aimed at understanding hypertension and its implication over the life span is essential in promoting patient and family compliance with both nonpharmacologic and pharmacologic therapies (see Compliance, Chapter 45).

Home BP measurements can facilitate surveillance in youngsters with chronic hypertension and can document effectiveness of therapy. A family member can be instructed in how to take and record accurate BP measurements, thus decreasing the number of trips to a health care facility. This individual needs to understand when to contact the practitioner regarding elevated values. The school nurse can often be a valuable resource in monitoring BP. The nurse plays an important role in assessing individual families and providing targeted information regarding nonpharmacologic modes of intervention, such as diet, weight loss, smoking cessation, and exercise programs. If extensive dietary counseling is required, the child should be referred to a nutritionist with expertise in working with children and adolescents. Exercise regimens should be individualized. Schoolchildren and young adolescents generally prefer team sports rather than individual training, which they may view as a burden rather than an enjoyable activity. If peers and family members can be encouraged to participate in any of the management strategies, the child's compliance is likely to be greater.

Young hypertensive women should avoid oral contraceptives because of their pressor effects. Other options need to be presented before this form of birth control is discontinued (see Contraception, Chapter 7).

If drug therapy is prescribed, the nurse needs to provide information to the family regarding the reasons for it, how the drug works, and possible side effects. General instructions for antihypertensive drugs include:

- Rise slowly from a horizontal position and avoid sudden position changes.
- Take drug as prescribed.
- Maintain adequate hydration.
- Notify practitioner if unpleasant side effects occur, but do not discontinue drug.
- Avoid alcohol and stay on prescribed diet.

The need for follow-up is stressed, especially because antihypertensive therapy can sometimes be safely discontinued if BP remains under control over time.

Kawasaki Disease (Mucocutaneous Lymph Node Syndrome)

KD is an acute systemic vasculitis of unknown cause. It is seen in every racial group, and about 75% of the cases occur in children younger than the age of 5 years, with peak incidence in the toddler age group. The acute disease is self-limited. However, without treatment approximately 15% to 25% of children with KD develop coronary artery aneurysms (Belay et al, 2006). Infants younger than 1 year of age are most seriously affected by KD and are at the greatest risk for heart involvement.

The etiology of KD is unknown. Although it is not spread by person-to-person contact, several factors support infectious etiologic factors. It is often seen in geographic and seasonal outbreaks, with most cases reported in the late winter and early spring (Newburger et al, 2004).

Pathophysiology

The principal area of involvement is the cardiovascular system. During the initial stage of the illness, extensive inflammation of the arterioles, venules, and capillaries occurs. In addition, segmental damage to the medium-size muscular arteries, mainly the coronary arteries, can occur, causing the formation of coronary artery aneurysms in some children. When death occurs (in less than 0.05% of cases), it is usually the result of myocardial ischemia from coronary thrombosis or, over time, severe scar formation and stenosis in coronary aneurysms (Wilder et al, 2007).

BOX 48-11 Diagnostic Criteria for Kawasaki Disease

Child must have fever for more than 5 days along with four of five clinical criteria (diagnosis may be made on day 4 by an experienced clinician if child has all the clinical criteria):

1. Changes in the extremities: in the acute phase, edema and erythema of the palms and soles, and in the subacute phase, periungual desquamation (peeling) of the hands and feet
2. Bilateral conjunctival injection (inflammation) without exudation
3. Changes in the oral mucous membranes, such as erythema of the lips, oropharyngeal reddening, or "strawberry tongue" (large papillae are exposed)
4. Polymorphous rash
5. Cervical lymphadenopathy (one lymph node larger than 1.5 cm)

NOTE: Kawasaki disease can be diagnosed with fewer clinical criteria when coronary artery changes are noted.

Clinical Manifestations

Because no specific diagnostic test exists for KD, the diagnosis is established on the basis of clinical findings and associated laboratory results (Box 48-11). These criteria should be used as guidelines. It is important to note that many children with KD do not fulfill standard diagnostic criteria and infants often have an incomplete presentation. Therefore it is important to consider KD as a possible diagnosis in any infant or child with prolonged elevated temperature that is unresponsive to antibiotics and not attributable to another cause.

KD manifests in three phases: acute, subacute, and convalescent. The *acute phase* begins with the abrupt onset of high fever that is unresponsive to antibiotics and antipyretics. The child then develops the remaining diagnostic symptoms. During this stage he or she is typically *very* irritable. The *subacute phase* begins with resolution of the fever and lasts until all clinical signs of KD have disappeared. During this phase the child is at greatest risk for the development of coronary artery aneurysms. Echocardiograms are used to monitor myocardial and coronary artery status. A baseline echocardiogram should be obtained at the time of diagnosis for comparison with future studies. Irritability persists during this phase. In the *convalescent phase,* all the clinical signs of KD have resolved, but the laboratory values have not returned to normal. This phase is complete when all blood values are normal (6 to 8 weeks after onset). At the end of this stage the child has regained his or her usual temperament, energy, and appetite.

Cardiac Involvement

Long-term complications of KD include the development of coronary artery aneurysms, disrupting blood flow. In children with aneurysms, there is the potential for myocardial infarction, which can result from thrombotic occlusion of a coronary aneurysm. Over time, as the damaged vessel tries to heal, stenosis of the aneurysm may develop and may lead to myocardial ischemia. Most of the morbidity and mortality occurs in children affected with the largest aneurysms (giant aneurysms larger than 8 mm). Symptoms of acute myocardial infarction in children may include abdominal pain, vomiting, restlessness, inconsolable crying, pallor, and shock.

Therapeutic Management

The current treatment of KD includes high-dose IV γ-globulin along with salicylate therapy. γ-Globulin has been demonstrated to be effective at reducing the incidence of coronary artery abnormalities when given within the first 10 days of the illness. A single large infusion of 2 g/kg over 10 to 12 hours is recommended. Retreatment with IV γ-globulin is indicated in patients who continue with fever after treatment.

Aspirin is given initially in an antiinflammatory dose (80 to 100 mg/kg/day in divided doses every 6 hours) to control fever and symptoms of inflammation. After fever has subsided, it is continued at an antiplatelet dose (3 to 5 mg/kg/day). Low-dose aspirin is continued in patients without echocardiographic evidence of coronary abnormalities until the platelet count has returned to normal (6 to 8 weeks). If the child develops coronary abnormalities, salicylate therapy is continued indefinitely. Additional anticoagulation (e.g., clopidogrel [Plavix], enoxaparin [Lovenox], or warfarin) may be indicated in children who have medium-size or giant coronary artery aneurysms.

Prognosis

Most children with KD recover fully after treatment. However, when cardiovascular complications occur, serious morbidity may result. Death occurs rarely but almost always results from coronary thrombosis.

Nursing Care Management

In the initial phase the nurse must monitor the child's cardiac status carefully. Intake and output and daily weight measurements are recorded. Although the child may be reluctant to eat and therefore may be partially dehydrated, fluids need to be administered with care because of the usual finding of myocarditis. The child should be assessed frequently for signs of CHF, including decreased urinary output, gallop rhythm (an additional heart sound), tachycardia, and respiratory distress.

Administration of γ-globulin should follow the same guidelines as for any blood product, with frequent monitoring of vital signs. Patients must be watched for allergic reactions. Cardiac status must be monitored because of the large volume being administered to patients with myocarditis and diminished left ventricular function.

Most nursing care focuses on symptomatic relief. To minimize skin discomfort, cool cloths; unscented lotions; and soft, loose clothing are helpful. During the acute phase, mouth care, including lubricating ointment to the lips, is important for mucosal inflammation. Clear liquids and soft foods can be offered.

Patient irritability is perhaps the most challenging problem. These children need a quiet environment that promotes adequate rest. Their parents need to be supported in their efforts to comfort an often inconsolable child. They may need time away from their child, and nurses can often provide respite care for the family. Parents need to understand that irritability is a hallmark of KD and that they need not feel guilty or embarrassed about their child's behavior.

Discharge Teaching

Parents need accurate information about the progression of KD, including the importance of follow-up monitoring and when they should contact their practitioner (see Patient Teaching box). Irritability is likely to persist for up to 2 months after the onset of symptoms. Peeling of the hands and feet is painless and occurs primarily in the second and third weeks. Arthritis, especially of the larger weight-bearing joints, may persist for several weeks. Children are typically most stiff in the mornings, during cold weather, and after naps. Passive range-of-motion exercises in the bathtub are often helpful in increasing flexibility. Any live immunizations (e.g., measles-mumps-rubella, varicella) should be deferred for 11 months after the administration of γ-globulin because the body might not produce the appropriate amount of antibodies (American Academy of Pediatrics, Committee on Infectious Diseases, 2006). The decision to give the varicella (chickenpox) vaccine while the child is receiving aspirin therapy is made individually by the practitioner. Temperature should be recorded after discharge until the child has been afebrile for several days.

PATIENT TEACHING Concerns for Myocardial Infarction

All parents should understand the unlikely but real possibility of myocardial infarction and the signs and symptoms of cardiac ischemia in a child. At discharge the ultimate cardiac sequela is generally not known because vessels do not reach their maximum diameter until 4 to 6 weeks after the onset of Kawasaki disease. In addition, the parents of children with known severe coronary artery sequelae may be taught cardiopulmonary resuscitation.

Shock

Shock, or *circulatory failure*, is a complex clinical syndrome characterized by inadequate tissue perfusion to meet the metabolic demands of the body, resulting in cellular dysfunction and eventual organ failure. Although the causes are different, the physiologic consequences are the same: hypotension, tissue hypoxia, and metabolic acidosis. Circulatory failure in children is a result of hypovolemia, altered peripheral vascular resistance, or pump failure. Types of shock are listed in Table 48-6.

Pathophysiology

A healthy child's circulatory system is able to transport oxygen and metabolic substrates to body tissues, which require a constant source for these essential needs. The cardiac output and distribution to the various body tissues can change rapidly in response to intrinsic (myocardial and intravascular) or extrinsic (neuronal) control mechanisms. In shock states these mechanisms are altered or challenged.

Reduced blood flow, as in hypovolemic shock, causes diminished venous return to the heart, low CVP, low cardiac output, and hypotension. Vasomotor centers in the medulla are signaled, causing a compensatory increase in the force and

Table 48-6 Types of Shock

CHARACTERISTICS	MOST FREQUENT CAUSES
Hypovolemic	
Reduction in size of vascular compartment Falling blood pressure Poor capillary filling Low central venous pressure	Blood loss (hemorrhagic shock)—Trauma, gastrointestinal bleeding, intracranial hemorrhage Plasma loss—Increased capillary permeability associated with sepsis and acidosis, hypoproteinemia, burns, peritonitis Extracellular fluid loss—Vomiting, diarrhea, glycosuric diuresis, sunstroke
Distributive	
Reduction in peripheral vascular resistance Profound inadequacies in tissue perfusion Increased venous capacity and pooling Acute reduction in return blood flow to the heart Diminished cardiac output	Anaphylaxis (anaphylactic shock)—Extreme allergy or hypersensitivity to a foreign substance Sepsis (septic shock, bacteremic shock, endotoxic shock)—Overwhelming sepsis and circulating bacterial toxins Loss of neuronal control (neurogenic shock)—Interruption of neuronal transmission (spinal cord injury) Myocardial depression and peripheral dilation—Exposure to anesthesia or ingestion of barbiturates, tranquilizers, opioids, antihypertensive agents, or ganglionic blocking agents
Cardiogenic	
Decreased cardiac output	After surgery for congenital heart disease Primary pump failure—Myocarditis, myocardial trauma, biochemical derangements, congestive heart failure Dysrhythmias—Supraventricular tachycardia, atrioventricular block, and ventricular dysrhythmias; secondary to myocarditis or biochemical abnormalities (occasionally)

rate of cardiac contraction and constriction of arterioles and veins, thereby increasing peripheral vascular resistance. Simultaneously the lowered blood volume leads to the release of large amounts of catecholamines, antidiuretic hormone, adrenocorticosteroids, and aldosterone in an effort to conserve body fluids. This causes reduced blood flow to the skin, kidneys, muscles, and viscera to shunt the available blood to the brain and heart. Consequently, the skin feels cold and clammy, there is poor capillary filling, and glomerular filtration rate and urinary output are significantly reduced.

As a result of impaired perfusion, oxygen is depleted in the tissue cells, causing them to revert to anaerobic metabolism, producing lactic acidosis. The acidosis places an extra burden

BOX 48-12 Clinical Manifestations of Shock

Compensated
Apprehensiveness
Irritability
Unexplained tachycardia
Normal blood pressure
Narrowing pulse pressure
Thirst
Pallor
Diminished urinary output
Reduced perfusion of extremities

Decompensated
Confusion and somnolence
Tachypnea
Moderate metabolic acidosis
Oliguria
Cool, pale extremities
Decreased skin turgor
Poor capillary filling

Irreversible
Thready, weak pulse
Hypotension
Periodic breathing or apnea
Anuria
Stupor or coma

on the lungs as they attempt to compensate for the metabolic acidosis by increasing respiratory rate to remove excess carbon dioxide. Prolonged vasoconstriction results in fatigue and atony of the peripheral arterioles, which leads to vessel dilation. Venules, less sensitive to vasodilator substances, remain constricted for a time, causing massive pooling in the capillary and venular beds, which further depletes blood volume.

Complications of shock create further hazards. Central nervous system hypoperfusion may eventually lead to cerebral edema, cortical infarction, or intraventricular hemorrhage. Renal hypoperfusion causes renal ischemia with possible tubular or glomerular necrosis and renal vein thrombosis. Reduced blood flow to the lungs can interfere with surfactant secretion and result in acute respiratory distress syndrome (ARDS), characterized by sudden pulmonary congestion and atelectasis with formation of a hyaline membrane. Gastrointestinal tract bleeding and perforation are always a possibility after splanchnic ischemia and necrosis of intestinal mucosa. Metabolic complications of shock may include hypoglycemia, hypocalcemia, and other electrolyte disturbances.

Diagnostic Evaluation

The etiology of shock can be discerned from the history and physical examination. The severity of the shock is determined by measurements of vital signs, including CVP and capillary filling (Box 48-12). Shock can be regarded as a form of compensation for circulatory failure. Because of its progressive nature, it can be divided into the following three stages or phases:

1. **Compensated shock**—Vital organ function is maintained by intrinsic compensatory mechanisms;

blood flow is usually normal or increased but generally uneven or maldistributed in the microcirculation.

2. **Decompensated shock**—Efficiency of the cardiovascular system gradually diminishes until perfusion in the microcirculation becomes marginal despite compensatory adjustments. The outcomes of circulatory failure that progress beyond the limits of compensation are tissue hypoxia, metabolic acidosis, and eventual dysfunction of all organ systems.
3. **Irreversible, or terminal, shock**—Damage to vital organs, such as the heart or brain, is of such magnitude that the entire organism will be disrupted regardless of therapeutic intervention. Death occurs even if cardiovascular measurements return to normal levels with therapy.

At all stages the principal differentiating signs are observed in the (1) degree of tachycardia and perfusion to extremities, (2) level of consciousness, and (3) BP. Additional signs or modifications of these more universal signs may be present, depending on the type and cause of the shock. Initially the child's ability to compensate is effective; therefore early signs are subtle. As the shock state advances, signs are more obvious and indicate early decompensation.

Additional signs may be present, depending on the type and cause of the shock. In early septic shock there are chills, fever, and vasodilation, with increased cardiac output that results in warm, flushed skin (hyperdynamic, or "hot," shock). A later and ominous development is disseminated intravascular coagulation (see Chapter 49), the major hematologic complication of septic shock. Anaphylactic shock is frequently accompanied by urticaria and angioneurotic edema, which is life threatening when it involves the respiratory passages (see Anaphylaxis, p. 1485).

Laboratory tests that assist in assessment are blood gas measurements, pH, and sometimes liver function tests. Coagulation tests are evaluated when there is evidence of bleeding, such as oozing from a venipuncture site, bleeding from any orifice, or petechiae. Cultures of blood and other sites are indicated when there is a high suspicion of sepsis. Renal function tests are performed when impaired renal function is evident.

Therapeutic Management

Treatment of shock consists of three major interventions: (1) ventilation, (2) fluid administration, and (3) improvement of the pumping action of the heart (vasopressor support). The first priority is to establish an airway and administer oxygen. After the airway is ensured, circulatory stabilization is the major concern. Establishment of adequate IV access, ideally with multilumen central lines, is essential to deliver fluids and medications.

Ventilatory Support

The lung is the organ most sensitive to shock. Decreased distribution or redistribution of blood flow to respiratory muscles plus the increased work of breathing can rapidly lead to respiratory failure. Critically ill patients are unable to maintain an adequate airway. To place the lung at rest and improve ventilation, tracheal intubation is initiated early with positive-pressure ventilation. Supplemental oxygen is always given as soon as possible. Blood gases and pH are monitored frequently.

Increased extravascular lung water caused by edema contributes to the development of respiratory complications. Therapy is directed toward maintaining normal arterial blood gas measurements, normal acid-base balance, and circulation. Efforts are made to remove fluid and prevent its accumulation with the use of diuretics.

Cardiovascular Support

In most cases rapid restoration of blood volume is all that is needed for resuscitation of the child in shock. An isotonic crystalloid solution (normal saline or Ringer's lactate) is the fluid of choice; colloids such as albumin are also used. Successful resuscitation is reflected by an increase in BP and a reduction in heart rate; increased cardiac output results in improved capillary circulation and skin color. CVP measurements of right atrial pressure help guide fluid therapy, and urinary output measurement is an important indicator of adequacy of circulation. Correction of acidosis, hypoxemia, hypoglycemia, hypothermia, and any metabolic derangements is mandatory.

Temporary pharmacologic support may be required to enhance myocardial contractility, reverse metabolic or respiratory acidosis, and/or maintain arterial pressure. The principal agents used to improve cardiac output and circulation are catecholamines, such as dopamine (Intropin) or epinephrine (Adrenalin). Vasodilators that are sometimes used include nitroprusside (Nipride) or milrinone.

Nursing Care Management

The child who is in shock requires intensive observation and care. *The initial action is to ensure adequate tissue oxygenation.* The nurse should be prepared to administer oxygen by the appropriate route and assist with any intubation and ventilatory procedures indicated. Other procedures and activities that require immediate attention are establishing an IV line, weighing the child, obtaining baseline vital signs, placing an indwelling catheter, obtaining blood gases and other measurements, and administering medications as indicated. The child is best positioned flat with the legs elevated.

NURSING ALERT Early clinical signs of shock include apprehension, irritability, normal BP, narrowing pulse pressure (difference between diastolic and systolic BP), thirst, pallor, diminished urinary output, unexplained mild tachycardia, and decreased perfusion of the hands and feet.

The nurse's responsibilities are to monitor the IV infusion, intake and output, vital signs (including CVP), and general systems assessments on a routine basis. IV medications are titrated according to patient responses, and vital signs are taken every 15 minutes during the critical periods and thereafter as needed. Urinary output is measured hourly; blood gases, hematocrit, pH, and electrolytes are monitored frequently to assess the child's status and the efficacy of therapy. An apnea and cardiac monitor is attached and monitored continuously. In the initial stages of acute shock, more than one nurse is often needed to manage all the necessary activities that must be carried out simultaneously (see Emergency box).

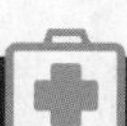

EMERGENCY

Shock

Ventilation

Establish airway; be prepared for intubation.

Administer oxygen, usually 100% by mask.

Fluid Administration

Obtain vascular access (preferably intravenous [IV]; intraosseous in emergency).

Restore fluid volume as ordered (initial volume resuscitation is 20 ml/kg of isotonic crystalloid [normal saline or Ringer's lactate] over 5 to 20 minutes).

Cardiovascular Support

Administer vasopressors, especially IV epinephrine (dose: 0.01 mg/kg = 0.1 ml/kg of 1 : 10,000 solution).

This may be repeated every 3 to 5 minutes for patients in cardiac arrest.

General Support

Provide continuous electrocardiographic monitoring.

Monitor pulse oximetry.

Keep child warm and calm.

In Addition:

Septic Shock—Administer broad-spectrum antibiotics intravenously.

Anaphylaxis—Remove allergen if possible; provide intramuscular epinephrine and corticosteroids as ordered.

Anaphylaxis

Anaphylaxis is the acute clinical syndrome resulting from the interaction of an allergen and a patient who is hypersensitive to that allergen. When the antigen enters the circulatory system, a generalized reaction rapidly takes place. Vasoactive amines (principally histamine or a histamine-like substance) are released and cause vasodilation, bronchoconstriction, and increased capillary permeability.

Severe reactions are immediate in onset; are often life threatening; and frequently involve multiple systems, primarily the cardiovascular, respiratory, gastrointestinal, and integumentary systems. Exposure to the antigen can be by ingestion, inhalation, skin contact, or injection. Examples of common allergens associated with anaphylaxis include drugs (e.g., antibiotics, chemotherapeutic agents, radiologic contrast media), latex, foods, venom from bees or snakes, and biologic agents (antisera, enzymes, hormones, blood products).

NURSING ALERT Penicillin allergy is associated with immediate (within an hour of administration) or accelerated (1 to 72 hours after administration) onset of skin eruption, especially a urticarial rash, or more serious symptoms such as laryngeal edema or anaphylactic shock.

Clinical Manifestations

The onset of clinical symptoms usually occurs within seconds or minutes of exposure to the antigen, and the rapidity of the reaction is directly related to its intensity: the sooner the onset, the more severe the reaction. The reaction may be preceded by symptoms of uneasiness, restlessness, irritability, severe anxiety, headache, dizziness, paresthesia, and disorientation. The patient may lose consciousness. Cutaneous signs of flushing and urticaria are common early signs, followed by angioedema, most notable in the eyelids, lips, tongue, hands, feet, and genitalia.

Bronchiolar constriction may follow, causing narrowing of the airway; pulmonary edema and hemorrhage also may occur. Laryngeal edema with severe acute upper airway obstruction may be life threatening and requires rapid intervention. Shock occurs as a result of mediator-induced vasodilation, which causes capillary permeability and loss of intravascular fluid into the interstitial space. Sudden hypotension and impaired cardiac output with poor perfusion are seen.

Therapeutic Management

Successful outcome of anaphylactic reactions depends on rapid recognition and institution of treatment. The goals of treatment are to provide ventilation, restore adequate circulation, and prevent further exposure by identifying and removing the cause when possible.

A mild reaction with no evidence of respiratory distress or cardiovascular compromise can be managed with subcutaneous administration of antihistamines, such as diphenhydramine (Benadryl) and epinephrine.

Moderate or severe distress presents a potentially life-threatening emergency. Establishing an airway is the first concern, as with all shock states. Epinephrine is given subcutaneously or intravenously as an antihistamine and to support the cardiovascular system and increase BP. Other routes for giving epinephrine are intramuscular and via the airway, either nebulized or injected through an ET tube. In severe anaphylaxis, epinephrine by any route is better than none. Fluids are given to restore blood volume. Additional vasopressors may be given to improve cardiac output.

Prevention of a reaction is preferable. Preventing exposure is more easily accomplished in children known to be at risk, including those with (1) a history of previous allergic reaction to a specific antigen; (2) a history of atopy; (3) a history of severe reactions in immediate family members; and (4) a reaction to a skin test, although skin tests are not available for all allergens. Desensitization may be recommended in certain cases.

Nursing Care Management

When an anaphylactic reaction is suspected, both immediate intervention and preparation for medical therapy are nursing responsibilities. Ventilation is ensured by placing the child in a head-elevated position, unless contraindicated by hypotension, to facilitate breathing and administer oxygen. If the child is not breathing, CPR is initiated and emergency medical services are summoned.

If the cause can be determined, measures are implemented to slow the spread of the offending substance. An IV infusion is established immediately. Emergency medications are given intravenously whenever possible; however, epinephrine may be given subcutaneously (see Emergency box). Vital signs and urinary output are monitored frequently. Medications are administered as prescribed, with regular assessment to monitor effectiveness and detect signs of side effects of medication and fluid overload.

To prevent an anaphylactic reaction, parents are always asked about possible allergic responses to foods, latex, medications, and environmental conditions. These are displayed prominently on the patient's chart. The specific allergen is noted, as is the type and severity of the reaction. Parents are excellent historians, especially when the child has displayed a pronounced reaction to a substance. Drugs, including related drugs (e.g., penicillin, nafcillin), and other items such as latex that have produced a reaction previously are *never* used. If the child is allergic to insect venom, the family is instructed to purchase an emergency kit to be kept with him or her at all times. If the child is old enough, both the family and the child are taught how to use the equipment. The patient should carry medical identification at all times.

Septic Shock

Sepsis and septic shock are caused by an infectious organism (Maar, 2004). Normally an infection triggers an inflammatory response in a local area, which results in vasodilation, increased capillary permeability, and eventually elimination of the infectious agent. The widespread activation and systemic release of inflammatory mediators is called the *systemic inflammatory response syndrome* (SIRS). Box 48-13 provides the exact definitions for SIRS, infection, sepsis, and severe sepsis. SIRS can occur in response to both infectious and noninfectious (e.g., trauma, burns) causes. When caused by infection, it is called *sepsis*. Septic shock is defined as sepsis with organ dysfunction and hypotension.

Most of the physiologic effects of shock occur because the exaggerated immune response triggers more than 30 different mediators that result in diffuse vasodilation, increased capillary permeability, and maldistribution of blood flow. This impairs oxygen and nutrient delivery to the cells, resulting in cellular dysfunction. If the process continues, multiple organ dysfunction occurs and may result in death. Table 48-7 includes the age-specific vital signs and laboratory values reflective of septic shock in children.

The incidence of septic shock is increasing in adults and children (Arnal & Stein, 2003), possibly as a result of greater numbers of immunosuppressed patients, more widespread use of invasive devices in the seriously ill, increased awareness of the diagnosis, and a growing number of resistant microorganisms.

Three stages have been identified in septic shock. In early septic shock the patient has chills; fever; and vasodilation with increased cardiac output, which results in warm, flushed skin that reflects vascular tone abnormalities and hyperdynamic, warm, or hyperdynamic-compensated responses. BP and urinary output are normal. The patient has the best chance for survival in this stage. The second stage—the normodynamic, cool, or hyperdynamic-decompensated stage—lasts only a few hours. The skin is cool, but pulses and BP are still normal. Urinary output diminishes, and the mental state becomes depressed. With advancing disease, certain signs of circulatory decompensation that deteriorate to signs of circulatory collapse are indistinguishable from late shock of any cause. In the hypodynamic, or cold, stage of shock, cardiovascular function progressively deteriorates, even with aggressive therapy. The patient has hypothermia, cold extremities, weak pulses, hypotension, and oliguria or anuria. Patients are severely lethargic or comatose. Multiorgan failure is common. This is the most dangerous stage of shock.

Management of septic shock involves measures to provide hemodynamic stability and adequate oxygenation to the tissues and the use of antimicrobials to treat the infectious organism. As with other forms of shock, hemodynamic stability is achieved with fluid volume resuscitation and inotropic agents as needed. Providing adequate oxygenation often

BOX 48-13 Definitions of Systemic Inflammatory Response Syndrome, Infection, Sepsis, and Severe Sepsis

Systemic inflammatory response syndrome (SIRS)—The presence of at least two of the following four criteria, one of which must be abnormal temperature or leukocyte count:

1. Core temperature of more than 38.5° C (101.3° F) or less than 36° C (96.8° F)
2. Tachycardia, defined as a mean heart rate more than 2 SD above normal for age in the absence of external stimulus, chronic drugs, or painful stimuli; or otherwise unexplained persistent elevation over a 0.5- to 4-hour period; or, for children less than 1 year old: bradycardia, defined as a mean heart rate less than the 10th percentile for age in the absence of external vagal stimulus, β-blocker drugs, or congenital heart disease; or otherwise unexplained persistent depression over a 0.5-hour period
3. Mean respiratory rate more than 2 SD above normal for age or mechanical ventilation for an acute process not related to underlying neuromuscular disease or the receipt of general anesthesia
4. Leukocyte count elevated or depressed for age (not secondary to chemotherapy-induced leukopenia) or more than 10% immature neutrophils

Infection—A suspected or proven (by positive culture, tissue stain, or polymerase chain reaction test) infection caused by any pathogen; or a clinical syndrome associated with a high probability of infection. Evidence of infection includes positive findings on clinical examination, imaging, or laboratory tests (e.g., white blood cells in a normally sterile body fluid, perforated viscus, chest radiograph consistent with pneumonia, petechial or purpuric rash, or purpura fulminans)

Sepsis—SIRS in the presence of or as a result of suspected or proven infection

Severe sepsis—Sepsis plus cardiovascular organ dysfunction or acute respiratory distress syndrome; or two or more other organ dysfunctions

From Goldstein B et al: International Pediatric Sepsis Consensus Conference: definitions for sepsis and organ dysfunction in pediatrics, *Pediatr Crit Care Med* 6(1):2-8, 2005; used with permission.

Table 48-7 Age-Specific Vital Signs and Laboratory Variables in Septic Shock*

AGE GROUP	Heart Rate (beats/min) TACHYCARDIA	BRADYCARDIA	RESPIRATORY RATE (breaths/min)	LEUKOCYTE COUNT (leukocytes × $10^3/mm^3$)	SYSTOLIC BLOOD PRESSURE (mm Hg)
0 days-1 wk	>180	<100	>50	>34	<65
1 wk-1 mo	>180	<100	>40	>19.5 or <5	<75
1 mo-1 yr	>180	<90	>34	>17.5 or <5	<100
2-5 yr	>140	N/A	>22	>15.5 or <6	<94
6-12 yr	>130	N/A	>8	>13.50 or <4.5	<105
13-<18 yr	>110	N/A	>4	>11 or <4.5	<117

From Goldstein B et al: International pediatric sepsis consensus conference: definitions for sepsis and organ dysfunction in pediatrics, *Pediatr Crit Care Med* 6(1):2-8, 2005; used with permission.
N/A, Not applicable.
*Lower values for heart rate, leukocyte count, and systolic blood pressure are for 5th percentile, and upper values for heart rate, respiratory rate, or leukocyte count are for 95th percentile.

requires intubation and mechanical ventilation, supplemental oxygen, sedation, and paralysis to decrease the work of breathing. Septic shock involves activation of complement proteins that promote clumping of the granulocytes in the lung. The granulocytes can release chemicals that can cause direct lung injury to the pulmonary capillary endothelium. This causes a fluid leak into the alveoli, which causes stiff, noncompliant lungs. Disseminated intravascular coagulation and multiorgan dysfunction may also occur and require prompt assessment and management.

Newer therapies are being developed to modify the host immune response by attempting to block various mediators, thereby interrupting the inflammatory cascade.

Early identification of the symptoms of septic shock is critical to patient survival. A high index of suspicion is required in all critically ill patients who are at greater risk for sepsis because of multiple invasive lines and devices, poor nutrition, and impaired immune function. Subtle alterations in tissue perfusion and unexplained tachypnea and tachycardia often are early warning signs. Identification of the infectious agent and prompt treatment are also critical to patient survival. Broad-spectrum antibiotics should be given, and the site of infection should be removed if possible (e.g., drain abscesses, remove indwelling lines). Patients should be managed in an ICU, in which continuous monitoring and sophisticated cardiac and respiratory support are available. Multidisciplinary collaboration is essential in managing these critically ill patients.

Key Points

- CHD is the most common form of cardiac disease in children.
- Major categories to investigate in the cardiac history are poor weight gain, poor feeding habits, and fatigue during feeding; frequent respiratory tract infections and difficulties; and evidence of exercise intolerance.
- The most common tests used in assessing cardiac function are radiography, ECG, echocardiography, and cardiac catheterization.
- Cardiac catheterization procedures can be divided into three groups: (1) diagnostic procedures, including angiography, that measure pressures and saturations to establish cardiac diagnosis; (2) interventional procedures, in which catheters or balloon devices are used to correct cardiac defects; and (3) electrophysiology studies, in which catheters with electrodes are used to evaluate dysrhythmias.
- Diagnostic cardiac catheterization provides important information about oxygen saturation of blood within the chambers and great vessels, pressure changes, changes in cardiac output or stroke volume, and anatomic abnormalities.

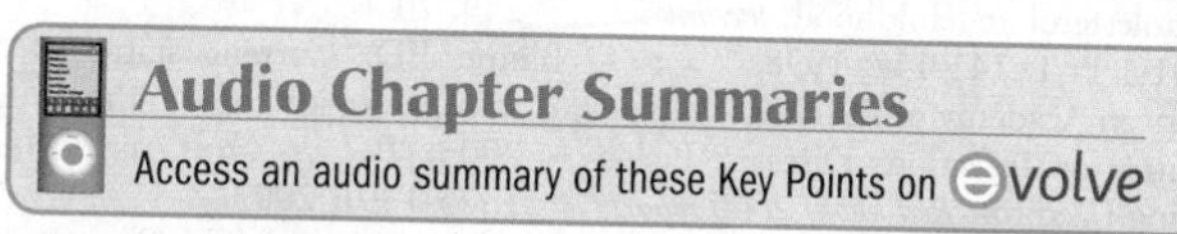
Audio Chapter Summaries
Access an audio summary of these Key Points on evolve

- Several prenatal factors may predispose children to CHD: maternal rubella during pregnancy, maternal alcoholism, maternal age older than 40 years, and maternal type 1 diabetes.
- Congenital heart defects can be divided into four main groups, as determined by hemodynamic patterns: (1) defects that result in increased pulmonary blood flow, (2) obstructive defects, (3) defects that result in decreased pulmonary blood flow, and (4) mixed defects.
- Clinical consequences of congenital heart defects include CHF and hypoxemia. A child can have both hypoxemia and CHF, although usually they occur independently.
- Clinical manifestations of CHF are impaired myocardial function (tachycardia, cardiomegaly), pulmonary congestion (dyspnea, tachypnea, orthopnea, cyanosis), and systemic congestion (hepatosplenomegaly, edema, distended veins).

- Nursing measures in the care of a child with CHF are to assist in improving cardiac function, decrease cardiac demands, reduce respiratory distress, maintain nutritional status, promote fluid loss, and provide family support.
- Clinical manifestations of hypoxemia are cyanosis, polycythemia, clubbing, and delayed growth and development. The child is at increased risk for hypercyanotic spells, CVAs, brain abscess, and bacterial endocarditis.
- Caring for the child with CHD and the family requires helping them to adjust to the disorder and cope with the effects of the defect and fostering growth-promoting family relationships.
- Preoperative care of the child with a congenital heart defect involves introducing the child and family to the hospital and preparing them for preoperative and postoperative procedures.
- Providing postoperative care includes observing vital signs and arterial and venous pressures, maintaining respiratory status, allowing maximum rest, providing comfort, monitoring fluids, planning for progressive activities, giving emotional support, observing for complications of surgery, and planning for discharge and home care.
- Acquired cardiovascular disorders include bacterial endocarditis, RF, hyperlipidemia (hypercholesterolemia), and cardiac dysrhythmias.
- Prevention of bacterial endocarditis in certain children with CHD involves administration of prophylactic antibiotics when specific procedures are performed.
- Acute RF is a systemic inflammatory disease that can damage the cardiac valves and is associated with previous GABHS infection. Its incidence has increased in some areas of the United States.
- Cholesterol screening in children is controversial; currently, children with known risk factors for hyperlipidemia are screened and treated as needed. The influence of childhood cholesterol levels on later development of coronary artery disease is under investigation.
- Common dysrhythmias in children include slow (bradycardias, heart block) and fast (sinus tachycardia, SVT) rhythms.
- Heart transplantation has been extended to infants and children with cardiomyopathy and complex congenital heart defects involving ventricular dysfunction, such as hypoplastic left heart syndrome.
- Education of the child with hypertension and the family focuses on drug therapy, diet control, and appropriate exercise.
- KD is an extensive inflammation of small vessels and capillaries that may progress to involve the coronary arteries, causing aneurysm formation. The administration of γ-globulin is an important aspect of treatment.
- Emergency treatment for shock includes ensuring ventilation; administering vasopressors, fluids, blood, and antibiotics as needed; and providing supportive measures such as correct positioning, warmth, and psychologic reassurance to the child and family.
- Persons at risk for anaphylaxis may be identified by a history of previous allergic reaction, history of atopy, history of severe reactions in family, and positive skin test to the allergen.

References

American Academy of Pediatrics: Cholesterol in childhood, *Pediatrics* 101(1 Pt 1):141-147, 1998.

American Academy of Pediatrics, Committee on Infectious Diseases, Pickering L, editor: *Red book: 2006 report of the Committee on Infectious Diseases*, ed 27, Elk Grove Village, Ill, 2006, The Academy.

Arnal LE, Stein F: Pediatric septic shock: why has mortality decreased? The utility of goal-directed therapy, *Semin Pediatr Infect Dis* 14(2):165-172, 2003.

Arnold R et al: Outcome after mechanical aortic valve replacement in children and young adults, *Ann Thorac Surg* 85(2): 604-610, 2008.

Barst RJ: Recent advances in the treatment of pediatric pulmonary artery hypertension, *Pediatr Clin North Am* 46(2):333-345, 1999.

Beekman RH: Coarctation of the aorta. In Allen HD et al (editors): *Moss and Adams' heart disease in infants, children and adolescents*, ed 6, Philadelphia, 2001, Lippincott Williams & Wilkins.

Belay E et al: Kawasaki syndrome and risk factors for coronary artery abnormalities, *Pediatr Infect Dis* 25(3):245-249, 2006.

Blume ED: Current status of heart transplantation in children: update 2003, *Pediatr Clin North Am* 50: 1375-1391, 2003.

Boucek MM et al: The Registry of the International Society for Heart and Lung Transplantation: tenth official pediatric heart transplantation report—2007, *J Heart Lung Transplant* 26(8):796-807, 2007.

Carapetis JR, McDonald M, Wilson NJ: Acute rheumatic fever, *Lancet* 366:155-168, 2005.

Dodds KM, Merle C: Discharging neonates with congenital heart disease after cardiac surgery: a practical approach, *Clin Perinatol* 32:1031-1042, 2005.

Freed MD: Aortic stenosis. In Allen HD et al (editors): *Moss and Adams' heart disease in infants, children, and adolescents*, ed 6, Philadelphia, 2001, Lippincott Williams & Wilkins.

Gentles T et al: Left ventricular mechanics during and after acute rheumatic fever: contractile dysfunction is closely related to valve regurgitation, *J Heart Lung Transplant* 37(1):201-207, 2001.

Goldmuntz E et al: Frequency of 22q11 deletion in patients with conotruncal defects, *J Am Coll Cardiol* 32:492-498, 1998.

Hoffman JIE, Kaplan S: The incidence of congenital heart disease, *J Am Coll Cardiol* 39:1890-1900, 2002.

Jacobs JP et al: Lessons learned from the data analysis of the second harvest (1998-2001) of the Society of Thoracic Surgeons (STS) Congenital Heart Surgery Database, *J Am Coll Cardiol* 26(1):18-37, 2004.

Latson LA: Critical pulmonic stenosis, *J Interv Cardiol* 14(3):345-350, 2001.

LeRoy S et al: Recommendations for preparing children and adolescents for invasive cardiac procedures: AHA Scientific Statement, *Circulation* 108:2550-2564, 2003.

Maar SP: Emergency care in pediatric septic shock, *Pediatr Emerg Care* 20(9):617-624, 2004.

Majnemer A, Limperopoulos C: Developmental progress of children with congenital heart defects requiring open heart surgery, *Semin Pediatr Neurol* 6:12-19, 1999.

Maron BJ: Hypertrophic cardiomyopathy. In Allen HD et al (editors): *Moss and Adams' heart disease in infants, children, and adolescents*, ed 6, Philadelphia, 2001, Lippincott Williams & Wilkins.

McCrindle BW et al: Drug therapy of high-risk lipid abnormalities in children and adolescents: a scientific statement from the American Heart Association Atherosclerosis, Hypertension, and Obesity in Youth Committee, Council of Cardiovascular Disease in the Young, with the Council on Cardiovascular Nursing, *Circulation* 115:1948-1967, 2007.

National High Blood Pressure Education Program Working Group on High Blood Pressure in Children and Adolescents: The fourth report on the diagnosis, evaluation, and treatment of high blood pressure in children and adolescents, *Pediatrics* 114(2):555-576, 2004.

Newburger JW et al: Diagnosis, treatment, and long-term management of Kawasaki disease: a statement for health professionals from the

Committee on Rheumatic Fever, Endocarditis and Kawasaki Disease, Council on Cardiovascular Disease in the Young, American Heart Association, *Circulation* 110(17):2747-2771, 2004.

Park MK: *Pediatric cardiology handbook*, ed 3, St Louis, 2003, Mosby.

Rome JJ, Kreutzer J: Pediatric interventional catheterization: reasonable expectations and outcomes, *Pediatr Clin North Am* 51:1589-1610, 2004.

Rosenthal D et al: International Society for Heart and Lung Transplantation: practice guidelines for management of heart failure in children, *J Heart Lung Transplant* 23(12):1313-1333, 2004.

Shanmugam G, MacArthur K, Pollock J: Mechanical aortic valve replacement: long-term outcomes in children, *J Heart Valve Dis* 14(2):166-171, 2005.

Smith P: Primary care in children with congenital heart disease, *J Pediatr Nurs* 16(5):308-319, 2001.

Stetzler M, Rudd N, Pick B: Nutrition care for newborns with congenital heart disease, *Clin Perinatol* 32:1017-1030, 2005.

Tweddell JS et al: Improved survival of patients undergoing palliation of hypoplastic left heart syndrome: lessons learned from 115 consecutive patients, *Circulation* 106(12 Suppl 1):182-189, 2002.

Uzark K: Therapeutic cardiac catheterization for congenital heart disease: a new era in pediatric care, *J Pediatr Nurs* 16(5):300-307, 2001.

Van Horn L et al: Children's adaptations to a fat-reduced diet: the dietary intervention study in children, *Pediatrics* 115(60):1723-1733, 2005.

Wilder M et al: Delayed diagnosis by physicians contributes to the development of coronary artery aneurysms in children with Kawasaki syndrome, *Pediatr Infect Dis* 26(3):256-260, 2007.

Wilson W et al: Prevention of infective endocarditis: guidelines from the American Heart Association, *Circulation* 116(15):1736-1754, 2007.

Unit 11

49 Hematologic or Immunologic Dysfunction

Learning Objectives

On completion of this chapter the reader will be able to:

- Distinguish between the various categories of anemia.
- Describe the prevention of iron deficiency anemia and the care of the child with iron deficiency anemia.
- Compare sickle cell anemia and β-thalassemia major in relation to pathophysiology and nursing care.
- Describe the mechanisms of inheritance and nursing care of the child with hemophilia.
- Relate the pathophysiology and clinical manifestations of leukemia.
- Demonstrate an understanding of the rationale of therapies for neoplastic disease.
- Outline a plan of care for the child with neoplastic disease and the family.
- Contrast the pathophysiology and management of the immunodeficiency disorders.
- List nursing precautions and responsibilities during blood transfusion.
- Describe the types of hematopoietic stem cell transplants.

Electronic Resources

Additional information related to the content in Chapter 49 can be found on

evolve the Companion Website at

http://evolve.elsevier.com/Perry/maternal/

- NCLEX Review Questions
- Animation—Hemophilia A
- Animation—Platelets and Blood Clotting
- Animation—Sickle Cell Anemia
- Case Study—Acute Lymphoid Leukemia
- Case Study—Sickle Cell Anemia
- Critical Thinking Exercise—Bleeding
- Critical Thinking Exercise—Bone Marrow Test
- Critical Thinking Exercise—HIV Testing in Children
- Nursing Care Plan—The Child with Anemia
- Nursing Care Plan—The Child with Cancer
- Nursing Care Plan—The Child with HIV Infection
- Nursing Care Plan—The Child with Sickle Cell Disease

Hematologic and Immunologic Dysfunction

Several tests can be performed to assess hematologic function, including additional procedures to identify the cause of the dysfunction. The following discussion is limited to a description of the most common and one of the most valuable tests, the *complete blood cell count (CBC)*. Other procedures, such as those related to iron, coagulation, and immune status, are discussed throughout the chapter as appropriate. The nurse should be familiar with the significance of the findings from the CBC (Table 49-1) and aware of normal values for age, which are listed in Appendix D.

As with any disorder, the history and physical examination are essential to identify hematologic dysfunction, and the nurse is often the first person to suspect a problem based on information from these sources. Comments by the parent regarding the child's lack of energy, food diary of poor sources of iron, frequent infections, and bleeding that is difficult to control offer clues to the more common disorders affecting the blood. A careful physical appraisal, especially of the skin, can reveal findings (e.g., pallor, petechiae, bruising) that may indicate minor or serious hematologic conditions. Nurses need to be aware of the clinical manifestations of blood diseases to assist in recognizing symptoms and establishing a diagnosis.

Red Blood Cell Disorders

Anemia

The term *anemia* describes a condition in which the number of red blood cells (RBCs) or the hemoglobin (Hgb or Hb) concentration is reduced below normal values for age. This diminishes the oxygen-carrying capacity of the blood, causing a reduction in the oxygen available to the tissues. Anemia is the most common hematologic disorder of infancy and childhood and is not a disease itself but an indication or manifestation of an underlying pathologic process.

Classification

Anemias are classified in relation to (1) *etiology* or *physiology*, manifested by erythrocyte or Hgb depletion; and (2) *morphol-*

Table 49-1 Tests Performed as Part of the Complete Blood Cell Count

TEST (AVERAGE VALUE)*	DESCRIPTION AND COMMENTS
Red blood cell (RBC) count (4.5-5.5 million/mm^3)	Number of RBCs/mm^3 of blood Indirectly estimates Hgb content of blood Reflects function of bone marrow
Hemoglobin (Hgb) determination (11.5-15.5 g/dl)	Amount of Hgb (g)/dl of whole blood Total blood Hgb primarily dependent on number of circulating RBCs but also on amount of Hgb in each cell
Hematocrit (Hct) (35%-45%)	Percent volume of packed RBCs in whole blood Indirectly measures Hgb content Is approximately three times Hgb content
RBC indexes	
Mean corpuscular volume (MCV) (77-95 fl)	Average or mean volume (size) of a single RBC MCV values are expressed as femtoliters (fl) or cubic microns (μm^3)
Mean corpuscular hemoglobin (MCH) (25-33 pg/cell)	Average or mean quantity (weight) of Hgb in a single RBC MCH values are expressed as picograms (pg) or micromicrograms (μmcg) MCV and MCH depend on accurate counts of RBCs, whereas MCHC does not; therefore MCHC is often more reliable All indexes depend on average cell measurements and do not show individual RBC variations (anisocytosis)
Mean corpuscular hemoglobin concentration (MCHC) (31%-37% Hgb [g]/dl RBC)	Average concentration of Hgb in a single RBC MCHC values are expressed as percent Hgb (g)/cell or Hgb (g)/dl RBC
RBC volume distribution width (RDW) (13.4% ± 1.2%)	Average size of RBCs Differentiates some types of anemia
Reticulocyte count (0.5%-1.5% erythrocytes)	Percent reticulocytes in RBCs Index of production of mature RBCs by bone marrow Decreased count indicates depressed bone marrow function Increased count indicates erythrogenesis in response to some stimulus When reticulocyte count is extremely high, other forms of immature RBCs (normoblasts, even erythroblasts) may be present Indirectly estimates hypochromic anemia Usually elevated in patients with chronic hemolytic anemia
White blood cell (WBC) count (4.5-13.5 × 10^3 cells/mm^3)	Number of WBCs/mm^3 of blood Total number of WBCs less important than differential count
Differential WBC count	Inspection and quantification of WBC types present in peripheral blood Values are expressed as percentages; to obtain absolute number of any type of WBC, multiply its respective percentage by total number of WBCs
Neutrophils (polys) (54%-62%) (3-5.8 × 10^3 cells/mm^3)	Primary defense in bacterial infection; capable of phagocytizing and killing bacteria
Bands (3%-5%) (0.15-0.4 × 10^3 cells/mm^3)	Immature neutrophil Increased numbers in bacterial infection Also capable of phagocytosis and killing
Eosinophils (1%-3%) (0.05-0.25 × 103 cells/mm^3)	Named for their staining characteristics with eosin dye Increased in allergic disorders, parasitic diseases, certain neoplasms, and other diseases
Basophils (0.075%) (0.015-0.030 cells/mm^3)	Named for their characteristic basophilic stippling Contain histamine, heparin, and serotonin; believed to cause increased blood flow to injured tissues while preventing excessive clotting
Lymphocytes (25%-33%) (1.5-3.0 × 103 cells/mm^3)	Involved in development of antibody and delayed hypersensitivity
Monocytes (3%-7%)	Large phagocytic cells that are involved in early stage of inflammatory reaction
Absolute neutrophil count (ANC) (>1000)	Percent neutrophils/bands times WBC count Indicates capability of body to handle bacterial infections
Platelet count (150-400 ×103/mm^3)	Number of platelets/mm^3 of blood Cellular fragments that are necessary for clotting to occur
Stained peripheral blood smear	Visual estimation of amount of Hgb in RBCs and overall size, shape, and structure of RBCs Various staining properties of RBC structures may be evidence of immature forms of erythrocytes Shows variation in size and shape of RBCs: microcytic, macrocytic, poikilocytic (variable shapes)

*See Appendix D for normal values according to ages.

evolve Animation–Platelets and Blood Clotting

ogy, the characteristic changes in RBC size, shape, or color (Box 49-1). Although the morphologic classification is more useful in terms of laboratory evaluation of anemia, the etiologic approach provides direction for planning nursing care. For example, anemia with reduced Hgb concentration may be caused by a dietary depletion of iron, and the principal intervention is replenishing iron stores. The classification of anemias is found in Fig. 49-1.

Consequences of Anemia

The basic physiologic defect caused by anemia is a decrease in the oxygen-carrying capacity of blood and consequently a reduction in the amount of oxygen available to the cells. When the anemia has developed slowly, the child usually adapts to the declining Hgb level.

The effects of anemia on the circulatory system can be profound. Because the viscosity of blood depends almost entirely on the concentration of RBCs, the resulting hemodilution of severe anemia decreases peripheral resistance, causing greater quantities of blood to return to the heart. The increased circulation and turbulence within the heart may produce a murmur. Because the cardiac workload is greatly increased, especially during exercise, infection, or emotional stress, cardiac failure may ensue.

Children seem to have a remarkable ability to function well despite low levels of Hgb. *Cyanosis* (the result of the quantity of deoxygenated Hgb in arterial blood) is typically not evident. Growth retardation, resulting from decreased cellular metabolism and coexisting anorexia, is a common finding in chronic severe anemia and is frequently accompanied by delayed sexual maturation in the older child.

BOX 49-1 Red Blood Cell Morphology

Size (Cell Size)

Variation in red blood cell (RBC) sizes (anisocytosis)

- Normocytes (normal cell size)
- Microcytes (smaller than normal cell size)
- Macrocytes (larger than normal cell size)

Shape (Cell Shape)

Variation in RBC shapes (poikilocytosis)

- Spherocytes (globular cells)
- Drepanocytes (sickle-shaped cells)
- Numerous other irregularly shaped cells

Color (Cell Staining Characteristics)

Variation in hemoglobin concentration in the RBCs

- Normochromic (sufficient or normal amount of hemoglobin per RBC)
- Hypochromic (reduced amount of hemoglobin per RBC)
- Hyperchromic (increased amount of hemoglobin per RBC)

Diagnostic Evaluation

In general, anemia may be suspected based on findings in the history and physical examination, such as lack of energy, easy fatigability, and pallor; however, unless the anemia is severe, the first clue to the disorder may be alterations in the CBC, such as decreased RBCs, and decreased Hgb and hematocrit (Hct) levels (see Fig. 49-1). Although anemia is sometimes defined as an Hgb level below 10 or 11 g/dl, this arbitrary cutoff is inappropriate for all children, because Hgb levels normally vary with age (see Table 49-1 and Appendix D).

Other tests specific to a particular type of anemia are used to determine the underlying cause of anemia. These are discussed in relation to the particular disorder.

Therapeutic Management

The objectives of medical management are to reverse the anemia by treating the underlying cause and to make up for

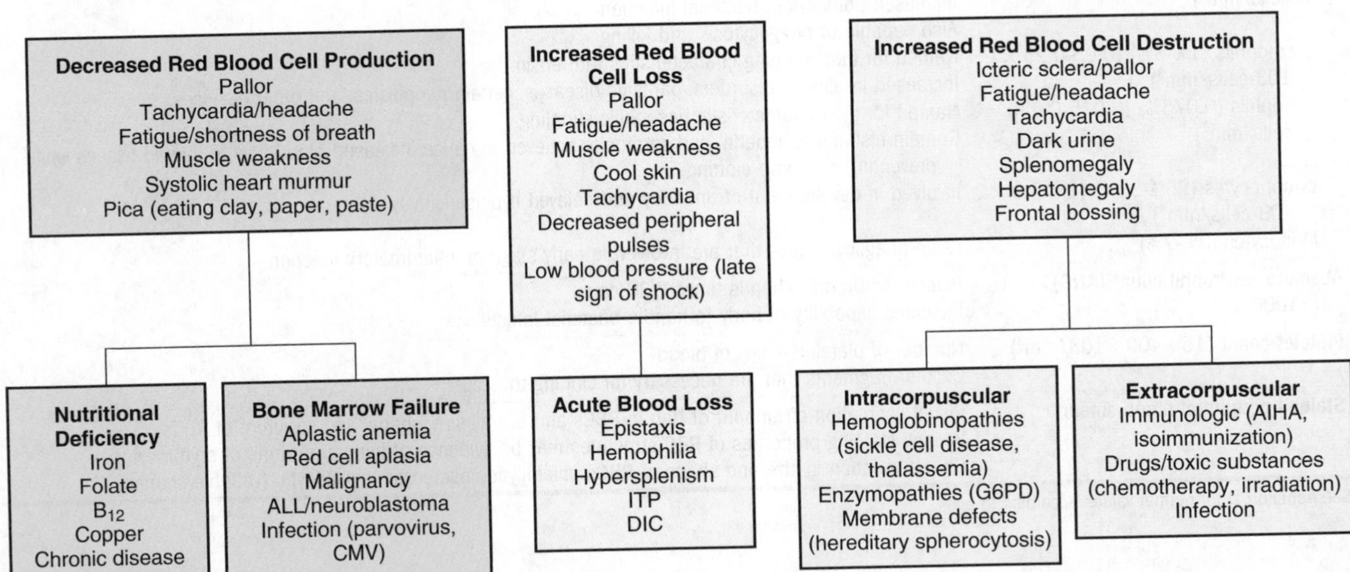

Fig. 49-1 Classifications of anemias. *AIHA,* Autoimmune hemolytic anemia; *ALL,* acute lymphoid leukemia; *CMV,* cytomegalovirus; *DIC,* disseminated intravascular coagulation; *G6PD,* glucose-6-phosphate dehydrogenase; *ITP,* idiopathic thrombocytopenic purpura.

any deficiency of blood, blood component, or substance the blood needs for normal functioning. For example, blood or blood cells are replaced after hemorrhage; in nutritional anemias the specific deficiency is replaced.

In patients with severe anemia, supportive medical care may include oxygen therapy, bed rest, and replacement of intravascular volume with intravenous (IV) fluids. The prognosis for anemia depends on the correction of the cause.

Nursing Care Management

The assessment of anemia includes the basic techniques that are applicable to any condition. The age of the infant or child provides some clues regarding the possible etiology of the anemia. For example, iron deficiency anemia occurs more frequently in the toddler between 12 and 36 months of age and during the growth spurt of adolescence.

Racial or ethnic background is significant. For example, the anemias related to abnormal Hgb levels are found in Southeast Asians and persons of African or Mediterranean ancestry. These same groups may be genetically deficient in the enzyme lactase after the period of infancy. Affected individuals are unable to tolerate lactose in the diet, with consequent intestinal irritation and chronic blood loss.

Special emphasis is placed on a careful history to elicit any information that might help identify the cause of the anemia. For example, a statement such as "My child drinks lots of milk" is a frequent finding in toddlers with iron deficiency anemia. An episode of diarrhea may have precipitated temporary lactose intolerance in a young child.

Stool examination for occult (microscopic) blood (Hemoccult test) can identify chronic intestinal bleeding that results from a primary or secondary lactase deficiency. It is also important to understand the significance of various blood tests (see Table 49-1).

Prepare Child and Family for Laboratory Tests

Usually several blood tests are ordered; because they are generally done sequentially rather than at one time, the child is subjected to multiple finger or heel punctures or venipunctures. Laboratory technicians frequently are not aware of the trauma that repeated punctures represent to a child. However, these invasive procedures need not be painful (see Blood Specimens, Chapter 45). For example, the topical application of an eutectic mix of lidocaine and prilocaine (EMLA) or 4% lidocaine (Ela-Max) before needle punctures can eliminate pain (see Pain Management, Chapter 35). Therefore the nurse is responsible for preparing the child and family for the tests by:

- Explaining the significance of each test, particularly why the tests are not all done at one time
- Encouraging parents or another supportive person to be with the child during the procedure
- Allowing the child to play with the equipment on a doll or participate in the actual procedure (e.g., by cleansing the finger with an alcohol swab)

Older children may appreciate the opportunity to observe the blood cells under a microscope or in photographs. This experience is especially important if a serious blood disorder, such as leukemia, is suspected because it serves as a foundation for explaining the pathophysiology of the disorder.

Bone marrow aspiration is not a routine hematologic test but is essential for definitive diagnosis of the leukemias, lymphomas, and certain anemias.

NURSING ALERT The following are suggested explanations for teaching children about blood components:

Red blood cells (RBCs)–Carry the oxygen you breathe from your lungs to all parts of your body

White blood cells (WBCs)–Help keep germs from causing infection

Platelets–Small parts of cells that help make bleeding stop by forming a clot (scab) over the hurt area

Plasma–The liquid portion of blood, which has clotting factors that help make bleeding stop

Decrease Tissue Oxygen Needs

Because the basic pathologic process in anemia is a decrease in oxygen-carrying capacity, an important nursing responsibility is to assess the child's energy level and minimize excess demands. The child's level of tolerance for activities of daily living and play is assessed, and adjustments are made to allow as much self-care as possible without undue exertion. During periods of rest the nurse takes vital signs and observes behavior to establish a baseline of nonexertion energy expenditure. During periods of activity the nurse repeats these measurements and observations to compare them with resting values.

Prevent Complications

Children who are so severely anemic that they are hospitalized may require oxygen to prevent or reduce tissue hypoxia. Because these children are susceptible to infection, every effort is expended to prevent exposure to infectious agents. All the usual precautions are taken to prevent infection, such as practicing thorough hand washing, selecting an appropriate room in a noninfectious area, restricting visitors or hospital personnel with active infection, and maintaining adequate nutrition. The nurse also observes for signs of infection, particularly temperature elevation and leukocytosis.

Iron Deficiency Anemia

Anemia caused by an inadequate supply of dietary iron is the most prevalent nutritional disorder in the United States and the most common mineral disturbance. Children 12 to 36 months of age are at risk for anemia as a result of cow's milk being a major staple of the child's diet (Richardson, 2007; Segel, Hirsh, & Feig, 2002). The prevalence of iron deficiency anemia has decreased, probably in part because of families' participation in the Women, Infants, and Children (WIC) program, which provides iron-fortified formula for the first year of life and routine screening of Hgb levels during early childhood (Bogen, Krause, & Serwint, 2001). Preterm infants are especially at risk because of their reduced fetal iron supply. Adolescents are also at risk because of their rapid growth rate combined with poor eating habits.

evolve Nursing Care Plan—The Child with Anemia

Pathophysiology

Iron deficiency anemia can be caused by any number of factors that decrease the supply of iron, impair its absorption, increase the body's need for iron, or affect the synthesis of Hgb. Although the clinical manifestations and diagnostic evaluation are similar regardless of the cause, the therapeutic and nursing care management depend on the specific reason for the iron deficiency. The following discussion is limited to iron deficiency anemia resulting from inadequate iron in the diet.

During the last trimester of pregnancy, iron is transferred from mother to fetus. Most of the iron is stored in the circulating erythrocytes of the fetus, with the remainder stored in the fetal liver, spleen, and bone marrow. These iron stores are usually adequate for the first 5 to 6 months in a full-term infant but for only 2 to 3 months in preterm infants or multiple births. If dietary iron is not supplied to meet the infant's growth demands after the fetal iron stores are depleted, iron deficiency anemia results. Physiologic anemia should not be confused with iron deficiency anemia resulting from nutritional causes.

Although most toddlers with iron deficiency anemia are underweight, many infants are overweight because of excessive milk ingestion (known as *milk babies*). These children become anemic for two reasons: milk, a poor source of iron, is given almost to the exclusion of solid foods; and 50% of iron-deficient infants fed cow's milk have an increased fecal loss of blood.

Therapeutic Management

After the diagnosis of iron deficiency anemia is made, therapeutic management focuses on increasing the amount of supplemental iron the child receives. This is usually done through dietary counseling and the administration of oral iron supplements.

In formula-fed infants the most convenient and best sources of supplemental iron are iron-fortified commercial formula and iron-fortified infant cereal. Iron-fortified formula provides a relatively constant and predictable amount of iron and is not associated with an increased incidence of gastrointestinal (GI) symptoms, such as colic, diarrhea, or constipation. Infants younger than 12 months of age should *not* be given fresh cow's milk because it may increase the risk of GI blood loss occurring from allergy to the milk protein or from GI mucosal damage resulting from a lack of cytochrome iron (heme protein) (Richardson, 2007; Segel, Hirsh, & Feig, 2002). If GI bleeding is suspected, the child's stool should be guaiac tested on at least four or five occasions to identify any intermittent blood loss.

Dietary addition of iron-rich foods is usually inadequate as the sole treatment of iron deficiency anemia, since the iron is poorly absorbed and thus provides insufficient supplemental quantities of iron. If dietary sources of iron cannot replace body stores, oral iron supplements are prescribed for approximately 3 months. Ferrous iron, more readily absorbed than ferric iron, results in higher Hgb levels. Ascorbic acid (vitamin C) appears to facilitate absorption of iron and may be given as vitamin C–enriched foods and juices with the iron preparation.

If the Hgb level fails to rise after 1 month of oral therapy, it is important to assess for persistent bleeding, iron malabsorption, noncompliance, improper iron administration, or other causes for the anemia. Parenteral (IV or intramuscular [IM]) iron administration is safe and effective but painful, expensive, and occasionally associated with regional lymphadenopathy or allergic reaction (Andrews, 2003; McKenzie, 2004). Therefore parenteral iron is reserved for children who have iron malabsorption or chronic hemoglobinuria. Transfusions are indicated for the most severe anemia and in cases of serious infection, cardiac dysfunction, or surgical emergency when anesthesia is required. Packed RBCs (2 to 3 ml/kg), not whole blood, are used to minimize the chance of circulatory overload. Supplemental oxygen is administered when tissue hypoxia is severe.

Prognosis

The prognosis for a child with this condition is very good. However, there is some evidence that, if the iron deficiency anemia is severe and long-standing, cognitive, behavioral, and motor impairment may result (Burden et al, 2007; Andrews, 2003).

Nursing Care Management

An essential nursing responsibility is instructing parents in the administration of iron. Oral iron should be given as prescribed in two divided doses between meals, when the presence of free hydrochloric acid is greatest, since more iron is absorbed in the acidic environment of the upper GI tract. Citrus fruit or juice taken with the medication aids in absorption.

NURSING ALERT Cow's milk contains substances that bind the iron and interfere with absorption. Iron supplements should not be administered with milk or milk products (Carley, 2003).

An adequate dosage of oral iron turns the stools a tarry green color. The nurse advises parents of this normally expected change and inquires about its occurrence on follow-up visits. Absence of the greenish black stool may be a clue to poor administration of iron, in either schedule or dosage. Vomiting or diarrhea can occur with iron therapy. If the parents report these symptoms, the iron can be given with meals and the dosage reduced and then gradually increased until tolerated.

Liquid preparations of iron may temporarily stain the teeth. If possible, the medication should be taken through a straw or given through a syringe or medicine dropper placed toward the back of the mouth. Brushing the teeth after administration of the drug lessens the discoloration.

If parenteral iron preparations are prescribed, iron dextran must be injected deeply into a large muscle mass using the Z-track method. The injection site is *not* massaged after injection to minimize skin staining and irritation. Because no more than 1 ml should be given in one site, the IV route should be considered to avoid multiple injections. Careful observation is required because of the risk of adverse reactions, such as anaphylaxis, with IV administration. A test dose is recommended before routine use.

Diet

A primary nursing objective is to prevent nutritional anemia through family education. Because breast milk is a poor iron source after 5 months of lactation, the nurse must reinforce the importance of administering iron supplementation to the exclusively breastfed infant by 6 months of age (Andrews, 2003; Chandran & Gelfer, 2006; Richardson, 2007).

The American Academy of Pediatrics (2005) recommends that preterm and low-birth-weight infants or infants with inadequate iron stores at birth receive iron supplements before 6 months of age.

For the formula-fed infant, the nurse discusses with parents the importance of using iron-fortified formula and introducing solid foods at the appropriate age during the first year of life. Traditionally, cereals are one of the first semisolid foods to be introduced into the infant's diet at approximately 6 months of age (Chandran & Gelfer, 2006; Glader, 2007). The best solid-food source of iron is commercial iron-fortified cereals. It may be difficult at first to teach the infant to accept foods other than milk. The same principles are applied as those for introducing new foods (see Nutrition, Chapter 36), especially feeding the solid food before the milk. Predominantly milk-fed infants rebel against solid foods, and parents are cautioned about this and the need to be firm in not relinquishing control to the child. It may require intense problem solving on the part of both the family and the nurse to overcome the child's resistance.

A difficulty encountered in discouraging the parents from feeding milk to the exclusion of other foods is dispelling the popular myth that milk is a "perfect food." Many parents believe that milk is best for the infant and equate the weight gain with a "healthy child" and "good mothering." The nurse can also stress that overweight is not synonymous with good health.

Sickle Cell Anemia

Sickle cell anemia (SCA) is one of a group of diseases collectively termed *hemoglobinopathies,* in which normal adult Hgb (Hgb A [HbA]) is partly or completely replaced by abnormal sickle Hgb (HbS). *Sickle cell disease (SCD)* includes all the hereditary disorders with clinical, hematologic, and pathologic features that are related to the presence of HbS. Even though the term *SCD* is sometimes used to refer to SCA, this use is incorrect. Other correct terms for SCA are *SS* and *homozygous SCD.*

The following are the most common forms of SCD in the United States:

SCA, the homozygous form of the disease (HbSS or SS)

Sickle cell–C disease, a heterozygous variant of SCD, including both HbS and HbC (SC)

Sickle cell–Hgb E disease, a variant of SCD in which glutamic acid has been substituted for lysine in the number-26 position of the β-chain (SE)

Sickle thalassemia disease, a combination of sickle cell trait and β-thalassemia trait (Sβ-thal); β+ refers to the ability to still produce some normal HbA; β^0 indicates that there is no ability to produce HbA

Of the SCDs, SCA is the most common form in African-Americans, followed by sickle cell–C disease and sickle thalassemia. Sickle syndromes exist when the HbS is paired with other mutant globins.

SCA is found primarily in 1 in 375 births of African-Americans, 1 in 1200 births of Hispanics, with lower incidence in the other ethnic groups (Driscoll, 2007). The incidence of the disease varies in different geographic locations. Among African-Americans the incidence of sickle cell trait is about 9%. In West Africa the incidence is reported to be as high as 40% among native Africans. The high incidence of sickle cell trait in West Africans is believed by some to be the result of selective protection afforded trait carriers against one type of malaria.

The gene that determines the production of HbS is situated on an autosome and, when present, is always detectable and therefore dominant. Heterozygous persons who have both normal HbA and abnormal HbS are said to have *sickle cell trait.* Persons who are homozygous have predominantly HbS and have SCA. The inheritance pattern is essentially that of an autosomal recessive disorder. Therefore, when both parents have sickle cell trait, there is a 25% chance with each pregnancy of producing an offspring with SCA.

Although the defect is inherited, the sickling phenomenon is usually not apparent until later in infancy because of the presence of fetal Hbg (HbF). As long as the child has predominantly HbF, sickling does not occur because there is less HbS. The newborn with SCA is generally asymptomatic because of the protective effect of HbF (60% to 80% HbF), but this rapidly decreases during the first year; thus the child is at risk for sickle cell–related complications (Dover & Platt, 2003; Driscoll, 2007).

evolve Animation—Sickle Cell Anemia

Pathophysiology

The clinical features of SCA are primarily the result of (1) *obstruction* caused by the sickled RBCs, and (2) increased RBC *destruction* (Fig. 49-2). The abnormal adhesion, entanglement, and enmeshing of rigid sickle-shaped cells with one another intermittently block the microcirculation, causing vasoocclusion. The resultant absence of blood flow to adjacent tissues causes local hypoxia, leading to tissue ischemia and infarction (cellular death). Most of the complications seen in SCA can be traced to this process and its impact on various organs of the body. The effect of sickling and infarction on organ structures occurs in the following sequence (Box 49-2):

1. Stasis with enlargement
2. Infarction with ischemia and repeated destruction
3. Replacement with fibrous tissue (scarring)

Clinical Manifestations

The clinical manifestations of SCA vary greatly in severity and frequency. The most acute symptoms of the disease occur during periods of exacerbation called *crises.* There are several types of episodic crises: vasoocclusive, acute splenic sequestration, aplastic, hyperhemolytic, cerebrovascular accident (CVA), chest syndrome, and infection. The crises may occur individually or concomitantly with one or more other crises. The episode may be a *vasoocclusive crisis,* preferably called a "painful episode," characterized by distal ischemia and pain; *sequestration crisis,* a pooling of blood in the liver and spleen with decreased blood volume and shock; *aplastic crisis,* diminished RBC production resulting in profound anemia; or *hyperhemolytic crisis,* an accelerated rate of RBC destruction characterized by anemia, jaundice, and reticulocytosis.

Another serious complication is *acute chest syndrome (ACS),* which is clinically similar to pneumonia. It is the presence of a new pulmonary infiltrate and is associated with chest

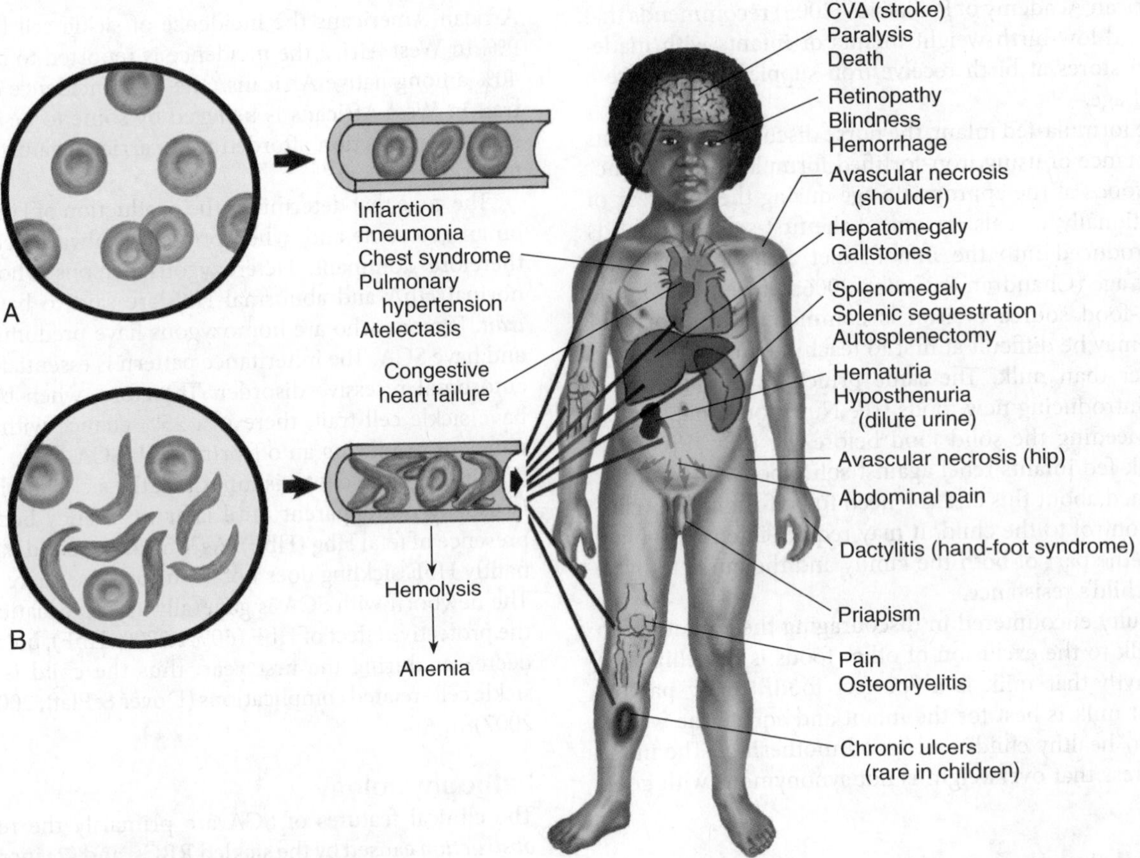

Fig. 49-2 Differences between effects of normal (A) and sickled (B) red blood cells on circulation with related complications. *CVA*, Cerebrovascular accident.

evolve Case Study—Sickle Cell Anemia

BOX 49-2 Clinical Manifestations of Sickle Cell Anemia

General

Possible growth retardation
Chronic anemia (hemoglobin level of 6 to 9 g/dl)
Possible delayed sexual maturation
Marked susceptibility to sepsis

Vasoocclusive Crisis

Pain in area(s) of involvement
Manifestations related to ischemia of involved areas

- **Extremities**—Painful swelling of hands and feet (sickle cell dactylitis, or hand-foot syndrome), painful joints
- **Abdomen**—Severe pain resembling acute surgical condition
- **Cerebrum**—Stroke, visual disturbances
- **Chest**—Symptoms resembling pneumonia, protracted episodes of pulmonary disease
- **Liver**—Obstructive jaundice, hepatic coma
- **Kidney**—Hematuria
- **Genitalia**—Priapism (painful, constant penile erection)

Sequestration Crisis

Pooling of large amounts of blood

- Hepatomegaly
- Splenomegaly
- Circulatory collapse

Effects of Chronic Vasoocclusive Phenomena

Heart—Cardiomegaly, systolic murmurs
Lungs—Altered pulmonary function, susceptibility to infections, pulmonary insufficiency
Kidneys—Inability to concentrate urine, enuresis, progressive renal failure
Liver—Hepatomegaly, cirrhosis, intrahepatic cholestasis
Spleen—Splenomegaly, susceptibility to infection, functional reduction in splenic activity progressing to autosplenectomy
Eyes—Intraocular abnormalities with visual disturbances; sometimes progressive retinal detachment and blindness
Extremities—Avascular necrosis of hip or shoulder; skeletal deformities, especially lordosis and kyphosis; chronic leg ulcers; susceptibility to osteomyelitis
Central nervous system—Hemiparesis, seizures

pain, fever, cough, tachypnea, wheezing, and hypoxia. A *CVA (stroke)* is a sudden and severe complication, often with no related illnesses. Sickled cells block the major blood vessels in the brain, resulting in cerebral infarction, which causes variable degrees of neurologic impairment. The current treatment for SCD children who have experienced a stroke is chronic transfusion therapy. Repeat CVAs causing progressively greater brain damage occur in approximately 70% of untreated children who have experienced one stroke (Dover & Platt, 2003).

Diagnostic Evaluation

Newborn screening for SCA is mandatory in most of the United States so that infants can be identified before symptoms occur. At birth the infant has up to 80% of HbF, which does not carry the defect. Because levels of HbS are low at birth, Hgb electrophoresis or other tests that measure Hgb concentrations are indicated. Early diagnosis (before 3 months of age) enables initiation of appropriate interventions to minimize complications. The family is taught to administer prophylactic antibiotics and identify early signs of infection to seek medical therapy as soon as possible.

If SCA is not diagnosed in early infancy, it is likely to manifest symptoms during the toddler and preschool years. SCA is occasionally first diagnosed during a crisis that follows an acute respiratory tract or GI infection. Routine hematologic tests are done to evaluate the anemia. Several specific tests detect the presence of the abnormal Hgb in the heterozygote or the homozygote. For *screening* purposes the *sickle-turbidity test (Sickledex)* is frequently used because it can be performed on blood from a finger stick and yields accurate results in 3 minutes. However, if the test is positive, Hgb electrophoresis is necessary to distinguish between children with the trait and those with the disease. *Hgb electrophoresis* ("fingerprinting" of the protein) is an accurate, rapid, and specific test for detecting the homozygous and heterozygous forms of the disease and the percentages of the various types of Hgb.

Therapeutic Management

The aims of therapy are (1) to prevent the sickling phenomena, which are responsible for the pathologic sequelae; and (2) to treat the medical emergencies of sickle cell crisis. The successful achievement of the aims depends on prompt nursing interventions, medical therapies, patient and family preventive measures, and use of innovative treatments.

Medical management of a crisis is usually directed toward supportive and symptomatic treatment. The main objectives are to provide (1) rest to minimize energy expenditure and oxygen use; (2) hydration through oral and IV therapy; (3) electrolyte replacement because hypoxia results in metabolic acidosis, which also promotes sickling; (4) analgesics for the severe pain from vasoocclusion; (5) blood replacement to treat anemia and reduce the viscosity of the sickled blood; and (6) antibiotics to treat any existing infection.

Administration of pneumococcal and meningococcal vaccines is recommended for these children because of their susceptibility to infection as a result of a functional asplenia. In addition to routine immunizations, the child with SCD should receive an annual influenza vaccination. Oral penicillin prophylaxis is also recommended by 2 months of age to reduce the chance of pneumococcal sepsis (see Evidence-Based Practice box) (American Academy of Pediatrics, Section on Hematology/Oncology, Committee on Genetics, 2002; National Institutes of Health, National Heart, Lung, and Blood Institute, 2002; Redding-Lallinger & Knoll, 2006).

Short-term oxygen therapy may be helpful if a child has symptoms of respiratory difficulty. Severe hypoxia must be prevented because this causes massive systemic sickling that can be fatal. Although oxygen may prevent more sickling, it usually is not effective in reversing sickling because the oxygen is unable to reach the enmeshed sickled erythrocytes in clogged vessels (Perkins, 2001; Chiocca, 1996). In addition, prolonged administration can depress bone marrow, further aggravating the anemia (Khoury & Grimsley, 1995; Dover & Platt, 2003).

Exchange transfusion, which reduces the number of circulating sickle cells and slows down the vicious circle of hypoxia, thrombosis, tissue ischemia, and injury, has been successful. The procedure is sometimes advocated as a possible preventive technique. A transcranial Doppler (TCD) test identifies the child with SCD who is at high risk for developing a CVA by monitoring the intracranial vascular flow (American Academy of Pediatrics, Section on Hematology/Oncology, Committee on Genetics, 2002; Bulas, 2005; Driscoll, 2007). The TCD is performed annually on children from 2 to 16 years of age. If the TCD is abnormal, the recommended treatment is chronic transfusion therapy (Driscoll, 2007; Segel, Hirsh, & Feig, 2002). However, multiple transfusions carry the risk of transmission of viral infection, hyperviscosity, transfusion reactions, alloimmunization, and hemosiderosis (Redding-Lallinger & Knoll, 2006; Orkin & Nathan, 2003; Driscoll, 2007). After a CVA, blood transfusions are usually given every 3 to 4 weeks to help prevent a repeat stroke. To reduce iron overload from chronic transfusion therapy, chelation therapy may be started (see p. 1501).

In children with recurrent life-threatening splenic sequestration, splenectomy may be a lifesaving measure. However, the spleen usually atrophies on its own through progressive fibrotic changes *(functional asplenia)* by 6 years of age. Prophylactic penicillin postsplenectomy and pneumococcal vaccines have decreased the incidence of pneumococcal sepsis. Packed RBC transfusions are recommended for treatment of splenic sequestration and stroke and preoperatively for most surgical procedures in the child with SCD.

The most frequent problem for patients with SCA is *vasoocclusive pain.* The chronic nature of this pain can greatly affect the child's development. *Priapism (continuous* or *intermittent)* is defined as painful erection of the penis. As a vasoocclusive crisis, the priapism event is caused by sickling in sinusoids of the corpora cavernosa and is treated with aspiration of the corpora cavernosa only when conventional approaches fail (Redding-Lallinger & Knoll, 2006). A multidisciplinary approach is best for vasoocclusive pain management that includes pharmacologic treatment, hydration, physical therapy, and complementary treatment (e.g., prayer, spiritual healing, massage, herbs, relaxation, acupuncture, and biofeedback) (Redding-Lallinger & Knoll, 2006; Yoon & Black, 2006). When mild to moderate pain is reported, ibuprofen or acet-

EVIDENCE-BASED PRACTICE Sickle Cell Anemia and Penicillin Prophylaxis

Ask the Question

In children with sickle cell anemia, does prophylaxis with penicillin prevent pneumococcal infection?

Search for Evidence

Search Strategies

Search selection criteria included English language, publication within the past 25 years, research-based articles (level 3 or lower), and child populations.

Databases Used

PubMed, Cochrane Collaboration, MD Consult

Critically Analyze the Evidence

Administration of oral prophylactic penicillin was compared with the 14-valent pneumococcal vaccine in preventing pneumococcal infection in 242 children between the ages of 6 months and 3 years with homozygous sickle cell disease. In the first 5 years of the trial, there were 11 pneumococcal infections in the pneumococcal vaccine group and higher infection rates in those given the vaccine before 1 year of age. No pneumococcal isolates were found in the group receiving penicillin, although four pneumococcal isolates were found in this group within 1 year of stopping the penicillin prophylaxis at age 3 years. This study supported the use of penicillin prophylaxis to prevent pneumococcal infection in children younger than 3 years of age (John et al, 1984).

In a multicenter, randomized, double-blind, placebo-controlled clinical trial, 105 children received penicillin twice daily; a control group of 110 children received a placebo twice daily. The trial was terminated 8 months early when an 84% reduction in the incidence of pneumococcal infections was observed in the group treated with penicillin compared with the placebo group. There were no deaths in the penicillin group, but three deaths from infection occurred in the placebo group. Researchers stressed the importance of screening children during the neonatal period and prescribing prophylactic penicillin to decrease the morbidity and mortality associated with pneumococcal infection (Gaston et al, 1986).

Zarkowsky and colleagues (1986) conducted a retrospective analysis of 178 episodes of bacteremia in children with sickle hemoglobinopathies that occurred during 13,771 patient-years of follow-up ($N = 3451$). The predominant pathogen in patients younger than 6 years of age was *Streptococcus pneumoniae* (66%), and gram-negative organisms were responsible for 50% of the bacteremias in patients 6 years and older. The incidence of pneumococcal bacteremia in children with sickle cell anemia younger than 3 years of age was 6.1 events per 100 patient-years. The results of this study supported prophylactic administration of penicillin for prevention of pneumococcal bacteremia in children younger than 3 years of age.

A cohort study of 315 patients with homozygous sickle cell disease who lived in Jamaica was conducted between June 1973 and December 1981. The patients were divided into three groups to determine whether interventions such as penicillin prophylaxis, parental education in early diagnosis of acute splenic sequestration, and close monitoring in a sickle cell clinic improved survival. A significant decline in deaths from acute splenic sequestration and pneumococcal septicemia and meningitis was found. The research indicated that early detection of sickle cell disease and prophylactic measures could significantly reduce deaths associated with homozygous sickle cell disease (Lee et al, 1995).

In a retrospective longitudinal study conducted from January 1995 through December 1999, 261 children under 4 years of age with sickle cell disease who did not have adequate health insurance were found to have received inadequate refills for antibiotic prophylaxis that placed them at increased risk of developing pneumococcal infection. Study findings showed that an increased number of outpatient visits for preventive care was associated with improved dispensing of prophylactic antibiotic refills (Sox et al, 2003).

Riddington and Owusu-Ofori (2002) conducted a systematic review of randomized controlled trials evaluating the effectiveness of prophylactic antibiotic administration in preventing pneumococcal infection in children with sickle cell disease. The review of published research found that penicillin prophylaxis significantly reduced the risk of pneumococcal infection in children with homozygous sickle cell disease with minimal adverse reactions.

Apply the Evidence: Nursing Implications

The evidence demonstrated that penicillin prophylaxis significantly reduces the risk of pneumococcal infection in children with sickle cell anemia. The epidemiologic studies strongly suggest that all children with sickle cell anemia should be started on prophylactic penicillin at 2 months of age. Parents and children with sickle cell anemia should be instructed in the importance of taking the prophylactic penicillin twice daily and seeking medical attention immediately for acute illness, especially if the temperature exceeds 38.3° C (101° F), regardless of the use of prophylaxis.

References

Gaston MH et al: Prophylaxis with oral penicillin in children with sickle cell anemia: a randomized trial, *N Engl J Med* 314(25):1593-1599, 1986.

John AB et al: Prevention of pneumococcal infection in children with homozygous sickle cell disease, *BMJ* 288(6430):1567-1570, 1984.

Lee A et al: Improved survival in homozygous sickle cell disease: lessons from cohort study, *BMJ* 311(7020):1600-1602, 1995.

Riddington C, Owusu-Ofori S: *Prophylactic antibiotics for preventing pneumococcal infection in children with sickle cell disease*, 2002. Available at www.cochrane.org/reviews/en/ab003427.html (accessed August 19, 2005).

Sox CM et al: Provision of pneumococcal prophylaxis for publicly insured children with sickle cell disease, *JAMA* 290(8):1057-1061, 2003.

Zarkowsky HS et al: Bacteremia in sickle hemoglobinopathies, *J Pediatr* 109(4):579-585, 1986.

aminophen (Tylenol) is used initially. If these drugs are not effective alone, codeine can be added. The dosages of both drugs are titrated (adjusted) to a therapeutic level. Opioids such as immediate- and sustained-release morphine, oxycodone, hydromorphone (Dilaudid), and methadone are administered intravenously or orally for severe pain and given around the clock. Patient-controlled analgesia (PCA) has been used successfully for sickle cell–related pain. PCA reinforces the patient's role and responsibility in managing the pain and provides flexibility in dealing with pain, which may vary in severity over time (see Pain Management, Chapter 35).

Prognosis

The prognosis varies, but most patients live into the fifth decade. Most of the time, children are without symptoms and participate in normal activities without restrictions. The greatest risk is usually in children younger than 5 years of age, and the majority of deaths in these children are caused by overwhelming infection. Consequently, SCA is a chronic illness with a potentially terminal outcome. Physical and sexual maturation are delayed in adolescents with SCA. Although adults achieve normal height, weight, and sexual function, the delay may present problems to the adolescent (Dover & Platt, 2003; Redding-Lallinger & Knoll, 2006).

SCD individuals with higher levels of HbF tend to have a milder disease with fewer complications than those with lower levels (Anderson, 2006; Driscoll, 2007). Hydroxyurea is a U.S. Food and Drug Administration–approved medication that increases the production of HbF, reduces endothelial adhesion of sickle cells, and improves the sickle cell hydration (National Institutes of Health, National Heart, Lung, and Blood Institute, 2002). Long-term follow-up of patients taking hydroxyurea alone revealed a 40% reduction in mortality and decreased frequency of vasoocclusive crisis, ACS, hospital admissions, and need for transfusions, thus making SCD crises milder (Anderson, 2006; Steinberg et al, 2003). Pediatric studies have shown that hydroxyurea can be safely used in children (Miller et al, 2001; Zimmerman et al, 2004).

Hematopoietic stem cell transplantation (HSCT) offers the only cure for some children, although the mortality rate is approximately 8% and graft failures after transplantation range from 9% to 14% (Dover & Platt, 2003; Driscoll, 2007) (see p. 1522).

Nursing Care Management

Educate Family and Child

Family education begins with an explanation of the disease and its consequences. After this explanation, the most important issues to teach the family are to (1) seek early intervention for problems such as fever of 38.5° C (101.3° F) or greater, (2) give penicillin as ordered, (3) recognize signs and symptoms of splenic sequestration and respiratory problems that can lead to hypoxia, and (4) treat the child normally. The nurse tells the family that the child is normal but can get sick in ways that other children cannot.

The nurse emphasizes the importance of adequate hydration to prevent sickling and to delay the adhesion-stasis-thrombosis-ischemia cycle in a crisis. It is not sufficient to advise parents to "force fluids" or "encourage drinking." They need specific instructions on how many daily glasses or bottles of fluid are required. Many foods are also a source of fluid, particularly soups, flavored ice pops, ice cream, sherbet, gelatin, and puddings.

Increased fluids combined with impaired kidney function result in the problem of *enuresis.* Parents who are unaware of this fact frequently use the usual measures to discourage bed-wetting, such as limiting fluids at night, and may resort to punishment and shame to force bladder control. Enuresis is treated as a complication of the disease, such as joint pain or some other symptom, to alleviate parental pressure on the child.

Promote Supportive Therapies During Crises

The success of many of the medical therapies relies heavily on nursing implementation. Management of pain is an especially difficult problem and often involves experimenting with various analgesics, including opioids, and schedules before relief is achieved. Unfortunately, these children tend to be undermedicated, resulting in their "clock watching" and demands for additional doses sooner than might be expected. Often this incorrectly raises suspicions of drug addiction, when in fact the problem is one of improper dosage (see Family-Centered Care box). In choosing and scheduling analgesics, the goal should be *prevention* of pain.

FAMILY-CENTERED CARE

Fear of Addiction

Although the pain during a sickle cell crisis is usually severe and opioids are needed, many families fear that their child will become addicted to the narcotic. Unfortunately, misinformed health professionals may foster this unfounded fear, which results in needless suffering. Very few children who receive opioids for severe pain become behaviorally addicted to the drug (American Pain Society, 1999; National Institutes of Health, National Heart, Lung, and Blood Institute, 2002). Families and older children, especially adolescents, need to be reassured that opioids are medically indicated, high doses may be needed, and children rarely become addicted.

NURSING ALERT Advise parents to be particularly alert to situations such as hot weather in which dehydration may be a possibility and to recognize early signs of reduced intake such as decreased urinary output (e.g., fewer wet diapers) and increased thirst.

Any pain program should be combined with psychologic support to help the child deal with the depression, anxiety, and fear that may accompany the disease. This includes regular visits with the child to discuss any concerns during the hospitalization and positive reinforcement of coping skills, such as successful methods of dealing with the pain and compliance with treatment prescriptions. To reduce the negative connotation associated with the term *crisis,* it is best to say *pain episode.*

Frequently, heat to the affected area is soothing. Cold compresses are not applied because this enhances sickling and vasoconstriction. Bed rest is usually well tolerated during a

evolve Nursing Care Plan–The Child with Sickle Cell Disease

crisis, although actual rest depends greatly on pain alleviation and organized schedules of nursing care. Some activity, particularly passive range-of-motion exercises, is beneficial to promote circulation. Usually the best course of action is to let children dictate their activity tolerance.

If blood transfusions or exchange transfusions are given, the nurse has the responsibility of observing for signs of transfusion reaction (see Table 49-5). Because hypervolemia from too-rapid transfusion can increase the workload of the heart, the nurse also is alert to signs of cardiac failure.

In splenic sequestration the size of the spleen is gently measured by abdominal palpation (see Abdomen, Chapter 34). The nurse should be aware of spleen size because increasing splenomegaly is an ominous sign. A decreasing spleen size denotes response to therapy. Vital signs and blood pressure are also closely monitored for impending shock. Anemia is typically not a presenting complication in vasoocclusive crises but is a critical problem in other types of crises. The nurse monitors for evidence of increasing anemia and institutes appropriate nursing interventions (see p. 1499). Oxygen is not beneficial in vasoocclusive episodes unless hypoxemia is present (Dover & Platt, 2003; Karayalcin, 2000). It does not reverse sickled RBCs, and if used in the nonhypoxic patient, it decreases erythropoiesis (Khoury & Grimsley, 1995). Because prolonged use of oxygen can aggravate the anemia, signs of lack of therapeutic benefit, such as restlessness, increased pallor, and continued pain, are reported.

Intake, especially of IV fluids, and output are recorded. The child's weight should be taken on admission to serve as a baseline for evaluating hydration. Because diuresis can result in electrolyte loss, the nurse also observes for signs of hypokalemia and should be familiar with normal serum electrolyte values to report changes.

Recognize Other Complications

Nurses also need to be aware of the signs of ACS and CVA, both potentially fatal complications. It is essential to educate parents about these symptoms.

Support Family

Families need the opportunity to discuss their feelings regarding transmitting a potentially fatal, chronic illness to their child. Because of the widely publicized prognosis for children with SCA, many parents express their prevalent fear of the child's death. Three manifestations of SCD that may appear in the first 2 years of life (dactylitis, severe anemia, leukocytosis) can be predictors of disease severity (Platt et al, 1994; Ohls & Christensen, 2007). However, nursing care for the family should be the same as for any family with a child with a life-threatening illness. Particular emphasis is placed on the siblings' reactions, the stress on the marital relationship, and the childrearing attitudes displayed toward the child (see Chapter 31). Several resources are available to the family with a sickling disorder.

β-Thalassemia (Cooley Anemia)

The term *thalassemia,* which is derived from the Greek word *thalassa,* meaning "sea," is applied to a variety of inherited blood disorders characterized by deficiencies in the rate of production of specific globin chains in Hgb. The name appropriately refers to descendants of or people living near the Mediterranean Sea, who have the highest incidence of the disease (i.e., Italians, Greeks, and Syrians). Evidence suggests that the high incidence of the disorders among these groups is a result of the selective advantage the trait confers in relation to malaria, as is postulated in SCD. However, the disorder has a wide geographic distribution, probably as a result of genetic migration through intermarriage or possibly as a result of spontaneous mutation.

β-Thalassemia is the most common of the thalassemias and occurs in four forms:

- Two heterozygous forms, *thalassemia minor,* an asymptomatic silent carrier, and *thalassemia trait,* which produces a mild microcytic anemia
- *Thalassemia intermedia,* which is manifested as splenomegaly and moderate to severe anemia
- A homozygous form, *thalassemia major* (also known as *Cooley's anemia*), which results in a severe anemia that would lead to cardiac failure and death in early childhood without transfusion support

Pathophysiology

Normal postnatal Hgb is composed of two α- and two β-polypeptide chains. In β-thalassemia there is a partial or complete deficiency in the synthesis of the β-chain of the Hgb molecule. Consequently, there is a compensatory increase in the synthesis of α-chains, and γ-chain production remains activated, resulting in defective Hgb formation. This unbalanced polypeptide unit is very unstable; when it disintegrates, it damages RBCs, causing severe anemia.

To compensate for the hemolytic process, an overabundance of erythrocytes is formed unless the bone marrow is suppressed by transfusion therapy. Excess iron from hemolysis of supplemental RBCs in transfusions and from the rapid destruction of defective cells is stored in various organs *(hemosiderosis).*

Diagnostic Evaluation

The onset of thalassemia major may be insidious and not recognized until the latter half of infancy. The clinical effects of thalassemia major are primarily attributable to (1) defective synthesis of HbA, (2) structurally impaired RBCs, and (3) shortened life span of erythrocytes (Box 49-3).

Hematologic studies reveal the characteristic changes in RBCs (i.e., microcytosis, hypochromia, anisocytosis, poikilocytosis, target cells, and basophilic stippling of various stages). Low Hgb and Hct levels are seen in severe anemia, although they are typically lower than the reduction in RBC count because of the proliferation of immature erythrocytes. Hgb electrophoresis confirms the diagnosis, and radiographs of involved bones reveal characteristic findings.

Therapeutic Management

The objective of supportive therapy is to maintain sufficient Hgb levels to prevent bone marrow expansion and the resulting bony deformities and to provide sufficient RBCs to support normal growth and normal physical activity. Transfusions are the foundation of medical management. Recent studies have evaluated the benefits of maintaining the child's Hgb level above 9.5 g/dl, a goal that may require transfusions as often as

BOX 49-3 Clinical Manifestations of β-Thalassemia

Anemia (Before Diagnosis)
Pallor
Unexplained fever
Poor feeding
Enlarged spleen or liver

Progressive Anemia
Signs of chronic hypoxia
- Headache
- Precordial and bone pain
- Decreased exercise tolerance
- Listlessness
- Anorexia

Other Features
Small stature
Delayed sexual maturation
Bronzed, freckled complexion (if not receiving chelation therapy)

Bone Changes (Older Children If Untreated)
Enlarged head
Prominent frontal and parietal bosses
Prominent malar eminences
Flat or depressed bridge of the nose
Enlarged maxilla
Protrusion of the lip and upper central incisors and eventual malocclusion
Generalized osteoporosis

every 3 to 5 weeks. The advantages of this therapy include (1) improved physical and psychologic well-being because of the ability to participate in normal activities, (2) decreased cardiomegaly and hepatosplenomegaly, (3) fewer bone changes, (4) normal or near-normal growth and development until puberty, and (5) fewer infections.

One of the potential complications of frequent blood transfusions is iron overload. Because the body has no effective means of eliminating the excess iron, the mineral is deposited in body tissues. To minimize the development of hemosiderosis, the oral iron chelator deferasirox has been shown to be equivalent to *deferoxamine (Desferal),* a parenteral iron-chelating agent, and more tolerable by patients and families (Morris, Singer, & Walters, 2006; Okpala, 2005).

In some children with severe splenomegaly who demonstrate increased transfusion requirements, a splenectomy may be necessary to decrease the disabling effects of abdominal pressure and to increase the life span of supplemental RBCs. Over time, the spleen may accelerate the rate of RBC destruction and thus increase transfusion requirements. After a splenectomy, children generally require fewer transfusions, although the basic defect in Hgb synthesis remains unaffected. A major postsplenectomy complication is severe and overwhelming infection. Therefore these children continue to receive prophylactic antibiotics with close medical supervision for many years and should receive the pneumococcal and meningococcal vaccines in addition to the regularly scheduled immunizations.

NURSING ALERT Ensure that the family and patient understand the need to notify the health professional of all fevers of 38.5° C (101.3° F) or greater because of the risk of sepsis in a child with asplenia.

Prognosis

Most children treated with blood transfusion and early chelation therapy survive well into adulthood. The most common cause of death is iron-induced heart disease, multiple organ failure, postsplenectomy sepsis, liver disease, and malignancy (Paley, 2000). HSCT has the best results in the least symptomatic pediatric patients, with an 85% to 90% rate of complication-free survival (Morris, Singer, & Walters, 2006; Orkin & Nathan, 2003; Richardson, 2007).

Nursing Care Management

The objectives of nursing care are to (1) promote compliance with transfusion and chelation therapy, (2) assist the child in coping with the anxiety-provoking treatments and the effects of the illness, (3) foster the child's and family's adjustment to a chronic illness, and (4) observe for complications of multiple blood transfusions. Basic to each of these goals is explaining to parents and older children the defect responsible for the disorder, its effect on RBCs, and the potential effects of untreated iron overload (such as diabetes and heart disease). Because the prevalence of this condition is high among families of Mediterranean descent, the nurse also inquires about the family's previous knowledge about thalassemia. All families with a child with thalassemia should be tested for the trait and referred for genetic counseling.

As with any chronic illness, the family's needs must be met for optimal adjustment to the stresses imposed by the disorder (see Chapter 41). Sources of information for the family include the Cooley's Anemia Foundation* and the Northern California Comprehensive Thalassemia Center.† Genetic counseling for the parents and fertile offspring is mandatory, and both prenatal diagnosis using amniocentesis at 20 weeks of gestation or fetal blood sampling at 10 weeks and screening for thalassemia trait are available.

Aplastic Anemia

Aplastic anemia (AA) refers to a bone marrow failure condition in which the formed elements of the blood are simultaneously depressed. The peripheral blood smear demonstrates pancytopenia or the triad of profound anemia, leukopenia, and thrombocytopenia. *Hypoplastic anemia* is characterized by a profound depression of RBCs but normal or slightly decreased WBCs and platelets.

Etiology

AA can be *primary (congenital,* or present at birth) or *secondary (acquired).* The best-known congenital disorder of which AA is an outstanding feature is *Fanconi syndrome,* a rare hereditary disorder characterized by pancytopenia, hypopla-

---

**330 Seventh Ave., No. 900, New York, NY 10001; 800-522-7222; fax: 212-279-5999;* www.cooleysanemia.org.

†747 52nd St., Oakland, CA 94609; 510-428-3885, ext. 4398; www.thalassemia.com.

BOX 49-4 Common Causes of Acquired Aplastic Anemia

- Human parvovirus infection, hepatitis, or overwhelming infection
- Irradiation
- Immune disorders such as eosinophilic fasciitis and hypoimmunoglobulinemia
- Drugs such as certain chemotherapeutic agents, anticonvulsants, and antibiotics
- Industrial and household chemicals, including benzene and its derivatives, which are found in petroleum products, dyes, paint remover, shellac, and lacquers
- Infiltration and replacement of myeloid elements, such as in leukemia or the lymphomas
- Idiopathic (In most cases no identifiable precipitating cause can be found.)

sia of the bone marrow, and patchy brown discoloration of the skin resulting from the deposit of melanin and associated with multiple congenital anomalies of the musculoskeletal and genitourinary systems. The syndrome appears to be inherited as an autosomal recessive trait with varying penetrance; therefore affected siblings may demonstrate several different combinations of defects.

Several etiologic factors contribute to the development of acquired hypoplastic anemia; however, most of the cases are considered idiopathic (Box 49-4). Acquired AA is classified as either severe acquired AA or moderate acquired AA. The following discussion focuses on severe acquired AA, which carries a poorer prognosis and follows a more rapidly fatal course than the primary types.

Diagnostic Evaluation

The onset of clinical manifestations, which include anemia, leukopenia, and decreased platelet count, is usually insidious. Definitive diagnosis is determined from bone marrow aspiration, which demonstrates the conversion of red bone marrow to yellow, fatty bone marrow. Severe AA is defined as less than 25% bone marrow cellularity with at least two of the following findings: absolute granulocyte count less than 500/mm^3, platelet count less than 20,000/mm^3, and absolute reticulocyte count less than 40,000/mm^3 (Hord, 2007; Shimamura & Guinan, 2003). Moderate AA is defined as more than 25% bone marrow cellularity with the presence of mild or moderate cytopenia (Shimamura & Guinan, 2003; Shende, 2000).

Therapeutic Management

The objectives of treatment are based on the recognition that the underlying disease process is failure of the bone marrow to carry out its hematopoietic functions. Therefore therapy is directed at restoring function to the marrow and involves two main approaches: (1) immunosuppressive therapy to remove the presumed immunologic functions that prolong aplasia or (2) replacement of the bone marrow through transplantation. Bone marrow transplantation is the treatment of choice for severe AA when a suitable donor exists (see p. 1522).

Antilymphocyte globulin (ALG) or *antithymocyte globulin (ATG)* is the principal drug treatment used for AA. The rationale for using ATG is based on the theory that AA may be a result of autoimmunity. ATG and cyclosporine suppress T cell–dependent autoimmune responses but do not cause bone marrow suppression. Cyclosporine is administered orally for several weeks to months. ATG usually is administrated intravenously over 12 to 16 hours for 4 days, after a test dose to check for hypersensitivity. A course may be repeated, depending on the reduction in circulating lymphocytes and the patient's response. Because of the hypersensitivity response associated with ATG (i.e., fever, chills, myalgias), methylprednisolone is given intravenously to prevent these side effects. Colony-stimulating factor (CSF) and granulocyte-macrophage colony-stimulating factor (GM-CSF) given parenterally may be used to enhance bone marrow production. Androgens may be used with ATG to stimulate erythropoiesis if the AA is unresponsive to initial therapies.

HSCT should be considered early in the course of the disease if a compatible donor can be found. Transplantation is more successful when performed before multiple transfusions have sensitized the child to leukocyte and *human leukocyte antigens (HLAs)*. HSCT is associated with an 85% survival rate in untransfused patients compared with a 70% survival rate in transfused patients (Marsh, 2005; Shende, 2000).

Nursing Care Management

The care of the child with AA is similar to that of the child with leukemia (see p. 1509)—specifically, preparing the child and family for the diagnostic and therapeutic procedures, preventing complications from the severe pancytopenia, and emotionally supporting them in the face of a potentially fatal outcome. Information and support are available from the Aplastic Anemia and MDS International Foundation, Inc.*

Because the aspects of nursing care are discussed in the section on leukemia, only the exceptions are presented here. The drug ATG is usually administered by way of a central vein. If not, vigilant care must be directed to the IV infusion to prevent extravasation. Meticulous care of the venous access is essential because of the child's susceptibility to infection. CSFs are usually given by subcutaneous injection over several days. Chemotherapeutic agents have been reported in the treatment of the relapsed patient with AA after ATG and CSF therapy. Many of the side effects associated with chemotherapy such as nausea and vomiting, alopecia, and mucositis are experienced by children receiving treatment for AA. Specialized care is required for children who have HSCT (see p. 1522).

Defects in Hemostasis

Hemostasis is the process that stops bleeding when a blood vessel is injured. Vascular and plasma clotting factors, as well as platelets, are required. A complex system of clotting, anticlotting, and clot breakdown *(fibrinolysis)* mechanisms exists in equilibrium to ensure clot formation only in the presence of blood vessel injury and to limit the clotting process to the

**PO Box 310, Churchton, MD 20733 USA; 800-747-2820, 410-867-0242; fax: 410-867-0240; e-mail: help@aamds.org; www.aamds.org.*

site of vessel wall injury. Dysfunction in these systems leads to bleeding or abnormal clotting. Although the coagulation process is complex, clotting depends on three factors: (1) vascular influence, (2) platelet role, and (3) clotting factors.

Hemophilia

The term *hemophilia* refers to a group of bleeding disorders in which there is a deficiency of one of the factors necessary for coagulation of the blood. Although the symptomatology is similar regardless of which clotting factor is deficient, the identification of specific factor deficiencies allows definitive treatment with replacement agents.

In about 80% of all cases of hemophilia, the inheritance pattern is demonstrated as X-linked recessive. The two most common forms of the disorder are *factor VIII deficiency (hemophilia A,* or *classic hemophilia)* and *factor IX deficiency (hemophilia B,* or *Christmas disease). Von Willebrand disease (vWD)* is another hereditary bleeding disorder characterized by a deficiency, abnormality, or absence of the protein called von Willebrand factor (vWF) and a deficiency of factor VIII. Unlike hemophilia, vWD affects both males and females. The following discussion is primarily concerned with factor VIII deficiency, which accounts for 80% to 85% of all hemophilia cases.

Pathophysiology

The basic defect of hemophilia A is a deficiency of *factor VIII (antihemophilic factor [AHF])*. AHF is produced by the liver and is necessary for the formation of thromboplastin in phase I of blood coagulation. The less AHF found in the blood, the more severe the disease. Individuals with hemophilia have two of the three factors required for coagulation: vascular influence and platelets. Therefore they may bleed for longer periods but not at a faster rate.

Bleeding into subcutaneous and IM tissue is common. Hemarthrosis, which is bleeding into a joint space, is the most frequent type of internal bleeding. Bony changes and crippling deformities occur after repeated bleeding episodes over several years. Signs of hemarthrosis are swelling, warmth, redness, pain, and loss of movement. Bleeding in the neck, mouth, or thorax is serious because the airway can become obstructed. Intracranial hemorrhage can have fatal consequences and is one of the major causes of death. Hemorrhage anywhere along the GI tract can lead to anemia, and bleeding into the retroperitoneal cavity is especially hazardous because of the large space for blood to accumulate. Hematomas in the spinal cord can cause paralysis.

Diagnostic Evaluation

Overt, prolonged hemorrhage is readily apparent; bleeding into tissues is less apparent (Box 49-5). The diagnosis is usually made from a history of bleeding episodes, evidence of X-linked inheritance (only one third of the cases are new mutations), and laboratory findings. The tests specific for hemophilia plasma depend on specific factors for a reaction to occur, such as the partial thromboplastin time (PTT). Specific determination of factor deficiencies requires assay procedures normally performed in specialized laboratories. Carrier detection is possible in classic hemophilia using deoxyribonucleic acid (DNA) testing and is an important consideration in families in which female offspring may have inherited the trait.

BOX 49-5 Clinical Manifestations of Hemophilia

- Prolonged bleeding anywhere from or in the body
- Hemorrhage from any trauma—Loss of deciduous teeth, circumcision, cuts, epistaxis, injections
- Excessive bruising, even from a slight injury such as a fall
- Subcutaneous and intramuscular hemorrhages
- Hemarthrosis (bleeding into the joint cavities), especially the knees, ankles, and elbows
- Hematomas—Pain, swelling, and limited motion
- Spontaneous hematuria

Therapeutic Management

The primary therapy for hemophilia is replacement of the missing clotting factor. The products available are *factor VIII concentrate* from pooled plasma or a genetically engineered recombinant, to be reconstituted with sterile water immediately before use, and *DDAVP (1-deamino-8-D-arginine vasopressin)*, a synthetic form of vasopressin that increases plasma factor VIII and vWF levels and is the treatment of choice in mild hemophilia and vWD if the child shows an appropriate response. DDAVP is not effective in the treatment of severe hemophilia A, severe vWD, or any form of hemophilia B. Vigorous therapy is instituted to prevent chronic crippling effects from joint bleeding.

evolve Animation—Hemophilia A

Other drugs may be included in the therapy plan, depending on the source of the hemorrhage. Corticosteroids are given for hematuria, acute hemarthrosis, and chronic synovitis. Nonsteroidal antiinflammatory drugs (NSAIDs), such as ibuprofen, are effective in relieving pain caused by synovitis; however, they must be used with caution because they inhibit platelet function (Curry, 2004; National Hemophilia Foundation, Bleeding Disorders Information Center, 2006). Oral administration or local application of ε-aminocaproic acid (Amicar) prevents clot destruction; however, its use is limited to mouth or trauma surgery, and a dose of factor concentrate must be given first.

A regular program of exercise and physical therapy is an important aspect of management. Physical activity within reasonable limits strengthens muscles around joints and may decrease the number of spontaneous bleeding episodes.

Treatment without delay results in more rapid recovery and a decreased likelihood of complications; therefore most children are treated at home. The family is taught the technique of venipuncture and to administer the AHF to children older than 2 to 3 years of age. The child learns the procedure for self-administration at 8 to 12 years of age. Home treatment is highly successful; and the rewards, in addition to the immediacy, are less disruption of family life, fewer school or work days missed, and enhancement of the child's self-esteem and independence.

Primary prophylaxis in hemophilia patients has proved to be effective in preventing bleeding complications by administrating periodic factor replacement. Primary prophylaxis involves the infusion of factor VIII concentrate on a regular basis before the onset of joint damage. Secondary prophylaxis involves the infusion of factor VIII concentrate on a regular basis after the child experiences his or her first joint bleed. The infusions are given three times a week. Aggressive factor replacement may be a cost-effective alternative to primary prophylaxis. This involves the infusion of a high dose of factor VIII concentrate when a joint bleed occurs, followed by 2 days of more standard doses of factor VIII concentrate, with consideration of additional treatment every other day for one week (Montgomery, Gill, & Scott, 2003).

Prognosis

Although there is no cure for hemophilia, its symptoms can be controlled, and its potentially crippling deformities greatly reduced or even avoided. Today many children with hemophilia function with minimal or no joint damage. They are normal children with an average life expectancy in every respect but one: they have a tendency to bleed, which is a significant inconvenience but not necessarily a life-threatening event.

Gene therapy may prove to be a treatment option in the future. This therapy involves introducing a working copy of the factor VIII gene into a patient who has a flawed copy of the gene. Problems exist with appropriate selection of the vector, identification of the cell for gene expression, and control of side effects (Montgomery, Gill, & Scott, 2003).

evolve Critical Thinking Exercise—Bleeding

Nursing Care Management

The earlier a bleeding episode is recognized, the more effectively it can be treated. Signs that indicate internal bleeding are especially important to recognize. Children are aware of internal bleeding and are reliable in telling the examiner where an internal bleed is. In addition to the manifestations described (see Box 49-5), the nurse maintains a high level of suspicion when a child with hemophilia demonstrates signs such as headache, slurred speech, loss of consciousness (from cerebral bleeding), and black tarry stools (from GI bleeding).

Prevent Bleeding

The goal of prevention of bleeding episodes is directed toward decreasing the risk of injury. Prevention of bleeding episodes is geared mostly toward appropriate exercises to strengthen muscles and joints and to allow age-appropriate activity. During infancy and toddlerhood the normal acquisition of motor skills creates innumerable opportunities for falls, bruises, and minor wounds. Restraining the child from mastering motor development can foster more serious long-term problems than allowing the behavior. However, the environment should be made as safe as possible, with close supervision during playtime to minimize incidental injuries.

The family usually needs assistance in preparing older children for school. A nurse who knows the family can be instrumental in discussing the situation with the school nurse and jointly planning an appropriate activity schedule. Because almost all persons with hemophilia are boys, the physical limitations in regard to active sports may be a difficult adjustment, and activity restrictions must be tempered with sensitivity to the child's emotional and physical needs. Use of protective equipment, such as padding and helmets, is particularly important; noncontact sports, especially swimming, walking, jogging, tennis, golf, fishing, and bowling, are encouraged (National Hemophilia Foundation, Bleeding Disorders Information Center, 2006).

To prevent oral bleeding, some readjustment in terms of dental hygiene may be needed to minimize trauma to the gums, such as use of a water irrigating device, softening the toothbrush in warm water before brushing, or using a sponge-tipped disposable toothbrush. A regular toothbrush should be small and have soft bristles.

Because any trauma can lead to a bleeding episode, all persons caring for these children must be aware of their disorder. The children should wear medical identification, and older children should be encouraged to recognize situations in which disclosing their condition is important, such as during dental extraction or injections. Health personnel need to take special precautions to prevent the use of procedures that may cause bleeding, such as IM injections. The subcutaneous route is substituted for IM injections whenever possible. Venipunctures for blood samples are usually preferred for these children. There is usually less bleeding after the venipuncture than after finger or heel punctures. Neither aspirin nor any aspirin-containing compound should be used. Acetaminophen is a suitable aspirin substitute, especially for controlling pain at home.

Recognize and Control Bleeding

As noted, the earlier a bleeding episode is recognized, the more effectively it can be treated. Factor replacement therapy should be instituted according to established medical protocol, and supportive measures—such as *RICE*, which stands for *R*est, *I*ce, *C*ompression, and *E*levation—may be implemented. When parents and older children are taught such measures beforehand, they can be prepared to initiate immediate treatment. Plastic bags of ice or cold packs should be kept in the freezer for such emergencies. However, such measures do not take the place of factor replacement.

Prevent Crippling Effects of Bleeding

As a result of repeated episodes of hemarthrosis, incompletely absorbed blood in the joints, and limitation of motion, bone and muscle changes occur that result in flexion contractures and joint fixation. During bleeding episodes the joint is elevated and immobilized. Active range-of-motion exercises are usually instituted after the acute episode. This allows the child to control the degree of exercise and discomfort. If an exercise program is instituted in the home, a physical therapist or public health nurse may need to supervise compliance with the regimen. Rarely, orthopedic intervention, such as casting, application of traction, or aspiration of blood, may be necessary to preserve joint function. Diet is also an important consideration because excessive body weight can increase the strain on affected joints, especially the knees, and predispose the child to hemarthrosis. Consequently, calories need to be supplied in accordance with energy requirements.

Support Family and Prepare for Home Care

Genetic counseling is essential as soon as possible after diagnosis. Unlike many other disorders in which both parents carry the trait, the feeling of responsibility for this condition usually rests with the mother. Without an opportunity to discuss her feelings, the marital relationship can suffer. Technology is now available to identify carriers in approximately

80% of cases and may reduce the anxiety regarding childbearing in women who may be at risk of carrying the defective gene, such as sisters or maternal aunts of an affected male. The discovery of factor concentrates has greatly changed the outlook for these children. Bleeding can be minimized, and the child can live a much more normal, unrestricted life. Children are taught to take responsibility for their disease at an early age. They learn their limitations, other preventive measures, and self-administration of the prophylactic AHF.

The needs of families who have children with hemophilia are best met through a comprehensive team approach of physicians (pediatrician, hematologist, orthopedist), nurse practitioner, nurse, social worker, and physical therapist. Parent-group discussions are beneficial in meeting the needs often best met by similarly affected families. For example, with the improved prognosis for these children, parents and adolescents with hemophilia face vocational and financial problems, in addition to concern over future childbearing. After children reach 21 years of age, many insurance companies will no longer carry them. This can be disastrous in terms of the cost of treatment. The National Hemophilia Foundation* and the Canadian Hemophilia Society† provide numerous services and publications for both health providers and families. Financial support is particularly important. A person with severe hemophilia may require factor replacement therapy and other medical treatments that cost in excess of $70,000 to $90,000 a year.

Children who have become infected with HIV through transfusions and factor replacement products are faced with the consequences of this dreaded disease. Consequently, they need the support of health professionals, especially in the areas of safe sexual practices, to avoid disease transmission and public education regarding acquired immunodeficiency syndrome (AIDS) and ways to deal with public reactions to persons who have AIDS (see p. 1516).

Idiopathic Thrombocytopenic Purpura

Idiopathic thrombocytopenic purpura (ITP) is an acquired hemorrhagic disorder characterized by (1) *thrombocytopenia,* excessive destruction of platelets; (2) *purpura,* a discoloration caused by petechiae beneath the skin; and (3) *normal bone marrow with normal or increased number of immature platelets (megakaryocytes) and eosinophils.* Although the cause is unknown, it is believed to be an autoimmune response to disease-related antigens. It is the most frequently occurring thrombocytopenia of childhood. The greatest frequency of occurrence is between 2 and 10 years of age.

The disease occurs in one of two forms: an acute, self-limiting course or a chronic condition (greater than 6 months' duration). The acute form is most often seen after upper respiratory tract infections; after the childhood diseases measles, rubella, mumps, and chickenpox; or after infection with parvovirus B19.

BOX 49-6 Clinical Manifestations of Idiopathic Thrombocytopenic Purpura

Easy bruising
- Petechiae
- Ecchymoses
- Most often over bony prominences

Bleeding from mucous membranes
- Epistaxis
- Bleeding gums
- Internal hemorrhage evidenced by hematuria, hematemesis, melena, hemarthrosis, or menorrhagia

Hematomas over lower extremities

Diagnostic Evaluation

The diagnosis is suspected on the basis of clinical manifestations (Box 49-6). In ITP the platelet count is reduced to below 20,000/mm^3; therefore tests that depend on platelet function, such as the tourniquet test, bleeding time, and clot retraction, are abnormal. Although there is no definitive test on which to establish a diagnosis of ITP, several are usually performed to rule out other disorders in which thrombocytopenia is a manifestation, such as systemic lupus erythematosus, lymphoma, or leukemia.

Therapeutic Management

Management of ITP is primarily supportive because the course of the disease is self-limited in most cases. Activity is restricted at the onset while the platelet count is low and while active bleeding or progression of lesions is occurring. Treatment for acute presentation is symptomatic and has included prednisone, IV immune globulin (IVIG), and anti-D antibody. These are not curative therapies. *Anti-D antibody* is a relatively new therapy for ITP. Its infusion causes a transient hemolytic anemia in the patient. Along with the clearance of antibody-coated RBCs, there is prolonged survival of platelets resulting from the blockade of the Fc receptors of the reticuloendothelial cells. The platelet count does not increase until 48 hours after an infusion of anti-D antibody; therefore it is not appropriate therapy for patients who are actively bleeding. The benefits of choosing anti-D antibody therapy over prednisone or IVIG is that anti-D antibody can be given in one dose over 5 to 10 minutes and is significantly less expensive than IVIG. Historically, patients who are treated with prednisone must first undergo a bone marrow examination to rule out leukemia. Therefore the use of anti-D antibody alleviates the need for a bone marrow examination. Patients must meet certain criteria before it is administered (Box 49-7). Premedication with acetaminophen 5 to 10 minutes before infusion is recommended.

NURSING ALERT After administration of anti-D antibody, observe the child for a minimum of 1 hour and maintain a patent IV line. Obtain baseline vital signs before the infusion and again 5, 20, and 60 minutes after beginning the infusion.

*116 W. 32nd St., 11th Floor, New York, NY 10001; 800-42-HANDI, 212-328-3700; fax: 212-328-3777; e-mail: handi@hemophilia.org; www.hemophilia.org.

†625 President Kennedy Ave., Suite 505, Montreal, Quebec H3A 1K2; 800-668-2686, 514-848-0503; fax: 514-848-9661; e-mail: chs@hemophilia.ca; www.hemophilia.ca.

BOX 49-7 Criteria for Anti-D Antibody Therapy

- Age between 1 and 19 years; Rh(D)-positive blood type
- Normal white blood count and hemoglobin level for age; platelet count of 20,000/mm³
- No active mucosal bleeding
- No history of reaction to plasma products
- No known immune globulin A deficiency
- No concurrent infection
- Absence of Evans syndrome (characterized by the combination of idiopathic thrombocytopenic purpura and autoimmune hemolytic anemia)
- No suspicion of lupus erythematosus or other collagen-vascular disorder
- No splenectomy

Fever, chills, and headache may occur during or shortly after the infusion. If so, diphenhydramine (Benadryl) and hydrocortisone (Solu-Cortef) should be given, and the patient observed for an additional hour.

Splenectomy is reserved for patients in whom ITP has persisted for 1 year or longer. It is the only treatment associated with long-term remission for 60% to 90% of children. Splenectomy removes the risk of hemorrhage but increases the risk of septicemia (Buchanan, 2005; Scott & Montgomery, 2007). Before considering splenectomy, it is generally recommended to wait until the child is older than 5 years of age because of the increased risk of bacterial infection. Pneumococcal and meningococcal vaccines are recommended before splenectomy. The child also receives penicillin prophylaxis after splenectomy. The length of prophylactic therapy is controversial, but in general, a minimum of 3 years is recommended.

Prognosis

Most children have a self-limited course without major complications. Some develop chronic ITP and require ongoing therapy. A splenectomy may modify the disease process, and the child will be asymptomatic.

Nursing Care Management

Nursing care is largely supportive and should include teaching regarding possible side effects of therapy and limitation in activities while the child's platelet count is 50,000 to 100,000/mm³. Children with ITP should not participate in *any* contact sports, bike riding, skateboarding, in-line skating, gymnastics, climbing, or running. Parents are encouraged to engage their children in quiet activities and prevent any injuries to the child's head. The harmful effects of using aspirin and NSAIDs to control pain are critical for these children; therefore salicylate substitutes (such as acetaminophen) are always used. As in any condition with an uncertain outcome, the family needs emotional support.

Disseminated Intravascular Coagulation

Disseminated intravascular coagulation (DIC), also known as *consumption coagulopathy,* is characterized by diffuse fibrin deposition in the microvasculature, consumption of coagulation factors, and endogenous generation of thrombin and plasmin. DIC is a secondary disorder of coagulation that occurs as a complication of a number of pathologic processes, such as hypoxia, acidosis, shock, and endothelial damage. It can result from many severe systemic diseases, such as congenital heart disease, necrotizing enterocolitis, gram-negative bacterial sepsis, rickettsial infections, and some severe viral infections.

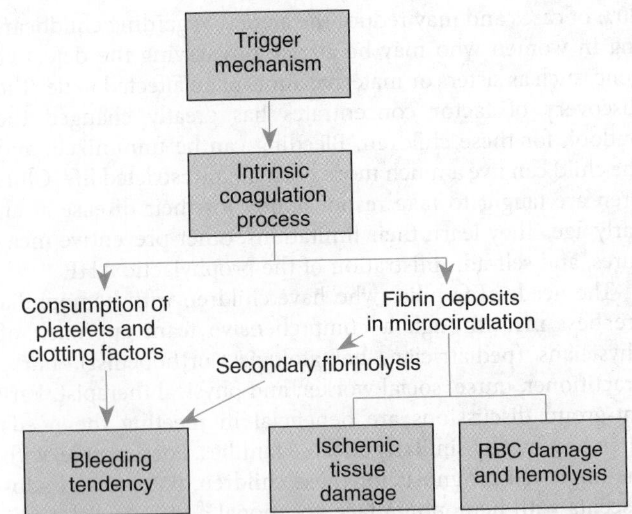

Fig. 49-3 Effects of disseminated intravascular coagulation. *RBC,* Red blood cell.

Pathophysiology

DIC occurs when the first stage of the coagulation process is abnormally stimulated. Although no well-defined sequence of events occurs, two distinct phases can be identified. First, when the clotting mechanism is triggered in the circulation, thrombin is generated in greater amounts than can be neutralized by the body. Consequently, there is rapid conversion of fibrinogen to fibrin, with aggregation and destruction of platelets. If local and widespread fibrin deposition in blood vessels takes place, obstruction and eventual necrosis of tissues occur. Second, the fibrinolytic mechanism is activated, causing extensive destruction of clotting factors. With a deficiency of clotting factors, the child is vulnerable to uncontrollable hemorrhage into vital organs. An additional complication is damage and hemolysis of RBCs (Fig. 49-3).

Diagnostic Evaluation

DIC is suspected when the patient has an increased tendency to bleed (Box 49-8). Hematologic findings include prolonged prothrombin time (PT), PTT, and thrombin time (TT). There is a profoundly depressed platelet count, fragmented RBCs, and depleted fibrinogen.

Therapeutic Management

Treatment of DIC is directed toward control of the underlying or initiating cause, which in most instances stops the coagulation problem spontaneously. Platelets and fresh-frozen plasma may be needed to replace lost plasma components, especially in the child whose underlying disease remains uncontrolled. The extremely ill newborn infant may require exchange transfusion with fresh blood. The IV administration of heparin to

BOX 49-8 Clinical Manifestations of Disseminated Intravascular Coagulation

Petechiae
Purpura
Bleeding from openings in the skin
- Venipuncture site
- Surgical incision

Bleeding from umbilicus, trachea (newborn)
Evidence of gastrointestinal bleeding
Hypotension
Organ dysfunction from infarction and ischemia

inhibit thrombin formation is most often restricted to patients who have not responded to treatment of the underlying disease or replacement of coagulation factors and platelets.

Nursing Care Management

The goals of nursing care are to be aware of the possibility of DIC in the severely ill child and to recognize signs that might indicate its presence. The skills needed to monitor IV infusion and blood transfusions and to administer heparin are the same as for any child receiving these therapies (see p. 1520). (See Chapter 41 for care of the child with a life-threatening illness.)

Epistaxis (Nosebleeding)

Isolated and transient episodes of epistaxis, or nosebleeding, are common in childhood. The nose, especially the septum, is a highly vascular structure, and bleeding usually results from direct trauma, including blows to the nose, foreign bodies, and nose picking, or from mucosal inflammation associated with allergic rhinitis and upper respiratory tract infections. The bleeding ordinarily stops spontaneously or with minimal pressure and requires no medical evaluation or therapy.

Recurrent epistaxis and severe bleeding may indicate an underlying disease, particularly vascular abnormalities, leukemia, thrombocytopenia, and clotting factor deficiency diseases (e.g., hemophilia, vWD). Nosebleeds are sometimes associated with administration of aspirin, even in normal amounts. Persistent episodes of epistaxis require medical evaluation.

Nursing Care Management

In the event of a nosebleed, an essential intervention is to remain calm. Otherwise, the child will become more agitated, the blood pressure will increase, and he or she will not cooperate. Although in most instances a nosebleed is not serious, it can be upsetting to family members as well. They need reassurance that the loss of blood is not serious and that the bleeding usually stops within 10 to 15 minutes.

To control the bleeding, the child is instructed to sit up and lean forward (not lie down) to avoid aspiration of blood. Most nosebleeding originates in the anterior part of the nasal septum and can be controlled by applying pressure to the soft lower portion of the nose with the thumb and forefinger (see Emergency box). During this time the child breathes through the mouth.

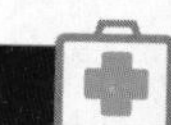

EMERGENCY

Epistaxis

- Have child sit up and lean forward (not lie down).
- Apply continuous pressure to nose with thumb and forefinger for at least 10 minutes.
- Insert cotton or wadded tissue into each nostril, and apply ice or cold cloth to bridge of nose if bleeding persists.
- Keep child calm and quiet.

In the event that hemorrhage continues, the child should be evaluated by a practitioner, who may pack the nose with epinephrine-soaked gauze. After a nosebleed, petroleum or water-soluble jelly can be inserted into each nostril to prevent crusting of old blood and to lessen the likelihood of the child's picking at the nose and restarting the hemorrhage. If a child has numerous nosebleeds, factors believed to increase the likelihood of bleeds are eliminated, such as discouraging nose picking or altering the household humidity by placing a cool-mist humidifier in the child's room. Repeated bleeding episodes lasting longer than 30 minutes may be an indication to refer the child for evaluation for the possibility of a bleeding disorder.

Neoplastic Disorders

Neoplastic disorders are the leading cause of death from disease in children past infancy, and almost half of all childhood cancers involve the blood or blood-forming organs. Leukemias and lymphomas are discussed here. Malignant solid tumors of childhood are discussed elsewhere in relation to the tissues or organs involved.

Leukemias

Leukemia, cancer of the blood-forming tissues, is the most common form of childhood cancer. The annual incidence is 3 to 4 cases per 100,000 Caucasian children younger than 15 years of age (Margolin, Steuber, & Poplack, 2006; Pearce & Sills, 2005). It is more common in males and Caucasians, with the peak onset between 2 and 5 years of age (Margolin, Steuber, & Poplack, 2006; Pearce & Sills, 2005). It is one of the forms of cancer that has demonstrated dramatic improvements in survival rates. Long-term disease-free survival for children with acute lymphoid leukemia approaches 80% (Pui, Relling, & Downing, 2004; Pearce & Sills, 2005), whereas acute non-lymphoid leukemia has a nearly 50% survival rate (Pearce & Sills, 2005). (See also Prognosis, p. 1509.)

Classification

Leukemia is a broad term given to a group of malignant diseases of the bone marrow and lymphatic system. Research has revealed that it is a complex disease of varying heterogeneity. Consequently, classification has become increasingly complex, sophisticated, and essential, since identification of the subtype of leukemia has therapeutic and prognostic implications. The following is a brief overview of the major classification systems currently being used.

evolve Case Study—Acute Lymphoid Leukemia

Morphology

Two forms are generally recognized in children: *acute lymphoid leukemia (ALL)* and *acute nonlymphoid (myelogenous) leukemia (ANLL or AML)*. Synonyms for ALL include lymphatic, lymphocytic, lymphoblastic, and lymphoblastoid leukemia. Usually the terms *stem cell* or *blast cell leukemia* also refer to the lymphoid type. Synonyms for the AML type include granulocytic, myelocytic, monocytic, myelogenous, monoblastic, and monomyeloblastic.

Cytochemical markers—Several chemical stains (e.g., terminal deoxynucleotidyl transferase [TdT]) aid in differentiation between ALL and ANLL.

Chromosome studies—Chromosome analysis has become an important tool in the diagnosis of ALL. For example, children with trisomy 21 have 20 times the risk of other children for developing ALL. Children with more than 50 chromosomes on the leukemic cells (hyperdiploid) have the best prognosis (Margolin, Steuber, & Poplack, 2006). Translocations of chromosomes also found on the leukemic cells can denote a good prognosis, as in the trisomies 4 and 10, or a poor prognosis, as in the t(9:22) or Philadelphia chromosome.

Cell-surface immunologic markers—Cell-surface antigens have permitted differentiation of ALL into three broad classes: non-T, non-B ALL; B-cell ALL; and T-cell ALL. Children with non-T, non-B ALL have the best prognosis, especially if they have the common ALL antigen, known as CALLA positive (or CD10+), on their cell surfaces (Margolin, Steuber, & Poplack, 2006).

Pathophysiology

Leukemia is an unrestricted proliferation of immature WBCs in the blood-forming tissues of the body. Although not a "tumor" as such, the leukemic cells demonstrate the same neoplastic properties as solid cancers. Therefore the resulting pathologic condition and clinical manifestations are caused by infiltration and replacement of any tissue of the body with nonfunctional leukemic cells. Highly vascular organs, such as the spleen and liver, are the most severely affected.

To understand the pathophysiology of the leukemic process, it is important to clarify two common misconceptions. First, although leukemia is an overproduction of WBCs, most often in the acute form the leukocyte count is low (thus the term *leukemia*). Second, these immature cells do not deliberately attack and destroy the normal blood cells or vascular tissues. Cellular destruction takes place by infiltration and subsequent competition for metabolic elements (Table 49-2).

In all types of leukemia the proliferating cells depress the production of formed elements of the blood in bone marrow by competing for and depriving the normal cells of the essential nutrients for metabolism. The most frequent presenting signs and symptoms of leukemia are a result of infiltration of the bone marrow. The three main consequences are (1) *anemia* from decreased RBCs, (2) *infection* from neutropenia, and (3) *bleeding* from decreased platelet production. The invasion of the bone marrow with leukemic cells gradually causes a weakening of the bone and a tendency toward fractures. As leukemic cells invade the periosteum, increasing pressure causes severe pain.

Diagnostic Evaluation

Leukemia is usually suspected based on the history, physical manifestations (see Table 49-2), and a peripheral blood smear that contains immature forms of leukocytes, frequently combined with low blood counts. Definitive diagnosis is based on flow cytometry of the cells obtained in the bone marrow aspi-

Table 49-2 Pathology and Related Clinical Manifestations of Leukemia

ORGAN OR TISSUE	CONSEQUENCES	MANIFESTATIONS
Bone marrow dysfunction	Decreased red blood cells–Anemia Neutropenia–Infection Decreased platelets–Bleeding tendencies Invasion of bone marrow–Bone weakness; invasion of periosteum	Pallor, fatigue Fever Hemorrhage (petechiae) Tendency toward fractures Pain
Liver	Infiltration, enlargement, eventual fibrosis	Hepatomegaly
Spleen		Splenomegaly
Lymph glands		Lymphadenopathy
Central nervous system–Meninges	Increased intracranial pressure, ventricular enlargement Meningeal irritation	Severe headache Vomiting Irritability, lethargy Papilledema Eventual coma Pain Stiff neck and back
Hypermetabolism	Cell deprivation of nutrients by invading cells	Muscle wasting Weight loss Anorexia Fatigue

ration or biopsy. Flow cytometry identifies the specific type of blast cell. Typically, the bone marrow is hypercellular, with primarily blast cells. After the diagnosis is confirmed, a lumbar puncture is performed to determine whether there is any central nervous system (CNS) involvement. A few children have CNS involvement at diagnosis, although most are asymptomatic.

Therapeutic Management

Treatment of leukemia involves the use of chemotherapeutic agents, with or without cranial irradiation, in four phases: (1) *induction therapy,* which achieves a complete remission or less than 5% leukemic cells in the bone marrow; (2) *CNS prophylactic therapy,* which prevents leukemic cells from invading the CNS; (3) *intensification therapy* (consolidation), which eradicates residual leukemia cells, followed by delayed intensification, which prevents emergence of resistant leukemic clones; and (4) *maintenance therapy,* which serves to maintain the remission phase. Although the combination of drugs and radiation may vary according to institutions, the prognostic or risk characteristics of the patient, and the type of leukemia being treated, the following general principles for each phase are consistently used.

Hematopoietic Stem Cell Transplantation

HSCT has been used successfully for treating children who have ALL and AML. It is *not* recommended for children with ALL during the first remission because of the excellent results possible with chemotherapy. Because of the poorer prognosis in children with AML, HSCT may be considered during the first remission when a suitable donor is available (Bollard, Krance, & Heslop, 2006).

HSCT may be not only from antigen-matched related donors but also from matched unrelated or mismatched donors. Peripheral blood stem cell transplants are capable of differentiating into specialized cells of the hematologic system and can be obtained from related or unrelated donors or from umbilical cord blood. Regardless of the type of transplant, it is accompanied by significant morbidity and mortality, including graft-vs-host disease (GVHD), overwhelming infection, or severe organ damage.

Prognosis

The most important prognostic factors for determining long-term survival for children with ALL (in addition to treatment) are (1) the initial WBC count, (2) the child's age at the time of diagnosis, (3) the type of cell involved, (4) the sex of the child, and (5) karyotype analysis. Children with a normal or low WBC count and who have non-T, non-B ALL and are CALLA positive have a much better prognosis than those with a high count or other cell types. Children diagnosed between 2 and 9 years of age have consistently demonstrated a better outlook than those diagnosed before 2 or after 10 years of age, and girls appear to have a more favorable prognosis than boys. Children with a DNA index greater than 1.16 (hyperdiploid) and translocation of chromosomes 4 and 10 have a better prognosis (Margolin, Steuber, & Poplack, 2006).

Late Effects of Treatment

Although vigorous treatment of childhood cancers has resulted in dramatically improved survival rates, increasing concern surrounds late effects—adverse changes related to treatment modalities—and recurrence of the disease process. Almost no organ is exempt, and almost every antineoplastic agent, especially irradiation, is responsible for some adverse effect.

The most devastating late effect is development of a second malignancy. Children who received cranial irradiation at age 5 years or younger are most susceptible to developing brain tumors (Silverman & Sallan, 2003; Bhatia, 2004). Treatment with an anthracycline is associated with cardiomyopathy; cranial irradiation and intrathecal chemotherapy are associated with cognitive and neuropsychologic deficits, which are just a few of the long-term sequelae. Consequently, close monitoring for late effects is essential, especially with the advent of additional clinical trials.

Nursing Care Management

Nursing care of the child with leukemia is directly related to the therapeutic regimen. The Nursing Care Plan for the Child with Cancer is found on pp. 1510-1512.

Prepare Child and Family for Diagnostic and Therapeutic Procedures

From the time before diagnosis to cessation of therapy, children must undergo several tests; the most traumatic are bone marrow aspiration, bone marrow biopsy, and lumbar punctures. Multiple finger sticks and venipunctures for blood analysis and drug infusion are common occurrences. Therefore the child needs an explanation of each procedure and what can be expected. In addition, effective pharmacologic measures, including conscious and unconscious sedation, and nonpharmacologic strategies are used to reduce discomfort associated with these painful procedures.

Relieve Pain

The effective use of analgesia is especially important when the malignant process is uncontrolled and causes acute pain. Dosages of opioids (narcotics) are adjusted, or *titrated,* to the child's needs and administered *around the clock* for optimal pain control. Nonpharmacologic strategies should be implemented as needed but are not substitutes for pharmacologic management. The reader is encouraged to review the principles of pain assessment and management presented in Chapter 35 and Preparation for Diagnostic and Therapeutic Procedures, Chapter 45, when caring for a child with leukemia.

Prevent Complications of Myelosuppression

The leukemic process and most of the chemotherapeutic agents cause myelosuppression. The reduced numbers of blood cells result in secondary problems of infection, bleeding tendencies, and anemia. Supportive care involves both medical and nursing management. Because these are so closely linked, they are discussed together.

Infection A frequent complication of treatment for childhood cancer is overwhelming infection secondary to neutropenia. The child is most susceptible to overwhelming infection during three phases of the disease: (1) at the time of diagnosis and relapse when the leukemic process has replaced normal leukocytes; (2) during immunosuppressive therapy; and (3) after prolonged antibiotic therapy, which predisposes the child to the growth of resistant organisms. However, the use of granulocyte colony-stimulating factor (GCSF) has reduced the incidence and duration of infection in children receiving treatment for cancer.

The first defense against infection is prevention. When the child is hospitalized, the nurse uses all measures to control transfer of infection. These typically include the use of a private room, restriction of all visitors and health personnel with active infection, and strict handwashing technique with an antiseptic solution. In some research centers special germ-free environments are available during complete myelosuppression from intensive chemotherapy or for bone marrow transplant.

NURSING ALERT Because the usual viral infections of childhood are particularly dangerous, the child is not immunized against these diseases (measles, rubella, mumps, and polio) until the immune system is capable of responding appropriately to the vaccine. If given when the immune system is depressed, the attenuated virus can result in an overwhelming infection. The child can receive the Salk (inactivated) vaccine for poliomyelitis. Children with cancer should not routinely receive the varicella vaccine. Siblings and other

NURSING CARE PLAN ✤ The Child with Cancer

Nursing Diagnosis	Expected Patient Outcomes	Nursing Interventions	Rationale
Risk for injury related to chemotherapy treatment	Child will exhibit no complications of chemotherapy.	Administer chemotherapeutic agents using established guidelines.	To minimize inappropriate administration techniques
	Child will receive prompt, appropriate treatment of complications.	Assist with procedures for administration of chemotherapeutic agents.	To promote safer cancer treatment
Child's/Family's Defining Characteristics	**The Following NOC Concept Applies to These Outcomes**	Administer medications around the clock to prevent nausea and vomiting before chemotherapy.	To minimize side effects of nausea and vomiting
(Subjective and Objective Data)	Risk Control	Administer IV fluid as prescribed.	To maintain hydration
Anaphylaxis—Wheezing, hypotension, urticaria, cyanosis		Encourage frequent intake of fluids in small amounts.	To promote hydration
Nausea, vomiting		Observe for signs of infiltration of IV site: pain, stinging, swelling redness.	To prevent infiltration when possible
Intravenous (IV) infiltration—Pain, redness, swelling at IV infusion site		Institute policies to treat infiltration if it occurs.	To prevent complications
		Observe child for 20 minutes after infusion of drugs that are associated with risk of anaphylaxis.	To prevent anaphylaxis
		Stop infusion of drug and flush IV line with normal saline if reaction is suspected.	To prevent further reaction
		Have emergency equipment and emergency drugs readily available.	To prevent delay in treatment
		The Following NIC Concepts Apply to These Interventions	
		Chemotherapy Management	
		Nausea Management	

Nursing Diagnosis	Expected Patient Outcomes	Nursing Interventions	Rationale
Risk for infection related to depressed body defenses	Child will not exhibit signs of infection.	Use good handwashing technique.	To minimize exposure to infective organisms
	Child will not come in contact with infected persons.	Screen all visitors and staff for signs of infection.	To decrease exposure to possible infective organisms
Child's/Family's Defining Characteristics	**The Following NOC Concepts Apply to These Outcomes**	Use aseptic technique for all invasive procedures.	To decrease chance of infection spread
(Subjective and Objective Data)	Risk Control	Monitor temperature.	To detect possible infection
Fever	Immune Status	Evaluate child for any potential sites of infection: needle puncture sites, mucosa for ulceration, minor abrasions.	To detect signs of possible infection
Altered vital signs	Infection Severity	Provide nutritionally complete diet.	To support body's natural defenses
Lethargy		Avoid giving live attenuated virus vaccines.	To prevent overwhelming infection
Change in behavior		Give inactivated virus vaccines.	To prevent specific infections and to avoid placing the child at risk for acquiring the illness
Septic shock		Administer antibiotics as prescribed.	To treat a specific infection
		Administer granulocyte colony-stimulating factor (G-CSF) as prescribed.	To promote production of infection-fighting cells
		The Following NIC Concepts Apply to These Interventions	
		Infection Protection	
		Infection Control	
		Immunization/Vaccination Management	

NURSING CARE PLAN ✤ The Child with Cancer—cont'd

Nursing Diagnosis	Expected Patient Outcomes	Nursing Interventions	Rationale
Imbalanced nutrition: less than body requirements related to loss of appetite **Child's/Family's Defining Characteristics** ***(Subjective and Objective Data)*** Weight loss Lack of appetite Nausea	Child's nutritional intake will be adequate. **The Following NOC Concepts Apply to These Outcomes** Nutritional Status: Food and Fluid Intake Nutritional Status: Nutrient Intake	Encourage parents to relax pressure placed on child concerning eating. Allow child any food tolerated; selections can improve once appetite increases. Explain expected increase in appetite if child will be taking steroids. Fortify foods with nutritious supplements. Allow child to be involved in food preparation and selection. Make food appealing. Monitor child's weight. **The Following NIC Concepts Apply to These Interventions** Nutrition Management Nutrition Therapy	To educate that loss of appetite is a consequence of chemotherapy To encourage child to eat To prepare child and family for this change To maximize quality of intake To encourage eating To encourage eating To evaluate for weight change

Nursing Diagnosis	Expected Patient Outcomes	Nursing Interventions	Rationale
Pain (specify: acute, chronic) related to diagnosis, treatment, physiologic effects of cancer **Child's/Family's Defining Characteristics** ***(Subjective and Objective Data)*** Crying Withdrawal Fear of procedures Reluctance to move Change in vital signs	Child will experience no pain or reduction of pain to level acceptable to the child. **The Following NOC Concepts Apply to These Outcomes** Pain Level Pain: Disruptive Effects Pain Control	Use pharmacologic and nonpharmacologic interventions before painful procedures. Assess pain with each vital sign measurement. Evaluate effectiveness of pain relief. Administer analgesics as prescribed on preventive schedule (around the clock) when needed. **The Following NIC Concept Applies to These Interventions** Pain Management	To minimize discomfort To determine level of pain To determine effectiveness To prevent pain from recurring

Nursing Diagnosis	Expected Patient Outcomes	Nursing Interventions	Rationale
Fear related to diagnostic tests, procedures, treatment **Child's/Family's Defining Characteristics** ***(Subjective and Objective Data)*** Worry and anxiety before procedures Withdrawal Lack of control Outbursts, anger Lack of cooperation	Child will have reduced fear related to diagnostic procedures and treatment. **The Following NOC Concepts Apply to These Outcomes** Fear Self-Control Pain Control	Explain procedures carefully at child's level of understanding. Explain what will take place and what child will feel, see, and hear. Listen to special requests of child when possible. Provide child with some means of involvement with procedures (e.g., holding a piece of equipment, helping put on bandage, counting). Implement distraction techniques and pain reduction interventions. **The Following NIC Concept Applies to These Interventions** Pain Management	To reduce fear of unknown To provide sense of control To encourage cooperation To provide sense of control, encourage cooperation, and support child's coping skills To reduce pain

Nursing Diagnosis	Expected Patient Outcomes	Nursing Interventions	Rationale
Disturbed body image related to changes caused by cancer and treatment **Child's/Family's Defining Characteristics** ***(Subjective and Objective Data)*** Sadness Depression Withdrawal Anger	Child will exhibit positive coping skills. **The Following NOC Concept Applies to These Outcomes** Body Image	Encourage child to decide how he or she will cope with hair loss (e.g., wig, cap, scarf). Provide adequate covering during exposure to sunlight, wind, or cold. Explain that hair begins to regrow in 3 to 6 months and may be a different color and texture. Encourage good hygiene and grooming. Encourage rapid return to peer group and friends. Encourage visits from friends before discharge. **The Following NIC Concepts Apply to These Interventions** Counseling Body Image Enhancement	To promote early adjustment and preparation for hair loss To prevent exposure Natural hair protection is lost with alopecia To reduce risk of infection To prepare child for reactions of others To support child

Continued

NURSING CARE PLAN ✤ The Child with Cancer—cont'd

Nursing Diagnosis	Expected Patient Outcomes	Nursing Interventions	Rationale
Interrupted family processes related to having a child with a life-threatening disease **Child's/Family's Defining Characteristics** ***(Subjective and Objective Data)*** Lack of understanding of disease and treatment ✤ Inability to identify side effects of treatment Inability to understand child's treatment plan Lack of family support	Child and family will demonstrate understanding of the disease and treatment. **The Following NOC Concepts Apply to These Outcomes** Family Functioning Family Coping Family Normalization Knowledge: Illness Care	Teach parents and child about the disease, and explain all procedures. Advise family of expected side effects and toxicities; clarify which demand medical evaluation. Reassure family that reactions are complications of treatment. Prepare family for what to do when side effects occur. Interpret prognostic statistics carefully, realizing family's level of understanding. Schedule time for family to be together without interruptions. Help family plan for future. Encourage family to discuss feelings regarding child's disease. **The Following NIC Concepts Apply to These Interventions** Counseling Family Support	To promote understanding To prevent delay in treatment To provide support To prevent delay in treatment To promote understanding To encourage communication and expression of feelings To promote child's development To promote expression of feelings

family members can receive the varicella vaccine without risk to the child with cancer (American Academy of Pediatrics, Committee on Infectious Diseases, 2006; Walsh, Roilides, & Groll, 2006).

The child is evaluated for potential sites of infection (e.g., mucosal ulceration, skin abrasion, skin tear such as a hangnail) and observed for any elevation in temperature. To identify the source of infection, chest radiographs and blood, stool, urine, and nasopharyngeal cultures are taken. IV antibiotics are administered; if this therapy is prolonged, a venous access device, such as a peripherally inserted central catheter, intermittent infusion device (saline lock or PRN adaptor), is used to maintain IV access.

Prevention of infection continues to be a priority after discharge from the hospital. Ordinarily, the child is allowed to return to school when the WBC count is at a satisfactory level, usually an absolute neutrophil count (ANC) greater than 500/mm^3. At all times, family members are encouraged to practice good hand washing to prevent introducing pathogens into the home. The child may need to be isolated from school contacts in the event of an outbreak of a childhood disease, especially chickenpox.

Nutrition is another important component of infection prevention. An adequate protein-caloric intake provides the child with better host defenses against infection and increased tolerance to chemotherapy and irradiation. However, providing optimal nutrition during periods of anorexia and vomiting from chemotherapy is a tremendous challenge (see Feeding the Sick Child, Chapter 45).

Hemorrhage Before the use of transfused platelets, hemorrhage was a leading cause of death in patients with leukemia. Now most bleeding episodes can be prevented or controlled with the administration of platelet concentrates or platelet-rich plasma.

Because infection increases the tendency toward hemorrhage and bleeding sites become more easily infected, skin punctures are avoided whenever possible. When finger sticks, venipunctures, IM injections, and bone marrow aspirations are performed, aseptic technique must be used, along with continued observation for bleeding. Meticulous mouth care is essential, since gingival bleeding with resultant mucositis is a frequent problem. Because the rectal area is prone to ulceration from various drugs, feces and urine are removed immediately, and the perianal area is washed. Using rectal temperatures is avoided to prevent trauma. Children are advised to avoid activities that might cause injury or bleeding, such as riding bicycles or skateboards, climbing trees or playground equipment, and playing contact sports.

Platelet transfusions are generally reserved for active bleeding episodes that do not respond to local treatment and that may occur during induction or relapse therapy. Epistaxis and gingival bleeding are the most common. The nurse teaches parents and older children measures to control nosebleeding (see p. 1507). Pressure at the site without disturbing clot formation is the general rule.

Anemia Initially, anemia may be profound from complete replacement of the bone marrow by leukemic cells. During induction therapy, blood transfusions may be necessary. The usual precautions in caring for the child with anemia are instituted (see p. 1493).

Use Precautions in Administering and Handling Chemotherapeutic Agents

In addition to the nurse's many responsibilities in regard to the child and family, nurses must also use safeguards to protect themselves. Handling chemotherapeutic agents may present risks to handlers and their offspring, although the exact degree of risk is not known. Many chemotherapeutic agents are vesicants (sclerosing agents) that can cause severe cellular damage if even minute amounts of the drug infiltrate surrounding tissue. Only nurses experienced with chemotherapeutic agents should administer vesicants. Guidelines are available* and must be followed exactly to prevent tissue damage to patients. Interventions for extravasation vary, but each nurse should be aware of the institution's policies and implement them at once.

In addition to extravasation, a potentially fatal complication is anaphylaxis, especially from L-asparaginase, teniposide (VM-26), etoposide (VP-16), bleomycin, and cisplatin. Nursing responsibilities include prevention of, recognition of, and preparation for serious reactions. Prevention begins with a careful history for known allergies.

Most children with cancer have a venous access device, which facilitates administration of IV drugs. During treatment and remission, many drugs are taken orally at home. Compliance with the medication schedule is essential, and nurses play an important role in educating the family about the drugs and encouraging adherence to the plan.

NURSING ALERT Chemotherapeutic drugs must be given through a free-flowing IV line. The infusion is stopped immediately if any sign of infiltration (pain, stinging, swelling, or redness at the cannulation site) occurs.

NURSING ALERT When chemotherapeutic and immunologic agents are given, the child must be observed for 20 minutes after the infusion for signs of anaphylaxis (cyanosis, hypotension, wheezing, severe urticaria). Emergency equipment (especially blood pressure monitor and bag-valve-mask) and emergency drugs (especially oxygen, epinephrine, antihistamine, aminophylline, corticosteroids, and vasopressors) must be available. If a reaction is suspected, the drug is discontinued, the IV line is flushed with saline, and the child's vital signs and subsequent responses are monitored.

Manage Problems of Drug Toxicity

Chemotherapy presents several nursing challenges. The complexity of the treatment protocols is often overwhelming to families. In addition, each therapy is associated with a number of predictable side effects. Nurses must be aware of these side effects and use judgment in recognizing reactions and toxicities.

Nausea and Vomiting The nausea and vomiting that occur shortly after administration of several of the drugs and from cranial or abdominal radiation can be profound. The serotonin-receptor antagonists (e.g., ondansetron, granisetron) are effective in the control of nausea and vomiting occurring after emetogenic chemotherapy and radiotherapy. When combined with dexamethasone, these agents are the treatment of choice in the prevention of delayed emesis (Berde, Billett, & Collins, 2006).

The most beneficial regimen for antiemetic control has been the administration of the antiemetic *before* the chemotherapy begins. The goal is to prevent the child from ever experiencing nausea or vomiting, thus preventing development of anticipatory symptoms (the conditioned response of developing nausea and vomiting before receiving the drug).

Anorexia Loss of appetite is a direct consequence of the chemotherapy or irradiation. It is a major problem for parents because it is the one area they feel responsible for, particularly when so many other facets of care are outside their control. There are no universally successful techniques for encouraging a sick child to eat. However, the guidelines in Chapter 45 can be helpful during the anorexic period and can prevent additional problems during the remission.

Some children still do not eat despite these approaches. When loss of appetite and weight persist, the nurse should investigate the family situation to determine whether any factors (e.g., conditioned aversion to food, environmental stress related to eating, controlling behavior, anger) might be contributing to the problem. Nasogastric tube feedings or total parenteral nutrition may be implemented for children with significant nutritional problems.

Mucosal Ulceration One of the most distressing side effects of several drugs is GI mucosal cell damage, which can produce ulcers anywhere along the alimentary tract. Oral ulcers greatly compound anorexia because eating is extremely uncomfortable, but the following interventions may be helpful: (1) provide a bland, moist, soft diet appropriate for the child's age and preferences; (2) use a soft sponge toothbrush (Toothettes) or cotton-tipped applicator; (3) provide frequent mouthwashes with normal saline (using a solution of 1 tsp of table salt and 1 pint of water) or sodium bicarbonate mouth rinses (using a solution of 1 tsp of baking soda in 1 qt of water); and (4) use local anesthetics (e.g., Chloraseptic lozenges) or nonprescription preparations without alcohol (e.g., hydrocortisone dental paste [Orabase], antiseptic mouth rinse [UlcerEase], diphenhydramine [Benadryl], and aluminum and magnesium hydroxide [Maalox] solution). Although local anesthetics are effective in temporarily relieving the pain, many children dislike the taste and numb feeling they produce.

NURSING ALERT Viscous lidocaine is not recommended for young children; if applied to the pharynx, it may depress the gag reflex, increasing the risk of aspiration. Seizures rarely have been associated with the use of oral viscous lidocaine (Berde, Billett, & Collins, 2006; Cho, Cheng, & Cheng, 2000).

Other preparations that may be used to prevent or treat mucositis include chlorhexidine gluconate (Peridex) because of its dual effectiveness against candidal and bacterial infections, antifungal troches (lozenges) or mouthwash, and lip balm (e.g., Aquaphor) to keep the lips moist. Agents that should not be used include lemon glycerin swabs (irritate eroded tissue and can decay teeth), hydrogen peroxide (delays healing by breaking down protein), and milk of magnesia (dries mucosa).

Stomatitis may cause such difficulty with eating that the child may require hospitalization for hydration, parenteral nutrition, and pain control (often with IV morphine). The child will usually choose the foods that are best tolerated, and the nurse should encourage parents to relax any eating

**Cancer Chemotherapy Guidelines can be obtained from the Oncology Nursing Society, 125 Enterprise Drive, Pittsburgh, PA 15275; 866-257-4ONS, 412-859-6100; fax: 877-369-5497; e-mail: customer.service@ons.org; www.ons.org.*

pressures. Because the stomatitis is a temporary condition, the child can resume good food habits after the ulcers heal. Dental hygiene can become a serious problem for children with orthodontic appliances. Sometimes it may be necessary to remove the braces to allow chemotherapy to continue.

Rectal ulcers are managed by meticulous toilet hygiene, warm sitz baths after each bowel movement, and use of an occlusive ointment or dressing applied to the ulcerated area to promote epithelialization. Stool softeners are necessary to prevent further discomfort. Parents are advised to record bowel movements because the child may voluntarily avoid defecation to prevent discomfort. Rectal thermometers and suppositories are contraindicated because insertion may further traumatize the area.

Neuropathy Vincristine and, to a lesser extent, vinblastine can cause various neurotoxic effects. Nursing interventions for management of these effects include (1) administering stool softeners or laxatives for severe constipation caused by decreased bowel innervation; (2) maintaining good body alignment and, if patient is on bed rest, using a footboard or high-top shoes to minimize or prevent footdrop; (3) carrying out safety measures during ambulation because of weakness and numbing of the extremities, which may cause difficulty in walking or fine hand movement; and (4) providing a soft or liquid diet for severe jaw pain.

Hemorrhagic Cystitis Sterile hemorrhagic cystitis, a side effect of chemical irritation to the bladder from cyclophosphamide, can be decreased and often prevented by (1) promoting a liberal fluid intake (at least one and a half times the recommended daily fluid requirement); (2) frequent voiding immediately after feeling the urge, before bed, and after arising; (3) administering the drug early in the day to allow for sufficient oral intake and voiding; and (4) administering mesna (an agent that provides protection to the bladder) as ordered. If oral home administration is prescribed, the family needs *specific* instructions regarding exactly how much fluid the child must have.

Alopecia Hair loss is a common side effect of several chemotherapeutic drugs and cranial irradiation, although not all children lose their hair during drug therapy. It is better to warn children and parents of this side effect than to allow them to think that it is only a remote possibility. A soft cotton cap is the most comfortable head wear for children. Polyester increases perspiration and causes itching. Other options include scarves, hats, or a wig.

The nurse should also inform the family that hair regrows in 3 to 6 months and may be of a different color and texture. Frequently the hair is darker, thicker, and curlier than before. If the child chooses not to wear a wig, attention to some type of head covering, especially in cold climates and during exposure to sun, and scalp hygiene are important. The scalp should be washed like any other body part.

Moon Face Short-term steroid therapy produces no acute toxicities and two beneficial reactions: increased appetite and a sense of well-being. However, it does produce alterations in appearance, which, although not clinically significant, can be extremely distressing to older children. One of these is moon face, in which the child's face becomes rounded and puffy. It is helpful to reassure the child that, after cessation of the drug, the facial shape will return to normal. Unlike hair loss, little can be done to camouflage this obvious change. If the child resumes activity early in the course of treatment, the change may be less noticeable to peers than after a long absence.

Mood Changes Shortly after beginning steroid therapy, children experience a number of mood changes that range from feelings of well-being and euphoria to depression and irritability. If parents are unaware of these drug-induced changes, they may become unduly concerned. Therefore the nurse should warn them of the reactions and encourage them to discuss the behavioral changes with each other and the child.

Provide Emotional Support

An important aspect of continued emotional support involves the prognosis. Although leukemia is no longer invariably fatal, it must be remembered that survival statistics are only average estimates and apply to children treated with the latest protocols since diagnosis. For the low risk child the chances may be better, but for the high risk child they may be significantly poorer. Of those who do survive after discontinuing therapy, some relapse. Therefore at present only the passage of time is positive confirmation of the child's being ultimately "cured" of the disease. Remission, even in excess of 5 years, cannot be equated with a cure. With increasing concern regarding late effects of treatment, continued surveillance of the child's health status is needed. The nurse who is working with family members must individualize information regarding the "numbers" and the potential risks. An understanding of each member's emotional needs, as well as competent care of physical ones, is essential to the positive, growth-promoting support of the family. Comprehensive emotional support for the family of the child with a potentially fatal illness is discussed in Chapter 41.

Lymphomas

Pediatric lymphomas are the third most common group of malignancies in children and adolescents. The lymphomas, a group of neoplastic diseases that arise from the lymphoid and hematopoietic systems, are divided into Hodgkin's disease and non-Hodgkin's lymphoma (NHL). These diseases are further subdivided according to tissue type and extent of disease. NHL is more prevalent in children younger than 14 years of age, whereas Hodgkin's disease is prevalent in adolescence and the young adult period, with a striking increase between ages 15 and 19 years.

Hodgkin's Disease

Hodgkin's disease is a neoplastic disease that originates in the lymphoid system and primarily involves the lymph nodes. It predictably metastasizes to nonnodal or extralymphatic sites, especially the spleen, liver, bone marrow, and lungs, although no tissue is exempt from involvement (Fig. 49-4). It is classified according to four histologic types: (1) lymphocytic predominance, (2) nodular sclerosis, (3) mixed cellularity, and (4) lymphocytic depletion. Accurate staging of the extent of disease is the basis for treatment protocols and expected prognoses.

The Ann Arbor staging system assigns a stage based on the number of sites of lymph node involvement, presence of extra-

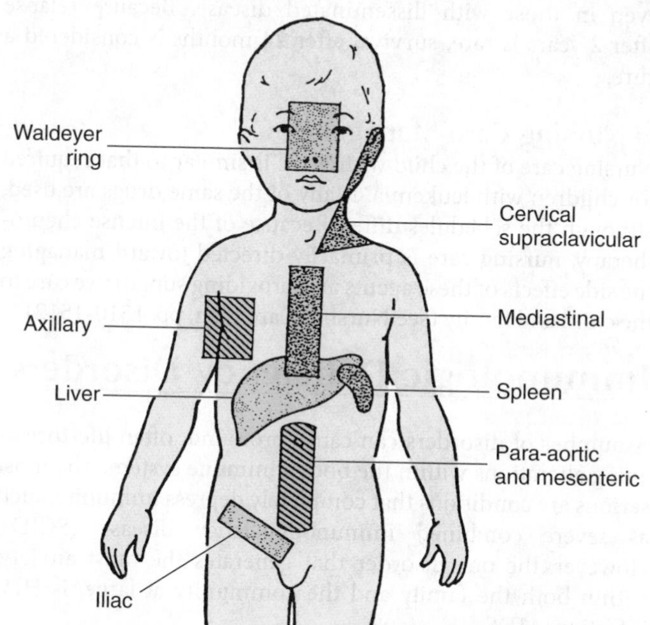

Fig. 49-4 Main areas of lymphadenopathy and organ involvement in Hodgkin's disease.

nodal disease, and history of any symptoms. Patients are classified as A if asymptomatic and as B if they have the following symptoms: temperature of 38° C (100.4° F) or higher for 3 consecutive days, drenching night sweats, or unexplained loss of body weight (10% or more) over the preceding 6 months (Hudson, Onciu, & Donaldson, 2006).

Asymptomatic enlarged cervical or supraclavicular lymphadenopathy is the most common presentation of Hodgkin's disease. Other systemic symptoms may be manifested, including fever, weight loss, night sweats, cough, abdominal discomfort, anorexia, nausea, and pruritus. Because multiple organs may be involved, diagnosis is based on several tests and the extent of metastatic disease. Tests include a CBC, erythrocyte sedimentation rate, serum copper, ferritin level, fibrinogen, immune globulins, uric acid level, liver function tests, T-cell function studies, and urinalysis. Radiographic tests include computed tomography (CT) scans of the neck, chest, abdomen, and pelvis; a gallium scan (identifies metastatic or recurrent disease); a chest x-ray film; and, if clinically indicated, a bone scan to identify metastatic disease.

Although used rarely, *lymphangiography* may be performed. This is visualization of the lymphatic circulation of the lower extremities, groin, ileopelvic and abdominal-aortic regions, and thoracic duct by way of a radiopaque medium injected in the feet or hands.

A lymph node biopsy is essential to establish histologic diagnosis and staging. The presence of Reed-Sternberg cells is characteristic of Hodgkin's disease. These large cells, which are multilobed and nucleated with abundant cytoplasm and a typically halolike clear zone around the nucleolus, are often described as having an "owl's eyes" appearance (Hudson, Oncui, & Donaldson, 2006). A bone marrow aspiration or biopsy is usually performed. With the advent of CT and gallium scans to identify metastatic disease and multiagent chemotherapy to eradicate it, a laparotomy without splenectomy is avoided except in a few selected cases.

Therapeutic Management

The primary modalities of therapy are radiation and chemotherapy. Each may be used alone or in combination based on the clinical staging. Radiation may involve only the involved field (IF), an extended field (EF) (involved areas plus adjacent nodes), or total nodal irradiation (TNI), depending on the extent of involvement.

An effective combination of chemotherapy widely used is MOPP (mechlorethamine, vincristine [Oncovin], procarbazine, prednisone) or ABVD (doxorubicin [Adriamycin], bleomycin, vinblastine, dacarbazine). However, this therapy combination has caused severe late effects, especially secondary malignancies. Other drug combinations such as COPP (cyclophosphamide, vincristine, prednisone, procarbazine) as a substitute for MOPP have minimized late effects.

Follow-up care of children no longer receiving therapy is essential to identify relapse and secondary cancers. In children with splenectomy resulting from laparotomy or splenic irradiation, prophylactic antibiotics are administered for an indefinite period. Immunizations against pneumococci and meningococci are also recommended before the splenectomy.

Prognosis

Long-term survival for all stages of Hodgkin's disease is excellent. Early-stage disease can have survival rates greater than 90%, with advanced stages having rates between 65% and 75%.

Nursing Care Management

Nursing care involves the same objectives as for patients with other types of cancer, specifically: (1) preparation for diagnostic and operative procedures, (2) explanation of treatment side effects, and (3) child and family support (see Chapter 41). Because this is most often a disease of adolescents and young adults, the nurse must have an appreciation of their psychologic needs and reactions during the diagnostic and treatment phases (see Nursing Care Plan, pp. 1510-1512).

The most common side effect of irradiation is fatigue. This is particularly difficult for active, outgoing school-age children and adolescents because it prevents them from keeping up with their peers. Sometimes adolescents push themselves to the point of physical exhaustion rather than admit and succumb to the decreased activity tolerance. The nurse cautions parents to observe for behavior such as extreme fatigue at the end of the day, falling asleep at the dinner table, inability to concentrate on homework, or an increased susceptibility to infection. A regular bedtime and scheduled rest periods are important for these children, especially during chemotherapy, when myelosuppression increases the risk of infection and debilitation. Before discharge the nurse should discuss a feasible school schedule with the parents and child.

An area of concern for adolescents is the high risk of sterility from irradiation and chemotherapy. Both drugs, particularly procarbazine and alkylating agents, and irradiation to the gonads can lead to infertility. Adolescents should be informed of these side effects early in the course of the diagnosis and treatment. Sperm banking is now offered at many cancer centers before the initiation of treatment in adolescent boys. Sexual function is not altered, although the appearance of secondary sexual characteristics and menstruation may be delayed in the pubescent child. Delayed sexual maturation may be an extremely sensitive and stressful issue for children.

Non-Hodgkin's Lymphoma

NHL occurs more frequently in children than Hodgkin's disease. NHL is diagnosed in approximately 750 to 800 children each year in the United States (Link & Weinstein, 2006). Histologic classification of childhood NHL is strikingly different from that of Hodgkin's disease, as demonstrated in the following statements:

- The disease is usually diffuse rather than nodular.
- The cell type is either undifferentiated or poorly differentiated.
- Dissemination occurs early, more often, and rapidly.
- Mediastinal involvement and invasion of meninges are common.

NHL exhibits a variety of morphologic, cytochemical, and immunologic features, not unlike the diversity seen in leukemia. Classification is based on the histologic pattern: (1) lymphoblastic, (2) Burkitt or non-Burkitt, or (3) large cell. Immunologically these cells are also classified as T cells; B cells; or non-T, non-B cells (lacking immunologic properties). The clinical staging system used in Hodgkin's disease is of little value in NHL, although it has been modified and other systems have been developed.

Diagnostic Evaluation

Because the clinical presentation of most children with NHL is widespread disseminated disease, thorough pathologic staging is unnecessary. Clinical manifestations depend on the anatomic site and extent of involvement. These manifestations include many of those seen in Hodgkin's disease and leukemia, as well as organ symptoms related to pressure from enlargement of adjacent lymph nodes, such as intestinal or airway obstruction, cranial nerve palsies, and spinal paralysis.

Recommendations for staging include a surgical biopsy of an enlarged node, histopathologic confirmation of disease with cytochemical and immunologic evaluation, bone marrow examination, radiographic studies (especially tomograms of the lungs and GI organs), and lumbar puncture.

Therapeutic Management

The treatment protocols for NHL include aggressive use of irradiation and chemotherapy. Similar to leukemic therapy, the protocols include induction, consolidation, and maintenance phases, some with intrathecal chemotherapy. Several antineoplastic agents used in the treatment of NHL include vincristine, prednisone, L-asparaginase, methotrexate, 6-mercaptopurine, cytarabine, cyclophosphamide, anthracyclines, and teniposide or etoposide (Link & Donaldson, 2003; Link and Weinstein, 2006).

Prognosis

The prognosis is excellent for children with localized disease, and long-term remissions are possible in many patients, even in those with disseminated disease. Because relapse after 2 years is rare, survival after 24 months is considered a cure.

Nursing Care Management

Nursing care of the child with NHL is similar to that required for children with leukemia. Many of the same drugs are used, although the schedules differ. Because of the intense chemotherapy, nursing care is primarily directed toward managing the side effects of these agents and providing supportive care to the child and family (see Nursing Care Plan, pp. 1510-1512).

Immunologic Deficiency Disorders

A number of disorders can cause profound, often life-threatening alterations within the body's immune system. The most serious are conditions that completely depress immunity, such as severe combined immunodeficiency disease (SCID). However, the one disorder that generates the most anxiety, within both the family and the community at large, is HIV infection/AIDS.

Several classifications of immune dysfunction exist. *AIDS*, SCID, and *Wiskott-Aldrich syndrome (WAS)* are syndromes wherein the body is unable to mount an immune response. The immune response can also be misdirected. In *autoimmune disorders* antibodies, macrophages, and lymphocytes attack healthy cells.

Human Immunodeficiency Virus Infection and Acquired Immunodeficiency Syndrome

Since the first cases of AIDS were identified in the early 1980s, HIV infection has generated intense medical investigation. Research has led to early diagnosis of and improved medical treatments for HIV infection, changing this disease from a rapidly fatal one to a chronic, but terminal, disease of childhood.

Epidemiology

The first AIDS cases in the pediatric population in the United States were identified in children born to HIV-infected mothers and in children who received blood products. More than 90% of these children acquired the disease perinatally from their mothers. Smaller numbers of children were infected through the transfusion of contaminated blood or blood products before 1985 or were infected through sexual abuse. In contrast, sexual activity and IV drug use are major sources of HIV infection in adolescents.

The estimated number of children with perinatally acquired AIDS peaked in 1992; subsequent years have seen significant declines. This trend is a result of implementation of recommended HIV counseling and voluntary testing practices and the use of highly active antiretroviral therapy (HAART) to prevent perinatal transmission. HAART, typically a combination of two nucleoside analog reverse transcriptase inhibitors and a protease inhibitor, is the current standard in the United States for the treatment of HIV-infected pregnant women, and it has significantly reduced the transmission of HIV (Cibulka, 2006; Perinatal HIV Guidelines Working Group, Public Health Service Task Force, 2007).

evolve Nursing Care Plan—The Child with HIV Infection

Etiology

HIV is a retrovirus that is transmitted by lymphocytes and monocytes. It is found in the blood, semen, vaginal secretions, and breast milk. It has an incubation period of months to years (Ezekowitz & Stockman, 2003). There are different strains of HIV. HIV-2 is prevalent in Africa, whereas HIV-1 is the dominant strain in the United States and elsewhere. *Horizontal transmission* of HIV occurs through intimate sexual contact or parenteral exposure to blood or body fluids containing visible blood. *Perinatal (vertical) transmission* occurs when an HIV-infected pregnant woman passes the infection to her infant. There is no evidence that *casual* contact between infected and uninfected individuals can spread the virus.

Pathophysiology

HIV primarily infects a specific subset of T lymphocytes, the CD4+ T cells. The virus takes over the machinery of the CD4+ lymphocyte, using it to replicate itself, rendering the CD4+ cell dysfunctional. The CD4+ lymphocyte count gradually decreases over time, leading to progressive immunodeficiency. The count eventually reaches a critical level below which there is substantial risk of opportunistic illnesses, followed by death.

Clinical Manifestations

Common clinical manifestations of HIV infection in children are varied (Box 49-9). The diagnosis of AIDS is associated with certain illnesses or conditions. The most common AIDS-defining conditions observed among American children are listed in Box 49-10. Other problems in these children may include short stature, malnutrition, and cardiomyopathy. CNS abnormalities resulting from HIV infection may include neuropsychologic deficits; developmental disabilities; and deficits in motor skills, communication, and behavioral functioning.

Diagnostic Evaluation

For children 18 months of age and older, the HIV enzyme-linked immunosorbent assay (ELISA) and Western blot immunoassay are performed to determine HIV infection. In infants born to HIV-infected mothers, these assays will be positive because of the presence of maternal antibodies derived transplacentally. Maternal antibodies may persist in the infant up to 18 months of age. Therefore other diagnostic tests are used, most commonly the HIV polymerase chain reaction (PCR) for detection of proviral DNA. With this technique, more than 95% of infected infants can be diagnosed by 1 to 4 months of age (Ezekowitz & Stockman, 2003; Goldschmidt & Fogler, 2006).

The Centers for Disease Control and Prevention (1994) has developed a classification system to describe the spectrum of HIV disease in children (Table 49-3). The system indicates the severity of clinical signs and symptoms and the degree of immunosuppression. Mild signs and symptoms include lymphadenopathy, parotitis, hepatosplenomegaly, and recurrent or persistent sinusitis or otitis media. Moderate signs and symptoms include lymphoid interstitial pneumonitis (LIP) and a variety of organ-specific dysfunctions or infections. Severe signs and symptoms include AIDS-defining illnesses with the exception of LIP. Children with LIP have a better prognosis than those with other AIDS-defining illnesses. In children whose HIV infection is not yet confirmed, the letter *E* (vertically exposed) is placed in front of the classification. The immune categories are based on CD4+ lymphocyte counts and percentages. Age adjustment of these numbers is

BOX 49-9 Common Clinical Manifestations of Human Immunodeficiency Virus Infection in Children

- Lymphadenopathy
- Hepatosplenomegaly
- Oral candidiasis
- Chronic or recurrent diarrhea
- Failure to thrive
- Developmental delay
- Parotitis

BOX 49-10 Common Defining Conditions for Acquired Immunodeficiency Syndrome in Children

- *Pneumocystis carinii* pneumonia
- Lymphoid interstitial pneumonitis
- Recurrent bacterial infections
- Wasting syndrome
- Candidal esophagitis
- Human immunodeficiency virus encephalopathy
- Cytomegalovirus disease
- *Mycobacterium avium-intracellulare* complex infection
- Pulmonary candidiasis
- Herpes simplex disease
- Cryptosporidiosis

Table 49-3 Pediatric Human Immunodeficiency Virus Infection Classification*

IMMUNOLOGIC CATEGORY	N: NO SIGNS/ SYMPTOMS	A: MILD SIGNS/ SYMPTOMS	B: MODERATE SIGNS/ SYMPTOMS†	C: SEVERE SIGNS/ SYMPTOMS†
No evidence of suppression	N1	A1	B1	C1
Evidence of moderate suppression	N2	A2	B2	C2
Severe suppression	N3	A3	B3	C3

From Centers for Disease Control and Prevention: 1994 Revised classification system for human immunodeficiency virus infection in children less than 13 years of age, *MMWR Recomm Rep* 43(RR-12):1-10, 1994.

*Children whose human immunodeficiency virus infection status is not confirmed are classified by using the above table with the letter *E* (for perinatally exposed) placed before the appropriate classification code (e.g., EN2).

†Both category C and lymphoid interstitial pneumonitis in category B are reportable to state and local health departments as acquired immunodeficiency syndrome.

evolve Critical Thinking Exercise—HIV Testing in Children

Table 49-4 Immunologic Categories Based on Age-Specific CD4+ T-Lymphocyte Counts and Percent of Total Lymphocytes

	Age of Child					
	<12 Mo		1-5 Yr		6-12 Yr	
IMMUNOLOGIC CATEGORY	μl	(%)	μl	(%)	μl	(%)
No evidence of suppression	≥1500	(≥25)	≥1000	(≥25)	≥500	(≥25)
Evidence of moderate suppression	750-1499	(15-24)	500-999	(15-24)	200-499	(15-24)
Severe suppression	<750	(<15)	<500	(<15)	<200	(<15)

From Centers for Disease Control and Prevention: 1994 Revised classification system for human immunodeficiency virus infection in children less than 13 years of age, *MMWR Recomm Rep* 43(RR-12):1-10, 1994.

necessary because normal counts, which are relatively high in infants, decline steadily until 6 years of age, when they reach adult norms (Table 49-4).

Therapeutic Management

The goals of therapy for HIV infection include slowing the growth of the virus, preventing and treating opportunistic infections, and providing nutritional support and symptomatic treatment. *Antiretroviral drugs* work at various stages of the HIV life cycle to prevent reproduction of functional new virus particles. Although not a cure, these drugs can suppress viral replication, preventing further deterioration of the immune system, and thus delay disease progression. Classes of antiretroviral agents include nucleoside reverse transcriptase inhibitors (e.g., zidovudine, didanosine, stavudine, lamivudine, abacavir), nonnucleoside reverse transcriptase inhibitors (e.g., nevirapine, delavirdine, efavirenz), nucleotide reverse transcriptase inhibitors (e.g., adefovir), protease inhibitors (e.g., indinavir, saquinavir, ritonavir, nelfinavir, amprenavir), and adjunctive antiretrovirals (e.g., hydroxyurea). Combinations of these drugs are used to forestall the emergence of drug resistance. Antiretroviral therapy regimens and guidelines are continually evolving. Therapy is lifelong, making adherence difficult. Laboratory markers (CD4+ lymphocyte count, viral load) assist in monitoring both disease progression and response to therapy.

Pneumocystis carinii pneumonia (PCP) is the most common opportunistic infection of children infected with HIV. It occurs most frequently between 3 and 6 months of age. All infants born to HIV-infected women should receive prophylaxis during the first year of life, according to guidelines from the Centers for Disease Control and Prevention (1995) and the American Academy of Pediatrics, Committee on Pediatric AIDS (2000a). Trimethoprim-sulfamethoxazole (TMP-SMZ) is the agent of choice. If adverse effects are experienced with TMP-SMZ, dapsone or pentamidine can be used.

Prophylaxis is often used for other opportunistic infections, such as disseminated *Mycobacterium avium-intracellulare* complex (MAC), candidiasis, or herpes simplex. IVIG has been helpful in preventing recurrent or serious bacterial infections in some HIV-infected children.

Immunization against common childhood illnesses is recommended for all children exposed to and infected with HIV (American Academy of Pediatrics, Committee on Pediatric AIDS, 2000b). Varicella (chickenpox) vaccine and measles-mumps-rubella (MMR) vaccine can be administered if there is no evidence of severe immunocompromise. Because antibody production to vaccines may be poor or decrease over time, immediate prophylaxis after exposure to several vaccine-preventable diseases (e.g., measles, varicella) is warranted. It should be recognized that children receiving IV γ-globulin prophylaxis may not respond to the MMR vaccine (Centers for Disease Control and Prevention, 2003).

HIV infection often leads to marked failure to thrive and multiple nutritional deficiencies. Nutritional management may be difficult because of recurrent illness, diarrhea, and other physical problems. Intensive nutritional interventions should be instituted when the child's growth begins to slow or weight begins to decrease.

Prognosis

Early recognition and improved medical care have changed HIV disease from a rapidly fatal illness to a chronic disease. After the introduction of combination antiretroviral therapy, the numbers of new AIDS cases and deaths declined substantially. Between 1995 and 1998, the annual number of AIDS cases declined by 38%, and deaths declined by 63% (Centers for Disease Control and Prevention, 2003; 2007). The annual number of AIDS cases has remained stable in children younger than 13 years of age since 1998 (Klause & Johnson, 2007).

Nursing Care Management

Education concerning transmission and control of infectious diseases, including HIV infection, is essential for children with HIV infection and anyone involved in their care. The basic tenets of Standard Precautions should be presented in an age-appropriate manner, with careful consideration of the educational levels of the individuals (see Infection Control, Chapter 45). Safety issues, including appropriate storage of special medications and equipment (e.g., needles and syringes), are emphasized.

Unfortunately, relatives, friends, and the general public may be fearful of contracting HIV infection, and the child and family may be criticized and ostracized. In an effort to protect the child, the family may limit his or her activities outside the home. Although certain precautions are justified in limiting exposure to sources of infections, they must be tempered with concern for the child's normal developmental needs. Both the family and the community need ongoing education about HIV to dispel many of the myths that have been perpetuated by uninformed persons.*

**Additional information is available from the AIDS Hotline: 800-342-2437 (342-AIDS).*

Prevention is a key component of HIV education. Educating adolescents about HIV is essential in preventing HIV infection in this age group. It should include the routes of transmission, the hazards of IV and other recreational drug use, and the value of sexual abstinence and safe sex practices. Such education should be a part of anticipatory guidance provided to all adolescent patients. Nurses can also encourage adolescents at risk to undergo HIV counseling and testing. In addition to identifying infected teenagers and getting them into care, such counseling affords adolescents an opportunity to learn about, and possibly change, their risky behaviors.

The multiple complications associated with HIV disease are potentially painful (Ezekowitz & Stockman, 2003; Sullivan & Woda, 2003). Aggressive pain management is essential for these children to have an acceptable quality of life. Their pain may be caused by infections (e.g., otitis media, dental abscess), encephalopathy (e.g., spasticity), adverse effects of medications (e.g., peripheral neuropathy), or an unknown source (e.g., deep musculoskeletal pain). Sources of pain are related not only to disease processes but also to various treatments these children often undergo, including venipunctures, lumbar punctures, biopsies, and endoscopies. Ongoing assessment of pain is crucial and is most easily accomplished in older children who are able to communicate. Nonverbal and developmentally delayed children are more difficult to assess. The nurse should be alert for signs of pain such as emotional detachment, lack of interactive play, irritability, and depression. Effective pain management depends on the appropriate use of pharmacologic agents, including EMLA cream, acetaminophen, NSAIDs, muscle relaxants, and opioids. Tolerance to opioids may indicate increased dosing; monitored use ensures safety. Nonpharmacologic interventions (e.g., guided imagery, hypnosis, relaxation, and distraction techniques) are useful adjuncts.

Common psychosocial concerns include disclosing the diagnosis to the child, making custody plans when the parent is infected, and anticipating the loss of a family member. Other stressors may include financial difficulties, HIV-associated stigma, efforts to keep the diagnosis secret, other infected family members, and the multiple losses associated with HIV. Most mothers of these children are single mothers who are also HIV infected. As primary caretakers, they often attend to the needs of their child first, neglecting their own health in the process (see Family-Centered Care box). The nurse can encourage the mother to receive regular health care. Family members are often involved in the care of the child, particularly if the mother has symptomatic illness. After the mother's death, a grandparent or other relative typically assumes responsibility for care of the child. The nurse can provide support and encouragement for the new surrogate parent, particularly during the transition phase. If no family member is available, the child may be placed in a foster or group home. Nursing is an integral part of the multidisciplinary team necessary for the successful management of the complex medical and social problems of these families.

Children with HIV infection attend day care centers and schools. It is well established that the risk of HIV transmission in these settings is minimal. These institutions are required to follow Centers for Disease Control and Prevention and Occupational Safety and Health Administration (OSHA) guidelines for infection control measures. Standard Precautions describing proper management of blood and body fluids should also be followed. It is recommended that school personnel receive current HIV information and include it in the health education curriculum for kindergarten through twelfth grade (American Academy of Pediatrics, Committee on Pediatric AIDS, 2000a; American Academy of Pediatrics, Committee on Pediatric AIDS and Committee on Infectious Diseases, 1999). School nurses play a vital role in educating the school staff, students, and parents. They are also invaluable in monitoring the needs of known affected children.

Confidentiality is a major issue in day care or school attendance. Parents and legal guardians have the right to decide whether to inform these agencies of their child's HIV diagnosis. Unfortunately, myths about HIV infection continue to exist, and the family often wishes to avoid any potential criticism or ostracism of the child.

FAMILY-CENTERED CARE

Caregivers and the Infant with Human Immunodeficiency Virus Infection

Unlike other fatal pediatric diseases, human immunodeficiency virus (HIV) infection is associated with special family alterations. The infant infected in utero faces multiple physical and parental problems. Because the mother is infected, she may be ill or dying and therefore unable to care for the child. If possible, grandparents or other relatives may assume care. Foster care is often difficult to arrange because of the nature of the disease, especially in relation to the social stigma and the child's multiple medical needs. When these children are hospitalized, the importance of consistent caregivers, especially primary nurses who attend to the youngsters' physical, developmental, and emotional needs, cannot be overemphasized. However, primary nurses may face the risk of overinvolvement and must be aware of the boundaries of a therapeutic relationship.

Severe Combined Immunodeficiency Disease

SCID is a defect characterized by absence of both humoral and cell-mediated immunity. The terms *Swiss-type lymphopenic agammaglobulinemia* (an autosomal recessive form of the disease) and *X-linked lymphopenic agammaglobulinemia* have been used to describe this disorder, which, as the names imply, can follow either mode of inheritance.

Susceptibility to infection occurs early, most often in the first month of life. The child suffers from chronic infection, fails to completely recover from an infection, is frequently reinfected, and is infected with unusual agents. Failure to thrive is a consequence of the persistent illnesses.

Diagnosis is usually based on a history of recurrent, severe infections from early infancy; a familial history of the disorder; and specific laboratory findings, which include lymphopenia, lack of lymphocyte response to antigens, and absence of plasma cells in the bone marrow. Documentation of immune globulin deficiency is difficult during infancy because of the normally delayed response of infants in producing their own immune globulins and material transfer of immune globulin G (IgG).

Therapeutic Management

The definitive treatment for SCID is HSCT from a histocompatible donor, a haplo-identical donor (usually a parent), or a matched unrelated donor. IVIG infusions and PCP prophylaxis are used to augment the humoral immunity until the transplant is performed. Several investigators are attempting gene therapy with some success, but there is a potential complication of insertional mutagenesis (Buckley, 2007).

Nursing Care Management

Nursing care focuses on preventing infection and supporting the child and family. The care is consistent with that needed for HSCT for any condition (see p. 1523). Because the prognosis for SCID is very poor if a compatible bone marrow donor is not available, nursing care is directed at supporting the family in caring for a child with a life-threatening illness (see Chapter 41). Genetic counseling is essential because of the modes of transmission in either form of the disorder.

Wiskott-Aldrich Syndrome

WAS is an X-linked recessive disorder characterized by a triad of abnormalities: (1) thrombocytopenia, (2) eczema, and (3) immunodeficiency of selective functions of B and T lymphocytes. A defective gene has been identified and designated the WAS protein (Bonilla & Geha, 2003; Fleisher, 2006). At birth the presenting symptoms may be bloody diarrhea as a result of thrombocytopenia. As the child grows older, recurrent infection and eczema become more severe, and the bleeding becomes less frequent.

Eczema is typical of the allergic type and easily becomes superinfected. Chronic infection with herpes simplex is a frequent problem and may lead to chronic keratitis of the eye with loss of vision. Chronic pulmonary disease, sinusitis, and otitis media result from repeated infections. In children who survive the bleeding episodes and overwhelming infections, malignancy presents an additional risk to survival. Medical treatment involves:

- Counteracting the bleeding tendencies with platelet transfusions.
- Using IV γ-globulin to provide passive immunity.
- Administering prophylactic antibiotics to prevent and control infection.

The only curative therapy is HSCT from a matched donor (Buckley, 2007).

Nursing Care Management

Because of the poor prognosis for these children, the main nursing consideration is supporting the family in the care of a fatally ill child (see Chapter 41). Physical care is directed at controlling the problems imposed by the disorder. The measures used to control bleeding are similar to those for hemophilia and vWD (see previous discussions). Another major goal is prevention or control of infection. Because eczema is a troublesome problem, nursing measures specific to this condition are especially important (see Chapter 53). The genetic implications of this X-linked recessive disorder differ little from those of any other X-linked disorder.

Technologic Management of Hematologic and Immunologic Disorders

Blood Transfusion Therapy

Technologic advances in blood banking and transfusion medicine enable the administration of only the blood component needed by the child, such as packed RBCs in anemia or platelets for bleeding disorders. However, regardless of the blood component infused, all transfusions have some risks. Therefore nurses need to be aware of the possible complications and the appropriate interventions. Table 49-5 summarizes the major hazards of transfusions, the signs and symptoms typically associated with each, and nursing responsibilities. General guidelines that apply to all transfusions include:

- Take vital signs, including blood pressure, *before* administering blood to establish baseline data for intratransfusion and posttransfusion comparison and then every 15 minutes for 1 hour while blood is infusing and on completion of transfusion.
- Check the identification of the recipient with the donor's blood group and type, regardless of the blood product being used.
- Administer the first 50 ml of blood or 20% of the volume (whichever is smaller) *slowly* and stay with the child.
- Administer with normal saline on a piggyback setup or have normal saline available.
- Administer blood through an appropriate filter to eliminate particles in the blood and prevent the precipitation of formed elements; gently shake the container frequently.
- Use blood within 30 minutes of its arrival from the blood bank; if it is not used, return to the blood bank—do not store in the regular unit refrigerator.
- Infuse a unit of blood (or the specified amount) within 4 hours. If the infusion will exceed this time, the blood should be divided into appropriately sized quantities by the blood bank, and the unused portion refrigerated under controlled conditions.
- If a reaction of any type is suspected, take vital signs, stop the transfusion, maintain a patent IV line with normal saline and new tubing, notify the practitioner, and do not restart the transfusion until the child's condition has been medically evaluated.

Although hemolytic reactions are rare, ABO incompatibility remains the most common cause of death from blood transfusion, and human error is usually responsible (administration of the wrong type to the patient or mislabeling of the blood product) (Norville & Bryant, 2002; Bell, 2007). Hemolysis can also cause the release of large quantities of phospholipids, which are capable of stimulating DIC (see p. 1506). Acute kidney shutdown and eventual renal failure are the results of renal vasoconstriction from antigen-antibody complexes derived from the RBC surface.

Blood is usually administered to children by infusion pump; therefore the usual precautions and management related to pumps apply. When the blood is started with a

Table 49-5 Nursing Care of the Child Receiving Blood Transfusions

COMPLICATION	SIGNS AND SYMPTOMS	PRECAUTIONS AND NURSING RESPONSIBILITIES
Immediate Reactions		
Hemolytic Reactions		
Most severe type, but rare Incompatible blood Incompatibility in multiple transfusions	Sudden severe headache Chills Shaking Fever Pain at needle site and along venous tract Nausea and vomiting Sensation of tightness in chest Red or black urine Flank pain Progressive signs of shock or renal failure	Identify donor and recipient blood types and groups before transfusion is begun; verify with another nurse or practitioner. Transfuse blood slowly for first 15-20 min and/or initial 20% of blood volume; remain with patient. Stop transfusion immediately in event signs or symptoms occur, maintain patent intravenous line, and notify practitioner. Save donor blood to recrossmatch with patient's blood. Monitor for evidence of shock. Insert urinary catheter and monitor hourly outputs. Send sample of patient's blood and urine to laboratory for presence of hemoglobin (indicates intravascular hemolysis). Observe for signs of hemorrhage resulting from disseminated intravascular coagulation. Support medical therapies to reverse shock.
Febrile Reactions		
Leukocyte or platelet antibodies Plasma protein antibodies	Fever Chills	Acetaminophen may be given for prophylaxis. Leukocyte-poor red blood cells (RBCs) are less likely to cause reaction. Stop transfusion immediately; report to practitioner for evaluation.
Allergic Reactions		
Recipient reaction to allergens in donor's blood	Urticaria Pruritus Flushing Asthmatic wheezing Laryngeal edema	Give antihistamines for prophylaxis to children with tendency to allergic reactions. Stop transfusion immediately. Administer epinephrine for wheezing or anaphylactic reaction.
Circulatory Overload		
Too rapid transfusion (even a small quantity) Transfusion of excessive quantity of blood (even slowly)	Precordial pain Dyspnea Rales Cyanosis Dry cough Distended neck veins Hypertension	Transfuse blood slowly. Prevent overload by using packed RBCs or administering divided amounts of blood. Use infusion pump to regulate and maintain flow rate. Stop transfusion immediately if signs of overload. Place child upright with feet in dependent position to increase venous resistance.
Air Emboli		
May occur when blood is transfused under pressure	Sudden difficulty in breathing Sharp pain in chest Apprehension	Normalize pressure before container is empty when infusing blood under pressure. Clear tubing of air by aspirating it with syringe at nearest Y connector if it is observed in tubing; disconnect tubing and allow blood to flow until air has escaped only if a Y connector is not available.
Hypothermia	Chills Low temperature Irregular heart rate Possible cardiac arrest	Allow blood to warm at room temperature (<1 hr). Use approved mechanical blood warmer or electric warming coil to warm blood rapidly; never use microwave oven. Take temperature if patient complains of chills; if subnormal, stop transfusion.
Electrolyte Disturbances		
Hyperkalemia (in massive transfusions or in patients with renal problems)	Nausea, diarrhea Muscle weakness Flaccid paralysis Paresthesia of extremities Bradycardia Apprehension Cardiac arrest	Use washed RBCs or fresh blood if patient is at risk.

Continued

Table 49-5 Nursing Care of the Child Receiving Blood Transfusions—cont'd

COMPLICATION	SIGNS AND SYMPTOMS	PRECAUTIONS AND NURSING RESPONSIBILITIES
Delayed Reactions		
Transmission of Infection		
Hepatitis Human immunodeficiency virus (HIV) infection Malaria Syphilis Other bacterial or viral infection	Signs of infection (e.g., jaundice) Toxic reaction–High fever, severe headache or substernal pain, hypotension, intense flushing, vomiting or diarrhea	Blood is tested for antibodies to HIV, hepatitis C virus, and hepatitis B core antigen; in addition, it is tested for hepatitis B surface antigen and alanine aminotransferase, and a serologic test is performed for syphilis; units that test positive are destroyed; individuals at risk for carrying certain viruses are deterred from donation. Report any sign of infection and, if it occurs during transfusion, stop transfusion immediately, send sample for culture and sensitivity testing, and notify practitioner.
Alloimmunization Antibody formation Occurs in patients receiving multiple transfusions	Increased risk of hemolytic, febrile, and allergic reactions	Use limited number of donors. Observe carefully for signs of reactions.
Delayed Hemolytic Reaction	Destruction of RBCs and fever 5-10 days after transfusion	Observe for posttransfusion anemia and decreasing benefit from successive transfusion.

standard transfusion set, the filter chamber is filled to allow the total filter to be used. The drip chamber is partially filled with blood to permit counting of the drops. In adjusting the flow rate, it is important to remember that blood administration sets do not use microdrops (60 drops/ml) but regular drops (usually 10 or 15 drops/ml).

Hematopoietic Stem Cell Transplantation

HSCT is used to establish healthy hemopoiesis in both malignant and nonmalignant disease. Candidates for transplantation are children who have disorders that are unlikely to be cured by other means. Most HSCT patients undergo intensive ablative therapy using high-dose combination chemotherapy with or without total body irradiation (Bollard, Krance, & Heslop, 2006). After the immune system is suppressed to prevent rejection of the transplanted marrow, the stem cells harvested from the bone marrow, peripheral blood, or umbilical vein of the placenta are given to the patient by IV transfusion. The newly transfused stem cells will begin to repopulate the ablative bone marrow. In essence, a new blood-forming organ will be accepted by the recipient.

The selection process for a suitable donor and the potential complications in transplantation are related to the *HLA system complex.* Some of the major HLAs are A, B, C, D, and DR. There is a wide diversity for each of these HLA loci. There are more than 20 different HLA-As that can be inherited and more than 40 different HLA-Bs.

The genes are inherited as a single unit or *haplotype.* A child inherits one unit from each parent; thus a child and each parent have one identical and one nonidentical haplotype. Because the possible haplotype combinations among siblings follow the laws of Mendelian genetics, there is a one-in-four chance that two siblings have two identical haplotypes and are perfectly matched at the HLA loci.

The importance of HLA matching is to prevent the serious complication known as *GVHD.* Because the child's immune system is essentially rendered nonfunctional, there is little difficulty with bone marrow rejection by the recipient. However, the donor's marrow may contain antigens not matched to the recipient's antigens, which begin attacking body cells. The more closely the HLA systems match, the less likely GVHD is to develop. However, it can occur even with a perfect HLA match because there are as yet unidentified and thus unmatched histocompatibility antigens (Bollard, Krance, & Heslop, 2006).

Different types of HSCT are now performed in children with cancer. *Allogeneic HSCT* involves matching a histocompatible donor with the recipient. However, allogeneic HSCT is limited by the presence of a suitable marrow donor.

Because of the limited numbers of patients having HLA-identical siblings, other types of allogeneic transplants have evolved. *Umbilical cord blood stem cell transplantation* is an established, rich source of hematopoietic stem cells for use in children with cancer. Because stem cells can be found with high frequency in the circulation of newborns, cord blood transplantation has become an alternative for some children. The benefit of using umbilical cord blood is the blood's relative immunodeficiency at birth, allowing for partially matched unrelated cord blood transplants to be successful, with a lower risk of GVHD-related problems (Bollard, Krance, & Heslop, 2006; Ryan et al, 2002).

Autologous HSCTs use the patient's own marrow that was collected from disease-free tissue, frozen, and sometimes treated to remove malignant cells. Children with solid tumors such as neuroblastoma, Hodgkin's disease, NHL, rhabdomyosarcoma, Ewing sarcoma, and Wilms tumor have been treated with autologous HSCTs.

Peripheral stem cell transplants (PSCTs) are also used in children with cancer. PSCT, a type of autologous transplant, differs in the way stem cells are collected from the patient. CSF is first given to stimulate the production of many stem cells (Ryan et al, 2002). After the WBC count is high enough, the stem cells are collected by an apheresis machine. This machine filters out peripheral stem cells from whole blood, returning the remainder of the blood cells and plasma to the child. Stem cells have been collected in very small children without problems (Lipton, 2003). The peripheral stem cells are then frozen until the patient is ready for the PSCT.

Nursing Care Management

The care of children undergoing HSCT is similar to that of any child receiving chemotherapy and radiotherapy. The hospitalization is typically 3 to 6 weeks in an isolated environment, during which time the child is subjected to numerous procedures and side effects of therapy. Throughout this long ordeal the family is concerned with successful engraftment and fear of fatal complications (see Family-Centered Care box). Consequently, nurses involved with the child and family need to provide sensitive care and maintain a supportive attitude during the many crises that may arise. If the procedure is not successful, the families need care consistent with that required by the family of any child with a life-threatening disorder (see Chapter 41).

FAMILY-CENTERED CARE

The Decision for a Hematopoietic Stem Cell Transplant

A family's decision for a child to undergo hematopoietic stem cell transplantation (HSCT) may be fraught with challenges. Often the child is facing certain death from the malignancy. The preparation of the child for the transplant also places the patient at great medical risk.

Once the preparatory regimen is begun and the child's immune system is destroyed, there is no turning back. Unlike kidney transplantation, HSCT does not have a "rescue" procedure, such as dialysis, for supportive therapy. If the donor is a sibling, the issue of his or her marrow "saving" the brother or sister can be a concern, especially if the transplant fails. Parents often must leave the home to stay at the transplant center and encounter additional stressors such as arranging child care, taking a leave from work, and managing finances. The patient faces the greatest stress—fear of HSCT failure or life-threatening complications.

Apheresis

Apheresis is the removal of blood from an individual, separation of the blood into its components, retention of one or more of these components, and reinfusion of the remainder of the blood into the individual. It is most often used to remove large quantities of platelets from healthy adult donors. These transfusion products have greatly prolonged the survival of patients with hematologic and oncologic diseases.

This technique is used to remove peripheral blood stem cells (PBSCs) from children before they receive HSCT or high-dose chemotherapy or radiotherapy, which is severely toxic to the bone marrow. These PBSCs can then be used to restore the child's bone marrow. Apheresis is also used as a therapeutic modality. The blood component that is diseased or toxic is separated from the blood, and the remainder is returned to the individual. Therapeutic apheresis is considered part of standard therapy for many diseases. Plasma is selectively removed from individuals with hyperviscosity, life-threatening complications of myasthenia gravis, Guillain-Barré syndrome, thrombotic thrombocytopenic purpura, and certain drug overdoses. WBCs are removed from individuals with high–WBC count leukemia.

Nursing Care Management

Difficult venous access and small blood volume can limit the ability to use this therapy in the infant and young child. Education of the family and child includes the purposes of the therapy and the technology.

Specially trained individuals perform the apheresis procedure. Attention focuses on rate of removal, blood component separation, and reinfusion of blood into the child. Vital signs are monitored, and the child is continuously observed for any adverse reactions secondary to the circulatory volume changes and the anticoagulant used.

When apheresis components are infused, nursing measures differ depending on whether the product is autologous (blood component from the child) or allogeneic (blood component from another individual). Autologous components are the child's own blood; therefore a major precaution is proper identification to ensure the correct component. The rate of infusion should be adjusted to the child's tolerance. If the product is allogeneic, all precautions for blood transfusions apply.

Key Points

- Anemia is defined as reduction of RBCs or Hgb concentration to levels below normal for age; disorders are classified either by etiology and physiology or by morphology.
- The nurse's role in treatment of anemia is to assist in establishing a diagnosis, prepare the child for laboratory tests, administer prescribed medications, decrease tissue oxygen needs, implement safety precautions, and observe for complications.
- The main nursing goal in prevention of nutritional anemia is parent education regarding correct feeding practices.
- SCA is a hereditary hemoglobinopathy caused by normal adult Hgb (HbA) being partly or completely replaced by sickle Hgb (HbS).
- Nursing care of the child with SCA focuses on teaching the family how to prevent and recognize sickle cell

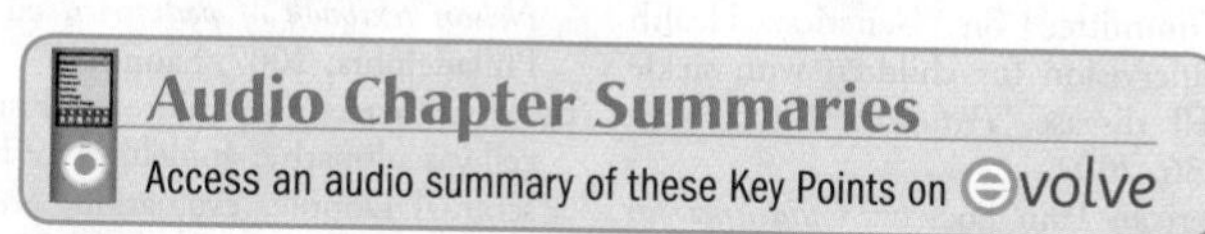
Audio Chapter Summaries
Access an audio summary of these Key Points on evolve

problems; managing pain during crises; and helping the child and parents adjust to a lifelong chronic disease.
- Nursing care of the child with β-thalassemia includes observing for complications of multiple blood transfusions, assisting the child in coping with the effects of illness, and fostering parent-child adjustment to long-term illness.
- Causes of acquired AA include irradiation, drugs, industrial and household chemicals, infections, and infiltration and replacement of myeloid elements; however, most cases are idiopathic.

- Clotting depends on three processes: vascular spasm, platelet aggregation, and coagulation and clot formation.
- Nursing care of the child with hemophilia involves preventing bleeding by decreasing the risk of injury, recognizing and managing bleeding with factor replacement, preventing the crippling effects of joint degeneration, and preparing and supporting the child and family for home care.
- Goals in the care of the child with leukemia are to prepare the family for diagnostic and therapeutic procedures, prevent complications of myelosuppression, manage problems of irradiation and drug toxicity, and provide continued emotional support.
- The lymphomas include Hodgkin's lymphoma and NHL and are disorders involving the lymphoid system.
- Immunodeficiency disorders render the affected individual unable to fight infectious organisms.
- HIV infection is primarily acquired in infants during pregnancy or birth from an infected mother and in adolescents from engaging in high risk behaviors.
- Blood transfusions supply needed blood components.
- HSCT replaces the diseased or malfunctioning bone marrow with viable blood stem cells.
- Apheresis is the selective removal of a blood component. It can be used to supply cellular elements needed for therapy (i.e., platelets or stem cells) or to remove diseased components.

References

American Academy of Pediatrics: Breastfeeding and the use of human milk, *Pediatrics* 115(2):496-506, 2005.

American Academy of Pediatrics, Committee on Infectious Diseases, Pickering L, editor: *Red book: 2006 report of the Committee on Infectious Diseases*, ed 27, Elk Grove Village, Ill, 2006, The Academy.

American Academy of Pediatrics, Committee on Pediatric AIDS: Identification and care of HIV-exposed and HIV-infected infants, children, and adolescents in foster care, *Pediatrics* 106(1):149-153, 2000a.

American Academy of Pediatrics, Committee on Pediatric AIDS: Technical report: perinatal human immunodeficiency virus testing and prevention of transmission, *Pediatrics* 106(6):1-12, 2000b.

American Academy of Pediatrics, Committee on Pediatric AIDS and Committee on Infectious Diseases: Issues related to human immunodeficiency virus transmission in schools, child care, medical settings, the home, and community, *Pediatrics* 104(2):318-324, 1999.

American Academy of Pediatrics, Section on Hematology/Oncology, Committee on Genetics: Health supervision for children with sickle cell disease, *Pediatrics* 109(3):526-536, 2002.

American Pain Society: *Guidelines for the management of acute and chronic pain in sickle-cell disease*, Glenview, Ill, 1999, The Society.

Anderson N: Hydroxyurea therapy: improving the lives of patients with sickle cell disease, *Pediatr Nurs* 32(6):541-543, 2006.

Andrews NC: Disorders of iron metabolism and sideroblastic anemia. In Nathan D et al, editors: *Nathan and Oski's hematology of infancy and childhood*, ed 6, Philadelphia, 2003, Saunders.

Bell MD: Red blood cell transfusions, *Pediatr Rev* 28(8):299-304, 2007.

Berde CB, Billett AM, Collins JJ: Symptom management in supportive care. In Pizzo PA, Poplack DG, editors: *Principles and practice of pediatric oncology*, ed 5, Philadelphia, 2006, Lippincott.

Bhatia S: Epidemiology. In Wallace WHB, Green DM, editors: *Late effects of childhood cancer*, London, 2004, Arnold.

Bogen DL, Krause JP, Serwint JR: Outcome of children identified as anemic by routine screening in an inner-city clinic, *Arch Pediatr Adolesc Med* 155:366-371, 2001.

Bollard CM, Krance RA, Heslop HE: Hematopoietic stem cell transplantation in pediatric oncology. In Pizzo PA, Poplack DG, editors: *Principles and practice of pediatric oncology*, ed 5, Philadelphia, 2006, Lippincott.

Bonilla FA, Geha RS: Primary immunodeficiency diseases. In Nathan D et al, editors: *Nathan and Oski's hematology of infancy and childhood*, ed 6, Philadelphia, 2003, Saunders.

Buchanan GR: Thrombocytopenia during childhood: what the pediatrician needs to know, *Pediatr Rev* 26(11):401-409, 2005.

Buckley RH: Evaluation of the immune system. In Behrman RE et al, editors: *Nelson textbook of pediatrics*, ed 18, Philadelphia, 2007, Saunders.

Bulas D: Screening children for sickle cell vasculopathy: guidelines for transcranial Doppler evaluation, *Pediatr Radiol* 35:235-241, 2005.

Burden MJ et al: An event-related potential study of attention and recognition memory in infants with iron-deficiency anemia, *Pediatrics* 120(2):336-345, 2007.

Carley A: Anemia: when is it iron deficiency? *Pediatr Nurs* 29(2):127-133, 2003.

Centers for Disease Control and Prevention: *HIV/AIDS surveillance report—2005* (revised edition) 17:1-54, 2007.

Centers for Disease Control and Prevention: Advancing HIV prevention: new strategies for a changing epidemic—United States, *MMWR* 52(15):329-332, 2003.

Centers for Disease Control and Prevention: 1995 revised guidelines for prophylaxis against *Pneumocystis carinii* pneumonia for children infected with or perinatally exposed to human immunodeficiency virus, *MMWR* 44(RR-4):1-11, 1995.

Centers for Disease Control and Prevention: 1994 revised classified system for human immunodeficiency virus infection in children less than 13 years of age, *MMWR* 43(RR-12):1-10, 1994.

Chandran L, Gelfer P: Breastfeeding: the essential principles, *Pediatr Rev* 27(11):409-417, 2006.

Chiocca EM: Sickle cell crisis: severe pain and potential tissue necrosis are the major concerns, *Am J Nurs* 96(9):49, 1996.

Cho S, Cheng AC, Cheng MCK: Oral care for children with leukemia, *Hong Kong Med J* 6(2):203-208, 2000.

Cibulka NJ: Mother-to-child transmission of HIV in the United States, *Am J Nurs* 106(7):56-63, 2006.

Curry H: Bleeding disorder basics, *Pediatr Nurs* 30(5):402-405, 2004.

Dover GJ, Platt OS: Sickle cell disease. In Nathan D et al, editors: *Nathan and Oski's hematology of infancy and childhood*, ed 6, Philadelphia, 2003, Saunders.

Driscoll MC: Sickle cell disease, *Pediatr Rev* 28(7):259-267, 2007.

Ezekowitz RAB, Stockman III JA: Hematologic manifestations of systemic diseases. In Nathan D et al, editors: *Nathan and Oski's hematology of infancy and childhood*, ed 6, Philadelphia, 2003, Saunders.

Fleisher TA: Primary immune deficiencies: windows into the immune system, *Pediatr Rev* 27(10):363-373, 2006.

Glader B: Anemias of inadequate production. In Behrman RE et al, editors: *Nelson textbook of pediatrics*, ed 18, Philadelphia, 2007, Saunders.

Goldschmidt RH, Fogler JA: Opportunities to prevent HIV transmission to newborns, *Pediatrics* 117(1):208-209, 2006.

Hord JD: The acquired pancytopenia. In Behrman RE et al, editors: *Nelson textbook of pediatrics*, ed 18, Philadelphia, 2007, Saunders.

Hudson MM, Onciu M, Donaldson SS: Hodgkin's disease. In Pizzo PA, Poplack DG, editors: *Principles and practice of pediatric oncology*, ed 4, Philadelphia, 2006, Lippincott.

Karayalcin G: Hemolytic anemia (sickle cell anemia). In Lanzkowsky P, editor: *Manual of pediatric hematology and oncology*, ed 3, San Diego, 2000, Academic Press.

Khoury H, Grimsley E: Oxygen inhalation in nonhypoxic sickle cell patients during vaso-occlusive crisis, *Blood* 86(10):3998, 1995.

Klause BD, Johnson M: Paradigm shift: new testing guidelines for HIV, *Adv Nurse Pract* 15(3):59-93, 2007.

Link MP, Donaldson SS: The lymphomas and lymphadenopathy. In Nathan D et al, editors: *Nathan and Oski's hematology of infancy and childhood*, ed 6, Philadelphia, 2003, Saunders.

Link MP, Weinstein HJ: Malignant non-Hodgkin lymphomas in children. In Pizzo PA, Poplack DG, editors: *Principles and practice of pediatric oncology*, ed 5, Philadelphia, 2006, Lippincott.

Lipton JM: Peripheral blood as a stem cell source for hematopoietic cell transplantation in children: is the effort in vein? *Pediatr Transplant* 7(Suppl 3):65-70, 2003.

Margolin JF, Steuber CP, Poplack DG: Acute lymphoblastic leukemia. In Pizzo PA, Poplack DG, editors: *Principles and practice of pediatric oncology*, ed 4, Philadelphia, 2006, Lippincott.

Marsh JCW: Management of acquired aplastic anemia, *Blood Rev* 19:143-151, 2005.

McKenzie SB: Anemias of disordered iron metabolism and heme synthesis. In McKenzie SB, editor: *Clinical laboratory hematology*, Upper Saddle River, NJ, 2004, Pearson Prentice Hall.

Miller M et al: Hydroxyurea therapy for pediatric patients with hemoglobin SC disease, *J Pediatr Hematol Oncol* 23(5):306-308, 2001.

Montgomery RR, Gill JC, Scott JP: Hemophilia and von Willebrand disease. In Nathan D et al, editors: *Nathan and Oski's hematology of infancy and childhood*, ed 6, Philadelphia, 2003, Saunders.

Morris CR, Singer ST, Walters MC: Clinical hemoglobinopathies: iron, lungs and new blood, *Curr Opin Hematol* 13:407-418, 2006.

National Hemophilia Foundation, Bleeding Disorders Information Center: *Newly diagnosed: parents FAQ*, 2006. Available at www.hemophilia.org/bdi/bdi_newly7c.htm (accessed March 25, 2008).

National Institutes of Health, National Heart, Lung, and Blood Institute, Division of Blood Disease and Resources: *The management of sickle cell disease*, NIH Pub No 02-2117, Bethesda, Md, 2002, NHLBI Health Information Network.

Norville R, Bryant R: Blood component deficiencies. In Baggott CR et al, editors: *APON nursing care of children and adolescents with cancer*, ed 3, Philadelphia, 2002, Saunders.

Ohls R, Christensen RD: Hemoglobin disorders. In Behrman RE et al, editors: *Nelson textbook of pediatrics*, ed 18, Philadelphia, 2007, Saunders.

Okpala I: New therapies for sickle cell disease, *Hematol Oncol Clin North Am* 19:975-987, 2005.

Orkin SH, Nathan DG: The thalassemias. In Nathan D et al, editors: *Nathan and Oski's hematology of infancy and childhood*, ed 6, Philadelphia, 2003, Saunders.

Paley C: Hemolytic anemia (thalassemias). In Lanzkowsky P, editor: *Manual of pediatric hematology and oncology*, ed 3, San Diego, 2000, Academic Press.

Pearce JM, Sills RH: Childhood leukemia, *Pediatr Rev* 26(3):96-104, 2005.

Perinatal HIV Guidelines Working Group, Public Health Service Task Force: *Recommendations for use of antiretroviral drugs in pregnant HIV-infected women for maternal health and interventions to reduce perinatal HIV transmission in the United States*, 2007. Available at www.aidsinfo.nih.gov/ContentFiles/PerinatalGL.pdf (accessed March 24, 2008).

Perkins S: Disorders of hematopoiesis. In Collins RD, Swerdlow SH, editors: *Pediatric hematopathology*, Philadelphia, 2001, Churchill Livingstone.

Platt OS et al: Mortality in sickle cell disease: life expectancy and risk factors for early death, *N Engl J Med* 330:1639-1644, 1994.

Pui CH, Relling MV, Downing JR: Acute lymphoblastic leukemia, *N Engl J Med* 350:1535-1548, 2004.

Redding-Lallinger R, Knoll C: Sickle cell disease—pathophysiology and treatment, *Curr Probl Pediatr Adolesc Health Care* 36(10):346-376, 2006.

Richardson M: Microcytic anemia, *Pediatr Rev* 28(1):5-13, 2007.

Ryan LG et al: Hematopoietic stem cell transplantation. In Baggott CR et al, editors: *Nursing care of children and adolescents with cancer*, ed 3, Philadelphia, 2002, Saunders.

Scott JP, Montgomery RR: Platelet and blood vessel disorder. In Behrman RE et al, editors: *Nelson textbook of pediatrics*, ed 18, Philadelphia, 2007, Saunders.

Segel GB, Hirsh MG, Feig SA: Managing anemia in a pediatric office practice, part I, *Pediatr Rev* 23(3):75-83, 2002.

Shende A: Bone marrow failure. In Lanzkowsky P, editor: *Manual of pediatric hematology and oncology*, ed 3, San Diego, 2000, Academic Press.

Shimamura A, Guinan EC: Acquired aplastic anemia. In Nathan D et al, editors: *Nathan and Oski's hematology of infancy and childhood*, ed 6, Philadelphia, 2003, Saunders.

Silverman LB, Sallan SE: Acute lymphoblastic leukemia. In Nathan D et al, editors: *Nathan and Oski's hematology of infancy and childhood*, ed 6, Philadelphia, 2003, Saunders.

Steinberg MH et al: Effect of hydroxyurea on mortality and morbidity in adult sickle cell anemia: risks and benefits up to 9 years of treatment, *JAMA* 289(13):1645-1651, 2003.

Sullivan JL, Woda BA: Lymphohistiocytic disorders. In Nathan D et al, editors: *Nathan and Oski's hematology of infancy and childhood*, ed 6, Philadelphia, 2003, Saunders.

Walsh TJ, Roilides E, Groll AH: Infectious complications in pediatric cancer patients. In Pizzo PA, Poplack DG, editors: *Principles and practice of pediatric oncology*, ed 4, Philadelphia, 2006, Lippincott

Yoon SL, Black S: Comprehensive, integrative management of pain for patients with sickle-cell disease, *J Altern Complement Med* 12(10):995-1001, 2006.

Zimmerman S et al: Sustained long-term hematologic efficacy of hydroxyurea at maximum tolerated dose in children with sickle cell disease, *Blood* 103(6):2039-2045, 2004.

Unit 11

50 Genitourinary Dysfunction

Learning Objectives

On completion of this chapter the reader will be able to:

- Describe the various factors that contribute to urinary tract infections in infants and children.
- Discuss the preoperative preparation of the child and parents when the child has a structural defect of the genitourinary tract.
- Demonstrate an understanding of the causes and mechanisms of edema formation in nephrotic syndrome.
- Outline a nursing care plan for a child with nephrotic syndrome.
- Compare the child with minimal-change nephrotic syndrome and the child with acute glomerulonephritis in terms of clinical manifestations and nursing care.
- Contrast the causes, complications, and management of acute and chronic renal failure.
- List the types of renal dialysis.
- Recognize signs of kidney transplant rejection.

Electronic Resources

Additional information related to the content in Chapter 50 can be found on

evolve the Companion Website at

http://evolve.elsevier.com/Perry/maternal/

- NCLEX Review Questions
- Animation—Bladder
- Animation—Kidney Function
- Nursing Care Plan—The Child with Chronic Renal Failure

Genitourinary Dysfunction

Assessment of kidney and urinary tract integrity and diagnosis of renal or urinary tract disease are based on several evaluative tools. Physical examination, history taking, and observation of symptoms are the initial procedures. In suspected urinary tract diseases or disorders, further assessment by laboratory, radiologic, and other evaluative methods is carried out.

Clinical Manifestations

As in most disorders of childhood, the incidence and type of kidney or urinary tract dysfunction change with the child's age and maturation. In addition, the presenting complaints and the significance of these complaints vary with maturation. For example, a complaint of enuresis has greater significance at age 8 years than at age 4. In the newborn, urinary tract disorders are associated with a number of obvious malformations of other body systems, including the curious and unexplained but frequent association between malformed or low-set ears and urinary tract anomalies.

Many of the clinical manifestations of renal disease are common to a variety of childhood disorders, but their presence is an indication to obtain further information from the child's history, family history, and laboratory studies as part of a complete physical examination. Suspected renal disease can be further evaluated by means of radiographic studies and renal biopsy (Table 50-1).

Laboratory Tests

Both urine and blood studies contribute vital information for detection of renal problems. The single most important test is probably routine urinalysis. Specific urine and blood tests provide additional information. Because nurses are usually the persons who collect the specimens for examination and who often perform many of the screening tests, they should be familiar with the tests, their functions, and factors that can alter or distort the results of the tests. The major urine and blood tests are outlined in Tables 50-2 and 50-3.

Nursing Care Management

Nursing responsibilities in assessment of genitourinary disorders or diseases begin with observation of the child for any manifestations that might indicate dysfunction. Many conditions have specific characteristics that distinguish them from other disorders. These are discussed as appropriate throughout the chapter.

The nurse is generally responsible for preparing infants, children, and parents for tests and for collecting urine and

Table 50-1 Radiologic and Other Tests of Urinary System Function

TEST	PROCEDURE	PURPOSE	COMMENTS AND NURSING RESPONSIBILITIES
Urine culture and sensitivity	Collection of sterile specimen	Determines presence of pathogens and the drugs to which they are sensitive	Does not require specific parental permission. Send specimen to laboratory immediately after collection. Use catheterization, clean-catch, or suprapubic specimen.
Renal and bladder ultrasound	Transmission of ultrasonic waves through renal parenchyma, along ureteral course, and over bladder	Allows visualization of renal parenchyma and renal pelvis without exposure to external beam radiation or radioactive isotopes Visualization of dilated ureters and bladder wall also possible	Noninvasive procedure.
Testicular (scrotal) ultrasound	Transmission of ultrasonic waves through scrotal contents and testis	Allows visualization of scrotal contents, including testis Testicular ultrasound is used to identify masses, and Doppler-enhanced ultrasound is used to differentiate hyperemia of epididymo-orchitis from ischemia or torsion	Noninvasive procedure.
Scout film	Flat plate roentgenogram of abdomen and pelvis for kidney, ureters, bladder (KUB)	Detects and establishes renal outlines, presence of calculi, or opaque foreign bodies in bladder	Prepare as for routine x-ray film.
Voiding cystourethrography	Contrast medium injected into bladder through urethral catheter until bladder is full; films taken before, during, and after voiding	Visualizes bladder outline and urethra, reveals reflux of urine into ureters, and shows complications of bladder emptying	Prepare child for catheterization.
Radionuclide (nuclear) cystogram	Radionuclide-containing fluid injected through urethral catheter until bladder is full; images generated before, during, and after voiding	Alternative to voiding cystourethrography in children with allergy to intravesical contrast material Allows evaluation of reflux, although visualization of anatomic details is relatively poor	Prepare child for catheterization. Reassure patient and parents that allergic response to contrast materials is avoided by use of radionuclide.
Radioisotope imaging studies	Contrast medium injected intravenously; computer analysis to measure uptake or washout (excretion) for analysis of organ function	DTPA radioisotope used to measure glomerular filtration rate; estimate of differential renal function and renal washout to determine presence and location of upper urinary tract obstruction DMSA radioisotope used to visualize renal scars and differential renal function; does not visualize ureters and bladder MAG3 radioisotope combines features of DTPA (evaluation of upper urinary tract obstruction) with features of DMSA radioisotope (differential renal function)	Insert or assist with insertion of intravenous infusion. Monitor intravenous infusion. Urethral catheterization may accompany DTPA radioisotope scan; prepare child for catheterization when indicated.
Intravenous pyelography (IVP) (intravenous urogram; excretory urogram)	Intravenous injection of a contrast medium Medium secreted and concentrated by tubules X-ray films made 5, 10, and 15 minutes after injection; delayed films (30, 60 minutes, etc.) are obtained if obstruction suspected	Defines urinary tract Provides information about integrity of kidneys, ureters, and bladder Retroperitoneal masses visualized when they shift position of ureters	Preparation for test: **Infants <2 yr of age**—Give no solid food, omit one bottle on morning of examination; perform studies early to avoid withholding of fluids. **Children 2-14 yr of age**—Give cathartic evening before examination, nothing orally after midnight, enema (soapsuds) morning of examination.
Computed tomography (CT)	Narrow-beam x-rays and computer analysis providing precise reconstruction of area	Visualizes vertical or horizontal cross section of kidney Especially valuable to distinguish tumors and cysts	Noncontrast scan is noninvasive. Contrast-enhanced CT scan preparation similar to that for IVP.

Continued

evolve Animation—Kidney Function

Table 50-1 Radiologic and Other Tests of Urinary System Function—cont'd

TEST	PROCEDURE	PURPOSE	COMMENTS AND NURSING RESPONSIBILITIES
Cystoscopy	Direct visualization of bladder and lower urinary tract through small scope inserted via urethra	Investigation of bladder and lower tract lesions; visualizes ureteral openings, bladder wall, trigone, and urethra	Give nothing orally after midnight. Carry out preoperative preparations. Prepare the child for cystoscopy.
Retrograde pyelography	Contrast medium injected through ureteral catheter	Visualizes pelvic calyces, ureters, and bladder	Give cathartic if ordered. Give preoperative medication if ordered. Observe for reaction to contrast medium. Monitor vital signs after procedure.
Renal angiography	Contrast medium injected directly into renal artery via catheter placed in femoral artery (or umbilical artery in newborn) and advanced to renal artery	Visualizes renal vascular system, especially for renal arterial stenosis	Prepare child for insertion of a spinal needle or perfusion catheter in renal pelvis (anesthetic often required).
Whitaker perfusion test	Injection of contrast material through renal pelvis and ureters Measures pressures in renal pelvis and urinary bladder	Determine presence of obstruction causing upper urinary tract dilation	Give nothing orally 4-6 hr before test. Premedicate as ordered. Prepare setup for procedure. Assist with procedure. Take vital signs. Apply pressure to area with pressure dressing and, if feasible, a sandbag. Place on bed rest for 24 hr. Observe for abdominal pain, tenderness. Monitor input and output; surgical incision may be required in infants.
Renal biopsy	Removal of kidney tissue by open or percutaneous technique for study by light, electron, or immunofluorescent microscopy	Yields histologic and microscopic information about glomeruli and tubules; helps distinguish between types of nephritic syndromes Distinguishes other renal disorders	Prepare child for catheterization. Insertion of a rectal tube produces feelings of rectal fullness or pressure. Insertion of needles may be required for sphincter electromyography.
Urodynamics	Set of tests designed to measure bladder filling, storage, and evacuation functions **Uroflowmetry**—Test to determine efficiency of urination **Cystometrogram**—Graphic comparison of bladder pressure as a function of volume **Voiding pressure study**—Comparison of detrusor contraction pressure, sphincter electromyelogram, and urinary flow	Determine characteristic of voiding dysfunction Used to identify type (cause) of incontinence or urinary retention Especially valuable for voiding dysfunction complicated by urinary tract infection, urinary retention, or neurogenic bladder dysfunction	Prepare child for urinary catheterization. The bladder will be filled with saline solution and filling pressures will be recorded; the child may experience fullness, coolness from the saline fluid, and urine leakage during the study.

DMSA, Dimercaptosuccinic acid; *DTPA,* diethylenetriamine pentaacetic acid; *MAG3,* mercaptoacetyltriglycine.

(sometimes) blood specimens for observation and laboratory analysis (see Preparation for Diagnostic and Therapeutic Procedures, and Collection of Specimens, Chapter 45). An important nursing responsibility is to maintain careful *intake and output* and *blood pressure* measurements on most children with genitourinary dysfunction and those who might be at risk for developing renal complications (e.g., children in shock, postoperative patients). For example, any significant degree of renal disease can diminish the glomerular filtration rate, a measure of the amount of plasma from which a given substance is totally cleared in 1 minute. A number of substances can be used, but the most useful clinical estimation of glomerular filtration is the clearance of *creatinine,* an end product of protein metabolism in muscle and a substance that is freely filtered by the glomerulus and secreted by renal tubular cells. The nurse's responsibility in this test is collection of urine, usually a 12- or 24-hour specimen.

Table 50-2 Urine Tests of Renal Function

TEST	NORMAL RANGE	DEVIATIONS	SIGNIFICANCE OF DEVIATIONS
Physical Tests			
Volume	Age-related Newborn–30-60 ml Children–Bladder capacity (oz) = Age (yr) + 2	Polyuria Oliguria Anuria	Osmotic factors (urinary glucose level in diabetes mellitus) Retention caused by obstructive disease Inadequate bladder emptying caused by neurogenic bladder or obstructive disorder Obstruction of urinary tract; acute renal failure
Specific gravity	With normal fluid intake–1.016-1.022 Newborn–1.001-1.020 Others–1.001-1.030	High Low	Dehydration Presence of protein or glucose Presence of radiopaque contrast medium after radiologic examinations Excessive fluid intake Distal tubular dysfunction Insufficient antidiuretic hormone Diuresis
Osmolality	Newborn–50-600 mOsm/L Thereafter–50-1400 mOsm/L	Fixed at 1.010 High or low	Chronic glomerular disease Same as for specific gravity More sensitive index than specific gravity
Appearance	Clear pale yellow to deep gold	Cloudy Cloudy reddish pink to reddish brown Light Dark Red	Contains sediment Blood from trauma or disease Myoglobin after severe muscle destruction Dilute Concentrated Trauma
Chemical Tests			
pH	Newborn–5-7 Thereafter–4.8-7.8 Average–6	Weak acid or neutral Alkaline	If associated with metabolic acidosis, suggests tubular acidosis If associated with metabolic alkalosis, suggests potassium deficiency Urinary infection Metabolic alkalosis
Protein level	Absent	Present	Abnormal glomerular permeability (e.g., glomerular disease, changes in blood pressure) Most kidney disease Orthostatic in some individuals
Glucose level	Absent	Present	Diabetes mellitus Infusion of concentrated glucose-containing fluids Glomerulonephritis Impaired tubular reabsorption
Ketone levels	Absent	Present	Conditions of acute metabolic demand (stress) Diabetic ketoacidosis
Leukocyte esterase	Absent	Present	Can identify both lysed and intact white blood cells via enzyme detection
Nitrites	Absent	Present	Most species of bacteria convert nitrates to nitrites in the urine
Microscopic Tests			
White blood cell count	<1 or 2	>5 polymorphonuclear leukocytes/field Lymphocytes	Urinary tract inflammatory process Allograft rejection Malignancy
Red blood cell count	<1 or 2	4-6/field in centrifuged specimen	Trauma Stones Glomerular injury Infection Neoplasms
Presence of bacteria	Absent to a few	>100,000 organisms/ml in centrifuged specimen	Urinary tract infection

Continued

Table 50-2 Urine Tests of Renal Function—cont'd

TEST	NORMAL RANGE	DEVIATIONS	SIGNIFICANCE OF DEVIATIONS
Microscopic Tests—cont'd			
Presence of casts	Occasional	Granular casts	Tubular or glomerular disorders Degenerative process in advanced renal disease
		Cellular casts White blood cell Red blood cell Hyaline casts	Pyelonephritis Glomerulonephritis Proteinuria; usually transient

Table 50-3 Blood Tests of Renal Function

TEST	NORMAL RANGE (mg/dl)	DEVIATIONS	SIGNIFICANCE of Deviations
Blood urea nitrogen (BUN)	Newborn–4-18 Infant, child–5-18	Elevated	Renal disease–acute or chronic (the higher the BUN, the more severe the disease) Increased protein catabolism Dehydration Hemorrhage High protein intake Corticosteroid therapy
Uric acid	Child–2.0-5.5	Increased	Severe renal disease
Creatinine	Infant–0.2-0.4 Child–0.3-0.7 Adolescent–0.5-1.0	Increased	Severe renal impairment

Genitourinary Tract Disorders and Defects

Urinary Tract Infection

Infection of the genitourinary tract is one of the most common conditions of childhood. Up to 10% of children will have a febrile urinary tract infection (UTI) during the first 2 years of life (Kanellopoulos et al, 2006). Among febrile males, circumcision status is important in determining risk for UTI. Uncircumcised male infants less than 3 months of age had the highest prevalence of UTI (20.1%) of any group, male or female (Shaikh et al, 2008). Circumcision status should be assessed in male infants with unexplained fever. UTI may involve the urethra and bladder (lower urinary tract) or the ureters, renal pelvis, calyces, and renal parenchyma (upper urinary tract). Because it is often impossible to localize the infection, the broad designation *UTI* is applied to the presence of significant numbers of microorganisms anywhere within the urinary tract, except the distal third of the urethra, which is usually colonized with bacteria.

Classification

Infection of the urinary tract may be present with or without clinical symptoms. As a result, the site of infection is often difficult to pinpoint with any degree of accuracy. Various terms used to describe urinary tract disorders include:

Bacteriuria—Presence of bacteria in the urine

Asymptomatic bacteriuria—Significant bacteriuria (usually defined as more than 100,000 colony-forming units) with no evidence of clinical infection

Symptomatic bacteriuria—Bacteriuria accompanied by physical signs of UTI (dysuria, suprapubic discomfort, hematuria, fever)

Recurrent UTI—Repeated episode of bacteriuria or symptomatic UTI

Persistent UTI—Persistence of bacteriuria despite antibiotic treatment

Febrile UTI—Bacteriuria accompanied by fever and other physical signs of UTI; presence of a fever typically implies a pyelonephritis

Cystitis—Inflammation of the bladder

Urethritis—Inflammation of the urethra

Pyelonephritis—Inflammation of the upper urinary tract and kidneys

Urosepsis—Febrile UTI coexisting with systemic signs of bacterial illness; blood culture reveals presence of urinary pathogen

Etiology

A variety of organisms can be responsible for UTI. *Escherichia coli* (80% of cases) and other gram-negative enteric organisms are most frequently implicated; these organisms are usually found in the anal and perineal region. Other organisms associated with UTI include *Proteus, Pseudomonas, Klebsiella, Staphylococcus aureus, Haemophilus,* and coagulase-negative *Staphylococcus* organisms. Several factors contribute to the development of UTI in childhood.

Anatomic and Physical Factors

The structure of the lower urinary tract is believed to account for the increased incidence of bacteriuria in females (Rosenthal, 2004). The short urethra, which measures about 2 cm (¾ inch) in young girls and 4 cm (1⅗ inches) in mature women, provides a ready pathway for invasion of organisms. In addition, the closure of the urethra at the end of micturition may return contaminated bacteria to the bladder. The longer male urethra (as long as 20 cm [8 inches] in an adult) and the antibacterial properties of prostatic secretions inhibit the entry and growth of pathogens.

NURSING ALERT Considerable evidence suggests there are fewer UTIs among circumcised male infants than among uncircumcised male infants, but the difference is not significant enough to recommend routine circumcision in newborns (American Academy of Pediatrics, 1999).

The single most important host factor influencing the occurrence of UTI is *urinary stasis.* Ordinarily, urine is sterile, but at 37° C (98.6° F) it provides an excellent culture medium. Under normal conditions the act of completely and repeatedly emptying the bladder flushes away any organisms before they have an opportunity to multiply and invade surrounding tissue. However, urine that remains in the bladder allows bacteria from the urethra to rapidly become established in the rich medium. Incomplete bladder emptying (stasis) may result from *reflux* (see Vesicoureteral Reflux, p. 1532), anatomic abnormalities (especially those involving the ureters), dysfunction of the voiding mechanism, or extrinsic ureteral or bladder compression that may be caused by constipation. The key to preventing UTI is to maintain adequate blood supply to the bladder wall by avoidance of overdistention and high bladder pressure.

Altered Urine and Bladder Chemistry

Several mechanical and chemical characteristics of the urine and bladder mucosa help maintain urinary sterility. An increased fluid intake promotes flushing of the normal bladder and lowers the concentration of organisms in the infected bladder. Diuresis also seems to enhance the antibacterial properties of the renal medulla.

Most pathogens favor an alkaline medium. Normally, urine is slightly acidic with a median pH of 6.0. A urine pH of about 5 hampers but does not eliminate bacterial multiplication. Much has been reported about the use of cranberry products to increase urine acidity in an effort to prevent UTI. Studies done in adults offer limited evidence for the value of cranberry products in promoting urinary tract health (Jepson, Mihaljevic, & Craig, 2004; Bailey et al, 2007). Further research that controls for type of cranberry product used, dosing regimens, and patient selection based on age and underlying medical condition is required to clarify unanswered questions before recommendations can be made regarding the use of this supplement, especially in the pediatric population.

Diagnostic Evaluation

The clinical manifestations of UTI depend on the child's age (Box 50-1). Diagnosis of UTI is confirmed by detection of bacteriuria in urine culture, but urine collection is often difficult, especially in infants and very small children. Several factors may alter a urine specimen, and contamination of a specimen by organisms from sources other than the urine, such as perineal and perianal flora in bag specimens, is the most frequent cause of false-positive results. Unless the specimen is a first morning sample, a recent high fluid intake may indicate a falsely low organism count. Therefore children should not be encouraged to drink large volumes of water in an attempt to obtain a specimen quickly.

BOX 50-1 Clinical Manifestations of Urinary Tract Disorders or Disease

Neonatal Period (Birth to 1 Month)
Poor feeding
Vomiting
Failure to gain weight
Rapid respiration (acidosis)
Respiratory distress
Spontaneous pneumothorax or pneumomediastinum
Frequent urination
Screaming on urination
Poor urine stream
Jaundice
Seizures
Dehydration
Other anomalies or stigmata
Enlarged kidneys or bladder

Infancy (1 to 24 Months)
Poor feeding
Vomiting
Failure to gain weight
Excessive thirst
Frequent urination
Straining or screaming on urination
Foul-smelling urine
Pallor
Fever
Persistent diaper rash
Seizures (with or without fever)
Dehydration
Enlarged kidneys or bladder

Childhood (2 to 14 Years)
Poor appetite
Vomiting
Growth failure
Excessive thirst
Enuresis, incontinence, frequent urination
Painful urination
Swelling of face
Seizures
Pallor
Fatigue
Blood in urine
Abdominal or back pain
Edema
Hypertension
Tetany

evolve Animation—Bladder

NURSING ALERT A child who exhibits the following should be evaluated for UTI:

- Incontinence in a toilet-trained child
- Strong-smelling urine
- Frequency or urgency

More accurate estimates of bacterial content are obtained from *suprapubic aspiration* (in children younger than 2 years of age) and properly performed bladder catheterization (as long as the first few milliliters are excluded from collection). The specimen should be taken directly to the laboratory for immediate culture.

Tests to detect bacteriuria are being used with increased frequency in screening for UTI. The dipstick tests for leukocyte esterase or nitrite are quick and inexpensive methods for detecting infection before obtaining final culture results.

Localization of the infection site may involve more specific tests, including percutaneous kidney taps and bladder washout procedures. Other tests such as ultrasonography, voiding cystourethrogram (VCUG), intravenous pyelogram, and DMSA (dimercaptosuccinic acid) scan may be performed after the infection subsides to identify anatomic abnormalities contributing to the development of infection and existing kidney changes from recurrent infection.

Therapeutic Management

The objectives of treatment of children with UTI are (1) to eliminate current infection, (2) to identify contributing factors to reduce the risk of recurrence, (3) to prevent systemic spread of the infection, and (4) to preserve renal function. Antibiotic therapy should be initiated on the basis of identification of the pathogen, the child's history of antibiotic use, and the location of the infection. Several antimicrobial drugs are available for treating UTI, but all of them can occasionally be ineffective because of resistance of organisms. Common antiinfective agents used for UTI include the penicillins, sulfonamide (including trimethoprim and sulfisoxazole in combination), the cephalosporins, and nitrofurantoin.

If anatomic defects such as primary reflux or bladder neck obstruction are present, surgical correction of these abnormalities may be necessary to prevent recurrent infection. Follow-up study is an important component of medical management, since the relapse rate is high and infection tends to recur 1 to 2 months after termination of treatment. The aim of therapy and careful follow-up is to reduce the chance of renal scarring. However, recurrent infection of the urinary bladder predisposes the individual to transient episodes of vesicoureteral reflux (VUR).

Vesicoureteral Reflux

VUR refers to the abnormal retrograde flow of bladder urine into the ureters. During voiding, urine is swept up the ureters and then flows back into the empty bladder, where it acts as a reservoir for bacterial growth until the next void. *Primary reflux* results from congenitally abnormal insertion of ureters into the bladder; *secondary reflux* occurs as a result of an acquired condition.

It is not clear that reflux necessarily causes infections. What is clear is that reflux is more likely to be associated with recurring kidney infections rather than simple bladder infections (cystitis). In the presence of reflux, infected urine (bacteria) from the bladder has access to the kidney, resulting in kidney infections (pyelonephritis). These children are usually very symptomatic with high fevers, vomiting, and chills. Reflux, when associated with UTI, is the most common cause of renal scarring in children. Renal scarring may occur with the first episode of febrile UTI. Reflux in the presence of sterile urine does not cause renal damage. Therefore the most important concept in managing VUR is preventing bacteria from reaching the kidneys. VUR is managed conservatively with daily low-dose antibiotic therapy. A urine culture should be done every 2 to 3 months and any time the child has a fever. This method of management requires a motivated, reliable, and cooperative family. Many children will outgrow the reflux over a period of years. An annual VCUG is done to assess the status of the reflux.

For children with mild to moderate reflux, a minimally invasive endoscopic option (subtrigonal injection, or STING) is an alternative to daily antibiotics or open surgical intervention. A bulking agent—dextranomer–hyaluronic acid polymer (Deflux)—is injected into the mucous membrane of the ureter, making retrograde flow of urine more difficult. Overall cure rates relate to degree of reflux and range from 72% to 84% (Kirsch, Perez-Brayfield, & Scherz, 2003; Lavelle, Conlin, & Skoog, 2005).

Indications for open surgical intervention include significant anatomic abnormality at the ureterovesical junction, recurrent UTIs, severe forms of VUR, noncompliance with medical therapy, intolerance to antibiotics, and VUR after puberty in females.

Prognosis

With prompt and adequate treatment at the time of diagnosis, the long-term prognosis for UTI is usually excellent. However, the hazard of progressive renal injury is greatest when infection occurs in young children (especially those younger than 2 years of age) and is associated with congenital renal malformations and reflux. Therefore early diagnosis of children at risk is particularly important.

Nursing Care Management

Nurses should instruct parents to observe regularly for clues suggesting UTI. Unfortunately, the signs of UTI are not as evident as those of upper respiratory tract infection. Therefore many cases go undetected because no one thought to investigate this very common problem.

Because infants and young children often are unable to express their feelings and sensations verbally, it is difficult to detect discomfort they may be experiencing from dysuria. A careful history regarding voiding habits, stooling pattern, and episodes of unexplained irritability may assist in detecting less obvious cases of UTI. Consequently, parents should be cautioned to observe for specific clues of UTI in suspected cases.

When infection is suspected, collecting an appropriate specimen is essential. It is the nurse's responsibility to take every precaution to obtain acceptable clean-voided specimens to avoid the use of other, more invasive collecting procedures except when absolutely indicated. Because of the unreliability of a specimen obtained via a urine collection bag, suprapubic aspiration of urine or sterile catheterization should be done in the infant or young child who is seen with fever.

Frequently, additional tests are performed to detect anatomic defects. Children are prepared for these tests as appropriate for their age. This includes an explanation of the procedure, its purpose, and what the children will experience (see Preparation for Diagnostic and Therapeutic Procedures, Chapter 45). Sometimes a simple description of the urinary system is helpful. Especially for preschool children, the nurse must clarify that the urinary tract is separate from any sexual function and that the test is for a problem that they did not cause. Children may associate blame for perceived wrongdoing (e.g., masturbation) or unacceptable thoughts with the reason for the illness or the tests. For children younger than 3 to 4 years of age, the procedure can be explained on a doll. For those who are older, a simple drawing of the bladder, urethra, ureters, and kidneys makes the procedure more understandable.

Handling actual equipment when feasible can be helpful in allaying anxiety in children of all ages. Anticipatory instruction on distraction techniques such as deep breathing, storytelling, and imagery may help the child relax and be more cooperative during the actual procedures. If surgery is indicated, facts and understanding of the procedure will help decrease the child's fear and anxiety concerning more extensive medical-surgical intervention.

Because antibacterial drugs are indicated in UTI, the nurse advises parents of proper dosage and administration. When antiseptics such as nitrofurantoin are used for prolonged therapy to maintain urine sterility, parents need an explanation of the drug's continued necessity when no signs of infection are present. For all children an adequate or increased fluid intake is encouraged.

Prevention

Prevention is the most important goal in both primary and recurrent infection, and most preventive measures are simple hygienic habits that should be a routine part of daily care (see Guidelines box). For example, parents are taught to cleanse their infant's genital areas from front to back to avoid contaminating the urethral area with fecal organisms. Girls are taught to wipe from front to back after voiding or defecating. Children should void as soon as they feel the urge (see Critical Thinking Exercise).

Sexually active adolescent girls are advised to urinate as soon as possible after they have intercourse to flush out bacteria introduced during the activity. Children who have recurrent UTIs or neurogenic bladder are frequently maintained on daily low-dose antibiotics. Giving the dose at bedtime allows the drug to remain in the bladder overnight. The nurse should reinforce the importance of compliance to parents and older children.

GUIDELINES Prevention of Urinary Tract Infection

Factors Predisposing to Development

Short female urethra close to vagina and anus
Incomplete emptying (reflux) and overdistention of bladder
Concentrated urine
Constipation

Measures of Prevention

Practice perineal hygiene: wipe from front to back.
Avoid tight clothing or diapers; wear cotton panties rather than nylon.
Check for vaginitis or pinworms, especially if child scratches between legs.
Avoid "holding" urine; encourage child to void frequently, especially before long trip or other circumstances in which toilet facilities are not available.
Empty bladder completely with each void. Have the child "double void" (void, wait a few minutes, and void again). Severe cases may require clean, intermittent catheterization or biofeedback instruction.
Avoid straining during defecation and avoid constipation.
Encourage generous fluid intake.

CRITICAL THINKING EXERCISE

Urinary Tract Infection and Constipation

During your assessment of Lisa, a 5-year-old admitted to the hospital for a severe urinary tract infection (UTI), her mother tells you that Lisa has bowel movements every third or fourth day. They are usually large, hard-formed stools, and Lisa sometimes has trouble evacuating the stool.

1. Evidence—Is there sufficient evidence to draw conclusion about Lisa's UTI and constipation?
2. Assumptions—Describe an underlying assumption about each of the following:
   a. UTIs and females
   b. Normal bowel patterns for 5-year-old children
   c. Association between UTIs and constipation
3. What priorities for nursing care should be established for Lisa?
4. Does the evidence support your nursing intervention?
5. What alternative perspectives might you have?

Obstructive Uropathy

Structural or functional abnormalities of the urinary system that obstruct the normal flow of urine can produce renal disorders. When there is interference with urine flow, the backup of urine above the obstruction causes *hydronephrosis* (dilation of the renal pelvis from distention) with eventual pressure destruction of renal parenchyma, although the dilating ureters form a reservoir that reduces the effect on the kidneys for a long time.

Obstruction may be congenital or acquired, unilateral or bilateral, complete or incomplete, with acute or chronic manifestations. The obstruction can occur at any level of the upper or lower urinary tract (Fig. 50-1). Partial obstruction may not be symptomatic unless there is a water or solute diuresis. Boys are affected more frequently than girls, and malformations should be suspected when patients have some other congenital defects (e.g., prune belly syndrome, chromosomal anomalies, anorectal malformations, defects of the pinna of the ear).

Damage to distal nephrons in chronic uropathy alters the ability to concentrate urine, contributing to increased urine flow and metabolic acidosis occurring from decreased excre-

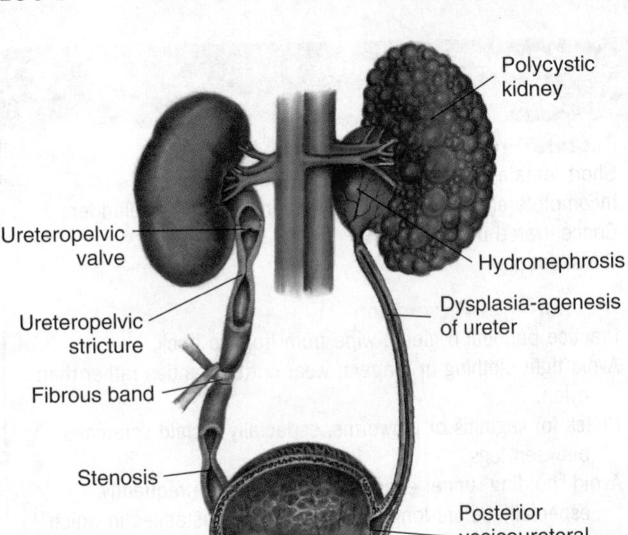

Fig. 50-1 Major sites of urinary tract obstruction.

tion of acid secondary to impaired ability of the distal nephron to secrete hydrogen ions. Partial obstruction results in progressive loss of renal function as a result of irreversible damage to the nephrons. Pooled urine serves as a medium for bacterial growth; therefore UTIs further increase the extent of renal damage.

Early diagnosis and surgical correction or procedures that divert the flow of urine to bypass the obstruction, such as placement of a temporary percutaneous nephrostomy tube or cutaneous ureterostomy, are essential to prevent progressive renal damage. Medical complications of acute or chronic renal failure (CRF) or infection are managed as described for those disorders.

Nursing Care Management

Nursing goals in urinary tract obstruction include helping to identify cases, assisting with diagnostic procedures, and caring for children with complications (described elsewhere). Preparing parents and children for procedures is a major nursing responsibility. Preparation for urinary diversion procedures is of special importance (see Preparation for Diagnostic and Therapeutic Procedures, Chapter 45).

Parents and children need emotional support and counseling during the lengthy management of these disorders. Many children are discharged with ureteral drainage systems in place that must be protected from damage, and the danger of infection is a constant concern. Parents are taught to care for the equipment and recognize the signs of possible obstruction or infection within the system. Maintaining adequate urine flow is imperative. Fluids should be encouraged. The tube should be observed frequently for indications of obstruction resulting from sediment, small blood clots, or kinking. The physician should inspect any drainage from around the tube.

Children with external diversional systems need psychologic support and guidance, especially as they reach adolescence and body image concerns assume more prominence. Those with progressive renal deterioration may face the prospect of dialysis or transplantation and the emotions that accompany these procedures.

External Defects

Defects of the external genitourinary tract are serious conditions primarily because of the psychologic impact on the child. Satisfactory surgical repair is successful for the more common disorders and is carried out or initiated as early as possible. The major anomalies of the lower genitourinary tract, their description, and their management are outlined in Table 50-4.

Psychologic Problems Related to Genital Surgery

Surgery involving sexual organs can be particularly disruptive to children, especially preschoolers fearing punishment, retaliation, body mutilation, or castration. Some of the problems of hospitalization, separation, and anxiety can be eased by hospital practices that are sensitive to the child's needs (see Chapter 44).

A child's body image is largely derived as a result of feedback from the primary caregivers, and parental anxiety regarding an acceptable physical appearance and adequate future sexual competency is readily communicated to an affected child. Therefore children with birth defects are at risk for developing a distorted body image that reflects the caregiver's subtly communicated evaluation of their bodies. The trend toward repair of visible genital defects is based in large part on these psychologic variables. The earlier a repair can be achieved, the more likely it is that the child will develop a normal body image.

During the years from 3 to 6, the phallic-oedipal period, children show a strong interest and concern about the genital area, sex differences, and genital normality or its lack. It is also a time when children are frightened of what they perceive to be threats to their body and bodily function. They also view any untoward happening as a punishment for real or imagined wrongdoing or unacceptable sexual feelings, such as masturbation, sex play, or erotic feelings. Surgical repair is recommended before these fears and anxieties develop. After extensive review of the emotional, cognitive, and body-image problems that may occur in children undergoing surgical reconstruction of a genital deformity, Kass (1996) recommended that surgery be accomplished between the ages of 6 and 15 months to minimize the psychologic effects of surgery and anesthesia.

Nursing Care Management

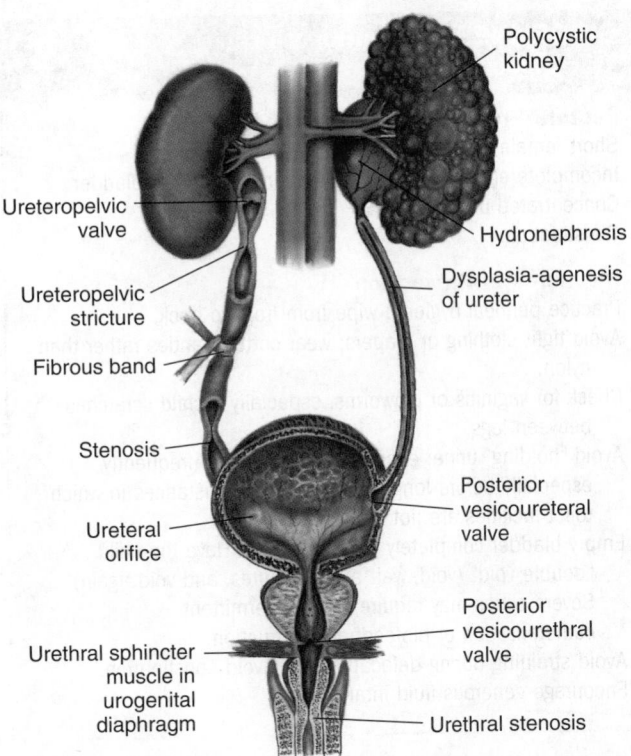

Preparing children and their families for diagnostic and surgical procedures (see Preparation for Diagnostic and Therapeutic Procedures, Chapter 45) and for home care is a major nursing function. Most postoperative care involves care of the surgical site. Tub baths are discouraged for 1 week after simple surgeries. The surgical site is kept clean and otherwise pro-

Table 50-4 Defects of the Genitourinary Tract

DEFECT	THERAPEUTIC MANAGEMENT
Inguinal hernia—Protrusion of abdominal contents through inguinal canal into scrotum	Detected as painless inguinal swelling of variable size Surgical closure of inguinal defect
Hydrocele—Fluid in scrotum	Surgical repair indicated if spontaneous resolution not accomplished in 1 yr
Phimosis—Narrowing or stenosis of preputial opening of foreskin	Mild cases—manual retraction of foreskin and proper cleansing of area Severe cases—circumcision or vertical division and transverse suturing of foreskin
Hypospadias—Urethral opening located behind glans penis or anywhere along ventral surface of penile shaft	Objectives of surgical correction: Enable child to void in standing position and direct stream voluntarily in usual manner Improve physical appearance of genitalia Produce a sexually adequate organ
Chordee—Ventral curvature of penis, often associated with hypospadias	Surgical release of fibrous band causing the deformity
Epispadias—Meatal opening located on dorsal surface of penis	Surgical correction, usually including penile and urethral lengthening and bladder neck reconstruction (if necessary)
Cryptorchidism—Failure of one or both testes to descend normally through inguinal canal	Detected by inability to palpate testes within scrotum Medical—Administration of human chorionic gonadotropin (older child) Surgical—Orchiopexy Objectives of therapy— Prevent damage to undescended testicle Decrease incidence of malignant tumor formation Avoid trauma and torsion Close inguinal canal Prevent cosmetic and psychologic disability from empty scrotum
Exstrophy of bladder—Eversion of posterior bladder through anterior bladder wall and lower abdominal wall; associated with open pubic arch (a severe defect)	Potential objectives of surgical correction: Preserve renal function Attain urinary control Perform adequate reconstructive repair Improve sexual function (especially in males)
Ambiguous genitalia	
Masculinized female (female pseudohermaphrodite)	Assign gender as female; assign gender while avoiding irreversible surgery, realizing some children may change gender later in life; family participation essential
Incompletely masculinized male (male pseudohermaphrodite)	Assign gender while avoiding irreversible surgery, realizing some children may change gender later in life; family participation essential
True hermaphrodite (both ovaries and testes)	Assign gender while avoiding irreversible surgery, realizing some children may change gender later in life; gender assignment depends on predominant characteristics; family participation essential
Mixed gonadal dysgenesis	Assign gender while avoiding irreversible surgery, realizing some children may change gender later in life; gender assignment depends on predominant characteristics; family participation essential

tected from infection and is inspected for signs of infection. Dressings, if any, are inspected regularly. More complex surgeries require additional care and observation (e.g., catheter care for urethral reconstruction and care of urinary diversion stomas and collection devices).

Some older children's activities, such as pushing, lifting, playing with straddle toys or in sandboxes, swimming, and engaging in rough activities, may be restricted after some types of surgical repairs. Precise restrictions depend on the specific type of surgery. Activities of infants and toddlers are not limited.

In most cases the results of surgery are satisfactory. However, in some of the more severe defects, such as exstrophy and those that require stomas, additional emotional interventions may be needed. A major concern of parents and children is related to surgery affecting the genitalia directly. Concerns about penis size, appearance of the genitalia, potential ability to procreate, and rejection by peers (especially the opposite sex) are potential fears that require psychologic adjustment, particularly during adolescence.

Glomerular Disease

Nephrotic Syndrome

Nephrotic syndrome is a clinical state that includes massive proteinuria, hypoalbuminemia, hyperlipidemia, and edema. The disorder can occur as (1) a primary disease known as *idiopathic nephrosis, childhood nephrosis, or minimal-change nephrotic syndrome (MCNS);* (2) a secondary disorder that occurs as a clinical manifestation after or in association with glomerular damage that has a known or presumed cause; or (3) a congenital form inherited as an autosomal recessive disorder. The disorder is characterized by increased glomerular permeability to plasma protein, which results in massive urinary protein loss. The glomerulus is responsible for the initial step in the formation of urine, and the filtration rate depends on an intact glomerular membrane. This discussion is devoted to MCNS because it constitutes 80% of nephrotic syndrome cases.

Pathophysiology

The onset of MCNS can occur at any age but predominantly occurs in children between 2 and 7 years of age. It is rare in children younger than 6 months of age, uncommon in infants younger than 1 year of age, and unusual after the age of 8. Patients with MCNS are twice as likely to be male.

The pathogenesis of MCNS is not understood. There may be a metabolic, biochemical, physiochemical, or immune-mediated disturbance that causes the basement membrane of the glomeruli to become increasingly permeable to protein, but the cause and mechanisms are only speculative.

The glomerular membrane, normally impermeable to albumin and other proteins, becomes permeable to proteins, especially albumin, which leak through the membrane and are lost in urine *(hyperalbuminuria)*. This reduces the serum albumin level *(hypoalbuminemia)*, decreasing the colloidal osmotic pressure in the capillaries. As a result, the vascular hydrostatic pressure exceeds the pull of the colloidal osmotic pressure, causing fluid to accumulate in the interstitial spaces *(edema)* and body cavities, particularly in the abdominal cavity *(ascites)*. The shift of fluid from the plasma to the interstitial spaces reduces the vascular fluid volume *(hypovolemia)*, which in turn stimulates the renin-angiotensin system and the secretion of antidiuretic hormone and aldosterone. Tubular reabsorption of sodium and water is increased in an attempt to increase intravascular volume. The elevation of serum lipids is not fully understood. The sequence of events in nephrotic syndrome is diagrammed in Fig. 50-2.

NURSING ALERT A child who exhibits the following should be evaluated for the possibility of nephrotic syndrome:

- Weight gain over that expected based on previous pattern
- Parent observation that the child's clothes fit tightly
- Decreased urine output
- Pallor, fatigue

Diagnostic Evaluation

The disease is suspected on the basis of clinical manifestations (Box 50-2), especially when weight gain in a previously well child increases slowly over days or weeks. The generalized edema may develop rapidly or gradually but eventually prompts the family to seek medical attention. Parents usually give a history of the child being well but steadily gaining weight; appearing edematous; and then becoming anorexic, irritable, and less active.

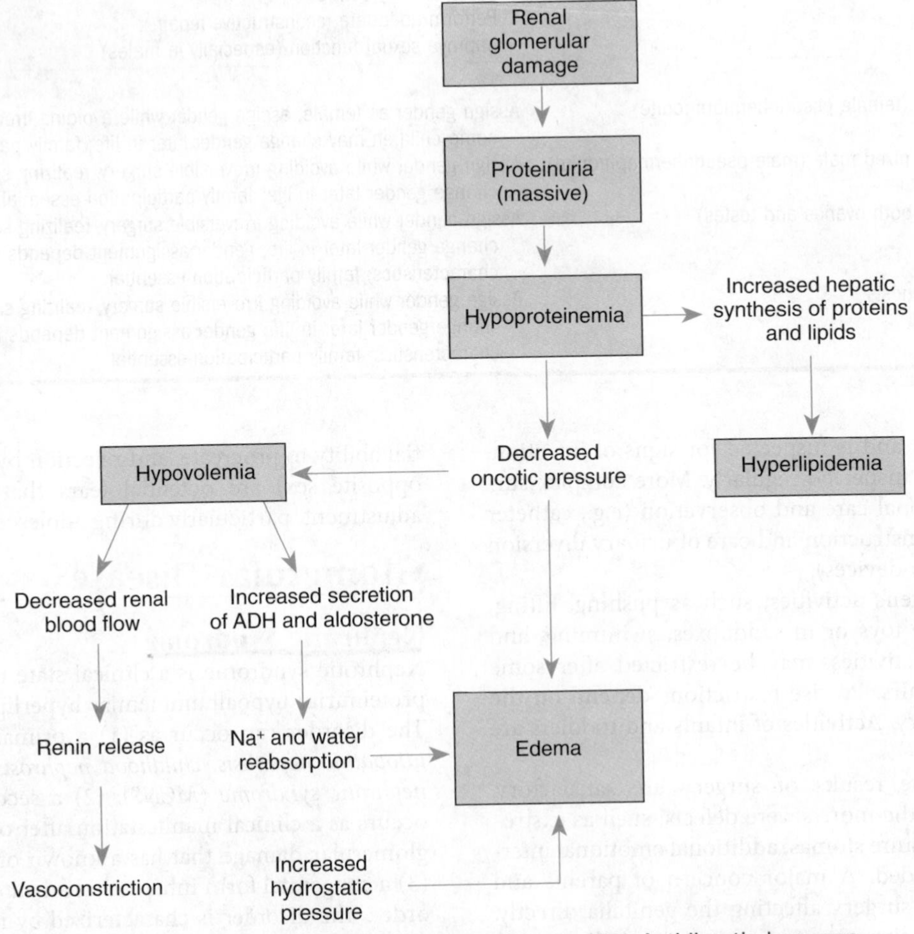

Fig. 50-2 Sequence of events in nephrotic syndrome. *ADH*, Antidiuretic hormone.

BOX 50-2 Clinical Manifestations of Nephrotic Syndrome

Weight gain
Puffiness of face (facial edema):
- Especially around the eyes
- Apparent on arising in the morning
- Subsides during the day

Abdominal swelling (ascites)
Pleural effusion
Labial or scrotal swelling
Edema of intestinal mucosa, possibly causing:
- Diarrhea
- Anorexia
- Poor intestinal absorption

Ankle or leg swelling
Irritability
Tendency to fatigue easily
Lethargy
Blood pressure normal or slightly decreased
Susceptibility to infection
Urine alterations:
- Decreased volume
- Frothy

The diagnosis of MCNS is suspected on the basis of the history and clinical manifestations (edema, proteinuria, hypoalbuminemia, and hypercholesterolemia in the absence of hematuria and hypertension) in children between the ages of 2 and 8 years. The hallmark of MCNS is massive proteinuria (higher than 3+ on urine dipstick). Hyaline casts, oval fat bodies, and a few red blood cells can be found in the urine of some affected children, although there is seldom gross hematuria. The glomerular filtration rate is usually normal or high.

Total serum protein concentration is low, with the serum albumin significantly reduced and plasma lipids elevated. Hemoglobin and hematocrit are usually normal or elevated as a result of hemoconcentration. The platelet count may be elevated. Serum sodium concentration may be low. If the patient does not respond to a 4- to 8-week course of steroids, a renal biopsy may be needed to distinguish between other types of nephrotic syndrome. The biopsy results of children with MCNS are remarkable for effacement of the foot processes of the epithelial cells lining the basement membrane, but otherwise the kidney tissue is normal.

Therapeutic Management

Objectives of therapeutic management include (1) reducing excretion of urinary protein, (2) reducing fluid retention in the tissues, (3) preventing infection, and (4) minimizing complications related to therapies. Dietary restrictions include a low-salt diet and, in more severe cases, fluid restriction. If complications of edema develop, diuretic therapy may be initiated to provide temporary relief from edema. Sometimes infusions of 25% albumin are used. Acute infections are treated with appropriate antibiotics.

Corticosteroids are the first line of therapy for MCNS. The starting dosage for prednisone is usually 2 mg/kg body weight/day, in one or more divided doses. Most children respond within 7 to 21 days. The medication is then tapered over a period of several months and eventually stopped if the child remains asymptomatic. About two thirds of children with MCNS have a relapse, heralded first by increased urine protein. Relapses can be diagnosed early if parents are taught routine home monitoring of urine protein by dipstick. Relapses are treated with a repeated course of high-dose steroid therapy. Side effects of the steroids include weight gain, rounding of the face, behavior changes, and increased appetite. Long-term therapy may result in hirsutism, growth retardation, cataracts, hypertension, gastrointestinal bleeding, bone demineralization, infection, and hyperglycemia. Children who do not respond to steroid therapy, those who have frequent relapses, and those in whom the side effects threaten their growth and general health may be considered for a course of therapy using other immunosuppressant medications (cyclophosphamide, chlorambucil, or cyclosporine).

MCNS episodes, both the first episode and the relapse, often happen in conjunction with a viral or bacterial infection. Relapses can also be triggered by allergies and immunizations. Relapses in children with MCNS may continue over many years.

Complications of nephrotic syndrome include infection, circulatory insufficiency secondary to hypovolemia, and thromboembolism. Infections that may be seen in children with nephrotic syndrome include peritonitis, cellulitis, and pneumonia and require prompt recognition and vigorous treatment with appropriate antibiotic therapy.

Prognosis

The prognosis for ultimate recovery in most cases is good. It is a self-limiting disease, and in children who respond to steroid therapy the tendency to relapse decreases with time. With early detection and prompt implementation of therapy to eradicate proteinuria, progressive basement membrane damage is minimized, so that when the tendency to relapse is past, renal function is usually normal or near normal. It is estimated that approximately 80% of affected children have this favorable prognosis.

Nursing Care Management

Continuous monitoring of fluid retention or excretion is an important nursing function. Strict intake and output records are essential but may be difficult to obtain from very young children. Application of collection bags is irritating to edematous skin that is readily subject to breakdown. Applying diapers or weighing wet pads may be necessary.

NURSING ALERT Another strategy for obtaining a daily urine protein is to place cotton balls in the diaper at night before bedtime and then squeeze them out in the morning.

Other methods of monitoring progress include urine examination for albumin, daily weight, and measurement of abdominal girth. Assessment of edema (e.g., increased or decreased swelling around the eyes and dependent areas), the degree of pitting, and the color and texture of skin are part of nursing care. Vital signs are monitored to detect any early signs of complications such as shock or an infective process.

Infection is a constant source of danger to edematous children and those receiving corticosteroid therapy. These children are particularly vulnerable to upper respiratory tract infection; therefore they must be kept warm and dry, active, and protected from contact with infected individuals (e.g., roommates, visitors, and personnel). Vital signs are monitored to detect any early signs of an infective process.

Loss of appetite accompanying active nephrosis creates a perplexing problem for nurses. During this time the combined efforts of nurse, dietitian, parents, and child are needed to formulate a nutritionally adequate and attractive diet. Salt is usually restricted (but not eliminated) during the edema phase and while the child is on steroid therapy. Fluid restriction (if prescribed) is limited to short-term use during massive edema. Every effort should be made to serve attractive meals with preferred foods and a minimum of fuss, but it usually requires considerable ingenuity to entice the child to eat (see Feeding the Sick Child, Chapter 45).

Children usually adjust activities according to their tolerance level. However, they may require guidance in selecting play activities. Suitable recreational and diversional activities are an important part of their care. Irritability and mood swings that accompany steroid therapy are not unusual in these children and may create an additional challenge for the nurse and family.

Family Support and Home Care

Continuous support of the child and family is one of the major nursing considerations. Many children are treated at home during relapses. Parents are taught to detect signs of relapse and to call for changes in treatment at the earliest indications. Unless the edema and proteinuria are severe or the parents, for some reason, are unable to care for the ill child, *home care is preferred.* Parents are instructed in testing urine for albumin, administering medications, and providing general care. Parents are also instructed regarding avoiding contact with infected playmates, but the child should attend school.

The prolonged course of the relapsing form of nephrotic syndrome is taxing to both the child and the family. The up-and-down course of remissions and exacerbations with periodic disruption of family life by hospitalization places a severe strain on the child and the family, both psychologically and financially. Reassurance regarding this characteristic of the course of the disease, with emphasis on the importance of long-term care, needs to be provided to parents and children to gain their cooperation. A satisfactory response is more likely when relapses are detected and therapy is instituted early, and remissions are prolonged when instructions are carried out faithfully.

Acute Glomerulonephritis

Acute glomerulonephritis (AGN) may be a primary event or a manifestation of a systemic disorder that can range from minimal to severe. Common features include oliguria, edema, hypertension and circulatory congestion, hematuria, and proteinuria. Most cases are postinfectious and have been associated with pneumococcal, streptococcal, and viral infections. *Acute poststreptococcal glomerulonephritis (APSGN)* is the most common of the postinfectious renal diseases in childhood and the one for which a cause can be established in the majority of cases. APSGN can occur at any age but affects primarily early school-age children, with a peak age of onset of 6 to 7 years. It is uncommon in children younger than 2 years of age, and males outnumber females 2 : 1.

Etiology

APSGN is an immune-complex disease that occurs after an antecedent streptococcal infection with certain strains of the group A β-hemolytic streptococcus. Most streptococcal infections *do not* cause APSGN. A latent period of 10 to 21 days occurs between the streptococcal infection and the onset of clinical manifestations. Disease secondary to streptococcal pharyngitis is more common in the winter or spring, but when APSGN is associated with pyoderma (principally *impetigo*), it may be more prevalent in later summer or early fall, especially in warmer climates. Second episodes of AGN are rare.

Pathophysiology

The pathophysiology of APSGN is still uncertain. Immune complexes are deposited in the glomerular basement membrane. The glomeruli become edematous and infiltrated with polymorphonuclear leukocytes, which occlude the capillary lumen. The resulting decrease in plasma filtration results in an excessive accumulation of water and retention of sodium that expands plasma and interstitial fluid volumes, leading to circulatory congestion and edema. The cause of the hypertension associated with AGN cannot be completely explained by fluid retention. Excess renin may also be produced.

Diagnostic Evaluation

Typically, affected children are in good health until they experience the streptococcal infection. In some instances they have a history of only a mild cold or no previous infection at all. The onset of nephritis appears after an average latency period of about 10 days (Box 50-3). Because the child appears to be well during the latency period, parents do not recognize the association. The edema is relatively moderate and may not be appreciated by someone unfamiliar with the child's normal appearance.

Urinalysis during the acute phase characteristically shows hematuria and proteinuria. Proteinuria generally parallels the hematuria and may be 3+ or 4+ in the presence of gross hematuria. Gross discoloration of the urine reflects red blood cell and hemoglobin content. Microscopic examination of the sediment shows many red blood cells, leukocytes, epithelial cells, and granular and red blood cell casts. Bacteria are not seen.

Azotemia that results from impaired glomerular filtration is reflected in elevated blood urea nitrogen (BUN) and creatinine levels in at least 50% of cases. Occasionally proteinuria is excessive and the patient may have nephrotic syndrome (i.e., hypoproteinemia and hyperlipidemia).

Cultures of the pharynx are rarely positive for streptococci, since the renal disease occurs weeks after the infection.

Some serologic tests are necessary to make the diagnosis of AGN. Circulating serum antibodies to streptococci indicate the presence of a previous infection. The antistreptolysin O (ASO) titer is the most familiar and readily available test for

BOX 50-3 Clinical Manifestations of Acute Poststreptococcal Glomerulonephritis

Edema:
- Especially periorbital
- Facial edema more prominent in the morning
- Spreads during the day to involve extremities and abdomen

Anorexia
Urine:
- Cloudy, smoky brown (resembles tea or cola)
- Severely reduced volume

Pallor
Irritability
Lethargy
Child appearing ill
Child seldom expressing specific complaints
Older children complaining of:
- Headaches
- Abdominal discomfort
- Dysuria

Vomiting possible
Mild to moderately elevated blood pressure

streptococcal infection. Other antibodies that may aid in diagnosis are elevated antihyaluronidase (AHase), antideoxyribonuclease B (ADNase-B), and streptozyme.

All patients with APSGN have reduced serum complement (C3) activity in the early stages of the disease. Rising C3 levels are used as a guide to indicate improvement of the disease and should be normal in almost all patients 8 weeks after the disease onset.

Studies that may be useful include chest x-ray examination, which generally shows cardiac enlargement, pulmonary congestion, or pleural effusion during the edematous phase of acute disease. Renal biopsy for diagnostic purposes is seldom required but may be useful in the diagnosis of atypical cases.

Therapeutic Management

Management consists of general supportive measures and early recognition and treatment of complications. Children who have normal blood pressure and a satisfactory urine output can generally be treated at home. Those with substantial edema, hypertension, gross hematuria, or significant oliguria should be hospitalized because of the unpredictability of complications.

Dietary restrictions depend on the stage and severity of the disease, especially the extent of edema. Moderate sodium restriction and even fluid restriction may be instituted for children with hypertension and edema. Foods with substantial amounts of potassium are generally restricted during the period of oliguria.

Regular measurement of vital signs, body weight, and intake and output is essential to monitor the progress of the disease and to detect complications that may appear at any time during the course of the disease. *A record of daily weight is the most useful means for assessing fluid balance.* Rarely, children with AGN will develop acute renal failure (ARF) with oliguria that significantly alters the fluid and electrolyte balance (resulting in hyperkalemia, acidosis, hypocalcemia, and/or hyperphosphatemia). These children require careful management. Peritoneal dialysis or hemodialysis is seldom needed.

Acute hypertension must be anticipated and identified early. Blood pressure measurements are taken every 4 to 6 hours. A variety of antihypertensive medications and diuretics are used to control hypertension. Antibiotic therapy is indicated only for those children with evidence of persistent streptococcal infections. It is used to prevent transmission of nephritogenic streptococci to other family members.

Prognosis

Almost all children correctly diagnosed as having APSGN recover completely, and specific immunity is conferred, so that subsequent recurrences are uncommon. Some of these children have been reported to develop chronic disease, but most of these cases are now believed to be different glomerular diseases misdiagnosed as poststreptococcal disease.

Nursing Care Management

Nursing care of the child with glomerulonephritis involves careful assessment of the disease status, with regular monitoring of vital signs (including frequent measurement of blood pressure), fluid balance, and behavior.

Vital signs provide clues to the severity of the disease and early signs of complications. They are carefully measured, and any deviations are reported and recorded. The volume and character of urine are noted, and the child is weighed daily. Children with restricted fluid intake, especially those who are not severely edematous or those who have lost weight, are observed for signs of dehydration.

Assessment of the child's appearance for signs of cerebral complications is an important nursing function, since the severity of the acute phase is variable and unpredictable. The child with edema, hypertension, and gross hematuria may be subject to complications, and anticipatory preparations such as seizure precautions and intravenous (IV) equipment are included in the nursing care plan.

For most children a regular diet is allowed, but it should contain no added salt. Foods high in sodium and salted treats are eliminated, and parents and friends are advised not to bring snacks such as potato chips or pretzels. However, the total amount of salt ingested is usually less than prescribed because of the child's poor appetite. Fluid restriction, if prescribed, is more difficult, and the amount permitted should be evenly divided throughout the waking hours. Meal preparation and service require special attention, since the child is indifferent to meals during the acute phase. Again, collaboration with parents and the dietitian and special consideration for food preferences facilitate meal planning.

During the acute phase children are generally content to lie in bed. As they begin to feel better and their symptoms subside, they will want to be up and about. Activities should be planned to allow for frequent rest periods and avoidance of fatigue. Children who have mild edema and no hypertension, as well as convalescent children who are being treated at home, need follow-up care. Parents are instructed regarding general measures, including diet and prevention of infection.

Health supervision is continued, with weekly, followed by monthly, visits for evaluation and urinalysis. Parent education and support in preparation for discharge and home care include education in home management and the need for follow-up care and health supervision.

Miscellaneous Renal Disorders

Hemolytic Uremic Syndrome

Hemolytic uremic syndrome (HUS) is an uncommon, acute renal disease that occurs primarily in infants and small children between the ages of 6 months and 5 years. HUS is one of the most frequent causes of acquired ARF in children (Davis & Avner, 2004). The clinical features of the disease include acquired hemolytic anemia, thrombocytopenia, renal injury, and central nervous system symptoms. The etiology of HUS is thought to be associated with bacterial toxins, chemicals, and viruses. The appearance of the disease has been associated with *Rickettsia* organisms, viruses (especially coxsackievirus, echovirus, and adenovirus), *E. coli*, pneumococci, shigellae, and salmonellae and may represent an unusual response to these infections. Multiple cases of HUS caused by enteric infection of the *E. coli* O157:H7 serotype have been traced to undercooked meat, especially ground beef. Other sources are unpasteurized milk or fruit juice, especially apple; alfalfa sprouts; lettuce; and salami. Drinking or swimming in sewage-contaminated water can also cause infection. The clinical presentation is usually a history of a prodromal illness (most often gastroenteritis or an upper respiratory tract infection) followed by the sudden onset of hemolysis and renal failure.

Pathophysiology

The primary site of injury appears to be the endothelial lining of the small glomerular arterioles, which become swollen and occluded with deposits of platelets and fibrin clots (intravascular coagulation). Red blood cells are damaged as they attempt to move through the partially occluded blood vessels. These damaged cells are removed by the spleen, causing acute hemolytic anemia. The platelet aggregation within the damaged blood vessels or the damage and removal of platelets produce the characteristic thrombocytopenia.

Diagnostic Evaluation

The triad of anemia, thrombocytopenia, and renal failure is sufficient for diagnosis (Box 50-4). Renal involvement is evidenced by proteinuria, hematuria, and urinary casts; BUN and serum creatinine levels are elevated. A low hemoglobin and hematocrit and a high reticulocyte count confirm the hemolytic nature of the anemia.

BOX 50-4 Clinical Manifestations of Hemolytic Uremic Syndrome

Vomiting
Irritability
Lethargy
Marked pallor
Hemorrhagic manifestations:
- Bruising
- Petechiae
- Jaundice
- Bloody diarrhea

Oliguria or anuria
Central nervous system involvement:
- Seizures
- Stupor or coma

Signs of acute heart failure (sometimes)

Therapeutic Management

The goals of therapy are early diagnosis and aggressive, supportive care of the ARF and hemolytic anemia. The most consistently effective treatment of HUS is hemodialysis or peritoneal dialysis, which is instituted in any child who has been anuric for 24 hours or who demonstrates oliguria with uremia or hypertension and seizures. Other treatments include use of pharmacologic agents, fresh-frozen plasma, and plasmapheresis. Blood transfusions with fresh, washed packed cells are administered for severe anemia but are used with caution to prevent circulatory overload from added volume.

Prognosis

With prompt treatment the recovery rate is about 95%, but residual renal impairment ranges from 10% to 50%. Long-term complications include CRF, hypertension, and central nervous system disorders. Death is usually caused by residual renal impairment or central nervous system injury.

Nursing Care Management

Nursing care is the same as that provided in ARF and, for children with continued impairment, includes management of chronic disease. Because of the sudden and life-threatening nature of the disorder in a previously well child, parents are often ill prepared for the impact of hospitalization and treatment. Therefore support and understanding are especially important aspects of care.

Wilms' Tumor

Wilms' tumor, or nephroblastoma, is the most common malignant renal and intraabdominal tumor of childhood. Its frequency is estimated to be 7.6 cases per million in Caucasian children younger than 15 years (Dome et al, 2006). Wilms' tumor occurs about three times more often in African-Americans than in East Asians in the United States. The peak age at diagnosis is approximately 3 years, and occurrence is slightly more frequent in boys than in girls. The majority of patients with Wilms' tumor are diagnosed at younger than 5 years of age, with 1% to 2.5% of cases having a familial origin. Unfortunately, there is no method of identifying gene carriers at this time.

Etiology

Wilms' tumor probably arises from a malignant, undifferentiated cluster of primordial cells capable of initiating the regeneration of an abnormal structure. Its occurrence slightly favors the left kidney, which is advantageous because surgically this kidney is easier to manipulate and remove. In about 10% of cases both kidneys are involved. Studies have shown that development of Wilms' tumor is frequently associated with

BOX 50-5 Clinical Manifestations of Wilms' Tumor

Abdominal swelling or mass:
- Firm
- Nontender
- Confined to one side

Hematuria (less than one fourth of cases)
Fatigue and malaise
Hypertension (occasionally)
Weight loss
Fever
Manifestations resulting from compression of tumor mass
Secondary metabolic alterations from tumor or metastasis
If metastasis, symptoms of lung involvement:
- Dyspnea
- Cough
- Shortness of breath
- Chest pain (sometimes)

aniridia, hemihypertrophy, Beckwith-Wiedemann syndrome, or genitourinary anomalies (Kline & Sevier, 2003; Dome et al, 2006).

Diagnostic Evaluation

In a child suspected of having Wilms' tumor, special emphasis is placed on the history and physical examination for the presence of congenital anomalies, a family history of cancer, and signs of malignancy (e.g., weight loss, size of liver and spleen, indications of anemia, lymphadenopathy). Most children with Wilms' tumor are brought to the practitioner because of abdominal swelling or an abdominal mass (Box 50-5). Specific tests include radiographic studies, including abdominal ultrasound and abdominal and chest computed tomography scan; hematologic studies; biochemical studies; and urinalysis. Studies to demonstrate the relationship of the tumor to the ipsilateral kidney and the presence of a normal functioning kidney on the contralateral side are essential. If a large tumor is present, an inferior venacavagram is necessary to demonstrate possible tumor involvement adjacent to the vena cava. A bone marrow aspiration may be performed to rule out metastasis, which is rare in children with Wilms' tumor.

NURSING ALERT To reinforce the need for caution, it may be necessary to post a sign on the bed that reads "DO NOT PALPATE ABDOMEN." Careful bathing and handling are also important in preventing trauma to the tumor site.

Therapeutic Management

Combined treatment with surgery and chemotherapy with or without radiation is based on the histologic pattern and clinical stage. Surgery is scheduled as soon as possible after confirmation of a renal mass, usually within 24 to 48 hours of admission. A large transabdominal incision is performed for optimal visualization of the abdominal cavity. The tumor, affected kidney, and adjacent adrenal gland are removed. Great care is taken to keep the encapsulated tumor intact, since rupture can seed cancer cells throughout the abdomen, lymph channel, and bloodstream. The contralateral kidney is carefully inspected for evidence of disease or dysfunction. Regional lymph nodes are inspected, and a biopsy is performed when indicated. Any involved structures, such as part of the colon, diaphragm, or vena cava, are removed. Metal clips are placed around the tumor site for exact marking during radiotherapy.

If both kidneys are involved, the child may be treated with radiotherapy or chemotherapy before surgery to decrease the size of the tumor, allowing more conservative surgery. It may be possible to perform a partial nephrectomy on the less affected kidney, with a total nephrectomy on the opposite side. When a transplant is feasible, such as from a twin, sibling, or parent, bilateral nephrectomy is considered as a last resort.

Postoperative radiotherapy is indicated for children with large tumors, metastasis, residual postoperative disease, unfavorable histologic characteristics, or recurrence. Chemotherapy is indicated for all stages. The most effective agents for treating Wilms' tumor are actinomycin D (dactinomycin), vincristine, and adriamycin, with the addition of cyclophosphamide for unfavorable histologic characteristics or advanced disease (Dome et al, 2006). The duration of therapy ranges from 6 to 15 months.

Prognosis

Survival rates for Wilms' tumor are the highest among all childhood cancers. Children with localized tumor (stages I and II) have a 90% chance of cure with multimodal therapy. Factors that favorably affect the success of further therapy include initial treatment with only vincristine and dactinomycin, relapse to the lungs only, relapse in the abdomen of a patient who received no prior abdominal irradiation, and relapse more than 12 months after diagnosis. Wilms' tumor may recur, especially in the lungs. Both chemotherapy and radiotherapy can induce second malignancies, usually in areas that have been irradiated (Dome et al, 2006).

Nursing Care Management

Nursing care of the child with Wilms' tumor is similar to that of children with other cancers treated with surgery, irradiation, and chemotherapy. However, there are some significant differences; these are discussed for each phase of nursing intervention.

Preoperative Care

The preoperative period is one of swift diagnosis. The nurse faces the challenge of preparing the child and parents for all laboratory and operative procedures within 24 to 48 hours of admission. Because of the minimal preparatory time, explanations should be simple, repetitive, and focused on the child's actual experiences. In addition to the usual preoperative observations, blood pressure is monitored, since hypertension from excess renin production is a possibility.

There are several special preoperative concerns, the most important of which is that the *tumor is not palpated unless absolutely necessary* because manipulation of the mass may cause dissemination of cancer cells to adjacent and distant sites.

Because radiotherapy and chemotherapy are usually begun immediately after surgery, parents need an explanation of what to expect, such as major benefits and side effects. The timing of the information should be considered to avoid overwhelming the family. Ideally, the nurse should be present during physic … questions as they arise. It … ng the child about these si … ia, usually of most concern … ntil approximately 2 weel … n. Therefore the child can … peratively.

Postopera …

Despite th … necessary in many childre … ry is usually rapid. The ma … ame as those after any abdominal surgery (see Surgical Procedures, Chapter 45). Because these children are at risk for intestinal obstruction from vincristine-induced ileus, radiation-induced edema, and postsurgical adhesion formation, the nurse carefully monitors gastrointestinal activity, such as bowel movements, bowel sounds, distention, vomiting, and pain. The nurse also monitors blood pressure, urine output, and signs of infection, as well as instituting pulmonary hygiene to prevent postoperative pulmonary complications.

Family Support

The postoperative period is frequently difficult for parents. The shock of seeing their child immediately after surgery may be the first realization of the seriousness of the diagnosis. It also marks the confirmation of the stage of the tumor. During this period, the nurse should be with the parents to assure them of the child's recovery after surgery and to assess the parents' understanding of the total experience. Older children need an opportunity to deal with their feelings concerning the many procedures to which they have been subjected in rapid succession. Play therapy with dolls or puppets or through drawing can be extremely beneficial in helping them adjust. It is not unusual for children to feel angry because of the extent of surgery, the need for additional therapy, or the seriousness of the disorder.

NURSING ALERT Because the child is left with one kidney, certain precautions, such as avoiding contact sports, are recommended to prevent injury to the remaining organ. Prompt detection and treatment of any genitourinary signs or symptoms are mandatory.

Renal Failure

Renal failure is the inability of the kidneys to excrete waste material, concentrate urine, and conserve electrolytes. It can occur suddenly *(ARF)* in response to inadequate perfusion, kidney disease, or urinary tract obstruction, or it can develop slowly *(CRF)* as a result of longstanding kidney disease or an anomaly.

Azotemia and *uremia* are terms often used in relation to renal failure. *Azotemia* is the accumulation of nitrogenous waste within the blood. *Uremia* is a more advanced condition in which retention of nitrogenous products produces toxic symptoms. Azotemia is not life threatening, whereas uremia is a serious condition that often involves other body systems.

Acute Renal Failure

ARF is said to exist when the kidneys suddenly are unable to regulate the volume and composition of urine appropriately in response to food and fluid intake and the needs of the organism. The principal feature of ARF is oliguria* associated with azotemia, metabolic acidosis, and diverse electrolyte disturbances. ARF is not common in childhood, but the outcome depends on the cause, associated findings, and prompt recognition and treatment.

BOX 50-6 Clinical Manifestations of Acute Renal Failure

Specific:
- Oliguria
- Anuria uncommon (except in obstructive disorders)

Nonspecific (may develop):
- Nausea
- Vomiting
- Drowsiness
- Edema
- Hypertension

Manifestations of underlying disorder or pathologic condition

The pathologic conditions that produce ARF caused by glomerulonephritis and HUS are discussed in relation to those disorders. ARF can also develop as a result of a large number of related or unrelated clinical conditions: poor renal perfusion; urinary tract obstruction; acute renal injury; or the final expression of chronic, irreversible renal disease. The most common cause in children is transient renal failure resulting from severe dehydration or other causes of poor perfusion that may respond to restoration of fluid volume.

Pathophysiology

ARF is usually reversible, but the deviations of physiologic function can be extreme, and mortality in the pediatric age group remains high. There is severe reduction in the glomerular filtration rate, an elevated BUN level, and a significant reduction in renal blood flow.

The clinical course is variable and depends on the cause. In reversible ARF there is a period of severe oliguria, or a low-output phase, followed by an abrupt onset of diuresis, or a high-output phase, and then a gradual return to (or toward) normal urine volumes.

Diagnostic Evaluation

In many instances of ARF the infant or child is already critically ill with the precipitating disorder, and the explanation for development of oliguria may or may not be readily apparent (Box 50-6). When a previously well child develops ARF without obvious cause, a careful history is taken to reveal symptoms that may be related to glomerulonephritis, obstructive uropathy, or exposure to nephrotoxic chemicals (e.g., ingestion of heavy metals, inhalation of carbon tetrachloride or other organic solvents, or medications such as nonsteroidal antiinflammatory drugs [Krause et al, 2005] known to be toxic to the kidneys). Significant laboratory measurements during renal shutdown that serve as a guide for therapy are BUN, serum creatinine, pH, sodium, potassium, and calcium.

**The definition of oliguria varies extensively in the literature, from 1.8 to 4 dl/m²/24 hr.*

NURSING ALERT Diminished urine output and lethargy in a child who is dehydrated, is in shock, or has recently undergone surgery should be evaluated for possible ARF.

NURSING ALERT Any of the following signs of hyperkalemia constitute an emergency and are reported immediately:

- Serum potassium concentrations in excess of 7 mEq/L
- Electrocardiographic abnormalities, such as prolonged QRS complex, depressed ST segment, high peaked T waves, bradycardia, or heart block

Therapeutic Management

Treatment of ARF is directed toward (1) treatment of the underlying cause, (2) management of the complications of renal failure, and (3) provision of supportive therapy within the constraints imposed by the renal failure.

Treatment of poor perfusion resulting from dehydration consists of volume restoration, as described in Chapter 47 in treatment of dehydration. If oliguria persists after restoration of fluid volume or if the renal failure is caused by intrinsic renal damage, the physiologic and biochemical abnormalities that have resulted from kidney dysfunction must be corrected or controlled. Initially a Foley catheter is inserted to rule out urine retention, to collect available urine for analysis, and to monitor results of diuretic administration. The catheter may or may not be removed during the oliguric phase.

The amount of exogenous water provided should not exceed the amount needed to maintain zero water balance. It is calculated on the basis of estimated endogenous water formation and losses from sensible (primarily gastrointestinal) and insensible sources. No allotment is calculated for urine as long as oliguria persists.

When the output begins to increase, either spontaneously or in response to diuretic therapy, the intake of fluid, potassium, and sodium must be monitored and adequate replacement provided to prevent depletion and its consequences. Some patients pass enormous amounts of electrolyte-rich urine.

Complications

The child with ARF has a tendency to develop water intoxication and hyponatremia, which makes it difficult to provide calories in sufficient amounts to meet the child's needs and reduce tissue catabolism, metabolic acidosis, hyperkalemia, and uremia. If the child is able to tolerate oral foods, food sources high in concentrated carbohydrate and fat but low in protein, potassium, and sodium may be provided. However, many children have functional disturbances of the gastrointestinal tract, such as nausea and vomiting; therefore the IV route is generally preferred and usually consists of essential amino acids or a combination of essential and nonessential amino acids administered by the central venous route.

Control of water balance in these patients requires careful monitoring of feedback information, such as accurate intake and output, body weight, and electrolyte measurements. In general, during the oliguric phase, no sodium, chloride, or potassium is given unless there are other large, ongoing losses. Regular measurement of plasma electrolyte, pH, BUN, and creatinine levels is required to assess the adequacy of fluid therapy and to anticipate complications that require specific treatment.

Hyperkalemia is the most immediate threat to the life of the child with ARF. Hyperkalemia can be minimized and sometimes avoided by eliminating potassium from all food and fluid, by reducing tissue catabolism, and by correcting acidosis. Measures to reduce serum potassium levels are oral or rectal administration of an ion-exchange resin such as sodium polystyrene sulfonate (Kayexalate) and peritoneal dialysis or hemodialysis (p. 1547). The resin produces its effect by exchange of its sodium for the potassium, thus binding potassium for removal from the body. This increased sodium concentration may contribute to fluid overload, hypertension, and cardiac failure. Dialysis removes potassium and other waste products from the serum by diffusion through a semipermeable membrane.

Hypertension is a frequent and serious complication of ARF, and to detect it early, blood pressure measurements are made every 4 to 6 hours. The most common cause of hypertension in ARF is overexpansion of extracellular fluid and plasma volume together with activation of the renin-angiotensin system. Hypertension is controlled with antihypertensive drugs. Other measures that may be used include limiting fluids and salt.

Anemia is frequently associated with ARF, but transfusion is not recommended unless the hemoglobin drops below 6 g/dl. Transfusions, if used, consist of fresh, packed red blood cells given slowly to reduce the likelihood of increasing blood volume, hypertension, and hyperkalemia.

Seizures occur often when renal failure progresses to uremia and are also related to hypertension, hyponatremia, and hypocalcemia. Treatment is directed to the specific cause when known. More obscure causes are managed with antiepileptic drugs.

Cardiac failure with pulmonary edema is almost always associated with hypervolemia. Treatment is directed toward reduction of fluid volume, with water and sodium restriction and administration of diuretics.

Prognosis

The prognosis of ARF depends largely on the nature and severity of the causative factor or precipitating event and the promptness and competence of management. The outcome is least favorable in children with rapidly progressive nephritis and cortical necrosis. Children in whom ARF is a result of HUS or AGN recover completely, but residual renal impairment or hypertension is more often the rule. Complete recovery is usually expected in children whose renal failure is a result of dehydration, nephrotoxins, or ischemia. ARF after cardiac surgery is less favorable. It is often impossible to assess the extent of recovery for several months.

Nursing Care Management

Meticulous attention to fluid intake and output is mandatory and includes all of the physical measurements discussed previously in relation to problems of fluid balance. Monitoring fluid balance and vital signs is a continuous process, and observers are constantly on the alert for signs of complications so that appropriate interventions can be implemented. Because these children require intensive observation and often specialized treatment, such as dialysis, they are usually admitted to an intensive care unit in which needed equipment and trained personnel are available (see Nursing Care Plan).

NURSING CARE PLAN ✤ The Child with Acute Renal Dysfunction

Nursing Diagnosis	Expected Patient Outcomes	Nursing Interventions	Rationale
Risk for injury related to accumulated electrolytes and waste products	Child will exhibit no evidence of waste product accumulation.	Assist with renal dialysis.	To maintain renal excretory function
	The Following NOC Concept Applies to This Outcome	Administer sodium polystyrene sulfate (Kayexalate).	To reduce serum potassium levels
	Risk Control	Provide diet low in potassium, sodium, and phosphorus.	To reduce excretory demand on kidneys
Child's/Family's Defining Characteristics *(Subjective and Objective Data)*		Observe for evidence of accumulated waste products.	To ensure prompt treatment
Excesses in potassium, sodium, and phosphorus		Increase water intake.	To increase waste excretion by kidneys
Evidence of hyperkalemia, hyperphosphatemia, uremia		**The Following NIC Concepts Apply to These Interventions**	
Excess blood urea nitrogen		Risk Identification Medication Administration Surveillance Teaching: Disease Process	

Nursing Diagnosis	Expected Patient Outcomes	Nursing Interventions	Rationale
Imbalanced nutrition: less than body requirements related to restricted diet	Child will consume an adequate amount of appropriate foods. Child will show no evidence of deficiencies or weight loss.	Provide dietary instructions for foods that reduce excretory demands on kidney and provide sufficient calories and protein for growth.	To provide an appropriate diet that can reduce kidney demands
	The Following NOC Concepts Apply to These Outcomes	Limit phosphorus, salt, and potassium as prescribed.	To prevent mineral excess
Child's/Family's Defining Characteristics *(Subjective and Objective Data)*	Nutritional Status: Nutrient Intake Nutritional Status: Food and Fluid Intake Weight Control	Encourage intake of carbohydrates and foods high in calcium.	To provide calories for growth and calcium to prevent bone demineralization
Weight loss Inadequate growth Poor nutritional intake		Arrange for renal dietitian to meet with family to review allowable foods and assist in dietary planning.	To promote understanding of the child's dietary needs
		Help hemodialysis patient to fill out menu requests for meals.	To promote appropriate food choice decisions
		The Following NIC Concepts Apply to These Interventions	
		Teaching: Prescribed Diet Vital Signs Monitoring Fluid Management Nutrition Management Nutrition Therapy Nutritional Monitoring	

Limiting fluid intake requires ingenuity on the part of caregivers to cope with the child who is thirsty. Rationing the daily intake in small amounts of fluid served in containers that give the impression of larger volumes is one strategy. Older children who understand the rationale of fluid limits can help determine how their daily ration should be distributed.

Meeting nutritional needs is sometimes a problem; the child may be nauseated, and encouraging concentrated foods without fluids may be difficult. When nourishment is provided by the IV route, careful monitoring is essential to prevent fluid overload. In addition, nursing measures such as maintaining an optimal thermal environment, reducing any elevation of body temperature, and reducing restlessness and anxiety are employed to decrease the rate of tissue catabolism.

The nurse must be continually alert for changes in behavior that indicate the onset of complications. Infection from reduced resistance, anemia, and general morbidity is a constant threat. Fluid overload and electrolyte disturbances can precipitate cardiovascular complications such as hypertension and cardiac failure. Fluid and electrolyte imbalances, acidosis, and accumulation of nitrogenous waste products can produce neurologic involvement manifested by coma, seizures, or alterations in sensorium.

Although children with ARF are usually quite ill and voluntarily diminish their activity, infants may become restless and irritable, and children are often anxious and frightened. Frequent, painful, and stress-producing treatments and tests must be performed. A supportive, empathetic nurse can provide comfort and stability in a threatening and unnatural environment.

Family Support

Providing support and reassurance to parents is among the major nursing responsibilities. The seriousness of ARF and its emergency nature are stressful to parents, and most feel some degree of guilt regarding the child's condition, especially when the illness is a result of ingestion of a toxic substance, dehydration, or a genetic disease. They need reassurance and a sympathetic listener. They also need to be kept informed of the child's progress and provided explanations regarding the therapeutic regimen. The equipment and the child's behavior are sometimes frightening and anxiety provoking. Nurses can do much to help parents comprehend and deal with the stresses of the situation.

Chronic Renal Failure

The kidneys are able to maintain the chemical composition of fluids within normal limits until more than 50% of functional renal capacity is destroyed by disease or injury. Chronic renal insufficiency or failure begins when the diseased kidneys can no longer maintain the normal chemical structure of body fluids under normal conditions. Progressive deterioration over months or years produces a variety of clinical and biochemical disturbances that culminate in the clinical syndrome known as *uremia*.

A variety of diseases and disorders can result in CRF. The most frequent causes are congenital renal and urinary tract malformations, VUR associated with recurrent UTI, chronic pyelonephritis, hereditary disorders, chronic glomerulonephritis, and glomerulonephropathy associated with systemic diseases such as anaphylactoid purpura and lupus erythematosus.

Pathophysiology

Early in the course of progressive nephrotic destruction, the child remains asymptomatic with only minimal biochemical abnormalities. Unless the presence of CRF is detected in the process of routine assessment, signs and symptoms that indicate advanced renal damage frequently emerge only late in the course of the disease. Midway in the disease process, as increasing numbers of nephrons are totally destroyed and most others are damaged to varying degrees, the few that remain intact are hypertrophied but functional. These few normal nephrons are able to make sufficient adjustments to stresses to maintain reasonable degrees of fluid and electrolyte balance. Definitive biochemical examination at this time will reveal limited tolerance to excesses or restrictions. As the disease progresses to the end stage, because of a severe reduction in the number of functioning nephrons, the kidneys are no longer able to maintain fluid and electrolyte balance, and the features of uremic syndrome appear.

The accumulation of various biochemical substances in the blood, those that result from diminished renal function, produces complications such as the following:

Retention of waste products, especially BUN and creatinine

Water and sodium retention, which contributes to edema and vascular congestion

Hyperkalemia of dangerous levels

Metabolic acidosis of a sustained nature because of continual hydrogen ion retention and bicarbonate loss

Calcium and phosphorus disturbances, resulting in altered bone metabolism, which in turn causes growth arrest or retardation, bone pain, and deformities known as *renal osteodystrophy*

Anemia caused by hematologic dysfunction, including shortened life span of red blood cells, impaired red blood cell production related to decreased production of erythropoietin, prolonged bleeding time, and nutritional anemia

Growth disturbance, probably caused by such factors as renal osteodystrophy, poor nutrition associated with dietary restrictions and loss of appetite, and biochemical abnormalities

Children with CRF seem to be more susceptible to infection, especially pneumonia, UTI, and septicemia, although the reason for this is unclear. These children become extraordinarily sensitive to changes in vascular volume that may cause pulmonary overload, central nervous system symptoms, hypertension, and cardiac failure.

Diagnostic Evaluation

The diagnosis of CRF is usually suspected on the basis of any number of clinical manifestations, a history of prior renal disease, or biochemical findings. The onset is usually gradual, and the initial signs and symptoms are vague and nonspecific (Box 50-7).

Laboratory and other diagnostic tools and tests are of value in assessing the extent of renal damage, biochemical disturbances, and related physical dysfunction (see Tables 50-1 to 50-3). Often they can help establish the nature of the underlying disease and differentiate between other disease processes and the pathologic consequences of renal dysfunction.

Therapeutic Management

In irreversible renal failure the goals of medical management are to (1) promote maximum renal function, (2) maintain body fluid and electrolyte balance within safe biochemical limits, (3) treat systemic complications, and (4) promote as active and normal a life as possible for the child for as long as possible. The child is allowed unrestricted activity and is allowed to set his or her own limits regarding rest and extent of exertion. School attendance is encouraged as long as the child is able. When the effort is too great, home tutoring is arranged.

Diet regulation is the most effective means, short of dialysis, for reducing the quantity of materials that require renal excretion. The goal of diet management in renal failure is to provide sufficient calories and protein for growth while limiting the excretory demands made on the kidney, to minimize metabolic bone disease *(osteodystrophy)*, and to minimize fluid and electrolyte disturbances. Dietary protein intake is limited only to the reference daily intake (RDA) for the child's age. Restriction of protein intake below the RDA is believed to negatively affect growth and neurodevelopment. Malnutrition may develop in patients with CRF even before they need dialysis (Nailescu, Kaskel, & Kaskel, 2004).

Sodium and water are not usually limited unless there is evidence of edema or hypertension, and potassium is not usually restricted. However, restrictions of any or all three may be imposed in later stages or at any time that abnormal serum concentrations are evident.

Dietary phosphorus is controlled through reduction of protein and milk intake to prevent or correct the calcium/phosphorus imbalance. Phosphorus levels can be further reduced by oral administration of calcium carbonate preparations or other phosphate-binding agents that combine with

evolve Nursing Care Plan—The Child with Chronic Renal Failure

BOX 50-7 Clinical Manifestations of Chronic Renal Failure

Early signs:
- Loss of normal energy
- Increased fatigue on exertion
- Pallor, subtle (may not be noticed)
- Elevated blood pressure (sometimes)

As the disease progresses:
- Decreased appetite (especially at breakfast)
- Less interest in normal activities
- Increased or decreased urine output with compensatory intake of fluid
- Pallor more evident
- Sallow, muddy appearance of skin

Child may complain of:
- Headache
- Muscle cramps
- Nausea

Other signs and symptoms:
- Weight loss
- Facial edema
- Malaise
- Bone or joint pain
- Growth retardation
- Dryness or itching of the skin
- Bruised skin
- Sensory or motor loss (sometimes)
- Amenorrhea (common in adolescent girls)

Uremic syndrome (untreated):
- Gastrointestinal symptoms: anorexia, nausea and vomiting
- Bleeding tendencies: bruises, bloody diarrheal stools, stomatitis, bleeding from lips and mouth
- Intractable itching
- Uremic frost (deposits of urea crystals on skin)
- Unpleasant "uremic" breath odor
- Deep respirations
- Hypertension
- Congestive heart failure
- Pulmonary edema
- Neurologic involvement: progressive confusion, dulled sensorium, coma (ultimately), tremors, muscular twitching, seizures

the phosphorus to decrease gastrointestinal absorption and thus the serum levels of phosphate. Treatment with 25-OH vitamin D is begun to increase calcium absorption and suppress elevated parathyroid hormone levels.

Metabolic acidosis is alleviated through administration of alkalizing agents such as sodium bicarbonate or a combination of sodium and potassium citrate.

Growth failure is one major consequence of CRF, especially in the preadolescent. These children grow poorly both before and after the initiation of hemodialysis. The use of recombinant human growth hormone to accelerate growth in children with growth retardation secondary to CRF has been successful (Mehls et al, 2002; Vimalachandra et al, 2006). *Osseous deformities* that result from renal osteodystrophy, especially those related to ambulation, are troublesome and require correction if they occur. *Dental defects* are common in children with CRF, and the earlier the onset of the disease, the more severe are the dental manifestations (including hypoplasia, hypomineralization, tooth discoloration, alteration in size and shape of teeth, malocclusion, and ulcerative stomatitis). Therefore regular dental care is especially important in these children.

Anemia in children with CRF is related to decreased production of erythropoietin. Recombinant human erythropoietin is being offered to these children as thrice-weekly or weekly subcutaneous injections and is replacing the need for frequent blood transfusions. The drug corrects the anemia and in turn increases appetite, activity, and general well-being.

Hypertension of advanced renal disease may be managed initially by cautious use of a low-sodium diet, fluid restriction, and perhaps diuretics such as hydrochlorothiazide or furosemide. Severe hypertension requires the use of antihypertensive agents, singly or in combination.

Intercurrent infections are treated with appropriate antimicrobials at the first sign of infection; however, any drug eliminated through the kidneys is administered with caution. Other complications are treated symptomatically (e.g., central-acting antiemetics for *nausea,* antiepileptics for *seizures*, and diphenhydramine [Benadryl] for *pruritus*).

Once evidence of *end-stage renal disease (ESRD)* appears in a child, the disease runs its relentless course and results in death in a few weeks, unless waste products and toxins are removed from body fluids by dialysis or kidney transplantation. These techniques have been adapted for infants and small children and are implemented in most cases of renal failure after conservative management is no longer effective (see Technologic Management of Renal Failure, p. 1547).

Prognosis

Dialysis and transplantation are the only treatments currently available for children with ESRD. Although children may survive on dialysis, it is not an ideal long-term modality. Complications include infection of access sites, growth failure, and disruption of normal socialization. Many pediatric centers encourage families of children with ESRD to consider kidney transplantation. The North American Renal Transplantation in Children Report of the North American Pediatric Renal Trials and Collaborative Studies reports a graft survival of 90% at 1 year and 74% at 6 years for living donor kidneys, and 80% at 1 year and 58% at 6 years for cadaver kidneys (Benfield et al, 2003).

Posttransplant complications include infection, hypertension, steroid toxicity, hyperlipidemia, aseptic necrosis, malignancy, and growth retardation (Benfield, 2003). Long-term graft survival is not guaranteed, and many children require a second or third transplant. Successful kidney transplantation does improve rehabilitation of children with CRF, both educationally and psychologically. Increasing use of primary or preemptive kidney transplants is becoming the optimal form of renal replacement therapy, leading to substantial improvement in quality of life (Goldstein et al, 2006).

Nursing Care Management

The multiple complications of ESRD are managed according to evidence-based clinical practice guidelines such as the ESRD Clinical Performance Measures Project (Fadrowski et al, 2007). However, progressive disease places a number of stresses on the child and family, including those of a potentially fatal illness (see Chapter 44). There is a continuing need for repeated examinations that often entail painful procedures, side effects, and frequent hospitalizations. Diet therapy becomes progressively more restricted and intense, and the child is required to take a variety of medications. Ever present in all aspects of the treatment regimen is the agonizing realization that without treatment, death is inevitable.

Some specific stresses related to ESRD and its treatment are predictable. When it first becomes apparent that ESRD is inevitable, both parents and child experience depression and anxiety. Acceptance is particularly difficult if renal failure progresses rapidly after diagnosis. Denial and disbelief are usually pronounced, especially among the parents. After renal failure is established and symptoms become progressively more distressing, the initiation of dialysis is usually perceived as a positive experience, and after experiencing initial concerns regarding the treatment, the child begins to feel better and parental anxiety is relieved for a time.

Initiating a dialysis regimen is a traumatic and anxiety-provoking experience for most children because it involves surgery for implantation of a graft, fistula, or peritoneal catheter. The initial experience with the dialysis procedure is frightening to most children. They need reassurance about the nature of the preparations for dialysis and the conduct of the treatment.

Both the graft and the fistula require needle insertions at each dialysis. The goal is to perform pain-free venipuncture. Using buffered lidocaine with a small-gauge needle (30 gauge) to anesthetize the area before venipuncture of the graft or fistula is one method. Using an anesthetizing topical preparation such as EMLA (eutectic mixture of local anesthetics [lidocaine and prilocaine]) 1 hour before venipuncture is another approach (see Pain Management, Chapter 35). External dual-lumen venous access devices eliminate the need for needles but are more prone to infection and other central line complications.

Adolescents, with their increased need for independence and their urge for rebellion, usually adapt less well than younger children. They resent the control and enforced dependence imposed by the rigorous and unrelenting therapy program. They resent being dependent on hemodialysis technology, their parents, and the professional staff. Depression or hostility is common in adolescents undergoing hemodialysis.

The availability of home peritoneal dialysis has offered a greater degree of freedom for persons undergoing long-term dialysis. The nurse is responsible for teaching the family about (1) the disease, its implications, and the therapeutic plan; (2) the possible psychologic effects of the disease and the treatment; and (3) the technical aspects of the procedure. The family learns how to manage the various aspects of the dialysis procedure, how to maintain accurate records, and how to observe for signs of complications that need to be reported to the proper persons.

Body changes related to the disease process, such as pale or ashen skin color, growth retardation, and lack of sexual maturation, are stress provoking. Dietary restrictions are particularly burdensome for both children and parents. Children feel deprived when they are unable to eat foods previously enjoyed and that are unrestricted for other family members. Consequently, they may fail to cooperate. Diet restrictions may be interpreted as punishment. Some children, unable to fully understand the purpose of restrictions, will sneak forbidden food items at every opportunity. Allowing children, especially adolescents, maximum participation in and responsibility for their own treatment program is helpful.

After months or years of dialysis, the parents and child feel anxiety associated with the prognosis and continued pressures of the treatment. The relentless need for treatment interferes with family plans. The time spent in transportation to and from the dialysis unit and the time spent undergoing dialysis treatments cut into time for outside activities, including school. Graft and fistula problems, as well as peritoneal catheter exit site infections, may develop and present a common source of aggravation.

The possibility of kidney transplantation often provides hope for relief from the rigors of hemodialysis and peritoneal dialysis. Most children and families respond well to a kidney transplant, and most children can be successfully rehabilitated.

The National Kidney Foundation* and other agencies provide a number of services and information for families of children with renal disease.

Technologic Management of Renal Failure

Dialysis

Dialysis is the process of separating colloids and crystalline substances in solution by the difference in their rate of diffusion through a semipermeable membrane. Methods of dialysis currently available for clinical management of renal failure are *peritoneal dialysis*, wherein the abdominal cavity acts as a semipermeable membrane through which water and solutes of small molecular size move by osmosis and diffusion according to their respective concentrations on either side of the membrane, and *hemodialysis*, in which blood is circulated outside the body through artificial membranes that permit a similar passage of water and solutes. A third type of dialysis is *hemofiltration*, in which blood filtrate is circulated outside the body by hydrostatic pressure exerted across a semipermeable membrane with simultaneous infusion of a replacement solution. Types of hemofiltration include *continuous venovenous hemofiltration*, *continuous venovenous hemodialysis*, and *continuous venovenous hemodiafiltration*. These continuous renal replacement therapies are used in ARF, severe fluid overload, and inborn errors of metabolism or after bone marrow transplant (Goldstein, 2003).

Peritoneal dialysis is the preferred form of dialysis for infants, for children and parents who wish to remain independent, for families who live a long distance from the medical center, and for children who prefer fewer dietary restrictions and a gentler form of dialysis. Chronic peritoneal dialysis is

**30 E. 33rd St., New York, NY 10016; 212-889-2210 or 800-622-9010;* www.kidney.org. *In Canada: Kidney Foundation of Canada, 300-5165 Sherbrooke St. West, Montreal QC H4A 1T6; 514-369-4806 or 800-361-7494;* www.kidney.ca.

most often performed at home. The two types of peritoneal dialysis are *continuous ambulatory peritoneal dialysis* and *continuous cycling peritoneal dialysis*. In both methods, commercially available sterile dialysis solution is instilled into the peritoneal cavity through a surgically implanted indwelling catheter tunneled subcutaneously and sutured into place. The warmed solution is allowed to enter the peritoneal cavity by gravity and remains a variable length of time according to the rate of solute removal and glucose absorption in individual patients. The care and management of the procedure are the responsibility of the parents of young children. Some centers have initiated use of home health nurses to give parents respite from care. Older children and adolescents can carry out the procedure themselves, which provides them with some control and less dependency. This is especially important for adolescents.

NURSING ALERT Observe for changes in the color of the dialysate draining from the child. The spent solution should be clear. If the color is cloudy, notify the practitioner immediately (Schaefer, 2003).

Hemodialysis requires the creation of a vascular access and the use of special dialysis equipment—the hemodialyzer, or so-called artificial kidney. Vascular access may be one of three types: fistulas, grafts, or external vascular access devices. An *arteriovenous fistula* is an access in which a vein and artery are connected surgically. The preferred site is the radial artery and a forearm vein that produces dilation and thickening of the superficial vessels of the forearm to provide easy access for repeated venipuncture. An alternative is the creation of a subcutaneous (internal) *arteriovenous graft* by anastomosing artery and vein, with a synthetic prosthetic graft for circulatory access. The most commonly used material is expanded polytetrafluoroethylene (ePTFE). Both the graft and the fistula require needle insertions with each dialysis treatment.

For external vascular access devices, percutaneous catheters are inserted in the femoral, subclavian, or internal jugular veins, even in very small children. A more permanent form of external access is available via a central catheter inserted surgically into the internal jugular vein. This catheter has a dual lumen, which allows a larger volume of blood flow with minimum recirculation. Catheters eliminate the need for skin punctures but may require some home care.

Hemodialysis is best suited to children who do not have someone in the family who is able to perform home peritoneal dialysis and to those who live close to a dialysis center. The procedure is usually performed three times per week for 4 to 6 hours, depending on the child's size. Hemodialysis achieves rapid correction of fluid and electrolyte abnormalities but can cause problems in association with this rapid change, such as muscle cramping and hypotension. Disadvantages include school absence during dialysis and strict fluid and dietary restrictions between dialysis sessions. Boredom for the child and family is often a problem during dialysis, and planned activities should be introduced (Fig. 50-3).

Most children show rapid clinical improvement with the implementation of dialysis, although it is directly related to the duration of uremia before dialysis and good nutrition.

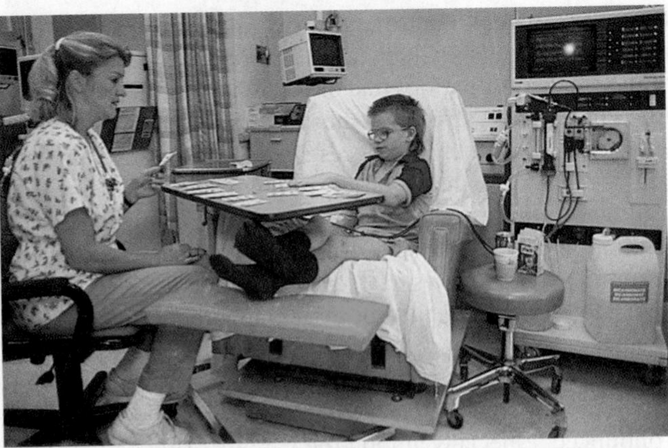

Fig. 50-3 Diversional activities help lessen the boredom children can experience during hemodialysis.

Growth rate and skeletal maturation improve, but recovery of normal growth is infrequent. In many cases, sexual development, although delayed, progresses to completion.

Transplantation

Kidney transplantation is now an acceptable and effective means of therapy in the pediatric age group. Although peritoneal dialysis and hemodialysis are life preserving, both require major alterations in lifestyle. Transplantation offers the opportunity for a relatively normal life and is the preferred form of treatment for children with ESRD. Primary or preemptive transplants maintain the greatest amount of normalcy in the family's life.

Kidneys for transplant are available from two sources: a *living related donor*, usually a parent or a sibling, or a *cadaver donor*, a dead or brain-dead patient whose family consents to donation of a healthy kidney. Retransplantation occurs frequently.

The primary goal in transplantation is the long-term survival of grafted tissue by securing tissue that is antigenically similar to that of the recipient and by suppressing the recipient's immune mechanism. The immunosuppressant therapy of choice has been corticosteroids (prednisone) in conjunction with cyclosporine or tacrolimus and mycophenolate mofetil. Other therapies include antilymphoblast globulin or monoclonal antibodies. New immunosuppressant medications are rapidly coming into clinical trials and into use in large transplant centers. It is important for the nurse to learn about the medications used in the antirejection protocol(s) and about their side effects. Because the immunosuppressant medications are taken indefinitely, transplant patients experience many side effects of the drugs, including hypertension, growth retardation, cataracts, risk of infection, obesity, characteristics of Cushing's syndrome, and hirsutism (Smith, Nemeth, & McDonald, 2003).

NURSING ALERT The child with a kidney transplant who exhibits any of the following should be evaluated immediately for possible rejection:

- Fever
- Swelling and tenderness over graft area
- Diminished urine output

- Elevated blood pressure
- Elevated serum creatinine

Rejection of the transplanted kidney is the most common cause of transplant failure. Rejection is treated aggressively with immunosuppressant medications and can often be reversed. Some patients do not respond to treatment of acute rejection or develop chronic rejection and must eventually return to dialysis or undergo another kidney transplant.

Key Points

- Common inflammatory disorders of the genitourinary tract include UTI, nephrotic syndrome, and AGN.
- Management of UTIs is directed at eliminating infection, detecting and correcting functional or anatomic abnormalities, preventing recurrences, and preserving renal function.
- VUR is the retrograde flow of bladder urine into the ureters.
- Obstructive uropathy is a result of structural or functional abnormalities of the urinary system that obstruct the normal flow of urine.
- The more common defects of the genitourinary tract include phimosis, cryptorchidism, inguinal hernia, hydrocele, and hypospadias.
- Body-image concerns and castration anxiety are particularly intense in children with defects in the genital area.
- Nephrotic syndrome is characterized by increased glomerular permeability to protein, with massive urinary loss of protein resulting in hypoproteinemia and edema.
- Management of nephrotic syndrome is aimed at reducing excretion of protein, reducing or preventing fluid retention by tissues, and preventing infection and other complications.
- Common features of AGN are oliguria, edema, hypertension, circulatory congestion, hematuria, and proteinuria.
- Therapeutic management of AGN involves maintenance of fluid balance, treatment of hypertension, and antibiotic therapy.

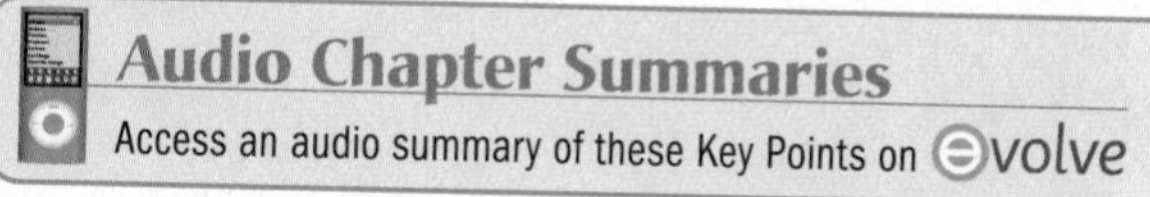
Audio Chapter Summaries
Access an audio summary of these Key Points on evolve

- Management of HUS is aimed at control of complications and hematologic manifestations of renal failure.
- Wilms' tumor is the most common malignant neoplasm of the kidney in infants and children.
- In ARF, management is directed at determining treatment of the underlying cause, managing complications of renal failure, and providing supportive therapy.
- Abnormalities in CRF are waste product retention, water and sodium retention, hyperkalemia, acidosis, calcium and phosphorus disturbance, anemia, and growth disturbances.
- The types of dialysis used in ESRD are peritoneal dialysis and hemodialysis.
- When the child will need home dialysis, the nurse educates the family about the disease, its implications, the therapeutic plan, possible psychologic effects of the disease, and the treatment and technical aspects of the procedure.
- The major concerns in kidney transplantation are tissue matching and prevention of rejection; psychologic concerns involve self-image as related to possible body changes as a result of the effects of corticosteroid therapy.

References

American Academy of Pediatrics: Task Force on Circumcision, *Pediatrics* 103(3):686-693, 1999.

Bailey DT et al: Can a concentrated cranberry extract prevent recurrent urinary tract infections in women? A pilot study, *Phytomedicine* 14(4):237-241, 2007.

Benfield MR: Current status of kidney transplant: update 2003, *Pediatr Clin North Am* 50(6):1301-1334, 2003.

Benfield MR et al: Changing trends in pediatric transplantation: 2001 annual report of the North American Pediatric Renal Transplant Cooperative Study, *Pediatr Transplant* 7(4): 321-335, 2003.

Davis ID, Avner ED: Conditions particularly associated with hematuria. In Behrman RE, Kliegman RM, Jenson HB (editors): *Nelson textbook of pediatrics*, ed 17, Philadelphia, 2004, Saunders.

Dome JS et al: Renal tumors. In Pizzo PA, Poplack DP (editors): *Principles and practices of pediatric oncology*, ed 5, Philadelphia, 2006, Lippincott.

Fadrowski JJ et al: Children on long-term dialysis in the United States: findings from the 2005 ESRD clinical performance measures project, *Am J Kidney Dis* 50(6):958-966, 2007.

Goldstein SL: Overview of pediatric renal replacement therapy in acute renal failure, *Artif Organs* 27(9):781-785, 2003.

Goldstein SL et al: Health-related quality of life in pediatric patients with ESRD, *Pediatr Nephrol* 21(6): 846-850, 2006.

Jepson RG, Mihaljevic L, Craig J: Cranberries for preventing urinary tract infections, *Cochrane Database Syst Rev* (2):CD001321, 2004.

Kanellopoulos TA et al: First urinary tract infection in neonates, infants and young children: a comparative study, *Pediatr Nephrol* 21(8):1131-1137, 2006.

Kass E: Timing of elective surgery on the genitalia of male children with particular reference to the risks, benefits, and psychological effects of surgery and anesthesia, *Pediatrics* 97(4):590-594, 1996.

Kirsch AJ, Perez-Brayfield MR, Scherz HC: Minimally invasive treatment of vesicoureteral reflux with endoscopic injection of dextranomer/hyaluronic acid copolymer: the Children's Hospital of Atlanta experience, *J Urol* 170(1):211-215, 2003.

Kline NE, Sevier N: Solid tumors in children, *J Pediatr Nurs* 18(2):96-102, 2003.

Krause I et al: Acute renal failure, associated with non-steroidal anti-inflammatory drugs in healthy children, *Pediatr Nephrol* 20(9):1295-1298, 2005.

Lavelle MT, Conlin MJ, Skoog SJ: Subureteral injection of Defluz for correction of reflux: analysis of factors predicting success, *Urology* 65(3):564-567, 2005.

Mehls O et al: Effectiveness of growth hormone treatment in

short children with chronic renal failure, *J Pediatr* 141(1):147-148, 2002.

Nailescu C, Kaskel PJ, Kaskel FJ: Nutrition and metabolism. In Avner ED, Harmon WE, Niaudet P (editors): *Pediatric nephrology*, ed 5, Philadelphia, 2004, Lippincott Williams & Wilkins.

Rosenthal M: Current concept in managing UTIs in children, *Infect Dis Child* 17(3):30-31, 2004.

Schaefer F: Management of peritonitis in children receiving chronic peritoneal dialysis, *Paediatr Drugs* 5(5): 315-325, 2003.

Shaikh N et al: Prevalence of urinary tract infection in childhood: a meta-analysis, *Pediatr Infect Dis J* 27(4): 302-308, 2008.

Smith JM, Nemeth TL, McDonald RA: Current immunosuppressive agents: efficacy, side effects, and utilization, *Pediatr Clin North Am* 50(6):1283-1300, 2003.

Vimalachandra D et al: Growth hormone for children with chronic kidney disease, *Cochrane Database Syst Rev* (3):CD003264, 2006.

Unit 11

51

Cerebral Dysfunction

Learning Objectives

On completion of this chapter the reader will be able to:

- Describe the various modalities for assessment of cerebral function.
- Differentiate between the stages of consciousness.
- Formulate a care plan for the unconscious child.
- Distinguish between the types of head injuries and the serious complications.
- Describe the nursing care of a child with a tumor of the central nervous system.
- Outline a care plan for the child with bacterial meningitis.
- Differentiate between the various types of seizure disorders.
- Demonstrate an understanding of the manifestations of a seizure disorder and the management of a child with such a disorder.
- Describe the preoperative and postoperative care of a child with hydrocephalus.

Electronic Resources

Additional information related to the content in Chapter 51 can be found on

evolve the Companion Website at http://evolve.elsevier.com/Perry/maternal/

- NCLEX Review Questions
- Animation—Brain Lobes
- Animation—Seizure, Generalized
- Animation—Subdural Hematoma
- Animation—Ventriculoperitoneal Shunt
- Case Study—Meningitis
- Case Study—Hydrocephalus with Myelomeningocele
- Critical Thinking Exercise—Seizures
- Nursing Care Plan—The Unconscious Child
- Nursing Care Plan—The Child with Bacterial Meningitis
- Nursing Care Plan—The Child with Seizure Disorder

Assessment of Cerebral Function

Most of the information about the status of the brain is obtained by indirect measurements. Some of these measurements are discussed elsewhere in relation to numerous aspects of child care (e.g., as part of assessments of health [Chapter 34], newborn status [Chapter 36], cognitive impairment [Chapter 42], hypoxic injury [cerebral palsy, Chapter 55], and attainment of developmental milestones at each stage of development). Since increased intracranial pressure (ICP) and altered states of consciousness have such prominent places in neurologic dysfunction, they are described here, followed by techniques for neurologic assessment and diagnostic tests.

General Aspects

Children younger than 2 years of age require special evaluation, since they are unable to respond to directions designed to elicit specific neurologic responses. Early neurologic responses in infants are primarily reflexive; these responses are gradually replaced by meaningful movement in the characteristic cephalocaudal direction of development. This evidence of progressive maturation reflects more extensive myelinization and changes in neurochemical and electrophysiologic properties.

Most information about infants and small children is gained by observing their spontaneous and elicited reflex responses as they develop increasingly complex locomotor and fine motor skills and by eliciting progressively sophisticated communicative and adaptive behaviors. Delay or deviation from expected milestones helps identify high-risk children. Persistence or reappearance of reflexes that normally disappear indicates a pathologic condition. In evaluating the infant or young child, it is also important to obtain the pregnancy and delivery history to determine the possible impact of intrauterine environmental influences known to affect the orderly maturation of the central nervous system (CNS). These influences include maternal infections, chemicals, trauma, and metabolic insults.

General aspects of assessment that provide clues to the etiology of dysfunction include:

Family history—Sometimes offers clues regarding possible genetic disorders with neurologic manifestations

Health history—May provide valuable clues regarding the cause of dysfunction (e.g., an injury, short febrile illness, encounter with an animal or insect, ingestion of neurotoxic substances, inhalation of chemicals, a past illness, or known diabetes mellitus)

Physical evaluation of infants—Includes observation of:

- Size and shape of the head
- Spontaneous activity and postural reflex activity
- Sensory responses
- Attitude—normal flexed posture, extreme extension, opisthotonos, hypotonia
- Symmetry in movement of extremities
- Excessive tremulousness or frequent twitching movements
- Altered expiratory cycle—prolonged apnea, ataxic breathing, paradoxic chest movement, and hyperventilation
- Skin and hair texture
- Distinctive facial features
- A high-pitched, piercing cry
- Abnormal eye movements
- Inability to suck or swallow
- Lip smacking
- Asymmetric contraction of facial muscles
- Yawning (may indicate cranial nerve involvement)
- Muscular activity and coordination
- Level of development

Increased Intracranial Pressure

The brain, tightly enclosed in the solid bony cranium, is well protected but highly vulnerable to pressure that may accumulate within the enclosure. The cranium's total volume—brain (80%), cerebrospinal fluid (CSF) (10%), and blood (10%)—must remain approximately the same at all times. A change in the proportional volume of one of these components (e.g., increase or decrease in intracranial blood) must be accompanied by a compensatory change in another. In this way the volume and pressure normally remain constant. Examples of compensatory changes are reduction in blood volume, decrease in CSF production, increase in CSF absorption, or shrinkage of brain mass by displacement of intracellular and extracellular fluid. Children with open fontanels compensate by skull expansion and widened sutures. However, at any age the capacity for spatial compensation is limited. An increase in ICP may be caused by tumors or other space-occupying lesions, accumulation of fluid within the ventricular system, bleeding, or edema of cerebral tissues. Once compensation is exhausted, any further increase in volume will result in a rapid rise in ICP.

Early signs and symptoms of increased ICP are often subtle and assume many patterns (Box 51-1). As pressure increases, signs and symptoms become more pronounced and the level of consciousness (LOC) deteriorates.

Altered States of Consciousness

Consciousness implies awareness—the ability to respond to sensory stimuli and have subjective experiences. Consciousness has two components: *alertness,* an arousal-waking state, including the ability to respond to stimuli; and *cognitive power,* which includes the ability to process stimuli and produce verbal and motor responses.

An altered state of consciousness usually refers to varying states of unconsciousness that may be momentary or may extend for hours, for days, or indefinitely. *Unconsciousness* is depressed cerebral function—the inability to respond to sensory stimuli and have subjective experiences. *Coma* is defined as a state of unconsciousness from which the patient cannot be roused even with powerful stimuli.

Levels of Consciousness

Assessment of LOC remains the earliest indicator of improvement or deterioration in neurologic status. LOC is determined by observations of the child's responses to the environment. Other diagnostic tests, such as motor activity, reflexes, and vital signs, are more variable and do not necessarily directly parallel the depth of the comatose state. The most consistently used terms are described in Box 51-2.

Coma Assessment

Several scales have been devised in an attempt to standardize the description and interpretation of the degree of depressed

BOX 51-1 Clinical Manifestations of Increased Intracranial Pressure in Infants and Children

Infants

Tense and/or bulging fontanel
Separated cranial sutures
Macewen sign (cracked-pot sound on percussion)
Irritability
High-pitched cry
Increased occipitofrontal circumference
Distended scalp veins
Changes in feeding habits
Crying when disturbed
Setting-sun sign

Children

Headache
Nausea
Vomiting
Diplopia, blurred vision
Seizures

Personality and Behavioral Signs

Irritability, restlessness
Indifference, drowsiness
Decline in school performance
Diminished physical activity and motor performance
Increased sleeping
Memory loss
Inability to follow simple commands
Lethargy and drowsiness

Late Signs

Bradycardia
Lowered level of consciousness
Decreased motor response to commands
Decreased sensory response to painful stimuli
Alterations in pupil size and reactivity
Flexion or extension posturing
Cheyne-Stokes respirations
Papilledema
Coma

evolve Animation—Brain Lobes

BOX 51-2 Levels of Consciousness

Full consciousness—Awake and alert; oriented to person, place, and time; behavior appropriate for age

Confusion—Impaired decision making

Disorientation—Disorientation to time and place, decreased level of consciousness

Lethargy—Limited spontaneous movement, sluggish speech, drowsiness

Obtundation—Arousable with stimulation

Stupor—Remaining in a deep sleep, responsive only to vigorous and repeated stimulation

Coma—No motor or verbal response to noxious (painful) stimuli

Persistent vegetative state (PVS)—The permanently lost function of the cerebral cortex; eyes following objects only by reflex or when attracted to the direction of loud sounds, all four limbs spastic but can withdraw from painful stimuli, hands showing reflexive grasping and groping, face grimacing, some food may be swallowed, groaning or crying but without uttering any words

Modified from Seidel HM et al (editors): *Mosby's guide to physical examination,* ed 6, St Louis, 2006, Mosby.

consciousness. The most popular of these is the *Glasgow Coma Scale (GCS),* which consists of a three-part assessment: eye opening, verbal response, and motor response (Fig. 51-1). When LOC is being assessed in young children, it is often useful to have a parent present to help elicit a desired response. An infant or child may not respond in an unfamiliar environment or to unfamiliar voices. Children older than 3 years of age should be able to give their name, although they may not be cognizant of place or time.

Numeric values of 1 through 5 are assigned to the levels of response in each category. The sum of these numeric values provides an objective measure of the patient's LOC. The lower the score, the deeper the coma. A person with an unaltered LOC would score the highest, 15; a score of 8 or below is generally accepted as a definition of coma; the lowest score, 3, indicates deep coma. The Task Force for the Determination of Brain Death in Children (1987) has established physical examination criteria for cases of irreversible coma.

NURSING ALERT Lack of response to painful stimuli is abnormal and should be reported immediately.

Neurologic Examination

The purpose of the neurologic examination is to establish an accurate, objective baseline of neurologic information. It is essential that the neurologic examination be documented in a fashion that is able to be reproduced by others. This allows for a comparison of the findings so the observer can detect subtle changes in the neurologic status that might not otherwise be evident. Descriptions of behaviors should be simple, objective, and easily interpreted: "Drowsy but awake and conversationally rational/oriented"; "Sleepy but arousable with vigorous physical stimuli. Pressure to nail base of right hand results in upper extremity flexion/lower extremity extension."

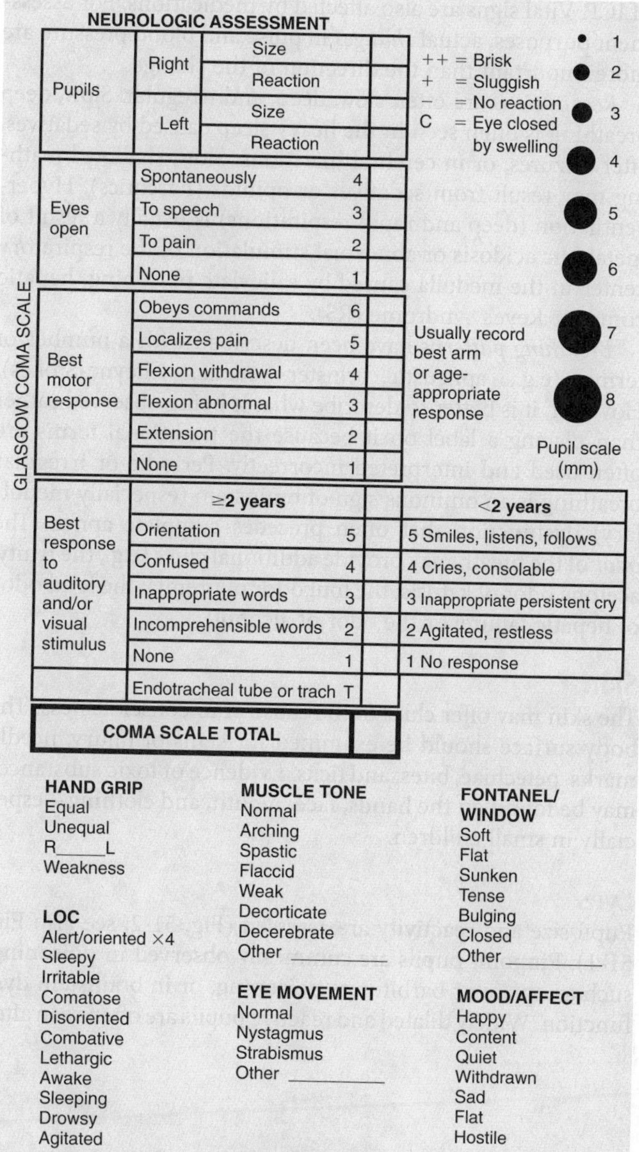

NEUROLOGIC ASSESSMENT

Pupils	Right	Size	
		Reaction	
	Left	Size	
		Reaction	

++ = Brisk
\+ = Sluggish
− = No reaction
C = Eye closed by swelling

Pupil scale (mm): 1, 2, 3, 4, 5, 6, 7, 8

GLASGOW COMA SCALE

Eyes open	Spontaneously	4
	To speech	3
	To pain	2
	None	1
Best motor response	Obeys commands	6
	Localizes pain	5
	Flexion withdrawal	4
	Flexion abnormal	3
	Extension	2
	None	1

Usually record best arm or age-appropriate response

	≥2 years		<2 years
Best response to auditory and/or visual stimulus	Orientation	5	5 Smiles, listens, follows
	Confused	4	4 Cries, consolable
	Inappropriate words	3	3 Inappropriate persistent cry
	Incomprehensible words	2	2 Agitated, restless
	None	1	1 No response
	Endotracheal tube or trach	T	

COMA SCALE TOTAL

HAND GRIP
Equal
Unequal
R_____L
Weakness

MUSCLE TONE
Normal
Arching
Spastic
Flaccid
Weak
Decorticate
Decerebrate
Other

FONTANEL/ WINDOW
Soft
Flat
Sunken
Tense
Bulging
Closed
Other

LOC
Alert/oriented ×4
Sleepy
Irritable
Comatose
Disoriented
Combative
Lethargic
Awake
Sleeping
Drowsy
Agitated

EYE MOVEMENT
Normal
Nystagmus
Strabismus
Other ________

MOOD/AFFECT
Happy
Content
Quiet
Withdrawn
Sad
Flat
Hostile

Fig. 51-1 Pediatric coma scale.

Vital Signs

Pulse, respiration, and blood pressure provide information regarding the adequacy of circulation and the possible underlying cause of altered consciousness. Autonomic activity is most intensively disturbed in cases of deep coma or brainstem lesions.

Body temperature is often elevated, and sometimes the elevation may be extreme. High temperature is most frequently a sign of an acute infectious process or heat stroke but may be caused by ingestion of some drugs (especially salicylates, alcohol, and barbiturates) or by intracranial bleeding, especially subarachnoid hemorrhage. Hypothalamic involvement may cause elevated or decreased temperature. Coma of a toxic origin may produce hypothermia.

The *pulse* is variable and may be rapid, slow and bounding, or feeble. *Blood pressure* may be normal, elevated, or at shock levels. The Cushing reflex, or pressor response, which causes a slowing of the pulse and an increase in blood pressure, is uncommon in children; when it occurs, it is a very late sign of ICP. Vital signs are also affected by medications. For assessment purposes, actual *changes* in pulse and blood pressure are more important than the direction of the change.

Respirations are often slow, deep, and irregular. Slow, deep breathing is often seen in the heavy sleep caused by sedatives, after seizures, or in cerebral infections. Slow, shallow breathing may result from sedatives or opioids (narcotics). Hyperventilation (deep and rapid respirations) is usually a result of metabolic acidosis or abnormal stimulation of the respiratory center in the medulla caused by salicylate poisoning, hepatic coma, or Reye's syndrome (RS).

Breathing patterns have been described with a number of terms (e.g., apneustic, cluster, ataxic, Cheyne-Stokes). However, it is better to describe what is being observed rather than placing a label on it because the traditional terms are often used and interpreted incorrectly. Periodic or irregular breathing is an ominous sign of brainstem (especially medullary) dysfunction that often precedes complete apnea. The *odor* of the breath may provide additional clues (e.g., the fruity, acetone odor of ketosis; the foul odor of uremia; the fetid odor of hepatic failure; or the odor of alcohol).

Skin

The skin may offer clues to the cause of unconsciousness. The body surface should be examined for signs of injury, needle marks, petechiae, bites, and ticks. Evidence of toxic substances may be found on the hands, face, mouth, and clothing—especially in small children.

Eyes

Pupil size and reactivity are assessed (Fig. 51-2; see also Fig. 51-1). Pinpoint pupils are commonly observed in poisoning, such as opiate or barbiturate poisoning, or in brainstem dysfunction. Widely dilated and reactive pupils are often seen after seizures and may involve only one side. Dilated pupils may also be caused by eye trauma. Widely dilated and fixed pupils suggest paralysis of cranial nerve III secondary to pressure from herniation of the brain through the tentorium. A unilateral fixed pupil usually suggests a lesion on the same side. If pupils are fixed bilaterally for more than 5 minutes, brainstem damage is usually implied. Dilated and nonreactive pupils are also seen in hypothermia, anoxia, ischemia, poisoning with atropine-like substances, or prior instillation of mydriatic drugs.

NURSING ALERT The sudden appearance of a fixed and dilated pupil(s) is a neurosurgical emergency.

The description of eye movements should indicate whether one or both eyes are involved and how the reaction was elicited. The parents should be asked about preexisting strabismus, which will cause the eyes to appear normal under compromise. Posttraumatic strabismus indicates cranial nerve VI damage.

Special tests, usually performed by qualified persons, include:

Doll's head maneuver—Elicited by rotating the child's head quickly to one side and then to the other. Conjugate (paired, or working together) movement of the eyes in the direction opposite to the head rotation is normal. Absence of this response suggests dysfunction of the brainstem or oculomotor nerve (cranial nerve III).

NURSING ALERT Any tests that require head movement are not attempted until after cervical spine injury has been ruled out.

Caloric test, or oculovestibular response—Elicited with the child's head up (head of bed is elevated 30 degrees) by irrigating the external auditory canal with 10 ml of

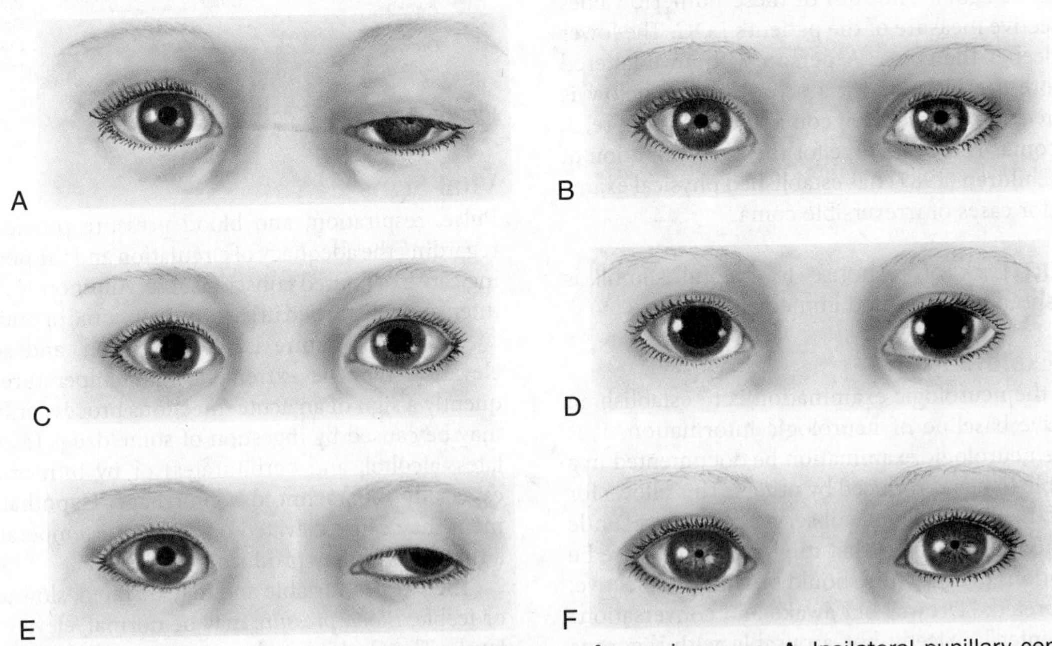

Fig. 51-2 Variations in pupil size with altered states of consciousness. **A,** Ipsilateral pupillary constriction with slight ptosis. **B,** Bilateral small pupils. **C,** Midposition, light fixed to all stimuli. **D,** Bilateral dilated and fixed pupils. **E,** Dilated pupils, left eye abducted with ptosis. **F,** Pinpoint pupils.

ice water for 20 seconds, which normally causes conjugate movement of the eyes toward the side of stimulation. This movement is lost when the pontine centers are impaired, thus providing important information in assessment of the comatose patient.

NURSING ALERT The caloric test is painful and is never performed on a child who is awake or on an individual with a ruptured tympanic membrane.

Funduscopic examination—Reveals additional clues. Papilledema will not be evident early in the course of unconsciousness because it takes 24 to 48 hours to develop, if it develops at all. Papilledema is characterized by optic disc swelling, indistinct optic disc margins, hemorrhage, tortuosity of vessels, and absence of venous pulsations. The presence of preretinal (subhyaloid) hemorrhages in children is almost invariably a result of acute trauma with intracranial bleeding, usually subarachnoid or subdural hemorrhage.

Motor Function

Observing spontaneous activity, posture, and response to painful stimuli provides clues to the location and extent of cerebral dysfunction. Even subtle movements (e.g., the outward rotation of a hip) should be noted and the child observed for other signs. Asymmetric movements of the limbs or absence of movement suggests paralysis. In hemiplegia the affected limb lies in external rotation and will fall uncontrollably when lifted and allowed to drop. These observations should be described rather than labeled.

In the deeper comatose states there is little or no spontaneous movement, and the musculature tends to be flaccid. There is considerable variability in the motor behavior in lesser degrees of coma. For example, the child may be relatively immobile or restless and hyperkinetic; muscle tone may be increased or decreased. Tremors, twitching, and spasms of muscles are common observations. The patient may display purposeless plucking or tossing movements. Combative or negativistic behavior is not uncommon. Hyperactivity is more common in acute febrile and toxic states than in cases of increased ICP. Seizures are common in children and may be present in coma from any cause. Any repetitive or seizure movements should be described.

Posturing

Primitive postural reflexes emerge as cortical control over motor function is lost in brain dysfunction. These reflexes are evident in posturing and motor movements directly related to the area of the brain involved. Posturing reflects a balance between the lower exciting and the higher inhibiting influences, and strong muscles overcome weaker ones. *Flexion posturing* (Fig. 51-3, *A*) is seen with severe dysfunction of the cerebral cortex or with lesions to corticospinal tracts above the brainstem. Typical flexion posturing includes rigid flexion, with arms held tightly to the body; flexed elbows, wrists, and fingers; plantar flexed feet; legs extended and internally rotated; and possibly fine tremors or intense stiffness. *Extension posturing* (see Fig. 51-3, *B*) is a sign of dysfunction at the level of the midbrain or lesions to the brainstem. It is characterized by rigid extension and pronation of the arms and legs, flexed wrists and fingers, clenched jaw, extended neck, and possibly an arched back. Unilateral extension posturing is often caused by tentorial herniation.

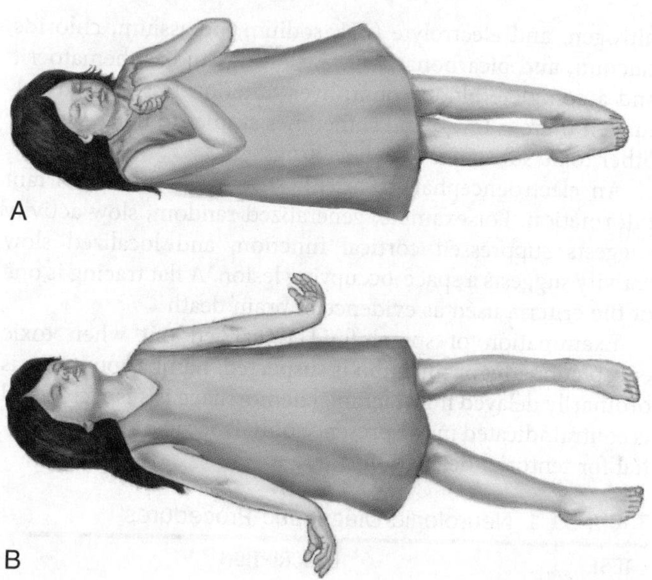

Fig. 51-3 A, Flexion posturing. B, Extension posturing.

Posturing may not be evident when the child is quiet but can usually be elicited by applying painful stimuli, such as a blunt object pressed on the base of the nail. Nurses should avoid applying thumb pressure to the supraorbital region of the frontal bone (risk of orbital damage). Noxious stimuli (e.g., suctioning) will elicit a response, as may turning or touching. When the nurse is describing posturing, the stimulus needed to provoke the response is as important as the reaction.

Reflexes

Testing of some reflexes may be of limited value. In general, the corneal, pupillary, muscle-stretch, superficial, and plantar reflexes tend to be absent in deep coma. The state of reflexes is variable in lighter grades of unconsciousness and depends on the underlying pathologic process and the location of the lesion. Absence of corneal reflexes and presence of a tonic neck reflex are associated with severe brain damage. The Babinski reflex (see Extremities, Chapter 34) may be of value if it is found to be present consistently in children older than 18 months. A positive Babinski reflex is significant in assessment of pyramidal tract lesions when it is unilateral and associated with other pyramidal signs.

NURSING ALERT Three key reflexes that demonstrate neurologic health in young infants are the Moro, tonic neck, and withdrawal reflexes.

Special Diagnostic Procedures

Numerous diagnostic procedures are used for assessment of cerebral function. Laboratory tests that may help delineate the cause of unconsciousness include blood glucose, urea nitrogen, and electrolyte (pH, sodium, potassium, chloride, calcium, and bicarbonate) tests; clotting studies, hematocrit, and a complete blood count; liver function tests; blood cultures if there is fever; and sometimes studies to detect lead or other toxic substances, such as drugs.

An electroencephalogram (EEG) may provide important information. For example, generalized random, slow activity suggests suppressed cortical function, and localized slow activity suggests a space-occupying lesion. A flat tracing is one of the criteria used as evidence of brain death.

Examination of spinal fluid is carried out when toxic encephalopathy or infection is suspected. Lumbar puncture is ordinarily delayed if intracranial hemorrhage is suspected and is contraindicated in the presence of ICP because of the potential for tentorial herniation.

Auditory and visual evoked potentials are sometimes used in neurologic evaluation of very young children. Brainstem auditory evoked potentials are useful for evaluating the continuity of brainstem auditory tracts and are particularly useful for detecting demyelinating disease and neoplasms of the brainstem and distinguishing between brainstem and cortical lesions. For example, a normal evoked potential in a comatose patient suggests involvement of the cerebral hemispheres.

Highly sophisticated tests are carried out with specialized equipment. Two imaging techniques, computed tomography (CT) and magnetic resonance imaging (MRI), assist in diagnosis by scanning both soft tissues and solid matter. Most of these tests are outlined in Table 51-1. Because such tests can be threatening to children, the nurse needs to prepare patients for the tests and provide support and reassurance during the

Table 51-1 Neurologic Diagnostic Procedures

TEST	DESCRIPTION	PURPOSE	COMMENTS
Lumbar puncture (LP)	Spinal needle is inserted between L3-L4 or L4-L5 vertebral spaces into subarachnoid space; cerebrospinal fluid (CSF) pressure is measured, and sample is collected for examination.	Diagnostic–Measures spinal fluid pressure, obtains CSF for laboratory analysis Therapeutic–Injection of medication	Contraindicated in patients with increased intracranial pressure (ICP) or infected skin over puncture site
Subdural tap	Needle is inserted into anterior fontanel or coronal suture (midline to pupil).	Helps rule out subdural effusions Removes CSF to relieve pressure	Place infant in semierect position after subdural tap to minimize leakage from site; prevent child from crying if possible Check site frequently for evidence of leakage
Ventricular puncture	Needle is inserted into lateral ventricle via coronal suture (midline to pupil).	Removes CSF to relieve pressure	Risk of intracerebral or ventricular hemorrhage
Electroencephalography (EEG)	EEG records changes in electrical potential of brain. Electrodes are placed at various points to assess electrical function in a particular area. Impulses are recorded by electromagnetic pen or digitally.	Detects spikes, or bursts of electrical activity that indicate the potential for seizures Used to determine brain death	Patient should remain quiet during procedure; may require sedation Minimize external stimuli during procedure
Nuclear brain scan	Radioisotope is injected intravenously, then counted and recorded after fixed time intervals. Radioisotope accumulates in areas where blood-brain barrier is defective.	Identifies focal brain lesions (e.g., tumors, abscesses) Positive uptake of material with encephalitis and subdural hematoma Visualizes CSF pathways	Requires intravenous (IV) access; patient may require sedation In normal children or noncommunicating hydrocephalus, no retrograde filling of ventricles occurs Areas of concentrated uptake of material are termed *hot spots*
Endocephalography	Pulses of ultrasonic waves are beamed through head; echoes from reflecting surfaces are recorded graphically.	Identifies shifts in midline structures from their normal positions as a result of intracranial lesions May show ventricular dilation	Simple, safe, rapid procedure Fontanel must be patent
Real-time ultrasonography (RTUS)	RTUS is similar to CT but uses ultrasound instead of ionizing radiation.	Allows high-resolution anatomic visualization in variety of imaging planes	Produces images similar to CT scan Especially useful in neonatal central nervous system problems Anterior fontanel must be patent
Radiography	Skull films are taken from different views–lateral, posterolateral, axial (submentoventricular), half-axial.	Shows fractures, dislocations, spreading suture lines, craniosynostosis Shows degenerative changes, bone erosion, calcifications	Simple, noninvasive procedure

Table 51-1 Neurologic Diagnostic Procedures—cont'd

TEST	DESCRIPTION	PURPOSE	COMMENTS
Computed tomography (CT) scan	Pinpoint x-ray beam is directed on horizontal or vertical plane to provide series of images that are fed into computer and assembled in image displayed on video screen. CT uses ionizing radiation.	Visualizes horizontal and vertical cross section of brain in three planes (axial, coronal, sagittal) Distinguishes density of various intracranial tissues and structures–congenital abnormalities, hemorrhage, tumors, demyelinating and inflammatory processes, calcification	Requires IV access if contrast agent is used Patient may require sedation Rapid
Magnetic resonance imaging (MRI)	MRI produces radiofrequency emissions from elements (e.g., hydrogen, phosphorus), which are converted to visual images by computer.	Permits visualization of morphologic feature of target structures Permits tissue discrimination unavailable with many techniques	MRI is noninvasive procedure except when IV contrast agent is used No exposure to radiation occurs Patient may require sedation Parent or attendant can remain in room with child MRI does not visualize bone detail or calcifications No metal can be present in scanner
Positron emission tomography (PET)	PET involves IV injection of positron-emitting radionucleotide; local concentrations are detected and transformed into visual display by computer.	Detects and measures blood volume and flow in brain, metabolic activity, biochemical changes within tissue	Requires lengthy period of immobility Minimum exposure to radiation occurs Patient may require sedation
Digital subtraction angiography (DSA)	Contrast dye is injected intravenously; computer "subtracts" all tissues without contrast medium, leaving clear image of contrast medium in vessels studied.	Visualizes vasculature of target tissue Visualizes finite vascular abnormalities	Safe alternative to angiography Patient must remain still during procedure; may require sedation
Single-photon emission computed tomography (SPECT)	SPECT involves IV injection of photon-emitting radionuclide; radionuclides are absorbed by healthy tissue at different rate than by diseased or necrotic tissue; data are transferred to computer, which converts image to film.	Provides information regarding blood flow to tissues; analyzing blood flow to organ may help determine how well it is functioning	Requires lengthy period of immobility Minimum exposure to radiation occurs Patient may require sedation

tests (see Preparation for Diagnostic and Therapeutic Procedures, Chapter 45). Children who are old enough to understand require careful explanation of the procedure, why it is being done, what they will experience, and how they can help. School-age children usually appreciate a more detailed description of why contrast material is injected. The importance of lying still for tests, particularly CT, needs to be stressed. Children unfamiliar with the machines can be shown a picture beforehand. Although radiographic examinations are not painful, the machinery is often so frightening in appearance that the child protests because of anxiety.

This is especially true of CT and MRI, both of which require that the child's head be placed within a special immobilizing device. Chin and cheek pads are sometimes used to prevent the slightest head movement, and straps are applied to the body to prevent a slight change in body position. The nurse can explain these events to a frightened child by comparing them to an astronaut's preparation for a space flight. It is important to emphasize to the child that at no time is the procedure painful.

The nurse should not expect cooperation from a young child. Sedation may be required. Many different agents are currently used for sedation of children undergoing neurologic diagnostic procedures. Chloral hydrate or benzodiazepines have been used for decades as short-term sedative agents and remain safe methods of pediatric outpatient sedation (Kao et al, 1999; Wetzell, 2007). Chloral hydrate is used alone for sedating children for procedures such as MRI. In recent years other sedative agents have been used safely, alone and in combination, for children in the outpatient setting. These include intravenous (IV) sodium pentobarbital (Nembutal), IV fentanyl (Sublimaze), IV midazolam (Versed) (Wetzell, 2007), and intranasal midazolam (Ljungman et al, 2000; Lloyd, Alredy, & Lloyd, 2000) (see Pain Management, Chapter 35).

Physical preparation for the diagnostic test may involve administration of a sedative. If so, children should be helped through the preparation and administration and assured that someone will remain with them (if possible). Children need continual support and reinforcement during procedures in which they remain conscious. Vital signs and physiologic responses to the procedure are monitored throughout. Many diagnostic procedures performed on an outpatient basis require sedation, and children need recovery time and observation. The nurse should review written instructions with parents if the child is discharged after a procedure. Children who have undergone a procedure with a general anesthetic require postanesthesia care, including positioning to prevent aspiration of secretions and frequent assessment of vital signs and LOC. In addition, other neurologic functions such as pupillary responses, motor strength, and movement are tested at regular intervals. Any surgical wound resulting from the test is checked for bleeding, CSF leakage, and other complications. Children who undergo repeated subdural taps should have their hematocrit monitored to detect excessive blood loss from the procedure.

Nursing Care of the Unconscious Child

evolve Nursing Care Plan—The Unconscious Child

The unconscious child requires nursing attendance, with observation, recording, and evaluation of changes in objective signs. These observations provide valuable information regarding the patient's progress. Often they serve as a guide to diagnosis and treatment. Therefore careful and detailed observations are essential for the patient's welfare. In addition, vital functions must be maintained and complications prevented through conscientious and meticulous nursing care. The outcome of unconsciousness may be early and complete recovery, death within a few hours or days, persistent and permanent unconsciousness, or recovery with varying degrees of residual mental or physical disability. The outcome and recovery of the unconscious child may depend on the level of nursing care and observational skills.

Emergency measures are directed toward ensuring a patent airway, treatment of shock, and reduction of ICP (if it is increased). Delayed treatment often leads to increased damage. As soon as emergency measures have been implemented—and in many cases concurrently—therapies for specific causes are begun. Because nursing care is closely related to medical management, both are considered here.

Continual observation of LOC, pupillary reaction, and vital signs is essential to manage CNS disorders. Regular assessment of neurologic signs is a vital part of nursing comatose children. Vital signs are measured and recorded regularly. The frequency depends on the cause of coma, the status, and the progression of cerebral involvement. Intervals may be as short as every 15 minutes or as long as every 2 hours. Significant alterations are reported immediately. Temperature is taken every 2 to 4 hours, depending on the patient's condition.

An elevated temperature may occur in children with CNS dysfunction; therefore a light covering is sufficient. Vigorous efforts, such as tepid sponge baths or application of a hypothermia blanket, are needed to prevent brain damage if temperature exceeds 40° C (104° F) rectally.

The LOC is assessed periodically, including size, equality, and reaction of pupils to light. Signs of meningeal irritation such as nuchal rigidity are also assessed. Other aspects of LOC assessment include response to vocal commands, spontaneous behavior, resistance to care, and response to painful stimuli. Motions of any type, changes in muscle tone or strength, and body position are noted. Seizure activity is described according to the type and length of seizure and body areas involved. An antiepileptic drug such as phenytoin (Dilantin) or phenobarbital is ordered for control of seizure activity.

Pain management for the comatose child requires astute nursing observation and management. Signs of pain include changes in behavior (e.g., increased agitation and rigidity, alterations in physiologic parameters); increased heart rate, respiratory rate, and blood pressure; and decreased oxygen saturation. Since these findings are not specific for pain, the nurse should observe for their appearance during times of induced or suspected pain and their disappearance after the end of the inciting procedure or the administration of analgesia. A pain assessment record should be used to document indications of pain and the effectiveness of interventions (see Pain Assessment, Chapter 35).

The use of opioids, such as morphine, to relieve pain is controversial because they may mask signs of altered consciousness or depress respirations. However, unrelieved pain activates the stress response, which can elevate ICP. To block the stress response, some authorities advocate the use of analgesics, sedatives, and, in some cases such as head injury, paralyzing agents via continuous IV infusion. A frequently used combination is fentanyl, midazolam, and vecuronium (Norcuron). If there are concerns about assessing the LOC or respiratory depression, naloxone (Narcan) can be used to reverse the opioid effects. Acetaminophen (Tylenol) and codeine may also be effective analgesics for mild to moderate pain. Regardless of which drugs are used, adequate dosage and regular administration are essential to provide optimal pain relief (see Pain Management, Chapter 35).

Other measures to relieve discomfort include providing a quiet, dimly lit environment; limiting visitors; preventing any sudden, jarring movement, such as banging into the bed; and preventing an increase in ICP. The last is most effectively achieved by proper positioning and prevention of straining, such as during coughing, vomiting, or defecating.

NURSING ALERT When opioids are used, bowel elimination must be closely monitored because of the potential constipating effect. Stool softeners should be given with laxatives as needed to prevent constipation.

Respiratory Management

Respiratory effectiveness is the primary concern in the care of the unconscious child, and establishment of an adequate airway is *always* the first priority. Carbon dioxide has a potent vasodilating effect and will increase cerebral blood flow (CBF) and ICP. Cerebral hypoxia that lasts longer than 4 minutes nearly always causes irreversible brain damage.

NURSING ALERT Respiratory obstruction and subsequent compromise lead to cardiac arrest. Maintaining an adequate, patent airway is of the utmost importance.

Children in lighter states of coma may be able to cough and swallow, but those in deeper states are unable to handle secretions, which tend to pool in the throat and pharynx. Dysfunction of cranial nerves IX and X places the child at risk for aspiration and cardiac arrest; therefore the child is positioned to prevent aspiration of secretions, and the stomach is emptied to reduce the likelihood of vomiting. In infants, blockage of air passages from secretions can happen in seconds. In addition, upper airway obstruction from laryngospasm is a frequent complication in comatose children.

An oral airway can be used for the child who is suffering a temporary loss of consciousness, such as after a contusion, seizure, or anesthesia. For children who remain unconscious for a longer time, a nasotracheal or orotracheal tube is inserted to maintain the open airway and facilitate removal of secretions. A tracheostomy is performed in cases in which laryngoscopy for introduction of an endotracheal tube would be difficult or dangerous. Suctioning is used only as needed to clear the airway, exerting care to prevent increasing ICP. Respiratory status is observed and evaluated regularly. Signs of respiratory embarrassment may be an indication for ventilatory assistance.

When the respiratory center is involved, mechanical ventilation is usually indicated (see Chapter 46). Blood gas analysis is performed regularly, and oxygen is administered when indicated. Moderately severe hypoxia and respiratory acidosis are often present but are not always evident from clinical manifestations. Hyperventilation frequently accompanies unconsciousness and may lead to respiratory alkalosis, or it may represent the body's attempt to compensate for metabolic acidosis. Therefore blood gas and pH determinations are essential guides for electrolyte therapy. Chest physical therapy is carried out on a regular basis, and the child's position is changed at least every 2 hours to prevent pulmonary complications.

Intracranial Pressure Monitoring

Management of the child with increased ICP is possibly the most formidable task and the most controversial subject in pediatric critical care. It appears that the outcome in pediatric neurologic injury may reflect the initial cerebral damage more than the subsequent intracranial hypertension. Of note, ICP gives little indication of the severity of the initial insult (Bayir, Kochanek, & Clark, 2003).

When increased ICP is a result of accumulation of CSF from obstruction of CSF flow, a ventricular tap will provide relief quickly and effectively. Evacuation of a hematoma reduces pressure from this source. Indications for inserting an ICP monitor are as follows:

- GCS evaluation of 8
- GCS evaluation of less than 8 with respiratory assistance
- Deterioration of condition
- Subjective judgment regarding clinical appearance and response

Four major types of ICP monitors are

1. Intraventricular catheter with fibroscopic sensors attached to a monitoring system
2. Subarachnoid bolt (Richmond screw)
3. Epidural sensor
4. Anterior fontanel pressure monitor

Transducers for both ventricular and subarachnoid monitoring should be set up without the use of a flush device. Direct ventricular pressure measurement remains the gold standard of ICP monitoring.

The catheter method involves introduction of a catheter into the lateral ventricle on the nondominant side, if known, or placement in the subdural space. The catheter has the advantage of providing a means of extraventricular (or continuous) drainage to reduce pressure. A drainage bag attached to the system is kept at the level of the ventricles and can be lowered to decrease ICP (see Critical Thinking Exercise).

CRITICAL THINKING EXERCISE

Hydrocephalus

Three-year-old Emma is 5 days postoperative for removal of a posterior fossa tumor. Although an external ventricular drain (EVD) was placed to treat her hydrocephalus, she continues to demonstrate signs of increased intracranial pressure (ICP), including holding the back of her head, anorexia, crying when moved or when strangers enter the room, and intermittent lethargy. On examination, fluid drainage is noted on the mother's clothes, and Emma is experiencing repetitive, rapid eyelid blinking.

1. Evidence—Is there sufficient evidence to draw conclusions about Emma's behavior, physical assessment findings, and ICP?
2. Assumptions—Describe any underlying assumption about each of the following:
   a. A preschool-age child who had a posterior fossa tumor removed 5 days ago
   b. A preschool-age child who has an EVD placed to treat the hydrocephalus
   c. A preschool-age child with an EVD who continues to demonstrate physical signs associated with increased ICP after recent surgery
3. What priorities for nursing care should be established?
4. Does the evidence support your nursing intervention?
5. What alternative perspectives might you have?

NURSING ALERT If the external ventricular drain (EVD) is unclamped for CSF drainage, carefully monitor the level of the collection container. If the container is too low, improper CSF decompression could lower ICP too rapidly, causing bleeding and pain.

With the bolt method the end of the bolt is placed into the subarachnoid space. The bolt cannot be adequately secured in a small child's pliant skull, although special modifications have been developed for children younger than 6 years of age.

NURSING ALERT The bolt is stabilized with dressings, but these are not changed or disturbed, even to check the site.

The placement of the bolt is not adjusted by anyone except the neurosurgeon who placed the device. The neurosurgeon is notified if a satisfactory waveform is not observed.

An epidural sensor can be placed between the dura and the skull through a burr hole and connected to a stopcock assembly and a transducer, which provides a readout of the pressure. Correlation of pressure readings is less invasive but may be inconsistent. In infants a fontanel transducer can be used to detect impulses from a pressure sensor and convert them to electrical energy. The electrical energy is then converted to visible waves or numeric readings on an oscilloscope. ICP measurement from the anterior fontanel is noninvasive but may prove to be inaccurate if the equipment is poorly placed or inconsistently recalibrated. The intraparenchymal pressure monitoring device (e.g., Camino) is a result of fiberoptic technology and performs reliably.

ICP can be increased by instillation of solutions; therefore antibiotics are administered systemically if a positive CSF culture is obtained. However, IV ICP monitoring rarely causes infection. Since CSF is a body fluid, Standard Precautions are implemented according to hospital policy (see Infection Control, Chapter 45).

Nurses caring for patients with intracranial monitoring devices must be acquainted with the system, assist with insertion, interpret the monitor readings, and be able to distinguish between danger signals and mechanical dysfunction.

For increased ICP resulting from cerebral edema, several medical measures are available. Osmotic diuretics may provide rapid relief in emergency situations. Although their effect is transient, lasting only about 6 hours, they can be lifesaving in emergencies. These substances are rapidly excreted by the kidneys and carry with them large quantities of sodium and water. Mannitol (or sometimes urea) administered intravenously is the drug most frequently used for rapid reduction. The infusion is generally given slowly but may be pushed rapidly in cases of herniation or impending herniation. Because of the profound diuretic effect of the drug, an indwelling catheter is inserted to ensure bladder emptying. Adrenocorticosteroids are not recommended for cerebral edema secondary to head trauma. $Paco_2$ should be maintained at 25 to 30 mm Hg to produce vasoconstriction, which reduces CSF, thereby decreasing ICP.

Nursing Activities

In cases of high levels of increased ICP, nursing procedures tend to trigger reactive pressure waves in many patients. For example, increased intrathoracic or abdominal pressure will be transmitted to the cranium. Particular care should be taken in positioning these patients to avoid neck vein compression, which may further increase ICP by interfering with venous return.

The child can be propped to one side or the other, and the use of an alternating-pressure mattress reduces the chance of prolonged pressure to vulnerable areas. Frequent clinical assessment of the child cannot be replaced by an ICP monitoring device.

NURSING ALERT The head of the bed is elevated to 30 degrees, and the child is positioned so that the head is maintained in midline to facilitate venous drainage and avoid jugular compression (Palmer, 2000). Turning side to side is contraindicated because of the risk of jugular compression.

It is important to avoid activities that may increase ICP by causing pain or emotional stress. Gentle range-of-motion exercises can be carried out but should not be performed vigorously. Nontherapeutic touch can cause an increase in ICP. Any disturbing procedures to be performed should be scheduled to take advantage of therapies that reduce ICP, such as osmotherapy and sedation. Efforts are taken to minimize or eliminate environmental noise. Assessment and intervention to relieve pain are important nursing functions to decrease ICP. Individualizing nursing activities and minimizing environmental stimuli by decreasing noxious procedures help control ICP (El Bashir, Laundy, & Booy, 2003; Vernon-Levett, 1998).

Suctioning

Suctioning and percussion are poorly tolerated and are therefore contraindicated unless concurrent respiratory problems exist. Hypoxia and Valsalva's maneuver associated with cough both acutely elevate ICP. Vibration, which does not increase ICP, accomplishes excellent results and should be tried first if treatment is needed. If suctioning is necessary, it should be brief and preceded by hyperventilation with 100% oxygen, which can be monitored during suctioning with a pulse oxygen sensor reading to determine oxygen saturation.

Nutrition and Hydration

Fluids and calories are supplied initially by the IV route (see Chapter 45). An IV infusion is started early, and the type of fluid administered is determined by the patient's general condition. Fluid therapy requires careful monitoring and adjustment based on neurologic signs and electrolyte determinations. Often, comatose children are unable to cope with the same amounts of fluid they could tolerate at other times, and overhydration must be avoided to prevent fatal cerebral edema.

Hydration is maintained in the same manner (initially by IV and later by feeding tube). When cerebral edema is a threat, fluids may be restricted to reduce the chance of fluid overload. Skin and mucous membranes are examined for signs of dehydration. Observation for signs of altered fluid balance related to abnormal pituitary secretions is a part of nursing care.

Altered Pituitary Secretion

An altered ability to handle fluid loads is attributed in part to the syndrome of inappropriate antidiuretic hormone secretion (SIADH) and diabetes insipidus (DI) resulting from hypothalamic dysfunction (see Chapter 52). SIADH frequently accompanies CNS diseases such as head injury, meningitis, encephalitis, brain abscess, brain tumor, and subarachnoid hemorrhage. In the patient with SIADH, scant quantities of urine are excreted, electrolyte analysis reveals hyponatremia and hyposmolality, and manifestations of overhydration are evident. It is important to evaluate all parameters, since the reduced urine output might be erroneously interpreted as a sign of dehydration.

The treatment of SIADH consists of restriction of fluids until serum electrolytes and osmolality return to normal levels. Since SIADH frequently occurs with meningitis in children, fluid restriction is often prescribed. Likewise, DI may occur after intracranial trauma. There is increased urine volume and the accompanying danger of dehydration. Adequate replacement of fluids is essential, and observation of electrolyte balance is necessary to detect signs of hypernatremia and hyperosmolality. Exogenous vasopressin may be administered.

Medications

The cause of unconsciousness determines specific drug therapies. Children with infectious processes are given antibiotics appropriate to the disease and the infecting organism, and corticosteroids are prescribed for inflammatory conditions and edema. Cerebral edema is an indication for osmotherapy with osmotic diuretics. Sedatives or antiepileptics are prescribed for seizure activity (see p. 1585). Sedation in the combative child provides amnesic and anxiolytic properties in conjunction with a paralytic agent. The combination decreases ICP and allows treatment of cerebral edema. Usual drugs include morphine, midazolam, and pancuronium (Pavulon). Midazolam is attractive because of its short half-life.

Deep coma, induced by administration of barbiturates, is controversial in the management of ICP. Barbiturates are currently reserved for the reduction of increased ICP when all else has failed. Barbiturates decrease the cerebral metabolic rate for oxygen and protect the brain during times of reduced cerebral perfusion pressure. Barbiturate coma requires extensive monitoring, cardiovascular and respiratory support, and ICP monitoring to assess response to therapy. Paralyzing agents such as pancuronium also may be needed to aid in performing diagnostic tests, improving effectiveness of therapy, and reducing risks of secondary complications. Elevation of ICP and/or heart rate of patients who are being given paralyzing agents or are under sedation may indicate the need for another dose of either or both medications.

Thermoregulation

Hyperthermia often accompanies cerebral dysfunction; if it is present, measures are implemented to reduce the temperature to prevent brain damage and to reduce metabolic demands generated by the increased body temperature. Medically induced hypothermia assists in controlling ICP and may result in an improved outcome (Palmer, 2000). Antipyretics are the method of choice for fever reduction; cooling devices are used to induce hypothermia. Laboratory tests and other methods are used in an attempt to determine the cause, if any, of the hyperthermia.

Elimination

A retention catheter is usually inserted in the acute phase, although diapers may be used and weighed to record urine output. The child who formerly had bowel and bladder control is generally incontinent. If the child remains comatose for a long period, the indwelling catheter may be removed and periodic bladder emptying accomplished by intermittent catheterization. Stool softeners are usually sufficient to maintain bowel function, but suppositories or enemas may be needed occasionally for adequate elimination and to prevent an impaction. The passage of liquid stool after a period of no bowel activity is usually a sign of an impaction. To avoid this preventable problem, daily recording of bowel activity is essential.

Hygienic Care

Routine measures for cleansing and maintaining skin integrity are an integral part of nursing care of the unconscious child (see Maintaining Healthy Skin, Chapter 45).

Mouth care is performed at least twice daily, since the mouth tends to become dry or coated with mucus. The teeth are carefully brushed with a soft toothbrush or cleaned with gauze saturated with saline. Commercially prepared cleansing devices, such as Toothettes, are convenient for cleansing the mouth and teeth. Lips are coated with ointment or other preparations to protect them from drying, cracking, or blistering.

The deeply comatose child is also prone to eye irritation. The corneal reflexes are absent; therefore the eyes are easily irritated or damaged by linen, dust, or other substances that may come in contact with them. There is excessive dryness as a result of incomplete closure of the eyes and/or decreased secretions, especially if the child is undergoing osmotherapy to reduce or prevent brain edema.

NURSING ALERT The eyes should be examined regularly and carefully for early signs of irritation or inflammation. Artificial tears (methylcellulose) are placed in the eyes every 1 to 2 hours. Eye dressings may sometimes be needed to protect the eyes from possible damage.

Positioning and Exercise

The unconscious child is positioned to prevent aspiration of saliva, nasogastric secretions, and vomitus and to minimize ICP. The head of the bed is elevated, and the child is placed in a side-lying or semiprone position. A small, firm pillow is placed under the head, and the uppermost limbs are flexed and supported with pillows. The weight of the body should not rest on the dependent arm. In the semiprone position the child lies with the dependent arm at the side behind the body, the opposite side supported on pillows, and the uppermost arm and leg flexed and resting on the pillows. This position prevents undue pressure on the dependent extremities. The dependent position of the face encourages drainage of secretions and prevents the flaccid tongue from obstructing the airway.

Normal range-of-motion exercises help maintain function and prevent contractures of joints. Exercises should be done gently and with full range of motion. A small rolled pad can be placed in the palms to help maintain proper position of fingers; footboards or boots can be used to help prevent footdrop; and splinting may be needed to prevent severe contractures of the wrist, knee, or ankle in decerebrate children.

Stimulation

Sensory stimulation is important in the care of the unconscious child, just as it is in the care of the alert child. For the temporarily unconscious or semiconscious child, sensory stimulation helps arouse the child to the conscious state and orient the child in terms of time and place. Auditory and tactile stimulation are especially valuable. Tactile stimulation is not appropriate for the child in whom it may elicit an undesirable response. However, for other children tactile contact often has a relaxing and calming effect. When the child's condition permits, holding or rocking has a soothing effect and provides the body contact needed by young children.

The auditory sense is often present in a state of coma. Hearing is the last sense to be lost and the first one to be regained; therefore the child should be spoken to as any other child. Conversation around the child should not include thoughtless or derogatory remarks. A radio playing soft music or a music box or CD player is frequently used to provide auditory stimulation. Singing the child's favorite songs or reading a favorite story is a tactic used to maintain the child's contact with a familiar world. Playing songs or stories recorded in the parents' voices can provide a continuous source of familiar stimulation.

Regaining Consciousness

Awakening from a coma is a gradual process; however, sometimes children regain consciousness within a short time. Regaining orientation involves knowing person, place, and time, in that order.

Certain behaviors have been observed when children awaken from the unconscious state. The stress and anxiety they appear to feel in a strange and unfamiliar environment are consistently expressed in silent and withdrawn behavior. Children respond to basic questioning but usually do not display their prehospitalization personality and social behavior until they are transferred from the critical care area.

Family Support

Helping parents of an unconscious child cope with the situation is especially difficult. They may demonstrate all the guilt, fear, hostility, and anxiety of any parent of a seriously ill child (see Chapter 44). In addition, these parents are faced with the uncertain outcome of the cerebral dysfunction. The fear of death, intellectual disability, or other permanent disability is present. Nursing intervention with parents depends on the nature of the pathologic condition, the parents' personality, and the parent-child relationship before the injury or illness.

If there is little or no residual effect, the child will be dismissed to home care fairly soon. The parents need the most intensive nursing intervention during the period of crisis and uncertainty. During the recovery phase they are given information, information is clarified, and they are encouraged to become involved in the child's care. Often the child's hospitalization is brief; however, some children require extended hospitalization for intensive therapy and rehabilitation.

Like parents who lose a child through death, the parents of the child lost to their world attempt to reconstitute a representation of the child. They bring items that belong to the child, such as favorite toys, music, and other objects cherished by the child. This is interpreted as an attempt to provide stimulation for the child in the hope of eliciting a response, to let the hospital staff know the child as the unique individual he or she was so that the parents' distress can be better appreciated, and to reconstitute an image of the child "lost" to them and for whom they mourn. An awareness of these behaviors and coping mechanisms provides nurses with the understanding that helps them support the parents in their grief process.

Superimposed on the process of grieving for the "lost" child, parents may be faced with difficult decisions. When the child's brain is so severely damaged that vital functions must be maintained by artificial means, the parents must make the final decision of whether to remove life support systems. Since the decision is so difficult for parents, the practitioner is frequently placed in a position of making the decision indirectly. After providing the parents with all of the information, the practitioner will suggest that the child be removed from the life support to "see if the child can make it without help." The approach relieves the parents of the decision and can be effective, but it is based on an evaluation of the parents' intellectual level and emotional state. Sometimes parents may even choose to refuse treatment if they believe it to be best for the child and the family (informed dissent). At other times parents request that "everything possible" be done for the child.

When the child has survived the cerebral insult and is not comatose, but physical and/or mental capacity is limited, either minimally or severely, families must cope with the long and tedious rehabilitation process and the uncertain outcome (see Patient Teaching box). The drain on financial, emotional, and social resources can be enormous.

PATIENT TEACHING Preparation for Discharge

- For parents who choose to care for their child at home, planning for home care begins early in the recovery process.
- The family should become involved with the child's care as soon as they indicate an interest and ability to do so.
- They need education and support in learning to care for the child, regular follow-up observation and assessment of the home management, and planning for some respite care of the child.
- Parents need to understand that it is important to plan for periodic relief from the continual care of the child.

Cerebral Trauma

Head Injury

Head injury is a pathologic process involving the scalp, skull, meninges, or brain as a result of mechanical force. According to national statistics and Safe Kids Worldwide,* injuries are the number one health risk for children and the leading cause of death in children older than 1 year of age. Yearly, one in four children in the United States will suffer an injury serious enough to require medical attention. Tragically, 8000 children are killed every year by injuries. It has been estimated that 300 per 100,000 children per year have a traumatic brain injury and that 10 per 100,000 children per year die as a result of the brain injury. Studies indicate that as many as three fourths of the childhood deaths caused by mechanical trauma are the direct result of a brain injury. There is evidence to demonstrate

1301 Pennsylvania Ave., NW, Suite 1000, Washington, DC 20004-1707; 202-662-0600; www.safekids.org.

that a previous head injury increases a child's risk of having a subsequent head injury (Swaine et al, 2007).

Etiology

The three major causes of brain damage in childhood, in order of importance, are falls, motor vehicle injuries, and bicycle injuries. Neurologic injury accounts for the highest mortality rate, with boys affected twice as often as girls. In motor vehicle accidents children younger than 2 years of age are almost exclusively injured as passengers, whereas older children may also be injured as pedestrians or cyclists. The majority of deaths from brain trauma caused by bicycle injuries occur between the ages of 5 and 19 years. Bicycle helmet laws have been effective in reducing the risk of head injury by 85% and brain injury by 88% (Rivara & Grossman, 2007).

The exposed nature of the head renders it particularly vulnerable to external violence, and many of the physical characteristics of children predispose them to craniocerebral trauma. For example, infants are frequently left unattended on beds, in high chairs, and in other places from which they can fall. Because the head of an infant or toddler is proportionately larger and heavier in relation to other body parts, it is the most likely to be injured. Incomplete motor development contributes to falls at young ages, and children's natural curiosity and exuberance also increase their risk of injury.

Pathophysiology

The pathology of brain injury is directly related to the force of impact. Intracranial contents (brain, blood, CSF) are damaged because the force is too great to be absorbed by the skull and musculoligamentous support of the head. The elastic, pliable skull of the infant and young child absorbs much of the direct energy of physical impact to the head and affords some protection to intracranial structures. Although nervous tissue is delicate, it usually requires a severe blow to cause significant damage.

A child's response to head injury is different from that of an adult. The larger head size and insufficient musculoskeletal support render the very young child particularly vulnerable to acceleration-deceleration injuries.

Primary head injuries are those that occur at the time of trauma and include skull fracture, contusions, intracranial hematoma, and diffuse injury. Subsequent complications include hypoxic brain damage, increased ICP, infection, and cerebral edema. The predominant feature of a child's brain injury is the amount of diffuse swelling that occurs. Hypoxia and hypercapnia threaten the energy requirements of the brain and increase CBF. The added volume across the blood-brain barrier, along with the loss of autoregulation, exacerbates cerebral edema. Pressure inside the skull that is greater than arterial pressure results in inadequate perfusion.

Cerebral hyperemia occurs more often in children than adults, and this volume expansion may account for their tendency to develop intracranial hypertension. However, because the cranium of very young children has the ability to expand and the thin skull is more compliant, they may tolerate increases in ICP better than older children and adults do. Children have a significantly higher percentage of good outcomes, a lower mortality rate, and a lower incidence of surgical mass lesions after severe head trauma. However, their thinner, softer skull may sustain greater long-term damage than previously suggested.

Physical forces act on the head through *acceleration, deceleration,* or *deformation.* Acceleration or deceleration is more descriptive of the circumstances responsible for most head injuries. When the stationary head receives a blow, the sudden acceleration causes deformation of the skull and mass movement of the brain. Continued movement of the intracranial contents allows the brain to strike parts of the skull (e.g., the sharp edges of the sphenoid or the irregular surface of the anterior fossa) or the edges of the tentorium.

Although the brain volume remains unchanged, significant distortion takes place as the brain changes shape in response to the force of impact to the skull. This movement can cause bruising at the point of impact *(coup)* and/or at a distance as the brain collides with the unyielding surfaces far removed from the point of impact *(contrecoup)* (Fig. 51-4). Thus a blow to the occipital region can cause severe injury to the frontal and temporal areas of the brain. Sudden deceleration, such as takes place during a fall, causes the greatest cerebral injury at the point of impact. Children with an acceleration-deceleration injury demonstrate diffuse generalized cerebral swelling produced by increased blood volume or a redistribution of cerebral blood volume (cerebral hyperemia) rather than by increased water content (edema), as seen in adults.

Another effect of brain movement is shearing stresses, which may tear small arteries and cause subdural hemorrhages. Damage can also occur when severe compression of the skull forces the brain through the tentorial opening. This can produce irreparable damage to the brainstem (Fig. 51-5).

Concussion

The most common head injury is *concussion,* a transient and reversible neuronal dysfunction, with instantaneous loss

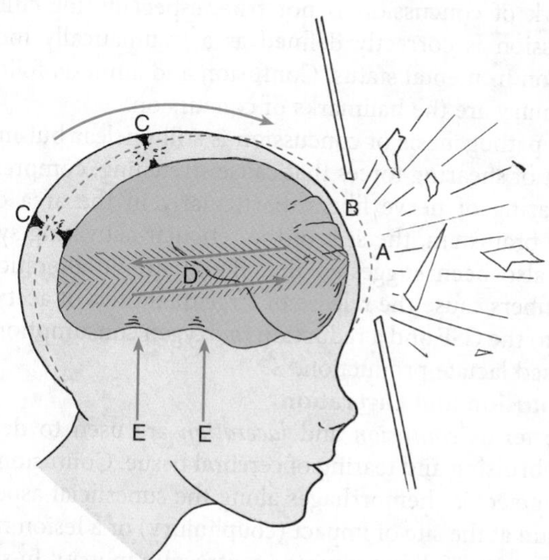

Fig. 51-4 Mechanical distortion of cranium during closed head injury. *A,* Preinjury contour of skull. *B,* Immediate postinjury contour of skull. *C,* Torn subdural vessels. *D,* Shearing forces. *E,* Trauma from contact with floor of cranium. (Redrawn from Grubb RL, Coxe WS: Central nervous system trauma: cranial. In Eliasson SG, Presky AL, Hardin Jr WB (editors): *Neurological pathophysiology,* New York, 1974, Oxford University Press.)

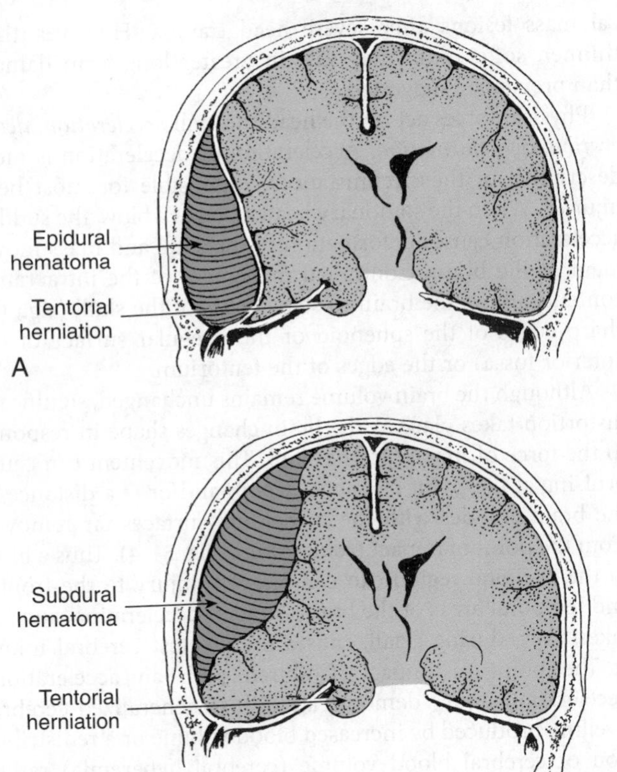

Fig. 51-5 **A,** Epidural (extradural) hematoma and compression of temporal lobe through tentorial hiatus. **B,** Subdural hematoma.

of awareness and responsiveness, that results from trauma to the head and persists for a relatively short time, usually minutes or hours. It is generally followed by amnesia for the moment of the injury and a variable period after the injury. The common misconception that loss of consciousness is the hallmark of concussion is not true, especially for children. Concussion is correctly defined as a traumatically induced alteration in mental status. Confusion and amnesia following head injury are the hallmarks of concussion.

The pathogenesis of concussion is still unclear but may be a result of shearing forces that cause stretching, compression, and tearing of nerve fibers, particularly in the area of the central brainstem, the seat of the reticular activating system. It has also been suggested that the anatomic alterations of nerve fibers cause the release of large quantities of acetylcholine into the CSF and a reduction in oxygen consumption with increased lactate production.

Contusion and Laceration

The terms *contusion* and *laceration* are used to describe visible bruising and tearing of cerebral tissue. Contusions represent petechial hemorrhages along the superficial aspects of the brain at the site of impact (coup injury) or a lesion remote from the site of direct trauma (contrecoup injury). In serious accidents there may be multiple sites of injury.

The major areas of the brain susceptible to contusion or laceration are the occipital, frontal, and temporal lobes. Also, the irregular surfaces of the anterior and middle fossae at the base of the skull are capable of producing bruises or lacerations on forceful impact. Contusions may cause focal disturbances in strength, sensation, or visual awareness. The degree of brain damage in the contused areas varies according to the extent of vascular injury. Signs will vary from mild, transient weakness of a limb to prolonged unconsciousness and paralysis. However, the signs and symptoms may be clinically indistinguishable from those of concussion.

The lower incidence of cerebral contusion in infancy has been attributed to the infant's pliable skull with less convolutional markings of the inner space between brain tissue and bone. In addition, the infant's brain tissue has a softer consistency, which also reduces surface injury. However, infants who are roughly shaken (shaken baby syndrome) can sustain profound neurologic impairment, seizures, retinal hemorrhages, and intracranial subarachnoid or subdural hemorrhages. In addition to these classic injuries, high cervical spinal cord hemorrhages and contusions can occur.

Cerebral lacerations are generally associated with penetrating or depressed skull fractures. However, they may occur without fracture in small children. When brain tissue is actually torn, with bleeding into and around the tear, usually more severe and prolonged unconsciousness and paralysis occur, leaving permanent scarring and some degree of disability.

Fractures

Because of its flexibility, the immature skull is able to sustain a greater degree of deformation than the adult skull before it incurs a fracture. A great deal of force is required to produce a fracture in an infant's skull. However, the undersurface of the skull contains grooves in which the meningeal arteries lie. A fracture that runs through one of these grooves may tear the artery and produce severe and damaging hemorrhage. Hypovolemic hypotension can occur in infants with skull fractures.

The types of fractures that occur are as follows:

Linear fractures are those in which the lines of the fracture are predetermined by the site and velocity of the impact, as well as by the strength of the bone. These are uncommon before 2 to 3 years of age but constitute the majority of childhood skull fractures. Most linear skull fractures are associated with an overlying hematoma or soft-tissue swelling (Schutzman & Greenes, 2001).

Depressed fractures are those in which the bone is locally broken, usually into several irregular fragments that are pushed inward, causing pressure on the brain. The inner portion of the bone is more extensively fragmented than the outer portion, which almost invariably produces tears in the dura. These are uncommon before 2 to 3 years of age. In infants and very young children, the soft, malleable bone may become dented in a peculiar rounded or "Ping-Pong ball" depression, without laceration of either skin or dura.

Comminuted fractures consist of multiple associated linear fractures. They usually result from intense impact. These types of fractures often result from repeated blows against an object and may suggest child abuse.

Basilar fractures involve the basilar portion of the frontal, ethmoid, sphenoid, temporal, or occipital bones. Because of the proximity of the fracture line to structures surrounding the brainstem, this is a serious head injury. Approximately 80% of the cases may include clinical features such as subcutaneous bleeding in the posterior neck area and over the mastoid process (battle sign). Bleeding around the eyes (raccoon eyes) or bleeding behind the tympanic membrane (hemotympanum) may occur.

Open fractures cause communication between the skull and the scalp or the surfaces of the upper respiratory tract. Open fractures increase the risk of CNS infection. They may have an overlying laceration called a *compound fracture.* Open fractures can also create an opening in the paranasal sinuses or middle ear that can lead to CSF rhinorrhea or otorrhea. Facial paralysis, vertigo, tinnitus, or hearing loss may develop.

Diastatic fractures are traumatic separations of the cranial sutures. These most frequently affect the lambdoid suture and are rarely seen beyond the first 3 years of life. They require no specific treatment but should be observed for "growing fractures."

Growing fractures are skull fractures associated with an underlying dural tear that may be caused by a leptomeningeal cyst, dilated ventricles, or a herniated brain. Neurologic symptoms include headache, seizures, and asymmetric cranial growth (Schutzman & Greenes, 2001). Infants and young children who have isolated skull fractures should be evaluated for growing skull fractures from 1 to 2 months after the injury (Schutzman & Greenes, 2001).

Complications

The major complications of trauma to the head are hemorrhage, infection, edema, and herniation through the tentorium. Infection is always a hazard in open injuries, and edema is related to tissue trauma. Vascular rupture may occur even in minor head injuries, causing hemorrhage between the skull and cerebral surfaces. Compression of the underlying brain produces effects that can be rapidly fatal or insidiously progressive.

NURSING ALERT Posttraumatic meningitis should be suspected in children with increasing drowsiness and fever who also have basilar skull fractures.

Epidural Hemorrhage

The blood accumulates between the dura and the skull to form a hematoma, which, because of the difficulty with which dura is stripped from bone, forces the underlying brain contents downward and inward as the brain expands (see Fig. 51-5, *A*). Since bleeding is generally arterial, brain compression occurs rapidly. Most often the expanding hematoma is located in the parietotemporal region, forcing the medial portion of the temporal lobe under the edge of the tentorium, where it causes pressure on nerves and blood vessels. The lower incidence of epidural hematoma in childhood has been attributed to the fact that the middle meningeal artery is not embedded in the bone surface of the skull until approximately 2 years of age. Therefore a fracture of the temporal bone is less likely to lacerate the artery. Second, the dura closely adheres to the inner table of the skull, especially at the level of the sutures, making separation from bleeding less likely. However, a child's skull can be indented with sufficient force to tear the middle meningeal artery and rebound intact without causing a fracture. Hemorrhage can also derive from dural veins or the dural sinuses, especially in infants and small children, in whom fracture is less likely to occur. In 20% to 40% of children a skull fracture is not detectable. The classic clinical picture of epidural hemorrhage (momentary unconsciousness followed by a normal period, then lethargy or coma) is seldom evident in children (see Box 51-3 for clinical manifestations). The period of impaired consciousness is frequently lacking, and the symptom-free period is atypical because of nonspecific complaints such as irritability, headache, and vomiting. When it does occur, the symptom-free period frequently lasts longer than 48 hours.

Clinically significant epidural hematomas are uncommon in children younger than 4 years of age. These differences may be caused by the decreased tendency of the resilient skull to fracture; the ability of blood to escape through widened sutures, an open fontanel, or a fracture; bleeding from smaller vessels with less rapid and massive bleeding; lower systolic blood pressure in children; and possibly the decreased susceptibility of the child's brain to pressure changes.

Subdural Hemorrhage

A subdural hemorrhage is bleeding between the dura and the cerebrum, usually as a result of rupture of cortical veins

BOX 51-3 Clinical Manifestations of Acute Head Injury

Minor Injury
May or may not lose consciousness
Transient period of confusion
Somnolence
Listlessness
Irritability
Pallor
Vomiting

Signs of Progression
Altered mental status (e.g., difficulty rousing child)
Mounting agitation
Development of focal lateral neurologic signs
Marked changes in vital signs

Severe Injury
Signs of increased intracranial pressure (see Box 51-1)
Increased head size (infant)
Bulging or full fontanel (infant)
Retinal hemorrhage
Extraocular palsies (especially cranial nerve VI)
Hemiparesis
Quadriplegia
Elevated temperature
Unsteady gait (older child)
Papilledema (older child)
Retinal hemorrhages

Associated Signs
Scalp trauma
Other injuries (e.g., to extremities)

evolve Animation—Subdural Hematoma

that bridge the subdural space (see Fig. 51-5, *B*). Subdural hematomas are 10 times more frequent than epidural hematomas, occurring most often in infancy, with a peak incidence at 6 months.

Unlike epidural hemorrhage, which develops inwardly against the less resistant brain tissue, subdural hemorrhage tends to develop more slowly and spreads thinly and widely until it is limited by the dural barriers—the falx and tentorium. Subdural hematoma is fairly common in infants, frequently as a result of birth trauma, falls, assaults, or violent shaking. The small subdural space and dura firmly attached to the skull in this area are highly vulnerable to increased ICP.

NURSING ALERT Children with a subdural hematoma and retinal hemorrhages should be evaluated for the possibility of child abuse, especially shaken baby syndrome.

Repeated subdural taps often provide relief in the infant, as revealed by follow-up CT scans, improved neurologic status, and a flat anterior fontanel. Surgical evacuation of the hematoma is the treatment of choice in the older child and is frequently required in infants.

Cerebral Edema

Some degree of brain edema is expected, especially 24 to 72 hours after craniocerebral trauma. Cerebral edema caused by direct cellular injury or vascular injury induces vascular stasis, anoxia, and further vasodilation. If the progression continues unchecked, ICP exceeds arterial pressure and fatal anoxia ensues, and/or the pressure causes herniation of a portion of the brain over the edge of the tentorium, compressing the brainstem and occluding the posterior cerebral arteries. Diffuse cerebral swelling and changes in CBF are common patterns after head injury in children.

NURSING ALERT If a child loses consciousness or vomits more than three times, medical attention should be sought.

Diagnostic Evaluation

A detailed history, especially a health history, both past and present, is essential in evaluating the child with a craniocerebral trauma. Certain disorders, such as drug allergies, hemophilia, diabetes mellitus, or epilepsy, may produce similar symptoms. Furthermore, even minor traumatic injury can aggravate a preexisting disease process. Events surrounding the injury often supply significant data. It must be determined whether the infant or child exhibited alterations in consciousness; any other signs and behaviors exhibited by the child must be noted. Since head injuries are frequently accompanied by injuries in other areas, the examination is performed with care to avoid further damage.

NURSING ALERT Stabilize a child's spine after head injury until a spinal cord injury is ruled out.

Initial Assessment

Priorities in the initial stabilization phase of a child with a head injury include assessment of the ABCs (airway, breathing, circulation); evaluation for shock; a neurologic examination, especially LOC; assessment of pupillary symmetry and response to light; and observation for seizures (Bayir, Kochanek, & Clark, 2003). The assessment is carried out quickly in relation to vital signs (see Emergency box). Excited and irritable children may have a rapid pulse, hyperventilate, appear pale, and feel clammy shortly after an injury.

EMERGENCY

Head Injury

Assess child:

- A—Airway (with cervical-spine immobilization)
  - Use jaw thrust to open airway
- B—Bleeding
- C—Circulation

Clean any abrasions with soap and water.

- Apply clean dressing.
- If bleeding, apply ice to relieve pain and swelling.

Keep NPO (nothing by mouth) until instructed otherwise.

Assess pain, but do not give analgesics or sedatives.

Check pupil reaction every 4 hours (including twice during night) for 48 hours.

Awaken twice during the night to check level of consciousness.

Seek medical attention if any of the following apply:

- Injury sustained:
  - At high speed (e.g., automobile)
  - Fall from a significant distance (e.g., roof, tree, or height greater than that of the child)
  - From great force (e.g., baseball bat)
  - Under suspicious circumstances
- Loss of consciousness
- Amnesia
- Discomfort (crying) more than 10 minutes after injury
- Headache that is severe, worsening, interferes with sleep
- Fluid leak from ears or nose
- Vomiting three or more times
- Swelling in front of or above earlobe or increased swelling
- Confusion or abnormal behavior
- Difficult to arouse from sleep
- Difficulty speaking
- Blurred vision or seeing double
- Unsteady gait
- Difficulty using extremities
- Neck pain
- Pupils dilated, unequal, or fixed
- Infant with full or bulging fontanel
- Bruising below the eyes

NURSING ALERT Signs of brainstem involvement include deep, rapid, periodic, or intermittent and gasping respirations; wide fluctuations or noticeable slowing of the pulse; and widening pulse pressure or extreme fluctuations in blood pressure. Note that marked hypotension may represent internal injuries.

Ocular signs such as fixed and dilated pupils, fixed and constricted pupils, and pupils that are poorly reactive or nonreactive to light and accommodation indicate increased ICP or brainstem involvement. It is important to remain with the child who demonstrates fixed and dilated pupils, since these are ominous signs, with the probability of respiratory arrest. Dilated, nonpulsating blood vessels indicate increased ICP before the appearance of papilledema. Retinal hemorrhages are seen in acute head injuries.

NURSING ALERT Observation of asymmetric pupils or one dilated, nonreactive pupil in a comatose child is a neurosurgical emergency.

Less urgent but important additional assessments include examination of the scalp for lacerations and palpation for other abnormalities. A significant amount of blood loss can occur from scalp lacerations.

NURSING ALERT Bleeding from the nose or ears needs further evaluation, and a watery discharge from the nose (rhinorrhea) that is positive for glucose (as tested with Dextrostix) suggests leaking of CSF from a skull fracture.

An accurate assessment of clinical signs provides baseline information. Serial evaluations, preferably by a single observer, help to detect changes in the neurologic status. Alterations in mental status, evidenced by increased difficulty in rousing the child, mounting agitation, development of focal lateral neurologic signs, or marked changes in vital signs, usually indicate extension or progression of the basic pathologic process.

Special Tests

After a thorough clinical examination, a variety of diagnostic tests are helpful in providing a more definitive diagnosis of the type and extent of the trauma. The severity of a head injury may not be apparent on clinical examination of a child, but it will be detectable on a CT scan. Whenever the child has a history consistent with a serious head injury (e.g., unrestrained occupant in a severe motor vehicle accident or a fall from a significant height), it is important that a scan be performed even if the child initially appears alert and oriented. All children with head injuries who have any alteration of consciousness, headache, vomiting, skull fracture, seizure, or a predisposing medical condition should also undergo CT scanning.

MRI and neurobehavioral assessment after early head injury may be useful in documenting cognitive impairment in relation to structural alterations in the young brain. MRI provides details of soft tissues better than any other noninvasive device. Electroencephalography is not particularly helpful for early diagnosis but is useful for defining seizure activity or focal destructive lesions after the acute phase of illness. Lumbar puncture is rarely used in craniocerebral trauma and is contraindicated in the presence of increased ICP because of the possibility of herniation. In some centers monitoring ICP is part of the assessment.

Posttraumatic Syndromes

Posttraumatic syndromes can be clinically manifested because of structural complications resulting from a head injury and through the signs and symptoms demonstrated by the child. Structural complications can include hydrocephalus and focal deficits such as optic atrophy, cranial nerve palsies, motor deficits, DI, aphasia, and seizures. Behavioral disturbances include sleep disturbances, phobias, emotional lability, altered school performance, and changes related to aggressiveness or withdrawal. *Postconcussion syndrome* is a common sequela to brain injury and can occur within minutes to an hour after a head injury. The manifestations vary with the child's age. The syndrome occurs frequently in children younger than 1 year of age. The syndrome in adolescents is similar to that in adults. The duration of manifestations can vary from several days to several months. Death from concussion is preventable unless overwhelming secondary brain injury has occurred (Durkin et al, 1998; Gennarelli, 1999).

Posttraumatic seizures occur in a number of children who survive a head injury and are more common in children than in adults. Seizures are more likely to occur within the first few days of the head injury (Chiaretti et al, 2000). *Structural complications* (e.g., hydrocephalus) may occur after a head injury. The type of residual effect depends on the location and nature of the disorder. True intellectual disability occurs only after severe injuries.

Therapeutic Management

The majority of children with mild to moderate concussion who have not lost consciousness can be cared for and observed at home after careful examination reveals no serious intracranial injury. Nurses should provide parents with clear explanations and instructions and should encourage them to ask questions both before and after leaving the medical facility if clarification is needed (see Family-Centered Care box).

FAMILY-CENTERED CARE

Maintaining Contact

Maintaining contact with parents for continued observation and reevaluation of the child, when indicated, facilitates early diagnosis and treatment of possible complications from head injury, such as hematoma, hydrocephalus, cysts, and posttraumatic seizures. Children are generally hospitalized for 24 to 48 hours' observation if their family lives far from medical facilities or lacks transportation or a telephone that would provide access to immediate help. Other circumstances such as language or other communication barriers, or even emotional trauma, may hinder learning and make it difficult for families to feel confident in caring for their child at home.

The parents are instructed to check the child every 2 hours to determine any changes in responsiveness. The sleeping child should be wakened to see if he or she can be roused normally. Parents are advised to maintain contact with the health professional, who usually wishes to examine the child again in 1 or 2 days. The manifestations of epidural hematoma in children do not generally appear until 24 hours or more after injury.

Children with severe injuries, those who have lost consciousness for more than a few minutes, and those with prolonged and continued seizures or other focal or diffuse neurologic signs must be hospitalized until their condition is stable and their neurologic signs have diminished.

The child is maintained on nothing by mouth (NPO) or restricted to clear liquids, if able to take fluids by mouth, until it is determined that vomiting will not occur. IV fluids are indicated in the child who is comatose or displays dulled sensorium and in the child with persistent vomiting. Fluid balance is closely monitored by daily weights; accurate intake and output measurements; and serum osmolality to detect early signs of water retention, excessive dehydration, and states of hypertonicity or hypotonicity.

The volume of IV fluid is carefully monitored to avoid aggravating any cerebral edema and to minimize the possibility of overhydration in case of SIADH. However, damage to the hypothalamus or pituitary gland may produce DI with its accompanying hypertonicity and dehydration.

Restlessness can be satisfactorily managed, if necessary, with mild sedation, and headache is usually controlled with acetaminophen. Antiepileptics are used for seizure control and frequently in cases of suspected contusion or laceration. Antibiotics may be administered if lacerations, CSF leakage, or excessive cerebral tissue damage is present. Prophylactic tetanus toxoid is given as appropriate. Cerebral edema is managed as described for the unconscious child. Hyperthermia is controlled with tepid sponges or a hypothermia blanket.

Surgical Therapy

Scalp lacerations are sutured after the underlying bone is carefully examined. Depressed fractures require surgical reduction and removal of bone fragments. Torn dura is sutured. Ping-Pong ball skull fractures in very young infants ordinarily correct themselves within a few weeks and do not require specific treatment, although they can be reduced by pressure against the bone.

Prognosis

The outcome of craniocerebral trauma depends on the extent of injury and complications. However, the outlook is generally more favorable for children than for adults (Faillace, 2002; Masson et al, 2003). More than 90% of children with concussions or simple linear fractures recover without symptoms after the initial period. The incidence of fatalities and neurologic sequelae is lower in children than in adults, even in those with severe head injuries. The prognosis for recovery is primarily related to the duration of coma and the degree of injury. The combination of impaired consciousness and skull fracture carries the highest risk of complication.

The concern regarding outcome is increasingly focused on cognitive, emotional, and mental problems. Children experience a higher frequency of psychologic disturbances after head injury, whereas adults are more prone to physical complaints. Children may be more vulnerable than adults to long-term cognitive and behavioral dysfunction after diffuse brain injury. Even with recovery, the effects of brain injury on a child's potential can never be known.

True coma (not obeying commands, eyes closed, and not speaking) usually does not last more than 2 weeks. A child's eventual outcome can range from brain death to a persistent vegetative state to complete recovery. However, even the best recovery may be associated with personality changes, including mood lability and loss of confidence; impaired short-term memory; headaches; and subtle cognitive impairments. Many children are left with significant disabilities after a head injury that appear months later as learning difficulties, behavioral changes, or emotional disturbances (Faillace, 2002). Generally, within 6 months to 1 year after the injury, 90% of the long-term neurologic outcome has been achieved.

Nursing Care Management

The hospitalized child requires careful neurologic assessment and evaluation (including vital signs) repeated at frequent intervals to provide information needed to establish a correct diagnosis, reveal signs and symptoms of increased ICP, determine clinical management, prevent many complications, and provide support to the child and family during the recovery phases.

The child is placed on bed rest, usually with the head of the bed elevated slightly. Appropriate safety measures, such as side rails kept up and seizure precautions for children of all ages, are implemented. For the extremely restless child, hard surfaces may have to be padded and restraints used to prevent the possibility of further injury. Care is individualized according to the child's specific needs. The unconscious child is managed as described in the previous section, but most childhood head injuries are those causing momentary stunning or temporary unconsciousness. Children may be restless and irritable, but more often their reaction is to fall asleep when left undisturbed. A quiet environment helps reduce restlessness and irritability. Shining bright lights directly into the child's face is irritating and often aggravates the child, making assessment of ocular responses difficult.

Frequent examinations of vital signs, neurologic signs, and LOC are extremely important nursing observations. When possible, they should be performed by a single observer to better detect subtle changes that may indicate worsening neurologic status. Pupils are checked for size, equality, reaction to light, and accommodation. After the initial elevations usually seen following injury, the vital signs generally return to normal unless there is brainstem involvement. An axillary measurement of temperature is the safest method, since seizures are not uncommon and vomiting is a frequent response in children, especially when the child is disturbed.

The most important nursing observation is assessment of the child's LOC. Alterations in consciousness appear earlier in the progression of an injury than alterations of vital signs or focal neurologic signs. Some expected responses may be misinterpreted as deviations from the normal. Frequent examinations of alertness are fatiguing to the child; therefore the child often desires to fall asleep, which may be confused with depressed consciousness. When left alone, the child goes to sleep. It is not uncommon to observe ocular divergence through the partially closed eyelids.

A key nursing role is to provide sedation and analgesia for the child. The conflict between the need to promote comfort and relieve anxiety in the child vs. the need to assess for neurologic changes presents a dilemma. However, both goals can be achieved with close observation of the child's LOC and response to analgesics, use of a pain assessment record, and effective communication with the practitioner. To differentiate between sedation from an opioid and sedation from the injury, naloxone can be given *slowly* to reverse the opioid's sedative effect. Decreasing restlessness after administration of an analgesic most likely reflects pain control rather than a declining LOC.

Observations of position and movement provide additional information. Any abnormal posturing is noted, as well as whether it occurs continuously or intermittently. Are the child's handgrips strong and equal in strength? Are there any signs of flexion-extension posturing? What is the child's response to stimulation? Is movement purposeful, random, or absent? Are movement and sensation equal on both sides or restricted to one side only?

The child may complain of headache or other discomfort. The child who is too young to describe a headache will be fussy and resist being handled. The child who suffers from vertigo will often assume a position of comfort and vigorously resist efforts to be moved. Forcible movement causes the child to vomit and display spontaneous nystagmus. Seizures, relatively common in children with craniocerebral trauma, may be of any type but are more often generalized, regardless of the type of injury. Any seizure activity should be carefully observed and described in detail. Children in postictal (postseizure) states are lethargic, with sluggish pupils.

Drainage from any orifice is noted. Bleeding from the ear suggests the possibility of a basal skull fracture. The amount and characteristics of the drainage are observed, and since the auditory canal may be a source of infection, dry, sterile cotton can be placed loosely at the orifice and changed when soiled.

Head trauma is frequently accompanied by other undetected injuries; therefore any bruises, lacerations, or evidence of internal injuries or fractures of the extremities are noted and reported. Associated injuries are evaluated and treated appropriately.

The child with normal LOC is usually allowed clear liquids unless fluid is restricted. If the child has an IV infusion, it is maintained as prescribed. The diet is advanced to that appropriate for the child's age as soon as the condition permits. Intake and output are measured and recorded, and any incontinence of bowel or bladder is noted in the child who has been toilet trained.

The child should be observed for any unusual behavior, but behavior should be interpreted in relation to the child's normal behavior. For example, urinary incontinence during sleep would be of no consequence in a child who routinely wets the bed but would be highly significant for one who is always dry. In addition, a child who is subject to nightmares might cry out and demonstrate agitated behavior at night. There would be less concern about a child who falls asleep several times during the day if this were consistent with the child's usual behavior. Parents are valuable resources. Information obtained from parents at or shortly after admission is helpful in evaluating the child's behavior (e.g., the ease with which the child is roused normally, the usual sleeping position, how much the child sleeps during the day, motor activity the child is capable of [rolling over, sitting up, climbing], hearing and visual acuity, appetite, and manner of eating [spoon, bottle, cup]).

Family Support

The emotional and educational support of the family of children who have suffered head injury presents a formidable, challenging aspect to nursing care. Witnessing the parents' ordeal of grief and helplessness on seeing their child in an altered state, connected to monitoring equipment in an intensive care unit, evokes empathy. The nurse can encourage the family to be involved in the child's care, to bring in familiar belongings, or to make a tape recording of familiar voices and sounds. Parents may need a demonstration on how to touch or cuddle their child and may want to talk about their grief. The nurse can listen attentively, reinforce what is being done to assist the child, and direct parents toward signs and symptoms of recovery to instill hope without promises. A common phenomenon is for families to seek information from all health care providers, asking, "What will she be like? What do you know?" as they search for some clue that the child is recovering. Honesty and kindness, along with competent care, distinguish excellent nursing abilities.

When the child is discharged, the parents are advised of probable posttraumatic symptoms that may be expected, such as behavioral changes, sleep disturbances, phobias, and seizures. They should understand observations they need to make and how to contact the physician, nurse, or health facility in case the child develops any unusual signs or symptoms. The importance of follow-up evaluation should be emphasized. It is often advisable to refer the family to a public health agency for home follow-through to be certain that the child receives posthospital evaluation.

Rehabilitation

The rehabilitation and management of the child with permanent brain injury are essential aspects of care. Rehabilitation of brain-injured children is begun as soon as feasible and usually involves the family and a rehabilitation team. Careful assessment of the child's capabilities, limitations, and probable potential is made as early as possible, and appropriate interventions are implemented to maximize the residual capacities. The Brain Injury Association of America* provides information and listings of rehabilitation services and support groups throughout the country.

Pediatric trauma rehabilitation is a national concern. Coordinating care and services for early rehabilitation involves identifying the child and family's response to the traumatic injury and disability, securing available resources, and recognizing the parental role in the process.

The child with a disability resulting from head trauma requires assessment on a physical, cognitive, emotional, and social level. The child has experienced separation, pain, sensory deprivation and overload, changes in circadian cycle, and fear of the unknown. Recovery and transition require new coping strategies at the same time that regressive and acting-out behavior may start. Parents and children need honest communication for decision making. A rehabilitation facility or home rehabilitation is advocated when the child has progressed beyond what can be provided in a hospital setting. The Rancho Los Amigos Scale provides a systematic assessment of the possible progress a child may achieve after a severe head injury.

Prevention

Tremendous strides have been taken in the prevention of cerebral damage after head injury in children. New developments requiring research point to the prevention of cellular

**1608 Spring Hill Road, Suite 110, Vienna, VA 22182; 703-761-0750; fax: 703-761-0755;* www.biausa.org.

injury or the primary insult. However, the greatest benefit lies in prevention of head injuries. Nurses can exert a valuable influence on behalf of children through education. The reason injuries remain preventable is that unnecessary risks go unchecked. Inadequate supervision combined with a child's natural sense of indestructibility and exploration can lead to lethal results. Nurses are in the unique position of influencing caregivers in terms of growth and development. Banning the use of infant walkers is an example. This equipment does not help develop motor skills and places infants at risk for head and neck injuries from falls, especially down steps. Public education, coupled with legislative support, can prevent childhood injuries. (For extensive discussions of childhood injuries and prevention, see Chapters 36 to 40. See also Childhood Mortality, Chapter 29.)

Near-Drowning

Drowning is a major cause of accidental death in children over 1 year of age. Most cases of drowning are accidental, usually involving the following individuals:

- Children who are helpless in water, such as inadequately attended children in or near swimming pools or infants in bathtubs
- Small children who fall into ponds, streams, and flooded excavations, usually near home
- Occupants of pleasure boats who fail to wear life preservers
- Children who have diving accidents
- Children who are able to swim but overestimate their endurance

Accidental drowning occurs five times more often in boys than in girls; almost 40% of children are younger than age 5, and 90% of cases occur in private swimming pools (Kallas, 2004). Drowning can take place in any body of water, including such unlikely ones as a pail of water. Top-heavy toddlers fall head first into a pail of water, their arms become trapped, and they are unable to free themselves. Hot tubs and whirlpool spas have been implicated in childhood drowning injury. The suction created at the outlet is strong enough to trap even larger children underwater. Drowning as a form of fatal child abuse has also been recognized as a problem. Homicidal drownings are unwitnessed, they usually occur in the home, and the victims are either infants or toddlers. With expeditious treatment many children are being saved.

For purposes of this discussion, two terms need clarification:

1. **Drowning**—Death from asphyxia while submerged, regardless of whether fluid has entered the lungs
2. **Near-drowning**—Survival at least 24 hours after submersion in a fluid medium

Pathophysiology

The major pulmonary changes that occur in drowning are directly related to the length of submersion (regardless of the type and amount of fluid aspirated), the victim's physiologic response, and the development and degree of immersion hypothermia. In addition, cerebral recovery depends on the effectiveness of initial resuscitation and subsequent critical care measures to support cerebral salvage.

Physiologic factors that influence the extent of damage from immersion include resistance to asphyxia and anoxia, which shows some individual variation. There is greater resistance with diminishing age; young children can withstand longer periods of submersion. More important is the drowning, or diving, reflex. This neurologic response is triggered by immersion of the face in cold water. Blood is shunted away from the periphery, and the flow is concentrated in the brain and heart predominantly.

The problems created by near-drowning are (1) hypoxia and asphyxiation, (2) aspiration, and (3) hypothermia (except for near-drowning in hot tubs). Cardiopulmonary arrest is secondary to asphyxiation.

Hypoxia is the primary problem because it results in global cell damage, and different cells tolerate variable lengths of anoxia. Neurons, especially cerebral cells, sustain irreversible damage after 4 to 6 minutes of submersion. The heart and lungs can survive up to 30 minutes. Regardless of the amount of water aspirated, there is arterial hypoxemia (resulting from atelectasis with shunting of blood through the nonventilated alveoli) and a combined respiratory acidosis (resulting from retained carbon dioxide) and metabolic acidosis (caused by buildup of acid metabolites from anaerobic metabolism). The pathologic events are directly related to the duration of submersion. The major difficulty is acute ventilatory insufficiency. Approximately 10% of drowning victims die without aspirating fluid but succumb from acute asphyxia as a result of prolonged reflex laryngospasm.

Aspiration of fluid occurs in the majority of drownings. The aspirated fluid results in pulmonary edema, atelectasis, airway spasm, and pneumonitis, which aggravates the hypoxia. It was previously thought that submersion in salt water vs. fresh water altered the physiologic response to near-drowning. However, there is no clinically significant difference in the response of human survivors, and the type of water does not alter the therapy or outcome.

Hypothermia occurs rapidly in infants and children, partly because of their large surface area relative to body mass and partly as a result of the cold water itself. Water is an excellent heat conductor, and contact with the skin is increased by struggling. Hypothermia may make resumption or maintenance of cardiac function possible if body temperature is less than 30° C (86° F). Profound hypothermia is usually evidence of lengthy submersion.

Therapeutic Management

Resuscitative measures should begin at the scene of a drowning, and the victim should be transported to the hospital with maximal ventilatory and circulatory support. Many victims need care for some time after aspiration of fluid. In the hospital, intensive pulmonary care is implemented and continued according to the patient's needs.

In general, the management of the near-drowning victim is based on the degree of cerebral insult (Box 51-4). The first priority is to restore oxygen delivery to the cells and prevent further hypoxic damage. A spontaneously breathing child will do well in an oxygen-enriched atmosphere; the more severely affected child will require endotracheal intubation and mechanical ventilation. Blood gases and pH are moni-

BOX 51-4 Clinical Manifestations of Near-Drowning

Category A
Awake, minimal injury
Fully conscious; may have mild hypothermia, mild chest radiograph changes, mild arterial blood gas abnormalities

Category B
Blunted sensorium, moderate injury
Obtund, stuporous, purposeful response to painful stimuli, mild to moderate hypothermia, frequent respiratory distress, abnormal chest radiographs, arterial blood gas abnormalities

Category C
Comatose, severe anoxia
Unarousable, abnormal response to pain, abnormal respiratory pattern, seizures, shock, marked arterial blood gas abnormalities, abnormal chest radiographs, arrhythmias, metabolic acidosis, hyperkalemia, hyperglycemia, disseminated intravascular coagulation
C1—Decorticate posturing, Cheyne-Stokes respirations
C2—Decerebrate posturing, central hyperventilation
C3—Flaccid, apneic, or cluster breathing
C4—Flaccid, apneic, no detectable circulation

tored frequently as a guide to oxygen, fluid, and electrolyte therapies.

NURSING ALERT All children who have a near-drowning experience should be admitted to the hospital for observation. Although many patients do not appear to have suffered adverse effects from the event, complications (e.g., respiratory compromise, cerebral edema) may occur 24 hours after the incident.

Aspiration pneumonia is a frequent complication that occurs about 48 to 72 hours after the episode. Bronchospasm, alveolocapillary membrane damage, atelectasis, abscess formation, and acute respiratory distress syndrome are other complications that occur after aspiration of fluid.

Prognosis

Studies report that the best predictors of a good outcome were length of submersion in nonicy water (more than 5° C [41° F]) for less than 5 minutes and the presence of sinus rhythm, reactive pupils, and neurologic responsiveness at the scene. The worst prognoses—for death or severe neurologic impairment—were in children submerged for more than 10 minutes and not responding to advanced life support within 25 minutes. All children without spontaneous, purposeful movement and normal brainstem function 24 hours after near-drowning suffered severe neurologic deficits or death (Zuckerman, Gregory, & Santos-Damiani, 1998; Kallas, 2004) (see Guidelines box).

Nursing Care Management

Nursing care depends on the child's condition. A child who survives may need intensive respiratory nursing care with attention to vital signs, mechanical ventilation and/or tracheostomy, blood gas determination, chest therapy, and IV infusion. Frequently the child is comatose for an indefinite period and requires the same care as an unconscious child. A difficult aspect in the care of the child victim of near-drowning is helping the parents cope with severe guilt reactions. The magnitude of the event is so great that efforts to provide comfort and support are of only limited success. Parents need to hear that everything possible is being done to treat the child, and this message needs to be repeated often.

The parents of the child who is saved from death are also faced with the anxiety of not knowing what the outcome will be. The situation generates such intense feelings of loneliness, it is important for families to know that they are not alone.

GUIDELINES Establishing Brain Death in Children

1. Coma and apnea must coexist. Child must exhibit complete loss of consciousness, vocalization, and volitional activity.
2. Brainstem function must be absent, as defined by:
   a. Midposition or fully dilated pupils that do not respond to light. Drugs may influence and invalidate pupillary assessment.
   b. Absence of spontaneous eye movements and those induced by oculocephalic and caloric (oculovestibular) testing.
   c. Absence of movement of bulbar musculature, including facial and oropharyngeal muscles. The corneal, gag, cough, sucking, and rooting reflexes are absent.
   d. Absence of respiratory movements when child is removed from respirator. Apnea testing using standardized methods can be performed but is done after other criteria are met.
3. Child must not be significantly hypothermic or hypotensive for age.
4. Flaccid tone and absence of spontaneous or induced movements, including spinal cord events such as reflex withdrawal or spinal myoclonus, should exist.
5. Examination should remain consistent with brain death throughout the observation and testing period.
6. Observation periods according to age:
   Seven days to 2 months–Two separate examinations and two electroencephalograms (EEGs), separated by at least 48 hours
   Two months to 1 year–Two separate examinations and two EEGs, separated by at least 24 hours
   Over 1 year–Two separate examinations separated by at least 12 hours; if irreversible cause exists, no laboratory testing needed; if difficult to assess extent of reversibility of brain damage, observation indicated for at least 24 hours

Modified from Task Force for the Determination of Brain Death in Children: Guidelines for the determination of brain death in children, *Ann Neurol* 21:616, 1987; Janakiraman N: Brain death, *Indian J Pediatr* 65:525-527, 1998; and Lutz-Dettinger N, de Jaeger A, Kerremanas I: Care of the potential pediatric organ donor, *Pediatr Clin North Am* 48:715-749, 2001.

They need to be reminded frequently that there are caring people to assist them both during the crisis and later. Additional sources of support that can be recommended are psychiatric and social work consultants, community services, and religious support. Self-help groups are excellent if these are available in the community.

Nurses often have difficulty relating to the parents if obvious neglect has precipitated the accident and subsequent problems; therefore it is important for those who care for these children and their families to assess their own feelings about the situation, as well as the family's coping abilities and resources. Caring for near-drowning victims and their families requires nurses to be sensitive to the needs of the child and family and to recognize their own reactions and emotions.

Prevention

Most drownings, particularly of infants or small children, can be prevented with adequate supervision. Water safety and survival training should be required for all school-age children, and nurses can be active advocates in their communities. Nurses are also in a position to emphasize the importance of adequate adult supervision when children are in the water. Aquatic programs for infants and toddlers do not decrease the risk of drowning; young children should never be left unattended when in or near the water (American Academy of Pediatrics, Committee on Sports Medicine and Fitness and Committee on Injury and Poison Prevention, 2000; Kallas, 2004). Parents with pools should know cardiopulmonary resuscitation techniques. (See also Injury Prevention, Chapters 36 to 40.)

Nervous System Tumors

Brain tumor and neuroblastoma are two major forms of childhood cancer derived from neural tissue. CNS tumors account for approximately 20% of all childhood cancers, and approximately 3.3 cases per 100,000 occur in children under 15 years of age (Blaney et al, 2006). Both of these tumors are difficult to treat and have not demonstrated the dramatic improvements in survival seen in other forms of childhood cancer.

Brain Tumors

Brain tumors are the most common solid tumors in children and are the second most common childhood cancer. The majority of tumors (about 60%) are *infratentorial* (below the tentorium cerebelli), which means that they occur in the posterior third of the brain, primarily in the cerebellum or brainstem. This anatomic distribution accounts for the frequency of symptoms resulting from increased ICP. The other tumors are *supratentorial*, or within the anterior two thirds of the brain, mainly the cerebrum.

Brain tumors, whether benign or malignant, can arise from any cell within the cranium. Consequently, the cranial cells' origin provides a histologic classification for major tumors. For instance, astrocytes (cells that form the supportive tissue for neurons) may form a common glial tumor called an astrocytoma. The major infratentorial tumors are medulloblastomas, cerebellar astrocytomas, brainstem gliomas, and ependymomas, and the major supratentorial tumors are astrocytomas, hypothalamic tumors, optic pathway tumors, and craniopharyngiomas.

Diagnostic Evaluation

The signs and symptoms of brain tumors are directly related to their anatomic location and size and, to some extent, the child's age. In infants, whose cranial sutures are still open, virtually no early detectable symptoms develop. It is not until spinal fluid obstruction causes markedly increased head size that a lesion may be suspected. Even in older children, clinical manifestations are nonspecific. However, the most common symptoms are headache, especially on awakening, and vomiting that is not related to feeding. Vomiting occurs from increased ICP that compresses the brainstem, directly stimulating the vomiting center in the medulla (Blaney et al, 2006).

Diagnosis of a brain tumor is based subjectively on presenting clinical signs and objectively on neurologic tests and histologic diagnosis via surgery. Because the signs and symptoms are vague and easily overlooked, early diagnosis relies on a high index of suspicion during history taking. A number of tests may be used in the neurologic evaluation, but the most common diagnostic procedure is MRI, which determines the location and extent of the tumor. Other tests that may be used include CT, angiography, electroencephalography, and lumbar puncture. Lumbar puncture is dangerous in the presence of increased ICP because of the possibility of brainstem herniation following a sudden release of pressure. The definitive diagnosis is based on brain tissue specimens obtained during surgery.

Therapeutic Management

Treatment may involve the use of surgery, radiotherapy, and chemotherapy. All three may be used, depending on the type of tumor. The treatment of choice is total removal of the tumor without residual neurologic damage. Patients with the most complete tumor removal have the greatest chance of survival. Radiotherapy is used to treat most tumors and to shrink the size of the tumor before attempting surgical removal. Chemotherapy has emerged in the past decade to delay radiation in children younger than 3 years of age because of the rapid brain development occurring in the first 3 years of life (Blaney et al, 2006; Murray-Ryan & Petriccione, 2002). Chemotherapy is also used as adjunct therapy for residual tumor, nonresectable tumor, or recurrent tumor. Water-soluble agents are able to penetrate the disrupted blood-brain barrier and attack brain tumor cells (Blaney et al, 2006; Murray-Ryan & Petriccione, 2002). Typically, the most commonly used chemotherapy agents are cisplatin, carboplatin, vincristine, cyclophosphamide, lomustine, carmustine, etoposide, ifosfamide, and topotecan. Surgery (biopsy, resection, laser, or stereotactic), radiotherapy (hyperfractionated, fractionated, or stereotactic), and multiagent chemotherapy are all instrumental in the treatment of brain tumors.

Prognosis

The prognosis for the child with a brain tumor depends on the type of brain tumor, the tumor's size, the extent of the disease, and the child's age. Problems associated with treatment and a relatively poor prognosis, primarily in infants and young children, are compounded by serious late effects of therapy. A decline in incidence of children with medulloblastoma has been significantly linked with a protective effect of maternal folate, iron, and multivitamin supplementation. Along with the recent advances in surgical instrumentation allowing aggressive surgical intervention (e.g., stereotactic surgery, radiosurgery), modifications in radiation (e.g., hyperfractionation, brain mapping) and use of chemotherapy (e.g., intrathecal, intratumoral) have increased the long-term survival rates for many children with brain tumors (Alston et al, 2003; Blaney et al, 2006; Gupta & Berger, 2003; Murray-Ryan & Petriccione, 2002).

Nursing Care Management

A brain tumor is often suspected in a child admitted to the hospital with neurologic dysfunction, although the actual diagnosis may not yet be confirmed. Establishing a baseline of data with which to compare preoperative and postoperative changes is an essential step toward planning physical care and preventing complications. It also allows the nurse to assess the degree of physical incapacity and the family's emotional reaction to the diagnosis.

Vital signs, including blood pressure and pulse pressure (the difference between systolic and diastolic pressures), are taken routinely and more often when any change is noted. Any sudden variations are reported immediately. It is especially important to note a change in vital signs during or after diagnostic procedures. A routine neurologic assessment is also performed at the same time as vital signs, and head circumference is measured on infants and very young children.

The child is observed for evidence of headache, vomiting, and any seizure activity. The location, severity, and duration of the headache are noted, as well as its relationship to activity and time of day. Behaviors such as lying flat and facing away from light or refusing to engage in play are clues to discomfort in the nonverbal child. The child's gait is observed at least once daily. Head tilt and other changes in posturing are always noted.

Prevent Postoperative Complications

Usually the surgeon will prescribe specific orders for vital signs, neurologic checks, positioning, fluid regulation, and medication. These vary somewhat, depending on the location of the craniotomy. The following are general principles of care for infratentorial or supratentorial surgery. Additional aspects of care that are discussed elsewhere may include care of the child with seizures and neurologic assessment of the unconscious child.

Vital signs are taken as frequently as every 15 to 30 minutes until the child is stable. Temperature measurement is particularly important because of hyperthermia resulting from surgical intervention in the hypothalamus or brainstem and from some types of general anesthesia. To prepare for this reaction, a cooling blanket should be placed on the bed *before* the child returns to the unit so that it is ready for use when needed. The temperature is monitored carefully when any cooling measures are taken because hypothermia can occur suddenly. Recognizing signs of other complications such as increased ICP, meningitis, and respiratory tract infection is imperative.

Neurologic checks are an essential aspect of care and include pupillary reaction to light, LOC, sleep patterns, and response to stimuli. Although children may be comatose for a few days, once they regain consciousness, there should be a steady increase in alertness. Regression to a lethargic, irritable state indicates increasing pressure, possibly caused by meningitis or cerebral edema.

NURSING ALERT Sluggish, dilated, or unequal pupils are reported immediately because they may indicate increased ICP and potential brainstem herniation, a medical emergency.

Observations for function are not instituted until the child regains consciousness. However, as soon as possible the nurse should begin testing reflexes, handgrip, and functioning of the cranial nerves. Muscle strength is usually diminished as a result of general weakness after surgery but should improve daily. Ataxia may be significantly worse with cerebellar intervention, but it will slowly improve. Edema near the cranial nerves may depress important functions such as the gag, blink, or swallowing reflex.

Dressings are observed for evidence of drainage. If soiled, the dressing is not removed but is reinforced with dry sterile gauze. The approximate amount of drainage is estimated and recorded. A drain may be placed in the operative site.

NURSING ALERT To keep an accurate account of drainage, the soiled area is circled with a pen every hour or so. In this way, continuous bleeding is easily recognized. The presence of colorless drainage is reported immediately, since it most likely is CSF from the incisional area. A foul odor from the dressing may indicate an infection. Such a finding is reported, and a culture is taken.

Correct positioning after surgery is critical to prevent pressure against the operative site, reduce ICP, and avoid the danger of aspiration. If a large tumor was removed, the child is not placed on the operative side, since the brain may suddenly shift to that cavity, causing trauma to the blood vessels, linings, and the brain itself. The nurse confers with the surgeon to be certain of the correct position, including degree of neck flexion. The first 24 to 48 hours after brain surgery are critical. If the child's position is restricted, notice of this is posted above the head of the bed. When the child is turned, every precaution is used to prevent jarring or malalignment to prevent undue strain on the sutures. Two nurses are needed—one supporting the head and the other supporting the body. The use of a turning sheet may facilitate turning a heavy child.

The child with an infratentorial procedure is usually positioned on either side with the bed flat. When a supratentorial craniotomy is performed, the head of bed is elevated 20 to 30 degrees with the child on either side or on the back. In a supratentorial craniotomy the head elevation facilitates CSF drainage and decreases excessive blood flow to the brain to prevent hemorrhage. Pillows should be placed against the child's back, not head, to maintain the desired position. Ordinarily the head and neck are kept in midline with the body, and the neck should not be flexed (Curley & Moloney-Harmon, 2001).

NURSING ALERT Trendelenburg's position is contraindicated in both infratentorial and supratentorial surgeries because it increases ICP and the risk of hemorrhage. If shock is impending, the practitioner is notified immediately, before the head is lowered.

With an infratentorial craniotomy the child is allowed nothing by mouth for at least 24 hours, or longer if the gag and swallowing reflexes are depressed or the child is comatose. With a supratentorial operation, clear fluids may be resumed soon after the child is alert, sometimes within 24 hours. If the child vomits, oral liquids are stopped. Vomiting not only predisposes the child to aspiration, but also increases ICP and the potential for incisional rupture.

The child should be fed to conserve energy and minimize movement. If there is any sign of facial paralysis, the child is fed slowly to prevent choking or aspiration. Sometimes gavage feeding is necessary when body functions are too depressed to permit safe oral feedings or when the child refuses to eat or drink. IV fluids are continued until oral fluids are well tolerated. Because of the postoperative cerebral edema and danger of increased ICP, fluids are carefully monitored.

Headache may be severe and is largely a result of cerebral edema. Measures to relieve some of the discomfort include providing a quiet, dimly lit environment; restricting visitors; preventing any sudden jarring movement, such as banging into the bed; and preventing an increase in ICP. Avoiding increased ICP is most effectively achieved by proper positioning and prevention of straining, such as during coughing, vomiting, or defecating. The use of opioids, such as morphine, to relieve pain is controversial because it is thought that they may mask signs of altered consciousness or depress respirations. However, they can be given safely, since naloxone can be used to reverse opioid effects, such as sedation or respiratory depression. Acetaminophen and codeine are also effective analgesics for mild to moderate pain. Regardless of the drugs used, adequate dosage and regular administration are essential to providing optimal pain relief (see also Pain Assessment; Pain Management, Chapter 35). Placing an ice bag on the forehead may also provide some headache relief, especially if facial edema is severe.

Support Child and Family

The family's emotional needs are immense when the diagnosis is a brain tumor, and feelings are influenced by the extent of surgery, any neurologic deficits, the expected prognosis, and additional therapy.* Since few definitive answers can be given before surgery, the surgeon's report is a significant finding that can vary from a completely benign, resected neoplasm to a highly malignant, invasive, and only partially removed tumor. Although parents try to prepare themselves for a potentially fatal diagnosis, it is a shock for them.

Parents should be encouraged to verbalize their feelings about the diagnosis. Often they express tremendous guilt for viewing the insidious onset of symptoms, such as ataxia, visual difficulty, or headache, as "minor complaints" by the child. Any comments that insinuate that the parents should have sought medical advice sooner are avoided, since such remarks only add to the parents' guilt feelings.

During this period the nurse should also discuss with parents what they plan to tell the child. If the child was prepared honestly, the diagnosis can be expressed in a similar manner. During recovery the child will need additional explanation about the treatment and the reason for any residual neurologic effects, such as ataxia or blindness.

Neuroblastoma

Neuroblastomas are the most common malignant extracranial solid tumors in children, accounting for 8% to 10% of all childhood cancers (Brodeur & Maris, 2006). They occur in about 1 per 10,000 live births, with a slightly higher incidence in boys. The majority of children with neuroblastoma manifest the disease before 10 years of age, with the median age of occurrence at 22 months (Brodeur & Maris, 2006). These tumors originate from embryonic neural crest cells that normally give rise to the adrenal medulla and the sympathetic ganglia. Consequently, the majority of tumors develop in the adrenal gland or the retroperitoneal sympathetic chain. Other sites may be in the head, neck, chest, or pelvis.

Neuroblastoma is a "silent" tumor. In more than 70% of cases, diagnosis is made after metastasis occurs, with the first signs caused by involvement in the nonprimary site, usually the lymph nodes, bone marrow, skeletal system, skin, or liver.

Diagnostic Evaluation

The objective of diagnosis is to locate the primary site and areas of metastasis. The signs and symptoms of neuroblastoma depend on the location and stage of the disease. Most presenting signs are caused by compression of adjacent structures. Skeletal survey; skull, neck, chest, abdominal, and bone CT scans; and bilateral bone marrow aspirations and biopsies are used to locate a tumor mass and metastasis. A metaiodobenzylguanidine (MIBG) scan is used to determine involvement of bone or tissue; however, it is only available at certain centers.

Urinary excretion of catecholamines is detected in approximately 95% of children with adrenal or sympathetic tumors. Analyzing the breakdown products excreted in the urine, namely vanillylmandelic acid, homovanillic acid, dopamine, and norepinephrine, permits detection of suspected tumor before and after medical-surgical intervention (Brodeur & Maris, 2006; Kline & Sevier, 2003). Amplification of proto-oncogene, known as the *N-myc* gene, and chromosomal abnormalities correlates strongly with advanced-stage disease, rapid tumor progression, and a poor prognosis (Brodeur & Maris, 2006).

Therapeutic Management

Accurate clinical staging is important for establishing initial treatment. Therefore surgery is used both to remove as much of the tumor as possible and to obtain biopsies. In early stages, complete surgical removal of the tumor is the treatment of

**Excellent publications are available from the National Brain Tumor Society, 22 Battery St., Suite 612, San Francisco, CA 94111-5520; 800-934-2873 (patient line) or 800-770-8287;* www.braintumor.org. *The pamphlet* When Your Child Is Ready to Return to School *is available from the American Brain Tumor Association, 2720 River Road, Des Plaines, IL 60018; 847-827-9910; fax: 847-827-9918;* www.abta.org.

choice. If the tumor is large, partial resection is attempted, with a course of irradiation postoperatively to shrink the tumor in the hope of complete removal at a later date. Surgery is usually limited to biopsy in stages III and IV because of the extensive metastasis, although the use of additional surgery to assess tumor regression or remove a regressed tumor is not unlikely.

Radiotherapy provides emergency management of a massive neuroblastoma that is causing spinal cord compression (Kline & Sevier, 2003; Nguyen et al, 2000). Radiotherapy also offers palliation for metastatic lesions in the bones, lung, liver, or brain.

Chemotherapy is the mainstay of therapy for extensive local or disseminated disease. Agents used in various combinations include cyclophosphamide, doxorubicin, cisplatin, etoposide, vincristine, ifosfamide, carboplatin, topotecan, and teniposide. In children with high risk disease or recurrent disease, retinoic acid, radiotherapy, and myeloablative chemotherapy with peripheral stem cell rescue may be used to obtain a longer remission, even though the overall survival rate is poor (Brodeur & Maris, 2006; Kline & Sevier, 2003).

Prognosis

If all stages are grouped together, the 5-year disease-free survival rates range from 88% to 90% for children in the low risk stage, and from 22% to 30% in children in the high risk stage (Brodeur & Maris, 2006). Generally, the younger the child at diagnosis (especially younger than 1 year of age), the better the survival rate. Neuroblastoma is one of the few tumors that demonstrate spontaneous regression (especially stage IV-S), possibly as a result of maturity of the embryonic cell or the development of an active immune system.

Nursing Care Management

Nursing considerations are similar to those discussed for leukemia and brain tumors, including psychologic and physical preparation for diagnostic and operative procedures; prevention of postoperative complications for abdominal, thoracic, or cranial surgery; and explanation of chemotherapy, radiotherapy, and their side effects.

Since this tumor carries a poor prognosis for many children, every consideration must be given the family in terms of coping with a life-threatening illness (see Chapter 41). Because of the high degree of metastasis at the time of diagnosis, many parents suffer substantial guilt for not having recognized signs earlier. Parents need much support in dealing with these feelings and expressing them to the appropriate people.

Intracranial Infections

The nervous system is subject to infection by the same organisms that affect other organs of the body. However, the nervous system is limited in the ways in which it responds to injury. Laboratory studies are needed to identify the causative agent. The inflammatory process can affect the meninges (meningitis) or brain (encephalitis).

Meningitis can be caused by a variety of organisms, but the three main types are (1) bacterial, or pyogenic, caused by pus-forming bacteria, especially meningococci, pneumococci, and *Haemophilus* organisms; (2) viral, or aseptic, caused by a wide variety of viral agents; and (3) tuberculous, caused by the tuberculin bacillus. The majority of children with acute febrile encephalopathy have either bacterial meningitis or viral meningitis as the underlying cause.

Bacterial Meningitis

Bacterial meningitis is an acute inflammation of the meninges and CSF. The advent of antimicrobial therapy has had a marked effect on the course and prognosis, although the introduction of conjugate vaccines against *Haemophilus influenzae* type b (Hib vaccine) in 1990 has led to the most dramatic change in the epidemiology of bacterial meningitis (Centers for Disease Control and Prevention, 2002; Prober, 2007; Scheifele et al, 2005). In 1993 the incidence of *H. influenzae* was 2 cases per 100,000 children younger than 5 years, whereas in 1987 the incidence was 41 per 100,000 (Centers for Disease Control and Prevention, 2002). Today, *H. influenzae* type b infection has been virtually eradicated among young children in areas of the world where the Hib vaccine is administered routinely (Centers for Disease Control and Prevention, 2002; Yogev & Guzman-Cottrill, 2005). Routine use of the conjugated pneumococcal vaccine introduced in 2000 may lead to world trends in young children similar to those experienced with the Hib vaccine (Yogev & Guzman-Cottrill, 2005). Practitioners are optimistic that the use of the new pneumococcal conjugate vaccine will produce a rapid and adequate antibody response in young children. Bacterial meningitis from *Streptococcus pneumoniae* will soon be on the decline (Prober, 2007).

Bacterial meningitis remains a significant cause of illness in the pediatric age groups because of the residual damage caused by undiagnosed and untreated or inadequately treated cases. The majority of reported cases occur in children between 1 month and 5 years of age, with an increased mortality risk in the adolescent and young adult (Saez-Llorens & McCracken, 2003; Sotir et al, 2005).

Bacterial meningitis can be caused by a variety of bacterial agents. Currently *H. influenzae* type b, *S. pneumoniae,* and *Neisseria meningitidis* (meningococcus) are responsible for bacterial meningitis in 95% of children older than 2 months.

Other organisms are β-hemolytic streptococci, *Staphylococcus aureus*, and *Escherichia coli*. The leading causes of neonatal meningitis are group B streptococci, *E. coli*, and *Listeria monocytogenes*. *E. coli* infection is seldom seen beyond infancy. Meningococcal meningitis occurs in epidemic form and is the only type readily transmitted by droplet infection from nasopharyngeal secretions. Although this condition may develop at any age, the risk of meningococcal infection increases with the number of contacts; therefore it occurs predominantly in school-age children and adolescents.

There appear to be some seasonal variations. Meningitis caused by *H. influenzae* primarily occurs in autumn or early winter. Pneumococcal and meningococcal infections can occur at any time but are more common in later winter or early spring.

Pathophysiology

The most common route of infection is vascular dissemination from a focus of infection elsewhere. For example, organisms from the nasopharynx invade the underlying blood vessels

evolve Case Study—Meningitis

and enter the cerebral blood supply or form local thromboemboli that release septic emboli into the bloodstream. Invasion by direct extension from infections in the paranasal and mastoid sinuses is less common. Organisms also gain entry by direct implantation after penetrating wounds, skull fractures that provide an opening into the skin or sinuses, lumbar puncture or surgical procedures, anatomic abnormalities such as spina bifida, or foreign bodies such as an internal ventricular shunt or an external ventricular device. Once implanted, the organisms spread into the CSF, by which the infection spreads throughout the subarachnoid space.

The infective process is like that seen in any bacterial infection: inflammation, exudation, white blood cell accumulation, and varying degrees of tissue damage. The brain becomes hyperemic and edematous, and the entire surface of the brain is covered by a layer of purulent exudate that varies with the type of organism. For example, meningococcal exudate is most marked over the parietal, occipital, and cerebellar regions; the thick, fibrinous exudate of pneumococcal infection is confined chiefly to the surface of the brain, particularly the anterior lobes; and the exudate of streptococcal infections is similar to that of pneumococcal infections, but thinner.

As infection extends to the ventricles, thick pus, fibrin, or adhesions may occlude the narrow passages and obstruct the flow of CSF.

Clinical Manifestations

The clinical manifestations of acute bacterial meningitis depend to a large extent on the child's age. The picture is also influenced to some degree by the type of organism, the effectiveness of therapy for antecedent illness, and whether it occurs as an isolated entity or as a complication of another illness or injury. The onset of illness is likely to be abrupt, with fever, chills, headache, and vomiting that are associated with or quickly followed by alterations in sensorium. See Box 51-5 for clinical manifestations of bacterial meningitis.

NURSING ALERT Any child who is ill and develops a purpuric or petechial rash may have (overwhelming) meningococcemia and must receive medical attention immediately.

Diagnostic Evaluation

A lumbar puncture is the definitive diagnostic test. The fluid pressure is measured, and samples are obtained for culture, Gram stain, blood cell count, and determination of glucose and protein content. The findings are usually diagnostic. Culture and sensitivity testing are needed to identify the causative organism. Spinal fluid pressure is usually elevated, but interpretation is often difficult when the child is crying. Sedation with fentanyl and midazolam can alleviate the child's pain and fear associated with this procedure. If there is evidence or suspicion of increased ICP (papilledema, focal neurologic deficits, bulging fontanel), a CT scan of the head may be warranted before the procedure.

The patient generally has an elevated white blood cell count, often predominantly polymorphonuclear leukocytes. The glucose level is reduced, generally in proportion to the duration and severity of the infection. The relationship between the CSF glucose and serum glucose levels is important in evaluating the glucose content of CSF; therefore a serum glucose sample is drawn approximately one half hour before the lumbar puncture. Protein concentration is usually increased.

A blood culture is advisable for all children suspected of having meningitis and occasionally will be positive when CSF culture is negative. Nose and throat cultures may provide helpful information in some cases.

Therapeutic Management

Acute bacterial meningitis is a medical emergency that requires early recognition and immediate institution of therapy to prevent death or residual disabilities. The initial therapeutic management includes:

- Isolation precautions
- Initiation of antimicrobial therapy
- Maintenance of hydration
- Maintenance of ventilation
- Reduction of increased ICP
- Management of systemic shock
- Control of seizures
- Control of temperature
- Treatment of complications

The child is isolated from other children, usually in an intensive care unit for close observation. An IV infusion is started to facilitate the administration of antimicrobial agents, fluids, antiepileptic drugs, and blood, if needed. The child is placed on a cardiac monitor and in respiratory isolation.

Drugs

Until the causative organism is identified, the choice of antibiotic is based on the known sensitivity of the organism most likely to be the infective agent. After identification of the organism, antimicrobial agents are adjusted accordingly.

Dexamethasone may play a role in the initial management of increased ICP and cerebral herniation, but its ability to reduce long-term complications of bacterial meningitis remains controversial. There is evidence that dexamethasone therapy decreases the risk of neurologic sequelae in children with *H. influenzae* type b meningitis and should be considered for use in other bacterial types of meningitis (American Academy of Pediatrics, Committee on Infectious Diseases, 2006; Prober, 2007). It should not be used if aseptic or nonbacterial meningitis is suspected (Bonthius & Karacay, 2002).

Signs of gastrointestinal hemorrhage or secondary infection may complicate steroid administration. Antibiotic treatment with cephalosporins demonstrates superiority for promptly sterilizing the CSF and reducing the incidence of severe hearing impairment.

Nonspecific Measures

Maintaining hydration is a prime concern, and IV fluids and the type and amount of fluid are determined by the patient's condition. The optimum hydration involves correction of any fluid deficits followed by fluid restriction as ordered to prevent cerebral edema. Cerebral edema and electrolyte disturbances are associated with poor neurologic outcome following bacterial meningitis (Bonthius & Karacay, 2002). Children with bacterial meningitis must be monitored for signs of increased ICP. If needed, measures to decrease ICP are implemented (see p. 1559).

BOX 51-5 Clinical Manifestations of Bacterial Meningitis

Children and Adolescents

Usually abrupt onset
Fever
Chills
Headache
Vomiting
Alterations in sensorium
Seizures (often the initial sign)
Irritability
Agitation
May develop:

- Photophobia
- Delirium
- Hallucinations
- Aggressive behavior
- Drowsiness
- Stupor
- Coma

Nuchal rigidity

- May progress to opisthotonos

Positive Kernig and Brudzinski signs
Hyperactive but variable reflex responses
Signs and symptoms peculiar to individual organisms:

- Petechial or purpuric rashes (meningococcal infection), especially when associated with a shocklike state
- Joint involvement (meningococcal and *Haemophilus influenzae* infection)
- Chronically draining ear (pneumococcal meningitis)

Infants and Young Children

Classic picture (above) rarely seen in children between 3 months and 2 years of age
Fever
Poor feeding
Vomiting
Marked irritability
Frequent seizures (often accompanied by a high-pitched cry)
Bulging fontanel
Nuchal rigidity (may or may not be present)
Brudzinski and Kernig signs not helpful in diagnosis
Difficult to elicit and evaluate in this age group
Subdural empyema (*H. influenzae* infection)

Neonates: Specific Signs

Extremely difficult to diagnose
Manifestations vague and nonspecific
Well at birth but within a few days begins to look and behave poorly
Refusal of feedings
Poor sucking ability
Vomiting or diarrhea
Poor tone
Lack of movement
Weak cry
Full, tense, and bulging fontanel sometimes appearing late in course of illness
Neck usually supple

Neonates: Nonspecific Signs That May Be Present

Hypothermia or fever (depending on the infant's maturity)
Jaundice
Irritability
Drowsiness
Seizures
Respiratory irregularities or apnea
Cyanosis
Weight loss

Complications are treated appropriately, such as aspiration of subdural effusion in infants and treatment for disseminated intravascular coagulation syndrome. Shock is managed by restoration of circulating blood volume and maintenance of electrolyte balance. Seizures can occur during the first few days of treatment. These are controlled with the appropriate antiepileptic drug. Hearing loss is not uncommon. The patient should undergo auditory evaluation 6 months after the illness has resolved.

Lumbar puncture is carried out as needed to determine the effectiveness of therapy. The patient is evaluated neurologically during the convalescent period.

Prognosis

Ten percent to 15% of cases of bacterial meningitis are fatal (Centers for Disease Control and Prevention, 2000). The child's age, duration of illness before antibiotic therapy, rapidity of diagnosis after onset, type of organism, and adequacy of therapy are important in the prognosis for bacterial meningitis. Bacterial meningitis can result in brain damage, hearing loss, or learning disability (Centers for Disease Control and Prevention, 2000; Prober, 2007).

Neonatal meningitis carries the highest mortality. However, with the development of new antibiotics and the advent of aggressive supportive care measures, the mortality rate for bacterial meningitis in children caused by *H. influenzae* type b, *S. pneumoniae*, and *N. meningitidis* is less than 10% in most studies (Prober, 2007).

The sequelae of bacterial meningitis are seen most often when the disease occurs in the first 2 months of life and least often in children with meningococcal meningitis. The residual deficits in infants are primarily a result of communicating hydrocephalus and the greater effects of cerebritis on the immature brain. In older children the residual effects are related to the inflammatory process itself or result from vasculitis associated with the disease. Bacterial meningitis continues to cause substantial morbidity in infants and children. The mortality rate and incidence of poor neurologic outcome are highest in patients with pneumococcal meningitis (Saez-Llorens & McCracken, 2003; Prober, 2007).

Hearing impairment is the most common sequela of this disease. Evaluation of cranial nerve VIII is needed for at least a 6-month follow-up period to assess for possible hearing loss.

Prevention

Vaccines are available for types A, C, Y, and W-135 meningococci and *H. influenzae* type b. Routine meningococcal polysaccharide vaccination of children is licensed for use only in children 2 years and older (Pichichero, 2005). The new quadrivalent meningococcal conjugate vaccine (Menactra) was licensed by the U.S. Food and Drug Administration (FDA) in January 2005 for children and adults from 11 to 55 years (Pichichero, 2005). However, routine vaccinations for *H. influenzae* type b are recommended for all children beginning at 2 months of age (see Immunizations, Chapter 36). Pneumococcal conjugate vaccine is now recommended for all children beginning at 2 months of age (American Academy of Pediatrics, 2000).

NURSING ALERT A major priority of nursing care of a child suspected of having meningitis is to administer antibiotics as soon as they are ordered. The child is placed on respiratory isolation for at least 24 hours after initiation of antimicrobial therapy.

Nursing Care Management

evolve Nursing Care Plan—The Child with Bacterial Meningitis

The room is kept as quiet as possible, and environmental stimuli are kept to a minimum because most children with meningitis are sensitive to noise, bright lights, and other external stimuli. Most children are more comfortable without a pillow and with the head of the bed slightly elevated. A side-lying position is more often assumed because of nuchal rigidity. The nurse should avoid actions that cause pain or increase discomfort, such as lifting the child's head. Evaluating the child for pain and implementing appropriate relief measures are important during the initial 24 to 72 hours. Acetaminophen with codeine is often used. Measures are used to ensure safety because the child is often restless and subject to seizures.

The nursing care of the child with meningitis is determined by the child's symptoms and treatment. Observation of vital signs, neurologic signs, LOC, urine output, and other pertinent data is carried out at frequent intervals. The child who is unconscious is managed as described previously (see p. 1558), and all children are observed carefully for signs of the complications just described, especially increased ICP, shock, or respiratory distress. Frequent assessment of the open fontanels is needed in the infant because subdural effusions and obstructive hydrocephalus can develop as a complication of meningitis.

Fluids and nourishment are determined by the child's status. The child with dulled sensorium is usually given nothing by mouth. Other children are allowed clear liquids initially and, if these are tolerated, progress to a diet suitable for their age. Careful monitoring and recording of intake and output are needed to determine deviations that might indicate impending shock or increasing fluid accumulation, such as cerebral edema or subdural effusion.

One of the most difficult problems in the nursing care of children with meningitis is maintaining IV infusion for the length of time needed to provide adequate antimicrobial therapy (usually 10 days). Because continuous IV fluids are usually not necessary, an intermittent infusion device is used. In some cases children who are recovering uneventfully are sent home with the device, and the parents are taught IV drug administration.

Family Support

The sudden nature of the illness makes emotional support of the child and parents extremely important. Parents are upset and concerned about their child's condition and often feel guilty for not having suspected the seriousness of the illness sooner. They need much reassurance that the natural onset of meningitis is sudden and that they acted responsibly in seeking medical assistance when they did. The nurse encourages the parents to openly discuss their feelings to minimize blame and guilt. They also are kept informed of the child's progress and of all procedures, results, and treatments. In the event that the child's condition worsens, they need the same psychologic care as parents who face the possible death of their child (see Chapter 41).

Nonbacterial (Aseptic) Meningitis

Aseptic meningitis is caused by many different viruses. The onset may be abrupt or gradual. The initial manifestations are headache, fever, malaise, and gastrointestinal symptoms. Signs of meningeal irritation develop 1 or 2 days after the onset of illness. Onset is more insidious in infants and toddlers. Signs and symptoms are vague and are often thought to be associated with a minor illness.

Diagnosis is based on clinical features and CSF findings. Variations in CSF values in bacterial and viral meningitis are listed in Table 51-2. It is important to differentiate this self-limiting disorder from the more serious forms of meningitis.

Treatment is primarily symptomatic, such as acetaminophen for headache and muscle pain, maintenance of hydration, and positioning for comfort. Until a definitive diagnosis is made, antimicrobial agents may be administered and isolation enforced as a precaution against the possibility that the disease might be of bacterial origin. Nursing care is similar to the care of the child with bacterial meningitis.

Encephalitis

Encephalitis is an inflammatory process of the CNS that is caused by a variety of organisms, including bacteria, spirochetes, fungi, protozoa, helminths, and viruses. Most infections are associated with viruses, and this discussion is limited to those agents.

Etiology

Encephalitis can occur as a result of (1) direct invasion of the CNS by a virus or (2) postinfectious involvement of the CNS after a viral disease. Often the specific type of encephalitis may not be identified. The cause of more than half the cases

Table 51-2 Variation of Cerebrospinal Fluid Analysis in Bacterial and Viral Meningitis

MANIFESTATIONS	BACTERIAL*	VIRAL
White blood cell count	Elevated; increased polys	Slightly elevated; increased lymphs
Protein content	Elevated	Normal or slightly increased
Glucose content	Decreased	Normal
Gram stain; bacteria culture	Positive	Turbid or cloudy
Color	Negative	Clear or slightly cloudy

*Results may vary in the neonate.

reported in the United States is unknown. The majority of cases of known etiology are associated with the childhood diseases of measles, mumps, varicella, and rubella and, less often, with the enteroviruses, herpesviruses, and West Nile virus.

Herpes simplex encephalitis is an uncommon disease, but 30% of cases involve children. The initial clinical findings are nonspecific (fever, altered mental status), but most cases evolve to demonstrate focal neurologic signs and symptoms. Children may experience focal seizures. The CSF is abnormal in most cases. Because of a rise in the number of children with herpes simplex encephalitis, suspected cases require prompt attention, especially because the diagnosis can be difficult. The clinical diagnosis can be confirmed by the rapid appearance of immunoglobulin M antibody to herpes simplex virus type 1 in CSF and serum. The early use of IV acyclovir reduces mortality and morbidity. Empiric therapy with acyclovir is given before precise virologic diagnosis has been established. CSF should be sent for viral titers.

The multiplicity of causes of viral encephalitis makes diagnosis difficult. Most are those involved with arthropod vectors (togaviruses and bunyaviruses) and those associated with hemorrhagic fevers (arenaviruses, filoviruses, and hantaviruses). In the United States the vector reservoir for most agents pathogenic for humans is the mosquito (St. Louis or West Nile encephalitis); therefore most cases of encephalitis appear during the hot summer months and subside during the autumn.

The clinical features of encephalitis are similar regardless of the agent involved. Manifestations can range from a mild benign form that resembles aseptic meningitis, lasts a few days, and is followed by rapid and complete recovery, to a fulminating encephalitis with severe CNS involvement. The onset may be sudden or may be gradual with malaise, fever, headache, dizziness, apathy, nuchal rigidity, nausea and vomiting, ataxia, tremors, hyperactivity, and speech difficulties (Box 51-6). In severe cases the patient has high fever, stupor, seizures, disorientation, spasticity, and coma that may proceed to death. Ocular palsies and paralysis also may occur.

BOX 51-6 Clinical Manifestations of Encephalitis

Onset: Sudden or Gradual

Malaise
Fever
Headache
Dizziness
Apathy
Lethargy
Neck stiffness
Nausea and vomiting
Ataxia
Tremors
Hyperactivity
Speech difficulties: mutism
Altered mental status

Severe Cases

High fever
Stupor
Seizures
Disorientation
Spasticity
Coma (may proceed to death)
Ocular palsies
Paralysis

Diagnostic Evaluation

The diagnosis is made on the basis of clinical findings and, where possible, identification of the specific virus. Early in the course of encephalitis, CT scan results may be normal. Later, hemorrhagic areas in the frontotemporal region may be seen. Togaviruses (some of which were formerly labeled arboviruses) are rarely detected in the blood or spinal fluid, but viruses of herpes, mumps, measles, and enteroviruses may be found in the CSF. Serologic testing may be required. The first blood sample should be drawn as soon as possible after onset, with the second sample drawn 2 or 3 weeks later.

Therapeutic Management

Patients suspected of having encephalitis are hospitalized promptly for observation. Treatment is primarily supportive and includes conscientious nursing care, control of cerebral manifestations, and adequate nutrition and hydration, with observation and management as for other cerebral disorders. Viral encephalitis can cause devastating neurologic injury. Cerebral hyperemia occurs in severe viral encephalitis, and ICP monitoring to reduce the pressure may be needed (Prober, 2007). Follow-up care with periodic reevaluation and rehabilitation is important for patients who develop residual effects of the disease.

The prognosis for the child with encephalitis depends on the child's age, the type of organism, and residual neurologic damage. Very young children (younger than 2 years of age) may exhibit increased neurologic disability, including learning difficulties and seizure disorders.

Nursing Care Management

Nursing care of the child with encephalitis is the same as for any unconscious child and for the child with meningitis. Additional nursing interventions include observation for deterioration in consciousness. Isolation of the child is not necessary; however, good handwashing technique must be followed. A main focus of nursing management is the control of rapidly rising ICP. Neurologic monitoring, administration of medications, and support of the child and parents are the major aspects of care.

Rabies

Rabies is an acute infection of the nervous system caused by a virus that is almost invariably fatal if left untreated. It is transmitted to humans by the saliva of an infected mammal and is introduced through a bite or skin abrasion. After entry into a new host, the virus multiplies in muscle cells and is spread through neural pathways without stimulating a protective host immune response.

Approximately 88% of rabies cases come from wild animals and 12% from domestic animals. Carnivorous wild animals (skunks, raccoons, and bats) are the animals most often infected with rabies and the cause of most indigenous cases of human rabies in the United States (Centers for Disease Control and Prevention, 2001; Toltzis, 2007). The likelihood of human exposure to a rabid domestic animal has decreased greatly.

The circumstances of a biting incident are important. An unprovoked attack is more likely than a provoked attack to indicate a rabid animal. Bites inflicted on a child attempting to feed or handle an apparently healthy animal can generally be regarded as provoked. Any child bitten by a wild animal is assumed to be exposed to rabies.

NURSING ALERT Unusual behavior in an animal is cause for suspicion; children should be warned to beware of wild animals that appear to be friendly.

Although rabies is common among wildlife species, human rabies is rarely acquired. Modern-day prophylaxis is nearly 100% successful. The highest incidence occurs in children under age 15 years. The incubation period usually ranges from 1 to 3 months but may be as short as 10 days or as long as 8 months. Only 10% to 15% of persons bitten develop the disease, but once symptoms are present, rabies progresses to a fatal outcome. In the United States, human fatalities associated with rabies occur in people who fail to seek medical attention, usually because they are unaware of their exposure.

The disease is characterized by a period of general malaise, fever, and sore throat followed by a phase of excitement that features hypersensitivity and increased reaction to external stimuli, convulsions, maniacal behavior, and choking (Box 51-7). Attempts at swallowing may cause such severe spasm of respiratory muscles that apnea, cyanosis, and anoxia are produced—the characteristics from which the term *hydrophobia* was derived.

Diagnosis is made on the basis of history and clinical features. Treatment is of little avail once symptoms appear, but the long incubation period allows time for the induction of active and passive immunity before the onset of illness.

Therapeutic Management

Two types of immunizing products are available for use in humans: (1) the inactivated rabies vaccines, which induce an active immune response; and (2) the globulins, which contain preformed antibodies. The two types of products should be used concurrently for rabies postexposure treatment when prophylaxis is indicated.

The current therapy for a rabid animal bite consists of thorough cleansing of the wound and passive immunization with human rabies immunoglobulin as soon as possible after exposure to provide rapid, short-term passive immunity (Centers for Disease Control and Prevention, 1999; Toltzis, 2007).

Postexposure active immunity is conferred by administration of the human diploid cell rabies vaccine. The first intramuscular injection of the vaccine is given at the same time as the immunoglobulin (day 0) and is followed by injections at 3, 7, 14, and 28 days after the first dose (Centers for Disease Control and Prevention, 1999; Toltzis, 2007). Before antirabies prophylaxis is initiated, the local or state health department should be consulted.

BOX 51-7 Clinical Manifestations of Rabies

Initial Signs
General malaise
Fever
Sore throat

Excitement Phase
Hypersensitivity
Increased reaction to external stimuli
Seizures
Maniacal behavior
Choking

Severe Spasm of Respiratory Muscles*
Apnea
Cyanosis
Anoxia

*From attempts at swallowing (characteristics from which the term *hydrophobia* was derived).

Nursing Care Management

Parents and children are frightened by the urgency and seriousness of the situation. They need anticipatory guidance for the therapy and support and reassurance regarding the efficacy of the preventive measures for this dreaded disease. The vaccine is well tolerated by children, although they need preparation for the series of injections. Mass immunization is unnecessary and unlikely to be implemented. In areas in which rabies is rare, the schedule given is sufficient. However, certain circumstances may warrant preexposure vaccination, such as when a child is being taken to an area of the world where rabies in stray dogs is still a problem.

Reye's Syndrome

RS is a disorder defined as toxic encephalopathy associated with other characteristic organ involvement (Kamienski, 2003). It is characterized by fever, profoundly impaired consciousness, and disordered hepatic function.

The etiology of RS is not well understood, but most cases follow a common viral illness, most commonly influenza or varicella. RS is a condition characterized pathologically by cerebral edema and fatty changes of the liver. The onset of RS is notable for profuse vomiting and varying degrees of neurologic impairment, including personality changes and deterioration in consciousness (Carey & Balistreri, 2007). The cause of RS is a mitochondrial insult induced by different viruses, drugs, exogenous toxins, and genetic factors. Elevated serum ammonia levels tend to correlate with the clinical manifestations and prognosis.

Definitive diagnosis is established by liver biopsy. The staging criteria for RS are based on liver dysfunction and on neurologic signs that range from lethargy to coma (Box 51-8). As a result of improved diagnostic techniques, children who in the past would have been diagnosed with RS are now diag-

BOX 51-8 Staging Criteria for Reye's Syndrome

Stage I—Vomiting, lethargy, and drowsiness; liver dysfunction; type I electroencephalogram (EEG); follows commands; pupillary reaction brisk

Stage II—Disorientation, combativeness, delirium, hyperventilation, hyperactive reflexes, appropriate responses to painful stimuli; evidence of liver dysfunction; type I EEG; pupillary reaction sluggish

Stage III—Obtunded, coma, hyperventilation, decorticate rigidity, preservation of pupillary light reaction and oculovestibular reflexes (although sluggish); type II EEG

Stage IV—Deepening coma, decerebrate rigidity, loss of oculocephalic reflexes, large and fixed pupils, loss of doll's eye reflex, loss of corneal reflexes; minimal liver dysfunction; type III or IV EEG; evidence of brainstem dysfunction

Stage V—Seizures, loss of deep tendon reflexes, respiratory arrest, flaccidity; type IV EEG; usually no evidence of liver dysfunction

nosed with other illnesses such as viral or metabolic diseases. Cases of unrecognized, drug-induced encephalopathy by antiemetics given to children during viral illnesses have symptoms similar to those of RS.

The potential association between aspirin therapy for the treatment of fever in children with varicella or influenza and the development of RS precludes its use in these patients. However, by the time the FDA required aspirin product labeling in 1986, most of the decline in RS incidence had already occurred.

Therapeutic Management

The most important aspect of successful management of the child with RS is early diagnosis and aggressive therapy. Rapid progression through coma stages and high peak ammonia concentrations are associated with a more serious prognosis. Cerebral edema with increased ICP represents the most immediate threat to life. Recovery from RS is rapid and usually without sequelae if diagnosis is determined early and therapy is initiated promptly.

Prognosis

Although the incidence of RS has markedly decreased, health professionals must remind parents and caregivers to avoid using both aspirin and non-aspirin–containing salicylates during febrile illnesses in children (Bhutta, Van Savell, & Schexnayder, 2003; Kamienski, 2003). Survivors may have subtle neuropsychologic deficits. Generally, recovery is good given the gravity of the disease (Bhutta, Van Savell, & Schexnayder, 2003; Kamienski, 2003).

Nursing Care Management

The most important aspect of successful management of the child with RS is early diagnosis and aggressive therapy (Bhutta, Van Savell, & Schexnayder, 2003). Cerebral edema with increased ICP represents the most immediate threat to life. Recovery from RS is rapid and usually without sequelae given early diagnosis and implementation of therapy. In about one third of patients, RS causes death or long-term neurologic sequelae.

Care and observations are implemented as for any child with an altered state of consciousness (see p. 1552) and increasing ICP. Accurate and frequent monitoring of intake and output is essential for adjusting fluid volumes to prevent both dehydration and cerebral edema. Because of related liver dysfunction, laboratory studies to determine impaired coagulation, such as prolonged bleeding time, should be monitored.

Parents of children with RS need to be kept informed of the child's progress, to have diagnostic procedures and therapeutic management explained, and to be given concerned and sympathetic support.* Families need to be aware that salicylate, the alleged offending ingredient in aspirin, is contained in other products (e.g., Pepto-Bismol). They should refrain from administering any product for influenza-like symptoms without first checking the label for "hidden" salicylates.

Seizure Disorders

Seizures are caused by excessive and disorderly neuronal discharges in the brain. The manifestation of seizures depends on the region of the brain in which they originate and may include unconsciousness or altered consciousness; involuntary movements; and changes in perception, behaviors, sensations, and posture. Seizures are the most common treatable neurologic disorder in children and can occur with a wide variety of conditions involving the CNS.

Epilepsy

Epilepsy is a condition characterized by two or more unprovoked seizures and can be caused by a variety of pathologic processes in the brain. Seizures are a symptom of an underlying disease process. A single seizure event should not be classified as epilepsy and is generally not treated with long-term antiepileptic drugs. Some seizures may result from an acute medical or neurologic illness and cease once the illness is treated. In other cases, children may have a single seizure without the cause ever being known. Once it is determined that the child has had a seizure, it is important to classify the seizure, according to the Classification of Epileptic Seizures, and assign it to the appropriate epilepsy syndrome, according to the Classification of Epilepsies and Epileptic Syndromes. Optimum treatment and prognosis require an accurate diagnosis and a determination of the cause whenever possible.

Etiology

Seizures in children have many different causes. Seizures are classified not only according to type, but also according to etiology. Acute symptomatic seizures are associated with an acute insult such as head trauma or meningitis. Remote symptomatic seizures are those without an immediate cause but with an identifiable prior brain injury such as major head trauma, meningitis or encephalitis, hypoxia, stroke, or a static

*National Reye's Syndrome Foundation, 800-233-7393 (United States only) or 419-924-9000; fax: 419-924-9999; e-mail: nrsf@reyessydrome.org; www.reyessyndrome.org.

BOX 51-9 Etiology of Seizures in Children

Nonrecurrent (Acute)
Febrile episodes
Intracranial infection
Intracranial hemorrhage
Space-occupying lesions (cyst, tumor)
Acute cerebral edema
Anoxia
Toxins
Drugs
Tetanus
Lead encephalopathy
Shigella, Salmonella organisms
Metabolic alterations:
- Hypocalcemia
- Hypoglycemia
- Hyponatremia or hypernatremia
- Hypomagnesemia
- Alkalosis
- Disorders of amino acid metabolism
- Deficiency states
- Hyperbilirubinemia

Recurrent (Chronic)
Idiopathic epilepsy
Epilepsy secondary to:
- Trauma
- Hemorrhage
- Anoxia
- Infections
- Toxins
- Degenerative phenomena
- Congenital defects
- Parasitic brain disease
- Hypoglycemia injury

Epilepsy—sensory stimulus
Epilepsy-stimulating states:
- Narcolepsy and catalepsy
- Psychogenic
- Tetany from hypocalcemia, alkalosis

Hypoglycemic states:
- Hyperinsulinism
- Hypopituitarism
- Adrenocortical insufficiency
- Hepatic disorders

Uremia
Allergy
Cardiovascular dysfunction or syncopal episodes
Migraine

encephalopathy such as intellectual disability or cerebral palsy. Cryptogenic seizures are those occurring with no clear cause. Idiopathic seizures are genetic in origin. A partial list of causative factors is presented in Box 51-9.

Pathophysiology

evolve Animation—Seizure, Generalized

Regardless of the etiologic factor or type of seizure, the basic mechanism is the same. Abnormal electrical discharges (1) may arise from central areas in the brain that affect consciousness; (2) may be restricted to one area of the cerebral cortex, producing manifestations characteristic of that particular anatomic focus; or (3) may begin in a localized area of the cortex and spread to other portions of the brain and, if sufficiently extensive, produce generalized seizure activity.

In response to physiologic stimuli, such as cellular dehydration, severe hypoglycemia, electrolyte imbalance, sleep deprivation, emotional stress, and endocrine changes, these hyperexcitable cells activate normal cells in surrounding areas and distant, synaptically related cells. A generalized seizure develops when the neuronal excitation from the epileptogenic focus spreads to the brainstem, particularly the midbrain and reticular formation. These centers within the brainstem, known as the *centrencephalic system,* are responsible for the spread of the epileptic potentials. The discharges can originate spontaneously in the centrencephalic system or be triggered by a focal area in the cortex. On the basis of these characteristic neuronal discharges (as recorded by the EEG), seizures are designated as partial, generalized, and unclassified epileptic seizures (Menkes & Sankar, 2000). In a large proportion of children focal seizures spread to other areas, ultimately becoming generalized with loss of consciousness.

Seizure Classification and Clinical Manifestations

There are many different types of seizures, and each has unique clinical manifestations. Seizures are classified into three major categories:

1. Partial seizures, which have a local onset and involve a relatively small location in the brain
2. Generalized seizures, which involve both hemispheres of the brain and are without local onset
3. Unclassified epileptic seizures

Descriptions of the different types of seizures are found in Box 51-10 and Table 51-3.

Diagnostic Evaluation

Establishing a diagnosis is critical for establishing a prognosis and planning the proper treatment. The process of diagnosis in a child suspected of having epilepsy includes (1) determining whether epilepsy or seizures exist and not an alternative diagnosis, and (2) defining the underlying cause, if possible. The assessment and diagnosis rely heavily on a thorough history, skilled observation, and several diagnostic tests.

It is especially important to differentiate epilepsy from other brief alterations in consciousness or behavior. Clinical entities that mimic seizures include migraine headaches, toxic effects of drugs, syncope (fainting), breath-holding spells in infants and young children, movement disorders (tics, tremor, chorea), prolonged QT syndrome, sleep disturbances (sleepwalking, night terrors), psychogenic seizures, rage attacks, and transient ischemic attacks (rare in children) (Browne & Holmes, 2004). Cocaine intoxication should be considered in the differential diagnosis of new-onset seizure activity in newborn infants.

BOX 51-10 Classification and Clinical Manifestations of Seizures

Partial Seizures

Simple Partial Seizures with Motor Signs

Characterized by:

- Localized motor symptoms
- Somatosensory, psychic, autonomic symptoms
- Combination of these
- Abnormal discharges remaining unilateral

Manifestations:

- Aversive seizure (most common motor seizure in children)—Eye or eyes and head turn away from the side of the focus; awareness of movement or loss of consciousness
- Rolandic (Sylvan) seizure—Tonic-clonic movements involving the face, salivation, arrested speech; most common during sleep
- Jacksonian march (rare in children)—Orderly, sequential progression of clonic movements beginning in a foot, hand, or face and moving, or "marching," to adjacent body parts

Simple Partial Seizures with Sensory Signs

Characterized by various sensations, including:

- Numbness, tingling, prickling, paresthesia, or pain originating in one area (e.g., face or extremities) and spreading to other parts of the body
- Visual sensations or formed images
- Motor phenomena such as posturing or hypertonia

Uncommon in children younger than 8 years of age

Complex Partial Seizures (Psychomotor Seizures)

Observed more often in children from 3 years through adolescence

Characterized by:

- Period of altered behavior
- Amnesia for event (no recollection of behavior)
- Inability to respond to environment
- Impaired consciousness during event
- Drowsiness or sleep usually following seizure
- Confusion and amnesia possibly prolonged
- Complex sensory phenomena (aura)—Most frequent sensation is a strange feeling in the pit of the stomach that rises toward the throat; often accompanied by:
  - — Odd or unpleasant odors or tastes
  - — Complex auditory or visual hallucinations
  - — Ill-defined feelings of elation or strangeness (e.g., déjà vu, a feeling of familiarity in a strange environment)
  - — Strong feelings of fear and anxiety; distorted sense of time and self
  - — In small children, emission of a cry or attempt to run for help

Patterns of motor behavior:

- Stereotypic
- Similar with each subsequent seizure
- May suddenly cease activity, appear dazed, stare into space, become confused and apathetic, and become limp or stiff or display some form of posturing
- May be confused
- May perform purposeless, complicated activities in a repetitive manner (automatisms), such as walking, running, kicking, laughing, or speaking incoherently, most often followed by postictal confusion or sleep
- May exhibit oropharyngeal activities, such as smacking, chewing, drooling, swallowing, and nausea or abdominal pain followed by stiffness, a fall, and postictal sleep
- Rarely manifests actions such as rage or temper tantrums; aggressive acts uncommon during seizure

Generalized Seizures

Tonic-Clonic Seizures (Formerly Known as Grand Mal)

Most common and most dramatic of all seizure manifestations

Occur without warning

Tonic Phase

Lasts approximately 10 to 20 seconds

Manifestations:

- Eyes roll upward
- Immediate loss of consciousness
- If standing, falls to floor or ground
- Stiffens in generalized, symmetric tonic contraction of entire body musculature
- Arms usually flexed
- Legs, head, and neck extended
- May utter a peculiar piercing cry
- Apneic; may become cyanotic
- Increased salivation and loss of swallowing reflex

Clonic Phase

Lasts about 30 seconds but can vary from only a few seconds to a half hour or longer

Manifestations:

- Violent jerking movements as the trunk and extremities undergo rhythmic contraction and relaxation
- May foam at the mouth
- May be incontinent of urine and feces

As event ends, movements less intense, occurring at longer intervals, then ceasing entirely

Status Epilepticus

Series of seizures at intervals too brief to allow the child to regain consciousness between the time one event ends and the next begins

- Requires emergency intervention
- Can lead to exhaustion, respiratory failure, and death

Postictal State

Manifestations:

- Appears to relax
- May remain semiconscious and difficult to arouse
- May awaken in a few minutes
- Remains confused for several hours
- Poor coordination
- Mild impairment of fine motor movements
- May have visual and speech difficulties
- May vomit or complain of severe headache
- When left alone, usually sleeps for several hours
- On awakening is fully conscious

Continued

BOX 51-10 Classification and Clinical Manifestations of Seizures—cont'd

Generalized Seizures—cont'd

Tonic-Clonic Seizures (Formerly Known as Grand Mal)—cont'd

Postictal State–cont'd

- Usually feels tired and complains of sore muscles and headache
- No recollection of entire event

Absence Seizures (Formerly Called Petit Mal or Lapses)

Characterized by:

- Onset usually between 4 and 12 years of age
- More common in girls than in boys
- Usually cease at puberty
- Brief loss of consciousness
- Minimum or no alteration in muscle tone
- May go unrecognized because of little change in child's behavior
- Abrupt onset; suddenly develops 20 or more attacks daily
- Event often mistaken for inattentiveness or daydreaming
- Events possibly precipitated by hyperventilation, hypoglycemia, stresses (emotional and physiologic), fatigue, or sleeplessness

Manifestations:

- Brief loss of consciousness
- Appear without warning or aura
- Usually last about 5 to 10 seconds
- Slight loss of muscle tone may cause child to drop objects
- Ability to maintain postural control; seldom falls
- Minor movements such as lip smacking, twitching of eyelids or face, or slight hand movements
- Not accompanied by incontinence
- Amnesia for episode
- May need to reorient self to previous activity

Atonic and Akinetic Seizures (Also Known as Drop Attacks)

Characterized by:

- Onset usually between 2 and 5 years of age
- Sudden, momentary loss of muscle tone and postural control
- Events recurring frequently during the day, particularly in the morning hours and shortly after awakening

Manifestations:

- Loss of tone causing child to fall to the floor violently; unable to break fall by putting out hand; may incur a serious injury to the face, head, or shoulder
- Loss of consciousness only momentary

Myoclonic Seizures

A variety of seizure episodes

May be isolated as benign essential myoclonus

May occur in association with other seizure forms

Characterized by:

- Sudden, brief contractures of a muscle or group of muscles
- Occur singly or repetitively
- No postictal state
- May or may not be symmetric
- May or may not include loss of consciousness

Infantile Spasms

Also called infantile myoclonus, massive spasms, hypsarrhythmia, salaam episodes, or infantile myoclonic spasms

Most commonly occur during the first 6 to 8 months of life

Twice as common in boys as in girls

Numerous seizures during the day without postictal drowsiness or sleep

Poor outlook for normal intelligence

Manifestations:

- Possible series of sudden, brief, symmetric, muscular contractions
- Head flexed, arms extended, and legs drawn up
- Eyes sometimes rolling upward or inward
- May be preceded or followed by a cry or giggling
- May or may not include loss of consciousness
- Sometimes flushing, pallor, or cyanosis

Infants who are able to sit but not stand:

- Sudden dropping forward of the head and neck with trunk flexed forward and knees drawn up—the *salaam* or *jackknife* seizure

Less often: alternate clinical forms:

- Extensor spasms rather than flexion of arms, legs, and trunk, and head nodding
- Lightning events involving a single, momentary, shocklike contraction of the entire body

The history of the seizure should be equally detailed, including the type of seizure or description of the child's behavior during the event, the age at onset, and the time at which the seizure occurs (e.g., early morning, before meals, while awake, or during sleep). Any factors that may have precipitated the seizure are important, including fever, infection, head trauma, anxiety, fatigue, sleep deprivation, menstrual cycle, alcohol, and activity (e.g., hyperventilation or exposure to strong stimuli such as bright flashing light or loud noises). If the child can describe any sensory phenomena, these are recorded. The duration and progression of the seizure (if any) and the postictal feelings and behavior (e.g., confusion, inability to speak, amnesia, headache, and sleep) are recorded. It is important to determine whether more than one seizure type exists. It is often more informative to ask parents to mime the seizure rather than relying on their oral description. Miming often reveals features, such as head turning, that would otherwise go unrecognized. Some seizures are overlooked by parents. For example, some parents may not identify brief head nods or brief single jerks as seizures unless specifically asked whether their child has these symptoms. The family history should include whether other family members have had a seizure, intellectual disability, cerebral palsy, or other neurologic disorders. A family history can offer clues to

Table 51-3 Comparison of Simple Partial, Complex Partial, and Absence Seizures

CLINICAL MANIFESTATIONS	SIMPLE PARTIAL	COMPLEX PARTIAL	ABSENCE
Age of onset	Any age	Uncommon before age 3 yr	Uncommon before age 3 yr
Frequency (per day)	Variable	Rarely >1-2 times	Multiple
Duration	Usually <30 sec	Usually >60 sec, rarely <10 sec	Usually <10 sec, rarely >30 sec
Aura	May be sole manifestation of seizure	Frequent	Never
Impaired consciousness	Never	Always	Always; brief loss of consciousness
Automatisms	Never	Frequent	Frequent
Clonic movements	Frequent	Occasional	Occasional
Postictal impairment	Rare	Frequent	Never
Mental disorientation	Rare	Common	Unusual

paroxysmal disorders such as migraine headaches, breath-holding spells, febrile seizures, or neurologic diseases.

A complete physical and neurologic examination, including developmental assessment of language, learning, behavior, and motor abilities, may provide clues to the cause of the seizures. A number of laboratory and neuroimaging tests may be ordered depending on the child's age, whether this is a new onset seizure, characteristics of the seizure, and the history. Laboratory studies that may prove to be of value include a venous lead level if the history warrants or white blood cell count (for signs of infection). Blood glucose may give evidence of hypoglycemic episodes, and serum electrolytes, blood urea nitrogen, calcium, serum amino acids, lactate, ammonia, and urine organic acids may indicate metabolic disturbances. Blood for chromosomal analysis may also be tested if a genetic etiology is suspected. A toxic screen may be done if alcohol or drug abuse or withdrawal is suspected. Lumbar puncture can confirm a suspected diagnosis of meningitis. CT may be done to detect a cerebral hemorrhage, infarctions, and gross malformations. MRI provides greater anatomic detail and is used to detect developmental malformations, tumors, and cortical dysplasias (Kuzniecky, 2001).

The EEG is obtained for all children with seizures and is the most useful tool for evaluating a seizure disorder. The EEG confirms the presence of abnormal electrical discharges and provides information on the seizure type and the focus. The EEG is carried out under varying conditions—with the child asleep, awake, awake with provocative stimulation (flashing lights, noise), and hyperventilating. Stimulation may elicit abnormal electrical activity, which is recorded on the EEG. Various seizure types produce characteristic EEG patterns: high-voltage spike discharges are seen in tonic-clonic seizures, with abnormal patterns in the intervals between seizures; a three-per-second spike and wave pattern is observed in an absence seizure; and absence of electrical activity in an area suggests a large lesion, such as an abscess or subdural collection of fluid.

A normal EEG does not rule out seizures because the EEG is only a surface recording and only represents approximately 1 hour of time and therefore may show normal interictal activity. If there is concern about whether a child has seizures or the seizure type cannot be determined, then a long-term video EEG may be done to record the child during wakefulness and sleep. The full body image is recorded on video, with selected EEG channels displayed on the same screen for simultaneous recording and viewing. EEG monitoring is also available in digital EEG and digital video imaging, which allows for greater selection of EEG channels and is available in both routine and long-term EEGs. Polygraph equipment may also be used to monitor physiologic data such as respiratory effort, eye movements, heart rate, and systemic blood pressure. These techniques can be used concurrently and are especially valuable in differentiating epileptic activity from paroxysmal behavior or nonepileptic motor events.

evolve Critical Thinking Exercise—Seizures

Therapeutic Management

The goal of treatment of seizure disorders is to control the seizures or to reduce their frequency and severity, discover and correct the cause when possible, and help the child live as normal a life as possible. If the seizure activity is a manifestation of an infectious, traumatic, or metabolic process, the seizure therapy is instituted as part of the general therapeutic regimen. Management of epilepsy has four treatment options: drug therapy, the ketogenic diet, vagus nerve stimulation, and epilepsy surgery.

Drug Therapy

It is known that persons predisposed to epilepsy have seizures when their basal level of neuronal excitability exceeds a critical point; no event occurs if the excitability is maintained below this threshold. The administration of antiepileptic drugs serves to raise this threshold and prevent seizures. Consequently, the primary therapy for seizure disorders is the administration of the appropriate antiepileptic drug or combination of drugs in a dosage that provides the desired effect without causing undesirable side effects or toxic reactions. Antiepileptic drugs are believed to exert their effect primarily by reducing the responsiveness of normal neurons to the sudden, high-frequency nerve impulses that arise in the epileptogenic focus. Thus the seizure is effectively suppressed; however, the abnormal brain waves may or may not be altered. Complete control can be achieved in 75% of children with epilepsy; good control can be achieved in another 15% (Shafer, 1999).

Therapy is begun with a single drug known to be effective and have the lowest toxicity, that is, the safest side effect profile for the child's particular type of seizure. The dosage is gradually increased until the seizures are controlled or the child develops side effects. If the drug is effective but does not sufficiently control the seizures, a second drug is added in gradually increasing doses. Once seizures are controlled, the first drug may be tapered to reduce the potential adverse effects of polytherapy. However, this decision is individualized for each child (Browne & Holmes, 2004). Monotherapy remains the treatment method of choice for epilepsy, but polypharmacy may be a viable alternative for children who cannot attain seizure control with only one agent (Leppik, 2000).

Measurement of blood levels of the drug is important if the seizures continue once the child is on a therapeutic dose of medication, to adjust the dosage, and to assist in determining which medication may be causing the side effects if the child is on multiple antiepileptic medications. Some possible causes of low serum blood concentrations are noncompliance, poor absorption, and drug interactions. The dosage needs to be increased as the child grows. Blood cell counts, urinalysis, and liver function tests are obtained at frequent intervals in children receiving particular antiepileptic medications that can affect organ function.

If complete seizure control is maintained on an anticonvulsant drug for 2 years, it is safe to discontinue the drug for patients with no risk factors. Risk factors include children over 12 years of age at onset, history of neonatal seizures, numerous seizures before control is achieved, and the presence of a neurologic dysfunction (e.g., motor handicap or intellectual disability). Up to 25% of children whose medications are discontinued will experience seizure recurrence. Recurrence occurs most frequently within 6 months of discontinuation (Johnston, 2007).

When seizure medications are discontinued, the dosage is decreased gradually over several weeks. Sudden withdrawal of a drug is not recommended because it can cause an increase in the number and severity of seizures.

NURSING ALERT Fosphenytoin is often used to treat seizures instead of IV phenytoin because of possible complications and drug interactions associated with IV phenytoin. If IV phenytoin is used, it should be administered via slow IV push at a rate that does not exceed 50 mg/min. Because phenytoin precipitates when mixed with glucose, only normal saline is used to flush the tubing or catheter. Fosphenytoin may be given in saline or glucose solutions at a rate of up to 150 mg PE (phenytoin equivalent)/min, and it may be given intramuscularly if necessary.

Ketogenic Diet

The ketogenic diet is a high-fat, low-carbohydrate, and adequate protein diet (Lefevre & Aronson, 2000). Consumption of such a diet forces the body to shift from using glucose as the primary energy source to using fat, and the individual develops a state of ketosis. The diet is rigorous. All foods and liquids the child consumes must be carefully weighed and measured. The diet is deficient in vitamins and minerals; therefore vitamin supplements are necessary. Potential side effects of the diet are constipation, weight loss, lethargy, and kidney stones. It is unknown whether long-term effects such as increased blood lipids will occur (Levy & Cooper, 2003).

The ketogenic diet has been shown to be an efficacious and tolerable treatment for difficult-to-control seizures (Freeman, Kossoff, & Hartman, 2007). Outcomes of 150 children with uncontrollable seizures revealed that 7% of the children were seizure free and another 20% had a 90% decrease in seizures 1 year after instituting the ketogenic diet (Freeman et al, 1998). Three to 6 years later, 27% of these children had few or no seizures while on the ketogenic diet (Hemingway et al, 2001).

Vagus Nerve Stimulation

Vagus nerve stimulation uses an implantable device that reduces seizures in individuals who have not had effective control with drug therapy. It is currently indicated as adjunct therapy in patients 12 years and older with partial onset seizures (with or without secondary generalization). A programmable signal generator is implanted subcutaneously in the chest. Electrodes tunneled underneath the skin deliver electrical impulses to the left vagus nerve (cranial nerve X). The device is programmed noninvasively to deliver a precise pattern of stimulation to the left vagus nerve. The patient or caregiver can activate the device using a magnet at the onset of a seizure. Studies show that about one third of patients have a 50% or greater reduction in seizures after 1 year of therapy (Morris, Mueller, & Vagus Nerve Stimulation Study Group E01-E05, 1999).

Surgical Therapy

When seizures are determined to be caused by a hematoma, tumor, or other cerebral lesion, surgical removal is the treatment. In children with epilepsy, surgery is reserved for those who suffer from incapacitating, refractory seizures. Refractory seizures are usually defined as the persistence of seizures despite adequate trials of three antiepileptic medications, alone or in combination (Browne & Holmes, 2004). The epileptogenic area should be in a surgically removable and functionally silent region of the brain. Early removal of the symptomatic area is associated with seizure control and decreased use of antiepileptic drugs (Mathern et al, 1999). An extensive medical (e.g., invasive EEG monitoring), psychosocial, and psychoneurologic evaluation is required.

Status Epilepticus

Status epilepticus is a continuous seizure that lasts more than 30 minutes or a series of seizures from which the child does not regain a premorbid LOC (Shorvon & Walker, 2005; Treiman & Walker, 2006). The duration required for seizures to be considered status epilepticus continues to be debated (Chen & Wasterlain, 2006). The initial treatment is directed toward support and maintenance of vital functions, that is, attending to the ABCs of life support, administering oxygen, and gaining IV access, immediately followed by IV administration of antiepileptic agents.

Rectal diazepam is a simple, effective, and safe treatment for home or prehospital management (Pellock & Shinnar, 2005). It is available in a prefilled rectal gel syringe (Diastat) for easy administration. Rectal diazepam is not associated with respiratory depression when used as recommended (Pellock & Shinnar, 2005). Midazolam has been given successfully by intranasal route for treatment of acute epileptic seizures (Fisgin et al, 2000; Kutlu et al, 2000). Intranasal midazolam is not only safe and effective for stopping seizures, but is easier to administer that rectal diazepam (Harbord et al, 2004).

For in-hospital management of status epilepticus, IV diazepam or lorazepam (Ativan) is the first-line drug of choice (Browne & Holmes, 2004). Lorazepam may be replacing IV diazepam as the drug of choice. It has a longer duration of action and causes less respiratory depression in children over 2 years of age. Concurrent IV loading with fosphenytoin is usually necessary for sustained control of seizures. Valproic acid has also been reported to be effective in status epilepticus when given rectally or intravenously (Yamamoto & Yim, 2000). The child must be closely monitored during administration to detect early alterations in vital signs that may indicate impending respiratory depression. When diazepam is ineffective, fosphenytoin or phenobarbital is given intravenously as the next line of treatment. This combination of therapy places the child at high risk for apnea, and therefore respiratory support is generally necessary. Children who continue to have seizures despite the above drug treatment may be given anesthetizing doses of midazolam, propofol, or pentobarbital. In this situation, continuous EEG monitoring is typically done to monitor for and treat electrographic seizures.

NURSING ALERT Diazepam is incompatible with many drugs. To give intravenously, inject slowly and directly into the vein or through tubing as close as possible to the vein insertion site.

Nursing care of a child with status epilepticus includes, in addition to the ABCs of life support, monitoring blood pressure and body temperature. During the first 30 to 45 minutes of the seizure the blood pressure may be elevated. Thereafter the blood pressure typically returns to normal but may be decreased depending on the medications being administered for seizure control. Hyperthermia requiring treatment may occur as a result of increased motor activity.

Prognosis

Most children who experience a second seizure will experience additional seizures. Therefore a history of two seizures is sufficient to diagnose epilepsy (Shinnar et al, 2000). Epidemiologic studies using population- or community-based cohorts show that the etiology and specific epilepsy syndromes are the most important factors affecting prognosis. Children who have intellectual disability or cerebral palsy are at the highest risk for developing epilepsy. Seizures will remit in more than two thirds of children with childhood onset of seizure. Mortality is increased in children with epilepsy; those with neurologic abnormalities or seizures that are refractory to treatment are at the highest risk (Browne & Holmes, 2004).

Nursing Care Management

An important nursing responsibility is to observe the seizure episode and accurately document the events. Any alterations in behavior preceding the seizure and the characteristics of the episode, such as sensory-hallucinatory phenomena (e.g., an aura), motor effects (e.g., eye movements, muscular contractions), alterations in consciousness, and postictal state, are noted and recorded (Box 51-11). The nurse should describe only what is observed, rather than trying to label a seizure type. He or she notes the time that the seizure began and the duration of the seizure.

Based on a thorough assessment, several nursing diagnoses are identified. The more common diagnoses for the child with a seizure disorder are included in the Nursing Care Plan.

The child must be protected from injury during the seizure. Nursing observations made during the event provide valuable information for diagnosis and management of the disorder (see Emergency box). It is impossible to halt a seizure once it has begun, and no attempt should be made to do so. The nurse must remain calm, stay with the child, and prevent the child from sustaining any harm during the seizure. If possible, the child should be isolated from the view of others by closing a door or pulling screens. A seizure can be upsetting to the child, other visitors, and their families. If other persons are present, they should be assured that everything is being done for the child. After the seizure, they can be given a simple explanation about the event as needed.

If the nurse is able to reach the child in time, a child who is standing or seated in a chair (including a wheelchair) is eased to the floor immediately. During (and sometimes after) the tonic-clonic seizure, the swallowing reflex is lost, salivation increases, and the tongue is hypotonic. Therefore the child is at risk for aspiration and airway occlusion. Placing the child on the side facilitates drainage and helps maintain a patent airway. Suctioning the oral cavity and posterior oropharynx may be necessary. Vital signs should be taken. The child is allowed to rest if at school or away from home. When feasible, the child is integrated into the environment as soon as possible. Sending a child with a chronic seizure disorder home from school is not necessary unless requested by the parents.

Seizure precautions are required for children who are known to have seizures or who are under observation for seizures. The extent of these measures depends on the type and frequency of the seizure (Box 51-12).

NURSING ALERT Do not move or forcefully restrain the child during a tonic-clonic seizure, and do not place a solid object between the teeth.

Long-Term Care

Care of the child with a recurrent seizure disorder involves physical care and instruction regarding the importance of the drug therapy and, probably more significant, the problems related to the emotional aspects of the disorder. Few diseases generate as much anxiety among relatives as epilepsy. Fears and misconceptions about the disease and its treatment abound in the layperson's mind. For many, it represents the archetype of severe hereditary affliction. Nursing care is directed toward educating the child and family about epilepsy and helping them develop strategies to cope with the psychologic and sociologic problems related to epilepsy.

Children with epilepsy are prescribed antiepileptic medications. These medications are administered at regular intervals to maintain adequate levels in the blood. The most convenient times for administration seem to be with meals or at bedtime. It is important to impress on the family the necessity of giving

NURSING CARE PLAN ✤ The Child with Seizure Disorder

Nursing Diagnosis

Risk for injury related to central nervous system (CNS) dysfunction and inability to control self (motor) secondary to type of seizure

Child's/Family's Defining Characteristics

(Subjective and Objective Data)

- Change in level of consciousness (LOC)
- Disorientation
- Clonic movements
- Automatisms
- Aura
- Postictal impairment (dependent on the type of seizure)

Expected Patient Outcomes

Child will not experience physical injury as a result of seizure activity.

The Following NOC Concepts Apply to These Outcomes

- Risk Control
- Personal Safety Behavior
- Safe Home Environment
- Falls Occurrence

Nursing Interventions and Rationale

Nursing Interventions	Rationale
Administer antiepileptic medication (AED).	To prevent seizure activity
Teach family and child, as appropriate, the purpose of AED medication, action, potential side effects, and administration of medications.	To prevent seizure activity and encourage self-care
Monitor for side effects of AED and therapeutic levels according to child's growth, illness factors that affect metabolism, and effects of drug.	To prevent secondary effects of AED and prevent seizure from subtherapeutic drug levels
Stress importance of compliance with medication regimen even if child has no evidence of seizure activity.	To prevent seizure activity
Advise family and child to avoid situations that are known to precipitate a seizure (e.g., blinking lights, fatigue, excess activity or exercise, physical factors).	To prevent exposure to situations that may cause a seizure
Assess home care environment for risk factors that may produce childhood physical injury: loose rugs; unprotected stairway; access to water buckets, pool, or standing water.	To prevent physical harm
Teach parents by anticipatory guidance risk factors for injury in environment based on child's developmental age and type of seizure (e.g., not leaving child in bathtub without adult supervision).	
Counsel female patients of childbearing age taking AEDs about contraception and birth defects associated with AEDs.	To prevent birth defects in offspring of women taking AEDs
In the event of a tonic-clonic seizure: ✤ Place child on side. ✤ Time seizure. ✤ Protect child during seizure. ✤ Do not attempt to restrain child or use force. ✤ If child is standing or sitting in wheelchair at beginning of episode, ease child to floor. ✤ Do not put anything in child's mouth. ✤ Place small cushion or blanket under child's head. ✤ Remove child's eyeglasses. ✤ Loosen clothing. ✤ Prevent child from hitting head on objects. ✤ Remove hazards. ✤ Pad objects such as crib, side rails, or wheelchair. ✤ Keep side rails raised when child is sleeping, resting, or having a seizure. ✤ Allow seizure to end without interference.	To prevent injury and trauma To prevent aspiration and maintain a patent airway
Teach parents or caregiver how to care for child during seizure and in postictal state.	To protect child and caregiver from injury
Protect child after seizure (postictal period). Time the period. Maintain child in a side-lying or recovery position. Call emergency medical services as necessary or ensure child receives medical evaluation after seizure.	To prevent trauma and implement therapeutic intervention

The Following NIC Concepts Apply to These Interventions

- Surveillance: Safety
- Environmental Management: Safety
- Medication Administration
- Teaching: Disease Process
- Neurologic Monitoring
- Seizure Precautions

NURSING CARE PLAN ✤ The Child with Seizure Disorder—cont'd

Nursing Diagnosis	Expected Patient Outcomes	Nursing Interventions	Rationale
Risk for aspiration and ineffective breathing pattern related to impaired motor activity, loss of consciousness, and loss of airway protection (tonic-clonic seizure)	Child's airway will remain patent. Child will have effective ventilations. **The Following NOC Concepts Apply to These Outcomes** Aspiration Prevention Respiratory Status: Airway Patency Respiratory Status: Ventilation	In the event of a seizure, place child in a side-lying position on a flat surface such as floor or bed.	To prevent aspiration and protect airway
		Remain with child.	To determine need for emergency care
		Remove secretions, food, and liquids from mouth when seizure subsides.	To prevent choking, aspiration
Child's/Family's Defining Characteristics ***(Subjective and Objective Data)*** Reduced LOC Depressed cough reflex Apnea Decreased inspiratory pressure		If child has emesis, place on side.	To prevent choking, aspiration
		In postictal state monitor oxygenation status.	To determine need for oxygen
		Administer oxygen as necessary to maintain pulse oximeter over 89%.	To prevent hypoxia
		Suction oropharynx once seizure subsides as necessary to clear mucus or food.	To prevent aspiration
		Administer medications intended to stop seizure (rectal diazepam [Diastat], rectal phenytoin, intravenous phenytoin). **The Following NIC Concepts Apply to These Interventions** Risk Identification Aspiration Precautions Oxygen Therapy Medication Administration	To prevent continued seizure activity

Nursing Diagnosis	Expected Patient Outcomes	Nursing Interventions	Rationale
Risk for injury related to impaired consciousness and automatisms	Child will not experience physical injury and will remain calm. **The Following NOC Concepts Apply to These Outcomes** Risk Control Safe Home Environment Personal Safety Behavior Physical Injury Severity Falls Occurrence	Time seizure.	To establish duration and possible need for emergency care
		Protect child during seizure. Do not attempt to restrain child or use force.	To prevent injury to child or self
Child's/Family's Defining Characteristics ***(Subjective and Objective Data)*** Immediate loss of consciousness Tonic rigidity replaced by intense jerking movements May become incontinent of urine and feces Postictal impairment Change in vital signs, respiratory status, color Vomiting		Remove hazards in immediate environment.	To prevent injury
		Redirect child to safe area, especially away from windows, stairs, heating elements, or sources of water.	To prevent injury from falls, burns, and drowning
		Talk in calm voice and reassuring manner.	To prevent further agitation
		Watch to see whether seizure generalizes into a tonic-clinic seizure.	To determine type of seizure
		Protect child after seizure (postictal period). Time the period. Stay with child until fully alert. **The Following NIC Concepts Apply to These Interventions** Risk Identification Environmental Management: Safety Surveillance Seizure Precautions	To provide support, because child may be confused and frightened

Continued

NURSING CARE PLAN ✤ The Child with Seizure Disorder—cont'd

Nursing Diagnosis	Expected Patient Outcomes	Nursing Interventions	Rationale
Anxiety/fear (parent), related to child having life-threatening and incapacitating seizure activity*	Parent will cope with child's condition and receive adequate support.	Allow parent(s) to remain with child during seizure.	To decrease fear of unknown and allow parent to see measures taken to protect child
	The Following NOC Concepts Apply to These Outcomes Anxiety Self-Control Coping Fear Self-Control	Instruct parent on proper protection interventions during child's seizure activity: positioning, safety, airway maintenance, reassurance techniques, emergency medication administration.	To promote parent participation and to promote sense of control over situation
Child's/Family's Defining Characteristics ***(Subjective and Objective Data)*** Anguish Fright Feelings of inadequacy and hopelessness Worry, apprehension Panic Excitement		Provide information regarding nature (type) of seizure, therapeutic interventions, and lifestyle modifications.	To promote knowledge of condition, parental intervention, sense of control
		Encourage family involvement in daily care of child, with goal of normalization and promotion of optimal growth and development of child.	To provide hope and promote family functioning and coping
		Involve parents in discussion of fears and anxieties; discuss resource and support options available to family.	To promote family integrity and functioning
		The Following NIC Concepts Apply to These Interventions Support Group Coping Enhancement Anxiety Reduction Family Process Maintenance Active Listening Counseling Decision-Making Support Family Involvement Promotion	

*Nursing diagnosis may also apply to child in the postictal phase, depending on type of seizure and child's understanding and cognitive level.

BOX 51-11 General Observations: The Child During a Seizure

Observations During Seizure

General Description

Order of events (before, during, and after)
Duration of seizure

- Tonic-clonic—from first signs of event until jerking stops
- Absence—from loss of consciousness until consciousness is regained
- Complex partial—from first sign of unresponsiveness, motor activity, automatisms until there are signs of responsiveness to environment

Onset

Time of onset
Significant precipitating events—missed medication dosage, illness, stress, sleep deprivation, menses

Behavior

Change in facial expression
Cry or other sound
Stereotypic or automatous movements
Random activity (wandering)
Position of eyes, head, body, extremities
Unilateral or bilateral posturing of one or more extremities

Movement

Change of position, if any
Site of commencement—hand, thumb, mouth, generalized
Tonic phase—length, parts of body involved
Clonic phase—twitching or jerking movements, parts of body involved, sequence of parts involved, generalized, change in character of movements
Lack of movement or muscle tone of body part or entire body

Face

Color change—pallor, cyanosis, flushing
Perspiration
Mouth—position, deviation to one side, teeth clenched, tongue bitten, frothing at mouth, flecks of blood or bleeding
Lack of expression
Asymmetric expression

Eyes

Position—straight ahead, deviation upward or outward, conjugate or divergent gaze
Pupils—change in size, equality, reaction to light

BOX 51-11 General Observations: The Child During a Seizure—cont'd

Observations During Seizure—cont'd

Respiratory Effort

Presence and length of apnea

Other

Incontinence

Postictal Observations

Duration of postictal period

State of consciousness

Orientation

Arousability

Motor ability:

- Any change in motor function
- Ability to move all extremities
- Paresis or weakness

Speech

Sensations:

- Complaint of discomfort or pain
- Any sensory impairment

Recollection of preseizure sensations (aura)

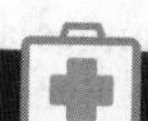

EMERGENCY

Seizures

Tonic-Clonic Seizure

During the Seizure

Remain calm.

Time seizure episode.

If child is standing or seated, ease child down to the floor.

Place pillow or folded blanket under child's head.

Loosen restrictive clothing.

Remove eyeglasses.

Clear area of any hazards or hard objects.

Allow seizure to end without interference.

If vomiting occurs, turn child to one side.

Do not:

- Attempt to restrain child or use force
- Put anything in child's mouth
- Give any food or liquids

After the Seizure

Time postictal period.

Check for breathing. Check position of head and tongue.

Reposition if head is hyperextended. If child is not breathing, give rescue breathing and call emergency medical services (EMS).

Keep child on side.

Remain with child.

Do not give food or liquids until child is fully alert and swallowing reflex has returned.

Call EMS when necessary.

Look for medical identification, and determine what factors occurred before onset of seizure that may have been triggering factors.

Check head and body for possible injuries.

Check inside of mouth to see if tongue or lips have been bitten.

Complex Partial Seizure

During the Seizure

Do not restrain.

Remove harmful objects from area.

Redirect to safe area.

Do not agitate; instead, talk in calm, reassuring manner.

Do not expect child to follow instructions.

Watch to see if seizure generalizes.

After the Seizure

Stay with child and reassure until fully conscious.

Call Emergency Medical Services If

Child stops breathing.

There is evidence of injury or child is diabetic or pregnant.

Seizure lasts for more than 5 minutes (unless duration of seizure is typically longer than 5 minutes) and written medical order is present.

Status epilepticus occurs.

Pupils are not equal after seizure.

Child vomits continuously 30 minutes after seizure has ended (sign of possible acute problem).

Child cannot be awakened and is unresponsive to pain after seizure has ended.

Seizure occurs in water.

This is child's first seizure.

Modified from Epilepsy Foundation: *Seizure recognition and first aid*, 2001. Available at www.epilepsyfoundation.org (accessed March 5, 2007).

the antiepileptic medication regularly and for as long as required. In general, antiepileptic medications are continued until the child has been seizure free for 2 years (Johnston, 2007). The medication is then slowly tapered over a period of weeks to avoid the possibility of precipitating a seizure. It is sometimes easy to skip doses or omit them for a variety of reasons, especially when the child is free of seizures most of the time. This is particularly so when the child is older and assumes responsibility for his or her medication. The seizure threshold may be lowered during any illness, but particularly with fever. Therefore parents should be aware that if their child has an illness, he or she is at increased risk for seizures. Parents should contact their health professional if their child misses medications during an illness because of vomiting.

Rectal preparations of some antiepileptic medications are highly effective when a child is unable to take oral medications because of repeated vomiting, gastrointestinal surgery, or status epilepticus. Parents can learn to administer rectal antiepileptic medication for home treatment. Rectal diazepam is a useful adjunctive home treatment for children at risk for

BOX 51-12 Seizure Precautions

The extent of precautions depends on type, severity, and frequency of seizures. They may include:

- Side rails raised when child is sleeping or resting
- Side rails and other hard objects padded
- Waterproof mattress or pad on bed or crib

Appropriate precautions during potentially hazardous activities may include:

- Swimming with a companion
- Taking showers; bathing only with close supervision
- Using protective helmet and padding during bicycle riding, skateboarding, in-line skating
- Supervising child during use of hazardous machinery or equipment

Have child carry or wear medical identification.

Alert other caregivers to need for any special precautions.

Child may not drive or operate hazardous machinery or equipment unless seizure free for designated period (varies by state).

prolonged seizures or clusters of seizures. Hospitalization is minimized, and parental confidence is enhanced.

NURSING ALERT Children taking phenobarbital or phenytoin should receive adequate vitamin D and folic acid, since deficiencies of both have been associated with these drugs. Phenytoin should not be taken with milk.

Nurses should educate the child and parents about the possible adverse reactions to the medications used to treat seizures. Parents should understand the common side effects and be encouraged to report their observations to their health care provider. Parents should understand that the child needs periodic physical assessment and laboratory studies. Possible adverse effects on the hematopoietic system, liver, and kidneys may be reflected in symptoms such as fever, sore throat, enlarged lymph nodes, jaundice, and bleeding (e.g., easy bruising, petechiae, ecchymoses, epistaxis). A common factor in status epilepticus is inadequate blood levels of antiepileptic drugs.

Although children with epilepsy are at increased risk for injury, limitations on activities should be relatively few. The degree to which activities are restricted is individualized for each child and depends on the type, frequency, and severity of the seizures; the child's response to therapy; and the length of time the seizures have been controlled. To prevent head injuries, children should always wear appropriate safety devices, such as helmets, and should avoid activities involving heights. Although bike riding is safe for most children, children with frequent seizures and impairment of consciousness should avoid it. Skating, in-line skating, and skateboarding should be restricted only in children with frequent seizures. Helmets must be worn while participating in these activities.

Children with epilepsy are at higher risk for drowning than children without epilepsy. Young children should never be left alone in the bathtub, even for a few seconds. Older children and adolescents should be encouraged to use a shower and reminded not to lock the bathroom door when showering. They should never swim unsupervised.

Because the child is encouraged to attend school, camp, and other normal activities, the school nurse and teachers should be made aware of the child's condition and therapy. They can help ensure regularity of medication administration and provision of any special care the child might need. Teachers, child care providers, camp counselors, youth organization leaders, coaches, and other adults who assume responsibility for children should be instructed regarding care of the child during a seizure so that they can act calmly for the child's welfare and influence the attitude of the child's peers.

Triggering Factors

Careful and detailed documentation of seizures over time may indicate a pattern. When this occurs, the nurse or responsible adult may intervene to identify the triggering factors and make changes in the environment that may prevent seizures or decrease their frequency. Often the necessary changes are simple but can make an enormous difference in the lives of the child and family.

The most common factors that may trigger seizures in children include emotional stress, sleep deprivation, fatigue, fever, and illness (Frucht et al, 2000; Nakken et al, 2005). Other precipitating factors include sleep, flickering lights, menstrual cycle, alcohol, heat, hyperventilation, and fasting (Frucht et al, 2000). Some individuals have pattern-sensitive epilepsy, that is, seizures precipitated by changes in dark-light patterns, such as those that occur with a flash on a camera, automobile headlights, reflections of light on snow or water, or rotating blades on a fan. A study by Radhakrishnan and colleagues (2005) showed that most of these individuals had absence, myoclonic, or generalized tonic-clonic seizures. Some children have seizures while playing video games. These children are sensitive to intermittent photic stimulation that can trigger an epileptic episode (Fylan et al, 1999; Ricci & Vigevano, 1999). However, the overwhelming majority of children with epilepsy can play video or computer games and watch television without the risk of seizures.

Febrile Seizures

The International League Against Epilepsy defines a febrile seizure as "a seizure in association with a febrile illness in the absence of a central nervous system infection or acute electrolyte imbalance in children older than 1 month of age without prior afebrile seizures" (Baram & Shinnar, 2002). Febrile seizures are one of the most common neurologic conditions of childhood, affecting approximately 3% to 8% of children (Sadleir & Scheffer, 2007). Most febrile seizures occur between 6 months and 3 years of age, with the average age of onset between 12 and 30 months. They are unusual after 5 years of age. Boys are affected about twice as often as girls, and there appears to be an increased familial susceptibility.

The cause of febrile seizures is still uncertain. Both animal and human studies demonstrate that there is an age-specific susceptibility to seizures induced by fever and that it is the peak temperature that is important, not the rapidity of the temperature elevation (Baram & Shinnar, 2002). The temperature usually exceeds 38.8° C (101.8° F), and the seizure occurs during the temperature rise rather than after a prolonged elevation. Sometimes it constitutes the dramatic beginning of an illness, often an upper respiratory tract or gastrointestinal infection.

Most febrile seizures have stopped by the time the child is taken to a medical facility. However, if the seizure continues, treatment consists of controlling the seizure with IV or rectal diazepam and reducing the temperature with acetaminophen. Antiepileptic prophylaxis is not indicated. Parental education and emotional support are important interventions. Parents need reassurance regarding the benign nature of febrile seizures. Several large studies show no difference in intelligence, behavior, or academic performance in children with febrile seizures compared with either population or sibling controls (Verity, Greenword, & Golding, 1998). Parents also need education on how to protect the child from harm and observe exactly what happens to the child during the event. Attempts to lower the temperature will not prevent a seizure. Tepid sponge baths are not recommended for several reasons: they are ineffective in significantly lowering the temperature, the shivering effect further increases metabolic output, and cooling causes discomfort to the child.

Long-term antiepileptic therapy is usually not required for children with simple febrile seizures. Antipyretic therapy during febrile illness offers symptomatic relief for fever-associated symptoms but appears to be ineffective in preventing a seizure (Sadleir & Scheffer, 2007).

NURSING ALERT If a febrile seizure lasts more than 5 minutes, parents should seek medical attention right away. Instruct them to call for emergency assistance (911) and not to place the child who is actively having a seizure in the car.

Cerebral Malformations

Cranial Deformities

In the normal newborn the cranial sutures are separated by membranous seams several millimeters wide. For the first few hours to 1 to 2 days after birth, the cranial bones are highly mobile, which allows them to mold and slide over one another, adjusting the circumference of the head to accommodate to the changing shape and character of the birth canal. The principal sutures in the infant's skull are the sagittal, coronal, and lambdoidal sutures, and the major soft areas at the juncture of these sutures are the anterior and posterior fontanels.

After birth, growth of the skull bones occurs in a direction *perpendicular* to the line of the suture, and normal closure occurs in a regular and predictable order. Although there are wide variations in the age at which closure takes place in individual children, normally all sutures and fontanels are ossified by the following ages:

Eight weeks—Posterior fontanel closed
Six months—Fibrous union of suture lines and interlocking of serrated edges
Eighteen months—Anterior fontanel closed
After 12 years—Sutures unable to be separated by increased ICP

Solid union of all sutures is not completed until late childhood. Closure of a suture before the expected time inhibits the perpendicular growth. Since normal increase in brain volume requires expansion, the skull is forced to grow in a direction *parallel* to the fused suture. This alteration in skull growth always produces a distortion of the head shape when the underlying brain growth is normal. The small head with closed and normal shape is a result of deficient brain growth. The suture closure is secondary to this brain growth failure; failure of brain growth is not secondary to suture closure.

Various types of cranial deformities are encountered in early infancy. These include the enlarged head with frontal protrusion (*bossing;* characteristic of hydrocephalus), the parietal bossing that is seen in chronic subdural hematoma, the small head, and a variety of skull deformities. Some occur during prenatal development; in others, head circumference is usually within normal limits at birth, and the deviation from normal development becomes apparent with advancing age.

Prognosis

The majority of infants with craniosynostosis have normal brain development. The exceptions are those with genetic disorders that involve brain pathologic conditions.

Nursing Care Management

Nursing care of families in which there is a child with a cranial defect involves identifying children with deformities and referring them for evaluation. Since no therapy is available for children with microcephaly, nursing care is directed toward helping parents adjust to rearing a child with brain damage (see Chapter 42).

Caring for infants who benefit from surgery requires special emphasis on observation for signs of decreased hematocrit and hemoglobin because of the large blood loss during surgery. A cardiac monitor may demonstrate a resting heart rate of 200 beats/min. Nursing care includes observation for signs of hemorrhage, infection, pain, and swelling, as well as parental education for suture care and safety. Surgical sutures should remain dry and intact. Parents need to observe for any signs of redness, drainage, or swelling and report any temperature greater than 38.4° C (101° F).

Early surgical management of craniosynostosis allows proper expansion of the brain and the creation of an acceptable appearance. Parents require special support and education during this time, especially from the health care team (Stal, Chebret, & McElroy, 1998).

Hydrocephalus

Hydrocephalus is a condition caused by an imbalance in the production and absorption of CSF in the ventricular system. When production is greater than absorption, CSF accumulates within the ventricular system, usually under increased pressure, producing passive dilation of the ventricles.

Pathophysiology

The causes of hydrocephalus are varied, but the result is either (1) impaired absorption of CSF fluid within the subarachnoid space, obliteration of the subarachnoid cisterns, or malfunction of the arachnoid villi (*nonobstructive* or *communicating hydrocephalus*); or (2) obstruction to the flow of CSF through the ventricular system (*obstructive* or *noncommunicating hydrocephalus*) (Kinsman & Johnston, 2007). The terms *communicating* and *noncommunicating hydrocephalus* traditionally referred to obstructive and nonobstructive types of hydrocephalus when pneumoencephalography was used to establish the diagnosis; because other diagnostic methods are now used, the terms may be used only as a reference point in the diagnosis. Other authorities suggest that hydrocephalus be

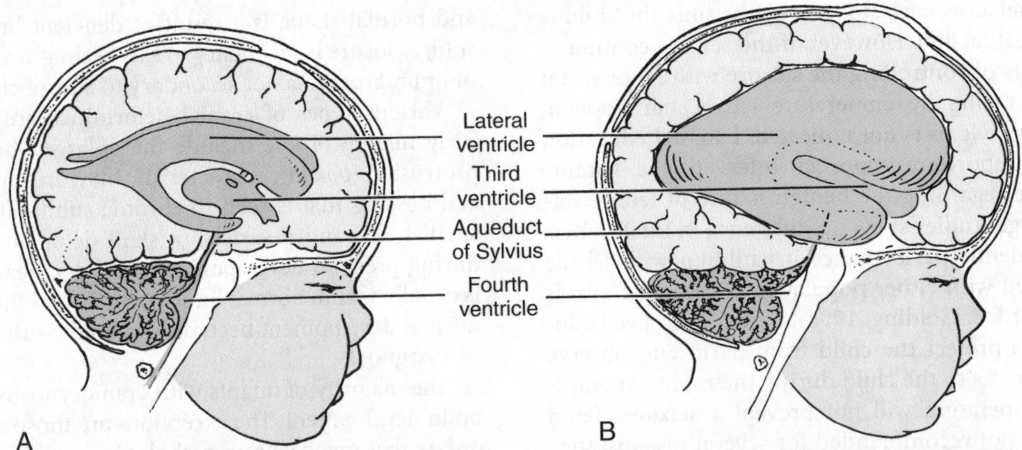

Fig. 51-6 Hydrocephalus: a block in flow of cerebrospinal fluid. **A,** Patent cerebrospinal fluid circulation. **B,** Enlarged lateral and third ventricles caused by obstruction of circulation—stenosis of aqueduct of Sylvius.

evolve Case Study—Hydrocephalus with Myelomeningocele

classified according to the cause and therefore refer to either congenital or acquired hydrocephalus (Rudy, 2005). Rarely, a tumor of the choroid plexus causes increased CSF secretion. Any imbalance of secretion and absorption causes an increased accumulation of CSF in the ventricles, which become dilated (ventriculomegaly) and compress the brain substance against the surrounding rigid bony cranium. When this occurs before fusion of the cranial sutures, it causes enlargement of the skull and dilation of the ventricles (Fig. 51-6). In children younger than 10 to 12 years of age, partially closed suture lines, especially the sagittal suture, may become diastatic or opened. After 12 years of age the sutures are fused and will not open.

Most cases of noncommunicating hydrocephalus are a result of developmental malformations. Although the defect usually is apparent in early infancy, it may become evident at any time from the prenatal period to late childhood or early adulthood. Other causes include neoplasms, infections, and trauma. An obstruction to the normal flow can occur at any point in the CSF pathway to produce increased pressure and dilation of the pathways proximal to the site of obstruction.

Developmental defects (e.g., Arnold-Chiari malformations, aqueduct stenosis, aqueduct gliosis, and atresia of the foramina of Luschka and Magendie [Dandy-Walker syndrome]) account for most cases of hydrocephalus from birth to 2 years of age. Hydrocephalus is so often associated with myelomeningocele that all infants with this condition should be observed for its development. In the remainder of cases there is a history of intrauterine infection, perinatal hemorrhage, and neonatal meningoencephalitis. In older children hydrocephalus is most often a result of space-occupying lesions, intracranial infections, hemorrhage, or preexisting developmental defects, such as aqueduct stenosis or the *Arnold-Chiari malformation* (a congenital anomaly in which the cerebellum and medulla oblongata extend down through the foramen magnum).

Diagnostic Evaluation

The two factors that influence the clinical picture in hydrocephalus are the time of onset and preexisting structural lesions. In infancy, before closure of the cranial sutures, head enlargement is the predominant sign, whereas in older infants and children the lesions responsible for hydrocephalus produce other neurologic signs through pressure on adjacent structures before causing CSF obstruction (Box 51-13).

In infancy the diagnosis of hydrocephalus is based on head circumference that crosses one or more grid lines on the measurement chart within a period of 2 to 4 weeks and on associated neurologic signs that are present and progressive. However, other diagnostic studies are needed to localize the site of CSF obstruction. Routine daily head circumference measurements are carried out in infants with myelomeningocele and intracranial infections. In evaluation of a preterm infant, specially adapted head circumference charts are consulted to distinguish abnormal head growth from rapid head growth that takes place normally.

The signs and symptoms in early to late childhood are caused by increased ICP, and specific manifestations are related to the focal lesion. Most commonly resulting from posterior fossa neoplasms and aqueduct stenosis, the clinical manifestations are primarily those associated with space-occupying lesions.

The primary diagnostic tools for detecting hydrocephalus are CT and MRI. Sedation is required, since the child must remain absolutely still for an accurate picture to be produced. Diagnostic evaluation of children who have symptoms of hydrocephalus after infancy is similar to that used in those with suspected intracranial tumor. In the neonate, echoencephalography is useful in comparing the ratio of lateral ventricle to cortex.

Therapeutic Management

The treatment of hydrocephalus is directed toward relief of the hydrocephalus, treatment of complications, and management of problems related to the effect of the disorder on psychomotor development. The treatment is, with few exceptions, surgical. This is accomplished by direct removal of an obstruction (such as a tumor) or placement of a shunt that provides primary drainage of the CSF from the ventricles to an extracranial compartment, usually the peritoneum *(ventriculoperitoneal [VP] shunt)* (Fig. 51-7).

BOX 51-13 Clinical Manifestations of Hydrocephalus

Infancy (Early)

Abnormally rapid head growth
Bulging fontanels (especially anterior) sometimes without head enlargement:
- Tense
- Nonpulsatile

Dilated scalp veins
Separated sutures
Macewen sign (cracked-pot sound on percussion)
Thinning of skull bones

Infancy (Later)

Frontal enlargement, or bossing
Depressed eyes
Setting-sun sign (sclera visible above the iris)
Pupils sluggish, with unequal response to light

Infancy (General)

Irritability
Lethargy
Infant crying when picked up or rocked and quieting when allowed to lie still
Early infantile reflex acts may persist
Normally expected responses failing to appear
May display:
- Change in level of consciousness
- Opisthotonos (often extreme)
- Lower extremity spasticity
- Vomiting

Advanced cases:
- Difficulty in sucking and feeding
- Shrill, brief, high-pitched cry
- Cardiopulmonary embarrassment

Childhood

Headache on awakening; improvement following emesis or upright posture
Papilledema
Strabismus
Extrapyramidal tract signs (e.g., ataxia)
Irritability
Lethargy
Apathy
Confusion
Incoherence
Vomiting

Most shunt systems consist of a ventricular catheter, a flush pump, a unidirectional flow valve, and a distal catheter. In all models the valves are designed to open at a predetermined intraventricular pressure and close when the pressure falls below that level, thus preventing backflow of secretions.

The initial shunt is placed when necessary to relieve CSF obstruction, and revisions are needed when signs of malfunction appear. In all mechanisms the initial success rate is relatively high; however, shunts are associated with complications that interfere with continued shunt function or threaten the child's life.

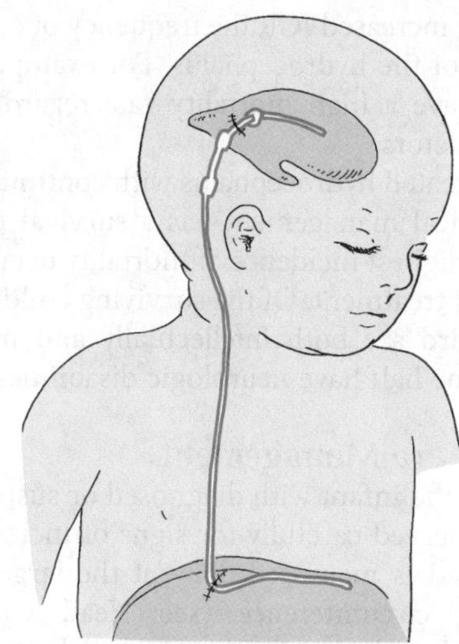

Fig. 51-7 Ventriculoperitoneal shunt. Catheter is threaded beneath the skin.

The major complications of VP shunts are infection and malfunction. All shunts are subject to mechanical difficulties, such as kinking, plugging, or separation or migration of the tubing. Malfunction is most often caused by mechanical obstruction either within the ventricles from particulate matter (tissue or exudate) or at the distal end from thrombosis or displacement as a result of growth. The child with a shunt obstruction is often first seen in an emergency department with clinical manifestations of increased ICP, frequently accompanied by worsening neurologic status.

The most serious complication, shunt infection, can occur at any time, but the period of greatest risk is 1 to 2 months after placement. The infection is generally a result of intercurrent infections at the time of shunt placement. Infections include septicemia, bacterial endocarditis, wound infection, shunt nephritis, meningitis, and ventriculitis. Meningitis and ventriculitis are of greatest concern, since any complicating CNS infection is a significant predictor of poor intellectual outcome. Infection is treated with massive doses of antibiotics administered by the IV route. A persistent infection requires removal of the shunt until the infection is controlled. External ventricular drainage (EVD) is used until CSF is sterile. The EVD allows for removal of CSF through a tube that is placed in the child's ventricle and flows by gravity into a collection device.

An alternative to shunt placement is the endoscopic third ventriculostomy in children with noncommunicating hydrocephalus. In this procedure, an endoscope is used to make a small opening in the floor of the third ventricle that allows the CSF to flow freely through the previously blocked ventricle. Aldana and colleagues (2003) have shown that endoscopic septal fenestration has an overall patency rate of 81%, which may eliminate the need for a CSF shunt. The complication rate of the endoscopic septal fenestration procedure was 9.3% and included intraventricular hemorrhage, sterile meningitis, and septostomy failure.

Prognosis

The prognosis for children with treated hydrocephalus depends largely on the rate at which hydrocephalus develops,

evolve Animation—Ventriculoperitoneal Shunt

the duration of increased ICP, the frequency of complications, and the cause of the hydrocephalus. For example, malignant tumors may have a high mortality rate regardless of other complicating factors.

Surgically treated hydrocephalus with continued neurosurgical and medical management has a survival rate of about 80%, with the highest incidence of mortality occurring within the first year of treatment. Of the surviving children, approximately one third are both intellectually and neurologically normal, and one half have neurologic disabilities.

Nursing Care Management

Preoperatively the infant with diagnosed or suspected hydrocephalus is observed carefully for signs of increasing ICP. In infants the head is measured daily at the largest point, the occipitofrontal circumference (see Head Circumference, Chapter 34, for technique). Fontanels and suture lines are gently palpated for size, signs of bulging, tenseness, and separation. An infant with normal ICP will display bulging under certain circumstances such as straining or crying; therefore such accompanying behavior should be noted. Irritability, lethargy, or seizure activity, as well as altered vital signs and feeding behavior, may indicate an advancing pathologic condition.

In older children, who are usually admitted to the hospital for elective or emergency shunt revision, the most valuable indicator of increasing ICP is an alteration in the child's LOC and the way in which the child interacts with the environment. Changes are identified by observation and by comparison of present behavior with customary behavior, sleep patterns, developmental capabilities, and habits, all obtained through a detailed history and a baseline assessment. This baseline information serves as a guide for postoperative assessment and evaluation of shunt function.

General nursing care of the infant with hydrocephalus may present special problems. Maintaining adequate nutrition often requires flexible feeding schedules to accommodate diagnostic procedures, since feeding before or after handling can precipitate an episode of vomiting. Small feedings at more frequent intervals are often better tolerated than larger ones spaced further apart. These infants are often difficult to feed and require extra time and innovation.

The nurse is responsible for preparing the child for diagnostic tests such as tomography and for assisting the practitioner with procedures such as a ventricular tap, which is often performed to relieve excessive pressure during the preoperative period and for CSF examination. Sedation is required, since the child must remain absolutely still during diagnostic testing. IV pentobarbital or oral chloral hydrate is commonly used for these procedures (see Preparation for Diagnostic and Therapeutic Procedures, Chapter 45).

NURSING ALERT If surgery is anticipated, IV lines should not be placed in a scalp vein on a child with hydrocephalus.

Postoperative Care

Routine postoperative care and observation are instituted. In addition, the infant or child is positioned carefully on the unoperated side to prevent pressure on the shunt valve and pressure areas. The child is kept flat to avoid complications resulting from too-rapid reduction of intracranial fluid. When the ventricular size is reduced too rapidly, the cerebral cortex may pull away from the dura and tear the small interlacing veins, producing a subdural hematoma. This is not a problem in children with elective shunt revision, since their intraventricular size and pressure have been normal. The surgeon indicates the position to be maintained and the extent of activity allowed. If there is increased ICP, the surgeon will prescribe elevation of the head of the bed and allow the child to sit up to enhance gravity flow through the shunt. Pain management can usually be achieved with acetaminophen with or without codeine for mild to moderate pain and opioids for severe pain (see Pain Management, Chapter 35).

Observation is continued for signs of increased ICP, which indicates obstruction of the shunt. Neurologic assessment includes evaluation of pupillary dilation (pressure causes compression or stretching of the oculomotor nerve, producing dilation on the same side as the pressure) and blood pressure (hypoxia to the brainstem causes variability in these vital signs).

NURSING ALERT Arbitrary pumping of the shunt may cause obstruction or other problems and should not be performed unless indicated by the neurosurgeon.

The child is also observed for abdominal distention, since CSF may cause peritonitis or a postoperative ileus as a complication of distal catheter placement. In addition, intake and output are carefully monitored. Children may be placed on fluid restriction with nothing by mouth for 24 hours. The IV infusion is closely monitored to prevent fluid overload. Routine feeding is resumed after the prescribed NPO period, but the presence of bowel sounds is determined before feeding a child with a VP shunt.

Since infection is the greatest hazard of the postoperative period, nurses are continually on the alert for the usual manifestations of CSF infection, such as elevated vital signs, poor feeding, vomiting, decreased responsiveness, and seizure activity. There may be signs of local inflammation at the operative sites and along the shunt tract. The child's diaper should be kept off the peritoneal dressing site or suture line. Antibiotics are administered by the IV route as ordered, and the nurse may also need to assist the practitioner with intraventricular instillation. The incision site is inspected for leakage, and any suspected drainage is tested for glucose, an indication of CSF.

Meticulous skin care is continued postoperatively, with extra care taken to prevent tissue damage from pressure. A pressure-reducing mattress or overlay pad underneath the child helps prevent pressure on prominent areas. Skin is inspected regularly for any signs of pressure, irritation, or infection.

Family Support

Specific needs and concerns of parents during periods of hospitalization are related to the reason for the child's hospitalization (shunt revision, infection, diagnosis) and the diagnostic and surgical procedures to which the child is subjected. Often parents have little understanding of anatomy; therefore they need further exploration and reinforcement of information that was given to them by the physician and neurosurgeon, as well as information about what they can expect. They are especially frightened of any procedure that involves the brain, and the fear of intellectual disability or brain damage is real and pervasive. Nurses can do much to allay their anxiety by explaining the rationale underlying the various nursing and medical activities, such as positioning or testing, and by simply being available and willing to listen to their concerns.

To prepare for the child's discharge and home care, the parents are instructed on how to recognize signs that indicate shunt malfunction or infection and how to pump the shunt, if necessary. Active children may have accidents, such as a fall, that can damage the shunt, and the tubing may pull out of the distal insertion site or become disconnected during normal growth.

Safe transportation is an essential issue to discuss with parents. The tendency for the enlarged head to fall forward and to turn to the side, combined with poor head control, influences the type of child restraint system needed. Small infants can be restrained reclining in an approved car-restraint bed.

The management of hydrocephalus in a child is a demanding task for both family and health professionals, and helping a family cope with the child is an important nursing responsibility. It is important to emphasize that hydrocephalus is a lifelong problem and that the child will require evaluation on a regular basis. The overall aim is to establish realistic goals and an appropriate educational program that will help the child to achieve his or her optimal potential.

Families can be referred to community agencies for support and guidance. The National Hydrocephalus Foundation* and the Hydrocephalus Association† provide information on the condition for families and assist interested groups in establishing local organizations. Helpful booklets are available from these and other sources.

*12413 Centralia Road, Lakewood, CA 90715-1653; 562-924-6666 or 888-857-3434; www.nhfonline.org.

†870 Market St., Suite 705, San Francisco, CA 94102; 415-732-7040 or 888-598-3789; www.hydroassoc.org. *A booklet titled* About Hydrocephalus: A Book for Parents *is available in English or Spanish.*

Key Points

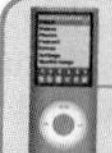

Audio Chapter Summaries

Access an audio summary of these Key Points on evolve

- LOC is the most important indicator of neurologic health; altered levels include full consciousness, confusion, disorientation, lethargy, obtundation, stupor, coma, and persistent vegetative state.
- Complete neurologic examination includes LOC; posture; motor, sensory, cranial nerve, and reflex testing; and vital signs.
- Nursing care of the unconscious child focuses on ensuring respiratory management; performing neurologic assessment; monitoring ICP; supplying adequate nutrition and hydration; providing drug therapy; promoting elimination, hygienic care, proper positioning, exercise, and stimulation; and providing family support.
- Fractures resulting from head injuries may be classified as depressed, compound, basilar, and diastatic.
- Primary head injury involves features that occur at the time of trauma, including fractured skull, contusions, intracranial hematoma, and diffuse injury. Secondary complications include hypoxic brain damage, increased ICP, infection, cerebral edema, and posttraumatic syndromes.
- The young child's response to head injury is different because of the following features: larger head size; expandable skull; larger blood volume to the brain; small subdural spaces; and thinner, softer brain tissue.
- Problems resulting from near-drowning include hypoxia and asphyxiation, aspiration, and hypothermia.
- Nursing care of the child with a brain tumor includes observing for signs and symptoms related to the tumor, preparing the child and family for diagnostic tests and operative procedures, preventing postoperative complications, planning for discharge, and promoting a return to optimal health.
- Nursing care of the child with meningitis includes administering antibiotics, taking isolation precautions, removing environmental stimuli, ensuring correct positioning, monitoring vital signs, administering IV therapy, promoting adequate fluid and nutritional status, and providing supportive care to the family.
- Routine immunization of infants with *H. influenzae* type b and pneumococcal conjugate vaccines has reduced the incidence of bacterial meningitis.
- Encephalitis may result from direct invasion of the CNS by a virus or from involvement of the CNS after viral disease.
- A seizure is a symptom of an underlying pathologic condition and may be manifested by sensory-hallucinatory phenomena, motor effects, sensorimotor effects, or loss of consciousness.
- Partial seizures are categorized as simple (without associated impairment of consciousness) or complex (with impaired consciousness); both types may become generalized.
- Generalized seizures are categorized as tonic-clonic convulsive, absence, atonic and akinetic, myoclonic, and infantile spasms.
- Long-term care of the child with recurrent seizure disorders includes physical care and education regarding the importance of drug therapy and problems related to emotional aspects of the disorder.
- Febrile seizures are the most common type of childhood seizure.
- Many cranial deformities are amenable to surgical correction.
- Hydrocephalus is a symptom of underlying brain pathologic condition demonstrated by impaired

absorption of CSF or obstruction to the flow of CSF within the ventricles.

- Therapy for hydrocephalus involves relief of the hydrocephalus, treatment of the underlying brain disorder if possible, prevention or treatment of complications, and management of problems related to psychomotor development.

References

Aldana PR et al: Results of endoscopic septal fenestration in the treatment of isolated ventricular hydrocephalus, *Pediatr Neurosurg* 38(6):286-294, 2003.

Alston RD et al: Childhood medulloblastoma in northwest England, 1954 to 1977: incidence and survival, *Dev Med Child Neurol* 45(5):308-314, 2003.

American Academy of Pediatrics: Recommendations for the prevention of pneumococcal infections, including the use of pneumococcal conjugant vaccine, pneumococcal polysaccharide vaccine and antibiotic prophylaxis, *Pediatrics* 106(2):362-366, 2000.

American Academy of Pediatrics, Committee on Infectious Diseases, Pickering L (editor): *Red book: 2006 report of the Committee on Infectious Diseases*, ed 27, Elk Grove Village, IL, 2006, The Academy.

American Academy of Pediatrics, Committee on Sports Medicine and Fitness and Committee on Injury and Poison Prevention: Swimming programs for infants and toddlers, *Pediatrics* 105:868-870, 2000.

Baram TZ, Shinnar S: *Febrile seizures*, San Diego, 2002, Academic Press.

Bayir H, Kochanek PM, Clark RS: Traumatic brain injury in infants and children: mechanisms of secondary damage and treatment in the intensive care unit, *Crit Care Clin* 19(3):529-549, 2003.

Bhutta AT, Van Savell H, Schexnayder SM: Reye's syndrome: down but not out, *South Med J* 96(1):43-45, 2003.

Blaney SM et al: Tumors of the central nervous system. In Pizzo PA, Pollack DG (editors): *Principles and practice of pediatric oncology*, ed 5, Philadelphia, 2006, Lippincott-Raven.

Bonthius DJ, Karacay B: Meningitis and encephalitis in children: an update, *Neurol Clin* 20(4):1013-1038, 2002.

Brodeur GM, Maris JM: Neuroblastoma. In Pizzo PA, Pollack DG (editors): *Principles and practice of pediatric oncology*, ed 5, Philadelphia, 2006, Lippincott-Raven.

Browne TR, Holmes GL: *Handbook of epilepsy*, ed 3, Philadelphia, 2004, Lippincott Williams & Wilkins.

Carey RG, Balistreri W: Mitochondrial hepatopathies. In Behrman RE et al (editors): *Nelson textbook of pediatrics*, ed 18, Philadelphia, 2007, Saunders.

Centers for Disease Control and Prevention: Progress toward elimination of *Haemophilus influenzae* type b invasive disease among infants and children—United States, 1998-2000, *Morbid Mortal Wkly Rep* 51:234-239, 2002.

Centers for Disease Control and Prevention: Compendium of animal rabies prevention and control, 2001, National Association of State Public Health Veterinarians, Inc., *Morbid Mortal Wkly Rep* 50(RR-8):1-9, 2001.

Centers for Disease Control and Prevention: *Meningococcal disease*, 2000. Available at www.cdc.gov/ncidod/dbmd/diseaseinfo/meningococcal_t.htm (accessed March 5, 2007).

Centers for Disease Control and Prevention: Human rabies prevention—United States, 1999, *Morbid Mortal Wkly Rep* 48(RR-1):1-21, 1999.

Chen JWY, Wasterlain CG: Status epilepticus: pathophysiology and management in adults, *Lancet Neurol* 5:246-256, 2006.

Chiaretti A et al: Early post-traumatic seizures in children with head injury, *Childs Nerv Syst* 16(12):862-866, 2000.

Curley MAQ, Moloney-Harmon PA: *Critical care nursing of infants and children*, ed 2, Philadelphia, 2001, Saunders.

Durkin MS et al: The epidemiology of urban pediatric neurological trauma: evaluation of, and implications for, injury prevention programs, *Neurosurgery* 42(2):300-310, 1998.

El Bashir H, Laundy M, Booy R: Diagnosis and treatment of bacterial meningitis, *Arch Dis Child* 88(7):814-819, 2003.

Faillace WJ: Management of childhood neurotrauma, *Surg Clin North Am* 82(2):349-363, 2002.

Fisgin T et al: Nasal midazolam effects on childhood acute seizures, *J Child Neurol* 15(12):833-835, 2000.

Freeman JM, Kossoff ER, Hartman AL: The ketogenic diet: one decade later, *Pediatrics* 119(3):535-543, 2007.

Freeman JM et al: The efficacy of the ketogenic diet: 1998—a prospective evaluation of intervention in 150 children, *Pediatrics* 102(6):1358-1363, 1998.

Frucht MM et al: Distribution of seizure precipitants among epilepsy syndromes, *Epilepsia* 41(12):1543-1549, 2000.

Fylan F et al: Mechanisms of video game epilepsy, *Epilepsia* 40(Suppl 4):28-30, 1999.

Gennarelli TA: Trauma to the head: general considerations. In Schwartz GR (editor): *Principles and practices of emergency medicine*, ed 4, Philadelphia, 1999, Lippincott Williams & Wilkins.

Gupta N, Berger MS: Brain mapping for hemispheric tumors in children, *Pediatr Neurosurg* 38(6):302-306, 2003.

Harbord JG et al: Use of intranasal midazolam to treat acute seizures in paediatric community settings, *J Pediatr Child Health* 40(9-10):556-558, 2004.

Hemingway C et al: The ketogenic diet: a 3-to-6-years follow up of 150 children enrolled prospectively, *Pediatrics* 108(4):898-905, 2001.

Johnston MV: Seizures in childhood. In Behrman RE et al (editors): *Nelson textbook of pediatrics*, ed 18, Philadelphia, 2007, Saunders.

Kallas HJ: Drowning and near-drowning. In Behrman RE, Kliegman RM, Jenson HTS (editors): *Nelson textbook of pediatrics*, ed 17, Philadelphia, 2004, Saunders.

Kamienski MC: Reye syndrome, *Am J Nurs* 103(7):54-57, 2003.

Kao SC et al: A survey of post-discharge side-effects of conscious sedation using chloral hydrate in pediatric CT or MR imaging, *Pediatr Radiol* 29(4):287-290, 1999.

Kinsman SL, Johnston MV: Congenital anomalies of the central nervous system. In Behrman RE et al (editors): *Nelson textbook of pediatrics*, ed 18, Philadelphia, 2007, Saunders.

Kline NE, Sevier N: Solid tumors in children, *J Pediatr Nurs* 18(2):96-102, 2003.

Kutlu NO et al: Intranasal midazolam for prolonged convulsive seizures, *Brain Dev* 22(6):359-361, 2000.

Kuzniecky RI: Neuroimaging in pediatric epilepsy. In Pellock JM, Dodson WE, Bourgeois BFD (editors): *Pediatric epilepsy: diagnosis and therapy*, New York, 2001, Demos Medical Publishing.

Lefevre F, Aronson N: Ketogenic diet for the treatment of refractory epilepsy in children: a systematic review of efficacy, *Pediatrics* 105(4):e46, 2000. Available at www.pediatrics.org/cgi/content/full/105/4/e46 (accessed March 5, 2007).

Leppik IE: Monotherapy and polypharmacy, *Neurology* 55(Suppl 3):525-529, 2000.

Levy R, Cooper P: Ketogenic diet for epilepsy, *Cochrane Database Syst Rev* (3):CD001903, DOI:10.1002/14651858.CD001903, 2003.

Ljungman G et al: Midazolam nasal spray reduces procedural anxiety in children, *Pediatrics* 105(1 Pt 1):73-78, 2000.

Lloyd CJ, Alredy T, Lloyd JC: Intranasal midazolam as an alternative to general anaesthesia in the management of children with oral and maxillofacial trauma, *Br J Oral Maxillofac Surg* 38(6):593-595, 2000.

Masson F et al: Epidemiology of traumatic comas: a prospective population-based study, *Brain Inj* 17(4):279-293, 2003.

Mathern GW et al: Postoperative seizure control and antiepileptic drug use in pediatric epilepsy surgery patients: the UCLA experience, 1986-1997, *Epilepsia* 40(12):1740-1749, 1999.

Menkes JH, Sankar R: Paroxysmal disorders. In Menkes JH, Sarnat HB (editors): *Child neurology*, Philadelphia, 2000, Lippincott Williams & Wilkins.

Morris GL, Mueller WM, Vagus Nerve Stimulation Study Group E01-E05: Long term treatment with vagus nerve stimulation in patients with refractory epilepsy, *Neurology* 53:1731-1735, 1999.

Murray-Ryan J, Petriccione MM: Central nervous system tumors. In Baggott CR et al (editors): *Nursing care of children and adolescents with cancer*, ed 3, Philadelphia, 2002, Saunders.

Nakken KO et al: Which seizure-precipitating factors do patients with epilepsy most frequently report? *Epilepsy Behav* 6(1):85-89, 2005.

Nguyen NP et al: Neuroblastoma producing spinal cord compression: rapid relief with low dose of radiation, *Anticancer Res* 20(6c):4687-4690, 2000.

Palmer J: Management of raised intracranial pressure in children, *Intens Crit Care Nurs* 16:319-327, 2000.

Pellock JM, Shinnar S: Respiratory adverse events associated with diazepam rectal gel, *Neurology* 64(10):1768-1770, 2005.

Pichichero M: Meningococcal conjugate vaccine in adolescents and children, *Clin Pediatr* 44(6):479-489, 2005.

Prober CG: Central nervous system infections. In Behrman RE et al (editors): *Nelson textbook of pediatrics*, ed 18, Philadelphia, 2007, Saunders.

Radhakrishnan K et al: Pattern-sensitive epilepsy: electroclinical characteristics, natural history, and delineation of the epileptic syndrome, *Epilepsia* 46(1):48-58, 2005.

Ricci S, Vigevano F: The effect of video-game software in video-game epilepsy, *Epilepsia* 40(Suppl 4):31-37, 1999.

Rivara FP, Grossman D: Injury control. In Behrman RE et al (editors): *Nelson textbook of pediatrics*, ed 18, Philadelphia, 2007, Saunders.

Rudy C: Hydrocephalus, *J Pediatr Health Care* 19(2):111, 127-128, 2005.

Sadleir LG, Scheffer IE: Febrile seizures, *BMJ* 334:307-311, 2007.

Saez-Llorens X, McCracken Jr GH: Bacterial meningitis in children, *Lancet* 361(9375):2139-2148, 2003.

Scheifele D et al: Invasive *Haemophilus influenzae* type b infections in vaccinated and unvaccinated children in Canada, 2001-2003, *CMAJ* 172(1): 53-56, 2005.

Schutzman SA, Greenes DS: Pediatric minor head trauma, *Ann Emerg Med* 37(1):65-74, 2001.

Shafer PO: Epilepsy and seizures: advances in seizure assessment, treatment, and self-management, *Nurs Clin North Am* 34(3):743-759, 1999.

Shinnar S et al: Predictors of multiple seizures in a cohort of children prospectively followed from the time of their first unprovoked seizure, *Ann Neurol* 48(2), 140-147, 2000.

Shorvon S, Walker M: Status epilepticus in idiopathic generalized epilepsy, *Epilepsia* 46(Suppl 9):73-79, 2005.

Sotir MJ et al: Meningococcal disease incidence and mortality in Wisconsin, 1993-2002, *Wisc Med J* 104(3):38-44, 2005.

Stal S, Chebret L, McElroy C: The team approach in the management of congenital and acquired deformities, *Clin Plast Surg* 25(4):485-491, 1998.

Swaine BR et al: Previous head injury is a risk factor for subsequent head injury in children: a longitudinal cohort study, *Pediatrics* 119(4):749-758, 2007.

Task Force for the Determination of Brain Death in Children: Guidelines for the determination of brain death in children, *Arch Neurol* 44(6):587-588, 1987.

Toltzis P: Rabies. In Behrman RE et al (editors): *Nelson textbook of pediatrics*, ed 18, Philadelphia, 2007, Saunders.

Treiman DM, Walker MC: Treatment of seizure emergencies: convulsive and non-convulsive status epilepticus, *Epilepsy Res* 68S:S77-S82, 2006.

Verity CM, Greenword R, Golding J: Longterm intellectual and behavioral outcomes of children with febrile convulsions, *N Engl J Med* 338(24):1723-1728, 1998.

Vernon-Levett P: Neurologic system. In Slota MC (editor): *Core curriculum for pediatric critical care nursing*, Philadelphia, 1998, Saunders.

Wetzell RC: Anesthesia and perioperative care. In Behrman RE et al (editors): *Nelson textbook of pediatrics*, ed 18, Philadelphia, 2007, Saunders.

Yamamoto LG, Yim GK: The role of intravenous valproic acid in status epilepticus, *Pediatr Emerg Care* 16(4):296-298, 2000.

Yogev R, Guzman-Cottrill J: Bacterial meningitis in children: critical review of current concepts, *Drugs* 65(8):1097-1112, 2005.

Zuckerman GB, Gregory PM, Santos-Damiani SM: Predictors of death and neurologic impairment in pediatric submersion injuries: the pediatric risk of mortality score, *Arch Pediatr Adolesc Med* 152:134-140, 1998.

Unit 11

52 Endocrine Dysfunction

Learning Objectives

On completion of this chapter the reader will be able to:

- Differentiate between the disorders caused by hypopituitary and hyperpituitary dysfunction.
- Describe the manifestations of thyroid hypofunction and hyperfunction and the management of children with the disorders.
- Distinguish between the manifestations of adrenal hypofunction and hyperfunction.
- Differentiate among the various categories of diabetes mellitus.
- Discuss the management and nursing care of the child with diabetes mellitus in the acute care setting.
- Distinguish between a hypoglycemic and a hyperglycemic reaction.
- Design a teaching plan for a child with diabetes mellitus.
- Formulate a teaching plan for the parents of a child with diabetes mellitus.

Electronic Resources

Additional information related to the content in Chapter 52 can be found on

evolve the Companion Website at

http://evolve.elsevier.com/Perry/maternal/

- NCLEX Review Questions
- Animation—Adrenal Function
- Case Study—Diabetes Mellitus
- Critical Thinking Exercise—Hypothyroidism
- Nursing Care Plan—The Child with Diabetes Mellitus
- Nursing Care Plan—The Child with Diabetic Ketoacidosis

Disorders of Pituitary Function

Deficiencies of the anterior pituitary hormones may be due to organic defects or have an idiopathic etiology and may occur as a single hormonal problem or in combination with other hormonal deficiencies. The clinical manifestations depend on the hormones involved and the age of onset. If the tropic hormones are involved, the resulting disorder reflects the altered stimulus to the target gland. For example, if thyroid-stimulating hormone (TSH) is deficient, thyroid hormone (TH) is also deficient and the child displays the manifestations of hypothyroidism.

An overproduction of the anterior pituitary hormones can result in gigantism (caused by excess growth hormone [GH] production during childhood), hyperthyroidism, hypercortisolism (Cushing's syndrome), and precocious puberty from excessive gonadotropins. Overproduction may be caused by hyperplasia of the pituitary cells—which may eventually progress to a tumor (adenoma)—or a primary hypothalamic defect that results in an excess of the hormone's releasing factor. Although the initial clinical manifestations are a result of pituitary oversecretion, eventually pituitary insufficiency occurs, and the signs of panhypopituitarism become evident.

NURSING ALERT Children with panhypopituitarism should wear medical identification, such as a bracelet.

Hypopituitarism

Hypopituitarism is diminished or deficient secretion of pituitary hormones. The consequences of the condition depend on the degree of dysfunction and lead to gonadotropin deficiency with absence or regression of secondary sex characteristics; GH deficiency, in which children display retarded somatic growth; TSH deficiency, which produces hypothyroidism; and corticotropin deficiency, which results in manifestations of adrenal hypofunction. Hypopituitarism can result from any of the conditions listed in Box 52-1. The most common organic cause of pituitary undersecretion is tumors in the pituitary or hypothalamic region, especially the craniopharyngiomas.

Constitutional growth delay refers to individuals (usually boys) with delayed linear growth, generally beginning as a toddler, and skeletal and sexual maturation that is behind that of age-mates (Miller & Zimmerman, 2004; Halac & Zimmerman, 2004). Typically these children will reach normal adult height. Often one of the child's parents or another family member has a history of a similar pattern of growth. The untreated child will proceed through normal changes as

BOX 52-1 Clinical Manifestations of Hypopituitarism

Presenting complaint—short stature
- Usually normal growth first year
- Growth during second year drops below established percentile
- Growth measurements below 5th percentile

Premature aging common in later life
Height may be retarded more than weight
Appear well nourished
Skeletal proportions normal
Tend to be relatively inactive
Less likely to participate in aggressive, sporting-type activities
Bone age nearly always retarded but closely related to height age
Primary teeth usually appear at expected age; eruption of permanent teeth delayed
Teeth overcrowded and malpositioned (because of underdeveloped jaw)
Sexual development usually delayed but normal

expected on the basis of bone age. These changes, although occurring later than in the average child, will appear in normal sequence and manner, and treatment with GH is not usually indicated. However, its use has become controversial, especially in relation to parental and child requests for treatment to accelerate growth.

Diagnostic Evaluation

Only a small number of children with delayed growth or short stature have hypopituitary dwarfism. In the majority of instances the cause is constitutional delay. Diagnostic evaluation is aimed at isolating organic causes, which, in addition to GH deficiency, may include hypothyroidism, oversecretion of cortisol, gonadal aplasia, chronic illness, nutritional inadequacy, Russell-Silver dwarfism, or hypochondroplasia.

A complete diagnostic evaluation should include a family history, a history of the child's growth patterns and previous health status, physical examination, psychosocial evaluation, radiographic surveys, and endocrine studies. Accurate measurement of height (using a calibrated stadiometer) and weight and comparison with standard growth charts are essential. Multiple height measures reflect a more accurate assessment of abnormal growth patterns (Box 52-2) (Hall, 2000).

A skeletal survey in children less than 3 years of age and radiographic examination of the hand-wrist for centers of ossification (bone age) (Box 52-3) in older children are important in evaluating growth.

Definitive diagnosis is based on absent or subnormal reserves of pituitary GH. Because GH levels are normally so low in children that differentiation from abnormal concentrations is unreliable, GH secretion should be stimulated, followed by measurement of blood levels. Exercise is a natural and benign stimulus for GH release, and elevated levels can be detected after 20 minutes of strenuous exercise in normal

BOX 52-2 Evaluating the Growth Curve

Ensure reliability of measurements—Accurately obtain and plot height and weight measurements.

Determine absolute height—The child's absolute height bears some relationship to the likelihood of a pathologic condition. However, the majority of children who have a height below the lowest percentile (either 3rd or 5th percentile on the height curve) do not have a pathologic growth problem.

Assess height velocity—The most important aspect of a growth evaluation is the observation of a child's height over time, or height velocity. Accurate determination of height velocity requires at least 4 and preferably 6 months of observation. A substantial deceleration in height velocity (crossing several percentiles) between 3 and 12 or 13 years of age indicates a pathologic condition until proven otherwise.

Determine weight-to-height relationship—Determination of the weight-to-height ratio has some diagnostic value in ascertaining the cause of growth retardation in a short child.

Project target height—The height of a child can be judged inappropriately short only in the context of his or her genetic potential. Determine the target height of the child with the formula:

[Father's height (cm) + Mother's height (cm) + 13]/2 for boys

or

[Father's height (cm) + Mother's height (cm) − 13]/2 for girls

Most children achieve an adult stature within approximately 10 cm (4 inches) of the target height.

Modified from Vogiatzi MG, Copeland KC: The short child, *Pediatr Rev* 19(3):92-99, 1998.

children. Also, GH levels are elevated 45 to 90 minutes after the onset of sleep.

Initial assessment of the serum insulin-like growth factor-I (IGF-I) and IGF binding protein 3 (IGFBP3) indicates a need for further evaluation of GH dysfunction if levels are less than −1 SD below the mean for age. It is recommended that GH stimulation tests be reserved for children with low serum IGF-I and IGFBP3 levels and poor growth (Hochberg, 1999).

Studies have shown that traditional GH stimulation tests can yield inaccurate results and be impacted by a child's body type or response to stimuli (Hilczer, Smyczynska, & Lewinski, 2006; Guyda, 2000; Mauras et al, 2000). GH-dependent growth factors may be more sensitive indicators of GH deficiency than GH stimulation tests. Increasingly sensitive radioimmunoassays for GH levels have been developed.

Therapeutic Management

Treatment of GH deficiency caused by organic lesions is directed toward correction of the underlying disease process (e.g., surgical removal or irradiation of a tumor). The definitive treatment of GH deficiency is replacement of GH, which is successful in 80% of affected children. A Cochrane Review of nine randomized controlled trials confirmed that GH

BOX 52-3 Bone Age for Evaluating Growth Disorders

Bone age refers to a method of assessing skeletal maturity by comparing the appearance of representative epiphyseal centers obtained on x-ray examination with age-appropriate published standards.

Most conditions that cause poor linear growth also cause a delay in skeletal maturation and a retarded bone age. Observation of even a profoundly delayed bone age is never diagnostic or even indicative of a specific diagnosis. A delayed bone age merely indicates that the associated short stature is to some extent "partially reversible," since linear growth will continue until epiphyseal fusion is complete. In comparison, a bone age that is not delayed in a short child is of much greater concern and may, in fact, be of some diagnostic value under certain circumstances.

Modified from Vogiatzi MG, Copeland KC: The short child, *Pediatr Rev* 19(3):92-99, 1998.

therapy can increase short-term grown and improve final height (Bryant, Cave, & Milne, 2003). Reiter and colleagues (2006) found final height within the midparental height range in 1258 patients with idiopathic GH deficiency treated at an early age.

The decision to stop GH therapy is made jointly by the child, family, and health care team. Radiologic evidence of epiphyseal closure is a criterion for ending therapy. Dosage is increased as the time of epiphyseal closure nears to optimize use of the GH. Children with other hormone deficiencies require replacement therapy to correct the specific disorders. This may involve administration of thyroid extract, cortisone, testosterone, or estrogens and progesterone. Treatment with the sex hormones is usually begun during adolescence to promote normal sexual maturation.

Nursing Care Management

The principal nursing consideration is identifying children with growth problems. Despite the fact that the majority of growth problems are not a result of organic causes, any delay in normal growth and sexual development poses special emotional adjustments for these children.

The nurse may be a key person in helping establish a diagnosis. For example, if serial height and weight records are not available, the nurse can question parents about the child's growth compared with that of siblings, peers, or relatives. Investigating clothing sizes is often helpful in determining growth at different ages. Parents may comment that the child wears out clothes before growing out of them or that, if the clothing fits the body, it often is too long in the sleeves or legs.

Because the behavioral or physical changes that suggest a tumor are insidious, they are frequently overlooked. It is important to correlate the onset of any positive findings with the initial evidence of growth retardation. For example, visual problems and headache are not uncommon in school-age children and can coincidentally occur after a growth problem is recognized. In fact, headache may represent the emotional trauma caused by short stature rather than be a symptom of a tumor. This line of questioning should be pursued cautiously to avoid alarming parents unduly about the possibility of a brain tumor.

Part of a nurse's role in helping establish a diagnosis is assisting with diagnostic tests. Preparation of the child and family is especially important if a number of tests are being performed, and the child requires particular attention during provocative testing. Blood samples are usually taken every 30 minutes for a 3-hour period. Children also have difficulty overcoming hypoglycemia generated by tests with insulin, so they must be observed carefully for signs of hypoglycemia, whereas those receiving glucagon are at risk of nausea and vomiting.

NURSING ALERT Optimum dosing is often achieved when GH is administered at bedtime. Physiologic release is more normally stimulated as a result of pituitary release of GH during the first 45 to 90 minutes after the onset of sleep.

Pituitary Hyperfunction

Excess GH before closure of the epiphyseal shafts results in proportional overgrowth of the long bones until the individual reaches a height of 2.4 m (8 feet) or more. Vertical growth is accompanied by rapid and increased development of muscles and viscera. Weight is increased but is usually in proportion to height. Proportional enlargement of head circumference also occurs and may result in delayed closure of the fontanels in young children. Children with a pituitary-secreting tumor may also demonstrate signs of increasing intracranial pressure, especially headache.

If oversecretion of GH occurs after epiphyseal closure, growth is in the transverse direction, producing a condition known as *acromegaly.* Typical facial features include overgrowth of the head, lips, nose, tongue, jaw, and paranasal and mastoid sinuses; separation and malocclusion of the teeth in the enlarged jaw; disproportion of the face to the cerebral division of the skull; increased facial hair; thickened, deeply creased skin; and increased tendency toward hyperglycemia and diabetes mellitus (DM).

Diagnostic Evaluation

Diagnosis is based on a history of excessive growth during childhood and evidence of increased levels of GH. Radiographic studies may reveal a tumor in an enlarged sella turcica, normal bone age, enlargement of bones (such as the paranasal sinuses), and evidence of joint changes. Endocrine studies to confirm excess of other hormones, specifically thyroid, cortisol, and sex hormones, should also be included in the differential diagnosis.

Therapeutic Management

If a lesion is present, surgical treatment by cryosurgery or hypophysectomy is performed to remove the tumor when feasible. Other therapies aimed at destroying pituitary tissue include external irradiation and radioactive implants. Depending on the extent of surgical extirpation and degree of pituitary insufficiency, hormone replacement with thyroid extract, cortisone, and sex hormones may be necessary.

Nursing Care Management

The primary nursing consideration is early identification of children with excessive growth rates. Although medical management is unable to reduce growth already attained, further growth can be retarded. The earlier the treatment, the more control there is in predetermining a normal adult height. Nurses in ambulatory settings who are frequently involved in growth screening should refer children who demonstrate excessive linear growth for a medical evaluation. They should also observe for signs of a tumor, especially headache, and evidence of concurrent hormonal excesses, particularly the gonadotropins, which cause sexual precocity.

Children with excessive growth rates require as much emotional support as those with short stature. Children and their parents need an opportunity to express their thoughts. A compassionate nurse can be supportive to these children, especially before adolescence when they are larger than their peers. The nurse can emphasize to a tall girl that as boys grow older, they become taller and she will not always be looking down at them.

Precocious Puberty

Manifestations of sexual development before age 9 years in boys or age 8 years in girls have traditionally been considered precocious development, and these children were recommended for further evaluation (Midyett, Moore, & Jacobson, 2003; Kempers & Otten, 2002). Recent examination of the age limit for defining when puberty is precocious reveals that the onset of puberty in girls is occurring earlier than previous studies have documented (Slyper, 2006; Biro et al, 2006). Mean onset of puberty was 10.2 and 9.6 years in Caucasian and African-American girls, respectively. Based on these findings, precocious puberty evaluation for a pathologic cause should be performed for Caucasian girls younger than 7 years of age or for African-American girls younger than 6 years of age. No change in the guidelines for evaluation of precocious puberty in boys is recommended. However, recent data suggest that boys may be beginning maturation earlier as well (Slyper, 2006; Herman-Giddens, 2006).

Normally the hypothalamic-releasing factors stimulate secretion of the gonadotropic hormones from the anterior pituitary at the time of puberty. In the male, interstitial cell–stimulating hormone stimulates Leydig's cells of the testes to secrete testosterone; in the female, follicle-stimulating hormone (FSH) and luteinizing hormone stimulate the ovarian follicles to secrete estrogens (Nebesio & Eugster, 2007). This sequence of events is known as the *hypothalamic-pituitary-gonadal axis.* If for some reason the cycle undergoes premature activation, the child will display evidence of advanced or precocious puberty. Causes of precocious puberty are found in Box 52-4.

Isosexual precocious puberty is more common among girls than boys. Approximately 80% of children with precocious puberty have *central precocious puberty (CPP),* in which pubertal development is activated by the hypothalamic gonadotropin-releasing hormone (GnRH) (Greiner & Kerrigan, 2006). This produces early maturation and development of the gonads with secretion of sex hormones, development of secondary sex characteristics, and sometimes production of mature sperm and ova (Lee, 1999; Root, 2000). CPP may be the result of congenital anomalies; infectious, neoplastic, or traumatic insults to the central nervous system (CNS); or treatment of longstanding sex hormone exposure (Trivin et al, 2006). CPP occurs more frequently in girls and is usually idiopathic, with 95% demonstrating no causative factor (Nebesio & Eugster, 2007; Greiner & Kerrigan, 2006; Root, 2000). A CNS insult or structural abnormality is found in more than 90% of boys with CPP (Root, 2000).

BOX 52-4 Causes of Precocious Puberty

Central Precocious Puberty

Idiopathic, with or without hypothalamic hamartoma

Secondary

- Congenital anomalies
- Postinflammatory—Encephalitis, meningitis, abscess, granulomatous disease
- Radiotherapy
- Trauma
- Neoplasms

After effective treatment of longstanding pseudoisosexual precocity

Peripheral Precocious Puberty

Familial male-limited precocious puberty

Albright's syndrome

Gonadal or extragonadal tumors

Adrenal

- Congenital adrenal hyperplasia
- Adenoma, carcinoma
- Glucocorticoid resistance

Exogenous sex hormones

Primary hypothyroidism

Incomplete Precocious Puberty

Premature thelarche

Premature menarche

Premature pubarche or adrenarche

Modified from Root AW: Precocious puberty, *Pediatr Rev* 21(1):10-19, 2000.

Peripheral precocious puberty (PPP) includes early puberty resulting from hormone stimulation other than the hypothalamic GnRH–stimulated pituitary gonadotropin release. Isolated manifestations that are usually associated with puberty may be seen as variations in normal sexual development (Greiner & Kerrigan, 2006). They appear without other signs of pubescence and are probably caused by unusual end-organ sensitivity to prepubertal levels of estrogen or androgen. Included are premature thelarche (development of breasts in prepubertal girls), premature pubarche (premature adrenarche, early development of sexual hair), and premature menarche (isolated menses without other evidence of sexual development).

Therapeutic Management

Treatment of precocious puberty is directed toward the specific cause when known. Precocious puberty of central (hypothalamic-pituitary) origin is managed with monthly injections of a synthetic analog of *luteinizing hormone–releasing hormone,* which regulates pituitary secretions (Greiner & Kerrigan, 2006; Muir, 2006). The available preparation, leuprolide acetate (Lupron Depot), is given in a dosage of 0.2 to 0.3 mg/kg intramuscularly once every 4 weeks. Breast development regresses or does not advance, and growth returns to normal rates, enhancing predicted height. Studies suggest that not all patients attain adult targeted heights and the addition of GH therapy may be warranted (Walvoord & Pescovitz, 1999). Treatment is discontinued at a chronologically appropriate time, allowing pubertal changes to resume. Psychologic management of the patient and family is an important aspect of care. Both parents and the affected child should be taught the injection procedure.

Nursing Care Management

Psychologic support and guidance of the child and family are the most important aspects of management. Parents need anticipatory guidance, support and information resources, and reassurance of the benign nature of the condition (Greiner & Kerrigan, 2006; O'Sullivan & O'Sullivan, 2002). Dress and activities for the physically precocious child should be appropriate to the chronologic age. Sexual interest is not usually advanced beyond the child's chronologic age, and parents need to understand that the child's mental age is congruent with the chronologic age and that the child's normal, overt manifestations of affection are age-appropriate and do not represent sexual advances.

Although the child's heterosexual behavior is appropriate for the chronologic age, the nurse should emphasize to parents that the child is fertile. Usually no form of contraception is necessary unless the child is sexually active. In this situation proper counseling is important because hormonal forms of birth control, such as estrogen pills, will prematurely initiate epiphyseal closure, resulting in stunted linear growth.

Diabetes Insipidus

The principal disorder of posterior pituitary hypofunction is diabetes insipidus (DI), also known as *neurogenic DI,* resulting from undersecretion of *antidiuretic hormone (ADH),* or *vasopressin* (Pitressin), and producing a state of uncontrolled diuresis (Wong & Verbalis, 2002). This disorder is not to be confused with nephrogenic DI, a rare hereditary disorder affecting primarily males and caused by unresponsiveness of the renal tubules to the hormone.

Neurogenic DI may result from a number of different causes. Primary causes are familial or idiopathic; of the total cases, approximately 45% to 50% are idiopathic. Secondary causes include trauma (accidental or surgical), tumors, granulomatous disease, infections (meningitis or encephalitis), and vascular anomalies (aneurysm). Certain drugs, such as alcohol or phenytoin (diphenylhydantoin), can cause a transient polyuria.

The cardinal signs of DI are polyuria and polydipsia. In the older child, signs such as excessive urination accompanied by a compensatory insatiable thirst may be so intense that the child does little more than go to the toilet and drink fluids (Cheetham & Baylis, 2002). Frequently the first sign is enuresis. In the infant the initial symptom is irritability that is relieved with feedings of water but not milk. The infant is also prone to dehydration, electrolyte imbalance, hyperthermia, azotemia, and potential circulatory collapse.

Dehydration is usually not a serious problem in older children, who are able to drink larger quantities of water. However, any period of unconsciousness, such as after trauma or anesthesia, may be life threatening because the voluntary demand for fluid is absent. During such instances careful monitoring of urine volumes, blood concentration, and intravenous (IV) fluid replacement is essential to prevent dehydration.

NURSING ALERT The child with DI complicated by congenital absence of the thirst center must be encouraged to drink sufficient quantities of liquid to prevent electrolyte imbalance.

Diagnostic Evaluation

The simplest test used to diagnose this condition is restriction of oral fluids and observation of consequent changes in urine volume and concentration. Normally, reducing fluids results in concentrated urine and diminished volume. In DI, fluid restriction has little or no effect on urine formation but causes weight loss from dehydration. Accurate results from this procedure require strict monitoring of fluid intake and urine output, measurement of urine concentration (specific gravity or osmolality), and frequent weight checks. A weight loss between 3% and 5% indicates significant dehydration and requires termination of the fluid restriction.

NURSING ALERT Small children require close observation during fluid deprivation to prevent them from drinking, even from toilet bowls, flower vases, or other unlikely sources of fluid.

If this test is positive, the child should be given a test dose of injected *aqueous vasopressin,* which should alleviate the polyuria and polydipsia. Unresponsiveness to exogenous vasopressin usually indicates nephrogenic DI. An important diagnostic consideration is to differentiate DI from other causes of polyuria and polydipsia, especially DM. DI may be the early sign of an evolving cerebral process (De Buyst et al, 2007).

Therapeutic Management

The usual treatment is hormone replacement, either with an intramuscular or subcutaneous injection of vasopressin tannate in peanut oil or with a nasal spray of aqueous lysine vasopressin (Verbalis, 2003). The injectable form has the advantage of lasting 48 to 72 hours, which affords the child a full night's sleep. However, it has the disadvantage of requiring frequent injections and proper preparation of the drug.

NURSING ALERT To be effective, vasopressin must be thoroughly resuspended in the oil by being held under warm running water for 10 to 15 minutes and shaken vigorously before being drawn into the syringe. If this is not done, the oil may be injected minus the ADH. Small brown particles, which indicate drug dispersion, must be seen in the suspension.

Nursing Care Management

The initial objective is identification of the disorder. Because an early sign may be sudden enuresis in a child who is toilet trained, excessive thirst with bed-wetting is an indication for further investigation. Another clue is persistent irritability and crying in an infant that is relieved only by bottle-feedings of water. After head trauma or certain neurosurgical procedures, the development of DI can be anticipated; therefore these patients must be closely monitored.

Assessment includes measurement of body weight, serum electrolytes, blood urea nitrogen, hematocrit, and urine specific gravity taken before surgery and every other day after the procedure. Fluid intake and output should be carefully measured and recorded. Alert patients are able to adjust intake to urine losses, but unconscious or very young patients require closer fluid observation. In children who are not toilet trained, collection of urine specimens may require application of a urine-collecting device.

After confirmation of the diagnosis, parents need a thorough explanation regarding the condition with specific clarification that DI is a different condition from DM. They must realize that treatment is lifelong. If children are to receive the injectable vasopressin, ideally two caregivers should be taught the correct procedure for preparation and administration of the drug. Once children are old enough, they should be encouraged to assume full responsibility for their care.

For emergency purposes, these children should wear medical alert identification. Older children should carry the nasal spray with them for temporary relief of symptoms. School personnel need to be aware of the problem so they can grant children unrestricted use of the lavatory. Failure to permit this may result in embarrassing accidents that often lead to a child's unwillingness to attend school.

Syndrome of Inappropriate Antidiuretic Hormone

The disorder that results from oversecretion of the posterior pituitary hormone, or ADH, is known as syndrome of inappropriate antidiuretic hormone (SIADH). It is observed with increased frequency in a variety of conditions, especially those involving infections, tumors, or other CNS disease or trauma (Lin, Liu, & Lim, 2005).

The manifestations are directly related to fluid retention and hypotonicity. Excess ADH causes most of the filtered water to be reabsorbed from the kidneys back into central circulation. Serum osmolality is low, and urine osmolality is inappropriately elevated. When serum sodium levels are diminished to 120 mEq/L, affected children display anorexia, nausea (and sometimes vomiting), stomach cramps, irritability, and personality changes. With progressive reduction in sodium, other neurologic signs, stupor, and convulsions may be evident. The symptoms usually disappear when the underlying disorder is corrected.

The immediate management consists of restricting fluids. Subsequent management depends on the cause and severity. Fluids continue to be restricted to one-fourth to one-half maintenance. When there are no fluid abnormalities but SIADH can be anticipated, fluids are often restricted expectantly at two-thirds to three-fourths maintenance.

Nursing Care Management

The first goal of nursing management is recognizing the presence of SIADH from symptoms described in patients at risk, especially those in the pediatric intensive care unit.

NURSING ALERT Nausea, vomiting, and malaise may precede the onset of more severe stages such as disorientation, confusion, coma, and seizures (Majzoub & Muglia, 2003).

Accurately measuring intake and output, noting daily weight, and observing for signs of fluid overload are primary nursing functions, especially in the child receiving IV fluids. Seizure precautions are implemented, and the child and family need education regarding the rationale for fluid restrictions. The rare child with chronic SIADH will be placed on long-term ADH-antagonizing medication, and the child and family will require instructions for its administration.

Disorders of Thyroid Function

The thyroid gland secretes two types of hormones: *TH,* which consists of the hormones *thyroxine (T_4)* and *triiodothyronine (T_3);* and *calcitonin.* The secretion of thyroid hormones is controlled by TSH from the anterior pituitary, which in turn is regulated by thyrotropin-releasing factor (TRF) from the hypothalamus as a negative feedback response. Consequently, hypothyroidism or hyperthyroidism may result from a defect in the target gland or from a disturbance in the secretion of TSH or TRF. Because the functions of T_3 and T_4 are qualitatively the same, the term *TH* is used throughout the discussion.

The synthesis of TH depends on available sources of dietary iodine and tyrosine. The thyroid is the only endocrine gland capable of storing excess amounts of hormones for release as needed. During circulation in the bloodstream, T_4 and T_3 are bound to carrier proteins (thyroxine-binding globulin). They must be unbound before they are able to exert their metabolic effect.

The main physiologic action of TH is to regulate the basal metabolic rate and thereby control the processes of growth and tissue differentiation. Unlike GH, TH is involved in many more diverse activities that influence the growth and development of body tissues. Therefore a deficiency of TH exerts a more profound effect on growth than that seen in hypopituitarism.

Calcitonin helps maintain blood calcium levels by decreasing the calcium concentration. Its effect is the opposite of parathyroid hormone (PTH) in that it inhibits skeletal demineralization and promotes calcium deposition in the bone.

Juvenile Hypothyroidism

evolve Critical Thinking Exercise—Hypothyroidism

Hypothyroidism is one of the most common endocrine problems of childhood. It may be either congenital or acquired and represents a deficiency in secretion of TH (Foley, 2001). Hypothyroidism from dietary insufficiency of iodine is now rare in the United States, since iodized salt is a readily available source of the nutrient.

Beyond infancy, primary hypothyroidism may be caused by a number of defects. For example, a congenital hypoplastic thyroid gland may provide sufficient amounts of TH during the first year or two but be inadequate when rapid body growth increases demands on the gland. A partial or complete thyroidectomy for cancer or thyrotoxicosis can leave insufficient thyroid tissue to furnish hormones for body requirements. Radiotherapy for Hodgkin's disease or other malignancies may lead to hypothyroidism (Pizzo & Poplack, 2006). Infectious processes may cause hypothyroidism. It can also occur when dietary iodine is deficient.

Clinical manifestations depend on the extent of dysfunction and the child's age at onset. Primary congenital hypothyroidism is characterized by low levels of circulating thyroid hormones and raised levels of TSH at birth (Macchia, 2000). The GnRH test and baseline measurement of gonadotropin and sex hormone serum concentrations at 3 months of age are promising options for assessment of hypothalamic-pituitary-gonadal function in infants with congenital hypothyroidism (van Tijn et al, 2007). The presenting symptoms are decelerated growth from chronic deprivation of TH or thyromegaly. Impaired growth and development are less severe when hypothyroidism is acquired at a later age, and, because brain growth is nearly complete by 2 to 3 years of age, intellectual disability and neurologic sequelae are not associated with juvenile hypothyroidism. Other manifestations are myxedematous skin changes (dry skin, puffiness around the eyes, sparse hair), constipation, sleepiness, and mental decline (Box 52-5).

Therapy is TH replacement, the same as for hypothyroidism in the infant, although the prompt treatment needed in the infant is not required in the child. In children with severe symptoms, the restoration of euthyroidism is achieved more gradually with administration of increasing amounts of L-thyroxine over a period of 4 to 8 weeks to avoid symptoms of hyperthyroidism, which can occur with treatment of chronic hypothyroidism. Researchers have found that children treated early continue to have mild delays in reading, comprehension, and arithmetic but catch up by grade six (Rovet & Ehrlich, 2000). However, adolescents may demonstrate problems with memory, attention, and visuospatial processing.

Nursing Care Management

The importance of early recognition in the infant is discussed in Chapter 28. Growth cessation or retardation in a child whose growth has previously been normal should alert the observer to the possibility of hypothyroidism. After diagnosis and implementation of thyroxine therapy, the importance of compliance and periodic monitoring of response to therapy should be stressed to parents. Children should learn to take responsibility for their own health as soon as they are old enough, at about 9 or 10 years of age.

BOX 52-5 Clinical Manifestations of Juvenile Hypothyroidism

Decelerated growth
- Less when acquired at later age

Myxedematous skin changes
- Dry skin
- Puffiness around eyes
- Sparse hair
- Constipation
- Sleepiness
- Mental decline

Goiter

A goiter is an enlargement or hypertrophy of the thyroid gland. It may occur with deficient (hypothyroid), excessive (hyperthyroid), or normal (euthyroid) TH secretion. It can be congenital or acquired. Congenital disease usually occurs as a result of maternal administration of antithyroid drugs or iodides during pregnancy. Acquired disease can result from increased secretion of pituitary TSH in response to decreased circulating levels of TH or from infiltrative neoplastic or inflammatory processes. In areas where dietary iodine (essential for TH production) is deficient, goiter can be endemic.

Enlargement of the thyroid gland may be mild and noticeable only when there is an increased demand for TH (e.g., during periods of rapid growth). Where iodine deficiency is severe, a large percentage of the population displays goiters. Enlargement of the thyroid at birth can be sufficient to cause severe respiratory distress. Sporadic goiter is usually caused by lymphocytic thyroiditis, and intrinsic biochemical defects in synthesis of the hormones are associated with goiters. TH replacement is necessary to treat the hypothyroidism and reverse the TSH effect on the gland.

Nursing Care Management

Large goiters are identified by their obvious appearance. Smaller nodules may be evident only on palpation. Nurses in ambulatory settings need to be aware of the possibility of goiters and report such findings. Benign enlargement of the thyroid gland may occur during adolescence and should not be confused with pathologic states. Nodules rarely are caused by a cancerous tumor but always require evaluation. Questions regarding exposure to radiation should be included in the assessment.

NURSING ALERT If an infant is born with a goiter, immediate precautions are instituted for emergency ventilation, such as supplemental oxygen and a tracheostomy set nearby. Hyperextension of the neck often facilitates breathing. Immediate surgery to remove part of the gland may be lifesaving in infants born with a goiter.

Lymphocytic Thyroiditis

Lymphocytic thyroiditis *(Hashimoto's disease, juvenile autoimmune thyroiditis)* is the most common cause of thyroid disease in children and adolescents and accounts for the largest percentage of juvenile hypothyroidism (Szymborska & Staroszczyk, 2000). It accounts for many of the enlarged thyroid glands formerly designated *thyroid hyperplasia of adolescence* or *adolescent goiter*. Although it can occur during the first 3 years of life, it occurs more frequently after age 6. It reaches a peak incidence during adolescence, and there is evidence that the disease is self-limiting. The presence of a goiter and elevated thyroglobulin antibody with progressive increase in both thyroid peroxidase antibody and TSH may be predictive factors for future development of hypothyroidism (Radetti et al, 2006).

The presence of the enlarged thyroid gland is usually detected by the practitioner during a routine examination,

BOX 52-6 Clinical Manifestations of Lymphocytic Thyroiditis

Enlarged Thyroid Gland
Usually symmetric
Firm
Freely movable
Nontender

Tracheal Compression
Sense of fullness
Hoarseness
Dysphagia

Hyperthyroidism (Possible)
Nervousness
Irritability
Increased sweating
Hyperactivity

although it may be noted by parents when the youngster swallows. In most children the entire gland is enlarged symmetrically (though it may be asymmetric) and is firm, freely movable, and nontender. There may be manifestations of moderate tracheal compression (sense of fullness, hoarseness, and dysphagia), but it is extremely rare for a nontoxic diffuse goiter to enlarge to the extent that it causes mechanical obstruction. Most children are euthyroid, but some display symptoms of hypothyroidism. Other signs suggestive of hyperthyroidism are found in Box 52-6.

Diagnostic Evaluation

Thyroid function tests are usually normal, although TSH levels may be slightly or moderately elevated. With progressive disease the T_4 decreases, followed by a decrease in T_3 levels and an increase in TSH. A variety of abnormalities in radioactive iodine uptake may be noted. The majority of children have serum antibody titers to thyroid antigens, but fewer children have a positive red blood cell hemagglutination test result. When both tests are used, almost all children with thyroid autoimmunity are detected. However, levels in children are lower than in adults; therefore repeated measurements may be needed in doubtful cases, since titers may increase later in the disease.

Therapeutic Management

In many cases the goiter is transient and asymptomatic and regresses spontaneously within a year or two. Therapy of a nontoxic diffuse goiter is usually simple, uncomplicated, and effective. Oral administration of TH decreases the size of the gland significantly and provides the feedback needed to suppress TSH stimulation, and the hyperplastic thyroid gland gradually regresses in size. Surgery is contraindicated in this disorder. Untreated patients should be evaluated periodically.

Nursing Care Management

Nursing care consists of identifying the youngster with thyroid enlargement, reassuring the child that the condition is probably only temporary, and reinforcing instructions for thyroid therapy.

Hyperthyroidism

The largest percentage of hyperthyroidism in childhood is caused by *Graves' disease*, which is usually associated with an enlarged thyroid gland and exophthalmos (Ma et al, 2006; Streetman & Khanderia, 2004; Thompson, 2002). Most cases of Graves' disease in children occur between ages 6 and 15, with a peak incidence at 12 to 14 years of age, but the disease may be present at birth in children of thyrotoxic mothers. The incidence is five times higher in girls than in boys.

The hyperthyroidism of Graves' disease is apparently caused by an autoimmune response to TSH receptors, but no specific etiology has been identified. There is definitive evidence for familial association, with a high concordance incidence in twins. Patients with Graves' disease possess the histocompatibility antigens A1, B8, and DR3 (Dallas & Foley, 2003; Simmonds et al, 2005).

The development of manifestations is highly variable. Signs and symptoms develop gradually, with an interval between onset and diagnosis of approximately 6 to 12 months. The principal clinical features are excessive motion—irritability, hyperactivity, short attention span, tremors, insomnia, and emotional lability. Clinical manifestations are presented in Box 52-7.

Exophthalmos (protruding eyeballs), observed in many children, is accompanied by a wide-eyed staring expression, increased blinking, lid lag, lack of convergence, and absence of wrinkling of the forehead when looking upward. As protrusion of the eyeball increases, the child may not be able to completely cover the cornea with the lid. Visual disturbances may include blurred vision and loss of visual acuity. Ophthalmopathy can develop long before or after the onset of hyperthyroidism. A consistent pathogenic link between them has not been identified. It is now thought that Graves' ophthalmopathy is a disorder of autoimmune origin caused by a complex interplay of endogenous and environmental factors (Bartalena et al, 2003).

Diagnostic Evaluation

The presence of a thyroid mass in a child requires a thorough history, including inquiry into prior irradiation to the head and neck and exposure to a goitrogen. The diagnosis is established on the basis of increased levels of T_4 and T_3. TSH is suppressed to unmeasurable levels (Ma et al, 2006). Other tests are rarely indicated.

Therapeutic Management

Therapy for hyperthyroidism is controversial, but all methods are directed toward retarding the rate of hormone secretion. The three acceptable modes available are the antithyroid drugs, including propylthiouracil (PTU) and methimazole (MTZ, Tapazole), which interfere with the biosynthesis of TH; subtotal thyroidectomy; and ablation with radioiodine (^{131}I iodide) (Streetman & Khanderia, 2004; Rivkees & Cornelius, 2003). Each is effective, but each has advantages and disadvantages.

Thyrotoxicosis (thyroid *crisis* or thyroid *storm*) may occur from sudden release of the hormone. Although thyrotoxicosis is unusual in children, a crisis can be life threatening. These "storms" are evidenced by the acute onset of severe irritability and restlessness, vomiting, diarrhea, hyperthermia, hyperten-

BOX 52-7 Clinical Manifestations of Hyperthyroidism (Graves' Disease)

Cardinal Signs
Emotional lability
Physical restlessness, characteristically at rest
Decelerated school performance
Voracious appetite with weight loss in 50% of cases
Fatigue

Physical Signs
Tachycardia
Widened pulse pressure
Dyspnea on exertion
Exophthalmos (protruding eyeballs)
Wide-eyed, staring expression with lid lag
Tremor
Goiter (hypertrophy and hyperplasia)
Warm, moist skin
Accelerated linear growth
Heat intolerance (may be severe)
Hair fine and unable to hold a curl
Systolic murmurs

Thyroid Storm
Acute onset:
- Severe irritability and restlessness
- Vomiting
- Diarrhea
- Hyperthermia
- Hypertension
- Severe tachycardia
- Prostration

May progress rapidly to:
- Delirium
- Coma
- Death

sion, severe tachycardia, and prostration. There may be rapid progression to delirium, coma, and even death. A crisis may be precipitated by acute infection, surgical emergencies, or discontinuation of antithyroid therapy. Treatment, in addition to antithyroid drugs, is administration of β-adrenergic blocking agents (propranolol), which provide relief from the adrenergic hyperresponsiveness that produces the disturbing side effects of the reaction. Therapy is usually required for 2 to 3 weeks.

The American Thyroid Association* has an extensive website with information related to prevention, treatment, and cure of thyroid disease.

Nursing Care Management

The initial nursing objective is identification of children with hyperthyroidism. Because the clinical manifestations often appear gradually, the goiter and ophthalmic changes may not be noticed, and the excessive activity may be attributed to behavioral problems. Nurses in ambulatory settings, particularly schools, need to be alert to signs that suggest this disorder, especially weight loss despite an excellent appetite, academic difficulties resulting from a short attention span and inability to sit still, unexplained fatigue and sleeplessness, and difficulty with fine motor skills such as writing. Exophthalmos may develop long before the onset of signs and symptoms of hyperthyroidism and may be the only presenting sign (Thompson, 2002). Exophthalmos is less common in adults than children (Jospe, 2001).

Much of these children's care is related to treating physical symptoms before a response to drug therapy is achieved. These children need a quiet, unstimulating environment that is conducive to rest. Sometimes hospitalization is necessary during the immediate treatment phase to remove a child from a troubled home. A regular routine is beneficial in providing frequent rest periods, minimizing the stress of coping with unexpected demands, and meeting the children's needs promptly. Physical activity is restricted. For example, school physical education classes are discontinued.

Emotional lability is often manifested by sudden episodes of crying or elation. Such behavior, coupled with irritability, disrupts interpersonal relationships, creating difficulties within and outside the home. Parents need help in understanding the uncontrollable nature of these outbursts and ways of minimizing them through decreased environmental stimulation, stress, and frustration. The child should be encouraged to express feelings about behavior and its effect on others. The nurse can encourage the child to concentrate on friendship with one special peer rather than a group until the condition is stabilized.

Heat intolerance may produce considerable family conflict. Preferring a cooler environment than others, the child is likely to open windows, complain about the heat, wear minimum clothing, and remove blankets while sleeping. Although the child should dress in accordance with climatic conditions, the use of light cotton clothing in the home, good ventilation, air conditioning or fans, frequent baths, and adequate hydration is helpful in providing comfort. Hygiene should be stressed because of excessive sweating.

Dietary requirements should be adjusted to meet the child's increased metabolic rate. Although the need for calories is increased, these should be provided in wholesome foods rather than "junk" foods. The child may require vitamin supplements to meet daily requirement. Rather than three large meals, the child's appetite may be better satisfied by five or six moderate meals throughout the day. Family members should refrain from making remarks about the child's appetite because the child may voluntarily restrict his or her eating to avoid such attention.

Once therapy is instituted, the nurse explains the drug regimen, emphasizing the importance of observing for side effects of antithyroid drugs. Untoward effects of propylthiouracil and related compounds include urticarial rash, fever, arthritis, or arthralgia. There may be enlargement of the salivary and cervical lymph glands, a diminished sense of taste, hepatitis, and edema of the lower extremities. Parents should also be aware of the signs of hypothyroidism, which can occur

**6066 Leesburg Pike, Suite 550, Falls Church, VA 22041; 800-THYROID; e-mail: thyroid@thyroid.org;* www.thyroid.org.

from overdose of the drugs. The most common indications are lethargy and somnolence.

NURSING ALERT Children being treated with propylthiouracil or methimazole must be carefully monitored for side effects of the drug. Because sore throat and fever accompany the grave complication of leukopenia, these children should be seen by a practitioner if such symptoms occur. Parents and children should be taught to recognize and report symptoms immediately.

Disorders of Parathyroid Function

The parathyroid glands secrete *PTH,* the main function of which, along with vitamin D and calcitonin, is homeostasis of serum calcium concentration (Perheentupa, 2003). The effect of PTH on calcium is opposite that of calcitonin. The net result of the integrated action of PTH and vitamin D is maintenance of serum calcium levels within a narrow normal range and the mineralization of bone. Secretion of PTH is controlled by a negative feedback system involving the serum calcium ion concentration. Low ionized calcium levels stimulate PTH secretion, causing absorption of calcium by the target tissues; high ionized calcium concentrations suppress PTH.

Hypoparathyroidism

Hypoparathyroidism is a spectrum of disorders that result in deficient PTH. *Congenital hypoparathyroidism* may be caused by a specific defect in the synthesis or cellular processing of PTH or by aplasia or hypoplasia of the gland (Perheentupa, 2003).

Hypoparathyroidism can also occur secondary to other causes. Postoperative hypoparathyroidism may follow thyroidectomy with acute or gradual onset and be transient or permanent. Two forms of transient hypoparathyroidism may be present in the newborn, both of which are the result of a relative PTH deficiency. One type is caused by maternal hyperparathyroidism or maternal DM. A more common, later form appears almost exclusively in infants fed a milk formula with a high phosphate-to-calcium ratio.

Clinical signs of hypoparathyroidism are found in Box 52-8. Muscle cramps are an early symptom, progressing to numbness, stiffness, and tingling in the hands and feet. A positive Chvostek's or Trousseau's sign or laryngeal spasms may be present. Convulsions with loss of consciousness may occur. These episodes may be preceded by abdominal discomfort, tonic rigidity, head retraction, and cyanosis. Headaches and vomiting with increased intracranial pressure and papilledema may occur and may suggest a brain tumor (Behrman, Kliegman, & Jenson, 2004).

Diagnostic Evaluation

The diagnosis of hypoparathyroidism is made on the basis of clinical manifestations associated with *decreased serum calcium* and *increased serum phosphorus.* Levels of plasma PTH are low in idiopathic hypoparathyroidism but high in pseudohypoparathyroidism. End-organ responsiveness is tested by the administration of PTH with measurement of urinary cyclic adenosine monophosphate (cAMP). Kidney function tests are included in the differential diagnosis to rule out renal insufficiency. Although bone radiographs are usually normal, they may demonstrate increased bone density and suppressed growth.

BOX 52-8 Clinical Manifestations of Hypoparathyroidism

Pseudohypoparathyroidism
Short stature
Round face
Short, thick neck
Short, stubby fingers and toes
Dimpling of skin over knuckles
Subcutaneous soft tissue calcifications
Intellectual disability a prominent feature

Idiopathic Hypoparathyroidism
None of the above physical characteristics observed
May include papilledema
May have intellectual disability

Both Types
Dry, scaly, coarse skin with eruptions
Hair often brittle
Nails thin and brittle with characteristic transverse grooves
Dental and enamel hypoplasia
Muscle contractions:
- Tetany
- Carpopedal spasm
- Laryngospasm (laryngeal stridor)
- Muscle cramps and twitching
- Positive Chvostek's sign or Trousseau's sign (see Nursing Alert below)
- Paresthesias, tingling

Neurologic:
- Headache
- Seizures (generalized, absence, or focal)
- Swings of emotion
- Loss of memory
- Depression
- Confusion possible

Gastrointestinal:
- Muscle cramps
- Diarrhea
- Vomiting

Retarded skeletal growth

NURSING ALERT The earliest indication of hypoparathyroidism may be anxiety and mental depression, followed by paresthesia and evidence of heightened neuromuscular excitability, such as:

Chvostek's sign—Facial muscle spasm elicited by tapping the facial nerve in the region of the parotid gland
Trousseau's sign—Carpal spasm elicited by pressure applied to nerves of the upper arm
Tetany—Carpopedal spasm (sharp flexion of wrist and ankle joints), muscle twitching, cramps, seizures, and stridor

Therapeutic Management

The objective of treatment is to maintain normal serum calcium and phosphate levels with minimum complications. Acute or severe tetany is corrected immediately by IV and oral administration of calcium gluconate and follow-up daily doses to achieve normal levels. Twice-daily serum calcium measurements are taken to monitor the efficacy of therapy and prevent hypercalcemia. When diagnosis is confirmed, *vitamin D therapy* is begun. Vitamin D therapy is somewhat difficult to regulate because the drug has a prolonged onset and a long half-life (see Patient Teaching box).

PATIENT TEACHING Vitamin D Toxicity

After initiating treatment for hypoparathyroidism, the nurse discusses with the parents the need for continuous daily administration of calcium salts and vitamin D. Because vitamin D toxicity can be a serious consequence of therapy, parents are advised to watch for signs that include weakness, fatigue, lassitude, headache, nausea, vomiting, and diarrhea. Early renal impairment is manifested by polyuria, polydipsia, and nocturia.

Long-term management consists of administration of massive doses of vitamin D, and oral calcium supplementation may be useful in maintaining adequate serum calcium levels, although it is not essential. Blood calcium and phosphorus are monitored frequently until the levels have stabilized; they are then monitored monthly and less often until the child is seen at 6-month intervals. Renal function, blood pressure, and serum vitamin D levels are measured every 6 months. Serum magnesium levels are measured every 3 to 6 months to permit detection of hypomagnesemia, which may raise the requirement for vitamin D.

Nursing Care Management

The initial objective is recognition of hypocalcemia. Unexplained convulsions, irritability (especially to external stimuli), gastrointestinal symptoms (diarrhea, vomiting, cramping), and positive signs of tetany should lead the nurse to suspect this disorder. Much of the initial nursing care is related to the physical manifestations and includes institution of seizure and safety precautions; reduction of environmental stimuli (e.g., avoiding sudden or loud noise, bright lights, stimulating activities); and observation for signs of laryngospasm such as stridor, hoarseness, and a feeling of tightness in the throat. A tracheostomy set and injectable calcium gluconate should be located near the bedside for emergency use. The administration of calcium gluconate requires precautions against extravasation of the drug and tissue destruction.

Hyperparathyroidism

Hyperparathyroidism is rare in childhood but can be primary or secondary. The most common cause of primary hyperparathyroidism is adenoma of the gland (Behrman, Kliegman, & Jenson, 2004). The most common causes of secondary hyperparathyroidism are chronic renal disease, renal osteodystrophy, and congenital anomalies of the urinary tract. The common factor is hypercalcemia. The clinical signs of hyperparathyroidism are listed in Box 52-9.

BOX 52-9 Clinical Manifestations of Hyperparathyroidism

Gastrointestinal
- Nausea
- Vomiting
- Abdominal discomfort
- Constipation

Central Nervous System
- Delusions
- Confusion
- Hallucinations
- Impaired memory
- Lack of interest and initiative
- Depression
- Varying levels of consciousness

Neuromuscular
- Weakness
- Easy fatigability
- Muscle atrophy (especially proximal muscles of lower limbs)
- Tongue twitching
- Paresthesias in extremities

Skeletal
- Vague bone pain
- Subperiosteal resorption of phalanges
- Spontaneous fractures
- Absence of lamina dura around teeth

Renal
- Polyuria
- Polydipsia
- Renal colic
- Hypertension

Diagnostic Evaluation

Blood studies to identify *elevated calcium* and *decreased phosphorus levels* are routinely performed. Measurement of PTH, as well as several tests to isolate the cause of the hypercalcemia, such as renal function studies, should be included. Other procedures used to substantiate the physiologic consequences of the disorder include electrocardiography and radiographic bone surveys.

Therapeutic Management

Treatment depends on the cause of hyperparathyroidism. The treatment of primary hyperparathyroidism is surgical removal of the tumor or hyperplastic tissue. Treatment of secondary hyperparathyroidism is directed at the underlying contributing cause, which subsequently restores the serum calcium balance. However, in some instances such as in chronic renal failure the underlying disorder is irreversible. In this case treatment is aimed at raising serum calcium levels to inhibit the stimulatory effect of low levels on the parathyroids. This includes oral administration of calcium salts, high doses of vitamin D to enhance calcium absorption, a low-phosphorus diet, and administration of a phosphorus-mobilizing aluminum hydroxide to reduce phosphate absorption.

Nursing Care Management

The initial nursing objective is recognition of the disorder. Because secondary hyperparathyroidism is a consequence of chronic renal failure, the nurse is always alert to signs that suggest this complication, especially bone pain and fractures. Because urinary symptoms are the earliest indication, assessment of other body systems for evidence of high calcium levels is indicated when polyuria and polydipsia coexist. Clues to the possibility of hyperparathyroidism include change in behavior, especially inactivity; unexplained gastrointestinal symptoms; and cardiac irregularities.

Disorders of Adrenal Function

The *adrenal cortex* secretes three main groups of hormones collectively called *steroids* and classified according to their biologic activity: (1) *glucocorticoids* (cortisol, corticosterone), (2) *mineralocorticoids* (aldosterone), and (3) *sex steroids* (androgens, estrogens, and progestins). Alterations in the levels of these hormones produce significant dysfunction in a variety of body tissues and organs. Because the adrenocortical cells are capable of producing any of the steroids, pathologic conditions may result in a deficiency or an excess of more than one type of hormone. However, most are rare in children.

The *adrenal medulla* secretes the *catecholamines epinephrine* and *norepinephrine*. Both hormones have essentially the same effects on various organs as those caused by direct sympathetic stimulation, except that the hormonal effects last several times longer. Catecholamine-secreting tumors are the primary cause of adrenal medullary hyperfunction.

Acute Adrenocortical Insufficiency

The acute form of adrenocortical insufficiency *(adrenal crisis)* may have a number of causes during childhood. Although a rare disorder, some of the more common etiologic factors include hemorrhage into the gland from trauma, which may be caused by a prolonged, difficult labor; fulminating infections, such as meningococcemia, which result in hemorrhage and necrosis (Waterhouse-Friderichsen syndrome); abrupt withdrawal of exogenous sources of cortisone or failure to increase exogenous supplies during stress; or congenital adrenogenital hyperplasia of the salt-losing type.

Early symptoms of adrenocortical insufficiency include increased irritability, headache, diffuse abdominal pain, weakness, nausea and vomiting, and diarrhea. Other clinical signs are found in Box 52-10. In the newborn, adrenal crisis is accompanied by extreme hyperpyrexia (high temperature), tachypnea, cyanosis, and seizures. Usually there is no evidence of infection or purpura. However, hemorrhage into the adrenal gland may be evident as a palpable retroperitoneal mass.

BOX 52-10 Clinical Manifestations of Acute Adrenocortical Insufficiency

Early Symptoms

Increased irritability
Headache
Diffuse abdominal pain
Weakness
Nausea and vomiting
Diarrhea

Generalized Hemorrhagic Manifestations (Waterhouse-Friderichsen Syndrome)

Fever (increases as condition worsens)
Central nervous system signs:
- Nuchal rigidity
- Seizures
- Stupor
- Coma

Shocklike State

Weak, rapid pulse
Decreased blood pressure
Shallow respirations
Cold, clammy skin
Cyanosis
Circulatory collapse (terminal event)

Newborn

Hyperpyrexia
Tachypnea
Cyanosis
Seizures
Gland evident as palpable retroperitoneal mass (hemorrhagic)

Diagnostic Evaluation

There is no rapid, definitive test for confirmation of acute adrenocortical insufficiency. Routine procedures such as measurement of plasma cortisol levels are too time-consuming to be practical. Therefore diagnosis is usually made based on clinical presentation, especially when a fulminating sepsis is accompanied by hemorrhagic manifestations and signs of circulatory collapse despite adequate antibiotic therapy. Because there is no real danger in administering a cortisol preparation for a short period, treatment should be instituted immediately. Improvement with cortisol therapy confirms the diagnosis.

Therapeutic Management

Treatment involves replacement of cortisol, replacement of body fluids to combat dehydration and hypovolemia, administration of glucose solutions to correct hypoglycemia, and specific antibiotic therapy in the presence of infection. Initially IV hydrocortisone (Solu-Cortef) is administered. Normal saline containing 5% glucose is given parenterally to replace lost fluid, electrolytes, and glucose. If hemorrhage has been severe, whole blood may be replaced. In the event that these measures do not reverse the circulatory collapse, vasopressors are used for immediate vasoconstriction and elevation of blood pressure.

Once the child's condition is stabilized, oral doses of cortisone, fluids, and salt are given, similar to the regimen used for

evolve Animation—Adrenal Function

chronic adrenal insufficiency. To maintain sodium retention, aldosterone is replaced by synthetic salt-retaining steroids.

Nursing Care Management

Because of the abrupt onset and potentially fatal outcome of this condition, prompt recognition is essential. Vital signs and blood pressure are taken every 15 minutes to monitor the hyperpyrexia and shocklike state. Seizure precautions are instituted, since convulsions from the elevated temperature are not uncommon. As soon as therapy is instituted, the nurse should monitor the child's response to fluid and cortisol replacement. Too rapid administration of fluids can precipitate cardiac failure, whereas overdosage with cortisol produces hypotension and a sudden fall in temperature.

Once the acute phase is over and the hypovolemia is corrected, the child is given oral fluids, such as small quantities of ginger ale, fruit juice, or salted broth. Too rapid ingestion of oral fluids may induce vomiting, which increases dehydration. Therefore the nurse should plan a gradual schedule for reintroducing liquids. For children who refuse to drink, the prospect of having the IV infusion removed once oral fluids are increased is often a motivating factor.

NURSING ALERT Monitor serum electrolyte levels and observe for signs of hypokalemia or hyperkalemia (e.g., weakness, poor muscle control, paralysis, cardiac dysrhythmias, and apnea). The condition is rapidly corrected with IV or oral potassium replacement.

NURSING ALERT When an oral potassium preparation is given, it should be mixed with a small amount of strongly flavored fruit juice to disguise its bitter taste.

The sudden, severe nature of this disorder necessitates a great deal of emotional support for the child and family. The child may be placed in an intensive care unit where the surroundings are strange and frightening. Despite the need for emergency intervention, the nurse must be sensitive to the family's psychologic needs and prepare them for each procedure, even if this is a brief statement such as "The intravenous infusion is necessary to replace fluid that the child is losing." Because recovery within 24 hours is often dramatic, the nurse should keep the parents apprised of the child's condition, emphasizing signs of improvement, such as a lowered temperature and elevated blood pressure. If paralysis occurs, the nurse should assure them that this condition is temporary and quickly reversed.

Chronic Adrenocortical Insufficiency (Addison's Disease)

Chronic adrenocortical insufficiency is rare in children. When it does occur, it is usually caused by a destructive lesion of the adrenal gland or neoplasms, or the cause is idiopathic. At one time, generalized tuberculosis was the leading cause of adrenal gland destruction.

Evidence of this disorder is usually gradual in onset, since 90% of adrenal tissue must be nonfunctional before signs of insufficiency are manifested. However, during periods of stress, when demands for additional cortisol are increased, symptoms of acute insufficiency may appear in a previously well child (Box 52-11).

BOX 52-11 Clinical Manifestations of Chronic Adrenocortical Insufficiency

Neurologic Symptoms
Muscular weakness
Mental fatigue
Irritability, apathy, and negativism
Increased sleeping, listlessness

Pigmentary Changes
Previous scars
Palmar creases
Mucous membranes
Hair
Hyperpigmentation over pressure points (elbows, knees, or waist)
Less frequently, vitiligo (loss of pigmentation)

Gastrointestinal Symptoms
Dehydration
Anorexia
Weight loss

Circulatory Symptoms
Hypotension
Small heart size
Dizziness
Syncopal (fainting) attacks

Hypoglycemia
Headache
Hunger
Weakness
Trembling
Sweating

Other Signs (Seen in Some Children)
Recurrent, unexplained seizures
Intense craving for salt
Acute abdominal pain
Electrolyte imbalances

Definitive diagnosis is based on measurements of functional cortisol reserve. The cortisol and urinary 17-hydroxycorticosteroid levels are low and fail to rise, while plasma *adrenocorticotropic hormone (ACTH)* levels are elevated with corticotropin (ACTH) stimulation, the definitive test for the disease.

Therapeutic Management

Treatment involves replacement of *glucocorticoids (cortisol)* and *mineralocorticoids (aldosterone)*. Some children are able to be maintained solely on oral supplements of cortisol (cortisone or hydrocortisone preparations) with a liberal intake of salt. During stressful situations, such as fever, infection, emotional upset, or surgery, the dosage must be tripled to accommodate the body's increased need for glucocorticoids. Failure to meet this requirement will precipitate an acute crisis. Overdosage produces appearance of cushingoid signs.

Children with more severe states of chronic adrenal insufficiency require mineralocorticoid replacement to maintain fluid and electrolyte balance. Other forms of therapy include monthly injections of desoxycorticosterone acetate or implantation of desoxycorticosterone acetate pellets subcutaneously every 9 to 12 months.

Nursing Care Management

Once the disorder is diagnosed, parents need guidance concerning drug therapy. They must be aware of the continuous need for cortisol replacement. Sudden termination of the drug because of inadequate supplies or inability to ingest the oral form because of vomiting places the child in danger of an acute adrenal crisis. Therefore parents should always have a spare supply of the medication in the home. Ideally they will have a prefilled syringe of hydrocortisone and be instructed in proper technique for intramuscular administration of the drug in case of crisis. Unnecessary administration of cortisone will not harm the child, but if it is needed, it may be lifesaving. Any evidence of acute insufficiency should be reported to the practitioner immediately.

Parents also need to be aware of side effects of the drugs. Undesirable side effects of cortisone include gastric irritation, which is minimized by ingestion with food or the use of an antacid; increased excitability and sleeplessness; weight gain, which may require dietary management to prevent obesity; and, rarely, behavioral changes, including depression or euphoria. Parents should be aware of signs of overdose and report these to the practitioner. In addition, the drug has a bitter taste, which creates a challenge for nurses and parents in its administration.

Because the body cannot supply endogenous sources of cortical hormones during times of stress, the home environment should be stable and relatively unstressful. Parents need to be aware that during periods of emotional or physical crisis the child requires additional hormone replacement. The child should wear medical identification, such as a bracelet, to permit medical personnel to adjust requirements during emergency care.

Cushing's Syndrome

Cushing's syndrome is a characteristic group of manifestations caused by excessive circulating free cortisol. It can result from a variety of causes, which generally fall into one of five categories (Box 52-12). Cushing's syndrome in young children may be due to an adrenal tumor (Moshang, 2003).

Cushing's syndrome is uncommon in children. When seen, it is often caused by excessive or prolonged steroid therapy that produces a cushingoid appearance (Fig. 52-1). This condition is reversible once the steroids are gradually discontinued. Abrupt withdrawal will precipitate acute adrenal insufficiency. Gradual withdrawal of exogenous supplies is necessary to allow the anterior pituitary an opportunity to secrete increasing amounts of ACTH to stimulate the adrenals to produce cortisol.

Clinical Manifestations

Because the actions of cortisol are widespread, clinical manifestations are equally profound and diverse. Those symptoms that produce changes in physical appearance occur early in the disorder and are of considerable concern to school-age and older children. The physiologic disturbances, such as hyperglycemia, susceptibility to infection, hypertension, and hypokalemia, may have life-threatening consequences unless recognized early and treated successfully. Children with

BOX 52-12 Etiology of Cushing's Syndrome

Pituitary—Cushing's syndrome with adrenal hyperplasia, usually attributed to an excess of adrenocorticotropic hormone (ACTH)

Adrenal—Cushing's syndrome with hypersecretion of glucocorticoids, generally a result of adrenocortical neoplasms

Ectopic—Cushing's syndrome with autonomous secretion of ACTH, most often caused by extrapituitary neoplasms

Iatrogenic—Cushing's syndrome, frequently a result of administration of large amounts of exogenous corticosteroids

Food dependent—Inappropriate sensitivity of adrenal glands to normal postprandial increases in secretion of gastric inhibitory polypeptide

Adapted from Magiakou MA et al: Cushing's syndrome in children and adolescents: presentation, diagnosis, and therapy, *N Engl J Med* 331(10):629-636, 1994.

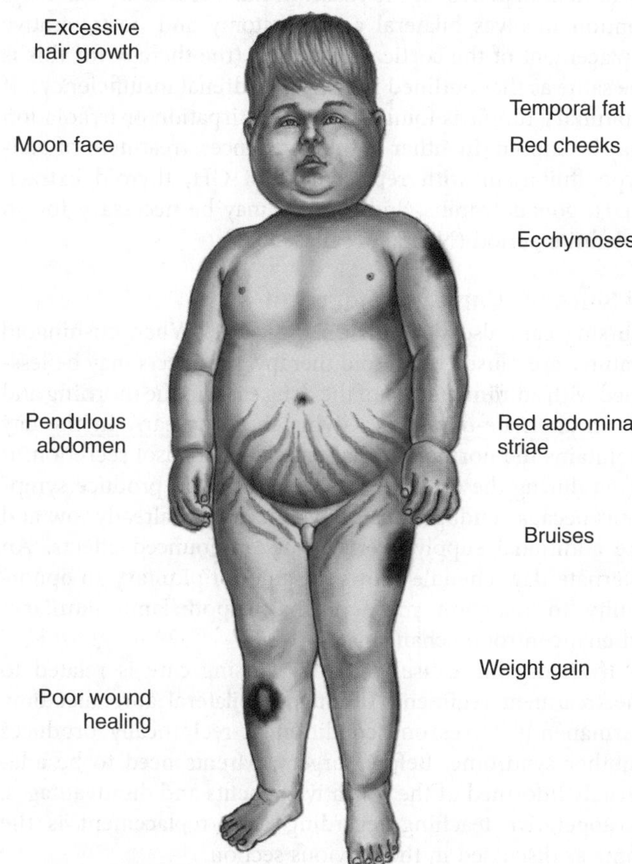

Fig. 52-1 Characteristics of Cushing's syndrome.

short stature may be responding to increased cortisol levels, resulting in Cushing's syndrome. Cortisol inhibits the action of GH.

Diagnostic Evaluation

Several tests are helpful in confirming excess cortisol levels. They include fasting blood glucose levels for hyperglycemia, serum electrolyte levels for hypokalemia and alkalosis, 24-hour urinary levels of elevated 17-hydroxycorticoids and 17-ketosteroids, and radiographic studies of bone for evidence of osteoporosis and of the skull for enlargement of the sella turcica. Another procedure used to establish a more definitive diagnosis is the dexamethasone (cortisone) suppression test (Nieman & Ilias, 2005). Administration of an exogenous supply of cortisone normally suppresses ACTH production. However, in individuals with Cushing's syndrome, cortisol levels remain elevated. This test is helpful in differentiating between children who are obese and those who appear to have cushingoid features.

Therapeutic Management

Treatment depends on the cause. In most cases surgical intervention involves bilateral adrenalectomy and postoperative replacement of the cortical hormones (the therapy for this is the same as that outlined for chronic adrenal insufficiency). If a pituitary tumor is found, surgical extirpation or irradiation may be chosen. In either of these instances, treatment of panhypopituitarism with replacement of GH, thyroid extract, ADH, gonadotropins, and steroids may be necessary for an indefinite period (Nieman & Ilias, 2005).

Nursing Care Management

Nursing care also depends on the cause. When cushingoid features are caused by steroid therapy, the effects may be lessened with administration of the drug early in the morning and on an alternate-day basis. Giving the drug early in the day maintains the normal diurnal pattern of cortisol secretion. If given during the evening, it is more likely to produce symptoms because endogenous cortisol levels are already low and the additional supply exerts more pronounced effects. An alternate-day schedule allows the anterior pituitary an opportunity to maintain more normal hypothalamic-pituitary-adrenal control mechanisms.

If an organic cause is found, nursing care is related to the treatment regimen. Although a bilateral adrenalectomy permanently solves one condition, it reciprocally produces another syndrome. Before surgery, parents need to be adequately informed of the operative benefits and disadvantages. Postoperative teaching regarding drug replacement is the same as discussed in the previous section.

NURSING ALERT Postoperative complications of adrenalectomy are related to the sudden withdrawal of cortisol. Observe for shocklike symptoms (e.g., hypotension, hyperpyrexia).

Anorexia, nausea, and vomiting are common and may be improved with the use of nasogastric decompression. Muscle and joint pain may be severe, requiring use of analgesics. The psychologic depression can be profound and may not improve for months. Parents should be aware of the physiologic reasons behind these symptoms in order to be supportive of the child.

Congenital Adrenal Hyperplasia

Congenital adrenal hyperplasia (CAH) is a family of disorders caused by decreased enzyme activity required for cortisol production in the adrenal cortex. The most common defect is *21-hydroxylase deficiency,* which constitutes more than 90% of all cases of CAH (American Academy of Pediatrics, Section on Endocrinology and Committee on Genetics, 2000; Levine, 2000). This deficiency occurs in approximately 1 per 12,000 to 15,000 births and causes overproduction of the adrenal androgens, resulting in virilization of the female fetus.

Excessive androgens cause masculinization of the urogenital system at approximately the tenth week of fetal development. The most pronounced abnormalities occur in the girl, who is born with varying degrees of ambiguous genitalia. Masculinization of external genitalia causes the clitoris to enlarge so that it appears as a small phallus. Fusion of the labia produces a saclike structure resembling the scrotum without testes. However, no abnormal changes occur in the internal sexual organs, although the vaginal orifice is usually closed by the fused labia. The label *ambiguous genitalia* should be applied to any infant with hypospadias or micropenis and no palpable gonads, and a diagnostic evaluation for CAH should be contemplated. Boys do not display genital abnormalities at birth (New & Ghizzoni, 2003).

Diagnostic Evaluation

Clinical diagnosis is initially based on congenital abnormalities that lead to difficulty in assigning sex to the newborn and on signs and symptoms of adrenal insufficiency or hypertension. Definitive diagnosis is confirmed by evidence of increased 17-ketosteroid levels in most types of CAH (Levine, 2000). Usually the level of 17-hydroxycorticoids is low or near normal. In complete 21-hydroxylase deficiency, blood electrolytes demonstrate loss of sodium and chloride and elevation of potassium. In older children bone age is advanced, and linear growth is increased. Chromosome typing for positive sex determination and to rule out any other genetic abnormality (e.g., Turner's syndrome) is always done in any case of ambiguous genitalia.

Another test that can be used to visualize the presence of pelvic structures is ultrasonography, a noninvasive, painless imaging technique that does not require anesthesia or sedation. It is especially useful in CAH because it readily identifies the absence or presence of female reproductive organs in a newborn or child with ambiguous genitalia. Because ultrasonography yields immediate results, it has the advantage of determining the child's gender long before the more complex laboratory results for chromosome analysis or steroid levels are available.

Therapeutic Management

The initial medical objective is to confirm the diagnosis and assign a sex to the child, usually according to the genotype. In both sexes cortisone is administered to suppress the abnormally high secretions of ACTH. If cortisone is begun early enough, it is very effective. Cortisone depresses the secretion of ACTH by the adenohypophysis, which in turn inhibits the secretion of adrenocorticosteroids and thus stems the progressive virilization. The signs and symptoms of masculinization in the female gradually disappear, and excessive early linear growth is slowed. Puberty occurs normally at the appropriate age.

The recommended oral dosage is divided to simulate the normal diurnal pattern of ACTH secretion. Because these children are unable to produce cortisol in response to stress, it is necessary to increase the dosage during episodes of infection, fever, or other stresses. Acute emergencies require immediate IV or intramuscular administration. Emergency situations include bacterial and viral infections, vomiting, surgery, fractures, major injuries, and sometimes insect stings.

Children with the salt-losing type of CAH require aldosterone replacement, as outlined under chronic adrenal insufficiency, and supplementary dietary salt. Frequent laboratory tests are conducted to assess the effects on electrolytes, hormonal profiles, and renin levels. The frequency of testing is individualized to the child.

Depending on the degree of masculinization in the female, reconstructive surgery may be required to reduce the size of the clitoris, separate the labia, and create a vaginal orifice (Miranda et al, 2004). Surgery is performed when the infant is physically able to withstand the procedure but before she is old enough to be aware of the abnormal genitalia. Plastic surgery is generally done in stages and yields excellent cosmetic results. Reports concerning sexual satisfaction after partial clitoridectomy indicate that the capacity for orgasm and sexual gratification is not necessarily impaired.

Unfortunately, not all children with CAH are diagnosed at birth and raised in accordance with their genetic sex. Particularly in the case of affected girls, masculinization of the external genitalia may have led to sex assignment as a male. In boys, diagnosis is usually delayed until early childhood, when signs of virilism appear. In these situations it is advisable to continue rearing the child as a male in accordance with assigned sex and phenotype. Hormone replacement may be required to permit linear growth and to initiate male pubertal changes. Surgery is usually indicated to remove the female organs and reconstruct the phallus for satisfactory sexual relations. These individuals are not fertile.

Nursing Care Management

Of major importance is recognition of ambiguous genitalia in newborns. If there is any question regarding assignment of sex, the parents need to be told immediately to prevent the embarrassing situation of informing family members of the child's sex and then having to change the announcement.

As soon as the sex is determined, parents should be informed of the findings and encouraged to choose an appropriate name, and the child should be identified as a male or female, with no reference to ambiguous sex. If the appearance of the enlarged genitalia in a girl concerns the parents, they should be encouraged to discuss their feelings. Suggesting ways to avoid questioning remarks from visitors, such as diapering the child in a separate room, is also helpful. If surgery is anticipated, showing parents before-and-after photographs of reconstruction helps to reinforce the expected cosmetic benefits.

In general, rearing the genetically female child as a girl is preferred because of the success of surgical intervention and the satisfactory results with hormones in reversing virilism and providing a prospect of normal puberty and the ability to conceive. This is in contrast to the choice of rearing the child as a boy, in which case the child is sterile and may never be able to function satisfactorily in heterosexual relationships. If the parents persist in their decision to assign a male sex to a genetically female child, a psychologic consultation should be requested to explore their motivations and ensure their understanding of the future consequences for the child.

Nursing care management regarding cortisol and aldosterone replacement is the same as that discussed for chronic adrenocortical insufficiency. Because infants are especially prone to dehydration and salt-losing crises, parents need to be aware of signs of dehydration and the urgency of immediate medical intervention to stabilize the child's condition. Parents should have injectable hydrocortisone available and know how to prepare and administer the intramuscular injection (see Chapter 45).

In the unfortunate situation in which the sex is erroneously assigned and the correct sex determined later, parents need a great deal of help in understanding the reason for the incorrect sex identification and the options for sex reassignment or medical-surgical intervention. Because children become aware of their sexual identity by 18 months to 2 years of age, it is believed that any reassignment after this period can cause tremendous psychologic conflicts in the child. Therefore sex rearing should be continued as previously established with medical-surgical intervention as required.

Pheochromocytoma

Pheochromocytoma is a rare tumor characterized by secretion of catecholamines. The tumor most commonly arises from the chromaffin cells of the adrenal medulla but may occur wherever these cells are found, such as along the paraganglia of the aorta or thoracolumbar sympathetic chain (Pacak et al, 2007). Approximately 10% of these tumors are located in extraadrenal sites. In children they are frequently bilateral or multiple and are generally benign. Often there is a familial transmission of the condition as an autosomal dominant trait (Behrman, Kliegman, & Jenson, 2004).

The clinical manifestations of pheochromocytoma are caused by an increased production of catecholamines, producing hypertension, tachycardia, headache, decreased gastrointestinal activity with resultant constipation, increased metabolism with anorexia, weight loss, hyperglycemia, polyuria, polydipsia, hyperventilation, nervousness, heat intolerance, and diaphoresis. In severe cases, signs of congestive heart failure are evident.

Diagnostic Evaluation

The clinical manifestations mimic those of other disorders, such as hyperthyroidism or DM.

Therapeutic Management

Definitive treatment consists of surgical removal of the tumor. In children the tumors may be bilateral, requiring a bilateral adrenalectomy and lifelong glucocorticoid and mineralocorticoid therapy.

Nursing Care Management

An initial nursing objective is identification of children with this disorder. Outstanding clues are hypertension and hypertensive attacks. Because of behavioral changes (nervousness, excitability, overactivity, even psychosis), increased cardiac and respiratory activity may appear to be related to an acute anxiety attack. Therefore a careful history of the onset of symptoms and association with stressful events is helpful in distinguishing between an organic and a psychologic cause for the symptoms.

Preoperative nursing care involves frequent monitoring of vital signs and observation for evidence of hypertensive attacks and congestive heart failure. Therapeutic effects are evidenced by normal vital signs and absence of glycosuria. Daily blood glucose levels, urine acetone, and any signs of hyperglycemia are noted and reported immediately.

NURSING ALERT Do not palpate the mass. Preoperative palpation of the mass releases catecholamines, which can stimulate severe hypertension and tachyarrhythmias.

The environment is made conducive to rest and free of emotional stress. This requires adequate preparation during hospital admission and before surgery. Parents are encouraged to room-in with their child and to participate in care. Play activities need to be tailored to the child's energy level without being overly strenuous or challenging because these can increase metabolic rate and promote frustration and anxiety.

After surgery the child is observed for signs of shock from removal of excess catecholamines. If a bilateral adrenalectomy was performed, the nursing interventions are those discussed for chronic adrenocortical insufficiency.

Disorders of Pancreatic Hormone Secretion: Diabetes Mellitus

evolve Case Study–Diabetes Mellitus

DM is a chronic disorder of metabolism characterized by a partial or complete deficiency of the hormone *insulin.* It is the most common metabolic disease, resulting in metabolic adjustment or physiologic change in almost all areas of the body. Approximately one in three children born in the United States will develop diabetes. The odds are higher for African-American and Hispanic children: nearly 50% of them will develop diabetes (Urrutia-Rojas & Menchaca, 2006). DM in children can occur at any age but has a peak incidence between ages 10 and 15 years, with 75% diagnosed before 18 years of age. The incidence in boys is slightly higher than in girls (1:1 to 1.2:1).

Traditionally DM had been classified according to the type of treatment needed. The old categories were insulin-dependent diabetes mellitus (IDDM), or type I; and non-insulin-dependent diabetes mellitus (NIDDM), or type II. In 1997 these terms were eliminated because treatment can vary (some people with NIDDM require insulin) and because the terms do not indicate the underlying problem. The new terms are *type 1* and *type 2,* using Arabic symbols to avoid confusion (e.g., type II could be read as type eleven) (American Diabetes Association, 2001). The characteristics of type 1 DM and type 2 DM are outlined in Table 52-1.

Type 1 DM is more prominent in Caucasians, with an incidence of 20 per 100,000; the incidence in African-Americans is 11 per 100,000; the incidence in Hispanics is 15.2 per 100,000; and the incidence in Cubans is 2.6 per 100,000. Native Americans tend to develop type 2 DM rather than type 1 DM even when diagnosed in childhood. The Pima Tribe reports a greater than 55% incidence of type 2 DM. Type 1 diabetes is characterized by destruction of the pancreatic β cells, which produce insulin; this usually leads to absolute insulin deficiency. Type 1 diabetes has two forms. Immune-mediated DM results from an autoimmune destruction of the β-cells; it typically starts in children or young adults who are slim, but it can arise in adults of any age. *Idiopathic type 1* refers to rare forms of the disease that have no known cause.

Type 2 diabetes usually arises because of insulin resistance, in which the body fails to use insulin properly, combined with relative (rather than absolute) insulin deficiency. People with type 2 can range from predominantly insulin resistant with relative insulin deficiency to predominantly deficient in insulin secretion with some insulin resistance. It typically occurs in those who are over 45, are overweight and sedentary, and have a family history of diabetes.

The symptomatology of diabetes is more readily recognizable in children than in adults, so it is surprising that the diagnosis may sometimes be missed or delayed. Diabetes is a great imitator; influenza, gastroenteritis, and appendicitis are the conditions most often diagnosed when it turns out that the disease is really diabetes (Box 52-13).

Pathophysiology

Insulin is needed to support the metabolism of carbohydrates, fats, and proteins, primarily by facilitating the entry of these substances into the cell, with the exception of nerve cells and vascular tissue. With a deficiency of insulin, glucose is unable to enter the cell, and its concentration in the bloodstream *(hyperglycemia)* increases. The increased concentration of glucose produces an osmotic gradient that causes the movement of body fluid from the intracellular space to the extracellular space; from there the body fluid is excreted by the kidneys. When the serum glucose level exceeds the renal threshold (±180 mg/dl), glucose "spills" into the urine *(glycosuria),* along with an osmotic diversion of water *(polyuria),* a cardinal sign of diabetes. The urinary fluid losses cause the excessive thirst *(polydipsia)* observed in diabetes. As might be expected, this water washout results in a depletion of other essential chemicals.

Protein is also wasted during insulin deficiency. Because glucose is unable to enter the cells, protein is broken down and converted to glucose by the liver *(glucogenesis);* this glucose then contributes to the hyperglycemia. Without the use of carbohydrates for energy, fat and protein stores are depleted as the body attempts to meet its energy needs. The hunger mechanism is triggered, but the increased food intake *(polyphagia)* enhances the problem by further elevating the blood glucose.

Table 52-1 Characteristics of Types 1 and 2 Diabetes Mellitus

CHARACTERISTIC	TYPE 1	TYPE 2
Age at onset	<20 yr	Increasingly occurring in younger children
Type of onset	Abrupt	Gradual
Sex ratio	Affects males slightly more than females	Females outnumber males
Percentage of diabetic population	5%-8%	85%-90%
Heredity:		
Family history	Sometimes	Frequently
Human leukocyte antigen	Associations	No association
Twin concordance	25%-50%	90%-100%
Ethnic distribution	Primarily Caucasians	Increased incidence in Native Americans, Hispanics, African-Americans
Presenting symptoms	Three P's common: polyuria, polydipsia, polyphagia	May be related to long-term complications
Nutritional status	Underweight	Overweight
Insulin (natural):		
Pancreatic content	Usually none	>50% normal
Serum insulin	Low to absent	High or low
Primary resistance	Minimum	Marked
Islet cell antibodies	80%-85%	<5%
Therapy:		
Insulin	Always	20%-30% of patients
Oral agents	Ineffective	Often effective
Diet only	Ineffective	Often effective
Chronic complications	>80%	Variable
Ketoacidosis	Common	Infrequent

BOX 52-13 Clinical Manifestations of Type 1 Diabetes Mellitus

Polyphagia
Polyuria
Polydipsia
Weight loss
Enuresis or nocturia
Irritability; "not himself" or "herself"
Shortened attention span
Lowered frustration tolerance
Dry skin
Blurred vision
Poor wound healing
Fatigue
Flushed skin
Headache
Frequent infections
Hyperglycemia
- Elevated blood glucose levels
- Glucosuria

Diabetic ketosis
- Ketones and glucose in urine
- Dehydration in some cases

Diabetic ketoacidosis
- Dehydration
- Electrolyte imbalance
- Acidosis
- Deep, rapid breathing (Kussmaul's)

Ketoacidosis

When insulin is absent or insulin sensitivity is altered, glucose is unavailable for cellular metabolism, and the body chooses alternate sources of energy, principally fat. Consequently fats break down into fatty acids, and glycerol in the fat cells is converted by the liver to ketone bodies (β-hydroxybutyric acid, acetoacetic acid, acetone). Any excess is eliminated in the urine *(ketonuria)* or the lungs *(acetone breath)*. The ketone bodies in the blood (ketonemia) are strong acids that lower serum pH, producing *ketoacidosis.*

Ketones are organic acids that readily produce excessive quantities of free hydrogen ions, causing a fall in plasma pH. Then chemical buffers in the plasma, principally bicarbonate, combine with the hydrogen ions to form carbonic acid, which readily dissociates into water and carbon dioxide. The respiratory system attempts to eliminate the excess carbon dioxide by increased depth and rate—*Kussmaul's respirations,* or the hyperventilation characteristic of metabolic acidosis. The ketones are buffered by sodium and potassium in the plasma. The kidney attempts to compensate for the increased pH by increasing tubular secretion of hydrogen and ammonium ions in exchange for fixed base, thus depleting the base buffer concentration.

With cellular death, potassium is released from the cell (intracellular fluid) into the bloodstream (extracellular fluid) and excreted by the kidney, where the loss is accelerated by osmotic diuresis. The total body potassium is then decreased, even though the serum potassium level may be elevated as a result of the decreased fluid volume in which it circulates. Alteration in serum and tissue potassium can lead to cardiac arrest.

If these conditions are not reversed by insulin therapy in combination with correction of the fluid deficiency and electrolyte imbalance, progressive deterioration occurs, with dehydration, electrolyte imbalance, acidosis, coma, and death. *Diabetic ketoacidosis (DKA)* should be diagnosed promptly in a seriously ill patient and therapy instituted in an intensive care unit.

Long-Term Complications

Long-term complications of diabetes involve both the microvasculature and the macrovasculature. The principal microvascular complications are *nephropathy, retinopathy,* and *neuropathy.* Microvascular disease develops during the first 30 years of diabetes, beginning in the first 10 to 15 years after puberty, with renal involvement evidenced by proteinuria and clinically apparent retinopathy.

With poor diabetic control, vascular changes can appear as early as 2½ to 3 years after diagnosis; however, with good to excellent control, changes can be postponed for 20 or more years. Intensive insulin therapy appears to delay the onset and slow the progression of clinically important retinopathy, including vision-threatening lesions, nephropathy, and neuropathy. Hypertension and atherosclerotic cardiovascular disease are also major causes of morbidity and mortality in patients with DM (Karnik, Fields, & Shannon, 2007). The postpubertal duration, not the total duration, of type 1 DM is implicated as a risk factor for the development of microvascular disease (Schultz et al, 1999). The process appears to be one of glycosylation, wherein proteins from the blood become deposited in the walls of small vessels (e.g., glomeruli), where they become trapped by "sticky" glucose compounds (glycosyl radicals). The buildup of these substances over time causes narrowing of the vessels, with subsequent interference with microcirculation to the affected areas (Beisswenger, Szwergold, & Yeo, 2001). Macrovascular disease develops after 25 years of diabetes and creates the predominant problems in patients with type 2 DM.

Other complications have been observed in children with type 1 DM. Hyperglycemia appears to influence thyroid function, and altered function is frequently observed at the time of diagnosis and in poorly controlled diabetes. Limited mobility of small joints of the hand occurs in 30% of 7- to 18-year-old children with type 1 DM and appears to be related to changes in the skin and soft tissues surrounding the joint as a result of glycosylation.

Diagnostic Evaluation

Three groups of children who should be considered as candidates for diabetes are (1) children who have glycosuria, polyuria, and a history of weight loss or failure to gain despite a voracious appetite; (2) those with transient or persistent glycosuria; and (3) those who display manifestations of metabolic acidosis, with or without stupor or coma. In every case diabetes must be considered if there is glycosuria, with or without ketonuria, and unexplained hyperglycemia.

Glycosuria by itself is not diagnostic of diabetes. Other sugars, such as galactose, can produce a positive result with certain test strips, and a mild degree of glycosuria can be caused by other conditions, such as infection, trauma, emotional or physical stress, hyperalimentation, and some renal or endocrine diseases.

An 8-hour fasting blood glucose level of 126 mg/dl or more, a random blood glucose value of 200 mg/dl or more accompanied by classic signs of diabetes, or an oral glucose tolerance test (OGTT) finding of 200 mg/dl or more in the 2-hour sample is almost certain to indicate diabetes (American Diabetes Association, 2005; Hoffman, 2003). Postprandial blood glucose determinations and the traditional OGTTs have yielded low detection rates in children and are not usually necessary for establishing a diagnosis. Serum insulin levels may be normal or moderately elevated at the onset of diabetes; delayed insulin response to glucose indicates impaired glucose tolerance.

Ketoacidosis must be differentiated from other causes of acidosis or coma, including hypoglycemia, uremia, gastroenteritis with metabolic acidosis, salicylate intoxication encephalitis, and other intracranial lesions. DKA is a state of relative insulin insufficiency and may include the presence of hyperglycemia (blood glucose level 330 mg/dl or greater), ketonemia (strongly positive), acidosis (pH less than 7.30 and bicarbonate less than 15 mmol/L), glycosuria, and ketonuria (Magee & Bhatt, 2001). Tests used to determine glycosuria and ketonuria are the glucose oxidase tapes (Keto-Diastix).

Therapeutic Management

The management of the child with type 1 DM consists of a multidisciplinary approach involving the family; the child (when appropriate); and professionals, including a pediatric endocrinologist, diabetes nurse educator, nutritionist, and exercise physiologist. Often psychologic support from a mental health professional is also needed. Communication among the team members is essential and extends to other individuals in the child's life, such as teachers, school nurse, school guidance counselor, and coach.

The definitive treatment is replacement of insulin that the child is unable to produce. However, insulin needs are also affected by emotions, nutritional intake, activity, and other life events such as illnesses and puberty. The complexity of the disease and its management requires that the child and family incorporate diabetes needs into their lifestyle. Medical and nutritional guidance are primary, but management also includes continuing diabetes education, family guidance, and emotional support.

Insulin Therapy

Insulin replacement is the cornerstone of management of type 1 DM. Insulin dosage is tailored to each child based on home blood glucose monitoring. The goal of insulin therapy is maintaining near-normal blood glucose values while avoiding too frequent episodes of hypoglycemia. The goals of treatment are to maintain near-normal glucose levels of less than 126 mg/dl, and glycosylated hemoglobin (hemoglobin A_{1c}) of 7% or less (Hannon, Gungor, & Arslanian, 2006). Glycemic control decreases the likelihood of long-term complications in patients with DM (Petitti et al, 2007). Insulin is administered as two or more injections per day or as continuous subcutaneous infusion using a portable insulin pump.

Healthy pancreatic cells secrete insulin at a low but steady basal rate with superimposed bursts of increased secretion that coincide with intake of nutrients. Consequently insulin levels in the blood increase and decrease coincidentally with rises and falls in blood glucose levels. In addition, insulin is secreted directly into the portal circulation; therefore the liver, which is the major site of glucose disposal, receives the largest concentration of insulin. No matter which method of insulin replacement is used, this normal pattern cannot be duplicated. Subcutaneous injection results in absorption of the drug into the general circulation, thus reducing the concentrations of insulin to which the liver is exposed.

Insulin Preparations Insulin is available in highly purified pork preparations and in human insulin biosynthesized by and extracted from bacterial or yeast cultures. Most clinicians suggest human insulin as the treatment of choice. Insulin is available in rapid-, intermediate-, and long-acting preparations, and all are packaged in the strength of 100 units/ml. Some insulins are available as premixed insulins, such as 70/30 and 50/50 ratios, the first number indicating the percentage of intermediate-acting and the second number the percentage of rapid-acting insulin. The different types of insulin are found in Box 52-14.

NURSING ALERT The human insulins from various manufacturers may be interchangeable, but human insulin and pork insulin or pure pork insulin should never be substituted for one another.

Dosage Conventional management has consisted of a *twice-daily insulin* regimen of a combination of *rapid-acting* and *intermediate-acting* insulin drawn up into the same syringe and injected before breakfast and before the evening meal. The amount of morning regular insulin is determined by patterns in the late morning and lunchtime blood glucose values. The morning intermediate-acting dose is determined by patterns in the late afternoon and supper blood glucose values. Fasting blood glucose patterns at breakfast help determine the evening dose of intermediate insulin, and the blood glucose patterns at bedtime help determine the evening dose of rapid-acting (regular) insulin. For some children, better morning glucose control is achieved by a later (bedtime) injection of intermediate-acting insulin.

Regular insulin is best administered at least 30 minutes before meals. This allows sufficient time for absorption and results in a significantly greater reduction in the postprandial rise in blood glucose than if the meal were eaten immediately after the insulin injection. Intensive therapy consists of multiple injections throughout the day with a once- or twice-daily dose of long-acting (Ultralente) insulin to simulate the basal insulin secretion and injections of rapid-acting insulin before each meal. A multiple daily injection program reduces microvascular complications of diabetes in young, healthy patients who have type 1 DM.

BOX 52-14 Types of Insulin

There are four types of insulin, based on the following criteria:

- How soon the insulin starts working (onset)
- When the insulin works the hardest (peak time)
- How long the insulin lasts in the body (duration)

However, each person responds to insulin in his or her own way. That is why onset, peak time, and duration are given as ranges.

Rapid-acting insulin (e.g., NovoLog) reaches the blood within 15 minutes after injection. The insulin peaks 30 to 90 minutes later and may last as long as 5 hours.

Short-acting (regular) insulin (e.g., Novolin R) usually reaches the blood within 30 minutes after injection. The insulin peaks 2 to 4 hours later and stays in the blood for about 4 to 8 hours.

Intermediate-acting insulins (e.g., Novolin N) reach the blood 2 to 6 hours after injection. The insulins peak 4 to 14 hours later and stay in the blood for about 14 to 20 hours.

Long-acting insulin (e.g., Lantus) takes 6 to 14 hours to start working. It has no peak or a very small peak 10 to 16 hours after injection. The insulin stays in the blood between 20 and 24 hours.

Some insulins come mixed together (e.g., Novolin 70/30). For example, you can buy regular insulin and NPH (intermediate) insulins already mixed in one bottle, which makes it easier to inject two kinds of insulin at the same time. However, you cannot adjust the amount of one insulin without also changing how much you get of the other insulin.

Adapted from American Diabetes Association: *Resource guide 2005*, 2005. Available at www.diabetes.org/rg2005/insulin.jsp (accessed April 10, 2009).

The precise dosage of insulin needed cannot be predicted. Therefore the total dosage and percentage of regular- to intermediate-acting insulin should be determined empirically for each child. Usually 60% to 75% of the total daily dose is given before breakfast, and the remainder before the evening meal. Furthermore insulin requirements do not remain constant but change continuously during growth and development; the need varies according to the child's activity level and pubertal status. For example, less insulin is required during spring and summer months, when the child is more active. Illness also alters insulin requirements. Some children require more frequent insulin administration. This includes children with difficult-to-control diabetes and children during the adolescent growth spurt.

Methods of Administration Daily insulin is administered subcutaneously by twice-daily injections, by multiple-dose injections, or by means of an insulin infusion pump. The *insulin pump* is an electromechanical device designed to deliver fixed amounts of regular or lispro insulin continuously (basal rate), thereby more closely imitating the release of the hormone by the islet cells (Olohan & Zappitelli, 2003).

Table 52-2 Plasma Blood Glucose and Hemoglobin A_{1c} Goals for Type 1 Diabetes Mellitus by Age Group

AGE	VALUE* BEFORE MEALS (mg/dl)	VALUE* AT BEDTIME, OVERNIGHT (mg/dl)	HEMOGLOBIN A_{1c} (%)	IMPLICATIONS
Toddlers and preschoolers (<6 yr)	100-180	110-200	≤8.5% (but ≥7.5%)	High risk and vulnerability to hypoglycemia
School age (6-12 yr)	90-180	100-180	<8%	Risk of hypoglycemia and relatively low risk of complications before puberty
Adolescents (>12 yr) and young adults	90-130	90-150	<7.5%	Risk of hypoglycemia Developmental and psychologic issues

Modified from American Diabetes Association: Standards of medical care in diabetes, *Diabetes Care* 28(Suppl):S4-S36, 2005.
*Plasma blood glucose goal range.

Although the pump delivers a programmed amount of basal insulin, the child or parent must program a dose for the pump to deliver before each meal.

The system consists of a syringe to hold the insulin, a plunger, and a computerized mechanism to drive the plunger. The insulin flows from the syringe through a catheter to a needle inserted into subcutaneous tissue (the abdomen or thigh), and the lightweight device is worn on a belt or a shoulder holster. The needle and catheter are changed every 48 to 72 hours by the child or parent, using aseptic technique, and then taped in place.

Although the pump provides more consistent insulin delivery, it has certain disadvantages. Pump therapy is expensive and requires commitment from the parent and child. A certain level of math skills is required to calculate infusion rates. It should also not be removed for more than 1 hour at a time, which may limit some activities. Skin infections are common; and, as with any other mechanical device, it is subject to malfunction. However, the pumps are equipped with alarms that signal problems, such as a depleted battery, an occluded needle or tubing, or a microprocessor malfunction.

Monitoring

Daily monitoring of blood glucose levels is an essential aspect of appropriate DM management. Plasma blood glucose and hemoglobin A_{1c} goal ranges are found in Table 52-2.

Blood Glucose *Self-monitoring of blood glucose (SMBG)* has improved diabetes management and is used successfully by children from the onset of their diabetes. By testing their own blood, children are able to change their insulin regimen to maintain their glucose level in the euglycemic (normal) range of 80 to 120 mg/dl. Diabetes management depends to a great extent on SMBG. In general, children tolerate the testing well.

Glycosylated Hemoglobin The measurement of hemoglobin A_{1c} levels is a satisfactory method for assessing control of the diabetes. As red blood cells circulate in the bloodstream, glucose molecules gradually attach to the hemoglobin A molecules and remain there for the lifetime of the red blood cell, approximately 120 days. The attachment is not reversible; therefore this glycosylated hemoglobin reflects the average blood glucose levels over the previous 2 to 3 months. The test is a satisfactory method for assessing control, detecting incorrect testing, monitoring effectiveness of changes in treatment, defining patients' goals, and detecting nonadherence. Nondiabetic hemoglobin A_{1c} values are generally between 4% and 6% but can vary by laboratory. Diabetes control for children depends on age, with hemoglobin A_{1c} levels of 6.5% to 8% indicating a slightly elevated but acceptable range (American Diabetes Association, 2005). Hemoglobin A_{1c} levels of less than 7% are a well-established goal at most care centers.

Urine Urine testing for glucose is no longer used for diabetes management; there is poor correlation between simultaneous glycosuria and blood glucose concentrations. However, urine testing can be carried out to detect evidence of ketonuria.

NURSING ALERT It is recommended that urine be tested for ketones every 3 hours during an illness or whenever the blood glucose level is over 240 mg/dl when illness is not present.

Nutrition

Essentially the nutritional needs of children with diabetes are no different from those of healthy children. Children with diabetes need no special foods or supplements. They need sufficient calories to balance daily expenditure for energy and to satisfy the requirement for growth and development. Unlike the child without diabetes, whose insulin is secreted in response to food intake, insulin injected subcutaneously has a relatively predictable time of onset, peak effect, duration of action, and absorption rate depending on the type of insulin used. Consequently the timing of food consumption must be regulated to correspond to the timing and action of the insulin prescribed.

Meals and snacks must be eaten according to peak insulin action, and the total number of calories and proportions of basic nutrients must be consistent from day to day. The constant release of insulin into the circulation makes the child prone to hypoglycemia between the three daily meals unless a snack is provided between meals and at bedtime. The distribution of calories should be calculated to fit each child's activity pattern. For example, a child who is more active in the afternoon will need a larger snack at that time. This larger snack might also be split to allow some food at school and some food after school. Food intake should be altered to balance food, insulin, and exercise. Extra food is needed for increased activity.

Concentrated sweets are discouraged, and because of the increased risk for atherosclerosis in persons with DM, fat is reduced to 30% or less of the total caloric requirement. Dietary fiber has become increasingly important in dietary planning because of its influence on digestion, absorption, and metabolism of many nutrients. It has been found to diminish the rise in blood glucose after meals.

Correctly used, the diet allows for flexibility and the incorporation of preferred foods in most instances. For the growing child, food restriction should never be used for diabetes control, although caloric restrictions may be imposed for weight control if the child is overweight. In general, the child's appetite should be the guide for the amount of calories needed, with the total caloric intake adjusted to appetite and activity.

Exercise

Exercise is encouraged and never restricted unless indicated by other health conditions. Exercise lowers blood glucose levels, depending on the intensity and duration of the activity. Consequently exercise should be included as part of diabetes management, and the type and amount of exercise should be planned around the child's interests and capabilities. However, in most instances children's activities are unplanned, and the resulting decrease in blood glucose can be compensated for by providing extra snacks before (and, if the exercise is prolonged, during) the activity. In addition to a feeling of well-being, regular exercise aids in utilization of food and often results in a reduction of insulin requirements.

Hypoglycemia

Occasional episodes of hypoglycemia are an integral part of insulin therapy, and an objective of diabetes management is to achieve the best possible glycemic control while minimizing the frequency and severity of hypoglycemia. Even with good control, a child may frequently experience mild symptoms of hypoglycemia. If the signs and symptoms are recognized early and promptly relieved by appropriate therapy, the child's activity should be interrupted for no more than a few minutes.

NURSING ALERT Hypoglycemic episodes most commonly occur before meals, or when the insulin effect is peaking.

The signs and symptoms of hypoglycemia are caused by both increased adrenergic activity and impaired brain function. The increased adrenergic nervous system activity plus increased secretion of catecholamines produces nervousness, pallor, tremulousness, palpitations, sweating, and hunger. Weakness, dizziness, headache, drowsiness, irritability, loss of coordination, seizures, and coma are more severe responses and reflect CNS glucose deprivation and the body's attempts to elevate the serum glucose levels.

It is often difficult to distinguish between hyperglycemia and a hypoglycemic reaction (Table 52-3). Because the symptoms are similar and usually begin with changes in behavior, the simplest way to differentiate between the two is to test the blood glucose level. The blood glucose level is low in hypoglycemia, whereas in hyperglycemia the glucose level is significantly elevated. Urinary ketones may be present after hypoglycemia as a result of starvation ketone production. In doubtful situations it is safer to give the child some simple carbohydrate. This will help alleviate the symptoms in the case of hypoglycemia but will do little harm if the child is hyperglycemic.

Children are usually able to detect the onset of hypoglycemia, but some are too young to implement treatment. Parents should become adept at recognizing the onset of symptoms—for example, a change in a child's behavior, such as tearfulness or euphoria. In the majority of cases, 10 to 15 g of simple carbohydrate, such as 1 tbsp of table sugar, will elevate the blood glucose level and alleviate the symptoms. The simpler the carbohydrate, the more rapidly it will be absorbed (8 oz of milk equals 15 g of carbohydrate). The rapid-releasing sugar is followed by a complex carbohydrate such as a slice of bread or a cracker and by a protein such as peanut butter or milk.

For a mild reaction, milk or fruit juice is a good food to use in children. Milk supplies them with lactose or milk sugar, as well as a more prolonged action from the protein and fat (aids in decreased absorption). Other glucose sources include Insta-Glucose (cherry-flavored glucose), carbonated drinks (not sugarless), sherbet, gelatin, or cake icing. All children with diabetes should carry with them glucose tabs, Insta-Glucose, sugar cubes, or sugar-containing candy such as LifeSavers or Charms. A difficulty with candies or icing is that the child may learn to fake a reaction to get the sweets; therefore commercial treatment products such as Insta-Glucose or glucose tabs may be preferred.

Glucagon is sometimes prescribed for home treatment of hypoglycemia. It is available as an emergency kit that must be mixed at the time of use and is administered intramuscularly or subcutaneously. Glucagon functions by releasing stored glycogen from the liver and requires about 15 to 20 minutes to elevate the blood glucose level.

NURSING ALERT Vomiting may occur after administration of glucagon; therefore precautions against aspiration must be taken (e.g., placing the child on the side), since the child often becomes unconscious.

Once the child is responsive, the lost glycogen stores are replaced by small amounts of sugar-containing fluid administered frequently until the child feels comfortable trying solid foods.

Morning Hyperglycemia

The management of elevated morning blood glucose levels depends on whether the increase is a true dawn phenomenon, insulin waning, or a rebound hyperglycemia (the *Somogyi effect*). *Insulin waning* is a progressive rise in blood glucose levels from bedtime to morning. It is treated by increasing the nocturnal insulin dose. The true dawn phenomenon shows a relatively normal blood glucose level until about 3 AM, when the level begins to rise. The Somogyi effect may occur at any time but often entails an elevated blood glucose level at bedtime and a drop at 2 AM with a rebound rise following. The treatment for this phenomenon is decreasing the nocturnal insulin dose to prevent the 2 AM hypoglycemia. The rebound rise in the blood glucose level is a result of counterregulatory hormones (epinephrine, GH, and corticosteroids), which are stimulated by hypoglycemia. More frequent blood monitoring (especially at times of anticipated peak insulin action) will usually identify these conditions. Trace

Table 52-3 Comparison of Manifestations of Hypoglycemia and Hyperglycemia

VARIABLE	HYPOGLYCEMIA	HYPERGLYCEMIA
Onset	Rapid (minutes)	Gradual (days)
Mood	Labile, irritable, nervous, weepy	Lethargic
Mental status	Difficulty concentrating, speaking, focusing, coordinating Nightmares	Dulled sensorium Confusion
Inward feeling	Shaky feeling Hunger Headache Dizziness	Thirst Weakness Nausea and vomiting Abdominal pain
Skin	Pallor Sweating	Flushed Signs of dehydration
Mucous membranes	Normal	Dry, crusty
Respirations	Shallow, normal	Deep, rapid (Kussmaul's)
Pulse	Tachycardia, palpitations	Less rapid, weak
Breath odor	Normal	Fruity, acetone
Neurologic	Tremors	Diminished reflexes Paresthesia
Ominous signs	Late—Hyperreflexia, dilated pupils, seizure Shock, coma	Acidosis, coma
Blood:		
Glucose	Low: <60 mg/dl	High: ≥250 mg/dl
Ketones	Negative	High, large
Osmolarity	Normal	High
pH	Normal	Low (≤7.25)
Hematocrit	Normal	High
Bicarbonate	Normal	<20 mEq/L
Urine:		
Output	Normal	Polyuria (early) to oliguria (late)
Glucose	Negative	Enuresis, nocturia
Ketones	Negative or trace	High
Vision	Diplopia	Blurred vision

amounts of urinary ketones aid in identifying undetected hypoglycemia.

Illness Management

Illness alters diabetes management, and maintaining control is usually related to the seriousness of the illness. In the well-controlled child an illness will run its course as it does in the unaffected child. The goals during an illness are to restore euglycemia, treat urinary ketones, and maintain hydration. Blood glucose levels and urinary ketones should be monitored every 3 hours. Some hyperglycemia and ketonuria are expected in most illnesses, even with diminished food intake, and are an indication for increased insulin. Insulin should never be omitted during an illness, although dosage requirements may increase, decrease, or remain unchanged, depending on the severity of the illness and the child's appetite. Often the child will need supplemental insulin between usual dose times. If the child vomits more than once, if blood glucose levels remain above 240 mg/dl, or if urinary ketones remain high, the health care practitioner should be notified. Simple carbohydrates may be substituted for carbohydrate-containing exchanges in the meal plan. Although insulin and diet are important tools in sick-day care, fluids are the most important intervention. Fluids must be encouraged to prevent dehydration and to flush out ketones.

Therapeutic Management of Diabetic Ketoacidosis

DKA, the most complete state of insulin deficiency, is a life-threatening situation. Management consists of rapid assessment, adequate insulin to reduce the elevated blood glucose level, fluids to overcome dehydration, and electrolyte replacement (especially potassium).

Because DKA constitutes an emergency situation, the child should be admitted to an intensive care facility for management. The priority is to obtain a venous access for administration of fluids, electrolytes, and insulin. The child should be weighed, measured, and placed on a cardiac monitor. Blood glucose and ketone levels are determined at the bedside, and samples are obtained for laboratory measurement of glucose, electrolytes, blood urea nitrogen, arterial pH, Po_2, Pco_2,

evolve Nursing Care Plan—The Child with Diabetic Ketoacidosis hemoglobin, hematocrit, white blood cell count and differential, calcium, and phosphorus.

Oxygen may be administered to patients who are cyanotic and in whom arterial oxygen is less than 80%. Gastric suction is applied to unconscious children to avoid the possibility of pulmonary aspiration. Antibiotics may be administered to febrile children after appropriate specimens are obtained for culture. A Foley catheter may or may not be inserted for urine samples and measurement. Unless the child is unconscious, a collection bag is usually sufficient for accurate assessments.

Fluid and Electrolyte Therapy

All patients with DKA suffer from dehydration (10% of total body weight in severe ketoacidosis) because of the osmotic diuresis, accompanied by depletion of electrolytes, sodium, potassium, chloride, phosphate, and magnesium. Serum pH and bicarbonate reflect the degree of acidosis. Prompt and adequate fluid therapy restores tissue perfusion and suppresses the elevated levels of stress hormones.

The initial hydrating solution is 0.9% saline solution. Traditionally deficits have been replaced at a rate of 50% over the first 8 to 12 hours and the remaining 50% over the next 16 to 24 hours. Current trends suggest more cautious fluid management to reduce the risk of cerebral edema. The fluid deficit is replaced evenly over a period of 24 to 48 hours.

Serum potassium levels may be normal on admission, but after fluid and insulin administration the rapid return of potassium to the cells can seriously deplete serum levels, with the attendant risk of cardiac arrhythmias. As soon as the child has established renal function (is voiding at least 25 ml/hr) and insulin has been given, vigorous potassium replacement is implemented. The cardiac monitor is used as a guide to therapy, and configuration of T waves should be observed every 30 to 60 minutes to determine changes that might indicate alterations in potassium concentration (widening of the QT interval and the appearance of a U wave following a flattened T wave indicate hypokalemia; an elevated and spreading T wave and shortening of the QT interval indicate hyperkalemia).

Insulin should not be given until urinary ketones and a blood glucose level have been obtained. Continuous IV regular insulin is given at a dosage of 0.1 units/kg/hr. Insulin therapy should be started after the initial rehydration bolus, since serum glucose levels fall rapidly after volume expansion. Blood glucose levels should decrease by 50 to 100 mg/dl/hr. When blood glucose levels fall to 250 to 300 mg/dl, dextrose is added to the IV solution. The goal is to maintain blood glucose levels between 120 and 240 mg/dl by adding 5% to 10% dextrose. Sodium bicarbonate is used conservatively; it is used for pH less than 7.0, severe hyperkalemia, or cardiac instability. Because sodium bicarbonate has been associated with increased risk for cerebral edema, children receiving this substance must be carefully monitored for changes in level of consciousness (Glaser et al, 2001).

When the critical period is over, the task of regulating insulin dosage in relation to diet and activity is started. Children should be actively involved in their own care and are given responsibility according to their ability and the guidance of the nurse.

NURSING ALERT Because insulin can chemically bind to plastic tubing and in-line filters, thereby reducing the amount of medication reaching the systemic circulation, an insulin mixture is run through the tubing to saturate the insulin-binding sites before the infusion is started.

Nursing Care Management

Children with DM may be admitted to the hospital at the time of their initial diagnosis; during illness or surgery; or for episodes of ketoacidosis, which may be precipitated by any of a variety of factors. Many children are able to keep the disease under control with periodic assessment and adjustment of insulin, diet, and activity as needed under the supervision of a practitioner. Under most circumstances these children can be managed well at home and require hospitalization only for a serious illness or upset.

However, a small number of children with diabetes exhibit a degree of metabolic lability and have repeated episodes of DKA that require hospitalization, which interferes with education and social development. These children appear to display a characteristic personality structure. They tend to be unusually passive and nonassertive and to come from families that are inclined to smooth over conflicts without resolution. Children in this type of setting experience emotional arousal with little, if any, opportunity or ability to resolve it. Other children from psychosocially dysfunctional families display behavioral and personality problems. This emotional stress causes an increased production of endogenous catecholamines, which stimulate fat breakdown, leading to ketonemia and ketonuria.

Hospital Management

The child with DKA requires intensive nursing care (see Nursing Care Plan). Vital signs should be observed and recorded frequently. Hypotension caused by the contracted blood volume of the dehydrated state may cause decreased peripheral blood flow, which can be particularly hazardous to the heart, lungs, and kidneys. An elevated temperature may indicate infection and should be reported so that treatment can be implemented immediately.

Careful and accurate records should be maintained, including vital signs (pulse, respiration, temperature, blood pressure), weight, IV fluids, electrolytes, insulin, blood glucose level, and intake and output. A urine collection device or retention catheter is used to obtain the urine measurements, which include volume, specific gravity, and glucose and ketone values. The volume relative to the glucose content is important because 5% glucose in a 300-ml sample is a significantly greater amount than a similar reading from a 75-ml sample. A diabetic flow sheet maintained at the bedside provides an ongoing record of the vital signs, urine and blood tests, amount of insulin given, and intake and output. The level of consciousness is assessed and recorded at frequent intervals. The comatose child generally regains consciousness fairly soon after initiation of therapy but is managed like any unconscious child until then.

When the critical period is over, the task of regulating insulin dosage to diet and activity is begun. The same meticulous records of intake and output, urine glucose and acetone levels, and insulin administration are maintained. Capable children should be actively involved in their own care and are given responsibility for keeping the intake and output record, testing the blood and urine, and, when appropriate, administering their own insulin—all under the nurse's supervision and guidance (see Patient Teaching box).

Medical Identification

One of the first things the nurse should call to the parents' attention is the need for the child to wear some means of medical identification. Usually recommended is the Medic-Alert identification, a stainless steel or silver- or gold-plated identification bracelet that is visible and immediately recognizable. It contains a collect telephone number that medical personnel can call around the clock for medical records and personal information.

Meal Planning

Normal nutrition is a major aspect of the family education program. Diet instruction is usually conducted by the nutritionist, with reinforcement and guidance from the nurse. The emphasis is on adequate intake for age, consistent menus, complex carbohydrates, and consistent eating times. The family

NURSING CARE PLAN ✤ The Child with Diabetes Mellitus

Nursing Diagnosis	Expected Patient Outcomes	Nursing Interventions	Rationale
Risk for injury related to insulin deficiency	Child will demonstrate normal blood glucose levels.	Obtain blood glucose level.	To determine most appropriate dosage of insulin
	The Following NOC Concepts Apply to These Outcomes Blood Glucose Control Nutritional Status: Nutrient Intake	Administer insulin as prescribed.	To maintain normal blood glucose level
		Understand the action of insulin: differences in composition, time of onset, and duration of action for the various preparations.	To ensure accurate insulin administration
Child's/Family's Defining Characteristics ***(Subjective and Objective Data)*** Polyphagia Polydipsia Polyuria Weight loss Enuresis or nocturia Abnormal blood profile—glucose, insulin Irritability Shortened attention span Fatigue Dry skin Blurred vision Headache Frequent infections Hyperglycemia Flushed skin		Employ aseptic techniques when preparing and administering insulin.	To prevent infection
		Rotate sites.	To enhance absorption of insulin
		The Following NIC Concepts Apply to These Interventions Health Education Hyperglycemia Management Hypoglycemia Management Nutritional Management Medication Administration	

Nursing Diagnosis	Expected Patient Outcomes	Nursing Interventions	Rationale
Risk for injury related to hypoglycemia	Child will exhibit no evidence of hypoglycemia.	Recognize signs of hypoglycemia early. Be alert at times when blood glucose levels are lowest (before meals and snacks; 2-4 AM; after bursts of physical activity without additional food; or with delayed, omitted, or incompletely consumed meal or snack).	To prevent hypoglycemia
Child's/Family's Defining Characteristics ***(Subjective and Objective Data)*** Shaky feeling Hunger Headache Dizziness Difficulty concentrating, speaking, or focusing Tremors Tachycardia Shallow respirations Can lead to convulsion, shock, and coma	**The Following NOC Concept Applies to These Outcomes** Blood Glucose Control	Test blood glucose.	To evaluate glucose level
		Offer 10-15 g of readily absorbed carbohydrates, such as orange juice, hard candy, or milk.	To elevate blood glucose level and alleviate symptoms of hypoglycemia
		Follow with complex carbohydrate and protein, such as bread or cracker spread with peanut butter or cheese.	To maintain blood glucose level
		Administer glucagons to unconscious or combative child; position child to minimize risk of aspiration because vomiting may occur.	To elevate blood glucose level
		The Following NIC Concepts Apply to These Interventions Health Education Hypoglycemia Management	

NURSING CARE PLAN ✤ The Child with Diabetes Mellitus—cont'd

Nursing Diagnosis	Expected Patient Outcomes	Nursing Interventions	Rationale
Deficient knowledge (diabetes management) related to care of a child with newly diagnosed diabetes mellitus	Child and family will have attitude conducive to learning.	Select methods, vocabulary, and content appropriate to learners' level.	To maximize learning
		Allow time for family and child to begin to adjust to initial impact of the diagnosis.	To allow child and family to set pace
		Select an environment conducive to learning.	To promote learning
Child's/Family's Defining Characteristics ***(Subjective and Objective Data)***		Involve all senses and employ a variety of teaching strategies, especially participation.	To promote effective learning
Lack of understanding		Provide pamphlets or other supplementary materials.	To promote learning
Inability to prepare and administer insulin	Child and family will demonstrate understanding of meal planning	Emphasize relationship between normal nutritional needs and the disease.	To encourage sense of normalcy
Inability to follow meal planning guidelines		Become familiar with family's culture and food preferences.	To include culture preferences in meal planning
Difficulty describing treatment plan		Teach or reinforce learners' understanding of the basic food groups and the prescribed meal plan.	To reinforce existing knowledge base
		Help child and family estimate portion sizes by volume.	To provide a more practical method than weighing food
		Suggest low-carbohydrate snack items.	To promote appropriate food choices
		Guide family in assessing labels of food products for carbohydrate content.	To reinforce that consistency in carbohydrate portions is essential
	Child and family will demonstrate knowledge of and ability to administer insulin.	Teach child and family the characteristics of the insulins prescribed.	To increase understanding that there are several insulin preparations
		Teach proper mixing of insulins.	To prevent contaminating the vials
		Teach injection procedure.	To promote appropriate administration
		Teach basic techniques using an orange or similar item.	To build confidence
		Use demonstration and return demonstration techniques on another adult before injecting child.	To minimize stress for the child
		Help families and child work out a set rotational pattern.	To ensure maximum absorption of insulin and prevent hypertrophy at injection site
		Teach proper care of insulin and equipment.	To prevent contamination and minimize complications
	Child and family will demonstrate ability to test blood glucose level.	Teach family and child, if old enough, blood glucose monitoring or use of equipment, interpretation of results, and care and maintenance of equipment.	To ensure that child and family learn how to adjust insulin based on blood glucose level
	Child and family will demonstrate knowledge of management of hyperglycemia and hypoglycemia.	Instruct learners in how to recognize signs of hyperglycemia and hypoglycemia.	To prevent delay of treatment
		Explain relationship of insulin needs to illness, activity, and intense emotion.	To ensure appropriate treatment
		Teach how to adjust food, activity, and insulin at times of illness and during other situations that alter blood glucose levels.	To ensure appropriate treatment
		Suggest carrying source of carbohydrate, such as sugar cubes or hard candy, in pocket.	To prevent delay in treatment
		Instruct parents and child in how to treat hypoglycemia with food, simple sugars, or glucagons.	To establish health practices that last a lifetime
	Child and family will demonstrate understanding of proper hygiene.	Emphasize importance of personal hygiene.	To promote child's general health
		Encourage regular dental care and yearly ophthalmologic examinations.	To minimize risk of infection and check for retinopathy.
		Teach proper care of cuts and scratches; teach proper foot care.	To prevent infection

The Following NOC Concepts Apply to These Outcomes
Blood Glucose Control
Knowledge: Medication
Knowledge: Treatment Regimen

The Following NIC Concepts Apply to These Interventions
Health Education
Hyperglycemia Management
Hypoglycemia Management

PATIENT TEACHING Teaching About Diabetes

The better the parents understand the pathophysiology of diabetes and the function and action of insulin and glucagon in relation to caloric intake and exercise, the better they will understand the disease and its effects on the child. Parents need answers to a number of questions (voiced or unvoiced) to increase their confidence in coping with the disease. For example, they may want to know about the various procedures performed on their child and treatment rationale, such as what is being put in the intravenous bottle and the expected effect.

is taught how the meal plan relates to the requirements of growth and development, the disease process, and the insulin regimen. Meals and snacks are modified based on the child's preferences and current menu, preserving cultural patterns and preferences as much as possible. Extensive exchange lists are available that include foods compatible with most lifestyles.

Learning about foods within specific food groups helps in making choices. Weights and measures of foods are used as eye-training devices for defining serving sizes and should be practiced for about 3 months, with gradual progression to estimation of food portions. Even when the child and family become competent in estimating portion sizes, reassessment should take place weekly or monthly and when there is any change of brands.

Family members should also be guided in reading labels for the nutritional value of foods and food content. They need to become familiar with the carbohydrate content of food groups. Substitution with foods of equal carbohydrate content is the skill needed for successful carbohydrate counting. Substitution might be necessary if a food is not available in sufficient quantity or if the teenager wishes to eat fast food with peers. The use of a multiple daily injection program lends flexibility to the timing of meals.

Children should use sugar substitutes in moderation in items such as soft drinks. Artificial sweeteners have been shown to be safe, but if there is any question about amounts, the physician, dietitian, or nurse specialist can provide guidelines based on body weight. Sugar-free chewing gum and candies made with sorbitol may be used in moderation by children with DM. Although sorbitol is less cariogenic than other varieties of sugar substitutes, it is an alcohol sugar that is metabolized to fructose and then to glucose. Furthermore, large amounts can cause osmotic diarrhea. Most dietetic foods contain sorbitol. They are more expensive than regular foods. Also, while a product may be sugar free, it is not necessarily carbohydrate free.

Traveling

Traveling requires planning, especially when a trip involves crossing time zones. A number of tips are included in pamphlets available free of charge. Suggestions for traveling encompass what will be needed from the practitioner before leaving, what and how much to take along, needs in transit, what to consider at the destination, and planning for when the child returns home. Planning is needed no matter what type of travel is considered—automobile, plane, bus, or train.

Insulin

Families need to understand the treatment method and the insulin prescribed, including the effective duration, onset, and peak action. They also need to know the characteristics of the various types of insulins, the proper mixing and dilution of insulins, and how to substitute another type when their usual brand is not available (insulin is a nonprescription drug). Insulin need not be refrigerated but should be maintained at a temperature between 15° and 29.4° C (59° and 85° F). Freezing renders insulin inactive.

Insulin bottles that have been "opened" (i.e., the stopper has been punctured) should be stored at room temperature or refrigerated for up to 28 to 30 days. After 1 month these vials should be discarded. Unopened vials should be refrigerated and are good until the expiration date on the label. Diabetic supplies should not be left in a hot environment.

Injection Procedure

Learning to give insulin injections is a source of anxiety for both parents and children. It is helpful for the learner to know that this important aspect of care will become as routine as brushing the teeth. First, the basic injection technique is taught, using an orange or similar item and sterile normal saline for practice.

Insulin can be injected into any area in which there is adipose (fat) tissue over muscle; the drug is injected at a 90-degree angle. Newly diagnosed children may have lost adipose tissue, and care should be exerted not to inject intramuscularly. The pinch technique is the most effective method for tenting the skin to allow easy entrance of the needle to subcutaneous tissues in children. The site selected will sometimes depend on whether children or parents administer the insulin. The arms, thighs, hips, and abdomen are usual injection sites for insulin. The children can reach the thighs, abdomen, and part of the hip and arm easily but may require help to inject other sites. For example, a parent can pinch a loose fold of skin of the arm while the child injects the insulin.

The parents and child are helped to work out a rotation pattern to various areas of the body to enhance absorption, since insulin absorption is slowed by fat pads that develop in overused injection areas. The most efficient rotation plan involves giving about four to six injections in one area (each injection about 2.5 cm [1 inch] apart, or the diameter of the insulin vial from the previous injection) and then moving to another area.

It is important to remember that the absorption rate varies in different parts of the body (Table 52-4). The methodical use of one anatomic area and then movement to another (as described in the previous paragraph) minimizes variations in absorption rates. However, absorption is also altered by

Table 52-4 Insulin's Onset and Duration of Action Related to Injection Site

	Site of Injection			
	ABDOMEN	ARM	LEG	BUTTOCK
Rate	Very fast	Fast	Slow	Very slow
Duration	Very short	Short	Long	Very long

From Albisser AM, Sperlich M: Adjusting insulins, *Diabetes Educ* 18(3):211-218, 1992.

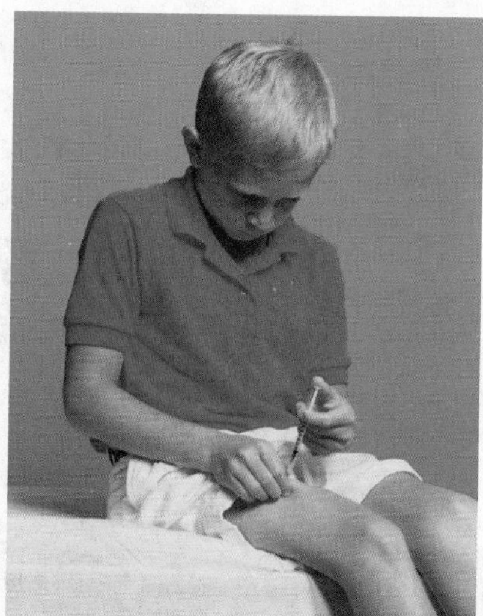

Fig. 52-2 School-age children are able to administer their own insulin.

vigorous exercise, which enhances absorption from exercised muscles; therefore it is recommended that a site be chosen other than the exercising extremity (e.g., avoiding legs and arms when playing in a tennis tournament).

Injection sites for an entire month can be determined in advance on a simple chart. For example, a "paper doll" (body outline) can be constructed and insulin sites marked by the child. After injection, the child places the date on the appropriate site. To keep in practice, it is a good idea for the parent to give two or three injections a week in areas that are difficult for the child to reach. The same basic methodology is used when teaching children to give their own insulin injections (Fig. 52-2). They should practice first on an orange or a doll, building courage gradually. Other devices are available for insulin injection and may offer advantages to some children. Children who do not wish to give themselves injections can be taught to use a syringe-loaded injector (Inject-Ease). With the device, puncture is always automatic. Adolescents respond well to a self-contained and compact device resembling a fountain pen (NovoPen), which eliminates conventional vials and syringes. Preloaded pens may also cause less pain, since the needle is not blunted by piercing the rubber top of the insulin vial (Lteif & Schwenk, 1999).

Continuous Subcutaneous Insulin Infusion Some children are considered candidates for use of a portable insulin pump, and even some young children with unsatisfactory metabolic control can benefit from its use. The child and the parents are taught to operate the device, including the mechanics of the pump, battery changes, and alarm systems. A number of devices are on the market that vary in the basal rates they are able to deliver and in the cost of the equipment. Families can investigate the various devices and select the model that best suits their needs. Product information is available from pump manufacturers and distributors.*

Parents and children learn (1) the technical aspects of the pump and self-monitoring of blood glucose; (2) prevention and treatment for hyperglycemia, sick-day management, and meal planning; (3) the effects of exercise, stress, and diet on blood glucose levels; and (4) decision-making strategies to evaluate blood glucose patterns and make adjustments in all aspects of the regimen.

Numerous blood glucose measurements (at least four times per day) are an essential part of infusion pump use. Intensive education and supervision are critical to obtaining maximum efficiency and control. This is particularly important if the family has been accustomed to a conventional insulin regimen. They must realize that simply wearing the pump will not normalize blood glucose. The pump is merely an insulin delivery device, and frequent, routine blood glucose determinations are necessary to adjust the insulin delivery rate.

The major problem with use of the insulin pump is inflammation from irritation or infection at the insertion site. The site should be cleaned thoroughly before the needle is inserted and then covered with a transparent dressing. The site is changed and rotated every 48 to 72 hours (this may vary) or at the first sign of inflammation. Nurses working where pumps are part of the therapeutic regimen should become familiar with the operation of the specific device being used and the protocol of disease management. Others should be aware of this management technique and be prepared to assist patients using the pump.

Monitoring

Nurses should also be prepared to teach and supervise blood glucose monitoring. SMBG is associated with few complications, and although it does not necessarily lead to improved metabolic control, it provides a more accurate assessment of blood glucose levels than can be obtained with the historical urine testing. Blood glucose monitoring has the added advantage that it can be performed anywhere (see Atraumatic Care box).

ATRAUMATIC CARE

Minimizing Pain of Blood Glucose Monitoring

- To enhance blood flow to the finger, hold it under warm water for a few seconds before the puncture.
- When obtaining blood samples, use the ring finger or thumb (blood flows more easily to these areas), and puncture the finger just to the side of the finger pad (more blood vessels and fewer nerve endings).
- To prevent a deep puncture, press the platform of the lancet device lightly against the skin and avoid steadying the finger against a hard surface.
- Use lancet devices with adjustable-depth tips. Begin with the shallowest setting.
- Use glucose monitors that require small blood samples (e.g., Ascensia Elite) to avoid repeated punctures.

Blood for testing can be obtained by two different methods: manually or with a mechanical bloodletting device. A mechanical device is recommended for children, although the child and family should learn to use both methods in the event of

**Medtronic MiniMed,* www.minimed.com; *Disetronic,* www.disetronic-usa.com; *Animas,* www.animascorp.com.

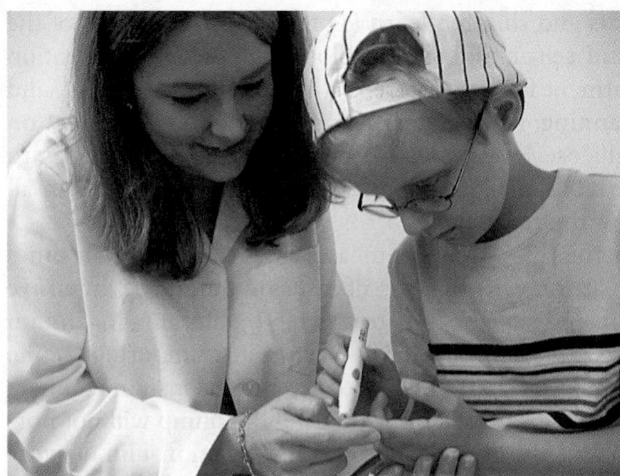

Fig. 52-3 Child using finger-stick device to obtain blood sample.

mechanical failure. Several lancet devices are available, and each provides a means for obtaining a large drop of blood for testing (Fig. 52-3).

NURSING ALERT Caution children not to allow anyone else to use their lancet because of the risk of contracting hepatitis B virus or human immunodeficiency virus infection.

The blood sample may be obtained from fingertips or alternate sites such as the forearm. Alternate site testing requires a meter that can test a small volume of blood. Not all meters are capable of this.

Signs of redness and soreness at the site of finger puncture should be examined by the practitioner. It may be evidence of poor technique, poor hygiene, or poor skin healing relative to poor control. Many types of blood-testing meters are available for home use. Newer technology has brought about improvements in meter size and ease of use. The family should be shown features of several meters, including advantages and disadvantages, and allowed to choose equipment that best meets their needs.

The least expensive testing method uses a reagent strip to which blood is applied (Fig. 52-4). After blotting, the color change is compared against a color scale for an estimation of the blood glucose level. The strips can be cut in half (although not all professionals recommend this) to obtain two readings per strip. This method is not accepted practice but may be necessary for some families or situations.

Urine Testing Testing for urinary ketones is recommended during times of illness or when blood glucose values are elevated. Information on a specific ketone-testing product should include correct procedure, storage, and product expiration. Families need a clear understanding of home management of ketones: fluids and additional insulin as directed by the health care team.

Signs of Hyperglycemia

Severe hyperglycemia is most often caused by illness, growth, emotional upset, or missed insulin doses. Emotional stress from school examinations or physical response to immunizations are examples of causes of hyperglycemia. With careful glucose monitoring, any elevation can be managed by

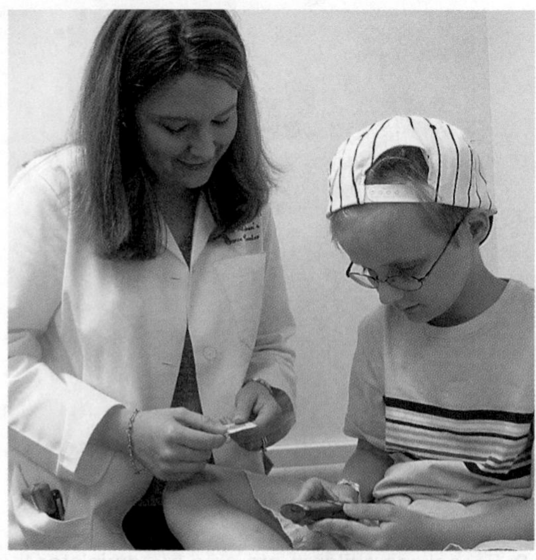

Fig. 52-4 Child using blood glucose monitor and reagent strips to test blood for glucose.

adjustment of insulin or food intake. Parents should understand how to adjust food, activity, and insulin at the time of illness or when the child is treated for an illness with a medication known to raise the blood glucose level (e.g., steroids). The hyperglycemia is managed by increasing insulin soon after the increased glucose level is noted. Health care professionals should be aware that adolescent girls often become hyperglycemic around the time of their menses and should be advised to increase insulin dosages if necessary.

Signs of Hypoglycemia

Hypoglycemia is caused by imbalances of food intake, insulin, and activity. Ideally hypoglycemia should be prevented, and parents need to be prepared to prevent, recognize, and treat the problem. They should be familiar with the signs of hypoglycemia and instructed in treatment, including care of the child with seizures. Early signs are adrenergic, including sweating and trembling, which help raise the blood glucose level, much like the reaction when an individual is startled or anxious. The second set of symptoms that follow an untreated adrenergic reaction is neuroglycopenic (also called *brain hypoglycemia*). These symptoms typically include difficulty with balance, memory, attention, or concentration; dizziness or lightheadedness; and slurred speech. Severe and prolonged hypoglycemia leads to seizures, coma, and possible death (Cryer, 2000). Hypoglycemia can be managed effectively, as outlined in the Emergency box.

It is advisable for parents to plan for anticipated excitement or exercise. In addition, gastroenteritis may decrease insulin needs slightly as a result of poor appetite, vomiting, or diarrhea. If the blood glucose level is low but urinary ketones are present, the family should be aware of the increased need for simple carbohydrates and liquids.

Hygiene

All aspects of personal hygiene should be emphasized for the child with diabetes. The child should be cautioned against wearing shoes without socks, wearing sandals, or walking barefoot. Correct nail and extremity care tailored to the individual child (with the guidance of a podiatrist) can begin

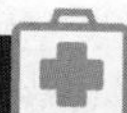

EMERGENCY

Hypoglycemia

Mild Reaction—Adrenergic Symptoms

Give child 10 to 15 g of a simple, high-carbohydrate substance (preferably liquid, e.g., 3 to 6 oz of orange juice).

Follow with starch-protein snack.

Moderate Reaction—Neuroglycopenic Symptoms

Give child 10 to 15 g of a simple carbohydrate as above.

Repeat in 10 to 15 minutes if symptoms persist.

Follow with larger snack.

Watch child closely.

Severe Reaction—Unresponsive, Unconscious, or Seizures

Administer glucagon as prescribed.

Follow with planned meal or snack when child is able to eat, or add a snack of 10% of daily calories.

Nocturnal Reaction

Give child 10 to 15 g of a simple carbohydrate.

Follow with snack of 10% of daily calories.

health practices that last a lifetime. Eyes should be checked once a year unless the child wears glasses, and then as directed by the ophthalmologist. Regular dental care is emphasized, and cuts and scratches should be treated with plain soap and water unless otherwise indicated. Diaper rash in infants and candidal infections in teens may indicate poor diabetes control.

Exercise

Exercise is an important component of the treatment plan. If the child is more active at one time of the day than at another time, food or insulin can be altered to meet that activity pattern. Food should be increased in the summer, when children tend to be more active. Decreased activity on return to school may require a decrease in food intake or increase in insulin dosage. The child who is active in team sports will need a snack about a half hour before the anticipated activity. Races or other competition may call for a slightly higher food intake than at practice times.

Food intake will usually need to be repeated for prolonged activity periods, often as frequently as every 45 minutes to 1 hour. Families should be informed that if increased food is not tolerated, decreased insulin is the next course of action. If the timing of the exercise is changed so that the supper meal is delayed, the insulin in the second or third dose of the day may be moved back to precede the mealtime. Sugar may sometimes be needed during exercise periods for quick response. Elevated blood glucose levels after extreme activity may represent the body's adrenergic response to exercise. If the blood glucose level is elevated (240 mg/dl or higher) before planned exercise, urinary ketones should be checked and the activity may need be postponed until the blood glucose is controlled.

Record Keeping

Home records are an invaluable aid to diabetes self-management. The nurse and family devise a method to chart insulin administered, blood glucose values, urine ketone results, and other factors and events that affect diabetes control. The child and family are encouraged to observe for patterns of blood glucose responses to events such as exercise. If lapses in management occur (such as eating a candy bar), the child should be encouraged to note this and not be criticized for the transgression.

Self-Management

Self-management is the key to close control. Being able to make changes when they are needed rather than waiting until the next contact with health care professionals is important for self-management and gives the individual and family the feeling they have control over the disease. Psychologically this helps family members feel they are useful and participating members of the team. Allowing the child to learn to look at records objectively promotes independence in self-management. As children grow and assume more responsibility for self-management, they develop confidence in their ability to manage their disease and confidence in themselves as persons. They learn to respond to the disease and to make more accurate interpretations and changes in treatment when they become adults.

Puberty is associated with decreased sensitivity to insulin that normally would be compensated for by an increased insulin secretion. Health care professionals should anticipate that pubertal patients will have more difficulty maintaining glycemic control. Insulin doses commonly need to be increased, often dramatically (McConnell et al, 2001). Patients should be taught to give themselves additional doses of rapid-acting insulin (5% to 10% of their daily dose) when their blood glucose levels are increased. The use of supplemental rapid-acting insulin is preferred to withholding food in the adolescent.

Child and Family Education and Support

For all families, daily compliance with numerous procedures and structured living schedules is difficult. Maintaining good blood glucose control requires ongoing motivation. Nurses can encourage families to adhere to treatment regimens and lifestyle adjustments by emphasizing the benefits of preventing complications such as hypoglycemia. When children are able to accept the difference as a part of life—in other words, that each person is different in some way—then, with adequate parental support, they should be able to adjust well (see Critical Thinking Exercise).

Camping and other special group activities are useful. At diabetes camp, children learn that they are not alone. As a result, they become more independent and resourceful in other settings. Useful information about such camps and organizations can be obtained from the American Diabetes Association. A list of accredited camps specifically for children and teenagers with diabetes is also available from the American Camping Association.*

Several organizations are prepared to assist with education and dissemination of knowledge and support for diabetes. The

**5000 State Road 67 N., Martinsville, IN 46151; 765-342-8456; www.*acacamps.org.

CRITICAL THINKING EXERCISE

Type 1 Diabetes Mellitus

Rebecca, a 15-year-old with a 3-year history of type 1 diabetes mellitus (DM), has been admitted to the pediatric intensive care unit for treatment of diabetic ketoacidosis (DKA). This is her fifth hospital admission for DKA in the past year. Rebecca's parents are divorced, and she has four younger siblings, none of whom has diabetes. Rebecca's mother has maintained two jobs for the past 5 years and frequently leaves Rebecca in charge of the household. In anticipation of her discharge, you are planning a patient education program for Rebecca and her mother. What important issues regarding Rebecca's unstable diabetes management must you consider to plan the education program?

1. Evidence—Is there sufficient evidence to draw conclusions about Rebecca's recurrent episodes of DKA?
2. Assumptions—Describe an underlying assumption about each of the following:
   a. Type 1 DM in adolescence
   b. Type 1 DM and menses
   c. Emotional stress and elevated blood glucose levels
   d. Blood glucose monitoring for insulin management
3. What priorities for nursing care should be established for Rebecca?
4. Does the evidence support your nursing intervention?
5. What alternative perspectives might you have?

American Diabetes Association,* Canadian Diabetes Association,† Juvenile Diabetes Research Foundation International,‡ and American Association of Diabetes Educators§ are valuable resources for a wide variety of educational materials. The National Institute of Diabetes and Digestive and Kidney Diseases¶ publishes a number of comprehensive annotated bibliographies, including "Educational Materials for and About Young People with Diabetes," a compilation of resource materials for children, siblings, parents, teachers, and health professionals; and "Sports and Exercise for People with Diabetes."

**1701 N. Beauregard St., Alexandria, VA 22311; 800-342-2383;* www.diabetes.org.

†1400-522 University Ave., Toronto, ON M5G 2R5; 800-226-8464; www.diabetes.ca.

‡120 Wall St., New York, NY 10005; 800-533-CURE; www.jdrf.org.

§200 W. Madison St., Suite 800, Chicago, IL 60606; 800-338-3633; e-mail: education@aadenet.org; www.diabeteseducator.org.

¶Office of Communications and Public Liaison, NIDDK, NIH, Building 31, Room 9A06, 31 Center Drive, MSC 2560, Bethesda, MD 20892-2560; 301-496-3583; www.niddk.nih.gov.

Key Points

- Pituitary dysfunction is manifested primarily by growth disturbance.
- The main physiologic action of TH is to regulate the basal metabolic rate and control the processes of growth and tissue differentiation.
- Disorders of thyroid function include hypothyroidism, autoimmune thyroiditis, goiter, and hyperthyroidism.
- Therapy for hyperthyroidism is directed at retarding the rate of hormone secretion and may include drug therapy, thyroidectomy, or radioiodine therapy.
- Classic forms of hypoparathyroidism in childhood are idiopathic (deficient production of PTH) and pseudohypoparathyroidism (increased PTH production with end-organ unresponsiveness to PTH).
- The adrenal cortex secretes three important groups of hormones: glucocorticoids, mineralocorticoids, and sex steroids.
- Disorders of adrenal function include acute adrenocortical insufficiency, chronic adrenocortical insufficiency, Cushing's syndrome, and CAH.

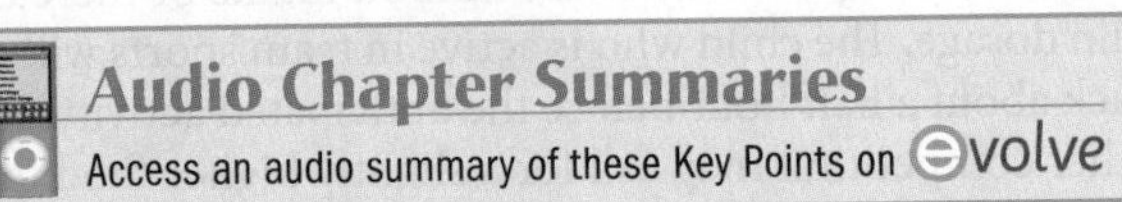
Audio Chapter Summaries
Access an audio summary of these Key Points on evolve

- Five categories of Cushing's syndrome are pituitary, adrenal, ectopic, iatrogenic, and food dependent.
- Management of CAH includes assignment of a sex according to genotype, administration of cortisone, and, possibly, reconstructive surgery.
- DM is categorized as type 1 diabetes and type 2 diabetes.
- The focus of treatment for type 1 DM is insulin replacement, diet, and exercise.
- Education of families includes explanation of diabetes, meal planning, administering insulin injections, monitoring general hygienic practices, promoting exercise, record keeping, and observing for complications.

References

American Academy of Pediatrics, Section on Endocrinology and Committee on Genetics: Technical report: congenital adrenal hyperplasia, *Pediatrics* 106(6):1511-1518, 2000.

American Diabetes Association: Care of children and adolescents with type 1 diabetes, *Diabetes Care* 28:186-212, 2005.

American Diabetes Association: Report of the Expert Committee on the Diagnosis and Classification of Diabetes Mellitus, *Diabetes Care* 24(Suppl 1):S5-S20, 2001.

Bartalena L et al: Oxidative stress and Graves' ophthalmopathy: in vitro studies and therapeutic implications, *Biofactors* 19(3-4):155-163, 2003.

Behrman RE, Kliegman RM, Jenson HB: *Nelson textbook of pediatrics*, ed 17, Philadelphia, 2004, Saunders.

Beisswenger P, Szwergold B, Yeo K: Glycated proteins in diabetes, *Clin Lab Med* 21(10):53-78, 2001.

Biro FM et al: Pubertal correlates in black and white girls, *J Pediatr* 148(2):234-240, 2006.

Bryant J, Cave C, Milne R: Recombinant growth hormone for idiopathic short stature in children and adolescents, *Cochrane Database Syst Rev* (2):CD004440, DOI:10.1002/14651858.CD004440, 2003.

Cheetham T, Baylis PH: Diabetes insipidus in children: pathophysiology, diagnoses and management, *Paediatr Drugs* 4(12):785-796, 2002.

Cryer P: Glucose counterregulatory hormones: physiology, pathophysiology, and relevance to clinical hypoglycemia. In Le Roith D, Taylor S, Olefsky J (editors): *Diabetes mellitus: a fundamental and clinical text*, ed 5, Philadelphia, 2000, Lippincott Williams & Wilkins.

Dallas JS, Foley TP: Hyperthyroidism. In Lifshitz F (editor): *Pediatric endocrinology*, ed 4, New York, 2003, Marcel Dekker.

De Buyst J et al: Clinical, hormonal and imaging findings in 27 children with central diabetes insipidus, *Eur J Pediatr* 166(1):43-49, 2007.

Foley TP: Hypothyroidism. In Hoekelman RA et al (editors): *Primary pediatric care*, ed 4, St Louis, 2001, Mosby.

Glaser N et al: Risk factors for cerebral edema in children with diabetic ketoacidosis: the Pediatric Emergency Medicine Collaborative Research Committee of the American Academy of Pediatrics, *N Engl J Med* 344(4):264-269, 2001.

Greiner MV, Kerrigan JR: Puberty: timing is everything, *Pediatr Ann* 35(12):916-922, 2006.

Guyda HJ: Growth hormone testing and the short child, *Pediatr Res* 48(5):579-580, 2000.

Halac I, Zimmerman D: Evaluating short stature in children, *Pediatr Ann* 33(3):171-176, 2004.

Hall DMB: Growth monitoring, *Arch Dis Child* 82(1):10-15, 2000.

Hannon TS, Gungor N, Arslanian SA: Type 2 diabetes in children and adolescents: review for the primary care provider, *Pediatr Ann* 35(12):880-887, 2006.

Herman-Giddens ME: Recent data on pubertal milestones in United States children: the secular trend toward earlier development, *Int J Androl* 29(1):241-246, 2006.

Hilczer M, Smyczynska J, Lewinski A: Limitations of clinical utility of growth hormone stimulating tests in diagnosing children with short stature, *Endocrinol Regul* 40(3):69-75, 2006.

Hochberg Z: *Practical algorithms in pediatric endocrinology*, Basel, Switzerland, 1999, Karger.

Hoffman RP: Juvenile diabetes: avoiding problems during therapy, *Clin Advisor* May 2003, pp 70-75.

Jospe N: Hyperthyroidism. In Hoekelman RA et al (editors): *Primary pediatric care*, ed 4, St Louis, 2001, Mosby.

Karnik AA, Fields AV, Shannon RP: Diabetic cardiomyopathy, *Curr Hypertens Rep* 9(6):467-473, 2007.

Kempers MJ, Otten BJ: Idiopathic precocious puberty versus puberty in adopted children: auxological response to gonadotrophin-releasing hormone agonist treatment and final height, *Eur J Endocrinol* 147(5):609-616, 2002.

Lee PA: Central precocious puberty: an overview of diagnosis, treatment, and outcome, *Endocrinol Metab Clin North Am* 28(4):901-918, 1999.

Levine LS: Congenital adrenal hyperplasia, *Pediatr Rev* 21(5):159-170, 2000.

Lin M, Liu SJ, Lim IT: Disorders of water imbalance, *Emerg Med Clin North Am* 23(3):749-770, 2005.

Lteif AN, Schwenk WF: Accuracy of pen injectors versus insulin syringes in children with type 1 diabetes, *Diabetes Care* 22(10):137-140, 1999.

Ma C et al: Radioiodine treatment for pediatric Graves' disease (protocol), *Cochrane Database Syst Rev* (4):CD006294, DOI:10.1002/14651858, 2006.

Macchia PE: Recent advances in understanding the molecular basis of primary congenital hypothyroidism, *Mol Med Today* 6(1):36-42, 2000.

Magee MF, Bhatt BA: Management of decompensated diabetes: diabetic ketoacidosis and hyperglycemic hyperosmolar syndrome, *Crit Care Clin* 17(1):75-106, 2001.

Majzoub JA, Muglia LJ: Disorders of water homeostasis. In Lifshitz F (editor): *Pediatric endocrinology*, ed 4, New York, 2003, Marcel Dekker.

Mauras N et al: Growth hormone stimulation testing in both short and normal statured children: use of an immunofunctional assay, *Pediatr Res* 48(5):614-618, 2000.

McConnell EM et al: Achieving optimal diabetic control in adolescence: the continuing enigma, *Diabetes Metab Res Rev* 17(10):67-74, 2001.

Midyett LK, Moore WV, Jacobson JD: Are pubertal changes in girls before age 8 benign? *Pediatrics* 111(1):47-51, 2003.

Miller BS, Zimmerman D: Idiopathic short stature in children, *Pediatr Ann* 33(3):177-181, 2004.

Miranda ML et al: Labioscrotal island flap in feminizing genitoplasty, *J Pediatr Surg* 39(7):1030-1033, 2004.

Moshang T: Cushing's disease, 70 years later … and the beat goes on (editorial), *J Clin Endocrinol Metab* 88(1):31-33, 2003.

Muir A: Precocious puberty, *Pediatr Rev* 27(10):373-381, 2006.

Nebesio TD, Eugster EA: Current concepts in normal and abnormal puberty, *Curr Prob Pediatr Adolesc Health Care* 37(2):50-72, 2007.

New MI, Ghizzoni L: Update on congenital adrenal hyperplasia. In Lifshitz F (editor): *Pediatric endocrinology*, ed 4, New York, 2003, Marcel Dekker.

Nieman LK, Ilias I: Evaluation and treatment of Cushing's syndrome, *Am J Med* 118(12):1340-1346, 2005.

Olohan K, Zappitelli D: The insulin pump, *Am J Nurs* 103(4):48-56, 2003.

O'Sullivan E, O'Sullivan M: Precocious puberty: a parent's perspective, *Arch Dis Childhood* 86:320-321, 2002.

Pacak K et al: Pheochromocytoma: recommendations for clinical practice from the First International Symposium, *Natl Clin Pract Endocrinol Metab* 3(2):92-102, 2007.

Perheentupa J: Hypoparathyroidism and mineral homeostasis. In Lifshitz F (editor): *Pediatric endocrinology*, ed 4, New York, 2003, Marcel Dekker.

Petitti BD et al: Serum lipids and glucose control: the SEARCH for Diabetes in Youth study, *Arch Pediatr Adolesc Med* 161(2):159-165, 2007.

Pizzo PA, Poplack DG (editors): *Principles and theories of pediatric oncology*, Philadelphia, 2006, Lippincott Williams & Wilkins.

Radetti G et al: The natural history of euthyroid Hashimoto's thyroiditis in children, *J Pediatr* 149(6):827-832, 2006.

Reiter EO et al: Effect of growth hormone (GH) treatment on the near-final height of 1258 patients with idiopathic GH deficiency: analysis of a large international database, *J Clin Endocrinol Metab* 91(6):2047-2054, 2006.

Rivkees SA, Cornelius EA: Influence of iodine-131 dose on the outcome of hyperthyroidism in children, *Pediatrics* 111(4):745-748, 2003.

Root AW: Precocious puberty, *Pediatr Rev* 21(1):10-19, 2000.

Rovet JF, Ehrlich R: Psychoeducational outcome in children with early-treated congenital hypothyroidism, *Pediatrics* 105(3):515-522, 2000.

Schultz CJ et al: Microalbuminuria prevalence varies with age, sex, and puberty in children with type 1 diabetes followed from diagnosis in a longitudinal study, *Diabetes Care* 22(3):495-502, 1999.

Simmonds MJ et al: Regression mapping of association between the human leukocyte antigen region and Graves disease, *Am J Human Genet* 76(1):157-163, 2005.

Slyper AH: The pubertal timing controversy in the USA, and a review of possible causative factors for the advance in timing of onset of puberty, *Clin Endocrinol (Oxf)* 65(1):1-8, 2006.

Streetman DD, Khanderia U: Diagnosis and treatment of Graves disease, *Am J Nurse Pract* 8(1):27-36, 2004.

Szymborska M, Staroszczyk B: Thyroiditis in children, *Med Wieku Rozwoj* IV(4):383-391, 2000.

Thompson GB: Surgical management in Graves' disease, *Panminerva Med* 44(4):287-293, 2002.

Trivin C et al: Presentation and evolution of organic central precocious puberty according to the type of CNS lesion, *Clin Endocrinol (Oxford)* 65(2):239-245, 2006.

Urrutia-Rojas X, Menchaca J: Prevalence of risk for type 2 diabetes in school children, *J Sch Health* 76(5):189-194, 2006.

van Tijn DA et al: Early assessment of hypothalamic-pituitary-gonadal function in patients with congenital hypothyroidism of central origin, *J Clin Endocrinol Metab* 92(1):104-109, 2007.

Verbalis JG: Diabetes insipidus, *Rev Endocr Metab Disord* 4(2):177-185, 2003.

Walvoord EC, Pescovitz OH: Combined use of growth hormone and gonadotropin-releasing hormone analogues in precocious puberty: theoretic and practical considerations, *Pediatrics* 104(4 Pt 2):1010-1014, 1999.

Wong LL, Verbalis JG: Systemic diseases associated with disorders of water homeostasis, *Endocrinol Metab Clin North Am* 31(1):121-140, 2002.

Unit 11

53 Integumentary Dysfunction

Learning Objectives

On completion of this chapter the reader will be able to:

- Describe the distribution and configuration of the various skin lesions.
- List the benefits of a moist environment for wound healing.
- Discuss the nursing care related to therapies for skin disorders.
- Contrast the manifestations of and therapies for bacterial, viral, and fungal infections of the skin.
- Compare the skin manifestations related to age in children.
- Outline a care plan to prevent and treat diaper dermatitis.
- Outline a care plan for a child with atopic dermatitis.
- Formulate a teaching plan for an adolescent with acne.
- Describe the methods for assessing a burn wound.
- Discuss the physical and emotional care of a child with a severe burn wound.

Electronic Resources

Additional information related to the content in Chapter 53 can be found on

Evolve the Companion Website at http://evolve.elsevier.com/Perry/maternal/

- NCLEX Review Questions
- Animation—Burns in Children
- Case Study—Acne Vulgaris
- Case Study—Burns
- Case Study—Impetigo
- Case Study—Poison Ivy
- Nursing Care Plan—The Child with Burns

Integumentary Dysfunction

Skin Lesions

Lesions of the skin result from a variety of etiologic factors. Skin lesions originate from (1) contact with injurious agents (infective organisms, toxic chemicals, and physical trauma), (2) hereditary factors, (3) external factors (e.g., allergens), or (4) systemic diseases (e.g., measles, lupus erythematosus, nutritional deficiency diseases). Responses to these agents or factors are highly individualized. An agent that is harmless to one individual may be damaging to another, and a single agent may produce varying degrees of response.

An important factor in the etiology of skin manifestations is the child's age. Infants are subject to "birthmark" malformations and atopic dermatitis (AD) that appear early in life; the school-age child is susceptible to ringworm of the scalp; and acne is a characteristic skin disorder of puberty. Contact dermatitis, such as poison ivy, is seen only when the noxious agent is found in the environment. Tension and anxiety may produce, modify, or prolong skin conditions.

Skin of Younger Children

The major skin layers arise from different embryologic origins. Early in the embryonic period, a single layer of epithelium forms from the ectoderm, while simultaneously the corium develops from the mesenchyme. In the infant and small child the epidermis is loosely bound to the dermis. This poor adherence causes the layers to separate easily during an inflammatory process to form blisters. This is especially true in preterm infants, who have a propensity to blister formation and separation of the skin with minor trauma such as the removal of adhesive tape. In contrast, the skin of the older child is thinner, and the cells of all the strata are more compressed.

Pathophysiology of Dermatitis

More than half of the dermatologic problems in children are forms of dermatitis. This implies a sequence of inflammatory changes in the skin that are grossly and microscopically similar but diverse in course and causation. Acute responses produce intercellular and intracellular edema, the formation of intradermal vesicles, and an initial infiltration of inflammatory cells into the epidermis. In the dermis there is edema, vascular dilation, and early perivascular cellular infiltration. The location and manner of these reactions produce the lesions characteristic of each disorder. The changes are usually reversible, and the skin ordinarily recovers without blemish unless complicating factors such as ulceration from the primary irritant, scratching, and infection are introduced or underlying vascular disease develops. In chronic conditions permanent effects are seen that vary according to the disorder, the general condition of the affected individual, and the available therapy.

Diagnostic Evaluation

Although this chapter explores the history and subjective symptoms of skin lesions first, the obvious objective characteristics of the lesions are often noted simultaneously. Many skin lesions are easily diagnosed after careful inspection.

History and Subjective Symptoms

Many cutaneous lesions are associated with local symptoms. The most common local symptom is itching *(pruritus),* which varies in intensity. Pain or tenderness often accompanies some skin lesions. Other skin sensations such as burning, prickling, stinging, or crawling are also described. Alterations in local feeling include absence of sensation *(anesthesia);* excessive sensitiveness *(hyperesthesia);* diminished sensation *(hypesthesia* or *hypoesthesia);* or abnormal sensation, such as burning or prickling *(paresthesia).* These symptoms may remain localized or migrate; may be constant or intermittent; and may be aggravated by a specific activity, such as exposure to sunlight.

It is important to determine whether the child has an allergic condition such as asthma or hay fever or history of a previous skin disease. AD, often associated with allergies, frequently begins in infancy. Important questions for the parent include when the lesion or symptom first appeared; whether it occurred with ingestion of a food or other substance, including any medication; and whether the condition was related to activity such as contact with plants, insects, or chemicals.

Objective Findings

The distribution, size, morphologic characteristics, and arrangement of skin lesions provide significant information. Extrinsic causes usually result from physical, chemical, or allergic irritants or from an infectious agent such as bacteria, fungi, viruses, or animal parasites. Skin manifestations are also produced by intrinsic causes such as an infection (measles or chickenpox), drug sensitization, or other allergic phenomena.

Types of Lesions

Skin lesions assume distinct characteristics that are related to the pathologic process. Nurses should become familiar with the common terms that are applied to skin lesions because these terms are used in the processes of record keeping and communication. These terms include:

Erythema—A reddened area caused by increased amounts of oxygenated blood in the dermal vasculature

Ecchymoses (bruises)—Localized red or purple discolorations caused by extravasation of blood into dermis and subcutaneous tissues

Petechiae—Pinpoint, tiny, and sharp circumscribed spots in the superficial layers of the epidermis

Primary lesions—Skin changes produced by a causative factor; common primary lesions in pediatric skin disorders are macules, papules, and vesicles (Fig. 53-1)

Secondary lesions—Changes that result from alteration in the primary lesions, such as those caused by rubbing, scratching, medication, or involution and healing (Fig. 53-2)

Distribution pattern—The pattern in which lesions are distributed over the body, whether local or generalized, and the specific areas associated with the lesions

Configuration and arrangement—The size, shape, and arrangement of a lesion or groups of lesions (e.g., *discrete, clustered, diffuse,* or *confluent*)

Laboratory Studies

If a skin problem is related to a systemic disease (e.g., collagen or immunodeficiency disease), laboratory studies are performed to identify the condition. Diagnostic techniques include microscopic examination, cultures, skin scrapings or biopsy, cytodiagnosis, patch testing, Wood light examination, allergic skin testing, and other laboratory tests such as blood count and sedimentation rate.

Wounds

Wounds are structural or physiologic disruptions of the skin that activate normal or abnormal tissue repair responses. Wounds are classified as acute or chronic. *Acute wounds* are those that heal uneventfully within 2 to 3 weeks. *Chronic wounds* are those that do not heal in the expected time frame or are associated with complications. Cofactors that disrupt or delay wound healing include compromised perfusion, malnutrition, and infection. In children, most wounds are acute and can be prevented from becoming chronic wounds through appropriate nursing care. Wounds are also classified as surgical and nonsurgical and then further classified in the same manner as burns: superficial, partial thickness, or full thickness (complex wounds that include muscle or bone).

Epidermal Injuries

Abrasions are the most common epidermal wounds in children, usually in the form of a skinned knee or elbow. In most injuries the margins of the abraded area are superficial, involving only the outer layers of epidermis, although the central portion may extend into the dermis. Epithelial tissue is composed of labile cells, which are constantly destroyed and replaced throughout the life span. Therefore epidermal injuries usually result in rapid, uneventful healing and recovery.

Injury to Deeper Tissues

Tissues composed of *permanent cells* such as muscle and nerve cells are unable to regenerate. These tissues repair themselves by substituting fibrous connective tissue for the injured tissue. This fibrous tissue, or *scar,* serves as a patch to preserve or restore the continuity of the tissue. Wounds involving permanent cells include surgical incisions, lacerations, ulcers, evulsions, and full-thickness burns.

Process of Wound Healing

When the skin is injured, its normal protective barrier function is broken. In the healthy immunocompetent individual,

Macule—flat; nonpalpable; circumscribed; less than 1 cm in diameter; brown, red, purple, white, or tan in color
Examples: Freckles; flat moles; rubella; rubeola

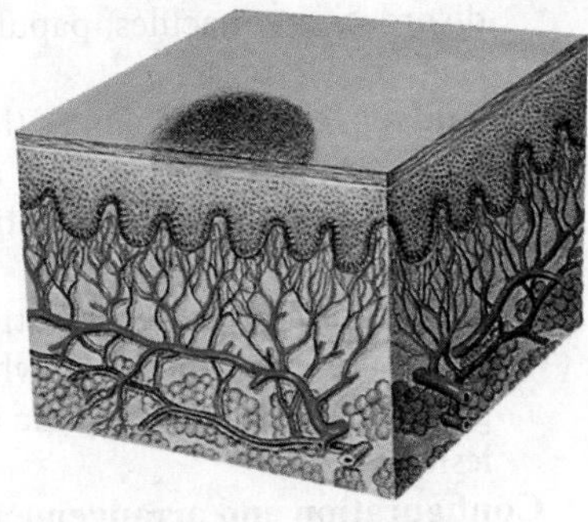

Plaque—elevated; flat topped; firm; rough; superficial papule greater than 1 cm in diameter; may be coalesced papules
Examples: Psoriasis; seborrheic and actinic keratoses

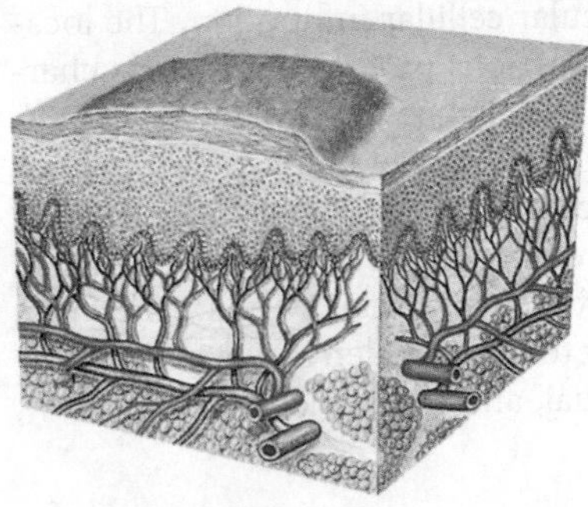

Patch—flat; nonpalpable; irregular in shape; macule that is greater than 1 cm in diameter
Examples: Vitiligo; port-wine marks

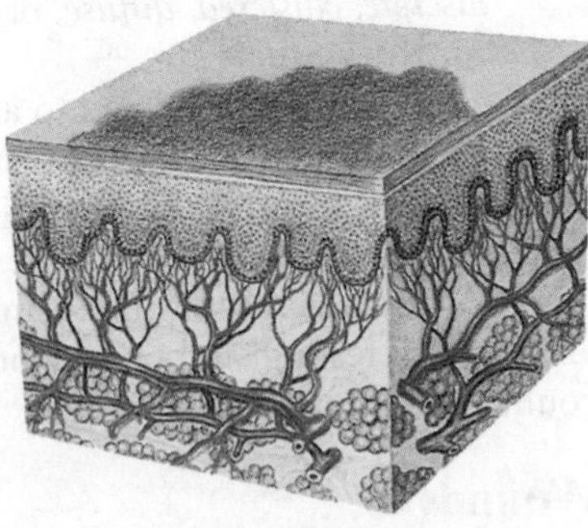

Wheal—elevated, irregularly shaped area of cutaneous edema; solid, transient, changing, variable diameter; pale pink with lighter center
Examples: Urticaria; insect bites

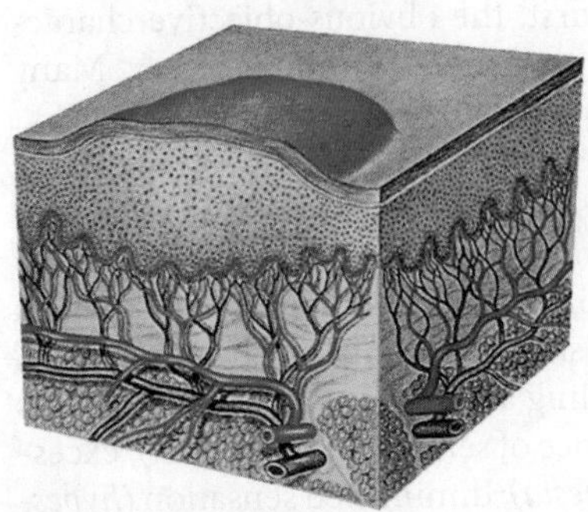

Papule—elevated; palpable; firm; circumscribed; less than 1 cm in diameter; brown, red, pink, tan, or bluish red in color
Examples: Warts; drug-related eruptions; pigmented nevi

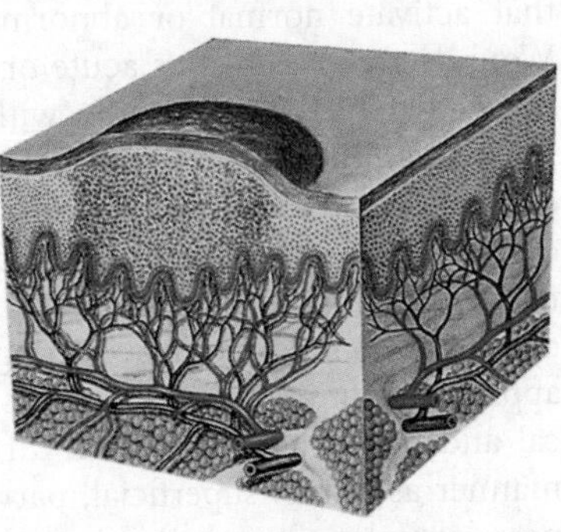

Nodule—elevated; firm; circumscribed; palpable; deeper in dermis than papule; 1 to 2 cm in diameter
Examples: Erythema nodosum; lipomas

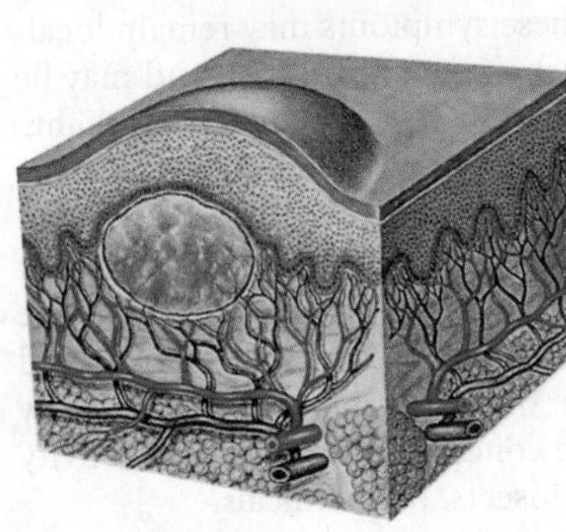

Vesicle—elevated; circumscribed; superficial; filled with serous fluid; less than 1 cm in diameter
Examples: Blister; varicella

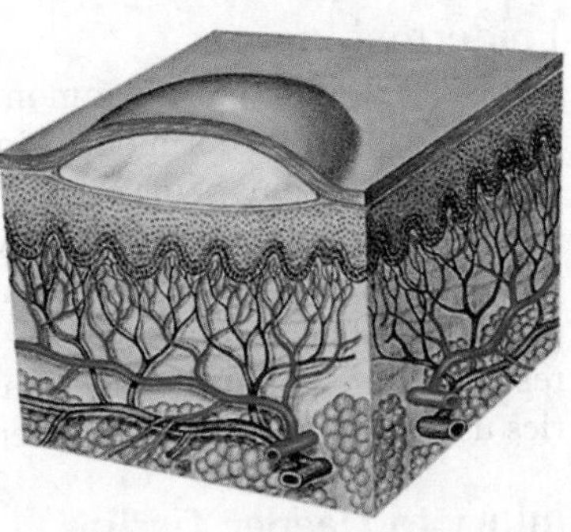

Pustule—elevated; superficial; similar to vesicle but filled with purulent fluid
Examples: Impetigo; acne; variola

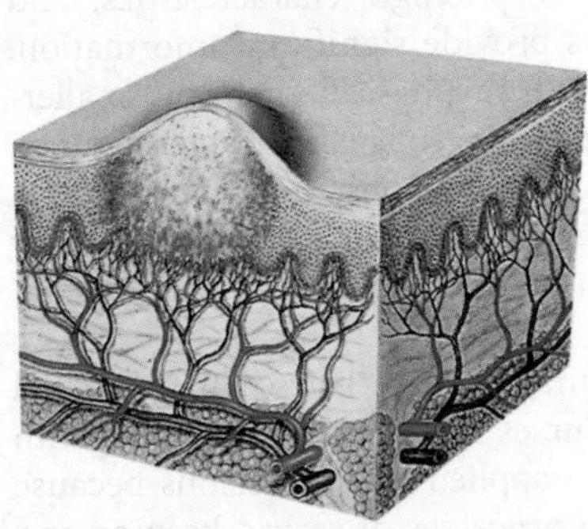

Bulla—vesicle greater than 1 cm in diameter
Examples: Blister; pemphigus vulgaris

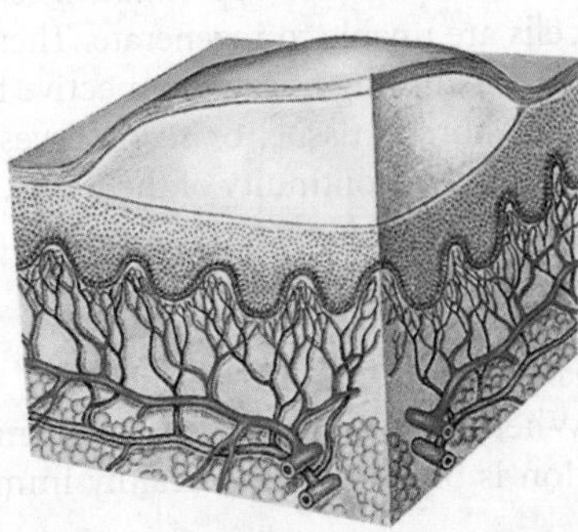

Cyst—elevated; circumscribed; palpable; encapsulated; filled with liquid or semisolid material
Example: Sebaceous cyst

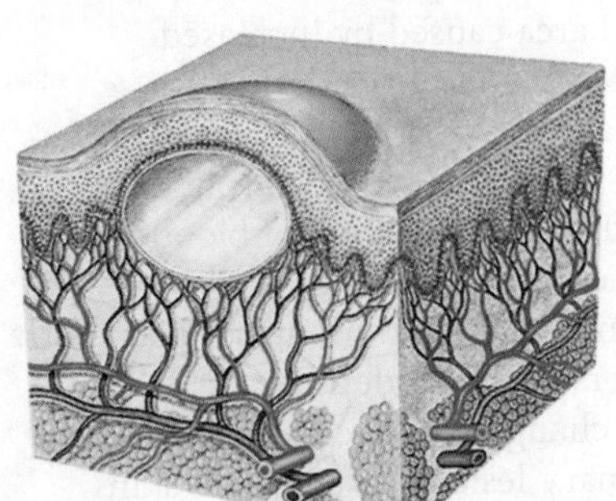

Fig. 53-1 Primary skin lesions. (From Seidel HM et al: *Mosby's guide to physical examination,* ed 6, St Louis, 2006, Mosby.)

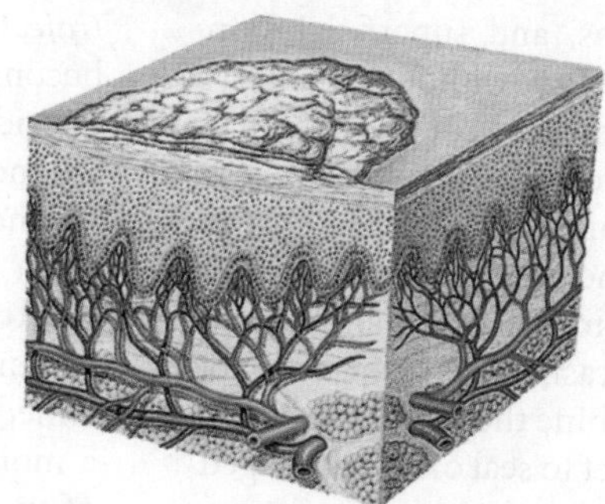

Scale—heaped-up keratinized cells; flaky exfoliation; irregular; thick or thin; dry or oily; varied size; silver, white, or tan in color
Examples: Psoriasis; exfoliative dermatitis

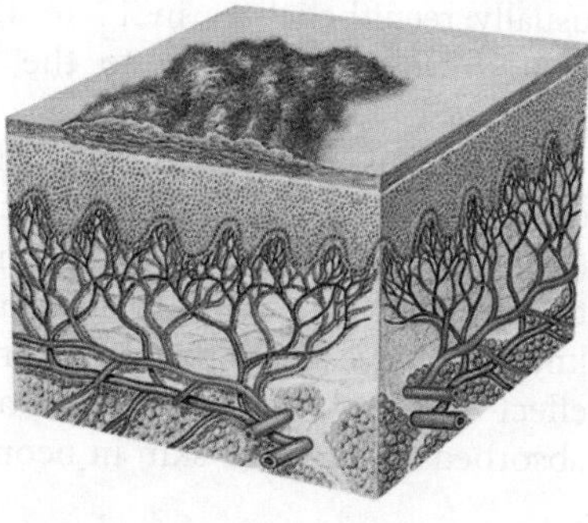

Crust—dried serum, blood, or purulent exudate; slightly elevated; size varies; brown, red, black, tan, or straw in color
Examples: Scab on abrasion; eczema

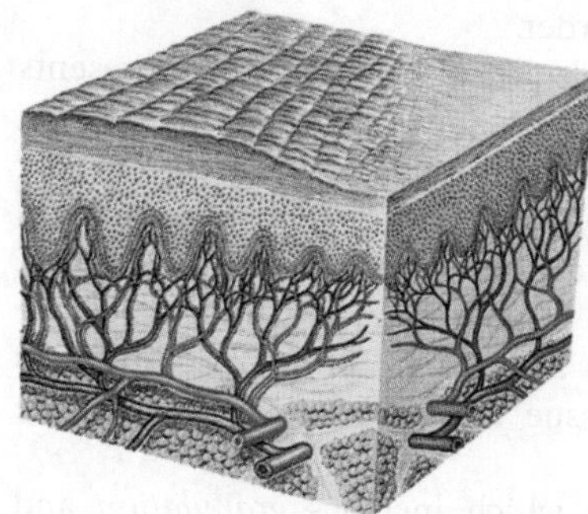

Lichenification—rough, thickened epidermis; accentuated skin markings caused by rubbing or irritation; often involves flexor aspect of extremity
Example: Chronic dermatitis

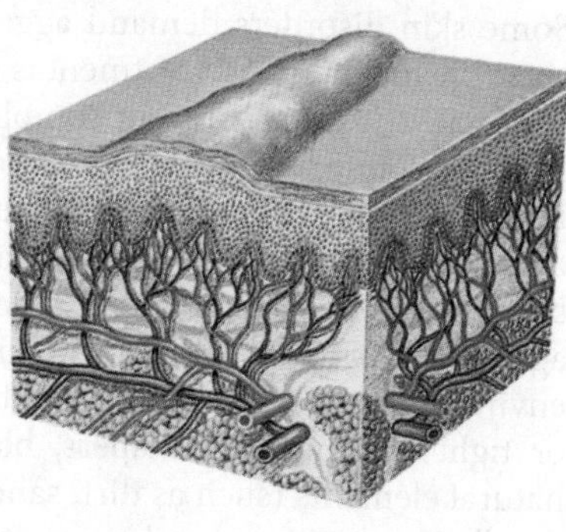

Scar—thin to thick fibrous tissue replacing injured dermis; irregular; pink, red, or white in color; may be atrophic or hypertrophic
Example: Healed wound or surgical incision

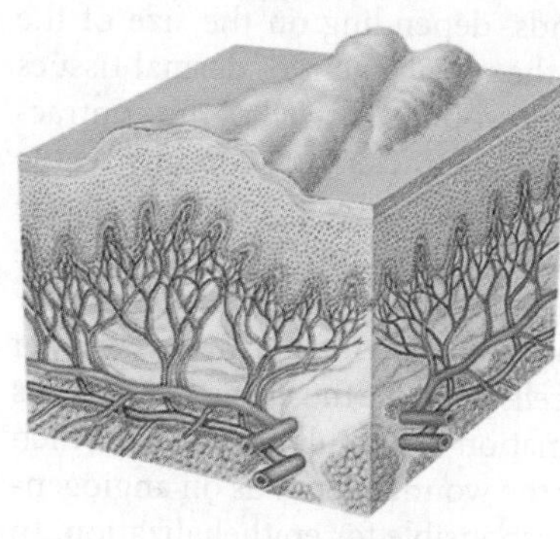

Keloid— irregularly shaped, elevated, progressively enlarging scar; grows beyond boundaries of wound; caused by excessive collagen formation during healing
Example: Keloid from ear piercing or burn scar

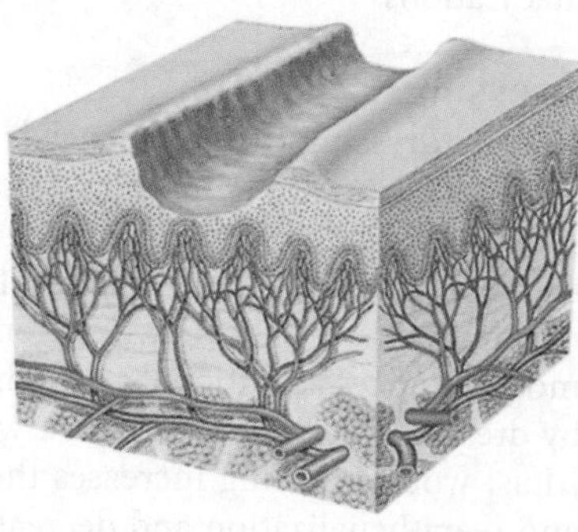

Excoriation—loss of epidermis; linear or hollowed-out crusted area; dermis exposed
Examples: Abrasion; scratch

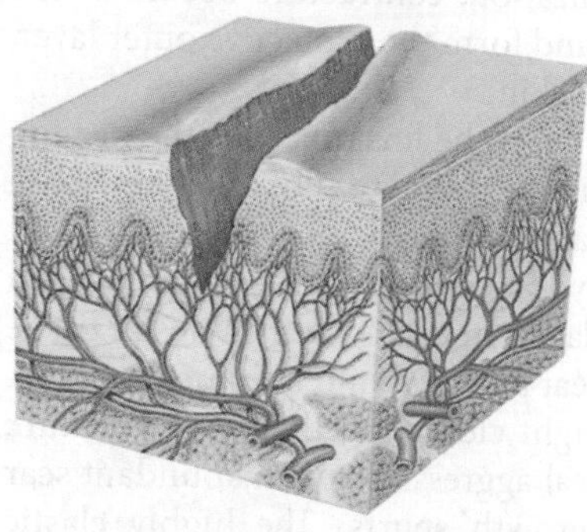

Fissure—linear crack or break from epidermis to dermis; small; deep; red
Examples: Athlete's foot; cheilosis

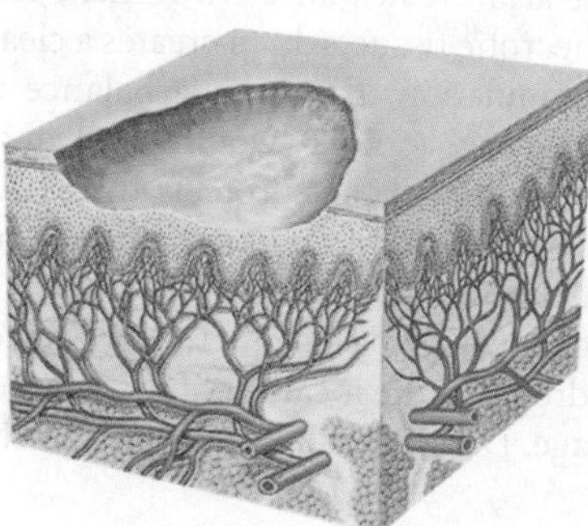

Erosion—loss of all or part of epidermis; depressed; moist; glistening; follows rupture of vesicle or bulla; larger than fissure
Examples: Varicella; variola following rupture

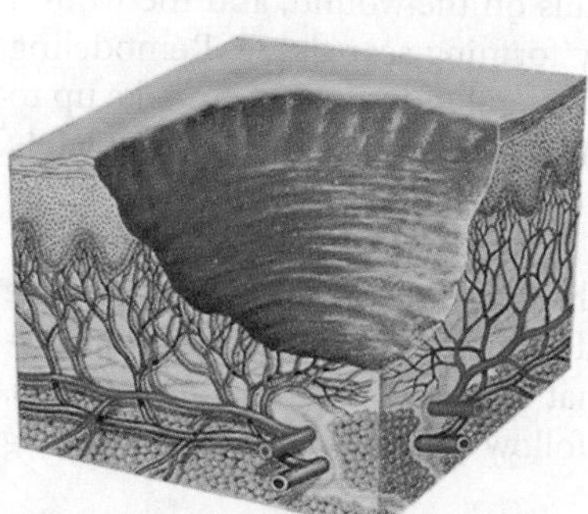

Ulcer—loss of epidermis and dermis; concave; varies in size; exudative; red or reddish blue
Examples: Decubiti; stasis ulcers

Fig. 53-2 Secondary skin lesions. (From Seidel HM et al: *Mosby's guide to physical examination,* ed 6, St Louis, 2006, Mosby.)

acute traumatic abrasions, lacerations, and superficial skin and soft-tissue injuries heal spontaneously without complications. The process of tissue healing involves complex cellular interactions and biochemical reactions. The healing process is segregated into four phases that are characterized by the particular cells involved and the chemicals produced. The four stages of wound healing are hemostasis, inflammation, proliferation, and remodeling (Krasner, Rodeheaver, & Sibbald, 2001). Some authorities combine the first two phases.

In the *hemostasis* phase, platelets act to seal off the damaged blood vessels and to form a stable clot. Hemostasis occurs within minutes of the initial injury to the skin unless there is an underlying clotting disorder.

Inflammation, the second stage of wound healing, presents a clinical picture that involves erythema, swelling, and warmth, often associated with pain at the wound site. This stage usually lasts up to 4 days after injury. The inflammation phase involves white blood cells such as the neutrophils, monocytes, and macrophages. These cells mount an initial defense against microbial invasion and secrete proteolytic enzymes that destroy nonviable tissue and microorganisms in the wound area.

The *proliferative* phase, which includes *granulation* and *contracture,* is the third stage of healing. This phase lasts from 4 to 21 days in acute wounds, depending on the size of the wound. The phase involves the replacement of dermal tissues and subdermal tissues in deep wounds, as well as the contraction of the wound. The phase is characterized clinically by the presence of granulation tissue, the "beefy," pebbled red tissue in the wound base. Fibroblasts, or immature connective tissue cells, secrete collagen, which provides the foundation for dermal regeneration. Angiocytes regenerate the outer layers of capillaries, and endothelial cells produce the lining in a process called *angiogenesis.* The formation of granulation tissue, which provides the foundation for the wound, depends on angiogenesis. The keratinocytes are responsible for epithelialization. In the final stage of epithelialization, contracture occurs as the keratinocytes differentiate and form the protective outer layer, or stratum corneum, of the skin.

Remodeling, or *maturation,* is the final phase of the healing process. This phase occurs in the dermis as fibroblasts increase the tissue tensile strength and gradually replace type 3 collagen in the scar tissue with type 1 collagen, thicken the collagen fibers, and reorient the collagen fibers along the lines of tissue tension. Fibroblasts disappear as the wound becomes stronger. The wound edges are brought closer together, and a mature scar is formed. Children heal aggressively with abundant scar tissue, especially during growth spurts. The highly elastic quality of children's skin pulls on the wound, and the wound defends against this pull by forming scar tissue. Remodeling and maturation occur over several months and can take up to 2 years. Thus some wounds that appear to be completely healed can break down suddenly if attention is not paid to the initial causative factors.

The phases of wound healing are complex and may be interrupted by disease conditions, medications, and other systemic and local factors that influence the healing process. When a wound does not follow the "*normal wound healing trajectory,*" it may become stuck in one of the stages and become a chronic wound. It is important that health care providers understand and address the factors that influence wound healing and prevent the development of chronic wounds.

Factors That Influence Healing

Wound care management has shifted from interventions aimed at maintaining a dry environment to those that promote a moist, crust-free environment that enhances the migration of epithelial cells across the wound and facilitates remodeling. An acute full-thickness wound kept in a moist environment usually reepithelializes in 12 to 15 days, whereas the same wound when kept open to the air heals in about 25 to 30 days.

Numerous factors can delay healing (Table 53-1). For example, traditional practices, such as the use of antiseptics (hydrogen peroxide and povidone-iodine [Betadine] solutions), which were once thought to prevent infection, are now known to have a cytotoxic effect on healthy cells and minimal effect on controlling infections. Povidone-iodine may also be absorbed through the skin in neonates and young children.

General Therapeutic Management

Some skin disorders demand aggressive therapy, but by and large the major aim of treatment is to prevent further damage, eliminate the cause, prevent complications, and provide relief from discomfort while tissues undergo healing (McCord & Levy, 2006). Factors that contribute to the development of dermatitis and that prolong the course of the disease should be eliminated when possible. The most common causative agents of dermatitis in infants, children, and adolescents are environmental factors (soaps, bubble baths, shampoos, rough or tight clothing, wet diapers, blankets, and toys) and the natural elements (such as dirt, sand, heat, cold, moisture, and wind). Dermatitis may also result from home remedies and medications.

Dressings

No one dressing meets the needs of all wounds. The traditional *dry* gauze dressing should not be used on open wounds, since it allows the wound surface to dry, does little to prevent bacterial invasion, and adheres to the dried scab so that removal disturbs the newly regenerating epithelial cells. In most instances, traditional gauze dressings have been replaced by dressings that promote moist wound healing (Table 53-2). Moist wound healing increases the rate of collagen synthesis and reepithelialization and decreases pain and inflammation. It also creates an environment for autolytic debridement of necrotic tissue, which creates a clean wound bed and enhances granulation. However, a balance must be achieved between creating a moist wound bed and maintaining a dry periwound area that protects the skin and wound from maceration. The dressing type and frequency of dressing changes help to achieve this balance. The frequency of dressing changes is based on the presence of infection, the type of dressing, the location of the wound, and the amount of drainage. Dressings should always be changed when they are loose

Table 53-1 Factors That Delay Wound Healing

FACTOR	EFFECT ON HEALING
Dry wound environment	Allows epithelial cells to dry out and die; impairs migration of epithelial cells across wound surface
Nutritional deficiencies	
Vitamin A	Results in inadequate inflammatory response
Vitamin B_1	Results in decreased collagen formation
Vitamin C	Inhibits formation of collagen fibers and capillary development
Protein	Reduces supply of amino acids for tissue repair
Zinc	Impairs epithelialization
Immunocompromise	Results in inadequate or delayed inflammatory response
Impaired circulation	Inhibits inflammatory response and removal of debris from wound area Reduces supply of nutrients to wound area
Stress (pain, poor sleep)	Releases catecholamines that cause vasoconstriction
Antiseptics	
Hydrogen peroxide	Toxic to fibroblasts; can cause subcutaneous gas formation (mimics gas-forming infection)
Povidone-iodine	Toxic to white and red blood cells and fibroblasts
Chlorhexidine	Toxic to white blood cells
Medications	
Corticosteroids	Impair phagocytosis Inhibit fibroblast proliferation Depress formation of granulation tissue Inhibit wound contraction
Chemotherapy	Interrupts the cell cycle; damages DNA or prevents DNA repair
Antiinflammatory drugs	Decrease the inflammatory phase
Foreign bodies	Increase inflammatory response Inhibit wound closure
Infection	Increases inflammatory response Increases tissue destruction
Mechanical friction	Damages or destroys granulation tissue
Fluid accumulation in area	Inhibits tissues from approximating
Radiation	Inhibits fibroblastic activity and capillary formation May cause tissue necrosis
Diseases	
Diabetes mellitus	Inhibits collagen synthesis Impairs circulation and capillary growth Hyperglycemia impairs phagocytosis
Anemia	Reduces oxygen supply to tissues
Peripheral vascular disease	Reduces oxygen supply to wounds
Uremia	Decreases collagen and granulation tissue

DNA, Deoxyribonucleic acid.

or soiled. They should be changed more frequently in areas where contamination is likely (e.g., the sacral area, the buttocks, the tracheal area) or when wound infection is suspected or present.

Topical Therapy

Several agents and methods are available for treatment. In selecting a therapeutic regimen, the practitioner considers (1) the active ingredient, (2) the proper vehicle or base, (3) the cosmetic effect, (4) the cost, and (5) instructions for use. Several basic concepts must also be considered. Overtreatment is avoided. For example, when the dermatitis is acute, topical applications should be mild and bland to avoid further irritation. Broken or inflamed skin, especially in children, is more absorbent than intact skin, and chemicals that are nonirritating to intact skin may be quite irritating to inflamed skin.

Topical applications may be applied to treat the disorder, reduce itching, decrease external stimuli, or apply external heat or cold. The emollient action of soaks, baths, and lotions provides a soothing film over the skin surface that reduces external stimuli. Ordinarily, lukewarm, tepid, or cool applications offer the greatest relief.

NURSING ALERT Application of heat tends to aggravate most conditions, and its use is usually reserved for reducing specific inflammatory processes, such as folliculitis and cellulitis.

Table 53-2 Common Wound Care Products

TYPE OF PRODUCT	INDICATIONS	FUNCTION	DRESSING CHANGE FREQUENCY	COMMENTS
Transparent film (e.g., Tegaderm)	Skin tears, IV and tube sites, partial-thickness wounds, primary and secondary dressings	Provides moist wound healing; impermeable to fluid and bacteria; promotes autolytic debridement; nonabsorptive	Daily, up to 7 days	Seals wound from contaminants
Hydrocolloid (e.g., DuoDERM)	Pressure ulcers, partial- and full-thickness wounds, skin tears, tape anchor	Occlusive; impermeable to bacteria and contaminants; promotes autolytic debridement; minimal absorption	Up to 7 days	Do not place over infected or heavily draining wounds
Alginates-hydrofibers—calcium, collagen, and silver (e.g., Aquacel, Fibracol)	Moderate to large drainage, partial- and full-thickness wounds, dehiscence, infection, bleeding	Absorptive	Daily, but depends on amount of drainage; silver impregnated, 3-7 days	Excellent for packing, tunneling, and undermining; trauma-free removal
Barrier dressings (e.g., Stomahesive wafer, Coloplast wafer)	Protect periwound, tube and tape anchor	Protect skin from drainage or adhesive stripping	Up to once weekly	Excellent around G tube sites; apply around wounds or on skin to attach tape
Barrier cream or ointment (e.g., Sensi-Care, Critic-Aid, Laniseptic)	Perineal and diaper areas	Protects skin from moisture	With each diaper change	Some impregnated with antifungals; choose those formulated to stick to moist lesions
Foam (e.g., Lyofoam, Mepilex, Allevyn, PolyMem)	Moderate to heavy drainage, partial- and full-thickness wounds	More absorptive than gauze	Depends on drainage; up to 7 days	Excellent around leaking tubes and tracheostomies; available with fenestration; comfortable; nonadherent; trauma-free removal
Silver (e.g., SilvaSorb dressing and gel, Arglaes powder)	Infected or colonized full- and partial-thickness wounds	Depends on dressing type; available in foam, hydrocolloid, hydrofiber, alginate, and powder	Depends on dressing type; usually 3-7 days	Consider in wounds recalcitrant to previous treatments; controls odor
Wound gels (e.g., Flaminal)	Dry, partial- and full-thickness wounds and burns	Adds moisture; promotes epithelialization; fills up dead space	Once or twice daily	Easy to use; base frequency on wound moisture
Hydrogel dressing (CarraGauze, CarraDres)	Burns, partial- and full-thickness wounds, painful wounds	Adds moisture; aids autolytic debridement; minimal to moderate absorption	Daily	Nonadherent; trauma- and pain-free removal
Becaplermin gel (Regranex)	Ulcers	Promotes granulation	Daily	Contraindicated in infected and necrotic wounds; refrigerate; expensive
Enzymatic debrider (Accuzyme)	Necrotic wounds in patients who are not surgical candidates	Selectively dissolves necrotic tissue	Once or twice daily	Cross-hatch eschar with a scalpel for enzyme penetration; cover with moist N/S gauze to activate; avoid use with silver or mercury
Gauze	All wound types	Minor absorption; mild debridement	3-4 times per day	Dries out; poor absorbency; can macerate periwound; increased labor costs and supplies secondary to dressing change frequency

From McCord SS, Moise L: Practical guide to pediatric wound care, *Semin Plast Surg* 20(3):192-199, 2006.
G tube, Gastrostomy tube; *IV*, intravenous; *N/S*, normal saline.

Ointments in a petrolatum base provide protection from moisture. Therefore this type of ointment is indicated around gastrostomy tubes, in skin folds, and in the diaper area. Creams are absorbed by the skin and are used for areas where a nongreasy "feel" is desired (e.g., face, hands).

Topical Corticosteroid Therapy

Glucocorticoids are the therapeutic agents used most frequently for skin disorders. Their local antiinflammatory effects are merely palliative, so the medication must be applied until the condition undergoes a remission or the causative agent is eliminated. Corticosteroids are applied directly to the affected area, are essentially nonsensitizing, and have only minor side effects. As with the use of any steroids, their use in large amounts may mask signs of infection, and symptoms may be exacerbated after termination of the drug. Families are cautioned that the medication cannot be used for all skin disorders. The concentrations available without prescription are not adequate for stubborn skin conditions (e.g., psoriasis) and may further aggravate inflammation caused by fungus or bacteria. Most parents and children apply too much topical hydrocortisone; therefore they should be counseled that it is both effective and economical to apply only a thin film and to massage it into the skin. Parents and children should also be advised to use the application for no more than 5 to 7 days because these agents may cause depigmentation and other changes in the skin.

Other Topical Therapies

Other topical treatments include chemical cautery (especially useful for warts), cryosurgery, electrodesiccation (chiefly used for warts, granulomas, and nevi), ultraviolet (UV) therapy (primarily used in psoriasis and acne), laser therapy (especially for birthmarks), and acne therapies such as dermabrasion and chemical peels. New drugs called *topical immunomodulators* are effective in reducing the itching of AD (eczema) and preventing "flares."

Systemic Therapy

Systemic drugs may be used as an adjunct to topical therapy in some dermatologic disorders. The drugs most frequently used are corticosteroids, antibiotics, and antifungal agents. Corticosteroids are valuable because of their capacity to inhibit inflammatory and allergic reactions. Dosage is carefully adjusted and gradually tapered to the minimum dosage that is effective and tolerated. In infants and children, the dosage is larger than is usually calculated from body weight ratios. However, prolonged use may temporarily suppress growth.

Antibiotics are used in severe or widespread skin infections. However, because these drugs tend to produce hypersensitivity in some patients, they are used with caution. Antifungal agents are the only means for treating systemic fungal infections.

Nursing Care Management

The child's subjective symptoms and the parent's history provide valuable information to help establish a diagnosis. Older children often describe the condition as painful, itching, or tingling or in other descriptive terms. However, much can be determined by also observing the younger child's behavior. Does the child scratch? Is the child restless or irritable? Does the child favor or avoid using a body part? A careful history provides important clues. Has the child had access to chemicals or been in the woods or around a woodpile? Has the child eaten a new food? Is the child taking medication? Has the child any known allergy? Do siblings or playmates have similar lesions? What soap or bubble bath is used for bathing?

It is important for nurses to not only describe but also assess skin lesions and wounds. The color, shape, and distribution of lesions and wounds are important. Individual lesions are described according to standard terminology. Sometimes two descriptors are used for a particular characteristic (e.g., maculopapular rash). To confirm or amplify the findings made by inspection, the nurse may gently palpate the skin to detect characteristics such as temperature, moisture, texture, elasticity, and edema. Wounds are assessed for depth of tissue damage, evidence of healing, and signs of infection.

NURSING ALERT Signs of wound infection are:

- Increased erythema, especially beyond the wound margin
- Edema
- Purulent exudate
- Pain
- Increased temperature

The frequency of wound assessment depends on the severity and complexity of the wound. For example, simple or chronic wounds are assessed weekly; infected or complex wounds are assessed daily. Wounds are measured at least weekly (height, width, and depth). The wound bed is assessed for color, drainage, odor, necrosis, granulation tissue, fibrin slough, undermining and condition of the wound edges, and the color and condition of the surrounding skin.

Therapeutic programs are designed to include general measures such as rest, protection, and relief of discomfort and specific treatments such as medication and physical techniques. Only a few skin diseases are contagious; therefore it is usually not necessary to isolate the affected child, except from persons in danger of acquiring a secondary infection (e.g., a child receiving large doses of corticosteroids or other immunosuppressant drugs or a child with an immunologic deficiency disorder). However, if the skin manifestation is caused by a viral exanthema, such as measles or chickenpox, the child is prevented from exposing other susceptible children.

Wound Care

Parents can generally manage small skin lesions or wounds at home. The parents are instructed to wash their hands and then wash the wound gently with mild soap and water or normal saline. They are cautioned to avoid povidone-iodine, alcohol, and hydrogen peroxide because these products are toxic to wounds.

NURSING ALERT Do not put anything in a wound that you would not put in the eye. The safest solution is normal saline.

Open wounds are covered with a dressing, such as a commercial adhesive bandage, although larger wounds may benefit from the use of occlusive dressings (see Table 53-2). If occlusive dressings are applied, parents should learn how to apply and remove the dressings correctly. For example, hydrocolloid dressings adhere best if a wide margin is left around the wound and the dressing is pressed against intact skin until it adheres. If a dressing needs to be secured, a nonalcohol skin barrier can be applied to protect the skin, or the wound can be "picture framed" with hydrocolloid dressing and dressing tape can be secured to the hydrocolloid. This method of securing the dressing protects the skin when the tape is removed. Montgomery straps or stretch netting can also be used to secure dressings and to avoid the use of tape.

NURSING ALERT Advise parents that the yellow gel forming under hydrocolloid dressings may look like pus and has a distinct odor (somewhat fruity) but is normal leakage.

Dressings are removed carefully to protect intact skin and the epithelial surface of the wound. When removing transparent or hydrocolloid dressings, the nurse or parent should raise one edge of the dressing and pull *parallel* to the skin to loosen the adhesive. The longer the dressings are left on, the easier they are to remove. Less frequent dressing changes decrease wound contamination.

Lacerations present a special challenge. The injured child and family are usually distressed by the bleeding. In particular, scalp lacerations tend to bleed profusely. Parental guilt and shock usually accompany the injury. The initial nursing intervention is to apply pressure to the area and to attempt to calm the child before further examination. Unless there is bleeding from a severed artery, the wound is cleansed with a forced jet of sterile tepid water or saline (via syringe) and examined for extent; depth; and presence of foreign material such as dirt, glass, or fabric fragments.

The location of the wound facilitates assessment. Wounds over bony areas may contain bone chips, and clear fluid seeping from severe head wounds may indicate cerebrospinal fluid. A pressure dressing is applied for transfer to medical care. After the child is in a medical facility, he or she is prepared for suturing.

Puncture wounds that do not require a tetanus booster are soaked in warm water and soap for several minutes. Causing the wound to rebleed may be helpful. An adhesive bandage can be applied if desired. Puncture wounds of the head, chest, or abdomen or those that could still contain a portion of the puncturing object must be evaluated carefully.

Parents are cautioned against opening blisters or kissing a wound "to make it better." The wound can easily become contaminated from germs in the human mouth. If scabs form, they are allowed to slough off without assistance; picking or early removal may cause scarring and secondary infection. Parents are advised to seek medical help if there is evidence of infection.

Relief of Symptoms

Most therapeutic regimens for skin lesions are directed toward relief of pruritus, the most common subjective complaint. Cooling the affected area and increasing the skin pH with cool baths or compresses and alkaline applications (e.g., baking soda baths) are helpful in reducing the itching. Clothing and bed linen should be soft and lightweight to decrease irritation from friction and stimulation.

During treatment, both the affected and unaffected skin is protected from damage and secondary infection. Preventing scratching is important. Older children can cooperate, although they may need to be reminded to stop scratching or rubbing. However, small or uncooperative children may require the use of devices such as mittens (especially during sleep) or special coverings. Keeping fingernails clean, short, and trimmed reduces the risk of secondary infection.

Antipruritic medications, such as diphenhydramine (Benadryl) or hydroxyzine (Atarax), may be prescribed for severe itching, especially if it disturbs the child's rest. Pain and discomfort are usually managed with nonpharmacologic measures and mild analgesia. Severe pain requires more potent medication. Occlusive dressings over wounds reduce pain. For suturing wounds a topical anesthetic or intradermal buffered lidocaine should be used (see Pain Management, Chapter 35).

Topical Therapy

The specific type of topical therapy and the mode of application depend on the nature and location of the lesion. It is especially important to wash the hands before and after application of any topical therapy. The skin is assessed before the application and reassessed after treatment. Any observed changes are noted and described.

Wet compresses or *dressings* cool the skin by evaporation, relieve itching and inflammation, and cleanse the area by loosening and removing crusts and debris. A variety of ingredients, such as plain water or Burow's solution (available without a prescription), can be applied on Kerlix gauze; plain gauze; or (preferably) soft cotton cloths such as freshly laundered handkerchiefs or strips from diaper, sheeting, or pillowcase material.

Dressings immersed in the desired solution are wrung out slightly and applied to the affected area wet but not dripping. They are applied flat and smooth in such a way that motion is not totally restricted—fingers are wrapped separately, and arms and legs are wrapped so that elbows and knees can bend. Dressings are held in place by Kerlix or other cotton wrap, tubular stockinette, mittens, and socks (two pairs—one to hold the dressings in place, the other to protect from movement). When evaporation begins to dry them, the dressings are removed, rewet in the solution, and reapplied using aseptic technique. The solution is *not* poured or applied with a syringe directly over the dressings. As fluid evaporates, the solution becomes more concentrated, and this could damage sensitive lesions.

Fresh solution at room temperature is applied at 2-, 3-, or 4-hour intervals and allowed to remain on the lesion from 20 to 90 minutes. Wet dressings are seldom continued after about 48 hours. The child is protected against chilling during treatment, and no more than 20% of the body is covered with a dressing at one time to avoid the risk of hypothermia. After treatment, the skin is dried thoroughly by patting with a towel. Lotion or other medication (if prescribed) is applied at this time.

When children are uncooperative in the use of wet dressings, *soaks* are often used for removal of crusts and for their mild astringent action. The same solutions are used as for wet compresses. Gaining young children's cooperation for hand or foot soaks is difficult unless the procedure is accompanied by play. Older infants and toddlers delight in playing with brightly colored objects or poker chips scattered over the bottom of the receptacle, and preschoolers can be challenged to hold a floating item beneath the water's surface. However, these activities require supervision; infants and small children place items in their mouths, and children easily lose control with water play. Washing dishes, cars, dolls, or doll clothes will also occupy time during soaks.

Although older children can cooperate, they, too, need something to do during the procedure, such as listening to music or a story or watching television. Placing the solution and the extremity in a plastic sealable bag is an effective method to soak a hand or foot.

Baths are useful in the treatment of widespread dermatitis by evenly distributing the soothing antipruritic and antiinflammatory effects of the solution, usually oatmeal or mineral oil preparations. The solution is added to a tub of lukewarm water. The temperature of the bath is tepid, and the treatment usually lasts 15 to 53 minutes. Therapeutic baths are more interesting when toy boats or other items for water play accompany the procedure.

Topical applications are applied to skin lesions to ease discomfort, prevent further injury, and facilitate healing. A thin application of the ointment or cream may be covered with a plastic film and anchored with adhesive, covered with a commercial transparent dressing, or wrapped in Kerlix gauze and held in place by a stretchy net dressing. Topical preparations are applied systematically with the contour of the body surface (not simply up and down). Children love to be "painted," and lotion applications can be fun when an ordinary paintbrush is used. Regardless of the type of preparation used, parents need detailed information on how to apply it and how long the preparation should remain on the skin.

NURSING ALERT Provide written instructions and demonstrate to parents the correct amount of topical medication to apply (e.g., size of a pea; thin film to cover). If more than one preparation is applied, mark the containers with numbers so the parents remember the correct order of application. Stress that more is not necessarily better with some medications, such as steroids.

Home Care and Family Support

Dermatologic conditions always involve the family, but few situations require hospitalization and most care is delivered at home. Because the family members must carry out the treatment plan, their cooperation is essential. Regimens that are simple to accomplish in the clinic, hospital, or primary care provider's office may be frustrating and baffling at home. The family may also need assistance in adapting equipment available for home therapy.

It is important that the child and family be given as detailed explanations as possible about both the expected and unexpected results of treatment, including any ill effects that might occur. If unexplained reactions develop, the family is directed to discontinue treatment and report the reactions to the appropriate person. The use of over-the-counter medicines is discouraged unless the preparations have been discussed with the health care provider and have received approval.

Because the skin is the most visible portion of the body, defects in its surface alter its appearance and cause distress for the child. Skin problems may also result in rejection by others. Parents of other children may fear that their children will "catch" the disorder. Occasionally the affected child's own family members reduce their interaction or physical contact with the child. This is seldom a problem with dermatitis of short duration, but chronic conditions can frequently create problems and affect the child's self-esteem.

Infections of the Skin

Bacterial Infections

Normally, the skin harbors a variety of bacterial flora, including the major pathogenic varieties of staphylococci and streptococci. The degree of pathogenicity of the organism depends on its invasiveness and toxicity, the integrity of the skin, and the immune and cellular defenses of the host. Children with congenital or acquired immunodeficiency disorders (such as acquired immunodeficiency syndrome [AIDS]), those in a debilitated condition, those receiving immunosuppressant therapy, and those with a generalized malignancy such as leukemia or lymphoma are at risk for developing bacterial infections.

evolve Case Study–Impetigo

Because of the characteristic "walling-off" process of the inflammatory reaction (abscess formation), staphylococci are more difficult to treat, and the local infected area is associated with an increase in bacteria all over the skin surface that serves as a source of continuing infection. In previous years, methicillin-resistant *Staphylococcus aureus* (MRSA) infections were primarily seen in nursing homes and hospitals. In recent years, the number of community-acquired MRSA infections has risen (Kaplan, 2006). All these factors underline the importance of careful handwashing and cleanliness when caring for infected children and their lesions to prevent the spread of infection and as an essential prophylactic measure when caring for infants and small children. Common bacterial skin disorders are outlined in Table 53-3.

Nursing Care Management

The major nursing interventions related to bacterial skin infections are to prevent the spread of infection and to prevent complications. Impetigo contagiosa and MRSA infection can easily spread by self-inoculation; therefore the child must be cautioned against touching the involved area. Handwashing is mandatory before and after contact with an affected child, and this practice is emphasized to all those who care for the child. Many children with AD are colonized with MRSA in the nares and under the fingernails. For many bacterial infections, and for MRSA infection in particular, the child should be provided with washcloths and towels separate from those of other family members. Pajamas, underwear, and other clothes should be changed daily and washed in hot water. Razors used for shaving should be discarded after each use and not shared. To prevent recurrence, some infectious disease specialists recommend bathing in a chlorine bath twice weekly with 1 tsp of chlorine per gallon of water.

Table 53-3 Bacterial Infections

DISORDER AND ORGANISM	MANIFESTATIONS	MANAGEMENT	COMMENTS
Impetigo contagiosa (Fig. 53-3)—Staphylococci	Begins as a reddish macule Becomes vesicular Ruptures easily, leaving superficial, moist erosion Tends to spread peripherally in sharply marginated irregular outlines Exudate dries to form heavy, honey-colored crusts Pruritus common *Systemic effects*—Minimal or asymptomatic	Careful removal of undermined skin, crusts, and debris by softening with 1:20 Burow's solution compresses Topical application of bactericidal ointment Systemic administration of oral or parenteral antibiotics (penicillin) in severe or extensive lesions	Tends to heal without scarring unless secondary infection Autoinoculable and contagious Common in toddler, preschooler May be superimposed on eczema
Pyoderma—Staphylococci, streptococci	Deeper extension of infection into dermis Tissue reaction more severe *Systemic effects*—Fever, lymphangitis	Soap and water cleansing Wet compresses Bathing with antibacterial soap as prescribed Do not share washcloths or towels Mupirocin to nares and lesions as prescribed Systemic antibiotics	Autoinoculable and contagious May heal with or without scarring
Folliculitis (pimple), furuncle (boil), carbuncle (multiple boils)—*Staphylococcus aureus*	Folliculitis—Infection of hair follicle Furuncle—Larger lesion with more redness and swelling at a single follicle Carbuncle—More extensive lesion with widespread inflammation and "pointing" at several follicular orifices *Systemic effects*—Malaise, if severe	Skin cleanliness Local warm, moist compresses Topical application of antibiotic agents Systemic antibiotics in severe cases Incision and drainage of severe lesions, followed by wound irrigation with antibiotics or suitable drain implantation	Autoinoculable and contagious Furuncle and carbuncle tend to heal with scar formation Never squeeze a lesion
Cellulitis—Streptococci, staphylococci, *Haemophilus influenzae* (Fig. 53-4)	Inflammation of skin and subcutaneous tissues with intense redness, swelling, and firm infiltration Lymphangitis "streaking" frequently seen Involvement of regional lymph nodes common May progress to abscess formation *Systemic effects*—Fever, malaise	Oral or parenteral antibiotics Rest and immobilization of both affected area and child Hot, moist compresses to area	Hospitalization may be necessary for child with systemic symptoms Otitis media may be associated with facial cellulitis
Staphylococcal scalded skin syndrome—*S. aureus*	Macular erythema with "sandpaper" texture of involved skin Epidermis becoming wrinkled (in 2 days or less), and large bullae appearing	Systemic administration of antibiotics Gentle cleansing with saline, Burow's solution, or 0.25% silver nitrate compresses	Infant subject to fluid loss; impaired body temperature regulation; and secondary infection, such as pneumonia, cellulitis, and septicemia Heals without scarring

Children and parents are often tempted to squeeze follicular lesions. They must be warned that squeezing will not hasten the resolution of the infection and may make the lesion worse or spread the infection. No attempt should be made to puncture the surface of the pustule with a needle or sharp instrument. A child with a sty may waken with the eyelids of the affected eye sealed shut with exudate. The child or the parents are instructed to gently wipe the lid from the inner to the outer edge with warm water and a clean washcloth until the exudate is removed.

The child with limited cellulitis of an extremity is usually managed at home on a regimen of oral antibiotics and warm compresses. Children with more extensive cellulitis, especially around a joint with lymphadenitis or on the face, are usually admitted to the hospital for parenteral antibiotics, followed by continued treatment at home. Nurses are responsible for teaching the family to administer the medication and apply compresses.

Viral Infections

Viruses are intracellular parasites that produce their effect by using the intracellular substances of the host cells. Composed of only a deoxyribonucleic acid (DNA) or ribonucleic acid (RNA) core enclosed in an antigenic protein shell, viruses are unable to provide for their own metabolic needs or to reproduce themselves. After a virus penetrates a cell of the host

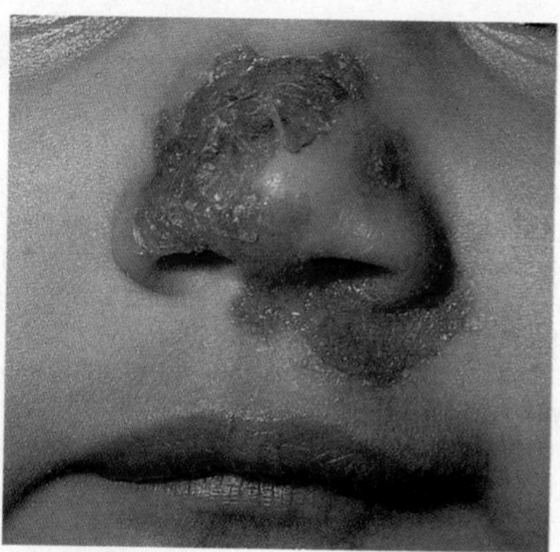

Fig. 53-3 Impetigo contagiosa. (From Weston WL, Lane AT, Morelli JG: *Color textbook of pediatric dermatology,* ed 3, St Louis, 2002, Mosby.)

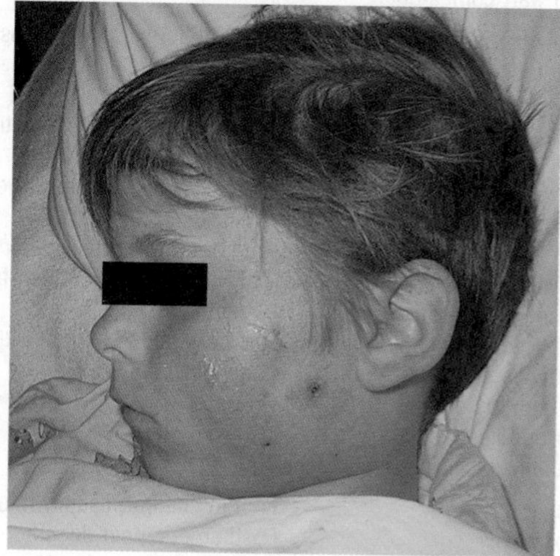

Fig. 53-4 Cellulitis of cheek from puncture wound. (From Weston WL, Lane AT, Morelli JG: *Color textbook of pediatric dermatology,* ed 4, St Louis, 2007, Mosby.)

organism, it sheds the outer shell and disappears within the cell, where the nucleic acid core stimulates the host cell to form more virus material from its intracellular substance. In a viral infection the epidermal cells react with inflammation and vesiculation (as in herpes simplex) or by proliferating to form growths (warts).

Many of the communicable viral diseases of childhood are associated with rashes, and each rash is characteristic. Other common viral disorders of the skin are outlined in Table 53-4.

Dermatophytoses (Fungal Infections)

The dermatophytoses (ringworm) are infections caused by a group of closely related filamentous fungi that invade primarily the stratum corneum, hair, and nails. These are superficial infections that live on, not in, the skin. They are confined to the dead keratin layers and are unable to survive in the deeper layers. Because the keratin is desquamated constantly, the fungus must multiply at a rate that equals the rate of keratin production to maintain itself; otherwise the infection would be shed with the discarded skin cells. Common dermatophytoses are outlined in Table 53-5.

Dermatophytoses are designated by the Latin word *tinea,* with further designation related to the area of the body where they are found (e.g., tinea capitis [ringworm of the scalp]). Dermatophyte infections are most often transmitted from one person to another or from infected animals to humans. Diagnosis is made from microscopic examination of scrapings taken from the advancing periphery of the lesion, which almost always produces a scale.

Nursing Care Management

When teaching families how to care for ringworm, the nurse should emphasize good health and hygiene. Because of the infectious nature of the disease, affected children should not exchange with other children grooming items, headgear, scarves, or other articles of apparel that have been in proximity to the infected area. Affected children are provided their own towels and directed to wear a protective cap at night to avoid transmitting the fungus to bedding, especially if they sleep with another person. Because the infection can be acquired by animal-to-human transmission, all household pets should be examined for the disorder. Other sources of infection are seats with headrests (such as theater seats), seats in public transportation vehicles, helmets, and gymnasium mats.

Both 2% ketoconazole and 1% selenium sulfide shampoos may reduce colony counts of dermatophytes. These shampoos can be used in combination with oral therapy to reduce the transmission of disease to others. The shampoo should be applied to the scalp for 5 to 10 minutes at least three times per week. The child may return to school once the therapy is initiated.

Alternately, if the child is treated with the drug griseofulvin, the therapy frequently continues for weeks or months, and because subjective symptoms subside, children or parents may be tempted to decrease or discontinue the drug. The nurse should emphasize to family members the importance of maintaining the prescribed dosage schedule and of taking the medication with high-fat foods for best absorption. They are also instructed regarding possible drug side effects, such as headache, gastrointestinal upset, fatigue, insomnia, and photosensitivity. For children who take the drug over many months, periodic testing is required to monitor leukopenia and assess liver and renal function. Newer antifungal medications such as terbinafine, itraconazole, and fluconazole may be used when there are adverse reactions to griseofulvin. Currently, these drugs are being studied to determine their efficacy and safety in treating tinea capitis in children but are not approved by the U.S. Food and Drug Administration (FDA) for this indication.

Systemic Mycotic (Fungal) Infections

Mycotic (systemic or deep fungal) infections have the capacity to invade the viscera, as well as the skin. The most common infections are the lung diseases, which are usually acquired by inhalation of fungal spores. These fungi produce a variable spectrum of disease, and some are common in certain geographic areas. They are not transmitted from person to person but appear to reside in the soil, from which their spores are airborne. The cutaneous lesions caused by deep fungal infections are granulomatous and appear as ulcers, plaques,

Table 53-4 Viral Infections

INFECTION	MANIFESTATIONS	MANAGEMENT	COMMENTS
Verruca (warts) **Cause**—Human papillomavirus (various types)	Usually well-circumscribed, gray or brown, elevated, firm papules with a roughened, finely papillomatous texture Occur anywhere, but usually appear on exposed areas such as fingers, hands, face, and soles May be single or multiple Asymptomatic	Not uniformly successful Local destructive therapy, individualized according to location, type, and number—surgical removal, electrocautery, curettage, cryotherapy (liquid nitrogen), caustic solutions (lactic acid and salicylic acid in flexible collodion, retinoic acid, salicylic acid plasters), x-ray treatment, laser	Common in children Tend to disappear spontaneously Course unpredictable Most destructive techniques tend to leave scars Autoinoculable Repeated irritation will cause to enlarge Apply topical anesthetic EMLA
Verruca plantaris (plantar wart)	Located on plantar surface of feet and, because of pressure, is practically flat; may be surrounded by a collar of hyperkeratosis	Apply caustic solution to wart Wear foam insole with hole cut to relieve pressure on wart Soak 20 minutes after 2-3 days; repeat until wart comes out	Destructive techniques tend to leave scars, which may cause problems with walking Apply topical anesthetic EMLA
Herpes simplex virus Type I (cold sore, fever blister) Type II (genital)	Grouped, burning, and itching vesicles on inflammatory base, usually on or near mucocutaneous junctions (lips, nose, genitalia, buttocks) Vesicles dry, forming a crust, followed by exfoliation and spontaneous healing in 8-10 days May be accompanied by regional lymphadenopathy	Avoidance of secondary infection Burow's solution compresses during weeping stages Topical therapy (penciclovir) to shorten duration of cold sores Oral antiviral (acyclovir) for initial infection or to reduce severity in recurrence Valacyclovir (Valtrex), an oral antiviral, used for episodic treatment of recurrent genital herpes; reduces pain, stops viral shedding, and has a more convenient administration schedule than acyclovir	Heal without scarring unless secondary infection Type I cold sores prevented by using sunscreens protecting against ultraviolet A and ultraviolet B light to prevent lip blisters Aggravated by corticosteroids Positive psychologic effect from treatment May be fatal in children with depressed immunity
Varicella-zoster virus (herpes zoster; shingles)	Caused by same virus that causes varicella (chickenpox) Virus has affinity for posterior root ganglia, posterior horn of spinal cord, and skin; crops of vesicles usually confined to dermatome following along course of affected nerve Usually preceded by neuralgic pain, hyperesthesias, or itching May be accompanied by constitutional symptoms	Symptomatic Analgesics for pain Mild sedation sometimes helpful Local moist compresses Drying lotions sometimes helpful Ophthalmic variety: use systemic corticotropin (adrenocorticotropic hormone) or corticosteroids Acyclovir Lidocaine (Lidoderm) topical anesthetic	Pain in children usually minimal Postherpetic pain does not occur in children Chickenpox may follow exposure; isolate affected child from other children in a hospital or school May occur in children with depressed immunity; can be fatal
Molluscum contagiosum **Cause**—Pox virus Small, benign tumors	Flesh-colored papules with a central caseous plug (umbilicated) Usually asymptomatic	Cases in well children resolve spontaneously in about 18 mo Treatment reserved for troublesome cases Apply topical anesthetic EMLA and remove with curette Use tretinoin gel 0.01% or cantharidin (Cantharone) liquid* Curettage or cryotherapy	Common in school-age children Spread by skin-to-skin contact, including autoinoculation and fomite-to-skin contact

EMLA, Eutectic mix of lidocaine and prilocaine.
*Not available in the United States, but can be purchased in Canada.

Table 53-5 Dermatophytoses (Fungal Infections)

DISEASE AND ORGANISM	MANIFESTATIONS	MANAGEMENT	COMMENTS
Tinea capitis—*Trichophyton tonsurans, Microsporum audouinii, Microsporum canis* (Fig. 53-5, *A*)	Lesions in scalp but may extend to hairline or neck Characteristic configuration of scaly, circumscribed patches or patchy, scaling areas of alopecia Generally asymptomatic, but severe, deep inflammatory reaction may occur that manifests as boggy, encrusted lesions (kerions) Pruritic Microscopic examination of scales is diagnostic	Oral griseofulvin Oral ketoconazole for difficult cases Selenium sulfide shampoos Topical antifungal agents (e.g., clotrimazole, haloprogin, miconazole)	Person-to-person transmission Animal-to-person transmission Rarely, permanent loss of hair *M. audouinii* transmitted from one human being to another directly or from personal items; *M. canis* usually contracted from household pets, especially cats Atopic individuals more susceptible
Tinea corporis—*Trichophyton rubrum, Trichophyton mentagrophytes, M. canis, Epidermophyton* organisms (see Fig. 53-5, *B*)	Generally round or oval, erythematous scaling patch that spreads peripherally and clears centrally; may involve nails (tinea unguium) *Diagnosis*—Direct microscopic examination of scales Usually unilateral	Oral griseofulvin Local application of antifungal preparation such as tolnaftate, haloprogin, miconazole, clotrimazole; apply 1 in beyond periphery of lesion; continual application 1-2 wk after no sign of lesion	Usually of animal origin from infected pets Majority of infections in children caused by *M. canis* and *M. audouinii*
Tinea cruris ("jock itch")—*Epidermophyton floccosum, T. rubrum, T. mentagrophytes*	Skin response similar to that in tinea corporis Localized to medial proximal aspect of thigh and crural fold; may involve scrotum in males Pruritic *Diagnosis*—Same as for tinea corporis	Local application of tolnaftate liquid Wet compresses or sitz baths may be soothing	Rare in preadolescent children Health education regarding personal hygiene
Tinea pedis ("athlete's foot")—*T. rubrum, Trichophyton interdigitale, E. floccosum*	On intertriginous areas between toes or on plantar surface of feet Lesions vary: Maceration and fissuring between toes Patches with pinhead-sized vesicles on plantar surface Pruritic *Diagnosis*—Direct microscopic examination of scrapings	Oral griseofulvin Local applications of tolnaftate liquid and antifungal powder containing tolnaftate *Acute infections*—Compresses or soaks followed by application of glucocorticoid cream Elimination of conditions of heat and perspiration by clean, light socks and well-ventilated shoes; avoidance of occlusive shoes	Most frequent in adolescents and adults; rare in children, but occurrence increases with wearing of plastic shoes Transmission to other individuals rare despite general opinion to contrary Ointments not successful
Candidiasis (moniliasis)—*Candida albicans*	Grows in chronically moist areas Inflamed areas with white exudate, peeling, and easy bleeding Pruritic *Diagnosis*—Characteristic appearance	Amphotericin B, nystatin ointment, or other antifungal preparations to affected areas	Common form of diaper dermatitis (see Fig. 53-9) Oral form common in infants Vaginal form in older females May be disseminated in immunosuppressed children

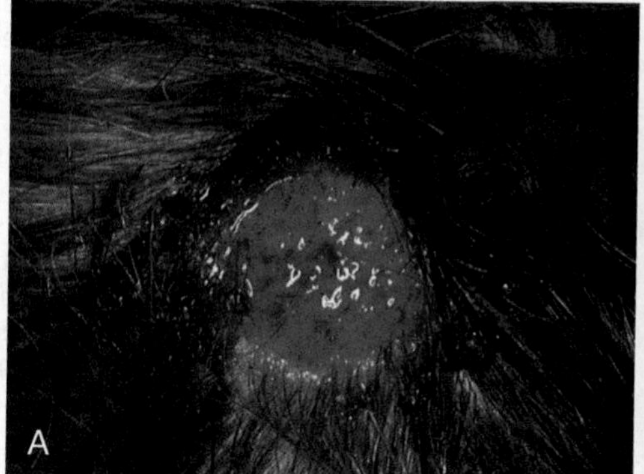

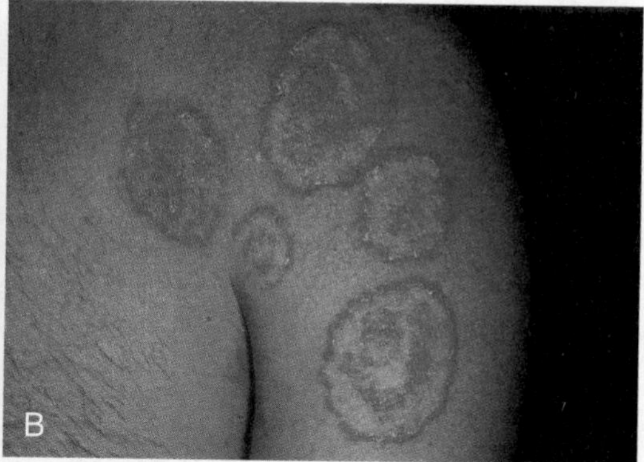

Fig. 53-5 A, Tinea capitis. **B,** Tinea corporis. Both infections are caused by *Microsporum canis,* the "kitten" or "puppy" fungus. (From Habif TP: *Clinical dermatology: a color guide to diagnosis and therapy,* ed 4, St Louis, 2004, Mosby.)

nodules, fungating masses, and abscesses. The course of deep fungal diseases is chronic with slow progression that favors sensitization (Table 53-6).

Skin Disorders Related to Chemical or Physical Contacts

Contact Dermatitis

Contact dermatitis is an inflammatory reaction of the skin to chemical substances, natural or synthetic, that evoke a hypersensitivity response or direct irritation. The initial reaction occurs in an exposed region, most commonly the face and neck, backs of the hands, forearms, male genitalia, and lower legs. Early in the reaction, there is usually a sharp delineation between inflamed and normal skin that ranges from a faint, transient erythema to massive bullae on an erythematous swollen base. Itching is a constant symptom.

The cause may be a primary irritant or a sensitizing agent. A *primary irritant* is one that irritates any skin. A *sensitizing agent* produces an irritation on those individuals who have met the irritant or something chemically related to it, have undergone an immunologic change, and have become sensitized. Prior exposure is not necessarily a factor in the reaction. A sensitizer irritates in relatively low concentrations only persons who are allergic to it.

In infants, contact dermatitis occurs on the convex surfaces of the diaper area (see Diaper Dermatitis, p. 1655). Other agents that produce contact dermatitis include plants (poison ivy, oak, or sumac), animal irritants (wool, feathers, and furs), metal (nickel found in jewelry and the snaps on sleepers and denim), vegetable irritants (oleoresins, oils, and turpentine), synthetic fabrics (e.g., shoe components), dyes, cosmetics, perfumes, and soaps (including bubble baths). The list is endless.

The major goal in treatment is to prevent further exposure of the skin to the offending substance. Provided there is no

Table 53-6 Systemic Mycoses

DISORDER AND ORGANISM	SKIN MANIFESTATIONS	SYSTEMIC MANIFESTATIONS	MANAGEMENT	COMMENTS
North American blastomycosis—*Blastomyces dermatitidis*	Chronic granulomatous lesions and microabscesses in any part of body Initial lesion a papule; undergoes ulceration and peripheral spread	Pulmonary symptoms, such as cough, chest pain, weakness, and weight loss May have skeletal involvement, with bone destruction and formation of cutaneous abscesses	Intravenous (IV) administration of amphotericin B	Usual portal of entry is lungs Source of infection unknown Noninfectious Pulmonary infections may be mild and self-limiting and require no treatment Progressive disease often fatal
Cryptococcosis—*Cryptococcus neoformans (Torula histolytica)*	Usually on face; acneiform, firm, nodular, painless eruption	*Central nervous system (CNS) manifestations*—Headache, dizziness, stiff neck, and signs of increased intracranial pressure Low-grade fever, mild cough, lung infiltration	IV amphotericin B; may be administered intrathecally for CNS involvement 5-Fluorocytosine for meningitis Excision and drainage of local lesions	Acquired by inhalation of dust but may enter through skin Prognosis serious Noninfectious Increased incidence in persons receiving corticosteroids with lymphoreticular malignancies, or type 2 diabetes
Histoplasmosis—*Histoplasma capsulatum*	Not distinctive or uniform, but most appear as punched-out or granulomatous ulcers	General systemic symptoms may include pallor, diarrhea, vomiting, irregular spiking temperature, hepatosplenomegaly, and pulmonary symptoms Any tissue of body may be involved with related symptoms	IV amphotericin B for severe cases Oral ketoconazole	Organism cultured from soil, especially where contaminated with fowl droppings Fungus enters through skin or mucous membranes of mouth and respiratory tract Endemic in Mississippi and Ohio River valleys Disseminated diseases most common in infants and children
Coccidioidomycosis (valley fever)—*Coccidioides immitis*	Erythema nodosum Erythema multiforme Erythematous maculopapular rash	Primary lung disease usually asymptomatic May be sign of acute febrile illness Disseminated disease is serious	IV amphotericin B IV miconazole (synthetic imidazole) Intraventricular miconazole plus oral ketoconazole for CNS involvement Surgical resection of persistent pulmonary cavities	Inhalation of aerospores from soil Endemic in southwestern United States Usually resolves spontaneously Increased incidence in dark-skinned races (Filipino, African-American, Mexican, Asian)

further irritation, the skin's normal recuperative powers will often produce healing without treatment. Otherwise, treatment of contact dermatitis is based on severity. Mild cases are treated with topical steroids. Mild to moderately severe cases may require a 2-week course of strong topical corticosteroids. Very severe cases require systemic corticosteroids (Kronemyer, 2003).

Nursing Care Management

Nurses frequently detect evidence of contact dermatitis during routine physical assessments. Skin manifestations in specific areas suggest limited contact, such as around the eyes (mascara), areas of the body covered by clothing but not protected by undergarments (wool), or areas of the body not covered by clothing (UV injury). Generalized involvement is more likely to be caused by bubble bath or soap. Often nurses can determine the offending agent and counsel families regarding management. However, if the lesions persist, are extensive, or show evidence of infection, medical evaluation is indicated.

Poison Ivy, Oak, and Sumac

Contact with the dry or succulent portions of any of three poisonous plants (ivy, oak, and sumac) produces localized, streaked or spotty, oozing, and painful impetiginous lesions. The offending substance in these plants is an oil, *urushiol*, that is extremely potent. Sensitivity to urushiol is not inborn but is developed after one or two exposures and may change over a lifetime. All parts of the plants contain the oil, including dried leaves and stems. Even smoke from burning brush piles can produce a reaction.

Animals do not seem to be affected by the oil; however, dogs or other animals that have run or played in the plants may carry the sap on their fur, and animals that eat the plants can transfer the oil in their saliva. Shoes, tools, and toys can transfer the oil. Golf balls that have been in the rough are another source of contact.

Urushiol takes effect as soon as it touches the skin. It penetrates through the epidermis and bonds with the dermal layer, where it initiates an immune response. The full-blown reaction is evident after about 2 days, with redness, swelling, and itching at the site of contact. Several days later, streaked or spotty blisters oozing serum from damaged cells produce the characteristic impetiginous lesions (Fig. 53-6). The lesions dry and heal spontaneously, and itching stops by 10 to 14 days.

Therapeutic Management

As soon as an exposure is realized, there is no time to waste. The earlier the skin is cleansed, the greater the chance of removing the urushiol before it attaches to the skin. The exposed skin can be cleansed with isopropyl alcohol followed by water. A shower with soap and warm water should follow. Clothes, tools, shoes, and any other objects that had contact with the plants should be cleaned with alcohol and then water.

Treatment of the lesions includes calamine lotion, soothing Burow's solution compresses, or Aveeno baths to relieve discomfort. Topical corticosteroid gel is effective for prevention or relief of inflammation, especially when applied before blisters form. Oral corticosteroids may be needed for severe

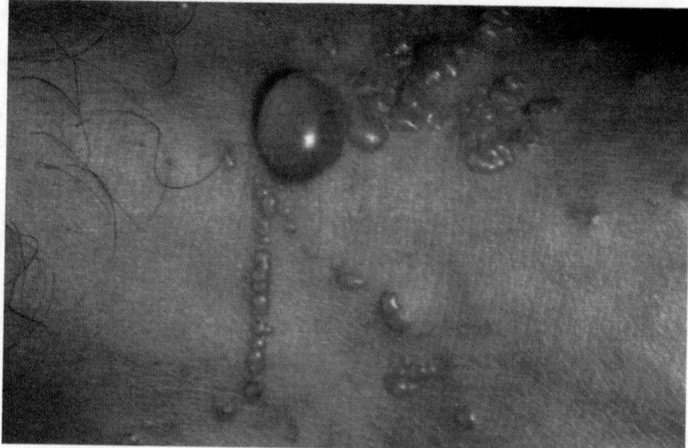

Fig. 53-6 Poison ivy lesions. Note "streaked" blisters surrounding one large blister. (From Habif TP: *Clinical dermatology: a color guide to diagnosis and therapy,* ed 4, St Louis, 2004, Mosby.)

evolve Case Study–Poison Ivy

CRITICAL THINKING EXERCISE

Poison Ivy

While at an overnight camp near a stream, Billy, age 9, runs up to the campfire and shows the nurse some leaves he has picked in the woods. The nurse recognizes the leaves as poison ivy. One of the adolescent assistants wants to throw the leaves on the campfire and scrub Billy's hands vigorously with soap. Billy's cabin mates ask the nurse: "Is poison ivy catching? Are we going to get it too?" What nursing actions should the camp nurse implement?

1. Evidence—Is there sufficient evidence to draw any conclusions at this time?
2. Assumptions—Describe some underlying assumptions about the following:
   a. The agent that causes poison ivy
   b. Effects of poison ivy on the skin
   c. Immediate treatment for poison ivy
   d. Contraindicated treatments for poison ivy
3. What implications and priorities for nursing care can be drawn at this time?
4. Does the evidence support this conclusion?
5. Are there alternative perspectives to your arguments?

reactions, and a sedative such as diphenhydramine may be ordered.

Nursing Care Management

When it is known that the child has made contact with the plant, the area is immediately flushed (preferably within 15 minutes) with *cold* running water to neutralize the urushiol not yet bonded to the skin. If there is a stream nearby, an effective method is to have the child enter the water (clothes and all) and allow the water to rinse the oil from both skin and clothing. Harsh soap is contraindicated because it removes protective skin oils and dilutes the urushiol, allowing it to spread; hard scrubbing irritates the skin. All clothing that has come in contact with the plant is removed with care and thoroughly laundered in hot water and detergent. Every effort is made to prevent the child from scratching the lesions. Although the lesions do not spread by contact with the blister serum or from scratching, they can become secondarily infected.

Prevention

Prevention is best accomplished by avoiding contact and removing the plant from the environment. All children, especially those known to be sensitive, should be taught to recognize the plant. Information regarding means for destroying plants can be obtained from the U.S. Department of Agriculture or U.S. Forestry Service If poisonous plants are growing in public community area, the local authorities should be contacted to remove the plants. A cream that protects exposed skin from poison oak and ivy is Ivy Block.

Drug Reactions

Adverse reactions to drugs are seen more often in the skin than in any other organ, although any organ of the body can be affected. The reaction may be a result of toxicity related to drug concentration, individual intolerance to the average dosage of the drug, or an allergic or idiosyncratic response. The manifestations may be associated with side effects or secondary effects of a drug, either of which are unrelated to its primary pharmacologic actions.

Although any drug is capable of producing a reaction in the susceptible individual, some drugs have a tendency to produce a particular reaction consistently, and others are more likely to produce an untoward effect. Many are allergenic responses that occur after a previous administration of the drug, even a topical application. Other factors influence a drug response in a particular individual. For example, the incidence increases with the amount and number of drugs given.

NURSING ALERT Intravenous (IV) drugs are more likely to cause a reaction than oral drugs. Stop the drug, but maintain the infusion with normal saline.

Manifestations of drug reactions may be delayed or immediate. A period of 7 days is usually required for a child to develop sensitivity to a drug that has never been administered previously. With prior sensitivity the manifestations appear almost immediately. Rashes are the most common manifestation of adverse drug reactions in children. However, individual drug reactions may vary from a single lesion to extensive, generalized epidermal necrosis such as that seen in Stevens-Johnson syndrome. Cutaneous manifestations can resemble almost any skin disease and can appear in almost any degree of severity. With few exceptions, the distribution of a drug eruption is widespread because it results from a circulating agent; appears as an inflammatory response with itching; is sudden in onset; and may be associated with constitutional symptoms such as fever, malaise, gastrointestinal upsets, anemia, or liver and kidney damage.

In most cases treatment for simple cutaneous reactions consists of discontinuing the drug. Sometimes a decision is made to continue the drug (such as an antibiotic in an infant or small child) until the cause of the rash is clearly indicated. In urticarial-type eruptions antihistamines may be ordered, and for widespread and severe lesions corticosteroids are beneficial. Severe anaphylactic reactions are a medical emergency (see Anaphylaxis, Chapter 48).

Nursing Care Management

The most effective means of management is prevention. Parents always remember a severe reaction. A careful history will elicit evidence of a previous drug reaction. The history should include the drug's name, nature of the reaction, drug dosage, and how soon after administration the reaction occurred (see Chapter 34).

Nurses who suspect that a rash is caused by a medication should withhold any further dose and report the eruption to the practitioner. Frequent offenders in drug reactions are penicillin and sulfonamides, and nurses must be alert to this possibility. However, even commonplace drugs, including aspirin, barbiturates, chemical agents in some foods, flavoring agents, and preservatives, are capable of producing an undesired response. Persons who have severe reactions should wear a medical identification bracelet or necklace in case of emergency or inadvertent administration of the offending drug.

Foreign Bodies

Parents can remove small wooden splinters with a needle and tweezers that have been sterilized with alcohol or a flame. The area around the sliver is washed with soap and water before removal is attempted. The sliver is exposed with the needle, then grasped firmly by the tweezers and pulled out. Some foreign bodies, such as a fishhook, pieces of glass, a difficult-to-see object, or a deeply embedded object (such as a needle in a foot or near a joint), require medical evaluation.

Small cactus prickles or spines are troublesome to remove, but the following methods may prove helpful:

- Apply a thin layer of water-soluble household glue and cover with gauze; when the glue dries, peel off the gauze.
- Apply hair removal wax or body sugar, let dry, and remove.
- Place cellophane tape, sticky side down, over the spines and lift off.

Skin Disorders Related to Animal Contacts

Arthropod Bites and Stings

Bites and stings account for a significant amount of mild to moderate discomfort in children. Most bites and stings are managed by simple symptomatic measures, such as compresses, calamine lotion, and prevention of secondary infection. *Arthropods* include insects and arachnids, such as mites, ticks, spiders, and scorpions. Most arthropods in the United States, including tarantulas, are relatively harmless. Although all spiders produce venom that is injected via fangs, some are unable to pierce the skin and others produce venom that is insufficiently toxic to be harmful. Only scorpions and two spiders—the brown recluse and the black widow—inject venom deadly enough to require immediate attention. Children bitten by these arachnids must receive medical attention as soon as possible. Major offending creatures, their manifestations, and management are outlined in Table 53-7.

When a hymenopteran (bees in particular) stings, its barbed stinger penetrates the skin. As long as the stinger

Table 53-7 Skin Lesions Caused by Arthropods

MECHANISM AND CHARACTERISTIC	MANIFESTATIONS	MANAGEMENT
Insect Bites—Flies, Gnats, Mosquitoes, Fleas		
Mechanism—Foreign protein in insects' saliva introduced when skin is penetrated for a blood-sucking meal Distribution: Almost everywhere—Fleas, mosquitoes, ants Suburbs and rural areas—Bees Urban areas—Hornets, wasps, yellow jackets	Hypersensitivity reaction Papular urticaria Firm papules; may be capped by vesicles or excoriated Little or no reaction in nonsensitized person	Treatment: Use antipruritic agents and baths. Administer antihistamines. Prevent secondary infection. Prevention: Avoid contact. Remove focus, such as treating furniture, mattresses, carpets, and pets, where insects may live. Apply insect repellent when exposure is anticipated.
Chiggers—Harvest Mites		
Mechanism—Attach with claws and secrete a digestive substance that liquefies the host's epidermis Manifestations: Erythematous papules Intense itching	Same as insect bites Favor warm areas of body, especially intertriginous areas and areas covered with clothing	Avoid contact, especially in areas of tall grass and underbrush. Apply insect repellant when exposure is anticipated. Administer systemic steroids for extensive bites.
Hymenopterans—Bees, Wasps, Hornets, Yellow Jackets, Fire Ants		
Mechanism: Injection of venom through stinging apparatus Venom contains histamine; allergenic proteins; and often a spreading factor, hyaluronidase Severe reactions caused by hypersensitivity or multiple stings	*Local reaction*—Small red area, wheal, itching, and heat *Systemic reactions*—May be mild to severe, including generalized edema, pain, nausea and vomiting, confusion, respiratory embarrassment, and shock	Treatment: Carefully scrape off stinger or pull out stinger as quickly as possible. Cleanse with soap and water. Apply cool compresses. Apply common household product (e.g., lemon juice, paste made with aspirin or baking soda). Administer antihistamines. *Severe reactions*—Administer epinephrine, corticosteroids; treat for shock. Prevention: Teach child to wear shoes; to avoid wearing bright clothing, flowery prints, shiny jewelry, or perfumed grooming products (cologne, scented hairspray), which might attract the insect; and to avoid places where the insect may be contacted. Hypersensitive children should wear medical identification to indicate allergy and therapy needed; family should keep emergency medication and be taught its administration.
Black Widow Spider		
Mechanism—Venom injected through a clawlike appendage; has neurotoxic action Characteristics: Shiny black spider, with a body about 1.25 cm (½ inch) long and a red or orange hourglass-shaped marking on underside Avoids light and bites in self-defense	Mild sting at time of bite Area becomes swollen, painful, and erythematous Dizziness, weakness, and abdominal pain May produce delirium, paralysis, seizures, and (if large amount of venom absorbed) death	Treatment: Cleanse wound with antiseptic. Apply cool compresses. Administer antivenin. Administer muscle relaxant, such as calcium gluconate; analgesics or sedatives; hydrocortisone or diazepam intravenously. *Prevention*—Teach children to avoid places that harbor the spider (e.g., woodpiles).
Brown Recluse Spider		
Mechanism: Venom injected via fangs Venom contains powerful necrotoxin Characteristics: Slender spider, with long legs and body length of 1-2 cm; color is fawn to dark brown; recognized by fiddle-shaped mark on head Shy; bites only when annoyed or surprised Prefers dark areas where seldom disturbed	Mild sting at time of bite Transient erythema followed by bleb or blister; mild to severe pain in 2-8 hr; purple, star-shaped area in 3-4 days; necrotic ulceration in 7-14 days Systemic reactions may include fever, malaise, restlessness, nausea, vomiting, and joint pain Generalized petechial eruption Wounds heal with scar formation	Treatment: Apply cool compresses locally. Administer antibiotics, corticosteroids. Relieve pain. Wound may require skin graft. *Prevention*—Teach children to avoid possible nesting sites.

Continued

Table 53-7 Skin Lesions Caused by Arthropods—cont'd

MECHANISM AND CHARACTERISTIC	MANIFESTATIONS	MANAGEMENT
Scorpions Mechanism: Sting by means of a hooked caudal stinger that discharges venom Venom of more venomous species contains hemolysins, endotheliolysins, and neurotoxins *Characteristics*—Usual habitat southwestern United States	Intense local pain, erythema, numbness, burning, restlessness, vomiting Ascending motor paralysis with seizures, weakness, rapid pulse, excessive salivation, thirst, dysuria, pulmonary edema, coma, and death Some species produce only local tissue reaction with swelling at puncture site (distinctive) Symptoms subside in a few hours Deaths occur among children <4 yr of age, usually in first 24 hr	Treatment: Delay absorption of venom by keeping child quiet; place involved area in dependent position. Administer antivenin. Relieve pain. Admit to pediatric intensive care unit for surveillance. *Prevention*—Teach children to avoid possible nesting sites.
Ticks *Mechanism*—In process of sucking blood, head and mouth parts are buried in skin Characteristics: Feed on blood of mammals Significant in humans because of pathologic organism carried May be vectors of various infectious diseases, such as Rocky Mountain spotted fever, Q fever, tularemia, relapsing fever, Lyme disease, tick paralysis Must attach and feed for 1-2 hr to transmit disease Usual habitat is wooded area	Tick usually attached to skin, head embedded Produce firm, discrete, intensely pruritic nodules at site of attachment May cause urticaria or persistent localized edema	Treatment: Grasp tick with tweezers (forceps) as close as possible to point of attachment. Pull straight up with steady, even pressure; if bare hands, use a tissue to touch tick during removal; wash hands thoroughly with soap and water. Remove any remaining part (e.g., head) with sterile needle. Cleanse wounds with soap and disinfectant. Prevention: Teach children to avoid areas where prevalent. Inspect skin (especially scalp) after being in wooded areas. See discussion on p. 1653.

remains in the skin, the muscles push the stinger deeper and the venom is pumped into the wound. The best approach is to remove the stinger as quickly as possible and to get away from the vicinity of other insects to prevent further injury. Children who have become sensitized to hymenopteran bites may demonstrate a severe systemic response that can be life threatening. One sting can produce generalized urticaria, respiratory difficulty (from laryngeal edema), hypotension, and death. Intramuscular administration of epinephrine provides immediate relief and must be available for emergency use.

Hypersensitive children should wear a medical identification bracelet. They should also have a kit that contains epinephrine and a hypodermic syringe. Families are reminded to check the expiration date on the kit and to replace an outdated one. They should determine whether a nurse is available at the school and the school policy regarding administration of drugs. If a school nurse is not present, someone at the school should be designated to inject the epinephrine in case of an emergency.

Scabies

Scabies is an endemic infestation caused by the scabies mite, *Sarcoptes scabiei*. Lesions are created as the impregnated female burrows into the stratum corneum of the epidermis (never into living tissue) to deposit her eggs and feces. The inflammatory response and intense itching occur after the host becomes sensitized to the mite, approximately 30 to 60 days after initial contact. If the person has been previously sensitized to the mite, the response occurs within 48 hours after exposure. After this time, the areas over which the mite has traveled will begin to itch and develop the characteristic eruption (Box 53-1). Consequently, mites will not necessarily be located at all sites of eruption.

The types of lesions demonstrate great variability. Infants often develop an eczematous eruption; therefore the observer must look for discrete papules, burrows, or vesicles.

BOX 53-1 Clinical Manifestations of Scabies

Lesion

Children—Minute grayish brown, threadlike (mite burrows), pruritic
- Black dot at end of burrow (mite)

Infants—Eczematous eruption, pruritic

Distribution

Generally in intertriginous areas—Interdigital, axillary-cubital, popliteal, inguinal

Children older than 2 years of age—Primarily hands and wrists

Children younger than 2 years—Primarily feet and ankles

Nursing Care Management

The treatment of scabies is the application of a scabicide. Currently, permethrin 5% cream (Elimite) is the drug of choice. Alternative drugs are 1% lindane cream or lotion and 10%

crotamiton. Permethrin is preferred because it is safer, it avoids the risk of neurotoxicity, and it is more effective than lindane. Nurses instructing families in the use of scabicides should emphasize the importance of following directions carefully. Lindane should not be used immediately after a bath or shower. Permethrin is applied to all skin surfaces from the neck down to the toes (not just areas with rash, but also areas between the fingers and toes, the umbilicus, and the cleft of the buttocks). The cream should remain on the skin for 8 to 14 hours and then be removed by bathing. Lindane is removed by bathing after 8 to 12 hours. A second treatment with the same lotion may be required 7 to 10 days later. Lindane should not be used for preterm infants, young infants, people with known seizure disorders, people with hypersensitivity to the product, patients with crusted scabies, or patients with extensive dermatitis. Pregnant women and younger children are often treated with milder scabies medications. Crotamiton is applied once a day for 2 days, followed by a cleansing bath 48 hours after the last application. All clothes, bedding, and towels used by the infested person 3 days before treatment should be washed in hot water and dried in a hot dryer (Centers for Disease Control and Prevention, Division of Parasitic Diseases, 2008).

Another prescription drug used to treat scabies is ivermectin (Frankowski & Weiner, 2002). Ivermectin is administered orally in a single dose for treatment of severe or crusted scabies. It should be considered for patients whose infestation is refractory or those who cannot tolerate topical scabicides. However, the safety and efficacy of ivermectin for pediatric patients younger than 5 years of age or children weighing less than 15 kg (33 lb) is not established. This drug is not currently licensed for treatment of scabies by the FDA (American Academy of Pediatrics, Committee on Infectious Diseases, 2006). Families need to know that although this treatment will kill the mite that causes scabies, it will not eliminate the rash and the itch until the stratum corneum is replaced in approximately 2 to 3 weeks. Soothing ointments or lotions can be applied for itching. Antibiotics may be given for secondary infection.

Pediculosis Capitis

Pediculosis capitis (head lice) is an infestation of the scalp by *Pediculus humanus capitis,* a common parasite in school-age children. The adult louse lives only about 48 hours when away from a human host, and the life span of the average female is 1 month. The female lays her eggs at night at the junction of a hair shaft and close to the skin because the eggs need a warm environment. The *nits,* or eggs, hatch in approximately 7 to 10 days. Itching is usually the only symptom. Common areas involved are the occipital area, behind the ears, and the nape of the neck (Box 53-2).

BOX 53-2 Clinical Manifestations of Pediculosis

Pruritus (caused by crawling insects and insect saliva on skin)
Nits observable on hair shaft (see Fig. 53-7)

Distribution

Occipital area
Behind ears
Nape of neck
Eyebrows and eyelashes (occasionally) (caused by pubic lice)

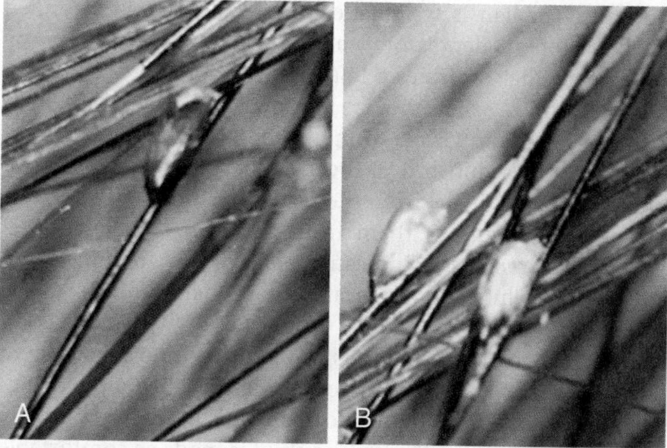

Fig. 53-7 A, Empty nit case. B, Viable nits. (From *The contemporary approach to the control of head lice in schools and communities,* Pittsburgh, 1991, SmithKline Beecham.)

Diagnostic Evaluation

Diagnosis is made by observation of the white eggs (nits) firmly attached to the hair shafts (Fig. 53-7). Because of their brief life span and mobility, adult lice are more difficult to locate. Nits must be differentiated from dandruff, lint, hair spray, and other items of similar size and shape. Scratch marks or inflammatory papules, caused by secondary infection, may also be found on the scalp in the vulnerable areas.

Therapeutic Management

Treatment consists of the application of pediculicides and manual removal of nit cases. The drug of choice for infants and children is permethrin 1% cream rinse (Nix), which kills adult lice and nits. This product and preparations of pyrethrin with piperonyl butoxide (RID or A-200 Pyrinate) can be obtained without a prescription and are more effective and safer than lindane (Strong & Johnstone, 2008). The FDA has issued a warning regarding the use of lindane because of the potential for neurotoxicity (US Food and Drug Administration, 2003). Although the FDA believes that the benefits of lindane outweigh the risks when used as directed, patients should be treated with these medications when other treatments are not tolerable or have failed. Another product approved for treatment of head lice, malathion 0.5% (Ovide), is available only by prescription. However, malathion contains flammable alcohol, must remain on the hair for 8 to 12 hours, and is not recommended for children younger than 6 years of age.

Because of concerns that head lice may be developing resistance to chemical shampoos and that repeated exposure of children to strong chemicals on the scalp may be unwise, effective nonchemical control measures are essential. Daily removal of nits from the child's hair with a metal nit comb at least every 2 or 3 days is a control measure after treatment with a pediculicide (Mumcuoglu et al, 2007).

Nursing Care Management

An important nursing role is educating the parents about pediculosis. Nurses should emphasize that *anyone* can get pediculosis; it has no respect for age, socioeconomic level, or cleanliness. The louse does not jump or fly, but it can be transmitted from one person to another on personal items. Lice are more likely to infest Caucasian children, those with straight hair, and girls. Children are cautioned against sharing combs, hair ornaments, hats, caps, scarves, coats, and other items used on or near the hair. Children who share lockers are more likely to become infested, and slumber parties place children at risk. Lice are not carried or transmitted by pets.

Nurses or parents should carefully inspect children who scratch their head more than usual for bite marks, redness, and nits. The hair is systematically spread with two flat-sided sticks or tongue depressors, and the scalp is observed for any movement that indicates a louse. Nurses should wear gloves when examining the hair. Lice are small and grayish tan, have no wings, and are visible to the naked eye. The nits, or eggs, appear as tiny whitish oval specks adhering to the hair shaft about 6 mm (¼ inch) from the scalp. The adherent nature of the nits distinguishes them from dandruff, which falls off readily. *Empty nit cases*, indicating hatched lice, are translucent rather than white and are located more than 6 mm from the scalp (see Fig. 53-7).

If evidence of infestation is found, it is important to treat the child according to the directions on the label of the pediculicide. Parents are advised to read the directions carefully before beginning treatment. The child is made as comfortable as possible during the application process because the pediculicide must remain on the scalp and hair for several minutes. Playing "beauty parlor" during the shampoo is a useful strategy. The child lies supine, with the head over a sink or basin, and covers the eyes with a dry towel or washcloth. This prevents medication, which can cause chemical conjunctivitis, from splashing into the eyes. If eye irritation occurs, the eyes must be flushed well with tepid water. It is not necessary to remove the nits after treatment because only live lice cause infestation. However, because none of the pediculicides is 100% effective in killing all the eggs, the makers of some pediculicides recommend manual removal of the nits after treatment (Centers for Disease Control, Division of Parasitic Diseases, 2005). An extra-fine-tooth comb that is included in many commercial pediculicides or is available at community pharmacies facilitates manual removal. If the comb is ineffective in removing the nit cases, the examiner should remove them by scraping them off the strands of hair with his or her fingernails.

Live lice survive for up to 48 hours away from the host, but nits are shed into the environment and are capable of hatching in 7 to 10 days; retreatment may be required (Centers for Disease Control, Division of Parasitic Diseases, 2005). Therefore measures must be taken to prevent further infestation (see Patient Teaching box). Spraying with insecticide is not recommended because of the danger to children and animals. Families should also be advised that the pediculicide is relatively expensive, especially when several members of the household require treatment. Families may be inclined to try home remedies to treat the lice. A study by (Lee and colleagues (2004) showed that home remedies such as petroleum jelly, oils, vinegar, butter, alcohol, and mayonnaise did little to kill louse eggs but increased the risk for skin infection with *S. aureus.* Another study by Pearlman (2004) showed that dry-on pediculicide lotions may effectively treat lice without the use of current shampoos with neurotoxins, nit removal, or extensive housecleaning. Another study (Goates et al, 2006) demonstrated that one 3-minute application of hot air has the potential to eliminate lice infestations.

PATIENT TEACHING Preventing the Spread and Recurrence of Pediculosis

- Machine wash all washable clothing, towels, and bed linens in hot water, and dry in a hot dryer for at least 20 minutes. Dry clean nonwashable items.
- Thoroughly vacuum carpets, car seats, pillows, stuffed animals, rugs, mattresses, and upholstered furniture.
- Seal nonwashable items in plastic bags for 14 days if unable to dry clean or vacuum.
- Soak combs, brushes, and hair accessories in lice-killing products for 1 hour or in boiling water for 10 minutes.
- In day care centers, store children's clothing items such as hats and scarves and other headgear in separate cubicles.
- Discourage the sharing of items such as hats, scarves, hair accessories, combs, and brushes among children in group settings such as day care centers.
- Avoid physical contact with infested individuals and their belongings, especially clothing and bedding.
- Inspect children in a group setting regularly for head lice.
- Provide educational programs on the transmission of pediculosis, its detection, and treatment.

Modified from Chin J (editor): *Control of communicable diseases manual,* Washington, DC, 2000, American Public Health Association.

Prevention

The increasing incidence of pediculosis in schoolchildren is a serious concern for school nurses, parents, and community health agencies. However, school head lice screening programs have not proven to have a significant effect on the incidence of head lice in the school setting; parent education programs may be more helpful in the management of head lice. Children with head lice should be allowed to return to school after proper treatment. Both the American Academy of Pediatrics and the National Association of School Nurses discourage a "no nit" policy for schools (Frankowski & Weiner, 2002).

Rickettsial Diseases

Rickettsiae, the organisms responsible for a number of disorders (Table 53-8), are transmitted to human beings via arthropods. Mammals become infected only through the bites of infected lice, fleas, ticks, and mites, all of which serve as both infectors and reservoirs. Rickettsiae are intracellular parasites, similar in size to bacteria that inhabit the alimentary tract of a wide range of natural hosts. Rickettsial diseases are more common in temperate and tropical climates where humans live in association with arthropods. Infection in humans is

Table 53-8 Eruptions Caused by Rickettsiae

DISORDER, ORGANISM, AND HOST	MANIFESTATIONS	MANAGEMENT	COMMENTS
Rocky Mountain spotted fever—*Rickettsia rickettsii* *Arthropod*—Tick *Transmission*—Tick *Mammal source*—Wild rodents, dogs	*Gradual onset*—Fever, malaise, anorexia, myalgia *Abrupt onset*—Rapid temperature elevation, chills, vomiting, myalgia, severe headache Maculopapular or petechial rash primarily on extremities (ankles and wrists) but may spread to other areas, characteristically on palms and soles	*Control*—Protection from tick bite by wearing proper apparel, tick repellent Tetracycline or chloramphenicol Vigorous supportive therapy	Usually self-limiting in children Onset in children may resemble any infectious disease Severe disease rare in children Inspect children and dogs regularly if they play in wooded areas See Table 53-7 for management of ticks
Epidemic typhus—*Rickettsia prowazekii* *Arthropod*—Body louse *Transmission*—Infected feces into broken skin *Mammal source*—Humans	Abrupt onset of chills, fever, diffuse myalgia, headache, malaise Maculopapular rash becoming petechial 4-7 days later, spreading from trunk outward	*Control*—Immediate destruction of vectors Tetracycline or chloramphenicol Supportive treatment	Patient should be isolated until deloused See discussion on p. 1651 for management of pediculosis Excreta from infected lice also in dust; disinfect patient's clothing, bedding, and possessions and wash in hot water
Endemic typhus—*Rickettsia typhi* *Arthropod*—Rat fleas or lice *Transmission*—Flea bite; inhaling or ingesting flea excreta *Mammal source*—Rats	Headache, arthralgia, backache followed by fever; may last 9-14 days Maculopapular rash after 1-8 days of fever; begins in trunk and spreads to periphery; rarely involves face, palms, soles	*Control*—Eliminate rat reservoir, insect vectors, or both Tetracycline or chloramphenicol Supportive treatment	Fairly common in United States Shorter duration than epidemic typhus Mild, seldom fatal illness Difficult to distinguish from epidemic typhus
Rickettsialpox—*Rickettsia akari* *Arthropod*—Mouse mite *Transmission*—Mite *Mammal source*—House mouse	Maculopapular rash following primary lesion; eschar at site of bite; fever, chills, headache	*Control*—Eradication of rodent reservoir and mite vector Tetracycline or chloramphenicol Supportive treatment	Self-limiting nonfatal disease Endemic in New York City Found in many cities in United States

incidental (except epidemic typhus) and not necessary for the survival of the rickettsial species. However, after the organism invades a human, it causes a disease that varies in intensity from a benign, self-limiting illness to a disease that is fulminating and fatal.

Lyme Disease

Lyme disease is the most common tick-borne disorder in the United States. It is caused by the spirochete *Borrelia burgdorferi,* which enters the skin and bloodstream through the saliva and feces of ticks, especially the deer tick. Most cases of Lyme disease are reported in the Northeast from southern Maine to northern Virginia. The disease may initially appear in any of three stages:

1. *Stage 1* consists of the tick bite at the time of inoculation, followed in 3 to 31 days by the development of *erythema migrans* at the site of the bite (Fig. 53-8).
2. *Stage 2,* the most serious stage of the disease, is characterized by systemic involvement of neurologic, cardiac, and musculoskeletal systems that appears several weeks after the cutaneous phase is completed.
3. *Stage 3,* or the late stage, includes musculoskeletal pain that involves the tendons, bursae, muscles, and synovia. Arthritis may occur, and late neurologic problems include deafness and chronic encephalopathy.

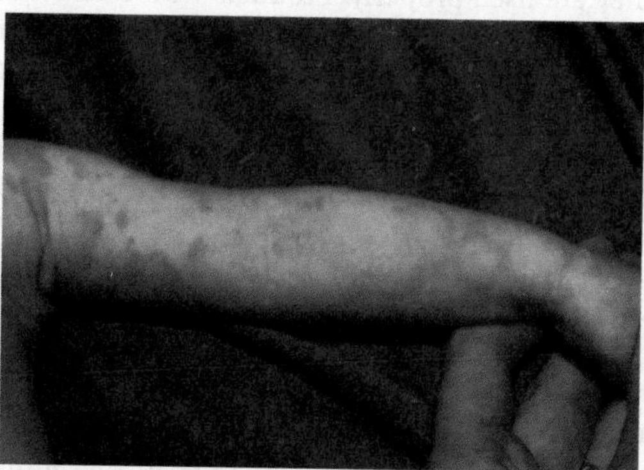

Fig. 53-8 Lyme disease. Note annular red rings in erythema chronicum migrans. (From Weston WL, Lane AT: *Color textbook of pediatric dermatology,* ed 4, St Louis, 2007, Mosby.)

Diagnostic Evaluation

Diagnosis is best made clinically during the early stages by recognizing the characteristic rash, erythema migrans. Serologic testing may be used to establish the diagnosis in later stages of the disease.

Therapeutic Management

Early and appropriate treatment is essential to prevent complications. Children older than 8 years of age are treated with oral doxycycline; amoxicillin is recommended for children younger than 8 years of age (American Academy of Pediatrics, Committee on Infectious Diseases, 2006). For patients allergic to penicillin, alternative drugs include cefuroxime or erythromycin (Wade, 2000). Most experts treat individuals with early Lyme disease for 14 to 21 days. Persons who have removed ticks from themselves should be monitored closely for signs and symptoms of tick-borne diseases for 30 days; in particular they should be monitored for erythema migrans, a red expanding skin lesion at the site of the tick bite that may suggest Lyme disease. People who develop a skin lesion or viral infection–like illness within 1 month of an attached tick should seek prompt medical attention (Wormser et al, 2006). Treatment of erythema migrans most often prevents development of later stages of Lyme disease.

Nursing Care Management

The major thrust of nursing care should be educating parents to protect their children from exposure to ticks. Children should avoid tick-infested areas or wear light-colored clothing so that ticks can be spotted easily, tuck pant legs into socks, and wear a long-sleeved shirt tucked into pants when in wooded areas. Parents and children need to perform regular tick checks when they are in infested areas (with special attention to the scalp, neck, armpits, and groin areas). Parents should also be alert for signs of the skin lesion, especially if their children have been in tick-infested areas. Insect repellents containing diethyltoluamide (DEET) and permethrin can protect against ticks, but parents should use these chemicals cautiously. Although there have been reports of serious neurologic complications in children resulting from frequent and excessive application of DEET repellants, the risk is low when they are used properly. Products with DEET should be applied sparingly according to label instructions and not applied to a child's face or hands or to any areas of irritated skin. After the child returns indoors, treated skin should be washed with soap and water. Information about Lyme disease can be obtained from the American Lyme Disease Foundation, Inc.*

Mammal Bites and Scratches

Pet and Wild Animal Bites

Animal bites are common in childhood. However, children are bitten more often by animals belonging to the family or to neighbors than by stray animals. The majority of victims of dog bites are boys between the ages of 5 and 9 years (Centers for Disease Control and Prevention, 2003; Bernardo et al, 2000). Most dog or cat injuries are to the upper extremities. Small children are likely to be bitten or scratched on the head, face, and neck because they tend to put their heads near the animal's head and flail their arms rather than protecting their heads. Animal bites are potentially serious because of the likelihood of significant infection. Injuries vary in intensity from small puncture wounds to complete evulsion of tissue that is associated with significant crush injury.

*PO Box 466, Lyme, CT 06371; e-mail: inquire@aldf.com; www.aldf.com.

Therapeutic Management

General wound care consists of rinsing the wound with copious amounts of saline or Ringer's lactate under pressure via a large syringe and of washing the surrounding skin with mild soap. A clean pressure dressing is applied, and the extremity is elevated if the wound is bleeding. Medical evaluation is advised because of the danger of tetanus and rabies, although dogs in most urban areas must be immunized against rabies. Bites from wild animals, such as squirrels, bats, raccoons, foxes, and skunks, are also dangerous.

Prophylactic antibiotics are indicated for puncture wounds and wounds in areas that may prove to be cosmetically or functionally impaired if infected. Extensive lacerations are debrided and loosely sutured to allow drainage in the event of infection. Tetanus toxoid is administered according to standard guidelines (see Immunizations, Chapter 36), and rabies protocol is followed (see Rabies, Chapter 51). Injuries to poorly vascularized areas, such as the hands, are more likely to become infected than those in more vascularized areas, such as the face; puncture wounds are more likely to become infected than lacerations.

Nursing Care Management

The most important aspect related to animal bites is prevention. Children should understand animal behavior and develop respect for animals (see Patient Teaching box). Parents should monitor their children's behavior with a dog and instruct them not to tease or surprise a dog, invade its territory, interfere with its feeding or sleeping, take its toy, or interact with a sick or injured dog or a dog with pups. Parents who are considering getting a pet, especially a dog, for themselves or their children should select a dog that has a high level of sociability with, and is unlikely to be a danger to, children.

Human Bites

Children often acquire lacerations from the teeth of other humans in rough play, during fights, or as victims of child abuse. Many preschool children bite others out of frustration or anger. Because human dental plaque and gingiva harbor pathogenic organisms, all human bites should receive attention. Delayed treatment increases the risk of infection.

If the laceration is less than 6 mm (¼ inch) in length, the wound can be treated at home. The wound is washed vigorously with soap and water, and a pressure dressing is applied to stop bleeding. Ice applications minimize discomfort and swelling. Increased pain or redness at the wound site is an indication that the child should receive medical attention for antibiotic therapy. Tetanus toxoid is needed if the child is insufficiently immunized. Wounds larger than 6 mm should receive medical attention.

Cat-Scratch Disease

Cat-scratch disease is the most common cause of regional lymphadenitis in children and adolescents. It usually follows the scratch or bite of an animal (a cat or kitten in 99% of cases). The disease is usually a benign, self-limiting illness that resolves spontaneously in about 2 to 4 months. Diagnosis is

PATIENT TEACHING Animal Safety

- Teach children to avoid all strange animals, especially wild, sick, or injured ones, who may be carriers of rabies (use the same techniques employed in teaching children not to talk to strangers).
- Teach children to avoid dangerous and nervous animals in the neighborhood.
- Vaccinate your own dog against rabies.
- Never permit children to break up an animal fight, even when their own pet is involved. Use a rake, broom, or garden hose to separate animals.
- Teach children the danger of mistreating or teasing pets (animals will bite if mauled, annoyed, or frightened).
- Spay or neuter your pets (spaying or neutering reduces aggression, not protectiveness).
- Avoid direct eye contact with a threatening dog, and remain motionless until the dog leaves the area.
- Never hold your face close to an animal.
- Teach children not to disturb an animal that is eating; sleeping; or caring for young puppies, kittens, etc.
- Never tease; pull the tail; or take away food, a bone, or a toy with which an animal is playing.
- Never approach a strange dog that is confined or restrained; do not keep animals confined with short ropes or chains (this can make them aggressive or vicious, especially when teased).
- Do not run, ride a bicycle, or skate in front of a dog (it will startle the dog); teach children the importance of avoiding bike routes where dogs are known to chase vehicles.
- Do not allow an inexperienced child or adult to feed a dog (if the person pulls back when the animal moves to take the food, this can frighten and startle the animal).
- If a dog is asleep or unaware of your presence or has not seen you approach, speak to the animal to make it aware of your presence to avoid startling the animal.
- Allow a dog to see and sniff a child before the child attempts to pet the animal.
- Do not permit a child to lead a large dog.
- Train or socialize a dog for appropriate behavior; avoid aggressive play with pets.
- Do not adopt pets for children until children demonstrate their maturity and ability to handle and care for pets.

From Humane Society of the United States: *Preventing and avoiding dog bites*, Washington, DC, 1998, The Society.

made on the basis of (1) history of contact with a cat or kitten, (2) the presence of regional lymphadenopathy for several days, and (3) serologic identification of the causative organism by indirect fluorescent antibody assay or polymerase chain reaction test. The disease may persist for several months before gradual resolution. In some children, especially those who are immunocompromised, the adenitis may progress to suppuration and serious complications. Treatment is primarily supportive, but antibiotic therapy may hasten the resolution of adenopathy in the disease (Centers for Disease Control and Prevention, 2002).

Miscellaneous Skin Disorders

A number of miscellaneous skin lesions occur in children. Some occur as a result of congenital disorders and are inherited as an autosomal dominant trait. *Ichthyoses* are a heterogeneous group of disorders characterized by scaling that create challenging problems in treatment. These disorders are not discussed in detail here because of their wide variability.

Skin Disorders Associated with Specific Age Groups

Several common dermatologic conditions are confined to children in specific age groups. These conditions include diaper, atopic, and seborrheic dermatitis, which occurs predominantly in infants, and acne, which is most common in adolescence.

Diaper Dermatitis

Diaper dermatitis is common in infants and is one of several acute inflammatory skin disorders caused either directly or indirectly by wearing diapers. The peak age of occurrence is 9 to 12 months of age, and the incidence is greater in bottle-fed infants than in breast-fed infants.

Pathophysiology and Clinical Manifestations

Diaper dermatitis is caused by prolonged and repetitive contact with an irritant (e.g., urine, feces, soaps, detergents, ointments, friction). Although the irritant in the majority of cases is urine and feces, a combination of factors contributes to irritation.

Prolonged contact of the skin with diaper wetness produces higher friction, greater abrasion damage, increased transepidermal permeability, and increased microbial counts. Healthy skin is less resistant to potential irritants.

Although ammonia was once thought to cause diaper rash because of its association with the strong odor on diapers and dermatitis, ammonia alone is not sufficient. The irritant quality of urine is related to an increase in pH from the breakdown of urea in the presence of fecal urease. The increased pH promotes the activity of fecal enzymes, principally the proteases and lipases, which act as irritants. Fecal enzymes also increase the permeability of skin to bile salts, another potential irritant in feces.

The eruption of diaper dermatitis is manifested primarily on convex surfaces or in folds. The lesions represent a variety of types and configurations. Eruptions involving the skin in most intimate contact with the diaper (e.g., the convex surfaces of buttocks, inner thighs, mons pubis, scrotum) but sparing the folds are likely to be caused by chemical irritants, especially from urine and feces (Fig. 53-9). Other causes are detergents or soaps from inadequately rinsed cloth diapers or the chemicals in disposable wipes. Perianal involvement is usually the result of chemical irritation from feces, especially diarrheal stools. *Candida albicans* infection produces perianal inflammation and a maculopapular rash with satellite lesions that may cross the inguinal fold (Fig. 53-10). It is seen in up

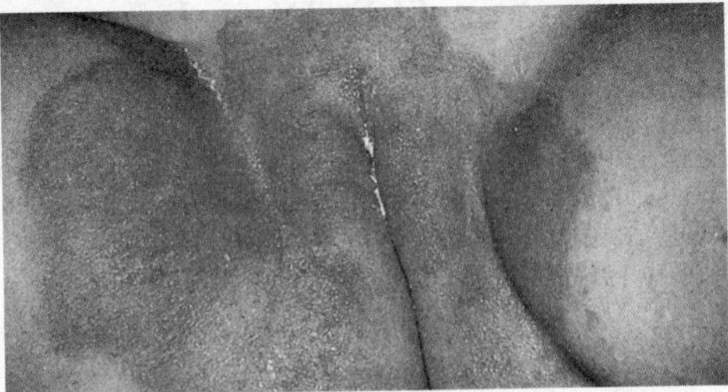

Fig. 53-9 Irritant diaper dermatitis. Note sharply demarcated edges. (From Habif TP: *Clinical dermatology: a color guide to diagnosis and therapy,* ed 4, St Louis, 2003, Mosby.)

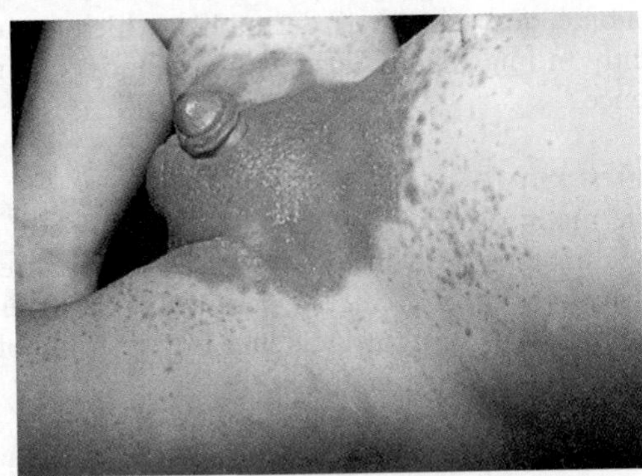

Fig. 53-10 Candidiasis of diaper area. Note beefy red central erythema with satellite pustules. (From Weston WL, Lane AT, Morelli JG: *Color textbook of pediatric dermatology,* ed 4, St Louis, 2007, Mosby.)

to 90% of infants with chronic diaper dermatitis and should be considered in diaper rashes that are recalcitrant to treatment.

Nursing Care Management

Nursing interventions are aimed at altering the three factors that produce dermatitis: wetness, pH, and fecal irritants. The most significant factor amenable to intervention is the moist environment created in the diaper area. Changing the diaper as soon as it becomes wet eliminates a large part of the problem, and removing the diaper to expose healthy skin to air facilitates drying. The use of a hair dryer or heat lamp is not recommended because these devices can cause burns.

Diaper construction has a significant impact on the incidence and severity of diaper dermatitis. Superabsorbent disposable paper diapers reduce diaper dermatitis. They contain an absorbent gelling material that binds water tightly to decrease skin wetness, maintains pH control by providing a buffering capacity, and decreases skin irritation by preventing mixing of urine and feces in the diaper. Another advance in diapers is the addition of an inner layer or top sheet that is impregnated with petrolatum (as in Pampers Swaddler with Absorb Away Liner).

Guidelines for controlling diaper rash are presented in the Patient Teaching box. A common misconception about using cornstarch on skin is that it promotes the growth of *C. albicans.* Neither cornstarch nor talc promotes the growth of fungi under conditions normally found in the diaper area. Cornstarch is more effective in reducing friction and tends to cake less than talc when the skin is wet. On the basis of these properties and its safety in terms of inhalation injury, cornstarch is the preferred product. Talc should not be used.

PATIENT TEACHING Controlling Diaper Rash

Keep skin dry.*

- Use superabsorbent disposable diapers to reduce skin wetness.
- If using cloth diapers, use only overwraps that allow air to circulate; avoid rubber pants.
- Change diapers as soon as soiled—especially with stool—whenever possible, preferably once during the night.
- Expose healthy or only slightly irritated skin to air, not heat, to dry completely.

Apply ointment, such as zinc oxide or petrolatum, to protect skin, especially if skin is very red or has moist, open areas.

- Avoid removing skin barrier cream with each diaper change; remove waste material and reapply skin barrier cream.
- To completely remove ointment, especially zinc oxide, use mineral oil; do not wash vigorously.

Avoid overwashing the skin, especially with perfumed soaps or commercial wipes, which may be irritating.

- You may use a moisturizer or nonsoap cleanser, such as cold cream or Cetaphil, to wipe urine from skin.
- Gently wipe stool from skin using water and mild soap, such as Dove.
- When traveling, fill an old baby wipe container with soft paper towels and warm water.

*Powder helps keep the skin dry, but talc is dangerous if breathed into the lungs. Plain cornstarch or cornstarch-based powder is safer. When using any powder product, first shake it into your hand, then apply it to the diaper area. Store the container away from the infant's reach; keep the container closed when not in use.

Atopic Dermatitis (Eczema)

Eczema or eczematous inflammation of the skin refers to a descriptive category of dermatologic diseases and not to a specific etiology. AD is a type of pruritic eczema that usually begins during infancy and is associated with allergy with a hereditary tendency *(atopy).* AD manifests in three forms based on the child's age and the distribution of lesions:

1. *Infantile (infantile eczema)*—Usually begins at 2 to 6 months of age; generally undergoes spontaneous remission by 3 years of age
2. *Childhood*—May follow the infantile form; occurs at 2 to 3 years of age; 90% of children have manifestations by age 5 years
3. *Preadolescent and adolescent*—Begins at about 12 years of age; may continue into the early adult years or indefinitely

The diagnosis of AD is based on a combination of history and morphologic findings (Box 53-3). Children with AD have

BOX 53-3 Clinical Manifestations of Atopic Dermatitis

Distribution of Lesions

Infantile form—Generalized, especially cheeks, scalp, trunk, and extensor surfaces of extremities (see Fig. 53-11)

Childhood form—Flexural areas (antecubital and popliteal fossae, neck), wrists, ankles, and feet

Preadolescent and adolescent form—Face, sides of neck, hands, feet, face, and antecubital and popliteal fossae (to a lesser extent)

Appearance of Lesions

Infantile Form

Erythema
Vesicles
Papules
Weeping
Oozing
Crusting
Scaling
Often symmetric

Childhood Form

Symmetric involvement
Clusters of small erythematous or flesh-colored papules or minimally scaling patches
Dry and may be hyperpigmented
Lichenification (thickened skin with accentuation of creases)
Keratosis pilaris (follicular hyperkeratosis) common

Adolescent or Adult Form

Same as childhood manifestations
Dry, thick lesions (lichenified plaques) common
Confluent papules

Other Physical Manifestations

Intense itching
Unaffected skin dry and rough
African-American children likely to exhibit more papular or follicular lesions than are Caucasian children
May exhibit one or more of the following:

- Lymphadenopathy, especially near affected sites
- Increased palmar creases (many cases)
- Atopic pleats (extra line or groove of lower eyelid)
- Prone to cold hands
- Pityriasis alba (small, poorly defined areas of hypopigmentation)
- Facial pallor (especially around nose, mouth, and ears)
- Bluish discoloration beneath eyes ("allergic shiners")
- Increased susceptibility to unusual cutaneous infections (especially viral)

a lower threshold for cutaneous itching than do other children, and many authorities believe the dermatologic manifestations appear subsequent to scratching from the intense pruritus. For example, infants rub their faces against bed linen, and their crawling (a form of scratching) results in irritation of knees and elbows. Lesions disappear if the scratching is stopped (Fig. 53-11).

The majority of children with infantile AD have a family history of eczema, asthma, food allergies, or allergic rhinitis, which strongly supports a genetic predisposition. The cause is unknown but appears to be related to abnormal function of the skin, including alterations in perspiration, peripheral vascular function, and heat tolerance. Manifestations of the chronic disease improve in humid climates and get worse in the fall and winter, when homes are heated and environmental humidity is lower. The disorder can be controlled but not cured.

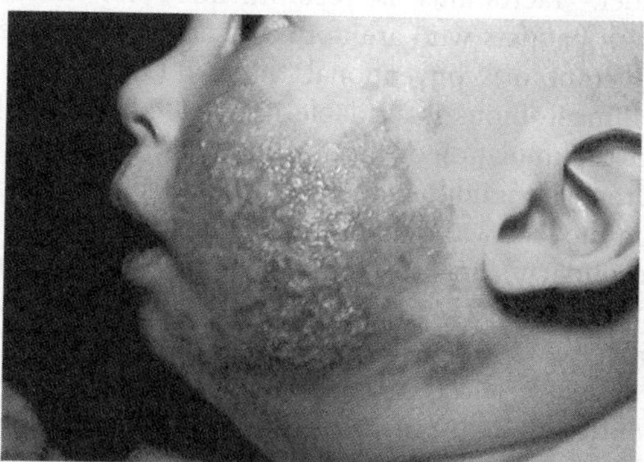

Fig. 53-11 Infantile atopic dermatitis with oozing and crusting of lesions. (From Weston WL, Lane AT, Morelli JG: *Color textbook of pediatric dermatology,* ed 4, St Louis, 2002, Mosby.)

Therapeutic Management

The major goals of management are to (1) hydrate the skin, (2) relieve pruritus, (3) reduce flare-ups or inflammation, and (4) prevent and control secondary infection. The general measures for managing AD focus on reducing pruritus and other aspects of the disease. Management strategies include avoiding exposure to skin irritants or allergens; avoiding overheating; and administrating medications such as antihistamines, topical immunomodulators, topical steroids, and (sometimes) mild sedatives as indicated.

Enhancing skin hydration and preventing dry, flaky skin are accomplished in a number of ways, depending on the child's skin characteristics and individual needs. A tepid bath with a mild soap (Dove or Neutrogena), no soap, or an emulsifying oil, followed immediately by application of an emollient (within 3 minutes), assists in trapping moisture and preventing its loss. Bubble baths and harsh soaps should be avoided. The bath may need to be repeated once or twice daily, depending on the child's status; excessive bathing without emollient application only dries out the skin. Some lotions are not effective, and emollients should be chosen carefully to prevent excessive skin drying. Aquaphor, Cetaphil, and Eucerin are acceptable lotions for skin hydration. A nighttime bath, followed by emollient application and dressing in soft cotton pajamas, may help alleviate most nighttime pruritus.

Sometimes colloid baths, such as the addition of 2 cups of cornstarch to a tub of warm water, provide temporary relief of itching and may help the child sleep if given before bedtime. Cool wet compresses are soothing to the skin and provide antiseptic protection.

Oral antihistamine drugs such as hydroxyzine or diphenhydramine usually relieve moderate or severe pruritus. Nonsedating antihistamines such as loratadine (Claritin) or fexofenadine (Allegra) may be preferred for daytime pruritus relief. Because pruritus increases at night, a mildly sedating antihistamine may be needed.

Occasional flare-ups require the use of topical steroids to diminish inflammation. Low-, moderate-, or high-potency topical corticosteroids are prescribed, depending on the degree of involvement, the area of the body to be treated, the child's age, the potential for local side effects (striae, skin atrophy, and pigment changes), and the type of vehicle to be used (e.g., cream, lotion, ointment). Patients receiving topical corticosteroid therapy for chronic conditions should be evaluated for risk factors for suboptimal linear growth and reduced bone density (American Academy of Dermatology, 2003). Topical immunomodulators, a new nonsteroidal treatment for AD, are best used at the beginning of a flare-up just as the skin becomes red and itches. Two new immunomodulator medications used in children with AD are tacrolimus and pimecrolimus (Kronemyer, 2003). Tacrolimus is available in two ointment strengths (0.03% and 0.1%); the 0.03% concentration has been approved for use in children 2 years of age and older. Tacrolimus is recommended for intermittent therapy in patients who are not adequately responsive to, or are intolerant of, conventional therapy (Yetman & Parks, 2002). Pimecrolimus is available in a 1% cream that has no systemic accumulation or effects. This drug is approved for use in children with mild to moderate AD. Both drugs can be used freely on the face without worrying about steroid side effects.

If secondary skin infections occur in children with AD, these infections are managed with appropriate systemic antibiotics.

✻ Nursing Care Management

Assessment of the child with AD includes a family history for evidence of atopy, a history of previous involvement, and any environmental or dietary factors associated with the present and previous exacerbations. The skin lesions are examined for type, distribution, and evidence of secondary infection. Parents are interviewed regarding the child's behavior, especially in relation to scratching, irritability, and sleeping patterns. Exploration of the family's feelings and methods of coping is also important.

The nursing care of the child with AD is challenging. Controlling the intense pruritus is imperative if the disorder is to be successfully managed, since scratching leads to new lesions and may cause secondary infection. In addition to the medical regimen, other measures can be taken to prevent or minimize the scratching. Fingernails and toenails are cut short, kept clean, and filed frequently to prevent sharp edges. Gloves or cotton stockings can be placed over the hands and pinned to shirtsleeves. One-piece outfits with long sleeves and long pants also decrease direct contact with the skin. If gloves or socks are used, the child needs time to be free from such restrictions. An excellent time to remove gloves, socks, or other protective devices is during the bath or after receiving sedative or antipruritic medication.

Conditions that increase itching are eliminated when possible. Woolen clothes or blankets, rough fabrics, and furry stuffed animals are removed from the child's environment. Because heat and humidity cause perspiration (which intensifies itching), proper dress for climatic conditions is essential. Pruritus is often precipitated by exposure to the irritant effects of certain components of common products such as soaps, detergents, fabric softeners, perfumes, and powders. Most children experience less itching when soft cotton fabrics are worn next to the skin. During cold months, synthetic fabrics (not wool) should be used for overcoats, hats, gloves, and snowsuits. Exposure to latex products, such as gloves and balloons, should also be avoided.

Clothes and sheets are laundered in a mild detergent and rinsed thoroughly in clear water (without fabric softeners or antistatic chemicals). Putting the clothes through a second complete wash cycle without using detergent reduces the amount of residue remaining in the fabric.

Preventing infection is usually accomplished by preventing scratching. Baths are given as prescribed, the water is kept tepid, and soaps (except as indicated) and bubble baths are avoided, as are oils or powders. Skin folds and diaper areas need frequent cleansing with plain water. A room humidifier or vaporizer may benefit children with extremely dry skin. The skin lesions are examined for signs of infection—usually honey-colored crusts or pustules with surrounding erythema. Any signs of infection are reported to the practitioner.

NURSING ALERT If the child is being treated with baths for hydration, it is imperative that the emollient preparation be applied immediately after bathing (while the skin is still slightly moist) to prevent drying.

Wet soaks and compresses are applied and medications for pruritus or infection are administered as directed. The family is given explicit instructions on the preparation and use of soaks; special baths; and topical medications, including the order of application if more than one is prescribed. It is important to emphasize that one thick application of topical medication is *not* equivalent to several thin applications, and that excessive use of an agent (particularly steroids) can be hazardous. If children have difficulty remaining still for a 10- or 15-minute soak, bath, or dressing application, these can be carried out at naptime or when the child is engrossed in watching television, listening to a story, or playing with tub toys.

Diet modification is another source of frustration to parents. When a hypoallergenic diet is prescribed, parents need help to understand the reason for the diet and the guidelines for avoiding hyperallergenic foods (see Guidelines box). Because hypoallergenic diets take time before effects are apparent, parents need reassurance that results may not be seen immediately. If airborne allergens make eczema worse, the family is counseled about "allergy proofing" the home (see Asthma, Chapter 46).

GUIDELINES Preventing Atopy in Children

Identify Children at Risk

Family history of allergy

Increased immunoglobulin E in cord blood and postnatal serum

Dry, flaky skin

Prenatal Precautions (Last Trimester)

Avoiding any known food allergens

Avoiding milk and other dairy products, peanuts, and eggs

Minimizing ingestion of other hyperallergenic foods

Postnatal Precautions

Breast milk or casein-whey hydrolysate formula (e.g., Nutramigen, Pregestimil, Alimentum) exclusively for at least 6 months

No solid food for first 6 months

No cow's milk or soy formula for 12 months

No eggs, fish, corn, citrus, peanuts, nuts, or chocolate for 12 to 18 months

One new food added at 5- to 7-day intervals to identify possible reaction

Environmental Control

Limited exposure to dust, molds, furry animals, and cigarette smoke

Data from Johnstone D: Strategy for intervention of food allergy in infants, *Int Pediatr* 4(4):319-325, 1989; Zeiger R et al: Effectiveness of dietary manipulation in the prevention of food allergy in infants, part II, *J Allergy Clin Immunol* 78(1 Pt 2):224-238, 1986; Wood RA: Prospects for the prevention of allergy in children, *Curr Opin Pediatr* 8(6):601-605, 1995.

Family Support

Parents are assured that the lesions will not produce scarring (unless secondarily infected) and that the disease is not contagious. However, the child may have repeated exacerbations and remissions. Spontaneous and permanent remission takes place at approximately 2 to 3 years of age in most children with the infantile disorder.

During acute phases, emotional stress can become intense for the family. They need time to discuss negative feelings and to be reassured that these feelings are normal. Stress tends to aggravate the severity of the condition. Therefore efforts to relieve anxiety in both the parents and the child have a beneficial emotional and physical effect.

Seborrheic Dermatitis

Seborrheic dermatitis is a chronic, recurrent, inflammatory reaction of the skin. It occurs most commonly on the scalp (cradle cap) but may involve the eyelids (blepharitis), external ear canal (otitis externa), nasolabial folds, and inguinal region. The cause is unknown, although it is more common in early infancy, when sebum production is increased. The lesions are characteristically thick, adherent, yellowish, scaly, oily patches that may or may not be mildly pruritic. Unlike AD, seborrheic dermatitis is not associated with a positive family history for allergy and is common in infants shortly after birth and in adolescents after puberty. Diagnosis is made primarily on the basis of the appearance and the location of the crusts or scales.

Nursing Care Management

Cradle cap may be prevented with adequate scalp hygiene. Not infrequently, parents omit shampooing the infant's hair for fear of damaging the "soft spots," or fontanels. The nurse should discuss how to shampoo the infant's hair and emphasize that the fontanel is like skin anywhere else on the body—it does not puncture or tear with mild pressure.

When seborrheic lesions are present, the treatment is directed at removing the crusts. Parents are taught the appropriate procedure to clean the scalp. Education may need to include a demonstration. Shampooing should be done daily with a mild soap or commercial baby shampoo; medicated shampoos are not necessary, but an antiseborrheic shampoo containing sulfur and salicylic acid may be used. Shampoo is applied to the scalp and allowed to remain on the scalp until the crusts soften. Then the scalp is thoroughly rinsed. A fine-tooth comb or a soft facial brush helps remove the loosened crusts from the strands of hair after shampooing.

Acne

Acne vulgaris is the most common skin problem treated by physicians during patients' adolescence. Acne is not caused by dirt but by testosterone, a hormone present in males and females that increases during puberty. It stimulates the sebaceous glands of the skin to enlarge, or produce oil, and plug the pores. Whiteheads, blackheads, and pimples are present in teenage acne (American Academy of Dermatology, 2006).

One half of the adolescent population experiences acne by the end of the teenage years. Although the disorder can appear before the age of 10 years, the peak incidence occurs in middle to late adolescence (at age 16 to 17 years in girls and 17 to 18 years in boys). It is more common in boys than in girls. The degree to which an individual is affected may range from nothing more than a few isolated comedones to a severe inflammatory reaction. Although the disease is self-limiting and not life threatening, it has great significance to the adolescent. Health professionals should not underestimate the impact that acne has on teens.

Numerous factors affect the development and course of acne. Its distribution in families and a high degree of concordance in identical twins suggest hereditary factors. Premenstrual flares of acne occur in nearly 70% of adolescent girls, suggesting a hormonal cause. Studies do not indicate a clear association between stress and acne, but adolescents commonly cite stress as a cause for acne outbreaks. Cosmetics containing lanolin, petrolatum, vegetable oils, lauryl alcohol, butyl stearate, and oleic acid can increase comedone production. Exposure to oils in cooking grease can be a precursor in adolescents who work over fast-food restaurant hot oils. There is no known link between dietary intake and the development or worsening of acne.

Pathophysiology

Acne is a disease that involves the *pilosebaceous follicles* (the hair follicle and sebaceous gland complex) of the face, neck, chest, and upper back. Three pathophysiologic factors are involved in the development of acne: excessive sebum production, comedogenesis, and the overgrowth of *Propionibacterium acnes* (Mancini, 2000).

evolve Case Study—Acne Vulgaris

Comedogenesis (formation of comedones) results in a noninflammatory lesion that may be either an *open comedone* ("blackhead") or a *closed comedone* ("whitehead"). Inflammation occurs with the proliferation of *P. acnes,* which draws in neutrophils, causing inflammatory papules, pustules, nodules, and cysts.

Therapeutic Management

Successful management of acne depends on a cooperative effort between the health care provider, the adolescent, and the parents. Unlike many other dermatologic conditions, acne lesions resolve slowly, and improvement may not be apparent for at least 6 weeks. Individual comedones can take several weeks to months to resolve, and papules and pustules usually resolve in about 1 week. The multifactorial causes of acne necessitate a combined approach for successful treatment. Treatment consists of general measures of care and specific treatments determined by the type of lesions involved.

General Measures

Improvement of the adolescent's overall health status is part of the general management. Adequate rest, moderate exercise, a well-balanced diet, reduction of emotional stress, and elimination of any foci of infection are all part of general health promotion.

Cleansing

Dirt or oil on the surface of the skin does not cause acne. Gentle cleansing with a mild cleanser once or twice daily is usually sufficient. Antibacterial soaps are ineffective and may be too drying when used in combination with topical acne medications. For some adolescents hygiene of the hair and scalp appears to be related to the clinical activity of the acne. Acne on the forehead may improve with brushing the hair away from the forehead and more frequent shampooing.

Medications

Treatment success depends on commitment from the adolescent. Before prescribing treatment, the practitioner should determine the adolescent's level of comfort and readiness to begin treatment.

Tretinoin (Retin-A) is the only drug that effectively interrupts the abnormal follicular keratinization that produces microcomedones, the invisible precursors of the visible comedones. Tretinoin alone is usually sufficient for management of comedonal acne (Russell, 2000). Tretinoin is available as a cream, gel, or liquid. This drug can be extremely irritating to the skin and requires careful patient education for optimal usage. The patient should be instructed to begin with a pea-sized dot of medication, which is divided into the three main areas of the face and then gently rubbed into each area. The medication should not be applied for at least 20 to 30 minutes after washing to decrease the burning sensation. The avoidance of sun and the daily use of sunscreen must be emphasized, since sun exposure can result in severe sunburn. Adolescents should be advised to apply the medication at night and to use a sunscreen with a sun protection factor (SPF) of at least 15 in the daytime.

Topical *benzoyl peroxide* is an antibacterial agent that inhibits the growth of *P. acnes* organisms. It is effective against both inflammatory and noninflammatory acne and is an effective first-line agent. This medication is available as a cream, lotion, gel, or wash. The patient should be informed that the medication may have a bleaching effect on sheets, bedclothes, and towels. The adolescent can be reassured that skin bleaching will not occur. Accommodation to the medication can be gained with a gradual increase in the strength and frequency of application.

When inflammatory lesions accompany the comedones, a *topical antibacterial agent* may be prescribed. These agents are used to prevent new lesions and to treat preexisting acne. Clindamycin, erythromycin, metronidazole, azelaic acid, and the combination of either benzoyl peroxide and erythromycin (Benzamycin) or benzoyl peroxide and glycolic acid are all choices for topical antibacterial therapy. The combination of 5% benzoyl peroxide and 3% erythromycin is especially beneficial, although the exact mechanism of action is not understood (Burkhart, Specht, & Neckers, 2000). Tretinoin improves the penetration of other topical agents, and combination therapy with tretinoin and an antibacterial treatment is the only way to address three of the pathogenic causes of acne: keratinization, *P. acnes,* and inflammation (Laude, 2000).

Systemic antibiotic therapy is used when moderate to severe acne does not respond to topical treatments. Oral antibiotics such as tetracycline, erythromycin, minocycline, and doxycycline are considered safe to use (American Academy of Dermatology, 2006).

Females with mild to moderate acne may respond well to topical treatment and the addition of an *oral contraceptive pill (OCP).* OCPs reduce the endogenous androgen production and decrease the bioavailability of the woman's circulating androgens. Both of these actions result in decreased acne.

Isotretinoin, 13-cis-retinoic acid (Accutane), is a potent and effective oral agent that is reserved for severe cystic acne that has not responded to other treatments. Isotretinoin is the only agent available that affects factors involved in the development of acne. However, treatment with isotretinoin should be managed *only* by a dermatologist. Adolescents with multiple, active, deep dermal or subcutaneous cystic and nodular acne lesions are treated for 20 weeks. Multiple side effects can occur, including dry skin and mucous membranes, nasal irritation, dry eyes, decreased night vision, photosensitivity, arthralgia, headaches, mood changes, aggressive or violent behaviors, depression, and suicidal ideation. Adolescents on this drug should be monitored for depression, depressive symptoms, and suicidal ideation (Jacobs, Deutsch, & Brewer, 2001). The drug should be given only at the recommended doses for no longer than the recommended duration. The most significant side effects of this drug are the teratogenic effects. Isotretinoin is absolutely contraindicated in pregnant women. Sexually active young women must be using an effective contraceptive method during treatment and for 1 month after treatment. Patients receiving isotretinoin should also be monitored for elevated cholesterol and triglyceride levels. Significant elevation may require discontinuation of the medication.

Nursing Care Management

Because acne is so common and its appearance may seem so mild, the health care provider may underestimate the relative importance of the disease to the adolescent. The nurse should assess the individual adolescent's level of distress, current management, and perceived success of any regimen before initiating a referral. If adolescents do not perceive the acne to be a problem, they may lack motivation to follow the treatment plan.

The nurse can provide ongoing support for the adolescent when a treatment plan is initiated. The family is also encouraged to support the adolescent in his or her efforts. Use of medications and basic skin care information should be discussed in detail with the adolescent. Written instructions should accompany the verbal discussion. Information to dispel myths regarding the use of abrasive cleansing products can prevent unnecessary costs and trauma to the skin.

Teenagers need education about the factors that aggravate and damage the skin, such as too vigorous scrubbing. In addition, picking, squeezing, and manual expression with fingernails break down the ductal walls of lesions and cause the acne to worsen. Mechanical irritation, such as vinyl helmet straps that rub areas predisposed to acne, can also cause the development of lesions.

Thermal Injury

Burns

Burn injuries are usually attributed to extreme heat sources but may also result from exposure to cold, chemicals, electricity, or radiation. Most burns are relatively minor and do not require definitive medical treatment. However, burns involving a large body surface area, critical body parts, or the geriatric or pediatric population often benefit from treatment in specialized burn centers. The American Burn Association has established criteria to guide decisions regarding the severity of injury and the need for transfer for specialized care.*

When burns are characterized by patients' age and type of injury, the following patterns become apparent: (1) hot-water scalds are most frequent in toddlers, (2) flame-related burns are more common in older children, (3) 10% to 20% of documented cases of child abuse include burn injuries (Herndon, 2007), and (4) children playing with matches or lighters account for 1 in 10 house fires.

The extent of tissue destruction is determined by the intensity of the heat source, the duration of contact or exposure, the conductivity of the tissue involved, and the rate at which the heat energy is dissipated by the skin. A brief exposure to high-intensity heat from a flame can produce burn injuries similar to those induced by long exposure to less intense heat in hot water.

Characteristics of Burn Injury

The physiologic responses, therapy, prognosis, and disposition of the injured child are all directly related to the *amount of tissue destroyed.* Therefore the severity of the burn injury is assessed on the basis of the percentage of *total body surface area (TBSA)* burned and depth of the burn. Among children in the school-age group or younger age groups, a burn that is 10% of TBSA can be life threatening if not treated correctly. Other important factors in determining the seriousness of the injury are the location of the wounds, the child's age and general health, the causative agent, the presence of respiratory involvement, and any associated injury or condition.

Type of Injury

The majority of burns result from contact with thermal agents such as a flame, hot surfaces, or hot liquids. Electrical injuries caused by household current have the greatest incidence in young children, who insert conductive objects into electrical outlets and bite or suck on connected electrical cords (Herndon, 2007). These burns occur most commonly during the spring and summer months and are also associated with risk-taking behaviors in boys. Direct contact with high- or low-voltage current, as well as lightning strikes, is the most frequent mechanism of injury. The resistance of the tissue and the path of the electric current are responsible for the damage incurred. Electric current travels through the body following the path of least resistance, which involves the tissues, fluid, blood vessels, and nerves. A more localized burn is produced if skin resistance is high at the area of contact, and a more systemic pattern of injury is produced if skin resistance is low. Often compared with a crush injury, serious electrical trauma results from current passing through vital organs, muscle compartments, and nerve or vascular pathways. Loss of limbs, cardiac fibrillation, respiratory collapse, and burns are common occurrences after exposure to electrical energy. Criteria for admission, as derived from evidence-based practice for electrical burn injuries, include a history of loss of consciousness, electrocardiographic (ECG) changes, 10% TBSA affected, or the need for monitoring an affected extremity. Cardiac monitoring is therefore included in standard burn care when ECG changes are identified on admission (Arnoldo, Klein, & Gibran, 2006).

evolve Animation—Burns in Children

Chemical burns are seen in the pediatric population and can cause extensive injury. The severity of injury is related to the chemical agent (acid, alkali, or organic compound) and the duration of contact. The mechanism of injury differs from that in other burns in that there is a chemical disruption and alteration of the physical properties of the exposed body area. Noxious agents exist in many cleaning products commonly found in the home. In addition to concern for localized damage, the potential for systemic toxicity must be addressed. Of particular concern is the exposure of the eyes to chemical agents, the ingestion of caustic substances, and inhalation of toxic gases produced from chemicals.

Extent of Injury

The extent of a burn is expressed as a percentage of the TBSA. This is most accurately estimated by using specially designed age-related charts (Fig. 53-12). It is more efficient to use a chart designed to assign body proportions to children of different ages.

Depth of Injury

A thermal injury is a three-dimensional wound that is also assessed in relation to depth of injury. Traditionally the terms *first-*, *second-*, and *third-degree* have been used to describe the depth of tissue injury. However, with the current emphasis on wound healing, these have been replaced by more descriptive terms based on the extent of destruction to the epithelializing elements of the skin (Fig. 53-13).

Superficial (first-degree) burns are usually of minor significance. With these burns, there is often a latent period followed

**The American Burn Association offers an Advanced Burn Life Support program;* www.ameriburn.org/ablsnow.php.

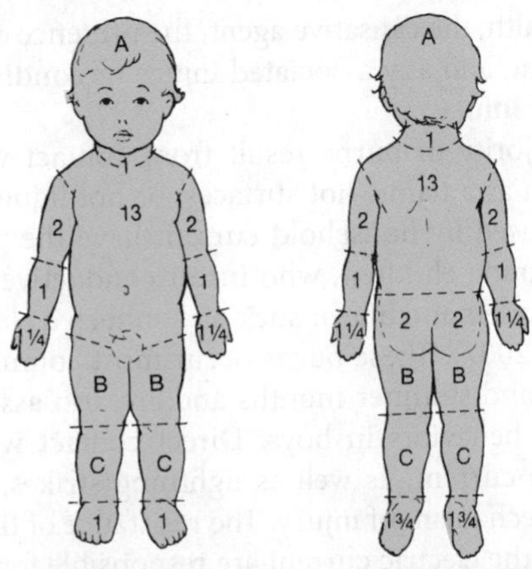

RELATIVE PERCENTAGES OF AREAS AFFECTED BY GROWTH

AREA	BIRTH	AGE 1 YR	AGE 5 YR
A = ½ of head	9½	8½	6½
B = ½ of one thigh	2¾	3¼	4
C = ½ of one leg	2½	2½	2¾

A

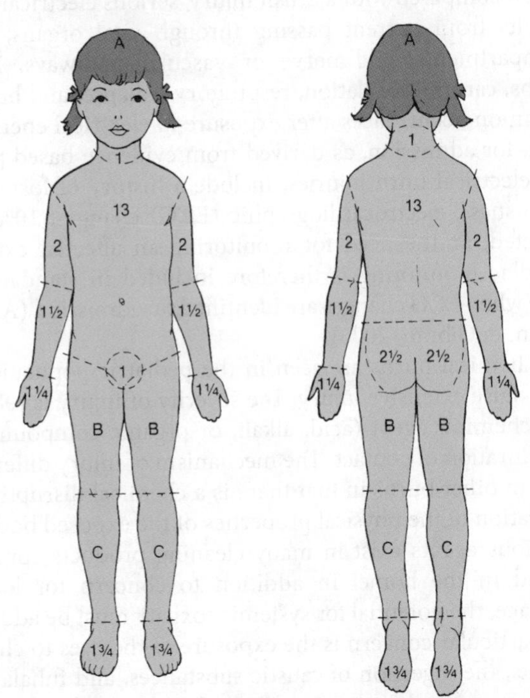

RELATIVE PERCENTAGES OF AREAS AFFECTED BY GROWTH

AREA	AGE 10 YR	AGE 15 YR	ADULT
A = ½ of head	5½	4½	3½
B = ½ of one thigh	4½	4½	4¾
C = ½ of one leg	3	3¼	3½

B

Fig. 53-12 Estimation of distribution of burns in children. **A**, Children from birth to age 5 years. **B**, Older children.

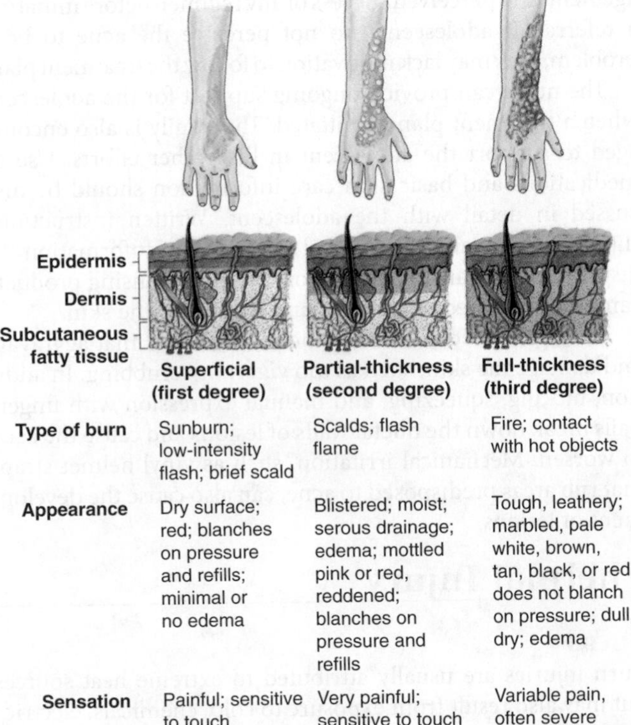

	Superficial (first degree)	Partial-thickness (second degree)	Full-thickness (third degree)
Type of burn	Sunburn; low-intensity flash; brief scald	Scalds; flash flame	Fire; contact with hot objects
Appearance	Dry surface; red; blanches on pressure and refills; minimal or no edema	Blistered; moist; serous drainage; edema; mottled pink or red, reddened; blanches on pressure and refills	Tough, leathery; marbled, pale white, brown, tan, black, or red; does not blanch on pressure; dull, dry; edema
Sensation	Painful; sensitive to touch	Very painful; sensitive to touch	Variable pain, often severe

Fig. 53-13 Classification of burn depth. (Redrawn from Grant HD, Murray RH: *Emergency care,* ed 7, Upper Saddle River, NJ, 1995, Prentice-Hall.)

by erythema. Tissue damage is minimal, the protective functions of the skin remain intact, and systemic effects are rare. Pain is the predominant symptom, and the burn heals in 5 to 10 days without scarring. Mild sunburn is an example of a superficial burn.

Partial-thickness (second-degree) injuries involve the epidermis and varying degrees of the dermis. These wounds are painful, moist, red, and blistered. Superficial partial-thickness burns involve the epidermis and part of the dermis. Dermal elements are intact, and the wound should heal in approximately 14 days with variable amounts of scarring (Fig. 53-14). The wound is extremely sensitive to temperature changes, exposure to air, and light touch. Although classified as partial-thickness (or second-degree) burns, deep dermal burns resemble full-thickness injuries in many respects. Sweat glands and hair follicles remain intact. The burn may appear mottled, with pink, red, or waxy white areas exhibiting blisters and edema formation. Systemic effects are similar to those encountered with full-thickness burns. Although many of these wounds heal spontaneously, healing time may be extended beyond 14 days. These burn wounds often heal with extensive scarring.

Full-thickness (third-degree) burns are serious injuries that involve the entire epidermis and dermis and extend into subcutaneous tissue (see Fig. 53-13). Nerve endings, sweat glands, and hair follicles are destroyed. The burn varies in color from red to tan, waxy white, brown, or black and is distinguished by a dry, leathery appearance (Fig. 53-15). Normally, full-thickness burns lack sensation in the area of injury because of the destruction of nerve endings. However, most full-thickness burns have superficial and partial-thickness burned areas at the periphery of the burn, where nerve endings are intact and exposed. Excised eschar and donor sites also cause exposed nerve fibers. As the peripheral fibers regenerate, painful sensations return. Consequently, children often experience severe pain related to the size and depth of the burn. Full-thickness wounds are not capable of reepithelialization and require surgical excision and grafting to close the wound.

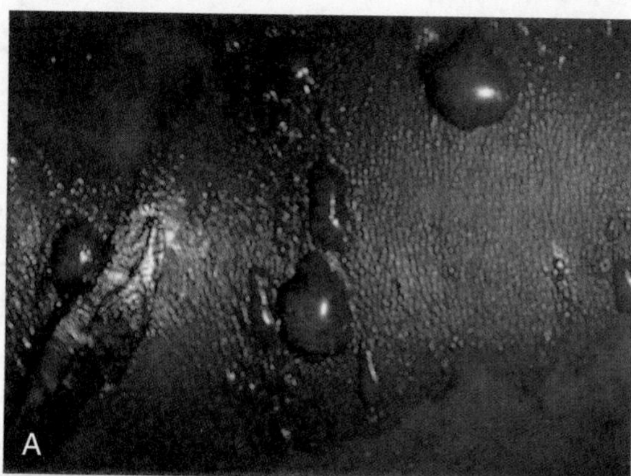

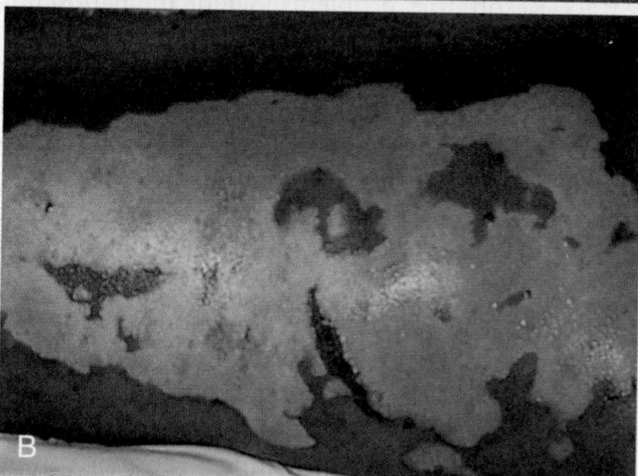

Fig. 53-14 Superficial partial-thickness burns on an African-American child. **A,** Blisters intact. **B,** Blisters removed. *(Courtesy Hillcrest Medical Center, Tulsa, OK.)*

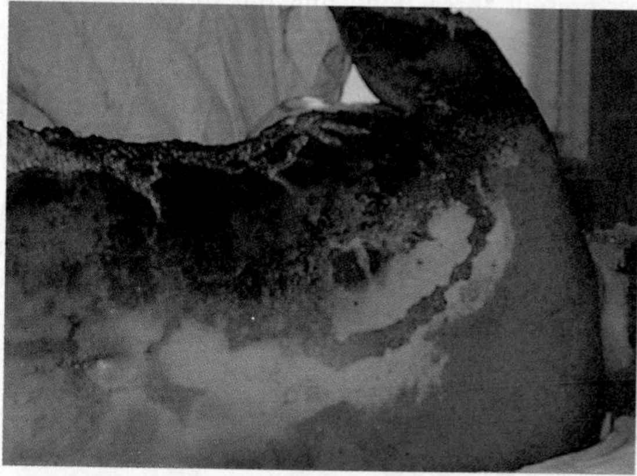

Fig. 53-15 *Bottom to top:* Deep partial-thickness burn *(red area)*; full-thickness burn *(white area)*; full-thickness burn with eschar *(brown area)*. *(Courtesy Hillcrest Medical Center, Tulsa, OK.)*

Fourth-degree burns are full-thickness injuries that involve underlying structures such as muscle, fascia, and bone. The wound appears dull and dry, and ligaments, tendons, and bone may be exposed (Fig. 53-16).

Severity of Injury

Burns are classified as minor, moderate, or major, which is useful in determining the disposition of the patient for treatment. Burn patients are categorized as (1) those with a *major burn injury,* who require the services and facilities of a specialized burn center; (2) those with a *moderate burn,* who may be treated in a hospital with expertise in burn care; and (3) those with *minor injuries,* who may be treated on an outpatient basis. The extent and depth of the burn (Table 53-9), the causative agent, the body area involved, the patient's age, and concomitant injuries and illnesses determine the severity of the injury.

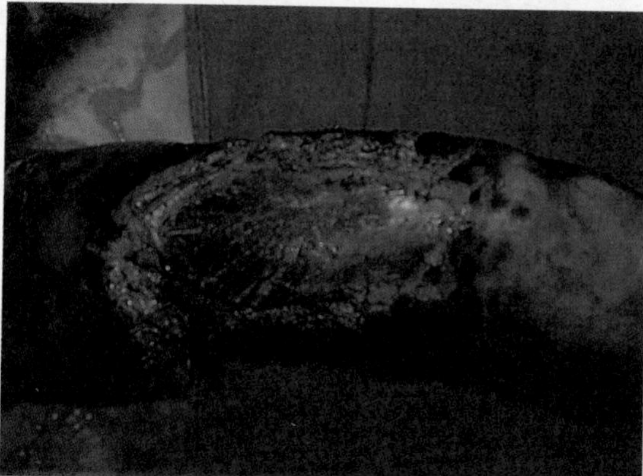

Fig. 53-16 Full-thickness burn with muscle and fascia involved. *(Courtesy Hillcrest Medical Center, Tulsa, OK.)*

Because the skin of infants is so thin, it is likely to sustain deeper injuries compared with older children. Children younger than 2 years of age, especially 6 months or younger, have a significantly higher mortality rate than older children with burns of similar magnitude. Acute or chronic illnesses or superimposed injuries also complicate burn care and response to treatment.

Inhalation Injury

Trauma to the tracheobronchial tree often follows inhalation of the heated gases and toxic chemicals produced during combustion. Although direct thermal injury to the upper airway may occur, heat damage below the vocal cords is rare. Inspired heated air is cooled in the upper airway before reaching the trachea. Reflex closure of the cords and laryngospasm also prevent full inhalation. However, evidence of direct thermal injury to the upper airway includes burns of the face and lips, singed nasal hairs, and laryngeal edema. Clinical manifestations may be delayed as long as 24 to 48 hours. Wheezing, increasing secretions, hoarseness, wet rales, and carbonaceous secretions are signs of respiratory tract involvement. Upper airway obstruction is often associated with burn shock and fluid resuscitation. In such situations, endotracheal intubation may also be necessary to preserve a patent airway.

Inhalation of carbon monoxide is suspected when the injury has occurred in an enclosed space. Mucosal erythema and edema followed by sloughing of the mucosa are manifestations of respiratory tract injury. A mucopurulent membrane replaces the mucosal lining and seriously compromises respiration and ventilation.

Early in the postburn period most pulmonary infections result from nosocomial exposure, immobility, and abdominal distention. The hematogenous variety occurs later and is related to the septic burn wound or other foci, such as phlebitis at the site of an invasive IV line. A significant increase in mortality has been observed when inhalation injury and pneumonia are both present.

Table 53-9 Severity Grading System Adopted by the American Burn Association

	MINOR*	MODERATE	MAJOR
Partial-thickness burns	<10% of total body surface area (TBSA)	>10%-20% TBSA	>20% TBSA
Full-thickness burns	—	—	All
Treatment	Usually outpatient; may require 1- to 2-day admission	Admission to hospital, preferably one with expertise in burn care	Admission to a burn center

From Vaccaro P, Trofino RB: Care of the patient with minor to moderate burns. In Trofino RB (editor): *Nursing care of the burn-injured patient,* Philadelphia, 1991, Davis.
*Minor burns exclude any burn involving the face, hands, feet, perineum, or crossing joints; electrical burns; any injury complicated by the presence of inhalation injury or concomitant trauma; and children with psychosocial factors affecting the injury.

Deep burns, especially those circling the thorax, may cause restriction of chest excursion as a result of edema and inelastic eschar formation. Young children are particularly at risk because of the pliability of the skeletal structure. Restriction of the chest is relieved by an escharotomy incision, which allows expansion of the chest wall to facilitate ventilation.

Pathophysiology

Thermal injuries produce both local and systemic effects that are related to the extent of tissue destruction. In superficial burns the tissue damage is minimal. In partial-thickness burns there is considerable edema and more severe capillary damage. With a major burn greater than 30% TBSA, there is a systemic response involving an increase in capillary permeability, allowing plasma proteins, fluids, and electrolytes to be lost. Maximum edema formation in a small wound occurs about 8 to 12 hours after injury. After a larger injury, hypovolemia, associated with this phenomenon, will slow the rate of edema formation, with maximum effect at 18 to 24 hours.

evolve Case Study—Burns

Another systemic response is anemia, caused by direct heat destruction of red blood cells, hemolysis of injured red blood cells, and trapping of red blood cells in the microvascular thrombi of damaged cells. A long-term decrease in the number of red blood cells may occur as a result of increased red blood cell fragility. Initially there is an increased blood flow to the heart, brain, and kidneys, with decreased blood flow to the gastrointestinal tract. There is an increase in metabolism to maintain body heat, providing for the body's increased energy needs.

Complications

Thermally injured children are subject to a number of serious complications, both from the wound and from systemic alterations resulting from the injury. The immediate threat to life is related to airway compromise and profound shock. During healing, infection—both local and systemic sepsis—is the primary complication. Mortality associated with thermal trauma in children increases with the severity of injury and decreases as age advances. In children older than 3 years, the mortality rate is similar to that of adults. Below this age, the survival rate with burns and their associated complications lessens considerably.

A less apparent respiratory tract injury is inhalation of carbon monoxide. Carbon monoxide has a greater affinity for hemoglobin than does oxygen, thereby depriving peripheral tissues and oxygen-dependent organs (such as the heart and brain) of the oxygen needed for survival. Treatment for either of these two problems is 100% oxygen, which reverses the situation rapidly.

Pulmonary problems are a major cause of fatality in children with either thermal burns or complications in the respiratory tract. Respiratory problems include inhalation injuries, aspiration in unconscious patients, bacterial pneumonia, pulmonary edema, pulmonary embolus, posttraumatic pulmonary insufficiency, and atelectasis. The most common cause of respiratory failure in the pediatric age group is bacterial pneumonia, which requires prolonged intubation and sometimes a tracheostomy. Tracheostomies increase the incidence of serious complications and are performed only in extreme cases.

A less common complication is pulmonary edema resulting from fluid overload or acute respiratory distress syndrome (ARDS) in association with gram-negative sepsis. ARDS results from pulmonary capillary damage and leakage of fluid into the interstitial spaces of the lung. A loss of compliance and interference with oxygenation are the consequences of pulmonary insufficiency in conjunction with systemic sepsis.

Wound Sepsis

Sepsis is a critical problem in the treatment of burns and an ever-present threat following the shock phase. Initially, burn wounds are relatively pathogen free unless they are contaminated with potentially infectious material, such as dirt or polluted water. However, dead tissue and exudate provide a fertile field for bacterial growth. On approximately the third postburn day, early colonization of the wound surface by a preponderance of gram-positive organisms (primarily staphylococci) changes to predominantly gram-negative opportunistic organisms, particularly *Pseudomonas aeruginosa.* By the fifth postburn day, bacterial invasion is well under way beneath the surface of the burn wound. Early surgical excision of eschar together with placement of autograft reduces the incidence of sepsis.

Therapeutic Management

Emergency Care

The initial management of the burn patient begins at the scene of injury. The first priority is to stop the burning process (see Emergency box). The child should then be transported immediately to the nearest medical facility for treatment and evaluation. The child and the family are usually extremely frightened and anxious; sensitivity to their emotional state and reassurance should be provided during the transport process.

Stop the Burning Process The chief aim of rescue in flame burns is to smother the fire, not fan it. Children tend to panic and run, which spreads the flames and makes assistance more difficult. The injured child should be placed in a horizontal position and rolled in a blanket, rug, or similar article, with

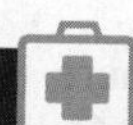

EMERGENCY

Burns

Minor Burns

Stop the burning process:

- Apply cool water to the burn or hold the burned area under cool running water.
- Do not use ice.

Do not disturb any blisters that form, unless the injury is from a chemical substance.

Do not apply anything to the wound.

Cover with a clean cloth if risk of damage or contamination.

Remove burned clothing and jewelry.

Major Burns

Stop the burning process:

- Flame burns—smother the fire.
- Place victim in the horizontal position.
- Roll victim in a blanket or similar object; avoid covering the head.

Assess for an adequate airway and breathing.

If child is not breathing, begin mouth-to-mouth resuscitation.

Remove burned clothing and jewelry.

Cover wound with a clean cloth.

Keep victim warm.

Transport to medical aid.

Begin intravenous and oxygen therapy as prescribed.

care taken not to cover the head and face because of the danger of inhalation of toxic fumes. If nothing is available, the victim should lie down and roll over slowly to extinguish the flames. Remaining in the vertical position may cause the hair to ignite or the inhalation of flames, heat, or smoke.

Major burns with large amounts of denuded skin should not be cooled. Heat is rapidly lost from burned areas, and additional cooling leads to a drop in core body temperature and potential circulatory collapse. Wet dressings also promote vasoconstriction because of cooling, resulting in impaired circulation to the burned area and increased tissue damage. Chemical burns require continuous flushing with large amounts of water before transport to a medical facility. The use of neutralizing agents on the skin is contraindicated, since a chemical reaction is initiated and further injury may result. If the chemical is in powder form, the addition of water may spread the caustic agent. The powder should be brushed off if possible.

Burned clothing is removed to prevent further damage from smoldering fabric and hot beads of melted synthetic materials. Jewelry is removed to eliminate the transfer of heat from the metal and constriction resulting from edema formation. This also provides access to the wound and prevents painful removal later.

Assess the Victim's Condition As soon as the flames are extinguished, the child is assessed. Airway, breathing, and circulation are the primary concerns. Cardiopulmonary complications may result from exposure to electric current, inhalation of toxic fumes and smoke, hypovolemia, and shock. Emergency measures are instituted as appropriate.

Cover the Burn The burn wound should be covered with a clean cloth to prevent contamination, decrease pain by eliminating air contact, and prevent hypothermia. No attempt should be made to treat the burn. Application of topical ointments, oils, or other home remedies is contraindicated.

Transport the Child to Medical Aid The child with an extensive burn is not given anything by mouth to avoid aspiration in the presence of paralytic ileus and upper airway edema and to prevent water intoxication. The child is transported to the nearest medical facility. If this cannot be accomplished within a relatively short period, IV access should be established, if possible, with a large-bore catheter. Oxygen is administered, if available, at 100%. A report of the initial assessment and any interventions implemented is given to the medical facility assuming care of the child.

Provide Reassurance Providing reassurance and psychologic support to both the family and the child helps immeasurably during the period of postinjury crisis. Reducing anxiety conserves energy the family and child will need to cope with the physiologic and emotional stress of injury.

Minor Burns

Treatment of burns classified as minor can usually be managed adequately on an outpatient basis when it is determined that the parent can be relied on to carry out instructions for care and observation. Patients with less than optimum circumstances may require close follow-up to ensure adherence with treatment.

The wound is cleansed with a mild soap and tepid water. Debridement of the wound includes removal of any embedded debris, chemicals, and devitalized tissue. Removal of intact blisters remains controversial. Some authorities argue that blisters provide a barrier against infection; others maintain that blister fluid is an effective medium for the growth of microorganisms. However, blisters should be broken if the injury is due to a chemical agent to control absorption. Most practitioners favor covering the wound with an antimicrobial ointment to reduce the risk of infection and to provide some form of pain relief. The dressing consists of nonadherent fine-mesh gauze placed over the ointment and a light wrap of gauze dressing that avoids interference with movement. This helps keep the wound clean and protect it from trauma. The caregiver is instructed to wash the wound, reapply the dressing, and return the child to the office or clinic as directed for wound observation. The frequency of dressing changes may vary from every other day to once a day.

Some practitioners prefer an occlusive dressing, such as a hydrocolloid, which is placed over the wound after cleansing. Hydrogel dressings, which are soothing and nonadherent, may also be used. The dressing is changed when leakage occurs—at regular intervals or at least weekly. This method eliminates the discomfort associated with frequent dressing changes but impairs visualization of the wound surface.

If there is a high probability of infection or other complications or if there is doubt about the ability to carry out instructions, the caregiver may be directed to bring the patient in daily for dressing changes and inspection. Another option is have a nurse make a home visit to inspect the wound and perform the dressing change. Frequent removal of the dressing is an effective mode of debridement. Soaking the dressing in tepid water or normal saline before removal helps loosen the dressing and debris and reduce discomfort. Burns of the face are usually treated by an open method. The wound is washed and debrided in the same manner, and a thin film of antimicrobial ointment is applied.

A tetanus history is obtained on admission. If there is no history of immunization, or if more than 5 years have passed since the last immunization, tetanus prophylaxis is administered. There is no evidence that systemic antibiotic prophylaxis decreases the incidence of infection in small burn wounds (Herndon, 2007). Therefore antibiotics should be used only when there is evidence of infection. A mild analgesic such as acetaminophen is usually sufficient to relieve discomfort; the antipyretic effect of the drug also alleviates the sensation of heat.

Most minor burns heal without difficulty, but if the wound margin becomes erythematous, gross purulence is noted, or the child develops evidence of systemic reaction, such as fever or tachycardia, hospitalization is indicated. The child should also be evaluated for functional impairment, and the caregiver should be instructed in the exercise and ambulation program. After wound healing, an evaluation of scar maturation and range of motion will indicate any need for further therapy.

Major Burns

The first priority is airway maintenance. The inhalation of noxious agents or respiratory burns are suggested when there is a history of injury in an enclosed space; edema of the oral and nasal membranes; thermal injury to the face, nares, and upper torso; hyperemia; and blisters or evidence of trauma to the upper respiratory passages. When respiratory involvement is suspected or evident, 100% oxygen is administered and blood gas values, including carbon monoxide levels, are determined.

If the child exhibits changes in sensorium, air hunger, or other signs of respiratory distress, an endotracheal tube is inserted to maintain the airway. When severe edema of the face and neck is anticipated, intubation is performed before swelling makes intubation difficult or impossible. Controlled intubation is preferred to an emergency procedure. Intubation allows for the delivery of humidified oxygen, the removal of secretions from respiratory passages, and the provision of ventilatory support.

When full-thickness burns encircle the chest, constricting eschar may limit chest wall excursion, and ventilation of the child becomes more difficult. Escharotomy of the chest relieves this constriction and improves ventilation.

Fluid Replacement Therapy The objectives of fluid therapy are to (1) compensate for water and sodium lost to traumatized areas and interstitial spaces, (2) reestablish sodium balance, (3) restore circulating volume, (4) provide adequate perfusion, (5) correct acidosis, and (6) improve renal function.

Fluid replacement is required during the first 24 hours because of fluid shifts that occur after the injury. Various formulas are used to calculate fluid needs, and the one adopted depends on practitioner preference. Crystalloid solutions are used during this initial phase of therapy. Parameters such as vital signs (especially heart rate), urine output, adequacy of capillary filling, and state of sensorium determine adequacy of fluid resuscitation.

After the initial 24-hour period, theoretically there is a capillary seal, and capillary permeability is restored. Colloid solutions such as albumin, Plasma-Lyte, or fresh frozen plasma are useful in maintaining plasma volume. However, children with burn injuries usually require fluids in excess of their calculated maintenance and replacement volume. Reasons for this may include underestimation of burn size (particularly in pediatric patients), pulmonary injury that sequesters resuscitation fluid in the lung, electrical injury with greater tissue destruction than that which is visible, and a delay in the initiation of fluid resuscitation. Irreversible burn shock that persists despite aggressive fluid resuscitation remains a significant cause of death in the immediate postburn period. Fluid balance may continue to be a problem throughout the course of treatment, especially when there is considerable evaporative loss from the wound.

Nutrition The enhanced metabolic requirements and catabolism in severe burns make nutritional needs of paramount importance and often difficult to satisfy. The diet must provide sufficient calories to meet the increased metabolic needs and enough protein to avoid protein breakdown. Hypoglycemia can result from the stress of the burn injury because the liver glycogen stores are rapidly depleted.

A high-protein, high-calorie diet is encouraged. Many children have poor appetites and are unable to meet energy requirements solely by oral feeding. Most children with burns in excess of 25% TBSA require supplementation with tube feeding. Early and continued nutritional support is an important part of therapy for seriously burned patients. Enteral feeding provides direct nourishment to the gastrointestinal tract and helps reverse the defective gut barrier that accompanies burn shock (Purdue, 2007).

If nutritional requirements cannot be met entirely by the enteral route, parenteral hyperalimentation is used to supplement intake. However, enteral feeding increases blood flow in the intestinal tract, preserves gastrointestinal function, and minimizes bacterial translocation by decreasing mucosal atrophy of the intestines. These factors make enteral feeding the preferred route of nutritional support (Herndon, 2007).

To facilitate growth and proliferation of epithelial cells, administration of vitamins A and C is begun early in the postburn period. Zinc is also supplemented because of its important role in wound healing and epithelialization.

Medication Antibiotics are usually not administered prophylactically. The administration of systemic antibiotics to control wound colonization is not indicated, since decreased circulation to the injured area prevents delivery of the medication to areas of deepest injury. Surveillance cultures and monitoring of the clinical course provide the most reliable indicators of developing infection. Appropriate antibiotics are instituted to treat the specific identified organism. Otitis media should not be overlooked as a source of fever in the pediatric population.

Some form of sedation and analgesia is required in the care of burned children. Morphine sulfate is the drug of choice for severe burn injuries. Morphine has extensive distribution but is metabolized rapidly; continuous infusion or frequent administration is needed for pain management in burns. Morphine is administered intravenously and titrated to individual need. The unstable circulatory status and edema formation preclude intramuscular or subcutaneous administration. When combined, midazolam (Versed) and fentanyl (Sublimaze) also provide excellent IV sedation and analgesia to control procedural pain in children with burns (Herndon, 2007). The oral form of fentanyl, Oralet, provides effective analgesia in a convenient form that the child can suck. Dosage monitoring is important because tolerance to opioids may develop. IV analgesics are most effective when they are administered just before the onset of procedural pain.

The use of short-acting anesthetic agents, such as propofol (Diprivan) and nitrous oxide, has proved beneficial in eliminating procedural pain. Pharyngeal reflexes remain intact, thus ensuring a patent airway. Propofol is an IV sedative hypnotic agent that produces sedation in less than 1 minute and lasts only a few minutes. Nitrous oxide is a useful short-term analgesic when given in a mixture of gases on a fixed ratio of 50% nitrous oxide and 50% oxygen (Annequin et al, 2000). Initiation of action is approximately 1 minute, with peak effect reached in 3 to 5 minutes. Nitrous oxide is useful to alleviate anxiety and raise the threshold of pain during procedures. The child may self-administer the nitrous oxide mixture with assistance. For any conscious or unconscious sedation, the child must be monitored continuously during the procedure (see Preoperative Care, Chapter 45; and Pain Assessment and Pain Management, Chapter 35).

Management of the Burn Wound After the initial period of shock and the restoration of fluid balance, the primary concern is the burn wound. The objectives of wound management include prevention of infection, removal of devitalized tissue, and closure of the wound. The application of dressings and topical antimicrobial therapy reduce pain by minimizing the exposure to air.

Primary Excision In children with large, full-thickness burn wounds, excision is performed as soon as the patient is hemodynamically stable after initial resuscitation. Because the burn wound precipitates an exaggerated physiologic response, many complications do not resolve until the eschar is excised and the wound is closed. Early excision of deep partial- and full-thickness burns reduces the incidence of infection and the threat of sepsis.

Debridement Partial-thickness wounds require debridement of devitalized tissue to promote healing. Debridement is painful and requires analgesia and a sedative before the procedure. Medications given for pain need to be readily available during this procedure and may need to be titrated upward during the procedure. Hydroxyzine and diphenhydramine are often needed for itching that occurs after whirlpool and debridement. The itching becomes particularly bothersome as the burns heal.

Hydrotherapy is employed to cleanse the wound and involves soaking in a tub or showering at least once a day for no more than 20 minutes. The water loosens and removes sloughing tissue, exudate, and topical medications. Hydrotherapy helps to cleanse not only the wound but the entire body and aids in maintenance of range of motion. Mesh gauze entraps the exudative slough and is readily removed during hydrotherapy. Any loose tissue is carefully trimmed away before the wound is redressed.

Topical Antimicrobial Agents Methods used for managing the burn wound include:

Exposure—Wounds are left open to air; crust forms on partial-thickness wounds, and eschar forms on full-thickness burns.

Open—Topical antimicrobial agent is applied directly to the wound surface and the wound is left uncovered.

Modified—Antimicrobial agent is applied directly or impregnated into thin gauze and applied to the wound; gauze or net secures the area.

Occlusive—Antimicrobial agent is impregnated in gauze or applied directly to the wound; multiple layers of bulky gauze are placed over the primary layer and secured with gauze or net.

All these methods provide wound coverage and employ some type of topical agent. Topical agents do not eliminate organisms from the wound but can effectively inhibit bacterial growth. To be effective, a topical application must be nontoxic, capable of diffusing through eschar, harmless to viable tissue, inexpensive, and easy to apply. A topical ointment should not encourage the development of resistant strains of bacteria and should produce minimal electrolyte derangement. A comparison of commonly used agents is summarized in Table 53-10.

Biologic Skin Coverings Permanent coverage of extensive burns is a prolonged process that requires repeated operative procedures using general anesthesia for atraumatic care in debridement and grafting. Early closure shortens the period of metabolic stress and decreases the likelihood of burn wound sepsis. In the acute phase, biologic dressings cover and protect the wound from contamination, reduce fluid and protein loss, increase the rate of epithelialization, reduce pain, and facilitate movement of joints to retain range of motion.

Allograft (homograft) skin is obtained from human cadavers that are screened for communicable diseases. Allograft is particularly useful in the coverage of surgically excised deep partial- and full-thickness wounds in extensive burns when available donor sites are limited. Severe immunosuppression occurs in massively burned children, and the allograft becomes adherent. The allograft can remain in place until suitable donor sites become available. Typically, rejection is seen approximately 3 to 4 weeks after application (Herndon, 2007). The insufficient availability of tissue banks and suitable donors limits the use of allografts.

Xenograft from a variety of species, most notably pigs, is commercially available. In large burns, the porcine xenograft is commonly applied when extensive early debridement is indicated to cover a partial-thickness burn; this provides a temporary covering for the wound until an available autograft can be applied to the full-thickness areas (Herndon, 2007). Pigskin dressings are replaced every 1 to 3 days. They are particularly effective in children with partial-thickness scald burns of the hands and face because they allow relatively pain-free movement, which reduces contracture formation and has the added benefit of improving appetite and morale.

When applied early to a superficial partial-thickness injury, biologic dressings stimulate epithelial growth and faster wound healing. However, biologic dressings must be applied to clean wounds. If the dressing covers areas of heavy microbial contamination, infection occurs beneath the dressing. In

Table 53-10 Comparison of Common Topical Preparations

AGENT	DRESSINGS	ADVANTAGES	DISADVANTAGES
Silver nitrate 0.5% ($AgNO_3$)	Open, modified or occlusive; impedes joint movement; dressings changed twice daily; keep dressing moist (rewet at least every 2 hr)	Greatly reduces evaporative losses; does not interfere with wound healing; bacteriostatic action against major burn flora, including *Pseudomonas* and *Staphylococcus* organisms; inexpensive	Does not penetrate eschar; ineffective on established burn wound infections; little effect on *Klebsiella* and *Aerobacter* groups; stains skin, clothing, linens; makes assessment of the wound difficult because of staining; hypotonicity pulls electrolytes from the wound, depleting sodium, potassium, chloride, and magnesium; stings on application
Silver sulfadiazine 1% (AgSD)	Occlusive; motion of joints maintained; applied twice daily; do not use in patients with a history of allergy to sulfa	Little pain on application; bactericidal by altering DNA and cell metabolism; effective against gram-positive and gram-negative bacteria; easy to apply; nontoxic	Transient neutropenia; does not penetrate eschar; forms proteinaceous gel on wound surface that is painful to remove; occasional rashes and pruritus; decreases granulocyte formation
Mafenide acetate 10% (Sulfamylon)	*Cream*—Usually open; do not apply to face; apply twice daily *Solution*—Occlusive; keep dressing moist (rewet at least every 2 hr); protect solution from light	Penetrates eschar and diffuses rapidly into burn wound and underlying tissues; effective in deep flame, electrical, and infected wounds; biostatic against many gram-positive and gram-negative organisms, including *Pseudomonas* and *Clostridium*	Difficult and painful to remove cream; pain on application; metabolic acidosis, hypercapnia, and carbonic anhydrase inhibition; inhibits wound healing; hypersensitivity in some patients
Bacitracin	Open, modified; motion of joints maintained; change dressing twice daily	Bactericidal and bacteriostatic against gram-positive organisms; low toxicity; painless application; easy to apply	Limited activity against gram-negative organisms; allergic reaction in sensitive individuals

the case of partial-thickness burns, such infection may convert the wound to a full-thickness injury.

Synthetic skin coverings are available for the management of partial-thickness burn wounds. Ideally, the dressing should provide the properties of human skin: adherence, elasticity, durability, and hemostasis. Synthetic skin substitutes are readily available, have an indefinite shelf life, and are relatively inexpensive.

Synthetic dressings are composed of a variety of materials and can be used successfully in the management of superficial partial-thickness burns and donor sites. Examples include adherent elastic films; hydroactive materials; or colloidal suspensions that are usually permeable to air, vapor, and fluids.

Biobrane is a flexible silicone-nylon membrane bonded to collagenous peptides of porcine skin. Calcium alginate is another treatment for donor sites. As with biologic dressings, it is important that the wound be free of debris before the dressing is applied. Body temperature elevation or evidence of purulence, erythema, or cellulitis around the wound edges may indicate that the wound has become infected beneath the dressing. If this occurs, prompt discontinuance of the synthetic dressing is indicated. All synthetic dressings are reputed to hasten wound healing and reduce discomfort.

Permanent Skin Coverings Permanent coverage of deep partial- and full-thickness burns is usually accomplished with a split-thickness skin graft. This graft consists of the epidermis and a portion of the dermis removed from an intact area of skin by a special instrument, the *dermatome* (Fig. 53-17). With extensive burns it is often difficult to find enough viable skin to cover the wounds; therefore available donor sites and special techniques are used. Split-thickness skin grafts may be sheet graft or mesh graft.

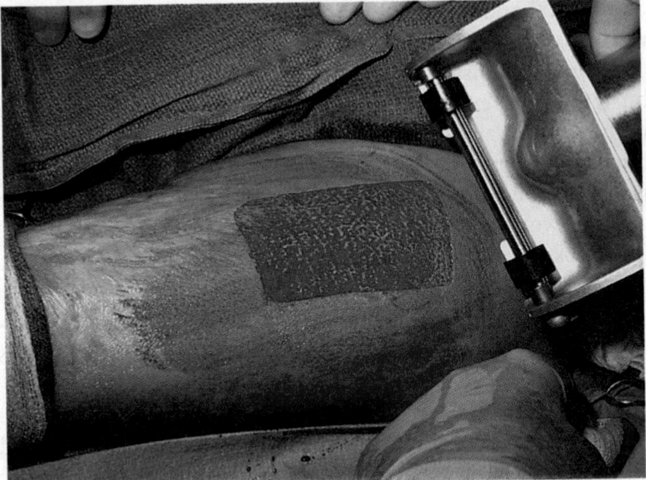

Fig. 53-17 Removal of split-thickness skin graft with a dermatome.

Sheet Graft A sheet of skin, removed from the donor site, is placed intact over the recipient site and sutured in place; this is used in areas where cosmetic results are most visible.

Mesh Graft A sheet of skin is removed from the donor site and passed through a mesher, which produces tiny slits in the

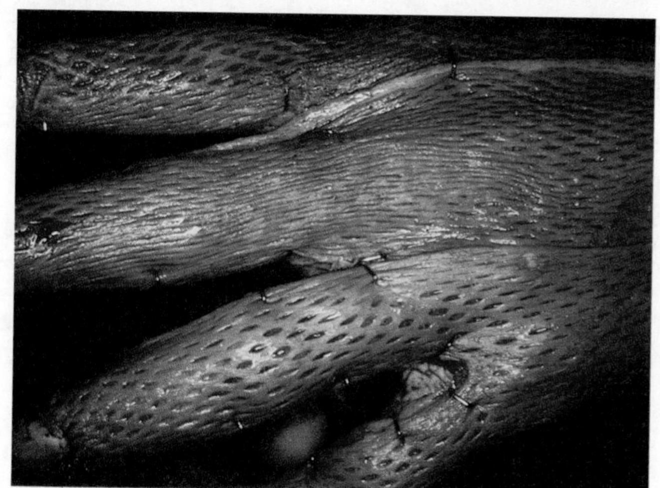

Fig. 53-18 Mesh graft.

skin that allow the skin to cover 1.5 to 9 times the area of the sheet graft; this results in a less desirable cosmetic and functional outcome (Fig. 53-18).

The donor site is dressed with synthetic wound coverings or fine-mesh gauze until the dressing separates at 10 to 14 days, when the wound is healed. Dressings are not changed on donor sites to avoid damage to newly healed, delicate epithelium. Healed donor sites are available for reharvesting in patients with extensive burns and limited undamaged skin, but the quality of skin is decreased when multiple grafts are taken.

Artificial Skin The development of Integra, a product that allows the dermis to regenerate, has produced significant improvement in burn wound healing and decreased scar formation. It is applied to partial- and full-thickness burns. The two-layer membrane is made of collagen (a fibrous protein from animal tendons and cartilage) and silicone rubber (i.e., Silastic). The Silastic layer is peeled off after the dermis is formed. The application of artificial skin does not replace the grafting procedure, but it prepares the burn wound to accept an ultrathin autograft. Advantages include faster healing of the burn wound when integrity of the dermis is restored, faster healing of donor sites with the use of ultrathin grafts, and restoration of sweat glands and hair follicles. A disadvantage is its high cost.

Cultured Epithelium When burns are extensive and donor sites for split-thickness skin grafting are limited, it is possible to culture cells from a full-thickness skin biopsy and produce coherent sheets that can be applied to clean, excised full-thickness wounds. Epithelial cell culture grafts offer the possibility of an unlimited source of autografts in patients with extensive burns. Cultured epithelial autografts are effective in early wound closure. The child's own skin is fractionated and cultured in a porcine media to form a thin epithelial layer that is applied to the burn wound. This technique offers an improved rate of survival in patients with extensive burns and limited donor sites.

Prognosis

Children differ from adults in their responses to thermal injury, and the mortality rates in young children are significantly higher than those in older children and adults. Mortality is greatest for children younger than 48 months of age. Many children who do survive have long-term functional and cosmetic impairments.

Nursing Care Management

Because the care of burned children encompasses a broad range of skills, nursing care has been divided into segments that correspond with the major phases of burn treatment. The *acute phase*, also referred to as the *emergent* or *resuscitative* phase, involves the first 24 to 48 hours. The *management phase* extends from the completion of adequate resuscitation through wound coverage. The *rehabilitative phase* begins once the majority of the wounds have healed and rehabilitation has become the predominant focus of the care plan. This phase continues until all reconstructive procedures and corrective measures are accomplished (often a period of months or years).

evolve Nursing Care Plan—The Child with Burns

Acute Phase

The primary emphasis during the emergent phase is the treatment of burn shock and the management of pulmonary status. Monitoring vital signs, output, fluid infusion, and respiratory parameters are ongoing activities in the hours immediately after injury. IV infusion is begun immediately and is regulated to maintain a urine output of at least 1 to 2 ml/kg in children weighing less than 30 kg (66 lb); an output of 30 to 50 ml/hr is expected in children weighing more than 30 kg. Urine output and specific gravity, vital signs, laboratory data, and objective signs of adequate hydration guide the rate of fluid administration.

Children who are hospitalized with burns require constant observation and assessment for complications. Alterations in electrolyte balance produce clinical symptoms of confusion, weakness, cardiac irregularities, and seizures. Changes in respiratory function and gas exchange are reflected clinically by restlessness, irritability, increased work of breathing, and alterations in blood gas values. The loss of protective function of the skin exposes burned children to increased risk of hypothermia. Edema formation and circulatory impairment result in the loss of sensation and deep throbbing pain.

NURSING ALERT Evaluate the burned extremity and check the pulse every hour. If unable to palpate, use Doppler to ascertain loss of circulation and pulse. If the pulse is lost, escharotomy may be necessary to relieve the edema causing pressure on blood vessels, to restore adequate circulation.

Burn units maintain a pictorial record of the wound to record progress and for legal purposes (if child abuse is suspected). The burn wound is treated according to the protocol of the specific burn facility. The burn team monitors infection control procedures and ensures that staff and visitors comply with established protocols to prevent cross-contamination in the burn unit.

Throughout the acute phase of care, the psychosocial needs of the children and their families should not be overlooked. The child is frightened, uncomfortable, and often confused. Children may be isolated from familiar persons and surroundings; the overwhelming physical needs at this time are the primary focus of the staff and parents. In addition to feeling concern for their child, the family experiences guilt, which may be related to the fact that the parents did not or could not protect their child from injury. Consistency in the information presented and in the staff's attitude creates a sense of familiarity and stability during the acute phase of care. Consistent caregivers can also help decrease the patient and family's anxiety and provide coordination of care. For example, when many teams of consultants and specialists are involved in the child's care, appointing one "spokesperson" decreases the confusion and enhances communication regarding the child's care.

Management and Rehabilitative Phases

After the patient's condition is stabilized, the management phase begins. The multidisciplinary team concentrates on preventing wound infections, closing the wound as quickly as possible, and managing the numerous complications. Although the rehabilitative phase begins when permanent wound closure has been achieved, rehabilitation issues are identified on admission and are included in the care plan throughout the hospital course.

NURSING ALERT Disorientation in the burned patient is one of the first signs of overwhelming sepsis and may indicate inadequate hydration. Assessment of the sensorium is another important indicator of the adequacy of hydration. With inadequate hydration, a spiking fever and diminished bowel sounds accompanied by paralytic ileus are noted and progressively increase over 48 to 72 hours, after which the temperature falls to subnormal limits. At this time the wound deteriorates, the white blood cell count is depressed, and septic shock becomes manifest.

Comfort Management

The severe pain of the wound and resultant therapies, the anxiety generated by these experiences, sleep deprivation, itching related to wound healing, and the conscious and unconscious interpretations of traumatic events contribute to the psychologic behaviors commonly observed in children with burns. It is always difficult to deal with a child in pain, and inflicting pain on a helpless child is contrary to the empathic nature of nursing. Interventions to promote comfort may include medications (including IV morphine or midazolam and short-term anesthetics such as propofol), relaxation techniques, distraction therapy, behavioral techniques, operant conditioning (e.g., tokens, star chart), and family participation.

Children need age-appropriate explanations before all procedures. When children appear to accept pain with little or no response, psychologic consultation may be needed. Consistency in caregivers is important. If this is not possible, a carefully developed, multidisciplinary care plan is necessary to provide consistency.

Care of the Burn Wound

The nurse has a major responsibility for cleansing, debriding, and applying topical medications and dressings to the burn wound. Pain medication should be administered so that the peak effect of the drug coincides with the procedure. Children who have an understanding of the procedure to be performed and some perceived control demonstrate less maladaptive behavior. Children also respond well to participating in decisions (see Atraumatic Care box).

ATRAUMATIC CARE

Reducing the Stress of Burn Care Procedures

- Have all materials ready before beginning.
- Administer appropriate analgesics and sedatives.
- Remind the child of the impending procedure to allow sufficient time to prepare.
- Allow the child to test and approve the temperature of the water.
- Allow the child to select the area of the body on which to begin.
- Allow the child to request a short rest period during the procedure.
- Allow the child to remove the dressings if desired.
- Provide something constructive for the child to do during the procedure (e.g., holding a package of dressings or a roll of gauze).
- Inform the child when the procedure is near completion.
- Praise the child for cooperation.

Outer dressings are removed. Any dressings that have adhered to the wound can be more easily removed by applying tepid water or normal saline. Loose or easily detached tissue is debrided during the cleansing process. In dressing the wound, it is important that all areas be clean, that medication be amply applied, and that no two burned surfaces touch each other (e.g., fingers or toes; ears touching the side of the head). If they are touching, the burned surfaces will heal together, causing deformity or dysfunction.

Topical medications may be applied directly to the wound with a tongue blade or gloved hand or impregnated into fine-mesh gauze before application. Dressings are then applied to assist in exudate absorption, wound debridement, and increased patient comfort. All dressings applied circumferentially should be wrapped in a distal-to-proximal manner. The dressing is applied with sufficient tension to remain in place but not so tightly as to impair circulation or limit motion. Elastic bandages are applied over dressings to prevent epithelial breakdown, decrease edema, stimulate circulation, and improve mobility. A stable dressing is especially important when the child is ambulatory.

Standard Precautions, including the use of protective garb and barrier techniques, should be followed when caring for patients with thermal injuries. Frequent handwashing and forearm washing are the single most important elements of the infection control program. Strict policies for cleaning the environment and patient care equipment should be implemented to minimize the risk of cross-contamination. All visitors and members of other departments should be oriented to the infection control policies, including the importance of handwashing and forearm washing and use of protective garb. Visitors should be screened for infection and contagious diseases before patient contact.

Nutrition

Oral feedings are encouraged unless the child is intubated or paralytic ileus persists. Because children with burns often lack an appetite, the child needs encouragement, help, and patience. Consultation between the caregiver and the dietitian helps determine food preferences. Children who are old enough to participate should be included in meal planning. In addition, many children prefer an atmosphere more nearly like that provided at home. Therefore, when possible, many children enjoy sitting at a table and interacting with other children at mealtimes. Painful procedures should not be scheduled near mealtimes, since most children will be too physically exhausted and emotionally upset to eat.

Children who require enteral supplementation must be monitored for feeding intolerance and tube malposition. The nurse should also monitor and report any abdominal distention, diarrhea, or electrolyte and metabolic deviations.

Prevention of Complications

Acute Care

The maintenance of body temperature is important to the child with burns. Core body temperature is supported when energy is conserved with an environmental temperature of 28° to 33° C (82.4° to 91.4° F). Large areas of the body should not be exposed simultaneously during dressing changes. Warmed solutions, linens, occlusive dressings, heat shields, a radiant warmer, and warming blankets assist in preventing hypothermia.

The chief danger during acute care is infection—wound infection, generalized sepsis, or bacterial pneumonia. Accurate and ongoing assessments of all parameters that provide clues to the early diagnosis and treatment of infection are essential. Symptoms of sepsis include a change in the level of consciousness, a rising or falling white blood cell count, hypothermia or hyperthermia, a loss of the progression of wound healing, increasing fluid requirements, hypoactive or absent bowel sounds, a rising or falling blood glucose level, tachycardia, tachypnea, and thrombocytopenia.

Children are reluctant to move if movement causes pain, and they are likely to assume a position of comfort. Unfortunately, the most comfortable position often encourages the formation of contractures and loss of function. Ongoing efforts to prevent contractures include maintaining proper body alignment, positioning and splinting involved extremities in extension, providing active and passive physical therapy, and encouraging spontaneous movement when feasible. Frequent position changes are important to promote adequate bronchopulmonary hygiene and capillary perfusion to common pressure areas. Low-air loss beds are beneficial for the morbidly obese or children with posterior grafts. Special attention should be given to areas at risk for increased pressure, such as the posterior scalp, heels, sacrum, and areas exposed to mechanical irritation from splints and dressings.

Long-Term Care

The rehabilitative phase of care begins once wound coverage is achieved. Scar formation becomes a major problem as burn wounds heal (Fig. 53-19). Contractile properties of the scar tissue can result in disabling contractures, deformity, and disfigurement.

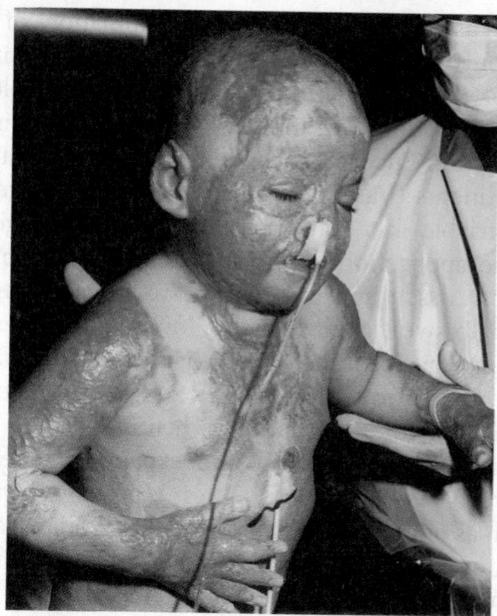

Fig. 53-19 Extensive scars from flame burn. *(Courtesy The Paul and Carol David Foundation Burn Institute, Akron, Ohio.)*

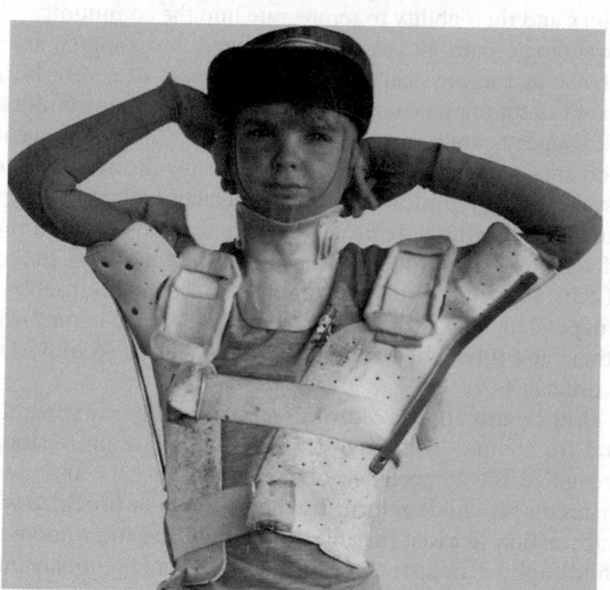

Fig. 53-20 Child in elasticized (Jobst) garment and "airplane" splints.

Uniform pressure applied to the scar decreases the blood supply. When pressure is removed, blood supply to the scar is immediately increased; therefore periods without pressure should be brief to avoid nourishment of the hypertrophic tissue. Continuous pressure to areas of scarring can be achieved by elastic bandages or commercially available pressure garments. Because these custom-made garments are often worn for months, revisions may be required as the child grows. It is much easier to prevent scarring and contracture of the wound than to resolve an existing problem. Splints and appliances may also be needed until wound maturation is achieved (Fig. 53-20).

Scar tissue has certain significant properties, particularly for growing children. Intense itching occurs in healing burn wounds and scar tissue until the scar is no longer active.

Itching is usually treated with a combination of H_1 and H_2 antagonists such as cetirizine (Zyrtec) and cimetidine (Tagamet) (Baker et al, 2001); an H_1 antagonist alone; and frequent applications of a moisturizer, such as Vaseline, Cetaphil, Aquaphor, Eucerin, cocoa butter, or Nivea. Petrolatum-based ointments (Vaseline, Aquaphor) seem to spread more easily on friable skin than thick creams do. Massage therapy during the application of moisturizers is also beneficial to stretch scar tissue and aid in contracture prevention. Scar tissue has no sweat glands, and children with extensive scarring may experience difficulty during hot weather. Caregivers should be alerted to this possibility and be prepared to institute alternate methods of cooling when necessary.

Scar tissue does not grow and expand, as does normal tissue, which may create difficulties, especially in functional areas such as on the hands and over joints. Additional surgery is sometimes required to allow independent functioning in daily activities, to improve cosmetic appearance, or to restore anatomic integrity.

The nursing activities in the rehabilitative phase of treatment focus on the child and family's adaptation to the burn injury and their ability to reintegrate into the community. The psychologic pain and sequelae of severe burn injury are as intense as the physical trauma. The impact of severe burns taxes the coping mechanisms at all ages. Very young children, who suffer acutely from separation anxiety, and adolescents, who are developing an identity, are probably the most affected psychologically. Toddlers cannot understand why the parents they love and who have protected them can leave them in such a frightening and unfamiliar place. Adolescents, in the process of achieving independence from the family, find themselves in a dependent role with a damaged body. Being different from others at a time when conformity with peers is so important is difficult to accept.

Anticipation of the return to school can be overwhelming and frightening. It is essential that health care professionals recognize the importance of preparing teachers and classmates for the child's return. Teachers need to be provided with information to assist the child and family and to promote the child's optimal adjustment. Hospital-sponsored school reentry programs use a variety of methods to provide education and information about the implications of the injury, the garments and appliances, and the need for support and acceptance. Telephone calls, videotapes, information packets, and visits by members of the health care team offer opportunities to help with reintegration into the school environment—a focal point of the child's life.

Psychosocial Support of the Child

Children should begin early to do as much for themselves as possible and to be active participants in their care. Loss of control and perceived helplessness may result in acting-out behaviors. During illness, children regress to a previous developmental level that allows them to deal with stress. As children begin to participate in their care, they gain confidence and self-esteem. Fears and anxieties diminish with accomplishment and self-confidence. If the child demonstrates nonadherence in the rehabilitative phase, a behavior modification program can be initiated to promote or reward the child's accomplishment in care.

Children need to know that their injury and the treatments are not punishment for real or imagined transgressions and that the nurse understands their fear, anger, and discomfort. They also need body contact. This is often difficult to arrange for the child with massive burns. Stroking areas of unburned skin is comforting. Even older children enjoy sitting on the parent's lap and being cuddled and hugged. This can be a reward or a comfort in times of stress, but most of all it should be kept in mind that it is a natural part of childhood.

Psychosocial Support of the Family

Recognizing and respecting each family's strengths, differences, and methods of coping allow the nurse to respond to their unique needs by implementing a family-centered approach to care. In the acute phase, all attention is focused on the child, and the parents feel powerless and ineffectual. Most parents feel overwhelming guilt, whether or not the guilt is justified. They feel responsible for the injury. These feelings may impede the child's rehabilitation. Parents may indulge the child and allow nonadherent behaviors that affect physical and emotional recovery. Parents need to be informed of the child's progress and helped to cope with their feelings while supporting their child. The nurse can help them understand that it is not selfish to look after themselves and their own needs to meet their child's needs. It is important to recognize the parents' need to grieve the change in their child's normal appearance as part of the grieving process. Definitive professional help may be needed for parents whose response to the injury is severe or whose response to stress is manifested in destructive behavior.

The parents are members of the multidisciplinary team and participate in the development of the care plan. It is important to facilitate their input; to consider all aspects of the physical, emotional, social, and cultural factors affecting the child and family; and to establish a realistic home therapy program. The family's willingness to assume responsibility for care and their ability to implement the therapeutic regimen are assessed. Home, school, and other environmental factors are explored; financial concerns and available community resources are discussed; and a specific care plan for the child, with an anticipated follow-up program, is developed.

Prevention of Burn Injury

The best intervention is to prevent burns from occurring. Hot liquids in the kitchen and bathroom most commonly injure infants and toddlers. Hot liquids should be kept out of reach; tablecloths and dangling appliance cords are often pulled by toddlers, who spill hot grease and liquids on themselves. Electrical cords and outlets represent a potential risk to small children, who may chew on accessible cords and insert objects into outlets.

The Consumer Product Safety Commission recommends a reduction of water heater thermostats to a maximum of 48.9° C (120° F). The "dial-down" recommendation has been suggested by utility companies, burn treatment centers, medical personnel, and others interested in public safety. However, many water heaters continue to remain set at levels well above the safe level. Small children are especially at risk for scald injuries from hot tap water because of their decreased reaction time and agility, their curiosity, and the thermal sensitivity of their skin. Caregivers should never leave a child unattended in a bath and without adult supervision. Water should always be tested before a child is placed in the tub or shower.

The increased use of microwave ovens has resulted in burn injuries from the extremely hot internal temperatures generated in heated items. Baby formula, jelly-filled pastries, and hot liquids and dishes may result in cutaneous scalds or the ingestion of overheated liquids. Parents should use caution when removing items from the microwave oven and should always test the food before giving it to children.

As children mature, risk-taking behaviors increase. Matches and lighters are dangerous in the hands of the young. Adults must remember to keep potentially hazardous items out of the reach of children; a lighter, like a match, is a tool for adult use.

Education related to fire safety and survival should begin with the very young. They can practice "stop, drop, and roll" to extinguish a fire. The fire escape route, including a safe meeting place away from the home in case of fire, also should be practiced.

Community activities are also helpful in supporting burn survivors and preventing burns. The Aluminum Cans for Burned Children (ACBC) is an exemplary effort based at the Paul and Carol David Foundation Burn Institute, Akron, Ohio.* Activities funded by ACBC include Burn Survivors Support Group, Burn Camp, and meetings of Juvenile Firestoppers (for children with fire-setting behavior). Adult weekend retreats and school and family education sessions are a part of this program. The burn center and fire department provide the personnel to present programs.

Additional information on burn care and prevention can be obtained from the American Burn Association† and the National Safety Council.‡ The Alisa Ann Ruch Burn Foundation§ provides assistance to burn victims and burn centers. The Shriners Burn Institutes are staffed to treat pediatric patients after acute burn injuries and those requiring rehabilitative and reconstructive services as a result of scarring and functional impairment. Information can be obtained from local Shrine Temples and Shrine Clubs, from Shriners Hospitals, or by contacting Shriners International.¶ The Alisa Ann Ruch Foundation and Shriners Hospitals for Children support research to improve burn care and treatment and promote public education in burn prevention.

Sunburn

Sunburn is a common skin injury caused by overexposure to UV light waves. The sun emits a continuous spectrum of visible and nonvisible light rays that range in length from very short to very long. The shorter, higher-frequency waves are more damaging than longer wavelengths, but much of the light is filtered out as it travels through the atmosphere. Of the light that does filter through, *ultraviolet A (UVA) waves* are the longest and cause only minimum burning, but play a significant role in photosensitive and photoallergic reactions. They are also responsible for premature aging of the skin and potentiate the effects of *ultraviolet B (UVB)* waves. UVB waves are shorter and are responsible for tanning, burning, and most of the harmful effects attributed to sunlight, especially skin cancer.

Numerous factors influence the amount of UVB exposure. Maximum exposure occurs at midday (10 AM to 3 PM), when the distance from the sun to a given spot on the earth is shortest. There is more exposure at higher altitudes and near the equator, and less when the sky is hazy (although the amount of UV radiation that does penetrate is easily underestimated). Window glass effectively screens out UVB but not UVA rays. Fresh snow, water, and sand reflect UV rays, especially when the sun is directly overhead.

Sunburn is usually an epidermal burn, although severe sunburn can be a partial-thickness burn with blister formation. Treatment of sunburn involves stopping the burning process, decreasing the inflammatory response, and rehydrating the skin. Local application of cool tap water soaks, or immersion in a tepid-water bath (temperature slightly below 36.7° C [98° F]) for 20 minutes or until the skin is cool, limits tissue destruction and relieves the discomfort. After the cool applications, a bland oil-in-water moisturizing lotion can be applied. Partial-thickness burns are treated the same as those from any heat source (see earlier discussion on burns).

Nursing Care Management

Protection from sunburn is the major goal of management, and the harmful effects of the sun on the delicate skin of infants and children are currently receiving increased attention. To protect skin exposed to the sun for extended periods, skin should be covered with clothing, and FDA-approved sun protection agents should be applied.

Two types of products are available for sun protection: *topical sunscreens*, which partially absorb UV light, and *sun blockers*, which block out UV rays by reflecting sunlight. The most frequently recommended sun blockers are zinc oxide and titanium dioxide ointments. Sunscreens are products containing an *SPF* based on evaluation of effectiveness against UV rays. The SPF is a number, such as 15, which indicates that if individuals normally burn in 10 minutes without a sunscreen, use of a sunscreen with SPF 15 allows them to remain in the sun 15 times 10, or 150 minutes (2½ hours) before acquiring the same degree of burns. The most effective sunscreens against UVB are *p*-aminobenzoic acid (PABA) and *PABA-esters*. However, many individuals are allergic to PABA, and sunscreens without PABA are encouraged to prevent these reactions in children.

Sunscreens are applied evenly to all exposed areas, with special attention to skin folds and areas that might become exposed as clothing shifts. Parents are directed to read labels of sunscreen products carefully for the SPF and follow the manufacturer's directions for application.

**Akron Children's Hospital, One Perkins Square, Akron, OH 44308-1062; 330-543-8224;* www.akronchildrens.org.

†625 N. Michigan Ave., Suite 2550, Chicago, IL 60611; 312-642-9260; fax: 312-642-9130; e-mail: info@ameriburn.org; www.ameriburn.org.

‡1121 Spring Lake Drive, Itasca, IL 60143-3201; 630-285-1121, e-mail: info@nsc.org; www.nsc.org.

§2501 W. Burbank Blvd., Suite 201, Burbank, CA 91505; 800-242-BURN; www.aarbf.org.

¶2900 Rocky Point Drive, Tampa, FL 33607; 813-281-0300; Shriners International website: www.shrinershq.org; *Shriners Hospitals for Children website:* www.shrinershq.org.

NURSING ALERT Sunscreens are not recommended for infants younger than 6 months of age. However, infants younger than 6 months of age may have sunscreen applied over small areas of skin such as the back of hands that may not be adequately covered by clothing when they are in the sun (American Academy of Pediatrics, Committee on Environmental Health, 1999). Infants should be kept out of the sun or physically shaded from it. Fabric with a tight weave, such as cotton, offers good protection.

Individuals who work in the community, such as teachers, day care workers, coaches, and youth-group leaders, and relatives should all be made aware of sun safety for children. Sunscreens must be applied *liberally*.

Cold Injury

Cold injuries are most commonly seen in very cold regions. The nature of the body's heat-regulating mechanisms are such that the inner portion of the body, or core, produces heat, and the periphery, or outer area, conserves or dissipates heat. When the body attempts to conserve heat, the outer tissues are subjected to low temperatures, and local trauma may result.

Chilblain, redness and swelling of the skin, occurs when extremities, usually the hands, are exposed intermittently to temperatures of −1.1° to 15.5° C (30° to 60° F). The response may vary but is characterized by intense vasodilation that increases the temperature of involved tissues above that of unaffected tissue and produces edematous, reddish blue patches that itch and burn. As warming takes place, the sensations become more intense, but ordinarily they subside in a few days.

Frostbite is the term used to describe tissue damage caused when excessive heat loss to local tissues allows ice crystals to form in tissues. The frostbitten part appears white or blanched, feels solid, and is without sensation. Rapid rewarming is associated with less tissue necrosis than slow thawing. It restores blood flow and shortens the period of cellular damage. Rewarming produces a flush (sometimes deep purple) and a return of sensation, which is extremely painful. Large blisters may appear in 24 to 48 hours after rewarming and begin to reabsorb within 5 to 10 days, followed by the formation of a hard black eschar. Superficial injury often heals without incident. Rewarming is accomplished by immersing the part in well-agitated water at 37.8° to 42.2° C (100° to 108° F). Discomfort is managed with analgesics and sedatives. Care of blistered skin is similar to that described for burns. It is seldom possible to estimate the extent of tissue loss until new skin layers are revealed after the eschar layer separates.

Key Points

- A variety of factors can produce lesions of the skin.
- It is important for nurses to be able to describe skin lesions accurately.
- The process of wound healing consists of hemostasis, inflammation, proliferation, and remodeling.
- A moist environment promotes wound healing.
- Bacterial, viral, and fungal infections are common in childhood.
- Some skin diseases are transmitted by arthropod vectors, especially ticks.
- The most common skin infestations of childhood—scabies and pediculosis capitis—affect children of any age and from any social class.
- Contact dermatitis may involve a primary irritant or a sensitizing agent.
- Adverse reactions to drugs are manifested more often in the skin than in any other body organ.
- The most common skin disorders of infancy are diaper dermatitis, seborrheic dermatitis, and AD.
- Acne, a disorder affecting many adolescents, is related to hormonal fluctuation, stimulation of the sebaceous glands, excessive sebum production, the formation of comedones, and the overgrowth of the *P. acnes* organism.
- Medication and gentle facial cleansing are the treatments of choice for acne.

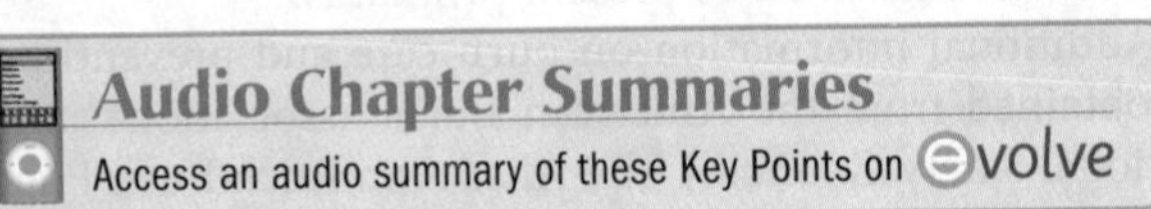
Audio Chapter Summaries
Access an audio summary of these Key Points on evolve

- Burns are caused by thermal, chemical, electric, or radioactive agents.
- Burns are assessed on the extent, depth, and severity of the wound.
- Essentials of emergency care of burn injury include stopping the burning process, covering the burn, transporting the injured child to medical aid, and providing reassurance to the child and family.
- Management of minor burns consists of facilitating wound healing, relieving discomfort, and preventing complications.
- Management of major burns consists of facilitating wound healing, relieving discomfort, replacing destroyed skin, preventing or treating complications, and providing rehabilitation.
- Sunscreen is recommended for use when the skin is exposed to the damaging effects of the sun's rays.
- Thermal injuries to the skin can result from exposure to extreme cold.

References

American Academy of Dermatology: *Acne*, 2006. Available at www.aad.org/public/Publications/pamphlets/Acne.htm (accessed February 1, 2007).

American Academy of Dermatology: *Guidelines for the care of atopic dermatitis*, 2003. Available at www.aad.org/professionals/guidelines/AtopicDermatitis.htm (accessed February 2, 2007).

American Academy of Pediatrics, Committee on Environmental Health: Ultraviolet light: a hazard to children, *Pediatrics* 104(2):328-333, 1999.

American Academy of Pediatrics, Committee on Infectious Diseases, Pickering L (editor): *Red book: 2006 report of the Committee on Infectious Diseases*, ed 27, Elk Grove Village, Ill, 2006, The Academy.

Annequin D et al: Fixed 50% nitrous oxide oxygen mixture for painful procedures: a French survey, *Pediatrics* 105(4):E47, 2000.

Arnoldo B, Klein M, Gibran NS: Practice guidelines for the management of electrical injuries, *J Burn Care Res* 27(4):439-447, 2006.

Baker RAU et al: Burn wound itch control using H_1 and H_2 antagonists, *J Burn Care Rehabil* 22(4):263-268, 2001.

Bernardo LM et al: Dog bites in children treated in a pediatric emergency department, *J Spect Pediatr Nurs* 5(2):87-95, 2000.

Burkhart CN, Specht K, Neckers D: Synergistic activity of benzoyl peroxide and erythromycin, *Skin Pharmacol Appl Skin Physiol* 13(5):292-296, 2000.

Centers for Disease Control and Prevention: Nonfatal dog bite–related injuries treated in hospital emergency departments—United States, 2001, *Morbid Mortal Wkly Rep* 52(26):605-610, 2003.

Centers for Disease Control and Prevention: Cat-scratch disease in children—Texas, September 2000–August 2001, *Morbid Mortal Wkly Rep* 51(10):212-214, 2002.

Centers for Disease Control and Prevention, Division of Parasitic Diseases: *Scabies*, February 4, 2008. Available at www.cdc.gov/ncidod/dpd/parasites/scabies/factsht_scabies.htm (accessed April 22, 2008).

Centers for Disease Control and Prevention, Division of Parasitic Diseases: *Treating head lice infestation*, August 19, 2005. Available at www.cdc.gov/ncidod/dpd/parasites/lice/factsht_head_lice_treating.htm (accessed April 22, 2008).

Frankowski BL, Weiner LB: Head lice, *Pediatrics* 110(3):638-643, 2002.

Goates BM et al: An effective nonchemical treatment for head lice: a lot of hot air, *Pediatrics* 188(5):1962-1970, 2006.

Herndon DN (editor): *Total burn care*, ed 3, London, 2007, Saunders.

Jacobs DG, Deutsch NL, Brewer M: Suicide, depression, and isotretinoin: is there a causal link? *J Am Acad Dermatol* 45(5):S168-S175, 2001.

Kaplan SL: Community-acquired methicillin-resistant *Staphylococcus aureus* infections in children, *Semin Pediatr Infect Dis* 17(3):113-119, 2006.

Krasner DL, Rodeheaver GT, Sibbald RG: *Chronic wound care: a clinical source book for healthcare professionals*, ed 3, Wayne, PA, 2001, HMP Communications.

Kronemyer B: Scratching the surface of atopic and contact dermatitis, *Infect Dis Child* 16(3):40, 2003.

Laude TA: Acne in childhood and adolescence: update on treatment choices, *Consultant* 3:457-465, 2000.

Lee MC et al: Management and outcome of children with skin and soft tissue abscesses caused by community-acquired methicillin-resistant *Staphylococcus aureus*, *Pediatr Infect Dis J* 23(2):123-127, 2004.

Mancini AJ: Acne vulgaris: a treatment update, *Contemp Pediatr* 17(12):122-133, 2000.

McCord SS, Levy ML: Practical guide to pediatric wound care, *Semin Plast Surg* 20(3):92-199, 2006.

Mumcuoglu KY et al: International guidelines for effective control of head louse infestations, *J Drugs Dermatol* 6(4):409-414, 2007.

Pearlman DL: A simple treatment for head lice: dry on, suffocation based pediculicide, *Pediatrics* 114(3):e275-e279, 2004.

Purdue GF: American Burn Association presidential address 2006 on nutrition: yesterday, today, and tomorrow, *J Burn Care Res* 28(1):1-5, 2007.

Russell JJ: Topical therapy for acne, *Am Fam Physician* 61(2):357-366, 2000.

Strong M, Johnstone PW: Interventions for treating scabies, *Cochrane Database Syst Rev* 18(3):CD000320, 2008.

US Food and Drug Administration: FDA issues health advisory regarding labeling changes for lindane products, *HealthInfo Tx Rep* April 2003. Available at www.fda.gov/bbs/topics/ANSWERS/2003/ANS01205.html (accessed March 4, 2007).

Wade CF: Keeping Lyme disease at bay: an integrated approach to prevention, *Am J Nurs* 100(7):26-31, 2000.

Wormser GP et al: The clinical assessment, treatment, and prevention of Lyme disease, human granulocytic anaplasmosis, and babesiosis: clinical practice guidelines by the Infections Diseases Society of America, *Clin Infect Dis* 43:1089-1134, 2006.

Yetman RJ, Parks D: Diagnosis and management of atopic dermatitis, *J Pediatr Health Care* 16(3):143-145, 2002.

Unit 11

54 Musculoskeletal or Articular Dysfunction

Learning Objectives

On completion of this chapter the reader will be able to:

- Outline a care plan for a child immobilized with an injury or a degenerative disease.
- Formulate a teaching plan for the parents of a child in a cast.
- Explain the functions of the various types of traction.
- Differentiate among the various congenital skeletal defects.
- Design a teaching plan for the parents of a child with a congenital skeletal deformity.
- Describe the therapies and nursing care of a child with scoliosis.
- Outline a care plan for a child with osteomyelitis.
- Differentiate between osteosarcoma and Ewing's sarcoma.
- Describe the nursing care of a child with rheumatoid arthritis.
- Demonstrate an understanding of the management of systemic lupus erythematosus.

Electronic Resources

Additional information related to the content in Chapter 54 can be found on

evolve the Companion Website at http://evolve.elsevier.com/Perry/maternal/

- NCLEX Review Questions
- Animation—Bone Fractures
- Animation—Spine Structure
- Assessment Video
- Case Study—Developmental Dysplasia of the Hip
- Case Study—Fractures
- Case Study—Osteomyelitis
- Critical Thinking Exercise—Osteogenic Sarcoma
- Nursing Care Plan—The Child Who Is Immobilized
- Skill—Monitoring Neurovascular Status

The Immobilized Child

One of the most difficult aspects of illness in children is the immobility it imposes. Children by nature are usually active, and immobility, however temporary, may have lasting effects on the child's developmental progress. The most frequent reasons for immobility are congenital defects (e.g., spina bifida); degenerative disorders (e.g., muscular dystrophy); and infections or injuries that impair the integumentary system (severe burns), the musculoskeletal system (e.g., multiple fractures, osteomyelitis), or the neurologic system (e.g., spinal cord injury, Guillain-Barré syndrome, head injury). At times therapies such as traction and spinal fusion are responsible for prolonged immobilization, although the increasing trends in health care are early mobilization and discharge and outpatient treatment.

Physiologic Effects of Immobilization

Many clinical studies, including space program research, have documented predictable consequences that occur after immobilization and the absence of gravitational force. Functional and metabolic responses to restricted movement can be noted in most of the body systems. Each has a direct influence on the child's growth and development because homeostatic mechanisms thrive on normal use and need feedback to maintain dynamic equilibrium. Inactivity leads to a decrease in the functional capabilities of the whole body as dramatically as the lack of physical exercise leads to muscle weakness.

Disuse from illness, injury, or a sedentary lifestyle can limit function and potentially delay age-appropriate milestones. Most of the pathologic changes that occur during immobilization arise from decreased muscle strength and mass, decreased metabolism, and bone demineralization, which are closely interrelated, with one change leading to or affecting the other. Some results of immobilization are primary and produce a direct effect; other pathophysiologic consequences occur frequently but seem to be more indirect and are therefore secondary effects. Many pathophysiologic changes affect more than one body system, with the primary or secondary effect being demonstrated in both systems.

The major effects of immobilization are outlined briefly in Table 54-1 and are related directly or indirectly to decreased muscle activity, which produces numerous primary changes in the musculoskeletal system with secondary alterations in the cardiovascular, respiratory, metabolic, and renal systems. The musculoskeletal changes that occur during disuse are a result of alterations in gravity and stress on the muscles, joints,

Table 54-1 Summary of Physical Effects of Immobilization*

PRIMARY EFFECTS	SECONDARY EFFECTS
Muscular System	
Decreased muscle strength, tone, and endurance	Decreased venous return and decreased cardiac output Decreased metabolism and need for oxygen Decreased exercise tolerance Bone demineralization
Disuse atrophy and loss of muscle mass	Catabolism Loss of strength
Loss of joint mobility	Contractures, ankylosis of joints
Weak back muscles	Secondary spinal deformities
Weak abdominal muscles	Impaired respiration
Skeletal System	
Bone demineralization—osteoporosis, hypercalcemia	Negative calcium balance Pathologic fractures Calcium deposits Extraosseous bone formation, especially at hip, knee, elbow, and shoulder Renal calculi
Negative calcium balance	Life-threatening electrolyte imbalance
Metabolism	
Decreased metabolic rate	Slowing of all systems Decreased food intake
Negative nitrogen balance	Decline in nutritional state Impaired healing
Hypercalcemia	Electrolyte imbalance
Decreased production of stress hormones	Decreased physical and emotional coping capacity
Cardiovascular System	
Decreased efficiency of orthostatic neurovascular reflexes	Inability to adapt readily to upright position Pooling of blood in extremities in upright posture
Diminished vasopressor mechanism	Orthostatic hypotension (intolerance) with syncope—hypotension, decreased cerebral blood flow, tachycardia
Altered distribution of blood volume	Decreased cardiac workload Decreased exercise tolerance
Venous stasis	Systemic embolus or thrombus development, pulmonary emboli
Dependent edema	Tissue breakdown and susceptibility to infection
Respiratory System	
Decreased need for oxygen	Altered oxygen–carbon dioxide exchange and metabolism
Decreased chest expansion and diminished vital capacity	Diminished oxygen intake Dyspnea and inadequate arterial oxygen saturation; acidosis
Poor abdominal tone and distention	Interference with diaphragmatic excursion Hypostatic pneumonia
Mechanical or biochemical secretion retention	Bacterial and viral pneumonia Atelectasis
Loss of respiratory muscle strength	Poor cough Upper respiratory tract infection
Gastrointestinal System	
Distention caused by poor abdominal muscle tone	Interference with respiratory movements
No specific primary effect	Difficulty in feeding in prone position; gravitation effect on feces through ascending colon, or weakened smooth muscle tone causing constipation Decreased appetite Anorexia
Urinary System	
Alteration of gravitational force	Difficulty in voiding in prone position
Impaired ureteral peristalsis	Urinary retention in calyces and bladder Infection Renal calculi
Integumentary System	
No specific primary effect	Decreased circulation and pressure leading to tissue injury and decreased healing capacity Difficulty with personal hygiene

*Not all problems will apply in every situation.

and bones. Muscle disuse leads to tissue breakdown and loss of muscle mass *(atrophy)*. Muscle atrophy causes decreased strength and endurance, which may take weeks or months to restore.

During immobilization a joint contracture begins when the arrangement of collagen, the main structural protein of connective tissues, is altered, resulting in a denser tissue that does not glide as easily. Eventually muscles, tendons, and ligaments can shorten and reduce joint movement, ultimately producing contractures that restrict function. The daily stresses on bone created by motion and weight bearing maintain the balance between bone formation (osteoblastic activity) and bone resorption (osteoclastic activity). During immobilization, increased calcium leaves the bone, causing osteopenia (demineralization of the bones), which may predispose bone to pathologic fractures. The major musculoskeletal consequences of immobilization are (1) significant decrease in muscle size, strength, and endurance; (2) bone demineralization leading to osteoporosis; and (3) contractures and decreased joint mobility. The larger the portion of the body immobilized and the longer the immobilization, the greater the hazards of immobility.

Prolonged immobilization also causes venous stasis, particularly in the lower extremities; this may lead to thrombus formation, which in turn may obstruct vessels in organs such as the lungs, kidneys, or brain. Pulmonary embolus is a life-threatening complication of immobilization.

Psychologic Effects of Immobilization

For children, one of the most difficult aspects of illness is immobilization. Throughout childhood, physical activity is an integral part of daily life and is essential for physical growth and development. The activity helps children deal with a variety of feelings and impulses and provides a mechanism by which they can exert control over inner tensions. Children respond to anxiety with increased activity. Removal of this power deprives them of necessary input and a natural outlet for their feelings and fantasies.

When children are immobilized by disease or as part of a treatment regimen, they experience diminished environmental stimuli with a loss of tactile input and an altered perception of themselves and their environment. Sudden or gradual immobilization narrows the amount and variety of environmental stimuli children receive by means of all of their senses: touch; sight; hearing; taste; smell; and proprioception, or the feeling of where they are in their environment. This sensory deprivation commonly leads to feelings of isolation and boredom, and of being forgotten, especially by peers.

Physical interference with the activity of young children gives them a feeling of frustration and helplessness. Even speech and language skills require sensorimotor activity and experience. For the toddler, exploration and imitative behaviors are essential to developing a sense of autonomy; the preschooler's expression of initiative is evidenced by the need for vigorous physical activity; the school-age child's development is strongly influenced by physical achievement and competition; and the adolescent relies on mobility to achieve independence. The quest for mastery at every stage of development is related to mobility.

The monotony of immobilization can lead to sluggish intellectual and psychomotor responses, decreased communication skills, increased fantasizing, and even hallucinations and disorientation. Children are likely to become depressed over their loss of ability to function or any marked changes in body image. They may seek the attention of others by reverting to earlier developmental behaviors, such as wanting to be fed or bed-wetting.

Limbs in casts or traction transmit less than normal sensory data. Children who have limited ability to feel others touching them not only experience less tactile stimuli in a physical sense, but are also deprived of warm, loving feelings that arise from being touched. The loss of feeling derived from touch can further add to their sense of being isolated and unwanted.

Children may react to immobility by active protest, anger, and aggressive behavior; or they may become quiet, passive, and submissive. They may believe the immobilization is a justified punishment for misbehavior. Children should be allowed to express their feelings, but it should be within the limits of safety to their self-esteem and not damaging to the integrity of others. For example, providing an inanimate object to attack rather than a person or a valued possession is safe and therapeutic. When children are unable to express anger and frustration, aggression is often displayed inappropriately through regressive behavior and outbursts of crying or temper tantrums.

Effect on Families

Even brief periods of immobilization may disrupt family function, and sudden catastrophic illness or chronic disability may severely tax their resources and coping abilities.

The family's needs often must be met by the services of a multidisciplinary team, and nurses play a key role in anticipating the services they will need and in coordinating conferences to plan care. In preparation for discharge, home visits are advisable, and home management is commonly planned weeks in advance of the actual discharge. Such planning includes special considerations for cultural, economic, physical, and psychologic needs. A child with a severe disability is very dependent, and caregivers need rest periods to revitalize themselves. Individual and group counseling is beneficial for solving problems in advance and provides an emotional support system. Parent groups may also be helpful and often allow nonthreatening social contact. The families of children with permanent disabilities need long-term resources because some of the most difficult problems arise as they try to sustain high-quality care for many years (see Chapter 41).

Nursing Care Management

Physical assessment of the child who is immobilized as a result of an injury or a degenerative disease focuses not only on the injured part (e.g., fracture or damaged joint) but also on the functioning of other systems that may be affected secondarily (e.g., the circulatory, renal, respiratory, muscular, and gastrointestinal systems). With long-term immobilization there may also be neurologic impairment and changes in electrolytes (especially calcium), nitrogen balance, and the general metabolic rate. The psychologic impact of immobilization should also be assessed.

Children who require prolonged total immobility and are unable to move themselves in bed should be placed on a special surface to prevent skin breakdown. Frequent position changes also help prevent dependent edema and stimulate circulation, respiratory function, gastrointestinal motility, and neurologic sensation. Children at greater risk for skin breakdown include those with prolonged immobilization; orthotic and prosthetic devices, including wheelchairs; and plaster casts (Samaniego, 2003). Additional risk factors include poor nutrition, friction (from bed linen with traction), and moist skin (from urine or perspiration). In critically ill children factors associated with increased skin breakdown included requirement for mechanical ventilation, age less than 2 years, length of stay of 4 days or more, and a respiratory diagnosis on admission (Schindler et al, 2007). In neonates and infants, skin breakdown is more likely to occur on the occiput and on the nasal septum when nasal continuous positive airway pressure devices are used (McCord et al, 2004; Razmus, Roberts, & Curley, 2001).

Nursing care of children at risk includes proactive strategies for preventing skin breakdown when such conditions are present. On admission to the acute care facility, each child should have a skin assessment and a skin score documented in the medical record. The Modified Braden Q Scale is a reliable, objective tool that may be used in the assessment for pressure ulcer development in children who are acutely ill or who are at risk for skin breakdown from neurologic conditions and immobilization (Curley et al, 2003). Frequent position changes help prevent dependent edema and stimulate circulation, respiratory function, gastrointestinal motility, and neurologic sensations. Antiembolism stockings or sequential compression devices (SCDs) also help minimize or prevent dependent edema in the lower extremities.

The child should be allowed as much activity as possible within the limitations of the illness or treatment; any functional mobility, however minimal, is preferred to total immobility. This poses few problems for most children, whose innate ingenuity and natural inclination toward mobility provide them with the impetus for physical activity. They need the opportunity, the materials or objects to stimulate activity, and the encouragement and participation of others. Those who are unable to move need passive exercise and movement, often in consultation with a physical therapist.

When possible, transporting the child by stretcher, stroller, or wagon outside the confines of the room increases environmental stimuli and provides social contact with others. While hospitalized, children benefit from same-age visitors, computers, books, interactive video games, and other items brought from their own room at home, all of which help them function in a more normal way. An activity center or tray that slants can be particularly helpful for the child with limited mobility to use for drawing, coloring, writing, and playing with small toys such as trucks and cars. A play therapist or child life specialist should be consulted for recreational planning. The use of play (see Chapter 44) and any activity that is tolerated (e.g., turning in bed or changing the location of the bed within the room) help alter the monotony of immobilization and decrease tension and frustration.

Using dolls, stuffed animals, or puppets to illustrate and explain the immobilization is a valuable tool for small children. Placing a cast, tubing, or other restraining equipment on the doll offers the child a nonthreatening opportunity to express, through the doll, feelings concerning the restrictions and feelings toward the nurse and other health care providers.

As soon as possible, hospitalized children should be allowed to wear their own clothes (street clothes, especially in preadolescent and adolescent girls) and resume school and previous activities. A parent or siblings should be allowed to stay overnight and room in with the hospitalized child to minimize the effects of family disruption from hospitalization. Visits from significant persons, such as family members and friends, offer occasions for emotional support and also provide opportunities for learning how to care for the child. If a traumatic incident caused the child's disability, guilt feelings may be displayed overtly or masked behind regressive or aggressive behavior. The feeling that "I must have been bad for this to happen" is common, and honest feedback stating, "It just happened—it was an accident," needs to be repeated many times.

Some privacy is needed, particularly by the teenager, and most long-term health care facilities recognize that private or semiprivate rooms shared by one or two children, rather than large wards, are better environments for habilitation or rehabilitation. Within the framework of family-centered care, institutions are placing more emphasis on providing a room wherein the child's parent may stay overnight and significant others may visit.

High-protein, high-calorie foods are encouraged to prevent negative nitrogen balance, which may be difficult to correct by diet, especially if there is anorexia as a result of immobility and decreased gastrointestinal function (decreased motility and possibly constipation). Stimulating the appetite with small servings of attractively arranged, preferred foods may be sufficient. Children typically dislike hospital food, which is usually not tailored to their age. In some institutions food services are geared toward children's preferences with child-friendly menus and smaller food portions served. Parents and friends are allowed to bring in favorite foods from home or other sources such as fast food places, provided they meet necessary requirements for the illness. Allowing such choices enables children to exert more healthy control of their environment and subsequently decreases resistance to treatments and schedules, which is common behavior evidenced when adults and children are not given any choices in an acute care setting. Sometimes, supplementary nasogastric or gastrostomy feedings or intravenous (IV) fluids may be needed, but these are reserved for serious disability in which oral intake is impossible.

One of the most useful interventions to help children cope with immobility is participation in their own care. Self-care is usually well received by children. They can help plan their daily routine; select their diet (when possible); and choose clothes, including innovative adornments such as baseball caps, brightly decorated sunglasses, or brightly colored stockings, to express their autonomy and individuality. They are encouraged to do as much as they are able to for themselves to keep muscles active and their interest alive. Most of children's activity of daily living is play; therefore therapies that incorporate this concept are more apt to gain their cooperation.

With the increased trend toward early mobilization, early discharge, and home health care, many children are discharged home within a few hours or days of hospitalization. Follow-up treatment may take place in the home setting or an outpatient ambulatory facility. Although most of the suggestions discussed relate to hospital care, the same consultations (physical therapist, occupational therapist, child life specialist, and speech therapist) and environment may be considered in the home as well to help the child and family achieve independence and normalization.

Family Support and Home Care

The needs of a child with severe or chronic disabilities can be complex, and although the optimal situation is for family members to have time to assimilate the teachings and demonstrations needed to understand the child's situation and care, this is often shortened considerably by moving the child to a rehabilitation facility or even to the home within a matter of days. Even the child who is confined on a short-term basis can be a challenge for the family, which is usually unprepared for the problems imposed by the child's special needs. Home modification is usually needed for facilitating care, especially when it involves traction, large casts, or extended confinement (see Chapter 43). Suitable child care may be needed for times when all family members work.

Just as in the hospital, the child at home is encouraged to be as independent as possible and to follow a schedule that approximates his or her normal lifestyle as nearly as possible, such as continuing school lessons, regular bedtime, and suitable recreational activities.

Traumatic Injury

Soft-Tissue Injury

Injuries to the muscles, ligaments, and tendons are common in children (Fig. 54-1). In young children, soft-tissue injury usually results from mishaps during play. In older children and adolescents, participation in sports is the more common cause.

Contusions

A contusion is damage to the soft tissue, subcutaneous structures, and muscle. The tearing of these tissues and small blood vessels and the inflammatory response lead to hemorrhage, edema, and associated pain when the child attempts to move the injured part. The escape of blood into the tissues is observed as *ecchymosis,* a black-and-blue discoloration.

Large contusions cause gross swelling, pain, and disability, and those sustained while the child is participating in sports usually receive immediate attention from health personnel. The less spectacular, smaller injuries may go unnoticed, allowing continued participation; however, they can become disabling after rest because of pain and muscle spasm. The young athlete is commonly instructed to "walk it off" or disregard the pain. Instead of this approach, first a qualified health care worker or certified athletic trainer should carry out an assessment of the affected area because further damage to the site may result if the area is severely traumatized. Immediate treatment consists of cold application, as described in the section on sprains. Return to participation is allowed when the strength and range of motion of the affected extremity are equal to those of the opposite extremity. *Myositis ossificans* may occur from deep contusions to the biceps or quadriceps muscles; this condition may result in a restriction of flexibility of the affected limb.

Contusions are crush injuries that occur in children when they slam their fingers (in doors, folding chairs, or equipment) or hit their fingers (as when hammering a nail). A severe crush injury involves the bone, with swelling and bleeding beneath the nail (subungual) and sometimes laceration of the pulp of the distal phalanx. The *subungual hematoma* can be released by creating a hole at the proximal end of the nail with a battery-operated microcautery device or a heated sterile 18-gauge needle.

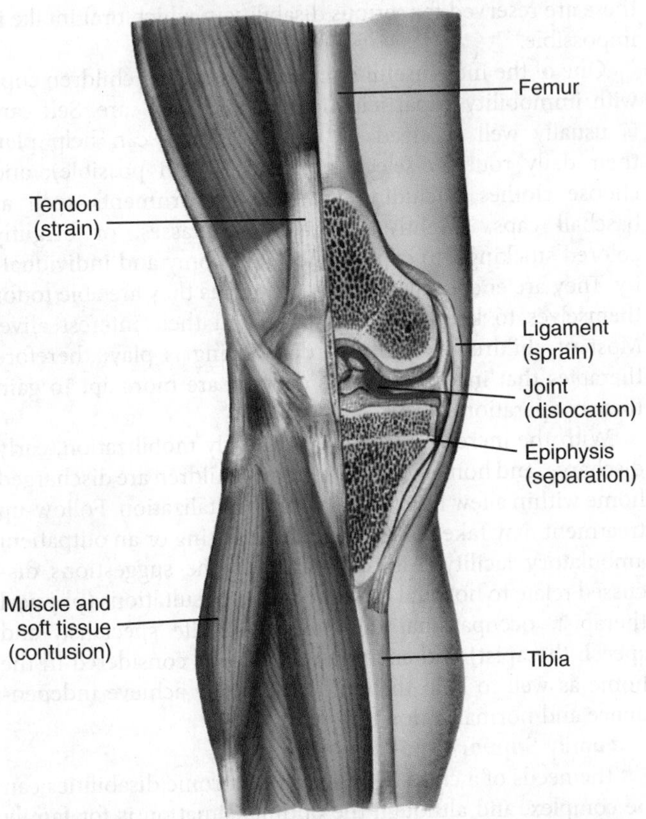

Fig. 54-1 Sites of injuries to bones, joints, and soft tissues.

Dislocations

Long bones are held in approximation to one another at the joint by ligaments. A dislocation occurs when the force of stress on the ligament is so great as to displace the normal position of the opposing bone ends or to displace the bone end from its socket. The predominant symptom is pain that increases with attempted passive or active movement of the extremity. In dislocations there may be an obvious deformity and inability to move the joint. Dislocation of the phalanges is the most common type seen in children, followed by elbow dislocation. One of the most common injuries in young children is subluxation of the annular ligament, also called "pulled elbow" or "*nursemaids' elbow.*" With this injury the annular ligament slips proximally off the radial head into the joint between the radial head and ulna, causing immediate pain and limited supination (Cornwall, 2007). In the majority of cases the injury occurs in a child younger than 5 years who receives a sudden longitudinal pull or traction at the wrist while the arm is fully extended and the forearm pronated. It usually occurs when an adult or older sibling who is holding the child by the hand or wrist gives a sudden pull or jerk to prevent a fall or attempts to lift the child by pulling the wrist, or when the child pulls away by dropping to the floor or ground. The child often cries, appears anxious, and refuses to use the affected limb. The practitioner manipulates the arm by applying firm finger pressure to the head of the radius, then supinates and flexes the forearm to return the ligament to its place. A click may be heard or felt, and functional use of the arm returns within minutes. However, the longer the subluxation is present, the longer it takes for the child to recover mobility after treatment. No anesthetic is usually required but a mild pain reliever such as acetaminophen may be given. In an older child, severe elbow injury or dislocation should be carefully evaluated by a practitioner immediately; likewise, a traumatic elbow injury in the younger child that is not a subluxation should be carefully evaluated.

In children younger than 5 years of age, the hip can be dislocated by a fall. The greatest risk after this injury is the potential loss of blood supply to the head of the femur. Relocation of the hip within 60 minutes after the injury provides the best chance for prevention of damage to the femoral head.

Shoulder dislocations occur most often in older adolescents and are often sports related. Temporary restriction of the joint, with a sling or bandage that secures the arm to the chest, in a shoulder dislocation, can provide sufficient comfort and immobilization until medical attention is received.

Simple dislocations should be reduced as soon as possible with the child under mild (procedural) sedation and often local anesthesia. Anesthetics such as IV ketamine (Ketalar), midazolam (Versed), IV propofol (Diprivan), or fentanyl (Sublimaze) can be used to produce partial or complete analgesia. An unreduced dislocation will be complicated by increased swelling, making reduction difficult and increasing the risk of neurovascular problems. Treatment depends on the severity of the injury.

Sprains

A sprain occurs when trauma to a joint is so severe that a ligament is partially or completely torn or stretched by the force created as a joint is twisted or wrenched, often accompanied by damage to associated blood vessels, muscles, tendons, and nerves.

The presence of joint laxity is the most valid indicator of the severity of a sprain. In a severe injury the child complains of the joint "feeling loose" or as if "something is coming apart," and may describe hearing a "snap," "pop," or "tearing." Pain is seldom the principal subjective symptom. There is a rapid onset with swelling (often diffuse), accompanied by immediate disability and appreciable reluctance to use the injured joint.

Strains

A strain is a microscopic tear to the musculotendinous unit and has features in common with sprains. The area is painful to touch and swollen. Most strains are incurred over time rather than suddenly, and the rapidity of the appearance provides clues regarding severity. In general, the more rapidly the strain occurs, the more severe the injury. When the strain involves the muscular portion, there is more bleeding, often palpable soon after injury and before edema obscures the hematoma.

Therapeutic Management

The first minutes to 12 hours are the most critical period for virtually all soft-tissue injuries. Basic principles of managing sprains and other soft-tissue injuries are summarized in the acronyms *RICE* and *ICES:*

RICE	ICES
R—Rest	**I**—Ice
I—Ice	**C**—Compression
C—Compression	**E**—Elevation
E—Elevation	**S**—Support

Soft-tissue injuries should be iced immediately. This is best accomplished with crushed ice wrapped in a towel or encased in a screw-top ice bag or resealable storage bag. A wet elastic wrap, which transfers cold better than dry wrap, is applied to provide compression and to keep the ice pack in place. Chemical-activated ice packs are also effective for immediate treatment but are not reusable and must be closely monitored for leakage. A cloth barrier should be used between the ice container and the skin to prevent trauma to the tissues. Ice has a rapid cooling effect on tissues and reduces the pain threshold. However, ice should never be applied for more than 30 minutes at a time because of the body's homeostatic response to cold, which may trigger a decrease in vascularization at the injury site. A plastic bag of frozen vegetables, such as peas, serves as a convenient ice pack for soft-tissue injuries. It is clean, watertight, and easily molded to the injured part. When available, snow placed in a plastic bag may serve as an ice bag.

Elevating the extremity uses gravity to facilitate venous return and to reduce edema formation in the damaged area. The point of injury should be kept several inches above the level of the heart for therapy to be effective. Several pillows can be used for elevation. Allowing the extremity to be dependent causes excessive fluid accumulation in the area of injury, delaying healing and causing painful swelling.

Torn ligaments, especially those in the knee, are usually treated by immobilization with a knee immobilizer or range-of-motion brace until the child is able to walk without a limp. Crutches are used for mobility to rest the affected extremity. Passive leg exercises, gradually increased to active ones, are begun as soon as sufficient healing has taken place. Parents and children are cautioned against using any form of liniment or other heat-producing preparation before examination. If the injury requires casting or splinting, the heat generated in the enclosed space can cause extreme discomfort and may even cause tissue damage. In some cases torn knee ligaments are managed with arthroscopy and ligament repair or reconstruction as necessary, depending on the extent of the tear, the ligaments involved, and the child's age. Surgical reconstruction of the anterior cruciate ligament may be performed in young athletes who wish to continue in active sports.

Fractures

Bone fractures occur when the resistance of bone against the stress being exerted yields to the stress force. Fractures are a common injury at any age but are more likely to occur in children and older adults. Because childhood is a time of rapid bone growth, the pattern of fractures, problems of diagnosis, and methods of treatment differ in the child and the adult. In children fractures heal much faster than in adults. Consequently, children may not require as long a period of immobilization of the affected extremity as an adult with a fracture.

Fracture injuries in children are most often a result of traumatic incidents at home, at school, in a motor vehicle, or in association with recreational activities. Children's everyday

evolve Animation—Bone Fractures

activities include vigorous play that predisposes them to injury—climbing, falling down, running into immovable objects, skateboarding, and receiving blows to any part of their bodies.

Aside from automobile accidents or falls from heights, true injuries that cause fractures rarely occur in infancy; therefore bone injury in children of that age group warrants further investigation. In any small child, radiographic evidence of fractures at various stages of healing is, with few exceptions, a result of physical abuse. Any investigation of fractures in infants, particularly multiple fractures, should include consideration of *osteogenesis imperfecta.*

The clavicle is probably the bone most commonly broken in childhood, with approximately half of clavicle fractures occurring in children under 10 years of age. Common mechanisms of injury include a fall with an outstretched hand or direct trauma to the bone.

Fractures in school-age children are often a result of bicycle, automobile, or skateboard injuries. Adolescents are vulnerable to multiple and severe trauma because they are active in sports and mobile on bicycles, all-terrain vehicles, skateboards, skis, snowboards, bicycles, and motorcycles.

Epiphyseal (or Physeal) Injuries

The weakest point of long bones is the cartilage growth plate, or epiphyseal plate. Consequently this is a common site of damage during trauma. Detection of epiphyseal injuries is sometimes difficult, but it is critical. Fractures involving the epiphysis or epiphyseal plate present special problems in determining whether bone growth will be affected. Treatment of these fractures may include open reduction and internal fixation to prevent or reduce growth disturbances.

Types of Fractures

A fractured bone consists of fragments—the fragment closer to the midline, or the proximal fragment; and the fragment farther from the midline, or the distal fragment. When fracture fragments are separated, the fracture is *complete;* when fragments remain attached, the fracture is *incomplete.* The fracture line can be any of the following:

- **Transverse**—Crosswise, at right angles to the long axis of the bone
- **Oblique**—Slanting but straight, between a horizontal and a perpendicular direction
- **Spiral**—Slanting and circular, twisting around the bone shaft

The twisting of an extremity while the bone is breaking results in a spiral break. If the fracture does not produce a break in the skin, it is a *simple,* or *closed, fracture. Open,* or *compound, fractures* are those with an open wound through which the bone is or has protruded. If the bone fragments cause damage to other organs or tissues (such as the lung or bladder), the injury is said to be a *complicated fracture.* When small fragments of bone are broken from the fractured shaft and lie in the surrounding tissue, the injury is a *comminuted fracture.* This type of fracture is rare in children. The types of fractures seen most often in children are described in Box 54-1 and in Fig. 54-2.

Immediately after a fracture occurs, the muscles contract and physiologically splint the injured area. This phenomenon accounts for the muscle tightness observed over a fracture site and the deformity that is produced as the muscles pull the bone ends out of alignment. This muscle response must be overcome by traction or complete muscle relaxation (e.g., with anesthesia) in order to realign the distal bone fragment to the proximal bone fragment.

BOX 54-1 Types of Fractures in Children

Plastic deformation—Occurs when the bone is bent but not broken. A child's flexible bone can be bent 45 degrees or more before breaking. However, if bent, the bone will straighten slowly, but not completely, to produce some deformity but without the angulation seen when the bone breaks. Bends occur most commonly in the ulna and fibula, often in association with fractures of the radius and tibia.

Buckle, or torus, fracture—Produced by compression of the porous bone; appears as a raised or bulging projection at the fracture site. These fractures occur in the most porous portion of the bone near the metaphysis (the portion of the bone shaft adjacent to the epiphysis) and are more common in young children.

Greenstick fracture—Occurs when a bone is angulated beyond the limits of bending. The compressed side bends, and the tension side fails, causing an incomplete fracture similar to the break observed when a green stick is broken.

Complete fracture—Divides the bone fragments. These fragments often remain attached by a periosteal hinge, which can aid or hinder reduction.

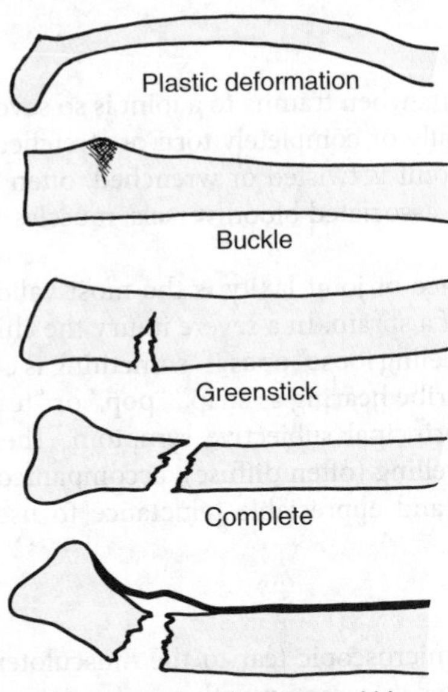

Fig. 54-2 Types of fractures in children.

Bone Healing and Remodeling

Bone healing is characteristically rapid in children because of the thickened periosteum and generous blood supply. When there is a break in the continuity of bone, the osteoblasts are stimulated to maximum activity. New bone cells are formed in immense numbers almost immediately after the injury and, in time, are evidenced by a bulging growth of new bone tissue between the fractured bone fragments. This is followed by deposition of calcium salts to form a *callus*.

Fractures heal in less time in children than in adults. The approximate healing times for a femoral shaft are as follows:

Neonatal period—2 to 3 weeks
Early childhood—4 weeks
Later childhood—6 to 8 weeks
Adolescence—8 to 12 weeks

Diagnostic Evaluation

A history is often lacking in childhood injuries. Infants are unable to communicate, and older children seldom volunteer information (even under direct questioning) when the injury occurred during suspicious activities. Unless they are witnesses to the injury, parents may misinterpret what the child is trying to say. In cases of child abuse, parents may give false information to protect themselves.

The child may exhibit the same manifestations seen in adults (Box 54-2). However, often a fracture is remarkably stable because of intact periosteum. The child may even be able to use an affected arm or walk on a fractured leg. In some cases, however, a fracture may not be apparent on radiographs. A fracture should be strongly suspected in a small child who refuses to bear weight or walk.

Radiographic examination is the most useful diagnostic tool for assessing skeletal trauma. The calcium deposits in bone make the entire structure radiopaque. Radiographic films are taken after fracture reduction and, in some cases, may be taken during the healing process to determine satisfactory progress.

Therapeutic Management

The majority of children's fractures heal well, and nonunion is rare. Most fractures are readily reduced by simple traction and immobilization until healing takes place. However, the position of the bone fragments in relation to one another influences the rapidity of healing and the residual deformity. Healing is prompt and complete with end-to-end apposition, but a gap between fragments delays (or prevents) healing. The goals of fracture management are:

- To regain alignment and length of the bony fragments (reduction)
- To retain alignment and length (immobilization)
- To restore function to the injured parts
- To prevent further injury

In children the bone fragments are usually realigned and immobilized by traction or by closed manipulation and casting until an adequate callus is formed. Weight bearing on lower extremity fractures and active movement for the purpose of regaining function can begin after the fracture site is stable. The child's natural tendency to be active is usually sufficient to restore normal mobility, and physical therapy is rarely needed. In most cases children's fractures can be managed by closed reduction and cast immobilization, which is most often provided on an outpatient basis with reevaluation in 7 to 10 days.

Children are most frequently hospitalized for fractures of the femur and the supracondylar area of the distal humerus, which may require internal fixation and pinning; displaced supracondylar fractures in children should be treated surgically (Do & Herrera-Soto, 2003; Shrader, 2008). Fractures of the humerus, which usually result from a fall with the arm in extension, frequently involve the supracondylar portion. These fractures especially place the patient at risk for nerve damage and angulation deformities; therefore most children with a fractured humerus are taken to surgery for either a closed or open reduction with a percutaneous pinning of the fractured bone segments. Preoperatively the fracture is reduced with adequate analgesia and a temporary splint for immobilization.

If simple reductions cannot be achieved or if a neurovascular problem is detected after injury, observation in a hospital is indicated. Severe contusions with profound swelling cannot be treated with a cast, which would act as a tourniquet on the extremity. A badly malaligned fracture requires traction for a period before a cast is applied.

Wrist buckle fractures are common in a child who falls and extends the arm forward to break the fall. There are reports of radius and/or ulna buckle fractures in children treated with a removable splint for 3 to 4 weeks instead of a short arm cast (Plint et al, 2006). The children treated with removable splints had better wrist function, had adequate bone healing, and experienced less inconvenience for bathing compared with the group of children placed in a short arm cast.

The major methods for immobilizing a fracture—casting and traction—are described in the following sections.

Nursing Care Management

Nurses are frequently the persons who make the initial assessment of a child with a suspected fracture (see Emergency box). The child and parents may be frightened and upset, and the child is often in pain. Therefore, if the child is alert and there is no evidence of hemorrhage, the initial nursing interventions are directed toward calming and reassuring the child and parents so that a more extensive assessment can be more easily accomplished.

The child may arrive with the limb supported in some manner; if not, careful support or immobilization may be provided to the affected site. In the event that the limb is supported or immobilized, it may be best not to touch the child but to ask him or her to point to the painful area and to wiggle the fingers or toes. By this time the child may feel

BOX 54-2 Clinical Manifestations of a Fracture

Signs of injury:
- Generalized swelling
- Pain or tenderness
- Diminished functional use of affected part

May be:
- Bruising
- Severe muscular rigidity
- Crepitus (grating sensation at fracture site)

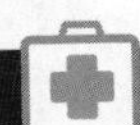

EMERGENCY

Fracture

Assess the extent of injury—Five *Ps*:
1. Pain and point of tenderness
2. Pulses—Distal to the fracture site
3. Pallor
4. Paresthesia—Sensation distal to the fracture site
5. Paralysis—Movement distal to the fracture site

Determine the mechanism of injury.
Move the injured part as little as possible.
Cover open wounds with a sterile or clean dressing.
Immobilize the limb, including joints above and below the fracture site; do not attempt to reduce the fracture or push protruding bone under the skin.
- Soft splint (pillow or folded towel)
- Rigid splint (rolled newspaper or magazine)
- Uninjured leg can serve as a splint for a leg fracture if no splint available

Reassess neurovascular status.
Apply traction if circulatory compromise is present.
Elevate the injured limb if possible.
Apply cold to the injured area.
Call emergency medical services or transport to medical facility.

relatively safe and will allow someone to gently touch the area just enough to feel the pulse and test for sensation. A child's anxiety is greatly influenced by previous experiences with injury and with health personnel; however, he or she needs to be told what will happen and what to do to help. The affected limb need not be palpated, and it should not be moved unless properly splinted. If the child is at home or if the practitioner is not present to examine the child, some type of splint is applied carefully for transport to the medical facility. Parental anxiety may be heightened by the child's pain reaction and fear, and possibly other events surrounding the accident; thus it is important to communicate to the parents that the child will receive the necessary care, including pain management.

NURSING ALERT The "five P's" of ischemia from a vascular injury should be included in an assessment of the injury:
1. Pain
2. Pallor
3. Pulselessness
4. Paresthesia
5. Paralysis

The Child in a Cast

The completeness of the fracture, the type of bone involved, and the amount of weight bearing influence how much of the extremity must be included in the cast to immobilize the fracture site completely. In most cases the joints above and below the fracture are immobilized to eliminate the possibility of movement that might cause displacement at the fracture site. Four major categories of casts are used for fractures: *upper extremity* to immobilize the wrist or elbow, *lower extremity* to immobilize the ankle or knee, *spinal* and *cervical* for immobilization of the spine, and *spica casts* to immobilize the hip and knee.

The Cast

Casts are constructed from gauze strips and bandages impregnated with plaster of paris or, more commonly, from synthetic lighter weight and water-resistant materials (e.g., fiberglass and polyurethane resin).

Both types of casting produce heat from chemical reaction activated by water immediately after application. Plaster casts mold closely to the body part, take several hours to dry, have a smooth exterior, and are inexpensive. The newer synthetic casting material is lighter, dries in 5 to 30 minutes, permits earlier weight bearing, and is water resistant. The disadvantage of synthetic casting is its inability to mold closely to body parts; its rough exterior, which may scratch surfaces; and increased cost.

Synthetic casts have special advantages for children. They come in different colors and with designs (e.g., cartoons, stripes); they are lightweight, durable, easy to clean, and relatively water resistant, depending on the type of inner lining used; only those with a Gore-Tex inner lining may be immersed in water without affecting the cast integrity. Bathing with a synthetic cast may be accomplished by covering the cast with a plastic bag; if the synthetic cast gets wet, it should be dried thoroughly. One drawback to immersion is the time necessary to completely dry the cast. The synthetic casts are difficult to write on. A waterproof marker or color markers may be used for writing on the cast.

Cast Application

The child's developmental age should be considered before the cast is applied. For preschoolers who fear bodily harm and fantasize about the loss of an extremity, it may be helpful to use a plastic doll or stuffed animal to explain the procedure beforehand. Toddlers and preschoolers do not have easily defined body boundaries; if an extremity is wrapped in a bandage, cast or splint, to the young child the extremity often ceases to exist. It is also helpful to explain that some synthetic cast material will become warm but will not burn. During the application of the cast various distraction methods can be used, including discussing favorite pets or activities at school, blowing bubbles, and so forth. In this age group explanations such as "This will help your arm get better" are futile because the child has no concept of causality.

Before the cast is applied, the extremities are checked for any abrasions, cuts, or other alterations in the skin surface and for the presence of rings or other items that might cause constriction from swelling; such objects are removed. The skin may be protected by cloth stockinette or cotton batting, which is applied liberally to the area to be casted. Particular attention is given to bony prominences, which are padded with extra cotton batting. Some practitioners use a Gore-Tex liner under a hip spica cast to prevent continuous exposure to moisture and possible skin breakdown. Dry rolls of plaster casting material are immersed in a pail of water. The (plaster) wet rolls are put on in bandage fashion and molded to the extremity. During application of the plaster cast, the underlying stockinette or cotton batting is pulled over the rough edges of the cast and secured with a layer of wet plaster ½ to 1 inch below the rim to form a smooth, padded edge to protect the skin. Alternatively a roll of thin cotton gauze may be wrapped over the plaster cast before it dries; this makes the cast edges smoother. Synthetic casts usually do not require additional padding on the edges because they do not crack like plaster material.

Nursing Care Management

The complete evaporation of the water from a hip spica cast can take 24 to 48 hours when older types of plaster materials are used. Fiberglass cast material dries within minutes. The cast must remain uncovered to allow it to dry from the inside out. Turning the child in a plaster cast at least every 2 hours will help dry a body cast evenly and prevent complications related to immobility. A regular fan or cool-air hair dryer to circulate air may be helpful when the humidity is high.

Heated fans or dryers are not used because they cause the cast to dry on the outside and remain wet beneath or cause burns from heat conduction by way of the cast to the underlying tissue.

A wet plaster cast should be supported by a pillow that is covered with plastic and handled by the palms of the hands to avoid indenting the cast, which can create pressure areas. A dry plaster-of-paris cast produces a hollow sound when it is tapped with the finger. If "hot spots" are felt on the cast surface (usually indicating infection beneath the area), this should be reported so that a window can be made in the cast to observe the site.

During the first few hours after a cast is applied, the chief concern is that the extremity may continue to swell to the extent that the cast becomes a tourniquet, shutting off circulation and producing neurovascular complications. To reduce the likelihood of this potential problem, the body part can be elevated, thereby increasing venous return. If edema is excessive, casts are bivalved (i.e., cut to make anterior and posterior halves that are held together with an elastic bandage). The cast and the involved extremity are observed frequently for neurovascular integrity and any signs of compromise. Permanent muscle and tissue damage can occur within 6 to 8 hours.

NURSING ALERT Observations such as pain (unrelieved by pain medication 1 hour after administration), swelling, discoloration (pallor or cyanosis) of the exposed portions, decreased pulses, decreased temperature, or the inability to move the distal exposed part(s) should be reported immediately.

When an extremity that has sustained an open fracture is casted, a window is often left over the wound area to allow for observation and for dressing of the wound. In some cases a cast may not be applied for days to permit access to the wound for observation; instead, a temporary immobilization device such as a splint may be applied. For the first few hours after surgery, there may be substantial bleeding that will soak through the cast. Periodically the circumscribed blood-stained area should be outlined with a ball-point pen or pencil and the time indicated to provide a guide for assessing the amount of bleeding.

Usually the child is discharged to home care after a cast is applied in the emergency department or clinic. Parents need instructions on drying and caring for the cast and on checking for signs and symptoms that indicate the cast is too tight (see Patient Teaching box). They should also be told to take the child to the health professional for attention if the cast becomes too loose, since a loose cast no longer serves its purpose. A cast is a badge of honor for the child and serves as visible evidence of an otherwise invisible injury.

PATIENT TEACHING Cast Care

Keep the casted extremity elevated on pillows or similar support for the first day, or as directed by the health professional.

Avoid denting the plaster cast with fingertips (use palms of hand to handle) while it is still wet to avoid creating pressure points.

Observe the extremities (fingers or toes) for any evidence of swelling or discoloration (darker or lighter than a comparable extremity), and contact the health professional if noted.

Check movement and sensation of the visible extremities frequently.

Follow health professional's orders regarding any restriction of activities.

Restrict strenuous activities for the first few days.

- Engage in quiet activities but encourage use of muscles.
- Move the joints above and below the cast on the affected extremity.

Encourage frequent rest for a few days, keeping the injured extremity elevated while resting.

Avoid allowing the affected limb to hang in a dependent position for any length of time.

- Keep an injured upper extremity elevated (e.g., in a sling) while upright.
- Elevate a lower limb when sitting and avoid standing for too long.

Do not allow the child to put anything inside the cast. Keep small items that might be placed inside the cast away from small children.

Keep a clear path for ambulation. Remove toys, hazardous floor rugs, pets, or other items the child might stumble over.

Use crutches appropriately if lower limb fracture requires non–weight bearing on affected extremity.

The crutches should fit properly, have a soft rubber tip to prevent slipping, and be well padded at the axilla.

With crutch walking the child's body weight is supported on the hand grips, not the axilla.

Nurses can help families adapt the child's home environment to meet the temporary encumbrance of a cast. Home care creates problems of various magnitudes, especially for children in large casts (e.g., a hip spica). Commonplace situations become problematic (e.g., transporting a child safely and comfortably in a car). Standard seat belts and car seats may not be readily adapted for use by children in some casts.

Specially designed car seats and restraints that meet safety requirements are available.* Alterations to standard car seats to accommodate the cast are not recommended because the structure may be adversely altered and fail to properly restrain the child.

Parents are taught the proper care of the cast (or immobilization device) and are helped to devise means for maintaining cleanliness. With a hip spica cast, a superabsorbent disposable diaper (newborn size) may be tucked beneath the entire perineal opening of the cast. A larger (toddler size) diaper can be applied and fastened over the small diaper and cast.

For tightly fitting casts, transparent film dressings can be cut into strips as for petaling, and one edge applied to the cast edge and the other directly to the perineum; this forms a continuous, waterproof bridge between the perineum and the cast to prevent leakage. An additional advantage to the use of this transparent dressing is that it keeps both the skin and the cast dry while allowing for observation of skin beneath the dressing.

Older infants and small children may stuff bits of food, small toys, or other items under the cast; parents should be alerted to this possibility so that suitable preventive measures can be initiated.

Feeding the infant in a hip spica cast offers problems in positioning. Very young infants can be fed in the supine position with the head elevated; with the infant's hips and legs supported on a pillow at the side, the parent can cuddle the infant in his or her arms during feeding. A somewhat similar position can be used for breastfeeding (i.e., with the infant supported on pillows or held in a "football" hold facing the mother with the legs behind her).

Children in spica casts may find the prone position easier for self-feeding from a small table placed next to the dining table. The use of a conventional toilet is almost impossible. Small bedpans or other containers offer alternatives for elimination. The nurse may suggest waterproofing methods, using plastic wraps that can help with elimination and showers. Baths are possible only if the plaster cast is kept out of the water and covered to prevent it from becoming wet from splashes.

Cast Removal

Cutting the cast to remove it or to relieve tightness is frequently a frightening experience for children. They fear the sound of the cast cutter and are terrified that their flesh, as well as the cast, will be cut. The oscillating blade vibrates rapidly back and forth and will not cut when placed *lightly* on the skin. Children have described it as producing a "tickly" sensation. The vibration also generates heat that may be felt by the child. Both of these feelings should be explained. Many young children come to regard the cast as part of themselves, which intensifies their fear of removal (Fig. 54-3). Preparation for the procedure will help reduce anxiety, especially if a trusting relationship has been established between the child and the nurse. Using the analogy of having fingernails trimmed or a haircut sometimes helps reduce their anxiety. They need continual reassurance that all is going well and that their behavior is accepted.

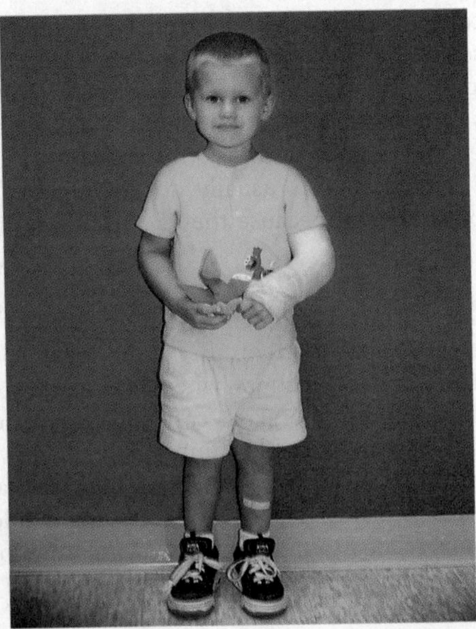

Fig. 54-3 Young children usually adapt well to a cast but often fear the removal.

After the cast is removed, the skin surface will be caked with desquamated skin and sebaceous secretions. Simple soaking in a bathtub is usually sufficient for their removal, but several days may be required to eliminate the accumulation completely. Application of oil or skin lotion may provide comfort. The parents and child should be instructed not to pull or forcibly remove this material with vigorous scrubbing because it may cause excoriation and bleeding.

The Child in Traction

The ever-changing health care arena has witnessed the demise of many long-term treatments involving lengthy hospitalization; one such change is in the area of traction. Most balanced skeletal traction is applied in children after a severe or complex injury to allow physiologic stabilization, align bone fragments, and permit closer evaluation of the injured site. Newer technology has produced orthopedic fixation devices that allow partial or full mobility, thus preventing long-term immobilization and its consequences. In many situations, surgical intervention may be carried out within a matter of days; therefore skeletal traction devices described herein may be used infrequently or only for very short periods.

Purposes of Traction

The three essential components of traction management are traction, countertraction, and friction (Fig. 54-4). To reduce or realign a fracture site, *traction* (forward force) is produced by attaching weight to the distal bone fragment; body weight provides *countertraction* (backward force); and the patient's contact with the bed constitutes the *frictional* force. These forces are used to align the distal and proximal bone fragments

**For information on specially adapted molded-plastic chairs for children who have spica casts, contact Britax Hippo by SnugSeat, 800-336-7684; www.snugseat.com. The E-Z-On vest is a special safety harness for larger children with poor trunk control. Additional safety restraints and a listing of distributors are available from SafetyBeltSafe U.S.A.,* www.carseat.org

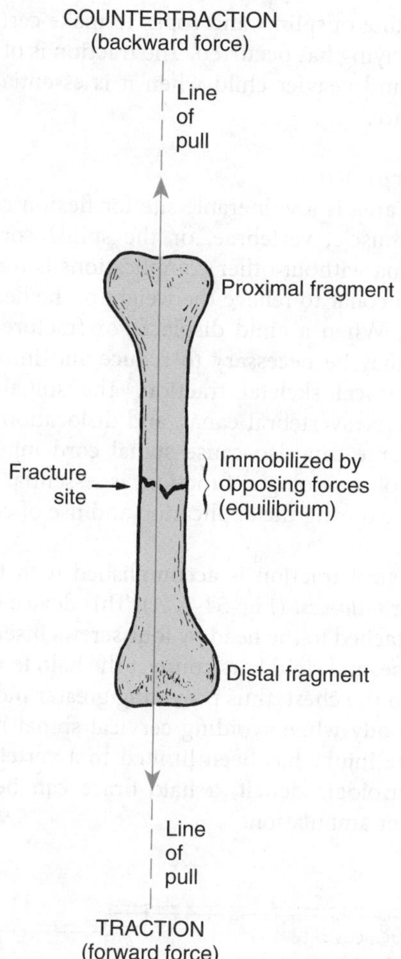

Fig. 54-4 Application of traction for maintaining equilibrium.

by adjusting the line of pull upward or downward and adducting or abducting the extremity.

To attain equilibrium, the amount of forward force is adjusted by adding weight to or subtracting weight from the traction, and/or countertraction can be increased by elevating the foot of the bed to create a greater gravitational pull to the backward force.

The four primary purposes of traction for reduction of fractures are to:

1. Fatigue the involved muscle and reduce muscle spasm so that bones can be realigned
2. Position the distal and proximal bone ends in desired realignment to promote satisfactory bone healing
3. Immobilize the fracture site until realignment has been achieved and sufficient healing has taken place to permit casting or surgical fixation
4. Allow preoperative and/or postoperative positioning and alignment

The *all-or-none law,* characteristic of muscle contractibility, influences the complete relaxation. When muscle is stretched, muscle spasm ceases and permits the realignment of the bone ends. The continuous maintenance of traction is important during this phase because releasing the traction allows the normal contracting ability of the muscle to again cause a malpositioning of the bone ends.

BOX 54-3 Types of Traction

Manual traction—Applied to the body part by the hands placed distal to the fracture site. Manual traction may be provided during application of a cast but more commonly when a closed reduction is performed.

Skin traction—Applied directly to the skin surface and indirectly to the skeletal structures. The pulling mechanism is attached to the skin with adhesive material or an elastic bandage. Both types are applied over soft, foam-backed traction straps to distribute the traction pull.

Skeletal traction—Applied directly to the skeletal structure by a pin, wire, or tongs inserted into or through the diameter of the bone distal to the fracture.

The realignment of the fragments is a gradual process that is achieved more rapidly in infants, who have limited muscle tone, than in muscular teenagers. The desired line of pull and callus formation are checked periodically by radiographic examination. The traction pull to some degree immobilizes the fracture site; however, adjunctive immobilizing devices such as splints or casts are sometimes used with skeletal traction. In injuries in which there is severe soft-tissue swelling or vascular and nerve damage, traction may be used until these complications have been resolved and it is safe to apply a cast or to perform surgical fixation. Immobilization with traction will be maintained until the bone ends are in satisfactory realignment, after which a less-confining type of immobilization—a cast, pins, or external stabilization device—will be applied.

Types of Traction (General)

The pull needed for traction can be applied to the distal bone fragment in several ways (Box 54-3). The type of traction applied is determined primarily by the child's age, the condition of the soft tissues, and the type and degree of displacement of the fracture. Fractures most commonly treated by application of traction are those involving the femur and vertebrae. The major types of traction for specific fractures are discussed in the following sections.

Upper Extremity Traction

The use of upper extremity traction in children is uncommon. Newer surgical techniques allow for early mobilization and optimal results without traction. Nursing care of the child with upper extremity traction is the same as that for lower extremity traction, which is discussed below.

Lower Extremity Traction

The severity of the fracturing force and the ability of the muscles to hold the fracture out of alignment will determine the fracture type and the amount of overriding of the fragments. The periosteum may remain intact, which helps maintain alignment. A fracture in the middle third of the shaft of the femur results in significant overriding but minimal displacement. In a fracture in the lower third of the shaft, the pull of the gastrocnemius muscle causes the distal fragment to become downwardly displaced.

Fractures of the femur can often be reduced with immediate application of a hip spica cast in young children. When traction is required, several types may be used, based on the initial assessment.

Bryant's traction is a type of running traction in which the pull is in only one direction. Skin traction is applied to the legs, which are flexed at a 90-degree angle at the hips. The child's trunk (with the buttocks raised slightly off the bed) provides countertraction.

Buck's extension is a type of skin traction with the legs in an extended position. Except for fracture cases, turning from side to side with care is permitted to maintain the involved leg alignment. Buck's extension is used primarily for short-term immobilization, preoperatively with dislocated hips, for correcting contractures, or for bone deformities such as Legg-Calvé-Perthes disease.

Russell traction uses skin traction on the lower leg and a padded sling under the knee. Two lines of pull, one along the longitudinal line of the lower leg and one perpendicular to the leg, are produced. This combination of pulls allows realignment of the lower extremity and immobilizes the hip and knee in a flexed position. The hip flexion must be kept at the prescribed angle to prevent fracture malalignment, since there is no direct support under the fracture and the skin traction may slip. Special nursing measures include carefully checking the position of the traction so that the amount of desired hip flexion is maintained and damage to the common peroneal nerve under the knee does not produce footdrop.

One of the most common types of skeletal traction is *90-degree–90-degree* traction (90-90 traction) (Fig. 54-5). The lower leg is supported by a boot cast or a calf sling, and a skeletal Steinmann pin or Kirschner's wire is placed in the distal fragment of the femur, resulting in a 90-degree angle at both the hip and the knee. From a nursing standpoint, this traction facilitates position changes, toileting, and prevention of complications related to traction.

Balance suspension traction (Fig. 54-6) may be used with or without skin or skeletal traction. Unless used with another traction, the balanced suspension merely suspends the leg in a desired flexed position to relax the hip and hamstring muscles and does not exert any traction directly on a body part. A *Thomas ring splint* extends from the groin to midair above the foot, and a *Pearson attachment* supports the lower leg. When the child is lifted off the bed, the traction lifts with the child without loss of alignment. This traction requires very careful checking of splints and ropes to make certain that no slippage or fraying has occurred. The traction is of great value in an older and heavier child when it is essential to lift the patient for care.

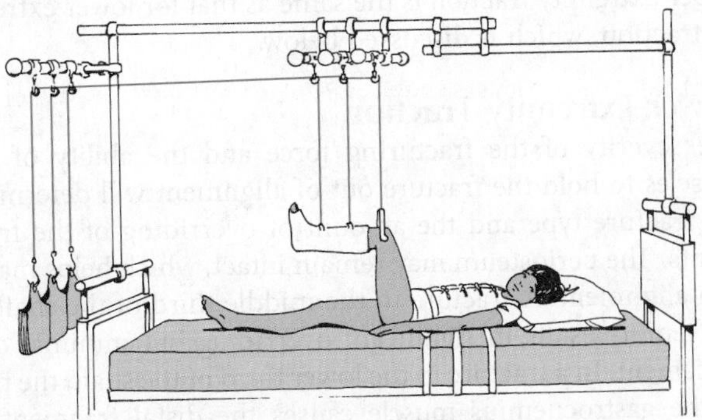

Fig. 54-5 "Ninety-ninety" traction.

Cervical Traction

The cervical area is a vulnerable site for flexion or extension injuries to muscle, vertebrae, or the spinal cord. Cervical muscle trauma without other complications is treated with a cervical hard collar to relieve the weight of the head from the fracture site. When a child displaces or fractures a cervical vertebra, it may be necessary to reduce and immobilize the site with cervical skeletal traction. The spinal cord runs through the intravertebral canal, and dislocation or fracture of the vertebrae can also cause spinal cord injury. Nursing assessment of neurologic function is essential to prevent further injury during the application and use of cervical skeletal traction.

Most cervical traction is accomplished with the use of a *halo brace* or *halo vest* (Fig. 54-7, *A*). This device consists of a steel halo attached to the head by four screws inserted into the outer skull; several rigid bars connect the halo to a vest that is worn around the chest, thus providing greater mobility of the rest of the body while avoiding cervical spinal motion altogether. If the injury has been limited to a vertebral fracture without neurologic deficit, a halo brace can be applied to permit earlier ambulation.

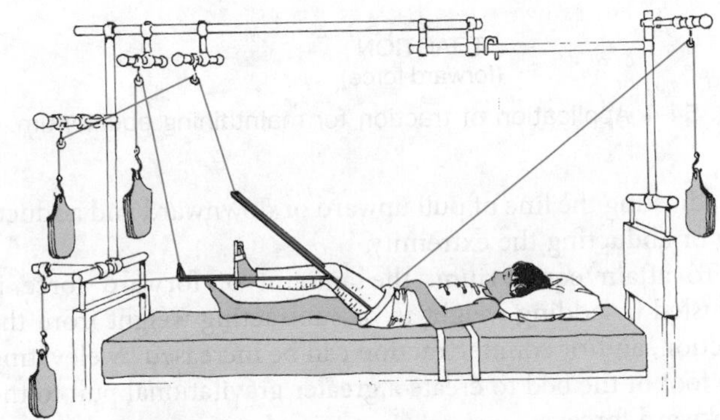

Fig. 54-6 Balance suspension with Thomas ring splint and Pearson attachment.

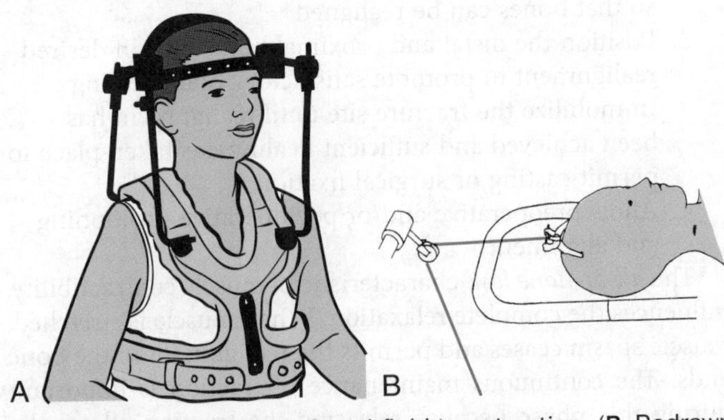

Fig. 54-7 A, Halo vest. B, Crutchfield tong traction. (B, Redrawn from Hilt NE, Schmitt EW: *Pediatric orthopedic nursing*, St Louis, 1975, Mosby.)

Cervical traction may also be accomplished by the insertion of *Crutchfield, Barton,* or *Gardner-Wells tongs* through burr holes in the skull and weights attached to the hyperextended head (see Fig. 54-7, *B*). As the neck muscles fatigue with constant traction pull, the vertebral bodies gradually separate so that the cord is no longer pinched between the vertebrae. Immobilization until fracture healing or surgical fixation can occur is an essential goal of cervical traction.

Nursing Care Management

To assess the child in traction, it is essential to know the purpose for which the traction is applied and to understand the basic principles of traction. Regular assessment of both the child and the traction apparatus is required (see Guidelines box). Many of the nursing problems associated with a child in traction are related to immobility or improper maintenance and care of the traction device, which may lead to complications.

Skeletal traction, when used, should be maintained as originally set by the practitioner. When the child needs to be moved in the bed or the traction needs to be adjusted or released for any other reason, an orthopedist is consulted. For skeletal traction to be effective, ensure that the weights are hanging freely at all times.

GUIDELINES Traction Care

Understand Therapy

Understand purposes of traction.

Understand function of traction in each specific situation.

Maintain Traction

Check desired line of pull and relationship of distal fragment to proximal fragment. Check whether fragment is being directed upward, adducted, or abducted.

Check function of each component.

- Position of bandages, frames, splints, specialized boot
- Ropes—In center track of pulley, taut, no fraying, knots tied securely
- Pulleys—In original position on attachment bar; have not been displaced from original site
- Wheels freely moveable
- Weights—Correct amount of weight, hanging freely, in safe location

Check bed position; head or foot should be elevated as directed for desired amount of pull and countertraction.

Do not remove skeletal traction or adhesive traction straps on skin traction.

Maintain Alignment

Observe for correct body alignment with emphasis on alignment of shoulder, hip, and leg.

Check after child has moved.

Maintain correct angles at joints.

Skin Traction

Replace nonadhesive straps and/or elastic bandage on skin traction *when permitted* and/or absolutely necessary, but make certain that traction on limb is maintained by someone during procedure.

Assess straps or bandages to ascertain whether they are correctly applied (diagonal or spiral), not too loose or too tight, which could cause slippage and malalignment of traction.

Assess traction boot to ensure it has not slipped and is not causing compression of the foot, thus impairing the circulation.

Skeletal Traction

Check pin sites frequently for signs of bleeding, inflammation, or infection.

Cleanse and dress pin sites per institution protocol or as ordered.

Apply topical antiseptic or antibiotic to pin sites daily as ordered.

Cover ends of pins with protective rubber or padding to prevent child's being scratched by pin.

Note pull of traction on pin; pull should be even.

Check pin screws to be certain that screws are tight in metal clamp that attaches traction apparatus to pin.

Prevent Skin Breakdown

Provide foam overlay or alternating-pressure mattress underneath hips and back.

Make total-body skin checks for redness or breakdown, especially over areas that receive greatest pressure.

Wash and dry skin at least daily.

Inspect pressure points daily or more often if risk of breakdown is observed.

Use a skin breakdown assessment scale such as Modified Braden Q.

Stimulate circulation with gentle massage over pressure areas.

Change position at least every 2 hours to relieve pressure.

Encourage increased intake of oral fluids.

Provide and encourage patient to eat a balanced diet, including vegetables and fruits.

Prevent Complications

Check pulses in affected area and compare with pulses in contralateral site.

Assess circular dressings for excessive tightness.

Assess restrictive bandages or devices used to maintain traction on affected limb.

- Make certain that they are not too loose or too tight.
- Remove periodically and check for pressure areas.

Encourage deep breathing frequently with maximum inspiratory chest expansion. Note any neurovascular changes, such as:

- Changes in color in skin and nail beds
- Alterations in sensation, increased pain
- Alterations in motor ability

Take immediate action to correct problem or report to practitioner if neurovascular changes are found.

Record findings of neurovascular changes.

Carry out passive, active, or active-with-resistance exercises of uninvolved joints.

Note if any tightness, weakness, edema, or contractures are developing in uninvolved joints and muscles.

Take measures to correct or prevent further development of weakness, such as applying footboard or foot orthoses to prevent footdrop.

evolve Skill—Monitoring Neurovascular Status

In addition to routine skin observation and care, the child in skeletal traction will need special skin care at the pin site according to hospital policy or practitioner preference. Pin sites should be frequently assessed and cleaned to prevent infection; after the first 48 to 72 hours pin site care may be performed once daily or weekly for mechanically stable pins (Holmes, Brown, & Pin Site Care Expert Panel, 2005). Use of a 2 mg/ml chlorhexidine solution has been recommended as best-practice care for skeletal pin sites by the National Association of Orthopaedic Nurses (Holmes, Brown, & Pin Site Care Expert Panel, 2005). Before the child's discharge, the family is taught pin site care, including how to observe for infection or pin instability, using a return demonstration method. A pressure reduction device, such as a special mattress, decreases the chance of skin breakdown.

When the child is first placed in traction, an increase in discomfort is common as a result of the traction pull fatiguing the muscle. Orthopedic conditions are associated with a higher-than-average number of painful events and a higher percentage of bodily symptoms than other common conditions. IV opioids, including analgesics and muscle relaxants, help during this phase of care and should be administered liberally.

The specific nursing responsibilities for the patient in traction are outlined in the Guidelines box.

Distraction

Unlike traction, which helps bones realign and fuse properly, distraction is the process of separating opposing bone to encourage regeneration of new bone in the created space. Distraction can also be used when limbs are of unequal lengths and new bone is needed to elongate the shorter limb.

External Fixation

The *Ilizarov external fixator (IEF)* is a common external fixation device. The IEF uses a system of wires, rings, and telescoping rods that permits limb lengthening to occur by manual distraction. In addition to lengthening bones, the device can be used to correct angular or rotational defects or to immobilize fractures. The device is attached surgically by securing a series of external full or half rings to the bone with wires. External telescoping rods connect the rings to each other. Manual distraction is accomplished by manipulating the rods to increase the distance between the rings. A percutaneous osteotomy is performed when the device is applied to create a "false" growth plate. A special osteotomy or corticotomy involves cutting only the cortex of the bone while preserving its blood supply, bone marrow, endosteum, and periosteum. Capillary blood flow to the transected area is essential for proper bone growth. Cut bone ends typically grow at a rate of 1 cm/month. The IEF can result in up to a 15-cm (6-inch) gain in length.

Nursing Care Management

Success of the IEF depends on the child's and family's cooperation; therefore before surgery they must be fully informed of the appearance of the device, how it accomplishes bone growth, needed alterations in activities, and home and follow-up care. Children are involved in learning to adjust the

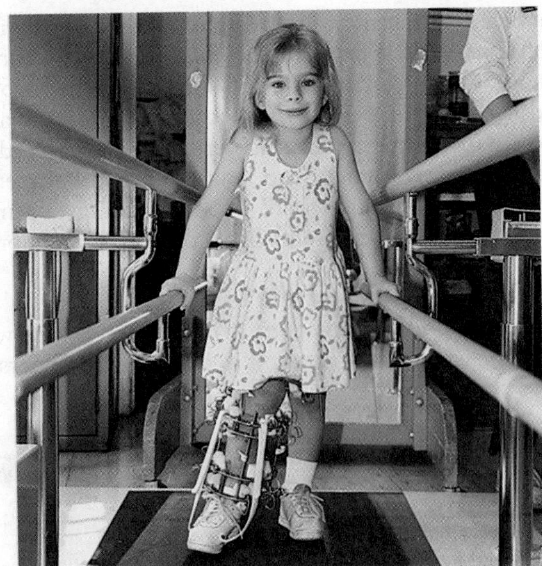

Fig. 54-8 Child with Ilizarov external fixator (right leg) during physical therapy on parallel bars.

device to accomplish distraction. Children, as well as parents, should be instructed in pin care, including observation for infection and loosening of the pins. Cleaning routines for the pin sites vary among practitioners but should not traumatize the skin.

Children who participate actively in their care report less discomfort. Because the device is external and bulky, the child and family may need to modify clothing for increased comfort and accessibility (Fig. 54-8). Partial weight bearing is allowed, and the child needs to learn to walk with crutches. Alterations in activity include modifications at school and in physical education. Full weight bearing is not allowed until the distraction is completed and bone consolidation has occurred. Follow-up care is essential to maintaining appropriate distraction until the desired leg length is achieved. The device is removed surgically after the bone has consolidated, and the child may need to use crutches or have a cast for 4 to 6 weeks after removal.

Amputation

A child may be born with the congenital absence of a body part, have a traumatic loss of an extremity, or need a surgical amputation for a pathologic condition such as *osteosarcoma* (see p. 1705). With today's surgical technology and the quick thinking of bystanders who save a traumatically amputated body part, children have had fingers and arms reattached with variable degrees of functional use regained.

NURSING ALERT For an amputated limb or body part that may be reattached, do the following:

1. Rinse limb gently with normal saline.
2. Loosely wrap limb in sterile gauze.
3. Place wrapped limb in a watertight bag.
4. Cool (without freezing) bag in ice water (do not pack in ice because this may harm tissue).
5. Label with child's name, date, and time, and transport with the child to the hospital.

Surgical amputation or the surgical repair of a permanently severed limb focuses on constructing an adequately nourished stump. A smooth, healthy, padded stump, free of nerve endings, is important in prosthesis fitting and subsequent ambulation. In some situations in which there is no vascular or neurologic deficit, a cast is applied to the stump immediately after the procedure, and a pylon, metal extension, and artificial foot are attached so that the patient can walk on the temporary prosthesis within a few hours.

Nursing Care Management

Stump shaping is performed postoperatively with special elastic bandaging using a figure-8 bandage, which applies pressure in a cone-shaped fashion. This technique decreases stump edema, controls hemorrhage, and aids in developing desired contours so that the child will bear weight on the posterior aspect of the skin flap rather than on the end of the stump. Stump elevation may be used during the first 24 hours, but after this time the extremity should not be left in this position because contractures will develop in the proximal joint and seriously hamper ambulation. Monitoring proper body alignment will further decrease the risk of flexion contractures.

For older children and adolescents, arm exercises (as well as parallel bars, which are used in prosthesis-training programs) help build up the arm muscles necessary for walking with crutches. Full range-of-motion exercises of joints above the amputation must be performed several times daily using active and isotonic exercises.

Depending on the child's age, children or their parents will need to learn stump hygiene, including careful soap and water washing every day and checking for skin irritation, breakdown, or infection. A tube of stockinette or powder is used to slide the prosthesis on more easily. Skin must be checked carefully every time the prosthesis is removed, and prosthesis tolerance time must be adjusted to prevent skin breakdown.

For children who have had an amputation, *phantom limb sensation* is an expected experience because the nerve-brain connections are still present. Gradually these sensations fade, although in many amputees they persist for years. Preoperative discussion of this phenomenon will aid a child in understanding these "unusual feelings" and in not hiding the experiences from others. Limb pain, especially pain that increases with ambulation, should be evaluated for the possibility of a neuroma at the free nerve endings in the stump, or other problems such as a poorly fitting prosthesis or joint instability.

Congenital Defects

Some skeletal defects may be diagnosed at birth or within days, weeks, or months after birth. In other cases the deviation may be difficult to detect without careful inspection. Therefore it is imperative that nurses become acquainted with signs of these defects and understand the principles of therapy in order to direct others in the care and management of these children.

Developmental Dysplasia of the Hip

The broad term *developmental dysplasia of the hip (DDH)* describes a spectrum of disorders related to abnormal development of the hip that may develop at any time during fetal life, infancy, or childhood. A change in terminology from *congenital hip dysplasia* and *congenital dislocation of the hip* to DDH more properly reflects a variety of hip abnormalities in which there is a shallow acetabulum, subluxation, or dislocation.

The incidence of hip instability of some kind is approximately 10 per 1000 live births. The incidence of frank dislocation or a dislocatable hip is 1 per 1000 live births (Wall, 2000), and approximately 16% to 25% of infants with DDH are born breech (Hosalkar et al, 2007). The left hip is involved in 60% of cases, the right hip in 20%, and both hips in 20%. Sixty percent of the patients are girls. Caucasian children have a higher incidence of developmental dysplasia than other groups (Maher, Salmond, & Pellino, 2002).

Pathophysiology

The cause of DDH is unknown but certain factors such as gender, birth order, family history, intrauterine position, delivery type, joint laxity, and postnatal positioning are believed to affect the risk of DDH. Predisposing factors associated with DDH may be divided into three broad categories:

1. Physiologic factors, which include maternal hormone secretion and intrauterine positioning.
2. Mechanical factors, which involve breech presentation, multiple fetuses, oligohydramnios, and large infant size. Other mechanical factors may include continued maintenance of the hips in adduction and extension, which will in time cause a dislocation (see Cultural Awareness box).
3. Genetic factors, which entail a higher incidence (6%) of DDH in siblings of affected infants, and an even greater incidence (36%) of recurrence if a sibling and one parent were affected.

Some experts categorize DDH into two major groups: (1) *typical,* in which the infant is neurologically intact; and (2) *teratologic,* which involves a neuromuscular defect such as arthrogryposis or myelodysplasia. The teratologic forms usually occur in utero and are much less common.

CULTURAL AWARENESS

Developmental Dysplasia of the Hip

A striking relationship exists between the development of the dislocation and methods of handling infants. Among the cultures with the highest incidence of dislocation, newly born infants are tightly wrapped in blankets or other swaddling material or are strapped to cradle boards. In cultures such as the Far East, where mothers traditionally carry infants on their backs or hips in the widely abducted straddle position, the disorder is virtually unknown.

Three degrees of DDH are illustrated in Fig. 28-18 (p. 774):

1. **Acetabular dysplasia (or preluxation)**—This is the mildest form of DDH, in which there is neither

BOX 54-4 Clinical Manifestations of Developmental Dysplasia of the Hip

Infant

Shortening of limb on affected side
Restricted abduction of hip on affected side
Unequal gluteal folds (infant prone)
Positive Ortolani test
Positive Barlow test

Older Infant and Child

Affected leg shorter than the other
Telescoping or piston mobility of joint—Head of femur felt to move up and down in buttock when extended thigh is pushed first toward child's head and then pulled distally
Trendelenburg's sign—When child stands first on one foot and then on the other (holding onto a chair, rail, or someone's hands) bearing weight on affected hip, pelvis tilts downward on normal side instead of upward, as it would with normal stability
Greater trochanter prominent and appearing above a line from anterosuperior iliac spine to tuberosity of ischium
Marked lordosis (bilateral dislocations)
Waddling gait (bilateral dislocations)

subluxation nor dislocation. Acetabular development is delayed, as evidenced by osseous hypoplasia of the acetabular roof that is oblique and shallow, although the cartilaginous roof is comparatively intact. The femoral head remains in the acetabulum.

2. **Subluxation**—The largest percentage of DDH, subluxation, implies incomplete dislocation of the hip and is sometimes regarded as an intermediate state in the development from primary dysplasia to complete dislocation. The femoral head remains in contact with the acetabulum, but a stretched capsule and ligamentum teres cause the head of the femur to be partially displaced. Pressure on the cartilaginous roof inhibits ossification and produces a flattening of the socket.
3. **Dislocation**—The femoral head loses contact with the acetabulum and is displaced posteriorly and superiorly over the fibrocartilaginous rim. The ligamentum teres is elongated and taut.

Diagnostic Evaluation

DDH is often not detected at the initial examination after birth; thus all infants should be carefully monitored for hip dysplasia at follow-up visits throughout the first year of life. In the newborn period dysplasia usually appears as hip joint laxity rather than as outright dislocation. The clinical manifestations of DDH are outlined in Box 54-4.

The Ortolani and Barlow tests must be performed by an experienced clinician to prevent further damage to the hip. If these tests are performed too vigorously in the first 2 days of life, when the hip subluxates freely, persistent dislocation may occur (see Fig. 24-8, p. 620).

Radiographic examination in early infancy is not reliable, since ossification of the femoral head does not normally take place until the third to sixth month of life. However, the cartilaginous head can be visualized directly by ultrasonography. Widespread newborn screening with ultrasound has been proposed; however, numerous studies reveal this approach has a high rate of false positives and subsequent overtreatment. Therefore ultrasound is recommended as an adjunct to other diagnostic procedures (American Academy of Pediatrics, Committee on Quality Improvement and Subcommittee on Developmental Dysplasia of the Hip, 2000). In infants older than age 4 months and in children, radiographic examination is useful in confirming the diagnosis. An upward slope in the roof of the acetabulum (the acetabular angle) greater than 40 degrees with upward and outward displacement of the femoral head is a frequent finding in older children. Computed tomography (CT) scan may be useful to assess the position of the femoral head relative to the acetabulum after closed reduction and casting. The American Academy of Pediatrics, Committee on Quality Improvement and Subcommittee on Developmental Dysplasia of the Hip (2000), has published extensive clinical guidelines for the early detection of DDH. The U.S. Preventive Services Task Force (2006) has expressed concerns regarding the benefit of routine screening for DDH in early infancy, citing a lack of evidence-based studies to support early screening and subsequent surgical and nonsurgical treatments.

Therapeutic Management

Treatment is begun as soon as the condition is recognized because early intervention is more favorable to the restoration of normal bony architecture and function. The longer treatment is delayed, the more severe the deformity, the more difficult the treatment, and the less favorable the prognosis. The treatment varies with the child's age and the extent of the dysplasia. The goal of treatment is to obtain and maintain a safe, congruent position of the hip joint to promote normal hip joint development.

Newborn to Age 6 Months

The hip joint is maintained by splinting with the proximal femur centered in the acetabulum in an attitude of flexion. Of the numerous devices available, the *Pavlik harness* is the most widely used, and with time, motion, and gravity, the hip works into a more abducted, reduced position (see Fig. 28-19). The harness is worn continuously until the hip is clinically and radiographically stable, usually in about 3 to 6 months. After the age of 6 months the Pavlik harness tends to lose its effectiveness because of the child's increasing mobility and strength (Hosalkar et al, 2007).

When adduction contracture is present, skin traction may be used to slowly and gently stretch the hip to full abduction, after which wide abduction is maintained until stability is attained. When maintaining stable reduction is difficult, a hip spica cast is applied and changed periodically to accommodate the child's growth. After 3 to 6 months, sufficient stability is acquired to allow transfer to a removable protective abduction brace. The duration of treatment depends on development of the acetabulum but is usually accomplished within the first year.

Ages 6 to 18 Months

In this age group the dislocation is not recognized until the child begins to stand and walk, when attendant shortening of the limb and contractures of hip adductor and flexor muscles become apparent (see Fig. 24-8). Gradual reduction by traction is used for approximately 3 weeks. An individualized home traction program may be developed for the child preoperatively to decrease the length of hospitalization and maintain the home environment. The child then undergoes an attempted closed reduction of the hip under general anesthesia if the hip is not reducible and open reduction is performed. After reduction, the child is placed in a hip spica cast for 2 to 4 months until the hip is stable, at which time a flexion-abduction brace is applied.

Older Child

Correction of the hip deformity in older children is inherently more difficult than in the preceding age groups, because secondary adaptive changes and other etiologic factors (such as juvenile idiopathic arthritis or nonambulatory cerebral palsy) complicate the condition. Operative closed reduction, which may involve preoperative traction, tenotomy of contracted muscles, and any one of several innominate osteotomy procedures designed to construct an acetabular roof, is usually required. After cast removal and before weight bearing is permitted, range-of-motion exercises help restore movement. Successful reduction and reconstruction become increasingly difficult after the age of 4 years and are usually impossible or inadvisable in children older than 6 years of age because of severe shortening and contracture of muscles and deformity of the femoral and acetabular structures.

Nursing Care Management

Nurses are in a unique position to detect DDH in early infancy. During the infant assessment process and routine nurturing activities, the hips and extremities are inspected for any deviations from normal. These observations are reported to the attending practitioner, and the ambulatory child who displays a limp or an unusual gait should be referred for evaluation. This may indicate an orthopedic or neurologic problem. Nonambulatory children with cerebral palsy should also be assessed for evidence of dislocation.

The major nursing problems in the care of an infant or child in a cast or other device are related to maintenance of the device and adaptation of nurturing activities to meet his or her needs. Generally, treatment and follow-up care of these children are carried out in a clinic, practitioner's office, or outpatient unit. Hospitalization may be necessary for cast application or brace fitting but seldom exceeds 24 to 48 hours. Longer hospitalization is required for open reduction.

The former practice of double- or triple-diapering for DDH is not recommended because it promotes hip extension, thus worsening proper hip development.

The primary nursing goal is teaching parents to apply and maintain the reduction device. The Pavlik harness allows for easy handling of the infant and usually produces less apprehension in the parent than heavy braces and casts. Because of the infant's rapid growth, the straps should be checked in the beginning of therapy every week for possible adjustments (Hart et al, 2006). It is important that parents understand the correct use of the appliance, which may or may not allow for its removal during bathing. Unbuckling or removing the harness is determined individually on the basis of the family's level of understanding and the degree of hip deformity. Parents are instructed not to adjust the harness without medical supervision. The child should be examined by the practitioner before any adjustment is attempted to make certain the hips are in correct placement before the harness is resecured.

Skin care is an important aspect of the care of an infant in a harness. The following instructions for preventing skin breakdown are stressed:

- Always put an undershirt (or a shirt with extensions that close at the crotch) under the chest straps, and put knee socks under the foot and leg pieces to prevent the straps from rubbing the skin.
- Check frequently (at least two or three times a day) for red areas under the straps and the clothing.
- Gently massage healthy skin under the straps once a day to stimulate circulation. In general, avoid lotions and powders because they can cake and irritate the skin.
- Always place the diaper under the straps.

Parents are encouraged to hold the infant with a harness and continue care and nurturing activities. The nurse can assist by being available for parents' questions about the necessary adaptations to daily care to decrease the parent's anxiety and possible feelings about the child being hurt by routine caring.

Casts and orthotics devices (harness) offer more challenging nursing problems because they cannot be removed for routine care, although sometimes a brace may be removed for bathing. Care of an infant or small child with a cast requires nursing innovation to reduce skin pressure or friction and to maintain cleanliness of both the child and the cast, particularly in the diaper area. (See p. 1685 for care of the child in a cast.)

It is important for nurses, parents, and other caregivers to understand that children in corrective devices need to be involved in all the activities of any child in the same age group. Play and diversion activities are chosen that can be used in a prone position on the floor or in the seats devised for feeding and other activities. Confinement in a cast or appliance should not exclude children from play activities.

Congenital Clubfoot

Congenital *clubfoot* is a complex deformity of the ankle and foot that includes forefoot adduction, midfoot supination, hindfoot varus, and ankle equinus. Deformities of the foot and ankle are described according to the position of the ankle and foot. The more common positions involve the following variations:

Talipes varus—An inversion or a bending inward
Talipes valgus—An eversion or bending outward
Talipes equinus—Plantar flexion, in which the toes are lower than the heel
Talipes calcaneus—Dorsiflexion, in which the toes are higher than the heel

Most cases of clubfoot are a combination of these positions, and the most commonly occurring type of clubfoot (approximately 95%) is the composite deformity *talipes equinovarus*

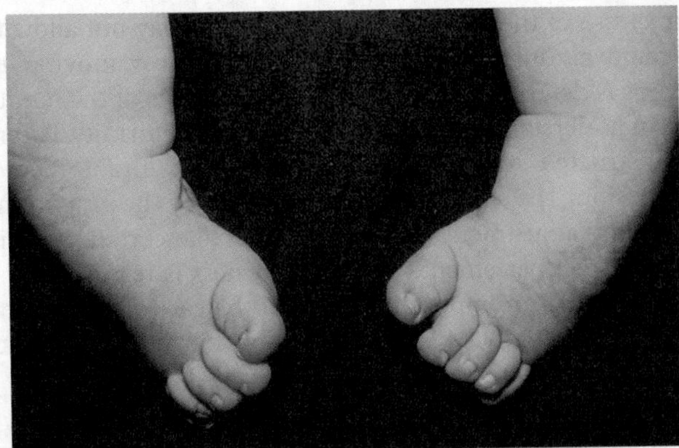

Fig. 54-9 Bilateral congenital talipes equinovarus (congenital clubfoot) in 2-month-old infant. (From Zitelli BJ, Davis HW: *Atlas of pediatric physical diagnosis*, ed 4, St Louis, 2002, Mosby.)

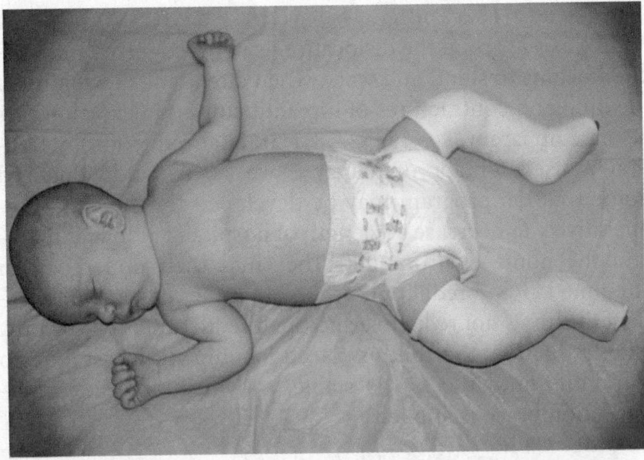

Fig. 54-10 Feet casted for correction of bilateral congenital talipes equinovarus.

(TEV), in which the foot is pointed downward and inward in varying degrees of severity (Fig. 54-9). Unilateral clubfoot is somewhat more common than bilateral clubfoot and may occur as an isolated defect or in association with other disorders or syndromes, such as chromosomal defects, arthrogryposis (a generalized immobility of the joints), cerebral palsy, or spina bifida.

The incidence of clubfoot in the general population is 1 to 2 per 1000 live births, with boys affected twice as often as girls. Bilateral clubfeet occur in 50% of the cases (Hosalkar, Spiegel, & Davidson, 2007). The cause of clubfoot is believed to be multifactorial. Some authorities attribute the defect to abnormal positioning and restricted movement in utero, although the evidence is not conclusive. Other experts implicate arrested or abnormal embryonic development. Arrested development during this early stage tends to result in a rigid deformity, whereas mechanical pressures from intrauterine positioning are likely causes of more flexible deformities.

Classification

The literature describes three major categories of clubfoot: (1) positional clubfoot (also called transitional, mild, or postural clubfoot), which is believed to occur primarily from intrauterine crowding and responds to simple stretching and casting; (2) syndromic (or teratologic) clubfoot, which is associated with other congenital anomalies such as myelomeningocele or arthrogryposis and is a more severe form of clubfoot that is often resistant to treatment; (3) congenital clubfoot, also referred to as idiopathic, which may occur in an otherwise normal child and has a wide range of rigidity and prognosis. The third category may be detected in utero by ultrasonography and is the most common type of TEV seen.

The mild, or postural, clubfoot may correct spontaneously or may require passive exercise or serial casting. There is no bony abnormality, but there may be tightness and shortening of the soft tissues medially and posteriorly. The teratologic clubfoot is associated with other congenital anomalies such as myelodysplasia or arthrogryposis. These feet usually require surgical correction and have a high incidence of recurrence. The congenital idiopathic clubfoot, or "true clubfoot," almost always requires surgical intervention because there is bony abnormality.

Diagnostic Evaluation

The deformity is often readily apparent and easily detected prenatally through ultrasonography or at birth. However, it must be differentiated from some positional deformities that can be passively corrected or overcorrected. Radiographic examination is recommended by some clinicians, whereas others may postpone radiographs in infancy (Hosalkar, Spiegel, & Davidson, 2007). Paralytic changes in the lower extremity of children with neuromuscular involvement often produce equinovarus deformity. An increased risk of hip dysplasia is associated with clubfoot deformities.

Therapeutic Management

The goal of treatment for clubfoot is to achieve a painless, plantigrade, and stable foot. Treatment of clubfoot involves three stages: (1) correction of the deformity, (2) maintenance of the correction until normal muscle balance is regained, and (3) follow-up observation to avert possible recurrence of the deformity. Some feet respond to treatment readily; some respond only to prolonged, vigorous, and sustained efforts; and the improvement in others remains disappointing even with maximum effort on the part of all concerned.

Serial casting is begun shortly after birth, before discharge from the nursery. Successive casts allow for gradual stretching of skin and tight structures on the medial side of the foot (Fig. 54-10). Manipulation and casting are repeated frequently (every few days for 1 to 2 weeks, then at 1- to 2-week intervals) to accommodate the rapid growth of early infancy. The extremity or extremities are casted until maximum correction is achieved, usually within 8 to 12 weeks. A Denis Browne splint may be used to manage feet that correct with casting and manipulation. A radiograph or ultrasound is then evaluated to see the relationship of the bones to each other. Failure to achieve normal alignment by 3 months indicates the need for surgical intervention, which may take place between 6 and 12 months of age. The foot (or feet) is immobilized postoperatively for approximately 6 to 12 weeks, and the child is allowed to walk after the cast is removed.

Surgical intervention for clubfoot involves pin fixation and the release of tight joints and tendons. Casting of the affected foot and leg is performed, and after 2 or 3 months, a varus-prevention brace is used to maintain correction. With severe deformities, repeated surgical tendon or joint releases may be necessary.

In recent years several nonsurgical approaches to clubfoot have been reintroduced. These methods involve daily or weekly manipulation and stretching of tissues with either casting (Ponseti's manipulation) or taping and splinting of the affected extremity (French physical therapy). A percutaneous calcaneal tendon (Achilles tendon) lengthening may be performed before the final casting at 6 to 7 weeks to correct the equinus deformity. With French physical therapy treatment, a continuous passive motion machine may be used several hours daily to stretch and strengthen muscle groups involved (Faulks & Luther, 2005).

Nursing Care Management

Nursing care of the child with clubfoot is the same as for any child who has a cast (see p. 1685). Because the child will spend considerable time in a corrective device, nursing care plans include both long- and short-term goals. Conscientious observation of the skin and circulation is particularly important in young infants because of their normally rapid growth rate. Because treatment and follow-up care are handled in the orthopedist's office, clinic, or outpatient department, parent education and support are important in nursing care of these children.

Parents need to understand the overall treatment program and the importance of regular cast changes in the long-term effectiveness of the therapy. Reinforcing and clarifying the orthopedist's explanations and instructions, teaching parents about care of the cast or appliance (including vigilant observation for potential problems), and encouraging parents to facilitate normal development within the limitations imposed by the deformity or therapy are all part of nursing responsibilities.

Metatarsus Adductus (Varus)

Metatarsus adductus, or metatarsus varus, is probably the most common congenital foot deformity. In most instances it is a result of abnormal intrauterine positioning, particularly in the firstborn child, and is usually detected at birth. The deformity is characterized by medial adduction of the toes and forefoot, frequently in association with inversion, and by convexity of the lateral border of the foot. Metatarsus adductus may be divided into three categories: type I, in which the forefoot is flexible and corrects easily with manipulation; type II, in which there is only partial flexibility in the forefoot, and it corrects passively past neutral position but only to neutral position with active manipulation; and type III, in which the forefoot is rigid and will not stretch to neutral position with manipulation. Unlike TEV, with which it is often confused, the angulation occurs at the tarsometatarsal joint, whereas the heel and ankle remain in a neutral position. Ankle range of motion is normal. This deformity often causes a pigeon-toed gait in the child.

Therapeutic management depends on the rigidity and type of the deformity. Correction with types I and II can usually be accomplished by gentle manipulation and passive stretching of the foot, which the parent is taught to perform. Repeated and consistent stretching is continued for the first 6 weeks, after which the treatment is based on the flexibility of the foot. With type III, the child will usually require serial manipulation and casting to correct the defect. Casting is performed every 1 to 2 weeks for 6 to 8 weeks after which a corrective shoe or orthosis may be used. Surgical correction is rarely required for the condition unless there is residual deformity at 4 to 6 years of age, at which time soft-tissue release and serial casting are performed. Older children with deformity may require more extensive surgery (Hosalkar, Spiegel, & Davidson, 2007).

Nursing Care Management

The nursing role primarily involves identifying the defect, so that early therapy and instruction of the parents can be initiated. The nurse teaches the parents how to hold the heel firmly and to stretch only the forefoot; otherwise, undue force on the heel may produce a valgus deformity. If casting or orthosis is required, the nurse instructs the parents in cast care and observation of the corrective device (see p. 1685).

Skeletal Limb Deficiency

Congenital limb deficiencies, or reduction malformations (disruption defects), are manifested by a variety of degrees of loss of functional capacity. They are characterized by underdevelopment of skeletal elements of the extremities. The range of malformation can extend from minor defects of the digits to serious abnormalities such as *amelia,* absence of an entire extremity; or *meromelia,* partial absence of an extremity that includes *phocomelia* (seal limbs), interposed deficiency of long bones with relatively good development of hands and feet attached at or near the shoulder or the hips. Most reduction defects are primary defects of development of the limb, but prenatal destruction of the limb can occur, such as the amputation of a limb in utero from constriction of an amniotic band (amniotic band disruption sequence).

Pathophysiology

Limb deficiencies can be attributed to both heredity and environment and can originate at any stage of limb development. Formation of limbs may be suppressed at the time of limb bud formation, or there may be interference in later stages of differentiation and growth. Heredity appears to play a prominent role, and prenatal environmental insults have been implicated in a number of cases. The latter includes the well-publicized thalidomide tragedy of the 1950s and early 1960s, which demonstrated a clear relationship between the time of exposure of the pregnant woman to the antiemetic drug and the presence and type of limb deformity in the newborn. Many drugs may still have similar *teratogenic* effects in the first trimester of pregnancy; therefore medication administration during this period should be carefully evaluated by the practitioner. Unfortunately, during this period, the woman may not realize her pregnant condition unless the event is anticipated, and she may inadvertently consume harmful medications. Deletion or shortening of digits or limbs may also be associated with *chorionic villus sampling,* especially before 10 to 12 weeks of gestation; however, the incidence and relationship remain uncertain.

Therapeutic Management

Children with congenital limb deficiencies should be fitted with prosthetic devices whenever possible, and the devices should be applied at the earliest possible stage of development in an attempt to match the infant's motor readiness. This favors natural progression of prosthetic use. For example, a young infant with an upper extremity deficiency is fitted with a simple passive device, such as a mitten prosthesis, to encourage limb exploration, sitting (with the extremities needed for support), and bilateral hand activities.

Lower limb prostheses are applied when the infant begins sitting up and can maintain balance. In preparation for prosthetic devices, surgical modification may be necessary to ensure the most favorable use of the device, since severe deformity can interfere with its effective use. Phocomelic digits are preserved for controlling switches of externally powered appliances in upper extremities. Digits (in both upper and lower extremities) provide the child with surfaces for tactile exploration and stimulation. Prostheses are replaced to accommodate the child's growth and increasing capabilities.

Nursing Care Management

Prosthetic application training and habilitation are most successfully carried out in a center that specializes in meeting the special needs of these children, especially very young children and those with amputations or missing limbs. Therapeutic management involves a *prosthetist*, who specializes in the development, fitting, and maintenance of prosthetic limbs, and other health care workers such as physical and occupational therapists. Parents need special attention and support and are encouraged to assist the child in making age-commensurate adjustments to the environment.

Osteogenesis Imperfecta

Osteogenesis imperfecta (OI) is the most common osteoporosis syndrome in children, characterized by excessive fractures and bone deformity. There are at least six types of OI, accounting for significant disease variability. Clinical features may include varying degrees of bone fragility, deformity, and fracture; blue sclerae; hearing loss; and dentinogenesis imperfecta (hypoplastic discolored teeth). The inheritance pattern is autosomal dominant in the majority of cases, although the most severe form demonstrates autosomal recessive inheritance (Box 54-5).

Most types of OI have defects in the *COL1A1* or *COL1A2* genes, which code for polypeptide chains in type 1 procollagen, a precursor of type 1 collagen, a major structural component of bone. The error results in faulty bone mineralization, abnormal bone architecture, and increased susceptibility to fracture.

Classifications for OI are based on clinical features and patterns of inheritance (see Box 54-5). Clinically, type I is the most common, with wide variability of bone fragility; some affected family members have significant deformity and disability, whereas others lead agile, active lives. Type II variants are the most severe and are considered lethal in infancy. Type III OI is characterized by multiple fractures, bone deformity, and severe disability; affected individuals rarely live to 30 years of age. Type IV is similar to type I with blue or white sclerae.

BOX 54-5 Classification of Osteogenesis Imperfecta

Type I*
- A—Mild bone fragility; blue sclerae; normal teeth; hearing loss (occurs between ages 20 and 30 years); autosomal dominant inheritance
- B—Same as A except dentinogenesis imperfecta instead of normal teeth
- C—Same as B but no bone fragility

Type II—Lethal; stillborn or die in early infancy; severe bone fragility, multiple fractures at birth; 10% of cases of osteogenesis imperfecta (OI); autosomal recessive inheritance

Type III—Severe bone fragility leading to severe progressive deformities; normal sclerae; marked growth failure; most autosomal recessive inheritance, with a few autosomal dominant inheritance

Type IV
- A—Mild to moderate bone fragility; normal sclerae; normal teeth; short stature; variable deformity; autosomal dominant inheritance
- B—Same as A except dentinogenesis imperfecta instead of normal teeth; approximately 6% of cases of OI

Type V—Clinically similar to type IV; hyperplastic callus; collagen mutation is negative

Type VI—Sclerae and dentition normal; moderate to severe bone fragility; diagnosis by bone biopsy because of similarities to other types; only identified in eight persons to date (Land et al, 2007)

*Two thirds of cases are type I.

Another variant, or type V, has been described in which those affected have a hyperplastic callus, a radiodense metaphyseal band and calcification of the interosseous membrane of the forearm; no collagen mutations are noted in this group (Marini, 2007). A type VI has been described with a characteristic mineralization defect, which does not respond to pamidronate therapy as do types I to V (Land et al, 2007). Children affected with this type have no dental involvement and normal sclerae; a bone biopsy is the only way to establish a diagnosis because of the similarities to other types.

Therapeutic Management

The treatment for OI is primarily supportive, although patients and families are optimistic about new research advances. Bone marrow transplant for severe OI was first reported in 1999 with positive results; however, this is still considered an experimental treatment. Bisphosphonate therapy with pamidronate, olpadronate, neridronate, or alendronate to promote increased bone density and prevent fractures has become standard therapy for many children with OI. Bisphosphonate therapy reportedly is more beneficial for increasing vertebral bone density but is considered less effective for long bones (Marini, 2007). Bachrach and Ward (2009) suggest data are inadequate to recommend the use of bisphosphonate therapy in children with OI for sole treatment of BMD reduction.

The goals of a rehabilitative approach to management are directed to preventing (1) positional contractures and deformities, (2) muscle weakness and osteoporosis, and (3) malalignment of lower extremity joints prohibiting weight bearing. Lightweight braces and splints help support limbs, prevent fractures, and aid in ambulation. Physical therapy helps prevent disuse osteoporosis and strengthens muscles, which in turn improves bone density. Surgery is sometimes used to help treat the manifestations of the disease. Surgical techniques are used to correct deformities that interfere with bracing, standing, or walking. For the child with recurrent fractures, inserting an intramedullary rod provides stability to bones.

Because there is a 50% risk of an affected individual passing the gene to an offspring, genetic counseling is recommended.

Nursing Care Management

Infants and children with this disorder require careful handling to prevent fractures. They must be supported when they are being turned, positioned, moved, and held. Even changing a diaper may cause a fracture in severely affected infants. These children should never be held by the ankles when being diapered but should be gently lifted by the buttocks or supported with pillows. Children with current fractures or healing fractures should be screened for osteogenesis imperfecta—the assumption that abuse or neglect is the cause of fractures in children must be carefully evaluated by a multidisciplinary team.

Both parents and the affected child need education regarding the child's limitations and guidelines in planning suitable activities that promote optimum development and protect the child from harm. Realistic occupational planning and genetic counseling are part of the long-term goals of care. Educational materials and information can be obtained from the Osteogenesis Imperfecta Foundation,* which also has a network that can put a family in contact with other families with a similar problem.

OI is a differential diagnosis that must be ruled out in the event of multiple fractures that may be attributed to nonaccidental injury. A detailed history, no evidence of associated soft-tissue injury, and the presence of other symptoms related to OI help determine the diagnosis.

Acquired Defects

Legg-Calvé-Perthes Disease

Legg-Calvé-Perthes disease, sometimes called *coxa plana* or *osteochondritis deformans juvenilis,* is a self-limiting disorder in which there is aseptic necrosis of the femoral head. The disease affects children ages 2 to 12 years, but most cases occur in boys between 4 and 8 years of age as an isolated event. In approximately 10% of cases the involvement is bilateral; most of the affected children have a skeletal age significantly below their chronologic age (Hosalkar et al, 2007). The male/female ratio is 4:1 or 5:1. Caucasian children are affected 10 times more frequently than African-American children.

804 W. Diamond Ave., Suite 210, Gaithersburg, MD 20878; 800-981-2663; www.oif.org.

BOX 54-6 Radiographic Stages of Legg-Calvé-Perthes Disease

Stage I: initial or avascular stage—Aseptic necrosis or infarction of the capital femoral epiphysis with degenerative changes producing flattening of the upper surface of the femoral head.

Stage II: fragmentation or revascularization stage—Capital bone resorption and revascularization with fragmentation (vascular resorption of the epiphysis) that gives a mottled appearance on radiographs.

Stage III: reossification or reparative stage—New bone formation, which is represented on radiographs as calcification and ossification or increased density in the areas of radiolucency. This filling-in process appears to take place from the periphery of the head centrally.

Stage IV: residual or regenerative stage—Gradual reformation of the head of the femur without radiolucency and, it is hoped, to a spherical form.

Pathophysiology

The cause of the disease is unknown, but there is a disturbance of circulation to the femoral capital epiphysis that produces an ischemic aseptic necrosis of the femoral head. During middle childhood, circulation to the femoral epiphysis is more tenuous than at other ages and can become obstructed by trauma, inflammation, coagulation defects, and a variety of other causes. The pathologic events seem to take place in four stages (Box 54-6). The entire process may encompass as little as 18 months or continue for several years. The reformed femoral head may be severely altered or appear entirely normal.

Clinical Manifestations and Diagnostic Evaluation

The onset of Legg-Calvé-Perthes disease is usually insidious, and the history may reveal only intermittent appearance of a limp on the affected side or a symptom complex including hip soreness, ache, or stiffness that can be constant or intermittent. The parents may report seeing the child limping, and the limp becomes more pronounced with increased activity. The pain may be experienced in the hip, along the entire thigh, or in the vicinity of the knee joint. The pain and limp are usually most evident on arising and at the end of a long day of activities. The pain is usually accompanied by joint dysfunction and limited range of motion. There may be a vague history of trauma. The diagnosis is established by radiographic examination, with the definitive diagnosis being magnetic resonance imaging (MRI), which demonstrates osteonecrosis.

Therapeutic Management

Because deformity occurs early in the disease process, the aims of treatment are to eliminate hip irritability; restore and maintain adequate range of hip motion; prevent capital femoral epiphyseal collapse, extrusion, or subluxation; and ensure a well-rounded femoral head at the time of healing. Treatment varies according to the child's age at the time of diagnosis and the appearance of the femoral head vasculature and position within the acetabulum. Nonsurgical containment of the femoral head may be accomplished with abduction casts, whereas a pelvic or femoral osteotomy may be used to contain the femoral head. Activity causes microfractures of the soft ischemic epiphysis, which tend to induce synovitis, stiffness, and adductor contracture. The initial therapy is rest and non–weight bearing, which helps reduce inflammation and restore motion. Later, active motion is encouraged. In some cases traction is applied to stretch tight adductor muscles.

Containment can be accomplished in several ways. One is the use of non–weight-bearing devices, such as an abduction brace (e.g., Atlanta Scottish Rite orthosis), leg casts, or a leather harness sling, which prevent weight bearing on the affected limb. Another includes the use of various weight-bearing appliances, such as abduction-ambulation braces or casts after a period of bed rest and traction. A third option consists of surgical reconstruction and containment procedures. Conservative therapy must be continued for 2 to 4 years, although braces constructed from lightweight materials allow the child to maintain a nearly normal activity level. Surgical correction, although subjecting the child to additional risks (e.g., from anesthesia, infection, blood transfusion), returns the child to normal activities in 3 to 4 months. The use of home traction has also been explored.

Prognosis

The disease is self-limiting, but the ultimate outcome of therapy depends on early and efficient treatment and the child's age at the onset of the disorder. Children 5 years and younger, whose epiphyses are more cartilaginous, have the best prognosis for complete recovery. Children over 9 years old have a significant risk for degenerative arthritis, especially with femoral head deformity at the time of diagnosis (Hosalkar et al, 2007). The later the diagnosis is made, the more femoral damage will have occurred before treatment is implemented. In many cases, with good patient compliance, the prognosis is excellent.

✱Nursing Care Management

Nurses may be the first health professionals to identify affected children and to refer them for medical evaluation. They are also persons on whom the child and the family can rely to help them understand and adjust to the therapeutic measures. Because most of the child's care is conducted on an outpatient basis, the major emphasis of nursing care is teaching the family the care and management of the corrective appliance selected for therapy. The family needs to learn the purpose, function, application, and care of the corrective device and the importance of compliance to achieve the desired outcome (see Family-Centered Care box).

One of the most difficult aspects associated with the disorder is coping with a normally active child who feels well but must remain relatively inactive. Suitable activities must be devised to meet the needs of the child in the process of developing a sense of initiative or industry. Activities that meet the creative urges are well received.

Slipped Capital Femoral Epiphysis

Slipped capital femoral epiphysis (SCFE), or coxa vara, refers to the spontaneous displacement of the proximal femoral epiphysis in a posterior and inferior direction. It develops most frequently shortly before or during accelerated growth and the onset of puberty (children between the ages of 10 and 16 years; median age, 13 for boys, 12 for girls) and is most frequently observed in boys and obese children. Bilateral involvement occurs in up to 60% of cases. Osteonecrosis is a common complication of SCFE and is reported to occur in 17% to 47% of all patients (Hosalkar et al, 2007).

FAMILY-CENTERED CARE

Legg-Calvé-Perthes Disease

A family with five healthy children was one day startled to learn that their 2-year-old son could no longer walk. He was diagnosed with Legg-Calvé-Perthes disease. Through several years of prosthetic devices and numerous physician visits, hospitalizations, and surgeries, this family turned a potentially devastating experience into one with cherished memories.

Today, the parents reflect on how their family coped with the reality of a debilitating disease. It was difficult for the parents to observe an eager, energetic child watch other children riding bicycles, running, or playing outdoor games. But they are warmed by memories of watching their other children make the difference for their sibling. They all developed a strong bond through caring and sharing with one another. Coping as a family was an easy adjustment and, most of all, therapeutic. Today, more than 20 years later, the parents believe that each family member has grown with feelings of faith and trust. The experience proved to them that life will go on, and that life is what you make it!

—Shona Swenson Lenss, MS, RN, FNP
Cheyenne, WY

Pathophysiology

Most cases of SCFE are idiopathic, although it can be associated with endocrine disorders, renal osteodystrophy, and radiotherapy. The cause of idiopathic SCFE is multifactorial and includes obesity, physeal architecture and orientation, and pubertal hormone changes that affect physeal strength. Approximately 65% of patients with SCFE are above the 90th percentile in weight-for-age profiles; therefore obesity is believed to play a significant role in the development of the condition (Hosalkar et al, 2007). Although obesity stresses the physeal plate, SCFE can also occur in children who are not obese. Radiographs show medial displacement of the epiphysis and uncovered upper portion of the femoral neck adjacent to the physis. There is a widened growth plate and irregular metaphysis. The capital femoral epiphysis remains in the acetabulum, but the femoral neck slips, deforming the femoral head and stretching blood vessels to the epiphysis.

Diagnostic Evaluation

The disorder is suspected when an adolescent or preadolescent displays clinical signs or complains of thigh pain; hip pain may be referred to the knee as a result of the distribution of sensory nerves (Hart, Grottkau, & Albright, 2007) (Box 54-7). The diagnosis is confirmed by radiographic examination.

Therapeutic Management

Treatment goals are to prevent further slippage and provide stability for the epiphysis (Hart, Grottkau, & Albright, 2007). Once the diagnosis is established, the child should be made completely non–weight bearing with either crutches and a wheelchair to prevent further slippage. Surgical treatment varies with the degree of displacement. Traditional methods included presurgery bed rest and traction followed by surgical pinning. Surgical pinning involves the placement of a single pin through the femoral neck into the proximal femoral epiphysis to prevent further slippage (Hart, Grottkau, & Albright, 2007). Postsurgical care includes non–weight-bearing crutch ambulation (or wheelchair use if bilateral) for 6 to 8 weeks. SCFE is an emergency and requires early diagnosis and treatment to increase the likelihood of a satisfactory cure. The two most severe complications of SCFE are avascular necrosis of the proximal femoral physis and chondrolysis, which involves the loss of articular cartilage, decreased range of motion, and pain (Hart, Grottkau, & Albright, 2007).

BOX 54-7 Clinical Manifestations of Slipped Capital Femoral Epiphysis

Limp on affected side
Pain in hip
- Continuous or intermittent
- Frequently referred to groin, anteromedial aspect of thigh, or knee

Restricted internal rotation on adduction with external rotation deformity
Loss of abduction and internal rotation as severity increases
Shortening of lower extremity

✱ Nursing Care Management

Nursing care is the same as that for a child in a cast or a child in traction, as discussed earlier in this chapter. Postoperative care involves hemodynamic stabilization and assessment for complications. The adolescent is taught the proper use of crutches and the importance of a avoiding any weight bearing on the affected hip (if unilateral). The adolescent may be involved in building upper body strength during the convalescent period to increase mobility from bed to wheelchair, as appropriate. Self-care and performance of activities of daily living to capability are encouraged to promote confidence and decrease a sense of helplessness.

Kyphosis and Lordosis

The spine, consisting of numerous segments, can acquire deformity curves of three types: kyphosis, lordosis, and scoliosis (Fig. 54-11).

Kyphosis is an abnormally increased convex angulation in the curvature of the thoracic spine (see Fig. 54-11, *B*). It can occur secondary to disease processes such as tuberculosis, chronic arthritis, osteodystrophy, or compression fractures of the thoracic spine. The most common form of kyphosis is "postural." Children, especially during the time when skeletal growth outpaces growth of muscle, are prone to exaggeration of a normal kyphosis. They assume abnormal sitting and standing positions. This is particularly common in self-conscious adolescent girls who assume a round-shouldered slouching posture in an attempt to hide their developing breasts. *Scheuermann's kyphosis* is a thoracic curve greater than 45 degrees with wedging greater than 5 degrees of at least three adjacent vertebral bodies and vertebral irregularity.

Postural kyphosis is almost always accompanied by a compensatory postural lordosis, an abnormally exaggerated concave lumbar curvature. Treatment of kyphosis consists of exercises to strengthen shoulder and abdominal muscles and bracing for more marked deformity. With adolescents who are significantly self-conscious about their appearance, the best approach is to emphasize the cosmetic value of corrective

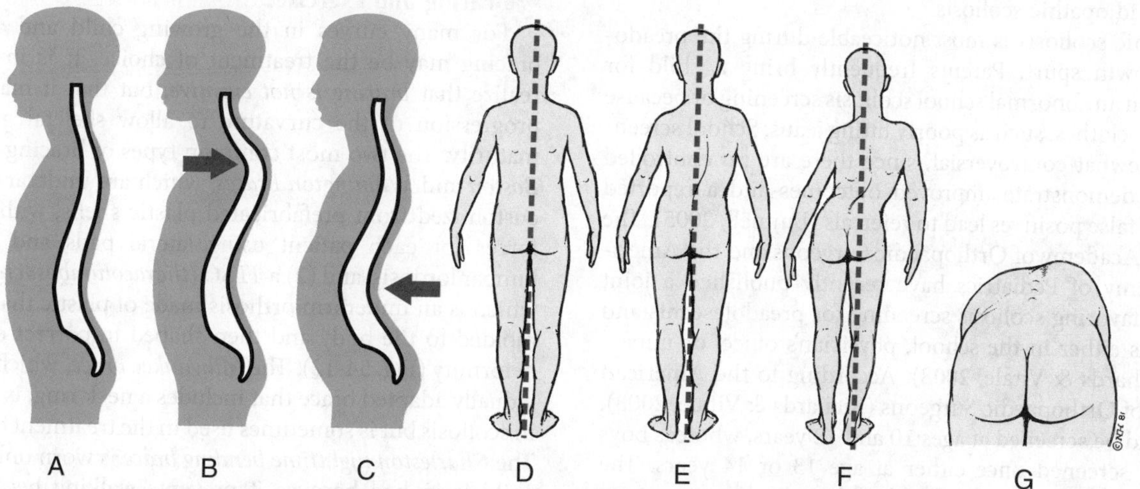

Fig. 54-11 Spinal column curvatures. **A**, Normal spine. **B**, Kyphosis. **C**, Lordosis. **D**, Normal spine in balance. **E**, Mild scoliosis in balance. **F**, Severe scoliosis not in balance. **G**, Rib hump and flank asymmetry seen in flexion caused by rotary component. (Redrawn from Hilt NE, Schmitt EW: *Pediatric orthopedic nursing*, St Louis, 1975, Mosby.)

evolve Animation—Spine Structure

therapy and to place the responsibility on the adolescent for carrying out an exercise program at home, with regular visits to and assessments by a therapist. Treatment with a brace may be indicated until skeletal maturity; surgical spinal fusion may be considered for severe, painful, or progressive deforming thoracic curves such as Scheuermann's kyphosis.

Lordosis is an accentuation of the cervical or lumbar curvature beyond physiologic limits (see Fig. 54-11, *C*). It may be a secondary complication of a disease process, a result of trauma, or idiopathic. It is often seen in association with flexion contractures of the hip, scoliosis, obesity, developmental dysplasia of the hip, and slipped capital femoral epiphysis. During the pubertal growth spurt, lordosis of varying degrees is observed in teenagers, especially girls. Unlike kyphosis, severe lordosis is usually accompanied by pain.

Treatment involves management of the predisposing cause when possible, such as weight loss and correction of deformities. Postural exercises or support garments are helpful in relieving symptoms in some cases; however, these do not usually effect a permanent cure.

Idiopathic Scoliosis

Scoliosis is a complex spinal deformity in three planes, usually involving lateral curvature, spinal rotation causing rib asymmetry, and thoracic hypokyphosis. It is the most common spinal deformity and can be further classified according to age of onset: *congenital,* during fetal development; *infantile,* at birth or up to 3 years of age; *childhood (juvenile),* in children 4 to 10 years of age; or *adolescent,* during the growth spurt of early adolescence (the most common type). Scoliosis can be caused by a number of conditions and may occur alone or in association with other diseases, particularly neuromuscular conditions (neuromuscular scoliosis). In most cases, however, there is no apparent cause, and thus the name *idiopathic scoliosis.* The following discussion involves the adolescent type, which is often called *adolescent idiopathic scoliosis.* There appears to be a genetic component to the etiology of idiopathic scoliosis; however, the exact relationship has yet to be established. The following section is limited to a discussion of adolescent idiopathic scoliosis.

Idiopathic scoliosis is most noticeable during the preadolescent growth spurt. Parents frequently bring a child for follow up on an abnormal school scoliosis screening or because of ill-fitting clothes, such as poorly fitting jeans. School screening is somewhat controversial, since there are no controlled studies to demonstrate improved outcomes and a reported number of false positives lead to referrals (Bunnell, 2005). The American Academy of Orthopaedic Surgeons and the American Academy of Pediatrics have recently published a joint statement favoring scoliosis screening for preadolescents and adolescents either in the school, physician's office, or nurses' clinic (Richards & Vitale, 2008). According to the American Academy of Orthopaedic Surgeons (Richards & Vitale, 2008), girls should be screened at ages 10 and 12 years, whereas boys should be screened once either at age 13 or 14 years. The benefits of early detection, referral, and medical treatment are considered to be significant, but the persons performing the screenings must be educated in the detection of spinal deformity.

Diagnostic Evaluation

Observation is performed behind an undressed (in undergarments) standing child, noting asymmetry of shoulder height, scapular or flank shape, or hip height and alignment. When the child bends forward at the waist (the Adams test) with hanging arms, asymmetry of the ribs and flanks may be noted. A scoliometer is also used in the initial screening to measure truncal rotation (also measured by the Adams test). Often a primary curve and a compensatory curve will place the head in alignment with the gluteal cleft. However, in the uncompensated curve the head and hips are not aligned (see Fig. 54-11, *E* and *F*). (See Spine, Chapter 34, for additional information.) Definitive diagnosis is made by radiographs of the child in the standing position and use of the Cobb technique (standard measurement of angle curvature), which establishes the degree of curvature. The Risser scale is used to evaluate skeletal maturity on the radiographs; the scale assists in making a determination of the likely progression of the spinal angulature as the child's bones mature. The Tanner maturity rating is also used to evaluate the risk of curve progression in adolescents. Not all spinal curvatures are scoliosis. A curve of less than 10 degrees is considered a postural variation. Curves of less than 20 degrees are mild and, if nonprogressive, do not require treatment.

Intraspinal conditions or other disease processes that can cause scoliosis must be ruled out. The presence of pain, sacral dimpling or hairy patches, cutaneous vascular changes, absent or abnormal reflexes, bowel or bladder incontinence, or left thoracic curve may indicate an intraspinal abnormality such as syringomyelia, diastematomyelia, or tethered cord syndrome. An MRI scan should be obtained for evaluation.

Therapeutic Management

Current management options include observation with regular clinical and radiographic evaluation, orthotic intervention (bracing), and surgical spinal fusion. Treatment decisions are based on the magnitude, location, and type of curve; the age and skeletal maturity of the child or adolescent; and any underlying or contributing disease process.

Bracing and Exercise

For many curves in the growing child and adolescent, bracing may be the treatment of choice. It is important to realize that *bracing is not curative,* but that it may slow the progression of the curvature to allow skeletal growth and maturity. The two most common types of bracing are (1) the *Boston* and *Wilmington braces,* which are underarm orthoses customized from prefabricated plastic shells, with corrective forces for each patient using lateral pads and decreasing lumbar lordosis; and (2) a *TLSO (thoracolumbosacral orthotic),* which is an underarm orthosis made of plastic that is custom molded to the body and then shaped to correct or hold the deformity (Fig. 54-12). The *Milwaukee brace,* which is an individually adapted brace that includes a neck ring, is rarely used in scoliosis but is sometimes used in the treatment of kyphosis. The *Charleston nighttime bending brace* is worn only when the child is in bed because it prevents walking because of the severity of the trunk bend. Bracing, although used as the gold standard treatment for mild to moderate curvatures, has not proved to be entirely effective in the treatment of scoliosis

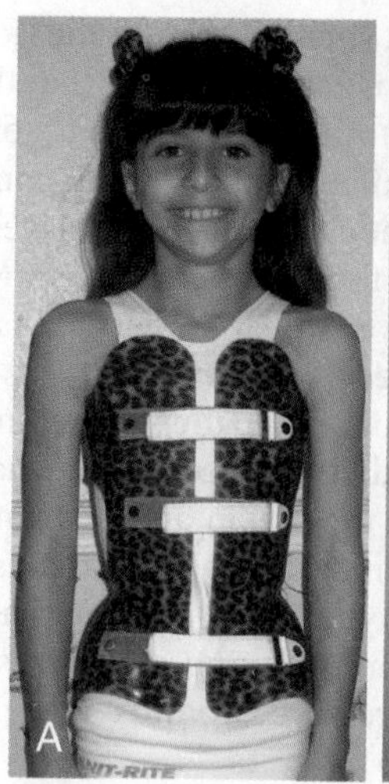
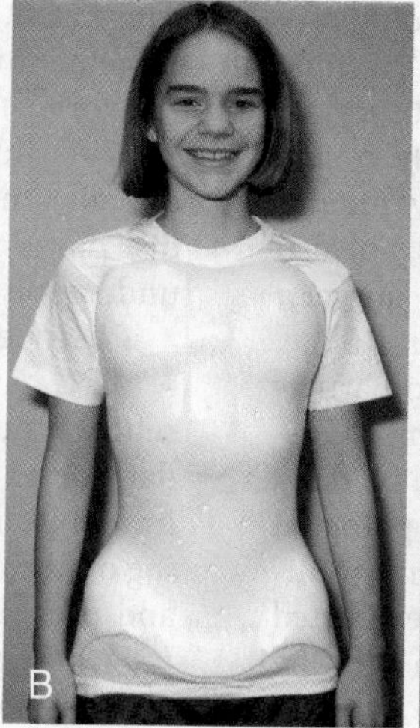
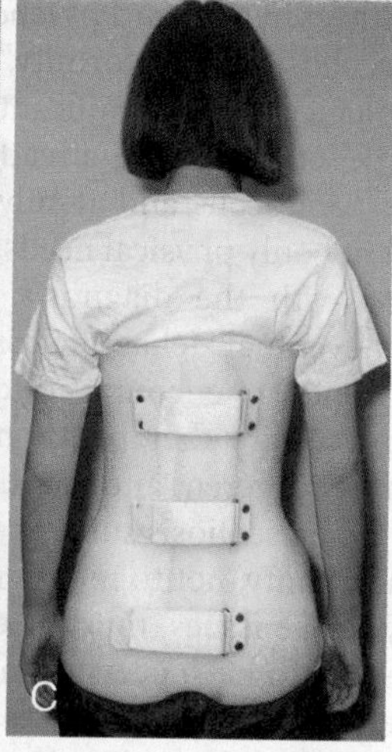

Fig. 54-12 **A,** Standard thoracolumbosacral (TLSO) brace for idiopathic scoliosis. Note the color and design incorporated into the brace to make it more acceptable to children and adolescents. **B,** Variation of a standard TLSO that fastens in the back **(C)** to provide needed support for the spine curvature.

(Newton & Wenger, 2001). Compliance in wearing the brace is difficult because of the adolescent's age and preoccupation with body image and appearance. Experts recognize that brace treatment in some children with significant scoliosis may help avoid surgical intervention by slowing curve progression; however, further studies are needed to clarify the effectiveness of bracing (Richards & Vitale, 2008).

Exercises alone and chiropractic treatment are rarely of value in managing scoliosis; transcutaneous electrical nerve stimulation has also proved to be an ineffective treatment for this condition. Exercises are of benefit when used in conjunction with bracing to maintain and increase the strength of spinal and abdominal muscles during treatment.

Surgical Management

Surgical intervention may be required for correction of severe curves (usually 45 degrees or more in skeletally immature patients and 50 to 55 degrees or more in the skeletally mature [Spiegel, Hosalkar, & Dormans, 2007]). The degree of curvature and the cause guide the decision to have surgery. Bracing and exercise have been universally disappointing in curves greater than 40 degrees, and paralytic and congenital curves, which will eventually progress, are best treated with early surgical stabilization if the child's health status will allow major surgery. The child's age and location of the curvature influence the decision for surgery, and any progressive or severe curve that does not respond to more conservative orthotic measures requires surgical correction. Difficulties with balance or seating, respiratory excursion, or pain are also considered.

The surgical technique consists of realignment and straightening with internal fixation and instrumentation combined with bony fusion *(arthrodesis)* of the realigned spine. The goals of surgical intervention are to correct the curvatures on the sagittal and coronal planes and to have a solid, pain-free fusion in a well-balanced torso, with maximum mobility of the remaining spinal segments.

Many instrumentation systems, including Harrington, Dwyer, Zielke, Luque, Cotrel-Dubousset, Isola, TSRH (Texas Scottish Rite Hospital), and Moss Miami, are available. Selection of the system is individualized according to the patient's needs and surgeon's preference. Posterior or anterior surgical approaches can be used.

The Harrington system, the first internal spinal instrumentation device, consists of distraction and compression rods, hooks, and nuts. The posterior elements are decorticated, and bone from the iliac crest or donor bone is placed across the vertebrae to provide fusion. Postoperatively the child is logrolled to prevent spinal motion, and a molded plastic jacket is used to stabilize the spine until the fusion is solid.

The Luque-rod segmental spinal instrumentation provides segmental stability by the use of wires and L-shaped rods. By way of a posterior approach, the wires are threaded beneath the lamina of each vertebra and tightened around the rods resting along the transverse processes to stabilize the spine. Bone from the iliac crest or donor bone is used to fuse the spine. The advantage of this method is that the patient can be mobile within a few days and requires no postoperative immobilization. The disadvantage is the risk of nerve damage.

The Cotrel-Dubousset instrumentation combines the Harrington and L-rod approaches by using bilateral rods and hooks at many sites. Anterior approaches using the Dwyer or Zielke instrumentation involve screws into the vertebral bodies connected by a cable or rod. These systems require postoperative immobilization with a custom-fitted plastic jacket.

Advances in surgical technology are currently being evaluated, including thoracoscopic spinal fusion and placement of implants; metallic staples may also be placed into the vertebral bodies to achieve spinal fusion and to correct the deformity (Spiegel, Hosalkar, & Dormans, 2007).

Nursing Care Management

Treatment for scoliosis extends over a significant portion of the affected child's period of growth. In adolescents this period is the one in which their identity, physical and psychologic, is formed. The identification of scoliosis as a "deformity," in combination with unattractive appliances and a significant surgical procedure, can have a negative effect on the already fragile adolescent body image. The adolescent and family require excellent nursing care to meet not only physical needs, but also psychologic needs associated with the diagnosis, surgery, postoperative recovery, and eventual rehabilitation (Slote, 2002). Although these adolescents are encouraged to participate in most peer activities, necessary therapeutic modifications are likely to make them feel different and apart. Nursing care of the adolescent who is facing scoliosis surgery, potential social isolation, pain, and uncertainty, not to mention misunderstood emotions and body image issues, must be evaluated from the adolescent's perspective to be successful in meeting the individual's needs (Napierkowski, 2007).

When a child or adolescent first faces the prospect of a prolonged period in a brace, jacket, or other device, the therapy program and the nature of the device must be explained thoroughly to both the child and the parents so that they will understand the anticipated results, how the appliance corrects the defect, the freedoms and constraints imposed by the device, and what they can do to help achieve the desired goal. The management involves the skills and services of a team of specialists, including the orthopedist, physical therapist, orthotist (a specialist in fitting orthopedic braces), nurse, social worker, and sometimes a thoracic or pulmonary specialist.

It is difficult for a child to be restricted at any phase of development, but the adolescent needs continual positive reinforcement, encouragement, and as much independence as can be safely assumed during this time. Guidance and assistance regarding anticipated problems, such as selection of clothing and participation in social activities, are appreciated by adolescents. Socialization with peers is strongly encouraged, and every effort is expended to help the adolescent feel attractive and worthwhile.

Preoperative Care

The preoperative workup usually involves a radiographic series, including bending and traction films, pulmonary function studies, and a number of routine laboratory studies (including prothrombin, partial thromboplastin, and bleeding times; blood count; electrolyte levels; urinalysis and urine culture; and blood levels of any medications). Because spinal surgery usually involves considerable blood loss, several options are considered preoperatively to maintain or replace blood volume. These options include autologous blood donations obtained from the patient before the surgery; intraoperative blood salvage; intraoperative hemodilution; erythropoietin administration; and controlled induced hypotension, which must be carefully monitored at all times to prevent physiologic instability (Newton & Wenger, 2001).

Surgery for spinal fusion is complex, and often adolescents who require the procedure because of idiopathic scoliosis are not familiar with medical terms, procedures, or experiences. Preoperative teaching is critical for the adolescent to be able to cooperate and participate in his or her treatment and recovery. Because the surgery is extensive, the patient is taught how to manage his or her own patient-controlled analgesia (PCA) pump; how to log-roll; and the use and function of other equipment, such as a chest tube (for anterior repair) and Foley catheter. It is recommended that the child or adolescent bring a favorite toy (age dependent) or personal items such as a favorite stuffed animal, laptop computer (for web surfing and e-mails), movie player, MP3 player, iPod, or portable compact disc player for postoperative use. Meeting with a peer who has undergone a similar surgery is also valuable (Slote, 2002).

Postoperative Care

After surgery, patients are monitored in an acute care setting and log rolled when changing position to prevent damage to the fusion and instrumentation. In some cases an immobilization brace or cast is used postoperatively depending on the type of surgical intervention. Skin care is important, and pressure-relieving mattresses or beds may be needed to prevent pressure wounds (see Maintaining Healthy Skin, Chapter 45).

In addition to the usual postoperative assessments of wound, circulation, and vital signs, the neurologic status of the patient's extremities requires special attention. Prompt recognition of any neurologic impairment is imperative because delayed paralysis may develop that requires surgical intervention. Common postoperative problems after spinal fusion include neurologic injury or spinal cord injury, hypotension from acute blood loss, wound infection, syndrome of inappropriate secretion of antidiuretic hormone, atelectasis, pneumothorax, ileus, delayed neurologic injury, and implanted hardware complications (Freeman, 2007; Newton & Wenger, 2001). Superior mesenteric artery (SMA) syndrome may occur several days after spinal surgery; this involves duodenal compression by the aorta and SMA and may result in acute partial or complete duodenal obstruction. Clinical manifestations include epigastric pain, nausea, copious vomiting, and eructation; symptoms are aggravated in the supine position and often relieved with the patient in a left lateral decubitus or prone position.

The adolescent usually has considerable pain for the first few days after surgery and requires frequent administration of pain medication, preferably opioids administered intravenously on a regular schedule. For children able to understand the concept, PCA is recommended (see Pain Assessment; Pain Management, Chapter 35). In most cases the patient begins walking as soon as possible. Depending on the instrumentation used and the surgical approach, most patients are walking by the second or third postoperative day and are discharged by 1 week. In addition to pain management, the patient is evaluated for skin integrity, adequate urine output, fluid and electrolyte balance, and ileus (Slote, 2002). Discharge planning should include a timetable for follow-up with the practitioner and resumption of regular activities.

All patients are started on physical therapy as soon as they are able, beginning with range-of-motion exercises on the first postoperative day, and many of the activities of daily living in the following days. Self-care, such as washing and eating, is always encouraged. Throughout the hospitalization, age-appropriate activities and contact with family and friends are important parts of nursing care and planning (see The Immobilized Child, p. 1676).

The family is encouraged to become involved in the patient's care to facilitate the transition from hospital to home management. An organization that provides education and services to both families and professionals is the National Scoliosis Foundation.* The American Academy of Orthopaedic Surgeons† and Scoliosis Research Society,‡ an organization of physicians and scientists, have published an excellent book, *Scoliosis,* and the Scoliosis Research Society has educational information available on its website.

Infections of Bones and Joints

Osteomyelitis

Osteomyelitis, an infectious process in the bone, can occur at any age but most frequently is seen in children 10 years of age or younger. *Staphylococcus aureus* is the most common causative organism. *Acute hematogenous osteomyelitis* results when a bloodborne bacterium causes an infection in the bone. Common foci include infected lesions, upper respiratory tract infections, otitis media, tonsillitis, abscessed teeth, pyelonephritis, and infected burns. *Exogenous osteomyelitis* is acquired from direct inoculation of the bone from a puncture wound, open fracture, surgical contamination, or adjacent tissue infection. *Subacute osteomyelitis* has a longer course and may be caused by less virulent microbes with a walled-off abscess or Brodie's abscess, typically in the proximal or distal tibia. *Chronic osteomyelitis* is a progression of acute osteomyelitis and is characterized by dead bone, bone loss, and drainage and sinus tracts.

Generally, healthy bone is not likely to become infected. Factors that contribute to infection include inoculation with a large number of organisms, presence of a foreign body, bone injury, high virulence of an organism, immunosuppression, and malnutrition; certain types and locations of bone are also more vulnerable to infection.

Typically children with acute hematogenous osteomyelitis are seen with a 2- to 7-day history of pain, warmth, tenderness, and decreased range of motion in the affected limb, along with systemic symptoms of fever, irritability, and lethargy (Box 54-8). Symptoms often resemble those observed in other diseases involving bones such as arthritis or leukemia.

Pathophysiology

Osteomyelitis can be acquired exogenously by direct inoculation of bone during trauma or surgery; the hand and foot are commons sites. Hematogenous osteomyelitis is seeded by organisms from a preexisting infection such as tonsillitis or impetigo or from a contiguous source such as an adjacent infected bone or joint. Hematogenous osteomyelitis usually occurs in the metaphyses of long bones such as the femur or tibia. The infecting organism travels from the site of infection to the small end-artery capillary loops in the bone metaphyses, causing obstruction and initiating infection, with complications of bone destruction and abscess formation. In infants the diagnosis is challenging because of difficulty localizing symptoms and the increased likelihood of multiple bone involvement.

BOX 54-8 Clinical Manifestations of Acute Osteomyelitis

General Manifestations

- History of trauma to affected bone (frequent)
- Child appears very ill
- Irritability
- Elevated temperature
- Restlessness
- Rapid pulse
- Dehydration

Local Manifestations

- Tenderness
- Increased warmth
- Diffuse swelling over involved bone
- Involved extremity painful, especially on movement
- Involved extremity held in semiflexion
- Surrounding muscles tense and resistant to passive movement

Diagnostic Evaluation

Organism identification and antibiotic susceptibility testing are essential for effective therapy. Cultures of aspirated subperiosteal pus along with cultures of blood, joint fluid, and infected skin samples should be obtained. Bone biopsy is indicated if blood culture results and radiographic findings are not consistent with osteomyelitis. Supporting evidence for osteomyelitis includes leukocytosis and elevated erythrocyte sedimentation rate. Radiographic signs, except for soft-tissue swelling, are evident only after 2 to 3 weeks. A three-phase technetium bone scan can show areas of increased blood flow, such as occurs in early stages in infected bone, and is useful in locating multiple sites; however, it is not a diagnostic test. CT can detect bone destruction, and MRI provides anatomic details useful in delineating the area of involvement, especially if surgical intervention is planned. Sometimes the osteomyelitis may be unrecognized if it occurs as a complication of a severe toxic and debilitating disease.

Therapeutic Management

After culture specimens are obtained, empiric therapy is started with IV antibiotics covering the mostly likely organisms. For *S. aureus,* nafcillin or clindamycin is generally used; methicillin-resistant *S. aureus* may require vancomycin. When the infective agent is identified, administration of the appropriate antibiotic is initiated and continued for at least 4 weeks, but the length of therapy is determined by the duration of the symptoms, the response to treatment, and the organism's sensitivity. In selected cases oral antibiotic therapy may follow a shorter IV course. Because of the prolonged duration of high-dose antibiotic therapy, it is important to monitor for hematologic, renal, hepatic, ototoxic, and other potential side effects.

evolve Case Study–Osteomyelitis

*Five Cabot Place, Stoughton, MA 02072; 800-673-6922; www.scoliosis.org.

†6300 N. River Road, Rosemont, IL 60018-4262; 847-823-7186; www.aaos.org.

‡611 E. Wells St., Suite 1100, Milwaukee, WI 53202; 414-289-9107; www.srs.org.

Surgery may be indicated if there is no response to specific antibiotic therapy, persistent soft-tissue abscess is seen, or the infection spreads to the joint. Opinions differ regarding surgical intervention, but many advocate sequestrectomy and surgical drainage to decompress the metaphyseal space before pus erupts and spreads to the subperiosteal space, forming abscesses that strip the periosteum from bone or form draining sinuses. When these complications occur, a chronic infection usually persists. When surgical drainage is carried out, polyethylene tubes are placed in the wound; one tube instills an antibiotic solution directly into the infected area by gravity, and the other, connected to a suction apparatus, provides drainage.

Nursing Care Management

During the acute phase of illness any movement of the affected limb will cause discomfort; therefore the child is positioned comfortably with the affected limb supported. Moving and turning are carried out carefully and gently to minimize pain. The child may require pain medication or sedation. Vital signs are taken and recorded frequently, and measures are implemented to reduce a significant temperature elevation.

Antibiotic therapy requires careful observation and monitoring of the IV equipment and site. Because more than one antibiotic is usually administered, the compatibility of the drugs is determined and care is taken to avoid mixing incompatible drugs. For long-term antibiotic therapy, an intermittent infusion device or peripherally inserted central catheter is used (see Parenteral Fluid Therapy, Chapter 45). Antibiotic therapy is often continued at home.

Standard Precautions are put in effect for children with open wounds, depending on the institution's policies. The wound is managed according to the practitioner's directions. Administration of antibiotic solution directly into the wound is most efficiently accomplished using a regular infusion setup that is prepared and regulated in the same manner as for any IV infusion. Intake and output are measured and recorded, and the character of both the wound and drainage is noted. The amount and character of drainage on the wound dressing are also noted.

Casts are sometimes used for immobilization, and, if so, routine cast care is carried out. The extremity is examined for sensation, circulation, and pain, and the area over the inflammation is usually left open for observation. The affected area, casted or uncasted, is assessed for color, swelling, heat, and tenderness.

The child usually has a poor appetite and may be prone to vomiting. The appetite returns as the acute symptoms recede. During convalescence, adequate nutrition must be maintained to aid healing and formation of new bone.

When the acute stage subsides, children begin to feel better, appetite improves, and they become interested in their surroundings and relationships. Weight bearing on the affected limb is not permitted until healing is well under way in order to avoid pathologic fractures. Provision of diversional and constructive activities becomes an important nursing intervention. Children are usually confined to bed for some time after the acute phase but may be allowed to move about on a stretcher or in a wheelchair when isolation and bed rest are no longer necessary. At this stage the continuous IV infusion may be replaced by a heparin lock system to allow greater freedom.

As the infection subsides, physical therapy is instituted to ensure restoration of optimum function. The child is usually discharged on a regimen of oral antibiotics, and progress is followed closely for some time.

Septic Arthritis

Septic arthritis is a bacterial infection in the joint. It usually results from hematogenous spread or from direct extension of an adjacent cellulitis or osteomyelitis. Direct inoculation from trauma accounts for 15% to 20% of septic arthritis cases. The most common causative organism is *S. aureus*. Community-acquired methicillin-resistant *S. aureus* is commonly a cause of septic arthritis (Gutierrez, 2005). In addition to *S. aureus*, pathogens seen in neonates include group B streptococci, *Escherichia coli*, and *Candida albicans*. In children 2 months to 5 years of age, *S. aureus, Streptococcus pyogenes, Streptococcus pneumoniae*, and *Kingella kingae* are the primary organisms causing infection, whereas children older than 5 years are more likely to be infected by *S. aureus* and *S. pyogenes*; sexually active adolescents may be infected by *Neisseria gonorrhoeae* (Gutierrez, 2005).

Knees, hips, ankles, and elbows are the most common joints affected. Clinical manifestations include severe joint pain, swelling, warmth of overlying tissue, and occasionally erythema. The child is resistant to any joint movement. Features of systemic illness such as fever, malaise, headache, nausea, vomiting, and irritability may also be present.

Therapeutic Management and Nursing Care Management

The affected joint is aspirated and the specimen evaluated by Gram stain; culturing (including separate cultures for *Haemophilus influenzae* and *N. gonorrhoeae*); and determination of leukocyte count and glucose, lactate, and protein levels. An infection involving the hip, however, is considered a surgical emergency to prevent compromised blood supply to the head of the femur (Lampe, 2007). In addition, blood culture should be performed, and complete blood count with differential and erythrocyte sedimentation rate or C-reactive protein level should be obtained. Early radiographic findings are limited to soft-tissue swelling but may reveal a foreign body, and such films always provide a baseline for comparison. Technetium scans reveal areas of increased blood flow but will not differentiate between sites. MRI and CT scans provide more detailed images of cartilage loss, joint narrowing, erosions, and ankylosis of progressive disease.

Surgical intervention may also be required if there was a penetrating wound or a possible involvement of a foreign object. Physical therapy may be initiated for the child who is immobilized in a cast or traction to prevent flexion contractures.

Treatment is IV antibiotic therapy based on Gram stain results and the clinical presentation. The benefits of serial aspirations to demonstrate sterility of synovial fluid and reduce pressure or pain are controversial. Pain management is an important aspect of nursing care, particularly with involvement of a large joint such as the hip. Additional nursing care is the same as for osteomyelitis.

Skeletal Tuberculosis

In children tubercular infection of the bones and joints is acquired by lymphohematogenous spread at the time of primary infection. Occasionally it is from chronic pulmonary tuberculosis. Skeletal tubercular infection is not common in the United States but should be considered in communities with high tuberculosis case rates. The infection is most likely to involve the vertebrae, causing tubercular spondylitis. If the infection is progressive, it causes Pott's disease with destruction of the vertebral bodies and results in kyphosis. Symptoms are insidious. The child may report persistent or intermittent pain. Other findings include joint swelling and stiffness; fever and weight loss are not common. Tubercular arthritis can also affect single joints such as a knee or hip and tends to cause severe destruction of adjacent bone. Infection in the fingers causes spina ventosa, a tuberculous dactylitis.

As with pulmonary tuberculosis, the index case should be located. A family and environmental history needs to be obtained and tuberculin skin tests (TSTs) performed. Results of TSTs are positive for the majority of children with tuberculous arthritis; however, the results are not diagnostic, and the clinical and laboratory features do not differentiate tubercular arthritis from a nontubercular septic arthritis. Diagnosis requires isolation of *Mycobacterium tuberculosis* from the site. Patients with the susceptible organism start treatment with combined antituberculosis chemotherapy (isoniazid, rifampin, and pyrazinamide); directly observed therapy is preferred (see also Chapter 46).

Nursing Care Management

Nursing care depends on the site and extent of infection. Tuberculous spondylitis and hip infection may require immobilization, casting, and fusion. Nursing care is the same as for osteomyelitis and septic arthritis.

Bone and Soft-Tissue Tumors

General Concepts: Bone Tumors

Malignant bone tumors represent less than 5% of all malignant neoplasms, but 85% of all primary malignant bone tumors in children are either osteogenic sarcoma or Ewing's sarcoma. The peak ages during childhood are 15 to 19 years. The sexes are affected equally until puberty, at which time the ratio approaches 2:1 in favor of males. This propensity for males with a peak incidence during adolescence is thought to result from the accelerated growth rate of osseous tissue.

Neoplastic disease can arise from any tissues involved in bone growth, such as osteoid matrix, bone marrow elements, fat, blood and lymph vessels, nerve sheath, and cartilage. They have several characteristics in common, which are discussed in the following sections, along with specific information about each tumor.

Most malignant bone tumors produce localized pain in the affected site, which may be severe or dull and may be attributed to trauma or the vague complaint of "growing pains." The pain is often relieved by a flexed position, which relaxes the muscles overlying the stretched periosteum. Frequently it draws attention when the child limps, curtails physical activity, or is unable to hold heavy objects (Box 54-9).

BOX 54-9 Clinical Manifestations of Bone Tumors

Pain localized at affected site
- May be severe or dull
- Often relieved by position of flexion

Frequently brought to attention when child:
- Limps
- Curtails own physical activity
- Is unable to hold heavy objects

Diagnostic Evaluation

Diagnosis begins with a thorough history and physical examination. A primary objective is to rule out causes such as trauma or infection. Careful questioning regarding pain is essential in determining the duration and rate of tumor growth. Physical assessment focuses on functional status of the affected area; signs of inflammation; size of the mass; involvement of regional lymph nodes; and any systemic indication of generalized malignancy, such as anemia, weight loss, and frequent infection.

Definitive diagnosis is based on radiologic studies, such as CT to determine the extent of the lesion; MRI to assess soft tissue, tumor boundaries, and nerve and vessel involvement; radioisotope bone scans to evaluate metastasis; and either needle or surgical bone biopsy to determine the histologic pattern. Radiologic findings are characteristic for each type of tumor. In osteogenic sarcoma, needlelike new bone formation growing at right angles to the diaphysis (shaft) produces a "sunburst" appearance. In Ewing's sarcoma the deposits of new bone in layers under the periosteum produce an "onion skin" appearance. In both types of bone tumors, soft-tissue infiltration may be apparent.

At present there is no reliable biochemical test for bone cancers. Elevated alkaline phosphatase levels may occur in osteoid tumors. Several tests may be done for differential diagnosis in terms of secondary bone metastasis from Wilms' tumor, neuroblastoma, retinoblastoma, rhabdomyosarcoma, lymphoma, or leukemia. Lung CT is usually a standard procedure, since pulmonary metastasis is the most common complication of primary bone tumors. Bone marrow aspiration is helpful in diagnosing Ewing's sarcoma in the rare event that the child has bone marrow metastasis.

Osteosarcoma

Osteosarcoma (osteogenic sarcoma) is the most common bone cancer in children. Its peak incidence is between 10 and 25 years of age (Link, Gebhardt, & Myers, 2006). It presumably arises from bone-forming mesenchyme, which gives rise to malignant osteoid tissue. Most primary tumor sites are in the metaphysis (wider part of the shaft, adjacent to the epiphyseal growth plate) of long bones, especially in the lower extremities. More than half occur in the femur, particularly the distal portion, with the rest involving the humerus, tibia, pelvis, jaw, and phalanges.

evolve Critical Thinking Exercise—Osteogenic Sarcoma

Therapeutic Management

Optimum treatment of osteosarcoma is surgery and chemotherapy. The surgical approach consists of surgical biopsy followed by either limb salvage or amputation. Depending on the tumor site, surgery includes amputation of the affected extremity at least 7.5 cm (3 inches) above the proximal tumor margin or above the joint proximal to the involved bone. With tumors of the distal femur, preservation of the hip joint may be possible. Other procedures include an above-the-knee amputation for tumors of the tibia or fibula, a hemipelvectomy for tumors of the innominate (hip) bone, and a forequarter amputation (removal of arm, scapula, and portion of the clavicle on the affected side) for tumors of the upper humerus.

The other surgical approach for selected patients is the *limb salvage procedure,* which involves en bloc resection of the primary tumor with prosthetic replacement of the involved bone. For example, with osteosarcoma of the distal femur, a total femur and joint replacement is performed. Frequently children undergoing a limb salvage procedure will receive preoperative chemotherapy in an attempt to decrease the tumor size and make surgery more manageable (Link, Gebhardt, & Myers, 2006).

Chemotherapy plays a vital role in treatment of osteosarcoma. Antineoplastic drugs, such as high-dose methotrexate with citrovorum factor rescue, doxorubicin, bleomycin, actinomycin D, cyclophosphamide, ifosfamide, and cisplatin, may be administered singly or in combination and may be employed both before and after surgery. When pulmonary metastasis is found, thoracotomy and chemotherapy have resulted in prolonged survival and potential cure. These combined-modality approaches have significantly improved the survival rates for osteosarcoma to approximately 60% to 70% in nonmetastatic patients (Heare, Hensley, & Dell'orfano, 2009; Ta et al, 2009). New trials have recently been completed using muramyl tripeptide phosphatidylethanolamine to eradicate micrometastases by stimulating macrophages to kill tumor cells not eliminated by chemotherapy (Link, Gebhardt, & Myers, 2006).

✽ Nursing Care Management

Nursing care depends on the type of surgical approach. Obviously the family may have more difficulty adjusting to an amputation than a limb salvage procedure. In either instance, preparation of the child and family is critical. Straightforward honesty is essential in gaining the child's cooperation and trust. The diagnosis of cancer should not be disguised with falsehoods such as "infection." To accept the need for radical surgery, the child must be aware of the lack of alternatives for treatment. Although the responsibility of telling the child is generally left to the physician, the nurse should be present at the discussion or be aware of exactly what is said. The child should be told a few days before surgery to allow him or her time to think about the diagnosis and consequent treatment and to ask questions.

Sometimes children have many questions about the prosthesis, limitations on physical ability, and prognosis in terms of cure. At other times they react with silence or with a calm manner that belies their concern and fear. Either response must be accepted, since it is part of the grieving process of a loss. For those who desire information, it may be helpful to introduce them to another amputee before surgery or to show them pictures of the prosthesis.* However, the nurse must be careful not to overwhelm children with information. A sound approach is to answer questions without offering additional information. For those who do not pursue additional information, the nurse expresses a willingness to talk.

The child is also informed of the need for chemotherapy and its side effects before surgery. Caution must be exercised about offering too much information at one time. It is wise to discuss hair loss with an emphasis on positive aspects, such as wearing a wig. Because bone tumors affect adolescents and young adults, it is not unusual for them to become angry over all the radical body alterations.

If an amputation is performed, the child is usually fitted with a temporary prosthesis immediately after surgery, which permits early functioning and fosters psychologic adjustment. If this is not done, the child requires stump care, which is the same as for any amputee. A permanent prosthesis is usually fitted within 6 to 8 weeks. During hospitalization the child begins physical therapy to become proficient in the use and care of the device.

Phantom limb pain may develop after amputation. This symptom is characterized by sensations such as tingling, itching, and, more frequently, pain felt in the amputated limb. The child and family need to know that the sensations are real, not imagined. Amitriptyline (Elavil) has been used successfully in children to decrease the pain (Olsson, 1999).

Discharge planning must begin early in the postoperative period. Once the child has begun physical therapy, the nurse should consult with the therapist and practitioner to evaluate the child's physical and emotional readiness to reenter school. It is an opportune time to involve a community nurse in the child's home care. Every effort is made to promote normalcy and gradual resumption of realistic preamputation activities.† Role-playing is beneficial in preparing the child for the inevitable confrontation by others. Environmental barriers, such as stairs, are assessed in terms of the accessibility in the school and home, especially because the child may need to use crutches or a wheelchair before complete healing and prosthetic competency are achieved.

The nurse encourages the child to select clothing that best camouflages the prosthesis, such as pants or long-sleeved shirts. Well-fitted prostheses are so natural looking that girls can usually wear sheer stockings without revealing the device. Emphasizing feminine or masculine apparel helps the child regain a feeling of self-identity. Even during the postoperative period, encouraging the child to wear blue jeans and a T-shirt may distract attention from the deformity and focus it on familiar aspects of appearance.

The family and child need much support in adjusting not only to a life-threatening diagnosis but also to alteration in

---

**Information about prostheses can be obtained from the National Amputation Foundation, 40 Church St., Malverne, NY 11565; 516-887-3600; www.nationalamputation.org.*

†Information about special programs for children with amputations is available from the Candlelighters Childhood Cancer Foundation, PO Box 498, Kensington, MD 20895; 800-366-2223 or 301-962-3520; fax: 301-962-3521; www.candlelighters.org.

body form and function. Because loss of a limb entails a grieving process, those caring for the child need to recognize that the reactions of anger and depression are normal and necessary. Often parents view the anger as a direct affront to them for allowing the amputation to occur, or they see the depression as rejection. These are not personal attacks but the child's attempts to cope with a loss.

Ewing's Sarcoma (Primitive Neuroectodermal Tumor)

Ewing's sarcoma, classified as a primitive neuroectodermal tumor, is the second most common malignant bone tumor (after osteosarcoma) in childhood. Ewing's sarcoma arises in the marrow spaces of the bone rather than from osseous tissue. The tumor originates in the shaft of long and trunk bones, most often affecting the femur, tibia, fibula, humerus, ulna, vertebrae, scapula, ribs, pelvic bones, and skull (Link, Gebhardt, & Myers, 2006). It occurs almost exclusively in individuals under age 30, with the majority being between 4 and 25 years of age.

Therapeutic Management

Surgical amputation is not routinely recommended but may be considered when the results of radiotherapy render the extremity useless or deformed (e.g., from restricted growth in young children). The treatment of choice is intensive irradiation of the involved bone combined with chemotherapy. A widely used drug regimen includes vincristine, actinomycin D, cyclophosphamide or ifosfamide, etoposide, and doxorubicin. The addition of ifosfamide and etoposide has increased the 3-year survival to 80% (Lanzkowsky, 2000).

Nursing Care Management

The psychologic adjustment to Ewing's sarcoma is typically less traumatic than it is to osteosarcoma because of the preservation of the affected limb. Many families accept the diagnosis with relief in knowing that this type of bone cancer does not necessitate amputation, and initially they may not be aware of the damaging effects on the irradiated site. Consequently they need preparation for the various diagnostic tests, including bone marrow aspiration and surgical biopsy, and adequate explanation of the treatment regimen. High-dose radiotherapy often causes a skin reaction of dry or moist desquamation followed by hyperpigmentation. The child should wear loose-fitting clothes over the irradiated area to minimize additional skin irritation. Because of increased sensitivity, the area is protected from sunlight and sudden changes in temperature, such as from heating pads or ice packs. The child is encouraged to use the extremity as tolerated. Occasionally the physical therapist may plan an active exercise program to preserve maximum function.

The child needs the same considerations for adjusting to the effects of chemotherapy as any other patient with cancer. The drug regimen usually results in hair loss, severe nausea and vomiting, peripheral neuropathy, and possibly cardiotoxicity. Every effort should be made to outline a treatment plan that allows the child maximum resumption of a normal lifestyle and activities (Kline & Sevier, 2003) (see also Nursing Care Plan: The Child with Cancer, Chapter 49).

Rhabdomyosarcoma

Soft-tissue sarcomas are the fourth most common type of solid tumors in children. These malignant neoplasms originate from undifferentiated mesenchymal cells in muscles, tendons, bursae, and fascia, or in fibrous, connective, lymphatic, or vascular tissue. They derive their name from the specific tissue(s) of origin, such as myosarcoma (*myo*, muscle). Rhabdomyosarcoma (*rhabdo*, striated) is the most common soft-tissue sarcoma in children. Striated (skeletal) muscle is found almost anywhere in the body, so these tumors occur in many sites, the most common of which are the head and neck, especially the orbit (eye). The disease occurs in children in all age groups but is most common in children younger than 5 years of age. Its incidence is approximately 8.5 per 1 million for Caucasian children but only 4.0 per 1 million for African-American children from 2 to 19 years (Lanzkowsky, 2000). Rhabdomyosarcoma arises from embryonic mesenchyme.

The initial signs and symptoms are related to the site of the tumor and compression of adjacent organs (Box 54-10). Some tumor locations, particularly the orbit, produce symptoms early in the course of the illness and contribute to rapid diagnosis and an improved prognosis. Other tumors, such as those of the retroperitoneal area, produce no symptoms until they are large, invasive, and widely metastasized. Unfortunately, many of the signs and symptoms attributable to rhabdomyosarcoma are vague and frequently suggest a common childhood illness, such as "earache" or "runny nose." In some instances a primary tumor site is never identified.

Diagnostic Evaluation

Diagnosis begins with a careful examination of the head and neck area, particularly palpation of a nontender, hard mass. The nasopharynx and oropharynx are inspected for any evidence of a visible mass. Radiographic studies to isolate a tumor site are performed, accompanied by chest radiographs, CT, MRI, bone surveys, and bone marrow aspiration to rule out metastasis. A lumbar puncture is indicated for head and neck tumors to examine the cerebrospinal fluid for malignant cells. An excisional biopsy is done to confirm the histologic type.

Careful staging is extremely important for planning treatment and determining the prognosis. The Intergroup Rhabdomyosarcoma Study Group has established clinical staging (Wexler, Meyer, & Helman, 2006).

With the change in treatment from radical surgery or radiotherapy to a multimodal approach, survival rates for all stages have increased considerably. Five-year survival rates are approximately 65% (Lanzkowsky, 2000; Wexler, Meyer, & Helman, 2006). Data suggest that children who remain disease free for 2 years are probably cured; however, if relapse occurs, the prognosis for long-term survival is extremely poor.

Therapeutic Management

Because this tumor is highly malignant, with metastasis frequently occurring at the time of diagnosis, aggressive multimodal therapy is recommended. In the past, radical surgical removal of the tumor was the treatment of choice, but with improved survival from combined chemotherapy and irradiation, surgery plays a lesser role. Complete removal of the

BOX 54-10 Clinical Manifestations of Rhabdomyosarcoma According to Tumor Site

Central Nervous System
- Headaches
- Morning vomiting
- Diplopia

Orbit
- Rapidly developing unilateral proptosis
- Ecchymosis of conjunctiva
- Loss of extraocular movements (strabismus)
- Orbital cellulitis

Nasopharynx
- Stuffy nose (earliest sign)
- Nasal obstruction-dysphagia, nasal voice (obstruction of posterior nasal conchae)
- Pain (sore throat and ear)
- Epistaxis
- Palpable neck nodes
- Visible mass in oropharynx (late sign)

Paranasal Sinuses
- Nasal obstruction
- Local pain, swelling
- Discharge (may be unilateral)
- Sinusitis
- Swelling

Middle Ear
- Signs of chronic serous otitis media
- Pain, swelling
- Mass in external canal
- Sanguinopurulent drainage
- Facial nerve palsy

Retroperitoneal Area
- Usually a "silent" tumor
- Abdominal mass
- Pain
- Signs of intestinal or genitourinary obstruction

Perineum
- Visible superficial mass (scrotum, vaginal, or cervical areas)
- Bowel or bladder dysfunction (from tumor compression)
- Vaginal bleeding or mucosanguineous discharge

Extremity
- Pain
- Palpable fixed mass
- Regional lymph enlargement

primary tumor is advocated whenever possible. However, only biopsy is required in certain tumor locations, such as those of the orbit, when followed by irradiation and chemotherapy. This is a fortunate change, since it avoids the devastating effects of enucleation, amputation, or pelvic exenteration.

High-dose irradiation to the primary tumor is recommended, except in group I tumors. Chemotherapy plays a major role in treatment of all groups. Drugs that are cytotoxic for rhabdomyosarcoma are vincristine, actinomycin D, ifosfamide, cisplatin, carboplatin, etoposide, cyclophosphamide, topotecan, melphalan, and doxorubicin, which are administered for 1 to 2 years, depending on the stage of the disease (Lanzkowsky, 2000).

Nursing Care Management

The nursing responsibilities are similar to those for other types of cancer, especially the solid tumors when surgery is employed. Specific objectives include (1) careful assessment for signs of the tumor, especially during well-child examinations; (2) preparation of the child and family for the multiple diagnostic tests; and (3) supportive care during each stage of multimodal therapy (Kline & Sevier, 2003).

Disorders of Joints

Juvenile Idiopathic Arthritis (Juvenile Rheumatoid Arthritis)

Juvenile idiopathic arthritis (JIA) is a new name replacing *juvenile rheumatoid arthritis (JRA)* in the research literature and more slowly in clinical practice. The JRA nomenclature revision to JIA was due in part to the minimally applicable reference to "rheumatoid" in JRA. Only a small percentage of children have a positive rheumatoid factor, yet the name burdens the family with images of adult disfiguring rheumatoid arthritis. Furthermore, the JRA classification system focuses more on disease at onset vs. disease progression, which is more important (Warren et al, 2001). In 2004 the International League of Associations for Rheumatology further refined the definitions for JIA to provide improved categorization and treatment of the disease (Petty et al, 2004).

Semantics aside, JIA is a chronic autoimmune inflammatory disease causing inflammation of joints and other tissue with an unknown cause. JIA starts before age 16 years with peak onset between 1 and 3 years of age. Twice as many girls as boys are affected. The incidence is reported to be approximately 13.9 per 100,000 children per year among Caucasian children with an overall prevalence of approximately 113 per 100,000 children (Miller & Cassidy, 2007). The cause is unknown, but two factors are hypothesized: immunogenic susceptibility and an environmental or external trigger such as a virus (e.g., rubella, Epstein-Barr virus, parvovirus B19) (Miller & Cassidy, 2007).

Pathophysiology

The disease process is characterized by chronic inflammation of the synovium with joint effusion and eventual erosion, destruction, and fibrosis of the articular cartilage. Adhesions between joint surfaces and ankylosis of joints occur if the inflammatory process persists.

Clinical Manifestations

The outcome of JIA is variable and unpredictable. The disease, even in severe forms, is rarely life threatening but can cause significant disability. The arthritis tends to wax and wane and eventually becomes inactive in approximately 70% of the cases; however, these children may have severe or minimal joint damage remaining when active arthritis abates.

Approximately 30% of the children will have progressive arthritis into adulthood. Their arthritis can cause significant joint deformity and functional disability, requiring medication, physical therapy, and perhaps future joint replacement. Chronic and acute uveitis can cause permanent vision loss if undiagnosed and not aggressively treated.

Classification of Juvenile Idiopathic Arthritis

JIA is not a single disease, but a heterogeneous group of diseases. The universal Durban classification of JIA, revised and published in 1998, lists several disease categories, each with its own set of criteria and exclusions, which continue to be revised (Petty et al, 2004; Petty et al, 1998):

Systemic arthritis is arthritis in one or more joints associated with at least 2 weeks of fever, rash, lymphadenopathy, hepatosplenomegaly, and serositis.

Oligoarthritis (or pauciarticular arthritis) is arthritis in one to four joints for the first 6 months of disease. It is subdivided to *persistent oligoarthritis* if it remains in four joints or less, and becomes *extended oligoarthritis* if it involves more than four joints after 6 months.

Polyarthritis rheumatoid factor negative affects five or more joints in the first 6 months with a negative rheumatoid factor.

Polyarthritis rheumatoid factor positive also affects five or more joints in first 6 months, but these children have a positive rheumatoid factor.

Psoriatic arthritis is arthritis with psoriasis or an associated dactylitis, nail pitting, or onycholysis or psoriasis in a first-degree relative.

Enthesitis-related arthritis is arthritis and/or enthesitis (inflammation at the tendon insertion site) associated with at least two of the following: sacroiliac or lumbosacral pain, HLA-B27 antigen, arthritis in male older than 6 years, acute anterior uveitis, inflammatory bowel disease, Reiter's syndrome, or acute anterior uveitis in a first-degree relative.

The JIA classification is replacing the JRA classification, which had three subtypes: pauciarticular, polyarticular, and systemic JRA.

Diagnostic Evaluation

JIA is a diagnosis of exclusion; there are no definitive tests. Classifications are based on the clinical criteria of age of onset before 16 years, arthritis in one or more joints for 6 weeks or longer, and exclusion of other causes. Laboratory tests may provide supporting evidence of disease. Sedimentation rate may or may not be elevated. Leukocytosis is frequently present during exacerbations of systemic JIA. Antinuclear antibodies are common in JIA but are not specific for arthritis; however, they help identify children who are at greater risk for uveitis. Plain radiographs are the best initial imaging studies and may show soft-tissue swelling and joint space widening from increased synovial fluid in the joint. Later films can reveal osteoporosis, narrow joint space, erosions, subluxation, and ankylosis. A slit lamp eye examination is necessary to diagnose uveitis, inflammation in the anterior chamber of the eye, which is most common in antinuclear antibody–positive young girls with oligoarthritis. Routine examinations are necessary for early diagnosis and treatment to avoid sight-threatening disease (Kump et al, 2006).

Therapeutic Management

There is no cure for JIA. The major goals of therapy are to control pain, preserve joint range of motion and function, minimize effects of inflammation such as joint deformity, and promote normal growth and development. Outpatient care is the mainstay of therapy; lengthy hospitalizations are infrequent in this era of managed care. The treatment plan can be exhaustive and intrusive for the child and family, including medication administration, physical and occupational therapy, ophthalmologic slit lamp examinations, splints, comfort measures, dietary management, school modifications, and psychosocial support.

Medications

Many arthritis medications are available, and most are effective in suppressing the inflammatory process and relieving pain. These drugs may be given alone or in combination and are prescribed in a stepwise manner dependent on disease response to each level.

Nonsteroidal antiinflammatory drugs (NSAIDs) are the first drugs used. Naproxen, ibuprofen, and tolmetin are approved for use in children. They are effective with few common side effects other than gastrointestinal irritation and bruising; with naproxen, skin fragility is a possible side effect. NSAIDs must be taken with food. There is unofficial use of other NSAIDs approved for arthritis in adults but not yet children. Aspirin, once the drug of choice, has been replaced by NSAIDs because they have fewer side effects and easier administration schedules.

Methotrexate is the second-line medication used in children who have failed with NSAIDS alone. It is started in combination with an NSAID. It is effective, with acceptable toxicity, which requires monitoring of complete blood cell counts and liver function tests. Patient education about possible side effects, including discussions with teens about birth defects and avoiding alcohol, is essential. Methotrexate is considered the safest and most effective second-line drugs for the treatment of JIA (Miller & Cassidy, 2007).

Corticosteroids are potent immunosuppressives used for life-threatening complications, incapacitating arthritis, and uveitis. They are administered at the lowest effective dose for the briefest period and discontinued on a tapering schedule. They may be administered orally, as intraarticular joint injections, as IV pushes, or in eye drop form for uveitis. A single intraarticular injection may provide effective relief for children with pauciarticular disease unresponsive to NSAIDs (Padeh & Passwell, 1998). Prolonged use of systemic steroids is associated with significant side effects, including Cushing's syndrome, osteoporosis, increased infection risk, glucose intolerance, cataracts, and growth suppression.

Etanercept is a tumor necrosis factor (inhibitor) α-receptor blocker and an effective drug for children with JIA who are nonresponsive to methotrexate (Lovell et al, 2003). It is given as twice per week via subcutaneous injections. Possible side effects include transient allergic reaction at injection site, increased infection risk, and rare reports of demyelinating disease and pancytopenia. The risk of malignancy is unknown.

Parents and patients should be informed that biologic drugs are new therapies and more will be learned about potential side effects in the postmarketing period. Infliximab, a tumor necrosis factor blocker, may also be used but is reported to have more side effects than etanercept.

Slow-acting antirheumatic drugs (SAARDs) may require months to be effective and typically work in combination with NSAIDs. SAARDs include sulfasalazine, hydroxychloroquine, gold, and D-penicillamine. SAARDs are used less often because methotrexate has been recognized as the most effective second-line therapy drug.

Physical and Occupational Therapy

Programs of physical management are individualized for each child and designed to reach the ultimate goal: preserving function or preventing deformity. Physical therapy is directed toward specific joints, focusing on strengthening muscles, mobilizing restricted joint motion, and preventing or correcting deformities. Occupational therapy assumes responsibility for generalized mobility and performance of activities of daily living.

General treatment or maintenance programs vary; physical therapists may be involved several times weekly to monthly in management of a home program, or their visits may be limited to infrequent review of the home program for compliance, effectiveness, and need. Normal activities of daily living and the child's natural tendency to be active are usually sufficient to maintain muscle strength and joint mobility.

Exercising in a pool is excellent therapy, since it allows freedom of movement with support and minimal gravitational pull. If there is pain on motion, a hot pack or warm bath before therapy may help.

Practitioners may recommend nighttime splinting to help minimize pain and reduce flexion deformity. Joints most frequently splinted are the knees, wrists, and hands. Positioning during rest is also important. The child rests on a firm mattress with no pillow or a very low one and has no support under the knee. Loss of extension in the knee, hip, and wrist causes special problems and requires vigilance to detect the earliest signs of involvement and vigorous attention to prevent deformity with specialized passive stretching, positioning, and resting splints.

❋ Nursing Care Management

Nursing the child with JIA involves assessment of the child's general health, the status of involved joints, and the child's emotional response to all ramifications of the disease—discomfort, physical restrictions, therapies, and self-concept.

The effects of JIA are manifest in every aspect of the child's life, including physical activities, social experiences, and personality development. Although children with severe disease may have more physical barriers to overcome, studies show that emotional and behavioral functioning is most closely linked with maternal depression and parental distress, not with physical disability (Frank et al, 1998). Nursing interventions to support the parents may foster successful adaptation for the entire family. Parental concerns about the disease prognosis, financial and insurance issues, spouse and sibling relationships, and job and schedule conflicts must all be addressed. Referral to social workers, counselors, or support groups may be needed.

Relieve Pain

The pain of JIA is related to several aspects of the disease: disease severity, functional status, individual pain threshold, family variables, and psychologic adjustment. The aim is to provide as much relief as possible with medication and other therapies to help children tolerate the pain and cope as effectively as possible. Nonpharmacologic modalities such as behavioral therapy and relaxation techniques have proved effective in modifying pain perception (see Pain Management, Chapter 35) and activities that aggravate pain. Opioid analgesics are typically avoided in juvenile arthritis; however, for children immobilized with refractory pain, short-term opioid analgesics can be part of a comprehensive plan that uses multiple pain relief techniques (Connelly & Schanberg, 2006).

Promote General Health

The child's general health must be considered. A well-balanced diet with sufficient calories to maintain growth is essential. If the child is relatively inactive, caloric intake should match energy needs to avoid excessive weight gain, which places additional stress on affected joints. Sleep and rest are essential for children with JIA. Some children require rest during the day; however, daytime napping that interferes with nighttime sleepiness should be avoided. A bedtime routine that involves comfort measures can help induce sleep. A firm mattress, heated water bed, electric blanket, or sleeping bag helps provide warmth, comfort, and rest. Nighttime splints needed to maintain range of motion might initially be a source of bedtime conflict. The family needs to be instructed on how to use the splint appropriately; the splint should not be painful or impede sleep. Behavior modification programs that reward splint and exercise compliance may be helpful in reducing compliance barriers. Well-child care to assess growth, development, and immunization requirements needs to be coordinated between the primary care provider and the rheumatologist. Common childhood illnesses, such as upper respiratory tract infections, may cause arthritis to worsen; consequently, medical attention must be sought quickly for relatively minor illness to prevent arthritis flares. Effective communication between the family, the primary care provider, and the rheumatology team is essential for care coordination.

Children are encouraged to attend school, even on days when there may be some pain or discomfort. The school nurse's assistance is enlisted so that a child is permitted to take the prescribed medication at school and to arrange for rest in the nurse's office during the day. Split days or half days may help a child remain involved in school. Permitting the child to come to school late allows time to gain joint movement and reduces the time at school to avoid exhaustion. It is important that the child attend school to learn skills and engage in social interaction, especially if the JIA continues to limit physical skills. Arranging for two sets of textbooks eliminates the need to carry books to and from school, thus reducing discomfort and difficulty walking. A formal school hearing may be necessary to obtain an individualized education plan, ensured by public law, which includes intensive school modifications.

Facilitate Compliance

The child and family are involved in the therapeutic plan. They need to know the purpose and correct use of any splints and appliances and the medication regimen. The family is instructed regarding administration of medications and the value of a regular schedule of administration to maintain a satisfactory drug level in the body. They need to know that NSAIDs should not be given on an empty stomach and to be alert for signs of medication toxicity. If evidence of drug toxicity is noted, the family is instructed to notify the health professional and follow that person's instructions.

Encourage Heat and Exercise

Heat has been shown to be beneficial to children with arthritis. Moist heat is best for relieving pain and stiffness, and the most efficient and practical method is in the bathtub with warm water. In some cases a daily whirlpool bath, paraffin bath, or hot packs may be used as needed for temporary relief of acute swelling and pain. Hot packs are easily applied using a bath towel wrung out after being immersed in hot water or heated in a microwave oven, applied to the area, and covered with plastic for 20 minutes. Commercial pads that warm in only a few minutes in the microwave are also available. Painful hands or feet can be immersed in a pan of warm water for 10 minutes two or three times daily in addition to tub baths. Another method of supplying warmth before the child arises is to plug an electric blanket into an appliance timer. Set the blanket to medium or high and adjust the timer to turn on the blanket 1 hour before the child awakens (McIlvain-Simpson & Singsen, 1997).

Pool therapy is the easiest method for exercising a large number of joints. Swimming activities strengthen muscles and maintain mobility in larger joints. Very small children who are frightened of the water can carry out their exercises in the bathtub. Small children love to splash, kick, and throw things in the water. Remember, adult supervision is necessary for all water activities.

Activities of daily living provide satisfactory exercise for older children to maintain maximal mobility with minimal pain. These children are encouraged in their efforts to be independent and patiently allowed to dress and groom themselves, to assume daily tasks, and to care for their belongings. It is often difficult for children to manipulate buttons, comb or brush hair, and turn faucets, but unless there is an acute flare, parents and other caregivers should not offer assistance. In addition, children should learn and understand why others do not help them. Many helpful devices, such as self-adhering fasteners, tongs for manipulating difficult items, and grab bars installed in bathrooms for safety, can be used to facilitate tasks. A raised (higher) toilet seat often makes the difference between dependent and independent toileting, since weak quadriceps muscles and sore knees inhibit the ability to raise the body from a low sitting position.

A child's natural affinity for play offers many opportunities for incorporating therapeutic exercises. Throwing or kicking a ball and riding a tricycle (with the seat raised to achieve maximum leg extension) are excellent moving and stretching exercises for a very young child whose daily living activities are physically limited.

An effective approach to beginning the day's activities is to awaken children early to give them their medication and then to allow them to sleep for an hour. On arising, children take a hot bath (or shower) and perform a simple ritual of limbering-up exercises, after which they commence the day's activities, such as going to school. Exercise, heat, and rest are spaced throughout the remainder of the day according to the child's individual needs and schedules. Parents are instructed in exercises that meet the child's needs.

The Arthritis Foundation* and the American Juvenile Arthritis Organization (a council of the Arthritis Foundation)† provide services for both parents and professionals. Nurses should refer families to these agencies as an added resource.

Support Child and Family

JIA affects every aspect of life for the child and family. Physical limitations may interfere with self-care, school participation, and recreational activities. The intensive treatment plan, including multiple medications, physical therapy, comfort measures, and medical appointments, is intrusive and disruptive to the parents' work schedule and the family routine. To prevent isolation and foster independence, the family is encouraged to pursue their normal activities. Unfortunately, the adaptations necessary require resourcefulness and commitment from all family members. At diagnosis and throughout the span of JIA, it is essential to recognize signs of stress and counterproductive coping and provide the necessary support to maximize adaptation. The problems and needs of these families are discussed in Chapter 41, and the reader is directed to that chapter for guidance in planning care. (See also Nursing Care Plan, The Child with Arthritis.)

Systemic Lupus Erythematosus

Systemic lupus erythematosus (SLE) is a chronic, multisystem, autoimmune disease of the connective tissues and blood vessels characterized by inflammation in potentially any body tissue. Its course and symptoms are variable and unpredictable, with mild to life-threatening complications. In addition to SLE, there are other forms of lupus, such as neonatal lupus, which occurs when maternal autoantibodies cross the placenta and cause transient lupuslike symptoms in the newborn, with the potential serious complication of heart block. The remaining discussion focuses on SLE.

Reports suggest that survival rates in children with SLE have significantly improved; 5-year survival rates are said to be almost 100%, and 10-year survival rates are close to 90% (Ravelli, Ruperto, & Martini, 2005). SLE is more common in girls, with an approximate 5 : 1 female-to-male ratio, and typically occurs between the ages of 10 and 19 years. There is a familial tendency, although many newly diagnosed patients are unaware of other affected family members. SLE has been reported in all cultures, but within the United States there has been a disproportionately higher incidence in African-American, Asian, and Hispanic children.

The cause of SLE is not known. It appears to result from a complex interaction of genetics with an unidentified trigger

**PO Box 7669, Atlanta, GA 30357-0669; 800-283-7800;* www.arthritis.org. *In Canada, the Arthritis Society may be contacted for locations of all local Canadian province offices:* www.arthritis.ca.
†http://arthritis.about.com/od/jra/p/ajao.htm

NURSING CARE PLAN ✤ The Child with Arthritis

Nursing Diagnosis	Expected Patient Outcome	Nursing Interventions	Rationale
Chronic pain related to joint inflammation	Child is able to move (joints) and complete activities of daily living with no discomfort or minimal discomfort.	Use pain rating scale to evaluate pain (discomfort) level.	To provide objective assessment of pain level
		Administer antiinflammatory medications (nonsteroidal antiinflammatory drugs [NSAIDs]) promptly on report of pain and around the clock when discomfort is acute.	To manage pain and prevent breakthrough pain
Child's/Family's Defining Characteristics *(Subjective and Objective Data)* Verbal report of pain Guarding behavior Change in sleep pattern	**The Following NOC Concepts Apply to These Outcomes** Comfort Level Pain Control Anxiety Self-Control Coping	Administer other rheumatic drugs such as methotrexate or slow-acting antirheumatic drugs (SAARDs).	To provided relief from inflammation
		Schedule routine rest periods throughout the day.	
		Encourage child to eat a well-balanced diet and exercise daily.	To prevent obesity and promote wellness
		Help child set up a routine of daily exercise.	To prevent further joint stiffness
		Encourage nonpharmacologic pain relief remedies such as use of heat pad, moist heat, and pool therapy.	To promote mobility of joints and relieve painful stiff joints To prevent excessive weight gain
		Encourage child to discuss effect of pain on lifestyle and activities.	To provide outlet for emotions such as anger, frustration, depression at having a chronic illness
		The Following NIC Concepts Apply to These Interventions Analgesic Administration Sleep Enhancement Exercise Promotion Medication Management Environmental Management: Comfort	

Nursing Diagnosis	Expected Patient Outcome	Nursing Interventions	Rationale
Impaired physical mobility related to pain and swelling in joints	Child engages in activities of daily living.	Encourage ambulation and performance of activities of daily living to maximum potential every day.	To keep joints limber and prevent disuse contractures
	The Following NOC Concepts Apply to These Outcomes Ambulation Body Mechanics Performance Rest Joint Movement: Ankle Joint Movement: Spine Joint Movement: Wrist Joint Movement: Knee Joint Movement: Hip Joint Movement: Elbow Joint Movement: Fingers	Assist with range-of-motion exercises for child who is severely limited.	To promote muscle movement and keep joints limber
Child's/Family's Defining Characteristics *(Subjective and Objective Data)* Limited ability to perform fine and gross motor skills Limited range of motion Verbal report of pain Measurable pain on pain scale		Encourage child to be as active as tolerated.	To promote independence
		Assist with planning and encourage rest periods during the day.	To prevent fatigue
		Encourage taking pain medication such as NSAIDs before ambulation and activity.	To promote activity with minimum pain
		Use nonpharmacologic pain adjuncts such as heat pad and hydrotherapy.	To decrease pain and encourage mobility of joints
		Encourage child to be active in self-care activities to maximum potential.	To enhance self-worth and independence
		The Following NIC Concepts Apply to These Interventions Energy Management Exercise Promotion: Stretching Exercise Therapy: Joint Mobility Self-Care Assistance Teaching: Prescribed Activity/Exercise	

that activates the disease. Suspected triggers include exposure to ultraviolet light, estrogen, pregnancy, infections, and drugs. Patients with JIA have been known to develop SLE symptoms as a result of the use of tumor necrosis factor drugs such as etanercept. Genetic predisposition to SLE is evidenced in an increased concordance rate in twins (tenfold), increased incidence within family members (10% to 16%), and increased frequency of certain gene alleles in population-based studies.

Clinical Manifestations and Diagnostic Evaluation

The child with SLE may have any clinical manifestation with mild to life-threatening severity (Box 54-11). The diagnosis is established when 4 of the 11 diagnostic criteria in Box 54-12 are met; however, children with fewer than 4 criteria who are suspected of having lupus should receive appropriate medical treatment (Klein-Gitelman & Miller, 2007). Kidney involve-

BOX 54-11 Clinical Manifestations of Systemic Lupus Erythematosus Related to Tissues Involved

Constitutional—Fever, fatigue, weight loss, anorexia
Cutaneous—Erythematous butterfly rash over bridge of nose and across cheeks, discoid rash, photosensitivity, mucocutaneous ulceration, alopecia, periungual telangiectasias
Musculoskeletal—Arthritis, arthralgia, myositis, myalgia, tenosynovitis
Neurologic—Headache, seizure, forgetfulness, behavior change, change in school performance, psychosis, chorea, stroke, cranial and peripheral neuropathy, pseudotumor cerebri
Pulmonary and cardiac—Pleuritis, basilar pneumonitis, atelectasis, pericarditis, myocarditis, endocarditis
Renal—Glomerulonephritis, nephrotic syndrome, hypertension
Gastrointestinal—Abdominal pain, nausea, vomiting, blood in stool, abdominal crisis, esophageal dysfunction, colitis
Hepatic, splenic, and nodal—Hepatomegaly, splenomegaly, lymphadenopathy
Hematologic—Anemia, cytopenia
Ophthalmologic—Cotton wool spots, papilledema, retinopathy
Vascular—Raynaud's phenomenon, thrombophlebitis, livedo reticularis

BOX 54-12 Classification Criteria for Systemic Lupus Erythematosus

Four of the following 11 criteria must be met for diagnosis:

1. **Malar rash**—Fixed malar erythema
2. **Discoid rash**—Patchy erythematous lesions
3. **Photosensitivity**—Rash with sun exposure
4. **Oral ulcers**—Painless ulcers in mouth, nose
5. **Arthritis**—Swelling, tenderness, or effusion in two or more peripheral joints (nonerosive)
6. **Serositis**—Pleuritis, pericarditis
7. **Renal disorder**—Proteinuria, casts
8. **Neurologic disorder**—Psychosis, seizures
9. **Hematologic disorder**—Hemolytic anemia, thrombocytopenia, leukopenia, lymphopenia
10. **Immunologic disorder**—Anti-dsDNA, anti-SM, antiphospholipid antibodies, lupus anticoagulant, false-positive syphilis test (RPR)
11. **Antinuclear antibody**

ment heralds progressive disease and the need for rigorous therapeutic management.

Therapeutic Management

The goal of treatment is to ensure the child's health by balancing the medications necessary to avoid exacerbation and complications while preventing or minimizing treatment-associated morbidity. Therapy involves the use of specific medications and general supportive care. The drugs used to control inflammation are corticosteroids administered in doses sufficient to control inflammation, then tapered to the lowest suppressive dose. Other drugs include antimalarial preparations, which are useful for rash and arthritis; NSAIDs, which relieve muscle and joint inflammation; and immunosuppressive agents, such as cyclophosphamide, for renal and central nervous system disease. Rituximab, a chimeric anti-CD20 monoclonal antibody, is used to treat SLE in adults and has recently been shown to be effective in children. The combined use of rituximab and cyclophosphamide has also been shown to be effective for decreasing symptoms in children with SLE (Lehman, 2008). Antihypertensives, aspirin, and antibiotics are just a few of the additional drugs that may be necessary to treat or avoid complications.

General supportive care includes sufficient nutrition, sleep and rest, and exercise. Exposure to the sun and ultraviolet B (UVB) light is limited because of its association with SLE exacerbation.

Nursing Care Management

The principal nursing goal is to help the child and family positively adjust to the disease and therapy. The child and family must learn to recognize subtle signs of disease exacerbation and potential complications of medication therapy and to communicate these concerns to their care provider. Consequently, patient and family education is an ongoing process initiated at diagnosis and tailored to the patient's individual needs. Referral to a social worker, psychologist, or support group may help the child and family make a successful adjustment. Support groups are associated with the Lupus Foundation of America* and the Arthritis Foundation.†

Key issues include therapy compliance; body-image problems associated with rash, hair loss, and steroid therapy; school attendance; vocational activities; social relationships; sexual activity; and pregnancy. (See Chapter 41 for a discussion on adjusting to a chronic illness.) Specific instructions for avoiding exposure to the sun and UVB light, such as using sunscreens, wearing sun-resistant clothing, and altering outdoor activities, must be provided with great sensitivity to ensure compliance while minimizing the associated feeling of being different from peers (see Sunburn, Chapter 53). Patients need to be instructed to maintain regular medical supervision and seek attention quickly during illness or before elective surgical procedures, such as dental extraction, because of potential needs for increased steroids or prophylactic antibiotics. People with SLE should carry medical identification for their disease and steroid dependence.

*2000 L St. NW, Suite 710, Washington, DC 20036; 202-349-1155 or 800-558-0121; www.lupus.org.
†*See footnote on p. 1711.*

Key Points

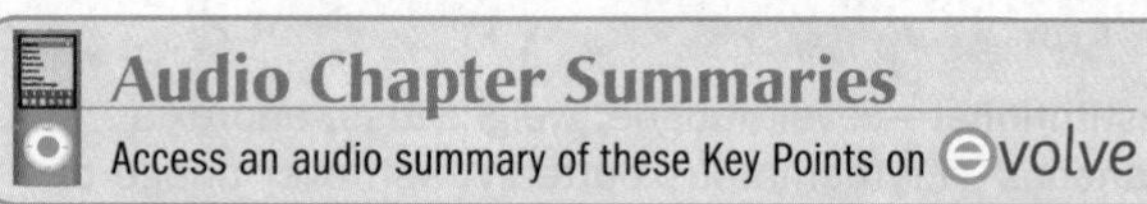
Audio Chapter Summaries
Access an audio summary of these Key Points on evolve

- Immobility has a profound effect on all aspects of growth and development.
- The major physical consequences of immobilization are loss of muscle strength, endurance, and muscle mass; bone demineralization; loss of joint mobility; and contractures.
- Features of children's fractures not observed in the adult include presence of growth plate, thicker and stronger periosteum, bone porosity, more rapid healing, and less joint stiffness.
- The goals of fracture management are to regain alignment and length of bony fragments, retain alignment and length, and restore function to injured parts.
- The method of fracture reduction is determined by the child's age, degree of displacement, amount of overriding, amount of edema, condition of the skin and soft tissues, sensation, and circulation distal to the fracture.
- The primary purposes of traction are to fatigue involved muscles and reduce muscle spasm, position bone ends in desired realignment, and immobilize the fracture site until realignment has been achieved to permit casting or splinting.
- The etiology of DDH appears to be related to intrauterine, genetic, and cultural factors.
- Treatment of clubfoot consists of manipulation and casting to correct the deformity, maintenance of the correction, and prevention of possible recurrence of the deformity.
- Acquired hip deformities are managed with non–weight-bearing devices (Legg-Calvé-Perthes disease) or surgical stabilization (SCFE).
- Observation for idiopathic scoliosis is an important part of an adolescent's routine physical assessment.
- Idiopathic scoliosis is managed by observation, bracing, and exercise or surgical correction.
- Bone infections are managed with vigorous antibiotic therapy, immobilization of the affected part, and (sometimes) surgical drainage.
- Osteosarcoma is a neoplasm of bone-forming tissues; Ewing's sarcoma is a neoplasm that arises from bone marrow spaces.
- Rhabdomyosarcoma may occur almost anywhere in the body, but the most common sites are the head and neck.
- Nursing care of the child with juvenile arthritis consists of promoting general health, relieving discomfort, preventing deformity, and preserving function.
- SLE is a chronic autoimmune disorder that affects the collagen tissues of the body.

References

American Academy of Pediatrics, Committee on Quality Improvement and Subcommittee on Developmental Dysplasia of the Hip: Clinical practice guideline: early detection of developmental dysplasia of the hip, *Pediatrics* 105(4):896-905, 2000.

Bachrach LK, Ward LM: Clinical review 1: bisphosphonate use in childhood osteoporosis, *J Clin Endocrinol Metab* 94(2):400-409, 2009.

Bunnell WP: Selective screening for scoliosis, *Clin Orthop Relat Res* 434:40-45, 2005.

Connelly M, Schanberg L: Opioid therapy for the treatment of refractory pain in children with juvenile rheumatoid arthritis, *Natl Clin Pract Rheumatol* 2(12):636-637, 2006.

Cornwall R: Bone and joint disorders: upper limb. In Kliegman RM et al (editors): *Nelson textbook of pediatrics*, ed 18, Philadelphia, 2007, Saunders.

Curley MA et al: Predicting pressure ulcer risk in pediatric patients: the Braden Q Scale, *Nurs Res* 52(1):22-33, 2003.

Do T, Herrera-Soto J: Elbow injuries in children, *Curr Opin Pediatr* 15(1):68-73, 2003.

Faulks S, Luther B: Changing paradigm for the treatment of clubfeet, *Orthop Nurs* 24(1):25-30, 2005.

Frank RG et al: Disease and family contributors to adaptation in juvenile rheumatoid arthritis and juvenile diabetes, *Arthritis Care Res* 11(3):166-176, 1998.

Freeman BL III: Scoliosis and kyphosis. In Canale ST, Beaty JH, editors: *Campbell's operative orthopaedics*, ed 11, Philadelphia, 2007, Mosby.

Gutierrez K: Bone and joint infections in children, *Pediatr Clin North Am* 52(3):779-794, 2005.

Hart ES, Grottkau BE, Albright MB: Slipped capital femoral epiphysis: don't miss this pediatric hip disorder, *Nurs Pract* 32(3):14, 16-18, 21, 2007.

Hart ES et al: Developmental dysplasia of the hip: nursing implications and anticipatory guidance for parents, *Orthop Nurs* 25(2):100-109, 2006.

Heare T, Hensley MA, Dell'orfano S: Bone tumors: osteosarcoma and Ewing's sarcoma, *Curr Opin Pediatr* 21(3):365-372, 2009.

Holmes SB, Brown SJ, Pin Site Care Expert Panel: Skeletal pin site care: National Association of Orthopaedic Nurses guidelines for orthopaedic nursing, *Orthop Nurs* 24(2):99-107, 2005.

Hosalkar HS, Spiegel DA, Davidson RS: Bone and joint disorders: the foot and toes. In Kliegman RM et al (editors): *Nelson textbook of pediatrics*, ed 18, Philadelphia, 2007, Saunders.

Hosalkar HS et al: The hip. In Kliegman RM et al (editors): *Nelson textbook of pediatrics*, ed 18, Philadelphia, 2007, Saunders.

Klein-Gitelman MS, Miller ML: Systemic lupus erythematosus. In Kliegman RM et al, editors: *Nelson textbook of pediatrics*, ed 18, Philadelphia, 2007, Saunders.

Kline NE, Sevier N: Solid tumors in children, *J Pediatr Nurs* 18(2):96-102, 2003.

Kump LI et al: Visual outcomes in children with juvenile idiopathic arthritis–associated uveitis, *Ophthalmology* 113(10):1874-1877, 2006.

Lampe RM: Osteomyelitis and suppurative arthritis. In Kliegman RM et al (editors): *Nelson textbook of pediatrics*, ed 18, Philadelphia, 2007, Saunders.

Land C et al: Osteogenesis imperfecta type VI in childhood and adolescence: effects of cyclical intravenous pamidronate treatment, *Bone* 40(3):638-644, 2007.

Lanzkowsky P: *Manual of pediatric hematology and oncology*, San Diego, 2000, Academic Press.

Lehman TJA: Systemic lupus erythematosus in children, *UpToDate*, 2008. Available at www.uptodate.com (accessed July 25, 2008).

Link MP, Gebhardt MC, Myers PA: Osteosarcoma. In Pizzo PA, Poplack DG (editors): *Principles and practices of pediatric oncology*, ed 5, Philadelphia, 2006, Lippincott.

Lovell DJ et al: Long-term efficacy and safety of etanercept in children with polyarticular-course juvenile rheumatoid arthritis: interim results from an ongoing multicenter, open-label, extended-treatment trial, *Arthritis Rheum* 48(1):218-226, 2003.

Maher AB, Salmond SW, Pellino TA: *Orthopaedic nursing*, ed 3, Philadelphia, 2002, Saunders.

Marini JC: Osteogenesis imperfect. In Kliegman RM et al (editors): *Nelson textbook of pediatrics*, ed 18, Philadelphia, 2007, Saunders.

McCord S et al: Risk factors associated with pressure ulcers in the pediatric intensive care unit, *JWOCN* 31(4):179-183, 2004.

McIlvain-Simpson G, Singsen B: Decreasing morning stiffness, *Small Talk* 3(6):8, 1997.

Miller ML, Cassidy JT: Juvenile rheumatoid arthritis. In Kliegman RM et al (editors): *Nelson textbook of pediatrics*, ed 18, Philadelphia, 2007, Saunders.

Napierkowski DB: Scoliosis: a case study in an adolescent boy, *Orthop Nurs* 26(3):147-153, 2007.

Newton PO, Wenger DR: Idiopathic and congenital scoliosis. In Morrissy RT, Weinstein SL (editors): *Lovell and Winter's pediatric orthopaedics*, Philadelphia, 2001, Williams & Wilkins.

Olsson GL: Neuropathic pain in children. In McGrath PJ, Finley GA (editors): *Chronic and recurrent pain in children and adolescents*, Seattle, 1999, IASP Press.

Padeh S, Passwell P: Intraarticular corticosteroid injection in the management of children with chronic arthritis, *Arthritis Rheum* 41(7):1210-1214, 1998.

Petty RE et al: International League of Associations for Rheumatology classification of juvenile idiopathic arthritis: second revision, Edmonton, 2001, *J Rheumatol* 31(2):390-392, 2004.

Petty RE et al: Revision of the proposed classification criteria for juvenile idiopathic arthritis: Durban, 1997, *J Rheumatol* 25(10):1991-1994, 1998.

Plint AC et al: A randomized, controlled trial of removable splinting versus casting for wrist buckle fractures in children, *Pediatrics* 117(3): 691-697, 2006.

Ravelli A, Ruperto N, Martini A: Outcome in juvenile onset lupus erythematosus, *Curr Opin Rheumatol* 17(5):568-573, 2005.

Razmus IS, Roberts KE, Curley MA: Pressure ulcers in critically ill children: incidence and associated factors (abstract), *Crit Care Med* 29(Suppl): A148, 2001.

Richards BS, Vitale MG: Screening for idiopathic scoliosis in adolescents: an information statement, *J Bone Joint Surg* 90(1):195-198, 2008.

Samaniego IA: A sore spot in pediatrics: risk factors for pressure ulcers, *Pediatr Nurs* 29(4):278-283, 2003.

Schindler CA et al: Skin integrity in critically ill and injured children, *Am J Crit Care* 16(6):568-574, 2007.

Shrader MW: Pediatric supracondylar fractures and pediatric physeal elbow fractures, *Orthop Clin North Am* 39(2):163-171, 2008.

Slote RJ: Psychological effects of caring for the adolescent undergoing spinal fusion for scoliosis, *Orthop Nurs* 21(6):19-28, 2002.

Spiegel DA, Hosalkar HS, Dormans JP: Bone and joint disorders: the spine. In Kliegman RM et al (editors): *Nelson textbook of pediatrics*, ed 18, Philadelphia, 2007, Saunders.

Ta HT et al: Osteosarcoma treatment: state of the art, *Cancer Metastasis Rev* 28(1):247-263, 2009.

US Preventive Services Task Force: Screening for developmental dysplasia of the hip: recommendation statement, *Am Fam Physician* 73(11): 1992-1996, 2006.

Wall EJ: Practical primary pediatric orthopaedics, *Nurs Clin North Am* 35(1):95-113, 2000.

Warren RW et al: Juvenile idiopathic arthritis (juvenile rheumatoid arthritis). In Koopman WJ (editor): *Arthritis and allied conditions*, Philadelphia, 2001, Lippincott Williams & Wilkins.

Wexler LH, Meyer WH, Helman LJ: Rhabdomyosarcoma and the undifferentiated sarcomas. In Pizzo PA, Poplack DG (editors): *Principles and practices of pediatric oncology*, ed 5, Philadelphia, 2006, Lippincott.

55 Neuromuscular or Muscular Dysfunction

Learning Objectives

On completion of this chapter the reader will be able to:

- Discuss the nursing role in helping parents cope with a child with cerebral palsy.
- Formulate a nursing care plan for the preoperative and postoperative care of a child with myelomeningocele.
- Outline a plan of care for a child with Duchenne muscular dystrophy.
- Discuss the prevention and treatment of tetanus.
- Identify the causes of botulism in infants and children.
- List three causes of spinal cord injury in children.

Electronic Resources

Additional information related to the content in Chapter 55 can be found on

evolve the Companion Website at

http://evolve.elsevier.com/Perry/maternal/

- NCLEX Review Questions
- Animation—Guillain-Barré Syndrome
- Critical Thinking Exercise—Guillain-Barré Syndrome
- Critical Thinking Exercise—Myelomeningocele
- Nursing Care Plan—The Child with Cerebral Palsy

Congenital Neuromuscular or Muscular Disorders

Cerebral Palsy

A new definition recently proposed describes cerebral palsy (CP) as a "group of permanent disorders of the development of movement and posture, causing activity limitation, that are attributed to nonprogressive disturbances that occurred in the developing fetal or infant brain" (Rosenbaum et al, 2007). In addition to motor disorders, the condition often involves disturbances of sensation, perception, communication, cognition, and behavior; secondary musculoskeletal problems; and epilepsy (Rosenbaum et al, 2007). The etiology, clinical features, and course are variable and are characterized by abnormal muscle tone and coordination as the primary disturbances. CP is the most common permanent physical disability of childhood, and the incidence is reported to be between 1.5 and 3 in every 1000 live births in the United States (Ashwal et al, 2004; Dabney, Lipton, & Miller, 1997; Winter et al, 2002). Since the 1960s the prevalence of CP has risen approximately 20%, which most likely reflects the improved survival of extremely-low-birth-weight and very-low-birth-weight infants.

Although the prevalent traditional hypothesis has been that CP results from perinatal problems, especially birth asphyxia, it is now believed that some types of CP result more often from existing *prenatal* brain abnormalities; however, the exact cause of these abnormalities remains elusive. It has been estimated that as many as 80% of CP cases are caused by unknown prenatal factors (Krigger, 2006). Intrauterine exposure to maternal chorioamnionitis is associated with an increased risk of CP in infants of normal birth weight and preterm infants (Gibson et al, 2003; Volpe, 2008); however, not all term infants exposed to chorioamnionitis develop CP (Grether et al, 2003; Wu et al, 2003). The prevalence of CP in infants born before 36 weeks of gestation and weighing less than 2000 g (4.4 lb) has been reported to be 12%; the strongest independent risk factor for development of CP was periventricular leukomalacia (Han et al, 2002). Damage occurring as a result of shaken baby syndrome may also result in CP in survivors (Smith, 2003). Additional factors that may contribute to the development of CP *postnatally* include bacterial meningitis, viral encephalitis, motor vehicle accidents, and child abuse (Krigger, 2006). A significant percentage (15% to 60%) of children with CP will also have epilepsy, thus compromising issues of self-care and progression to normalization.

Pathophysiology

It is difficult to establish a precise location of neurologic lesions based on etiology or clinical signs because no characteristic pathologic pattern exists. Some patients have gross malformations of the brain; others may have evidence of vascular occlusion, atrophy, loss of neurons, and degeneration. A few exceptions occur and are related to anatomic areas such as spastic diplegia (associated with preterm birth), caused by hypoxic infarction or hemorrhage in the area adjacent to the lateral ventricles. Ataxic CP may occur in relation to cerebral hypoplasia and, in some cases, severe hypoglycemia (Volpe, 2008). The American Academy of Pediatrics, in conjunction with the American College of Obstetricians and Gynecologists (2003), published a report that defines neonatal encephalopathy. The report affirms that approximately 70% of cases of neonatal encephalopathy occur as a result of events before the onset of labor; it establishes criteria to define events sufficiently capable of causing intrapartum asphyxia and CP. Evidence indicates that the majority of CP cases occur not as a result of intrapartum asphyxia, but as a result of other causes that have been discussed previously (American Academy of Pediatrics & American College of Obstetricians and Gynecologists, 2003).

CP has been classified in several ways. A functional classification is based on the nature and distribution of neuromuscular dysfunction (Box 55-1). Additional classifications describe the area of the brain involved, the degree of motor involvement, accompanying impairments, anatomic distribution, and cause of CP (Rosenbaum et al, 2007).

Diagnostic Evaluation

Infants at risk according to known etiologic factors associated with CP warrant careful assessment during early infancy to identify the signs of muscular dysfunction as early as possible. The neurologic examination and history are the primary modalities for diagnosis. Neuroimaging of the child with suspected brain abnormality and CP is now recommended for diagnostic assessment, with magnetic resonance imaging (MRI) preferred to computed tomography (CT) scan. Metabolic and genetic testing is recommended if no structural abnormality is identified by neuroimaging; laboratory tests are no longer recommended in the diagnostic process for CP (Ashwal et al, 2004).

Early recognition is made more difficult by the lack of reliable neonatal neurologic signs. However, infants with known etiologic risk factors should be monitored and evaluated closely in the first 2 years of life. The alert observer may be suspicious when a child demonstrates some of the manifestations outlined in Box 55-2. Because cortical control of movement does not occur until later in infancy, motor impairment associated with voluntary control is usually not apparent until after 2 to 4 months of age at the earliest. More often the diagnosis cannot be confirmed until the age of 2 years because motor tone abnormalities may be indicative of another neuromuscular illness.

Diagnosis may also be assisted by identification of persistent primitive reflexes: (1) either the asymmetric tonic neck reflex or persistent Moro reflex (beyond 4 months of age), and (2) the crossed extensor reflex. The tonic neck reflex normally disappears between 4 and 6 months of age. An "obligatory" response is considered abnormal. Hand preference in the first 2 years of life is reported to be a sign of hemiplegic CP (Berker & Yalçin, 2008). The crossed extensor reflex, which normally disappears by 4 months, is elicited by applying a noxious stimulus to the sole of one foot with the knee extended. Normally the contralateral foot responds with extensor, abduction, and then adduction movements. The possibility of CP is suggested if these reflexes are found after the age at which they should have disappeared.

BOX 55-1 Clinical Classification of Cerebral Palsy

Spastic (Pyramidal)—70% to 80% of All Cases of Cerebral Palsy

Characterized by persistent primitive reflexes, positive Babinski, ankle clonus, exaggerated stretch reflexes, eventual development of contractures

- **Diplegia**—All extremities affected; lower more than upper (30% to 40% of spastic cerebral palsy [CP])
- **Quadriplegia**—All four extremities involved: legs and trunk, mouth, pharynx, and tongue (10% to 15% of spastic CP)
- **Triplegia**—Three limbs involved
- **Monoplegia**—Only one limb involved
- **Hemiplegia**—Motor dysfunction on one side of the body; upper extremity more affected than lower (20% to 30% of spastic CP)

Other features:

- Hypertonicity with poor control of posture, balance, and coordinated motion
- Impairment of fine and gross motor skills

Dyskinetic (Nonspastic, Extrapyramidal)

Athetoid—Chorea (involuntary, irregular, jerking movements); characterized by slow, wormlike, writhing movements that usually involve the extremities, trunk, neck, facial muscles, and tongue

Dystonic—Slow, twisting movements of the trunk or extremities; abnormal posture

Involvement of the pharyngeal, laryngeal, and oral muscles causing drooling and dysarthria (imperfect speech articulation)

Ataxic (Nonspastic, Extrapyramidal)

Wide-based gait

Rapid, repetitive movements performed poorly

Disintegration of movements of the upper extremities when the child reaches for objects

Mixed Type

Combination of spastic CP and dyskinetic CP

May be labeled *mixed* when no specific motor pattern is dominant; however, this term losing favor to more precise descriptions of motor function and affected area of brain involved (Rosenbaum et al, 2007)

Data from Nehring W: Cerebral palsy. In Allen PJ, Vessey JA (editors): *Primary care of the child with a chronic condition*, St Louis, 2004, Mosby; Jones MW et al: Cerebral palsy: introduction and diagnosis, part 1, *J Pediatr Health Care* 21(3):146-152, 2007; and National Institute of Neurologic Disorders and Stroke: *Cerebral palsy: hope through research*, 2006. Available at www.ninds.nih.gov/disorders/cerebral_palsy/detail_cerebral_palsy.htm (accessed July 9, 2007).

Therapeutic Management

The goals of therapy for children with CP are early recognition and promotion of optimal development to enable affected children to attain normalization and their potential within the limits of their existing health problems. The disorder is permanent, and therapy is primarily preventive and symptomatic.

Therapy has five broad aims:

BOX 55-2 Clinical Signs and Symptoms of Cerebral Palsy

Spastic Type
Increased muscle tone (hypertonicity)
Increased deep tendon reflexes and *clonus* (sudden dorsiflexion of the ankle or rapid distal movement of the patella resulting in alternating spasm and relaxation of the muscles being stretched)
Flexor, adductor, and internal rotator muscles more involved than extensor, abductor, and external rotator muscles
Difficulty with fine and gross motor skills
Most common contracture: that of the heel cord
Hip adductor contractures leading to progressive subluxation and dislocation
Knee contractures
Scoliosis common
Typical gait crouched, intoeing, scissoring
Elbow, wrist, and fingers in flexed position with thumb adducted
Motor weakness of antagonist muscle groups

Dyskinetic Type
Purposeless, involuntary, uncontrollable movements of face and extremities
Increased movements with stress and voluntary movements; absent during sleep
Contractures rare
Normal deep tendon reflexes

Ataxic Type
Disturbed coordination
Lack of equilibrium
Unsteady gait
Few orthopedic problems
Hyporeflexia
Loss of ability to gauge distance, speed, power of movement
Muscles hypotonic
Speech slurred, jerky, explosive
Nystagmus common

Other Manifestations
Visual deficits (most common in spastic type)
Hearing impairment (most common in dyskinetic type)
Oral motor involvement resulting in drooling and feeding problems
Developmental delay (40% to 60%; most common in spastic quadriplegia)
Sensory impairment
Seizures (approximately 40% of those with spastic hemiplegia affected)

From Maher AB, Salmond SW, Pellino TA: *Orthopaedic nursing,* ed 3, Philadelphia, 2002, Saunders.

1. To establish locomotion, communication, and self-help skills
2. To gain optimal appearance and integration of motor functions
3. To correct associated defects as effectively as possible

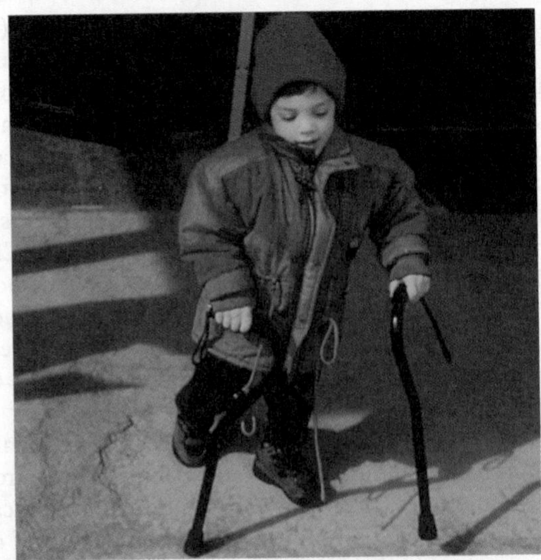

Fig. 55-1 Mobilization device for child.

4. To provide educational opportunities adapted to the child's needs and capabilities
5. To promote socialization experiences with other affected and unaffected children

Each child is evaluated and managed on an individual basis. The scope of the child's needs requires multidisciplinary planning and care coordination among professionals and the child's family. The outcome for the child and family with CP is normalization and promotion of self-care activities that empower the child and family to achieve maximum potential.

Ankle-foot orthoses (AFOs, braces) are worn by many of these children and are used to help prevent or reduce deformity, increase the energy efficiency of gait, and control alignment. Other mobilization devices include wheeled scooter boards that allow children to propel themselves while on the abdomen, wheeled go-carts that provide sitting balance and serve as early "wheelchair" experience for young children, bicycle walkers, and special devices that leave the upper extremities free (Figs. 55-1 and 55-2). Strollers can be equipped with custom seats for dependent mobilization.

Orthopedic surgery may be required to correct contracture or spastic deformities, to provide stability for an uncontrollable joint, and to provide balanced muscle power. This includes tendon-lengthening procedures (especially heel-cord lengthening), release of spastic wrist flexor muscles, and correction of hip and adductor muscle spasticity or contracture to improve locomotion. Selective dorsal rhizotomy has provided marked improvement in some children with CP. The procedure involves selectively cutting dorsal column sensory rootlets that have an abnormal response to electrical stimulation. Achieving the benefits from the surgery requires intensive physical therapy and family commitment. Because the procedure results in flaccid muscles, the child must be retaught to sit, stand, and walk.

Surgical intervention is usually reserved for the child who does not respond to the more conservative measures, but it is also indicated for the child whose spasticity causes progressive deformities. Surgery is primarily used to improve function

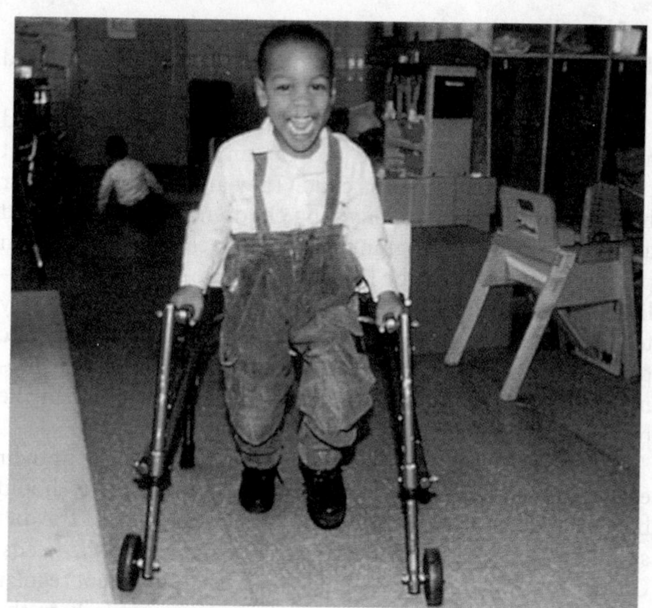

Fig. 55-2 Child ambulating with use of assistive device.

rather than for cosmetic purposes and is followed by physical therapy.

Intense pain may occur with muscle spasms in patients with CP. Pharmacologic agents given orally (dantrolene sodium, baclofen [Lioresal], and diazepam [Valium]) have had little effectiveness in improving muscle coordination in children with CP; however, they are effective in decreasing overall spasticity. The most common side effects of these agents include hepatotoxicity (dantrolene), drowsiness, fatigue, and muscle weakness; less commonly, diaphoresis and constipation may be seen with baclofen. Diazepam is used frequently but should be restricted to older children and adolescents.

Botulinum toxin A (Botox) is also used to reduce spasticity in targeted muscles. Botulinum toxin A is injected into a selected muscle (commonly the quadriceps, gastrocnemius, or medial hamstrings) after a topical anesthetic is applied. The drug acts to inhibit the release of acetylcholine into a specific muscle group, thereby preventing muscle movement. When it is administered early in the course of the illness, affected muscle contractures may be prevented, particularly in lower extremities, thus avoiding surgical procedures with possible adverse effects. The goal is to allow stretching of the muscle as it relaxes and permit ambulation with an AFO. The major reported adverse effect of botulinum toxin A injection is pain at the injection site (Roscigno, 2002). Prime candidates for botulinum toxin A injections are children with spasticity confined to the lower extremities; the drug weakens spasticity so the muscles can be stretched and the child may ambulate with or without orthoses. The onset of action occurs within 24 to 72 hours, with a peak effect observed at 2 weeks and a duration of action of 3 to 6 months (Green, Greenberg, & Hurwitz, 2003).

Children with CP may also experience pain as a result of surgical procedures intended to reduce contracture deformities, position and gastroesophageal reflux, and physical therapy (McKearnan et al, 2004). Therefore pain management is an important aspect of care of the child with CP.

Neurosurgical and pharmacologic approach to managing the spasticity associated with CP involves the implantation of a pump to infuse baclofen directly into the intrathecal space surrounding the spinal cord to provide relief of spasticity. Intrathecal baclofen therapy is best suited for children with severe spasticity that interferes with activities of daily living (ADLs) and ambulation. Patients are screened before pump placement by the infusion of a "test dose" of intrathecal baclofen delivered via a lumbar puncture. Close monitoring for side effects (hypotonia, somnolence, seizures, nausea, vomiting, headache, and catheter- or pump-related problems [Albright et al, 2003]) and relief of spasticity occurs for several hours after the infusion. If a positive effect is noted, the patient is considered a candidate for pump placement.

The implantation procedure is done in the operating room by a neurosurgeon. The pump, which is approximately the size of a hockey puck, is placed in the subcutaneous space of the midabdomen. An intrathecal catheter is tunneled from the lumbar area to the abdomen and connected to the pump. The pump is filled with baclofen and, using a telemetry wand and a computer, is programmed to provide a set dose. Benefits of intrathecal baclofen include fewer systemic side effects than oral medication, dosage titration for maximizing effects, and reversibility of therapy with removal of the pump if so desired (Jacobs, 2001). The patient may remain hospitalized for 3 to 7 days to adjust the dosage and ensure proper healing. Outpatient visits to refill the pump and make dosage adjustments occur about every 4 to 6 weeks, depending on the patient's response to the treatment. This procedure is most suited for a multidisciplinary setting where rehabilitation specialists are readily available and consistently involved in the patient's ongoing care. Abrupt withdrawal of intrathecal baclofen, especially at high doses, may result in adverse effects such as rebound spasticity, pruritus, hyperthermia, rhabdomyolysis, disseminated intravascular coagulation, multiorgan failure, and death. In some cases intrathecal baclofen withdrawal may mimic sepsis.

Antiepileptic drugs (AEDs) such as carbamazepine (Tegretol) and divalproex (valproate sodium and valproic acid; Depakote) are prescribed routinely for children who have seizures. Gabapentin (Neurontin) has been used in adults with spinal cord injury (SCI) to decrease spasticity with success; no studies are available on the effectiveness of the drug in children. The α_2-adrenergic agonists clonidine (Catapres) and tizanidine (Zanaflex) have been used to decrease spasticity in adults with SCI and multiple sclerosis; however, their use in children does not appear to have gained widespread acceptance in the United States. The effectiveness of oral tizanidine given in conjunction with botulinum type A has been reported to be more effective than oral baclofen and botulinum type A in one study of children with CP (Dai, Wasay, & Awan, 2008). All medications should be monitored for maintenance of therapeutic levels and avoidance of subtherapeutic or toxic levels.

Dental hygiene is especially important. Regular visits to the dentist and prophylaxis, including brushing, fluoride, and flossing, should be instituted as soon as the teeth erupt. Dental care is especially important for children being given phenytoin, since they often develop gum hyperplasia. Additional problems common among children with CP include constipation caused by neurologic deficits and lack of exercise; poor bladder control and urinary retention; chronic respiratory tract infections and aspiration pneumonia, which occur as a result of gastroesophageal reflux, abnormal muscle tone, immobility, and altered positioning; and skin problems as a result of altered positioning, poor nutrition, and immobility.

A wide variety of technical aids is available to improve the functioning of children with CP. These include electromechanical toys that employ the concept of biofeedback and operate from a head unit. The toy is manipulated only when the head and trunk are in correct alignment. Eye-hand coordination can also be enhanced by computerized toys and games. Microcomputers combined with voice synthesizers help children with speech difficulties to "speak." These and other devices print messages onto screen monitors and paper.

Many other electronic devices allow independent functioning. Sensors can be activated and deactivated by using a headstick or tongue, or other voluntary muscle movement over which the child has control. Voice-activated computer technology may also allow increased mobility and ambulation with specially designed devices such as wheelchairs. The application of this technology makes it possible for persons with CP to function eventually in their own residences and can be extended into the workplace.

Physical therapy is one of the most frequently used conservative treatment modalities. It requires the specialized skills of a qualified therapist with an extensive repertoire of exercise methods who can design a program to stimulate each child to achieve his or her functional goals. An active therapy program involves the family; the physical therapist; and often other members of the health team, including the nurse. The most common approach employs traditional types of therapeutic exercises that consist of stretching, passive, active, and resistive movements applied to specific muscle groups or joints to maintain or increase range of motion, strength, and endurance.

Prognosis

In general, the more severe the functional disability, the worse the prognosis. Children with a severe physical disability, cognitive impairment, tube feedings, and severe seizures are known to have a shortened life expectancy. According to available data, approximately 30% to 50% of individuals with CP have cognitive impairment, and an even higher percentage have mild cognitive and learning deficits (Green, Greenberg, & Hurwitz, 2003); however, many children with severe spastic quadriplegic CP have normal intelligence. Growth is affected in children with spastic quadriplegia, and many children remain below the 5th percentile for age and gender. As children with CP transition to adulthood, about 30% remain in the home and are cared for by a parent or caregiver; 50% of individuals with spastic quadriplegia live in independent settings and function at appropriate social levels considering their disability (Green, Greenberg, & Hurwitz, 2003). Vocational rehabilitation and higher education are possible for adults with CP, and one study found that 53% of all persons with CP were able to work outside the home in regular jobs; one third of the severely disabled adults with CP worked outside the home (Murphy, Molnar, & Lankasky, 2000).

Nursing Care Management

The nursing process in the care of the child with CP is outlined in the Nursing Process box.

Because children with CP are being identified and treated at an earlier age, parents are participating earlier in treatment programs for their disabled child. They are taught the proper handling and home care of young children with CP and need a carefully planned program so that their change of role from parent to caregiver can be incorporated into the already established relationship. Close work with other multidisciplinary team members is essential. Nurses reinforce the therapeutic plan and assist the family in devising and modifying equipment and activities to continue the therapy program in the home (see Nursing Care Plan).

Because children with CP expend so much energy in their efforts to accomplish ADLs, more frequent rest periods should be arranged to avoid taxing their limited capabilities. The diet should be tailored to the child's activity and metabolic needs. Gastrostomy feedings may be necessary to supplement regular feedings and ensure adequate weight gain, particularly in the child who is at risk for growth failure and chronic malnutrition. In children with severe CP and subsequent oral feeding difficulties, a feeding gastrostomy should be considered (Rogers, 2004). Gastrostomy feeding as a supplement to oral feeding is often recommended, especially when illness and decreased fluid or medication intake affect the child's well-being (Rogers, 2004). Oral feedings may be continued to maintain oral motor skills. Weight gain is perceived as an important measure of adequate oral feeding efficiency.

Parents may need assistance and advice with medication administration through a gastrostomy tube to prevent clotting of the device. A skin-level gastrostomy is particularly suited for the child with CP.

Because jaw control is often compromised, more normal control can be achieved if the feeder provides stability of the oral mechanism from the side or front of the face. When directed from the front, the middle finger of the nonfeeding hand is placed posterior to the body portion of the chin, the thumb is placed below the bottom lip, and the index finger is placed parallel to the child's mandible (Fig. 55-3). Manual jaw control from the side assists with head control, correction of

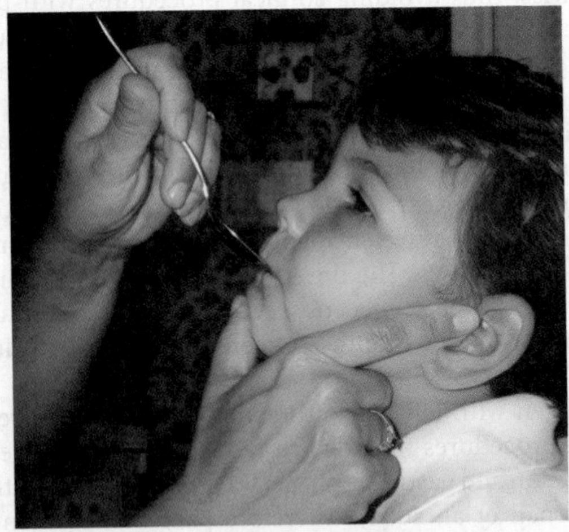

Fig. 55-3 Manual jaw control provided anteriorly.

NURSING PROCESS: CEREBRAL PALSY

Assessment

Nursing assessment includes risk identification of infants with etiologic factors that are associated with cerebral palsy (CP). Early recognition of CP is important so early interventions may be implemented (Box 55-3). Ongoing assessment of infants for abnormal muscle tone, inability to achieve developmental milestones, and persistence of neonatal reflexes alerts the nurse to investigate further.

Nursing Diagnoses

After a thorough assessment a number of nursing diagnoses are evident (see Nursing Care Plan, pp. 1722-1723). Other nursing diagnoses include:

Imbalanced nutrition: less than body requirements related to
- decreased oral intake of nutrients
- uncoordinated oral motor function

Delayed growth and development related to
- inadequate caloric intake
- energy expenditure that exceeds caloric intake

Interrupted family processes related to
- level of care required in caring for the chronically ill child (e.g., medication administration, special feeding methods, physical therapy, assistive devices [AFOs, wheelchair, braces])

Risk for aspiration related to
- uncoordinated oral motor function resulting in swallowing difficulty
- muscle spasticity

Planning

Expected outcomes for the child with CP include:

- Child will receive adequate nutrient intake for body growth (weight gain).
- Child will achieve developmental milestones to maximum potential.
- Family will cope with child's illness and functions to maximum potential.
- Child's airway will remain patent.

Implementation

Numerous intervention strategies for the child with CP are found on pp. 1720-1724.

Evaluation

The effectiveness of nursing interventions for the family and child with CP is determined by continual reassessment and evaluation of care based on the following observational guidelines:

- Child's movements and use of mobilization devices
- Child's speech and ability to use communication devices
- Child's activities, especially those related to self-care
- Family perception regarding child's activities and school attendance
- Child's interactions with others and choice of activities; child's feelings and concerns
- Family feelings, concerns, and interaction with the child
- Child's behavior and responses during hospitalization

BOX 55-3 Early Signs of Cerebral Palsy

- Failure to meet any developmental milestones such as rolling over, raising head, sitting up, crawling
- Persistent primitive reflexes such as Moro, atonic neck
- Poor head control (head lag) and clenched fists after 3 months of age
- Stiff or rigid arms or legs; scissoring legs
- Pushing away or arching back; stiff posture
- Floppy or limp body posture, especially while sleeping
- Inability to sit up without support by 8 months
- Using only one side of the body, or only the arms to crawl
- Feeding difficulties
- Persistent gagging or choking when fed
- After 6 months of age, tongue pushing soft food out of the mouth
- Extreme irritability or crying
- Failure to smile by 3 months
- Lack of interest in surroundings
- Hand preference in first 2 years of life

Data from Pathways Awareness Foundation: *Parents . . . if you see any of these warning signs . . . don't delay,* Chicago, 1991, The Foundation; Nehring W: Cerebral palsy. In Allen PJ, Vessey JA (editors): *Primary care of the child with a chronic condition*, St Louis, 2004, Mosby; and Jones MW et al: Cerebral palsy: introduction and diagnosis, part 1, *J Pediatr Health Care* 21(3):146-152, 2007.

neck and trunk hyperextension, and jaw stabilization. The middle finger of the nonfeeding hand is placed posterior to the bony portion of the chin, the index finger is placed on the chin below the lower lip, and the thumb is placed obliquely across the cheek to provide lateral jaw stability (Fig. 55-4).

Safety precautions are implemented, such as having children wear protective helmets if they are subject to falls or capable of injuring their heads on hard objects. Because the child with CP is at risk for altered proprioception and subsequent falls, the home and play environment should be adapted to the child's needs to prevent bodily harm. Appropriate immunizations should be administered to prevent childhood illnesses and protect against respiratory tract infections such as influenza. Depending on the level of involvement, dental problems may be more common in children with CP, which creates a need for meticulous attention to all aspects of dental care.

The involvement of physical therapy, speech therapy, and occupational therapy is particularly important in establishment and maintenance of muscle function, development of adequate speech and phonation, and identification of modifications necessary for the child's environment so that ADLs can be performed to the child's satisfaction.

As in all aspects of care, educational requirements are determined by the child's needs and potential. Children with mild to moderate involvement are generally able to participate, for varying amounts of time, in regular classes. Resource rooms are available in most schools to provide more individualized attention. Integration of children with CP into regular classrooms should be the initial goal. For those who are unable to benefit from formal education, a vocational training program may be appropriate. At adolescence, prevocational and vocational counseling and guidance are arranged. At any phase or in any setting, education is geared toward the child's assets.

Recreational outlets and after-school activities should be considered for the child who is unable to participate in the regular athletic programs and other peer activities. Some children can compete in athletic and artistic endeavors, and many games and pastimes are suited to their capabilities. Competitive sports are also becoming increasingly available to children with disabilities and offer an added dimension to physical activities. For more information access the United Cerebral Palsy website *(www.ucp.org)* and go to the Sports and Leisure link.

Recreational activities serve to stimulate children's interest and curiosity, help them adjust to their disability, improve their functional abilities, and build self-esteem. Any accomplishment that helps children approach a "normal" way of life enhances their self-concept.

NURSING CARE PLAN ✤ The Child with Cerebral Palsy

Nursing Diagnosis	Patient Outcomes	Nursing Interventions	Rationale
Impaired physical mobility related to neuromuscular impairment **Child's/Family's Defining Characteristics** ***(Subjective and Objective Data)*** Postural instability during performance of routine activities of daily living Limited ability to perform gross motor skills Limited range of motion Limited ability to perform fine motor skills Gait changes Movement-induced tremor Persistence of primitive reflexes	The infant or toddler will demonstrate active joint movement. The child will have adequate mobility to perform activities of daily living to maximum potential. **The Following NOC Concepts Apply to These Outcomes** Body Mechanics Performance Ambulation: Wheelchair Joint Movement: Elbow, wrist, neck, knee, hip, ankle Mobility	Carry out and teach family to perform stretching exercises on affected joints. Use assistive devices such as wheelchair, ankle-foot orthoses (AFOs), and wrist splints. Administer medications intended to decrease muscle spasticity. Encourage and teach parent(s) to use jaw control during feedings. Position child semiupright during feedings. Encourage play exercises that involve joint movement and promote fine and gross motor skill acquisition and repetition. **The Following NIC Concepts Apply to These Interventions** Exercise Therapy: Joint Mobility Exercise Promotion: Stretching Self-Care Assistance	To prevent muscle contractures To increase mobility To minimize pain and decrease spasticity To facilitate eating To decrease chance of aspiration and facilitate mobilization of food and fluids through esophagus To promote joint movement To promote achievement of developmental milestones
Risk for injury related to mobility limitation, neuromuscular impairment, and perception and cognition impairment **Child's/Family's Defining Characteristics** ***(Subjective and Objective Data)*** Physical factors: altered mobility Neuromuscular factors: ✤ Limited perception of danger ✤ Uncontrollable muscular movements	Child will remain injury free. Home physical environment will be safe. **The Following NOC Concepts Apply to These Outcomes** Personal Safety Behavior Falls Occurrence	Educate family regarding child's physical limitations that place him or her at greater risk for injury. Instruct family in steps to avoid injury: padded furniture, lowered bed or side rails as appropriate, gates on stairs, avoidance of throw rugs, thick carpeting. Position child in semiupright position after feedings. Use jaw support as needed during feedings. Use appropriate mobilization devices and ensure they are safe for child's age. Encourage mobilization and play activities that stretch muscles. Teach child which activities of daily living are safe and appropriate to perform without assistance of another person. **The Following NIC Concepts Apply to These Interventions** Risk Identification Environmental Management: Safety Surveillance: Safety Physical Restraint Parent Education: Childrearing Family	To prevent accidental injury during mobilization To promote family involvement in injury prevention To prevent aspiration To prevent choking To prevent muscle contractures To promote personal safety To promote self-care

NURSING CARE PLAN ✤ The Child with Cerebral Palsy—cont'd

Nursing Diagnosis	Patient Outcomes	Nursing Interventions	Rationale
Pain (chronic) related to involuntary muscle movements (spasticity) and treatments for muscle spasticity	Child's optimum comfort level will be maintained.	Administer medications to control spasticity.	To prevent muscle spasm pain
	The Following NOC Concepts Apply to These Outcomes	Perform stretching exercises after pain medication has been administered (60 minutes for oral medications).	To control pain impulses during exercises
Child's/Family's Defining Characteristics	Comfort Level	Administer pain medications such as nonsteroidal antiinflammatory drugs.	To minimize pain
(Subjective and Objective Data)	Pain: Disruptive Effects	For treatments such as botulinum toxin A (Botox) injections, apply topical analgesic such as EMLA (an eutectic mix of lidocaine and prilocaine) or LMX4 (4% lidocaine).	To decrease pain of injection at site
Observed evidence of guarded behavior, grimace, crying, restlessness	Depression Level		
Atrophy of involved muscle group			
Altered ability to continue previous activities			
		For postoperative pain, administer pain medications on an around-the-clock schedule for 48 to 72 hours; use patient-controlled analgesia pump as child's cognitive and motor skills allow.	To promote personal physical comfort
		Use objective pain scale to assess pain level.	To provide objective measure of pain for intervention
		Encourage child to verbalize effects of pain on activities of daily living.	To provide outlet for frustration related to chronic pain experience
		Use assistive devices such as AFOs.	To decrease muscle spasticity and contractures.
		Teach parent(s) and child appropriate positions to assume while sitting and recumbent to minimize effects of muscle spasticity.	To promote self-care
		The Following NIC Concepts Apply to These Interventions	
		Medication Administration	
		Analgesic Administration	
		Emotional Support	
		Splinting	
		Environmental Management: Comfort	
		Exercise Promotion	

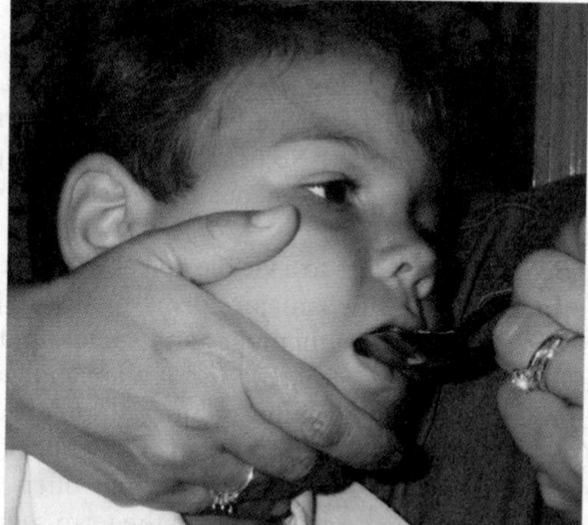

Fig. 55-4 Manual jaw control provided from the side.

Support Family

Probably the nursing interventions most valuable to the family are support and help in coping with the emotional aspects of the disorder, many of which are discussed in relation to the child with a disability (see Chapter 41). Initially the parents need supportive counseling directed toward understanding the implications of the diagnosis and all of the feelings that it engenders. Later they need clarification regarding what they can expect from the child and from health professionals. Educating families in the principles of family-centered care and parent-professional collaboration is essential. The family may require assistance in modifying the home environment for care of the child (see also Chapter 43). Transportation to the practitioner's office and other health care agencies often requires special considerations.

Care management for the child and family with CP is an important nursing role. In many cases the family assumes complete care of the child and becomes adept at meeting his or her individual needs. The home health nurse or care manager has an important role in support and encouragement for families who assume the primary care of a child with CP. Having a child with CP implies numerous problems of daily management and changes in family life, and the nurse can stress principles of normalization.

The nurse needs to support the parents in their frustration, problem solving, concerns, approaches to helping the child, and lack of gratification, as well as the positive approaches they use. All these aspects must be explored and discussed. Parents and other family members require much support and counseling. Siblings of a child with a disability are affected and may respond to the child's presence with overt or less evident behavioral problems. The family needs a relationship with nurses who can provide continued contact, support, and encouragement through the long process of habilitation.

Parents may also find help and comfort from parent groups, with whom they can share problems and concerns and from whom they can derive comfort and practical information. Parent support groups are most helpful through sharing experiences and accomplishments. For example, parents can learn from others what it is like to have a child with CP, which is generally not possible from professionals (see Family-Centered Care box). The national organization United Cerebral Palsy* has branches in most communities that provide a variety of services for children and families. A number of excellent books also are available to guide parents and nurses who work with the child with CP.

FAMILY-CENTERED CARE

The Reality of Acceptance of Cerebral Palsy

Acceptance is rarely achieved in the length of time implied in the literature.

In the first place, what is it? To me, it is the end of comparing my son with every other child I see. I focus on *his* gains, not society's expectations.

It is also being able to laugh periodically *at* his "clumsiness." It is "gallows humor" as he achieves adulthood; jokes about CP can be funny now.

The bitterness is gone; I am now happy for people who have children without CP.

I no longer feel sorry for my son, but rather for the people who cannot see him for the great person he is; the CP does *not* come first.

He is now a young man of 25 years and I am learning to accept his independence.

It is a "never-ending story."

–Elaine A. Dunham, RN, Shriners Hospitals for Children Springfield, MA

Support Hospitalized Child

CP is not a disorder that requires hospitalization; therefore, when children with CP are hospitalized, they are usually admitted for another reason or for corrective surgery. Nursing care for the child with CP is the same as for any other child with a disability. Children with CP should be approached the same as any child in the hospital. Speech impairment is common in children with CP. To facilitate the care and management of these children, the therapy program should be continued, insofar as their condition allows, during the time they are hospitalized. This should be incorporated into the nursing care plan with every effort expended to make certain that the ground that has been so laboriously gained is not lost. Encouraging the parent to room-in and actively participate in the child's care facilitates a continuation of the home therapy program and helps the child adjust to an unfamiliar environment. However, it is equally important to remember that hospitalization may be the first time a parent can defer care to a nurse and not be the primary caregiver. This respite may be crucial to the parent's well-being.

1660 L St., NW, Suite 700, Washington, DC 20036; 800-872-5827; fax: 202-776-0414; e-mail: info@ucp.org; www.ucp.org. *The website also has links to each state's United Cerebral Palsy organization.*

Spina Bifida (Myelomeningocele)

Abnormalities that derive from the embryonic neural tube *(neural tube defects [NTDs])* constitute the largest group of congenital anomalies that are consistent with multifactorial inheritance. Normally the spinal cord and cauda equina are encased in a protective sheath of bone and meninges (Fig. 55-5, *A*). Failure of neural tube closure produces defects of varying degrees (Box 55-4). They may involve the entire length of the neural tube or may be restricted to a small area.

In the United States, rates of NTDs have declined from 1.3 per 1000 births in 1970, to 0.3 per 1000 births after the introduction of mandatory food fortification with folic acid in 1998 (Honein, 2001). Further data indicate that the incidence of NTDs showed a 23% decline from 1996 to 2001 (Matthews, Honein, & Erickson, 2002). Maternal periconceptual intake of folic acid may reduce the incidence of NTDs in pregnancies at risk by as much as 50% (Kinsman & Johnston, 2007). Increased use of prenatal diagnostic techniques and termination of pregnancies have also affected the overall incidence of NTDs (see also Prevention, p. 1728).

Myelodysplasia refers broadly to any malformation of the spinal canal and cord. Midline defects involving failure of the osseous (bony) spine to close are called *spina bifida (SB)*, the most common defect of the central nervous system. SB is categorized into two types: spina bifida occulta and spina bifida cystica.

Spina bifida occulta refers to a defect that is not visible externally. It occurs most frequently in the lumbosacral area (L5 and S1) (see Fig. 55-5, *B*). SB occulta may not be apparent unless there are associated cutaneous manifestations or neuromuscular disturbances.

Spina bifida cystica refers to a visible defect with an external saclike protrusion. The two major forms of SB cystica are *meningocele,* which encases meninges and spinal fluid but no neural elements (see Fig. 55-5, *C*), and *myelomeningocele* (or *meningomyelocele*), which contains meninges, spinal fluid, and nerves (see Fig. 55-5, *D*). Meningocele is not associated with neurologic deficit, which occurs in varying, often serious, degrees in myelomeningocele. Clinically the term *spina bifida* is used to refer to myelomeningocele.

Pathophysiology

Most authorities believe that the primary defect in NTDs is a failure of neural tube closure during the embryo's early develop-

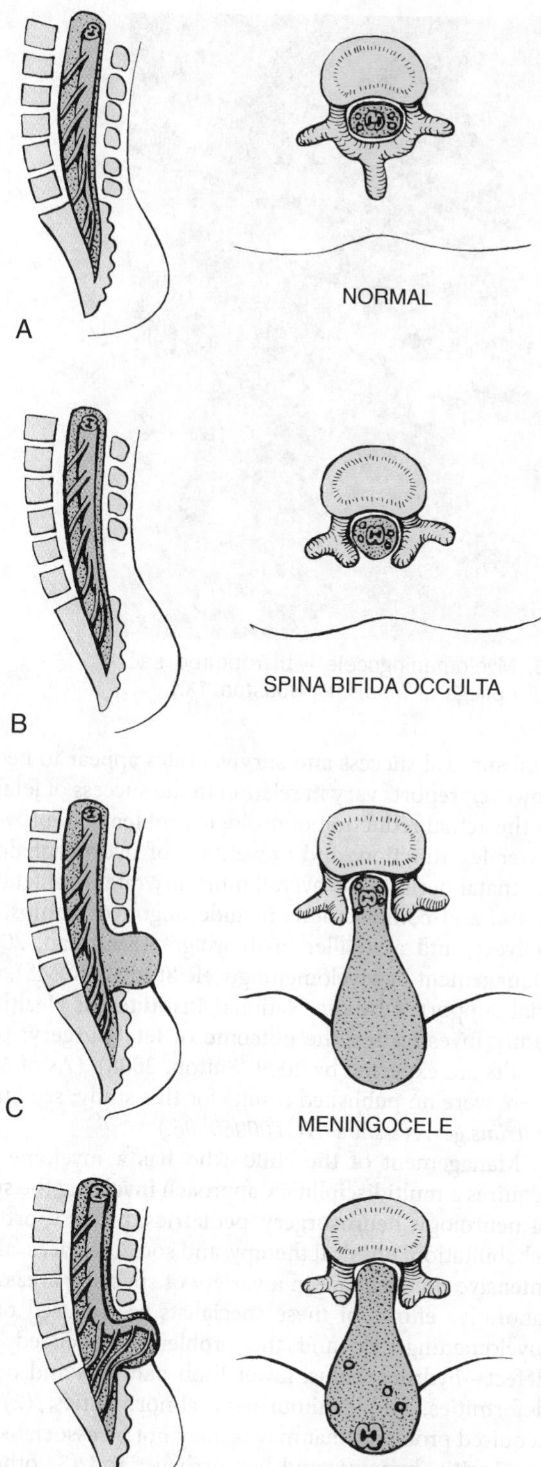

Fig. 55-5 **A** through **D**, Midline defects of osseous spine with varying degrees of neural herniations.

ment (the first 3 to 5 weeks). However, evidence also implicates a multifactorial etiology, including drugs, radiation, maternal malnutrition, chemicals, and possibly a genetic mutation in folate pathways in some cases, which may result in abnormal development. There is also evidence of a genetic component in the development of SB; myelomeningocele may occur in association with syndromes such as trisomy 18, PHAVER syndrome, and Meckel-Gruber syndrome (Shaer, Chescheir, & Schulkin, 2007). Additional factors predisposing children to an increased risk of NTDs include prepregnancy maternal obesity, maternal diabetes mellitus, previous NTD pregnancy, low maternal vitamin B_{12} status, maternal hyperthermia, and the use of AEDs (e.g., valproic acid) in pregnancy.

The degree of neurologic dysfunction depends on where the sac protrudes through the vertebrae, the anatomic level of the defect, and the amount of nerve tissue involved. Most myelomeningoceles involve the lumbar or lumbosacral area (Fig. 55-6). Hydrocephalus with a type II Chiari defect develops in 80% of the children (Kinsman & Johnston, 2007).

BOX 55-4 Neural Tube Defects

Cranioschisis—A skull defect through which various tissues protrude

Exencephaly—Brain totally exposed or extruded through an associated skull defect; fetus usually aborted

Anencephaly—If fetus with exencephaly survives, degeneration of the brain to a spongiform mass with no bony covering; incompatible with life usually beyond a few days

Encephalocele—Herniation of brain and meninges through a defect in the skull producing a fluid-filled sac

Rachischisis or **spina bifida**—Fissure in the spinal column that leaves the meninges and spinal cord exposed

Meningocele—Hernial protrusion of a saclike cyst of meninges filled with spinal fluid (see Fig. 55-5, *C*)

Myelomeningocele (meningomyelocele) —Hernial protrusion of a saclike cyst containing meninges, spinal fluid, and a portion of the spinal cord with its nerves (see Fig. 55-5, *D*)

Diagnostic Evaluation

The diagnosis of SB is made on the basis of clinical manifestations (Box 55-5) and examination of the meningeal sac (see Fig. 55-6, *A*). Diagnostic measures used to evaluate the brain and spinal cord include MRI, ultrasound, CT, and myelography. Laboratory examinations are used primarily to determine causative organisms for common complications associated with myelomeningocele: meningitis and urinary tract infections.

Prenatal Detection

It is possible to determine the presence of some major open NTDs prenatally. Ultrasonographic scanning of the uterus and elevated maternal concentrations of alpha-fetoprotein (AFP, or MS-AFP), a fetal-specific γ_1-globulin, in amniotic fluid may indicate anencephaly or myelomeningocele. The optimum time for performing these diagnostic tests is between 16 and 18 weeks of gestation, before AFP concentrations normally diminish and in sufficient time to permit a therapeutic abortion. It is recommended that such diagnostic procedures and genetic counseling be considered for all mothers who have borne an affected child, and testing is offered to all pregnant women (Kirkham, Harris, & Grzybowski, 2005). In addition, elective prelabor cesarean birth may result in less motor dysfunction. Chorionic villus sampling is also a method for prenatal diagnosis of NTDs; however, it carries certain risks (skeletal limb depletion) and is not recommended before 10 weeks of gestation.

evolve Critical Thinking Exercise–Myelomeningocele

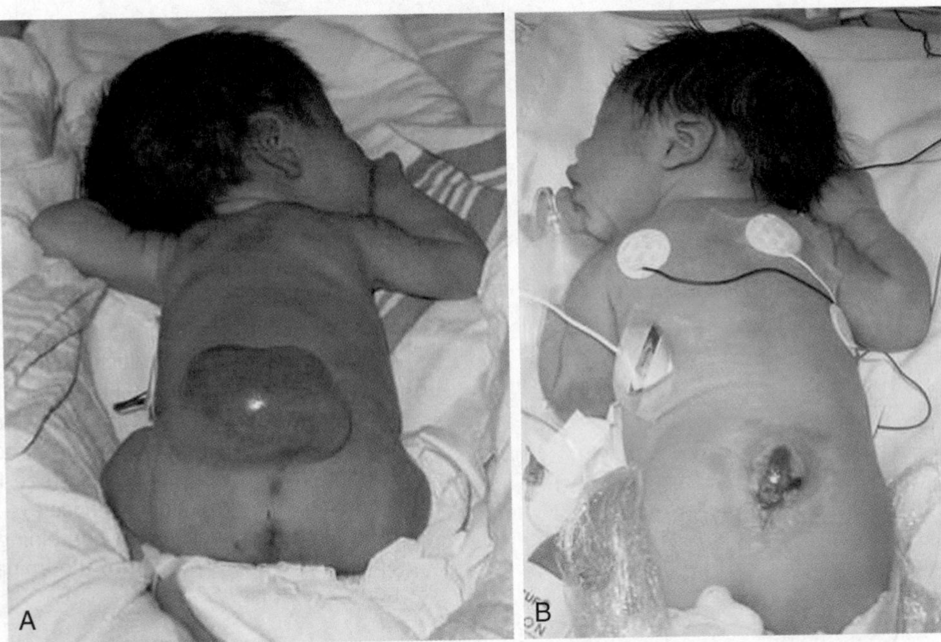

Fig. 55-6 A, Myelomeningocele with intact sac. **B,** Myelomeningocele with ruptured sac. *(Courtesy Dr. Robert C. Dauser, Neurosurgery, Baylor College of Medicine, Houston, TX.)*

BOX 55-5 Clinical Manifestations of Spina Bifida

Spina Bifida Cystica

Sensory disturbances usually parallel to motor dysfunction

- Below second lumbar vertebra—Flaccid, partial paralysis of lower extremities, varying degrees of sensory deficit, overflow incontinence with constant dribbling of urine, lack of bowel control, rectal prolapse (sometimes)
- Below third sacral vertebra—No motor impairment, may have saddle anesthesia with bladder and anal sphincter paralysis

Associated deformities (sometimes produced in utero):

- Talipes valgus or varus contractures
- Kyphosis
- Lumbosacral scoliosis
- Hip dislocation or subluxation

Spina Bifida Occulta

Frequently no observable manifestations

May be associated with one or more cutaneous manifestations:

- Skin depression or dimple
- Port-wine angiomatous nevi
- Dark tufts of hair
- Soft, subcutaneous lipomas

May have neuromuscular disturbances:

- Progressive disturbance of gait with foot weakness
- Bowel and bladder sphincter disturbances

Therapeutic Management

Early surgical closure of the myelomeningocele sac through fetal surgery has been evaluated in relation to prevention of injury to the exposed spinal cord tissue and improvement of neurologic and urologic outcomes in the affected child. Initial fetal surgical success and survival rates appear to be positive; however, reports vary in relation to the success of fetal surgery in the actual reduction of urologic problems, improvement of lower leg function, and prevention of hydrocephalus in the postnatal period. The overall mortality rate from fetal surgery is 4%, and complications include oligohydramnios, preterm delivery, and a smaller birth weight (Kaufman, 2004). The Management of Myelomeningocele Study (MOMS), a clinical trial supported by the National Institutes of Health, is currently investigating the outcome of fetal surgery; published results are expected by 2009 (Sutton, 2008). (As of May 2009 there were no published results for this study; see *http://clinicaltrials.gov/ct2/show/NCT00060606*.)

Management of the child who has a myelomeningocele requires a multidisciplinary approach involving the specialties of neurology, neurosurgery, pediatrics, urology, orthopedics, rehabilitation, physical therapy, and social services, along with intensive nursing care in a variety of specialty areas. The collaborative efforts of these specialists are focused on (1) the myelomeningocele and the problems associated with the defect—hydrocephalus, lower limb paralysis and orthopedic deformities, and genitourinary abnormalities; (2) possible acquired problems that may or may not be associated, such as meningitis, hypoxia, and hemorrhage; and (3) other conditions, such as cardiac or gastrointestinal malformations. Early neurologic management of myelomeningocele has demonstrated improved upper urinary tract function and a reduction in the need for surgery (Kessler et al, 2006).

Postnatal Management

Initial care of the newborn involves preventing infection; performing a neurologic assessment, including observing for associated anomalies; and dealing with the impact of the anomaly on the family. Although meningoceles are repaired early, especially if there is danger of rupture of the sac, the opinion regarding skin closure of myelomeningocele varies.

Most authorities believe that early closure, within the first 24 to 72 hours, offers the most favorable outcome. Early closure, preferably in the first 12 to 18 hours, not only prevents local infection and trauma to the exposed tissues, but also avoids stretching of other nerve roots (which may occur as the meningeal sac expands during the first hours after birth), thus preventing further motor impairment. Broad-spectrum antibiotics are initiated, and neurotoxic substances such as povidone-iodine are avoided at the malformation.

Associated problems are assessed and managed by appropriate surgical and supportive measures. Shunt procedures provide relief from imminent or progressive hydrocephalus (see Chapter 51). Meningitis, urinary tract infection, and ventriculitis are treated with vigorous antibiotic therapy and supportive measures. Surgical intervention for Chiari malformation (a downward herniation of the brain into the brainstem) or for tethered cord (scar tissue binding the spinal cord) is indicated only when the child is symptomatic.

Improved surgical techniques do not alter the major physical disability, spinal defect, or chronic urinary tract infections that affect the quality of life for these children. Superimposed on the physical problems are the effects that the disorder has on family life and finances, including the need for long-term specialized school and health care services.

Orthopedic Management

Most orthopedists recommend early evaluation and treatment (where indicated) of musculoskeletal problems that will affect later locomotion. Neurologic assessment will determine the neurosegmental level of the lesion and enable recognition of spasticity and progressive paralysis, potential for deformity, and functional expectations. Orthopedic management includes prevention of joint contractures, correction of the existing deformity, prevention or minimization of the effects of motor and sensory deficits, prevention of skin breakdown, and acquisition of the best possible function of affected lower extremities. Common orthopedic problems requiring attention in SB include deformities of the knees, hips (subluxation), feet (clubfeet), and spine; fractures and insensate skin further complicate orthopedic care. Other problems that may occur later include kyphosis and scoliosis (Brown, 2001). Because children with this condition often have decreased sensitivity in lower extremities, preventive skin care is important. A high percentage (60%) of children seen in a wound clinic for skin breakdown had spina bifida (Samaniego, 2003). The status of the neurologic deficit remains the most important factor in determining the child's ultimate functional abilities.

With technologic advances, a variety of lightweight orthoses, including braces, special "walking" devices, and custom-built wheelchairs, are available to provide mobility to children with spinal cord lesions (see also Chapter 42). Early in infancy, intervention with passive range-of-motion exercises, positioning, and stretching exercises may help decrease the incidence of muscle contractures (Brown, 2001). Corrective surgical procedures, when indicated, are best initiated at an early age so that the child will not lag significantly behind age-mates in developmental progress. Where there is little hope for lower extremity functioning, surgery is seldom recommended unless it will improve sitting position in a wheelchair and function for ADLs and mobility.

Management of Genitourinary Function

Myelomeningocele is one of the most common causes of *neuropathic (neurogenic) bladder dysfunction* among children. In infants the goal of treatment is to preserve renal function. In older children the goal is to preserve renal function and achieve optimal urinary continence. Urinary incontinence is a chronic, often debilitating problem for the child. In addition, the neuropathic bladder may produce *urinary system distress,* characterized by symptomatic urinary tract infections, ureterohydronephrosis, and vesicoureteral reflux or renal insufficiency. The characteristics of bladder dysfunction in children vary according to the level of the neurologic lesion and the influence of bony growth and development on the spine. Therefore ongoing urologic monitoring is essential. Evidence is growing that early intervention, based on evaluation during the neonatal period and before complications occur, serves to improve bladder function, reduces the risk of subsequent urinary system distress, and decreases the need for reconstructive surgery of the lower urinary tract (Snodgrass & Adams, 2004; Tarcan et al, 2006; Kessler et al, 2006).

Treatment of renal problems includes (1) regular urologic care with prompt and vigorous treatment of urinary tract infections; (2) a method of regular emptying of the bladder, such as *clean intermittent catheterization (CIC)* taught to and performed by parents and self-catheterization taught to children; (3) medications to improve bladder storage and continence, such as oxybutynin chloride (Ditropan) and tolterodine (Detrol); and (4) surgical procedures such as *vesicostomy* (bladder surgically brought out to the abdominal wall, allowing continuous urinary drainage) and *augmentation enterocystoplasty* (using a segment of bowel or stomach to increase bladder capacity, thereby reducing high bladder pressures).

However, despite the combined efforts of CIC, medication, and surgical intervention, some children with myelodysplasia may continue to experience debilitating urinary incontinence. Many of these children are able to attain social continence with a continent *urinary diversion* commonly referred to as Mitrofanoff's procedure. In this procedure, a catheterizable channel is surgically created from appendix, ureter, or tapered bowel. The proximal end of the channel is connected to the bladder with the distal end brought out as a small stoma on the abdominal wall, usually at the umbilicus or suprapubic area (Gray & Moore, 2009). The bladder neck may be sutured to prevent urinary leakage from the urethra. CIC through the easily accessible abdominal route fosters greater independence in children, especially in those unable to transfer from wheelchair to toilet to perform CIC.

Bowel Control

Some degree of fecal continence can be achieved in most children with myelomeningocele with diet modification, regular toilet habits, and prevention of constipation and impaction. It is frequently a lengthy process. Dietary fiber supplements (recommended 10 g/day), laxatives, stool softeners, suppositories, or enemas aid in producing regular evacuation. Older children and adolescents seeking more independence may attain bowel continence and higher quality of life after undergoing an antegrade continence enema procedure (Doolin, 2006). In a procedure similar to Mitrofanoff's, the appendix or ileum is used to create a catheterizable channel with attachment of the proximal end to the colon. The distal end of the channel exits through a small abdominal stoma. Every 1 or 2 days, a catheter is passed through the stoma, allowing enema solution to be instilled directly into the colon. After administration of the enema solution, the child sits on the toilet for 30 to 60 minutes as stool is flushed out through the rectum. Frequency of enemas and volume of solution used to completely evacuate the bowel vary among individuals.

Prognosis

The early prognosis for the child with myelomeningocele depends on the neurologic deficit present at birth, including motor ability, bladder innervation, and associated neurologic anomalies. Early surgical repair of the spinal defect, antibiotic therapy to reduce the incidence of meningitis and ventriculitis, prevention of urinary system dysfunction, and early detection and correction of hydrocephalus have significantly increased the survival rate and quality of life in such children. Overall mortality rate in those children treated aggressively is approximately 10% to 15%, and most deaths occur before age 4; as many as 70% of survivors will have normal intelligence (Kinsman & Johnston, 2007). Multidisciplinary follow up is required for life. Many children with SB achieve partial independent living and gainful employment. Reports of survival rates vary, and many include adults who were born before medical advances and surgical techniques seen in the past 25 years.

Researchers have noted that as adolescents with SB transition to young adulthood, they have increased difficulty obtaining centralized health care for the different health problems associated with SB (Lazzaretti & Pearson, 2004). This chronic condition has an array of associated complications, including hydrocephalus and shunt malfunctions, scoliosis, bowel and bladder management issues, latex allergy, and epilepsy. However, based on current medical knowledge and ethical considerations, aggressive, early management for the child with myelomeningocele improves the prognosis.

Prevention

The widespread use of folic acid among women of childbearing age has significantly decreased the incidence of SB. It has been estimated that a daily intake of 0.4 mg of folic acid in women of childbearing age will prevent 50% to 70% of all cases of NTDs (Centers for Disease Control and Prevention, 2004). A 24% decrease in cases of SB occurred between 1996 and 2001 (Matthews, Honein, & Erickson, 2002). While the incidence of SB decreased only 10% between 1999 to 2000 and 2003 to 2004, the decrease in anencephaly was significant (20%) (Boulet et al, 2008). Although folic acid intake increased in 1999 to 2000 (compared with intake from 1988 to 1994), recent data indicate that serum folate concentrations among women of childbearing age decreased 16% from 2003 to 2004 in all ethnic groups studied. Lowest serum folate levels were seen in non-Hispanic Caucasians in 2003 to 2004; however, overall serum folate levels remained below recommended levels in non-Hispanic African-Americans during all three periods studied (Centers for Disease Control and Prevention, 2007). Data from the years 1995 to 2002 indicate that highest prevalence rates of SB and anencephaly occurred among Hispanic births, followed by non-Hispanic Caucasian births (Williams et al, 2005). These results indicate that nurses and other health care workers have an important task in disseminating information that may decrease the incidence of birth defects in children by promoting maternal consumption of folic acid.*

Because approximately half of all pregnancies in the United States are unplanned (Henshaw, 1998), adolescent girls and women of childbearing age need to be educated about the necessity of folic acid to prevent NTDs. The daily dose of 0.4 mg (400 mcg) is most easily obtained from a multivitamin supplement. For women who have had a previous pregnancy affected by NTDs, folic acid intake is increased to 4 mg/day under supervision of a practitioner beginning 1 month before a planned pregnancy and continuing during the first trimester. Supplementation of 4 mg of folate should not be given in multivitamin preparations because of the risk of overdose of other vitamins.

To ensure adequate daily intake of the recommended amount of folic acid, women must take a folic acid supplement, eat a fortified breakfast cereal containing 100% of the recommended dietary allowance of folic acid (e.g., Kellogg's Product 19, General Mills Total, Multigrain Cheerios Plus), or increase their consumption of other fortified foods (cereal, bread, rice, grits, pasta) and foods naturally rich in folate (green leafy vegetables and citrus fruits). The only population in which folic acid has *not proved* to be effective in decreasing the incidence of NTDs is epileptic women taking AEDs during pregnancy.

Nursing Care Management

At birth an examination is performed to assess the intactness of the membranous cyst. During transport to the nursery, every effort is made to prevent trauma to this protective covering. In addition to the routine assessment of the newborn (see Chapter 24), the infant is assessed for the level of neurologic involvement. Movement of extremities or skin response, especially an anal reflex, that might provide clues to the degree of motor or sensory impairment is noted. It is important to observe the infant's behavior in conjunction with the stimulus, since limb movements can be induced in response to spinal cord reflex activity that has no connection with the higher centers. Observation of urine output, especially if a diaper remains dry, may indicate urinary retention. Abdominal assessment revealing bladder distention, even with a wet diaper, may indicate urinary overflow in a retentive bladder. The head circumference is measured daily, and the fontanels are examined for signs of tension or bulging.

Care of the Myelomeningocele Sac

The infant is usually placed in an incubator or warmer so that temperature can be maintained without clothing or covers that might irritate the spinal defect. When an overhead warmer is used, the dressings over the defect require more frequent moistening because of the dehydrating effect of the radiant heat.

**Information is available from Division of Birth Defects and Pediatric Genetics, NCBDDD, CDC, 1600 Clifton Road NE, Mailstop E-86, Atlanta, GA 30333; 800-232-4636; e-mail: cdcinfo@cdc.gov;* www.cdc.gov/ncbddd/folicacid; *and also from March of Dimes Resource Center, 1275 Mamaroneck Ave., White Plains, NY 10605;* www.marchofdimes.com.

Before surgical closure the myelomeningocele is prevented from drying by the application of a sterile, moist, nonadherent dressing over the defect. The moistening solution is usually sterile normal saline. Dressings are changed frequently (every 2 to 4 hours), and the sac is closely inspected for leaks, abrasions, irritation, or any signs of infection. The sac must be carefully cleansed if it becomes soiled or contaminated. Sometimes the sac ruptures during delivery or transport, and any opening in the sac greatly increases the risk of infection to the central nervous system (see Fig. 55-6, *B*).

NURSING ALERT Avoid measuring rectal temperatures in infants with SB. Because bowel sphincter function is frequently affected, the thermometer can cause irritation and rectal prolapse.

One of the most important and challenging aspects in the early care of the infant with myelomeningocele is positioning. Before surgery the infant is kept in the prone position to minimize tension on the sac and the risk of trauma. The prone position allows for optimal positioning of the legs, especially in cases of associated hip subluxation. The infant is placed prone with the hips slightly flexed and supported to reduce tension on the defect. The legs are maintained in abduction with a pad between the knees to counteract hip subluxation, and a small roll is placed under the ankles to maintain a neutral foot position. A variety of aids, including diaper rolls, pads, small foam pads, or specially designed frames and appliances, can be used to maintain the desired position.

Prevent Complications

The prone position affects other aspects of the infant's care. For example, in this position the infant is more difficult to keep clean, pressure areas are a constant threat, and feeding becomes a problem. The infant's head is turned to one side for feeding. Fortunately, most defects are repaired early, and the infant can be held for feeding soon after surgery. Special care must be taken to avoid pressure on the operative site.

Diapering the infant may be contraindicated until the defect has been repaired and healing is well advanced or epithelialization has taken place. The padding beneath the diaper area is changed as needed to keep the skin dry and free of irritation. When urinary retention is detected, CIC is employed. Because the bowel sphincter is frequently affected, there is continual passage of stool, often misinterpreted as diarrhea, which is a constant irritant to the skin and a source of infection to the spinal lesion.

Areas of sensory and motor impairment are subject to skin breakdown and therefore require meticulous care. Placing the infant on a special mattress or mattress overlay reduces pressure on the knees and ankles. Periodic cleansing and gentle massage aid circulation.

Gentle range-of-motion exercises are carried out to prevent contractures, and stretching of contractures is performed when indicated. However, these exercises may be restricted to the foot, ankle, and knee joint. When the hip joints are unstable, stretching against tight hip flexors or adductor muscles, which act much like bowstrings, may aggravate a tendency toward subluxation. Consultation with a physical therapist is an important aspect of the short- and long-term management of infants with myelomeningocele.

Infants with unrepaired myelomeningocele may be held in the arms and cuddled as unaffected infants are, so their need for tactile stimulation is met by caressing, stroking, and other comfort measures. One method to protect the sac while the parent is holding is to place a pillow on the parent's lap and lay the infant on its side on the pillow. Individualized developmental care with age-appropriate stimulation is provided (see Developmental Outcome, Chapter 27).

Observe for early signs of infection, such as temperature instability (axillary), irritability, and lethargy, and for signs of increased intracranial pressure, which might indicate developing hydrocephalus.

Provide Postoperative Care

Postoperative care of the infant with myelomeningocele involves the same basic care as that of any postsurgical infant: monitoring vital signs, monitoring intake and output, providing nourishment, observing for signs of infection, and managing pain as needed. Care of the operative site is carried out under the direction of the surgeon and includes close observation for signs of leakage of cerebrospinal fluid (CSF). General care is continued as preoperatively.

The prone position is maintained after surgical closure, although many neurosurgeons allow a side-lying or partial side-lying position unless it aggravates a coexisting hip subluxation or permits undesirable hip flexion. This offers an opportunity for position changes, which reduces the risk of pressure sores and facilitates feeding. If permitted, the infant can be held upright against the body, with care taken to avoid pressure on the operative site. After the effects of anesthesia have subsided and the infant is alert, feedings may be resumed unless there are other anomalies or associated complications.

Support Family and Educate About Home Care

As soon as the parents are able to cope with the infant's condition, they are encouraged to become involved in care. They need to learn how to continue at home the care that has been initiated in the hospital—positioning, feeding, skin care, and range-of-motion exercises when appropriate. They are taught CIC technique when it is prescribed. Parents also need to know the signs of complications (urinary, neurologic, orthopedic) and how to obtain assistance when needed.

The mother who wishes to breastfeed the infant is encouraged to do so, since this will be beneficial. Shortly after delivery the mother is started on a program of pumping to initiate and maintain milk supply until the infant is stable enough to begin breastfeeding (Hurtekant & Spatz, 2007). This process may require considerable support from nurses, physicians, and family members because of separation from the infant for surgical care and recovery.

The long-range planning with and support of the parents and newborn begin in the hospital and continue throughout childhood and even into young adulthood. The life expectancy of children with SB extends well into adulthood; therefore planning should involve long-term goals and plans for optimum function as an adult. Discussion about aspects of adulthood such as receiving educational or vocational training and education, living independently, having a mate, having sexual relationships, and bearing and rearing children is important and should not be overlooked. The unique service needs of adolescents with SB as they attempt to gain independence from family and establish a life of their own have not been adequately addressed in the literature (Buran, McDaniel, & Brei, 2002). Nurses assume an important role as a central member of the health team. As a care manager and coordinator, the nurse reviews information with the family, takes responsibility for family teaching, and acts as a liaison between inpatient and outpatient services. The child will need numerous hospitalizations over the years, and each one will be a source of stress to which the younger child is especially vulnerable (see Chapter 41 for a discussion of care of the child with a disability).

Habilitation involves not only solving problems of self-help and locomotion, but also solving the most distressing problem of urinary or bowel incontinence, which threatens the child's social acceptability. Assistance in preparing the child and the school regarding the child's special needs helps provide a better initial adjustment to this broader social experience. The Spina Bifida Association of America* is organized to provide services and support for families of children with spinal lesions.

Latex Allergy

Latex allergy was identified as a serious health hazard when a report linked intraoperative anaphylaxis with latex in children with SB. The high prevalence of latex allergy (up to 80%) in children with SB has been attributed to the repeated exposure to latex products during surgery and numerous bladder catheterizations and possible disease-associated factors. Some evidence suggests that children with SB are at increased risk for latex allergy as a result of the disease itself rather than repeated latex exposures (Eiwegger et al, 2006). Allergic reactions range from urticaria, wheezing, watery eyes, and rashes to anaphylactic shock. More severe reactions tend to occur when latex comes in contact with mucous membranes, wet skin, the bloodstream, or an airway. There also can be cross-reactions to a number of foods (e.g., banana, avocado, kiwi, chestnut). Latex allergy has been diagnosed in infants; symptoms include wheezing, facial swelling, facial rash, and anaphylaxis (Kimata, 2004). In addition to patients with SB, high risk populations include patients with urogenital anomalies or multiple surgeries and health care workers (see Box 55-6 for medical conditions associated with risk of latex allergy).

The most important goals are prevention of latex allergy and identification of children with a known hypersensitivity (see Guidelines box). High risk and latex-allergic individuals must be managed in a *latex-free* environment. Care must be taken so that they do not come in direct or secondary contact with products or equipment containing latex *at any time* during medical treatment. Allergy testing has been used to identify latex allergy with varying success. Skin prick testing and provocation testing carry the risk of allergic reaction or anaphylaxis. The radioallergosorbent test (RAST) has been used to measure the serum level of latex-specific immunoglobulin E. The RAST has been shown to be 90% to 95% sensitive (Kellett, 1997). Pretreatment with an antihistamine and steroids (dexamethasone) before and after surgery to reduce the possibility of a serious reaction remains controversial, since it may interfere with healing.

BOX 55-6 Medical Conditions Associated with Risk of Latex Allergy

- Spina bifida
- Urogenital anomalies
- Imperforate anus
- Tracheoesophageal fistula
- VATER association (vertebral defects, imperforate *a*nus, *t*racheoesophageal fistula, and *r*adial and renal dysplasia)
- Preterm infants
- Ventriculoperitoneal shunt
- Cognitive impairment
- Cerebral palsy
- Quadriplegia
- Multiple surgeries
- Atopy

GUIDELINES Identifying Latex Allergy

- Does your child have any symptoms, such as sneezing, coughing, rashes, or wheezing, when handling rubber products (e.g., balloons, tennis or Koosh balls, adhesive bandage strips) or when in contact with rubber hospital products (e.g., gloves, catheters)?
- Has your child ever had an allergic reaction during surgery?
- Does your child have a history of rashes, asthma, or allergic reactions to medication or foods, especially milk, kiwi, bananas, or chestnuts?
- How would you identify or recognize an allergic reaction in your child?
- What would you do if an allergic reaction occurred?
- Has anyone ever discussed latex or rubber allergy or sensitivity with you?
- Has your child had any allergy testing?
- When did your child last come in contact with any type of rubber product? Were you present?

Modified from Romanczuk A: Latex use with infants and children: it can cause problems, *MCN* 18(4):208-212, 1993.

Because children who have SB are prone to develop an allergy to latex, reducing exposure, from birth on, may decrease the chance of allergy development. Many health care facilities are establishing latex-safe environments when patients and health care workers are at risk. In the health care arena it is important to use products with the lowest potential risk of sensitizing patients and staff members.

Lists have been published of products, such as vinyl gloves, that may be substituted for latex. The U.S. Food and Drug

4590 MacArthur Blvd. NW, Suite 250, Washington, DC 20007-4226; 202-944-3285 or 800-621-3141; www.spinabifidaassociation.org.

BOX 55-7 Clinical Manifestations of Spinal Muscular Atrophy

Type 1 (Werdnig-Hoffmann Disease)

Disease acquired in utero or during first 2 months of life
Hypotonia and inactivity most prominent features
Infant lying in the frog position with legs externally rotated, abducted, and flexed at knees
Weakness
Absent deep tendon reflexes
Limited movements of shoulder and arm muscles
Active movement usually limited to fingers and toes
Diaphragmatic breathing with intercostal retractions (diaphragmatic paralysis may occur)
Abnormal tongue movements
Weak cry and cough
Secretions tending to pool in oropharynx
Alert facies
Normal sensation and intellect
Tiring quickly during feedings (if breastfed, may lose weight before noticeable)
Affected infants failing to progress to sitting alone, rolling over, or walking
Early death (usually by 2 years of age) from respiratory failure or infection

Type 2 (Intermediate Spinal Muscular Atrophy)

Symptoms manifest between 2 and 12 months of age
Early—Weakness confined to arms and legs
Later—Becomes generalized
Legs usually involved to greater extent than arms
Prominent pectus excavatum
Movements absent during complete relaxation or sleep
Some infants able to sit if placed in position
Failure to walk is common
Life span varies from 7 months to 7 years or even longer in some cases

Type 3 (Kugelberg-Welander Disease)

Onset of symptoms in late childhood or adolescence (may be initially misdiagnosed as muscular dystrophy [limb-girdle])
Normal head control and ability to sit unassisted by 6 to 8 months of age
Thigh and hip muscles weak
In those who manage to walk:

- Lumbar lordosis
- Waddling gait
- Genu recurvatum
- Protuberant abdomen
- Ambulation increasingly difficult
- Age of onset influences ambulatory difficulty—the later (after 2 years) the onset, the better the prognosis
- Confined to a wheelchair by second decade (may vary)

Deep tendon reflexes may be present early but disappear
Scoliosis common

NOTE: These classifications are general, and experts suggest there may be variations in life span and other characteristics (Iannaccone & Burghes, 2002; Russman, 1996; Russman et al, 1992).

Administration has proposed user labeling for latex-containing devices that come into contact, directly or indirectly, with live human tissue.*

NURSING ALERT Ask all patients, not only those at risk, about allergic reactions to latex during the health interview with the parent or child. Be certain that this is a routine part of all preoperative and preprocedural histories. Stress the importance of the allergy history to all personnel (e.g., phlebotomists).

The identification of those sensitive to latex is best accomplished through careful screening of *all* patients (see Guidelines box for questions related to latex allergy). Children with latex allergy should carry or wear some form of medical identification; those who have had serious reactions should also carry an injectable epinephrine pen and a pair of latex-free gloves for emergencies. Education programs regarding latex hypersensitivity are aimed at those who care for high risk groups, such as children with SB, and may include relatives, school nurses, teachers, child care workers, and baby-sitters. In addition to educating caregivers about the child's exposure to medical products that contain latex, nurses need to inform them of common nonmedical latex objects. Parents should also be given literature explaining signs and symptoms of latex hypersensitivity and appropriate emergency treatment (see Anaphylaxis, Chapter 48).

**Additional information regarding latex allergy may be found at* www.latex-allergy.org, *and* http://latexallergylinks.tripod.com. *For a list of latex products and alternative products, see Latex List on the Spina Bifida Association home page,* www.spinabifidaassociation.org.

Spinal Muscular Atrophy

Spinal muscular atrophy (SMA) is a group of disorders characterized by a progressive degeneration of motor neurons, which eventually results in muscle fiber atrophy. The disorder may be manifested early—often at birth—and almost always before 2 years of age; death may occur as a result of respiratory failure by age 2 years (Iannaccone & Burghes, 2002). The manifestations (Box 55-7) and prognosis are categorized according to the age of onset, severity of weakness, and clinical course; for some children, clinical function may fluctuate between exhibiting symptoms of types 1 and 2, or types 2 and 3 (Sarnat, 2007). A severe rare fetal form of SMA, classified as type 0, is reported to be lethal in the perinatal period (Sarnat, 2007).

Spinal Muscular Atrophy Type 1 (Werdnig-Hoffmann Disease)

SMA type 1 (Werdnig-Hoffmann disease) is a disorder characterized by progressive weakness and wasting of skeletal muscles caused by degeneration of anterior horn cells. It is inherited as an autosomal recessive trait and is the most common and most severe paralytic form of the *floppy infant syndrome (congenital hypotonia).* The sites of the pathologic condition are the anterior horn cells of the spinal cord and the motor nuclei of the brainstem, but the primary effect is atrophy of skeletal muscles. The age of onset is variable, but the earlier the onset, the more disseminated and severe the motor weakness.

Diagnostic Evaluation and Therapeutic Management

The diagnosis is based on the molecular genetic marker for the *SMN* (survival motor neuron) gene, which is located on chromosome 5q13. Prenatal diagnosis may be made by genetic analysis of circulating fetal cells in maternal blood (Beroud et al, 2003) or circulating fetal cells in amniotic fluid. The risk of subsequent affected offspring in carriers of the mutant gene or in families with known cases of SMA may also be evaluated genetically. Further diagnostic studies include muscle electromyography (EMG), which demonstrates a denervation pattern, and muscle biopsy; however, genetic analysis has become the gold standard for diagnosis of the condition.

There is no cure for the disease, and treatment is symptomatic and preventive, primarily preventing joint contractures and treating orthopedic problems, the most serious of which is scoliosis. Hip subluxation and dislocation may also occur. Many children benefit from powered chairs, lifts, special pressure-adjustable mattresses, and accessible environmental controls. Muscle and joint contractures require careful attention and care to prevent further complications. Nutritional growth failure (failure to thrive) may occur in infants and toddlers as a result of poor feeding; supplemental gastrostomy feedings may be required to maintain adequate nutritional status and maintain weight gain. The use of lower extremity orthoses may assist with ambulation, but eventually the child may be confined to a wheelchair as muscle atrophy progresses. Sleep-disordered breathing is common in children with SMA and often requires nocturnal mechanical ventilation. Noninvasive ventilation methods such as bilevel positive airway pressure (BiPAP) have decreased the morbidity and increased the survival rate of children with SMA types 1 and 2. Upper respiratory tract infections may occur and are treated with antibiotic therapy.

Prognosis

Prognosis varies according to age of onset or group as described in Box 55-7. Individuals with SMA type 1 may succumb to respiratory tract infections or failure between 1 and 24 months of age (Iannaccone & Burghes, 2002); however, some may live into their third or fourth decade of life. A significant number of infants with SMA require a tracheotomy, and associated medical conditions in survivors include gastroesophageal reflux, scoliosis, early onset puberty, hip dysplasia, and recurrent oral candidiasis (Bach, 2007).

❋ Nursing Care Management

The infant or small child with progressive muscle weakness requires nursing care similar to that of the immobilized patient (see Chapter 54). However, the underlying goal of treatment should be to assist the child and family in dealing with the illness while progressing toward a life of normalization within the child's capabilities. Special attention should be directed to preventing muscle and joint contractures, promoting independence in performance of ADLs, and incorporating the child into the mainstream of school when possible. In addition, parents need support and resources to be able to provide for the child and remain an intact family. Because children with neuromuscular disease have abnormal breathing patterns that often contribute to early death, it is important to assess adequate oxygenation, especially during the sleep phase when shallow breathing occurs and hypoxemia may develop. Home pulse oximetry may be used to assess the child during sleep and provide noninvasive ventilation as necessary (Young et al, 2007; Bush et al, 2005) (see Duchenne [Pseudohypertrophic] Muscular Dystrophy, p. 1733, for respiratory management). Supportive care also includes management of orthoses and other orthopedic equipment as required. Because children with SMA are intellectually normal, verbal, tactile, and auditory stimulation are important aspects of developmental care. Supporting them so that they can see the activities around them and transporting them in appropriate conveyances (e.g., wagon, power wheelchair) for a change of environment provide stimulation and a broader scope of contacts.

Children who are able to sit require proper support and attention to alignment to prevent deformities and other complications. Children who survive beyond infancy will need attention to educational needs and opportunities for social interaction with other children. The parents of a child who is chronically ill require much support and encouragement* (see Chapter 41). Parents who have not sought genetic counseling should be encouraged to do so to evaluate further risk potential.

Spinal Muscular Atrophy Type 3 (Kugelberg-Welander Disease)

SMA type 3 (Kugelberg-Welander disease) is a result of anterior horn cell and motor nerve degeneration. The disease is characterized by a pattern of muscular weakness similar to that of type 1 SMA (see Box 55-7). Several modes of inheritance have been reported for the disease: autosomal recessive, autosomal dominant, and X-linked recessive.

The onset occurs from younger than 1 year of age into adulthood, with symptoms resembling those of type 1 SMA. Proximal muscle weakness (especially of the lower limbs) and muscular atrophy are the predominant features. The disease runs a slowly progressive course. Some children lose the ability to walk 8 to 9 years after the onset of symptoms, but many can still walk after 30 years or more. Many affected persons have a normal life expectancy (Iannaccone, 1998).

**Family resources for SMA include Families of Spinal Muscular Atrophy, PO Box 196, Libertyville, IL 60048; 800-886-1762;* www.fsma.org; *and Muscular Dystrophy Association–USA, 3300 E. Sunrise Drive, Tucson, AZ 85718; 800-572-1717;* www.mda.org. *In Canada: Families of Spinal Muscular Atrophy Canada, PO Box 97, Rivers, MB R0K 1X0; 800-866-0016;* www.curesma.ca.

Therapeutic Management and Nursing Care Management

The management is primarily symptomatic and supportive and is related to maintaining mobility as long as possible, preventing complications such as skin breakdown, optimizing and maintaining respiratory function, and providing support to the child and family.

Muscular Dystrophies

Muscular dystrophies (MDs) constitute the largest and most important single group of muscle diseases of childhood. The MDs have a genetic origin in which there is gradual degeneration of muscle fibers, and they are characterized by progressive weakness and wasting of symmetric groups of skeletal muscles, with increasing disability and deformity. In all forms of MD there is insidious loss of strength, but each type differs in regard to muscle groups affected (Fig. 55-7), age of onset, rate of progression, and inheritance pattern. The most common form, *Duchenne muscular dystrophy (DMD),* is considered separately in the next section.

Facioscapulohumeral (Landouzy-Dejerine) MD is inherited as an autosomal dominant disorder with onset in early adolescence. It is characterized by difficulty in raising the arms over the head, lack of facial mobility, and a forward slope of the shoulders. The progression is slow, and the life span is usually unaffected.

Limb-girdle muscular dystrophy is an autosomal recessive disease of later childhood, adolescence, or early adulthood with variable but usually slow progression. It is characterized by weakness of proximal muscles of the pelvic and shoulder girdles.

Treatment of the MDs consists mainly of supportive measures, including physical therapy, orthopedic procedures to minimize deformity, ventilation support, and assistance for the affected child in meeting the demands of daily living.

Duchenne (Pseudohypertrophic) Muscular Dystrophy

DMD is the most severe and the most common MD of childhood. It is inherited as an X-linked recessive trait, and the single-gene defect is located on the short arm of the X chromosome. DMD has a reportedly high mutation rate, with a positive family history in 65% of all cases (Thompson & Berenson, 2001); therefore genetic counseling is an important aspect of the care of the family.

As in all X-linked disorders, males are affected almost exclusively. At the genetic level, both DMD and Becker's MD (a milder variant) result from mutations of the gene that encodes dystrophin, a protein product in skeletal muscle. Dystrophin is absent from the muscle of children with DMD and is reduced or abnormal in children with Becker's MD. Children with Becker's MD have a later onset of symptoms, which are usually not as severe as those seen in DMD. The incidence is approximately 1 in 3600 male births for the Duchenne form and approximately 1 in 30,000 live births for the Becker type (Sarnat, 2007; Thompson & Berenson, 2001). Box 55-8 describes the characteristics of DMD.

Most children with DMD reach the appropriate developmental milestones early in life, although they may have mild, subtle delays. Evidence of muscle weakness usually appears during the third to seventh year, although there may have been a history of delay in motor development, particularly walking. Difficulties in running, riding a bicycle, and climbing stairs are usually the first symptoms noted. Later, abnormal gait on a level surface becomes apparent. In the early years, rapid developmental gains may mask the progression of the disease.

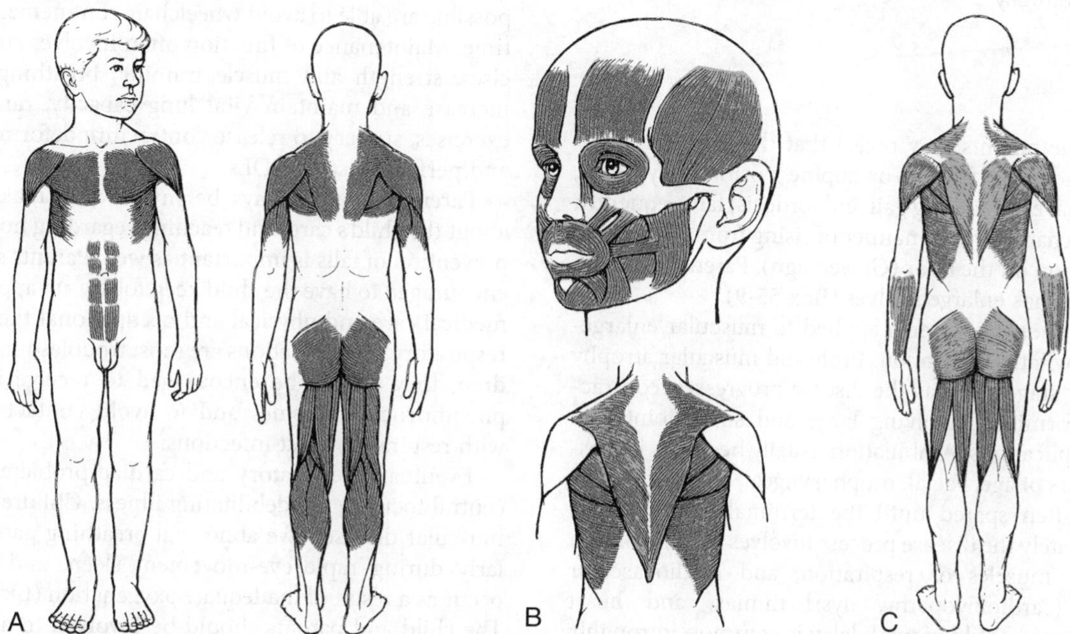

Fig. 55-7 Initial muscle groups involved in muscular dystrophies. A, Pseudohypertrophic. B, Facioscapulohumeral. C, Limb-girdle.

BOX 55-8 Characteristics of Duchenne Muscular Dystrophy

- Early onset, usually between 3 and 5 years of age
- Progressive muscular weakness, wasting, and contractures
- Calf muscle hypertrophy in most patients
- Loss of independent ambulation by 9 to 11 years of age
- Slowly progressive, generalized weakness during teenage years
- Relentless progression until death from respiratory or cardiac failure

BOX 55-9 Clinical Manifestations of Duchenne Muscular Dystrophy

Waddling gait
Lordosis
Frequent falls
Gower sign (child turning onto side or abdomen, flexing knees to assume a kneeling position, then with knees extended gradually pushing torso to an upright position by "walking" the hands up the legs)
Enlarged muscles (especially thighs and upper arms); feel unusually firm or woody on palpation
Later stages: profound muscular atrophy
Cognitive impairment (common)

- Mild (about 20 IQ points below normal)
- Cognitive impairment present in 25% to 30% of patients

Complications:

- Contracture deformities of hips, knees, and ankles
- Disuse atrophy
- Obesity

Questioning the parents may reveal that the child has difficulty in rising from a sitting or supine position. Typically, affected boys have a waddling gait and lordosis, fall frequently, and develop a characteristic manner of rising from a squatting or sitting position on the floor (Gower sign). Parents may also notice the child has enlarged calves (Box 55-9).

Pseudohypertrophy is a term applied to muscular enlargement caused by fatty infiltration. Profound muscular atrophy occurs in later stages, and as the disease progresses, contractures and deformities involving large and small joints are common complications. Ambulation usually becomes impossible by 12 years of age. Facial, oropharyngeal, and respiratory muscles are often spared until the terminal stages of the disease. Ultimately the disease process involves the diaphragm and auxiliary muscles of respiration, and cardiovascular involvement (cardiomyopathy, dysrhythmias, and heart failure) is common. Mild mental delay is common in roughly 30% of all individuals with MD, and many will have permanent learning disabilities; however, children with DMD should be involved in early learning programs and eventually moved into regular classrooms as much as possible. The eventual cause of death is usually respiratory tract infection or cardiac failure; however, much progress has been made in providing ventilatory methods to prolong and maintain quality of life.

Diagnostic Evaluation

The diagnosis of DMD is primarily established by blood polymerase chain reaction (PCR) for the dystrophin gene mutation (Sarnat, 2007). Prenatal diagnosis is also possible as early as 12 weeks of gestation. Serum enzyme measurement, muscle biopsy, and EMG may also be used in establishing the diagnosis. Serum creatine kinase levels are extremely high in the first 2 years of life, before the onset of clinical weakness. If the child demonstrates the usual characteristics, has a positive family history for DMD, and the PCR is positive, the muscle biopsy may be deferred.

Therapeutic Management

No effective treatment exists for childhood MD. The use of the corticosteroids prednisone and deflazacort has been evaluated as a treatment for DMD. Several clinical trials demonstrated increased muscle strength and improved performance and pulmonary function, with significant decrease in the progression of weakness, when prednisone was administered for 6 months. The American Academy of Neurology has published a practice parameter for the administration of corticosteroids in the treatment of DMD (Moxley et al, 2005). Major side effects in these studies included weight gain and a cushingoid facial appearance. Deflazacort caused less weight gain than prednisone and was effective in decreasing muscle wasting in some children (Angelini, 2007). Deflazacort is not available in the United States but is in Canada.

Maintaining optimum function in all muscles for as long as possible is the primary goal; secondary is the prevention of contractures. Children with DMD who remain as active as possible are able to avoid wheelchair confinement for a longer time. Maintenance of function often involves stretching exercises, strength and muscle training, breathing exercises to increase and maintain vital lung capacity, range-of-motion exercises, surgery to release contracture deformities, bracing, and performance of ADLs.

Parents should always be involved in making decisions about the child's care, and teaching regarding home safety and prevention of falls is important as well. Parents should also be encouraged to have the child keep follow-up appointments for medical care and physical and occupational therapy. Because respiratory tract infections are most troublesome in these children, they should be encouraged to receive influenza and pneumococcal vaccines and to avoid contact with persons with respiratory tract infections.

Eventually respiratory and cardiac problems become the central focus of the debilitating illness. Children with neuromuscular disease have abnormal breathing patterns, particularly during rapid-eye-movement sleep, and hypoxia may occur as a result of inadequate oxygenation (Birnkrant, 2002). The child and parents should be involved in a discussion of long-term ventilation options. Cardiac and respiratory assessment during wake-sleep cycles is imperative. Respiratory care for children with neuromuscular conditions such as SMA and

DMD may involve the use of noninvasive ventilation with BiPAP on a temporary or full-time basis, mechanically assisted coughing (MAC), or tracheotomy and relief of airway obstruction with coughing and suctioning devices; the tracheotomy, however, is associated with more complications (Simonds, 2006; Young et al, 2007). Home pulse oximetry may be used to monitor oxygenation during sleep or to aid in decision making regarding the use of MAC to clear the airways.

Several devices are available for children with neuromuscular disease to assist in clearing the airway when the cough reflex is ineffective or diminished. The mechanical cough in-exsufflator (MIE) has been evaluated and found to be safe and effective in the daily management of respiratory function (Miske et al, 2004). The MIE delivers positive inspiratory pressures at a set rate, followed by negative pressure exsufflation coordinated with the patient's own breathing rhythm; the exsufflation is designed to mimic a cough reflex so mucus can be effectively cleared. Airway suctioning after exsufflation is accomplished as necessary to clear the airways. In children the MIE may be connected directly to a tracheostomy or used with a mouthpiece or face mask.

Survival in individuals with DMD may be prolonged several years with the use of noninvasive ventilation and MAC as alternatives to tracheotomy and airway suctioning (Simonds, 2006). The American Thoracic Society (2004) has published extensive guidelines for respiratory monitoring and care of children and adults with DMD.

The American Academy of Pediatrics (2005) recommends an extensive cardiac evaluation of the child diagnosed with either DMD or Becker MD. Patients with neuromuscular conditions may not have the typical signs and symptoms of cardiac dysfunction. Therefore symptoms such as weight loss, nausea and vomiting, cough, increased fatigue on performance of ADLs, and orthopnea should be carefully evaluated to detect early signs of cardiomyopathy.

Genetic counseling is also recommended for parents, sisters, and maternal aunts and their daughters. Long-term care, end-of-life directives, and palliative care options are issues that must be discussed with the child and family affected by MD. Professional counseling may be required to allow frank discussion of these issues in some cases, and referrals should be made as appropriate.

Research evaluating a number of treatments for DMD is in progress. These include clinical trials with glutamine and creatine monohydrate to preserve muscle strength; utrophin, a protein that is similar to dystrophin and in large quantities may counteract the effects of the deficiency of dystrophin (Chakkalakal et al, 2005); and the enzyme CT GalNAc transferase, which blocks muscle wasting in mice (Metules, 2002).

Nursing Care Management

The major emphasis of nursing care is to help the child and family cope with a chronic, progressive, incapacitating disease; to help design a program that will afford maximal independence and reduce the predictable and preventable disabilities associated with the disorder; and to help the child and family deal constructively with the limitations the disease imposes on their daily lives. Because of advances in technology, children with MD may live into early adulthood; therefore the goals of care should also involve decisions regarding quality of life, achievement of independence, and transition to adulthood.

Working closely with other team members, nurses assist the family in developing the child's self-help skills to give the child the satisfaction of being as independent as possible for as long as possible. This requires continual evaluation of the child's capabilities, which are often difficult to assess. Fortunately, most children with MD instinctively recognize the need to become as independent as possible and strive to do so.

Practical difficulties faced by families are physical limitations of housing and mobility. Some families live in houses or apartments that are unsuited to wheelchairs. Transportation may also be a barrier for families of children with MD. Assisting with these challenges requires team problem solving. Diet, nutritional needs, and nutrition modification are discussed according to the needs of the individual child and family.

The parents' social activities are also restricted, and the family's activities must be continually modified to accommodate the needs of the affected child. When the child becomes increasingly incapacitated, the family may consider home-based care, an assisted living facility, or respite care. Unless the child is severely incapacitated, he should also be involved in the decisions regarding such care. Nurses can assist with decision making by exploring all available options and resources and supporting the child and family in the decision. Older boys with MD may also need psychiatric or psychologic counseling to deal with issues such as depression, anger, and quality of life. Parents also need to be encouraged to become involved in support groups because adequate social support from family, community, and other parents is crucial to appropriate coping in families with children with chronic illness.

Regardless of how successful the program or how well the family adapts to the disorder, superimposed on the physical and emotional problems associated with a child with a long-term disability is the constant knowledge of the ultimate outcome of the disease. All the manifestations seen in the child with a chronic fatal illness are encountered in these families (see Chapter 41).

Nurses are especially valuable health professionals as they come to know the family and the family's problems. Nurses can be alert to the family's problems and needs and make necessary referrals when supplementary services are indicated. The Muscular Dystrophy Association–USA* has branches in most communities to assist families in which there is a member with MD.

Acquired Neuromuscular Disorders

Guillain-Barré Syndrome (Infectious Polyneuritis)

Guillain-Barré syndrome (GBS), also known as infectious polyneuritis, is an uncommon acute demyelinating polyneuropathy with a progressive, usually ascending flaccid paralysis.

*See footnote, p. 1732. In Canada: Muscular Dystrophy Canada, 2345 Yonge St., Suite 900, Toronto, ON M4P 2E5; 866-MUSCLE-8; fax: 416-488-7523; www.muscle.ca.

evolve Animation—Guillain-Barré Syndrome

Children are affected less often than adults; among children, those between ages 4 and 10 years have higher susceptibility. The male/female ratio is reported to be 1.5:1. Two peak time periods have been identified with an increased incidence of GBS: late adolescence and young adulthood. The incidence is also increased in pregnant and postpartum women (Newswanger & Warren, 2004).

Congenital GBS is rare yet may be seen in the neonatal period and consists of hypotonia, weakness, and decreased or absent reflexes; maternal neuromuscular disease may or may not be present. Diagnosis is established by the same criteria as in older children, but the symptoms gradually subside over the first few months of life and disappear by 12 months (Sarnat, 2007).

Pathophysiology

GBS is an immune-mediated disease often associated with a number of viral or bacterial infections or the administration of certain vaccines. It has been associated with infectious mononucleosis, measles, mumps, *Campylobacter jejuni* (gastroenteritis), cytomegalovirus, *Borrelia burgdorferi* (Lyme disease), Epstein-Barr virus, *Helicobacter pylori,* and *Mycoplasma* and *Pneumocystis* infections. Onset of GBS symptoms usually occurs within 10 days of the primary infection. Pathologic changes in spinal and cranial nerves consist of inflammation and edema with rapid, segmented demyelination and compression of nerve roots within the dural sheath. Nerve conduction is impaired, producing ascending partial or complete paralysis of muscles innervated by the involved nerves. GBS has three phases (Sulton, 2002):

1. *Acute*—Phase starts when symptoms begin and continues until new symptoms stop appearing or deterioration ceases; it may last as long as 4 weeks.
2. *Plateau*—Symptoms remain constant without further deterioration; it may last from days to weeks.
3. *Recovery*—Patient begins to improve and progress to optimum recovery; it usually lasts a few weeks to months depending on the deficits incurred by the illness.

Diagnostic Evaluation

Diagnosis of GBS is based on clinical manifestations (Box 55-10), CSF analysis, and EMG findings. CSF analysis reveals an increased protein concentration, and EMG shows evidence of acute muscle denervation; other laboratory studies are usually noncontributory. The symmetric nature of the paralysis helps differentiate this disorder from spinal paralytic poliomyelitis, which usually affects sporadic muscles.

Therapeutic Management

Treatment of GBS is primarily supportive. In the acute phase patients are hospitalized because respiratory and pharyngeal involvement may require assisted ventilation, sometimes with a temporary tracheotomy. Treatment modalities include aggressive ventilatory support, intravenous administration of immunoglobulin (IVIG), and steroids; plasmapheresis and immunosuppressive drugs may also be used. Plasmapheresis has been shown to decrease the length of recovery in patients with severe GBS yet is expensive, and side effects include hypotension, fever, bleeding disorders, chills, urticaria, and bradycardia. Further evidence reports equal benefits to treatment of GBS with IVIG administration or plasmapheresis; both sped up recovery time in studies reviewed (Hughes & Cornblath, 2005). Corticosteroids alone did not decrease the symptoms or shorten the duration of the disease. CSF filtration has been used in patients with GBS with some success; CSF is removed, filtered, and replaced into the patient. This process presumably removes toxins and bacteria; however, further studies are needed to evaluate this treatment modality (Atkinson et al, 2006).

Medications that may be administered during the acute phase include a low-molecular-weight heparin to prevent deep vein thrombosis, a mild laxative or stool softener to prevent constipation, pain medication such as acetaminophen, and a histamine-antagonist to prevent stress ulcer formation. Chronic neuropathic pain following GBS may be treated with gabapentin, which is reported to be more effective than carbamazepine (Sarnat, 2007).

Course and Prognosis

Better outcomes are associated with younger age, no requirement for mechanical respiratory assistance, slower progression of disease, normal peripheral nerve function on EMG, and treatment with either IVIG or plasmapheresis. Recovery usually begins within 2 to 3 weeks, and most patients regain full muscle strength. The recovery of muscle strength progresses in the reverse order of onset of paralysis, with lower extremity strength being the last to recover. Poor prognosis with subsequent residual effects in children is reportedly associated with cranial nerve involvement, extensive disability at time of presentation, and intubation.

Most deaths associated with GBS are caused by respiratory failure; therefore early diagnosis and access to respiratory

BOX 55-10 Clinical Manifestations of Guillain-Barré Syndrome

Initial Symptoms

Muscle tenderness
Paresthesia and cramps (sometimes)
Proximal symmetric muscle weakness

Paralysis

Ascending bilateral paralysis from lower extremities
Frequent involvement of muscles of trunk and upper extremities and those supplied by cranial nerves (especially facial)
Flaccid paralysis with loss of reflexes
May involve facial, extraocular, labial, lingual, pharyngeal, and laryngeal muscles
Intercostal and phrenic nerves:
- Breathlessness in vocalizations
- Shallow, irregular respirations

Other Manifestations

Tendon reflexes depressed or absent
Variable degrees of sensory impairment
Muscle tenderness or sensitivity to slight pressure
Urinary incontinence or retention and constipation

support are especially important. The rate of recovery is usually related to the degree of involvement and may extend from a few weeks to months. The greater the degree of paralysis, the longer the recovery phase.

Nursing Care Management

Nursing care is essentially supportive and is the same as that required for the child with immobilization and respiratory depression. The emphasis of care is on close observation to assess the extent of paralysis and on prevention of complications, including autonomic dysfunction (hypertension, orthostatic hypotension, syndrome of inappropriate antidiuretic hormone secretion, life-threatening dysrhythmias), respiratory dysfunction, fear and anxiety, and pain.

During the acute phase of GBS the child's condition should be carefully observed for possible difficulty in swallowing and respiratory involvement. The child's respiratory function is closely monitored, and oxygen source, appropriate-sized resuscitation bag and mask, endotracheal intubation and suctioning equipment, tracheotomy tray, and vasoconstrictor drugs are kept available. Vital signs, including neurologic signs and level of consciousness, are monitored frequently. For the child who develops respiratory impairment, the care is the same as that for any child with respiratory distress requiring mechanical ventilation.

Throughout the recovery phase, special emphasis is placed on prevention of complications, including proper postural alignment, frequent change of position, assessment of skin at pressure points, and passive range-of-motion exercises. Respiratory care, should intubation be required, requires close monitoring of oxygenation status, usually by pulse oximetry and arterial blood gases; maintenance of an open airway with suctioning; and postural changes to prevent pneumonia. Children with oral and pharyngeal involvement may be fed via a nasogastric tube to ensure adequate feeding. Immobilization, which occurs with GBS, decreases gastrointestinal function; therefore problems such as decreased gastric emptying and constipation require nursing assessment and appropriate collaborative interventions.

Prevention of deep vein thrombosis is accomplished with sequential compression (antiembolism) devices, administration of a low-molecular-weight heparin, and early mobilization and ambulation. Temporary urinary catheterization may be required; urinary retention is not uncommon, and appropriate assessment of urine output is vital. Sensory impairment and paralysis in the lower extremities make the child susceptible to skin breakdown; therefore attention should be given to meticulous skin care. Although the child may have a generalized paralysis, cognitive function remains intact; therefore it is important for nursing care to involve communication with the child regarding procedures and treatments that may be frightening, especially if mechanical ventilation is required. Parents are encouraged to talk to the child and make eye and physical contact as much as possible to reassure the child during the illness. Psychosocial care of the child with GBS focuses on dealing with the child's anxiety and fear related to the disease itself and the unknown prognosis. In addition, the child's parents are allowed to express feelings and are encouraged to be involved in the child's daily care.

Pain management is essential in the care of children with GBS. Although neuromuscular impairment may make pain perception more difficult to accurately evaluate, objective pain scales should be used.

Physical therapy is limited to passive range-of-motion exercises during the evolving phase of the disease. Later, as the disease stabilizes and recovery begins, an active physical therapy program is implemented to prevent contracture deformities and facilitate muscle recovery. This may include active exercise, gait training, and bracing.

Throughout the course of the illness, support of the child and parents is paramount. The usual rapidity of the paralysis and the long period of recovery greatly tax the emotional reserves of all family members. The parents and child benefit from repeated reassurance that recovery is occurring and from realistic information regarding the possibility of permanent disability. In the event of a residual disability, the family needs assistance in accepting and adjusting to the loss of function (see Chapter 41). The GBS/CIDP Foundation International* is a nonprofit organization devoted to support, education, and research. It provides support to families from recovered persons, publishes informational literature and a newsletter, and maintains a list of practitioners experienced with the disease.

Tetanus

Tetanus, or lockjaw, is an acute, preventable, but often fatal disease caused by an exotoxin produced by the anaerobic spore-forming, gram-positive bacillus *Clostridium tetani*. It is characterized by painful muscular rigidity primarily involving the masseter and neck muscles. There are four requirements for the development of tetanus: (1) presence of tetanus spores or vegetative forms of the bacillus, (2) injury to the tissues, (3) wound conditions that encourage multiplication of the organism, and (4) a susceptible host.

Tetanus spores are found in soil; dust; and the intestinal tracts of humans and animals, especially herbivorous animals. The organisms are more prevalent in rural areas but are readily carried to urban areas by the wind. The organisms are not invasive but enter the body by way of wounds, particularly a puncture wound, burn, or crushed area. They may enter through a minor, unnoticed break in the skin, such as a thorn or needle prick, bee sting, or scratch. In the newborn, infection may occur through the umbilical cord, usually in situations in which infants are delivered in severely contaminated surroundings or the mother is not adequately immunized. The disease has the greatest incidence in months when persons are more involved in outdoor activities.

Pathophysiology

When prevention efforts are not effective and conditions are favorable, the organisms proliferate and form potent exotoxins, one of which is tetanospasmin. Tetanospasmin affects the central nervous system to produce the clinical manifestations of the disease. The ideal conditions for the organisms' growth are devitalized tissues without access to air, such as wounds

The Holly Building, 104½ Forrest Ave., Narberth, PA 19072; 610-667-0131 or 866-224-3301; http://gbs-cidp.org.

that have not been washed or kept clean and those that have crusted over, trapping pus beneath. The exotoxin appears to reach the central nervous system by way of either the neuron axons or the vascular system. The toxin becomes fixed on nerve cells of the anterior horn of the spinal cord and the brainstem. The toxin acts at the myoneural junction to produce muscular stiffness and lower the threshold for reflex excitability.

The incubation period for tetanus varies from 2 days to months and averages 8 days; most cases occur within 14 days. In neonates it is usually 5 to 14 days. Shorter incubation periods have been associated with more heavily contaminated wounds, more severe disease, and a worse prognosis (American Academy of Pediatrics, Committee on Infectious Diseases, 2009).

The manner of onset varies, but the initial symptoms are usually a progressive stiffness and tenderness of the muscles in the neck and jaw. Eventually all voluntary muscles are affected (Box 55-11). As the child recovers from the disease, the paroxysms become less frequent and gradually subside. Survival beyond 4 days usually indicates recovery, but complete recovery may require weeks.

Therapeutic Management

Preventive measures are based on the child's immune status and the nature of the injury. Specific prophylactic therapy after trauma is administration of *tetanus toxoid* (equine tetanus antitoxin is not available in the United States) (see Immunizations, Chapter 36, for age-specific recommendations).

The unprotected or inadequately immunized child who sustains a "tetanus-prone" wound (including wounds contaminated with dirt, feces, soil, and saliva; puncture wounds; avulsions; and wounds resulting from missiles, crushing, burns, and frostbite) should receive *tetanus immunoglobulin (TIG)*. Concurrent administration of both TIG and tetanus toxoid at separate sites is recommended both to provide protection and to initiate the active immune process. Once the individual has received primary tetanus immunization, antitoxin (human) is believed to provide protection for at least 10 years and for a longer period after booster immunization (American Academy of Pediatrics, Committee on Infectious Diseases, 2009). Completion of active immunization is carried out according to the usual pattern. Antibiotic treatment with oral or intravenous metronidazole (Flagyl) (alternatively parenteral penicillin G) is important in the management of tetanus as an adjunct against vegetative forms of clostridia (American Academy of Pediatrics, Committee on Infectious Diseases, 2009).

Aggressive supportive care is necessary to treat tetanus in the acute phase. The acutely ill child is best treated in an intensive care facility where close and constant observation and equipment for monitoring and respiratory support are readily available. A quiet environment is desirable to reduce the amount of stimuli on the central nervous system.

General supportive care is indicated, including maintaining adequate airway and fluid and electrolyte balance, managing pain, and ensuring adequate caloric intake. Indwelling oral or nasogastric feedings may be required to maintain adequate fluid and caloric intake; continued laryngospasm may necessitate total parenteral nutrition or gastrostomy feeding. Severe or recurrent laryngospasm or excessive secretions may require advanced airway management such as endotracheal intubation.

TIG therapy to neutralize toxins is the most specific therapy for tetanus. Antibiotics are administered to control the proliferation of the vegetative forms of the organism at the site of infection. Local care of the wound by surgical debridement and cleansing helps reduce the numbers of proliferating organisms at the site of injury. The cleansing should be repeated several times during the first 48 hours, and deep, infected lacerations are usually exposed and debrided.

Diazepam is the drug of choice for seizure control and muscle relaxation (Arnon, 2007b), but lorazepam (Ativan) may be used in some cases. Other AEDs may be administered as well. Intrathecal baclofen, magnesium sulfate, dantrolene sodium, and midazolam may also be used in the management of tetanus. Patients with severe tetanus and those who do not respond to other muscle relaxants may require the administration of a neuromuscular blocking agent, such as rocuronium or vecuronium; intrathecal baclofen may be used as a muscle relaxant but only in the intensive care unit, since it often induces apnea. Because of their paralytic effect on respiratory muscles, use of these drugs requires mechanical ventilation with endotracheal intubation or tracheotomy and constant cardiopulmonary monitoring. Endotracheal tube insertion or tracheostomy should be performed before severe respiratory

BOX 55-11 Clinical Manifestations of Tetanus

Initial Symptoms

Progressive stiffness and tenderness of muscles in neck and jaw

Characteristic difficulty in opening the mouth (trismus)

Risus sardonicus (sardonic smile) caused by facial muscle spasm

Progressive Involvement

Opisthotonic positioning

Boardlike rigidity of abdominal and limb muscles

Difficulty swallowing

High sensitivity to external stimuli (slight noise, gentle touch, or bright light):

- Trigger paroxysmal muscular contractions that last seconds to minutes
- Contractions recur with increased frequency until almost continuous (sustained tetanic)

Laryngospasm and tetany of respiratory muscles:

- Accumulated secretions
- Respiratory arrest
- Atelectasis
- Pneumonia

Other Aspects

Mentation unaffected; patient alert

Pain and distress are reflected in:

- Rapid pulse
- Sweating
- Anxious expression

Fever usually absent or only mild

distress develops. Despite the absence of pain manifestation with these drugs, it is important to administer adequate analgesia. The administration of corticosteroids has met with success in some cases.

Nursing Care Management

The care of the child with tetanus requires supportive management with particular attention to airway and breathing. Respiratory status is carefully evaluated for any signs of distress, and appropriate emergency equipment is kept available at all times. The location, extent, and severity of muscle spasms are important nursing observations. Muscle relaxants, opioids, and sedatives that may be prescribed can also cause respiratory depression; therefore the child must be assessed for excessive central nervous system depression. Attention to hydration and nutrition involves monitoring an intravenous infusion, monitoring nasogastric or gastrostomy feedings, and suctioning oropharyngeal secretions when indicated.

In caring for the child with tetanus during the acute phase, the nurse makes every effort to control or eliminate stimulation from sound, light, and touch. Although a darkened room is ideal, sufficient light is essential so that the child can be carefully observed; light appears to be less irritating than vibratory or auditory stimuli. The infant or child is handled as little as possible, and extra effort is expended to avoid any sudden or loud noise to prevent seizures.

If a potent muscle relaxant such as vecuronium is used, the total paralysis makes oral communication impossible. The drug is not a sedative, however, and anxiety should be considered in children who are intubated. Therefore all the child's needs must be anticipated and procedures carefully explained beforehand.

Because their mental status is clear, children are aware of what is happening to them and are often extremely anxious. They should not be left alone, and all efforts should be made to reduce anxiety, which can contribute to muscle spasms. Parents are encouraged to stay with the child to offer security and support. They also need support, information and reassurance from the nurse.

Botulism

Botulism is an acute flaccid paralysis caused by the preformed toxin produced by the anaerobic bacillus *Clostridium botulinum*. In classic, or foodborne, botulism the most common source of the toxin is a contaminated food source. In addition to foodborne botulism, other forms include wound botulism; infant botulism; and man-made botulism, usually a result of bioterrorism (Arnon, 2007a). In foodborne illness, central nervous system symptoms appear abruptly within a few hours or gradually over several days after ingestion of contaminated food and may not be preceded by acute digestive disturbance (Box 55-12).

Treatment consists of intravenous administration of botulism antitoxin and general supportive measures, primarily respiratory and nutritional. Toxins vary in protein-binding capacity. Some have a relatively short half-life and do not bind to tissues firmly; therefore therapy is continued until paralysis abates. Other toxins appear to bind irreversibly to nerve endings and are therefore not amenable to neutralization.

BOX 55-12 Clinical Manifestations of Botulism

General Signs
- Weakness
- Dizziness
- Headache
- Difficulty talking and speaking
- Diplopia
- Vomiting
- Progressive, life-threatening respiratory paralysis

Infant Botulism*
- Constipation (a common symptom)
- Generalized weakness
- Decrease in spontaneous movements
- Diminished or absent deep tendon reflexes
- Loss of head control
- Difficulty feeding
- Weak cry
- Reduced gag reflex
- Progressive respiratory paralysis

*Most commonly diagnosed as a "rule out sepsis" in the acute phase because of clinical presentation.

Infant Botulism

Infant botulism, unlike the disease in older persons, is caused by ingestion of spores or vegetative cells of *C. botulinum* and the subsequent release of the toxin from organisms colonizing the gastrointestinal tract. *C. botulinum* types A and B are the most common causative strains of infant botulism. This form of botulism has become more prevalent than any other form. Many cases of infant botulism occur in breastfed infants who are being introduced to nonhuman milk substances (American Academy of Pediatrics, Committee on Infectious Diseases, 2009). There appears to be no common food or drug source of the organisms; however, the *C. botulinum* organisms have been found in honey. Botulism may occur in infants as young as 1 week of age up to 12 months of age with peak incidence between 2 and 4 months of age.

The severity of the disease varies widely, from mild constipation to progressive sequential loss of neurologic function and respiratory failure (see Box 55-12). The affected infant is usually well before the onset of symptoms. Constipation is a common presenting symptom, and almost all infants exhibit generalized weakness and a decrease in spontaneous movements. Deep tendon reflexes are usually diminished or absent. Cranial nerve deficits are common, as evidenced by loss of head control, difficulty in feeding, weak cry, and reduced gag reflex. SMA type 1 and metabolic disorders are often mistaken for infant botulism in the initial diagnostic phase because of the similarities in clinical manifestations of hypotonia, lethargy, and poor feeding (Francisco & Arnon, 2007). Presenting clinical signs also often mimic those of sepsis in young infants. Botulism toxin exerts its effect by inhibiting the release of acetylcholine at the myoneural junction, thereby impairing motor activity of muscles innervated by affected nerves.

Diagnosis is made on the basis of the clinical history, physical examination, and laboratory detection of the organism in the patient's stool and, less commonly, blood. However, isolation of the organism may take several days; therefore suspicion of botulism by clinical presentation should require emergent treatment (Arnon, 2007a). EMG may be helpful in establishing the diagnosis; however, results may be normal early in the course of the illness.

Treatment consists of immediate administration of botulism immune globulin intravenously (BIG-IV [BabyBIG]) (Francisco & Arnon, 2007), without waiting for laboratory diagnosis. Early administration of BIG-IV neutralizes the toxin and stops the progression of the disease. The human-derived botulism antitoxin (BIG-IV) has been evaluated and is now available nationwide for use only in infant botulism. Infants treated with BIG-IV experienced a mean length of hospitalization decrease from 5.7 to 2.6 weeks and also had decreased time spent in intensive care, decreased mean duration of mechanical ventilation, and decreased mean duration of tube or intravenous feeding. In addition, the infants did not experience any adverse events related to BIG-IV. Most infants received BIG-IV treatment within 3 to 18 days of hospitalization for botulism (Arnon et al, 2006). Approximately 50% of affected infants will require intubation and mechanical ventilation; therefore respiratory support is crucial, as is nutritional support, since the infant is unable to feed. Trivalent equine botulinum antitoxin and bivalent antitoxin, used in adults and older children, is not administered to infants. Antibiotic therapy is not part of the management because the botulinum toxin is an intracellular molecule and antibiotics would not be effective; aminoglycosides in particular should not be administered because they may potentiate the blocking effects of the neurotoxin (Arnon, 2007a).

The prognosis is generally good if the patient is adequately treated, although recovery may be slow, requiring a few weeks after severe illness. The average length of stay for infant botulism is 44 days, and the fatality rate is reported to be less than 2%. Untreated patients may require a longer hospitalization.

NURSING ALERT Although the precise source of *C. botulinum* spores has not been identified as originating from honey in many cases of infant botulism, it is still recommended that honey not be given to infants less than 12 months of age because the spores have been found in honey (Centers for Disease Control and Prevention, 2008).

Nursing Care Management

Nursing responsibilities include observing for and reporting signs of neuromuscular weakness or impairment and providing intensive nursing care when the infant is hospitalized (see Chapter 27). Parental support and reassurance are important. Most infants recover when the disorder is recognized and therapy is implemented. Parents should be aware that, during recovery, patients tire easily when muscular action is sustained. This has important implications for timing the resumption of feedings because of the risk of aspiration. Parents should also be advised that normal bowel activity may not return for several weeks; therefore a stool softener can be beneficial.

Spinal Cord Injuries

SCIs with major neurologic involvement traditionally have not been a common cause of physical disability in children. However, a sufficient number of children with these injuries are admitted to major medical centers, and because of the increased survival rate as a result of improved management, nurses are often involved in the care and rehabilitation of children with SCI.

Mechanisms of Injury

The most common cause of serious spinal cord damage in children is trauma involving motor vehicle crashes (MVCs) (including automobile-bicycle, all-terrain vehicles, and snowmobiles), sports injuries (especially from diving, trampoline activities, gymnastics, and football), birth trauma, and nonaccidental trauma. The increased use of recreational activities involving motorized vehicles such as jet water skis, all-terrain vehicles, and motorcycles has also increased the incidence of SCIs in children. Congenital defects of the spine such as myelomeningocele also may in some cases produce the effects of SCI.

Transverse myelitis (inflammation of the spinal cord) has also been reported to develop from inadvertent intraarterial administration of long-acting penicillin injected into the buttocks. Damage can be extensive enough to result in paraplegia or even lower limb amputation.

In MVCs most SCIs in children are a result of indirect trauma caused by sudden hyperflexion or hyperextension of the neck, often combined with a rotational force. Trauma to the spinal cord without evidence of vertebral fracture or dislocation (SCIWORA) is particularly likely to occur in an MVC when proper safety restraints are not used. An unrestrained child becomes a projectile during sudden deceleration and is subject to injury from contact with a variety of objects inside and outside the vehicle. Individuals who use only a lap seat belt restraint are at greater risk of SCI than those who use a combination lap and shoulder restraint. High cervical spine injuries have been reported in children younger than 2 years of age who are improperly restrained in forward-facing car seats. Infants who are improperly restrained in an infant car seat may experience cervical trauma in a car crash. Small children may also be severely injured by deploying front seat air bags.

Falling from heights occurs less often in children than in adults, but vertebral compression from blows to the head or buttocks can occur in water sports (diving and surfing), falls from horses, or other athletic activities. Birth injuries may occur in breech deliveries from traction force on the spinal cord during delivery of the head and shoulders. When shaken, infants commonly sustain cervical cord damage, as well as subdural hematoma and retinal hemorrhage; cognitive impairment and death may occur subsequent to the traumatic event. Infants have weak neck muscles, and during vigorous shaking their large and heavy heads rapidly wobble back and forth. A significant number of adolescents receive SCIs secondary to gunshot wounds, stabbings, or other violent inflicted injury.

The injury sustained can affect any of the spinal nerves, and the higher the injury, the more extensive the damage. The child can be left with complete or partial paralysis of the lower extremities *(paraplegia)* or with damage at a higher level and without functional use of any of the four extremities *(quadriplegia)*. A high cervical cord injury that affects the phrenic nerve paralyzes the diaphragm and leaves the child dependent on mechanical ventilation.

A mild but equally frightening form of cord trauma is *spinal cord compression,* a temporary neural dysfunction without visible damage to the cord. Complete quadriplegia can result but initially may not be differentiated from serious cord injury.

Therapeutic Management

The management of the child with SCI has changed dramatically in the past two decades as a result of improved technology, surgical procedures, and research into the complexity of the spinal cord and its neurologic components. Initial care begins at the scene of the accident; therefore education and training of first responder personnel in spinal immobilization, stabilization, and transfer techniques to prevent or reduce the severity of injury are critically important. Because of the complexity of these injuries, it is usually recommended that those with injuries be transported to a spinal injury center for care by specially trained health care personnel as soon as possible after the injury for appropriate diagnostic evaluation and intervention.

A number of special pediatric immobilization devices are now available that are physiologically appropriate for children's unique characteristics. A large head (proportionately), weak neck musculature, and weak tracheal cartilage predispose small children to airway compromise if placed supine; hence a spinal board with a built-in head drop may serve to protect the child's spine and neck and provide better airway management than the traditional flat board (DeBoer & Seaver, 2004).

Treatment with *functional electrical stimulation* (an implantable electrical stimulator with leads attached to the paralyzed muscles or nerves) has allowed children with certain SCIs greater mobility and functional use of paralyzed muscles to sit; stand; and walk with the aid of crutches, a walker, or other orthoses. Administration of pharmacologic agents such as clonidine hydrochloride may improve ambulation in patients with partial SCI, and exercise therapy through interactive locomotor training has been beneficial in helping some individuals with SCI regain ambulatory function.

In recent years patients with acute incomplete SCI have benefited from body weight supported treadmill training, which enhances ambulation and gait training (Barker, 2005). This treatment has enabled some wheelchair-bound SCI patients to walk for short distances.

SCI management guidelines and standards of care have recently been published for adult and pediatric patients with spinal injuries by the American Association of Neurological Surgeons and the Congress of Neurological Surgeons. The reader is referred to the Barker and Saulino (2002) reference for a synopsis of the guidelines and a more in-depth review of SCI care, or see "Guidelines for the Management of Acute Cervical Spine and Spinal Cord Injuries" by Hadley and colleagues (2002).

Nursing Care Management

The nursing care of the paraplegic or quadriplegic child is complex and challenging. A multidisciplinary SCI team is equipped to manage the acute phase of the injury, and some members, including the nurse, may follow the patient to eventual recovery. Nursing management is concerned with ensuring adequate initial stabilization of the entire spinal column with a rigid cervical collar with supportive blocks on a rigid backboard. During the acute phase of the injury it is imperative that airway patency be maintained and respiratory function monitored. It is important to evaluate the extent of the neurologic damage early to establish a baseline for neurologic functioning; continual assessment of function should occur to prevent further deterioration of neurologic status as a result of spinal cord edema. The American Spinal Injury Association Impairment Scale may be used to assess neurologic function on a routine basis during the patient's recovery (Barker & Saulino, 2002). Once the patient is admitted, further evaluation of the patient's abilities to perform ADLs can be made with the Functional Independence Measure scale; this scale measures the patient's abilities during recovery and need for assistance (Barker & Saulino, 2002).

In any situation in which SCI is suspected or a possibility, the child should be calmed, reassured, and told not to move; no one should be allowed to move the child unless he or she is able to stabilize the entire spine. A rigid cervical collar is used to immobilize the cervical spine, and the child is placed supine on a rigid immobilization board. Infants and small children may be removed in their car seats; no attempt should be made to take them out of the seat.

The nursing care of the child with an SCI is, in most respects, the same as that of any immobilized child (see The Immobilized Child, Chapter 54). Additional aspects of care that should be addressed on an individual basis include hypercalcemia in adolescent males, deep vein thrombosis, latex sensitization, and sleep-disordered breathing (Vogel et al, 2004).

Respiratory care often focuses on maintaining an adequate airway and effective ventilation. The child with a high-level cervical injury (C3 and above) requires continuous ventilatory assistance. In most instances a tracheostomy is the method of choice for greater ease in clearing secretions and for less trauma to tissues during long-term ventilatory dependence. In some children breathing pacemaker devices (phrenic nerve stimulators) are implanted to stimulate the phrenic nerve and produce diaphragmatic contractions and lung expansion without assisted ventilation. In the child who does not require mechanical ventilation, special attention to clearance of secretions is vital because of decreased pulmonary function. In addition to chest physiotherapy, the child may require a cough-assist device to clear secretions effectively (see Duchenne [Pseudohypertrophic] Muscular Dystrophy: Therapeutic Management).

Temperature is often poorly regulated in children with SCI; therefore body temperature must be monitored closely for fluctuations. Response to environmental temperature changes may be slow or absent, and the ability to dissipate heat through the process of shivering may be compromised.

Children with SCI have unique needs in relation to skin care. Because of decreased sensation and impaired mobility, they depend on others to assess and assist in the management of intact skin. Skin care practices are the same as those for any child who is immobilized. A skin score scale such as the

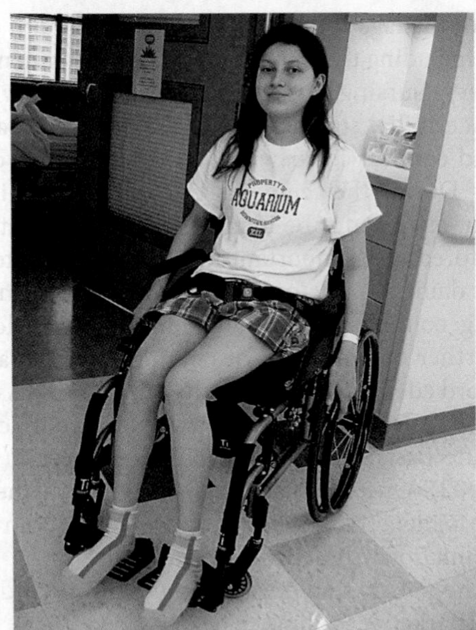
AQUARIUM

Fig. 55-8 Wheelchair allows adolescent mobility and independence. *(Courtesy Texas Children's Hospital, Houston.)*

Braden Q Scale should be used to objectively evaluate risks for skin breakdown and skin conditions (Curley et al, 2003). An alternating-pressure mattress or other pressure relief or reduction device is kept underneath the child, and the skin is thoroughly inspected at least once a day (or more often if there is increased risk) for signs of pressure and breakdown, especially over bony prominences.

Bowel and bladder function is often affected in the child with SCI. CIC may be required to regularly empty the neurogenic bladder and prevent urinary tract infections. A regular bowel management program is tailored to the child's needs.

All adaptive devices help children increase their mobility, function, and endurance. The child with some lower extremity function progresses to parallel bars and then to a walker; the child with quadriplegia learns to use a wheelchair—among the most valuable aids available to the child with an SCI (Fig. 55-8). The wheelchair should be selected carefully in relation to where it will be used, the architectural barriers, and the child's functional capacity. For children with severe upper extremity paralysis, a variety of motorized wheelchairs are used; however, the more complex they are, the greater their cost, weight, and tendency to break down. Wheelchair tolerance is gained over time and is accompanied by measures to prevent orthostatic hypotension and pressure ulcers.

A variety of orthoses and other appliances can be adapted for use by many children. The primary purpose of lower extremity bracing in the child with an SCI is for ambulation, although correction of deformities may be attempted.

During the recovery and rehabilitation phase, patients with SCI must be carefully monitored for complications of immobility such as deep vein thrombosis and pulmonary embolus.

The child and family with SCI are prepared for the eventual discharge from the acute care facility to a rehabilitation center. The major aims of physical rehabilitation are to prepare the child and family to achieve normalization and resume life at home and in the community. Additional goals of rehabilitation in children with SCI are to promote independence in mobility and self-care skills, academic achievement, independent living, and employment.

The nurse is a crucial member of the health care team in helping the family cope with the magnitude of the injury and disability, understand the extent of the disability, verbalize expected outcomes, and move toward eventual rehabilitation and normalization within the child's capabilities. The goals of rehabilitation include preparing the child and family to live at home and function as independently as possible.

Key Points

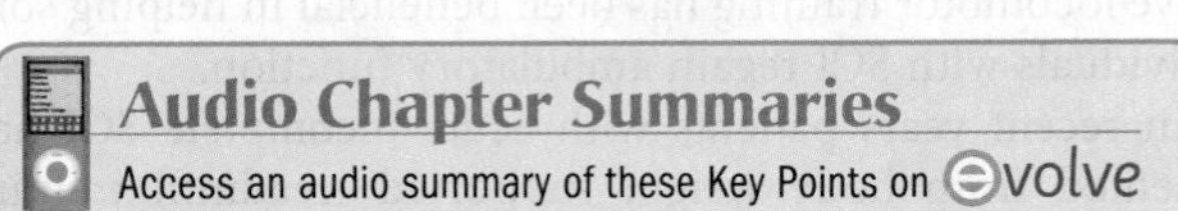
Audio Chapter Summaries
Access an audio summary of these Key Points on evolve

- Clinical manifestations of CP include delayed gross motor development; abnormal motor performance; alterations of muscle tone; abnormal postures; reflex abnormalities; and associated disabilities such as cognitive impairment, seizures, and sensory impairment.
- Therapy for CP takes into account the nature of the physical disability, defects associated with the disorder, and interpersonal and social influences encountered by the affected child.
- Care of the infant and child with myelomeningocele is directed toward protecting the meningeal sac, preventing infection and skin breakdown, observing for signs of urologic and bowel complications, and planning appropriate interventions to optimize the child's development.
- SMA is characterized by progressive weakness and wasting of skeletal muscles caused by degeneration of anterior horn cells of the spinal cord.
- MDs are the greatest and most important cause of muscular dysfunction of childhood.
- Major complications of DMD include joint contractures, disuse atrophy, obesity, and respiratory and cardiac problems.
- Nursing care of the child with GBS consists of monitoring vital signs, providing respiratory support and physical therapy, providing reassurance, and providing support to the child and family.
- Tetanus occurs when tetanus spores or vegetative bacilli enter a wound and multiply in a susceptible host.
- Infant botulism results from the release of toxins from *C. botulinum* colonizing the gastrointestinal tract.

- Therapeutic management of SCI is directed toward immobilizing the entire spinal column at the scene of the traumatic event, safely transporting the patient by health care personnel trained to transport possible spinal trauma victims, evaluating neurologic damage, preventing further neurologic damage, and implementing an aggressive rehabilitation program designed to help achieve independence and movement.

References

Albright AL et al: Long-term intrathecal baclofen therapy for severe spasticity of cerebral origin, *J Neurosurg* 98(2):291-295, 2003.

American Academy of Pediatrics: Cardiovascular health supervision for individuals affected by Duchenne or Becker muscular dystrophy, *Pediatrics* 116(6):1569-1573, 2005.

American Academy of Pediatrics, Committee on Infectious Diseases, Pickering L (editor): *2009 red book: report of the Committee on Infectious Diseases*, ed 28, Elk Grove Village, Ill, 2009, The Academy.

American Academy of Pediatrics, American College of Obstetricians and Gynecologists: *Neonatal encephalopathy and cerebral palsy: defining the pathogenesis and pathophysiology*, Washington, DC, 2003, The College.

American Thoracic Society: Respiratory care of the patient with Duchenne muscular dystrophy, *Am J Respir Crit Care Med* 170(4):456-465, 2004.

Angelini C: The role of corticosteroids in muscular dystrophy: a critical appraisal, *Muscle Nerve* 36(4):424-435, 2007.

Arnon SS: Anaerobic bacterial infections: botulism *(Clostridium botulinum)*. In Kliegman RM et al (editors): *Nelson textbook of pediatrics*, ed 18, Philadelphia, 2007a, Saunders.

Arnon SS: Tetanus *(Clostridium tetani)*. In Kliegman RM et al (editors): *Nelson textbook of pediatrics*, ed 18, Philadelphia, 2007b, Saunders.

Arnon SS et al: Human botulism immune globulin for the treatment of infant botulism, *N Engl J Med* 354(5):462-471, 2006.

Ashwal S et al: Practice parameter: diagnostic assessment of the child with cerebral palsy: report of the Quality Standards Subcommittee of the American Academy of Neurology and the Practice Committee of the Child Neurology Society, *Neurology* 62(6):851-863, 2004.

Atkinson SB et al: The challenge of managing and treating Guillain-Barré syndrome during the acute phase, *Dimensions Crit Care Nurs* 25(6):256-263, 2006.

Bach JR: Medical considerations of long-term survival of Werdnig-Hoffmann disease, *Am J Phys Med Rehabil* 86(5):349-355, 2007.

Barker E: SCI patients take a big step forward, *RN* 68(7):30-34, 2005.

Barker E, Saulino MF: Special report: first-ever guidelines for spinal cord injuries, *RN* 65(10):32-37, 2002.

Berker AN, Yalçin MS: Cerebral palsy: orthopedic aspects and rehabilitation, *Pediatr Clin North Amer* 55(5):1209-1225, 2008.

Beroud C et al: Prenatal diagnosis of spinal muscular atrophy by genetic analysis of circulating fetal cells, *Lancet* 361(9362):1013-1014, 2003.

Birnkrant DJ: The assessment and management of the respiratory complications of pediatric neuromuscular diseases, *Clin Pediatr* 41(5):301-308, 2002.

Boulet SL et al: Trends in the postfortification prevalence of spina bifida and anencephaly in the United States, *Birth Defects Res A Clin Mol Teratol* 82(7):527-532, 2008.

Brown JP: Orthopaedic care of children with spina bifida: you've come a long way, baby! *Orthop Nurs* 20(4):51-58, 2001.

Buran CF, McDaniel AM, Brei TJ: Needs assessment in a spina bifida program: a comparison of the perceptions by adolescents with spina bifida and their parents, *Clin Nurs Spec* 16(5):256-262, 2002.

Bush A et al: Respiratory management of the infant with type 1 spinal muscular atrophy, *Arch Dis Child* 90(7):709-711, 2005.

Centers for Disease Control and Prevention: *Botulism*, 2008. Available at www.cdc.gov/nczved/dfbmd/disease_listing/botulism_gi.html (accessed May 11, 2009).

Centers for Disease Control and Prevention: Folate status in women of childbearing age, by race/ethnicity—United States, 1999-2000, 2001-2002, and 2003-2004, *Morbid Mortal Wkly Rep* 55(51):1377-1380, 2007.

Centers for Disease Control and Prevention: Spina bifida and anencephaly before and after folic acid mandate—United States, 1995-1996 and 1999-2000, *MMWR* 53(17):362-365, 2004.

Chakkalakal JV et al: Molecular, cellular, and pharmacological therapies for Duchenne/Becker muscular dystrophies, *FASEB J* 19(8):880-891, 2005.

Curley MAQ et al: Predicting pressure ulcer risk in pediatric patients: the Braden Q Scale, *Nurs Res* 52(1):22-33, 2003.

Dabney KW, Lipton GE, Miller F: Cerebral palsy, *Curr Opin Pediatr* 9(1):81-88, 1997.

Dai AI, Wasay M, Awan S: Botulinum toxin type A with oral baclofen versus oral tizanidine: a randomized pilot comparison in patients with cerebral palsy and equines foot deformity, *J Child Neurol* 23(12):1464-1466, 2008.

DeBoer SL, Seaver M: Pediatric spinal immobilization: C-spines, car seats, and color-coded collars, *J Emerg Nurs* 30(5):481-484, 2004.

Doolin E: Bowel management for patients with myelodysplasia, *Surg Clin North Am* 86(2):505-514, 2006.

Eiwegger T et al: Early exposure to latex products mediates latex sensitization in spina bifida but not in other diseases with comparable latex exposure rates, *Clin Exp Allergy* 36(10):1242-1246, 2006.

Francisco AM, Arnon SS: Clinical mimics of infant botulism, *Pediatrics* 119(4):826-828, 2007.

Gibson CS et al: Antenatal causes of cerebral palsy: associations between inherited thrombophilias, viral and bacterial infection, and inherited susceptibility to infection, *Obstet Gynecol Surv* 58(3):209-220, 2003.

Gray M, Moore KN: *Urologic disorders: adult and pediatric care*, St Louis, 2009, Mosby.

Green L, Greenberg GM, Hurwitz E: Primary care of children with cerebral palsy, *Clin Fam Pract* 5(2):1-21, 2003.

Grether JK et al: Intrauterine exposure to infection and risk of cerebral palsy in very preterm infants, *Arch Pediatr Adolesc Med* 157(1):26-32, 2003.

Hadley MN et al: Guidelines for management of acute cervical spine and spinal cord injuries, *Neurosurgery* 50(3 Suppl):S21-S29, 2002.

Han TR et al: Risk factors of cerebral palsy in preterm infants, *Am J Phys Med Rehabil* 81(4):297-303, 2002.

Henshaw SK: Unintended pregnancy in the United States, *Fam Plan Perspect* 30:24-29, 1998.

Honein MA: Impact of folic acid fortification of the US food supply and occurrence of neural tube defects, *JAMA* 285(23):2981-2986, 2001.

Hughes RA, Cornblath DR: Guillain-Barré syndrome, *Lancet* 366(9497):1653-1666, 2005.

Hurtekant KM, Spatz DL: Special considerations for breastfeeding the infant with spina bifida, *J Perinat Neonatal Nurs* 21(1):69-75, 2007.

Iannaccone ST: Spinal muscular atrophy, *Semin Neurol* 18(1):19-26, 1998.

Iannaccone ST, Burghes A: Spinal muscular atrophies, *Adv Neurol* 88:83-98, 2002.

Jacobs JM: Management options for the child with spastic cerebral palsy, *Orthop Nurs* 20(3):53-59, 2001.

Kaufman BA: Neural tube defects, *Pediatr Clin North Am* 51(2):389-419, 2004.

Kellett PB: Latex allergy: a review, *J Emerg Nurs* 23(1):27-36, 1997.

Kessler TM et al: Early proactive management improves upper urinary tract function and reduces the need for surgery in patients with myelomeningocele, *Neurourol Urodyn* 25(7):758-762, 2006.

Kimata H: Latex allergy in infants younger than 1 year, *Clin Exp Allergy* 34(12):1910-1915, 2004.

Kinsman SL, Johnston MV: Congenital anomalies of the central nervous system. In Kliegman RM et al (editors): *Nelson textbook of pediatrics*, ed 18, Philadelphia, 2007, Saunders.

Kirkham C, Harris S, Grzybowski S: Evidence-based prenatal care, part I, General prenatal care and counseling issues, *Am Fam Physician* 71(7):1307-1316, 2005.

Krigger KW: Cerebral palsy: an overview, *Am Fam Physician* 73(1):91-100, 101-102, 2006.

Lazzaretti CC, Pearson C: Myelodysplasia. In Allen PJ, Vessey JA (editors): *Primary care of the child with a chronic condition*, ed 4, St Louis, 2004, Mosby.

Matthews TJ, Honein MA, Erickson JD: Spina bifida and anencephaly prevalence—United States, 1991-2001, *Morbid Mortal Wkly Rep Recomm Rep* 51(RR-13):9-11, 2002.

McKearnan KA et al: Pain in children with cerebral palsy: a review, *J Neurosci Nurs* 36(5):252-259, 2004.

Metules T: Duchenne muscular dystrophy, *RN* 65(10):39-47, 2002.

Miske LJ et al: Use of the mechanical in-exsufflator in pediatric patients with neuromuscular disease and impaired cough, *Chest* 125(4):1406-1412, 2004.

Moxley RT et al: Practice parameter: corticosteroid treatment of Duchenne dystrophy, *Neurology* 64(1):13-20, 2005.

Murphy KP, Molnar GE, Lankasky K: Employment and social issues in adults with cerebral palsy, *Arch Phys Med Rehabil* 81:807-811, 2000.

Newswanger DI, Warren CR: Guillain-Barré syndrome, *Am Fam Physician* 69(10):2405-2410, 2004.

Rogers B: Feeding method and health outcomes of children with cerebral palsy, *J Pediatr* 145(2 Suppl):S28-S32, 2004.

Roscigno CI: Addressing spasticity-related pain in children with spastic cerebral palsy, *J Neurosci Nurs* 34(3):123-131, 2002.

Rosenbaum P et al: A report: the definition and classification of cerebral palsy April 2006, *Dev Med Child Neurol* 49(S109):1-44, 2007.

Russman BS: Function changes in spinal muscular atrophy II and III: the DCN/SMA group, *Neurology* 47(4):973-976, 1996.

Russman BS et al: Spinal muscular atrophy: new thoughts on the pathogenesis and classification schema, *J Child Neurol* 7(4):347-353, 1992.

Samaniego IA: A sore spot in pediatrics: risk factors for pressure ulcers, *Pediatr Nurs* 29(4):278, 2003.

Sarnat HB: Neuromuscular disorders. In Kliegman RM et al (editors): *Nelson textbook of pediatrics*, ed 18, Philadelphia, 2007, Saunders.

Shaer CM, Chescheir N, Schulkin J: Myelomeningocele: a review of the epidemiology, genetics, risk factors for conception, prenatal diagnosis, and prognosis for affected individuals, *Obstet Gynecol Surv* 62(7):471-479, 2007.

Simonds AK: Recent advances in respiratory care for neuromuscular disease, *Chest* 130(6):1879-1886, 2006.

Smith J: Shaken baby syndrome, *Orthop Nurs* 22(3):196-203, 2003.

Snodgrass WT, Adams R: Initial urologic management of myelomeningocele, *Urol Clin North Am* 31(3):427-434, viii, 2004.

Sulton LL: Meeting the challenge of Guillain-Barré syndrome, *Nurs Manage* 33(7):25-30, 2002.

Sutton LN: Fetal surgery for neural tube defects, *Best Pract Res Clin Obstet Gynaecol* 22(1):175-188, 2008.

Tarcan T et al: The timing of primary neurosurgical repair significantly affects neurogenic bladder prognosis in children with myelomeningocele, *J Urol* 176(3):1161-1165, 2006.

Thompson GH, Berenson FR: Other neuromuscular disorders. In Morrissy RT, Weinstein SL (editors): *Lovell and Winter's pediatric orthopaedics*, ed 5, Philadelphia, 2001, Lippincott Williams & Wilkins.

Vogel LC et al: Unique issues in pediatric spinal cord injury, *Orthop Nurs* 23(5):300-308, 2004.

Volpe JJ: *Neurology of the newborn*, ed 5, Philadelphia, 2008, Saunders.

Williams LJ et al: Decline in the prevalence of spina bifida and anencephaly by race/ethnicity, *Pediatrics* 116(3):580-586, 2005.

Winter S et al: Trends in the prevalence of cerebral palsy in a population-based study, *Pediatrics* 110(6):1220-1225, 2002.

Wu YW et al: Chorioamnionitis and cerebral palsy in term and near-term infants, *JAMA* 290(20):2677-2684, 2003.

Young HK et al: Outcome of noninvasive ventilation in children with neuromuscular disease, *Neurology* 68(3):198-201, 2007.

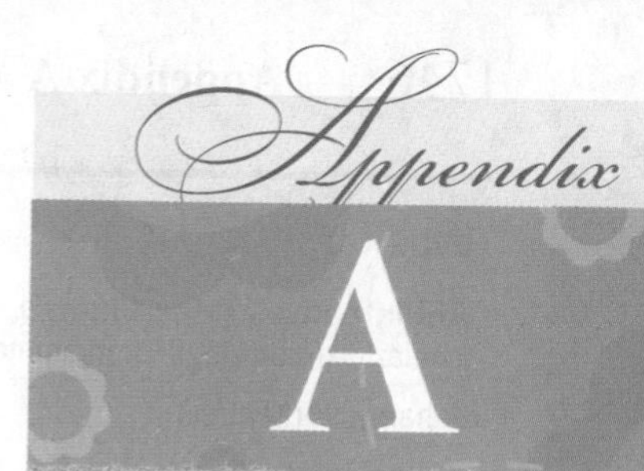

Relationship of Drugs to Breast Milk and Effect on Infant

The drugs listed in this appendix have been categorized by their major use. The ratings given are those published by the American Academy of Pediatrics (AAP) Committee on Drugs. These ratings label drugs that transfer into human milk. Drugs without a rating were not included in the AAP list. The ratings are described as follows:

- Drugs that are contraindicated during breastfeeding
- Drugs of abuse that are contraindicated during breastfeeding
- Radioactive compounds that require temporary cessation of breastfeeding
- Drugs with unknown effects on breastfeeding but may be of concern
- Drugs that have been associated with significant effects on some breastfeeding infants and should be given to breastfeeding mothers with caution
- Maternal medication usually compatible with breastfeeding
- Food and environmental agents that have an effect on breastfeeding

DRUG	EXCRETED IN MILK	% ADULT DOSE IN MILK	AAP RATING	COMMENTS
Analgesics and Antiinflammatory Drugs (Nonnarcotic)				
Acetaminophen (Datril, Tylenol, Darvocet, Comtrex, Excedrin)	Yes	0.04-1.85	6	Drug found in milk; drug and metabolite found in infant's urine
Aspirin (Bayer, Anacin, Bufferin, Excedrin, Fiorinal, Empirin, etc.)	Yes	0.5-21	5	Metabolized in liver
Ibuprofen (Advil, Nuprin, Motrin, etc.)	Yes	<0.8	6	Metabolites are inert; food slows absorption
Indomethacin (Indocin)	Yes	0.07-0.98	6	Food delays absorption
Ketorolac tromethamine (Toradol)	Yes	0.16-0.4	6	Food decreases rate but not amount of absorption
Mefenamic acid (Ponstel)	Yes	0.036-0.8	6	Infant able to excrete via urine
Nalbuphine (Nubain)	Yes	<1	NR	Has active metabolites
Naproxen (Anaprox, Naprosyn, Aleve)	Yes	0.26-1.1	6	Food delays absorption
Propoxyphene (Darvon, Wygesic)	Yes	Unknown	6	Metabolized in liver
Antiinfectives (May Change Intestinal Flora of Infant and Sensitize for Later Allergic Reaction)				
Acyclovir (Zovirax)	Yes	5.6 ± 4.4	6	Minimal absorption through skin
Amoxicillin (Amoxil, Augmentin)	Yes	0.7	6	Dose-dependent oral availability
Ampicillin (Polycillin, Amcill, Omnipen, Penbritin, Unasyn)	Yes	0.05-0.4	NR	In neonates, up to 12% plasma protein bound; oral availability increases
Carbenicillin (Pyopen, Geopen, Geocillin)	Yes	0.001	NR	Drug is given to neonate; not well absorbed from gastrointestinal (GI) tract
Cefazolin (Ancef, Kefzol)	Yes	0.075	6	Detected in milk if given intravenously (IV)
Cephalexin (Keflex)	Yes	0.85 ± 0.35	NR	Completely gone by 8 hours; absorption less in first few months
Cephalothin (Keflin)	Yes	0.4	NR	Higher volume of distribution in infant
Chloramphenicol (Chloromycetin)	Yes	1.3-7.4	4	Possible idiosyncratic bone marrow depression
Colistin (Coly-Mycin)	Yes	0.07	NR	Not absorbed orally
Demeclocycline (Declomycin)	Yes		NR	Drug remains in milk 3 days after dose
Erythromycin (Ilosone, E-Mycin, Erythrocin, Benzamycin)	Yes	0.1-2.1	6	Should not be given to infants under 1 mo of age because of risk of jaundice
Gentamicin (Garamycin, G-Myticin)	Yes	Unknown	NR	Appreciable absorption in neonate

Continued

DRUG	EXCRETED IN MILK	% ADULT DOSE IN MILK	AAP RATING	COMMENTS
Antiinfectives (May Change Intestinal Flora of Infant and Sensitize for Later Allergic Reaction)—cont'd				
Isoniazid (Nydrazid, INH, Rifamate)	Yes	2.3	6	Not detected in infant's blood but in urine
Kanamycin (Kantrex)	Yes	0.95	6	Serum half-life in infant is inversely related to age
Metronidazole (Flagyl, MetroGel, Protostat)	Yes	0.13-36	4	AAP says to discard milk for 12 hr if mother takes 2-g dose
Nitrofurantoin (Furadantin, Macrodantin)	Yes	0.6	6	Caution needed in infants with glucose-6-phosphate dehydrogenase (G6PD) deficiency
Novobiocin (Albamycin, Cathomycin)	Yes	0.15	NR	Can be given to infant directly
Nystatin (Mycostatin)	No	Not absorbed orally	NR	Can be given to infant directly
Oxacillin (Prostaphlin, Bactocill)	Yes	Trace	NR	Displaces bilirubin from albumin in infants
Penicillin G, benzathine (Bicillin)	Yes	0.8	NR	Best on empty stomach; increased in neonate
Streptomycin	Yes	0.5	6	Is given to infants directly
Sulfisoxazole (Gantrisin, Pediazole)	Yes	0.45	6	Jaundice may develop; avoid in infants with G6PD
Tetracycline HCl (Achromycin, Panmycin, Sumycin)	Yes	0.03-4.8	6	Probably chelated by calcium in milk
Anticoagulants				
Dicumarol (bishydroxy-coumarin), warfarin (Panwarfin)	Yes	0.5	NR	Not measurable in all milk samples; has been associated with bleeding in breastfed infants
Heparin	No	None	NR	Heparin ineffective orally
Anticonvulsants and Sedatives (Barbiturates May Pass into Milk but Do Not Sedate Infant)				
Magnesium sulfate (Eldertonic, Vicon Forte)	Yes	0.5	6	May produce sedation in infant
Pentobarbital (Nembutal)	Yes	Traces	NR	Depends on liver for detoxification so may accumulate in newborn
Phenobarbital (Luminal, Donnatal, Tedral)	Yes	1.5	5	Sleepiness and decreased sucking possible
Phenytoin (Dilantin)	Yes	1.4-7.2	6	No problem if mother's plasma concentration is in therapeutic range
Antihistamines (May Suppress Lactation; Administer After Breastfeeding; All Pass into Breast Milk)				
Brompheniramine maleate (Dimetane, Dristan)	Yes	Unknown	NR	Well absorbed from GI tract
Diphenhydramine (Benadryl)	Yes	Unknown	NR	Metabolism shows ethnic variation; volume of distribution is greater in Asians than in Caucasians
Promethazine (Phenergan, Mepergan)	Yes	Unknown	NR	Passage into human milk is expected; increases serum prolactin level
Autonomic Drugs				
Amphetamine (Adderall)	Yes	6.1 ± 0.1	2	Jitteriness, irritability, and sleepiness may be seen in nursing infants
Atropine sulfate* (Donnatal, Lomotil, Urised)	Yes	Unknown	6	May inhibit lactation
Ergotamine (Cafergot)	Yes	Unknown	5	May inhibit lactation; vomiting, diarrhea, convulsions in infant
Neostigmine (Prostigmin)	No	None	NR	Poorly absorbed from GI tract
Propantheline bromide (Pro-Banthine)	No	Uncontrolled data indicate no measurable levels	NR	Activity of long-acting dose not studied
Propranolol (Inderal)	Yes	0.05-1	6	Risk of effect almost nonexistent; some Caucasians poor absorbers
Cardiovascular Drugs				
Diazoxide (Hyperstat)	Unknown	Unknown	NR	Antihypertensive
Digoxin (Lanoxin)	Yes	0.07-14	6	Not detected in infant's plasma
Hydralazine (Apresoline)	Yes	0.8	6	Antihypertensive
Methyldopa (Aldomet, Aldoril, Aldoclor)	Yes	0.02-0.09	6	Antihypertensive
Nifedipine (Procardia)	Yes	0.00163 ± 0.00125	6	Calcium channel blocker; minimal amount in milk
Quinidine (Quinaglute)	Yes	4.1	6	May suppress prolactin secretion

DRUG	EXCRETED IN MILK	% ADULT DOSE IN MILK	AAP RATING	COMMENTS
Diuretics				
Chlorothiazide (Aldochlor, Diupres, Diuril)	Yes	Minimal	6	Absorption from GI tract is incomplete and dose dependent
Furosemide (sulfamoyl anthranilic acid) (Lasix)	Possible	Not found in all samples	NR	Drug is given to neonates under medical management
Spironolactone (Aldactazide, Aldactone)	Yes	Unknown	6	80% of drug converted to canrenone
Gastrointestinal Agents				
Casanthranol (Peri-Colace)	Yes	Low	NR	Can cause diarrhea and colic in infant
Cascara sagrada (Milk of Magnesia)	Yes	Low	6	May increase bowel activity in infant
Senna (Senokot)	No	None	6	None
Hormones and Contraceptives				
Cortisone (Cortone)	Yes	Significant amounts	NR	Probably OK to use as replacement therapy in Addison's disease
Epinephrine (Adrenalin, EpiPen)	Yes	Unknown	NR	Destroyed in GI tract of infant
Estradiol (Emcyt, Estrace)	Yes	0.004-<10	6	
Estrogen	Yes	0.1	6	May alter quality and quantity of milk
Insulin	No	None	NR	Not excreted in human milk
Levonorgestrel (Norplant, Levlen, Triphasil)	Yes	1.1	6	Does not affect milk production
Medroxyprogesterone acetate (Amen, Cycrin, Depo-Provera)	Yes	0.86-5	6	Increased prolactin level before and after sucking; 6-mo injection may affect milk supply; 3-mo injection should not decrease supply
Prednisone (Deltasone)	Yes	0.15 ± 0.11	6	
Progesterone (Crinone, Prometrium, Cyclogest, Gesterol, Gestone)	Unknown	Unknown	6	In low doses, progesterone-only oral contraceptives are OK
Propylthiouracil	Yes	0.03-2.6	6	Get baseline levels of T_3, T_4, and TSH in infant before and 6 wk after mother starts taking medication
Thyroid and thyroxine (T_4)	Yes	0.3-2.0	6	Appears to protect breastfed infants of hypothyroid mothers
Tolbutamide (Orinase)	Yes	18	6	Watch for jaundice
Narcotics				
Cocaine	Yes	Significant levels in milk	2	No metabolites or drug found in milk after 36 hr or in infant's urine after 60 hr
Codeine	Yes	5 ± 2	6	Chinese metabolize less drug than Caucasians do
Heroin	Yes	Significant	2	Level in milk enough to cause addiction in infant
Marijuana (*Cannabis sativa* L.)	Yes	Unknown	2	Shown in laboratory animals to produce structural changes in nursling's brain cells; infant at risk of inhaling smoke during feeding or when held by person who is smoking
Meperidine (Demerol, Mepergan)	Yes	Unknown	6	Renal excretion of drug and metabolite is pH dependent
Methadone	Yes	2.2	6	No signs in infant if mother getting <20 mg/24 hr; if more than that, withdrawal may be a problem; suggest mother take daily dose after evening feeding and supplement with formula at next feeding
Morphine	Yes	0.8-1.2	6	Amounts in breast milk too variable to consider breastfeeding as means of treating withdrawal symptoms; may cause galactorrhea and prolactin increase
Oxycodone	Yes	Unknown	NR	
Psychotropic and Mood-Changing Drugs				
Alcohol (ethanol)	Yes	1-19.5	6	Milk may smell like alcohol; high amounts cause depression of milk-ejection reflex (dose dependent); infant cannot metabolize ethanol

Continued

DRUG	EXCRETED IN MILK	% ADULT DOSE IN MILK	AAP RATING	COMMENTS
Psychotropic and Mood-Changing Drugs—cont'd				
Amitriptyline (Elavil, Etrafon, Triavil)	Yes	0.8 ± 0.2	4	Galactorrhea or prolactin increase
Caffeine	Yes	0.66-2.3	6	Caffeine present in many hot and cold drinks; consider if infant very wakeful
Chlordiazepoxide (Librium)	Yes	Unknown	NR	May contribute to jaundice; may cause drowsiness
Chlorpromazine (Thorazine)	Yes	0.07-0.2	4	May cause drowsiness and lethargy in infants
Desipramine (Norpramin, Pertofrane)	Yes	1	4	Neither drug nor metabolite recovered from nursing infant's serum or urine; some Caucasians are poor metabolizers
Diazepam (Valium)	Yes	2-12	4	Sedation if fed 4 hr but not 8 hr after dose; more in evening milk
Haloperidol (Haldol)	Yes	0.15-2	4	Causes prolactin increase; in animals, nurslings have behavioral abnormalities; these effects not seen in humans
Imipramine (Tofranil)	Yes	0.1	4	Causes galactorrhea and prolactin increase
Lithium carbonate (Eskalith, Lithane, Lithonate)	Yes	1.8	5	Measurable lithium in infant's serum; inhibits cAMP, which is significant for brain growth; cyanosis, poor muscle tone, and ECG changes seen in breastfeeding infant
Meprobamate (Miltown, Equanil)	Yes	Unknown	NR	Galactorrhea seen in some women
Phencyclidine (PCP)	Yes	Unknown	2	Animal studies show PCP in milk even after drug has been discontinued for 40 days
Theobromine	Yes	20	NR	Chocolate the most common cause of exposure; if mother consumes >1 lb/day, may see irritability or increased bowel activity
Thioridazine (Mellaril)	Yes	Unknown	NR	Galactorrhea reported in some women
Trifluoperazine (Stelazine)	Yes	Unknown	4	Excretion into milk not significant after therapeutic doses; galactorrhea reported in some women; increase in serum prolactin levels
Miscellaneous				
DPT	Yes	Minimum	NR	Does not interfere with immunization schedule
Methotrexate (Folex, Rheumatrex)	Yes	0.93	1	Food delays absorption; peaks at 19 hr in milk
Nicotine	Yes	Unknown	NR	May suppress lactation decreased response of prolactin and oxytocin to suckling; smoke exposure may be a concern
Poliovirus vaccine	No	None	NR	Live vaccine taken orally; not necessary to withhold breastfeeding
Rh antibodies	Yes	Unknown	NR	Inactivated by gastric juices; not a contraindication for breastfeeding
Rubella virus vaccine	Yes	Minimum		Will not confer passive immunity
Theophylline (Marax, Quibron, Theolair)	Yes	<1-15	6	Extremely low clearance in infants <6 mo of age
Tuberculin test	Yes	Unknown	NR	Tuberculin-sensitive mothers can immunize their infants through breast milk; immunity may last several years

Compiled from Lawrence RA, Lawrence RM: *Breastfeeding: a guide for the medical profession*, ed 6, St Louis, 2005, Mosby.
DPT, Diphtheria, pertussis, tetanus; *NR*, not rated.
*Atropine sulfate is an ingredient in many prescription and nonprescription drugs.

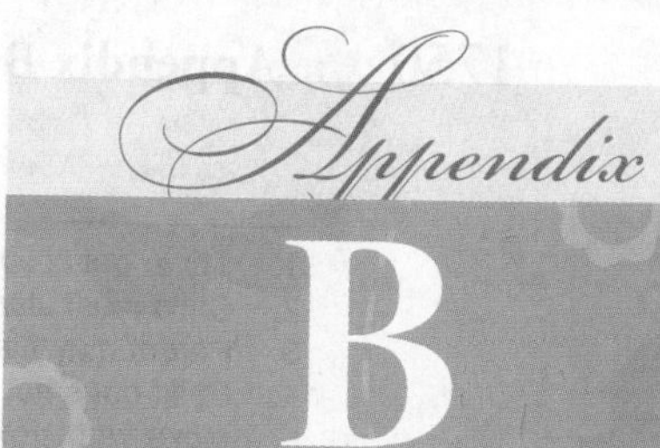

Developmental/Sensory Assessment

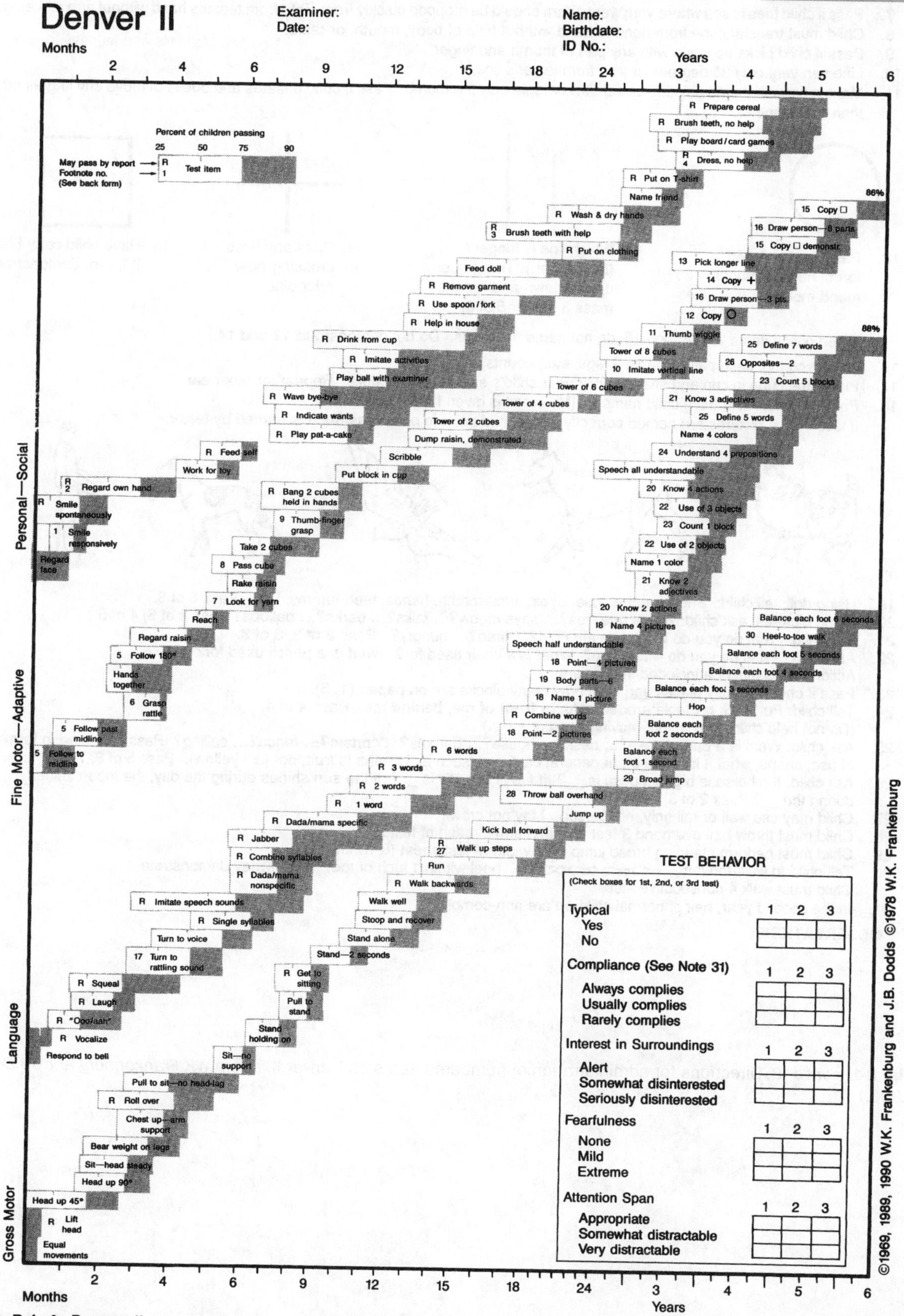

Denver II

Examiner:
Date:

Name:
Birthdate:
ID No.:

Months: 2, 4, 6, 9, 12, 15, 18, 24 — Years: 3, 4, 5, 6

Percent of children passing: 25, 50, 75, 90

May pass by report → R
Footnote no. (See back form) → 1
Test item

Personal—Social

- R Prepare cereal
- R Brush teeth, no help
- R Play board/card games
- R 4 Dress, no help
- R Put on T-shirt
- Name friend
- R Wash & dry hands
- R 3 Brush teeth with help
- R Put on clothing
- Feed doll
- R Remove garment
- R Use spoon/fork
- R Help in house
- R Drink from cup
- R Imitate activities
- Play ball with examiner
- R Wave bye-bye
- R Indicate wants
- R Play pat-a-cake
- R Feed self
- Work for toy
- R 2 Regard own hand
- R Smile spontaneously
- 1 Smile responsively
- Regard face

Fine Motor—Adaptive

- 15 Copy □ (86%)
- 16 Draw person—6 parts
- 15 Copy □ demonstr.
- 13 Pick longer line
- 14 Copy +
- 16 Draw person—3 pts.
- 12 Copy ○
- 11 Thumb wiggle
- Tower of 8 cubes
- 10 Imitate vertical line
- Tower of 6 cubes
- Tower of 4 cubes
- Tower of 2 cubes
- Dump raisin, demonstrated
- Scribble
- Put block in cup
- R Bang 2 cubes held in hands
- 9 Thumb-finger grasp
- Take 2 cubes
- 8 Pass cube
- Rake raisin
- 7 Look for yarn
- Reach
- Regard raisin
- 5 Follow 180°
- Hands together
- 6 Grasp rattle
- 5 Follow past midline
- 5 Follow to midline

Language

- 25 Define 7 words (88%)
- 26 Opposites—2
- 23 Count 5 blocks
- 21 Know 3 adjectives
- 25 Define 5 words
- Name 4 colors
- 24 Understand 4 prepositions
- Speech all understandable
- 20 Know 4 actions
- 22 Use of 3 objects
- 23 Count 1 block
- 22 Use of 2 objects
- Name 1 color
- 21 Know 2 adjectives
- 20 Know 2 actions
- 18 Name 4 pictures
- Speech half understandable
- 18 Point—4 pictures
- 19 Body parts—6
- 18 Name 1 picture
- R Combine words
- 18 Point—2 pictures
- R 6 words
- R 3 words
- R 2 words
- R 1 word
- R Dada/mama specific
- R Jabber
- R Combine syllables
- R Dada/mama nonspecific
- R Imitate speech sounds
- R Single syllables
- Turn to voice
- 17 Turn to rattling sound
- R Squeal
- R Laugh
- R "Ooo/aah"
- R Vocalize
- Respond to bell

Gross Motor

- Balance each foot 6 seconds
- 30 Heel-to-toe walk
- Balance each foot 5 seconds
- Balance each foot 4 seconds
- Balance each foot 3 seconds
- Hop
- Balance each foot 2 seconds
- Balance each foot 1 second
- 29 Broad jump
- 28 Throw ball overhand
- Jump up
- Kick ball forward
- R 27 Walk up steps
- Run
- R Walk backwards
- Walk well
- Stoop and recover
- Stand alone
- Stand—2 seconds
- R Get to sitting
- Pull to stand
- Stand holding on
- Sit—no support
- Pull to sit—no head-lag
- R Roll over
- Chest up—arm support
- Bear weight on legs
- Sit—head steady
- Head up 90°
- Head up 45°
- R Lift head
- Equal movements

TEST BEHAVIOR

(Check boxes for 1st, 2nd, or 3rd test)

Typical	1	2	3
Yes			
No			

Compliance (See Note 31)	1	2	3
Always complies			
Usually complies			
Rarely complies			

Interest in Surroundings	1	2	3
Alert			
Somewhat disinterested			
Seriously disinterested			

Fearfulness	1	2	3
None			
Mild			
Extreme			

Attention Span	1	2	3
Appropriate			
Somewhat distractable			
Very distractable			

A

Fig. B-1 A, Denver II.

Continued

DIRECTIONS FOR ADMINISTRATION

1. Try to get child to smile by smiling, talking or waving. Do not touch him/her.
2. Child must stare at hand several seconds.
3. Parent may help guide toothbrush and put toothpaste on brush.
4. Child does not have to be able to tie shoes or button/zip in the back.
5. Move yarn slowly in an arc from one side to the other, about 8" above child's face.
6. Pass if child grasps rattle when it is touched to the backs or tips of fingers.
7. Pass if child tries to see where yarn went. Yarn should be dropped quickly from sight from tester's hand without arm movement.
8. Child must transfer cube from hand to hand without help of body, mouth, or table.
9. Pass if child picks up raisin with any part of thumb and finger.
10. Line can vary only 30 degrees or less from tester's line.
11. Make a fist with thumb pointing upward and wiggle only the thumb. Pass if child imitates and does not move any fingers other than the thumb.

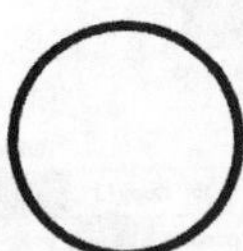

12. Pass any enclosed form. Fail continuous round motions.

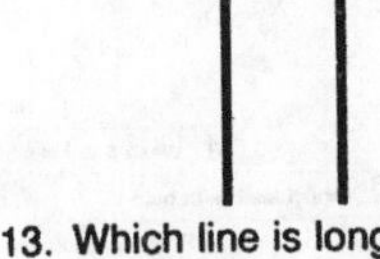

13. Which line is longer? (Not bigger.) Turn paper upside down and repeat. (pass 3 of 3 or 5 of 6)

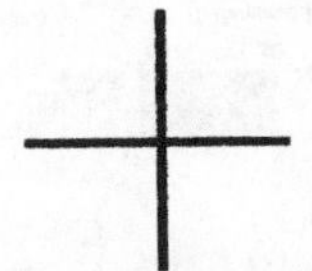

14. Pass any lines crossing near midpoint.

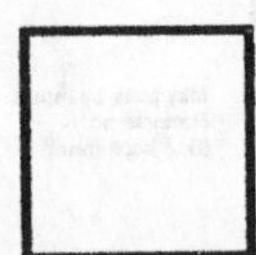

15. Have child copy first. If failed, demonstrate.

When giving items 12, 14, and 15, do not name the forms. Do not demonstrate 12 and 14.

16. When scoring, each pair (2 arms, 2 legs, etc.) counts as one part.
17. Place one cube in cup and shake gently near child's ear, but out of sight. Repeat for other ear.
18. Point to picture and have child name it. (No credit is given for sounds only.) If less than 4 pictures are named correctly, have child point to picture as each is named by tester.

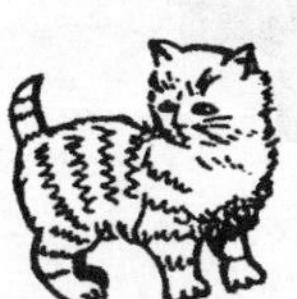
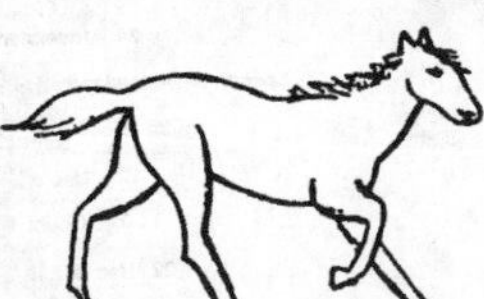
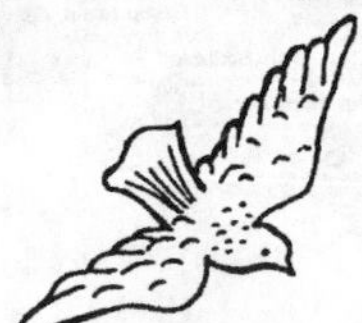
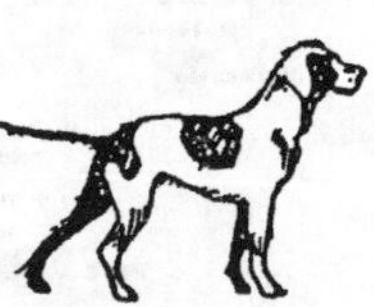
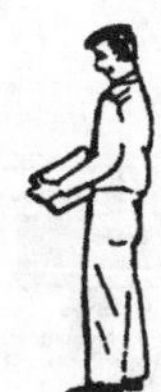

19. Using doll, tell child: Show me the nose, eyes, ears, mouth, hands, feet, tummy, hair. Pass 6 of 8.
20. Using pictures, ask child: Which one flies?... says meow?... talks?... barks?... gallops? Pass 2 of 5, 4 of 5.
21. Ask child: What do you do when you are cold?... tired?... hungry? Pass 2 of 3, 3 of 3.
22. Ask child: What do you do with a cup? What is a chair used for? What is a pencil used for? Action words must be included in answers.
23. Pass if child correctly places and says how many blocks are on paper. (1, 5).
24. Tell child: Put block **on** table; **under** table; **in front of** me, **behind** me. Pass 4 of 4. (Do not help child by pointing, moving head or eyes.)
25. Ask child: What is a ball?... lake?... desk?... house?... banana?... curtain?... fence?... ceiling? Pass if defined in terms of use, shape, what it is made of, or general category (such as banana is fruit, not just yellow). Pass 5 of 8, 7 of 8.
26. Ask child: If a horse is big, a mouse is __? If fire is hot, ice is __? If the sun shines during the day, the moon shines during the __? Pass 2 of 3.
27. Child may use wall or rail only, not person. May not crawl.
28. Child must throw ball overhand 3 feet to within arm's reach of tester.
29. Child must perform standing broad jump over width of test sheet (8 1/2 inches).
30. Tell child to walk forward, → heel within 1 inch of toe. Tester may demonstrate. Child must walk 4 consecutive steps.
31. In the second year, half of normal children are non-compliant.

B **OBSERVATIONS:**

Fig. B-1, cont'd B, Directions for administration of numbered items on Denver II. *(From WK Frankenburg and JB Dodds, 1990.)*

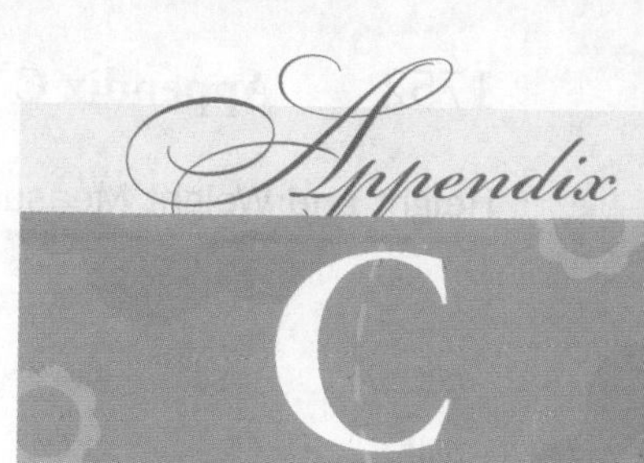

Growth Measurements

Height and Weight Measurements for Boys

	Height by Percentiles						Weight by Percentiles					
	5		50		95		5		50		95	
AGE*	cm	inches	cm	inches	cm	inches	kg	lb	kg	lb	kg	lb
Birth	46.4	18¼	50.5	20	54.4	21½	2.54	5½	3.27	7¼	4.15	9¼
3 mo	56.7	22¼	61.1	24	65.4	25¾	4.43	9¾	5.98	13¼	7.37	16¼
6 mo	63.4	25	67.8	26¾	72.3	28½	6.20	13¾	7.85	17¼	9.46	20¾
9 mo	68.0	26¾	72.3	28½	77.1	30¼	7.52	16½	9.18	20¼	10.93	24
1	71.7	28¼	76.1	30	81.2	32	8.43	18½	10.15	22½	11.99	26½
1½	77.5	30¼	82.4	32½	88.1	34¾	9.59	21¼	11.47	25¼	13.44	29½
2†	82.5	32½	86.8	34¼	94.4	37¼	10.49	23¼	12.34	27¼	15.50	34¼
2½†	85.4	33½	90.4	35½	97.8	38½	11.27	24¾	13.52	29¾	16.61	36½
3	89.0	35	94.9	37¼	102.0	40¼	12.05	26½	14.62	32¼	17.77	39¼
3½	92.5	36½	99.1	39	106.1	41¾	12.84	28¼	15.68	34½	18.98	41¾
4	95.8	37¾	102.9	40½	109.9	43¼	13.64	30	16.69	36¾	20.27	44¾
4½	98.9	39	106.6	42	113.5	44¾	14.45	31¾	17.69	39	21.63	47¾
5	102.0	40¼	109.9	43¼	117.0	46	15.27	33¾	18.67	41¼	23.09	51
6	107.7	42½	116.1	45¾	123.5	48½	16.93	37¼	20.69	45½	26.34	58
7	113.0	44½	121.7	48	129.7	51	18.64	41	22.85	50¼	30.12	66½
8	118.1	46½	127.0	50	135.7	53½	20.40	45	25.30	55¾	34.51	76
9	122.9	48½	132.2	52	141.8	55¾	22.25	49	28.13	62	39.58	87¼
10	127.7	50¼	137.5	54¼	148.1	58¼	24.33	53¾	31.44	69¼	45.27	99¾
11	132.6	52¼	143.3	56½	154.9	61	26.80	59	35.30	77¾	51.47	113½
12	137.6	54¼	149.7	59	162.3	64	29.85	65¾	39.78	87¾	58.09	128
13	142.9	56¼	156.5	61½	169.8	66¾	33.64	74¼	44.95	99	65.02	143¼
14	148.8	58½	163.1	64¼	176.7	69½	38.22	84¼	50.77	112	72.13	159
15	155.2	61	169.0	66½	181.9	71½	43.11	95	56.71	125	79.12	174½
16	161.1	63½	173.5	68¼	185.4	73	47.74	105¼	62.10	137	85.62	188¾
17	164.9	65	176.2	69¼	187.3	73¾	51.50	113½	66.31	146¼	91.31	201¼
18	165.7	65¼	176.8	69½	187.6	73¾	53.97	119	68.88	151¾	95.76	211

Modified from National Center for Health Statistics, Health Resources Administration, Department of Health, Education and Welfare, Hyattsville, Md.
Conversion of metric data to approximate inches and pounds by Ross Laboratories.
*Years unless otherwise indicated.
†Height data include some recumbent length measurements, which make values slightly higher than if all measurements had been of stature (standing height).

Height and Weight Measurements for Girls

	Height by Percentiles						Weight by Percentiles					
	5		50		95		5		50		95	
AGE*	cm	inches	cm	inches	cm	inches	kg	lb	kg	lb	kg	lb
Birth	45.4	17¾	49.9	19¾	52.9	20¾	2.36	5¼	3.23	7	3.81	8½
3 mo	55.4	21¾	59.5	23½	63.4	25	4.18	9¼	5.4	12	6.74	14¾
6 mo	61.8	24¼	65.9	26	70.2	27¾	5.79	12¾	7.21	16	8.73	19¼
9 mo	66.1	26	70.4	27¾	75.0	29½	7.0	15½	8.56	18¾	10.17	22½
1	69.8	27½	74.3	29¼	79.1	31¼	7.84	17¼	9.53	21	11.24	24¾
1½	76.0	30	80.9	31¾	86.1	34	8.92	19¾	10.82	23¾	12.76	28¼
2†	81.6	32¼	86.8	34¼	93.6	36¾	9.95	22	11.8	26	14.15	31¼
2½†	84.6	33¼	90.0	35½	96.6	38	10.8	23¾	13.03	28¾	15.76	34¾
3	88.3	34¾	94.1	37	100.6	39½	11.61	25½	14.1	31	17.22	38
3½	91.7	36	97.9	38½	104.5	41¼	12.37	27¼	15.07	33¼	18.59	41
4	95.0	37½	101.6	40	108.3	42¾	13.11	29	15.96	35¼	19.91	44
4½	98.1	38½	105.0	41¼	112.0	44	13.83	30½	16.81	37	21.24	46¾
5	101.1	39¾	108.4	42¾	115.6	45½	14.55	32	17.66	39	22.62	49¾
6	106.6	42	114.6	45	122.7	48¼	16.05	35½	19.52	43	25.75	56¾
7	111.8	44	120.6	47½	129.5	51	17.71	39	21.84	48¼	29.68	65½
8	116.9	46	126.4	49¾	136.2	53½	19.62	43¼	24.84	54¾	34.71	76½
9	122.1	48	132.2	52	142.9	56¼	21.82	48	28.46	62¾	40.64	89½
10	127.5	50¼	138.3	54½	149.5	58¾	24.36	53¾	32.55	71¾	47.17	104
11	133.5	52½	144.8	57	156.2	61½	27.24	60	36.95	81½	54.0	119
12	139.8	55	151.5	59¾	162.7	64	30.52	67¼	41.53	91½	60.81	134
13	145.2	57¼	157.1	61¾	168.1	66¼	34.14	75¼	46.1	101¾	67.3	148¼
14	148.7	58½	160.4	63¼	171.3	67½	37.76	83¼	50.28	110¾	73.08	161
15	150.5	59¼	161.8	63¾	172.8	68	40.99	90¼	53.68	118¼	77.78	171½
16	151.6	59¾	162.4	64	173.3	68¼	43.41	95¾	55.89	123¼	80.99	178½
17	152.7	60	163.1	64¼	173.5	68¼	44.74	98¾	56.69	125	82.46	181¾
18	153.6	60½	163.7	64½	173.6	68¼	45.26	99¾	56.62	124¾	82.47	181¾

Modified from National Center for Health Statistics, Health Resources Administration, Department of Health, Education and Welfare, Hyattsville, Md. Conversion of metric data to approximate inches and pounds by Ross Laboratories.

*Years unless otherwise indicated.

†Height data include some recumbent length measurements, which make values slightly higher than if all measurements had been of stature.

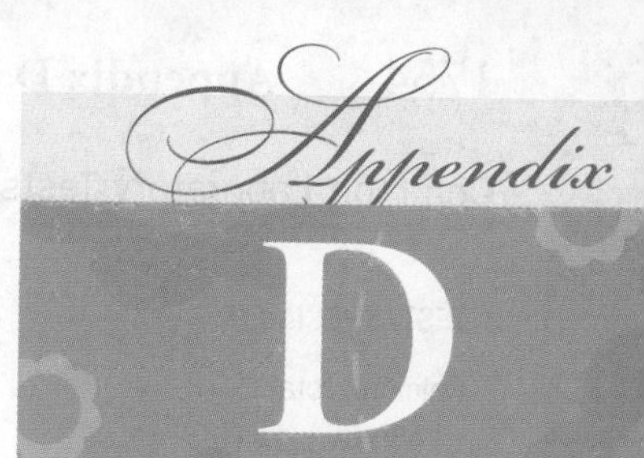

Common Laboratory Tests

Common Laboratory Tests and Tests Results*

TEST/SPECIMEN	AGE/GENDER/REFERENCE	Normal Ranges: CONVENTIONAL UNITS		Normal Ranges: INTERNATIONAL UNITS (SI)	
Acetaminophen					
Serum or plasma	Therap. conc.	10-30 mcg/ml		66-200 μmol/L	
	Toxic conc.	>200 mcg/ml		>1300 μmol/L	
Ammonia nitrogen					
Plasma or serum	Newborn	90-150 mcg/dl		64-107 μmol/L	
	0-2 wk	79-129 mcg/dl		56-92 μmol/L	
	>1 mo	29-70 mcg/dl		21-50 μmol/L	
	Thereafter	0-50 mcg/dl		0-35.7 μmol/L	
Antistreptolysin O titer (ASO)					
Serum	2-4 yr	<160 Todd units			
	School-age children	170-330 Todd units			
Base excess					
Whole blood	Newborn	(−10)-(−2) mEq/L		(−10)-(−2) mmol/L	
	Infant	(−7)-(−1) mEq/L		(−7)-(−1) mmol/L	
	Child	(−4)-(+2) mEq/L		(−4)-(+2) mmol/L	
	Thereafter	(−3)-(+3) mEq/L		(−3)-(+3) mmol/L	
Bicarbonate (HCO_3)					
Serum	Arterial	21-28 mEq/L		21-28 mmol/L	
	Venous	22-29 mEq/L		22-29 mmol/L	
Bilirubin, total		**Premature** (mg/dl)	**Full term** (mg/dl)	**Premature** (μmol/L)	**Full term** (μmol/L)
Serum	Cord	<2.0	<2.0	<34	<34
	0-1 d	<8.0	<6.0	<137	<103
	1-2 d	<12.0	<8.0	<205	<137
	2-5 d	<16.0	<12.0	<274	<205
	Thereafter	<20.0	<10.0	<340	<171
Bilirubin, direct (conjugated)					
Serum		0.0-0.2 mg/dl		0-3.4 μmol/L	
Bleeding time					
Blood from skin puncture					
Ivy	Normal	2-7 min		2-7 min	
	Borderline	7-11 min		7-11 min	
Simplate (G-D)		2.75-8 min		2.75-8 min	
Blood volume					
Whole blood	Male	52-83 ml/kg		0.052-0.083 L/kg	
	Female	50-75 ml/kg		0.050-0.075 L/kg	
C-reactive protein (CRP)					
Serum	Cord	52-1330 ng/ml		52-1330 mcg/L	
	2-12 yr	67-1800 ng/ml		67-1800 mcg/L	
Calcium, ionized					
Serum, plasma, or whole blood	Cord	5.0-6.0 mg/dl		1.25-1.50 mmol/L	
	Newborn, 3-24 hr	4.3-5.1 mg/dl		1.07-1.27 mmol/L	
	24-48 hr	4.0-4.7 mg/dl		1.00-1.17 mmol/L	
	Thereafter	4.8-4.92 mg/dl or 2.24-2.46 mEq/L		1.12-1.23 mmol/L	

Continued

Common Laboratory Tests and Tests Results—cont'd

TEST/SPECIMEN	AGE/GENDER/REFERENCE	Normal Ranges: CONVENTIONAL UNITS	Normal Ranges: INTERNATIONAL UNITS (SI)
Calcium, total			
Serum	Cord	9.0-11.5 mg/dl	2.25-2.88 mmol/L
	Newborn, 3-24 hr	9.0-10.6 mg/dl	2.3-2.65 mmol/L
	24-48 hr	7.0-12.0 mg/dl	1.75-3.0 mmol/L
	4-7 d	9.0-10.9 mg/dl	2.25-2.73 mmol/L
	Child	8.8-10.8 mg/dl	2.2-2.70 mmol/L
	Thereafter	8.4-10.2 mg/dl	2.1-2.55 mmol/L
Carbon dioxide, partial pressure (Pco_2)			
Whole blood, arterial	Newborn	27-40 mm Hg	3.6-5.3 kPa
	Infant	27-41 mm Hg	3.6-5.5 kPa
	Thereafter: Male	35-48 mm Hg	4.7-6.4 kPa
	Female	32-45 mm Hg	4.3-6.0 kPa
Carbon dioxide, total (tCO_2)			
Serum or plasma	Cord	14-22 mEq/L	14-22 mmol/L
	Premature (1 wk)	14-27 mEq/L	14-27 mmol/L
	Newborn	13-22 mEq/L	13-22 mmol/L
	Infant, child	20-28 mEq/L	20-28 mmol/L
	Thereafter	23-30 mEq/L	23-30 mmol/L
Cerebrospinal fluid (CSF)			
Pressure		70-180 mm H_2O	70-180 mm H_2O
Volume	Child	60-100 ml	0.06-0.10 L
	Adult	100-160 ml	0.10-0.16 L
Chloride			
Serum or plasma	Cord	96-104 mEq/L	96-104 mmol/L
	Newborn	97-110 mEq/L	97-110 mmol/L
	Thereafter	98-106 mEq/L	98-106 mmol/L
Sweat	Normal (homozygote)	<40 mEq/L	<40 mmol/L
	Marginal (e.g., asthma, Addison disease, malnutrition)	45-60 mEq/L	45-60 mmol/L
	Cystic fibrosis	>60 mEq/L	>60 mmol/L
Cholesterol, total			
Serum or plasma†	Acceptable	<170 mg/dl	<4.4 mmol/L
	Borderline	170-199 mg/dl	4.4-5.1 mmol/L
	High	≥200 mg/dl	≥5.2 mmol/L
Clotting time (Lee-White)			
Whole blood		5-8 min (glass tubes)	5-8 min
		5-15 min (room temp)	5-15 min
		30 min (silicone tube)	30 min
Creatine kinase (CK, CPK)			
Serum	Cord	70-380 U/L	70-380 U/L
	5-8 hr	214-1175 U/L	214-1175 U/L
	24-33 hr	130-1200 U/L	130-1200 U/L
	72-100 hr	87-725 U/L	87-725 U/L
	Adult	5-130 U/L	5-130 U/L
Creatinine			
Serum	Cord	0.6-1.2 mg/dl	53-106 μmol/L
	Newborn	0.3-1.0 mg/dl	27-88 μmol/L
	Infant	0.2-0.4 mg/d	18-35 μmol/L
	Child	0.3-0.7 mg/dl	27-62 μmol/L
	Adolescent	0.5-1.0 mg/dl	44-88 μmol/L
	Adult: Male	0.6-1.2 mg/dl	53-106 μmol/L
	Female	0.5-1.1 mg/dl	44-97 μmol/L
Urine, 24 hr	Premature	8.1-15.0 mg/kg/24 hr	72-133 μmol/kg/24 hr
	Full term	10.4-19.7 mg/kg/24 hr	92-174 μmol/kg/24 hr
	1.5-7 yr	10-15 mg/kg/24 hr	88-133 μmol/kg/24 hr
	7-15 yr	5.2-41 mg/kg/24 hr	46-362 μmol/kg/24 hr

Common Laboratory Tests and Tests Results—cont'd

TEST/SPECIMEN	AGE/GENDER/REFERENCE	Normal Ranges CONVENTIONAL UNITS	INTERNATIONAL UNITS (SI)
Creatinine clearance (endogenous)			
Serum or plasma and urine	Newborn	40-65 ml/min/1.73 m^2	
	<40 yr: Male	97-137 ml/min/1.73 m^2	
	Female	88-128 ml/min/1.73 m^2	
Digoxin			
Serum, plasma; collect at least 12 hr after dose	Therap. conc.		
	CHF	0.8-1.5 ng/ml	1.0-1.9 nmol/L
	Arrhythmias	1.5-2.0 ng/ml	1.9-2.6 nmol/L
	Toxic conc.		
	Child	>2.5 ng/ml	>3.2 nmol/L
	Adult	>3.0 ng/ml	>3.8 nmol/L
Eosinophil count			
Whole blood, capillary blood		50-250 cells/mm^3 (µl)	50-250 × 10^6 cells/L
Erythrocyte (RBC) count			
Whole blood	Cord	3.9-5.5 million/mm^3	3.9-5.5 × 10^{12} cells/L
	1-3 d	4.0-6.6 million/mm^3	4.0-6.6 × 10^{12} cells/L
	1 wk	3.9-6.3 million/mm^3	3.9-6.3 × 10^{12} cells/L
	2 wk	3.6-6.2 million/mm^3	3.6-6.2 × 10^{12} cells/L
	1 mo	3.0-5.4 million/mm^3	3.0-5.4 × 10^{12} cells/L
	2 mo	2.7-4.9 million/mm^3	2.7-4.9 × 10^{12} cells/L
	3-6 mo	3.1-4.5 million/mm^3	3.1-4.5 × 10^{12} cells/L
	0.5-2 yr	3.7-5.3 million/mm^3	3.7-5.3 × 10^{12} cells/L
	2-6 yr	3.9-5.3 million/mm^3	3.9-5.3 × 10^{12} cells/L
	6-12 yr	4.0-5.2 million/mm^3	4.0-5.2 × 10^{12} cells/L
	12-18 yr: Male	4.5-5.3 million/mm^3	4.5-5.3 × 10^{12} cells/L
	Female	4.1-5.1 million/mm^3	4.1-5.1 × 10^{12} cells/L
Erythrocyte sedimentation rate (ESR)			
Whole blood			
Westergren (modified)	Child	0-10 mm/hr	0-10 mm/hr
	<50 yr: Male	0-15 mm/hr	0-15 mm/hr
	Female	0-20 mm/hr	0-20 mm/hr
Wintrobe	Child	0-13 mm/hr	0-13 mm/hr
	Adult: Male	0-9 mm/hr	0-9 mm/hr
	Female	0-20 mm/hr	0-20 mm/hr
Fibrinogen			
Plasma	Newborn	125-300 mg/d	1.25-3.00 g/L
	Thereafter	200-400 mg/dl	2.00-4.00 g/L
Galactose			
Serum	Newborn	0-20 mg/dl	0-1.11 mmol/L
	Thereafter	<5 mg/dl	<0.28 mmol/L
Urine	Newborn	≤60 mg/dl	≤3.33 mmol/L
	Thereafter	<14 mg/24 hr	<0.08 mmol/d
Glucose			
Serum	Cord	45-96 mg/dl	2.5-5.3 mmol/L
	Newborn, 1 d	40-60 mg/dl	2.2-3.3 mmol/L
	Newborn, >1 d	50-90 mg/dl	2.8-5.0 mmol/L
	Child	60-100 mg/dl	3.3-5.5 mmol/L
	Thereafter	70-105 mg/dl	3.9-5.8 mmol/L
Whole blood	Adult	65-95 mg/dl	3.6-5.3 mmol/L
CSF	Adult	40-70 mg/dl	2.2-3.9 mmol/L
Urine (quantitative)		<0.5 g/d	<2.8 mmol/d
Urine (qualitative)		Negative	Negative

Continued

Common Laboratory Tests and Tests Results—cont'd

TEST/SPECIMEN	AGE/GENDER/REFERENCE	CONVENTIONAL UNITS (Normal Ranges)		INTERNATIONAL UNITS (SI) (Normal Ranges)	
Glucose tolerance test (GTT), oral					
Serum					
Dosages		Normal	Diabetic	Normal	Diabetic
Adult: 75 g	Fasting	70-105 mg/dl	≥126 mg/dl	3.9-5.8 mmol/L	≥7.0 mmol/L
Child: 1.75 g/kg of ideal	60 min	120-170 mg/dl	≥200 mg/dl	6.7-9.4 mmol/L	≥11 mmol/L
weight up to maximum of	90 min	100-140 mg/dl	≥200 mg/dl	5.6-7.8 mmol/L	≥11 mmol/L
75 g	120 min	70-120 mg/dl	≥200 mg/dl	3.9-6.7 mmol/L	≥11 mmol/L
Growth hormone (GH, somatotropin)					
Plasma	1 d	5-53 ng/ml		5-53 mcg/L	
	1 wk	5-27 ng/ml		5-27 mcg/L	
	1-12 mo	2-10 ng/ml		2-10 mcg/L	
	Fasting child/adult	<0.7-6.0 ng/ml		<0.7-6.0 mcg/L	
Hematocrit (HCT, Hct)					
Whole blood	1 d (cap)	48%-69%		0.48-0.69 vol fraction	
	2 d	48%-75%		0.48-0.75 vol fraction	
	3 d	44%-72%		0.44-0.72 vol fraction	
	2 mo	28%-42%		0.28-0.42 vol fraction	
	6-12 yr	35%-45%		0.35-0.45 vol fraction	
	12-18 yr: Male	37%-49%		0.37-0.49 vol fraction	
	Female	36%-46%		0.36-0.46 vol fraction	
Hemoglobin (Hb)					
Whole blood	1-3 d (cap)	14.5-22.5 g/dl		2.25-3.49 mmol/L	
	2 mo	9.0-14.0 g/dl		1.40-2.17 mmol/L	
	6-12 yr	11.5-15.5 g/dl		1.78-2.40 mmol/L	
	12-18 yr: Male	13.0-16.0 g/dl		2.02-2.48 mmol/L	
	Female	12.0-16.0 g/dl		1.86-2.48 mmol/L	
Hemoglobin A					
Whole blood		>95% of total		>0.95 fraction of Hb	
Hemoglobin F					
Whole blood	1 d	63%-92% HbF		0.63-0.92 mass fraction HbF	
	5 d	65%-88% HbF		0.65-0.88 mass fraction HbF	
	3 wk	55%-85% HbF		0.55-0.85 mass fraction HbF	
	6-9 wk	31%-75% HbF		0.31-0.75 mass fraction HbF	
	3-4 mo	<2%-59% HbF		<0.02-0.59 mass fraction HbF	
	6 mo	<2%-9% HbF		<0.02-0.09 mass fraction HbF	
	Adult	<2.0% HbF		<0.02 mass fraction HbF	
Immunoglobulin A (IgA)					
Serum	Cord	1.4-3.6 mg/dl		14-36 mg/L	
	1-3 mo	1.3-53 mg/dl		13-530 mg/L	
	4-6 mo	4.4-84 mg/dl		44-840 mg/L	
	7-12 mo	11-106 mg/dl		110-1060 mg/L	
	2-5 yr	14-159 mg/dl		140-1590 mg/L	
	6-10 yr	33-236 mg/dl		330-2360 mg/L	
	Adult	70-312 mg/dl		700-3120 mg/L	
Immunoglobulin D (IgD)					
Serum	Newborn	None detected		None detected	
	Thereafter	0-8 mg/dl		0-80 mg/L	
Immunoglobulin E (IgE)					
Serum	Male	0-230 IU/ml		0-230 kIU/L	
	Female	0-170 IU/ml		0-170 kIU/L	
Immunoglobulin G (IgG)					
Serum	Cord	636-1606 mg/dl		6.36-16.06 g/L	
	1 mo	251-906 mg/dl		2.51-9.06 g/L	
	2-4 mo	176-601 mg/dl		1.76-6.01 g/L	
	5-12 mo	172-1069 mg/dl		1.72-10.69 g/L	
	1-5 yr	345-1236 mg/dl		3.45-12.36 g/L	
	6-10 yr	608-1572 mg/dl		6.08-15.72 g/L	
	Adult	639-1349 mg/dl		6.39-13.49 g/L	

Common Laboratory Tests and Tests Results—cont'd

TEST/SPECIMEN	AGE/GENDER/REFERENCE	Normal Ranges: CONVENTIONAL UNITS		Normal Ranges: INTERNATIONAL UNITS (SI)
Immunoglobulin M (IgM)				
Serum	Cord	6.3-25 mg/dl		63-250 mg/L
	1-4 mo	17-105 mg/dl		170-1050 mg/L
	5-9 mo	33-126 mg/dl		330-1260 mg/L
	10-12 mo	41-173 mg/dl		410-1730 mg/L
	2-8 yr	43-207 mg/dl		430-2070 mg/L
	9-10 yr	52-242 mg/dl		520-2420 mg/L
	Adult	56-352 mg/dl		560-3520 mg/L
Iron				
Serum	Newborn	100-250 mcg/dl		18-45 μmol/L
	Infant	40-100 mcg/dl		7-18 μmol/L
	Child	50-120 mcg/dl		9-22 μmol/L
	Thereafter: Male	65-170 mcg/dl		12-30 μmol/L
	Female	50-170 mcg/dl		9-30 μmol/L
	Intoxicated child	280-2550 mcg/dl		50.12-456.5 μmol/L
	Fatally poisoned child	>1800 mcg/dl		>322.2 μmol/L
Iron-binding capacity, total (TIBC)				
Serum	Infant	100-400 mcg/dl		17.90-71.60 μmol/L
	Thereafter	250-400 mcg/dl		44.75-71.60 μmol/L
Lead				
Whole blood	Child	<10 mcg/dl		<0.48 μmol/L
Urine, 24 hr		<80 mcg/L		<0.39 μmol/L
Leukocyte count (WBC count)		×1000 cells/mm^3 (μl)		×10^9 cells/L
Whole blood	Birth	9.0-30.0		9.0-30.0
	24 hr	9.4-34.0		9.4-34.0
	1 mo	5.0-19.5		5.0-19.5
	1-3 yr	6.0-17.5		6.0-17.5
	4-7 yr	5.5-15.5		5.5-15.5
	8-13 yr	4.5-13.5		4.5-13.5
	Adult	4.5-11.0		4.5-11.0
		×1000 cells/mm^3 (μl)		×10^6 cells/L
CSF (cell count)	Premature	0-25 mononuclear		0-25
		0-10 polymorphonuclear		0-10
		0-1000 RBC		0-1000
	Newborn	0-20 mononuclear		0-20
		0-10 polymorphonuclear		0-10
		0-800 RBC		0-800
	Neonate	0-5 mononuclear		0-5
		0-10 polymorphonuclear		0-10
		0-50 RBC		0-50
	Thereafter	0-5 mononuclear		0-5
Leukocyte differential count				
Whole blood	Myelocytes	0%	0 cells/mm^3 (μl)	Number fraction 0
	Neutrophils–"bands"	3%-5%	150-400 cells/mm^3 (μl)	Number fraction 0.03-0.05
	Neutrophils–"segs"	54%-62%	3000-5800 cells/mm^3 (μl)	Number fraction 0.54-0.62
	Lymphocytes	25%-33%	1500-3000 cells/mm^3 (μl)	Number fraction 0.25-0.33
	Monocytes	3%-7%	285-500 cells/mm^3 (μl)	Number fraction 0.03-0.07
	Eosinophils	1%-3%	50-250 cells/mm^3 (μl)	Number fraction 0.01-0.03
	Basophils	0%-0.75%	15-50 cells/mm^3 (μl)	Number fraction 0-0.0075

Continued

Common Laboratory Tests and Tests Results—cont'd

TEST/SPECIMEN	AGE/GENDER/REFERENCE	Normal Ranges: CONVENTIONAL UNITS	Normal Ranges: INTERNATIONAL UNITS (SI)
Mean corpuscular hemoglobin (MCH)			
Whole blood	Birth	31-37 pg/cell	0.48-0.57 fmol/cell
	1-3 d (cap)	31-37 pg/cell	0.48-0.57 fmol/cell
	1 wk–1 mo	28-40 pg/cell	0.43-0.62 fmol/cell
	2 mo	26-34 pg/cell	0.40-0.53 fmol/cell
	3-6 mo	25-35 pg/cell	0.39-0.54 fmol/cell
	0.5-2 yr	23-31 pg/cell	0.36-0.48 fmol/cell
	2-6 yr	24-30 pg/cell	0.37-0.47 fmol/cell
	6-12 yr	25-33 pg/cell	0.39-0.51 fmol/cell
	12-18 yr	25-35 pg/cell	0.39-0.54 fmol/cell
	18-49 yr	26-34 pg/cell	0.40-0.53 fmol/cell
Mean corpuscular hemoglobin concentration (MCHC)			
Whole blood	Birth	30%-36% Hb/cell or g Hb/dl RBC	4.65-5.58 mmol Hb/L RBC
	1-3 d (cap)	29%-37% Hb/cell or g Hb/dl RBC	4.50-5.74 mmol Hb/L RBC
	1-2 wk	28%-38% Hb/cell or g Hb/dl RBC	4.34-5.89 mmol Hb/L RBC
	1-2 mo	29%-37% Hb/cell or g Hb/dl RBC	4.50-5.74 mmol Hb/L RBC
	3 mo–2 yr	30%-36% Hb/cell or g Hb/dl RBC	4.65-5.58 mmol Hb/L RBC
	2-18 yr	31%-37% Hb/cell or g Hb/dl RBC	4.81-5.74 mmol Hb/L RBC
	>18 yr	31%-37% Hb/cell or g Hb/dl RBC	4.81-5.74 mmol Hb/L RBC
Mean corpuscular volume (MCV)			
Whole blood	1-3 d (cap)	95-121 μm^3	95-121 fl
	0.5-2 yr	70-86 μm^3	70-86 fl
	6-12 yr	77-95 μm^3	77-95 fl
	12-18 yr: Male	78-98 μm^3	78-98 fl
	Female	78-102 μm^3	78-102 fl
Osmolality			
Serum	Child, adult	275-295 mOsm/kg H_2O	
Urine, random		50-1400 mOsm/kg H_2O, depending on fluid intake; after 12-hr fluid restriction: >850 mOsm/kg H_2O	
Urine, 24 hr		≅300-900 mOsm/kg H_2O	
Oxygen, partial pressure (Po_2)			
Whole blood, arterial	Birth	8-24 mm Hg	1.1-3.2 kPa
	5-10 min	33-75 mm Hg	4.4-10.0 kPa
	30 min	31-85 mm Hg	4.1-11.3 kPa
	>1 hr	55-80 mm Hg	7.3-10.6 kPa
	1 d	54-95 mm Hg	7.2-12.6 kPa
	Thereafter (decreased with age)	83-108 mm Hg	11-14.4 kPa
Oxygen saturation (Sao_2)			
Whole blood, arterial	Newborn	85%-90%	Fraction saturated 0.85-0.90
	Thereafter	95%-99%	Fraction saturated 0.95-0.99
Partial thromboplastin time (PTT)			
Whole blood (Na citrate)			
Nonactivated		60-85 s (Platelin)	60-85 s
Activated		25-35 s (differs with method)	25-35 s
pH			H^+ concentration
Whole blood, arterial (must be corrected for body temperature)	Premature (48 hr)	7.35-7.50	31-44 nmol/L
	Birth, full term	7.11-7.36	43-77 nmol/L
	5-10 min	7.09-7.30	50-81 nmol/L
	30 min	7.21-7.38	41-61 nmol/L
	>1 hr	7.26-7.49	32-54 nmol/L
	1 d	7.29-7.45	35-51 nmol/L
	Thereafter	7.35-7.45	35-44 nmol/L
Urine, random	Newborn/neonate	5-7	0.1-10 µmol/L
	Thereafter	4.5-8 (average ≅6)	0.01-32 µmol/L (average ≅1.0 µmol/L)
Stool		7.0-7.5	31-100 nmol/L

Common Laboratory Tests and Tests Results—cont'd

TEST/SPECIMEN	AGE/GENDER/REFERENCE	Normal Ranges CONVENTIONAL UNITS	INTERNATIONAL UNITS (SI)
Phenylalanine			
Serum	Premature	2.0-7.5 mg/dl	120-450 μmol/L
	Newborn	1.2-3.4 mg/dl	70-210 μmol/L
	Thereafter	0.8-1.8 mg/dl	50-110 μmol/L
Urine, 24 hr	10 d–2 wk	1-2 mg/d	6-12 μmol/d
	3-12 yr	4-18 mg/d	24-110 μmol/d
	Thereafter	Trace–17 mg/d	Trace–103 μmol/d
Plasma volume			
Plasma	Male	25-43 ml/kg	0.025-0.043 L/kg
	Female	28-45 ml/kg	0.028-0.045 L/kg
Platelet count (thrombocyte count)			
Whole blood (EDTA)	Newborn (after 1 wk, same as adult)	84-478 × 10^3/mm^3 (μl)	84-478 × 10^9/L
	Adult	150-400 × 10^3/mm^3 (μl)	150-400 × 10^9/L
Potassium			
Serum	Newborn	3.0-6.0 mEq/L	3.0-6.0 mmol/L
	Thereafter	3.5-5.0 mEq/L	3.5-5.0 mmol/L
Plasma (heparin)		3.4-4.5 mEq/L	3.4-4.5 mmol/L
Urine, 24 hr		2.5-125 mEq/d (varies with diet)	2.5-125 mmol/L
Protein			
Serum, total	Premature	4.3-7.6 g/dl	43-76 g/L
	Newborn	4.6-7.4 g/dl	46-74 g/L
	1-7 yr	6.1-7.9 g/dl	61-79 g/L
	8-12 yr	6.4-8.1 g/dl	64-81 g/L
	13-19 yr	6.6-8.2 g/dl	66-82 g/L
Total			
Urine, 24 hr		1-14 mg/dl	10-140 mg/L
		50-80 mg/d (at rest)	50-80 mg/d
		<250 mg/d (after intense exercise)	<250 mg/d (after intense exercise)
CSF		Lumbar: 8-32 mg/dl	80-320 mg/L
Prothrombin time (PT)			
One-stage (Quick)			
Whole blood (Na citrate)	In general	11-15 s (varies with type of thromboplastin)	11-15 s
	Newborn	Prolonged by 2-3 s	Prolonged by 2-3 s
Two-stage modified (Ware and Seegers)			
Whole blood (sodium citrate)		18-22 s	18-22 s
RBC count: see Erythrocyte (RBC) count			
Red blood cell volume			
Whole blood	Male	20-36 ml/kg	0.020-0.036 L/kg
	Female	19-31 ml/kg	0.019-0.031 L/kg
Reticulocyte count			
Whole blood	Adults	0.5%-1.5% of erythrocytes or 25,000-75,000/mm^3 (μl)	0.005-0.015 (number fraction) or 25,000-75,000 × 10^6/L
Capillary	1 d	0.4%-6.0%	0.004-0.060 (number fraction)
	7 d	<0.1%-1.3%	<0.001-0.013 (number fraction)
	1-4 wk	<0.1%-1.2%	<0.001-0.012 (number fraction)
	5-6 wk	<0.1%-2.4%	<0.001-0.024 (number fraction)
	7-8 wk	0.1%-2.9%	0.001-0.029 (number fraction)
	9-10 wk	<0.1%-2.6%	<0.001-0.026 (number fraction)
	11-12 wk	0.1%-1.3%	0.001-0.013 (number fraction)
Salicylates			
Serum, plasma	Therap. conc.	15-30 mg/dl	1.1-2.2 mmol/L
	Toxic conc.	>30 mg/dl	>18.5 mmol/L

Continued

Common Laboratory Tests and Tests Results—cont'd

TEST/SPECIMEN	AGE/GENDER/REFERENCE	Normal Ranges: CONVENTIONAL UNITS		Normal Ranges: INTERNATIONAL UNITS (SI)	
Sedimentation rate: see Erythrocyte sedimentation rate (ESR)					
Sodium					
Serum or plasma	Newborn	134-146 mEq/L		134-146 mmol/L	
	Infant	139-146 mEq/L		139-146 mmol/L	
	Child	138-145 mEq/L		138-145 mmol/L	
	Thereafter	136-146 mEq/L		136-146 mmol/L	
Urine, 24 hr		40-220 mEq/L (diet dependent)		40-220 mmol/L	
Sweat	Normal	<40 mEq/L		<40 mmol/L	
	Indeterminate	45-60 mEq/L		45-60 mmol/L	
	Cystic fibrosis	>60 mEq/L		>60 mmol/L	
Specific gravity					
Urine, random	Adult	1.002-1.030		1.002-1.030	
	After 12-hr fluid restriction	>1.025		>1.025	
Urine, 24 hr		1.015-1.025			
Theophylline					
Serum, plasma	Therap. conc.				
	Bronchodilator	10-20 mcg/ml		56-110 μmol/L	
	Premature apnea	5-10 mcg/ml		28-56 μmol/L	
	Toxic conc.	>20 mcg/ml		>110 μmol/L	
Thrombin time					
Whole blood (Na citrate)		Control time ±2 s when control is 9-13 s		Control time ±2 s when control is 9-13 s	
Thyroxine, total (T_4)					
Serum	Cord	8-13 mcg/dl		103-168 nmol/L	
	Newborn	11.5-24 mcg/dl (lower in low-birth-weight infants)		148-310 nmol/L	
	Neonate	9-18 mcg/dl		116-232 nmol/L	
	Infant	7-15 mcg/dl		90-194 nmol/L	
	1-5 yr	7.3-15 mcg/dl		94-194 nmol/L	
	5-10 yr	6.4-13.3 mcg/dl		83-172 nmol/L	
	Thereafter	5-12 mcg/dl		65-155 nmol/L	
	Newborn screen (filter paper)	6.2-22 mcg/dl		80-284 nmol/L	
Triglycerides (TG)		**Male** (mg/dl)	**Female** (mg/dl)	**Male** (g/L)	**Female** (g/L)
Serum, after ≥2-hr fast	Cord	10-98	10-98	0.10-0.98	0.10-0.98
	0-5 yr	30-86	32-99	0.30-0.86	0.32-0.99
	6-11 yr	31-108	35-114	0.31-1.08	0.35-1.14
	12-15 yr	36-138	41-138	0.36-1.38	0.41-1.38
	16-19 yr	40-163	40-128	0.40-1.63	0.40-1.28
Triiodothyronine (T_3), free					
Serum	Cord	20-240 pg/dl		0.3-3.7 pmol/L	
	1-3 d	200-610 pg/dl		3.1-9.4 pmol/L	
	6 wk	240-560 pg/dl		3.7-8.6 pmol/L	
	Adults (20-50 yr)	230-660 pg/dl		3.5-10.0 pmol/L	
Triiodothyronine, total (T_3-RIA)					
Serum	Cord	30-70 ng/dl		0.46-1.08 nmol/L	
	Newborn	72-260 ng/dl		1.16-4 nmol/L	
	1-5 yr	100-260 ng/dl		1.54-4 nmol/L	
	5-10 yr	90-240 ng/dl		1.39-3.70 nmol/L	
	10-15 yr	80-210 ng/dl		1.23-3.23 nmol/L	
	Thereafter	115-190 ng/dl		1.77-2.93 nmol/L	
Urea nitrogen					
Serum or plasma	Cord	21-40 mg/dl		7.5-14.3 mmol/L	
	Premature (1 wk)	3-25 mg/dl		1.1-9 mmol/L	
	Newborn	3-12 mg/dl		1.1-4.3 mmol/L	
	Infant/child	5-18 mg/dl		1.8-6.4 mmol/L	
	Thereafter	7-18 mg/dl		2.5-6.4 mmol/L	

Common Laboratory Tests and Tests Results—cont'd

TEST/SPECIMEN	AGE/GENDER/REFERENCE	Normal Ranges CONVENTIONAL UNITS	INTERNATIONAL UNITS (SI)
Urine volume			
Urine, 24 hr	Newborn	50-300 ml/d	0.05-0.3 L/d
	Infant	350-550 ml/d	0.35-0.5 L/d
	Child	500-1000 ml/d	0.5-1 L/d
	Adolescent	700-1400 ml/d	0.7-1.4 L/d
	Thereafter: Male	800-1800 ml/d	0.8-1.8 L/d
	Female	600-1600 ml/d (varies with intake and other factors)	0.6-1.6 L/d
WBC: see Leukocyte count (WBC count)			

Modified from Kliegman RM, Behrman RE, Jenson HB, and others, editors: *Nelson textbook of pediatrics*, ed 18, Philadelphia, 2007, Saunders; McMillan JA, Deangelis CD, Feigin RD, and others, editors: *Oski's pediatrics: principles and practice*, ed 3, Philadelphia, 1999, Lippincott Williams & Wilkins; and Fischbach F: *A manual of laboratory and diagnostic tests*, ed 6, Philadelphia, 2000, Lippincott Williams & Wilkins.

*For a description of abbreviations, see below.

†From National Cholesterol Education Program: Report of the expert panel on blood cholesterol levels in children and adolescents, *Pediatrics* 89(3 pt 2):527, 1992.

Abbreviations Used in Laboratory Tests

ABBREVIATION	TERM	ABBREVIATION	TERM
cap	capillary	mol	mole
CHF	congestive heart failure	mOsm	milliosmole
conc.	concentration	Na	sodium
CSF	cerebrospinal fluid	Pa	pascal
d	day; diem	RBC	red blood cells
EDTA	ethylenediaminetetraacetate	s	second
g	gram	temp	temperature
H^+	hydrogen ion	therap.	therapeutic
Hb	hemoglobin	U	international unit of enzyme activity
hr	hour	vol	volume
IU	International unit	WBC	white blood cells
L	liter	wk	week
m	meter	yr	year
mEq	milliequivalent	>	greater than
min	minute	≥	greater than or equal to
mm	millimeter	<	less than
mm Hg	millimeters of mercury	≤	less than or equal to
mm H_2O	millimeters of water	±	plus/minus
mm^3	cubic millimeter	≅	approximately equal to
mo	month		

Prefixes Denoting Decimal Factors

PREFIX	SYMBOL	AMOUNT
deci	d	one tenth (10^{-1})
centi	c	one hundredth (10^{-2})
milli	m	one thousandth (10^{-3})
micro	mc, μ	one millionth (10^{-6})
nano	n	one billionth (10^{-9})
pico	p	one trillionth (10^{-12})
femto	f	one quadrillionth (10^{-15})

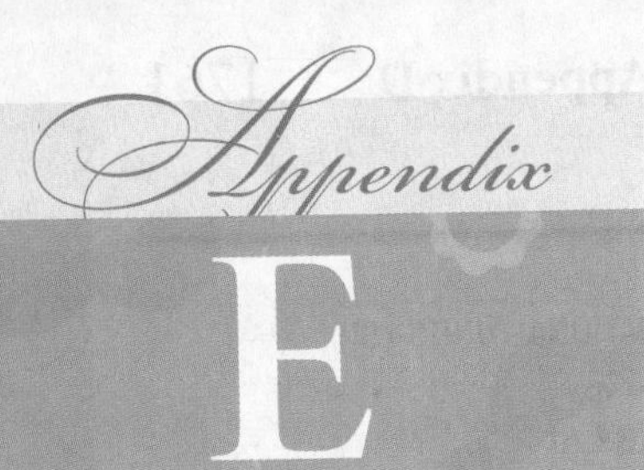

Pediatric Vital Signs and Parameters

Centigrade to Fahrenheit Temperature Conversions

°C	°F	°C	°F	°C	°F
35.0	**95.0**	**37.0**	**98.6**	**39.0**	**102.2**
35.2	95.4	37.2	99.0	39.2	102.6
35.4	95.7	37.4	99.3	39.4	102.9
35.6	96.1	37.6	99.7	39.6	103.3
35.8	96.4	37.8	100.0	39.8	103.6
36.0	**96.8**	**38.0**	**100.4**	**40.0**	**104.0**
36.2	97.2	38.2	100.8	40.2	104.4
36.4	97.5	38.4	101.1	40.4	104.7
36.6	97.9	38.6	101.5	40.6	105.1
36.8	98.2	38.8	101.8	40.8	105.4
				41.0	**105.8**

Conversion Formulas

°F = (°C × $\frac{9}{5}$) + 32 or (°C × 1.8) + 32
°C = (°F − 32) +$\frac{5}{9}$ or (°F − 32) + 0.55

Normal Heart Rates for Infants and Children

	Rate (beats/min)		
AGE	RESTING (AWAKE)	RESTING (SLEEPING)	EXERCISE (FEVER)
Newborn	100-180	80-160	Up to 220
1 wk to 3 mo	100-220	80-200	Up to 220
3 mo to 2 yr	80-150	70-120	Up to 200
2 yr to 10 yr	70-110	60-90	Up to 200
10 yr to adult	55-90	50-90	Up to 200

From Gillette PC: Dysrhythmias. In Adams FH, Emmanoulides GC, Riemenschneider TA, editors: *Moss' heart disease in infants, children, and adolescents*, ed 4, Baltimore, 1989, Williams & Wilkins.

Normal Temperatures in Children

	Temperature	
AGE	°F	°C
3 mo	99.4	37.5
6 mo	99.5	37.5
1 yr	99.7	37.7
3 yr	99.0	37.2
5 yr	98.6	37.0
7 yr	98.3	36.8
9 yr	98.1	36.7
11 yr	98.0	36.7
13 yr	97.8	36.6

Modified from Lowrey GH: *Growth and development of children*, ed 8, St Louis, 1986, Mosby.

Normal Respiratory Rates for Children

AGE	RATE (breaths/min)
Newborn	35
1 to 11 mo	30
2 yr	25
4 yr	23
6 yr	21
8 yr	20
10 yr	19
12 yr	19
14 yr	18
16 yr	17
18 yr	16-18

Blood Pressure (BP) Levels for Boys by Age and Height Percentile

		Systolic BP (mm Hg) Percentile of Height							Diastolic BP (mm Hg) Percentile of Height						
AGE (yr)	BP PERCENTILE	5th	10th	25th	50th	75th	90th	95th	5th	10th	25th	50th	75th	90th	95th
1	50th	80	81	83	85	87	88	89	34	35	36	37	38	39	39
	90th	94	95	97	99	100	102	103	49	50	51	52	53	53	54
	95th	98	99	101	103	104	106	106	54	54	55	56	57	58	58
	99th	105	106	108	110	112	113	114	61	62	63	64	65	66	66
2	50th	84	85	87	88	90	92	92	39	40	41	42	43	44	44
	90th	97	99	100	102	104	105	106	54	55	56	57	58	58	59
	95th	101	102	104	106	108	109	110	59	59	60	61	62	63	63
	99th	109	110	111	113	115	117	117	66	67	68	69	70	71	71
3	50th	86	87	89	91	93	94	95	44	44	45	46	47	48	48
	90th	100	101	103	105	107	108	109	59	59	60	61	62	63	63
	95th	104	105	107	109	110	112	113	63	63	64	65	66	67	67
	99th	111	112	114	116	118	119	120	71	71	72	73	74	75	75
4	50th	88	89	91	93	95	96	97	47	48	49	50	51	51	52
	90th	102	103	105	107	109	110	111	62	63	64	65	66	66	67
	95th	106	107	109	111	112	114	115	66	67	68	69	70	71	71
	99th	113	114	116	118	120	121	122	74	75	76	77	78	78	79
5	50th	90	91	93	95	96	98	98	50	51	52	53	54	55	55
	90th	104	105	106	108	110	111	112	65	66	67	68	69	69	70
	95th	108	109	110	112	114	115	116	69	70	71	72	73	74	74
	99th	115	116	118	120	121	123	123	77	78	79	80	81	81	82
6	50th	91	92	94	96	98	99	100	53	53	54	55	56	57	57
	90th	105	106	108	110	111	113	113	68	68	69	70	71	72	72
	95th	109	110	112	114	115	117	117	72	72	73	74	75	76	76
	99th	116	117	119	121	123	124	125	80	80	81	82	83	84	84
7	50th	92	94	95	97	99	100	101	55	55	56	57	58	59	59
	90th	106	107	109	111	113	114	115	70	70	71	72	73	74	74
	95th	110	111	113	115	117	118	119	74	74	75	76	77	78	78
	99th	117	118	120	122	124	125	126	82	82	83	84	85	86	86
8	50th	94	95	97	99	100	102	102	56	57	58	59	60	60	61
	90th	107	109	110	112	114	115	116	71	72	72	73	74	75	76
	95th	111	112	114	116	118	119	120	75	76	77	78	79	79	80
	99th	119	120	122	123	125	127	127	83	84	85	86	87	87	88
9	50th	95	96	98	100	102	103	104	57	58	59	60	61	61	62
	90th	109	110	112	114	115	117	118	72	73	74	75	76	76	77
	95th	113	114	116	118	119	121	121	76	77	78	79	80	81	81
	99th	120	121	123	125	127	128	129	84	85	86	87	88	88	89
10	50th	97	98	100	102	103	105	106	58	59	60	61	61	62	63
	90th	111	112	114	115	117	119	119	73	73	74	75	76	77	78
	95th	115	116	117	119	121	122	123	77	78	79	80	81	81	82
	99th	122	123	125	127	128	130	130	85	86	86	88	88	89	90
11	50th	99	100	102	104	105	107	107	59	59	60	61	62	63	63
	90th	113	114	115	117	119	120	121	74	74	75	76	77	78	78
	95th	117	118	119	121	123	124	125	78	78	79	80	81	82	82
	99th	124	125	127	129	130	132	132	86	86	87	88	89	90	90

Continued

		Systolic BP (mm Hg)							Diastolic BP (mm Hg)						
		Percentile of Height							Percentile of Height						
AGE (yr)	BP PERCENTILE	5th	10th	25th	50th	75th	90th	95th	5th	10th	25th	50th	75th	90th	95th
12	50th	101	102	104	106	108	109	110	59	60	61	62	63	63	64
	90th	115	116	118	120	121	123	123	74	75	75	76	77	78	79
	95th	119	120	122	123	125	127	127	78	79	80	81	82	82	83
	99th	126	127	129	131	133	134	135	86	87	88	89	90	90	91
13	50th	104	105	106	108	110	111	112	60	60	61	62	63	64	64
	90th	117	118	120	122	124	125	126	75	75	76	77	78	79	79
	95th	121	122	124	126	128	129	130	79	79	80	81	82	83	83
	99th	128	130	131	133	135	136	137	87	87	88	89	90	91	91
14	50th	106	107	109	111	113	114	115	60	61	62	63	64	65	65
	90th	120	121	123	125	126	128	128	75	76	77	78	79	79	80
	95th	124	125	127	128	130	132	132	80	80	81	82	83	84	84
	99th	131	132	134	136	138	139	140	87	88	89	90	91	92	92
15	50th	109	110	112	113	115	117	117	61	62	63	64	65	66	66
	90th	122	124	125	127	129	130	131	76	77	78	79	80	80	81
	95th	126	127	129	131	133	134	135	81	81	82	83	84	85	85
	99th	134	135	136	138	140	142	142	88	89	90	91	92	93	93
16	50th	111	112	114	116	118	119	120	63	63	64	65	66	67	67
	90th	125	126	128	130	131	133	134	78	78	79	80	81	82	82
	95th	129	130	132	134	135	137	137	82	83	83	84	85	86	87
	99th	136	137	139	141	143	144	145	90	90	91	92	93	94	94
17	50th	114	115	116	118	120	121	122	65	66	66	67	68	69	70
	90th	127	128	130	132	134	135	136	80	80	81	82	83	84	84
	95th	131	132	134	136	138	139	140	84	85	86	87	87	88	89
	99th	139	140	141	143	145	146	147	92	93	93	94	95	96	97

The 90th percentile is 1.28 SD, the 95th percentile is 1.645 SD, and the 99th percentile is 2.326 SD over the mean.

Blood Pressure (BP) Levels for Girls by Age and Height Percentile

		Systolic BP (mm Hg) Percentile of Height							Diastolic BP (mm Hg) Percentile of Height						
AGE (yr)	BP PERCENTILE	5th	10th	25th	50th	75th	90th	95th	5th	10th	25th	50th	75th	90th	95th
1	50th	83	84	85	86	88	89	90	38	39	39	40	41	41	42
	90th	97	97	98	100	101	102	103	52	53	53	54	55	55	56
	95th	100	101	102	104	105	106	107	56	57	57	58	59	59	60
	99th	108	108	109	111	112	113	114	64	64	65	65	66	67	67
2	50th	85	85	87	88	89	91	91	43	44	44	45	46	46	47
	90th	98	99	100	101	103	104	105	57	58	58	59	60	61	61
	95th	102	103	104	105	107	108	109	61	62	62	63	64	65	65
	99th	109	110	111	112	114	115	116	69	69	70	70	71	72	72
3	50th	86	87	88	89	91	92	93	47	48	48	49	50	50	51
	90th	100	100	102	103	104	106	106	61	62	62	63	64	64	65
	95th	104	104	105	107	108	109	110	65	66	66	67	68	68	69
	99th	111	111	113	114	115	116	117	73	73	74	74	75	76	76
4	50th	88	88	90	91	92	94	94	50	50	51	52	52	53	54
	90th	101	102	103	104	106	107	108	64	64	65	66	67	67	68
	95th	105	106	107	108	110	111	112	68	68	69	70	71	71	72
	99th	112	113	114	115	117	118	119	76	76	76	77	78	79	79
5	50th	89	90	91	93	94	95	96	52	53	53	54	55	55	56
	90th	103	103	105	106	107	109	109	66	67	67	68	69	69	70
	95th	107	107	108	110	111	112	113	70	71	71	72	73	73	74
	99th	114	114	116	117	118	120	120	78	78	79	79	80	81	81
6	50th	91	92	93	94	96	97	98	54	54	55	56	56	57	58
	90th	104	105	106	108	109	110	111	68	68	69	70	70	71	72
	95th	108	109	110	111	113	114	115	72	72	73	74	74	75	76
	99th	115	116	117	119	120	121	122	80	80	80	81	82	83	83
7	50th	93	93	95	96	97	99	99	55	56	56	57	58	58	59
	90th	106	107	108	109	111	112	113	69	70	70	71	72	72	73
	95th	110	111	112	113	115	116	116	73	74	74	75	76	76	77
	99th	117	118	119	120	122	123	124	81	81	82	82	83	84	84
8	50th	95	95	96	98	99	100	101	57	57	57	58	59	60	60
	90th	108	109	110	111	113	114	114	71	71	71	72	73	74	74
	95th	112	112	114	115	116	118	118	75	75	75	76	77	78	78
	99th	119	120	121	122	123	125	125	82	82	83	83	84	85	86
9	50th	96	97	98	100	101	102	103	58	58	58	59	60	61	61
	90th	110	110	112	113	114	116	116	72	72	72	73	74	75	75
	95th	114	114	115	117	118	119	120	76	76	76	77	78	79	79
	99th	121	121	123	124	125	127	127	83	83	84	84	85	86	87
10	50th	98	99	100	102	103	104	105	59	59	59	60	61	62	62
	90th	112	112	114	115	116	118	118	73	73	73	74	75	76	76
	95th	116	116	117	119	120	121	122	77	77	77	78	79	80	80
	99th	123	123	125	126	127	129	129	84	84	85	86	86	87	88
11	50th	100	101	102	103	105	106	107	60	60	60	61	62	63	63
	90th	114	114	116	117	118	119	120	74	74	74	75	76	77	77
	95th	118	118	119	121	122	123	124	78	78	78	79	80	81	81
	99th	125	125	126	128	129	130	131	85	85	86	87	87	88	89

Continued

		Systolic BP (mm Hg)							*Diastolic BP (mm Hg)*						
		Percentile of Height							*Percentile of Height*						
AGE (yr)	**BP PERCENTILE**	**5th**	**10th**	**25th**	**50th**	**75th**	**90th**	**95th**	**5th**	**10th**	**25th**	**50th**	**75th**	**90th**	**95th**
12	50th	102	103	104	105	107	108	109	61	61	61	62	63	64	64
	90th	116	116	117	119	120	121	122	75	75	75	76	77	78	78
	95th	119	120	121	123	124	125	126	79	79	79	80	81	82	82
	99th	127	127	128	130	131	132	133	86	86	87	88	88	89	90
13	50th	104	105	106	107	109	110	110	62	62	62	63	64	65	65
	90th	117	118	119	121	122	123	124	76	76	76	77	78	79	79
	95th	121	122	123	124	126	127	128	80	80	80	81	82	83	83
	99th	128	129	130	132	133	134	135	87	87	88	89	89	90	91
14	50th	106	106	107	109	110	111	112	63	63	63	64	65	66	66
	90th	119	120	121	122	124	125	125	77	77	77	78	79	80	80
	95th	123	123	125	126	127	129	129	81	81	81	82	83	84	84
	99th	130	131	132	133	135	136	136	88	88	89	90	90	91	92
15	50th	107	108	109	110	111	113	113	64	64	64	65	66	67	67
	90th	120	121	122	123	125	126	127	78	78	78	79	80	81	81
	95th	124	125	126	127	129	130	131	82	82	82	83	84	85	85
	99th	131	132	133	134	136	137	138	89	89	90	91	91	92	93
16	50th	108	108	110	111	112	114	114	64	64	65	66	66	67	68
	90th	121	122	123	124	126	127	128	78	78	79	80	81	81	82
	95th	125	126	127	128	130	131	132	82	82	83	84	85	85	86
	99th	132	133	134	135	137	138	139	90	90	90	91	92	93	93
17	50th	108	109	110	111	113	114	115	64	65	65	66	67	67	68
	90th	122	122	123	125	126	127	128	78	79	79	80	81	81	82
	95th	125	126	127	129	130	131	132	82	83	83	84	85	85	86
	99th	133	133	134	136	137	138	139	90	90	91	91	92	93	93

The 90th percentile is 1.28 SD, the 95th percentile is 1.645 SD, and the 99th percentile is 2.326 SD over the mean.
Downloaded from www.pediatrics.org at HAM/TMC Library on April 4, 2005.

Index

A

AAMR Adaptive Behavior Scale, 1178
AAP. *See* American Academy of Pediatrics (AAP).
Abbreviations
  in laboratory tests, 1761t
  list of "do not use", 14t
Abdomen
  of newborn, 626t-636t, 645-646
  nutritional status and, 884t-886t
  physical assessment of, 917-919, 917f-919f, 918b-919b
  postpartum changes in, 527, 528f
  trauma during pregnancy and, 373
    blunt, 371-372, 371b
    penetrating, 372
Abdominal breathing, 249f, 545f
Abdominal circumference
  of acutely ill child, 1393
  of infant, 891f
  ultrasound measurement of, 196, 197f
Abdominal ectopic pregnancy, 353, 357f
Abdominal hernias, 1418t
Abdominal pain
  in abruptio placentae, 365
  in colic, 1001-1002, 1002b, 1003f
  in pregnancy, 227
  recurrent, in school-age child, 1101-1102
  respiratory infections and, 1305b
Abdominal palpation. *See* Leopold maneuvers.
Abdominal surgery during pregnancy, nonobstetric, 368-369, 369b
Abducens nerve (cranial nerve VI), 925t
Abduction of newborns, 9, 540, 662
Abilify. *See* Aripiprazole.
Abnormal breath sounds in newborns, 648b
Abnormal labor patterns in dystocia, 501-502, 502t, 503f
Abnormal uterine bleeding (AUB), 95-96, 95b
ABO incompatibility, 766-767
Aborted SIDS death. *See* Apparent life-threatening events (ALTE).
Abortion, 156-159
  counseling about, 157, 157b
  emotional considerations in, 158
  laws regarding
    in Canada, 156
    in the United States, 4b, 156, 156b
  nurses' rights and responsibilities related to, 156-157, 157b
  signs of complications, 157, 158b
Abortus, definition of, 7b

Page numbers followed by f *indicate figures;* t, *tables;* b, *boxes.*

Abruptio placentae, 360, 360f, 362t, 365-366, 365f
  trauma-related, 371, 371b, 373-374
Absence seizures, 1583b-1584b, 1585t
Absolute neutrophil count, 1491t, 1512
Absolute standard of poverty, 825
Absorptive defects, 1423
Abstinence, periodic. *See* Natural family planning (NFP).
Abstract thinking, 1110-1111
Abuse
  child, 1066
    child neglect and, 1066, 1070b
    child support in, 1073
    clinical manifestations of, 1071b-1072b
    family support in, 1073-1074
    nursing care plan for, 1069-1074
      caregiver-child interaction and, 1070
      history and interview and, 1069b, 1071b-1072b
      nurse biases and, 1069b
      physical assessment and, 1072-1073, 1072b
      talking with children who reveal abuse and, 1069b
    physical abuse and, 1066-1068, 1067b
    plan for discharge in, 1074
    prevention of, 1074, 1075b
    protection from further abuse, 1073, 1073b
    sexual abuse and. *See* Sexual abuse.
    warning signs of, 1070b
  high risk pregnancy and, 191b
  of woman
    health assessment and, 76, 77f, 79
    history of, 240
    during pregnancy, 370
    prevention of, 58-59
Abuse assessment screen, 76, 77f
Acceleration head injuries, 1563
Accelerations of fetal heart rate, 429-430, 430b, 430f
Accessory nerve (cranial nerve XI), 925t
Accidental decannulation, 1294
Accountability in standards of care, 13b
Acculturation, 21, 828
Accutane. *See* Isotretinoin.
Acesulfame potassium, 280, 281b
Acetabular dysplasia, 774-775, 774f, 1691-1692
Acetabulum, 69f
Acetaminophen
  breastfeeding and, 1745t-1748t
  children and, 938-939, 939t, 942t
  normal test ranges for, 1753t-1761t
  overdose of, 1428b-1429b
Achilles reflex, 924f
Acid indigestion during pregnancy, 254t-256t
Acid poisoning, 1428b-1429b
Acid-base balance during pregnancy, 222
Acidemia, 437t
Acidosis
  ketoacidosis, 299, 1617-1618
  metabolic, 1546
  pregnancy and, 370
Acini, 69-70, 70f
ACLS protocol. *See* Advanced cardiac life support (ACLS) protocol.
Acne, 224, 254t-256t, 325, 325b, 1659-1661
ACOG. *See* American College of Obstetrics and Gynecologists (ACOG).
Acoustic feedback, 1187-1188
Acoustic nerve. *See* Vestibulocochlear nerve (cranial nerve VIII).
Acquaintance, 555
Acquired immunodeficiency syndrome (AIDS)
  in children
    clinical manifestations of, 1517, 1517b
    diagnostic evaluation of, 1517-1518, 1518t
    epidemiology of, 1516
    in industrialized vs. resource-poor parts of the world, 12
    therapeutic management of, 1518-1519
  perinatal transmission of, 328
  pregnancy and, 328-330
Acrodynia, 1432
Acroesthesia, 225-226
Acromegaly, 1602
Acrosome, 172
Across-the-lap position. *See* Cross cradle position.
Activated charcoal, 1430
Active phase of labor, 388
Actives of daily living, special needs children and, 1160
Activity
  adolescents and, 1113, 1113f, 1119-1120, 1119f
  after pediatric heart surgery, 1471
  infants and, 976-978, 977t
  preschoolers and, 1054-1055
  restriction in home care of mild preeclampsia, 342, 343b
  school-age children and, 1090-1091, 1090f
  toddlers and, 1031
Actualizing perinatal loss, 601-602, 601b-602b, 602f-603f
Acupressure
  for nausea during pregnancy, 290-291, 291f
  for pain management during labor, 403-404, 405f
  perinatal education and, 270
Acupuncture
  for cocaine abuse in pregnancy, 50-51
  for pain management during labor, 404
Acute adrenocortical insufficiency, 1611-1612, 1611b-1612b
Acute appendicitis, 1398-1400, 1399b
Acute chest syndrome, 1495-1497
Acute cholecystitis, 325
Acute epiglottitis, 1318-1319, 1318b-1319b, 1318t
Acute glomerulonephritis, 1538-1540, 1539b
Acute hepatitis, 1406-1409, 1407t
Acute illness, definition of, 791
Acute infectious diarrhea, 1383
Acute laryngitis, 1319
Acute laryngotracheobronchitis (LTB), 1318t, 1320-1321, 1320b
Acute lung injury (ALI), 1331-1332
Acute lymphoid anemia, 1492f
Acute lymphoid leukemia, 1508
Acute nonlymphoid leukemia, 1508
Acute otitis media, 1314b-1315b
Acute poststreptococcal glomerulonephritis, 1538
Acute renal failure (ARF), 1542-1545, 1542b-1544b
Acute respiratory distress syndrome (ARDS), 1331-1332
Acute spasmodic laryngitis, 1318t, 1321
Acute supraglottitis. *See* Acute epiglottitis.
Acute tracheitis, 1318t
Acute wounds, 1633
Acyanotic defects, 1447, 1447f
Acyclovir, 105, 1057
  breastfeeding and, 1745t-1748t
  during pregnancy, 106
Adalimumab, 1402
Adaptation to grandparenthood, 571-573, 572b, 572f-573f
Adaptation to labor
  fetal, 390
  maternal, 390-392, 391b
Adaptation to parenthood, 548, 554, 559
  maternal, 561-562, 561t, 562b, 563f
  paternal, 564-565, 564t, 565f
  preterm infants and, 710-726, 711f, 712b
Adaptation to pregnancy
  family, 230-232, 231b, 232f
  grandparent, 231-232, 232f, 234-235, 236f, 237b, 264-265
  maternal, 230
    accepting the pregnancy, 230-231, 231b
    establishing a relationship with the fetus, 232, 235b
    identifying with the mother role, 231
  physiologic, 212, 212b, 227-228, 338b
    after trauma, 370, 370b, 371t
    breasts and, 217, 217f
    cardiovascular system and, 218-219, 218f-219f, 219b, 220t-221t, 338b

Adaptation to pregnancy *(Continued)*
endocrine system and, 227, 227t, 338b
gastrointestinal system and, 226-227, 226f
hematologic system and, 338b
integumentary system and, 223-224, 223f, 224b
musculoskeletal system and, 224-225, 225f
neurologic system and, 225-226, 225f
renal system and, 217f, 222-223, 223t, 338b
respiratory system and, 218f, 219-222, 222t
signs of pregnancy and, 212, 213t
uterus and, 212-216, 214f-216f
vagina and vulva and, 216-217, 216f-217f
preparing for childbirth, 232-233
reordering personal relationships, 231-232, 232f
paternal, 233-234, 233b, 233f, 235b
sexual, 256-258, 257b, 258f
sibling, 234, 235b-236b, 236f, 264-265
Addiction, 756
Addison's disease. *See* Chronic adrenocortical insufficiency.
Adenohypophysis, 1106
Adenoidectomy, 1312, 1316
Adenoids, 1311-1312, 1312f
Adenosine, 1359t
Adequate dietary intake, 288-290, 290b
ADHD. *See* Attention deficit hyperactivity disorder (ADHD).
Adherence. *See* Compliance.
Adherent retained placenta, 578
Adhesives, newborn skin and, 720-721, 721b-722b
Adjuvant analgesics for children, 939, 941t
Adjuvant chemotherapy for breast cancer, 122
Administration of medications
home care and, 39-40
induction of labor with oxytocin, 509b
during labor
intramuscular, 418
intravenous, 418
pain management, 418-420, 419f
pediatric
in cardiopulmonary resuscitation, 1358, 1359t
checking dosage and, 1273
determination of drug dosage and, 1273
family teaching and home care and, 1284, 1284b
insulin, 1619-1620
intramuscular, 1275-1278, 1276t-1277t, 1277f, 1278b

Administration of medications *(Continued)*
newborns and, 663-665, 663f, 665b
intravenous, 1279-1282, 1280b-1281b, 1281f, 1282t
nasogastric, orogastric, or gastrostomy, 1282, 1283b
optic, otic, and nasal, 1282-1284, 1282b-1284b, 1283f-1284f
oral, 1273-1275, 1274b, 1275f, 1284b
rectal, 1282
routes of analgesic administration in, 943b-944b, 945-946, 946b, 947f
subcutaneous and intradermal, 1278-1279, 1279b
unconscious child and, 1561
Admission assessment of child, 1225, 1226b-1228b
Admission data, 443-444
Admission to labor unit, 443, 443b, 443f
Adnexa, 68f
Adolescence, 843b, 1105
Adolescent Pediatric Pain Tool (APPT), 931
Adolescent pregnancy
health risks in, 48
intimate partner violence during, 62, 240
nursing care plan for, 260-261, 261f, 262b
nutrition needs in, 52, 279, 285
prevention programs for, 7b
rate of, 32-33, 260-261
Adolescents, 1144
acne and, 1659-1661
amenorrhea in, 1125
anorexia nervosa and, 52, 52b, 1132, 1133b-1135b
anticipatory guidance and, 1124-1125, 1125b
approaches to physical examination of, 888t
bacterial meningitis in, 1577b
biologic development of, 1105-1109, 1106b, 1107f-1108f
body image of, 853, 1115
bulimia and, 52-53, 1132, 1134b
class on the process of childbirth for, 387b
cognitive development of, 1110-1111, 1116t
cognitively impaired, 1182
communication with, 872, 872b, 1112b
contraception for, 141b
dental health of, 1120
divorce and, 817b
dysmenorrhea in, 88, 1125-1126
effects of adoption on, 816
exercise and activity of, 1119-1120, 1119f
female reproductive physical assessment of, 70t
growth and development of, 845, 845t, 1107-1109, 1116t
gynecomastia in, 1127
health assessment of, 78, 78b
health promotion and, 33, 1116-1117, 1117b

Adolescents *(Continued)*
health risks of, 47-48, 48b
high risk behaviors of, 32-33
hormonal changes of puberty, 1106
hospitalization of, 1221. *See also* Hospitalization: pediatric.
bathing during, 1258
developmentally appropriate activities and, 1232, 1232b
loss of control and, 1223, 1230-1231, 1231b
urine specimen collection and, 1267-1270
immunizations for, 1117-1118
improving immunization rates among, 990b
injury prevention and, 78, 1122-1124, 1123b
interests and activities of, 1113, 1113f
major tasks for, 78
male reproductive disorders in, 1126-1127, 1127b
moral development of, 1111
morbidity and mortality and, 1116
nutrition and, 1118-1119, 1118f
obesity and, 1119, 1127-1132, 1128f, 1131b-1132b
parenthood and, 566-567, 566b
pelvic examination of, 81, 81f
personal care and, 1120-1121
physical growth of, 1107-1109
premenstrual syndrome in, 90b
privacy of, 1117b, 1246
psychologic preparation for procedures, 1248b-1249b
psychosocial development of, 1109-1110, 1110b, 1116t
relationship with parents, 1111-1112, 1112b, 1116t
relationship with peers, 1112-1113, 1113f, 1116t
responses to puberty, 1115
self-concept and, 852-853, 1115
sexual history in health history and, 878, 878b
sexual maturation of, 1106-1107, 1106b, 1107f-1108f
sexuality activity of, 32-33, 48, 55
sexuality and, 48b, 878b, 1113-1115, 1114f, 1115b, 1116t
sexuality education and guidance for, 48, 48b, 1122
sleep and rest and, 1119
smoking and, 1136-1137, 1137b-1138b
social development of, 1111-1113, 1112b, 1113f
special needs, 1161t-1162t, 1163
spiritual development of, 1111
sports injuries and, 1096-1097, 1124
stress reduction and, 1121, 1121b, 1121f
substance abuse and, 1137-1140, 1137b
suicide and, 1140-1143, 1140b-1142b
understanding and reaction to death, 1167t-1168t
vaginitis in, 1126

Adoption, 138, 138f
acquaintance period in, 555
parenting of adopted child, 815-816, 815b-816b, 815f
Adrenal cortex, 182, 1611
Adrenal disorders, 1611
acute adrenocortical insufficiency, 1611-1612, 1611b-1612b
chronic adrenocortical insufficiency, 1612-1613, 1612b
congenital adrenal hyperplasia, 1614-1615
Cushing's syndrome, 1613-1614, 1613b-1614b, 1613f
pheochromocytoma, 1615-1616, 1616b
Adrenal medulla, 1611
Adrenalectomy, 1614b
Adrenalin. *See* Epinephrine.
Adrenarche, 1106, 1108f
Adrenocorticotropic hormone
chronic adrenocortical insufficiency and, 1612
Cushing's syndrome and, 1613b
Adult lactase deficiency, 49
Adulthood, health risks in, 48
Advanced cardiac life support (ACLS) protocol, 319
Advanced life support, 1355
Adventitious sounds, 915-916
Adverse drug reactions, 1648
Advil. *See* Ibuprofen.
Aerobic exercise, 53, 53f
Aerosol therapy, 1290-1291
AFE. *See* Amniotic fluid embolism (AFE).
Affect, infants and, 960
AFI. *See* Amniotic fluid index (AFI).
African-American culture
expression of pain in childbirth in, 396b
food patterns of, 292t-293t
health beliefs and practices in, 833, 838t-840t
pica and, 284-285
African-Americans, 827b
breast cancer in, 117, 117f, 120b
childbearing and parenting beliefs and practices of, 25t-26t
insurance coverage and, 47
maternal mortality rates of, 8, 28-29
morbidity/mortality rates of, 6
sickle cell anemia in, 49, 322
Afterpains, 526
AFV. *See* Amniotic fluid volume (AFV).
AGA infants. *See* Appropriate-for-gestational-age (AGA) infants.
Age
abruptio placentae and, 365
adaptation to pregnancy and, 260-261, 261f, 262b
breast cancer and, 117
health risks in childbearing years and, 45, 47-49, 48b
high risk pregnancy and, 191b
insurance coverage and, 47
invasive prenatal testing and, 202b
normal blood pressure levels in boys and, 1763

Age (Continued)
normal blood pressure levels in girls and, 1765
respiratory infections and, 1304
transitions to parenthood and, 566-567, 566b, 568b
Age of majority, 1246
Agency for Healthcare Research and Quality, 6
Age-specific death rate, 801b
Aggression, preschoolers and, 1052-1053
Agnosia, 1187
Agonal breaths, 915b
Agranulocytosis, 309-310
AIDS. *See* Acquired immunodeficiency syndrome (AIDS).
Air embolism, 1521t-1522t
Air travel during pregnancy, 252
Airborne precautions, 1263, 1263b
Airway obstruction
in children, 1320b, 1358-1360, 1358b, 1358f, 1360f
in newborns at birth, 646-648, 647f, 648b
in pregnant women, 319b, 320, 320f
Akinetic seizures, 1583b-1584b
Alaskan Natives, 827b
breast cancer in, 117f
intimate partner violence and, 61
morbidity/mortality rates of, 6, 32
Alcohol
abuse of, 57
adolescents and, 1137b, 1138
children and, 789
maternal, 755
breastfeeding and, 1745t-1748t
cessation of intake of, 57-58
fetal and neonatal effects of, 50, 191b, 755-758, 756t, 757f, 758b
health risks of, 50
intake during lactation, 286
intake during pregnancy, 50, 252-253, 330, 331b
Alcoholism, 50, 252-253
Alcohol-related neurodevelopmental disorder (ARND), 756-757, 756t
Aldactone. *See* Spironolactone.
Aldomet. *See* Methyldopa.
Aldosterone, 227t
Alertness, definition of, 1552
Aleve. *See* Naproxen.
Alfalfa leaf, 582t
Algerian mothers, 569
Alginates, 1638t
ALI. *See* Acute lung injury (ALI).
Alkali poisoning, 1428b-1429b
All fours position. *See* Hands-and-knees position during labor and birth.
Alleles, 166
Allen card test, 905-906
Allergen avoidance, asthma and, 1342-1343, 1343b
Allergen control, asthma and, 1337, 1338b
Allergic reactions
to analgesia and anesthesia, 409, 418-419
to blood transfusion, 1521t-1522t
Allergies, 1370
breastfeeding and, 679
food, 286-287, 1370-1373, 1370b, 1372b
health history in, 877, 877b
latex, spina bifida and, 1730-1731, 1730b-1731b
penicillin, 1485b
Allevyn tracheostomy dressing, 1292-1293
Allograft skin, 1667
Alloimmunization, 1521t-1522t
All-or-none law, 1687
All-terrain vehicles (ATVs), 1094
Alopecia, chemotherapy-related, 1514
Alpha-fetoprotein assay, 200t, 203-204
Alpha-thalassemia, 161
ALTE. *See* Apparent life-threatening events (ALTE).
Alterations in cyclic bleeding, 93-94, 94b
Altered states of consciousness, 1552-1553, 1553b, 1553f
Alternate cover test, 905, 905b, 905f
Alternative child care arrangements, 965-970
Alternative therapies. *See* Complementary and alternative therapies.
Alveolus, 69-70, 70f, 682, 682f
Ambiguous genitalia, 776-777, 776f, 1535t
Amblyopia, 904, 1192b-1193b
Ambulation
after cesarean birth, 516
first stage of labor and, 457t, 459-460, 460f
play activities and, 1255b
Ambulatory setting, 1239
Amelia, 171f, 1695
Amenorrhea, 86-87
in adolescents, 1125
exercise-associated, 87
hypogonadotropic, 87
management of, 87
substance abuse and, 330-331
American Academy of Pediatrics (AAP), 487
American College of Nurse-Midwives, 9
American College of Obstetrics and Gynecologists (ACOG), 487
American Nurses Association (ANA)
ANA's Health System Reform Agenda, 5
Code of Ethics for Nurses, 794, 795b, 1165
American Sign Language, 1190
American Society for Psychoprophylaxis in Obstetrics (ASPO/ Lamaze), 4b
Amino acid infant formulas, 702
Amiodarone, 1359t
Amitriptyline, breastfeeding and, 1745t-1748t
Ammonia nitrogen, 1753t-1761t
Amniocentesis, 197-198, 200t, 201, 201f
Amnioinfusion, 436
Amnion, development of, 175, 175f
Amniotic fluid, 175-176
assessment during first stage of labor, 455t
meconium in, 200t, 202, 474
Amniotic fluid embolism (AFE), 479, 522-523, 523b
Amniotic fluid index (AFI), 519
Amniotic fluid volume (AFV), 198
Amniotic infection syndrome, 100
Amniotic membranes, 455, 455b
Amniotomy, 505-507, 506b-507b
Amoxicillin
breastfeeding and, 1745t-1748t
for chlamydia during pregnancy, 99
Amphetamines, 51
adolescents and, 1139
breastfeeding and, 1745t-1748t
Ampicillin, breastfeeding and, 1745t-1748t
Ampulla of uterine tube, 68f, 173
Amputation, 1690-1691, 1690b, 1706
Amylase, 954
ANA. *See* American Nurses Association (ANA).
Anaclitic depression. *See* Separation anxiety.
Anaerobic exercise, 53
Anal reflex, 921
Anal sphincter, 67f
Anal stage of psychosexual development, 848-849
Anal-digital activity, 98
Anal-genital intercourse, 98
Analgesia
breastfeeding and, 1745t-1748t
for children, 938-940, 939b, 940t-942t, 943b-944b
for burns, 1666-1667
during circumcision, 668-669, 670b
epidural, 945, 945f
evaluation of effectiveness of, 948-950
routes of administration, 943b-944b, 945-946, 946b, 947f
timing of, 946-947
in immediate postpartum period, 543, 543b
during labor, 406, 406b, 420-421
general anesthesia, 415-416, 416f
maternal hypothermia after, 420
myasthenia gravis and, 328
nerve block analgesia and anesthesia, 409
allergic reactions to, 409
combined spinal-epidural, 414
epidural, 412-415, 412b-413b, 413f
local infiltration anesthesia, 409
nitrous oxide, 415
paracervical, 415
pudendal, 409, 410f
spinal, 409-412, 411b, 411f-412f, 420
nursing care management in, 416, 417b
administration of medication, 418-420, 419f
informed consent and, 416-418, 416b-418b
Analgesia (Continued)
self-assessment of pain and, 416
obese women and, 420
preparation of patient for, 418
safety and general care in, 419-420, 419f
sedatives, 406
signs of potential problems in, 418-419
systemic analgesia, 406-409, 407b-409b
timing of administration of, 418
patient-controlled. *See* Patient-controlled analgesia.
Anaphylactoid syndrome of pregnancy, 479, 522-523, 523b
Anaphylaxis, 1485-1486, 1485b
in food allergy, 1370-1371
during pain management in labor, 419
Anaprox. *See* Naproxen.
Androgens
adolescence and, 1106
ovaries and production of, 68
Android pelvis, 381, 383t
Anemia, 1490-1493, 1491t, 1493b
in acute renal failure, 1543
aplastic, 1501-1502, 1502b
in chronic renal failure, 1545-1546
classification of, 1490-1492, 1492b, 1492f
delayed wound healing and, 1637t
in high risk pregnancy, 320-322, 320b, 332-333
folic acid deficiency anemia, 322
iron deficiency anemia, 321-322
sickle cell hemoglobinopathy, 322, 323t
thalassemia, 322
iron deficiency, 1493-1494, 1494b
in leukemia, 1512
sickle cell, 1495-1500, 1496b, 1496f, 1498b-1499b
Anencephaly, 44-45, 768, 1725b
Anesthesia
in cesarean birth, 513
in children, 1252
for burns, 1666-1667
during circumcision, 668-669, 670b
during labor, 406, 406b, 420-421
general anesthesia, 415-416, 416f
maternal hypothermia after, 420
nerve block analgesia and anesthesia, 409
allergic reactions to, 409
combined spinal-epidural, 414
epidural, 412-415, 412b-413b, 413f
local infiltration, 409
nitrous oxide, 415
paracervical, 415
pudendal, 409, 410f
spinal, 409-412, 411b, 411f-412f, 420
nursing care management in, 416, 417b
administration of medication, 418-420, 419f

Anesthesia (Continued)
informed consent and, 416-418, 416b-418b
self-assessment of pain and, 416
obese woman and, 420
preparation of patient for, 418
safety and general care in, 419-420, 419f
signs of potential problems in, 418-419
timing of administration of, 418
obstetric recovery from, 480-483, 483b
surgery during pregnancy and, 368
Aneuploidy, 166
Angel dust. *See* Phencyclidine (PCP).
Angioedema, 1485
Angiogenesis, 1636
Angiomas, 223-224, 254t-256t
Angle of Louis, 912
Animal bites, 1654, 1655b
Animism, 1021b, 1052
Anion gap, 657b
Anisometropia, 1192b-1193b
Ankle clonus, 341-342, 341f
Ankle edema during pregnancy, 254t-256t
Ankle-foot orthoses, 1718, 1718f-1719f
Ann Arbor staging system, 1514-1515
Anorectal malformations, 774, 774f, 1422-1423, 1422b
Anorexia
chemotherapy-related, 1513
pediatric respiratory infections and, 1305b
Anorexia nervosa, 52
in adolescents, 52, 52b, 1132, 1133b-1135b
amenorrhea and, 87
screening for, 52, 52b
Anovulation in dysfunctional uterine bleeding, 95
Anovulatory bleeding, 88
Antenatal glucocorticoids, 496, 496b
Antepartal hemorrhage, 350
Antepartum care. *See* Prenatal care.
Antepartum testing. *See* Prenatal testing.
Anterior fontanel, 376, 377f
Anterior ligament, 67f
Anterior pituitary glands, 74
Anthropoid pelvis, 381, 383t
Anthropometry, 886
Antiarrhythmias during pregnancy, 317t
Antibiotics
cystic fibrosis and, 1349
inflammatory bowel disease and, 1402
otitis media and, 1315
pharyngitis and, 1311
yeast infections and, 111, 205b
Antibody testing for human immunodeficiency virus, 108
Anticholinergics, asthma and, 1339
Anticipatory grief, 1172
Anticipatory guidance
adolescents and, 878b, 1124-1125, 1125b
communication with parents and, 869
disease prevention and, 793
for health promotion and prevention, 57-63, 57b-58b
health screening schedule and, 58, 59t
intimate partner violence and. *See* Intimate partner violence (IPV).
in lead poisoning, 1435
preschoolers and, 1055, 1056b
substance use cessation and, 57-58, 58b
terminally ill children and, 1172
toddlers and, 1040, 1041b
Anticoagulants
breastfeeding and, 1745t-1748t
for deep venous thrombosis, 584-585, 585b
during pregnancy, 317, 317t
Anticonvulsants
breastfeeding and, 1745t-1748t
oral contraceptives and, 326b
Anti-D antibody therapy, 1505-1506, 1505b-1506b
Antidepressants
anorexia nervosa and, 1135
children and, 939, 941t, 1103
for postpartum depression, 597
Antidiuretic hormone, 1604
Antiepileptic drugs, 939, 941t, 1585-1591, 1592b
cerebral palsy and, 1719
teratogenicity of, 326
vitamin K deficiency and, 326
Antihistamines
breastfeeding and, 1745t-1748t
children and, 1308
Antihypertensives for severe preeclampsia, 346, 346b, 348t
Antiinfectives, breastfeeding and, 1745t-1748t
Antiinflammatory drugs, breastfeeding and, 1745t-1748t
Antilymphocyte globulin, 1502
Antipsychotic medications for postpartum depression, 594, 597, 597t
Antipyretic drugs, 1259-1260
Antiretroviral drugs, 109, 1518
Antistreptolysin O titer, 1473, 1753t-1761t
Anus, 66f-67f
assessment of, 81, 921
imperforate, 774f
of newborn, normal findings, 626t-636t
Anxiety
about cesarean birth, 515
about childbirth, 232-233, 404b, 458b-459b
about high risk infants, 737b
about preeclampsia, 344b
about preterm labor, 490b
in childbirth, 318, 391b, 394, 396
dystocia and, 499b
postpartum hemorrhage and, 580b
Anxiety (Continued)
related to hyperemesis gravidarum, 351b
during trial of labor, 518
Aortic stenosis, 1451b-1453b
Aortic valve stenosis, 313
Apgar, Virginia, 4b
Apgar scoring, 4b, 625
initial assessment of newborn and, 643-646, 644b, 644t, 645f-646f, 647b
Aphasia, 1187
Apheresis, 1523
Apical impulse
of newborns, 610, 637
during pregnancy, 218
Aplastic anemia, 1501-1502, 1502b
Aplastic crisis, 1495
Apnea, 915b, 1354
of infancy, 1010-1012, 1011b-1012b, 1012f
pregnancy and, 370
Apparent life-threatening events (ALTE), 1010-1012, 1011b-1012b, 1012f
Appendectomy during pregnancy, 368
Appendicitis
in children, 1398-1400, 1399b
during pregnancy, 226f, 227, 368
Appetite
after birth, 529, 538b
obesity and, 1128
during pregnancy, 226
Approach behaviors in coping, 1152, 1152b
Appropriate-for-gestational-age (AGA) infants, 651, 707b
APPT. *See* Adolescent Pediatric Pain Tool (APPT).
Apresoline. *See* Hydralazine.
Apt test, 203b, 365
ARDS. *See* Acute respiratory distress syndrome (ARDS).
Areolae, 69, 217, 223, 224b
Areolar reconstruction, 122
ARF. *See* Acute renal failure (ARF).
Aripiprazole, 597, 597t
Arm circumference, measurement of, 892
Arm raises, 545f
Arm recoil, 651b
Arm restraints, 1266
ARND. *See* Alcohol-related neurodevelopmental disorder (ARND).
Arnold-Chiari malformation, 768-769, 1594
Aromatase inhibitors, 123
Aromatherapy for pain management, 405, 405b
Arousal, 74
Arterial blood gases in newborns, 657b, 730t
Arterial blood sample, 1271
Arteriovenous fistulas, 1548
Arteriovenous graft, 1548
Arthritis
juvenile idiopathic, 1708-1711, 1712b
septic, 1704
Arthropod bites and stings, 1648-1650, 1649t-1650t
pediculosis capitis, 1651-1652, 1651b-1652b, 1651f
Arthropod bites and stings (Continued)
Rickettsial diseases, 1652-1653, 1653t
scabies, 1650, 1650b
Artificial airways, 1291
Artificial skin, 1669
Artificial sweeteners during pregnancy, 280, 281b
Artificial ventilation, 1291-1294, 1291f-1292f, 1292b-1294b, 1294f
ARTs. *See* Assisted reproductive therapies (ARTs)
Ascariasis, 1396t
Ascorbic acid. *See* Vitamin C.
ASDs. *See* Autism spectrum disorders (ASDs).
Aseptic meningitis, 1578, 1578t
Ashkenazi Jews, 49, 161, 829
Asian-American culture
breastfeeding and, 559b
childbearing and parenting beliefs and practices of, 25t-26t
communication and, 832
health beliefs and practices in, 835b
nutrition after childbirth and, 546f
parenting beliefs in, 568-569
Asian-Americans
breast cancer in, 117f, 120b
morbidity/mortality rates of, 6
ASKED model of cultural competence, 838, 838b
Aspartame during pregnancy, 280, 281b
Asphyxia
fetal responses to, 204-205
perinatal, 734, 736
Aspiration
of baby powder, 991
of foreign objects, 991
in near-drowning, 1570
suprapubic, 1270, 1532
toddlers and, 1034t-1035t, 1040
Aspiration abortion, 157, 158b
Aspiration pneumonia, 1330-1331
Aspirin
anticoagulant therapy and, 585b
breastfeeding and, 1745t-1748t
children and, 942t
overdose of, 1428b-1429b
Asplenia, 1501b
ASPO/Lamaze. *See* American Society for Psychoprophylaxis in Obstetrics (ASPO/Lamaze).
Asset mapping approach, community, 30
Assimilation, 21
Assisted hatching, 137t
Assisted reproductive therapies (ARTs), 136, 136b, 137f, 137t
Assisted suicide. *See* Euthanasia.
Association of Ontario Midwives, 9
Association of Women's Health, Obstetric and Neonatal Nurses (AWHONN)
campaign to address problems of preterm birth, 487
definition of home care, 35-36
on fetal heart rate assessment, 424
history of, 4b

Association of Women's Health, Obstetric and Neonatal Nurses (AWHONN) *(Continued)*
position on nurses' role in abortion, 156-157
research priorities for women's and neonatal health, 12b
research-based practice projects of, 11, 11b
standards of practice and education for perinatal nurses, 12-13, 13b
Associative play, 855-856, 855f, 1047
Asthma, 1334, 1337
acute care in, 1344-1345, 1345f
allergen avoidance and, 1342-1343, 1343b
allergen control in, 1337, 1338b
bronchospasm in, 1343-1344, 1343b-1344b, 1343f
chest physiotherapy for, 1340
classification of, 1334, 1334b
diagnostic evaluation in, 1335-1337, 1335b-1337b
drug therapy in, 1337-1340
etiology of, 1334, 1335b
exercise-induced, 1340
family and child support in, 1345-1346
high risk pregnancy and, 322-324, 324t
hyposensitization and, 1340
nursing care plan for, 1341-1342, 1342b
pathophysiology of, 1335, 1335f
prognosis in, 1340-1341
severity classification of, 324t
status asthmaticus and, 1341
Astigmatism, 1192b-1193b
Asymmetric intrauterine growth restriction, 707b
Asymptomatic bacteriuria, 1530
Asynclitism, 388, 389f
Ataxic cerebral palsy, 1717b
Atelectasis, 1470b
Athlete's foot, 1645t
Atlantoaxial instability, 1183-1184
Atonic seizures, 1583b-1584b
Atopic dermatitis, 1656-1659, 1657b-1659b, 1657f
Atopy, 1371, 1371b, 1656
Atresia
biliary, 1410-1411, 1410b
choanal, 770, 770f
esophageal, 772-773, 772f
Atrial septal defects, 1448b-1450b
pregnancy and, 313
teratogens and, 171f
Atrioventricular canal defects, 1448b-1450b
Atrophy, 1676-1677
Atropine sulfate
breastfeeding and, 1745t-1748t
for cardiopulmonary resuscitation, 1359t
Attachment
infants and, 961-962
newborns and, 638b
parent-infant, 548, 554-558, 555t-556t, 557b, 557f
Attention deficit hyperactivity disorder (ADHD), 789, 1099-1100
Attitude, fetal, 377, 378f-380f
ATVs. *See* All-terrain vehicles (ATVs).
Atypical pneumonia, primary, 1324
AUB. *See* Abnormal uterine bleeding (AUB).
Auditory acuity, infants and, 955
Auditory brainstem response, 910t
Auditory evoked potentials, 1556
Auditory nerve. *See* Vestibulocochlear nerve (cranial nerve VIII).
Auditory stimulation
play during infancy and, 964t
unconscious child and, 1561-1562
Auditory testing, 910t
Augmentation enterocystoplasty, 1727
Augmentation of labor, 505, 507-510, 508b-509b, 508f
Augmentin. *See* Amoxicillin.
Aural temperature, 894t-895t, 895b-896b
Auricle, 907
Auscultation
for bowel sounds, 918
in cardiac assessment, 1443
of chest, 914-915, 914b-915b
for heart sounds, 916-917, 916b, 916f, 917t
of maternal heart rate during labor, 451b
Authoritarian parents, 812
Authoritative parents, 812
Autism spectrum disorders (ASDs), 1198-1201, 1199b-1200b
Autoimmune disorders
during pregnancy, 327, 332-333
myasthenia gravis, 327-328, 327b
systemic lupus erythematosus, 327
systemic lupus erythematosus, 1711-1713, 1713b
Autoimmune hemolytic anemia, 1492f
Autologous flap reconstruction, 122
Autonomic drugs, breastfeeding and, 1745t-1748t
Autonomy vs. shame and doubt in psychosocial development, 849-850, 1019
AutoPap test, 83b
Autopsy
of newborns, 603
of terminally ill children, 1172
Autosomal dominant inheritance disorders, 163, 169, 169f
Autosomal recessive inheritance disorders, 163, 169-170, 169f
Autosome abnormalities, 166-167
Autosomes, 165-166
Avian influenza virus, 1313
Avoidance behaviors in coping, 1152, 1152b
Avulsed permanent tooth, 1092, 1092b
AWHONN. *See* Association of Women's Health, Obstetric, and Neonatal Nurses (AWHONN).
Axillary lymph nodes, 121-122, 121f
Axillary sensors, 897b
Axillary temperature, 626t-636t, 636, 894t-895t, 895b-896b
Azithromycin, 99
Azotemia, 1538, 1542

B

Babinski reflex, 620, 621t-625t
Baby foods, commercially prepared, 975
Baby Friendly Hospital Initiative, 557-558
Baby powder aspiration, 991
Baby-Friendly Hospital Initiative (BFHI), 699-700
Baby-napping, 9, 540, 662
Bacille Calmette-Guerin vaccine, 1328
Back
of children, 921, 921b
of newborns, 626t-636t
Back blows, 1358, 1358f
Back labor, 403
Back pain
occiput posterior position of fetus and, 500, 500b
during pregnancy, 247, 249f, 250b, 387
Back to Sleep campaign, 1009
Bacterial infections
acute diarrhea and, 1384t-1386t
chlamydia, 32-33, 99, 754, 755b
in endocarditis, 1472-1473, 1472b-1473b
gonorrhea, 32-33, 99-100, 100b, 749
group B streptococcus, 112, 754
in meningitis, 1575-1578, 1576b-1578b, 1578t
neonatal, 745-746, 745t, 754
pelvic inflammatory disease and, 101-103
in pneumonia, 1324-1326, 1326f
prevention of, in herpes lesions, 105
of the skin, 1641, 1642t, 1643f
syphilis, 100-101, 101b, 101f, 749-750, 750b, 750f
tuberculosis, 754, 1326-1329, 1327b-1329b, 1705
Bacterial overgrowth in short-bowel syndrome, 1425
Bacterial tracheitis, 1321
Bacterial vaginosis, 110-111, 110t
Bacteriuria, 1530
Balance, concept of, 834
Balance suspension traction, 1688, 1688f
Ballard scale. *See* New Ballard scale.
Balloon atrioseptostomy, 1444t
Balloon catheters, 505
Balloon dilation, 1444t
Balloon valvuloplasty, 313
Ballottement, 215, 216f
Bandl ring, 498
Barbiturate coma, 1561
Barbiturates during labor, 406
Bariatric surgery for adolescents, 1130
Barlow test, 775, 775b, 1692
Barrel chest, 671-672
Barrier dressings, 1638t
Barrier methods of contraception, 145
cervical cap, 146f, 150, 150b
condoms, 146, 146b-147b, 146f
contraceptive sponge, 146f, 150
diaphragms, 146-150, 146f, 148b-150b
Barrier methods of contraception *(Continued)*
maternal diabetes mellitus and, 306
spermicides, 145-146, 145f-146f
Barrier protection, 1262-1263
Bartholin glands, 65-66, 66f
Basal body temperature (BBT), 133b, 133t, 142, 142b, 142f
Basal metabolic rate (BMR)
changes during pregnancy, 221-222
fluid loss in infants and, 1381
Base excess, 657b
Baseline fetal heart rate, 427-429, 428t, 429f, 430t
Basilar skull fractures, 1564-1565
Bathing
during hospitalization, 1257-1258
during labor, 403, 403f, 443, 457t
of newborns, 674, 675b, 721b-722b
during pregnancy, 246
for skin lesion relief, 1641
Battered woman. *See* Intimate partner violence (IPV).
Batteries, ingestion of, 996
Battledore placenta, 366, 367f
Beanbag chairs, labor and, 469
Beans during pregnancy, 280t
Bearing-down efforts, 384-385, 468-471, 471b
Becaplermin gel, 1638t
Bed rest
adverse effects of, 492b
in cardiovascular disorders during pregnancy, 314
coping with, 342, 343b-344b
elimination during labor and, 457t
in preterm labor, 36f, 37, 490b, 491-492, 492b
Bed-wetting, 1100
Bee stings, 1649t-1650t
Behavior
attention-deficit hyperactivity disorder and, 1099
child maltreatment and, 1071b-1072b
in childhood depression, 1102, 1102b
distress, 929, 930f, 931t
in first stage of labor, 467t
minimizing misbehavior of children, 812, 813b
in parent and infant attachment, 555t
in pediatric physical assessment, 900
television-influenced, 862b
Behavior modification theory, 814
Behavioral characteristics
in high risk pregnancies, 190, 191b
of newborns, 637-641, 638b
response to environmental stimuli and, 640-641
sensory behaviors and, 639-640, 640f
sleep-wake states and, 637-639, 638f, 639b
Behavioral contracting, 937b
Behavioral genetics, 170-172
Behavioral pain assessment scales for children, 931t

Behavioral repertoires, 560f, 565-566
Behavioral therapy for treating obesity, 1131, 1132b
Belching
 during labor, 392
 during pregnancy, 254t-256t
BELIEF framework, 836b
Bell's palsy, 327
Benadryl. *See* Diphenhydramine.
Benchmarking, 1209
Beneficence, 794
Benign breast disease, 115
Benzamycin. *See* Erythromycin.
Benzodiazepines, 406
Benzoyl peroxide, 1660
Bereavement. *See* Grief.
Best practices, 29
Beta-adrenergic agonists
 asthma and, 1339
 preterm labor and, 494, 494b-495b
Beta-adrenergic blockers, hyperthyroidism and, 310
Beta-blockers during pregnancy, 317t
Beta-endorphins, pain and, 396
Beta-thalassemia
 in children, 1500-1501, 1501b
 ethnicity and, 49, 161
BFHI. *See* Baby-Friendly Hospital Initiative (BFHI).
Bibliotherapy, 873b-874b
Bicarbonate during pregnancy, 370
Bicarbonate serum, 1753t-1761t
Biceps reflex, 340-341, 341f, 923f
Bicornuate uterus, 132f, 135-136
Bicycle injuries, 787-788, 1094, 1094b, 1094f
Bidirectional Glenn shunts, 1466t
Biliary atresia, 1410-1411, 1410b
Biliary tract, fetal, 181
Bilious vomiting, 1393
Bilirubin
 conjugation of, 653
 jaundice in newborn at birth and, 614, 616f, 653-656, 654b, 654f, 655t, 656b
 pregnancy versus nonpregnancy values of, 220t-221t
 standard laboratory values in newborns, 657b, 1753t-1761t
Billings method. *See* Cervical mucus ovulation-detection method.
Bimanual palpation, 83-84, 84f
Binge eating. *See* Bulimia nervosa.
Binocularity, 955
Binuclear families, 16
Biobrane, 1668
Biochemical assessment, 200-201, 200t
 alpha-fetoprotein assay in, 203-204
 amniocentesis in, 200t, 201, 201f
 chorionic villus sampling in, 203, 203b, 204f
 Coombs' test in, 204
 indications for, 201-202, 202b
 percutaneous umbilical blood sampling in, 202-203, 203f
Biochemical markers in preterm labor, 487
Biofeedback
 for pain management during labor, 405
 perinatal education and, 270
Biographic data, 78
Biologic therapies, inflammatory bowel disease and, 1402
Biologic development, 844-846, 844f-845f, 845b, 845t
 of adolescents, 1105-1109, 1106b, 1107f-1108f
 of infants, 953
  fine motor development and, 955, 955f
  gross motor development and head control, 955-956, 956b, 956f
   locomotion, 957, 957b, 959f
   rolling over, 956, 957f
   sitting, 956-957, 958f
  maturation of systems and, 954-955
  proportional changes in, 953-954
 of preschoolers, 1043-1044, 1044f
 of school-age children, 1077-1079, 1078f
 of toddlers, 1017-1018, 1018f
Biologic skin coverings, 1667-1668
Biophysical profile (BPP), 198-199, 199t, 519
Biopsy
 bone marrow, 1267, 1267b
 endometrial, 59t, 133t
 lymph node, 1515
 renal, 1527t-1528t
Biorhythmicity, parent-infant communication and, 559, 559f, 565
Biosynthetic human insulin preparations, 303
Biot respiration, 915b
Biotinidase deficiency, 658t
Biparietal cephalometry, 196, 197f
Birth. *See* Childbirth.
Birth balls, 460, 462f, 469
Birth canal. *See* Passageway.
Birth centers, 268-269, 269f
 free-standing, 9, 268-269
Birth control. *See also* Contraception.
 cultural beliefs about, 550b
 definition of, 138
 Supreme Court ruling on, 4b
Birth history, 876
Birth plans, 267-268, 398, 398b, 445
Birth settings, 268
 birth centers, 268-269, 269f
 home births, 269, 270b
 labor, delivery, recovery, and postpartum rooms, 268, 268f, 443, 473
Birth trauma
 maternal
  cystocele and rectocele in, 588-589, 589f, 592
  genital fistulas and, 589-592, 590f
  urinary incontinence and, 589, 590f, 592
  uterine displacement and prolapse in, 587-588, 588f, 592
 neonatal, 652-653, 653f, 742-743, 743t
Birth trauma *(Continued)*
  central nervous system injuries in, 745
  diabetic mothers and, 736
  nursing care management in, 743
  peripheral nervous system injuries in, 743-745, 744f
  skeletal injuries in, 743, 743f
Birth weight
 classification of newborn by, 651-652, 652f
 mortality and, 790
Birthing beds, 469, 470f, 480
Birthing chairs, 469, 470f
Birthing From Within, 401
Birthing rooms, 471-473, 472f
Birthing stools, 469
Birthing tables, 480
Birthrate
 among adolescents, 32-33, 260-261
 definition of, 7b
Birthrate trends, 6, 7b, 8, 28-29
Bishop score, 504-505, 505t
Bismuth compounds, 1406
Biting, infants and, 957
Bittersweet grief, 600
Black cohosh root, 90t
Black eye (hematoma), 1193b
Black haw, 90t
Black widow spiders, 1649t-1650t
Blackheads, 1660
Bladder, 67f
 catheterization of
  during labor, 457t, 459
  pediatric, 1269-1270, 1269b-1270b, 1269t
 changes during pregnancy, 217f, 222, 223t, 387
 exstrophy of, 776, 776f, 1535t
 postpartum assessment of, 483b
 postpartum care of, 544
 postpartum changes in, 528-529
 prevention of postpartum distention of, 542
 in spina bifida, 1727
 trauma during pregnancy and, 370
Bladder capacity of school-age children, 1078
Bladder ultrasound, 1527t-1528t
Blalock-Taussig shunt, 1466t
Blanket swaddling, 723
Blastocyst, 173-174, 174f
Blastocyst cavity, 173-174, 174f, 176
Blastomeres, 173-174, 174f
Blastomycosis, 1646t
Bleeding
 after first-trimester abortion, 157
 after tonsillectomy, 1313b
 hemophilia and, 1504
 postpartum, 479, 580b
  bladder and, 529
  definition and incidence of, 576
  etiology and risk factors for, 577-581, 577b
  hemorrhagic shock and, 581-583, 582b-583b
  nursing care management of, 579-580, 579b
   bleeding with a contracted uterus and, 581
   herbal remedies and, 581, 582t
Bleeding *(Continued)*
   hypotonic uterus and, 580-581
   medications in, 580, 580b-581b
  prevention of, 540-541, 540b-542b, 540f
 during pregnancy, 350
  abruptio placentae and, 360, 360f, 365-366, 365f
  clotting disorders and, 366-368
  cord insertion and placental variations and, 366, 367f
  early part of pregnancy and, 350-351
  ectopic pregnancy and
   clinical manifestations of, 357
   collaborative care for, 357-358, 357b-358b
   incidence and etiology of, 356-357, 356f
   nursing care management in, 353-354, 353b-355b
  gestational trophoblastic disease and, 358
   gestational trophoblastic neoplasia, 349, 358
   hydatidiform mole, 358-359, 359b, 359f
  late part of pregnancy and, 360, 360f
  miscarriage and, 351-354, 352f, 353t
  placenta previa and
   clinical manifestations of, 361-362, 362t
   diagnosis of, 362, 363b
   home care in, 364
   hospital care in, 363-364
   incidence and etiology o, 361, 361b
   maternal and fetal outcomes in, 362
   nursing care plan for, 364b
   types of, 361, 361f
   vaginal examination in, 362, 364
  recurrent premature dilation of cervix and, 355-356, 355b, 356f
 trauma and, 373
Bleeding time, normal ranges for, 1753t-1761t
Blended families, 16, 819
Blind parents, 570, 570b
Blindisms, 1194
Blindness in children, trauma and, 1191-1194
Blissymbols, 1181
Blisters, 1647f
Bloating during pregnancy, 254t-256t
Blood cholesterol, 59t
Blood glucose
 fetal concentration of, 178, 657b
 during labor, 391b
 monitoring of
  in gestational diabetes mellitus, 308-309
  in myasthenia gravis, 327-328
  in pediatric diabetes mellitus, 1620, 1620t, 1627-1628, 1627b-1628b, 1628f
 during preconceptional period, 298b

Blood glucose *(Continued)*
in pregestational diabetes mellitus, 299-306, 300b-301b, 301f, 304b, 304f
during antepartum period, 304-305, 304b-305b
during intrapartum period, 305-306
during postpartum period, 306
normal test ranges for, 1753t-1761t
pregnancy versus nonpregnancy values of, 220t-221t
Blood groups, 611
Blood loss
in abruptio placentae, 366
in placenta previa, 363
postpartal, 540-541, 540b-542b, 540f
Blood pressure
maternal
adaptation to labor, 390-391, 391b, 449-451, 451b, 451f
after childbirth, 483b, 530t, 538b
changes during pregnancy, 218-219, 219b, 219f, 221t
health screening recommendations for, 59t
hypertensive disorders and, 339, 339b
measurement in prenatal follow-up visits, 242-243, 242b
preeclampsia and, 335-336, 336t
severe preeclampsia and, 346, 346b, 348t
sexual response and, 74t
pediatric
cerebral dysfunction and, 1553-1554
of infants, 954
of newborns, 611, 626t-636t, 637
normal levels, 1763, 1765
physical assessment of, 897-900, 898f-899f, 898t-899t, 899b-900b
postoperative, 1254t
of preterm infants, 709
Blood replacement
in abruptio placentae, 366
in hemorrhagic shock, 583
in trauma during pregnancy, 373
Blood sampling, fetal scalp, 436
Blood specimen, pediatric, 1271-1272, 1271b-1272b, 1271f
heel stick and, 659, 659f, 660b, 1271
venipuncture and, 659-660, 660b
Blood tests
during first stage of labor, 454-455
normal ranges in, 1753t-1761t
before planned cesarean birth, 514
for renal function, 1530t
Blood transfusion therapy, 1520-1522, 1521t-1522t
Blood typing in prenatal period, 241t
Blood urea nitrogen (BUN), 1530t
changes during pregnancy, 223t, 241t
postpartum changes in, 528
Blood urea nitrogen (BUN) *(Continued)*
pregnancy versus nonpregnancy values of, 220t-221t
Blood volume
after birth, 529, 530b
increase during pregnancy, 218-219, 220t-221t
of newborn at birth, 611
normal test ranges for, 1753t-1761t
trauma during pregnancy and, 370
Blood-patch therapy, 412, 412f
Blue cohosh, 582t
Blue spells. *See* Hypercyanotic spells.
Blunt abdominal trauma during pregnancy, 371-372, 371b
BMI. *See* Body mass index (BMI).
BMR. *See* Basal metabolic rate (BMR).
BNBAS. *See* Brazelton Neonatal Behavioral Assessment Scale (BNBAS).
Bodily damage
adolescents and, 1123b
infants and, 992b-993b, 998
school-age children and, 1095t
toddlers and, 1034t-1035t, 1040
Body art, 1120-1121
Body image
adolescents and, 853, 1115
development of, 853
infants and, 960-961, 961f
preschoolers and, 1045
school-age children and, 1084-1085
toddlers and, 1022
Body language
first stage of labor and, 446
during health assessment interviews, 75
Body mass index (BMI), 1127
childhood obesity and, 1129-1130
definition of, 52
ideal body weight with, 52b, 277
Body mass index-for-age charts, 889-890, 890b
Body mechanics during pregnancy, 248b-250b, 249f
Body surface area and fluid loss in infant, 1381
Body temperature
of children
cerebral dysfunction and, 1553
maturation and, 847
normal ranges for, 1762
physical assessment of, 893, 893b-897b, 894t-895t
postoperative, 1254t
fever and
in hospitalized children, 1259-1260
in infants and children, 893b
in respiratory infections, 1306, 1306b
maternal
after childbirth, 530t, 538b
during labor, 391b
postpartum assessment of, 483b
of newborns
at birth, 636, 648
discharge teaching in, 671
in late-preterm infants, 708t
normal findings, 626t-636t
Body temperature *(Continued)*
phototherapy and, 666
transition to extrauterine life and, 612-613, 612f
in preterm infants, 709, 713, 728b-730b
Body weight. *See* Weight.
Bolt method, 1559, 1559b
Bonding, 554, 556
cultural influences on, 559b
parent-infant, 649
Bone age for evaluating growth disorders, 1602b
Bone marrow aspiration in children, 1267, 1267b
Bone marrow dysfunction in leukemia, 1508t
Bone meal, lead and, 283b
Bone mineral density testing, 59t
Bones
fetal, 183, 376, 377f
fracture of, 1681-1684, 1682b, 1682f, 1684b, 1686f
casting for, 1684-1686, 1685b, 1686f
stress, 1096
traction for, 1686-1690, 1687b, 1687f-1688f, 1689b
growth and maturation of, 846
healing and remodeling of, 1682-1683
newborn transition to extrauterine life and, 619-620, 619f-620f, 621t-625t
osteogenesis imperfecta and, 1682, 1696-1697, 1696b
osteomyelitis and, 1703-1704, 1703b
in school-age children, 1078
soft-tissue injuries and, 1680-1681, 1680f
tumors of, 1705, 1705b
Ewing's sarcoma and, 1707
osteosarcoma and, 1705-1707
Bony pelvis, 68, 69f
labor process and, 378-381, 380f-381f, 382t-383t
Booster seats, 1036
Bordetella pertussis, 983
Borrelia burgdorferi, 1653
Boston brace, 1700-1701
Bottle-mouth caries, 701, 1033, 1033f
Bottles, 701. *See also* Formula feeding.
Botulinum toxin A, 1719
Botulism, 1739-1740, 1739b-1740b
Botulism immune globulin, 1740
Bowel elimination
during labor, 457t, 459
postpartum changes in, 529
promotion in postpartum period, 544
spina bifida and, 1727-1728
Bowel injuries, 370
Bowel sounds, 918
Bowlegs
in newborns, 619-620, 620f
in toddlers, 921, 922f
BPP. *See* Biophysical profile (BPP).
Brachial palsy, 744
Brachial pulse in infants, 1357f
Bracing in scoliosis, 1700-1701, 1701f
Bradley, Robert, 400
Bradley method of childbirth, 399-400
Bradycardia
fetal, 429, 430t
during pregnancy, 254t-256t
Bradydysrhythmias, 1476-1477, 1477b
Bradypnea, 915b
Braille, 1195
Brain
altered states of consciousness and, 1552-1553, 1553b, 1553f
aseptic meningitis and, 1578, 1578t
bacterial meningitis and, 1575-1578, 1576b-1578b, 1578t
cranial deformities and, 1593
encephalitis and, 1578-1579, 1579b
epilepsy and, 1581
classification and clinical manifestations of, 1582, 1583b-1584b, 1585t
etiology of, 1581-1582, 1582b
nursing care management in, 1587-1592, 1587b-1592b
pathophysiology of, 1582
during pregnancy, 326, 326b
prognosis, 1587
therapeutic management of, 1585-1587, 1586b-1587b
febrile seizures and, 1260, 1592-1593, 1593b
fetal, 182
head injuries and, 1562-1563
complications of, 1565-1566, 1565b-1566b
diagnostic evaluation of, 1566-1567, 1566b-1567b
etiology of, 1563
nursing care management in, 1566, 1568-1570
pathophysiology of, 1563-1565, 1563f-1564f
therapeutic management of, 1567-1570, 1567b
hydrocephalus and, 1559b, 1593-1597, 1594f-1595f, 1595b-1596b
increased intracranial pressure and, 1552, 1552b
near-drowning and, 1570-1572, 1571b
neuroblastomas and, 1574-1575
of newborns, 620
rabies and, 1579-1580, 1580b
Reye's syndrome and, 1580-1581, 1581b
tumors of, 1572-1574, 1573b-1574b
unconscious child and, 1558-1562
elimination and, 1561
family support in, 1562, 1562b
hygienic care of, 1561, 1561b
intracranial pressure monitoring in, 1559-1560, 1559b-1560b
medications and, 1561
nutrition and hydration for, 1560-1561
positioning and exercise for, 1561
regaining consciousness, 1562

Brain *(Continued)*
respiratory management of, 1558-1559, 1558b
sensory stimulation and, 1561-1562
thermoregulation and, 1561
Bras, maternity, 251
BRATT diet, 1388b
Braxton Hicks contractions, 213-214, 387, 489
Brazelton Neonatal Behavioral Assessment Scale (BNBAS), 637, 638b, 760
BRCA1 gene, 4b, 117
BRCA2 gene, 4b, 117
BRCA1/BRCA2 mutation testing, 164-165
Breakthrough bleeding, 94
Breast cancer, 113-115, 127
care management in, 124-127, 126b
exercise after mastectomy, 124-126, 125b-126b
home care after mastectomy, 124, 125b
Reach to Recovery program, 124b
chemoprevention of, 118
clinical manifestations and diagnosis of, 118-120, 119f, 119t, 120b
cultural awareness in screening, 119, 120b, 127
relative location of malignant lesions, 118-119, 119f
ethical considerations of genetic testing for, 117-118
etiology of, 117-118, 117b, 117f
hormone replacement therapy and, 118
medical management of, 121
adjuvant chemotherapy, 122
breast implants, 122
breast reconstruction, 122
chemotherapy, 123-124
hormone therapy, 122-123, 123b
radiation therapy, 122
surgery, 121-122, 121f
pathophysiology of, 118
prognosis of, 120-121, 120f
susceptibility, 164
Breast Cancer Risk Assessment Tool, 118
Breast implants, 122
Breast milk
energy provided by, 680-681
expressing and storing, 691-693, 692f-693f, 693b, 973
nutritional value of, 678, 681-682, 973
preterm infants and, 717
protective mechanisms in, 747-748
uniqueness of, 684
Breast pumps, 692, 693f
Breast reconstruction, surgical, 122
Breast self-examination, 12f, 69-70, 71b, 85, 695
Breast shells, 247, 247f, 694-695, 695f
Breastfeeding, 529, 663, 676b
after cesarean birth, 516-517
after delivery, 483
Breastfeeding *(Continued)*
Baby Friendly Hospital Initiative and, 557-558
benefits of, 678-679, 747-748, 786
breast care in, 694-695, 695f
breastfeeding education and, 698-700, 699b
in cleft deformities, 772
contraception and, 145, 695
contraindications to, 246, 679
cultural influences on, 559b, 680
diabetic mothers and, 306, 695-696
drugs and, 543, 597-598, 696, 1745t-1748t
duration of, 678, 687-689
engorgement and, 696-698
exercise and, 694
expressing and storing breast milk and, 691-693, 692f-693f, 693b, 973
follow-up after hospital discharge and, 691
food sensitivity and, 1371
frequency of feedings and, 687
fussy newborns and, 689-690
guidelines for support in, 680b
hepatitis B and C and, 698
HIV-infected women and, 109, 751-752
infant assessment and, 685, 685b
jaundice and, 656, 691
latch-on and, 686-687, 688f, 699b
mastitis and, 698
maternal assessment and, 685
maternal care and, 694-696, 695f
maternal cystic fibrosis and, 325
maternal diet and, 694-696
maternal employment and, 693, 973
maternal heart disease and, 318
maternal phenylketonuria and, 311
maternal systemic lupus erythematosus and, 327
maternal weight loss during, 694
menstruation and, 695
milk banking and, 694
milk ejection and, 687
milk production and, 682-700, 682f-683f
monilial infections and, 697-698
nursing care management in, 685, 686b
nursing caries and, 1033, 1033f
plugged milk ducts and, 698
positioning for, 543-544, 685-686, 687f-688f
during pregnancy, 695
preparation for, 246-247, 247f, 266b, 679-680
of preterm infants, 691, 717
promotion of, 546, 546b, 698-700, 699b
sexual sensations during, 695
sleepy newborns and, 689-691
slow weight gain in infants and, 690-691
sore nipples and, 694-695, 695f, 697, 697b
substance-dependent mothers and, 332, 766
supplements, bottles, and pacifiers and, 689, 690b
twins and, 691, 692f
Breastfeeding *(Continued)*
uniqueness of human milk, 684
weaning from, 693, 957-958, 976
in workplace, 10
Breasts
anatomy of, 68-70, 70f
assessment across the life cycle, 70t
care during breastfeeding, 694-695, 695f
changes during pregnancy, 217, 217f, 254t-256t, 258
development of, 68, 914, 1107f
fibroadenomas of, 115, 116t
fibrocystic changes in, 115, 116t
health screening recommendations for, 59t
intraductal papilloma of, 116-117, 116t
lipomas of, 115, 116t
malignant conditions of. *See* Breast cancer.
mammary duct ectasia of, 116, 116t
masses in, 113-115, 116t
mastitis and, 586-587, 586f, 698
in newborn at birth, 619
nipple discharge and, 115-116
pain during menstrual cycles, 90t
physical examination of, 80
postpartum changes in, 529, 538b
engorgement and, 528-529, 539b-540b, 543, 546
problems of, 113-127
review of systems and, 79
self-examination of, 12f, 69-70, 71b, 85
sexual response of, 74t
tenderness before menstruation, 69-70
yeast infections of, 697-698
Breath sounds, 914, 915b
Breathing
cardiopulmonary resuscitation of pregnant women and, 319b
cerebral dysfunction and, 1554
newborn at birth and, 480, 609-610, 648b, 709
pain management during labor and, 270, 402, 402b, 402f
during second stage of labor, 470
Breech presentation, 377, 379f, 500-501
external cephalic version for, 500-503, 505f
fetal heart rate in, 451
neonatal birth trauma and, 652-653, 653f
prolapsed umbilical cord and, 520-522, 521f
types of, 500, 500f
Brethine. *See* Terbutaline.
British Sign Language, 1190
Broad ligaments, 66-68, 68f
Brompheniramine maleate, breastfeeding and, 1745t-1748t
Bronchial breath sounds, 915b
Bronchial drainage, 1291
Bronchiolitis, 1272, 1321-1324, 1322t
Bronchitis, 1321, 1322t
Bronchopneumonia, 1324
Bronchopulmonary dysplasia, 732-733
Bronchospasm, 1343-1344, 1343b-1344b, 1343f
Bronchovesicular breath sounds, 915b
Broom devices, 83b
Brow presentation, 380f, 501
Brown, Louise, 4b
Brown recluse spiders, 1649t-1650t
Bruising, 652-653, 653f, 1633
Bryant's traction, 1688
Bubble stability test, 202
Buckle fractures, 1682b, 1682f
Buck's extension traction, 1688
Buddhist religion, 836t-837t
Bugleweed, 90t
Bulb syringes, 481f, 646-648, 647f
Bulbar conjunctiva, 903
Bulimia nervosa, 52-53
in adolescents, 52-53, 1132, 1134b
screening for, 52b
Bulla, 1634f
Bullet wounds during pregnancy, 372-373
Bullying, 1082-1083
BUN. *See* Blood urea nitrogen (BUN).
Burning, 835b
Burns, 1661
acute care and, 1671
adolescents and, 1123b
child mortality and, 788
complications in, 1664
depth of injury in, 1661-1663, 1662f-1663f
emergency care in, 1664-1665, 1665b
extent of injury in, 1661, 1662f
family support in, 1672
infants and, 788, 992b-993b, 997-998, 997f-998f
inhalation injury in, 1663-1664
long-term care in, 1671-1672, 1671f
major, 1663, 1664t, 1665-1669, 1668f-1669f, 1668t
management of burn wounds, 1667
minor, 1663, 1664t, 1665-1666
nursing care plan for, 1669-1670, 1669b-1670b
nutrition and, 1666, 1671
pain management in, 1666-1667, 1670
pathophysiology of, 1664
prevention of, 1672-1673
prevention of complications in, 1671-1673, 1671f
prognosis, 1669
psychosocial support in, 1672
school-age children and, 1095t
severity of injury in, 1663, 1664t
toddlers and, 1034t-1035t, 1038-1039, 1038f
types of, 1661
wound sepsis in, 1664
Burping of newborn, formula feeding and, 701, 702f
Burping position, 672f
Butorphanol, 408, 408b
Buttocks, neonatal birth trauma and, 652-653, 653f
Buttocks lift, 545f

C

CAD. *See* Computer-aided detection and diagnosis (CAD).
Cadaver donors, 1548
Caffeine
fetal and neonatal effects of, 761
health risks of, 50
intake during lactation, 286, 696
intake during pregnancy, 50, 253, 280
CAGE test, 330
Calcitonin, 1605
Calcium
fertility and, 135
intake during lactation, 289
intake during pregnancy, 226, 275t-276t, 280-282, 283b
nutritional significance of, 1377t-1379t
osteoporosis and, 52
premenstrual syndrome and, 91
supplementation of, 87
Calcium channel blockers during pregnancy, 317t
Calcium gluconate, 346b
Calendar rhythm method, 141
Calgary Family Assessment Model (CFAM), 19, 19f
Caloric intake
of adolescents, 1118
of infants, 680-681
Caloric test, 1554-1555, 1555b
Campylobacter, 1383-1386, 1384t-1386t
Cancer
breast, 113-115, 127
care management in, 124-127, 126b
exercise after mastectomy, 124-126, 125b-126b
home care after mastectomy, 124, 125b
Reach to Recovery program, 124b
chemoprevention of, 118
clinical manifestations and diagnosis of, 118-120, 119f, 119t, 120b
cultural awareness in screening, 119, 120b, 127
relative location of malignant lesions, 118-119, 119f
ethical considerations of genetic testing for, 117-118
etiology of, 117-118, 117b, 117f
hormone replacement therapy and, 118
medical management of, 121
adjuvant chemotherapy, 122
breast implants, 122
breast reconstruction, 122
chemotherapy, 123-124
hormone therapy, 122-123, 123b
radiation therapy, 122
surgery, 121-122, 121f
pathophysiology of, 118
prognosis of, 120-121, 120f
susceptibility, 164
cervical
genital herpes and, 104-105, 986, 990b
screening for, 214
Hodgkin's disease, 1514-1516, 1515f
Cancer *(Continued)*
leukemia, 1507
chemotherapy in, 1510b-1513b, 1512-1513
classification of, 1507-1508
diagnostic evaluation in, 1508-1509, 1508t
drug toxicity and, 1513-1514, 1513b
late effects of treatment, 1509
nursing care plan for, 1510b-1512b
pain management in, 1509
pathophysiology of, 1508, 1508t
preparing child and family for procedures, 1509
prevention of complications and myelosuppression in, 1509-1512, 1510b-1512b
therapeutic management of, 1509
osteosarcoma, 1705-1707
smoking and, 49
testicular, 1126
Candida albicans, 111, 216-217, 1655-1656
Candidiasis, 111-112, 1645t
diaper, 672-673, 721b-722b, 1655-1656, 1656b, 1656f
management of, 112
neonatal, 754-755, 755b
patient teaching on, 111b
screening and diagnosis of, 110t, 111-112
vulvovaginal, 110t, 111-112, 111b, 697-698
Capacity, community, 30
Capillary blood sample
in children, 1271
in newborns, 660b
Capillary hemangiomas, 618
Capillary refill time, 915-916, 916b
CAPPA. *See* Childbirth and Postpartum Professional Association (CAPPA).
Caput succedaneum, 511f, 615-616, 617f
Car seats
for infants, 994-995, 995b, 995f
for newborns, 673, 673b, 673f, 738, 738b
for toddlers, 1035-1036, 1035f, 1036b
Carbamazepine, 597t
Carbenicillin, breastfeeding and, 1745t-1748t
Carbohydrates
newborns and, 614, 615b, 681
pregestational diabetes mellitus and, 302
Carbon dioxide partial pressure, normal test ranges for, 1753t-1761t
Carboprost tromethamine, 354
Carbuncles, 1642t
Cardiac arrest
in children, 1355-1358, 1356f-1357f, 1359t
during pregnancy, 319
Cardiac catheterization, 1368-1370, 1374t-1379t
postprocedural care and, 1445, 1445b
preprocedural care and, 1444-1445
Cardiac disease. *See* Heart disease.
Cardiac dysrhythmias, 1476-1477, 1477b
Cardiac failure in acute renal failure, 1543
Cardiac output
cardiovascular disease during pregnancy and, 313, 321b
changes during pregnancy, 218-219, 221t
during labor, 385, 391b
maternal, during the immediate postbirth period, 318b
placenta previa and, 364b
postpartum changes in, 530-531, 530t
in postpartum hemorrhage, noninvasive assessments of, 579b
trauma during pregnancy and, 370
Cardiac tamponade, 1470b
Cardinal ligament, 66, 67f-68f
Cardinal positions of gaze, 924f
Cardiogenic shock, 1483t
Cardiomyopathy
in infants of diabetic mothers, 736
pediatric, 1478
peripartum, 312
Cardiopulmonary resuscitation (CPR)
certification in, 672
parent education on, 727
pediatric, 1355-1358, 1356f-1357f, 1359t
of pregnant women, 319-320, 319b, 320f
Cardiotocography (CTG). *See* Electronic fetal monitoring (EFM).
Cardiovascular drugs, breastfeeding and, 1745t-1748t
Cardiovascular dysfunction
in children, 1442, 1487-1488
anaphylaxis and, 1485-1486, 1485b
bacterial endocarditis and, 1472-1473, 1472b-1473b
cardiac catheterization and, 1443t-1444t, 1444
postprocedural care and, 1445, 1445b
preprocedural care and, 1444-1445
cardiac dysrhythmias and, 1476-1477, 1477b
cardiomyopathy and, 1478
congenital heart disease and. *See* Congenital heart disease (CHD).
diagnostic evaluation of, 1443-1445, 1443b, 1443t-1444t
echocardiography in, 1443t, 1444
electrocardiography in, 1443, 1444t
exercise and, 53
heart transplantation and, 1478-1479
history and physical examination in, 1442-1443
hyperlipidemia and, 1474-1476, 1475t
Cardiovascular dysfunction *(Continued)*
Kawasaki disease and, 1481-1482, 1481b-1482b
pulmonary artery hypertension and, 1477-1478
rheumatic fever and, 1473-1474, 1474b
septic shock and, 1486-1487, 1486b, 1487t
shock and, 1482-1484, 1483b-1485b, 1483t
systemic hypertension and, 1479-1481, 1480b
classification of, 311-312
high risk pregnancy and, 311-319, 311b-312b, 332-333
atrial and ventricular septal defects in, 313
Eisenmenger's syndrome in, 312b, 313
heart transplantation and, 314
intrapartum care in, 312
Marfan syndrome in, 313-314
mitral and aortic valve stenosis in, 313
mitral valve prolapse in, 313
nursing care management in, 314, 315b-316b
abnormal/normal signs and symptoms and, 314, 314t, 316b
cultural awareness and, 314
peripartum cardiomyopathy in, 312
plan of care and implementation in, 314-319, 321b
heart surgery and, 317
intrapartum period, 317-318, 318b
medication and, 316, 317t
postpartum period, 315b-316b, 318-319, 318b
rheumatic heart disease in, 247, 312-313
tetralogy of Fallot in, 313
opioid analgesics and, 407b
Cardiovascular system
maternal
adaptation to labor, 390-391
adaptations to pregnancy, 218-219, 218f-219f, 219b, 220t-221t, 338b, 371t
nutritional status and, 884t-886t
postpartum adaptation of, 529-531, 530b, 530t
review of systems and, 79
pediatric
congenital anomalies of, 769-770
effects of immobilization on, 1677t
preterm infants and, 709
review of systems and, 882b
signs of neonatal sepsis, 747t
transition to extrauterine life, 610-611
Care coordination. *See* Case management.
Care paths
home care and, 1208
for newborns, 661
in prenatal care, 244-245, 256-259, 257b, 258f

Caregivers
childbirth and, 397
home care and, 40b
Caring, pediatric nursing and, 793
Carotid pulse, 916b
Carpal tunnel syndrome during pregnancy, 225-226, 254t-256t
Caruncle, 903f, 921
Casanthranol, breastfeeding and, 1745t-1748t
Cascara sagrada, breastfeeding and, 1745t-1748t
Case management, 1208, 1208b
Casein-based infant formulas, 702
Casting
in clubfoot, 775
for fractures, 1684-1686, 1685b, 1686f
for osteomyelitis, 1704
Casts, renal, 1529t-1530t
Cataracts, 171f, 1192b-1193b
Catecholamines, 416
Catharsis, 1427-1430
Catheterization
cardiac, 1443t-1444t, 1444
postprocedural care and, 1445, 1445b
preprocedural care and, 1444-1445
during labor, 457t, 459
urinary, 1269-1270, 1269b-1270b, 1269t
clean intermittent, 1727
in spina bifida, 1727
Cat-scratch disease, 1654-1655
Caucasians, 827b
breast cancer in, 117, 117f
insurance coverage and, 47
Caudal regression, 299
Cause-specific death rate, 801b
Cavities. *See* Dental caries.
CDC. *See* Centers for Disease Control and Prevention (CDC).
CDH. *See* Congenital diaphragmatic hernia (CDH).
Cefazolin, breastfeeding and, 1745t-1748t
Cefixime, 100
Ceftriaxone, 100
Celiac disease, 1423, 1424b
Cell division, 172
Cell-surface immunologic markers, 1508
Cellulitis, 1642t, 1643f
Census data, 31, 827, 827b
Centering pregnancy approach, 237, 238b
Centers for Disease Control and Prevention (CDC)
promotion of safe motherhood, 9
reporting of local and state health data, 31
Centigrade to Fahrenheit temperature conversion, 1762
Central auditory imperception, 1187
Central nervous system (CNS). *See also* Neurologic system.
birth-related injuries of, 745
congenital anomalies of, 768
encephalocele and anencephaly, 768
hydrocephalus, 769
Central nervous system (CNS) *(Continued)*
microcephaly, 769
spina bifida, 768-769, 768f
development of, 171f
neonatal abstinence syndrome and, 762t
of preterm infants, 709-710, 728b-730b
signs of neonatal sepsis, 747t
Central nervous system depressants, adolescents and, 1139
Central nervous system stimulants, adolescents and, 1139
Central precocious puberty, 1603
Central shunts, 1466t
Central venous access devices, 1279-1282, 1281b, 1281f, 1282t
Centration, 1021b
Cephalexin, breastfeeding and, 1745t-1748t
Cephalhematoma, 616, 616b, 617f
Cephalic presentations, 377, 378f
Cephalocaudal development, 843, 845
Cephalopelvic disproportion, 499
Cephalothin, breastfeeding and, 1745t-1748t
Cerclage, cervical, 355-356
Cereal, infant nutrition and, 974
Cerebellar function, pediatric physical assessment of, 922-923, 923b
Cerebral cortex, 182
Cerebral dysfunction, 1597-1598
aseptic meningitis and, 1578, 1578t
assessment of cerebral function in, 1551-1552
altered states of consciousness and, 1552-1553, 1553b, 1553f
increased intracranial pressure and, 1552, 1552b
neurologic examination and, 1553-1555, 1554b-1555b, 1554f-1555f
special diagnostic procedures in, 1555-1558, 1556t-1557t
bacterial meningitis and, 1575-1578, 1576b-1578b, 1578t
brain tumors and, 1572-1574, 1573b-1574b
cranial deformities and, 1593
encephalitis and, 1578-1579, 1579b
epilepsy and, 1581
classification and clinical manifestations of, 1582, 1583b-1584b, 1585t
diagnostic evaluation of, 1582-1585
etiology of, 1581-1582, 1582b
nursing care management in, 1587-1592, 1587b-1592b
pathophysiology of, 1582
prognosis, 1587
therapeutic management of, 1585-1587, 1586b-1587b
febrile seizures and, 1260, 1592-1593, 1593b
head injuries and, 1562-1563
Cerebral dysfunction *(Continued)*
complications of, 1565-1566, 1565b-1566b
diagnostic evaluation of, 1566-1567, 1566b-1567b
etiology of, 1563
nursing care management in, 1566, 1568-1570
pathophysiology of, 1563-1565, 1563f-1564f
therapeutic management of, 1567-1570, 1567b
hydrocephalus and, 1559b, 1593-1597, 1594f-1595f, 1595b-1596b
near-drowning and, 1570-1572, 1571b
neuroblastomas and, 1574-1575
rabies and, 1579-1580, 1580b
Reye's syndrome and, 1580-1581, 1581b
unconscious child and, 1558-1562
elimination and, 1561
family support in, 1562, 1562b
hygienic care of, 1561, 1561b
intracranial pressure monitoring in, 1559-1560, 1559b-1560b
medications and, 1561
nutrition and hydration for, 1560-1561
positioning and exercise for, 1561
regaining consciousness, 1562
respiratory management of, 1558-1559, 1558b
sensory stimulation and, 1561-1562
thermoregulation and, 1561
Cerebral edema, 1566, 1566b
Cerebral hyperemia, 1563
Cerebral palsy, 1716
diagnostic evaluation of, 1717, 1718b
early signs of, 1721b
education and, 1721-1722
family support in, 1723-1724, 1724b
hospitalization in, 1724
increase in, 422
nursing care management of, 1720, 1720f, 1721b-1723b, 1723f
pathophysiology of, 1716-1717, 1717b
therapeutic management of, 1717-1724, 1718f-1719f
Cerebrospinal fluid (CSF), 1552, 1753t-1761t
Cerebrovascular accident
after pediatric heart surgery, 1470b
cyanotic cardiac defects and, 1465
sickle cell disease and, 1495, 1496f
Certified nurse-midwives, 9
Certified professional midwives, 267
Cerumen, 908
Cervical cancer
genital herpes and, 104-105, 986, 990b
screening for, 214
Cervical cap, 146f, 150, 150b
Cervical cerclage, 355-356
Cervical lacerations, 577-578
Cervical mucous assessment, 133-134, 133b, 133t
Cervical mucus ovulation-detection method, 142-143, 143b
Cervical ripening methods
amniotomy, 505-507, 506b-507b
chemical agents, 505, 506b-507b
mechanical agents, 505
Cervical traction, 1688-1689, 1688f
Cervicitis, 104-105
Cervidil insert, 507b
Cervix, 66-67, 67f-68f
adaptations to pregnancy, 214-215, 214f
anomalies of, 82, 83b
bimanual palpation of, 84
childbirth-related injury of, 476
effacement and dilation of, 384-385, 384f, 387-388, 453, 464t
examination of, 82, 82f, 519
infertility and, 130b
outer, 67
postpartum changes in, 527
recurrent premature dilation of, 355-356, 355b, 356f
sexual response of, 74t
in true labor vs. in false labor, 442b
Cesarean birth, 511-517, 515f
in abruptio placentae, 366
anesthesia in, 513
breastfeeding after, 516-517
in cardiovascular disorders during pregnancy, 318
complications and risks in, 513
cystic fibrosis and, 325
on demand, 513
epidural block and, 412-413
forced, 513
general anesthesia and, 415
immediate postoperative care in, 516
incidence of, 8-9, 28-29, 422, 512
indications for, 512-513
intraoperative care in, 515-516, 515f-516f, 516b
management approaches to reduce the rate of, 512, 512b
maternal human immunodeficiency virus and, 328
maternal systemic lupus erythematosus and, 327
multifetal births and, 501
penetrating wounds and, 373
percent of women receiving, 8t
perimortem, 374
in placenta previa, 363-364
placental variations and, 366
postpartum care in, 516-517, 517b
pregestational diabetes mellitus and, 305-306
prenatal preparation for, 270-271, 514
preoperative care in, 514-515
scheduled, 513-514
surgical techniques in, 513, 513f
unplanned, 514
vaginal birth after. *See* Vaginal birth after cesarean (VBAC).
CFAM. *See* Calgary Family Assessment Model (CFAM).

Chadwick sign, 216
Chair method, 148b-149b
Chalmers, Iain, 11
Chancre, 100-101, 101f
Charleston nighttime bending brace, 1700-1701
Chaste tree fruit, 90t
CHD. *See* Congenital heart disease (CHD).
Cheating, school-age children and, 1088
Chelation therapy
in beta-thalassemia, 1501
for lead poisoning, 1436, 1436b
Chemical burns, 1193b, 1661
Chemical dot thermometers, 897b
Chemoprevention of breast cancer, 118
Chemotherapy
in brain tumors, 1572
in breast cancer, 122-124
delayed wound healing and, 1637t
in gestational trophoblastic neoplasia, 360
in Hodgkin's disease, 1515
in leukemia, 1510b-1513b, 1512-1513
in neuroblastomas, 1575
in non-Hodgkin lymphoma, 1516
in osteosarcoma, 1706
in Wilms' tumor, 1541-1542
Chest
of infants, 954
of newborns, 610, 626t-636t, 645-646
nutritional status and, 884t-886t
physical assessment of, 912-914, 913f
review of systems and, 882b
trauma during pregnancy, 372
Chest circumference of toddlers, 1017
Chest compressions, 1357-1358, 1357f
Chest physical therapy, 1291
Chest physiotherapy, 1340
Chest radiography, 1443t
Chest thrusts, 1358, 1358f
Chest wall stretch, 125b-126b
Cheyne-Stokes respiration, 915b
CHF. *See* Congestive heart failure (CHF).
Chickenpox. *See* Varicella.
Chief complaints, 875-876
Chiggers, 1649t-1650t
Child. *See* Children.
Child care arrangements, alternative, 965-970
Child center-based care, 965
Child maltreatment
child behaviors in, 1071b-1072b
child neglect in, 1066, 1070b
child support in, 1073
clinical manifestations of, 1071b-1072b
family support in, 1073-1074
nursing care plan for, 1069-1074
caregiver-child interaction and, 1070
history and interview and, 1069b, 1071b-1072b
nurse biases and, 1069b
physical assessment and, 1072-1073, 1072b
Child maltreatment *(Continued)*
protection from further abuse, 1073, 1073b
talking with children who reveal abuse and, 1069b
physical abuse in, 1066-1068, 1067b
plan for discharge in, 1074
prevention of, 1074, 1075b
sexual abuse in. *See* Sexual abuse.
warning signs of, 1070b
Child pornography, 1068
Child prostitution, 1068
Child spacing, 46, 46b
Childbearing families
beliefs and practices of, 22, 22b-23b, 25t-26t
obtaining cultural expectations about childbearing from, 24b
personal space and, 23-24
preparation for newborn, 20
time orientation of, 24
use of interpreters and, 22-23, 23b
Childbed fever, 4b
Childbirth, 392, 484-485
abruptio placentae and, 366
anesthesia for. *See* Anesthesia: during labor.
anxiety about, 232-233, 458b-459b
augmentation of labor and, 508-510
bearing-down efforts and, 384-385, 468-471, 471b
cardiovascular disorders during pregnancy and, 317-318, 318b
care during pregnancy and, 8-10
childbirth practices, 9, 9f
health literacy, 10
international concerns, 10
involving consumers and promoting self-management, 10
safe motherhood, 9
view of women, 8-9
cesarean. *See* Cesarean birth.
chronic hypertension and, 349
circulatory changes in infants at, 1446, 1446f
class for adolescents on the process of, 387b
cultural considerations in, 25t-26t
cystic fibrosis and, 325
dystocia and, 497
abnormal labor patterns in, 501-502, 502t, 503f
dysfunctional labor and, 497-498, 499b
fetal causes of, 498-501, 500b, 500f
maternal position and, 501
multifetal pregnancy and, 501
nursing care management in, 504b
psychologic responses to, 501
emergency, 477, 478b
fathers' participation in, 9, 9f, 463-464, 464t, 465b
cultural factors in, 448-449
during second stage of labor, 471, 472t
fetal assessment during. *See* Fetal assessment.
Childbirth *(Continued)*
forceps-assisted, 377, 510-511, 510b, 510f-511f
gestational diabetes mellitus and, 309
HIV-infected women and, 329
at home, 237b, 269, 270b
immediate assessment and care of newborn and, 475
induction of labor and, 504-505, 505t, 518
cervical ripening methods and, 505
amniotomy, 505-507, 506b-507b
chemical agents, 505, 506b-507b
oxytocin and, 505, 507-508, 508b-510b, 508f
labor and. *See* Labor.
in LDR or LDRP room, 268, 268f, 443, 473
live vs. cesarean, 9
maternal preparation for, 232-233
nonpharmacologic pain management in, 397-406, 420-421
acupressure and acupuncture in, 403-404, 405f
aromatherapy in, 405, 405b
biofeedback in, 405
birth plans and, 398, 398b
childbirth education and, 398-401, 398b-399b
conscious breathing in, 402, 402b, 402f
effleurage and counterpressure in, 402-403
energy work in, 402
heat and cold application in, 404-405
hypnosis in, 405
imagery and visualization techniques in, 401
intradermal water block in, 405-406, 405f
music in, 401-402
nursing care plan for, 404b
relaxation in, 399b, 401, 401f
touch and massage in, 402
transcutaneous electrical nerve stimulation in, 403, 404b, 404f
water therapy in, 403, 403f
normal vaginal delivery in, 481b-482b
obstetric emergencies and
amniotic fluid embolism, 479, 522-523, 523b
prolapsed umbilical cord, 520, 521f, 522b
shoulder dystocia, 519, 520f
uterine rupture, 372, 522
options for care providers, 266-267, 267b
parental role after
maternal adjustment and, 561-562, 561t, 562b, 563f
parental tasks and responsibilities in, 560-561
paternal adjustment and, 561-562, 561t, 562b, 563f
transition to parenthood and, 548-549, 549f
paternal preparation for, 234
Childbirth *(Continued)*
perineal trauma related to, 475-477, 476f
pharmacologic pain management in, 406, 420-421
analgesia and anesthesia, 406, 406b
nerve block analgesia and anesthesia. *See* Nerve block analgesia and anesthesia.
systemic, 406-409, 407b-409b
general anesthesia, 415-416, 416f
maternal hypothermia after, 420
nursing care management in, 416, 417b
administration of medication, 418-420, 419f
informed consent and, 416-418, 416b-418b
self-assessment of pain and, 416
obese woman and, 420
preparation of patient for, 418
safety and general care in, 419-420, 419f
sedatives in, 406
signs of potential problems in, 418-419
timing of administration of, 418
postterm, 518-519, 519b
premature rupture of membranes and, 496, 746
premature separation of placenta and, 360, 360f, 362t, 365-366, 365f
preterm, 486, 523-524
causes of, 487-488, 488b
home care and, 35b, 36f, 37, 40-41, 257b, 263b
incidence of, 487
inevitable, 496, 496b
low birth weight versus, 486-487
nursing care management in, 488-489, 489b, 496, 496b
bed rest and, 37, 491-492, 492b
early recognition and diagnosis in, 491
home care and, 492-493, 492b-493b, 493f
lifestyle modifications and, 491
prevention strategies and, 489-490, 491b
promotion of fetal lung maturity and, 496, 496b
uterine activity suppression and, 493-496, 494b-495b
nursing care plan for, 490b
risk factors for, 192b, 487, 487b-488b
signs and symptoms of, 489-490, 491b, 491f
socioeconomic factors in, 487
sequelae of trauma in
cystocele and rectocele in, 588-589, 589f, 592
genital fistulas and, 589-592, 590f
urinary incontinence and, 589, 590f, 592

Childbirth (Continued)
uterine displacement and prolapse in, 587-588, 588f, 592
settings for, 268-269, 268f-269f
Standard Precautions during, 449, 450b
supplies, instruments, and equipment for, 471, 471f-472f
supportive care during, 460-466, 462b, 463f, 464t, 465b
systemic lupus erythematosus and, 327
trial of labor and, 503-504
vacuum-assisted, 377, 510b, 511, 511f
version and, 502-503, 505f
vertex presentation and, 380f, 473-474, 474f
emergency birth in, 478b
fetal heart rate in, 451
prolapsed umbilical cord and, 520-522, 521f
Childbirth and Postpartum Professional Association (CAPPA), 401
Childbirth education, 263-271
on cesarean birth, 514
current practices in, 265
establishment of, 4b
nonpharmacologic pain management and, 398-401, 398b-399b
early methods of, 399-400
Bradley method, 399-400
Dick-Read method, 399
Lamaze method, 399-400
new methods of, 400-401
Birthing From Within, 401
Childbirth and Postpartum Professional Association and, 401
Coalition to Improve Maternity Services method, 400-401
HypnoBirthing, 401
outcomes of, 401
role of fathers and/or partners in, 464
strategies for, 265-266
Childbirth practices, 9
Childhood depression, 1102-1103, 1102b
Childhood hysteria, 1102
Childhood nephrosis, 1535-1536
Childhood schizophrenia, 1103
Children
administration of medications
checking dosage and, 1273
determination of drug dosage and, 1273
family teaching and home care and, 1284, 1284b
intramuscular, 1275-1278, 1276t-1277t, 1277f, 1278b
intravenous, 1279-1282, 1280b-1281b, 1281f, 1282t
nasogastric, orogastric, or gastrostomy, 1282, 1283b
optic, otic, and nasal, 1282-1284, 1282b-1284b, 1283f-1284f
oral, 1273-1275, 1274b, 1275f, 1284b
Children (Continued)
rectal, 1282
subcutaneous and intradermal, 1278-1279, 1279b
airway obstruction in, 1358-1360, 1360f
chronic illness and. *See* Chronic illness.
communication with, 870-872, 870b, 871f-872f, 873b-874b, 891f
community-based health care for, 799-802, 800b-801b, 801f
compliance and, 1253-1256, 1256b
cultural influences on, 822-829, 840-841
community and, 826
cultural relativism and, 830-831
cultural shock and cultural competence and, 828-829, 828b-829b
ethnicity and, 824, 824f
food customs and, 832-833, 833f
health beliefs and practices and, 833-835, 835b
hereditary factors and, 829
homelessness and, 825, 830
immigrant children and, 825, 830
migrant farmworker families and, 825, 830
minority-group membership and, 827-828, 827b-828b
peer cultures and, 826-827
poverty and, 825, 830
relationships with health care providers and, 831-832, 831b-833b, 831f
religion and, 825-826, 826f, 835, 836b, 836t-837t
schools and, 826
social roles and, 823-824
socioeconomic class and, 824-825, 829-830
subcultures and, 824-827, 824f, 826f
death of. *See* Death.
developmental assessment of, 923-927, 926b
developmental influences on. *See* Growth and development.
dietary reference intakes for, 881-883, 883b
end-of-life care, 1164, 1174-1175
child's understanding and reaction to death, 1167t-1168t
decision making and, 1164-1169, 1166b, 1167t-1168t
fear and, 1169-1171, 1170b-1171b, 1170f
grief and mourning and, 1172-1174, 1173b
home care and, 1168
nurses' reactions to caring for terminally ill children, 1174, 1174b
nursing care plan for, 1147b, 1169-1174, 1170f, 1173b
organ/tissue donation and autopsy and, 1172
Children (Continued)
pain and symptom management in, 1165b, 1169-1170, 1170b
parental support in, 1170
principles of palliative care, 1164
treatment options in, 1168-1169
family influences on, 806, 821
divorce and, 816-818, 817b
dual-earner family and, 819
employer accommodation of parenting situations and, 819
family nursing interventions and, 806-807, 806b-807b
family size and configuration and, 807-808, 808f
foster parenting and, 819
parental roles and, 807
parenting and, 810-814, 811f-812f, 813b-814b
parenting the adopted child and, 815-816, 815b-816b, 815f
reconstituted family and, 819
role learning and, 807-810, 808f-809f, 809b-810b
sibling interactions and, 808-809, 809f
single parenting and, 818-819
spacing of children and ordinal position and, 808-810, 809b, 809f
fever in, 893b
health history and, 875, 875b
chief complaints, 875-876
family history, 879
family structure, 879, 879b-881b
history, 876-878, 877b-878b
identifying information, 875
present illness, 876, 876b
review of systems, 881, 882b
sexual history, 878, 878b
health problems of, 786
injuries, 787-788, 788f-789f, 788t
mental health problems, 789-790
obesity and type 2 diabetes, 786-787, 787f
substance abuse, 789
violence, 788-789
Healthy People 2010 and, 785-786
hearing impairment in, 1189, 1189b
hospitalization of. *See* Hospitalization: pediatric.
immobilized, 1676-1680, 1677t, 1704
informed consent and, 1245-1247
mental health issues and, 786, 789-790
morbidity and, 786, 791
mortality and, 788t, 790-791, 790t-791t
nutritional assessment and, 881-886, 883b, 884t-886t
nutritional disturbances in delayed wound healing and, 1637t
food sensitivity and, 1370-1374, 1370b-1373b
Children (Continued)
mineral imbalances and, 1365, 1377t-1379t
protein-energy malnutrition and, 1368-1370
vegetarian diets and, 1365-1366, 1366b
vitamin imbalances, 1363-1365, 1374t-1377t
pain assessment in, 929, 930b
behavioral measures and, 929, 930f, 931t
chronic illness and complex pain and, 935
cultural awareness in, 934-935
multidimensional measures and, 931
physiologic measures and, 929-930
self-report measures and, 930-931, 932t-933t
pain management in, 950
complementary, 938
nonpharmacologic, 935-938, 936f, 937b, 938f
pharmacologic, 938-950
calculation of dosage in, 939-940, 939t-941t
epidural analgesia, 945, 945f
evaluation of effectiveness of, 948-950
monitoring side effects in, 947-948, 947b-948b, 949f
NSAIDs, 938-939, 939t
opioids, 938-940, 939b, 940t-942t
patient-controlled analgesia, 942-945, 942f, 943b-944b, 945t
routes of analgesic administration in, 943b-944b, 945-946, 946b, 947f
timing of, 946-947
physical assessment of, 888-889, 889f, 927
abdomen and, 917-919, 917f-919f, 918b-919b
age-specific approaches to, 888t
anus and, 921
blood pressure in, 897-900, 898f-899f, 898t-899t, 899b-900b
body temperature in, 893, 893b-897b, 894t-895t
cerebellar function and, 922-923, 923b
chest and, 912-914, 913f
cranial nerves and, 923, 924f, 925t
ears and, 907-910, 907f-909f, 910t, 923f
extremities and, 921-922, 922f
eyes and, 903-907, 903f-905f, 905b, 906t, 907b
general appearance in, 900-901
genitalia and, 919-921, 919f-920f, 921b
growth measurements in, 889-892, 890b, 891f-892f
head and neck and, 902-903, 902b-903b
heart and, 915-917, 915f-916f, 916b, 917t
joints and, 922

Children *(Continued)*
lungs and, 914-915, 914b-915b, 914f
lymph nodes and, 902, 902f
mouth and throat and, 911-912, 911b, 911f-912f
muscles and, 922
nose and, 910-911, 911f
preparation of child for, 886-888, 887b, 887f, 888t, 889f
pulse in, 893-897, 897t
reflexes and, 923, 923f-924f
respiration in, 897
sequence of examination in, 886
skin and, 886, 892, 901-902, 901t, 902f
spine and, 921, 921b
postoperative care of, 1252-1253, 1253b, 1254t
preoperative care for, 1251-1252, 1251f, 1252t
preschooler. *See* Preschoolers.
psychologic preparation before procedures, 1247-1250, 1247b-1249b
school-age. *See* School-age children.
supportive care during procedures for, 1250, 1250b
unconscious, 1558-1562
elimination and, 1561
family support in, 1562, 1562b
hygienic care of, 1561, 1561b
intracranial pressure monitoring in, 1559-1560, 1559b-1560b
medications and, 1561
nutrition and hydration for, 1560-1561
positioning and exercise for, 1561
regaining consciousness, 1562
respiratory management of, 1558-1559, 1558b
sensory stimulation and, 1561-1562
thermoregulation and, 1561
Chilblain, 1674
Chin lift maneuver, 1355, 1356f, 1357
Chinese culture
birth practices and, 447-449, 448b
expression of pain in childbirth in, 396b
food patterns and, 292t-293t
health beliefs and practices in, 833, 838t-840t
postpartum period and, 550b, 559b
Chlamydia, 99
among adolescents, 32-33
neonatal, 754, 755b
Chloasma, 223, 531
Chloramphenicol, breastfeeding and, 1745t-1748t
Chlordiazepoxide, breastfeeding and, 1745t-1748t
Chloride
normal test ranges for, 1753t-1761t
nutritional significance of, 1377t-1379t
Chlorothiazide
breastfeeding and, 1745t-1748t
for congestive heart failure, 1460t
Chlorpromazine, 597t, 1745t-1748t
Choanal atresia, 770, 770f
Choking, 646-648, 647f, 648b
Cholecalciferol. *See* Vitamin D3.
Cholecystitis, 325, 325b
Cholelithiasis, 325, 325b
Cholestasis, 226-227
Cholesterol, 59t, 1475, 1475t, 1753t-1761t
Choline magnesium trisalicylate, 939t
Chordee, 1535t
Chorea, 1474
Chorioamnionitis, 496-497
Choriocarcinoma, 359, 359b
Chorion, 175, 175f
Chorionic membrane, 175f
Chorionic villi, 174-176, 179
Chorionic villus sampling (CVS), 197-198, 203, 203b, 204f
Christian Science, 836t-837t
Chromosomal abnormalities, 166-169, 167f
in autosome chromosomes, 166-167
incidence of, 160
risk factors for, 192b
sex chromosome abnormalities, 167-169
Chromosome studies, 1508
Chromosomes, 165-166, 167f, 172
Chronic active hepatitis, 1408-1409
Chronic adrenocortical insufficiency, 1612-1613, 1612b
Chronic diarrhea, 1383
Chronic hypertension in pregnancy, 334, 335t, 336, 348-349, 362t
Chronic illness, 1174-1175
coping with, 1151-1152, 1152b, 1157-1159, 1158b-1159b
definition of, 1147b
developmental focus in, 1147
end-of-life care in, 1164, 1174-1175
child's understanding and reaction to death, 1167t-1168t
decision making and, 1164-1169, 1166b, 1167t-1168t
fear and, 1169-1171, 1170b-1171b, 1170f
grief and mourning and, 1172-1174, 1173b
home care and, 1168
nurses' reactions to caring for terminally ill children, 1174, 1174b
nursing care plan for, 1147b, 1169-1174, 1170f, 1173b
organ/tissue donation and autopsy and, 1172
pain and symptom management in, 1165b, 1169-1170, 1170b
parental support in, 1170
principles of palliative care, 1164
treatment options in, 1168-1169
establishing realistic future goals for, 1163-1164
Chronic illness *(Continued)*
family education in, 1159-1160
family-centered care in, 1147, 1149, 1149b
assessment of family's adjustment, 1156-1157, 1156t, 1157b
cultural awareness and, 1148
family-health care provider communication and, 1147
shared decision making and, 1148, 1148b
therapeutic relationships and, 1147-1148
fear and, 1169-1171, 1170b-1171b, 1170f
impact on child, 1154-1156, 1155b, 1155f
impact on parents, 1149-1150, 1150b
impact on siblings, 1150-1151, 1151b, 1159
managed care in, 1149
normalization in, 1148-1149, 1159, 1159b
pain assessment in, 935
promotion of normal development for, 1160-1163, 1161t-1162t, 1162f-1163f
scope of problem, 1146, 1147b
support for family at time of diagnosis, 1152-1154, 1153b, 1157, 1157b, 1157f
support systems for families of, 1154, 1154b
Chronic lung disease
in preterm infants, 732-733
smoking and, 49
Chronic nonspecific diarrhea, 1383
Chronic otitis media, 1315b
Chronic renal failure (CRF), 1542, 1545-1547, 1546b
Chronic wounds, 1633
Church of Christ Scientist, 836t-837t
Church of Jesus Christ of Latter-day Saints, 836t-837t
Chvostek's sign, 1609b
Cigarette smoking. *See* Smoking.
CIMS. *See* Coalition to Improve Maternity Services (CIMS).
Circulatory failure. *See* Shock.
Circulatory overload, blood transfusions and, 1521t-1522t
Circulatory system
developmental milestones of, 184t-186t
fetal, 179-181, 180f
changes at birth, 1446, 1446f
during labor and birth process, 390
Circumcision, 667-669
community focus on, 667b
home care after, 669, 669b, 676b
pain management during, 668-669, 670b
procedure, 667-668, 667f-668f
urinary tract infections and, 1531b
Cirrhosis in children, 1409-1410, 1410b
Citrovorum factor, 1374t-1377t
Clarification in health assessment interviews, 75
Classic hemophilia, 1503
Classification skills, 1081
Clavicle, birth-related fracture of, 743, 743f
Clean intermittent catheterization, 1727
Clean-catch urine specimen
in first stage of labor, 454
during follow-up prenatal visits, 244
pediatric, 1269
Cleansing breath, 402b
Cleavage, 173-174, 174f
Cleft lip and palate, 771-772, 771f-772f, 1411-1414, 1413f, 1414b-1415b
teratogens and, 171f
Climacteric, menopause and, 74
Clinical benchmarking, 12-13
Clinical nurse specialists, 10
Clitoris, 65, 66f, 74t
Cloaca, 1422
Cloacal exstrophy, 1422
Clonazepam, 597t
Cloned embryos, human, 4b
Closed captioning, 1190
Closed fractures, 1682
Closed-Glottis pushing, 402b
Clostridium botulinum, 1384t-1386t
Clostridium difficile, 1384t-1386t, 1386
Clostridium perfringens, 1384t-1386t
Clothing
of home care nurses, 41
for infants, 991, 998
for newborns, 673
during pregnancy, 251, 252f, 260
Clotrimazole, 112
Clotting disorders
postpartum
disseminated intravascular coagulation, 583-584
von Willebrand disease and, 583
in pregnancy, 366-368, 374
nursing care management in, 368
von Willebrand disease and, 368
Clotting time, normal test ranges for, 1753t-1761t
Clozapine, 597t
Clozaril. *See* Clozapine.
Clubbing, 1465, 1465f
Clubfoot, 775, 1693-1695, 1694f
Coagulase negative staphylococcus, 1530
Coagulation factors
after birth, 531
in newborns at birth, 614
normal clotting and, 366-367
pregnancy values of, 220t-221t
Coagulopathies
in abruptio placentae and placenta previa, 362t, 366
postpartum, 583
disseminated intravascular coagulation, 583-584
idiopathic thrombocytopenic purpura, 583
von Willebrand disease, 583
Coalition to Improve Maternity Services (CIMS), 265, 400-401
Coanalgesics for children, 939, 941t

Coarctation of the aorta, 1451b-1453b
Cobalamin. *See* Vitamin B12.
Cobedding, 724
Cocaine, 50-51
abruptio placentae and, 365
adolescents and, 1138-1139
fetal and neonatal effects of, 756t, 759-760
use during pregnancy, 50-51, 331, 759-760
Coccidioidomycosis, 1646t
Coccyx, 68, 69f
Cochlear implants, 1188
Cochrane Pregnancy and Childbirth Database, 11-12
Cockscomb, 82
Codeine
breastfeeding and, 1745t-1748t
for children, 938-939, 940t, 942t
Cognition, definition of, 850
Cognitive development
of adolescents, 1110-1111, 1116t
of infants, 958-960, 960f, 966t-968t
of preschoolers, 1044-1045, 1045b, 1050t
of school-age children, 1079-1081, 1080f
theory of, 849t, 850-851
of toddlers, 1019-1021, 1020f, 1021b
Cognitive impairments, 1201
communication and, 1181, 1181f
discipline and, 1181
in Down syndrome, 1183-1185, 1183f, 1184b-1185b
education of child and family in, 1178-1180, 1180f
in fragile X syndrome, 1185-1186, 1186b
general concepts of, 1177-1178, 1178b, 1179t
hospitalization and, 1182-1183
optimal development and, 1180
pain assessment in children with, 934
play and exercise and, 1180-1181, 1180f-1181f
prevention of, 1183
self-care skills and, 1180
sexuality and, 1182
socialization and, 1181-1182
support for family at time of diagnosis, 1182
Cognitive power, 1552
Cognitive restructuring, 230
Cognitive strategies for pain management, 399b
Coil occlusion, 1444t
Coining, 835b
Coitus interruptus, 139-140
Cold and heat application, 404-405
Cold injuries, 1674
Cold sores, 1644t
Cold stress in newborns, 612-613, 612f
Colectomy-ileostomy, 1404
Colic, 1001-1002, 1002b, 1003f
Colistin, breastfeeding and, 1745t-1748t
Collaboration
of families in health care, 17-18
pediatric nursing and, 794
in standards of care, 13b
Collaborative care
for abruptio placentae, 366
for ectopic pregnancy, 357-358, 357b-358b
for hydatidiform mole, 359, 359b
for hyperemesis gravidarum, 349-350
for recurrent premature dilation of cervix, 355-356, 356f
Collaborative caring, 1211
College of Midwives of Ontario, 9
Collegiality, 13b
Colon cancer screening, 59t
Color pain tool, 932t-933t
Color vision, 907
Colostrum, 217, 684
Coma, 1558-1562
elimination and, 1561
family support in, 1562, 1562b
hygienic care of, 1561, 1561b
intracranial pressure monitoring in, 1559-1560, 1559b-1560b
medications and, 1561
nutrition and hydration for, 1560-1561
positioning and exercise for, 1561
regaining consciousness, 1562
respiratory management of, 1558-1559, 1558b
sensory stimulation and, 1561-1562
thermoregulation and, 1561
Combined estrogen-progestin contraceptives, 151-152, 151t
flowchart for missed tablets, 152f
potential complications, signs of, 151b
transdermal contraceptive system, 152
vaginal contraceptive ring, 152
Combined spinal-epidural analgesia (CSEA) technique, 414
Comedogenesis, 1660
Comedones, 1660
Comic books, 861
Commercial infant formulas, 701-704, 717-718, 974
Comminuted fractures, 1564-1565, 1682
Common cold, 1307
Common roundworm, 1396t
Communicable diseases, 1055-1056, 1058t-1064t
comfort measures in, 1057-1066, 1066b
complications of, 1057, 1057b
family support in, 1066, 1066b
nursing care management for, 1056
prevention of spread of, 1056-1057, 1056b-1057b
Communicating hydrocephalus, 1577, 1593-1594
Communication
with adolescents, 872, 872b, 1112b
with childbearing families, 22, 22b
with children, 870-872, 870b, 871f-872f, 873b-874b, 891f
cognitive impairment and, 1181, 1181f
cultural considerations in, 831-832, 832b-833b, 838t-840t, 868-869
Communication *(Continued)*
death of newborn and, 601-605, 601b-602b
actualizing the loss, 601-602, 601b-602b, 602f-603f
creating memories for parents to take home, 604-605, 605f
helping in acknowledgement and expression of feelings, 603-604
helping parents with decision making, 602-603
normalizing the grief process and facilitating positive coping, 604
physical needs of postpartum bereaved mother and, 604
providing sensitive care at and after discharge, 606
within families, 17
gender considerations in, 47
guidelines for, 866-867, 867b-868b, 867f
between health care providers and families of needs children, 1147
with hearing impaired women, 76
hearing impairment and, 1190
history taking and. *See* History taking.
home health care and, 35-36, 1211, 1211b
between parent and infant, 558-559, 558f-560f, 559b
with parents, 867-870, 869b-870b
regarding condom use, 99b
techniques in, 873b-874b, 875
variations in health assessment interviews, 75-76, 76b
Communication impairment, 934
Community
definition of, 43, 799
influence on child health promotion, 826
obesity and, 1129
Community assessment, 29-32, 30f, 32b
Community asset mapping approach, 30
Community capacity, 30
Community evaluation, 804-805
Community intervention, 804
Community needs assessment, 802-803, 803b
Community nursing process, 802-805, 802b-804b
Community planning, 803, 803b-804b
Community resources for postpartum women, 552
Community walk-throughs, 31, 32b
Community-based health care, 9, 10b, 29
assessment of community in, 29-32, 30f, 32b
challenges in, 34
for children and families, 799-802, 800b-801b, 801f, 805
community evaluation and, 804-805
community intervention and, 804
community needs assessment and, 802-803, 803b
Community-based health care *(Continued)*
community planning and, 803, 803b-804b
data collection and, 30-32, 30f, 32b, 43
demography and, 800
epidemiology and, 800-801, 801b, 801f
health promotion and, 29
levels of preventive care in, 29
nursing process in, 802-805, 802b-804b
vulnerable populations and, 32-34
Compensated shock, 1483-1484
Competitive games, 854
Complementary and alternative therapies, 5
calcium sources and, 283b
hospitalized child and, 1228b
infant nutrition and, 972-973
overuse of vitamins in, 1364-1365
for pediatric pain management, 938
for postpartum depression, 598, 598b
during pregnancy, 253b
Complete atrioventricular block, 1476
Complete blood cell count, 1490, 1491t
pregnancy values of, 220t-221t
Complete breech, 379f, 500, 500f
Complete fractures, 1682b, 1682f
Complete heart block, 1476
Complete miscarriage, 352, 352f, 353t
Complete rupture of uterus, 522
Complex partial seizures, 1583b-1584b, 1585t, 1591b
Compliance
children and, 1253-1256, 1256b
juvenile rheumatoid arthritis and, 1710-1711
Complicated fractures, 1682
Compound fractures, 1682
Computed tomography
in acute appendicitis, 1399
in cerebral assessment, 1556-1557, 1556t-1557t
in head injuries, 1567
Computer-aided detection and diagnosis (CAD), 120b
Computers
impact on child, 864
privacy issues and, 867
Conception, 172-174
definition of, 172
folic acid deficiency anemia during, 322
nutrient needs before, 273, 274b
Conceptual thinking, 1079-1080
Concha, 911, 911f
Concrete operations stage of cognitive development, 850-851, 1079
Concussion, 1563-1564
Condoms, 146, 146b, 146f
female, 4b, 98, 146, 146f
herpes simplex virus and, 106
male, 98, 146, 146f, 147b
for prevention of sexually transmitted infections, 98, 99b
safer sex practices and, 46b, 146b

Conduction disturbances, 1476
Conduction heat loss in newborns, 612
Conductive hearing loss, 1187-1188, 1188b, 1188f
Condylomata acuminate, 103-110, 103f
Condylomata lata, 101, 101f, 104
Confidentiality
  adolescents and, 872
  in human immunodeficiency virus infection, 1519
  interview and, 866-867, 867b
Confrontation in health assessment interviews, 75
Congenital adrenal hyperplasia, 658t, 1614-1615
Congenital aganglionic megacolon, 1391
Congenital anomalies, 742, 767-768, 779
  ambiguous genitalia, 776-777, 776f
  anorectal malformations, 774, 774f
  choanal atresia, 770, 770f
  cleft lip and palate, 771-772, 771f-772f
  clubfoot, 775, 1693-1695, 1694f
  congenital diaphragmatic hernia, 770-771, 771f
  developmental dysplasia of hip
    in children, 1691-1693, 1691b-1692b
    in newborns, 774-776, 774f-775f, 775b
  encephalocele and anencephaly, 768
  esophageal atresia and tracheoesophageal fistula, 772-773, 772f
  exstrophy of bladder, 776, 776f
  genetic diagnosis of, 777
  genetic evaluation and counseling and, 778
  gestational diabetes mellitus and, 308
  heart defects, 769-770
  hydrocephalus, 769
  hypertrophic pyloric stenosis in, 1372b, 1417-1420, 1419b
  hypospadias and epispadias, 776, 776f
  imperforate anus in, 774f, 1422
  intestinal obstruction, 773
  maternal diabetes mellitus and, 299, 735
  maternal substance abuse and, 330
  microcephaly, 769
  neonatal death and, 190
  newborn screening for, 777-778
  nursing care in, 777-779
  omphalocele and gastroschisis, 773, 773f
  polydactyly, 775-776
  spina bifida. *See* Spina bifida.
  teratogens and, 171f
  teratomas, 777
  twins and, 263
Congenital diaphragmatic hernia (CDH), 770-771, 771f
Congenital disability, definition of, 1147b
Congenital heart disease (CHD), 769-770, 1442, 1445-1446
  altered hemodynamics in, 1446-1447
  circulatory changes at birth and, 1446, 1446f
  classification of defects in, 1447-1450, 1447f
    decreased pulmonary blood flow defects, 1450, 1453f, 1454b-1455b
    increased pulmonary blood flow defects, 1447, 1447f, 1448b-1450b
    mixed defects, 1450, 1455b-1458b
    obstructive defects, 1447-1450, 1450f, 1451b-1453b
  congestive heart failure in. *See* Congestive heart failure (CHF).
  discharge and home care in, 1468-1469, 1471-1472, 1472b
  family adjustment to, 1467-1468, 1467b
  family education in, 1468
  hypoxemia in, 1464-1467, 1465b, 1465f-1466f, 1466t, 1467b
  postoperative care in, 1469-1471, 1470b-1471b
  preprocedural preparation in, 1469
Congenital hypoparathyroidism, 1609
Congenital hypothyroidism, 182, 658t
Congenital hypotonia, 1731-1732
Congenital lactase deficiency, 1377t-1379t
Congenital malformations
  genetic transmission of, 169-170, 169f
  nongenetic factors in, 170, 170b, 171f
Congestive heart failure (CHF), 1442, 1453
  afterload reduction in, 1463
  child and family support in, 1464
  diagnostic evaluation in, 1453
  nursing care plan for, 1461b-1462b
  nutritional status and, 1463-1464
  pathophysiology of, 1453, 1458f, 1459b
  respiratory distress and, 1463
  therapeutic management of, 1453-1460
    accumulation of fluids and sodium and, 1459, 1459b, 1460t, 1464
    cardiac demands and, 1459, 1463
    cardiac function and, 1459-1461, 1459b-1463b
    tissue oxygenation and, 1459-1460, 1460b
Conjoined twins, 183-186
Conjunctiva, 903
Conjunctivitis, 1194
Connecting stalk, 175f, 176
Conscience, 1044
Conscious breathing, 270, 402, 402b, 402f
Conscious relaxation, 250, 251b
Consciousness, altered states of, 1552-1553, 1553b, 1553f
Consent. *See* Informed consent.
Conservation
  school-age children and, 1080-1081, 1080f
  toddlers and, 1021b
Consolability, newborns and, 641
Constipation
  in children, 1389-1391, 1391b
  opioid-related, 947
  during pregnancy, 226, 254t-256t, 291
  urinary tract infections and, 1533b
Constitutional delay, 1097
Consumption coagulopathy. *See* Disseminated intravascular coagulation (DIC).
Contact between parents and infants, 548, 557-558, 557f
Contact dermatitis, 1646-1647
Contact lenses, 1196
Contact precautions, 1263b-1264b, 1264
Containment tucking, 723, 936
Continuous ambulatory peritoneal dialysis, 1547-1548
Continuous combined hormone therapy, 93
Continuous cycling peritoneal dialysis, 1547-1548
Continuous distending pressure, 714-715, 714f
Continuous epidural block, 413-414
Continuous positive airway pressure (CPAP), 714-715, 714f, 715t
Continuous venovenous hemodiafiltration, 1547
Continuous venovenous hemodialysis, 1547
Continuous venovenous hemofiltration, 1547
Continuum of care, 36f
Contraception, 138, 159
  for adolescents, 141b
  barrier methods of, 145
    cervical cap, 146f, 150, 150b
    condoms, 146, 146b-147b, 146f
    contraceptive diaphragms, 146-150, 146f, 148b-150b
    contraceptive sponge, 146f, 150
    spermicides, 145-146, 145f-146f
  breastfeeding and, 695, 1745t-1748t
  chronic hypertension and, 349
  coitus interruptus, 139-140
  cultural beliefs about, 550b
  education on, 138b
  effectiveness of, 138-139, 140b
  emergency, 153, 153b
  fertility awareness methods of, 140-145
    basal body temperature method, 142, 142b, 142f
    calendar rhythm method, 141
    cervical mucus ovulation-detection method, 142-143, 143b
    home predictor test kits for ovulation, 144-145, 145f
    lactational amenorrhea method, 145
    natural family planning, 141
Contraception *(Continued)*
    Standard Days Method, 141-142, 142f
    symptothermal method, 143-144, 144f
    two day method of family planning, 145
  gestational trophoblastic neoplasia and, 360
  health promotion and, 46, 46b
  hormonal methods of, 150-151, 151t
    combined estrogen-progestin contraceptives, 151-152, 151b, 151t, 152f
    transdermal contraceptive system, 152
    vaginal contraceptive ring, 152
    progestin-only contraception, 151t, 152-153, 152b
    vaginal contraceptive ring, 152
  intrauterine devices, 153-154, 154b, 154f
  maternal diabetes mellitus and, 306
  nursing care management for, 138-156, 139b-140b, 139f
  optimal birth spacing, 140b
  postpartum, 551
  sterilization procedures, 154-156, 154f-155f, 155b
Contraceptive diaphragms, 146-150, 146f
  toxic shock syndrome and, 147-150, 150b
  use and care of, 148b-149b
Contraceptive sponge, 146f, 150
Contraction stress test (CST), 204, 206-207, 206b
  indications for, 205b
  interpretation of, 206-207, 207f, 207t
Contractions. *See* Uterine contractions.
Contracture, wound healing and, 1636
Contrecoup head injuries, 1563
Contusions, 1564, 1680
Convection heat loss in newborns, 612
Conventional audiometry, 910t
Conventional level of moral development, 851-852
Conversion reaction, 1102
Convulsions
  in eclampsia, 346, 346f, 347b
  in severe preeclampsia, 343-344
Cool compresses, 405
Cool mist therapy, 1304
Cooley anemia, 322
Cooperative play, 855-856, 855f
Cooper's ligaments, 69, 70f, 118
Coordination, cerebellar functioning and, 922-923
Coordination of secondary schema, 960
Coping
  with separation and stranger fear, 965
  with special needs child, 1151-1152, 1152b, 1157-1159, 1158b-1159b

Coping *(Continued)*
stress in childhood and, 860-861
transition to parenthood and, 811-812
Copper, 1377t-1379t
Copper intrauterine device, 153-154, 154f
Copycat suicides, 1142
Cordocentesis, 202
Cords, strangulation and, 994
Core body temperature, 893
Cornea, 903
Corneal light reflex test, 904-905, 904f
Cornstarch ingestion during pregnancy, 284-285
Corona radiate, 172, 173f
Coronal suture, 377f
Corporal punishment, 814
Corpus luteum
ovarian cycle and, 72f, 73
placenta and, 177
Corpus of uterus, 66, 67f-68f
Corrosive poisoning, 1428b-1429b
Corticosteroids
for asthma, 1338-1339
delayed wound healing and, 1637t
for juvenile idiopathic arthritis, 1709
topical, 1639
Cortisol
changes during pregnancy, 227t
fetal, 182
Cortisone, breastfeeding and, 1745t-1748t
Corynebacterium diphtheriae, 1058t-1065t
Cosleeping, 1006-1007, 1007b
Costal angle, 912-913, 913f
Cotrel-Dubousset instrumentation, 1701
Cotton root bark, 582t
Cotyledons, 176, 177f
Cough, 1305b
Cough etiquette, 113b-114b
Cough suppressants for children, 1308
Coumadin. *See* Warfarin.
Counseling
about abortion, 157, 157b
about iron supplementation, 290, 290b
about ultrasound, 199-200
genetic, 162-163, 162f, 163b, 778
in human immunodeficiency virus testing, 108-109
pediatric nurse role in, 794
preconception, 44-45, 45b, 63
telephone, 867, 868b
Counterpressure, 403
Countertraction, 1686-1687
Coup head injuries, 1563
Couplet care, 649-650
Couvelaire uterus, 365
Cover tests, 904-905, 905b, 905f, 906t
Cow's milk
allergy to, 1372-1373, 1372b
iron-deficiency anemia and, 1494b
Cow's milk-based infant formulas, 702, 974
for preterm infants, 717-718
CPAP. *See* Continuous positive airway pressure (CPAP).
CPPD. *See* Cyclic perimenstrual pain and discomfort (CPPD).
Crack, 50, 1138
Crackles, 915
Cradle cap, 1659
Cradling hold, 672f, 685, 687f
Cranial deformities, 1593
Cranial nerve I. *See* Olfactory nerve (cranial nerve I).
Cranial nerve II. *See* Optic nerve (cranial nerve II).
Cranial nerve III. *See* Oculomotor nerve (cranial nerve III).
Cranial nerve IV. *See* Trochlear nerve (cranial nerve IV).
Cranial nerve V. *See* Trigeminal nerve (cranial nerve V).
Cranial nerve VI. *See* Abducens nerve (cranial nerve VI).
Cranial nerve VII. *See* Facial nerve (cranial nerve VII).
Cranial nerve VIII. *See* Vestibulocochlear nerve (cranial nerve VIII).
Cranial nerve IX. *See* Glossopharyngeal nerve (cranial nerve IX).
Cranial nerve X. *See* Vagus nerve (cranial nerve X).
Cranial nerve XI. *See* Accessory nerve (cranial nerve XI).
Cranial nerve XII. *See* Hypoglossal nerve (cranial nerve XII).
Cranial nerves
birth injury of, 743t
physical assessment of, 923, 924f, 925t
Cranioschisis, 1725b
Craniosynostosis, 1593
Craniotomy, 1574
CRASH Course in Cultural Competency, 24, 26b
Crawling reflex of newborn, 621t-625t
C-reactive protein, 1753t-1761t
Creatine kinase, 1753t-1761t
Creatinine, 223t, 1530t, 1753t-1761t
Creatinine clearance, 1753t-1761t
Creative expression, hospitalized child and, 1234, 1234f
Creativity, play and, 856
Creighton model ovulation method. *See* Cervical mucus ovulation-detection method.
Cremasteric reflex, 920, 920f
CRF. *See* Chronic renal failure (CRF).
Cribs, 994
hospital, 1261, 1262f
toddlers and, 1039-1040
Cricoid pressure before intubation, 416, 416f
CRIES neonatal postoperative pain scale, 934, 934t
Critical thinking, 794-795
Crohn's disease, 1401-1404, 1401t, 1404b
Cromolyn sodium, 1339
Cross cradle position, 685
Crossed extension reflex, 621t-625t
Cross-racial adoption, 816, 816b
Croup syndromes, 1318-1321, 1318b-1320b, 1318t
Crowning, 473, 474f, 478b, 481f
Crude birth rate, 801b
Crude death rate, 801b
Crush injuries, 1680
Crust, 1635f
Crutchfield tong traction, 1688f, 1689
Crying
infants and, 871
newborn and, 641
night, 977t
Cryopreservation of embryos, 136b
Cryptorchidism, 1535t
Cryptococcosis, 1646t
Cryptorchidism, 1535t
Cryptosporidium infection, 1383-1386
CSEA technique. *See* Combined spinal-epidural analgesia (CSEA) technique.
CSF. *See* Cerebrospinal fluid (CSF).
CST. *See* Contraction stress test (CST).
Cuddliness, newborns and, 641
Cued speech, 1190
Cuff selection for measurement of pediatric blood pressure, 898-899, 898f-899f, 899b, 899t
Cul-de-sac of Douglas, 66, 67f
Cultural awareness
in access to epidural analgesia in labor, 413b
in bladder catheterization, 1270b
in breast cancer screening, 119, 120b
in cardiovascular disorders during pregnancy, 314
in care and disposal of placenta, 479
in care and handling of newborns, 484
in child health promotion, 822-829, 840-841
community and, 826
cultural relativism and, 830-831
cultural shock and cultural competence and, 828-829, 828b-829b
ethnicity and, 824, 824f
food customs and, 832-833, 833f
health beliefs and practices and, 833-835, 835b
hereditary factors and, 829
immigrant children and, 825, 830
migrant farmworker families and, 825, 830
minority-group membership and, 827-828, 827b-828b
peer cultures and, 826-827
poverty and, 825, 830
relationships with health care providers and, 831-832, 831b-833b, 831f
religion and, 825-826, 826f, 835, 836b, 836t-837t
schools and, 826
social roles and, 823-824
socioeconomic class and, 824-825, 829-830
subcultures and, 824-827, 824f, 826f
in communication, 868-869
Cultural awareness *(Continued)*
death of newborn and, 601b-602b, 603, 605
in developmental dysplasia of hip, 1691b
in eye contact, 558, 570
family bed and, 1007b
in family-centered care, 1148
in fertility and infertility, 131b
first stage of labor and, 447-449, 448b, 448f
in food practices, 883b
in fostering bonding, 559b
in health assessment, 75-76, 76b
in home care, 1210-1211, 1210b
in infant feeding, 680
in intimate partner violence, 61
in lead poisoning, 1434b
in learning sociocultural mores, 1044b
in nutrition
during lactation, 291-293, 292t-293t
postpartum, 544, 546f
during pregnancy, 284-285, 285f
in pain, 396, 396b, 446t
assessment and management, 934-935
expression of, 395
perception of, 395
in parenting behaviors, 568-569
in parent-newborn interactions, 484
in postpartum care, 549-550, 549b-550b
in prenatal care, 192b, 259-260, 260b, 260f
questions to ask to obtain cultural expectations about childbearing, 24b
in religious orientation, 1081b
in social interactions during neonatal period, 662, 662b-663b, 662f
Cultural competence, 24, 828-829, 829b-830b
assessment and, 26-27, 75
community-based health care and, 34
development of, 22b, 24-27, 24b, 26b
in the Emergency Department, 22b
evaluation and, 27
expected outcomes and, 27
in health assessment interviews, 75-76, 76b
importance to nurses, 837-840, 838b, 838t-840t, 840b
integration with the nursing care plan, 26
nursing care plan and, 40
nursing diagnoses and, 27
Cultural diversity, 827
Cultural relativism, 22, 830-831
Cultural sensitivity. *See* Cultural competence.
Cultural shock, 828-829, 828b-829b
Culture, 822
definition of, 822
families and, 16-17, 17f, 20-22
family roles and, 24, 25t-26t, 26
genetics testing and, 164
health care access and, 47

Culture *(Continued)*
health risks and, 49
personal space and, 23-24
time orientation and, 24
Cultured epithelium, 1669
Cunnilingus, 232
Cupping, 835b
Cushing's syndrome, 1613-1614, 1613b-1614b, 1613f
Custody after divorce, 818
Cutaneous disorders. *See also* Skin lesions; Wounds.
acne, 224, 254t-256t, 325, 325b, 1659-1661
animal bites and, 1654, 1655b
arthropod bites and stings and, 1648-1650, 1649t-1650t
pediculosis capitis, 1651-1652, 1651b-1652b, 1651f
Rickettsial diseases, 1652-1653, 1653t
scabies, 1650, 1650b
bacterial infections and, 1641, 1642t, 1643f
burns. *See* Burns.
cold injuries, 1674
contact dermatitis, 1646-1647
diaper dermatitis, 672-673, 721b-722b, 1655-1656, 1656b, 1656f
eczema, 1656-1659, 1657b-1659b, 1657f
foreign bodies and, 1648
fungal infections and dermatophytoses, 1643, 1645t
systemic mycotic, 1643-1646, 1646t
high risk pregnancy and, 325-326, 325b
human bites and, 1654
Lyme disease and, 1653-1654, 1653f
poison ivy, oak, and sumac exposure and, 1647-1648, 1647b, 1647f
seborrheic dermatitis and, 1659
sunburn and
in children, 1673, 1674f-1675f
infants and, 997
topical therapy for, 1637-1641, 1637b, 1641b
viral infections and, 1642-1643, 1644t
Cutaneous stimulation for pain management, 399b
CVS. *See* Chorionic villus sampling (CVS).
Cyanosis
in anemia, 1492
in congenital heart defects, 1464-1466
differences in color changes and, 901t
in esophageal atresia, 1416, 1416b
in pediatric congestive heart failure, 1446-1447
Cyanotic heart defects, 1447, 1447f
Cycle-Beads necklace, 141-142, 142f
Cyclic perimenstrual pain and discomfort (CPPD), 87-88
dysmenorrhea, 88
primary, 88-89, 88f, 89t-90t
secondary, 89-90
Cyclic perimenstrual pain and discomfort (CPPD) *(Continued)*
endometriosis, 91-93, 92f
premenstrual syndrome, 90-91, 90b
Cystic fibrosis
ethnicity and, 49, 161, 829
maternal, 241, 324-325
pediatric, 1346-1353, 1346f, 1347b, 1348f, 1349b
Cystitis, hemorrhagic, 1514
Cystocele, 588-589, 589f, 592
Cystoscopy, 1527t-1528t
Cysts
breast, 115
ovarian, 369
Cytobrush, 83b, 84f
Cytochemical markers, 1508
Cytomegalovirus infection, 329, 752-753, 752f
Cytotec. *See* Misoprostol.

D

Dactinomycin, 360
Daily fetal movement count (DFMC), 191-192, 192b-193b, 195f
in postterm pregnancy, 519
in preterm premature rupture of membranes and, 497, 497b
Daily food guide, 280t, 290
Danazol, 93
Dandy-Walker syndrome, 1594
Data collection, community assessment and, 30-32, 30f, 32b, 43
Day care, 820b, 1048-1049, 1049f
DDH. *See* Developmental dysplasia of hip (DDH).
DDST. *See* Denver II.
D&E. *See* Dilation and evacuation (D&E).
Dead space, injection and, 1275
Deaf, definition of, 1186-1187
Deaf parents, 570
Deaf-blind children, 1196-1197
Deafness, teratogens and, 171f
Death
of child
end-of-life care and, 1164, 1174-1175
child's understanding and reaction to death, 1167t-1168t
decision making and, 1164-1169, 1166b, 1167t-1168t
fear and, 1169-1171, 1170b-1171b, 1170f
grief and mourning and, 1172-1174, 1173b
home care and, 1168
nurses' reactions to caring for terminally ill children, 1174, 1174b
nursing care plan for, 1147b, 1169-1174, 1170f, 1173b
organ/tissue donation and autopsy and, 1172
pain and symptom management in, 1165b, 1169-1170, 1170b
parental support in, 1170
Death *(Continued)*
principles of palliative care, 1164
treatment options in, 1168-1169
injuries and, 787-788, 788f-789f, 788t
of fetus, 190, 195
maternal, 189, 606-607, 606b
of newborn, 190, 598-600
acute distress in, 598-599
communicating and caring techniques and, 601-605, 601b-602b
actualizing the loss, 601-602, 601b-602b, 602f-603f
creating memories for parents to take home, 604-605, 605f
helping in acknowledgement and expression of feelings, 603-604
helping parents with decision making, 602-603
normalizing the grief process and facilitating positive coping, 604
physical needs of postpartum bereaved mother and, 604
providing sensitive care at and after discharge, 606
community resources and, 598b
cultural and spiritual needs of parents and, 605
documentation in, 605-606
family aspects of grief in, 600-601
funeral arrangements in, 603
intense grief in, 599-600
postmortem care of newborn and, 605, 605f
reorganization and, 600, 600b
Debridement of burn wounds, 1667
Decannulation, accidental, 1294
Deceleration head injuries, 1563
Decelerations of fetal heart rate, 430-433, 431b-433b, 431f
Decibels, 1187, 1187t
Decidua basalis, 174, 175f, 176
Decidua capsularis, 174-175, 175f
Decidua vera, 174, 175f
Decimal prefixes, 1761t
Decision making
death of newborn and, 602-603
at end of life, 1164-1169, 1166b, 1167t-1168t
ethical, pediatric nursing and, 794, 795b
in families, 17
families' role in, 17-18
in family-centered care, 1148, 1148b
Decompensated shock, 1483-1484
Deep breathing in children, 1255b
Deep tendon reflexes
in hypertension, 340, 341f, 341t
newborns and, 621t-625t
physical assessment of, 923, 923f-924f
Deep venous thrombosis, postpartum, 584-585, 585b
DEET. *See* Diethyltoluamide (DEET).
Defibrillation, 319b
Deformation head injuries, 1563
Dehydration
pediatric, 1380-1383, 1381b, 1382t
in acute diarrhea, 1387-1388, 1387b
in acute renal failure, 1543-1545
hospitalized child and, 1258
hypoxemic child and, 1466-1467
during pregnancy, 279-280
Delayed developmental milestones, 1178
Delayed gratification, 957
DeLee-Hillis fetoscope, 423, 423f
Delivery rooms, 471-473, 472f
Demeclocycline, breastfeeding and, 1745t-1748t
Demerol. *See* Meperidine.
Democratic parents, 812
Demographic factors in preterm labor and birth, 487b
Demography, 800
Demerol. *See* Meperidine.
Dental caries
school-age children and, 1092
toddlers and, 1031, 1033f
Dental health
of adolescents, 1120
of children, 786
chronic renal failure and, 1546
of infants, 978
during pregnancy, 247
of preschoolers, 1055
of school-age children, 1091-1092, 1091f, 1092b
of toddlers, 1031-1033, 1032f-1033f, 1032t
Dental hygiene
in children with cerebral palsy, 1719-1720
high risk pregnancy and, 191b
Denver II, 924-926, 926b, 1749f-1750f
Dependent edema, 222-223
Depo-Provera. *See* Depot medroxyprogesterone acetate (DMPA).
Depot medroxyprogesterone acetate (DMPA), 151t, 152, 152b, 306
Depressed skull fractures, 1564-1565
Depression
in adolescents and suicide, 1142
anorexia and, 52
postpartum, 562, 592-593
assessment of, 593b
newborn death and, 599
nursing care management in, 594-595, 595b
complementary and alternative therapies and, 598, 598b
home visits and, 596
postpartum unit and, 595-596, 596b
psychiatric hospitalization and, 596-597, 596b
psychotropic medications and, 597-598, 597t
referral and, 596
suicidal thoughts and, 596, 596b
with psychotic features, 594-595, 595b, 597t
risk factors for, 592, 592b

Depression (*Continued*)
without psychotic features, 593-594
in school-age children, 1102-1103, 1102b
treatment of, 50
Depth perception, 955
Dermatitis
atopic, 1656-1659, 1657b-1659b, 1657f
contact, 1646-1647
diaper, 1655-1656, 1656b, 1656f
pathophysiology of, 1632-1633, 1636
seborrheic, 1659
Dermatologic disorders. *See* Integumentary disorders.
Dermatome, 1668-1669, 1668f
Dermatophytosis, 1643, 1645f, 1645t
DES. *See* Diethylstilbestrol (DES).
Descent of labor, 388, 389f, 450t, 466, 468t, 469, 472t
Desensitization, preschoolers and, 1052
Desipramine, breastfeeding and, 1745t-1748t
Deslanoside, 318
Desmopressin, 368
Desquamation in newborn, 617
Deuteranomaly, 907
Development, definition of, 842
Development, growth and. *See* Growth and development.
Development, human
developmental milestones of, 184t-186t
first few weeks of, 174f
sensitive/critical periods in, 171f
Developmental age periods, 843b
Developmental assessment, 923-927, 926b, 1749f-1750f
Developmental care
of preterm infants, 723-726, 724f, 725b
of special needs children, 1160-1163, 1161t-1162t, 1162f-1163f
Developmental delay, definition of, 1147b, 1177-1178
Developmental disability, 1147b
Developmental dysplasia of hip (DDH)
in children, 1691-1693, 1691b-1692b
in newborns, 619-620, 620f, 774-776, 774f-775f, 775b
Developmental lactase deficiency, 1373
Developmental pace, 844
Developmental task, 842
Developmental theory, 20
Dexamethasone, 1576
DFMC. *See* Daily fetal movement count (DFMC).
Diabetes insipidus, 1604-1605, 1604b
Diabetes mellitus, 295-296, 298, 332-333
age and, 48
maternal
breastfeeding and, 306, 695-696
classification of, 296, 297t
family planning and contraception in, 306
fetal and neonatal risks and complications in, 299
Diabetes mellitus (*Continued*)
gestational, 179, 296, 306-309
cystic fibrosis and, 324
interventions in, 308-309
maternal and fetal risks in, 307-308
screening for, 308, 308f
intrapartum interventions in, 300b-301b, 305-306
metabolic changes associated with pregnancy and, 296-298, 297f
monitoring of blood glucose in, 299-306, 300b-301b, 301f, 304b, 304f
mortality rate in, 296
nursing care plan for, 307b
pathogenesis of, 296
postpartum interventions in, 300b-301b, 306
preconception counseling and, 298, 298b
prenatal care and, 299-305, 300b-301b, 301t
complications requiring hospitalization and, 305
determination of birth date and mode of delivery, 305
diet, 302, 303b
exercise, 302
insulin therapy, 302-304, 303b, 303t, 304f
monitoring blood glucose levels, 304-305, 304b-305b
risks and complications in, 298-299
target blood glucose levels in, 301t
pediatric, 1616
classification of, 1616, 1617t
delayed wound healing and, 1637t
diabetic ketoacidosis in, 1622-1630, 1623b
diagnostic evaluation in, 1616, 1618
family support in, 1629-1630, 1630b
hospitalization in, 1623-1624, 1626b
hygiene and, 1628-1629
infants of diabetic mothers and, 735-737, 736f, 737b
injection procedures and, 1626-1627, 1626t, 1627f
meal planning and, 1624-1626
medical identification and, 1624
nursing care plan for, 1624b-1625b
obesity and type 2 diabetes, 786-787, 787f
pathophysiology of, 1616-1618
record keeping and, 1629
self-management of, 1629
therapeutic management of, 1618
exercise and, 1621, 1629
hyperglycemia and, 1621-1622, 1622t, 1628
hypoglycemia and, 1621, 1621b, 1622t, 1628, 1629b
illness management and, 1622
insulin therapy and, 1618-1620, 1619b, 1626
Diabetes mellitus (*Continued*)
monitoring in, 1620, 1620t, 1627-1628, 1627b-1628b, 1628f
nutrition and, 1620-1621
travel and, 1626
Diabetic ketoacidosis (DKA), 299, 1618
therapeutic management of, 1622-1630, 1623b
Diagnosis, nursing. *See* Nursing process.
Dialysis, 1547-1548, 1548b, 1548f
in end-stage renal disease, 1546-1547
Diamond-shaped position, 76, 77f
Diaper dermatitis, 672-673, 721b-722b, 1655-1656, 1656b, 1656f
Diaphragmatic hernias, 770-771, 771f, 1418t
Diaphragms, contraceptive. *See* Contraceptive diaphragms.
Diarrhea
in children, 1383-1389
acute, 1383, 1384t-1386t
diagnostic evaluation in, 1386-1387
etiology of, 1383-1386
nursing care plan for, 1388-1389, 1389b-1390b
pathophysiology of, 1386
prevention of, 1387-1388, 1388b
respiratory infections and, 1305b
therapeutic management of, 1387-1388, 1387b
onset of labor and, 392
Diastasis recti abdominis, 527
Diastatic skull fractures, 1564-1565
Diastolic blood pressure (DBP)
in children, 898t, 899
in infants, 954
during labor, 451b
during pregnancy, 218, 219b, 221t, 242b, 243
Diazepam
breastfeeding and, 1745t-1748t
for children, 939, 941t
tetanus and, 1738-1739
Diazoxide, breastfeeding and, 1745t-1748t
DIC. *See* Disseminated intravascular coagulation (DIC).
Dick-Read, Grantly, 4b, 399, 401
Dick-Read method of childbirth, 399
Diclofenac, 89t
Dictatorial parents, 812
Dicumarol, breastfeeding and, 1745t-1748t
Diet
in acute glomerulonephritis, 1539
atopic dermatitis and, 1658
breastfeeding and, 694
burns and, 1666
cardiovascular disorders and, 316
chronic renal failure and, 1545-1546
in cystic fibrosis, 1351
diabetes mellitus and, 1624-1626
during diabetic pregnancy, 302, 303b
gestational diabetes mellitus and, 308
for high cholesterol, 1476
Diet (*Continued*)
iron supplementation and, 1494-1495
ketogenic, 1586
menstrual discomfort and, 88
mild preeclampsia and, 285, 342-343, 343b
obese child and, 1130
premenstrual syndrome and, 91
Dietary Guidelines for Americans 2005, 51
Dietary history, 286-288, 288b, 289t, 877, 883b
Dietary Reference Intakes (DRIs), 1366-1368, 1367f
children and, 881-883, 883b
for infants, 972t
during pregnancy and lactation, 274-275, 275t-276t
Diethylstilbestrol (DES), 82, 83b, 130, 355, 355b
Diethyltoluamide (DEET), 1654
Differentiation, 842-844
Difficult child, 640, 848
Digestion
defects in, 1423
infants and, 954
newborns at birth and, 614
toddlers and, 1018
Digital subtraction angiography, 1556t-1557t
Digital thermometers, 897b
Digital-anal activities, 98
Digoxin
for pediatric congestive heart failure, 1460-1461, 1461b-1463b
during pregnancy, 317t
toxicity of, 1460b, 1461
Dilated cardiomyopathy, 312b, 1478
Dilation and curettage
after miscarriage, 354
home care after, 354, 355b
Dilation and evacuation (D&E), 156, 158, 354
Dilation of cervix
during labor, 384-385, 384f, 387-388
recurrent premature, 355-356, 355b, 356f
Dilaudid. *See* Hydromorphone.
Dinoprostone, 507b
Diphenhydramine, 1745t-1748t
Diphtheria, 1058t-1064t
tetanus, pertussis vaccine. *See* Tetanus-diphtheria-acellular pertussis (Tdap) vaccine.
Direct-contact transmission, 1264
Directed pushing, 402b
Direct-entry midwives, 267
Directional trends in growth and development, 843-844, 843f
Disabilities
in children, 1174-1175
coping with, 1151-1152, 1152b, 1157-1159, 1158b-1159b
developmental focus in, 1147
family education in, 1159-1160
family-centered care in, 1147, 1149, 1149b
assessment of family's adjustment, 1156-1157, 1156t, 1157b

Disabilities (Continued)
cultural awareness and, 1148
family-health care provider communication and, 1147
shared decision making and, 1148, 1148b
therapeutic relationships and, 1147-1148
impact on child, 1154-1156, 1155b, 1155f
impact on parents, 1149-1150, 1150b
impact on siblings, 1150-1151, 1151b, 1159
injuries and, 787-788, 788f-789f, 788t
managed care in, 1149
normalization in, 1148-1149, 1159, 1159b
promotion of normal development, 1160-1163, 1161t-1162t, 1162f-1163f
realistic future goals and, 1163-1164
scope of problem, 1146, 1147b
support for family at time of diagnosis, 1152-1154, 1153b, 1157, 1157b, 1157f
support systems for families, 1154, 1154b
definition of, 1147b
end-of-life care in, 1164, 1174-1175
child's understanding and reaction to death, 1167t-1168t
decision making and, 1164-1169, 1166b, 1167t-1168t
fear and, 1169-1171, 1170b-1171b, 1170f
grief and mourning and, 1172-1174, 1173b
home care and, 1168
nurses' reactions to caring for terminally ill children, 1174, 1174b
nursing care plan for, 1147b, 1169-1174, 1170f, 1173b
organ/tissue donation and autopsy and, 1172
pain and symptom management in, 1165b, 1169-1170, 1170b
parental support in, 1170
principles of palliative care, 1164
sibling support in, 1170
treatment options in, 1168-1169
tertiary prevention and, 29
Discharge after birth, 534, 552-553
advantages and disadvantages of, 535b
after cesarean birth, 517, 517b
cardiovascular disorders during pregnancy and, 319
criteria for, 534-535, 535b, 536f, 537b
death of newborn and, 606
discharge teaching and, 550-552, 551b
follow-up after, 552
laws relating to, 534
Discharge after birth (Continued)
nursing care management of physical needs in, 535-537, 538b
breastfeeding and, 546, 546b
exercise and, 544, 545f
maintenance of uterine tone and, 542, 542f
normal bladder function and, 544
normal bowel function and, 544
nutrition and, 544, 546f
pain management and, 542-543, 543b
plan of care and implementation, 537-540, 539b-540b
prevention of bladder distention and, 542
prevention of excessive bleeding and, 540-541, 540b-542b, 540f
prevention of infection and, 540, 541b
prevention of Rh isoimmunization and, 546-547, 547b
rest and, 543-544, 543b
rubella vaccination and, 546, 546b
signs of potential problems, 538b
suppression of lactation and, 546
nursing care management of psychosocial needs in, 547, 547f, 548b, 549-552
adaptation to parenthood and parent-infant interactions and, 548
birth experience and, 548
cultural diversity and, 549-550, 549b-550b
family structure and functioning and, 549, 549f
maternal self-image and, 548
Discharge planning and teaching, 550-552, 551b
after lead poisoning, 1437
after pediatric heart surgery, 1471-1472, 1472b
after trauma in pregnancy, 374
in cesarean birth, 517, 517b
in child maltreatment, 1074
high risk newborns and, 737-738, 738b
home care and, 369, 369b, 1205-1206, 1206b-1207b, 1207f
in Kawasaki disease, 1482, 1482b
in newborn care, 669
body temperature and, 671
care seats and, 673, 673b, 673f
clothing and, 673
elimination and, 671
immunizations and, 674
infant follow-up care and, 674
nonnutritive sucking and, 673-674, 674f
positioning and holding and, 671-672, 671b, 672f
rashes and, 672-673
respirations and, 671
sponge bathing, cord care, skin care and, 674, 675b
Discharge planning and teaching (Continued)
in osteosarcoma, 1706
in pediatric hospitalization, 1238-1239
Discipline
cognitively impaired child and, 1181
infants and, 970
parenting and, 812-814, 813b-814b
school-age children and, 1087
Discomfort. *See* Pain.
Disease
delayed wound healing and, 1637t
epidemiology and, 800-801, 801b, 801f
influence on child development, 859-860
prevention of, 29, 793
Dishonest behavior school-age children and, 1087-1089
Dislocations
in children, 1680-1681
in developmental dysplasia of hip, 774-775, 774f, 1691-1692
Disorientation in burn patients, 1670b
Disseminated intravascular coagulation (DIC), 1492f, 1506-1507, 1506f, 1507b
postpartum, 583-584
during pregnancy, 367-368
Distal intestinal obstruction syndrome, 1347
Distance visual acuity, 906t
Distraction
musculoskeletal, 1690, 1690f
for pain management, 397
during pediatric procedures, 937b, 1250
Distress behaviors, 929, 930f, 931t
Distributive shock, 1483t
Diuresis
magnesium sulfate and, 345
postpartum, 528
Diuretics
breastfeeding and, 1745t-1748t
congestive heart failure and, 1459, 1460t
during pregnancy, 317t
Diuril. *See* Chlorothiazide.
Diversional activities for hospitalized child, 1233, 1233f
Diversity, respect for, 1210-1211, 1210b
Diverticulum, Meckel's, 1400-1401, 1400b
Divorce
children and, 16, 816-818, 817b
parenting and, 816-818
preschoolers and, 1045b
Dizygotic twins, 183, 187f, 810, 810b
DKA. *See* Diabetic ketoacidosis (DK).
DMPA. *See* Depot medroxyprogesterone acetate (DMPA).
DNA replication in meiosis, 172
DNR orders. *See* Do-not-resuscitate (DNR) orders.
"Do not use" list, 13, 14t
Documentation
of gravidity and parity, 210-211, 211t
in home care, 41
during labor, 424, 424b, 434b, 437-438, 438f, 449, 449f, 471b, 509b
of newborn death, 605-606
in pediatric nursing, 796
transfer from recovery area and, 533, 534t
vacuum extraction and, 511
Dog bites, 1654
Doll's head maneuver, 1554-1555, 1554b
Dolophine. *See* Methadone.
Domestic abuse. *See* Intimate partner violence (IPV).
Domestic mimicry, 1020, 1020f
Domestic violence. *See* Intimate partner violence (IPV).
Donald, Ian, 4b
Dong quai, 90t
Donnatal. *See* Phenobarbital.
Donor embryos, 137t
Donor oocytes, 137t
Do-not-resuscitate (DNR) orders, 1166
Doppler blood flow analysis, 198, 199f
Doppler effect, 198
Doppler ultrasound, 898
Dorsal penile nerve block (DPNB), 668-669, 670b
Dorsal rhizotomy, 1718
Double effect, principle of, 1169-1170, 1170b
Double hip squeeze, 500b
Double knee rolls, 545f
Doubt and shame vs. autonomy in psychosocial development, 849-850, 1019
Doulas, 9, 267
labor support by, 464-465
questions to ask when choosing, 267b
Down syndrome
diagnosis of, 1183, 1183f, 1184b, 1185
early studies of, 4b
etiology of, 1183
growth and development and, 845
maternal serum alpha-fetoprotein and, 204
nursing care plan in, 168b, 1184-1185, 1185b
risk of, 167
therapeutic management in, 1183-1184, 1184b
Doxycycline, 99
DPNB, dorsal penile nerve block (DPNB)
DPT, breastfeeding and, 1745t-1748t
Dramatic play, 854
hospitalized child and, 1234-1235, 1235b
preschoolers and, 1047, 1047f
Drawing, 873b-874b, 1234, 1234f
Dreams, 873b-874b
Dressings, 1636-1637, 1638t, 1639-1640
DRIs. *See* Dietary Reference Intakes (DRIs).
Drop attacks, 1583b-1584b

Droplet precautions, 1263-1264, 1263b
Droppers, 1274
Dropping. *See* Lightening.
Drowning, 1570
adolescents and, 1123b
children and, 788, 788f
infants and, 788, 788f, 992b-993b, 998
school-age children and, 1095t
toddlers and, 1034t-1035t, 1038
Drug history in initial prenatal care interview, 239
Drug testing during pregnancy, 49b, 239b
Drug therapy
administration of. *See* Administration of medications.
adverse cutaneous reactions to, 1648, 1648b
in asthma, 1337-1340
breastfeeding and, 543, 597-598, 696, 1745t-1748t
for cardiopulmonary resuscitation, 1358, 1359t
for cardiovascular disorders, 316, 317t
for childhood depression, 1103
for endometriosis, 92-93
for enterobiasis, 1398
for enuresis, 1100
for epilepsy, 1585-1586, 1586b
for female infertility, 135
for giardiasis, 1397
for hemophilia, 1503
home care and, 39-40
for hypertension in pregnancy, 348t
for infant experiencing withdrawal, 762
for inflammatory bowel disease, 1402
for juvenile rheumatoid arthritis, 1709-1710
for neonatal eye prophylaxis, 648-649, 649b, 649f
for peptic ulcer disease, 1405-1406
during pregnancy, 252
for premenstrual syndrome, 91
for primary dysmenorrheal, 88-89, 89t
for systemic hypertension, 1480
Drug toxicity, leukemia and, 1513-1514, 1513b
Drug-exposed newborns, 756
Dual-earner families, 819
DUB. *See* Dysfunctional uterine bleeding (DUB).
Duchenne muscular dystrophy, 1733-1735, 1733f, 1734b
Ductal carcinoma, 118
Ductule, 70f
Ductus arteriosus, 180, 180f, 730, 1446, 1446f
Ductus venosus, 180f
Duncan mechanism, 479
Duodenal ulcers in children, 1404
Duragesic. *See* Fentanyl.
Dwarfism, 1097
Dying children. *See* Terminally ill children.
Dysacusis, 1187
Dysfunctional labor, dystocia and, 497-498, 499b
Dysfunctional swallowing, 1380b
Dysfunctional uterine bleeding (DUB), 95
Dyskinetic cerebral palsy, 1717b
Dyslalia, 1053
Dysmenorrhea, 88
in adolescents, 88, 1125-1126
pain during childbirth and, 395-396
primary, 88-89, 88f, 89t-90t
in adolescents, 1125
complementary and alternative therapies for, 89, 90t
medications for, 88-89, 89t
secondary, 89-90
Dyspareunia, 93
Dysphagia, 1380b
Dysplasia
acetabular, 774-775, 774f, 1691-1692
bronchopulmonary, 732-733
developmental dysplasia of hip
in children, 1691-1693, 1691b-1692b
in newborns, 619-620, 620f, 774-776, 774f-775f, 775b
Dyspnea, 254t-256t, 915b
Dysrhythmias, 1476-1477, 1477b
Dystocia, 497
abnormal labor patterns in, 501-502, 502t, 503f
dysfunctional labor and, 497-498, 499b
fetal causes of, 498-501, 500b, 500f
maternal position and, 501
multifetal pregnancy and, 501
nursing care management in, 504b
psychologic responses to, 501
trauma secondary to, 652
Dystrophin, 1733

E

Ear drops, 1283-1284
Ear-based temperature sensors, 894t-895t, 895b-897b
Early adolescence, 1105, 1116t
Early childhood, 843b
communication and, 871, 872f
developmental aspects of special needs in, 1160-1162, 1161t-1162t, 1162f
hospitalization during, 1221
Early decelerations of fetal heart rate, 430-431, 431b, 431f
Early discharge after birth
advantages and disadvantages of, 535b
criteria for, 534-535, 535b, 536f, 537b
legal considerations in, 534
newborn home care after, 676b
Early intervention programs, 1149, 1179-1180
Early pregnancy bleeding, 94, 350-351
miscarriage and, 351-354, 352f, 353t
Ears
development of, 171f
of newborns, 626t-636t
otitis media and, 1314-1317, 1314b-1315b
physical assessment of, 80, 907-910, 907f-909f, 910t, 923f
review of systems and, 79, 882b
Easy children, 640, 848
Eating disorder not otherwise specified (EDNOS), 1133
Eating disorders
anorexia nervosa, 52, 52b, 87, 1132, 1133b-1135b
bulimia nervosa, 52-53, 52b, 1132, 1134b
eating disorder not otherwise specified, 1133
obesity and, 8, 52, 278-279, 309, 420, 786-787, 787f, 1119, 1127-1132, 1128f, 1131b-1132b
Eating habits
of adolescents, 1118-1119, 1118f
of children, 786
Ecchymoses, 1633
differences in color changes and, 901t
neonatal birth trauma and, 652
Echocardiography, 1443t, 1444
Eclampsia, 374
classification of, 335t, 336
convulsions in, 346, 346f
epilepsy versus, 326
immediate care in, 346-347, 347b, 374
morbidity and mortality in, 335
postpartum nursing care in, 347-348, 347b
pregestational diabetes mellitus and, 298
ECMO. *See* Extracorporeal membrane oxygenation (ECMO).
Ecomaps, 20, 21f
Economics of health care, 802
Ectoderm, 174, 174f
Ectopic pregnancy, 374
abdominal, 353, 357f
assisted reproductive therapies and, 136
clinical manifestations of, 357
collaborative care for, 357-358, 357b-358b
incidence and etiology of, 356-357, 356f
nursing care management in, 353-354, 353b-355b
pelvic inflammatory disease and, 102
ECV. *See* External cephalic version (ECV).
Eczema, 1656-1659, 1657b-1659b, 1657f
EDB. *See* Estimating date of birth (EDB).
Edema
angioedema, 1485
ankle, 254t-256t
cerebral, 1566, 1566b
dependent, 222-223, 339-340
in hypertension, 339-340, 341f
laryngeal, 1485, 1485b
in legs, position for reducing, 251f
pitting, 340, 341f
pulmonary, 480
EDNOS. *See* Eating disorder not otherwise specified (EDNOS).
Educable cognitive impairment, 1178
Education
attention-deficit hyperactivity disorder and, 1099
cerebral palsied children and, 1721-1722
cognitively impaired children and, 1178-1180, 1180f
for contraceptive use, 138b
disparities in, 6
hospitalized children and, 1235
prenatal. *See* Prenatal education.
visually impaired children and, 1195
Education of the Handicapped Act Amendments, 923-924, 1149
Edwards' syndrome, 167
EEC. *See* External anal sphincter (EEC).
EEG. *See* Electroencephalography (EEG).
Effacement of cervix, 384-385, 384f, 387-388, 453, 464t
Effleurage, 402-403
Eggs during pregnancy, 280t
Ego, 848, 1084
Egocentrism, 1021b
Eisenmenger's syndrome, 312b, 313
Elbow restraints, 1266
Elbow winging, 125b-126b
ELBW infants. *See* Extremely-low-birth-weight (ELBW) infants.
Elective abortion, 156-158, 158b, 203b
Electrical burns, 997-998, 997f-998f, 1661
in toddlers, 1038-1039, 1038f
Electrocardiography, pediatric, 1443, 1444t
Electroencephalography (EEG)
in cerebral dysfunction, 1556, 1556t-1557t
in seizures, 1585
Electrolyte balance. *See* Fluid and electrolyte balance.
Electrolyte disturbances, blood transfusion-related, 1521t-1522t
Electronic continuous thermometers, 893
Electronic fetal monitoring (EFM), 422-427, 426t
after maternal trauma, 373-374, 373b
contraction stress test and. *See* Contraction stress test (CST).
documentation of, 424, 424b, 434b, 437-438, 438f
evidence-based practice on, 425b
external, 425-426, 426f, 426t
fetal heart rate patterns and, 422
fetal heart rate variability and, 205
fetal responses to hypoxia and asphyxia and, 204-205
indications for, 204, 205b
internal, 426-427, 426t, 427f
intrapartal meconium-stained amniotic fluid and, 202
nonstress test and. *See* Nonstress test (NST).
nursing care management in, 433, 433b, 435f
care plan for, 434b
legal considerations in, 434b

Electronic fetal monitoring (EFM) *(Continued)*
patient and family teaching and, 437, 437b
pattern recognition and, 433-438
additional methods of assessment and intervention in, 435-437, 437t
nonreassuring patterns, 434-435, 435b
vibroacoustic stimulation and, 205-206
Electronic intermittent thermometers, 893
Electronic thermometers, 893, 897b
Electrophysiologic cardiac catheterization, 1476
Elimination
after childbirth, 538b
in children
enemas and, 1299, 1299b
family teaching and home care and, 1300
ostomies and, 1299-1300
unconscious child and, 1561
during labor, 457t, 459
newborns and, 671
preterm infants and, 718
ELISA. *See* Enzyme-linked immunosorbent assay (ELISA).
ELSIs of human genome research. *See* Ethical, Legal, and Social Implications (ELSIs) of human genome research.
Emancipated minors, 1246
Embolism
air, 1521t-1522t
amniotic fluid, 479, 522-523, 523b
pulmonary, 584
thromboembolism, 584-585, 585b
Embryo
amniotic fluid and, 175-176
critical periods in embryogenesis, 756f
cryopreservation of, 136b
development of, 171f, 175
developmental milestones of, 184t-186t
membranes of, 175, 175f
placenta and
functions of, 177-179, 178b, 178f
structure of, 176-179, 177f-178f
sex differentiation in, 182-183
umbilical cord and, 175f, 176
yolk sac and, 174f-175f, 176, 181
Embryo adoption, 136, 137t
Embryo hosting, 136, 137t
Embryoblast, 173-174
Emergency admission of children, 1239-1242, 1241b
Emergency care
in acute renal failure, 1543b
in amniotic fluid embolism, 479, 522-523, 523b
in avulsed tooth, 1092b
in burns, 1664-1665, 1665b
in cardiac arrest
in children, 1355-1358, 1356f-1357f, 1359t
during pregnancy, 317b, 319b
culturally competent, 22b
Emergency care *(Continued)*
in eclampsia, 346-347, 347b, 374
in epistaxis, 1507b
in eye injuries, 1193b
during first stage of labor, 466, 467b
in fractures, 1684b
in head injuries, 1573b
in hemorrhagic shock, 582b-583b
in hypoglycemia, 1629b
in hypovolemic shock, 542b
in induction of labor with oxytocin, 509b
in maternal hypotension with decreased placental perfusion, 411b
in pediatric airway obstruction, 1358-1360, 1358b, 1358f, 1360f
in poisoning, 1426-1432, 1430b
assessment and, 1427
gastric decontamination and, 1427-1431, 1431b
poison control center and, 997b, 1039b, 1426-1427, 1426b-1427b
prevention of recurrence and, 1431-1432, 1432b
in prolapsed umbilical cord, 520, 521f, 522b
in respiratory failure, 1354-1355, 1354b
in rupture of uterus, 372, 522
in second stage of labor, 477, 478b
in seizures, 1591b
in shock, 1485b
in shoulder dystocia, 519, 520f
in tracheostomy tube occlusion, 1294, 1294b
in uterine inversion, 578
in vertex presentation, 478b
Emergency cesarean birth, 514
Emergency childbirth, 477, 478b
Emergency contraception, 4b, 153, 153b
Emergency Medical Treatment and Active Labor Act (EMTALA), 443b
EMLA. *See* Eutectic mixture of local anesthetics (EMLA).
Emollients for newborn skin care, 721, 721b-722b
Emotional abuse, 1066, 1071b-1072b
clinical manifestations of, 1071b-1072b
history and interview and, 1070
physical assessment and, 1072
Emotional attachment
maternal-paternal-fetal, 232, 234, 235b
parent-infant, 554-557, 555t-556t, 557b
Emotional bank, 860
Emotional deprivation, 859
Emotional disabilities, 76
Emotional lability, 230, 1608
Emotional responses, cultural influences on, 259-260, 260b
Emotionality, 1110
Empathy, 75, 869
Employment
breastfeeding and, 693
employer accommodation of parenting situations, 819
pregnancy and, 250-251
Empowerment, parental, 1152, 1159
EMTALA. *See* Emergency Medical Treatment and Active Labor Act (EMTALA).
Enamel hypoplasia, 171f
Encephalitis, 1578-1579, 1579b
Encephalocele, 768, 1725b
Encephalopathy, 1580-1581, 1581b
Encopresis, 1100, 1389
Endemic typhus, 1653t
Endocarditis, 1472-1473, 1472b-1473b
Endocephalography, 1556t-1557t
Endocervical canal, 68f
Endocervical length, 487
Endocervical sampling devices, 83b, 84f
Endocrine dysfunction, 1630-1631
adrenal disorders and, 1611
acute adrenocortical insufficiency, 1611-1612, 1611b-1612b
chronic adrenocortical insufficiency, 1612-1613, 1612b
congenital adrenal hyperplasia, 1614-1615
Cushing's syndrome, 1613-1614, 1613b-1614b, 1613f
pheochromocytoma, 1615-1616, 1616b
in cystic fibrosis, 1350
diabetes mellitus and. *See* Diabetes mellitus.
Graves disease and, 309, 1607, 1608b
parathyroid disorders and, 1609
hyperparathyroidism, 1610-1611, 1610b
hypoparathyroidism, 1609-1610, 1609b-1610b
pituitary disorders and, 1600
diabetes insipidus, 1604-1605, 1604b
hypopituitarism, 1600-1602, 1601b-1602b
pituitary hyperfunction, 1602-1603
precocious puberty, 1603-1604, 1603b
syndrome of inappropriate antidiuretic hormone, 1605, 1605b
thyroid disorders and, 1605
goiter, 1606, 1606b
hyperthyroidism. *See* Hyperthyroidism.
juvenile hypothyroidism, 1605-1606, 1606b
lymphocytic thyroiditis, 1606-1607, 1607b
Endocrine system
adaptation to labor, 392
adaptations to pregnancy, 227, 227t, 338b
fetal, 182
pediatric, 882b
postpartum adaptation of, 528
review of systems and, 79
Endoderm, 174f, 175
End-of-life care, 1164, 1174-1175
child's understanding and reaction to death, 1167t-1168t
decision making and, 1164-1169, 1166b, 1167t-1168t
End-of-life care *(Continued)*
fear and, 1169-1171, 1170b-1171b, 1170f
grief and mourning and, 1172-1174, 1173b
home care and, 1168
nurses' reactions to caring for terminally ill children, 1174, 1174b
nursing care plan for, 1147b, 1169-1174, 1170f, 1173b
organ/tissue donation and autopsy and, 1172
pain and symptom management in, 1165b, 1169-1170, 1170b
parental support in, 1170
principles of palliative care, 1164
treatment options in, 1168-1169
Endometrial ablation, 94
Endometrial biopsy
health screening recommendations for, 59t
in impaired fertility, 133t
Endometrial cycle, 72-73, 72f
Endometriosis, 91-93, 92f, 127
management of, 92-93, 135
during postpartum period, 585, 587
Endometritis, 585
Endometrium, 66, 68f, 135-136
fetal, 183
Endorphins, pain and, 396
End-stage liver disease, 1409-1410, 1410b
End-stage renal disease (ESRD), 1546-1547
Enemas
during labor, 459
pediatric, 1299, 1299b
Energy needs
of infants, 680-681
during lactation, 275t-276t, 286
during pregnancy, 275-277, 275t-276t
diabetes mellitus and, 302
hazards of restricting adequate weight gain and, 277-279, 278t, 279b
pattern of weight gain and, 277, 278f
weight gain and, 277, 281b
of toddlers, 1029
Energy work, 270, 402
Enforced dependency, 1222
Engagement, birth process and, 378, 388, 389f
Engerix-B. *See* Hepatitis B vaccine (HepB).
Engorgement during breastfeeding, 696-698
Engrossment, 564, 565f
Enteral feeding
necrotizing enterocolitis and, 732
parenteral therapy and, 1294b
Enterobacter sakazakii, 718b
Enterobiasis, 1397-1398, 1398b
Enterocolitis, 1392
Enthesitis-related arthritis, 1709
Entrainment, parent-infant communication and, 559
Enucleation in retinoblastoma, 1197
Enuresis, 1100

Environment
attention-deficit hyperactivity disorder and, 1099
hospitalized children and, 1261-1262, 1261f-1262f
influence on child development, 860, 860b
during labor and birth, 397
newborns and, 639-641, 661-662, 662b
obesity and, 1128-1129
parent-infant attachment and, 556t
physical abuse and, 1068
preterm infants and, 712-713, 722-723, 723f
Environmental and workplace hazards, 56-57
Environmental contaminants, breastfeeding and, 696
Environmental tobacco smoke exposure, 1333, 1333b
Enzymatic debrider, 1638t
Enzyme-linked immunosorbent assay (ELISA), 212, 1517
Eosinophil count, normal test ranges for, 1753t-1761t
Epicanthal folds, 904-905, 904f
Epidemic typhus, 1653t
Epidemiologic triangle, 801, 801f
Epidemiology, 800-801, 801b, 801f
Epidermal injuries, 1257, 1633
Epidermal stripping, 1257
Epidermis, 183
Epididymis, 919f
Epidural and intrathecal opioids, 414-415
Epidural anesthesia/analgesia, 410f, 412-414, 412b-413b, 413f, 466
in cesarean births, 513
in children, 943b-944b, 945, 945f
contraindications to, 415
neonates and, 415
obesity and, 420
Epidural blood patch, 412, 412f
Epidural hematomas, 1564f
Epidural hemorrhage, 1565, 1565b
Epiglottitis, acute, 1318-1319, 1318b-1319b, 1318t
Epilepsy, 1581
classification and clinical manifestations of, 1582, 1583b-1584b, 1585t
diagnostic evaluation of, 1582-1585
etiology of, 1581-1582, 1582b
nursing care management in, 1587-1592, 1587b-1592b
pathophysiology of, 1582
during pregnancy, 326, 326b
prognosis, 1587
therapeutic management of, 1585-1587, 1586b-1587b
Epinephrine
for anaphylactic reactions, 1371b
breastfeeding and, 1745t-1748t
for cardiopulmonary resuscitation, 1359t
Epiphyseal injuries, 1682
Epiphysis, 846
Episiotomy, 476-477, 476f, 480
in crowning, 473
healing of, 527
infection of, 540
Episiotomy *(Continued)*
in nulliparous women, 469
postpartum care of, 539b-541b, 540
pudendal nerve blocks and, 409, 410f
Epispadias, 776, 1535t
Epistaxis, 254t-256t
in children, 1507, 1507b
during pregnancy, 254t-256t
Epithelium, cultured, 1669
Epoophoron, 68f
Epstein-Barr virus (EBV), 1317
Epulis, 224, 226, 254t-256t
Equianalgesia, 940, 942t
Equilibrium, concept of, 834
Equipment
for childbirth, 471, 472f
home care and, 1206b, 1207f
Erb-Duchenne paralysis, 743-744, 744f
Ergocalciferol. *See* Vitamin D2.
Ergonovine, 354, 580, 580b
Ergotamine, breastfeeding and, 1745t-1748t
Ergotrate. *See* Ergonovine.
Erikson's psychosocial development theory, 849-850, 849t, 850f
adolescents and, 1109-1110, 1110b
infants and, 957-958
school-age children and, 1079, 1079f
toddlers and, 1019
Erosion, 1635f
Erythema, 901t, 1633
Erythema infectiosum, 1058t-1064t
Erythema migrans, 1653, 1653f
Erythema toxicum, 618, 618f
Erythroblastosis fetalis, 766
Erythrocyte (RBC) count. normal test ranges for, 1753t-1761t
Erythrocyte sedimentation rate
normal test ranges for, 1753t-1761t
pregnancy values of, 220t-221t
Erythromycin
breastfeeding and, 1745t-1748t
for chlamydia during pregnancy, 99
Erythromycin opthalmic ointment, 649, 649b
Escherichia coli
acute diarrhea and, 1384t-1386t
in neonatal sepsis, 755-761
urinary tract infections and, 1530
Esophageal atresia, 772-773, 772f, 1414-1417, 1415b-1416b
Esophageal replacement surgery, 1417
Esophagus during pregnancy, 226
ESRD. *See* End-stage renal disease (ESRD).
Essential hypertension, 1479
Essential oils, 405, 405b
Estimating date of birth (EDB), 230, 244
Estradiol, 177, 1745t-1748t
Estriol, 177
Estrogen
adolescence and, 1106
benign breast disease and, 115
breastfeeding and, 1745t-1748t
changes during pregnancy, 219, 227t
deprivation at menopause, 66
Estrogen *(Continued)*
hyperemesis gravidarum and, 349
influence on breasts, 68-70
menarche and, 71
ovaries and production of, 68
placental, 177
postpartum changes in, 66, 528
Estrogen-progestin contraceptives, 151-152, 151t
emergency contraception, 153
flowchart for missed tablets, 152f
potential complications, signs of, 151b
transdermal contraceptive system, 152
vaginal contraceptive ring, 152
Etanercept, 1709-1710
Ethical, Legal, and Social Implications (ELSIs) of human genome research, 165
Ethical decision making, 794, 795b
Ethical issues
in end-of-life decision making, 1165
extremely-low-birth-weight infants and, 707
in genetics, 117-118, 165
Human Genome Project and, 165
in perinatal nursing, 14
Ethnic considerations
in child health promotion, 822, 824, 824f, 829
in communication, 831-832, 832b-833b
in food customs, 832-833, 833f
in genetic disorders, 829
in growth and development, 890
in skin assessment during pregnancy, 224b
Ethnic diversity within North America, 4-5, 16
Ethnic stereotyping, 824
Ethnicity
anemia and, 1493
definition of, 822, 824
genetic disorders and, 161
genetics testing and, 164
health outcomes and, 4-5, 32
health risks and, 49
high risk pregnancy and, 191b
infant mortality rates and, 28-29
insurance coverage and, 47
intimate partner violence and, 61
prenatal care and, 9
second stage of labor and, 388
Ethnocentrism, 21-22, 824
Euglycemia, 301
Euploidy, 166
European-Americans, 25t-26t, 448-449
Eutectic mixture of local anesthetics (EMLA), 945
during circumcision, 668-669, 670b
lumbar puncture and bone marrow test and, 1267b
Euthanasia, 1165
Evaporative heat loss in newborns, 612
Evidence-based practice, 11-12, 11b-12b, 794
on autism spectrum disorders and, 1199b
on continuous labor support, 462b
Evidence-based practice *(Continued)*
on day care, 820b
on early discharge after birth, 537b
on exercise and work during pregnancy, 54b
on fetal monitoring, 425b
on gastric lavage in children, 1431b
on glucose water feedings in the newborn period, 664b
home care and, 1209
on hypoglycemia monitoring, 615b
on kangaroo care, 725b
on nasogastric tube placement in children, 1297b
nursing process and, 795, 796t
on nutrition supplements, 282b
on optimal birth spacing, 140b
on pain and symptom management at the end of life, 1165b
on peripherally inserted central catheters, 1280b
on postpartum depression, 593b
on prenatal breastfeeding education, 266b
on sickle cell anemia and penicillin prophylaxis, 1498b
on temperature measurement in pediatrics, 895b-896b
on tracheostomy suctioning, 1293b
Evoked otoacoustic emissions, 910t
Ewing's sarcoma, 1707
Exanthem subitum, 1058t-1064t
Exchange transfusion, 767, 1497
Excitement phase of sexual response cycle, 74, 74t
Excoriation, 1635f
Exencephaly, 1725b
Exercise
adolescents and, 1119-1120, 1119f, 1132
after breast surgery, 124-126, 125b-126b
asthma and, 1340
breastfeeding and, 694
cognitively impaired child and, 1180-1181, 1180f-1181f
cystic fibrosis and, 1349
diabetic children and, 1621, 1629
gestational diabetes mellitus and, 309
health promotion and, 53-54, 53b, 53f
in juvenile idiopathic arthritis, 1711
postpartum, 544, 545f
pregestational diabetes mellitus and, 302
during pregnancy, 54, 54b, 54f, 248b
cultural influences on, 260
nutrition and, 285
patient teaching in, 247-249, 249f
premenstrual syndrome and, 91
to relieve menstrual discomfort, 88
school-age children and, 1090-1091, 1090f
unconscious children and, 1561

Exercise stress test, 1443t
Exercise-associated amenorrhea, 87
Exercise-induced asthma, 1340
Exercise-induced bronchospasm, 1340
Exhibitionism, 1068
Exophthalmos, 1607
Experiential history, 240
Expiratory volume during pregnancy, 222t
Expressive activities, hospitalized child and, 1234
Expulsion, birth process and, 390
Exstrophy of bladder, 776, 776f, 1535t
Extended families, 16-17, 17f
Extension, birth process and, 389f, 390
Extension posturing, 1555, 1555f
External anal sphincter (EEC), 67f
External cephalic version (ECV), 500-503, 505f
External electronic fetal monitoring, 425-426, 426f, 426t
External fixation, 1690
External genital organs
  anatomy of, 65-66, 66f
  development of, 171f
  inspection and palpation of, 81, 81f
  in newborns at birth, 618-619, 619f
External iliac vessels, 67f
External os of cervix, 66-67, 68f
External rotation, birth process and, 389f, 390
External ventricular drains, 1559b
Extracellular fluid, 955, 1380
Extracorporeal membrane oxygenation (ECMO), 716
Extrahepatic biliary atresia, 1410b
Extravasation, 1288, 1288b-1289b
Extremely-low-birth-weight (ELBW) infants, 707b
  body temperature and, 713
  environmental concerns of, 722-723
  ethical issues in resuscitation of, 707
  hydration and, 718
  hyperglycemia and, 734-735
  nutrition and, 717
  respiratory distress syndrome and, 709
  retinopathy of prematurity in, 732
Extremities, 80
  of children, 921-922, 922f
  of newborns, 626t-636t
Extremity venipuncture, 1266-1267
Extrusion reflex of newborn, 621t-625t
Eye contact
  as communication between parent and infant, 558, 558f
  cultural variations in, 76b, 570
  visually impaired parents and, 570
Eye protection
  infection control and, 113b-114b
  phototherapy and, 666, 666f
Eyelids, 903
Eyes
  cerebral dysfunction and, 1554, 1554b-1555b, 1554f
  of children, 903-907, 903f-905f, 905b, 906t, 907b
Eyes *(Continued)*
    unconscious, 1561, 1561b
  development of, 171f
  of fetus, 182
  of newborns, 639
    facial paralysis and, 744
    normal findings, 626t-636t
    prophylaxis in, 648-649, 649b, 649f
  nutritional status and, 884t-886t
  physical examination of, 80
  review of systems and, 79, 882b

F

Face
  of newborns, 619, 619f, 626t-636t
  nursing care during labor, 457t
Face presentation, 501, 652-653, 653f
Face shields, 113b-114b
FACES Pain Rating Scale, 930-931, 932t-933t
Facial melasma, 223
Facial nerve (cranial nerve VII), 744, 744f, 925t
Facies, 900
Facilitated tucking, 723, 936
Facilitation
  in health assessment interviews, 75
  in shared decision making in family-centered care, 1148, 1148b
Facilitative response, 873b-874b
Facioscapulohumeral muscular dystrophy, 1733
Factor IX deficiency, 1503
Factor VIII concentrate, 1503-1504
Factor VIII deficiency, 368, 1503
Fahrenheit to centigrade temperature conversion, 1762
Failure to rescue, 14
Failure to thrive (FTT), 1003-1005, 1004b-1005b, 1005f
  chronic renal failure and, 1546
Fainting during pregnancy, 225-226, 254t-256t
Fairy tales, 861
Faith healing, 835
Fallopian tubes. *See* Uterine tubes.
Falls
  hospitalized children and, 1262
  infants and, 992b-993b, 995-996
  spinal cord injuries in, 1740-1741
  toddlers and, 1034t-1035t, 1039-1040
False labor, 442, 442b
False pelvis, 68, 69f, 380
Famciclovir, 105
Families, 27
  adaptation to pregnancy, 230-232, 231b, 232f
  antepartal hospitalizations and, 35
  assessment of
    framework for, 18, 20
    in the history-taking process, 879, 879b-881b
  binuclear, 16
  blended, 16, 819
  childbearing beliefs and practices of, 22, 22b-23b, 25t-26t
  cognitive impairment and, 1182
  communication and interaction of, 17, 19-20
Families *(Continued)*
  communication with
    children and, 870-872, 870b, 871f-872f, 873b-874b, 891f
    interpreters and, 869-870, 869b
    parents and, 867-870, 869b-870b
    techniques for, 873b-874b, 875
  community and, 16-17, 17f, 29
  community-based health care and, 799-802, 800b-801b, 801f
  cultural competence and, 22b, 24-27, 24b, 26b, 838t-840t
  cultural context of, 16-17, 17f, 20-22, 827
  definition of, 806
  dynamics of, 17
  end-of-life care and, 1164, 1174-1175
    child's understanding and reaction to death, 1167t-1168t
    decision making and, 1164-1169, 1166b, 1167t-1168t
    fear and, 1169-1171, 1170b-1171b, 1170f
    grief and mourning and, 1172-1174, 1173b
    home care and, 1168
    nurses' reactions to caring for terminally ill children, 1174, 1174b
    nursing care plan for, 1147b, 1169-1174, 1170f, 1173b
    organ/tissue donation and autopsy and, 1172
    pain and symptom management in, 1165b, 1169-1170, 1170b
    parental support in, 1170
    principles of palliative care, 1164
    sibling support in, 1170
    treatment options in, 1168-1169
  extended, 16-17, 17f
  home care and, 492
  homosexual, 17
  immobilized child and, 1678
  influences on child health promotion, 806, 821
    divorce and, 816-818, 817b
    dual-earner family and, 819
    employer accommodation of parenting situations and, 819
    family nursing interventions and, 806-807, 806b-807b
    family size and configuration and, 807-808, 808f
    foster parenting and, 819
    obesity and, 1131
    parental roles and, 807
    parenting and, 810-814, 811f-812f, 813b-814b
    parenting the adopted child and, 815-816, 815b-816b, 815f
    reconstituted family and, 819
    role learning and, 807-810, 808f-809f, 809b-810b
    sibling interactions and, 808-809, 809f
    single parenting and, 818-819
Families *(Continued)*
    spacing of children and ordinal position and, 808-810, 809b, 809f
  interaction with newborn, 662, 662b-663b, 662f
  maternal death and, 606-607
  nuclear, 16-17, 17f
  organization and structure of, 16-17, 17f, 27
  perinatal loss and, 600-601
  preschoolers' relationships with, 1050t
  role in health care, 17-18, 24, 25t-26t, 26
  school-age children and, 1083, 1084b
  single-parent, 17
  social context of, 16
  special needs child and, 1174-1175
    coping with, 1151-1152, 1152b, 1157-1159, 1158b-1159b
    developmental focus in, 1147
    establishing realistic future goals for, 1163-1164
    family education in, 1159-1160
    family-centered care and, 1147, 1149, 1149b
      assessment of family's adjustment, 1156-1157, 1156t, 1157b
      cultural awareness and, 1148
      family-heath care provider communication, 1147
      shared decision making and, 1148, 1148b
      therapeutic relationships and, 1147-1148
    impact on child, 1154-1156, 1155b, 1155f
    impact on parents, 1149-1150, 1150b
    impact on siblings, 1150-1151, 1151b, 1159
    managed care in, 1149
    normalization in, 1148-1149, 1159, 1159b
    promotion of normal development, 1160-1163, 1161t-1162t, 1162f-1163f
    scope of problem, 1146, 1147b
    support for family at time of diagnosis, 1152-1154, 1153b, 1157, 1157b, 1157f
    support systems for families, 1154, 1154b
  substance abuse and, 1140
  support for. *See* Family support.
  theoretic approaches to, 18-20, 18t, 19f-21f, 27
  transition to parenthood and, 548-549, 549f
    adolescent father and, 567
    adolescent mother and, 566-567, 566b
    communication between parent and infant in, 558-559, 558f-560f, 559b
    culture and, 568-569
    grandparent adaptation and, 571-573, 572b, 572f-573f
    hearing-impaired parent and, 570

Families *(Continued)*
infant-parent adjustment in, 559f-560f, 565-566
maternal adjustment in, 561-562, 561t, 562b, 563f
older fathers and, 567
older mothers and, 566b, 567, 568b
parental attachment, bonding, and acquaintance in, 554-557, 555t-556t, 557b
parental tasks and responsibilities in, 560-561
parent-infant contact and, 548, 557-558, 557f
paternal adjustment in, 561-562, 561t, 562b, 563f
sibling adaptation and, 484, 484f, 549, 549f, 570-571, 571f, 572b
social support and, 567-568
socioeconomic conditions and, 569
visually impaired parent and, 570, 570b
weight and, 1128
Family and Medical Leave Act, 4b, 819
Family assessment, 879, 879b-881b, 1212b
Family bed. *See* Cosleeping.
Family genograms, 20, 20f
Family history, 879
in the health assessment, 79
in initial prenatal care interview, 240
Family integrity promotion, 556t
Family Life Cycle (Developmental) Theory, 18t
Family nursing, 17-18
Family planning, 46, 46b, 48b, 138. *See also* Contraception.
maternal diabetes mellitus and, 306
Family Stress Theory, 18t
Family structure, 879, 879b
Family support
acute diarrhea in children and, 1389
in acute renal failure, 1544-1545
after tonsillectomy, 1313
in asthma, 1345-1346
in atopic dermatitis, 1659
autism spectrum disorders and, 1200-1201
in bacterial meningitis, 1578
in biliary atresia, 1411
in brain tumors, 1574
in burns, 1672
in cerebral palsy, 1723-1724, 1724b
chronically ill children and, 1012
in communicable diseases, 1066, 1066b
in congestive heart failure, 1464
in cystic fibrosis, 1352-1353
in diabetes mellitus, 1629-1630, 1630b
in head injuries, 1569
in hydrocephalus, 1596-1597
immobilization and, 1679-1680
inflammatory bowel disease in children and, 1404
in integumentary disorders, 1641
Family support *(Continued)*
in juvenile idiopathic arthritis, 1711
in nephrotic syndrome, 1538
in osteosarcoma, 1706-1707
in pediatric respiratory infections, 1307, 1310, 1310b
in sickle cell anemia, 1500
in spina bifida, 1729-1730
in substance abuse, 1140
unconscious child and, 1562, 1562b
in Wilms' tumor, 1542
Family systems theory, 18-19
Family teaching
on administration of medications, 1284, 1284b
on alternative feedings, 1298
on elimination procedures, 1300
on fetal assessment during labor, 437, 437b
on induction of labor with oxytocin, 509b
on sickle cell anemia, 1499
Family violence. *See* Intimate partner violence (IPV).
Family-centered care, 9
cesarean birth and, 514
elements of, 792, 792b
home care and, 1209-1217
family-to-family support in, 1216-1217
nursing process and, 1212-1214, 1212b-1214b
parent-professional collaboration in, 1211-1212, 1211b-1212b
promotion of optimal development, self-care, and education in, 1214-1215, 1214b, 1215f
respect for diversity in, 1210-1211, 1210b
safety issues in, 1215-1216, 1215b-1216b
in hospitalization of children, 1228-1230, 1230f, 1243b
supporting siblings, 1237b
labor and childbirth and, 443
special needs children and, 1147, 1149, 1149b
assessment of family's adjustment, 1156-1157, 1156t, 1157b
cultural awareness and, 1148
family-health care provider communication and, 1147
shared decision making and, 1148, 1148b
therapeutic relationships and, 1147-1148
Family-controlled analgesia, 943b-944b
Family-newborn relationships, 484, 484f
Family-to-family support, home care and, 1216-1217
Fanconi syndrome, 1501-1502
Fantasy child, 235b
FAS. *See* Fetal alcohol syndrome (FAS).
FASD. *See* Fetal alcohol spectrum disorder (FASD).
Fasting blood glucose
assessment of, 299, 301f
in diagnosis of diabetes mellitus, 1618
health screening recommendations for, 59t
Fasting recommendations in pediatric surgery, 1252t
Father-child attachment, 234
Fathers. *See also* Paternal adaptations.
adolescent, 567
coping with special needs child, 1150
older than 35 years, 567
participation in labor and birth, 9, 9f, 448-449, 463-464, 464t, 465b, 471, 472t
relationship with infants, 564-565, 564t, 565f, 811, 811f
relationship with newborns, 557
single, 818-819
stress during labor, 447
Fatigue
after childbirth, 543-544, 543b
during labor, 397, 456-459, 458b-459b
during pregnancy, 254t-256t
Fats
nutrient needs of newborns and, 681
pregestational diabetes mellitus and, 302
Fat-soluble vitamins, 275t-276t, 283-284
Faucial tonsils, 1311-1312, 1312f
Fear
of gynecologic examination, 80, 80b
hospitalized child and, 1231-1232
of pain in labor, 270
preschoolers and, 1052
school-age children and, 1089
terminally ill children and, 1169-1170, 1170b
Febrile seizures, 1260, 1592-1593, 1593b
Fecal incontinence in spina bifida, 1727-1728
Feeding. *See also* Nutrition.
cerebral palsied child and, 1720, 1720f, 1723f
cleft deformities and, 771f-772f, 772, 1413, 1413f
failure to thrive and, 1003-1005, 1004b-1005b, 1005f
gastrostomy, 720, 1296-1298, 1298f
gavage
of children, 1295, 1295b-1297b, 1295f, 1295t
of preterm infants, 718-720, 719b, 719f
during hospitalization, 1258, 1259b, 1264
hypertrophic pyloric stenosis and, 1419-1420
late-preterm infants and, 708t
of newborns, 663, 664b, 679. *See also* Breastfeeding; Formula feeding.
Feeding *(Continued)*
in pediatric congestive heart failure, 1463-1464
regurgitation and spitting up and, 999-1001
Female athlete triad, 1133
Female condoms, 4b, 98, 146, 146f
Female genital mutilation (FGM), 10, 56, 56b, 835b
Female genitalia
formation of, 183
masculinization of, 171f
of newborns, 626t-636t
physical assessment of, 920-921, 920f, 921b
Female reproductive system, 65, 85
bony pelvis, 68, 69f
breasts. *See* Breasts.
external structures, 65-66, 66f
internal structures, 65-68, 67f-68f
in newborn at birth, 618, 619f
physical assessment across the life cycle, 70t
Female sterilization, 154, 154f-155f, 155b
Femoral hernias, 918, 918f
Femoral pulses, 919, 919b, 919f
Femoral venipuncture, 1266, 1267f
Fencing reflex, 621t-625t
Fenoprofen, 89t
Fentanyl
for children, 939, 940t, 942t, 945, 945t, 1252
for pain management in labor, 407-408, 408b, 414, 418
Fenugreek, 1364
Ferning, 445b
Fertility
cultural awareness in, 131b
findings favorable to, 133b
health promotion and, 46, 46b
smoking and, 50
trends in, 6, 7b
Fertility awareness methods (FAMs) of contraception, 140-145
basal body temperature method, 142, 142b, 142f
calendar rhythm method, 141
cervical mucus ovulation-detection method, 142-143, 143b
home predictor test kits for ovulation, 144-145, 145f
lactational amenorrhea method (LAM), 145
natural family planning, 141
Standard Days Method, 141-142, 142f
symptothermal method, 143-144, 144f
two day method of family planning, 145
Fertility rate, 6, 7b
Fertilization, 72f, 73, 173-174, 173f-174f, 188
gametogenesis and, 172, 173f
Fetal acoustic stimulation test, 205-206
Fetal activity monitoring, 191-192, 192b-193b, 195f
Fetal alcohol effects, 755-758, 756t, 757f, 758b
Fetal alcohol spectrum disorder (FASD), 50

Fetal alcohol syndrome (FAS), 50, 756-758, 756t, 757f, 758b
Fetal assessment, 190-191, 194b, 422, 438-439
  electronic, 422-427, 426t
    after maternal trauma, 373-374, 373b
    evidence-based practice on, 425b
    external, 425-426, 426f, 426t
    internal, 426-427, 426t, 427f
    nursing care plan for, 434b
    vibroacoustic stimulation and, 205-206
  during labor and birth, 423
    accelerations of fetal heart rate and, 429-430, 430b, 430f
    amnioinfusion and, 436
    baseline fetal heart rate and, 427-429, 428t, 429f, 430t
    basis for, 422-423
    decelerations of fetal heart rate and, 430-433, 431b-433b, 431f
    documentation of, 424, 424b, 434b, 437-438, 438f
    fetal heart rate patterns and, 427-438, 428b
    fetal heart rate response to stimulation and, 436
    fetal oxygen saturation monitoring in, 436
    fetal scalp blood sampling in, 436
    intermittent auscultation in, 423-424, 423f, 424b
    nursing care management in, 433, 433b, 435f
      documentation of, 424, 424b, 434b, 437-438, 438f
      legal considerations in, 434b
      patient and family teaching and, 437, 437b
      pattern recognition and, 433-438, 435b, 437t
    tocolytic therapy and, 436
    umbilical cord acid-base determination and, 436-437, 437t
  during prenatal follow-up visits, 243-244, 245f
Fetal circulation during labor and birth process, 390
Fetal deaths
  abruptio placentae and, 366, 371
  confirmation of, 195
  definition of, 707b
  heroin withdrawal and, 760
  maternal trauma and, 369-372
  placenta previa and, 362
  reduction of, 28
  as a result of injury, 251-252
Fetal fibronectins, 387, 487, 491
Fetal growth, ultrasound and, 196-197, 197f
Fetal heart rate (FHR), 181, 422
  abruptio placentae and, 365-366
  amniotomy and, 506b-507b
  assessment of, 244, 245f
  diabetic mother and, 305
  external cephalic version and, 502-503
  during labor and birth, 390, 423, 438-439
Fetal heart rate (FHR) *(Continued)*
  accelerations of, 429-430, 430b, 430f
  baseline rate and, 427-429, 428t, 429f, 430t
  categorization of, 427-438, 428b
  decelerations of, 430-433, 431b-433b, 431f
  electronic fetal monitoring and, 422-427, 426t
    evidence-based practice on, 425b
    external, 425-426, 426f, 426t
    internal, 426-427, 426t, 427f
    nursing care plan for, 434b
  first stage of labor and, 451, 453f
  intermittent auscultation of, 423-424, 423f, 424b
  late decelerations and, 431-432, 431f, 432b
  maternal positioning and, 437
  nonreassuring patterns in, 434-435, 435b, 467b
    fundal pressure and, 475
  nursing care management in, 433, 433b, 435f
    documentation of, 424, 424b, 434b, 437-438, 438f
    legal considerations in, 434b
    patient and family teaching and, 437, 437b
    pattern recognition and, 433-438, 435b, 437t
  prolonged decelerations and, 432-433, 433b
  response to stimulation, 436
  second stage of labor and, 471
  variable decelerations and, 431f, 432, 432b
  water therapy and, 403, 403f
  variability and, 205, 427-429, 428t, 429f, 430t
Fetal heart tones (FHTs), 243
Fetal hemoglobin, 181
Fetal hemolytic disease, 202
Fetal lung maturity, 496, 496b
Fetal maturity, 200t, 202
Fetal membranes, development of, 175, 175f
Fetal movement chart, 195f
Fetal movements, 192b
Fetal nuchal translucency (FNT) screening, 198f
Fetal oxygen saturation monitoring, 436
Fetal pulse oximetry (FPO), 436
Fetal respiration, 390
Fetal risks in postterm pregnancy, labor, and birth, 518
Fetal scalp blood sampling, 436
Fetal waste products, 181
Fetopelvic disproportion, 499, 587
Fetoscopes, 244, 245f, 422-423, 423f
Fetus, 179, 522
  abruptio placentae and placenta previa and, 362, 362t
  amniotic fluid and, 175-176
  circulatory system of, 179-181, 180f
  critical organ development, 44
  death of, 190
  developmental milestones of, 184t-186t
Fetus *(Continued)*
  dystocia and, 498-501, 500b, 500f
  endocrine system of, 182
  gastrointestinal system of, 181
  gestational diabetes mellitus and, 307-309
  hematopoietic system of, 181
  hepatic system of, 181
  hepatitis B virus and, 750-751
  immunologic system of, 183, 184t-186t
  integumentary system of, 183
  labor process and
    adaptation in, 390
    attitude in, 377, 378f-380f
    basis for monitoring of, 422-423
    fetal assessment during. *See* Fetal assessment.
    fetal position in, 377-378, 378f-380f
    head size and, 376-377, 377f, 379f, 392
    lie in, 377, 378f-379f
    presentation in, 377-378, 378f-379f
    in true labor vs. in false labor, 442b
  malposition of, 500, 500b
  malpresentation of, 500-501, 500f, 511f
  maternal adaptation and, 232, 235b
  maternal diabetes mellitus and, 299
  maternal hypothyroidism and, 310
  maternal physiologic adaptations to, 215-216, 216f
  maternal substance abuse and, 755-756
    alcohol and, 330, 331b, 755-758, 756t
    cocaine and, 50-51, 331, 759-760
    heroin and, 760
    marijuana and, 756t, 759
    methamphetamines and, 756t, 761
    phencyclidine and, 760
    phenobarbital, 761
    tobacco and, 756t, 758-759, 759b
  maternal trauma and, 370-372
  metabolic waste products of, 178-179
  musculoskeletal system of, 183
  neurologic system of, 182
  parental relationship with, 554
  paternal adaptation and, 234, 235b
  postconception age of, 174
  postterm pregnancy and, 519
  preeclampsia and, 336t, 342
  renal system of, 181-182
  reproductive system of, 182-183
  respiratory system of, 179
  rights of, 203b
  sensory awareness of, 182
  severe preeclampsia and, 343
  ultrasound of, 196f, 503-504
  viability of, 179
Fever
  definition of, 1259
  in hospitalized children, 1259-1261, 1261b
Fever *(Continued)*
  in infants and children, 893b
  respiratory infections and, 1305b
FGM. *See* Female genital mutilation (FGM).
FHR. *See* Fetal heart rate (FHR).
FHTs. *See* Fetal heart tones (FHTs).
Fiber intake during pregnancy and lactation, 275t-276t
Fiberoptic blankets, 666f, 667
Fibrinogen, 220t-221t, 531, 1753t-1761t
Fibrinolysis, 583-584, 1502-1503
Fibrinolytic activity during pregnancy, 220t-221t, 366-367
Fibroadenomas, 115, 116t
Fibrocystic changes in breasts, 115, 116t
Fibronectin, fetal, 387
Fifth disease, 1057, 1058t-1064t
Filipino culture
  birth practices and, 449
  food patterns in, 292t-293t
  pregnancy beliefs and practices in, 260
Fimbriae, 68f
Financial issues in health care, 46-47
Fine motor development
  during infancy, 955, 955f, 966t-968t
  preschoolers and, 1044, 1050t
  toddlers and, 1018, 1018f, 1025t-1026t
Fine-needle aspiration of breast mass, 115
Finger spelling, 1196
Finger sweeps, 1358b
Fingernails
  fetal, 183
  of nurses, 747b
Finger-to-nose test, 923b
Fire ants, 1649t-1650t
Firearms
  adolescent injury and, 1124
  child mortality and, 788
  suicide and, 1141, 1141b-1142b
First period of reactivity in transition to extrauterine life, 609
First stage of labor, 387-388, 392
  cervical effacement, dilation, and fetal descent in, 384-385, 384f, 387-388, 453, 464t
  expected maternal progress in, 450t
  in normal vaginal childbirth, 481b-482b
  nursing care management in, 440-455
    admission data and, 443-444
    admission to labor unit and, 443, 443b, 443f
    cultural factors and, 447-449, 448b, 448f
    interview and, 444-446, 445b
    laboratory and diagnostic tests and, 444, 454-455, 455b-456b, 455t
    physical examination and, 449-454
      expected maternal progress and, 450t

First stage of labor *(Continued)*
fetal heart rate and pattern and, 451, 453f
general systems assessment and, 449
Leopold's maneuvers and, 451, 452b, 452f
Standard Precautions and, 449, 450b
uterine contractions and, 392, 394, 440-441, 450t, 451-453, 453b
vaginal examination and, 454, 454f
vital signs and, 449-451, 451b, 451f
prenatal data and, 444
psychosocial factors and, 446-447, 446t
stress in, 416, 447
nursing care plan in, 456-460, 457t, 458b-459b
ambulation and positioning and, 459-460, 460f-462f, 461b
elimination and, 457t, 459
emergency interventions and, 466, 467b
general hygiene and, 456, 457t
nutrient and fluid intake and, 456-459, 457b-459b, 457t
standards of care and, 455-456
supportive care and, 460-466, 462b, 463f, 464t, 465b
pain during, 394, 395f
phases of, 388, 440-441
First trimester, 229
abortion in, 156-158, 158b
discomforts during, 254t-256t
insulin production during, 297, 297f
miscarriage in, 354
nutrition during, 273-277
signs and symptoms of potential complications during, 243b
ultrasound in, 196b
Firstborn children, 809b
First-degree burns. *See* Superficial burns.
First-pass effect, 940
Fish during pregnancy, mercury and, 279, 279b, 280t
Fissure, 1635f
Fistulas
arteriovenous, 1548
genital, 589-592, 590f
omphalomesenteric, 1400
tracheoesophageal, 772-773, 772f
Fixed splitting, 916b
FLACC scale, 929, 931t
Flagyl. *See* Metronidazole.
Flame burns, 1038
Flatulence during pregnancy, 254t-256t
Flea bites, 618, 618f, 1649t-1650t
Flexion, birth process and, 388-390, 389f
Flexion posturing, 1555, 1555f
Flies, 1649t-1650t
Floppy infant syndrome, 1731-1732
Flu. *See* Influenza.
Fluid and electrolyte balance
changes during pregnancy, 222-223, 223t
cystic fibrosis and, 325
Fluid and electrolyte balance *(Continued)*
measurement of intake and output and, 1285, 1285b
in newborns at birth, 613
parenteral fluid therapy and complications in, 1288-1289, 1288b-1289b
infusion pumps in, 1287
removal of peripheral intravenous lines in, 1288, 1288b
safety catheters and needleless systems in, 1286-1287, 1287b, 1287f
securement of peripheral intravenous lines in, 1287-1288, 1287f
site and equipment in, 1285-1286, 1285b-1286b, 1286f
postpartum hemorrhage and, 580b
Fluid intake
during labor, 456-459, 457b-459b, 457t
during lactation, 286
during pregnancy, 279-280
requirements during infancy, 1381, 1381b
use of play activities in, 1255b
Fluid replacement therapy
in abruptio placentae, 366
in burn injuries, 1666
in diabetic ketoacidosis, 1623, 1623b
in hemorrhagic shock, 583
newborns and, 721b-722b
Fluid restriction
after heart surgery, 1471, 1471b
in congestive heart failure, 1459, 1464
Fluid retention, delayed wound healing and, 1637t
Flunitrazepam, 1139
Fluoride
infant nutrition and, 682
intake during pregnancy, 283
nutritional significance of, 1377t-1379t
supplementation of, 978, 1032-1033, 1032t, 1120
Fluphenazine, 597t
Flush. *See* Reactive hyperemia.
FNT screening. *See* Fetal nuchal translucency (FNT) screening.
Foam test, 202
Folate, 1374t-1377t
food sources of, 274b
intake during lactation, 275t-276t, 285-286
intake during pregnancy, 275t-276t, 284
neural tube defects and, 52
in the periconceptual period, 273
Folex. *See* Methotrexate.
Folic acid deficiency anemia, 322
Folk healers and remedies, 834-835, 835b
Follicle-stimulating hormone (FSH)
analysis of, 132-133
hypothalamic-pituitary cycle and, 72f, 73
Follicular phase of the ovarian cycle, 72f, 73
Folliculitis, 1642t
Follow-up care, 9, 552
anorectal malformations and, 1423
in breastfeeding, 691
in hyperemesis gravidarum, 350
of newborns, 551
Fontanels
labor and, 376-377, 377f
physical assessment of, 626t-636t
Food
aspiration of, 991
baby, commercially prepared, 975
cravings during pregnancy, 254t-256t, 284-285, 285f
daily guide for pregnancy and lactation, 280t
high fiber, 1391b
for infants, 974-975, 976b
Food allergies, 286-287, 1370-1373, 1370b, 1372b
Food and Nutrition Board of the National Academy of Sciences, 274-275, 275t-276t
Food customs, 832-833, 833f, 883b
Food diary, 882-883
Food frequency questionnaire, 883
Food guide pyramid, 51
Food intake questionnaire, 288b
Food intolerance, 1370
Food sensitivity, 1370-1374, 1370b-1373b
Food stamp program, 288
Foot
clubfoot, 775, 1693-1695, 1694f
heel stick for newborn blood specimen, 659, 659f
physical assessment of, 922
Football hold, 672f, 685, 687f
Foramen ovale, 180, 180f, 1446
Forced cesarean birth, 513
Forced kneeling, 835b
Forceps delivery, 8t
Forceps injuries in newborns, 652
Forceps-assisted birth, 377, 510-511, 510b, 510f-511f
Forebrain, 182
Foreign bodies
airway obstruction
in children, 1358-1360, 1358b, 1358f, 1360f
in pregnant women, 320, 320f
aspiration, 991, 1330, 1330b
cutaneous, 1648
delayed wound healing and, 1637t
Formal games, 854
Formal operational thought, 1110-1111
Formal operations stage of cognitive development, 850-851
Formula feeding, 676b, 974
iron-fortified formula and, 974, 1494-1495
microwave heating of, 973b, 997
parent education on, 700-704, 701f-702f, 703b
for preterm infants, 717-718, 718b
rationale for, 700
weaning from, 704
Fornices, 66, 67f-68f
Fosphenytoin, 1586b
Foster parenting, 819
Fourchette, 65, 66f
Fourth stage of labor, 388, 480
assessment during, 480, 483b
breastfeeding and, 480
family-newborn relationships in, 484, 484f
interactions with newborn in, 483
nutrition and, 480
postanesthesia recovery during, 480-483, 483b
tremors during, 480
Fourth trimester. *See* Postpartum period.
Fourth-degree burns, 1663, 1663f
Fovea centralis, 904
Fowler's spiritual development theory, 849t, 852
FPO. *See* Fetal pulse oximetry (FPO).
Fractures, 1681-1684, 1682b, 1682f, 1684b, 1686f
birth-related, 743, 743f
casting for, 1684-1686, 1685b, 1686f
skull, 371-372
stress, 1096
traction for, 1686-1690, 1687b, 1687f-1688f, 1689b
Fragile X syndrome, 1185-1186, 1186b
Frank breech, 379f, 500, 500f
Frank prolapse, 520, 521f
Frankenburg, William, 924
Fraternal twins. *See* Dizygotic twins.
Free-standing birth centers, 9
Frenulum, 65
Freud's psychosexual development theory, 848-849, 849t
Friction, pressure ulcers and, 1257
Frontal suture, 377f
Frostbite, 1674
Fruit during pregnancy, 280t
Fruit juices
infant nutrition and, 975
preschooler nutrition and, 1054
toddler nutrition and, 975
FSH. *See* Follicle-stimulating hormone (FSH).
FTT. *See* Failure to thrive (FTT).
Full consciousness, 1553b
Full-field digital mammography, 120b
Full-thickness burns, 1661-1662, 1662f-1663f, 1664t, 1667
Fulminant hepatitis, 1408-1409
Functional asplenia, 1497
Functional electrical stimulation, 1741
Functional hearing loss, 1187
Fundal height, 213, 214f, 242-244, 243f
abruptio placentae and, 366
Fundal massage, 542, 542f
Fundal pressure, 475, 475b
Funduscopic examination, 904, 904b, 904f
Fundus of uterus, 66, 68f
height by weeks of normal gestation, 214f
postpartum assessment of, 483b
Funduscopic examination, 1554-1555
Funeral arrangements, death of newborn and, 603

Fungal infections
cutaneous
dermatophytoses, 1643, 1645t
systemic mycotic, 1643-1646, 1646t
neonatal, 746, 754-755, 755b
Furosemide
breastfeeding and, 1745t-1748t
for congestive heart failure, 1459, 1460t
during pregnancy, 317t, 318
Furuncles, 1642t
Fussiness, newborns and, 689-690

G

Gabapentin, 597t
Gait
during pregnancy, 224
of toddlers, 922
Galactorrhea, 116
Galactose, normal test ranges for, 1753t-1761t
Galactosemia, 658t, 777-778
Galant reflex, 621t-625t
Gallbladder
disorders during pregnancy, 325, 325b
of newborns, 614
Games, 854
Gamete intrafallopian transfer (GIFT), 136, 137f, 137t
Gametogenesis, 172, 173f
Gamulin Rh, 547b
Gardasil, 986
Gardnerella, 110-111, 110t
Gardner-Wells tongs, 1688f, 1689
Garlic application, 835b
Gas pain, postpartum, 544
Gastric decontamination, 1427-1431, 1431b
Gastric lavage, 1430, 1431b
Gastric ulcers, 1404
Gastric washings, 1272
Gastroenteritis, neonatal, 746
Gastroesophageal reflux disease (GERD), 1394-1395, 1394b, 1395f
Gastroesophageal reflux (GER), 1394-1395, 1394b, 1395f
Gastrointestinal agents, breastfeeding and, 1745t-1748t
Gastrointestinal dysfunction
maternal, 325
cholelithiasis and cholecystitis, 325, 325b
inflammatory bowel disease, 325
pediatric, 1380, 1438-1439
clinical manifestations of, 1380b
in cystic fibrosis, 1349-1350
dehydration and, 1380-1383, 1381b, 1382t
hepatic disorders
acute hepatitis, 1406-1409, 1407t
biliary atresia, 1410-1411, 1410b
cirrhosis, 1409-1410, 1410b
inflammatory disorders
acute appendicitis, 1398-1400, 1399b
inflammatory bowel disease, 1401-1404, 1401t, 1404b
Meckel's diverticulum, 1400-1401, 1400b

Gastrointestinal dysfunction *(Continued)*
peptic ulcer disease, 1404-1406, 1405b
intestinal parasitic diseases, 1395-1398, 1396t, 1397b-1398b, 1397f
malabsorption syndromes and, 1423-1426, 1424b
motility disorders
constipation, 1389-1391, 1391b
diarrhea. *See* Diarrhea.
Hirschsprung disease, 1389-1393, 1392b, 1392f
vomiting, 1393-1394
nutritional disturbances
food sensitivity and, 1370-1374, 1370b-1373b
mineral imbalances and, 1365, 1377t-1379t
protein-energy malnutrition and, 1368-1370
vegetarian diets and, 1365-1366, 1366b
vitamin imbalances and, 1363-1364, 1374t-1377t
obstructive disorders and, 1417, 1419b
anorectal malformations, 774, 774f, 1422-1423, 1422b
hypertrophic pyloric stenosis, 1372b, 1417-1420, 1419b
intussusception, 1420-1421, 1420b-1421b, 1421f
malrotation and volvulus, 1422
poisoning and. *See* Poisoning.
structural defects and
cleft lip and palate, 771-772, 771f-772f, 1411-1414, 1413f, 1414b-1415b
esophageal atresia with tracheoesophageal fistula, 772-773, 772f, 1414-1417, 1415b-1416b
hernias, 918, 918f, 1417, 1418t
Gastrointestinal obstruction
anorectal malformations in, 774, 774f, 1422-1423, 1422b
congenital anomalies and, 773
distal intestinal obstruction syndrome in, 1347
hypertrophic pyloric stenosis in, 1372b, 1417-1420, 1419b
intussusception in, 1420-1421, 1420b-1421b, 1421f
malrotation and volvulus in, 1422
Gastrointestinal system
of children
congenital anomalies of, 771-774, 771f-774f
review of systems and, 882b
developmental milestones of, 184t-186t
effects of immobilization on, 1677t
of fetus, 181
maternal
adaptation to labor, 392
adaptation to pregnancy, 226-227, 226f, 370
after trauma, 370, 370b, 371t

Gastrointestinal system *(Continued)*
postpartum period and, 529
neonatal
neonatal abstinence syndrome and, 762t
signs of sepsis, 747t
transition to extrauterine life and, 613-614, 614b
Gastroschisis, 773
Gastrostomy feeding, 1282, 1283b
of children, 1296-1298, 1298f
of preterm infants, 720
Gate-control theory of pain, 397
Gauze, 1638t
Gavage feeding
in children, 1295, 1295b-1297b, 1295f, 1295t
of preterm infants, 718-720, 719b, 719f
Gaze, cardinal positions of, 924f
GBS. *See* Guillain-Barré syndrome.
GDM. *See* Gestational diabetes mellitus (GDM).
Gender identity, 1022
Gender issues in access to health care, 47
Gene therapy (gene transfer), 165
General anesthesia
in cesarean birth, 513-514, 516
during labor and birth, 415-416, 416f, 444, 483
General appearance
in maternal physical examination, 80
of newborns, 636, 637f
in pediatric physical assessment, 900-901
General flexion, 377, 378f
General hygiene in first stage of labor, 456, 457t
General systems assessment during the first stage of labor, 449
Generalized seizures, 1583b-1584b
Generation gap, 572, 572b
Generational continuity, 811
Genes, 165, 188
Genetic counseling, 162-163, 162f, 163b, 778
in breast cancer, 118
in Down syndrome, 1185
in Duchenne muscular dystrophy, 1735
Genetic disorders, 188
chromosomal abnormalities and, 160, 166-169, 167f
ethnicity and, 161
genetic testing and, 160-161, 164-165
history-taking and counseling services in, 162-163, 162f, 163b
inborn errors of metabolism in, 170, 202
potential impact on family and community, 161b
prenatal biochemical assessment for, 200-201, 200t
alpha-fetoprotein assay in, 203-204
amniocentesis in, 200t, 201, 201f
chorionic villus sampling in, 203, 203b, 204f
Coombs' test in, 204
indications for, 201-202, 202b

Genetic disorders *(Continued)*
percutaneous umbilical blood sampling in, 202-203, 203f
risk factors for, 162, 162f
Genetic factors in high risk pregnancies, 190, 191b
Genetic testing
for breast cancer, ethical considerations of, 117-118
for cystic fibrosis, 324
factors influencing the decision to undergo, 164-165
genetic disorders and, 160-161, 164-165
Genetics, 160, 188
behavioral, 170-172
breast cancer and, 117
chromosomal abnormalities and, 160, 166-169, 167f
dominance and recessivity in, concepts of, 166
Human Genome Project and, 163-165
internet resources on, 163b
patterns of genetic transmission in, 165, 169-170, 169f
relevance to nursing, 161-162, 161b
role of genes and chromosomes in, 165-166
Genetics/Genomics Nursing, 161
Genital fistulas, 589-592, 590f
Genital herpes. *See* Herpes simplex virus (HSV).
Genital stage of psychosexual development, 848-849
Genital surgery, psychologic problems related to, 1534
Genital system, developmental milestones of, 184t-186t
Genital tract infections
among adolescents, 32-33
chlamydia, 32-33, 99, 754, 755b
gonorrhea, 32-33, 99-100, 100b, 749
herpes simplex virus, 104-106, 105f
human papillomavirus, 85, 103-110, 103f
pelvic inflammatory disease, 101-103
prevention of, 98b
syphilis, 100-101, 101b, 101f
trichomoniasis, 110t, 112
Genital warts. *See Condylomata acuminate.*
Genitalia
ambiguous, 776-777, 776f
of children, physical assessment of, 919-921, 919f-920f, 921b
of newborn, 618-619, 619f
cleansing of, 675b
neonatal birth trauma and, 652-653, 653f
normal findings, 626t-636t
Genitourinary dysfunction, 1490, 1549
acute glomerulonephritis and, 1538-1540, 1539b
acute renal failure and, 1542-1545, 1542b-1544b
chronic renal failure and, 1542, 1545-1547, 1546b

Genitourinary dysfunction (Continued)
clinical manifestations of, 1526, 1527t-1528t
dialysis and, 1547-1548, 1548b, 1548f
external defects and, 1534-1535, 1535t
hemolytic uremic syndrome and, 1540, 1540b
laboratory tests and, 1526, 1529t-1530t
nephrotic syndrome and, 1535-1538, 1536b-1537b, 1536f
obstructive uropathy and, 1533-1534, 1534f
urinary tract infection and, 1530-1533, 1531b-1533b
Wilms' tumor and, 1540-1542, 1541b-1542b
Genitourinary system
congenital anomalies of, 776-779, 776f
neonatal, 645-646
review of systems and, 79, 882b
Genograms, family, 20, 20f
Genotype, 166
Gentamicin, breastfeeding and, 1745t-1748t
Genu valgum, 921
Genu varum, 921
Geodon. *See* Ziprasidone.
Geographic location
family history and, 879
high risk pregnancy and, 191b
Germ layers
formation of, 174f
primary, 174-175, 174f
German measles. *See* Rubella.
Gestational age, 229
assessment of, 244, 645f-646f, 650, 651b, 707-708
behavior of newborn and, 639
classification of newborn by, 651-652, 652f
ultrasound and, 195-196, 197f
Gestational carrier, 137t
Gestational diabetes mellitus (GDM), 179, 296, 306-309
cystic fibrosis and, 324
interventions in, 308-309
maternal and fetal risks in, 307-308
screening for, 308, 308f
Gestational hypertension, 335, 335t, 362t
Gestational trophoblastic disease (GTD), 358
gestational trophoblastic neoplasia, 349, 358
hydatidiform mole, 358-359, 359b, 359f
Gestational trophoblastic neoplasia (GTN), 349, 358
GFR. *See* Glomerular filtration rate (GFR).
Giardia, 1383-1386
Giardiasis, 1396-1397, 1397b, 1397f
GIFT. *See* Gamete intrafallopian transfer (GIFT).
Ginger, 90t
Gingivitis, 254t-256t, 1092
Glabellar reflex, 621t-625t
Glans clitoris, 67f, 74
Glasgow Coma Scale, 1552, 1553f
Glass mercury thermometers, 893b
Glasses, 1196
Glaucoma, 171f, 1192b-1193b
Glenn shunt, 1466t
Global Health eLearning Center, 12, 13b
Glomerular disease, 1535-1540, 1536b-1537b, 1536f, 1539b
Glomerular filtration rate (GFR), 222, 223t
Glomerulonephritis, 1538-1540, 1539b
Glossopharyngeal nerve (cranial nerve IX), 925t
Gloves
home care and, 42
infection control and, 113b-114b, 450b
Glucagon, 1621, 1621b
Glucocorticoids, 496, 496b, 1611, 1639
Glucogenesis, 1616
Glucometers, 304
Glucose. *See* Blood glucose.
Glucose tolerance tests, 241t, 1753t-1761t
Glucose water feedings in the newborn period, 663, 664b
Glucose-6-phosphate dehydrogenase deficiency (G6PD), 767, 1492f
Glucosuria, 223
Gluten-induced enteropathy. *See* Celiac disease.
Gluten-sensitive enteropathy. *See* Celiac disease.
Glyburide, 309
Glycemic control, 298-306, 300b-301b. *See also* Blood glucose.
Glycogen, fetal, 181
Glycosuria, 1618
Glycosylated hemoglobin, 1620
Glycosylation, 1618
Gnat bites, 1649t-1650t
GnRH. *See* Gonadotropin-releasing hormone (GnRH).
GnRH agonists. *See* Gonadotropin-releasing hormone (GnRH) agonists.
Goggles, 113b-114b
Goiter, 1606, 1606b
Gomco clamp, 667-668, 668f
Gonadotropin
analysis of, 132-133
menarche and, 71
Gonadotropin-releasing hormone (GnRH), 72f, 73
Gonadotropin-releasing hormone (GnRH) agonists, 92-93
Gonorrhea, 99-100
among adolescents, 32-33
management of, 100
neonatal, 749
reporting, 100b
Goodell sign, 214
Gowns
infection control and, 113b-114b, 450b
nursing care during labor, 457t
G6PD. *See* Glucose-6-phosphate dehydrogenase deficiency (G6PD).
Graafian follicles, 72f, 73
Grafts
arteriovenous, 1548
skin, 1668-1669, 1668f-1669f
Grains during pregnancy, 280t
Grandparents
adaptation to newborns, 571-573, 572b, 572f-573f
adaptation to pregnancy, 231-232, 232f, 234-235, 236f, 237b, 264-265
grief after death of grandchildren, 600-601
support during first stage of labor, 465
Granulation, wound healing and, 1636
Grasp reflex, 620, 621t-625t
Grasping, 955, 957
Grave's disease, 309, 1607, 1608b
Gravida, 210
Gravidity, 210-211, 211t
Greenstick fractures, 1682b, 1682f
Grief
death of newborn and, 523, 598-600
communicating and caring techniques and, 601-605, 601b-602b
actualizing the loss, 601-602, 601b-602b, 602f-603f
creating memories for parents to take home, 604-605, 605f
helping in acknowledgement and expression of feelings, 603-604
helping parents with decision making, 602-603
normalizing the grief process and facilitating positive coping, 604
physical needs of postpartum bereaved mother and, 604
providing sensitive care at and after discharge, 606
community resources and, 598b
cultural and spiritual needs of parents and, 605
family aspects of grief in, 600-601
postmortem care of newborn and, 605, 605f
dying child and, 1172-1174, 1173b
Gross motor development
infants and, 966t-968t
head control, 955-956, 956b, 956f
locomotion, 957, 957b, 959f
rolling over, 956, 957f
sitting, 956-957, 958f
preschoolers and, 1043-1044, 1044f, 1050t
toddlers and, 1018, 1018f, 1025t-1026t
Group B streptococcus, 112, 754
neonatal, 112, 754
Group identity, 1109-1110
Growing skull fractures, 1564-1565
Growth, definition of, 842
Growth and development, 842, 864
during adolescence, 845, 1107-1109, 1116t
altered maturation and, 1097-1099, 1098t
Growth and development (Continued)
biologic growth and physical development in. *See* Biologic development.
body image and, 853
infants and, 960-961, 961f
preschoolers and, 853, 1045
school-age children and, 1084-1085
toddlers and, 1022
cognitive development, 849t, 850-851
adolescents and, 1110-1111
infants and, 958-960, 960f
preschoolers and, 1044-1045, 1045b
school-age children and, 1079-1081, 1080f
toddlers and, 1019-1021, 1020f, 1021b
disease and, 859-860
embryonic, 171f, 175, 184t-186t
environmental hazards and, 860, 860b
ethnicity and, 890
health history in, 877
heredity and, 857
individual differences in, 844
during infancy, 966t-968t
interpersonal relationships and, 857-859, 859f
of language, 851
lymphoid tissues and, 844f, 846
mass media and, 861-864, 862b-863b
measurements of, 889-892, 890b, 891f-892f
height and weight measurements for boys, 1751t
height and weight measurements for girls, 1752t
moral development, 849t, 851-852
of adolescents, 1111
of preschoolers, 1045
of school-age children, 1081
neuroendocrine factors in, 857
neurologic maturation in, 846
nutrition and, 857, 859b, 884t-886t
of organ systems, 846
patterns of, 842-844, 843f, 1107-1109
physiologic changes and, 846-847
of preschoolers, 1050t
of preterm infants, 726-727
psychosexual development, 848-849, 849t
psychosocial development, 849-850, 849t, 850f
of adolescents, 1109-1110, 1110b, 1116t
of infants, 957-958
of preschoolers, 1044, 1044b
of school-age children, 1079, 1079f
of toddlers, 1019
role of play in, 853
classification of play, 853
content of play, 854, 854f
functions of play, 856-857, 856f
infants and, 960-963, 964t
preschoolers and, 1047-1048, 1047f

Growth and development (Continued)
school-age children and, 1083-1084, 1085f
social character of play, 855-856, 855f
toddlers and, 1023-1024, 1024f
toys and, 857, 858b
of school-age children, 1086t-1087t
of self-concept, 852-853, 1084-1085
self-esteem and, 853
sex differences in, 1107-1109
skeletal growth and maturation in, 846
socioeconomic level and, 859
spiritual development, 849t, 852
adolescents and, 1111
school-age children and, 1081, 1081b
toddlers and, 1021-1022
stages of, 842, 843b
stress and, 860-861
temperament and, 847-848, 847b-848b, 963-965, 966t-968t
during toddler years, 1025t-1026t
Growth charts, 889-890, 890b, 891f
Growth failure. *See* Failure to thrive (FTT).
Growth hormone
deficiency of, 1601-1602, 1601b-1602b
excess of, 1602-1603
normal test ranges for, 1753t-1761t
Growth spurt, 1107
GTD. *See* Gestational trophoblastic disease (GTD).
GTN. *See* Gestational trophoblastic neoplasia (GTN).
GTPAL acronym, 211
Guide to Effective Care in Pregnancy and Childbirth, 400
Guided imagery for pain management, 937b
Guidelines for Perinatal Care, 424
Guillain-Barré syndrome, 1735-1737, 1736b
Guilt vs. initiative in psychosocial development, 849-850, 850f
Gum hypertrophy, 224
Gums
changes during pregnancy, 226
of children, 912
Gunshot wounds during pregnancy, 372-373
Gynecoid pelvis, 381, 383t
Gynecologic health assessment, 75, 85
abused women and, 76, 77f
of adolescents, 78, 78b
cultural competence and, 75
female reproductive system and. *See* Female reproductive system.
health history in, 78-79
interview in, 75-76, 75f, 76b
laboratory and diagnostic procedures in, 85
mammography in, 59t, 118-120, 119f, 119t, 120b
menstruation and, 71-74, 77f
Gynecologic health assessment (Continued)
physical examination in, 79-85. *See also* Pelvic examination.
referral resources in, 75b
sexual response and, 74, 74t
woman with disabilities and, 76, 77f
Gynecologic history, 239
Gynecomastia, 1127

H

HAART. *See* Highly active antiretroviral therapy (HAART).
Habits, health history and, 877-878, 878b
Habitual miscarriage, 353
Habituation, 638b, 640-641
Haemophilus influenzae type B vaccine, 984-985, 987t-988t, 1575
Haemophilus vaginitis. *See* Bacterial vaginosis.
Hair
of children
hospitalization and, 1258
nutritional status and, 884t-886t
physical assessment of, 901
pubertal development and, 1108f, 1109
color of, 166
fetal, 183
maternal, 224, 457t, 531
Haitian culture
beliefs about naming babies, 559b
health beliefs and practices in, 838t-840t
postpartum care and, 550b
Haldol. *See* Haloperidol.
Hallucinogens, 51, 1139
Halo brace, 1688, 1688f
Halo vest, 1688, 1688f
Haloperidol, 597t, 1745t-1748t
Hand expression of breast milk, 692
Hand hygiene, 113b-114b, 449, 450b
Handheld nebulizers, 1290-1291
Handicap, definition of, 1147b
Hands, Down syndrome and, 902, 902f
Hands-and-knees position during labor and birth, 385, 386f, 459-460, 461b, 461f, 469, 500b
Hands-on approach to vertex presentation, 473
Hands-poised (hands-off) approach to vertex presentation, 473-474
Handwashing
home care and, 42
nursing care during labor, 457t
standard precautions and, 662, 662b, 1264b
Haploids, 172
Haplotype, 1522
Hard-of-hearing, definition of, 1186-1187
Hardy-Rand-Rittler test, 907
Harrington system, 1701
Harvest mites, 1649t-1650t
Hashimoto's disease, 310
HAV. *See* Hepatitis A virus (HAV).
HBIG. *See* Hepatitis B immune globulin (HBIG).
HBV. *See* Hepatitis B virus (HBV).
HCG. *See* Human chorionic gonadotropin (hCG).
HCS. *See* Human chorionic somatomammotropin (hCS).
HCV. *See* Hepatitis C virus (HCV).
Head
of children
nutritional status and, 884t-886t
review of systems and, 882b
of infants, 954
maternal, 79-80
of newborns, 637
labor and, 376-377, 377f
normal findings, 626t-636t
Head circumference
measurement of, 891f, 892
microcephaly and, 769
of newborns, 626t-636t, 637
of school-age children, 1078
of toddlers, 1017
ultrasound measurement of, 196, 197f
Head control, infants and, 955-956, 956b, 956f
Head injuries
in children
complications of, 1565-1566, 1565b-1566b
diagnostic evaluation of, 1566-1567, 1566b-1567b
etiology of, 1563
nursing care management in, 1566, 1568-1570
pathophysiology of, 1563-1565, 1563f-1564f
therapeutic management of, 1567-1570, 1567b
during pregnancy, 369-370
Head lice, 1651-1652, 1651b-1652b, 1651f
Headaches
after craniotomy, 1574
after dural puncture, 412
in preeclampsia, 336t
during pregnancy, 225-226, 254t-256t
Healing of bone, 1682-1683
Healing touch, 270
Health assessment, 75, 85
abused women and, 76, 77f
of adolescents, 78, 78b
cultural competence and, 75
female reproductive system and. *See* Female reproductive system.
health history in, 78-79
interview in, 75-76, 75f, 76b
laboratory and diagnostic procedures in, 85
menstruation and, 71-74, 77f
physical examination in, 79-85
referral resources in, 75b
sexual response and, 74, 74t
woman with disabilities and, 76, 77f
Health Belief Model, 18t, 20
Health care
access to, 3-4
as a measure of community health, 31
race/ethnicity and, 4-5
vulnerable populations and, 32-34
Health care (Continued)
barriers to receiving, 6
cultural issues, 47
financial issues, 46-47
gender issues, 47
during pregnancy, 236-237
for children, 785-786
economics of, 6, 35, 802
efforts to reduce disparities in, 6
families' role in, 17-18
integrative, 5, 5f
preconception counseling and, 44-45, 45b
regionalization of, 190
shifts in delivery of, 28
special needs child and, 1160
standards of practice in, 12-14, 13b, 14t
structure of delivery, 5
Health Care for the Homeless Program, 33-34
Health departments, data collection and, 31
Health Disparities Collaboratives, 6
Health history. *See* History; History taking.
Health Insurance Portability and Accountability Act (HIPAA), 867b, 1246
Health literacy, 10, 34
Health promotion and prevention, 44, 63, 85
adolescents and, 33, 1116-1117, 1117b
anticipatory guidance for, 57-63, 57b
health protection and, 58-60
health risk prevention and, 58, 58b
health screening schedule and, 58, 59t
intimate partner violence. *See* Intimate partner violence (IPV).
substance use cessation and, 57-58, 58b
of bacterial meningitis, 1577-1578, 1578b
of burns, 1672-1673
child, 785, 889f
of childhood injuries. *See* Injury prevention.
cognitive impairment and, 1183
community-based, 29, 801
cultural influences on child health and, 822-829, 840-841
community and, 826
cultural relativism and, 830-831
cultural shock and cultural competence and, 828-829, 828b-829b
ethnicity and, 824, 824f
food customs and, 832-833, 833f
health beliefs and practices and, 833-835, 835b
hereditary factors and, 829
homelessness and, 825, 830
immigrant children and, 825, 830
migrant farmworker families and, 825, 830
minority-group membership and, 827-828, 827b-828b
peer cultures and, 826-827

Health promotion and prevention (Continued)
poverty and, 825, 830
relationships with health care providers and, 831-832, 831b-832b, 831f
religion and, 825-826, 826f, 835, 836b, 836t-837t
schools and, 826
social roles and, 823-824
socioeconomic class and, 824-825, 829-830
subcultures and, 824-827, 824f, 826f
of diarrhea in children, 1387-1389, 1388b
of disease, 793
of drowning, 1572
environmental and workplace hazards and, 56-57
family influences on child health and, 806, 821
divorce and, 816-818, 817b
dual-earner family and, 819
employer accommodation of parenting situations and, 819
family nursing interventions and, 806-807, 806b-807b
family size and configuration and, 807-808, 808f
foster parenting and, 819
parental roles and, 807
parenting and, 810-814, 811f-812f, 813b-814b
parenting the adopted child and, 815-816, 815b-816b, 815f
reconstituted family and, 819
role learning and, 807-810, 808f-809f, 809b-810b
sibling interactions and, 808-809, 809f
single parenting and, 818-819
spacing of children and ordinal position and, 808-810, 809b, 809f
fertility control and, 46, 46b
of head injuries, 1569-1570
health risks in childbearing years and, 47
age and, 45, 47-49, 48b
gynecologic conditions and, 56
medical conditions and, 56
of hepatitis, 1409
herpes simplex virus and, 106
home care and, 36-37, 1214-1215, 1214b, 1215f
human papillomavirus and, 104
juvenile rheumatoid arthritis and, 1710
nutrition and, 51-53, 52b
adolescents and, 1118-1119, 1118f
during infancy, 972-976, 972t, 973b, 976b
preschoolers and, 1053-1054, 1054b, 1054f
school-age children and, 1089-1090
toddlers and, 1029-1031, 1030b
of obesity, 1132
of pediculosis, 1652
physical fitness and exercise and, 53-54, 53b, 53f-54f

Health promotion and prevention (Continued)
of poisoning, 1431-1432, 1432b
preconception counseling and care, 44-45, 45b
of preterm labor and birth, 489-490, 491b
of sexual abuse, 1075b
sexual practices and, 55-56, 56b
of spina bifida, 1728
stress and, 54-55, 55b
of substance abuse, 1140
of urinary tract infection, 1533, 1533b
of visual impairment, 1196, 1196b
well-woman care and, 45-46
Health Resources and Services Administration (HRSA)
Health Care for the Homeless Program, 33-34
Health Disparities Collaboratives of, 6
Health screening schedule, 58, 59t
Health teaching, 793-794
Healthy People 2010, 5, 5b, 28
breastfeeding and, 678
health care for children and, 785-787
infant mortality rates and, 28-29
maternal death and, 8, 189
Hearing
of fetus, 182
of newborns at birth, 640, 640f
screening recommendations for, 59t
Hearing aids, 1187-1188, 1188b-1189b, 1188f
Hearing impairments, 1186
adolescents and, 1120
clinical manifestations of, 1189b
communication and, 76
cued speech and, 1190
definition and classification of, 1186-1187, 1187t-1188t
health assessment and women with, 76
hospitalization and, 1190-1191
lipreading and, 1189, 1189b
neonatal rubella and, 752
in newborns at birth, 640, 640f
nursing care plan for, 1188-1189
parents with, 570
prevention of, 1191, 1191b
sign language and, 1190
socialization and, 1190
speech language therapy and, 1190
therapeutic management of, 1187-1191, 1188b, 1188f
Hearing-impaired parents, 570
Heart
in children
congenital defects of, 171f, 769-770
physical assessment of, 915-917, 915f-916f, 916b, 917t
in school-age children, 1078
fetal, 195
maternal, 80, 218, 218f
Heart disease
classification of, 311-312
maternal, 311-319, 311b-312b
atrial and ventricular septal defects, 313
Eisenmenger's syndrome, 312b, 313

Heart disease (Continued)
heart transplantation and, 314
intrapartum care in, 312
Marfan syndrome, 313-314
mitral and aortic valve stenosis, 313
mitral valve prolapse, 313
nursing care management in, 314, 315b-316b
abnormal/normal signs and symptoms and, 314, 314t, 316b
cultural awareness and, 314
nursing care plan for, 314-319, 321b
heart surgery and, 317
intrapartum period, 317-318, 318b
medication and, 316, 317t
postpartum period, 315b-316b, 318-319, 318b
peripartum cardiomyopathy, 312
rheumatic heart disease, 247, 312-313
smoking and, 49
tetralogy of Fallot, 313
pediatric
cardiac dysrhythmias and, 1476-1477, 1477b
cardiomyopathy and, 1478
congenital. *See* Congenital heart disease (CHD).
echocardiography in, 1443t, 1444
heart transplantation for, 1478-1479
hyperlipidemia and, 1474-1476, 1475t
Kawasaki disease and, 1481-1482, 1481b-1482b
pulmonary artery hypertension and, 1477-1478
rheumatic fever and, 1473-1474, 1474b
shock and, 1482-1484, 1483b-1485b, 1483t
systemic hypertension and, 1479-1481, 1480b
Heart rate
changes in labor, 221t, 391b, 395
changes in pregnancy, 221t
fetal. *See* Fetal heart rate (FHR).
of infants, 954
of newborns at birth, 610-611, 626t-636t
normal ranges for, 1762
postoperative, 1254t
sexual response and, 74t
Heart sounds
auscultation of, 916-917, 916b, 916f, 917t
of newborns at birth, 610-611
Heart surgery during pregnancy, 317
Heart transplantation
in children, 1478-1479
pregnancy after, 314
Heartburn during pregnancy, 254t-256t
Heat
to relieve arthritis discomfort, 1711
to relieve menstrual discomfort, 88
Heat and cold application, 404-405

Heat loss
in newborns at birth, 612, 648
in small-for-gestational-age infants, 735
Heavy metal poisoning, 1432, 1432b
Heel sticks
for newborns, 659, 659f, 660b
pain management during, 938, 938f, 1272b
for preterm infants, 720-721, 930f
Heel-to-shin test, 923b
Hegar sign, 213, 216f
Height
of adolescents, 1107
growth charts for boys, 1751t
growth charts for girls, 1752t
health screening recommendations for, 59t
of infants, 953-954
normal blood pressure levels in boys and, 1763
normal blood pressure levels in girls and, 1765
in pediatric physical assessment, 891, 891f
of preschoolers, 1043
of school-age children, 1077-1078, 1097-1098
of toddlers, 1017
trends during childhood, 842, 845b, 845t
Heimlich maneuver in pregnant women, 320, 320f
Helicobacter pylori, 1404-1405
HELLP syndrome, 338, 343, 344b, 374
Helplines, postpartum, 552
Hemarthrosis, 1503
Hematemesis, 1380b
Hematochezia, 1380b
Hematocrit, 1491t
after childbirth, 530
of newborns at birth, 657b
normal ranges of, 320, 1753t-1761t
during pregnancy, 221t, 241t, 320
Hematologic dysfunction, 1523-1524
apheresis and, 1523
assessment of hematologic function in, 1490, 1491t
blood transfusion therapy in, 1520-1522, 1521t-1522t
disseminated intravascular coagulation and, 1506-1507, 1506f, 1507b
epistaxis and, 1507, 1507b
hematopoietic stem cell transplantation for, 1522, 1523b
hemophilia and, 1503-1505, 1503b
idiopathic thrombocytopenic purpura and, 1505-1506, 1505b-1506b
in immunologic deficiency disorders, 1516
human immunodeficiency virus infection and acquired immunodeficiency syndrome, 1516-1519, 1517b, 1517t-1518t, 1519b
severe combined immunodeficiency disease, 1519-1520
Wiskott-Aldrich syndrome, 1520

Hematologic dysfunction (Continued)
in leukemia, 1507
chemotherapy in, 1510b-1513b, 1512-1513
classification of, 1507-1508
diagnostic evaluation in, 1508-1509, 1508t
drug toxicity and, 1513-1514, 1513b
late effects of treatment, 1509
nursing care plan for, 1510b-1512b
pain management in, 1509
pathophysiology of, 1508, 1508t
preparing child and family for procedures, 1509
prevention of complications and myelosuppression in, 1509-1512, 1510b-1512b
therapeutic management of, 1509
in lymphomas, 1514
Hodgkin's disease, 1514-1516, 1515f
non-Hodgkin's lymphoma, 1516
red blood cell disorders and anemia in, 1490-1493, 1491t, 1492b-1493b, 1492f
aplastic anemia in, 1501-1502, 1502b
beta-thalassemia in, 1500-1501, 1501b
iron deficiency anemia in, 1493-1494, 1494b
sickle cell anemia in, 1495-1500, 1496b, 1496f, 1498b-1499b
Hematologic system
physiologic adaptations to pregnancy, 338b, 371t
of preterm infants, 710
review of systems and, 79
Hematomas, 1193b
postpartum hemorrhage and, 577-578
subdural, 745, 1566b
subungual, 1680
Hematopoietic stem cell transplantation, 1522, 1523b
in leukemia, 1509
in sickle cell disease, 1499
Hematopoietic system
fetal, 181
transition to extrauterine life and, 611
Hemodialysis, 1547-1548, 1548f
Hemodynamic monitoring, 721b-722b
Hemofiltration, 1547
Hemoglobin, 1491t
after childbirth, 530
fetal, 181
in infants, 954
of newborns at birth, 611, 657b
normal test ranges for, 1753t-1761t
during pregnancy, 219, 220t-221t, 241t
Hemoglobin electrophoresis, 241t
Hemoglobinopathies, 1495
Hemolytic disease of the newborn, 766-767
Hemolytic reaction to blood transfusion, 1521t-1522t
Hemolytic uremic syndrome, 1540, 1540b
Hemophilia
in children, 1503-1505, 1503b
von Willebrand disease, 368
Hemorrhage
epidural, 1565, 1565b
intracranial, 745
in leukemia, 1512
postpartum, 479
definition and incidence of, 576
etiology and risk factors for, 577-581, 577b
hemorrhagic shock and, 581-583, 582b-583b
nursing care management of, 579-580, 579b
bleeding with a contracted uterus and, 581
herbal remedies and, 581, 582t
hypotonic uterus and, 580-581
medications in, 580, 580b-581b
nursing care plan in, 580b
nursing process in, 579b
subarachnoid, 745
subdural, 1565-1566, 1566b
subgaleal, 616-617, 617f
Hemorrhagic cystitis, 1514
Hemorrhagic disorders in pregnancy, 350
early pregnancy bleeding, 350-354, 352f, 353t
ectopic pregnancy
clinical manifestations of, 357
collaborative care for, 357-358, 357b-358b
incidence and etiology of, 356-357, 356f
nursing care management in, 353-354, 353b-355b
gestational trophoblastic disease, 358
gestational trophoblastic neoplasia, 349, 358
hydatidiform mole, 358-359, 359b, 359f
late pregnancy bleeding, 360, 360f
abruptio placentae and, 360, 360f, 365-366, 365f
clotting disorders and, 366-368
cord insertion and placental variations and, 366, 367f
placenta previa and
clinical manifestations of, 361-362, 362t
diagnosis of, 362, 363b
home care in, 364
hospital care in, 363-364
incidence and etiology of, 361, 361b
maternal and fetal outcomes in, 362
nursing care plan for, 364b
types of, 361, 361f
vaginal examination in, 362, 364
recurrent premature dilation of cervix, 355-356, 355b, 356f
Hemorrhagic shock
postpartum hemorrhage and, 581-583, 582b-583b
during pregnancy, 369-370
Hemorrhoids
postpartum, 527, 539b-541b
during pregnancy, 218-219, 219f, 226
Hemostasis, 366-367, 525, 1502-1503, 1636
Hemostatic system, 366-367
Heparin
breastfeeding and, 1745t-1748t
for deep venous thrombosis, 584-585
during pregnancy, 317t
Heparin lock, 1279
Hepatic disorders
acute hepatitis, 1406-1409, 1407t
biliary atresia, 1410-1411, 1410b
cirrhosis, 1409-1410, 1410b
Hepatic portoenterostomy, 1411
Hepatic system
fetal, 181
in newborns at birth, 614, 615b, 616f
Hepatitis A virus (HAV), 106, 982, 1406, 1407t
Hepatitis A virus (HAV) vaccine, 106, 982, 1117-1118
Hepatitis B immune globulin (HBIG), 663, 665b
Hepatitis B vaccine (HepB), 107, 982, 987t-988t
adolescents and, 1117-1118
health screening recommendations for, 59t
newborns and, 663, 665b, 674
Hepatitis B virus (HBV), 106-107, 982-985
in children, 1406-1408, 1407t
in newborns, 750-751
Hepatitis C virus (HCV), 107-108
breastfeeding and, 698
in children, 1407t, 1408
Hepatitis D virus, 1408
Hepatitis E virus, 1408
Hepatitis G virus, 1408
HepB. *See* Hepatitis B vaccine (HepB).
HER2. *See* Human epidermal growth factor receptor 2 (HER2).
Herbal preparations
breastfeeding and, 684, 696
children and, 1365
hyperemesis gravidarum and, 350
in initial prenatal care interview, 239
for menstrual disorders, 89, 90t
for postpartum hemorrhage, 581, 582t
during pregnancy, 252
to promote fertility, 135
Heredity
breast cancer and, 117-118, 117b
influence on child health, 829
influence on development, 857
Hernias
in children, 918, 918f, 1417, 1418t
congenital diaphragmatic, 770-771, 771f
femoral, 918, 918f
hiatal, 1418t
inguinal, 1535t
Heroin, 51
breastfeeding and, 1745t-1748t
fetal and neonatal effects of, 756t, 760, 760b
Herpes gestationis, 224b
Herpes simplex encephalitis, 1579
Herpes simplex virus (HSV), 104-106, 105f
in cutaneous infection, 1644t
in newborns, 106, 748-749, 753, 753f
Hiatal hernias, 1418t
High chairs for infants, 996
High risk infants, 740
ABO incompatibility in, 766-767
assessment of, 707-708
birth trauma and, 742-743, 743t
central nervous system injuries in, 745
nursing care management in, 743
peripheral nervous system injuries in, 743-745, 744f
skeletal injuries in, 743, 743f
classification of, 706, 707b
congenital anomalies in, 742, 767-768, 779
ambiguous genitalia, 776-777, 776f
anorectal malformations, 774, 774f
choanal atresia, 770, 770f
cleft lip and palate, 771-772, 771f-772f
clubfoot, 775
congenital diaphragmatic hernia, 770-771, 771f
developmental dysplasia of hip, 774-776, 774f-775f, 775b
encephalocele and anencephaly, 768
esophageal atresia and tracheoesophageal fistula, 772-773, 772f
exstrophy of bladder, 776, 776f
genetic diagnosis of, 777
heart defects, 769-770
hydrocephalus, 769
hypospadias and epispadias, 776, 776f
intestinal obstruction, 773
microcephaly, 769
nursing care in, 777-779
omphalocele and gastroschisis, 773, 773f
polydactyly, 775-776
screening for, 777-778
spina bifida, 768-769, 768f
teratomas, 777
diabetic mothers and, 735-737, 736f, 737b
discharge planning for, 737-738, 738b
factors in, 193b
hemolytic disease in, 766-767
infections and
perinatally acquired, 748-755, 749b
candidiasis, 754-755, 755b
chlamydia, 754, 755b
cytomegalovirus, 752-753, 752f
Escherichia coli, 755-761
gonorrhea, 749
group B streptococcus, 754

High risk infants (Continued)
hepatitis B virus, 750-751
herpes simplex virus, 753, 753f
human immunodeficiency virus, 751
parvovirus B19, 753-754
rubella, 752
syphilis, 749-750, 750b, 750f
toxoplasmosis, 749
tuberculosis, 754
varicella-zoster virus, 750
rubella, 752
sepsis, 745-748, 745t, 747b-748b, 747t
intrauterine growth restriction and, 707b, 734-735
large-for-gestational-age, 707b, 735
maternal substance abuse and, 755-761, 756f, 756t
alcohol and, 755-758, 756t, 757f, 758b
caffeine and, 761
cocaine and, 756t, 759-760
heroin and, 756t, 760, 760b
marijuana and, 756t, 759
methadone and, 760-761
methamphetamines and, 756t, 761
neonatal assessment and nursing care plan in, 761-762, 762b, 762t, 763f, 764b-765b
phencyclidine and, 760
phenobarbital and, 761
tobacco and, 756t, 758-759, 759b
postterm, 707b, 733-734, 733f
meconium aspiration syndrome and, 733, 733f
persistent pulmonary hypertension and, 733-734
preterm, 706-733, 740
assessment of, 707-708
body temperature maintenance in, 709, 713, 728b-730b
bronchopulmonary dysplasia in, 732-733
cardiovascular function of, 709
central nervous system function in, 709-710, 728b-730b
developmental care of, 723-726, 724f, 725b
environmental concerns of, 712-713, 722-723, 723f
evaluation of, 727, 728b-730b
growth and development potential of, 726-727
hematologic status of, 710
infection and, 710, 711b
late-preterm, 707, 708t
necrotizing enterocolitis in, 731-732, 732b
nursing process in care of, 712, 712b, 728b-730b
nutrition and, 710, 712b, 717-720, 718b, 720f, 724f, 728b-730b
oxygen therapy for, 713-717, 714f, 715t
parental adaptation to, 710-726, 711f, 712b
parental support and, 726-727, 726b, 726f

High risk infants (Continued)
patent ductus arteriosus in, 730-731
periventricular-intraventricular hemorrhage in, 731
physical care of, 712-713
renal function of, 710
respiratory distress syndrome and, 727-730, 730t
respiratory function of, 708-709
retinopathy of prematurity in, 732
skin care for, 720-721, 721b-722b, 728b-730b
weaning from respiratory assistance, 716-717
Rh incompatibility in, 766-767
small-for-gestational-age, 707b, 734-735
transport of
from regional tertiary care centers, 739, 739f
to regional tertiary care centers, 738-739, 739b, 739f
High risk pregnancy, 189, 208, 332-333
acquired immunodeficiency syndrome in, 328-330
anemia in, 320-322, 320b, 332-333
folic acid deficiency anemia, 322
iron deficiency anemia, 321-322
sickle cell hemoglobinopathy, 322, 323t
thalassemia, 322
autoimmune disorders in, 327, 332-333
myasthenia gravis, 327-328, 327b
systemic lupus erythematosus, 327
cardiopulmonary resuscitation and, 319-320, 319b, 320f
cardiovascular disorders in, 311-319, 311b-312b, 332-333
atrial and ventricular septal defects, 313
classification of, 311-312
Eisenmenger's syndrome, 312b, 313
heart transplantation, 314
intrapartum care in, 312
Marfan syndrome, 313-314
mitral and aortic valve stenosis, 313
mitral valve prolapse, 313
peripartum cardiomyopathy, 312
plan of care and implementation in, 314-319, 321b
heart surgery and, 317
intrapartum period, 317-318, 318b
medication and, 316, 317t
postpartum period, 315b-316b, 318-319, 318b
rheumatic heart disease, 247, 312-313
tetralogy of Fallot, 313
definition of, 189
diabetes mellitus in, 295-296, 298
classification of, 296, 297t
family planning and contraception in, 306

High risk pregnancy (Continued)
fetal and neonatal risks and complications in, 299
gestational, 179, 296, 306-309
interventions in, 308-309
maternal and fetal risks in, 307-308
screening for, 308, 308f
intrapartum interventions and, 300b-301b, 305-306
maternal risks and complications in, 298-299
metabolic changes associated with pregnancy and, 296-298, 297f
mortality rate in, 296
nursing care plan for, 307b
pathogenesis of, 296
postpartum interventions and, 300b-301b, 306
preconception counseling and, 298, 298b
prenatal care and, 299-305, 300b-301b, 301t
complications requiring hospitalization and, 305
determination of birth date and mode of delivery, 305
diet, 302, 303b
exercise, 302
insulin therapy, 302-304, 303b, 303t, 304f
monitoring blood glucose levels, 304-305, 304b-305b
monitoring blood glucose levels in, 299-306, 300b-301b, 301f, 304b, 304f
target blood glucose levels in, 301t
gastrointestinal disorders in, 325
cholelithiasis and cholecystitis, 325, 325b
inflammatory bowel disease, 325
hemorrhagic disorders in, 350
abruptio placentae and, 360, 360f, 365-366, 365f
clinical manifestations of, 357
clotting disorders and, 366-368
collaborative care for, 357-358, 357b-358b
cord insertion and placental variations and, 366
early pregnancy bleeding, 350-354, 352f, 353t
ectopic pregnancy
clinical manifestations of, 357
collaborative care for, 357-358, 357b-358b
incidence and etiology of, 356-357, 356f
nursing care management in, 353-354, 353b-355b
gestational trophoblastic disease, 358
gestational trophoblastic neoplasia, 349, 358
hydatidiform mole, 358-359, 359b, 359f
gestational trophoblastic neoplasia, 349, 358
hydatidiform mole, 358-359, 359b, 359f

High risk pregnancy (Continued)
incidence and etiology of, 356-357, 356f
late pregnancy bleeding, 360, 360f
abruptio placentae and, 360, 360f, 365-366, 365f
clotting disorders and, 366-368
cord insertion and placental variations and, 366
placenta previa and. *See* Placenta previa.
nursing care management in, 353-354, 353b-355b
placenta previa and. *See* Placenta previa.
recurrent premature dilation of cervix, 355-356, 355b, 356f
human immunodeficiency virus infection in, 328-330, 328b-329b
hyperemesis gravidarum in, 349-350, 351b
hypertension in, 243, 374
classification of, 335, 335t
chronic hypertension, 334, 335t, 336
chronic hypertension with superimposed preeclampsia, 334, 335t, 336
eclampsia, 335t, 336
gestational hypertension, 335, 335t
preeclampsia, 335, 335t-336t, 336b
severe preeclampsia, 336
HELLP syndrome and, 338
morbidity and mortality in, 335
nursing care management in, 340b
blood pressure assessment and, 339, 339b
chronic hypertension and, 348-349
deep tendon reflexes and, 340, 341f, 341t
eclampsia and, 346-348, 346f, 347b
edema and, 339-340, 341f
hyperactive reflexes and, 340-341, 341f
mild preeclampsia and home care and, 342-343, 342b-344b
pharmacologic therapy and, 348t
severe preeclampsia or HELLP syndrome and, 343-346, 344b-345b, 347b, 348t
preeclampsia and, 337-338, 337b-338b, 337f, 339f
significance and incidence of, 334
hyperthyroidism and, 309-310, 310b
hypothyroidism and, 310, 310b
integumentary disorders in, 325-326, 325b
maternal phenylketonuria and, 311

High risk pregnancy (Continued)
pulmonary disorders in, 322
asthma, 322-324, 324t
cystic fibrosis, 324-325
substance abuse in, 49, 253, 330-332, 330b-332b
travel during, 251
High-density lipoproteins, 1474-1475
High-fiber foods, 1391b
High-frequency jet ventilation (HFJV), 715t, 716
Highly active antiretroviral therapy (HAART), 329, 332-333
High-technology care, 8, 8t, 40-41
Hindu religion, 836t-837t
HIPAA. *See* Health Insurance Portability and Accountability Act (HIPAA).
Hips
developmental dysplasia of
in children, 1691-1693, 1691b-1692b
in newborns, 619-620, 620f, 774-776, 774f-775f, 775b
Legg-Calve-Perthes disease and, 1697-1698, 1697b-1698b
Hirschsprung disease, 1389-1393, 1392b, 1392f
Hirsutism, 224
Hispanic culture
breastfeeding and, 559b
childbearing and parenting beliefs and practices in, 25t-26t
communication and, 832
expression of pain in childbirth in, 396b
food patterns in, 292t-293t
infant feeding practices and, 680
parenting and, 568-569
Hispanics
breast cancer and, 117f, 120b
insurance coverage and, 47
morbidity/mortality rates of, 6, 28-29
Histoplasmosis, 1646t
History, 78-79, 1551-1552. *See also* History taking.
in child maltreatment, 1069b, 1071b-1072b
in dystocia, 504b
in mild preeclampsia, 340b
in obesity, 1129
pediatric, 876-878, 877b-878b
in pharmacologic pain management during labor, 417b
in pregestational diabetes mellitus, 300b-301b
prenatal data and, 444
of present illness, 78
preterm labor and, 489b
History taking
genetic, 162-163, 162f
gravidity and parity information obtained during, 210-211, 211t
pediatric, 875, 875b
cardiac assessment and, 1442-1443
chief complaints, 875-876
family history, 879
family structure, 879, 879b-881b
History taking (Continued)
history, 876-878, 877b-878b
identifying information, 875
present illness, 876, 876b
psychosocial history, 879-881
review of systems, 881, 882b
sexual history, 878, 878b
HIV. *See* Human immunodeficiency virus (HIV).
HLA system complex, 1522
Hmong women, 550b
Hodgkin's disease, 1514-1516, 1515f
Ho-Ku acupressure point, 405f
Holistic prenatal care, 235
Home birth, 237b, 269, 270b
Home care, 9, 1217
in abruptio placentae, 366
administration of medications and, 39-40, 1284, 1284b
after cesarean birth, 517b
after circumcision, 669, 669b
after dilation and curettage, 354, 355b
after mastectomy, 124, 125b
after tonsillectomy, 1313
in alternative feedings, 1298
anorectal malformations and, 1423
assessment phase, 39, 40b
availability of, 37b
case management and, 1208, 1208b
communication and technology applications in, 35-36, 36f, 43
in the community, 34-41
congenital heart disease and, 1468-1469, 1471-1472
in cystic fibrosis, 1352
definition of, 35-36, 1203
discharge planning and selection of home care agency, 1205-1206, 1206b-1207b, 1207f
documentation in, 41
in ectopic pregnancy, 358
effectiveness of, 1205, 1205b-1206b
elimination procedures and, 1300
family-centered, 1209-1217
family-to-family support in, 1216-1217
nursing process and, 1212-1214, 1212b-1214b
parent-professional collaboration in, 1211-1212, 1211b-1212b
promotion of optimal development, self-care, and education in, 1214-1215, 1214b, 1215f
respect for diversity in, 1210-1211, 1210b
safety issues in, 1215-1216, 1215b-1216b
first home care visit, 39
formula preparation and feeding and, 703b
guidelines for nursing practice and, 35-36
high-technology, 40-41
hydatidiform moles and, 349-350
of immobilized child, 1680
infection control and, 41-42
maternity, 34-35
Home care (Continued)
medical emergencies and, 41
in mild preeclampsia, 342-343, 342b-344b
nephrotic syndrome and, 1538
of newborns, 675b-676b
nonobstetric surgery during pregnancy and, 369, 369b
nursing process and, 37, 38b, 40b
nutrition counseling for cholecystitis or cholelithiasis in pregnancy, 325b
patient selection and referral, 37
perinatal continuum of care in, 35, 35b, 36f
perinatal services and, 36-37, 43
in placenta previa, 364
in postpartum depression, 596
in postterm pregnancy, 519b
posture and body mechanics and, 250b
preparation for home visits, 37-38, 38b
preterm labor and, 35b, 36f, 37, 40-41, 257b, 263b
nursing care management in, 492-493, 492b-493b, 493f
in preterm premature rupture of membranes, 497, 497b
recurrent premature dilation of cervix and, 356
regulation of, 37
respiratory infections and, 1307
on resumption of sexual intercourse, 551b
role of nurse and standards of care in, 1208-1209, 1209b
safety issues for nurses, 41-42
in sexuality in pregnancy, 257b
in sexually transmitted infections, 113b
in skin lesions, 1641
telephone nursing care in, 35, 43
for terminally ill children, 1168
trends in, 1203-1205
for the unconscious child, 1562b
Home deaths, 1170-1171, 1171b
Home predictor test kits for ovulation, 144-145, 145f
Home pregnancy test kits, 4b, 211-212, 211b, 211f
Home uterine activity monitoring (HUAM), 356, 493
Home visits, postpartum, 552
Homeless women as a vulnerable population, 33-34
Homelessness, child health and, 825, 830
Homocystinuria, 658t
Homograft skin, 1667
Homologous chromosomes, 165-166
Homosexual families, 17
Homozygous sickle cell disease, 1495
Hon, Edward, 4b
Hookworm disease, 1396t
Hopefulness, special needs children and, 1155
Horizontal fetal lie, 377, 379f
Hormonal methods of contraception, 150-151, 151t
combined estrogen-progestin contraceptives, 151-152, 151b, 151t, 152f
Hormonal methods of contraception (Continued)
transdermal contraceptive system, 152
vaginal contraceptive ring, 152
progestin-only contraception, 151t, 152-153, 152b
Hormone therapy, 118, 122-123, 123b
Hormones
changes during pregnancy, 216, 223, 227t, 230
changes in puberty, 1106, 1109
infertility and, 130b, 132-133
onset of labor and, 387
ovaries and production of, 68
placental, 177, 179
postpartum changes in, 528
Hornet stings, 1649t-1650t
Hospice care for terminally ill children, 1168-1169, 1203
Hospital births, 9
Hospital deaths, terminally ill children and, 1171, 1171b
Hospitalization
financial burden of, 28
maternal
in abruptio placentae, 366
for complications in diabetes mellitus, 305
in ectopic pregnancy, 358
negative effect on families, 35
in placenta previa, 363-364
postpartum psychosis and, 596-597, 596b
psychologic considerations in, 208
in severe preeclampsia or HELLP syndrome, 343, 344b-345b
surgery during pregnancy and, 369, 369b
pediatric, 1219, 1243-1244, 1300-1301
admission assessment and, 1225, 1226b-1228b
altered family roles and, 1224-1225
alternative feeding techniques and, 1294b
family teaching and home care and, 1298
gastrostomy feeding, 1296-1298, 1298f
gavage feeding, 1295, 1295b-1297b, 1295f, 1295t
nasoduodenal and nasojejunal tubes, 1298
total parenteral nutrition, 1298
ambulatory or outpatient setting and, 1239, 1240b
bathing during, 1257-1258
beneficial effects of, 1224
cerebral palsied child and, 1724
cognitively impaired child and, 1182-1183
controlling elevated temperature and, 1259-1260
in cystic fibrosis, 1351
developmentally appropriate activities and, 1232, 1232b
diabetes mellitus and, 1623-1624, 1626b

Hospitalization *(Continued)*
elimination and
enemas and, 1299, 1299b
ostomies and, 1299-1300
emergency admission and, 1239-1242, 1241b
family education during, 1260-1261
fears of bodily injury and pain and, 1231-1232
feeding and, 1258, 1259b
hair care and, 1258
head injuries and, 1566, 1568-1569
hearing impaired child and, 1190-1191
individual risk factors and, 1223-1224, 1223b
intensive care unit and, 1241b-1243b, 1242-1243, 1242f
isolation room and, 1239, 1239b
loss of control and, 1221-1223, 1230-1231, 1231b, 1231f
maintaining respiratory function and
artificial ventilation, 1291-1294, 1291f-1292f, 1292b-1294b, 1294f
bronchial drainage, 1291
inhalation therapy, 1289-1291, 1289b-1290b, 1289f-1290f
maximizing potential benefits of, 1235-1236, 1236f
measurement of intake and output and, 1285, 1285b
oral hygiene and, 1258
parent education during, 1237
parental participation and, 1237-1238
parental reactions to, 1224, 1224b
parent-child relationship and, 1235
parenteral fluid therapy and complications in, 1288-1289, 1288b-1289b
infusion pumps in, 1287
removal of peripheral intravenous lines in, 1288, 1288b
safety catheters and needleless systems in, 1286-1287, 1287b, 1287f
securement of peripheral intravenous lines in, 1287-1288, 1287f
site and equipment in, 1285-1286, 1285b-1286b, 1286f
play and expressive activities and, 1232-1235, 1233b, 1233f-1234f, 1235b
preparation for discharge and home care, 1238-1239
preparing child for admission, 1225-1228, 1225b, 1228f, 1229b
preventing or minimizing separation during, 1228-1230, 1229f-1230f
safety and, 1261
environmental factors in, 1261-1262, 1261f-1262f

Hospitalization *(Continued)*
infection control and, 1261f, 1262-1264, 1263b-1264b
positioning for procedures and, 1266-1267, 1267b, 1267f
restraining methods and therapeutic holding and, 1265-1266, 1266f
transporting infants and children, 1264-1265, 1264f
separation anxiety and, 1219-1221, 1220b, 1220f-1221f
sibling reactions to, 1224
skin care during, 1256-1257, 1257b
specimen collection and
blood, 1271-1272, 1271b-1272b, 1271f
respiratory secretions, 1272-1273
stool, 1270-1271, 1270b
urine, 1267-1270, 1268b-1270b, 1268f, 1269t
support of family during, 1236, 1237b
terminally ill children and, 1168
visually impaired child and, 1195-1196
pelvic inflammatory disease and, 102
Host factors in disease, 801
HPV. *See* Human papillomavirus (HPV).
HPV vaccine, 4b, 104
HRSA. *See* Health Resources and Services Administration (HRSA).
HSV. *See* Herpes simplex virus (HSV).
HUAM. *See* Home uterine activity monitoring (HUAM).
Humalog. *See* Lispro insulin.
Human bites, 1654
Human chorionic gonadotropin (hCG)
changes during pregnancy, 227t
as marker in pregnancy tests, 177, 211
miscarriage and, 354
during postpartum period, 528
Human chorionic somatomammotropin (hCS), 177, 227t
Human Developmental Ecology theory, 18t
Human epidermal growth factor receptor 2 (HER2), 121
Human Genome Project, 163-165
Human immunodeficiency virus (HIV), 108-110
assessing risk behaviors for, 97b
breastfeeding and, 246
in children, 1516-1519
clinical manifestations of, 1517, 1517b
diagnostic evaluation of, 1517-1518, 1517t-1518t
epidemiology of, 1516
etiology of, 1517
in industrialized vs. resource-poor parts of the world, 12
pathophysiology of, 1517

Human immunodeficiency virus (HIV) *(Continued)*
therapeutic management of, 1518-1519
management of, 110
perinatal transmission of, 108, 328, 329b, 751
preconception counseling and, 328
pregnancy and, 109-110, 328-330, 328b
prevention of, 46b, 55-56, 56b, 98-99
screening and diagnosis of, 108, 109b
counseling for HIV testing, 108-109
for pregnant women, 241, 242b, 329
for pregnant women and their infants, 109b
Human leukocyte antigens, 1502
Human milk
energy provided by, 680-681
expressing and storing, 691-693, 692f-693f, 693b, 973
nutritional value of, 678, 681-682, 973
preterm infants and, 717
protective mechanisms in, 747-748
uniqueness of, 684
Human papillomavirus (HPV), 85, 103-110, 103f
Human papillomavirus (HPV) vaccine, 986, 1117
Human placental lactogen (hPL). *See* Human chorionic somatomammotropin (hCS).
Humira. *See* Adalimumab.
Huntington's disease, 164-165
Hydatid of Morgagni, 68f
Hydatidiform mole, 358-359, 359b, 359f
Hydralazine
breastfeeding and, 1745t-1748t
for hypertension, 346, 348t
during pregnancy, 317t
Hydramnios, 298-299
Hydration
bacterial meningitis and, 1576
preterm infants and, 718, 718b
respiratory infections and, 1306-1307
unconscious child and, 1560-1561
Hydrocarbons poisoning, 1428b-1429b
Hydrocele, 1535t
Hydrocephalus, 769, 1559b, 1593-1597, 1594f-1595f, 1595b-1596b
Hydrocodone, 940t, 942t
Hydrocolloids, 1638t, 1640b
Hydrogel dressings, 1638t
Hydromorphone, 408, 939, 940t, 942t, 945t
Hydronephrosis, 1533
Hydrops fetalis, 766
Hydrotherapy. *See* Water therapy.
Hydroxyzine, 406
Hygiene
of children
diabetic mellitus and, 1628-1629

Hygiene *(Continued)*
ears and, 908
during hospitalization
bathing and, 1257-1258
family education and, 1260-1261
hair care and, 1258
maintaining healthy skin and, 1256-1257, 1257b
oral hygiene and, 1258
unconscious child and, 1561, 1561b
in first stage of labor, 456, 457t
odor in cystoceles and rectoceles and, 592
patient teaching in, 246
Hygroscopic dilators, 505
Hymen, 65-66, 66f
Hyperactive reflexes (clonus) at the ankle joint, 341-342, 341f
Hyperbilirubinemia
breastfeeding and, 691
home care and, 37
in infants of diabetic mothers, 737
neonatal indirect, 655t
therapy for, 644b, 665-667, 666f
Hypercholesterolemia, 1474
Hypercyanotic spells, 1465, 1465b
Hyperemesis gravidarum, 309, 349
clinical manifestations of, 349
collaborative care for, 349-350
etiology of, 349
infusion therapy for, 39-41
nursing care plan for, 351b
nutrition and, 291
Hyperemia, cerebral, 1563
Hyperemia, reactive, 1256
Hyperglycemia, 296
diabetic children and, 1621-1622, 1622t, 1628
fetal, 182, 457-459
in high risk infants, 734-735
identification of, 304b
morning, 1621-1622, 1622t
pregestational diabetes mellitus and, 305, 305b
Hyperhemolytic crisis, 1495
Hyperinsulinemia
fetal, 182, 457-459
in infants of diabetic mothers, 735
Hyperkalemia, acute renal failure and, 1543, 1543b
Hyperlipidemia, 1474-1476, 1475t
Hypermenorrhea. *See* Menorrhagia.
Hyperopia, 1192b-1193b
Hyperparathyroidism, 1610-1611, 1610b
Hyperpigmentation during pregnancy, 223
Hyperpnea, 915b
Hyperpyrexia. *See* Fever.
Hypertension
abruptio placentae and, 365
in acute glomerulonephritis, 1539
in acute renal failure, 1543
in chronic renal failure, 1546
home care and, 37
pediatric, 1479-1481, 1480b
in pregestational diabetes mellitus, 298
in pregnancy, 243, 374
classification of, 335, 335t
chronic hypertension, 334, 335t, 336

Hypertension (Continued)
chronic hypertension with superimposed preeclampsia, 334, 335t, 336
eclampsia, 335t, 336
gestational hypertension, 335, 335t
preeclampsia, 335, 335t-336t, 336b
severe preeclampsia, 336
HELLP syndrome and, 338
morbidity and mortality in, 335
nursing care management in, 340b
blood pressure assessment and, 339, 339b
chronic hypertension and, 348-349
deep tendon reflexes and, 340, 341f, 341t
eclampsia and, 346-348, 346f, 347b
edema and, 339-340, 341f
hyperactive reflexes and, 340-341, 341f
mild preeclampsia and home care and, 342-343, 342b-344b
pharmacologic therapy and, 348t
severe preeclampsia or HELLP syndrome and, 343-346, 344b-345b, 347b, 348t
preeclampsia and, 337-338, 337b-338b, 337f, 339f
significance and incidence of, 334
pulmonary artery, 1477-1478
sodium and, 52
Hyperthermia
automobile-related, 1038
cerebral dysfunction and, 1561
definition of, 1259
pediatric, 1253, 1260
Hyperthyroidism
high risk pregnancy and, 309-310, 310b
nursing care in, 310
pediatric, 1607-1609, 1608b-1609b
Hypertonic dehydration, 1381-1382
Hypertonic uterine dysfunction, 498, 502
Hypertrophic cardiomyopathy (HCM), 736, 1478
Hypertrophic pyloric stenosis, 1372b, 1417-1420, 1419b
Hyperventilation, 391, 395, 915b
Hypervolemia, pregnancy-induced, 529
HypnoBirthing, 401
Hypnosis, 405
Hypocalcemia
diabetic mothers and, 736
in newborns, 657
during pregnancy, 225-226
Hypoglossal nerve (cranial nerve XII), 925t
Hypoglycemia
diabetic children and, 1621, 1621b, 1622t, 1628, 1629b
evidence-based practice on monitoring for, 615b
in high risk infants, 734
Hypoglycemia (Continued)
in late-preterm infants, 708t
in newborns, 656-657
pregestational diabetes mellitus and, 299, 304-305, 736
treatment for, 302b
Hypogonadotropic amenorrhea, 87
Hypomagnesemia, 736
Hypomenorrhea, 93
Hyponatremic dehydration, 1381
Hypoparathyroidism, 1609-1610, 1609b-1610b
Hypopituitarism, 1600-1602, 1601b-1602b
Hypoplastic anemia, 1501
Hypoplastic left heart syndrome, 1455b-1458b
Hyposensitization, 1340
Hypospadias, 776, 776f, 1535t
Hypotension, 414
Hypotension with decreased placental perfusion, 411b
Hypothalamic-pituitary cycle, 72f, 73
Hypothalamic-pituitary-gonadal axis, 1603
Hypothalamus, 74
Hypothermia
after anesthesia and analgesia, 420
blood transfusion-related, 1521t-1522t
in near-drowning, 1570
in newborns, 611-613, 648
in preterm infants, 713
Hypothyroidism
congenital, 182, 658t, 778
high risk pregnancy and, 310, 310b
juvenile, 1605-1606, 1606b
nursing care in, 310
Hypotonic dehydration, 1381
Hypotonic uterus, 498, 499b, 580-581
Hypoventilation, 915b
Hypovolemia
during labor, 457b-459b
during pregnancy, 222, 373
in preterm infants, 709
Hypovolemic shock
in children, 1482-1483, 1483t
emergency care in, 542b
postpartum hemorrhage and, 581-583, 582b-583b
Hypoxemia, 1464-1467, 1465b, 1465f-1466f, 1466t, 1467b
Hypoxia, 1464-1465
fetal responses to, 204-205
in near-drowning, 1570
pregnancy and, 370
HypRho-D, 547b
Hysterectomy
for endometriosis, 93
for gestational trophoblastic neoplasia, 360
for hydatidiform moles, 359
pelvic examination after, 85
Hysterical conversion reaction, 1102
Hysterosalpingography, 133t, 135, 135f

I

"I" messages, 873b-874b
IA. See Intermittent auscultation (IA).
IBD. See Inflammatory bowel disease (IBD).
Ibuprofen, 939t
breastfeeding and, 1745t-1748t
to treat dysmenorrhea, 89t
ICH. See Intracranial hemorrhage (ICH).
Ichthyoses, 1655
Id (unconscious mind), 848
Ideal body weight, 52b
Identical twins. See Monozygotic twins.
Identifying information, 875
Identity, adolescence and, 1109-1110, 1110b, 1113, 1116t
Identity vs. role confusion in psychosocial development, 849-850
Idiopathic facial paralysis. See Bell's palsy.
Idiopathic hypoparathyroidism, 1609b
Idiopathic nephrosis, 1535-1536
Idiopathic scoliosis, 1700-1703, 1701f
Idiopathic thrombocytopenic purpura (ITP), 583, 1492f
in children, 1505-1506, 1505b-1506b
IgA. See Immunoglobulin A (IgA).
IgG. See Immunoglobulin G (IgG).
IgM. See Immunoglobulin M (IgM).
IgM antibody. See Immunoglobulin M (IgM) antibody.
Ileostomy, 1403-1404
Iliac crest, 69f
Iliac spines, 69f
Ilium, 68, 69f
Ilizarov external fixator, 1690
Illicit drugs, 49-51, 789
Illness
acute, 791
chronic. See Chronic illness.
Illocutionary stage of communicative development, 870-871, 871b
Imagery for pain management
in children, 935-936, 937b
during labor, 270, 401
Imaginary playmates, 1048
Imaginative play, 1047, 1047f
Imipramine, breastfeeding and, 1745t-1748t
Imitative games, 854
Imitative play, 960, 1047, 1047f
Immediate postoperative care in cesarean birth, 516
Immigrant children, 825, 830
Immigrants, 34, 235-236
Immobilization, 1676-1680, 1677t, 1704
Immune system
of newborns at birth, 614-615
postpartum changes in, 531
of school-age children, 1078
Immunization Coalition, 990
Immunizations
for adolescents, 1117-1118
health history of, 786, 877
health screening recommendations for, 59t, 889f
for infants, 786, 978
administration of, 986-991, 989b-990b
Immunizations (Continued)
contraindications and precautions for, 986, 987t-988t
reactions to, 986
routine, 982-985
schedule for, 978-982, 979f-981f
selected, 985-986
for newborns, 674
during pregnancy, 252
Immunoglobulin A (IgA)
fetal, 183
normal test ranges for, 1753t-1761t
Immunoglobulin G (IgG), 183
Immunoglobulin M (IgM), 183
Immunoglobulin M (IgM) antibody, 106
Immunologic deficiency disorders, 1516, 1523-1524
blood transfusion therapy in, 1520-1522, 1521t-1522t
hematopoietic stem cell transplantation and, 1522, 1523b
human immunodeficiency virus infection and acquired immunodeficiency syndrome, 1516-1519, 1517b, 1517t-1518t, 1519b
severe combined immunodeficiency disease, 1519-1520
Wiskott-Aldrich syndrome, 1520
Immunologic system
of fetus, 183, 184t-186t
of infants, 955
Immunomodulators, 1402
Impairment, sensory. See Sensory impairments.
Imperforate anus, 774f, 1422
Impetigo contagiosa, 1642t, 1643f
Implanon, 153, 695
Implantable progestins, 152-153
Implantation, 73, 174, 174f-175f
In vitro fertilization
insurance coverage for, 132b
multifetal pregnancies and, 188
In vitro fertilization–embryo transfer (IVF-ET), 136, 137t
Inactivated poliovirus vaccine, 983, 987t-988t
Inborn errors of metabolism, 170, 202, 777-778
Incarcerated women as a vulnerable population, 33
Incest, 1068
Incidence of disease, 800-801, 801b
Incisional pain, 517b
Incisions in cesarean birth, 513, 513f
Incompetent cervix. See Recurrent premature dilation of cervix.
Incomplete breech, 500, 500f
Incomplete miscarriage, 352, 352f, 353t, 354
Incomplete rupture of uterus, 522
Incontinence, urinary, 589, 590f, 592
Increased intracranial pressure, 1552, 1552b
Incubators, preterm Infants and, 713, 723, 723f
Independent midwives, 267
Inderal. See Propranolol.

Indian culture
birth practices and, 448b, 449
family planning beliefs in, 550b
infant feeding practices and, 680
Individual family service plan (IFSP), 1215
Individual identity, adolescents and, 1110, 1110b
Individuating-reflexive stage of spiritual development, 852
Indomethacin
breastfeeding and, 1745t-1748t
preterm labor and, 493-496, 495b
Induced abortion. *See* Abortion.
Induction of labor, 504-505, 518
Bishop score and, 504-505, 505t
in cardiovascular disorders during pregnancy, 318
cervical ripening methods and amniotomy, 505-507, 506b-507b
chemical agents, 505, 506b-507b
mechanical agents, 505
diabetic pregnancy and, 305
oxytocin and, 505, 507-508, 508b-510b, 508f
percent of women receiving, 8t
Industry vs. inferiority in psychosocial development, 849-850, 1079, 1079f
Inevitable miscarriage, 352, 352f, 353t, 354
Inevitable preterm birth, 496, 496b
Infancy period, 843b, 966t-968t
Infant abduction from hospitals, 9, 540, 662
Infant botulism, 1739-1740, 1739b
Infant formulas, 676b, 680-682, 701-704, 703b, 974
iron-fortified, 974, 1494-1495
microwave heating of, 973b, 997
for preterm infants, 717-718, 718b
Infant mortality rate, 790, 790t
definition of, 7b, 790
international trends in, 7
prenatal care and, 7
race/ethnicity and, 32, 190
in the United States, 7, 28-29, 190, 598
Infant walkers, falls and, 996
Infantile spasms, 1583b-1584b
Infant-parent adjustment, 559f-560f, 565-566
Infants
ABO incompatibility in, 766-767
airway obstruction in, 1358, 1358b, 1358f, 1360f
alternative child care arrangements and, 965-970
apnea of infancy and, 1010-1012, 1011b-1012b, 1012f
approaches to physical examination of, 888t
attachment process and, 961-962
mother-to-infant attachment, 554-557, 555t-556t, 557b
parent-infant contact, 548, 557-558, 557f
bacterial meningitis in, 1577b
biologic development of, 953
fine motor development and, 955, 955f
gross motor development and

Infants *(Continued)*
head control, 955-956, 956b, 956f
locomotion, 957, 957b, 959f
rolling over, 956, 957f
sitting, 956-957, 958f
maturation of systems and, 954-955
proportional changes in, 953-954
birth trauma and, 742-743, 743t
central nervous system injuries in, 745
nursing care management in, 743
peripheral nervous system injuries in, 743-745, 744f
skeletal injuries in, 743, 743f
body image and, 853, 960-961, 961f
cognitive development of, 958-960, 960f
colic in, 1001-1002, 1002b, 1003f
communication between parents and, 558-559, 558f-560f, 559b
congenital anomalies in, 742, 767-768, 779
ambiguous genitalia, 776-777, 776f
anorectal malformations, 774, 774f
choanal atresia, 770, 770f
cleft lip and palate, 771-772, 771f-772f
clubfoot, 775
congenital diaphragmatic hernia, 770-771, 771f
developmental dysplasia of hip, 774-776, 774f-775f, 775b
encephalocele and anencephaly in, 768
esophageal atresia and tracheoesophageal fistula, 772-773, 772f
exstrophy of bladder, 776, 776f
genetic diagnosis of, 777
heart defects, 769-770
hydrocephalus, 769
hypospadias and epispadias, 776, 776f
intestinal obstruction, 773
microcephaly, 769
newborn screening for, 777-778
nursing care in, 777-779
omphalocele and gastroschisis, 773, 773f
polydactyly, 775-776
spina bifida in, 768-769, 768f
teratomas, 777
constipation and, 1390
death of, 190, 598-600
acute distress in, 598-599
communicating and caring techniques and, 601-605, 601b-602b
actualizing the loss, 601-602, 601b-602b, 602f-603f
creating memories for parents to take home, 604-605, 605f
helping in acknowledgement and expression of feelings, 603-604

Infants *(Continued)*
helping parents with decision making, 602-603
normalizing the grief process and facilitating positive coping, 604
physical needs of postpartum bereaved mother and, 604
providing sensitive care at and after discharge, 606
community resources in, 598b
cultural and spiritual needs of parents and, 605
documentation of, 605-606
family aspects of grief in, 600-601
funeral arrangements in, 603
intense grief in, 599-600
mortality rate and, 28
postmortem care of newborn and, 605, 605f
dental health of, 978
of diabetic mothers, 735-737, 736f, 737b
divorce and, 817b
failure to thrive and, 1003-1005, 1004b-1005b, 1005f
father-infant relationship, 564-565, 564t, 565f
fever in, 893b
growth and development of, 845, 845t, 966t-968t
guidance during first year of, 1001b
hearing impairment in, 1189, 1189b
hemolytic disease in, 766-767
high risk. *See* High risk infants.
hospitalization of
bathing during, 1257-1258
individual risk factors and, 1223
loss of control and, 1222, 1230
separation anxiety and, 1221
transporting during, 1264-1265, 1264f
urine specimen collection and, 1267-1270, 1268b-1270b, 1268f, 1269t
immunizations for, 786, 978
administration of, 986-991, 989b-990b
contraindications and precautions for, 986, 987t-988t
reactions to, 986
routine, 982-985
schedule for, 978-982, 979f-981f
selected, 985-986
infections and
perinatally acquired, 748-755, 749b
candidiasis, 754-755, 755b
chlamydia, 754, 755b
cytomegalovirus, 752-753, 752f
Escherichia coli, 755-761
gonorrhea, 749
group B streptococcus, 754
hepatitis B virus, 750-751
herpes simplex virus, 753, 753f
human immunodeficiency virus, 751
parvovirus B19, 753-754
rubella, 752

Infants *(Continued)*
syphilis, 749-750, 750b, 750f
toxoplasmosis, 749
tuberculosis, 754
varicella-zoster virus, 750
sepsis, 745-748, 745t, 747b-748b, 747t
injury prevention and. *See* Injury prevention.
language development in, 962, 962b
large-for-gestational-age, 707b, 735
late preterm, 651
limit setting and discipline of, 970
mortality. *See* Infant mortality rate.
nonverbal communication and, 871
nutrition and, 643, 678, 704, 786, 972-976. *See also* Breastfeeding.
benefits of breastfeeding and, 678-679
contraindications to breastfeeding and, 246, 679
cultural influences on, 680
dietary reference intakes for, 972t
during the first 6 months, 973-974, 973b
guidelines for breastfeeding support, 680b
introduction of solid foods and, 975, 976b
lactation and breastfeeding in, 682-700, 682f-683f
nursing care management and, 685, 686b
breastfeeding complications and, 689-691, 692f
duration of feedings in breastfeeding and, 687-689
expressing and storing breast milk and, 691-693, 692f-693f, 693b
frequency of feedings in breastfeeding and, 687
infant assessment and, 685, 685b
latch-on in breastfeeding and, 686-687, 688f
maternal assessment before breastfeeding and, 685
maternal employment and, 693
milk banking and, 694
milk ejection in breastfeeding and, 687
positioning in breastfeeding and, 543-544, 685-686, 687f-688f
supplementation of breastfeeding in, 689, 690b
weaning from breastfeeding and, 693
nutrient needs and, 680-682
parent education on formula-feeding and, 700-704, 701f-702f, 703b
during the second 6 months, 974
selection and preparation of solid foods and, 974-975
pain assessment in, 933-934, 934t

Infants (Continued)
peptic ulcer disease and, 1405b
play and, 960-963, 964t
postterm, 707b, 733-734, 733f
meconium aspiration syndrome and, 733, 733f
persistent pulmonary hypertension and, 733-734
preterm. See Preterm infants.
psychologic preparation for procedures, 1248b-1249b
psychosocial development of, 957-958
regurgitation and spitting up and, 999-1001
respiratory infections in, 1304, 1305b
response to pain, 930b, 930f
Rh incompatibility in, 766-767
self-concept and, 852-853
separation anxiety in, 959, 962, 965
shoes for, 972
sleep and activity of, 976-978, 977t
small-for-gestational-age, 707b, 734-735
social development of, 961-963, 962b, 962f, 964t
special needs. See Special needs children.
spina bifida in, 1727, 1729
stranger fear in, 962, 962f, 965-972
sudden infant death syndrome and, 1005-1010, 1006t, 1009f
swallow reflex in, 1274b
teething and, 971-972, 971f, 972b
temperament of, 963-965, 966t-968t
thumb-sucking and use of pacifiers in, 970-971
understanding and reaction to death, 1167t-1168t
urinary tract disorders in, 1531b
vital signs of, 893
vitamin D supplementation and, 1363-1364
water balance in, 1380-1381, 1381b
Infection control
in care of newborns, 662, 662b
home care and, 41-42
hospitalized children and, 1261f, 1262-1264, 1263b-1264b
for neonatal sepsis, 746-748, 747b-748b, 747t
in postpartum period, 540, 541b
preterm infants and, 710, 711b
in preterm premature rupture of membranes, 497
Standard Precautions in, 113, 113b-114b
Infections
of burn wounds, 1671
chronic renal failure-related, 1546
cutaneous
bacterial, 1641, 1642t, 1643f
dermatophytoses, 1643, 1645f, 1645t
systemic mycotic, 1643-1646, 1646t
viral, 1642-1643, 1644t
definition of, 1486b
delayed wound healing and, 1637t
Infections (Continued)
during first stage of labor, 467b
intracranial, 1575
aseptic meningitis in, 1578, 1578t
bacterial meningitis in, 1575-1578, 1576b-1578b, 1578t
encephalitis in, 1578-1579, 1579b
rabies in, 1579-1580, 1580b
Reye's syndrome in, 1580-1581, 1581b
leukemia and, 1509-1512, 1510b-1512b
monilial, 697-698
neonatal
late-preterm infants and, 708t
perinatally acquired, 748-755, 749b
bacterial infections, 754
candidiasis, 754-755, 755b
chlamydia, 754, 755b
cytomegalovirus, 752-753, 752f
Escherichia coli, 755-761
gonorrhea, 749
group B streptococcus, 754
hepatitis B virus, 750-751
herpes simplex virus, 753, 753f
human immunodeficiency virus, 751
parvovirus B19, 753-754
rubella, 752
syphilis, 749-750, 750b, 750f
toxoplasmosis, 749
tuberculosis, 754
varicella-zoster virus, 750
sepsis, 745-747, 745t, 747t
signs and symptoms of, 710, 711b
ocular, 1194
in osteomyelitis, 1703-1704, 1703b
postpartum, 540, 541b, 585-587
endometritis, 585, 587
mastitis, 586-587, 586f
prevention of, 586-587, 587b
risk factors for, 585, 586b
urinary tract infections, 586-587
in wounds, 585-587
during pregnancy, 299, 455
after membranes rupture, 455
pregestational diabetes mellitus and, 299
preterm labor and birth and, 488
respiratory
in children, 1303
clinical manifestations of, 1304, 1305b
comfort during, 1304-1305
croup syndromes, 1318-1321, 1318b-1320b, 1318t
easing respiratory efforts in, 1304
etiology and characteristics of, 1303-1304
family support and home care and, 1307
hydration and, 1306-1307
lower respiratory tract. See Lower respiratory tract infections.
Infections (Continued)
nursing care plan for, 1308b-1309b
nursing process in, 1306b
nutrition and, 1307
pertussis, 1326
preventing spread of, 1305-1306
reducing temperature in, 1306, 1306b
respiratory function assessment in, 1307b
rest and, 1304
severe acute respiratory syndrome, 1329
tuberculosis, 1326-1329, 1327b-1329b
upper respiratory tract. See Upper respiratory tract infections.
sexually transmitted. See Sexually transmitted infections (STIs).
vaginal, 110-112, 110t
bacterial vaginosis, 110-111, 110t
candidiasis, 111-112, 111b
group B streptococcus, 112
trichomoniasis, 112
Infectious mononucleosis, 1317-1318, 1317b-1318b
Infectious polyneuritis. See Guillain-Barré syndrome.
Infective endocarditis, 1472-1473, 1472b-1473b
Inferiority vs. industry in psychosocial development. See Industry vs. inferiority in psychosocial development.
Infertility, 159
assessment of
the couple, 133-134
female infertility, 130-132, 132f, 133b, 133t
male infertility, 132-133, 134b
nurse's role in, 130, 131b
cultural awareness in, 131b
factors associated with, 129-130, 130b
female, 129-130, 130b
health promotion and, 46, 46b
incidence of, 129
insurance coverage for, 132b
male, 129-130, 130b
plan of care and implementation in
assisted reproductive therapies, 136, 136b, 137f, 137t
medical, 135
nonmedical, 134-136
preimplantation genetic diagnosis, 136-138
psychosocial, 134, 134b
surgical, 135-136, 135f-136f
religious considerations of, 132b
treatment of, 129
Infiltration, 1288, 1288b-1289b
Inflammation
chronic, 136
wound healing and, 1636
Inflammatory bowel disease (IBD)
in children, 1401-1404, 1401t, 1404b
during pregnancy, 325
Inflammatory disorders
acute appendicitis, 1398-1400, 1399b
inflammatory bowel disease, 1401-1404, 1401t, 1404b
Meckel's diverticulum, 1400-1401, 1400b
peptic ulcer disease, 1404-1406, 1405b
Influenza, 985, 1313-1314
Influenza vaccine
health screening recommendations for, 59t
in infants, 985, 987t-988t
Informants, pediatric health history and, 875
Informed consent
for contraceptive sterilization, 155b
external cephalic version and, 502
for induction or augmentation of labor with oxytocin, 508
for pediatric surgery or procedures, 1245-1247
for pharmacologic pain management during labor, 416-418, 416b-418b
for rubella vaccination, 546b
Infrared thermometers, 893, 897b
Infundibulopelvic ligament, 67f
Infundibulum of uterine tube, 67-68, 68f
Infusion pumps, 1287
Infusion therapy, 39-41
Inguinal hernia, 1535t
Inhalant abuse, 1139
Inhalation administration of analgesics, 943b-944b
Inhalation burn injuries, 1663-1664
Inhalation therapy, 1289-1291, 1289b-1290b, 1289f-1290f
Inhaled nitric oxide (INO) therapy, 716
Inheritance patterns, 169
multifactorial inheritance, 169, 188
unifactorial inheritance, 169-170, 169f
In-home child care, 965
Initiative vs. guilt in psychosocial development, 849-850, 850f
Injectable progestins, 151t, 152, 152b
Injections
children and, 1255b
newborns and, 663-665, 663f, 665b
safe practices, infection control and, 113b-114b
Injuries
in children
amputation and, 1690-1691, 1690b
blindness and, 1191-1194
distraction for, 1690, 1690f
fractures and, 1681-1684, 1682b, 1682f, 1684b, 1686f
head. See Head injuries.
mortality and, 787-788, 788f-789f, 788t
soft-tissue injuries and, 1680-1681, 1680f
traction for, 1686-1690, 1687b, 1687f-1688f, 1689b

Injuries *(Continued)*
maternal birth-related
cystocele and rectocele in, 588-589, 589f, 592
genital fistulas and, 589-592, 590f
uterine displacement and prolapse in, 587-588, 588f, 592
newborn birth-related, 652-653, 653f, 742-743, 743t
central nervous system injuries in, 745
nursing care management in, 743
peripheral nervous system injuries in, 743-745, 744f
skeletal injuries in, 743, 743f
Injury prevention
adolescents and, 78, 1122-1124, 1123b
infants and, 991, 992b-993b
aspiration of foreign objects and, 991, 992b-993b
bodily damage and, 992b-993b, 998
burns and, 992b-993b, 997-998, 997f-998f
child safety home checklist and, 1000b
drowning and, 992b-993b, 998
falls and, 992b-993b, 995-996
motor vehicle injuries and, 787, 788f, 994-995, 995b, 995f
nurse's role in, 998-999, 1000b
poisoning and, 992b-993b, 996-997, 997b, 997f
suffocation and, 992b-993b, 993-994
preschoolers and, 1055
school-age children and, 1093-1094, 1094b, 1094f, 1095t, 1096b
toddlers and, 1033, 1034t-1035t
aspiration and suffocation and, 1034t-1035t, 1040
bodily damage and, 1034t-1035t, 1040
drowning and, 1034t-1035t, 1038
falls and, 1034t-1035t, 1039-1040
motor vehicle injuries and, 1033-1038, 1034t-1035t, 1036b, 1037f
poisoning and, 1034t-1035t, 1039, 1039b, 1039f
Inlet contracture, 498
In-line skate safety, 1096b
INO therapy. *See* Inhaled nitric oxide (INO) therapy.
Insect bites, 1649t-1650t
Insensible water loss, 1381
Insomnia during pregnancy, 254t-256t
Inspection
of abdomen of child, 918, 918b, 918f
in cardiac assessment, 1443
Inspiratory capacity changes during pregnancy, 222t
Instruments for childbirth, 471, 471f
Insulin, 227t, 296-297, 297f
breastfeeding and, 1745t-1748t
Insulin pumps, 303-304, 304f
Insulin therapy
in diabetes mellitus, 1618-1620, 1619b, 1626-1627, 1626t, 1627f
in gestational diabetes mellitus, 309
in pregestational diabetes mellitus, 302-304, 303b, 303t, 304f
Insulin waning, 1621-1622
Insurance
coverage for infertility, 132b
financial issues in, 47
nurse-midwives and, 6
Intake and output
in acute renal failure, 1543-1544
after heart surgery, 1471, 1471b
in assessment of dehydration, 1383
in hyperemesis gravidarum, 350
measurement of, 1285, 1285b
Integrative health care, 5, 5f
Integumentary disorders, 1674-1675
acne and, 1659-1661
arthropod bites and stings and, 1648-1650, 1649t-1650t
Lyme disease and, 1653-1654, 1653f
pediculosis capitis and, 1651-1652, 1651b-1652b, 1651f
Rickettsial diseases and, 1652-1653, 1653t
scabies, 1650, 1650b
atopic dermatitis and, 1656-1659, 1657b-1659b, 1657f
burns and. *See* Burns.
cold injuries and, 1674
contact dermatitis and, 1646-1647
diaper dermatitis and, 1655-1656, 1656b, 1656f
drug reactions and, 1648, 1648b
foreign bodies and, 1648
home care and family support of, 1641
mammal bites and scratches and, 1654-1655, 1655b
poison ivy, oak, and sumac exposure and, 1647-1648, 1647b, 1647f
during pregnancy, 325-326, 325b
seborrheic dermatitis and, 1659
skin infections
bacterial, 1641, 1642t, 1643f
dermatophytoses, 1643, 1645f, 1645t
systemic mycotic, 1643-1646, 1646t
viral, 1642-1643, 1644t
skin lesions. *See* Skin lesions.
sunburn and, 1673, 1674f-1675f
wounds. *See* Wounds.
Integumentary system
adaptation to labor, 391
adaptations to pregnancy, 223-224, 223f, 224b
effects of immobilization on, 1677t
fetal, 183
postpartum adaptation of, 531
review of systems and, 882b
signs of neonatal sepsis, 747t
transition to extrauterine life and, 615-618, 616b, 617f-618f
Intellectual development, play and, 856
Intensive care unit, 1241b-1243b, 1242-1243, 1242f
Intercultural effectiveness. *See* Cultural competence.
Interferon alfa-2b, 108
Intermenstrual bleeding. *See* Metrorrhagia.
Intermittent auscultation (IA), 423-424, 423f, 424b
Intermittent epidural block, 413-414
Intermittent infusion device, 1279
Intermittent mandatory ventilation (IMV), 715t
Intermittent skilled nursing visit, 1205, 1205b
Internal ballottement, 215, 216f
Internal cervical os, 361
Internal electronic fetal monitoring, 426-427, 426t, 427f
Internal genital organs
anatomy of, 65-68, 67f-68f
physical examination of, 82, 82f, 83b
Internal os of cervix, 66-67, 68f
Internal rotation, birth process and, 389f, 390
Internal version, 503
International adoption, 816
International Childbirth Education Association, 4b
International Confederation of Midwives, 9
International Confederation of Midwives' Vision for Women and Their Health, 3, 3b
International medical outreach, 12, 12f
International Society of Nurses in Genetics (ISONG), 161
Internet
home health care and, 35
impact on children, 864
resources on genetics, 163b
Interpersonal relationships, child development and, 857-859, 859f
Interpregnancy interval (IPI), 140b
Interpretation, 75
Interpreters, 22-23, 23b, 449, 869-870, 869b
Interstitial pneumonia, 1324
Interview
adolescents and, 872, 1117b
child maltreatment and, 1069b, 1071b-1072b
in dystocia, 504b
in early discharge after birth, 538b
in family assessment, 879b-881b
first stage of labor and, 444-446, 445b
in follow-up prenatal visits, 242
guidelines for communication in, 866-867, 867b-868b, 867f
in health assessment, 75-76, 75f, 76b
in initial prenatal visit, 237-239, 239f
in pharmacologic pain management during labor, 417b
in pregestational diabetes mellitus, 300b-301b
in preterm labor, 489b
Intestinal gas after cesarean birth, 516, 517b
Intestinal obstruction
anorectal malformations, 774, 774f, 1422-1423, 1422b
congenital anomalies and, 773
hypertrophic pyloric stenosis in, 1372b, 1417-1420, 1419b
intussusception in, 1420-1421, 1420b-1421b, 1421f
malrotation and volvulus in, 1422
during pregnancy, 368-369
Intestinal parasitic diseases, 1395-1398, 1396t, 1397b-1398b, 1397f
Intimate partner violence (IPV), 60-63, 61b
cultural considerations in, 61
cycle of, 61-62
legal options in, 62, 63b
mandatory reporting of, 63b
myths and facts about, 61t
pattern of, 60, 60f
during pregnancy, 62-63, 62b-63b, 76, 240
prevention of, 63
signs of, 60b
Intracellular fluid, 1380-1381
Intracranial hemorrhage (ICH), 745
Intracranial infections, 1575
aseptic meningitis in, 1578, 1578t
bacterial meningitis in, 1575-1578, 1576b-1578b, 1578t
encephalitis in, 1578-1579, 1579b
rabies in, 1579-1580, 1580b
Reye's syndrome in, 1580-1581, 1581b
Intracranial pressure monitoring, unconscious child and, 1559-1560, 1559b-1560b
Intractable diarrhea of infancy, 1383
Intracytoplasmic sperm injections, 137t
Intradermal administration, 943b-944b, 946, 1278-1279
Intradermal water block, 405-406, 405f
Intraductal papilloma, 116-117, 116t
Intramuscular administration of medication
of analgesics, 418, 943b-944b, 1275-1278, 1276t-1277t, 1277f, 1278b
of magnesium sulfate, 345
newborns and, 663-665, 663f, 665b
Intranasal administration of analgesics, 943b-944b
Intraoperative care in cesarean birth, 515-516, 515f-516f, 516b
Intraosseous infusion, 1286
Intrapartum care
cardiovascular disorders and, 312, 317-318, 318b
gestational diabetes mellitus and, 309
in pregestational diabetes mellitus, 300b-301b, 305-306
Intrathecal administration of analgesics, 943b-944b
Intrauterine devices (IUDs), 153-154, 154f
diabetes mellitus and, 306
for emergency contraception, 153

Intrauterine devices (IUDs) (*Continued*)
intermenstrual bleeding and, 94
signs of potential complications, 154b
Intrauterine growth curves, 651
Intrauterine growth restriction (IUGR), 707b, 734-735
caffeine and, 761
cigarette smoking and, 253
fundal height and, 243-244
risk factors for, 192b
Intrauterine pressure catheter (IUPC), 426, 426t, 427f, 436
Intrauterine resuscitation, 434-435
Intravaginal spermicides, 145-146, 145f
Intravenous administration
of analgesics during labor, 407, 418
in children, 1279-1282, 1280b-1281b, 1281f, 1282t
analgesics and, 943b-944b
parenteral fluid therapy and complications in, 1288-1289, 1288b-1289b
removal of peripheral intravenous lines in, 1288, 1288b
safety catheters and needleless systems in, 1286-1287, 1287b, 1287f
securement of peripheral intravenous lines in, 1287-1288, 1287f
site and equipment in, 1285-1286, 1285b-1286b, 1286f
in hyperemesis gravidarum, 350
Intravenous fluid intake
during labor, 456-457, 457b-459b, 457t
in preterm labor, 494b
Intravenous pyelogram, 220t-221t
Intubation in general anesthesia, 416
Intuitive thought, 1044
Intuitive-projective stage of spiritual development, 852
Intussusception, 1420-1421, 1420b-1421b, 1421f
Invasive ductal carcinoma, 118
Inversion of uterus, 578
Inverted nipples, breastfeeding and, 246-247, 247f, 694-695, 695f
Invisible poverty, definition of, 825
Involution process, 525, 526f
Iodine
intake during pregnancy and lactation, 275t-276t
nutritional significance of, 1377t-1379t
Ipecac, syrup of, 1427-1430
IPV. *See* Intimate partner violence (IPV).
Iran, birth practices and, 448b
Iris, 903
Iron
absorption of, 1366, 1366b
intake during lactation, 275t-276t, 285-287, 290b
intake during pregnancy, 275t-276t, 280
Iron (*Continued*)
normal test ranges for, 1753t-1761t
nutritional significance of, 1377t-1379t
overdose of, 1428b-1429b
storage in newborn liver, 614
Iron deficiency anemia
in children, 1493-1494, 1494b
during pregnancy, 321-322
Iron-binding capacity, total, 1753t-1761t
Iron-fortified formula, 974, 1494-1495
Irradiation, 1515-1516
Irreversible shock, 1483-1484
Irritability
in newborns, 641
severe versus mild preeclampsia and, 336t
Ischial spines, 68, 69f
Ischial tuberosities, 68, 69f, 380-381, 380f
Ischium, 68, 69f
Ishihara test, 907
Islam. *See* Muslim culture.
Islets of Langerhans, 182
Isolation room, hospitalized child and, 1239, 1239b
ISONG. *See* International Society of Nurses in Genetics (ISONG).
Isoniazid, breastfeeding and, 1745t-1748t
Isotonic dehydration, 1381
Isotretinoin, 224b, 283-284, 325b, 1660
Isthmus, uterine, 66, 68f, 213, 216f
Italian culture, food patterns in, 292t-293t
Itching
skin lesion and, 1633
vaginal, 111
IUDs. *See* Intrauterine devices (IUDs).
IUGR. *See* Intrauterine growth restriction (IUGR).
IUPC. *See* Intrauterine pressure catheter (IUPC).
Ivermectin, 1651
IVF-ET. *See* In vitro fertilization-embryo transfer (IVF-ET).

J

Jacket restraint, 1265-1266
Japanese culture
birth practices in, 447-448, 448b
expression of pain in childbirth in, 396b
food patterns in, 292t-293t
health beliefs and practices in, 838t-840t
Jarisch-Herxheimer reaction, 101b
Jaundice
breastfeeding and, 656, 691
differences in color changes and, 901t
in late-preterm infants, 708t
in newborns at birth, 614, 626t-636t, 653-656, 654b, 654f, 655t, 656b, 676b
JBI. *See* Joanna Briggs Institute (JBI).
Jehovah's Witness, 547b, 836t-837t
Jet hydrotherapy, 403, 403f, 404b
Jewish culture
circumcision and, 667
infant feeding practices and, 680
Jewish Orthodox culture
birth practices and, 449
food patterns and, 292t-293t
laws on marital relations, 132b
Joanna Briggs Institute (JBI), 12
Joint Commission
criteria for home care operations, 35-36
description of a sentinel event, 13-14
list of abbreviations, acronyms, and symbols not to use, 13, 14t
Joint physical custody, 818
Joints
juvenile idiopathic arthritis and, 1708-1711, 1712b
pain during pregnancy, 254t-256t
physical assessment of, 922
systemic lupus erythematosus and, 1711-1713, 1713b
Jones criteria, modifications of, 1473
Jordanian mothers, 568-569
Juvenile hypothyroidism, 1605-1606, 1606b
Juvenile idiopathic arthritis, 1708-1711, 1712b
Juvenile rheumatoid arthritis. *See* Juvenile idiopathic arthritis.

K

Kanamycin, breastfeeding and, 1745t-1748t
Kangaroo mother care (KMC), 847
for low-birth-weight infants, 557
during pain procedures, 936, 938, 938f
for preterm infants, 723-724, 724f, 725b
Karmel, Marjorie, 4b, 399
Karyotypes, 166, 167f
Karyotyping, 176, 201
Kawasaki disease, 1481-1482, 1481b-1482b
Kegel exercises, 53, 53b, 84, 246, 544
perineal muscles and, 477
Keloids, 1635f
Kenya, 12f
Kernicterus, 655
Ketoacidosis
pediatric diabetes mellitus and, 1617-1618
pregestational diabetes mellitus and, 299
Ketogenic diet, 1586
Ketone levels, 1529t-1530t
Ketonemia, 278-279
Ketonuria, 243, 528
Ketoprofen, 89t
Ketorolac tromethamine, breastfeeding and, 1745t-1748t
Kick counts. *See* Daily fetal movement count (DFMC).
Kidney transplantation, 1547-1549, 1548b-1549b
Kidneys
fetal, 181-182
genitourinary dysfunction and acute glomerulonephritis and, 1538-1540, 1539b
Kidneys (*Continued*)
acute renal failure and, 1542-1545, 1543b-1544b
chronic renal failure and, 1545-1547, 1546b
dialysis and, 1546-1547
hemolytic uremic syndrome, 1540, 1540b
nephrotic syndrome and, 1535-1538, 1536b-1537b, 1536f
obstructive uropathy and, 1533-1534, 1534f
renal transplantation and, 1547-1549, 1548b-1549b
urinary tract infection and. *See* Urinary tract infections (UTIs).
Wilms' tumor and, 1540-1542, 1541b-1542b
maternal, 222-223, 528
of newborns, 613
water balance and, 1381
Kindergarten experience, 1048-1049, 1049f
Kinetic stimulation, 964t
Kleihauer-Betke stain, 365
Klinefelter's syndrome, 169, 1098-1099, 1098t
Klonopin. *See* Clonazepam.
Klumpke palsy, 743-744
KMC. *See* Kangaroo mother care (KMC).
Knee jerk reflex, 924f
Knee press, 500b
Knee-chest position, 1466f
prolapsed umbilical cord and, 520-522, 521f
retroverted uterus and, 590-592
Knock-knee, 921, 922f
Kohlberg's moral development theory, 849t, 851-852
adolescents and, 1111
preschoolers and, 1045
school-age children and, 1081
Korean culture, 550b
Kugelberg-Welander disease, 1731b, 1732
Kussmaul respirations, 915b
Kwashiorkor, 1368-1369
Kyphosis, 1699-1700, 1699f

L

Labetalol hydrochloride, 348t
Labia majora, 65, 66f-67f
assessment across the life cycle, 70t
pediatric physical assessment of, 921
Labia minora, 65, 66f-67f, 70t
Labor, 387, 392
anxiety about, 232-233, 458b-459b
augmentation of, 505, 507-510, 508b-509b, 508f
cesarean birth and. *See* Cesarean birth.
cultural considerations in, 25t-26t
diabetes mellitus and, 305
distinguishing true labor from false labor, 442, 442b
documentation during, 449, 449f, 471b
dystocia and, 497
abnormal labor patterns in, 501-502, 502t, 503f

Labor *(Continued)*
dysfunctional labor and, 497-498, 499b
fetal causes of, 498-501, 500b, 500f
maternal position and, 501
multifetal pregnancy and, 501
nursing care management in, 504b
psychologic responses to, 501
factors affecting, 376
passageway, 378
bony pelvis and, 378-381, 380f-381f, 382t-383t
soft tissues and, 381-384, 383f
passenger, 376
attitude and, 377, 378f-380f
fetal lie and, 377, 378f-379f
fetal position and, 377-378, 378f-380f
head size and, 376-377, 377f
presentation and, 377-378, 378f-379f
position, 385, 386f
powers, 384
primary, 384-385, 384f
secondary, 384-385
fathers' participation in, 9, 9f, 463-464, 464t, 465b
cultural factors in, 448-449
during second stage of labor, 471, 472t
fetal assessment during. *See* Fetal assessment.
forceps-assisted birth and, 377, 510-511, 510b, 510f-511f
gestational diabetes mellitus and, 309
induction of, 504-505, 505t, 518
Bishop score and, 504-505, 505t
in cardiovascular disorders during pregnancy, 318
cervical ripening methods and
amniotomy, 505-507, 506b-507b
chemical agents, 505, 506b-507b
mechanical agents, 505
diabetic pregnancy and, 305
oxytocin and, 505, 507-508, 508b-510b, 508f
mechanism of, 388-390, 389f, 392
and memories of sexual abuse, 446-447
myasthenia gravis and, 328
non–English-speaking women in, 449
nonpharmacologic pain management in, 397-406, 420-421
acupressure and acupuncture in, 403-404, 405f
aromatherapy in, 405, 405b
biofeedback in, 405
birth plans and, 398, 398b
childbirth education and, 398-401, 398b-399b
conscious breathing in, 402, 402b, 402f
effleurage and counterpressure in, 402-403
energy work in, 402
heat and cold application in, 404-405

Labor *(Continued)*
hypnosis in, 405
imagery and visualization techniques in, 401
intradermal water block in, 405-406, 405f
music in, 401-402
nursing care plan for, 404b
relaxation in, 399b, 401, 401f
touch and massage in, 402
transcutaneous electrical nerve stimulation in, 403, 404b, 404f
water therapy in, 403, 403f
obstetric emergencies and
amniotic fluid embolism, 479, 522-523, 523b
prolapsed umbilical cord, 520, 521f, 522b
shoulder dystocia, 519, 520f
uterine rupture, 372, 522
onset of, 387-388
pain during
anxiety about, 394
expression of, 395
factors influencing response to, 395-397, 396b
neurologic origins of, 394-395, 395f
pharmacologic pain management in, 406, 420-421
analgesia and anesthesia, 406, 406b
nerve block analgesia and anesthesia. *See* Nerve block analgesia and anesthesia.
systemic, 406-409, 407b-409b
general anesthesia, 415-416, 416f
maternal hypothermia after, 420
nursing care management in, 416, 417b
administration of medication, 418-420, 419f
informed consent and, 416-418, 416b-418b
self-assessment of pain and, 416
obese woman and, 420
preparation of patient for, 418
safety and general care in, 419-420, 419f
sedatives in, 406
signs of potential problems in, 418-419
timing of administration of, 418
physiologic adaptations to, 390-392, 391b
postterm pregnancy and, 518-519, 519b
precipitous, 502
premature rupture of membranes and, 496, 746
preterm, 486, 523-524
causes of, 487-488, 488b
home care and, 35b, 36f, 37, 40-41, 257b, 263b
incidence of, 487
inevitable, 496, 496b
low birth weight versus, 486-487

Labor *(Continued)*
nursing care management in, 488-489, 489b, 496, 496b
bed rest and, 37, 491-492, 492b
early recognition and diagnosis in, 491
home care and, 492-493, 492b-493b, 493f
lifestyle modifications and, 491
prevention strategies and, 489-490, 491b
promotion of fetal lung maturity and, 496, 496b
uterine activity suppression and, 493-496, 494b-495b
nursing care plan for, 490b
recognition of, 253-256, 257f
risk factors for, 192b, 487, 487b-488b
signs and symptoms of, 489-490, 491b, 491f
socioeconomic factors in, 487
signs of potential complications in, 456b
signs preceding, 387, 387b
stages of, 387, 440, 484-485
first stage. *See* First stage of labor.
fourth stage, 388, 480
assessment during, 480, 483b
breastfeeding and, 480
family-newborn relationships in, 484, 484f
interactions with newborn in, 483
nutrition and, 480
postanesthesia recovery during, 480-483, 483b
tremors during, 480
second stage. *See* Second stage of labor.
third stage, 388, 477-480, 477f, 479f
maternal physical status in, 479-480
in normal vaginal childbirth, 481b-482b
pain during, 394-395
telephone interview with women in latent phase of, 442-443, 442b
trial of, 503-504
vacuum-assisted birth and, 377, 510b, 511, 511f
version and, 502-503, 505f
water birth and, 473, 473f
Labor, delivery, and recovery (LDR) rooms, 268, 268f, 443, 473
Labor, delivery, recovery, and postpartum (LDRP) rooms, 268, 268f, 443, 473
Labor beds. *See* Birthing beds.
Laboratory tests, 1753t-1761t
abbreviations used in, 1761t
for breast cancer, 120
in cerebral dysfunction, 1555-1556
in disseminated intravascular coagulation, 367
eclampsia and, 347
in ectopic pregnancy, 357-358
in first stage of labor, 444, 454-455, 455b-456b, 455t

Laboratory tests *(Continued)*
in follow-up prenatal visits, 244
in genitourinary dysfunction, 1526, 1529t-1530t
in health assessment, 85
health screening recommendations for, 59t
in hyperemesis gravidarum, 349
in initial prenatal visit, 241, 241t, 242b
for newborns, 657, 657b, 658t
heel stick and, 659, 659f, 660b
sepsis and, 746-747
urine specimen collection and, 660-661, 661f
venipuncture and, 659-660, 660b
before planned cesarean birth, 514
in pregestational diabetes mellitus, 300b-301b
in skin disorders, 1633
Laboring down method. *See* Open-glottis pushing.
Lacerations, 1640
cerebral, 1564
of the genital tract, 577, 581b
neonatal birth trauma and, 653
related to childbirth, 475-477, 476f, 480, 541b
Lactase deficiency, 49, 161
Lactation. *See also* Breastfeeding.
counseling in, 556t
milk production and, 682-700, 682f-683f
nutrition during, 274-275, 275t-276t, 285-286
adequate dietary intake and, 288-290, 290b
cultural influences and, 291-293, 292t-293t
diet history and, 286-288, 288b, 289t
energy needs and, 286
iron supplementation and, counseling about, 290, 290b
nursing care management and, 286-293, 287b
psychotropic medications and, 597-598
suppression of, 546
weight loss and, 289-290
Lactation consultants, 10
Lactation rooms, 10, 10f
Lactational amenorrhea method (LAM), 145
Lactiferous duct, 70f
Lactiferous sinuses, 69, 70f
Lacto-ovo vegetarians, 1365
Lactose intolerance, 281-282, 283b, 286-287, 1373-1374, 1373b
Lactovegetarians, 1365
Lady's mantle, 582t
Laissez-faire parents, 812
LAM. *See* Lactational amenorrhea method (LAM).
Lamaze education, 237b
Lamaze Institute for Normal Birth (LINB), 400-401
Lamaze method, 399-400
Lamictal. *See* Lamotrigine.
Laminaria tents, 505
Lamotrigine, 597t
Landouzy-Dejerine muscular dystrophy, 1733

Language
autism and, 1198
barriers in, 34, 47
development of, 851
home care and, 40b
infants and, 962, 962b
preschoolers and, 1044, 1046, 1046f, 1050t
toddlers and, 1023, 1025t-1026t
Lanolin for nipple soreness, 694
Lanoxin. *See* Digoxin.
Lanugo, 183, 626t-636t
Laos, birth practices in, 448b
Lap belts, 251-252, 252f
Laparoscopy
for female infertility, 133b, 135, 136f
in gamete intrafallopian transfer, 137f
for ovarian cysts during pregnancy, 369
Laparotomy
in advanced ectopic pregnancy, 358
for ovarian cysts during pregnancy, 369
Large-for-gestational-age (LGA) infants, 707b, 735
Laryngitis, acute, 1319
Laryngotracheobronchitis, acute, 1318t, 1320-1321, 1320b
Larynx, 1109
Lasix. *See* Furosemide.
LATCH system, 1036-1037, 1037f
Latchkey children, 1087
Latch-on, 686-687, 688f, 699b
Late adolescence, 1105, 1116t
Late decelerations of fetal heart rate, 431-432, 431f, 432b
Late pregnancy bleeding, 360, 360f
abruptio placentae and, 360, 360f, 365-366, 365f
clotting disorders and, 366-368
cord insertion and placental variations and, 366, 367f
placenta previa and, 360, 360f
clinical manifestations of, 361-362, 362t
diagnosis of, 362, 363b
home care and, 364
hospital care and, 363-364
incidence and etiology of, 361, 361b
maternal and fetal outcomes in, 362
nursing care plan for, 364b
types of, 361, 361f
vaginal examination and, 362, 364
Late preterm infants, 651
Late reproductive age, health risks in, 48-49
Latency period of psychosexual development, 848-849, 1079
Latent phase of labor, 388, 466, 468t, 472t
Latent tuberculosis infection, 1310
Late-onset lactase deficiency, 1373
Late-preterm (near-term) infants, 707, 707b, 708t, 712b
Later childhood, 843b, 1221
Lateral abdominal stroking, 500b
Lateral position. *See* Side-lying position.
Latex allergy, 146b, 1730-1731, 1730b-1731b
Latex condoms, 146, 146b
Lay midwives, 267
LBW infants. *See* Low-birth-weight (LBW) infants.
LDR rooms. *See* Labor, delivery, and recovery (LDR) rooms.
LDRP rooms. *See* Labor, delivery, recovery, and postpartum (LDRP) rooms.
Lead, normal test ranges for, 1753t-1761t
Lead poisoning, 1432-1437
anticipatory guidance and, 1435
causes of, 1433, 1433b-1434b
diagnostic evaluation of, 1435
nursing care management in, 1436-1437, 1436b-1437b
pathophysiology and clinical manifestations of, 1433-1435, 1434f, 1435b
screening for, 1435
therapeutic management of, 1435-1437
Lead remedies, 835b
Learning disability, 1099-1100
Lecithin, 179
Lecithin/sphingomyelin (L/S) ratio, 179
Leff scope, 423
Left-sided heart failure, 1453
Leg cramps, 251, 252f, 254t-256t
Leg restraints, 1266
Leg rolls, 545f
Legal blindness, 1191
Legal considerations
in bleeding emergencies, 583b
in cardiac emergencies, 317b
in commitment for psychiatric care, 596b
in cryopreservation of embryos, 136b
in defining live birth, 603b
in delivery of care, 12-14, 13b, 14t
in documentation during childbirth, 471b
in drug testing during pregnancy, 239b, 330b
in early discharge after birth, 534, 535b
in electronic fetal monitoring during labor, 434b
Human Genome Project and, 165
in informed consent, 416b-418b, 546b
in intimate partner violence, 62, 63b
in mandatory reporting of domestic violence, 63b
in minor trauma during pregnancy, 373b
in obstetric triage, 443b
in reporting gonorrhea, 100b
in sterilization, 155, 155b
in substance abuse during pregnancy, 49, 239b, 330, 330b
in ultrasound examination, 200b
Legal guardians, informed consent and, 1246-1247
Legg-Calvé-Perthes disease, 1697-1698, 1697b-1698b
Legs
position for reducing edema and varicosities in, 251f
postpartum, 538b
Leg-up method, 148b-149b
Length
of newborns, normal findings, 626t-636t
in pediatric assessment, 890-891, 891f
Leopold maneuvers, 244, 245f, 423, 451, 452b, 452f
Lesbians, 47, 564
Let-down reflex, 687
Leukemia, 1507
chemotherapy in, 1510b-1513b, 1512-1513
classification of, 1507-1508
diagnostic evaluation in, 1508-1509, 1508t
drug toxicity and, 1513-1514, 1513b
late effects of treatment, 1509
nursing care plan for, 1510b-1512b
pain management in, 1509
pathophysiology of, 1508, 1508t
preparing child and family for procedures, 1509
prevention of complications and myelosuppression in, 1509-1512, 1510b-1512b
therapeutic management of, 1509
Leukocyte count, normal test ranges for, 1753t-1761t
Leukocyte esterase, 1529t-1530t
Leukocytosis
after childbirth, 530
in newborns at birth, 611
Leukokoria, 1197
Leukorrhea, 216, 254t-256t
Leukotrienes, 1339
Leuprolide, 92-93
Levator ani muscle, 67f
Levo-Dromoran. *See* Levorphanol.
Levonorgestrel, 153, 1745t-1748t
Levonorgestrel intrauterine system, 153, 154f
Levorphanol, 940t
Levothyroxine, 310, 310b
Lice, 1651-1652, 1651b-1652b, 1651f
Lichenification, 1635f
Lidocaine powder, 945
LidoSite Topical System, 946
Lie, fetal, 377, 378f-379f
Life cycle phases, 20
Life-limiting illness, 1147b
Lifestyle changes, preterm labor and, 491
Lift sheets, 1257
Ligaments, dislocation of, 1680-1681
Lightening, 387
Limb deficiency, 1695-1696
Limb salvage procedures, 1706
Limb-girdle muscular dystrophy, 1733
Limit setting
infants and, 970
parenting and, 812-814, 813b-814b
school-age children and, 1087
LINB. *See* Lamaze Institute for Normal Birth (LINB).
Linea nigra, 223, 223f
Linear growth, 845, 845t
Linear skull fractures, 1564-1565
Lingual tonsils, 1311-1312, 1312f
Lipase, 954
Lipomas, 115, 116t
Liposomal lidocaine cream (LMX), 945, 946b
Lipreading, 76, 1189, 1189b
Lips
physical assessment of, 911
upper, 171f
Liquid crystal skin contact thermometers, 897b
Lispro insulin, 303, 303t
Listening, 868-869
Listening to Mothers, 400
Lithium, 594, 597t
Lithium carbonate, breastfeeding and, 1745t-1748t
Lithotomy position
for childbirth, 385, 386f, 470f, 472-473
for pelvic examination, 77f, 80
for women with disabilities, 76, 77f
Live birth laws, 603b
Live births
definition of, 707b
race and, 790
rate of, 9
Liver
acute hepatitis and, 1406-1409, 1407t
biliary atresia and, 1410-1411, 1410b
changes during pregnancy, 226-227
cirrhosis and, 1409-1410, 1410b
fetal, 181
of infants, 954
newborn transition to extrauterine life and, 614
palpation of, 919b
transplantation of, 1409-1410
Living related donors, 1548
L-lysine, 105
LMX. *See* Liposomal lidocaine cream (LMX).
Lobar pneumonia, 1324
Lobular carcinoma, 118
Lobules of breasts, 69
Local infiltration anesthesia, 409
Lochia, 483b, 526-527, 527b, 538b
Lockjaw. *See* Tetanus.
Locomotion, infants and, 957, 957b, 959f
Locutionary stage of communicative development, 870-871, 871b
Longitudinal fetal lie, 377, 378f
Long-term care
in burns, 1671-1672, 1671f
in epilepsy, 1587-1592, 1592b
Long-term central venous access devices, 1281, 1281f
Lordosis
in children, 1699-1700, 1699f
during pregnancy, 224, 225f
Loss and grief. *See* Grief.
Low forceps, 510
Low income, definition of, 825
Low-birth-weight (LBW) infants, 707b
body temperature and, 713
caffeine and, 761
high cost of health care for, 6

Low-birth-weight (LBW) infants *(Continued)*
incidence of, 7, 28-29
kangaroo care and, 557, 723-724, 724f, 725b
maternal nutrition and, 273, 277
maternal substance abuse and, 755-756
mortality and, 790
preterm birth versus, 486-487
socioeconomic status and, 49
Low-cariogenic diet, 1033, 1033f
Low-density lipoproteins, 1474-1475
Lower extremity traction, 1687-1688, 1688f
Lower limb prosthesis, 1696
Lower limbs, development of, 171f
Lower reproductive tract infections, 95b
Lower respiratory tract, 1303
Lower respiratory tract infections, 1321, 1322t
bronchitis, 1321, 1322t
pneumonias, 1324-1326, 1324b, 1326f
respiratory syncytial virus and bronchiolitis, 1272, 1321-1324, 1322b, 1322t
Lower-segment cesarean birth, 513, 513f
Low-lying placenta, 361-362, 361f
Loxapine, 597t
Loxitane. *See* Loxapine.
L/S ratio. *See* Lecithin/sphingomyelin (L/S) ratio.
LTB. *See* Acute laryngotracheobronchitis (LTB).
Lumbar curve, restriction of, 250b
Lumbar puncture
bacterial meningitis and, 1576-1577
cerebral dysfunction and, 1556, 1556t-1557t
infection control practices for, 113b-114b
positioning of child for, 1267, 1267b, 1267f
Luminal. *See* Phenobarbital.
Lumpectomy, 121-122, 121f
Lungs
fetal, 180, 180f
maternal, 80, 222t, 500b
newborn transition to extrauterine life and, 610
pediatric assessment of, 914-915, 914b-915b, 914f
Luque-rod segmental spinal instrumentation, 1701
Luteal phase of the ovarian cycle, 72f, 73, 133b, 135
Luteinizing hormone (LH)
analysis of, 132-133
hypothalamic-pituitary cycle and, 72f, 73
Lying, school-age children and, 1088
Lyme disease, 1653-1654, 1653f
Lymph nodes
biopsy in Hodgkin's disease, 1515
breast cancer and, 120-122, 120f-121f
of children, 902, 902f
review of systems and, 79
Lymphadenopathy in Hodgkin's disease, 1515, 1515f
Lymphangiography, 1515
Lymphatics
of breast, 69
physical examination of, 80
Lymphocytes, pregnancy values of, 220t-221t
Lymphocytic thyroiditis, 1606-1607, 1607b
Lymphoid tissues, 844f, 846
Lymphomas, pediatric, 1514
Hodgkin's disease, 1514-1516, 1515f
non-Hodgkin's lymphoma, 1516
Lyon hypothesis, 166

M

Mackenrodt ligament. *See* Cardinal ligament.
Macrobiotics, 1365
Macrominerals, 1365
Macrosomia
fetal, 196-197, 298, 307-308, 499
in newborns, 735-736, 736f
Macules, 1634f
Magic as communication technique, 873b-874b
Magical thinking, 1021b, 1045
Magnesium
fertility and, 135
intake during pregnancy and lactation, 275t-276t, 282
nutritional significance of, 1377t-1379t
for pediatric cardiopulmonary resuscitation, 1359t
premenstrual syndrome and, 91
Magnesium sulfate, 374
breastfeeding and, 1745t-1748t
preterm labor and, 327b, 493-494, 495b
severe preeclampsia and, 343-346, 344b, 346b
signs of toxicity, 346b
tocolytic effects of, 347b
Magnet reflex, 621t-625t
Magnetic resonance imaging (MRI), 200
for breast cancer screening, 120b
in cardiac diagnosis, 1443t
in cerebral assessment, 1556-1557, 1556t-1557t
in head injuries, 1567
Mainstreaming, special needs child and, 1149
Major burn injuries, 1663, 1664t, 1665-1669, 1668f-1669f, 1668t
Malabsorption syndromes, 1423-1426, 1424b
Male condoms, 98, 146, 146f, 147b
Male genitalia
formation of, 182-183, 1108f
of newborns, 626t-636t
physical assessment of, 919-920, 919f-920f
Male reproductive system
disorders of, 1126-1127, 1127b
in newborns at birth, 618-619, 619f
Male sterilization, 154-155, 154f
Malformations
anorectal, 774, 774f, 1422-1423, 1422b
in cleft lip and cleft palate, 771-772, 771f-772f, 1411-1414, 1413f, 1414b-1415b
Malformations *(Continued)*
cranial, 1593
in esophageal atresia with tracheoesophageal fistula, 772-773, 772f, 1414-1417, 1415b-1416b
hydrocephalus and, 769, 1559b, 1593-1597, 1594f-1595f, 1595b-1596b
in skeletal limb deficiency, 1695-1696
type 1 diabetes mellitus and, 44-45
Malignant hyperthermia, 1253
Malignant lesions, 95b
Malnutrition
during pregnancy, 277-278
protein-energy, 1368-1370
Malocclusion, 971, 1092
Malposition of fetus, 500, 500b
Malpresentation of fetus, 500-501, 500f, 511f
Malrotation of intestine, 1422
Mammal bites and scratches
human bites, 1654
pet and wild animal bites, 1654, 1655b
Mammary duct ectasia, 116, 116t
Mammary glands. *See* Breasts.
Mammography, 59t, 118-120, 119f, 119t, 120b
Manual jaw control, cerebral palsy and, 1720, 1720f, 1723f
MAP. *See* Mean arterial pressure (MAP).
Maple syrup urine disease, 658t
Marasmus, 1369
Marax. *See* Theophylline.
March of Dimes Birth Defects Foundation, 31, 190b, 487
Marfan syndrome
with aortic root dilation, 312b
pregnancy and, 313-314
Marginal placenta previa, 361, 361f, 363
Marijuana, 50
breastfeeding and, 1745t-1748t
children's use of, 789
fetal and neonatal effects of, 50, 756t, 759
Marital status
high risk pregnancy and, 191b
insurance coverage and, 47
Masked deprivation, 859
Masks, infection control and, 113b-114b
Mass media, influence of, 861-864, 862b-863b
Massage
for pain management during labor, 270, 402, 443
to relieve menstrual discomfort, 88
of uterine fundus, 542, 542f
MAST. *See* Michigan Alcoholism Screening Test (MAST).
Mastectomy, 121-122, 121f
exercise after, 124-126, 125b-126b
home care after, 124, 125b
Mastitis, 586-587, 586f, 698
Mastodynia, 90t
Masturbation, 258
preschoolers and, 1052
toddlers and, 1022
Maternal adaptations
to labor, 390-392, 391b
to parenthood, 561-562, 561t, 562b, 563f
postpartum physiologic changes and, 525, 531-532
abdomen and, 527, 528f
breasts and, 529
cardiovascular system and
blood volume and, 529, 530b
cardiac output and, 530-531, 530t
varicosities and, 531
endocrine system and, 528
gastrointestinal system and, 529
immune system and, 531
integumentary system and, 531
musculoskeletal system and, 531
neurologic system and, 531
reproductive system and, 525-527, 526f, 527b, 528f
cervix and, 527
uterus and, 525-527, 526f, 527b
vagina and perineum and, 527
urinary system and, 528-529
to pregnancy. *See* Adaptation to pregnancy: maternal.
Maternal hypotension with decreased placental perfusion, 411b
Maternal hypothermia after anesthesia and analgesia, 420
Maternal mortality, 9, 189
in abruptio placentae, 365
antepartal hemorrhage and, 350
asthma and, 323
cystic fibrosis and, 324
in diabetes mellitus, 296
in ectopic pregnancy, 356
heart disease and, 311-312
hypertensive disorders and, 335
injuries and, 251-252
physical trauma and, 369-370, 372, 374
postpartum, 606-607, 606b
Maternal mortality rate, 7-8, 7b, 28-29, 49, 606
Maternal Role Attainment, 4b, 230, 231b, 561
Maternal self-image, postpartum, 548
Maternal sensitization, 766
Maternal serum alpha-fetoprotein (MSAFP), 203-204, 244
Maternal serum screening, definition of, 164
Maternal substance abuse, 755-761, 756f, 756t
alcohol and, 755-758, 756t, 757f, 758b
caffeine and, 761
cocaine and, 756t, 759-760
heroin and, 756t, 760, 760b
marijuana and, 756t, 759
methadone and, 760-761
methamphetamines and, 756t, 761
neonatal assessment and nursing care plan in, 761-762, 762b, 762t, 763f, 764b-765b
phencyclidine and, 760

Maternal substance abuse (Continued)
phenobarbital and, 761
tobacco and, 756t, 758-759, 759b
Maternal-fetal conflict, 513
Maternal-infant biostatistical terminology, 7b
Maternal-paternal-fetal relationship, 235b, 662f
Maternity bras, 251
Maternity nursing, 3, 15
access to health care and, 6
biostatistical terminology in, 7b
breastfeeding in workplace and, 10, 10f
and care during pregnancy and childbirth, 8-10
certified nurse-midwives, 9
childbirth practices and, 9, 9f
in community settings, 20, 29, 34
ethical issues in, 14
health care costs and, 6
Healthy People 2010 goals and, 5, 5b
high risk pregnancies and, increase in, 8
high-technology care and, 8, 8t
historic milestones in, 3-4, 4b
home care and. *See* Home care.
integrative health care and, 5, 5f
maternal mortality and, 7-8
Millennium Development Goals and, 5, 5b
model for, 3, 3b
reducing medical errors in, 6, 6b
research in, 14-15
standards of practice in, 12-14, 13b, 14t
trends in nursing practice, 10-12, 11b-13b, 12f
Maternity support hose, 251
Maturation, definition of, 842
Maturation of systems
infants and, 954-955
school-age children and, 1078
toddlers and, 1018
Mature minors, 1246
Mazzanti technique, 519, 520f
McBurney point, 226f, 227, 1399
McDonald procedure, 355, 356f
McGill Model of Nursing, 18t
McRoberts maneuver, 519-520, 520f
MDG. *See* Millennium Development Goals (MDGs).
Meal planning for diabetes mellitus, 1624-1626
Mean arterial pressure (MAP)
changes during pregnancy, 218, 219b
in pediatric physical assessment, 897-898, 898t
severe versus mild preeclampsia and, 336t
Mean corpuscular hemoglobin
normal test ranges for, 1753t-1761t
pregnancy values of, 220t-221t
Mean corpuscular hemoglobin concentration, 1753t-1761t
Mean corpuscular volume, 1753t-1761t
Measles, 983-984, 1058t-1064t
mumps, rubella vaccine. *See* Measles-mumps-rubella (MMR) vaccine.
Measles-mumps-rubella (MMR) vaccine, 983-984, 987t-988t
adolescents and, 1117
autism and, 1198
health screening recommendations for, 59t
Meat during pregnancy, 280t
Meatus
nasal, 911, 911f
urethral, 920-921
Mechanical methods for cervical ripening, 505
Mechanical ventilation for preterm infants, 714f, 715, 715t
Mechanism of labor, 388-390, 389f, 392
Meckel's diverticulum, 181, 1400-1401, 1400b
Meclofenamate, 89t
Meconium, 181, 202
in infant's stool, 614, 614b
Meconium aspiration syndrome, 474-475, 475b
postterm infants and, 733, 733f
Meconium ileus, 1346, 1347b, 1350, 1390
Meconium-stained infants, 474-475, 475b
Medicaid, 46
Medical abortion, early, 157-158
Medical history. *See* History; History taking.
Medical nutrition therapy, 290
Medical outreach, international, 12, 12f
Medication administration. *See* Administration of medications.
Medication history, current, 877
Medicine cups, 1274
Mediolateral episiotomy, 476, 476f
Medroxyprogesterone acetate, 1745t-1748t
Mefenamic acid, 89t, 1745t-1748t
Meiosis, 172
Melanotropin, 223
Melasma, facial, 223
Mellaril. *See* Thioridazine.
Menarche, 71, 1106
Meningismus, 1305b
Meningitis
aseptic, 1578, 1578t
bacterial, 1575-1578, 1576b-1578b, 1578t
posttraumatic, 1565b
Meningocele, 768-769, 1725b
Meningococcal vaccine, 985, 987t-988t
Menomune, 985
Menopause, 74
estrogen deprivation at, 66
FDA's approval of Premarin for symptoms of, 4b
smoking and, 50
Menorrhagia, 94
Menorrhea, 90t
Menstrual cycle, 71-73, 72f, 86
Menstrual disorders, 46, 86, 127
abnormal uterine bleeding, 95-96, 95b
alterations in cyclic bleeding, 93-94, 94b
amenorrhea in, 86-87
care management in, 96b
Menstrual disorders (Continued)
complementary and alternative therapies for, 89, 90t
cyclic perimenstrual pain and discomfort, 87-88
dysmenorrhea, 88-90, 88f, 89t
endometriosis, 91-93, 92f, 127
premenstrual syndrome, 90-91, 90b, 127
Menstruation
after childbirth, 528
breastfeeding and, 695
climacteric and menopause, 74
discomfort during, 88, 88f
menarche and puberty, 71, 1106
menstrual cycle, 71-73, 72f, 86
prostaglandins and, 73-74
Mental development, 849t, 850-852, 1086t-1087t
Mental health disorders in children, 789-790
Mental representation, 959-960
Mental retardation
alcohol exposure during pregnancy and, 50
aneuploidy and, 166
maternal phenylketonuria and, 311
teratogens and, 171f
Menu planning, 290
Meperidine
breastfeeding and, 1745t-1748t
for children, 942t
for pain management in labor, 407-408, 407b
Meperidine hydrochloride, 407
Meprobamate, breastfeeding and, 1745t-1748t
Mercury levels in fish, 279, 279b
Mercury toxicity, 1432, 1432b
Mercy killing. *See* Euthanasia.
Meromelia, 1695
Mesh grafts, 1668-1669, 1669f
Mesoderm, 174, 174f
Metabolic acidosis, 424, 1546
Metabolic disorders
diabetes mellitus. *See* Diabetes mellitus.
gestational diabetes mellitus and, 179, 296, 306-309
interventions in, 308-309
maternal and fetal risks in, 307-308
screening for, 308, 308f
hyperthyroidism, 309-310, 310b, 1607-1609, 1608b-1609b
hypothyroidism, 182, 310, 310b, 658t, 778, 1605-1606, 1606b
maternal phenylketonuria, 311
Metabolism
of child, 846-847
effects of immobilization on, 1677t
Metatarsus adductus, 1695
Metatarsus varus, 1695
Metered-dose inhalers, 1290-1291, 1337-1338, 1344b
Methergine. *See* Methylergonovine.
Methadone
breastfeeding and, 1745t-1748t
for children, 940t, 942t
fetal and neonatal effects of, 760-761
treatment during pregnancy, 51, 331
Methamphetamines, 51
adolescents and, 1139
fetal and neonatal effects of, 756t, 761
infants and, 996-997
Methergine. *See* Methylergonovine.
Methicillin-resistant *Staphylococcus aureus* (MRSA) infections, 1641
Methimazole, 1609b
Methotrexate
analgesics and, 357b
breastfeeding and, 1745t-1748t
ectopic pregnancy and, 356-358, 357b-358b
for gestational trophoblastic neoplasia, 360
for juvenile idiopathic arthritis, 1709
medical abortion and, 157-158
Methyldopa
breastfeeding and, 1745t-1748t
for treatment of hypertension, 348t
Methylergonovine, 580, 580b-581b
Metoprolol, 317t
MetroGel. *See* Metronidazole.
Metronidazole
for bacterial vaginosis, 111
breastfeeding and, 1745t-1748t
for giardiasis, 1397
for trichomoniasis, 112
Metrorrhagia, 90t, 93-94, 94b
Mexican culture
birth practices and, 448b, 449
clothing and, 260
eye contact and, 558
food patterns in, 292t-293t
health beliefs and practices in, 834, 838t-840t
infant feeding practices and, 680
nutrition and, 285
postpartum care and, 550b
MG. *See* Myasthenia gravis (MG).
Michigan Alcoholism Screening Test (MAST), 330
Miconazole, 112
Microcephaly, 769
Microminerals, 1365
Microphthalmia, 171f
Microwave heating of infant formula, 973b, 997
Midazolam, 939, 1252
Midcycle bleeding, 73. *See also* Metrorrhagia.
Middle adolescence, 1105, 1116t
Middle adulthood, 48
Middle childhood. *See* School-age children.
Middle children, 809b
Middle Eastern culture
expression of pain in childbirth in, 396b
food patterns in, 292t-293t
Middle-ear hearing loss, 1187
Midforceps, 510
Midline episiotomy, 476, 476f
Midpelvis, labor process and, 380-381, 381f
Midplane contracture, 498
Midwifery
health care costs and, 6, 47
Strategic Directions for Nursing and Midwifery Services of, 12, 12b

Midwives
certification of, 9
influence on maternal position in childbirth, 469
Mifepristone, 157-158
Migrant Clinicians Network, 34
Migrant workers, 33-34, 825, 830
Milk banking, 694
Milk ducts, plugged, 698
Milk ejection reflex, 687
Milk intake during pregnancy, 280t, 281-282
Milk stool, 614b
Millard rotational advancement technique, 1412
Millennium Development Goals (MDGs), 5, 5b, 7-8
Milwaukee brace, 1700-1701
Mind-altering drugs, 1139
Mineralocorticoids, 1611
Minerals
imbalances of, 1365, 1377t-1379t
infant nutrition and, 682
intake during pregnancy and lactation, 275t-276t, 280
calcium, 275t-276t, 280-282, 283b
fluoride, 283
iron, 275t-276t, 280
magnesium, 275t-276t, 282
potassium, 283
sodium, 282-283
zinc, 275t-276t, 283
Minilaparotomy in tubal ligation, 154, 155f
Minimal-change nephrotic syndrome, 1535-1536
Minipills, 151t, 152
Minor burn injuries, 1663, 1664t, 1665-1666
Minority-group membership and child health, 827-828, 827b-828b
Misbehavior, minimizing, 812, 813b
Miscarriage, 177, 351, 601
alcohol and, 252-253
caffeine consumption and, 253
clinical manifestations of, 352-353, 352f, 353t
complementary and alternative therapies and, 253b
disposition of fetal remains after, 354, 354b
heart disease during pregnancy and, 312
home care after, 354, 355b
incidence and etiology of, 351-352
laboratory findings in, 354
medical management of, 353t, 354
nursing care in, 354, 354b
types of, 352, 352f, 353t
Misoprostol
cervical ripening and, 506b
medical abortion and, 157-158, 354
for postpartum hemorrhage, 581b
Missed miscarriage, 352-354, 352f, 353t
Mitosis, 172
Mitral valve prolapse (MVP), 313
Mitral valve stenosis, 313
Mittelschmerz, 73
Mittelstaining, 93-94
Mixed conductive-sensorineural hearing loss, 1187
Mixed congenital heart defects, 1450, 1455b-1458b
MMR vaccine. *See* Measles-mumps-rubella (MMR) vaccine.
Modeling, preschoolers and, 1053
Moderate burn injuries, 1663, 1664t
Modified Blalock-Taussig shunt, 1466t
Modified radial mastectomy, 121, 121f
Modified Ritgen maneuver, 473, 474f
Modified Sims' position, 520-522, 521f
Modified-paced breathing, 402b
Molar pregnancy. *See* Hydatidiform mole.
Molding of newborn head, 619, 619f
Molestation, definition of, 1068
Molluscum contagiosum, 104, 1644t
Mongan Method of childbirth. *See* HypnoBirthing.
Mongolian spots, 617, 617f
Monilial infections, 697-698
Monitoring
of blood glucose levels
in diabetic children, 1620, 1620t, 1627-1628, 1627b-1628b, 1628f
during diabetic pregnancy, 304-305, 304b-305b
fetal, 423, 438-439
accelerations of fetal heart rate and, 429-430, 430b, 430f
amnioinfusion and, 436
baseline fetal heart rate and, 427-429, 428t-429f, 430t
basis for, 422-423
decelerations of fetal heart rate and, 430-433, 431b-433b, 431f
diabetic mother and, 305
documentation of, 424, 424b, 434b, 437-438, 438f
electronic, 422-427, 426t
documentation of, 424, 424b, 434b
evidence-based practice on, 425b
external, 425-426, 426f, 426t
internal, 426-427, 426t, 427f
nursing care plan for, 434b
fetal heart rate patterns and, 427-438, 428b
fetal heart rate response to stimulation and, 436
fetal oxygen saturation monitoring in, 436
fetal scalp blood sampling in, 436
intermittent auscultation in, 423-424, 423f, 424b
nursing care management in, 433, 433b, 435f
legal considerations in, 434b
patient and family teaching and, 437, 437b
pattern recognition and, 433-438, 435b, 437t
tocolytic therapy and, 436
umbilical cord acid-base determination and, 436-437, 437t
Monogenic disorders, 163
Mononucleosis, infectious. *See* Infectious mononucleosis.
Monosomies, 166-167
Monosomy X. *See* Turner's syndrome.
Monospot. *See* Spot test.
Monozygotic twins, 183-186, 187f, 810, 810b
Mons pubis, 65, 66f
Montgomery tubercles, 69, 217
Mood changes
chemotherapy-related, 1514
during pregnancy, 230
Mood disorders, postpartum. *See* Postpartum depression (PPD).
Mood stabilizers, 594, 597, 597t
Moon face, 1514
Moral development, 849t, 851-852
of adolescents, 1111
of preschoolers, 1045
of school-age children, 1081
Moral value of play, 856-857
Morbidity rates, 6
child, 786, 791
types of, 800-801, 801b
Morbidity statistics, definition of, 791
Mormon religion, 836t-837t
Morning sickness, 226, 254t-256t
Moro reflex, 621t-625t, 1555b
Morphine
breastfeeding and, 1745t-1748t
for children, 939, 940t, 945t
for burns, 1666-1667
unconscious, 1558
for pain management in labor, 414
Mortality rates, 6, 800-801, 801b
infant. *See* Infant mortality rate.
maternal. *See* Maternal mortality.
Mortality statistics, definition of, 790
Mosaicism, 167
Mosquito bites, 1649t-1650t
Mother-to-infant attachment, 554-557, 555t-556t, 557b
Motherwort, 582t
Motility disorders
in children
constipation, 1389-1391, 1391b
diarrhea, 1383-1389
acute, 1383, 1384t-1386t
diagnostic evaluation in, 1386-1387
etiology of, 1383-1386
gastrointestinal dysfunction and, 1394-1395, 1394b, 1395f
nursing care plan for, 1388-1389, 1389b-1390b
pathophysiology of, 1386
prevention of, 1387-1388, 1388b
therapeutic management of, 1387-1388, 1387b
Hirschsprung disease, 1389-1393, 1392b, 1392f
vomiting, 1393-1394
Motor function, cerebral dysfunction and, 1555
Motor vehicle injuries
abruptio placentae and, 365, 373
adolescents and, 1123-1124, 1123b
children and, 787, 788f
infants and, 787, 788f, 994-995, 995b, 995f
during pregnancy, 369-370, 373
school-age children and, 1095t
Motor vehicle injuries *(Continued)*
spinal cord injury in, 1740
toddlers and, 1033-1038, 1034t-1035t, 1036b, 1037f
Mouth
of children
care in unconscious child, 1561
nutritional status and, 884t-886t
physical assessment of, 911-912, 911b, 911f-912f
review of systems and, 882b
maternal
changes during pregnancy, 226
physical examination of, 80
review of systems and, 79
of newborns, 626t-636t
protection, infection control and, 113b-114b
Movies, influence on child development, 861
MRI. *See* Magnetic resonance imaging (MRI).
MRSA infections. *See* Methicillin-resistant *Staphylococcus aureus* (MRSA) infections.
MSAFP. *See* Maternal serum alpha-fetoprotein (MSAFP).
MSBP. *See* Munchausen syndrome by proxy (MSBP).
M-shaped position, 76, 77f
Mucocutaneous lymph node syndrome. *See* Kawasaki disease.
Mucosal protective agents, 1406
Mucosal ulceration, chemotherapy-related, 1513-1514, 1513b
Multichanneled implants, 1188
Multiculturalism. *See* Cultural competence.
Multidimensional measures and pain assessment in children, 931
Multifactorial conditions, 163
Multifactorial inheritance, 169, 188
Multifetal pregnancy, 183-188, 187f
dystocia and, 501
internal version and delivery in, 503
parental adjustment and, 810
prenatal care and, 261-263, 263b
sibling relationship and, 810, 810b
weight gain in, 277
Multigravida, definition of, 210
Multipara, definition of, 210
Multiparous women, 261
breast tenderness in the first trimester, 258
first stage of labor and, 440-441
full dilation in, 387-388
nutrition and, 286
older than 35 years of age, 261
pain management during labor for, 414
preeclampsia and, 337
pregnancy lightening in, 387
recognition of fetal movements, 215-216
second stage of labor and, 388, 466
sensory pain during labor of, 397
Multiple births. *See* Multifetal pregnancy; Twins.
Multiple sclerosis during pregnancy, 326-327

Multisystem, trauma and, 370, 374
Multivitamin-multimineral supplements, 284
Mummy restraint, 1266, 1266f
Mumps, 984, 1058t-1064t
Mumps vaccine, 59t, 984, 987t-988t
Munchausen syndrome by proxy (MSBP), 1067
Murmurs, 917, 917t
Muscle spasm in legs, 251, 252f
Muscles
fetal, 183
physical assessment of, 922
pubertal growth in, 1109
Muscular dysfunction, 1742-1743
botulism and, 1739-1740, 1739b-1740b
cerebral palsy and, 1716
diagnostic evaluation of, 1717, 1718b
early signs of, 1721b
education and, 1721-1722
family support in, 1723-1724, 1724b
hospitalization in, 1724
nursing care management of, 1720, 1721b-1723b
feeding and, 1720, 1720f, 1723f
pathophysiology of, 1716-1717, 1717b
therapeutic management of, 1717-1724, 1718f-1719f
Guillain-Barré syndrome and, 1735-1737, 1736b
muscular dystrophies and, 1733, 1733f
Duchenne, 1733-1735, 1733f, 1734b
spina bifida and, 1724-1731, 1725b, 1725f
complications in, prevention of, 1729
diagnostic evaluation of, 1725, 1726b, 1726f
family support and home care in, 1729-1730
latex allergy and, 1730-1731, 1730b-1731b
myelomeningocele sac care in, 1728-1729, 1729b
pathophysiology of, 1724-1725, 1726f
therapeutic management of, 1726-1730
spinal cord injuries and, 1740-1742, 1742f
spinal muscular atrophy and, 1731, 1731b
tetanus and, 1737-1739, 1738b
Muscular dystrophies, 1733, 1733f
Duchenne, 1733-1735, 1733f, 1734b
Musculoskeletal dysfunction, 1714
bone and soft-tissue tumors and, 1705, 1705b
osteosarcoma and, 1705-1707
clubfoot and, 775, 1693-1695, 1694f
developmental dysplasia of hip and
in children, 1691-1693, 1691b-1692b
in newborns, 774-776, 774f-775f, 775b
Musculoskeletal dysfunction *(Continued)*
Ewing's sarcoma and, 1707
idiopathic scoliosis and, 1700-1703, 1701f
immobilization and, 1676-1680, 1677t
juvenile idiopathic arthritis and, 1708-1711, 1712b
kyphosis and lordosis and, 1699-1700, 1699f
Legg-Calvé-Perthes disease and, 1697-1698, 1697b-1698b
metatarsus adductus and, 1695
osteogenesis imperfecta and, 1682, 1696-1697, 1696b
osteomyelitis and, 1703-1704, 1703b
rhabdomyosarcoma and, 1707-1708, 1708b
septic arthritis and, 1704
skeletal limb deficiency and, 1695-1696
skeletal tuberculosis and, 1705
slipped femoral capital epiphysis and, 1698-1699, 1699b
systemic lupus erythematosus and, 1711-1713, 1713b
traumatic injury and
amputation and, 1690-1691, 1690b
distraction for, 1690, 1690f
fractures and, 1681-1684, 1682b, 1682f, 1684b, 1686f
casts for, 1684-1686, 1685b, 1686f
soft-tissue injuries and, 1680-1681, 1680f
traction for, 1686-1690, 1687b, 1687f-1688f, 1689b
Musculoskeletal system
developmental milestones of, 184t-186t
of fetus, 183
maternal
adaptation to labor, 391
adaptations to pregnancy, 224-225, 225f, 371t
physical examination of, 80
postpartum adaptation of, 531
pediatric
congenital anomalies of, 774-776, 774f-775f, 775b
effects of immobilization on, 1677t
nutritional status and, 884t-886t
review of systems and, 882b
review of systems and, 79
Music for pain management during labor, 270, 401-402
Muslim culture, 836t-837t
birth practices and, 449
infant feeding practices and, 680
infertility management and, 132b
postpartum period and family planning in, 550b
Mutual play, 1048
Mutual storytelling, 873b-874b
MVP. *See* Mitral valve prolapse (MVP).
Myasthenia gravis (MG)
neonatal, 328
during pregnancy, 327-328, 327b
Mycotic stomatitis, 755
Myelodysplasia, 1724
Myelomeningocele, 768-769, 768f, 1725b, 1725f-1726f. *See also* Spina bifida.
Myelosuppression, 1509-1512
Myerson reflex, 621t-625t
Myocardial infarction, 1482b
Myoclonic seizures, 1583b-1584b
Myoepithelium of breasts, 69
Myomectomy, 94
Myometrium, 66, 68f, 85
Myopia, 1192b-1193b
Myositis ossificans, 1680
Myotonia, sexually stimulated, 74, 74t
MyPyramid, 288, 886, 1366
MyPyramid for Kids, 882, 1030b, 1054, 1366, 1367f
Myringotomy, 1316
Mythical-literal stage of spiritual development, 852

N

NAACOG. *See* Nurses Association of the American College of Obstetricians and Gynecologists (NAACOG).
NAEPP. *See* National Asthma Education and Prevention Program (NAEPP).
Nafarelin, 92-93
Nägele's rule, 230
Nails
changes during pregnancy, 224
of children, 901-902
fetal, 183
Naive instrumental orientation, 1045
Nalbuphine
breastfeeding and, 1745t-1748t
for pain management in labor, 408, 408b
intravenous administration of, 418
Naloxone
infants and, 760b
for pain management in labor, 409, 409b
for pediatric cardiopulmonary resuscitation, 1359t
Naming in perinatal loss, 601, 601b-602b
NANN. *See* National Association of Neonatal Nurses (NANN).
Naprosyn. *See* Naproxen.
Naproxen
breastfeeding and, 1745t-1748t
for children, 939t
to treat dysmenorrhea, 89t
Naproxen sodium, 89t
Narcan. *See* Naloxone.
Narcissism, 957
Narcotic agonist analgesics. *See* Opioid agonist analgesics.
Narcotic agonist-antagonist analgesics. *See* Opioid agonist-antagonist analgesics.
Narcotic antagonists. *See* Opioid antagonists.
Narcotics, breastfeeding and, 1745t-1748t
NAS. *See* Neonatal abstinence syndrome (NAS).
NAS system. *See* Neonatal abstinence syndrome (NAS) system.
Nasal administration of medication, 1282-1284, 1282b-1284b, 1284f
Nasal blockage in respiratory infection, 1305b
Nasal cannula
for preterm infant, 714, 714f, 1289
Nasal discharge, 1305b
Nasal stuffiness during pregnancy, 254t-256t
Nasoduodenal tubes, 1298
Nasogastric administration of medication, 1282, 1283b
Nasogastric tube feeding, 1295, 1295b-1297b, 1295f, 1295t
Nasojejunal tubes, 1298
Nasopharyngitis, 1307-1310, 1310b
National Association of Neonatal Nurses (NANN), 12-13
National Asthma Education and Prevention Program (NAEPP), 323, 324t
National Center for Health Statistics (NCHS), 31
National Childhood Vaccine Injury Act, 990-991
National Children's Study, 785
National Health Survey, 31
National Institute of Nursing Research, 6
National Institutes of Health, 6
National Migrant Resource Program, 34
National Quality Forum, 6, 6b
Native American culture
breastfeeding and, 559b
childbearing and parenting and, 25t-26t, 260, 447-448, 448f
communication and, 832
expression of pain in childbirth in, 396b
food patterns in, 292t-293t
health beliefs and practices in, 834, 838t-840t
umbilical amulets and, 260f
Native Americans, 827b
intimate partner violence and, 61
morbidity/mortality rates of, 6, 32
Natural family planning (NFP), 141
Nausea
chemotherapy-related, 1513
in hyperemesis gravidarum, 349-350
during labor, 392
during pregnancy, 226, 254t-256t, 290-291, 291f
Navane. *See* Thiothixene.
NCHS. *See* National Center for Health Statistics (NCHS).
Near-drowning, 1570-1572, 1571b
Near-miss SIDS. *See* Apparent life-threatening events (ALTE).
Near-term infants. *See* Late-preterm (near-term) infants.
Nebulizers, handheld, 1290-1291
NEC. *See* Necrotizing enterocolitis (NEC).
Neck
of children
nutritional status and, 884t-886t
physical assessment of, 902-903, 903b
review of systems and, 882b
hyperextension of, 921b

Neck *(Continued)*
maternal
physical examination of, 80
review of systems and, 79
of newborns, 626t-636t
Necrotizing enterocolitis (NEC), 731-732, 732b
Needleless system for parenteral fluid therapy, 1286-1287, 1287b, 1287f
Needles
intramuscular administration and, 1275
safe infection practices and, 113b-114b, 1264
Needlestick injuries, 1261f
Negativism, toddlers and, 1028-1029
Neglect, child, 1066, 1070b
clinical manifestations of, 1071b-1072b
nursing care plan for
history and interview and, 1070
physical assessment and, 1072
Negotiation in families, 17
Neisseria gonorrhoeae, 100, 241t
Neisseria meningitidis, 985
Neonatal abstinence syndrome (NAS), 760b, 762, 762t, 764
Neonatal abstinence syndrome (NAS) system, 763f
Neonatal deaths, definition of, 707b
Neonatal herpes simplex virus (HSV), 106
Neonatal intensive care units (NICUs)
parental support and, 726-727
preterm infants and
environmental concerns in, 712-713, 722-723, 723f
sepsis and infants in, 747
Neonatal mortality rate, definition of, 7, 7b, 790
Neonatal security in the hospital setting, 9
Neonates. *See* Newborns.
Neopresol. *See* Hydralazine.
Neostigmine, breastfeeding and, 1745t-1748t
Neotame during pregnancy, 281b
Nephritis, 247
Nephroblastoma. *See* Wilms' tumor.
Nephrotic syndrome, 1535-1538, 1536b-1537b, 1536f
Nerve block analgesia and anesthesia, 409
administration of, 418
allergic reactions to, 409
in children, 943b-944b
combined spinal-epidural, 414
epidural, 412-414, 412b-413b, 413f
intrathecal opioids and, 414-415
obesity and, 420
local infiltration, 409
nitrous oxide, 415
paracervical, 415
pudendal, 409, 410f
spinal, 409-412, 411b, 411f-412f, 420
Nerve deafness, 1187
Nervous system. *See* Neurologic system.
Nesting, 723
Nettle, 582t
Neural tissues, 844f
Neural tube defects (NTDs), 768-769, 768f, 1725b
folate and, 52, 273
prevention of, 44-45
screening for, 203-204
spina bifida. *See* Spina bifida.
teratogens and, 171f
Neuroblastomas, 1574-1575
Neurogenic diabetes insipidus. *See* Diabetes insipidus.
Neurologic assessment
in cerebral dysfunction, 1553-1555, 1554b-1555b, 1554f-1555f
of newborn reflexes, 637, 645-646
pediatric, 922-923, 923b, 923f-924f, 925t
Neurologic disorders during pregnancy, 326
Bell's palsy, 327
epilepsy, 326, 326b
multiple sclerosis, 326-327
Neurologic system
adaptation to labor, 391-392
adaptations to pregnancy, 225-226, 225f
brain tumors and, 1572-1574, 1573b-1574b
developmental milestones of, 184t-186t
of fetus, 182
of infants, 954
late-preterm infants and, 708t
maturation of, 846
neuroblastomas and, 1574-1575
physical examination of, 80
postpartum adaptation of, 531
review of systems and, 79
transition to extrauterine life and, 620-625, 621t-625t
Neuromuscular dysfunction, 1742-1743
botulism and, 1739-1740, 1739b-1740b
cerebral palsy and, 1716
diagnostic evaluation of, 1717, 1718b
education and, 1721-1722
family support in, 1723-1724, 1724b
hospitalization in, 1724
nursing care management of, 1720, 1721b-1723b
early signs of, 1721b
feeding and, 1720, 1720t, 1723t
pathophysiology of, 1716-1717, 1717b
therapeutic management of, 1717-1724, 1718f-1719f
Guillain-Barré syndrome and, 1735-1737, 1736b
muscular dystrophies and, 1733, 1733f
Duchenne, 1733-1735, 1733f, 1734b
spina bifida and, 1724-1731, 1725b, 1725f
complications in, prevention of, 1729
diagnostic evaluation of, 1725, 1726b, 1726f
family support and home care in, 1729-1730
Neuromuscular dysfunction *(Continued)*
latex allergy and, 1730-1731, 1730b-1731b
myelomeningocele sac care in, 1728-1729, 1729b
pathophysiology of, 1724-1725, 1726f
therapeutic management of, 1726-1730
spinal cord injuries and, 1740-1742, 1742f
spinal muscular atrophy and, 1731, 1731b
tetanus and, 1737-1739, 1738b
Neurontin. *See* Gabapentin.
Neuropathic bladder dysfunction, 1727
Neuropathy, chemotherapy-related, 1514
Neutral thermal environment (NTE), 709, 713, 730
Neutrophils, 220t-221t
Nevi, 618, 618f
New Ballard scale, 645f-646f, 650
New morbidity. *See* Pediatric social illness.
New York Heart Association (NYHA) classification of heart disease, 311-312
Newborns, 641
abduction from hospitals, 540
ABO incompatibility in, 766-767
assessment after delivery of, 480, 482f
bacterial meningitis in, 1577, 1577b
behavioral characteristics of, 637-641, 638b
response to environmental stimuli and, 640-641
sensory behaviors and, 639-640, 640f
sleep-wake states and, 637-639, 638f, 639b
birth trauma and, 742-743, 743t
central nervous system injuries in, 745
nursing care management in, 743
peripheral nervous system injuries in, 743-745, 744f
skeletal injuries in, 743, 743f
care of, after cesarean birth, 515-516, 516f
congenital anomalies in, 742, 767-768, 779
ambiguous genitalia, 776-777, 776f
anorectal malformations, 774, 774f
choanal atresia, 770, 770f
cleft lip and palate, 771-772, 771f-772f
clubfoot, 775
congenital diaphragmatic hernia, 770-771, 771f
developmental dysplasia of hip, 774-776, 774f-775f, 775b
encephalocele and anencephaly in, 768
esophageal atresia and tracheoesophageal fistula, 772-773, 772f
exstrophy of bladder, 776, 776f
Newborns *(Continued)*
genetic diagnosis of, 777
heart defects, 769-770
hydrocephalus, 769
hypospadias and epispadias, 776, 776f
intestinal obstruction, 773
microcephaly, 769
nursing care in, 777-779
omphalocele and gastroschisis, 773, 773f
polydactyly, 775-776
screening for, 777-778
spina bifida in, 768-769, 768f
teratomas, 777
constipation in, 1390
death of, 190, 598-600
acute distress in, 598-599
communicating and caring techniques and, 601-605, 601b-602b
actualizing the loss, 601-602, 601b-602b, 602f-603f
creating memories for parents to take home, 604-605, 605f
helping in acknowledgement and expression of feelings, 603-604
helping parents with decision making, 602-603
normalizing the grief process and facilitating positive coping, 604
physical needs of postpartum bereaved mother and, 604
providing sensitive care at and after discharge, 606
community resources in, 598b
cultural and spiritual needs of parents and, 605
documentation of, 605-606
family aspects of grief in, 600-601
funeral arrangements in, 603
intense grief in, 599-600
postmortem care of newborn and, 605, 605f
reorganization and, 600, 600b
with Down syndrome, nursing care plan for families with, 168b
early discharge of, 535b
effects of epidural block on, 415
family-newborn relationships and, 484, 484f
communication between parent and newborn in, 558-559, 558f-560f, 559b
early contact and, 557
grandparent adaptation in, 571-573, 572b, 572f-573f
parental attachment, bonding, and acquaintance in, 554-557, 555t-556t, 557b
paternal adjustment in, 564-565, 564t, 565f
sibling adaptation in, 484, 484f, 549, 549f, 570-571, 571f
follow-up checkup of, 551
growth and development of, 845
hemolytic disease in, 766-767
immediate assessment and care after birth, 475

Newborns *(Continued)*
infant-parent adjustment and, 559f-560f, 565-566
infections and
measures to control, 662, 662b
perinatally acquired, 748-755, 749b
candidiasis, 754-755, 755b
chlamydia, 754, 755b
cytomegalovirus, 752-753, 752f
Escherichia coli, 755-761
gonorrhea, 749
group B streptococcus, 754
hepatitis B virus, 750-751
herpes simplex virus, 753, 753f
human immunodeficiency virus, 751
screening for, 109b
parvovirus B19, 753-754
rubella, 752
syphilis, 749-750, 750b, 750f
toxoplasmosis, 749
tuberculosis, 754
varicella-zoster virus, 750
sepsis, 745-748, 745t, 747b-748b, 747t
maternal diabetes mellitus and, 299
maternal interactions after childbirth with, 483
maternal substance abuse and, 755-761, 756f, 756t
alcohol and, 755-758, 756t, 757f, 758b
caffeine and, 761
cocaine and, 756t, 759-760
heroin and, 756t, 760, 760b
marijuana and, 756t, 759
methadone and, 760-761
methamphetamines and, 756t, 761
neonatal assessment and nursing care plan in, 761-762, 762b, 762t, 763f, 764b-765b
phencyclidine and, 760
phenobarbital and, 761
tobacco and, 756t, 758-759, 759b
meconium aspiration syndrome and, 474-475, 475b
myasthenia gravis in, 328
nursing care of
from 2 hours after birth until discharge, 649-650
assessment of gestational age in, 645f-646f, 650, 651b
classification by gestational age and birth weight in, 651-652
umbilical cord care in, 651-652, 652f
from birth through the first 2 hours, 643, 647b
airway maintenance in, 646-648, 647f, 648b
body temperature maintenance in, 648
eye prophylaxis in, 648-649, 649b, 649f
initial assessment and Apgar scoring in, 643-646, 644b, 644t, 645f-646f, 647b

Newborns *(Continued)*
parent-infant bonding and, 649
vitamin K prophylaxis in, 649, 649b
care path for, 661
circumcision and, 667-669
community focus on, 667b
home care after, 669, 669b
pain management during, 668-669, 670b
procedure, 667-668, 667f-668f
conjugation of bilirubin and, 653
discharge planning and teaching in, 669, 676b
body temperature and, 671
care seats and, 673, 673b, 673f
clothing and, 673
elimination and, 671
immunizations and, 674
infant follow-up care and, 674
nonnutritive sucking and, 673-674, 674f
positioning and holding and, 671-672, 671b, 672f
rashes and, 672-673
respirations and, 671
sponge bathing, cord care, skin care and, 674, 675b
hyperbilirubinemia and, 644b, 665-667, 666f
hypocalcemia and, 657
hypoglycemia and, 656-657
infant feeding and, 663, 664b
infection control and, 662, 662b
intramuscular injection and, 663-665, 663f, 665b
jaundice associated with breastfeeding and, 656
laboratory and diagnostic tests in, 657, 657b, 658t
heel stick and, 659, 659f, 660b
urine specimen collection and, 660-661, 661f
venipuncture and, 659-660, 660b
physical injuries and, 652-653, 653f
physiologic jaundice and, 653-656, 654b, 654f, 655t, 656b
protective environment and, 661-662, 662b
safety factors and, 662
social interactions and, 662, 662b-663b, 662f
nutrition and feeding of, 643, 678, 704. *See also* Breastfeeding.
benefits of breastfeeding and, 678-679
contraindications to breastfeeding and, 246, 679
cultural influences on, 680
guidelines for breastfeeding support, 680b
lactation and breastfeeding in, 682-700, 682f-683f
nursing care management and, 685, 686b

Newborns *(Continued)*
breastfeeding complications and, 689-691, 692f
duration of feedings in breastfeeding and, 687-689
expressing and storing breast milk and, 691-693, 692f-693f, 693b
frequency of feedings in breastfeeding and, 687
infant assessment and, 685, 685b
latch-on in breastfeeding and, 686-687, 688f
maternal assessment before breastfeeding and, 685
maternal employment and, 693
milk banking and, 694
milk ejection in breastfeeding and, 687
positioning in breastfeeding and, 543-544, 685-686, 687f-688f
supplementation of breastfeeding in, 689, 690b
weaning from breastfeeding and, 693
nutrient needs and, 680-682
parent education on formula-feeding and, 700-704, 701f-702f, 703b
opioid antagonists and, 409
pain assessment in, 933-934, 934t
peptic ulcer disease in, 1405b
physical assessment of, 625-636
abdomen and, 645-646
baseline measurements of physical growth and, 637
from birth through the first 2 hours, 644b, 645-646
chest and, 645-646
general appearance and, 636, 637f
genitalia and, 645-646
initial, 644b, 645-646
neurologic assessment and, 637, 645-646
normal findings in, 626t-636t
vital signs and, 626t-636t, 636-637
preterm. *See* Preterm infants.
Rh incompatibility in, 766-767
shoulder dystocia and, 520
spina bifida in, 1726-1728
standards of care for, 13b
transition to extrauterine life, 609-625
cardiovascular system and, 610-611
gastrointestinal system and, 613-614, 614b
hematopoietic system and, 611
hepatic system and, 614, 615b, 616f
immune system and, 614-615
integumentary system and, 615-618, 616b, 617f-618f
neuromuscular system and, 620-625, 621t-625t
reflexes and, 620, 621t-625t, 625
renal system and, 613
reproductive system and, 618-619, 619f
respiratory system and, 609-625

Newborns *(Continued)*
skeletal system and, 619-620, 619f-620f, 621t-625t
thermogenic system and, 611-613, 612f
urinary tract disorders in, 1531b
visual acuity testing in, 906-907
Newborns' and Mothers' Health Protection Act, 4b, 517, 534
Niacin, 1374t-1377t
Nicotine, 49, 1745t-1748t
NICU Network Neurobehavioral Scale (NNNS), 762
NICUs. *See* Neonatal intensive care units (NICUs).
Niemann-Pick disease, 161
Nifedipine
breastfeeding and, 1745t-1748t
during pregnancy, 317t
preterm labor and, 493-494, 495b
for treatment of hypertension, 348t
Night crying, 977t
Nightmares, preschoolers and, 1055
Nighttime fears, 977t
Nighttime feeding, 977t
Ninety-degree–ninety-degree traction, 1688, 1688f
Nipple carcinoma, 118
Nipple pores, 70f
Nipple reconstruction, 122
Nipples, 69, 70f
breastfeeding and, 684
preparation for, 246-247, 247f
soreness during, 694-695, 695f, 697, 697b
changes during pregnancy, 217, 223
of children, 913
discharge from, 69, 115-116
breast cancer and, 119
mammary duct ectasia and, 116
intraductal papilloma and, 116-117, 116t
postpartum changes in, 539b-540b
sexual response of, 74t
Nipple-stimulation contraction test, 206
Nissen fundoplication, 1395, 1395f
Nitrazine test for pH, 445b
Nitrites, 1529t-1530t
Nitrofurantoin, 1745t-1748t
Nitrous oxide
for analgesia during labor, 415-416
for burn injuries, 1667
Nits, 1651-1652, 1651b-1652b, 1651f
NNNS. *See* NICU Network Neurobehavioral Scale (NNNS).
Nodules, 1634f
Noise, hearing loss and, 1191, 1191b
Nolvadex. *See* Tamoxifen.
Nomogram, 654f, 655-656
Nonadherent retained placenta, 578
Nonbreastfeeding jaundice, 656
Non-communicating Children's Pain Checklist, 934
Noncommunicating hydrocephalus, 1593-1595
Nondirectiveness, principle of, 163
Non–English-speaking women in labor, 449
Non-Hodgkin's lymphoma, 1516

Noninfectious irritants, pulmonary dysfunction caused by
aspiration pneumonia and, 1330-1331
environmental tobacco smoke exposure and, 1333, 1333b
foreign body aspiration and, 1330, 1330b
smoke inhalation injuries and, 1332-1333, 1332b
Nonnutritive sucking
discharge planning and teaching in, 673-674, 674f
during painful procedures, 936-938, 936f
preterm infants and, 720, 720f
Nonoxynol-9 (N-9)–based spermicides, 98, 130, 146
Nonpharmacologic pain management
during childbirth and labor, 397-406, 420-421
acupressure and acupuncture in, 403-404, 405f
aromatherapy in, 405, 405b
biofeedback in, 405
birth plans and, 398, 398b
conscious breathing in, 402, 402b, 402f
effleurage and counterpressure in, 402-403
energy work in, 402
heat and cold application in, 404-405
hypnosis in, 405
imagery and visualization techniques in, 401
intradermal water block in, 405-406, 405f
music in, 401-402
nursing care plan for, 404b
relaxation in, 399b, 401, 401f
touch and massage in, 402
transcutaneous electrical nerve stimulation in, 403, 404b, 404f
water therapy in, 403, 403f
in children, 935-938, 936f, 937b, 938f
after pediatric heart surgery, 1471
during circumcision, 668-669, 670b
for immediate postpartum period, 543
Nonreassuring fetal heart rate patterns, 434-435, 435b, 467b
fundal pressure and, 475
Nonspecific vaginitis. *See* Bacterial vaginosis.
Nonsteroidal antiinflammatory drugs (NSAIDs)
for children, 938-939, 939t
for juvenile idiopathic arthritis, 1709
preterm labor and, 494-496
for primary dysmenorrhea, 88-89, 89t
Nonstress test (NST), 204-205
before external cephalic version, 502
indications for, 205b
interpretation of, 205, 205f-206f, 206t
Nontunneled catheters, 1279
Nonverbal communication
with children, 873b-874b
culturally sensitive, 833b
infants and, 871
preschoolers and, 1046f
Normalization, special needs child and, 1148-1149, 1159, 1159b, 1204
Normodyne. *See* Labetalol hydrochloride.
Normoglycemia. *See* Euglycemia.
North America, cultural influence on child health in, 827-828, 827b-828b
North American blastomycosis, 1646t
Nose
of children
nutritional status and, 884t-886t
physical assessment of, 910-911, 911f
review of systems and, 882b
of newborns, 626t-636t
physical examination of, 79
protection, infection control and, 113b-114b
Nosebleeding. *See* Epistaxis.
Novobiocin, 1745t-1748t
NPO status, 1285, 1285b
NSAIDs. *See* Nonsteroidal antiinflammatory drugs (NSAIDs).
NST. *See* Nonstress test (NST).
NTDs. *See* Neural tube defects (NTDs).
NTE. *See* Neutral thermal environment (NTE).
Nubain. *See* Nalbuphine.
Nuchal cord, 176, 481f
Nuclear brain scan, 1556t-1557t
Nuclear families, 16-17, 17f
Nulligravida, definition of, 210
Nullipara, definition of, 210
Nulliparous women
episiotomy rate for, 469
first stage of labor and, 440-441
hyperemesis gravidarum and, 349
older than 35 years of age, 261
pain management during labor for, 414
recognition of fetal movements, 215-216
second stage of labor and, 388, 466
sensory pain during labor of, 397
Numbness during pregnancy, 254t-256t
Numeric pain scale, 932t-933t
Nurse-activated analgesia, 943b-944b
Nurse-family system, 19
Nursemaid's elbow, 1680-1681
Nurse-midwives, 9, 266-267
Nurses. *See* Maternity nursing; Pediatric nursing.
Nurses Association of the American College of Obstetricians and Gynecologists (NAACOG), 4b
Nursing bottle caries, 1033, 1033f
Nursing care plan
cultural competence and, 26-27, 40
integrating cultural competence with, 26
Nursing care plan *(Continued)*
maternal
for adolescent pregnancy, 260-261, 261f, 262b
breast cancer and, 126b
in breastfeeding, 699b
for cardiovascular disorders during pregnancy, 314-319
for dysfunctional labor, 499b
for electronic fetal monitoring during labor, 434b
for first stage of labor, 456-460, 457t, 458b-459b
ambulation and positioning and, 459-460, 460f-462f, 461b
elimination and, 457t, 459
emergency interventions and, 466, 467b
general hygiene and, 456, 457t
nutrient and fluid intake and, 456-459, 457b-459b, 457t
standards of care and, 455-456
supportive care and, 460-466, 462b, 463f, 464t, 465b
in home health care, 39
for pain management during labor, 404b
for placenta previa, 364b
for postpartum care in vaginal birth, 537, 539b-540b, 549-552
for postpartum hemorrhage, 580b
for postpartum women, postpartum care
for pregnancy complicated by pregestational diabetes, 307b
for preterm labor, 490b
pediatric
for arthritis, 1712b
for asthma, 1341-1342, 1342b
for burns, 1669-1670, 1669b-1670b
for cerebral palsy, 1722b-1723b
for cleft lip or palate, 1415b
for congestive heart failure, 1461b-1462b
for diabetes mellitus, 1624b-1625b
for drug-exposed newborns, 765b
for end-of-life care, 1147b, 1169-1174, 1170b-1171b, 1170f, 1173b
for families with neonates with Down syndrome, 168b
for high risk infants, 728b-730b, 737b
for leukemia, 1510b-1512b
for seizure disorders, 1588b-1590b
Nursing caries, 1033, 1033f
Nursing diagnoses, definition of, 796
Nursing practice
cultural competence and, 40
home care and guidelines for, 35-36
standards of practice in, 12-14, 13b, 14t
trends in, 10-12, 11b-13b, 12f
Nursing process
in acute pediatric respiratory infections, 1306b
in breastfeeding, 686b
in cardiac disease during pregnancy, 315b-316b
in cerebral palsy, 1721b
in community nursing, 802-805, 802b-804b
in contraception, 131b
drug-exposed newborns and, 764b
in dystocia, 504b
in early discharge after birth
physical needs and, 538b
psychosocial needs and, 548b
in family-centered home care, 1212-1214, 1212b-1214b
in fetal monitoring, 433b
in home care, 40b
in infertility, 131b
in labor, 441b
in late-preterm and preterm infant care, 712b
in menstrual disorders, 96b
in mild preeclampsia, 340b
in neonatal sepsis, 748b
in newborn care, 647b
in nursing care during pregnancy, 238b
in nutrition during pregnancy, 287b
in overweight children or adolescents, 1131b
in pain during labor, 417b
in pediatric diarrhea, 1390b
in pediatric nursing, 795-796
critical thinking and, 794-795
documentation and, 796
evidence-based thinking and, 795, 796t
health care planning and, 796-797
in placental previa, 363b
in postpartum depression, 595b
in postpartum hemorrhage, 579b
in postpartum structural disorders of the uterus and vagina, 579
in pregestational diabetes, 300b-301b
in preterm labor and birth, 489b
in transition to parenthood, 573b
Nursing shortage, 1205
Nutrition
assessment of, during fourth stage of labor, 480
fertility and, 135
health promotion and, 51-53, 52b
high risk pregnancy and, 191b
during lactation, 285-286
adequate dietary intake and, 288-290, 290b
cultural influences and, 291-293, 292t-293t
diet history and, 286-288, 288b, 289t
energy needs and, 286
nursing care management and, 286-293, 287b
neonatal, 643, 678, 704. *See also* Breastfeeding.
benefits of breastfeeding and, 678-679
contraindications to breastfeeding and, 246, 679

Nutrition (Continued)
cultural influences on, 680
formula feeding and, 700-704, 701f-702f, 703b
guidelines for breastfeeding support, 680b
lactation and breastfeeding in, 682-700, 682f-683f
nursing care management and, 685, 686b
breastfeeding complications and, 689-691, 692f
duration of feedings in breastfeeding and, 687-689
expressing and storing breast milk and, 691-693, 692f-693f, 693b
frequency of feedings in breastfeeding and, 687
infant assessment and, 685, 685b
latch-on in breastfeeding and, 686-687, 688f
maternal assessment before breastfeeding and, 685
maternal employment and, 693
milk banking and, 694
milk ejection in breastfeeding and, 687
positioning and, 543-544, 685-686, 687f-688f
supplementation of breastfeeding in, 689, 690b
weaning from breastfeeding and, 693
nutrient needs and, 680-682
nutrient intake during labor, 456-459, 457b-459b, 457t
pediatric
acute renal failure and, 1544
adolescents and, 1118-1119, 1118f
assessment of, 881-886, 883b, 884t-886t
burns and, 1666, 1671
congestive heart failure and, 1463-1464
diabetes mellitus and, 1620-1621
infants and, 972-976, 972t, 973b, 976b
inflammatory bowel disease and, 1403
influence on growth, 857, 859b
preschoolers and, 1053-1054, 1054b, 1054f
preterm infants and, 710, 712b, 717-720, 718b, 720f, 724f, 728b-730b
respiratory infections and, 1307
school-age children and, 1089-1090
short-bowel syndrome and, 1425
toddlers and, 1029-1031, 1030b
unconscious child and, 1560-1561
during pregnancy, 52, 273-274, 274f, 281b, 294
adequate dietary intake and, 288-289, 290b
adolescent pregnancy and, 52, 262b, 285

Nutrition (Continued)
cardiovascular disorders and, 316
cholecystitis and cholelithiasis and, 325b
constipation and, 291
counseling on, 286b
cultural influences on, 260
energy needs and, 275-277, 275t-276t
hazards of restricting adequate weight gain and, 277-279, 278t, 279b
pattern of weight gain and, 277, 278f
weight gain and, 277, 281b
exercise and, 285
fluid intake and, 279-280
hyperemesis gravidarum and, 350
mild preeclampsia and, 285, 342-343, 343b
minerals, vitamins, electrolytes and, 275t-276t, 280-284, 281b-283b
nausea and vomiting and, 290-291, 291f
nutrient needs before conception and, 273, 274b
patient teaching in, 245
pica and food cravings and, 284-285, 285f
preeclampsia and, 285
promotion in postpartum period, 544, 546f
protein intake and, 279, 279b, 280t
recommendations for daily intakes of nutrients, 274-275, 275t-276t
vegetarian diet and, 293
Nutrition therapy for anorexia nervosa and bulimia nervosa, 1134-1135
Nutritional assessment, pediatric, 881-886, 883b, 884t-886t
Nutritional counseling for obese adolescents, 1130-1131
Nutritional deficiencies, 52
Nutritional disturbances
delayed wound healing and, 1637t
food sensitivity and, 1370-1374, 1370b-1373b
mineral imbalances and, 1365, 1377t-1379t
protein-energy malnutrition and, 1368-1370
vegetarian diets and, 1365-1366, 1366b
vitamin imbalances, 1363-1365, 1374t-1377t
Nutritional history, 239
Nuts during pregnancy, 280t
NYHA classification of heart disease. *See* New York Heart Association (NYHA) classification of heart disease.
Nystatin, 755b, 1745t-1748t

O

OASIS. *See* Outcome and Assessment Information Set (OASIS).

Obesity
adolescents and, 1119, 1127-1132, 1128f, 1131b-1132b
childhood, 786-787, 787f, 1054b
definition of, 1127
gestational diabetes mellitus and, 309
health risks and, 52
high risk pregnancy and, 8
pharmacologic pain management during labor and, 420
during pregnancy, 52, 277-279
Object permanence, 959, 960f
Objective information, assessment and, 802
Oblique fetal lie, 377, 379f
Oblique fractures, 1682
Obstetric emergencies
amniotic fluid embolism, 479, 522-523, 523b
Emergency Medical Treatment and Active Labor Act, 443b
prolapsed umbilical cord in, 455b, 467b, 520, 521f, 522b
rupture of uterus, 372, 522
shoulder dystocia, 519, 520f
Obstetric history, 239
Obstetric measurements, 382t
Obstipation, 1389
Obstruction, airway
in children, 1320b, 1358-1360, 1358b, 1358f, 1360f
in newborns at birth, 646-648, 647f, 648b
in pregnant women, 319b, 320, 320f
Obstructive congenital heart defects, 1447-1450, 1450f, 1451b-1453b
Obstructive sleep-ordered breathing, 1353
Obstructive uropathy, 1533-1534, 1534f
Obturator foramen, 69f
Occipitoposterior position, 500, 500b
Occiput, 390
Occult prolapse, 520, 521f
Occupational hazards, high risk pregnancy and, 191b
Occupational history, 240
Occupational therapy, 1710
Occurrence risk, 163
OCPs. *See* Oral contraceptive pills (OCPs).
Ocular alignment, 904-905, 904f-905f, 905b, 906t
Ocular media clarity, 906t
Oculomotor nerve (cranial nerve III), 925t
Odor
in cystoceles and rectoceles, 592
parent-infant communication and, 559
response of newborn to, 640
Office of Research on Women's Health, 4b
Olanzapine, 597, 597t
Older fathers (older than 35 years), 567
Older mothers (older than 35 years), 48, 566b, 567, 568b
Olfactory nerve (cranial nerve I), 925t
Oligoarthritis, 1709

Oligohydramnios, 181-182, 192b, 198, 518
Oligomenorrhea, 93
Omalizumab, 1339-1340
Omphalocele, 181, 773, 773f
Onlooker play, 855-856
Only children, 809-810, 809b
Oocytes, 172, 173f
Oogenesis, 172, 173f, 183
Open fractures, 1682
Open skull fractures, 1564-1565
Open wounds, 1639-1640
Open-Glottis pushing, 402b
Open-glottis pushing, 402b
Ophthalmia neonatorum, 648-649
Ophthalmic ointment, 649, 649b
Ophthalmoscopic examination, 903-904, 904b, 904f
Opiates, 51
Opioid agonist analgesics, 407, 407b-408b
Opioid agonist-antagonist analgesics, 408, 408b
Opioid antagonists, 408-409, 409b
Opioids
after cesarean birth, 516
for children, 938-940, 939b, 940t-942t
monitoring side effects in, 947-948, 947b-948b, 949f
unconscious, 1558, 1558b
fear of addiction in, 936b
in immediate postpartum period, 543b
intrathecal, epidural and, 414-415
for pain management in labor, 406
obesity and, 420
respiratory depression and, 948b
side effects of, 415, 947b
Opisthotonos, 921b
Optic administration, 1282-1284, 1282b-1284b, 1283f
Optic nerve (cranial nerve II), 925t
Optimal birth spacing, 140b
Opt-out approach to HIV screening, 329
Oral administration of medication, 943b-944b, 1273-1275, 1274b, 1275f, 1284b
Oral candidiasis, 755
Oral contraceptive pills (OCPs), 87, 326b
breakthrough bleeding and, 94
chronic hypertension and, 349
combined estrogen-progestin pills, 151-152, 151t
flowchart for missed tablets, 152f
potential complications, signs of, 151b
diabetes mellitus and, 306
fibrocystic changes and, 115
gestational trophoblastic neoplasia and, 360
for primary dysmenorrhea, 89
progestin-only pills, 151t, 152
Oral hygiene, nursing care during labor, 457t
Oral intake during labor, 456-457, 457t
Oral poliovirus vaccine, 983
Oral progestins, 151t, 152
Oral rehydration therapy, 1387-1388, 1387b

Oral sex. *See* Cunnilingus.
Oral stage of psychosexual development, 848-849
Oral temperature, 894t-895t, 895b-896b
Ordinal position, 809-810, 809b, 809f
Organ donation
newborn death and, 603
terminally ill children and, 1172
Organ systems, development of, 846
Orgasm during pregnancy, 258
Orgasmic phase of sexual response cycle, 74, 74t
Orifice of urethra, 66f
Orifice of vagina, 66f
Orogastric administration of medication, 1282, 1283b
Orogastric tube feeding of preterm infants, 719, 719b
Oropharynx, 912, 912f
Orthodontic treatment, 1120
Orthopedic surgery, 1718-1719
Orthostatic hypotension
in children, 899-900, 900b
during pregnancy, 254t-256t
Ortolani maneuver, 619-620, 620f
Ortolani test, 775, 775b, 1692
Oscillometers, 897-898
Osmolality, normal ranges for, 1529t-1530t, 1753t-1761t
Ossification, 846
fetal, 183
pelvic, 68
Osteogenesis imperfecta, 1682, 1696-1697, 1696b
Osteomyelitis, 1703-1704, 1703b
Osteoporosis
calcium and, 52
smoking and, 50
Osteosarcoma, 1705-1707
Ostomies, 1299-1300
Otic administration of medication, 1282-1284, 1282b-1283b
Otitis media, 1314-1317, 1314b-1315b
Otitis media with effusion, 1314b, 1315-1316
Otoscopic examination, 908-910, 908b, 908f-909f
Oucher Pain Scale, 932t-933t, 935
Outcome and Assessment Information Set (OASIS), 1209
Outlet contracture, 498
Outlet forceps, 510, 510f
Out-of-hospital births, 9
Ova, 67-68
conception and, 172, 173f
fertilization of, 141
formation of, 172, 173f
stage of, 174-175, 174f
viability of, 129-130
Ovarian cycle, 72f, 73
Ovarian cysts during pregnancy, 369
Ovarian ligament, 67f-68f
Ovarian tumors, 135
Ovaries, 67f-68f, 68
assessment across the life cycle, 70t
hormone secretion from, 74
infertility and, 130b
Over-the-counter medication
for colds in children, 1306b
during pregnancy, 252
to treat dysmenorrhea, 89
Over-the-counter pregnancy tests, 211-212, 211b, 211f
Over-the-counter urinary tract infection detection kits, 246, 246f
Overuse syndromes in school-age children, 1096
Overweight, 52
children and, 1127
definition of, 1127
during pregnancy, 278-279, 279b
Ovulation, 68, 141
after birth, 528
breasts during, 69-70
dysfunction, 135
home predictor test kits for, 144-145, 145f
mammary gland tissue and, 68
prostaglandins and, 73-74
Ovum. *See* Ova.
Oxacillin, breastfeeding and, 1745t-1748t
Oxford Database of Perinatal Trials. *See* Cochrane Pregnancy and Childbirth Database.
Oximetry, 1290, 1290b, 1290f
Oxycodone
breastfeeding and, 1745t-1748t
for children, 938-939, 940t, 942t
OxyContin. *See* Oxycodone.
Oxygen consumption changes during pregnancy, 222t
Oxygen hoods, 714, 714f, 1289, 1289f
Oxygen saturation, 1332b, 1753t-1761t
Oxygen tents, 1289-1291, 1289f
Oxygen therapy
in hemorrhagic shock, 582
pediatric, 1289-1290, 1289b, 1289f
for preterm infants, 713-717, 714f, 715t
Oxygen-induced carbon dioxide narcosis, 1289-1290
Oxytocin
changes during pregnancy, 227t
for induction or augmentation of labor, 505, 507-508, 508b-509b, 508f
magnesium sulfate and, 346b
in myasthenia gravis, 328
lactation and, 683, 683f
for postpartum hemorrhage, 581b
for postpartum uterine contractions, 525
uterine tachysystole with, 508, 508b-510b
Oxytocin-stimulated contraction test, 206

P

Paced breathing. *See* Conscious breathing.
Pacemakers, pediatric, 1476-1477, 1477b
Pacific Islanders, 827b
Pacifiers, 673-674, 674f, 689, 970-971
aspiration of, 991
breastfeeding and, 690b
sudden infant death syndrome and, 689
Pain
in abruptio placentae and placenta previa, 362t, 365-366
acute postpartum, 539b-540b
in appendicitis, 368
in cerebral palsy, 1719, 1722b-1723b
child's response to, 930b
expression of, 395
history of, 876b
during labor and childbirth
anxiety about, 394
factors influencing response to, 395-397, 396b
neurologic origins of, 394-395, 395f
management of. *See* Pain management.
neonatal, 933-934, 934t
perception of, 395
Pain assessment
in children, 929, 930b
behavioral measures and, 929, 930f, 931t
with chronic illness and complex pain, 935
with communication and cognitive impairment, 934
cultural awareness in, 934-935
multidimensional measures and, 931
physiologic measures and, 929-930
self-report measures and, 930-931, 932t-933t
in newborns, 933-934, 934t
Pain Indicator for Communicatively Impaired Children (PICIC), 934
Pain management
nonpharmacologic
during childbirth and labor, 397-406, 420-421
acupressure and acupuncture in, 403-404, 405f
aromatherapy in, 405, 405b
biofeedback in, 405
birth plans and, 398, 398b
childbirth education and, 398-401, 398b-399b
conscious breathing in, 402, 402b, 402f
effleurage and counterpressure in, 402-403
energy work in, 402
heat and cold application in, 404-405
hypnosis in, 405
imagery and visualization techniques in, 401
intradermal water block in, 405-406, 405f
music in, 401-402
nursing care plan for, 404b
relaxation in, 399b, 401, 401f
touch and massage in, 402
transcutaneous electrical nerve stimulation in, 403, 404b, 404f
water therapy in, 403, 403f
in immediate postpartum period, 543
pediatric, 950
after heart surgery, 1471
Pain management *(Continued)*
in burns, 1666-1667, 1670
in cerebral palsy, 1719
during circumcision, 668-669, 670b
for comatose child, 1558
complementary, 938
in juvenile rheumatoid arthritis, 1710
in leukemia, 1509
nonpharmacologic, 935-938, 936f, 937b, 938f
pharmacologic, 938-950
calculation of dosage in, 939-940, 939t-941t
epidural analgesia, 945, 945f
evaluation of effectiveness of, 948-950
monitoring side effects in, 947-948, 947b-948b, 949f
NSAIDs, 938-939, 939t
patient-controlled analgesia, 942-945, 942f, 943b-944b, 945t
postoperative, 1253
routes of analgesic administration in, 943b-944b, 945-946, 946b, 947f
timing of, 946-947
in sickle cell disease, 1499-1500, 1499b
for terminally ill children, 1165b, 1169-1170, 1170b
perinatal education and, 270
pharmacologic. *See* Pharmacologic pain management.
Pain rating scales for children, 930-931, 932t-933t
Painting, hospitalized children and, 1234, 1234f
Palate, cleft, 771-772, 771f-772f
Palate, development of, 171f
Palatine tonsils, 1311-1312, 1312f
Palivizumab, 1323
Palliative care, 1164, 1165b
Pallor
during childbirth, 395
racial groups and differences in, 901t
Palmar erythema, 224, 224b, 254t-256t
Palmar grasp reflex, 621t-625t, 955
Palms, 902
Palpations
of abdomen
in fetal assessment, 423-424
in first stage of labor, 451, 452b, 452f
in pediatric physical assessment, 918-919, 918b-919b, 919f
in cardiac assessment, 1443
of external genitalia, 81, 81f
Palpitations during pregnancy, 254t-256t
Pancreas
cystic fibrosis and, 324-325
fetal, 182
Pancreatic fibrosis, 1346-1347
Panhypopituitarism, 1600b
Pant-blow breathing, 402b
Papanicolaou test, 59t, 83
after hysterectomy, 85
introduction of, 4b

Papanicolaou test *(Continued)*
during pregnancy, 84-85
in prenatal period, 241t
procedure, 83b, 84f
Paper-doll technique, 886, 887f
PapNet test, 83b
Papules, 1634f
Paracervical block, 415
Paracetamol. *See* Acetaminophen.
Parachute reflex, 956, 957f
Paradoxic respirations, 915b
Parallel play, 855-856, 855f
Paralysis, birth-related, 743-745, 744f
Paraplegia, 1741
Parathyroid disorders, 1609
hyperparathyroidism, 1610-1611, 1610b
hypoparathyroidism, 1609-1610, 1609b-1610b
Parathyroid hormone, 227t
Parent education
on cardiopulmonary resuscitation, 727
on formula feeding, 700-704, 701f-702f, 703b
on hyperbilirubinemia, 667
parent-infant attachment and, 556t
Parental empowerment, 1152, 1159
Parental overprotection, 1153b
Parent-child relationship, 17, 1235
Parenteral fluid therapy
complications in, 1288-1289, 1288b-1289b
enteral feeding and, 1294b
infusion pumps in, 1287
removal of peripheral intravenous lines in, 1288, 1288b
safety catheters and needleless systems in, 1286-1287, 1287b, 1287f
securement of peripheral intravenous lines in, 1287-1288, 1287f
site and equipment in, 1285-1286, 1285b-1286b, 1286f
Parenthood. *See also* Parent-infant relationship; Parents.
adolescent fathers and, 567
adolescent mothers and, 566-567, 566b
adopted child and, 815-816, 815b-816b, 815f
attachment, bonding, acquaintance and, 554-557, 555t-556t, 557b
communication between parent and infant in, 558-559, 558f-560f, 559b
culture and, 568-569
divorce and, 816-818, 817b
dual-earner family and, 819
employer accommodation of, 819
family size and configuration and, 807-808, 808f
foster parenting and, 819
infant-parent adjustment in, 559f-560f, 565-566
lesbian couple's adjustment to, 564
limit setting and discipline and, 812-814, 813b-814b
maternal adaptation to, 561-562, 561t, 562b, 563f
motivation for, 810-811
older fathers and, 567
Parenthood *(Continued)*
older mothers and, 48, 566b, 567, 568b
parental sensory impairment and, 569-570
hearing-impaired parent and, 570
visual impairment and, 570, 570b
parent-infant contact and, 548, 557-558, 557f
paternal adaptation to, 564-565, 564t, 565f
personal aspirations and, 569
preparation for, 811
preterm infants and, 710-726, 711f, 712b
reconstituted family and, 819
roles in, 807
single parenting and, 818-819
social support and, 567-568
socioeconomic conditions and, 569
spacing of children and ordinal position and, 808-810, 809b, 809f
styles of control in, 812
tasks and responsibilities in, 560-561
transition to, 548, 554, 559-560, 574-575, 811-812, 811f-812f
nursing care management, 573-574, 573b-574b
working mother and, 819
Parent-infant contact, 548, 557-558, 557f
phototherapy for hyperbilirubinemia and, 666b
Parent-infant relationship, 649
attachment, bonding, acquaintance and, 554-557, 555t-556t, 557b
communication and, 558-559, 558f-560f, 559b
contact and, 548, 557-558, 557f
Parenting, cultural considerations in, 25t-26t
Parent-professional partnership, 1211-1212, 1211b-1212b
Parents
adjustment to multiple births, 810
adolescents and, 1111-1112, 1112b, 1116t
communicating with, 867-870, 869b-870b
communication between infants and, 558-559, 558f-560f, 559b
dying child and, 1170, 1172-1173
in end-of-life decision making, 1166, 1166b
of hearing impaired children, 1190
of hospitalized child
information for, 1237
participation in child's care, 1237-1238
reactions to hospitalization, 1224, 1224b
relationship with child, 1235
impact of preterm labor and birth on, 496b
impact of special needs child on, 1149-1150, 1150b
Parents *(Continued)*
parenting process and. *See* Parenthood.
presence during pediatric procedure, 1249-1250
Parent-to-parent support, special needs children and, 1158
Parity, 210-211, 211t
Paroxysmal abdominal pain in infants, 1001-1002, 1002b, 1003f
Partial bicornuate uterus, 132f
Partial mastectomy, 121, 121f
Partial seizures, 1583b-1584b
Partial thromboplastin time, normal test ranges for, 1753t-1761t
Partially sighted, 1191
Partial-thickness burns, 1642t, 1661-1662, 1662f-1663f, 1664t
Parvovirus B19, 753-754
Passageway, 475
Passageway, birth process and, 378
bony pelvis and, 378-381, 380f-381f, 382t-383t
soft tissues and, 381-384, 383f
Passenger, birth process and, 376
attitude and, 377, 378f-380f
fetal lie and, 377, 378f-379f
fetal position and, 377-378, 378f-380f
head size and, 376-377, 377f
presentation and, 377-378, 378f-379f
Past health history, 78-79
Patau's syndrome, 167
Patch, 1634f
Patellar reflexes, 341, 341f, 924f
Patent ductus arteriosus (PDA), 716, 730-731, 1448b-1450b
Paternal adaptations
to parenthood, 564-565, 564t, 565f
to pregnancy, 233-234, 233b, 233f, 235b
Pathologic jaundice, 655
Patient-controlled analgesia
in children, 942-945, 942f, 943b-944b, 945t
during labor, 407
Patient-controlled epidural anesthesia, 413-414
Patterned-paced breathing, 402b
Pavlik harness, 775f, 778
PCP. *See* Phencyclidine (PCP).
PCV. *See* Pneumococcal conjugate vaccine (PCV).
PDA. *See* Patent ductus arteriosus (PDA).
PDQ II. *See* Prescreening Developmental Questionnaire (PDQ II).
Peak expiratory flow meters (PEFMs), 1336, 1343-1344, 1343b
Peak expiratory flow rate (PEFR), 1336, 1336b
Pearson attachment, 1688
Pectoralis major muscle, 70f
Pedestrian injuries, 787, 1037
Pediatric nursing, 797-798
atraumatic care and, 792
community-based, 799-802, 800b-801b, 801f, 805
nursing process in, 802-805, 802b-804b
Pediatric nursing *(Continued)*
family-centered care and, 792, 792b
future trends in, 797, 797b
Healthy People 2010 and, 785-786
nursing process in, 795-796
critical thinking and, 794-795
documentation and, 796
evidence-based practice and, 795, 796t
health care planning and, 796-797
philosophy of care in, 791
role of pediatric nurse in, 792-794, 793b, 795b
Pediatric Pain Questionnaire (PPQ), 931
Pediatric procedures, 1300-1301
alternative feeding techniques and, 1294b
family teaching and home care and, 1298
gastrostomy feeding, 1296-1298, 1298f
gavage feeding, 1295, 1295b-1297b, 1295f, 1295t
nasoduodenal and nasojejunal tubes, 1298
total parenteral nutrition, 1298
artificial ventilation, 1291-1294, 1291f-1292f, 1292b-1294b, 1294f
bronchial drainage, 1291
compliance after, 1253-1256, 1256b
informed consent for, 1245-1247
inhalation therapy, 1289-1291, 1289b-1290b, 1289f-1290f
measurement of fluid intake and output and, 1285, 1285b
parenteral fluid therapy in
complications in, 1288-1289, 1288b-1289b
infusion pumps in, 1287
removal of peripheral intravenous lines in, 1288, 1288b
safety catheters and needleless systems in, 1286-1287, 1287b, 1287f
securement of peripheral intravenous lines in, 1287-1288, 1287f
site and equipment in, 1285-1286, 1285b-1286b, 1286f
positioning for, 1266-1267, 1267b, 1267f
postprocedural support and, 1250-1251, 1251f
psychologic preparation for, 1247-1250, 1247b-1249b
related to elimination
enemas and, 1299, 1299b
family teaching and home care and, 1300
ostomies and, 1299-1300
specimen collection in
blood, 1271-1272, 1271b-1272b, 1271f
respiratory secretions, 1272-1273
stool, 1270-1271, 1270b
urine, 1267-1270, 1268b-1270b, 1268f, 1269t

Pediatric procedures *(Continued)*
supportive care during, 1250, 1250b
surgery
postoperative care, 1252-1253, 1253b, 1254t
preoperative care, 1251-1252, 1251f, 1252t
tracheostomy, 1291-1294, 1291f-1292f, 1292b-1294b, 1294f
Pediatric social illness, 786
Pediatric specula, 81
Pediatric surgery
in cerebral palsy, 1718-1719
for cleft lip, 1412
for cleft palate, 1412
in congenital heart disease, 1470b
in epilepsy, 1586
in esophageal atresia, 1416
in head injuries, 1568
hypertrophic pyloric stenosis and, 1419
in inflammatory bowel disease, 1403
informed consent for, 1245-1247
limb salvage procedures, 1706
postoperative care in. *See* Postoperative care.
preoperative care in. *See* Preoperative care.
in scoliosis, 1701
in Wilms' tumor, 1541-1542
Pediatric undernutrition. *See* Failure to thrive (FTT).
Pediculosis capitis, 1651-1652, 1651b-1652b, 1651f
Pedophilia, definition of, 1068
Peer groups
adolescents and, 1112-1113, 1113f, 1116t
influence on child health, 826-827
of school-age children, 1081-1083, 1082f
Pelvic dystocia, 498
Pelvic examination, 80-85
of adolescents, 78, 78b, 81
after hysterectomy, 85
assisting with, 80, 80b
collection of specimens in, 83, 83b, 84f
equipment for, 81, 81f
external inspection in, 81
external palpation in, 81, 81f
fear of, 80, 80b
health screening recommendations for, 59t
internal examination in, 82, 82f, 83b
in placenta previa, 362
during pregnancy, 84-85
relaxation techniques during, 80-81, 80b
vaginal wall examination in, 83-85, 84f
vulvar self-examination, 81-82
and women with disabilities, 76, 77f
Pelvic floor, 217f
Kegel exercises for, 246
labor process and, 382-384
Pelvic hematomas, 577-578
Pelvic inflammatory disease (PID), 101-103
Pelvic inlet, 69f, 380
Pelvic joints during pregnancy, 224
Pelvic muscle exercises. *See* Kegel exercises.
Pelvic outlet, labor process and, 380-381, 380f
Pelvic rocking, 249f, 250b, 545f
Pelvis, 68, 69f
fracture during pregnancy, 371
labor process and, 378-381, 380f-381f, 382t-383t
Penetrating abdominal trauma, 372
Penetrating wounds, ocular damage and, 1191-1193
Penicillin
allergic reaction to, 1485b
during pregnancy, 318
sickle cell anemia and, 1498b
for streptococcal sore throat infection, 1311
for syphilis, 101
Penicillin G, breastfeeding and, 1745t-1748t
Penis
hypospadias and epispadias of, 776, 776f
pediatric physical assessment of, 919, 919f
sexual response of, 74t
Pentobarbital, breastfeeding and, 1745t-1748t
Peptic ulcers
pediatric, 1404-1406, 1405b
during pregnancy, 226
Perceptive deafness, 1187
Perceptual abilities, first stage of labor and, 446
Percocet. *See* Oxycodone.
Percodan. *See* Oxycodone.
Percussion in cardiac assessment, 1443
Percutaneous umbilical blood sampling (PUBS), 197-198, 202-203, 203f
Pericardium 6 acupressure, 290-291, 291f
Perimenopause, 46, 74
Perimetrium, 68f
Perimortem cesarean delivery, 374
Perinatal asphyxia, 734, 736
Perinatal care choices, 265-267, 267b
Perinatal continuum of care, 35, 35b, 36f
Perinatal education, 263-271, 264b
Perinatal loss, grief and, 598-600
acute distress in, 598-599
community resources and, 598b
family aspects of grief in, 600-601
intense grief in, 599-600
nursing care management in, 601
communicating and caring techniques and, 601-605, 601b-602b
actualizing the loss, 601-602, 601b-602b, 602f-603f
creating memories for parents to take home, 604-605, 605f
helping in acknowledgement and expression of feelings, 603-604
helping parents with decision making, 602-603
normalizing the grief process and facilitating positive coping, 604
Perinatal loss, grief and *(Continued)*
physical needs of postpartum bereaved mother and, 604
providing sensitive care at and after discharge, 606
cultural and spiritual needs of parents and, 605
postmortem care of newborn and, 605, 605f
reorganization and, 600, 600b
Perinatal mortality
in abruptio placentae, 366
cystic fibrosis and, 324
definition of, 707b
in diabetic mellitus, 296
postterm infants and, 733
socioeconomic status and, 49
Perinatal mortality rate, definition of, 7, 7b
Perinatal services, home care and, 36-37, 43
Perinatal transmission of human immunodeficiency virus, 109, 328, 329b
Perinatally acquired infections, 748-755, 749b
candidiasis, 754-755, 755b
chlamydia, 754, 755b
cytomegalovirus, 752-753, 752f
Escherichia coli, 755-761
gonorrhea, 749
group B streptococcus, 754
hepatitis B virus, 750-751
herpes simplex virus, 753, 753f
human immunodeficiency virus, 751
parvovirus B19, 753-754
rubella, 752
syphilis, 749-750, 750b, 750f
toxoplasmosis, 749
tuberculosis, 754
varicella-zoster virus, 750
Perineal body, 66f
Perineum, 66, 66f
adaptations to pregnancy, 217
assessment of, 81
laceration during birth process, 475-476, 476f, 577
nursing care during labor, 457t
postpartum assessment of, 483b
postpartum care of, 540, 541b
postpartum changes in, 527, 538b
Periodic abstinence. *See* Natural family planning (NFP).
Periodic breathing, 709
Periodontal disease
high risk pregnancy and, 191b
school-age children and, 1092
toddlers and, 1031
Periodontal infections, preterm birth and labor and, 247, 488
Peripartum cardiomyopathy (PPCM), 312
Peripheral intermittent infusion device, 1279
Peripheral intravenous lines (PIVs), 1281b
removal of, 1288, 1288b
securement of, 1287-1288, 1287f
Peripheral lock, 1245, 1279
Peripheral nerve, birth injury of, 743t
Peripheral nervous system, birth-related injuries of, 743-745, 744f
Peripheral precocious puberty, 1603
Peripheral pulses, 626t-636t
Peripheral stem cell transplantation, 1522
Peripheral vascular disease, delayed wound healing in, 1637t
Peripheral vascular system
physical examination of, 80
review of systems and, 79
Peripheral vision, 907
Peripherally inserted central catheters (PICC), 1279-1281, 1281b
Peritoneal dialysis, 1547
Peritoneal lavage and trauma during pregnancy, 373
Peritoneum, 66
Periventricular-intraventricular hemorrhage (PV-IVH), 731
Perlocutionary stage of communicative development, 870-871, 871b
Permanency planning, 1204-1205
Permissive parents, 812
Perphenazine, 597t
PERRLA acronym, 903
Persistent pulmonary hypertension (PPHN), 733-734
Persistent urinary tract infection, 1530
Personal aspirations and parenthood and, 569
Personal protective equipment (PPE)
home care and, 42
infection control and, 113b-114b
Personal relationships during pregnancy, 231-234, 231b, 232f
Personal space, cultural traditions and, 23-24, 76b
Personality development, 848-850, 849t, 850f
Personal-social behavior
of preschoolers, 1046-1047, 1047f
of school-age children, 1086t-1087t
of toddlers, 1023
Pertussis, 983, 1058t-1064t, 1326
Pertussis vaccine. *See* Tetanus-diphtheria-acellular pertussis (Tdap) vaccine.
Pessaries, 590-592, 591f
PET. *See* Positron emission tomography (PET).
Pet and wild animal bites, 1654, 1655b
Petechiae, 1633
differences in color changes and, 901t
neonatal birth trauma and, 652
Pethidine. *See* Meperidine hydrochloride.
PGD. *See* Preimplantation genetic diagnosis (PGD).
PGF2α *See* Prostaglandin F2α (PGF2α).
PGs. *See* Prostaglandins (PGs).
PH
normal test ranges for, 1753t-1761t
urine, 1529t-1530t
Phallic stage of psychosexual development, 848-849

Phantom limb pain, 1691, 1706
Pharmacologic pain management
after cesarean birth, 516
during childbirth and labor, 406, 420-421
analgesia and anesthesia, 406, 406b
nerve block analgesia and anesthesia. *See* Nerve block analgesia and anesthesia.
systemic, 406-409, 407b-409b
general anesthesia, 415-416, 416f
in immediate postpartum period, 543, 543b
maternal hypothermia after, 420
nursing care management in, 416, 417b
administration of medication, 418-420, 419f
informed consent and, 416-418, 416b-418b
self-assessment of pain and, 416
obese woman and, 420
preparation of patient for, 418
safety and general care in, 419-420, 419f
sedatives in, 406
signs of potential problems in, 418-419
timing of administration of, 418
pediatric, 938-950
after pediatric heart surgery, 1471
for burns, 1666-1667
calculation of dosage in, 939-940, 939t-941t
in cerebral palsy, 1719
during circumcision, 668-669, 670b
epidural analgesia, 945, 945f
evaluation of effectiveness of, 948-950
monitoring side effects in, 947-948, 947b-948b, 949f
NSAIDs, 938-939, 939t
opioids, 938-940, 939b, 940t-942t
patient-controlled analgesia, 942-945, 942f, 943b-944b, 945t
postoperative, 1253
routes of analgesic administration in, 943b-944b, 945-946, 946b, 947f
timing of, 946-947
Pharyngeal tonsils, 1311-1312, 1312f
Phencyclidine (PCP)
breastfeeding and, 1745t-1748t
fetal and neonatal effects of, 51, 760
Phenobarbital
breastfeeding and, 1745t-1748t
fetal and neonatal effects of, 761
for seizures, 1592b
Phenothiazines, 406
Phenotype, 166
Phenylalanine, 280, 332-333, 1753t-1761t
Phenylketonuria (PKU)
ethnicity and, 161
maternal, 311
newborn screening for, 658t, 777
Phenytoin, breastfeeding and, 1745t-1748t
Pheochromocytoma, 1615-1616, 1616b
Phimosis, 1535t
Phobia, school, 1101
Phocomelia, 1695
Phosphorus
chronic renal failure and, 1545-1546
nutritional significance of, 1377t-1379t
Photoscreening, 905
Phototherapy
home care and, 37, 40-41
hyperbilirubinemia and, 644b, 665-667, 666f
Phrenic nerve paralysis, birth-related, 745
Physical abuse
of child
clinical manifestations of, 1071b-1072b
nursing care plan for
history and interview and, 1070
physical assessment and, 1072, 1072b
of children, 1066-1068, 1067b
history of, 240
Physical activity. *See* Exercise.
Physical assessment
from birth through the first 2 hours, 644b, 645-646
in child maltreatment, 1072-1073, 1072b
of children, 888-889, 889f, 927
abdomen and, 917-919, 917f-919f, 918b-919b
age-specific approaches to, 888t
anus and, 921
blood pressure in, 897-900, 898f-899f, 898t-899t, 899b-900b
body temperature in, 893, 893b-897b, 894t-895t
cardiac disease and, 1443
cerebellar function and, 922-923, 923b
cerebral function and, 1551
chest and, 912-914, 913f
cranial nerves and, 923, 924f, 925t
ears and, 907-910, 907f-909f, 910t, 923f
extremities and, 921-922, 922f
eyes and, 903-907, 903f-905f, 905b, 906t, 907b
general appearance in, 900-901
genitalia and, 919-921, 919f-920f, 921b
growth measurements in, 889-892, 890b, 891f-892f
head and neck and, 902-903, 902b-903b
heart and, 915-917, 915f-916f, 916b, 917t
joints and, 922
lungs and, 914-915, 914b-915b, 914f
lymph nodes and, 902, 902f
mouth and throat and, 911-912, 911b, 911f-912f
muscles and, 922
nose and, 910-911, 911f
Physical assessment *(Continued)*
preparation of child for, 886-888, 887b, 887f, 888t, 889f
pulse in, 893-897, 897t
reflexes and, 923, 923f-924f
respiration in, 897
sequence of examination in, 886
skin and, 886, 892, 901-902, 901t, 902f
spine and, 921, 921b
health screening recommendations for, 59t
of newborn, 625-636
baseline measurements of physical growth and, 637
general appearance and, 636, 637f
initial, 644b, 645-646
neurologic assessment and, 637
normal findings in, 626t-636t
vital signs and, 626t-636t, 636-637
of woman
nutritional status and, 287-288, 289t
in pregestational diabetes mellitus, 300b-301b
Physical disabilities, health assessment and, 76, 77f
Physical examination, 79-85
in abruptio placentae, 366
in cardiovascular disorders during pregnancy, 315b-316b
in dystocia, 504b
in early discharge after birth, 538b
in the first stage of labor, 449-454
expected maternal progress and, 450t
fetal heart rate and pattern and, 451, 453f
general systems assessment and, 449
Leopold's maneuvers and, 451, 452b, 452f
Standard Precautions and, 449, 450b
uterine contractions and, 392, 394, 440-441, 450t, 451-453, 453b
vaginal examination and, 454, 454f
vital signs and, 449-451, 451b, 451f
in follow-up prenatal visits, 241-242, 242b-243b, 243f
gynecologic portion of. *See* Pelvic examination.
in initial prenatal care visit, 240-241
in mild preeclampsia, 340b
in pharmacologic pain management during labor, 417b
in preterm labor, 489b
Physical fitness, health promotion and, 53-54, 53b, 53f-54f
Physical growth
of adolescents, 1107-1109
of school-age children, 1086t-1087t
Physical injuries in newborns, 652-653, 653f
Physical punishment, 814
Physical therapy
cerebral palsy and, 1720-1721
juvenile rheumatoid arthritis and, 1710
Physician-health care team decision making in end-of-life care, 1166
Physicians, 9, 266
Physiologic adaptations
to labor
fetal adaptation, 390
maternal adaptation, 390-392, 391b
postpartum, 525, 531-532
abdomen and, 527, 528f
breasts and, 529
cardiovascular system and
blood volume and, 529, 530b
cardiac output and, 530-531, 530t
varicosities and, 531
endocrine system and, 528
gastrointestinal system and, 529
immune system and, 531
integumentary system and, 531
musculoskeletal system and, 531
neurologic system and, 531
reproductive system and, 525-527, 526f, 527b, 528f
afterpains and, 526
cervix and, 527
uterus and, 525-527, 526f, 527b
vagina and perineum and, 527
urinary system and, 528-529
to pregnancy, 212, 212b, 227-228, 338b
after trauma, 212, 213t
breasts and, 217, 217f
cardiovascular system and, 218-219, 218f-219f, 219b, 220t-221t, 338b
endocrine system and, 227, 227t, 338b
gastrointestinal system and, 226-227, 226f
hematologic system and, 338b
integumentary system and, 223-224, 223f, 224b
musculoskeletal system and, 224-225, 225f
neurologic system and, 225-226, 225f
renal system and, 217f, 222-223, 223t, 338b
respiratory system and, 218f, 219-222, 222t
signs of pregnancy and, 212, 213t
uterus and, 212-216, 214f-216f
vagina and vulva and, 216-217, 216f-217f
Physiologic anemia of pregnancy, 320, 954
Physiologic anorexia, toddlers and, 1029
Physiologic jaundice, 653-656, 654b, 654f, 655t, 656b
Piaget's cognitive development theory, 849t, 850-851
adolescents and, 1110-1111
infants and, 958-960, 960f

Piaget's cognitive development theory *(Continued)*
preschoolers and, 1044-1045, 1045b
school-age children and, 1079-1081, 1080f
toddlers and, 1019-1021, 1020f, 1021b
Pica during pregnancy, 284-285, 285f
PICC. *See* Peripherally inserted central catheters (PICC).
PICIC. *See* Pain Indicator for Communicatively Impaired Children (PICIC).
PID. *See* Pelvic inflammatory disease (PID).
Piercing and tattooing, 1120-1121
Pigeon toe, 922
Pigmentation during pregnancy, 223, 223f, 254t-256t
Pinard fetoscopes, 244, 245f, 423
Pinch test for inverted nipple, 247, 247f
Pinna, 907, 909, 909f
Pinocytosis, 178
Pinworms, 1397-1398, 1398b
Pioneering, siblings and, 809
Piper forceps, 500
PIPP. *See* Premature Infant Pain Profile (PIPP).
Pitocin. *See* Oxytocin.
Pitting edema, 340, 341f
Pituitary dysfunction, 1600
in comatose child, 1560-1561
diabetes insipidus and, 1604-1605, 1604b
hypopituitarism and, 1600-1602, 1601b-1602b
pituitary hyperfunction and, 1602-1603
precocious puberty and, 1603-1604, 1603b
syndrome of inappropriate antidiuretic hormone and, 1605, 1605b
Pituitary hormones, postpartum changes in, 528
PKU. *See* Phenylketonuria (PKU).
Placebos, 939
Placenta
care after delivery of, 480
functions of, 177-179, 178b, 178f, 181
postpartum healing and, 526
postterm pregnancy and, 518
premature separation of. *See* Abruptio placentae.
retained, 578
separation and expulsion of, 477-480, 477f, 479f, 482f
severe versus mild preeclampsia and, 336t
structure of, 176-179, 177f-178f
ultrasound of, 197
uteroplacental blood flow and, 214
variations in, 366, 367f
Placenta accreta, 366, 578
Placenta increta, 366, 578
Placenta percreta, 366, 578
Placenta previa, 360, 360f
clinical manifestations of, 361-362, 362t
incidence and etiology of, 361, 361b
Placenta previa *(Continued)*
maternal and fetal outcomes in, 362
nursing care management in, 363b
diagnosis and, 362, 363b
home care and, 364
hospital care and, 363-364
vaginal examination and, 362, 364
nursing care plan for, 364b
types of, 361, 361f
Placental abruption. *See* Abruptio placentae.
Placental hormones, postpartum changes in, 528
Plagiocephaly, 1009-1010, 1009f
Plan B emergency contraception, 153
Plantar grasp reflex, 620, 620f, 621t-625t
Plantar reflex, 621t-625t
Plants, poisonous and nonpoisonous, 996, 1427b-1429b
Plaque, skin, 1634f
Plasma volume
after childbirth, 530
increase during pregnancy, 220t-221t
normal test ranges for, 1753t-1761t
PlastiBell, 667-668, 668f
Plastic bags, strangulation and, 994
Plateau phase of sexual response cycle, 74, 74t
Platelet count
of newborn at birth, 611
normal ranges for, 1491t, 1753t-1761t
pregnancy values of, 220t-221t
Platelet transfusion in leukemia, 1512
Platypelloid pelvis, 381, 383t
Play
after pediatric procedures, 1255b
blind children and, 1194
cognitively impaired child and, 1180-1181, 1180f-1181f
as communication technique, 873b-874b
hospitalized child and, 1232-1235, 1233b, 1233f-1234f, 1235b
infants and, 960-963, 964t
during pediatric procedures, 1251
preschoolers and, 1047-1048, 1047f
role in child development, 853
classification of play, 853
content of play, 854, 854f
functions of play, 856-857, 856f
social character of play, 855-856, 855f
toys and, 857, 858b
school-age children and, 1083-1084, 1085f
toddlers and, 1023-1024, 1024f
Playpens, 994
Plesiomonas, 1383-1386
Plexus, birth injury of, 743-744, 743t
PMDD. *See* Premenstrual dysphoric disorder (PMDD).
PMI. *See* Point of maximum impulse (PMI).
PMS. *See* Premenstrual syndrome (PMS).
Pneumococcal conjugate vaccine (PCV), 984, 987t-988t, 1316
Pneumocystis carinii pneumonia, 108, 329, 1518
Pneumonias
aspiration, 1330-1331
in children, 1324-1326, 1324b, 1326f
in newborns, 746
Pneumothorax, 1349b
Point of maximum impulse (PMI), 449, 451, 452b
Poison control center, 997b, 1039b, 1426-1427, 1426b-1427b
Poison ivy, oak, and sumac, 1647-1648, 1647b, 1647f
Poisoning, 1426-1437, 1428b-1429b
child mortality and, 788, 789f
emergency treatment in, 1426-1432, 1430b
assessment and, 1427
gastric decontamination and, 1427-1431, 1431b
poison control center and, 997b, 1039b, 1426-1427, 1426b-1427b
prevention of recurrence, 1431-1432, 1432b
heavy metal, 1432, 1432b
infants and, 788, 789f, 992b-993b, 996-997, 997b, 997f
lead, 1432-1437
anticipatory guidance and, 1435
causes of, 1433, 1433b-1434b
diagnostic evaluation of, 1435
nursing care management in, 1436-1437, 1436b-1437b
pathophysiology and clinical manifestations of, 1433-1435, 1434f, 1435b
screening for, 1435
therapeutic management of, 1435-1437
poisonous and nonpoisonous plants and, 996, 1427b-1429b
school-age children and, 1095t
toddlers and, 1034t-1035t, 1039, 1039b, 1039f
Poker chip pain tool, 932t-933t
Poliomyelitis, 1058t-1064t
Poliovirus vaccine, 983, 987t-988t, 1745t-1748t
Polyarthritis rheumatoid factor negative, 1709
Polyarthritis rheumatoid factor positive, 1709
Polycythemia
chronic hypoxemia and, 1465
in infants of diabetic mothers, 737
Polydactyly, 775-776
Polydipsia, 296
Polyhydramnios, 198
abruptio placentae and, 365
neonatal gastrointestinal obstruction and, 772
risk factors for, 192b
Polyploidy, 166
Polyuria, 166
Ponstel. *See* Mefenamic acid.
Popliteal angle, 651b
Populations, vulnerable, 32-34
Pornography, child, 1068
Portable telemetry monitor, 425-426
Port-wine stains, 618
Position, fetal, 377-378, 378f-380f
Positional plagiocephaly, 1009-1010, 1009f
Positioning
for breastfeeding, 543-544, 685-686, 687f-688f
in cesarean birth, 515
of children
after surgery for brain tumors, 1573, 1574b
for circumcision, 667, 667f
for hospital procedures, 1266-1267, 1267b, 1267f
for otoscopic examination, 908-910, 908b, 908f-909f
during painful procedures, 936
preterm infants and, 723
unconscious child and, 1560b, 1561
for epidural blocks, 413, 413f
for labor and birth, 385, 386f
dystocia and, 501
electronic fetal monitoring and, 425-426, 426f
fetal heart rate and, 437
first stage of labor and, 459-460, 460f-462f, 461b
second stage of labor and, 385, 386f, 461f-463f, 469-471, 470f
bearing-down efforts and, 468-471, 471b
fetal heart rate and pattern and, 471
of newborns, 671-672, 671b, 672f
for spinal anesthesia, 410, 411f, 413f, 419, 419f
Positive reinforcement, 1251
Positive self-talk, 937b
Positive signs of pregnancy, 212, 213t
Positron emission tomography (PET), 1556t-1557t
Postanesthesia recovery period, 480-483, 483b
Postcoital test, 133-134, 133t
Postconventional level of moral development, 851-852
Postdate, definition of, 210
Posterior fontanel, 376, 377f
Posthospital behaviors in children, 1223b
Postmature infants. *See* Postterm infants.
Postmortem care in death of newborn, 605, 605f
Postneonatal mortality, definition of, 790
Postoperative care
in appendectomy, 1399-1400
in brain tumors, 1573-1574, 1573b-1574b
in cesarean birth, 516-517, 517b
in cleft lip and palate, 1414, 1414b
in congenital heart disease, 1469-1471, 1470b-1471b
in esophageal atresia, 1416-1417
in Hirschsprung disease, 1393
in pediatric surgery, 1252-1253, 1253b, 1254t
in pyloromyotomy, 1420
in scoliosis, 1702-1703
in Wilms' tumor, 1542
Postpartum blues, 559f, 562, 562b

Postpartum care, 533, 552-553
  in cesarean birth, 516-517, 517b
  cultural considerations in, 25t-26t
  early postpartum discharge and, 534
    advantages and disadvantages of, 535b
    criteria for, 534-535, 535b, 536f, 537b
    discharge teaching and, 550-552, 551b
    follow-up after, 552
    laws relating to, 534
    nursing care management of physical needs in, 535-537, 538b
      breastfeeding and, 546, 546b
      exercise and, 544, 545f
      maintenance of uterine tone and, 542, 542f
      normal bladder function and, 544
      normal bowel function and, 544
      nutrition and, 544, 546f
      pain management and, 542-543, 543b
      plan of care and implementation, 537-540, 539b-540b
      prevention of bladder distention and, 542
      prevention of excessive bleeding and, 540-541, 540b-542b, 540f
      prevention of infection and, 540, 541b
      prevention of Rh isoimmunization and, 546-547, 547b
      rest and, 543-544, 543b
      rubella vaccination and, 546, 546b
      signs of potential problems, 538b
      suppression of lactation and, 546
    nursing care management of psychosocial needs in, 547, 547f, 548b, 549-552
      adaptation to parenthood and parent-infant interactions and, 548
      birth experience and, 548
      cultural diversity and, 549-550, 550b
      family structure and functioning and, 549, 549f
      maternal self-image and, 548
      signs of potential psychosocial complications, 549, 549b
  in eclampsia, 347-348, 347b
  gestational diabetes mellitus and, 309
  in maternal cardiovascular disorders, 315b-316b, 318-319, 318b
  pregestational diabetes mellitus and, 300b-301b, 306
  preterm labor and birth and, 496b
  systemic lupus erythematosus and, 327
  transfer from recovery area and, 533, 534t
Postpartum care *(Continued)*
  for vaginal birth without complications and, 537, 539b-540b
Postpartum depression (PPD), 562, 592-593
  assessment of, 593b
  nursing care management in, 594-595, 595b
    complementary and alternative therapies and, 598, 598b
    home visits and, 596
    postpartum unit and, 595-596, 596b
    psychiatric hospitalization and, 596-597, 596b
    psychotropic medications and, 597-598, 597t
    referral and, 596
    suicidal thoughts and, 596, 596b
  with psychotic features, 594-595, 595b, 597t
  risk factors for, 592, 592b
  without psychotic features, 593-594
Postpartum discharge, early. *See* Postpartum care: early postpartum discharge and.
Postpartum hemorrhage (PPH), 479
  definition and incidence of, 576
  etiology and risk factors for, 577-581, 577b
  hemorrhagic shock and, 581-583, 582b-583b
  nursing care management of, 579-580, 579b
    bleeding with a contracted uterus and, 581
    herbal remedies and, 581, 582t
    hypotonic uterus and, 580-581
    medications in, 580, 580b-581b
    nursing care plan in, 580b
    nursing process in, 579b
Postpartum period, 525
  complications in, 607
    coagulopathies, 583
      disseminated intravascular coagulation, 583-584
      idiopathic thrombocytopenic purpura, 583
      von Willebrand disease, 583
    infections, 585-587
      endometritis, 585, 587
      mastitis, 586-587, 586f
      prevention of, 586-587, 587b
      risk factors for, 585, 586b
      urinary tract infections, 586-587
      in wounds, 585-587
    maternal death and, 606-607, 606b
    newborn death and. *See* Death: of newborn.
    postpartum depression. *See* Postpartum depression (PPD).
    postpartum hemorrhage. *See* Postpartum hemorrhage (PPH).
    structural disorders of the uterus and vagina, 587
      cystocele and rectocele, 588-589, 589f, 592
      genital fistulas, 589-592, 590f
Postpartum period *(Continued)*
      nursing process in, 590-592, 591b, 591f
      urinary incontinence, 589, 590f, 592
      uterine displacement and prolapse, 587-588, 588f, 592
    thromboembolic disease, 584-585, 585b
  dealing with visitors during, 551
  fatigue in, 543-544
  nutrition during, 289-290
  physiologic changes during, 525-527, 526f, 527b, 528f
    breasts and, 529
    cardiovascular system and blood volume and, 529, 530b
      cardiac output and, 530-531, 530t
      varicosities and, 531
    cervix and, 527
    endocrine system and, 528
    gastrointestinal system and, 529
    immune system and, 531
    integumentary system and, 531
    musculoskeletal system and, 531
    neurologic system and, 531
    urinary system and, 528-529
    uterine contractions and, 525
    uterus and, 525-527, 526f, 527b
      afterpains and, 526
      involution process and, 525, 526f
      lochia and, 526-527, 527b
      placental site healing and, 526
    vagina and perineum and, 527
  routine mother and baby checkups during, 551
  self-management and signs of complications in, 550-551
  sexual activity and contraception during, 551, 551b, 562-564
  transition to parenthood and, 548, 554, 559-560, 574-575
    adolescent fathers and, 567
    adolescent mothers and, 566-567, 566b
    attachment, bonding, and acquaintance in, 554-557, 555t-556t, 557b
    communication between parent and infant in, 558-559, 558f-560f, 559b
    culture and, 568-569
    grandparent adaptation and, 571-573, 572b, 572f-573f
    infant-parent adjustment in, 559f-560f, 565-566
    lesbian couple's adjustment in, 564
    maternal adjustment in, 561-562, 561t, 562b
    older fathers and, 567
    older mothers and, 566b, 567, 568b
    parental sensory impairment and, 569-570
      hearing-impaired parent and, 570
      visual impairment and, 570, 570b
Postpartum period *(Continued)*
    parent-infant contact and, 548, 557-558, 557f
    paternal adjustment in, 564-565, 564t, 565f
    personal aspirations and, 569
    sibling adaptation and, 570-571, 571f, 572b
    social support and, 567-568
    socioeconomic conditions and, 569
    tasks and responsibilities in, 560-561
Postprocedural support for children, 1250-1251, 1251f
Postpubescence, 1105
Postterm infants, 707b, 733-734, 733f
  meconium aspiration syndrome and, 733, 733f
  persistent pulmonary hypertension and, 733-734
Postterm pregnancy, 192b, 518-519, 519b
Posttraumatic seizures, 1567
Posttraumatic stress disorder (PTSD), 1101
Postural drainage. *See* Bronchial drainage.
Postural hypotension. *See* Orthostatic hypotension.
Postural tone of newborn, 621t-625t
Posture
  adolescents and, 1120
  in assessing gestational age, 651b
  of newborn, 626t-636t
  in pediatric physical assessment, 900
  during pregnancy, 224, 225f, 248b-250b, 249f
Posturing, cerebral dysfunction and, 1555, 1555f
Potassium
  intake during pregnancy, 283
  normal test ranges for, 1753t-1761t
  nutritional significance of, 1377t-1379t
Potentilla, 90t
Poultry during pregnancy, 280t
Poverty
  child health and, 825, 830
  minority women and, 32
Powers, birth process and, 384
  primary, 384-385, 384f
  secondary, 384-385
PPCM. *See* Peripartum cardiomyopathy (PPCM).
PPD. *See* Postpartum depression (PPD).
PPE. *See* Personal protective equipment (PPE).
PPH. *See* Postpartum hemorrhage (PPH).
PPHN. *See* Persistent pulmonary hypertension (PPHN).
PPQ. *See* Pediatric Pain Questionnaire (PPQ).
PPROM. *See* Preterm premature rupture of membranes (PPROM).
Preadolescence, 1078-1079
Precipitous labor, 502
Precocious puberty, 71, 1603-1604, 1603b

Precolostrum, 217
Preconception counseling, 44-45, 45b, 63
  chronic hypertension and, 336
  in cystic fibrosis, 324
  diabetes mellitus and, 298, 298b
  human immunodeficiency virus and, 109, 328
  Marfan syndrome and, 313-314
Preconception education, 264, 264b
Preconventional level of moral development
  preschoolers and, 851-852, 1045
Precordial activity, 610
Predictive genetics testing, 164
Prednisone, breastfeeding and, 1745t-1748t
Preeclampsia
  classification of, 335, 335t-336t, 336b
  etiology of, 337, 337b, 337f
  home care in, 342-343, 342b-344b
  morbidity and mortality in, 335
  nutrition and, 285, 342-343, 343b
  pathophysiology of, 338, 338b, 339f
  periodontal infections and, 247
  pregestational diabetes mellitus and, 298
  prevention of, 337, 337b
  severe. *See* Severe preeclampsia.
  superimposed on chronic hypertension, 334, 335t, 336, 374
Preexisting conditions, 332-333
  acquired immunodeficiency syndrome, 328-330
  anemia, 320-322, 320b, 332-333
    folic acid deficiency anemia, 322
    iron deficiency anemia, 321-322
    sickle cell hemoglobinopathy, 322, 323t
    thalassemia, 322
  autoimmune disorders, 327, 332-333
    myasthenia gravis, 327-328, 327b
    systemic lupus erythematosus, 327
  cardiopulmonary resuscitation and, 319-320, 319b, 320f
  cardiovascular disorders, 311-319, 311b-312b, 332-333
    atrial and ventricular septal defects, 313
    classification of, 311-312
    Eisenmenger's syndrome, 312b, 313
    heart transplantation, 314
    intrapartum care in, 312
    Marfan syndrome, 313-314
    mitral and aortic valve stenosis, 313
    mitral valve prolapse, 313
    peripartum cardiomyopathy, 312
    plan of care and implementation in, 314-319, 321b
      heart surgery and, 317
      intrapartum period, 317-318, 318b
      medication and, 316, 317t
      postpartum period, 315b-316b, 318-319, 318b
Preexisting conditions *(Continued)*
    rheumatic heart disease, 247, 312-313
    tetralogy of Fallot, 313
  diabetes mellitus, 295-296, 298
    classification of, 296, 297t
    family planning and contraception in, 306
    fetal and neonatal risks and complications in, 299
    intrapartum interventions in, 300b-301b, 305-306
    maternal risks and complications in, 298-299
    metabolic changes associated with pregnancy and, 296-298, 297f
    monitoring maternal blood glucose levels in, 299-306, 300b-301b, 301f, 304b, 304f
    mortality rate in, 296
    nursing care plan for, 307b
    pathogenesis of, 296
    postpartum interventions in, 300b-301b, 306
    preconception counseling and, 298, 298b
    prenatal care and, 299-305, 300b-301b, 301t
      complications requiring hospitalization and, 305
      determination of birth date and mode of delivery, 305
      diet, 302, 303b
      exercise, 302
      insulin therapy, 302-304, 303b, 303t, 304f
      monitoring blood glucose levels, 304-305, 304b-305b
    target blood glucose levels in, 301t
  gastrointestinal disorders, 325
    cholelithiasis and cholecystitis, 325, 325b
    inflammatory bowel disease, 325
  human immunodeficiency virus infection, 328-330, 328b-329b
  hyperthyroidism, 309-310, 310b
  hypothyroidism, 310, 310b
  integumentary disorders in, 325-326, 325b
  maternal phenylketonuria, 311
  neurologic disorders, 326
    Bell's palsy, 327
    epilepsy, 326, 326b
    multiple sclerosis, 326-327
  pulmonary disorders, 322
    asthma, 322-324, 324t
    cystic fibrosis, 324-325
  substance abuse in, 49, 253, 330-332, 330b-332b
Prefixes denoting decimal factors, 1761t
Pregestational diabetes mellitus. *See* Diabetes mellitus.
Pregnancy
  acquired immunodeficiency syndrome in, 328-330
  adaptation to. *See* Adaptation to pregnancy.
  adolescent
    health risks in, 48
Pregnancy *(Continued)*
    intimate partner violence during, 62, 240
    nursing care plan for, 260-261, 261f, 262b
    nutrition needs in, 52, 279, 285
    prevention programs for, 7b
    rate of, 32-33, 260-261
  after age 35, 48
  alcohol use during, 50, 330, 331b, 755-758, 756t
  among homeless women, 33-34
  anemia in, 320-322, 320b, 332-333
    folic acid deficiency anemia, 322
    iron deficiency anemia, 321-322
    sickle cell hemoglobinopathy, 322, 323t
    thalassemia, 322
  appendicitis during, 226f, 227, 368
  autoimmune disorders in, 327, 332-333
    myasthenia gravis, 327-328, 327b
    systemic lupus erythematosus, 327
  breastfeeding during, 695
  caffeine consumption during, 50, 761
  cardiopulmonary resuscitation in, 319-320, 319b, 320f
  cardiovascular disorders in, 311-319, 311b-312b, 332-333
    atrial and ventricular septal defects, 313
    classification of, 311-312
    Eisenmenger's syndrome, 312b, 313
    heart transplantation, 314
    intrapartum care in, 312
    Marfan syndrome, 313-314
    mitral and aortic valve stenosis, 313
    mitral valve prolapse, 313
    peripartum cardiomyopathy, 312
    plan of care and implementation in, 314-319, 321b
      heart surgery and, 317
      intrapartum period, 317-318, 318b
      medication and, 316, 317t
      postpartum period, 315b-316b, 318-319, 318b
    rheumatic heart disease, 247, 312-313
    tetralogy of Fallot, 313
  care during childbirth and, 8-10
  cocaine during, 50-51, 331, 759-760
  cultural considerations in, 25t-26t
  dating of, ultrasound for, 176b
  diabetes mellitus in, 295-296, 298, 332-333
    classification of, 296, 297t
    family planning and contraception in, 306
    fetal and neonatal risks and complications in, 299
    intrapartum interventions in, 300b-301b, 305-306
    maternal risks and complications in, 298-299
Pregnancy *(Continued)*
    metabolic changes associated with pregnancy and, 296-298, 297f
    monitoring blood glucose levels in, 299-306, 300b-301b, 301f, 304b, 304f
    mortality rate in, 296
    nursing care plan for, 307b
    pathogenesis of, 296
    postpartum interventions in, 300b-301b, 306
    preconception counseling and, 298, 298b
    prenatal care and, 299-305, 300b-301b, 301t
      complications requiring hospitalization and, 305
      determination of birth date and mode of delivery, 305
      diet, 302, 303b
      exercise, 302
      insulin therapy, 302-304, 303b, 303t, 304f
      monitoring blood glucose levels, 304-305, 304b-305b
    target blood glucose levels in, 301t
  diagnosis of, 230
  drug testing during, 49b
  exercise during, 54, 54b, 54f, 248b
  fourth trimester of. *See* Postpartum period.
  gastrointestinal disorders in, 325
    cholelithiasis and cholecystitis, 325, 325b
    inflammatory bowel disease, 325
  gestational diabetes mellitus in, 179, 296, 306-309
    interventions in, 308-309
    maternal and fetal risks in, 307-308
    screening for, 308, 308f
  gonococcal infections during, 100
  hemorrhagic disorders in, 350
    early pregnancy bleeding, 350-351
      miscarriage and, 351-354, 352f, 353t
        nursing care management in, 353-354, 353b-355b
      ectopic pregnancy
        clinical manifestations of, 357
        collaborative care for, 357-358, 357b-358b
        incidence and etiology of, 356-357, 356f
      gestational trophoblastic disease, 358
        gestational trophoblastic neoplasia, 349, 358
        hydatidiform mole, 358-359, 359b, 359f
    late pregnancy bleeding, 360, 360f
      abruptio placentae and, 360, 360f, 365-366, 365f
      clotting disorders and, 366-368
      cord insertion and placental variations and, 366
      placenta previa and. *See* Placenta previa.

Pregnancy *(Continued)*
recurrent premature dilation of cervix, 355-356, 355b, 356f
high risk. *See* High risk pregnancy.
human immunodeficiency virus infection in, 109-110, 328-330, 328b-329b
screening for, 109b
hyperemesis gravidarum in, 349-350, 351b
hypertension in, 243, 374
classification of, 335, 335t
chronic hypertension, 334, 335t, 336
chronic hypertension with superimposed preeclampsia, 334, 335t, 336
eclampsia, 335t, 336
gestational hypertension, 335, 335t
preeclampsia, 335, 335t-336t, 336b
severe preeclampsia, 336
HELLP syndrome and, 338
morbidity and mortality in, 335
nursing care management in, 340b
blood pressure assessment and, 339, 339b
chronic hypertension and, 348-349
deep tendon reflexes and, 340, 341f, 341t
eclampsia and, 346-348, 346f, 347b
edema and, 339-340, 341f
hyperactive reflexes and, 340-341, 341f
mild preeclampsia and home care and, 342-343, 342b-344b
pharmacologic therapy and, 348t
severe preeclampsia or HELLP syndrome and, 343-346, 344b-345b, 347b, 348t
preeclampsia and, 337-338, 337b-338b, 337f, 339f
significance and incidence of, 334
hyperthyroidism in, 309-310, 310b
hypothyroidism in, 310, 310b
illicit drug use during, 50-51
integumentary disorders in, 325-326, 325b
intestinal obstruction during, 368-369
intimate partner violence during, 62-63, 62b-63b, 76
length of, 174, 229
marijuana during, 756t, 759
maternal phenylketonuria in, 311
multifetal. *See* Multifetal pregnancy.
neurologic disorders in, 326
Bell's palsy, 327
epilepsy, 326, 326b
multiple sclerosis, 326-327
nursing care during. *See* Prenatal care.
nutrition during, 52, 273-274, 274f, 281b, 294

Pregnancy *(Continued)*
adequate dietary intake and, 288-289, 290b
adolescent pregnancy and, 52, 285
constipation and, 291
counseling on, 286b
energy needs and, 275-277, 275t-276t
hazards of restricting adequate weight gain and, 277-279, 278t, 279b
pattern of weight gain and, 277, 278f
weight gain and, 277, 281b
exercise and, 285
fluid intake and, 279-280
minerals, vitamins, electrolytes and, 275t-276t, 280-284, 281b-283b
nausea and vomiting and, 290-291, 291f
nutrient needs before conception and, 273, 274b
pica and food cravings and, 284-285, 285f
preeclampsia and, 285
protein intake and, 279, 279b, 280t
recommendations for daily intakes of nutrients, 274-275, 275t-276t
vegetarian diet and, 293
obesity and, 52
optimal birth spacing, 140b
ovarian cysts during, 369
pelvic examination during, 84-85
personal relationships during, 231-232, 231b, 232f
postterm, 192b, 518-519, 519b
preexisting conditions and. *See* Preexisting conditions.
pulmonary disorders in, 322
asthma, 322-324, 324t
cystic fibrosis, 324-325
sexual activity during, 232, 257b
signs and symptoms of, 230
signs and symptoms of potential complications, 243, 243b, 253
smoking cessation during, 49b, 759b
smoking during, 49, 57, 756t, 758-759
substance abuse during
heroin and, 760
methamphetamines and, 756t, 761
phenobarbital, 761
substance abuse in, 49, 253, 330-332, 330b-332b
surgery during, nonobstetric, 368-369, 369b
trauma during, 369-374
fetal physiologic characteristics and, 370-371
maternal physiologic characteristics and, 370, 370b, 371t
mechanisms of, 371-372, 371b
nursing care management in immediate stabilization and, 372-374, 372b-373b
perimortem cesarean delivery and, 374

Pregnancy *(Continued)*
significance of, 369-372
work during, 54b
Pregnancy Risk Assessment Monitoring System (PRAMS), 193b
Pregnancy tests, 211-212, 211b, 211f
human chorionic gonadotropin and, 177
Pregnancy-induced hypertension. *See* Gestational hypertension.
Pregnancy-induced hypervolemia, 529
Pregnancy-Unique Quantification of Emesis, 350
Pregnant Patient's Bill of Rights, 4b
Preimplantation genetic diagnosis (PGD), 136-138
Premarin, 4b
Premature Infant Pain Profile (PIPP), 934
Premature rupture of membranes (PROM), 496, 746
Premature separation of placenta. *See* Abruptio placentae.
Prematurity. *See* Preterm labor and birth.
Premenstrual dysphoric disorder (PMDD), 91
Premenstrual syndrome (PMS), 90-91, 127
in adolescents, 90b
Prenatal assessment for postterm pregnancy, 518
Prenatal care, 45, 45b, 229, 235, 238b
adaptation to pregnancy and. *See* Adaptation to pregnancy.
age differences and, 260-261, 261f, 262b
barriers to receiving, 236-237
cardiovascular disorders and
mitral and aortic valve stenosis, 313
nursing process in, 315b-316b
care paths in, 244-245
education during. *See* Prenatal education.
psychosocial support, 259
sex counseling, 256-258, 257b, 258f
centering pregnancy approach, 237, 238b
childbirth and perinatal education and, 263-271, 264b, 398
cultural influences on, 192b, 259-260, 260b, 260f
culturally appropriate and adequate, 10b
failure to seek, 191b
follow-up visits in, 241-242
fetal assessment, 243-244, 245f
interview, 242
physical examinations, 241-242, 242b-243b, 243f
review of systems, 242
gestational diabetes mellitus and, 179, 296, 306-309
interventions in, 308-309
maternal and fetal risks in, 307-308
screening for, 308, 308f
initial visit in
drug/herbal preparations history, 239, 239b

Prenatal care *(Continued)*
family history, 240
history of physical abuse, 240
interview, 237-239, 239f
laboratory tests in, 241, 241t, 242b
medical history, 239
nutritional history, 239
obstetric and gynecologic history, 239
physical examination, 240-241
reason for seeking care in, 239
review of systems, 240
social, experiential, and occupational history, 240
maternal human immunodeficiency virus and, 328-330
maternal mortality rates and, 28-29
multifetal pregnancy and, 261-263, 263b
nursing diagnoses in, 238b
nutrition and, 52, 273-274, 274f, 281b, 294
adequate dietary intake and, 288-289, 290b
adolescent pregnancy and, 52, 285
constipation and, 291
counseling on, 286b
energy needs and, 275-277, 275t-276t
hazards of restricting adequate weight gain and, 277-279, 278t, 279b
pattern of weight gain and, 277, 278f
weight gain and, 277, 281b
exercise and, 285
fluid intake and, 279-280
minerals, vitamins, electrolytes and, 275t-276t, 280-284, 281b-283b
nausea and vomiting and, 290-291, 291f
nutrient needs before conception and, 273, 274b
pica and food cravings and, 284-285, 285f
preeclampsia and, 285
protein intake and, 279, 279b, 280t
recommendations for daily intakes of nutrients, 274-275, 275t-276t
vegetarian diet and, 293
pain management and, 398
pregestational diabetes mellitus and, 299-305, 300b-301b, 301t
complications requiring hospitalization and, 305
determination of birth date and mode of delivery, 305
diet, 302, 303b
exercise, 302
insulin therapy, 302-304, 303b, 303t, 304f
monitoring blood glucose levels, 304-305, 304b-305b
risks and complications in, 298-299
target blood glucose levels in, 301t

Prenatal care *(Continued)*
pregnancy outcomes and, 9, 235-236
signs and symptoms of potential complications, 243, 243b
Prenatal data first stage of labor and, 444
Prenatal education, 245
about maternal and fetal changes, 245
in alcohol, cigarette smoke, caffeine, and drugs, 252-253
in breastfeeding, 246-247, 247f, 266b, 679-680, 698
in clothing, 251, 252f
in dental health, 247
in employment, 250-251
in immunizations, 252
in Kegel exercises, 246
in medications and herbal preparations, 252
in normal discomforts, 253, 253b, 254t-256t
in nutrition, 245
in personal hygiene, 246
in physical activity, 247-249, 249f
in posture and body mechanics, 248b-250b, 249f
in prevention of urinary tract infections, 246, 246f
in recognition of potential complications, 243b, 253
in recognition of preterm labor, 253-256, 257b, 257f
in rest and relaxation, 250, 250f, 251b
in travel, 251-252, 252f
Prenatal interview, 237, 239f
Prenatal period, 229, 843b
Prenatal testing, 164, 190-191, 194b
biochemical assessment in, 200-201, 200t
alpha-fetoprotein assay in, 203-204
amniocentesis in, 200t, 201, 201f
chorionic villus sampling in, 203, 203b, 204f
Coombs' test in, 204
Coombs' test in, 204
indications for, 201-202, 202b
percutaneous umbilical blood sampling in, 202-203, 203f
daily fetal movement count in, 191-192, 192b-193b, 195f
electronic fetal monitoring in. *See* Electronic fetal monitoring (EFM).
magnetic resonance imaging in, 200
nursing role in, 207-208, 208b
psychologic considerations in, 207-208, 208b
ultrasound in, 192-199
amniotic fluid volume and, 198
biophysical profile and, 198-199, 199t
Doppler blood flow analysis and, 198, 199f
fetal anatomy and, 197
fetal face at 20 weeks, 196f
fetal genetic disorders and physical anomalies and, 197, 198f

Prenatal testing *(Continued)*
fetal growth and, 196-197, 197f
fetal heart activity and, 195
gestational age and, 195-196, 197f
indications for, 194-195, 196b
levels of, 194-195
nursing role in, 199-200, 200b
placental position and function and, 197
spina bifida and, 1725
umbilical cord at 26 weeks, 196f
Preoperational phase of cognitive development
preschoolers and, 1044-1045, 1045b
toddlers and, 1020-1021, 1021b
Preoperative care
in cesarean birth, 514-515
in cleft lip and palate, 1413
in Hirschsprung disease, 1392-1393
in pediatric surgery, 1251-1252, 1251f, 1252t
for pregnant women, 369, 374
in pyloromyotomy, 1420
in scoliosis, 1702
in Wilms' tumor, 1541-1542
Preoperative sedation of children, 1252
Preovulatory phase, 72f, 73
Prepackaged formula, postpartum discharge and, 551b
Prepubescence, 843b, 1078-1079, 1105
Prepuce, 66f, 618-619
Preschoolers, 843b, 1043, 1075-1076
aggression and, 1052-1053
anticipatory guidance for, 1055, 1056b
approaches to physical examination of, 888t
biologic development of, 1043-1044, 1044f
body image of, 853, 1045
child maltreatment and, 1066
child neglect in, 1066, 1070b
child support in, 1073
clinical manifestations of, 1071b-1072b
family support in, 1073-1074
nursing care plan for, 1069-1074
caregiver-child interaction and, 1070
history and interview and, 1069b, 1071b-1072b
nurse biases and, 1069b
physical assessment and, 1072-1073, 1072b
protection from further abuse, 1073, 1073b
talking with children who reveal abuse and, 1069b
physical abuse in, 1066-1068, 1067b
plan for discharge in, 1074
prevention of, 1074, 1075b
sexual abuse in, 1068-1069, 1069b, 1075b
warning signs of, 1070b
cognitive development of, 1044-1045, 1045b, 1050t
communicable diseases and, 1055-1056, 1058t-1064t

Preschoolers *(Continued)*
comfort measures in, 1057-1066, 1066b
complications of, 1057, 1057b
family support in, 1066, 1066b
nursing care management for, 1056
prevention of spread of, 1056-1057, 1056b-1057b
day care for, 820b
dental health of, 1055
Denver II and, 926
family relationships of, 1050t
fears of, 1052
gross and fine motor behavior of, 1043-1044, 1044f, 1050t
growth and development of, 1050t
trends in height and weight, 845t
hospitalization of. *See also* Hospitalization: pediatric.
fears of bodily injury and pain and, 1231-1232
individual risk factors and, 1223
loss of control and, 1222, 1230
preparation for admission, 1225-1228, 1225b
preventing or minimizing separation during, 1229, 1229f
separation anxiety and, 1221
specimen collection and, 1268-1269
injury prevention and, 1055
language and, 1044, 1046, 1046f, 1050t
moral development of, 1045
nutrition and, 1053-1054, 1054b, 1054f
peptic ulcer disease and, 1405b
play and, 1047-1048, 1047f
preschool and kindergarten experience of, 1048-1049, 1049f
psychologic preparation for procedures, 1248b-1249b
psychosocial development of, 1044, 1044b
self-esteem and, 853
sex education for, 1049-1052
sexuality and, 1045-1046
sleep and activity and, 1054-1055
social development of, 1046-1048, 1046f-1047f
special needs, 1161t-1162t
speech problems of, 1053
spiritual development of, 1045
stress and, 1052
understanding and reaction to death, 1167t-1168t
Prescreening Developmental Questionnaire (PDQ II), 926-927
Prescription medications, 50
abuse of, 49
misuse of, 50
Present health status, 78
Present illness, history of, 78
pediatric, 876, 876b
Presentation in labor, fetal, 377-378, 378f-379f
face, 652-653, 653f
vertex, 380f, 473-474, 474f

Presentation in labor, fetal *(Continued)*
emergency birth in, 478b
fetal heart rate in, 451
prolapsed umbilical cord and, 520-522, 521f
Pressure ulcers, 1256-1257
Pressure-reduction devices, 1256-1257
Pressure-relief devices, 1256-1257
Presumptive signs of pregnancy, 212, 213t
Presymptomatic genetics testing, 164
Pretend play, 854
Preterm, definition of, 210
Preterm infants, 706-733, 707b, 740
assessment of, 707-708
body temperature maintenance in, 709, 713, 728b-730b
breastfeeding of, 691
bronchopulmonary dysplasia in, 732-733
cardiovascular function of, 709
central nervous system function in, 709-710, 728b-730b
developmental care of, 723-726, 724f, 725b
environmental concerns of, 712-713, 722-723, 723f
evaluation of, 727, 728b-730b
growth and development potential of, 726-727
hematologic status of, 710
incidence of, 7, 28-29
infection and, 710, 711b
late-preterm, 707, 708t
maternal nutrition and, 273
necrotizing enterocolitis in, 731-732, 732b
nursing process in care of, 712, 712b, 728b-730b
nutrition and, 710, 712b, 717-720, 718b, 720f, 724f, 728b-730b
oxygen therapy for, 713-717, 714f, 715t
parental adaptation to, 710-726, 711f, 712b
parental support and, 726-727, 726b, 726f
patent ductus arteriosus in, 730-731
periventricular-intraventricular hemorrhage in, 731
physical care of, 712-713
renal function of, 710
respiratory distress syndrome and, 727-730, 730t
respiratory function of, 708-709
response to pain, 930f
retinopathy of prematurity in, 732
skin care for, 720-721, 721b-722b, 728b-730b
vitamin deficiencies and, 1364
weaning from respiratory assistance, 716-717
Preterm labor and birth, 486, 523-524
causes of, 487-488, 488b
home care and, 35b, 36f, 37, 40-41, 257b, 263b
incidence of, 487
inevitable, 496, 496b
intravenous fluid intake in, 494b
low birth weight versus, 486-487

Preterm labor and birth *(Continued)*
myasthenia gravis and, 327b
nursing care management in, 488-489, 489b
bed rest and, 37, 491-492, 492b
early recognition and diagnosis in, 491
home care and, 492-493, 492b-493b, 493f
lifestyle modifications and, 491
prevention strategies and, 489-490, 491b
promotion of fetal lung maturity and, 496, 496b
uterine activity suppression and, 493-496, 494b-495b
nursing care plan for, 490b
pregestational diabetes mellitus and, 298
premature rupture of membranes and. *See* Preterm premature rupture of membranes (PPROM).
recognition of, 253-256, 257b, 257f
risk factors for, 192b, 487, 487b-488b
signs and symptoms of, 489-490, 491b, 491f
socioeconomic factors in, 49, 487-488
Preterm premature rupture of membranes (PPROM), 488, 496-497
nursing care management in, 497, 497b
symptoms of, 496
Prevalence of disease, 800-801, 801b
Prevention. *See* Health promotion and prevention.
Preventive care, 29
Previous illness, injuries, and operations, pediatric health history and, 877
Priapism, 1497-1499
Primary amenorrhea, 1125
Primary atypical pneumonia, 1324
Primary care providers, 9
Primary circular reactions, 960
Primary dysmenorrhea, 88-89, 88f, 89t-90t
in adolescents, 1125
complementary and alternative therapies for, 89, 90t
medications for, 88-89, 89t
Primary germ layers, 174-175, 174f
Primary lactase deficiency, 1373
Primary powers, 384-385, 384f
Primary prevention, 29, 801
in pelvic inflammatory disease, 102
Primary skin lesions, 1633, 1634f
Primary social group, 823
Primary survey in trauma during pregnancy, 372-373, 372b
Primigravida, definition of, 210
Primipara, definition of, 210
Primitive neuroectodermal tumor, 1707
Privacy
adolescents and, 1117b
culture and, 47
interview and, 866-867, 867b
Private-duty nursing, 1205
Probable signs of pregnancy, 212, 213t
Procainamide, 317t
Procardia. *See* Nifedipine.
Progesterone
breastfeeding and, 1745t-1748t
changes during pregnancy, 221-222, 226, 227t
influence on breasts, 68-70
ovaries and production of, 68
placental, 177
postpartum changes in, 528
preterm labor prevention and, 491b
Progestin-only contraceptive methods, 151t, 152-153, 152b
breastfeeding and, 695
diabetes mellitus and, 306
emergency contraception, 153
Prolactin
breast milk production and, 683-684
drawing blood to determine level of, 116
postpartum changes in, 528
Prolapse
of rectum, 1347, 1350
uterine, 587-588, 588f, 592
Prolapsed umbilical cord, 455b, 467b, 520, 521f, 522b
Proliferative phase
of endometrial cycle, 72-73, 72f
of wound healing, 1636
Prolixin. *See* Fluphenazine.
Prolonged decelerations of fetal heart rate, 432-433, 433b
PROM. *See* Premature rupture of membranes (PROM).
Promethazine, breastfeeding and, 1745t-1748t
Prone position
spina bifida and, 1729
sudden infant death syndrome and, 671
Propantheline bromide, breastfeeding and, 1745t-1748t
Prophylactic therapy
for hemophilia patient, 1503-1504
in leukemia, 1509
Propofol for burns, 1667
Proportional changes, 845f
in infants, 953-954
in preschoolers, 1043
in school-age children, 1077-1078, 1078f
in toddlers, 1017
Propoxyphene, breastfeeding and, 1745t-1748t
Propranolol
breastfeeding and, 1745t-1748t
during pregnancy, 317t
Propylthiouracil, breastfeeding and, 1745t-1748t
Propylthiouracil (PTU), 309-310, 1609b
Prostaglandin E_1, 505, 506b
Prostaglandin E_2, 505, 507b
Prostaglandin $F_{2\alpha}$ ($PGF_{2\alpha}$)
postpartum hemorrhage and, 580, 580b-581b
primary dysmenorrhea and, 88
Prostaglandin (PGE2), 354
Prostaglandins (PGs)
induction of labor and, 505, 506b-507b
menstruation and, 73-74
primary dysmenorrhea and, 88
Prosthesis, lower limb, 1696
Prostitution, child, 1068
Protective environment, 661-662, 662b
Protein
adolescent intake of, 1118
intake during lactation, 275t-276t
intake during pregnancy, 275-277, 275t-276t, 279, 279b, 280t
diabetes mellitus and, 302
normal test ranges for, 1753t-1761t
nutrient needs of newborns and, 681
Protein-energy malnutrition, 1368-1370
Proteinuria
during labor, 391b
in preeclampsia, 335-336, 336b, 336t
during pregnancy, 223
Protestant denominations, 132b
Prothrombin time, normal test ranges for, 1753t-1761t
Protostat. *See* Metronidazole.
Proximodistal development, 843
Prurigo of pregnancy, 224b
Pruritic folliculitis of pregnancy, 224b
Pruritic urticarial papules and plaques of pregnancy (PUPPP), 224b, 326, 326f
Pruritus
opioid-related, 947
during pregnancy, 224, 224b, 254t-256t, 326, 326f
Pseudoephedrine, 51
Pseudohypertrophic muscular dystrophy, 1733-1735, 1733f, 1734b
Pseudohypoparathyroidism, 1609b
Psoriatic arthritis, 1709
Psychologic disorders, postpartum. *See* Postpartum depression (PPD).
Psychologic preparation for pediatric procedures, 1247-1250, 1247b-1249b
Psychologic responses to dystocia, 501
Psychoprophylactic method (PPM). *See* Lamaze method.
Psychosexual development, 848-849, 849t
Psychosocial care
after miscarriage, 354
in burns, 1672
in first stage of labor, 446-447, 446t
in hyperemesis gravidarum, 349-350
in infertility, 134, 134b
in postpartum period, 547, 547f, 548b
Psychosocial development, 849-850, 849t, 850f
of adolescents, 1109-1110, 1110b, 1116t
of infants, 957-958
of preschoolers, 1044, 1044b
Psychosocial development *(Continued)*
of school-age children, 1079, 1079f
of toddlers, 1019
Psychosocial history, 879-881
Psychosocial stressors, 191b
Psychosocial support during pregnancy, 259
Psychotherapy for anorexia nervosa and bulimia nervosa, 1135
Psychotropic medications, 597-598, 597t, 1745t-1748t
PTSD. *See* Posttraumatic stress disorder (PTSD).
Ptyalism, 226, 254t-256t
Pubertal delay, 1106-1107
Puberty, 1105
adolescent responses to, 1115
hormonal changes of, 1106
menarche and, 71
precocious. *See* Precocious puberty.
Pubic hair, 1108f
Pubis, 68, 69f
PUBS. *See* Percutaneous umbilical blood sampling (PUBS).
Pudendal nerve block, 409, 410f
Pudendum, 920-921, 920f
Puerperal fever, 4b
Puerperium. *See* Postpartum period.
Puerto Rican culture
food patterns of, 282, 1745t-1748t
health beliefs and practices in, 838t-840t
Pull-to-sit reflex, 621t-625t
Pulmonary artery hypertension, 1477-1478
Pulmonary dysfunction, 1360-1361
acute epiglottitis and, 1318-1319, 1318b-1319b, 1318t
acute laryngitis and, 1319
acute laryngotracheobronchitis and, 1318t, 1320-1321, 1320b
acute respiratory distress syndrome/acute lung syndrome and, 1331-1332
acute spasmodic laryngitis and, 1318t, 1321
aspiration pneumonia and, 1330-1331
asthma and, 1334, 1337
acute care in, 1344-1345, 1345f
allergen avoidance and, 1342-1343, 1343b
allergen control in, 1337, 1338b
bronchospasm in, 1343-1344, 1343b-1344b, 1343f
chest physiotherapy for, 1340
classification of, 1334, 1334b
diagnostic evaluation in, 1335-1337, 1335b-1337b
drug therapy in, 1337-1340
etiology of, 1334, 1335b
exercise-induced, 1340
family and child support in, 1345-1346
hyposensitization and, 1340
nursing care plan for, 1341-1342, 1342b
pathophysiology of, 1335, 1335f
prognosis in, 1340-1341
status asthmaticus and, 1341

Pulmonary dysfunction *(Continued)*
bronchiolitis and, 1272, 1321-1324, 1322t
bronchitis and, 1321, 1322t
environmental tobacco smoke exposure and, 1333, 1333b
foreign body aspiration and, 1330, 1330b
high risk pregnancy and, 322
asthma in, 322-324, 324t
cystic fibrosis in, 324-325
influenza and, 985, 1313-1314
nasopharyngitis and, 1307-1310, 1310b
pharyngitis and, 1310b
respiratory failure and, 1354-1355, 1354b
respiratory syncytial virus and, 1272, 1321-1324, 1322b
smoke inhalation injuries and, 1332-1333, 1332b
tonsillitis and, 1311-1313, 1311f-1312f, 1313b
tuberculosis and, 1326-1329, 1327b-1329b
Pulmonary edema after childbirth, 480
Pulmonary embolism, 584
Pulmonary function during pregnancy, 221, 222t
Pulmonary function tests, 1336
Pulmonary surfactants, 179
Pulmonary vascular resistance (PVR), 714-715
Pulmonic stenosis, 1451b-1453b
Pulse
of children
cardiopulmonary resuscitation and, 1357, 1357f
cerebral dysfunction and, 1553-1554
in physical assessment, 893-897, 897t, 915, 916f
maternal
after childbirth, 483b, 530t, 538b
cardiac emergency and, 318b
of newborns, 626t-636t, 637
Pulse oximetry, 1290, 1290b, 1290f
of newborn, 637
Pumping of breast milk, 692, 692f
Punishment and obedience orientation, 1045
Pupils
brain tumors and, 1573b
cerebral dysfunction and, 1554, 1554b, 1554f
in pediatric eye examination, 903
Purging, 1132-1133
Pushing efforts during labor, 385, 463f. *See also* Bearing-down efforts.
Pustules, 1634f
PV-IVH. *See* Periventricular-intraventricular hemorrhage (PV-IVH).
PVR. *See* Pulmonary vascular resistance (PVR).
Pyelonephritis, 1530
Pyloric stenosis, hypertrophic, 1372b, 1417-1420, 1419b
Pyloromyotomy, 1419
Pyoderma, 1642t
Pyridoxine, 275t-276t, 284, 1374t-1377t
Pyrosis, 254t-256t, 291

Q

Qi, 404
Quadriplegia, 1741
Quadruplets, 188
Quality improvement program, 1209
Quetiapine, 597, 597t
Quibron. *See* Theophylline.
Quickening, 182, 215-216, 244
Quiet games and activities, school-age children and, 1083-1084, 1085f
Quinidine
breastfeeding and, 1745t-1748t
during pregnancy, 317t
Quintuplets, 188

R

Rabies, 1579-1580, 1580b
Race
anemia and, 1493
definition of, 822
health care access and, 46-47
health outcomes and, 4-5, 32
hereditary health problems and, 829
infant mortality rate and, 7, 28-29, 190, 790
influence on child health promotion, 827-828, 827b
insurance coverage and, 47
intimate partner violence and, 61
live births and, 790
low birth weight infants and, 7
low birth weight/preterm birth and, 7
maternal mortality rate and, 8, 189
obesity and, 8
pregnancy-associated hypertension and, 334
prenatal care and, 9
skin color changes and, 901t
Rachischisis, 1725b
Racial diversity within North America, 4-5, 16
Radial pulse, maternal, 423
Radiation heat loss in newborns, 612
Radiation therapy for breast cancer, 122
Radical mastectomy, 4b, 121f, 122
Radiofrequency ablation, 1444t, 1477
Radiography, 1556t-1557t
abdominal, 719b
cerebral function and, 1556t-1557t
chest, 1348
developmental dysplasia of the hip and, 1692
Radiologic studies of genitourinary system function, 1527t-1528t
Radionuclide cystogram, 1527t-1528t
Radiotherapy
in brain tumors, 1572
in neuroblastomas, 1575
Raloxifene
breast cancer and, 123, 123b
role in prevention of breast cancer, 118
Range of motion
of pediatric joints, 922
in spina bifida, 1729
use of play activities in, 1255b
Rape awareness, 48b
Rapprochement, 1022
Rashes
diaper, 672-673
in erythema toxicum, 618, 618f
neonatal, 672-673
Raspberry leaves, red, 582t
Rating game, 873b-874b
RBCs. *See* Red blood cells (RBCs).
RDAs. *See* Recommended Dietary Allowances (RDAs).
RDS. *See* Respiratory distress syndrome (RDS).
Reach for the knees exercise, 545f
Reach to Recovery program, 124b
Reactive attachment disorder, 961-962
Reactive hyperemia, 1256
Reading ability, school-age child and, 1081
Reading materials, influence on child development, 861
Real-time ultrasonography, 1556t-1557t
Reason for seeking care
in the health history, 78
in prenatal care, 239
Reciprocity, parent-infant communication and, 559, 560f
Reclining in insertion of contraceptive diaphragms, 148b-149b
Recombivax HB. *See* Hepatitis B vaccine (HepB).
Recommended Dietary Allowances (RDAs), 274-275, 881-882
Reconstituted families. *See* Blended families.
Record keeping, diabetes mellitus and, 1629
Recovery area, transfer from, 533, 534t
Recovery nurse's report, 533, 534t
Recovery records, 484
Rectal administration of medication, 943b-944b, 1282
Rectal gonorrhea, 100
Rectal prolapse, 1347, 1350
Rectal smear, 241t
Rectal temperature, 894t-895t, 895b-896b, 1729b
Rectocele, 588-589, 589f, 592
Rectovaginal fistulas, 592
Rectovaginal palpation, 84, 84f
Rectum, 67f
imperforate anus and, 774f, 1422
physical examination of, 80, 84, 84f
prolapse of, 1347, 1350
Rectus abdominis muscle, 224-225, 225f
Recumbent length, 890-891
Recurrence risk, genetic disease and, 163
Recurrent abdominal pain, 1101-1102
Recurrent early miscarriage, 353, 353t
Recurrent premature dilation of cervix, 355-356, 355b, 356f
Recurrent spontaneous abortion. *See* Habitual miscarriage.
Recurrent urinary tract infection, 1530
Red blood cell count, 1491t
after childbirth, 530
normal test ranges for, 1753t-1761t
Red blood cell disorders
anemia in, 1490-1493, 1491t, 1492b-1493b, 1492f
aplastic anemia in, 1501-1502, 1502b
beta-thalassemia in, 1500-1501, 1501b
iron deficiency anemia in, 1493-1494, 1494b
sickle cell anemia in, 1495-1500, 1496b, 1496f, 1498b-1499b
Red blood cell indexes, 1491t
Red blood cell volume, 1753t-1761t
Red blood cells (RBCs)
increase during pregnancy, 219, 220t-221t
of newborn at birth, 611
Red raspberry leaves, 582t
Refeeding syndrome, 1134
Referral
to home care, 37
postpartum depression and, 596
resources in health assessment, 75b
Referred pain during labor, 394
Reflection in health assessment interviews, 75
Reflexes
cerebral dysfunction and, 1555, 1555b
infant use of, 960
in newborn at birth, 620, 621t-625t, 625, 637
pediatric physical assessment of, 923, 923f-924f
severe versus mild preeclampsia and, 336t
Refractive errors, 1191, 1192b-1193b
Refrigerant sprays, 945
Refugees, 34
Regional anesthesia
in cesarean birth, 513
in children, 943b-944b
Regression, toddlers and, 1029
Regurgitation, 999-1001
Rehabilitation
after burns, 1670
after head injuries, 1569
Rehydration in acute diarrhea, 1387-1388, 1387b
Relationships during pregnancy, personal, 231-234, 231b, 232f
Relaxation techniques
for amenorrhea, 87
biofeedback, 405
for pain management during labor and childbirth, 399b, 401-402, 401f, 463, 463f
during pelvic examination, 80-81, 80b
perinatal education and, 270
during pregnancy, patient teaching in, 250, 250f, 251b
Relaxin, 224

Religious considerations
in child health promotion, 825-826, 826f, 835, 836b, 836t-837t
in death of newborn, 601b-602b, 603, 605
food customs and, 833
in health care, 47, 49
home health care and, 1210, 1210b
in infertility, 132b
in pain during childbirth, 396
Remodeling
of bone, 1682-1683
of skin, 1636
Renal angiography, 1527t-1528t
Renal biopsy, 1527t-1528t
Renal dysfunction
in children
acute glomerulonephritis and, 1538-1540, 1539b
acute renal failure and, 1542-1545, 1542b-1544b
chronic renal failure and, 1542, 1545-1547, 1546b
dialysis and, 1547-1548, 1548b, 1548f
hemolytic uremic syndrome and, 1540, 1540b
nephrotic syndrome and, 1535-1538, 1536b-1537b, 1536f
Wilms' tumor and, 1540-1542, 1541b-1542b
Renal function tests
pediatric, 1529t-1530t
in prenatal period, 241t
Renal plasma flow, 220t-221t, 222, 223t
Renal system
developmental milestones of, 184t-186t
of fetus, 181-182
maternal
adaptation to labor, 391
adaptation to pregnancy, 217f, 222-223, 223t, 338b, 371t
of newborns, 613
of preterm infants, 710
Renal ultrasound, 1527t-1528t
Repetitive microtrauma, 1096
Reproductive system
adaptations to pregnancy, 212-217, 214f-217f, 371t
fetal, 182-183
in newborns at birth, 618-619, 619f
postpartum adaptations of, 525-527, 526f, 527b, 528f
cervix and, 527
uterus and, 525-527, 526f, 527b
vagina and perineum and, 527
Rescue, failure to, 14
Research
pediatric nursing and, 794
in perinatal nursing, 14-15
in standards of care, 13b
Resolution phase of sexual response cycle, 74, 74t
RESOLVE, 129
Respiration
after childbirth, 530t
fetal, 390
Respiration *(Continued)*
pediatric
cerebral dysfunction and, 1554
newborns and, 671
normal rates in, 626t-636t
patterns of, 915b
physical assessment of, 897
respiratory infections and, 1307b
sexual response and, 74t
Respiratory arrest, 1354
Respiratory depression, opioid-induced, 948b
Respiratory distress
in late-preterm infants, 708t
in newborns, 610
in pediatric congestive heart failure, 1463
Respiratory distress syndrome (RDS)
in infants of diabetic mothers, 736
in preterm infants, 709, 727-730, 730t
Respiratory dysfunction, 1360-1361. *See also* Respiratory infections.
acute epiglottitis and, 1318-1319, 1318b-1319b, 1318t
acute laryngitis and, 1319
acute laryngotracheobronchitis and, 1318t, 1320-1321, 1320b
acute respiratory distress syndrome/acute lung syndrome and, 1331-1332
acute spasmodic laryngitis and, 1318t, 1321
airway obstruction and, 1558b
aspiration pneumonia and, 1330-1331
asthma and, 1334, 1337
acute care in, 1344-1345, 1345f
allergen avoidance and, 1342-1343, 1343b
allergen control in, 1337, 1338b
bronchospasm in, 1343-1344, 1343b-1344b, 1343f
chest physiotherapy for, 1340
classification of, 1334, 1334b
diagnostic evaluation in, 1335-1337, 1335b-1337b
drug therapy in, 1337-1340
etiology of, 1334, 1335b
exercise-induced, 1340
family and child support in, 1345-1346
hyposensitization and, 1340
nursing care plan for, 1341-1342, 1342b
pathophysiology of, 1335, 1335f
prognosis in, 1340-1341
status asthmaticus and, 1341
asthma and high risk pregnancy and, 322-324, 324t
bronchiolitis and, 1272, 1321-1324, 1322t
bronchitis and, 1321, 1322t
cystic fibrosis and, 324-325
environmental tobacco smoke exposure and, 1333, 1333b
foreign body aspiration and, 1330, 1330b
influenza and, 985, 1313-1314
nasopharyngitis and, 1307-1310, 1310b
opioid analgesics and, 407b
Respiratory dysfunction *(Continued)*
pharyngitis and, 1310b
respiratory failure and, 1354-1355, 1354b
respiratory syncytial virus and, 1272, 1321-1324, 1322b
smoke inhalation injuries and, 1332-1333, 1332b
tuberculosis and, 1326-1329, 1327b-1329b
Respiratory failure, 1354-1355, 1354b
Respiratory hygiene, 113b-114b
Respiratory infections, 1303
in bronchiolitis, 1272, 1321-1324, 1322t
clinical manifestations of, 1304, 1305b
comfort during, 1304-1305
croup syndromes, 1318-1321, 1318b-1320b, 1318t
easing respiratory efforts in, 1304
etiology and characteristics of, 1303-1304
family support and home care and, 1307
hydration and, 1306-1307
lower respiratory tract, 1321, 1322t
bronchitis, 1321, 1322t
pneumonias, 1324-1326, 1324b, 1326f
respiratory syncytial virus and bronchiolitis, 1272, 1321-1324, 1322b, 1322t
nursing care plan for, 1308b-1309b
nursing process in, 1306b
nutrition and, 1307
pertussis, 1326
postoperative, 1253
preventing spread of, 1305-1306
reducing temperature in, 1306, 1306b
respiratory function assessment in, 1307b
rest and, 1304
severe acute respiratory syndrome, 1329
tuberculosis, 1326-1329, 1327b-1329b
upper respiratory tract
infectious mononucleosis, 1317-1318, 1317b-1318b
influenza, 1313-1314
nasopharyngitis, 1307-1310, 1310b
otitis media, 1314-1317, 1314b-1315b
pharyngitis, 1310-1311, 1310b, 1311f
tonsillitis, 1311-1313, 1311f-1312f, 1313b
Respiratory insufficiency, 1354
Respiratory rate
maternal
cardiac emergency and, 318b
changes during pregnancy, 221, 222t
during labor, 391b, 395
pediatric
newborn at birth and, 636
normal rates for, 1762
postoperative, 1254t
Respiratory secretion collection, 1272-1273
Respiratory syncytial virus (RSV), 1272, 1321-1324, 1322b
Respiratory system
developmental milestones of, 184t-186t
of fetus, 179
maternal
adaptation to labor, 391
adaptation to pregnancy, 218f, 219-222, 222t
after trauma, 371t
obesity and, 420
review of systems and, 79
pediatric
congenital anomalies of, 770-771, 770f-771f
effects of immobilization on, 1677t
infants and, 954
neonatal abstinence syndrome and, 762t
preterm infants and, 708-709
review of systems and, 882b
signs of neonatal sepsis and, 747t
transition to extrauterine life and, 609-625
Respite care, 1205
Responsivity, infant-parent adjustment and, 566
Rest
adolescents and, 1119
after childbirth, 538b, 543-544, 543b
after pediatric heart surgery, 1471
breastfeeding and, 694
cultural influences on, 260
growth and development and, 847
during pregnancy, 250, 250f, 251b
in respiratory infection, 1304
school-age children and, 1090
Restitution, birth process and, 389f, 390
Restless legs syndrome (RLS), 320b
Restraining methods for child, 1265-1266, 1266f
Restrictive cardiomyopathy, 1478
Retained placenta, 578
Retention catheter in comatose child, 1561
Reticulocyte count, 1491t, 1753t-1761t
Retinoblastoma, 1197-1198, 1197b
Retinopathy of prematurity, 4b, 732
Retrograde pyelography, 1527t-1528t
Retroperitoneal hematomas, 578
Review of systems
in child, 881, 882b
during the health assessment, 79
during pregnancy, 240, 242
Revised Infant Temperament Questionnaire (RITQ), 963
Reye's syndrome, 1580-1581, 1581b
Rh antibodies, breastfeeding and, 1745t-1748t
Rh immune globulin, 546-547, 547b
Rh incompatibility, 766-767
Rh isoimmunization, 546-547, 547b
Rhabdomyosarcoma, 1707-1708, 1708b
Rheumatic fever, 312-313, 1473-1474, 1474b

Rheumatic heart disease, 247, 312-313, 1473
Rheumatrex. *See* Methotrexate.
RhoGam, 547b
Rhophylac, 547b
Rhythm and infant-parent interactions, 559, 559f-560f, 565
Rib cage, 912, 913f
Ribavirin
for hepatitis C virus, 108
for respiratory syncytial virus, 1323
Riboflavin. *See* Vitamin B_2.
Rickets, 1363
Rickettsial diseases, 1652-1653, 1653t
Right-sided heart failure, 1453
Right-to-left shunt, 1446-1447
Rimantadine, 1314
Ringworm, 1643, 1645t
Risk factor assessment, 190
antepartum testing in, 190-191, 194b
biochemical assessment, 200-201, 200t
alpha-fetoprotein assay in, 203-204
amniocentesis in, 200t, 201, 201f
chorionic villus sampling in, 203, 203b, 204f
Coombs' test in, 204
indications for, 201-202, 202b
percutaneous umbilical blood sampling in, 202-203, 203f
daily fetal movement count in, 191-192, 192b-193b, 195f
electronic fetal monitoring in. *See* Electronic fetal monitoring (EFM).
fetal and neonatal health problems and, 190
magnetic resonance imaging in, 200
maternal health problems and, 189-190
nursing role in, 207-208, 208b
preconception care and, 45b
psychologic considerations in, 207-208, 208b
regionalization of health care services in, 190
ultrasound in, 192-199
amniotic fluid volume and, 198
biophysical profile and, 198-199, 199t
Doppler blood flow analysis and, 198, 199f
fetal anatomy and, 197
fetal face at 20 weeks, 196f
fetal genetic disorders and physical anomalies and, 197, 198f
fetal growth and, 196-197, 197f
fetal heart activity and, 195
gestational age and, 195-196, 197f
indications for, 194-195, 196b
levels of, 194-195
nursing role in, 199-200, 200b
Risk factor assessment *(Continued)*
placental position and function and, 197
umbilical cord at 26 weeks, 196f
preconception care and, 264b
Risk management, 13, 14t
Risperdal. *See* Risperidone.
Risperidone, 597, 597t
Ritgen maneuver, 481f
Ritodrine, 493-494
RITQ. *See* Revised Infant Temperament Questionnaire (RITQ).
Ritualism, toddlers and, 1019, 1029
Rocking chairs
after cesarean birth, 516
labor and, 469
Rocky Mountain spotted fever, 1653t
Role confusion vs. identity in psychosocial development, 849-850
Role continuity, 807
Role discontinuity, 807
Role learning in families, 807-810, 808f-809f, 809b-810b
Role pairing in families, 17
Rolling over, 956, 957f
Roman Catholic Church
contraception permitted by, 141
on infertility procedures, 132b
nursing care and, 836t-837t
prohibition of abortion by, 156
Romberg test, 923, 923b
Rooming-in facilities, 557, 557f
Rooting reflex, 621t-625t
Roseola. *See* Exanthem subitum.
Rotarix, 985-986, 1387-1388
RotaTeq, 985-986, 1387-1388
Rotavirus, 1383, 1384t-1386t
Rotavirus vaccine, 985-986, 987t-988t, 1387-1388
Round ligament, 66, 67f
pain during pregnancy, 254t-256t
Roundworms, 1396t
Roxicodone. *See* Oxycodone.
Royal College of Midwives, 9
RSL. *See* Restless legs syndrome (RSL).
RSV. *See* Respiratory syncytial virus (RSV).
Rubella, 984, 1058t-1064t
neonatal, 752
in prenatal period, 241t
Rubella vaccine, 4b, 752, 984, 987t-988t
breastfeeding and, 1745t-1748t
health screening recommendations for, 59t
HIV-infected women and, 329
during postpartum period, 546, 546b
Rubeola. *See* Measles.
Rubin, Reva, 4b, 230, 231b
Rubin technique, 519, 520f
Rugae, 66
Rupture
of appendix, 1399
of membranes, 445b
of uterus, 372, 522
Rural areas, access to health care in, 31-32
Russell traction, 1688

S

Saccharin during pregnancy, 281b
Sacral promontory, 67f, 69f
Sacroiliac joint, 69f
Sacrosciatic notch, 69f
Sacrum, 68, 69f
Safe infection practices, 113b-114b
Safe Motherhood Initiative, 4b
Safety
in care of newborn, 662
home care and, 41-42, 1215-1216, 1215b-1216b
pediatric hospitalization and, 1261
environmental factors in, 1261-1262, 1261f-1262f
infection control and, 1261f, 1262-1264, 1263b-1264b
positioning for procedures and, 1266-1267, 1267b, 1267f
restraining methods and therapeutic holding and, 1265-1266, 1266f
transporting infants and children, 1264-1265, 1264f
in pharmacologic pain management during labor, 419-420, 419f
toy, 857, 858b, 994, 1262
Salicylates, 1753t-1761t
Saline lock, 1279
Salmeterol, 1339
Salmonella, 1383-1386, 1384t-1386t
Salpingostomy, 357
Sandifer syndrome, 1394
Sanger, Margaret, 4b
Sarcoma
Ewing's, 1707
osteosarcoma, 1705-1707
rhabdomyosarcoma, 1707-1708, 1708b
Sarcoptes scabiei. See Scabies.
SARS. *See* Severe acute respiratory syndrome (SARS).
Saudi Arabian culture, 550b
SBS. *See* Shaken baby syndrome (SBS).
Scabies, 1650, 1650b
Scald burns, 997, 1039
Scales, cutaneous, 1635f
Scalp
assessment in child, 901
birth injury of, 743t
Scandinavian culture, 292t-293t
Scarf sign, 651b
Scarlet fever, 1058t-1064t
Scars, 1635f
burn-related, 1671-1672, 1671f
Scheduled cesarean birth, 513-514
Scheuermann's kyphosis, 1699
Schizophrenia, childhood, 1103
School phobia, 1101
School vision, 1191
School-age children, 1077, 1103-1104
adaptation to pregnancy, 236b
altered growth and maturation in, 1097-1099, 1098t
approaches to physical examination of, 888t
attention-deficit hyperactivity disorder in, 1099-1100
biologic development of, 1077-1079, 1078f
School-age children *(Continued)*
body image of, 853, 1084-1085
cognitive development of, 1079-1081, 1080f
communication with, 871-872
constipation in, 1390-1391
conversion reaction in, 1102
dental health of, 1091-1092, 1091f, 1092b
depression in, 1102-1103, 1102b
dishonest behavior in, 1087-1089
divorce and, 817b
encopresis in, 1100
enuresis and, 1100
exercise and activity and, 1090-1091, 1090f
growth and development of, 845t, 1086t-1087t
hospitalization of. *See also* Hospitalization: pediatric.
bathing during, 1258
developmentally appropriate activities and, 1232
loss of control and, 1222-1223, 1230-1231
preventing or minimizing separation during, 1229-1230, 1230f
separation anxiety and, 1221
specimen collection and, 1267-1268
injury prevention and, 1093-1094, 1094b, 1094f, 1095t, 1096b
latchkey, 1087
limit setting and discipline of, 1087
moral development of, 1081
nutrition and, 1089-1090
overuse syndromes in, 1096
peptic ulcer disease and, 1405b
play and, 1083-1084, 1085f
posttraumatic stress disorder in, 1101
psychologic preparation for procedures, 1248b-1249b
psychosocial development of, 1079, 1079f
recurrent abdominal pain in, 1101-1102
response to pain, 930b
schizophrenia in, 1103
school experience and, 1085-1087, 1088b
school health and, 1093
school phobia and, 1101
self-concept and, 852-853, 1084-1085
self-esteem and, 853
sex chromosome abnormalities in, 1098-1099, 1098t
sex education and, 1092-1093
sleep and rest and, 1090
social development of, 1081-1084, 1082f, 1084b, 1085f
special needs, 1161t-1162t, 1162-1163, 1163f
spiritual development of, 1081, 1081b
sports injuries and, 1096-1097
stress and fear and, 1089, 1089b
tall or short stature in, 1097-1098
understanding and reaction to death, 1167t-1168t

Schools
attention-deficit hyperactivity disorder and, 1099
influence on child health promotion, 826
Schultze mechanism, 479
SCID. *See* Severe combined immunodeficiency disease (SCID).
SCOFF questionnaire, 52-53, 52b
Scoliosis, idiopathic, 1700-1703, 1701f
Scope and Standards of Pediatric Nursing, 796-797
Scorpion stings, 1649t-1650t
Scout film, 1527t-1528t
Screen-film mammography, 120b
Screening
for abuse, 79
for bacterial vaginosis, 110-111, 110t
for candidiasis, 110t, 111-112
for chlamydia, 99
for gestational diabetes mellitus, 308, 308f
for gonorrhea, 100
for hepatitis B, 107
for herpes simplex virus, 105
for human immunodeficiency virus, 108, 109b
for human papillomavirus, 103-104
for lead poisoning, 1435
newborn, 777-778
for pelvic inflammatory disease, 102
secondary prevention and, 29, 801
for sickle cell anemia, 1497
for syphilis, 101
for trichomoniasis, 110t, 112
Scrotum
pediatric physical assessment of, 920
sexual response of, 74t
ultrasound of, 132-133
Scurvy, 1364
Seat belts, 251-252, 252f, 370, 1036
Sebaceous glands
of breast, 69
during pregnancy, 246
Seborrheic dermatitis, 1659
Secobarbital sodium, 406
Seconal. *See* Secobarbital sodium.
Second stage of labor, 388, 466-477
birth in delivery room or birthing room and, 471-473, 472f
birth in LDR or LDRP room and, 473
breathing during, 402b
duration of, 419, 466-468
emergency childbirth and, 477, 478b
expected maternal progress in, 468t
fundal pressure and, 475, 475b
immediate assessment and care of newborn and, 475
macrosomic infants and, 305
maternal position in, 385, 386f, 461f-463f, 469-471, 470f
bearing-down efforts and, 468-471, 471b
fetal heart rate and pattern and, 471
Second stage of labor *(Continued)*
meconium aspiration syndrome and, 474-475, 475b
in normal vaginal childbirth, 481b-482b
nursing care management in, 468-469, 468t
pain during, 394, 395f
perineal trauma related to childbirth and, 475-477, 476f
phases of, 388, 466
supplies, instruments, and equipment for, 471, 471f-472f
support of father or partner in, 471, 472t
Valsalva maneuver during, 437
vertex presentation and, 473-474, 474f
Second trimester, 229
abortion in, 156, 158
discomforts during, 254t-256t
insulin production during, 297, 297f
nutrition during, 275
signs and symptoms of potential complications during, 243b
ultrasound in, 196b
Secondary amenorrhea, 1125
Secondary circular reactions, 960
Secondary dysmenorrhea, 89-90
Secondary hypertension, 1479-1480
Secondary lactase deficiency, 1373
Secondary powers, 384-385
Secondary prevention, 29, 801
Secondary skin lesions, 1633, 1635f
Secondary social group, 823
Secondary survey in trauma during pregnancy, 373
Second-degree burns. *See* Partial-thickness burns.
Secretory phase of endometrial cycle, 72f, 73
Security in neonatal hospital settings, 9, 540
Sedatives
breastfeeding and, 1745t-1748t
for pain management during labor, 406
Seesaw respiration, 915b
Seizures, 1581
in acute renal failure, 1543
in eclampsia, 346, 346f, 347b
epilepsy and, 1581
classification and clinical manifestations of, 1582, 1583b-1584b, 1585t
diagnostic evaluation of, 1582-1585
etiology of, 1581-1582, 1582b
nursing care management in, 1587-1592, 1587b-1592b
pathophysiology of, 1582
during pregnancy, 326
prognosis, 1587
therapeutic management of, 1585-1587, 1586b-1587b
febrile, 1260, 1592-1593, 1593b
Selenium, 1377t-1379t
Self-assessment of pain during labor, 416
Self-awareness, play and, 856
Self-care
cognitively impaired children and, 1180
hospitalized children and, 1231
special needs children and, 1155
Self-concept
adolescents and, 852-853, 1115
development of, 852-853
school-age children and, 1084-1085
Self-esteem
after childbirth, 548
of children, 853
cultural influences on, 823-824
during labor, 416
Self-family learning checklist, 536f
Self-management
diabetic children and, 1629
postpartum discharge and, 550-551, 551b
promotion of, 10
Self-mastery, hospitalized child and, 1235-1236
Self-monitoring of glucose levels, 298b
Self-report measures, pain assessment in children and, 930-931, 932t-933t
Semen analysis, 132-133, 133b-134b
Semirecumbent position during labor and birth, 385, 386f, 461b
Semivegetarian diet, 1365
Semmelwies, Ignaz, 4b
Senna, 1745t-1748t
Sense-pleasure play, 854, 854f
Sensitive periods of growth, 844
Sensitization
food, 1370
maternal, 766
Sensorimotor stage of development, 850-851
infants and, 958-960, 960f, 966t-968t
play and, 856
toddlers and, 1019-1021, 1020f, 1021b, 1025t-1026t
Sensorineural hearing loss, 1187-1188
Sensory assessment, 1749f-1750f
Sensory awareness of fetus, 182
Sensory behaviors of newborns, 639-640, 640f
Sensory development of toddlers, 1018
Sensory impairments, 1201
autism spectrum disorders, 1198-1201, 1199b-1200b
hearing impairments, 1186
clinical manifestations of, 1189b
cued speech and, 1190
definition and classification of, 1186-1187, 1187t-1188t
hospitalization and, 1190-1191
lipreading and, 1189, 1189b
nursing care plan for, 1188-1189
prevention of, 1191, 1191b
sign language and, 1190
socialization and, 1190
speech language therapy and, 1190
therapeutic management of, 1187-1191, 1188b, 1188f
Sensory impairments *(Continued)*
parental, 569-570
hearing impairment and, 570
visual impairment and, 570, 570b
visual impairments, 1191
assessment of children for, 1184, 1194, 1194b
deaf-blind children and, 1196-1197
definition and classification of, 1191
development and independence and, 1194
education and, 1195
etiology of, 1191-1196, 1193b
hospitalization and, 1195-1196
optimum development and, 1194
parent-child attachment and, 1194
play and socialization and, 1194
prevention of, 1196, 1196b
in retinoblastoma, 1197-1198, 1197b
trauma-related, 1191-1194
types of, 1192b-1193b
Sensory organs, developmental milestones of, 184t-186t
Sensory stimulation
pain management and, 399b
unconscious child and, 1561-1562
Sentence completion, 873b-874b
Sentinel events, 13-14
Separation anxiety
hospitalized children and, 1219-1221, 1220b, 1220f-1221f
infants and, 959, 962, 965
Separation-individuation process, 1046
Sepsis
in children, 1486, 1486b
neonatal, 745-748, 745t, 747b-748b, 747t
during pregnancy, 247
wound, 1664
Septic arthritis, 1704
Septic miscarriage, 353, 353t
Septic shock, 1486-1487, 1486b, 1487t
Septum, nasal, 911
Sequential trends in growth and development, 844
Sequestration crisis, 1495
Serevent. *See* Salmeterol.
Seroquel. *See* Quetiapine.
Serum albumin, 220t-221t
Serum alkaline phosphatase, 220t-221t
Serum bicarbonate, 657b
Serum cholesterol
normal test ranges for, 1753t-1761t
pregnancy versus nonpregnancy values of, 220t-221t
Serum creatinine
normal test ranges for, 1753t-1761t
pregnancy versus nonpregnancy values of, 220t-221t
severe versus mild preeclampsia and, 336t
Serum globulin, 220t-221t
Serum osmolality, 1753t-1761t

Serum prolactin, 227t, 543
Serum proteins
normal test ranges for, 1753t-1761t
pregnancy versus nonpregnancy values of, 220t-221t
Serum uric acid, 220t-221t
Severe acute respiratory syndrome (SARS), 1329
Severe combined immunodeficiency disease (SCID), 1519-1520
Severe preeclampsia
classification of, 336
control of blood pressure and, 346, 346b, 348t
hospital care in, 343, 344b-345b
magnesium sulfate and, 343-346, 344b, 346b
Sex chromosome abnormalities, 167-169, 1098-1099, 1098t
Sex chromosomes, 166, 167f, 172
Sex counseling of expectant couples, 256-258, 257b, 258f
Sex differentiation, 182-183
Sex education
adolescents and, 48, 48b, 1122
preschoolers and, 1049-1052
school-age children and, 1092-1093
Sex-role identity, 1110
Sextuplets, 188
Sex-typing, 1045-1046
Sexual abuse
adolescents and, 48b, 878b, 1113-1115, 1114f, 1115b
of children, 1068-1069, 1069b
clinical manifestations of, 1071b-1072b
nursing care plan for
history and interview and, 1070-1072, 1072b
physical assessment and, 1072-1073
prevention of, 1075b
memories during labor of, 446-447
Sexual activity
of adolescents, 32-33, 48, 48b, 55
after childbirth, 551, 551b, 562-564
after perinatal loss, 600
cultural influences on, 260
health risks and, 55-56, 56b
high risk, 98
during pregnancy, 232
Sexual history
health history and, 878, 878b
sexually transmitted infections and, 97-98, 97b
Sexual intercourse
after childbirth, 551, 551b, 562-564
during pregnancy, 256-258, 257b, 258f
Sexual maturation, 1106
in boys, 1106-1107, 1106b, 1108f
in girls, 1106, 1106b, 1107f-1108f
Sexual orientation
adolescents and, 1113-1115, 1115b
suicide and, 1141b
health care access and, 47
Sexual response, 74, 74t
Sexuality
adolescents and, 878b, 1116t
after perinatal loss, 600
Sexuality *(Continued)*
cognitively impaired child and, 1182
postpartum, 548
in pregnancy, 257-258, 257b
preschoolers and, 1045-1046
Sexually transmitted infections (STIs), 96-99, 96b
and access to health care, 3-4
among adolescents, 32-33, 55
chlamydia, 99
among adolescents, 32-33
neonatal, 754, 755b
gonorrhea, 99-100
among adolescents, 32-33
management of, 100
neonatal, 749
reporting, 100b
hepatitis, 106-108
herpes simplex virus, 104-106, 105f
in cutaneous infection, 1644t
in newborns, 106, 748-749, 753, 753f
home care in, 113b
human immunodeficiency virus. *See* Human immunodeficiency virus (HIV).
human papillomavirus, 85, 103-110, 103f
pelvic inflammatory disease, 101-103
prevention of, 46b, 55-56, 56b, 97-99, 97b-99b
screening for, 59t
sexual practices and, 55-56
substance abuse and, 331
syphilis, 100-101, 101b, 101f
Jarisch-Herxheimer reaction in patients treated for, 101b
neonatal, 749-750, 750b, 750f
SGA infants. *See* Small-for-gestational-age (SGA) infants.
Shake test, 202
Shaken baby syndrome (SBS), 1067, 1067b
Shame and doubt vs. autonomy in psychosocial development. *See* Autonomy vs. shame and doubt in psychosocial development.
Sharps containers, 42
Shear, pressure ulcers and, 1257
Sheet grafts, 1668
Shepherd's purse, 90t, 582t
Shigella, 1383-1386, 1384t-1386t
Shingles. *See* Varicella zoster.
Shirodkar procedure, 355
Shivering after birth, 480
Shock
in abruptio placentae and placenta previa, 362t
pediatric, 1482-1484, 1483b-1485b, 1483t
postpartum hemorrhage and, 581-583, 582b-583b
in preterm infants, 709
Shoes
for infants, 972
during pregnancy, 251
Short stature, 1097-1098
Short-bowel syndrome, 1425-1426
Short-term catheters, 1279
Shoulder blade squeeze after breast surgery, 125b-126b
Shoulder blade stretch after breast surgery, 125b-126b
Shoulder dystocia, 307-308, 519, 520f
Shoulder presentation in labor, 377, 379f
Cesarean birth in, 501
external cephalic version for, 500-503, 505f
Shoulder stretch after breast surgery, 125b-126b
Shouldering, 432
Shoulder-lap safety belts, 1036
Showering
during labor, 457t
for pain management during labor, 403, 403f, 443
Shunt procedures for cardiac defects, 1466f, 1466t
Shunts
congenital heart anomalies and, 1446-1447
hydrocephalus and, 1594-1595, 1595f
SIADH. *See* Syndrome of inappropriate antidiuretic hormone secretion (SIADH).
Siamese twins. *See* Conjoined twins.
Sibling rivalry, 571, 1027-1028, 1028f
Siblings
adaptation of to newborn, 484, 484f, 549, 549f, 570-571, 571f, 572b
adaptation to pregnancy, 234, 235b-236b, 236f, 264-265
first stage of labor and, 465-466
grief after death of infant, 601
of hospitalized child, 1224-1225, 1236, 1237b
impact of special needs child on, 1146, 1150-1151, 1151b, 1159
influence on child development, 859
interactions between, 808-809, 809f
spacing of children and ordinal position and, 808-810, 809b, 809f
of terminally ill children, 1170, 1173-1174
Sick-child care, 965
Sickle cell anemia, 1495-1500, 1496b, 1496f, 1498b-1499b
ethnicity and, 49, 161, 829
newborn screening for, 658t
prenatal screening for, 241
Sickle cell disease, 1495
Sickle cell hemoglobinopathy, 322, 323t
Sickle cell thalassemia disease, 1495
Sickle cell trait, 1495
Sickle-turbidity test, 1497
Side bending after breast surgery, 125b-126b
Side-lying position
for breastfeeding, 543-544, 685, 687f
for childbirth, 385, 459-460, 460f, 461b, 463f, 469
disseminated intravascular coagulation and, 368
Side-lying position *(Continued)*
to facilitate rotation of fetal head, 500b
oxytocin and, 508f, 509b
for rest and relaxation, 250, 250f
for women with disabilities, 76, 77f
SIDS. *See* Sudden infant death syndrome (SIDS).
Sign language, 1190
Silence, communication and, 869
Silicone breast implants, 122
Simple partial seizures, 1583b-1584b, 1585t
Simpson, James Young, 4b
Sinciput presentation, 380f
Single fathers, 818-819
Single footling breech, 379f
Single knee rolls, 545f
Single mothers, poverty and perinatal outcomes of, 17
Single-parent families, 17, 818-819, 1150
Single-photon emission computed tomography (SPECT), 1556t-1557t
Single-room maternity care (SRMC), 649-650
Sinus tachycardia, 1477
Sinuses, 79
SIRS. *See* Systemic inflammatory response syndrome (SIRS).
Sitting, infants and, 956-957, 958f
head control and, 956b, 956f
Sitting/leaning position for labor, 386f
Sitz bath, 540, 541b
Skateboard safety, 1096b
Skeletal limb deficiency, 1695-1696
Skeletal system
birth-related injuries of, 743, 743f
effects of immobilization on, 1677t
growth and maturation of, 846
transition to extrauterine life and, 619-620, 619f-620f, 621t-625t
Skeletal traction, 1687b, 1689b
Skeletal tuberculosis, 1705
Skene glands, 65-66, 81
Skill play, 854, 854f
Skills acquisition, school-age children and, 1091
Skin
adaptations to pregnancy, 223-224, 224b
arthropod bites and stings and Lyme disease and, 1653-1654, 1653f
pediculosis capitis and, 1651-1652, 1651b-1652b, 1651f
Rickettsial diseases and, 1652-1653, 1653t
scabies, 1650, 1650b
burns of. *See* Burns.
care during hospitalization, 1256-1257, 1257b
cold injuries and, 1674
covering breasts, 69
disorders of. *See* Integumentary disorders.
drug reactions and, 1648, 1648b
fetal, 183
foreign bodies and, 1648

Skin *(Continued)*
health screening recommendations for, 59t
infections of
bacterial, 1641, 1642t, 1643f
dermatophytoses, 1643, 1645f, 1645t
systemic mycotic, 1643-1646, 1646t
viral, 1642-1643, 1644t
of newborns, 615-618, 616b, 617f-618f, 626t-636t, 674, 675b
nutritional assessment and, 884t-886t
physical assessment of, 80, 886, 892, 901-902, 901t, 902f
preterm infants and, 720-721, 721b-722b, 728b-730b
pubertal development and, 1109
review of systems and, 79
sunburn and, 1673, 1674f-1675f
traction care and, 1689b
unconscious child and, 1554
Skin color, changes in, 901, 901t
Skin fold thickness, 892
Skin grafts, 1668-1669, 1668f-1669f
Skin lesions, 1632-1633, 1655
acne and, 1659-1661
atopic dermatitis and, 1656-1659, 1657b-1659b, 1657f
contact dermatitis and, 1646-1647
diaper dermatitis and, 1655-1656, 1656b, 1656f
nursing care management of, 1639, 1639b
pathophysiology of, 1632-1633, 1636
poison ivy, oak, and sumac exposure and, 1647-1648, 1647b, 1647f
primary, 1633, 1634f
relief of symptoms in, 1640
seborrheic dermatitis and, 1659
secondary, 1633, 1635f
systemic therapy for, 1639
topical therapy for, 1637-1641, 1637b, 1641b
Skin testing in asthma, 1336-1337, 1337b
Skin traction, 1687b, 1689b
Skin-level gastrostomy device, 1296-1297, 1298f
Skin-to-skin contact (SSC)
with infant, 557
preterm infants and, 723-724, 724f, 725b
Skull
birth injury of, 743, 743t
of child, 903
fetal, 183
fracture of, 371-372
labor and size of, 376-377, 377f
of newborn, 619, 619f
SLE. *See* Systemic lupus erythematosus (SLE).
Sleep
adolescents and, 1119
after childbirth, 538b-540b
disturbed patterns related to infant demands, 574b
growth and development and, 847
infants and, 976-978, 977t
newborns and, 637-639, 638f, 639b, 676b
Sleep *(Continued)*
preschoolers and, 1054-1055
school-age children and, 1090
toddlers and, 1031
Sleep deprivation, 397
Sleep-wake states of newborns, 637-639, 638f, 639b
Slipped femoral capital epiphysis, 1698-1699, 1699b
Slow exhalation pushing, 402b
Slow-paced breathing, 402b
Slow-to-warm-up child, 640, 848, 965
SMA. *See* Spinal muscular atrophy (SMA).
Small-for-gestational-age (SGA) infants, 277, 707b, 734-735
Smegma, 618-619
Smell, response of newborn to, 640
Smoke inhalation injuries, 1332-1333, 1332b
Smokeless tobacco, 1136
Smoking
abruptio placentae and, 365
adolescents and, 1136-1137, 1137b-1138b
breastfeeding and, 696
cessation of, 57-58, 58b, 759b
during pregnancy, 49b
fetal and neonatal effects of, 756t, 758-759
health risks of, 49-50
high risk pregnancy and, 191b
during lactation, 286
during pregnancy, 49, 57, 253, 330
sudden infant death syndrome and, 1006
Snellen letter chart, 905, 906t
Soaks, children and, 1255b
Social development
of adolescents, 1111-1113, 1112b, 1113f
of infants, 961-963, 962b, 962f, 964t
of preschoolers, 1046-1048, 1046f-1047f
of school-age children, 1081-1084, 1082f, 1084b, 1085f
of toddlers, 1022-1024, 1023f-1024f
Social history in initial prenatal care interview, 240
Social interactions in neonatal period, 662, 662b-663b, 662f
Social roles
cultural influences on child health and, 823-824
in families, 17
Social support for new parents, 567-568
Social-affective play, 854
Socialization
blind children and, 1194
cognitively impaired child and, 1181-1182
definition of, 822
families and, 17
hearing impaired child and, 1190
hospitalized child and, 1236, 1236f
during infancy, 966t-968t
preschoolers and, 1050t
toddlers and, 1025t-1026t
Society, families and, 16
Society for Advancement of Women's Health Research, 4b
Society of Obstetricians and Gynaecologists of Canada (SOGC), 513
Socioeconomic factors
in health care, 46, 824-825, 829-830
health risks and, 49
influence on child development, 859
influence on child health promotion, 786
in preterm birth, 49, 487-488
in transition to parenthood, 569
Socioeconomic status
dietary practices and, 287
high risk pregnancy and, 191b
prenatal care and, 235-236
Sodium
hypertension and, 52
intake during pregnancy, 282-283
normal test ranges for, 1753t-1761t
nutritional significance of, 1377t-1379t
retention during pregnancy, 222
Sodium bicarbonate
for pediatric cardiopulmonary resuscitation, 1359t
pregnancy versus nonpregnancy values of, 220t-221t
Sodium pentothal, 4b
Sodium restriction, 1459
Soft tissues
injury in pediatric trauma, 1680-1681, 1680f
labor process and, 381-384, 383f
neonatal birth trauma and, 475-477, 476f, 652-653, 653f
tumors of, 1707-1708, 1708b
Soft-tissue dystocia, 498
SOGC. *See* Society of Obstetricians and Gynaecologists of Canada (SOGC).
Solid foods for infants
introduction to infants of, 975, 976b
selection and preparation of, 974-975
Solitary play, 855-856
Somatic pain
during labor, 394
sensory quality of, 395
Somogyi effect, 1621-1622
Sore throat
after tonsillectomy, 1312
pediatric respiratory infections and, 1305b
Sound
in decibels, 1187, 1187t
frequency of, 192-193
South Korea, 448b
Southeast Asian culture
care and handling of newborns in, 484
expression of pain in childbirth in, 396b
food patterns in, 292t-293t
postpartum care beliefs in, 550b
pregnancy beliefs in, 550
Soy-based infant formulas, 702
Spacer devices, 1290-1291
Spasmodic laryngitis, acute, 1318t, 1321
Spastic cerebral palsy, 1717b
Special needs, women with
abused women and, 76, 77f
adolescents and, 78, 78b
women with disabilities and, 76, 77f
Special needs children, 1174-1175
car safety restraints for, 1037
coping with, 1151-1152, 1152b, 1157-1159, 1158b-1159b
developmental focus in, 1147
end-of-life care and, 1164, 1174-1175
child's understanding and reaction to death, 1167t-1168t
decision making and, 1164-1169, 1166b, 1167t-1168t
fear and, 1169-1171, 1170b-1171b, 1170f
grief and mourning and, 1172-1174, 1173b
home care and, 1168
nurses' reactions to caring for terminally ill children, 1174, 1174b
nursing care plan for, 1147b, 1169-1174, 1170f, 1173b
organ/tissue donation and autopsy and, 1172
pain and symptom management in, 1165b, 1169-1170, 1170b
parental support in, 1170
principles of palliative care, 1164
sibling support in, 1170
treatment options in, 1168-1169
establishing realistic future goals for, 1163-1164
family education in, 1159-1160
family-centered care in, 1147, 1149, 1149b
assessment of family's adjustment, 1156-1157, 1156t, 1157b
cultural awareness and, 1148
family-health care provider communication and, 1147
shared decision making and, 1148, 1148b
therapeutic relationships and, 1147-1148
impact on child, 1154-1156, 1155b, 1155f
impact on parents, 1149-1150, 1150b
impact on siblings, 1150-1151, 1151b, 1159
managed care in, 1149
normalization in, 1148-1149, 1159, 1159b
promotion of normal development for, 1160-1163, 1161t-1162t, 1162f-1163f
scope of problem, 1146, 1147b
support for family at time of diagnosis, 1152-1154, 1153b, 1157, 1157b, 1157f
support systems for families of, 1154, 1154b

Special Supplemental Food Program for Women, Infants, and Children (WIC), 4b, 288
Specific gravity, 1529t-1530t, 1753t-1761t
Specimen collection
home care and, 42
pediatric
blood, 1271-1272, 1271b-1272b, 1271f
respiratory secretions, 1272-1273
stool, 1270-1271, 1270b
urine, 1267-1270, 1268b-1270b, 1268f, 1269t
during pelvic examination, 83, 83b, 84f
SPECT. *See* Single-photon emission computed tomography (SPECT).
Speculum examination, 81-82, 82f
Speech
autism and, 1198
development of, 851
problems in preschoolers, 1053
Speech language therapy, 1190
Sperm, 141
conception and, 172, 173f
fertilization and, 173, 173f
immunologic reactions to, 135
viability of, 129-130, 133b
Sperm immobilization antigen-antibody reaction, 133t
Sperm penetration assay, 132-133, 133t
Spermatocytes, 172, 173f
Spermatogenesis, 172, 173f
Spermicides, 98, 145-147, 145f-146f
Sphingomyelin, 179
Sphygmomanometers, 451b
Spica casts, 1684, 1686
Spider bites, 1649t-1650t
Spider nevi, 254t-256t
Spina bifida, 768-769, 768f, 1724-1731, 1725b, 1725f
complications in, prevention of, 1729
diagnostic evaluation of, 1725, 1726b, 1726f
family support and home care in, 1729-1730
latex allergy and, 1730-1731, 1730b-1731b
myelomeningocele sac care in, 1728-1729, 1729b
pathophysiology of, 1724-1725, 1726f
prevention of, 44-45
therapeutic management of, 1726-1730
Spina bifida cystica, 1724, 1725f, 1726b
Spina bifida occulta, 1724, 1725f, 1726b
Spinal anesthesia
in cesarean birth, 513
for pain management during labor, 409-412, 411b, 411f-412f
administration of, 418
obesity and, 420
safety and general care in, 419-420, 419f
Spinal cord, fetal, 182
Spinal cord injuries
birth injury of, 743t
in children, 1740-1742, 1742f
Spinal muscular atrophy (SMA), 1731, 1731b
type 1, 1731-1732, 1731b
type 3, 1731b, 1732
Spine
head injuries and, 1566b
of newborns, 620
physical assessment of, 921, 921b
Spinnbarkeit, 73
Spiral electrode for fetal heart rate, 426, 426t, 427f
Spiral fractures, 1682
Spiritual development, 849t, 852
of adolescents, 1111
of preschoolers, 1045
of school-age children, 1081, 1081b
of toddlers, 1021-1022
Spirituality, 835, 836b
Spironolactone
breastfeeding and, 1745t-1748t
for congestive heart failure, 1460t
Spitting up, 999-1001
Splenectomy, 1506
Sponge, contraceptive, 146f, 150
Sponge bathing of newborn, 674, 675b
Spontaneous abortion. *See* Miscarriage.
Spontaneous pushing, 402b, 471b
Sports
adolescents and, 1119-1120
school-age children and, 1090-1091, 1090f
Sports injuries
adolescents and, 1096-1097, 1124
school-age children and, 1096-1097
Spot test, 1317
Spouse abuse. *See* Intimate partner violence (IPV).
Sprains, 1681
Square window method in assessing gestational age, 651b
Squatting
in childbirth, 385, 386f, 419, 419f, 461f, 469
in insertion of contraceptive diaphragms, 148b-149b
for muscle relaxation, 250, 250f
SRMC. *See* Single-room maternity care (SRMC).
SSC. *See* Skin-to-skin contact (SSC).
St. John's wort, 598b
Stab wounds during pregnancy, 372
Stabilization in trauma during pregnancy, 372-374, 372b-373b
Stadol. *See* Butorphanol.
Stained peripheral blood smear, 1491t
Stairs, infants and, 996
Stammering, 1053
Standard Days Method (SDM), 141-142, 142f
Standard of care, 13, 13b
Standard Precautions
burn care and, 1670
during childbirth, 449, 450b
home care and, 42
in infection control, 113, 113b-114b, 747
Standard Precautions *(Continued)*
hospitalized child and, 1261f, 1262-1264, 1263b-1264b
osteomyelitis and, 1704
Standards of care
in first stage of labor, 455-456
in home care, 1208-1209, 1209b
Standards of practice
definition of, 796-797
and legal issues in delivery of care, 12-14, 13b, 14t
Standing position for labor, 386f, 469
Staphylococcal scalded skin syndrome, 1642t
Staphylococcus, 1384t-1386t
Startle reflex, 621t-625t
Starvation jaundice, 656
State modulation, 637-639
Station, fetal, 378, 380f
Status asthmaticus, 1341
Status epilepticus, 1586-1587, 1587b
Stealing, school-age children and, 1088-1089
Stelazine. *See* Trifluoperazine.
Stem cell, 1508
Stem cell transplantation, 1509, 1522, 1523b
Stenosis
aortic, 1451b-1453b
hypertrophic pyloric, 1372b, 1417-1420, 1419b
pulmonic, 1451b-1453b
Stent placement, 1444t
Stepping reflex of newborn, 621t-625t
Stereopsis, infants and, 955
Stereotyping, ethnic, 824
Sterilization
female, 154, 154f-155f, 155b
laws and regulations on, 155, 155b
male, 154-155, 154f
nursing considerations in, 155-156
Sternum, 912, 913f
Stethoscopes
blood pressure assessment and, 451b
contamination and, 1264b
fetal assessment and, 422
Stevia, 280
Stillbirth
definition of, 7b
maternal diabetes mellitus and, 299
Stimulation
of infants, 957, 963
of preterm infants, 723-726, 724f, 725b
of unconscious child, 1561-1562
STIs. *See* Sexually transmitted infections (STIs).
Stomach
changes during pregnancy, 226
of newborns at birth, 614
Stomatitis, chemotherapy-related, 1513-1514
Stool specimens, 1270-1271, 1270b
Stools of newborns, 614, 614b, 626t-636t, 666
Stork bites, 618f, 626t-636t
Storytelling, 873b-874b
Strabismus, 1192b-1193b
Strains, 1681
Stranger fear, 962, 962f, 965-972
Strangulation
infant, 994
precautions against, 1216b
Strategic Directions for Nursing and Midwifery Services of, 12, 12b
Strawberry hemangiomas, 618
Streptococcal sore throat infection, 1311
Streptococcus B, 110
Streptococcus pneumoniae conjugate vaccine, 984
Streptomycin, 1745t-1748t
Stress
adolescents and, 1121, 1121f, 1121b
delayed wound healing and, 1637t
dystocia and, 501
families and, 20
family relationships and, 18t
and health promotion and prevention, 54-55
home care and, 40b
influence on child development, 860-861
in labor, 416, 447
management of, 55
preschoolers and, 1052
school-age children and, 1089, 1089b
special needs child and, 1149-1150, 1150b, 1152
symptoms of, 54-55, 55b
Stress fractures, 1096
Stress incontinence, 414
Stress ulcers in children, 1404
Stress urinary incontinence, 589, 590f
Stress-reduction techniques, 53, 87, 91
Striae gravidarum, 217, 223, 223f
Strongyloidiasis, 1396t
Stuttering, 1053
Subacute bacterial endocarditis, 1472
Subarachnoid hemorrhage, birth-related, 745
Subcultures, 20-21, 823
influence on child health, 824-827, 824f, 826f
Subcutaneous administration of medication, 943b-944b, 1278-1279, 1279b
Subdiaphragmatic abdominal thrusts, 1358-1360, 1360f
Subdural hematomas, 745, 1564f, 1566b
Subdural hemorrhage, 1565-1566, 1566b
Subdural tap, 1556t-1557t
Subgaleal hemorrhage in newborn, 616-617, 617f
Subinvolution of uterus, 578
Subjective information, assessment and, 802
Sublimaze. *See* Fentanyl.
Sublingual administration of analgesics, 943b-944b
Subluxation of hip, 774-775, 774f, 1691-1692
Subpopulations
census data and, 31
definition of, 799
Subpubic angle, 381, 381f, 382t

Substance abuse, 49
adolescents and, 1137-1140, 1137b
cessation of, 57-58, 58b
children and, 789
definition of, 330
high risk pregnancy and, 191b
male fertility and, 130b
during pregnancy, 49, 253, 330-332, 330b-332b, 755-756
alcohol and, 330, 331b, 755-758, 756t
barriers to treatment in, 330
breastfeeding and, 332
caffeine and, 761
cocaine and, 331, 756t
heroin and, 760
HIV-infected women and, 329
legal considerations in, 330, 330b
marijuana and, 756t, 759
methadone and, 331, 760-761
methamphetamines and, 756t, 761
phencyclidine and, 760
phenobarbital and, 761
smoking and, 330
tobacco and, 756t, 758-759, 759b
sexually transmitted infections and, 331
Subtotal colectomy, 1403
Subtotal thyroidectomy, 310
Subungual hematomas, 1680
Succenturiate placenta, 366, 367f
Sucking
newborns at birth and, 613, 673-674, 674f
preterm infants and, 720, 720f
Sucking reflex, 621t-625t, 954-955
Sucralose, 281b
Suction curettage abortion, 157, 158b
Suctioning
in comatose child, 1560
of newborn at birth, 450b
tracheostomy, 1292, 1292b, 1292f
Sudden infant death syndrome (SIDS), 1005-1010, 1006t, 1009f
cardiopulmonary resuscitation in, 727
etiology of, 727
heroin and, 760
newborn positioning and, 671, 671b
pacifiers and, 689, 971
Sufenta. *See* Sufentanil.
Sufentanil, 407, 408b, 414
Suffocation
children and, 788, 789f
infants and, 992b-993b, 993-994
toddlers and, 1034t-1035t, 1040
Sugar alcohols during pregnancy, 281b
Suicidal ideation, 1140-1141
Suicidal thoughts and postpartum depression, 596, 596b
Suicide
adolescents and, 1140-1143, 1140b-1142b
children and, 789-790
warning signs of, 1142b
Sulfisoxazole, 1745t-1748t
Sulfonamides, 4b
Sun blockers, 1673
Sun protection, 860b
Sunburn
in children, 1673, 1674f-1675f
infants and, 997
Sunscreen, 1673-1674, 1674b
Superego, 1019, 1044
Superficial burns, 1661-1662, 1662f
Superficial venous thrombosis, 584-585, 585b
Supernatural forces, cultural beliefs about, 833-834
Supine hypotension, 242
effect on fetus, 437
first stage of labor and, 391, 451f
during pregnancy, 218, 254t-256t
signs and symptoms of, 85, 242b
Supine position
trauma during pregnancy and, 370, 473
Supplies for childbirth, 471, 471f-472f
Support groups
for breastfeeding, 546b
for parents of high risk infants, 726
for parents of special needs children, 1158
for postpartum women, 552
for women with endometriosis, 93
Support hose, maternity, 251
Support systems
effects of bed rest on, 492b
for family of child with apnea, 1012
for family of child with autism, 1200-1201
for family of special needs child, 1154, 1154b
for transition to parenthood, 811-812, 812f
Supportive care
for families. *See* Family support.
during first stage of labor, 460-466, 462b, 463f, 464t, 465b
pediatric nurse's role in, 794
during second stage of labor, 471, 472t
Suprapubic aspiration, 1270, 1532
Suprapubic pressure in shoulder dystocia, 519-520, 520f
Surfactant replacement therapy, 715-716
Surgery
for breast cancer, 121-122, 121f, 126b
in cerebral palsy, 1718-1719
in congenital heart disease, 1470b
in epilepsy, 1586
in esophageal atresia, 1416
in head injuries, 1568
in Hirschsprung disease, 1392-1393
for infertility, 135-136, 135f-136f
in inflammatory bowel disease, 1403
limb salvage procedures, 1706
pediatric
for cleft lip, 1412
for cleft palate, 1412
hypertrophic pyloric stenosis and, 1419
postoperative care, 1252-1253, 1254t
Surgery *(Continued)*
preoperative care, 1251-1252, 1251f, 1252t
during pregnancy, 368-369, 369b
nursing care management in, 369, 369b
in scoliosis, 1701
in Wilms' tumor, 1541-1542
Surgi-Gator, 541b
Surrogate mothers, 137t
Surrogate parenting, 136
Sutures of fetal head, 376-377, 377f, 626t-636t
Swaddling, blanket, 723, 936
Swaddling of infant, 1266, 1266f
Swallowing reflex
of infants, 1274b
of newborn, 621t-625t
Sweat glands in newborn at birth, 617
Swiss-type lymphogenic agammaglobulinemia, 1519
Symbolic play, 854
Symmetric intrauterine growth restriction, 707b
Sympathetic nervous system, 395
Symphysis pubis, 67f, 69f
Symptomatic bacteriuria, 1530
Symptothermal method of contraception, 143-144, 144f
Synchronized intermittent mandatory ventilation (SIMV), 715t
Synchrony, parent-infant communication and, 559, 560f
Synclitism, 389f
Syncope during pregnancy, 225-226
Syndrome of inappropriate antidiuretic hormone secretion (SIADH), 1560-1561, 1605, 1605b
Synthetic skin coverings, 1668
Synthetic-convention stage of spiritual development, 852
Syphilis, 100-101, 101b, 101f
Jarisch-Herxheimer reaction in patients treated for, 101b
neonatal, 749-750, 750b, 750f
Syrian culture, birth practices and, 449
Syringes and needles, intramuscular administration and, 1275
Syrup of ipecac, 1427-1430
Systemic analgesia during labor, 406-409, 407b-409b
Systemic arthritis, 1709
Systemic hypertension, 1479-1481, 1480b
Systemic inflammatory response syndrome (SIRS), 1486, 1486b
Systemic lupus erythematosus (SLE)
pediatric, 1711-1713, 1713b
during pregnancy, 327
Systemic mycotic infections, 1643-1646, 1646t
Systolic blood pressure (SBP)
in children, 898t-899t, 899
in infants, 954
during labor, 391b, 451b
during pregnancy, 218, 219b, 221t, 242b, 243
T
T-ACE test, 330, 331b
Tachycardia, fetal, 429, 430t
Tachydysrhythmias, 1476-1477
Tachypnea, 915b
Tachysystole with oxytocin, uterine, 508, 508b-510b
Tacrolimus, 1658
Tactile play, 1024
Tactile sense. *See* Touch.
Tactile stimulation, infants and, 957, 964t
Tail of Spence, 68
Tailor sitting position for labor, 386f
Taiwanese culture, 568-569
Talipes calcaneus, 775, 1693
Talipes equinovarus, 1693, 1694f
Talipes equinus, 775
Talipes valgus, 775, 1693
Talipes varus, 775, 1693
Tall stature, 1097-1098
Tamoxifen
breast cancer and, 122-123, 123b
role in prevention of breast cancer, 118
Tampon, 4b
Tandem nursing, 695
Tanner stages, 1106
Tanning, 1121
Tape, skin and, 1257
Tape test, 1398
Tapping method, 1194
Target populations, definition of, 799
Task analysis, 1179
Taste
cravings during pregnancy, 226
response of newborn to, 640
TAT. *See* Temporal artery temperature (TAT).
Tattoos, 1121
Tay-Sachs disease, 49, 161, 829
TcB monitors. *See* Transcutaneous bilirubinometry (TcB) monitors.
Tdap vaccine. *See* Tetanus-diphtheria-acellular pertussis (Tdap) vaccine.
TDI. *See* Therapeutic donor insemination (TDI).
Teachers' influence on children, 1085-1087
Teaching Patients with Low Literacy Skills, 10
Team play, 1083
Technology-dependent child
definition of, 1147b
predischarge assessment for, 1207b
Tedral. *See* Phenobarbital.
Teenage pregnancy. *See* Adolescent pregnancy.
Teenagers. *See* Adolescents.
Teeth
changes during pregnancy, 226
development of, 171f, 613
of preschoolers, 1055
during school-age years, 1091-1092, 1091f, 1092b
toddlers and, 1031-1032, 1032f
Teething, 971-972, 971f, 972b
Tegretol XR. *See* Carbamazepine.
Telangiectatic nevi, 618f, 626t-636t
Telecommunication, 36
Telecommunications devices for the deaf, 1190

Telehealth, 36
Telemedicine, 8, 36
Telephone follow-up, postpartum, 552, 606, 700
Telephone interview with women in latent phase of labor, 442-443, 442b
Telephone triage, 867, 868b, 1213-1214
Telephonic nursing care, 35, 43
Teletypewriters, 1190
Television
impact on child development, 861-863, 862b-863b
preschoolers and, 1047-1048
Temper tantrums
toddlers and, 1028
Temperament, 847-848, 847b-848b
of infants, 963-965, 966t-968t
of newborn, 640
Temperature. *See* Body temperature.
Temporal artery temperature (TAT), 894t-895t, 895b-896b
Tennison-Randall triangular flap, 1412
Tension headaches, 225-226
Teratogens, 170, 171f, 249b
Teratomas, 777
Terbutaline
external cephalic version and, 502
for preterm labor, 493-494, 495b
Term, definition of, 210
Terminal shock, 1483-1484
Terminally ill children, 1164, 1174-1175
child's understanding and reaction to death, 1167t-1168t
decision making and, 1164-1169, 1166b, 1167t-1168t
fear and, 1169-1171, 1170b-1171b, 1170f
grief and mourning and, 1172-1174, 1173b
home care and, 1168
nurses' reactions to caring for, 1174, 1174b
nursing care plan for, 1147b, 1169-1174, 1170f, 1173b
organ/tissue donation and autopsy and, 1172
pain and symptom management in, 1165b, 1169-1170, 1170b
parental support in, 1170
principles of palliative care, 1164
sibling support in, 1170
treatment options in, 1168-1169
Tertiary care centers, regional
transport of high risk infants from, 739, 739f
transport of high risk infants to, 738-739, 739b, 739f
Tertiary circular reactions, 1019-1020
Tertiary prevention, 29, 801
Testes
in newborn at birth, 618, 619f
sexual response and, 74t
tumors of, 1126
Testicular biopsy, 132-133
Testicular cancer, 1126
Testicular self-examination, 1127b
Testicular ultrasound, 1527t-1528t
Testosterone, 132-133
Tetanus, 983, 1737-1739, 1738b
Tetanus immunoglobulin, 1738
Tetanus-diphtheria-acellular pertussis (Tdap) vaccine, 982-983, 987t-988t
adolescents and, 1117
health screening recommendations for, 59t
Tetany, 1609b
Tetracycline, 1745t-1748t
Tetracycline opthalmic ointment, 649, 649b
Tetralogy of Fallot, 313, 1454b-1455b
TEWL. *See* Transepidermal water loss (TEWL).
Thalamus, 182
Thalassemia, 322, 1500
Thalidomide, 4b
Thelarche, 1106, 1107f
Theobromine, 1745t-1748t
Theolair. *See* Theophylline.
Theophylline, 1339
breastfeeding and, 1745t-1748t
normal test ranges for, 1753t-1761t
Therapeutic abortion, 156
Therapeutic donor insemination (TDI), 136, 137t
Therapeutic holding, 1265, 1266f
Therapeutic play, 856, 856f, 1234, 1250-1251, 1251f
Therapeutic relationships
pediatric nursing and, 793
special needs children and, 1147-1148
Therapeutic touch, 270
Thermal injuries. *See* Burns.
Thermogenesis in newborn at birth, 612
Thermogenic system, 611-613, 612f
Thermometers
chemical dot, 897b
glass mercury, 893b
mercury, 1432b
types of, 893, 897b
Thermoregulation
infants and, 955
in newborn at birth, 611-613, 612f
preterm infants and, 728b-730b
unconscious child and, 1561
Thiamin. *See* Vitamin B1.
Thiazides, 317t
Thimerosal-containing vaccines, 1198, 1199b
ThinPrep Pap Test, 83b
Thiopental, 416
Thioridazine, 597t, 1745t-1748t
Thiothixene, 597t
Third person technique in communication, 873b-874b
Third stage of labor, 388, 477-480, 477f, 479f
maternal physical status in, 479-480
care after placental delivery, 480
signs of potential problems, 479-480
in normal vaginal childbirth, 481b-482b
pain during, 394-395
Third trimester, 229
abortion in, 156
discomforts during, 233, 254t-256t
Third trimester (*Continued*)
insulin production during, 297, 297f
nutrition during, 273-275
prenatal care during, 241-242
signs and symptoms of potential complications during, 243b
ultrasound in, 196b
Third-degree burns. *See* Full-thickness burns.
Thirst
in early pregnancy, 222-223
vomiting and, 1394
Thomas ring splint, 1688
Thoracic cavity, 914, 914f
Thoracic trauma during pregnancy, 372
Thoracolumbosacral orthosis, 1700-1701
Thorazine. *See* Chlorpromazine.
Thought processes, communication related to development of, 870-872, 871f-872f, 872b-874b, 891f
Thought stopping, 937b
Threadworms, 1396t
Threatened miscarriage, 352, 352f, 353t, 354
Three wishes communication technique, 873b-874b
Throat
of children
physical assessment of, 912, 912f
review of systems and, 882b
maternal
physical examination of, 80
review of systems and, 79
Thrombin time, 1753t-1761t
Thrombocytopenia
in idiopathic thrombocytopenic purpura, 583
severe versus mild preeclampsia and, 336t
Thromboembolism after childbirth, 584-585, 585b
Throne position, 419, 419f
Thrush, 755
Thumb-sucking, 970-971
Thymectomy, 327-328
Thyroid and thyroxine (T4), 1745t-1748t
Thyroid disorders, 332-333, 1605
goiter in, 1606, 1606b
hyperthyroidism. *See* Hyperthyroidism.
hypothyroidism and, 310, 310b
juvenile hypothyroidism in, 1605-1606, 1606b
lymphocytic thyroiditis in, 1606-1607, 1607b
nursing care in, 310
Thyroid gland, fetal, 182
Thyroid hormones, 310
Thyroid storm, 310b, 1607-1608
Thyroidectomy, 310
Thyroiditis, lymphocytic, 1606-1607, 1607b
Thyrotoxicosis, 1607-1608
Thyroxine, 1605
changes during pregnancy, 227t
fetal, 182
normal test ranges for, 1753t-1761t
Thyroxine-binding globulin, 227t
Tick bites, 1649t-1650t
Tidal volume, changes during pregnancy, 222t
Time orientation, cultural variations in, 24, 76b
Time-out discipline strategy, 814, 814b
Tinea infections, 1645f, 1645t
Tissue oxygenation
anemia and, 1493
in pediatric heart failure, 1459-1460, 1460b
shock and, 1484
Tobacco. *See also* Smoking.
adolescents and, 1136-1137, 1137b-1138b
fetal and neonatal effects of, 756t, 758-759, 759b
health risks of, 49-50
Tocolysis, 8t, 436
Tocolytic therapy, 436
contraindication to, 494b
external cephalic version and, 502
for preterm labor, 40-41, 299
for preterm labor and birth, 493-496, 494b-495b
for recurrent premature dilation of cervix, 356
Tocopherol. *See* Vitamin E.
Tocotransducer, 425, 426t, 427f
Toddlers, 843b, 1017, 1041-1042
anticipatory guidance and, 1040, 1041b
approaches to physical examination of, 888t
biologic development of, 1017-1018, 1018f
body image and, 853, 1022
cognitive development of, 1019-1021, 1020f, 1021b
dental health of, 1031-1033, 1032f-1033f, 1032t
Denver II and, 926
gait of, 922
gender identity and, 1022
growth and development of, 845t, 1025t-1026t
hospitalization of. *See also* Hospitalization: pediatric.
fears of bodily injury and pain and, 1231-1232
loss of control and, 1222, 1230
preventing or minimizing separation during, 1229, 1229f
separation anxiety and, 1221
urine specimen collection and, 1267-1270, 1268b-1270b, 1268f, 1269t
injury prevention and, 1033, 1034t-1035t
aspiration and suffocation and, 1034t-1035t, 1040
bodily damage and, 1034t-1035t, 1040
burns and, 1034t-1035t, 1038-1039, 1038f
drowning and, 1034t-1035t, 1038
falls and, 1034t-1035t, 1039-1040
motor vehicle injuries and, 1033-1038, 1034t-1035t, 1036b, 1037f

Toddlers *(Continued)*
poisoning and, 1034t-1035t, 1039, 1039b, 1039f
negativism and, 1028-1029
nutrition and, 1029-1031, 1030b
psychologic preparation for procedures, 1248b-1249b
psychosocial development of, 1019
regression and, 1029
self-esteem and, 853
sibling rivalry and, 1027-1028, 1028f
sleep and activity and, 1031
social development of, 1022-1024, 1023f-1024f
special needs, 1161t-1162t
spiritual development of, 1021-1022
temper tantrums and, 1028
toilet training and, 1024-1029, 1026b, 1027f
understanding and reaction to death, 1167t-1168t
Toeing in, 922
Toenails, 183
Toilet training, 1024-1029, 1026b, 1027f
TOL. *See* Trial of labor (TOL).
Tolbutamide, 1745t-1748t
Tolectin. *See* Tolmetin.
Tolerance, opioid, 948
Tolmetin, 939t
Tongue, 912
Tonic neck reflex, 621t-625t, 1555b
Tonic-clonic seizures
in eclampsia, 347b
in epilepsy, 1583b-1584b, 1587b, 1591b
Tonsillectomy, 1312
Tonsillitis, 1311-1313, 1311f-1312f, 1313b
Toothbrushing
school-age children and, 1091
toddlers and, 1031-1032, 1032f
Topamax. *See* Topiramate.
Topical administration of analgesics, 943b-944b
Topical garlic application, 835b
Topical therapy
for burns, 1667, 1668t, 1670
for skin lesions, 1637-1641, 1637b, 1641b
Topiramate, 597t
TORCH infections, 748, 749b
cytomegalovirus, 752-753, 752f
gonorrhea, 749
hepatitis B virus, 750-751
herpes simplex virus, 753, 753f
human immunodeficiency virus, 751
parvovirus B19, 753-754
rubella, 752
syphilis, 749-750, 750b, 750f
toxoplasmosis, 749
varicella-zoster virus, 750
Torticollis, 1009-1010
Torus fractures, 1682b
Total anomalous pulmonary venous connection, 1455b-1458b
Total body fluid, 955
Total body surface area, burns and, 1661
Total lung capacity changes during pregnancy, 222t
Total mastectomy, 121f, 122
Total parenteral nutrition (TPN)
for inflammatory bowel disease, 1403, 1404b
pediatric, 1298
preterm infants and, 717
Touch
as communication between parent and infant, 558, 558f
cultural variations in, 76b
for pain management during labor, 402
response of newborn to, 640
sensitivity to, during labor, 463
Touchpoints, 1029
Toxic shock syndrome (TSS)
cervical cap and, 150
contraceptive diaphragms and, 147-150, 150b
Toxocara canis, 1396t
Toxoplasmosis, 241t, 329, 749
Toys
cognitively impaired child and, 1180-1181, 1181f
hospitalized children and, 1233-1234, 1234b
play during infancy and, 964t
role in development, 857
safety issues, 857, 858b, 994
hospitalized children and, 1262
Trace elements, 1365
Tracheitis, bacterial, 1321
Tracheobronchitis. *See* Bronchitis.
Tracheoesophageal fistula, esophageal atresia with, 772-773, 772f, 1414-1417, 1415b-1416b
Tracheostomy, 1291-1294, 1291f-1292f, 1292b-1294b, 1294f
Traction, 1686-1690, 1687b, 1687f-1688f, 1689b
Trainable cognitive impairment, 1178
Trained night crying, 977t
Transcatheter device closure, 1444t
Transcutaneous bilirubinometry (TcB) monitors, 655
Transcutaneous electrical nerve stimulation (TENS), 403, 404b, 404f
Transcutaneous monitoring of oxygen therapy, 1290
Transdermal administration of analgesics, 943b-944b, 945-946, 946b, 947f
Transdermal contraceptive system, 152
Transductive reasoning, 1021b
Transepidermal water loss (TEWL), 713, 718, 721b-722b
Transesophageal recording, 1476
Transfer from recovery area, 533, 534t
Transfer report, 533, 534t
Transformation zone, 67
Transfusion in hemorrhagic shock, 583
Transient hypertension in pregnancy, 335t
Transilluminator, 1286f
Transition phase of labor, 388, 466, 468t, 472t
Transition to extrauterine life, 609-625
cardiovascular system and, 610-611
Transition to extrauterine life *(Continued)*
gastrointestinal system and, 613-614, 614b
hematopoietic system and, 611
hepatic system and, 614, 615b, 616f
immune system and, 614-615
integumentary system and, 615-618, 616b, 617f-618f
neuromuscular system and, 620-625, 621t-625t
renal system and, 613
reproductive system and, 618-619, 619f
respiratory system and, 609-625
skeletal system and, 619-620, 619f-620f, 621t-625t
thermogenic system and, 611-613, 612f
Transitional stools, 614b
Translocation chromosomes, 163
Transmission-based Precautions, 1056b-1057b, 1263
Transmucosal administration of analgesics, 945-946, 946b, 947f
Transplantation
heart
pediatric, 1478-1479
pregnancy after, 314
kidney, 1547-1549, 1548b-1549b
liver, 1409-1410
stem cell, 1509, 1522, 1523b
Transport
of high risk infants from regional tertiary centers, 739, 739f
of high risk infants to regional tertiary centers, 738-739, 739b, 739f
of hospitalized child, 1264-1265, 1264f
Transportation special needs child and, 1160, 1216
Transposition of great arteries, 1455b-1458b
Transrectal ultrasound, 132-133
Transvaginal ultrasound, 194, 357
Transverse fetal lie, 377, 379f
Transverse fractures, 1682
Transverse incisions in cesarean birth, 513, 513f
Trauma
in children
amputation and, 1690-1691, 1690b
blindness and, 1191-1194
distraction for, 1690, 1690f
fractures and, 1681-1684, 1682b, 1682f, 1684b, 1686f
casts for, 1684-1686, 1685b, 1686f
head injuries and. *See* Head injuries.
soft-tissue injuries and, 1680-1681, 1680f
traction for, 1686-1690, 1687b, 1687f-1688f, 1689b
newborn birth-related, 742-743, 743t
central nervous system injuries in, 745
nursing care management in, 743
Trauma *(Continued)*
peripheral nervous system injuries in, 743-745, 744f
skeletal injuries in, 743, 743f
during pregnancy, 369-374
fetal physiologic characteristics and, 370-371
maternal physiologic characteristics and, 370, 370b, 371t
mechanisms of, 371-372, 371b
nursing care management in immediate stabilization and, 372-374, 372b-373b
perimortem cesarean delivery and, 374
significance of, 369-372
Travel
pediatric diabetes mellitus and, 1626
during pregnancy, 251-252, 252f
Tremors after birth, 480
Trendelenburg's position, 1574b
Treponema pallidum. See Syphilis.
Tretinoin, 283-284, 1660
Trexall. *See* Methotrexate.
Triage, telephone, 867, 868b
Trial of labor (TOL), 503-504, 517-518
Triceps reflex, 923f
Trichomoniasis, 110t, 112
Trichuriasis, 1396t
Tricuspid atresia, 1454b-1455b
Trifluoperazine, 597t, 1745t-1748t
Trigeminal nerve (cranial nerve V), 925t
Triglycerides, 1753t-1761t
Triiodothyronine, 1605
changes during pregnancy, 227t
normal test ranges for, 1753t-1761t
Trilafon. *See* Perphenazine.
Trilisate. *See* Choline magnesium trisalicylate.
Triple X syndrome, 1098t
Triplets, 188
Trisomies, 166-167
Trisomy 13. *See* Patau's syndrome.
Trisomy 18. *See* Edwards' syndrome.
Trisomy 21. *See* Down syndrome.
Trisomy XXY. *See* Klinefelter's syndrome.
Trochlear nerve (cranial nerve IV), 925t
Trophoblasts, 173-174, 176
Trousseau's sign, 1609b
True labor, 387, 442, 442b
True pelvis, 68, 69f, 380, 387
Truncal incurvation of newborn, 621t-625t
Truncus arteriosus, 313, 1455b-1458b
Trust vs. mistrust in psychosocial development, 849-850, 957-958
Trypsin, 954
TSS. *See* Toxic shock syndrome (TSS).
Tsubos, 403-404
Tubal ligation, 154, 155b, 155f, 159
Tubal reconstruction
female, 154
male, 155
Tubal tonsils, 1311-1312, 1312f

Tuberculin skin test
  in children, 1326-1327, 1327b-1328b
  health screening recommendations for, 59t
  HIV-infected women and, 329
  in prenatal period, 241t
Tuberculosis
  in children, 1326-1329, 1327b-1329b
  neonatal, 754
  skeletal, 1705
Tucking, facilitated, 723
Tug-of-war position, 419
Tumors
  brain, 1572-1574, 1573b-1574b
  in Ewing's sarcoma, 1707
  in gestational trophoblastic neoplasia, 349, 358
  neuroblastomas, 1574-1575
  in osteosarcoma, 1705-1707
  retinoblastoma, 1197-1198, 1197b
  rhabdomyosarcoma, 1707-1708, 1708b
  Wilms', 1540-1542, 1541b-1542b
Tunneled catheters, 1281b
Turgor, 901
Turner's syndrome, 167-169, 1098-1099, 1098t
Twenty-four-hour collection, 1269
Twin birth rate, 8, 501
Twins
  breastfeeding of, 691, 692f
  cobedding of, 724
  congenital anomalies and, 263
  dizygotic, 183, 187f
  incidence of, 183
  maternal weight gain and, 277
  monozygotic, 183-186, 187f
  sibling relationship and, 810, 810b
Two day method of family planning, 145
Tylectomy, 121, 121f
Tylenol. *See* Acetaminophen.
Tympanic membrane
  landmarks of, 909f
  pediatric ear examination and, 909f
Tympanostomy tubes, 1316
Type 1 diabetes mellitus. *See also* Diabetes mellitus.
  in children, 1616, 1617b, 1617t
    therapeutic management of, 1618
      exercise and, 1621, 1629
      hyperglycemia and, 1621-1622, 1622t, 1628
      hypoglycemia and, 1621, 1621b, 1622t, 1628, 1629b
      illness management and, 1622
      insulin therapy and, 1618-1620, 1619b, 1626
      monitoring in, 1620, 1620t
      nutrition and, 1620-1621
  maternal, 296, 298
Type 2 diabetes mellitus, 296, 298. *See also* Diabetes mellitus.
  in children, 1616, 1617t
    obesity and, 786-787, 787f

U

UA. *See* Uterine activity (UA).
Ulcerative colitis, 1401-1404, 1401t, 1404b
Ulcers
  chemotherapy-related, 1514
  peptic, 1404-1406, 1405b
  pressure, 1256-1257
Ultrasound, 192-199
  in abruptio placentae and placenta previa, 362t
  amniotic fluid volume and, 198
  biophysical profile and, 198-199, 199t
  for breast cancer screening, 120b
  for dating of pregnancy, 176b
  Doppler blood flow analysis and, 198, 199f
  before external cephalic version, 502
  fetal anatomy and, 197
  fetal face at 20 weeks, 196f
  fetal genetic disorders and physical anomalies and, 197, 198f
  fetal growth and, 196-197, 197f
  fetal heart activity and, 195
  gestational age and, 195-196, 197f, 244
  in impaired fertility, 133t
  indications for, 194-195, 196b
  levels of, 194-195
  nursing role in, 199-200, 200b
  in percutaneous umbilical blood sampling, 202, 203f
  in placenta previa, 364
  placental position and function and, 197
  transvaginal, 194, 357
  before trial of labor, 503-504
  umbilical cord at 26 weeks, 196f
Ultrasound fetoscopes, 423, 423f
Ultrasound transducer, 425, 426f, 426t
Ultraviolet burns, 1193b
Umbilical amulet, 260f
Umbilical cord, 175f, 176
  compression of, 176, 510b
  home care after birth, 673, 675b-676b
  prolapse, 455b, 467b, 520, 521f, 522b
  routine cord care of, 651-652, 652f
  ultrasound of, 196f
  variations in insertion of, 366, 367f
  vertex presentation and, 474
Unconscious child, 1558-1562
  elimination and, 1561
  family support in, 1562, 1562b
  hygienic care of, 1561, 1561b
  intracranial pressure monitoring in, 1559-1560, 1559b-1560b
  medications and, 1561
  nutrition and hydration for, 1560-1561
  positioning and exercise for, 1561
  regaining consciousness, 1562
  respiratory management of, 1558-1559, 1558b
  sensory stimulation and, 1561-1562
  thermoregulation and, 1561
Undifferentiated stage of spiritual development, 852
Unicornuate uterus, 132f
Unifactorial inheritance, 169-170, 169f
Unintentional injuries among children, 787
United Nations Millennium Summit. *See* Millennium Development Goals (MDGs).
Unoccupied behavior, 854
Unplanned cesarean birth, 514
Upper airway. *See* Upper respiratory tract.
Upper extremity traction, 1687
Upper respiratory tract, 219-221, 1303
Upper respiratory tract infections
  infectious mononucleosis, 1317-1318, 1317b-1318b
  influenza, 1313-1314
  nasopharyngitis, 1307-1310, 1310b
  otitis media, 1314-1317, 1314b-1315b
  pharyngitis, 1310-1311, 1310b, 1311f
  tonsillitis, 1311-1313, 1311f-1312f, 1313b
Upright position during labor and birth, 385, 419, 461b, 469
Uremia, 1542, 1545, 1637t
Urethra, 65-66, 67f, 528-529
Urethral meatus, 920-921
Urethrovesical angle, 590f
Uric acid, 1530t
Urinalysis, 1529t-1530t
  in acute glomerulonephritis, 1538
  for ketones, 1620, 1628
  before planned cesarean birth, 514
  in prenatal period, 241, 241t
  screening for illicit drug use, 330
Urinary catheterization, 1269-1270, 1269b-1270b, 1269t
  clean intermittent, 1727
  in spina bifida, 1727
Urinary frequency during pregnancy, 222, 254t-256t
Urinary incontinence
  postpartum, 589, 590f, 592
  in spina bifida, 1727
Urinary retention, 414
Urinary stasis, 1531
Urinary system
  effects of immobilization on, 1677t
  postpartum changes in, 528-529
Urinary system distress, 1727
Urinary tract infections (UTIs)
  in children, 1530-1533, 1531b-1533b
  constipation and, 1533b
  postpartum, 586-587
  pregestational diabetes mellitus and, 299
  prevention of, 1533b
    patient teaching in, 246, 246f
Urine
  postpartum changes in, 528
  during pregnancy, 222
Urine collection bags, 1268, 1268b, 1268f
Urine glucose, 220t-221t
Urine protein, 336b
Urine specific gravity, 1387
Urine specimen, 1267-1270, 1268b-1270b, 1268f, 1269t
  neonatal, 660-661, 661f
Urine volume, 1753t-1761t
Urobilinogen, 653
Urodynamics, 1527t-1528t
Urogenital diaphragm, 67f
Urosepsis, 1530
USAID Global Health eLearning Center, 12, 13b
Uterine activity (UA), 423
  electronic fetal monitoring and, 424-427, 426t
    external, 425-426, 426f, 426t
    internal, 426-427, 426t, 427f
  intermittent auscultation and, 423-424, 423f, 424b
  preterm labor and suppression of, 493-496, 494b-495b
Uterine atony, 539b-540b, 540, 577
Uterine contractions
  augmentation of labor and, 508-510
  changes in, 213-214
  dysfunction of, 497-498
    hypertonic, 498
    hypotonic, 498, 499b
  induction of labor and, 503-504
    oxytocin and, 505, 507-508, 508b-509b, 508f
  involuntary. *See* Primary powers.
  during labor, 385, 390
    fetal circulation and, 390
    fetal monitoring and, 423-424
    first stage of labor and, 392, 394, 440-441, 450t, 451-453, 453b, 464t
    pain and, 458b-459b
    postpartum, 525
    second stage of labor and, 388, 468t
  late decelerations, 206b
  placental circulation and, 179
  in true labor vs. in false labor, 442b
Uterine fibroids, 94
Uterine leiomyomas, 94
Uterine tachysystole with oxytocin, 508, 508b-510b
Uterine tubes, 67-68, 68f
Uterine tumors, 135-136
Uterine vessels, 68f
Uteroplacental blood flow, 214
Uterosacral block, 415
Uterosacral ligament, 66, 67f
Uterus, 66, 67f-68f
  adaptations to pregnancy, 212-216, 214f-216f, 387
  after trauma, 370
  bimanual palpation of, 84, 84f
  cesarean birth and incisions into, 513, 513f
  hypertonic, 498, 499b, 580-581
  infertility and, 130, 130b, 132f, 133b
  inversion of, 578
  postpartum displacement or prolapse of, 587-588, 588f, 592
  postpartum period and, 525-527, 526f, 527b
    afterpains and, 526
    involution process and, 525, 526f
    lochia and, 526-527, 527b
    maintenance of uterine tone and, 542, 542f
    placental site healing and, 526
  rupture of, 372, 522

Uterus *(Continued)*
sexual response of, 74t
stages of labor and, 383f
subinvolution of, 578
wall of, 66, 68f, 175f
UTIs. *See* Urinary tract infections (UTIs).

V

Vaccine Compensation Amendments, 990-991
Vaccines. *See* Immunizations.
Vacuum aspiration abortion, 157, 158b
Vacuum extraction
in cardiovascular disorders during pregnancy, 318
percent of women receiving, 8t
Vacuum-assisted birth, 377, 510b, 511, 511f
Vagina, 66, 67f-68f. *See also* Vaginal wall.
adaptations to pregnancy, 216-217, 216f-217f
assessment across the life cycle, 70t
childbirth-related laceration of, 475-476
hematoma-related postpartum hemorrhage and, 577-578
infertility and, 130b
postpartum changes in, 527
sexual response of, 74t
Vaginal birth. *See* Childbirth.
Vaginal birth after cesarean (VBAC), 517-518
decline in, 512-513
percent of women receiving, 8t
promotion of, 512b
Vaginal bleeding
in abruptio placentae, 362t, 365
after chorionic villus sampling, 203, 203b
early in pregnancy, 353, 353b
in ectopic pregnancy, 357
epileptic mother and, 326
during labor, 467b
in miscarriage, 353
in placenta previa, 361, 362t
postpartum, 527
Vaginal contraceptive ring, 152
Vaginal discharge, 110
during pregnancy, 216, 243, 387
in preterm labor, 491b
Vaginal examination
in first stage of labor, 454, 454f
in placenta previa, 362, 364
Vaginal infections, 110-112
bacterial vaginosis, 110-111, 110t
candidiasis, 111-112, 111b
group B streptococcus, 112
pregestational diabetes mellitus and, 299
trichomoniasis, 112
wet smear tests for, 110t
Vaginal orifice, 67f, 921
Vaginal smear, 241t
Vaginal speculum. *See* Speculum examination.
Vaginal vestibule, 65-66, 66f
Vaginal wall, 81, 83-85, 84f
Vaginitis, 110, 1126
Vagus nerve (cranial nerve X), 925t, 1586
Valacyclovir, 105
Valium. *See* Diazepam.
Valsalva maneuver, 312, 318, 391, 437
Variable decelerations of fetal heart rate, 431f, 432, 432b
Varicella, 1058t-1064t
Varicella vaccine, 329, 985, 987t-988t
Varicella zoster, 750, 1057, 1644t
Varicose veins
after childbirth, 531
during pregnancy, 251f, 254t-256t
VAS. *See* Visual analogue scale (VAS).
Vasa previa, 361, 366
Vascular spiders, 223-224
Vasectomy, 154-155, 154f, 159
Vasoocclusive crisis, 1495
Vasoocclusive pain, 1497-1499
Vasopressin, 1604, 1604b
VBAC. *See* Vaginal birth after cesarean (VBAC).
Vegans, 1365
Vegetarian diets, 1365-1368, 1366b
food pyramid for, 1366
nutritional disturbances and, 1365-1366, 1366b
during pregnancy, 282, 293
Velamentous insertion of cord, 366, 367f
Vena cava syndrome, 254t-256t
Venereal diseases. *See* Sexually transmitted infections (STIs).
Venipuncture
in newborns, 659-660, 660b
positioning child for, 1266-1267, 1267f
Venography, 584
Venous access devices, central, 1279-1282, 1281b, 1281f, 1282t
Venous blood samples, 659-660, 660b
Venous thromboembolism (VTE), 584
Ventricular septal defects, 1448b-1450b
pregnancy and, 313
teratogens and, 171f
Ventriculoperitoneal shunts, 1594-1595, 1595f
Verapamil, 317t
Verbal communication
with children, 873b-874b
culturally sensitive, 833b
first stage of labor and, 446
Vernix caseosa, 617
Version, 502-503, 505f
Vertex presentation, 380f, 473-474, 474f
emergency birth in, 478b
fetal heart rate in, 451
prolapsed umbilical cord and, 520-522, 521f
Vertical incisions in cesarean birth, 513, 513f
Very-low-birth-weight (VLBW) infants, 707b
body temperature and, 713
environmental concerns of, 722-723
hyperglycemia and, 734-735
kangaroo care and, 723-724, 724f, 725b
necrotizing enterocolitis and, 732
Very-low-birth-weight (VLBW) infants *(Continued)*
nutrition and, 717
rates of, 28-29
respiratory distress syndrome and, 709
retinopathy of prematurity in, 732
Vesicular breath sounds, 915b
Vestibulocochlear nerve (cranial nerve VIII), 925t
Viability
definition of, 210
of fetus, 179
Vibrio cholerae, 1384t-1386t
Vibroacoustic stimulation, 205-206
Video games, influence on child development, 863-864
Vietnamese culture
birth practices and, 449
communication and, 832
food patterns of, 292t-293t
health beliefs and practices in, 838t-840t
postpartum practices in, 549b, 569
pregnancy beliefs and practices in, 260
Violence
children and, 787-789, 791
high risk pregnancy and, 191b, 370
intimate partner. *See* Intimate partner violence (IPV).
Viral infections
acute diarrhea and, 1384t-1386t
cutaneous, 1642-1643, 1644t
hepatitis, 106-108
herpes simplex virus, 104-106, 105f
human immunodeficiency virus. *See* Human immunodeficiency virus (HIV).
human papillomavirus, 103-110, 103f
in pneumonia, 1324, 1324b
Virtual reality for pain management, 936
Visceral larva migrans, 1396t
Visceral pain
during labor, 394
sensory quality of, 395
Vision of newborns, 639-640
Vision testing
during adolescence, 1120
health screening recommendations for, 59t
pediatric, 904-907, 904f-905f, 905b, 906t, 907b
Visual acuity, toddlers and, 1018
Visual analogue scale (VAS), 932t-933t
Visual evoked potentials, 1556
Visual impairments, 1191, 1201
assessment of children for, 1184, 1194, 1194b
deaf-blind children and, 1196-1197
definition and classification of, 1191
development and independence and, 1194
education and, 1195
etiology of, 1191-1196, 1193b
health assessment and women with, 76
Visual impairments *(Continued)*
hospitalization and, 1195-1196
optimum development and, 1194
parent-child attachment and, 1194
parents with, 570, 570b
play and socialization and, 1194
prevention of, 1196, 1196b
in retinoblastoma, 1197-1198, 1197b
severe versus mild preeclampsia and, 336t
trauma-related, 1191-1194
types of, 1192b-1193b
Visualization for pain management during labor, 401
perinatal education and, 270
Vital capacity, changes during pregnancy, 222t
Vital signs
after cesarean birth, 516
after surgery for congenital heart disease, 1469-1470
blood pressure. *See* Blood pressure.
body temperature. *See* Body temperature.
brain tumors and, 1573
of children, 1254t
in first stage of labor, 449-451, 451b, 451f
in gynecologic physical examination, 80
heart rate. *See* Heart rate.
of infants, 893
in neurologic examination, 1553-1554
of newborn, 626t-636t, 636-637, 676b
postpartum changes in, 530, 530t
respiratory rate. *See* Respiratory rate.
taking, blood pressure cuff and, 124b
Vital statistics, definition of, 790
Vitamin A
deficiency of, 1364, 1374t-1377t
intake during pregnancy and lactation, 275t-276t, 283-284
measles and, 1057
toxicity, 1057b
Vitamin B_1, 1374t-1377t
Vitamin B_2, 1374t-1377t
Vitamin B_6, 1374t-1377t
intake during pregnancy and lactation, 275t-276t
Vitamin B_{12}, 275t-276t, 284, 293, 1374t-1377t
Vitamin C, 1374t-1377t
children and, 1364
fertility and, 135
intake during pregnancy and lactation, 275t-276t, 284
iron supplementation and, 290b
toddlers and, 1031
Vitamin D
infant nutrition and, 682, 973
intake during pregnancy and lactation, 275t-276t, 283-284
supplementation of, 1363-1364
toddlers and, 1031
Vitamin D_2, 1374t-1377t
Vitamin D_3, 1374t-1377t
Vitamin D deficiency, 284

Vitamin D deficiency rickets, 1363
Vitamin D toxicity, 682, 973, 1610b
Vitamin E
fertility and, 135
for fibrocystic changes, 115
intake during pregnancy and lactation, 275t-276t, 283-284
premenstrual syndrome and, 91
1377t, 1374t-1377t
Vitamin K, 1374t-1377t
antiepileptic drug-associated deficiency of, 326
infant nutrition and, 682
intake during pregnancy and lactation, 275t-276t, 283-284
newborn and, 649, 649b, 663
Vitamins
fat-soluble, 275t-276t, 283-284
formula feeding and, 704
imbalances, 1363-1364, 1374t-1377t
infant nutrition and, 682
intake during pregnancy and lactation, 275t-276t, 280
megadoses of, 52
water-soluble vitamins, 275t-276t, 284
VLBW infants. *See* Very-low-birth-weight (VLBW) infants.
Vocal cords, 1109
Vocalization during infancy, 962, 962b, 966t-968t
Voice, 559
Voiding
after childbirth, 528-529, 539b-540b
during labor, 457t, 459
during pregnancy, urgency and frequency of, 254t-256t
Voiding cystourethrography, 1527t-1528t
Volume guarantee ventilation, preterm infants and, 715t
Volvulus, 1422
Vomiting
chemotherapy-related, 1513
children and, 1393-1394
pediatric respiratory infections and, 1305b
during pregnancy, 226, 243, 254t-256t, 349-350
Von Willebrand disease, 368, 583, 1503
VSE. *See* Vulvar self-examination (VSE).
V-shaped position, 76, 77f
VTE. *See* Venous thromboembolism (VTE).
Vulnerable child syndrome, 1216
Vulnerable populations, 32-34, 43
Vulva, 65-66, 66f
adaptations to pregnancy, 216-217, 216f-217f, 223
hematoma of, 577-578
nursing care for, after third stage of labor, 480
self-examination of, 81-82
Vulvar self-examination (VSE), 81-82
Vulvovaginal candidiasis, 110t, 111-112, 111b
Vulvovaginitis, 110

W
Waldeyer tonsillar ring, 1311-1312, 1312f
Walk-in clinics, 31
Walking epidural analgesia, 414, 419
Walking position for labor, 386f
Walking reflex of newborn, 621t-625t
Walking surveys, 31, 32b
Wand exercise, 125b-126b
Warfarin, 584-585, 585b
Warm compresses, 404-405, 477
Warm lines, 552
Warm mist therapy, 1304
Warts, 1644t
Wasp stings, 1649t-1650t
Water aerobics, 53f
Water birth, 473, 473f
Water imbalance in infants, 1380-1381, 1381b
Water intake
of infants, 681
during pregnancy and lactation, 275t-276t
Water intoxication, 1543
Water therapy, 403, 403f
Water-soluble vitamins, 275t-276t, 284
Weaning
from breastfeeding, 693, 957-958, 976
from formula feeding, 704
of newborns, 949f
from respiratory assistance, 716-717
to solid foods, 976
Weight
of adolescents, 1107
classification of newborns by, 651-652, 652f
growth charts and, 889
growth charts for boys, 1751t
growth charts for girls, 1752t
health screening recommendations for, 59t
Weight *(Continued)*
of infants, 953-954
of newborn, 637
in pediatric physical assessment, 891-892, 892f
of preschoolers, 1043
of school-age children, 1077-1078
of toddlers, 1017
trends during childhood, 845t, 846
Weight gain
during pregnancy, 277-279, 278t, 279b, 329
in sick preterm infants, 718, 718b
Weight loss
maternal, 286, 289-290, 694
in sick preterm infants, 718, 718b
Well-woman care, 45-46
Werdnig-Hoffmann disease, 1731-1732, 1731b
Wet compresses, 1640
Wet smear tests, 110-111, 110t
Wharton's jelly, 176
Wheals, 1634f
Wheelchairs, 1742, 1742f
Whey-hydrolysate infant formulas, 702
Whipworms, 1396t
Whitaker perfusion test, 1527t-1528t
White, Priscilla, 296, 297t
White blood cell count, 1491t
adaptation to labor, 391, 391b
after childbirth, 530
increase during pregnancy, 219, 220t-221t
normal test ranges for, 1753t-1761t
urine, 1529t-1530t
Whooping cough. *See* Pertussis.
WIC. *See* Special Supplemental Food Program for Women, Infants, and Children (WIC).
Wife battering. *See* Intimate partner violence (IPV).
Wild animal bites, 1654, 1655b
Wilmington brace, 1700-1701
Wilms' tumor, 1540-1542, 1541b-1542b
Wiskott-Aldrich syndrome, 1520
Witch hazel, 582t
Withdrawal
in infants
heroin and, 760
methadone and, 760-761
patient teaching on, 762b
opioid, 408, 408b, 948, 949f
Women for Sobriety, 331
Wong-Baker Faces Pain Rating Scale, 930-931, 932t-933t
Word association game, 873b-874b
Word-graphic pain rating scale, 932t-933t
Work-based group care, 965
Workplace, breastfeeding in, 10
Workplace hazards, 56-57
Wounds, 1633
care of, 1639-1640, 1639b-1640b
dressings for, 1636-1637, 1638t
healing of, 1633-1636, 1637t
mammal bites and scratches and
human bites, 1654
pet and wild animal bites, 1654, 1655b
postpartum infection in, 585-587
stab, 372
Wrist buckle fractures, 1683

X
X chromosomes, 166
Xenograft skin, 1667
X-inactivation, 166
X-linked disorders, 166
X-linked dominant inheritance disorders, 170
X-linked lymphopenic agammaglobulinemia, 1519
X-linked recessive inheritance disorders, 170
Xolair. *See* Omalizumab.
XYY males, 1098t

Y
Yeast infections. *See* Vulvovaginal candidiasis.
Yellow jacket stings, 1649t-1650t
Yersinia, 1383-1386
Yersinia enterocolitica, 1384t-1386t
Yoga, 88, 88f
Yolk sac, 174f-175f, 176, 181
Young adulthood, 48
Youngest children, 809b
Yutopar. *See* Ritodrine.

Z
Zanamivir, 1314
ZIFT. *See* Zygote intrafallopian transfer (ZIFT).
Ziprasidone, 597, 597t
Zollinger-Ellison syndrome, 1405
Zona pellucida, 172-174, 173f
Zona reaction, 173
Zovirax. *See* Acyclovir.
Zygote, 173f
Zygote intrafallopian transfer (ZIFT), 136, 137t
Zyprexa. *See* Olanzapine.